Vaccines

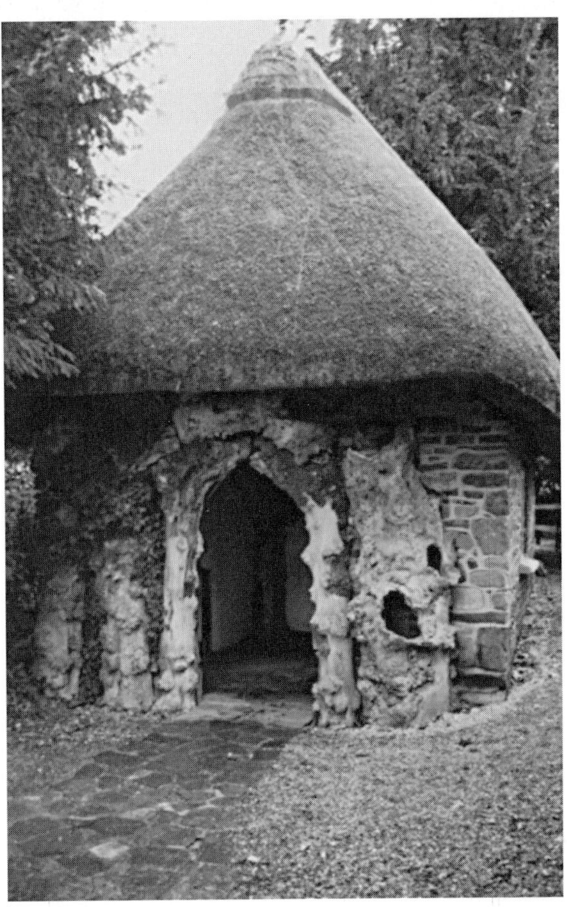

"Vaccination cottage" near the home of Edward Jenner in Berkeley, England, where he administered smallpox vaccine to thousands of the rural poor.

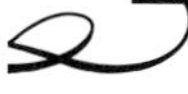

Vaccines

Third Edition

Stanley A. Plotkin, M.D.

Former Medical and Scientific Director, Pasteur Mérieux Connaught
Marnes-la-Coquette, France
Emeritus Professor of Pediatrics, University of Pennsylvania
Emeritus Professor, Wistar Institute
Former Chief, Division of Infectious Diseases
The Children's Hospital of Philadelphia
Philadelphia, Pennsylvania

Walter A. Orenstein, M.D.

Director, National Immunization Program
Centers for Disease Control and Prevention
Atlanta, Georgia

W.B. SAUNDERS COMPANY
A Division of Harcourt Brace & Company
Philadelphia London Toronto Montreal Sydney Tokyo

W.B. SAUNDERS COMPANY
A Division of Harcourt Brace & Company

The Curtis Center
Independence Square West
Philadelphia, Pennsylvania 19106

Library of Congress Cataloging-in-Publication Data

Vaccines / [edited by] Stanley A. Plotkin, Walter A. Orenstein.—3rd ed.

p. cm.

Includes bibliographical references and index.

ISBN 0–7216–7443–7

1. Vaccines. I. Plotkin, Stanley A. II. Orenstein, Walter A.
[DNLM: 1. Vaccines. 2. Vaccination. 3. Immunization Programs.
QW 805 V1163 1999]

QR189.V268 1999 615′.372—dc21

DNLM/DLC 98–31650

VACCINES ISBN 0–7216–7443–7

Printed in the United States of America.

Last digit is the print number: 9 8 7 6 5 4 3 2 1

Acknowledgments

Sincere appreciation to Grace Fries, Frederic Medina, and Denise Derhy for their invaluable secretarial help, and to Marie-Laure Remusat and Claire Soldaini for bibliographic research. We are grateful to Richard Zorab of W.B. Saunders for supervising the transformation of the manuscript to a finished book.

S.A.P.

Many thanks to Mrs. Gwen Nunnally for her assistance in preparing, revising, and tracking submission of manuscripts, Dr. David Satcher for allowing me to work full-time on the book, and Dr. José Cordero and the staff of the National Immunization Program, who continued to provide leadership and support in our efforts to control vaccine-preventable diseases during the period I spent on this project.

W.A.O.

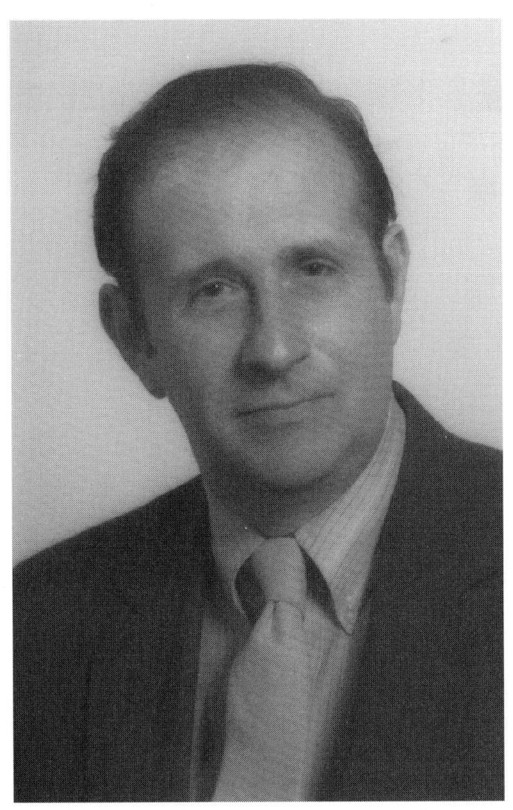

Stanley A. Plotkin, M.D.

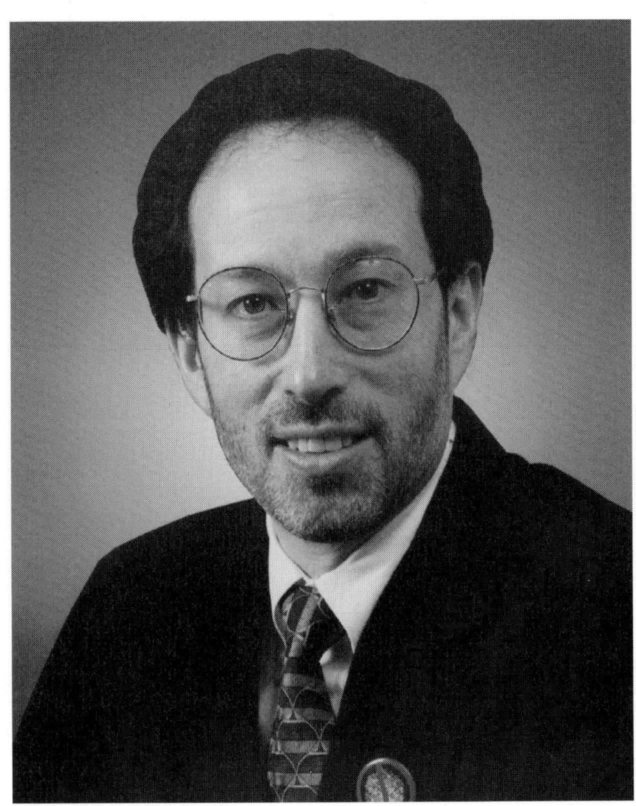

Walter A. Orenstein, M.D.

To Susan, the love of my life.
S.A.P.

To my loving and supportive wife, Diane, and our children, Eleza and Evan.
W.A.O.

Contributors

Gordon Ada, D.Sc.
Visiting Fellow, Division of Immunology and Cell Biology, John Curtin School of Medical Research, Australian National University, Canberra City, Australia.
The Immunology of Vaccination

Nancy H. Arden, M.N.
Research Associate, Baylor College of Medicine, Houston, Texas.
Inactivated Influenza Vaccines

Elizabeth Day Barnett, M.D.
Assistant Professor of Pediatrics, Boston University School of Medicine; Assistant Professor of Pediatrics, Maxwell Finland Laboratory for Infectious Diseases, Boston Medical Center, Boston, Massachusetts.
Vaccines for International Travel

P. Noel Barrett, Ph.D.
Vice-President, Research and Development of Vaccines, Baxter-Immuno Biomedical Research Center, Orth/Donau, Austria.
Tick-Borne Encephalitis Vaccine

Philip S. Brachman, M.D.
Professor, Department of International Health, Emory University, Rollins School of Public Health, Atlanta, Georgia.
Anthrax

Martin L. Bryant, Ph.D., M.D.
Vice-President of Research, Aviron, Mountain View, California.
Live Influenza Virus Vaccine

Michel Cadoz, M.D.
Clinical Research Director, Pasteur Mérieux Connaught, Marcy L'Etoile, France.
Cholera Vaccines

Gwong-Jen J. Chang, D.V.M., Ph.D.
Team Leader, Molecular Epidemiology and Immunochemistry Laboratory, Arbovirus Diseases Branch, Division of Vectorborne Infectious Diseases, Centers for Disease Control and Prevention, Fort Collins, Colorado.
Japanese Encephalitis Vaccines

Robert T. Chen, M.D.
Chief, Vaccine Safety and Development Activity, National Immunization Program, Centers for Disease Control and Prevention, Atlanta, Georgia.
Vaccines for International Travel; Safety of Vaccines

H. Fred Clark, D.V.M., Ph.D.
Research Professor of Pediatrics, School of Medicine; Adjunct Associate Professor, School of Veterinary Medicine, University of Pennsylvania, Philadelphia, Pennsylvania.
Rotavirus Vaccines

Stephen L. Cochi, M.D., M.P.H.
Director, Vaccine Preventable Disease Eradication Division, National Immunization Program, Centers for Disease Control and Prevention, Atlanta, Georgia.
Live Attenuated Poliovirus Vaccines

Felicity T. Cutts, M.D., M.Sc.
Reader in International Health and Epidemiology, London School of Hygiene and Tropical Medicine, London, England, United Kingdom.
Vaccination Programs in Developing Countries

Michael D. Decker, M.D., M.P.H.
Associate Professor, Departments of Preventive Medicine and Medicine (Infectious Diseases), Vanderbilt University School of Medicine, Nashville, Tennessee.
Pertussis Vaccine; Combination Vaccines

David T. Dennis, M.D., M.P.H., D.C.M.T.
Faculty Affiliate, Department of Environmental Health, Colorado State University; Chief, Bacterial Zoonoses Branch, Division of Vectorborne Infectious Diseases, National Center for Infectious Disease, Centers for Disease Control and Infection, Fort Collins, Colorado.
Plague

Sieghart Dittman, M.D.
Coordinator, Communicable Disease and Immunization Programme, World Health Organization, Regional Office for Europe, Copenhagen, Denmark.
Immunization in Europe

Friedrich Dorner, Ph.D.
Professor, Institute for Applied Microbiology, Vienna; General Manager/Vice-President of Vaccines, Baxter-Immuno Biomedical Research Center, Orth/Donau, Austria.
Tick-Borne Encephalitis Vaccine

Gary B. Ebbert, Ph.D.
Corporate Vice President, Technology, Pasteur Mérieux Connaught, Swiftwater, Pennsylvania.
Overview of Vaccine Manufacturing and Quality Assurance

Kathryn M. Edwards, M.D.
Professor of Pediatrics, Vanderbilt University School of Medicine, Division of Pediatric Infectious Disease, Nashville, Tennessee.
Pertussis Vaccine; Combination Vaccines

Stephen Eley, B.Sc. (Hons.)
Principal Scientist, Defence Evaluation and Research Agency, Salisbury, Wiltshire, United Kingdom.
Plague

Ronald W. Ellis, Ph.D.
Vice-President, Vaccine Development, General Manager, Biochem Pharma, Inc., Northborough, Massachusetts.
New Technologies for Making Vaccines

Juhani Eskola, M.D.
Research Professor, Director, Division of Infectious Diseases, National Public Health Institute, Helsinki, Finland.
Pneumococcal Vaccine

Geoffrey Evans, M.D.
Medical Director, National Vaccine Injury Compensation Program, Health Resources and Services Information, Rockville, Maryland.
U.S. Law

Janine Evans, M.D.
Associate Professor of Medicine, Section of Rheumatology, Yale University School of Medicine, New Haven, Connecticut.
Lyme Disease Vaccine

Jean-Louis Excler, M.D.
Medical Officer, Pasteur Mérieux Connaught, Marnes-La-Coquette, France.
Human Immunodeficiency Virus

David S. Fedson, M.D.
Former Harry T. Peters, Jr., Professor of Internal Medicine, University of Virginia School of Medicine, Charlottesville, Virginia; Director, Medical Affairs, Pasteur Mérieux MSD, Lyon, France.
Pneumococcal Vaccine

Stephen M. Feinstone, M.D.
Chief, Laboratory of Hepatitis Viruses, Center for Biologics Evaluation and Research, U.S. Food and Drug Administration, Bethesda, Maryland.
Hepatitis A Vaccine

Erol Fikrig, M.D.
Associate Professor, Yale School of Medicine, New Haven, Connecticut.
Lyme Disease Vaccine

George R. French, Ph.D.
Former General Manager of the Salk Institute, Government Services Division, Swiftwater, Pennsylvania.
Miscellaneous Limited-Use Vaccines

Arthur M. Friedlander, M.D.
US Army Medical Research Institute, Fort Detrick, Maryland.
Anthrax

Charlotte A. Gaydos, M.P.H., Dr.P.H.
Assistant Professor, Infectious Diseases Division, Johns Hopkins University School of Medicine, Baltimore, Maryland.
Adenovirus Vaccines

Joel C. Gaydos, M.D., M.P.H.
Adjunct Associate Professor of Preventive Medicine and Biometrics, F. Edward Hébert School of Medicine, Uniformed Services University of the Health Sciences, Bethesda, Maryland; Coordinator, United States Department of Defense, Global Emerging Infections System, The Henry M. Jackson Foundation, Rockville, Maryland; The Walter Reed Army Institute of Research, Washington, D.C.
Adenovirus Vaccines

Anne A. Gershon, M.D.
Professor of Pediatrics, Columbia University, College of Physicians and Surgeons; Attending Physician, Babies and Children's Hospital, New York, New York.
Varicella Vaccine

Marc P. Girard, D.V.M., D.Sc.
Professor, Institut Pasteur, Paris, France.
Human Immunodeficiency Virus

Roger I. Glass, M.D., Ph.D.
Chief, Viral Gastroenteritis Section, National Center for Infectious Diseases, Centers for Disease Control and Prevention; Clinical Professor, Department of Pediatrics, Emory University School of Medicine; Adjunct Professor of International Health, Emory University, Rollins School of Public Health, Atlanta, Georgia.
Rotavirus Vaccines

Robyn Gopin, J.D.
Office of the General Counsel, US Department of Health and Human Services, Rockville, Maryland.
U.S. Law

Ian D. Gust, M.D.
Professor of Clinical Virology, University of Melbourne, Honorary Professor of Microbiology, Monash University, Director, Research and Development, CSL, Ltd., Melbourne, Victoria, Australia.
Hepatitis A Vaccine

M. Carolyn Hardegree, M.D.
Director, Office of Vaccines Research and Review, Center for Biologics Evaluation and Research, Food and Drug Administration, Bethesda, Maryland.
Regulation and Testing of Vaccines

Donald A. Henderson, M.D., M.P.H.
University Distinguished Service Professor, The Johns Hopkins School of Hygiene and Public Health, Baltimore, Maryland.
Smallpox and Vaccinia

M. Louise Herlocher, M.S., Ph.D.
Assistant Research Scientist, Department of Epidemiology, University of Michigan, School of Public Health, Ann Arbor, Michigan.
Live Influenza Virus Vaccine

Alan R. Hinman, M.D., M.P.H.
Adjunct Professor of Epidemiology, Rollins School of Public Health, Emory University, Atlanta; Senior Consultant for Public Health Programs, Task Force for Child Survival and Development, Decatur, Georgia.
Public Health Considerations—United States; Cost-Benefit and Cost-Effectiveness Analysis of Vaccine Policy

Peter J. Hotez, M.D., Ph.D.
Associate Professor, Departments of Epidemiology and Public Health and Pediatrics (Infectious Diseases Division), Yale University School of Medicine; Associate Physician, Children's Hospital at Yale–New Haven, New Haven, Connecticut.
Parasitic Disease Vaccines

Patricia A. Hughes, D.O.
Assistant Professor of Pediatrics and Infectious Disease, Albany Medical College, Albany, New York.
Meningococcal Vaccines

Mark Kane, M.D.
Medical Officer, Expanded Program on Immunization, Global Program for Vaccines and Immunization, World Health Organization, Geneva, Switzerland.
Hepatitis B Vaccine

Samuel L. Katz, M.D.
Wilburt C. Davison Professor and Chairman Emeritus, Department of Pediatrics, Duke University Medical Center, Durham, North Carolina.
Measles Vaccine

Edwin D. Kilbourne, M.D.
Research Professor, Department of Microbiology and Immunology, New York Medical College, Valhalla, New York.
Inactivated Influenza Vaccines

Edmund W. Kitch, J.D.
Joseph M. Hartfield Professor of Law, University of Virginia, Charlottesville, Virginia.
U.S. Law

Hilary Koprowski, M.D.
Professor, Department of Microbiology and Immunology, Head, Center of Neurovirology, President, Biotechnology Foundation, Inc., Thomas Jefferson University, Philadelphia, Pennsylvania.
Rabies Vaccine

Martha L. Lepow, M.D.
Professor of Pediatrics, Albany Medical College, Attending Physician, Albany Medical Center Hospital, Albany, New York.
Meningococcal Vaccines

Myron M. Levine, M.D., D.T.P.H.
Professor, Departments of Medicine and Pediatrics, Director, Center for Vaccine Development, University of Maryland School of Medicine, Baltimore, Maryland.
Typhoid Fever Vaccines

Per Ljungman, M.D., Ph.D.
Associate Professor of Hematology, Department of Medicine, Head, Department of Hematology, Huddinge University Hospital, Karolinska Institute, Huddinge, Sweden.
Immunization in the Immunocompromised Host

Hunein F. Maassab, M.P.H., Ph.D.
Professor, Department of Epidemiology, University of Michigan School of Public Health, Ann Arbor, Michigan.
Live Influenza Virus Vaccine

Francis J. Mahoney, M.D.
Medical Epidemiologist, Chief, Hepatitis Prevention Unit, Centers for Disease Control and Prevention, Atlanta, Georgia.
Hepatitis B Vaccine

Lauri E. Markowitz, M.D.
Scientific Director, Department of Retrovirology, AFRIMS, Bangkok, Thailand.
Measles Vaccine

Eugene D. Mascolo, B.S.
Director, Business Resource Planning, Pasteur Mérieux Connaught, Swiftwater, Pennsylvania.
Overview of Vaccine Manufacturing and Quality Assurance

Joseph L. Melnick, Ph.D.
Distinguished Service Professor—Emeritus Faculty, Division of Molecular Virology, Baylor College of Medicine, Houston, Texas.
Live Attenuated Poliovirus Vaccines

Mark A. Miller, M.D.
Medical Officer, Children's Vaccine Initiative, World Health Organization, Geneva, Switzerland.
Cost-Benefit and Cost-Effectiveness Analysis of Vaccine Policy

Thomas P. Monath, M.D.
Vice-President, Research and Medical Affairs, OraVay, Inc., Cambridge, Massachusetts; Adjunct Professor, Department of Tropical Public Health, Harvard School of Public Health, Boston, Massachusetts.
Yellow Fever

Edward A. Mortimer, Jr., M.D.
Elisabeth Severance Prentiss Professor of Epidemiology Emeritus, Case Western Reserve University School of Medicine, Associate Pediatrician, University Hospitals, Cleveland, Ohio.
Diphtheria Toxoid; Pertussis Vaccine

Bernard Moss, M.D., Ph.D.
Chief, Laboratory of Viral Diseases, National Institutes of Health, Bethesda, Maryland.
Smallpox and Vaccinia

Andrew D. Murdin, Ph.D.
Section Head, Molecular Vaccines, Pasteur Mérieux Connaught, North York, Ontario, Canada.
Inactivated Polio Vaccine

Daniel M. Musher, M.D.
Professor of Medicine, Professor of Microbiology and Immunology, Head of Infectious Diseases, Baylor College of Medicine, Chief, Infectious Disease Section, Veterans Affairs Medical Center, Houston, Texas.
Pneumococcal Vaccine

Paul A. Offit, M.D.
Associate Professor, University of Pennsylvania School of Medicine; Chief, Section of Infectious Diseases, Henle Professor of Immunologic and Infectious Diseases, The Children's Hospital of Philadelphia, Philadelphia, Pennsylvania.
Rotavirus Vaccines

Jean-Marc Olivé, M.D., M.P.H.
Medical Officer, Expanded Programe on Immunization, Global Programe for Vaccine and Immunization, World Health Organization, Geneva, Switzerland.
Vaccination Programs in Developing Countries

Walter A. Orenstein, M.D.
Director, National Immunization Program, Centers for Disease Control and Prevention, Atlanta, Georgia.
Tetanus Toxoid; Public Health Considerations—United States

Paul D. Parkman, M.D.
President, Parkman Associates, Kensington, Maryland.
Regulation and Testing of Vaccines

Bradley A. Perkins, M.D.
Chief, Meningitis and Special Pathogens Branch, Division of Bacterial and Mycotic Diseases, Centers for Disease Control and Prevention, Atlanta, Georgia.
Meningococcal Vaccines

Georges Peter, M.D.
Professor of Pediatrics, Brown University School of Medicine; Director, Division of Pediatric Infectious Diseases, Rhode Island Hospital (Hasbro Children's Hospital), Providence, Rhode Island.
General Immunization Practices

Stanley A. Plotkin, M.D.
Former Medical and Scientific Director, Pasteur Mérieux Connaught, Marnes-la-Coquette, France; Emeritus Professor of Pediatrics, University of Pennsylvania,

Emeritus Professor, Wistar Institute, Former Chief, Division of Infectious Diseases, The Children's Hospital of Pennsylvania, Philadelphia, Pennsylvania.
A Short History of Vaccination; Mumps Vaccine; Inactivated Polio Vaccine; Rubella Vaccine; Miscellaneous Limited-Use Vaccines; Rabies Vaccine; Cytomegalovirus Vaccines; Tick-Borne Encephalitis Vaccine

Susan L. Plotkin, M.S.L.S.
Doylestown, Pennsylvania.
A Short History of Vaccination

Jan T. Poolman, Ph.D.
Associate Director, Head, Preclinical Bacteriology—Immunology Research and Development, SmithKline Beecham, Rixensart, Belgium.
Meningococcal Vaccines

Stephen C. Redd, M.D.
Chief, Air Pollution and Respiratory Health Branch, National Center for Environmental Health, Former Chief, Measles Elimination Activity, National Immunization Program, Centers for Disease Control and Prevention, Atlanta, Georgia.
Measles Vaccine

Michel Rey, M.D.
Professor Emeritus, Professor of Infectious and Tropical Diseases, School of Medicine, Clermont-Ferrand, France.
Vaccines for International Travel

Frederick C. Robbins, M.D.
University Professor Emeritus, Department of Epidemiology and Biostatistics, Case Western Reserve University School of Medicine, Cleveland, Ohio.
The History of Polio Vaccine Development

Lance E. Rodewald, M.D.
Associate Director for Science, Immunization Services Division, National Immunization Program, Centers for Disease Control and Prevention, Atlanta, Georgia.
Public Health Considerations—United States

Charles E. Rupprecht, V.M.D., M.S., Ph.D.
Centers for Disease Control and Prevention, Atlanta, Georgia.
Rabies Vaccine

William A. Rutala, Ph.D., M.P.H.
Professor of Medicine, Adult Infectious Disease Division, Department of Epidemiology, University of North Carolina School of Medicine, Chapel Hill, North Carolina.
Vaccines for Healthcare Workers

David A. Sack, M.D.
Professor, Department of International Health, Johns Hopkins University, Baltimore, Maryland.
Cholera Vaccines

David M. Salisbury, M.B., F.R.C.P., M.F.P.H.M.
Honorary Senior Lecturer, Child Health, Kings College, University of London; Principal Medical Officer, Department of Health, London, England, United Kingdom.
Immunization in Europe

Howard R. Six, Ph.D.
Senior Vice-President, Research and Development, Pasteur Mérieux Connaught, Swiftwater, Pennsylvania.
Overview of Vaccine Manufacturing and Quality Assurance

Kim Connelly Smith, M.D., M.P.H.
Associate Professor of Pediatrics, University of Texas-Houston Medical School, Director, Children's Tuberculosis Clinics, Hermann Children's Hospital, Lyndon B. Johnson Hospital, Houston, Texas.
Bacille Calmette-Guérin Vaccine

Jeffrey R. Starke, M.D.
Associate Professor of Pediatrics, Baylor College of Medicine, Director, Children's Tuberculosis Clinics, Ben Taub General Hospital, Houston, Texas.
Bacille Calmette-Guérin Vaccine

Roland W. Sutter, M.D., M.P.H., T.M.
Acting Chief, Technical Services Branch, Vaccine Preventable Disease Eradication Division, National Immunization Program, Centers for Disease Control and Prevention, Atlanta, Georgia.
Live Attenuated Poliovirus Vaccines; Tetanus Toxoid

Michiaki Takahashi, M.D.
Emeritus Professor of Osaka University, Director, Research Foundation for Microbial Diseases of Osaka University, Suita City, Osaka, Japan.
Varicella Vaccine

Richard W. Titball, B.Sc., Ph.D.
Head of Microbiology, Defence Evaluation and Research Agency, Salisbury, Wiltshire, United Kingdom.
Plague

Theodore F. Tsai, M.D., M.P.H.
Medical Officer, Division of Vectorborne Infectious Diseases, Centers for Disease Control and Prevention, Fort Collins, Colorado.
Japanese Encephalitis Vaccines

Emmanuel Vidor, M.D.
Direction Médicale, Pasteur Mérieux Connaught, Lyon, France.
Inactivated Polio Vaccine

Joel I. Ward, M.D.
Professor of Pediatrics, University of California, Los Angeles School of Medicine, Harbor-UCLA Medical Center, UCLA Center for Vaccine Research, Los Angeles; Chief, Pediatric Infectious Diseases, Harbor–UCLA Medical Center, Torrance, California.
Haemophilus influenzae *Vaccines*

Steven G. F. Wassilak, M.D.
Medical Epidemiologist, Vaccine Preventable Disease Eradication Division, National Immunization Program, Centers for Disease Control and Prevention, Atlanta, Georgia; Communicable Diseases and Immunization Unit, World Health Organization, Regional Office for Europe, Copenhagen, Denmark.
Tetanus Toxoid

John C. Watson, M.D., M.P.H.
Medical Epidemiologist, National Immunization Program, Centers for Disease Control and Prevention, Atlanta, Georgia.
General Immunization Practices

David J. Weber, M.D., M.P.H.
Associate Professor of Medicine, Pediatrics, and Epidemiology, UNC Schools of Medicine and Public Health; Associate Chief of Staff, Medical Director, Hospital of Epidemiology and Occupational Health, UNC Hospitals, Chapel Hill, North Carolina.
Vaccines for Healthcare Workers

Kristen Weigle, M.D., M.P.H.
Associate Professor, Departments of Epidemiology and Pediatrics, University of North Carolina Schools of Public Health and Medicine; Chapel Hill, North Carolina.
Vaccines for Healthcare Workers

Melinda Wharton, M.D., M.P.H.
Chief, Child Vaccine Preventable Diseases Branch, Epidemiology and Surveillance Division, National Immunization Program, Centers for Disease Control and Prevention, Atlanta, Georgia.
Diphtheria Toxoid; Mumps Vaccine

C. Jo White, M.D.
Senior Vice-President, Medical Affairs, Aviron, Mountain View, California.
Varicella Vaccine

E. Diane Williamson, B.Sc., Ph.D.
Principal Scientist, Defence Evaluation and Research Agency, Salisbury, Wiltshire, United Kingdom.
Plague

Yong Xin Yu
Professor, Former Chief, First Division of Viral Vaccines, National Institute for Control of Pharmaceutical and Biological Products, Temple of Heaven, Beijing, China.
Japanese Encephalitis Vaccines

Kenneth M. Zangwill, M.D.
Assistant Professor of Pediatrics, Harbor-UCLA Medical Center, University of California at Los Angeles, Member, Division of Infectious Diseases and UCLA Center for Vaccine Research, Harbor-UCLA Medical Center, Los Angeles, California.
Haemophilus influenzae *Vaccines*

Preface

The third edition of this book appears at a time when vaccines are very popular: biotechnology is churning out new candidate antigens, the pharmaceutical industry now views biologicals as potentially lucrative, and vaccination has taken on a political dimension reflected in declarations by heads of state. Recent commemoration of the 200th anniversary of Jenner's first smallpox vaccination in 1796 and the 100th anniversary of Pasteur's death in 1895 both served to augment publicity about vaccines. Moreover, the escalating costs of curative medicine make prevention in general, and vaccines in particular, attractive to economists.

Thus, it seemed appropriate to enlarge the book considerably, all the more so in view of the signal advances in vaccination that have been made since the last edition, including the plummeting incidence of poliomyelitis, the dramatic success of vaccination against *Haemophilus influenzae* type b disease, the increasing use of varicella vaccine, the adoption of acellular pertussis vaccines by a number of countries, and the efflorescence of combination vaccines. Although all of these developments are covered, this new edition is not merely an updated version of the previous one. We have added new chapters on general aspects of vaccination (immunology, vaccine production, general immunization practices, cost-benefit analyses, vaccine safety, immunization of healthcare workers, immunization for foreign travel, and immunization of the immunocompromised) and on specific vaccines (combinations, plague, Lyme disease, parasitic diseases, and miscellaneous arbovirus and rickettsial vaccines).

The list of authors shows that the participation of the Centers for Disease Control and Prevention, Atlanta, has materially increased and strengthened the book with regard to public health issues. We have also emphasized international public health through the addition of chapters on concerns specific to Europe and the developing world.

In accomplishing this task, we had to do without the help of Ted Mortimer, who was co-editor for the first two editions, and whose efforts were crucial to their success. Although illness has lowered the volume of Ted's voice and caused him to bow out as co-editor, his figurative voice and his influence continue unabated in the world of vaccines.

As we enter the 21st century, a paradox exists in the world of vaccines: never have so many children benefited from vaccination, and yet many children and adults throughout the world still do not receive recommended vaccines, leading to unnecessary infectious disease burdens. The gap in the use of new vaccines between the developing world and the developed world is large. Means must be found to assure that poorer countries can also benefit from the new but more costly technologies. Economic and organizational issues interfere with improvement in extension of preventive medicine to the poorer countries, although on the positive side the growing economies in many such nations make improvement in vaccination quite feasible.

In the rich countries, antivaccinationists still thrive, often becoming stronger as vaccines reduce the occurrence of a disease to the point that, to the unsophisticated, it appears that vaccines offer little benefit, only risk. These groups advocate individual rights over protection of the community and frequently mistake a temporal relationship to vaccination as causal. In that regard, one cannot overemphasize the importance of nascent epidemiological studies using linked databases that enable objective assessment of risk and association with vaccination.

Finally, we propose a new definition of a vaccine, inasmuch as former definitions, such as "a preparation of killed microorganisms or living attenuated organisms that is administered to produce or artificially increase immunity to a particular disease" are too vague. The following is a modern definition:

> Vaccines are proteins, polysaccharides, or nucleic acids of pathogens that are delivered to the immune system as single entities, as part of complex particles, or by living attenuated agents or vectors, thereby inducing specific responses that inactivate, destroy, or suppress the pathogen.

Stanley A. Plotkin, M.D.
Walter A. Orenstein, M.D.

Contents

PUBLIC HEALTH AND REGULATORY ISSUES

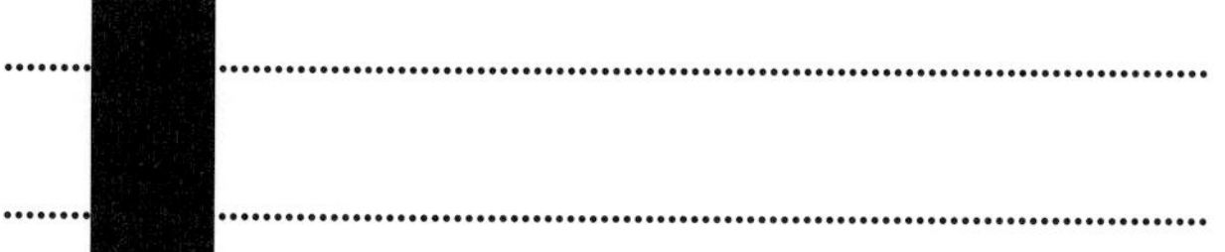

INTRODUCTION

chapter 1

A Short History of Vaccination

Susan L. Plotkin
Stanley A. Plotkin

Vaccination as a deliberate attempt to protect humans against disease has a long history, although only in the 20th century has the practice flowered into the routine vaccination of large populations. During the last 200 years, since the time of Edward Jenner (Fig. 1–1), vaccination has controlled the following 10 major diseases, at least in parts of the world: smallpox, diphtheria, tetanus, yellow fever, pertussis, *Haemophilus influenzae* type b disease, poliomyelitis, measles, mumps, and rubella. In the case of smallpox, the dream of eradication has been fulfilled, as this disease has disappeared from the world.[1] Poliomyelitis is targeted by the World Health Organization for eradication by the year 2000. Vaccinations against influenza, hepatitis B, and pneumococcal infection have made major headway against those diseases, although much remains to be done, even in developed countries.

The impact of vaccination on the health of the world's peoples is hard to exaggerate. With the exception of safe water, no other modality, not even antibiotics, has had such a major effect on mortality reduction and population growth.

EARLY DEVELOPMENTS

Attempts to vaccinate did not begin with Edward Jenner. In the 7th century, some Indian Buddhists drank snake venom in an attempt to become immune to its effect. They may have been inducing toxoid-like immunity.[2] Writings citing the use of inoculation and variolation in 10th-century China[3–5] make interesting reading but apparently cannot be verified.[6] There is, however, 17th-century documentation of variolation in China with reference to its use in the 16th century. A Chinese medical text printed in 1742, *The Golden Mirror of Medicine*, listed four forms of inoculation against smallpox practiced in China at least since 1695: (1) the nose plugged with powdered scabs laid on cotton wool, (2) powdered scabs blown into the nose, (3) the undergarments of an infected child put on a healthy child for several days, and (4) a piece of cotton smeared with the

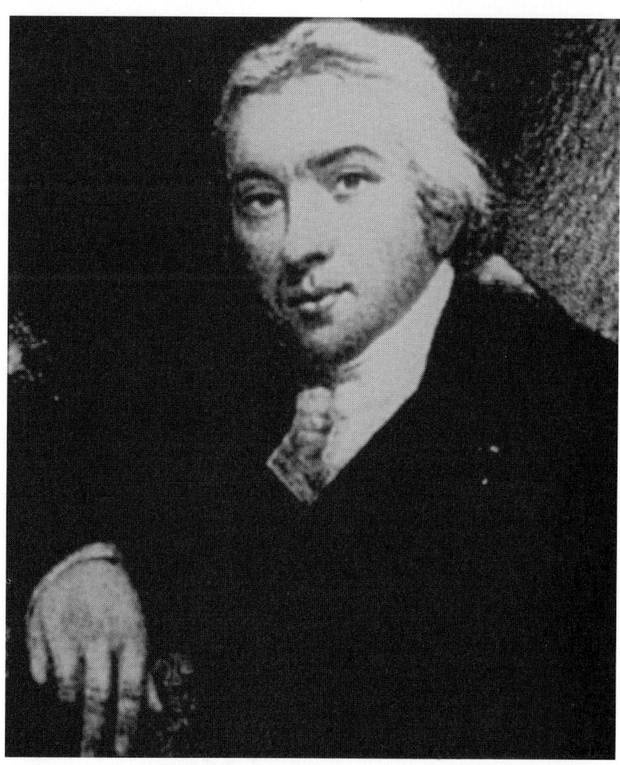

Figure 1–1. Edward Jenner. (Photo courtesy of the Institute of the History of Medicine, The Johns Hopkins University, Baltimore, MD.)

contents of a vesicle and stuffed into the nose.[3,6] Another text on Chinese medicine stated that white cow fleas were used for smallpox prevention a century before Jenner.[4] The fleas were ground into powder and made into pills, which may have been the first attempt at an oral vaccine.

Variolation, the introduction of dried pus from smallpox pustules into the skin of the patient, was practiced at regular intervals by the Brahmin caste of Hindus in India in the 16th century. Some claim that a description of variolation can be found in the *Atharva Veda* (a pre-Hindu Indian religious text circa 1000 BC), but this is probably exaggerated enthusiasm.[7] Vaccination for smallpox with cowpox did not begin to be used in India until after Jenner's discovery, although when "vaccination" arrived in India, attempts were made to alter some Indian religious documents to make it appear to be an earlier Indian practice.[7]

Similarly, in the mid-18th century, several treatises were written on inoculation or vaccination against measles, and the Scottish physician Francis Home actively inoculated humans against measles and published the results of his work.[8–10]

To protect against smallpox, variolation was introduced into England by Lady Mary Wortley Montagu in 1721, when she returned from Constantinople, where she had observed Muslims use the technique. Although the treatment was often effective, results were erratic, and 2 to 3% of those treated died of smallpox obtained from the variolation itself.[11] In 1774 in Yetminster, England (Dorset County), a cattle breeder named Benjamin Jesty, himself immune to smallpox after contracting cowpox from his herd, deliberately inoculated his wife and two children with cowpox to avoid a smallpox epidemic. His experiment succeeded; the two children remained immune even 15 years later, when they were deliberately inoculated with smallpox.[11]

Thus, the precise origin of variolation remains unknown, but it appears to have developed somewhere in Central Asia in the early part of the second millennium and then spread east to China and west to Turkey and Europe.

Despite these antecedents, Edward Jenner's work with cowpox vaccination holds title to the first scientific attempt to control an infectious disease by means of deliberate systematic inoculation.[12]

Cowpox was not a widespread disease. It appeared sporadically in certain rural counties of England. Thus, the local wisdom that those who contracted cowpox "did not take the smallpox" was not widely known. Jenner took this village folklore and experimented with it. Eventually, he proved that cowpox could be passed directly from one infected person to another, thereby providing "large-scale" inoculation without depending on the sporadic outbreaks of natural cowpox. When Jenner published his work *Variolae Vaccinae* in 1798, he brought to the attention of the entire medical community the merits of inoculation with the relatively obscure animal disease, cowpox, to prevent one of humankind's deadliest scourges. Years after his own successful experiments had been published and his reputation secured, Jenner acknowledged Jesty's early work.

During the 87 years that elapsed between Jenner's *Variolae Vaccinae* treatise and Louis Pasteur's (Fig. 1–2) first human vaccination against rabies (1885), the field was far from dormant. The ideas of attenuation and virulence were developing, and the necessity of revaccination was discussed.[12a] By 1810, Jenner realized that immunity was not lifelong, but he did not know why.[11] The concept of *passages* of the immunizing agent (transmission from one human or animal to another) was well formed. In 1836, Edward Ballard discussed the problems of choosing new strains of cowpox for vaccination because the old strains were too weak from so many passages. He recommended that the lymph (vesicle fluid) be passed back through a calf to regain strength.[13]

The "lymph" obtained from the cow itself came under scrutiny.[14] Concern had long been expressed that other diseases, such as syphilis, sometimes were transmitted along with the vaccinia virus. German scientists in about 1850 began to use glycerin to kill bacteria and also to preserve the lymph.[15] That process made available a ready supply of a stable vaccine of consistent potency.[11]

Pasteur's work on the attenuation of the chicken cholera bacterium in the latter half of the 1870s was the first major advance after Jenner's *Variolae Vaccinae*. Pasteur drew on concepts that had been developing for at least 40 years: attenuation; modification through passage; renewed virulence; and, most important, the need to replace person-to-person (or animal-to-animal) vaccination with something safer, more consistent, and less likely to transmit other diseases.

In the summer of 1879, Pasteur left a chicken cholera culture (*Pasteurella multocida*), exposed to air over a long holiday. On his return, he noticed that the culture, weakened by its exposure to the air, provided immunity

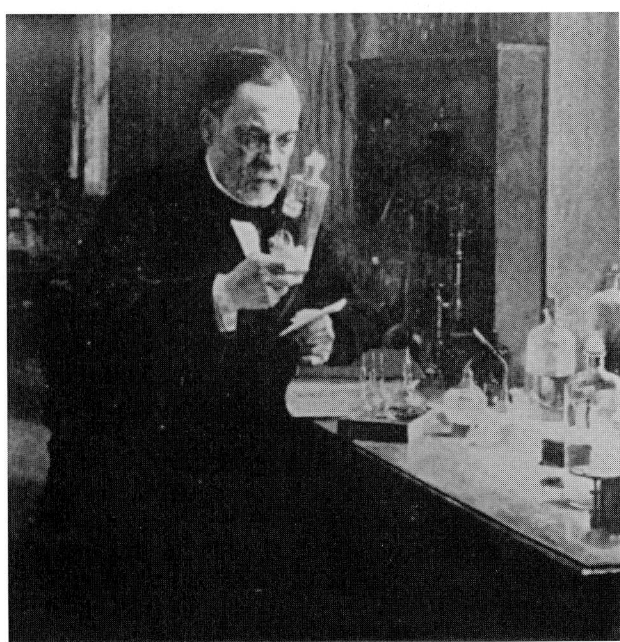

Figure 1–2. Louis Pasteur. (Photo courtesy of the Pasteur Institute, Paris.)

against a challenge with virulent organisms. He was quick to perceive that the principle was the same as Jenner's (i.e., using a weakened form of a virus to provide immunity), although attenuation had been achieved in a different manner.[15] Pasteur thought it might be preferable to use a weakened form of chicken cholera rather than a related organism to prevent the disease, as in Jenner's use of vaccinia to prevent smallpox. Thus, it would be less likely to transmit other diseases. Publication of his results to the Academy of Sciences in 1880 generated considerable interest.[16] In a sense, Pasteur's chicken cholera vaccine harkened back to Lady Montagu's variolation technique, which used a weakened form of smallpox to inoculate against smallpox. Therefore, the modern sense of vaccination, involving the development of vaccines in the laboratory, was really introduced with Pasteur's chicken cholera vaccine, 5 years before the famous vaccination of Joseph Meister against rabies.

Pasteur's research on anthrax began in 1877 and overlapped with his work on chicken cholera. In 1876, Robert Koch had demonstrated the anthrax bacillus and described its capability to survive indefinitely in the form of spores.[17] Although Casimir Davaine had seen the bacillus in 1850, and had even postulated it as the cause of anthrax,[18, 19] Koch was the first to obtain pure cultures of anthrax bacillus. He transmitted it to several laboratory animals and proved that there was a causal relationship between this bacillus and the disease anthrax.

Pasteur was aware of Davaine's and Koch's work, as well as that of a veterinarian named Henri Toussaint.[20] Indeed, he was in a neck and neck competition with Toussaint to find the first anthrax vaccine. The first public controlled experiment of anthrax vaccine took place at Pouilly-le-Fort on May 5, 1881.[21] It was initiated by Pasteur in an effort to silence his many critics who doubted that vaccination could be done systematically. Pasteur inoculated 24 sheep, 1 goat, and 6 cows with attenuated anthrax bacilli. On May 17, these same animals were inoculated again with more virulent but still attenuated anthrax bacilli. At the same time, 24 sheep, 1 goat, and 4 cows were kept as controls and given no inoculations. On May 31, both groups were inoculated with virulent anthrax, from spores that Pasteur had kept in his laboratory since 1877.

By June 2, 21 of the nonvaccinated sheep and the nonvaccinated goat were dead. Two more nonvaccinated sheep died before the spectators' eyes, and the last one succumbed before the day's end. All the vaccinated sheep, the vaccinated goat, and the six cows remained healthy. (The nonvaccinated cows did not die but showed clear evidence of having contracted anthrax. Their size perhaps had saved them.)

At the end of this experiment, the triumphant Pasteur wrote that he had shown that humans could now have vaccines, cultivatable at will by a method that could be generalized.

Recently, it has been documented that Pasteur's results with chicken cholera and anthrax were not as clear cut as was previously thought. It appears that Pasteur deliberately withheld critical data in his communications to the Academie de Medicine.[22–24] However, this in no way detracts from the significance of his findings, which proved that one could "create" standardized, reproducible vaccines at will. Pasteur's experiments with chicken cholera and anthrax[21] announced to the world that a new, scientific era in vaccination had begun.

By the time the rabies vaccine was first administered to humans in 1885,[25] the general public as well as the scientific community was well aware of the "new vaccination," but only in relation to animals. With the vaccination of Joseph Meister and Jean Baptiste Jupille, an outcry went forth. The thought of deliberately introducing a deadly agent—in any form—into a human being was met with horror and outrage. The concept of attenuation did not appease the general public or many of the medical community; those cases of rabies that occurred in vaccinees were attributed to the vaccine and were viewed as medical murders. Even Émile Roux, one of Pasteur's staunchest allies and a collaborator in the rabies experiments, was appalled at the vaccination of Joseph Meister, which he thought was unjustified by the experiments conducted up to that point. An examination of Pasteur's laboratory notebooks indicates that Roux was right to object.[23] These same notebooks also tell us that before vaccinating Joseph Meister, Pasteur had vaccinated two other people who had little chance of survival after having been seriously bitten by rabid animals. One of the two had died.[23] Roux, although he was a physician, did not give the injections to Joseph Meister. He left Pasteur's laboratory in protest and did not return for many months.[23, 26] The fact that hundreds of people were saved from rabies—many more than those who allegedly died from vaccination—did not lessen the opposition to rabies vaccination in humans. After all, 45 years earlier, variolation had been made a felony in England for the very same reason: It introduced the actual virus into a human being.[11]

The next major step in vaccine development took place in the United States shortly after Pasteur's administration of the chemically attenuated rabies vaccine. This step involved a new concept that was as important as Pasteur's: killed vaccines. In 1886, Edmund Salmon and Theobald Smith (Fig. 1–3) published their work on a killed hog cholera "virus" vaccine.[27, 28] The virus, killed by heat, immunized pigeons against the disease. The vaccine that they developed was actually a bacterial vaccine against a cholera-like salmonellosis,[29] but the term *virus* in the latter half of the 19th century did not have the specific meaning it has today. These events show that the ideas of live and killed vaccines developed almost simultaneously. The seminal work of Salmon and Smith bore fruit for humans 15 years later, when killed vaccines were developed for typhoid, cholera, and plague.

In 1888, Salmon read a paper to the American Association for the Advancement of Science defending their (Salmon and Smith's) priority in developing the first killed vaccine.[30] Ironically, their competitors were Charles Chamberland and Roux from Pasteur's laboratory, who had published on the same topic in December 1887,[31] 16 months after Salmon and Smith's original paper. The Institut Pasteur had just been established in

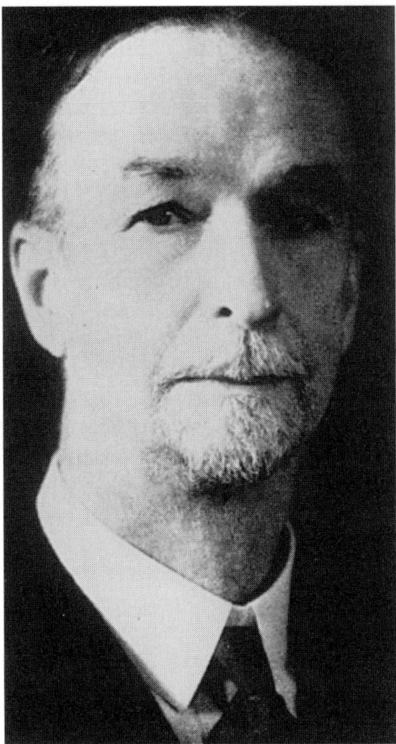

Figure 1–3. Theobald Smith. (From Cohen B (ed). Chronicles of the Society of American Bacteriologists, 1899–1950. Baltimore, Society of American Bacteriologists, 1950, p 36.)

1887; Pasteur was at the height of his fame and worldwide prestige. Not surprisingly, Salmon and Smith's claim was lost in the aura surrounding Pasteur and his associates. Salmon and Smith were working for the U.S. Department of Agriculture at the time of their discovery. Thus, even 100 years ago, the Institut Pasteur and the U.S. government were involved in disputations over discovery rights—similar to the more recent controversy over the discovery of the human immunodeficiency virus.

In parallel with the focused research on vaccines, important work on immunity was also being pursued at the end of the 19th century. Elie Metchnikoff, another Pasteur protégé, first published his theory of cellular immunity in 1884.[11, 32] He named those body cells that ingested and destroyed invading microorganisms and other foreign bodies *phagocytes*. Although he did not appreciate the role of serum and plasma in immunity at this early date, his work was truly pioneering, and for this he shared the Nobel Prize with Paul Ehrlich in 1908 for research in immunity.

Ehrlich's receptor theory of immunity was an equally strong contribution to vaccine development. When he developed this theory in 1897, it was used mainly to explain toxin-antitoxin interactions. But as the theory gradually expanded to meet various objections, it soon became one of the cornerstones of 20th-century immunology.[33] Ehrlich's other major contribution during this period was to point out the difference between active and passive immunity.[11, 34]

At the end of the century, we begin to see the practical results of the creative period of the 1870s and 1880s in the development of killed vaccines for typhoid, plague, and cholera. Richard Pfeiffer and Wilhelm Kolle in Germany and Almroth Wright in England worked independently on killed typhoid vaccines.[35–38] To this day, the debate continues as to exactly who inoculated the first human with killed typhoid vaccine. In truth, all three individuals deserve credit, as it is now clear that several groups were working on typhoid vaccine at that time.[39]

Shibasaburo Kitasato and Alexandre Yersin, each working independently, in 1894 discovered the causative bacillus of the plague, *Pasteurella pestis*.[11, 40, 41] With Albert Calmette and Amédée Borelle, Yersin went on to develop a killed vaccine for animals,[42] but it was Waldemar Haffkine who was given the task of developing a vaccine against human plague.[43, 44] He was in India working on cholera vaccine, but when bubonic plague developed in Bombay, he switched to studies of plague immunization. Haffkine was the first to be injected with his new killed plague vaccine. More than 8000 people were then vaccinated within a few weeks. For a while, Haffkine was considered a hero. However, subsequent evaluation of the vaccine by the Indian Plague Commission and the Mulkowal incident of 1902, when 19 people died from contaminated vaccine, seemed to indicate that the vaccine was far from perfect. Haffkine was removed from his post by the Indian government. His scientific career and reputation were severely damaged; he never fully recovered from the incident and retired early from science at the age of 55 years. Later, with the wisdom of hindsight, the Indian government renamed the Plague Research Laboratory where he had worked as The Haffkine Institute. Perhaps as important as his development of the plague vaccine was Haffkine's contribution to the literature on the proper way to conduct clinical trials.[45]

John Snow had shown from 1848 to 1849 that cholera was transmitted by contaminated water,[46] although he did not know the identity of the contaminant. That answer was supplied by Robert Koch, when he isolated *Vibrio cholerae* as the causal organism in 1883.[47] Early attempts at a vaccine were made by Jaime Ferrán, a pupil of Pasteur's, and by Haffkine. Both used live cultures, and both vaccines were given up because of severe reactions.[11]

Kolle developed a heat-killed cholera vaccine in 1896.[48, 49] He grew the vibrios in agar, suspended them in saline solution, heated them at 50°C for a few minutes (later changed to 56°C for 1 hour), and then added 0.5% phenol.

Thus, at the turn of the century, there were two human virus vaccines: Jenner's original variola vaccine and Pasteur's rabies vaccine (both live). Three human bacterial vaccines also existed, for typhoid, cholera, and plague (all killed). The century's end also saw the end of the use of arm-to-arm lymph inoculation as a vehicle for smallpox vaccine. This technique was replaced by glycerinated calf lymph in 1898.[11] The majority of the fundamental concepts of vaccinology had been introduced by the end of the 19th century; the work of the early 20th century would bring refinements to these theoretical underpinnings. Not until the advent of tissue culture would the field again become so dramatically fertile (Table 1–1).

Table 1–1. **OUTLINE OF THE DEVELOPMENT OF HUMAN VACCINES**

LIVE ATTENUATED	KILLED WHOLE ORGANISM	PURIFIED PROTEIN OR POLYSACCHARIDE	GENETICALLY ENGINEERED
	18th Century		
Smallpox, 1798			
	19th Century		
Rabies, 1885	Typhoid, 1896 Cholera, 1896 Plague, 1897		
	Early 20th Century		
Bacille Calmette-Guérin, 1927 (tuberculosis) Yellow fever, 1935	Pertussis, 1926 (whole cell) Influenza, 1936 Rickettsia, 1938	Diphtheria, 1923 Tetanus, 1927	
	After World War II (Cell Culture)		
Polio (oral) Measles Mumps Rubella Adenovirus Typhoid (salmonella Ty21a) Varicella Rotavirus (reassortants)	Polio (injected) Rabies (new) Japanese encephalitis Hepatitis A	Pneumococcus Meningococcus *Haemophilus influenzae* PRP Hepatitis B (plasma derived) Tick-borne encephalitis *H. influenzae* PRP-protein (conjugate) Typhoid (Vi) Acellular pertussis	Hepatitis B recombinant (yeast or mammalian cell derived) Pertussis toxoid

PRP, polyribosylribitol phosphate.

EARLY 20TH CENTURY

After the introduction of typhoid vaccines, Almroth Wright proceeded with a field trial among 4000 volunteers from the Indian Army that gave encouraging results. He proposed mass immunization of British troops during the Boer War (1899), but because of opposition by influential people, he was able to vaccinate only 14,000 volunteers. In fact, opposition ran so high that consignments of vaccine were dumped overboard from transport ships in Southampton. The results were catastrophic: more than 58,000 cases of typhoid and 9000 deaths in the British Army.[36] A bitter battle over the merits of the vaccine took place in the *British Medical Journal* between Wright and the statistician Karl Pearson. The scientific community itself was divided on the value of vaccination; one could expect no more from the general public. Ultimately, the War Board initiated a broad-based trial that showed the overwhelming effectiveness of the vaccine. Wright was then knighted. By the time World War I broke out, general vaccination was conducted in the British Army, although it was still not mandatory.[36, 50]

Roux and Yersin had demonstrated in 1888 that the diphtheria bacillus produced a powerful toxin.[11, 51] Two years later, Emil von Behring and Kitasato, following up on preliminary work by their colleague Karl Fraenkel, published results that showed the presence of powerful antitoxins in the serum of animals previously infected with low doses of diphtheria bacilli.[52, 53] This antitoxin neutralized diphtheria toxin in culture. Further experiments showed that the antitoxin provided protection in animals against challenge with the diphtheria bacillus itself. Progress occurred so rapidly after von Behring's discovery that the first child was treated with diphtheria antitoxin just a year later, in December 1891. Shortly thereafter, the commercial production of antitoxin began.

In the early 20th century, the chemical inactivation of diphtheria and other bacterial toxins led to the development of the first toxoids: diphtheria and tetanus. Here also, Theobald Smith played a significant role. In 1907, he determined that "toxoids" provided immunity in guinea pigs. In 1909, reporting on long-lasting immunity against diphtheria in guinea pigs immunized with toxoid, he suggested that the method of making toxoids "invites further regard to its ultimate applicability to the human body."[29, 54]

In 1923, Alexander Glenny and Barbara Hopkins showed that diphtheria toxin could be transformed into a toxoid by formalin.[55] The discovery came about when the containers in which the batches of diphtheria toxin were kept were cleaned with formalin; they were too large to be autoclaved. The residual formalin in the vats rendered the batch of toxin so weak that 1000 times the normal dose did not kill the guinea pigs. Although using this "toxoid" was certainly safer than using toxin, it could be administered only in conjunction with antitoxin. In that same year, Gaston Ramon developed a diphtheria toxoid that could be used on its own (i.e., without antitoxin) by adding formalin and incubating the mixture at 37°C for several weeks.[56]

Ramon and Christian Zoeller went on to use a tetanus toxoid developed in the same manner for the first human vaccinations against tetanus in 1926.[57, 58]

The vaccine against tuberculosis, bacille Calmette-Guérin (BCG), was the first live vaccine for humans to be produced since Pasteur's rabies vaccine in 1885. Albert Calmette was a Pasteur protégé and founder of the Pasteur Institutes at Lille and in Indochina.[11] In 1906, Calmette and Camille Guérin started subculturing a strain of mycobacteria obtained from a bovine, which they perhaps thought was the tubercle bacillus. After 13 years of attenuation by 230 passages in beef bile, this strain eventually became the BCG strain. Clinical trials in children began in 1921, and the vaccine became available for human use in 1927.[11, 59–63]

In 1931, E. W. Goodpasture introduced the use of the chorioallantoic membrane of the fertile hen's egg as a medium for growing viruses.[26, 64] This technique represented a major advance, because until then human viruses could be grown only in animals such as ferrets and mice. Ferrets were very expensive, and mouse brain could produce allergic brain encephalitis. The chick embryo proved to be a cheaper and safer medium for the cultivation of viruses. S. Monkton Copeman had made an earlier attempt to use hens' eggs to grow a virus. In the Milroy Lectures for 1898, he mentioned conducting such an experiment while studying the relationship between vaccinia and variola, but he had little success at that time.[65]

Yellow fever virus was isolated in 1927 by two independent groups: researchers at the Rockefeller Foundation working in Nigeria, who isolated the Asibi strain,[66–68] and those at the Pasteur Institute in Senegal, who isolated the French strain.[69, 70] The French strain was given to various research groups for study.[70] In 1928, A. W. Sellards at the Harvard Medical School began collaborative research on the French strain with Jean Laigret at the Pasteur Institute in Senegal. Max Theiler, working for Sellards, developed an animal model to study the virus.[71] Using mouse brain tissue as a medium, others were able to "fix" the neurovirulence of the strain,[72] which then was used as a vaccine. Theiler left Harvard after this work to join the Rockefeller Institute.

The French strain yellow fever vaccine that resulted from Theiler's work at Harvard was a live vaccine derived from mouse brain passage.[73] It was used first in humans without immune serum by Sellards and Laigret in 1932.[74] However, the neurovirulence of the French strain, owing to the strain's passage through mouse brain tissue, presented grave dangers.

The Rockefeller group, deciding to pursue a vaccine that would contain no residual neurovirulence, switched to the Asibi strain. Theiler then developed the 17D strain from Asibi in fertile hen's egg membrane per Goodpasture's method. Although not as potent as the French strain, the 17D strain was much safer.[26, 70, 75–77]

The French strain certainly saved many lives, especially in French West Africa, where it was used extensively. That vaccine (in modified form) remained in production until 1982; however, safety concerns about the use of mouse brain tissue overrode its proven efficacy, and 17D won out as the vaccine strain of choice.[70]

Wilson Smith, Christopher Andrewes, and Patrick Laidlaw isolated influenza A virus in ferrets in 1933.[78] Frank Horsfall, Alice Chenoweth, and colleagues developed a vaccine in mouse lung tissue in 1936.[79, 80] A live virus was used in the vaccine that, Chenoweth claimed, became inactivated when it was administered parenterally.[80, 81] That same year, 1936, saw the development of two killed influenza A vaccines in embryonated eggs, one by Wilson Smith[82] and the other by Thomas Francis and Thomas Magill.[83, 84] Even though these two vaccines were considered safer because they were developed in embryonated eggs, Chenoweth's mouse lung vaccine had a higher virus yield and was the first to demonstrate true protection in humans, albeit transient.

In 1937, Anatol Smorodintsev and colleagues in the Soviet Union reported on the administration of the Wilson Smith strain to humans, using dosages that were lethal when given to mice.[85] This vaccine is considered to be the first live human influenza virus vaccine, and although it would not receive a passing grade by today's standards (20% of vaccinees developed febrile influenza), it absolutely demonstrated the role of the virus in the development of influenza.[81, 86]

Once rickettsiae were discovered by Charles Nicolle in 1909 to be the cause of typhus, many attempts were made to develop vaccines against these organisms.[11] The first truly successful vaccine was developed in 1938 by Herald Cox,[87] who used the yolk sac of the chick embryo to grow *Rickettsia rickettsii.* Although Cox worked on Rocky Mountain spotted fever, once he found a method to cultivate the rickettsia, vaccines for typhus and Q fever quickly followed. There was a heavy demand for the typhus vaccine during World War II.[11, 88, 89]

Jules Bordet and Octave Gengou first observed the causal agent of pertussis in 1900 and cultivated it by 1907.[11] The production and testing of several vaccines were attempted without formal trials. Thorvald Madsen later carried out the first controlled clinical trials of a pertussis vaccine (i.e., whole killed organisms) on the Faeroe Islands from 1923 to 1924 and again in 1929.[90, 91] During the 1923 to 1924 epidemic, Madsen reported that the vaccine did not prevent disease but greatly reduced mortality and the severity of illness among vaccinated individuals. By the 1929 epidemic, the vaccine had been considerably improved.[92] Several whole-cell pertussis vaccines were in use by the late 1940s.[93, 94] However, adverse reactions made public acceptance a problem.

AFTER WORLD WAR II

The golden age of vaccine development began in 1949 with virus propagation in stationary cell culture. Goodpasture's method using chick embryo membrane was successful, but most searches for improved techniques centered around the flask culture technique of Maitland and Maitland.[11, 29] They grew vaccinia virus in sterile cultures of minced chicken kidney in media composed of chicken serum and mineral salts. Gey improved the virus yield of this method by continually rolling the tubes and thus increasing the oxygenation of the cells.[29]

Enders, Weller, and Robbins took up research on cell culture at Boston Children's Hospital in the late 1940s. After using cultures of the Maitland type, they decided to try to grow viruses in human cells using fibroblasts grown from the skin and muscle tissue of infants who had died soon after birth. Their first success was to grow Lansing type II poliovirus in human cell culture.[95] The ability to grow human viruses outside a living host, in a relatively easy and safe manner, led to an explosion of creativity in vaccinology, which continues unabated (see Table 1–1).

The first live polio vaccine, developed with a variant virus strain grown in mice, was tested in humans in 1950 by Koprowski.[96] The first licensed product developed using the tissue culture technique of Enders, Weller, and Robbins was the trivalent, formalin-inactivated polio vaccine of Salk.[97] Eventually, live poliovirus vaccines grown in monkey kidney cell culture by Sabin came into wide use.[98] Thanks to the use of these vaccines, polio has been eradicated from the Western Hemisphere, and the World Health Organization has targeted the year 2000 to efface the disease from the entire world.

During the late 1950s, Katz, Enders, and colleagues developed the Edmonston strain of measles vaccine, grown in chick embryo cell culture,[99] which was attenuated further by Schwarz[100] and Hilleman and colleagues.[101] Hilleman also attenuated the Jeryl Lynn strain of mumps virus in the hen's egg and obtained licensure in 1967.[102] Cell culture was also used to attenuate rubella virus, and by 1970 several strains had been developed by Meyer and Parkman,[103] Prinzie, Huygelen, and colleagues,[104] and Plotkin.[105] The last strain (Wistar-RA27/3), grown in human fibroblasts, is now the sole rubella vaccine in wide use.

When inactivated adenovirus vaccine proved unreliable, attention turned to the production of live attenuated vaccines. Several orally administered adenovirus vaccines were tested by Top and colleagues, including types 4, 7, and 21, which caused epidemics among military recruits.[106–108] Use of the adenovirus vaccines remains restricted to the military.

The live attenuated Oka strain of varicella vaccine was developed in the 1970s by Takahashi[109, 110] and underwent extensive clinical trials before being licensed in Japan and several European countries.[111, 112] After a long and convoluted development, licensure was obtained in the United States in 1995.[113]

Subsequent to the early work on killed typhoid vaccine, a variety of heat-phenol–killed or acetone-killed, parenteral typhoid vaccines became available.[114–117] All were subject to high rates of adverse reactions and were never considered quite satisfactory. An important advance was made by Germanier and Fürer when they developed an attenuated strain of the Gal E mutant Ty21a of *Salmonella typhi*.[118] Based on the results from preliminary vaccine studies in a volunteer group in the United States,[119] large trials were conducted successfully in Egypt [120] and in Chile.[121, 122] Protection rates varied; however, there were few adverse reactions, and oral formulation of this vaccine made it less expensive to produce and distribute.[123, 124]

A purified Vi polysaccharide component vaccine against typhoid was developed by Landy, Webster, and colleagues[125–127] and later improved on by Wong and associates[128] and Robbins and Robbins.[129]

The adaptation of rabies virus to human diploid cell culture permitted the development of a potent inactivated rabies vaccine by Koprowski, Wiktor, and associates.[130] Since then, many other cell culture rabies vaccines have been developed, including a vaccinia-recombinant rabies vaccine for veterinary use.[131]

The development of a Japanese encephalitis vaccine was attempted during World War II,[132] but the current vaccine, consisting of formalin-inactivated whole virus harvested from mouse brain, was developed in Japan in 1965.[133] It was put into use almost immediately to vaccinate Japanese children, although few data regarding its efficacy had been published.

After two Americans who had traveled in Asia died from Japanese encephalitis, the U.S. Department of Defense conducted a vaccine trial in northern Thailand,[134] which showed an efficacy of 91%. A bivalent vaccine was developed using both the Nakayama-NIH strain (from the original vaccine) and the Beijing-1 strain, because the researchers thought that there were at least two strains of virus that caused disease. Japanese encephalitis vaccine has been available for distribution in the United States and other countries since that trial.[134–136] Yu and coworkers have developed an inactivated vaccine and a live attenuated vaccine against Japanese encephalitis, both in primary hamster kidney cells.[137–141] Both of these vaccines are manufactured and available for use only in the People's Republic of China.

A vaccine against hepatitis A virus (HAV) remained elusive until relatively recently. In 1979, Provost and Hilleman[142] were able to grow HAV in cell culture, thus opening the path for the development of a vaccine. Provost and coworkers developed the first inactivated HAV vaccine in 1986[143]; however, the cell culture used to produce the HAV antigen was not suitable for use in humans. Formaldehyde-inactivated, whole-virion HAV vaccines grown in human fibroblasts were later developed and licensed.[113, 144, 145]

During the 1970s and 1980s, bacterial vaccines consisting of purified capsular polysaccharides were developed. These included meningococcal group A and C vaccines, developed by Artenstein,[146] Gotschlich,[147] and associates; pneumococcal vaccine, by Austrian and associates[148]; and the first generation *H. influenzae* type b vaccine, by Anderson,[149] Schneerson,[150] and associates.

In the 1920s and 1930s, Pittman had determined that of the six different polysaccharides of *H. influenzae*, organisms encapsulated with type b caused the largest proportion of serious disease in children. She identified the composition of the capsule as a polymer of ribosyl ribitol phosphate, now called polyribosylribitol phosphate (PRP).[151] In the 1970s, several teams began research and efficacy studies on an *H. influenzae* type b vaccine, primarily in Finland and North Carolina.[149–150, 152–154] This work ultimately culminated in the 1985 licensure of the PRP vaccine.[155] However, the vaccine was not effective for children younger than 18 months, those most at risk for bacterial meningitis, and it had limited efficacy in older children. Vaccines against *H. influenzae* type b bacteria have advanced rapidly to a second and third generation.

As Avery and Goebel had shown (in relation to pneumococcus) that the immunogenicity of a capsular polysaccharide could be increased by binding it to a carrier protein,[156, 157] Schneerson and Robbins linked PRP to diphtheria toxoid and developed the first conjugate polysaccharide vaccine.[158] This vaccine had improved immunogenicity and efficacy and was licensed in 1987 for children older than 15 months. Younger children still remained at risk, but three more immunogenic conjugates soon followed, using nontoxic diphtheria toxoid (HbOC) derived from a mutant strain, an outer membrane protein of *Neisseria meningitidis* (PRP-OMP), or tetanus toxoid.[155, 158]

The first killed tick-borne encephalitis (TBE) vaccine, produced in mouse brain, was developed in the Soviet Union in 1939 only 2 years after the virus had been identified and the tick vector verified.[159, 160] In the 1960s, based on the work of Benda and Danes,[161, 162] Levkovich in the USSR[163] and Kunz in Austria[164] used chick embryo cell culture to develop a second, less reactogenic, formalin-inactivated vaccine. The current subunit vaccine was developed by Heinz, Kunz, and Fauma in 1980[165] and appears to be effective against different isolates of the TBE virus that all share a homologous envelope glycoprotein.[166–168] Since the collapse of the Soviet Union and the opening of Eastern Europe, the geographical range of TBE has been shown to be large.

The discovery that the particles of hepatitis B surface antigen (HBsAg) found in infected people are immunogenic and protective but noninfectious[169–171] provided the basis for efforts to purify these particles from the blood of chronic carriers. Hilleman and colleagues succeeded in licensing a plasma-derived vaccine in the United States in 1981.[172] Although the vaccine was safe and effective,[173] the acquired immunodeficiency syndrome (AIDS) epidemic arrived about the same time as licensure of the vaccine; products made from the derivatives of human blood came to be considered potentially dangerous. Despite rigorous safety testing and many inactivation processes to kill any foreign living particle in the vaccine, the manufacturer could not overcome the reluctance of the public and physicians to use a product that had even a remote risk of containing the human immunodeficiency virus. Also, because the vaccine depended on human serum, sources of antigen were limited.

These obstacles prompted the formulation of the first recombinant DNA vaccine, which was licensed in 1986. Development was accomplished by cloning the gene for HBsAg in yeast (*Saccharomyces cerevisiae*) and in mammalian cells. HBsAg was produced by the cells and then made into vaccine through adsorption on an alum adjuvant.[174–177] In yeast, the surface antigen aggregated into particles very similar to the extensively purified surface region antigen from the plasma-derived vaccine.[178] Initial trials and subsequent studies have shown the recombinant vaccine to be as effective as the plasma-derived vaccine.[176, 179, 180] In addition, because it is derived from a gene, it does not bear the stigma of possible contamination with undetected foreign agents.

Whole-cell pertussis vaccine continued to cause a number of adverse reactions. By 1975, after two infants died in Japan following pertussis vaccination, public rejection of the vaccine reached such proportions that the Japanese Ministry of Health suspended its use. An astronomical increase in the incidence of pertussis followed: 206 reported cases in 1971 grew to 13,105 cases by 1979.[181] This increase in turn led to the development of an acellular pertussis vaccine based on the isolated main protective antigens of *Bordetella pertussis*: toxin and filamentous hemagglutinin.[181, 182] Other components contained in the vaccine may also be important. Acellular pertussis vaccines that are less reactogenic than whole-cell pertussis vaccine have been licensed for use in Japan since 1981 and were licensed in the United States in 1996 for children 2 months and older.

An orally administered live rotavirus vaccine is about to be licensed, consisting of a mixture of a type 3 virus of monkeys and reassortants between single genes derived from types 1, 2, and 4 of human rotaviruses and 10 genes derived from the same monkey virus. The mixture, which is attenuated for infants but protective against disease caused by wild virus, was developed by Midthun and colleagues working at the National Institutes of Health under the direction of A. Z. Kapikian.[183]

The majority of vaccines now being developed use new technologies. The focus is on subunit (purified protein or polysaccharide), genetically engineered, or vectored antigens, because *new* is more interesting and exciting and also appears to offer greater safety with regard to the ability to screen out unwanted and often unknown living organisms. However, older methods continue to yield new vaccines, such as a live virus vaccine against influenza, which is likely to be licensed.

The early 21st century may well mirror the 40 years after Pasteur's momentous and controversial rabies trial; public reaction will compel scientists to find ever more ingenious and secure ways to protect humans against disease. If the new technologies succeed, the golden age will turn to platinum.

REFERENCES

1. Global Commission for the Certification of Smallpox Eradication. The achievement of the global eradication of smallpox. Geneva, World Health Organization, 1979.
2. deBary WT (ed). The Buddhist Tradition in India, China and Japan. New York, Vintage Books, 1972.
3. Hume EH. The Chinese Way in Medicine. Baltimore, Johns Hopkins University Press, 1940.
4. Wong KC, Wu LT. History of Chinese Medicine. Tientsin, China, Tientsin Press, 1932.
5. Huard PA, Wong K. Chinese Medicine. New York, McGraw-Hill, 1968.
6. Leung AK. Variolation and vaccination in late imperial China, ca 1570–1911. In Plotkin SA, Fantini B (eds). Vaccinia, Vaccination, Vaccinology: Jenner, Pasteur, and Their Successors. Paris, Elsevier, 1996, pp 65–71.
7. Major RH. A History of Medicine. Springfield, IL, Charles C Thomas, 1954.
8. Huygelen C. The long prehistory of modern measles vaccination. In Plotkin SA, Fantini B (eds). Vaccinia, Vaccination, Vaccinology: Jenner, Pasteur, and Their Successors. Paris, Elsevier, 1996, pp 257–263.
9. Plotkin SA. Vaccination against measles in the 18th century. Clin Pediatr (Phila) 6:312–315, 1967.
10. Enders JF. Francis Home and his experimental approach to medicine. Bull Hist Med 38:101–112, 1964.
11. Parish HJ. A History of Immunization. London, E & S Livingstone, 1965.
12. Jenner E. An Inquiry into the Causes and Effects of the *Variolae Vaccinae*. London, Low, 1798.

12a. DuMesnil O. Nécessité de la révaccination des ouvriers venants prendre du travail à Paris. Ann Hyg Paris 3(suppl.)1:444, 1879.

13. Ballard E. On Vaccination, Its Value and Alleged Dangers. London, Longmans, 1868.

14. Dudgeon JA. Development of smallpox vaccine in England in the eighteenth and nineteenth centuries. BMJ 1:1367–1372, 1963.
15. Copeman SM. Vaccination, Its Natural History and Pathology. London, Macmillan, 1899.
16. Pasteur L. De l'atténuation du virus du choléra des poules. C R Acad Sci Paris 91:673–680, 1880.
17. Koch R. The aetiology of anthrax based on the ontogeny of the anthrax bacillus. Med Classics 2:787, 1937. (Original publication, Beitr Biol Pflanz 2:277, 1877.)
18. Davaine C. Researches into infusoria of the blood in the disease known as sang de rate. In Nicolle J (ed). Louis Pasteur: A Master of Scientific Enquiry. London, Hutchinson, 1961, pp 172–178.
19. Besredka A. Local Immunisation. Plotz H, English trans. London, Ballière, 1927.
20. Toussaint H. Sur quelques points relatifs à l'immunité charbonneuse. C R Acad Sci Paris 93:163, 1881.
21. Pasteur L, Chamberland C-E, Roux E. Sur la vaccination charbonneuse. C R Acad Sci Paris 92:1378–1383, 1881.
22. Cadeddu A. Pasteur et le choléra des Poules: Révision critique d'un récit historique. Hist Phil Life Sci 7:87–104, 1985.
23. Geison GL. The Private Science of Louis Pasteur. Princeton, NJ, Princeton University Press, 1995.
24. Cadeddu A. Pasteur et la vaccination contre le charbon: Une analyse historique et critique. Hist Phil Life Sci 9:255–276, 1987.
25. Pasteur L. Méthode pour prévenir la rage après morsure. C R Acad Sci Paris 101:765–772, 1885.
26. Williams G. Virus Hunters. London, Hutchinson, 1960.
27. Salmon DE, Smith T. On a new method of producing immunity from contagious diseases. Am Vet Rev 10:63–69, 1886.
28. Salmon DE. The theory of immunity from contagious diseases. Proc Am Assoc Adv Sci 35:262–266, 1886.
29. Chase A. Magic Shots: A Human and Scientific Account of the Long and Continuing Struggle to Eradicate Infectious Diseases by Vaccination. New York, William Morrow & Co, 1982.
30. Salmon DE. Discovery of the production of immunity from contagious diseases by chemical substances formed during bacterial multiplication. Proc Am Assoc Adv Sci 37:275–280, 1888.
31. Roux E, Chamberland C-E. Immunité contre la septicémie conferée par des substances solubles. Ann Inst Pasteur Paris 1:561–572, 1887.
32. Metchnikoff E. Immunity in the Infective Diseases (English trans). Cambridge, UK, Cambridge University Press, 1905.
33. Ehrlich P. Die Werthbemessung des diphtherie Heil-serum und deren theoretische Grundlagen. Klin Jahrb Jena 6:299–326, 1897.
34. Ehrlich P. On immunity with special reference to cell life. [From Proc R Soc, 1900.] In Himmelweit F (ed). The Collected Papers of Paul Ehrlich. Vol. 2. London, Pergamon Press, 1957, pp 178–195.
35. Kolle W, Hetsch H. Experimental Bacteriology. Eyre J (ed); Erikson D, trans 7th German ed. London, Allen and Unwin, 1929.
36. Colebrook L. Almroth Wright. Provocative Doctor and Thinker. London, Heinemann, 1954.
37. Wright AE, Semple D. Remarks on vaccination against typhoid fever. BMJ 1:256–259, 1897.
38. Pfeiffer R, Kolle W. Experimentelle Untersuchungen zur Frage der Schutzimpfung des Menschen gegen Typhus adbdominalis. Dtsch Med Wochenschr 22:735–737, 1896.
39. Sansonetti PJ. Vaccination against typhoid fever: A century of research. End of the beginning or beginning of the end? In Plotkin SA, Fantini B (eds). Vaccinia, Vaccination, Vaccinology: Jenner, Pasteur, and Their Successors. Paris, Elsevier, 1996, pp 115–120.
40. Kitasato S. The bacillus of bubonic plague. Lancet 2:428–430, 1894.
41. Yersin A. La peste bubonique à Hong Kong. Ann Inst Pasteur Paris 8: 662–667, 1894.
42. Yersin A, Calmette A, Borrel A. La peste bubonique: Deuxième note. Ann Inst Pasteur Paris 9:589–592, 1895.
43. Haffkine WM. Remarks on the plague prophylactic fluid. BMJ 1:1461, 1897.
44. Haffkine WM. Protective inoculation against plague and cholera [editorial]. BMJ i:35–36, 1899.
45. Löwy I. Producing a trustworthy knowledge: Early field trials of anticholera vaccines in India. In Plotkin SA, Fantini B (eds). Vaccinia, Vaccination, Vaccinology: Jenner, Pasteur, and Their Successors. Paris, Elsevier, 1996, pp 121–126.
46. Snow J. Snow on Cholera; Being a Reprint of Two Papers, Together with a Bibliographic Memoir by B. W. Richardson. New York, Commonwealth Fund, 1936.
47. Koch R. Der Seitens des Dr. Koch an den Staatssecretari des Innern Herrn Staatsminster von Boetticher Excellenz erstettete Bericht von Alexandrie, 17 September 1883. Dtsch Med Wochenschr 9:615, 743–744, 1883.
48. Kolle W. Zur aktiven Immunisierung der Menschen gegen Cholera. Zentralbl Bakteriol Abt Jena 19:97–104, 1896.
49. Kolle W. Die aktive Immunisierung der Menschen gegen Cholera, nach Haffkine's Verfahren in Indien ausgefuhrt. Zentralbl Bakteriol Abt Jena 19:217–221, 1896.
50. Fleming A, Petrie GF. Recent Advances in Vaccine and Serum Therapy. Philadelphia, Blakiston, 1934.
51. Roux E, Yersin A. Contribution à l'étude de la diphtérie. Ann Inst Pasteur Paris 2:629–661, 1888.
52. Behring E von, Kitasato S. Über das Zustandekommen der Diphtherie—Immunität und der Tetanus—Immunität bie Tieren. Dtsch Med Wochenschr 16:1113–1114, 1890.
53. Behring von E. Untersuchungen über das Zustandekommen der Diphtherie—Immunität bei Tieren. Dtsch Med Wochenschr 16:1145–1148, 1890.
54. Smith T. Degree and duration of passive immunity to diphtheria toxin transmitted by immunized female guinea-pigs to their immediate offspring. J Med Res 16:359–379, 1907.
55. Glenny AT, Hopkins BE. Diphtheria toxoid as an immunising agent. Br J Exp Pathol 4:283–288, 1923.
56. Ramon G. Sur le pouvoir floculant et sur les propriétés immunisantes d'une toxine diphtérique rendue anatoxique (anatoxine). C R Acad Sci Paris 177:1338–1340, 1923.
57. Ramon G, Zoeller C. De la valeur antigénique de l'anatoxine tétanique chez l'homme. C R Acad Sci Paris 182:245–247, 1926.
58. Ramon G, Zoeller C. L'anatoxine tétanique et l'immunisation active de l'homme vis-à-vis du tétanos. Ann Inst Pasteur Paris 41:803–833, 1927.
59. Calmette A, Guérin C. Origine intestinale de la tuberculose pulmonaire et mécanism de l'infection tuberculose: 2ème et 3ème memoires. Ann Inst Pasteur Paris 20:353–363, 609–624, 1906.
60. Calmette A, Guérin C, Breton M. Contribution à l'étude de la tuberculose expérimentale du cobaye (infection et essais de vaccination par la voie digestive). Ann Inst Pasteur Paris 21:401–416, 1907.
61. Calmette A, Guérin C. Contribution à l'étude de l'immunité antituberculose chez les bovidés. Ann Inst Pasteur Paris 28:329–337, 1914.
62. Calmette A. La Vaccination Préventive Contre la Tuberculose par le B.C.G. Paris, Masson, 1927.
63. Calmette A. L'Infection Bacillaire et la Tuberculose (4th ed). Paris, Masson, 1936.
64. Woodruff AM, Goodpasture EW. The susceptibility of the chorio-allantoic membrane of chick embryos to infection with the fowl-pox virus. Am J Pathol 7:209–222, 1931.
65. Wilkinson L. The development of the virus concept as reflected in corpora of studies on individual pathogens. 5. Smallpox and the evolution of ideas on acute (viral) infections. Med Hist 23:1–28, 1979.
66. Warren AJ. Landmarks in the conquest of yellow fever. In Strode G (ed). Yellow Fever. New York, McGraw-Hill, 1951, pp 5–37.
67. Stokes A, Bauer JH, Hudson NP. Transmission of yellow fever to *Macacus rhesus*, preliminary note. JAMA 90:253–254, 1928.
68. Sawyer WA, Lloyd WDM, Kitchen SF. Preservation of yellow fever virus. J Exp Med 50:1–13, 1929.
69. Mathis C, Sellards AW, Laigret J. Sensibilité du *Macacus rhesus* au virus de la fièvre jaune. C R Acad Sci Paris 186:604–606, 1928.
70. Monath TP. Yellow fever vaccines: The success of empiricism, pitfalls of application, and transition to molecular vaccinology. In Plotkin SA, Fantini B (eds). Vaccinia, Vaccination, Vaccinology: Jenner, Pasteur, and Their Successors. Paris, Elsevier, 1996, pp 157–182.
71. Theiler M. Susceptibility of white mice to virus of yellow fever. Science 71:367, 1930.
72. Lloyd W, Penna HA, Mahaffy AF. Yellow fever virus encephalitis in rodents. Am J Hyg 18:323–344, 1933.

73. Sawyer WA, Kitchen SF, Lloyd W. Vaccination of humans against yellow fever with immune serum and virus fixed for mice. Proc Soc Exp Biol Med 29:62–64, 1931.
74. Sellards AW, Laigret J. Vaccination de l'homme contre la fièvre jaune. C R Acad Sci Paris 194:1609–1611, 1932.
75. Theiler M, Smith HH. The use of yellow fever virus by in vitro cultivation for human immunization. J Exp Med 65:787–800, 1937.
76. Lloyd W, Theiler M, Ricci NI. Modification of virulence of yellow fever virus by cultivation in tissues in vitro. Trans R Soc Trop Med Hyg 29:481–529, 1936.
77. Theiler M, Smith HH. Effect of prolonged cultivation in vitro upon pathogenicity of yellow fever virus. J Exp Med 65:767–786, 1937.
78. Smith W, Andrewes CH, Laidlaw PP. A virus obtained from influenza patients. Lancet 2:66–68, 1933.
79. Horsfall FL Jr, Lennette EH, Rickard ER, Hirst GK. Studies on the efficacy of a complex vaccine against influenza A. Public Health Rep 56:1863–1875, 1941.
80. Chenoweth A, Waltz AD, Stokes J Jr, Gladen RG. Active immunization with the viruses of human and swine influenza. Am J Dis Child 52:757, 1936.
81. Kilbourne ED. A race with evolution—a history of influenza vaccines. In Plotkin SA, Fantini B (eds). Vaccinia, Vaccination, Vaccinology: Jenner, Pasteur, and Their Successors. Paris, Elsevier, 1996, pp 183–188.
82. Smith W. The complement-fixation reaction in influenza. Lancet 2:1256–1259, 1936.
83. Francis T Jr, Magill TP. Vaccination of human subjects with virus of human influenza. Proc Soc Exp Biol Med 33:604–606, 1936.
84. Francis T Jr, Magill TP. The antibody response of human subjects vaccinated with the virus of human influenza. J Exp Med 65:251–259, 1937.
85. Smorodintsev AA, Tushinsky MD, Drobyshevskaya AI, Korovin AA. Investigation on volunteers infected with the influenza virus. Am J Med Sci 194:159–170, 1937.
86. Kilbourne, ED. A history of influenza virology. In Koprowski H, Oldstone MBA (eds). Microbe Hunters—Then and Now. Bloomington, IL, Medi-Ed Press, 1996, pp 187–204.
87. Cox HR. Use of yolk sac of developing chick embryo as medium for growing rickettsiae of Rocky Mountain spotted fever and typhus groups. Public Health Rep 53:2241–2247, 1938.
88. Weindling P. Victory with vaccines: The problem of typhus vaccines during World War II. In Plotkin SA, Fantini B (eds). Vaccinia, Vaccination, Vaccinology: Jenner, Pasteur, and Their Successors. Paris, Elsevier, 1996, pp 341–347.
89. Harden VK. Rocky Mountain Spotted Fever. History of a Twentieth-Century Disease. Baltimore, Johns Hopkins University Press, 1990.
90. Madsen T. Whooping cough: Its bacteriology, diagnosis, prevention and treatment. Boston Med Surg J 192:50–60, 1925.
91. Madsen G. Vaccination against whooping cough. JAMA 101:187–188, 1933.
92. Granström M. The history of pertussis vaccination: From whole-cell to subunit vaccines. In Plotkin SA, Fantini B (eds). Vaccinia, Vaccination, Vaccinology: Jenner, Pasteur, and Their Successors. Paris, Elsevier, 1996, pp 107–114.
93. Burnette WN, Mar VL, Bartley TD, et al. The molecular engineering of pertussis toxoid. Dev Biol Stand 73:75–79, 1991.
94. Lapin JH. Whooping Cough. Springfield, IL, Charles C Thomas, 1943.
95. Enders JF, Weller TH, Robbins FC. Cultivation of the Lansing strain of poliomyelitis virus in cultures of various human embryonic tissues. Science 109:85–87, 1949.
96. Koprowski H, Jervis GA, Norton TW. Immune responses in human volunteers upon oral administration of a rodent-adapted strain of poliomyelitis virus. Am J Hyg 55:108–126, 1952.
97. Salk JE, Krech U, Youngner JS, et al. Formaldehyde treatment and safety testing of experimental poliomyelitis vaccines. Am J Public Health 44:563–570, 1954.
98. Sabin AB, Hennessen WA, Winsser J. Studies on variants of poliomyelitis virus. I. Experimental segregation and properties of avirulent variants of three immunological types. J Exp Med 99:551–576, 1954.
99. Katz SL, Kempe CH, Black FL, et al. Studies on an attenuated measles virus vaccine. VIII. General summary and evaluation of results of vaccine. N Engl J Med 263:180–184, 1960.
100. Schwarz AJF. Preliminary tests of a highly attenuated measles vaccine. Am J Dis Child 103:386–389, 1962.
101. Hilleman MR, Buynak EB, Weibel RE, et al. Development and evaluation of the Moraten measles virus vaccine. JAMA 206:587–590, 1968.
102. Hilleman MR, Buynak EB, Weibel RE, Stokes J Jr. Live attenuated mumps-virus vaccine. N Engl J Med 278:227–232, 1968.
103. Meyer HM, Parkman PD. Rubella vaccination: A review of practical experience. JAMA 215:613–619, 1971.
104. Prinzie A, Huygelen C, Gold J, et al. Experimental live attenuated rubella virus vaccine: Clinical evaluation of Cendehill strain. Am J Dis Child 118:172–177, 1969.
105. Plotkin SA, Farquhar JD, Katz M, Buser F. Attenuation of RA27/3 rubella virus in WI-38 human diploid cells. Am J Dis Child 118:178–185, 1969.
106. Top FH Jr, Buescher EL, Bancroft WH, et al. Immunization with live types 7 and 4 adenovirus vaccines. II. Antibody response and protective effect against acute respiratory disease due to adenovirus type 7. J Infect Dis 124:155–160, 1971.
107. Top FH Jr, Dudding BA, Russell PK. Control of respiratory disease in recruits with types 4 and 7 adenovirus vaccines. Am J Epidemiol 84:141–146, 1971.
108. Top FH Jr, Grossman RA, Bartelloni PJ. Immunization with live types 7 and 4 adenovirus vaccines. I. Safety, infectivity, and potency of adenovirus type 7 vaccine in humans. J Infect Dis 124:148–154, 1971.
109. Takahashi M, Otsuka T, Okuno Y, et al. Live vaccine used to prevent the spread of varicella in children in hospitals. Lancet 2:1288–1290, 1974.
110. Takahashi M, Okuno Y, Otsuka T, et al. Development of a live attenuated varicella vaccine. Biken J 18:25–33, 1975.
111. Weibel RE, Neff BJ, Kuter B, et al. Live attenuated varicella virus vaccine efficacy trial in healthy children. N Engl J Med 310:1409–1415, 1984.
112. Arbeter AM, Starr SE, Weibel R, Plotkin SA. Live attenuated varicella vaccine: Immunization of healthy children with the OKA strain. J Pediatr 100:886–893, 1982.
113. Galambos L, Sewell JE. Networks of Innovation. Vaccine Development at Merck, Sharp & Dohme, and Mulford, 1895–1995. New York, Cambridge University Press, 1995.
114. Yugoslav Typhoid Commission. A controlled field trial of the effectiveness of acetone-dried and inactivated and heat-phenol–inactivated typhoid vaccines in Yugoslavia. Bull World Health Organ 30:623–630, 1964.
115. Ashcroft MT, Singh B, Nicholson CC, et al. A seven-year field trial of two typhoid vaccines in Guyana. Lancet 2:1056–1059, 1967.
116. Polish Typhoid Commission. Controlled field trials and laboratory studies on the effectiveness of typhoid vaccines in Poland 1961–64. Bull World Health Organ 34:211–222, 1966.
117. Hejfec LB, Samin LV, Lejtman MZ, et al. A controlled field trial and laboratory study of five typhoid vaccines in the USSR. Bull World Health Organ 34:321–339, 1966.
118. Germanier R, Fürer E. Isolation and characterization of Gal E mutant Ty21a of *Salmonella typhi*. A candidate for a live, oral typhoid vaccine. J Infect Dis 131:553–558, 1975.
119. Gilman RH, Hornick RB, Woodward WE, et al. Immunity in typhoid fever: Evaluation of Ty21a—an epimeraseless mutant of *S. typhi* as a live oral vaccine. J Infect Dis 136:717–723, 1977.
120. Wahdan MH, Sérié C, Cerisier Y, et al. A controlled field trial of live *Salmonella typhi* strain Ty21a oral vaccine against typhoid: Three-year results. J Infect Dis 145:292–295, 1982.
121. Levine MM, Black RE, Ferreccio C, et al. Large-scale field trial of Ty21a live oral typhoid vaccine in enteric-coated capsule formulation. Lancet 1:1049–1052, 1987.
122. Hackett J. Salmonella-based vaccines. Vaccine 8:5–11, 1990.
123. Black RE. Efficacy of one or two doses of Ty21a *Salmonella typhi* vaccine in enteric-coated capsules in a controlled field trial. Vaccine 8:81–84, 1990.
124. Ferreccio C, Levine M, Rodriguez H, et al. Comparative efficacy of two, three and four doses of Ty21a live oral typhoid vaccine in enteric-coated capsules: A field trial in an endemic area. J Infect Dis 159:766–769, 1989.

125. Landy J. Studies of Vi antigen. VI. Immunization of human beings with purified Vi antigen. Am J Hyg 50:52–62, 1954.
126. Landy M, Gaines S, Seal JP, et al. Antibody responses of man to three types of antityphoid immunizing agents. Am J Public Health 44:1572–1579, 1954.
127. Webster ME, Landy M, Freeman ME. Studies on Vi antigen. II. Purification of Vi antigen from *Escherichia coli* 5396/38. J Immunol 69:135–142, 1952.
128. Wong KH, Feeley JC, Northrup RS, et al. Vi antigen from *Salmonella typhosa* and immunity against typhoid fever. I. Isolation and immunologic properties in animals. Infect Immun 9:348–353, 1974.
129. Robbins JD, Robbins JB. Reexamination of the protective role of the capsular polysaccharide Vi antigen of *Salmonella typhi*. J Infect Dis 150:436–439, 1984.
130. Wiktor TJ, Fernandez MV, Koprowski H. Cultivation of rabies virus in human diploid cell strain WI-38. J Immunol 93:353–366, 1964.
131. Wiktor TJ, MacFarlane RI, Reagen KJ, et al. Protection from rabies by vaccinia virus recombinant containing the rabies virus glycoprotein gene. Proc Natl Acad Sci U S A 81:7194–7198, 1984.
132. Sabin AB. Encephalitis. In Coates JB Jr, Hoff EC, Hoff PM (eds). Preventive Medicine in WWII. Vol. 7. Washington, DC, Office of the Surgeon General, Department of the Army, 1964, pp 9–21.
133. Takaku K, Yamshita T, Osanai T, et al. Japanese encephalitis purified vaccine. Biken J 11:25–39, 1968.
134. Hoke CH, Nisalak A, Sangawhipa N, et al. Protection against Japanese encephalitis by inactivated vaccines. N Engl J Med 319:608–614, 1988.
135. Poland JD, Cropp CB, Craven RB, et al. Evaluation of the potency and safety of inactivated Japanese encephalitis vaccine in US inhabitants. J Infect Dis 161:878–882, 1990.
136. Centers for Disease Control. Japanese encephalitis with special reference to the low risk for travellers to the 1988 Olympics to be held in Korea. Advisory Memorandum No. 93. Atlanta, GA, Centers for Disease Control, 1988.
137. Gu PW, Ding ZF. Inactivated Japanese encephalitis (JE) vaccine made from hamster cell culture [review]. Jpn Encephalitis Hemorrhagic Fever Renal Syndrome Bull 2:15–26, 1987.
138. Yu YX, Wu PF, Ao J, et al. Selection of a better immunogenic and highly attenuated live vaccine virus strain of JE. I. Some biological characteristics of SA 14-14-2 mutant. Chin J Microbiol Immunol 1:77–84, 1981.
139. Ao J, Yu Y, Tang YS, et al. Selection of a better immunogenic and highly attenuated live vaccine strain of Japanese encephalitis. II. Safety and immunogenicity of live JBE vaccine SA14-14-2 observed in inoculated children. Chin J Microbiol Immunol 3(4):245–248, 1983.
140. Xin YY, Ming ZG, Peng GY, et al. Safety of a live-attenuated Japanese encephalitis virus vaccine (SA14-14-2) for children. Am J Trop Med Hyg 39:214–217, 1988.
141. Huang CH. Studies of Japanese encephalitis in China. Adv Virus Res 27:71–101, 1982.
142. Provost PJ, Hilleman MR. Propagation of human hepatitis A virus in cell culture in vitro. Proc Soc Exp Biol Med 160:213–221, 1979.
143. Provost PJ, Hughes JV, Miller WJ, et al. An inactivated hepatitis A vaccine of cell culture origin. J Med Virol 19:23–31, 1986.
144. Wiedermann M, Ambrosch F, Kollaritsch H, et al. Safety and immunogenicity of an inactivated hepatitis A candidate vaccine in healthy adult volunteers. Vaccine 8:581–584, 1990.
145. André FE, Hondt d'E, Delem AD, Safary A. Clinical assessment of the safety and efficacy of an inactivated hepatitis-A vaccine—rationale and summary of findings. Vaccine 10:S160–S168, 1992.
146. Artenstein MS, Gold R, Zimmerly JG, et al. Prevention of meningococcal disease by group C polysaccharide vaccine. N Engl J Med 282:417–420, 1970.
147. Gotschlich EC, Liu TY, Artenstein MS. Human immunity to the meningococcus. III. Preparation and immunochemical properties of the group A, group B and group C meningococcal polysaccharides. J Exp Med 129:1349–1365, 1969.
148. Austrian R, Douglas RM, Schiffman G, et al. Prevention of pneumococcal pneumonia by vaccination. Trans Assoc Am Physicians 89:184–192, 1976.
149. Anderson P, Peter G, Johnston RB Jr, et al. Immunization of humans with polyribophosphate, the capsular antigen of *Haemophilus influenzae* type b. J Clin Invest 51:39–44, 1972.
150. Schneerson R, Rodrigues LP, Parke JC Jr, et al. Immunity to disease caused by *H. influenzae* type b. II. Specificity and some biologic characteristics of "natural," infection-acquired, and immunization-induced antibodies to the capsular polysaccharide of *H. influenzae* type b. J Immunol 107:1081–1089, 1971.
151. Robbins JB, Schneerson R, Pittman M. *Haemophilus influenzae* type b infections. In Germanier R (ed). Bacterial Vaccines. Orlando, FL, Academic Press, 1984, pp 289–316.
152. Peltola H, Kayhty H, Sivonen A, et al. *Haemophilus influenzae* type b capsular polysaccharide vaccine in children: A double-blind field study of 100,000 vaccinees 3 months to 5 years of age in Finland. Pediatrics 60:730–737, 1977.
153. Peltola H, Kayhty H, Virtanen M, et al. Prevention of *Haemophilus influenzae* type b bacteremic infections with the capsular polysaccharide vaccine. N Engl J Med 310:1561–1566, 1984.
154. Parke JC Jr, Schneerson R, Robbins JB, et al. Interim report of a controlled field trial of immunization with capsular polysaccharides *of Haemophilus influenzae* type b and group C *Neisseria meningitidis* in Mecklenburg County, North Carolina. J Infect Dis 136:S51–S57, 1977.
155. Ward J. Prevention of invasive *Haemophilus influenzae* type b disease: Lessons from vaccine efficacy trials. Vaccine 9(suppl): S17–S24, 1991.
156. Avery OT, Goebel WF. Chemical-immunological studies on conjugated carbohydrate-proteins. II. Immunological specificity of synthetic sugar-protein antigens. J Exp Med 50:533–542, 1929.
157. Goebel WF. Studies on antibacterial immunity induced by artificial antigens. I. Immunity to experimental pneumococcal infection with an antigen containing cellobiuronic acid. J Exp Med 69:353–364, 1939.
158. Schneerson R, Barrera O, Sutton A, Robbins JB. Preparation, characterization and immunogenicity of *Haemophilus influenzae* type b polysaccharide-protein conjugates. J Exp Med 152:361–376, 1980.
159. Smorodinstev AA, Kagan UV, Levkovich EN, et al. Experimenteller und epidemiologischer Beitrag zur aktiven Immunisierung gegen die Frülin-Sommer-Zecken-Encephalitis. Arch Ges Virusforsch 3:1, 1941.
160. Smorodinstev AA. Tick-borne spring-summer encephalitis. Prog Med Virol 1:210–247, 1958.
161. Benda R, Danes L. Study of the possibility of preparing a vaccine against tick-borne encephalitis, using tissue culture methods. V. Experimental data for the evaluation of the efficiency of formol treated vaccines in laboratory animals. Acta Virol 5:37, 1961.
162. Benda R, Danes L. Evaluation of the immunogenic efficiency of tick-borne encephalitis virus vaccine. In Libikova H (ed). Biology of Viruses of the Tick-Borne Encephalitis Complex. Prague, Czechoslovak Academy of Sciences, 1962, p 245.
163. Levkovich EN. Experimental and epidemiological bases of the specific prophylaxis of tick-borne encephalitis. In Libikova H (ed). Biology of Viruses of the Tick-Borne Encephalitis Complex. Prague, Czechoslovak Academy of Sciences, 1962, p 317.
164. Kunz C. Aktiv und passive Immunoprophylaxe der Frühsommer-Meningoencephalitis (FSME). Arzneim Forsch 28:1806, 1962.
165. Heinz FX, Kunz C, Fauma H. Preparation of a highly purified vaccine against tick-borne encephalitis by continuous flow zonal ultra-centrifugation. J Med Virol 6:213–222, 1980.
166. Heinz FX, Kunz C. Homogeneity of the structural glycoprotein from European isolates of tick-borne encephalitis virus: Comparison with other flaviviruses. J Gen Virol 57:263–274, 1981.
167. Heinz FX, Berger R, Tuma W, et al. A topological and functional model of epitopes on the structural glycoprotein of tick-borne encephalitis virus defined by monoclonal antibodies. Virology 126:525–537, 1983.
168. Stephenson JR, Lee JM, Wilton-Smith PD. Antigenic variation among members of the tick-borne encephalitis complex. J Gen Virol 65:81–89, 1984.
169. Prince AM. An antigen detected in the blood during the incubation period of serum hepatitis. Proc Natl Acad Sci U S A 60:814, 1968.

170. Krugman S, Giles JP, Hammond J. Infectious hepatitis: Evidence for two distinctive clinical, epidemiological, and immunological types of infection. JAMA 200:365–373, 1967.
171. Krugman S, Giles JP, Hammond J. Viral hepatitis, type B (MS-2 strain): Studies on active immunization. JAMA 217:41–45, 1971.
172. Hilleman MR, Bertland VA, Bunyak EB, et al. Clinical and laboratory studies of HBsAg vaccine. In Vyas GN, Cohen SN, Schmid R (eds). Viral Hepatitis. Philadelphia, Franklin Institute Press, 1978, pp 525–527.
173. Krugman S. The newly licensed hepatitis B vaccine. Characteristics and indications for use. JAMA 247:2012–2015, 1982.
174. Valenzuela P, Medina A, Rutter WJ, et al. Synthesis and assembly of hepatitis B virus surface antigen particles in yeast. Nature 298:347–350, 1982.
175. McAleer WJ, Buynak EB, Maigetter RZ, et al. Human hepatitis B vaccine from recombinant yeast. Nature 307:178–180, 1984.
176. Skolnick EM, McLean AA, West DJ, et al. Clinical evaluation in healthy adults of a hepatitis B vaccine made by recombinant DNA. JAMA 251:2812–2815, 1984.
177. Michel M-L, Pontisso P, Sobczak E, et al. Synthesis in animal cells of hepatitis B surface antigen particles carrying a receptor for polymerized human serum albumin. Proc Natl Acad Sci U S A 81:7708–7712, 1984.
178. Emini EA, Ellis RW, Miller WJ, et al. Production and immunological analysis of recombinant hepatitis B vaccine. J Infect 13(suppl A):3–9, 1986.
179. Scheiermann N, Gesemann M, Mauer C, et al. Persistence of antibodies after immunization with a recombinant yeast-derived hepatitis B vaccine following two different schedules. Vaccine 8(suppl):S44–S46, 1990.
180. André FE. Overview of a 5-year clinical experience with a yeast-derived hepatitis B vaccine. Vaccine 8(suppl):S74–S78, 1990.
181. Sato Y, Izumiya K, Sato H, et al. Role of antibody to leukocytosis-promoting factor hemagglutinin and to filamentous hemagglutinin in immunity to pertussis. Infect Immun 31:1223–1231, 1981.
182. Sato Y, Kimura M, Fukimi H. Development of a pertussis component vaccine in Japan. Lancet 1:122–126, 1984.
183. Midthun K, Greenberg HB, Hoshino Y, et al. Reassortant rotaviruses as potential live rotavirus vaccine candidates. J Virol 53:949–954, 1985.

chapter

2 The History of Polio Vaccine Development

Frederick C. Robbins

Poliomyelitis viruses have probably been prevalent as infectious agents of humans from the time that humans gathered together in villages and groups large enough to facilitate the person-to-person spread of infectious agents. Paralytic disease, however, was not recognized to be a significant problem until late in the 19th century, when epidemics began to appear in northern Europe.[1] Heine provided one of the first descriptions of the clinical disease as we now know it.[2] The earliest and best description of an epidemic of any size is that of Medin from Stockholm in 1887.[3] From that time on, seasonal (summer and early fall in the Northern Hemisphere) epidemics of increasing severity occurred in the industrialized countries. The average age of patients also rose, with concomitant increases in the severity of disease and its mortality.[4] By 1953, the incidence of paralytic poliomyelitis in the United States was more than 20 per 100,000 population. Although this rate was not particularly high compared with that of other diseases such as measles, much public concern was generated by polio because of its mysterious seasonal incidence (an attribute that is still not adequately explained), its disfiguring nature, and its propensity for paralyzing the respiratory muscles. Paralyzed patients often required artificial assistance to breathe, usually through the use of that cumbersome and fearsome instrument, the "iron lung," or Drinker respirator.

PRE–TISSUE CULTURE ERA

Not long after polio had been recognized as an epidemic disease, Landsteiner and Popper were able to reproduce the disease in monkeys by intracerebral inoculation of a filtrate of central nervous system tissue from a fatal case.[5, 6] Although this discovery was of great importance, the monkey was not an experimental animal that lent itself well to the kind of research necessary to elucidate the characteristics and epidemiology of the poliovirus or to develop preventive measures. In 1939, Armstrong succeeded in adapting the Lansing strain of poliovirus to rodents, which made it possible to expand the scope of experimentation.[7] However, the usefulness of the rodent-adapted virus was limited because it was a single type, later found to be type 2. Many years later, Li and Schaeffer were able to adapt a type 1 strain to mice.[8]

In the 40-year interval from the isolation of the poliovirus in monkeys to the development of tissue culture techniques, considerable progress was made in understanding poliomyelitis.[4] Evidence was presented to suggest that the virus multiplied in the gastrointestinal tract and that infection could be transferred by the fecal-oral route.[9, 10] Monkeys were shown to develop immunity to challenge with active virus, and various efforts were made to prepare experimental vaccines. The starting material was central nervous system tissue from infected monkeys that had been treated in a variety of ways. Although some success was reported, the experiments were inconsistent, and the results were disappointing overall.[11, 12] In spite of the ambiguous animal data, in 1936 two investigators independently conducted field trials of vaccines prepared from monkey spinal cord, using children and some adults as subjects. Brodie and Park[13] used a formalin-treated preparation, whereas Kolmer[14] treated the spinal cord suspension with ricinoleate to "attenuate" the virus. Kolmer assumed that it was necessary to use live virus to achieve immunity.

By modern standards, these trials were ill conceived. The scientific base was woefully inadequate to justify human trials. Appropriate tests for safety and efficacy were lacking, and, indeed, there seems to have been little concern for the known risk attendant with the injection of central nervous system tissue. Furthermore, it was not yet known whether there was more than one type of poliovirus, and there was no readily available means to diagnose infection. Thousands of subjects received these vaccines, some of whom developed paralysis soon after inoculation, often in the inoculated limb. These findings raised the specter of persistence of live virulent virus in the vaccine, and the trials were terminated.[15, 16, 16a]

Another abortive attempt to prevent polio was by chemical treatment of the nasal mucosa, with the purpose of blocking viral invasion. Picric acid, sodium alum, and zinc sulfate were instilled into the nose. This rather bizarre procedure was based on the observation that certain species of monkeys could be infected by the nasopharyngeal route and that prior treatment with the aforementioned chemicals seemed to interfere with infection. Trials in humans were not promising, and this technique was soon abandoned.[17, 18]

In the effort to develop better methods for propagating the virus, various investigators[18] tried tissue culture without success, except for Sabin and Olitsky, who in 1936 reported the growth of poliovirus in cultures of human embryonic brain tissue.[19] However, they had no success with cells from non–nervous system tissues. These results tended to strengthen the idea that poliovirus was a strict neurotrope, in spite of the evidence that it was present in the nasopharynx and intestine in vivo.

Burnet and Jackson from the Walter and Eliza Hall Institute of Melbourne, Australia, mentioned in a paper published in 1940 that they had had suggestive success in propagating a local strain of poliovirus (Mars) in cultures of human fetal pharyngeal and intestinal tissues.[20] Unfortunately, they did not pursue these findings; otherwise, the vaccine might have been available almost a decade earlier. The techniques employed by Burnet and Jackson were not significantly different from those of Sabin. The discrepancy in results most likely can be attributed to differences in the viral strains employed, as is discussed subsequently.

A large-scale cooperative experiment in monkeys, reported in 1949, demonstrated conclusively that there were three, and only three, immunologically distinct strains of poliovirus; this was crucial information in compounding a fully protective vaccine.[21–24] Using children in a field trial of human serum γ-globulin as a prophylactic against polio, Hammon and colleagues demonstrated a significant level of protection against paralytic disease.[25] This finding—that relatively low levels of antibody could prevent invasion of the central nervous system—provided encouragement to those who were developing a means of active immunization. An excellent analysis of the pathogenesis of poliomyelitis and the implication for the success of preventive measures was published by Bodian in 1952 and is still applicable today.[26]

TISSUE CULTURE ERA

Although much had been learned about polio and its causative virus, there was no optimism in 1949 about the possibility of developing a practical means of preventing polio with the techniques at hand.[27, 28] That same year, however, Enders and colleagues (Fig. 2–1) published the paper in *Science* that described the successful cultivation of the Lansing strain of poliovirus in cultures of human non–nervous system tissues,[29] which provided the breakthrough that was so eagerly sought. There is no ready explanation as to why these experiments succeeded whereas those of Sabin and Olitsky did not. The principal technical difference was that in Enders's laboratory, the cultures were maintained for a longer time, with periodic changes of nutrient medium; the availability of antibiotics that were incorporated in the medium made this possible. Sabin did go back to the original virus (MV strain) used in the 1936 experiments and found it to be noncytopathic for monkey kidney cells.[30] The implication is that after many passages in monkey brain, it had lost its capacity to infect non–nervous system cells.

Poliovirus was soon found to propagate in cells from a variety of tissues from both humans and nonhuman primates.[31–36] The monkey kidney became the preferred source of tissue for much subsequent work, including the growth of virus for vaccine production. Because the virus was released into the tissue culture medium, the cell-free fluid component of the culture made an excellent source of virus, relatively free of extraneous proteinaceous material, from which the inactivated vaccine was prepared.

It was noted early in the course of poliovirus cultiva-

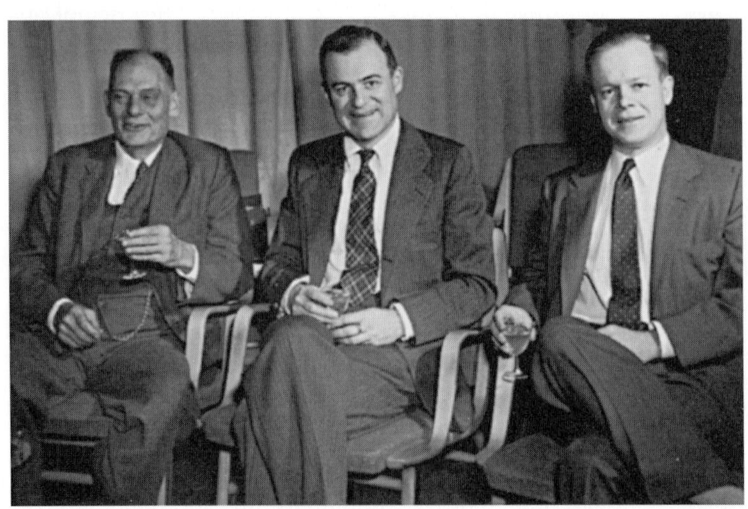

Figure 2–1. John Enders, Frederick Robbins, and Thomas Weller in Stockholm, 1954.

tion that infected cells were rapidly destroyed,[37] and this "cytopathic" effect was exploited as an indicator of viral replication. Thus, a single test tube, flask, or, later, well in a plastic plate could be used as the equivalent of an experimental animal. With some technical modifications, one could use tissue cultures for virus titration, antibody quantification, virus isolation from clinical specimens, and antigenic typing of virus isolates.[38–44] These relatively simple techniques greatly facilitated the development and testing of vaccines.

Dulbecco, adapting a technique that he had developed for producing plaques in monolayers of chick embryo cells in culture with western equine encephalitis and Newcastle disease viruses,[45] was able to do the same with polioviruses.[46] He prepared monolayers from suspensions of monkey kidney cells prepared by trypsinization. The plaquing techniques placed the study of poliovirus and other animal viruses on a quantitative basis comparable to the technique that had proved to be fruitful with bacteriophages. The ability to establish clones from single virus particles was invaluable in the development of lines of poliovirus suitable for use as live attenuated vaccines.

Trypsin had been used for preparing cells for transfer from plasma clot cultures since first described by Rous and Jones in 1916.[47] However, only after Dulbecco's work did trypsinization become widely used as the standard method of preparing cell suspensions for viral propagation in tissue cultures.[48] Homogeneous suspensions of kidney cells prepared by trypsinization proved to be a more practical source of cells than HeLa cells, which had been used by some investigators for tissue culture titration of poliovirus or its antibody.[49–53]

Although it was only after the observations of Enders, Robbins, and Weller that techniques based on the cytopathic effect of viruses on cells in tissue culture became widely used, many investigators had previously observed various kinds of effects of viruses on cells in tissue culture.[18] Sanders and Alexander isolated directly in tissue cultures a virus from cases of keratoconjunctivitis.[54] Huang performed titrations of western equine encephalitis virus and antibody to this virus, using cytopathology as the indicator of virus growth.[55] He also employed the interference phenomenon to titrate noncytopathic viruses (St. Louis encephalitis and Jungeblut-Sanders mouse viruses) in culture,[56] foreshadowing the techniques later employed for rubella virus. Huang also used pH change as an indicator of virus growth.[57] By incorporating sulfadiazine in the medium for bacteriostasis, Sanders and Huang were able to use tissue cultures in field studies.[58] Thus, the work of Huang and associates anticipated many of the practical applications of tissue cultures that were to prove valuable in the work with poliovirus and, later, with many other viruses.

With the availability of tissue culture techniques making a vaccine against poliomyelitis a realistic possibility, a number of laboratories began work toward this end. Salk and colleagues chose to pursue a formalin-inactivated vaccine, whereas Milzer and associates[59] pursued ultraviolet irradiation as a means of inactivation. Cox, Koprowski, and Sabin took the approach of a live attenuated vaccine.[79, 81–83]

INACTIVATED VACCINES

Milzer, Wolf, and colleagues pursued the ultraviolet irradiation–inactivated vaccine to the point of demonstrating immunogenicity in humans,[59, 60] but it was never adopted for general use.

Work on the formalinized vaccine proceeded apace in Salk's laboratory. Using virus grown in tissue cultures of monkey kidney as starting material, Salk and his colleagues determined the formalin inactivation curve; performed safety and immunogenicity studies in animals; and, by 1953, performed preliminary studies in humans.[61–64] Salk supported the hypothesis that once the host had been primed with an adequate dose of antigen, the booster response would occur on challenge with inactive antigen or live virus.[65] On live virus challenge, antibody would be elaborated rapidly enough to prevent viremia and thus paralysis. Although viremia had been demonstrated in monkeys,[26] it was sometime later that it was demonstrated in humans.[66, 67] In April 1953, a letter signed by Rivers and the members of the Vaccine Advisory Committee of the National Foundation for Infantile Paralysis was published in the *Journal of the American Medical Association*, suggesting some steps that should be taken before the inactivated vaccine could be considered for a large-scale field trial.[68, 69] By early 1954, the data were considered sufficient to warrant conducting such a trial, and the decision was made to proceed.

Francis of the University of Michigan School of Public Health was director of the project, which was the largest experiment of its kind up to that time.[70] Trial participants included a total of 1,829,916 children in communities from all parts of the United States, and several from Canada and Finland. The experiment involved both observed controls and, in some areas, placebo controls. The results were presented on April 12, 1955. The conclusions were that the vaccine was safe and effective at a level of approximately 70% and that effectiveness could be correlated with potency, as measured by antibody response in children. On the basis of the evidence from the trial and the data presented by the manufacturers, the products of six producers were licensed within a few days after the announcement of the field trial results.

The Cutter Episode

Interest in the vaccine was high, and many communities organized specific programs, which obtained widespread coverage. However, not long after the vaccine had become generally available, cases of paralytic disease were reported in recipients.[71–73] As the interval between vaccination and onset of disease corresponded to the incubation period of polio, and as the paralysis usually occurred in the inoculated limb, it was suspected that these cases were caused by residual active virus in the vaccine. Epidemiological investigation revealed that almost all the cases occurred in children who had received vaccine made by the same manufacturer—Cutter. On further investigation, it was established that certain lots of the Cutter vaccine were particularly implicated.

The Public Health Service immediately suspended vaccination, recalled the Cutter vaccine, and launched an intensive investigation, including a careful review of the regulations governing the manufacture of vaccine and the techniques employed by the companies.[74] Active virus was isolated from a number of vaccine lots. As a result, new requirements were introduced for safety testing along with a filtration step. With these relatively modest changes, the problem was solved, and no untoward reactions from the inactivated vaccine have since been observed.

Cutter produced the smallest amount of vaccine of any of the manufacturers, and the products of the other companies proved to be safe. Nonetheless, 260 cases of poliomyelitis were identified as being caused by the Cutter vaccine. Of these, 94 were in vaccinees, 126 were in family contacts, and 40 were in community contacts. Of the 260 cases, 192 were paralytic; there were no deaths. Surprisingly, the "Cutter incident" did not shake public confidence in the vaccine, and when vaccination was resumed, it was well accepted. The outcome might have been very different if the product of just one other manufacturer had proved to be unsafe.

One important outcome of the Cutter incident was the creation of the surveillance unit at the Centers for Disease Control (now the Centers for Disease Control and Prevention [CDC]), which has maintained excellent scrutiny of polio and other vaccination programs.

With the resumption of vaccination in the United States and many other countries, the impact on the incidence of disease soon became evident.[75, 76]

LIVE ATTENUATED VACCINES

The use of attenuated forms of organisms for the induction of active immunity dates back at least to Jenner's use of the cowpox virus to immunize against smallpox. Pasteur reduced the virulence of rabies virus by the desiccation of infected spinal cords, and bacille Calmette-Guérin was attenuated by passage in an unfavorable medium. However, the first demonstration of attenuation of a virus in tissue culture was that of Lloyd and Theiler and their associates[77, 78] with the yellow fever virus. The attenuated virus that resulted from prolonged passage in cultures of chick embryo tissue proved to be a safe and effective immunizing agent in humans.

The idea of attenuated vaccines as opposed to killed vaccines appealed to many investigators, because it was presumed that an active infection most nearly reproduced the natural situation and could be expected to give longer-lasting immunity and greater resistance of the bowel to reinfection.

It was demonstrated in Enders's laboratory that the polioviruses lost virulence for the central nervous system on passage in non–nervous system tissues.[44] The characteristics of strains suitable as vaccines would need to include the following:

1. The capacity to parasitize the gut and induce neutralizing antibody
2. An inability to infect the central nervous system and thus cause disease
3. Genetic stability such that the strains would not revert to neurovirulence after multiplication in the human host

The approaches were, of necessity, empirical and involved passage of virus in rodents, various types of tissue culture, and a combination of the two.[79–85] The first published report on the use of a live attenuated poliovirus in a human appeared in 1952 from Koprowski and coworkers.[79] They used virus attenuated by passage through cotton rats.

Three groups in the United States were the principal investigators working to develop a live attenuated polio vaccine. They were Cox at Lederle, Koprowski and associates at the Wistar Institute in Philadelphia, and Sabin in Cincinnati. Cox and Koprowski were working with strains of the same origin, whereas Sabin developed his own set of mutant viruses. During the 1950s, much work was conducted to test the immunogenicity and safety of the vaccine strains in the laboratory. An important point at issue was the genetic stability of the vaccine strains—would they revert to virulence after multiplying in the human host? Unfortunately, few in vitro markers of virulence, such as growth at higher temperature, were available, and these were not particularly precise. The most definitive test for neurovirulence was considered to be inoculation of monkeys intracerebrally or directly into the spinal cord. Although expensive and requiring expert interpretation, the monkey test was adopted as the definitive test for neurovirulence by the regulatory agencies. The literature from this period on attenuated vaccine viruses is voluminous, and no effort is made to provide a comprehensive bibliography here. However, a number of international conferences on poliomyelitis were held, some dealing specifically with the oral attenuated vaccines, and a perusal of the findings from these conferences can provide one with a reasonably complete picture of the development of the vaccines and their early use.[86–93]

Field trials of increasingly large size were conducted with the various candidate strains in different parts of the world. It was difficult to conduct large-scale trials in the United States because the Salk vaccine had been licensed and was being used widely; therefore, only a few trials were conducted there.[94–96] Originally, the different types of vaccines were fed separately because some degree of interference occurred among them. However, it was later found that by adjusting the amounts, virus interference could be overcome to a large extent; a trivalent vaccine thereby became possible. In 1957, a World Health Organization (WHO) committee recommended that field trials be conducted with Sabin's strains. The first large-scale trial of these strains occurred in 1958. In Singapore, 200,000 children received type 2 vaccine in an effort to abort, through interference, a type 1 epidemic. The vaccine virus did indeed appear to interfere with the wild virus and to be safe. In the same year, Sabin provided Professor Chumakov of Moscow a supply of his attenuated virus strains, which were used for early field trials and as seed for the manufacture of vaccine in what was then the USSR. The Soviets moved rapidly. In just over a year, approximately 15 million people were vaccinated without any recorded untoward event and with evident effectiveness. By 1960, about 100 million people in the USSR and Eastern European countries had received the three individual types of Sabin vaccine separately.[97, 98] This large success was presented as evidence to support an application for licensure in the United States of the Sabin live poliovirus vaccine. Dr. Dorothy Horstmann was asked to visit the USSR and Eastern European countries to evaluate the program and the reliability of the data. Her report in 1959 was favorable,[99] and, in part on the basis of her evaluation, the vaccine was licensed in 1960. Thus, within just over 10 years from the time that tissue culture techniques were first described, two effective and safe vaccines against poliomyelitis were available for general use.

ROLE OF THE NATIONAL FOUNDATION FOR INFANTILE PARALYSIS

An important element in the developments leading up to the achievement of poliovirus vaccines was the National Foundation for Infantile Paralysis. The foundation was established in 1938 as a goal-oriented voluntary organization. Its principal goal was to prevent polio, and thus a significant proportion of the money raised by voluntary contributions was used to support virus research and fellowships for investigators. The scientific program was led by Dr. Thomas Rivers, who enlisted as advisers the most knowledgeable individuals from the scientific community. Benison's book, *An Oral History Memoir*,[16] gives an interesting account of the conduct of the research effort. Once a vaccine became a possibility, the Foundation supported the developmental work by Salk and Sabin and financed a large-scale field trial of the inactivated vaccine. The way in which this program was conducted effectively illustrates how biomedical research can function in solving a practical problem. The first need is to establish a knowledge base, which is derived from basic explorations. Only when the scientific base has been laid can the practical goal—in this instance, the vaccine—be successfully pursued.[100]

THE SIMIAN VIRUS 40 EPISODE

In 1960, Sweet and Hilleman described the isolation of a virus that caused a typical vacuolation in cells from cynomolgus monkeys; the virus had been isolated from cultures of rhesus monkey kidney cells.[101] This virus, simian virus 40 (SV40), was found to cause an inapparent infection in rhesus monkeys in nature. It remained latent in the kidney cells until activated in tissue culture and could be detected only by testing in cultured cells from a susceptible species. It was found to be a contaminant of many lots of both inactivated and live vaccines. SV40's inactivation curve with formaldehyde was such that some active virus might survive an exposure that was fully adequate to inactivate poliovirus.[102]

Once the presence of the contaminating virus was recognized, proper measures were taken to ensure its exclusion from the vaccine. However, this finding did cause a great deal of concern, because SV40 was a DNA virus of the papovavirus family and had been shown to cause cancer in several species of animals and to transform cells in culture.[103, 104] Evidence was presented that some people who received contaminated poliovirus vaccines orally or parenterally developed antibodies to SV40[105–107] and that virus was occasionally isolated from the feces of recipients of oral poliovirus vaccine (OPV).[108] Similar findings were obtained with volunteer subjects who had received SV40 by the respiratory route.[109] In some populations, antibodies to SV40 were present in sera collected before poliovirus vaccines had been available, suggesting that the antibodies were evoked by natural infection with related viruses.[110, 111]

Two epidemiological approaches have been taken in assessing whether SV40-contaminated vaccine causes any deleterious effects in recipients. Fraumeni and associates compared the causes of mortality, particularly from cancer, between populations that had presumably received SV40-contaminated vaccine and those that had not.[112] No differences of any kind were found. In addition, during an observation period of 17 to 19 years, prospective surveillance of a cohort of approximately 1077 infants who received contaminated OPV in the first days of life and 150 who received inactivated (killed) poliovirus vaccine (IPV) that contained SV40 intramuscularly revealed no excessive incidence of cancer or mortality from any other cause.[113, 114] These findings, although not absolute proof of the benignity of SV40 in humans, are reassuring, and it seems highly unlikely that SV40 is carcinogenic or otherwise pathogenic for humans. However, the experience with SV40 has clearly demonstrated one of the problems associated with the use of primary cell cultures to produce vaccines and biologicals for use in humans.

KILLED POLIOVIRUS VACCINE VERSUS ORAL POLIOVIRUS VACCINE

The new availability of the live (OPV) vaccine prompted a comparison with the IPV already in use. The principal points raised were the following:

1. The IPV had been used widely for approximately 6 years and had proved to be safe and effective.
2. The OPV was less expensive and much simpler to administer. Thus, it was more suitable than the IPV for mass campaigns and programs directed at difficult-to-reach populations, as the IPV had to be administered by injection with a four-dose schedule.
3. The principal disadvantage of the OPV was its relative lability, compared with that of the IPV, at temperatures above freezing. There was also concern that it would not be effective in the presence of an enterovirus infection.

4. Early evidence indicated that whereas both vaccines gave satisfactory protection against paralytic disease, the active infection of the bowel that occurred with the OPV resulted in resistance to reinfection more similar to that resulting from natural infection. Conversely, the IPV seemed to produce little resistance to intestinal infection.[115, 116] Thus, the OPV could be expected to be more effective than the IPV in interrupting the spread of the virus within the community. A side benefit of OPV was thought to be the spread of the vaccine virus from vaccinees to susceptible contacts, thus amplifying its effect.[117–120]

5. In spite of the 1954 field trial's evidence of the effectiveness of IPV, there was some concern that outbreaks of paralytic disease were still occurring between 1955, when IPV was licensed, and 1961, when OPV became available. Thus, some questions were raised about the true effectiveness of IPV as it was produced and used in the United States; indeed, Berkovich and colleagues[121] presented evidence that the 1959 epidemic of polio in Boston was likely caused by the use of low-potency vaccine.

In 1962, Luther Terry, the Surgeon General of the U.S. Public Health Service, issued Public Health Service recommendations for the use of poliomyelitis vaccine for the 1962 poliomyelitis season.[122] The relative advantages of the OPV and the IPV were enumerated, but neither vaccine was recommended to the exclusion of the other. However, the OPV was soon being given almost exclusively in the United States. By 1964, the Committee on the Control of Infectious Diseases of the American Academy of Pediatrics[123] expressed a clear preference for the OPV: "Evaluation of the virtues and limitations of killed and live poliovaccines reveals a clearcut superiority of the OPV from the point of view of ease of administration, immunogenic effect, protective capacity, and potential for the eradication of poliomyelitis."

As already indicated, the USSR had previously determined to use the OPV exclusively, and most countries did the same. However, Sweden, Finland, and the Netherlands chose to administer only the IPV and thus provided an interesting population with which to compare the effectiveness of IPV and OPV. In the early years of OPV use, monotypic vaccines were used in sequence—vaccines 1, 3, and 2 at 6-week or 2-month intervals, followed 6 months later by a dose of trivalent vaccine. Later, the trivalent vaccine was found to be adequate, and a simplified regimen was adopted in the United States: three doses of trivalent vaccine at 2-month intervals beginning at 2 months of age, given simultaneously with the first inoculation of the diphtheria, pertussis, and tetanus vaccine. A fourth dose of trivalent OPV approximately 1 year later completed the series, and a fifth dose was administered on entry to school.[124]

In those countries that have been able to achieve a high level of immunization, whether with OPV or IPV, paralytic poliomyelitis has become almost unknown. This group encompasses most of the industrialized countries. Among less developed countries, Cuba and Costa Rica[125] appear to have achieved eradication. In the United States, the fall in incidence of paralytic polio that had begun with the introduction of IPV in 1955 continued at much the same rate after 1963, when OPV became the predominant vaccine in use. By 1969, only about a dozen cases were recorded in the entire country, and this average has continued up to the present, except that in more recent years all the cases have been vaccine associated. A total of 69 cases was reported from 1978 to 1983. Fifty-one cases were classified as vaccine associated, six of which occurred in immunodeficient children.[126] Furthermore, only one case of infection caused by a wild strain (nonvaccine) of poliovirus has been identified since 1980.

DISEASE ASSOCIATED WITH THE ORAL POLIOVIRUS VACCINE

Although the OPV has been highly effective, its benefits have been achieved at some cost, namely, vaccine-associated cases of paralysis. Largely because of the excellent surveillance system that had been set up by the CDC, it was recognized soon after the OPV became used on a large scale that cases of paralytic disease were occurring in vaccinees and their intimate contacts. Given the time of year when these cases occurred, the temporal association with vaccination, and the fact that the virus isolated from the cases had the characteristics of vaccine strains, there was a strong presumption that these cases of paralytic disease were caused by the vaccine virus.[127–129] As more data have accumulated, it is clear that only rarely do either vaccinees or contacts contract paralytic polio from the vaccine virus. A small proportion of these patients are immunodeficient, but most have no detectable immunological or other abnormality that might enhance their susceptibility to infection. It has also been shown that some normal vaccinees develop viremia, usually owing to type 2 virus, although this viremia does not seem to be associated with paralytic disease.[130–132]

In a 10-year multinational study conducted under the auspices of the WHO, it was found that vaccine-associated cases developed in all countries but that there was considerable variation in incidence, with a few countries having notably higher rates than others[133–135]; no reason for this variation was identified. Type 3 virus was isolated most often from cases in vaccinees, and type 2 from contact cases. From the data of the WHO study and additional data gathered in the United States by the CDC, rough estimates of the risk of paralysis to vaccinees and contacts can be made. Based on the number of doses of vaccine distributed, the risk to recipients and contacts is well below one case per 1 million doses. However, the risk from the first dose (one case per 500,000 doses administered for recipients and contacts) is considerably higher than that from subsequent doses (one case per 13 million doses). Thus, OPV does pose a small risk to recipients of the vaccine and their nonimmune intimate contacts, most of whom are adults. Obviously, the risk to contacts should be further reduced as the level of immunity in the community is increased. In most circumstances, the risk-benefit ratio is acceptable. However, in countries such as the United States, in which vaccine-associated cases account for all the indigenous cases of paralytic polio, even though few, consideration must be given to changing the policy so as to use IPV for primary immunization, which, as far as we know, carries no risk.[136–139] The pertinence of this consideration is enhanced by a number of developments.

Workers at the Rijks Institut voor de Volksgezardheid in Bilthoven, Netherlands, developed a more potent and more highly purified IPV[140] that requires only two doses—possibly one—for primary immunization.[141] Furthermore, poliovaccine can be successfully combined with the diphtheria, pertussis, and tetanus (DPT) vaccine, greatly simplifying the use of IPV.[142]

Data from those countries that have used only IPV[143–146] indicate unequivocally that poliomyelitis has been controlled and that the virus can no longer be recovered from the environment. In each instance, the percentage of the population immunized has been very high (approximately 90%), and herd immunity seems to have been achieved. It has been hypothesized that in societies in which fecal-oral spread is limited, the principal route of spread is from close contact and that pharyngeal virus is the most important source of infection. Infection of the pharyngeal cells is suppressed much more readily by circulating antibody than is infection of the lower bowel, which is relatively insensitive to antibody and where high titers are required to show any demonstrable effect.[146, 147] Even in highly immunized populations, however, small outbreaks of paralytic poliomyelitis resulting from wild viruses have occurred in groups of people who were not immunized. This type of outbreak occurred in the Netherlands among a religious sect that rejected vaccination.

In 1984, there was a small outbreak of type 3 polio in Finland.[148, 149] There had been no poliomyelitis in Finland for 20 years when, in October 1984, a few cases of clinical disease occurred. Type 3 virus of wild type was isolated from all the patients, 45% of 86 intimate contacts, and 15% of 700 well children in the vicinity. The same virus was also isolated from sewage at a number of sites in the country. Nine cases of paralysis and one of meningoencephalitis were reported. All but two of the patients had been immunized, and the one fatality, a 17-year-old male adolescent, had received five doses of IPV. In attempting to explain the reestablishment of wild poliovirus in a highly immunized population that had been virus free for many years, three factors were identified as possible contributing causes:

1. The vaccine that had been in use was found to be of marginal potency for type 3 virus.
2. There had been a drop in the percentage of infants and young children receiving vaccine.
3. There was a minor antigenic difference between the circulating wild virus and the virus in the vaccine.

It is probable that the most important factor was the poor potency of the vaccine, although the other factors may have played some role.

In response to the evidence of widespread infection, 1.5 million children younger than 19 years were given a dose of IPV, and in a mass campaign shortly thereafter, a dose of OPV was administered to approximately 94% of the entire population of 4.5 million. At present, the country is once again polio free, and the regular use of a more potent IPV has been resumed.

The Finnish experience is instructive in several ways. First, it emphasizes the value of an effective surveillance program. Second, it indicates that attention should be paid to monitoring the potency of the vaccines being used and again illustrates the relationship among vaccine potency, antibody response, and protection. However, it does not appear to support the hypothesis that prior experience with the antigen, even in the absence of detectable antibody, primes the immune system so that response to infection will be rapid enough to prevent disease. Third, even in the relatively small, homogeneous country of Finland, with its well-organized healthcare delivery system, there was some decrease in the percentage of vaccinated children in the population. This suggests that, as one might expect, with the disappearance of a disease for 20 years or more, it becomes more difficult to motivate both the public and the health providers to sustain immunization against a threat that seems purely theoretical. Finally, it is reassuring that in spite of considerable seeding of the population with a virulent strain of poliovirus, only a few cases of paralytic disease occurred; presumably, the high level of immunity in the community kept it in check.

Another experience that has been instructive is the 1982 epidemic of paralytic polio in Taiwan.[150] This epidemic, in which there were 1031 recorded cases of paralytic disease (and an overall attack rate of 5.8 per 100,000), was the largest outbreak in the history of Taiwan. The outbreak occurred although there had been only the occasional case of paralytic polio since 1975. Routine immunization with OPV had been conducted since 1967, and approximately 80% of infants had received at least two doses of trivalent OPV. Thus, the level of immunization was quite high, comparable with that in most of the industrialized countries. Approximately 66% of the cases had received no vaccine, and 19% had received only one dose. The evidence indicated that the epidemic was due primarily to a pool of nonimmunized susceptible people rather than to a failure of the vaccine. Indeed, vaccine efficacy was calculated to be 82% for one dose and more than 95% for two or more doses.

This experience reinforces the observation that polio can occur in nonimmunized susceptible people even when there is a high overall rate of vaccination. In spite of the widespread use of OPV for a number of years, spread from vaccinees to nonvaccinated susceptible people seems not to have been an important factor in supplementing immunity in the population. This result tends to conform with the observation of Fox and colleagues[118] and others that whereas vaccine strains disseminate readily to susceptible people within the family, spread to less intimate contacts is limited. It has also raised the question as to whether OPV induces intestinal immunity that is as effective and long-lasting as is generally believed.[151, 152]

POLIO IN DEVELOPING COUNTRIES

Poliomyelitis presents a special problem in developing countries, particularly those in the tropical zone. It is only recently that poliomyelitis has been recognized as a significant problem in these countries. With careful surveillance and the conducting of lameness surveys, a considerable reservoir of paralytic disease in children has been detected.[153, 154] Indeed, the incidence of crippling disease in those countries in which surveys were done was found to be as high as in industrialized countries before vaccine was available. Epidemiologically, the disease occurs in young children, and there is no seasonal peak.

It was expected that OPV would be the ideal vaccine in Third World countries.[155] Experience in Cuba and Costa Rica, in particular, indicated a high level of effectiveness, and paralytic disease has virtually disappeared.[125] However, in other developing countries, particularly those in the tropical zone, experience has not been so satisfactory. The problem is due in part to the lability of the vaccine (i.e., exposure to high temperatures leads to inactivation), so that the vaccine must be kept refrigerated at all times. This is not always easy to guarantee in tropical, underdeveloped countries. Even when the so-called *cold chain* has been well managed, however, the live vaccines have proved to be less effective in these environments than anticipated; the exact reason for this is not known. Speculation has included the possibility of (1) interference by other enteroviruses that tend to be prevalent in these populations, (2) interference in some nonspecific way owing to diarrhea that is common in infants in these countries, and (3) antibody in the breast milk. Although there does seem to be a difference in effectiveness in the tropical countries, in those situations in which the active vaccine has been delivered to a large proportion of the population, satisfactory control of the disease has been possible. Thus, the problem seems to be as much logistical as it is scientific.

Most of the successful programs in tropical or developing countries have employed the technique of mass campaigns. Sabin has been the principal proponent of this approach, and there is no question that when the logistics are well handled, this technique can be highly effective.[156–159] However, legitimate concern has been expressed that such targeted campaigns can absorb resources to the detriment of a broader sustained health-care program based on primary care, which few would disagree is the ultimate goal. In many countries, unfortunately, this goal is not realizable in the near future, and targeted campaigns should ideally be used to further this goal rather than retard it.

With the production of the more potent IPV, there has been increased interest in its use in developing and tropical countries.[160, 161] The IPV is more heat stable, has as good or better antibody response than the OPV, and has no untoward effects. In spite of these advantages, however, it still must be given parenterally, which requires needles and syringes. Jet injectors might overcome this need, but they present major problems of maintenance in the field. It may be that some prepackaged system (e.g., Ezeject), such as was developed by Hilleman and associates[162] for measles, will help solve the delivery problem. However, there are still the matters of cost and the safe disposal of used syringes.

Thus, for use in developing and tropical countries, both OPV and IPV have advantages and disadvantages. OPV is inexpensive, easy to administer, and ideally suited for use in mass campaigns and in situations lacking adequately trained health professionals. However, it is less effective in tropical climates for unknown reasons, and its sensitivity to heat makes it difficult to transport and store. It is doubtful that the greater intestinal immunity conferred by OPV, or its somewhat limited capacity to spread to unvaccinated people, is a major factor in its favor in the tropical environment.

IPV is more stable, seems to be fully effective in the tropics, and, with the development of more potent vaccines, requires no more doses than does OPV. However, it is still much more expensive than OPV and, because it must be injected, requires a more sophisticated delivery system.

Regardless of which vaccine is used, it would seem that if paralytic polio is to be controlled in tropical countries, a high rate of immunization (80–90%) in young infants must be achieved and maintained. The need for sustaining a high level of immunity in infants and young children is probably greater in the tropical zone, where viral dissemination occurs year round, than in the temperate zone, where dissemination is seasonal.[163] This immunity level demands political commitment and adequate infrastructure, both of which are often lacking.

MOLECULAR BIOLOGY OF POLIOMYELITIS AND IMPLICATIONS FOR THE FUTURE

Rapid advances in molecular biology have made it possible to learn more about the structure of the poliovirus and its genome. This information offers the prospect of manipulating virulence; preparing more stable, inexpensive, and safe vaccines; and accurately characterizing viral strains.[164–166]

Results of studies on the structure of the viral particle have shown that populations of virions are made up of infective particles—designated as D particles—and noninfective, or empty, particles—designated as C particles. These two types of particles are similar antigenically but have detectable differences that may be related to tertiary structure.

The viral capsid is composed of 60 copies of each of four polypeptides (V_1, V_2, V_3, V_4) that surround the single-stranded RNA genome of about 7450 nucleotides.[167]

A key observation that set the stage for exploration of the molecular biology of poliovirus was that of Racaniello and Baltimore,[168] who were able to prepare DNA complementary to the poliovirus RNA and to show that this DNA was infectious when introduced into mammalian cells. This finding has made possible genetic manipulation that was otherwise impossible.

The base sequence of poliovirus RNA and complementary DNA has been established. Progress has been rapid in determining the relationship between the genomic location and the polypeptide structure, including the identity of certain epitopes and their position on the genome; this information makes it possible to produce the specific peptides using cloning techniques. Purified or synthetic peptides are rarely very antigenic in themselves and require some form of adjuvant. Wimmer and colleagues, however, have shown that two relatively small peptides (VP1) derived from the polypeptides of type 1 poliovirus were capable of priming an animal so that a broad antibody response was obtained on reimmunization.[169] It is also possible to consider construction of a strain of poliovirus possessing the key epitopes of the three types.[166]

Rapid progress is being made in defining the molecular basis for virulence or the lack of it. Although the construction of stable avirulent strains is far from possible now, it is a reasonable goal. Avirulent types 1 and 2 have more base substitutions compared with wild strains than does type 3, which may explain the greater genetic instability of the type 3 virus.

At a less sophisticated level, the treatment of poliovirus RNA with ribonuclease T_1 produces a variety of oligonucleotides that when separated by two-dimensional electrophoresis, give a "fingerprint" that is characteristic for each viral strain.[170] This technique makes possible what is referred to as *molecular epidemiology*, by which the source of viral isolates can be defined with comparative ease. Vaccine strains can be distinguished from wild strains, and a particular virus can be tracked. This technique was used with the agent that infected people belonging to a religious sect in the Netherlands who transmitted it to contacts in Canada and the United States. With the use of oligonucleotide fingerprinting, the infectious agent was shown to be the same virus strain. The polymerase chain reaction is another means of rapid, accurate characterization of virus strain.

Thus, aside from their innate scientific interest, studies of the molecular biology of the poliovirus offer the prospect of practical outcomes, such as cheaper, more stable, and more effective vaccines, as well as new tools for epidemiological investigations and diagnosis.

ERADICATION OF POLIOMYELITIS

From the experiences in many countries, it is evident that paralytic disease caused by wild poliovirus can be eliminated. Elimination may be achieved with either IPV or OPV, provided that a high level of immunization is obtained and maintained in the population. With the present OPV strains, rare cases of paralysis resulting from the vaccine viruses will continue to occur in vaccinees and their contacts. With the available OPV, then, it does not appear that paralytic disease caused by polioviruses can be totally eliminated. However, it has been pointed out that this elimination has been achieved with the sole use of IPV or a combined regimen, such as was used in Denmark.[171]

If we define *control* of poliomyelitis as a reduction of poliovirus-induced paralytic disease to very low levels, such as exist in the United States, we can consider this level of control to have been achieved in most of the industrialized countries and in some developing countries. However, *eradication*, defined as an absence of the causative agent from the environment, has seldom been accomplished for any length of time. Even when eradication has been demonstrated, as in Finland, where for many years polioviruses could not be isolated from sewage samples, infection and disease can occur from wild viruses introduced from the outside; such infection can occur even when only a small group of susceptible people remains in the population. Thus, as long as wild polioviruses exist in the world, it will be necessary to maintain consistently high levels of immunization to control or eradicate poliomyelitis in a country or region.

Obviously, if worldwide eradication of polioviruses could be accomplished, as was done successfully with smallpox, it would no longer be necessary to continue vaccination. In reviewing whether diseases other than smallpox might be eradicated, Stetten[172] cited polio as a possibility, and it was considered further at the 1980 International Conference on the Eradication of Infectious Diseases.[173]

Certain features make the global eradication of poliomyelitis technically feasible.[174–176] These features include the following:

1. Immunity can be provided by two excellent vaccines, and viral transmission can be interrupted.
2. There is no animal reservoir.
3. There are only three immunological types of virus, and they are genetically stable.
4. The OPV is inexpensive and easy to administer in mass campaigns.
5. It is expected that the more potent IPV will require fewer doses for primary immunization and will be less expensive than the OPV.

The features of polio that militate against its easy eradication are as follows:

1. IPV is relatively inefficient in preventing the spread of virus.
2. Poliovirus is contagious, particularly by the fecal-oral route.
3. The use of OPV in tropical countries has had peculiar problems.
4. Eradication efforts are complicated by the technical issues concerning administration of the vaccine, such as monitoring a cold chain, particularly for OPV; the need to give IPV by injection; and cost factors, particularly for IPV.
5. Probably most important is whether, in many countries, the political will exists that is so necessary for a successful effort to be undertaken. There is continual tension between those who favor mass campaigns and those who emphasize the value of incorporating vaccination into primary care programs and consider mass cam-

paigns as distracting and as diverting resources from the development of ongoing basic health services.

6. Verification of success will be more difficult than was the case with smallpox. Inapparent infection occurs often (100–1000 people are infected for each paralytic case), requiring the use of methods such as sewage sampling and population surveys to demonstrate the absence of wild viruses. Furthermore, a number of other viruses and conditions can mimic paralytic poliomyelitis.[177–179] A particularly dramatic example of this was the 1982 epidemic of enterovirus 71 infection in Bulgaria, in which there were more than 700 nonparalytic cases, with 149 cases of paralysis and 44 deaths.[180] These cases could be distinguished from poliomyelitis only by virus isolation and antibody determination.

At the 1984 International Symposium on Poliomyelitis Control, it was concluded that whereas global eradication of poliomyelitis was probably technically feasible, a realistic goal for the near future should be the control of paralytic disease, with eradication in certain countries or regions.[181]

In spite of the difficulties that were anticipated, the Pan American Health Organization in 1985 began a major campaign to eradicate poliovirus from the Western Hemisphere. Support from the countries of the region has been remarkably strong, and various organizations have contributed resources, including Rotary International, which has provided considerable support in money and volunteer workers.

The program has required skilled management and organization, and a remarkable spirit of cooperation has been generated. Regional laboratories have been set up, surveillance systems organized, and volunteer participation enlisted. To a great extent, countries have relied on mass campaigns with oral vaccine. When suspicious cases have occurred in an area, house-to-house programs have been conducted to saturate the area. One of the most difficult problems has been to differentiate poliomyelitis cases from paralysis due to other causes. This process requires conducting a careful clinical evaluation, obtaining adequate specimens, and transporting these specimens to a laboratory in good time.[182] Another problem that has had to be solved is distinguishing between wild viruses and vaccine strains, the latter being widely disseminated in the environment. Molecular biological techniques such as polymerase chain reaction have been developed at the CDC and are highly sensitive and discriminating. The program has been remarkably successful, and most countries of the Americas have had no cases of infection caused by wild poliovirus for periods of years. The last case was diagnosed in Peru in September 1991, although compatible cases still occur in which polio cannot be ruled out.

Following these efforts, the problem then became that of proving that eradication had been achieved. An international commission for certification was established similar to the one that was created during the smallpox campaign. The commission stipulated certain criteria that must be met for certification to be provided[183]:

1. No cases of poliomyelitis caused by a wild virus for 3 years within the hemisphere
2. A satisfactory surveillance system, including adequate diagnostic procedures to distinguish poliovirus infection from other causes of acute flaccid paralysis
3. Environmental surveys (e.g., sewage, stool surveys) that demonstrate the absence of wild poliovirus

In 1994, the International Commission for Certification of Poliomyelitis Eradication in the Americas met to review the individual country reports. No cases caused by wild virus had occurred since the one in 1991. It was found that environmental surveys were not very useful but that the large number of specimens tested from suspect cases and their contacts, all of which were negative, provided adequate data. The commission concluded that the evidence was sufficient to declare that eradication had been achieved in the Western Hemisphere.[184]

The experience in the Americas has been instrumental in the WHO Assembly's initiation of a program of global eradication.[185] Eradication will not be an easy task; it would be expedited were a heat-stable vaccine available. Thus, the development of such a vaccine has been given priority by international bodies. In spite of the absence of a more stable vaccine, the global eradication of polio is proceeding remarkably well. There is reason to believe that eradication has been achieved in China, and mass immunization days are being conducted in many countries in Eastern Europe, Asia, and Africa. It will not be easy to reach the goal of global eradication by the year 2000, but there is reason to believe that it can occur in the not too distant future. (A summary of the status of the global program as of 1997 was reviewed in a special issue of the *Journal of Infectious Diseases*.[186]) Only when global eradication has been achieved will it be possible to cease routine vaccination—the eventual goal—and to relegate poliomyelitis and its causative virus to history.

VACCINATION REGIMENS

As has previously been indicated, different vaccines and different regimens are used in different countries. Much of the world uses OPV (i.e., trivalent oral poliovaccine) exclusively, whereas Sweden, Finland, France, and the Netherlands use only IPV, in most instances combined with DPT or with diphtheria and tetanus toxoids (DT). Certain countries in Africa, particularly the French-speaking countries, are also using IPV. Denmark employs IPV for primary immunization combined with DT, followed by three doses of OPV. Some countries use mass campaigns once or twice a year; in Brazil, for example, there is a 2-day period twice a year when every young child, regardless of previous history, is immunized. Neither the vaccine nor the regimen adopted seems to be critical, provided that adequate coverage is achieved.

In the United States, since the adoption of OPV as the preferred vaccine, the regimen recommended by the official bodies has been as follows: DPT and OPV at 2, 4, and 6 months of age, with another dose of OPV at

18 months and again on entry to school. The Advisory Committee on Immunization Practices has recommended that the 6-month dose of OPV be dropped.

In 1988, the Evaluation of Poliomyelitis Vaccine Policy Options Committee of the Institute of Medicine of the National Academy of Sciences[187] recommended that primary immunization in the United States should be with combined DPT-IPV, to be followed later by a dose of OPV. This recommendation was made because the only poliovirus-induced paralysis since 1980 was caused by the vaccine virus. The recommendation has not been implemented, however, because the four-component vaccine has not been licensed in the United States.

The Advisory Committee on Immunization practices has recommended a new vaccination schedule: IPV at 2 and 4 months of age followed by OPV at 6 to 12 months of age and an additional dose of OPV at 18 to 24 months of age. This regimen should prevent most vaccine cases and still provide intestinal immunity.[188]

An important issue is educating parents and vaccinees about the risk associated with the use of OPV. It is generally suggested that the person administering the vaccine, usually the physician, inform the parents or recipients of the small risk to vaccinees and intimate contacts. The vaccination histories of the parents or other adults in the family who are in intimate contact with the vaccinees should be determined. If they have not been vaccinated or there is doubt about the vaccination history, the adults should receive OPV at the same time as the infants, or vaccination of the infants can be delayed so that the adults can receive IPV. The recommendations of the Committee on Infectious Diseases of the American Academy of Pediatrics are as follows:

1. For those who have had a partial course of immunization, a booster dose of IPV can be given when the child receives OPV.
2. If there is no history of immunization or if the history is unknown, three doses of IPV a month apart can be given to the contact, and the child can receive the first dose of OPV simultaneously with the third IPV dose.

Although such a procedure is prudent, it has been stressed repeatedly that immunization of the adult should not be allowed to interfere with immunization of the infant. Only parents or others having comparable intimate contact with the infant are at risk, and mothers are at greater risk than fathers. Although such advice is not always mentioned in official recommendations, it would probably be wise to advise the contacts to wash their hands, particularly after changing diapers, and to educate them about properly disposing of soiled diapers.

Because practices are subject to change, one should be aware of the sources of information about current recommendations of the various official or quasi-official bodies. One such source is the package insert prepared by the vaccine manufacturer and approved by the Food and Drug Administration. Another is the *Red Book: Report of the Committee on Infectious Diseases*, which is revised every few years. The recommendations of the Advisory Committee on Immunization Practices serve as the basis for decisions by most governmental agencies and are usually in agreement with the *Red Book*. These recommendations are published in the *Morbidity and Mortality Weekly Report* of the CDC. Finally, there is the *Guide for Adult Immunization* of the American College of Physicians.

The OPV should not be given to a person with immunodeficiency syndrome, to one receiving immunosuppressive therapy, or to one who suffers from altered immune states due to diseases such as lymphoma, leukemia, and generalized malignancy. Furthermore, the OPV should not be given to household contacts of people with impaired immune responses, for any of the aforementioned reasons.

REFERENCES

1. Hutchin EF. Historical summary. In Poliomyelitis: A Survey Made Possible by a Grant from the International Committee for the Study of Infantile Paralysis. Baltimore, Williams & Wilkins, 1932, pp 1–22.
2. Heine J. Beobachtungen Über Lahmungs zustande der unteren Extremitatien und deren Behandlung. Stuttgart, Kohler, 1840.
3. Medin O. Über eine Epidemic von spinaler Kinderlahmung. Verh Int Med Kongr 2 Abt 6:37, 1891.
4. Paul JR. Poliomyelitis. In Clinical Epidemiology. Chicago, University of Chicago Press, 1966, pp 177–195.
5. Landsteiner K, Popper E. Mikroscopische Preparate von einem menschlichen and zwei Affenruckenmarken. Klin Wochenschr 21:1830, 1908.
6. Landsteiner K, Popper E. Übertragung der Poliomyelitis acuta auf Affen. Z Immunitaetsforsch Exp Ther 2:377, 1909.
7. Armstrong C. The experimental transmission of poliomyelitis to the eastern cotton rat. Public Health Rep 54:1719, 1939.
8. Li CP, Schaeffer M. Adaptation of type 1 poliomyelitis virus to mice. Proc Soc Exp Biol Med 82:477, 1953.
9. Melnick JL, Horstmann DM. Active immunity to poliomyelitis in chimpanzees following subclinical infection. J Exp Med 85:287, 1947.
10. Howe HA, Bodian D, Morgan IM. Subclinical poliomyelitis in the chimpanzee and its relation to alimentary reinfection. Am J Hyg 51:85, 1950.
11. Rivers TM. Immunity in virus diseases with particular reference to poliomyelitis. Am J Public Health 26:136, 1936.
12. Hammon WMcD. Possibilities of specific prevention and treatment of poliomyelitis. Pediatrics 6:696, 1950.
13. Brodie M, Park WH. Active immunization against poliomyelitis. Am J Public Health 26:119, 1936.
14. Kolmer JA. Vaccination against acute anterior poliomyelitis. Am J Public Health 26:126, 1936.
15. Leake JP. Poliomyelitis following vaccination against this disease. JAMA 105:2152, 1935.
16. Benison S. Tom Rivers: Reflections on a life in medicine and science. In Benison S (ed). An Oral History Memoir. Cambridge, MA, MIT Press, 1967, pp 184–190.

16a. Rivers TM. Discussion of papers on poliomyelitis by William M. Park, MD, and Maurice Brodie, MD, and John A. Kolmer, MD, October 1938. In Benison S (ed). An Oral History Memoir. Cambridge, MA, MIT Press, 1967, pp 599–601.

17. Van Rooyen CF, Rhodes AJ. Virus Diseases of Man. London, Oxford University Press, 1940.
18. Robbins FC, Enders JF. Tissue culture techniques in the study of animal viruses. Am J Med Sci 220:316, 1950.
19. Sabin AB, Olitsky PK. Cultivation of poliomyelitis virus in vitro in human embryonic nervous tissue. Proc Soc Exp Biol Med 31:357, 1936.
20. Burnet FM, Jackson AV. Poliomyelitis 4. The spread of poliomyelitis virus in cynomolgus monkeys with particular reference to infection by the pharyngeal-intestinal route. Aust J Exp Biol Med Sci 18:361, 1940.

21. Bodian D. Differentiation of types of poliomyelitis viruses. I. Reinfection experiments in monkeys (second attacks). Am J Hyg 49:200, 1949.
22. Morgan IM. Differentiation of types of poliomyelitis viruses. II. By reciprocal vaccination-immunity. Am J Hyg 49:225, 1949.
23. Bodian D, Morgan IM, Howe HA. Differentiation of types of poliomyelitis viruses. III. The grouping of fourteen strains into three basic immunological types. Am J Hyg 49:234, 1949.
24. Kessel JF, Pait CF. Immunologic groups of poliomyelitis viruses. Am J Hyg 51:76, 1950.
25. Hammon WM, Coriell LL, Wehrle PF, Stokes J. Evaluation of Red Cross gamma globulin as a prophylactic agent for poliomyelitis. 4. Final report of results based on clinical diagnoses. JAMA 151:1272, 1953.
26. Bodian D. A reconsideration of the pathogenesis of poliomyelitis. Am J Hyg 55:414, 1952.
27. Hammon WMcD. Immunity in poliomyelitis. Bacteriol Rev 13:135, 1949.
28. Burnet FM. Some aspects of the epidemiology of poliomyelitis. Proc R Aust Coll Physicians 4:95, 1949.
29. Enders JF, Weller TH, Robbins FC. Cultivation of the Lansing strain of poliomyelitis virus in cultures of various human embryonic tissues. Science 109:85, 1949.
30. Sabin AB. Non-cytopathic variants of poliomyelitis viruses and resistance to superinfection in tissue culture. Science 120:357, 1954.
31. Weller TH, Robbins FC, Enders JF. Cultivation of poliomyelitis virus in cultures of human foreskin and embryonic tissues. Proc Soc Exp Biol Med 72:153, 1949.
32. Weller TH, Enders JF, Robbins FC, Stoddard MB. Studies on the cultivation of poliomyelitis viruses in tissue culture. I. The propagation of poliomyelitis viruses in suspended cell cultures of various human tissues. J Immunol 69:645, 1952.
33. Robbins FC, Weller TH, Enders JF. Studies on the cultivation of poliomyelitis viruses in tissue culture. II. The propagation of poliomyelitis viruses in roller-tube cultures of various human tissues. J Immunol 69:673, 1952.
34. Smith WM, Chambers VC, Evans CA. Growth of neurotropic viruses in extraneural tissues: Preliminary report on propagation of poliomyelitis virus [Lansing and Hof strains] in cultures of human testicular tissue. Northwest Med 49:368, 1950.
35. Syverton JT, Scherer WF, Butorac G. Propagation of poliomyelitis virus in cultures of monkey and human testicular tissues. Proc Soc Exp Biol Med 77:23, 1951.
36. Smith WM, Chambers VC, Evans CA. Growth of neurotropic viruses in extraneural tissues. IV. Poliomyelitis virus in human testicular tissue in vitro. Proc Soc Exp Biol Med 76:696, 1951.
37. Robbins FC, Enders JF, Weller TH. Cytopathogenic effect of poliomyelitis viruses in vitro on human embryonic tissues. Proc Soc Exp Biol Med 75:370, 1950.
38. Robbins FC, Enders JF, Weller TH, Florentino GL. Studies on the cultivation of poliomyelitis viruses in tissue culture. V. The direct isolation and serologic identification of virus strains in tissue culture from patients with nonparalytic and paralytic poliomyelitis. Am J Hyg 54:286, 1951.
39. Ledinko N, Riordan JT, Melnick JL. Multiplication of poliomyelitis viruses in tissue cultures of monkey testes. I. Growth curves of type 1 (Brunhilde) and type 2 (Lansing) strains and description of a quantitative neutralization test. Am J Hyg 55:323, 1952.
40. Riordan JT, Ledinko N, Melnick JL. Multiplication of poliomyelitis viruses in tissue cultures of monkey testes. II. Direct isolation and typing of strains from human stools and spinal cords in roller tubes. Am J Hyg 55:339, 1952.
41. Youngner JS, Ward EN, Salk JE. Studies on poliomyelitis viruses in cultures of monkey testicular tissue. I. Propagation of virus in roller tubes. Am J Hyg 55:291, 1952.
42. Youngner JS, Ward EN, Salk JE. Studies on poliomyelitis viruses in cultures of monkey testicular tissue. II. Differences among strains in tissue culture infectivity with preliminary data on the quantitative estimation of virus and antibody. Am J Hyg 55:301, 1952.
43. Youngner JS, Lewis LJ, Ward EN, Salk JE. Studies on poliomyelitis viruses in cultures of monkey testicular tissue. III. Isolation and immunologic identification of poliomyelitis viruses from fecal specimens by means of roller-tube cultures. Am J Hyg 55:347, 1952.
44. Enders JF, Robbins FC, Weller TH. The cultivation of the poliomyelitis viruses in tissue culture. Les Prix Nobel 1954. Stockholm, 1955.
45. Dulbecco R. Production of plaques in monolayer tissue cultures by single particles of an animal virus. Proc Natl Acad Sci U S A 38:747, 1952.
46. Dulbecco R, Vogt M. Plaque formation and isolation of pure lines with poliomyelitis viruses. J Exp Med 99:167, 1954.
47. Rous P, Jones FS. A method for obtaining suspensions of living cells from the fixed tissue, and for the plating out of individual cells. J Exp Med 23:549, 1916.
48. Melnick JL. Tissue culture techniques and their application to original isolation, growth, and assay of poliomyelitis and orphan viruses. Ann N Y Acad Sci 61:754, 1955.
49. Youngner JS. Monolayer tissue cultures. I. Preparation and standardization of suspensions of trypsin-dispersed monkey kidney cells. Proc Soc Exp Biol Med 85:202, 1954.
50. Youngner JS. Monolayer tissue cultures. II. Poliomyelitis virus assay in roller-tube cultures of trypsin-dispersed monkey kidney. Proc Soc Exp Biol Med 85:527, 1954.
51. Salk JE, Youngner JS, Ward EN. Use of color change of phenol red as the indicator in titrating poliomyelitis or its antibody in a tissue culture system. Am J Hyg 60:214, 1954.
52. Lipton MM, Steigman AJ. A simple colorimetric test for poliomyelitis virus and antibody. Proc Soc Exp Biol Med 88:114, 1955.
53. Robertson HE, Brunner KT, Syverton JT. Propagation in vitro of poliomyelitis viruses. VII. pH change of HeLa cell cultures for assay. Proc Soc Exp Biol Med 88:119, 1955.
54. Sanders M, Alexander RC. Epidemic keratoconjunctivitis. I. Isolation and identification of a filterable virus. J Exp Med 77:71, 1943.
55. Huang CH. Further studies on the titration of the western strain of equine encephalomyelitis virus in tissue culture. J Exp Med 78:111, 1943.
56. Huang CH. Titration of St. Louis encephalitis virus and Jungeblut-Sanders mouse virus in tissue culture. Proc Soc Exp Biol Med 54:158, 1943.
57. Huang CH. A visible method for titration and neutralization of viruses on the basis of pH changes in tissue cultures. Proc Soc Exp Biol Med 54:160, 1943.
58. Sanders M, Huang CH. Tissue cultures for virus investigations in the field. Am J Public Health 34:461, 1944.
59. Milzer A, Levinson SO, Shaughnessy HJ, et al. Immunogenicity studies in human subjects of trivalent tissue culture poliomyelitis vaccine inactivated by ultraviolet irradiation. Am J Public Health 44:26, 1954.
60. Wolf AM, Shaughnessy HJ, Church RE, et al. Immunogenicity, in children, of ultraviolet-treated poliomyelitis vaccine. JAMA 161:775, 1956.
61. Salk JE, Bennett BL, Lewis LJ, et al. Studies in human subjects on active immunization against poliomyelitis. I. A preliminary report of experiments in progress. JAMA 151:1081, 1953.
62. Salk JE. Recent studies in immunization against poliomyelitis. Pediatrics 12:471, 1953.
63. Salk JE, Bennett BL, Lewis LJ, et al. Studies in human subjects on active immunization against poliomyelitis. II. A practical means of inducing and maintaining antibody formation. Am J Public Health 44:994, 1954.
64. Salk JE, Krech U, Youngner JS, et al. Formaldehyde treatment and safety testing of experimental poliomyelitis vaccines. Am J Public Health 44:563, 1954.
65. Salk JE. A concept of the mechanism of immunity for preventing paralyses in poliomyelitis. Ann N Y Acad Sci 61:1023, 1955.
66. Bodian D, Paffenbarger RS. Poliomyelitis infection in households: Frequency of viremia and specific antibody response. Am J Hyg 60:83, 1954.
67. Horstmann DM, McCollum RW, Mascola AD. Viremia in human poliomyelitis. J Exp Med 99:355, 1954.
68. Rivers TM. Vaccine for poliomyelitis [correspondence]. JAMA 151:1224, 1953.
69. Research on a vaccine for the prevention of poliomyelitis [editorial]. JAMA 151:1198, 1953.
70. Francis T, Napier JA, Voight RB, et al. Evaluation of the 1954 Field Trial of Poliomyelitis Vaccine. Final Report. Poliomyelitis Vaccine Evaluation Center, Department of Epidemiology, School of Public Health, University of Michigan, Ann Arbor, 1957.

71. Nathanson N, Langmuir AD. The Cutter incident: Poliomyelitis following formaldehyde-inactivated poliovirus vaccination in the United States during the spring of 1955. I. Background. Am J Hyg 78:16, 1963.
72. Nathanson N, Langmuir AD. The Cutter incident: Poliomyelitis following formaldehyde-inactivated poliovirus vaccination in the United States during the spring of 1955. II. Relationship of poliomyelitis to Cutter vaccine. Am J Hyg 78:29, 1963.
73. Nathanson N, Langmuir AD. The Cutter incident: Poliomyelitis following formaldehyde-inactivated poliovirus vaccination in the United States during the spring of 1955. III. Comparison of the clinical character of vaccinated and contact cases occurring after use of high-rate lots of Cutter vaccine. Am J Hyg 78:61, 1963.
74. US Public Health Service Technical Report on Salk Poliomyelitis Vaccine. US Department of Health, Education and Welfare, Public Health Service, June 1955.
75. Langmuir AD. Results obtained by means of vaccine composed of inactivated viruses. In Poliomyelitis, Proceedings of the Fourth International Poliomyelitis Conference. Philadelphia, JB Lippincott, 1958, p 86.
76. Langmuir AD. Inactivated virus vaccines: Protective efficacy. In Poliomyelitis, Proceedings of the Fifth International Poliomyelitis Conference. Philadelphia, JB Lippincott, 1961, p 105.
77. Lloyd W, Theiler M, Ricci NI. Modification of the virulence of yellow fever virus by cultivation in tissue in vitro. Trans R Soc Trop Med Hyg 29:481, 1936.
78. Theiler M, Smith HH. The effect of prolonged cultivation in vitro upon the pathogenicity of yellow fever virus. J Exp Med 65:767, 1937.
79. Koprowski H, Jervis GA, Norton TW. Immune responses in human volunteers upon oral administration of a rodent adapted strain of poliomyelitis virus. Am J Hyg 55:108, 1952.
80. Melnick JL. Variations in poliomyelitis virus on serial passage through tissue culture. Cold Spring Harb Symp Quant Biol 18:278, 1953.
81. Sabin AB, Hennessen WA, Winsser J. Studies on variants of poliomyelitis virus. Experimental segregation and properties of avirulent variants of three immunologic types. J Exp Med 99:551, 1954.
82. Sabin AB. Immunity in poliomyelitis with special reference to vaccination. WHO Monogr Ser No. 26:297, 1955.
83. Sabin AB. Characteristics and genetic potentialities of experimentally produced and naturally occurring variants of poliomyelitis virus. Ann N Y Acad Sci 61:924, 1955.
84. Roca-Garcia M, Jervis GA. Experimentally produced poliomyelitis variant in chick embryo. Ann N Y Acad Sci 61:911, 1955.
85. Li CP, Schaeffer M, Nelson DB. Experimentally produced variants of poliomyelitis virus combining in vivo and in vitro techniques. Ann N Y Acad Sci 61:902, 1955.
86. Poliomyelitis: Papers and discussion presented at the 1st International Poliomyelitis Congress. Philadelphia, JB Lippincott, 1948.
87. Poliomyelitis: Papers and discussion presented at the 2nd International Poliomyelitis Congress. Philadelphia, JB Lippincott, 1951.
88. Poliomyelitis: Papers and discussion presented at the 3rd International Poliomyelitis Congress. Philadelphia, JB Lippincott, 1954.
89. Poliomyelitis: Papers and discussion presented at the 4th International Poliomyelitis Congress. Philadelphia, JB Lippincott, 1957.
90. Poliomyelitis: Papers and discussion presented at the 5th International Poliomyelitis Congress. Philadelphia, JB Lippincott, 1961.
91. Live Poliovirus Vaccines. Papers presented and discussions held at the 1st International Conference on Live Poliovirus Vaccines. Washington, DC, Pan American Health Organization, 1959.
92. Live Poliovirus Vaccines. Papers presented and discussions held at the 2nd International Conference on Live Poliovirus Vaccines. Washington, DC, Pan American Health Organization, 1960.
93. Oral Live Poliovirus Vaccine. Papers presented at the 4th Scientific Conference of the Institute of Poliomyelitis and Virus Encephalitis and the International Symposium on Live Poliovirus Vaccine. Moscow, Academy of Medical Sciences of the USSR, 1961.
94. Sabin AB. Immunization of chimpanzees and human beings with avirulent strains of poliomyelitis virus. Ann N Y Acad Sci 61:1050, 1955.
95. Koprowski H. Historical aspects of the development of live virus vaccine in poliomyelitis. BMJ 2:5192, 1960.
96. Cabasso VJ, Jervis GA, Moyer AW, et al. Cumulative testing experience with consecutive lots of oral poliomyelitis vaccine. BMJ 1:373, 1960.
97. Benison S. International medical cooperation: Dr. Albert Sabin, live poliovirus vaccine and the Soviets. Bull Hist Med 56:460, 1982.
98. Sabin AB. Role of my cooperation with Soviet scientists in the conquest of polio: Some lessons and challenges. The 23rd Cosmos Club Award. Washington, DC, April 1986.
99. Hortsmann D. Report on live poliovirus vaccination in the Union of Soviet Socialist Republics, Poland and Czechoslovakia, August–October 1959. New Haven, CT, Yale University Press, 1960, pp 1–122.
100. Shannon JA. National Institutes of Health: Present and potential contribution to application of biomedical knowledge. Research in the Service of Man: Biomedical Knowledge, Development and Use. US Senate, 90th Congress, 1st Session, Document No. 55, 1967.
101. Sweet BH, Hilleman MR. The vacuolating virus, SV_{40}. Proc Soc Exp Biol Med 105:420, 1960.
102. Gerber P, Hottle GA, Grubbs RE. Inactivation of vacuolating virus (SV_{40}) by formaldehyde. Proc Soc Exp Biol Med 108:205, 1961.
103. Eddy BE. Simian virus (SV_{40}): An oncogenic virus. Prog Exp Tumor Res 4:1, 1964.
104. Schein HM, Enders JF. Transformation induced by simian virus 40 in human renal cell cultures. I. Morphology and growth characteristics. Proc Natl Acad Sci U S A 48:1164, 1962.
105. Gerber P. Patterns of antibodies to SV_{40} in children following the last booster with inactivated poliomyelitis vaccines. Proc Soc Exp Biol Med 125:1284, 1967.
106. Shah KV. Evidence for an SV_{40}-related papovavirus infection of man. Am J Epidemiol 95:199, 1972.
107. Shah K, Nathanson N. Human exposure to SV_{40}: Review and comment. Am J Epidemiol 103:1, 1976.
108. Melnick JL, Stinebaugh S. Excretion of vacuolating SV_{40} virus (papovavirus group) after ingestion as a contaminant of oral poliovaccine. Proc Soc Exp Biol Med 109:965, 1962.
109. Morris JA, Johnson KM, Aulisio CG, et al. Clinical and serologic responses in volunteers given vacuolating virus [SV_{40}] by respiratory route. Proc Soc Exp Biol Med 108:56, 1961.
110. Geissler F, Scherneek S, Prokoph H, et al. SV_{40} in human brain tumors: Risk factor or passenger? In Giraldo G, Beth E (eds). The Role of Viruses in Human Cancer. Vol. 2. New York, Elsevier, 1984, pp 265–279.
111. Geissler E, Konzer P, Scherneek S, Zimmerman W. Sera collected before introduction of contaminated polio vaccine contain antibodies against SV_{40}. Acta Virol 29:420, 1985.
112. Fraumeni JF, Ederer F, Miller RW. An evaluation of the carcinogenicity of simian virus 40 in man. JAMA 185:713, 1963.
113. Fraumeni JF, Stark CR, Gold E, Lepow ML. Simian virus 40 in polio vaccine: Follow-up of newborn recipients. Science 167:59, 1970.
114. Mortimer EA Jr, Lepow ML, Gold E, et al. Long-term follow-up of persons inadvertently inoculated with SV_{40} as neonates. N Engl J Med 305:1517, 1981.
115. Fox JP. Epidemiology of poliomyelitis in populations before and after vaccination with inactivated viruses. In Poliomyelitis, Proceedings of the Fourth International Poliomyelitis Conference. Philadelphia, JB Lippincott, 1958, pp 136–149.
116. Sabin AB. Present status of attenuated live-virus poliomyelitis vaccine. JAMA 162:1589, 1956.
117. Horstmann DM, Wiederman JC, Paul JR. Attenuated type 1 poliovirus vaccine: Its capacity to infect and to spread from vaccinees within an institutional population. JAMA 170:1, 1959.
118. Fox JP, LeBlanc DR, Gelfand HM, et al. Spread of a vaccine strain of poliovirus in southern Louisiana communities. Proceedings of the 2nd International Conference on Live Poliovirus Vaccines. Washington, DC, Pan American Health Organization, 1960.
119. Kimball AC, Barr RN, Bauer H, et al. Minnesota studies with oral poliomyelitis vaccine. Community spread of orally administered attenuated poliovirus vaccine strains. Proceedings of the 2nd International Conference on Live Poliovirus Vaccines. Washington, DC, Pan American Health Organization, 1960.

120. Paul JR. Poliomyelitis immunization—1963. Med Clin North Am 47:1219, 1963.
121. Berkovich S, Pickering JE, Kibrick S. Paralytic poliomyelitis in Massachusetts, 1959. A study of the disease in a well vaccinated population. N Engl J Med 264:1323, 1961.
122. US Public Health Service: Interim document gives advice on use of Salk and Sabin vaccines. JAMA 180:23, 1962.
123. Red Book: Report of the Committee on Infectious Diseases (14th ed). Elk Grove Village, IL, American Academy of Pediatrics, 1964.
124. Red Book: Report of the Committee on Infectious Diseases (20th ed). Elk Grove Village, IL, American Academy of Pediatrics, 1986.
125. Assaad F, Ljungars-Esteves K. World overview of poliomyelitis: Regional patterns and trends. Rev Infect Dis 6(suppl 2):S302, 1984.
126. Kim-Farley RJ, Bart KJ, Schonberger LB, et al. Poliomyelitis in the USA: Virtual elimination of disease caused by wild virus. Lancet 2:1315, 1984.
127. Henderson DA, Witte JJ, Morris L, et al. Paralytic disease associated with oral polio vaccines. JAMA 190:41, 1964.
128. Report of the Special Advisory Committee on Oral Poliomyelitis Vaccines to the Surgeon General of the Public Health Service. Oral poliomyelitis vaccines. JAMA 190:49, 1964.
129. Sabin AB. Commentary on oral poliomyelitis vaccines. JAMA 190:164, 1964.
130. McKay HW, Fodor AR, Kokko UP. Viremia following the administration of live poliovirus vaccines. Am J Public Health 53:274, 1963.
131. Horstmann DM, Opton EM, Klemperer R, et al. Viremia in infants vaccinated with oral poliovirus vaccine (Sabin). Am J Hyg 79:47, 1964.
132. Melnick JL, Proctor RO, Ocampo AR, et al. Free and bound virus in serum after administration of oral poliovirus vaccine. Am J Epidemiol 84:329, 1966.
133. World Health Organization Consultative Group. The relationship between acute persisting spinal paralysis and poliomyelitis vaccine (oral): Results of a WHO enquiry. Bull World Health Organ 53:319, 1976.
134. World Health Organization Consultative Group. The relationship between acute persisting spinal paralysis and poliomyelitis vaccine—results of a ten-year inquiry. Bull World Health Organ 60:231, 1982.
135. Division of Immunization, Centers for Disease Control, Public Health Service, Department of Health and Human Services. Risks of oral polio vaccine. Paper presented at the meeting of the Advisory Committee on Immunization Practices; Atlanta, GA; October 24, 1985.
136. Salk D. Eradication of poliomyelitis in the United States. I. Live virus vaccine–associated and wild poliovirus disease. Rev Infect Dis 2:228, 1980.
137. Salk D. Eradication of poliomyelitis in the United States. II. Experience with killed poliovirus vaccine. Rev Infect Dis 2:243, 1980.
138. Salk D. Eradication of poliomyelitis in the United States. III. Poliovaccines—practical considerations. Rev Infect Dis 2:258, 1980.
139. Fox JP. Eradication of poliomyelitis in the United States. A commentary on the Salk review. Rev Infect Dis 2:277, 1980.
140. Van Wezel AL, Van Steenis G, van der Marel P, Osterhaus ADME. Inactivated poliovirus vaccine: Current production methods and new developments. Rev Infect Dis 6(suppl 2):S335, 1984.
141. McBean AM, Thoms ML, Johnson RH, et al. A comparison of the serologic responses to oral and injectable trivalent poliovirus vaccines. Rev Infect Dis 6(suppl 2):S552, 1984.
142. Cohen H, Nagel J. Two injections of diphtheria-tetanus-pertussis polio vaccine as the backbone of a simplified immunization schedule in developing countries. Rev Infect Dis 6(suppl 2):S350, 1984.
143. Bijkerk H. Surveillance and control of poliomyelitis in the Netherlands. Rev Infect Dis 6(suppl 2):S451, 1984.
144. Lapinleimu K. Elimination of poliomyelitis in Finland. Rev Infect Dis 6(suppl 2):S457, 1984.
145. Bottiger M. Long-term immunity following vaccination with killed poliovirus vaccine in Sweden, a country with no circulating poliovirus. Rev Infect Dis 6(suppl 2):S548, 1984.
146. Fox JP. Modes of action of poliovirus vaccines and relation to resulting immunity. Rev Infect Dis 6(suppl 2):S352, 1984.
147. Chin TDY. Immunity induced by inactivated poliovirus vaccine and excretion of virus. Rev Infect Dis 6(suppl 2):S369, 1984.
148. Poliomyelitis—Finland. MMWR Morb Mortal Wkly Rep 34:5–6, 1985.
149. Update: Poliomyelitis outbreak—Finland. 1984–1985. MMWR Morb Mortal Wkly Rep 35:82–86, 1986.
150. Kim-Farley RJ, Rutherford G, Lichfield P, et al. Outbreak of paralytic poliomyelitis, Taiwan. Lancet 2:1322, 1984.
151. John TJ. Poliomyelitis in Taiwan: Lessons for developing countries [letter to the editor]. Lancet 1:872, 1985.
152. Division of Immunization, Centers for Disease Control, Public Health Service, Department of Health and Human Services. Community spread of poliovaccine virus. Paper presented at the meeting of the Advisory Committee on Immunization Practices; Atlanta, GA; October 24, 1985.
153. Bernier RH. Some observations on lameness surveys. Rev Infect Dis 6(suppl 2):S371, 1984.
154. Heymann DL. House-to-house and school lameness surveys in Cameroon: A comparison of two methods for estimating the prevalence and annual incidence of paralytic poliomyelitis. Rev Infect Dis 6(suppl 2):S376, 1984.
155. Cruz RR. Cuba: Mass polio vaccination program, 1962–1982. Rev Infect Dis 6(suppl 2):S408, 1984.
156. Sabin A. Vaccination against poliomyelitis in economically underdeveloped countries. Bull World Health Organ 58:141, 1980.
157. Montefiore DG. Problems of poliomyelitis immunization in countries with warm climates. International Conference on the Application of Vaccines Against Viral, Rickettsial, and Bacterial Diseases of Man. Pan American Health Organization Scientific Publ. No. 226. Washington, DC, Pan American Health Organization, World Health Organization, 1970.
158. Sabin AB. Strategy for rapid elimination and continuing control of poliomyelitis and other vaccine preventable diseases of children in developing countries. BMJ 292:531, 1986.
159. Robbins FC, Nightingale EO. Selective primary health care: Strategies for control of disease in the developing world. IX. Poliomyelitis. Rev Infect Dis 5:957, 1983.
160. Salk J. One-dose immunization against paralytic poliomyelitis using noninfectious vaccine. Rev Infect Dis 6(suppl 2):S444, 1984.
161. Stoeckel P, Schlumberger M, Parent G, et al. Use of killed poliovirus vaccine in a routine immunization program in West Africa. Rev Infect Dis 6(suppl 2):S463, 1984.
162. Hilleman MR, McAteer WJ, McLean AA, et al. Stabilized measles vaccine in a novel single-dose delivery system: A practical reality for the worldwide elimination of measles. Rev Infect Dis 5:511, 1983.
163. Nathanson N. Epidemiologic aspects of poliomyelitis eradication. Rev Infect Dis 6(suppl 2):S308, 1984.
164. Almond JW, Stanway G, Cann AJ, et al. New poliovirus vaccines: A molecular approach. Vaccine 2:179, 1984.
165. Baltimore D. Picornaviruses are no longer black boxes. Science 229:1366, 1985.
166. Minor PD, Schild GC, Cann AJ, et al. Studies on the molecular aspects of antigenic structure and virulence of poliovirus. Ann Inst Pasteur Paris 137:107, 1986.
167. Hogle JM, Chow M, Filman DJ. Three-dimensional structure of poliovirus at 2.9 Å resolution. Science 229:1358, 1985.
168. Racaniello VR, Baltimore D. Cloned poliovirus complementary DNA is infectious in mammalian cells. Science 214:916, 1981.
169. Wimmer E, Emini EA, Jameson BA. Peptide priming of poliovirus neutralizing antibody response. Rev Infect Dis 6(suppl 2):S505, 1984.
170. Kow OM, Nottay BK. Molecular epidemiology of polioviruses. Rev Infect Dis 6(suppl 2):S499, 1984.
171. Von Magnus H, Petersen I. Vaccination with inactivated poliovirus vaccine and oral poliovirus vaccine in Denmark. Rev Infect Dis 6(suppl 2):S471, 1984.
172. Stetten D. Eradication [editorial]. Science 210:1203, 1980.
173. Report on the International Conference on the Eradication of

Infectious Diseases. Can infectious diseases be eradicated? Rev Infect Dis 4:912, 1982.

174. Yekutiel P. Lessons from the big eradication campaigns. World Health Forum 2:465, 1981.
175. Chin J. Can poliomyelitis be eliminated? Rev Infect Dis 6(suppl 2):S581, 1984.
176. Melnick JL. Towards the eradication of poliomyelitis. In La Maza LM, Peterson EM (eds). Symposium on Medical Virology. Proceedings of the 1981 International Symposium on Medical Virology, Anaheim, CA. New York, Elsevier Biomedical, 1982, pp 261–299.
177. Sabin AB. Paralytic poliomyelitis: Old dogmas and new perspectives. Rev Infect Dis 3:543, 1981.
178. Gear JHS. Non-polio causes of polio-like paralytic syndromes. Rev Infect Dis 6(suppl 2):S379, 1984.
179. Grist NR, Bell EJ. Paralytic poliomyelitis and non-polio enteroviruses: Studies in Scotland. Rev Infect Dis 6(suppl 2):S385, 1984.
180. Melnick JL. Enterovirus type 71 infections: A varied clinical pattern sometimes mimicking paralytic poliomyelitis. Rev Infect Dis 6(suppl 2):S387, 1984.
181. Robbins FC. International Symposium on Poliomyelitis Control. Summary and recommendations. Rev Infect Dis 6(suppl 2):S596, 1984.
182. Andrus JK, de Quadros CA, Olive JM. The surveillance challenge: Final stages of eradication of poliomyelitis in the Americas. MMWR Morb Mortal Wkly Rep 41:21, 1992.
183. First Meeting of the International Commission for Certification of Poliomyelitis Eradication in the Americas. 9th Technical Advisory Group Meeting on Vaccine-Preventive Diseases, July 1990.
184. Robbins FC, deQuadros CA. Certification of the eradication of indigenous transmission of wild poliovirus in the Americas. J Infect Dis 175(suppl 1):S281, 1997.
185. Wright PF, Kim-Farley RJ, de Quadros CA, et al. Strategies for the global eradication of poliomyelitis by the year 2000. N Engl J Med 325:1774, 1991.
186. Cochi SL, Hull HF, Sutter RW, et al. Global poliomyelitis eradication initiative: Status report. J Infect Dis 175(suppl 1), 1997.
187. Report of a study: An evaluation of poliomyelitis vaccine policy options. Washington, DC, National Academy of Sciences, Institute of Medicine, 1988, pp 1–50.
188. Poliomyelitis prevention in the United States: Introduction of a sequential vaccination schedule of inactivated poliovirus vaccine followed by oral poliovirus vaccine. Recommendations of the Advisory Committee on Immunization Practices (ACIP). MMWR Morb Mortal Wkly Rep 46:1–25.

chapter 3

The Immunology of Vaccination

Gordon Ada

Many of the most successful vaccines that have been in general use for decades were developed without any, or with only a slight, knowledge of how the mammalian immune system operates and how that system can be manipulated to achieve different responses. In developing a live attenuated viral vaccine, for example, the essential criterion was that the product would be safe but effective at protecting against clinical disease if the vaccinee were later exposed to the wild-type agent. The need was great; exposure to measles, for example, caused considerable morbidity and mortality in a naive population.[1]

Two features characterize many of the agents for which current, successful viral and bacterial vaccines have been developed:

1. The agent causes an acute infection (e.g., many viral and all extracellular bacterial infections); or, if the agent has failed to rapidly cause death, the host's immune response clears the infection within approximately 1 week.
2. The agent is antigenically stable; or, if there are different serotypes in the field (e.g., measles virus and the three subtypes of poliovirus), they remain essentially antigenically stable.

The agent with the major exception to these features is influenza virus, for which a new vaccine with antigenic properties closely matching the prevailing circulating strains is made each year. For the former agents, the main requirement of a vaccine is to induce the formation of an antibody of sufficiently high titer to neutralize the infectivity of almost all the wild-type agent. The small proportion of wild-type agents that escapes neutralization by antibody will most likely cause only a subclinical infection. This feature of infectious agents led to the demonstration, with poliovirus vaccines, for example,[2] that a vaccine preparation would be successful if it induced in a recipient a certain titer of specific antibody. In such situations, a subunit or hapten-carrier conjugate containing the antigenic moiety that possesses major neutralizing epitopes would also likely be successful if its immunogenicity were sufficiently high.

The pressure to better understand the immune mechanisms involved in preventing or controlling an infection increases considerably when one is faced with the need to develop vaccines against agents that naturally cause persistent or chronic infections (e.g., parasites such as plasmodia, and some bacteria such as chlamydia), demonstrated substantial antigenic variation (e.g., human immunodeficiency virus [HIV]), or a combination of these. To a significant extent, such a need coincides with a much increased understanding of the properties and functions of components of the mammalian immune system, such that the 1990s especially have witnessed the involvement of more immunologists in the general area of vaccinology.

This chapter briefly outlines our current understanding of the adaptive immune system, new approaches to manipulating different components of that system, and the major requirements expected of a vaccine if it is to be effective. A more detailed account can be found elsewhere.[3]

NATURE OF THE MAMMALIAN IMMUNE SYSTEM

There are two immune systems—the innate (nonspecific, nonadaptive) and the acquired (specific, adaptive) systems. Both are necessary for survival in nature. The former consists of a series of specialized cells, such as macrophages, neutrophils, and natural killer (NK) cells; and different products, such as the cytokines, α-, β-, and γ-interferons (IFNs), chemokines, and larger proteins such as the C-reactive proteins and those of the complement cascade. Components of the innate system may be activated within minutes or hours after an infection is initiated. This process is a necessary requirement of the innate immune system, as it generally takes several days (sometimes much longer) for components of the adaptive system to acquire effector function. It was previously thought that the innate and adaptive systems were quite distinct, but it is now realized that there is considerable interaction as well as some overlap between these systems. Thus, γ-IFN, a critical cytokine, used to be called *immune interferon* because it was thought to be made only by effector T cells, but it is now known to be made also by NK cells. Another example is the classical and alternative complement pathways that share the later effector functions but also differ, in that antigen-antibody complexes are recognized in the former whereas a pathogen surface is recognized in the latter.

Adaptive Immune System

The adaptive immune system, which is thought to have been "superimposed" on the innate system during evolution, differs from the latter in two critical properties—great specificity and memory—both of which are the exclusive hallmarks of one cell type, the lymphocyte. Because the practice of vaccination depends utterly on these properties, the remainder of this chapter outlines our current knowledge of important features of the adaptive system. There are three major components of this system—two classes of lymphocytes as well as cells that specialize in antigen presentation, particularly dendritic cells and macrophages.

Two Classes of Lymphocytes

Humoral Response. Immunoglobulin (Ig) receptors on B lymphocytes recognize and interact with epitopes of antigens. The complex is endocytosed and then processed within the cell, thereby completing a first step that leads to activation and differentiation processes involved in the formation of a plasma cell. Plasma cells produce and secrete different subclasses of antibodies (IgM, IgG, IgA, IgE) with specificities closely related to those of the IgM and IgD receptors on the cell surface. Once secreted, the antibodies circulate around the body and hence act independently of the plasma cell. The epitopes may constitute a linear peptide or carbohydrate sequence or, quite frequently, a shape (about 25 × 25 Å) formed by adjacent sequences within a molecule or by adjacent molecules; this latter structure is called a *discontinuous epitope*. Both types of epitopes may have strict three-dimensional conformations, and even mutations outside the epitope can modify the epitope's conformation.[4, 5]

Cell-Mediated Immune Response. Responses mediated by T (thymus-derived) lymphocytes are referred to as *cell mediated*, even though many are actually mediated by secreted factors termed *cytokines* (also called interleukins [ILs] and referred to by IL numbers). In contrast to hormones, cytokines almost invariably act over very short distances. Many cells, including B cells, express receptors for cytokines and chemokines, but T cells are both major producers and responders to these factors. T cells are a more diverse group than B cells and express three different classes of receptors: (1) the specific T-cell receptor (TCR), which recognizes processed antigen that is presented by the antigen-presenting cell (APC, composed of α and β chains); (2) a receptor that is specific for the costimulator molecule expressed by the APC; and (3) receptors recognizing a range of cytokines.

The two main classes of T cells express either the CD4 or the CD8 differentiation antigens, which function as accessory molecules to the TCR. $CD4^+$ T cells and $CD8^+$ T cells are said to be class II or class I major histocompatibility complex (MHC)–restricted cells, respectively, because they recognize antigenic peptides complexed with class II MHC or class I MHC molecules at the surface of the APC. A major role of $CD4^+$ T cells is to help B cells make antibody; hence, they are called helper T (Th) cells. In both humans and mice, there are two subsets of Th cells—Th1 and Th2 cells—that are distinguished by the profiles of the cytokines produced and their effector functions (Table 3–1). In contrast, a major function of $CD8^+$ T cells is to recognize and lyse infected target cells; hence, they are called cytotoxic T lymphocytes (CTLs). This function of CTLs was first demonstrated with virus-infected cells but is also seen with cells infected with bacteria or parasites. CTLs secrete a panel of cytokines that resemble those secreted by Th1 cells, so there is an increasing tendency to refer to CTLs and Th1 cells as *type 1 cells* and Th2 cells as *type 2 cells*. More recently, there has been evidence, at least from in vitro work, that $CD8^+$ T cells convert to a form resembling Th2 cells after exposure to the cytokine IL-4, which is secreted by Th2 cells. These two subsets of $CD8^+$ T cells are now called cytotoxic T cell populations types 1 and 2 (Tc1 and Tc2), to bring the nomenclature into line with $CD4^+$ T-cell subsets.[6] Table 3–1 outlines some of the characteristics of $CD4^+$ and $CD8^+$ T cells with αβ-chain receptors. A second group of T cells with γδ-chain receptors has been described (see later).

T cells play a central role in immune responses. Because they are the first component of the adaptive system

Table 3–1. **CYTOKINES SECRETED BY AND EFFECTOR ACTIVITIES OF T-LYMPHOCYTE SUBSETS, AND THEIR INFLUENCE ON Ig ISOTYPES PRODUCED BY B CELLS HELPER ACTIVITIES)**

	$CD4^+$ T CELLS		$CD8^+$ T CELLS	
	Th1	**Th2**	**Tc1**	**Tc2**
Cytokines secreted				
IL-2	+	−	+	−
IL-3	+	−	−	−
IL-4	−	+	−	+
IL-5	−	+	−	+
IL-6	−	+	−	?
IL-10	−	+	−	?
IL-13	−	+	−	?
α-TNF	+	+	−	−
β-TNF	+	−	+	−
γ-IFN	+	−	+	−
Effector activity				
Cytotoxicity*	−	−	+	−
DTH	+	−	+/−	−
Helper activity				
Ig produced by B cells	IgG2a† IgG1‡	IgG1,† IgA† IgE†	−	+

+, activity produced; −, activity not produced; +/−, small level of activity produced; ?, unknown

*Class 1 major histocompatibility complex–restricted cytotoxic activity of primary (uncultured) cells.

†In mice.

‡In humans.

DTH, delayed-type hypersensitivity; IFN, interferon; Ig, immunoglobulin; IL, interleukin; Tc1 and Tc2, cytotoxic T cells types 1 and 2; Th1 and Th2, helper T cells types 1 and 2; TNF, tumor necrosis factor.

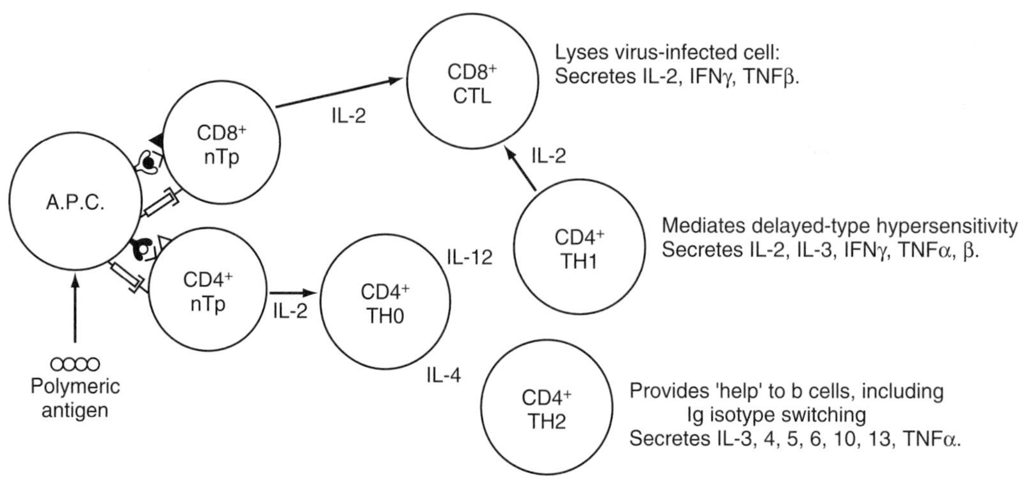

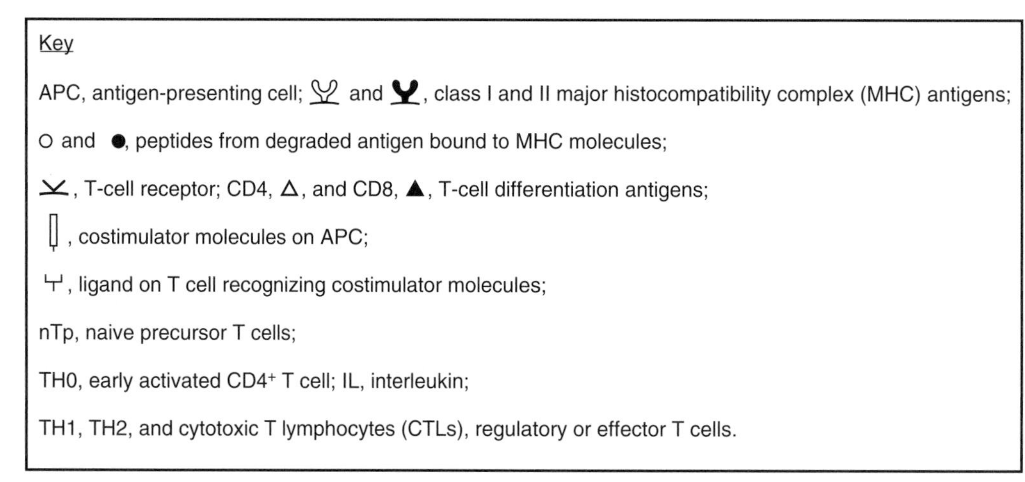

Figure 3–1. *A,* Antigen presentation and T-cell activation.

to achieve effector activity after infection, they must be able to circulate freely within the lymphoid system.

Antigen-Presenting Cells

Whereas the B-cell receptors (IgD and IgM, but principally the latter) often directly recognize a foreign antigen (which may vary from a portion of a protein to protein aggregates), the TCR recognizes an antigen that has been "processed" within an APC. Peptides derived from foreign antigens bind to a self-antigen, the MHC protein, to form a complex that is expressed at the cell surface. Generally, but not invariably, noninfectious material (e.g., a protein) enters a cell via the endosomal-lysosomal pathway. After this material degrades in lysosomes, an appropriate peptide forms a complex with a class II MHC molecule. In contrast, if an infectious agent enters the cytoplasm of the APC and replicates, some newly synthesized protein (as well as self-proteins) becomes degraded to peptides that may associate with a class I MHC molecule, and the complex is expressed at the cell surface. The separation of these pathways is not absolute. A protein may fuse with the cell membrane, or some protein may escape from a lysosome, such that in either case the protein enters the cytoplasmic pathway and a CD8+ T-cell response can occur. Furthermore, a number of adjuvant preparations are now available that promote a CD8+ T-cell response to an antigen preparation that otherwise would not induce such a response, as is described later. A second crucial property of an APC is to express a costimulator molecule for which a receptor is present on the naive T cell. Without this second signal, a naive T cell is not activated.

Cells that express high levels of MHC and costimulator molecules are often referred to as *professional APCs.* Chief among these are the different dendritic cells, originally called *veiled cells* because of the extensive folding of the plasma membrane. These cells are motile and are found especially in afferent lymph, as a major task is to rapidly transmit components of an infectious agent to a draining lymph node, where the opportunity to contact naive (or memory) T cells is greatest. Macrophages may also act as APCs, particularly for particulate material

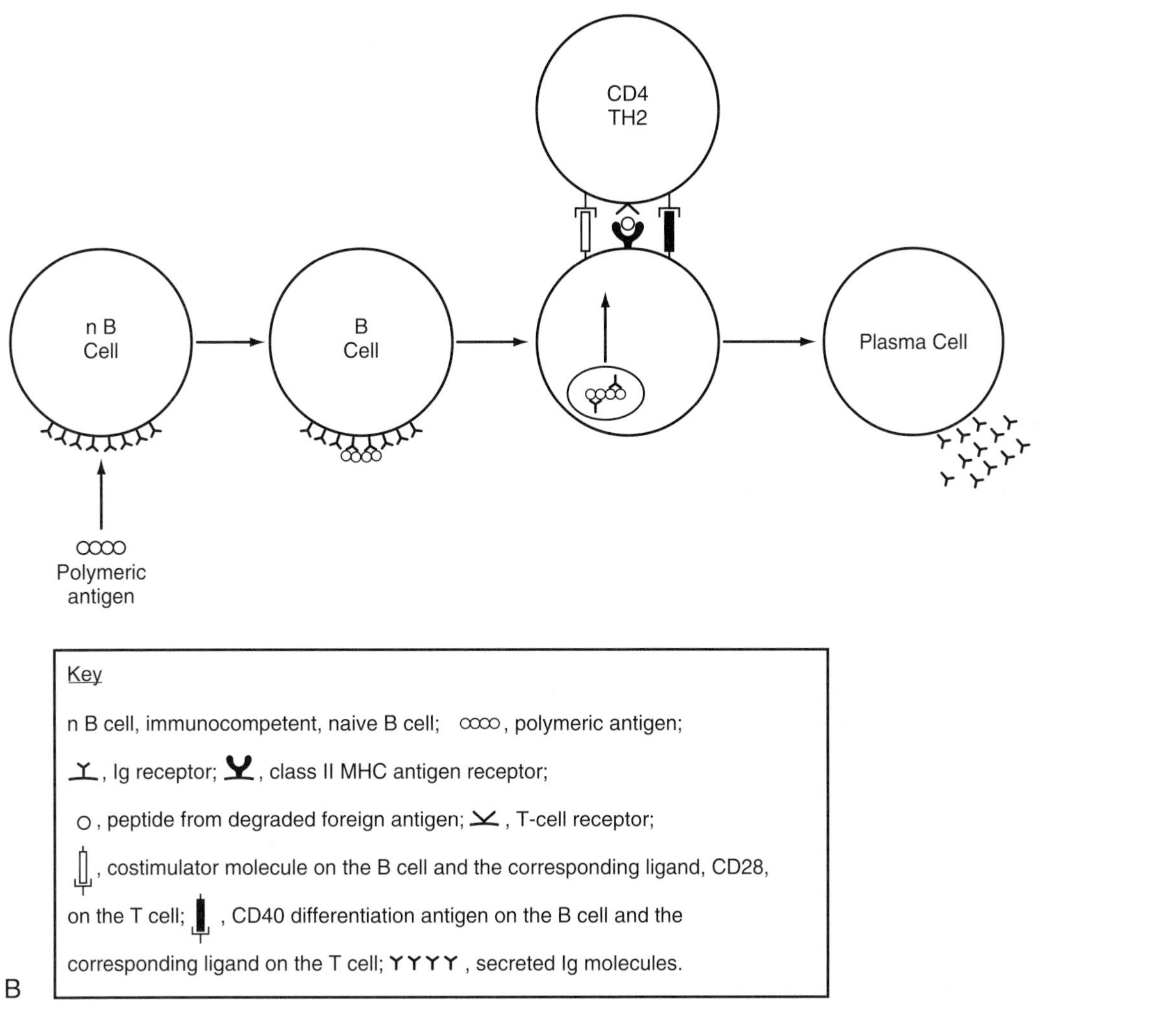

Figure 3–1 *Continued. B,* Antigen presentation and B-cell activation. (*A* and *B* adapted from Ada G, Ramsay A. Vaccines, Vaccination and the Immune Response. Philadelphia, Lippincott-Raven, 1977.)

(e.g., bacteria), and B cells present antigen especially to activated or memory T cells.

Figure 3–1 outlines the major cellular interactions that lead to T-cell and B-cell activation and differentiation to become effector cells. The formation of Tc2 cells is not illustrated in Figure 3–1A, as this pathway in vivo is not yet certain.

SEQUENCE OF RESPONSES DURING AN INFECTION

During an acute infection in mice, such as an influenza virus infection in the lung, the sequence of appearance of effector cells is as follows: (1) $CD4^+$ T cells, (2) $CD8^+$ T cells, followed by (3) antibody-secreting cells (ASCs) that produce first IgM (about day 6) and then IgG and IgA (some days later).[7] The decrease in lung virus titers begins at days 5 through 8 (depending on the size of the infecting dose). This decrease coincides with the increase in CTL activity and occurs before there are significant numbers of ASCs. About 3 days after the infectious virus disappears (days 10–12), CTL effector activity is no longer detected. Memory CTLs are then found and persist for many months, possibly for the life of the mouse. ASCs are present for at least 18 months, although in gradually decreasing numbers. Maximum levels of specific B memory cells are found about 3 months after infection.

In the case of human HIV infections, memory CTLs have been found in blood at the time of viremia,[8, 9] which may occur a few weeks after exposure to HIV. This CTL activity coincides with the subsequent decrease in viremia. Thereafter, in most infected individuals, effector CTLs are present in the blood for several years. This quite unusual occurrence is thought to result from the intense CTL response in the lymphoid tissues, where a high rate of viral replication occurs. Neutralizing antibody is often found shortly after viremia occurs; in some cases, however, such antibody may not be detected for months after the initiation of infection.[10] This observation is consistent with the murine influenza result that, in a naive host, CTLs are the major response for controlling and sometimes clearing a viral infection.[8, 9]

ROLE OF DIFFERENT IMMUNE RESPONSES

Table 3–2 summarizes the roles of different components of the immune response in preventing, controlling, and clearing an infectious agent. There are two types of infections—extracellular and intracellular. In the former, specific antibody is crucially important in preventing infection and at all subsequent stages. Cytokines secreted by CD4+ Th1 cells help activate phagocytic cells such as macrophages and thereby facilitate the uptake and destruction of the agent, either as such or complexed with antibody. Theoretically, at least, CTLs are unlikely to be formed, nor would they be expected to have a role in such situations. The remainder of this section provides evidence to support the assessment in Table 3–2.

Intracellular Infections: The Role of Antibody

Neutralization of the infectivity of the challenge agent is a critical role for specific antibody. If some infectious agent escapes neutralization and replicates in host cells, antibody may neutralize any progeny agent (e.g., prevent or limit viremia) and destroy infected cells through antibody-dependent cellular cytoxicity and complement-mediated lysis. There are reports of model systems in which antibody has cleared an intracellular infection. Certain monoclonal antibodies (MABs) to the fusion protein of respiratory syncytial virus (RSV) were found to clear an infection in mice.[11] These antibodies may have been endocytosed into an infected cell and thus prevented viral formation. It has also been shown that a preparation of anti-RSV Fab, made by the technique of combinatorial libraries expressed on phages, cleared the virus infection when it was instilled intranasally into the lungs of infected mice daily for 3 days.[12] In another example, MABs or hyperimmune serum specific for Sindbis virus was able to clear the virus from infected neurons in mice with severe combined immunodeficiency disease (SCID).[13] SCID mice infected with a low dose of egg-grown influenza virus that caused delayed death (occurring at about 18 days) were protected from death if transfused with specific antibody.[14] Although these examples are of considerable interest in demonstrating the potential properties of high-titer antibodies, they are atypical. There are many examples of an intracellular infection persisting in the presence of high titers of specific antibody.

Does specific antibody ever completely prevent an infection and thus induce so-called sterilizing immunity? Probably not, but we do not know. The difficulty of finding a correct answer is indicated by experiments of Ramphal and colleagues.[15] When mice were transfused with high-titer anti-influenza IgG and then infected by intranasal inoculation of virus of the correct specificity, only the surface epithelial cells became infected; the mice had tracheitis. However, when the mice were transfused with high-titer polymerized IgA (which is converted to secretory IgA [sIgA] on passage through the surface epithelial cells into the airways) and then inoculated with virus, most (but not all) mice were protected and showed no sign of infection when the surface layer of cells in the lung air passages were examined in detail.[16] Subsequent experiments showed that the protection was due to the sIgA.[17]

If a vaccine-induced neutralizing antibody titer is sufficiently high and closely matches the viral antigen specificity, nearly all the challenge virus should be neutralized; if this occurs, the vaccine may not need to additionally induce a strong type 1 T-cell response to control the minor infection caused by any escaped virus. A vaccine that induces the generation of type 1 effector T cells assumes greater relevance and importance as (1) the specificity of vaccine-induced neutralizing antibody increasingly diverges from the antigenic specificity of the challenge virus and (2) naive susceptible cells are infected by intimate contact with virus-producing cells (e.g., the formation of syncytia).

Table 3–2. **FUNCTIONS OF LYMPHOCYTE SUBSETS AFTER VACCINATION OF MICE AGAINST EXTRACELLULAR (BACTERIA) OR INTRACELLULAR (VIRUSES OR BACTERIA) INFECTIONS**

	TYPE OF RESPONSE			
	Prevents Infection	**Limits Infection**	**Reduces Infection**	**Clears/Controls Infection**
		Extracellular Infection		
Antibody	+ + +	+ + +	+ + +	+ + +
CD4+ Th2	–			
CD4+ Th1	–	+ +	+ +	+ +
CD8+ Tc1	–	–	–	–
		Intracellular Infection		
Antibody	+ + +	+ +	+ +	+/–
CD4+ Th2				
CD4+ Th1				
Bacterial infections	–	+ + +	+ + +	+ + +
Viral infections	–	+ +	+ +	+
CD8+ Tc1 (CTLs)	–	+ + +	+ + +	+ + +
CD8+ Tc2	–		Suppresses CTL activity	

+ + +, very important; + +, important; +, less important.
CTL, cytoxic T lymphocyte. See also Table 3–1 for abbreviations.

Intracellular Infections: The Role of Type 1 T-Cell Responses

The role of type 1 T-cell responses in viral and other intracellular infections is discussed sequentially. In viral infections, the evidence favoring a dominant role for CTLs has been reviewed[18]; the information is summarized in Table 3–3. Overall, the findings reported in this table support the dominant role of CTLs in controlling and frequently clearing viral infections.

It is difficult to find data that support a dominant role for $CD4^+$ Th1 cells in viral infections. In one special situation, the zosteriform spread model of a herpes type 2 infection in mice, Th1 cells were clearly protective against the cutaneous infection.[30] In contrast, CTLs mediated protection when the infection spread to the nervous system.[31] Especially in in vitro experiments, Th1 cells facilitate a CTL response; however, there are now a number of reports that confirm that in knockout (KO) mice lacking $CD4^+$ T cells, quite strong CTL responses can be generated to some viral infections.[32, 33] In one report, it was shown with a persistent viral infection (herpes in $CD4^+$ T-cell KO mice) that a strong CTL response was induced but that over time the CTL response in the KO mice decreased markedly compared with the response in control mice.[33a] The authors suggested that an effect like this might operate in those HIV infections that progress to acquired immunodeficiency syndrome.

In bacterial and other infections, the picture appears to be less clear-cut. In murine listeriosis, CTLs specific for a single nonamer peptide determinant of the bacterial protein listeriolysin are protective in vivo.[34] Further, it has since been shown that specific immune $CD8^+$ T cells, but not immune $CD4^+$ T cells, lyse *Listeria monocytogenes*–infected hepatocytes in a class I MHC–restricted fashion.[35] In contrast, depletion of $CD4^+$ T cells in mice infected with bacille Calmette-Guérin (BCG, consisting of attenuated *Mycobacterium bovis*), using specific antiserum to deplete both cell types, resulted in a large increase in the numbers of bacteria, whereas depletion of $CD8^+$ T cells apparently had little effect on the course of infection.[36] Other work using cell transfer also pointed to the importance of $CD4^+$ T cells in controlling the infection of mice with virulent *Mycobacterium tuberculosis*, although a role for $CD8^+$ T cells was not ruled out.[37] However, later work using β_2-microglobulin KO mice (which cannot make functional $CD8^+$ T cells) showed that CTLs were important in controlling a virulent *M. tuberculosis* infection but not important for controlling a BCG infection.[38] In a separate study in mice, both $CD4^+$ type 1 cells and CTLs were found to have a protective role in BCG infections,[39] with the former possibly being highly effective in containing the organism in granulomas. When mice were infected with mouse-passaged *M. tuberculosis*, $\gamma\delta$–T cells were found to have a protective role in the early stages of protection.[40]

Francisella tularensis infections cause the lethal disease tularemia.[41] An attenuated live vaccine strain is highly virulent for mice when given intraperitoneally but much less so when given intradermally. Using $CD8^+$ T-cell KO mice and $CD4^+$ T cell–negative mice, it was found that either cell class was sufficient to resolve a sublethal intradermal live vaccine strain infection and subsequently to protect against a lethal challenge of these bacteria.[42] This suggested that (1) whereas one cell type may have a stronger role than the other at different times during the infection or with different levels of infection, both were important; and (2) $\gamma\delta$–T cells also played a more subtle but still significant role in protection.

Chlamydia trachomatis is an obligate intracellular bacterium responsible for causing trachoma and genital infections. A study in an endemic area has tested the blood of children and adults of human leukocyte antigen B8 or B35 haplotype for the presence of CTLs reacting with nonapeptides from the major outer membrane and heat-shock proteins of the chlamydia. Although the number of positive reactions was not very high, CTL responses were observed only in children resolving a current infection and in adults lacking scarring of the conjunctiva, suggesting that these cells may be important in resolving a natural infection.[43]

The effect of genetic disruptions in mice on the progress of protozoal infections has been reviewed,[44] but

Table 3–3. SUMMARY OF EVIDENCE SUPPORTING A DOMINANT ROLE FOR CYTOTOXIC T LYMPHOCYTES IN THE CONTROL AND CLEARANCE OF MANY VIRAL INFECTIONS

GENERAL ARGUMENTS

1. Clearance of many viral infections is associated with the induction of a CTL response prior to the appearance of neutralizing antibody.
2. Nearly all mammalian cell types express class I MHC antigens. Exceptions include gametes, neurons, red blood cells, and cells of the trophoblast.
3. CTLs secrete potent cytokines with antiviral and macrophage-activating activities, such as γ-IFN and α-TNF.
4. Infected cells become susceptible to lysis by CTLs long before viral progeny are made.

MORE DIRECT EVIDENCE

1. Transfer of specific effector CTLs into an MHC-compatible host clears established infections in a specific organ or protects from death. In humans, CTLs have been shown to reconstitute specific CMV[19, 20] and EBV[21] immunity after allogeneic bone marrow transplants.
2. In infections of mice with LCMV, a noncytopathic virus, CTLs have been shown to lyse infected cells in vivo[22] as well as in vitro. Similarly, virus-specific CTLs transferred to transgenic mice expressing the hepatitis B surface antigen caused apoptosis of the hepatocytes.[23] The cytotoxicity of LCMV-specific CTLs is greatly impaired in perforin-deficient mice.[24]
3. In the case of HIV-1 infections, there are four situations in which virus- and antibody-negative individuals exposed to HIV have HIV-specific CTL activity in babies born of infected mothers,[25, 26] in long-term seronegative partners of infected people,[27] in long-term African prostitutes,[28] and in some healthcare workers exposed once to HIV.[29]

CMV, cytomegalovirus; CTL, cytotoxic T lymphocyte; EBV, Epstein-Barr virus; HIV-1, human immunodeficiency virus type 1; LCMV, lymphocyte choriomeningitis virus; MHC, major histocompatibility complex. See also abbreviations in Table 3–1.

Information in table reviewed in Ada GL, McElrath MJ. HIV-vaccine induced T cell response. Potential role in vaccine efficacy. AIDS Res Hum Retroviruses 13:243–248, 1996.

there are still too few examples to draw clear conclusions. Using β_2-microglobulin KO mice, for example, no difference was found with infection by *Plasmodium* spp. or *Leishmania major*, whereas the infection with *Trypanosoma cruzi* was exacerbated. It had been shown earlier that CD8+ T cells were important in protection in *Toxoplasma gondii*–infected normal mice.

Regional Immunity

The area of the mucosa is far greater than that of the skin, and with the exception of the female vagina, it is generally well endowed with draining lymphoid tissues. The main routes leading to infection are the gut, the rectum, the genitourinary tract, the respiratory tract, and the eye. Studies over many years led to the concept of a common mucosal system whereby infection at one mucosal site could result in protection at that and other mucosal sites.[45] When the adenovirus vaccine is administered orally, for example, protection is afforded against a respiratory infection. There is much to be learned about this system, however. For reasons that are as yet unclear, immunization via the respiratory tract rather than the oral route appears to be the more effective at affording some protection in the female genital tract.

The mucosal immune system has several characteristic features.[46] Foremost of these is the formation and secretion into the lumen of sIgA, of which there are two classes in humans, sIgA1 and sIgA2. Dimeric IgA, secreted from plasma cells, binds to a polymeric Ig receptor (pIgR) on the basolateral surface of the epithelial cells that line the mucous membrane. The complex is endocytosed, and the external domain of the pIgR is split off at the apical surface of the cells. The remaining portion, now termed the *secretory component*, remains attached to IgA to form sIgA, which is secreted into the mucosal lumen. sIgA is the first line of defense, because it binds to antigens, microbes, and their toxins and helps prevent especially viruses from attaching to or penetrating the mucosal surface.[16, 17] This function is enhanced by the resistance to many proteases, although sIgA1 is particularly susceptible to some bacterial proteases.

There is increasing evidence from in vitro studies with Sendai and influenza viruses[46, 47] that IgA in transit through an epithelial cell can contact and effectively neutralize a virus that may infect those cells; this function is supported by several in vivo studies.[48] There is additional evidence that the complexes so formed may be discharged into the lumen. In this particular circumstance, it has been suggested that IgA should be able to synergize with cell-mediated immune responses in controlling an intracellular infection.[48]

A diverse group of cells, the intraepithelial lymphocytes, are composed largely of CD8+ T cells. Some have the usual αβ-TCR, but others have γδ-TCR. Some are cytotoxic, and one of their roles may be to destroy infected epithelial cells. Antiviral CD8+ CTLs with αβ-TCRs have been found in the vaginal mucosa of simian immunodeficiency virus–infected monkeys[49] and in cytobrush specimens from the cervix of HIV-infected women.[50]

Commentary on the Roles of Different T-Cell Subsets in Intracellular Infections

It has become abundantly clear that varying results can be obtained using KO mice to elucidate the role of different T cells. In many situations, compensatory mechanisms such as greater activity of NK cells or primary CD4+ T cells assuming cytotoxic activity can contribute to controlling the infection. Nevertheless, a pattern is beginning to emerge that is most clearly seen with viral infections. There is significantly impaired clearance of lymphocytic choriomeningitis virus (LCMV),[24] Theiler's virus,[51] and ectromelia virus (G. Karupiah, personal communication) in CD8+ T cell–deficient mice. In contrast, such mice have survived infection with influenza virus (in mice with SCID[14, 52]), vaccinia virus (in nu-/nu- mice[53, 54]), and Sendai virus.[55] The most notable difference among these findings is that the former (i.e., LCMV, Theiler's, and ectromelia viruses) are natural mouse pathogens, whereas influenza and vaccinia viruses are not. The Sendai virus case is of special interest, as this virus behaves like a mouse pathogen. In Sendai virus–infected β_2-microglobulin mice, there is delayed clearance, but many mice survive. In such situations, however, the CD4+ T cells become cytotoxic. As the virus mainly infects the lung epithelial cells, which are class II MHC positive, the "unnaturally" cytotoxic CD4+ T cells "take over" the role of CD8+ CTLs. CD8+ T cells are also important in *Listeria* and virulent *Mycobacterium* infections, but they are less important in infections with the attenuated BCG strain. Thus, in some situations, CD4+ type 1 cells can contribute significantly to protection.

This review has illustrated one important message. Vaccines for human use are made to protect against natural human pathogens. Therefore, if there is reason for a vaccine to stimulate a type 1 T-cell response (as discussed earlier), the decision should be to choose a protocol for vaccine development that induces specific CD8+ and CD4+ type 1 T-cell responses. Conditions for stimulating a CD8+ CTL response frequently also stimulate a type 1 CD4+ T-cell response, whereas protocols for stimulating the latter response do not always induce a CTL response.

Pathogenesis of Infections and Vaccine Requirements

The interpretations expressed in Table 3–2 concerning the relative roles of different responses—antibody versus type 1 T-cell responses—in controlling an intracellular infection represent an "average" situation. The pathogenesis of a particular infection could influence the relative intensity of the responses that should be induced by a vaccine used to control that infection. Three different situations are possible:

1. Poliovirus infects the gut mucosa, and the viral progeny are secreted mainly into the gut. Oral poliovirus vaccine (OPV) induces IgM, IgG, and sIgA; however, it is sIgA that not only greatly limits the initial infection but also neutralizes much of the viral progeny. The IgM and IgG induced by the OPV and inactivated poliovirus vaccine prevent the viremia that can occur in some cases and that might otherwise result in infection of nerve cells. The importance of the antibody response is indicated by the ratings given in Table 3–4. Similarly, with diphtheria and tetanus, the overwhelming need is for the vaccines to induce sufficiently high levels of antibody to neutralize the secreted toxins.

2. In the case of measles, mumps, and, perhaps to a lesser extent, rubella, the initial infection leads to a primary viremia. After infections at other sites, a secondary viremia may follow. As the viremias do not appear to be cell associated, it is important for a vaccine to induce a strong antibody response as well as a type 1 T-cell response to limit the production of virus at both the primary and secondary sites. (This is the basis for the ratings given in Table 3–4.)

3. If, after the initial infection, viral progeny become largely (although not necessarily entirely) cell associated, being passed from cell to cell, then a desirable vaccine is one that induces a strong type 1 T-cell response to contain and clear a subsequent infection. Pox and rabies viral infections are in this category (see Table 3–4). Similarly, after exposure to *M. tuberculosis*, infected cells transport the organisms from the lung to other sites in the body, where fibrosis and encapsulation can occur. Here again, a vaccine is needed that induces a strong type 1 T-cell response (see Table 3–4), as illustrated by the discussion in the earlier section.

IMMUNOLOGICAL MEMORY

An essential role for a vaccine is to induce strong immunological memory; however, especially in the case of T cells, this has been one of the more difficult areas in which to elucidate mechanisms. Some aspects of this topic have been reviewed.[56]

B-Cell Memory

Memory B cells are formed in the germinal centers of lymphoid tissue. Foreign antigen, as antigen-antibody complexes and in the presence of complement (C′), attach via C′ receptors to the surface of follicular dendritic cells (FDCs). A rapidly dividing B cell, the centrocyte, in the germinal center undergoes somatic hypermutation. Subsequently, cells with Ig receptors of high affinity are selected by the retained antigen to undergo further differentiation. Some of these become ASCs such as plasma cells, most of which migrate to the bone marrow. Others become memory B cells, which circulate around the body. When these cells return to antigen-containing lymphoid tissue, the cycle of differentiation may begin again, resulting in the production of antibodies of increasingly high affinities. Even intact viral particles (e.g., HIV[57]) may attach to FDCs in this way, thereby assisting in the production of antibody that binds with high affinity to the intact virus, some of which would therefore be expected to neutralize infectivity (especially viral) effectively.

Memory B cells, having at an earlier stage interacted with Th cells, express receptors of other subtypes (e.g., IgA, IgG, IgE). There is some evidence that they express less of another B-cell marker.[3]

The purpose of a boosting dose is to generate further ASCs and B memory cells and to increase or replenish the antigen depot in the germinal centers and so enhance the recruitment of cells from the total memory B-cell pool. An early experiment demonstrated the importance of the size of the antigen dose.[58] Groups of rats were immunized with 10-fold graded doses of *Salmonella* flagella, varying from 100 pg to 10 μg. This antigen is polymeric and induces long-lasting antibody production. Six weeks later, each group of rats was challenged with a dose of *Salmonella* flagella varying from 1 ng to 10 μg. Antibody titers were subsequently measured at different times. The answer was clear-cut: An anamnestic response was not seen until the boosting dose was at least as high as the priming dose.

A second possibility is that some forms of antigen may be more effective at priming than boosting. For example, mice given DNA coding for influenza virus hemagglutinin were challenged 4 weeks later with a fowlpox virus–hemagglutinin construct. Three weeks later, antihemagglutinin antibody titers were measured: mice given 10 or 100 μg of DNA before the challenge had antibody titers 25- to 50-fold higher than controls.[59] It may be that antigens that persist (in a depot with adjuvant) on FDCs (e.g., polymers) or in cells (e.g., DNA) are more effective than soluble, monomeric antigens at priming an immune response.

Table 3–4. **RELATIVE ROLES OF ANTIBODY OR TYPE 1 T CELLS IN THE CONTROL OF SOME INFECTIONS FOR WHICH VACCINES ARE AVAILABLE**

DISEASE AGENT	ANTIBODY	TYPE 1 T CELL
Poliovirus, *Clostridium tetani*, *Corynebacterium diphtheriae*	+ + +	+
Measles virus, mumps virus	+ +	+ +
Poxvirus, rabies virus(?), *Mycobacterium tuberculosis*	+	+ + +

+ + +, very important; + +, important; +, less important.

T-Cell Memory

Less is known about the development of memory T cells. The TCR does not undergo somatic hypermutation. It is now generally recognized that persistence of specific antigen is not required for long-term CTL memory to occur[3]; and it is therefore not surprising that memory T-cell induction does not seem to be limited to any particular site. This type of development has made it more difficult to distinguish among activated, effector, and memory T cells. There is one particular cellular marker, an isoform of the CD45 molecule, that is expressed to a higher level in memory T cells.

To properly discharge their role, it is critical that T cells, especially memory T cells, migrate freely around the body. It was shown in 1973 that chronic thoracic duct drainage would remove virtually all T cells but only some B cells from a mouse (reviewed by Sprent[60]).

One feature generally observed is that after a priming dose of antigen, the relative number of precursor cells with that receptor specificity is increased, often 10- to 20-fold, most of which are memory cells. One important property of memory T cells is that the requirements for stimulation are less stringent than those for naive T cells.[61] Memory T cells, for example, can be stimulated by APCs that do not express the costimulator molecule.[62] The net result of such factors is that a memory T-cell response has shortened kinetics and is likely to be much more potent than a primary response—the hallmarks of a memory response. For example, CTLs to an infection with primary influenza virus (e.g., H1N1) are first detected about 4 days later in the lungs of mice infected intranasally with the virus and reach peak levels after 6 to 7 days. If mice receive a priming dose of influenza virus (H2N2) some weeks before challenge with H1N1 virus, CTLs are found 1 to 2 days earlier and reach higher levels more rapidly than in the primary response.[63] This time difference may not seem great but could be critical in the case of a virus such as influenza virus, which has an 8- to 10-hour replication cycle.

For a marked boosting effect such as this to occur, a sufficient quantity of the challenge virus must avoid neutralization by preexisting antibody to initiate a substantial infection. Antibodies to the H1N1 and H2N2 influenza viruses do not cross-neutralize.

IMMUNOMODULATION

Alum, first used in the 1940s, is still the only adjuvant regularly used in human vaccination. For many years, however, there have been great efforts to develop more effective preparations, especially by pharmaceutical companies.

The actions of adjuvants can be separated into three types[3, 64]:

1. The formation of a depot of antigen primarily at the site of application and from which the antigen is released during a period that can be varied
2. The increased uptake of antigen into APCs, particularly dendritic cells, macrophages, and B lymphocytes
3. The induction of synthesis and secretion of enhancing factors, such as cytokines, which act principally but not exclusively on cells of the immune system, especially T and B lymphocytes

In addition to achieving these goals, an adjuvant must be safe, stable, and affordable and should target particular cells of the immune system with reasonable specificity. By the nature of their role simply as immunomodulators, the development of preparations that fulfill all these criteria is a time-consuming and expensive task. Table 3–5 describes in general terms a variety of materials used as adjuvants and provides a general statement about their activities. Not surprisingly, initial studies have usually been in murine systems, as it is much more expensive to carry out clinical trials. Preparations that have showed promise in murine systems have often given less encouraging results in primates or humans.

Table 3–5. **MATERIALS WITH ADJUVANT ACTIVITY AND POSSIBLE SITES OF ACTION**

ACTIVITIES	MATERIALS
Delayed release of antigen	Depot formers: water-in-oil, oil-in-water emulsion; control release devices; carriers (e.g., alum)
Mobilization of helper T cell	Proteins as carriers; polyclonal activators of T cells, PPD, poly/A/poly U
Modulation of immunoglobulin receptors on B cells	B-cell mitogens; antigen-polymerizing factors
Localization of antigens in T cell–dependent areas	Hydrophobic antigens; addition of lipid tail to proteins
Stimulation of APCs	MDP derivatives; LPS; lipid A
Facilitate cell-cell interaction	Surface-acting materials (e.g., saponin, lysolecithin, Quil A, liposomes, pluronic polymers)
Focusing of antigen on cells with Fc receptors	Activators of alternative pathway of complement, inulin, zymosan, endotoxin

APCs, antigen-presenting cells; LPS, lipopolysaccharide; MDP, muramyl dipeptide; PPD, purified protein derivative.
From Ada G, Ramsay A. Vaccines, Vaccination and the Immune Response. Philadelphia, Lippincott-Raven, 1997.

Selective Induction of Different Immune Responses

As previously indicated, many adjuvants preferentially stimulate the production of certain cytokines, and some of these, at least in the mouse, can influence the production of different Ig isotypes (reviewed in Ada and Ramsay[3]). Of particular interest is the role of IL-6 in stimulating mucosal IgA and IgG responses. Two other cytokines, IL-4 and IL-12, have been shown to dominate the overall immune response: IL-4 induces a type 2 T-cell response characterized by strong Ig responses. When introduced early in the response to an infectious agent, IL-4 has been shown to greatly decrease a subsequent CTL response.[65] In contrast, transfer of IL-12 favors a type 1 T-cell response, of which there are now numerous reports. One report of special interest is that a single subcutaneous injection of recombinant IL-12 2 days before challenge with *Plasmodium cynomolgi* sporozoites protected all of seven rhesus monkeys.[66] Protection was associated particularly with high levels of γ-IFN, which may have contributed to the elimination of infected hepatocytes. In another example, coadministration of a DNA preparation to induce an anti-HIV response in mice together with DNA coding for IL-12 resulted in a "dramatic increase" in the specific CTL response.[67] This approach would need to be monitored carefully, because there are other reports showing that administration of IL-12 can lead to unwanted effects.

For example, IL-12 has been shown to exacerbate *Onchocerca volvulus* antigen–mediated corneal pathology by enhancing chemokine expression and recruitment of inflammatory cells.[68]

Table 3–6 presents an estimate of the effectiveness of different viral and bacterial preparations, viral antigens, and immunomodulators at inducing CTL responses. Attenuated preparations of viruses or bacteria that induce an acute infection have generally been highly effective at generating CTL responses. They are also effective when used as vectors of other antigens. Currently, DNA seems to be at least as effective as attenuated infectious agents at inducing CTL responses. The inclusion of DNA coding for many antigens into a vector or into a DNA construct should give a broader response. The responses to inactivated whole virus may vary. Influenza A virus inactivated by γ-irradiation but not ultraviolet irradiation induces a strong, cross-reactive influenza A CTL response. Feline immunodeficiency virus, inactivated with paraformaldehyde and administered with threonyl muramyl dipeptide and SAF-M, induced strong and long-lasting CTL responses. When this virus was used as a vaccine in cats, the protective immunity observed was associated with CTL activity.[72] Table 3–6 also indicates that although alum preferentially induces a strong antibody response, a variety of preparations or means of antigen formulation are now available that may induce medium to strong CTL responses.

A comparison of a number of different delivery systems for the induction of CTL responses showed that the three most immunogenic systems were DNA, recombinant Ty virus–like particles, and a recombinant vaccinia virus preparation, Ankara.[84] It would be of interest to see whether, as was done to improve antibody production,[59] enhanced CTL responses could be achieved using a sequential administration approach, such as priming with DNA followed by boosting with the recombinant vector or virus-like particles.

Table 3–6. **SELECTIVE INDUCTION OF CYTOTOXIC T-CELL RESPONSES**

PREPARATION	CTL INDUCTION	REFERENCE
Viruses, Bacteria		
Live attentuated viruses, bacteria	+ + +	
Recombinant, live attenuated viruses, bacteria	+ +	
DNA as immunogen	+ + +	69
Inactivated (ultraviolet irradiation) whole virus*	−	70
Inactivated (γ irradiation) whole virus*	+ +	71
Inactivated whole virus with adjuvants†	+ +	72
Immunomodulators		
Alum	−	73
IL-4	−	65
IL-12	+ + +	67
Lipid-associated antigens, liposomes, FCA, FIA, QS21, lipopeptides	+ +	74–78
Particulate antigens	+ +	79–82
ISCOMs, antigens on beads or aggregated, lipid-encapsulated antigen		
Oxidative conjugation to mannan	+ + +	83

+ + +, high levels; + +, medium levels; −, little, if any, generated.
*Influenza virus inactivated by ultraviolet or γ-irradiation.
†Feline immunodeficiency virus inactivated with paraformaldehyde and administered with threonyl muramyl dipeptide and SAF-M.
FCA, Freund's complete adjuvant; FIA, Freund's incomplete adjuvant; QS21, adjuvant derived from saponin; ISCOMs, immunostimulating complexes.

REQUIREMENTS FOR SUCCESSFUL VACCINATION

The requirements for successful vaccination can be described as follows (modified from Ada and Ramsay[3]):

1. Activation of APCs, involving processing of antigens by the lysosomal or cytoplasmic pathways, expression of costimulatory factors at the cell surface, and secretion of certain cytokines
2. Activation, replication, and differentiation of T and B lymphocytes, leading to the generation of large pools of both types of memory cells
3. Incorporation of B-cell epitopes sufficient to generate strong neutralizing antibody responses as well as of T-cell determinants that bind with high affinity to at least the major regional human leukocyte antigen haplotypes such that the complex is recognized by the T-cell receptor
4. Long-term persistence of conformationally intact antigen, preferably as aggregates complexed with antibody and held at the surface of follicular dendritic cells in lymphoid tissues; this persistence allows the continuing production of cells that secrete antibody of increasingly higher affinity and of memory B cells

There are two further considerations with regard to point 3. At times, one or a few T-cell determinants in an antigen may be dominant, in the sense that other determinants are not recognized as well—the concept of *immunodominance*. The infectious agent may escape control by CTLs if these determinants are in a variable region of the antigen. In this situation, attempts should be made to induce responses to less dominant determinants in conserved regions of the antigen.[85] Because of a phenomenon called *cross-tolerance*, all individuals expressing an MHC antigen of a given specificity may not respond to a determinant that is known to bind strongly to that molecule.[86] This again stresses the need for a vaccine to contain several T-cell determinants. These aspects and the evidence favoring the interpretation proposed in point 4 are discussed in greater detail elsewhere.[3]

Acknowledgment

The author thanks Stanley Plotkin for helpful comments on an early draft of this chapter.

REFERENCES

1. Panum PL. Observations made during the epidemic of measles on the Faroe Islands in the year 1846. Med Classics 3:839–886, 1939.

2. Salk J, Drucker JA, Malvy D. Noninfectious poliovirus vaccine. In Plotkin SA, Mortimer ER (eds). Vaccines (2nd ed). Philadelphia, WB Saunders, 1994, pp 205–228.
3. Ada G, Ramsay A. Vaccines, Vaccination and the Immune Response. Philadelphia, Lippincott-Raven, 1997.
4. Nara PL, Smit L, Dunlop N, et al. Emergence of viruses resistant to neutralization by V3-specific antibodies in experimental human immunodeficiency virus type IIIB infection of chimpanzees. J Virol 64:3779–3791, 1990.
5. Parry N, Fox G, Rowlands D, et al. Structural and serological evidence for a novel method of antigenic variation in foot and mouth disease virus. Nature 347:569–572, 1990.
6. Croft M, Carter L, Swain SL, Dutton RW. Generation of polarized antigen-specific CD8 effector populations: Reciprocal action of interleukins (IL)-4 and IL-12 in promoting type 2 instead of type 1 cytokine profiles. J Exp Med 180:1715–1725, 1994.
7. Ada GL, Jones PD. The immune response to influenza infection. Curr Top Microbiol Immunol 128:1–54, 1986.
8. Koup RA, Safrit JT, Cao Y, et al. Temporal association of cellular immune responses with the initial control of viremia in primary human immunodeficiency virus type-1 syndrome. J Virol 68:4650–4655, 1994.
9. Borrow P, Lewicki H, Hahn B, et al. Virus-specific $CD8^+$ cytotoxic T-lymphocyte activity associated with control of viremia in primary human immunodeficiency virus type-1 infection. Virology 68:6103–6110, 1994.
10. Imagawa DT, Lee MH, Wolinsky SM, et al. Human immunodeficiency virus type 1 infection in homosexual men who remain seronegative for prolonged periods. New Engl J Med 320:1458–1462, 1989.
11. Taylor G. The role of antibody in controlling and/or clearing virus infections. In Ada GL (ed). Strategies in Vaccine Design. Austin, TX, RG Landes, 1994, pp 17–34.
12. Chanock RM, Crowe JE, Murphy BR, Burton DR. Human monoclonal antibody Fab fragments cloned from combinatorial libraries: Potential usefulness in prevention and/or treatment of major human viral disease. Infect Agents Dis 2:118–131, 1993.
13. Griffin DE, Levine B, Tyor WB, Irani DN. The immune response in viral encephalovirus. Semin Immunol 4:111–119, 1992.
14. Scherle PA, Palladino G, Gerhardt W. Mice can recover from pulmonary influenza virus infection in the absence of class I–restricted cytotoxic T cells. J Immunol 148:212–221, 1992.
15. Ramphal R, Cogliano RB, Shands JW, Small PA Jr. Serum antibody prevents lethal murine influenza pneumonitis but not tracheitis. Infect Immun 25:992–997, 1979.
16. Renegar KB, Small PA. Passive transfer of local immunity to influenza virus infection by IgA antibody. J Immunol 146:1972–1978, 1991.
17. Renegar KB, Small PA. Immunoglobulin A mediates murine anti-influenza virus immunity. J Virol 65:2146–2148, 1992.
18. Ada GL, McElrath MJ. HIV-vaccine induced cytotoxic T cell response. Potential role in vaccine efficacy. AIDS Res Hum Retroviruses 13:243–248, 1996.
19. Riddell SR, Watanabe KS, Goodrich JM, et al. Restoration of viral immunity in immunodeficient humans by the adoptive transfer of T cell clones. Science 257:238–241, 1992.
20. Walter EA, Greenberg PD, Gilbert MJ, et al. Reconstitution of cellular immunity against cytomegalovirus in recipients of allogeneic bone marrow by transfer of T cell clones from the donor. N Engl J Med 333:1038–1044, 1995.
21. Rooney CM, Smith CA, Ng CY, et al. Use of gene-modified virus-specific T lymphocytes to control Epstein-Barr virus–related lymphoproliferation. Lancet 345:9–13, 1995.
22. Kyburz D, Speiser DE, Battegay M, et al. Lysis of infected cells in vivo by anti-viral cytotoxic T cells demonstrated by release of cell internal viral proteins. Eur J Immunol 23:1540–1545, 1993.
23. Ando K, Guidotti LC, Wirth S, et al. Class I–restricted cytotoxic T lymphocytes are directly cytopathic for their target cells in vivo. J Immunol 152:3245–3253, 1994.
24. Kagi D, Ledermann B, Burki K, et al. Cytotoxicity mediated by T cells and natural killer cells is greatly impaired in perforin-deficient mice. Nature 369:31–36, 1994.
25. Rowland-Jones S, Sutton J, Ariyoshi K, et al. HIV-specific CTL activity in an HIV-exposed but uninfected infant. Lancet 341:860–861, 1993.
26. Cheynier R, Langlade-Demoyen P, Marescot M, et al. CTL responses in the PBMC of children born to HIV-infected mothers. Eur J Immunol 22:2211–2217, 1992.
27. Langlade-Demoyen P, Ngo-Giang-Huong N, Ferchal F, Oksenhendler E. Human immunodeficiency virus (HIV) nef-specific cytotoxic T lymphocytes in noninfected heterosexual contact of HIV-infected patients. J Clin Invest 93:1293–1297, 1994.
28. Rowland-Jones S, Sutton J, Ariyoshi K, et al. HIV-specific cytotoxic T cells in HIV-exposed but uninfected Gambian women. Nature Med 1:59–64, 1995.
29. Pinto LA, Sullivan J, Berzofsky JA, et al. Env-specific cytotoxic T lymphocytes in HIV-seronegative health care workers occupationally exposed to HIV-contaminated body fluids. J Clin Invest 96:867–876, 1995.
30. Simmons A, Nash AA. Zosteriform spread of herpes simplex virus as a model of recrudescence and its use to investigate the role of immune cells in prevention of recurrent disease. J Virol 52:816–821, 1984.
31. Simmons A, Tscharke DC. Anti-CD8 impairs clearance of herpes simplex virus from the nervous system: Implications for the fate of virally infected neurones. J Exp Med 175:1337–1344, 1992.
32. Liu Y, Mullbacher A. Activated B cells can deliver help for the in vitro generation of antiviral cytotoxic T cells. Proc Natl Acad Sci U S A 86:4629–4633, 1989.
33. Cardin RD, Brooks JW, Sarawar SR, Doherty PC. Progressive loss of $CD8^+$ T cell–mediated control of a gamma-herpesvirus in the absence of $CD4^+$ T cells. J Exp Med 184:863–871, 1996.
33a. Cardin RD, Brooks JW, Sarawar SR, Doherty PC. Progressive loss of $CD8^+$ T cell–mediated control of a gamma-herpesvirus in the absence of $CD4^+$ T cells. J Exp Med 184:863–871, 1996.
34. Harty JT, Bevan MJ. $CD8^+$ T cells specific for a single nonamer epitope of *Listeria monocytogenes* are protective in vivo. J Exp Med 175:1531–1538, 1992.
35. Jiang X, Gregory SH, Wing EJ. Immune $CD8^+$ T lymphocytes lyse *Listeria monocytogenes*–infected hepatocytes by a classical class I–restricted mechanism. J Immunol 158:287–293, 1997.
36. Pedrazzini T, Hug K, Louis JA. Importance of $L3T4^+$ and $Lyt\text{-}2^+$ cells in the immunologic control of infection with *Mycobacterium bovis* strain bacillus Calmette-Guérin in mice. Assessment by elimination of T cell subsets in vivo. J Immunol 139:2032–2037, 1987.
37. Leveton C, Barnass S, Champion B, et al. T cell–mediated protection of mice against virulent *Mycobacterium tuberculosis*. Infect Immun 57:390–395, 1989.
38. Flynn JL, Goldstein MM, Triebold KJ, et al. Major histocompatibility class I–restricted T cells are required for resistance to *Mycobacterium tuberculosis* infection. Proc Natl Acad Sci U S A 89:12013–12017, 1993.
39. Ladel CH, Daugelat S, Kaufmann SHE. Immune response to *Mycobacterium bovis* bacille Calmette Guérin infection in major histocompatibility complex class I– and II–deficient knock-out mice: Contribution of CD4 and CD8 T cells to acquired resistance. Eur J Immunol 25:377–384, 1995.
40. Ladel CH, Blum C, Dreher A, et al. Protective role of γ/δ T cells and α/β T cells in tuberculosis. Eur J Immunol 25:2877–2881, 1995.
41. Tarnvic A. Nature of protective immunity to *Francisella tularensis*. Rev Infect Dis 11:440–450, 1989.
42. Yee D, Rhinehart-Jones TR, Elkins KL. Loss of either $CD4^+$ or $CD8^+$ T cells does not affect the magnitude of protective immunity to an intracellular pathogen, *Francisella tularensis* strain LVS. J Immunol 157:5042–5048, 1996.
43. Holland MJ, Conway DJ, Blanchard TJ, et al. Synthetic peptides based on *Chlamydia trachomatis* antigens identify cytotoxic T lymphocyte responses in subjects from a trachoma-endemic population. Clin Exp Immunol 107:44–49, 1997.
44. Arnoldi J, Kaufmann SHE. The contribution of $CD8^+$ cytolytic T cells to the control of bacterial and parasitic infections. In Ada GL (ed). Strategies in Vaccine Design. Austin, TX, RG Landes, 1994, pp 83–98.
45. Rudzik O, Clancy RL, Percy DYE, et al. Repopulation with IgA-containing cells of bronchial and intestinal lamina propria after transfer of homologous Peyer's patches and bronchial lymphocytes. J Immunol 114:1599–1604, 1975.
46. Mazanec MB, Coudret CL, Fletcher DR. Intracellular neutraliza-

tion of influenza virus by IgA anti-HA monoclonal antibodies. J Virol 69:1339–1343, 1995.
47. Mazanec MB, Kaetzel CS, Lamm ME, et al. Intracellular neutralization of virus by immunoglobulin A antibodies. Proc Natl Acad Sci U S A 89:6901–6905, 1992.
48. Lamm ME. Interaction of antigens and antibodies at mucosal surfaces. Annu Rev Microbiol 51:311–340, 1997.
49. Lohman BL, Miller CJ, McChesney MB. Antiviral cytotoxic T lymphocytes in vaginal mucosa of simian immunodeficiency virus–infected rhesus macaques. J Immunol 155:5855–5860, 1995.
50. Musey L, Hu Y, Eckert L, et al. HIV induces cytotoxic T lymphocytes in the cervix of infected women. J Exp Med 185:293–303, 1997.
51. Fiette L, Aubert C, Brahie M, Rossi CP. Theiler's virus infection of β_2-microglobulin–deficient mice. J Virol 67:589–592, 1993.
52. Eichelberger M, Allan W, Zijlstra M, et al. Clearance of influenza virus respiratory infection in mice lacking class I major histocompatibility complex–restricted $CD8^+$ T cells. J Exp Med 174:875–880, 1991.
53. Ramshaw IA, Andrew ME, Phillips SM, et al. Recovery of immunodeficient mice from a vaccinia virus/IL-2 recombinant infection. Nature 329:545–547, 1987.
54. Spriggs MK, Koller BH, Sato T, et al. β_2-microglobulin–, $CD8^+$ T-cell–deficient mice survive inoculation with high doses of vaccinia virus and exhibit altered IgG responses. Proc Natl Acad Sci U S A 89:6070–6074, 1992.
55. Hou S, Doherty PC, Zijlstra M, et al. Delayed clearance of Sendai virus in mice lacking class I MHC-restricted $CD8^+$ T cells. J Immunol 149:1319–1325, 1992.
56. Doherty PC, Ahmed R. Memory to viruses. In Nathanson N (ed). Viral Pathogenesis. Philadelphia, Lippincott-Raven, 1997, pp 141–162.
57. Heath SL, Tew JG, Tew JG, et al. Follicular dendritic cells and human immunodeficiency virus infectivity. Nature 377:740–744, 1995.
58. Nossal GJV, Austin CM, Ada GL. Antigens in immunity. VII. Analysis of immunological memory. Immunology 9:333–348, 1965.
59. Leong KH, Ramsay AJ, Morin MJ, et al. Generation of enhanced immune responses by consecutive immunization with DNA and recombinant fowlpox virus. In Brown F, Chanock R, Ginsberg H, Norrby E (eds). Vaccines 95. Cold Spring Harbor, NY, Cold Spring Harbor Laboratory Press, 1995, pp 327–321.
60. Sprent J. Circulating T and B lymphocytes in the mouse. 1. Migratory properties. Cell Immunol 7:10–39, 1973.
61. Byrne JA, Butler JL, Cooper MD. Differential activation requirements for virgin and memory T cells. J Immunol 141:3249–3257, 1988.
62. Mullbacher A, Flynn K. Aspects of cytotoxic T cell memory. Immunol Rev 150:113–128, 1996.
63. Yap KL, Ada GL. The recovery of mice from influenza A virus infection: Adoptive transfer of immunity with influenza virus–specific cytotoxic T cells recognizing a common virion antigen. Scand J Immunol 8:413–420, 1978.
64. Chedid L. Adjuvants of immunity. Ann Immunol Inst Pasteur 136D:283–291, 1985.
65. Sharma DP, Ramsay AJ, Maguire DJ, et al. Interleukin-4 mediates down regulation of antiviral cytokine expression and cytotoxic T lymphocyte responses and exacerbates vaccinia virus infection in vivo. J Virol 70:7103–7107, 1996.
66. Hoffman SL, Crutcher FM, Puri SK, et al. Sterile protection of monkeys against malaria after administration of interleukin-12. Nat Med 3:80–83, 1997.
67. Kim JJ, Ayyavoo V, Bagarazzi ML, et al. In vivo engineering of a cellular immune response by coadministration of IL-12 expression vector with a DNA immunogen. J Immunol 158:816–826, 1997.
68. Pearlman E, Lass JH, Bardenstein DS, et al. IL-12 exacerbates helminth-mediated corneal pathology by augmenting inflammatory cell recruitment and chemokine expression. J Immunol 158:827–833, 1997.
69. McDonnell WM, Askari FK. Molecular medicine. DNA vaccines. N Engl J Med 334:42–45, 1995.
70. Braciale TJ, Yap KL. Role of viral infectivity in the induction of influenza virus–specific cytotoxic T cells. J Exp Med 147:1236–1252, 1978.
71. Mullbacher A, Ada GL, Tha Hla R. Gamma-irradiated influenza A virus can prime for a cross-reactive and cross-protective immune response against influenza A virus. Immunol Cell Biol 66:153–158, 1988.
72. Flynn JN, Keating P, Hosie MJ, et al. Env-specific CTL predominate in cats protected from feline immunodeficiency virus infection by vaccination. J Immunol 157:3658–3665, 1996.
73. Bomford R. Relative adjuvant efficacy of $Al(OH)_3$ and saponin is related to the immunogenicity of the antigen. Int Arch Allergy Immunol 75:280–281, 1984.
74. Gupta RK, Relyveld EH, Lindblad EB, et al. Adjuvants—a balance between toxicity and adjuvanticity. Vaccine 11:293–306, 1993.
75. Yong K, Ying L, Kapp JA. Ovalbumin injected with complete Freund's adjuvant stimulates cytolytic responses. Eur J Immunol 25:549–553, 1995.
76. Blum-Tirouvanziam U, Beghdadi-Rais C, Roggero MA, et al. Elicitation of specific cytotoxic T cells by immunization with malaria soluble synthetic polypeptides. J Immunol 153:4134–4141, 1994.
77. Hancock GE, Speelman DJ, Frenchick PJ, et al. Formulation of the purified fusion protein of respiratory syncytial virus with the saponin QS21 induces protective immune responses in Balb/c mice that are similar to those generated by experimental infection. Vaccine 13:391–400, 1995.
78. Sauzet JP, Deprez B, Martinon F, et al. Long-lasting anti-viral cytotoxic T lymphocytes induced in vivo with chimeric-multirestricted lipopeptides. Vaccine 13:1339–1345, 1995.
79. Jones PD, Tha Hla R, Morein B, Ada GL. Cellular immune response in the murine lung to local immunization with influenza A virus glycoproteins in micelles and immunostimulating complexes (iscoms). Scand J Immunol 27:645–652, 1988.
80. Kovacsovics-Bankowski M, Clark K, Benacceraf B, Rock KL. Efficient major histocompatibility complex class I presentation of exogenous antigen upon phagocytosis by macrophages. Proc Natl Acad Sci U S A 90:4942–4946, 1993.
81. Bachmann MF, Kundig TM, Freer G, et al. Induction of protective cytotoxic T cells with viral proteins. Eur J Immunol 24:2228–2236, 1994.
82. Zhou F, Rouse BT, Huang L. Induction of cytotoxic T lymphocytes in vivo with protein entrapped in membranous vehicles. J Immunol 149:1599–1604, 1992.
83. Apostolopoulos V, Loveland BE, Pietersz GA, McKenzie IFC. CTL in mice immunized with human mucin 1 are MHC restricted. J Immunol 155:5089–5094, 1995.
84. Allsopp CEM, Plebanski M, Gilbert S, et al. Comparison of numerous delivery systems for the induction of cytolytic T lymphocytes. Eur J Immunol 26:1951–1959, 1996.
85. Good MF. Harnessing cytotoxic T lymphocytes for vaccine design. Lancet 345:1003–1007, 1995.
86. Hill AB, Mullbacher A, Blanden RV. Ir genes, peripheral cross-tolerance and immunodominance in MHC class I–restricted T-cell responses: An old quagmire revisited. Immunol Rev 133:75–92, 1993.

chapter 4

Overview of Vaccine Manufacturing and Quality Assurance

Gary B. Ebbert

Eugene D. Mascolo

Howard R. Six

One of the most significant accomplishments in medicine is the development of safe and effective vaccines for the prevention of infectious diseases that are associated with high mortality and morbidity. Although only one disease—smallpox—has been eradicated, a significant reduction in the number of childhood cases of diphtheria, tetanus, pertussis, poliomyelitis, measles, mumps, and rubella has been realized through modern immunizing agents.[1]

The success of a vaccine in preventing disease depends on several factors, including the quality of the immunizing agent, how it is handled, and how it is used by clinicians. This chapter focuses on the production of a quality immunizing agent. In the United States, new vaccines are subjected to a well-defined regulatory process for approval. The approval process consists of three principal elements[2]:

1. Testing for safety and effectiveness through nonclinical and clinical studies
2. Preparing and submitting data and other related information through the Investigational New Drug Application (IND)
3. Food and Drug Administration (FDA) reviews of the IND submissions

For each new product, the FDA decides what clinical testing and data submissions are necessary to satisfy the efficacy provisions of the law. The FDA writes and enforces federal regulations, which are compiled in the Code of Federal Regulations. The FDA describes what manufacturers must do to meet agency premarketing requirements and also outlines approval procedures and processes. The FDA publishes many guidelines, which, unlike regulations, are not legally binding but provide manufacturers informal guidance on specific methods through which FDA requirements can be satisfied. The FDA also maintains an active communication program with publication of information sheets, staff manual guides, and other pertinent materials, such as "Points to Consider" documents.[2]

Before the FDA allows a new product to be administered to humans, it requires evidence that the substance is reasonably safe. There are several ways a manufacturer can meet this requirement[2]:

1. Compile existing preclinical data derived from past animal studies of the new product
2. Compile data obtained from previous clinical testing or use of the vaccine in the United States or another country whose population is relevant to the U.S. population
3. Undertake new preclinical studies designed to provide the necessary evidence to support the safety of initial clinical trials

When a manufacturer satisfies the pretesting requirements and demonstrates that the vaccine is sufficiently safe to be used in initial clinical trials, the company prepares and submits an IND to the FDA.[2]

This chapter presents the regulations in place at the time of writing. The FDA is in the process of adopting new regulations specified in the FDA Modernization Act. The principal difference is that all data will be reviewed prior to acceptance of a license application.

INVESTIGATIONAL NEW DRUG APPLICATION

The IND is a proposal through which the manufacturer obtains the FDA's permission to begin testing a product in human subjects. The IND must provide information in two key areas. First, it must disclose the results of all preclinical testing and provide information on the vaccine's components, the manufacturing process, and quality control procedures used to produce the vaccine. Second, the IND must provide clinical protocols.

These are detailed descriptions of the clinical studies through which the manufacturer expects to prove the vaccine's safety and efficacy in preventing a specific disease in human subjects.[2]

The FDA has 30 days in which to review the application and decide whether the vaccine is sufficiently safe for initial administration to humans. If the FDA does not contact the applicant within 30 days of the IND submission, clinical trials can begin. If the agency decides that a certain clinical trial should not be initiated, a *clinical hold* is put on the start of clinical trials until the issue is resolved.[2]

Generally, clinical trials proceed in at least three stages or phases[2]:

Phase 1: Cautious use of a vaccine in a few (20–80) patients or normal human volunteers to gain basic safety and efficacy information.

Phase 2: Use of the vaccine in a small number (100–200) of subjects to give the first indication of the vaccine's effectiveness in its proposed use.

Phase 3: Use of the vaccine in a significantly larger group (several hundred to several thousand) of subjects to assess the vaccine's safety and effectiveness and to help determine the best dosage in a larger and more varied patient population. These trials may be conducted at several sites and may include both controlled and uncontrolled studies. The type and amount of clinical testing vary. Clinical vaccine development time averages 5 years but can range from 2 to 10 years.

GOOD CLINICAL PRACTICES

In addition to determining which clinical studies are necessary, the FDA sets minimum standards for conducting these tests. The FDA does this through a set of regulations called Good Clinical Practices (GCPs). In general, the GCPs outline the responsibilities of people who are involved in a clinical trial, including the manufacturer or sponsor, the investigator, the monitor, and the Institutional Review Board (IRB).[3]

Sponsor (Manufacturer). In general, the manufacturer or sponsor is responsible for selecting qualified investigators and providing them with the information they need to properly conduct an investigation. The sponsor ensures that the investigation is monitored and conducted in accordance with the general investigational plan and protocols contained in the IND. The sponsor is also responsible for maintaining an effective IND and keeping the FDA and investigators informed of any significant new adverse effects or risks related to the product.[3]

Investigators. The investigator is the person who actually conducts a clinical investigation. He or she is responsible for ensuring that an investigation is conducted according to the signed investigator statement, the investigational plan, and applicable regulations. In addition, the investigator has the responsibility of protecting the rights, safety, and welfare of the clinical subjects and controlling the product under investigation.[3]

Institutional Review Board. The IRB's function is to see that risks to clinical subjects are minimized and that the subjects are adequately informed about the clinical trial and its implications for their treatment. The IRB consists of at least five people, each member having the professional competence to review research activities. At least one board member must have a primary interest other than science, such as law, ethics, or religion.[3] The clinical investigator is responsible for obtaining IRB approval for each clinical study.

PRODUCT DEVELOPMENT

Vaccine development involves the process of taking a new antigen or immunogen identified in the research process and developing this substance into a final vaccine that can be evaluated through preclinical and clinical studies to determine the safety and efficacy of the resultant vaccine. During this process, the product's components, in-process materials, final product specifications, and the manufacturing process are defined. The manufacturing scale used during development is usually significantly smaller than that used in the final manufacturing process. Phase 1, and sometimes phase 2, clinical trial vaccines are typically produced in product development, but it is usually anticipated that at least one of the three or more consistency lots used for phase 3 clinical trials is manufactured at full-scale production volume. The vaccines used for these trials are usually derived from the consistency lots manufactured to support the Product License Application and the Establishment License Application. The product manufactured during the development phase is manufactured according to Current Good Manufacturing Practices (CGMPs).[4]

ESTABLISHMENT LICENSE APPLICATION AND PRODUCT LICENSE APPLICATION

There are two forms of licenses: establishment and product. The establishment license application involves licensing all locations where manufacturing takes place. An establishment license is issued only after inspection of the location and determination that the location complies with applicable standards. No establishment license is issued unless a product is available for examination during all phases of manufacturing, and a product license is requested and issued simultaneously.[4]

To obtain a product license, the manufacturer must submit data from nonclinical laboratory and clinical studies demonstrating that the manufactured product meets prescribed standards of safety, purity, and potency. (Applications for licenses are submitted to the Director, Center for Biologics Evaluation and Research [CBER].) Information contained in the product license and establishment license applications will now be combined in a single document, a Biologic License Application.

EXAMPLES OF VACCINE PRODUCTION

Live Vaccine (Oral Polio)

Poliovirus live oral trivalent vaccine is a mixture of three types of attenuated polioviruses (Sabin) prepared in *Macaca* or *Cercopithecus* monkey kidney cell cultures: type 1 (LS-C, 2ab/KP_2), type 2 (P712, Ch, 2ab/KP_2), and type 3 (Leon 12a, b/KP_3).[5]

The cells are grown in Eagle's basal medium, consisting of Earle's balanced salt solution containing amino acids, antibiotics, and calf serum. After cell growth, the medium is removed, inoculated with one of the attenuated polioviruses suspended in the same medium without calf serum. The resulting monovalent virus is pooled, tested, and filtered before being used for trivalent vaccine formulation.

Each human dose of the live oral trivalent vaccine is constituted to have infectivity titers in the final container material of $10^{6.0}$ to $10^{7.0}$ for type 1, $10^{5.1}$ to $10^{6.1}$ for type 2, and $10^{5.8}$ to $10^{6.8}$ for type 3 when assayed in Hep-2 cells. The final vaccine is a sterile suspension of poliovirus types 1, 2, and 3, unpreserved, normally containing antibiotics and stabilizers.[6]

The poliovirus live oral trivalent vaccine is made as follows.[7]

Criteria for Qualification of the Seed Virus. Each seed virus used in vaccine manufacturing is prepared from an acceptable strain in monkey kidney cell cultures. The seed virus must be demonstrated to be free of extraneous microbial agents except for unavoidable bacteriophage.[8] In addition, the neurovirulence of each of the first five consecutive monovalent virus pools prepared from the seed virus must meet the neurovirulence requirements.[9]

Manufacture of Live Poliovirus. The seed virus in vaccine manufacturing is prepared in a seed lot system from a master virus seed lot.[10] Virus in the final vaccine should represent no more than five tissue culture passages from the original strain.[11]

Kidneys are processed separately for each monkey. The resulting viral fluid is identified as a separate monovalent harvest and is kept separate from other monovalent harvests until all samples for testing are taken.[12] Prior to inoculation with the seed virus, and at least 3 days after complete formation of the tissue sheet, the tissue culture growth in vessels derived from each pair of kidneys is examined microscopically for cell degeneration. If such evidence is observed, the tissue cultures from that pair of kidneys must not be used for vaccine manufacturing.[13]

The tissue found free of cell degeneration is tested for further evidence of freedom from demonstrable, viable, microbial agents. If these tests indicate the presence of any viable microbial agent in the monkey kidney production vessels, the viral harvest from these tissue cultures is not used for poliovirus vaccine manufacture.[14]

Control Vessels. At least 25% of the cell suspension from each pair of kidneys is set aside and used to establish control cultures, which must be examined microscopically for cell degeneration for an additional 14 days. The culture fluids from such controls must be tested both at the time of the virus harvest and at the end of the observation period. In the culture systems just described, the control cell sheet is also examined for the presence of hemadsorbing viruses by the addition of guinea pig red blood cells.[15] At least 80% of the control vessels must be free of cell degeneration at the end of the observation period to qualify the kidneys for poliovirus vaccine manufacture. If any extraneous agent is present at the time of virus harvest, the virus harvest from that tissue culture preparation is not used for poliovirus vaccine manufacture. If any tests or observations demonstrate the presence of any microbial agent known to be capable of producing human disease, the virus grown in each tissue culture preparation is not used for vaccine production.[16]

Incubation. The temperature of the kidney tissue production vessels after inoculation with the virus is held at 33 to 35°C during the course of virus propagation.[17]

Virus Harvests. Virus harvests are conducted no later than 72 hours after virus inoculation. Virus harvested from kidney tissue from one monkey may be tested separately, or samples of viral harvest from more than one pair of kidneys may be combined, identified, and tested as a monovalent virus pool. The samples are withdrawn immediately after harvesting.[18]

Additional tests for safety are conducted on the monovalent virus pools. The pools must demonstrate no viable microbial agents except for unavoidable bacteriophage and the intended attenuated live poliovirus. The vaccine is tested for the absence of other infectious agents, including polioviruses of other types or strains.[19] After the harvest and removal of samples for safety testing, the pool is sterile filtered, yielding a sterile monovalent virus pool.[20] The sterile-filtered monovalent virus pool is then tested for potency.

Potency Testing. Concentrations of living virus in each monovalent virus pool are expressed as infectivity titer per mL for cell cultures, using the live attenuated reference poliovirus of the same type as a control. Titration of the monovalent virus pool is not a valid test unless the titration of the reference virus when tested in parallel is within $\pm 0.5 \log_{10}$ of its established titer.[21]

Neurovirulence Testing. After the monovalent virus pool is sterile filtered, a neurovirulence test is performed in *Macaca* monkeys.[22] In this test, the absence of neurovirulence of the monovalent pool is confirmed after intraspinal inoculation in monkeys shown not to have neutralizing antibodies.[23] As a control, monkeys are separately inoculated with a reference attenuated poliovirus. The monovalent virus pool may be used for poliovirus vaccines if a comparative analysis of the test results demonstrates that the numerical value assigned for neurovirulence of the monovalent virus pool is equal to or less than that of the corresponding type of reference attenuated poliovirus.[24] The monovalent virus pool is acceptable if (1) the numerical value assigned for neurovirulence of the monovalent virus pool is greater than that of the reference attenuated poliovirus and (2) the difference between these two values is not greater than that calculated by a mathematical method that is designed to reject vaccines with neurovirulence identical to the reference attenuated poliovirus.[25]

Additional Tests for Safety

Before Filtration. Tests are performed on the monovalent virus pools before filtration to demonstrate the absence of microbial agents except for unavoidable bacteriophage and the intended attenuated live poliovirus. The vaccine is tested for the absence of other infectious agents, including poliovirus of other types or strains. These tests include the following[26, 27]:

1. Inoculation of rabbits
2. Inoculation of adult mice
3. Inoculation of suckling mice
4. Inoculation of guinea pigs
5. Inoculation of monkey kidney tissue cultures
6. Inoculation of human cell cultures
7. Inoculation of a rabbit kidney tissue culture
8. Tests for in vitro markers

After Filtration. In addition to the required neurovirulence tests, the following safety tests are performed on each monovalent virus pool after the filtration process[28]:

1. In vitro marker tests
2. Final container sterility test, if needed

General Requirements. Each monovalent virus pool must (1) be manufactured by the same procedure, (2) meet the criteria for neurovirulence for monkeys,[29] (3) meet the criteria of in vitro markers,[30] and (4) be released for further manufacturing by the director of the CBER.[31]

Samples and Protocols. The following materials must be submitted to the director of the CBER: a protocol that consists of a summary of the history of manufacture of each monovalent virus pool,[32] including any test results requested by the director of the CBER; 20 mL of monovalent virus pool before filtration[33]; and 40 mL of monovalent virus pool after filtration.[34]

Formulation

The trivalent poliovirus vaccine is formulated from monovalent poliovirus vaccine pools consisting of the three types of polio attenuated viruses. The human dose of trivalent poliovirus vaccine must be constituted to have infectivity titers in the final container material of $10^{6.0}$ to $10^{7.0}$ for type 1, $10^{5.1}$ to $10^{6.1}$ for type 2, and $10^{5.8}$ to $10^{6.8}$ for type 3.[35]

General Requirements. No lot of trivalent vaccine may be released by the manufacturer unless each monovalent virus pool has met all the requirements and has been released by the CBER for further manufacturing.[36]

Labeling. The final container label must bear a statement indicating that liquid vaccine may not be used for more than 7 days after the container is opened.[37]

Samples and Protocols. For each trivalent vaccine, the following materials must be submitted in accordance with instructions from the director of the CBER[38]:

1. Protocol that consists of a summary of the history of manufacture of each trivalent lot, including any test results requested by the director of the CBER[39]
2. 20 mL of monovalent virus pool before filtration[40]
3. 40 mL of monovalent virus pool after filtration[41]
4. Total of at least 50 single doses of the trivalent vaccine[42]

The final vaccine is a sterile suspension of polioviruses types 1, 2, and 3, unpreserved, normally containing antibiotics and stabilizers.

Killed Vaccine (Influenza)

These vaccines contain two strains of influenza A viruses and a single influenza B virus. The two type A viruses are identified by their subtypes of hemagglutinin (H) and neuraminidase (N). Today's vaccines usually contain the influenza A virus H1N1 and the influenza A virus H3N2.

The trivalent subunit vaccine is the predominant influenza vaccine used today. This vaccine is produced from viral strains that are identified by the World Health Organization, the Centers for Disease Control and Prevention (CDC), and the CBER. For U.S.-licensed manufacturers, the viral strains are normally acquired from the CBER or the CDC. These suspensions are used to prepare the inoculum for vaccine production. The substrate most commonly used by producers of influenza vaccine is the 11-day-old embryonated egg. A certain quantity of eggs is inoculated with a certified monovalent viral inoculum that has been verified for infectivity titer, specificity, and sterility. The inoculation process is adjusted to instill a small volume of the viral suspension directly into the allantoic fluid. The inoculated eggs are then incubated using a predetermined time, temperature, and relative humidity.

After completion of the incubation process, the inoculated eggs are normally refrigerated to facilitate harvesting of the allantoic fluid. This fluid, which contains the live virus, is then withdrawn from the eggs, collected into a vessel, and held under refrigeration. The fluid is then clarified, and the virus is inactivated by adding a predetermined concentration of the prescribed inactivating agent; formalin is often used for this purpose. Fluid containing the inactivating agent may be further clarified and held under a predetermined temperature and time regimen to completely inactivate the virus; the regimen used may vary depending on the viral strain.

The inactivated fluids are further processed, usually via zonal ultracentrifugation. Sucrose gradient fractions are selected for further processing on the basis of sucrose content and the extent of hemagglutination. The selected fractions are then diluted, usually with phosphate-buffered saline. The detergent-splitting agent is added at a prescribed concentration for a predetermined exposure time. Further purification methods are applied, resulting in a purified, inactivated, monovalent virus concentrate. This final concentrate may contain a preservative and a stabilizer, depending on the specific product design.

Depending on the process steps involved in the manufacturing of an inactivated monovalent virus concentrate, several in-process tests may be incorporated. The final concentrate is normally tested for sterility, virus inactivation, potency, endotoxin concentration, protein content, stabilizer concentration, residuals, pH, sodium chloride concentration, identity, safety, and preservative concentration, if present.

Concentrates of the same strain can be pooled and tested per the testing regimen listed earlier or held as a single concentrate. For U.S.-licensed manufacturers, the CBER tests the concentrates or concentrate pools for potency and reports the result(s) to the manufacturer.

The final trivalent inactivated subunit vaccine is then formulated according to the approved vaccine formula. The resulting bulk vaccine is tested for potency, sterility, safety, sodium chloride concentration, residuals, protein concentration, preservative concentration, pH, virus inactivation, and endotoxin.

If the bulk vaccine meets the quality control and CBER release criteria, the vaccine is aseptically filled and closed into final containers, labeled, packaged, and stored under refrigeration. Only after the filled containers are tested for the attributes required by the license and also meet quality control and CBER release criteria is the product released for distribution.

Recombinant Vaccine

Recombinant vaccines use a piece of DNA derived from an organism that codes for a protective protein. The DNA is derived either directly from the genome of the organism or by transcription of messenger RNA or viral RNA into complementary DNA through reverse transcription. The protein can then be produced by insertion of the DNA into a variety of expression vehicles, such as *Escherichia coli*, baculovirus or poxvirus, or cell lines such as Chinese hamster ovary, or by direct injection into the muscle of a bacterial plasmid carrying the DNA. With the exception of the last technique, proteins produced by recombinant DNA must be purified after expression.

The manufacturer should describe the method used, including the cell type and the origin of the source material. The manufacturer should also include a detailed nucleotide sequence analysis and a restriction enzyme digestion map of the cloned segment. Construction of the vector used for expression of the cloned nucleotide segment into its respective product must be detailed, including an explanation of the source and function of the component parts of the vector. The component parts may include the origins of replication, antibiotic resistance genes, promoters, and enhancers.[43]

The host cell system should be described, including the relevant phenotype and genotype. The host cell should be thoroughly characterized if it is of mammalian origin, and the method of transfer (e.g., transfection, transduction, infection, or microinjection) from the vector to the host cell should be provided.[43]

Master Cell Bank. A seed lot consists of aliquots of a single culture, stored in a manner that gives a reasonable assurance of genetic stability. The master cell bank is a designated seed lot from which all subsequent seed lots are made. Maintaining the integrity of the master cell bank is critical for DNA vaccine production. In most instances, a single host cell containing the expression vector should be cloned to give rise to the master cell bank. If new master cell banks are generated periodically by expression vector transfer and clonal selection, acceptance criteria should be described for the new clones and the product produced by these clones. The stability of both the host cell and expression vector should be investigated. In particular, the fidelity of the nucleotide sequence encoding the expression product in the master cell bank should be certified. Whenever clonal selection is used to construct a new seed lot, DNA sequence analysis of the coding region should be performed.[43] The identity and purity of the cells in each seed lot should be assured by isoenzyme analysis, auxotrophy, antibiotic resistance, and karyology, as appropriate. Each seed lot is characterized for adventitious agents, including *Mycoplasma* or other bacteria, fungi, viruses, and virus-like particles.

Production. For each production run, the cells used should be characterized by analysis of relevant phenotypic or genotypic markers and then tested for adventitious agents in samples taken just before termination culture. For each master cell bank, a detailed restriction enzyme digestion map of the expression vector and the nucleotide sequence of the insert encoding the expression product should be determined at least once after full-scale culture. The procedures and materials used for cell growth and induction of product expression should be described in detail. Data should be maintained on the consistency of yield of the product from full-scale culture, and criteria should be established for the rejection of culture lots.

Penicillin and other β-lactam–containing antibiotics may derivatize proteins and generally should not be used in production runs because of the risk of hypersensitization in product recipients. Similarly, caution should be exercised in the use of such materials as phenylmethylsulfonyl fluoride (a protease inhibitor), β-propiolactone, formaldehyde, and other protein-derivatizing chemicals, since multiple exposure to derivatized proteins may lead to undesirable immune responses in recipients of the final product.[43]

Purification. The methodology of harvesting, extraction, and purification should be described in detail, and the removal of any undesirable chemicals introduced by these procedures should be demonstrated.[43]

Characterization of the Product. Evidence for identity, purity, and stability of the product in comparison with reference preparations may be derived from the results of a wide variety of tests.

Combination Vaccine

A combination vaccine consists of two or more live organisms, inactivated organisms, or purified antigens combined by the manufacturer or mixed immediately before administration.[44] A combination vaccine is intended to prevent multiple diseases or prevent one disease caused by different strains or serotypes of the same organism. Vectored vaccines and conjugated vaccines are considered to be combination vaccines if one of the combinations indicated is prevention of the disease caused by the vector organism or the carrier moiety.[44]

Regulatory Requirements. Regulations that pertain to biological products also apply to combination vaccines. The section on permissible combinations (Code of Federal Regulations, Title 21, Section 610.17) is important for combinations and states that licensed products may not be combined with other licensed or unlicensed products unless a license is obtained for the combined product.

Manufacturing Issues for Combination Vaccines. Combining monovalent vaccines may result in a combination that is less safe or effective than is desired. For example, the components of inactivated vaccines may adversely affect one or more of the active components. This occurred when whole-cell pertussis vaccine and inactivated poliovirus vaccine were combined, resulting in a combination with a decreased pertussis potency.[44]

When live vaccines are combined, immunological interference has been observed between vaccine viruses or virus subtypes. A weaker immune response or a component cross-reactivity may occur, and the recombination may also allow attenuated organism to be reconstituted to virulent forms. Consequently, validation of the compatibility of the components is important before the onset of clinical trials. The CBER advises that the combination should be characterized and its components assessed through a battery of physicochemical, biochemical, and biological assays.

The CBER also recommends conducting preclinical animal studies to determine the combination consequences on potency and immunogenicity. The manufacturer must evaluate some of the physical characteristics, including the combination vaccine's resuspension, and ensure container and closure suitability. If the combination vaccine is too large to be safely administered, the manufacturer may pursue the possibility of dose reduction for some or all its components. The effects of such changes should be assessed before clinical trials.[44]

ADJUVANTS, ANTIBIOTICS, PRESERVATIVES, AND STABILIZERS

Adjuvants. Adjuvants are sometimes incorporated into vaccines to enhance the immune response of the vaccine's antigen(s). This enhancing effect allows for added benefits such as the use of lesser quantities of costly antigens or, in the case of highly purified antigens produced through techniques using recombinant DNA, provides for the ability of these antigens to stimulate levels of antibody comparable to their more complex counterparts.

Although the use of adjuvants dates to the early 1900s, the precise mechanisms that control their mode of action are still not precisely defined. A diversity of substances possess adjuvant properties, and a wide range of these (e.g., aluminum compounds, oil emulsions, detoxified lipopolysaccharides, peptides, liposomes, purified saponin, and polymeric species) have been investigated for their adjuvant properties. At present, only aluminum-containing adjuvants are licensed by the FDA for human use.

Adjuvants can be placed into two major categories, vehicles and immunomodulators. Vehicles include liposomes, emulsions, and immunostimulating complexes that help carry the components of the vaccine and retain them in proximity with lymphoid tissues. Immunomodulators include muramyldipeptide and monophosphoryl lipid A, both of which stimulate local secretion of cytokines.[45, 46]

Antibiotics. Antibiotics can be used in the manufacture of some viral vaccines during the propagation phase to reduce or suppress the growth of any extraneous contaminants that may be introduced during various processing steps.

For vaccines produced through the use of purified preparations of plasmid DNA, antibiotic resistance is a commonly used selection marker. The FDA recommends that manufacturers of plasmid DNA vaccines avoid the use of penicillin or other β-lactam antibiotics, since severe reactions in certain individuals may occur. Antibiotics such as kanamycin and neomycin (aminoglycoside antibiotics) are commonly recommended by the FDA for plasmid DNA vaccines. Neomycin may be used in other viral vaccines as an antibacterial agent during the manufacturing phase.[47]

Preservatives. Preservatives are added to vaccines only when there is a risk of contamination, such as when the vaccine is prepared in multidose vials. For a combination vaccine, the preservative or stabilizer in one monovalent vaccine can affect the potency of the other vaccine. Thimerosal adversely affected the potency of the inactivated poliovirus vaccine combination with diphtheria and tetanus toxoids and adsorbed pertussis vaccine.[44] If single-dose vials are used, the use of preservatives can be avoided.

Whether or not a preservative is used, the manufacturer still needs to evaluate the vaccine for potency and reversion to toxicity for each of the active components. The manufacturer should also determine the levels of constituents or antimicrobials remaining in the vaccine and conduct studies on the preservative's ability to prevent contamination of the product.

Stabilizers. Vaccine stability is essential in being able to reliably deliver a safe, effective product to key target populations. In many areas of the globe, cold chains either are nonexistent or can be easily compromised; these areas therefore require vaccines with high thermal stability.

It is believed that the instability of vaccines can be attributed, at least in part, to the loss of antigenic properties or, as in the case of live viral vaccines, to the loss of infectivity. Work has been heavily focused on those factors that influence the structural and conformational integrity of vaccine epitopes, such as temperature and pH. Each vaccine category (i.e., live attenuated, inactivated viral or bacterial antigens, toxoids, or antitoxins) presents different challenges to the scientist. Bacterial vaccines, for example, can demonstrate instability because of the hydrolysis and aggregation of protein and carbohydrate molecules.

Research and development efforts in the global vaccine community have been focused heavily on developing oral polio vaccines with increased thermal stability in addition to improving other globally important vaccines. The stabilizer of choice for oral polio vaccine remains $MgCl_2$. Molar $MgSO_4$ has been demonstrated to stabilize viruses such as respiratory syncytial virus and measles virus, and other vaccines, such as the yellow fever vaccine, have been effectively stabilized through the use of lactose-sorbitol and sorbitol-gelatin combinations.

Because of growing concerns regarding the potential risks of using materials of bovine origin, which have been associated with bovine spongiform encephalopathy, development of alternative stabilizers containing mixtures of amino acids, polysaccharides, and salts in lieu of animal products (bovine, ovine, and porcine) should be considered.[48, 49]

REFERENCES

1. Casto DT, Brunell PA. Safe handling of vaccines. Pediatrics 87:108–112, 1991.
2. Mathieu M. The new drug approval process: A primer. In New Drug Development: A Regulatory Overview. Cambridge, MA, Parexel International Corporation, 1990, pp 1–12.
3. Mathieu M. Good clinical practices. In New Drug Development: A Regulatory Overview. Cambridge, MA, Parexel International Corporation, 1990, pp 105–118.
4. Mathieu M. Clinical testing of new drugs. In New Drug Development: A Regulatory Overview. Cambridge, MA, Parexel International Corporation, 1990, pp 83–104.
5. Code of Federal Regulations, Title 21, Sec. 630.10(a), April 1, 1996.
6. Code of Federal Regulations, Title 21, Sec. 630.12(a), April 1, 1996.
7. Code of Federal Regulations, Title 21, Sec. 630.10(c), April 1, 1996.
8. Code of Federal Regulations, Title 21, Sec. 630.11(c-1), April 1, 1996.
9. Code of Federal Regulations, Title 21, Sec. 630.11(c-2), April 1, 1996.
10. Code of Federal Regulations, Title 21, Sec. 630.11(c-4), April 1, 1996.
11. Code of Federal Regulations, Title 21, Sec. 630.13(a), April 1, 1996.
12. Code of Federal Regulations, Title 21, Sec. 630.13(b-2), April 1, 1996.
13. Code of Federal Regulations, Title 21, Sec. 630.13(b-3), April 1, 1996.
14. Code of Federal Regulations, Title 21, Sec. 630.13(b-3), April 1, 1996.
15. Code of Federal Regulations, Title 21, Sec. 630.13(b-4), April 1, 1996.
16. Code of Federal Regulations, Title 21, Sec. 630.13(b-5), April 1, 1996.
17. Code of Federal Regulations, Title 21, Sec. 630.13(b-6), April 1, 1996.
18. Code of Federal Regulations, Title 21, Sec. 630.13(b-7), April 1, 1996.
19. Code of Federal Regulations, Title 21, Sec. 630.18(a), April 1, 1996.
20. Code of Federal Regulations, Title 21, Sec. 630.13(b-8), April 1, 1996.
21. Code of Federal Regulations, Title 21, Sec. 630.15(a), April 1, 1996.
22. Code of Federal Regulations, Title 21, Sec. 630.16(a, b), April 1, 1996.
23. Code of Federal Regulations, Title 21, Sec. 630(b), April 1, 1996.
24. Code of Federal Regulations, Title 21, Sec. 630.16(b-2), April 1, 1996.
25. Code of Federal Regulations, Title 21, Sec. 630.16(b-2), April 1, 1996.
26. Code of Federal Regulations, Title 21, Sec. 630.18(a), April 1, 1996.
27. Code of Federal Regulations, Title 21, Sec. 630.18(a-1 to a-7), April 1, 1996.
28. Code of Federal Regulations, Title 21, Sec. 630.18(b, c), April 1, 1996.
29. Code of Federal Regulations, Title 21, Sec. 630.19(a-2), April 1, 1996.
30. Code of Federal Regulations, Title 21, Sec. 630.9(a-3), April 1, 1996.
31. Code of Federal Regulations, Title 21, Sec. 630.19(a-4), April 1, 1996.
32. Code of Federal Regulations, Title 21, Sec. 630.19(c-1), April 1, 1996.
33. Code of Federal Regulations, Title 21, Sec. 630.19(c-2), April 1, 1996.
34. Code of Federal Regulations, Title 21, Sec. 630.19(c-3), April 1, 1996.
35. Code of Federal Regulations, Title 21, Sec. 630.15(b), April 1, 1996.
36. Code of Federal Regulations, Title 21, Sec. 630.19(1-4), April 1, 1996.
37. Code of Federal Regulations, Title 21, Sec. 630.19(b), April 1, 1996.
38. Code of Federal Regulations, Title 21, Sec. 630.19(c), April 1, 1996.
39. Code of Federal Regulations, Title 21, Sec. 630.19(c-1), April 1, 1996.
40. Code of Federal Regulations, Title 21, Sec. 630.19(c-3), April 1, 1996.
41. Code of Federal Regulations, Title 21, Sec. 630.19(c-3), April 1, 1996.
42. Code of Federal Regulations, Title 21, Sec. 630.19(c-4), April 1, 1996.
43. Points to Consider in the Production and Testing of New Drugs and Biologicals Produced by Recombinant DNA Technology. Bethesda, MD, Office of Biologics Research and Review, Center for Drugs and Biologics, 1985, pp 4–7.
44. Guidance for Industry for the Evaluation of Combination Vaccines for Preventable Diseases: Production, Testing, and Clinical Studies. Washington, DC, U.S. Department of Health and Human Services, Food and Drug Administration, Center for Biologics Evaluation and Research, 1997, pp 1–4.
45. Adam A. Synthetic Adjuvants, Modern Concepts in Immunology. Vol. 1. Paris, University of Paris-Sud Orsay, Institute of Biochemistry, 1985.
46. Van Regenmortel M. Searching for safer, more potent, better-targeted adjuvants. ASM News 63:136–139, March 1997.
47. Glaser V. Adjuvants boost safety, efficacy while lowering costs of new vaccines. Genet Eng News June 1, 1995:6–7.
48. New approaches to stabilization of vaccines potency, developments in biological standardization. World Health Organization/International Association of Biological Standardization Symposium on Progress on the Stability of Vaccines; Vol. 87; Geneva; May 29–31, 1995.
49. Pharmaceutical products [draft proposal]. Pharmaceutical Research and Manufacturers of America Bovine Spongiform Encephalopathy Committee, May 21, 1997.

chapter

5 General Immunization Practices

John C. Watson

Georges Peter

Recommendations for immunization practices are based on scientific knowledge of vaccine characteristics, the principles of immunization, and the epidemiology of specific diseases. In addition, the experience and judgment of public health officials and specialists in clinical and preventive medicine play a key role in developing recommendations that maximize the benefits and minimize the risks and costs associated with immunization. General guidelines for immunization practices are based on evidence and expert opinion of the benefits, costs, and risks of vaccination as they apply to the current epidemiology of disease and use of vaccines in the United States. However, many of the principles are universal and are applicable to other countries with different public health infrastructures.

VACCINE STORAGE AND HANDLING

Vaccines must be properly shipped, stored, and handled to avoid loss of their biological activity. Recommended storage and handling requirements for each vaccine are given in the manufacturer's product label.[1] Correct shipping, storage, and handling practices are also published in the recommendations of the major vaccine policymaking committees, such as the Advisory Committee on Immunization Practices (ACIP) of the Centers for Disease Control and Prevention and the American Academy of Pediatrics (AAP) (see Chapter 42).[2–4] Failure to adhere to these requirements can lead to a loss of vaccine potency, resulting in an inadequate immune response in the vaccinee. Visible evidence of altered vaccine integrity may or may not be present. The manufacturer should be contacted when questions arise about the correct handling of a vaccine. New vaccines or new formulations of an existing vaccine may have different shipping, storage, and handling requirements. Table 5–1 gives recommended storage practices for the most commonly used vaccines in the United States.

Exposure to either higher or lower temperatures than recommended can inactivate a vaccine (see Table 5–1). For example, live virus vaccines such as oral poliovirus vaccine (OPV) and varicella are sensitive to temperatures above freezing and should be kept frozen until just before administration. Measles-mumps-rubella (MMR) vaccine and yellow fever vaccine should be kept frozen, although storage at below 8°C (46°F) and below 5°C (41°F), respectively, is acceptable.[3, 5] However, vaccines composed of purified antigens or inactivated microorganisms, such as hepatitis A, hepatitis B, *Haemophilus influenzae* type b (Hib), and influenza, can lose their potency if frozen and therefore should be kept at 2 to 8°C (36 to 46°F) and never frozen.[3, 4] Diluents should not be frozen.[3, 4]

Maintenance of a "cold chain" from vaccine production to use helps ensure vaccine potency at the time of administration.[3, 4] Temperature monitoring and control is important for all storage and handling, particularly during transport and field use. Temperatures should be monitored regularly, using a thermometer that records current, maximum, and minimum temperatures. Whereas maintenance of cold and freezing temperatures is a problem in tropical climates, recent data suggest that inappropriate freezing of inactivated vaccines is a problem in maintaining vaccine stability in cold and temperate climates.[6] Kendal and associates[4, 6] have suggested methods for packing and shipping vaccines based on tests conducted under representative conditions within the United States. Shipping containers should be sturdy and the correct size for the amount of vaccine to be shipped. Appropriate insulation (e.g., panels and boxes of polystyrene, isocyanurate, or polyurethane) and cold source (e.g., dry ice, gel packs, or bottles with frozen liquid) should be used to maintain the recommended temperature. Loose fillers do not provide reliable temperature insulation.

Vaccines should not be reconstituted until immediately before use. If it is not administered within the time interval recommended by the manufacturer, reconstituted vaccine should be discarded.[3] With the exception of OPV, live virus vaccines should not be refrozen after

Table 5–1. **RECOMMENDED STORAGE CONDITIONS FOR COMMONLY USED VACCINES***

VACCINE	RECOMMENDED TEMPERATURE	DURATION OF STABILITY†	NORMAL APPEARANCE
Diphtheria and tetanus toxoids and acellular pertussis vaccine, adsorbed (DTaP)	2–8°C. Do not freeze. As little as 24 hr at <2°C or >25°C may cause antigens to fall from suspension and be difficult to resuspend.	Not more than 18 mo from the time of issue from manufacturer's cold storage	Markedly turbid and whitish suspension. If product contains clumps of material that cannot be resuspended with vigorous shaking, it should *not* be used.
Diphtheria and tetanus toxoids and whole-cell pertussis vaccine, adsorbed (DTP)	2–8°C. Do not freeze. As little as 24 hr at <2°C or >25°C may cause antigens to fall from suspension and be difficult to resuspend.	Not more than 18 mo from the time of issue from manufacturer's cold storage	Markedly turbid and whitish suspension. If product contains clumps of material that cannot be resuspended with vigorous shaking, it should *not* be used.
Diphtheria and tetanus toxoids, whole-cell pertussis vaccine adsorbed, and *Haemophilus* b conjugate vaccine (DTP-HbOC)	2–8°C. Do not freeze. As little as 24 hr at <2°C or >25°C may cause antigens to fall from suspension and be difficult to resuspend.	Not more than 18 mo from the time of issue from manufacturer's cold storage	Markedly turbid, white suspension. If product contains clumps of material that cannot be resuspended with vigorous shaking, it should *not* be used.
Diphtheria toxoid, adsorbed	2–8°C. Do not freeze.	Not more than 2 yr from the time of issue from manufacturer's cold storage	Turbid and white, slightly gray, or slightly pink suspension
Haemophilus b conjugate vaccine: HbOC (diphtheria CRM197 protein conjugate)	2–8°C. Do not freeze.	Not more than 2 yr from date of issue from manufacturer's cold storage	Clear, colorless liquid
Haemophilus b conjugate vaccine: PRP-D (diphtheria toxoid conjugate)	2–8°C. Do not freeze.	Not more than 2 yr from date of issue from manufacturer's cold storage	Clear, colorless liquid
Haemophilus b conjugate vaccine: PRP-OMP (meningococcal protein conjugate)	Lyophilized formulation: 2–8°C. Do not freeze formulation or diluent.	Not more than 2 yr from date of issue from manufacturer's cold storage	
	Reconstituted formulation: 2–8°C. Do not freeze.	Discard reconstituted vials if not used within 24 hr	Reconstituted: after agitation, slightly opaque, white suspension
Haemophilus b conjugate vaccine: PRP-T (tetanus toxoid conjugate)	Lyophilized formulation: 2–8°C. Do not freeze formulation or diluent. May be reconstituted with DTP produced by Connaught Laboratories.	Not more than 2 yr from date of issue from manufacturer's cold storage	
	Reconstituted formulation: 2–8°C. Do not freeze.	Vaccine should be used immediately when reconstituted	Reconstituted: clear and colorless
Hepatitis A vaccine, inactivated	2–8°C. Do not freeze. Do not use if product has been frozen.	2 yr, if kept refrigerated	Opaque, white suspension
Hepatitis B virus vaccine, inactivated (recombinant)	2–8°C. Storage outside this temperature range may reduce potency. Freezing substantially reduces potency.	2 yr from date of issue from manufacturer's cold storage	After thorough agitation, a slightly opaque, white suspension
Influenza virus vaccine (subvirion)	2–8°C. Freezing destroys potency.	Vaccine is recommended only during the year for which it is manufactured; antigenic composition differs annually	Clear, colorless liquid

Measles-mumps-rubella virus (MMR) vaccine, live	Lyophilized formulation: 2–8°C, but may be frozen. Protect from light, which may inactivate virus. Diluent: store at room temperature or refrigerated, do not freeze. Reconstituted formulation: 2–8°C. Protect from light, which may inactivate virus.	Discard reconstituted vials if not used within 8 hr	Reconstituted: clean, yellow solution
Measles virus vaccine, live	See MMR	See MMR	See MMR
Mumps virus vaccine, live	See MMR	See MMR	See MMR
Rubella virus vaccine, live	See MMR	See MMR	See MMR
Pneumococcal vaccine, polyvalent	2–8°C. Freezing destroys potency.	See expiration date on vial	Clear, colorless, or slightly opalescent liquid
Poliovirus vaccine, inactivated (IPV)	2–8°C. Do not freeze.	Not more than 1 yr from date of issue from manufacturer's cold storage	Clear, colorless suspension. Vaccine that contains particulate matter, develops turbidity, or changes in color should *not* be used.
Poliovirus vaccine, live, oral (OPV)	Must be stored at <0°C. Because of sorbitol in the vaccine, it will remain fluid at temperatures above −14°C. Refreezing the thawed product is acceptable (maximum of 10 thaw-freeze cycles), if the temperature never exceeds 8°C, and the cumulative thawing time is <24 hr.	Not more than 1 yr from date of issue from manufacturer's cold storage	Clear solution, usually red or pink, from the phenol red (pH indicator) it contains; may have a yellow color if shipment was packed with dry ice. Color changes that occur during storage or thawing are unimportant, provided the solution remains clear.
Tetanus and diphtheria toxoids, adsorbed (DT and Td)	2–8°C. Do not freeze.	Not more than 2 yr from the time of issue from manufacturer's cold storage	Markedly turbid and white suspension. If product contains clumps of material that cannot be resuspended with vigorous shaking, it should *not* be used.
Varicella virus vaccine‡	Lyophilized formulation: keep frozen, at temperature of −15°C or colder. Protect from light.	Lyophilized formulation: 18 mo	Lyophilized formulation: whitish powder
	Diluent: store at room temperature or refrigerated. Reconstituted formulation: use immediately; do not store.	Discard reconstituted vials if not used within 30 min	Reconstituted formulation: clear, colorless to pale yellow liquid
	For temporary storage, unreconstituted vaccine may be stored at 2–8°C for a maximum of 72 hr.	Discard if not used within 72 hr (do not refreeze)	

*For recently licensed combination vaccines, see package inserts; instructions may be different from those for products listed in the table. Also, any changes in the formulation of currently available immunizing agents may alter their appearance, stability, and storage requirements.

†Questions regarding the stability of biologicals subjected to potentially harmful environmental conditions should be addressed to the manufacturer of the product in question.

‡For questions concerning stability, contact the manufacturer by calling 1-800-9-VARIVAX.

From American Academy of Pediatrics. Active immunization. In Peter G (ed). 1997 Red Book: Report of the Committee on Infectious Diseases (24th ed). Elk Grove Village, IL, American Academy of Pediatrics, 1997, pp 4–36.

thawing (see Table 5–1). Certain vaccines (e.g., MMR and varicella) must also be protected from light to prevent inactivation of the vaccine virus.

ADMINISTRATION OF VACCINES

Complete and accurate records documenting the administration of all vaccines should be maintained by both healthcare providers who administer vaccines and vaccine recipients (or their parents). For each immunization, the following information should be recorded: (1) date of vaccination; (2) product administered, manufacturer, lot number, and expiration date; (3) site and route of administration; and (4) name, address, and title of healthcare provider administering the vaccine.

Infection Control and Sterile Injection Technique

Infection resulting from administration of vaccines is unlikely if appropriate precautions are used. Hand washing before and after injecting vaccines is indicated to reduce the risk of bacterial contamination and transmission of infection between recipients and healthcare personnel. In general, the use of protective gloves is not necessary when administering vaccines unless the healthcare worker will have contact with potentially infectious body fluids or has open lesions on the hands.[2, 7]

Failure to follow relevant infection control guidelines can result in the transmission of bloodborne pathogens or bacterial infection and abscess formation. Contamination of an injection site can occur from bacteria on the skin at the site of injection. To prevent such contamination, the skin at the injection site should be prepared with isopropyl alcohol (70%) or another disinfecting agent and allowed to dry before injection.[8] Transmission of pathogens can also occur if needles, syringes, vaccines, or other equipment used to administer vaccines becomes contaminated.

To prevent such contamination, syringes and needles must be sterile. A separate needle and syringe should be used for each injection. Disposable needles and syringes should be discarded after a single use in a labeled, puncture-proof container to prevent inadvertent needle stick injury or reuse. Because recapping and removing a used needle from a syringe can result in injury to the user, needles should not be recapped after use.[2] The needle and syringe should be discarded as a single unit without removing the needle from the syringe. Single-use disposable needles and syringes should not be sterilized and reused.

If only reusable (i.e., nondisposable) needles and syringes are available, they must be thoroughly cleaned and sterilized after each injection to prevent transmission of bloodborne or other pathogens between patients. Reusable syringes are usually glass rather than plastic. Because of its inert characteristics, glass can be cleaned and sterilized more easily than plastic. Because hypodermic needles enter deep tissues, great care must be taken to ensure that all contaminant is removed from the needle and syringe.[8, 9] Liquid germicides alone are insufficient for needle sterilization because of the restricted access of the chemical agent to the narrow lumen of the needle.[9] Strict adherence to the recommended time and temperature for the sterilization procedure used must be observed.[8]

Route of Administration

One or more routes of administration (i.e., intramuscular, subcutaneous, intradermal, intranasal, or oral) are recommended for each vaccine and are listed both in the manufacturer's product label and in published recommendations of immunization advisory committees (Table 5–2).[2, 7] These routes are usually determined during prelicensure vaccine studies and are based on vaccine composition and immunogenicity. Vaccines should be administered in sites where they elicit the desired immune response and where the likelihood of local tissue, neural, or vascular injury is minimal.[2] To avoid unnecessary local and systemic adverse events and to ensure the appropriate immune response, persons administering vaccines should not deviate from the recommended route of administration in the product label unless specific data can be cited to justify an alternative route. A route of administration or anatomical site of injection different from that recommended can result in an inadequate immune response. For example, the immunogenicity of hepatitis B vaccine and rabies vaccine is substantially lower when the gluteal instead of the deltoid vaccination site is used.[10, 11] The reduced immunogenicity is presumably due to inadvertent injection into subcutaneous or deep fatty tissue rather than muscle.[12, 13]

Deep intramuscular injection is generally recommended for adjuvant-containing vaccines because subcutaneous or intradermal administration can cause marked local irritation, induration, skin discoloration, inflammation, and granuloma formation.[2, 7] However, subcutaneous injection can lessen the risk of local neurovascular injury and is recommended for vaccines, such as live virus vaccines, that are nonreactogenic and highly immunogenic when administered by this route. Intradermal administration is preferred for live bacille Calmette-Guérin (BCG) vaccine and is sometimes used for certain rabies and typhoid vaccines.[14–16]

Care should be taken to ensure that vaccines are not injected into a blood vessel. Accordingly, the needle should be inserted into the recommended site and the plunger should be pulled back before the vaccine is injected. If blood appears in the needle hub, the needle should be withdrawn and the injection made at another site. This procedure should be repeated until no blood appears in the needle hub, at which point the vaccine can be administered.

Subcutaneous Injections

Vaccines are usually administered into the thigh of infants and the deltoid region of older children and adults. A ⅝- to ¾-inch, 23- to 25-gauge needle is recommended in most situations.[2, 7] The needle is inserted into the tissues below the dermal layer of the skin. To avoid administering the vaccine into a muscle, the skin

Table 5–2. **LICENSED VACCINES AND TOXOIDS AVAILABLE IN THE UNITED STATES, BY TYPE AND RECOMMENDED ROUTES OF ADMINISTRATION**

VACCINE	TYPE	ROUTE
Adenovirus*	Live virus	Oral
Anthrax†	Inactivated bacteria	Subcutaneous
BCG (bacille Calmette-Guérin)	Live bacteria	Percutaneous (intradermal)
Cholera	Inactivated bacteria	Subcutaneous; intramuscular; intradermal‡
Diphtheria-tetanus-pertussis (DTP)	Toxoids; inactivated whole bacteria	Intramuscular
Diphtheria–tetanus–acellular pertussis (DTaP)	Toxoids; inactivated bacterial components	Intramuscular
Hepatitis A	Inactivated virus	Intramuscular
Hepatitis B	Inactivated viral antigen	Intramuscular
Haemophilus influenzae type b conjugate (Hib)	Bacterial polysaccharide conjugated to protein	Intramuscular
Hib-DTP	Bacterial polysaccharide conjugated to protein; toxoids; inactivated whole bacteria	Intramuscular
Hib-DTaP	Bacterial polysaccharide conjugated to protein; toxoids; inactivated bacterial components	Intramuscular
Hib–hepatitis B	Bacterial polysaccharide conjugated to protein; inactivated viral antigen	Intramuscular
Influenza	Inactivated whole virus or viral components	Intramuscular
Japanese encephalitis	Inactivated virus	Subcutaneous
Measles	Live virus	Subcutaneous
Measles-mumps-rubella (MMR)	Live virus	Subcutaneous
Meningococcal	Bacterial polysaccharide (serotypes A/C/Y/W-135)	Subcutaneous
Mumps	Live virus	Subcutaneous
Pertussis†	Inactivated whole bacteria	Intramuscular
Plague	Inactivated bacteria	Intramuscular
Pneumococcal	Bacterial polysaccharide (23 serotypes)	Intramuscular; subcutaneous
Poliovirus, inactivated (IPV)	Inactivated virus	Subcutaneous
Poliovirus, oral (OPV)	Live virus	Oral
Rabies	Inactivated virus	Intramuscular; intradermal§
Rubella	Live virus	Subcutaneous
Tetanus	Toxoid (inactivated toxin)	Intramuscular
Tetanus-diphtheria (Td or DT)‖	Toxoids (inactivated toxins)	Intramuscular
Typhoid		
Live oral/Ty21a	Live bacteria	Oral
Vi polysaccharide	Capsular polysaccharide	Intramuscular
Heat-phenol–inactivated	Inactivated whole bacteria	Subcutaneous¶
Varicella	Live virus	Subcutaneous
Yellow fever	Live virus	Subcutaneous

*Available only to the U.S. Armed Forces.
†Distributed by Michigan Biological Products Institute, Michigan Department of Public Health.
‡The intradermal dose is lower than the subcutaneous dose.
§The intradermal dose of rabies vaccine, human diploid cell (HDCV), is lower than the intramuscular dose and is used only for preexposure vaccination. Rabies vaccine, adsorbed, should not be used intradermally.
‖Td, tetanus and diphtheria toxoids for use in persons 7 years of age and older; DT, tetanus and diphtheria toxoids for use in children younger than 7 years.
¶Booster doses may be administered intradermally.

and subcutaneous tissue can be held gently between the thumb and fingers to raise it above the muscle layer. The needle is inserted into the resulting skinfold at about a 45-degree angle.[2]

Intramuscular Injections

Injection Site. Selection of the site of injection and needle size is based on the volume of vaccine to be administered, the thickness of the overlying subcutaneous tissue, the size of the muscle, and the desired depth below the muscle surface into which the material is to be injected. For most intramuscular injections, the quadriceps muscle mass in the anterolateral aspect of the upper thigh and the deltoid muscle of the upper arm are the preferred vaccination sites.[2, 7]

The quadriceps muscle mass in the anterolateral thigh is most commonly used for intramuscular injection in infants, whereas the upper arm is the usual recommended site for older children and adults.[12] After a child begins to walk, the upper arm is the preferred site.[12, 17] By this age, the child's deltoid muscle is usually large enough to be used for intramuscular injection. Although the anterolateral thigh is also an acceptable site, intramuscular injection into the thigh of 18-month-old children has been reported to cause transient limping.[12, 18, 19]

Because of the potential risk of injury to the sciatic nerve, the gluteal region is usually not recommended for routine vaccination.[2, 7, 20] This recommendation is primarily based on reported cases of sciatic nerve injury resulting from injection of antibiotics or antiserum into the buttocks.[12, 21–26] No reports of direct nerve injury resulting from gluteal injection of current childhood vaccines have been published.[27–29]

Because reports of sciatic nerve injury from intramuscular injection have involved administration of substances other than vaccines, some physicians continue to advocate the use of the gluteal region for routine vaccination.[30–32] When injections are given in the gluteal site, care must be taken to avoid nerve injury. The central region of the buttocks should be avoided. The needle should be inserted well into the upper, outer quadrant and directed anteriorly (i.e., not caudally or perpendicular to the skin surface). The ventrogluteal site (i.e., the center of the triangle bounded by the anterior superior iliac spine, the tubercle of the iliac crest, and the upper border of the greater trochanter of the femur) can also be used and is free of major neurovascular structures.[12] Because of the large volume that must be injected and the large muscle mass, the gluteal site is often used for passive immunization with immune globulin preparations.[7, 20]

Needle Size. A 22- to 25-gauge needle is appropriate for the intramuscular administration of most vaccines. The ideal needle length may depend on the vaccination technique.[33] The technique recommended for intramuscular injections in the United States consists of gently bunching the muscle in the free hand while the needle is inserted to help minimize injury to nearby neurovascular structures and bone.[7, 33] However, the technique recommended by the World Health Organization (WHO) when using the anterolateral thigh consists of using the thumb and index finger to stretch the skin flat over the injection site while inserting the needle and injecting the vaccine.[33, 34]

The subcutaneous tissue and muscle layer thickness of the anterolateral thigh and deltoid region has been determined by ultrasonography.[33, 35, 36] On the basis of the resulting data, a ⅝-inch (16-mm) needle used according to the WHO technique is estimated to be adequate for intramuscular injection in the thigh of infants and toddlers and in the deltoid of toddlers.[33] However, using the technique recommended in the United States, a ⅞- to 1-inch (22- to 25-mm) needle would be necessary for adequate intramuscular penetration of the thigh of a 4-month-old infant and the thigh and deltoid of toddlers and older children.[2, 7, 33, 35]

For adolescents and adults, the ideal needle length for intramuscular injection depends on the weight and sex of the vaccinee. Poland and colleagues[36] reported that women have a greater deltoid fat pad thickness by ultrasonography and a greater deltoid skinfold thickness than men of an equal body mass index. These authors recommend a 1-inch (25-mm) needle for men for all weight ranges studied (i.e., 59 to 118 kg); for women, a ⅝-inch (16-mm) needle is indicated for those weighing less than 60 kg, a 1-inch (25-mm) needle is sufficient for those weighing 60 to 90 kg, and a 1½ inch (38-mm) needle is recommended for those weighing more than 90 kg.

Bleeding Disorders. Persons with bleeding disorders such as hemophilia can be at increased risk for bleeding after intramuscular injection. When hepatitis B or other vaccines recommended for intramuscular injection are indicated, vaccination can be scheduled shortly after administration of clotting factor replacement or similar therapy.[7] A 23-gauge or smaller needle can be used, and firm pressure without rubbing should be applied to the injection site for several minutes.[37] Alternatively, vaccines recommended for intramuscular injection might be administered subcutaneously to persons with a bleeding diathesis if the immune response and clinical reaction to these vaccines are generally expected to be comparable by either route of injection.[2, 7] An example is Hib (PRP-T) conjugate vaccine.[38–40]

Intradermal Injections

The deltoid region of the upper arm or the volar surface of the forearm is used for most intradermal injections.[2, 7, 20, 41] A ⅜- to ¾-inch, 25- to 27-gauge needle is recommended.[2, 7] The needle is inserted into the epidermis at an angle parallel to the long axis of the forearm. Care should be taken that the needle is inserted such that the entire bevel penetrates the skin and the injected solution raises a small bleb, thus demonstrating intradermal rather than subcutaneous injection of the vaccine. Because the amount of injected antigen is small, inadvertent subcutaneous injection may result in a suboptimal immunological response.[2, 7, 20] BCG vaccine is usually administered near the middle of the upper arm, over the insertion of the deltoid muscle.[41a]

Oral Administration

For vaccines given orally, the vaccine must be swallowed and retained. If a patient spits out, fails to swallow, or regurgitates a vaccine immediately after administration, the dose should be repeated.[2, 7, 42] Vomiting within 10 minutes is also a reason to readminister the dose of vaccine. If a second dose of the vaccine also is not retained, the dose should be readministered at a later date.[2, 7, 42]

Jet Injectors

Multiple-use nozzle jet injectors use the same nozzle tip to administer vaccine to multiple individuals. They have been used most frequently during mass vaccination campaigns and by the military to vaccinate large numbers of persons in a short time interval.[43–46]

These jet injectors have generally been considered safe and effective when they are used correctly by trained personnel. However, because the multiple-use nozzle of these jet injectors can become contaminated with blood or other infectious agents during use, the potential for patient-to-patient transmission of bloodborne pathogens exists and is a cause for serious concern.[47–53] The multiple-use nozzle jet injector that has been most widely used in the United States (Ped-O-Jet, Keystone Industries, Cherry Hill, NJ) has not been implicated in such transmission of bloodborne pathogens.[7, 44, 45, 54, 55] However, an outbreak of hepatitis B attributed to noncompliant use of another multiple-use nozzle jet injector (Med-E-Jet, Med-E-Jet Corporation, Cleveland, OH) has been reported.[56, 57]

The potential risk of disease transmission associated with multiple-use nozzle jet injectors would be greatest when vaccinating groups or populations in which the prevalence of hepatitis B virus, human immunodeficiency virus (HIV), or other bloodborne pathogens is expected to be high because of behavioral or other risk factors.[58–60] Brito and coworkers[60] estimated the theoretical risk of patient-to-patient transmission of hepatitis B virus from use of a contaminated jet injector to be as high as 1 per 388 to 1 per 3367 injections in a population with a high seroprevalence of hepatitis B virus infection.

The potential risk of disease transmission can be minimized by effective training of healthcare workers on the proper care and use of jet injectors and by changing the injector tip or removing the jet injector from use until the nozzle is properly sterilized if contamination with blood or other body fluid is evident.[7] Swabbing the injector nozzle tip with alcohol or acetone between injections is recommended to reduce the risk of bloodborne disease transmission.[7, 61] However, results from one in vitro study of transmission of hepatitis B surface antigen (HBsAg) suggest that mechanical cleaning of a contaminated jet injector tip with a cotton ball moistened with acetone may reduce but not eliminate the potential risk of bloodborne disease transmission.[57]

Despite the potential risks, multiple-use nozzle jet injectors may be helpful for the rapid vaccination of large numbers of persons with the same vaccine when the use of needles and syringes is not practical. Public health authorities must assess whether the public health benefit from using a jet injector outweighs any potential risk of bloodborne disease transmission.[7] For example, because of the risks, the WHO no longer encourages the use of these jet injectors for mass vaccination campaigns.[62] To minimize vaccination-associated injury and disease, persons using jet injectors should be well trained in their use and maintenance. The manufacturer's guidelines for the use and maintenance of these devices should be strictly followed. Those with practical experience in the use of jet injectors, such as military recruit training centers, public health departments, and international organizations, can often advise on the use of these injectors in mass vaccination programs.

Unlike multiple-use nozzle jet injectors, recently developed jet injectors employ a single-use disposable nozzle.[62, 63, 63a] These needle-less jet injectors reduce the potential risk of bloodborne disease transmission both from vaccinee to vaccinee and from vaccinee to the person administering vaccine and thus are considered safer than either multiple-use nozzle jet injectors or needles with syringes.

ALLEVIATION OF PAIN AND DISCOMFORT ASSOCIATED WITH VACCINATION

Several methods have been reported to reduce the pain and discomfort associated with vaccination injection, but they have not been widely tested.[63a] Pretreatment with topical lidocaine-prilocaine emulsion 5% (Emla cream, Astra Pharmaceutical Products, Inc., Westborough, MA) can decrease the pain of diphtheria-tetanus-pertussis vaccination among infants by causing superficial anesthesia.[64] This cream is not licensed in the United States for use in infants younger than 1 month (i.e., neonates) or in infants younger than 12 months who are receiving treatment with methemoglobin-inducing agents because of a lack of safety data in neonates and concern about possible development of methemoglobinemia.[64, 64a, 65] Acetaminophen has been used in children to reduce the discomfort and fever associated with vaccination.[66] However, acetaminophen can cause formation of methemoglobin and, thus, may interact with lidocaine-prilocaine cream if it is used concurrently.[64] Use of a topical refrigerant spray can reduce the short-term pain associated with injections and may be as effective as lidocaine-prilocaine cream.[67–69] Oral administration of sweet-tasting fluid just before injection may cause a calming or analgesic effect in some infants.[70] Distraction techniques such as listening to music or "blowing away pain" may also help children cope with the discomfort associated with vaccination.[71, 72]

The Z-track method of injection may also decrease the pain associated with intramuscular injection. Traction is applied to the skin and subcutaneous tissues prior to insertion of the needle and is released after injection. The injection track superficial to the muscle is thus displaced in relation to the track within the muscle, thereby preventing leakage of the vaccine from the muscle into the overlying tissues.

AGES FOR ADMINISTRATION OF IMMUNOBIOLOGICALS

Recommendations for the age and timing of vaccination are based on multiple factors, and childhood immunization schedules in various countries differ. Factors include the epidemiology and age-specific risks of contracting the naturally occurring disease, the age-specific risks of complications from the naturally occurring disease, the age-specific immunogenicity of the vaccine, the duration of immunity, and the schedule of recommended health visits. Ideally, a vaccine is recommended for the youngest age group at risk for the disease that is capable of an immunological response to the vaccine. These principles are exemplified by the following examples.

The optimal timing for administration of measles vaccine depends on both the rate of disappearance of passively acquired maternal antibody and the risk of exposure to measles virus. At birth and in the first 6 months of life, most infants have passive immunity to measles because of transplacentally acquired maternal measles antibodies. These antibodies interfere with the immune response to live virus measles vaccine by limiting vaccine virus replication. In many developing countries, where measles is highly endemic and frequently affects infants, routine measles vaccination is recommended at age 9 months.[2, 73] However, in the United States, where measles is less common and usually does not occur in infants, measles vaccine is routinely recommended at age 12 to 15 months.[2]

Another example is the recommended age of pertussis vaccination. Early infancy is the time of greatest risk of serious complications from naturally occurring pertussis, but infants who are younger than 1 month do not respond as well immunologically to pertussis vaccine as older infants do.[74–80] Initiation of routine immunization with pertussis vaccine is recommended at age 2 months.[81] This scheduling represents a compromise between factors affecting the immune response and the epidemiology of the disease necessitating early protection against pertussis.[79, 82, 83]

Vaccines[1] are listed under the routinely recommended ages. **Bars** *indicate range of acceptable ages for immunization. Catch-up immunization should be done during any visit when feasible. Shaded* **ovals** *indicate vaccines to be assessed and given if necessary during the early adolescent visit.*

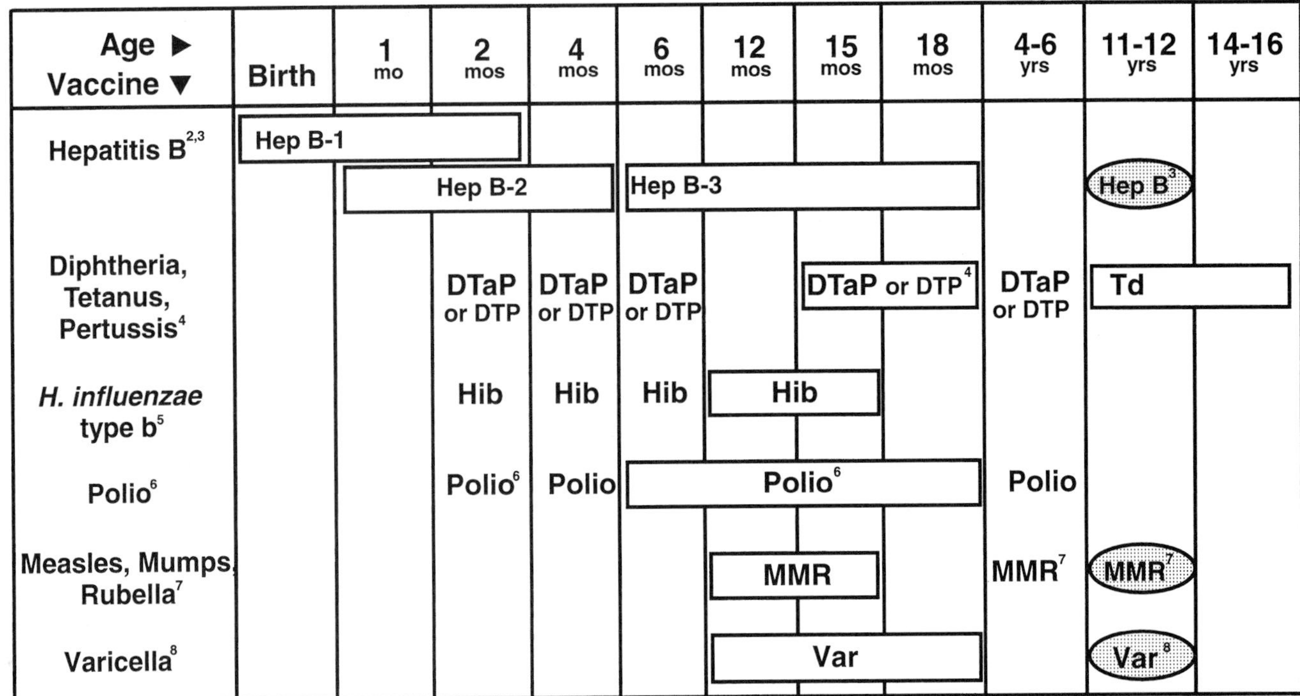

Age ▶ / Vaccine ▼	Birth	1 mo	2 mos	4 mos	6 mos	12 mos	15 mos	18 mos	4-6 yrs	11-12 yrs	14-16 yrs
Hepatitis B[2,3]	Hep B-1										
		Hep B-2			Hep B-3					Hep B[3]	
Diphtheria, Tetanus, Pertussis[4]			DTaP or DTP	DTaP or DTP	DTaP or DTP		DTaP or DTP[4]		DTaP or DTP	Td	
H. influenzae type b[5]			Hib	Hib	Hib	Hib					
Polio[6]			Polio[6]	Polio	Polio[6]				Polio		
Measles, Mumps, Rubella[7]						MMR			MMR[7]	MMR[7]	
Varicella[8]						Var				Var[8]	

Approved by the Advisory Committee on Immunization Practices (ACIP), the American Academy of Pediatrics (AAP), and the American Academy of Family Physicians (AAFP).

[1] This schedule indicates the recommended age for routine administration of currently licensed childhood vaccines. Combination vaccines may be used whenever any components of the combination is indicated and its other components are not contraindicated. Providers should consult the manufacturers' package inserts for detailed recommendations.

[2] ***Infants born to HBsAg-negative mothers*** should receive 2.5 μg of Merck vaccine (Recombivax HB®) or 10 μg of SmithKline Beecham (SB) vaccine (Engerix-B®). The 2nd dose should be administered at least 1 mo after the 1st dose. The 3rd dose should be given at least 2 mos after the second, but not before 6 mos of age.
Infants born to HBsAg-positive mothers should receive 0.5 mL hepatitis B immune globulin (HBIG) within 12 hrs of birth, and either 5 μg of Merck vaccine (Recombivax HB®) or 10 μg of SB vaccine (Engerix-B®) at a separate site. The 2nd dose is recommended at 1-2 mos of age and the 3rd dose at 6 mos of age.
Infants born to mothers whose HBsAg status is unknown should receive either 5 μg of Merck vaccine (Recombivax HB®) or 10 μg of SB vaccine (Engerix-B®) within 12 hrs of birth. The 2nd dose of vaccine is recommended at 1 to 2 mo of age and the 3rd dose at 6 mos of age. Blood should be drawn at the time of delivery to determine the mother's' HBsAg status; if it is positive, the infant should receive HBIG as soon as possible (no later than 1 wk of age). The dosage and timing of subsequent vaccine doses should be based upon the mother's HBsAg status.

[3] Children and adolescents who have not been vaccinated against hepatitis B in infancy may begin the series during any visit. Those who have not previously received 3 doses of hepatitis B vaccine should initiate or complete the series during the 11-12 year-old visit, and unvaccinated older adolescents should be vaccinated whenever possible. The 2nd dose should be administered at least 1 mo after the 1st dose, and the 3rd dose should be administered at least 4 mos after the 1st dose and at least 2 mos after the 2nd dose.

[4] DTaP (diphtheria and tetanus toxoids and acellular pertussis vaccine) is the preferred vaccine for all doses in the vaccination series, including completion of the series in children who have received 1 or more doses of whole-cell DTP vaccine. Whole-cell DTP is an acceptable alternative to DTaP. The 4th dose (DTP or DTaP) may be administered as early as 12 mos of age, provided 6 mos have elapsed since the 3rd dose and if the child is unlikely to return at age 15-18 mos. Td (tetanus and diphtheria toxoids) is recommended at 11-12 years of age if at least 5 years have elapsed since the last dose of DTP, DTaP or DT. Subsequent routine Td boosters are recommended every 10 years.

[5] Three *H. influenzae* type b (Hib) conjugate vaccines are licensed for infant use. If PRP-OMP (PedvaxHIB® [Merck]) is administered at 2 and 4 mos of age, a dose at 6 mos is not required.

[6] Two poliovirus vaccines are currently licensed in the US: inactivated poliovirus vaccine (IPV) and oral poliovirus vaccine (OPV). The following schedules are all acceptable to the ACIP, the AAP, and the AAFP. Parents and providers may choose among these options.

1) 2 doses of IPV followed by 2 doses of OPV.
2) 4 doses of IPV.
3) 4 doses of OPV.

The ACIP recommends 2 doses of IPV at 2 and 4 mos of age followed by 2 doses of OPV at 12-18 mos and 4-6 years of age. IPV is the only poliovirus vaccine recommended for immunocompromised persons and their household contacts.

[7] The 2nd dose of MMR is recommended routinely at 4-6 yrs of age but may be administered during any visit, provided at least 1 mo has elapsed since receipt of the 1st dose and that both doses are administered beginning at or after 12 mos of age. Those who have not previously received the second dose should complete the schedule no later than the 11-12 year visit.

[8] Susceptible children may receive Varicella vaccine (Var) at any visit after the first birthday, and those who lack a reliable history of chickenpox should be immunized during the 11-12 year-old visit. Susceptible children 13 years of age or older should receive 2 doses, at least 1 month apart.

Figure 5–1. Recommended childhood immunization schedule, United States, January–December 1998.

Vaccination too early in life may also affect the immune response to subsequent doses of vaccine. For example, neonatal administration of diphtheria and tetanus toxoids may result in the suppression of antibody responses to subsequent doses of Hib conjugate vaccines.[84] When children who receive measles vaccine before the age of 1 year are revaccinated, they develop vaccine-induced immunity against disease but may have a somewhat diminished antibody response compared with children vaccinated initially after their first birthday.[85]

Current immunization schedules in the United States are given in Figure 5–1 and Table 5–3.[2, 86] The minimum ages for initial administration of childhood vaccines and minimum acceptable intervals between doses in the United States are listed in Table 5–4. Other immunization schedules are discussed in Chapters 42 to 44.

SPACING OF VACCINE DOSES

Nonsimultaneous Administration of the Same Vaccine

Although administration of one dose of some vaccines usually induces a protective antibody response, many other vaccines require the administration of multiple doses in a primary series for development of immunity. Examples of the former are rubella, yellow fever, and pneumococcal vaccines; examples of the latter are poliovirus, hepatitis B, and pertussis vaccines. In addition, periodic revaccination with certain vaccines may be necessary to maintain immunity. Examples are yellow fever and pertussis vaccines and tetanus and diphtheria toxoids. Table 5–4 lists recommended minimum intervals between doses of the same vaccine.

Because of immunological memory, longer than routinely recommended intervals between doses do not impair the immunological response to live and killed vaccines that require more than one dose to achieve primary immunity.[2, 7] Similarly, delayed administration of recommended booster doses does not adversely affect the antibody response to such doses.[2, 7] Thus, the interruption of a recommended primary series or an extended lapse between booster doses does not necessitate reinitiation of the entire vaccination series.[2, 7] For example, lengthening the interval between two doses of inactivated poliovirus vaccine (IPV) may actually increase the antibody response to the second dose.[87–89] In the case of oral

Table 5–3. **RECOMMENDED IMMUNIZATION SCHEDULES FOR CHILDREN NOT IMMUNIZED IN THE FIRST YEAR OF LIFE***

RECOMMENDED TIME/AGE	IMMUNIZATION†‡	COMMENTS
	Younger than 7 Years	
First visit	DTaP (or DTP), Hib, HBV, MMR, OPV¶	If indicated, tuberculin testing may be done at the same visit. If child is 5 yr of age or older, Hib is not indicated in most circumstances.
Interval after first visit		
1 mo (4 wk)	DTaP (or DTP), HBV, Var**	The second dose of OPV may be given if accelerated poliomyelitis vaccination is necessary, such as for travelers to areas where polio is endemic.
2 mo	DTaP (or DTP), Hib, OPV¶	Second dose of Hib is indicated only if the first dose was received when younger than 15 mo.
≥8 mo	DTaP (or DTP), HBV, OPV¶	OPV and HBV are not given if the third doses were given earlier.
Age 4–6 yr (at or before school entry)	DTaP (or DTP), OPV,¶ MMR††	DTaP (or DTP) is not necessary if the fourth dose was given after the fourth birthday; OPV is not necessary if the third dose was given after the fourth birthday.
Age 11–12 yr	See Figure 5–1	
	7–12 Years	
First visit	HBV, MMR, Td, OPV¶	
Interval after first visit		
2 mo (8 wk)	HBV, MMR,†† Var,** Td, OPV¶	OPV may also be given 1 mo after the first visit if accelerated poliomyelitis vaccination is necessary.
8–14 mo	HBV,‡‡ Td, OPV¶	OPV is not given if the third dose was given earlier.
Age 11–12 yr	See Figure 5–1	

*The table is not completely consistent with all package inserts. For products used, also consult manufacturer's package insert for instructions on storage, handling, dosage, and administration. Biologicals prepared by different manufacturers may vary, and package inserts of the same manufacturer may change from time to time. Therefore, the physician should be aware of the contents of the current package insert.

†If all needed vaccines cannot be administered simultaneously, priority should be given to protecting the child against those diseases that pose the greatest immediate risk. In the United States, these diseases for children younger than 2 years are usually measles and *Haemophilus influenzae* type b infection; for children older than 7 years, they are measles, mumps, and rubella. Before 13 years of age, immunity against hepatitis B and varicella should be ensured.

‡DTaP, HBV, Hib, MMR, and Var can be given simultaneously at separate sites if failure of the patient to return for future immunizations is a concern.

¶IPV is also acceptable. However, for infants and children starting vaccination late (i.e., after 6 months of age), OPV is preferred to complete an accelerated schedule with a minimum number of injections.

**Varicella vaccine can be administered to susceptible children any time after 12 months of age. Unvaccinated children who lack a reliable history of chickenpox should be vaccinated before their 13th birthday.

††Minimal interval between doses of MMR is 1 month (4 weeks).

‡‡HBV may be given earlier in a 0-, 2-, and 4-month schedule.

HBV, hepatitis B virus vaccine; Var, varicella vaccine; DTP, diphtheria and tetanus toxoids and pertussis vaccine; DTaP, diphtheria and tetanus toxoids and acellular pertussis vaccine; Hib, *Haemophilus influenzae* type b conjugate vaccine; OPV, oral poliovirus vaccine; IPV, inactivated poliovirus vaccine; MMR, live measles-mumps-rubella vaccine; Td, adult tetanus toxoid (full dose) and diphtheria toxoid (reduced dose), for children 7 years of age and older and adults.

Adapted from American Academy of Pediatrics. Active immunization. In Peter G (ed). 1997 Red Book: Report of the Committee on Infectious Diseases (24th ed). Elk Grove Village, IL, American Academy of Pediatrics, 1997, p 20.

Table 5–4. **MINIMUM AGE FOR INITIAL VACCINATION AND MINIMUM INTERVAL BETWEEN VACCINE DOSES, BY TYPE OF VACCINE**

VACCINE	MINIMUM AGE FOR FIRST DOSE*	MINIMUM INTERVAL FROM DOSE 1 TO 2*	MINIMUM INTERVAL FROM DOSE 2 TO 3*	MINIMUM INTERVAL FROM DOSE 3 TO 4*
DTaP/DTP (DT)†	6 wk	4 wk	4 wk	6 mo
Hib (primary series)				
HbOC	6 wk	4 wk	4 wk	‡
PRP-T	6 wk	4 wk	4 wk	‡
PRP-OMP	6 wk	4 wk	‡	
Hib-DTP combination	6 wk	4 wk	4 wk	6 mo
Hepatitis B	Birth	4 wk	8 wk§	
Poliovirus				
IPV/OPV sequential	6 wk	4 wk	4 wk	4 wk
OPV only	6 wk	4 wk	4 wk	¶
IPV only	6 wk	4 wk	8 wk‖	¶
Measles-mumps-rubella	12 mo**	4 wk		
Varicella	12 mo	4 wk††		

*These minimum acceptable ages and intervals may not correspond with the *optimal* ages and intervals for vaccination recommended by the Advisory Committee on Immunization Practices, the American Academy of Pediatrics, and the vaccine manufacturer. Four weeks is considered to be 28 days.

†The total number of doses of diphtheria and tetanus toxoids should not exceed six each before the seventh birthday. Children who have received all four primary vaccination doses before their fourth birthday should receive a fifth dose at 4 to 6 years of age (i.e., before entering kindergarten or elementary school) *and* at least 6 months after the fourth dose.

‡The booster dose of Hib vaccine, which is recommended after the primary vaccination series, should be administered no earlier than 12 months of age *and* at least 2 months after the previous dose of Hib vaccine.

§This final dose is recommended at least 4 months after the first dose and no earlier than 6 months of age.

¶If the third dose is administered on or after the fourth birthday, the fourth dose is not required.

‖The preferred interval between the second and third doses of IPV is at least 6 months. If accelerated protection is needed because of increased risk of exposure to poliovirus (e.g., due to international travel), the interval between the second and third dose of IPV can be 4 weeks.

**Although the age for measles vaccination may be as young as 6 months in outbreak areas, where cases are occurring in children who are younger than 1 year, children initially vaccinated before the first birthday should be revaccinated at 12 to 15 months of age, and an additional dose of vaccine should be administered at the time of school entry or according to local policy. Doses of measles-mumps-rubella vaccine or other measles-containing vaccines should be separated by at least 4 weeks.

††Two doses of varicella vaccine are recommended only for people 13 years and older.

DT, diphtheria and tetanus toxoids vaccine; HbOC, *H. influenzae* oligosaccharide conjugate; PRP-T, polyribosylribitol phosphate–tetanus toxoid vaccine; PRP-OMP, polyribosylribitol phosphate outer membrane protein conjugate.

typhoid (Ty21a) vaccine, an exception has been proposed. Specifically, if the primary vaccination series is interrupted for longer than 3 weeks, the primary series should be started again (see Chapter 33).

Administration of doses of a vaccine at shorter intervals than recommended may result in a reduced immune response with diminished vaccine efficacy and should be avoided[2, 7] (see Table 5–4). Multiple doses of some live vaccines are recommended to stimulate an immune response to different types of the same virus, such as poliovirus types 1, 2, and 3, or to induce immunity in persons who failed to mount an immune response to an earlier dose of vaccine, such as measles.[42, 90] These multiple doses constitute a primary vaccination series and are not "booster doses."

Guidelines for spacing the administration of different vaccines are given in Table 5–5. The theoretical possibility that two doses of the same or different live virus vaccines administered within too short an interval may inhibit the immunological response to the second dose is based on evidence from both animal and human studies.[91–94] Although the potential for immune interference is the reason for the recommendation that doses of live virus vaccines not administered at the same time should be separated by at least 4 weeks, the biological reason for such interference is not known. Petralli and colleagues[93, 94] reported that the immune response to smallpox vaccination was affected by prior administration of live attenuated measles vaccine, and interferon produced in response to the initial dose of live virus vaccine has been postulated to inhibit replication of vaccine virus in the subsequent vaccine dose. Such interference remains theoretical and has not been reported between doses of currently licensed live virus vaccines. In addition, multiple studies have demonstrated that previous or intercurrent viral illness in a vaccinee does not appear to interfere with the immune response to live virus vaccines.[95–100] Such interference might be expected on the basis of the findings of Petralli and colleagues.[93, 94] These inconsistencies suggest that the question of interference between live virus vaccines should be re-examined.

Table 5–5. **GUIDELINES FOR SPACING THE ADMINISTRATION OF KILLED AND LIVE ANTIGENS**

ANTIGEN COMBINATION	RECOMMENDED MINIMUM INTERVAL BETWEEN DOSES
≥2 Killed antigens	None; may be given simultaneously or at any interval between doses
Killed and live antigens	None; may be given simultaneously or at any interval between doses (*exception: cholera and yellow fever vaccines**)
≥2 Live antigens	4 wk, if not administered simultaneously (*exception: oral poliovirus vaccine can be administered at any time before, with, or after measles-mumps-rubella and oral typhoid vaccines*)

*If time permits, cholera and yellow fever vaccines should not be administered simultaneously with each other; at least 3 weeks should elapse between administration of these vaccines. If these two vaccines must be administered simultaneously or within 3 weeks of each other, the antibody response may not be optimal.

Too frequent administration of some killed vaccines such as tetanus toxoid can result in increased rates of reactions in some vaccinees.[2, 101–103] Such reactions probably result from the formation of circulating antigen-antibody complexes.[2, 104–107]

Simultaneous Administration of Different Vaccines

Simultaneous administration of all indicated vaccines is an essential component of childhood vaccination programs.[2, 7] Simultaneous administration of different vaccines is also particularly important when return of the recipient for further vaccination is questioned, when imminent exposure to several vaccine-preventable diseases is expected, or when preparing for international travel on short notice. Unless specifically licensed for injection in the same syringe, different vaccines administered simultaneously should be injected separately and at different anatomical sites. If both upper and lower limbs must be used for simultaneous administration of different vaccines, the anterolateral thigh is often chosen for intramuscular injections and the deltoid region for subcutaneous injections. If more than one injection must be administered in a single limb, the thigh is usually preferred because of its large muscle mass. The distance separating two injections in the same limb should be sufficient (e.g., 1 to 2 inches) to minimize the chance of overlapping local reactions.[17, 18] In general, different vaccines, including live virus products, can be administered simultaneously without reducing their safety and effectiveness[108] (see Table 5–5). Studies of cortisol levels and behavioral responses of infants to vaccination indicate that responses are similar in infants who receive two inoculations during one visit and infants who receive a single inoculation, suggesting that a second injection does not increase stress.[109, 110]

Whereas simultaneous administration of vaccines associated with frequent local or systemic reactions could result in accentuation of these reactions, increased severity or incidence of adverse reactions has not been observed after simultaneous administration of the most widely used vaccines.[7] Similarly, simultaneous administration of vaccines does not generally cause immunological interference.[108] An exception is concurrent administration of yellow fever and cholera vaccines.[111, 112]

Nonsimultaneous Administration of Different Vaccines

With the exception of two live virus vaccines administered within an interval of 4 weeks of each other, vaccines can generally be administered at any time before or after a different vaccine[2, 7] (see Table 5–5). As previously noted, the immune response to a live virus vaccine theoretically might be impaired if it is administered nonsimultaneously within 4 weeks after another live virus vaccine.[93, 94] Whereas interference has not been observed for currently available live virus vaccines in the United States, to minimize the theoretical possibility of interference, live virus vaccines not administered at the same time should generally be separated by at least 4 weeks.[2, 7] However, OPV and MMR vaccines can be administered at any interval before or after each other.

INTERFERENCE BY IMMUNE GLOBULINS

Passively acquired antibodies can interfere with the immune response to certain vaccines, both live and inactivated, and toxoids. The result can be either the absence of seroconversion or a blunting of the immune response with lower final antibody concentrations in the vaccinee. Passively acquired antibody, however, does not affect the immune response to all vaccines.

Interference with Live Vaccines

To elicit an adequate immune response, live vaccine virus must replicate within the recipient. The probable mechanism by which passively acquired immune globulin blunts the immune response to live virus vaccines is by neutralization of vaccine virus resulting in inhibition of viral replication and insufficient antigenic mass.[113] For example, persisting transplacentally acquired maternal measles antibodies inhibit the response to live measles vaccine in infants for as long as 12 months and perhaps longer.[114–116] The age to which inhibition persists has been correlated with concentrations of maternal or cord blood antibodies.[117–119] Rubella vaccine virus may be less susceptible than measles vaccine virus to these transplacentally acquired maternal antibodies.[120]

Intramuscular or intravenous administration of immune globulin–containing preparations (e.g., serum immune globulin, hyperimmune globulins, intravenous immune globulin, and blood) before or simultaneous with certain vaccines can also affect the immune response to live virus vaccines. When partially attenuated Edmonston B measles vaccine, which is no longer used in the United States, was administered concurrently with measles immune globulin in an effort to reduce the incidence of adverse events associated with this vaccine, the rate of seroconversion was not affected but the geometric mean titer of serum measles antibody was diminished.[121–123] In one study, children who received an investigational bacterial polysaccharide immune globulin (BPIG) intramuscularly had a reduced immune response to live measles vaccine for as long as 5 months after receipt of BPIG.[124] The measles antibody seroconversion rate and geometric mean titer were lower among the children who received BPIG compared with those who received placebo. Blunting of the immune response to live rubella vaccine also occurred after receipt of BPIG but was less marked and of shorter duration.[124]

Although passively acquired antibodies can interfere with the response to rubella vaccine, the low doses of anti-Rh(D) globulin administered to postpartum women have not been demonstrated to inhibit the immune response to RA27/3 strain rubella vaccine.[125] Parenterally administered immune globulin preparations also do not appear to adversely affect the immune response to yellow fever vaccine.[126] Although high concentrations of passively acquired antibodies may reduce the serum antibody response to live poliovirus vaccine, they have little effect on the replication of vaccine virus and development of gastrointestinal tract immunity.[79, 126–128] Data are insufficient to determine the extent to which passively acquired antibodies interfere with the immune response to other live viral or bacterial vaccines, such as varicella, mumps, and typhoid (Ty21a strain).[129]

Interference with Inactivated (Killed) Vaccines

Interference with current inactivated and component vaccines is less marked than with live vaccines and requires exposure to large doses of passively acquired antibodies.[79, 128, 130, 131] The mechanism by which passively acquired antibodies interfere with the immunological response of inactivated and toxoid vaccines is not clear. Moderate doses of parenterally administered immune globulins have not inhibited the development of a protective immune response to diphtheria and tetanus toxoids and pertussis vaccine (DTP), tetanus toxoid, hepatitis B vaccines, Hib conjugate vaccines, and rabies vaccines.[131–133] For example, although the concurrent administration of inactivated hepatitis A vaccine and immune globulin can result in lower serum antibody concentrations than if vaccine alone is administered, seroconversion rates have not been diminished.[2, 134–136] In another study, infants with high concentrations of passively acquired maternal antibody to hepatitis A virus had seroconversion rates similar to those of vaccinated infants without maternal antibodies but lower serum antibody concentrations after receipt of hepatitis A vaccine.[137] Further studies are under way to determine if these findings are of clinical significance.

The manufacturer of respiratory syncytial virus immune globulin, intravenous (RSV-IGIV) has suggested that an additional dose of certain inactivated vaccines (i.e., diphtheria, tetanus, and acellular pertussis vaccine [DTaP]; DTP; Hib; and OPV) may be necessary to ensure a protective immune response from these vaccines in recipients of RSV-IGIV (RespiGam package insert). However, currently available data are inconclusive and do not support a recommendation for additional doses of these vaccines.[138]

Recommendations for Spacing Administration of Vaccines and Immune Globulins

Interference of immune globulins with the immune response to vaccines is dose related and, therefore, more likely to occur and to persist for a longer period after receipt of larger doses of immune globulins.[124, 139] The recommended interval between administration of immune globulin preparations and vaccines is based on the following considerations: (1) whether evidence suggests interference between immune globulin and the vaccine; (2) the dose of the immune globulin administered; and (3) the expected half-life of immunoglobulin G. Recommended intervals between administration of immune globulin preparations and various live and killed vaccines are listed in Tables 5–6 and 5–7.

Table 5–6. **GUIDELINES FOR SPACING THE ADMINISTRATION OF IMMUNE GLOBULIN PREPARATIONS* AND VACCINES**

SIMULTANEOUS ADMINISTRATION

Immunobiological Combination	Recommended Minimum Interval Between Doses
Immune globulin and killed antigen	None; may be administered simultaneously at different sites or at any time between doses
Immune globulin and live antigen	Should generally not be administered simultaneously (*exception: oral poliovirus vaccine, yellow fever vaccine, and oral typhoid [Ty21a] vaccine can be administered at any time before, after, or simultaneous with an immune globulin preparation*) If simultaneous administration of measles-mumps-rubella vaccine or its component vaccines or varicella vaccine in unavoidable, administer at different sites and test for seroconversion or revaccinate after the recommended interval.†

NONSIMULTANEOUS ADMINISTRATION

Immunobiological Administered: *First*	*Second*	Recommended Minimum Interval Between Administration of Immune Globulin Preparations and Vaccine Antigens: *Interval*	*Antigen*
Immune globulin	Killed antigen	None	
Killed antigen	Immune globulin	None	
Immune globulin	Live antigen	None	Oral poliovirus, yellow fever, oral typhoid (Ty21a)
		3 mo	Rubella, mumps
		5 mo	Varicella
		Dose related†	Measles
Live antigen	Immune globulin	2 wk	Measles, rubella, mumps
		3 wk	Varicella

*Blood products containing large amounts of immune globulin (e.g., serum immune globulin, specific immune globulins, immune globulin [intravenous], whole blood, packed red blood cells, plasma, or platelet products).

†Rubella and mumps vaccines, 3 months; varicella vaccine, 5 months; measles-containing vaccines, dose related. See Table 5–7.

Table 5–7. **SUGGESTED INTERVALS BETWEEN ADMINISTRATION OF IMMUNE GLOBULIN PREPARATIONS FOR VARIOUS INDICATIONS AND VACCINES CONTAINING LIVE MEASLES VIRUS***

INDICATIONS	DOSE (mg IgG/kg)	TIME INTERVAL (mo) BEFORE MEASLES VACCINATION
Tetanus prophylaxis (TIG)	250 units (10 mg IgG/kg) IM	3
Hepatitis A prophylaxis (IG)		
Contact prophylaxis	0.02 mL/kg (3.3 mg IgG/kg) IM	3
International travel	0.06 mL/kg (10 mg IgG/kg) IM	3
Hepatitis B prophylaxis (HBIG)	0.06 mL/kg (10 mg IgG/kg) IM	3
Rabies prophylaxis (HRIG)	20 IU/kg (22 mg IgG/kg) IM	4
Varicella prophylaxis (VZIG)	125 units/10 kg (20–40 mg IgG/kg) IM (maximum, 625 units)	5
Measles prophylaxis (IG)		
Standard (i.e., nonimmunocompromised contact)	0.25 mL/kg (40 mg IgG/kg) IM	5
Immunocompromised contact	0.50 mL/kg (80 mg IgG/kg) IM	6
Blood transfusion		
RBCs, washed	10 mL/kg (negligible IgG/kg) IV	0
RBCs, adenine-saline added	10 mL/kg (10 mg IgG/kg) IV	3
Packed RBCs (Hct 65%)†	10 mL/kg (60 mg IgG/kg) IV	6
Whole blood (Hct 35–50%)†	10 mL/kg (80–100 mg IgG/kg) IV	6
Plasma/platelet products	10 mL/kg (160 mg IgG/kg) IV	7
Replacement therapy for immune deficiencies	300–400 mg/kg IV‡ (as IGIV)	8
Respiratory syncytial virus prophylaxis	750 mg/kg IV (as RSV-IGIV)	9
Treatment of		
Immune thrombocytopenic purpura	400 mg/kg IV (as IGIV)	8
	1000 mg/kg IV (as IGIV)	10
Kawasaki disease	2 g/kg IV (as IGIV)	11

*This table is not intended for determining the correct indications and dosage for the use of immune globulin preparations. Unvaccinated persons may not be fully protected against measles during the entire suggested time interval, and additional doses of immune globulin or measles vaccine may be indicated after measles exposure. The concentration of measles antibody in a particular immune globulin preparation can vary by lot. The rate of antibody clearance after receipt of an immune globulin preparation can also vary. The recommended time intervals are extrapolated from an estimated half-life of 30 days for passively acquired antibody and an observed interference with the immune response to measles vaccine for 5 months after a dose of 80 mg IgG/kg.

†Assumes a serum IgG concentration of 16 mg/mL.

‡Measles vaccination is recommended for human immunodeficiency virus–infected children who do not have evidence of severe immunosuppression, but it is contraindicated for patients who have congenital disorders of the immune system.

HBIG, hepatitis B immune globulin; Hct, hematocrit; HRIG, human rabies immune globulin; IG, serum immune globulin; IGIV, immune globulin, intravenous; IM, intramuscularly; IV, intravenously; RBCs, red blood cells; RSV-IGIV, respiratory syncytial virus immune globulin, intravenous; TIG, tetanus immune globulin; VZIG, varicella-zoster immune globulin.

In the United States, killed (i.e., inactivated) vaccines may be administered simultaneously with or at any time before or after receipt of an immune globulin preparation.[2, 7, 20] The vaccine and immune globulin preparation should be administered at different sites, and the standard recommended doses of the corresponding vaccines should be used.[2, 7] Supplementary doses are not indicated.

Recommendations for administration of live virus vaccines vary on the basis of the aforementioned considerations. After receipt of an immune globulin preparation or other blood product, measles vaccine should be deferred during the intervals listed in Table 5–7.[128, 140] Immune globulin preparations also contain rubella, mumps, and varicella antibodies. Because high doses of passively acquired antibodies can inhibit the immune response to live rubella vaccine for as long as 3 months, administration of rubella vaccine should be postponed for at least 3 months after receipt of an immune globulin preparation or blood product.[7, 124, 141] Although the effect of immune globulin preparations on the response to live mumps and live varicella vaccines has not been defined, postponement of administration of mumps and varicella vaccines for 3 months and 5 months, respectively, after receipt of an immune globulin preparation is recommended because of possible interference.[7, 142–144]

Immune globulin preparations administered too soon after vaccination with MMR or varicella vaccines can interfere with the immune response. Therefore, according to current guidelines, if administration of an immune globulin preparation becomes necessary less than 2 weeks after receipt of MMR or its component vaccines or less than 3 weeks after receipt of varicella vaccine, readministration of the vaccine is recommended after the appropriate interval listed in Tables 5–6 and 5–7, unless serological testing indicates that a protective antibody response already occurred.[7, 140, 144] For example, if an immune globulin preparation is administered less than 3 weeks after receipt of varicella vaccine, vaccine should be readministered at least 5 months after the immune globulin preparation unless serological testing indicates an adequate immune response to the initial dose of varicella vaccine.

Because the immune response to OPV and yellow fever vaccines is not adversely affected by immune globulin preparations, these vaccines can be administered at any time in relation to the receipt of immune globulin preparations.[126] Live oral typhoid (Ty21a) vaccine is also recommended for administration at any time in relation to receipt of immune globulin preparations.[7, 15]

INTERCHANGEABILITY OF VACCINES OF DIFFERENT MANUFACTURERS

Combination and monovalent vaccines against the same diseases with similar antigens and produced by the same manufacturer are considered interchangeable in most situations.[2, 7] However, supporting data on the safety, immunogenicity, and efficacy of using comparable vaccines from different manufacturers for different doses of a vaccination series are frequently limited or unavailable. When the same vaccine cannot be used to complete an immunization series, similar vaccines produced by different manufacturers or produced by the same manufacturer in different countries have generally been considered acceptable to complete the immunization series as long as each vaccine is used as licensed and recommended.[2, 7]

Some diseases have serological correlates of immunity that can be used to evaluate vaccine interchangeability. For example, in studies in which one or more doses of hepatitis B vaccine produced by one manufacturer were followed by doses from another manufacturer, the immune response was comparable to that resulting from use of a single vaccine type.[145, 146] Whereas Hib conjugate vaccines differ in antigen composition, interchangeability of different products has been validated on the basis of the accepted serological correlate of immunity against *H. influenzae* type b invasive disease.[147–149]

Determination of vaccine interchangeability is more difficult for diseases without serological correlates of immunity. For example, in the absence of such a correlate for *Bordetella pertussis* infection, the interchangeability of acellular pertussis vaccines is difficult to assess. Thus, when feasible, acellular pertussis vaccine from the same manufacturer is preferred for the entire primary vaccination series.[2, 150] However, if this regimen is not feasible, any of the licensed products can be used to continue or complete the series.[2, 150]

HYPERSENSITIVITY TO VACCINE COMPONENTS

Types of Reactions

Hypersensitivity reactions after vaccination can be local or systemic. They can vary in severity from mild discomfort at the site of vaccination to severe anaphylaxis. Onset can be either immediate or delayed. Serious reactions are rare. Whether a specific hypersensitivity reaction is caused by a vaccine component or an unrelated environmental allergen can be difficult to determine. However, symptoms occurring immediately after vaccination that are suggestive of an anaphylactic reaction contraindicate further administration of that vaccine to the recipient.[2, 7]

Urticaria and anaphylactic reactions have been reported after the administration of DTP, diphtheria and tetanus toxoids (DT, Td), and tetanus toxoid.[151–154] Whereas immunoglobulin E–type antibodies to tetanus and diphtheria antigens have been identified in some patients with these symptoms, transient urticarial rashes are not a contraindication to subsequent vaccination, because they are unlikely to be anaphylactic unless they appear within minutes after vaccination.[2, 154–156] A serum sickness–type reaction caused by circulating complexes of vaccine antigen and previously acquired antibody is the likely cause of these reactions, and subsequent vaccination is unlikely to result in the necessary ratio of antigen to antibody concentration to form immune complexes.[154, 157]

Tetanus toxoid is contraindicated in persons who experienced an immediate anaphylactic reaction to tetanus toxoid–containing vaccine, unless the person can be desensitized to the toxoid.[2] Because of the importance of tetanus immunization and the uncertainty about which vaccine component might be the cause of the reaction, the patient may be referred to an allergist for evaluation and possible desensitization.[154, 158–161] On occasion, a history of a prior allergic reaction to tetanus vaccine may refer to a reaction to tetanus antiserum of equine origin that was used for tetanus prophylaxis before human-derived tetanus immune globulin became available in the 1960s. Thus, before use of tetanus toxoid is discontinued because of an alleged episode of anaphylaxis, skin testing and possible desensitization should be considered.[158, 159]

Local or systemic reactions, such as redness and soreness at the vaccination site and fever, have been associated with receipt of DTP, plague, cholera, and inactivated whole-cell typhoid vaccines.[107, 162–166] Such reactions are usually caused by a toxin in the vaccine rather than by hypersensitivity to a specific component.[7]

With some vaccines, such as Japanese encephalitis, immediate or delayed onset of generalized urticaria and angioedema that can progress to respiratory distress and hypotension has been reported after vaccination.[167–169] The pathogenesis of these reactions is not known.

Vaccine Components Causing Hypersensitivity

Proteins

Egg protein is a constituent of vaccines prepared with use of embryonated chicken eggs. Examples include influenza, yellow fever, measles, and mumps vaccines. On rare occasions, these vaccines can induce anaphylaxis or other immediate hypersensitivity reactions, and these reactions are sometimes attributed to egg protein antigen.[2, 5, 90, 170–175] As a result, some of these vaccines are contraindicated in persons with a history of anaphylactic reactions to egg ingestion unless desensitization has been successfully completed.[2, 5, 170, 171, 173, 176] For example, persons needing yellow fever vaccine who have a history of systemic anaphylactic-like symptoms (e.g., generalized urticaria, wheezing, and hypotension) after egg ingestion can be skin tested with yellow fever vaccine before vaccination and desensitized.[2, 5, 170] Although available, skin testing and desensitization with influenza vaccine are often precluded by the risk of reactions, the need for yearly vaccination, and the availability of chemoprophylaxis against influenza A with amantadine or rimantadine.[2, 171, 176, 177]

Although measles and mumps vaccines are produced by use of chick embryo fibroblast cell culture, persons with hypersensitivity to eggs are at low risk for anaphylactic reactions to these vaccines, and skin testing with vaccine is not predictive of allergic reaction after immunization.[2, 178–180] Therefore, neither skin testing nor administration of gradually increasing doses of vaccine is required when these vaccines are administered to persons who are allergic to eggs.[2, 90, 140, 142]

Live virus vaccines, such as measles, mumps, rubella, yellow fever, and varicella, contain gelatin as a stabilizer. Persons with a history of allergy to gelatin have rarely experienced an anaphylactic reaction after vaccination with such a vaccine.[181–183] Skin testing of persons with a history of systemic anaphylactic-like symptoms after gelatin ingestion may be useful to identify those at risk for severe hypersensitivity reactions to vaccination, but no protocol for such testing or desensitization has been published. Because gelatin used as a vaccine stabilizer may be of porcine origin whereas ingested food gelatin may be of bovine origin, the absence of a history of allergy to gelatin-containing foods does not eliminate the possibility of a gelatin-mediated reaction to vaccine.

Approximately 6% of persons who receive a booster dose of human diploid rabies vaccine develop a serum sickness–type illness.[184, 185] This reaction is thought to be caused by sensitization to human albumin that has been altered chemically by a virus-inactivating agent used in the production of the vaccine.[2, 186]

Antibiotics

Live virus vaccines frequently contain trace amounts of one or more antibiotics such as neomycin, streptomycin, and polymyxin B. Vaccine contents are listed in the manufacturer's product label for each vaccine. The most common allergic response to neomycin is a delayed-type (cell-mediated) local contact dermatitis consisting of an erythematous, pruritic papule that occurs 48 to 96 hours after vaccine administration.[2, 7, 187] Such delayed-type reactions are not contraindications for vaccination.[2, 7, 187, 188] However, persons who have experienced an anaphylactic reaction to neomycin or to another antibiotic vaccine constituent should not receive vaccines containing that antibiotic.[2, 90, 189, 190] No vaccines currently licensed in the United States contain penicillin or penicillin derivatives.

Mercury Compounds

Mercury hypersensitivity may be rarely elicited after receipt of vaccines containing the preservative thimerosal.[191–193] Many vaccines produced in the United States, such as diphtheria, tetanus, pertussis, hepatitis B, influenza, and Japanese encephalitis, contain this preservative. However, most patients do not react adversely to thimerosal as a vaccine component even if patch or intradermal skin test responses are positive.[194] Furthermore, hypersensitivity to this compound usually consists of local delayed-type reactions, and mercury hypersensitivity is not a contraindication to vaccinations.[2, 7, 159, 195, 196]

Recommended Management of Acute Vaccine Reactions

Although it is extremely rare after immunization, the immediate onset and life-threatening nature of an anaphylactic reaction require that personnel and facilities providing vaccination be capable of providing initial care for suspected anaphylaxis. Epinephrine and equipment for maintaining an airway should be available for immediate use.

Anaphylaxis usually begins within several minutes of administration of vaccine. Rapid recognition and initiation of treatment are required to prevent possible progression to cardiovascular collapse. If flushing, facial edema, urticaria, itching, swelling of the mouth or throat, wheezing, difficulty breathing, or other signs of anaphylaxis occur, the patient should be placed in a recumbent position with the legs elevated. Aqueous epinephrine (1:1000) should be administered and may be repeated within 10 to 20 minutes.[197] A dose of diphenhydramine hydrochloride may shorten the reaction, but it will have little immediate effect. Maintenance of any airway and oxygen administration may be necessary. Arrangements should be made for immediate transfer to an emergency facility for further evaluation and treatment. All patients should be observed for at least 12 hours after the onset of symptoms.[197]

Postvaccination syncope, unrelated to anaphylactic hypersensitivity, can also occur. In a report of 697 cases of syncope after vaccination, six patients suffered skull fracture, cerebral bleeding, or cerebral contusion from falls.[198] In this same study, almost 90% of the cases of syncope occurred within 15 minutes or less of vaccination, and 98% of cases occurred within 30 minutes. Because of the small risk of an anaphylactic reaction and the unrelated risk of postvaccination syncope, the AAP recommends observation for 15 to 20 minutes after immunization whenever possible.[2]

VACCINATION OF PRETERM INFANTS

The immune response to vaccination is a function of postnatal age rather than of gestational age.[199–202] Transplacentally acquired maternal antibody is present at lower concentrations and, thus, persists for a shorter interval in preterm infants than in gestationally mature infants.[201, 203–205] Because they have less transplacentally acquired maternal antibody, inhibition of the immune response in premature infants may be less than in full-term infants.[201, 206]

DTP, OPV, IPV, and Hib vaccines are generally immunogenic and safe for preterm infants when vaccination is initiated at the same chronological age (i.e., approximately 2 months) and administered according to the same routine schedule as for full-term infants.[207–218] However, some studies also suggest that the immune response to certain vaccines may be impaired when vaccination of extremely premature infants or those of very low birth weight is initiated at the usual time.[212, 213, 219–223] For example, D'Angio and colleagues[212] reported that a similar proportion of extremely premature infants (i.e., less than 29 weeks' gestation and birth weight less than 1000 g) and full-term infants had protective antibody concentrations to tetanus toxoid, Hib, and poliovirus serotypes 1 and 2 after a vaccination series of three doses of DTP and Hib vaccines and two doses of poliovirus vaccine (i.e., IPV followed by OPV) initiated at a chronological age of 2 months. However, the preterm infants were less likely to have detectable antibody to poliovirus serotype 3. Protective antibody titers were still present when the children were retested at 3 to 4 years of age.[223a] The initial immune response to diphtheria and pertussis vaccines was not determined. Munoz and coworkers[222] also reported that after administration of Hib vaccine at 2 and 4 months' postnatal age, the geometric mean concentration of serum Hib antibody was significantly lower among infants with a gestational age less than 28 weeks than in other infants.

Lau and colleagues[221] reported that the seroconversion rate to hepatitis B vaccine was lower in preterm infants weighing less than 2000 g who were vaccinated soon after birth than in preterm infants vaccinated at a later age or term infants vaccinated shortly after birth. Other investigators have observed a diminished immune response to hepatitis B vaccine among premature infants of lower gestational ages (e.g., less than 33 weeks) or of lower birth weights (e.g., less than 2000 g).[217, 224–226] As a result, administration of the first dose of hepatitis B vaccine for preterm infants born to HBsAg-negative mothers is recommended just before hospital discharge, if the infant already weighs 2000 g, or at age 2 months when other childhood vaccines are recommended.[7, 227, 228]

Several studies suggest that the incidence of adverse events after vaccination of preterm infants is the same as or lower than that of full-term infants vaccinated at the same chronological age.[207, 208, 212, 213] A temporal association between receipt of DTP and Hib vaccine and a transient increase or recurrence of apnea in premature infants has been reported, although the significance of this finding is unclear.[229]

Infants who are born prematurely should be immunized at the same postnatal chronological age and according to the same recommended schedule as full-term infants are.[7, 227] The one exception, as previously discussed, is hepatitis B vaccine. The recommended standard dose of each vaccine should be administered; divided or reduced doses are not indicated.[7, 227, 230–232] A preterm infant who is still hospitalized at age 2 months can receive the vaccines routinely scheduled at that age. However, because poliovirus vaccine strains are excreted after receipt of OPV, IPV instead of OPV should be administered to hospitalized infants to prevent the risk of poliovirus transmission in the hospital.[7, 227]

BREAST-FEEDING AND IMMUNIZATION

Neither killed nor live vaccines given to a mother or infant who is breast-feeding have adverse consequences.[2, 7] Because killed and inactivated vaccines do not multiply within the body, they pose no special risk for lactating mothers or their infants. Lactating mothers may also safely receive live vaccines, such as yellow fever, MMR, OPV, varicella, and rubella, without interruption of their breast-feeding schedule.[7, 90, 144, 227] Although live vaccines contain attenuated live viruses or bacteria that replicate within the vaccine recipient, most live vaccine strains are not known to be secreted in breast milk. An exception is attenuated rubella vaccine virus, which has been detected in breast milk and recovered from the nasopharynx and throat of some breast-fed infants after maternal immunization.[233–235] In one study, transient seroconversion to rubella virus without evidence of clinical disease was noted in 25% of the breast-fed infants.[233]

Breast-feeding of infants does not adversely affect their development of a protective immune response and is not a contraindication for any vaccine.[7, 144, 236–241] The antibody response to the components of DTP or Hib conjugate vaccines is not inhibited by breast-feeding.[79, 242–244] Vaccination of breast-fed infants results in protective immunity, although doses of OPV administered to these infants during the first 3 days of life may be somewhat less effective than doses administered to older breast-fed infants and infants who are not breast-fed.[79, 237, 238, 240, 245–254] Breast-fed infants who acquired rubella vaccine virus and rubella-specific antibodies from breast milk have a normal immune response to rubella vaccine administered at 15 to 18 months of age.[239]

Compared with infants who are formula fed, breast-fed infants may have an enhanced immune response to certain oral and parenteral vaccines such as conjugate Hib vaccine, OPV, and diphtheria and tetanus toxoids.[244, 255, 256] However, the significance of such an effect is unclear.

Oral rotavirus vaccine is a possible exception to the lack of inhibition by breast-feeding of the immune response to vaccines. Meta-analyses of studies using a single dose of rotavirus vaccines concluded that the immune response to these vaccines was reduced in breast-fed infants.[257, 258] However, the potential inhibitory effect is largely overcome by administration of three doses of vaccine, and no significant decrease in the protective efficacy of rotavirus vaccine is observed in breast-fed compared with non–breast-fed infants.[259, 260]

IMMUNIZATION AND PREGNANCY

Women usually should not receive vaccines during pregnancy unless specifically indicated. This recommendation is based on theoretical concern that a previously unrecognized teratogenic potential from the product administered may occur or that a birth defect unrelated to vaccine will be falsely attributed to the immunization. However, the benefits of vaccination to a pregnant woman in some circumstances outweigh any potential risks, such as if the risk of infection is high, if the infection can have serious consequences for the woman or her fetus, and if the vaccine is unlikely to be associated with an increased incidence of adverse events.[7, 236] Table 5–8 lists vaccines that are indicated and contraindicated during pregnancy.

Use of Live Vaccines

Live vaccines contain attenuated viruses or bacteria that multiply within the vaccine recipient. Because some of the diseases they prevent, such as rubella or varicella, are known to have teratogenic or other serious effects on the fetus, live virus vaccines are usually contraindicated during pregnancy.[7, 227, 236]

Based on a case of vaccine-like rubella virus transmission to a fetus conceived 7 weeks after rubella vaccination, women should be counseled to avoid becoming pregnant for 3 months after receipt of a rubella-containing vaccine.[90, 141, 260a, 260b] Pregnancy should be avoided for 1 month after the receipt of other non–rubella-containing parenteral live virus vaccines, by which time antibody production usually has occurred and vaccine-virus viremia is expected to have ceased.[90, 140, 142, 144] Other practices in dealing with women of childbearing age include asking if a woman is pregnant, not administering live virus vaccine if a woman states that she is pregnant, and explaining the potential risk for the fetus to the woman who states that she is not pregnant.[7, 90] Both OPV and yellow fever vaccine can be administered to pregnant women who are nonimmune and at substantial risk of imminent exposure to infection, such as from impending international travel.[5, 7, 42, 227]

Table 5–8. **VACCINATION DURING PREGNANCY**

VACCINE	TYPE	INDICATIONS FOR VACCINATION DURING PREGNANCY
Live Virus		
Measles-mumps-rubella	Live attenuated virus	Contraindicated
Poliomyelitis	Trivalent live attenuated virus (oral poliovirus vaccine)	Persons at substantial risk of exposure to polio
Varicella	Live attenuated virus	Contraindicated
Yellow fever	Live attenuated virus	Contraindicated, except if exposure to yellow fever virus is unavoidable
Live Bacterial		
Typhoid	Live attenuated bacteria (Ty21a)	Should reflect actual risks of disease and probable benefits of vaccine
Inactivated Virus		
Hepatitis A	Killed virus	Data on safety in pregnancy are not available; should weigh the theoretical risk of vaccination against the risk of disease
Hepatitis B	Recombinant produced, purified hepatitis B surface antigen	Pregnancy is not a contraindication
Influenza	Inactivated type A and type B virus vaccines	Recommended both for women who will be in the second or third trimester during influenza season and for patients with serious underlying disease; consult health authorities for current recommendations
Japanese encephalitis	Killed virus	Should reflect actual risks of disease and probable benefits of vaccine
Poliomyelitis	Killed virus (inactivated poliovirus vaccine)	Persons at substantial risk of exposure to polio
Rabies	Killed virus	Substantial risk of exposure
Inactivated Bacterial		
Cholera	Killed bacterial	Should reflect actual risks of disease and probable benefits of vaccine
Haemophilus influenzae type b conjugate	Polysaccharide-protein	Only for high-risk persons
Meningococcal	Polysaccharide	Only in unusual outbreak situations
Plague	Killed bacterial	Selective vaccination of exposed persons
Pneumococcal	Polysaccharide	Only for high-risk persons
Typhoid	Killed bacterial or polysaccharide	Should reflect actual risks of disease and probable benefits of exposure
Toxoids		
Tetanus-diphtheria	Combined tetanus-diphtheria toxoids, adult formulation (Td)	Lack of primary series, or no booster within last 10 yr (5 yr, if other than clean minor wounds)
Other		
Immune globulins, pooled or hyperimmune	Immune globulin or specific globulin preparations	Exposure or anticipated exposure to measles, hepatitis A, hepatitis B, rabies, tetanus

Despite precautions, some pregnant women may be inadvertently vaccinated with a live virus vaccine. Available data on these vaccines when they are administered to pregnant women have not demonstrated any serious risk to the mother or fetus.[261–269] Because of the existing safety data and because the risk to the fetus is largely theoretical, administration of a live vaccine during pregnancy is not a reason to consider interrupting the pregnancy.[90, 144] A Varicella Vaccination in Pregnancy Registry, like that which documented the apparent safety of inadvertent rubella vaccination during pregnancy, has been established to monitor prospectively maternal-fetal outcomes in pregnant women inadvertently vaccinated with varicella vaccine (telephone: 800-986-8999).[144, 227]

Use of Inactivated Vaccines

Killed and inactivated vaccines pose no special risk during pregnancy because they do not multiply within the body. Although one study reported an association between administration of IPV during pregnancy and malignant neoplasms of neural origin in offspring,[270] this finding has not been confirmed by other investigators, and IPV can be administered to a pregnant woman who requires immediate protection against poliomyelitis.[7, 42, 227] Other killed and inactivated vaccines and toxoids are not known to be deleterious when they are administered during pregnancy and are sometimes indicated to prevent infection with possible serious outcomes for both mother and fetus. For example, influenza vaccine has recently been recommended for women who will be in the second or third trimester of pregnancy during influenza season because influenza infection may cause increased morbidity in these women.[171, 271]

In some cases, vaccination during pregnancy is intended to protect the fetus or newborn infant from infection. For example, neonatal tetanus remains common in many developing countries where women are not adequately immunized before pregnancy and childbirth and protection of the newborn infant from neonatal tetanus is conferred by placental transfer of maternal antibody from the immune mother.[272, 273] Widespread vaccination of pregnant women in such areas has demonstrated the safety and efficacy of administering tetanus toxoid during pregnancy to prevent neonatal tetanus.[274] In the United States, administration of combined tetanus-diphtheria toxoid is recommended for pregnant women who have not completed a primary vaccination series or who need a booster dose.[7, 158, 236]

Some physicians prefer to wait until the second or third trimester of pregnancy to administer inactivated (killed) vaccines or toxoids.[236] However, no increased risk to the mother or fetus from vaccination during the first trimester has been proved, and vaccination in some cases may be indicated before the second or third trimester. Examples include influenza, hepatitis B, and tetanus-diphtheria vaccines.[7, 58, 171, 227, 236]

Vaccination of Household Contacts

Administration of both live and killed vaccines to household members does not present a known hazard to pregnant women who are not severely immunocompromised. Although transmission of varicella vaccine virus from a 12-month-old infant to his pregnant mother has been reported, no virus was detected in fetal tissue after an elective abortion.[275] Pregnancy of a mother is not a contraindication to administration of varicella vaccine to her child.[143, 144, 276] However, if a woman is known to be nonimmune to varicella-zoster virus, some physicians may prefer to defer administration of varicella vaccine to her children at least until her third trimester.[143] OPV is the only vaccine contraindicated for household contacts of severely immunocompromised pregnant women.[42, 227]

VACCINATION OF PEOPLE WITH A PERSONAL OR FAMILY HISTORY OF SEIZURES

Infants and young children with either a personal history of convulsions or a parent or sibling with a history of convulsions are at increased risk for a convulsion after receipt of whole-cell pertussis vaccine or MMR (or monovalent measles) vaccine.[277–279] In most cases, these convulsions are brief, self-limited, and associated with fever. Studies have not established a causal association between these convulsions and residual seizure disorders or permanent neurological sequelae.[280, 281] Because acellular pertussis vaccines are less frequently associated with fever than are whole-cell pertussis vaccines, DTaP vaccine is preferred for immunizing children in the United States against pertussis.[81, 150]

Because neurological disorders such as epilepsy or degenerative disorders marked by loss of developmental milestones often become manifest during infancy, DTP vaccination may coincide with onset or recognition of such disorders and cause confusion about the etiological role of pertussis vaccine. For infants with a personal history of a seizure, delaying pertussis vaccination is recommended until a progressive neurological disorder is excluded or the cause of the seizure has been established.[150, 227] Acetaminophen or ibuprofen can be administered at the time of pertussis vaccination and every 4 hours for 24 hours thereafter to reduce the possibility of postvaccination fever.[150] Because measles vaccine is administered at an age when a child's neurological status is likely to have been already established, deferring measles immunization of a child with a personal history of a seizure is not recommended.[90, 227]

Pertussis and measles vaccinations are not contraindicated in persons with a family history of convulsions. Even though children with a parent or sibling who has had a seizure are themselves at increased risk for a seizure, the benefits of administering pertussis and measles vaccine to children with a family history of convulsions substantially outweigh the small risks, because of the benign nature of these seizures.[90, 150, 227, 280, 281]

VACCINATION DURING ACUTE ILLNESS

The decision to administer or delay vaccination because of an intercurrent or recent illness depends on evaluation of the etiology of the disease and the severity of symptoms.[2, 7] Mild illness, either febrile (≥38°C) or afebrile, is not a contraindication to vaccination with live virus vaccines or inactivated (killed) vaccines.[2, 7] Although one study reported a lower rate of seroconversion to the measles but not to the rubella or mumps components of MMR vaccine in children with evidence of a recent or current upper respiratory infection compared with children without this history, a difference in seroconversion to measles vaccine in healthy children compared with those who are ill has not been found in other studies.[95, 97–100, 117, 282]

Acute minor illnesses, such as upper respiratory infection, diarrhea, and acute otitis media, are common during infancy and childhood.[283] Postponing vaccination in children with minor febrile or afebrile illness constitutes a missed opportunity to protect a child from disease, can contribute to outbreaks of vaccine-preventable disease, and can significantly impede efforts to immunize infants and young children on schedule.[284–288] Every opportunity should be used to provide indicated vaccines and to avoid missed vaccination opportunities in persons who may not return for medical care and administration of recommended vaccines.[2, 7, 289] The potential benefit of preventing disease by timely vaccination far outweighs any small possible risk of vaccine failure.[2]

Vaccination is usually deferred in persons who have moderate or severe illness. A person with signs or symptoms of moderate or severe illness at the scheduled time of vaccination should be requested to return as soon as the illness resolves so that vaccines can be administered at the recommended ages. Waiting until after a person has recovered from the acute phase of a moderate or severe illness avoids superimposing a reaction to vaccination on the underlying illness or mistakenly attributing a manifestation of the underlying illness to the vaccine.[2, 7]

ROUTINE CONTRAINDICATIONS AND PRECAUTIONS TO VACCINATION

Vaccine contraindications and precautions are described in the manufacturer's product labeling and in the recommendations on the use of vaccines developed by national advisory committees such as the ACIP and the Committee on Infectious Diseases of the AAP. In the United States, the content of the product label is regulated by the Food and Drug Administration on the basis of specific studies required of the manufacturer to prove the safety and efficacy of a specific product. Most recommendations of vaccine advisory committees are the same as those in the product label. However, differences sometimes exist because of advisory committees' assessments of the risks and benefits of a given recommendation, their goal to make immunization as practical as possible, and their responsibility to develop recommendations for the use of vaccines in circumstances in which specific safety and efficacy data may be limited but for which physicians, nurses, and public health officials need guidance. For example, the manufacturer's product label recommends that women vaccinated with live virus varicella vaccine avoid becoming pregnant for 3 months, whereas the ACIP and AAP advise waiting only 1 month.[1, 143, 144] Similarly, the AAP and ACIP advise that pregnancy should not be considered a contraindication to hepatitis B vaccination, whereas the manufacturer's product label states that hepatitis B vaccine should be administered to pregnant women only if it is clearly needed.[1, 290]

A contraindication indicates that a vaccine should not be administered. In contrast, a precaution specifies a situation in which vaccine may be indicated if, after careful assessment, the benefit of vaccination to the individual patient is judged to outweigh the risk.[7] Contraindications and precautions may be generic and apply to all vaccines, or they may be specific to one or more vaccines (Table 5–9). The following two guidelines apply to all vaccines: (1) an anaphylactic reaction to a vaccine or vaccine constituent contraindicates further use of that vaccine or vaccines containing that constituent (see *Hypersensitivity to Vaccine Components*), and (2) vaccination is generally contraindicated during moderate or severe acute illnesses regardless of the absence or presence of fever (see *Vaccination During Acute Illness*).

Immunosuppression resulting from underlying disease or therapy is a contraindication for receipt of most live vaccines.[90, 227] An exception is measles vaccine, which is recommended for HIV-infected persons who are not severely immunosuppressed.[90, 227, 291] Corticosteroid therapy can suppress the immune system of an otherwise healthy person, although the minimal dose and duration of therapy necessary to cause immunosuppression are not well defined. Underlying disease, concurrent therapies, and the frequency and route of administration of corticosteroids can also affect immunosuppression. Steroid therapy does not usually contraindicate administration of live virus vaccines when it consists of low to moderate doses administered daily or on alternate days; physiological maintenance doses; or doses administered topically, by aerosol, or by local (e.g., intra-articular) injection.[7, 90, 227] In most cases, persons receiving high doses of systemic corticosteroids (i.e., at least 2 mg per kg per day or 20 mg per day of prednisone or its equivalent) for less than 14 days can receive live virus vaccines immediately after discontinuation of therapy.[2, 7] However, live virus vaccines are not usually administered to persons who have received high doses of systemic corticosteroids for 14 days or more until at least 1 month after cessation of steroid therapy.[90, 227]

Most live virus vaccines are usually contraindicated for pregnant women because of a theoretical risk to the fetus (see *Immunization and Pregnancy*). However, the small theoretical risk from administration of a live vaccine to a pregnant woman is sometimes far outweighed by the risk of contracting a disease with serious consequences for mother and fetus.

Healthcare providers sometimes inappropriately consider a condition to be a contraindication or precaution to vaccination.[2, 7] Withholding vaccine in such instances results in a missed opportunity to administer needed vaccine. A concise summary of appropriate and inappropriate contraindications is given in Table 5–9, adapted from the national *Standards for Pediatric Immunization Practices* (see Chapter 42).

Table 5–9. GUIDE TO CONTRAINDICATIONS AND PRECAUTIONS TO VACCINATIONS*

TRUE CONTRAINDICATIONS AND PRECAUTIONS	NOT CONTRAINDICATIONS (VACCINES MAY BE ADMINISTERED)
General for All Vaccines (DTaP/DTP, OPV, IPV, MMR, Varicella, Hib, Hepatitis B)	
Contraindications Anaphylactic reaction to a vaccine contraindicates further doses of that vaccine Anaphylactic reaction to a vaccine constituent contraindicates the use of vaccines containing that substance Moderate or severe illnesses with or without a fever	*Not Contraindications* Mild to moderate local reaction (soreness, redness, swelling) after a dose of an injectable antigen Low-grade or moderate fever after a prior vaccine dose Mild acute illness with or without low-grade fever Current antimicrobial therapy Convalescent phase of illnesses Prematurity (same dosage and indications as for normal, full-term infants) Recent exposure to an infectious disease History of penicillin or other nonspecific allergies or fact that relatives have such allergies Pregnancy of mother or household contact Unvaccinated household contact
DTaP/DTP	
Contraindications Encephalopathy within 7 d of administration of previous dose of DTaP/DTP *Precautions*[1] Fever of ≥40.5°C (105°F) within 48 hr after vaccination with a prior dose of DTaP/DTP and not attributable to another identifiable cause Collapse or shock-like state (hypotonic-hyporesponsive episode) within 48 hr of receiving a prior dose of DTaP/DTP Convulsions within 3 d of receiving a prior dose of DTaP/DTP (see footnote 2 regarding management of children with a personal history of seizures at any time) Persistent, inconsolable crying lasting ≥3 hr, within 48 hr of receiving a prior dose of DTaP/DTP Guillain-Barré syndrome within 6 wk after a dose[3]	*Not Contraindications* Fever of <40.5°C (105°F) after a previous dose of DTaP/DTP Family history of convulsions[2] Family history of sudden infant death syndrome Family history of an adverse event after DTaP/DTP administration
OPV	
Contraindications Infection with HIV or a household contact with HIV infection Known immunodeficiency (hematological and solid tumors; congenital immunodeficiency; long-term immunosupprssive therapy) Immunodeficient household contact *Precaution*[1] Pregnancy	*Not Contraindications* Breast-feeding Current antimicrobial therapy Mild diarrhea
IPV	
Contraindication Anaphylactic reaction to neomycin, streptomycin, or polymyxin B *Precaution*[1] Pregnancy	
MMR	
Contraindications Anaphylactic reaction to neomycin or gelatin Pregnancy Known immunodeficiency (hematological and solid tumors; congenital immunodeficiency; long-term immunosuppressive therapy; HIV infection with evidence of severe immunosuppression) *Precautions*[1] Recent (within 3–11 mo, depending on product and dose) administration of a blood product or immune globulin preparation Thrombocytopenia[5] History of thrombocytopenic purpura[5]	*Not Contraindications* Tuberculosis or positive purified protein derivative test response Simultaneous tuberculin skin testing[4] Breast-feeding Pregnancy of mother or household contact of vaccine recipient Immunodeficient family member or household contact HIV infection without evidence of severe immunosuppression Allergic reaction to eggs[6] Nonanaphylactic reactions to neomycin
Hib	
Contraindications None *Precautions* None	

Table continued on opposite page

Table 5–9. **GUIDE TO CONTRAINDICATIONS AND PRECAUTIONS TO VACCINATIONS*** *(Continued)*

TRUE CONTRAINDICATIONS AND PRECAUTIONS	NOT CONTRAINDICATIONS (VACCINES MAY BE ADMINISTERED)
Hepatitis B	
Contraindication	*Not Contraindication*
Anaphylactic reaction to common baker's yeast	Pregnancy
Varicella	
Contraindications	*Not Contraindications*
Anaphylactic reaction to neomycin or gelatin	Immunodeficiency in a household contact
Pregnancy	HIV infection in a household contact
Infection with HIV	Pregnancy in the mother or other household contact of the recipient
Known immunodeficiency (hematological and solid tumors; congenital immunodeficiency; long-term immunosuppressive therapy)	
Precautions[1]	
Recent (within 5 mo) administration of an immune globulin preparation[7]	
Family history of immunodeficiency[8]	

*This information is based on the recommendations of the Advisory Committee on Immunization Practices (ACIP) and of the Committee on Infectious Diseases of the American Academy of Pediatrics (AAP). Sometimes these recommendations vary from those in the manufacturer's product label. For more detailed information, healthcare providers should consult the published recommendations of the ACIP, AAP, the American Academy of Family Physicians, and the manufacturer's product label. These guidelines have been adapted and updated from those published by the U.S. Public Health Service in January 1996.

[1]The events or conditions listed as precautions, although not contraindications, should be carefully reviewed. The benefits and risks of administering a specific vaccine to an individual under the circumstances should be considered. If the risks are believed to outweigh the benefits, the vaccine should be withheld; if the benefits are believed to outweigh the risks (e.g., during an outbreak or foreign travel), the vaccine should be administered. Whether and when to administer DTaP/DTP to children with proven or suspected underlying neurological disorders should be decided on an individual basis. Avoiding administration of certain vaccines to pregnant women is prudent on theoretical grounds. If immediate protection against poliomyelitis is needed, either OPV or IPV is recommended.

[2]Acetaminophen administered before DTaP or DTP vaccination and thereafter every 4 hours for 24 hours should be considered for children with a personal history or a family history of convulsions in siblings or parents.

[3]The decision to give additional doses of DTaP or DTP should be based on consideration of the benefit of further vaccination versus the risk of recurrence of Guillain-Barré syndrome. For example, completion of the primary vaccination series in children is justified.

[4]Measles vaccination may temporarily suppress tuberculin reactivity. MMR vaccine may be administered after, or on the same day as, tuberculin testing. If MMR has been given recently, postpone the tuberculin test until 4 to 6 weeks after administration of MMR. If administering MMR simultaneously with tuberculin skin test, use the Mantoux test and not multiple puncture tests, because the latter require confirmation if positive, which would have to be postponed 4 to 6 weeks.

[5]The decision to vaccinate should be based on consideration of the benefits of immunity to measles, mumps, and rubella versus the risk of recurrence or exacerbation of thrombocytopenia after vaccination, or from natural infections of measles or rubella. In most instances, the benefits of vaccination will be much greater than the potential risks and justify giving MMR, particularly in view of the even greater risk of thrombocytopenia after measles or rubella disease. However, if a prior episode of thrombocytopenia occurred in close temporal proximity to vaccination, it might be prudent to avoid a subsequent dose.

[6]Recent data suggest that most anaphylactic reactions to measles- and mumps-containing vaccines are associated with hypersensitivity not to egg antigens but to other components of the vaccines. Because the risk of anaphylactic reactions after administration of measles- or mumps-containing vaccines in persons who are allergic to eggs is extremely low and skin testing with vaccine is not predictive of allergic reactions to these vaccines, skin testing and desensitization are no longer required before administration of MMR vaccine to persons who are allergic to eggs.

[7]Varicella vaccine should not be administered for at least 5 months after administration of blood (except washed red blood cells) or plasma transfusions, immune globulin, or varicella-zoster immune globulin (VZIG). Immune globulin or VZIG should not be given for 3 weeks after vaccination unless the benefits exceed those of the vaccination. In such cases, the vaccinee should either be revaccinated 5 months later or tested for immunity 6 months later and revaccinated if seronegative.

[8]Varicella vaccine should not be administered to a member of a household with a family history of immunodeficiency until the immune status of the recipient and other children in the family is documented.

DTaP, diphtheria and tetanus toxoids and acellular pertussis vaccine; DTP, diphtheria and tetanus toxoids and whole-cell pertussis vaccine; Hib, *Haemophilus influenzae* type b vaccine; HIV, human immunodeficiency virus; IPV, inactivated poliovirus vaccine; MMR, measles-mumps-rubella virus vaccine; OPV, oral poliovirus vaccine.

REFERENCES

1. Physicians' Desk Reference. Montvale, NJ, Medical Economics Company, 1997.
2. American Academy of Pediatrics. Active immunization. In Peter G (ed). 1997 Redbook: Report of the Committee on Infectious Diseases (24th ed). Elk Grove Village, IL, American Academy of Pediatrics, 1997, pp 4–36.
3. Vaccine Management: Recommendations for Handling and Storage of Selected Biologicals. Atlanta, US Department of Health and Human Services, Public Health Service, Centers for Disease Control and Prevention, 1996.
4. Guidelines for Vaccine Packing and Shipping. Atlanta, US Department of Health and Human Services, Public Health Service, Centers for Disease Control and Prevention, 1997.
5. Centers for Disease Control. Yellow fever vaccine: Recommendations of the Immunization Practices Advisory Committee (ACIP). MMWR Morb Mortal Wkly Rep 39(RR-6):1–6, 1990.
6. Kendal AP, Synder R, Garrison PJ. Validation of cold chain procedures suitable for distribution of vaccines by public health programs in the USA. Vaccine 15:1459–1465, 1997.
7. Centers for Disease Control and Prevention. General recommendations on Immunization: Recommendations of the Advisory Committee on Immunization Practices (ACIP). MMWR Morb Mortal Wkly Rep 43(RR-1):1–38, 1994.
8. Fulginiti VA. Practical aspects of immunization practice. In Fulginiti VA (ed). Immunization in Clinical Practice. Philadelphia, JB Lippincott, 1982, pp 49–55.
9. Favero MS, Bond WW. Sterilization, disinfection, and antisepsis in the hospital. In Manual of Clinical Microbiology. Washington, DC, American Society for Microbiology, 1991, pp 183–200.
10. Shaw FE Jr, Guess HA, Roets JM, et al. Effect of anatomic injection site, age, and smoking on the immune response to hepatitis B vaccination. Vaccine 7:425–430, 1989.
11. Fishbein DB, Sawyer LA, Reid-Sanden FL, Weir EH. Administration of human diploid-cell rabies vaccine in the gluteal area [letter]. N Engl J Med 318:124–125, 1988.
12. Bergeson PS, Singer SA, Kaplan AM. Intramuscular injections in children. Pediatrics 70:944–948, 1982.
13. Lachman E. Applied anatomy of intragluteal injections. Am Surg 29:236–241, 1963.
14. Centers for Disease Control and Prevention. The role of BCG vaccine in the prevention and control of tuberculosis in the United States: A joint statement by the Advisory Council for the Elimination of Tuberculosis and the Advisory Committee on Immunization Practices. MMWR Morb Mortal Wkly Rep 45(RR-4):1–18, 1996.

15. Centers for Disease Control and Prevention. Typhoid immunization — recommendations of the Advisory Committee on Immunization Practices (ACIP). MMWR Morb Mortal Wkly Rep 43(RR-14):1–7, 1994.
16. Centers for Disease Control. Rabies prevention—United States, 1991: Recommendations of the Immunization Practices Advisory Committee (ACIP). MMWR Morb Mortal Wkly Rep 40(RR-3):1–19, 1991.
17. Scheifele D, Bjornson G, Barreto L, et al. Controlled trial of *Haemophilus influenzae* type B diphtheria toxoid conjugate combined with diphtheria, tetanus and pertussis vaccines, in 18-month-old children, including comparison of arm versus thigh injection. Vaccine 10:455–460, 1992.
18. Ipp MM, Gold R, Goldbach M, et al. Adverse reactions to diphtheria, tetanus, pertussis-polio vaccination at 18 months of age: Effect of injection site and needle length. Pediatrics 83:679–682, 1989.
19. Bergeson PS. Immunizations in the deltoid region [letter]. Pediatrics 85:134–135, 1990.
20. American College of Physicians Task Force on Adult Immunization and Infectious Diseases Society of America. General recommendations for adult immunization. In Guide for Adult Immunization (3rd ed). Philadelphia, American College of Physicians, 1994, pp 1–11.
21. Gilles FH, French JH. Postinjection sciatic nerve palsies in infants and children. J Pediatr 58:195–204, 1961.
22. Combes MA, Clark WK, Gregory CF, James JA. Sciatic nerve injury in infants. Recognition and prevention of impairment resulting from intragluteal injections. JAMA 173:1336–1339, 1960.
23. Curtiss PH, Tucker HJ. Sciatic palsy in premature infants: A report and follow-up study of ten cases. JAMA 174:1586–1588, 1960.
24. Brandt PA, Smith ME, Ashburn SS, Graves J. IM injections in children. Am J Nurs 72:1402–1406, 1972.
25. Gilles FH, Matson DD. Sciatic nerve injury following misplaced gluteal injections. J Pediatr 76:247–254, 1970.
26. Clark K, Williams PE Jr, Willis W, McGavran WL. Injection injury of the sciatic nerve. Clin Neurosurg 17:111–125, 1969.
27. MacDonald NE, Marcuse EK. Neurologic injury after vaccination: Buttocks as injection site [letter]. Can Med Assoc J 150:326, 1994.
28. Marcuse EK, MacDonald NE. Neurologic injury after vaccination in buttocks [letter]. Can Med Assoc J 155:374, 1996.
29. Marcuse EK, MacDonald NE. Vaccine injury—no reports [letter]. Pediatrics 99:144, 1997.
30. Thompson MK. Needling doubts about where to vaccinate. Br Med J 297:779–780, 1988.
31. Moss ALH. Re: Needling doubts about where to vaccinate [letter]. BMJ 297:980, 1988.
32. Thompson MK. Site for immunising infants [letter]. BMJ 304:1178, 1992.
33. Grosswasser J, Kahn A, Bouche B, et al. Needle length and injection technique for efficient intramuscular vaccine delivery in infants and children evaluated through an ultrasonographic determination of subcutaneous and muscle layer thickness. Pediatrics 100:400–403, 1997.
34. World Health Organization. Module 3: When and how to give vaccines. In Immunization in Practice—A Guide for Health Workers Who Give Vaccines. Geneva, World Health Organization, 1984. EPI/PHW/84/3 Rev 1.
35. Hick JF, Charbonneau JW, Brackke DM. Optimum needle length for diphtheria-tetanus-pertussis inoculation of infants. Pediatrics 84:136–137, 1989.
36. Poland GA, Borrud A, Jacobson RM. Determination of deltoid fat pad thickness. Implications for needle length in adult immunization. JAMA 277:1709–1711, 1997.
37. Evans DIK, Shaw A. Safety of intramuscular injection of hepatitis B vaccine in haemophiliacs. Br Med J 1694–1695, 1990.
38. Kristensen K. Antibody response to a *Haemophilus influenzae* type b polysaccharide tetanus toxoid conjugate vaccine in splenectomized children and adolescents. Scand J Infect Dis 24:629–632, 1992.
39. Granoff DM, Suarez BK, Pandey JP, Shackelford PG. Genes associated with the G2m(23) immunoglobulin allotype regulate the IgG subclass responses to *Haemophilus influenzae* type b polysaccharide vaccine. J Infect Dis 157:1142–1149, 1988.
40. *Haemophilus influenzae* B immunization. Drug Ther Bull 31:1–2, 1993.
41. American Academy of Pediatrics. Rabies. In Peter G (ed). 1997 Redbook: Report of the Committee on Infectious Diseases (24th ed). Elk Grove Village, IL, American Academy of Pediatrics, 1997, pp 435–442.
41a. Tuberculosis: BCG immunisation. In Salisbury DM, Begg NT (eds). 1996 Immunisation against infectious disease. London, Her Majesty's Stationery Office, 1996, pp 219–241.
42. Centers for Disease Control and Prevention. Poliomyelitis prevention in the United States: Introduction of a sequential vaccination schedule of inactivated poliovirus vaccine followed by oral poliovirus vaccine. MMWR Morb Mortal Wkly Rep 46(RR-3):1–25, 1997.
43. Spiegel A, Greindl Y, Lippeveld T, et al. Effect of two meningococcal vaccination strategies during the epidemic in N'Djamena, Chad, in 1988. Bull World Health Organ 71:311–315, 1993.
44. Hoke CH Jr, Egan JE, Sjogren MH, et al. Administration of hepatitis A vaccine to a military population by needle and jet injector and with hepatitis B vaccine. J Infect Dis 171(suppl 1):S53–S60, 1995.
45. Nuefield PD, Katz L. Comparative evaluation of three jet injectors for mass immunization. Can J Public Health 68:513–516, 1977.
46. Warren J, Ziherl FA, Kish AW, Ziherl LA. Large-scale administration of vaccines by means of an automatic jet injection syringe. JAMA 157:633–637, 1955.
47. Elisberg BL, McCown JM, Smadel JE. Vaccination against smallpox. II. Jet injection of chorio-allantoic membrane vaccine. J Immunol 77:340–351, 1956.
48. Lipson MJ, Carver DH, Eleff MG, et al. Antibody response to poliomyelitis vaccine administered by jet injection. Am J Public Health 48:599–603, 1958.
49. Anderson EA, Lindberg RB, Hunter DH. Report of a large-scale field trial of jet injection in immunization for influenza. JAMA 167:549–552, 1958.
50. Brink PRG, van Loon AM, Trommelen JCM, et al. Virus transmission by subcutaneous jet injection. J Med Microbiol 20:393–397, 1985.
51. Stanfield JP, Bracken PM, Waddell KM, Gall D. Diphtheria-tetanus-pertussis immunization by intradermal jet injection. BMJ 2:197–199, 1972.
52. Rosenthal SR. Transference of blood by various inoculation devices. Am Rev Respir Dis 96:815–819, 1967.
53. Zachoval R, Deinhardt F, Gurtler L, et al. Risk of virus transmission by jet injection [letter]. Lancet 1:189, 1988.
54. Abb J, Deinhardt F, Eisenburg J. The risk of transmission of hepatitis B virus using jet injection in inoculation. J Infect Dis 144:179, 1981.
55. Robertson JS. Jet injectors and infection. Public Health 101:147–148, 1987.
56. Canter J, MacKey K, Good LS, et al. An outbreak of hepatitis B associated with jet injections in a weight reduction clinic. Arch Intern Med 150:1923–1927, 1990.
57. Centers for Disease Control. Hepatitis B associated with jet gun injection—California. MMWR Morb Mortal Wkly Rep 35:446–447, 1986.
58. Centers for Disease Control. Hepatitis B virus: A comprehensive strategy for eliminating transmission in the United States through universal childhood vaccination. Recommendations of the Immunization Practices Advisory Committee (ACIP). MMWR Morb Mortal Wkly Rep 40(RR-13):1–25, 1991.
59. Aylward B, Kane M, McNair-Scott R, Hu DH. Model-based estimates of the risk of human immunodeficiency virus and hepatitis B virus transmission through unsafe injections. Int J Epidemiol 24:446–452, 1995.
60. Brito GS, Chen RT, Stefano CA, et al. The risk of transmission of HIV and other blood born diseases via jet injectors during immunization mass campaigns in Brazil [abstract PC0132]. In Abstracts from the Tenth International Conference on AIDS; Yokohama, Japan; August 7–12, 1994.
61. Aylward B, Lloyd J, Zaffran M, et al. Reducing the risk of unsafe injections in immunization programmes: Financial and

operational implications of various injection technologies. Bull World Health Organ 73:531–540, 1995.
62. Zaffran M, Lloyd J, Clements J, Stilwell B. A Drive to Safer Injections. Geneva, World Health Organization, 1997. WHOGPVSAGE.97/WP.05, 1997.
63. Parent du Chatelet I, Lang J, Schlumberger M, et al. Clinical immunogenicity and tolerance studies of liquid vaccines delivered by jet-injector and a new single-use cartridge (Imule): Comparison with standard syringe injection. Vaccine 15:449–458, 1997.
63a. Reis EC, Jacobson RM, Tarbell S, Weniger BG. Taking the sting out of shots: Control of vaccination-associated pain and adverse reactions. Pediatr Ann 27:375–385, 1998.
64. Taddio A, Nulman I, Goldbach M, et al. Use of lidocaine-prilocaine cream for vaccination pain in infants. J Pediatr 124:643–648, 1994.
64a. Uhari M. A eutectic mixture of lidocaine and prilocaine for alleviating vaccination pain in infants. Pediatrics 92:719–721, 1993.
65. Jakobson B, Nilsson A. Methemoglobinemia associated with a prilocaine-lidocaine cream and trimethoprim-sulphamethoxazole: A case report. Acta Anaesthesiol Scand 29:453–455, 1985.
66. Lewis K, Cherry JD, Sachs MH, et al. The effect of prophylactic acetaminophen administration on reactions to DTP vaccination. Am J Dis Child 142:62–65, 1988.
67. Abbott K, Fowler-Kerry S. The use of a topical refrigerant anesthetic to reduce injection pain in children. J Pain Symptom Manage 10:584–590, 1995.
68. Maikler VE. Effects of a skin refrigerant/anesthetic and age on the pain responses of infants receiving immunizations. Res Nurs Health 14:397–403, 1991.
69. Reis E, Holubkov R. Vapocoolant spray is equally effective as EMLA cream in reducing immunization pain in school-aged children. Pediatrics 100:e5, 1997. http://www.pediatrics.org/cgi/content/full/100/6/e5.
70. Allen KD, White DD, Walburn JN. Sucrose as an analgesic agent for infants during immunization injections. Arch Pediatr Adolesc Med 150:270–274, 1996.
71. French GM, Painter EC, Coury DL. Blowing away shot pain: A technique for pain management during immunization. Pediatrics 93:384–388, 1994.
72. Fowler-Kerry S, Lander JR. Management of injection pain in children. Pain 30:169–175, 1987.
73. Global Programme for Vaccines and Immunization. Basic immunization schedules and strategies. In Immunization Policy. Geneva, World Health Organization, 1997. http://www.who.ch/programmes/gpv/gEnglish/avail/gpvcatalog/policy.htm.
74. Evans DG, Smith JWG. Response of the young infant to active immunization. Br Med Bull 19:225–229, 1963.
75. Orenstein WA, Weisfeld JS, Halsey NA. Diphtheria and tetanus toxoids and pertussis vaccine, combined. In Halsey NA, de Quadros CA (eds). Recent Advances in Immunization: A Bibliographic Review. PAHO Scientific Publ. No. 451. Washington, DC, Pan American Health Organization, 1983, pp 30–51.
76. di Sant' Agnese PA. Combined immunization against diphtheria, tetanus and pertussis in newborn infants. I. Production of antibodies in early infancy. Pediatrics 3:20–33, 1949.
77. Butler NR, Wilson BD, Benson PF, et al. Response of infants to pertussis vaccines at one week and to poliomyelitis, diphtheria, and tetanus vaccine at six months. Lancet 2:112–114, 1962.
78. di Sant' Agnese PA. Combined immunization against diphtheria, tetanus and pertussis in newborn infants. III. Relationship of age to antibody protection. Pediatrics 3:333–344, 1949.
79. Halsey N, Galazka A. The efficacy of DPT and oral poliomyelitis immunization schedules initiated from birth to 12 weeks of age. Bull World Health Organ 63:1151–1169, 1985.
80. Wilkins J, Chan LS, Wehrle PF. Age and dose interval as factors in agglutinin formation to pertussis vaccine. Vaccine 5:49–54, 1987.
81. American Academy of Pediatrics. Pertussis. In Peter G (ed). 1997 Red Book: Report of the Committee on Infectious Diseases (24th ed). Elk Grove Village, IL, American Academy of Pediatrics, 1997, pp 394–407.
82. Galazka AM. Module 4: Pertussis. In The Immunologic Basis for Immunization Series. Global Programme for Vaccines and Immunization, Expanded Programme on Immunization. Geneva, World Health Organization, 1993, pp 1–20.
83. Funkhouser AW, Wassilak SG, Orenstein WA, et al. Estimated effects of a delay in the recommended vaccination schedule for diphtheria and tetanus toxoids and pertussis vaccine. JAMA 257:1341–1346, 1987.
84. Lieberman JM, Greenberg DP, Wong VK, et al. Effect of neonatal immunization with diphtheria and tetanus toxoids on antibody responses to *Haemophilus influenzae* type b conjugate vaccines. J Pediatr 126:198–205, 1995.
85. Markowitz LE, Katz SL. Measles vaccine. In Plotkin SA, Mortimer EA Jr (eds). Vaccines (2nd ed). Philadelphia, WB Saunders, 1994, pp 229–276.
86. American Academy of Pediatrics, Committee on Infectious Diseases. Recommended childhood immunization schedule—United States, January–December 1998. Pediatrics 101:154–157, 1998.
87. McBean AM, Thoms ML, Albrecht P, et al. Serologic response to oral polio vaccine and enhanced-potency inactivated polio vaccines. Am J Epidemiol 128:615–628, 1988.
88. Halsey NA, Blatter MM, Bader G. Safety and immunogenicity of a combination DTP/IPV vaccine administered to infants in a dual-chamber syringe. Protocol No. U93-3663-01. Final report. Swiftwater, PA, Connaught Laboratories, 1994.
89. Salk J. One-dose immunization against paralytic poliomyelitis using a noninfectious vaccine. Rev Infect Dis 6(suppl 2):S444–S450, 1984.
90. Centers for Disease Control. Measles, mumps, and rubella—vaccine use and strategies for measles, rubella, congenital rubella syndrome elimination and mumps control: Recommendations of the Advisory Committee on Immunizations. MMWR Morb Mortal Wkly Rep 47(RR-8):1–57, 1998.
91. Theiler M, Smith HH. The use of yellow fever virus modified by in vitro cultivation for human immunization. J Exp Med 65:787–800, 1937.
92. Smithburn KC, Mahaffy AF. Immunization against yellow fever: Studies on the time of development and the duration of induced immunity. Am J Trop Med 25:217–223, 1945.
93. Petralli JK, Merigan TC, Wilbur JR. Circulating interferon after measles vaccination. N Engl J Med 273:198–201, 1965.
94. Petralli JK, Merigan TC, Wilbur JR. Action of endogenous interferon against vaccinia infection in children. Lancet 2:401–405, 1965.
95. King GE, Markowitz LE, Heath J, et al. Antibody response to measles-mumps-rubella vaccine of children with mild illness at the time of vaccination. JAMA 275:704–707, 1996.
96. Halsey NA, Boulos R, Mode F, et al. Response to measles vaccine in Haitian infants 6 to 12 months old. N Engl J Med 313:544–549, 1985.
97. Ndikuyeze A, Munoz A, Stewart S, et al. Immunogenicity and safety of measles vaccine in ill African children. Int J Epidemiol 17:448–455, 1988.
98. Atkinson W, Markowitz L, Baughman A, et al. Serologic response to measles vaccination among ill children [abstract 422]. In Program and abstracts of the 32nd Interscience Conference on Antimicrobial Agents and Chemotherapy; Anaheim, CA; October 11–14, 1992.
99. Dennehy PH, Saracen CL, Peter G. Seroconversion rates to combined measles-mumps-rubella-varicella (MMRV) vaccine of children with upper respiratory tract infection. Pediatrics 94:514–516, 1994.
100. Ratnam S, West R, Gadag V. Measles and rubella antibody response after measles-mumps-rubella vaccination in children with afebrile upper respiratory tract infection. J Pediatr 127:432–434, 1995.
101. Myers MG, Beckman CW, Vosdingh RA, Hankins WA. Primary immunization with tetanus and diphtheria toxoids. Reaction rate and immunogenicity in older children and adults. JAMA 248:2478–2480, 1982.
102. Relihan M. Reactions to tetanus toxoid. J Irish Med Assoc 62:430–434, 1969.
103. White WG, Barnes GM, Barker E, et al. Reactions to tetanus toxoid. J Hyg (Lond) 71:283–297, 1973.
104. Eisen AH, Cohen JJ, Rose B. Reaction to tetanus toxoid. Report of a case with immunologic studies. N Engl J Med 269:1408–1411, 1963.
105. Schneider CH. Reactions to tetanus toxoid: A report of five cases. Med J Aust 1:303–305, 1964.

106. Edsall G, Elliot MW, Peebles TC, Eldred MC. Excessive use of tetanus toxoid boosters. JAMA 202:111–113, 1967.
107. Levine L, Edsall G. Tetanus toxoid: What determines reaction proneness? J Infect Dis 144:376, 1981.
108. King GE, Hadler SC. Simultaneous administration of childhood vaccines: An important public health policy that is safe and efficacious. Pediatr Infect Dis J 13:394–407, 1994.
109. Ramsay DS, Lewis M. Developmental change in infant cortisol and behavioral response to inoculation. Child Dev 65:1491–1502, 1994.
110. Lewis M, Ramsay DS, Suomi SJ. Validating current immunization practice with young infants. Pediatrics 90:771–773, 1992.
111. Felsenfeld O, Wolf RH, Gyr K, et al. Simultaneous vaccination against cholera and yellow fever. Lancet 1:457–458, 1973.
112. Gateff C. Influence de la vaccination anticholerique sur l'immunisation antiamarile associee. Bull Soc Pathol Exot 66:258–266, 1973.
113. Black FL. Measles active and passive immunity in a worldwide perspective. Prog Med Virol 36:1–33, 1989.
114. Albrecht P, Ennis FA, Saltzman EJ, Krugman S. Persistence of maternal antibody in infants beyond 12 months: Mechanism of measles vaccine failure. J Pediatr 91:715–718, 1977.
115. Wilkins J, Wehrle PF. Additional evidence against measles vaccine administration to infants less than 12 months of age: Altered immune response following active/passive immunization. J Pediatr 94:865–869, 1979.
116. Linnemann CC, Dine MS, Bloom JE, Schiff GM. Measles antibody in previously immunized children: The need for revaccination. Am J Dis Child 124:53–57, 1972.
117. Halsey NA, Boulos R, Mode F, et al. Response to measles vaccine in Haitian infants 6 to 12 months old. Influence of maternal antibodies, malnutrition, and concurrent illnesses. N Engl J Med 313:544–577, 1985.
118. Black FL, Berman LL, Borgono JM, et al. Geographic variation in infant loss of maternal measles antibody and in prevalence of rubella antibody. Am J Epidemiol 124:442–452, 1986.
119. Dagan R, Slater PE, Duvdevani P, et al. Decay of maternally derived measles antibody in a highly vaccinated population in southern Israel. Pediatr Infect Dis J 14:965–969, 1995.
120. Immunization of man against rubella. Discussion on sessions III and IV. Am J Dis Child 118:307–321, 1969.
121. Krugman S, Giles JP, Jacobs AM, Friedman H. Studies with a further attenuated live measles-virus vaccine. Pediatrics 31:914–928, 1963.
122. Lingham S, Miller CL, Clarke M, Pateman J. Antibody response and clinical reactions in children given measles vaccine with immunoglobulin. BMJ 292:1044–1045, 1986.
123. Benson PF, Butler NR, Goffe AP, et al. Vaccination of infants with living attenuated measles vaccine (Edmonston strain) with and without gamma-globulin. BMJ 2:851–853, 1964.
124. Siber GR, Werner BC, Halsey NA, et al. Interference of immune globulin with measles and rubella immunization. J Pediatr 122:204–211, 1993.
125. Black NA, Parsons A, Kurtz JB, et al. Postpartum rubella immunization: A controlled trial of two vaccines. Lancet 2:990–992, 1983.
126. Kaplan JE, Nelson DB, Schonberger LB, et al. The effect of immune globulin on the response to trivalent oral poliovirus and yellow fever vaccinations. Bull World Health Organ 62:585–590, 1984.
127. Simoes EAF, Padmini B, Steinhoff MC, et al. Antibody response of infants to two doses of inactivated poliovirus vaccine of enhanced potency. Am J Dis Child 139:977–980, 1985.
128. American Academy of Pediatrics, Committee on Infectious Diseases. Recommended timing of routine measles immunization for children who have recently received immune globulin preparations. Pediatrics 93:682–685, 1994.
129. Sato H, Albrecht P, Reynolds DW, et al. Transfer of measles, mumps, and rubella antibodies from mother to infant. Its effect on measles, mumps, and rubella immunization. Am J Dis Child 133:1240–1243, 1979.
130. Siber GR, Snydman DR. Use of immune globulin in the prevention and treatment of infections. In Remington J, Swartz M (eds). Current Clinical Topics in Infectious Diseases. Vol. 12. Oxford, UK, Blackwell Scientific Publications, 1992, pp 208–256.
131. Habig WH, Tankersley DL. Tetanus. In Cryz SJ (ed). Vaccines and Immunotherapy. New York, Pergamon Press, 1991, pp 13–19.
132. Plotkin SA, Koprowski H. Rabies vaccine. In Plotkin SA, Mortimer EA (eds). Vaccines. Philadelphia, WB Saunders, 1994, pp 649–670.
133. Letson GW, Santosham M, Reid R, et al. Comparison of active and combined passive/active immunization of Navajo children against *Haemophilus influenzae* type b. Pediatr Infect Dis J 7:747–752, 1988.
134. Leentvaar-Kuijpers A, Coutinho RA, Brulein V, Safary A. Simultaneous passive and active immunization against hepatitis A. Vaccine 10(suppl 1):S138–S141, 1992.
135. Wagner G, Lavanchy D, Darioli R, et al. Simultaneous active and passive immunization against hepatitis A studied in a population of travelers. Vaccine 11:1027–1032, 1993.
136. Green MS, Cohen D, Lerman Y, et al. Depression of the immune response to an inactivated hepatitis A vaccine administered concomitantly with immune globulin. J Infect Dis 168:740–743, 1993.
137. Shapiro CN, Letson GW, Huehn D, et al. Effect of maternal antibody on immunogenicity of hepatitis A vaccine in infants [abstract H61]. In Program and abstracts of the 35th Interscience Conference on Antimicrobial Agents and Chemotherapy (ICAAC); American Society for Microbiology; San Francisco, CA; September 17–20, 1995.
138. American Academy of Pediatrics. Respiratory syncytial virus immune globulin intravenous: Indications for use. Pediatrics 99:645–650, 1997.
139. Mason W, Takahashi M, Schneider T. Persisting passively acquired measles antibody following gamma globulin therapy for Kawasaki disease and response to live virus vaccination [abstract 311]. Presented at the 32nd meeting of the Interscience Conference on Antimicrobial Agents and Chemotherapy; Los Angeles, CA; October 11–14, 1992.
140. American Academy of Pediatrics. Measles. In Peter G (ed). 1997 Redbook: Report of the Committee on Infectious Diseases (24th ed). Elk Grove Village, IL, American Academy of Pediatrics, 1997, pp 344–357.
141. American Academy of Pediatrics. Rubella. In Peter G (ed). 1997 Redbook: Report of the Committee on Infectious Diseases (24th ed). Elk Grove Village, IL, American Academy of Pediatrics, 1997, pp 456–462.
142. American Academy of Pediatrics. Mumps. In Peter G (ed). 1997 Redbook: Report of the Committee on Infectious Diseases (24th ed). Elk Grove Village, IL, American Academy of Pediatrics, 1997, pp 366–369.
143. American Academy of Pediatrics. Varicella-zoster infections. In Peter G (ed). 1997 Redbook: Report of the Committee on Infectious Diseases (24th ed). Elk Grove Village, IL, American Academy of Pediatrics, 1997, pp 573–585.
144. Centers for Disease Control and Prevention. Prevention of varicella: Recommendations of the Advisory Committee on Immunization Practices (ACIP). MMWR Morb Mortal Wkly Rep 45(RR-11): 1–36, 1996.
145. Bush LM, Moonsammy GI, Boscia JA. Evaluation of initiating a hepatitis B vaccination schedule with one vaccine and completing it with another. Vaccine 9:807–809, 1991.
146. Chan CY, Lee SD, Tsai YT, Lo KJ. Booster response to recombinant yeast-derived hepatitis B vaccine in vaccinees whose anti-HBs responses were initially elicited by a plasma-derived vaccine. Vaccine 9:765–767, 1991.
147. Anderson EL, Decker MD, Englund JA, et al. Interchangeability of conjugated *Haemophilus influenzae* type b vaccines in infants. JAMA 273:849–853, 1995.
148. Bewley KM, Schwab JG, Ballanco GA, Daum RS. Interchangeability of *Haemophilus influenzae* type b vaccines in the primary series: Evaluation of a two-dose mixed regimen. Pediatrics 98:898–904, 1996.
149. Greenberg DP, Lieberman JM, Marcy SM, et al. Enhanced antibody response in infants given different sequences of heterogeneous *Haemophilus influenzae* type b conjugate vaccines. J Pediatr 126:206–211, 1995.
150. Centers for Disease Control and Prevention. Pertussis vaccination: Use of acellular pertussis vaccines among infants and young children. MMWR Morb Mortal Wkly Rep 46(RR-7):1–25, 1997.

151. Zaloga GP, Chernow B. Life-threatening anaphylactic reactions to tetanus toxoid. Ann Allergy 49:107–108, 1982.
152. Institute of Medicine. Evidence concerning pertussis vaccines and other illnesses and conditions. In Howson CP, Howe CJ, Fineberg HV (eds). Adverse Effects of Pertussis and Rubella Vaccines. Washington, DC, Institute of Medicine, 1991, pp 144–186.
153. Halpern SR, Halpern D. Reactions from DPT immunization and its relationship to allergic children. J Pediatr 47:60–67, 1955.
154. Mortimer EA, Sorensen RU. Urticaria following administration of diphtheria–tetanus toxoids–pertussis vaccine [letter]. Pediatr Infect Dis J 6:876–877, 1987.
155. Matuhasi T, Ikegami H. Elevation of levels of IgE antibody to tetanus toxin in individuals vaccinated with diphtheria-pertussis-tetanus vaccine. J Infect Dis 146:290, 1982.
156. Nagel J, Svec D, Waters T, Fireman P. IgE synthesis in man. I. Development of specific IgE antibodies after immunization with tetanus-diphtheria (Td) toxoids. J Immunol 118:334–341, 1977.
157. Lewis K, Jordan SC, Cherry JD, et al. Petechiae and urticaria after DTP vaccination: Detection of circulating immune complexes containing vaccine-specific antigens. J Pediatr 109:1009–1012, 1986.
158. American Academy of Pediatrics. Tetanus. In Peter G (ed). 1997 Redbook: Report of the Committee on Infectious Diseases (24th ed). Elk Grove Village, IL, American Academy of Pediatrics, 1997, pp 518–523.
159. Jacobs RL, Lowe RS, Lanier BQ. Adverse reactions to tetanus toxoid. JAMA 247:40–42, 1982.
160. Mansfield LE, Ting S, Rawls DO, Frederick R. Systemic reactions during cutaneous testing for tetanus toxoid hypersensitivity. Ann Allergy 57:135–137, 1986.
161. Facktor MA, Bernstein RA, Fireman P. Hypersensitivity to tetanus toxoid. J Allergy Clin Immunol 52:1–12, 1973.
162. Sisk CW, Lewis CE. Reactions to tetanus-diphtheria toxoid (adult). Arch Environ Health 11:34–36, 1965.
163. Beneson AS, Joseph PR, Oseasohn RO. Cholera vaccine field trials in East Pakistan. 1. Reaction and antigenicity studies. Bull World Health Organ 38:347–357, 1968.
164. Marshall JD Jr, Bartelloni PJ, Cavanaugh DC, et al. Plague immunization. II. Relation of adverse clinical reactions to multiple immunizations with killed vaccine. J Infect Dis 129(suppl): S19–S25, 1974.
165. Hejfec LB, Salmin LV, Lejtman MZ, et al. A controlled field trial and laboratory study of five typhoid vaccines in the USSR. Bull World Health Organ 34:321–339, 1966.
166. Ashcroft MT, Ritchie JM, Nicholson CC. Controlled field trial in British Guiana school children of heat-killed-phenolized and acetone-killed lyophilized typhoid vaccines. Am J Hyg 79:196–206, 1964.
167. Robinson HC, Russell ML, Csokonay WM. Japanese encephalitis vaccine and adverse effects among travelers. Can Dis Wkly Rep 17:173–177, 1991.
168. Anderson MM, Ronne T. Side effects with Japanese encephalitis vaccine. Lancet 337:1044, 1991.
169. Ruff TA, Eisen D, Fuller A, Kass R. Adverse reactions to Japanese encephalitis vaccine. Lancet 338:881–882, 1991.
170. Harvey RE, Posey WC, Jacobs RL. The predictive value of egg skin tests and yellow fever vaccine skin tests in egg-sensitive individuals [abstract 213]. J Allergy Clin Immunol 63:196–197, 1979.
171. Centers for Disease Control and Prevention. Prevention and control of influenza: Recommendations of the Advisory Committee on Immunization Practices. MMWR Morb Mortal Wkly Rep 46(RR-9):1–25, 1997.
172. Yamane N, Uemura H. Serological examination of IgE- and IgG-specific antibodies to egg protein during influenza virus immunization. Epidemiol Infect 100:291–299, 1988.
173. Bierman CW, Shapiro GG, Pierson WE, et al. Safety of influenza vaccination in allergic children. J Infect Dis 136:S652–S655, 1977.
174. Kamin PB, Fein BT, Britton HA. Use of live, attenuated measles virus vaccine in children allergic to egg protein. JAMA 193:1125–1126, 1965.
175. Brown FR, Wolfe HI. Chick embryo grown measles vaccine in an egg-sensitive child. J Pediatr 71:868–869, 1967.
176. Murphy KR, Strunk RC. Safe administration of influenza vaccine in asthmatic children sensitive to egg proteins. J Pediatr 106:931–933, 1985.
177. American Academy of Pediatrics. Influenza. In Peter G (ed). 1997 Redbook: Report of the Committee on Infectious Diseases (24th ed). Elk Grove Village, IL, American Academy of Pediatrics, 1997, pp 307–315.
178. Fasano MB, Wood RA, Cooke SK, Sampson HA. Egg hypersensitivity and adverse reactions to measles, mumps, and rubella vaccine. J Pediatr 120:978–981, 1992.
179. Kemp A, Van Asperen P, Mukhi A. Measles immunization in children with clinical reactions to egg protein. Am J Dis Child 144:33–35, 1990.
180. James JM, Burks AW, Roberson PK, Sampson HA. Safe administration of measles vaccine to children allergic to eggs. N Engl J Med 332:1262–1266, 1995.
181. Kelso JM, Jones RT, Yunginger JW. Anaphylaxis to measles, mumps, and rubella vaccine mediated by IgE to gelatin. J Allergy Infect Dis 91:867–872, 1993.
182. Sakaguchi M, Ogura H, Inouye S. IgE antibody to gelatin in children with immediate-type reactions to measles and mumps vaccines. J Allergy Infect Dis 96:563–565, 1995.
183. Sakaguchi M, Nakayama T, Inouye S. Food allergy to gelatin in children with systemic immediate-type reactions, including anaphylaxis, to vaccines. J Allergy Infect Dis 98:1058–1061, 1996.
184. Centers for Disease Control. Systemic allergic reactions following immunization with human diploid cell rabies vaccine. MMWR Morb Mortal Wkly Rep 33:185–188, 1984.
185. Dreeson DW, Bernard KW, Parker RA, et al. Immune complex–like disease in 23 persons following a booster dose of rabies human diploid cell vaccine. Vaccine 4:45–49, 1986.
186. Anderson MC, Baer H, Frazier DJ, Quinnan JV. The role of specific IgE and beta-propiolactone in reactions resulting from booster doses of human diploid cell rabies vaccine. J Allergy Clin Immunol 80:861–868, 1987.
187. Rietschel RL, Bernier R. Neomycin sensitivity and the MMR vaccine [letter]. JAMA 245:571, 1981.
188. Elliman D, Dhanraj B. Safe MMR vaccination despite neomycin allergy [letter]. Lancet 337:365, 1991.
189. Kwittken PL, Rosen S, Sweinberg SK. MMR vaccine and neomycin allergy [letter]. Am J Dis Child 147:128–129, 1993.
190. Goh CL. Anaphylaxis from topical neomycin and bacitracin. Aust J Dermatol 27:125–126, 1986.
191. Rietschel RL, Adams RM. Reactions to thimerosal in hepatitis B vaccines. Dermatol Clin 8:161–164, 1990.
192. Noel I, Galloway A, Ive FA. Hypersensitivity to thiomersal in hepatitis B vaccine [letter]. Lancet 338:705, 1991.
193. Forstrom L, Hannulksela M, Kousa M, Lehmuskallio E. Merthiolate hypersensitivity and vaccination. Contact Dermatitis 6:241–245, 1980.
194. Aberer W. Vaccination despite thimerosal sensitivity. Contact Dermatitis 24:6–10, 1991.
195. Kirkland LR. Ocular hypersensitivity to thimerosal: A problem with hepatitis vaccine? South Med J 83:497–499, 1990.
196. Reisman RE. Delayed hypersensitivity to merthiolate preservative. J Allergy 43:245–248, 1969.
197. American Academy of Pediatrics. Passive immunization. In Peter G (ed). 1997 Redbook: Report of the Committee on Infectious Diseases (24th ed). Elk Grove Village, IL, American Academy of Pediatrics, 1997, pp 36–47.
198. Braun MM, Patriarca PA, Ellenberg SS. Syncope after immunization. Arch Pediatr Adolesc Med 151:255–259, 1997.
199. Rothberg RM. Immunoglobulin and specific antibody synthesis during the first weeks of life of premature infants. J Pediatr 75:391–399, 1969.
200. Dancis J, Osborn JJ, Kunz HW. Studies of the immunology of the newborn infant. IV. Antibody formation in the premature infant. Pediatrics 12:151–157, 1953.
201. Bernbaum J, Anolik R, Polin RA, Douglas SD. Development of the premature infant's host defense system and its relationship to routine immunization. Clin Perinatol 11:73–84, 1984.
202. Wara DW, Barrett DJ. Cell-mediated immunity in the newborn: Clinical aspects. Pediatrics 64(suppl):822–828, 1979.
203. Evans HE, Akpata SO, Glass L. Serum immunoglobulin levels in premature and full-term infants. Am J Clin Pathol 56:416–418, 1971.

204. Whitelaw A, Parkin J. Development of immunity. Br Med Bull 44:1037–1051, 1988
205. Hyvarinen M, Zeltzer P, Oh W, Stiehm ER. Influence of gestational age on the newborn serum levels of alpha$_1$-fetoglobulin, IgG globulin and albumin. J Pediatr 82:430–437, 1973.
206. Linder N, Yaron M, Handsher R, et al. Early immunization with inactivated polioivirus vaccine in premature infants. J Pediatr 127:128–130, 1995.
207. Bernbaum JC, Daft A, Anolik R, et al. Response of preterm infants to diphtheria-tetanus-pertussis immunizations. J Pediatr 107:184–188, 1985.
208. Koblin BA, Townsend TR, Munoz A, et al. Response of preterm infants to diphtheria-tetanus-pertussis vaccine. Pediatr Infect Dis J 7:704–711, 1988.
209. Smolen P, Bland R, Heiligenstein E, et al. Antibody response to oral polio vaccine in premature infants. J Pediatr 103:917–919, 1983.
210. Conway SP, James JR, Smithells RW, et al. Immunization of the preterm baby [letter]. Lancet 2:1326, 1987.
211. Conway S, James J, Balfour A, Smithells R. Immunisation of the preterm baby. J Infect 27:143–150, 1993.
212. D'Angio CT, Maniscalco WM, Pinchichero ME. Immunologic response of extremely premature infants to tetanus, *Haemophilus influenzae*, and polio immunizations. Pediatrics 96:18–22, 1995.
213. Pullan CR, Hull D. Routine immunization of preterm infants. Arch Dis Child 64:1438–1441, 1989.
214. Pagano JS, Plotkin SA, Cornely D, et al. The response of premature infants to infection with attenuated poliovirus. Pediatrics 29:794–807, 1962.
215. Adenyi-Jones CA, Faden H, Ferdon MB, et al. Systemic and local immune responses to enhanced-potency inactivated poliovirus vaccine in premature and term infants. J Pediatr 120:686–689, 1992.
216. Linder N, Yaron M, Handsher R, et al: Early immunization with inactivated poliovirus vaccine in premature infants. J Pediatr 127:128–130, 1995.
217. Chirico G, Belloni C, Gasparoni A, et al. Hepatitis B immunization in infants from HbsAg negative mothers. Pediatrics 92:717–719, 1993.
218. Kristensen K, Gyhrs A, Lausen B, et al. Antibody response to *Haemophilus influenzae* type b capsular polysaccharide conjugated to tetanus toxoid in preterm infants. Pediatr Infect Dis J 15:525–529, 1996.
219. O'Shea TM, Dillard RG, Gillis DC, Abramson JS. Low rate of response to enhanced inactivated polio vaccine in preterm infants with chronic illness. Clin Res Reg Affairs 10:49–57, 1993.
220. Washburn LK, O'Shea TM, Gillis DC, et al. Response to *Haemophilus influenzae* type b conjugate vaccine in chronically ill premature infants. J Pediatr 123:791–794, 1993.
221. Lau Y, Tam AYC, Ng KW, et al. Response of preterm infants to hepatitis B vaccine. J Pediatr 121:962–965, 1992.
222. Munoz A, Salvador A, Brodsky NL, et al. Antibody response of low birth weight infants to *Haemophilus influenzae* type b polyribosylribitol phosphate–outer membrane protein conjugate vaccine. Pediatrics 96:216–219, 1995.
223. Kristensen K, Gyhrs A, Lausen B, et al. Antibody response to *Haemophilus influenzae* type b capsular polysaccharide conjugated to tetanus toxoid in preterm infants. Pediatr Infect Dis J 15:525–529, 1996.
223a. Khalak R, Pichichero ME, D'Angio CT. Three-year follow-up of vaccine response in extremely preterm infants. Pediatrics 101:597–603, 1998.
224. Chawareewong S, Jirapongsa A, Lokaphadhana K. Immune response to hepatitis B vaccine in premature neonates. Southeast Asian J Trop Med Public Health 22:39–40, 1991.
225. Losonsky GA, Stephens I, Mahoney F, et al. Preliminary results evaluating the immunogenicity of hepatitis B vaccination of premature infants starting in the first week of life [abstract 1752]. Pediatr Res 37:295a, 1995.
226. Patel DM, Butler J, Feldman S, et al. Immunogenicity of hepatitis B vaccine in healthy very low birth weight infants. J Pediatr 131:641–643, 1997.
227. American Academy of Pediatrics. Immunization in special clinical circumstances. In Peter G (ed). 1997 Redbook: Report of the Committee on Infectious Diseases (24th ed). Elk Grove Village, IL, American Academy of Pediatrics, 1997, pp 48–71.
228. American Academy of Pediatrics. Update on timing of hepatitis B vaccination for premature infants and for children with lapsed immunization. Pediatrics 94:403–404, 1994.
229. Sanchez PJ, Laptook AR, Fisher L, et al. Apnea after immunization of preterm infants. J Pediatr 130:746–751, 1997.
230. Bernbaum J, Daft A, Samuelson J, Polin RA. Half-dose immunization for diphtheria, tetanus, pertussis: Response of pre-term infants. Pediatrics 83:471–476, 1989.
231. Bernbaum J, Polin RA. Re: Half-dose immunization for diphtheria, tetanus, pertussis [letter]. Pediatrics 86144–145, 1990.
232. Plotkin SA. Re: Half-dose immunization for diphtheria, tetanus, pertussis [letter]. Pediatrics 86:145, 1990.
233. Losonsky GA, Fishaut JM, Strussenberg J, Ogra PL. Effect of immunization against rubella on lactation products. II. Maternal-neonatal interactions. J Infect Dis 145:661–666, 1982.
234. Losonsky GA, Fishaut JM, Strussenberg J, Ogra PL. Effect of immunization against rubella on lactation products. I. Development and characterization of specific immunologic reactivity in breast milk. J Infect Dis 145:654–660, 1982.
235. Tingle AJ, Chantler JK, Pot KH, et al. Postpartum rubella immunization: Association with development of prolonged arthritis, neurological sequelae, and chronic rubella viremia. J Infect Dis 152:606–612, 1985.
236. American College of Physicians Task Force on Adult Immunization and Infectious Diseases Society of America. Immunizations for special groups of patients. In Guide for Adult Immunization (3rd ed). Philadelphia, American College of Physicians, 1994, pp 25–41.
237. Kim-Farley R, Brink E. Orenstein W, Bart K. Vaccination and breast-feeding [letter]. JAMA 248:2451–2452, 1982.
238. Patriarca PA, Wright PF, John TJ. Factors affecting the immunogenicity of oral polio vaccine in developing countries: Review. Rev Infect Dis 13:926–939, 1991.
239. Krogh V, Duffy LC, Wong D, et al. Postpartum immunization with rubella virus vaccine and antibody response in breast-feeding infants. J Lab Clin Med 113:695–699, 1989.
240. John TJ, Devaranjan LV, Luther L, Vijayarathnam P. Effect of breast-feeding on seroresponse of infants to oral poliovirus vaccination. Pediatrics 57:47–53, 1976
241. Agarwal A, Sharma D, Kumari S, Khare S. Antibody response to three doses of standard and double dose of trivalent oral poliovaccine. Indian Pediatr 28:1141–1145, 1991.
242. Stephens S, Kennedy CR, Lakhani PK, Brenner MK. In vivo immune responses of breast- and bottle-fed infants to tetanus toxoid antigen and to normal gut flora. Acta Paediatr Scand 73:426–432, 1984.
243. Bell JA. Diphtheria immunization: Use of an alum-precipitated mixture of pertussis vaccine and diphtheria toxoid. JAMA 137:1009–1016, 1948.
244. Pabst HF, Spady DW. Effect of breast-feeding on antibody response to conjugate vaccine. Lancet 336:269–270, 1990.
245. Holguin AH, Reeves JS, Gelfand HM. Immunization of infants with the Sabin oral poliovirus vaccine. Am J Public Health 52:600–610, 1962.
246. Plotkin SA, Katz M, Brown RE, Pagano JS. Oral poliovirus vaccination in newborn African infants. The inhibitory effect of breast-feeding. Am J Dis Child 111:27–30, 1966.
247. Warren RJ, Lepow ML, Bartsch GE, et al. The relationship of maternal antibody, breast-feeding, and age to the susceptibility of newborn infants to infection with attenuated poliovirus. Pediatrics 34:4–13, 1964.
248. Katz M, Plotkin S. Oral polio immunization of the newborn infant: A possible method for overcoming interference by ingested antibodies. J Pediatr 73:267–270, 1968.
249. Katz M, Brown RE, Plotkin SA. Oral poliovirus vaccination in newborn African infants: Relative ineffectiveness of early feeding of vaccine. Trop Geogr Med 20:133–136, 1968.
250. Lepow ML, Warren RJ, Gray N, et al. Effect of Sabin type 1 poliomyelitis vaccine administered by mouth to newborn infants. N Engl J Med 264:1071–1078, 1961.
251. Lepow ML, Warren RJ, Ingram VG, et al. Sabin type 1 (LSc2ab) oral poliomyelitis vaccine. Effect of dose upon response of newborn infants. Am J Dis Child 104:67–71, 1962.
252. Sabin AB. Effect of oral poliovirus vaccine in newborn children. I. Excretion of virus after ingestion of large doses of type I or of

a mixture of all three types, in relation to level of placentally transmitted antibody. Pediatrics 31:623–640, 1963.
253. Deforest A, Parker PB, DiLiberti JH, et al. The effect of breast-feeding on the antibody response in infants to trivalent oral poliovirus vaccine. J Pediatr 83:93–95, 1973
254. Peradze T, Montefiiore D, Coker G. Oral poliovirus vaccination and breast-feeding. West Afr Med J 17:122–124, 1968.
255. Hahn-Zoric M, Fulconis F, Minoli I, et al. Antibody responses to parenteral and oral vaccines are impaired by conventional and low protein formulas as compared to breast-feeding. Acta Paediatr Scand 79:1137–1142, 1990.
256. Pabst HF, Godel J, Grace M, et al. Effect of breast-feeding on immune response to BCG vaccination. Lancet 1:295–297, 1989.
257. Pichichero ME. Effect of breast-feeding on oral rhesus rotavirus vaccine seroconversions: A metaanalysis. J Infect Dis 162:753–755, 1990.
258. Glass RI, Ing DJ, Stoll BJ, Ing RT. Immune response to rotavirus vaccines among breast-fed and non–breast-fed children. In Mestecky J (ed). Immunology of Milk and the Neonate. New York, Plenum Publishing, 1991, pp 249–253.
259. Rennels MB. Influence of breast-feeding and oral poliovirus vaccine on the immunogenicity and efficacy of rotavirus vaccines. J Infect Dis 174(suppl 1):S107–111, 1996.
260. Rennels MB, Wasserman SS, Glass RI, Keane VA. Comparison of immunogenicity and efficacy of rhesus rotavirus reassortment vaccines in breastfed and nonbreastfed children. Pediatrics 96:1132–1136, 1995.
260a. Fleet WF Jr, Benz EW Jr, Karzon DT, et al. Fetal consequences of maternal rubella immunization. JAMA 227:621–627, 1974.
260b. Modlin JF, Herrmann K, Brandling-Bennett AD, et al. Risk of congenital abnormality after inadvertent rubella vaccination of pregnant women. N Engl J Med 294:972–974, 1976.
261. Centers for Disease Control. Rubella vaccination during pregnancy—United States, 1971–1988. MMWR Morb Mortal Wkly Rep 38:289–293, 1989.
262. Sheppard S, Smithells RW, Dickson A, Holzel H. Rubella vaccination and pregnancy: Preliminary report of a national survey. Br Med J 292:727, 1986.
263. Enders G. Rubella antibody titers in vaccinated and nonvaccinated women and results of vaccination during pregnancy. Rev Infect Dis 7(suppl 1):S103–S107, 1985.
264. Markowitz LE, Katz SL. Measles vaccine. In Plotkin SA, Mortimer EA Jr (eds). Vaccines (2nd ed). Philadelphia, WB Saunders, 1994, pp 229–276.
265. Cochi SL, Wharton M, Plotkin SA. Mumps vaccine. In Plotkin SA, Mortimer EA Jr (eds). Vaccines (2nd ed). Philadelphia, WB Saunders, 1994, pp 277–301.
266. Yamauchi T, Wilson C, Geme JW Jr. Transmission of live, attenuated mumps virus to the human placenta. N Engl J Med 290:710–712, 1974.
267. Harjulehto-Mervaala T, Aro T, Hiilesmaa VK, et al. Oral polio vaccination during pregnancy: Lack of impact on fetal development and perinatal outcome. Clin Infect Dis 18:414–420, 1994.
268. Nasidi A, Monath TP, Vandenberg J, et al. Yellow fever vaccination and pregnancy: A four-year prospective study. Trans R Soc Trop Med Hyg 87:337–339, 1993.
269. Tsai TF, Paul R, Lynberg MC, Letson GW. Congenital yellow fever virus infection after immunization in pregnancy. J Infect Dis 168:1520–1523, 1993.
270. Heinonen OP, Shapiro S, Monson RR, et al. Immunization during pregnancy against poliomyelitis and influenza in relation to childhood malignancy. Int J Epidemiol 2:229–235, 1973.
271. Neuzil KM, Reed GW, Mitchel EF, Griffin MR. Influenza morbidity increases in late pregnancy [abstract 66]. In Program and abstracts of the Infectious Diseases Society of America 34th Annual Meeting; New Orleans, LA; September 18–20, 1996.
272. Stanfield JP, Galazka A. Neonatal tetanus in the world today. Bull World Health Organ 62:647–699, 1984.
273. Expanded programme on immunization. Progress towards neonatal tetanus elimination, 1988–1994. Wkly Epidemiol Rec 71:33–39, 1996.
274. Expanded Programme on Immunization. Issues in Neonatal Tetanus Control. Expanded Programme on Immunization, Global Advisory Group. Geneva, World Health Organization, 1987.
275. Salzman MB, Sharrar RG, Steinberg S, LaRusssa P. Transmission of varicella-vaccine virus from a healthy 12-month-old child to his pregnant mother. J Pediatr 131:151–154, 1997.
276. Long SS. Toddler-to-mother transmission of varicella-vaccine virus: How bad is that? J Pediatr 131:10–12, 1997.
277. Centers for Disease Control. Diphtheria, tetanus, and pertussis: Recommendations for vaccine use and other preventive measures—recommendations of the Immunization Practices Advisory Committee (ACIP). MMWR Morb Mortal Wkly Rep 40(RR-10):1–28, 1991.
278. Livengood JR, Mullen JR, White JW, et al. Family history of convulsions and use of pertussis vaccine. J Pediatr 115:527–531, 1989.
279. Centers for Disease Control. Adverse Events Following Immunization. Surveillance report No 3, 1985–1986. Atlanta, US Department of Health and Human Services, Public Health Service, Centers for Disease Control, 1989.
280. Institute of Medicine. Pertussis vaccines and evidence concerning pertussis vaccines and central nervous system disorders, including infantile spasms, hypsarrhythmia, aseptic meningitis, and encephalopathy. In Howson CP, Howe CJ, Fineberg HV (eds). Adverse Effects of Pertussis and Rubella Vaccines. Washington, DC, National Academy Press, 1991, pp 65–124.
281. Institute of Medicine. Measles and mumps vaccines. In Stratton KR, Howe CJ, Johnston RB Jr (eds). Adverse Events Associated with Childhood Vaccines: Evidence Bearing on Causality. Washington, DC, National Academy Press; 1994, pp 118–186.
282. Krober MS, Stracener CE, Bass JW. Decreased measles antibody response after measles-mumps-rubella vaccine in infants with colds. JAMA 265:2095–2096, 1991.
283. Wald ER, Dashefsky B, Byers C, et al. Frequency and severity of infections in day care. J Pediatr 112:540–546, 1988.
284. Centers for Disease Control. Measles—Dade County, Florida. MMWR Morb Mortal Wkly Rep 36:45–48, 1987.
285. Hutchins SS, Escolan J, Markowitz LE, et al. Measles outbreak among unvaccinated preschool-aged children: Opportunities missed by health care providers to administer measles vaccine. Pediatrics 83:369–374, 1989.
286. Farizo KM, Stehr-Green PA, Markowitz LE, Patriarca PA. Vaccination levels and missed opportunities for measles vaccination: A record audit in a public pediatric clinic. Pediatrics 89:589–592, 1992.
287. Lewis T, Osborn LM, Lewis K, et al. Influence of parental knowledge and opinions on 12-month diphtheria, tetanus, and pertussis vaccination rates. Am J Dis Child 142:283–286, 1988.
288. McConnochie KM, Roghmann KJ. Immunization opportunities missed among urban poor children. Pediatrics 89:1019–1026, 1992.
289. Centers for Disease Control and Prevention. Standards for pediatric immunization practices. MMWR Morb Mortal Wkly Rep 42(RR-5):1–13, 1993.
290. American Academy of Pediatrics. Hepatitis B. In Peter C (ed). 1997 Redbook: Report of the Committee on Infectious Diseases (24th ed). Elk Grove Village, IL, American Academy of Pediatrics, 1997, pp 247–260.
291. Centers for Disease Control and Prevention. Measles pneumonitis following measles-mumps-rubella vaccination of a patient with HIV infection, 1993. MMWR Morb Mortal Wkly Rep 45:603–606, 1996.

chapter

6 Smallpox and Vaccinia

Donald A. Henderson

Bernard Moss

Smallpox is now a disease of historical interest only, its eradication having been certified by the World Health Assembly on May 8, 1980.[1] An exanthematous viral disease, it was once prevalent throughout the world, existing as an endemic infection wherever concentrations of population were sufficient to sustain transmission. Outbreaks of variola major, the only known variety until the end of the 19th century, resulted in case-fatality rates of 20% or more. Most of those who survived had distinctive residual facial pockmarks, and some were blind. A second variety, variola minor, produced less severe illness and was associated with case-fatality rates of 1% or less. It was first described in South Africa by de Korte[2] and in the United States by Chapin[3] and subsequently became the prevalent variety throughout the United States, parts of South America, and Europe as well as some areas of eastern and southern Africa.[4]

Because there was no animal reservoir of smallpox and no human carriers, the virus had to spread continually from human to human to survive. Thus, historians speculate that it must have emerged sometime after the first agricultural settlements, about 10,000 BC.[5] The first certain evidence of smallpox in the ancient world comes from mummified remains of the 18th Egyptian dynasty (1580 to 1350 BC) and of the better known Ramses V (1157 BC).[6] Written descriptions of the disease, however, did not appear until the 4th century AD in China[7] and the 10th century in southwestern Asia.[8]

From northeastern Africa, smallpox was probably carried by Egyptian traders to India during the first millennium BC,[4] where it became established as an endemic infection. Whether smallpox persisted in Africa is uncertain. Although epidemics of disease are described in the Bible and in Greek and Roman literature, descriptions of clinical signs are sparse. Only one of these epidemics can be identified with some certainty as smallpox.[7] It occurred in Athens beginning in 430 BC and is described by Thucydides. There is, however, no original Greek or Latin word for smallpox despite its distinctive rash.[9] From the populated endemic areas of Asia and perhaps Africa, smallpox spread with increasing frequency into less populous areas of these continents and into Europe, becoming established as an endemic infection when populations increased sufficiently in number.

The name *variola* was first used during the 6th century by Bishop Marius of Avenches (Switzerland), the word being derived from the Latin *varius* (spotted) or *varus* (pimple).[10] Although Marius provides no clinical description of the disease concerned, there is little doubt that smallpox had already become endemic in some areas of Europe by this time.[7] In the Anglo-Saxon world, by the 10th century, the word *poc* or *pocca*, a bag or pouch, described an exanthematous disease, possibly smallpox, and English accounts began to use the word *pockes*. With the appearance of syphilis in Europe in the late 15th century, writers began to use the prefix *small* to distinguish variola, the smallpox, from syphilis, the great pox.[11]

In the early 16th century, smallpox began to be imported into the Western Hemisphere. Catastrophic epidemics followed, which literally decimated Amerindian tribes and resulted in the collapse of both the Aztec and Incan empires.[5] Central and southern Africa probably became endemic for smallpox about this time or soon thereafter.

The impact of smallpox on history and human affairs was profound.[7] Deities to smallpox became a part of the cultures of India, China, and parts of Africa. In Europe, as of the end of the 18th century, an estimated 400,000 persons died annually from smallpox, and survivors accounted for one third of all cases of blindness. During the 18th century alone, five reigning European monarchs died of smallpox, and the Austrian Hapsburg line of succession shifted four times in four generations.

A method for protection against naturally acquired smallpox infection appears to have been discovered in India sometime before AD 1000.[12, 13] There it became the practice to deliberately inoculate, either into the skin or by nasal insufflation, scabs or pustular material from lesions of patients. This practice resulted in an infection that was usually less severe than an infection acquired naturally by inhalation of droplets. From India, the practice spread to China, western Asia, and Africa and finally, in the early 18th century, to Europe and North America.[14] Case-fatality rates associated with variolation, as it was called, were about one tenth as great as when infection was naturally acquired, but those infected in this manner were capable of transmitting smallpox by

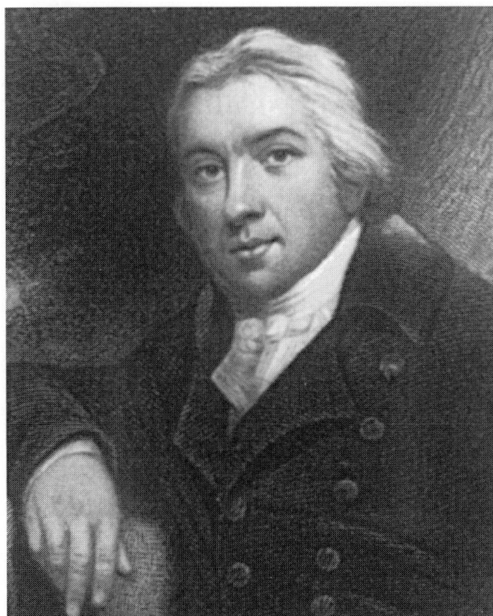

Figure 6–1. Edward Jenner (1749–1823) demonstrated that a person inoculated and infected with cowpox was protected against smallpox. The procedure, which he called vaccination, represented the first use of a vaccine in the prevention of disease. (Courtesy of the Institute of the History of Medicine, The Johns Hopkins University, Baltimore, MD.)

droplet inhalation to others. After cowpox began to be used as a protective vaccine, the practice of variolation diminished. Even as recently as the 1960s and 1970s, however, variolation continued to be performed among remote populations in some parts of Ethiopia, western Africa, Afghanistan, and Pakistan.[4]

In 1796, Edward Jenner (Fig. 6–1) demonstrated that material could be taken from a human pustular lesion caused by cowpox virus (i.e., an orthopoxvirus closely related to variola virus) and inoculated into the skin of another person, producing a similar infection.[15] He showed that the individual was protected from inoculation with smallpox after recovery. He called the material *vaccine*, from the Latin *vacca*, meaning cow, and the process *vaccination*. Pasteur,[16] in recognition of Jenner's discovery, later broadened the term to denote preventive inoculation with other agents. Jenner's discovery, one of the most important in medical history, was immediately recognized for its significance. Within 5 years, his paper had been translated into six other languages,[17] and the vaccine had begun to be employed widely in many countries of Europe; within a decade, it had been transported to countries throughout the world. The chronicles of the de Balmis expedition of 1803 to 1806 vividly describe the transport of the vaccine by sea to Spanish colonies in the Americas and Asia by arm-to-arm vaccination of orphaned children.[18, 19]

As the 19th century progressed, however, the initial wave of enthusiasm for vaccination subsided when difficulties were experienced in sustaining the virus through arm-to-arm inoculation and when it was found that, on some occasions, syphilis was transmitted in the process.[20, 21] Although vaccination material, dried on threads or ivory points, could be transported over long distances, it was often found, on receipt, to be noninfectious. When fresh material was sought, problems occurred in finding cows or horses with infections caused by cowpox or a related orthopoxvirus.[22] In some areas, significant opposition occurred among religious leaders and antivaccinationist societies who opposed the principle of infecting humans with an animal disease.[23] Confidence in the procedure was also diminished by the occurrence of smallpox in some who had previously been successfully vaccinated. Jenner had forcefully contended that protection was lifelong, as was the case after natural smallpox, but it soon became apparent that this was not so. Although the need for revaccination was demonstrated early in the century,[24] this practice was not widely accepted until many decades later.

Growth of the virus on the flank of a calf offered the prospect for provision of an adequate and safer supply of vaccine material. Although this approach was employed in Italy as early as 1805,[25] it appears to have been unknown elsewhere until it was more widely publicized at a medical congress in 1864.[26] Thereafter, the practice was gradually adopted in other countries, although arm-to-arm vaccination in England, for example, continued until it was finally banned in 1898.[27] With an ensured source of vaccinia, the numbers of vaccinations in Europe increased, and the incidence of smallpox in the more industrialized countries diminished more rapidly. Not until after World War I, however, did most of Europe become smallpox free, and not until after World War II was transmission stopped throughout Europe and North America.

In most other parts of the world, especially in tropical and semitropical areas and in the less developed countries, smallpox continued largely unabated until the middle of the 20th century. In these countries, continuing difficulties were experienced in sustaining the virus through arm-to-arm inoculation. After calves began to be used for vaccine production, the harvested vaccine remained viable for only 1 or 2 days at ambient temperatures, thus limiting its widespread application. The only control programs that were notably successful were those in Indonesia and in certain of the French colonies, which, in the 1920s, began using a specially prepared and more stable air-dried[28] or freeze-dried[29] vaccine.

In the late 1940s, a commercially feasible process for large-scale production of a stable freeze-dried vaccine was perfected by Collier.[30] This process offered vastly better possibilities for smallpox control. Recognizing the value of such a vaccine, the Pan American Sanitary Organization[31] decided, in 1950, to undertake a hemisphere-wide eradication program and by 1967 succeeded in eliminating smallpox from all countries of the Americas except Brazil. Meanwhile, in 1958, the Union of Soviet Socialist Republics proposed to the World Health Assembly that a global smallpox eradication program be undertaken,[32] and this was so decided the following year.[33] Some progress was made during the period from 1959 to 1966, but the results overall were disappointing. Finally, in 1966, the World Health Assembly decided to intensify the eradication program by providing additional funds specifically for this effort.[34]

During 1967, the year the Intensified Global Eradication Program began, an estimated 10 to 15 million smallpox cases[1] occurred in 31 countries in which the disease was endemic. The campaign was based on a twofold strategy: (1) mass vaccination campaigns in each country, using vaccine of ensured potency and stability that would reach at least 80% of the population and that would be assessed by independent teams, and (2) development of a system to detect and contain cases and outbreaks.[35] Numerous problems had to be surmounted, including deficient supervision and discipline in national health services, epidemic smallpox among refugees fleeing areas stricken by civil war and famine, shortages of funds and vaccine, and a host of other problems posed by difficult terrain, climate, and cultural beliefs.[36–38] Despite the problems, steady progress was made, and on October 26, 1977, the last known naturally occurring case of smallpox was recorded in Merka, Somalia.[39] Two further cases occurred in 1978 as a result of a laboratory infection in Birmingham, England,[40] but these cases were the last. Detailed accounts of national programs are provided in books dealing with those in India,[41, 42] Bangladesh,[43] Ethiopia,[44] and Somalia.[45]

An extensively illustrated volume entitled *Smallpox and Its Eradication*[4] provides a detailed account of the eradication campaign as well as an overall account of progress in smallpox control throughout history. It also gives a description of the virology, the clinical features, and the pathogenesis of the disease. Complementing this text is a historical record of smallpox, *Princes and Peasants*, by Hopkins.[7]

BACKGROUND

Clinical Description

Smallpox had an incubation period of about 12 days, with a range of 7 to 17 days. A 2- to 5-day period of high fever, malaise, and prostration with headache and backache was followed by the development of a maculopapular rash. The rash appeared first on the mucosa of the mouth and pharynx, the face, and the forearms and spread to the trunk and legs. Within 1 to 2 days, the rash became vesicular and then pustular. The pustules were characteristically round, tense, and deeply embedded in the dermis; crusts began to form about the eighth or ninth day. When they separated, they left pigment-free skin and, eventually, pitted scars. The eruption was characteristically more extensive on the face and distal parts of the arms and legs (Fig. 6–2), and lesions were occasionally found on the palms and soles. Death, when it occurred, was usually late in the first week or during the second week of the illness and was commonly due to the effects of an overwhelming viremia. On occasion, a severe and always fatal hemorrhagic form occurred, with extensive bleeding into the skin and gastrointestinal tract, followed by death within a few days.

Illness caused by variola major was generally more severe, with a more extensive rash, a higher fever, and a greater degree of prostration, than illness caused by variola minor. A milder form of disease was also seen among those who had previously been vaccinated; the rash in such persons tended to be more scant and atypical and the evolution of lesions more rapid.

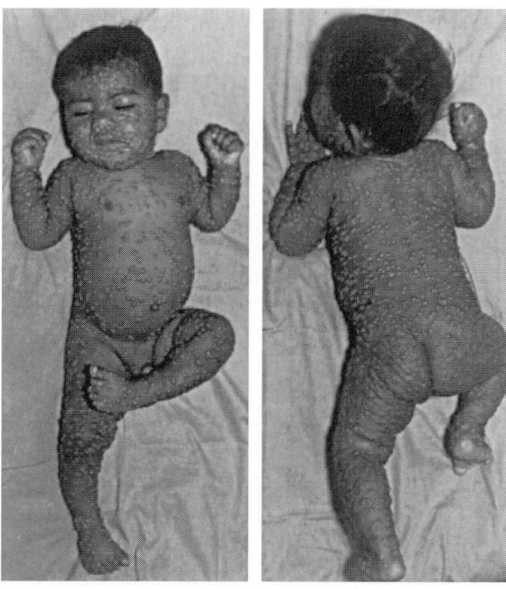

Figure 6–2. A typical case of variola major about 7 days after the onset of rash. (World Health Organization Smallpox Recognition Card.)

Cases of smallpox among pregnant women often resulted in spontaneous abortion of the fetus or a stillborn infant with evidence of lesions on the skin.

Virology

Variola virus belongs to the genus *Orthopoxvirus*, family Poxviridae, which includes the agents of vaccinia, monkeypox, cowpox, camelpox, and ectromelia.[46] All species exhibit extensive serological cross-reactivity, both in in vitro tests and in experimental animals. The poxvirus genome, the largest of all virions, is a brick-shaped structure with a diameter of about 200 nm, consisting of a single molecule of a double-stranded DNA. It differs from most other DNA viruses in that it multiplies in the cytoplasm rather than in the nucleus of susceptible cells.

The orthopoxviruses grow and produce a cytoplasmic effect in cultured cells derived from many species,[47, 48] although they generally grow best in cells from humans and other primates. The four that infect humans (variola, vaccinia, cowpox, and monkeypox viruses), however, cannot be differentiated readily from one another in most cell cultures. For diagnostic purposes, therefore, they are customarily grown on the chorioallantoic membrane of 10- to 12-day-old chick embryos on which they produce pocks characteristic of their species.[49]

Pathogenesis

Natural smallpox infection occurred by implantation of variola virus on the oropharyngeal or respiratory mucosa. Virions in droplets expressed from nasal and oropharyngeal secretions were far more infectious than those bound in the fibrin mesh of scabs. After migration to and multiplication in regional lymph nodes, an asymptomatic viremia developed about the third or fourth day, followed by multiplication of virus in the spleen, bone marrow, and lymph nodes. A secondary viremia began about the eighth day, accompanied by fever and toxemia. The virus, contained in leukocytes, then localized in small blood vessels of the dermis and beneath the oral and pharyngeal mucosa and subsequently infected adjacent cells. In the skin, this process resulted in the characteristic maculopapular lesions and, later, the vesicular and pustular lesions, which, for reasons unknown, were more extensive on the face and distal extremities. Lesions in the mouth and pharynx ulcerated quickly because of the absence of a stratum corneum, releasing large amounts of virus into the saliva about the time the cutaneous rash first became visible. Virus titers in saliva were highest during the first week of illness, corresponding with the period during which patients were most infectious.

Hemagglutinin-inhibiting (HI) and neutralizing antibodies could be detected beginning about the sixth day of illness, or about 18 days after infection, and complement-fixing (CF) antibodies approximately 2 days later.[50, 51] Neutralizing antibodies were long lasting, whereas HI antibodies declined to low levels within 5 years, and CF antibodies rarely persisted for longer than 6 months. Little is known about the development of cell-mediated immunity.

Vaccinia-induced antibody responses were more rapid. They could be detected as early as the 10th day[52] after primary vaccination and within a week of revaccination. This accelerated response was associated with complete or partial protection of persons vaccinated at or soon after exposure.

Except for the lesions in the skin and mucous membranes and reticulum cell hyperplasia, other organs were seldom involved in variola infection. Secondary bacterial infection was not common, and death, when it occurred, probably resulted from the toxemia associated with circulating immune complexes and soluble variola antigens.[53] Encephalitis sometimes ensued that was indistinguishable from the acute perivascular demyelination observed as a complication of infection due to vaccinia, measles, and varicella.

As the patient recovered, the scabs separated and the characteristic pitted scarring gradually developed (Fig. 6–3). The scars were most evident on the face and resulted from the destruction of sebaceous glands followed by shrinking of granulation tissue and fibrosis.

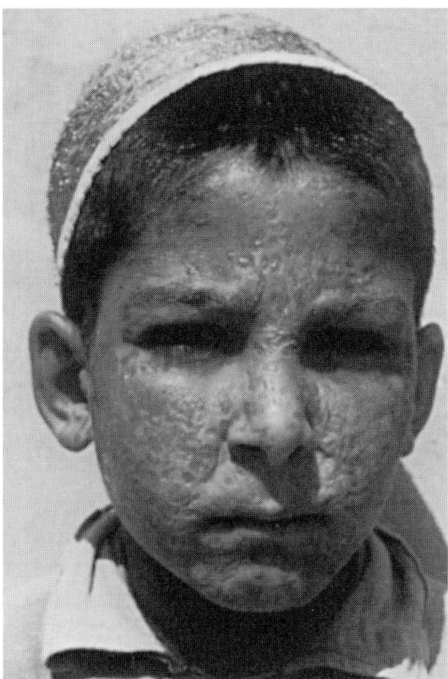

Figure 6–3. An Afghani boy with characteristic residual facial scars after smallpox. (Courtesy of the World Health Organization, Geneva, Switzerland.)

Diagnosis

Most cases of smallpox were able to be diagnosed readily by the appearance of the typical deep-seated rash, the centrifugal distribution of lesions, and the fact that all lesions were at the same stage of development on any given area of the body. The infrequent hemorrhagic cases were often initially misdiagnosed as meningococcemia, acute leukemia, or drug toxicity, but their identity was soon established by examination of other patients who were the source of infection or to whom disease had been transmitted. Varicella was by far the most frequent disease to be confused with smallpox. Smallpox patients who had previously been vaccinated and those with variola minor sometimes exhibited a sparse and sometimes atypical rash with minimal systemic symptoms that resembled varicella; severe cases of varicella in adults with extensive rash were also sometimes mistaken for smallpox.[54]

Diagnosis of a poxvirus infection can be rapidly confirmed by electron microscopic identification of virus particles in vesicular or pustular fluid or scabs. Differentiation as to which orthopoxvirus is the responsible agent is usually apparent from its characteristics of growth on the chorioallantoic membrane of chick embryos, although confirmation by other biological tests is sometimes necessary.

Recovered patients exhibit high titers of neutralizing, HI, and CF orthopoxvirus antibodies, but cross-absorption studies are required to identify which of the orthopoxvirus species is the agent responsible for illness. Characteristic residual facial scars are most useful in documenting prior cases of variola major,[55] but such scars were too infrequent to be of value in identifying recovered cases of variola minor.[56]

EPIDEMIOLOGY

Transmission

Transmission of variola virus, with few exceptions, resulted from droplets expressed by a patient from the oral, nasal, or pharyngeal mucosa that were inhaled by susceptible persons in close contact with the patient. Such transmission was possible from the time of onset of rash and was most frequent during the first week of the exanthem. Virus was also present in high titer in scabs that had separated from the skin lesions.[57] Epidemiological evidence showed that infected scabs played a negligible role in transmission of infection, presumably because the virus was tightly bound in its fibrin matrix. It was standard practice, nevertheless, during the global eradication program, to isolate patients until all scabs had separated from the skin. Airborne infection over longer distances was uncommon, although two outbreaks within hospitals demonstrated this to be possible.[58, 59] The infection of persons such as laundry workers who handled linen from patients has also been repeatedly documented.[9] However, various older accounts that purport to document transmission over great distances on other fomites, such as carpets, letters, and cotton rags, are suspect because the virus does not survive for long periods at customary ambient temperatures.[60]

Another method of transmission, the ancient practice of variolation (inoculation into the skin of material from pustules or scabs from patients), continued in a number of remote areas until August 1976 and was responsible for many cases in Afghanistan and Ethiopia. Those individuals so inoculated often developed extensive rash and transmitted infection to susceptible contacts by droplet infection.

Geographical Scope and Epidemiological Characteristics

Smallpox was once worldwide in scope, persisting as an endemic disease in areas where susceptible populations were sufficiently large to permit year-round transmission. In more remote or isolated areas, epidemics occurred when the disease was introduced, but because infection resulted in essentially permanent immunity, transmission eventually ceased when the number of susceptible contacts diminished to low numbers. Before vaccination was practiced, almost everyone eventually contracted the disease.

When a vaccine became available, its introduction followed a common pattern, at first being most extensively used among middle- and upper-income groups in or near cities where the vaccine was produced and in more prosperous countries. Thus, during recent years, smallpox incidence was highest among lower socioeconomic groups in urban areas and in the rural areas of developing countries.

The seasonal occurrence of smallpox was similar to that of varicella and measles, its incidence being highest during winter and spring. This factor was consonant with the observation that the duration of survival of the virus in the aerosolized form was inversely proportional to both temperature and humidity.[61] Such seasonal variation was undoubtedly amplified in many countries by social events, such as the congregation of large numbers of people during the dry season at festivals and marriage parties, and the movement of nomads during this period. Where there was less variation in temperature and humidity, as in equatorial areas of Indonesia and Zaire (now the Democratic Republic of Congo), there was little discernible fluctuation in incidence throughout the year.

There were also longer term trends in incidence in the endemic areas, which resulted in major epidemics at intervals of 4 to 7 years,[4, 62] presumably relating to an accumulation of susceptible persons and in part consequent to events, such as famine and civil war, that resulted in extensive refugee movements and widespread dissemination of the virus.

Within the household, smallpox was as infectious as chickenpox but less infectious than measles.[63–65] With few exceptions, however, smallpox spread less widely and rapidly than these diseases. This finding can be accounted for by the fact that transmission of variola virus did not occur until onset of rash, as attested by numerous epidemiological observations. By then, most patients were already confined to bed because of the high fever and malaise of the prodromal illness; secondary cases were usually restricted to the few who came in contact with them in the household or hospital. On average, a given case of smallpox seldom resulted in more than two to five cases in a subsequent generation, most of whom were relatives or friends. For this reason, smallpox outbreaks tended to be clustered in a segment of a town or village and in localized areas of a province or district.[66–69] Most outbreaks, therefore, could be contained successfully by vaccination of a comparatively small number of residents in and near the houses in which patients lived.

The age distribution of smallpox cases depended on the acquired immunity of the population, whether by vaccination or by infection. Cases among adults were regularly found, however, even as recently as 1974 to 1975 in India, where vaccination had been widely practiced and smallpox was endemic (Table 6–1). During this period, 21% of a carefully documented series of 23,546 patients were older than 20 years, and 2% or 412 of these patients were older than 50 years. In western Africa during the 1967 to 1969 period, most cases were in rural villages, and the age distribution of cases approximated the age profile of the population.[70] In all countries, males and females were equally affected.

Where the Asian form of variola major was prevalent, case-fatality rates were about 20% overall, but for those younger than 1 year, they ranged from 40 to 50%.

Table 6–1. **INDIA: CASES OF SMALLPOX, DEATHS, AND CASE-FATALITY RATES, BY AGE GROUP, 1974 TO 1975**

AGE GROUP (yr)	NUMBER OF CASES (% DISTRIBUTION BY AGE)	NUMBER OF DEATHS	CASE-FATALITY RATE (%)
<1	1373(6)	597	43.5
1–4	5867(25)	1436	24.5
5–9	5875(25)	783	13.3
10–19	5542(23)	432	7.8
≥20	4889(21)	855	17.5
Total	23,546(100)	4103	17.4

From Basu RN, Jesek Z, Ward NA. The eradication of smallpox from India. In History of International Public Health No. 2. New Delhi, World Health Organization, South-East Asia Regional Office, 1979, p 59.

Variola major in Africa was a somewhat milder disease, with age-standardized, case-fatality rates 20 to 30% lower. Variola minor, which after 1967 was present only in Brazil and southern and eastern Africa, resulted in case-fatality rates of 1% or less.

The Significance of Smallpox as a Public Health Problem

During recent centuries, smallpox was the most universally feared of all diseases. It could occur and spread in any country, and case-fatality rates were little altered by therapy. It was not dependent on a vector; thus, in contrast to malaria or yellow fever, it could occur anywhere in any season. Better sanitation and improved economic conditions diminished the concern for diseases such as cholera and typhoid, but such measures had little influence on smallpox.

Jenner's discovery of a protective inoculation was understandably lauded, and although it conferred a high level of protection, periodic revaccination was necessary. No country was able to sustain a vaccination program that ensured that everyone in the population was fully protected at all times; thus, all countries feared possible smallpox importations and subsequent spread. For this reason, through the mid-1970s, all countries required travelers to present certificates attesting to the fact that they had been vaccinated within the preceding 3 years. Even those countries that were smallpox free continued national vaccination programs in the belief that this practice would serve to impede the spread of disease, if it were introduced. When importations occurred, they were frequently accompanied by public hysteria and a demand for mass vaccination.

The costs of preventive measures for smallpox were substantial. Sencer and Axnick[71] documented activities and expenditures for smallpox control in the United States during 1968, nearly 20 years after its last case of smallpox. In all, nearly 15 million persons were vaccinated that year, and because of vaccine complications, 240 required hospitalization, 9 died, and 4 were permanently disabled. The total costs to the country, including the costs of quarantine services, were estimated to be $150 million. Other countries, such as the United Kingdom and the Federal Republic of Germany, maintained special buildings to be opened for the hospitalization of patients when imported cases of smallpox occurred. When importations occurred, extreme measures were frequently taken, such as in Yugoslavia in 1972 when the entire population was vaccinated, borders were closed to commerce, and thousands who had possibly been exposed were isolated in hotels coopted for this purpose.[72]

Although the concern was great, importations of smallpox into industrialized Europe, North America, and Japan were relatively infrequent after 1958. There was a total of only 36 episodes, with none after 1973.[4] These episodes resulted in 574 cases and 90 deaths, more than half being the result of exposure to patients in hospitals.[73] Most importations resulted from improperly vaccinated visitors returning from Bangladesh, India, and Pakistan, although importations from Africa and South America were also documented.

Countries in the endemic regions of the world experienced more frequent importations because of travelers and nomads moving freely across long open borders and serving to reinfect persons in countries that had become smallpox free. Relative to the extent and numbers of travelers, however, importations were comparatively few. This reflected the fact that smallpox outbreaks tended to remain localized, usually spread by relatives or friends to adjacent houses or villages in an area. Those who traveled were usually adults who were immune from smallpox as a result of past infections or immunizations; those who traveled long distances by plane tended to be fairly affluent and thus better vaccinated and with less contact with the lower socioeconomic groups and rural peoples, among whom most cases occurred.

ACTIVE IMMUNIZATION

Vaccine Strains

Strains of Vaccine and Their Passage. Many strains of vaccinia, known by different names, have been used by different producers during this and the past century, but little is known about their origins or passage histories. Characterization of strains is further complicated by the fact that a seed lot system for vaccine production was not used until the 1960s. Thus, even those strains with common names and ancestors have different passage histories, having been passed sequentially through a variety of vaccinifers, such as cows, sheep, and water buffalo, with periodic passages through rabbits, horses, and even humans. Indicative of the ignorance of vaccine technology until recent decades is a statement of the Ministry of Health of Great Britain, which, in 1928,[74] advised that seed lymph could be obtained from (1) "smallpox direct"; (2) cowpox; (3) horsepox, sheep-pox, or goatpox; and (4) vaccinia in the human body.

Jenner is believed to have used cowpox in vaccination, but the vaccinia virus strains used most recently are a different species of orthopoxvirus with distinctive DNA maps that are similar to each other but different from both cowpox and variola. That the vaccinia strains are not mutants of variola virus seems certain,[75] but where the present vaccinia species arose is unknown. It may have arisen either as a hybrid of cowpox and another orthopoxvirus or through thousands of serial passages under artificial conditions of culture. It is also possible that the species represents a laboratory survivor of a now naturally extinct species of orthopoxvirus.[76]

In 1958, a World Health Organization (WHO) Study Group first recommended that a seed lot system be employed in vaccine manufacture. Beginning in 1967, an increasing number of vaccine producers, encouraged by the WHO, began to use one of two strains. Most common was the Lister strain from the Lister Institute, England, which was propagated as seed virus by the National Public Health Institute of the Netherlands for distribution by the WHO. The second strain was the New York City Board of Health strain, propagated by

Wyeth Laboratories, Radnor, Pennsylvania, United States. Two of the largest countries, China and India, used other strains called, respectively, the Temple of Heaven strain and the Patwadanger strain.

During the 1930s, vaccinia strains began to be attenuated by serial passages in an effort to diminish the incidence of complications; the first was the Rivers strain, which was derived from the New York City Board of Health strain.[77] Three principal variants were developed that had been passed repeatedly through rabbit testis, chick embryo explants, and chorioallantoic membranes of embryonated hens' eggs.[78] Rivers and colleagues[79, 80] showed that the "second revived strain" produced less severe reactions in rabbits and humans than did the New York City Board of Health strain, especially if it was inoculated intradermally. This strain, administered with 2 mL of vaccinia immunoglobulin, was used for primary vaccination of 60,000 Dutch army recruits by van der Noordaa and colleagues.[81] One mild case of postvaccinal encephalitis occurred, but this was a lower incidence than that noted after administration of other strains. The resultant neutralizing antibody titers, however, were lower than those usually observed. This called into question the level of protection provided against smallpox, and the strain was not further employed.

Another variant of the Rivers vaccine, the CVI-78 strain, was also found to produce less severe local reactions, and although used to vaccinate children with eczema,[82] it was not thought likely to provide adequate protection against smallpox.[83] A large-scale comparative trial sponsored by the National Institutes of Health[84, 85] showed that the CVI-78 strain was 10-fold less infectious than the Lister strain and New York City Board of Health strains and produced smaller skin lesions and fewer febrile responses. Only 30% of children, however, exhibited neutralizing antibody, and after challenge vaccination with a standard strain, 25% still did not respond with neutralizing antibody.

Another attenuated vaccine, the modified vaccinia virus Ankara (MVA) strain produced by Stickl and collaborators[86] through passage in chick embryo fibroblast cells, had characteristics similar to those of the CVI-78 strain.[87] Some workers believed that a sequential vaccination schedule using the CVI-78 or MVA strain, followed after some months by application of a conventional strain, offered prospects for protection against smallpox with fewer complications. However, whether persons without neutralizing antibody response would be protected against natural challenge remained an unanswered question.

A more satisfactory attenuated strain, LC 16m8, was produced by Hashizume[88–90] through passage at low temperature in rabbit kidney cells. This strain produced a satisfactory immune response in humans (HI and neutralizing antibodies), and in a field trial of 50,000 persons, it was found to produce a markedly lower frequency of reactions than that noted for other strains.[91] However, the achievement of smallpox eradication precluded use of this vaccine under circumstances of natural challenge.

Dosage and Route. The vaccine is inoculated intradermally with use of a bifurcated needle. Vaccine, as reconstituted for use with the bifurcated needle, is required to have a titer of not less than 10^8 pock-forming units per milliliter when it is assayed on the chorioallantoic membranes of 12-day-old chick embryos. Approximately 0.0025 mL of vaccine adheres by capillarity to the tines of the needle when it is dipped into the vaccine. The needle is positioned vertically to the skin surface, usually the lateral surface of the upper arm (Fig. 6–4), and 5 to 15 rapid strokes are made. These strokes are sufficiently vigorous that within 20 to 30 seconds, a trace of blood appears at the vaccination site.

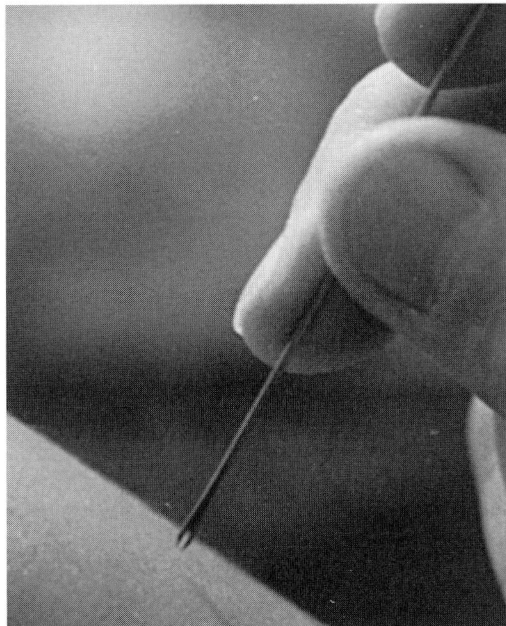

Figure 6–4. The bifurcated needle positioned to begin multiple puncture vaccination. (Courtesy of the World Health Organization, Geneva, Switzerland.)

Constituents of Vaccine. Most vaccine now available for use is grown on the skin of a calf and harvested after sacrifice of the animal. The vaccine is purified by the addition of fluorocarbon and differential centrifugation, and its bacterial content is reduced by the addition of phenol. Peptone is added as a stabilizing agent, and the vaccine is freeze-dried. Because of its source, the vaccine inevitably contains some bacteria, but properly prepared, the number of bacteria is 10/mL or less. Microbiological examination must confirm that none is a human pathogen. For reconstitution of the vaccine for multiple puncture vaccination, a solution of 50% (volume per volume) glycerin in McIlvaine solution is used; for vaccine intended for jet injection, saline is used.

Laboratories in Brazil, New Zealand, Sweden, and the United States (e.g., Texas State Health Department) harvested vaccinia virus from the chorioallantoic membranes of chick embryos, a simple process that permits production of a bacteria-free vaccine. However, vaccine from this source proved difficult to produce in a satisfactory thermostabile freeze-dried form, and as far as is known, only Sweden produced the vaccine in eggs that were free of avian leukosis virus.

Vaccinia virus grown in tissue culture also proved difficult to produce as a thermostabile freeze-dried product, but Hekker and colleagues[92] eventually achieved this result using primary rabbit kidney cells. In field trials, the vaccine was comparable to vaccine grown on calf skin,[93, 94] but because of the approaching conclusion of the smallpox eradication program, the WHO made no effort to introduce the method for use in other laboratories.

Producers. Because of the eradication of smallpox and the cessation of routine vaccination, the number of production laboratories diminished from 76 in 1977 to 11 in 1985. The few remaining laboratories are in the industrialized countries and are engaged only in the preparation of finished vaccine from bulk preparations harvested in quantity some years ago and preserved by freezing. Virus grown in tissue culture is available in the Netherlands (Lister strain) and Japan (LC 16m8 strain); other countries use vaccine grown on calf skin (primarily Lister and New York City Board of Health strains).

Storage Conditions. Freeze-dried smallpox vaccine is the most stable of currently available vaccines. The vaccine can be preserved indefinitely at −20°C and most batches are equally well preserved at 4°C. International standards require that the vaccine in its freeze-dried form maintain full potency when it is incubated at 37°C for 1 month. Studies of vaccine produced at the Lister Institute, however, demonstrated that the vaccine retained full potency for 64 weeks when it was incubated at temperatures of up to 45°C and for 104 weeks at 37°C.[95] Not all vaccines were this stable, but assay of vaccines produced in India and the former USSR and retrieved from the field revealed batches of vaccine that met potency standards after 6 to 9 months of exposure at high ambient summer temperatures. After reconstitution, the vaccine is much more sensitive both to temperature and to exposure to direct light. During the eradication program, unused reconstituted vaccine was routinely discarded at the end of each day, although it can be preserved in this form for at least 1 week at 4°C.

Results of Vaccination

Immune Response. After primary vaccination, neutralizing and HI antibodies develop about the 10th day and are present in almost all persons by the end of 2 weeks; CF antibodies develop in less than half of the vacinees.[52] Because the antibody response after primary vaccination usually occurs 4 to 8 days earlier than the response after naturally acquired smallpox infection,[96] primary vaccination even after exposure sometimes modified or aborted an overt attack of smallpox. The neutralizing antibodies are most persistent and may be detected for 20 years or more; HI and CF antibodies, however, are usually not detectable beyond 6 months. Little is known about the cell-mediated immunity that is induced, although Pincus and Flick[97] demonstrated the beginning development of delayed hypersensitivity, an index of cell-mediated immunity, as early as 2 days after vaccination. Antibody response after revaccination is more rapid, usually within 7 days, and antibody titers are generally higher. However, some persons who exhibit a substantial rise in neutralizing antibody titer after revaccination fail to exhibit a rise in either HI or CF antibody levels.

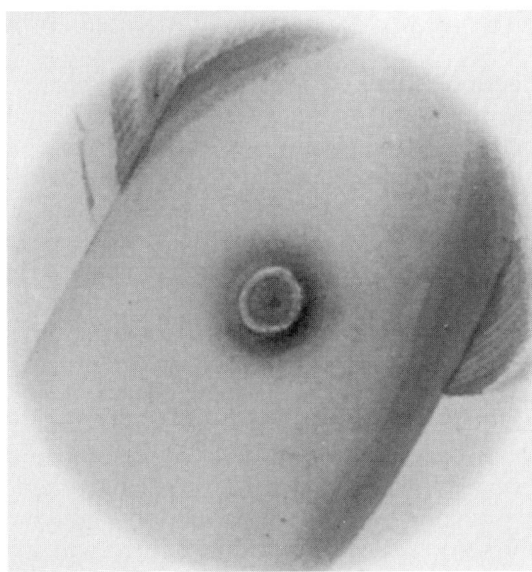

Figure 6–5. A primary vaccination response on the ninth day after inoculation shows erythema surrounding a pustular lesion. Although the picture is from a colored drawing made by Captain C. Gold in 1801, the lesion shown is indistinguishable from contemporary responses to primary vaccination. (Courtesy of the Library, London, Wellcome Institute for the History of Medicine.)

Successful primary vaccination results in virus proliferation in the basal cells of the epidermis, producing the typical jennerian vesicle (Fig. 6–5). A papule with surrounding erythema develops in 3 to 5 days, rapidly becoming a vesicle and later a pustule. It reaches its maximum size after 8 to 12 days. A scab forms that separates at 14 to 21 days, leaving a typical vaccination scar. A low-grade fever usually accompanies the development of the pustule, and swelling of the draining lymph nodes, associated with tenderness, is often observed. Viremia may occasionally occur[98] between the third and tenth days, and vaccinia virus can sometimes be isolated from tonsillar swabs.[99]

An individual's response to revaccination depends on the level of immunity. Erythema typically develops within 24 to 48 hours as a classic delayed hypersensitivity reaction. As Benenson[100] has shown, this reaction can be elicited with both live and inactivated vaccine. Persons with some residual cell-mediated immunity, but not enough to inhibit viral replication, develop erythema and sometimes a pustule at the site of a vesicle, both of which evolve in a sequence more rapid than that in a primary vaccination reaction. Those with substantial immunity may experience no more than the hypersensitivity reaction.

Because it is impossible to distinguish between a hypersensitivity reaction due to the use of impotent vaccine and a similar reaction due to a high level of immunity, the WHO Expert Committee on Smallpox[101] recommended that such a response be termed an *equivocal reaction*. For persons with equivocal reactions, repeated vaccinations were advised. Others who exhibited evidence of virus proliferation at 6 to 8 days, as manifested by a pustular lesion or an area of induration surrounding a central lesion, were said to have experienced a *major reaction*.

Protection Afforded by Vaccination. Reliable data are surprisingly sparse as to the efficacy and durability of protection afforded by vaccination. Before 1967, when the intensified global eradication program began, revaccination every 3 to 10 years was considered essential to ensure protection. In part, this practice was based on early data largely from the United Kingdom, such as those provided by Hanna,[102] and on more recent data from India,[103] which compared the frequency of cases among those with and without vaccination scars. However, the vaccine in use in the populations studied was far lower in titer than that used after 1967; most of the vaccine was heavily contaminated with bacteria. In India, the vaccination instrument that was used (i.e., the rotary lancet) was found to produce localized sepsis and an apparent scar, even when only the diluent was applied. Estimates of protection after successful vaccination were therefore almost certainly understated in these as in other early studies. Another observation that suggested that protection might persist for no more than 3 to 5 years was the increasing proportion of persons who exhibited a major reaction to revaccination beginning about this time. Mistakenly, resistance to intradermal inoculation with vaccinia virus was equated with resistance to variola virus acquired by droplet inhalation.

From studies conducted after 1967, it became apparent that vaccinial immunity was far more durable than most investigators believed. It was found that with the available higher titer vaccines, major reactions could be induced in persons successfully vaccinated as recently as 3 to 6 months before and, indeed, in almost all of those who had experienced smallpox only 1 year previously.[104] Because natural infection effectively confers permanent immunity, it was apparent that the ability of vaccinia virus to proliferate on inoculation into the basal cells of the dermis correlated poorly with the level of protection afforded against natural infection. Moreover, in most countries, 90% or more of cases were among individuals without vaccination scars. This finding led to surveys in the endemic countries that disclosed vaccine-efficacy ratios of 80% or more among those vaccinated 20 years previously. Heiner and colleagues,[65] however, showed that this protection could not be attributed solely to the vaccine. They discovered that previously vaccinated persons often developed inapparent infection with substantial increases in antibody levels. Immunity in the endemic countries was thus a composite of past experiences with both vaccinia and variola infections. Data from countries where smallpox was introduced after an absence of many years provide insufficient information to permit calculation of vaccine-efficacy ratios, but they do indicate that the vaccine provides substantial long-term protection against a fatal outcome.[73] Among 680 cases of variola major occurring after importations of smallpox into Europe, the case-fatality rate was 52% among those who had never been vaccinated, 1.4% among those vaccinated up to 10 years before exposure, and 11.1% among those vaccinated more than 20 years before.

Simultaneous Administration with Other Antigens. It has been shown that smallpox vaccine can be administered at the same time as a number of other antigens, usually at a different site, with levels of safety and efficacy comparable to those observed when the vaccines are given separately. Simultaneous administration of oral poliovirus and smallpox vaccines became a routine practice in many countries beginning in the 1960s.[105, 106] Smallpox and bacille Calmette-Guérin (BCG) vaccines began to be administered to newborns in Hong Kong in the 1960s[107]; this became a common practice in many African countries in the late 1960s. Yellow fever and smallpox vaccines were mixed and administered successfully in many French-speaking areas of western Africa,[108] and measles and smallpox vaccines were simultaneously administered in a program throughout western Africa from 1967 to 1972.[109] Mixing of smallpox, yellow fever, and measles vaccines for inoculation by jet injection resulted in a diminished immune response to yellow fever,[110] but responses were satisfactory when different sites of inoculation were used. Ruben and colleagues[111] extended the studies to the simultaneous administration by jet injection, but at different sites, of smallpox, yellow fever, measles, and diphtheria-pertussis-tetanus (DPT) vaccines. Systemic reactions were no more frequent or severe than those that occurred after measles or smallpox vaccination alone, but there was, in this study, a diminished immune response to measles. The last observation was not, however, confirmed in subsequent studies. From these and other observations, Foege and Foster[112] concluded that it was safe and efficacious to administer simultaneously all the vaccines (oral poliovirus, DPT, measles, and BCG) employed in the WHO Expanded Program of Immunization as well as smallpox and yellow fever vaccines.

Complications of Vaccination

Skin Infections. After vaccination, three types of abnormal skin reactions may occur as follows: (1) eczema vaccinatum and (2) progressive vaccinia, which are both associated with abnormal host reactions, and (3) generalized vaccinia. Vaccinia virus from a lesion may also be accidentally inoculated at other sites on the body or transferred to others. The approximate frequency of such complications and rates per million vaccinees are shown in Tables 6–2 and 6–3, based on a national survey by Lane and colleagues[113] in the United States, the only country in which comprehensive studies of this type were undertaken. More detailed prospective studies in 10 states[114] revealed higher rates for eczema vaccinatum, generalized vaccinia, and accidental infection as well as for other complications; the higher rates resulted from the detection of more minor complications.

Eczema vaccinatum occurs in both vaccinated persons and their unvaccinated contacts who have active or quiescent eczema. Either concurrently with or shortly after the development of the local vaccinial lesion or after an incubation period of 5 days in an unvaccinated eczematous contact, a vaccinial eruption occurs at sites that are eczematous or that had previously been so. The areas

Table 6–2. **COMPLICATIONS OF SMALLPOX VACCINATION IN THE UNITED STATES, 1968**

VACCINATION STATUS AND AGE (yr)	ESTIMATED NUMBER OF VACCINATIONS	NUMBER OF REPORTED CASES (deaths)					
		Postvaccinal Encephalitis	Progressive Vaccinnia	Eczema Vaccinatum	Generalized Vaccinia	Accidental Infection	Other
Primary vaccinations							
<1	614,000	4 (3)	—	5	43	7	10
1–4	2,733,000	6	1	31	47	91	40
5–9	1,553,000	5 (1)	1 (1)	11	20	32	8
10–19	406,000	—	1 (1)	3	5	3	1
≥20	288,000	1	2	7	13	4	5
Unknown		—	—	1	3	5	2
Total	5,594,000	16 (4)	5 (2)	58	131	142	66
Revaccinations							
<1	—	—	—	—	—	—	—
1–4	478,000	—	—	1	—	1	1
5–9	1,643,000	—	1 (1)	4	1	3	2
10–19	2,657,000	—	1	3	—	—	—
≥20	3,796,000	—	4 (1)	—	9	3	6
Total	8,574,000	—	6 (2)	8	10	7	9
Unvaccinated contacts		—	—	60 (1)	2	44	8
Total	14,168,000	16 (4)	11 (4)	126 (1)	143	193	83

From Lane JM, Ruben FL, Neff JM, Millar JD. Complications of smallpox vaccination, 1968. National surveillance in the United States. N Engl J Med 281:1201–1208, 1969.

become intensely inflamed, and the eruption sometimes spreads to normal skin. Constitutional symptoms are usually severe, with high temperature and generalized lymphadenopathy. Treatment with vaccinia immune globulin appears to reduce mortality.[115]

Progressive vaccinia occurs in persons who suffer from deficient immune mechanisms, such as agammaglobulinemia, defective cell-mediated immunity, or immune deficiency associated with tumors of the reticuloendothelial system or the use of immunosuppressive drugs. In such patients, the vaccinia lesion fails to heal; secondary lesions sometimes appear elsewhere on the body and then gradually spread. Methisazone (*N*-methylisatin β-thiosemicarbazone) is reported to be partially effective in treatment,[116] but one third of such patients die.[113]

With *generalized vaccinia*, one to many lesions develop in 6 to 9 days after vaccination at locations other than the vaccination site in otherwise healthy persons. The evolution of these lesions follows the same temporal course as that of the vaccination lesion itself. Although patients may experience high fever and malaise, an uneventful recovery without the need for specific therapy is usual.

Accidental inoculation of vaccinia virus, transferred from the lesion at the vaccination site, is by far the most common, although innocuous, complication. The most common sites for inoculation are the eyelids, vulva, and perineum. Such lesions evolve rapidly and heal at the same time as the primary lesion. Accidental infection of normal contacts may also occur.

Table 6–3. **COMPLICATIONS PER 1 MILLION SMALLPOX VACCINATIONS IN THE UNITED STATES DURING 1968**

VACCINATION STATUS AND AGE (yr)	POSTVACCINAL ENCEPHALITIS	PROGRESSIVE VACCINIA	ECZEMA VACCINATUM	GENERALIZED VACCINIA	ACCIDENTAL INFECTION	OTHER
Primary vaccination						
1	6.5	—	8.1	70.0	11.4	16.3
1–4	2.2	*	11.3	17.2	33.3	14.6
5–9	3.2	*	7.1	12.9	20.6	5.2
10–19	—	*	*	12.3	*	*
20	*	*	24.3	45.1	13.9	17.4
Total	2.9	0.9	10.4	23.4	25.4	11.8
Revaccination						
1	—	—	—	—	—	—
1–4	—	—	*	—	*	*
5–9	—	*	2.4	*	*	*
10–19	—	*	*	—	—	—
20	—	1.1	—	2.4	*	1.6
Total	—	0.7	0.9	1.2	0.8	1.0

*Fewer than 4 cases; rate not computed.

From Lane JM, Ruben FL, Neff JM, Millar JD. Complications of smallpox vaccination, 1968. National surveillance in the United States. N Engl J Med 281:1201–1208, 1969.

Postvaccinal Encephalopathy and Encephalitis. Among those without known contraindications to vaccination, postvaccinal encephalopathy and encephalitis are the most serious complications. The incidence of these related complications was substantially higher in Europe after the use of strains in common use at that time[117] than in the United States, where the New York City Board of Health strain was employed. Two pathological forms were distinguished by de Vries[118]: encephalopathy primarily in children younger than 2 years, and encephalitis or encephalomyelitis in those who were older. The encephalopathy is characterized by general hyperemia of the brain, lymphocytic infiltration of the meninges, widespread degenerative changes in ganglion cells, and perivascular hemorrhage. Severe symptoms begin abruptly within 6 to 10 days after vaccination,[119] with fever and convulsions, usually followed by hemiplegia and aphasia; death, when it occurs, follows within a few days. Recovery is seldom complete; the patient is left with mental impairment and some degree of paralysis. Postvaccinal encephalitis, characterized by perivenous demyelination and microglial proliferation, primarily afflicts persons older than 2 years and is similar to the form of encephalitis observed after vaccination against rabies or after measles infection. Illness usually begins between 11 and 15 days after vaccination and is accompanied by fever, vomiting, headache, malaise, and anorexia followed by disorientation and drowsiness and sometimes convulsions and coma. Death occurs in 10 to 35% of cases, usually within a week. Some survivors have residual paralysis or mental impairment. Paralysis, when it is present, tends to be of the upper motor neuron type. Among those patients who recover fully, symptoms and signs resolve within 2 weeks.[120–127]

Many reports document the frequency of cases of postvaccinal encephalopathy and encephalitis in Europe and the United States, but comparison of rates is difficult because of differing criteria for diagnosis and variability in the completeness of reporting (Table 6–4). The usual levels of incidence, such as those reported from the Netherlands, Germany, and Austria, were higher than those in the United Kingdom, and these rates in turn were higher than those in the United States.[113, 114, 128] Whatever the criteria and methods, differences between the rates appeared to be real, and this fact caused a number of countries, during the 1960s, to begin using the Lister strain, then in use in the United Kingdom. A dramatic reduction in the incidence of postvaccinal encephalitis subsequently occurred.[120, 129] The incidence in the Netherlands between 1964 and 1971 appeared to approach that in the United States; 10 of the 16 cases were fatal, however, compared with only 4 of 16 cases reported in the United States in 1968. The differences are not statistically significant, but the results

Table 6–4. **INCIDENCE OF POSTVACCINAL ENCEPHALOPATHY (IN INFANTS YOUNGER THAN 2 YEARS) AND POSTVACCINAL ENCEPHALOMYELITIS (IN PERSONS OLDER THAN 2 YEARS) AFTER PRIMARY VACCINATION, IN VARIOUS COUNTRIES AND AT VARIOUS TIMES**

	ENCEPHALOPATHY (age <2 yr)			ENCEPHALOMYELITIS (age >2 yr)		
COUNTRY AND INVESTIGATOR	Number of Cases	Number of Vaccinations	Cases per Million	Number of Cases	Number of Vaccinations	Cases per Million
Austria 1948–1953 (Berger and Puntigam,[121] 1954)	6	58,438	103	26	21,323	1219
England and Wales 1951–1960 (Conybeare,[122] 1964)	40	2,960,406	14	26	859,963	30
Germany						
Bavaria 1945–1953 (Herrlich,[123] 1954)	51	1,008,000	51	17	140,800	121
Dusseldorf 1948 (Stuart,[124] 1947; Femmer,[125] 1948)	0	28,768	0	14	67,068	209
Hamburg 1939–1958 (Seeleman,[126] 1960)	34	367,390	93	12	26,713	449
Netherlands						
1924–1928 (van den Berg,[127] 1946)	6	155,730	39	127	548,420	232
1940–1943 (Stuart,[124] 1947)	22	441,294	50	56	160,775	348
1959–1963 (Polak,[120] 1973)	34	1,033,000	33	—	—	—
1964–1971 (Polak,[120] 1973)	16	1,495,000	11	—	—	—
United States 1968						
National survey (Lane et al,[113] 1969)	4	614,000*	7	12	4,980,000†	2
10-state survey (Lane et al,[114] 1970)	3	71,000*	42	5	579,000†	9

*Age younger than 1 year.
†Age 1 year or older.
From Fenner F, Henderson DA, Arita I, et al. Smallpox and Its Eradication. Geneva, World Health Organization, 1988, p 307.

are consistent with other observations that suggest that the New York City Board of Health strain is somewhat less pathogenic than the Lister strain.

No single laboratory test correlates with strain virulence, but Marrenikova and colleagues,[130] as a result of a series of studies in mice and rats, provide a broad classification of a number of strains as follows: (1) least pathogenic: New York City Board of Health and EM-63 (a derivative of this strain); (2) moderately pathogenic: Lister, Berne, and Patwadanger (from India); and (3) highly pathogenic, Denmark, Tashkent (an older Russian strain), and Ikeda (an older Japanese strain).

Unusual Complications. In some laboratories, even during the present century, the vaccine was often contaminated with tetanus spores or other pyogenic bacteria that induced infections. With improved methods, however, such infections ceased to occur.

Vaccination during pregnancy did not appear to result in an increase in the incidence of abortions or stillbirths.[131–133] Fetal vaccinia is rare, having been documented on fewer than 20 occasions[134]; no studies have implicated vaccinia virus as a teratogen.[135]

A rare occurrence is the development of a malignant skin tumor, such as a melanoma, in the vaccination scar many years later,[136] and vaccinal osteomyelitis has occasionally been recorded and sometimes confirmed by recovery of vaccinia virus.[137]

Indications for Vaccination

In endemic countries, which, until after World War I, consisted of most of the world, vaccination was recommended for everyone, with revaccination to occur every 3 to 10 years. The only exceptions were infants, for whom primary vaccination was customarily delayed until they were 3 to 12 months of age, mainly because of more frequent vaccination failures at an earlier age. As higher titer vaccines became available in the 1920s, French and then German physicians showed that a high proportion of successful vaccinations could be achieved at birth, and in some hospitals, this became routine practice.[138] In at least one city in the United States, Detroit, neonatal vaccination was mandated in the mid-1920s.[139]

As time passed and smallpox incidence declined, it became increasingly common for smallpox-free countries to delay primary vaccination until children were older. This resulted in part from the demonstration that maternal antibody inhibited virus proliferation[140] and in part from the belief that older children could better cope with the fever and systemic symptoms of vaccinial infection.

Vaccination at a later age was also less likely to be associated mistakenly with other events. such as sudden infant death syndrome, which might be temporally but not causally related. Some European countries recommended that vaccination be delayed until the second year of life to avoid postvaccinal encephalopathy,[119] and the United States adopted the practice of vaccinating at 12 months of age when studies suggested a higher frequency of postvaccinal encephalitis among those vaccinated before 1 year of age than among those vaccinated between 1 and 4 years of age.[113] What these changes in policy may have achieved, however, is unknown, because no studies were performed to validate that complications were subsequently less frequent.

As a rule, most vaccination practices in the developing countries tended to parallel those in Europe and North America, and as of 1967, most countries, even those with endemic smallpox, delayed vaccination until the child was 3 to 9 months of age. Notable exceptions were Hong Kong,[107] where neonatal vaccination had been traditional at least since World War II, and Madras, India,[103] where neonatal vaccination was introduced in the late 1950s. During the late 1960s, it became apparent that vaccines that met international standards of potency consistently resulted in high levels of vaccination "takes" in newborns. Thus, newborn vaccination was recommended for all countries, although not all countries followed the practice. Unfortunately, there are no adequate studies that serve to compare the efficacy and durability of immunity provided at birth with that provided at older ages, nor is there information that permits a comparison to be made between the relative frequency of vaccination complications at this and older ages.

Primary vaccination was provided for adults if required, although many workers have considered it to be associated with a substantially higher incidence of postvaccinal encephalitis and other serious complications. Earlier European data suggest this to be the case,[117] but this was not borne out in studies conducted in the United States.[113, 128] Confirming this association was a review of United States military medical records between 1946 and 1962, conducted by the Centers for Disease Control and Prevention, which revealed no cases of central nervous system complications among an estimated 2 million recruits who were given primary vaccinations. The differences in experience in Europe and the United States almost certainly reflect differences in the pathogenicity of the strains employed.

Since 1980, routine vaccination has ceased in all countries, although a number of countries continue to provide vaccination to military forces as a protection in case variola virus is used as a biological warfare agent. Otherwise, vaccination is recommended only for those working in laboratories where orthopoxviruses are used.

Contraindications to Vaccination

During campaigns in areas that were endemic for smallpox, the WHO recognized no contraindications to vaccination for two reasons: first, the risk associated with smallpox infection was significantly greater than the risk of complications; second, most vaccinations were performed by individuals without medical training who could not be expected to recognize conditions such as eczema or to identify patients with immune deficiency syndromes. It was recommended that only those who were extremely sick not be vaccinated on the grounds that their subsequent death might be attributed mistakenly to vaccination.

In nonendemic areas, four conditions were generally accepted as contraindications.

Immune Disorders. Immune disorders included agammaglobulinemia, hypogammaglobulinemia, neoplasms affecting the reticuloendothelial system, and compromised immune status associated with the use of immunosuppressive drugs. Persons with such disorders, if vaccinated, were at substantial risk of developing the frequently fatal progressive vaccinia.

Eczema. Individuals with active eczema or a past history of eczema were at special risk of developing eczema vaccinatum, a serious and sometimes fatal complication. Because family members with eczema were also at risk from contact spread of vaccinia virus, it was recommended that either the healthy vaccinee or the eczematous family member live apart from the family until the lesion had fully scabbed over.

Pregnancy. Pregnant women were not vaccinated on the general principle that immunization of any sort should be avoided during pregnancy and because of the rare risk of fetal vaccinia.

Disorders of the Central Nervous System. Many countries recognized as contraindications disorders of the central nervous system in potential vaccinees and sometimes their families, hoping, in so doing, to minimize the risk of postvaccinal encephalitis. However, there is no evidence that the exclusion of such persons affected the incidence of that complication.

Some authorities recommended withholding vaccination from patients suffering from various acute or chronic illnesses of many other types, hypothesizing that the response to vaccination might be abnormal. There was no evidence for this occurrence except in the case of leprosy patients, some of whom developed erythema nodosum leprosum or neuritis after primary vaccination.[141, 142] In endemic areas, however, leprosy patients were vaccinated because the risk of smallpox substantially outweighed the risk of complications.

PUBLIC HEALTH

Epidemiological Effects of Vaccination

United States

Smallpox vaccination in the United States began in 1800, but its routine widespread use did not occur until this century. It was first demonstrated by Waterhouse in Boston in July 1800, with material provided by Jenner,[143] and its use was actively promoted by President Thomas Jefferson.[144] Because propagation of the virus at that time was primarily dependent on arm-to-arm transfer of material from a successful vaccinee to others, vaccination was practiced sporadically. Epidemics of variola major continued to occur at intervals, depending on population density and frequency of importations.

Toward the end of the 19th century in the United States, vaccinia virus began to be propagated on the flank of a calf, thus making vaccination more readily and widely available. By 1897, smallpox had largely been eliminated,[3] the result of vaccination and outbreak control. That summer, however, an outbreak of variola minor occurred in Pensacola, Florida, and within 4 years, this variety of smallpox had spread across the country.[145] Although outbreaks of variola major continued to occur until about 1927, most cases of smallpox were caused by variola minor. Because the disease was mild and the case-fatality rate was only 0.3 to 1.0%, interest in vaccination waned. To control the disease, public health authorities sought to compel vaccination as a requirement for school entry, an action upheld by the Supreme Court,[146] a highly effective measure.[147] However, antivaccinationist sentiment and antipathy toward compulsory measures prevailed in many states, most of which passed no legislation or prohibited compulsory vaccination. Reported cases of smallpox declined from 102,791 in 1921 to 30,151 in 1931, and between 1932 and 1939, 5000 to 15,000 cases were reported annually, with 23 to 52 deaths. During the following decade, reported cases steadily diminished, the last occurring in 1949. This progress occurred in the absence of any nationally coordinated smallpox control effort, and little is known about the extent of vaccination immunity in the country during the 1940s or about the epidemiology of smallpox. However, improved smallpox control, and eventually its elimination, is attributed by Leake[148] to the wider availability of better refrigeration and, consequently, better preservation of the vaccine. Routine vaccination continued in the United States until 1971 as a protection in case smallpox was imported and was enforced in most states by compelling vaccination as a requirement for school entry. Beginning in the 1960s, the Centers for Disease Control and Prevention urged the routine vaccination of hospital staff, a group at high risk if smallpox was imported, but few hospitals complied. After the global eradication of smallpox, distribution of vaccine was restricted to the military and to the few laboratories that were working with orthopoxviruses.

Other Industrialized Countries

Through the 1800s, the experience with vaccination in other industrialized countries was similar to that in the United States. After an initial surge of enthusiasm for vaccination in the early 1800s, vaccination was less uniformly and extensively practiced in most countries until near the close of the century, when the vaccinia virus began to be propagated on calves. By 1900, a number of countries in northern Europe became smallpox free, and by 1914, the incidence in most countries had decreased to comparatively low levels. Even so, during the period from 1910 to 1914, Russia experienced a reported 200,000 deaths, and nearly 25,000 deaths were recorded in other European countries.[149, 150] World War I led to a resurgence of smallpox in Russia and its spread from there to many other countries. During the 1920s, vaccination programs led to the interruption of smallpox transmission in many European countries, and by the mid-1930s, smallpox occurred only after importations except in Spain and Portugal. Endemic smallpox persisted in these countries until 1948 and 1953, respectively.

Of the other major industrialized countries, as they are often referred to today, Canada interrupted transmission of smallpox in the early 1940s and Japan about 1950. Vaccination continued in all the industrialized countries, as it did in the United States, until the mid to late 1970s as a protection in case smallpox was reintroduced. Australia and New Zealand were two notable exceptions. These countries, protected by distance and strict quarantine measures, never vaccinated widely but also never became endemic for smallpox.

Eradication from the World

The first commitment to smallpox eradication as such was made in 1950 by the Pan American Sanitary Organization, which decided that year on a hemisphere-wide effort.[151] Freeze-dried vaccine produced by an improved commercial process[30] was employed in mass vaccination campaigns, which during the succeeding decade eliminated smallpox from all countries except Argentina, Brazil, Colombia, and Ecuador.

In 1958, the Soviet Union proposed to the World Health Assembly that the WHO undertake a global eradication program,[32] a proposal that was agreed on in 1959.[33] During the succeeding 7 years, a number of countries embarked on mass vaccination campaigns, and several countries, including China, were successful in eliminating the disease (Fig. 6–6). Overall, however, progress was disappointing, especially in Africa and in the Indian subcontinent. Few countries voluntarily contributed resources, and the WHO, then preoccupied with a costly and disappointing global malaria eradication program, provided few of its own resources and little support.

Frustrated by lack of progress in the program, although skeptical about the feasibility of the concept of eradication itself, the World Health Assembly in 1966 decided, finally, to provide to the WHO a special allocation of $2.4 million annually for an intensified global smallpox eradication effort.[34] The hope was expressed that the task might be accomplished within a 10-year period, that is, by December 1976.[36]

In the intensified program, the strategy emphasized two principles that ultimately proved to be critical to its success. The first was to ensure, through the use of international vaccine testing centers, that all vaccine in the program met accepted standards and, likewise, to ensure, through concurrent sample surveys, that a satisfactory vaccination coverage had been achieved and that the vaccinations had been successful. The second principle was the identification of the absence of cases as the program's principal objective and the need to measure progress not in terms of numbers of vaccinations performed, as had been the practice, but in terms of declining incidence of smallpox. This principle required the development of an effective case notification system and focused attention on measures to reduce incidence.

During 1967, the first year of the program, 44 countries, 31 of which were endemic, reported 131,789 cases of smallpox. The endemic countries were Brazil, most countries of Africa south of the Sahara, and five countries in Asia: Afghanistan, India, Indonesia, Nepal, and Pakistan (see Fig. 6–6). Later surveys revealed that only about 1% of all cases were then being reported; thus, it is estimated that between 10 and 15 million cases occurred that year in countries whose population was about 1.2 billion people.

Provision of adequate supplies of fully potent vaccine was a critical first problem.[152, 153] Early surveys revealed that not more than 10% of the vaccine being produced in or provided to the endemic countries met accepted

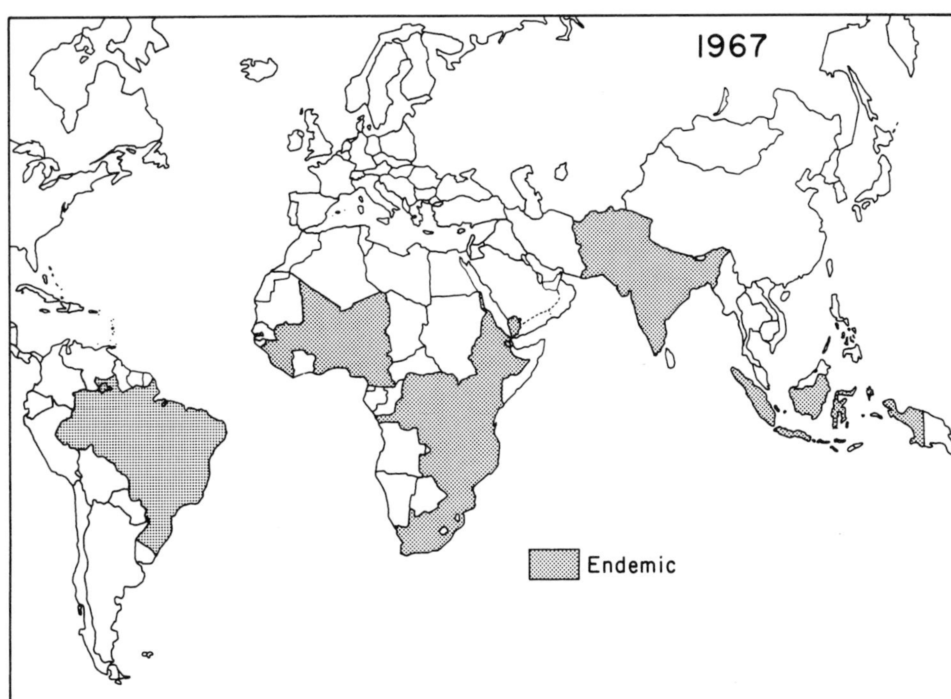

Figure 6–6. Countries with endemic smallpox in 1967 when the intensified program was initiated.

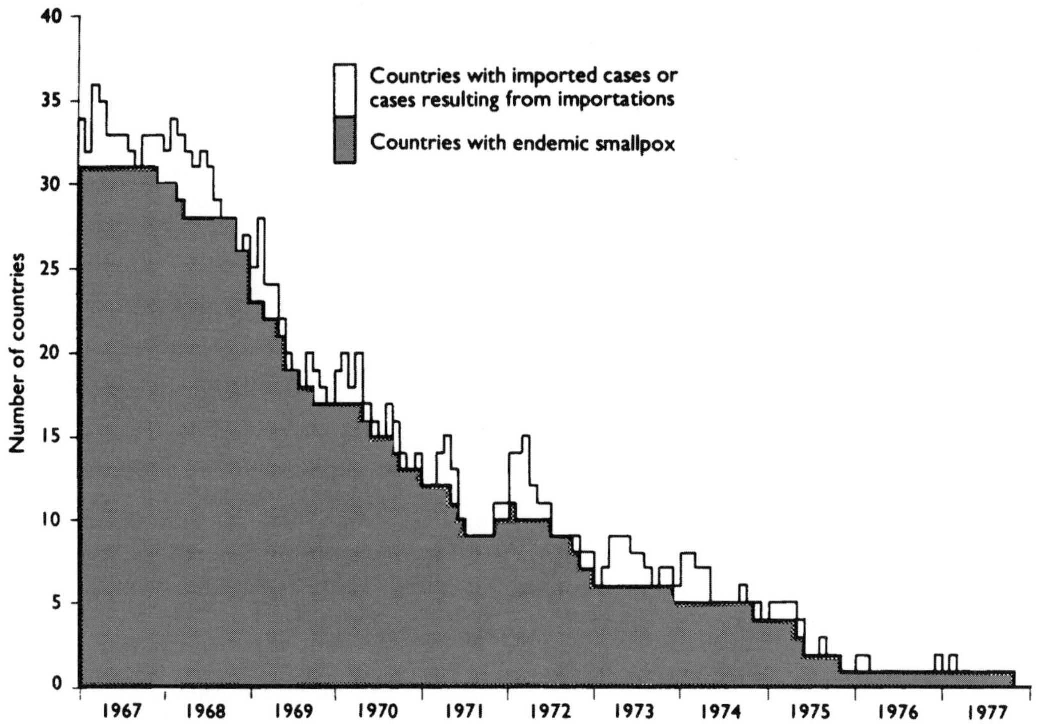

Figure 6–7. Number of countries experiencing smallpox each year from 1967 to 1978. (From Fenner F, Henderson DA, Arita I, et al. Smallpox and Its Eradication. Geneva, World Health Organization, 1988, pp 517–538.)

international standards. Laboratories in Canada and the Netherlands agreed to test samples of all vaccine to be used in the program, manufacturers collaborated in developing a detailed production manual, and consultants and equipment were provided to laboratories in the endemic countries. Donations of vaccine, primarily from the Soviet Union and the United States, met initial needs, but by 1973, more than 80% of all vaccine for the program was being produced in the developing countries.

The traditional method of vaccination by scarification was changed. In 1967, jet injectors were introduced for programs in Brazil and western and central Africa. One year later, a new instrument, the bifurcated needle, developed by Wyeth Laboratories, was found to be effective in multiple-puncture vaccinations[154]; by 1969, it was in use in all countries. Vaccination with the bifurcated needle required only one fourth as much vaccine, even illiterate village volunteers required less than an hour's training in its proper use, and workers could vaccinate as many as 1000 persons per day.

Vaccination programs were developed or strengthened in all endemic and neighboring countries, the last of them beginning in 1971. Although the strategy also called for the improvement of national reporting systems and containment of outbreaks by special teams, such activities were slow to begin. It quickly became apparent, however, that these activities, referred to as the surveillance-containment program, could serve to interrupt smallpox transmission more easily and quickly than anyone had imagined, even where vaccinial immunity was low.[69, 155, 156]

With increasingly greater emphasis on surveillance-containment activities, endemic smallpox steadily receded (Fig. 6–7; see also Fig. 6–6). It was eliminated from 20 countries of western and central Africa by 1970,[70] from Brazil in 1971, from Indonesia in 1972, and from the entire continent of Asia in 1975. Ethiopia stopped transmission in 1976 and Somalia on October 26, 1977. The last naturally occurring case of smallpox developed less than 1 year after the originally projected 10-year target date. WHO-organized international commissions visited each of the endemic countries and areas to confirm the fact of eradication, and in May 1980 the World Health Assembly, acting on the recommendation of a WHO Global Commission (Fig. 6–8), announced that worldwide eradication had been achieved and recommended that smallpox vaccination be used only for those working with orthopoxvirus in research laboratories.[1] The WHO established an international stockpile of vaccine in the unlikely event that its use would ever again be required and encouraged laboratories to destroy their stocks of variola virus. As of 1997, variola virus remained in only two research laboratories—one in the United States and one in Russia.

The overall cost of the program was estimated to be about $300 million, of which $98 million represented international assistance. The savings, as a result of cessation of vaccination and quarantine measures, was estimated to be in excess of $1 billion annually.[4]

With the eradication of smallpox, questions arose as to whether it might not be prudent to destroy the known remaining laboratory stocks of variola virus to provide added assurance that the virus might not accidentally or even deliberately be released into an unprotected world. This was considered in 1986 by a WHO Ad Hoc Committee on Orthopoxvirus Infections, which recommended a broader consultation with the international

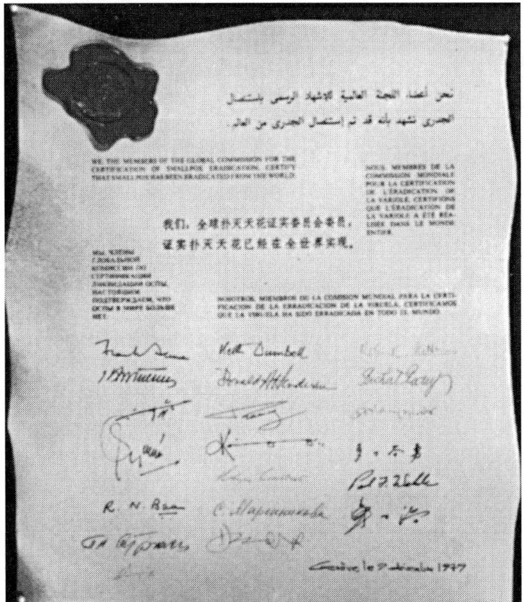

Figure 6–8. Document signed on December 9, 1979, by members of the World Health Organization Global Commission, certifying that smallpox had been eradicated. (From Fenner F, Henderson DA, Arita I, et al. Smallpox and Its Eradication. Geneva, World Health Organization, 1988, frontispiece.)

community and destruction of the virus if no serious objections were raised.[157] Meanwhile, in preparation for possible destruction, a library of cloned DNA restriction fragments of selected strains was prepared, and later the genomes of a number of prototype strains were fully or partially sequenced.[158]

Arguments were advanced both supporting[158] and objecting to[159] destruction of the virus stocks. In 1994, the question was again reviewed in depth by the WHO Committee, which again recommended to the WHO Director General that the considerations, on balance, strongly favored destruction of the virus.[160] It was ultimately decided in the 1996 World Health Assembly that destruction of the virus should take place on June 30, 1999.

RECOMBINANT VACCINIA VIRUS VACCINES

Shortly after the World Health Assembly resolution recommending cessation of smallpox vaccination, proposals were made to use recombinant vaccinia viruses for immunization against other infectious agents.[161, 162] The idea was to stably insert one or more genes of other pathogens into the genome of vaccinia virus while retaining the infectivity of the latter. Moreover, the large capacity of vaccinia virus for foreign DNA raised the possibility of polyvalent vaccines against multiple diseases.[163, 164] In principle, recombinant vaccinia viruses would have many of the properties of live attenuated virus vaccines and would present antigens in natural ways so as to stimulate humoral immunity to native protein conformation as well as cell-mediated immunity. Such vaccines might also retain the familiar advantages of smallpox vaccine: heat stability, low cost, ease of administration, and a scar as visible proof of vaccination. Although recombinant vaccinia viruses are still undergoing investigation for human and veterinary vaccination, their great value for vaccine research has been widely recognized.[165]

Construction of Recombinant Vaccinia Virus Vectors

The development of recombinant vaccinia viruses depended on a method of introducing a foreign gene into the vaccinia virus genome. Homologous recombination between poxviruses was well known and had been demonstrated by coinfecting cells with two viruses[166] and by infecting cells with one virus and transfecting them with genomic DNA[167, 168] or cloned DNA segments.[169] It is likely that DNA recombination occurs in the cytoplasm by enzymes encoded by vaccinia virus. Less well understood at the time was how to achieve expression of foreign genes. The recognition of vaccinia virus promoter elements provided a general method of preparing vaccinia virus expression vectors[161, 170, 171] that is illustrated in Figure 6–9. Insights achieved through basic studies of vaccinia virus promoters have led to substantial improvements in the level of gene expression.[172, 173] Other innovations, including alternative methods of selecting or identifying recombinant vaccinia viruses and the insertion of foreign genes by direct ligation, are summarized elsewhere.[174]

Selection of a Vaccinia Virus Strain

The WR strain of vaccinia virus, favored for basic poxvirus research in the United States and widely used to make recombinant viruses for laboratory studies, is unsuitable for vaccines. The four vaccinia virus strains administered most often for smallpox vaccination were EM-63, Lister, New York City Board of Health, and Temple of Heaven. Of these, the New York City Board of Health strain had relatively low pathogenicity[175] and was chosen to make a recombinant vaccinia virus intended for human use. Although the latter appeared to be safe in a small clinical trial,[176] further attenuation of recombinant vaccinia viruses seems prudent for large-scale administration. Several approaches have been taken to achieve a safer vector.

Although 50 or more of the nearly 200 genes of vaccinia virus are dispensable for replication in tissue culture cells, the deletion of some of these genes reduces virulence in animal models.[177–179] The deletional approach to making a safe vector was exemplified by the removal of 18 genes from the Copenhagen strain of vaccinia virus, thereby producing a highly attenuated derivative called NYVAC.[180] Several studies have indicated that NYVAC has good potential for human and veterinary vaccines.[181, 182] An alternative approach was to use one of several highly attenuated strains of vaccinia virus that were derived by serial passages in vitro and

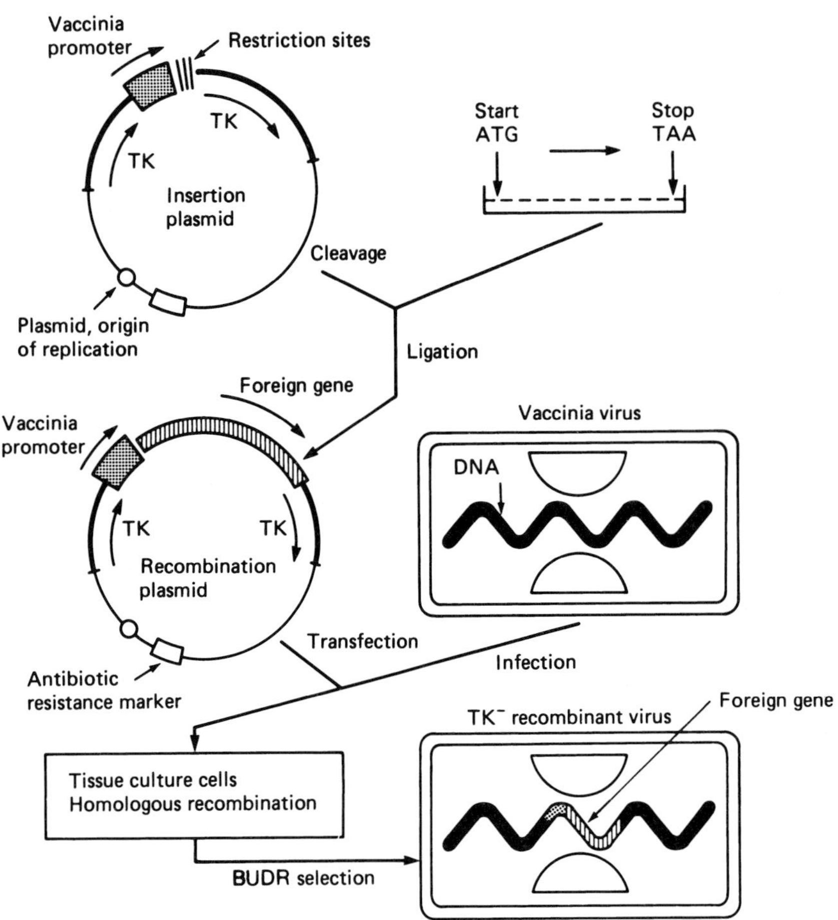

Figure 6–9. The insertion plasmid (or transfer vector) contains restriction endonuclease sites for ligation of the complete open reading frame (ATG---------TAA) of a foreign gene adjacent to a vaccinia virus promoter as well as flanking vaccinia virus DNA sequences (in this case from the thymidine kinase [TK] gene) to direct homologous recombinational insertion into the vaccinia virus genome. Tissue culture cells are infected with vaccinia virus and then transfected with the insertion plasmid, resulting in the formation of a stable recombinant virus. Because only about 0.1% of the progeny are recombinant viruses, selection techniques are frequently used. In the example shown here, the recombinant virus has an interrupted TK gene and can be selected by use of 5-bromodeoxyuridine (BuDR). Detailed protocols for constructing recombinant vaccinia viruses are available.[171]

had been tested in humans before the eradication of smallpox.[175] One of these strains, MVA, suffered multiple deletions and became severely host range restricted during more than 500 passages in chick embryo cells, providing a high degree of attenuation.[183, 184] Laboratory studies demonstrated unimpaired MVA gene expression in human cells and a block in virion morphogenesis.[185] The ability to achieve high expression of recombinant genes despite abortive replication is a remarkable feature of this mutant virus. Even though MVA probably does not replicate significantly in animal models, excellent immune responses to recombinant proteins were obtained; moreover, the dose required was similar to that of a standard replication-competent strain.[186–188]

Vaccinia Virus as a Tool for Vaccine Research

Recombinant vaccinia viruses provide a powerful means of dissecting the immune responses of humans and experimental animals to individual gene products of infectious agents. Only a few examples can be mentioned here. Thus, recombinant vaccinia viruses were used to demonstrate that the HA and NP proteins of influenza virus induced subtype-specific and cross-reactive cytotoxic T-cell responses, respectively.[189, 190] Evidence of human immunodeficiency virus type 1 (HIV-1)–specific cytotoxic T cells in patients with acquired immunodeficiency syndrome (AIDS) was first obtained by use of recombinant vaccinia viruses expressing the envelope or internal proteins to prepare target cells.[191, 192] Indeed, recombinant vaccinia viruses have become an important tool for cellular immunologists.[193] Because proteins expressed in mammalian cells by recombinant vaccinia viruses are folded, processed, and transported normally, they can be used to either induce or bind antibodies that recognize conformational epitopes.[194]

The wide host range of vaccinia virus makes it possible to determine protective immune responses against infectious agents in a variety of experimental animals from rodents to primates. For example, the F glycoprotein is most important for inducing protection to respiratory syncytial virus,[195] whereas the HN protein is better for parainfluenza virus type 3[196] and type 5.[197] Protection elicited by the respiratory syncytial virus M2 protein is due to $CD8^+$ T cells, whereas that induced by the F and G proteins is due to antibodies.[198] Similar results, with respect to the HA and NP proteins, have been obtained in studies with influenza virus.[199] In some cases, vaccination has a priming effect that is followed by an anamnestic antibody response, as indicated for the protection of chimpanzees after inoculation with a recombinant vaccinia virus expressing the hepatitis B surface antigen.[200] A list of viruses for which protective immune responses have been obtained may be found in a review.[201]

The induction of strong cytotoxic T-cell responses

elicited by recombinant vaccinia viruses has led to their evaluation as tumor vaccines in model systems.[202–205]

Other Poxvirus Vectors

The procedures developed for the construction of recombinant vaccinia viruses have been applied to members of other poxvirus genera including avian poxviruses[206] and capripoxviruses.[207] Although the avian poxviruses are naturally host range restricted, gene expression and protective immunity can be established in nonavian species.[208, 209] As nonreplicating vectors, avian poxviruses should be exceptionally safe recombinant vaccines.

Human Vaccines

Although vaccinia virus vectors have proved extremely useful for vaccine research as well as for research in many other fields, the potential for human vaccines is still under investigation. As for all vaccines, the critical factors include safety and efficacy as well as the facility for vaccine production, distribution, and administration. In addition, there are special questions regarding prior immunity to vaccinia virus acquired either through smallpox vaccination or through a recombinant vaccine and the design of polyvalent vaccines.

Safety issues have been minimized by the demonstration that host-restricted or "nonreplicating" vaccinia virus vectors, such as the MVA and NYVAC, are immunogenic. At the National Institutes of Health intramural laboratories in Bethesda, research with both of these strains is permitted at biosafety level 1 conditions, whereas level 2 and a recent smallpox vaccination are required for working with standard vaccinia virus strains.

Generic and specific factors are involved in vaccine efficacy. With regard to the former, great improvements in gene expression have been made so that present generation vectors produce many times more recombinant protein than the original vectors. In some instances, immunogenicity has been improved by altering the presentation of the recombinant protein so that it is plasma membrane associated rather than intracellular or secreted.[210, 211] Promising results have been obtained by constructing recombinant vaccinia viruses that coexpress an immunogen and an immunomodulatory cytokine.[212–214]

Although the use of live attenuated viruses as human vaccines may require no special knowledge regarding the targets of immunity, such specific information is needed for recombinant vectors. For many viruses, the membrane glycoproteins or capsids are targets of neutralizing antibody and the internal proteins provide good targets for cytotoxic T cells. Animal models may be helpful in identifying those targets that provide protective immunity. In addition, some infectious agents have special vaccine requirements such as those related to portal of entry, site of replication, antigenic variation, type of immune response needed, and presence of maternal antibodies, which may or may not be met by a recombinant vaccine.

The smallpox vaccine was most frequently prepared from vaccinia virus that was propagated in the skin of an animal, but an approved, stable, freeze-dried vaccine was produced in monolayer cultures of primary rabbit kidney cells.[215] Acceptable cultured cell lines or primary chick embryo fibroblasts would be alternative substrates for virus propagation. Thus, there should be no impediment to the preparation of vaccines that meet present standards of purity. Presumably, procedures for freeze-drying could be adapted to the production of recombinant vaccinia viruses, and it is hoped that such preparations would retain the excellent thermal stability that made a cold chain unnecessary for the smallpox vaccine.

The smallpox vaccine was generally administered by scarification of the skin or less commonly by a high-pressure jet injector.[175] The intradermal route was used for clinical testing of a recombinant virus made with the New York City Board of Health strain.[176] However, other routes (e.g., nasal, oral, subcutaneous, or intramuscular) may be preferred for nonreplicating strains of vaccinia virus.

Although it was based on a small sampling, prior smallpox vaccination appeared to diminish the immune response to a recombinant vaccine.[176] For children and the majority of individuals born during the past 20 years, who have not received a smallpox vaccination, this would not be a problem. However, a poxvirus may not be useful as a carrier for revaccination with a second gene because of the immune response to the vector. Whether prior immunity could be overcome by using vectors that express more recombinant protein or through alternative routes of administration is uncertain. Nevertheless, immunization with a single vector expressing multiple genes, simultaneously with a cocktail of vectors, or successively with distantly related poxvirus vectors might obviate such problems.

Accelerated efforts to develop an AIDS vaccine have led to the human testing of a first-generation recombinant vaccinia virus expressing the HIV-1 envelope gene.[176, 216] The modest immune response detected may be due in part to the relatively weak promoter used and the failure to eliminate poxvirus early transcriptional stop signals within the HIV-1 gene.[217] The HIV-1 neutralizing antibody response, however, was augmented by secondary immunization with a subunit HIV-1 envelope protein.[218, 219] There is considerable enthusiasm for such a prime-boost strategy because it can stimulate cell-mediated and humoral immunity. Prime-boost vaccinations carried out with a recombinant canarypox virus and recombinant HIV-1 envelope protein induced HIV-specific cytotoxic cells and neutralizing antibody in phase I clinical trials. Expanded phase II trials are in progress.[220–222]

A recombinant vaccinia virus that expresses the major Epstein-Barr virus membrane glycoprotein was immunogenic when it was administered to infants and young children and may have delayed or prevented natural infection for a period of 16 months.[223] A recombinant canarypox virus expressing the rabies virus glycoprotein was safe in humans, induced functional antibody to rabies glycoprotein, elicited cellular responses to rabies virus, and could be used successfully for boosting at a 6-month interval.[224, 225]

Veterinary and Wildlife Vaccines

Substantially different factors are involved in the applicability of vaccines for medical and veterinary practices.[226] Economic criteria, although of considerable importance for human vaccines in developing countries, are decisive for most veterinary vaccines. Also, there is far more latitude in the manufacture and use of veterinary vaccines than has been permitted by regulatory agencies for human vaccines. In addition, durable immunity is not important for livestock, and a small number of vaccine-associated illnesses can be tolerated in veterinary vaccines. Because live fowlpox virus vaccines are already used in the poultry industry to prevent fowlpox, recombinant poxvirus vaccines should be practical.

Recombinant vaccinia viruses have been shown to protect animals against diseases of veterinary importance including vesicular stomatitis virus[227] and rinderpest[228] in cattle, pseudorabies virus in swine,[229] and influenza virus in chickens.[230] A recombinant vaccinia virus expressing the rabies virus glycoprotein[231] has been successfully administered in bait form as a wildlife vaccine in both the United States and Europe.[232, 233]

Other poxviruses are also being tested as vectors for veterinary applications. Examples include a raccoon poxvirus vector for raccoons against rabies virus[234]; a capripoxvirus vector for cattle against rinderpest virus[235]; a swinepox virus vector for pigs against pseudorabies virus[236]; fowlpox vectors for chickens against influenza virus,[237] Newcastle disease virus,[238, 239] and infectious bursal disease virus[240]; and canarypox virus for cats against feline leukemia virus.[241]

REFERENCES

1. World Health Organization. The global eradication of smallpox. Final report of the global commission for the certification of smallpox eradication. In History of International Public Health No. 4. Geneva, World Health Organization, 1980.
2. de Korte WE. Amaas, or kaffir milk-pox. Lancet 1:1273–1276, 1904.
3. Chapin CV. Variation in type of infectious disease as shown by the history of smallpox in the United States 1895–1912. J Infect Dis 13:171–196, 1913.
4. Fenner F, Henderson DA, Arita I, et al. Smallpox and Its Eradication. Geneva, World Health Organization, 1988.
5. McNeill WH. Plagues and People. Garden City, NY, Anchor Press/Doubleday, 1976.
6. Ruffer MA. Pathological note on the royal mummies of the Cairo Museum. In Moodie RL (ed). Studies in the Paleopathology of Egypt. Chicago, University of Chicago Press, 1921, pp 175–176.
7. Hopkins DR. Princes and Peasants. Smallpox in History. Chicago, University of Chicago Press, 1983.
8. Rhazes (Al-Razi, Abu Bakr Muhammad ibn Zakariya). De Variolis et Morbillis Commentarius. Londini, G Bowyer, 1766. English translation: Med Class 4:22–84, 1939.
9. Dixon CW. Smallpox. London, Churchill, 1962.
10. Moore J. The History of the Smallpox. London, Longman, Hurst, Rees, Orme & Brown, 1815.
11. Creighton C. History of Epidemics in Britain. Cambridge, Cambridge University Press, 1894. Reprinted London, Cass, 1965.
12. Macgowan DJ. Report on the health of Wenchow for the half-year ended 31 March 1884. China, Imperial Maritime Customs Medical Reports 27:9–18, 1884.
13. Needham J. China and the origins of immunology. Centre of Asian Studies Occasional Papers and Monographs No. 41. University of Hong Kong, 1980.
14. Miller G. Putting Lady Mary in her place: A discussion of historical causation. Bull Hist Med 55:2–16, 1981.
15. Jenner E. An Inquiry into the Causes and Effects of the Variolae Vaccinae, a Disease Discovered in Some of the Western Counties of England, Particularly Gloucestershire and Known by the Name of the Cow Pox. London, 1798. Reprinted in Camac CNB (ed). Classics of Medicine and Surgery. New York, Dover, 1959.
16. Pasteur L. Vaccination in relation to chicken-cholera and splenic fever. Transactions of the International Medical Congress, Seventh Session; London; August 29, 1881, 1:85–90. Reproduced in Vallery-Radot P (ed). Oeuvres de Pasteur. Vol. 6. Paris, Masson, 1933, pp 370–378.
17. LeFanu W. A Bio-Bibliography of Edward Jenner 1749–1823. London, Harvey & Blythe, 1951.
18. del Castillo FF. Los Viajes de Don Francisco Xavier de Balmis. Mexico, Galas de Mexico, 1960.
19. Bowers JZ. The odyssey of smallpox vaccination. Bull Hist Med 55:17–33, 1981.
20. Nott JC. Smallpox epidemic in Mobile during the winter of 1865–6. Nashville J Med Surg 2:372–380, 1867.
21. Creighton C. The Natural History of Cow-Pox and Vaccinal Syphilis. London, Cassell, 1887.
22. Baxby D. The origins of vaccinia virus. J Infect Dis 136:453–455, 1977.
23. The History of Inoculation and Vaccination. London, Burroughs Wellcome Company, 1913.
24. Edwardes EJ. A Concise History of Small-Pox and Vaccination in Europe. London, Lewis, 1902.
25. Galbiati G. Memoria Sulla Inoculazione Vaccina coll'Umore Ricavato Immediatement dalla Vacca Precedentemente Inoculata. Napoli, 1810.
26. Congrès Médical de Lyon. Compterendu des travaux et des discussions. Gazette Med Lyon 19:449–471, 1864.
27. Dudgeon JA. Development of smallpox vaccine in England in the eighteenth and nineteenth centuries. BMJ 1:1367–1372, 1963.
28. Otten L. Trockenlymphe. Z Hyg Infektionskrankh 107:677–696, 1927.
29. Fasquelle R, Fasquelle A. A propos de l'histoire de la lutte contre la variole dans les pays d'Afrique francophone. Bull Soc Pathol Exot Filiales 64:734–756, 1971.
30. Collier LH. The development of a stable smallpox vaccine. J Hyg 53:76–101, 1955.
31. Pan American Sanitary Organization. Final Reports of the First, Second and Third Meetings of the Directing Council. Publication No. 247. Washington, DC, Pan American Sanitary Organization, 1950.
32. World Health Organization. Eradication of Smallpox. Official Records of the World Health Organization No. 87. Geneva, World Health Organization, 1958, pp 263–264, 508–512.
33. World Health Organization. Smallpox Eradication. Official Records of the World Health Organization No. 95. Geneva, World Health Organization, 1959, pp 572–588.
34. World Health Organization. Official Records of the World Health Organization No. 152. Geneva, World Health Organization, 1966, p 291.
35. World Health Organization. Handbook for Smallpox Eradication in Endemic Areas. Geneva, World Health Organization, 1967.
36. Henderson DA. The eradication of smallpox. Sci Am 235:25–33, 1976.
37. Henderson DA. Smallpox eradication. Proc R Soc Lond 199:83–97, 1977.
38. Henderson DA. The Deliberate Extinction of a Species. Philadelphia, American Philosophical Society, 1982.
39. Deria A, Jezek Z, Markvart K, et al. The world's last endemic case of smallpox: Surveillance and containment measures. Bull World Health Organ 58:279–283, 1980.
40. Shooter RA. Report of the Investigation into the Cause of the 1978 Birmingham Smallpox Occurrence. London, Her Majesty's Stationery Office, 1980.
41. Basu RN, Jezek Z, Ward NA. The eradication of smallpox from India. In History of International Public Health No. 2. New Delhi, World Health Organization, South-East Asia Regional Office, 1979.
42. Brilliant LB. The Management of Smallpox Eradication in India: A Case Study and Analysis. Ann Arbor, University of Michigan Press, 1985.

43. Joarder AK, Tarantola D, Tulloch J. The Eradication oF Smallpox from Bangladesh. World Health Organization Regional Publications South-East Asia Series No. 8. New Delhi, World Health Organization South-East Asia Regional Office, 1980.
44. Tekeste Y, Hailu A, do Amaral C, et al. Smallpox Eradication in Ethiopia. Brazzaville, World Health Organization, 1984.
45. Jezek Z, Al Aghbari M, Hatfield R, et al. Smallpox Eradication in Somalia. Alexandria, World Health Organization Eastern Mediterranean Regional Office and Ministry of Health, Somali Democratic Republic, 1981.
46. Nakano JH. Human poxvirus diseases. In Lennette EH (ed). Laboratory Diagnosis of Viral Infections. New York, Marcel Dekker, 1985, pp 401–423.
47. Hahon N. Cytopathogenicity and propagation of variola virus in tissue culture. J Immunol 81:426–432, 1958.
48. Pirsch JB, Mika LA, Purlson EH. Growth characteristics of variola virus in tissue culture. J Infect Dis 113:170–178, 1963.
49. World Health Organization. Guide to the Laboratory Diagnosis of Smallpox for Smallpox Eradication Programmes. Geneva, World Health Organization, 1969.
50. Downie AW, St Vincent L, Rao AR, Kempe CH. Antibody response following smallpox vaccination and revaccination. J Hyg 67:603–606, 1969.
51. Downie AW, St Vincent L, Goldstein L, et al. Antibody response in nonhaemorrhagic smallpox patients. J Hyg 67:609–618, 1969.
52. McCarthy K, Downie AW, Bradley WH. The antibody response in man following infection with viruses of the pox group. II. Antibody response following vaccination. J Hyg 56:466–478, 1958.
53. Downie AW, McCarthy K, Macdonald A, et al. Virus and virus antigen in the blood of smallpox patients. Their significances in early diagnosis and prognosis. Lancet 2:164–166, 1953.
54. White E. Chickenpox in Kerala. Indian J Public Health 22:141–151, 1978.
55. Jezek Z, Basu RN, Arya ZS. Problem of persistence of facial pock marks among smallpox patients. Indian J Public Health 22:95–101, 1978.
56. Jezek Z, Hardjotanojo W. Residual skin changes in patients who have recovered from variola minor. Bull World Health Organ 58:139–140, 1980.
57. Mitra AC, Sarkar JK, Mukherjee MK. Virus content of smallpox scabs. Bull World Health Organ 51:106–107, 1974.
58. Anders W, Posch J. Die Pockenausbrucke 1961/62 in Nordrhein-Westfalen. Bundesgesundheitbl 17:265–269, 1962.
59. Wehrle PF, Posch J, Richter KH, Henderson DA. An airborne outbreak of smallpox in a German hospital and its significance with respect to other recent outbreaks in Europe. Bull World Health Organ 43:669–679, 1970.
60. Huq F. Effect of temperature and relative humidity on variola virus in crusts. Bull World Health Organ 54:710–712, 1976.
61. Harper GJ. Airborne micro-organisms: Survival tests with four viruses. J Hyg 59:479–486, 1961.
62. Rogers L. Smallpox and vaccination in British India during the last seventy years. Proc R Soc Lond 38:135–139, 1944.
63. Hope Simpson RE. Infectiousness of communicable diseases in the household (measles, chickenpox and mumps). Lancet 2:549–554, 1952.
64. Carvalho Filho ES de, Morris L, Lavigne de Lemos A, et al. Smallpox eradication in Brazil, 1967–69. Bull World Health Organ 43:797–808, 1970.
65. Heiner GG, Fatima N, Daniel RW, et al. A study of inapparent infection in smallpox. Am J Epidemiol 94:252–268, 1971.
66. Henderson RH, Yekpe M. Smallpox transmission in southern Dahomey. A study of a village outbreak. Am J Epidemiol 90:423–428, 1969.
67. Thomas DB, McCormack WM, Arita I, et al. Endemic smallpox in rural East Pakistan. I. Methodology, clinical and epidemiologic characteristics of cases, and intervillage transmission. Am J Epidemiol 93:361–372, 1971.
68. Thomas DB, Arita I, McCormack WM, et al. Endemic smallpox in rural East Pakistan. II. Intravillage transmission and infectiousness. Am J Epidemiol 93:373–383, 1971.
69. Thomas DB, Mack TM, Ali A, Khan MM. Epidemiology of smallpox in West Pakistan. III. Outbreak detection and interlocality transmission. Am J Epidemiol 95:178–189, 1972.
70. Foege WH, Millar JD, Henderson DA. Smallpox eradication in west and central Africa. Bull World Health Organ 52:209–222, 1975.
71. Sencer DJ, Axnick NW. Cost-benefit analysis. In International Symposium on Vaccination Against Communicable Diseases. Symposia Series in Immunobiological Standardization 22:37–46, 1973.
72. Stojkovic L, Birtasevic B, Borjanovic S, et al (eds). Variola u Jugoslaviji 1972 Godine. Ljubljana, CCP Delo, 1974.
73. Mack TM. Smallpox in Europe, 1950–1971. J Infect Dis 125:161–169, 1972.
74. United Kingdom, Ministry of Health. Report of the Committee on Vaccination. London, His Majesty's Stationery Office, 1928.
75. Herrlich A, Mayr A, Mahnel H, Munz E. Experimental studies on transformation of the variola virus into the vaccinia virus. Arch Gesamte Virusforsch 12:579–599, 1963.
76. Baxby D. Jenner's Smallpox Vaccine. The Riddle of the Origin of Vaccinia Virus. London, Heinemann, 1981.
77. Rivers TM. Cultivation of vaccine virus for Jennerian prophylaxis in man. J Exp Med 54:453–461, 1931.
78. Barker LF. Further attenuated vaccinia virus: A possible alternative for primary immunization. In Sixth Annual Immunization Conference; Atlanta, GA; March 11–13, 1969, p 55.
79. Rivers TM, Ward SM. Jennerian prophylaxis by means of intradermal injections of cultured vaccine virus. J Exp Med 62:549–560, 1935.
80. Rivers TM, Ward SM, Baird RD. Amount and duration of immunity induced by intradermal inoculation of cultured vaccine virus. J Exp Med 69:857–866 1939.
81. van der Noordaa J, Dekking F, Posthuma J, Beunders BJW. Primary vaccination with an attenuated strain of vaccinia virus. Arch Gesamte Virusforsch 22:210–214, 1967.
82. Kempe CH, Fulginiti V, Minamitani M, Shinefeld H. Smallpox vaccination of eczema patients with a strain of attenuated live vaccinia (CV-I78). Pediatrics 42:980–989, 1968.
83. Tint H. The rationale for elective prevaccination with attenuated vaccine (CV-I78) in preventing some vaccination complications. In International Symposium on Smallpox Vaccine. Symposia Series in Immunobiological Standardization 19:281–292, 1973.
84. Galasso GJ, Karzon DT, Katz SL, et al (eds). Clinical and serological study of four smallpox vaccines comparing variations of dose and route of administration. J Infect Dis 135:131–186, 1977.
85. McIntosh K. A comparative study of four smallpox vaccines in children. In Quinnan GV Jr (ed). Vaccinia Viruses as Vectors for Vaccine Antigens. New York, Elsevier, 1985, pp 77–84.
86. Hochstein-Mintzel V, Hanichen T, Huber HC, et al. Vaccinia- und variolaprotektive Wirkung des modifizierten Vaccinia-Stammes MVA bei intramuskularer Immunisierung. Zentralbl Bakteriol Orig A 230:283–297, 1975.
87. Mayr A, Stickl H, Muller HK, et al. The smallpox vaccination strain MVA: Marker, genetic structure, experience gained with the parenteral vaccination and behavior in organisms with a debilitated defence mechanism. Zentralbl Bakteriol Orig B 167:375–390, 1978.
88. Hashizume S. A new attenuated strain of vaccinia virus, LC 16m8: Basic information [in Japanese]. J Clin Virol 3:229–235, 1975.
89. Hashizume S, Yoshizawa H, Morita M, Suzuki K. Properties of attenuated mutant of vaccinia virus, LC 16m8, derived from Lister strain. In Quinnan GV Jr (ed). Vaccinia Viruses as Vectors for Vaccine Antigens. New York, Elsevier, 1985, pp 87–99.
90. Kato S. Low neurovirulent variant of Lister strain of vaccinia virus. In Quinnan GV Jr (ed). Vaccinia Viruses as Vectors for Vaccine Antigens. New York, Elsevier, 1985, pp 85–86.
91. Japan, Ministry of Health. Report of Committee on Smallpox Vaccination. Investigation of treatment of complications caused by smallpox vaccination [in Japanese]. J Clin Virol 3:269–278, 1975.
92. Hekker AC, Bos JM, Smith L. A stable freeze-dried smallpox vaccine made in monolayer cultures of primary rabbit kidney cells. J Biol Stand 1:21–32, 1973.
93. Hekker AC, Huisman J, Polak MF, et al. Field work with a stable freeze-dried vaccine prepared in monolayers of rabbit kidney cells. In International Symposium on Smallpox Vaccine. Sympo-

sia Series in Immunobiological Standardization 19:187–195, 1973.
94. Hekker AC, Bos JM, Kumara Rai N, et al. Large-scale use of freeze-dried smallpox vaccine prepared in primary cultures of rabbit kidney cells. Bull World Health Organ 54:279–284, 1976.
95. Cross RM, Kaplan C, McClean D. The heat resistance of dried smallpox vaccine. Lancet 1:446–448, 1957.
96. Downie AW, McCarthy K. The antibody response in man following infection with viruses of the pox group. III. Antibody response in smallpox. J Hyg 56:479–487, 1958.
97. Pincus WB, Flick JA. The role of hypersensitivity in the pathogenesis of vaccinia virus infection in humans. J Pediatr 62:57–62, 1963.
98. Blattner RJ, Norman JO, Heys FM, Aksu I. Antibody response to cutaneous inoculation with vaccinia virus: Viremia and viruria in vaccinated children. J Pediatr 64:839–852, 1964.
99. Gins HA, Hackenthal H, Kamentzewa N. Experimentelle Untersuchungen über die Generalisierung des Vaccine-Virus beim Menschen und Versuchstier. Z Hyg Infectionskrankh 110:429–441, 1929.
100. Benenson AS. Immediate (so-called immune) reaction to smallpox vaccination. JAMA 143:1238–1249, 1950.
101. WHO Expert Committee on Smallpox. First report. WHO Technical Report Series No. 283. Geneva, World Health Organization, 1964.
102. Hanna W. Studies in Smallpox and Vaccination. Bristol, Wright, 1913.
103. Rao AR. Smallpox. Bombay, The Kothari Book Depot, 1972.
104. Zikmund V, Das N, Krishnayengar R, Kameswara Rao B. Contribution to the problem of challenge vaccination. Observations on vaccination of cured smallpox cases in India in 1971, 1972 and 1973. Indian J Public Health 22:102–106, 1978.
105. Winter PA, Mason JH, Kuhr E, et al. Combined immunization against poliomyelitis, diphtheria, whooping cough, tetanus and smallpox. S Afr Med J 37:513–515, 1963.
106. Karchmer AW, Friedman JP, Casey HL, et al. Simultaneous administration of live virus vaccines. Measles, mumps, poliomyelitis and smallpox. Am J Dis Child 121:382–388, 1971.
107. Lin HT. A study of the effect of simultaneous vaccination with BCG and smallpox vaccine in newborn infants. Bull World Health Organ 33:321–336, 1965.
108. Meers PD. Further observations on 17D–yellow fever vaccination by scarification, with and without simultaneous smallpox vaccination. Trans R Soc Trop Med Hyg 54:493–501, 1960.
109. Breman JG, Coffi E, Bomba-Ires KR, et al. Evaluation of a measles-smallpox vaccination campaign by a seroepidemiologic method. Am J Epidemiol 102:564–571, 1975.
110. Meyer HM Jr, Hostetler DD Jr, Bernheim BC, et al. Response of Volta children to jet inoculation of combined live measles, smallpox and yellow fever vaccines. Bull World Health Organ 30:783–794, 1964.
111. Ruben FL, Smith EA, Foster SO, et al. Simultaneous administration of smallpox, measles, yellow fever, and diphtheria-pertussis-tetanus antigens to Nigerian children. Bull World Health Organ 48:175–181, 1973.
112. Foege WH, Foster SO. Multiple antigen vaccine strategies in developing countries. Am J Trop Med Hyg 23:685–689, 1974.
113. Lane JM, Ruben FL, Neff JM, Millar JD. Complications of smallpox vaccination, 1968. National surveillance in the United States. N Engl J Med 281:1201–1208, 1969.
114. Lane JM, Ruben FL, Neff JM, Millar JD. Complications of smallpox vaccination, 1968: Results of ten statewide surveys. J Infect Dis 122:303–309, 1970.
115. Kempe CH. Studies on smallpox and complications of smallpox vaccination. Pediatrics 26:176–189, 1960.
116. Brainerd HD, Hanna L, Jawetz E. Methisazone in progressive vaccinia. N Engl J Med 276:620–622, 1967.
117. Wilson GS. The Hazards of Immunization. London, Athlone, 1967.
118. de Vries E. Post-vaccinal Perivenous Encephalitis. Amsterdam, Elsevier, 1960.
119. Weber G, Lange J. Zur Variationsbreite der "Inkubationszeiten" postvakzinaler zerebraler Erkrankungen. Dtsch Med Wochenschr 86:1461–1468, 1961.
120. Polak MF. Complications of smallpox vaccination in the Netherlands, 1959–1970. In International Symposium on Smallpox Vaccine. Symposia Series in Immunobiological Standardization 19:235–242, 1973.
121. Berger K, Puntigam F. Über die Erkrankungshaufigkeit verschiedener Altersklassen von Erstimpflingen an postvakzinaler Enzephalitis nachsubcutaner Pockenschutzimpfung. Wien Med 104:487–492, 1954.
122. Conybeare ET. Illnesses attributed to smallpox vaccination, 1951–1960. Part II. Illnesses reported as affecting the central nervous system. Monthly Bulletin of the Ministry of Health and the Public Health Laboratory Service 23:150–159, 1964.
123. Herrlich A. Probleme der Pocken und Pockenschutzimpfung. Munch Med Wochenschr 96:529–533, 1954.
124. Stuart G. Memorandum on postvaccinal encephalitis. Bull World Health Organ 1:36–53, 1947–1948.
125. Femmer J. Cited by Wilson GS. Hazards of Immunization. London, Athlone, 1967.
126. Seeleman K. Zerebrale Komplikationen nach Pock-enschutzimpfungen mit besonderer Berucksichtigung der Alterdisposition in Hamburg 1939 bis 1958. Dtsch Med Wochenschr 85:1081–1089, 1960.
127. van den Berg CA. L'encephalite post-vaccinale aux Pays-Bas. Bull Office Intern Hyg Publique 38:847–848, 1946.
128. Neff JM, Lane JM, Pert JH, et al. Complications of smallpox vaccination. I. National survey in the United States 1963. N Engl J Med 276:125–132, 1967.
129. Berger K, Heinrich W. Decrease in postvaccinal deaths in Austria after introducing a less pathogenic virus strain. In International Symposium on Smallpox Vaccine. Symposia Series in Immunobiological Standardization 19:199–203, 1973.
130. Marrenikova SS, Chimishkyan KL, Maltseva NN, et al. Characteristics of virus strains for production of smallpox vaccines. In Proceedings of the Symposium on Smallpox. Zagreb, Yugoslav Academy of Sciences and Arts, 1969, pp 65–79.
131. Bellows MT, Hyman MR, Merritt KK, et al. Effect of smallpox vaccination on outcome of pregnancy. Public Health Rep 64:319–323, 1949.
132. Abramowitz LJ. Vaccination and virus diseases during pregnancy. S Afr Med J 31:13, 1957.
133. Bourke GJ, Whitty RJ. Smallpox vaccination in pregnancy; a prospective study. BMJ 5364:1544–1546, 1964.
134. Communicable Disease Center. Manual of Operations: West and Central Africa Smallpox Eradication/Measles Control Program. Atlanta, Centers for Disease Control, 1966.
135. Tondury G, Foukas M. Die Gefahrdung des menschlichen Keimlings durch Pockenimpfung in Graviditate. Pathol Microbiol 27:602–623, 1964.
136. Marmelzat WL. Malignant tumors in smallpox vaccination scars. A report of 24 cases. Arch Dermatol 97:400–406, 1968.
137. Sewall S. Vaccinia osteomyelitis. Report of a case with isolation of the vaccinia virus. Bull Hosp Jt Dis 10:59–63, 1949.
138. Urner JA. Some observations of the vaccination of pregnant women and newborn infants. Am J Obstet Gynecol 13:70–76, 1927.
139. Lieberman BL. Vaccination of pregnant women and newborn infants. Am J Obstet Gynecol 14:217–220, 1927.
140. Donnally HH, Nicholson MM. A study of vaccination in five hundred newborn infants. JAMA 103:1269–1275, 1934.
141. Webster IM. The response of leprosy patients to smallpox vaccine. West Afr Med J 8:322–324, 1959.
142. Browne SG, Davis EM. Reaction in leprosy precipitated by smallpox vaccination. Lepr Rev 33:252–254, 1962.
143. Blake JB. Benjamin Waterhouse and the Introduction of Vaccination; a Reappraisal. Philadelphia, University of Pennsylvania Press, 1957.
144. Halsey RH. How the President, Thomas Jefferson and Dr. Benjamin Waterhouse established vaccination as a public health procedure. History of Medicine Series No. 5. New York, New York Academy of Medicine, 1936.
145. Chapin CV, Smith J. Permanency of the mild type of smallpox. J Preventive Med 6:273–320, 1932.
146. Vaughan VC. Smallpox before and after Edward Jenner. Hygeia 1:205–211, 1923.
147. Woodward SB, Feemster RF. The relation of smallpox morbidity to vaccination laws. N Engl J Med 208:317–318, 1933.

148. Leake JP. Questions and answers on smallpox vaccination. Public Health Rep 42:221–238, 1927.
149. Low RB. The Incidence of Small-pox Throughout the World in Recent Years. Reports to the Local Government Board on Public Health and Medical Subjects NS No. 117. London, His Majesty's Stationery Office, 1918.
150. Henneberg G. The distribution of smallpox in Europe 1919–1948. In Rodenwaldt E, Jusatz HJ (eds). World-Atlas of Epidemic Diseases, Part II. Hamburg, Falk-Verlag, 1956, pp 67–72.
151. Rodrigues BA. Smallpox eradication in the Americas. Bull Pan Am Health Organ 9:53–68, 1975.
152. Arita I, Henderson DA. Freeze-dried vaccine for the smallpox eradication programme. In Proceedings of the Symposium on Smallpox. Zagreb, Yugoslav Academy of Sciences and Arts, 1969, pp 39–50.
153. Arita I. The control of vaccine quality in the smallpox eradication programme. In International Symposium on Smallpox Vaccine. Symposia Series in Immunobiological Standardization 19:79–87, 1973.
154. Henderson DA, Arita I, Shafa E. Studies of the bifurcated needle and recommendations for its use. Unpublished document. Geneva, World Health Organization, 1969.
155. Mack TM, Thomas DB, Ali A, Khan MM. Epidemiology of smallpox in West Pakistan. I. Acquired immunity and the distribution of disease. Am J Epidemiol 95:157–168, 1972.
156. Foege WH, Millar JD, Lane JM. Selective epidemiologic control in smallpox eradication. Am J Epidemiol 94:311–315, 1971.
157. World Health Organization. Report of the WHO Ad Hoc Committee on Orthopoxvirus Infections. Wkly Epidemiol Rec 6:289, 1986.
158. Mahy BWJ, Almond JW, Berns KI, et al. The remaining stocks of smallpox virus should be destroyed. Science 262:1223–1224, 1993.
159. Roizman B, Joklik W, Fields B, Moss B. The destruction of smallpox virus stocks in national repositories: A grave mistake and a bad precedent. Infect Agents Dis 3:215–217, 1994.
160. World Health Organization. Report of the Ad Hoc Committee on Orthopoxvirus Infections. Executive Board Report EB 95/33 dated October 10, 1994.
161. Mackett M, Smith GL, Moss B. Vaccinia virus: A selectable eukaryotic cloning and expression vector. Proc Natl Acad Sci USA 79:7415–7419, 1982.
162. Panicali D, Paoletti E. Construction of poxviruses as cloning vectors: Insertion of the thymidine kinase gene from herpes simplex virus into the DNA of infectious vaccinia virus. Proc Natl Acad Sci USA 79:4927–4931, 1982.
163. Smith GL, Moss B. Infectious poxvirus vectors have capacity for at least 25,000 base pairs of foreign DNA. Gene 25:21–28, 1983.
164. Perkus ME, Piccini A, Lipinskas BR, Paoletti E. Recombinant vaccinia virus: Immunization against multiple pathogens. Science 229:981–984, 1985.
165. Moss B. Vaccinia virus: A tool for research and vaccine development. Science 252:1662–1667, 1991.
166. Fenner F, Comben BM. Genetic studies with mammalian poxviruses. I. Demonstration of recombination between two strains of poxviruses. Virology 5:530–548, 1958.
167. Sam CK, Dumbell KR. Expression of poxvirus DNA in coinfected cells and marker rescue of thermosensitive mutants by subgenomic fragments of DNA. Ann Virol 132E:135–150, 1981.
168. Nakano E, Panicali D, Paoletti E. Molecular genetics of vaccinia virus: Demonstration of marker rescue. Proc Natl Acad Sci USA 79:1593–1596, 1982.
169. Weir JP, Bajszar G, Moss B. Mapping of the vaccinia virus thymidine kinase gene by marker rescue and by cell-free translation of selected mRNA. Proc Natl Acad Sci USA 79:1210–1214, 1982.
170. Mackett M, Smith GL, Moss B. General method for production and selection of infectious vaccinia virus recombinants expressing foreign genes. J Virol 49:857–864, 1984.
171. Earl PL, Moss B. Generation of recombinant vaccinia viruses. In Ausubel FM, Brent R, Kingston RE, et al (eds). Current Protocols in Molecular Biology. New York, Greene Publishing Associates & Wiley Interscience, 1991, pp 16.17.11–16.17.16.
172. Davison AJ, Moss B. The structure of vaccinia virus early promoters. J Mol Biol 210:749–769, 1989.
173. Davison AJ, Moss B. The structure of vaccinia virus late promoters. J Mol Biol 210:771–784, 1989.
174. Moss B. Genetically engineered poxviruses for recombinant gene expression, vaccination, and safety. Proc Natl Acad Sci USA 93:11341–11348, 1996.
175. Fenner F, Henderson DA, Arita I, et al. Smallpox and Its Eradication. Geneva, World Health Organization, 1988.
176. Cooney EL, Collier AC, Greenberg PD, et al. Safety of and immunological response to a recombinant vaccinia virus vaccine expressing HIV envelope glycoprotein. Lancet 337:567–572, 1991.
177. Buller RML, Smith GL, Cremer K, et al. Decreased virulence of recombinant vaccinia virus expression vectors is associated with a thymidine kinase–negative phenotype. Nature 317:813–815, 1985.
178. Lee SL, Roos JM, McGuigan LC, et al. Molecular attenuation of vaccinia virus: Mutant generation and animal characterization. J Virol 66:2617–2630, 1992.
179. Buller RML, Palumbo GJ. Poxvirus pathogenesis. Microbiol Rev 55:80–122, 1991.
180. Tartaglia J, Perkus ME, Taylor J, et al. NYVAC—a highly attenuated strain of vaccinia virus. Virology 188:217–232, 1992.
181. Konishi E, Pincus S, Paoletti E, et al. A highly attenuated host range–restricted vaccinia virus strain, NYVAC, encoding the prM, E, and NS1 genes of Japanese encephalitis virus prevents JEV viremia in swine. Virology 190:454–458, 1992.
182. Stephenson CB, Welter J, Thaker SR, et al. Canine distemper virus (CDV) infection of ferrets as a model for testing *Morbillivirus* vaccine strategies: NYVAC- and ALVAC-based CDV recombinants protect against symptomatic infection. J Virol 71:1506–1513, 1997.
183. Mayr A, Hochstein-Mintzel V, Stickl H. Abstammung, Eigenschaften und Verwendung des attenuierten Vaccinia-stammes MVA. Infection 3:6–14, 1975.
184. Stickl H, Hochstein-Mintzel V, Mayr A, et al. MVA-Stufenimpfung gegen Pocken. Klinische Erprobung des attenuierten Pocken-lebendimpfstoffes, Stamm MVA. Dtsch Med Wochenschr 99:2386–2392, 1974.
185. Sutter G, Moss B. Non-replicating vaccinia vector efficiently expresses recombinant genes. Proc Natl Acad Sci USA 89:10847–10851, 1992.
186. Sutter G, Wyatt LS, Foley PL, et al. A recombinant vector derived from the host range–restricted and highly attenuated MVA strain of vaccinia virus stimulates protective immunity in mice to influenza virus. Vaccine 12:1032–1040, 1994.
187. Hirsch VM, Fuerst TR, Sutter G, et al. Patterns of viral replication correlate with outcome in simian immunodeficiency virus (SIV)–infected macaques: Effect of prior immunization with a trivalent SIV vaccine in modified vaccinia virus Ankara. J Virol 70:3741–3752, 1996.
188. Wyatt LS, Shors ST, Murphy BR, Moss B. Development of a replication-deficient recombinant vaccinia virus vaccine effective against parainfluenza virus 3 infection in an animal model. Vaccine 14:1451–1458, 1996.
189. Bennink JR, Yewdell JW, Smith JW, et al. Recombinant vaccinia virus primes and stimulates influenza virus HA-specific CTL. Nature 311:578–579, 1984.
190. Yewdell JW, Bennink JR, Smith GL, Moss B. Influenza A virus nucleoprotein is a major target for cross-reactive anti-influenza virus cytotoxic T lymphocytes. Proc Natl Acad Sci USA 82:1785–1789, 1985.
191. Walker BD, Chakrabarti S, Moss B, et al. HIV-specific cytotoxic T lymphocytes in seropositive individuals. Nature 328:345–348, 1987.
192. Walker BD, Flexner C, Paradis TJ, et al. HIV-1 reverse transcriptase is a target for cytotoxic T lymphocytes in infected individuals. Science 240:64–66, 1988.
193. Bennink JR, Yewdell JW. Recombinant vaccinia viruses as vectors for studying T lymphocyte specificity and function. Curr Top Microbiol Immunol 163:153–184, 1990.
194. Otteken A, Earl PL, Moss B. Folding, assembly, and intracellular trafficking of the human immunodeficiency virus type 1 envelope glycoprotein analyzed with monoclonal antibodies recognizing maturational intermediates. J Virol 70:3407-3415, 1996.
195. Olmsted RA, Elango N, Prince GA, et al. Expression of the F

glycoprotein of respiratory syncytial virus by a recombinant vaccinia virus: Comparison of the individual contributions of the F and G glycoproteins to host immunity. Proc Natl Acad Sci USA 83:7462–7466, 1986.

196. Spriggs MK, Murphy BR, Prince GA, et al. Expression of the F and HN glycoproteins of human parainfluenza virus type 3 by recombinant vaccinia viruses: Contributions of the individual proteins to host immunity. J Virol 61:3416–3423, 1987.

197. Paterson RG, Lamb RA, Moss B, Murphy BR. Comparison of the relative roles of the F and HN surface glycoproteins of the paramyxovirus simian virus 5 in inducing protective immunity. J Virol 61:1972–1977, 1987.

198. Connors M, Kulkarni AB, Collins PL, et al. Resistance to respiratory syncytial virus (RSV) challenge induced by infection with a vaccinia virus recombinant expressing the RSV M2 protein (VacM2) is mediated by $CD8^+$ T cells, while that induced by Vac-F or Vac-G recombinants is mediated by antibodies. J Virol 66:1277–1281, 1992.

199. Andrew ME, Coupar BEH, Boyle DB, Ada GL. The roles of influenza virus haemagglutinin and nucleoprotein as protective antigens against influenza virus infection in mice. Scand J Immunol 25:21–28, 1987.

200. Moss B, Smith GL, Gerin JL, Purcell RH. Live recombinant vaccinia virus protects chimpanzees against hepatitis B. Nature 311:67–69, 1984.

201. Flexner C, Moss B. New generation vaccines. In Levine MM, Woodrow GC, Kasper JB, Cobon GS (eds). New Generation Vaccines. New York, Marcel Dekker, 1997, pp 297–314.

202. Bernards R, Destree A, McKenzie S, et al. Effective tumor immunotherapy directed against an oncogene-encoded product using a vaccinia virus vector. Proc Natl Acad Sci USA 84:6854–6858, 1987.

203. Estin CD, Stevenson US, Plowman GD, et al. Recombinant vaccinia virus vaccine against the human melanoma antigen p97 for use in immunotherapy. Proc Natl Acad Sci USA 85:1052–1056, 1988.

204. Kantor J, Irvine K, Abrams S, et al. Immunogenicity and safety of a recombinant vaccinia virus vaccine expressing the carcinoembryonic antigen gene in a nonhuman primate. Cancer Res 52:6917–6925, 1992.

205. Carroll MW, Overwiijk WW, Chamberlain RS, et al. Highly attenuated modified vaccinia virus Ankara (MVA) as an effective recombinant vector: A murine tumor model. Vaccine 15:387–394, 1997.

206. Boyle DB, Coupar BEH. Construction of recombinant fowlpox viruses as vectors for poultry vaccines. Virus Res 10:343–356, 1988.

207. Romero CH, Barrett T, Evans SA, et al. Single capripoxvirus recombinant vaccine for the protection of cattle against rinderpest and lumpy skin disease. Vaccine 11:737–742, 1993.

208. Taylor J, Weinberg R, Languet B, et al. Recombinant fowlpox virus inducing protective immunity in non-avian species. Vaccine 6:497–503, 1988.

209. Somogyi P, Frazier J, Skinner MA. Fowlpox virus host range restriction: Gene expression, DNA replication, and morphogenesis in nonpermissive mammalian cells. Virology 197:439–444, 1993.

210. Langford DJ, Edwards SJ, Smith GL, et al. Anchoring a secreted plasmodium antigen on the surface of recombinant vaccinia virus infected cells increases its immunogenicity. Mol Cell Biol 6:3191–3199, 1986.

211. Both GW, Andrew ME, Boyle DB, et al. Relocation of antigens to the cell surface membrane can enhance immune stimulation and protection. Immunol Cell Biol 70:73–78, 1992.

212. Ramsay AJ, Ramsay AJ, Leong KH, et al. Vector-encoded interleukin-5 and interleukin-6 enhance specific mucosal immunoglobulin A reactivity in vivo. Adv Exp Med Biol 371A:35–42, 1995.

213. Chamberlain RS, Carroll MW, Bronte V, et al. Costimulation enhances the active immunotherapy effect of recombinant anticancer vaccines. Cancer Res 56:2832–2836, 1996.

214. Bronte V, Tsung K, Rao JB, et al. IL-2 enhances the function of recombinant poxvirus-based vaccines in the treatment of established pulmonary metastases. J Immunol 154:5282–5292, 1995.

215. Hekker AC, Bos JM, Smith L. A stable freeze-dried smallpox vaccine made in monolayer cultures of primary rabbit kidney cells. J Biol Stand 1:21–32, 1973.

216. Graham BS, Belshe RB, Clements ML, et al. Vaccination of vaccinia-naive adults with human immunodeficiency virus type-1 gp160 recombinant vaccinia virus in a blinded, controlled, randomized clinical trial. J Infect Dis 166:244–252, 1992.

217. Earl PL, Hügin AW, Moss B. Removal of cryptic poxvirus transcription termination signals from the human immunodeficiency virus type 1 envelope gene enhances expression and immunogenicity of a recombinant vaccinia virus. J Virol 64:2448–2451, 1990.

218. Cooney EL, McElrath MJ, Corey L, et al. Enhanced immunity to human immunodeficiency virus (HIV) envelope elicited by a combined vaccine regimen consisting of priming with a vaccinia recombinant expressing HIV envelope and boosting with gp160-protein. Proc Natl Acad Sci USA 90:1882–1886, 1993.

219. Graham BS, Matthews TJ, Belshe RB, et al. Augmentation of human immunodeficiency virus type-1 neutralizing antibody by priming with gp160 recombinant vaccinia and boosting with rgp160 in vaccinia-naive adults. J Infect Dis 167:533–537, 1993.

220. Pialoux G, Excler JL, Riviere Y, et al. A prime-boost approach to HIV preventive vaccine using a recombinant canarypox virus expressing glycoprotein 160 (MN) followed by a recombinant glycoprotein 160 (MN/LAI). AIDS Res Hum Retroviruses 11:373–381, 1995.

221. Egan M, Ravlat W, Tartaglia J, et al. Induction of human immunodeficiency virus type 1 (HIV-1)–specific cytolytic T lymphocyte responses in seronegative adults by a non-replicating, host-range-restricted canarypox vector (ALVAC) carrying the HIV-1_{MN} *env* gene. J Infect Dis 171:1623–1627, 1995.

222. Fleury B, Janvier G, Pialoux G, et al. Memory cytotoxic T lymphocyte responses in human immunodeficiency virus type 1 (HIV-1)–negative volunteers immunized with a recombinant canarypox expressing gp160 of HIV-1 and boosted with a recombinant gp160. J Infect Dis 174:734–738, 1996.

223. Gu SY, Huang TM, Ruan L, et al. First EBV vaccine trial in humans using recombinant vaccinia virus expressing the major membrane antigen. Dev Biol Stand 84:171–177, 1995.

224. Cadoz M, Strady A, Meignier B, et al. Immunization with canarypox virus expressing rabies glycoprotein. Lancet 339:1429–1432, 1992.

225. Fries LF, Tartaglia J, Taylor J, et al. Human safety and immunogenicity of a canarypox-rabies glycoprotein recombinant vaccine: An alternative poxvirus vector system. Vaccine 14:428–434, 1996.

226. Fenner F, Gibbs EPJ, Murphy FA, et al. Veterinary Virology (2nd ed). San Diego, CA, Academic Press, 1993.

227. Mackett M, Yilma T, Rose JK, Moss B. Vaccinia virus recombinants: Expression of VSV genes and protective immunization of mice and cattle. Science 227:433–435, 1985.

228. Giavedoni L, Jones L, Mebus C, Yilma T. A vaccinia virus double recombinant expressing the F and H genes of rinderpest virus protects cattle against rinderpest and causes no pock lesions. Proc Natl Acad Sci USA 88:8011–8015, 1991.

229. Brockmeier SL, Lager KM, Tartaglia J, et al. Vaccination of pigs against pseudorabies with highly attenuated vaccinia (NYVAC) recombinant viruses. Vet Microbiol 38:41–58, 1993.

230. Chambers TM, Kawaoka Y, Webster RG. Protection of chickens from lethal influenza infection by vaccinia-expressed hemagglutinin. Virology 167:414–421, 1988.

231. Wiktor TJ, Macfarlan RI, Reagan KJ, et al. Protection from rabies by a vaccinia virus recombinant containing the rabies virus glycoprotein gene. Proc Natl Acad Sci USA 81:7194–7198, 1984.

232. Rupprecht CE, Wiktor TJA, Johnston DH, et al. Oral immunization and protection of raccoons *(Procyon lotor)* with a vaccinia-rabies glycoprotein recombinant virus vaccine. Proc Natl Acad Sci USA 83:7947–7950, 1986.

233. Brochier B, Costy F, Pastoret PP. Elimination of fox rabies from Belgium using a recombinant vaccinia-rabies vaccine: An update. Vet Microbiol 46:269–279, 1995.

234. Esposito JJ, Knight JC, Shaddock JH, et al. Successful oral rabies vaccination of raccoons with raccoon poxvirus recombinants expressing rabies virus glycoprotein. Virology 167:313–316, 1988.

235. Romero CH, Barrett T, Chamberlain RW, et al. Recombinant capripoxvirus expressing the hemagglutinin protein gene of rinderpest virus: Protection of cattle against rinderpest and lumpy skin disease. Virology 204:425–429, 1994.

236. van der Leek ML, Feller JA, Sorenson G, et al. Evaluation of swinepox virus as a vaccine vector in pigs using an Aujeszky's disease (pseudorabies) virus gene insert coding for glycoproteins gp50 and gp63. Vet Rec 134:13–18, 1994.
237. Webster RG, Kawaoka Y, Taylor J, et al. Efficacy of nucleoprotein and haemagglutinin antigens expressed in fowlpox virus as vaccine for influenza in chickens. Vaccine 9:303–308, 1991.
238. Boursnell ME, Green PF, Samson AC, et al. A recombinant fowlpox virus expressing the hemagglutinin-neuraminidase gene of Newcastle disease virus (NDV) protects chickens against challenge by NDV. Virology 178:297–300, 1990.
239. Edbauer C, Weinberg R, Taylor J, et al. Protection of chickens with a recombinant fowlpox virus expressing the Newcastle disease virus hemagglutinin-neuraminidase gene. Virology 179:901–904, 1990.
240. Bayliss CD, Peters RW, Cook JKA, et al. A recombinant fowlpox virus that expresses the VP2 antigen of infectious bursal disease virus induces protection against mortality caused by the virus. Arch Virol 120:193–205, 1991.
241. Tartaglia J, Jarrett O, Neil JC, et al. Protection of cats against feline leukemia virus by vaccination with a canarypox virus recombinant, ALVAC-FL. J Virol 67:2370–2375, 1993.

chapter

7 Immunization in the Immunocompromised Host

Per Ljungman

Since the mid-1970s, the number of immunocompromised patients has increased rapidly. Patients can be immunocompromised, for example, by the immunosuppression given after solid organ transplantation; infection with the human immunodeficiency virus (HIV); and increased intensity of therapy for malignancies such as acute leukemia, which can include intensified chemotherapy protocols and allogeneic and autologous stem cell transplantation. Infections have been major obstacles to successful transplantations. In transplant patients, the highest risk for infection usually occurs soon after the transplantation. However, many of these patients remain immunosuppressed owing to either the interaction between the graft and the host, such as graft-versus-host disease (GVHD) after allogeneic bone marrow transplantation (BMT), or the immunosuppressive therapy given to prevent graft rejection. HIV-infected patients become progressively more immunosuppressed over time.

Immunizations of immunocompromised individuals are important from two points of view. Obviously, the most important need is that of protecting the patient against serious infections. However, the public health point of view is also important, as there is a need to prevent any increase in the number of individuals who are vulnerable to harmful infectious agents, such as poliovirus. Both priorities require an analysis of risks and benefits for the individual patient.[1]

PATIENTS INFECTED WITH HUMAN IMMUNODEFICIENCY VIRUS

HIV-infected patients are at risk for several different infections that can be prevented by immunization. Thus, the potential benefits of immunization are clear. The question of when immunizations should be performed in HIV-infected patients is complex, owing to progress of the disease that might influence both the risk for side effects and the effectiveness of immunization. In addition to the risks for severe complications from live attenuated vaccines in patients with more advanced HIV infection, there is the risk of activating the immune system by vaccination, which could potentially increase viral replication and thereby promote the HIV infection. None of the studies cited in this chapter has been performed in patients receiving modern combination antiretroviral therapy, a technique that might change the risks and benefits of vaccination with many of the vaccines discussed. Nevertheless, in general there is no harm in vaccinating HIV-infected patients with inactivated vaccines, and although efficacy is reduced in advanced disease, it does not appear wanting in patients early in infection.[1a] A summary of the recommendations for vaccination of HIV-infected people is shown in Table 7–1. Recommendations from a working group comprising the U.S. Public Health Service and the Infectious Disease Society of America are shown in Figure 7–1.

Activation of Virus Replication and Increased Viral Load Through Vaccination

One issue of importance in HIV-infected patients is the risk of activating T cells by vaccination; in addition, there can be an increase in susceptibility of $CD4^+$ T lymphocytes and a possibly associated increase in viral load. These risks have been studied by several investigators. O'Brien and colleagues showed a transient increase in plasma HIV type 1 (HIV-1) RNA levels after immunization with influenza vaccines that was more pronounced in patients with higher $CD4^+$ cell numbers.[1b] Similar results were found by other investigators after influenza vaccination[2–4] and after immunization with tetanus toxoid.[5] In a randomized trial, however, Glesby and colleagues found no difference between influenza vaccine and placebo recipients.[6] These conflicting results could depend on the number of $CD4^+$ cells in the studied recipients, since in two studies patients with higher $CD4^+$ cell numbers had more marked increases in viral load.[2, 3] Alternatively, the results could depend on the antiretroviral therapy given to the patients at the time of immunization.[4]

Table 7–1. **RECOMMENDATIONS FOR IMMUNIZATIONS IN HUMAN IMMUNODEFICIENCY VIRUS–INFECTED PATIENTS**

VACCINE	CHILDREN	ADULTS	COMMENTS
Pneumococcal	Yes	No	Early in the course of HIV infection
Conjugated *Haemophilus influenzae* type b virus	Yes	No	Children early in the course of HIV infection
Influenza	Yes	Yes	Seasonal
Hepatitis B virus	Yes	No	Children of HIV-infected mothers
Diphtheria toxoid	Yes	Yes	All children; adults in high-risk areas
Tetanus toxoid	Yes	No	All children; adults, same indications as in immunocompetent individuals
Inactivated poliovirus	Yes	No	All children; adults, same indications as in immunocompetent individuals
Measles	Yes	No	All children
Bacille Calmette-Guérin virus	In high-risk areas	No	Children in countries with high risk of tuberculosis

HIV, human immunodeficiency virus.

Killed Vaccines

Pneumococcal Vaccine. Patients infected with HIV have a high risk for infections with *Haemophilus influenzae* type b (Hib) and pneumococci, and thus immunizations against these infections have been studied extensively. Studies have documented that the antibody levels to pneumococci before vaccination are lower in HIV-infected patients than in healthy control subjects.[7, 8] The results of immunization studies have diverged regarding the influence of the duration and stage of HIV infection. Most studies have shown impaired immune responses with lower rates of seroconversion in patients with $CD4^+$ cell counts below 500 × 10^6/L,[9–11] whereas other studies have failed to find a correlation between immunoglobulin G (IgG) response and $CD4^+$ cell count.[8, 12–14] Several of these studies have reported other defects in the immune response to immunization, however, such as poor IgM responses,[8, 13] poor IgA responses in patients with fewer than 500 × 10^6/L $CD4^+$ cells,[13] or poor IgG2 responses.[15] Most evidence supports the idea that immunizations with pneumococcal vaccine should be given early in the course of HIV infection.

Nonresponders to polysaccharide-based pneumococcal vaccine do not benefit from reimmunization with a double dose of vaccine.[16] The new conjugate vaccines also may not influence the immune response in HIV-infected patients. King and colleagues found lower responses in HIV-infected children than in healthy control subjects to both the conjugated and standard pneumococcal vaccines, although slightly better responses were found with the conjugated vaccine.[7] In a randomized trial, Ahmed and colleagues also found similar responses to the two types of vaccines in HIV-infected individuals, whereas healthy control subjects responded with significantly higher titers to the T cell–dependent conjugated vaccine.[17]

***Haemophilus influenzae* Type b Vaccine.** Results similar to those obtained with pneumococcal vaccines have been found with conjugated vaccines against Hib. In a study of HIV-infected infants, Kale and colleagues found that patients with symptomatic HIV infection had lower responses to the conjugated Hib vaccine.[18] In a study by Peters and Sood, only 37% of children were found to be immune after receiving immunization.[19] Furthermore, Gibb and colleagues showed rapidly decreasing antibody levels in HIV-infected children after vertical HIV transmission.[20] Immunization of HIV-infected children should be performed early in the course of the HIV infection. Reimmunizations might be needed, but studies are presently lacking regarding the antibody response after reimmunization.

Influenza Vaccine. Because the immune response to influenza vaccine is T cell–dependent, it is logical to expect that patients with more advanced HIV infection and lower $CD4^+$ cell numbers will respond less than patients with early HIV infection. This result was obtained in a study by Kroon and colleagues, in which patients with levels of $CD4^+$ cells below 100 × 10^6/L were unable to respond with antibody formation to two doses of influenza vaccine.[12] Chadwick and colleagues showed that HIV-infected children produce lower antibody responses than age-matched control subjects and that children with acquired immunodeficiency syndrome (AIDS) responded poorly to immunization.[21] Influenza responses are inversely correlated with $CD4^+/CD8^+$ cell ratios in HIV-infected children.[21a] Influenza vaccinations must be given every year; however, because both the risk for severe infection and the likelihood for a poor response to immunization increase with more advanced HIV infection, the use of this vaccine has been questioned on a cost-effectiveness basis.[22] The benefit most likely exceeds the risk, however, and influenza vaccination should be considered in HIV-infected patients.

Tetanus Toxoid, Diphtheria Toxoid, and Inactivated Poliovirus Vaccine. In a study of HIV-infected patients' immune status to tetanus and diphtheria, the frequency of immunity against tetanus was similar to that expected for a normal population of the same age, whereas the immunity to diphtheria was lower than expected.[23] This means that reimmunization against diphtheria should be considered in areas where the risk for diphtheria is a reality as well as for HIV-infected patients traveling to such areas. The immune response to these antigens is T cell–dependent, and the response to vaccination is low in patients with more advanced HIV infection.[12, 24]

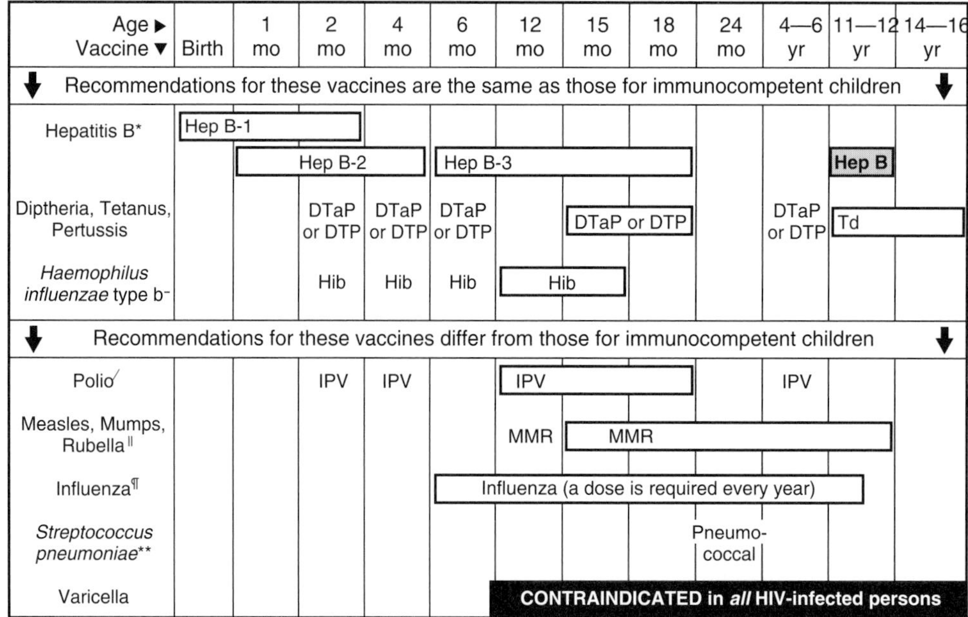

Figure 7–1. Recommended immunization schedule for human immunodeficiency virus (HIV)–infected children.

Note: Modified from the immunization schedule for immunocompetent children. This schedule also applies to children born to HIV-infected mothers whose HIV infection status has not been determined. Once it is known that a child is not infected with HIV, the schedule for immunocompetent children applies. This schedule indicates the recommended ages for routine administration of currently licensed childhood vaccines. Some combination vaccines are available and may be used whenever the administration of all components of the vaccine is indicated. Providers should consult the manufacturers' package inserts for detailed recommendations.

Vaccines are listed under the routinely recommended ages. Bars indicate the ranges of acceptable ages for vaccination. Shaded bars indicate catch-up vaccination: At 11 to 12 years of age, hepatitis B vaccine should be administered to children not previously vaccinated.

**Infants born to HBsAg (hepatitis B surface antigen)–negative mothers* should receive 2.5 μg of Merck vaccine (Recombivax HB) or 10 μg of SmithKline Beecham (SB) vaccine (Engerix-B). The second dose should be administered more than 1 month after the first dose.

Infants born to HBsAg-positive mothers should receive 0.5 mL of hepatitis B immune globulin at birth, in addition to either 5 μg of Merck vaccine (Recombivax) or 10 μg of SB vaccine (Engerix), followed by repeated vaccine doses at 1 to 2 months of age and the third dose at 6 months of age.

Infants born to mothers whose HBsAg status is unknown should receive either 5 μg of Merck vaccine (Recombivax) or 10 μg of SB vaccine (Engerix-B) within 12 hours of birth. The second dose of vaccine is recommended at 1 month of age, and the third dose at 6 months of age. Blood should be drawn at the time of delivery to determine the mother's HBsAg status; if it is positive, the infant should receive HBIG as soon as possible (no later than 1 week of age). The dosage and timing of subsequent vaccine doses should be based on the mother's HBsAg status.

Children and adolescents who have not been vaccinated against hepatitis B in infancy may begin the series at the 11- to 12-year-old visit. The second dose should be administered 1 or more months after the first dose, and the third dose should be administered 4 or more months after the first dose and 2 or more months after the second dose.

†DTaP (diphtheria and tetanus toxoids and acellular pertussis vaccine) is the preferred vaccine for all doses in the vaccination series, including completion of the series in children who have received more than 1 dose of whole-cell diphtheria, tetanus, and pertussis (DTP) vaccine. Whole-cell DTP is an acceptable alternative to DTaP. The fourth dose of DTaP may be administered as early as 12 months of age, provided that 6 months have elapsed since the third dose and the child is considered unlikely to return at 15 to 18 months of age. Td (tetanus and diphtheria toxoids, adsorbed, for adult use) is recommended for children 11 to 12 years of age if 5 or more years has elapsed since the last dose of DTP, DTaP, or DT. Subsequent routine Td boosters are recommended every 10 years.

‡Three *Haemophilus influenzae* type b (Hib) conjugate vaccines are licensed for infant use. If PedvaxHIB (Merck) is administered at 2 and 4 months of age, a dose at 6 months is not required. After the primary series has been completed, any Hib conjugate vaccine may be used as a booster.

§Inactivated poliovirus vaccine (IPV) is the only vaccine recommended for HIV-infected people and their household contacts. Although the third dose of IPV is generally administered at 12 to 18 months of age, the third dose of IPV has been approved to be administered as early as 6 months of age. Oral poliovirus vaccine should not be administered to HIV-infected people or their household contacts.

‖The measles, mumps, and rubella (MMR) vaccine should not be administered to severely immunocompromised children. HIV-infected children without severe immunosuppression should routinely receive their first dose of MMR as soon as possible after their first birthday. Consideration should be given to administering the second dose of MMR vaccine as soon as 1 month (i.e., 28 or more days) after the first dose, rather than waiting until school entry.

¶Influenza virus vaccine should be administered each year to all HIV-infected children older than 6 months. Children 6 months to 8 years of age who are receiving influenza vaccine for the first time should receive two doses of split-virus vaccine separated by at least 1 month. In subsequent years, a single dose of vaccine (split virus for people ≤12 years of age, whole or split virus for people >12 years of age) should be administered each year. The dose of vaccine for children aged 6 to 35 months is 0.25 mL; the dose for children 3 years and older is 0.5 mL.

**The 23-valent pneumococcal vaccine should be administered to HIV-infected children at 24 months of age. In general, revaccination should be offered to HIV-infected children younger than 10 years who were vaccinated 3 to 5 years earlier or to children older than 10 years who were vaccinated more than 5 years earlier.

(Adapted from U.S. Public Health Services and the Infectious Disease Society of America. Recommended immunization for HIV-infected children. USPHS/IDSA guidelines. Clin Infect Dis 25[suppl 3]:S330, 1997.)

Hepatitis B Virus Vaccine. Immunization against hepatitis B virus (HBV) has been studied in infants born to HIV-infected mothers. These studies have yielded similar results, namely, that children who become infected with HIV respond poorly to HBV vaccine, whereas children who are antibody positive against HIV but have not become infected respond well to the HBV vaccine.[25–27]

Other Vaccines. There is limited information regarding the response to other vaccines that might be considered in certain situations, such as before travel. The immune response to hepatitis A vaccine was found to be similar to the T cell–dependent vaccines in that patients with symptomatic HIV infection seroconverted at a lower frequency.[28] In a study of orally administered cholera toxin B subunit, HIV-infected patients developed good antibody responses after two doses of vaccine.[29] This study is of interest, since it illustrates that the mucosal route of immunization can be effective in immunocompromised subjects.

Live Attenuated Vaccines

The safety of immunization with live attenuated vaccines is a matter of concern in HIV-infected patients. The vaccines of importance include measles, bacille Calmette-Guérin (BCG), and oral poliovirus vaccines.

Measles Vaccine. Measles can be a life-threatening infection in immunocompromised hosts. Kaplan and colleagues reviewed 27 published cases of measles, of whom 20 (74%) developed pneumonitis and 8 (30%) died; previously vaccinated patients tended to have a lower mortality.[30] The number of measles cases has since increased in several countries, including the United States. In a series of 81 children, Arpadi and colleagues showed an overall serological response to immunization of 72%, with a better response if the children were immunized before 1 year of age.[31] However, there was a rapid loss of antibody, with only 52% of the children having detectable antibody to measles when studied more than 1 year after immunization. Poor and evanescent responses to measles vaccine were also reported by Krasinski and Borkowsky.[31a] Frenkel and colleagues studied 10 children with symptomatic HIV infection who were immunized with live attenuated measles, mumps, and rubella vaccine.[32] Although the serological response to immunization was poor, no child experienced symptoms thought to be related to the vaccine, and virus could not be recovered from blood cells or plasma.

Most HIV-infected adults are seropositive to measles. Wallace and colleagues found a 95% seropositivity rate in a survey of 210 HIV-infected adults.[33] Six seronegative HIV-infected adults were immunized, but only two of these responded. The rate of occurrence of side effects has been low, but a case of progressive vaccine-associated measles pneumonitis has been reported.[34] Thus, the prevention of measles in HIV-infected children could be beneficial and has been recommended by the American Academy of Pediatrics for all HIV-infected children.[35] This recommendation was based on the fact that no severe side effects were noted after vaccination in more than 100 HIV-infected children.[36]

Bacille Calmette-Guérin Vaccine. HIV-infected patients have a high risk of developing tuberculosis. The available BCG vaccine is live and attenuated, and several case reports have shown that HIV-infected patients can develop disseminated BCG infection.[37–39] In one patient with AIDS, a disseminated BCG infection was documented 30 years after the patient had received BCG vaccine.[40] Besnard and colleagues reported BCG-associated complications in 9 of 68 HIV-infected children who were vaccinated before being diagnosed with HIV infection.[41] The complications occurred as late as 35 months after immunization in children with rapidly progressing HIV infection. O'Brien and colleagues found an increased risk for BCG-associated complications in HIV-infected children who were given a higher than recommended dose of BCG.[42] Thus, most studies indicate an increased risk for complications in HIV-infected patients from BCG vaccine. Unfortunately no data exist regarding the protective efficacy of BCG in HIV-infected patients, making a risk-benefit assessment difficult. The World Health Organization currently recommends BCG immunization for all people in developing countries with a high risk for *Mycobacterium tuberculosis* infection and for HIV-infected children.[43] BCG immunization is not recommended in developed countries with a low risk for contracting tuberculosis.

Other Live Vaccines. The most commonly used live vaccine is probably oral poliovirus vaccine. It is generally not recommended for immunocompromised patients, as paralytic cases can occur. Little information exists about its use in HIV-infected individuals. Ryder and colleagues reported from Zaire that no severe side effects were seen in infants with HIV-1 infection who were given the trivalent oral Sabin vaccine.[44] However, use of the inactivated poliovirus vaccine is generally recommended because it is an effective alternative to the live vaccine and does not carry a risk for development of paralytic disease. No information is available regarding the risks of other live virus vaccines such as varicella-zoster virus (VZV) or yellow fever virus vaccines. VZV vaccine is not currently indicated in HIV-infected individuals, but studies are in progress. The decision regarding immunization with vaccine against yellow fever should be made after careful assessment of the vaccine's potential side effects in relation to the clinical status of the individual and his or her risk of contracting yellow fever.

Another potentially important issue is the immunization of hospital staff or family members with live virus vaccines that have the potential to cause secondary infection in HIV-infected patients. One situation in which this might be especially important is after immunization with the live oral poliovirus vaccine, which can be excreted by the vaccinees for an extended period.[45]

PATIENTS WITH CANCER

Most studies support the safety and efficacy of immunization of cancer patients. However, cancer chemotherapy and radiotherapy have been intensified substantially during the 1990s, and the results of earlier studies might not represent the true situation today. Few studies of immunity and vaccination have been published regarding adult solid tumor patients undergoing active anticancer therapy, and many studies have based their results on mixed study populations frequently not specified as to a type of cancer or intensity of given therapy. Moreover, most studies have concentrated on patients with hematological malignancies. Unless otherwise stated, the discussion in the remainder of this chapter refers to leukemia and lymphoma patients. A summary of the immunization recommendations is shown in Table 7–2.

Killed Vaccines

Pneumococcal Vaccine. Pneumococci are important causes of infection in patients with hematological malignancies. Patients with Hodgkin's disease are frequently splenectomized as a part of their diagnosis and therapy, making this group especially vulnerable to disseminated pneumococcal infections. Several studies have examined the effect of pneumococcal polysaccharide-based vaccines in patients with cancer. In children with leukemia, for example, the 14-valent vaccine gave suboptimal antibody responses.[46] The response in patients with Hodgkin's disease varied according to when in the course of therapy the immunization was performed. Patients who were immunized after chemotherapy, radiotherapy, or both had severely impaired antibody responses.[47, 48] In contrast, a good response can be obtained if immunizations are performed before therapy is initiated.[49, 50] The response in children with Hodgkin's disease was poorer if immunizations were performed after, rather than before, splenectomy.[51] However, although antibody responses can be elicited in splenectomized patients with non-Hodgkin's lymphoma and Hodgkin's disease[52]; the response is impaired for several years after the treatment of Hodgkin's disease.[50] Patients with carcinoma of the head or neck had poor antibody responses when immunizations were performed soon after radiotherapy.[53] Chan and colleagues showed that priming with a 7-valent conjugated pneumococcal vaccine could improve the response to the 23-valent polysaccharide vaccine in patients with previously treated Hodgkin's disease.[54] Immunization of patients with lymphoma against pneumococcal infections is recommended as early as possible after diagnosis and before chemotherapy or radiotherapy is initiated.

***Haemophilus influenzae* Type b Vaccine.** Compared with normal children, children with leukemia have a greater than sixfold risk of developing Hib disease.[55] Immunization with conjugated Hib vaccine resulted in lower antibody responses in children with leukemia than in normal children, and a booster dose was found to be ineffective; in these studies, longer duration and intensity of antileukemic chemotherapy were associated with a poor response to immunization.[55, 56] Children undergoing therapy for solid tumors also have lower than normal responses to vaccination with Hib vaccine.[57] One interesting approach that may improve the immunization results in patients with chronic lymphocytic leukemia is to add a histamine type 2 blocker—ranitidine—which in a randomized study was shown to improve the response to immunization with conjugated Hib vaccine.[58] Immunization with conjugated Hib vaccine is indicated in children with cancer, preferably early in the course of anticancer chemotherapy.

Influenza Vaccine. Influenza vaccination is recommended in immunocompromised patients.[59] The effect of influenza on morbidity and mortality varies in different types of cancer patients; the most severe consequences occur in acute leukemia patients undergoing induction chemotherapy,[60] whereas the morbidity in patients with other types of hematological malignancies is lower.[61] Kempe and colleagues reported that children with cancer had a duration of symptoms similar to that of healthy control subjects as well as too few clinical complications to analyze.[62] The responses to immunizations have been poorly studied in patients undergoing modern types of cancer chemotherapy. Two studies in children with leukemia and adult patients with lymphoma have shown responses of only approximately 40% after two doses of vaccine.[63, 64] Furthermore, titers that were protective in healthy control subjects reportedly failed to prevent influenza in 24% of children with cancer, although the severity of the infection may have been reduced in the vaccine failures.[62] Although influenza immunization is recommended in cancer patients, the protective effectiveness is likely to be low in those patients who have the highest risk for severe complication. Thus, other preventive strategies are needed. Elting and colleagues have reported that most influenza infections in acute leukemia patients undergoing chemotherapy are nosocomially acquired and that immunizations of family members and hospital staff members should therefore be considered.[60]

Tetanus Toxoid, Diphtheria Toxoid, and Inactivated Poliovirus Vaccine. The protection against tetanus toxoid, diphtheria toxoid, and poliovirus is fre-

Table 7–2. **RECOMMENDATIONS FOR IMMUNIZATIONS IN CANCER PATIENTS**

VACCINE	RECOMMENDATION	COMMENTS
Pneumococcal	Yes	Lymphoma patients
Conjugated *Haemophilus influenzae* type b virus	Yes	Children with cancer
Influenza	Yes	Seasonal
Varicella-zoster virus	Yes	Seronegative patients
Measles	No	Individual consideration, depending on local epidemiological situation

quently low in cancer patients undergoing chemotherapy. Hammarström and colleagues have shown that 41% of acute leukemia patients who had not had transplants were not protected against tetanus.[65] Risk factors for loss of immunity were acute lymphoblastic leukemia (compared with acute myeloblastic leukemia), more advanced disease, and increasing age. In addition, lymphoma patients were likely to be unprotected against these diseases. The immune responses to diphtheria toxoid and tetanus toxoid in children undergoing maintenance chemotherapy were similar to those of healthy individuals.[66] Similar results were obtained by a booster vaccination with inactivated poliovirus vaccine. Oral poliovirus vaccine can induce paralytic disease in immunocompromised patients and should not be used.[67] Furthermore, the vaccine strains can be transferred from healthy family members; the use of inactivated vaccine is therefore recommended for immunizing relatives. Because immunity to tetanus toxoid, diphtheria toxoid, and poliovirus is frequently deficient in cancer patients, booster immunizations should be considered in all patients with cancer.

Live Vaccines

Varicella-Zoster Virus Vaccine. Primary VZV infection has a high mortality in children with cancer. The existing vaccine is live attenuated and based on the Oka strain.[68] The vaccine was shown to be effective and safe in children with leukemia who were in remission.[69] In this study, the seroconversion rate was 88% after one dose and 98% after one or two doses. The rate of VZV infection was 8%, and all infected children had mild disease.[69] The frequency of side effects from the vaccine is low, and breakthrough vaccine disease can be treated effectively with acyclovir.[69, 70] The immunity is stable for at least 5 years after immunization. The risk for herpes zoster after vaccination was lower than in patients who had natural varicella.[71, 72] In a small randomized study, VZV vaccine was given to children with newly diagnosed cancer before starting chemotherapy. The vaccine produced a high rate of seroconversion and no severe side effects; however, the number of patients in the study was low.[73] Household exposure to VZV is associated with more severe varicella in secondary cases. An option with this type of exposure is to immunize healthy seronegative family members when the child with cancer is undergoing intensive therapy and vaccine cannot be given. Diaz and colleagues showed that the vaccine virus cannot be isolated from oropharyngeal secretions of the immunized siblings[74] and that none of the children with cancer showed clinical or serological evidence of vaccine virus transmission. Immunization with VZV vaccine is indicated in seronegative patients with cancer when the cancer chemotherapy schedule allows immunization.

Measles Vaccine. Measles virus has reemerged as an important infectious agent in many countries, and cancer patients who are infected have a high mortality rate.[30] Immunization with the live attenuated vaccine has been contraindicated, owing to the risk for severe side effects in cancer patients undergoing chemotherapy; however, it can be given 3 months after the cessation of cancer therapy.[35] It might be important to investigate the immune status of family members and, if necessary, to immunize siblings, for example. Measles immunization is not recommended in patients with cancer. However, immunization with measles vaccine can be considered in cancer patients not receiving active cancer chemotherapy when the epidemiological risk for measles is increased.

Other Live Vaccines. Few data exist on immunization with mumps, rubella, or BCG vaccine in cancer patients. However, the use of these vaccines is not recommended during active cancer therapy. A child with acute lymphoblastic leukemia demonstrated persistent infection with symptoms of rubella when given rubella vaccine during remission.[74a] As discussed earlier, live poliovirus vaccine should not be used in cancer patients because an effective inactivated vaccine exists. Live poliovirus vaccine should also be avoided in family members of patients undergoing cancer chemotherapy and in healthcare workers caring for severely immunocompromised patients.[45]

PATIENTS WITH BONE MARROW AND PERIPHERAL STEM CELL TRANSPLANTS

In recipients of allogeneic stem cell transplants, four components combine to produce the immunodeficient state of the patient: (1) the immunosuppressive activity of the primary disease and treatment, (2) the high doses of chemotherapy and radiotherapy used to eradicate the host's immune system, (3) the immunological reactivity between the graft and the host, and (4) the immunosuppressive therapy given after the transplantation. In autologous BMT recipients, only the first two components have to be considered. A summary of the recommendations is shown in Table 7–3.

Allogeneic Bone Marrow Transplantation

With allogeneic BMT, the immune system of the recipient is replaced by the immune system of the host. Immunity to infectious agents is transferred by the graft and can be detected in the patient soon after the BMT.[75–82] The transferred immunity is usually of a finite duration, and over time an increasing number of patients become susceptible to tetanus,[77, 83] polio,[84, 85] and measles,[86] for example. The immune status of the donor is important for the short-term transfer of immunity and can be improved by immunizing the donor before the transplant.[79, 87–89]

The transplantation period can be divided into three distinct phases, each with its unique combination of risks and benefits of immunization. The early posttransplant phase is characterized by neutropenia, and the characteristic infections are caused by bacteria and fungi, for which immunization is unlikely to be effective. During the intermediate posttransplant phase, the most common severe infections are caused by cytomegalovirus (CMV), VZV, *Streptococcus pneumoniae*, and *H. influenzae*.

Table 7–3. **RECOMMENDATIONS FOR IMMUNIZATIONS IN STEM CELL TRANSPLANT PATIENTS**

VACCINE	ALLOGENEIC BMT RECIPIENTS	AUTOLOGOUS BMT RECIPIENTS	COMMENTS
Tetanus toxoid + diphtheria toxoid	Yes	Yes	Two or three doses starting 6–12 mo after transplantation
Polio (inactivated polio virus)	Yes	Yes	Two or three doses starting 6–12 mo after transplantation; oral polio virus vaccine contraindicated
Measles	Children and adults in areas with epidemic measles	In children only	Not before 24 mo after BMT; not to be given in patients with graft-versus-host disease
Rubella	Individual consideration	Individual consideration	Females with pregnancy potential
Influenza	Yes	Yes	Seasonal, beginning 6–12 mo after BMT and continuing to at least 24 months after BMT; thereafter on individual indication in patients with graft-versus-host disease, pulmonary complications, or both
Conjugated *Haemophilus influenzae* type b virus	Yes	Yes	Two doses starting 6–12 mo after BMT
Hepatitis B virus	Regional	Regional	In countries where vaccination is recommended to the general population, starting 12 mo after transplantation
Pneumococcal	Yes	Individual consideration*	Efficacy poor in patients with chronic graft-versus-host disease
Varicella-zoster virus	No recommendation	Children and young adults	Not before 24 mo in seronegative patients and not in patients with chronic graft-versus-host disease

*Most patients retain antibodies to pneumococci.
BMT, bone marrow transplant.

The risk for infections is strongly influenced by the presence of GVHD. This pattern of infection is also characteristic of the late phase after BMT; however, additional long-term protection against other infections such as tetanus, diphtheria, polio, and measles should be considered. Several studies have shown a loss of immunity to tetanus, poliovirus, and diphtheria during extended follow-up after BMT.[83–85, 90]

Killed Vaccines

Pneumococcal Vaccine. Pneumococcal infections are significant causes of morbidity and mortality after allogeneic BMT. The risk for severe infections is increased in patients with chronic GVHD.[91–93] Immunization with the currently available pneumococcal vaccines can elicit good antibody responses 6 to 12 months after BMT in patients without GVHD, but it has failed to elicit adequate immune responses in patients with chronic GVHD.[89, 94–97] In particular, the specific IgG2 responses have been poor.[96, 98] The immune response in one study was not significantly improved by two doses of pneumococcal vaccine compared with one dose.[89] Thus, vaccination against pneumococci is indicated primarily in patients without GVHD and should be performed approximately 6 months after BMT. In a study in which the donors were immunized against pneumococci and the recipients were immunized with the same vaccines after transplantation, the recipients' immune responses were not improved against pneumococci when they were immunized 12 and 24 months after BMT.[99] The new conjugated vaccines might also improve immunization results in patients with chronic GVHD, but no results have been presented.

***Haemophilus influenzae* Type b Vaccine.** H. influenzae is also an important cause of infection in allogeneic BMT recipients. In contrast to the situation with pneumococci, immunization with Hib vaccine can elicit protective immune responses.[89, 97] A good immune response can be elicited when the donor is immunized before transplantation and the recipient at 3 months after transplantation. Immunization with Hib vaccine is indicated in allogeneic BMT recipients.

Influenza Vaccine. Influenza A and B can be severe and life threatening in BMT recipients.[61, 100, 101] Most severe infections occur early after BMT, when immunizations are ineffective. Studies have not examined whether pretransplant immunization of the marrow donor, the recipient, or both is protective. Another option for protecting the patient early after stem cell transplantation is to reduce the patient's risk of contracting influenza by immunizing family and hospital staff members, thereby reducing the risk of transmitting the infection to the patient. Immunization with two doses of influenza vaccine can elicit an immune response after BMT. One study showed that the time elapsed after BMT influenced the efficacy of the immunization.[102] No patient could respond when immunizations were given less than 6 months after BMT; approximately 25% of the patients responded when immunizations were given 6 months to 2 years after BMT; and more than 60% of the patients responded when immunizations were given more than 2 years after BMT.

Hepatitis B Virus Vaccine. Severe HBV infections are rare after BMT unless an HBV-positive donor is used with a seronegative recipient. Nevertheless, immunization of patients against HBV might be indicated in countries where the prevalence of HBV is high. Immunization early after BMT is likely to be ineffective.

Immunization of the donor marrow allows transfer of immunity to the recipient.[87, 88] Whether this transferred immunity can prevent infection in the recipient is presently unknown. Case reports suggest that the transfer of immunity from an HBV-immune donor can clear virus from a recipient who is positive for the HBV surface antigen and HBV DNA.[103, 104] Further studies are needed to assess the usefulness of donor vaccination as immune therapy against HBV.

Tetanus Toxoid, Diphtheria Toxoid, and Inactivated Poliovirus Vaccine. Most BMT patients lose immunity to tetanus toxoid, diphtheria toxoid, and poliovirus during extended follow-up. Several studies of immunization with these vaccines have been published.[83–85, 105] A new primary schedule with repeated doses of these vaccines is needed to obtain stable protective immunity.[83–85, 105] The inactivated poliovirus vaccine should be used to avoid vaccine-induced paralytic disease from the live vaccine. In most of the published studies, the immunization programs were initiated approximately 1 year after BMT. In a study by Gerritsen and colleagues, in which children were immunized before BMT and then revaccinated 6 weeks after BMT, only 30% of the patients responded to this early reimmunization.[106] However, one of the most recent studies showed that good and lasting immune responses can be obtained when immunizations are started 6 months after BMT.[107]

Live Attenuated Vaccines

Varicella-Zoster Virus Vaccine. Primary VZV infections can be very severe just following allogeneic transplantation. The existing vaccine is live and attenuated and therefore cannot be used early in the posttransplant period. A seronegative patient should probably be immunized before transplantation, providing that enough time can elapse between the vaccination and the transplant procedure. This strategy has not been tested in a clinical study, however, although children with acute leukemia who have been immunized with the VZV vaccine have subsequently undergone allogeneic stem cell transplantation. No data are available concerning the use of the VZV vaccine after BMT to prevent primary or reactivated VZV infection. This vaccine could be important in preventing primary VZV infections in seronegative BMT recipients. Moreover, because there are effective antiviral agents against VZV, the potential risk from the vaccine virus is probably low. Patients with GVHD and ongoing immunosuppression should not be immunized. A high proportion of BMT patients develop herpes zoster that occasionally becomes severe. No study has examined the live VZV vaccine as a booster to immunity. Redman and colleagues used heat-inactivated VZV vaccine and showed no reduction in the risk of developing herpes zoster but a reduced severity of the herpes zoster in the immunized group.[108]

Cytomegalovirus Vaccine. CMV is one of the most important pathogens after BMT. The vaccine currently available is live and attenuated based on the Towne strain[109] but has not been tested in BMT recipients. Other vaccines based on new vaccine technology, such as subcomponent vaccines and vaccines using other virus vectors, are currently in early clinical development.

Measles Vaccine. Most patients become seronegative to measles during extended follow-up.[86] Measles can cause severe disease in immunocompromised patients. There are documented cases of fatal measles in BMT recipients.[30] Immunization should be considered only in allogeneic BMT patients without chronic GVHD or ongoing immunosuppression. Existing data in such patients indicate that measles vaccine can be given without severe side effects 2 years after BMT.[110] No data exist as to whether it is safe to immunize earlier after transplantation. Measles immunization can be considered on an individual basis depending on the epidemiological situation in the community.

Other Live Vaccines. Other vaccines that may be considered after allogeneic stem cell transplantation are rubella, BCG, mumps, and yellow fever. These vaccines are live and attenuated, and the possible benefits must be weighed against the risk for side effects. Rubella vaccine may be indicated in female patients who have retained the potential for becoming pregnant. Data indicate that rubella vaccine can be given without severe side effects 2 years after BMT in patients without chronic GVHD or ongoing immunosuppression.[110] The same risks exist with the vaccine against mumps; although the risk for severe infections with mumps virus in BMT recipients is likely to be quite low, a case report of a fatal infection has been published.[111] Yellow fever is a life-threatening infection occurring primarily in South America and southern and central Africa. Rio and colleagues have presented three cases in which immunization occurred 5 years after BMT without severe side effects.[112] Immunization can be considered in patients who must visit areas where yellow fever is endemic. BCG vaccine can cause severe infections in patients with depressed T-cell function and is not recommended in BMT recipients.

Autologous Bone Marrow Transplantation

In autologous BMT recipients, there is obviously no immunological disparity between the graft and the host. In most patients, the immune regeneration is faster than after allogeneic BMT, and even more so after peripheral stem cell transplantation. Autologous BMT patients are usually not prone to severe infections that are preventable by immunization during the early posttransplant phase. However, several studies have shown that autologous BMT recipients lose protective immunity to tetanus, poliovirus, and measles during long-term follow-up.[85, 113, 114] No data have been published on long-term immunity in peripheral stem cell transplant recipients, although our own unpublished data (V. Hammarstrom and P. Ljungman) suggest a risk of losing immunity after autologous peripheral stem cell transplantation similar to that occurring after BMT.

Killed Vaccines

Influenza Vaccine. Influenza virus immunization is recommended during the first year after autologous stem cell transplantation. In a study of influenza immunization, however, no patient responded if the immunization was performed less than 6 months after autologous BMT.[102] Thus, the optimal timing of influenza vaccinations needs to be determined.

Pneumococcal Vaccine and Conjugated Hib Vaccine. Autologous BMT patients are less prone than allogeneic BMT patients to develop severe infections with Hib or pneumococcal vaccines. Most infections occur soon after the transplantation, when the response to immunization is poor. The immune response may be improved by immunizing the patient before the stem cell harvest. One study found that immunization with conjugated Hib vaccine before the harvest followed by immunization at 3, 6, 12, and 24 months after autologous BMT improved the antibody titers as early as 3 months after transplantation (when the second immunization was administered).[115] However, when immunizations with pneumococcal vaccines were given by the same schedule, there was no improvement in the response at any time after the autologous BMT. Immunization with conjugated Hib vaccine can be considered in autologous stem cell transplant recipients.

Tetanus Toxoid, Diphtheria Toxoid, and Inactivated Poliovirus Vaccine. Compared with the normal population, autologous BMT recipients have an increased risk of losing protective immunity to poliovirus and tetanus[85, 114] (Hammarström and Ljungman, unpublished data). Reimmunization with repeated-dose schedules of inactivated poliovirus vaccine and tetanus toxoid effectively restores protective immunity in autologous BMT recipients[85, 114] (Hammarström and Ljungman; unpublished data). The immune response that develops soon after the autologous BMT can be improved by immunizing the patient before the stem cell harvest and then repeatedly giving tetanus toxoid after the autologous BMT.[115]

Immunization with tetanus toxoid, diphtheria toxoid, and inactivated poliovirus is recommended after autologous stem cell transplantation.

Live Attenuated Vaccines

Measles Vaccine. Children who were immunized against measles before autologous BMT frequently become seronegative during follow-up, but adults who experienced natural measles disease before autologous BMT usually remain immune to measles at least 3 years after transplantation.[113] The risk for side effects after immunization seems to be low.[113] Measles immunization can be considered on an individual basis depending on the epidemiological situation in the community.

Varicella-Zoster Virus Vaccine. No studies have been conducted with the VZV vaccine specifically in autologous stem cell transplant patients. No real difference exists, however, in the immune status between autologous stem cell transplant patients and children with acute leukemia in remission; vaccination can therefore be considered before transplantation in seronegative autologous stem cell transplant recipients.

SOLID ORGAN TRANSPLANT RECIPIENTS

The need for immunization in solid organ transplant recipients can arise from three components, each causing a suppression of the immune system: (1) immunosuppressive activity of the underlying disease, such as chronic renal failure; (2) rejection of the organ graft; and (3) immunosuppressive therapy given after the transplantation. The different groups of organ transplant patients are discussed together in this section because there are no published data that distinguish different immunization efficacies in the separate solid organ transplant groups. Immunizations can be given either before solid organ transplantation, with the aim of preventing infections occurring during the early posttransplant phase, or after the transplantation, with the aim of preventing late infections. A summary of the recommendations for immunization is given in Table 7–4.

Killed Vaccines

HBV can be transferred to a solid organ transplant recipient either by a hepatitis B–positive organ graft or through blood transfusions. HBV vaccination is recommended in HBV-negative patients before the transplantation, as there is an increased risk for severe HBV infections in transplant patients. The efficacy of HBV vaccine is low in patients undergoing hemodialysis.[116, 117] The efficacy of vaccination is also low in patients with end-stage liver disease who are awaiting liver transplantation; one study found that an antibody response was produced in approximately 50% of the patients.[118] The response to immunization was better (73%) in children with biliary atresia.[119] The efficacy of HBV vaccination is low after solid organ transplantation, with response rates between 5 and 15%.[120, 121] Thus, pretransplant immunization is recommended.

Influenza can cause severe infections in renal trans-

Table 7–4. **RECOMMENDATIONS FOR IMMUNIZATIONS IN SOLID ORGAN TRANSPLANT RECIPIENTS**

VACCINE	RECOMMENDATION	COMMENTS
Hepatitis B virus	Yes	Before transplantation in seronegative patients
Varicella-zoster virus		Before transplantation in seronegative patients
Influenza	Yes	Seasonal
Conjugated *Haemophilus influenzae* type b virus	Yes	Children only
Pneumococcal	Yes	Children only

plant patients.[61, 100] Immunization is recommended by the Advisory Committee on Immunization Practices.[59] The reported results of immunization vary. Two studies have shown lower antibody responses in adults after solid organ transplantation compared with immunocompetent individuals.[122, 123] In contrast, two studies have shown normal responses to influenza immunization in children after organ transplantation.[124, 125]

Immunizations against *S. pneumoniae* and *H. influenzae* can be considered for patients—children, in particular—who are awaiting solid organ transplantation.[126, 127] Immunizations can also be considered after the transplantation. The efficacy of the 23-valent polysaccharide vaccine was similar to the response in normal immunocompetent control subjects.[128] There are no data concerning the need for or efficacy of immunization with tetanus toxoid or inactivated poliovirus vaccine in solid organ transplant recipients.

Live Attenuated Vaccines

Immunization with live vaccines has not been recommended after solid organ transplantation owing to the risk for vaccine-associated complications.

Varicella-Zoster Virus Vaccine. VZV can cause severe and fatal disease in patients after organ transplantation. Vaccination of seronegative patients awaiting organ transplantation should be considered. VZV vaccine given to uremic children awaiting renal transplantation has been shown to be safe and to reduce the posttransplant risk for varicella in prevaccination seronegative patients.[129] A follow-up study showed that the protection was of long duration, with 42% of patients still having antibodies more than 10 years after immunization. Furthermore, the risk for varicella was lower and the disease significantly less severe in immunized compared with nonimmunized patients.[130] A small study of VZV vaccination in children who had received renal transplants showed a good serological response and no severe side effects.[131] Further studies are needed, however.

CMV is an important pathogen after solid organ transplantation. The vaccine used until now is live attenuated and based on the Towne strain. Randomized studies have shown a reduction in the severity of CMV disease and a reduction in graft rejection primarily in seronegative patients receiving organs from seropositive donors.[109, 132] However, antiviral chemoprophylaxis is effective in preventing CMV disease, and the vaccine is not yet available for general use; ongoing work with new CMV vaccines may change this situation.

CHILDREN WITH CONGENITAL IMMUNE DEFICIENCIES

Many different types of congenital immune deficiencies exist, and different defects of the immune system influence both the effectiveness of immunization and the risk for side effects. Immunizations with live attenuated vaccines should be avoided in most children with congenital immune deficiencies. However, the immune deficiency is frequently unknown at the time of immunization with a live vaccine such as BCG, and the abnormal reaction to immunization might be the clue needed to diagnose an immune deficiency. In a French study, the prevalence of disseminated BCG infection was estimated at 0.59 case per 1 million immunized children.[133] Two different types of disseminated BCG infection have been described, presenting as either tuberculoid or lepromatous-like lesions that indicate different immunological defects.[134] Interferon-γ–receptor deficiency has been associated with fatal outcome after BCG infection.[135] Other live vaccines that should be avoided in children with immunodeficiencies include VZV and measles, mumps, and rubella.

Killed vaccines are safe but might be ineffective in children with congenital immune deficiencies. The response to immunization depends on the type of immune defect.

REFERENCES

1. Pirofski LA, Casadevall A. Use of licensed vaccines for active immunization of the immunocompromised host. Clin Microbiol Rev 11:1–26, 1998.

1a. Glesby MJ. Immunization during HIV infection. Curr Opin Infect Dis 11:17–21, 1998.

1b. O'Brien W, Grovit-Ferbas K, Namazi A, et al. Human immunodeficiency virus-type 1 replication can be increased in peripheral blood of seropositive patients after influenza vaccination. Blood 86:1082–1089, 1995.

2. Staprans S, Hamilton B, Follansbee S, et al. Activation of virus replication after vaccination of HIV-1-infected individuals. J Exp Med 182:1727–1737, 1995.

3. Rosok B, Voltersvik P, Bjerknes R, et al. Dynamics of HIV-1 replication following influenza vaccination of HIV+ individuals. Clin Exp Immunol 104:203–207, 1996.

4. Ramilo O, Hicks P, Borvak J, et al. T cell activation and human immunodeficiency virus replication after influenza immunization of infected children. Pediatr Infect Dis J 15:197–203, 1996.

5. Stanley S, Ostrowski M, Justement J, et al. Effect of immunization with a common recall antigen on viral expression in patients infected with human immunodeficiency virus type 1. N Engl J Med 334:1222–1230, 1996.

6. Glesby M, Hoover D, Farzadegan H, et al. The effect of influenza vaccination on human immunodeficiency virus type 1 load: A randomized, double-blind, placebo-controlled study. J Infect Dis 174:1332–1336, 1996.

7. King JC Jr, Vink PE, Farley JJ, et al. Comparison of the safety and immunogenicity of a pneumococcal conjugate with a licensed polysaccharide vaccine in human immunodeficiency virus– and non–human immunodeficiency virus–infected children. Pediatr Infect Dis J 15:192–196, 1996.

8. Carson P, Schut R, Simpson M, et al. Antibody class and subclass responses to pneumococcal polysaccharides following immunization of human immunodeficiency virus infected patients. J Infect Dis 172:340–345, 1995.

9. Rodrigues-Barradas M, Musher D, Lahart C, et al. Antibodies to capsular polysaccharides of *Streptococcus pneumoniae* after vaccination of human immunodeficiency virus–infected subjects with 23-valent pneumococcal vaccine. J Infect Dis 165:553–556, 1992.

10. Loeliger A, Rijkers G, Aerts P, et al. Deficient antipneumococcal polysaccharide responses in HIV-seropositive patients. FEMS Immunol Med Microbiol 12:33–41, 1995.

11. Weiss P, Wallace M, Oldfield E, et al. Response of recent human immunodeficiency virus seroconverters to the pneumococcal polysaccharide vaccine and *Haemophilus influenzae* type b conjugate vaccine. J Infect Dis 171:1217–1222, 1995.

12. Kroon F, van Dissel J, de Jong J, et al. Antibody response to influenza tetanus and pneumococcal vaccines in HIV-infected

individuals in relation to the number of CD4+ lymphocytes. AIDS 8:469–476, 1994.
13. Mascart-Lemone F, Gerard M, Libin M, et al. Differential effect of human immunodeficiency virus infection on the IgA and IgG antibody responses to pneumococcal vaccine. J Infect Dis 175:1253–1260, 1995.
14. Vanderbruaene M, Colebunders R, Mascart-Lemone F, et al. Equal IgG response to pneumococcal vaccination in all stages of human immunodeficiency virus disease. J Infect Dis 172:551–553, 1995.
15. Unsworth D, Rowen D, Carne C, et al. Defective IgG2 response to Pneumovax in HIV-seropositive patients. Genitourin Med 69:373–376, 1993.
16. Rodrigues-Barradas M, Groover J, Lacke C, et al. IgG antibody to pneumococcal capsular polysaccharide in human immunodeficiency virus–infected subjects: Persistence of antibody in responders, revaccination in nonresponders, and relation of immunoglobulin allotype to response. J Infect Dis 173:1347–1353, 1996.
17. Ahmed F, Steinhoff M, Rodrigues-Barradas M, et al. Effect of human immunodeficiency virus type 1 infection on the antibody response to a glycoprotein conjugate pneumococcal vaccine: Results from a randomized trial. J Infect Dis 173:83–90, 1996.
18. Kale K, King JJ, Farley J, et al. The immunogenicity of *Haemophilus influenzae* type b conjugate (HbOC) vaccine in human immunodeficiency virus–infected and uninfected infants. Pediatr Infect Dis J 14:350–354, 1995.
19. Peters V, Sood S. Immunity to *Haemophilus influenzae* type b polysaccharide capsule in children with human immunodeficiency virus infection immunized with a single dose of *Haemophilus* vaccine. J Pediatr 125:74–77, 1994.
20. Gibb D, Giacomelli A, Masters J, et al. Persistence of antibody responses to *Haemophilus influenzae* type b polysaccharide conjugate vaccine in children with vertically acquired human immunodeficiency virus infection. Pediatr Infect Dis J 15:1097–1101, 1996.
21. Chadwick EG, Chang G, Decker MD, et al. Serologic response to standard inactivated influenza vaccine in human immunodeficiency virus–infected children. Pediatr Infect Dis J 13:206–211, 1994.
21a. Jackson CR, Vavro CL, Valentine ME, et al. Effect of influenza immunization on immunologic and virologic characteristics of pediatric patients infected with human immunodeficiency virus. Pediatr Infect Dis J 16:200–294, 1997.
22. Rose D, Schechter C, Sacks H. Influenza and pneumococcal vaccination of HIV-infected patients: A policy analysis. Am J Med 94:160–168, 1993.
23. Kurtzhals J, Kjeldsen K, Heron I, et al. Immunity against diphtheria and tetanus in human immunodeficiency virus–infected Danish men born 1950–59. APMIS 100:803–808, 1992.
24. Kroon F, van Dissel J, Labadie J, et al. Antibody response to diphtheria, tetanus, and poliomyelitis vaccines in relation to the number of CD4+ T lymphocytes in adults infected with human immunodeficiency virus. Clin Infect Dis 21:1197–1203, 1995.
25. Arrazola M, de Juanes J, Ramos J, et al. Hepatitis B vaccination in infants of mothers infected with human immunodeficiency virus. J Med Virol 45:339–341, 1995.
26. Rutstein R, Rudy B, Codispoti C, et al. Response to hepatitis B immunization by infants exposed to HIV. AIDS 8:1281–1284, 1994.
27. Zuccotti G, Riva E, Flumine P, et al. Hepatitis B vaccination in infants of mothers infected with human immunodeficiency virus. J Pediatr 125:70–72, 1994.
28. Santatostino E, Gringeri A, Rocino A, et al. Patterns of immunogenicity of an inactivated hepatitis A vaccine in anti-HIV positive and negative hemophilic patients. Thromb Haemost 72:508–510, 1994.
29. Lewis D, Gilks C, Ojoo S, et al. Immune response following oral administration of cholera toxin B subunit to HIV-1 infected UK and Kenyan subjects. AIDS 8:779–785, 1994.
30. Kaplan L, Daum R, Smaron M, et al. Severe measles in immunocompromised patients. JAMA 267:1237–1241, 1992.
31. Arpadi S, Markowitz L, Baughman A, et al. Measles antibody in vaccinated human immunodeficiency type 1–infected children. Pediatrics 97:653–657, 1996.
31a. Krasinski K, Borkowsky W. Measles and measles immunity in children infected with human immunodeficiency virus. JAMA 261:2512–2516, 1989.
32. Frenkel LM, Nielsen K, Garakian A, et al. A search for persistent measles, mumps, and rubella vaccine virus in children with human immunodeficiency virus type 1 infection. Arch Pediatr Adolesc Med 148:57–60, 1994.
33. Wallace M, Hooper D, Graves S, et al. Measles seroprevalence and vaccine response in HIV-infected adults. Vaccine 12:1222–1224, 1994.
34. Anonymous. Measles pneumonitis following measles-mumps-rubella vaccination of a patient with HIV infection. MMWR Morbid Mortal Wkly Rep 45:603–606, 1996.
35. Peter G (ed). Report of the Committee on Infectious Diseases (Red Book, 24th ed.) Elk Grove Village, IL: American Academy of Pediatrics, 1997, pp 344–357.
36. McLaughlin M, Thomas P, Onorato I, et al. Live virus vaccines in human immunodeficiency virus–infected children: A retrospective survey. Pediatrics 82:229–233, 1988.
37. Boudes P, Sobel A, Deforges L, et al. Disseminated *Mycobacterium bovis* infection from BCG vaccination and HIV infection [letter: comment]. JAMA 262:2386, 1989.
38. Houde C, Dery P. *Mycobacterium bovis* sepsis in an infant with human immunodeficiency virus infection. Pediatr Infect Dis J 7:810–812, 1988.
39. Ninane J, Grymonprez A, Burtonboy G, et al. Disseminated BCG in HIV infection. Arch Dis Child 63:1268–1269, 1988.
40. Armbruster C, Junker W, Vetter N, et al. Disseminated bacille Calmette-Guérin infection in an AIDS patient 30 years after BCG vaccination [letter]. J Infect Dis 162:1216, 1990.
41. Besnard M, Sauvion S, Offredo C, et al. Bacillus Calmette-Guérin infection after vaccination of human immunodeficiency virus–infected children. Pediatr Infect Dis J 12:993–997, 1993.
42. O'Brien K, Ruff A, Louis M, et al. Bacillus Calmette-Guérin complications in children born to HIV-1–infected women with a review of the literature. Pediatrics 95:414–418, 1995.
43. Special Programme on AIDS and Expanded Programme on Immunization: Joint Statement. Consultation on human immunodeficiency virus (HIV) and routine childhood immunization. Wkly Epidemiol Rec 62, 1987, pp 297–299.
44. Ryder R, Oxtoby M, Mvula M, et al. Safety and immunogenicity of bacille Calmette-Guérin, diphtheria-tetanus-pertussis, and oral polio vaccines in newborn children in Zaire infected with human immunodeficiency virus type 1. J Pediatr 122:697–702, 1993.
45. Zuckerman MA, Brink NS, Kyi M, Tedder RS. Exposure of immunocompromised individuals to health-care workers immunised with oral poliovaccine [letter]. Lancet 343:985–986, 1994.
46. Feldman S, Malone W, Wilbur R, et al. Pneumococcal vaccination in children with leukemia. Med Pediatr Oncol 13:69–72, 1985.
47. Levine A, Overturf G, Field R, et al. Use and efficacy of pneumococcal vaccine in patients with Hodgkin's disease. Blood 54:1171–1175, 1979.
48. Siber G, Weitzman S, Aisenberg A, et al. Impaired antibody response to pneumococcal vaccine after treatment for Hodgkin's disease. N Engl J Med 299:442–448, 1978.
49. Addiego JJ, Ammann A, Schiffman G, et al. Response to pneumococcal polysaccharide vaccine in patients with untreated Hodgkin's disease. Lancet 2:450–452, 1980.
50. Frederiksen B, Specht L, Henrichsen J, et al. Antibody response to pneumococcal vaccine in patients with early stage Hodgkin's disease. Eur J Haematol 43:45–49, 1989.
51. Donaldson S, Vosti K, Berberich F, et al. Response to pneumococcal vaccine among children with Hodgkin's disease. Rev Infect Dis 3:S133–S143, 1981.
52. Grimfors G, Söderqvist M, Holm G, et al. A longitudinal study of class and subclass antibody response to pneumococcal vaccination in splenectomized individuals with special reference to patients with Hodgkin's disease. Eur J Haematol 45:101–108, 1990.
53. Ammann A, Schiffman G, Addiego J, et al. Immunization of immunosuppressed patients with pneumococcal polysaccharide vaccine. Rev Infect Dis 3:S160–S167, 1981.
54. Chan C, Molrine D, George S, et al. Pneumococcal conjugate vaccine primes for antibody responses to polysaccharide pneumo-

coccal vaccine after treatment for Hodgkin's disease. J Infect Dis 173:256–258, 1996.
55. Feldman S, Gigliotti F, Shenep J, et al. Risk of *Haemophilus influenzae* type b disease in children with cancer and response of immunocompromised leukemic children to a conjugate vaccine. J Infect Dis 161:926–931, 1990.
56. Ridgway D, Wolff L, Deforest A. Immunization response varies with intensity of acute lymphoblastic leukemia therapy. Am J Dis Child 145:887–891, 1991.
57. Shenep J, Feldman S, Gigliotti F, et al. Response of immunocompromised children with solid tumors to a conjugate vaccine for *Haemophilus influenzae* type b. J Pediatr 125:581–584, 1994.
58. Jurlander J, de Nully Brown P, Skov P, et al. Improved vaccination response during ranitidine treatment, and increased plasma histamine concentrations in patients with B cell chronic lymphocytic leukemia. Leukemia 9:1902–1909, 1995.
59. Prevention and control of influenza. Recommendations of the Advisory Committee on Immunization Practices (ACIP). MMWR Morbid Mortal Wkly Rep 41(RR-9):1–17, 1992.
60. Elting L, Whimbey E, Lo W, et al. Epidemiology in influenza A infection in patients with acute or chronic leukemia. Support Care Cancer 3:198–202, 1995.
61. Ljungman P, Andersson J, Aschan J, et al. Influenza A in immunocompromised patients. Clin Infect Dis 17:244–247, 1993.
62. Kempe A, Hall C, MacDonald N, et al. Influenza in children with cancer. J Pediatr 115:33–39, 1989.
63. Steinherz P, Brown A, Gross P, et al. Influenza immunization in children with neoplastic diseases. Cancer 45:750–756, 1980.
64. Lo W, Whimbey E, Elting L, et al. Antibody response to a two-dose influenza vaccine regimen in adult lymphoma patients on chemotherapy. Eur J Clin Microbiol Infect Dis 12:778–782, 1993.
65. Hammarström V, Pauksen K, Svensson H, et al. Tetanus immunity in patients with haematological malignancies. Support Care Cancer: in press.
66. van de Does-van der Berg A, Hermans J, Nagel J, et al. Immunity to diphtheria, pertussis, tetanus, and poliomyelitis in children with acute lymphocytic leukemia after cessation of chemotherapy. Pediatrics 67:222–229, 1981.
67. Löffel M, Meienberg O, Diem P, et al. Vaccine poliomyelitis in an adult undergoing chemotherapy for non-Hodgkin's lymphoma. Schweiz Med Wochenschr 112:419–421, 1982.
68. Takahashi M, Okuno Y, Otsuka T, et al. Development of a live attenuated varicella vaccine. Biken J 18:25–33, 1975.
69. Gershon A, Steinberg S. Persistence of immunity to varicella in children with leukemia immunized with live attenuated varicella vaccine. N Engl J Med 320:892–897, 1989.
70. Brunell P, Geiser C, Novelli V, et al. Varicella-like illness caused by live varicella vaccine in children with acute lymphocytic leukemia. Pediatrics 79:922–927, 1987.
71. Lawrence R, Gershon A, Holzman R, et al. The risk for zoster after varicella vaccination in children with leukemia. N Engl J Med 318:543–548, 1988.
72. Hardy I, Gershon A, Steinberg S, et al. The incidence of zoster after immunization with live attenuated varicella vaccine. A study in children with leukemia. Varicella Vaccine Collaborative Group. N Engl J Med 325:1545–1550, 1991.
73. Cristofani L, Weinberg A, Peixoto V, et al. Administration of live attenuated varicella vaccine to children with cancer before starting chemotherapy. Vaccine 9:873–876, 1991.
74. Diaz P, Au D, Smith S, et al. Lack of transmission of the live attenuated varicella vaccine virus to immunocompromised children after immunization of their siblings. Pediatrics 87:166–170, 1991.
74a. Geiger R, Fink FM, Sailer M, et al. Persistent rubella infection after erroneous vaccination in an immunocompromised patient with acute lymphoblastic leukemia in remission. J Med Virol 47:442–444, 1997.
75. Lum L, Seigneuret M, Storb R. The transfer of antigen-specific humoral immunity from marrow donors to marrow recipients. J Clin Immunol 6:389–396, 1986.
76. Lum L. The kinetics of immune reconstitution after human marrow transplantation. Blood 69:369–380, 1987.
77. Lum L, Noges J, Beatty P, et al. Transfer of specific immunity in marrow recipients given HLA-mismatched, T cell–depleted, or HLA-identical marrow grafts. Bone Marrow Transplant 3:399–406, 1988
78. Lum L. Effects of acute and chronic GVHD on immune recovery after BMT. In Burakoff SJ, Deeg HJ, Ferrara J, et al. (eds). Graft-Versus-Host Disease. New York, Marcel Dekker, 1990, pp 369–380.
79. Saxon A, Mitsuyaso R, Stevens R, et al. Transfer of specific immune responses after bone marrow transplantation. J Clin Invest 78:959–967, 1986.
80. Wahren B, Gahrton G, Linde A, et al. Transfer and persistence of viral antibody-producing cells in bone marrow transplantation. J Infect Dis 150:358–365, 1984.
81. Witherspoon R, Storb R, Ochs H, et al. Recovery of antibody production in human allogeneic marrow graft recipients: Influence of time posttransplantation, the presence or absence of chronic graft-versus-host disease, and antithymocyte globulin treatment. Blood 58:360–368, 1981.
82. Witherspoon R, Matthews D, Storb R, et al. Recovery of in vivo cellular immunity after human marrow grafting. Influence of time postgrafting and acute graft-versus-host disease. Transplantation 37:145–150, 1984.
83. Ljungman P, Wiklund HM, Duraj V, et al. Response to tetanus toxoid immunization after allogeneic bone marrow transplantation. J Infect Dis 162:496–500, 1990.
84. Ljungman P, Duraj V, Magnius L. Response to immunization against polio after allogeneic marrow transplantation. Bone Marrow Transplant 7:89–93, 1991.
85. Engelhard D, Handsher R, Naparstek E, et al. Immune responses to polio vaccination in bone marrow transplant recipients. Bone Marrow Transplant 8:295–300, 1991.
86. Ljungman P, Levensohn-Fuchs I, Hammarström V, et al. Long-term immunity to measles, mumps and rubella after allogeneic bone marrow transplantation. Blood 84:657–664, 1994.
87. Ilan Y, Nagler A, Adler R, et al. Adoptive transfer of immunity to hepatitis B virus after T cell–depleted allogeneic bone marrow transplantation. Hepatology 18:246–252, 1993.
88. Wimperis J, Brenner M, Prentice H, et al. Transfer of a functioning humoral immune system in transplantation of T-lymphocyte–depleted bone marrow. Lancet 1:339–343, 1986.
89. Guinan E, Molrine D, Antin J, et al. Polysaccharide conjugate vaccine response in bone marrow transplant recipients. Transplantation 57:677–684, 1994.
90. Lum L, Munn N, Schanfield M, et al. The detection of specific antibody formation to recall antigens after human bone marrow transplantation. Blood 67:582–587, 1986.
91. Cordonnier C, Bernaudin J, Bierling P, et al. Pulmonary complications occurring after allogeneic bone marrow transplantation. A study of 130 consecutive transplanted patients. Cancer 58:1047–1054, 1986.
92. Aucotourier P, Barra A, Intrator I, et al. Long lasting IgG subclass and antibacterial polysaccharide antibody deficiency after allogeneic bone marrow transplantation. Blood 70:779–785, 1987.
93. Winston D, Schiffman L, Wang D, et al. Pneumococcal infection after human bone marrow transplantation. Ann Intern Med 91:835–841, 1979.
94. Parkkali T, Kayhty H, Ruutu T, et al. A comparison of early and late vaccination with *Haemophilus influenzae* type B conjugate and pneumococcal polysaccharide vaccines after allogeneic BMT. Bone Marrow Transplant 18:961–967, 1996.
95. Avanzini M, Carra A, Macccario R, et al. Antibody response to pneumococcal vaccine in children receiving bone marrow transplantation. J Clin Immunol 15:137–144, 1995.
96. Hammarström V, Pauksen K, Azinge J, et al. The influence of graft versus host reaction on the response to pneumococcal vaccination in bone marrow transplant patients. J Support Care Cancer 1:195–199, 1993.
97. Barra A, Cordonnier C, Preziosi M, et al. Immunogenicity of *Haemophilus influenzae* type b conjugate vaccine in allogeneic bone marrow recipients. J Infect Dis 166:1021–1028, 1992.
98. Lortan J, Vellodi A, Jurges E, et al. Class- and subclass-specific pneumococcal antibody levels and response to immunization after bone marrow transplantation. Clin Exp Immunol 88:512–519, 1992.
99. Molrine D, Guinan E, Antin J, et al. Donor immunization with *Haemophilus influenzae* type B (HIB)-conjugate vaccine in allogeneic bone marrow transplantation. Blood 87:3012–3018, 1996.

100. Aschan J, Ringdén O, Ljungman P, et al. Influenza B in transplant patients. Scand J Infect Dis 21:349–350, 1989.
101. Whimbey E, Elting L, Couch R, et al. Influenza A virus infections among hospitalized adult bone marrow transplant recipients. Bone Marrow Transplant 13:437–440, 1994.
102. Engelhard D, Nagler A, Hardan I. Antibody response to a two-dose regimen of influenza vaccine in allogeneic T cell–depleted and autologous BMT recipients. Bone Marrow Transplant 11:1–5, 1993.
103. Brugger S, Oesterreicher C, Hofmann H, et al. Hepatitis B virus clearance by transplantation of bone marrow from hepatitis B immunized donor. Lancet 349:996–997, 1997.
104. Ilan Y, Nagler A, Adler R, et al. Ablation of persistent hepatitis B by bone marrow transplantation from a hepatitis B-immune donor. Gastroenterology 104:1818–1821, 1993.
105. Prager J, Baumert A, Thilo W, et al. Untersuchungen zur Kinetik der Impfantikörper gegen Tetanustoxoid, Diphterietoxoid, Masern-virus, Poliomyelitis-virus und Pneumokokken nach allogener und autologer Knochenmarktransplantaton und Wiederhholungsimpfung. Teil 3: Kinetik der Impfantikörper gegen Tetanustoxoid nach allogener und autologer Knochenmarktransplantation und kombinierter Wiederholungsimpfung gegen Diphterie and Tetanus. Kinderarztl Prax 60:230–238, 1992.
106. Gerritsen E, Van Tol M, Van't Veer M, et al. Clonal dysregulation of the antibody response to tetanus-toxoid after bone marrow transplantation. Blood 84:4374–4382, 1994.
107. Parkkali T, Ölander R-M, Ruutu T, et al. A randomized comparison between early and late vaccination with tetanus toxoid vaccine after allogeneic BMT. Bone Marrow Transplant 19:933–938, 1997.
108. Redman R, Nader S, Zerboni L, et al. Early reconstitution of immunity and decreased severity of herpes zoster in bone marrow transplant recipients immunized with inactivated varicella vaccine. J Infect Dis 176:187–200, 1997.
109. Plotkin S, Higgins R, Kurtz J, et al. Multicenter trial of Towne strain attenuated virus vaccine in seronegative renal transplant recipients. Transplantation 58:1176–1178, 1994.
110. Ljungman P, Fridell E, Lönnqvist B, et al. Efficacy and safety of vaccination of marrow transplant recipients with a live attenuated measles, mumps, and rubella vaccine. J Infect Dis 159:610–615, 1989.
111. Bakshi N, Lawson J, Hanson R, et al. Fatal mumps meningoencephalitis in a child with severe combined immunodeficiency after bone marrow transplantation. J Child Neurol 11:159–162, 1996.
112. Rio B, Marjanovic Z, Lévy V, et al. Vaccination for yellow fever after bone marrow transplantation. Bone Marrow Transplant 17(suppl 1):S95, 1996.
113. Pauksen K, Duraj V, Ljungman P, et al. Immunity to and immunization against measles, rubella and mumps in patients after autologous bone marrow transplantation. Bone Marrow Transplant 9:427–432, 1992.
114. Pauksen K, Hammarström V, Ljungman P, et al. Immunity to poliovirus and immunization with inactivated poliovaccine after autologous bone marrow transplantation. Clin Infect Dis 18:547–552, 1994.
115. Molrine D, Guinan E, Antin J, et al. *Haemophilus influenzae* type b (HIB)-conjugate immunization before bone marrow harvest in autologous bone marrow transplantation. Bone Marrow Transplant 17:1149–1155, 1996.
116. Crosnier J, Junges P, Courouce A-M, et al. Randomised placebo-controlled trial of hepatitis B surface antigen vaccine in French haemodialysis units: II. Haemodialysis patients. Lancet 2:797–800, 1981.
117. Stevens C, Alter H, Taylor P, et al. Hepatitis B virus vaccine in patients receiving hemodialysis: Immunogenicity and efficacy. N Engl J Med 311:496–501, 1984.
118. Van Thiel D, el-Ashmawy L, Love K, et al. Response to hepatitis B vaccination by liver transplant candidates. Dig Dis Sci 37:1245–1249, 1992.
119. Sokal E, Ulla L, Otte J. Hepatitis B vaccine response before and after transplantation in 55 extrahepatic biliary atresia children. Dig Dis Sci 37:1250–1252, 1992.
120. Wagner D, Wagenbreth I, Stachan-Kunstyr R, et al. Failure of vaccination against hepatitis B with Gen H-B-Vax-D in immunosuppressed heart transplant patients. J Infect Dis 166:1021–1028, 1992.
121. Wagner D, Wagenbroth J, Stachan-Kunstyr R, et al. Hepatitis B vaccination of immunosuppressed heart transplant recipients with the vaccine Hepa gene 3 containing pre-S1, pre-S2, and S gene products. Clin Invest 72:240–352, 1994.
122. Versluis D, Beyer W, Masurel N, et al. Impairment of the immune response to influenza vaccination in renal transplant recipients by cyclosporine, but not azathioprine. Transplantation 42:376–379, 1986.
123. Blumberg E, Albano C, Pruett T, et al. The immunogenicity of influenza virus in solid organ transplant recipients. Clin Infect Dis 23:295–302, 1996.
124. Mauch T, Crouch N, Freese D, et al. Antibody response of pediatric solid organ transplant recipients to immunization against influenza virus. J Pediatrics 127:957–960, 1995.
125. Furth S, Neu A, McColley S, et al. Immune response to influenza vaccination in children with renal disease. Pediatr Nephrol 9:566–568, 1995.
126. Linnemann C Jr, First M, Schiffman G. Response to pneumococcal vaccine in renal transplant and hemodialysis patients. Arch Intern Med 141:1637–1640, 1981.
127. Furth S, Neu A, Case B, et al. Pneumococcal polysaccharide vaccine in children with chronic renal disease: A prospective study of antibody response and duration. J Pediatr 128:99–101, 1996.
128. Dengler T, Strnad N, Zimmermann R, et al. Pneumococcal vaccination after heart and liver transplantation. Immune responses in immunosuppressed patients and in healthy controls. Dtsch Med Wochenschr 121:1519–1525, 1996.
129. Broyer M, Boudailliez B. Varicella vaccine in children with chronic renal insufficiency. Postgrad Med J 61(suppl 4):103–106, 1985.
130. Broyer M, Tete M, Guest G, et al. Varicella and zoster in children after kidney transplantation: Long-term results of vaccination. Pediatrics 99:35–39, 1997.
131. Zamora I, Simon J, Da Silva M, et al. Attenuated varicella virus vaccine in children with renal transplants. Pediatr Nephrol 8:190–192, 1994.
132. Plotkin SA, Starr S, Friedman H, et al. Effect of Towne live virus vaccine on cytomegalovirus disease after renal transplant. A controlled trial. Ann Intern Med 114:525–531, 1991.
133. Casanova J, Blanche S, Emile J, et al. Idiopathic disseminated bacillus Calmette-Guérin infection: A French national retrospective study. Pediatrics 98:774–778, 1996.
134. Emile J, Patey N, Altare F, et al. Correlation of granuloma structure with clinical outcome defines two types of idiopathic disseminated BCG infection. J Pathol 181:25–30, 1997.
135. Jouanguy E, Altare F, Lamhamedo S, et al. Interferon-gamma-receptor deficiency in an infant with fatal bacille Calmette-Guérin infection. N Engl J Med 335:1956–1961, 1996.

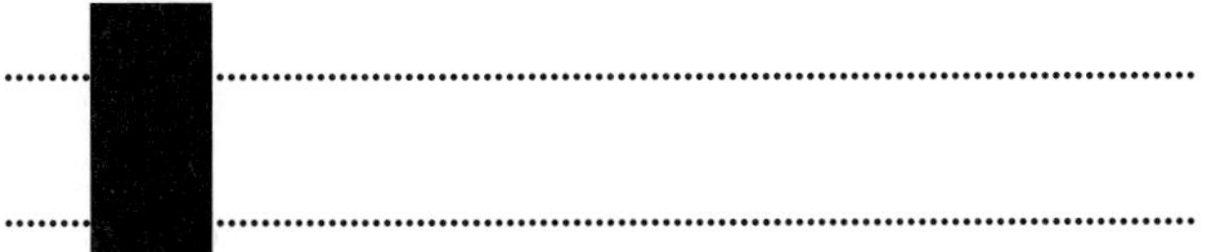

chapter 8

Bacille Calmette-Guérin Vaccine

Kim Connelly Smith
Jeffrey R. Starke

The bacille Calmette-Guérin (BCG) vaccines are the oldest of the vaccines currently used throughout the world.[1] They have been given to 4 billion people and have been used routinely since the 1960s in almost all countries of the world, with the exception of a few industrialized countries. The United States and the Netherlands are the only countries that have never routinely recommended BCG vaccination.[2] Yet, despite their widespread use, tuberculosis remains the single pathogen responsible for the most death and disease in the world.[3] It is estimated that one third of the world's current population is infected with *Mycobacterium tuberculosis* and that 8 million cases of disease and 2 to 3 million deaths can be attributed to this organism annually.[4, 5] Although most technologically advanced countries have managed to essentially control—although not eradicate—tuberculosis, the incidence of disease and infection is increasing in many poorer areas of the world. The economic and social consequences of tuberculosis in these developing countries are enormous, and only recently have they been fully recognized by governments, the World Bank, and the World Health Organization (WHO).[6]

There probably is no other widely used vaccine that is as controversial as BCG. Its effects in extremely large randomized, controlled, and case-control studies have been widely disparate, in some cases demonstrating a great degree of protection and in others offering no evidence that vaccination with BCG is beneficial. However, trials of BCG vaccines have provided some of the best and most complete information on tuberculosis in human populations and have played an important role in the development of vaccine trial methodology.[7] The BCG history contains aspects of folklore and superstition that often supersede facts in discussion and public health policy.[8] Many of the difficulties in evaluating the effectiveness of BCG vaccines are intrinsic to tuberculosis and the pathogenic and immunological events in the host that develop in response to infection with *M. tuberculosis*. The lack of reliable laboratory or serological markers for immunity to mycobacteria has hampered efforts to determine how BCG affects the host and what level of protection it provides, and it has limited studies of its efficacy to animal models of disease and field trials in humans.[9]

Many industrialized countries have decreased their use of BCG vaccination as tuberculosis rates have fallen. However, two developments in the clinical expression of tuberculosis have prompted a renewed interest in BCG vaccination in developed countries, especially within healthcare settings.[10, 11] First, the interaction between tuberculosis and infection with the human immunodeficiency virus (HIV) has been noted. People with HIV infection who were previously infected with *M. tuberculosis* develop tuberculosis disease at a rate of 5 to 10% per year, compared with the lifetime risk of 5 to 10% in immunocompetent adults.[12] The interaction of these infections is partly responsible for the resurgence of tuberculosis in the United States during the late 1980s and early 1990s. The safety and efficacy of BCG vaccination in adults and children with HIV infection are not yet well established.[13, 14] Second, outbreaks of tuberculosis caused by strains resistant to both isoniazid and rifampin have occurred in several areas in the United States.[15] The focal points of many outbreaks have been HIV-infected patients and their healthcare providers.[16, 17] Because no known chemotherapy regimen can prevent the progression of asymptomatic tuberculosis infection to tuberculosis disease in people infected with multidrug-resistant *M. tuberculosis*, some experts have suggested that a BCG vaccine should be used in carefully selected high-risk settings in the United States.[18]

HUMAN TUBERCULOSIS: A BRIEF HISTORY

Tuberculosis was probably the leading cause of death in Europe and the United States in recorded history.[19] The earliest known cases of tuberculosis were discovered in ancient Egyptian mummies, who suffered from tuberculosis of the spine, dating back to 4000 to 2000 BC.[20] Pulmonary tuberculosis was known in the time of Hippocrates as phthisis, which is derived from the Greek for "wasting away." The incidence of tuberculosis increased dramatically in Europe until the beginning of the 19th century, when rates peaked at 700 cases per 100,000 persons annually, then declined.

As industrialization, urbanization, and the accompanying social trends extended beyond Europe to the United States, tuberculosis followed. In the mid-19th century, annual tuberculosis mortality rates in eastern cities of the United States averaged 400 per 100,000 population. With improving socioeconomic conditions, the mortality rate fell to 200 per 100,000 around 1900 and to 26 per 100,000 by 1950.[21] These rates fell long before the availability of chemotherapy and without the use of BCG vaccine. It has long been recognized that stress in the forms of war, famine, population displacement, and crowded living and working conditions favors the spread of tuberculosis among humans and that periods of improvement in societal conditions favor its rapid decline. The influence of these and other societal conditions on tuberculosis case rates must be considered in BCG vaccine trials, which, by necessity, take place during a prolonged time.

In 1882, Koch identified the tubercle bacillus as the cause of human tuberculosis. The discovery that tuberculosis was an infectious disease led to the development of four basic disease control strategies.[19] First, the lack of effective treatment led to the creation of the sanatorium movement in 1854 in Europe and, in 1882, by Trudeau in the United States.[22] The measures used included exposure to fresh air and sunlight, community participation, and ordinances to improve sanitation and housing. The second development was the application of pasteurization to cow's milk, which virtually eliminated human disease caused by *Mycobacterium bovis*. The third development was the creation of BCG vaccine.[5] The final development was the discovery of antituberculosis drugs, which could cure established disease and prevent progression of tuberculosis infection to disease; the discovery of these drugs effectively closed the doors of sanatoria. In the United States, the combined use of curative chemotherapy and contact investigation for persons with infectious tuberculosis has been the cornerstone of tuberculosis control for the past four decades.

BACKGROUND

Clinical Description

The terminology used for the stages of tuberculosis can be confusing, but it follows the pathophysiology closely.[23] Tuberculosis infection is the preclinical stage of infection with *M. tuberculosis*. The result of the tuberculin skin test is positive, but findings on chest radiography are basically normal, and there are no signs or symptoms of illness. Tuberculosis disease occurs when clinical manifestations of pulmonary or extrapulmonary tuberculosis become apparent, either on the chest radiograph or in clinical signs and symptoms. The word *tuberculosis* usually refers to the disease. The time interval between the establishment of asymptomatic infection and the onset of disease may be several weeks or many decades. This variable, long-term period of dormant infection is one factor that makes BCG vaccine trials so difficult to perform and interpret.

The majority of adults and children who acquire primary infection with *M. tuberculosis* develop no signs or symptoms at any time, because the infection is held dormant by the host's immune system. On occasion, the initiation of infection is marked by several days of low-grade fever and mild cough that are indistinguishable from the symptoms of a viral respiratory infection. Some individuals experience fever and mild systemic symptoms at the onset of delayed hypersensitivity that resolve in 1 to 3 weeks.

When pulmonary tuberculosis disease occurs, the clinical presentation varies markedly by age. The physical signs and symptoms of primary intrathoracic tuberculosis in children are usually surprisingly meager considering the degree of radiographic changes that are often seen.[24]

Young infants and adolescents are more likely to have significant clinical findings than are older children.[22, 25] More than half of children with pulmonary tuberculosis have no symptoms or physical findings; they are discovered only by contact tracing of an adult with infectious tuberculosis.[26] Nonproductive cough, mild dyspnea, and low-grade fever are the most common symptoms in infants. Other systemic complaints such as night sweats, anorexia, and decreased activity (malaise) are less common. Pulmonary physical signs are even less common. Some infants and children with bronchial obstruction that is caused by inflamed hilar or peritracheal lymph nodes eroding through the bronchial wall develop signs of air trapping, such as localized wheezing or decreased breath sounds. These may be accompanied by tachypnea or frank respiratory distress.

A rare but serious complication of primary pulmonary tuberculosis occurs when the parenchymal focus enlarges and develops a large necrotic center. This complication is called *progressive primary pulmonary tuberculosis*, and its presentation resembles bacterial bronchopneumonia. The patient frequently experiences high spiking fevers, moderate to severe cough, night sweats, dullness to percussion, rales, and decreased breath sounds. The enlarging focus of infection may slough debris into an adjacent bronchus, which can result in intrapulmonary dissemination. Rupture of this cavity into the pleural space causes a bronchopleural fistula or pyopneumothorax; rupture into the pericardium causes acute pericarditis. Without appropriate treatment, the mortality rate of progressive primary pulmonary tuberculosis is 30 to 50%.

The chest radiograph is the cornerstone of diagnosis of primary pulmonary tuberculosis. The hallmark of this disease is the relatively large size and importance of the hilar or mediastinal adenopathy compared with the less significant size of the parenchymal lesion.[27–29] As the regional lymph nodes expand, they first cause partial obstruction of a bronchus, creating air trapping, hyperinflation, and even lobar emphysema. As the nodes erode into the bronchial wall, caseum may fill its lumen, causing complete obstruction. This leads to atelectasis of the lobar segment distal to the obstructed bronchial lumen. The resulting radiographic shadows are often called collapse-consolidation or segmental lesions. Several segmental lesions may occur simultaneously in different lobes. Patients occasionally have a radiographic picture of bronchopneumonia without impressive adenopathy. If the infection is progressively destructive, liquefaction of the lung parenchyma can result in formation of a thin-walled cavity.

The course of thoracic adenopathy and bronchial obstruction can follow several paths if antituberculosis chemotherapy is not given.[27] In many cases, the infection is controlled by the host, the segment or lobe re-expands, and the radiographic abnormalities resolve completely. Of course, the child still has infection with *M. tuberculosis* and is at risk of developing reactivation tuberculosis in the following months to years. In some cases, the segmental lesion resolves, but there is residual calcification of the parenchymal focus, regional lymph nodes, or both. These calcified foci contain live bacilli, and they may "break down" later, leading to reactivation disease. In addition, bronchial obstruction may cause scarring and progressive contraction of the segment or lobe, which is often associated with the formation of cylindrical bronchiectasis and chronic pyogenic infection.

Reactivation pulmonary tuberculosis occurs most often in adolescents and adults and has a wide spectrum of clinical manifestations. Often, until the disease is moderately or far advanced, symptoms are minimal and are usually attributed to other causes such as bronchitis or "smoker's cough."[30] The most common constitutional symptoms are low-grade fever, night sweats, malaise, irritability, fatigue, weakness, and weight loss.[31, 32] The patient may initially experience mild cough, but the respiratory symptoms become more pronounced with the development of caseous necrosis and the liquefaction of lung tissue. At this time, sputum production is usually apparent, often accompanied by mild hemoptysis. Chest pain may be localized and have a pleuritic quality. Dyspnea usually indicates either extensive disease or some form of bronchial obstruction. As with children, physical findings are usually less prominent than would be expected given the degree of radiographic change. Fine rales may be heard over the area of involvement, and egophony will occasionally be heard over a large cavity.

Although reactivation pulmonary tuberculosis may involve any lung segment, the disease occurs in the apical or posterior segment of the upper lobes or the superior segment of the lower lobes in 95% of cases.[31, 33, 34] The typical pattern is air space consolidation of a patchy or confluent nature. Cavitation is fairly common, but lymph node enlargement is rarely seen in the immunocompetent host. As the lesions become chronic, they become more sharply delineated and irregular in contour. The development of fibrosis leads to volume loss in the involved lung. The combination of patchy pneumonitis, fibrosis, and calcification is strongly suggestive of tuberculosis. Older adults are more prone to having unusual radiographic manifestations of tuberculosis, including lower lung field disease.[35]

Adults with HIV infection who develop pulmonary tuberculosis often have a clinical and radiographic presentation that differs from that of the classic disease.[36–38] The earlier tuberculosis develops with concomitant HIV infection, the more "usual" is its clinical presentation, whereas a later presentation often has atypical features.[39] The primary symptoms are usually nonspecific, including fever, cough, malaise, and weight loss. However, with advanced HIV infection, the radiographic presentation of tuberculosis often includes hilar or mediastinal adenopathy, diffuse or miliary pulmonary infiltrates, but an absence of cavitation.[40, 41] Lower lung field involvement and endobronchial tuberculosis are much more common in patients with HIV infection.[42] Disseminated or extrapulmonary tuberculosis occurs in more than half of the patients.[39, 43]

Extrapulmonary manifestations of disease occur in approximately 15% of immunocompetent adults and 25% of children with tuberculosis.[44] Virtually any organ of the body can be involved. Superficial lymph node disease in the cervical or supraclavicular regions is the most common manifestation, accounting for 67% of the cases of extrapulmonary tuberculosis in children. The affected nodes are typically enlarged and firm and are not tender but are fixed to underlying or overlying tissues.[45] Pleural tuberculosis accounts for almost one quarter of the cases of extrapulmonary tuberculosis, but it is uncommon in children and rare in infants. Other common sites of tuberculosis are the genitourinary system, the bones and joints, the peritoneum, and the pericardium.

The two forms of tuberculosis that are rapidly life threatening are disseminated or miliary disease and meningitis. The early clinical manifestations of miliary tuberculosis are protean, depending on the load of disseminated organisms and in what tissues they lodge. Lesions are usually largest in the lungs, spleen, liver, and bone marrow. The onset of clinical disease may be explosive, the patient becoming gravely ill during several days.[46] More often, the onset is insidious. Early systemic signs include malaise, anorexia, weight loss, and low-grade fever. Within several weeks, hepatosplenomegaly and generalized lymphadenopathy develop in about half of the patients. The lungs become filled with tubercles, accompanied by the onset of dyspnea, cough, rales, or wheezing. Signs or symptoms of meningitis or peritonitis are found in 20 to 40% of patients with advanced disease. Early diagnosis is often difficult because the signs and symptoms are nonspecific, classic radiographic findings are absent, and 40% of patients have a negative tuberculin skin test reaction. If untreated, the disease usually becomes fatal.

Central nervous system tuberculosis is the most serious complication, being uniformly fatal if effective treatment is not given.[47, 48] The meningeal exudate usually concentrates near the brain stem and may infiltrate the cortical or meningeal blood vessels, producing inflammation, obstruction, and subsequent infarction of the cerebral cortex. The brain stem inflammation accounts for the frequent involvement of cranial nerves III, VI, and VII, and it interferes with the normal flow of cerebrospinal fluid, which leads to hydrocephalus. The clinical progression of tuberculous meningitis may be rapid during several days but more commonly occurs in several weeks. The first stage is characterized by nonspecific symptoms such as fever, headache, malaise, irritability, and drowsiness. The second stage often begins abruptly with lethargy, nuchal rigidity, seizures, vomiting, hypertonia, and focal neurological findings. The third stage is marked by coma, hemiplegia, deterioration in vital signs, and, eventually, death. The prognosis of tuberculous meningitis correlates closely with the clinical stage of illness at the time that antituberculosis chemotherapy is started. Particularly in developing countries, the diagnosis is often delayed by the lack of available diagnostic tests, and death or profound handicap is a common outcome.

Bacteriology

In 1882, Robert Koch discovered the Koch bacillus—the etiological agent of human tuberculosis—now known as *M. tuberculosis*. All members of the genus *Mycobacterium* share the property of acid-fastness, which is related to the complex cell wall structure that contains derivatives of mycolic acid. Each species of mycobacteria has a unique pattern of mycolic acids that can be distinguished by high-performance liquid chromatography.[49] Several species of mycobacteria with similar growth characteristics and biochemical reactions are classified together into the *M. tuberculosis* complex. Three species—*M. tuberculosis*, *Mycobacterium africanum*, and *Mycobacterium ulcerans*—are primarily human pathogens. *Mycobacterium bovis*, the fourth member of this complex, causes tuberculosis primarily in cattle and other animals but can cause disease in humans who have extensive contact with infected animals or who drink animal milk laden with the organism. Veterinary control programs have all but eliminated *M. bovis* disease in the United States, but human infection still occurs in some countries with less stringent controls.[50] It has never been established with certainty why Calmette and Guérin chose a strain of *M. bovis* to develop their tuberculosis vaccine (but Guérin was a veterinarian!).

Although nontuberculous mycobacteria were discovered shortly after Koch's discovery of the tubercle bacillus, they were not recognized as human pathogens until the 1940s, about 20 years after the first use of BCG.[51] Currently, more than 55 species of these nontuberculous or environmental mycobacteria have been described, of which about half can be pathogenic in humans.[52] Many species of nontuberculous mycobacteria are present in soil, ground water, or aerosols throughout the world, with higher concentrations being present nearer the equator. The most ubiquitous species are those of the *Mycobacterium avium-intracellulare* complex. Although disease rates due to these environmental mycobacteria are low, they probably have other immunological effects on humans that are of significance in the prevention and control of tuberculosis. Their interactions with the effects of BCG vaccine are probably important and may explain some of the variability in reported clinical trials.

Pathogenesis as It Relates to Prevention

The primary complex of tuberculosis consists of local disease at the portal of entry—which is the lung in more than 95% of cases—and at the regional lymph nodes that drain the area of the primary focus. Tubercle bacilli within inhaled particles larger than 10 μ are usually caught by the mucociliary mechanisms of the bronchial tree and expelled. Smaller particles are inhaled beyond the clearance mechanisms.[53] The number of organisms required to establish infection is unknown, but it is likely that only several organisms are necessary. Most of the bacilli are ingested and killed, but in animal models, approximately 10% of the organisms survive.[54] These tubercle bacilli multiply first in the alveoli and alveolar ducts. They also multiply within macrophages and are released when these cells die. The released bacilli chemotactically attract inactivated monocytes and lymphocytes from the blood stream, creating the formation of an early primary tubercle.[55]

After several weeks of infection, great numbers of tubercle bacilli grow symbiotically within inactivated macrophages. The onset of delayed hypersensitivity and cell-mediated immunity greatly alters the pathogenic picture. The "incubation period" between the time the tubercle bacilli enter the body and the development of cutaneous hypersensitivity is usually between 2 and 12 weeks, most often between 3 and 8 weeks. At this time, the tissue reaction intensifies, and the primary complex may temporarily become visible on the chest radiograph. Caseous necrosis and eventual encapsulation of the primary complex usually occur. During the development of the primary complex and the accelerated caseation brought on by the development of delayed hypersensitivity, tubercle bacilli spread from the primary complex to many parts of the body through the blood stream and lymphatics. The tissues most commonly seeded are the liver, spleen, meninges, lymph nodes, kidneys, bone, and apices of the lungs. When this dissemination involves large numbers of bacilli in a susceptible host, disseminated tuberculosis follows. More commonly, small numbers of disseminated bacilli leave microscopic foci in these tissues, which may be the origin of either extrapulmonary tuberculosis or reactivation, adult-type pulmonary tuberculosis that occurs in some individuals.

Tuberculosis disease that occurs more than a year after infection is thought to be caused mainly by endogenous regrowth of persisting bacilli that remain from the primary infection and subclinical dissemination.[56] In some individuals, a temporary decline in the ability of their cell-mediated immunity to keep persisting bacilli dormant leads to massive replication of organisms and reactivation disease. In developed countries with low rates of tuberculosis, disease caused by exogenous reinfection from another person is rare.[57, 58] In countries in which tuberculosis rates remain high, exogenous reinfection may be a more common cause of disease. The reactivation form of pulmonary disease has also been called secondary, postprimary, adult-type, or reinfection tuberculosis. This is the most infectious form of tuberculosis. The most common form of reactivation tuberculosis is an infiltrate or cavity in the apex of the lung. Extrapulmonary forms of tuberculosis, including meningitis, can arise as reactivation disease, but dissemination during reactivation is rare among immunocompetent hosts.

If young children with tuberculosis infection do not suffer primary disease, their risk of developing reactivation tuberculosis later in life is low. Conversely, older children and adolescents rarely develop disease as a complication of the primary infection but have a higher risk of developing reactivation disease as an adolescent or adult. The timing of infection must be taken into account when vaccine efficacy is being determined, and vaccine effects on the occurrence of both primary and reactivation disease must be considered separately because vaccination may prevent one form but not the other.

The immunological reactions to *M. tuberculosis* are a critical determinant of clinical expression of infection and vaccine efficacy. Unfortunately, the exact immunological mechanisms that characterize human resistance to *M. tuberculosis* remain undetermined. The host response is determined by both delayed hypersensitivity, which kills bacilli-laden inactivated macrophages, and cell-mediated immunity, which amplifies the ability of macrophages to kill the bacilli they ingest.[59] Although both processes are associated with tuberculin reactivity and are transferable by lymphocytes, there is strong evidence that they are mediated by different mechanisms.[60, 61]

One component of immunity to *M. tuberculosis* is the activation of macrophages by cytokines derived from helper T cells. It also appears likely that cytolytic activity is involved in protection by facilitating destruction of immunologically effete, bacilli-laden cells, enabling immunocompetent activated macrophages to rephagocytose bacilli.[61, 62] In addition, there is evidence that apoptosis facilitates killing of intracellular bacilli, whereas simple necrosis does not.[63]

An important emerging concept is that differences in the maturation pathways of helper T cells may help explain why some mycobacterial challenges do not result in protection due to macrophage activation or cytolytic activity.[64] Helper T cells follow two distinct maturation pathways, resulting in Th1 and Th2 cells. The cell types can be identified by the cytokines they secrete or induce: Th1 cells produce interleukin-2 and γ-interferon, whereas Th2 cells produce or induce interleukins (-4, -6, and -10). Cytokines associated with one pathway may inhibit the other, leading to a locked-in immune response.[65] Certain antigenic challenges may "imprint" the immune system with a predisposition to mount either a Th1 or Th2 response to future challenges with the same or similar antigen.[66]

It appears that progressive tuberculosis is usually associated with a Th2 or a mixed Th1 and Th2 T-cell response, whereas a pure Th1 response mediates protection.[67, 68] In the presence of Th1 cytokines, tumor necrosis factor (TNF) facilitates macrophage activation and granuloma formation. However, some factor produced or induced by a Th2 response renders tissues sensitive to destruction by TNF, explaining, in part, the gross tissue necrosis most often seen in reactivation pulmonary tuberculosis.[69, 70] Obviously, genetic control over the responses is also important.

It appears that the immune system in tuberculosis is a "two-edged sword" capable of inflicting damage to either the invader or the host.[61] An effective vaccine should induce or boost protective immune responses (Th1) but not those that cause tissue necrosis (Th2). One explanation for the marked variation in the efficacy of BCG vaccines is the differing effect of sensitization of the population by saprophytic mycobacteria in the environment. In some regions or populations, an initial Th1 response may be produced by this sensitization that can be boosted by a BCG vaccine, whereas in others, an induced Th2 response may be boosted, with possible adverse effects.[61] It has been postulated that BCG vaccination of persons already infected with *M. tuberculosis* may actually promote reactivation of tuberculosis soon after vaccination by enhancing previously weak Th2 mechanisms.[71] In many countries, BCG vaccines are given to newborns before sensitization by environmental mycobacteria can occur. Again, genetic influences or maturational differences in the development of helper T-cell pathways could explain different responses to and efficacy of BCG vaccination. The specific cellular and cytokine responses to BCG vaccination in infants are basically unstudied.

Diagnosis

In looking at field trials of BCG vaccine, it is critically important to consider the diagnostic techniques used to define subsequent cases of tuberculosis within the study population. In some poor countries, the only diagnostic test is an acid-fast smear of the sputum; mycobacterial cultures and radiography are not available. The limitations of current diagnostic techniques are especially important in considering childhood or extrapulmonary tuberculosis.

Tuberculin Skin Test

A positive reaction to a tuberculin skin test is the hallmark of primary infection with *M. tuberculosis*. When tuberculin reactivity is due to infection by the tubercle bacillus, it usually remains for the individual's lifetime, even after chemotherapy is taken.[72, 73] Although multiple puncture techniques are available for tuberculin skin testing, they have many technical problems and should be avoided, especially as diagnostic tests or as screening tests among high-risk populations. The "gold standard" test is the Mantoux test, the intradermal injection of purified protein derivative (PPD) by use of a needle and syringe. Although experienced healthcare workers usually demonstrate good interobserver agreement on results, inexperienced observers frequently report results inaccurately.[74]

Unfortunately, a negative tuberculin skin test reaction never rules out tuberculosis because 10% of adults and children with tuberculous disease have anergy for tuberculin.[75, 76] A variety of host-related factors such as young or old age, poor nutrition, immunosuppression by disease or drugs, viral infections (particularly measles, varicella, and influenza), and overwhelming tuberculosis can lower tuberculin reactivity.[77] Many patients coinfected with HIV and *M. tuberculosis* have anergy for tuberculin with or without anergy to other skin test antigens.[78]

False-positive reactions to tuberculin also occur. Recent exposure to environmental mycobacteria can result in cross-sensitization and a false-positive reaction to a Mantoux test.[79] A study of U.S. naval recruits in the 1950s and 1960s showed that up to 70% of young adults from certain geographical regions (southeast United States) had some sensitization to mycobacterial antigens.[80] The reactions to tuberculin PPD in these individuals were usually transient and produced an induration of less than 12 mm, although larger reactions can occur.

The interpretation of the Mantoux tuberculin skin test reaction should be influenced by the purpose for which the test was given and by the consequences of false classification. The appropriate cutoff size indicating a positive reaction varies with the person being tested and with related epidemiological factors.[78, 81] The Centers for Disease Control and Prevention, the American Academy of Pediatrics, and the American Thoracic Society recommend varying cutoff points for a positive reaction by the risk of tuberculosis infection (Table 8–1). For adults and children at the highest risk for tuberculosis, a reactive area of 5 mm is classified as positive. For other groups at high risk for tuberculosis (Table 8–2), a reactive area of 10 mm is positive. In some locales in which tuberculosis is rare, the cutoff may be increased to 15 mm for individuals with no other risk factors for tuberculosis infection or disease.

Table 8–1. **SIZE OF INDURATION THAT DETERMINES A POSITIVE MANTOUX TUBERCULIN SKIN TEST REACTION**

≥5 mm	≥10 mm	≥15 mm
Contacts of infectious cases An abnormal finding on chest radiography Human immunodeficiency virus infection or other immunosuppression Clinical illness suggestive of tuberculosis	Other groups at high risk listed in Table 8–2	No risk factors

Table 8–2. **HIGH-RISK GROUPS FOR TUBERCULOSIS IN TECHNOLOGICALLY ADVANCED COUNTRIES**

INCREASED RISK OF EXPOSURE TO AN INFECTIOUS ADULT
Foreign-born persons from high-prevalence countries
Poor and medically indigent, especially city residents
Users of intravenous and other street drugs
Residents (present and former) of correctional institutions
Residents of nursing homes
Homeless persons
Healthcare workers in high-risk settings
INCREASED RISK OF DISEASE OCCURRING AFTER INFECTION
Persons who have coinfection with the human immunodeficiency virus
Persons who have other medical risk factors (e.g., diabetes mellitus, silicosis, carcinoma, gastrectomy)
Persons undergoing immunosuppressive therapies
Persons who are malnourished
Infants and the extreme elderly

Bacille Calmette-Guérin Vaccines and the Tuberculin Skin Test

The various BCG vaccines have an effect on the results of the tuberculin skin test. Unfortunately, the effect is variable, and no reliable method can distinguish tuberculin reactions caused by BCG vaccination from those caused by infection with *M. tuberculosis*. In various studies with different populations and characteristics, the proportion of previously BCG-vaccinated individuals with significant skin test reactions has ranged from 0 to 90%.[82–88] The size of the skin test reaction after BCG vaccination varies with the strain and dose of the vaccine,[85, 89] the route of administration,[88, 90] the age of the individual,[84, 87, 91] the nutritional status of the individual, the number of years since vaccination [84, 87, 91] and the frequency of skin testing.[92] Some studies have found that the size of the skin test reaction increases with repeated BCG vaccination,[93] whereas others have found no such correlation.[94]

In a large number of studies of children who received BCG vaccine, the mean reaction to a tuberculin skin test ranged from 0 to 19 mm, although many experts believe that reactions larger than 10 to 15 mm after vaccination are unusual. Several studies have shown that the intensity of tuberculin reactivity after BCG vaccination is similar among siblings and correlates most highly among twins, indicating a likely degree of genetic control over the response.[95, 96] Tuberculin reactivity then wanes rapidly during the next few years. Lifschitz[84] found that approximately 50% of infants given BCG vaccine shortly after birth were tuberculin negative at 6 months of age, and almost all children were tuberculin negative at 1 year after vaccination. A similar study found that only 18% of Sri Lankan children vaccinated with BCG at birth had significant reactions at 1 year of age, and none was significant at 5 years of age.[97] A study from Canada investigated older children and adults who had received BCG vaccine by the scarification method on the lower back either in infancy or as older children.[83] Among children with a mean age of 11 years at skin testing, 4.9% vaccinated in infancy had a positive tuberculin reaction compared with 12.5% of those vaccinated as older children. Among young adults with a mean age of 23 years at skin testing, 10.3% vaccinated in infancy had a positive skin test result compared with 25.5% of those vaccinated as older children. A similar study found that only 16% of U.S. naval recruits who had received BCG vaccine 8 to 15 years previously had a positive tuberculin skin test reaction at 10 mm or more.[86]

Interpretation of the tuberculin skin test in individuals previously vaccinated with BCG may be complicated by the booster phenomenon. The booster effect is the increase in reaction size to skin testing caused by repetitive testing in a person sensitized to mycobacterial antigens.[98, 99] This phenomenon is presumably caused by stimulation of a waned immunological response to mycobacterial antigens. Studies from Chile have shown that skin test reactions can be boosted significantly in both children and adults who previously received BCG vaccine.[100, 101] Boosting is an important cause of "positive" tuberculin skin test reactions among healthcare workers who previously received a BCG vaccine.[102] Repetition of the skin test in a short period of time (less than 1 year) should be avoided, or apparent conversions of the reaction from negative to positive may be created.

Severe reactions to a tuberculin skin test are extremely rare in individuals who have previously received BCG and are not infected with *M. tuberculosis*. Prior BCG vaccination is never a contraindication for tuberculin testing. A reaction to a skin test measuring 10 mm or more in an individual who has been vaccinated with BCG more than 3 years previously usually indicates infection with *M. tuberculosis*, especially if the individual has lived in an area of the world that has a high prevalence of tuberculosis. Menzies and Vissandjee[83] found that a significant tuberculin reaction among individuals who received BCG vaccine after infancy had a positive predictive value for infection with *M. tuberculosis* of 17% among a Canadian-born population and 78% among recent immigrants from an area endemic for tuberculosis. The probability that a skin test reaction has resulted from infection by *M. tuberculosis* increases (1) as the size of the reaction increases, (2) when a patient is a contact of a person with infectious tuberculosis, (3) if the person is in a high-risk group for tuberculosis, (4) when the patient's country of origin has a high prevalence of tuberculosis, and (5) as the length of time between vaccination and tuberculin testing increases.[94]

Microbiological Diagnosis

The most important laboratory test for the diagnosis of tuberculosis is the mycobacterial culture. Unfortunately, in many poor regions of the world where tuberculosis case rates are high, cultures are not available. The best culture specimen is freshly expectorated sputum, from which *M. tuberculosis* can be isolated in about 80% of cases of pulmonary tuberculosis in adults.[30] Most children with pulmonary tuberculosis cannot be induced to produce sputum. For them, the best culture material is an early morning gastric aspirate. Unfortunately, the yield from these cultures is less than 50%.[103] The yield from bronchoscopy cultures in children is usually lower than the yield from properly obtained gastric aspirate cultures.[104] The culture yield from body fluids or tissues of patients with various forms of extrapulmonary tuberculosis varies from 30 to 60%. The difficulty in microbiologically confirming the diagnosis of pulmonary tuberculosis in children and extrapulmonary tuberculosis is a limiting factor of many BCG vaccine efficacy trials.

The most rapid and widely available procedure to detect mycobacteria is microscopic observation with use of acid-fast stains of body fluids or tissues. The most common procedures used for acid-fast staining are the carbolfuchsin methods (Ziehl-Neelsen and Kinyoun stains) and the fluorochrome method (auramine-rhodamine dyes). Fluorochrome methods are more sensitive than carbolfuchsin techniques, but at least 10^4 acid-fast bacilli per milliliter of specimen are required for detection with either method. An acid-fast stain of sputum can identify 40 to 75% of adults with pulmonary tuberculosis.[105, 106] Although environmental mycobacteria can be present in sputum and create a false-positive smear, the specificity of the acid-fast smear of sputum is high, especially in locales in which tuberculosis is prevalent.[107] Unfortunately, the sensitivity of acid-fast smears of gastric aspirates from children is low, usually below 10% even in highly endemic areas.

The technique of polymerase chain reaction, which can amplify mycobacterial DNA from a specimen, has a specificity in adults of nearly 100% and a sensitivity similar to that of mycobacterial cultures, but results are available in 72 hours rather than the 3 to 6 weeks often required for conventional cultures.[108, 109] The polymerase chain reaction is less useful for diagnosing pulmonary tuberculosis in children because the sensitivity is only 60% and the specificity can be unacceptably low.[110, 111]

Clinical Diagnosis

In both developed and poorer nations, the majority of cases of pediatric tuberculosis are diagnosed on clinical grounds with use of one of several scoring systems based on symptoms, signs, and, when available, radiographic findings.[112] Although helpful, these systems have low sensitivity and specificity. One major unaddressed problem in virtually all reported BCG trials in children is the lack of uniformity of case definitions of pediatric tuberculosis; many study authors did not report a standardized case definition, and some variation of results among trials can probably be attributed to lack of standardization—exactly what was the vaccine preventing or not preventing?

Treatment and Prevention with Antibiotics

Since antituberculosis medications became available starting in the 1940s and continuing through the 1960s, tuberculosis has been treatable and preventable. Guidelines for treatment are published by the American Thoracic Society,[113] American Academy of Pediatrics,[81] and the Centers for Disease Control and Prevention.[114] In general, tuberculosis disease should be treated with three or four drugs—isoniazid, rifampin, pyrazinamide, and ethambutol or streptomycin—for 2 months followed by 4 months of isoniazid and rifampin. The choice of three versus four drugs depends on the prevalence of drug resistance in the community and the individual patient's risk of drug resistance. Four drugs are usually recommended for adults with active tuberculosis until culture and susceptibility results are available. For fully susceptible *M. tuberculosis*, isoniazid, rifampin, and pyrazinamide is the treatment of choice. Treatment for disseminated tuberculosis, complicated extrapulmonary disease, and multidrug-resistant tuberculosis usually requires more medications, longer treatment, and expert consultation. Adherence to therapy is essential for successful treatment, prevention of relapse, and prevention of drug resistance; therefore, directly observed therapy has become standard treatment for many health departments in the United States and the world.

Tuberculosis infection and disease are preventable with chemotherapy or chemoprophylaxis. Recommendations for treating exposure and infection vary by the patient's age, risk factors, and medical condition. For tuberculosis infection and no evidence of disease, 6 to 9 months of isoniazid has been shown to be efficacious in preventing the development of disease. Most experts recommend 9 months of isoniazid for children and adolescents and 6 months for adults younger than 35 years with tuberculosis infection. Treatment of infection in adults older than 35 years is recommended for individuals with medical conditions carrying increased risk for progression to disease such as immunosuppressive disorders, persons with documented recent tuberculin skin test conversion, or individuals with radiographic evidence of previous disease. Prophylactic therapy with isoniazid for close contacts to active pulmonary tuberculosis has been found effective in preventing infection and progression to disease. Isoniazid chemoprophylaxis is recommended in exposed children 4 years of age and younger because there is a higher risk of progression to disease after infection. Also, disease in this young age group is more likely to be disseminated and rapid in onset, sometimes before tuberculin skin test conversion. Once infection has been excluded by a negative skin test reaction 3 months after exposure, isoniazid can be discontinued, as long as exposure has been terminated by separation or treatment of the adult source case.

Public health practices of tuberculosis control such as timely contact investigation, treatment of infected contacts, and prophylaxis for young children exposed to tuberculosis are effective in preventing future cases. In developing countries where resources are limited, medications for treatment and prevention may not be available, much less funds to support public health investigative services. Despite the availability of treatment and technology to eliminate the disease, tuberculosis remains the leading infectious public health problem worldwide, which explains the continued reliance on BCG vaccine in developing countries.

EPIDEMIOLOGY

Developing Countries

Table 8–3 shows the estimated incidence of tuberculosis cases and mortality throughout the world.[4] Rates of infection and disease are highest throughout Asia and Africa. Disease rates are highest among young children and young adults in developing countries. Despite widespread use of BCG vaccination, disease incidence rates have increased in every region of the world except western Europe. It is estimated that slightly more than 300,000 annual cases are associated with HIV infection. In Africa, HIV-related tuberculosis has boosted the overall incidence of tuberculosis by 20%.[4] Many of these figures are estimates based on models of infectivity, because reported cases represent only a fraction of actual cases.[115] In developing nations, one third to one half of all individuals are infected with *M. tuberculosis*, despite widespread BCG vaccination programs.[4] The average annual incidence of new infection is 1 to 5%, and infection incidence rates are highest among young adults and children. The risk of new infection in these high-prevalence countries is fairly uniform across the population.

Table 8–3. **ESTIMATES OF GLOBAL TUBERCULOSIS INCIDENCE AND MORTALITY IN 1995**

WHO REGION	TUBERCULOSIS CASES	INCIDENCE RATE*	TUBERCULOSIS DEATHS	MORTALITY RATE*
Southeast Asia	3,499,000	241	1,225,000	84.4
Western Pacific†	2,045,000	140	716,000	49.0
Africa	1,467,000	242	581,000	95.8
Americas‡	606,000	123	121,000	24.6
Central Eastern Europe	202,000	47	30,000	7.0
Industrialized countries§	204,000	23	14,000	1.6
All regions	8,768,000	152	2,977,000	51.6

*Crude rate per 100,000 population.
†Includes all countries of western Pacific Region of the World Health Organization except Japan, Australia, and New Zealand.
‡Includes all countries of the American Region of the World Health Organization except the United States and Canada.
§Western European countries plus the United States, Canada, Israel, Japan, Australia, and New Zealand.
WHO, World Health Organization.
From Dolin PJ, Raviglione MC, Kochi A. Global tuberculosis incidence and mortality during 1990–2000. Bull World Health Organ 72:213–220, 1994.

Developed Countries

In contrast, tuberculosis in developed countries has been fairly well confined to large groups of high-risk individuals. Developed countries, including the United States, experienced a steady decline in tuberculosis case rates from the 1920s to the mid-1980s. In the United States, the annual number of tuberculosis cases increased about 20% between 1984 and 1992.[116] Some of this increase has been linked to the concurrent HIV epidemic, but the immigration of persons at high risk for tuberculosis, the decline in public health services in some communities, and transmission of *M. tuberculosis* in congregate settings (jails, hospitals, nursing homes, shelters) have also contributed to the relative resurgence of tuberculosis. In most Western countries, tuberculosis infection and disease rates among whites are highest among adults older than 50 years. However, among ethnic and racial minorities, who usually experience infection and disease rates that are substantially higher than those found in whites, the majority of infections and cases occur among young adults and children.[117] In Europe and North America, tuberculosis case rates are high among foreign-born immigrants from countries with a high prevalence of tuberculosis. Of foreign-born persons with tuberculosis, the majority are identified within the first 5 years after immigration.[118]

Certain environments in Western countries tend to contain large numbers of persons at high risk for tuberculosis. This disease occurs disproportionately among individuals who are poor, are undernourished, have poor access to healthcare, and live in crowded conditions. Tuberculosis case rates are 10 to 40 times higher within some prisons,[119] nursing homes,[120] homeless populations,[121] and migrant camps[122] than in the general community. In some areas, healthcare workers are at risk because of a high likelihood of exposure to infectious patients and improper infection control practices within hospitals and other healthcare institutions.[123]

Significance as a Public Health Problem

The significance of tuberculosis as a public health problem is self-evident. It remains, in 1998, the leading cause of morbidity and mortality in the world caused by a single pathogen. It remains the "Captain of the Men of Death" despite the availability of cheap and effective curative therapy, effective preventive therapy, and the use of BCG vaccine in 4 to 5 billion individuals. There is more tuberculosis afflicting mankind now than at any time in history. The inability to control tuberculosis throughout the world represents the most colossal failure of public health services in human history.

ACTIVE IMMUNIZATION WITH BACILLE CALMETTE-GUÉRIN

Prior Approaches that Have Been Abandoned

Organisms other than *M. bovis* have been considered candidates for vaccination of humans against tuberculosis through the years. A killed tubercle bacilli vaccine was studied in the 1930s and was found to have a protective efficacy of about 50% against disease in humans.[124] Avirulent environmental mycobacteria have also been evaluated as vaccine candidates against tuberculosis in humans with little success. The vole bacillus and BCG are the only vaccines that have been considered seriously for human use.[125]

The live attenuated BCG vaccine strain was first given orally to infants in Paris in 1921.[126] The peroral vaccine was used in France and other countries. In 1928, the League of Nations announced a declaration of safety for oral BCG vaccine. Unfortunately, in 1929 to 1930, 72 of 250 perorally vaccinated children died in Lübeck, Germany, of tuberculosis caused by laboratory contamination of an oral BCG preparation by virulent tubercle bacilli.[127] Despite this tragedy, BCG vaccination progressed, and new methods of administration were introduced—intradermal in 1927, multiple puncture in 1939, and scarification in 1947.[2]

History of Vaccine Development

A brief history of the development of BCG vaccine is summarized in Table 8–4. Two French scientists, Calmette, a physician, and Guérin, a veterinarian, began their studies on a tuberculosis vaccine in 1908.[128] The strain they selected for study was *M. bovis* from a cow with tuberculous mastitis. The isolate was cultured in a medium that contained glycerol, potato slices, and beef bile, the last to prevent contamination with *M. tuberculosis*. The organism was painstakingly subcultured every 3 weeks for 13 years, a total of 231 cycles. The genotypic changes that resulted at various stages cannot be determined because none of the original cultures or subcultures was preserved. This long process was marked by a loss of virulence first for calves and then for guinea pigs. Phenotypic changes in the organism occurred as well,

Table 8–4. **A BRIEF HISTORY OF BACILLE CALMETTE-GUÉRIN VACCINE**

1902	First isolation of *Mycobacterium bovis*
1908–1921	BCG developed from serial passage of *Nocardia* strain
1921	First human BCG vaccination
1928	League of Nations adopts BCG as standard vaccine
1929–1930	Lübeck disaster, 72 children die from oral BCG preparation contaminated with virulent strain
1939	Multiple puncture technique
1947	Scarification technique introduced
1948	First International BCG Congress concluded that BCG is effective; more than 10 million vaccinations carried out
1948–1974	WHO and UNICEF campaigns; 1.5 billion vaccinations carried out
1948–1997	Yearly increase of BCG vaccination estimated from 50 million to almost 100 million

BCG, bacille Calmette-Guérin; UNICEF, United Nations International Children's Emergency Fund; WHO, World Health Organization.

Adapted from Lugosi L. Theoretical and methodological aspects of BCG vaccine from the discovery of Calmette and Guérin to molecular biology. A review. Tuber Lung Dis 73:252–261, 1992.

colonies changing from rough, dry, and granular to viscous, moist, and smooth.

In 1948, the First International BCG Congress in Paris stated that BCG vaccine was effective and safe (despite the total lack of reported controlled trials or case-control studies). After World War II, the WHO and the United Nations International Children's Emergency Fund (UNICEF) organized campaigns to promote vaccination with BCG in several countries. The seed lot system for BCG was established in 1956,[128] and the WHO developed requirements for freeze-dried BCG vaccine in 1966.[129] Rates of BCG vaccination increased dramatically; by the end of 1974, more than 1.5 billion individuals had received the vaccine.

From 1974 to the present, BCG vaccination has been included in the WHO Expanded Programme on Immunization to strengthen the fight against infectious diseases among children in developing countries. Approximately 100 million children receive a BCG vaccine each year, expanding the total number of individuals who have received BCG to more than 4 billion. Only two countries—the Netherlands and the United States—have never used BCG vaccine on a national scale.

Different Strains and Their Relationship

The original strain of *M. bovis* used to make BCG was maintained by serial passage at the Pasteur Institute, until it was lost or discarded. Before its loss, it was distributed to dozens of laboratories in many countries. Each laboratory produced its own BCG and maintained it by serial passage. It became apparent that serial subculturing on various media under the different conditions maintained by the different laboratories resulted in the production of many daughter BCG strains that differed widely in colony morphology, growth characteristics, biochemical activity, ability to cause delayed hypersensitivity, and animal virulence[130–137] (Table 8–5). The patterns of large restriction fragments created by digestion of BCG DNA vary and can be used to accurately identify specific BCG substrains.[138] In an attempt to standardize production and vaccine characteristics, the production laboratories adopted a seed lot system in the mid-1950s. In the 1960s, the WHO recommended the stabilization of the biological characteristics of the daughter strains by lyophilization and storage of the samples at low temperature.[139] Interlaboratory studies showed unequivocally that the strains in use today vary widely in many characteristics.[140, 141] Some investigators have suggested grouping BCG substrains by certain properties.[142] Group 1 (Brazilian, Japanese, Swedish, and Russian) strains have secreted antigens, methoxymycolates, and two copies of the insertion sequence 6110. Group 2 (Dakar, Danish, Dutch, British, Pasteur, and Tice) strains have no secreted antigens or methoxymycolates and have only one copy of insertion sequence 6110.

Table 8–5. **RANKING OF SOME BACILLE CALMETTE-GUÉRIN STRAINS BY PROTECTION IN ANIMAL MODELS AND EFFECT ON THE TUBERCULIN REACTION IN CHILDREN**

STRAIN	MEAN SCORE
Rio de Janeiro (Moreau)	4.8
French (1173 P2)	4.3
Copenhagen (1331)	4.0
Moscow	4.0
Gothenburg	3.8
Madras	3.5
Tokyo	3.0
London	2.0
Prague	1.0

Adapted from Lagefoged A, Bunch-Christensen K, Guld J. Tuberculin sensitivity in guinea pigs after vaccination with varying doses of BCG of 12 different strains. Bull World Health Organ 53:435–443, 1976; and Vallishayee RS, Shashidhara AN, Bunch-Christensen K, Guld J. Tuberculin sensitivity and skin lesions in children after vaccination with 11 different BCG strains. Bull World Health Organ 51:489–494, 1974.

Laboratory studies and observations in humans have shown that some BCG strains can be called "strong" (Pasteur 1173 P2, Danish 1331), whereas others are "weak" (Glaxo 1077 and Tokyo 172). The strong strains are more immunogenic in various animal models, inducing a greater degree of cutaneous hypersensitivity and better protection from tuberculosis than weaker strains do.[143] Other measures of immunity such as local granuloma formation and residual virulence are more apparent after vaccination with the strong strains.[134, 140] In the guinea pig model of tuberculosis, which is probably the closest to the pathophysiology of tuberculosis in humans, the stronger strains provide better protection.

It is difficult to demonstrate that one strain of BCG is clearly superior to another in the protection of humans against tuberculosis.[139, 144] Results of BCG vaccination in case-control studies in children and in contacts of cases whose smears were positive suggest that the protection against tuberculosis differs among the major BCG strains. The WHO has estimated that immediate protection from severe forms of tuberculosis in children is about 60 to 80% for the Glaxo 1077 strain and 60 to 95% for the Tokyo 172 strain.[145] The protection against less severe forms of tuberculosis is 24 to 50% for the Glaxo 1077 strain, 39 to 53% for the Tokyo 172 strain, and 70 to 75% for the Pasteur 1173 P2 strain. Other studies from Hong Kong and Korea have also shown that the protection for children afforded by the Pasteur strain is higher than that of the Glaxo strain.[129] A problem with the interpretation of these data is that childhood tuberculosis is much more difficult to diagnose or confirm than disease in adults, and milder forms of tuberculosis in children may have gone unnoticed in these trials.

The incidence of side effects with BCG vaccination also differs between strong and weak strains.[146] The strong strains have been associated with a higher rate of lymphadenitis and osteitis, especially among neonates.[147–150] Reduction of the vaccination dose of the strong strains also reduces the incidence of lymphadenitis, probably with little effect on immediate vaccine efficacy.

It is apparent that there is no worldwide consensus about which strain of BCG is optimal for general use. The use of a weaker strain is tempting for both vaccine producers and users, because immediate results without side effects ensure few problems initially.[139] It also appears that various BCG strains have lost efficacy over time with serial passage.[151] It has been postulated that investigators have selected BCG strains by their desire to maximize tuberculin reactivity and minimize adenitis, which may actually create strains that are the inverse of an ideal vaccine. Local customs, history, and tradition have affected vaccine policy in many countries as much as vaccine efficacy and rates of adverse reactions. The past and continued use of both strong and weak vaccine strains makes interpretation and comparison of clinical trials extremely difficult.

Vaccine Production

Since the mid-1970s, an international system for the production and quality control of BCG vaccines has been centered at the WHO. Seed lots of the various BCG strains that have previously been subjected to laboratory testing and clinical efficacy studies are maintained by the WHO and the State Serum Institute in Copenhagen, which performs the following tasks[129]: (1) provides technical assistance to national BCG laboratories at the request of the WHO, (2) provides training in BCG production and quality control, (3) distributes reference and seed lots of BCG vaccine, (4) tests candidate BCG vaccines from providers, and (5) tests samples from BCG lots supplied to national immunization programs through UNICEF.

The seed lots are lyophilized bacilli that are part of the original harvest of the various BCG strains. In most laboratories, the bacilli are grown in liquid Sauton medium as a pedicle, the classical surface-grown culture. The organisms can be grown dispersed throughout the liquid media, which produces a slightly different colony morphology.[152] An early harvest of bacilli after 6 to 9 days of growth is essential for good survival of organisms after lyophilization. Even with these controls, the daughter strains are not homogeneous but contain more than one colony type; the proportion of these types in a vaccine can be altered profoundly by culture conditions.[130, 153] After filtering and pressing, the semidry mycobacterial mass is homogenized at controlled temperatures, diluted, and then freeze-dried. A stabilizer is added to the preparation. Vaccine stabilized with monosodium glutamate may be more difficult to reconstitute, whereas the presence of albumin may lead to the foaming of the product during reconstitution.[129]

Reconstituted vaccines contain both live bacilli that have pleomorphic coccal and bacillary forms and dead bacilli killed during lyophilization and reconstitution.[154] Studies conducted by the WHO have shown a wide range of culturable bacilli per dose of vaccine from various manufacturers (Table 8–6). The vaccines with relatively low numbers of bacilli per dose are the strong, more reactogenic strains.

The biochemical composition of BCG vaccines varies widely, even among preparations derived from the same parent strain. For example, MPB70, a unique BCG-specific antigen that elicits a delayed hypersensitivity reaction in guinea pigs sensitized with viable BCG cells,

Table 8–6. **CULTURABLE BACILLI IN BACILLE CALMETTE-GUÉRIN VACCINES**

PARENT STRAIN	NUMBER OF MANUFACTURERS	NUMBER OF CULTURABLE BACILLI PER DOSE
French 1173 P2	6	37,500–500,000
Danish 1331	3	150,000–300,000
Glaxo 1077	2	200,000–1,000,000
Tokyo 172	1	3,000,000
Montreal	2	200,000–3,200,000

Adapted from Milstien JB, Gibson JJ. Quality controls of BCG vaccine by WHO: A review of factors that may influence vaccine effectiveness and safety. Bull World Health Organ 68:93–108, 1990.

constitutes up to 10% of the total protein content of the culture medium of the Tokyo strain but only trace amounts of protein in other strains.[129, 155] The content of mycoside B, which is associated with colony morphology, varies with the production method.[153] It is not known how variations in these and other products in BCG vaccines correlate with the protective efficacy of or adverse reactions to BCG vaccine.[129] It is apparent, however, that the chemical composition of vaccine can vary widely among preparations.

Dosage and Route of Administration

It is generally accepted that the best method of BCG vaccination is intradermal injection with use of a syringe and needle. This is the most accurate method because the dose can be measured precisely and the administration can be controlled. Although many body sites can be used for vaccination, the most common site is the deltoid region of the arm. Unfortunately, intradermal injection can be difficult in newborns, especially if a large number of infants require vaccine fairly rapidly. The rate of local reactions, including ulcers and lymphadenitis, is higher with the intradermal method than with any other when other characteristics of the vaccine are controlled.[139] The intradermal method is relatively expensive, and in many poor countries, the needles and syringes are frequently reused, with the resulting danger of transmission of hepatitis viruses or HIV. Despite these problems, the intradermal method remains widely used throughout the world.

Other methods of administration were developed to address the problems created by intradermal administration. Subcutaneous injection gives adequate results in terms of induced tuberculin sensitivity but frequently produces abscesses and unsightly, retracted scars.[156] Other techniques such as scarification, jet injection, and use of bifurcated needles have yielded highly variable and, in some cases, inaccurate results.[156–158] The advantages of using these alternative techniques are a lower local complication rate and a choice of using a single-dose unit, which avoids cross-contamination among vaccine recipients. The multiple puncture technique was developed in the 1940s with good early success.[159–161] The Tice vaccine in the United States uses a multipuncture technique. A multipuncture technique has been used for more than 40 years in Japan with good apparent success and a low rate of adverse reactions.[139] There have been no conclusive reported trials that compared the various techniques of BCG administration for protection against subsequent tuberculosis, although local complication rates are generally lowest with multipuncture devices.

The recommended dosage of BCG vaccine differs by vaccine strain and age of the recipient. For each strain, the dosage is adjusted to maximize the protective effect and minimize the local reactions. The two factors that determine these results are the total mass of organisms and the viable bacilli count in the vaccine. In general, newborns are given half of the standard dose.

There is a wide disparity among nations concerning vaccine schedules. The official recommendation of the WHO is a single dose given in infancy. However, only three prospective community trials have evaluated the efficacy of BCG vaccine given at birth.[162] Studies of lymphocyte blastogenesis in response to PPD have shown much higher rates of immunogenic sensitization in children if BCG vaccination is delayed from the first week to 9 months of life.[162] However, even low-birth-weight newborns develop lymphocyte proliferation and interleukin-2 production in response to a BCG vaccine.[164] In the United Kingdom, a single dose of BCG is administered during adolescence.[165–167] Many countries give the first dose of BCG in infancy, then give repeated vaccinations throughout childhood. In some nations, repeated vaccination is universal; in others, it is based on either the lack of tuberculin sensitivity or the absence of a typical scar. Unfortunately, absence of a scar after BCG vaccination does not correlate with lack of tuberculin sensitivity or any specific immunological parameter. It is reasonable that the recommended schedules would vary with the local epidemiology of tuberculosis; age groups at highest risk of disease (young children versus adolescents or young adults) would be targeted for vaccination. However, these schedule differences reflect variation among countries in both the local epidemiology of tuberculosis and the opinions concerning the mechanism and duration of protection imparted by BCG. It must be concluded that the optimal age for administration and schedule (single versus multiple doses) has not been firmly established because adequate comparative trials have not been reported.

Preparations Available

The various strains of BCG are generally known by the name of the country or laboratory in which they are kept. Although many different strains are in use, four main strains account for more than 90% of the vaccines currently in use worldwide: (1) the French (Pasteur) strain 1173 P2, used in France and by 14 other countries for their production of vaccine[168]; (2) the Danish strain 1331; (3) the Glaxo strain 1077, derived from the Danish strain 1331 but differing from it substantially in biological characteristics[130, 141, 169] (the English "Evans" vaccine and the French "Mérieux" vaccine are the Glaxo 1077 strain); and (4) the Tokyo strain 172, selected for its high resistance to lyophilization. Other commonly used strains include the Moreau (Brazil), Montreal (Canada), Russia (former Soviet Union), and Tice (United States).

Currently in the United States, the only available BCG vaccine is the Tice strain, derived from the Pasteur strain 1173 P2 and developed at the University of Illinois. The Food and Drug Administration is considering another BCG vaccine for licensure in the United States that is produced by Connaught Laboratories and derived from the Montreal strain.

Vaccine Stability

For established BCG vaccines, repeated measurements of tuberculin sensitivity and lesion size as well as various in vitro tests on cultured BCG bacilli are used to verify that the vaccine lots are being reproduced satisfactorily.[129] In addition, the WHO suggests to the national programs that any change in manufacturing procedure be accompanied by field trials in tuberculin-negative humans to determine the optimal content of BCG bacilli. It is required that manufacturers conduct such studies in children on at least one batch of vaccine per year.

Several in vitro tests are used to verify consistency of BCG vaccines. A test for the number of viable bacilli is carried out by either colony growth in media or measurements of bioluminescence that are proportional to the adenosine triphosphate content of the vaccine. Growth in media is subject to considerable laboratory variability, and conditions must be controlled firmly. The viability of the vaccine is calculated by comparing the total bacterial mass as determined by dry weight or opacity with the count of viable bacilli. In general, the extent of the local reaction to BCG vaccination is proportional to the total bacterial mass, whereas the level of tuberculin sensitivity induced by the vaccine is related to the number of viable particles.[129] The thermal stability of each lot of BCG is tested. The WHO requires that the number of viable particles present after 28 days of incubation at 37°C must not be less than 20% of that in samples stored at 4°C. Differences in thermal stability can be attributed to the growth characteristics of the strain and the preparation, packaging, and storage of the lyophilized vaccine.[141, 170]

Other routine quality control procedures carried out by most production laboratories include a test of identity, a test for contamination, and a test for safety in guinea pigs.

RESULTS OF VACCINATION

Immune Responses to Bacille Calmette-Guérin Vaccine

The exact immune response elicited by BCG vaccination and its mechanism of action within the host are not well understood. Some information can be gleaned from field trials and autopsy studies in humans and protection studies in various animal models of tuberculosis.

Most of the major field trials and case-control trials of BCG vaccines have demonstrated that they afford a higher level of protection against the most serious forms of tuberculosis—such as meningitis and disseminated disease—than against the more moderate forms of disease.[171, 172] These observations have led to the hypothesis that the protective effect of BCG derives from its interference with the hematogenous spread of bacilli from the primary focus. That is, BCG vaccination does not prevent infection with *M. tuberculosis* but helps the host to retard the growth of organisms at the primary site of infection and prevent massive lymphohematogenous dissemination. This hypothesis is supported by autopsy studies in humans that have shown that virtually all infections with *M. tuberculosis* lead to the development of pulmonary foci irrespective of the BCG vaccination status of the individual.[173]

Experiments using animal models of tuberculosis have supported the results found in humans.[9] Studies in guinea pigs and mice inoculated with tubercle bacilli by the respiratory, intravenous, or subcutaneous routes have shown that tubercle bacilli multiply for several days equally well in BCG-vaccinated and unvaccinated animals.[174–176] In the guinea pig model, the number of tubercle bacilli recovered from the lung, spleen, and lymph nodes increases at the same rate in both vaccinated and unvaccinated animals until the 14th day after infection, when replication rates fall off in the vaccinated animals.[177] The obvious implication from these studies is that BCG vaccination does not result in the permanent creation of activated macrophages within the lung.[178, 179]

Studies of the immunological events that occur within the human host after BCG vaccination are almost totally lacking. Animal studies examining the immune responses to BCG in relation to infection with *M. tuberculosis* have been surprisingly infrequent.[9] From some of these studies, several broad conclusions can be made with some confidence: (1) protective immunity cannot be transferred with serum, indicating the lack of importance of antibodies in immunity; (2) protection can be transferred with T lymphocytes, the characteristics of the lymphocyte subpopulation required depending on the length of the interval after vaccination[180, 181]; (3) the immune response in animals with strong resistance to tuberculosis does not differ from that in susceptible animals until days after infection, implying that macrophages are not activated in an immune animal; and (4) the production of hydrogen peroxide and superoxide anion by activated macrophages is enhanced in animals that have been vaccinated with BCG, leading to a greater bactericidal effect against *M. tuberculosis*.[182] Both animal data and human clinical studies have provided information about the immune response to BCG, yet for no vaccine so widely used is so little known about its mechanisms of action.

A major difficulty in studying tuberculosis and BCG immunization is the lack of an accurate immunoassay that correlates with resistance to infection. There is no serological test for protective immunity after tuberculosis infection or BCG vaccination. Although most infectious diseases and commonly used vaccines cause a measurable serological response for an average known duration, BCG and tuberculosis do not.[183] The immunology is complicated, and development of an assay has been hampered by the lack of understanding of the protective response and the inability to identify specific antigens that stimulate immunity. Cellular immunity has been shown to play the major role in protection, but the specific antigenic determinants and the mechanisms involved in this response are not known. Although *M. tuberculosis* and BCG share many common antigens, it is unclear whether they share the specific antigenic determinants of immunity.

There has been much debate concerning which epitopes of BCG induce protective immunity. It has been assumed that species-specific antigens afford protection against tuberculosis, but recent evidence suggests that this notion is incorrect. Several studies have shown that BCG vaccine affords protection against *Mycobacterium leprae* infection that is as great as or even greater than that against tuberculosis.[184–186] The only epitopes shared by *M. tuberculosis* and *M. leprae* are common to all mycobacteria. There is also some epidemiological evidence that BCG protects children from lymphadenitis due to nontuberculous mycobacteria, especially those of the *M. avium* complex.[187, 188] It is likely that efficacy of BCG and other mycobacterial vaccines may depend on the manner in which common antigens are presented and the innate reactivity of the host immune system.[61]

Given our incomplete understanding of tuberculosis immunology, we are left with imperfect indicators of immunity. Tuberculin skin test conversion has long been used as evidence of mycobacterial infection or as a sign of adequate response to BCG vaccine. Many public health programs practice repeated vaccination until individuals become tuberculin positive, believing that reactivity indicates effective protection. The relationship between postvaccination delayed hypersensitivity and protective immunity is a controversial issue, with no clear relationship established.[189] Neither the presence nor the size of postvaccination tuberculin skin test reactions reliably predicts the degree of protection afforded by BCG.[190, 191] Animal studies evaluating this question have observed the following[9]: (1) no direct relationship between the size of the skin test reaction and the degree of acquired resistance was found; (2) some vaccinated animals whose skin test results remained negative were protected; and (3) tuberculin testing boosted a waning tuberculin reaction but did not boost a waning protective response. In humans, results of the Medical Research Council's BCG trial in Great Britain demonstrated a high level of protection against tuberculosis and showed that the degree of tuberculin sensitivity was independent of the degree of protection conferred by vaccination.[189] Other studies such as the Chingleput trial in southern India demonstrated poor protective efficacy yet had high levels of vaccine-induced tuberculin sensitivity.[192, 193] Other researchers have suggested a "two-pathway" theory, proposing that BCG vaccination may trigger either protective (Lister type) or antagonistic (tuberculin or Koch type) reactions, with the most protective vaccines producing little or no tuberculin-sensitizing reactions because the two pathways are competitive.[194–197] Although the skin test reaction does indicate a response of the immune system to mycobacterial infection or BCG vaccination in animals and humans, how this reaction is related to protective immunity remains unsettled. Most experts conclude that immunity and the presence of tuberculin sensitivity are related in some way but are not identical.

Results of Bacille Calmette-Guérin Vaccine Controlled Trials

The true effectiveness of BCG vaccine has been debated for decades. Large clinical trials conducted from the 1930s through the 1970s yielded wide-ranging and conflicting results, demonstrating efficacy from 0 to 80% (Fig. 8–1). The most recent trial in Chingleput, India, designed with hopes of settling the question of BCG's efficacy once and for all, had discouraging results and methodological difficulties that only served to continue the argument.[192] Experts have offered a number of explanations for the variation in results among trials, but no one theory has been proved.[156, 198–202] In recent years, researchers have studied BCG efficacy using case-control, cohort, and meta-analysis study designs, but conclusions still diverge. Even with years of study and debate, the question Does BCG work? cannot be answered definitively.

Despite these problems and uncertainties, BCG has enjoyed great success in one aspect—its widespread use. The success of the various national BCG vaccination programs is difficult to assess for a number of reasons. Many of these programs were instituted during times of social, economic, and public health improvements that may have effected a decrease in tuberculosis independent of BCG vaccination efforts. Most of the individuals vaccinated during the early programs are only now reaching the age at which tuberculosis is most important as a public health problem,[189] and the effects of BCG on them may not yet be apparent.

Major Field Trials of BCG Vaccine

Figure 8–1 contains a graphic display of eight representative field trials conducted between 1935 and 1975. These trials differed in a number of important aspects, including eligibility criteria, methods of disease surveillance, diagnostic criteria, vaccine strain and administration, and environmental factors. Dr. George Comstock[203] has published a comprehensive comparison of these eight trials as well as 11 additional controlled trials.

The randomized controlled trial is the ideal study design to address vaccine efficacy, but several considerations have complicated the evaluation of BCG vaccine with use of this method. First, the lack of a serological test for immunity precludes laboratory determination of protection, requiring long-term clinical observation of a large population. Second, the low incidence of tubercu-

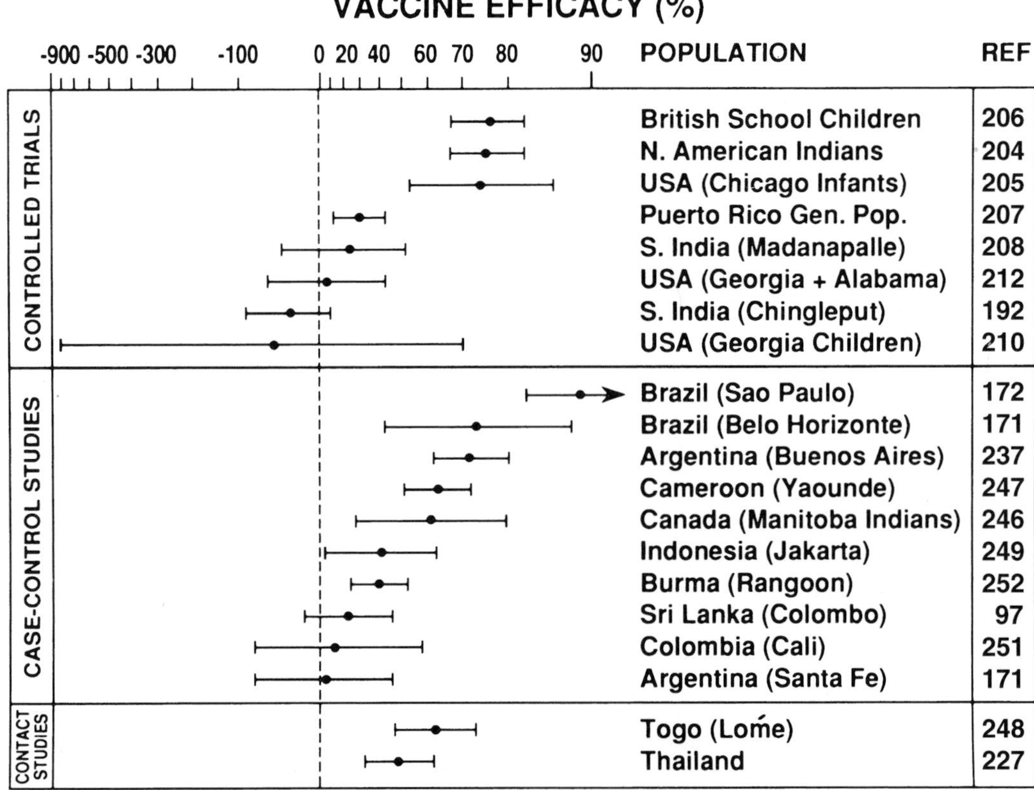

Figure 8–1. A summary of some reported trials of bacille Calmette-Guérin and their computed vaccine efficacy. These include the major controlled trials, case-control studies, and contact studies. Efficacy is expressed on a logarithmic scale, with bars indicating 95% confidence intervals. REF, reference numbers (in this chapter). (Adapted from Fine PE, Rodrigues LC. Modern vaccines: Mycobacterial diseases. Lancet 1:1016–1020, 1990. © The Lancet, 1990.)

losis and long incubation period for disease mean that huge study groups must be observed for long periods at great cost. Third, there is no gold standard for diagnosis of tuberculosis disease other than acid-fast stain and mycobacterial culture, which can have low sensitivity, especially among children. Also, many of these trials were conducted in developing countries in which resources for diagnosis, vaccination, follow-up, and tracking were inadequate. These challenges as well as the lack of understanding of the immunology involved in protection against tuberculosis make the design and execution of clinical trials extremely difficult.

The eight major BCG trials shown in Figure 8–1 can be grouped into three categories: those showing excellent, moderate, or poor to no protection. Three clinical trials demonstrated excellent protection. The first was conducted among North American Indians in the 1930s.[204] Eligibility for enrollment included persons from birth to 20 years of age who had a negative reaction to 250 tuberculin units (TU) of PPD. Approximately 1500 subjects each were in the vaccination and control groups, and the duration of follow-up was 9 to 11 years. The estimated efficacy in this trial was 80% with good statistical precision, calculated by subsequent investigators.[198] The second study was also conducted in the 1930s, in Chicago, among infants living in high-risk areas.[205] Study subjects were normal infants younger than 3 months whose family had normal findings on chest radiography. No baseline tuberculin tests were performed. Approximately 1700 subjects each were in the study and control groups, and follow-up ranged from 12 to 23 years. Among the control group, 65 cases of tuberculosis occurred compared with 17 cases among the vaccinated. The protective efficacy was 75% with good statistical precision. The third trial, which demonstrated excellent protection, was initiated in 1950 among British schoolchildren.[206] Eligibility criteria included an age of 14 to 15 years and a skin test response of less than 5 mm to 100 TU of old tuberculin, a form of skin test reagent. Approximately 13,000 subjects each were in the unvaccinated and BCG groups, and the duration of follow-up was around 15 years. There were 240 cases of tuberculosis among the control group and 56 cases among the vaccinated group. The protective efficacy was 76% with good statistical precision. These three trials that demonstrated excellent efficacy had two characteristics in common. First, they were conducted in geographical areas with a low prevalence of environmental mycobacteria. Second, the methodology and statistical precision of these three trials have been judged to be superior compared with those of the other major BCG trials.[198]

Two studies of BCG efficacy demonstrated moderate protective efficacy. The first was sponsored by the U.S. Public Health Service and conducted in Puerto Rico starting in 1949.[207] Eligibility criteria included an age of 1 to 18 years and a skin test reaction less than 6 mm to 10 TU of PPD. The trial enrolled approximately 27,000 control subjects and 51,000 children who had been vaccinated with BCG. Follow-up consisted of matching officially reported cases to study records and was conducted during 19 years. There were 73 cases of tuberculosis among the control subjects and 93 in the vaccinated group, resulting in an efficacy of 29%. The second study showing moderate protection was carried out in southern India (Madanapalle) and enrolled patients between 1950 and 1955.[208] Eligibility criteria included all ages and a skin test reaction of less than 5 mm to 5 TU of old tuberculin. The trial included approximately 6000 control subjects and 5000 vaccinated individuals, with follow-up at 2.5 to 7.0 years and then again at 15.0 years. The efficacy was originally estimated at 60%, but after 15 years of follow-up, the protective effect had decreased to 20% with wide confidence intervals.[209] The methodology of both of these trials had many potential biases and inadequate statistical precision.[198] Both were conducted in areas with a high prevalence of environmental mycobacteria.

Three major trials demonstrated poor protection or no protective effect of BCG vaccination. The first was conducted in Muscogee County, Georgia, beginning in 1947.[210, 211] Eligibility criteria included an age of 6 to 17 years and a skin test reaction of less than 5 mm to 100 TU of PPD. Approximately 2300 subjects were in the control group and 2500 in the BCG-vaccinated group, all of whom were observed for 20 years. Three cases of tuberculosis occurred in the control group and five in the vaccinated group, resulting in a negative protective efficacy and wide confidence intervals. The second study was carried out in Georgia and Alabama beginning in 1950.[212] Eligibility criteria included an age older than 5 years and a skin test reaction of less than 5 mm to 5 TU of PPD. The study groups included approximately 18,000 unvaccinated and 17,000 vaccinated individuals who were observed for up to 14 years. There were 32 cases of tuberculosis in the control group and 26 cases in the BCG group, resulting in a protective efficacy of 6% with wide confidence intervals. Both of the trials in Georgia and Alabama were conducted in areas with a high prevalence of environmental mycobacteria. Both trials had potential problems with methodology including a lack of random allocation of subjects, who were assigned by birth year, and passive follow-up surveillance for cases.

The eighth study was the largest BCG field trial ever conducted. The trial was cosponsored by the Indian Council of Medical Research, the WHO, and the U.S. Public Health Service. Intake began in 1968 in the Chingleput district of southern India and involved 260,000 participants from a population of 360,000.[192, 193] Children younger than 1 month were excluded, but all others were eligible regardless of age or skin test reaction. Participants were randomly divided into six groups, four to receive two different doses of two types of lyophilized vaccine and two groups to receive placebo. Ten years of follow-up were planned at 2.5-year intervals, using skin tests and chest radiographs. Sputum smears and cultures were to be collected if radiographs showed evidence of tuberculosis. Unfortunately, the follow-up varied among groups depending on size of the intake skin test reaction, age, and perception of risk. Chest radiographs were not obtained for persons younger than 10 years, and only those patients with symptoms or with previous radiographs that were suggestive of tuberculosis had repeated studies at follow-up in some of the surveys. Evaluation of interreader variation of radiographic interpretation found low agreement. Readers agreed in only 40 to 47% of radiographic categories ranging from most severe to probable or possible tuberculosis.[193] Bacteriological confirmation of cases diagnosed by radiography was obtained for only 22% of cases. Because of the wide range of disagreement in interpretation of chest radiographs and low yield of culture confirmation, radiographic diagnosis of tuberculosis was deemed unsatisfactory, and cases were defined only on the basis of sputum cultures that were positive for *M. tuberculosis*. Potential bias in the Chingleput study included both surveillance and diagnostic testing because of the method of follow-up. Cases among young children were probably missed because they did not routinely receive radiographs unless they were symptomatic, and symptoms are often subtle or absent in this age group. Also, case definition based on positive sputum culture is known to have poor yield in children, with only 40 to 50% testing positive under the best of circumstances. It is also noteworthy that the study was conducted in a geographical area in which environmental mycobacteria are endemic. The first results were published in 1979, after 7.5 years of follow-up. Neither of the two vaccines studied, in full or reduced dosage, showed any evidence of protection against pulmonary tuberculosis compared with that of placebo. Thus, the world's largest BCG field trial served only to create more uncertainties rather than to resolve issues about the efficacy of BCG.

Possible Factors Creating Variation in Field Trials of BCG

The protection demonstrated in the eight major controlled BCG field trials ranged from none to 80%. It is unclear why such a wide range of results has been found in these trials, and a number of theories attempting to explain these differences have been developed (Table 8–7). Some believe that this issue cannot be answered until we have a better understanding of the immune response to tuberculosis and BCG vaccine. It is unlikely that a single explanation can account for the variation among trials.

Table 8–7. THEORIES EXPLAINING DIFFERENT OUTCOMES IN CONTROLLED TRIALS OF BACILLE CALMETTE-GUÉRIN VACCINE

- Trial methodology
  - Subject assignment
  - Diagnostic surveillance
  - Case definition
  - Statistical precision
- Variations in vaccine
  - Strain
  - Administration
  - Potency
  - Dose
- Environmental mycobacteria
  - Protective effect
  - Vaccine interference
- Regional difference in strains of *Mycobacterium tuberculosis*
- Exogenous reinfection versus endogenous reactivation

Trial Methodology

Substantial variation in the quality of the methodology used in the BCG trials may have affected the outcomes. It is easy to understand the heterogeneity of methods used because the trials were conducted between 1935 and 1975 in nine different geographical areas in three different countries, and they were directed by a number of different investigators and organizations. Further difficulties in carrying out these trials included the large number of subjects and the long duration of follow-up that was required as well as the lack of resources in some of the regions in which the studies were conducted. Double-blind methods could not be used because BCG vaccination often leaves a cutaneous scar, making it difficult to conceal the vaccination status of subjects. Subject assignment, method of case definition, diagnostic surveillance, and statistical precision are all important aspects of study design that may affect outcome and introduce bias. The role of methodological and statistical variation among the eight major BCG trials has been critically evaluated. Some authors argue that methodological differences may have biased some of the trials and account for the variability in outcomes,[198] whereas others believe that none of the defects in methods could have appreciably affected the results.[202, 203] Unfortunately, none of the trials were conducted using all the standards of ideal experimental design.

Methodological problems leading to bias may arise if assignment of patients is not randomized. Vaccine assignment should be based on characteristics that are unrelated to tuberculosis susceptibility, such as the patient's registration number. Vaccine recipients and control subjects should have an equal distribution of known risk factors for tuberculosis, such as age, socioeconomic status, medical conditions, and exposure. These safeguards are essential in ensuring the choice of unbiased study groups.

Three of the major trials had methodological problems with subject assignment. The Chicago study lacked a systematic allocation scheme and used a haphazard method of BCG assignment in which infants were vaccinated alternately or in groups of 5 or 10. Personal familiarity with the patients was not considered in the distribution, so it is unlikely that the haphazard scheme created significant susceptibility bias. The Madanapalle trial had a high percentage of refusals (14%), and BCG assignment was made by the vaccinators. Although the potential for bias exists if refusals or vaccine assignments or both are systematically different from those used for the control group, it is difficult to ascertain the significance of these methodological flaws on the outcome of this trial. The Chingleput trial was the only trial to use double-blinded formally randomized vaccine allocation, but the distribution of susceptibility factors for tuberculosis was not considered. With systematic randomization, it is unlikely that there would be an unequal distribution of susceptibility factors, but this is a potential bias. The eight major BCG trials used different eligibility criteria, such as age, tuberculin sensitivity, and risk of exposure, making it even more difficult to compare the data.

Most of the trials revealed inconsistencies and problems with the methods of case surveillance and diagnosis. A difficult challenge in studying tuberculosis is the lack of a sensitive, objective, and reliable gold standard for case diagnosis. Clearly, any patient with culture-proven tuberculosis is a case. The problems with mycobacterial cultures include low sensitivity in some populations, especially in children, and their long incubation period. Because culture may not be a sensitive diagnostic test, a combination of epidemiological, historical, physical, radiographic, and laboratory findings must be considered for diagnosis. Clinical symptoms alone may be misleading in both adults and children because early cases may be asymptomatic. Results from some British trials showed that more than half the cases of tuberculosis were found during radiographic screening in asymptomatic patients.[124] Also, tuberculin skin test status was used as part of the diagnostic criteria for case finding in some of the trials. Because BCG vaccine can cause a positive result on a tuberculin skin test, cases may have been overestimated among the vaccinees, leading to an underestimation of the efficacy of the vaccine. If the examiners were not blinded to the patient's vaccination status, their beliefs about the vaccine might have influenced the interpretation of diagnostic tests. If follow-up evaluations were not scheduled routinely, the patient's motivation to seek medical care and the physician's diagnostic suspicion may have been influenced by knowledge of the patient's BCG status. Unequal surveillance of study groups may have led to underestimation or overestimation of disease. Both groups should have been observed equally to elicit symptoms and physical or radiographic findings that might have indicated tuberculosis. Diagnostic tests should have been ordered with use of the same criteria in both the vaccinated and control groups to ensure equal testing.

Five of the eight trials had methodological problems with surveillance and diagnostic testing. The Georgia, Puerto Rico, and Georgia-Alabama trials had no scheduled follow-up procedures, no blinded diagnostic review of radiographs, and no report of the frequencies and indications for chest radiographs. The Madanapalle and Chingleput trials also had flaws in diagnostic follow-up. Early in the Madanapalle trial, patients were observed actively and equally, and reviews were performed in a blinded fashion. With time, these safeguards were abandoned. In the Chingleput trial, the study population was actively observed, but the level of follow-up for children and tuberculin-negative patients is unclear. Cases were defined on the basis of sputum cultures that were positive for *M. tuberculosis* even though most children with tuberculosis do not produce sputum. Children younger than 10 years did not receive radiographs at intake, although all ages were included for vaccination, which may have led to inclusion of children who had disease at the time of enrollment. Adult patients may have been misclassified as well by the omission of radiographs, because follow-up radiographs were obtained only for patients with symptoms or a history of previously abnormal films. Radiographic blinding and reader verification were used in the Chingleput trial, but low agreement and poor correlation made these data useless in case definition.

In addition, statistical precision, which is based on the number of patients enrolled and the incidence of disease in the study population, is an important consideration in evaluating the accuracy of the results. The confidence interval estimates the precision of the results and is the range within which the true magnitude of effect lies 95% of the time. The statistical accuracy of the BCG trials has been compared in a number of publications and is illustrated in Figure 8–1.[198, 213] Three trials had narrow confidence intervals, indicating high statistical precision, including the North American Indian study, the British study, and the Chicago study. These trials also reported the highest protective efficacy and demonstrated the least biased methodology. The other five trials had wide confidence intervals, indicating poor precision, and lower reported protective efficacy. The poor precision of these trials failed to exclude the possibility of higher protective efficacy.

Variations in Vaccines

At least six different vaccines were used in the major BCG field trials. Fresh vaccine was used in all of the studies except the Chingleput trial, which used freeze-dried preparations. Some field trials have used different vaccines within the same trial and demonstrated equal efficacy. The Chingleput and some British studies used two different vaccines. British BCG and vole vaccine from Copenhagen Laboratory were used in a British trial and demonstrated a similar protective efficacy of 77% after 20 years of follow-up.[206] The Chingleput trial also used Copenhagen BCG as well as Madras BCG vaccine. Although the results of the Indian study were different from those of the British trial, the two vaccines had similar results within the Chingleput trial.[192, 193] In these examples, different vaccines have shown similar results when they are compared within the same trial and study populations.

Some vaccine strains have yielded inconsistent results among trials.[11] The Copenhagen BCG vaccine, used in the general population of southern India[208] and British schoolchildren,[206] demonstrated extremely variable efficacy between trials—0% in the Chingleput study compared with 77% in the British study. Three studies conducted in North America—the Chicago, Georgia, and Georgia-Alabama studies—used the Tice BCG vaccine yet found variable efficacy of 75%, 0%, and 14%, respectively.[205, 210, 212] Live BCG vaccine strains have changed over time, yet the trends in efficacy of BCG vaccination have not increased or decreased during almost 60 years of use.[201] On the basis of available information, definite conclusions cannot be drawn about the protective effect of the different BCG vaccines, although it is unlikely that a difference among vaccines is the only explanation for the variable results among trials.

Environmental Mycobacteria

The interaction between environmental mycobacteria and BCG vaccination has been considered a possible cause for variation in results among BCG trials.[200, 202, 214, 215] Exposure to environmental mycobacteria may lead to low-grade tuberculin sensitivity, which may be associated with immunity against tuberculosis. Sensitization to environmental mycobacteria has been shown to have specific geographical patterns of distribution, occurring primarily in the tropical and subtropical regions of the world. Europe and northern parts of North America have a low prevalence of environmental mycobacteria sensitivity. In southern areas of the United States and India, skin test surveys indicate a high level of sensitization to environmental mycobacteria. Three of the eight major BCG trials were conducted in geographical areas in which the prevalence of environmental mycobacteria is low, and these studies demonstrated the highest vaccine efficacy. Conversely, the five trials conducted in the southern United States and southern India, where the prevalence of environmental mycobacteria is high, demonstrated low vaccine efficacy. If sensitization to environmental mycobacteria induced any protective effect against tuberculosis, it could be more difficult to demonstrate a protective effect for a second agent, in this case BCG vaccine.

Evidence in animal and human studies indicates that sensitization to environmental mycobacteria provides protection against tuberculosis similar to that provided by BCG. A study of navy recruits in the United States found that those with low-grade tuberculin sensitivity had about half the incidence of tuberculosis of those with negative tuberculin skin test reactions, suggesting that sensitization to environmental mycobacteria provided some protective effect.[216] Animal studies have shown that infection with some environmental mycobacteria can induce as much protection against tuberculosis as BCG can.[217, 218] In addition, administration of BCG to guinea pigs previously infected with environmental mycobacteria did not boost their level of protection against tuberculosis. Obviously, sensitization to environmental mycobacteria does not provide a high level of protection against tuberculosis, because the disease continues to be prevalent in some areas with high environmental mycobacteria exposure, such as the Chingleput area of India. Some investigators have suggested that exposure to environmental mycobacteria might interfere with the response to BCG vaccination,[214, 215] but the results from clinical trials provide no support for this hypothesis.

Host Factors

Variation in clinical trials conducted in different populations has led to the hypothesis that genetic or nutritional factors might influence the immune response. Evidence from animal research suggests that genetic factors may determine the host's response to BCG vaccines.[54, 219–222] It is possible that vaccine efficacy may be lower in certain human populations owing to genetic, rather than environmental, factors. Some animal research has demonstrated that nutritional deficiencies can lower the immunological response to BCG vaccination.[223–225] However, studies in humans have found no evidence to support this concept.[212, 226, 227]

Regional Differences in *Mycobacterium tuberculosis* Strains

The theory that BCG vaccine did not protect against the regional strain of tuberculosis has been raised in respect to the Chingleput trial. The endemic strain of tuberculosis in that area is known as the south Indian variant, notable for its relatively low virulence in guinea pigs. However, studies in guinea pigs demonstrated that the Copenhagen BCG vaccine, used in the Chingleput trial, induced a high level of protection against the south Indian variant strain as well as other strains of *M. tuberculosis*.[228] Relatively new techniques that identify strains of tuberculosis by DNA fingerprinting may facilitate future studies of strain-related differences.

Exogenous Reinfection Versus Endogenous Reactivation

BCG vaccination does not prevent infection with *M. tuberculosis* but may prevent dissemination of disease. Also, in persons infected with *M. tuberculosis*, subsequent vaccination with BCG does not augment the level of immune response. Studies in guinea pigs demonstrated that previous infection with *M. tuberculosis* does not prevent reinfection with another strain in the lungs but does prevent dissemination of the second strain.[229] The majority of tuberculosis disease in adults in developed countries, such as the United States, is thought to arise from endogenous reactivation of organisms harbored within a previously infected host, as opposed to exogenous reinfection from contact with an infectious source case.[230] However, in areas in which the prevalence of tuberculosis is high, such as in many developing countries, exogenous reinfection may play a more significant role in disease transmission. Epidemiological studies of British and Eskimo populations have suggested that the declining incidence of tuberculous disease observed in all ages, including those who were previously infected, reflects a decrease in frequency of exogenous reinfection.[231]

Distinguishing between endogenous and exogenous infection is difficult without special laboratory techniques to distinguish the different strains of *M. tuberculosis*, and sensitive techniques, such as restriction fragment length polymorphism, have become available only in the past few years.[232, 233] It is difficult to estimate the effect of exogenous reinfection on previously reported clinical trials, although this issue could be addressed with currently available technology.

Other Evidence of Effectiveness: Case-Control, Contact, and Meta-Analysis Studies

The cost, extensive length of follow-up, and large numbers of subjects needed to conduct a large, randomized clinical trial, as well as the lack of consensus reached in previous studies, have led to the use of alternative methods for evaluating the efficacy of BCG vaccine.[234] In the 1980s, the WHO initiated a global study to evaluate programs in developing countries using a standardized case-contact protocol that evaluated children who were household contacts of cases with infectious disease. These children were evaluated by use of the WHO clinical scoring system and were observed during 3 months for development of tuberculosis disease. These methods as well as case-control studies have yielded results similar to those of the major controlled trials, with efficacy ranging from 0% to more than 80% (see Fig. 8–1).[171, 235]

Case-control and contact studies have the advantage of being fast and less expensive, but the potential for bias is increased. In retrospective studies, vaccine is not randomly allocated, so there is potential for confounding factors that may affect the outcome. Socioeconomic status is a potential confounding variable because persons with higher socioeconomic status are more likely to have access to and to use both preventive (vaccination) and curative healthcare and usually have a lower risk of exposure to tuberculosis. Studies that compare BCG scar rates in children who have tuberculosis with BCG scar rates within the community preclude analysis of many important potential confounding variables. Another disadvantage of retrospective studies is the decreased validity of historical information regarding vaccination status. Misclassification of vaccination status is less of a problem in BCG studies owing to the lasting scar formation that occurs in 90 to 95% of patients. Problems may arise if other marks are mistaken for BCG scars or if the vaccination does not leave a scar. Another consideration is the criteria for diagnosis of disease, especially in children. Safeguards to control for these potential problems must be strict in retrospective studies to avoid biased results. The quality of the case-control and cohort studies of BCG vaccine has varied from excellent to poor.

Findings from the case-control and cohort studies in children vary markedly, with a high level of protection of 70% or more found in many.[171, 172, 236–242] One study, looking at the efficacy of neonatal BCG vaccine during 20 years, found 82% protection in children younger than 15 years, 67% protection in the 15- to 24-year-old group, and 20% protection in persons 25 to 34 years of age, indicating better protection in younger age groups and waning immunity over time.[194] Most of the case-control and cohort studies have observed moderate protection of 30 to 66%.[227, 243–250] Few studies have shown efficacy less than 20%.[251–253] Studies that separately evaluated meningitis or miliary disease demonstrated that BCG offers good protection against these more serious forms of tuberculosis in young children.[171, 172, 254–257] These findings are consistent with the theory that BCG protects against hematogenous spread of disease but not against infection.

Understanding that there are limitations and potential biases in these retrospective studies, the best available information suggests that BCG provides some measure of protection to a substantial proportion of vaccinated infants and children living in places in which the risk of tuberculosis is high and that protection is highest against tuberculous meningitis and disseminated disease.

The technique of meta-analysis, in which results of similar studies with the same hypothesis are combined to increase the number of study subjects and improve interpretation of results, has been used to evaluate BCG vaccine.[255–257] Of course, one must question the validity of these analyses considering the grossly varied conditions of and variables within the trials. Investigators at the London School of Hygiene and Tropical Medicine found 10 randomized controlled trials and 8 case-control studies that met criteria for adequate methodology.[255] For meningeal and miliary disease, the protective effect was 86% in randomized controlled trials and 75% in case-control studies. For pulmonary tuberculosis, the degree of heterogeneity between studies precluded calculation of a summary estimate of protective efficacy. In other words, the findings were too divergent to simply average the results.

Investigators at the Harvard School of Public Health[257] found 15 prospective trials and 12 case-control studies that met their criteria for adequacy in study design and controls against potential bias. In the trials, the protective effect of BCG for tuberculosis disease was 51%. Among the case-control studies, protection by BCG was 50%. Analysis of eight studies involving only populations vaccinated as infants revealed a protective effect of 55% against tuberculosis among infant recipients of BCG. Seven trials reporting deaths from tuberculosis showed a BCG protective effect of 71%. The protective effect against tuberculous meningitis (five studies) was 64%, and protection against disseminated disease (three studies) was 72%.

The Harvard study used a random-effects regression model to examine variation in BCG efficacy among 13 prospective trials. Investigators found that the rate of tuberculosis in the unvaccinated group and the geographical latitude accounted for 85% of the between-study variance. Among the seven prospective trials that enrolled patients randomly, the estimated protective effect was 85% for BCG vaccination at birth, 73% for vaccination at age 10 years, and 50% for vaccination at 20 years of age. However, for the entire meta-analysis, mean age at vaccination accounted for less than 6% of the between-study variance ($P > .20$). Different strains of BCG were not consistently associated with more or less favorable results in the trials. Different BCG preparations and strains used in the same population gave similar levels of protection, whereas genetically identical BCG vaccines gave different levels of protection in different populations. The duration of protection from a single BCG vaccination and the role of booster doses could not be assessed owing to the inadequacy of the data.

The Harvard group also published a meta-analysis

evaluating the efficacy of BCG vaccination of newborns and infants.[256, 257] Five prospective trials and 11 case-control studies met the study criteria and were included in the analysis. The overall protective efficacy against all forms of tuberculosis for those vaccinated at birth or during infancy was 50% on average. Protection against death was 65%, meningitis 64%, and disseminated tuberculosis 78%.

In summary, there is no question that BCG vaccination has worked well in some situations but poorly in others. Because only a small fraction of the cases in the general population of contagious, smear-positive adult pulmonary tuberculosis is potentially preventable by BCG vaccination, it has had essentially no effect on the ultimate control of tuberculosis. The best use of BCG appears to be for the prevention of life-threatening forms of tuberculosis such as meningitis and disseminated disease in infants and young children. Vaccination with BCG remains the standard for tuberculosis prevention in most countries because it is available, is inexpensive, and requires only one encounter with the patient; in addition, it rarely causes serious complications, and systems for early diagnosis and effective treatment of tuberculosis are lacking in many areas of the world.

Duration of Immunity

The duration of immunity after BCG vaccination is not known. Estimates are based on data from clinical trials and case-control studies because there is no serological test to measure immunity to tuberculosis or the immune response after BCG vaccination. A case-control study by al-Kassimi and colleagues[194] compared BCG vaccine status in 537 cases of tuberculosis with 5756 normal control subjects. All subjects were vaccinated in the neonatal period, and protection was estimated by age group or years after vaccination. The study found decreasing protection with increasing age, demonstrating a waning immunity 20 years after vaccination. Experts speculate that protection declines over time and is probably nonexistent 10 to 20 years after vaccination.

Side Effects of Bacille Calmette-Guérin Vaccine

For more than 70 years, BCG vaccines have been administered safely to billions of individuals throughout the world. Complications are rare, but their rate varies depending on the skill and method of administration; the type, strength, and dose of the vaccine; and the age and immune status of the vaccinee.[258, 259]

Common Adverse Events

Localized adverse effects are common after BCG vaccination, but serious long-term complications are rare (Table 8–8). Ninety percent to 95% of patients vaccinated with BCG develop a local reaction followed by healing and scar formation within 3 months. Individuals with dormant tuberculosis infection often have an accelerated response to BCG vaccine characterized by induration within 1 to 2 days and scab formation and healing within 10 to 15 days. A study in healthy tuberculin-negative adults vaccinated with BCG found that all patients developed a local reaction with erythema, induration, and tenderness at the vaccination site; 75% developed muscle soreness; and 70% had local ulceration with drainage.[260] Only 2% developed tender regional adenopathy.

Table 8–8. **AGE-SPECIFIC ESTIMATED RISKS FOR COMPLICATIONS AFTER ADMINISTRATION OF BACILLE CALMETTE-GUÉRIN VACCINE**

COMPLICATION	INCIDENCE PER 1 MILLION VACCINATIONS	
	Age <1 yr	Age 1–20 yr
Local subcutaneous abscess, regional lymphadenopathy	387	25
Musculoskeletal lesions	0.39–0.89	0.06
Multiple lymphadenitis, nonfatal disseminated lesions	0.31–0.39	0.36
Fatal disseminated lesions	0.19–1.56	0.06–0.72

From Lotte A, Wasz-Hockert O, Poisson N, et al. Second IUATLD study on complications induced by intradermal BCG-vaccination. Bull Int Union Tuberc 63:47–59, 1988.

Local ulceration and regional lymphadenitis are the most common complications, following cutaneous reactions, occurring in less than 1% of immunocompetent recipients who receive intradermal administration.[261] Local cutaneous lesions and lymphadenitis usually occur within a few weeks to months after vaccination, but symptoms may be delayed for months in immunocompetent persons and for years in immunocompromised hosts.[262] Axillary, cervical, and supraclavicular nodes are usually involved on the ipsilateral side of vaccination. Certain BCG strains, especially the Tokyo strain and the Moreau strain in Brazil, are rarely associated with lymphadenitis, whereas the French (Pasteur) strain gives rise to a higher incidence.[258, 263, 264] Outbreaks of lymphadenitis after vaccination with BCG in certain countries or regions have frequently followed the introduction of a new BCG strain into the vaccination program.[265, 266] It is likely that an altered technique of administration has contributed to some of these outbreaks. A study in 291 Haitian infants reported an outbreak of complications after administration of 2.0 to 2.5 times the recommended dose of BCG vaccine.[267] The complications were mild to moderate with only a small increased risk of complications among HIV-infected children. There is no evidence that children who experience local complications are more likely to have immune deficits or to have enhanced or diminished protection against tuberculosis.[266] The risk of suppurative lymphadenitis is greater among newborns than among older infants and children, especially when a full dose of vaccine is given; therefore, the WHO recommends using a reduced dose in children younger than 30 days.

The treatment of local adenitis as a complication of

BCG vaccination is controversial and ranges from observation to surgical drainage to the administration of antituberculosis drugs to a combination of surgical management and medications.[268] Nonsuppurative lymph nodes usually improve spontaneously, although resolution may take several months.[269] The WHO recommends drainage and direct instillation of an antituberculosis drug into the lesion for adherent or fistulated lymph nodes.[270] Several studies have shown that some children with lymphadenitis respond to a course of isoniazid or erythromycin of several weeks' or months' duration.[271–273] However, a comparative study of 120 patients treated for 6 months showed that regimens of isoniazid, isoniazid plus rifampin, and erythromycin did not produce different results; that medical therapy was little better than observation; and that the rate of spontaneous drainage of the lymph nodes was higher among isoniazid-treated children than among the control subjects.[268]

Rare Adverse Events

Other complications of vaccination with BCG are much less frequent. The mean risk of osteitis after BCG vaccination has varied from 0.01 per million in Japan to 300 per million in Finland.[258, 274–277] As with lymphadenitis, osteitis rates have, on occasion, increased dramatically after introduction of a new vaccine strain into a region or country. Generalized BCG infection is extremely rare in immunocompetent patients.[278–282] A few autopsy studies of children who died of unrelated causes have demonstrated granulomas in various organs of vaccinated infants with apparently intact immune systems, suggesting that generalized nonfatal dissemination may occur in normal hosts.[280, 283, 284] Fatal disseminated BCG disease has been reported at a rate of 0.19 to 1.56 cases per 1 million vaccinated,[261] most occurring in patients with severe defects in cell-mediated immunity, such as chronic granulomatous disease, severe combined immunodeficiency, malnutrition, cancer, complete DiGeorge syndrome, γ-interferon receptor deficiency, or HIV infection.[285–290b] Disseminated BCG disease should be treated with antituberculosis medications, but pyrazinamide should not be included because all strains of BCG are resistant to this drug.[291]

Some experts have raised questions about a possible increased risk of certain types of cancer, especially lymphomas, among BCG-vaccinated individuals compared with unvaccinated persons.[202, 203] More studies may be indicated to evaluate this observation.

The safety of BCG vaccine in children and adults who are infected with HIV is unknown. Disseminated BCG infection has been described in an HIV-infected adult 30 years after he received BCG.[292] There have been other reports of disseminated BCG disease in infants and adults with HIV infection.[262, 286, 288, 293–295] Data derived soon after BCG vaccination from Zaire,[13, 296] Uganda,[297] Rwanda,[298] and the Congo[299] did not indicate an increased risk of serious adverse effects of BCG vaccination in infants of mothers infected with HIV. Long-term follow-up evaluations of these and other high-risk infants are not yet available. However, one French study showed that 9 of 68 HIV-infected children given BCG vaccine developed complications: 7 had large satellite adenopathy with or without skin fistulas, and 2 developed disseminated lesions.[300] The efficacy of BCG vaccine in HIV-infected infants is completely unknown. Currently, the WHO recommends giving BCG vaccine to asymptomatic HIV-infected infants who live in high-risk areas for tuberculosis. BCG is not recommended for symptomatic HIV-infected infants or for persons known to be or suspected of being HIV-infected if they are at minimal risk for infection with *M. tuberculosis*.[301] In reality, the lack of available HIV serodiagnosis in many regions of the world means that in some areas large numbers of HIV-infected infants and children are receiving BCG. Long-term studies of these children will be exceedingly important.

Recommendations for Use of Bacille Calmette-Guérin in the United States

In the United States, the general population is at low risk for infection with *M. tuberculosis*. Therefore, routine BCG vaccination of the United States population has not been recommended.[302] The most successful control measures include case detection, chemotherapy, and preventive chemotherapy. Vaccination may contribute to tuberculosis control in selected population groups. Vaccination with BCG should be considered for infants and children with negative tuberculin skin test reactions who (1) are continually exposed to a persistently untreated or ineffectively treated patient with infectious pulmonary tuberculosis, and the child cannot be removed from the source of exposure or prescribed long-term preventive therapy, or (2) are continually exposed to persons with tuberculosis who have bacilli resistant to isoniazid and rifampin, and the child cannot be separated from the infectious source case.

The emergence of multidrug-resistant strains of *M. tuberculosis* and subsequent nosocomial outbreaks in hospitals in some areas of the United States have led to consideration of the use of BCG vaccine for the prevention and control of tuberculosis among healthcare workers. Healthcare facilities at high risk are limited to a few geographical areas of the United States with high rates of multidrug-resistant tuberculosis in the population. In general, healthcare workers should be protected by infection control techniques, screening, and preventive treatment for infection. Even in high-risk settings, BCG should not be the major method of control or protection because it has unknown efficacy; does not protect unvaccinated patients or visitors; and confuses skin test, surveillance, and preventive treatment measures. Vaccination with BCG should be considered for healthcare workers only in areas that have a high risk of transmission of multidrug-resistant tuberculosis in which aggressive infection control measures have been implemented and have failed.[302] Even in these circumstances, the uncertain efficacy of BCG may make other control measures such as preventive chemotherapy preferable to vaccination alone.

The most frequent indication for use of BCG in the

United States today, which is unrelated to tuberculosis, is the treatment of bladder cancer by intravesicular administration.

Contraindications to Vaccination with Bacille Calmette-Guérin

BCG vaccine should not be given to persons (1) whose immunological responses are impaired because of HIV infection, congenital immunodeficiency, leukemia, lymphoma, or generalized malignant disease; (2) whose immunological responses have been suppressed by corticosteroids, alkylating agents, antimetabolites, or radiation; or (3) who are pregnant.[302] Persons in groups at high risk for HIV infection should be administered BCG with caution.

Simultaneous Administration with Other Vaccines

BCG vaccine can be administered safely with other childhood vaccines. It is impossible to measure whether simultaneous administration reduces the efficacy of BCG, because there is no serological test for the immune response. BCG vaccination does not appear to adversely affect the immune response to other childhood vaccinations given simultaneously, even in HIV-infected newborns.[13]

Future Vaccines for Tuberculosis

Tuberculosis will be eliminated only if new, more effective vaccines are developed.[303] Modern molecular genetics and biotechnology techniques should be applied rapidly to this problem. Because almost 2 billion people in the world are already infected with *M. tuberculosis*, vaccine research should address both preventing infection and halting progression of established infection to tuberculosis disease.

The varying effect of BCG vaccines may be, in part, due to our imperfect understanding of the determinants of protective immunity against tuberculosis. The significant antigens of *M. tuberculosis* are poorly defined and difficult to produce owing to the complex structure and chemistry of the mycobacterial cell wall. Our basic science knowledge of antigens, immune responses, and mediators must be expanded.

Because genetic factors may influence the response to BCG, environmental mycobacteria, and infection with *M. tuberculosis*, molecular genetic studies in animals and humans should be broadened. Animal studies have revealed that genetically determined susceptibility to mycobacteria infection in mice is regulated by a gene called *Bcg*, *Ity*, or *Lsh*. *Bcg* gene, which has been identified and characterized, codes for a membrane transport protein called Nramp.[304] The actual function of Nramp is not yet understood, but it appears to influence susceptibility to tuberculosis disease.

Innovative new approaches in tuberculosis vaccine development have emerged in recent years. These include (1) plasmid DNA vector-based vaccines, which deliver genes encoding antigens by use of vectors; (2) recombinant and mutant BCG vaccines, which use BCG as the delivery vehicle with improvements; (3) subunit vaccines, which use individual mycobacterial protein antigens to produce an immune response; and (4) attenuated *M. tuberculosis* vaccines, which lack the genes essential for virulence and contain the genes needed for protection.[305] All of these new strategies appear promising, and perhaps one of these techniques or a combination thereof will yield an effective new vaccine against tuberculosis.

Major field trials for BCG or any new tuberculosis vaccine would be a tremendous challenge given the necessary scope, duration, and expense of adequate trials. There is a pressing need for identification of some correlate of natural and vaccine-derived protective immunity, based on either an animal model or a measure of immune response in humans. Current animal models are inadequate, and human markers of protective immunity have not been determined. Tuberculin sensitivity after vaccination is not an adequate "assay." Continued research on operational variables such as the age of optimal vaccination and the role of booster vaccinations is needed. Finally, data on the safety and efficacy of BCG vaccines in HIV-infected children and adults should be sought vigorously.

PUBLIC HEALTH CONSIDERATIONS

For most infectious diseases, the expectation is that the availability of a potent vaccine can lead to the elimination of the disease from human populations if an effective, global program can be developed and implemented. Clearly, the BCG vaccines have not led to the elimination of tuberculosis from any country in the world. The distribution of these vaccines to 4 billion people has had almost no effect on the worldwide epidemiology of tuberculosis.[3] However, it is likely that millions of cases of meningeal and disseminated tuberculosis in children have been prevented by its widespread use.

Some of the confusion about the current role of BCG vaccines in the control of tuberculosis has occurred because the original intent for its use has been forgotten. In most developing countries, BCG was introduced as an emergency measure because it was the only inexpensive tuberculosis control measure that could be applied on a national scale.[156] With the advent of effective and inexpensive chemotherapy, a two-pronged approach to tuberculosis control became possible, consisting of (1) case finding and treatment and (2) BCG vaccination.[4, 6, 156] Prior receipt of BCG vaccination and chemotherapy of persons with reactive tuberculin skin test responses who have been close contacts of known cases are not mutually exclusive; this dual approach would prevent many cases of life-threatening disease in children and future cases of infectious reactivation disease. However, in developing countries, the impact of the current level of case finding and treatment programs on tuberculosis in young children may be small. Most transmission to children occurs before the adult source case is identified, and the short incubation period for meningeal and disseminated tuberculosis means that the time for intervention with the child has already passed.[306–308] The lack of sensitive diagnostic techniques for confirming tuberculosis in children often precludes early effective treatment of their disease. Under such conditions, only effective vaccination of the child can be expected to reduce the development of disease in children in a significant manner. Because the source of tuberculosis transmission to children in developing countries is usually within their household, a delay in vaccination after birth, although perhaps leading to a more vigorous and long-lasting immune response, may fail to prevent cases of childhood tuberculosis if a family member who has the disease is present.[156]

Vaccination of children with BCG probably will not prevent the majority of infectious pulmonary tuberculosis cases among adults in a population because the protection afforded by BCG appears to be of limited duration.[3] However, almost nothing is known about the efficacy for a short period of time of various BCG vaccines given to adults who have not been infected previously with *M. tuberculosis*. In developed countries, protecting high-risk adults, such as those who work with patients who have multidrug-resistant tuberculosis, is becoming a critical need when chemotherapy cannot be relied on. It is also completely unknown whether "booster" immunizations with BCG can maintain or even enhance protection against tuberculosis. It is remarkable that these basic questions about the effectiveness of BCG vaccine have never been answered or even addressed, despite the administration of more than 4 billion doses of vaccine.

The WHO has recommended that a single dose of BCG vaccine be given to newborns in developing countries with a high prevalence rate of infectious tuberculosis. This dosage schedule will have an economic impact and a short-term impact on mortality, although it will not contribute significantly to the control of tuberculosis. The United Kingdom adopted the strategy of a single dose of BCG in adolescence because the majority of cases were occurring in adolescents and young adults, and few occurred among infants and children. However, the optimal vaccine strain of BCG, the dosing schedule, the route of administration, and the age of the recipient have not been established firmly.

Many technologically advanced countries that have experienced great declines in the rate of tuberculosis either already have discontinued or are considering discontinuing BCG vaccination.[166, 167, 309] In the United Kingdom and Sweden, cessation of a generalized BCG vaccination program has led to a slight increase in childhood and adolescent cases of tuberculosis. However, in both areas, the majority of subsequent childhood cases have been from high-risk immigrant communities whose members lived previously in regions with high rates of tuberculosis. Fairly circumscribed groups such as these could be selectively targeted for BCG immunization or be subjected to increased surveillance and case-finding efforts.

Within the United States, there is no rational reason for the widespread use of BCG. However, it may be reasonable to consider its use in limited, well-controlled groups with high rates of tuberculosis when other control measures cannot be used or have failed. One possible group is healthcare workers and potential contacts of adults with infectious, multidrug-resistant tuberculosis.

The worldwide epidemic of HIV infection has had a profound effect on the epidemiology of tuberculosis and may have an impact on the optimal use of BCG. The safety and efficacy of BCG in HIV-infected children are really unknown at present. Epidemiology and autopsy studies will be particularly useful in establishing the role of mass BCG vaccination in developing countries at a time when the number of persons with acquired immunodeficiency syndrome is increasing.[14]

REFERENCES

1. Starke JR. Bacille Calmette-Guérin vaccine. Semin Pediatr Infect Dis 2:153–158, 1991.
2. Lugosi L. Theoretical and methodological aspects of BCG vaccine from the discovery of Calmette and Guérin to molecular biology. A review. Tuber Lung Dis 73:252–261, 1992.
3. Styblo K. Overview and epidemiologic assessment of the current global tuberculosis situation with an emphasis on control in developing countries. Rev Infect Dis 11(suppl 2):S339–S346, 1989.
4. Sudre P, ten Dam G, Kochi A. Tuberculosis: A global overview of the situation today. Bull World Health Organ 70:149–159, 1992.
5. Raviglione MC, Snider DE Jr, Kochi A. Global epidemiology of tuberculosis. Morbidity and mortality of a worldwide epidemic. JAMA 273:220–226, 1995.
6. Kochi A. The global tuberculosis situation and the new control strategy of the World Health Organization. Tubercle 72:1–6, 1991.
7. Comstock GW. The International Tuberculosis Campaign: A pioneering venture in mass vaccination and research. Clin Infect Dis 19:528–540, 1994.
8. Fine PEM. Bacille Calmette-Guérin vaccines: A rough guide. Clin Infect Dis 20:11–14, 1995.
9. Smith DW. Protective effect of BCG in experimental tuberculosis. Adv Tuberc Res 22:1–97, 1985.
10. Stevens JP, Daniel TM. Bacille Calmette-Guérin immunization of health care workers exposed to multidrug-resistant tuberculosis: A decision analysis. Tuber Lung Dis 77:315–321, 1996.
11. Brewer TF, Colditz GA. Bacille Calmette-Guérin vaccination for the prevention of tuberculosis in healthcare workers. Clin Infect Dis 20:136–142, 1995.
12. Selwyn PA, Hartel D, Lewis VA, et al. A prospective study of the risk of tuberculosis among intravenous drug users with human immunodeficiency virus infection. N Engl J Med 320:545–550, 1989.
13. Ryder RW, Oxtoby MJ, Mvula M, et al. Safety and immunogenicity of bacille Calmette-Guérin, diptheria-tetanus-pertussis, and oral polio vaccines in newborn children in Zaire infected with human immunodeficiency virus type 1. J Pediatr 122:697–702, 1993.
14. Braun MM, Cauthen G. Relationship of the human immunodeficiency virus epidemic to pediatric tuberculosis and bacillus Calmette-Guérin immunization. Pediatr Infect Dis J 11:220–227, 1992.
15. Bloch AB, Cauthen GM, Onorato IM, et al. Nationwide survey of drug-resistant tuberculosis in the United States. JAMA 271:665–671, 1994.
16. Dooley SW, Villarino ME, Lawrence M, et al. Nosocomial transmission of tuberculosis in a hospital unit for HIV-infected patients. JAMA 267:2632–2635, 1992.
17. Pearson ML, Jereb JA, Frieden TR, et al. Nosocomial transmission of multidrug-resistant *Mycobacterium tuberculosis*. A risk to

patients and healthcare workers. Ann Intern Med 117:191–196, 1992.
18. Taylor R. Saranac: America's Magic Mountain. Boston, Houghton-Mifflin, 1986.
19. Bloom BR, Murray CJL. Tuberculosis: Commentary on a reemergent killer. Science 257:1055–1064, 1992.
20. Morse D, Brothwell DR, Ucko PJ. Tuberculosis in ancient Egypt. Am Rev Respir Dis 90:524–541, 1964.
21. Starke JR, Smith MHD. Tuberculosis. In Feigin RD, Cherry JD (eds). Textbook of Pediatric Infectious Diseases (4th ed). Philadelphia, WB Saunders, 1998, pp 1196–1239.
22. Nemir RL. Perspectives in adolescent tuberculosis: Three decades of experience. Pediatrics 78:399–404, 1986.
23. Starke JR, Correa AG. Management of mycobacterial infection and disease in children. Pediatr Infect Dis J 14:455–470, 1995.
24. Smith MHD. Tuberculosis in children and adolescents. Clin Chest Med 10:381–395, 1989.
25. Vallejo JG, Ong LT, Starke JR. Clinical features, diagnosis and treatment of tuberculosis in infants. Pediatrics 94:1–7, 1994.
26. Perry S, Starke JR. Adherence to prescribed treatment and public health aspects of tuberculosis in children. Semin Pediatr Infect Dis 4:291–298, 1993.
27. Lincoln EM, Harris LC, Bovornkitti S, et al. The course and prognosis of endobronchial tuberculosis in childhood. Am Rev Tuberc 74:246–256, 1956.
28. Lorriman G, Bentley FJ. The incidence of segmental lesions in primary tuberculosis in childhood. Am Rev Tuberc 79:756–763, 1959.
29. Morrison JB. Natural history of segmental lesions in primary pulmonary tuberculosis. Arch Dis Child 48:90–98, 1973.
30. Rossman MD, Mayock RL. Pulmonary tuberculosis. In Schlossberg D (ed). Tuberculosis. Clinical Topics in Infectious Disease. New York, Springer-Verlag, 1988, pp 61–70.
31. Khan MA, Kovnat DM, Bachus B, et al. Clinical and roentgenographic spectrum of pulmonary tuberculosis in the adult. Am J Med 62:31–38, 1977.
32. Alvarez S, Shell C, Berk SL. Pulmonary tuberculosis in elderly men. Am J Med 82:602–606, 1987.
33. Gordin FM, Slutkin G, Schecter G, et al. Presumptive diagnosis and treatment of pulmonary tuberculosis based on radiographic findings. Am Rev Respir Dis 139:1090–1093, 1989.
34. Palmer PES. Pulmonary tuberculosis: Usual and unusual radiographic presentations. Semin Roentgenol 14:204–242, 1979.
35. Chang SC, Lee PY, Perng RP. Lower lung field tuberculosis. Chest 91:230–232, 1987.
36. Barnes PF, Bloch AB, Davidson PT, et al. Tuberculosis in patients with human immunodeficiency virus infection. N Engl J Med 324:1644–1650, 1991.
37. Jones BE, Young SMM, Antoniskis D, et al. Relationship of the manifestations of tuberculosis to CD4 cell counts in patients with human immunodeficiency virus infection. Am Rev Respir Dis 148:1292–1297, 1993.
38. Markowitz N, Hansen N, Hopewell PC, et al. Incidence of tuberculosis in the United States among HIV-infected patients. Ann Intern Med 126:123–132, 1997.
39. Hopewell PC. Tuberculosis in persons with human immunodeficiency virus infection: Clinical and public health aspects. Semin Respir Crit Care Med 18:471–484, 1997.
40. Pitchenik AE, Rubinson HA. The radiographic appearance of tuberculosis in patients with the acquired immune deficiency syndrome (AIDS) and pre-AIDS. Am Rev Respir Dis 131:393–396, 1985.
41. Long R, Maycher B, Scalcini M, Manfreda J. The chest roentgenogram in pulmonary tuberculosis patients seropositive for human immunodeficiency virus type 1. Chest 99:123–127, 1991.
42. Wasser LS, Shaw GW, Talvera W. Endobronchial tuberculosis in the acquired immunodeficiency syndrome. Chest 94:1240–1244, 1988.
43. Shafter RW, Kim DS, Weiss JP, et al. Extrapulmonary tuberculosis in patients with human immunodeficiency virus infection. Medicine (Baltimore) 70:384–397, 1991.
44. Rieder HL, Snider DE Jr, Cauthen GM. Extrapulmonary tuberculosis in the United States. Am Rev Respir Dis 141:347–351, 1990.
45. Schuitt KE, Powell DA. Mycobacterial lymphadenitis in childhood. Am J Dis Child 132:675–677, 1978.
46. Hussey G, Chisolm T, Kibel M. Miliary tuberculosis in children: A review of 94 cases. Pediatr Infect Dis J 10:832–836, 1991.
47. Doerr CA, Starke Jr, Ong LT. Clinical and public health aspects of tuberculous meningitis in children. J Pediatr 127:27–33, 1995.
48. Molavi A, Le Frock JL. Tuberculous meningitis. Med Clin North Am 69:315–331, 1985.
49. Floyd MM, Silcox VA, Jones WD Jr, et al. Separation of *Mycobacterium bovis* BCG from *Mycobacterium tuberculosis* and *Mycobacterium bovis* by using high-performance liquid chromatography of mycolic acids. J Clin Microbiol 30:1327–1330, 1992.
50. Sauret J, Jolis R, Ausina V, et al. Human tuberculosis due to *Mycobacterium bovis*: Report of 10 cases. Tuber Lung Dis 73:388–391, 1992.
51. Feldman WH, Davis R, Moses HE, et al. An unusual mycobacterium isolated from sputum of a man suffering from pulmonary disease of long duration. Am Rev Tuberc 48:82–93, 1943.
52. Wayne L. The atypical mycobacteria: Recognition and disease association. Crit Rev Microbiol 12:184–222, 1986.
53. Riley RL. The J. Burns Amberson lecture: Aerial dissemination of pulmonary tuberculosis. Am Rev Tuberc 76:931–941, 1957.
54. Lurie MB. Resistance to Tuberculosis: Experimental Studies in Native and Acquired Defensive Mechanisms. Cambridge, Harvard University Press, 1964.
55. Dannenberg AM Jr. Immune mechanisms in the pathogenesis of pulmonary tuberculosis. Rev Infect Dis 11(suppl 2):S369–S378, 1989.
56. Stead WW. Pathogenesis of a first episode of chronic pulmonary tuberculosis in man: Recrudescence of residual of the primary infection or exogenous reinfection? Am Rev Respir Dis 95:729–745, 1967.
57. Raleigh JW, Weichelhausen R. Exogenous reinfection with *Mycobacterium tuberculosis* confirmed by phage typing. Am Rev Respir Dis 108:639–642, 1973.
58. Nardell E, McInnis B, Thomas B, et al. Exogenous reinfection with tuberculosis in a shelter for the homeless. N Engl J Med 315:1570–1575, 1986.
59. Dannenberg AM Jr. Delayed-type hypersensitivity and cell-mediated immunity in the pathogenesis of tuberculosis. Immunol Today 12:228–236, 1991.
60. Orme IM. Characteristics and specificity of acquired immunologic memory to *Mycobacterium tuberculosis*. J Immunol 140:3589–3593, 1988.
61. Grange JM. Vaccination against tuberculosis: Past problems and future hopes. Semin Respir Crit Care Med 18:459–470, 1997.
62. Orme IM, Flynn JL, Bloom BR. The role of $CD8^+$ T cells in immunity to tuberculosis. Trends Microbiol 1:77–78, 1995.
63. Molloy A, Laochumroonvorapong P, Kaplan G. Apoptosis, but not necrosis, of infected monocytes is coupled with killing of intracellular bacillus Calmette-Guérin. J Exp Med 180:1499–1509, 1995.
64. Orme IM, Anderson P, Boom WH. T cell response to *Mycobacterium tuberculosis*. J Infect Dis 167:1481–1497, 1993.
65. Mosmann TR. Regulation of immune response by T cells with different cytokine secretor phenotypes: Role of a new cytokine, cytokine synthesis inhibitory factor (IL-10). Int Arch Allergy Appl Immunol 94:110–115, 1991.
66. Bretscher PA. A strategy to improve the efficacy of vaccination against tuberculosis and leprosy. Immunol Today 13:342–345, 1992.
67. Surcel HM, Troyer-Blomberg M, Paulie S, et al. Th1/Th2 profiles in tuberculosis based on proliferation and cytokine response of blood lymphocytes to mycobacterial antigens. Immunology 81:171–176, 1994.
68. Schauf V, Rom WN, Smith KA, et al. Cytokine gene activation and modified responsiveness to interleukin-2 in the blood of tuberculosis patients. J Infect Dis 168:1056–1059, 1993.
69. Rook GAW, Hernandez-Pando R. The pathogenesis of tuberculosis. Am Rev Microbiol 50:259–284, 1996.
70. Hernandez-Pando R, Rook GAW. The role of TNF in T cell–mediated inflammation depends on the Th1/Th2 cytokine balance. Immunology 82:591–595, 1994.
71. Springett VH, Sutherland I. A re-examination of the variations in the efficacy of BCG vaccination against tuberculosis in clinical trials. Tuber Lung Dis 75:227–233, 1994.
72. Hsu KHK. Tuberculin reaction in children treated with isoniazid. Am J Dis Child 137:1090–1092, 1983.

73. Hardy JB. Persistence of hypersensitivity to old tuberculin following primary tuberculosis in childhood: A long-term study. Am J Public Health 36:1417–1426, 1946.
74. Howard TP, Soloman DA. Reading the tuberculin skin test: Who, when and how? Arch Intern Med 148:2457–2459, 1988.
75. Steiner P, Rao M, Victoria MS, et al. Persistently negative tuberculin reactions: Their presence among children culture-positive for *Mycobacterium tuberculosis*. Am J Dis Child 134:747–750, 1980.
76. Kent DC, Schwartz R. Active pulmonary tuberculosis with negative tuberculin skin reactions. Am Rev Respir Dis 95:411–418, 1967.
77. American Thoracic Society. Diagnostic standards and classification of tuberculosis. Am Rev Respir Dis 142:725–735, 1990.
78. Huebner RE, Schein MF, Bass JB Jr. The tuberculin skin test. Clin Infect Dis 17:968–975, 1993.
79. O'Brien RJ, Geiter LJ, Snider DE Jr, et al. The epidemiology of nontuberculous mycobacterial diseases in the United States. Am Rev Respir Dis 135:1007–1014, 1987.
80. Edwards LB, Acquaviva FA, Livesay VT, et al. An atlas of sensitivity to tuberculin, PPD-B and histoplasmin in the United States. Am Rev Respir Dis 99:1–99, 1969.
81. American Academy of Pediatrics. Tuberculosis. In Peter G (ed). 1997 Red Book: Report of the Committee on Infectious Diseases (24th ed). Elk Grove Village, IL, American Academy of Pediatrics, 1997, p 541.
82. Nemir RL, Teichner A. Management of tuberculin reactions in children and adolescents previously vaccinated with BCG. Pediatr Infect Dis J 2:446–451, 1983.
83. Menzies R, Vissandjee B. Effect of bacille Calmette-Guérin vaccination on tuberculin reactivity. Am Rev Respir Dis 145:621–625, 1992.
84. Lifschitz M. The value of the tuberculin skin test as a screening test for tuberculosis among BCG-vaccinated children. Pediatrics 36:624–627, 1965.
85. Horwitz O, Bunch-Christensen K. Correlation between tuberculin sensitivity after 2 months and 5 years among BCG-vaccinated subjects. Bull World Health Organ 47:49–58, 1972.
86. Comstock GW, Edwards LB, Nabangxang H. Tuberculin sensitivity eight to fifteen years after BCG vaccination. Am Rev Respir Dis 103:572–575, 1971.
87. Margus JH, Khassis Y. The tuberculin sensitivity in BCG vaccinated infants and children in Israel. Acta Tuberc Pneumonol Scand 46:113–122, 1965.
88. Landi S, Ashley MJ, Grzybowski S. Tuberculin sensitivity following the intradermal and multiple puncture methods of BCG vaccination. Can Med Assoc J 97:222–225, 1967.
89. Ashley MJ, Siebenmann CO. Tuberculin skin sensitivity following BCG vaccination with vaccines of high and low viable counts. Can Med Assoc J 97:1335–1338, 1967.
90. Kemp EB, Belshe RB, Hoft DF. Immune responses stimulated by percutaneous and intradermal bacille Calmette-Guérin. J Infect Dis 174:113–119, 1996.
91. Joncas JH, Robitaille R, Gauthier T. Interpretation of the PPD skin test in BCG-vaccinated children. Can Med Assoc J 113:127–128, 1975.
92. Magnus K, Edwards LB. The effect of repeated tuberculin testing on post-vaccination allergy. Lancet 1:643–644, 1955.
93. Ildirim I, Hacimustafaoglu M, Ediz B. Correlation of tuberculin induration with the number of bacillus Calmette-Guérin vaccines. Pediatr Infect Dis J 14:1060–1063, 1995.
94. Young TK, Mirdad S. Determinants of tuberculin sensitivity in a child population covered by mass BCG vaccination. Tuber Lung Dis 73:94–100, 1992.
95. Sepulveda RL, Heiba IM, Naverrete C, et al. Tuberculin reactivity after newborn BCG immunization in mono- and dizygotic twins. Tuber Lung Dis 75:138–143, 1994.
96. Sepulveda RL, Heiba IM, King A, et al. Evaluation of tuberculin reactivity in BCG-immunized siblings. Am J Respir Crit Care Med 149:620–624, 1994.
97. Karalliede S, Katugha LP, Uragoda CG. The tuberculin response of Sri Lankan children after BCG vaccination at birth. Tubercle 68:33–38, 1987.
98. Thompson NJ, Glassroth JL, Snider DE, et al. The booster phenomenon in serial tuberculin testing. Am Rev Respir Dis 119:587–597, 1979.
99. Bass JB Jr, Serio RA. The use of repeat skin tests to eliminate the booster phenomenon in serial tuberculin testing. Am Rev Respir Dis 123:394–396, 1982.
100. Sepulveda RL, Burr C, Ferrer X, et al. Booster effect of tuberculin testing in healthy 6-year-old school children vaccinated with bacillus Calmette-Guérin at birth in Santiago, Chile. Pediatr Infect Dis J 7:578–581, 1988.
101. Sepulveda RL, Ferrer X, Latrach C, et al. The influence of Calmette-Guérin bacillus immunization on the booster effect of tuberculin testing in healthy young adults. Am Rev Respir Dis 142:24–28, 1990.
102. Horowitz HW, Luciano BB, Kadel JR, et al. Tuberculin skin test conversion in hospital employees vaccinated with bacille Calmette-Guérin: Recent *Mycobacterium tuberculosis* infection or booster effect? Am J Infect Control 23:181–187, 1995.
103. Starke JR, Taylor-Watts K. Tuberculosis in the pediatric population of Houston, Texas. Pediatrics 84:28–35, 1989.
104. Abadco DL, Steiner P. Gastric lavage is better than bronchoalveolar lavage for isolation of *Mycobacterium tuberculosis* in childhood pulmonary tuberculosis. Pediatr Infect Dis J 11:735–738, 1992.
105. Strumpf IJ, Tsang AY, Sayne JW. Reevaluation of sputum staining for the diagnosis of pulmonary tuberculosis. Am Rev Respir Dis 119:599–602, 1979.
106. Lipsky BA, Gates J, Tenover FC, et al. Factors affecting the clinical value of microscopy for acid-fast bacilli. Rev Infect Dis 6:214–222, 1984.
107. Gordin F, Slutkin G. The validity of acid-fast smears in the diagnosis of pulmonary tuberculosis. Arch Pathol Lab Med 114:1025–1027, 1990.
108. Eisenach KD, Sifford MD, Cane MD, et al. Detection of *Mycobacterium tuberculosis* in sputum samples using a polymerase chain reaction. Am Rev Respir Dis 144:1160–1163, 1991.
109. Noordhock A, Kolk A, Bjune G, et al. Sensitivity and specificity of polymerase chain reaction for detection of *Mycobacterium tuberculosis*: A blind comparison study among seven laboratories. J Clin Microbiol 32:277–284, 1994.
110. Pierre C, Oliver C, Lecoissier D, et al. Diagnosis of primary tuberculosis in children by amplification and detection of mycobacterial DNA. Am Rev Respir Dis 147:420–424, 1993.
111. Smith KC, Starke JR, Eisenach K, et al. Detection of *Mycobacterium tuberculosis* in clinical specimens from children using a polymerase chain reaction. Pediatrics 97:155–160, 1996.
112. Migliori AB, Borghesi A, Rossnigo P, et al. Proposal for an improved score method for the diagnosis of pulmonary tuberculosis in childhood in developing countries. Tuber Lung Dis 73:145–149, 1992.
113. American Thoracic Society. Treatment of tuberculosis and tuberculosis infection in adults and children. Am J Respir Crit Care Med 149:1359–1374, 1994.
114. Centers for Disease Control and Prevention. Core Curriculum on Tuberculosis: What a Clinician Should Know (3rd ed). Atlanta, Centers for Disease Control and Prevention, 1994.
115. Styblo K. The relationship between the risk of tuberculous infection and the risk of developing infectious tuberculosis. Bull Int Union Tuberc 60:117–119, 1985.
116. Cantwell MF, Snider DE Jr, Cauthen GM, et al. Epidemiology of tuberculosis in the United States, 1985 through 1992. JAMA 272:535–539, 1994.
117. Ussery XT, Valway SE, McKenna M, et al. Epidemiology of tuberculosis among children in the United States: 1985 to 1994. Pediatr Infect Dis J 15:697–704, 1996.
118. McKenna MT, McCray E, Onorato IM. The epidemiology of tuberculosis among foreign-born persons in the United States, 1986 to 1993. N Engl J Med 332:1071–1076, 1995.
119. Braun MM, Truman BI, Maguire B, et al. Increasing incidence of tuberculosis in a prison inmate population: Association with HIV infection. JAMA 261:393–397, 1989.
120. Stead WW. Special problems in tuberculosis. Clin Chest Med 10:397–405, 1989.
121. McAdam JM, Brickner PW, Scharer LL, et al. The spectrum of tuberculosis in a New York City men's shelter clinic (1982–1988). Chest 97:798–805, 1990.
122. Ciesielski SD, Seed JR, Esposito DH, et al. The epidemiology of tuberculosis among North Carolina migrant farm workers. JAMA 265:1715–1719, 1991.

123. Centers for Disease Control and Prevention. Nosocomial transmission of multidrug-resistant tuberculosis among HIV-infected persons—Florida and New York, 1988–1991. MMWR Morb Mortal Wkly Rep 40:585–591, 1991.
124. Wells CS, Flahiff EW, Smith HH. Results obtained in man with the use of a vaccine of heat-killed tubercle bacilli. Am J Hyg 40:116–126, 1944.
125. Great Britain Medical Research Council. BCG and vole bacillus vaccines in the prevention of tuberculosis in adolescence and early life. BMJ 2:379–396, 1959.
126. Weill-Halle B. Oral vaccination. In Rosenthal SR (ed). BCG Vaccination Against Tuberculosis. Boston, Little, Brown, 1957, pp 175–182.
127. Luelmo F. BCG vaccination. Am Rev Respir Dis 125(suppl):70–72, 1982.
128. International Union Against Tuberculosis. Phenotypes of BCG vaccines seed lot strains: Results of an international cooperative study. Tubercle 59:139–142, 1978.
129. Milstien JB, Gibson JJ. Quality control of BCG vaccine by WHO: A review of factors that may influence vaccine effectiveness and safety. Bull World Health Organ 68:93–108, 1990.
130. Osborn TW. Changes in BCG strains. Tubercle 64:1–13, 1983.
131. Jensen KA. Practice of the Calmette vaccination. Acta Tuberc Scand 20:1–45, 1946.
132. Jacox RF, Meade GM. Variation in the duration of tuberculin skin sensitivity produced by two strains of BCG. Am Rev Tuberc 60:541–546, 1949.
133. Dubos RJ, Pierce CH, Schaefer WB. Antituberculous immunity induced in mice by vaccination with living cultures of attenuated tubercle bacilli. J Exp Med 9:207–220, 1953.
134. Dubos RJ, Pierce CH. Differential characteristics in vitro and in vivo of several substrains of BCG. I. Multiplication and survival in vitro. Am Rev Tuberc 74:655–666, 1956.
135. Pierce CH, Dubos RJ. Differential characteristics in vitro and in vivo of several substrains of BCG. II. Morphologic characteristics in vitro and in vivo. Am Rev Tuberc 74:667–682, 1956.
136. Pierce CH, Dubos RJ, Schaefer WB. Differential characteristics in vitro and in vivo of several substrains of BCG. III. Multiplication and survival in vivo. Am Rev Tuberc 74:683–698, 1956.
137. Dubos RJ, Pierce CH. Differential characteristics in vitro and in vivo of several substrains of BCG. IV. Immunizing effectiveness. Am Rev Tuberc 74:699–717, 1956.
138. Zhang Y, Wallace RJ Jr, Mazurek GH. Genetic differences between BCG substrains. Tuber Lung Dis 76:43–50, 1995.
139. Gheorghiu M. The present and future role of BCG vaccine in tuberculosis control. Biologicals 18:135–141, 1990.
140. Sekuis VM, Freudenstein H, Sirks JL. Report on results of a collaborative assay of BCG vaccines organized by the International Association of Biological Standardization. J Biol Stand 5:85–109, 1977.
141. Gheorghiu M, Lagrange PH. Viability, heat stability and immunogenicity of four BCG vaccines prepared from four different BCG strains. Ann Immunol 134C:124–147, 1983.
142. Formukong NG, Dale JN, Osborn TW, et al. Use of gene probes based on the insertion sequence IS986 to differentiate between BCG vaccine strains. J Appl Bacteriol 72:126–133, 1992.
143. Smith D, Harding C, Chan J, et al. Potency of 10 BCG vaccines organized by the IABS. J Biol Stand 7:179–197, 1979.
144. Comstock GW. Identification of an effective vaccine against tuberculosis. Am Rev Respir Dis 138:479–480, 1988.
145. Tuberculosis Control Program and Expanded Program on Immunization. Efficacy of infant BCG immunization. Wkly Epidemiol Rec 28:216–218, 1986.
146. Pollock TM. BCG vaccination in man. Tubercle 40:339–412, 1959.
147. Lehman HG, Englehardt H, Freudenstein H, et al. BCG vaccination of neonates, infants, school children and adolescents. II. Safety of vaccine with strain 1331 Copenhagen. Dev Biol Stand 43:133–136, 1979.
148. Expanded Program on Immunization/Biologicals Unit. Lymphadenitis associated with BCG immunization. Wkly Epidemiol Rec 63:381–388, 1988.
149. Expanded Program on Immunization/Biologicals Unit. BCG-associated lymphadenitis in infants. Wkly Epidemiol Rec 30:231–232, 1989.
150. Kroger L, Brander E, Korppi M, et al. Osteitis after newborn vaccination with three different bacillus Calmette-Guérin vaccines: Twenty-nine years of experience. Pediatr Infect Dis J 12:113–116, 1994.
151. Behr MA, Small PM. Declining efficacy of BCG strains over time? A new hypothesis for an old controversy [abstract]. Am J Respir Crit Care Med 155:A222, 1997.
152. Gheorghiu M. The stability and immunogenicity of a dispersed-grown freeze-dried Pasteur BCG vaccine. J Biol Stand 15:15–26, 1988.
153. Abou-Zeid C, Rook GAW, Mannikin DE, et al. Effect of the method of preparation of bacille Calmette-Guérin vaccine on the properties of four daughter strains. J Appl Bacteriol 63:449–453, 1987.
154. Devadoss PO, Klegerman ME, Groves MJ. A scanning electron microscope study of mycobacterial developmental stages in commercial BCG vaccines. Curr Microbiol 22:247–252, 1991.
155. Harboe M, Nagel S. MPB70, a unique antigen of *Mycobacterium bovis* BCG. Am Rev Respir Dis 129:444–452, 1984.
156. ten Dam HG. Research on BCG vaccination. Adv Tuberc Res 21:79–106, 1984.
157. ten Dam HG, Fillastre C, Conge C, et al. The use of jet injectors in BCG vaccination. Bull World Health Organ 43:707–720, 1970.
158. Darmanger AM, Nekzad SM, Kuis M, et al. BCG vaccination by bifurcated needle in a pilot BCG vaccination programme. Bull World Health Organ 55:49–61, 1977.
159. Birkhaug K. An experimental and clinical investigation of a percutaneous (Rosenthal) method of BCG vaccination. Nord Med 10:1224–1231, 1941.
160. Briggs IL, Smith C. BCG vaccination by the multiple puncture method in northern Rhodesia. Tubercle 38:107–111, 1957.
161. Griffith AH. BCG vaccination by multiple puncture. Lancet 1:1170–1172, 1959.
162. ten Dam HG, Hitze KL. Does BCG vaccination protect the newborn and young infants? Bull World Health Organ 58:37–41, 1980.
163. Pabst HF, Godel JC, Spady DW, et al. Prospective trial of timing of bacillus Calmette-Guérin vaccination in Canadian Cree infants. Am Rev Respir Dis 140:1007–1011, 1989.
164. Ferreira AA, Bunn-Moreno MM, Sant'Anna CC, et al. BCG vaccination in low birth weight newborns: Analysis of lymphocyte proliferation, Il-2 generation and intradermal reaction to PPD. Tuber Lung Dis 77:476–481, 1996.
165. Hart PD. Efficacy and applicability of mass BCG vaccination in tuberculosis control. BMJ 1:587–592, 1967.
166. Sutherland I, Springett VH. The effects of the scheme for BCG vaccination of school children in England and Wales and the consequences of discontinuing the scheme at various dates. J Epidemiol Community Health 43:15–24, 1989.
167. Springett VH, Sutherland I. BCG vaccination of school children in England and Wales. Thorax 45:83–88, 1990.
168. Gheorghiu M, Augier J, Lagrange PH. Maintenance and control of the French BCG strain 1173P2 (primary and secondary seed lots). Bull Inst Pasteur 81:281–288, 1983.
169. Galbraith NS, Hall C. Comparative trials of British BCG vaccine double strength, and Danish BCG vaccine with standard strength British BCG vaccine. Tubercle 55:283–289, 1974.
170. Stainer DW, Landi S. Stability of BCG vaccines. Dev Biol Stand 58:119–125, 1986.
171. Smith PG. Case-control studies of the efficacy of BCG against tuberculosis. In International Union Against Tuberculosis. Proceedings of the XXVIth IUAT World Conference on Tuberculosis and Respiratory Diseases. Singapore, Japan, Professional Postgraduate Services International, 1987, pp 73–79.
172. Filho VW, de Castilho EA, Rodrigues LC, et al. Effectiveness of BCG vaccination against tuberculous meningitis: A case-control study in Sao Paulo, Brazil. Bull World Health Organ 68:69–74, 1990.
173. Sutherland I, Lindgren I. The protective effect of BCG vaccination as indicated by autopsy studies. Tubercle 60:225–231, 1979.
174. Smith DW, Harding G, Chan J, et al. Potency of 10 BCG vaccines as evaluated by their influence on the bacillemic phase of experimental airborne tuberculosis in guinea pigs. J Biol Stand 7:179–197, 1979.

175. Jensen KA, Bindsleu G, Holm J. Experimental studies on the development of tuberculous infection in allergic and non-allergic animals. I. Development of tuberculous infection in the lungs after inhalation of virulent tubercle bacilli. Acta Tuberc Scand 9:27–46, 1935.
176. Levy FM, Conge GA, Pasquier JF, et al. The effect of BCG-vaccination on the fate of virulent tubercle bacilli in mice. Am Rev Tuberc 84:28–36, 1961.
177. Smith DW, McMurray DN, Wiegeshaus EH, et al. Host-parasite relationship in experimental airborne tuberculosis. IV. Early events in the course of infection in vaccinated and nonvaccinated guinea pigs. Am Rev Respir Dis 102:937–949, 1970.
178. Dannenberg AM. Cellular hypersensitivity and cellular immunity in the pathogenesis of tuberculosis: Specificity, systemic and local nature, and associated macrophage enzymes. Bacteriol Rev 32:85–102, 1968.
179. Ho RS, Fok JS, Harding GE, et al. Host-parasite relationships in experimental airborne tuberculosis. VII. Fate of *Mycobacterium tuberculosis* in primary lung lesions and in primary lesion free lung tissue infected as a result of bacillemia. J Infect Dis 138:237–241, 1978.
180. Morrison NE, Collins FM. Restoration of T-cell responsiveness by thymosin: Development of antituberculosis resistance in BCG-infected animals. Infect Immun 13:554–563, 1976.
181. Lefford MJ, McGregor DD, Mackaness DB. Immune response to *Mycobacterium tuberculosis* in rats. Infect Immun 8:182–189, 1973.
182. Jackett PS, Aber VR, Mitchison DA, et al. The contribution of hydrogen peroxide resistance to virulence of *Mycobacterium tuberculosis* during the first six days after intravenous infection of normal and BCG-vaccinated guinea pigs. Br J Exp Pathol 62:34–40, 1980.
183. Workshop report. Summary, conclusions, and recommendations from the international workshop on Research Towards Global Control and Prevention of Tuberculosis: With an emphasis on vaccine development. J Infect Dis 158:248–253, 1988.
184. Browne JAK, Stone MM, Sutherland I. BCG vaccination of children against leprosy in Uganda. First results. Br Med J 1:7–14, 1966.
185. Ponninghaus JM, Fine PEM, Sterne JAC, et al. Efficacy of BCG vaccine against leprosy and tuberculosis in Northern Malawi. Lancet 339:636–639, 1992.
186. Karonga Prevention Trial Group. Randomized controlled trial of single BCG, repeated BCG, or combined BCG and killed *Mycobacterium leprae* vaccine for prevention of leprosy and tuberculosis. Lancet 348:17–24, 1996.
187. Trnka L, Dankova D, Svandova E. Six years' experience with the discontinuation of BCG vaccine. 4. Protective effect of BCG against *Mycobacterium avium-intracellulare* complex. Tuber Lung Dis 75:348–352, 1994.
188. Romanus V, Svensson A, Hollander HO. The impact of changing BCG coverage on tuberculosis in Swedish children between 1969 and 1989. Tuber Lung Dis 73:150–161, 1992.
189. Fine PEM. The BCG story: Lessons from the past and implications for the future. Rev Infect Dis 11(suppl 2):S353–S359, 1989.
190. Fine PEM, Ponnighaus JM, Maine NP. The relationship between delayed type hypersensitivity and protective immunity induced by mycobacterial vaccines in man. Lepr Rev 57(suppl 12):S274–S283, 1986.
191. Fine PEM, Sterne JAC, Ponnighaus JM, et al. Delayed type hypersensitivity, mycobacterial vaccines and protective immunity. Lancet 344:1245–1249, 1994.
192. Tuberculosis Prevention Trial. Trial of BCG vaccines in South India for tuberculosis prevention: First report. Bull World Health Organ 57:819–827, 1979.
193. Tripathy SP. Fifteen-year follow-up of the Indian BCG prevention trial. Bull Int Union Tuberc Lung Dis 62:69–73, 1987.
194. al-Kassimi FA, al-Hajjaj MS, al-Orainey IO, et al. Does the protective effect of neonatal BCG correlate with vaccine-induced tuberculin reaction? Am J Respir Crit Care Med 152:1575–1578, 1995.
195. Grange JM. Environmental mycobacteria and BCG vaccination. Tubercle 67:1–4, 1986.
196. Pithie AD, Rahelu M, Kumararatne DS, et al. Generation of cytolytic T cells in individuals infected with *Mycobacterium tuberculosis* and vaccinated with BCG. Thorax 47:695–701, 1992.
197. Fine PEM. Leprosy and tuberculosis: An epidemiological comparison. Tubercle 65:137–153, 1984.
198. Clemens JD, Chuong JJH, Feinstein AR. The BCG controversy: A methodological and statistical reappraisal. JAMA 249:2362–2369, 1983.
199. Fine PEM, Rodrigues LC. Modern vaccines: Mycobacterial diseases. Lancet 335:1016–1020, 1990.
200. Wilson ME, Fineberg HV, Colditz GA. Geographic latitude and the efficacy of bacillus Calmette-Guérin vaccine. Clin Infect Dis 20:982–991, 1995.
201. Brewer TF, Colditz GA. Relationship between bacille Calmette-Guérin (BCG) strains and the efficacy of BCG vaccine in the prevention of tuberculosis. Clin Infect Dis 20:126–135, 1995.
202. Fine PEM. Variation in protection by BCG: Implications of and for heterologous immunity. Lancet 346:1339–1345, 1995.
203. Comstock GW. Field trials of tuberculosis vaccines: How could we have done them better? Control Clin Trials 15:247–276, 1994.
204. Stein SC, Aronson JD. The occurrence of pulmonary lesions in BCG-vaccinated and unvaccinated persons. Am Rev Tuberc 68:695–712, 1953.
205. Rosenthal SR, Loewinsohn E, Graham ML, et al. BCG vaccination against tuberculosis in Chicago: A twenty-year study statistically analyzed. Pediatrics 28:622–641, 1961.
206. Hart PD, Sutherland I. BCG and vole bacillus vaccines in the prevention of tuberculosis in adolescence and early adult life. Final report to the Medical Research Council. Br Med J 2:293–295, 1977.
207. Palmer CE, Shaw LW, Comstock GW. Community trials of BCG vaccination. Am Rev Tuberc 177:877–907, 1958.
208. Frimodt-Moller J, Thomas J, Parthasanathy R. Observations on the protective effect of BCG vaccination in a south Indian rural population. Bull World Health Organ 30:545–574, 1964.
209. Frimodt-Moller J, Acharyulu G, Pillai K. Observations on the protective effect of BCG vaccination in a south Indian rural population: Fourth report. Bull Int Union Tuberc 48:40–52, 1973.
210. Comstock G, Shaw L. Controlled trial of BCG vaccination in a school population. Public Health Rep 75:583–594, 1960.
211. Comstock G, Webster R. Tuberculosis studies in Muscogee County, Georgia: VII. A 20 year evaluation of BCG vaccination in a school population. Am Rev Respir Dis 100:839–845, 1969.
212. Comstock G, Palmer C. Long-term results of BCG vaccination in the southern United States. Am Rev Respir Dis 93:171–183, 1966.
213. Comstock GW. Identification of an effective vaccine against tuberculosis. Am Rev Respir Dis 138:479–480, 1988.
214. Stanford JL, Shield MJ, Rook GAW. How environmental mycobacteria may predetermine the protective efficacy of BCG. Tubercle 62:55–62, 1981.
215. Rook GAW, Bahr GM, Stanford JL. The effect of two distinct forms of cell-mediated response to mycobacteria on the protective efficacy of BCG. Tubercle 62:63–68, 1981.
216. Edwards LB, Palmer CE. Identification of the tuberculous-infected by skin tests. Ann N Y Acad Sci 154:140–148, 1968.
217. Palmer CE, Hopwood L. Effect of previous infection with unclassified mycobacteria on survival of guinea pigs challenged with virulent tubercle bacilli. Bull Int Union Tuberc 32:389–391, 1962.
218. Edwards ML, Goodrich JM, Muller D, et al. Infection with *Mycobacterium avium-intracellulare* and the protective effects of bacilli Calmette-Guérin. J Infect Dis 145:733–741, 1982.
219. Fine PEM. Immunogenetics of susceptibility to leprosy, tuberculosis and leishmaniasis: An epidemiological perspective. Int J Lepr 49:437–454, 1981.
220. Schurr E, Buschman E, Gros P, et al. Genetic aspects of mycobacterial infections in mouse and man. In Melchers F (ed). Progress in Immunology. Vol. VII. New York, Springer-Verlag, 1990, pp 994–1001.
221. Skamene E. Genetic control of susceptibility to mycobacterial infections. Rev Infect Dis 11(suppl 2):S394–S399, 1989.
222. Vidal SM, Malo D, Vogan K, et al. Natural resistance to infection with intracellular parasites: Isolation of a candidate for *Bcg*. Cell 73:469–485, 1993.
223. Dubos R. Acquired immunity to tuberculosis. Am Rev Respir Dis 90:505–515, 1964.

224. Cohen MK, Bartow RA, Mintzer CL, et al. Effect of diet and genetics on *Mycobacterium bovis* BCG vaccine efficacy in inbred guinea pigs. Infect Immun 55:314–319, 1987.
225. McMurray DN, Kimball MS, Tetzlaff CL, et al. Effects of protein deprivation and BCG vaccination on alveolar macrophage function in pulmonary tuberculosis. Am Rev Respir Dis 133:1081–1085, 1986.
226. D'Arcy Hart P, Sutherland I. Acquired immunity to tuberculosis. Am Rev Respir Dis 91:939, 1965.
227. Padungchan S, Konjanart S, Kasiratta S, et al. The effectiveness of BCG vaccination of the newborn against childhood tuberculosis in Bangkok. Bull World Health Organ 64:247–258, 1986.
228. Hank JA, Chan JK, Edwards ML, et al. Influence of the virulence of *Mycobacterium tuberculosis* on protection induced by bacilli Calmette-Guérin in guinea pigs. J Infect Dis 143:734–738, 1981.
229. Ziegler JE, Edwards ML, Smith DW. Exogenous reinfection in experimental airborne tuberculosis. Tubercle 66:121–128, 1985.
230. Stead WW. The pathogenesis of pulmonary tuberculosis among older persons. Am Rev Respir Dis 91:811–822, 1965.
231. Styblo K. Recent advances in epidemiological research in tuberculosis. Adv Tuberc Res 20:1–63, 1980.
232. Eisenach KD, Crawford JT, Bates JH. Genetic relatedness among strains of the *Mycobacterium tuberculosis* complex. Am Rev Respir Dis 133:1065–1068, 1986.
233. Daley CL, Small PM, Schecter GF, et al. An outbreak of tuberculosis with accelerated progression among persons infected with the human immunodeficiency virus. An analysis using restriction-fragment-length polymorphisms. N Engl J Med 326:231–235, 1992.
234. Smith PG. Retrospective assessment of the effectiveness of BCG vaccination against tuberculosis using the case-control method. Tubercle 62:23–35, 1982.
235. Fine PEM. BCG vaccination against tuberculosis and leprosy. Br Med Bull 44:693–703, 1988.
236. Chavalittamrong B, Chearskul S, Tuchinda M. Protective value of BCG vaccination in children in Bangkok, Thailand. Pediatr Pulmonol 2:202–205, 1986.
237. Micheli I, de Kantor IN, Colaiacovo D, et al. Evaluation of the effectiveness of BCG vaccination using the case-control method in Buenos Aires, Argentina. Int J Epidemiol 17:629–634, 1988.
238. Sirinavin S, Chotpitayasunondh T, Suwanjutha S, et al. Protective efficacy of neonatal bacillus Calmette-Guérin vaccination against tuberculosis. Pediatr Infect Dis J 10:359–365, 1991.
239. Effectiveness of BCG vaccination in Great Britain in 1978: A report from the research committee of the British Thoracic Association. Br J Dis Chest 74:215–227, 1980.
240. Ferguson RG, Simes AB. BCG vaccination of Indian infants in Saskatchewan. Tubercle 30:5–11, 1949.
241. Curtis HM, Leck I, Bamford FN. Incidence of childhood tuberculosis after neonatal BCG vaccination. Lancet 1:145–148, 1984.
242. Shannon A, Kelly P, Lucey M, et al. Isoniazid resistant tuberculosis in a school outbreak: The protective effect of BCG. Eur Respir J 4:778–782, 1991.
243. Rodriques LC, Gill ON, Smith PG. BCG vaccination in the first year of life protects children of Indian subcontinent ethnic origin against tuberculosis in England. J Epidemiol Community Health 45:78–80, 1991.
244. Packe GE, Innes JA. Protective effect of BCG vaccination in infant Asians: A case-control study. Arch Dis Child 63:277–281, 1988.
245. Houston S, Fanning A, Soskolne CL, et al. The effectiveness of bacillus Calmette-Guérin (BCG) vaccination against tuberculosis: A case-control study in treaty Indians, Alberta, Canada. Am J Epidemiol 131:340–347, 1990.
246. Young TK, Hershfield ES. A case-control study to evaluate the effectiveness of mass neonatal BCG vaccination among Canadian Indians. Am J Public Health 76:783–786, 1986.
247. Blin P, Delolme HG, Heyraud JD, et al. Evaluation of the protective effect of BCG vaccination by a case-control study in Yaoundé, Cameroon. Tubercle 67:283–288, 1986.
248. Tidjani O, Amendome A, ten Dam HG. The protective effect of BCG vaccination of the newborn against childhood tuberculosis in an African community. Tubercle 67:269–281, 1986.
249. Putrali J, Sutrisna B, Rahayoe N, et al. A case-control study of effectiveness of BCG vaccination in children in Jakarta, Indonesia. Proceedings of the Eastern Regional Tuberculosis Conference of IUAT; Jakarta, Indonesia; November 20–25, 1983, pp 194–200.
250. Patel A, Schofield F, Siskind V, et al. Case-control evaluation of a school-age BCG vaccination programme in subtropical Australia. Bull World Health Organ 69:425–433, 1991.
251. Shapiro C, Cook N, Evans D, et al. A case-control study of BCG and childhood tuberculosis in Cali, Colombia. Int J Epidemiol 14:441–446, 1985.
252. Smith PG. Evaluating interventions against tropical diseases. Int J Epidemiol 16:159–166, 1987.
253. Sepulveda RL, Parcha C, Sorensen RU. Case-control study of the efficacy of BCG immunization against pulmonary tuberculosis in young adults in Santiago, Chile. Tuber Lung Dis 73:372–377, 1992.
254. Thilothammal N, Kirshnamurthy PV, Runyan DK, et al. Does BCG vaccine prevent tuberculous meningitis? Arch Dis Child 74:144–147, 1996.
255. Rodriques LC, Diwan VK, Wheeler JG. Protective effect of BCG against tuberculous meningitis and miliary tuberculosis: A meta-analysis. Int J Epidemiol 22:1154–1158, 1993.
256. Colditz GA, Berkey CS, Mosteller F, et al. The efficacy of bacillus Calmette-Guérin vaccination of newborns and infants in the prevention of tuberculosis: Meta-analyses of the published literature. Pediatrics 96:29–35, 1995.
257. Colditz GA, Brewer TF, Berkey CS, et al. Efficacy of BCG vaccine in the prevention of tuberculosis: Meta-analysis of the published literature. JAMA 271:698–702, 1994.
258. Lotte A, Wasz-Hockert O, Poisson N, et al. BCG complications: Estimates of the risks among vaccinated subjects and statistical analysis of their main characteristics. Adv Tuberc Res 21:107–193, 1984.
259. Victoria MS, Shah BR. Bacillus Calmette-Guérin lymphadenitis: A case report and review of the literature. Pediatr Infect Dis J 4:295–296, 1985.
260. Brewer MA, Edwards KM, Palmer PS, Hinson HP. Bacille Calmette-Guérin immunization in normal healthy adults. J Infect Dis 170:476–479, 1994.
261. Lotte A, Wasz-Hockert O, Poisson N, et al. Second IUATLD study on complications induced by intradermal BCG-vaccination. Bull Int Union Tuberc 63:47–59, 1988.
262. Reynes J, Perez C, Lamaury I, et al. Bacille Calmette-Guérin adenitis 30 years after immunization in a patient with AIDS [letter]. J Infect Dis 160:727, 1989.
263. Gheorghiu M. Potency and suppurative adenitis in BCG vaccination. Dev Biol Stand 41:79–84, 1978.
264. Muzy de Souza GR, Sant'Anna CC, Lapane Silva JR, et al. Intradermal BCG vaccination complications—analysis of 51 cases. Tubercle 64:23–27, 1983.
265. Helmick CG, D'Souza AJ, Goddard N. An outbreak of severe BCG axillary lymphadenitis in Saint Lucia, 1982–83. West Indies Med J 35:12–17, 1986.
266. Praveen KN, Smikle MF, Prabhakar P, et al. Outbreak of bacillus Calmette-Guérin–associated lymphadenitis and abscesses in Jamaican children. Pediatr Infect Dis J 9:890–893, 1990.
267. O'Brien KL, Ruff AJ, Louis MA, et al. Bacillus Calmette-Guérin complications in children born to HIV-1–infected women with a review of the literature. Pediatrics 95:414–418, 1995.
268. Caglayan S, Yegin O, Kayean K, et al. Is medical therapy effective for regional lymphadenitis following BCG vaccination? Am J Dis Child 141:1213–1214, 1987.
269. Oguz F, Mujgan S, Alper G, et al. Treatment of bacillus Calmette-Guérin–associated lymphadenitis. Pediatr Infect Dis J 11:887–888, 1992.
270. World Health Organization. BCG Vaccination of the Newborn: Rationale and Guidelines for Country Programs. Geneva, World Health Organization, 1986.
271. Hanley SP, Gumb J, MacFarlane JT. Comparison of erythromycin and isoniazid in treatment of adverse reactions to BCG vaccination. BMJ 290:970, 1985.
272. Murphy PM, Mayers DL, Brock NF, Wagner KF. Cure of bacille Calmette-Guérin vaccination abscess with erythromycin. Rev Infect Dis 11:335–337, 1989.
273. Power JT, Stewart IC, Ross JD. Erythromycin in the management of troublesome BCG lesions. Br J Dis Chest 78:192–193, 1984.

274. Kroger L, Korppi M, Brander E, et al. Osteitis caused by bacillus Calmette-Guérin vaccination: A retrospective analysis of 222 cases. J Infect Dis 172:574–576, 1995.
275. Bergdahl S, Fellander M, Robertson B. BCG osteomyelitis: Experience in the Stockholm region over the years 1961–1974. J Bone Joint Surg 58B:212–216, 1976.
276. Vanicek H. Complications after initial BCG vaccination in a 5-year period in the East Bohemia region. Cesk Pediatr 43:23–26, 1988.
277. Bottiger M. Osteitis and other complications caused by generalized BCGitis. Acta Paediatr Scand 71:471–478, 1982.
278. Rouillon A, Waaler H. BCG vaccination and epidemiological situation: A decision making approach to the use of BCG. Adv Tuberc Res 19:64–126, 1976.
279. Pedersen FK, Engbaek HC, Hertz H, Vergmann B. Fatal BCG infection in an immunocompetent girl. Acta Paediatr Scand 67:519–523, 1978.
280. Trevenen CL, Pagtakhan RD. Disseminated tuberculoid lesions in infants following BCG. Can Med J 15:502–504, 1982.
281. Lachaux A, Descos B, Mertani A, et al. Infection generalisée a BCG d'evolution favorable chez un nourrisson de 3 mois sans deficit immunitaire reconnu. Arch Fr Pediatr 43:807–809, 1986.
282. Tardieu M, Truffot-Pernot C, Carriere JP, et al. Tuberculosis meningitis due to BCG in two previously healthy children. Lancet 1:440–441, 1988.
283. Gormsen H. On the occurrence of epithelioid cell granulomas in the organs of BCG vaccinated human beings. Acta Pathol Microbiol Scand 39(suppl 111):117–120, 1956.
284. Casanova JL, Blanche S, Emile JF, et al. Idiopathic disseminated bacille Calmette-Guérin infection: A French national retrospective study. Pediatrics 98:774–778, 1996.
285. Gonzalez B, Moreno S, Burdach R, et al. Clinical presentation of bacillus Calmette-Guérin infections in patients with immunodeficiency syndromes. Pediatr Infect Dis J 8:201–206, 1989.
286. Boudes P, Sobel A, Deforges L. Disseminated *Mycobacterium bovis* infection from BCG vaccination and HIV infection [letter]. JAMA 262:2386, 1989.
287. Kobayashi Y, Komazawa Y, Kobayshi M, et al. Presumed BCG infection in a boy with chronic granulomatous disease. Clin Pediatr 23:586–589, 1984.
288. Houde C, Dery P. *Mycobacterium bovis* sepsis in an infant with human immunodeficiency virus infection. Pediatr Infect Dis J 11:810–811, 1988.
289. Sicevic S. Generalized BCG tuberculosis with fatal course in two sisters. Acta Paediatr Scand 61:178–184, 1972.
290. Talbot EA, Perkins MD, Silva SFM, et al. Disseminated bacille Calmette-Guérin disease after vaccination: Case report and review. Clin Infect Dis 24:1139–1146, 1997.
290a. Casanova JL, Blanche S, Emile JF, et al. Idiopathic disseminated bacillus Calmette-Guérin infection: A French national retrospective study. Pediatrics 98:774–778, 1996.
290b. Jouanguy E, Altare F, Lamhamedi S, et al. Interferon-gamma-receptor deficiency in an infant with fatal bacille Calmette-Guérin infection. N Engl J Med 335:1956–1961, 1996.
291. Konno K, Feldmann FM, McDermott W. Pyrazinamide susceptibility and amidase activity of tubercle bacilli. Am Rev Respir Dis 95:461–469, 1967.
292. Armbruster C, Junker W, Vetter N, Jaksch G. Disseminated bacille Calmette-Guérin infection in an AIDS patient 30 years after BCG vaccination [letter]. J Infect Dis 162:1216, 1990.
293. Ninane J, Grymonprez A, Burtonboy G, et al. Disseminated BCG in HIV infection. Arch Dis Child 63:1268–1269, 1988.
294. Centers for Disease Control and Prevention. Disseminated *Mycobacterium bovis* infection from BCG vaccination of a patient with acquired immunodeficiency syndrome. MMWR Morb Mortal Wkly Rep 34:227–228, 1985.
295. Edwards K, Kernodle DS. Possible hazards of routine bacillus Calmette-Guérin immunization in human immunodeficiency virus–infected children. Pediatr Infect Dis J 15:836–838, 1996.
296. Colebunders RL, Izaley L, Musampu M, et al. BCG vaccine abscesses are unrelated to HIV infection [letter]. JAMA 259: 352, 1988.
297. Carswell M. BCG immunization in the children of HIV-positive mothers. AIDS 1:258, 1987.
298. Dabis F, Lepage P, Nsengumuremyi F, et al. Infection par le virus V1HI et vaccination de routine de l'enfant: Une étude cohorte à Kigali, Rwanda—surveillance des effets indésirables de la vaccination [abstract C29]. Conference Internationale, Les Implications du SIDA pour la Mère et l'Enfant, Paris, 1989.
299. Lallemant–Le Coeur S, Cheynier D, Lallemant M, et al. Complications loco-régionales de la vaccination par le BCG chez des enfants nés de mères positive pour anti-HIV1: Étude cas-témoins à Brazzaville [abstract WG03]. In 5th International Conference on AIDS, Montreal, 1989. Ottawa, Canada, International Development Research Center, 1989, p 982.
300. Besnard M, Sauvion S, Offredo C, et al. Bacillus Calmette-Guérin infection after vaccination of human immunodeficiency virus–infected children. Pediatr Infect Dis J 12:993–997, 1993.
301. Special Program on AIDS and Expanded Programme on Immunization. Consultation on human immunodeficiency virus (HIV) and routine childhood immunization. Wkly Epidemiol Rec 62:297–304, 1987.
302. Centers for Disease Control and Prevention. The role of BCG vaccine in the prevention and control of tuberculosis in the United States. A joint statement by the Advisory Council for the Elimination of Tuberculosis and Advisory Committee on Immunization Practices. MMWR Morb Mortal Wkly Rep 45(RR-4):1–18, 1996.
303. Kaufmann SHE. Vaccines against tuberculosis: The impact of modern biotechnology. Scand J Infect Dis 75(suppl):54–59, 1990.
304. Harboe M, Andersen P, Colston MJ, et al. European Commission COST/STC Initiative. Report of the expert panel IX. Vaccines against tuberculosis. Vaccine 14:701–716, 1996.
305. Orme IM. Progress in the development of new vaccines against tuberculosis. Int J Tuberc Lung Dis 1:95–100, 1997.
306. Briggs B, Illingworth RS, Lorber J. The human source of tuberculous infection in children. Lancet 1:263–266, 1956.
307. Andrews RH, Devadatta S, Fox W, et al. Prevalence of tuberculosis among close family contacts of tuberculous patients in south India, and influence of segregation of the patient on the early attack rate. Bull World Health Organ 23:463–510, 1963.
308. Ramakrishnan CV, Andrews RH, Devadatta S, et al. Prevalence and early attack rate of tuberculosis among close family contacts of tuberculous patients in south India under domiciliary treatment with isoniazid plus PAS or isoniazid alone. Bull World Health Organ 25:361–407, 1964.
309. Romanus V. Tuberculosis in bacillus Calmette-Guérin–immunized and unimmunized children in Sweden: A ten year evaluation following the cessation of general bacillus Calmette-Guérin immunization of the newborn in 1975. Pediatr Infect Dis J 6:272–280, 1987.

chapter

9 Diphtheria Toxoid

Edward A. Mortimer Jr.
Melinda Wharton

Diphtheria is a bacterial respiratory infection caused by *Corynebacterium diphtheriae*, a gram-positive bacillus. The major manifestation is a membranous inflammation of the upper respiratory tract, usually of the pharynx but sometimes of the posterior nasal passages, larynx, and trachea, plus widespread damage to other organs including the myocardium, nervous system, and kidneys that is caused by the organism's exotoxin. A cutaneous form of diphtheria also occurs. The earliest description of a case of what was probably diphtheria is that of Hippocrates in the 5th century BC. Subsequent detailed descriptions of the clinical picture of the disease were provided by Aretaeus in the 2nd century AD and Aëtius in the 6th century.[1–3] However, it is clear in reading translations of the descriptions by the last two physicians that diphtheria was not distinguished from other infections with somewhat similar manifestations, including Ludwig angina and streptococcal tonsillitis, for the obvious reason that a definitive diagnostic method was unavailable. Aëtius termed the illness Egyptian and Syrian ulcers, indicating that it had probably been known in those two areas previously and reflecting the uncharitable tendency of the Greeks (among others) to blame pestilence on others, particularly the Egyptians. Although the disease has had many different names in various languages over the centuries, the term *diphtheria* is said to be derived from the Greek word for leather or tanned skin even though the disease was not so named until many years later.[1, 3]

Only isolated reports of the disease appeared until the 17th century, during which time devastating outbreaks occurred in Spain and were described in detail by several writers.[2] Indeed, in Spanish history, 1613 is known as the Year of Diphtheria (Año de Los Garrotillos).[1] Successive outbreaks occurred in southwestern Europe approximately every 12 years through the 18th century. The earliest definitive description of diphtheria in America was that of Samuel Bard in New York in 1771, although outbreaks had previously been noted in the American colonies.[1, 2, 4] In the early 19th century, Bretonneau provided detailed, accurate descriptions of the disease, including its contagiousness, course, and prognosis, and gave the disease its name.[1, 2] Bretonneau performed the first successful tracheotomy in 1825. A fascinating account of the horrors of diphtheria in childhood has been provided by Holt.[5]

During the 19th century, many efforts were made by bacteriologists to identify the causative agent. Progress was impeded by primitive methods for isolation of bacteria and the plethora of other organisms found in the pharynx, including streptococci. However, in 1883, Klebs first described the characteristic organisms in stained preparations of diphtheritic membranes, and Loeffler reported the successful growth of these organisms in culture a year later.[2] During the next 7 years, numerous investigators confirmed these observations and described the pathogenicity of the organism for guinea pigs.

In 1888, Roux and Yersin found that sterile broth filtrates of cultures of the organism, when injected into animals, produced death in a manner similar to that which occurred when virulent organisms were injected, thus demonstrating the presence of a potent exotoxin. Within the next few years, Behring produced antisera in guinea pigs by the injection of sublethal or inactivated broth cultures into these animals. These antisera were shown by Behring to prevent death in nonimmune animals that were challenged with virulent organisms.[1, 2] Behring named this preparation *antitoxin*. For his discovery, he received the Nobel Prize in 1901, after which he changed his name to von Behring.

Within a few years, the production and use of equine diphtheria antiserum was widespread. The concept of active immunization began with Theobald Smith in 1907, who noted that long-lasting immunity to diphtheria could be produced in guinea pigs by the injection of mixtures of diphtheria toxin and antitoxin. His suggestion that this procedure might be applicable to humans was followed up by von Behring with success.[1] Schick in 1913 introduced the well-known skin test for immunity that now goes by his name. The test consists of the injection of a small, measured amount of diphtheria toxin; in immune persons, circulating antibody neutralizes the toxin, and no local lesion is observed.[1] In the early 1920s, Ramon showed that diphtheria toxin, when treated with heat and formalin, lost its toxic properties but retained its ability to produce serological protection against the disease. Thus, the current immunizing preparation, diphtheria toxoid, came into being.[5a]

BACKGROUND

Clinical Description

Classic diphtheria has an insidious onset after an incubation period of 1 to 5 days, rarely longer. The gradual onset of diphtheria is in considerable contrast to the usually sudden, almost explosive manifestations of streptococcal pharyngitis. Symptoms of diphtheria are initially nonspecific and mild; throughout the course of the disease, fever does not usually exceed 38.5°C (101.3°F). Other early symptoms in children include diminished activity and some irritability. At first, the pharynx is injected on examination; but about a day after onset, small patches of exudate appear in the pharynx. Within 2 or 3 days, the patches of exudate spread and become confluent and may form a membrane that covers the entire pharynx, including the tonsillar areas, soft palate, and uvula. This membrane becomes grayish, thick, and firmly adherent. Efforts to dislodge the membrane result in bleeding. Anterior cervical lymph nodes become markedly enlarged and tender. These enlarged nodes feel soft and are associated with considerable inflammation and edema of the surrounding soft tissues, giving rise to the so-called bull neck appearance. Although fever is rarely high, the patient characteristically appears toxic and displays a rapid, thready pulse.

In untreated patients, the membrane begins to soften about a week after onset and gradually sloughs off, usually in pieces but sometimes as a single unit. As the membrane detaches, acute systemic symptoms, such as fever, begin to disappear.

Although pharyngeal diphtheria is by far the most common form of disease seen in unimmunized populations, other sites—respiratory tract and elsewhere—may be involved. Laryngeal diphtheria occurs in 25% of cases; in three fourths of these instances, the pharynx is also involved. Isolated nasal diphtheria is uncommon (about 2% of cases). Cutaneous, aural, vaginal, and conjunctival diphtheria together account for about 2% of cases and are often secondary to nasopharyngeal infection.

Laryngeal diphtheria may occur at any age but is particularly prone to occur in children younger than 4 years. It is marked by insidious onset with gradually increasing hoarseness and stridor. Fever is usually slight. The diagnosis is often missed or delayed when the pharynx is not simultaneously involved. The ensuing obstruction may lead to death.

Cutaneous diphtheria is an indolent skin infection that often occurs at sites of burns or other wounds and may act as a source of respiratory infection in others.[6] It is more common in warmer climates and in environments of poverty, overcrowding, and poor hygiene.[7]

Complications

The impact of diphtheria is largely measured by complications attributable to the local disease and to the effect of absorbed toxin on other organs, particularly on those of the cardiovascular and nervous systems. The major threat from laryngeal diphtheria is respiratory obstruction (croup). In the past, life-endangering obstruction was managed by the insertion of a small tube through the glottis, which was left in place for 4 days or more; intubation required considerable skill and experience.[8] Intubation was subsequently replaced by tracheostomy. Even with a tracheostomy tube in place, fatal acute respiratory obstruction occasionally occurs when a portion of a laryngeal membrane is dislodged and aspirated. The membrane may extend down into the tracheobronchial tree, resulting in pneumonia and expiratory respiratory obstruction. Because of edema of the upper respiratory tract, pharyngeal and nasal diphtheria are frequently associated with secondary otitis media and sinusitis. Deep tissue invasion and bacteremia, however, are extremely rare.

The majority of deaths from diphtheria are due to the effects of absorbed diphtheria toxin on various organs, particularly the myocardium. Almost all patients with diphtheria exhibit albuminuria, but severe nephritis is rare. Other than respiratory obstruction, severe complications of diphtheria are of three types: acute systemic toxicity; myocarditis; and neurological phenomena, usually peripheral neuritis. The frequency of these various complications appears to vary considerably among epidemics, for which no clear explanation is available. In the past, it was erroneously believed that the severity of the disease could be related to strains of the organism that were morphologically different on culture, being designated *gravis*, *intermedius*, and *mitis*.[9, 10] A possible explanation for variation in reported frequency of complications is the effect of therapy with diphtheria antitoxin. It is, however, clear that the severity of the remote complications of diphtheria parallels the extent of the local disease, presumably because more extensive local disease is associated with more production and absorption of toxin.

Severe cardiac toxicity usually occurs between the third and seventh day of the illness; many investigators classify this complication as early myocarditis.[11] Others, however, believe that the effects on the myocardium are only part of diffuse systemic toxicity, including fever, purpura, peripheral circulatory collapse, restlessness, somnolence, and disturbances of carbohydrate metabolism.[12, 13] This so-called early myocarditis is usually fatal.

In either early or late myocarditis, a wide variety of clinical and electrocardiographic findings may be noted.[12] Tachycardia, distant heart sounds, and a weak pulse may be observed. Electrocardiography most often shows conduction changes and alterations in T waves. Supraventricular and ventricular ectopic rhythms are common in severe diphtheria, even in the absence of evidence of heart failure.[14] The earlier the electrocardiographic changes appear, the worse is the prognosis. Complete heart block frequently occurs and is usually fatal; ventricular pacing may not improve survival.[15] Late myocarditis usually occurs in the second week after onset, occasionally later.

Neurological complications of diphtheria largely comprise toxic peripheral neuropathy and occur in approximately 20% of cases.[16] The manifestations are more motor than sensory and usually begin 2 to 8 weeks after onset of the illness. In severe cases, palatal paralysis with consequent nasal voice and nasal regurgitation of ingested fluids may occur during the acute membranous phase, particularly with extensive pharyngeal disease, and are believed to be attributable to local effects of the toxin. With milder disease, palatal paralysis is common as late as the third week. Symmetrical peripheral neuritis of the lower extremities is a frequent neurological complication, usually occurring 3 to 10 weeks after onset of the infection. Diaphragmatic paralysis occasionally occurs, usually a month or more after onset, and may require mechanical respiratory support. Ocular paralysis, involving either the extraocular muscles or those of accommodation, sometimes appears, usually 5 or 6 weeks after onset. Fortunately, recovery from these neuropathies is the rule. Rarely, hemiplegia is observed, sometimes with complete recovery.

Invasive disease due to *C. diphtheriae* occurs as well, most commonly due to nontoxigenic strains. Bacteremia, endocarditis, osteomyelitis, and arthritis have been reported.[17–20]

Biology of the Organism and Pathogenesis of Infection

C. diphtheriae is a slender gram-positive bacillus, usually with one end being wider, thus giving the often described club-shaped appearance. On culture, particularly under suboptimal conditions, characteristic bands or granules appear. On smear, the organisms often have a "pick-up sticks" relationship, assuming parallel (palisade-like), V- or L-type patterns. The organisms are resistant to environmental changes, such as freezing and drying. There are four biotypes of *C. diphtheriae (gravis, mitis, belfanti,* and *intermedius),* which historically were identified by colonial morphology and biochemical differences; however, in practice, only the *intermedius* biotype can be reliably distinguished by colonial morphology.[21] No consistent differences are found in severity of disease caused by different biotypes.

Identified features of *C. diphtheriae* that are important in the pathogenesis of the disease in humans comprise certain cell wall antigens and in particular the organism's exotoxin. The cell wall contains a heat-stable O antigen, which is found in all corynebacteria. The cell wall also contains K antigens, which are heat-labile proteins that differ among strains of *C. diphtheriae* and therefore permit categorization of the organism into a number of types.[22] The K antigens play two roles in relation to humans: first, they appear to be important in the establishment of infection; and second, they produce local type-specific immunity. Lack of immunity to K antigens appears to be responsible for the fact that local upper respiratory tract diphtheria can occur with non–toxin-producing organisms, and toxin-producing organisms may infect persons with ample serum antitoxin levels, but neither of these instances is associated with systemic manifestations, even though a faucial membrane is produced.[23] Another factor responsible for the local invasiveness of the organism is the so-called cord factor, which is a toxic glycolipid. This glycolipid has been shown to disrupt mitochondria, depress cell respiration, and interfere with oxidative phosphorylation.[24] The term *cord factor* is derived from a similar substance found in *Mycobacterium tuberculosis* that results in the growth of the organism in serpentine coils. Undoubtedly, there are other factors as well that help *C. diphtheriae* establish residence and provide nutritional substrates.

Diphtheria Toxin

By far the most important role in the pathogenesis of diphtheria is played by the organism's exotoxin. In recent years, the basic biology of diphtheria toxin, including its production and actions, has become reasonably well understood, although some gaps remain.[25]

In brief, like many bacteria, *C. diphtheriae* is susceptible to infection with a number of bacteriophages, one or more of which (but not all) results in toxin production by the bacterium. Lysis of the bacterium is not required for toxin production. The presence of the phage is thought to confer a survival advantage to the bacterium by increasing the probability of transmission in a susceptible population; transmission may be facilitated by local tissue damage resulting from the toxin.[26, 27] The sequence of diphtheria toxin has been demonstrated to be highly conserved in *C. diphtheriae* strains, suggesting that immunologically important differences among the toxins produced by different strains are unlikely to occur.[28] Synthesis of diphtheria toxin is regulated by an iron-binding regulatory protein, which is encoded by the bacterial chromosome; maximal synthesis of diphtheria toxin occurs only under conditions of low iron concentration.[29]

Diphtheria toxin is a polypeptide with a molecular weight of about 62,000. The whole toxin is a proenzyme that is relatively inactive until it is split into two components, designated A and B. Fragment B is responsible for attachment to and penetration of the host cell but appears to be nontoxic. However, it appears to be the antigen responsible for clinical immunity. The receptor domain of fragment B binds to a cell surface receptor, heparin-binding epidermal growth factor precursor,[30] and then undergoes receptor-mediated endocytosis.[31] After penetration of the cell, fragments A and B are detached. The released fragment A is the toxic moiety and acts by inhibiting protein synthesis, resulting in cell death.[27] Unless cell penetration occurs, fragment A is inactive. Differences in the tissue distribution of the receptor may account for the differential effects of diphtheria toxin on different organs.[32]

That toxin production is mediated by bacteriophages provides an explanation for the fact that, during outbreaks of diphtheria, both toxin-producing and non–toxin-producing strains of the organism may be isolated on culture surveys. Evidence indicates that the introduction of a toxin-producing strain of *C. diphtheriae* into a community may occasionally initiate an outbreak by transfer of phage to nontoxigenic strains of the organism carried in the respiratory tracts of community inhabitants, rather than a new strain being the responsible agent.[33]

On mucous membranes, the toxin causes local cellular destruction, and the accumulated debris and fibrin result in the characteristic membrane. More important, absorbed toxin is responsible for remote manifestations affecting various organs, including the myocardium, kidneys, nervous system, and others. Because the lethality of diphtheria is almost entirely determined by the organism's toxin, clinical immunity depends primarily on the presence of antibodies to the toxin. In the presence of small amounts of formaldehyde, diphtheria toxin loses its attachment and enzymatic activities while retaining its immunogenicity, thus becoming a toxoid. This process is the basis of active immunization against diphtheria.

Protective Levels of Antitoxin

On the basis of studies of diphtheria antitoxin levels early in the course of disease, persons with diphtheria antitoxin levels of less than 0.01 IU/mL are considered susceptible.[34, 35] Probably no level of circulating antitoxin confers absolute protection; Ipsen[34] reported two cases of fatal diphtheria in patients with antitoxin levels above 30 IU/mL the day after onset of symptoms. However, the data do allow some general conclusions regarding protective levels in most circumstances. An antitoxin level of 0.01 IU/mL is the lowest level giving some degree of protection, and 0.1 is considered a protective level of circulating antitoxin. Levels of 1.0 IU/mL and above are associated with long-term protection.[36]

Other Agents Producing Diphtheria Toxin

Some strains of two other closely related *Corynebacterium* species, *C. ulcerans* and *C. pseudotuberculosis*, have been demonstrated to produce diphtheria toxin,[37] and nontoxigenic strains can be converted to toxigenic strains by infection with β-corynebacteriophage.[38] Disease indistinguishable from that caused by toxigenic strains of *C. diphtheriae* has been associated with *C. ulcerans* infection.[39–41]

Diagnosis

The diagnosis of diphtheria in the United States is rapidly becoming a lost skill because of the infrequency of the disease in recent years. However, because it continues to exhibit high incidence in other parts of the world, particularly in developing countries, and has reappeared in epidemic form in the countries of the former Soviet Union, diphtheria remains an ever-present threat. Therefore, physicians should maintain a high index of suspicion and be aware of signs and symptoms suggestive of diphtheria.

Most often the disease appears as membranous pharyngitis; a patient with confluent pharyngeal exudate should be suspected of having diphtheria until proven otherwise. The onset is usually gradual, during a day or two, and is associated with only moderate fever. Although certain clinical characteristics of membranous pharyngitis due to diphtheria, such as the color, adherence, and odor of the membrane, can be recognized as being different from other forms of exudative pharyngitis by experienced clinicians, few physicians in the United States currently have such experience; thus, to attempt to make a differential diagnosis on the clinical appearance of the lesion is foolhardy indeed.

Because laryngeal diphtheria usually occurs concomitantly with pharyngeal involvement, membranous pharyngitis with stridor should be considered to be diphtheria until proven otherwise. However, about a quarter of all cases of laryngeal diphtheria do not display a pharyngeal lesion and accordingly may be readily misdiagnosed. The differential diagnosis includes epiglottitis caused by *Haemophilus influenzae* type b, spasmodic croup, the presence of a foreign body, and viral laryngotracheitis. There should be little confusion regarding the first three because the onset and clinical characteristics of each are well known and are different from diphtheritic croup, which ordinarily is associated with gradual onset and steady progression through hoarseness to stridor during a period of 2 or 3 days. Viral laryngotracheobronchitis may be more difficult to differentiate, and if diphtheria is suspected for epidemiological or other reasons, laryngoscopy is indicated.

Nasal diphtheria may be difficult to distinguish from many other causes of nasal discharge and accordingly is most likely to be suspected if the patient has been exposed to diphtheria, such as during an outbreak. Suspicion should be heightened if a serosanguineous discharge is present and if the upper lip is ulcerated, which also occurs with streptococcal infections. Any cutaneous or mucous membrane lesions at other sites should be considered suspicious if a membrane is noted.

The complications and mortality of diphtheria are inversely related to the alacrity with which the diagnosis is made and treatment is initiated. Thus, it is critical that the diagnosis be considered, appropriate clinical specimens be obtained, and a decision made regarding administration of antitoxin as early as possible in the course of illness. In instances in which diphtheria is suspected, treatment for the disease should be initiated immediately after bacteriological specimens are procured without waiting for results; procrastination, even for a few hours, can be fatal.

Swabs for culture should be obtained under direct visualization, preferably from the edge or beneath the edge of the membrane. Swabs should be inoculated promptly onto a Loeffler or Pai slant and tellurite media and onto blood agar.[25] Directly stained smears are usually grossly misleading even in experienced hands and should not be used. Cultures should be incubated promptly and interpreted by an experienced microbiologist. Not infrequently, characteristic organisms can be identified on smears from a Loeffler slant as early as 8 hours after inoculation. Because not all *C. diphtheriae* recovered on culture are toxigenic, testing for toxin production must be carried out by the Elek immunoprecipitation test or by cutaneous testing in guinea pigs.[36, 42] In addition, the diphtheria toxin gene can be detected by the polymerase chain reaction (PCR),[43–46] which can be performed directly on clinical specimens.[47]

Several approaches to typing of strains of *C. diphtheriae* as an adjunct to epidemiological investigations have been developed. During the 1960s, Saragea and Maximescu[48] developed a system of phage typing and demonstrated considerable diversity of circulating strains in different countries. Subsequently, the utility of molecular typing methods was demonstrated in analysis of outbreak-related strains in Sweden[49] and the United States.[50] More recently, ribotyping,[51, 52] pulsed-field gel electrophoresis,[51] and multilocus enzyme electrophoresis[52] have been used for molecular subtyping, as has PCR–single-stranded conformation polymorphism (SSCP) analysis.[53] A rapid ribotyping method using PCR-SSCP has been described.[54]

EPIDEMIOLOGY

The epidemiology of diphtheria has been markedly altered in the United States and other developed countries by active immunization. Indeed, diphtheria is now reported only rarely in the United States, with only 41 cases reported during the period 1980 to 1995.[55] In the developing world, however, diphtheria remains a major problem, and only in recent years has active immunization with diphtheria toxoid been sufficiently widespread to influence the disease's epidemiology.[56]

Humans are the only natural host for *C. diphtheriae.* Thus, transmission is person to person, most likely by intimate respiratory and physical contact. The organism is reasonably hardy and has been isolated from the environment of persons infected with *C. diphtheriae.*[57–60] Nonetheless, the occurrence of indirect transmission by airborne droplet nuclei, dust, or fomites has not been established. Evidence of outbreaks due to contaminated milk and milk products has been reported.[11, 61] There is also evidence that cutaneous lesions are important in transmission.[6]

Historically, peaks in incidence approximately every 10 years or so were observed. Because of these secular trends, doubts were expressed about the efficacy of developments in prevention and treatment during this century because the apparent effects of immunization might simply have reflected the natural epidemiology of the disease[62]; these doubts no longer exist.

In temperate climates, diphtheria occurs year-round but most often during colder months, probably because of the close contact of children indoors. In tropical climates, cutaneous diphtheria is more common and is unrelated to season. Preschool and school-aged children are most often affected by respiratory diphtheria. Even before the development of active immunization, diphtheria was rare in infants younger than 6 months, presumably because of the presence of maternal antibody. Although no differences in diphtheria incidence were noted by gender in the prevaccine era, an increased risk of diphtheria among women was reported in several outbreaks among adults in the 1940s and subsequently.[63–66]

Of interest is the fact that in the past, in the absence of immunization, most persons acquired immunity to diphtheria as measured by the Schick test without experiencing clinical diphtheria. This situation is in contrast to that with pertussis, measles, rubella, and mumps, diseases that every child was expected to experience before protective vaccines became available, but is somewhat analogous to patterns of natural immunity that are acquired against polioviruses and *H. influenzae* type b, to which most persons developed clinical and serological immunity without experiencing overt disease. Transplacental antitoxic immunity to diphtheria is present at birth in most infants but declines to nonprotective levels during the second 6 months of life. Thereafter, the proportion of immune children (Schick negative) in unimmunized populations gradually increased to 75% or more, presumably owing to subclinical infection with the organism, perhaps repeated infection.[67]

In the 1990s, it is difficult to comprehend what a major cause of morbidity and mortality diphtheria was in the past. For the United States before 1900, the best data stem from Massachusetts; during the years 1860 to 1897, death rates from diphtheria ranged between 46 and 196 per 100,000 annually, with a median of 78.[68] For 8 of those years, mortality exceeded 130 per 100,000, and the proportion of total deaths attributable to diphtheria annually ranged between 3 and 10% from 1860 to 1897. By 1900, a considerable fall in death rates had occurred, and the death rate continued to decline from 40 to 15 per 100,000 for the next 20 years, presumably owing to the therapeutic use of diphtheria antitoxin and, perhaps, other measures such as intubation. But even in 1900, more than half as many deaths from diphtheria were recorded in the United States as from cancer.[68] An interesting and readable history of diphtheria in the late 19th century has been published.[8]

Excellent data on morbidity, mortality, and case-fatality rates for diphtheria are available for the Province of Ontario for 1880 to 1940 and for several Canadian cities for some of those years.[69] Case-fatality rates from diphtheria were reported to be higher than 50% during most outbreaks before the advent of diphtheria antitoxin. Case-fatality rates subsequently declined to approximately 15% by World War I, although morbidity rates did not decline. With the widespread use of diphtheria toxoid beginning in the 1930s in Canada, the disease nearly disappeared.

Since introduction of vaccination with diphtheria toxoid, a number of diphtheria outbreaks have occurred in industrial countries. During World War II, a major outbreak, apparently originating in Germany, spread throughout western Europe; well above 1 million cases were reported.[70, 71] During World War II, outbreaks linked to Europe occurred in North America as well. A major outbreak that affected nearly 1% of the population of Halifax, Nova Scotia, during the winter of 1940 to 1941 was linked to disease imported by Norwegian sailors.[72] An outbreak occurred in Alabama in 1943 among German prisoners of war.[73]

Diphtheria Since the 1950s

By the late 1950s, diphtheria was markedly reduced in the United States, but disease continued to occur in some geographical areas. To better understand the epidemiology of diphtheria, the Diphtheria Surveillance Unit was begun in 1958 at the Communicable Diseases Center (later to become the Centers for Disease Control and Prevention). During the period 1959 to 1970, 5048 cases of diphtheria were reported in the United States, with the highest incidence rates reported in the southeast, south central, and northern plains states. Incidence rates were 20-fold higher for Native Americans and 7-fold higher for blacks compared with whites.[74] There were at least 10 outbreaks of more than 15 cases during the period, including outbreaks in Austin and San Antonio, Texas, between 1967 and 1970.[75, 76]

During the following decade, diphtheria incidence continued to decline (Fig. 9–1); during the period 1971 to 1981, 853 noncutaneous and 435 cutaneous cases were reported in the United States. Incidence rates exceeded 1 per million population in South Dakota, New Mexico, Alaska, Washington, Arizona, and Montana, and incidence rates were 100-fold greater for Native Americans than for whites and blacks. There were seven outbreaks with 15 or more cases.[77] From 1972 to 1982, a large outbreak of predominantly cutaneous diphtheria occurred among residents of Skid Road in Seattle, Washington.[50, 78]

In 1980, cutaneous diphtheria ceased being nationally notifiable, and during the period 1980 to 1995, only 41 cases of respiratory diphtheria were reported.[55] With so little disease reported in the United States, it seemed likely that toxigenic strains of *C. diphtheriae* were no longer circulating in this country. However, in 1996, surveillance revealed widespread circulation of the organism in one northern Plains Indian community. Strains were assayed by ribotyping and multilocus enzyme electrophoresis and found to be closely related to strains from the same area during the period 1979 to 1983, suggesting ongoing endemic circulation.[79] Similarly, although recognized cases of diphtheria remain rare, endemic transmission of *C. diphtheriae* continues to occur in some native communities in Canada[80–82] and among the aboriginal population in central Australia.[83] The common denominator in these communities is likely to be poverty, crowding, and poor hygiene.

Although diphtheria has become a rare disease in most developed countries, a major epidemic of diphtheria began in the Russian Federation in 1990 and subsequently spread throughout the countries of the former Soviet Union (Fig. 9–2). In 1993, more than 19,000 cases were reported from the new independent states. By 1994, incidence rates exceeded 1 per 100,000 population in all of the new independent states except for Estonia. Although the causes of the epidemic remain uncertain, contributing factors included inadequate population immunity among children and adults, delayed recognition and public health response, and social conditions that facilitated spread once the outbreak began.[84] In the Russian Federation, the emergence of an epidemic clone of *C. diphtheriae* biotype *gravis* was demonstrated.[52] However, many cases were due to biotype *mitis* strains as well, especially in the new independent states of Central Asia, suggesting that microbial factors alone cannot account for the epidemic.[85] The epidemic peaked in most countries in 1995, and with increasing levels of immunization coverage with diphtheria toxoid among both children and adults, the outbreak has now begun clearly to come under control in most of the countries of the former Soviet Union (see additional discussion in the *Results of Immunization* section).[86]

As noted earlier, the precise microbial events responsible for the transmission of diphtheria are unclear. Whether toxigenic bacteria are communicated from one individual to another, whether the mechanism comprises

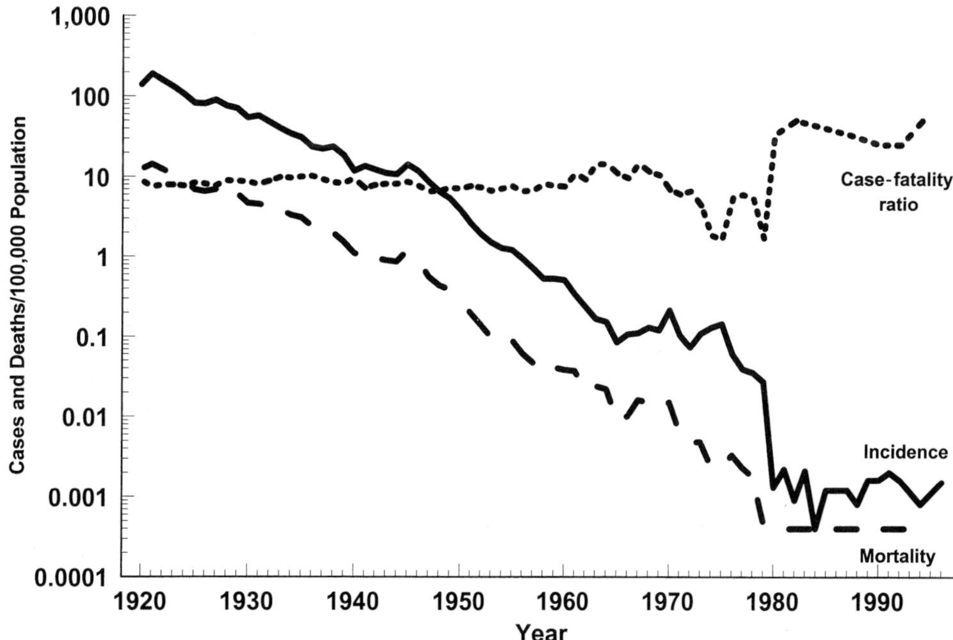

Figure 9–1. Diphtheria incidence, mortality rates, and case-fatality ratios in the United States, 1920 to 1996.

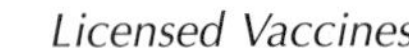

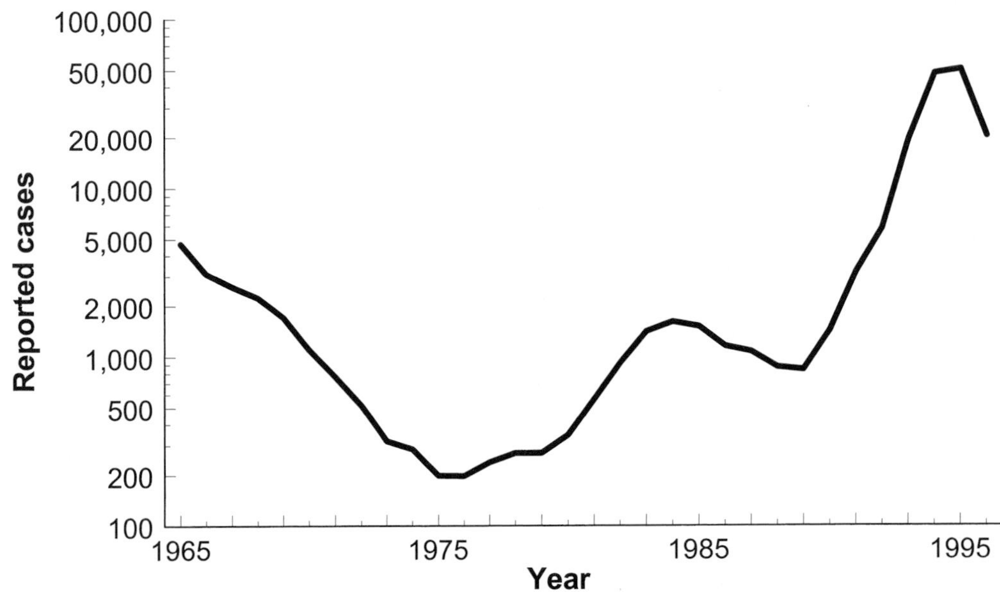

Figure 9–2. Reported cases of diphtheria, by year, Soviet Union (1965 to 1990) and new independent states of the former Soviet Union (1991 to 1996).

the transfer of bacteriophages governing toxin production from an infected person to carriers of nontoxigenic strains, or whether both mechanisms are important is unknown. Although no animal reservoir exists for *C. diphtheriae*, *C. ulcerans* may carry the β-corynebacteriophage that encodes diphtheria toxin,[87] and an animal reservoir does exist for this organism[88, 89]—and thus for the bacteriophage. Given the worldwide ubiquity of carriage of *C. diphtheriae* and the bacteriophages implicated in toxin production, prospects for eradication of diphtheria currently seem remote indeed. Therefore, continuing active immunization with diphtheria toxoid is the key to the control of diphtheria.

PASSIVE IMMUNIZATION

The history of the development of diphtheria antitoxin has been reviewed in detail by Andrewes and colleagues.[2] In brief, Roux and Yersin in 1888 reported their observation that bacteria-free filtrates of broth cultures of *C. diphtheriae*, when injected into animals, produced all of the manifestations of diphtheria except for the membranous local lesions.[89a] In rapid succession, other advances followed; von Behring showed that inactivated cultures of the organism injected into animals ultimately rendered them protected against living cultures, at first not recognizing the fact that the organisms themselves were unnecessary for immunity.[89b] Ultimately, von Behring demonstrated the transfer of protection from an immunized animal to another by serum. Diphtheria antitoxin was first given to a child in 1891, and antitoxin was commercially produced in Germany in 1892. The use of horses for the production of antitoxin began in 1894. Worthy of note is the fact that the lack of regulated standards for the production of equine diphtheria antitoxin, which resulted in the release of contaminated antisera and the inevitable appearance of charlatans who prepared and sold similar-appearing colored water, contributed to the development of the legislated predecessors of the present Center for Biologics Evaluation and Research of the United States Food and Drug Administration (FDA).[90, 91]

Equine diphtheria antitoxin is prepared by hyperimmunizing horses with diphtheria toxoid and toxin.[91] To diminish reactivity from horse serum, current preparations are semipurified by techniques that concentrate immunoglobulin G and remove as much extraneous protein as possible. There must be at least 500 units of antitoxin per milliliter, and sterility is attained by microfiltration. A cresol derivative is added as a preservative.

Diphtheria antitoxin is used for the treatment of diphtheria and occasionally, in the past, for the prevention in exposed persons. Its therapeutic efficacy is well established, although it is in no way a substitute for prior active immunization with diphtheria toxoid. No antiserum or hyperimmune globulin of human origin is currently available.

As of January 6, 1997, licensed diphtheria antitoxin with a valid expiration date was no longer available in the United States, and no manufacturer proposed to produce it. However, for treatment of the disease in the United States, the Centers for Disease Control and Prevention has a supply of European antitoxin (Pasteur Mérieux, Lyon, France) that can be distributed for treatment under an investigational new drug protocol.[92] This antitoxin is comparable to the prior U.S. product and may be requested by calling 404-639-8255 during working hours or 404-639-2889 at night and weekends.

Effectiveness of Antitoxin

The value of antitoxin in prophylaxis is dubious. Theoretically, it should be useful in preventing the establishment of infection in exposed, susceptible persons because the toxin plays a role in local invasiveness. However, there is no acceptable clinical evidence of prophylactic efficacy; all that exist are anecdotes and small, uncontrolled series of experiments.[2] Even if it were effective, antitoxin would be of little use in controlling community outbreaks because asymptomatic carriers, rather than persons with overt disease, are usually the major source of transmission.[93] For these reasons, antitoxin is not recommended for exposed, susceptible persons, particularly in view of the high rates of subsequent serum sickness and occasional anaphylaxis. The preferred treatment for exposed, unimmunized, asymptomatic persons is to obtain a throat culture, begin immunization with a preparation containing diphtheria toxoid that is appropriate for age, and institute prophylaxis with erythromycin or penicillin for 7 days, during which time the patient must be kept under surveillance.[94]

Many studies, too numerous to cite here, have demonstrated the efficacy of therapy with antitoxin in reducing mortality from diphtheria primarily by preventing cardiovascular toxicity.[3, 95] However, only a single controlled therapeutic trial is discussed in the literature.[96, 97] This nonblinded trial consisted of treating all patients admitted on alternate days with antitoxin and comparing their outcomes with those of patients admitted on nontreatment days. Eight (3.3%) of 242 patients treated with antitoxin died compared with 30 (12.2%) of 245 control subjects. In addition, many observations of the direct relationship between mortality and day of disease when antitoxin was administered provide ample evidence of its efficacy. Table 9–1 portrays two examples of such data.

Similarly, among 3558 patients observed by Ker,[95] 320 cases of paralysis occurred. There was a strong direct relationship between the frequency of postdiphtheritic paralysis and the number of days between onset of illness and administration of antitoxin. Only 4.8% of 1168 patients developed paralyses when antitoxin was administered no later than the second day of illness, in contrast to 12.1% of 1375 patients who received antitoxin on the fourth day of the disease or later.

Table 9–1. **RELATIONSHIP BETWEEN MORTALITY FROM DIPHTHERIA AND DAY OF ILLNESS WHEN ANTITOXIN WAS FIRST GIVEN**

DAY OF ILLNESS ANTITOXIN GIVEN	UNITED KINGDOM		LOS ANGELES	
	Cases	Deaths (%)	Cases	Deaths (%)
1	329	1.5	235	4.2
2	2269	3.4	249	5.2
3	2407	6.9	273	9.2
4	1612	10.9	203	10.8
5	911	14.9	157	13.4
6	416	13.0	64	12.3
7	320	16.6	112	12.5
Later	327	15.3	104	20.2
Total	8591	8.3	1397	9.6

Adapted by permission of Oxford University Press from Ker CB. Infectious Diseases, A Practical Textbook (3rd ed). London, Oxford University Press, 1929, p 423; and Naiditch MJ, Bower AG. Diphtheria. A study of 1,433 cases observed during a ten-year period at Los Angeles County Hospital. Am J Med 17:229–245, 1954.

Treatment of Diphtheria

Unfortunately, toxin that has already entered host cells is not affected by antitoxin; for this reason, the entire therapeutic dose should be administered at one time. Antitoxin is given intramuscularly or intravenously; many authorities prefer the intravenous route for at least part of the dose because a therapeutic blood level can be reached more rapidly.[98] The amount of antitoxin recommended varies between 20,000 and 120,000 units. Larger amounts are recommended for persons with extensive local lesions, because the amount of toxin produced depends on the size of the membrane. Further, the longer the interval since onset, the higher should be the dose of antitoxin.

Although diphtheria antitoxin is the mainstay of diphtheria therapy, penicillin or, alternatively, erythromycin should be given to hasten clearance of the organism[94]; antimicrobial agents are *not* a substitute for antitoxin. Treatment should be continued until at least three consecutive daily cultures fail to demonstrate *C. diphtheriae*. Before the development of antibiotic therapy, convalescent carriage of toxigenic organisms was a major problem. Up to 50 and 25% of patients continued to harbor the organism 2 and 4 weeks after onset, respectively. As late as 2 months after onset, reported carriage rates varied between 1 and 8%.[2] Long-term convalescent carriers were often subjected to tonsillectomy, probably with some effect.[99]

Although treatment with penicillin or erythromycin has no apparent effect on the clinical course of the disease, in most instances the organism can no longer be recovered on culture within a week; subsequent convalescent carriage is thus uncommon. Patients who continue to harbor the organism after treatment with either penicillin or erythromycin should receive an additional 10-day course of oral erythromycin, and specimens for follow-up cultures should be obtained.[94]

ACTIVE IMMUNIZATION

History

Subsequent to the investigations that led to the discovery of diphtheria toxin and the development of antitoxin in the 19th century, the development of current diphtheria toxoid was facilitated almost entirely by three important advances. The first of these was the discovery that balanced mixtures of toxin and antitoxin successfully immunized both animals and humans after injection.[100, 101] However, a preparation designed to provide active immunity against diphtheria would be of little utility unless some means of assessing the presence of such immunity were available. Fortunately, a reasonably simple and fairly accurate skin test (the Schick test) was developed almost simultaneously.[102] The third innovative step was the development of diphtheria toxoid a decade later.[103]

The combination preparation, toxin-antitoxin, was rapidly accepted as an active immunizing agent. It was widely used in the United States beginning in 1914 and was found to protect approximately 85% of recipients.[104]

There is little question that the toxin-antitoxin preparation developed by von Behring created active immunity against diphtheria, in spite of the absence of well-controlled studies, on the basis of the results of Schick testing and clinical observation.[2] Obviously, a major problem with active immunization with toxin-antitoxin is the likelihood of inducing sensitivity to horse serum, and undoubtedly many individuals in the United States and Europe, now in their 60s or older, are allergic to horse serum for this reason.

The Schick test consists of the intradermal injection of a minute amount of diphtheria toxin. The test result is ordinarily read after 48 hours; erythema and induration of 1 cm or more indicates susceptibility to diphtheria. Unfortunately, the results of the test are not that simple to interpret. Extraneous proteins in Schick test materials often produce false-positive reactions, and accordingly, a simultaneous injection of the same material, treated with heat to destroy the toxin, is required to assess sensitivity to extraneous proteins. Excellent descriptions of the Schick test and its interpretation are available in older texts.[2, 105] Because the correlation between results of the Schick test and clinical immunity to diphtheria is reasonable, although not perfect, the test served for many years as an acceptable surrogate for clinical immunity to diphtheria. It is rarely used in the United States at present.

The third major innovation was the development of diphtheria toxoid.[103] Ramon treated diphtheria toxin with small amounts of formalin and found that the product retained most of its immunizing capacity while losing its toxic properties. Ramon dubbed this preparation *anatoxine;* this name has since been replaced with the term *toxoid.* For primary immunization, the toxin-antitoxin preparation was gradually replaced by toxoid in the United States and Canada during the next 15 years and elsewhere thereafter. In 1926, Glenny and coworkers[106] found that alum-precipitated toxoid was more immunogenic, and by the mid-1940s, diphtheria toxoid was combined with tetanus toxoid and pertussis vaccine as the now-familiar diphtheria and tetanus toxoids and whole-cell pertussis vaccine (DTP). Adsorption of all three onto an aluminum salt followed shortly thereafter. It is clear that the immunogenicity of diphtheria toxoid, as well as that of tetanus toxoid, is enhanced by the adjuvant effects of both pertussis vaccine and the aluminum salt.[107–109] In recent years, diphtheria and tetanus toxoids with acellular pertussis components (DTaP) have been licensed, and various other combinations of DTaP with *H. influenzae* b (Hib) vaccine, inactivated poliovirus vaccine, and hepatitis B vaccine have been developed.[110]

Current Production

At present, diphtheria toxoid is produced worldwide in a standard fashion; in the United States, production and testing procedures are specified in the Code of Federal Regulations. Specifically, a strain of *C. diphtheriae* that is known to produce large amounts of toxin is grown in a liquid medium conducive to toxin production. After appropriate incubation, sterilization is achieved by centrifugation and filtration. After ascertainment of potency, the filtrate is incubated with formalin for conversion of toxin to toxoid. The product is then further purified and concentrated to achieve the necessary dosage. It is adsorbed onto an aluminum salt, usually aluminum phosphate, and thimerosal is added as a preservative. Appropriate tests for potency, toxicity, and sterility are conducted both by the manufacturer and by the FDA. Potency worldwide is ascertained by determining the content of flocculating units (Lf) in established fashion; 1 Lf is the amount of toxoid that flocculates 1 unit of a standard reference diphtheria antitoxin.

Currently in the United States, diphtheria toxoid is available in combination with tetanus toxoid and in combination with tetanus toxoid and pertussis vaccine. The product is available only in adsorbed form.

The preferred diphtheria toxoid preparation for children is now DTaP, although use of DTP remains acceptable. As of August 1998, DTaP vaccines from four manufacturers are licensed for use in infants in the United States (Tripedia, distributed by Connaught Laboratories, Inc.; ACEL-IMUNE, distributed by Wyeth-Lederle Vaccines and Pediatrics; Infanrix, distributed by SmithKline Beecham Pharmaceuticals; and Certiva, distributed by North American Vaccine, Inc). DTP vaccines from Connaught Laboratories, Inc., and Wyeth-Lederle Vaccines and Pediatrics continue to be distributed nationally. Until recently, the Massachusetts Public Health Biologic Laboratories and the Michigan Department of Public Health both manufactured DTP and its component vaccines, but both states have ceased production of DTP since licensure of DTaP vaccines for use in infants. One acellular DTP product combined with conjugated Hib vaccine is currently licensed (Connaught Laboratories, Inc.) for use as the fourth dose in the DTaP and Hib vaccine series, and two combined DTP-Hib products are still distributed (Tetramune, Wyeth-Lederle Vaccines and Pediatrics, and ActHIB, Connaught Laboratories, Inc.). The amounts of diphtheria toxoid in the DTaP vaccines currently licensed in the United States range from 6.7 to 25 Lf per 0.5 mL dose. They provide levels of serum antitoxin considerably lower than those after receipt of whole-cell DTP, probably reflecting the adjuvant effect of the whole-cell pertussis component.[111] However, the lower antitoxin levels induced by vaccination with DTaP are probably of no clinical consequence, being manyfold higher than protective levels.[110] For routine immunization of children, five doses are recommended (at 2, 4, 6, and 15 to 18 months and at school entry before the seventh birthday). The fourth dose should be administered at least 6 months after the third dose.[112]

DTaP or DTP is ordinarily not given to children younger than 6 weeks because responses to pertussis vaccine in the young infant are suboptimal; responses to tetanus and diphtheria toxoids, however, are satisfactory in such young infants regardless of the presence of maternally derived serum antibody and without induction of immunological tolerance.[113] The optimal age for immunization of premature infants cannot be stated with confidence, although one small study indicates that satisfactory responses are achieved by initiating the usual DTP series at 2 months of age regardless of pregnancy duration.[114] There is evidence that high titers of transplacental antibody to diphtheria toxin inhibit serological responses to the first two doses of diphtheria toxoid in infants; but after the third dose (administered in the Swedish schedule at 12 months of age), the effect is no longer evident.[115]

Diphtheria and tetanus toxoids, adsorbed, for pediatric use (DT) is recommended for the primary immunization of children younger than 7 years in whom pertussis vaccine is contraindicated. DT contains 10 to 12 Lf of diphtheria toxoid; infants who begin the series before 1 year of age should receive DT at 2, 4, 6, and 15 to 18 months of age. Satisfactory responses are obtained even in the absence of the adjuvant effect of pertussis vaccine.[116, 117] For unimmunized children 1 to 7 years of age, two doses 2 months apart and a third dose 6 to 12 months later constitute primary immunization.[118]

Tetanus and diphtheria toxoids, adsorbed, for adult use (Td) contains approximately the same amount of tetanus toxoid as do DTP and DT, but the amount of diphtheria toxoid is reduced to no more than 2 Lf per dose. This reduction minimizes reactivity in persons who may have been sensitized previously to diphtheria toxoid and is sufficient to provoke satisfactory anamnestic responses in previously immunized persons. In addition, in previously unimmunized older children and adults, Td is satisfactory for primary immunization,[119, 120] administered as a three-dose series, with the second dose given 4 to 8 weeks after the first dose and the third dose 6 to 12 months after the second dose.[118] Td should be administered approximately every 10 years after the completion of childhood immunization. Although Td is slightly more reactive than tetanus toxoid alone,[121] it is preferable to monovalent tetanus toxoid for prophylaxis of tetanus after wounds to maintain satisfactory population immunity against diphtheria. In the United States, DT and Td are distributed by three companies: Wyeth-Lederle, Pasteur Mérieux Connaught, and SmithKline Beecham. Monovalent diphtheria toxoid is no longer marketed in the United States.

Limited data regarding simultaneous administration of the first three doses of DTaP with other childhood vaccines indicate no interference with response to the diphtheria toxoid component. Data are available regarding administration of DTaP with other vaccines recommended at the same time as the fourth and fifth doses of the diphtheria, tetanus, and pertussis series (i.e., Hib conjugate vaccine, oral poliovirus vaccine, measles-mumps-rubella vaccine, and varicella vaccine) and regarding administration of whole-cell DTP (all doses in the series) with these vaccines.[122] DTaP may be administered simultaneously with hepatitis B vaccine, Hib vaccine, and inactivated or oral poliovirus vaccines to infants at ages 2, 4, or 6 months.[112]

Preparations containing diphtheria toxoid should always be injected intramuscularly, not subcutaneously. As with tetanus toxoid and pertussis vaccine, prolonging the interval between doses does not require restarting the series; indeed, immunity achieved after longer intervals between doses than those recommended is at least as good as that following the regular schedule, although the subject may be unprotected in the interim. Preparations containing diphtheria toxoid should be stored at usual refrigerator temperatures but not frozen.

In other countries, DTP is administered according to alternative schedules (see Chapters 43 and 44). According to the recommended schedule for the World Health Organization's Expanded Programme on Immunization (EPI), DTP is administered at 6, 10, and 14 weeks without additional doses. In a number of European countries, two doses of DTP or DTaP are administered early in the first year of life, followed by a third dose late in the first year or early in the second year of life. Recommendations regarding subsequent boosters vary by country. In response to the recent epidemic of diphtheria in the former Soviet Union, booster doses have been recommended or reinstated in a number of countries outside the former Soviet Union.

Results of Immunization

No controlled clinical trial, acceptable by today's scientific standards, of the efficacy of the toxoid in preventing diphtheria has ever been conducted for three reasons. First, given the serious nature of the disease and the clear perception of benefit first from the toxin-antitoxin combination and subsequently from the toxoid, its value seemed obvious to early investigators. Second, the development of surrogate approaches to assessing immunity (the Schick test and serological methods) made such trials unnecessary. Third, the early appearance of strong presumptive evidence that the toxin-antitoxin preparation and the toxoid were effective made such trials unethical.

In spite of the lack of a controlled clinical trial, ample evidence exists that diphtheria toxoid prevents clinical disease in the majority of recipients and controls the disease from the public health standpoint. First is the nearly complete disappearance of the disease in countries in which immunization has been widely employed. Second is the fact that during outbreaks of diphtheria, rates of disease are negligible among immunized persons. Third, when partially or, rarely, fully immunized individuals acquire diphtheria, the disease is milder and complications are fewer. Fourth, a good correlation has been established between clinical protection and the presence of serum antibody to the toxin, whether resulting from disease or immunization.

After three doses of diphtheria toxoid, virtually all infants develop diphtheria titers greater than 0.01 IU per mL.[122a] Geometric mean titers vary among vaccine preparations, with some DTaP products producing significantly lower geometric mean titers than those observed after vaccination with DTP[111]; however, these differences are unlikely to be clinically significant. When the toxoid is used for primary immunization of adults, data suggest that virtually all adults develop diphtheria antitoxin titers greater than 0.01 IU per mL after administration of three doses of diphtheria toxoid and that most develop titers greater than 0.1 IU per mL.[119]

There is solid circumstantial evidence, too vast to review here, that the introduction and widespread use of diphtheria toxoid immunization in populations are associated with a remarkable decline in morbidity and mortality from the disease.[3, 69, 77] These temporal trends and the near disappearance of diphtheria in developed countries are far too striking to be attributed to secular fluctuations in the disease or to better therapy.

Further, before the World Health Organization's EPI began, it was estimated that close to a million cases of diphtheria occurred annually in the Third World with 50,000 to 60,000 deaths.[123] From 1980 to 1996, reported cases of diphtheria globally decreased from 97,811 to 25,653. The reduction in morbidity during this period would have been more dramatic without the outbreak in the former Soviet Union; almost 80% of cases worldwide in 1996 were reported from the European Region[124] (Fig. 9–3). Under EPI, the goal is to achieve 90% or more immunization of 1-year-old children by the year 2000; by 1996, it was estimated that the proportion who had received three doses of diphtheria toxoid in combination with tetanus toxoid and pertussis vaccine had risen from negligible levels in the early 1970s to 80% worldwide, with Africa being the lowest at approximately 54%.[124]

Effectiveness in Epidemiological Studies

Although in most outbreaks of diphtheria the prevalence of prior immunization in persons who escape the disease is not known, a few studies have sufficient data to allow estimates of the degree of protection offered by the toxoid. Some evidence of the protective efficacy of diphtheria toxoid is provided by observations during the Halifax epidemic.[72] During the course of this outbreak, an intense effort was made to administer diphtheria toxoid to previously unimmunized individuals, and comparisons of the subsequent incidence of diphtheria in these children were made with the incidence in the unimmunized population during the next few months. Among those immunized, the monthly incidence of diphtheria fell to 24.5 per 100,000, about one seventh of the rate of 168.9 per 100,000 in the unimmunized during that same period. In Britain in 1943, the rate of clinical diphtheria among the unimmunized was 3.5 times that among the immunized, and mortality was 25-fold greater.[71] In an outbreak in Elgin, Texas, in 1970, only 2 of 205 fully immunized, exposed elementary schoolchildren acquired the disease.[125] In contrast, among 97 children who had received inadequate or no immunization, a 13% attack rate occurred.

In a household study during a diphtheria outbreak in San Antonio, Texas, in 1970, vaccine efficacy was estimated at only 54%.[76] However, because index cases were included and denominators of exposed individuals were unknown, the data are difficult to interpret. Further, any differences in attack rates between immunized and nonimmunized individuals might have been blunted by the institution of antibiotic therapy to all members of the household on recognition of a case. Thus, the apparent efficacy of 54% is probably low. In an outbreak in Yemen, the protective efficacy of diphtheria toxoid was determined to be 87% by the case-control method.[61]

The effectiveness of Russian-manufactured diphtheria toxoid was evaluated in several case-control studies during the recent epidemic in the former Soviet Union. Three or more doses of diphtheria toxoid were demonstrated to be highly effective in prevention of diphtheria among children younger than 15 years in a preliminary study in Ukraine in 1992 and a subsequent study performed in Moscow in 1993. In Moscow, the effectiveness of three or more doses was 95.5% (95% confidence interval, 92.1–97.4%), increasing to 98.4% for five or more doses (95% confidence interval, 96.5–99.3%).[126] In addition, administration of a booster dose of diphtheria toxoid within 2 years was shown to decrease risk of diphtheria among children 6 to 8 years of age compared with those who had received the last dose 3 to 4 or 5 to 7 years previously.[127]

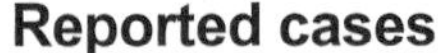

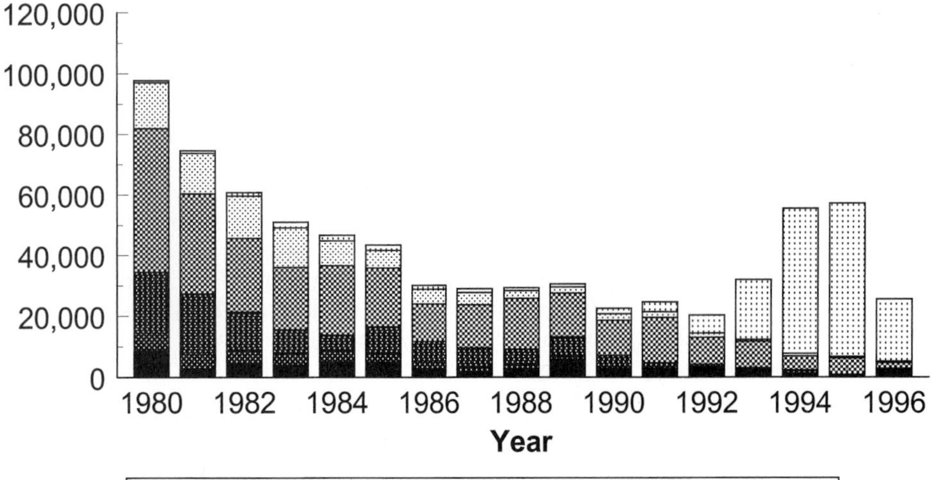

Figure 9–3. Reported cases of diphtheria, by year and by region, 1980 to 1996. AFR, African Region; AMR, American Region; EMR, Eastern Mediterranean Region; SEAR, Southeast Asia Region; WPR, Western Pacific Region; EUR, European Region. (From Expanded Programme on Immunization. EPI Information System. Global Summary, August 1997. Geneva, World Health Organization, 1997, p 14.)

Thus, it appears that the protective efficacy of diphtheria toxoid, as measured by incidence of the disease in immunized and unimmunized individuals during outbreaks, is high although not 100%. However, most reports indicate that the disease in previously immunized individuals is milder and less likely to be fatal.[69, 71, 77, 123, 125, 128–130] In Britain in 1943, case-fatality rates in unimmunized children were more than sevenfold greater than rates in those who had been immunized (6.4% versus 0.9%).[71] The failure to protect 100% of individuals on exposure indicates the importance of herd immunity in the disappearance of diphtheria from developed countries.[131]

No prospective study has been conducted of the incidence of diphtheria among persons who are Schick negative compared with those who are Schick positive during an epidemic. However, many studies have shown that the age-specific incidence of diphtheria, whether endemic or epidemic, is inversely related to the proportion of Schick-negative individuals by age. In addition, there is a correlation between Schick negativity and serum antitoxin levels; an antitoxin titer of 0.01 to 0.02 units/mL is usually associated with a negative Schick test response.

Duration of Immunity

Persistence of immunity after immunization with diphtheria toxoid has been of some concern in recent years, particularly in developed countries. This concern arose from the results of serological surveys for immunity to diphtheria that were conducted in response to localized outbreaks of the disease that occurred in Sweden in particular but also in England and elsewhere in Europe.[132, 133] The results of these serological studies, which suggest considerable susceptibility in adult populations, are difficult to assess and have yielded varying opinions about waning immunity and the necessity for booster doses beyond childhood.[133–147]

The reasons for difficulties in assessing and interpreting these studies from different regions include such factors as the lack of comparable data for the same or similar populations from the past, the varied immunization schedules among countries and for different time periods in the same nation, the effect of immunization during military service, and the unknown effects of natural exposure to toxigenic *C. diphtheriae.* In addition, uncertainties exist about the frequency of such exposure, the inclusion of immunized and unimmunized subjects (including the lack of information about prior immunization), dissimilar serological criteria for classifying persons as immune, and, in some instances, possible differences in laboratory methods.

In spite of these problems, a review of serological studies of adults from 1978 to the present indicates that approximately half of all adults in Europe and the United States are not optimally protected from diphtheria as indicated by antitoxin titers of less than 0.1 IU/mL. Indeed, in two areas (Los Angeles and Sweden), most or many of these subjects displayed titers of less than 0.01 IU/mL.[134, 141] There were striking variations among sites, undoubtedly owing to the factors listed previously. A distinct trend seems to be an increasing serosusceptibility with advancing age. Some studies also demonstrated less susceptibility among males, probably because of immunization during military service.

Nonetheless, it may be hypothesized that the reason that these low levels of immunity in adults have been associated only with small focal outbreaks of diphtheria in recent years is a form of herd immunity due to high levels of immunity in children. It has been generally accepted that 70% or more of a childhood population must be immune to diphtheria to prevent major community outbreaks,[97] but this is an oversimplification of a more complex issue.[131] Whether an epidemic of a given infectious disease occurs is influenced by a number of factors other than the proportion of susceptible persons in the population, including the age distribution of immune and susceptible persons, the extent of mixing of individuals and subgroups in the community, and the infectivity and routes of transmission of the organism. In countries with high rates of childhood immunization against diphtheria, it may well be that epidemics do not occur among adults, up to half of whom may be susceptible, because the reservoir of disease in the childhood population has been eliminated and because the strains of *C. diphtheriae* circulating in the community are less likely to be toxigenic. Nonetheless, although there is disagreement, the proportion of susceptible adults is of sufficient concern that most authorities recommend maintenance of diphtheria immunity by periodic reinforcement with use of Td.[148]

These concerns have been heightened by the recent epidemic of diphtheria in the former Soviet Union. A striking feature of this epidemic was the proportion of cases occurring among adults, varying from 38% in Azerbaijan to 82% in Latvia and Lithuania in 1994.[84] Before 1986, the last dose of diphtheria toxoid was routinely administered at 14 to 16 years of age in the Soviet Union; in response to an increase in reported cases of diphtheria in the early 1980s, targeted vaccination of certain occupational groups was initiated, but routine use of booster vaccinations among adults was not recommended. Immunogenicity studies in Russia and Ukraine demonstrated that some adults failed to develop a booster response to a single dose of diphtheria toxoid, suggesting that they may never have received an effective primary series in childhood.[149, 150] Childhood immunization coverage was low in some regions in the late 1980s and early 1990s, and this undoubtedly contributed to the epidemic.[151] For control of the epidemic, the World Health Organization recommended identification, isolation, and appropriate treatment of all cases; prevention of secondary cases by optimum management of close contacts of cases; and rapidly increasing population immunity by sustaining high coverage among children with four doses of DTP in all districts and administering a single dose of an age-appropriate formulation of diphtheria toxoid to the entire population.[84] By 1997, all countries had made significant progress in immunization of children and adults; in countries that had achieved high coverage, the declines in disease incidence were most dramatic.[86]

Although the factors that allowed this epidemic to occur are not completely understood, it is apparent that under the right combination of conditions, epidemic diphtheria can occur in industrialized countries. Notably, the outbreak occurred in spite of high vaccine coverage with a primary series among school-aged children. Many of the cases occurred among adults. A large proportion of the population of adults, although seronegative, was previously primed by prior immunization or infection with toxigenic *C. diphtheriae*, as evidenced by development of protective titers after a single booster dose of toxoid. Although the immunization histories of the adult cases were difficult to ascertain, the overall population data suggest that many probably had been immune but lost immunity over time. With implementation of booster vaccination for all age groups, the outbreak has come under control. The experience of this massive epidemic strongly suggests that sustaining high immunization coverage with a primary series of diphtheria toxoid among infants and administering booster doses at school entry and subsequently throughout life are important for maintenance of population immunity.

Untoward Effects of Diphtheria Toxoid

Initial efforts to administer recall doses of diphtheria toxoid to older children and adults more than 40 years ago were associated with unacceptably high rates of local and systemic reactions, sometimes sufficient to incapacitate the individual for several days.[152] Such individuals often reacted strongly on Schick testing to both the test and the control material; if the physician failed to include the control, such an individual would be deemed to be strongly Schick positive and therefore be given a booster dose of toxoid, usually with unpleasant results. These reactions appeared to be of the delayed hypersensitivity (tuberculin) type.

One approach to this problem was to try to identify hypersensitive persons by the so-called Moloney test, which consists of the injection of a small amount of diphtheria toxoid intradermally.[153] Local reactivity was interpreted as predictive of moderate to severe sensitivity to the toxoid and therefore deemed to be a contraindication. General use of the Moloney test before administration of a reinforcing dose is obviously impractical both logistically and economically, and it is no longer recommended and rarely, if ever, used.

The solution to the problem of hyperreactivity to diphtheria toxoid lay in three measures.[154] These were enhanced purification of the toxoid to remove extraneous proteins,[155–157] adsorption of the toxoid onto an aluminum salt,[158] and reduction of the amount of diphtheria toxoid per inoculation to 1 to 2 Lf, an amount shown to be sufficient as a reinforcing dose in a number of studies.[156, 159] Aluminum salts as adjuvants also enhance antibody production.[109] These and similar developments led to current recommendations for periodic reinforcement of diphtheria immunity in older children and adults.[148] Further, it has been shown that older children and adults respond satisfactorily to primary immunization with Td,[119, 120] and even the elderly respond well to small doses of diphtheria toxoid.[142] Almost all physicians are aware of the importance of tetanus prophylaxis for wounds. Fewer, however, are cognizant of the potential public health benefit from including a concomitant diphtheria booster when a tetanus booster is indicated for an injury. The use of Td, rather than monovalent tetanus toxoid, should be standard operating procedure in emergency departments, physicians' offices, and other situations in which tetanus-prone wounds are treated.[148, 160] There are essentially no indications for monovalent tetanus toxoid at present in the United States or elsewhere.

Extensive data on adverse reactions after administration of currently available preparations of diphtheria toxoid, adsorbed, are not available because the toxoid is usually administered in combination with tetanus toxoid and, in children, with pertussis vaccine as well. When it is given in combination with pertussis vaccine, local reactions are often ascribed to the pertussis-containing component. In several large clinical trials, the reactogenicity of DT was compared with that of DTaP for primary vaccination of infants. In general, the frequency of reported common systemic symptoms (i.e., temperature of 38°C or higher, crying for 1 hour or longer, irritability, drowsiness, loss of appetite, vomiting) and local reactions (i.e., redness, swelling, tenderness) after vaccination with DT or DTaP was comparable.[161–164] In clinical trials in Sweden and Italy, DT containing 15 or 25 Lf of diphtheria toxoid and 3.75 or 10 Lf of tetanus toxoid, respectively, were given to more than 7000 infants. The frequency of temperature of 38°C or higher after any vaccine dose was 35% in the Swedish trial and 9% in the Italian study. Other common systemic symptoms occurred with similar frequency in the two studies: crying for 1 hour or longer in 5% and 6%, irritability in 67% and 55%, drowsiness in 54% and 43%, loss of appetite in 22% and 26%, and vomiting in 15% and 9%. Redness and tenderness after any vaccine dose was reported in 42% and 22%, respectively, of infants in the Swedish trial, and in 19% and 9%, respectively, in the Italian trial; the frequency of marked redness or swelling was substantially lower in both studies, with redness and swelling of 2 cm or more reported in only 4% and 6% of infants in the Swedish trial.[161, 162, 165] The frequency of adverse reactions after DT increased with increasing dose number.[163, 164]

Available data suggest that both diphtheria and tetanus toxoids contribute to the reactogenicity of Td and DT. Among Swedish medical personnel with a history of receipt of previous primary immunization in childhood, adverse events (i.e., local tenderness and swelling >5 cm or general discomfort) were reported by 11% of those who received 2.5 Lf of diphtheria toxoid, compared with 20% of those who received 2.5 Lf of diphtheria toxoid combined with 0.75 Lf of tetanus toxoid, documenting the additive effects of the two toxoids.[166] Data from several controlled studies suggest that fever and local reactions are more common after administration of Td than after tetanus toxoid.[121, 167] Reports of adverse events to the Vaccine Adverse Events Reporting System are significantly higher after Td compared with tetanus toxoid, although the overall rate for either vaccine is low

(49.5 per million doses of Td and 23.7 per million doses of tetanus toxoid).[168] The highest rates were for local reactions, which were higher in Td recipients.

In some populations, large numbers of previously primed persons develop local reactions and fever to diphtheria toxoid, even at low doses. In a small study of Israeli military recruits who had been previously vaccinated in childhood, mild to moderate pain at the injection site was reported by 38% and severe pain by 20% after receipt of a booster dose of 2 Lf diphtheria toxoid without tetanus toxoid; limitation of abduction was reported by 8%. Systemic symptoms of mild to moderate or severe weakness were reported by 24% and 9%, respectively, and fever of 38°C or higher was reported by a single subject (<1%).[169] Similarly, a booster dose of 1.5 Lf was administered to 215 university students with prevaccination diphtheria antitoxin levels of less than 0.1 IU/mL. Eight percent reported tenderness at the injection site, and 13% reported pain with abduction, which was marked in 2% of subjects; none had erythema or swelling noted on examination.[170]

With current formulations of diphtheria toxoid, the frequency of reported adverse events varies by prior vaccination history, prevaccination diphtheria antitoxin level, and dose of diphtheria toxoid administered. Among 123 persons 30 to 70 years of age with diphtheria antitoxin levels of 0.05 IU/mL or less, adverse events after vaccination were more severe among those who received 12 Lf of diphtheria toxoid as a booster, compared with those who received doses of 5 Lf or 2 Lf, supporting the recommendation to administer reduced doses of diphtheria toxoid to adults. All vaccines were administered without tetanus toxoid.[171] A second study in military recruits 18 to 25 years of age, most of whom had documentation of receipt of a complete primary vaccination series in childhood, also showed no differences in adverse events between doses of 5 Lf and 2 Lf of diphtheria toxoid combined with tetanus toxoid.[172]

Use of adsorbed vaccine for primary immunization has been reported to result in higher rates of local adverse reactions after subsequent booster vaccination. A higher incidence of local reactions after booster vaccination with DT was observed among Swedish schoolchildren who received adsorbed DT for primary immunization in infancy compared with those who had received nonadsorbed fluid DTP. Seventy-three percent of children who had been primed with DT reported redness, 56% swelling, and 47% itching, compared with 23%, 15%, and 21%, respectively, among those who had received DTP.[173] In contrast, local reactions did not differ among children who had received adsorbed DT for the primary series and then were boosted with either adsorbed or nonadsorbed DT.[174, 175]

The potential for anaphylaxis exists with any protein antigen, but such has not been attributed to diphtheria toxoid. Curiously, the British National Childhood Encephalopathy Study, designed to examine the incidence of brain damage after the administeration of pertussis vaccine, showed a slight although statistically insignificant excess of acute encephalopathy in the first 7 days after a dose of DT.[176] It is likely, however, that this excess is attributable to the induction of inevitable manifestations of preexisting central nervous system disorders by the systemic effects of DT, as was observed with infantile spasms.[177]

Local reactions after administration of diphtheria toxoid (alone or in combination with tetanus toxoid or tetanus toxoid and pertussis vaccine) are common but usually minor; severe reactions are rare. Diphtheria toxoid is one of the safest vaccines in current use, and the benefit-to-risk ratio is therefore high.

Unresolved Problems

Diphtheria toxoid induces serological and clinical protection only against the exotoxin of *C. diphtheriae*.[25] Immunity to the exotoxin prevents the systemic manifestations of diphtheria, which are responsible for almost all of the morbidity and mortality from the disease. However, in rare instances, nontoxigenic strains may produce local disease[23]; infrequent instances of local disease may occur with toxigenic strains in persons with ample serological immunity. For this reason, there has been some interest in pursuing definition of the organism's somatic antigens and their relationship to infection in humans.[178]

It is also assumed that reactivity to diphtheria toxoid, usually only a nuisance but with the potential to be serious, stems largely from extraneous proteins present in the toxoid. This reactivity limits the amount of antigen that can be administered at one time, thus requiring that several doses be administered for protection. Alternatives in the future may include vaccination by the oral[179] or nasal[180] routes or use of a highly purified, less reactive antigen[181] or carrier systems[182] for diphtheria toxoid that would require fewer injections. Such products would be particularly useful in the developing world, where severe limitations in healthcare personnel and financial resources are major barriers.

Active immunization against diphtheria with use of current preparations represents a remarkable triumph of preventive medicine. Nonetheless, during the 1990s, a massive epidemic of diphtheria occurred in the countries of the former Soviet Union, with more than 140,000 cases reported. To prevent future epidemics, a high level of population immunity must be maintained among children, adolescents, and adults.

REFERENCES

1. Holmes WH. Diphtheria: History. Bacillary and Rickettsial Infections. New York, Macmillan, 1940, pp 291–305.
2. Andrewes FW, Bulloch W, Douglas SR, et al. Diphtheria. Its Bacteriology, Pathology and Immunology. London, His Majesty's Stationery Office, 1923.
3. English PC. Diphtheria and theories of infectious disease. Pediatrics 76:1–9, 1985.
4. Caulfield E. A true history of the terrible epidemic vulgarly called the throat distemper: Which occurred in His Majesty's New England colonies between the years 1735 and 1740. Yale J Biol Med 11:226–272, 1939.
5. Holt LE. Diphtheria. In Holt LE (ed). The Diseases of Infancy and Childhood. New York, D Appleton & Company, 1897, pp 951–1001.
5a. Ramon G. Sur le pouvoir floculant et sur les proprietes immuni-

santes d'une toxin diphterique rendue anatoxique (anatoxine). C R Acad Sci 177:1338–1340, 1923.
6. Belsey MA, Sinclair M, Roder MR, LeBlanc DR. *Corynebacterium diphtheriae* skin infections in Alabama and Louisiana. A factor in the epidemiology of diphtheria. N Engl J Med 280:135–141, 1969.
7. Höfler W. Cutaneous diphtheria. Int J Dermatol 30:845–847, 1991.
8. Metaxas Quiroga VA. Diphtheria and medical therapy in late 19th century New York City. N Y State J Med 90:256–262, 1990.
9. Anderson JS, Happold FC, McLeod JW, Thomson JG. On the existence of two forms of diphtheria bacillus—*B. diphtheriae gravis* and *B. diphtheriae mitis*—and a new medium for their differentiation and for the bacteriological diagnosis of diphtheria. J Pathol Bacteriol 34:667–681, 1931.
10. Robinson DT, Marshall FN. Investigations on the *gravis, mitis* and intermediate types of *C. diphtheriae* and their clinical significance. J Pathol Bacteriol 38:73–89, 1934.
11. Diphtheria. In Top FH (ed). Communicable and Infectious Diseases (4th ed). St. Louis, CV Mosby, 1960, pp 198–213.
12. Leete HM. The heart in diphtheria. Lancet 1:136–139, 1938.
13. Wesselhoeft C. Communicable diseases: Cardiovascular disease in diphtheria. N Engl J Med 223:57–66, 1940.
14. Bethell DB, Dung NM, Loan HT, et al. Prognostic value of electrocardiographic monitoring of patients with severe diphtheria. Clin Infect Dis 20:1259–1265, 1995.
15. Stockins BA, Lanas FT, Saavedra JG, Opazo JA. Prognosis in patients with diphtheritic myocarditis and bradyarrhythmias: Assessment of results of ventricular pacing. Br Heart J 72:190–191, 1994.
16. Ford FR. Diseases of the Nervous System in Infancy, Childhood and Adolescence (6th ed). Springfield, IL, Charles C Thomas, 1973, pp 716–721.
17. Afghani B, Stutman HR. Bacterial arthritis caused by *Corynebacterium diphtheriae.* Pediatr Infect Dis J 12:881–882, 1993.
18. Zuber PLF, Gruner E, Altwegg M, von Graevenitz A. Invasive infection with nontoxigenic *Corynebacterium diphtheriae* among drug users [letter]. Lancet 339:1359, 1992.
19. Poilane I, Fawaz F, Nathanson M, et al. *Corynebacterium diphtheriae* osteomyelitis in an immunocompetent child: A case report. Eur J Pediatr 154:381–383, 1995.
20. Patey O, Bimet F, Riegal P, et al and the Coryne Study Group. Clinical and molecular study of *Corynebacterium diphtheriae* systemic infections in France. J Clin Microbiol 35:441–445, 1997.
21. Funke G, von Graevenitz A, Clarridge JE, Bernard KA. Clinical microbiology of coryneform bacteria. Clin Microbiol Rev 10:125–159, 1997.
22. Lautrop H. Studies on the antigenic structure of *Corynebacterium diphtheriae.* Acta Pathol Microbiol Scand 27:443–447, 1950.
23. Edward DGF, Allison VD. Diphtheria in the immunized with observations on a diphtheria-like disease associated with nontoxigenic strains of *Corynebacterium diphtheriae.* J Hyg 49:205–219, 1951.
24. Kato M. Action of a toxic glycolipid of *Corynebacterium diphtheriae* on mitochondrial structure and function. J Bacteriol 101:709–716, 1970.
25. Willett HP. *Corynebacterium.* In Joklik WH, Willett HP, Amos DB, Wilfert CM (eds). Zinsser Microbiology (20th ed). East Norwalk, CT, Appleton & Lange, 1992, pp 487–496.
26. Pappenheimer AM, Gill DM. Diphtheria. Science 182:353–358, 1973.
27. Collier RJ. Diphtheria toxin: Mode of action and structure. Bacteriol Rev 39:54–85, 1975.
28. Nakao H, Mazurova IK, Glushkevich T, Popovic T. Analysis of heterogeneity of *Corynebacterium diphtheriae* toxin gene, *tox* and its regulatory element, *dtxR,* by direct sequencing. Res Microbiol 148:45–54, 1997.
29. Tao X, Schiering N, Zeng H, et al. Iron, DtxR, and the regulation of diphtheria toxin expression. Mol Microbiol 14:191–197, 1994.
30. Naglich JG, Metherall JE, Russell DW, Eidels L. Expression cloning of a diphtheria toxin receptor: Identity with a heparin-binding EGF-like growth factor precursor. Cell 69:1051–1061, 1992.
31. Morris RE, Gerstein AS, Bonventre PF, Saelinger CB. Receptor-mediated entry of diphtheria toxin into monkey kidney (Vero) cells: Electron microscopic evaluation. Infect Immun 50:721–727, 1985.
32. Vaughan TJ, Pascall JC, Brown KD. Tissue distribution of mRNA for heparin-binding epidermal growth factor. Biochem J 287:681–684, 1992.
33. Pappenheimer AM Jr, Murphy JR. Studies on the molecular epidemiology of diphtheria. Lancet 2:923–926, 1983.
34. Ipsen J. Circulating antitoxin at the onset of diphtheria in 425 patients. J Immunol 54:325–347, 1946.
35. Björkholm B, Böttiger M, Christensen B, Hagberg L. Antitoxin antibody levels and the outcome of illness during an outbreak of diphtheria among alcoholics. Scand J Infect Dis 18:235–239, 1986.
36. Efstratiou A, Maple PAC. Laboratory Diagnosis of Diphtheria. Copenhagen, The Expanded Programme on Immunization in the European Region of WHO, 1994.
37. Wong TP, Groman N. Production of diphtheria toxin by selected isolates of *Corynebacterium ulcerans* and *Corynebacterium pseudotuberculosis.* Infect Immun 43:1114–1116, 1984.
38. Maximescu P, Oprisan A, Pop A, Potorac E. Further studies on *Corynebacterium* species capable of producing diphtheria toxin *(C. diphtheriae, C. ulcerans, C. ovis).* J Gen Microbiol 82:49–56, 1974.
39. Meers PD. A case of classical diphtheria, and other infections due to *Corynebacterium ulcerans.* J Infect 1:139–142, 1979.
40. Hust MH, Metzler B, Schubert U, et al. Toxische Diphtherie durch *Corynebacterium ulcerans.* Dtsch Med Wochenschr 119:548–553, 1994.
41. Centers for Disease Control and Prevention. Respiratory diphtheria caused by *Corynebacterium ulcerans*—Terre Haute, Indiana, 1996. MMWR Morb Mortal Wkly Rep 46:330–332, 1997.
42. Engler KH, Glushkevich T, Mazurova IK, et al. A modified Elek test for detection of toxigenic corynebacteria in the diagnostic laboratory. J Clin Microbiol 35:495–498, 1997.
43. Pallen MJ. Rapid screening for toxigenic *Corynebacterium diphtheriae* by the polymerase chain reaction. J Clin Pathol 44:1025–1026, 1991.
44. Hauser D, Popoff MR, Kiredjian M, et al. Polymerase chain reaction assay for diagnosis of potentially toxinogenic *Corynebacterium diphtheriae* strains: Correlation with ADP-ribosylation activity assay. J Clin Microbiol 31:2720–2723, 1993.
45. Aravena-Román M, Bowman R, O'Neill G. Polymerase chain reaction for detection of toxigenic *Corynebacterium diphtheriae.* Pathology 27:71–73, 1995.
46. Mikhailovich VM, Melnikov VG, Mazurova IK, et al. Application of PCR for detection of toxigenic *Corynebacterium diphtheriae* strains isolated during the Russian diphtheria epidemic, 1990 through 1994. J Clin Microbiol 33:3061–3063, 1995.
47. Nakao H, Popovic T. Development of a direct PCR assay for detection of the diphtheria toxin gene. J Clin Microbiol 35:1651–1655, 1997.
48. Saragea A, Maximescu P. Phage typing of *Corynebacterium diphtheriae.* Bull World Health Organ 35:681–689, 1966.
49. Rappuoli R, Perugini M, Falsen E. Molecular epidemiology of the 1984–1986 outbreak of diphtheria in Sweden. N Engl J Med 318:12–14, 1988.
50. Coyle MB, Groman NB, Russell JQ, et al. The molecular epidemiology of three biotypes of *Corynebacterium diphtheriae* in the Seattle outbreak, 1972–1982. J Infect Dis 159:670–679, 1989.
51. De Zoysa A, Efstratiou A, George RC, et al. Molecular epidemiology of *Corynebacterium diphtheriae* from northwestern Russia and surrounding countries studied by using ribotyping and pulsed-field gel electrophoresis. J Clin Microbiol 33:1080–1083, 1995.
52. Popovic T, Kombarova SY, Reeves MW, et al. Molecular epidemiology of diphtheria in Russia, 1985–1994. J Infect Dis 174:1064–1072, 1996.
53. Nakao H, Pruckler JM, Mazurova IK, et al. Heterogeneity of diphtheria toxin gene, *tox,* and its regulatory element, *dxtR,* in *Corynebacterium diphtheriae* strains causing epidemic diphtheria in Russia and Ukraine. J Clin Microbiol 34:1711–1716, 1996.
54. Nakao H, Popovic T. Development of a rapid ribotyping method for *Corynebacterium diphtheriae* by using PCR single-strand conformation polymorphism: Comparison with standard ribotyping. J Microbiol Methods 31:127–134, 1998.

55. Bisgard KM, Hardy IRB, Popovic T, et al. Respiratory diphtheria in the United States, 1980–1995. Am J Public Health 88:787–791, 1998.
56. Galazka AM, Robertson SE. Diphtheria: Changing patterns in the developing world and the industrialized world. Eur J Epidemiol 11:107–117, 1995.
57. Wright HD, Shone HR, Tucker JR. Cross infection in diphtheria wards. J Pathol Bacteriol 52:111–128, 1941.
58. Crosbie WE, Wright HD. Diphtheria bacilli in floor dust. Lancet 1:656–659, 1941.
59. Belsey MA. Isolation of *Corynebacterium diphtheriae* in the environment of skin carriers. Am J Epidemiol 91:294–299, 1970.
60. Larsson P, Brinkhoff B, Larsson L. *Corynebacterium diphtheriae* in the environment of carriers and patients. J Hosp Infect 10:282–286, 1987.
61. Jones EE, Kim-Farley RJ, Algunaid M, et al. Diphtheria: A possible foodborne outbreak in Hodeida, Yemen Arab Republic. Bull World Health Organ 63:287–293, 1985.
62. Seckel HPG. Prevention of diphtheria. Am J Dis Child 58:512–526, 1939.
63. Mortensen V. Occurrence of diphtheria in recent years, with a special view to the influence of the antidiphtheric vaccination. Acta Med Scand 125:283–293, 1946.
64. Walker JV. Age and sex distribution of diphtheria in Oldenburg, Germany. Lancet 1:422–423, 1947.
65. Madsen S. II. Diphtheria immunization. Dan Med Bull 3:116–121, 1956.
66. Vitek C, Bisgard K, Lushniak B, et al. Diphtheria epidemic in the Russian Federation: Evidence for a decline in incidence [abstract G94]. Abstracts of the 36th Interscience Conference on Antimicrobial Agents and Chemotherapy; New Orleans, LA; September 15–18, 1996.
67. Burnet M, White DO. Natural History of Infectious Disease (4th ed). London, Cambridge University Press, 1972, pp 193–201.
68. US Bureau of the Census. Historical Statistics of the United States, Colonial Times to 1970, Bicentennial Edition, Part 1. Washington, DC, US Department of Congress, 1975, pp 58, 63.
69. McKinnon NE. Diphtheria prevented. In Cruickshank R (ed). Control of the Common Fevers. London, The Lancet Ltd, 1942, pp 41–56.
70. Stowman K. Diphtheria pandemic recedes. UN World Health Organ 1:60–67, 1947.
71. Stuart G. A note on diphtheria incidence in certain countries. Br Med J 2:613–615, 1945.
72. Wheeler SM, Morton AR. Epidemiological observations in the Halifax epidemic. Am J Public Health 32:947–956, 1942.
73. Fleck S, Kellam JW, Klippen AJ. Diphtheria among German prisoners of war. Bull US Army Med Dept 74:80–89, 1944.
74. Brooks GF, Bennett JV, Feldman RA. Diphtheria in the United States, 1959–1970. J Infect Dis 129:172–178, 1974.
75. Zalma VM, Older JJ, Brooks GF. The Austin, Texas, diphtheria outbreak. Clinical and epidemiological aspects. JAMA 211:2125–2129, 1970.
76. Marcuse EK, Grand MG. Epidemiology of diphtheria in San Antonio, Texas, 1970. JAMA 224:305–310, 1973.
77. Chen RT, Broome CV, Weinstein RA, et al. Diphtheria in the United States, 1971–1981. Am J Public Health 75:1393–1397, 1985.
78. Harnisch JP, Tronca E, Nolan CM, et al. Diphtheria among urban alcoholic adults. A decade of experience in Seattle. Ann Intern Med 111:71–82, 1989.
79. Centers for Disease Control and Prevention. Toxigenic *Corynebacterium diphtheriae*—northern plains Indian community, August–October 1996. MMWR Morb Mortal Wkly Rep 46:506–510, 1997.
80. Young TK. Endemicity of diphtheria in an Indian population in northwestern Ontario. Can J Public Health 75:310–313, 1984.
81. Wilson CR, Casson RI, Wherrett B, Fraser N. Toxigenic diphtheria in two isolated northern communities. Arctic Med Res Suppl: 346–347, 1991.
82. Cahoon FE, Brown S, Jamieson F. *Corynebacterium diphtheriae*—toxigenic isolations from northeastern Ontario [abstract K-171]. Abstracts of the 37th Interscience Conference on Antimicrobial Agents and Chemotherapy; Toronto, Ontario, Canada, September 28–October 1, 1997.
83. Patel M, Morey F, Butcher A, et al. The frequent isolation of toxigenic and non-toxigenic *Corynebacterium diphtheriae* at Alice Springs Hospital. Comm Dis Intell 18:310–311, 1994.
84. Hardy IRB, Dittman S, Sutter RW. Current situation and control strategies for resurgence of diphtheria in newly independent states of the former Soviet Union. Lancet 347:1739–1744, 1996.
85. Wharton M, Hardy IRB, Vitek C, et al. Epidemic diphtheria in the newly independent states of the former Soviet Union. In Scheld WM, Armstrong D, Hughes JM (eds). Emerging Infections. Vol. I. Washington, DC, ASM Press, 1998, pp 165–176.
86. Dittman S. Epidemic diphtheria in the newly independent states of the former USSR—situation and lessons learned. Biologicals 25:179–186, 1997.
87. Groman N, Schiller J, Russell J. *Corynebacterium ulcerans* and *Corynebacterium pseudotuberculosis* responses to DNA probes derived from corynephage and *Corynebacterium diphtheriae.* Infect Immun 45:511–517, 1984.
88. Hart RJC. *Corynebacterium ulcerans* in humans and cattle in North Devon. J Hyg Camb 92:161–164, 1984.
89. Bostock AD, Gilbert FR, Lewis D, Smith DCM. *Corynebacterium ulcerans* infection associated with untreated milk. J Infect 9:286–288, 1984.
89a. Roux E, Yersin A. Contribution à l'étude de la diphthérie. Ann Inst Pasteur 2:629–664, 1888.
89b. Behring E. Untersuchungen über das Zustandekommen der Diphtherie-Immunität bei Thieren. Dtsch Med Wochenschr 16:1145, 1890.
90. Kondratas RA. Death helped write the biologics law. FDA Consum 16:23–25, 1982.
91. US Food and Drug Administration. Biological products; bacterial vaccines and toxoids; implementation of efficacy review. Diphtheria antitoxin. Federal Register 50:51079–51082, 1985.
92. Centers for Disease Control and Prevention. Notice to Readers. Availability of diphtheria antitoxin through an investigational new drug protocol. MMWR Morb Mortal Wkly Rep 46:380, 1997.
93. Dowling HF. Diphtheria as a model. JAMA 226:550–553, 1973.
94. Farizo KM, Strebel PM, Chen RT, et al. Fatal respiratory disease due to *Corynebacterium diphtheriae:* Case report and review of guidelines for management, investigation, and control. Clin Infect Dis 16:59–68, 1993.
95. Ker CB. Infectious Diseases, A Practical Textbook (3rd ed). London, Oxford University Press, 1929.
96. Fibiger J. Om Serumbehandling of Difteri. Hosp-Tid 4.R. 6:309, 337, 1898.
97. Wilson G, Smith G. Diphtheria and other diseases due to corynebacteria. In Smith GR (ed). Topley and Wilson's Principles of Bacteriology, Virology and Immunity (7th ed). Baltimore, Williams & Wilkins, 1984, p 91.
98. Tasman A, Minkenhof JE, Vink HH, et al. Importance of intravenous injection of diphtheria antiserum. Lancet 1:1299–1304, 1958.
99. Weaver GH. Diphtheria carriers. JAMA 76:831–835, 1921.
100. Smith T. Active immunity produced by so-called balanced or neutral mixtures of diphtheria toxin and antitoxin. J Exp Med 11:241–256, 1909.
101. von Behring E. Über ein neues Diphtheries Schutzmittel. Dtsch Med Wochenschr 39:873–876, 1913.
102. Schick B. Die Diphtherietoxin-Hauktreation des Menschen als Vorprobe der prophylaktischen Diphtherieheilseruminjektion. Munch Med Wochenschr 60:2608–2610, 1913.
103. Ramon G. Sur le pouvoir floculant et sur les proprietes immunisantes d'une toxin diphterique rendue anatoxique (anatoxine). C R Acad Sci 177:1338–1340, 1923.
104. Park WH. Duration of immunity against diphtheria achieved by various methods. JAMA 109:1681–1684, 1937.
105. Harries EHR, Mitman M. Clinical Practice in Infectious Diseases. Diphtheria (3rd ed). Baltimore, Williams & Wilkins, 1947, pp 168–223.
106. Glenny AT, Pope CG, Waddington H, Wallace U. Immunological notes. XIII. The antigenic value of toxoid precipitated by potassium alum. J Pathol Bacteriol 29:38–39, 1926.
107. Greenberg L, Fleming DS. The immunizing efficacy of diphtheria toxoid when combined with various antigens. Can J Public Health 39:131–135, 1948.

108. Spiller V, Barnes JM, Holt LB, Cullington DE. Immunization against whooping-cough. Combined v. separate inoculations. Br Med J 2:639–642, 1955.
109. Aprile MA, Wardlaw AC. Aluminum compounds as adjuvants for vaccines and toxoids in man: A review. Can J Public Health 57:343–354, 1966.
110. Edwards KM, Decker MD. Combination vaccines consisting of acellular pertussis vaccines. Pediatr Infect Dis J 16(suppl):S97–S102, 1997.
111. Edwards KM, Meade BD, Decker MD, et al. Comparison of 13 acellular pertussis vaccines: Overview and serologic response. Pediatrics 96:548–557, 1995.
112. Pertussis vaccination: Use of acellular pertussis vaccines among infants and young children. Recommendations of the Advisory Committee on Immunization Practices (ACIP). MMWR Morb Mortal Wkly Rep 46(RR-7):1–25, 1997.
113. Dengrove J, Lee EJ, Heiner DC, et al. IgG and IgG subclass specific antibody responses to diphtheria and tetanus toxoids in newborns and infants given DTP immunization. Pediatr Res 20:735–739, 1986.
114. Bernbaum JC, Daft A, Anolik R, et al. Response of preterm infants to diphtheria-tetanus-pertussis immunization. J Pediatr 107:184–188, 1985.
115. Björkholm B, Granström M, Taranger J, et al. Influence of high titers of maternal antibody on the serologic response of infants to diphtheria vaccination at three, five and twelve months of age. Pediatr Infect Dis J 148:846–850, 1995.
116. Barkin AM, Pichichero ME, Samuelson JS, Barkin SZ. Pediatric diphtheria and tetanus toxoids vaccine: Clinical and immunologic response when administered as the primary series. J Pediatr 106:779–781, 1985.
117. Pichichero ME, Barkin RM, Samuelson JS. Pediatric diphtheria and tetanus toxoids-adsorbed vaccine: Immune response to the first booster following the diphtheria and tetanus toxoids vaccine primary series. Pediatr Infect Dis 5:428–430, 1986.
118. Centers for Disease Control and Prevention. Diphtheria, tetanus, and pertussis: Recommendations for vaccine use and other preventive measures: Recommendations of the Immunization Practices Advisory Committee (ACIP). MMWR Morb Mortal Wkly Rep 40(RR-10):1–28, 1991.
119. Myers MG, Beckman CW, Vosdingh RA, Hankins WA. Primary immunization with tetanus and diphtheria toxoids. Reaction rates and immunogenicity in older children and adults. JAMA 248:2478–2480, 1982.
120. Feery BJ, Benenson AS, Forsyth JRL, et al. Diphtheria immunization in adolescents and adults with reduced doses of adsorbed diphtheria toxoid. Med J Aust 1:128–130, 1981.
121. Macko MB, Powell CE. Comparison of the morbidity of tetanus toxoid boosters with tetanus-diphtheria toxoid boosters. Ann Emerg Med 14:33–35, 1985.
122. King GE, Hadler SC. Simultaneous administration of childhood vaccines: An important public health policy that is safe and efficacious. Pediatr Infect Dis J 13:394–407, 1994.
122a. Orenstein WA, Weisfeld JS, Halsey NA. Diphtheria and tetanus toxoids and pertussis vaccine, combined. In Halsey NA, de Quadros CA (eds). Recent Advances in Immunization: A Bibliographic Review. Washington, DC, Pan American Health Organization, 1983, pp 30–51.
123. Walsh JA, Warren KS. Selective primary health care. An interim strategy for disease control in developing countries [special article]. N Engl J Med 301:967–974, 1979.
124. Expanded Programme on Immunization. EPI Information System: Global Summary, August 1997. Geneva, World Health Organization, 1997.
125. Miller LW, Older JJ, Drake J, Zimmerman S. Diphtheria immunization. Effect upon carriers and the control of outbreaks. Am J Dis Child 123:197–199, 1972.
126. WHO Regional Office for Europe. Diphtheria Epidemic in Europe: Emergency and Response. Report on a WHO meeting. St. Petersburg, Russia, July 5–7, 1993. EUR/ICP/EPI 038, 1994.
127. Vitek C, Brennan M, Gotway C, et al. Risk for diphtheria among children associated with increasing time since last booster vaccination [abstract G-9]. Abstracts of the 37th Interscience Conference on Antimicrobial Agents and Chemotherapy; Toronto, Ontario, Canada; September 28–October 1, 1997.
128. Naiditch MJ, Bower AG. Diphtheria. A study of 1,433 cases observed during a ten-year period at Los Angeles County Hospital. Am J Med 17:229–245, 1954.
129. Brooks GF, Bennett JV, Feldman RA. Diphtheria in the United States, 1959–70. J Infect Dis 129:172–178, 1974.
130. Narkevich MI, Tymchakovskaia IM. Specific features of the spread of diphtheria in Russia in the presence of mass immunization of children. Zh Mikrobiol Epidemiol Immunobiol Mar-Apr:25–29, 1996.
131. Fox JP, Elveback L, Scott W, et al. Herd immunity: Basic concept and relevance to public health immunization practices. Am J Epidemiol 94:179–189, 1971.
132. Rappuoli R, Perugini M, Falsen E. Molecular epidemiology of the 1984–1986 outbreak of diphtheria in Sweden. N Engl J Med 318:12–14, 1988.
133. Kjeldsen K, Simonsen O, Heron I. Immunity against diphtheria 25 to 30 years after primary vaccination in childhood. Lancet 1:900–902, 1985.
134. Weiss BP, Strassburg MA, Feeley JC. Tetanus and diphtheria immunity in an elderly population in Los Angeles County. Am J Public Health 73:802–804, 1983.
135. Crossley K, Irvine P, Warren JB, et al. Tetanus and diphtheria immunity in urban Minnesota adults. JAMA 242:2298–2300, 1979.
136. Cellesi C, Zanchi A, Michelangeli C, et al. Immunity to diphtheria in a sample of adult population from central Italy. Vaccine 7:417–420, 1989.
137. Björkholm B, Wahl M, Granström M, Hagberg L. Immune status and booster effects of low doses of diphtheria toxoid in Swedish medical personnel. Scand J Infect Dis 21:429–434, 1989.
138. Galazka A, Kardymowicz B. Immunity against diphtheria in adults in Poland. Epidemiol Infect 103:587–593, 1989.
139. Koblin BA, Townsend TR. Immunity to diphtheria and tetanus in inner-city women of childbearing age. Am J Public Health 79:1297–1298, 1989.
140. Björkholm B, Olling S, Larsson P, Hagberg L. An outbreak of diphtheria among Swedish alcoholics. Infection 15:354–358, 1987.
141. Christenson B, Böttiger M. Serological immunity to diphtheria in Sweden in 1978 and 1984. Scand J Infect Dis 18:227–233, 1986.
142. Ruben FL, Nagel J, Fireman P. Antitoxin responses in the elderly to tetanus-diphtheria (Td) immunization. Am J Epidemiol 108:145–149, 1978.
143. Simonsen O, Kjeldsen K, Bentzon MW, Heron I. Susceptibility to diphtheria in populations vaccinated before and after elimination of indigenous diphtheria in Denmark. A comparative study of antitoxic immunity. Acta Pathol Microbiol Immunol Scand Sect C, 95:225–231, 1987.
144. Koizumi Y, Iseki M, Aoyama T, et al. Diphtheria antitoxin levels in Japanese adults (10–20 years after the last vaccination). Kansenshogaku Zasshi 64:1525–1529, 1990.
145. Sheffield FW, Dadswell JV, Rowlands DF, et al. Susceptibility to diphtheria. A survey by an ad-hoc working group. Lancet 1:428–430, 1978.
146. Maple PA, Efstratiou A, George RC, et al. Diphtheria immunity in UK blood donors. Lancet 345:963–965, 1995.
147. John C, Selzer G, Preiser W, Zielen S. Diphtheria immunity in health [letter]. Lancet 347:969, 1996.
148. Centers for Disease Control and Prevention. Update on adult immunization: Recommendations of the Immunization Practices Advisory Committee (ACIP). MMWR Morb Mortal Wkly Rep 40(RR-12):1–94, 1991.
149. Maksimova NM, Sukhorukova NL, Kostyuchenko GI, et al. Specific prophylaxis of diphtheria in adults in the focus of diphtheria infection. Zh Mikrobiol Epidemiol Immunobiol Aug:36–40, 1987.
150. Hardy I, Kozlova I, Tchoudnaia, et al. Immunogenicity of Td vaccine in Ukrainian adults [abstract G25]. Abstracts of the 35th Interscience Conference on Antimicrobial Agents and Chemotherapy; San Francisco, CA; September 17–20, 1995.
151. Galazka AM, Robertson SE, Oblapenko GP. Resurgence of diphtheria. Eur J Epidemiol 11:95–105, 1995.
152. Edsall G. Immunization of adults against diphtheria and tetanus. Am J Hyg 42:393–400, 1952.

153. Moloney PJ, Fraser CJ. Immunization with diphtheria toxoid (anatoxine Ramon). Am J Public Health 17:1027–1030, 1927.
154. Edsall G, Altman JS, Gaspar AJ. Combined tetanus-diphtheria immunization of adults: Use of small doses of diphtheria toxoid. Am J Public Health 44:1537–1545, 1954.
155. Pappenheimer AM Jr, Edsall G, Lawrence HS, et al. Study of reactions following administration of crude and purified diphtheria toxoid in an adult population. Am J Hyg 52:353–370, 1950.
156. Volk VK, Gottshall RY, Anderson HD, et al. Antibody response to booster dose of diphtheria and tetanus toxoids. Reactions in institutionalized adults and non-institutionalized children and young adults. Public Health Rep 78:161–164, 1963.
157. Smith JWG. Diphtheria and tetanus toxoids. Br Med Bull 25:177–182, 1969.
158. James G, Longshore WA Jr, Hendry JL. Diphtheria immunization studies of students in an urban high school. Am J Hyg 53:178–261, 1951.
159. Edsall G, Banton HJ, Wheeler RE. The antigenicity of single, graded doses of purified diphtheria toxoid in man. Am J Hyg 53:283–295, 1951.
160. Levin PL. Diphtheria immunization. Desirability of combined tetanus and diphtheria injection in wound management. Postgrad Med 79:139–140, 1986.
161. Greco D, Salmaso S, Mastrantonio P, et al and the Progetto Pertosse Working Group. A controlled trial of two acellular vaccines and one whole-cell vaccine against pertussis. N Engl J Med 334:341–348, 1996.
162. Gustafsson L, Hallander HO, Olin P, et al. A controlled trial of a two-component acellular, a five-component acellular, and a whole-cell pertussis vaccine. N Engl J Med 334:349–355, 1996.
163. Trollfors B, Taranger J, Lagergård, et al. A placebo-controlled trial of a pertussis-toxoid vaccine. N Engl J Med 333:1045–1050, 1995.
164. Schmitt-Grohé S, Stehr K, Cherry JD, et al and the Pertussis Vaccine Study Group. Minor adverse events in a comparative efficacy trial in Germany in infants receiving either the Lederle/Takeda acellular pertussis component DTP (DTaP) vaccine, the Lederle whole-cell component DTP (DTP) or DT vaccine. Dev Biol Stand 89:113–118, 1997.
165. Tozzi AE, Olin P. Common side effects in the Italian and Stockholm I trials. Dev Biol Stand 89:105–108, 1997.
166. Björkholm B, Wahl M, Granström M, Hagberg L. Immune status and booster effects of low doses of diphtheria toxoid in Swedish medical personnel. Scand J Infect Dis 21:429–434, 1989.
167. Wassilak SGF, Orenstein WA, Sutter RW. Tetanus toxoid. In Plotkin SA, Mortimer EA (eds). Vaccines (2nd ed). Philadelphia, WB Saunders, 1994, p 76.
168. Haber P, Lloyd J, Chen R. Adverse event reporting rates following tetanus-diphtheria (Td) and tetanus toxoid (TT) vaccinations, Vaccine Adverse Events Reporting System (VAERS), 1991–94 [abstract G58]. Abstracts of the 36th Interscience Conference on Antimicrobial Agents and Chemotherapy; New Orleans, LA; September 15–18, 1996.
169. Nahum E, Lerman Y, Cohen D, et al. The immune response to booster vaccination against diphtheria toxin at age 18–21 years. Isr J Med Sci 30:600–603, 1994.
170. Mortimer J, Melville-Smith M, Sheffield F. Diphtheria vaccine for adults. Lancet 2:1182–1183, 1986.
171. Simonsen O, Kjeldsen K, Vendborg H-A, Heron I. Revaccination of adults against diphtheria I: Responses and reactions to different doses of diphtheria toxoid in 30–70-year-old persons with low serum antitoxin levels. Acta Pathol Microbiol Immunol Scand Sect C 94:213–218, 1986.
172. Simonsen O, Klaerke M, Klaerke A, et al. Revaccination of adults against diphtheria II: Combined diphtheria and tetanus revaccination with different doses of diphtheria toxoid 20 years after primary vaccination. Acta Pathol Microbiol Immunol Scand Sect C 94:219–225, 1986.
173. Blennow M, Granström M, Strandell A. Adverse reactions after diphtheria-tetanus booster in 10-year-old schoolchildren in relation to the type of vaccine given for the primary vaccination. Vaccine 12:427–430, 1994.
174. Mark A, Granström M. The role of aluminum for adverse reactions and immunogenicity of diphtheria-tetanus booster vaccine. Acta Paediatr 83:159–163, 1994.
175. Mark A, Granström B, Granström M. Immunoglobulin E responses to diphtheria and tetanus toxoids after booster with aluminum-adsorbed and fluid DT-vaccines. Vaccine 13:669–673, 1995.
176. Alderslade R, Bellman MH, Rawson NSB, et al. The National Childhood Encephalopathy Study. In Whooping Cough: Reports from the Committee on the Safety of Medicines and the Joint Committee on Vaccination and Immunisation. London, Department of Health and Social Security, Her Majesty's Stationery Office, 1981, pp 79–154.
177. Bellman MH, Ross EM, Miller DL. Infantile spasms and pertussis immunisation. Lancet 1:1031–1034, 1983.
178. US Food and Drug Administration. Biological products; bacterial vaccines and toxoids; implementation of efficacy review. Generic statement on diphtheria toxoid. Federal Register 50:51013–51016, 1985.
179. Mirchamsy H, Hamedi M, Fateh G, Sassani A. Oral immunization against diphtheria and tetanus infections by fluid diphtheria and tetanus toxoids. Vaccine 12:1167–1172, 1994.
180. Aggerbeck H, Gizurarson S, Wantzin J, Heron I. Intranasal booster vaccination against diphtheria and tetanus in man. Vaccine 15:307–316, 1997.
181. Robbins FC, Robbins JB. Current status and prospects for some improved and new bacterial vaccines. Ann Rev Public Health 7:105–125, 1986.
182. Diwan M, Misra A, Khar RK, Talwar GP. Long-term high immune response to diphtheria toxoid in rodents with diphtheria toxoid conjugated to dextran as a single contact point delivery system. Vaccine 15:1867–1871, 1997.

chapter

10 Hepatitis B Vaccine

Francis J. Mahoney
Mark Kane

Viral hepatitis is a disease of multiple causes that was first described in the 5th century BC. When Hippocrates described epidemic jaundice, he was undoubtedly referring to people infected with acute hepatitis B virus (HBV) as well as with other agents capable of infecting the liver. Epidemics of jaundice have been described throughout history and were particularly common during various wars in the 19th and 20th century. In the U.S. Civil War, more than 70,000 cases occurred among Union troops; during World War II, hundreds of thousands of cases occurred among U.S., British, and French troops. Although many of these outbreaks were due to hepatitis A, it is likely that epidemic transmission of hepatitis B also occurred in settings where the use of blood-containing products was common.

The recognition of a form of hepatitis that was transmitted by direct inoculation of blood or blood products was first documented by Lurman in Bremen, Germany, in 1883, during a smallpox immunization campaign.[1] Thousands of people received smallpox vaccine that had been prepared from human lymph. Of 1289 shipyard workers who received this vaccine, 191 (15%) developed jaundice several weeks to 8 months after receiving vaccine, whereas jaundice did not occur among unvaccinated workers. In the first part of the 20th century, outbreaks of *long-incubation* hepatitis were described in a variety of risk groups, including people who attended clinics for venereal diseases, diabetes, and tuberculosis; patients who received blood transfusions; people inoculated with mumps or measles convalescent serum; and military personnel who received yellow fever vaccine during World War II.[2–5] The yellow fever outbreak was linked to a specific lot of vaccine that contained human serum. A follow-up study in the 1980s demonstrated that 97% of recipients of the serum-containing vaccine had serological evidence of HBV infection compared with 13% of people who received yellow fever vaccine that did not contain human serum, thus confirming that HBV was the cause of this outbreak.[6]

The discovery of the etiological agent for hepatitis B and the development of safe and effective vaccines for this virus are among the remarkable scientific achievements of the 20th century. In the 19th century, Virchow proposed that the pathogenesis of acute hepatitis was due to a plug of mucus in the ampulla of Vater.[7] This hypothesis was disputed when pathological studies revealed diffuse hepatic inflammation in people with acute jaundice, suggesting an infectious cause.[8, 9] Studies on human volunteers in the 1930s and 1940s provided convincing evidence of a viral cause with at least 2 etiological agents.[5, 10, 11] In 1947, MacCallum proposed the current nomenclature of hepatitis A for infectious hepatitis and hepatitis B for "homologous serum" hepatitis.[12] At that time, the epidemiology of the two diseases was known to be different. Hepatitis A was transmitted by the fecal-oral route, had an incubation period of 2 to 6 weeks, and was primarily a disease of younger children. In contrast, hepatitis B was transmitted by percutaneous exposure to blood products, had a longer incubation period of 2 to 6 months, and occurred more often in adults.

These observations were confirmed in a series of studies by Krugman and collaborators at the Willowbrook Institute in the 1960s and 1970s.[13–15] They described two types of viral hepatitis that were referred to as MS-1 and MS-2. MS-1 resembled what MacCallum had classified as hepatitis A. Studies in human volunteers confirmed it was transmitted by the fecal-oral route and had an incubation period of 30 to 38 days. MS-2 resembled hepatitis B in that it had a longer incubation period (41–108 d) and was transmitted by percutaneous exposure. These studies also confirmed the existence of homologous immunity after infection with hepatitis A virus or HBV.

Around the time of the Willowbrook studies, Blumberg and colleagues described an immunoprecipitin that was present in the serum of a leukemic patient and was detected in a gel diffusion experiment.[16] The subject was an Australia aborigine, and the antigen was named the Australia antigen. Subsequent studies revealed that the antigen had a variable distribution in different populations and occurred more commonly among patients who had received multiple transfusions and blood products. Extensive studies described the distribution of Australia antigen in various population groups and in patients whose diseases did not appear to be related to hepatitis. The association of the Australia antigen with acute hepatitis B was subsequently demonstrated and led to the development of specific tests for the identification of HBV infection.[17–19]

The viral cause of hepatitis B was firmly established by electron microscopy and the detection of several viral particles that reacted with antisera to Australia antigen.[20] It was demonstrated that the Dane particle was HBV, and its surface component was designated as hepatitis B surface antigen (HBsAg). The core component contained endogenous DNA and hepatitis B core antigen (HBcAg). The differential presence of HBsAg, antibodies to HBsAg (anti-HBs), and antibodies to HBcAg (anti-HBc) was used to classify patients as having acute or chronic infections. A third antigen related to infectivity, hepatitis B e antigen (HBeAg), was first described in 1972 by Magnius and Espmark.[21]

The development of sensitive and specific tests to detect HBV infection allowed investigators to define the natural history of HBV infection and develop strategies to prevent transmission. The development of assays to screen blood for HBsAg led to procedures to prevent transfusion-associated hepatitis B. In addition, units of blood that tested positive for anti-HBs were used for the preparation of hepatitis B immune globulin (HBIG). Early studies indicated that HBIG was effective in preventing or modifying the course of HBV infection.[22]

In 1970, in the course of studies on the natural history of HBV infection at Willowbrook, Krugman and colleagues boiled a preparation of MS-2 serum for 1 minute to determine the effect of heat on infectivity of the virus.[23] The 1-minute boil destroyed the infectivity of the preparation, but the heat-inactivated material proved to be antigenic. It was subsequently shown that the preparation was immunogenic and partially protective when volunteers were challenged with MS-2 serum after receiving the boiled preparation.[24] The description of this "inactivated" vaccine soon led to the development of plasma-derived subunit vaccines.[25]

The development of diagnostic assays to distinguish hepatitis A and hepatitis B soon led observers to recognize the existence of other agents that were the etiological agents of non-A, non-B hepatitis. In 1977, Rizzetto detected a new antigen in the sera of some patients with severe chronic liver disease.[26] The δ antigen was subsequently shown to be a core protein of a defective virus that has been classified as hepatitis D virus (HDV). HDV is defective in that it requires HBV to replicate. Thus, the prevention of HBV infection in turn prevents HDV transmission and associated morbidity and mortality. In the late 1980s, studies on patients with non-A, non-B hepatitis led to the discovery and development of serological assays for hepatitis C virus (HCV) and hepatitis E virus.[27–29]

BACKGROUND

Clinical Description

Acute Infection

The consequences of acute HBV infection are highly variable. The incubation period ranges from 6 weeks to 6 months, and the development of clinical manifestations of infection is highly age dependent. Newborns generally do not develop any clinical signs or symptoms, and infection produces typical illness in only 5 to 15% of children 1 to 5 years of age,[30] whereas 33 to 50% of infected older children and adults are symptomatic. Symptomatic infections vary in severity from mild to fulminant forms. Clinical signs and symptoms of acute HBV infection include anorexia, nausea, malaise, vomiting, jaundice, dark urine, clay-colored or light stools, and abdominal pain. Occasionally, extrahepatic manifestations occur and include rashes, arthralgias, and arthritis. Fulminant hepatitis occurs in approximately 1 to 2% of people with acute disease and has a case-fatality ratio of 63:100 to 93:100.

Chronic Infection

Chronic HBV infection is defined as the presence of HBsAg in serum for at least 6 months. The risk of developing chronic infection varies inversely with age and is highest (≤90%) for infants infected in the perinatal period.[30–32] Twenty-five to 50% of children infected between the ages of 1 and 5 years develop chronic infection, compared with 6 to 10% of acutely infected older children and adults (Fig. 10–1).

People with chronic HBV infection are at substantially increased risk of developing chronic liver disease, including cirrhosis of the liver or primary hepatocellular carcinoma. The age at which chronic infection occurs may alter the risk of developing disease. Prospective studies of people who acquire HBV infection as infants and young children indicate that 25% will die of either primary hepatocellular carcinoma or cirrhosis and that 15% of adolescents and young adults who acquire chronic HBV infection will develop chronic liver disease.[33, 34] Several host-related factors are associated with increased risk of developing chronic infection; factors include the presence of chronic diseases such as renal failure, human immunodeficiency virus (HIV) infection, and diabetes.[32, 35, 36]

People with chronic HBV infection are generally clas-

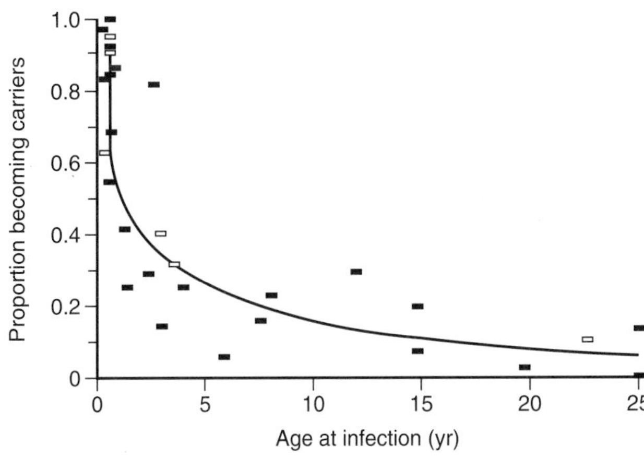

Figure 10–1. Studies evaluating the risk of chronic hepatitis B virus infection by age of infection. Filled squares represent data from developing countries; open squares represent data from developed countries. (From Edmunds WJ, Medley GF, Nokes DJ, et al. The influence of age on the development of the hepatitis B carrier state. Proc R Soc Lond B Biol Sci 253:197–201, 1993.)

sified as having one of three histological patterns on liver biopsy: chronic persistent hepatitis, chronic active hepatitis, or cirrhosis. The degree of histological injury is often not reflected by symptoms, and people with severe chronic liver disease are often asymptomatic until late in the course of their illness.[37] People with chronic active hepatitis develop fibrosis of the liver and are predisposed to the development of cirrhosis. Cirrhosis is an irreversible form of liver injury that can lead to the development of hepatocellular carcinoma through the promotional effect of hepatocyte regeneration.[38]

Virology

HBV is a double-stranded, enveloped, DNA virus of the Hepadnaviridae family that replicates in the liver and causes hepatic dysfunction. HBsAg is found on the surface of the virus and is also produced in excess amounts, circulating in the blood as 22-nm spherical and tubular particles (Fig. 10–2). The inner core of the virus contains HBcAg, HBeAg, a single molecule of partially double-stranded DNA, and a DNA-dependent DNA polymerase (Fig. 10–3). HBsAg can be identified in serum 30 to 60 days after exposure to HBV and persists for variable periods.

HBV is the smallest DNA virus known, having only 3200 base pairs in its genome. The genome is uniquely organized in a partly double-stranded, circular pattern.

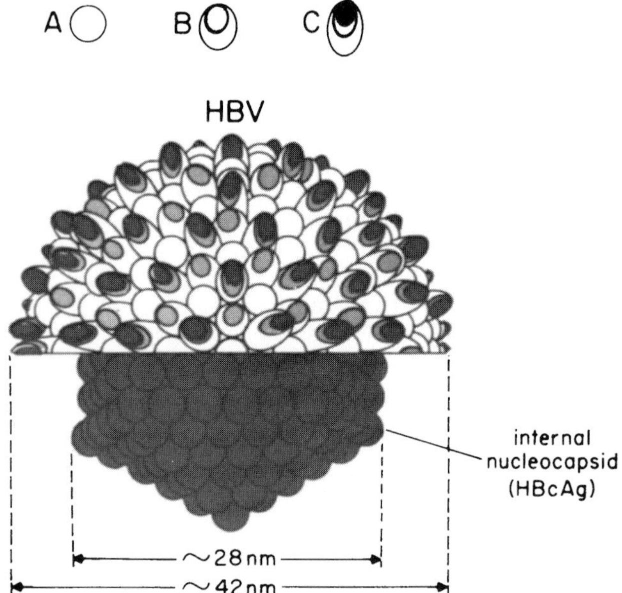

Figure 10–3. Schematic diagram of hepadnavirus particles. Individual subunits containing (*A*) S protein only, (*B*) S protein plus pre-S1, and (*C*) S protein plus pre-S1 and pre-S2 are shown at the top of the figure. S proteins correspond to the white areas, pre-S2 to the gray areas, and pre-S1 to the black areas. The virus particles contain an internal nucleocapsid shown in the bottom split-open section. (From Neurath AR, Thanavala Y. Hepadnaviruses. In von Regenmortel MHV, Neurath AR [eds]. Immunochemistry of Virus, II. The Basis for Serodiagnosis and Vaccines. New York, Elsevier Science, 1990, pp 403–458.)

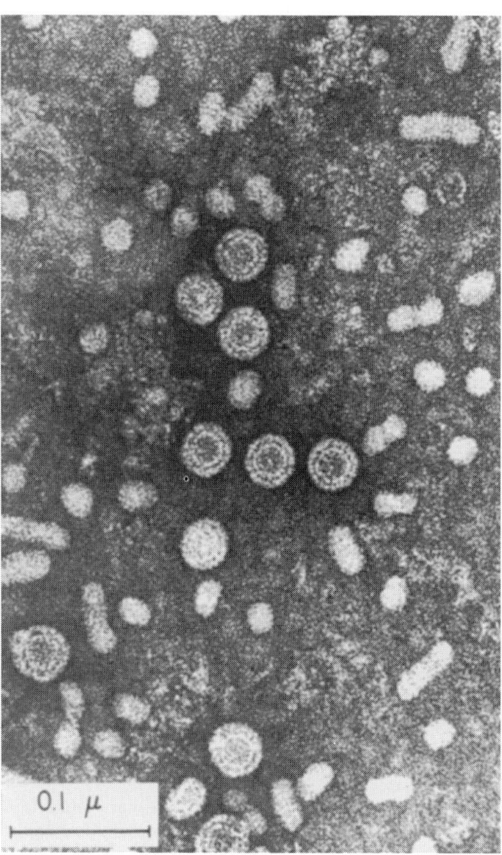

Figure 10–2. Electron micrograph of hepatitis B virus. Note Dane particles (43 nm) as well as spherical and tubular hepatitis B surface antigen particles (22 nm in diameter).

One strand of the DNA, known as the *minus strand,* is almost a complete circle and contains overlapping genes that encode structural proteins (pre-S, surface, core) and replicative proteins (polymerase, X). The *plus strand* of the DNA is shorter and variable in length.

Four messenger RNA transcripts of known function have been identified as being involved in HBV transcription and translation (Fig. 10–4).[39] The longest (3.5 kilobases [kb]) is the template for genome replication and the expression of precore/core and polymerase proteins. A 2.4-kb transcript encodes for pre-S1 and pre-S2 proteins and HBsAg, whereas a 2.1-kb transcript encodes for only pre-S2 protein and HBsAg. The smallest transcript (0.7 kb) encodes for the X protein.

HBcAg and HBeAg are translated from a common gene. When transcribed, HBcAg is targeted to endoplasmic reticulum, where it is cleaved and HBeAg (the precore fragment) is secreted. HBcAg is essential for viral packaging and is an integral part of the nucleocapsid. It is not detectable in serum by conventional techniques; however, it can be detected in liver tissue in patients with acute or chronic HBV infection. HBeAg is a soluble protein that can be detected in the serum of patients with high virus titers. It is not essential for viral replication.

The surface/pre-S gene encodes for the virus envelope. It is speculated that the pre-S proteins play an important role in the attachment of HBV to hepatocytes.[40] Liver-specific attachment sites have been identified in vitro for pre-S1 and pre-S2 proteins.[41–43] In addition, pre-S2 protein has been shown to attach to

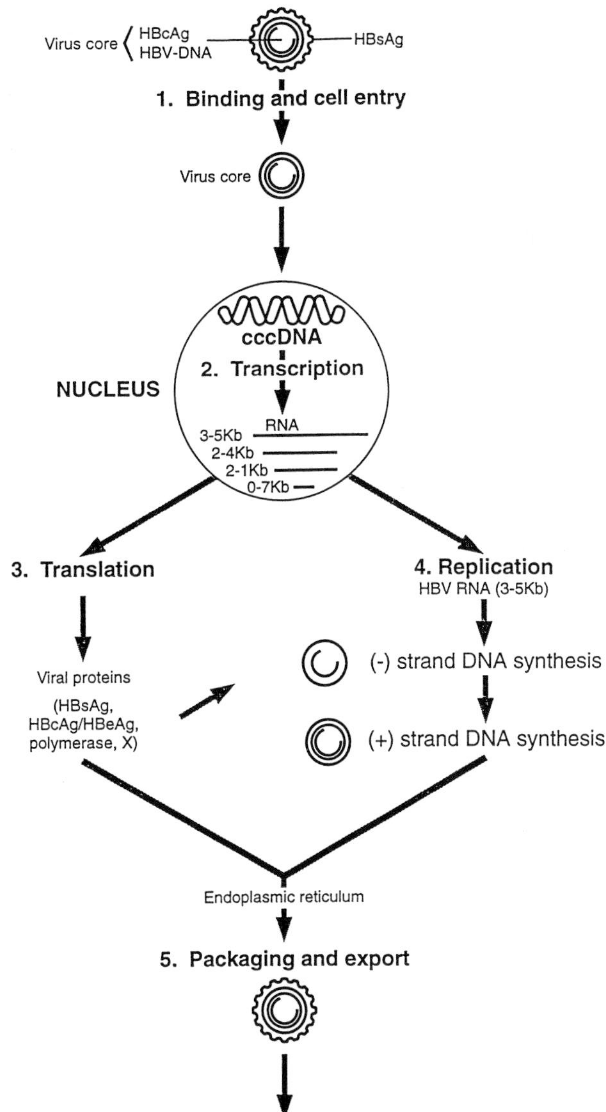

Figure 10–4. Binding and replication of hepatitis B virus (HBV). cccDNA, covalently closed circular DNA; HBcAg, hepatitis B core antigen; HBeAg, hepatitis B e antigen; HBsAg, hepatitis B surface antigen. (From Lau JYN, Wright TL. Molecular virology and pathogenesis of hepatitis B. Lancet 342:1335–1340, 1993.)

artificially polymerized human serum albumin.[42] Because binding of polymerized human serum albumin has also been observed on hepatocytes, it has been hypothesized that binding of HBV to its host cell might be mediated by a bridge of modified albumin.

At the molecular level, data supporting the hepatitis B surface protein (HBs) as the binding site for HBV to hepatocytes have been the subject of intense study and debate.[40] Studies have demonstrated the binding of HBs to Vero cells and recombinant HBs to hepatocytes.[44, 45] However, a direct interaction of natural HBs with hepatocytes or a role of HBs in the penetration of hepatocytes has not been convincingly demonstrated. Thus, the remarkable success of hepatitis B vaccines that do not contain pre-S components has been somewhat of an enigma.

One of the key reasons for the success of current vaccines is the existence of a neutralizing epitope on the HBs protein. This *a* determinant is found on the glycosolated form of HBs, which is cross-linked via disulfide bonds. Antibodies to the *a* determinant confer protection in adults to all the common subtypes of HBV, whereas antibodies to the subtype determinants do not.[46] The *a* determinants are located within the domains bordered by amino acids 120 to 147; these domains contain a predicted double-loop structure projecting from the surface of the virus. It is hypothesized that the major determinants are predominantly located on the second of these two loops, between amino acids 139 and 147 (Fig. 10–5).

Two other determinants of HBs have been described. One determinant has either *d* or *y* specificity, and the other has *w* or *r*. All combinations of these determinants have been found, resulting in four subtypes: adw, adr, ayw, ayr. The most common subtype among people with HBV infection in the United States is adw.[47]

HBV replication begins with binding of the virus to the cell surface and penetration.[39, 43] The virus is transported to the nucleus without processing, where the relaxed circular DNA is converted to a covalently closed circular DNA (cccDNA), which in turn acts as the template for viral RNA synthesis. HBV DNA does not integrate into the host genome during the normal course of replication. Transcription results in RNA of various sizes. The 3.5-kb genomic RNA serves as a template for reverse transcription and DNA synthesis, which produces an open circular DNA molecule. The mature core particles are packed into HBsAg/pre-S proteins in the endoplasmic reticulum and exported from the cell. A pool of cccDNA is maintained in the nuclei by transporting newly synthesized HBV DNA back to the nucleus. That HBsAg can inhibit formation of cccDNA may represent a negative feedback to HBV replication.[48]

Pathogenesis

The cellular and humoral immune responses to HBV infection are complex. Most studies suggest that HBV is not directly cytopathic to infected hepatocytes and that the cellular response to several viral proteins correlates with the severity of clinical disease and viral clearance.[49] It is believed that the antibody response to viral envelope antigens contributes to clearance of the virus and that the T-cell response to envelope, nucleocapsid, and polymerase antigens is responsible for eliminating infected cells. It is hypothesized that chronic infection is related to a weak T-cell response to viral antigens. Although neonatal immune tolerance to viral antigens appears to play an important role for viral persistence in patients infected at birth, the basis for poor T-cell response in adults is not well understood.

Diagnosis

Because the clinical symptoms of HBV infection are indistinguishable from those of other forms of viral hep-

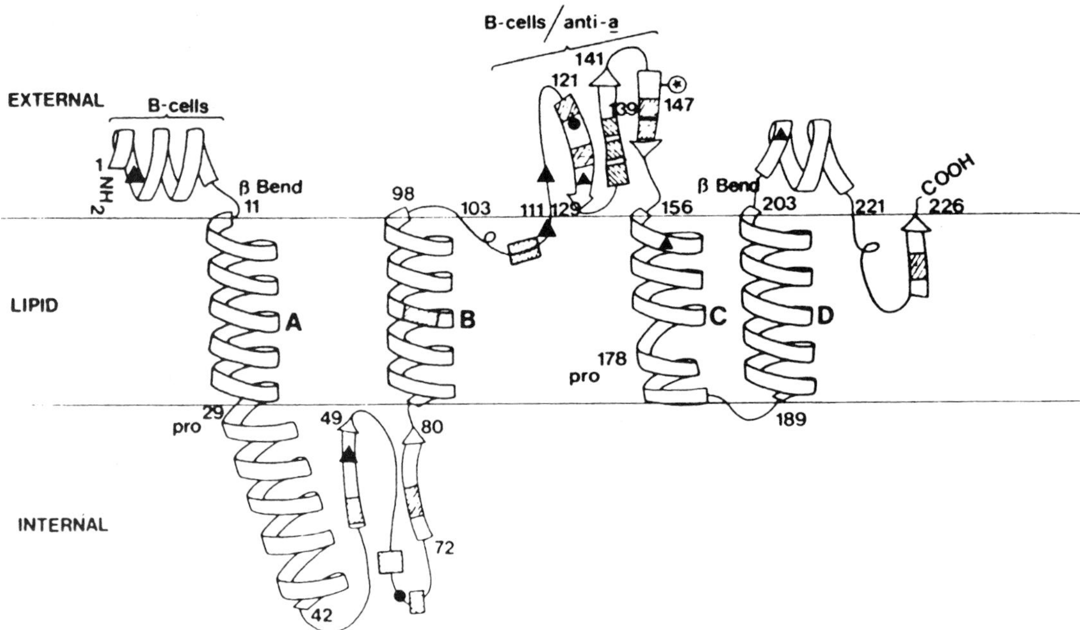

Figure 10–5. Secondary structure of hepatitis B virus s antigen in the lipid envelope as predicted by computer modeling. The shaded areas indicate the locations of sequence variations for *w/r* (▲) and *d/y* (●) subtypes. (From Howard C, Smith Stinh HJ, Brown SE, Steward MW. Towards the development of a synthetic hepatitis B vaccine. In Zuckerman A [ed]. Viral Hepatitis and Liver Disease. New York, Alan R Liss, 1988.)

atitis, definitive diagnosis is dependent on serological testing for HBV infection. Acute HBV infection is characterized by the presence of HBsAg in serum and the development of immunoglobulin M (IgM)–class antibody to HBcAg (IgM anti-HBc, Table 10–1). HBeAg is also detectable during acute infection. During convalescence, HBsAg and HBeAg are cleared, and IgG antibodies to HBsAg (anti-HBs), HBcAb (anti-HBc), and HBeAg develop (Fig. 10–6). Anti-HBs is a protective antibody that neutralizes the virus. The presence of anti-HBs following acute infection indicates recovery and immunity from reinfection. Anti-HBs is also detected among people who have received hepatitis B vaccine. Total anti-HBc includes both IgM- and IgG-class antibody to the core protein and indicates exposure to virus in the host and viral replication. Anti-HBc appears shortly after HBsAg among people with acute disease and generally persists for life. It is therefore not a good marker for people with acute disease. The detection of IgM anti-HBc is diagnostic of acute HBV infection.

In people with chronic HBV infection, HBsAg remains persistently detectable, generally for life (Fig. 10–7). HBeAg is variably present and IgM anti-HBc generally becomes undetectable 6 to 9 months after the development of acute infection.

Treatment

No specific treatment is available for people with acute HBV infection; supportive care and symptomatic care are the mainstays of therapy. Numerous antiviral agents have been investigated for the treatment of chronic HBV infection. In 1976, two studies, one with

Table 10–1. **INTERPRETATIONS OF AVAILABLE SEROLOGICAL TEST RESULTS FOR HEPATITIS B VIRUS***

HBsAg	IgM–ANTI-HBc	IgG–ANTI-HBc	ANTI-HBs	INTERPRETATION
+	−	−	−	Early HBV infection before anti-HBc response.
+	+	− or +	−	Early HBV infection. Because IgM anti-HBc is positive, the onset is within 6 months. IgG antibody usually appears shortly after IgM; therefore, both are usually positive when IgM is positive.
−	+	+	− or +	Recent acute HBV infection (within 4–6 mo) with resolution (i.e., HbsAg has already disappeared). Anti-HBs usually appears within a few weeks or months of HbsAg disappearance.
+	−	+	−	HBV infection, onset at least 6 months ago because IgM–anti-HBc has disappeared; probable chronic HBV infection.
−	−	+	+	Past HBV infection, recovered.

*+ and − indicate presence and absence of antibody, respectively.

HBV, hepatitis B virus; IgM–anti-HBs, immunoglobulin M antibody to hepatitis B surface antigen (HBsAg); IgG–anti-HBc, immunoglobulin G antibody to hepatitis B core antigen; IgM–anti-HBc, immunoglobulin M antibody to hepatitis B core antigen.

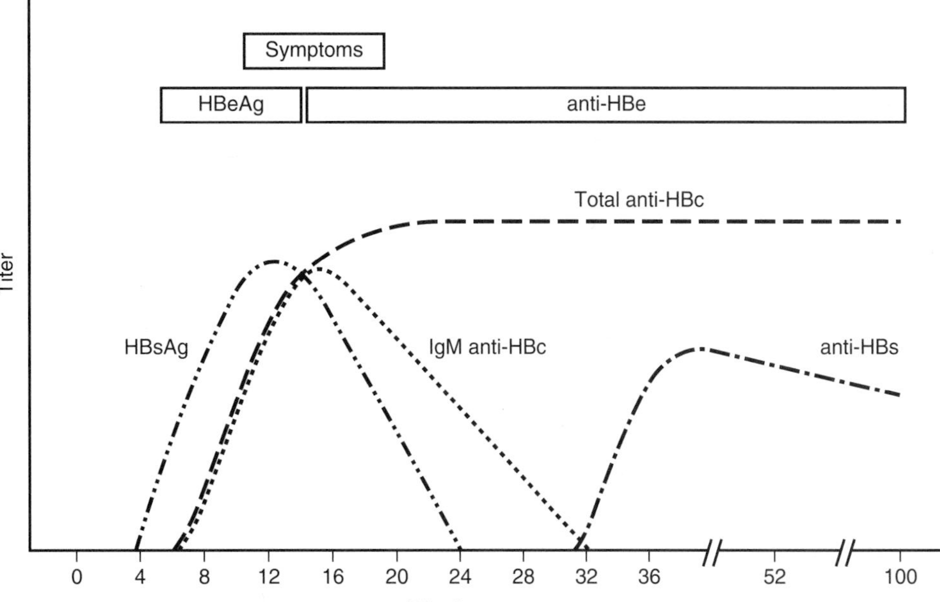

Figure 10–6. Titer of hepatitis B surface antigen (HBsAg), antibody to hepatitis B core antigen (anti-HBc), immunoglobulin M anti-HBc, and antibody to hepatitis B surface antigen (anti-HBs) in patients with acute hepatitis B with recovery.

leukocyte interferon and one with β-interferon, suggested that interferon can affect the serological profile of people with chronic HBV infection.[50, 51] Follow-up studies revealed the most promising agent to be interferon alfa-2b, which has been licensed for this purpose by the Food and Drug Administration (FDA). The goals of interferon treatment for patients with chronic HBV infection are to clear serological markers of HBV replication and improve the liver disease (normalization of alanine aminotransferase [ALT] levels and liver histology). In a meta-analysis of 15 clinical trials, the overall response rate (as measured by clearance of HBeAg from serum) was 33% among patients treated with interferon compared with 12% among control subjects.[52] Long-term follow-up of treated patients suggests that remission of chronic hepatitis induced by interferon alfa-2b is of long duration.[53]

Interferon alfa-2b treatment of patients with chronic hepatitis B is recommended for patients with persistent elevations in serum aminotransferase concentrations; detectable levels of HBsAg, HBeAg, and HBV DNA in serum; chronic hepatitis on liver biopsy; and compensated liver disease.[54] Patients with normal aminotransferase levels should not be treated. Biopsy of the liver should be performed before therapy to assess the degree of fibrosis present. The recommended regimen is either 5 million units daily or 10 million units three times weekly, given subcutaneously for 4 months. Patient characteristics associated with favorable response to therapy include low pretherapy HBV DNA levels, high prether-

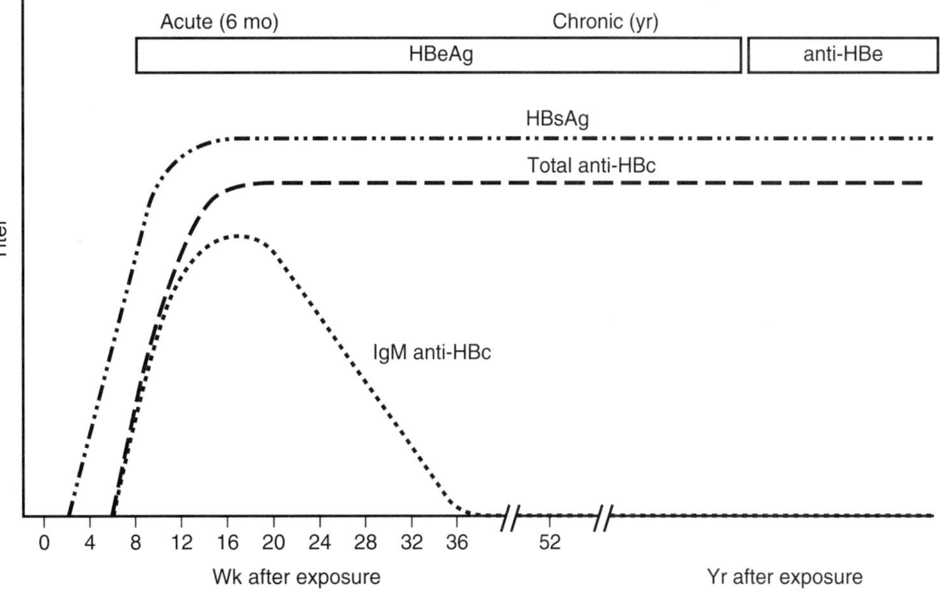

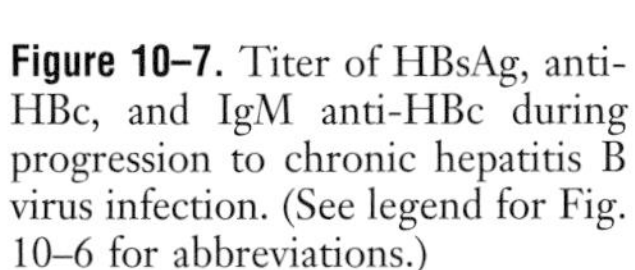
Figure 10–7. Titer of HBsAg, anti-HBc, and IgM anti-HBc during progression to chronic hepatitis B virus infection. (See legend for Fig. 10–6 for abbreviations.)

apy ALT levels, a short duration of infection, the acquisition of disease in adulthood, the presence of active inflammation on liver biopsy, and the absence of complicating diseases such as renal failure or HIV infection.

Because relatively few patients respond to interferon therapy, considerable research has been conducted on other antiviral and immune-modulating agents. Nucleoside analogues such as famciclovir and lamivudine have been extensively evaluated and shown to be well tolerated after oral administration.[55–57] Both drugs lead to rapid decreases in HBV DNA levels; clearance of HBeAg and decreases in serum aminotransferase levels have been observed in some patients. However, short courses of therapy have been followed by a rapid return of viral DNA to pretreatment levels and no sustained improvement in chronic liver disease. Clinical trials of long-term therapy are under way.

Combination therapies of hepatitis B vaccine with interferon and hepatitis B vaccine with anti-HBs have been shown to be effective in the treatment of chronic HBV infection[58, 59]; however, controlled trials have not been conducted. A placebo-controlled trial in transgenic mice has demonstrated that high-dose hepatitis B vaccine in adjuvant is effective in the treatment of chronic HBV infection.[60]

EPIDEMIOLOGY

HBV is transmitted by percutaneous or permucosal exposure to infectious body fluids, by sexual contact with an infected person, and perinatally from an infected mother to infant (Table 10–2). The frequency of HBV infection and patterns of HBV transmission vary markedly among different parts of the world. Approximately 45% of the world's population live in areas where the prevalence of chronic HBV infection is high (i.e., ≥8% of the population is HBsAg-positive); 43% live in areas where the prevalence is moderate (i.e., 2–7% of the population is HBsAg-positive); and 12% live in areas of low endemicity (i.e., <2% of the population is HBsAg-positive; Fig. 10–8).

Table 10–2. **MODES OF TRANSMISSION OF HEPATITIS B VIRUS**

Percutaneous transmission
Blood and transfusion products
Contaminated needles and syringes
Invasive medical procedures
Hemodialysis
Permucosal transmission
Perinatal
Sexual contact
Intimate physical contact

In areas of high endemicity, the lifetime risk of HBV infection is more than 60%, and most infections occur at birth or during early childhood, when the risk of chronic infection is greatest. Because most early childhood HBV infections are asymptomatic, there is little recognition of acute disease; however, rates of chronic liver disease and liver cancer are very high. Areas of high endemicity include most of Asia (except Japan and India), most of the Middle East, the Amazon basin, most Pacific Island groups, Africa, and other special

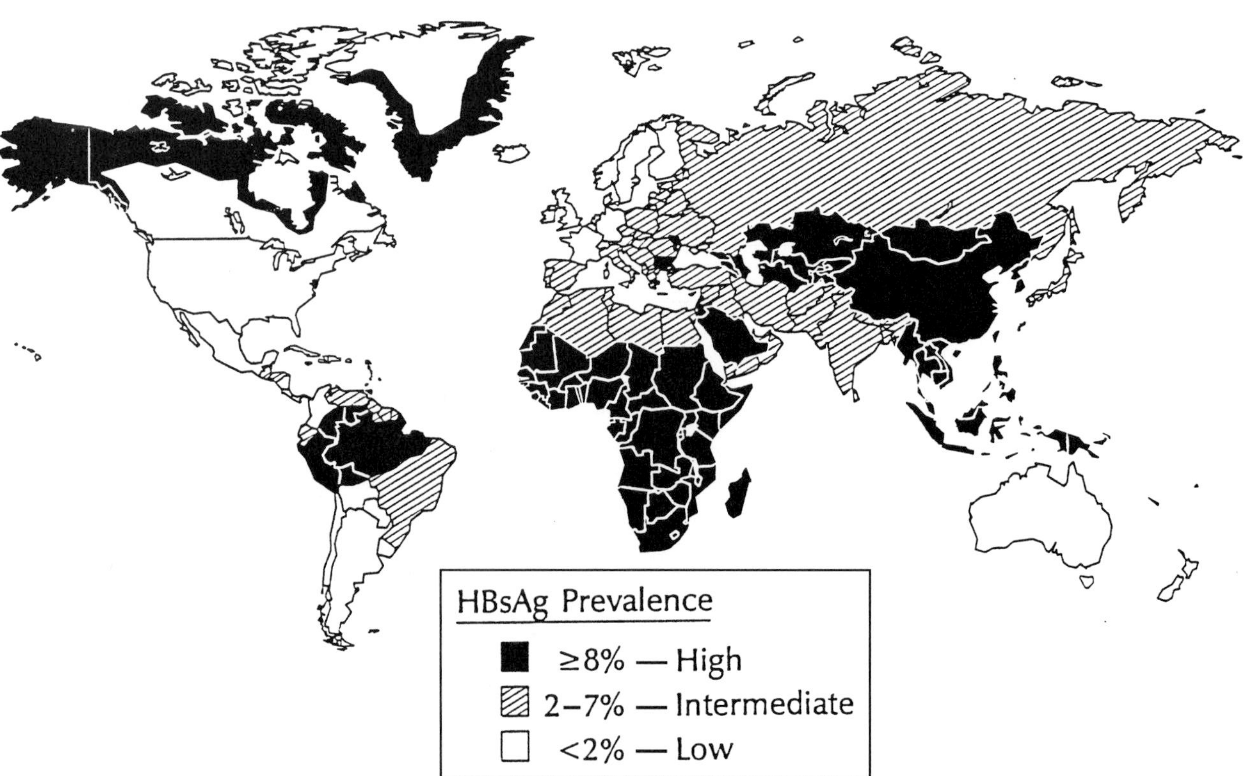

Figure 10–8. Geographical distribution of chronic hepatitis B virus infection.

populations such as Australian aborigines and Maoris in New Zealand.[30, 61–71]

The mechanisms of early childhood transmission in areas of high endemicity are variable. Generally, infections cluster in households of people with chronic infection.[72] The major determinants of infection include exposure to an HBsAg-positive mother or sibling. The contribution of perinatal transmission to the overall burden of disease is related to the prevalence of HBeAg among pregnant women. If a mother is HBsAg-positive and HBeAg-positive, 70 to 90% of infants become infected if not given immunoprophylaxis.[73, 74] Among infants born to HBsAg-positive mothers who are HBeAg-negative, approximately 5 to 20% are infected at birth. Infants of HBsAg-positive women who are not infected at birth are at increased risk of HBV infection during early childhood, owing to household contact with infected people.[75]

In east and southeast Asian countries as well as the Pacific, 35 to 50% of HBsAg-positive women are also HBeAg-positive.[67, 73–79] In these countries, it is estimated that 3 to 5% of all infants may develop chronic HBV infection at birth and that as many as 30 to 50% of all chronic infections among children result from perinatal transmission. In areas of high endemicity where the prevalence of HBeAg among pregnant women is low (i.e., Africa, South America, and the Middle East), perinatal HBV transmission contributes less to the pool of children with chronic infection than does postnatal person-to-person transmission.[61, 80–84] In general in these areas, 1 to 2% of infants develop chronic infection, and 10 to 20% of all chronic infections among children result from perinatal exposures.

In areas of moderate endemicity, the lifetime risk of HBV infection is 20 to 60%, and infections occur in all age groups. Recognition of acute disease is common because many infections occur in adolescents and young adults. In addition, high rates of HBV-related chronic liver disease also occur, owing to the high prevalence of chronic HBV infection. In general in areas of moderate endemicity, 2 to 7% of pregnant women are HBsAg-positive, and less than 20% of HBsAg-positive women are HBeAg-positive; thus, perinatal transmission accounts for a small proportion (10–20%) of the people with chronic infection. In these areas, early childhood HBV transmission may be quite variable in different regions or among different ethnic groups within a country. Acute disease among adults tends to occur in the same risk groups as in developed countries.

In areas of low endemicity, the lifetime risk of infection is less than 20%, and most infections occur among adults in well-defined risk groups. In the United States, the prevalence of chronic HBV infection is 0.35%, and 5% of the general population has evidence of prior HBV infection.[85, 86] In the United States, high-risk groups for HBV infection include injection drug users, homosexual men, people who have heterosexual contact with multiple partners, household contacts of people with chronic HBV infection, hemophiliacs, hemodialysis patients and staff, inmates of long-term correctional facilities, people with occupational exposure to blood and infectious body fluids, and institutionalized people with developmental disabilities.[87, 88]

Whereas most acute HBV infections in the United States occur among young adults, about one third of the chronic infections are acquired through perinatal and early childhood exposures.[85] It is estimated that 20,000 HBsAg-positive women give birth each year in the United States and that 9500 infants would become infected if prophylaxis were not provided.[89, 90] In addition, a number of well-defined populations with high rates of early childhood HBV transmission reside in the United States, including Alaskan Natives, children of Pacific Island communities, and children of first-generation immigrants from countries where HBV is of high or intermediate endemicity. Among U.S.-born children of first-generation immigrants during the first decade of life, infection rates average 1 to 2% per year, and the prevalence of chronic HBV infection ranges from 1 to 7%.[91–93] These infections are acquired through exposure to HBsAg-positive household members and exposures within the community.

In the United States, reports of acute hepatitis B increased by 37% from 1979 to 1985 but since 1986 declined to 1979 levels (Fig. 10–9).[87, 90] It is estimated that 100,000 to 150,000 people are infected each year and that 5000 people die each year owing to HBV-related liver disease. Three hundred of these deaths are due to fulminant hepatitis, 3000 to 4000 to cirrhosis, and 600 to 1000 to primary hepatocellular carcinoma.[85]

Worldwide, the consequences of acute and chronic HBV infection are major public health problems. Studies in Taiwan have demonstrated that people with chronic HBV infection are predisposed to developing chronic liver disease and have a more than 100-fold increased risk of hepatocellular carcinoma when compared with noninfected people.[94] Approximately 5% of the world's population (300 million people) has chronic HBV infection, which is the leading cause of chronic hepatitis, cirrhosis, and hepatocellular carcinoma worldwide.[77] Approximately 500,000 to 1 million people die annually owing to HBV-related liver disease.

PASSIVE IMMUNIZATION

The discovery that passively acquired anti-HBs could protect individuals from acute clinical hepatitis B and chronic HBV infection if given soon after exposure led to the development of a specific immune globulin containing high titers of anti-HBs. This HBIG was used before hepatitis B vaccines became available and is recommended, often in combination with hepatitis B vaccine, as postexposure prophylaxis following (1) perinatal exposure for an infant born to an HBsAg-positive mother, (2) percutaneous or mucous membrane exposure to HBsAg-positive blood, or (3) sexual exposure to an HBsAg-positive person (see *Indications for Vaccine, Postexposure Prophylaxis*). HBIG is also used to protect patients from severe recurrent HBV infection after liver transplantation.

HBIG is prepared by the Cohn Oncly fractionation procedure from serum containing high titers of anti-

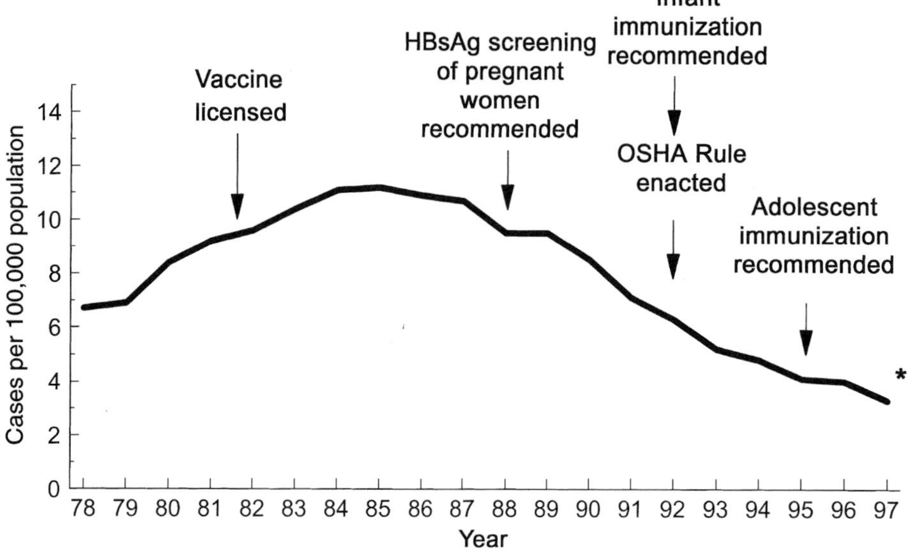

Figure 10–9. Reported cases of hepatitis B in the United States, 1978 to 1997. Case rate not adjusted for asymptomatic infections or for underreporting. HBsAg, hepatitis B surface antigen; OSHA, Occupational Safety and Health Administration. *Provisional data.

HBs and is standardized to 100,000 IU of anti-HBs per mL. Although HBIG is approximately 75% effective in preventing clinical hepatitis B or the development of the carrier state if used shortly after exposure to the virus,[95, 95a, 96] there are a number of drawbacks to its use. Protection afforded by HBIG lasts only several months, leaving the recipient susceptible to HBV infection after antibody titers decline. It is expensive and is usually not affordable in the developing world. Although HBIG is a plasma product that has never been linked to the transmission of HCV, HIV, or other bloodborne infections,[97, 98] other plasma products such as intravenous immunoglobulin have been rarely linked to HCV transmission,[99] and there may be some reluctance among healthcare providers and the public to use similar products.

One of the major uses of HBIG is as an adjunct to hepatitis B vaccine in preventing perinatal HBV transmission. Untreated, 70 to 90% of infants born to HBeAg-positive mothers become infected at birth and develop chronic HBV infection.[73, 74] A regimen of three doses of HBIG, if started within 48 hours of birth, is approximately 75% effective in preventing chronic infection in 1-year-old infants.[100] However, the child continues to live in a household with an infected mother and often becomes infected after the first year of life, so HBIG therapy alone is not sufficient for long-term protection of children born to HBsAg-positive mothers.

With the development of hepatitis B vaccines, it was shown that treatment with both HBIG and hepatitis B vaccine could increase the efficacy of preventing perinatal HBV transmission to 85 to 95% and provide long-term protection.[74, 101] More recent studies have shown that vaccine alone, when started at birth and at appropriate doses, provides as good protection as HBIG alone or HBIG plus vaccine.[102] In most industrialized countries, combination therapy with HBIG and vaccine is standard therapy to prevent perinatal HBV transmission. In these settings, pregnant women must be screened for HBsAg to identify which newborns receive immunoprophylaxis at birth. This strategy is not widely used in developing countries because the funds and infrastructure to screen pregnant women may not be available; HBIG may not be affordable; and, if all infants receive hepatitis B vaccine at birth, the incremental benefit of screening mothers and using HBIG plus vaccine in infants of carrier mothers is small.

HBIG is also indicated for postexposure prophylaxis of needle stick or other percutaneous injuries in susceptible individuals exposed to infectious body fluids from HBsAg-positive source-patients. Preexposure prophylaxis with hepatitis B vaccine has decreased the need for HBIG in this setting. The efficacy of HBIG alone in preventing acute clinical hepatitis B in needle stick recipients was demonstrated in two large, multicenter trials.[96] These trials demonstrated that, when untreated, approximately 30% of exposed people would develop clinical infection after needle stick exposure and that HBIG was approximately 75% effective in preventing clinical disease. With the availability of hepatitis B vaccine, postexposure prophylaxis protocols were developed that account for the vaccination and serological status of the exposed person (see under *Indications for Vaccine, Postexposure Prophylaxis*). These protocols use HBIG in nonvaccinated individuals or in vaccine nonresponders.

The efficacy of HBIG in preventing clinical hepatitis B or chronic HBV infection following sexual exposure to an acutely infected partner is approximately 75% if given within 7 days of exposure.[103] Current recommendations for postexposure prophylaxis following sexual exposure to an infected person include the use of HBIG and hepatitis B vaccine (see under *Indications for Vaccine, Postexposure Prophylaxis*).

ACTIVE IMMUNIZATION

Vaccines

Development of Vaccines

Safe, immunogenic, and effective hepatitis B vaccines have been commercially available since 1982. Hepatitis

B vaccines are composed of highly purified preparations of HBsAg. HBsAg is a glycoprotein that makes up the outer envelope of HBV and is also found as 22-nm spheres and tubular forms in the serum of people with acute or chronic infection. Vaccines are prepared by harvesting HBsAg from the plasma of people with chronic infection (plasma-derived vaccine) or by inserting plasmids containing the viral S gene, and in some cases the pre-S1 and/or pre-S2 gene, into yeast or mammalian cells; this insertion induces the cells to express HBsAg, which self-assembles into immunogenic particles (recombinant DNA vaccine). The vaccines undergo various inactivation steps and are highly purified; the adjuvant aluminum phosphate or aluminum hydroxide is then added to the vaccine, which is preserved with thymerosal.

Plasma-Derived Vaccines

Because it has not been possible to grow HBV in tissue culture and no animals except higher primates are susceptible to HBV infection, the development of hepatitis B vaccines is considered a major achievement in medicine. Plasma-derived vaccines are prepared by harvesting the 22-nm particles of HBsAg from plasma.[104] The particles are highly purified, and any residual infectious particles are inactivated by various combinations of urea, pepsin, formaldehyde, and heat. Plasma-derived vaccines are no longer produced by manufacturers in North America or western Europe, but several hundred million doses per year are produced by manufacturers in Asia, including several producers each in South Korea and China (Table 10–3).[104] New plasma-derived vaccines are under development in Indonesia, Vietnam, Myanmar, North Korea, and Iran.

Recombinant DNA Vaccines

Despite the licensure of highly effective plasma-derived vaccines in the early 1980s, vaccine use was limited because of the unfounded fears regarding the safety of plasma-derived products and the high cost of the vaccine. Subsequently, several vaccine manufacturers used recombinant DNA technology to express HBsAg in other organisms, which led to the development of recombinant DNA hepatitis B vaccines.[104–106] Although it was much more costly than the production of plasma-derived vaccines, recombinant DNA technology offered the potential to produce unlimited supplies of safe and effective vaccine that could eventually be produced at a lower price than plasma-derived vaccines. Despite this potential, plasma-derived vaccines have had equivalent safety and efficacy profiles and continue to remain less costly than recombinant DNA–derived vaccines.

Recombinant DNA vaccines are produced by inserting plasmids containing HBsAg genes into yeast or mammalian cells. All licensed vaccines consist of the 226-amino-acid S gene product (HBsAg protein), except for GENHEVAC B, which consists of the 281-amino-acid pre-S2 + S gene product. The yeast-produced vaccines, which are the most widely used, are obtained by inserting the gene for HBsAg into a plasmid downstream of three genes from *Saccharomyces cerevisiae* that serve to promote production of the antigen. A master seed of the transformed yeast is then made, from which working seeds are derived. Each time a lot of vaccine is needed, yeast from the working seed serves to start the fermentation in large vessels. The HBsAg must then be purified to eliminate yeast components. This is done by various physical separation techniques, including chromatography and filtration.

The expressed HBsAg polypeptide self-assembles into immunogenic spherical particles closely resembling the

Table 10–3. **HEPATITIS B VACCINES AVAILABLE INTERNATIONALLY***

MANUFACTURER	BRAND NAME†	COUNTRY	TYPE
Centro de Ingenieria Genetica Y Biotecnologia	Enivac-HB	Cuba	Recombinant DNA
Chiel Jedang	Hepaccine-B	South Korea	Plasma derived
Korea Green Cross	Hepavax B	South Korea	Plasma derived
Korea Green Cross	Hepavax-Gene	South Korea	Recombinant DNA
LG Chemical	Euvax B	South Korea	Recombinant DNA
Merck Sharp & Dohme	Recombivax H-B-Vax II	United States	Recombinant DNA
Merck Sharp & Dohme	Comvax	United States	Combined Hib and (recombinant)
Pasteur Mérieux Connaught	Genhevac B	France	Recombinant DNA (mammalian cell)
SmithKline Beecham	Engerix-B	Belgium	Recombinant DNA
SmithKline Beecham	Twinrix	Belgium	Combined hepatitis A and B (recombinant)
SmithKline Beecham	Tritanrix-HB	Belgium	Combined DTP and recombinant
SmithKline Beecham	Infanrix-HB	Belgium	Combined DTP (acellular P) and HB (recombinant)
Swiss Serum and Vaccines Institute	Heprecombe	Switzerland	Recombinant DNA (mammalian cell)

*Numerous producers who sell only in country of production are not listed. Presence on this list does not imply endorsement of these products by the World Health Organization.

†Brand names may vary in different countries.

DTP, diphtheria tetanus, and pertussis; HB, hepatitis B; Hib, *Haemophilus influenzae* type b.

natural 22-nm particles found in the serum of people with chronic HBV infection. The *a* epitope that is responsible for the most important immune response is exposed on the surface of the artificial HBsAg particle, as it is on the natural particle. The artificial particles differ from the natural ones only in the glycosylation of the HBsAg. The artificial particles may or may not contain pre-S1 or pre-S2 peptides attached to the surface antigen, depending on whether genetic information to code for these peptides was inserted into the expression vector. Recombinant DNA vaccines are produced in Belgium, China, Cuba, France, Japan, South Korea, and the United States, and new vaccines are under development in Brazil, China, Great Britain, Russia, and South Korea.

Combination Vaccines

Several vaccine manufacturers are working to produce combination vaccines containing a hepatitis B component. Diphtheria, tetanus, and pertussis–hepatitis B (DTP-Hep B) vaccine is licensed in Europe, and several other producers in a number of countries, including developing countries, are trying to produce this combination. Combination vaccines containing diphtheria, tetanus, and acellular pertussis (DTaP); hepatitis B (Hep B); *Haemophilus influenzae* type b (Hib); and inactivated polivirus are also under development. These include DTaP–Hep B, DTP–Hep B–Hib, and DTP–Hep B–Hib-IPV vaccines. An Hib-Hep B vaccine is licensed for use in the United States,[107] and a combination vaccine of hepatitis A virus and HBV is available in Europe (see Chapter 20).[108]

Stability of Hepatitis B Vaccine. Similar to DTP vaccine, hepatitis B vaccine should be shipped and stored at 2 to 8°C. As the adjuvant alum is added to the vaccine, freezing dissociates the antigen from the alum and interferes with the immunogenicity of the vaccine. The vaccine is quite thermostable, however, and heating of the vaccine at 45°C for 1 week or 37°C for 1 month altered neither reactogenicity nor immunogenicity of the vaccine.[109] In a study performed in Guangxi Province, China, the vaccine was taken out of the cold chain and stored for 1 to 2 months at an average temperature of 25°C without loss of immunogenicity.[110] This excellent stability may allow vaccine to be given by trained birth attendants during home deliveries where refrigeration is not available.

Route of Immunization and Dosage

Hepatitis B vaccine should be administered only in the deltoid muscle of adults, adolescents, and children or in the anterolateral thigh muscle of neonates, infants, and children in the second year of life. In adults, the immunogenicity of the vaccine is substantially lower when injections are given in the buttock.[111] For infants and children, vaccine should be administered using a ⅞- to 1-inch needle, whereas in adolescents and adults a 1- to 1½-inch needle is required to ensure delivery of vaccine into muscle tissue.

When hepatitis B vaccine is administered to infants at the same time as other vaccines, it is preferable to avoid administering two injections in the same limb, especially if DTP is the other product. If more than one injection is administered, the thigh is the preferred site; the injections should be sufficiently separated (1–2 inches apart) so that local reactions are unlikely to overlap. In older infants, the deltoid region and the anterolateral thigh can be used when giving multiple injections.

In the United States, vaccines are licensed for all age groups as a three-dose series consisting of two priming doses given 1 month apart and a third dose given 6 months after the third dose. The recommended dose varies by product; the recipient's age; and, for infants, the mother's HBsAg serological status (Tables 10–4 and 10–5). In general, the vaccine dose for infants and adolescents is 50% lower than that required for

Table 10–4. **RECOMMENDED DOSES OF CURRENTLY LICENSED HEPATITIS B VACCINES**

GROUP	RECOMBIVAX HB DOSE (μg)*	ENGERIX-B DOSE (μg)*
Infants of hepatitis B surface antigen (HBsAg)–negative mothers	5	10
Infants of HBsAg-positive mothers; prevention of perinatal infection	5	10
Children (1–10 yr)	5	10
Adolescents (11–19 yr)	5	10
Adults (≥20 yr)	10	20
Dialysis patients and other immunocompromised people	40†	40‡

*See Table 10–5 for dosage schedules.
†Special formulation in 1 mL.
‡Two 1-mL doses given at one site in a four-dose schedule at 0, 1, 2, and 6 mo.

Table 10–5. **RECOMMENDED SCHEDULE OF HEPATITIS B VACCINATION IN VARIOUS SETTINGS***

DOSE†	AGE INTERVAL
Infants born to HBsAg-negative mothers	
1	Birth–2 mo
2	1–4 mo
3	6–18 mo
Infants born to HBsAg-positive mothers	
1	Birth (within 12 hr)
HBIG‡	Birth (within 12 hr)
2	1–2 mo
3	6 mo
Children, Adolescents, and Adults§	
1	—
2	1–2 mo
3	4–6 mo

* The choice of schedule should be used to facilitate the highest rate of vaccination compliance.
† See Table 10–4 for appropriate vaccine dose.
‡ Hepatitis B immunoglobulin—0.5 mL given intramuscularly.
§ This age group should be vaccinated on a 0-, 1-, and 6-month schedule, although schedules of 0, 2, and 4 months and 0, 1, and 4 months have been shown to have comparable seroprotection rates.

adults. Among infants receiving preexposure vaccination, no differences in seroprotection exist between U.S.-licensed vaccines following the third vaccine dose, although some differences exist prior to complete vaccination.[112] However, there is little chance that HBV infection would occur prior to completion of the recommended vaccination schedule, making the early differences in immunogenicity of no practical significance.

Compared with three standard doses administered intramuscularly, a regimen of three low doses of plasma-derived or recombinant vaccine administered intradermally to adults usually results in lower seroconversion rates (55–81%) and lower final titers of anti-HBs. However, four doses of plasma-derived or recombinant vaccine administered intradermally have produced antibody responses comparable to vaccine administered by intramuscular injection.[113, 114] Routine intradermal vaccination is not recommended for a number of reasons, including poor immunogenicity in infants and young children, inconsistency of antibody response in older people, lack of experience by most healthcare providers in performing intradermal vaccination, and lack of data on the long-term protection afforded by this route of administration.

RESULTS OF VACCINATION

Immunogenicity

The protective efficacy of hepatitis B vaccination is directly related to the development of anti-HBs.[115–118] People who develop anti-HBs titers greater than 10 mIU per mL after a primary vaccination series are virtually 100% protected against clinical illness and chronic infection. Vaccine produced by each manufacturer has been evaluated in clinical trials to determine the age-specific dose that achieves the maximum seroprotection rate. The priming doses induce detectable levels of antibody in 70 to 90% of healthy infants, adolescents, and adults.[112, 119–125] The final dose induces protective levels of anti-HBs in more than 95% of infants of HBsAg-negative women and adolescents.

Currently licensed vaccines produce high rates of seroprotection (>95%) in a variety of vaccination schedules used to deliver childhood vaccines, including those beginning in the newborn period and those with a 2-month interval between vaccine doses. Increasing the interval between the first and second dose of hepatitis B vaccine has little effect on immunogenicity or final antibody titer. Longer intervals between the last two doses result in higher final antibody levels.

Infants born prematurely do not respond well to doses given at birth; if born to antigen-negative mothers, vaccination should be delayed (see under Indications for Vaccination).[125a]

The recommended series of three intramuscular doses of hepatitis B vaccine induces a protective antibody response in more than 90% of healthy adults younger than 40 years. After age 40 years, the cumulative age-specific decline in immunogenicity drops below 90%, and by age 60 years, only 65 to 75% of vaccinees develop protective levels of anti-HBs. Although other host factors, such as smoking, obesity, HIV infection, and the presence of a chronic disease, contribute to decreased immunogenicity of the primary vaccination series, age is the major determinant of poor vaccine response.[125–127]

Retrospective studies have suggested a difference in age-specific immunogenicity between the two vaccines licensed in the United States (Engerix-B and Recombivax HB) when given to adults.[126–127] However, a prospective study found no differences in immunogenicity for people younger than 55 years.[125] For people older than 55 years, the likelihood of nonresponse was approximately two times greater among people receiving Recombivax HB compared with people receiving Engerix-B. However, this difference in immunogenicity would result in only a marginal difference in disease prevention and does not warrant the preferential use of one vaccine. Routine postvaccination testing for antibody response is not indicated on the basis of age alone but must take into account the likelihood of the vaccinated person's risk of HBV infection and need for postexposure prophylaxis.

Results of Controlled Trials

The efficacy of hepatitis B vaccines has been demonstrated in clinical trials involving several high-risk groups, including homosexual men, healthcare workers, hemodialysis staff members, children living in areas of high endemicity, and infants of HBeAg-positive (highly infectious) mothers.[74, 101, 115–118] These studies demonstrated an overall efficacy of 85 to 95% and virtually complete protection among people who developed anti-HBs titers greater than 10 mIU following vaccination. Cases of clinical hepatitis B and rarely of chronic HBV infection were observed among people who developed anti-HBs responses less than 10 mIU. Studies among children living in areas of high endemicity have also demonstrated excellent vaccine efficacy among people who develop anti-HBs titers greater than 10 mIU per mL. For these reasons, an anti-HBs response greater than 10 mIU by commercial radioimmunoassay or enzyme immunoassay is considered to be the lower limit of adequate response to vaccine.

Among infants born to HBeAg-positive mothers, combined treatment with either plasma or recombinant vaccines and HBIG is 79 to 98% effective in preventing chronic HBV infection (Table 10–6).[130–141] One longitudinal study found significantly lower rates of chronic infection among infants treated with recombinant vaccines and HBIG (3.8%) compared with infants treated with plasma-derived vaccine and HBIG (10.5–13.9%).[142] Several studies have demonstrated high efficacy of vaccine alone in preventing perinatal HBV transmission, including reports in which the administration of HBIG provided no additional protection (see Table 10–6). However, lower doses of vaccine alone appear to be less effective in preventing perinatal HBV transmission when compared with vaccine and HBIG (Centers for Disease Control and Prevention [CDC], unpublished data).[140]

A Dutch study showed 92% efficacy of passive-active

Table 10–6. **STUDIES ON THE EFFICACY OF HEPATITIS B VACCINES IN NEONATES BORN TO HEPATITIS B e ANTIGEN–POSITIVE MOTHERS**

STUDY	VACCINE	DOSE (μg)	SCHEDULE (age in mo)	HBIG AT BIRTH	NO. PEOPLE STUDIED	HBsAg-POSITIVE (%)†	EFFICACY (%)
Beasley et al.[130]	MSD-P	20	0, 1, 6	Yes	159	2.0–8.6	91.4–98.0
Wong et al.[131]	DRC-P	3	0, 1, 2, 6	Yes	124	9.2–14.4	79.3–86.8
Lo et al.[133]	Pasteur	5	0, 1, 2, 12	Yes	72	8.1–11.4	85.5–89.7
Stevens et al.[142]	MSD-P	20	0, 1, 6	Yes	158	13.9	
	MSD-P	10	0, 1, 6	Yes	152	10.9	
	MSD-R	5	0, 1, 6	Yes	351	5.4	
Pongpipat et al.[136]	MSD-R	5	0, 1, 6	Yes	20	10.0	89.2
Lee et al.[137]	SKB	20	0, 1, 2, 12	Yes	54	7.4	91.6
	SKB	10	0, 1, 2, 12	Yes	56	1.8	98.0
	SKB	20	0, 1, 6	Yes	60	3.3	96.3
Poovorawan et al.[178a]	SKB	10	0, 1, 2, 12	Yes	65	1.5	97.6
	SKB	10	0, 1, 6	Yes	60	0	>97
Beasley et al.[130]	MSD-P	20	0, 1, 6	No	40	22.5	75.0
Wong et al.[131]	DRC-P	3	0, 1, 2, 6	No	64	24.3	65.1
Lo et al.[133]	Pasteur	5	0, 1, 2, 12	No	36	19.4	75.3
Poovorawan et al.[138]	SKB	10	0, 1, 2, 12	No	59	3.4	94.8
	SKB	10	0, 1, 6	No	59	3.4	94.8
Tin[139]	MSD-P	20	0, 1, 2, 6	No	113	17.7	70.4
	MSD-P	10	0, 1, 6	No	58	12.1	79.8
	MSD-R	5	0, 1, 6	No	60	5	91.6
Assateerawatt et al.[140]	MSD-R	2.5	0, 1, 2, 6	No	24	29	66.0
Moulia-Pelat et al.[141]	Pasteur-R	20	Mixed	No	16	6.2	93

DRC, Dutch Red Cross; HBIG, hepatitis B immune globulin; MSD, Merck Sharpe and Dohme; -P, plasma derived; -R, recombinant; SKB, SmithKline Beecham.

immunization of HBeAg-exposed neonates, unrelated to whether the first vaccine dose was given with the HBIG at birth or separately at 3 months of age. However, high maternal HBV DNA was associated with a failure to protect.

Population-Based Studies

Unlike the situation with other vaccine-preventable diseases, the efficacy of hepatitis B prevention programs is not based solely on surveillance of acute disease. Because most HBV infections in children younger than 10 years are asymptomatic, an evaluation based on surveillance data does not reliably measure the effectiveness of hepatitis B vaccination programs, especially those directed at infants. In areas of intermediate or high endemicity, assessments of infant vaccination programs are primarily evaluated by vaccination coverage surveys and population-based serological surveys. Because most of the HBV-associated morbidity and mortality is related to chronic infection, demonstrating a reduction in the prevalence of chronic infection is a major indicator of program success and disease reduction. Trends in disease incidence can be used to evaluate the effectiveness of programs directed at adolescents and adults who are more likely to have symptomatic infections after HBV exposure.[143, 144]

Between 1983 and 1989, hepatitis B vaccine was introduced into infant immunization schedules for Alaskan Natives and U.S.-affiliated Pacific Islander communities. Baseline studies revealed a high prevalence of chronic HBV infection (7–15%) among children in these com-

Table 10–7. **POPULATION-BASED STUDIES COMPARING THE PREVALENCE OF CHRONIC HEPATITIS B VIRUS INFECTION AMONG CHILDREN BEFORE AND AFTER THE INTRODUCTION OF HEPATITIS B VACCINE INTO INFANT IMMUNIZATION SCHEDULES**

STUDY	NO. TESTED*	AGE (yr)	VACCINE COVERAGE (%)	CHRONIC HEPATITIS B VIRUS INFECTION (%)	
				Before Program	After Program
Alaska†	268	1–10	96	16	0
Taiwan[146]	424	7–10	73	10	1.1
Samoa[90]	435	7–8	87	7	0.5
Lombok[147]	2519	4	>90	6.2	1.9
Saipan[67]	200	3–4	94	9	0.5
FSM[62]	364	3–4	82	NA	1.1
FSM[67]	544	2	37	12	3
Polynesia[141]	582	1–2	66	6.5	0.7

*Number of children tested of indicated age.
†R. Harpaz, unpublished data, 1997.
FSM, Federated States of Micronesia; NA, not available.

Table 10–8. **COHORT STUDIES DEMONSTRATING THE EFFICACY OF HEPATITIS B VACCINES AMONG CHILDREN LIVING IN AREAS OF HIGH ENDEMICITY***

COUNTRY	REFERENCE	HBsAg PREVACCINE (%)†	HBsAg POSTVACCINE (%)	REDUCTION (%)
Alaska Natives	149	5.2	0	100
Taiwan	150	9.8	0.7	93
Shanghai	110	8.8	0.3	97
Rural China	110	14.6	1.4	90
Gambia	148	12.0	0.9	94
Thailand	151	5.4	0.8	85
Senegal	152	19.0	2.0	89

*Percentages based on the prevalence of HBsAg before and after the institution of hepatitis B immunization.
†Prevalence of HBsAg in unvaccinated children or "historical" control subjects.
HBsAg, hepatitis B surface antigen.

munities. Population-based surveys have demonstrated a remarkable reduction in the prevalence of chronic HBV infection among children born after program implementation (Table 10–7).[67, 90, 145] In areas where vaccination coverage was high, the prevalence of chronic HBV infection declined to less than 1%, and residual transmission occurred among children who did not start the vaccination series at birth.[67] Similar studies in Taiwan, Indonesia, Polynesia, and the Gambia have demonstrated a similar reduction in the prevalence of chronic HBV infection.[146–152] Efficacy has also been demonstrated in cohort studies of children living in areas of high endemicity by showing that the prevalence of HBsAg in the serum decreases markedly after vaccination campaigns (Table 10–8).

The ultimate goal of hepatitis B vaccination programs is to decrease the incidence of HBV-related chronic liver disease and hepatocellular carcinoma. In areas of high endemicity, rates of chronic liver disease are relatively high among children. Studies in Taiwan have demonstrated a reduction in the incidence of primary liver cancer among children born after the implementation of routine infant hepatitis B vaccination programs (Fig. 10–10).[153, 153a]

Long-Term Protection

The duration of immunity after hepatitis B vaccination has been the subject of considerable study since vaccine licensure in 1982. Decline in anti-HBs titers after vaccination has been well quantified in several studies.[142, 154–164] In general, there is a rapid decline in protective antibody in the first 12 months after the third dose and a more gradual decline over time. Among adult vaccinees, anti-HBs levels declined to less than 10 mIU per mL in 7 to 50% of vaccinees 5 years after vaccination and in 30 to 60% of vaccinees by 9 to 11 years after vaccination. No studies reported acute cases of hepatitis B among vaccine responders; however, several studies detected asymptomatic infections through serological testing. Among 2708 people followed for 5 to 11 years, 70 (2.6%) became positive for anti-HBc, and none had evidence of chronic HBV infection. It is believed that these mild clinically inapparent infections will not produce sequelae associated with chronic HBV infections. These studies indicate that protection against serious HBV infection persists for at least 12 years despite the decline in antibody titer (Table 10–9).

Studies among infants and young children have shown

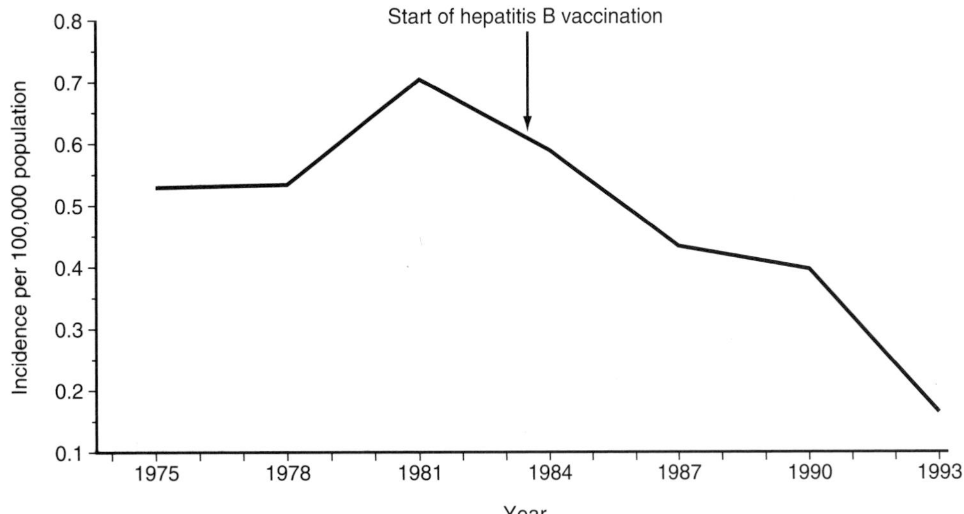

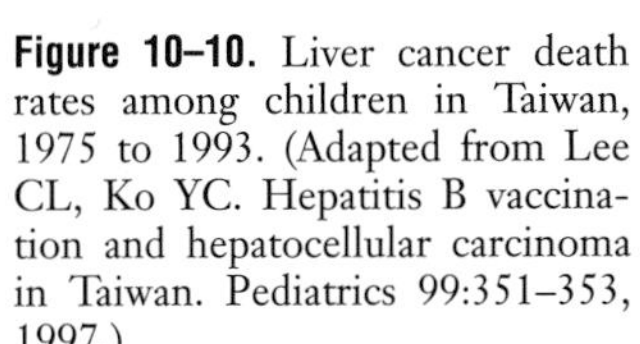
Figure 10–10. Liver cancer death rates among children in Taiwan, 1975 to 1993. (Adapted from Lee CL, Ko YC. Hepatitis B vaccination and hepatocellular carcinoma in Taiwan. Pediatrics 99:351–353, 1997.)

Table 10–9. **LONG-TERM PROTECTION AMONG ADULTS WHO RESPONDED* TO A PRIMARY HEPATITIS B VACCINATION SERIES**

GROUP	REFERENCE	NO. PEOPLE	FOLLOW-UP (yr)	ANTI-HBs LOSS (%)	LATE INFECTIONS (No).	
					All†	Chronic
Healthcare workers	156	144	11	31	0	0
Homosexual men	142	127	11	61	0	0
Alaska Natives	157‡	1194	9–10	24	13	0
Homosexual men	158§	634	9	54	48	0
Military personnel	159	190	6	45	4	0
Medical students	159	100	5	19	1	0
Healthcare workers	160	41	5	32	0	0
Healthcare workers	161	143	5	7	4	0
Healthcare workers	162	32	5	24	0	0
Healthcare workers	163	31	5–7	52	0	0
Healthcare workers	164	72	5	30	0	0

*Peak anti-HBs more than 10 mIU per mL.
†People who have antibody to hepatitis B core antigen.
‡Includes children.
§Includes follow-up unpublished data.
Anti-HBs, antibody to hepatitis B surface antigen.

excellent long-term protection among those who initially respond to hepatitis B vaccination, although breakthrough infections with viremia have been observed in several studies among vaccinated children born to HBsAg-positive women (Table 10–10).[119, 142, 155, 165–172] Data pooled from studies of 1993 infants who were born to chronically infected women and followed for 5 to 11 years indicated that 20 (1%) became HBsAg-positive more than 1 year after vaccination.

The proposed mechanism for continued protection against clinically significant HBV infection, despite declining antibody titers, is an anamnestic immune response after HBV exposure.[173] The phenomenon of immunological memory has been demonstrated by a rapid increase in anti-HBs following a booster dose of vaccine among people given a primary vaccination series several years earlier.[174–178] Booster dose studies among adults have shown that more than 90% of vaccines demonstrate such immune memory when challenged with hepatitis B vaccine and suggest that the immune system would be able to respond rapidly to HBV exposure. The long incubation period of HBV infection (60–120 d), coupled with excellent anamnestic antibody response to low levels of HBsAg among previously immunized people, appears to limit breakthrough infections to those that do not produce detectable viremia, symptomatic disease, or chronic infection.

The need for booster doses of hepatitis B vaccine after a primary vaccine series has been the subject of considerable debate. Among children living in areas of high endemicity, there was no difference in the prevalence of HBV infection at 8 to 12 years of age among

Table 10–10. **LONG-TERM PROTECTION FROM HEPATITIS B VIRUS INFECTION AFTER HEPATITIS B VACCINATION AMONG INFANTS AND CHILDREN WHO RESPONDED TO A PRIMARY VACCINATION SERIES**

GROUP AND LOCATION	NO. PEOPLE	FOLLOW-UP (yr)	ANTI-HBs LOSS (%)	CARRIERS (No.)	POSITIVE FOR HBsAg (No.)	POSITIVE FOR ANTI-HBc (No.)
Infants of HBeAg-positive mothers						
United States[142]*	315	4–11	12	0	0	30
China[165]	74	9	49	0	0	7
China[166]	536	9	44	14	14	NA
China[167]	50	5	17	1	3	NA
Taiwan[168]	199	6	3	0	0	0
Taiwan[169]	654	5	9	3	3	46
Taiwan[170]	165	5	17	0	0	11
Routine vaccinations in infancy and early childhood						
Senegal[171]	327	2–12	NA	NA	9	7
China[166]	536	8	39	3	3	NA
Venezuela[119]*	280	6	29	0	0	6

*Contains unpublished follow-up data.
Anti-HBs, antibody to hepatitis B surface antigen. See also abbreviations in Table 10–1.

children who received a booster dose of vaccine at school entry compared with those who did not.[171, 178a] At present, vaccine advisory groups in the United States do not recommend routine booster doses of hepatitis B vaccine for people who have responded to vaccination. European opinion is divided but often more cautious, with some experts recommending booster vaccination of individuals whose titers fall below 10 IU per mL, although no evidence for loss of efficacy yet supports this view.[178b] Ongoing studies should provide information on the need for booster doses during the second decade after vaccination.

Adverse Events

Numerous studies indicate that hepatitis B vaccines have an excellent safety profile and that serious adverse events after hepatitis B vaccination are exceedingly rare. Reactogenicity studies have shown that pain at the injection site (3–29%) and temperature greater than 37.7°C (1–6%) are the most frequently reported side effects among adults and children receiving vaccine.[179, 180] In placebo-controlled studies, these side effects were reported no more frequently among vaccines than among people receiving a placebo.[115, 116]

In the United States, data on adverse events associated with vaccination are available through the national Vaccine Adverse Event Reporting System (VAERS), a passive surveillance system. Case reports of anaphylaxis following hepatitis B vaccination have been reported in the medical literature and to VAERS.[181] Although none of the people who developed anaphylaxis died, anaphylaxis can be fatal, and hepatitis B vaccine may, in very rare instances, cause a life-threatening hypersensitivity reaction in certain individuals. Therefore, further vaccination with hepatitis B vaccine is contraindicated in people with a history of anaphylaxis after a previous dose of vaccine.

Other serious adverse events reported to occur after hepatitis B vaccination include Gullain-Barré syndrome and multiple sclerosis.[182–184] Establishing a causal relationship between these adverse events and hepatitis B vaccination is methodologically and logistically formidable. In general, these events (1) are rare, (2) occur in the absence of hepatitis B vaccination, and (3) have their peak incidence in the older age groups recommended to receive hepatitis B vaccine before the implementation of routine childhood hepatitis B vaccination.

In 1993, the Institute of Medicine reviewed case reports in the medical literature and those reported to VAERS from November 1990 to July 1992 and concluded that the evidence was insufficient to assess a causal link between serious neurological adverse events and hepatitis B vaccination.[185] A more recent review by the FDA of case reports in VAERS for the years 1991 to 1994 concluded that there were no unexpected adverse events in neonates and infants given hepatitis B vaccine, despite the use of at least 12 million doses of vaccine in these age groups.[186]

Grotto and colleagues reviewed the world's literature on reactions to yeast-derived recombinant vaccines and found them to be rare but consistent with immune complex–mediated diseases similar to those occurring after hepatitis B.[186a]

Large-scale infant hepatitis B immunization programs in Taiwan, Alaska, and New Zealand have observed no association between vaccination and the occurrence of severe adverse events, including seizures, Guillain-Barré syndrome, or anaphylaxis.[187, 188] However, systematic surveillance for adverse reactions in these populations has been limited, and the number of children who received recombinant DNA vaccine is limited. Any presumed risk of adverse events possibly causally associated with hepatitis B vaccination must be balanced with the expected risk of HBV-related liver disease.

INDICATIONS FOR VACCINATION

The epidemiology of HBV infection indicates that multiple age groups must be targeted to provide widespread immunity and to effectively prevent HBV transmission and HBV-related chronic liver disease. Beginning in the late 1980s, the Advisory Committee on Immunization Practices (ACIP) of the U.S. Public Health Service developed a comprehensive strategy to eliminate HBV transmission in the United States. The following indications for vaccination summarize recommendations by the ACIP for the prevention of HBV transmission in the United States.

Preexposure Vaccination to Prevent HBV Infection

Routine Vaccination of Infants

1. Hepatitis B vaccination is recommended for all infants. The first dose should be given during the newborn period and vaccination completed by 18 months of age. Infants born to HBsAg-positive mothers require special postexposure immunoprophylaxis to prevent HBV infection (see Table 10–4).

2. Vaccination in preterm infants born to HBsAg-negative women and weighing less than 1.5 kg should be delayed (1) until hospital discharge, if the infant then weighs 2 kg or more; or (2) until the infant is 2 months of age, when other routine vaccines are administered. Among infants weighing 1.5 to 2.0 kg, vaccination may be delayed until the child weighs at least 2.0 kg or is 2 months of age. However, if there is concern that an infant may not begin his or her vaccine series as an outpatient, the first dose should be administered prior to hospital discharge.

Preterm infants born to HBsAg-positive mothers or to mothers whose HBsAg status is unknown should receive postexposure immunoprophylaxis within 12 hours of birth, regardless of their gestational age.

3. Special efforts should be made to ensure that hepatitis B vaccination is started at birth and completed for all infants by 12 months of age in populations in which childhood HBV infection is highly endemic (i.e., Alaskan Natives, Pacific Islanders, and infants in immigrant or

refugee families from countries in which HBV is of intermediate or high endemicity) (see Fig. 10–8).

Catch-Up Vaccination of Children and Adolescents

All children and adolescents (≤18 years of age) not previously vaccinated with hepatitis B vaccine should be vaccinated with the age-appropriate dose of vaccine. Special efforts should be made to vaccinate children residing in households of Pacific Islander ethnicity or of first-generation immigrants from countries with an intermediate or high endemicity of HBV infection. To ensure comprehensive vaccination coverage of adolescents, it is recommended that providers offer hepatitis vaccine to all adolescents at 11 to 12 years of age (see Tables 10–4 and 10–5).

Vaccination of People in High-Risk Groups

People with the following risk factors for HBV infection should be vaccinated using the age-appropriate vaccine dose and schedule if not previously vaccinated as an infant, young child, or adolescent:

1. *Sexually active heterosexual adolescents and adults* diagnosed with a recently acquired sexually transmitted disease, identified as prostitutes, having more than one sexual partner in the previous 6 months, or seen in a clinic for sexually transmitted diseases
2. *Homosexual and bisexual adolescent and adult men*
3. *Household contacts and sexual partners of HBsAg-positive people,* including infants, children, adolescents, and adults
4. *Injection drug users*
5. *People at occupational risk of infection* through exposure to blood or blood-contaminated body fluid (i.e., healthcare workers, public safety workers), including trainees in healthcare fields in schools of medicine, dentistry, nursing, laboratory technology, and other allied health professions

   For those workers whose exposure to blood is infrequent, timely postexposure prophylaxis should be considered, rather than routine vaccination.
6. *Clients and staff of institutions for the developmentally disabled*

   Staff of nonresidential daycare programs for the developmentally disabled (e.g., schools, sheltered workshops) attended by people known to be HBsAg-positive should be vaccinated. Clients in these settings should be vaccinated if the HBsAg-positive classmate behaves aggressively or has special medical problems (e.g., exudative dermatitis, open skin lesions) that increase the risk of exposure to blood or serous secretions.

   The HBsAg or immunization status should be known for clients discharged from residential institutions into community residential programs.
7. *Hemodialysis patients* and patients with early renal failure before they require hemodialysis

   The need for booster doses of vaccine should be assessed by annual antibody testing and a booster dose given when antibody levels fall below 10 mIU per mL.
8. *Patients who receive clotting-factor concentrates,* as soon as their specific clotting disorder is identified
9. *Adoptees from countries where HBV infection is endemic*

   These individuals should be tested for HBsAg, and for those found to be HBsAg positive, all family members should be vaccinated.
10. *International travelers,* especially children, in areas with high or intermediate rates of HBV infection (see Fig. 10–8) who will have close contact with the local population or who are likely to have contact with blood (e.g., in a medical setting) or sexual contact with residents
11. *Inmates of long-term correctional facilities*

Postexposure Prophylaxis to Prevent HBV Infection

Prevention of Perinatal HBV Infection

1. All pregnant women should be routinely tested for HBsAg during an early prenatal visit in *each* pregnancy.
   a. HBsAg-negative women at high risk of HBV infection (e.g., injection drug users, those with intercurrent sexually transmitted diseases or multiple sexual partners) or who have had clinical hepatitis should have HBsAg testing repeated late in pregnancy.
   b. Household contacts and sexual partners of HBsAg-positive women should be vaccinated.
   c. HBsAg-positive women should be reported to local health departments in states with reporting requirements to ensure appropriate follow-up.
2. Infants born to mothers found to be HBsAg positive should have the following:
   a. Receive the appropriate dose of hepatitis B vaccine (see Tables 10–4 and 10–5) and HBIG (0.5 mL) within 12 hours of birth, administered concurrently but at different sites.
   b. Receive follow-up to ensure timely completion of vaccination with the appropriate vaccine dose according to the recommended schedule (see Tables 10–4 and 10–5).
   c. Be tested for anti-HBs and HBsAg following the completion of the vaccine series at 9 to 15 months of age. Infants found to be negative for anti-HBs should be revaccinated.
3. Women admitted for delivery without prenatal HBsAg testing should have blood drawn for testing. While test results are pending, the infant should receive hepatitis B vaccine within 12 hours of birth in a dose appropriate for infants born to *HBsAg-positive* mothers (see Table 10–4).
   a. If the mother is later found to be *HBsAg-positive,* her infant should receive the additional protection afforded by HBIG as soon as possible and within

7 days of birth. If HBIG has not been administered, it is important that the infant receive the second dose of hepatitis B vaccine (appropriate for an infant of an HBsAg-positive mother) at 1 month and not later than 2 months of age because of the high risk of infection. The last dose should be given at 6 months of age.

b. If the mother is found to be *HBsAg-negative*, her infant should receive hepatitis B vaccine as part of his or her routine vaccinations in the dose appropriate for infants born to *HBsAg-negative* mothers (see Table 10–4).

4. In populations in which it is not feasible to screen pregnant women for HBsAg, *all* infants should receive their first dose of hepatitis B vaccine within 12 hours of birth, their second dose at 1 to 2 months of age, and their third dose at 6 months of age as a part of their childhood vaccinations and well-child care. The vaccine dose used in this setting should be that used for infants of *HBsAg-positive* mothers (see Table 10–4); the use of HBIG is not indicated.

People with Accidental Percutaneous/ Permucosal Exposure to Blood

After a percutaneous (needle stick, laceration, bite) or permucosal (ocular, mucous membrane) exposure to blood that contains or might contain HBV, the following should be done:

1. Obtain a blood sample from the person who was the source of the exposure to determine their HBsAg status.
2. Review the vaccination and anti-HBs response status of the exposed person.

Prophylaxis for exposed people is dependent on the HBsAg status of the source-patient and the immunization status of the exposed person (Table 10–11).

Sexual Partners of People with Acute Hepatitis B Virus Infection

All susceptible sexual partners of people with acute HBV infection should receive a single dose of HBIG (0.06 mL/kg) and should begin the hepatitis B vaccine series if prophylaxis can be started within 14 days of the last sexual contact.

Household Contacts of People with Acute Hepatitis B Virus Infection

An unvaccinated infant whose mother or primary caregiver has acute HBV infection should receive HBIG (0.5 mL) and vaccination begun. For infants who have begun the hepatitis B vaccine series, no additional treatment is needed, and vaccination should be completed on schedule.

Prophylaxis for other household contacts of people with acute HBV infection is not indicated unless a blood exposure to the index patient is identified (e.g., sharing toothbrushes or razors). Such exposures should be treated similarly to sexual exposures. If the index patient becomes an HBV carrier, all household contacts should be vaccinated.

Contraindications to Vaccination

Hepatitis B vaccination is contraindicated for people with a history of allergic reactions to vaccine components including thimerosal. In addition, people with a history of serious adverse events after receipt of hepatitis B vaccine should not receive additional doses. There is a theoretical contraindication to vaccination in people with allergy to *Saccharomyces cerevisiae* (baker's yeast); however, there is little evidence documenting adverse reactions after vaccination of people with a history of

Table 10–11. **RECOMMENDATIONS FOR HEPATITIS B PROPHYLAXIS AFTER PERCUTANEOUS EXPOSURE**

STATUS OF EXPOSED PERSON	RECOMMENDATION IF SOURCE HBsAg POSITIVE	RECOMMENDATION IF SOURCE HBsAg NEGATIVE	RECOMMENDATION IF SOURCE NOT TESTED
Unvaccinated	HBIG × 1* plus initiate HB vaccine†	Initiate HB vaccine†	Initiate HB vaccine†
Previously vaccinated			
Known responder	No treatment; may consider booster	No treatment	No treatment
Known nonresponder	HBIG × 2 *or* HBIG × 1 plus 1 dose HB vaccine	No treatment	If known high-risk source, may treat as if source were HBsAg-positive
Response unknown	Test exposed person for anti-HBs 1. If inadequate,‡ HBIG × 1 plus HB vaccine booster dose 2. If adequate, no treatment	No treatment	Test exposed person for anti-HBs 1. If inadequate, HB vaccine booster dose 2. If adequate, no treatment

*Hepatitis B immune globulin (HBIG) dose 0.06 mL/kg intramuscularly.
†Hepatitis B (HB) vaccine dose—see Table 10–4.
‡Adequate anti-HBs is more than 10 IU by radioimmunoassay (RIA) or positive by enzyme immunoassay (EIA).
See abbreviations in Tables 10–1 and 10–10.

yeast allergy. On the basis of limited data, there is no apparent risk of adverse events to developing fetuses when hepatitis B vaccine is administered to pregnant women. The vaccine contains noninfectious HBsAg particles and should cause no risk to the fetus. HBV infection affecting a pregnant woman may result in severe disease for the mother and chronic infection for the newborn. Therefore, neither pregnancy nor lactation should be a contraindication to vaccination of women.

Mutant Viruses

HBV infection with molecular variants of the virus has been reported among vaccinated people in southern Italy, Singapore, the Gambia, and the United States and among liver transplant recipients who received HBIG for prophylaxis of relapse of HBV infection.[189–195] It has been proposed that these variants contain HBsAg that is not recognized by vaccine-induced antibodies and that acute HBV infection occurs in the presence of protective levels of anti-HBs. Several investigators have reported a mutation in the genome that causes a change in one amino acid in the *a* determinant of the HBs protein, which is the proposed conformational epitope essential for recognition and neutralization by anti-HBs antibodies. The most common alteration described is a replacement of glycine by arginine in amino acid 145; however, other mutations, such as the replacement of aspartic acid by alanine in amino acid 144, have also been described. Similar variants have been described in unvaccinated people with chronic HBV infection, suggesting that they occur naturally. The incidence of infection with variant strains of HBV among vaccinated infants has been reported in a population-based study of 1092 infants born to HBeAg-positive pregnant women between 1981 and 1993.[194] Overall, 94 (8.6%) of infants became infected, and HBV variant strains were isolated from 22 of the infected children. As found in other studies, the most common amino acid changes occurred in positions 143 to 145; however, mutations were also found across most of the region. Mixed infections of both wild-type and mutant viruses were often detected in both mothers and infants, suggesting that infants acquire their mutant strain from the mother and that the mutant is selected for by the pressure of antibodies against the standard epitope.

At present, the public health importance of the molecular variants of HBV is debatable. Studies of vaccinated household members living with people chronically infected with variants have not demonstrated intrahousehold transmission of the variant.[196] In addition, preexposure vaccination of chimpanzees with currently licensed vaccines (not containing pre-S epitopes) conferred protection following intravenous challenge with the 145-HBV mutant.[197] Further studies and enhanced surveillance to detect the emergence of these variants remain a high priority in evaluating the effectiveness of current immunization strategies.

Interaction of Hepatitis B Vaccines with Other Vaccines

Many studies demonstrate that there is no increase in adverse reactions or interference with antibody responses induced by any of the vaccines when hepatitis B vaccine and other vaccines are given simultaneously but at separate sites. Vaccines tested in simultaneous administration include bacille Calmette-Guérin,[198] DTP,[199, 200] inactivated and oral poliovirus vaccines,[201] and measles and yellow fever vaccines.[202] Several combined vaccines have been developed by manufacturers, notably DTP–Hep B,[203] Hep A–Hep B,[204] and Hib–Hep B.[107] In each case, the manufacturer has shown that the components remain sufficiently immunogenic. However, physicians should not attempt to make extemporaneous mixtures in the same syringe at point of use, as the results are unpredictable unless verified by the manufacturer and national control authorities.

PUBLIC HEALTH CONSIDERATIONS

Worldwide, the prevention of chronic HBV infection has become a high priority. In 1992, the Global Advisory Group (GAG) to the World Health Organization recommended that all countries integrate hepatitis B vaccine into national immunization programs by 1997. In countries where the prevalence of chronic HBV infection is more than 2%, the GAG recommended the incorporation of hepatitis B vaccine into infant immunization schedules. The strategy for low-endemicity countries could include routine adolescent immunization in addition to, or instead of, infant immunization.

At present, 80 countries have integrated hepatitis B vaccine into national immunization programs, and several others are planning to do so (Fig. 10–11). Infant vaccination programs have been implemented in highly endemic regions of Southeast Asia, China, the Pacific, and the Middle East, and there are plans to implement programs in several other endemic regions, including India. Most of the highly endemic countries in sub-Saharan Africa have not made plans to incorporate hepatitis B vaccine into Expanded Program of Immunization (EPI) schedules. The primary obstacle to implementing programs in these countries has been the high cost of vaccine when compared with other EPI antigens. Increased global production of vaccine has decreased the cost of vaccine during the 1990s. It is anticipated that increased production of vaccine and the development of combination vaccines containing hepatitis B vaccine will facilitate more widescale use of vaccine in economically disadvantaged countries.

In low-endemicity countries, the approach to the integration of hepatitis B vaccine into national immunization programs has been variable. The initially recommended strategy in the United States was selective vaccination of individuals with identified risk factors. However, programs to vaccinate high-risk people were not developed; most people with identified risk factors were difficult to target for vaccination; and many in-

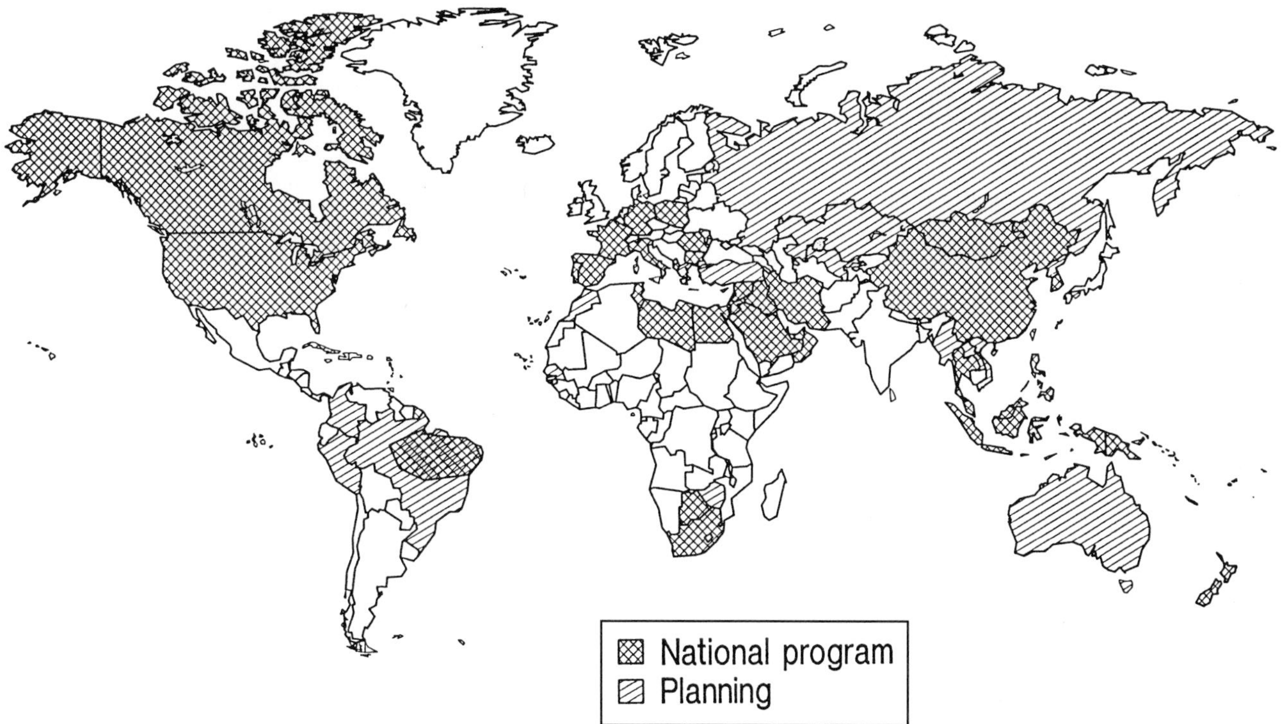

Figure 10–11. Countries that integrated hepatitis B vaccine into national immunization programs, 1996.

fected people had no identifiable risk factors. Thus, vaccinating people prior to exposure was generally not feasible, and the incidence of acute hepatitis B remained high during the first decade after vaccine licensure in 1982.

Recommendations to vaccinate all newborns were the subject of considerable debate among primary care providers in the United States, many of whom considered patients in their practice to be at low risk for acquiring HBV infection.[205, 206] Providers also expressed concerns about the cost-effectiveness of infant vaccination as well as long-term protection after hepatitis B vaccination of infants. It was proposed that routine adolescent vaccination would be a more effective primary immunization strategy.[207] However, cost-effectiveness analysis demonstrated that routine infant immunization was the most effective strategy to prevent HBV transmission in the United States because of the additional benefit in preventing early childhood transmission with infant immunization.[208] Despite the initial concerns of care providers, hepatitis B vaccination coverage of infants increased rapidly and reached levels as high as those observed for other childhood vaccines within 3 years of introduction.[90, 209] In 1997, more than 80% of children between 2 and 3 years of age had received three doses of hepatitis B vaccine.

The implementation of routine infant immunization will eventually produce broad population-based immunity to HBV infection and prevent HBV transmission among all age groups. However, because most HBV infections in the United States occur among young adults, it will take two to three decades before infant immunization affects the incidence of hepatitis B in the United States. To hasten the development of population-based immunity and to more rapidly decrease the incidence of hepatitis B, catch-up vaccination of 11- to 12-year-old adolescents was recommended by the ACIP in 1995. This strategy was expanded to include all adolescents in 1997. The strategy of routine infant and catch-up vaccination of adolescents has been implemented in several other countries, including France, Italy, and Germany.

Numerous studies have shown that routine infant immunization coupled with catch-up vaccination of older children can virtually eliminate HBV transmission in a community.[67, 143, 146] In fact, many long-term programs have demonstrated a greater than expected benefit in terms of disease reduction when compared with vaccination coverage. This effect could have a number of causes. Widescale use of vaccine creates immunized cohorts of children who no longer serve as reservoirs of virus. Thus, successive cohorts of children are less likely to be exposed to the HBV in early childhood, when the risk of chronic infection is greatest. Other prevention efforts have been implemented, such as safe injection practices, screening of blood products, and the use of universal precautions for infectious body fluid exposures. Finally, in settings where vaccination coverage is low, it appears that partial vaccination may provide some degree of protection in preventing HBV infection and chronic infection.

In comparison to the introduction of other vaccines, several features are unique to the introduction of hepatitis B vaccine into infant immunization schedules. Infections in children are asymptomatic, and routine disease surveillance may not reflect ongoing transmission in a community. Special studies are needed to assess ongoing transmission and to monitor the impact of vaccination programs. The serious adverse outcomes that are related to the acquisition of chronic HBV infection occur several decades after exposure; thus, the benefit of infant immunization will not be realized for several years. Commitment of public health resources to eliminate HBV transmission requires recognition of the importance of this disease, persistent efforts to ensure that populations are protected, and patience to realize the goals of disease reduction. Studies in Taiwan[153, 153a] demonstrating a reduction of liver cancer deaths in children provide assurance that the strategy of routine infant immunization is a well-conceived public health practice that will benefit generations to come.

REFERENCES

1. Lurman A. Eine icterus Epidemic. Berl Klin Woschenschr 22:20–23, 1855.
2. Flaum A, Malmros H, Persson E. Eine nosocomiale Ikterus—Epidemie. Acta Med Scand 16:544, 1926.
3. Findlay GM, MacCallum FO. Note on acute hepatitis and yellow fever immunization. Trans R Soc Trop Med Hyg 51:297–308, 1937.
4. Beeson PB. Jaundice occurring one to four months after transfusion of blood or plasma. Report of seven cases. JAMA 121:1332–1334, 1943.
5. Neefe JR, Gellis SS, Stokes J. Homologous serum hepatitis and infectious (epidemic) hepatitis: Studies in volunteers bearing on immunological and other characteristics of etiologic agents. Am J Med Sci 1:3–22, 1946.
6. Seefe LB, Beebe GW, Hoofnagle JH, et al. A serologic follow-up of the 1942 epidemic of post-vaccination hepatitis in the United States Army. N Engl J Med 316:965–970, 1987.
7. Virchow R. Uber das Vorkommen und den Nachweiss des hepatogenen, insebesondere des Katarrhalischen Ikterus. Virchows Arch A 32:117–125, 1865.
8. Eppinger H. Die pathogenesis des icterus. Verh Dtsch Ges Inn Med 34:15, 1922.
9. Rich AR. The pathogenisis of the forms of jaundice. Bull Johns Hopkins Hosp 47:338–377, 1930.
10. Havens WP. Period of infectivity of patients with experimentally induced infectious hepatitis. J Exp Med 83:251–258, 1946.
11. MacCallum FO, Bauer DJ. Homologous serum jaundice: Transmission experiments with human volunteers. Lancet 1:622–627, 1944.
12. MacCallum FO. Homologous serum hepatitis. Lancet 2:691–692, 1947.
13. Krugman S, Giles JP, Hammond J. Infectious hepatitis: Evidence for 2 distinctive clinical, epidemiological and immunological types of infection. JAMA 200:365–373, 1967.
14. Krugman S, Giles JP. Viral hepatitis, type B (MS-2 Strain): Further observations on natural history and prevention. N Engl J Med 288:755–760, 1973.
15. Giles JP, McCollum RW, Berndtson LW, Krugman S. Viral hepatitis: Relationship of Australia-SH antigen to the Willowbrook MS-2 strain. N Engl J Med 281:119–122, 1969.
16. Blumberg BS, Alter HJ, Visnich S. A "new" antigen in leukemia sera. JAMA 191:541–546, 1967.
17. Prince AM. An antigen detected in the blood of patients during the incubation period of serum hepatitis. Proc Natl Acad Sci U S A 60:814–821, 1968.
18. Blumberg BS. A serum antigen (Australia antigen) in Down's syndrome, leukemia, and hepatitis. Ann Intern Med 66:924–931, 1967.
19. Blumberg BS. Australia antigen and the biology of hepatitis B. Science 197:17–25, 1977.
20. Dane DS, Cameroon CH, Briggs M. Virus-like particles in the serum of patients with Australia-antigen–associated hepatitis. Lancet 1:695–698, 1970.
21. Magnius LO, Espmark JA. Specificities in Australia antigen-positive sera distinct from the Le Bouvier determinants. J Immunol 109:1017–1021, 1972.
22. Krugman S, Giles JP, Hammond J. Viral hepatitis type B: Prevention with specific hepatitis B immune serum globulin. JAMA 218:1665–1670, 1971.
23. Krugman S, Giles JP, Hammond JP. Viral hepatitis: Effect of heat on the infectivity and antigenicity of the MS-1 and MS-2 strains. J Infect Dis 122:432–436, 1970.
24. Krugman S, Giles JP, Hammond J. Viral hepatitis type B MS-2 strain: Studies on active immunization. JAMA 217:41–45, 1971.
25. Hilleman MR, Buynak EB, Roehm RR, et al. Purified and inactivated human hepatitis B vaccine. A progress report. Am J Med Sci 270:401–404, 1975.
26. Rizzetto M. The delta agent. Hepatology 3:729–737, 1983.
27. Choo QL, Kuo G, Weiner AJ, et al. Isolation of a cDNA clone derived from a blood-borne non-A, non-B viral hepatitis genome. Science 244:359–362, 1989.
28. Kuo G, Choo QL, Alter HJ, et al. An assay for circulating antibodies to a major etiologic virus of human non-A, non-B hepatitis. Science 244:362–364, 1989.
29. Bradley DW, Krawczynski K, Beach MJ, et al. Non-A, Non-B hepatitis: Toward the discovery of hepatitis C and E viruses. Semin Liver Dis 11:128–146, 1991.
30. McMahon BJ, Alward WL, Hall DB, et al. Acute hepatitis B virus infection: Relation of age to the clinical expression of disease and subsequent development of the carrier state. J Infect Dis 151:599–603, 1985.
31. Edmunds WJ, Medley GF, Nokes DJ, et al. The influence of age on the development of the hepatitis B carrier state. Proc R Soc Lond B Biol Sci 253:197–201, 1993.
32. Hyams KC. Risk of chronicity following acute hepatitis B virus infection: A review. Clin Infect Dis 20:992–1000, 1995.
33. Beasley RP, Hwang L-Y. Overview on the epidemiology of hepatocellular carcinoma. In Hollinger FB, Lemon SB, Margolis HS (eds). Viral hepatitis and Liver Disease. Baltimore, Williams & Wilkins, 1991, pp 532–535.
34. Hsieh CC, Tzonou A, Zavitsanos X, et al. Age at first establishment of chronic hepatitis B virus infection and hepatocellular carcinoma risk: A birth order study. Am J Epidemiol 136:1115–1121, 1992.
35. Halder SC, Judson FN, O'Malley PM, et al. Outcome of hepatitis B virus infection in homosexual men and its relation to prior human immunodeficiency virus infection. J Infect Dis 163:454–459, 1991.
36. Polish LB, Shapiro CN, Bauer F, et al. Nosocomial transmission of hepatitis B virus associated with the use of a spring-loaded fingerstick device. N Engl J Med 326:721–725, 1992.
37. Hoofnagle JH, Seef LB. Natural history of chronic type B hepatitis. Prog Liver Dis 7:469–479, 1982.
38. Di Bisceglie AM: Hepatocellular carcinoma. Ann Intern Med 108:390–401, 1988.
39. Lau JYN, Wright TL. Molecular virology and pathogenesis of hepatitis B. Lancet 342:1335–1340, 1993.
40. Gerlich WH, Bruss V. Functions of hepatitis B virus proteins and molecular targets for protective immunity. In Ellis RW (ed). Hepatitis B Vaccines in Clinical Practice. New York, Marcel Dekker, 1993, pp 41–82.
41. Neurath AR, Kent SB, Strick N, Parker K. Identification and chemical synthesis of a host cell receptor binding site on hepatitis B virus. Cell 46:429–436, 1986.
42. Pontisso P, Petit MA, Bankowski MJ, Peeples ME. Human liver plasma membranes contain receptors for the hepatitis B virus pre-S1 region and, via polymerized human serum albumin, for the pre-S2 region. J Virol 63:1981–1988, 1989.
43. Gerlich WH, Lu X, Heerman KH. Studies on the attachment and penetration of hepatitis B virus. J Hepatol 17:S10–S14, 1993.
44. Komani K, Peeples ME. Physiology and function of the Vero cell receptor for the hepatitis B small S protein. Virology 177:332–338, 1990.
45. Leenders WH, Glansbeek HL, Bruin WC, Yap S-H. Binding of the major and large HBsAg to human hepatocytes and liver plasma membranes: Putative external and internal receptors for infection and secretion of hepatitis B virus. Hepatology 12:141–147, 1990.

46. Prince AM, Ikram H, Hopp TP. Hepatitis B virus vaccine: Identification of HBsAg/a and HBsAg/d but not HBsAg/y subtype antigenic determinants on a synthetic immunogenic peptide. Proc Natl Acad Sci U S A 79:579–582, 1982.
47. Dodd RY, Holland PV, Ni LY, et al. Hepatitis B antigen: Regional variation in incidence and subtype ratio in the American Red Cross donor population. Am J Epidemiol 97:111–115, 1973.
48. Summers J, Smith PM, Horwich AL. Hepadnavirus envelope proteins regulate covalently closed circular DNA amplification. J Virol 64:2819–2824, 1990.
49. Chisari F, Ferrari C. Hepatitis B virus immunopathogenesis. Annu Rev Immunol 13:29–60, 1995.
50. Greenberg HB, Pollard RB, Lutwick LI, et al. Effect of human leukocyte interferon on hepatitis B virus infection in patients with chronic active hepatitis. N Engl J Med 295:517–522, 1976.
51. Desmyter J, De Groote J, Desmet VJ, et al. Administration of human fibroblast interferon in chronic hepatitis B infection. Lancet 2:645–647, 1976.
52. Wong DKH, Cheung AM, O'Rourke K, et al. Effect of alpha-interferon treatment in patients with B e antigen-positive chronic hepatitis B: A metaanalysis. Ann Intern Med 119:312–323, 1993.
53. Korenman J, Baker B, Wagonner J, et al. Long-term remission of chronic hepatitis B after alpha-interferon therapy. Ann Intern Med 114:629–634, 1991.
54. Hoofnagle JH, Di Bisceglie AM. The treatment of chronic viral hepatitis. N Engl J Med 336:347–356, 1997.
55. Doong S-L, Tsai C-H, Schinazi ER, et al. Inhibition of the replication of hepatitis B virus in vitro by 2′, 3′-dideoxy-3′-thiacytidine and related analogues. Proc Natl Acad Sci U S A 88:8495–8499, 1991.
56. Dienstag JL, Perrillo RP, Schiff ER, et al. A preliminary trial of lamivudine for chronic hepatitis B infection. N Engl J Med 333:1657–1661, 1995.
57. Boker KH, Ringe B, Kruger M, et al. Prostaglandin E plus famciclovir—a new concept for the treatment of severe hepatitis B after liver transplantation. Transplantation 57:1706–1708, 1994.
58. Pol S, Driss F, Michel ML, et al. Specific vaccine therapy in chronic hepatitis B infection. Lancet 344:342, 1994.
59. Wen YM, Wu XH, Hu DC, et al. Hepatitis B vaccine and anti-HBs complex as approach for vaccine therapy. Lancet 345:1575–1576, 1995.
60. Akbar SMF, Kajino K, Tanimoto K, et al. Placebo-controlled trial of vaccination with hepatitis B surface antigen in hepatitis B virus transgenic mice. J Hepatol 26:131–137, 1997.
61. Halder SC, Margolis HS. Epidemiology of Hepatitis B virus infection. In Ellis RW (ed). Hepatitis B Vaccines in Clinical Practice. New York, Marcel Dekker, 1993, pp 141–157.
62. Hu MD, Schenzle D, Dienhart F, Scheid R. Epidemiology of hepatitis A and B in Shanghai area: Prevalence of serum markers. Am J Epidemiol 120:404–413, 1984.
63. Tsega E, Mengesha B, Hansson B-G, et al. Hepatitis A, B, and delta infection in Ethiopia: A serologic survey with demographic data. Am J Epidemiol 123:344–351, 1986.
64. Hyams KC, Al-Arabi MA, Al-Tagani AA, et al. Epidemiology of hepatitis B in the Gezira region of Sudan. Am J Trop Med Hyg 40:200–206, 1989.
65. Toukan AU, Sharaiha ZK, Abu-El-Rub OA, et al. The epidemiology of hepatitis B virus among family members in the Middle East. Am J Epidemiol 132:220–232, 1990.
66. Bensebath G, Halder SC, Pereira Soares MC, et al. Epidemiologic and serologic studies of acute viral hepatitis in Brazil's Amazon Basin. Bull Pan Am Health Organ 21:16–27, 1987.
67. Mahoney F, Woodruff B, Auerbach S, et al. Progress on the elimination of hepatitis B virus transmission in Micronesia and American Samoa. Pacific Health Dialog 3:140–146, 1996.
68. Milne A, Allwood GK, Moyes CD, et al. Prevalence of hepatitis B infections in a multiracial New Zealand Community. N Z Med J 10:529–532, 1985.
69. Sung JL. Hepatitis B eradication strategy for Asia. Vaccine 8(suppl):96–99, 1990.
70. Barin F, Perrin J, Chotard J, et al. Cross-sectional and longitudinal epidemiology of hepatitis B in Senegal. Prog Med Virol 27:148–162, 1981.
71. Wong DC, Purcell RH, Rosen L. Prevelance of antibody to hepatitis A and B in selected Pacific populations of the South Pacific. Am J Epidemiol 110:227–236, 1979.
72. Lok ASF, Lai C, Wu PC, et al. Hepatitis B virus infection in Chinese families in Hong Kong. Am J Epidemiol 126:191–197, 1987.
73. Stevens CE, Neurath RA, Beasley RP, Szmuness W. HBeAg and anti-HBe detection with radioimmunoassay: Correlation with vertical transmission of hepatitis B virus in Taiwan. J Med Virol 3:237–241, 1979.
74. Xu Z-Y, Liu C-B, Francis DP, et al. Prevention of perinatal acquisition of hepatitis B virus carriage using vaccine: Preliminary report of a randomized, double-blind placebo-controlled and comparative trial. Pediatrics 76:713–718, 1985.
75. Beasley RP, Hwang L-Y. Postnatal infectivity of hepatitis B surface antigen–carrier mothers. J Infect Dis 147:185–190, 1983.
76. Hu MD, Schenzle D, Dienhart F, Scheid R. Epidemiology of hepatitis A and B in Shanghai area: Prevalence of serum markers. Am J Epidemiol 120:404–413, 1984.
77. Maynard JE, Kane MA, Alter MJ, Halder SC. Control of hepatitis B by immunization: Global perspectives. In Vyas GN, Dienstag JL, and Hoofnagle JH (eds). Viral Hepatitis and Liver Disease. New York, Grune & Stratton, 1988, pp 967–969.
78. Lingao AL, Domingo EO, West S, et al. Seroepidemiology of hepatitis B in the Philippines. Am J Epidemiol 123:473–480, 1986.
79. Lee SD, Lo KJ, Wu JC, et al. Prevention of maternal-infant hepatitis B transmission by immunization: The role of serum hepatitis B virus DNA. Hepatology 6:369–373, 1986.
80. Toukan AU, Sharaiha ZK, Abu-El-Rub OA, et al. The epidemiology of hepatitis B virus among family members in the Middle East. Am J Epidemiol 132:220–232, 1990.
81. Bensebath G, Halder SC, Pereira Soares MC, et al. Epidemiologic and serologic studies of acute viral hepatitis in Brazil's Amazon Basin. Bull Pan Am Health Organ 21:16–27, 1987.
82. Hyams KC, Osman NM, Khaled EM, et al. Maternal infant transmission of hepatitis B in Egypt. J Med Virol 24:191–197, 1988.
83. Toukan A, Al-Faleh F, Al-Kandari, et al. Strategy for control of hepatitis B virus infection in the Middle East and North Africa. Vaccine 8(suppl):117–121, 1990.
84. Marinier E, Barrios V, Larouze B, et al. Lack of perinatal hepatitis B virus infection in Senegal, West Africa. J Pediatr 106:843–849, 1985.
85. Margolis HS, Alter MJ, Hadler SC. Hepatitis B: Evolving epidemiology and implications for control. Semin Liver Dis 11:84–92, 1991.
86. McQuillan GM, Townsend TR, Fields HA, et al. Seroepidemiology of hepatitis B virus in the United States, 1976 to 1980. Am J Med 87:5S–10S, 1989.
87. Alter MJ, Hadler SC, Margolis HS, et al. The changing epidemiology of hepatitis B in the United States. JAMA 263:1218–1222, 1990.
88. Immunization Hepatitis B virus: A comprehensive Strategy for eliminating transmission in the United States through universal childhood vaccination. Recommendations of the Immunization Practices Advisory Committee (ACIP). MMWR Morb Mortal Wkly Rep 40(RR-13):1–25, 1991.
89. Margolis HS, Alter MJ, Hadler SC. Hepatitis B: Evolving epidemiology and implications for control. Semin Liver Dis 11:84–92, 1991.
90. Mahoney F, Smith N, Alter MJ, Margolis H. Progress towards the elimination of hepatitis B virus transmission in the United States. Viral Hepatitis Rev 3:105–119, 1997.
91. Franks AL, Berg CJ, Kane MA, et al. Hepatitis B infection among children born in the U.S. to southeast Asian refugees. N Engl J Med 321:1301–1305, 1989.
92. Hurie MB, Mast EE, Davis JP. Horizontal transmission of hepatitis B virus infection to U.S.-born children of Hmong refugees. Pediatrics 89:269–273, 1992.
93. Mahoney FJ, Lawrence M, McFarland L, et al. Continuing transmission of hepatitis B virus infection among US-born Southeast Asian children. Pediatrics 96:1113–1116, 1995.
94. Beasley RP. Hepatitis B virus: The major etiology of hepatocellular carcinoma. Cancer 61:1942–1956, 1988.
95. Seefe LB, Zimmerman HJ, Wright EL, et al. A randomized

controlled double blind trial of the efficacy of immune serum globulin for the prevention of post transfusion hepatitis. A Veterans Administration cooperative study. Gastroenterology 72:111–121, 1977.

95a. Palmovic D, Crnjakovic-Palmovic J. Prevention of hepatitis B virus infection in health care workers after accidental exposure: A comparison of two prophylactic schedules. Infection 21:42–45, 1993.

96. Grady GF, Lee VA, Prince AM, et al. Hepatitis B immune globulin for accidental exposures among medical personnel: Final report of a multicenter controlled trial. J Infect Dis 138:625–638, 1978.

97. Safety of therapeutic immune globulin preparations with respect to transmission for human T-lymphotrophic virus type III/lymphadenopathy-associated virus infection. MMWR Morb Mortal Wkly Rep 35:231–233, 1986.

98. Wells MA, Wittek AE, Epstein JS, et al. Inactivation and partition of human T-cell lymphotrophic virus, type III, during ethanol fractionation of plasma. Transfusion 26:210–213, 1986.

99. Bresee JS, Mast EE, Coleman PJ, et al. Hepatitis C virus infection associated with administration of intravenous immune globulin. JAMA 276:1563–1567, 1996.

100. Beasley RP, Hwang L-Y, Stevens CE, et al. Efficacy of hepatitis B immune globulin for prevention of perinatal transmission of the hepatitis B virus carrier state: Final report of a randomized double-blind, placebo-controlled trial. Hepatology 3:135–141, 1983.

101. Stevens CE, Toy P, Tong MJ, et al. Perinatal hepatitis B virus transmission in the United States; prevention with by passive-active immunization. JAMA 253:1740–1745, 1985.

102. Andre FJ, Zuckerman AJ. Review: Protective efficacy of hepatitis B vaccines in neonates. J Med Virol 44:144–151, 1994.

103. Redeker AG, Mosley JW, Gocke DJ, et al. Hepatitis B immune globulin as a prophylactic measure for spouses exposed to acute type B hepatitis. N Engl J Med 293:1055–1059, 1975.

104. Sitrin RD, Wampler DE, Ellis RW. Survey of licensed hepatitis B vaccines and their production processes. In Ellis RW (ed). Hepatitis B Vaccines in Clinical Practice. New York, Marcel Dekker, 1993, pp 83–101.

105. Emini EA, Eliis RW, Miller WJ, et al. Production and immunologic analysis of recombinant hepatitis B vaccine. J Infect 13(suppl A):3–9, 1986.

106. Stephenne J. Development and production aspects of a recombinant yeast-derived hepatitis B vaccine. Vaccine 8(suppl):S69–S73, 1990.

107. West D, Hesley T, Jonas L, et al. Safety and immunogenicity of a bivalent haemophilus influenzae type b/hepatitis B vaccine in healthy infants. Pediatr Infect Dis J 16:593–599, 1997.

108. Dedicoat M, Ellis C. New combined hepatitis A and B vaccine. BMJ 315:951, 1997.

109. Van Damme P, Cramm M, Safary A, et al. Heat stability of a recombinant DNA hepatitis B vaccine. Vaccine 10:366–367, 1992.

110. Xu ZY, Cao HL, Liu CB, et al. Control of hepatitis B in China. In Rizzetto M, Purcell PH, Gerin JL, Berme G (eds). Viral Hepatitis and Liver Disease. Turin, Italy, Edizioni Minerva Medica, 1997, pp 689–690.

111. Shaw FE, Guess HA, Roets JM, et al. Effect of anatomic injection site, age, and smoking on the immune response to hepatitis B vaccination. Vaccine 7:425–430, 1989.

112. West DJ. Clinical experience with hepatitis B vaccines. Am J Infect Contr 17:172–180, 1989.

113. Redfield RR, Innis BL, Scott RM, et al. Clinical evaluation of low-dose intradermally administered hepatitis B vaccine, a cost reduction strategy. JAMA 254:3203–3206, 1985.

114. Coleman PJ, Shaw FE, Serovich J, et al. Intradermal hepatitis B vaccination in a large hospital employee population. Vaccine 9:723–727, 1991.

115. Szmuness W, Stevens CE, Harley EJ, et al. Hepatitis B vaccine: Demonstration of efficacy in a controlled trial in a high risk population in the U.S. N Engl J Med 303:833–841, 1980.

116. Francis DP, Hadler SC, Thompson SE, et al. Prevention of hepatitis B with vaccine: Report from the Centers for Disease Control multi-center efficacy trial among homosexual men. Ann Intern Med 97:362–366, 1982.

117. Crosnier J, Jungers P, Courouce AM, et al. Randomised placebo-controlled trial of hepatitis B surface antigen vaccine in French haemodialysis units: I. Medical staff. Lancet 1:455–459, 1981.

118. Hadler SC, Francis DP, Maynard JE, et al. Long-term immunogenicity and efficacy of hepatitis B vaccine in homosexual men. N Engl J Med 315:209–214, 1986.

119. Hadler SC, Margolis HS. Hepatitis B immunization: Vaccine types, efficacy, and indications for immunization. In Remington JS, Swartz MN (eds). Current Clinical Topics in Infectious Diseases. Boston, Blackwell Scientific Publications, 1992, pp 282–308.

120. McLean AA, Hilleman MR, McAleer WJ, et al. Summary of worldwide experience with H-B-Vax (B, MSD). J Infect 7(suppl):95–104, 1983.

121. Andre FE. Summary of safety and efficacy data on a yeast-derived hepatitis B vaccine. Am J Med 87(suppl 3A):39–45, 1989.

122. West DJ, Calandra GB, Hesley TM, et al. Control of hepatitis B through routine immunization of infants: The need for flexible schedules and new combination vaccine formulations. Vaccine 11:S21–S27, 1993.

123. Greenberg DP, Vadheim CM, Wong VK, et al. Comparative safety and immunogenicity of two recombinant hepatitis B vaccines given to infants at two four and six months of age. Pediatr Infect Dis J 15:590–596, 1996.

124. Cassidy W, Watson B, Williams K, et al. Immunogenicity of alternative hepatitis B vaccination regimens in healthy adolescents [abstract 1177, AASLD]. Hepatology 22:401a, 1995.

125. Averhoff F, Mahoney FJ, Coleman P, et al. Risk factors for lack of response to hepatitis B vaccines: A randomized trial comparing the immunogenicity of recombinant hepatitis B vaccines in an adult population. Am J Prev Med 15:1–8, 1998.

125a. Patel D, Butler J, Feldman S, et al. Immunogenicity of hepatitis B vaccine in healthy very low birth weight infants. J Pediatr 131:641–643, 1997.

126. Roome AJ, Walsh SJ, Cartter ML, et al. Hepatitis B vaccine responsiveness in Connecticut Public Safety personnel. JAMA 270:2931–2934, 1993.

127. Wood RC, MacDonald KL, White KE, et al. Risk factors for lack of detectable antibody following hepatitis B vaccination of Minnesota Health Care Workers. JAMA 270:2935–2972, 1993.

128. Treadwell TL, Keeffe EB, Lake J, et al. Immunogenicity of two recombinant hepatitis B vaccines in older individuals. Am J Med 95:584–588, 1993.

129. Francis DP, Hadler SC, Thompson SE, et al. Prevention of hepatitis B with vaccine: Report from the Centers for Disease Control multi-center efficacy trial among homosexual men. Ann Intern Med 97:362–366, 1982.

130. Beasley RP, Hwang LY, Lee GC, et al. Prevention of perinatally transmitted hepatitis B virus with hepatitis B immune globulin and hepatitis B vaccine. Lancet 2:1099–1102, 1983.

131. Wong VCW, Ip HMP, Reesink HW, et al. Prevention of the HBsAg carrier state newborn infants of mothers who are chronic carriers of HBsAg and HBeAg by administration of hepatitis-B vaccine and hepatitis-B immunoglobulin. Double-blind randomised placebo-controlled study. Lancet 1:921–926, 1984.

132. Ip HMH, Lelie PN, Wong VCW, et al. Prevention of hepatitis B virus carrier state in infants according to maternal serum levels of HBV DNA. Lancet 1:406–409, 1989.

133. Lo K-W, Tsai Y-T, Lee S-D, et al. Immunoprophylaxis of infection with hepatitis B virus in infants born to hepatitis B surface antigen–positive carrier mothers. J Infect Dis 152:817–822, 1985.

134. Stevens CE, Taylor PE, Tong MJ, et al. Yeast-recombinant hepatitis B vaccine; efficacy with hepatitis B immune globulin in prevention of perinatal hepatitis B virus transmission. JAMA 257:2612–2616, 1987.

135. Stevens CE, Taylor PE, Tong MJ, et al. Prevention of perinatal hepatitis B virus infection with hepatitis B immune globulin and hepatitis B vaccine. In Zuckerman AJ (ed). Viral Hepatitis and Liver Disease. New York, Alan R Liss, 1988, pp 982–988.

136. Pongpipat D, Suvatte V, Assateerawats A. Hepatitis B immunization in high risk neonates born from HBsAg-positive mothers: Comparison between plasma derived and recombinant DNA vaccine. Asian Pac J Allergy Immunol 7:37–40, 1989.

137. Lee C-Y, Hwang L-Y, Beasley RP, et al. The protective efficacy of recombinant hepatitis B vaccine in newborn infants of hepati-

tis B e antigen–positive–hepatitis B surface antigen carrier mothers. Pediatr Inf Dis J 10:299–303, 1991.

137a. Del Canho R, Grosheide PM, Mazel JA, et al. Ten-year neonatal hepatitis B vaccination program, the Netherlands, 1982–1992: Protective efficacy and long-term immunogenicity. Vaccine 15:1624–1630, 1997.

138. Poovorawan Y, Sanpavat S, Pongpunlert W, et al. Long term efficacy of hepatitis B vaccine in infants born to hepatitis B e antigen positive mothers. Pediatr Inf Dis J 11:816–821, 1992.

139. Tin KM. Studies on the efficacy of hepatitis B vaccine in preventing perinatal HBV transmission in Burma. Presented at Symposium on Control of Hepatitis B in Infants and Children in High-Risk Areas of the World; Whakatane, New Zealand; November 12–14, 1987.

140. Assateerawatt A, Tanphaichitr VS, Suvatte V, In-ngarm L. Immunogenicity and protective efficacy of low dose recombinant DNA hepatitis B vaccine in normal and high-risk neonates. Asian Pac J Allergy Immunol 9:89–93, 1991.

141. Moulia-Pelat JP, Spiegel A, Martin PMV, et al. A 5-year immunization field trial against hepatitis B using a Chinese hamster ovary cell recombinant vaccine in French Polynesian newborns: Results at 3 years. Vaccine 12:499–502, 1994.

142. Stevens CE, Toy PT, Taylor PE, et al. Prospects for control of hepatitis B virus infection: Implications of childhood vaccination and long term protection. Pediatrics 90(suppl):170–173, 1992.

143. McMahon BJ, Rhoades ER, Heyward WL, et al. A comprehensive program to reduce the incidence of hepatitis B virus infection and its sequelae in Alaskan Natives. Lancet 2:1134–1136, 1987.

144. Mahoney F, Stewart K, Hu H, Alter MJ. Progress towards the elimination of hepatitis B virus transmission among health care workers in the United States. Arch Int Med 97:2601–2605, 1997.

145. Mahoney F, Woodruff B, Erben J, et al. Evaluation of a hepatitis B immunization program on the prevalence of hepatitis B virus infection. J Infect Dis 167:203–207, 1993.

146. Chen HL, Chang MH, Ni YH, et al. Seroepidemiology of hepatitis B virus infection in children: Ten years of mass vaccination in Taiwan. JAMA 276:906–908, 1996.

147. Ruff TA, Gertig DM, Otto BF, et al. Lombok Hepatitis B Model Immunization Project: Toward universal infant hepatitis B immunization in Indonesia. J Infect Dis 171:290–296, 1995.

148. Fortuin M, Chotard J, Jack AD, et al. Efficacy of hepatitis B vaccine in the Gambian expanded programme on Immunisation. Lancet 341:1129–1131, 1993.

149. Wainwright, Buklow LR, Parkinson AJ, et al. Protection provided by hepatitis B vaccine in a Yupik Eskimo population—results of a 10-year study. J Infect Dis 175:674–677, 1997.

150. Chen DS, Hsu HM, Chang MH, et al. Hepatitis B vaccines: Status report on long-term efficacy. In Rizzetto M, Purcell RH, Gerin JL, Verme G (eds). Viral Hepatitis and Liver Disease. Turin, Italy, Edizioni Minerva Medica, 1997, pp 635–637.

151. Xu ZY, Cao HL, Liu CB, et al. Control of hepatitis B in China. In Rizzetto M, Purcell RH, Gerin JL, Verme G (eds). Viral Hepatitis and Liver Disease. Turin, Italy, Edizioni Minerva Medica, 1997, pp 689–690.

152. Fortuin M, Chotard J, Jack AD, et al. Efficacy of hepatitis B vaccine in the Gambian expanded programme on immunisation. Lancet 341:1129–1131, 1993.

153. Lee C-L, Ko Y-C. Hepatitis B vaccination and hepatocellular carcinoma in Taiwan. Pediatrics 99:351–353, 1997.

153a. Chang MH, Chen CJ, Lai MS, et al. Universal hepatitis B vaccination in Taiwan and the incidence of hepatocellular carcinoma in children. Taiwan Childhood Hepatoma Study Group. N Engl J Med 336:1855–1859, 1997.

154. Chunsuttiwat S, Biggs BA, Maynard J, et al. Integration of hepatitis B vaccination into the Expanded Programme on Immunization in Chonburi and Chiangmai provinces, Thailand. Vaccine 15:769–774, 1997.

155. Coursaget P, Leboulleux D, Soumare M, et al. Twelve-year follow-up study of hepatitis B immunization of Senegalese infants. J Hepatol 21:250–254, 1994.

156. Myron Tong, unpublished data.

157. Wainwright RB, Bulkow LR, Parkinson AJ, et al. Protection provided by hepatitis B vaccine in a Yupik Eskimo Population—results of a 10-year study. J Infect Dis 175:674–677, 1997.

158. Hadler SC, Judson FN, O'Malley PM, et al. Studies of hepatitis B vaccine in homosexual men. In Coursaget P, Tong MJ (eds). Progress in Hepatitis B Immunization. Paris, John Libby Eurotest, 1990, pp 165–175.

159. Goh KT, Oon CJ, Heng BH, Lim GK. Long-term immunogenicity and efficacy of a reduced dose of plasma-based hepatitis B vaccine in young adults. Bull World Health Organ 73:523–527, 1995.

160. Taylor PE, Stevens CE. Persistence of antibody to hepatitis B surface antigen after vaccination in healthy adults. In Zuckermann AJ (ed). Viral Hepatitis and Liver Disease. New York, Alan R Liss, 1988.

161. Courouce AM, Loplanche A, Benhamou E, Jungers P. Long-term efficacy of hepatitis B vaccination in healthy adults. In Zuckermann AJ (ed). Viral Hepatitis and Liver Disease. New York, Alan R Liss, 1988, pp 1002–1005.

162. Gibas A, Watkins E, Hinkle C, Dienstag JL. Long-term persistence of protective antibody after hepatitis B vaccination of healthy adults. In Zuckermann AJ (ed). Viral Hepatitis and Liver Disease. New York, Alan R Liss, 1988, pp 998–1001.

163. Davidson M, Krugman S. Recombinant yeast hepatitis B vaccine compared with plasma-derived vaccine: Immunogenicity and effect of a booster dose. J Infect 13 (suppl):31–38, 1986.

164. Jilg W, Schmidt M, Deinhardt F. Persistence of specific antibodies after hepatitis B vaccination. J Hepatol 6:201–207, 1988.

165. Lieming D, Mintai Z, Yinfu W, et al. A 9-year follow-up study of the immunogenicity and long-term efficacy of plasma-derived hepatitis B vaccine in high-risk Chinese neonates. Clin Infect Dis 17:475–479, 1993.

166. Xia G, Liu C, Yan T, et al. Prevalence of hepatitis B virus markers in children vaccinated by hepatitis B vaccine in five hepatitis B vaccine experimental areas of China. Chin J Exp Clin Virol 9:17–23, 1995.

167. Xu ZY, Duan SC, Margolis H. Long term efficacy of postexposure immunization of infants for prevention of hepatitis B virus infection. United States–People's Republic of China Study Group on Hepatitis B. J Infect Dis 171:54–60, 1995.

168. Lo KJ, Lee SD, Tsai YT, et al. Long term immunogenicity and efficacy of hepatitis B vaccine in infants born to HBeAg-positive HBsAg-carrier mothers. Hepatology 8:1647–1650, 1988.

169. Hwang LY, Lee CY, Beasley RP. Five-year follow-up of HBV vaccination with plasma derived vaccine in neonates: Evaluation of immunogenicity and efficacy against perinatal transmission. In Hollinger FB, Lemon SM, Margolis HS (eds). Viral Hepatitis and Liver Disease. Baltimore, Williams & Wilkins, 1991, pp 759–761.

170. Lee PI, Lee CY, Huang LM, Chang MH. Long term efficacy of recombinant hepatitis B vaccine and risk of natural infection in infants born to mothers with hepatitis B e antigen. J Pediatr 126:716–721, 1995.

171. Coursaget P, Leboulleux D, Soumare M, et al. Twelve year follow-up of hepatitis B immunization of Senegalese infants. J Hepatol 21:25–54, 1994.

172. Coursaget P, Yvonne B, Chotard J, et al. Seven years study of hepatitis B vaccine efficacy in infants from an endemic area (Senegal). Lancet 2:1143–1145, 1986.

173. West DJ, Calandra GB. Vaccine induced memory for hepatitis B surface antigen: Implications for policy on booster vaccination. Vaccine 14:1019–1027, 1996.

174. Davidson M, Krugman S. Recombinant yeast hepatitis B vaccine compared with plasma-derived vaccine: Immunogenicity and effect of a booster dose. J Infect 13 (suppl):31–38, 1986.

175. Milne A, Waldon J. Recombinant DNA hepatitis B vaccination in teenagers: Effect of a booster dose at 51/2 years. J Infect Dis 166:942, 1992.

176. Milne A, Krugman S, Waldon JA, et al. Hepatitis B vaccination in children: Five year booster study. N Z Med J 26:336–338, 1992.

177. Horowitz MM, Ershler WB, McKinney WP, Battiola RJ. Duration of immunity after hepatitis B vaccination: Efficacy of low-dose booster vaccine. Ann Intern Med 108:185–189, 1988.

178. Chan CY, Lee SD, Tsai YT, Lo KJ. Booster response to recombinant yeast-derived hepatitis B vaccine in vaccinees whose anti-HBs response were elicited by a plasma-derived vaccine. Vaccine 9:765–767, 1991.

178a. Poovorawan Y, Sanpavat S, Chumdermpadetsuk S, Safary A. Long term hepatitis B vaccine in infants born to hepatitis B e antigen positive mothers. Arch Dis Child 77:F47–F51, 1997.
178b. Zannolli R, Morgese G. Hepatitis B vaccine: Current issues. Ann Pharmacother 31:1059–1067, 1997.
179. Zajac BA, West DJ, McAleer WJ, Scolnick EM. Overview of the clinical studies with hepatitis B vaccine made by recombinant DNA. J Infect 13(suppl A):39–45, 1986.
180. Andre FE. Summary of safety and efficacy data on a yeast-derived hepatitis B vaccine. Am J Med 87 (suppl 3A):39–45, 1989.
181. Lear JT, English JS. Anaphylaxis after hepatitis B vaccination [letter]. Lancet 345:1249, 1995.
182. Nadler JP. Multiple sclerosis and hepatitis B vaccination. Clin Infect Dis 17:928–929, 1993.
183. Herroelen L, de Keyser J, Ebinger G. Central nervous system demyelination after immunisation with recombinant hepatitis B vaccine. Lancet 338:1174–1175, 1991.
184. Waisbren BA. Perspectives on hepatitis B vaccination. JAMA 277:1124–1125, 1997.
185. Institute of Medicine, Stratton KR, Howe CJ, et al. (eds). Adverse Events Associated with Childhood Vaccines: Evidence Bearing on Causality. Washington, DC, National Academy Press, 1994.
186. Niu MT, Davis DM, Ellenberg S. Recombinant hepatitis B vaccination of neonates and infants: Emerging safety data from the Vaccine Adverse Event Reporting System. Pediatr Infect Dis J 15:771–776, 1996.
186a. Grotto I, Mandel Y, Ephrost M, et al. Major adverse reactions to yeast-derived hepatitis B vaccines—a review. Vaccine 16:329–334, 1998.
187. McMahon BJ, Helminiak C, Wainwright RB, et al. Frequency of adverse reactions to hepatitis B vaccine in 43,618 persons. Am J Med 92:254–256, 1992.
188. Centers for Disease Control and Prevention. Update: Vaccine side effects, adverse events, contraindications, and precautions; Recommendations of the Advisory Committee on Immunization Practices. MMWR Morb Mortal Wkly Rep 45(RR-12):1–35, 1996.
189. Zanetti AR, Tanzi E, Manzillo G, et al. Hepatitis B variants in Europe. Lancet 2:1132–1133, 1988.
190. Carman WF, Zanetti AR, Karayiannis P, et al. Vaccine-induced escape mutant of hepatitis B virus. Lancet 336:325–329, 1990.
191. Harrison TJ, Hopes EA, Oon CJ, et al. Independant emergence of a vaccine-induced escape mutant of hepatitis B virus. J Hepatol 13(suppl):S105–S107, 1991.
192. Zuckerman AJ, Harrison TJ, Oon CJ. Mutation in S region of hepatitis B virus. Lancet 343:737–738, 1994.
193. Howard CR. The structure of hepatitis B envelope and molecular variants of hepatitis B virus. J Viral Hepat 2:165–170, 1995.
194. Nainan OV, Stevens CE, Margolis HS. Hepatitis B virus (HBV) antibody resistant mutants: Frequency and significance [abstract 98]. Ninth Triennial International Symposium on Viral Hepatitis and Liver Disease; Rome, Italy; 1996.
195. McMahon G, Erlich PH, Moustapha ZA, et al. Genetic alterations in the gene encoding the major HBsAg: DNA and immunological analysis of recurrent HBsAg derived from monoclonal antibody–treated liver transplant patients. Hepatology 15:757–766, 1992.
196. Oon CJ, Lim GK, Zhao Y. Studies on the transmissability of HBV vaccine escape 145 GLY to ARG mutants in immune and hepatitis B carriers in the family [abstract C253]. Ninth Triennial International Symposium on Viral Hepatitis and Liver Disease; Rome, Italy; 1996.
197. Ogata N, Miller RH, Ishak KG, et al. Genetic and biologic characterization of two hepatitis B virus variants: A precore mutant implicated in fulminant hepatitis and a surface mutant resistant to immunoprophylaxis. In Nishioka K, Suzuki H, Mishiro S, Oda T (eds). Viral Hepatitis and Liver Disease. Tokyo, Springer-Verlag, 1993, pp 238–242.
198. Coursaget P, Relyveld E, Brizaard A, et al. Simultaneous injection of hepatitis B vaccine with BCG and killed poliovirus vaccine. Vaccine 10:319–321, 1992.
199. Coursaget P, Yvonnet B, Telyveld EH, et al. Simultaneous administration of diphtheria-tetanus-pertussis-polio and hepatitis B vaccines in a simplified immunization program: Immune response to diphtheria toxoid, tetanus toxoid, pertussis, and hepatitis B surface antigen. Infect Immun 51:784–787, 1986.
200. Aristegui J, Muniz J, Perez Legorburu A, et al. Newborn universal immunization against hepatitis B: Immunogenicity and reactogenicity of simultaneous administration of diphtheria/tetanus/pertussis (DPT) and oral polio vaccines with hepatitis B vaccine at 0, 2 and 6 months of age. Vaccine 13:973–977, 1995.
201. Barone P, Mauro L, Leonardi S, et al. Simultaneous administration of HB recombinant vaccine with diphtheria and tetanus toxoid and oral polio vaccines: A pilot study. Acta Paediatr Jpn 33:455–458, 1991.
202. Coursaget P, Fritzell B, Blondeau C, et al. Simultaneous injection of plasma-derived or recombinant hepatitis B vaccines with yellow fever and killed polio vaccines. Vaccine 13:109–111, 1995.
203. Diez-Delgado J, Dal-Re R, Llorente M, et al. Hepatitis B component does not interfere with the immune response to diphtheria, tetanus, and whole-cell *Bordetella pertussis* components of a quadrivalent (DPTw-HB) vaccine: A controlled trial in healthy infants. Vaccine 15:1418–1422, 1997.
204. Bruguera M, Bayas JM, Vilella A, et al. Immunogenicity and reactogenicity of a combined hepatitis A and B vaccine in young adults. Vaccine 15:1407–1411, 1996.
205. Freed GL, Bordley WC, Clark SJ, Konrad TR. Reactions of pediatricians to a new CDC recommendation for universal immunization of infants with hepatitis B vaccine. Pediatrics 91:699–702, 1993.
206. Deseda CC, Shapiro C, O'Connor K, Margolis H. Pediatricians attitudes, practices, and knowledge regarding universal infant vaccination against hepatitis B [abstract]. In Proceedings of Centers for Disease Control, Epidemic Intelligence Service 42nd Annual Conference; Atlanta GA; 1993, p 34.
207. Ganiats TR. Hepatitis B vaccination. Are we jumping on the bandwagon too early? J Fam Pract 36:147–149, 1993.
208. Margolis HS, Coleman PJ, Brown RE, et al. Prevention of hepatitis B virus transmission by immunization. An economic analysis of current recommendations. JAMA 274:1201–1208, 1995.
209. Freed GL, Konrad TR, DeFriese GH, Lohr JA. Adoption of new *Haemophilus influenzae* type b vaccine recommendation [letter]. Am J Dis Child 147:124–128, 1993.

chapter

11 *Haemophilus influenzae* Vaccines

Joel I. Ward

Kenneth M. Zangwill

Haemophilus influenzae is a respiratory pathogen of humans, and the infections it causes range from asymptomatic colonization of the upper respiratory tract to serious invasive disease, such as meningitis. It is an important pathogen, especially for children, causing considerable morbidity, mortality, and healthcare expense worldwide. Before the widespread use of effective vaccines in young infants, invasive *H. influenzae* disease was the leading cause of bacterial meningitis in the United States[1, 2] and many areas of the world. Great strides have been made in our understanding of its microbiology, immunology, pathogenesis, and epidemiology and in improved therapy for disease. Most significantly, the introduction of routine immunization in many countries of the world has nearly eliminated *H. influenzae* type b disease, providing important lessons for the prevention of other respiratory bacterial pathogens.

HISTORICAL BACKGROUND

During the 1889 influenza pandemic, Richard Pfeiffer (Fig. 11–1) first isolated the *H. influenzae* bacteria from sputum of patients who died of influenza, and he ascribed to the "Pfeiffer bacillus" the causation of this respiratory disease.[3, 4] The organism had also been recovered from the blood and cerebrospinal fluid (CSF) of young children with meningitis. Because the organism was difficult to grow on culture media (owing to the need for X and V factors as nutritional supplements), not until the great influenza pandemic of 1918 to 1919 did it become widely appreciated that the organism was a constituent of the normal bacterial flora of the human upper respiratory tract and not the cause of influenza. In 1920, Winslow and associates[5] renamed the organism *Haemophilus influenzae* to emphasize its requirement for blood factors (X and V factors) for growth (*haemophilus* meaning "blood-loving") and to acknowledge its historical association with influenza. Its name still causes confusion, particularly for lay persons trying to distinguish between the influenza and *H. influenzae* vaccines.

Our understanding of the microbiology and immunology of infections caused by *H. influenzae* was greatly enhanced by the pioneering work of Margaret Pittman (Fig. 11–2) in the early 1930s.[6, 7] She defined two major groupings of *H. influenzae:* encapsulated and unencapsulated strains. Among the encapsulated strains, she serologically characterized six antigenically distinct serotypes (designated a to f), which subsequently were shown to differ biochemically in the composition of the organism's polysaccharide capsule. Pittman also observed that *H. influenzae* type b strains were recovered primarily from the CSF and blood of young patients with meningitis and that unencapsulated strains were generally recovered from the upper respiratory tract secretions of adults. Pittman further demonstrated that antibody to the type b capsule conferred type-specific protection against lethal experimental *H. influenzae* type b infection in animals. This observation became the basis for serotherapy with horse and subsequently rabbit antiserum, which

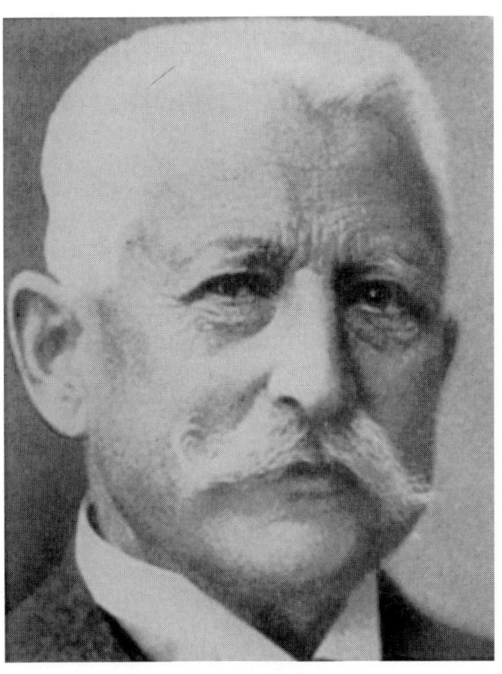

Figure 11–1. Richard Pfeiffer.

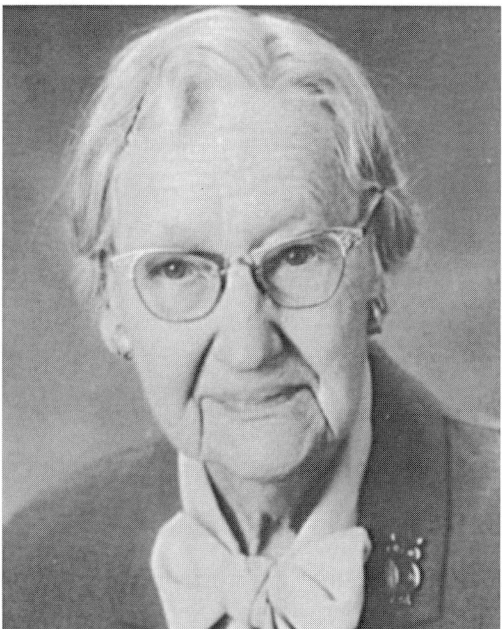

Figure 11–2. Margaret Pittman.

was the first effective therapy for invasive *H. influenzae* type b disease, a disease that previously was nearly always fatal.[8–10]

In 1933, Fothergill and Wright[11] described the fact that *H. influenzae* meningitis affected mostly children younger than 5 years, and they noted the correlation between the risk of disease and the absence of bactericidal antibodies. Later it was shown that the major antibody contributing to the protective activity of bactericidal serum was antibody to type b capsule.[12–14] These observations suggested that naturally acquired type b anticapsular antibody protects, and this remains the underlying premise for attempts to stimulate protective immunity with polysaccharide and polysaccharide-conjugate vaccines.

During most of the past 50 years, the advent of effective antibiotics for *H. influenzae* focused attention on treatment rather than prevention of disease. The appreciation that the morbidity and mortality of disease could never be completely eliminated by treatment, even with prompt diagnosis and use of highly effective antibiotics and other therapies, gave further impetus to the development of *H. influenzae* type b (Hib) vaccines. The first vaccine was the purified type b polysaccharide vaccine, which was followed by the more immunogenic polysaccharide-protein conjugate vaccines. Each of the Hib vaccines is reviewed in this chapter.

CLINICAL PRESENTATIONS

On the basis of disease pathogenesis, severity of disease, and microbiological differences, three categories of *H. influenzae* infections can be characterized (Table 11–1). First, the majority of *H. influenzae* infections involve asymptomatic infection or colonization of the upper respiratory tract.

Second, most common are mucosal infections, such as otitis media, sinusitis, and bronchitis. Although mucosal infections occur frequently, they do not result in bacteremia and therefore are rarely life threatening. The microbiological hallmark of mucosal infections is that they are caused by the same bacteria that normally colonize the oropharynx, usually unencapsulated strains of *H. influenzae*.[15] Extension of these organisms from colonized respiratory tract passages into contiguous body sites is enhanced by the compromise of normal defense mechanisms, such as the presence of eustachian tube reflux, foreign bodies, smoking damage to the bronchopulmonary epithelium, antecedent viral infection, or selected immune deficiencies.

Third and most important, invasive disease is characterized by the dissemination of bacteria, almost always *H. influenzae* type b, from the nasopharynx to the blood stream and subsequently to other body sites. The most serious manifestation of invasive *H. influenzae* type b disease is meningitis, which accounts for about half of all recognized cases of invasive *H. influenzae* type b infection.[16–19] Even with early diagnosis and the availability of effective antimicrobial therapy, about 5% of children with *H. influenzae* type b meningitis die.[20] Neurological sequelae of varying severity are relatively common after *H. influenzae* type b meningitis, occurring in 15 to 30% of survivors.[21–28] Neurological handicaps include hearing loss, language disorders or delay, mental retardation, learning disabilities, motor abnormalities, and seizure.

The clinical separation of invasive and mucosal disease is not absolute, inasmuch as type b strains can cause otitis media or sinusitis.[29] Likewise, other serotypes (especially type a) and nontypable strains occasionally cause bacteremia and meningitis. A notable example is neonatal sepsis or meningitis that occurs when nontypable strains, presumably acquired from the flora of the mother's genital tract, cause invasive disease.[30–32]

Pneumonia is another infection caused by either type b or nontypable strains. Reports from Africa and Papua New Guinea suggest that *H. influenzae* type b and non–type b *H. influenzae* are important causes of severe acute lower respiratory tract infections in developing countries.[33–37] *Haemophilus influenzae* type b pneumonia can be associated with bacteremia, empyema, or even pericarditis. Appearance on radiological examination includes lobar, bronchial, and interstitial patterns that are rarely specific for an etiological diagnosis.

Table 11–1. **SPECTRUM OF *Haemophilus influenzae* DISEASE**

	Invasive Disease (95% due to type b strains)	
Meningitis	Pneumonia	Empyema
Bacteremia	Septic arthritis	Osteomyelitis
Epiglottitis	Pericarditis	Cellulitis
	Abscesses	
	Mucosal Disease (predominantly due to nontypable strains)	
Otitis media	Bronchitis	Pneumonia
Sinusitis	Conjunctivitis	Urinary tract infections

Although not absolute, the distinction between invasive and mucosal disease is useful because there are many diagnostic, therapeutic, and prophylactic implications relating to the two types of infection. The vaccines available to control *H. influenzae* disease all have the type b polysaccharide as the primary immunogen and are therefore intended to prevent only *H. influenzae* type b disease. These vaccines have little or no impact on infections caused by non–type b strains. Therefore, most of this chapter concerns the prevention of invasive *H. influenzae* type b disease.

MICROBIOLOGY

Haemophilus influenzae is a small gram-negative coccobacillus that in clinical specimens appears filamentous or pleomorphic, especially when obtained from patients who have received antibiotics. It is a nonmotile, non–spore-forming, facultative anaerobe that requires two accessory factors for in vitro growth. The X factor, needed for aerobic growth, is a heat-stable, iron-containing protoporphyrin that is essential for activity of the electron transport chain. The V factor, a coenzyme, is a heat-labile factor supplied by nicotinamide adenine dinucleotide. Both factors are present within erythrocytes and are released by heat or enzyme lysis of the red blood cells, which permits growth on chocolate agar. The requirement of these factors for growth remains the primary basis for the laboratory differentiation of *H. influenzae* from other *Haemophilus* species; the organism grows in almost any enriched liquid or solid medium supplemented with X and V factors. Although it is not mandatory for growth, some strains grow better in 5 to 10% carbon dioxide. After overnight incubation on an enriched medium, colonies appear that are 0.5 to 1.5 mm in diameter and rough or granular. Encapsulated strains usually produce slightly larger colonies that are mucoid or glistening. Fermentation reactions and other metabolic activities are variable and therefore are not particularly useful for identification. However, a biotyping scheme, based on the metabolism of indole, urea, and ornithine decarboxylase activity, has been used to subtype strains.[38]

Several surface structures of *H. influenzae* appear to be important determinants of the organism's pathogenicity. As with many invasive pathogens, its outermost structure is a polysaccharide capsule. The type b capsule is of primary clinical and immunological importance inasmuch as type b organisms account for 95% of all strains that cause invasive disease (bacteremia and meningitis).[2, 16–19, 39] This polysaccharide consists of a repeating polymer of ribosyl and ribitol phosphate (polyribosylribitol phosphate [PRP]), which has a 1 to 1 linkage (Fig. 11–3). The other capsular serotypes are composed of hexose rather than pentose sugars and only occasionally cause invasive disease. Strains without capsules frequently cause infections of the respiratory tract and adjacent structures but rarely cause bacteremic infections.

Other important components of the *H. influenzae* cell envelope include lipopolysaccharide (endotoxin) and a number of proteins and lipids in the outer membrane. Some membrane proteins participate in cell transport

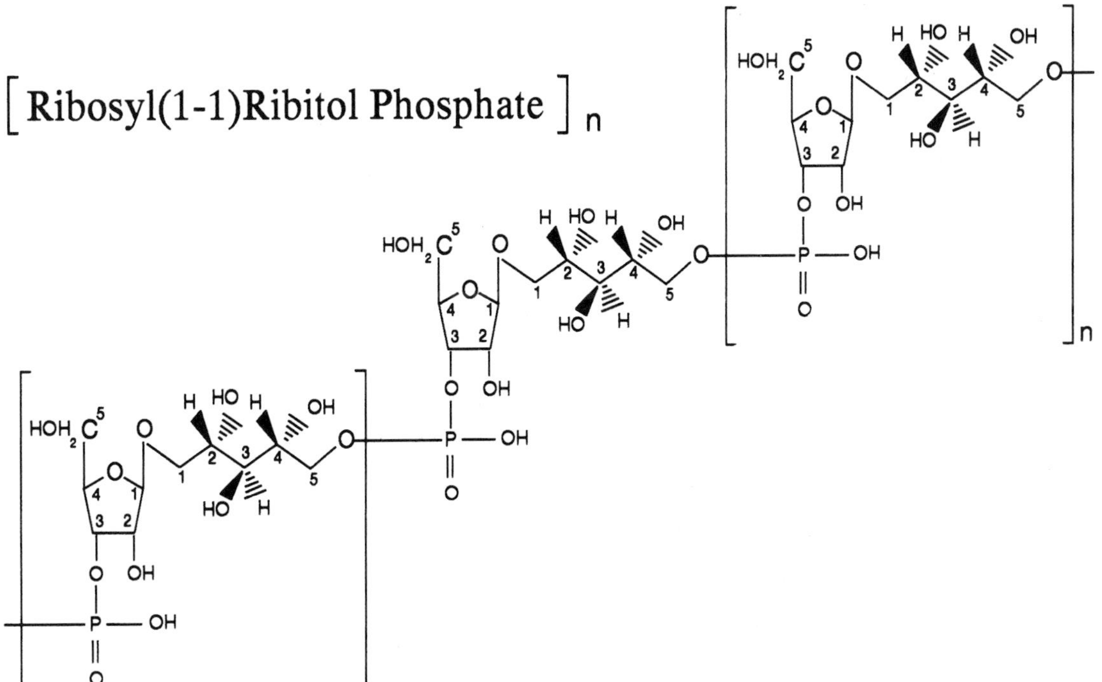

[Ribosyl(1-1)Ribitol Phosphate]$_n$

Figure 11–3. Repeating unit structure of *Haemophilus influenzae* type b capsular polysaccharide, shown in its protonated form: → 3)β-D Rib *f*-(1 → 1)-D-Ribol-5-(PO_2H →. (Adapted from Zon G, Robbins JD. ^{31}P- and ^{13}C-NMR–spectral and chemical characterization of the end-group and repeating-unit components of oligosaccharides derived by acid hydrolysis of *Haemophilus influenzae* type b capsular polysaccharide. Carbohydr Res 114:103–121, 1983.)

(porins) and others are adhesins; the functions of still others remain undefined. Pili or fimbriae are protein filaments extending from the outer membrane that appear to mediate attachment of the organism to epithelial cells.[40] Their expression appears to be reversible, but the importance of these structures in the pathogenesis of disease is unknown. The electrophoresis of a number of cytoplasmic enzymes has distinguished isoenzyme differences that have been useful in genetic analyses of *H. influenzae* strains.[41]

Another important microbiological feature of *H. influenzae* has been the development of antibiotic resistance. Resistance to a wide variety of antibiotics (e.g., sulfonamides, aminoglycosides, trimethoprim-sulfamethoxazole, erythromycin, tetracycline, penicillin) has been described, but these antibiotics are not essential for therapy. Of greater importance was resistance to ampicillin, first noted in the mid-1970s,[42–48] because it was the primary antibiotic used in therapy for disease. Since then, ampicillin resistance has been recognized worldwide.[49–54] The mechanism of resistance usually involves plasmid-mediated β-lactamase enzyme production,[55] and resistant strains are often characterized by their plasmid or β-lactamase enzyme content. Resistance to chloramphenicol is usually mediated by an enzyme, chloramphenicol acetyltransferase.[56, 57] Although chloramphenicol-resistant strains are rare in the United States, they are increasingly prevalent in some areas of the world,[53] and strains resistant to both ampicillin and chloramphenicol have been reported.[50, 57–61]

Third-generation cephalosporins, in particular ceftriaxone and cefotaxime, are currently the mainstays in therapy for invasive disease.[62] Concerns about the potential for the development of resistance to these highly effective agents emphasize the need for means to prevent disease.

PATHOGENESIS OF INFECTION AND DISEASE

To develop *H. influenzae* type b disease, an individual must experience a series of events, beginning with exposure to the organism and acquisition of infection (colonization of the mucosal membranes). Nearly all individuals are colonized with nontypable strains, and 1 to 5% of unimmunized persons carry type b strains asymptomatically.

Unfortunately, most of the factors that influence the efficiency of transmission and the ability of the organism to establish colonization are poorly understood.[63, 64] Carriage rates are lowest in adults and young infants and highest in preschool-aged children. In a prospective longitudinal study conducted at a daycare center in Dallas, Texas, where no invasive infections occurred, the average prevalence of colonization with *H. influenzae* type b was 10%.[65] During the 18 months of study, 71% of the children aged 18 to 35 months and 48% of the children aged 36 to 71 months were at some time colonized. Carriage rates can be as high as 58 to 91% in households or daycare centers in which a case has occurred.[66–70] Likewise, within families in which a case of invasive disease has occurred, rates of colonization of 60 to 70% among siblings and 20% among parents have been observed.[69–71] It is not clear whether the high carriage rates in these exposed, semiclosed populations are the cause or the result of disease.[64, 72–78] Close contact among exposed individuals, as occurs within families and daycare centers, increases the potential for transmission, and both larger families and attendance at large daycare centers increase the risk of colonization and disease.

Despite a low point prevalence of pharyngeal carriage (1 to 5%), most young children become colonized with *H. influenzae* type b during the first 2 to 5 years of life[72, 73, 75–77, 79] and consequently develop specific immunity.[14, 78, 80–84] Type b strains may persist in the nasopharynx for months[64, 65, 77] and often are not eliminated by treatment with antimicrobial agents that do not penetrate into respiratory secretions.[80, 85, 86]

The relationship between the carriage of type b organisms and the subsequent development of disease and immunity is not clearly understood. Two factors that may increase the potential for colonization and the risk of invasive disease are the size of the bacterial inoculum[87] and the presence of a concomitant viral infection.[88, 89] Invasive *H. influenzae* type b disease involves the bacteremic dissemination of the organism from the respiratory tract to distant body sites.[90, 91] As studied in animals, the initial stage of invasive infection involves attachment to respiratory epithelium and penetration through the mucosa, leading to bacteremia.[90–93] The organisms appear to enter the vascular system by breaking down the tight junctions between cells and invading intercellularly.[87] Local nasopharyngeal inflammation is generally absent.[90] The bacteremia is initially low grade but steadily increases during the passing hours.[90, 94] The dynamics between bacterial proliferation and clearance are influenced by antibody, complement, and the reticuloendothelial system and determine the magnitude of the bacteremia.[95–97] The type b polysaccharide capsule is antiphagocytic and therefore is a major determinant of the organism's invasiveness. The role of other bacterial virulence factors (e.g., attachment factors, toxins) in the pathogenesis of invasive disease, as well as that of the immune factors that mitigate infection, is also not well understood.

As infection proceeds and bacterial concentration in the blood mounts, metastatic seeding of serosal membranes occurs, especially to the meninges or to other sites including the lungs, pleura, joint synovium, or pericardium.[90] After a critical bacterial concentration is exceeded in the blood, *H. influenzae* type b organisms appear to enter the central nervous system through the choroid plexus.[90] Inflammation of the choroid plexus is a uniform feature of meningitis. Organisms then infect the CSF and the arachnoid villi of the leptomeninges, blocking the return of CSF and thereby increasing bacterial density and CSF pressure.[98] In general, the magnitude of bacteremia and the density of organisms in the CSF correlate with the severity of clinical illness.[99, 100]

DIAGNOSIS

The primary criterion for the diagnosis of *H. influenzae* infection is Gram stain and isolation of the organism from the infected focus (e.g., CSF, pleural fluid, sputum, or blood). The specimens must be processed immediately and appropriately because *H. influenzae* type b has several growth requirements, as described before. Selective media that suppress the growth of gram-positive organisms may increase the recovery of *H. influenzae* from upper respiratory tract specimens.[46, 101]

Other techniques are available that may assist in the microbiological diagnosis, including rapid antigen detection, staining techniques, and immunofluorescence. Such techniques are useful in the context of a patient whose cultures are sterile because of prior antibiotic therapy or to confirm the clinical diagnosis before bacterial growth occurs. The three most commonly used techniques for antigen detection are latex particle agglutination (LPA), countercurrent immunoelectrophoresis (CIE), and coagglutination (CoA). Overall, the LPA appears to be more sensitive than is CoA, and LPA and CoA are both more sensitive than is CIE in CSF, serum, urine, joint fluid, and pleural fluid.[102–104] False-positive results can be due to nonspecific agglutination (i.e., rheumatoid factors) or antigenic cross-reactivity with other organisms; false-positive results may also occur in the urine of children with nasopharyngeal carriage of the organism or, more commonly, for several days after immunization with Hib conjugate vaccine.[105, 106] Acridine orange fluorescent staining and immunofluorescence may be helpful in situations in which smaller bacterial concentrations are present.[107, 108] Several enzyme-linked immunosorbent assays for PRP detection are available, but these tests are generally used in the research setting and are not of substantial clinical value.

TREATMENT

Because bacteremia plays a central pathogenetic role in invasive *H. influenzae* type b disease, occult invasion of the central nervous system must always be considered in the context of any manifestation of invasive *H. influenzae* type b disease. Therefore, cure of *H. influenzae* type b bacteremia and its complications requires antimicrobial therapy that will (1) penetrate the blood-brain barrier to achieve bactericidal concentrations, (2) be of adequate duration to sterilize the primary and potential secondary foci, and (3) reflect the local antibiotic susceptibility patterns of invasive isolates. Resistance to several antimicrobials including ampicillin, chloramphenicol, trimethoprim-sulfamethoxazole, rifampin, and certain second-generation cephalosporins in *H. influenzae* type b has been increasing in several areas of the world.[54]

For proven or suspected *H. influenzae* type b meningitis, cefotaxime or ceftriaxone is recommended until the antibiotic susceptibility of the organism is known or an alternative diagnosis is established.[62] Cefuroxime no longer appears to have a role in the treatment of *H. influenzae* meningitis in that delayed sterilization may be at least twofold more common than with standard therapy of ampicillin, chloramphenicol, or the third-generation cephalosporins.[109, 110] Also, ampicillin, formerly a mainstay of therapy for this infection, should not be used alone to empirically treat infections due to *H. influenzae* type b because up to 50% of *H. influenzae* type b isolates in the United States are resistant by plasmid-mediated β-lactamase production.[54]

Children with occult *H. influenzae* type b bacteremia need to be carefully re-evaluated because 30 to 50% of such patients who are clinically well may develop focal disease.[111, 112] The duration of therapy is determined by the site of infection and the clinical response.

Equally important in the overall management of a child with invasive *H. influenzae* type b disease is supportive care. For *H. influenzae* type b meningitis, several studies have shown that adjunctive therapy with dexamethasone moderates the inflammatory cascade and may decrease the likelihood of hearing loss. The recommended dose is 0.6 mg/kg per day given every 6 hours for 4 days, with the first dose given just before or with the first antibiotic dose.[113] Management of the child with meningitis requires continuing careful evaluations for complications such as the development of shock, inappropriate secretion of antidiuretic hormone, seizures, subdural empyema, and secondary foci of infection.

EPIDEMIOLOGY

Invasive *H. influenzae* type b disease has been a leading infectious disease problem worldwide, one that primarily affects young children.[2, 114] Before the availability of vaccines, an estimated 20,000 to 25,000 persons developed invasive *H. influenzae* type b disease annually in the United States, and the estimated cumulative risk for *H. influenzae* type b disease was one episode in every 200 children during the first 5 years of life.[20, 115] Also, until 1992, *H. influenzae* type b was the most common cause of bacterial meningitis in the United States.[1, 2] In comparison, before the availability of Hib vaccines, the incidence and mortality of *H. influenzae* type b disease in the United States were similar to those for paralytic poliomyelitis during its peak epidemic year (1954) before the availability of poliovirus vaccines.

Humans are the only natural host for *H. influenzae* bacteria. Transmission occurs through respiratory droplets or contact with respiratory secretions, although there is limited evidence that contaminated fomites could play a role in transmission.[116] Colonization of the birth canal also occurs. The organism can be carried in the upper respiratory tract for prolonged periods and is usually transmitted from person to person through many transmission cycles before causing disease in a susceptible person. Owing to this asymptomatic carriage, it has not been possible to define an incubation period or pattern of transmission in endemic settings.

Incidence of Disease

Invasive *H. influenzae* type b disease occurs endemically, and community-wide epidemics have not been described. Because 85% of all invasive *H. influenzae* type b disease occurs in children younger than 5 years, epidemiological studies of invasive *H. influenzae* type b disease use disease rates for this age group.[117, 118]

Table 11–2. **AGE-SPECIFIC INCIDENCE* OF INVASIVE *Haemophilus influenzae* b DISEASE FROM UNITED STATES POPULATION-BASED STUDIES, 1976 TO 1984**

AGE (mo)	MENINGITIS ONLY		ALL INVASIVE DISEASE		CUMULATIVE PERCENTAGE OF DISEASE
	Median	Range	Median	Range	
0–5	101	59–141	148	98–197	10–15
6–11	179	143–279	275	218–452	37–43
12–17	146	88–184	223	123–248	60–61
18–23	62	20–64	92	57–107	64–68
24–35	31	18–39	50	37–70	75–78
36–47	17	5–26	31	7–39	80–83
48–59	4	2–16	11	7–41	84–86
≥60†	0.2	0.1–0.2	1.3	1.2–2.4	100

*Cases per 100,000 population per year. Range of point estimates from five studies, including Alaska, 1980–1982 (excluding Eskimos, Native Americans); Atlanta, 1983–1984; Fresno County, 1976–1978; Dallas, 1982–1984; and Minnesota, 1982–1984.

†Cumulative percentage and incidence data for ages ≥60 months are based on studies from Alaska, Atlanta, and Fresno County, where active surveillance for all age groups was conducted.

Although invasive *H. influenzae* type b disease is not reliably reported nationally or internationally, a number of population-based studies[119–132] have been conducted during the past 30 years that make it possible to define the incidence, epidemiological characteristics, and clinical spectrum of endemic *H. influenzae* type b disease (Table 11–2). Differences in the methods and rigor of case-finding efforts can explain, in part, the variability in incidence, as could differences in exposure or host susceptibility factors. The isolation of *H. influenzae* type b from a sterile body site is the basis for case detection, but not all infected children have cultures performed, or cultures may be negative owing to prior antimicrobial therapy. For these and other reasons, even the most carefully conducted surveillance studies inevitably underestimate the true incidence of disease.

A limited number of population-based studies of the incidence of *H. influenzae* disease have also been conducted outside of the United States (Table 11–3). Most of these studies were performed in Western industrialized nations and show an incidence of *H. influenzae* disease that is approximately one third to two thirds that in the United States. In Sweden,[133–136] Finland,[133, 137, 138] the Netherlands,[139] Australia,[140, 141] and Israel,[142, 143] *H. influenzae* type b was the most common cause of bacterial meningitis. It also ranked as the leading cause of bacterial meningitis in Canada, which had a disease incidence similar to that in the United States.[144, 145] In other parts of Europe, including the United Kingdom,[146, 147] and in most developing countries, meningococcal meningitis was reported to be more common than meningitis caused by *H. influenzae* type b. Population-based inci-

Table 11–3. **INCIDENCE* OF INVASIVE *Haemophilus influenzae* b DISEASE, SELECTED POPULATION-BASED STUDIES OUTSIDE THE UNITED STATES**

LOCATION	DATES	MENINGITIS		ALL INVASIVE INFECTIONS	
		<1 Year	<5 Years	<1 Year	<5 Years
Senegal (Dakar)[151]	1970–1979	132	36		
Scandinavia[133]	1974–1984	43	26	62	41
France[481] (Val-de-Marne and Haute-Garonne)	1975–1981		15		24
New Zealand (Auckland)[482]	1975–1981		27		41
Canada[144]	1981–1984				
Manitoba					
Native		126	35		
Nonnative		70	26		
Northwest Territories					
Inuit		2333	530		
The Gambia[149]	1985–1987	297	60		
Chile (Santiago)[483]	1985–1987	47	15	63	22
England (Oxford)[399]	1985–1988		24		33
Australia	1985–1988				
Northern Territory[140]					
Aborigines			159		529
Nonaborigines			53		92
Israel[143]	1988–1990		18		34

*Cases per 100,000 person-years.

dence data for developing countries are limited; however, *H. influenzae* appears to rank as the leading cause of bacterial meningitis in most countries.[148–153]

Investigators in Australia have reported an exceptionally high rate of invasive *H. influenzae* type b disease among aboriginal children in central Australia.[140, 141, 154] Populations with similar high risk include Navajo Indians, Native Alaskans (Indian and Eskimo), and Apache, Yakima, Athabascan, and Canadian Indians.[129, 155–161]

It has been difficult to adequately document the true incidence of invasive *H. influenzae* type b disease in Asia. Many studies of hospitalized patients with presumed bacterial meningitis throughout Asia (Indonesia, Singapore,[162] China, Hong Kong,[163] Philippines,[164] Taiwan,[165] Thailand, Vietnam, Korea, Japan) consistently show *H. influenzae* type b to be the leading cause of bacterial meningitis in children, but these studies have all shown a surprisingly high rate of negative bacterial cultures. The few population-based studies conducted (Taiwan, Hong Kong, Korea, and Japan) show incidence rates approximately one tenth that of North America and Europe before vaccines were in use. More recent investigations into reasons for this disparity indicate that multiple factors may have minimized the detection of invasive *H. influenzae* type b disease. These include (1) lack of clinical suspicion and evaluation of potential *H. influenzae* type b disease, (2) widespread antibiotic use before hospitalization and microbiological evaluations (often greater than 90%), (3) rarity of obtaining blood and CSF cultures, (4) few population-based studies with active surveillance, (5) microbiological methods suboptimal for culturing *H. influenzae* type b, (6) insufficient use of antigen detection methods to make a microbiological diagnosis in antibiotic-treated individuals, and (7) Hib vaccine use in the private sector. It is likely that *H. influenzae* type b disease occurs worldwide with similar incidence and epidemiological characteristics. Maintaining adequate case detection and surveillance is difficult and leads to underestimation of disease burden.

As discussed at the end of the chapter, the incidence of *H. influenzae* type b disease has fallen dramatically coincident with routine immunization of infants. In fact, *H. influenzae* type b disease has been eliminated in several well-immunized populations.

Seasonal Distribution

A characteristic bimodal seasonal pattern has been observed in several studies, with one peak occurring between September and December, a decrease in cases in January and February, and a second peak appearing between March and May.[1, 49, 129, 166] In contrast, the peak incidence of both pneumococcal and meningococcal meningitis is between January and March.[1, 2] The reason for these observations is unknown but may be related to the seasonality of births or the seasonal school attendance of older siblings who then introduce *H. influenzae* type b into the household.

Risk Factors

Age. The most important epidemiological feature of invasive *H. influenzae* type b disease is the age-related risk, a feature that has been appreciated for more than half a century.[11] Risk is usually highest between the ages of 6 and 12 months. The age-related incidence of *H. influenzae* type b disease has been evaluated with similar methods in several population-based surveillance studies[119, 126, 129] (see Table 11–2).

Invasive disease is relatively uncommon in infants younger than 6 months (<15% of cases), presumably because of reduced exposure, transplacental acquisition of maternal antibody, and protection conferred by breast-feeding. Figure 11–4 shows the cumulative proportion of disease by age during the first 5 years of life, which emphasizes the need to vaccinate young infants as early as possible. Each type of invasive infection has a characteristic age of occurrence.[17, 129] In most U.S. populations, the peak incidence of meningitis occurs in children 6 to 9 months of age and declines markedly after 2 years of age.[121–123, 132] *Haemophilus influenzae* type b cellulitis tends to occur during the first year of life, whereas epiglottitis generally occurs in children older than 2 years.

In populations with a high incidence of disease, such as Native Americans, the age-specific incidence is shifted to younger children.[129, 155–157, 161] Among Native Americans in southwestern Alaska, the incidence of *H. influenzae* type b disease peaks in children 4 to 7 months of age,[129] and similar peaks of meningitis are observed in Navajo Indian (4 to 5 months) and Apache Indian (4 to 6 months) children.[155, 157] The age shift is even more dramatic in the Gambia, where 83% of meningitis cases occur in children younger than 1 year.[149, 167] This age distribution contrasts with that in general U.S. populations, in which more than half of invasive disease occurs in children older than 12 months, and in Finland, where there is an even older spectrum of disease occurrence.[19]

Adults. In adults, meningitis accounts for a relatively small proportion of episodes of invasive disease; pneu-

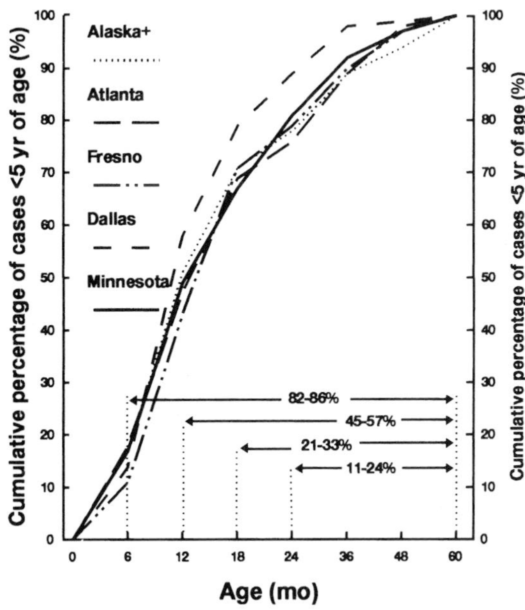

Figure 11–4. Age distribution of invasive *Haemophilus influenzae* disease in children younger than 5 years in the United States, 1976 to 1984 (population-based studies). +, excluding Eskimos, Native Americans.

monia is more common.[168] Most adults who develop invasive *H. influenzae* disease have an underlying condition such as chronic obstructive pulmonary disease, human immunodeficiency virus (HIV) infection, alcoholism, pregnancy, or malignant disease. About half of the invasive disease in older individuals is due to *H. influenzae* type b, with the remainder caused by other serotypes or nontypable strains.[167, 169] Most disease in adults is due to pneumonia.

Gender. Although most studies show approximately equal rates of disease in boys and girls, several population-based studies[119, 129, 170] and national surveillance data from passively reported cases of meningitis[1] find attack rates to be 1.2-fold to 1.5-fold higher in boys than in girls.

Race and Ethnicity. The incidence of *H. influenzae* type b meningitis has been shown consistently to be two to four times higher for black than for white children younger than 5 years.[120–122, 125, 130, 131, 170, 171] Also, the incidence of all invasive *H. influenzae* type b disease is 1.6-fold to 4-fold higher in blacks than in whites.[119] High incidence of invasive *H. influenzae* type b disease has also been described in Native Americans[129, 155–157, 159–161, 172] and in some Hispanics,[120] although studies in Dallas and Los Angeles found no difference in the incidence of *H. influenzae* type b disease between white and Hispanic children.[126, 171]

The hypothesis that racial or ethnic differences in incidence of *H. influenzae* type b disease are due to genetically determined differences in host susceptibility[173] is unproven, because of confounding social and economic variables that are associated both with race and ethnicity and with disease. In a study in Atlanta,[119] there was no increased risk in blacks, compared with that in whites, once the independent effects of household crowding, daycare, and family income on risk were accounted for by multivariate analysis, although in Los Angeles,[171] black maternal race was an independent risk factor.

Risk in Daycare Settings. Population-based studies have found that children who attend daycare are at significantly higher risk for invasive *H. influenzae* type b disease than are children who do not attend daycare.[119, 124, 127] One study estimated that up to 50% of all invasive *H. influenzae* type b disease may be attributable to daycare attendance.[119]

Socioeconomic Factors. The interplay of factors that affect exposure to the *H. influenzae* type b organism and host susceptibility appears to determine the overall risk of invasive *H. influenzae* type b disease.[174] Socioeconomic factors that may increase the likelihood of exposure among young children, and thereby increase the risk of *H. influenzae* type b disease, include large household size,[171, 175–177] crowding,[79] and increased population density. Other factors that are considered surrogates for increased exposure include low family income[121, 122, 130, 131, 170] and low parental education level.[121, 131, 177] Lack of access to vaccination is another socioeconomic factor in the United States that influences susceptibility.

Three studies have analyzed exposure-related risk factors, including socioeconomic factors, by multivariate analysis to assess the independent effects of each potential risk factor. In a case-control study in Atlanta,[119] household crowding (i.e., one or more persons per room) was significantly associated with *H. influenzae* type b disease, and a trend toward increased risk was associated with low family income and low maternal education level, although these were not independent risk factors. In a primarily white population in Colorado,[124] the risk of *H. influenzae* type b disease was increased in households with at least one member of elementary school age, suggesting that such children may introduce *H. influenzae* type b disease into a household with susceptible younger siblings. In Los Angeles,[171] the risk of *H. influenzae* type b disease was increased by living in a household consisting of more than six persons and by the presence of more than two smokers in the house.

Influence of Breast-feeding. Several case-control studies reveal that breast-feeding is associated with reduced risk of invasive *H. influenzae* type b disease in infants younger than 6 months.[119, 124, 178–181] Although the mechanism for protection is unknown, it may be the result of immune or nutritional factors present in human milk.[182] These hypotheses are biologically plausible and are based on studies demonstrating that human milk contains low levels of secretory antibody to the *H. influenzae* type b polysaccharide capsule that persist for 1 to 6 months after the onset of lactation.[183] In women immunized at 34 to 36 weeks' gestation with *H. influenzae* type b polysaccharide vaccine, both the colostrum and milk, measured 3 to 6 months after delivery, had anticapsular antibody levels more than 20 times higher than those observed in unimmunized women.[184]

Underlying Illness. Several hematological and immunological disorders are associated with increased risk for *H. influenzae* type b disease. These include HIV infection,[185–187] sickle cell anemia,[188–190] asplenia or splenectomy,[191] antibody[192, 193] and complement deficiency syndromes,[194, 195] and malignant neoplasms, especially Hodgkin disease during periods of chemotherapy.[196–198] The reasons for the increased susceptibility are not fully understood. Reduced reticuloendothelial clearance of bacteria in blood by macrophages in the spleen and liver may be involved. Clearly, complement and antibody are needed to clear bacteremia and to sustain bactericidal activity in blood.

Genetic Factors. Selected genetic markers (e.g., human leukocyte antigen, immunoglobulin allotypes) have been associated with an increased risk of invasive *H. influenzae* type b disease.[176, 199–208] However, the results of several of these studies have conflicted. Such studies have been limited, however, by potential confounding in that other known risk factors for disease were not independently evaluated; lack of control for multiple comparisons thereby increased the likelihood that a statistically significant result would be found by chance. Further, even in high-risk Alaskan Eskimos, in whom some genetic factors have been associated with disease risk (uridine monophosphate kinase 3), the majority of patients with *H. influenzae* type b disease do not possess the genetic marker in question and the degree of ethnic admixture does not correlate with disease risk.[204, 208] Therefore, it remains to be determined whether genetic factors play a significant role in risk of disease.

Role of Antecedent Viral Respiratory Infection. There is some evidence in experimental animal models[209, 210] and in children[88, 89] that respiratory viruses increase susceptibility to *H. influenzae* type b meningitis. Antecedent or concurrent viral respiratory infection could alter mucosal immunity or bacterial flora, thereby increasing host susceptibility to invasive *H. influenzae* type b disease. The difficulties of conducting prospective studies with appropriate controls have made it difficult to determine conclusively whether antecedent viral respiratory illness predisposes to invasive *H. influenzae* type b disease.

Summary of Risk Factors. The risk of developing invasive *H. influenzae* type b disease in a given individual is the consequence of a complex interaction of a variety of factors, including (1) exposure, (2) characteristics of the organism, and (3) characteristics of the host[132] (Fig. 11–5). In this discussion, we have enumerated some of the factors that affect exposure to the organism (exposure factors) and those that affect the host's susceptibility to disease (host susceptibility factors). Some exposure factors, such as household crowding and daycare attendance, are fairly direct measures of increased exposure to *H. influenzae* type b bacteria, whereas others, such as low family income and low parental education levels, are only indirect measures of increased exposure. Other risk factors cannot be categorized so easily, such as the association of black, Eskimo, or Native American race with increased risk for *H. influenzae* type b disease. Although abundant evidence suggests that more intense and early exposure to *H. influenzae* type b is the primary factor affecting risk in these high-risk populations, other lines of evidence suggest that susceptibility factors or genetic factors could also affect the response to *H. influenzae* type b.

Secondary Transmission

Although the direct contagiousness of invasive *H. influenzae* type b disease is limited, small outbreaks and direct secondary transmission of disease can occur. *Secondary* disease, that occurring after contact with a child with invasive *H. influenzae* type b disease, should be distinguished from *primary* or endemic disease, which occurs after contact with an asymptomatic carrier of *H. influenzae* type b. Instances of direct secondary transmission of *H. influenzae* type b disease have been reported since 1909,[211] but only since 1978 has the risk of secondary *H. influenzae* type b disease for contacts of a case been more accurately characterized and the potential been appreciated for invasive *H. influenzae* type b disease to be transmitted to contacts, particularly those younger than 2 years.[67, 212, 213]

Risk of Secondary Disease in Household Settings. A number of studies have estimated the risk of secondary disease in household contacts in the 30 days after onset of disease in an index case.[67, 71, 81, 214–216] Few data exist to determine the risk beyond 30 days. Overall, the attack rate for contacts of all ages was 0.3%, representing a risk about 600-fold higher than the age-adjusted risk in the general population.[215] However, attack rates varied significantly by age; the attack rate was more than 6% in contacts younger than 1 year, 3.3% in children younger than 2 years, 1.6% in children 24 to 47 months of age, 0.06% for children 4 to 5 years of age, and 0% for those 6 years of age or older. Among household contacts, 64% of secondary cases occurred within the first week after disease onset in the index patient, 20% during the second week, and 16% during the third and fourth weeks.[217] Thus, the risk of secondary disease in the household setting is confined almost exclusively to children younger than 4 years (especially those younger than 2 years) and is concentrated in the first 2 weeks after onset of disease in the index case.

Risk of Secondary Disease in Daycare Settings. Controversy exists about the degree of risk of secondary *H. influenzae* type b disease among daycare contacts exposed to a child with invasive *H. influenzae* type b disease. Five studies have estimated this risk for daycare classroom contacts of a case during the 30- to 60-day

HOST
Susceptibility Factors
Young age
Non breast-feeding (infants)
Underlying diseases
sickle cell anemia
asplenia/splenectomy
antibody deficiency syndromes
complement deficiencies
malignancies
Genetic factors
Race/ethnicity (?)
Antecedent viral infection (?)
ENVIRONMENT
Exposure Factors
Day care attendance
Large household size
Household crowding
School-age siblings
Low socioeconomic status
Low parental education levels
Race/ethnicity
AGENT
Pathogenicity Factors
Infectivity/Attachment
Invasive capability
Virulence

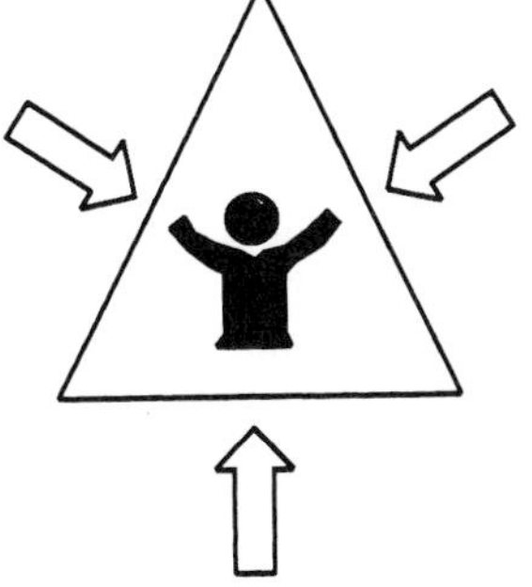

Figure 11–5. Risk factors for invasive *Haemophilus influenzae* type b disease.

period after onset of disease in the index case.[81, 216, 218–220] Three of the studies demonstrated a substantial risk—1.7 to 3.2%—for contacts younger than 24 months,[81, 216, 220] which is comparable to that of household contacts of a similar age. However, two other studies failed to demonstrate any increased risk for secondary disease in daycare contacts.[218, 219] There is no obvious explanation for the disparate findings, although there can be considerable variation in the risk of secondary *H. influenzae* type b disease over time, in different daycare settings, and perhaps by geographical region.[217, 221–223] Increased risk, when observed, has been largely confined to daycare classroom contacts younger than 24 months. This is in contrast to that of the household setting, in which substantial risk (an attack rate of 1.6%) exists in children 24 to 47 months of age. The secondary attack rates among children 24 to 47 months of age who attended daycare and who did not receive rifampin chemoprophylaxis were low: 0.5% (1 of 194) in Oklahoma,[218] 0.4% (1 of 226) in Dallas,[219] 0.0% (0 of 716) in Minnesota,[218] and 0.0% (0 of 379) in a multistate study by Fleming and colleagues.[216]

Risk of Secondary Disease in Other Institutional Settings. Transmission of secondary *H. influenzae* type b disease in chronic care institutions for children has been reported,[85, 224] as has nosocomial transmission among the elderly in a nursing home setting.[225] Only one instance of secondary transmission in children in an acute care hospital has been reported.[226] The lack of reports of hospital-acquired disease, despite the large number of *H. influenzae* type b cases that occurred yearly before routine immunization of infants, suggests that the risk of nosocomial transmission in acute care hospitals is low.

CHEMOPROPHYLAXIS

Chemoprophylaxis has been a means to prevent secondary transmission of *H. influenzae* type b disease. The goal of chemoprophylaxis is to protect the susceptible child from acquiring *H. influenzae* type b by eliminating *H. influenzae* type b colonization in close contacts (e.g., household or daycare contacts). Adults and older children who are colonized can transmit *H. influenzae* type b bacteria to susceptible children even though they are at little risk of developing invasive disease themselves.

Antimicrobials that are effective in the treatment of invasive *H. influenzae* type b disease, such as ampicillin[64] or chloramphenicol,[86] often do not eliminate the carrier state because they are not sufficiently concentrated in upper airway secretions. Rifampin, which achieves high concentrations in respiratory secretions,[227, 228] is the most effective antimicrobial agent for eradicating *H. influenzae* type b from the nasopharynx. Rifampin in a dosage of 20 mg/kg once daily (maximum daily dose 600 mg) for 4 days eradicates *H. influenzae* type b carriage in 95% or more of household[81, 214, 229] or daycare[67, 81, 85, 230–232] contacts of a case. Shorter or lower dose regimens of rifampin are less successful.[81, 233–236] The fluoroquinolone antibiotics, such as ciprofloxacin, may also be effective,[237] although they have not been evaluated sufficiently.

Both the U.S. Public Health Service Advisory Committee on Immunization Practices[217] and the American Academy of Pediatrics Committee on Infectious Diseases[238, 239] recommend rifampin prophylaxis for all household contacts, including adults, and for the index patient if there is a household contact younger than 4 years who is *not* fully immunized. In the daycare setting, there is no consensus concerning the need for rifampin prophylaxis because, as discussed earlier, the magnitude of risk of secondary transmission of *H. influenzae* type b disease in this setting is uncertain. Some authorities[217, 221–223] recommend chemoprophylaxis if there are classroom contacts younger than 2 years, whereas others[238, 239] believe that recommendations should be individualized. However, virtually all experts recommend prophylaxis if two or more cases of *H. influenzae* type b disease have occurred among attendees within 60 days.

In any case, secondary disease represents only a small proportion (less than 2%) of all cases of *H. influenzae* type b infection. With the availability of effective vaccines, routine immunization is a much more effective method of preventing secondary disease.

IMMUNOLOGY

Resistance to *H. influenzae* type b infection depends on the successful integration of a wide variety of host defenses, including (1) mucosal factors that prevent the organism from attaching and penetrating the respiratory epithelium; (2) activation of the alternative and classical complement pathways, which leads to killing of the organism and other inflammatory responses; (3) induction of antibodies; (4) phagocytosis and killing by macrophages and polymorphonuclear cells in tissues, the circulation, and the reticuloendothelial organs (e.g., the spleen); and (5) cell-mediated immunity. It is difficult to assess the role of each of these immunological mechanisms independently or to determine which mechanisms are most important in the host's defense. Although antibodies are not the sole defense against bacteremia, it has been the emphasis of vaccine research to induce antibodies that are bactericidal, opsonophagocytic, and ultimately protective.

Anticapsular Antibody

Initially, antibody activity was assessed by measuring agglutinin and bactericidal titers of serum. In 1933, Fothergill and Wright[11] suggested that bactericidal activity was responsible for immunity to *H. influenzae* type b meningitis and that acquisition of this antibody correlated with the age of the individual. Maternally acquired antibody, present in infants younger than 6 months, and the natural acquisition of antibodies by children between 2 and 5 years of age were proposed as the explanation for the increased risk for *H. influenzae* type b disease in children between 6 months and 2 years of age. The goal of vaccine development has been to find means to actively induce immunity by 6 months of age and thereby eliminate this window of age-related susceptibility.

Although antibodies to several surface antigens of *H. influenzae* play a role in conferring immunity,[12–14, 240–246] antibody to the type b capsular polysaccharide appears to be of primary importance.[247] By 5 years of age, most children have naturally acquired anticapsular antibody that appears to provide protection,[14, 83, 247, 248] although natural exposure also induces antibodies to outer membrane proteins, lipopolysaccharides, and other surface antigens of the bacteria that contribute to natural immunity. The evidence that anticapsular antibody protects humans from invasive *H. influenzae* type b disease is considerable; it activates complement,[249–254] it is opsonophagocytic,[255, 256] it is bactericidal,[11, 13, 255, 257–260] and it protects animals from lethal *H. influenzae* type b challenge.[209, 261, 262] Moreover, passive prophylaxis with serum preparations containing anticapsular antibody protects agammaglobulinemic patients[192, 247, 248] and high-risk Apache children from invasive *H. influenzae* type b disease.[263] Furthermore, in the preantibiotic era, the administration of immune sera was an effective therapy for *H. influenzae* type b disease.[7, 9, 10] Yet, the most compelling evidence for the protective efficacy of PRP antibody is the clinical protection achieved in older children vaccinated with purified PRP vaccine[138] and, more recently, in younger infants immunized with Hib conjugate vaccines.

Different exposures to the organism or its antigens (e.g., by vaccination or infection) induce anticapsular antibodies, although this response is markedly influenced by the age of the individual. In young infants, immunization with PRP vaccine induces antibody infrequently and poorly; young children respond a little better, but older children and adults demonstrate reasonably good antibody responses.[264–267] Even invasive *H. influenzae* type b disease does not reliably evoke an antibody response in young infants. Antibody to the type b capsule also develops after exposure to other bacteria that have immunologically cross-reactive antigens.[268, 269] The level of antibody induced is influenced by the type of exposure, the age of the individual, the duration of the exposure, and the rate of antigen clearance.

Protective Levels of Anticapsular Antibodies

A precise minimal level of anti-PRP antibody that is protective has not been established. Data from passive protection of agammaglobulinemic children, challenge experiments in infant rats, and studies of naturally acquired antibody levels in healthy individuals of various ages suggest that the minimum serum concentration of anti-PRP antibody that provides protection ranges from 0.05 μg/mL in animals[270] to 0.15 to 1.00 μg/mL in humans.[248, 271, 272] Such estimates are crude and do not take into account the different functional properties of different immunoglobulin isotypes and immunoglobulin G (IgG) subclasses or the contribution of antibodies to other *H. influenzae* type b antigens. Also, because vaccine-induced antibody levels decline over time, a given peak level may not predict long-term protection.[271–273] In the Finnish PRP vaccine field trial, an antibody level of higher than 1.0 μg/mL 1 month after immunization correlated with clinical protection for a minimum of 1 year.[138, 271, 272] However, this antibody level might not be readily extrapolated to immunogenicity data evaluated in different studies or with different Hib conjugate vaccines.

Class- and Subclass-Specific Antibody

A few studies have shown variable immunoglobulin isotype and IgG subclass responses to PRP polysaccharide after natural *H. influenzae* type b exposure, disease, and immunization. Several investigations have shown that IgG, IgM, and IgA antibodies to PRP are induced by infection and vaccination.[270, 274–276] Most individuals respond with IgG antibodies after PRP immunization, although some children have predominantly IgA or IgM responses.[275] The functional characteristics of these antibodies have been studied. Schreiber and associates[270] showed that IgG antibody is bactericidal, opsonic for polymorphonuclear neutrophil leukocytes in the presence of complement, and protective for animals. IgM antibody is equally protective and more bactericidal than IgG in the presence of complement, but it opsonizes poorly. IgA antibody is not bactericidal, opsonic, or protective for animals. Some investigators have hypothesized that IgA-specific antibody blocks the activity of other more functional antibodies and may thereby depress immunity.[275, 277–279]

Data from experiments in mice and humans suggest that polysaccharide antigens induce restricted IgG subclass responses.[280–283] The findings of increased susceptibility to *H. influenzae* type b disease in patients who are deficient in IgG subclasses (predominantly IgG2 and IgG4 deficiencies)[283–287] and the low levels of IgG2 in children younger than 2 years[288] suggest that there are differences in the role of subclass-specific anticapsular antibodies. In adults, natural exposure or immunization with PRP vaccine results in a predominantly IgG2 subclass response.[289, 290] Children develop IgG1 and IgG2 antibodies after immunization with PRP, but IgG1 antibodies predominate after immunization with Hib conjugate vaccines.[290, 291] After invasive disease, there is a significant IgG4 response.[289] However, the subclass response in individuals of different ages after different exposures has not yet been studied systematically.

Human anti-PRP antibodies express predominantly κ light chains[292, 293] and are resolvable by isoelectric focusing into a few restricted clonotypes. These clonotypes and antibody specificities have been characterized by idiotype analysis[294, 295] and amino acid sequencing of the immunoglobulin light chain.[296, 297] By idiotype analysis, Hibid-1 and Hibid-2 antibodies have been distinguished.[294, 295] By purification and amino acid sequencing, VKI, VKII (same as Hibid-1), VKIII, and V clonal antibodies have been distinguished.[296, 297] Individuals of different age produce different proportions or repertoires of antibody. Some differences in binding specificity, affinity, and avidity have been described with the different anti-PRP antibodies and different conjugate vaccines,[298] but it is not clear that the antibodies have different degrees of protective potency.

Table 11–4. **IMMUNOLOGICAL FEATURES OF THYMUS-DEPENDENT AND THYMUS-INDEPENDENT ANTIGENS**

	THYMUS DEPENDENT	THYMUS INDEPENDENT	
		Type 1	Type 2
Ontogeny of response	Present at birth	Early	3–18 mo after birth in humans
Responses in *xid* mice	Yes	Yes	No
Memory (booster)	Yes	No	
Affinity	Matures with immunization to high		Low, no maturation
Adjuvant	Enhances response		No effect on response
Class, subclass, and combining site	Heterogeneous (IgG)		Usually restricted (IgM)

Adapted from Stein KE. Thymus-independent and thymus-dependent responses to polysaccharide antigens. J Infect Dis 165(suppl 1):S49–S52, 1992.

T Cells

Most of our understanding of the interactions of B cells, T cells, and antigen-presenting cells (macrophages) derives from extensive research in mice.[247, 281–284, 299, 300] On the basis of T-cell involvement in antibody synthesis, antigens can be classified as T-dependent (thymus-dependent) or T-independent immunogens (Table 11–4). Most protein antigens induce helper T cell influence over antibody synthesis and are therefore considered T dependent. These antigens are first recognized and processed by macrophages and then presented to both T and B cells. The activated T cells induce proliferation and differentiation of specific antigen-reactive B-cell subpopulations. They also retain the memory necessary for subsequent booster responses.[282] Through the release of cytokines, helper T cells appear to regulate (1) the magnitude of the immune response, especially in young infants; (2) the switch in immunoglobulin classes (IgM to IgG); (3) the functional activity of antibody (avidity); and (4) the memory capacity.

Polysaccharides consist of repeating oligosaccharide units, which are relatively primitive antigenic units that elicit weak immune responses involving minimal T-cell influences.[282] These T-independent antigens elicit antibody responses primarily by direct stimulation of B cells. In general, polysaccharide vaccines have the following T-independent type 2 immunological characteristics: (1) delayed ontogeny of immune responsiveness in the young, (2) limited and variable quantitative immune responses, (3) restricted isotype (predominantly IgM) and IgG subclass responses, and (4) lack of booster or anamnestic response with secondary antigenic challenge.

The quest for an Hib vaccine that is immunogenic and protective for young infants has involved attempts to convert the capsular polysaccharide (PRP) antigen from a T-independent to a T-dependent antigen, employing the carrier-hapten principles first defined by Landsteiner[301] in the first half of this century. To achieve this purpose, PRP, which can be considered to be a hapten, is covalently linked to a T-dependent immunogen, a carrier, to form a conjugate vaccine.

Genetic Factors

Some studies have shown associations between immune responses to PRP vaccine and genetically determined factors, such as red blood cell antigens, human leukocyte antigen, or immunoglobulin allotypes.[173, 199–202, 204, 206, 302] However, it is difficult to know whether these associations have clinical relevance, because many factors influence immunogenicity, and it is difficult to control for these in most case-control studies. Furthermore, it is not known if the antibody differences, although statistically significant, are clinically important. No single genetic relationship regulating susceptibility or immune responses to polysaccharide antigens has yet been demonstrated convincingly. Fortunately, the responses to the polysaccharide-protein conjugate vaccines do not appear to be so variable.

Mucosal Immunity

The role of mucosal immunity in killing *H. influenzae* type b bacteria or inhibiting adherence or penetration of the mucosa is poorly understood, although there have been studies of secretory IgA antibody to the type b capsule.[279, 303–306] Moreover, *H. influenzae* type b strains produce an IgA protease that can inactivate mucosal antibody.[307] The observation of reduced carriage of *H. influenzae* type b in children given Hib conjugate vaccines,[308–311] as well as production of secretory IgA in saliva after vaccination,[312] suggests that mucosal immunity may be important in reducing transmission of disease.

Complement

The importance of complement components in host defense against *H. influenzae* type b is evidenced by the elimination of the bactericidal activity of serum by heat,[249–254] by the susceptibility of complement-depleted animals to *H. influenzae* type b disease,[252, 254] and by the increased susceptibility to *H. influenzae* type b disease of patients who have specific congenital complement deficiencies, such as C2, C3, C4, and C9 deficiencies.[195, 254]

Haemophilus influenzae type b bacteria are capable of activating both the classical and alternative complement pathways, thereby initiating opsonophagocytosis and cell killing and eliciting other inflammatory responses.[254]

Whereas the alternative pathway is probably most important early in the course of infection in the nonimmune host, the antibody-dependent classical complement pathway is more likely to predominate as a defense mechanism at a later stage of infection.[254] Both encapsulated and unencapsulated organisms activate complement, underscoring the importance of noncapsular antigens in host defense. Although the type b capsule is a poor activator of the alternative complement pathway, antibody to the capsule activates both the classical and alternative pathways.[253] Other cell wall antigens activate the alternative pathway, and antibody to these antigens activates the classical pathway.[249–254] Thus, antibodies to both capsular and noncapsular antigens activate the complement system, primarily through the classical pathway. Activation of the terminal complement components mediates the bactericidal activity of serum. Although the interaction among bacteria, antibody, and complement is complex, it is clear that complement plays an important role in host defense.

Phagocytosis

Opsonization leading to phagocytosis and killing of *H. influenzae* type b bacteria is also an important determinant of host defense. Impairment of phagocytic function or reduction in the numbers of phagocytes results in increased susceptibility to disease, as does the loss of the spleen or impairment of its function (e.g., hemoglobinopathies).[188–191, 196, 197, 255] The opsonic activity of serum is greatly influenced by the roles of complement and antibody. It appears that opsonization and phagocytosis of *H. influenzae* type b are dependent on (1) IgG binding, (2) antibody activation of the classical complement pathway with deposition of C3b on the bacterial surface, and (3) direct bacterial activation of the alternative complement pathway. Relatively little is known about direct cell-mediated killing of *H. influenzae* type b bacteria.[313]

PASSIVE IMMUNIZATION

Antibody to the type b polysaccharide is the immunological basis for both active and passive immunization against *H. influenzae* type b. Although active immunization is clearly preferred for the control of *H. influenzae* type b disease, before the availability of effective vaccines, passive prophylaxis was evaluated as a means of providing protection for selected high-risk groups. Passive prophylaxis was considered in high-risk settings (1) to prevent secondary disease in households, daycare centers, or institutions; (2) for selected racial groups (Eskimos or Native Americans) whose members are at high risk for disease soon after birth; (3) for functionally asplenic patients (patients with sickle cell disease or splenectomized patients); and (4) for immunocompromised patients.

A human hyperimmune globulin called bacterial polysaccharide immune globulin (BPIG) was prepared at the Massachusetts Biologic Laboratory[314–316] from the plasma of adult donors immunized with Hib, meningococcal, and pneumococcal polysaccharide vaccines. The preparation contains approximately 17 times the amount of PRP antibody found in standard immune serum globulin and has enhanced levels of antibody to selected meningococcal and pneumococcal serotypes. Pharmacological studies show that high levels of antibody (about 1 μg/mL) can be achieved within 4 days after an intramuscular injection (0.5 mL/kg), and levels considered to be protective against *H. influenzae* type b disease persist for as long as 4 months.[317]

Significant protective efficacy against invasive *H. influenzae* type b disease has been demonstrated in Apache children who were given three doses during the first year of life.[263] The hyperimmune globulin could be particularly useful in protecting young infants before they respond to vaccines. Protection lasts for 2 to 4 months after each dose, which means that repeated administrations are necessary. A more feasible approach is to employ a combined passive-active immunization schedule, which was studied in high-risk Navajo Indian infants who received simultaneous immunization with BPIG and an Hib conjugate vaccine at 2 months of age, followed by doses of vaccine at 4 and 6 months of age.[318] Infants who received concurrent passive immunization with BPIG had significantly higher anticapsular antibody concentrations at 4 months of age than did control children who received vaccine alone, maintained antibody concentrations of 0.15 mg/mL or more before 6 months of age, and appeared to respond to second and third doses of conjugate vaccine similarly to the control children.

Another possible approach to passive prophylaxis for infants is to immunize pregnant women so that their newborns might acquire higher levels of antibody transplacentally, thereby protecting them during early infancy.[319–321] In one study,[322] pregnant women were immunized with an Hib vaccine at 32 to 36 weeks' gestation. Infants of mothers who were given an Hib conjugate vaccine had high antibody levels at birth, and approximately 75% of infants were estimated to maintain protective levels of antibody through 6 months of age. This strategy has potential as an adjunct to active immunization of infants, but disadvantages include questions about the safety and acceptability of vaccinating pregnant women and the inability to immunize women who do not receive prenatal care.

Several case-control studies have demonstrated that breast-feeding confers passive protection against invasive *H. influenzae* type b disease.[119, 124, 178–180] However, breast-feeding does not ensure protection, and the mechanism for this effect is not understood. Breast milk may provide infants with immune or nutritional factors that reduce the acquisition, attachment, or invasion of *H. influenzae* type b organisms.[182, 303]

ACTIVE IMMUNIZATION

Polyribosylribitol Phosphate Polysaccharide Vaccine

The first vaccine available for the prevention of *H. influenzae* type b disease was the purified PRP polysac-

Table 11–5. ***Haemophilus influenzae* TYPE b VACCINES**

VACCINE	COMPANY	TRADE NAME	DATE LICENSED	AGE GROUP (mo)
PRP	Praxis	b-CAPSA 1*	April 1985	24–59
	Connaught	Hib-VAX*		18–24
	Lederle	Hib-IMUNE*		
PRP-D	Connaught	ProHIBiT	December 1987	18–59
			December 1989	15–59
HbOC	Lederle/Praxis	HibTITER	December 1988	18–59
			December 1989	15–59
			October 1990	2, 4, 6, and 12–15
HbOC-DTP	Lederle/Praxis	TETRAMUNE	March 1993	2, 4, 6, and 15–18
PRP-OMP	Merck & Co.	PedvaxHIB	December 1989	15–59
			December 1990	2, 4, and 12–15
PRP-T	Pasteur Mérieux/Connaught	ActHIB	March 1993	2, 4, 6, and 12–15
	Pasteur Mérieux/SmithKline Beecham	OmniHib	March 1993	2, 4, 6, and 12–15
DTaP–PRP-T	Connaught/Mérieux	TriHIBit	September 1996	15–18
PRP-OMP–Hep B	Merck & Co.	Comvax	October 1996	2, 4, 12–18

*No longer available.

DTaP, diphtheria and tetanus toxoids and acellular pertussis; DTP, diphtheria and tetanus toxoids and whole-cell pertussis; HbOC, *Haemophilus* b oligosaccharide conjugate; Hep B, hepatitis B; PRP, polyribosylribitol phosphate; PRP-D, PRP–diphtheria toxoid conjugate; PRP-OMP, PRP–outer membrane protein conjugate; PRP-T, PRP–tetanus toxoid conjugate.

charide vaccine licensed in the United States in April 1985 for use in older preschool-aged children (Table 11–5). This vaccine is mainly of historical significance, because its role was supplanted by the development and licensure of PRP-protein conjugate vaccines. The PRP vaccine was composed of an aqueous solution of the native capsular polysaccharide, polyribosylribitol phosphate (see Fig. 11–3), which was extracted and purified from the supernatant of *H. influenzae* type b broth cultures.[323–326] This vaccine is no longer available.

Immunogenicity

The response of children to PRP vaccine is strikingly age related. Young infants respond infrequently and with low antibody levels,[264, 266, 327] but the immune response improves with age. Less than 45% of 12- to 17-month-old children achieve antibody levels higher than 1 μg/mL,[138, 264] compared with approximately 50 to 75% of children 18 to 23 months of age[138, 264, 271, 327] and 90% of 24- to 35-month-old children. The duration of PRP vaccine–induced antibody is also age dependent. Mean antibody titers in children vaccinated at 18 to 23 months of age fall substantially in the months after immunization,[264] and antibody levels 1.5 years later are not significantly higher than those in unvaccinated control subjects. In 24- to 35-month-old children, significantly elevated mean antibody titers persist for at least 1.5 years, but not for 3.5 years. Among children who were vaccinated at 3 to 4 years of age, the mean serum antibody levels remained significantly higher than levels in unvaccinated control subjects for at least 3.5 years.[264] In summary, although the duration of the antibody response has not been precisely defined, it is doubtful that protective immunity is maintained beyond 2 to 3 years without repeated exposure to the antigen.[328, 329]

PRP vaccine induces the production of IgG, IgM, and IgA antibodies, although a disproportionate amount of IgM appears to be induced.[248, 270, 274, 275, 292] Differences in functional activity suggest that IgM antibody may be less active than IgG antibody, of shorter persistence, and less avid.[248, 270, 330] These studies suggest that PRP vaccine induces a relatively immature immune response, which may result in less protection than the measured antibody level might suggest.

Safety

Purified capsular polysaccharide vaccines are among the safest of all vaccines. Nearly 10 million net doses of PRP vaccine were distributed in the United States between 1985 and 1989, and no associations were established between the vaccine and serious reactions.[331] Minor reactions, such as fever and local reactions, were relatively uncommon, occurring in about 5% of vaccinees.

The only major concerns about safety were anecdotal reports of *H. influenzae* type b disease that occurred within 1 week of PRP vaccination.[332–339] An association was found in only one study.[335] These reports led some to believe that the PRP vaccine antigen absorbed out low levels of antibodies, but few if any immunized children of this age had detectable preexisting antibodies. Also, an epidemiological analysis[336] of each of 12 cases from different studies[332–335] of *H. influenzae* type b disease that occurred within 1 week of immunization indicated that most children were black, attended daycare facilities, had recent exposure to *H. influenzae* type b disease, or were thought to have increased susceptibility to disease (e.g., sickle cell disease, Down syndrome, recurrent *H. influenzae* type b disease). All of these factors suggested that the affected children were not comparable to those in the general population and that the increased relative risk was biased. Also, no increased risk of early disease was found in two of three studies examined.[332, 333]

Efficacy

There were two large-scale prospective clinical trials of the protective efficacy of Hib polysaccharide vaccine. One was conducted in Mecklenburg County, North Carolina, in which children 2 months to 5 years of age received the vaccine in a double-blind fashion.[340] Although the statistical power of this study was inadequate to assess the vaccine's efficacy accurately, it was clear that there was no substantial protective benefit for children younger than 2 years.

In a large-scale randomized clinical trial conducted in Finland,[138, 341] more than 98,000 children aged 3 to 71 months received either Hib polysaccharide vaccine or meningococcal group A polysaccharide vaccine in a double-blind fashion (children younger than 18 months of age received a second dose of vaccine 3 months after the first dose). Among children younger than 18 months, protective efficacy was not shown (Fig. 11–6). By contrast, among children aged 18 to 71 months at the time of immunization, the protective efficacy of PRP vaccine was 90% (95% confidence interval, 56 to 96%). Most cases in the control group occurred among children older than 30 months. This division at 18 months was not a precise indicator of the age at onset of protection.

In April 1985, the U.S. Food and Drug Administration (FDA) licensed Hib polysaccharide vaccine, and a single dose for all children at 24 months of age was recommended by the American Academy of Pediatrics[342] and the U.S. Public Health Service.[343] Although this age was beyond the period of highest risk for *H. influenzae* type b disease, this strategy was implemented as an interim measure in an effort to reduce the incidence of disease in children by as much as 11 to 24%, the proportion of disease that occurs in children 2 to 5 years of age (see Fig. 11–4). Soon thereafter, frequent reports of vaccine failures appeared, and questions arose about the vaccine's true efficacy.[344] A subsequent analysis of the data from the Finnish PRP trial revealed that the estimate of the protective efficacy of PRP vaccine for children 24 to 36 months of age (the ages at which routine immunization of U.S. children was recommended) was 80%, but the 95% confidence interval ranged from 7 to 95%.[336]

Case-control studies (Table 11–6) conducted to assess the efficacy of PRP vaccine yielded widely conflicting results in different geographical areas.[336–339] A particularly low estimate of efficacy (−55%) was reported from Minnesota[334]; however, the methods of the study were identical to those used for the multicenter study conducted in Connecticut, Pittsburgh, and Dallas, in which the vaccine was found to be highly efficacious (91%, 92%, and 81% at each of these sites, respectively).[332] The results from these studies were replicated in subsequent studies at the same sites.[345, 346] Careful evaluation has not definitively determined the reasons for the marked differences in these case-control studies, but methodological explanations are likely.

Haemophilus influenzae Type b Conjugate Vaccines

The limited immunogenicity of the plain polysaccharide PRP vaccine in infants and young children led to the development of the *H. influenzae* type b protein conjugate vaccines. These vaccines employ the carrier-hapten principles of antigen presentation first defined by Landsteiner in 1924.[301] The first successful bacterial polysaccharide conjugate vaccine was synthesized by Avery and Goebel[347, 348] in 1929. However, it was more than 50 years later that Schneerson and colleagues,[349] Gordon,[350] Anderson,[351] Tai and associates,[352] and others developed PRP conjugate vaccines. Basic to all conjugate

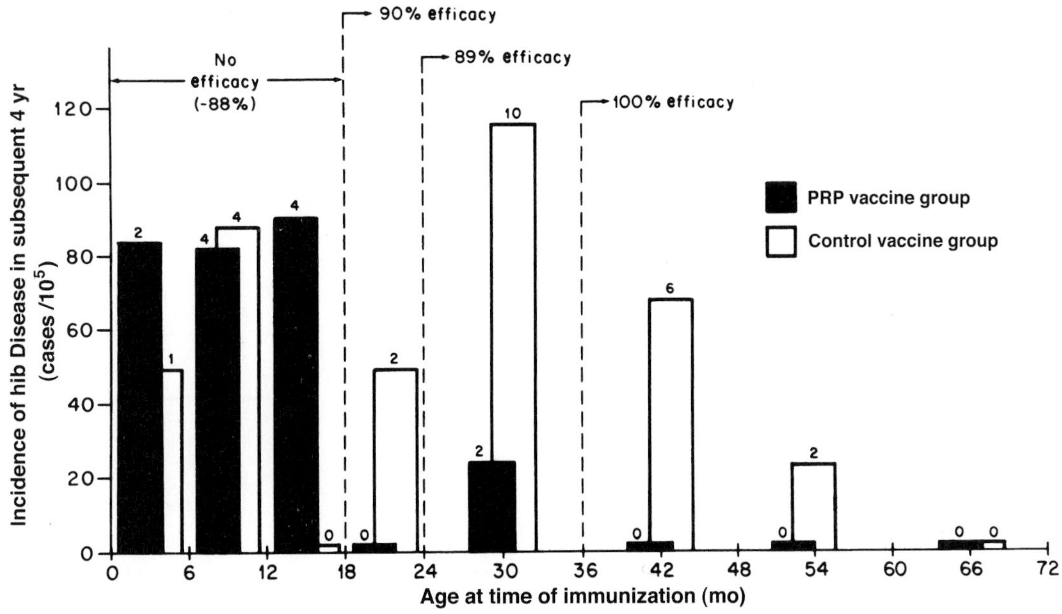

Figure 11–6. Efficacy of polyribosylribitol phosphate (PRP) vaccine and incidence of *Haemophilus influenzae* type b (Hib) disease in the vaccine and control groups in Finland, 1974 to 1978.

Table 11–6. **EFFICACY OF PRP VACCINE IN CASE-CONTROL STUDIES**

STUDY SITE	TIME PERIOD	PROTECTIVE EFFICACY*	95% CONFIDENCE INTERVAL
Multicenter†[332]	1985–1987	~88%	74 to 96%
Connecticut and Pittsburgh, PA[346]	1988–1990	~82%	38 to 94%
Centers for Disease Control‡[352a]	1986	~70%	17 to 89%
Kaiser Permanente, northern California[335]	1985–1987	~62%	−44 to 90%
Centers for Disease Control§[333]	1986	~45%	−1 to 70%
Massachusetts[373]	1988–1990	~18%	−487 to 89%
Minnesota[345]	1988–1989	−6%	−184 to 60%
Minnesota[334]	1985–1987	−55%	−238 to 29%
Los Angeles County, CA[369]	1988–1989	−58%	−309 to 39%

*Estimates of efficacy adjusted for confounders as reported.
†Conducted in Connecticut; Pittsburgh, PA; and Dallas, TX.
‡Subjects did not attend daycare and were from the same areas as reported by Harrison et al.[333]
§Subjects attended daycare centers. Children as young as 18.5 months were included. Subjects were from New Jersey, Los Angeles, Tennessee, Missouri, Washington, and Oklahoma.
PRP, polyribosyloribitol phosphate.

vaccines is the use of an immunogenic protein carrier that is recognized by T cells and macrophages and stimulates T-dependent (thymus-dependent) immunity. The protein carrier is covalently linked (conjugated) to the PRP polysaccharide, which, in principle, confers the immunological responsiveness of the protein carrier on the polysaccharide hapten.

As discussed in the section on immunology, conjugate

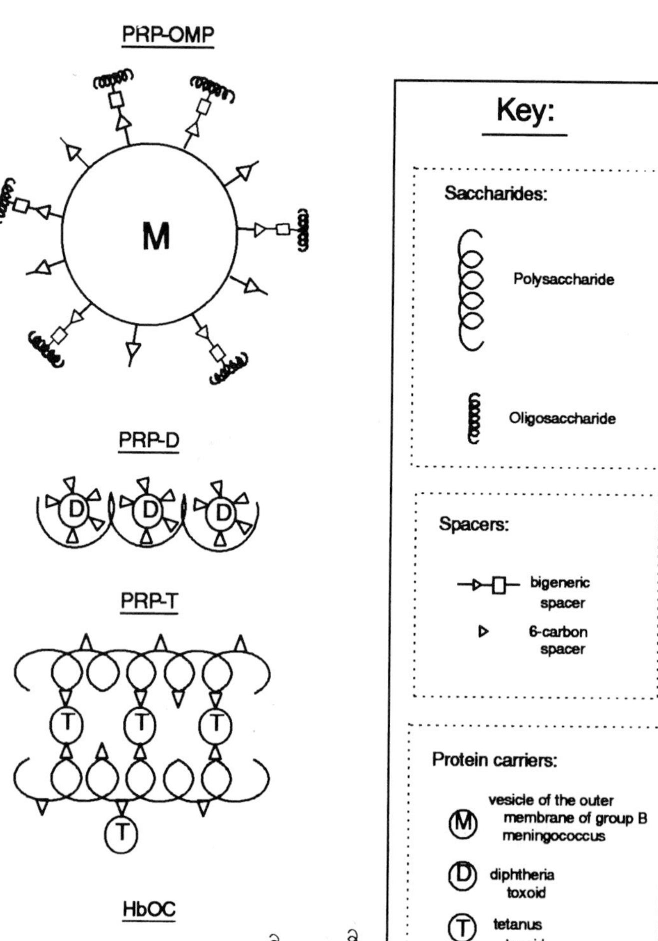

Figure 11–7. Configurations of polyribosylribitol phosphate (PRP)–protein conjugate vaccines. OMP, outer membrane protein; HbOC, *Haemophilus* b oligosaccharide conjugate. *CRM_{197}, diphtheria toxin mutant protein.

vaccines generally elicit an immune response that is characterized by helper T cell activation. The immune response induced by T-dependent antigens is quantitatively and qualitatively different from the response induced by T-independent antigens (e.g., PRP): (1) it is quantitatively enhanced, particularly in younger children; (2) repeated administrations elicit booster responses; (3) the immune response matures as evidenced by a predominance of IgG antibody; and (4) prior or concomitant administration of the carrier protein enhances the immune response (carrier priming).

Four Hib conjugate vaccines (see Table 11–5) have undergone extensive evaluation in humans. The vaccines (Fig. 11–7) all employ the same hapten (PRP) but otherwise differ in the size of the polysaccharide, the protein carrier, and the type of linkage as well as the type of immune response induced. Therefore, each of the conjugate vaccines is reviewed separately.

PRP–Diphtheria Toxoid Conjugate Vaccine

Composition

PRP–diphtheria toxoid conjugate (PRP-D) vaccine was developed by Schneerson and Robbins and their colleagues[349, 353] and later was modified and produced commercially by Connaught Laboratories (Swiftwater, PA). It contains medium-sized lengths of polysaccharide (heat sized) that are linked to a diphtheria toxoid carrier by a six-carbon spacer. There are no adjuvants or antibiotics added, and the vaccine is maintained refrigerated in the aqueous state. Thimerosal is added as a preservative, and the dose is 0.5 mL by intramuscular injection. Other vaccine characteristics are listed in Table 11–7.

Immunogenicity

PRP-D has been evaluated extensively in adults and children of all ages. A single vaccine dose elicits high levels of antibody (geometric mean titer 200 mg/mL) in nearly all adults. As with PRP, the response to PRP-D in children varies with age, although PRP-D induces higher antibody levels than does PRP at all ages. In children 15 months of age and older, high antibody concentrations are achieved with a single dose, and booster doses are not required to provide lasting protection.[354, 355] In older children and adults, there do not appear to be major differences in immunogenicity among PRP-D and other Hib conjugate vaccines.[355] Similarly, when PRP-D is given as the 15-month booster dose to children immunized with any of the other three Hib conjugate vaccines as infants, it induces an immune response at least as good as that induced by a booster dose with the primary vaccine.[356]

In children 9 to 15 months of age, PRP-D elicits a booster response (unlike plain PRP vaccine), and two doses of PRP-D achieve antibody levels greater than 1 mg/mL in all subjects.[357] These antibody levels fall in the following year, leaving a little more than half of vaccine recipients with antibody levels greater than 1 mg/mL. A booster dose induces a sharp rise in antibodies.[358]

In infants younger than 6 months, the immune response to PRP-D is limited and much less than that induced by the other three Hib conjugate vaccines (see Table 11–15). The antibody response to a first dose in infants 2 months of age is not measurable, and only a few infants respond to a second dose at 4 months of age. Even after a third dose at 6 months of age, less than half of all infants develop antibody levels greater than 1 μg/mL,[359–361] with decline of these meager antibody levels in the ensuing 3 to 12 months leaving many children without levels of antibody thought to be protective during the period of greatest disease risk.

PRP-D has also been evaluated in some high-risk populations. Splenectomized patients with Hodgkin disease respond to PRP-D, although their antibody response is less than that noted in normal hosts.[362] About 90% of children older than 18 months with sickle cell disease achieve an antibody level greater than 1 mg/mL in response to a single dose of PRP-D.[363] Children aged 2 to 6 years with acute leukemia respond less frequently and with lower antibody levels than do healthy children, although many attain protective levels of antibody (par-

Table 11–7. **CHARACTERISTICS OF *Haemophilus influenzae* b CONJUGATE VACCINES**

PROPERTIES	PRP-D	HbOC	PRP-OMP	PRP-T
Polysaccharide	Medium (heat size)	Small (periodate oxidized)	Medium (native)	Large (native)
Polymer size				
Content	25 mg	10 mg	15 mg	10 mg
Protein Carrier	Diphtheria toxoid	CRM_{197}	Mening group B OMP	Tetanus toxoid
Content	18 mg	20 mg	250 mg	20 mg
Linkage	Protein	PS	Protein and PS	PS
Activation reactants	ADH CNBr (protein)	Periodate Cyanoborohydrate	N-ABC (PS) N-AHC (protein)	ADH CNB (PS Carbodiimide HCl
Linkages	Amide/protein Iminocarbamate/PS	2° amino	Amide/protein Carbamate/PS Thioester/spacer	Amide/protein Iminocarbamate/PS
Spacer	6-carbon	None	Bigeneric 1. N-ABC (linked to PS) 2. N-AHC (linked to protein)	6-carbon

HbOC, *Haemophilus* b oligosaccharide conjugate; PRP, polyribosylribitol phosphate; PRP-D, PRP–diphtheria toxoid conjugate; PRP-OMP, PRP–outer membrane protein conjugate; PRP-T, PRP–tetanus toxoid conjugate; PS, polysaccharide; mening group B OMP, *Neisseria meningitidis* group B outer membrane protein; CRM_{197}, diphtheria toxin mutant protein; ADH, adipic dihydrazide: the completed reaction cleaves both hydrazide moieties, leaving a six-carbon linkage; CNBr, cyanogen bromide; N-ABC, *N*-acetylbutylcarbamate; N-AHC, *N*-acetylhomocysteine.

Table 11–8. **EFFICACY OF PRP-D IN OLDER CHILDREN IN 5 CASE-CONTROL STUDIES**

STUDY	IMMUNIZATION RATES Cases	Control Subjects	PROTECTIVE EFFICACY	95% CONFIDENCE INTERVAL
Minnesota[345]	1/75 (1%)	30/150 (20%)	96%	65–99%
Los Angeles[369]	3/62 (3%)	46/159 (29%)	84%	36–96%
Connecticut/Pittsburgh[346]	1/39 (3%)	39/156 (25%)	84%	28–97%
Centers for Disease Control[372]	9/75 (12%)	42/161 (26%)	74%	30–90%
Massachusetts[373]	2/24 (8%)	11/32 (34%)	88%	45–98%

PRP-D, polyribosylribitol phosphate–diphtheria toxoid conjugate vaccine.

ticularly among those receiving chemotherapy for less than a year).[364, 365]

Safety

Millions of doses of PRP-D were administered in the United States and Europe between 1988 and 1990 without reports of serious adverse consequences. Less than 2% of children 18 months of age and older develop fever with the administration of PRP-D.[366] Local reactions at the injection site are also infrequent and generally mild. Although an early anecdotal report associated three cases of Guillain-Barré syndrome with PRP-D administration in children 18 to 60 months of age,[367] subsequent evaluation has not confirmed an association.[368]

Efficacy

Before the 1987 licensure of PRP-D in the United States for children 18 months of age and older, its efficacy had not been documented. Subsequently, case-control studies (Table 11–8) determined that a single dose of vaccine was 74 to 96% efficacious in preventing disease in older children.[345, 346, 369–373]

Two clinical efficacy trials yielded disparate protective efficacy results. In Finland,[374, 375] more than 100,000 infants were enrolled in an open, randomized trial in which infants received study vaccine at 3, 4, 6, and 14 to 18 months of age. The protective efficacy of the PRP-D vaccine after three doses was 94% (95% confidence interval, 83 to 98%), and the calculated efficacy after four doses was 100% (95% confidence interval, 82 to 100%) (Table 11–9). In contrast, a randomized, double-blind, placebo-controlled trial conducted in Native Alaskan infants found no evidence of protection in that high-risk population.[376] More than 2100 infants were enrolled in the study and were vaccinated with PRP-D or saline placebo at approximately 2, 4, and 6 months of age. Even after three doses of vaccine, the protective efficacy was only 43% (95% confidence interval, −43 to 78%) (Table 11–10).

The discrepancy between the results of the two studies has not been fully explained, although it may be due to the higher rates of early infections in Alaska. The poor efficacy seen in the Native Alaskan infants paralleled its poor immunogenicity in these infants, and there was little, if any, difference in the immunogenicity of PRP-D between Finnish and Alaskan infants. The later ages of immunization with diphtheria and tetanus toxoids and whole-cell pertussis vaccine (DTP) and PRP-D in Finland may also have been a factor. Follow-up studies did reveal sustained efficacy of PRP-D in reducing incidence of disease,[377] as do data from Iceland.[378]

Recommendations

Although PRP-D has been used in infants in some European countries, it will not be licensed for use in U.S. infants because of concerns about its limited immunogenicity in young infants, its failure to protect high-risk infants, and the availability of much more immunogenic vaccines.

Haemophilus b Oligosaccharide Conjugate Vaccine

Composition

Haemophilus b oligosaccharide conjugate (HbOC) vaccine was developed by Porter Anderson at the University

Table 11–9. **EFFICACY TRIAL OF PRP-D IN FINNISH INFANTS**

DOSE	APPROXIMATE AGE (mo)	EPISODES OF Hib DISEASE/NUMBER OF SUBJECTS Vaccinees	Control Subjects	PROTECTIVE EFFICACY	95% CONFIDENCE INTERVAL
Post 1 or 2	2–6	4/58,000	8/56,000	43%	−95 to 83%
Post 3	6–13	4/58,000	37/56,000	89%	70 to 96%
Post 4	14–24	0/58,000	27/56,000	100%	82 to 100%
Post any	2–24	8/58,000	72/56,000	89%	78 to 95%

Hib, *Haemophilus influenzae* type b; PRP-D, polyribosylribitol phosphate–diphtheria toxoid conjugate vaccine.

From Eskola J, Kayhty H, Takala AK, et al. A randomized, prospective field trial of a conjugate vaccine in the protection of infants and young children against invasive *Haemophilus influenzae* type b disease. N Engl J Med 323:1381–1387, 1990; and Eskola, J, Peltola H, Takala AK, et al. Efficacy of *Haemophilus influenzae* type b polysaccharide–diphtheria toxoid conjugate vaccine in infancy. N Engl J Med 317:717–722, 1987. Used with permission from the New England Journal of Medicine, 1987, 1990.

Table 11–10. **EFFICACY TRIAL OF PRP-D IN NATIVE ALASKAN INFANTS**

DOSE	EPISODES OF Hib DISEASE/ NUMBER OF SUBJECTS		PROTECTIVE EFFICACY	95% CONFIDENCE INTERVAL
	Vaccinees	Placebo Recipients		
Post 1	3/1054	4/1048	25%	−233 to 83%
Post 2	2/991	3/966	35%	−288 to 89%
Post 3*	7/915	12/883	43%	−43 to 78%
Post any*	12/1054	19/1048	37%	−29 to 69%

*One vaccine had two episodes of Hib infection, the first between the first and second dose and the second after the third dose. In this tabulation, the case is counted once.

Hib, *Haemophilus influenzae* type b; PRP-D, polyribosylribitol phosphate–diphtheria toxoid conjugate vaccine.

From Ward J, Brenneman G, Letson GW, Heyward WL. The Alaska *H. influenzae* Vaccine Study Group. Limited efficacy of a *Haemophilus influenzae* type b conjugate vaccine in Alaska Native infants. N Engl J Med 323:1393–1401, 1990. Reprinted with permission from The New England Journal of Medicine, 1990.

of Rochester; it is manufactured and licensed by Praxis Laboratories and distributed by Ayerst-Wyeth-Lederle Laboratories (Pearl River, NY). HbOC differs significantly from other Hib conjugate vaccines. It consists of short oligosaccharides of approximately 20 PRP repeat units that are covalently linked, without a spacer, to the protein carrier CRM_{197}, which is a nontoxic variant of diphtheria toxin (see Table 11–7). It is a well-defined aqueous preparation without adjuvants or antibiotics and is available both as a monovalent product and as a combined vaccine with DTP. Thimerosal is added as a preservative, and the dose is 0.5 mL by intramuscular injection.

Immunogenicity

As with other Hib conjugate vaccines, a single dose of HbOC is highly immunogenic in children 18 to 24 months of age and older.[355, 379–381] In young infants, immunogenicity is age dependent, and two or three doses are required. An initial dose at 2 months of age does not induce an antibody response, but a significant number of infants respond to a second dose at 4 months of age. This enhanced response to the second dose may be due to the older age when it is administered, a booster response, or carrier priming as a result of prior administration of DTP. After a third dose at 6 months, high antibody levels are achieved in nearly all infants[361, 382, 383] (see Table 11–15). Interestingly, antibody levels in Finland induced after two doses at 4 and 6 months of age appear to be similar to those induced by three doses given at 2, 4, and 6 months of age.[384, 385] The antibody levels induced by three doses of HbOC are greater than the levels induced by PRP-D or PRP–outer membrane protein conjugate vaccine (PRP-OMP) and are roughly equivalent to those of PRP–tetanus toxoid conjugate (PRP-T).[361, 386] Preexisting maternally acquired antibody or passively administered hyperimmune globulin does not affect the immune response to HbOC.[318, 387] Antibody persists for at least a year in most infants; a booster is recommended between 12 and 15 months of age.

The antibody induced by HbOC is predominantly IgG1[291, 381] and is bactericidal.[383] Further, children deficient in IgG2[388, 389] or IgA,[388, 390] children with sickle cell disease[391–393] or prior *H. influenzae* type b disease,[394] and men infected with HIV[395] have good responses to HbOC. Diphtheria antibodies increase significantly after a dose of HbOC,[381, 396] and withholding DTP from young infants significantly inhibits the immune response to HbOC,[397, 398] indicating the importance of prior exposure to the carrier protein (carrier priming) in inducing an immune response to conjugate vaccines.

Safety

Experience with the administration of several million doses of HbOC supports a conclusion that the vaccine is safe. Local reactions, such as erythema or tenderness, occur significantly less often after vaccination with HbOC (2%) than with DTP (19%).[399] Fever and systemic reactions are described in 7 to 33% of infants who receive the two vaccines simultaneously at different sites, which is similar to the incidence with use of DTP alone.[383, 400] No serious reactions have been reported with HbOC. The safety profile of the combined HbOC-DTP vaccine is comparable to that of the vaccines coadministered at separate injection sites.[401, 402] The incidence of local and systemic reactions is similar, except for swelling after the first dose, which is more common with the combined product (8.0% combined versus 4.3% separate).[402]

Efficacy

Two prospective studies show that two or three doses of HbOC administered in the first 6 months of life provide a high degree of protective efficacy. In an unblinded, quasi-randomized study involving more than 60,000 infants in the Northern California Kaiser Permanente Health Plan,[403] HbOC was administered to 20,800 infants at 2, 4, and 6 months of age. Overall, only three cases of invasive *H. influenzae* type b disease occurred in the vaccinated group compared with 22 cases in the unimmunized population (Table 11–11). All three cases in the HbOC group occurred in children who had received only one immunization. Analysis of the data revealed that the vaccine provided no real protection after a single dose but was extremely effective after three doses, with a calculated efficacy of 100% (95% confidence interval, 68 to 100%). The limited duration of follow-up between the second and third doses precludes an accurate assessment of the vaccine's efficacy after only two doses. Long-term follow-up in the Northern California Kaiser Permanente Health Plan confirms HbOC's efficacy.[404] In the 4 years before January 31,

Table 11–11. **EFFICACY TRIAL OF HbOC IN NORTHERN CALIFORNIAN INFANTS**

DOSE	MEAN AGE (mo)	EPISODES OF Hib DISEASE/ SUBJECT-YEARS		PROTECTIVE EFFICACY	95% CONFIDENCE INTERVAL
		Vaccinees	Comparison Group*		
Post 1	2.6	3/6553	2/NP	26%	−166 to 80%
Post 2	4.9	0/5512	7/NP	100%	47 to 100%
Post 3	7.2	0/12,949	12/11,335	100%	68 to 100%
Post any	1.4–2.4	3/25,014	21/26,962	84%	60 to 100%

*The comparison group consists of concurrent children at the Kaiser Permanente study clinics who refused or were never offered HbOC vaccine. Because no placebo or alternative vaccine was administered to these control subjects, the number of cases of *Haemophilus influenzae* type b disease and subject-years of follow-up that are used for comparison with the vaccinated groups are estimated on the basis of their ages and periods of follow-up.

HbOC, *Haemophilus* b oligosaccharide conjugate vaccine; Hib, *Haemophilus influenzae* type b; NP, not presented in the published manuscript of the trial.

1992, more than 75,000 infants and children had been immunized with HbOC, and only six vaccine failures occurred. Five of these failures (including the three in the efficacy study) occurred in children who had received only a single dose of vaccine at 2 months, and one case occurred in a 3½-year-old child who had received three doses in infancy but had not received a booster dose.

The vaccine was also evaluated in Finland, where beginning in 1988 infants were randomized to receive either HbOC or PRP-D at 4, 6, and 14 to 18 months of age. During the subsequent 2 years, more than 50,000 infants were immunized with HbOC. Only 3 cases of invasive *H. influenzae* type b disease occurred in children vaccinated with HbOC compared with 11 cases in recipients of PRP-D (P = .04). One case occurred after a single HbOC dose and two cases after the second dose.[405]

Recommendations

In October 1990, HbOC became the first Hib conjugate vaccine to be licensed in the United States for use in infants at 2, 4, and 6 months of age with a booster dose at 12 to 15 months of age (Table 11–12).[406] In March 1993, a combined HbOC-DTP vaccine was licensed in the United States on the basis of its safety and its immunogenicity profile.[239, 407] This combined vaccine can be used for routine infant immunization and can be used to complete an immunization series begun with HbOC.

PRP–Outer Membrane Protein Conjugate Vaccine

Composition

PRP-OMP vaccine was developed and is marketed by Merck Sharp & Dohme (West Point, PA). PRP-OMP differs markedly in both composition and immunogenicity from the other Hib conjugate vaccines. It links medium lengths of PRP by a bigeneric spacer molecule to protein components of outer membrane vesicles of a strain of serogroup B *Neisseria meningitidis* (see Table 11–7). The vesicles are visible by light microscopy and contain lipopolysaccharides, outer membrane proteins, and other undefined constituents of the outer membrane of this gram-negative bacterium. The vaccine is a lyophilized preparation that is reconstituted just before administration in an aqueous buffer with aluminum adjuvant. Thimerosal is added as a preservative, lactose as a stabilizer, and the dose is 0.5 mL by intramuscular injection.

Immunogenicity

PRP-OMP induces an immune response that is less age dependent than is the response to the other Hib conjugate vaccines. Most adults and children respond to a single vaccine dose by producing high levels of antibody. A booster response is seen in older children who are given a repeated dose of PRP-OMP or PRP vaccine,[408] although a clear booster response is not seen with the second or third dose of a primary series in young infants.

PRP-OMP is unique among the Hib conjugate vaccines in its ability to induce a strong antibody response in young infants with the first dose. In young infants 6 weeks of age and older, a single injection of PRP-OMP induces a good antibody response (see Table 11–15), and 15 to 80% of infants achieve titers greater than 1 mg/mL.[386, 409–414] A second dose at 4 months of age increases the proportion of infants with an immune response, although a small percentage of infants (less than 6%) fails to respond to two doses of PRP-OMP.[412, 415] PRP-OMP does not elicit a classic booster response in most infants, but the titers achieved after two doses of PRP-OMP vaccine are higher than those achieved after two doses of HbOC, PRP-D, or PRP-T vaccines.[361, 386, 414] A third dose at 6 months of age does not boost levels or the proportion of responders,[387] and therefore only a two-dose primary series has been recommended for infants.

An additional concern relates to the decay of antibody levels between 4 and 12 months of age. Because the peak antibody levels are lower than those achieved after a primary series of HbOC or PRP-T vaccines and are achieved at an earlier age, the period of time with high antibody titers is less with PRP-OMP vaccine. To compensate, a booster dose was recommended at 12 months of age, earlier than for the other two infant vaccines. Admittedly, it is not clear what antibody level must be maintained to ensure protection, and it is possible that the initial response (i.e., priming) is as important as the level of antibody. However, a late vaccine failure in the

Table 11–12. **RECOMMENDED VACCINATION SCHEDULES FOR *Haemophilus influenzae* b CONJUGATE VACCINES**

VACCINE	ROUTINE SCHEDULE (mo) 2	4	6	12–15
HbOC*	Dose 1	Dose 2	Dose 3	Booster†
PRP-T	Dose 1	Dose 2	Dose 3	Booster†
PRP-OMP‡	Dose 1	Dose 2		Booster†

VACCINE	"CATCH-UP" SCHEDULE: Age at First Dose (mo)	Primary Series (Doses)	Booster§ (mo)
HbOC§ or PRP-T	2–6	3‡	12–15
	7–11	2‡	12–18
	12–14	1‡	15
	15–59	1	
PRP-OMP‖	2–6	2‡	12–15
	7–11	2‡	12–18
	12–14	1	15
	15–59	1	
PRP-D	12–14	1	12–15
	15–59	1	

*Or HbOC-DTP combined vaccine when both HbOC and DTP are due.
†Any licensed *Haemophilus influenzae* b conjugate vaccine is acceptable for the booster dose.
‡Or PRP-OMP–hepatitis B combined vaccine when both PRP-OMP and heaptitis B are due.
§At least 2 months after previous dose.
‖At least 2 months between doses.
HbOC, *Haemophilus* b oligosaccharide conjugate; PRP, polyribosylribitol phosphate; PRP-D, PRP–diphtheria toxoid conjugate; PRP-OMP, PRP–outer membrane protein conjugate; PRP-T, PRP–tetanus toxoid conjugate.

Navajo efficacy trial in a child with an initial antibody response[416] suggests that maintaining high levels is an important determinant of protection. About one fourth of vaccine recipients have levels less than 0.15 mg/mL a year after completing their primary immunization series.[417]

In postlicensure studies, PRP-OMP was also evaluated in newborns as a possible means to provide earlier protection in a high-risk population.[418] Surprisingly, the antibody levels achieved with three doses given at birth and at 2 and 6 months of age were markedly depressed throughout the first year of life, suggesting immune tolerance if the vaccine is given too early in life.

As with other Hib conjugate vaccines, responses to PRP-OMP are not affected by maternally acquired or passively administered antibody.[387] It is also immunogenic in high-risk individuals who had poor responses to PRP vaccine.[419] Children 27 to 61 months of age who had developed invasive *H. influenzae* type b disease despite previous immunization with PRP and were still without a protective level of antibody were immunized with either PRP or PRP-OMP.[420] All 14 children immunized with PRP-OMP responded with greater than fivefold increases in antibody levels, whereas just 6 of 20 children immunized with PRP responded with antibody levels greater than 1 mg/mL. Similarly, black children who are negative for the Km(1) allotype and do not respond as well to PRP vaccination (and may have a higher risk of invasive *H. influenzae* type b disease) do respond well to immunization with PRP-OMP.[200]

The antibody induced by PRP-OMP is primarily IgG1[291, 411, 421] and is opsonophagocytic[422] and bactericidal.[408, 411] Functional studies of the antibodies indicate that they are of lower avidity than those elicited by HbOC or PRP-T.[423] Some have concluded that PRP-OMP's immune profile suggests that it has T-independent type 1 immune characteristics (see Table 11–4).[424] Immunization results in increases in antibody to the carrier, but there is no evidence concerning the possible protective efficacy of these antibodies to the group B meningococcal outer membrane vesicles against this pathogen.

After licensure, a problem arose with the discovery that selected early lots of PRP-OMP were significantly less immunogenic than expected. Sixteen lots, representing approximately 23% of the lots distributed between August 1990 and May 1992, elicited lower than expected antibody levels in young children. The reason for the impaired immunogenicity has not been determined definitively but is thought to be associated with inadequate conjugation of the PRP. Revaccination of children who received these lots exclusively was recommended.[425]

Safety

Although PRP-OMP contains trace amounts of meningococcal endotoxin, local and systemic reactions are less than those that occur with DTP and range from 3 to 15%.[409, 411–413, 415, 426, 427] An earlier study showed higher rates of local and febrile reactions but also showed reduced rate of reactions with the addition of aluminum phosphate adjuvant. Presumably this slows the release of reactogenic components. More serious adverse reactions, specifically seizures, hospitalizations, early-onset *H. influenzae* type b disease, and sudden infant death syndrome, have not been associated with PRP-OMP vaccination.

Table 11–13. **EFFICACY TRIAL OF PRP-OMP IN NAVAJO INFANTS**

DOSE	APPROXIMATE AGE (mo)	EPISODES OF Hib DISEASE/ NUMBER OF SUBJECTS: Vaccinees	Placebo Recipients	PROTECTIVE EFFICACY	95% CONFIDENCE INTERVAL
Post 1	2	0/2588	8/2602	100%	41–100%
Post 2	4	1/1913	14/1929	93%	53–98%
Post any*	2–16	1/2588	22/2602	95%	72–99%

*A second vaccine failure was subsequently reported in a 7-month-old child who had received a single vaccine dose at 8 weeks of age.

PRP-OMP, polyribosylribitol phosphate–outer membrane protein conjugate vaccine; Hib, *Haemophilus influenzae* type b.

From Santosham M, Wolff M, Reid R, et al. The efficacy in Navajo infants of a conjugate vaccine consisting of *Haemophilus influenzae* type b polysaccharide and *Neisseria meningitidis* outer-membrane protein complex. N Engl J Med 324:1767–1772, 1991. Reprinted with permission from The New England Journal of Medicine, 1991.

Efficacy

PRP-OMP was evaluated in a randomized, double-blind, placebo-controlled trial in a high-risk Navajo Indian population.[416] More than 5000 infants were enrolled in the study and were vaccinated with PRP-OMP or placebo at approximately 2 and 4 months of age. Only 1 case of invasive *H. influenzae* type b disease occurred in an immunized child compared with 22 cases in the placebo group, yielding an overall efficacy of 95% (95% confidence interval, 72 to 99%) (Table 11–13). The one vaccine failure occurred at 15½ months of age in a child who had received two doses of vaccine. Consistent with its immunological profile, the vaccine appeared to provide protection after a single dose because no cases of *H. influenzae* type b disease occurred between the first and second injection in the vaccinated group; eight cases occurred in the placebo group. Late follow-up in this population revealed a second vaccine failure, a 7-month-old child who had received a single vaccine dose at 6 weeks of age.[428] Subsequently, PRP-OMP vaccine has proved to be effective in eliminating *H. influenzae* type b disease in participants in the Southern California Kaiser Health Plan.[429]

Recommendations

Previously licensed in December 1989 for use in children 15 months of age and older, PRP-OMP vaccine was licensed in the United States in December 1990 for use in infants.[406] It is recommended for administration at 2 and 4 months of age with a booster dose at 12 to 15 months of age (see Table 11–12). These recommendations are different from those for HbOC and PRP-T vaccines.

PRP–Tetanus Toxoid Conjugate Vaccine

Composition

PRP-T was among the first PRP-protein conjugate vaccines developed at the National Institutes of Health by Schneerson and associates.[349, 353] It is now manufactured by Pasteur Mèrieux Connaught (Lyon, France) and is marketed by that organization and also by SmithKline Beecham. The vaccine contains large polysaccharide polymers that are extracted from culture supernatants and linked by a six-carbon spacer to tetanus toxoid carrier (see Table 11–7). The process of conjugation is similar to that of PRP-D and results in many cross-linkages and a complex three-dimensional structure. For reasons of maintaining potency over time, it is prepared lyophilized and is reconstituted just before administration with aqueous buffer without adjuvants or antibiotics. The dose is 0.5 mL by intramuscular injection.

Immunogenicity

The pattern of immune response to PRP-T is similar to that of HbOC. A single dose of the vaccine is highly immunogenic in adults[430] and in older children.[431] In young infants first immunized between 2 and 4 months of age, no response is seen in most instances. One or two booster doses can be given to induce high antibody concentrations in even the youngest infants.[361, 386, 414, 432–435] After a second and third dose, 70 to 100% and 98 to 100% respond, respectively.[436] Some comparative immunogenicity studies show this vaccine to be the most immunogenic vaccine after three doses,[361, 414] although it is not clear that these differences result in improved protective efficacy. Geometric mean anti-PRP antibody concentrations of 5 to 10 μg/mL are generally achieved after a three-dose primary series, and good antibody levels usually persist a year after immunization.[437]

As with other Hib conjugate vaccines, the antibodies induced are primarily IgG1.[438] PRP-T is immunogenic in high-risk individuals, such as those who have had bone marrow transplantation,[439] children with sickle cell anemia or malignant neoplasms,[440] children with HIV infection,[441] or those who have had invasive *H. influenzae* type b disease.[440]

Safety

In prelicensure studies of safety and immunogenicity, the vaccine was administered to more than 115,000 children without serious side effects.[436] In children 18 to 23 months of age, local reactions were more frequent after vaccination with PRP-T than with PRP,[431] occurring in as many as 32% of recipients. These were thought to be due to Arthus-like reactions in older children who had high levels of tetanus immunity. In infants, only 7 to 15% had such reactions.[436, 437] None of the reactions was serious, and they were less likely to occur with subsequent doses. Temperature higher than 38°C occurs after 4.7 to 10.0% of PRP-T administrations, and this rate is less than that after vaccination with DTP, which is usually given concurrently.

There is discrepancy in the data on the simultaneous administration of PRP-T and DTP, especially when they are mixed in the same syringe. Some studies show an interference in immune response to other antigens[442] or to PRP,[443] although the possible clinical significance of these findings is unclear.

Efficacy

PRP-T was evaluated for its protective efficacy in two large, randomized, double-blind trials in infants in the United States[436] and one recent trial in the Gambia.[444] Both trials in the United States were discontinued before completion because of the October 1990 recommendation for use of HbOC in infants. In a trial in North Carolina, with more than 2000 randomized subjects, two cases of *H. influenzae* type b disease occurred among control subjects, whereas none occurred among PRP-T vaccinees. In another trial in southern California with more than 10,000 subjects, three cases of *H. influenzae* type b disease occurred among control subjects, whereas none occurred among PRP-T vaccinees.[445] These results suggested, but did not prove, that the vaccine is protective. In the Gambia,[444] more than 42,000 infants received either PRP-T mixed with DTP or DTP alone at 2, 3, and 4 months of age (Table 11–14). One case of *H. influenzae* type b disease occurred in a vaccinee compared with 19 cases among control subjects—a protective efficacy of 95% (95% confidence interval, 67 to 100%) against any invasive *H. influenzae* type b disease and 100% against *H. influenzae* type b pneumonia (95% confidence interval, 55 to 100%), and a reported 21% decrease in radiologically confirmed pneumonia of all types in vaccinees compared with control subjects. This is the only Hib conjugate vaccine efficacy trial to date that studied the incidence of pneumonia. PRP-T also proved to be effective in a British trial in which the vaccine was administered at 2, 3, and 4 months of age[446, 447] and a Chilean trial when it was given to infants at 2, 4, and 6 months of age.[448]

In addition to these studies, a nationwide immunization program with PRP-T vaccine has been implemented in Finland since January 1990.[449] All infants are given doses of PRP-T at 4 and 6 months of age and a booster dose at 14 to 18 months of age. During the first 22 months of the immunization program (January 1990 to October 1991), approximately 97,000 infants were immunized with two doses of PRP-T. Two cases of invasive *H. influenzae* type b disease occurred in vaccinees after one dose, at 4 days and 2 months, respectively, after immunization. No infant receiving two or more doses of the PRP-T vaccine in any study has had invasive *H. influenzae* type b disease.[436]

Recommendations

PRP-T was the last of the four Hib conjugate vaccines to complete clinical testing. In March 1993, it was licensed in the United States for use in infants.[239, 407] It is recommended for use in the United States at 2, 4, and 6 months of age with a booster dose at 12 to 15 months (see Table 11–12). In November 1993, the FDA approved the reconstitution of PRP-T with Connaught's DTP vaccine to allow simultaneous administration in a single injection whenever both vaccines are indicated.[450]

Additional Considerations Regarding Hib Conjugate Vaccines

Comparative Immunogenicity Studies

Comparing the immunogenicity of different vaccines among studies should be done with caution. Apparent differences in immunogenicity among studies may be due to differences in study design (e.g., age of each immunization, timing of postvaccination phlebotomies), differences in specific vaccine lots, differences in the laboratory assays used to measure antibody,[451] and differences in the statistical methods used to calculate mean levels and other analyses.

Several studies have directly compared the immunogenicity of the different Hib conjugate vaccines in trials with standardized vaccine schedules using uniform laboratory and statistical methods.[361, 386, 414, 434] Data from these four studies are summarized in Table 11–15. The data highlight some of the problems associated with comparisons of vaccine immunogenicity, because there are some significant differences in results among the studies.

In general, the studies show consistent results concerning immune responses by age and dose in infants. PRP-OMP is the only vaccine that induces a good immune response with a single dose in infants immunized

Table 11–14. **CASES OF CONFIRMED INVASIVE *Haemophilus influenzae* b DISEASE BY VACCINATION STATUS AND DIAGNOSIS IN THE GAMBIA[444]**

	PNEUMONIA*		MENINGITIS		OTHER		ALL	
DOSES	PRP-T	Control	PRP-T	Control	PRP-T	Control	PRP-T	Control
0	0	1	3	1	0	0	3	2
1	2	4	3	4	0	1	5	9
2	0	5	0	4	1	1	1	10
3	0	5	1	12	0	2	1	19
Total	2	15	7	21	1	4	10	40
2 or 3	0	10	1	16	1	3	2	29

*Children with pneumonia that occurred in association with proven *Haemophilus influenzae* type b meningitis were classified as meningitis.
PRP-T, polyribosylribitol phosphate–tetanus toxoid conjugate.

Table 11–15. **COMPARATIVE IMMUNOGENICITY OF DIFFERENT *Haemophilus influenzae* b CONJUGATE VACCINES IN INFANTS**

STUDY	AGE AT IMMUNIZATION	VACCINE	ANTIBODY LEVELS (mg/mL) AT AGE					
			4 Months		6 Months		7 Months	
			GMT	*% >1*	*GMT*	*% >1*	*GMT*	*% >1*
Vanderbilt[361]	(2, 4, 6)	PRP-D	0.06		0.08		0.28	29
		HbOC	0.09		0.13		3.08	75
		PRP-OMP	0.83		0.84	50	1.14	55
		PRP-T	0.05		0.30		3.64	83
U.S. multicenter[414]	(2, 4, 6)	HbOC	0.11		0.45	23	6.31	90
		PRP-OMP	2.69		4.00	85	5.21	88
		PRP-T	0.19	80	1.25	56	6.37	97
Finland[434]	(4, 6) 0	PRP-D			0.10	6	0.63	32
		HbOC			0.09	0	4.32	78
		PRP-T			0.82	50	6.10	96
Alaskan Native†[386]	(2, 4, 6)	PRP-D	0.04	2	0.06	11	0.55	45
		HbOC	0.07	0	0.59	43	13.72	94
		PRP-OMP*	1.37	57	2.71	79		
		PRP-T	0.08	3	0.51	41	4.38	75

*Only two doses of PRP-OMP administered at 2 and 4 months of age.

†Enrollment in this study was sequential by vaccine availability. Other studies were randomized trials.

GMT, geometric mean titer; HbOC, *Haemophilus* b oligosaccharide conjugate; PRP, polyribosylribitol phosphate; PRP-D, PRP–diphtheria toxoid conjugate; PRP-OMP, PRP–outer membrane protein conjugate; PRP-T, PRP–tetanus toxoid conjugate.

at 2 to 4 months of age. There is little if any boost with a second or third dose of PRP-OMP. HbOC and PRP-T each require two or three doses to achieve good antibody levels at this age; but after three doses, the levels achieved are higher than those achieved with PRP-OMP after two or three doses. The immune responses after two doses of HbOC or PRP-T are variable among studies. PRP-D is clearly the least immunogenic of the four vaccines. Last, the level of maternal antibody does not influence the ultimate immune response (data not shown).

Although these studies help to define the pattern of the immune response seen with each of the vaccines, they do not clearly indicate a "best" vaccine. Because PRP-OMP is the only vaccine that induces an antibody response in 2-month-old infants after a single dose, it may be advantageous for use in populations with incomplete immunizations and for high-risk populations in which there is early onset of disease (before 6 months of age). HbOC and PRP-T produce higher and more sustained antibody levels after completion of the primary immunization series; the duration of antibody levels appears to relate to peak level achieved.

There have not been any comparative efficacy trials, except for a comparison of PRP-D and HbOC in Finland, in which HbOC was shown to provide better protection.[452] Each of the three vaccines licensed in the United States for use in infants (HbOC, PRP-OMP, PRP-T) appears to be highly efficacious, and the available surveillance data cannot yet distinguish which vaccine is the most efficacious. Careful postlicensure case-control and cohort studies may determine if there are important differences in efficacy.

Schedules of Primary Immunization

Differences in the epidemiology of *H. influenzae* type b disease and in public health practices have led to the adoption of various national schedules of immunization. In countries where the peak of *H. influenzae* type b disease occurs in the second 6 months of life, three doses are given before 6 months of age. The United States, Canada, and Belgium are among the countries using a 2, 4, and 6 months schedule. To conform to the schedule of DTP administration, France and the United Kingdom recommend Hib vaccine at 2, 3, and 4 months of age. A more compressed schedule has been used in developing countries where considerable *H. influenzae* type b disease may occur before 6 months of age. On the other hand, in the Scandinavian countries in which the peak of *H. influenzae* type b disease occurred after 1 year of age, a two-dose schedule in the first year of life (5 and 7 months) followed by a booster third dose early in the second year of life is used.

Immunogenicity is influenced by the schedule used: intervals of 2 months between doses give better responses than intervals of 1 month, and the mean titers of antibody are directly correlated with increasing age at administration of the first dose of Hib vaccine.[436]

Mixed Administration of Hib Vaccines

The availability in many countries of more than one type of Hib vaccine generated concern that administration of different vaccines to the same child might reduce immunogenicity. In fact, several studies have shown that Hib vaccine conjugates are interchangeable, in that primary antibody responses remained excellent and booster responses were not impaired in the schedules that were studied.[453–455a]

Simultaneous Administration with Other Vaccines

In an attempt to reduce the number of injections necessary to vaccinate young infants, various formulations combining the Hib conjugate vaccines with other routine immunogens have been evaluated. Currently, three combination vaccines that include Hib are available and recommended for general use in the United States: DTP-HbOC, diphtheria and tetanus toxoids and acellular pertussis vaccine (DTaP)–PRP-T, and PRP-OMP–hepatitis B (see Chapter 20). Each Hib conjugate vaccine, PRP-D,[455] HbOC,[402] PRP-OMP,[456] and PRP-T,[442, 443, 457, 458] has been evaluated when it was combined in the same syringe as DTP. A reduction in the immune response to Hib[443] and to pertussis[442] has been shown compared with responses among children who were given the vaccines separately, but the significance of these findings is unknown. This emphasizes the importance of evaluating combination vaccines for immunogenicity as well as for safety. Other combination vaccines such as Hib combined with inactivated poliovirus vaccine or hepatitis A vaccine are under development or in various stages of evaluation.

Booster Immunizations and Duration of Immunity

Because antibody levels decline over time after completion of the primary immunization series in infants, a booster dose is currently recommended at 12 to 15 months of age. This booster dose elicits a brisk antibody response. Immunization with the Hib conjugate vaccines during infancy primes the immune system so that a booster immunization with PRP-D[356] or plain polysaccharide vaccine,[459] which is not very immunogenic in unprimed 12- to 15-month-old children, elicits a strong anamnestic response. The duration of immunity after a primary series varies with the age of the child and the vaccine. In several studies, more than 75% of infants had antibody levels above 1 μg/mL 3 to 5 years after the primary series with PRP-T or HbOC vaccine[460–462] compared with less than 50% of infants who received the PRP-OMP vaccine.[461, 463] The relative importance of absolute antibody levels versus immunological priming regarding maintenance of long-lasting immunity is not clear.

It is unclear whether a single booster immunization during the second year of life is sufficient for lifelong immunity, or conversely whether a booster dose is necessary at all. The United Kingdom has pursued a policy of not providing an Hib booster in the second year of life, which assumes long-term protection after three doses of PRP-T given at 2, 3, and 4 months of age. At a mean age of 4.5 years, 92% of a group of previously vaccinated children retained anti-Hib antibodies, with a geometric mean titer of 0.89 μg/mL. In addition, Hib pharyngeal carriage was still low.[463a] The British experience has been reviewed by Booy and colleagues,[464] who identified 43 true vaccine failures during a 3-year period. Protective efficacy declined slightly with time since vaccination: 99.1% in infants aged 5 to 11 months, 97.3% in infants aged 12 to 23 months, and 94.7% in infants aged 24 to 35 months. Continuing follow-up should show whether efficacy wanes and whether *H. influenzae* type b disease will become a problem in older children not given a booster.

Carrier Priming

Some studies have shown that an optimal response to immunization with conjugate vaccines requires prior or concomitant exposure to the carrier protein (carrier priming). Withholding immunization with diphtheria and tetanus toxoids (DT) from rhesus monkeys[397] and human infants[398] reduced the immune response to HbOC but not to PRP-OMP. It has been suggested that administration of carrier protein before immunization with Hib conjugate vaccines may prime T cells for an enhanced immune response to the subsequent immunization. The effect of carrier priming on the immune response is dependent on many variables,[398] and preliminary results from two studies show the complexity of the issue. Administration of DT at 1 month of age enhanced antibody responses to HbOC and PRP-T given at 2, 4, and 6 months of age,[465] but a similar study with DT given at birth did not show enhancement of the immune response.[466] In fact, immune responses to HbOC were suppressed in infants primed with DT at birth.

Contraindications and Precautions

There are no specific contraindications that are unique to Hib conjugate vaccines. Standard contraindications to vaccination in general, such as hypersensitivity to vaccine components, apply. A full description of such considerations is available from the American Academy of Pediatrics[238] and the U.S. Public Health Service.[217] All Hib vaccines may be given to immunocompromised individuals or other high-risk populations although immunogenicity may be suboptimal and protective efficacy has not been specifically demonstrated in these groups.

There have been rare reports of serious reactions such as urticaria, erythema multiforme, seizures, renal failure, and Guillain-Barré syndrome,[367] but a causal effect has not been established. In particular, seizures and sudden infant death syndrome do not appear to be more common in vaccinees than in control subjects.[331]

Candidate Noncapsular Vaccines

To date, essentially all *H. influenzae* vaccines are based on immunity to the type b capsule, because type b anticapsular antibodies are bactericidal, are opsonophagocytic, and induce protective efficacy. Antibodies to other components of the bacteria have also been shown to be bactericidal, opsonophagocytic, and protective in animal studies. Vaccines containing alternative antigens could provide supplemental protection against *H. influenzae* type b infection, although this does not appear to be necessary on the basis of the efficacy of the available Hib conjugate vaccines. More important, such alternative vaccines could provide immunity to non–type b strains, which commonly cause otitis media, sinusitis, chronic bronchitis, and pneumonia. Non–type b *H. influenzae* are ubiquitous colonizers of the upper respiratory tract of humans, and they constitute a diverse popu-

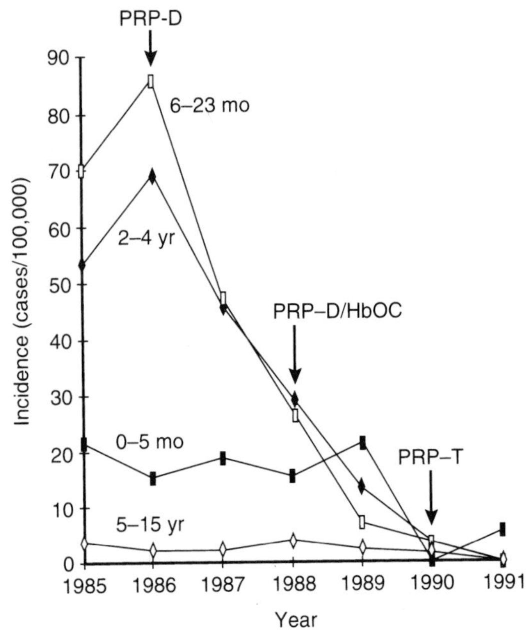

Figure 11–8. Eradication of *Haemophilus influenzae* type b disease in Finland. Half of the population received PRP-D vaccine between 1986 and 1988. PRP, polyribosylribitol phosphate; PRP-D, PRP–diphtheria toxoid conjugate; HbOC, *Haemophilus* b oligosaccharide conjugate; PRP-T, PRP–tetanus toxoid conjugate. (From Peltola H, Kilpi T, Anttila M. Rapid disappearance of *Haemophilus influenzae* type b meningitis after routine childhood immunisation with conjugate vaccines. Lancet 340:592–594, 1992. © The Lancet Ltd., 1992.)

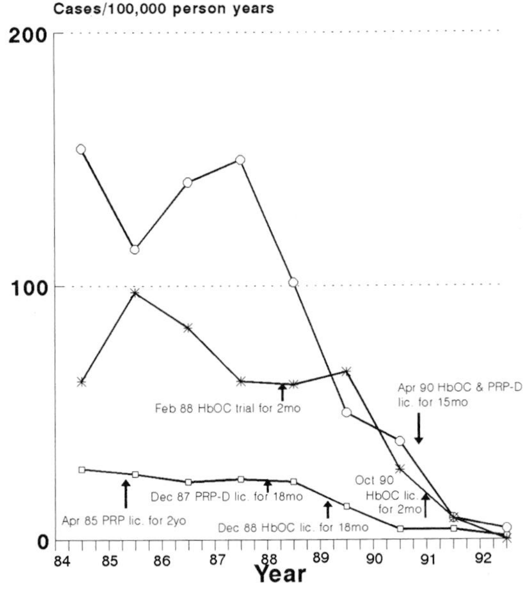

Figure 11–9. Incidence of *Haemophilus influenzae* type b disease in the Kaiser Permanente Medical Care Program in Northern California, January 1984 to December 1992. PRP, polyribosylribitol phosphate; HbOC, *Haemophilus* b oligosaccharide conjugate; PRP-D, PRP–diphtheria toxoid conjugate; mo, months old; yo, years old. (From Black SB, Shinefield HR. Immunization with oligosaccharide conjugate *Haemophilus influenzae* type b [HbOC] vaccine on a large health maintenance organization population. Pediatr Infect Dis J 11:610–613, 1992. © Williams & Wilkins, 1992.)

lation of bacteria with much phenotypic and genetic variability.[41]

The basic microbiological problem that hinders the development of such vaccines has been the diversity and instability of cell wall antigens among most *H. influenzae* strains. Studies have attempted to define outer membrane proteins, cell wall lipopolysaccharides, or fimbriae surface antigens of the organism.[68] Owing to the variability in these antigens among heterologous strains and even among homologous strains over time, it has been difficult to find an antigen that is relevant to all or the majority of strains. Also, not all bacterial antigens elicit protective immunity. The focus of most investigations has been to characterize outer membrane proteins. Of particular interest has been the P-6 lower molecular weight outer membrane protein (16.6 kDa) found in essentially all nontypable and *H. influenzae* type b isolates.[467, 468] Antibodies to the P-6 protein are bactericidal for homologous and heterologous strains and protect against experimental *H. influenzae* type b bacteremia in infant rats. The gene for the P-6 protein has been cloned and sequenced.[469] Other efforts have focused on selected higher molecular weight proteins,[470] lipopolysaccharides, or fimbrial antigens.[471] Immunity to these

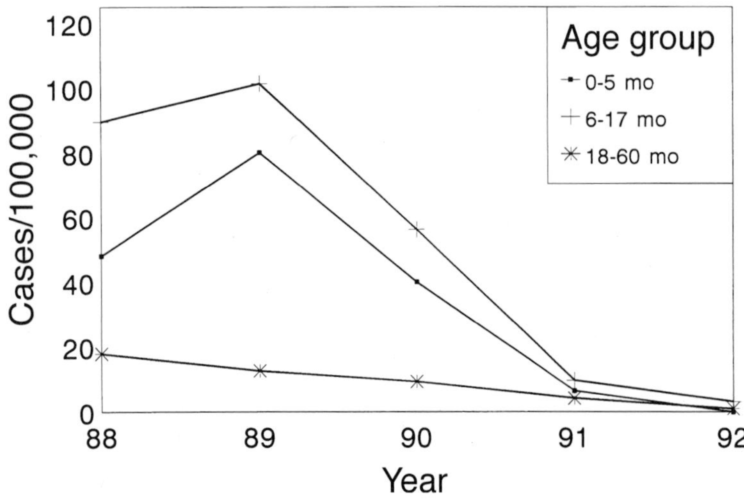

Figure 11–10. Incidence of *Haemophilus influenzae* type b disease in the Southern California Kaiser Health Plan. (From Vadheim CM, Greenberg DP, Eriksen E, et al. Eradication of *Haemophilus influenzae* type b disease in Southern California. Arch Pediatr Adolesc Med 148:51–56, 1994.)

other antigens has not been consistent against heterologous strains. Clinical trials have not yet been conducted and could prove to be difficult.

PUBLIC HEALTH CONSIDERATIONS

Impact of *Haemophilus influenzae* Type b Conjugate Vaccines on Disease and Carriage of the Organism

In several North American[428, 429, 472–475] and European[449, 476] countries, routine immunization with Hib conjugate vaccines has resulted in a dramatic decrease in the incidence of disease in the targeted populations. In general, the fall in incidence of disease has exceeded that predicted on the basis of the estimated proportion of the population that is completely immunized, suggesting an element of herd immunity. In addition, in essentially all of these populations, a significant fall in incidence of disease was observed among infants before the licensure and recommended use of vaccines in that age group.

These findings, which underline the importance of mucosal immunity to Hib, are probably explained by reductions in *H. influenzae* type b carriage caused by vaccination,[308–311] leading to decreased transmission from immunized children to unimmunized young children and infants.

Shown in Figures 11–8 to 11–11 are the experiences in four carefully studied populations. Data on the U.S. Army,[472] Native American,[428] and several European populations have also been evaluated. Each of the four selected studies highlights an important point. In Finland,[377, 449] three different vaccines were used in sequence, and high immunization levels were achieved (see Fig. 11–8). PRP-D vaccine, in use between 1987 and 1989, proved to be effective in eliminating the majority of all *H. influenzae* type b disease. Subsequently, the use of HbOC and PRP-T vaccine proved to be even more effective, and the routine immunization of Finnish infants has virtually eliminated *H. influenzae* type b disease among children younger than 5 years, making Finland the first population to essentially eliminate *H. influenzae* type b disease. Some disease continues to occur in adults and in infants younger than 4 months. With the introduction of Hib conjugate vaccines, similar changes in incidence of disease have occurred in other European countries, such as Iceland,[378] the United Kingdom, and Switzerland.

In the United States, the Northern California Kaiser Permanente Health Plan has used HbOC vaccine exclusively. In this population[404] (see Fig. 11–9), disease has been eliminated, except for a rare case in an unimmunized child and a few cases in children with incomplete immunizations. In the Southern California Kaiser Health Plan,[429] PRP-D and subsequently PRP-OMP vaccines were used in older children between 1987 and 1990. Since 1990, PRP-OMP vaccine has been used almost exclusively. There were a few PRP-D failures and only two PRP-OMP failures; disease has been essentially eliminated (see Fig. 11–10) even though complete age-appropriate immunization levels have not yet been achieved. Similar control of disease has been achieved with use of PRP-OMP vaccine in Alaska and Navajo Native American populations.[428]

In Los Angeles County,[429] Minnesota and Dallas,[473] and selected other U.S. sites under surveillance by the Centers for Disease Control and Prevention[474] (see Fig. 11–11), similar but less complete disease eradication has been achieved. In these areas, both HbOC and PRP-OMP vaccine have been used in varying proportions over time, and complete immunization is not yet achieved. In Los Angeles, it is estimated that only 50% of children receive three doses of HbOC or two doses of PRP-OMP vaccine by 12 months of age. Despite the incomplete immunization of children, dramatic decreases in the incidence of disease in Los Angeles have occurred.

Unresolved Issues

Despite the availability of several Hib conjugate vaccines and the tremendous advances in the control of *H.*

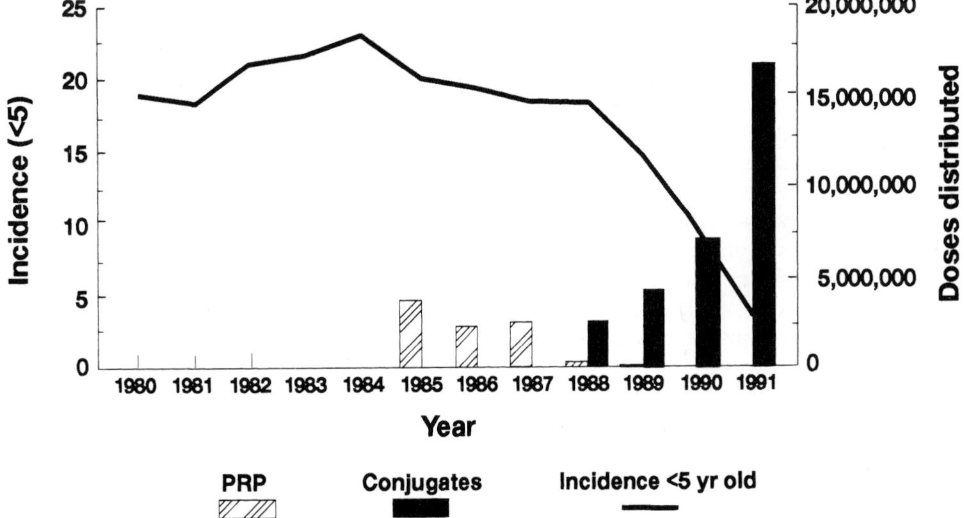

Figure 11–11. *Haemophilus influenzae* vaccine doses sold or distributed and incidence of *H. influenzae* meningitis in children younger than 5 years in the United States, 1980 to 1991. PRP, polyribosylribitol phosphate vaccine. (Data from the National Bacterial Meningitis Reporting System [20 continuously reporting states], 1980 to 1991.)

influenzae type b disease in vaccinated populations, several questions remain. Fundamental issues regarding the clinical burden and epidemiology of disease in several areas of the industrialized world and most areas of the developing world are completely unknown. Although several studies have been performed from such areas, frequently they are not population based or are limited in the study design and laboratory methods for detection of *H. influenzae* type b. Such studies underestimate the true burden of disease and therefore the potential impact of routine vaccination with an effective vaccine. In addition, in areas with routine *H. influenzae* type b vaccination, it is not yet known if other *Haemophilus* serotypes (non-b) will emerge as important pathogens.[477]

Basic questions about the protective efficacy of Hib conjugate vaccines remain unanswered, such as differences by vaccine, age, and population (i.e., Is the vaccine effective in all high-risk groups?); number of doses to be given; or duration of protection. Other issues of potential public health importance include availability, cost, lot-to-lot potency, formulation with other childhood immunizations, and long-term safety. Some differences among vaccines are already evident (i.e., protection after a single dose in infants), but the overall balance of advantages and disadvantages of each vaccine is not yet clear. The recent efficacy study in the Gambia[444] suggests that Hib vaccine significantly reduces the incidence of pneumonia. Confirmation and extension of these results in other areas of the world are awaited.

Should the recommended schedules for each vaccine be altered to optimize protection? Several studies have suggested that alternative vaccine schedules (such as receiving the first dose at birth[478]) do not compromise immunogenicity. Others have shown that an initial dose of PRP-OMP at 2 months of age followed by subsequent doses of HbOC or PRP-T at 4 and 6 months provides enhanced immunogenicity after the third dose compared with vaccination with three doses of the same vaccine.[453, 455] Could one induce earlier or greater immune responses with HbOC or PRP-T vaccine by the prior administration of diphtheria or tetanus toxoids so as to prime for the carrier proteins of these vaccines, through maternal immunization with subsequent transplacental transfer of antibody, as shown in one study,[479] or perhaps through subcutaneous rather than intramuscular injection?[480] Are current recommendations for booster immunization in the second year of life adequate to ensure lifelong protection?

Particularly important to delineate are the immunological determinants of protection, which include consideration of the levels of specific antibodies and the type of immunity elicited. This has relevance to evaluating the protective efficacy of Hib conjugate vaccines when detailed efficacy data may not be available and for better understanding of how to construct new polysaccharide-protein conjugate vaccines against other encapsulated bacterial pathogens. Furthermore, age is the most important risk factor for disease and determinant of the immune response, yet the immunological determinants of this susceptibility and immune maturation are not fully understood. Research on developmental immunology might explain why young infants and children are so uniquely susceptible to infection with encapsulated bacteria between 6 months and 2 years of age.

The differences in mucosal immunity induced by Hib conjugate vaccines[312] may be particularly relevant, because infection of mucosal membranes is undoubtedly the first step in the pathogenesis of disease. If the vaccines effectively eliminate carriage, as suggested by some studies,[308–311] or otherwise impede transmission of the organism, then there will be population-wide benefits in reduced disease risk, even for those who are not immunized.

From a public health perspective, additional characterization of the microbial factors that determine virulence would be useful in defining other potential vaccine immunogens as well as improving our understanding of disease pathogenesis. Current vaccines are based on the principle that anticapsular antibody alone is sufficient to prevent disease, but it is clear that other antigens of the organism also elicit antibodies that may be protective. In addition, anticapsular vaccines do not address the problem of mucosal infections caused by unencapsulated strains of *H. influenzae*. In this regard, the prevention of mucosal diseases will require vaccines that induce more diverse immunological stimulation.

Opportunities

Decades of clinical and laboratory work, begun more than 100 years ago, have led to the near-elimination of *H. influenzae* type b disease in several populations. Before this effort, *H. influenzae* type b was one of the most important bacterial pathogens of childhood. The degree of disease control has exceeded expectations and is in excess of what known levels of immunization coverage would have predicted. Unfortunately, Hib conjugate vaccines are used in relatively few countries worldwide, leaving most of the world's children still at risk. The World Health Organization has recently assigned evaluation and control of *H. influenzae* type b disease to high priority.

Although many unanswered questions remain, *H. influenzae* type b disease has joined a growing list of major pediatric diseases now preventable by routine immunization. Hib conjugate vaccine technology has been the prototype for vaccines to prevent disease caused by other important encapsulated bacteria, such as the pneumococcus, meningococcus, and group B streptococcus. The lessons learned in the quest to eliminate *H. influenzae* type b disease have important implications for the prevention of these and other bacterial diseases.

REFERENCES

1. Schlech WF, Ward JI, Band JD. Bacterial meningitis in the United States 1978–1981: The national bacterial meningitis surveillance study. JAMA 253:1749–1754, 1985.
2. Wenger JD, Hightower AW, Facklam RR, et al. Bacterial meningitis in the United States, 1986: Report of a multistate surveillance study. J Infect Dis 162:1316–1323, 1990.
3. Pfeiffer R. Vorlaufige mit Heilungen über die Erreger der Influenzae. Dtsch Med Wochenschr 18:28–34, 1892.

4. Pfeiffer R. Die Aetiologie der Influenza. Z Hyg Infektionskr 13:357–386, 1893.
5. Winslow CE, Broadhurst J, Buchanan RE, et al. The families and genera of the bacteria: Final report of the committee of the Society of American Bacteriologists on characterization and classification of bacterial types. J Bacteriol 5:191–229, 1920.
6. Pittman M. Variation and type specificity in the bacterial species *H. influenzae.* J Exp Med 53:471–495, 1931.
7. Pittman M. The action of type-specific *H. influenzae* antiserum. J Exp Med 58:683–706, 1933.
8. Alexander HE, Leidy G, MacPherson C. Production of types a, b, c, d, e, and f *H. influenzae* antibody for diagnostic and therapeutic purposes. J Immunol 54:207–211, 1946.
9. Alexander HE, Heidelberger M, Leidy G. The protective or curative element in type b *H. influenzae* rabbit serum. Yale J Biol Med 16:425–440, 1944.
10. Alexander HE. Experimental basis for treatment of *H. influenzae* infections. Am J Dis Child 66:160–171, 1943.
11. Fothergill LD, Wright J. Influenzal meningitis: The relation of age incidence to the bactericidal power of blood against the causal organism. J Immunol 24:273–284, 1933.
12. Johnston RB Jr, Anderson P, Rosen FS, Smith DH. Characterization of human immunity to polyribophosphate, the capsular antigen of *H. influenzae* type b. Clin Immunol Immunopathol 1:234–240, 1973.
13. Anderson P, Johnston RB Jr, Smith DH. Human serum activities against *H. influenzae* type b. J Clin Invest 51:31–38, 1972.
14. Schneerson R, Rodrigues LP, Parke JC Jr, Robbins JB. Immunity to disease caused by *H. influenzae* type b. II. Specificity and some biological characteristics of "natural" infection acquired and immunization induced antibody to the capsular polysaccharide. J Immunol 107:1081–1089, 1971.
15. Turk DC. Clinical importance of *H. influenzae*—1981. In Sell SH, Wright PF (eds). *Haemophilus influenzae.* New York, Elsevier Science Publishing, 1982, pp 3–9.
16. Todd JK, Bruhn FW. Severe *H. influenzae* infections: Spectrum of disease. Am J Dis Child 129:607–611, 1975.
17. Dajani AS, Asmar BI, Thirumoorthi MC. Systemic *H. influenzae* disease: An overview. J Pediatr 94:355–364, 1979.
18. Granoff DM, Basden M. *H. influenzae* infections in Fresno County, California: A prospective study of the effects of age, race and contact with a case on incidence of disease. J Infect Dis 140:40–46, 1980.
19. Peltola H, Virtanen M. Systemic *H. influenzae* infection in Finland. Clin Pediatr 5:275–280, 1984.
20. Cochi SL, Broome CV, Hightower AW. Immunization of U.S. children with *H. influenzae* type b polysaccharide vaccine: A cost-effectiveness model of strategy assessment. JAMA 253:521–529, 1985.
21. Taylor HG, Michaels RH, Mazur PM, Liden CB. Intellectual, neuropsychological and achievement outcomes in children six to eight years after recovery from *H. influenzae* meningitis. Pediatrics 74:198–205, 1984.
22. Feigin RD, Stechenberg BW, Chang MJ. Prospective evaluation of treatment of *H. influenzae* meningitis. J Pediatr 88:542–548, 1976.
23. Sell SHW, Merrill RE, Doyne EO, Zinsky EP. Long-term sequelae of *H. influenzae* meningitis. Pediatrics 42:206–217, 1972.
24. Sproles ET III, Azerrad J, Williamson C, Merrill RE. Meningitis due to *H. influenzae:* Long-term sequelae. J Pediatr 75:782–788, 1969.
25. Dodge PR, Swartz MN. Bacterial meningitis—a review of selected aspects. II. Special neurologic problems, postmeningitis complications and clinicopathological correlations. N Engl J Med 272:1003–1010, 1965.
26. Ferry PC, Culbetson JL, Cooper JA. Sequelae of *H. influenzae* meningitis. In Sell SH, Wright PF (eds). *Haemophilus influenzae.* New York, Elsevier Science Publishing, 1982, pp 111–117.
27. Pomeroy SL, Holmes SJ, Dodge PR, Feigin RD. Seizures and other neurologic sequelae of bacterial meningitis in children. N Engl J Med 323:1651–1657, 1990.
28. Taylor HG, Mills EL, Ciampi A, et al. The sequelae of *Haemophilus influenzae* meningitis in school-age children. N Engl J Med 323:1657–1663, 1990.
29. Harding AL, Anderson P, Howie VM, et al. *H. influenzae* isolated from otitis media. In Sell SH, Karzon DT (eds). *Haemophilus influenzae.* Nashville, TN, Vanderbilt University Press, 1973, pp 21–27.
30. Wallace RJ, Baker CJ, Quinones FJ. Nontypable *H. influenzae* (biotype 4) as a neonatal, maternal and genital pathogen. Rev Infect Dis 5:123–136, 1983.
31. Campognone P, Singer DB. Neonatal sepsis due to nontypable *H. influenzae.* Am J Dis Child 140:117–121, 1986.
32. Halla IJ, Dobson SRM, Crook DWM, et al. Population-based study of nontypable *Haemophilus influenzae* invasive disease in children and neonates. Lancet 341:851–854, 1993.
33. Greenwood B. Epidemiology of acute lower respiratory tract infections, especially those due to *Haemophilus influenzae* type b, in the Gambia, West Africa. J Infect Dis 165(suppl 1):S26–28, 1992.
34. Lehmann D. Epidemiology of acute respiratory tract infections, especially those due to *Haemophilus influenzae,* in Papua New Guinean children. J Infect Dis 165(suppl 1):S20–25, 1992.
35. Shann F, Graaten M, Germer S, et al. Aetiology of pneumonia in children in Goroka Hospital, Papua New Guinea. Lancet 2:537–541, 1984.
36. Wall RA, Corrah PT, Mabey DCW, Greenwood BM. The etiology of lobar pneumonia in the Gambia. Bull World Health Organ 64:553–558, 1986.
37. Shann F. Etiology of severe pneumonia in children in developing countries. Pediatr Infect Dis J 5:247–252, 1986.
38. Campos JM. Haemophilus. In Murray PR (ed). Manual of Clinical Microbiology (6th ed). Washington, DC, American Society for Microbiology, 1995, pp 556–565.
39. Mason EO, Kaplan SL, Lambeth LB. Serotype and ampicillin susceptibility of *H. influenzae* causing systemic infections in children: Three years of experience. J Clin Microbiol 15:543–546, 1982.
40. Van Ham SM, van Alphen L, Mooi FR. Fimbria-mediated adherence and hemagglutination of *Haemophilus influenzae.* J Infect Dis 165(suppl 1):S97–99, 1992.
41. Musser JM, Kroll JS, Moxon ER, Selander RK. Evolutionary genetics of the encapsulated strains of *Haemophilus influenzae.* Proc Natl Acad Sci USA 85:7758–7762, 1988.
42. Centers for Disease Control. Ampicillin-resistant *H. influenzae* meningitis—Maryland, Georgia. MMWR Morb Mortal Wkly Rep 23:77–78, 1974.
43. Centers for Disease Control. Ampicillin-resistant *H. influenzae*—Texas. MMWR Morb Mortal Wkly Rep 23:99, 1974.
44. Tomeh MO, Starr SE, McGowan JE. Ampicillin-resistant *H. influenzae* type b infection. JAMA 229:295–297, 1974.
45. Khan W, Ross S, Rodriguez W. *H. influenzae* type b resistant to ampicillin. JAMA 229:298–301, 1974.
46. Schiffer MS, MacLowry J, Schneerson R. Clinical, bacteriological and immunological characterization of ampicillin-resistant *H. influenzae* type b. Lancet 2:257–259, 1974.
47. American Academy of Pediatrics, Committee on Infectious Diseases. Ampicillin-resistant strains of *H. influenzae* type b. Pediatrics 55:145–146, 1975.
48. Jacobson JA, McCormick JB, Hayes P. Epidemiologic characteristics of infections caused by ampicillin-resistant *H. influenzae.* Pediatrics 58:388–391, 1976.
49. Istre GR, Conner JS, Glode MP, Hopkins RS. Increasing ampicillin-resistance rates in *H. influenzae* meningitis. Am J Dis Child 138:366–369, 1984.
50. Campos J, Garcia-Tornel S, Sanfeliu I. Susceptibility studies of multiply resistant *H. influenzae* isolated from pediatric patients and contacts. Antimicrob Agents Chemother 25:706–709, 1984.
51. Meyroritch J, Frand M, Altman G. Ampicillin-resistant *H. influenzae* type b infections in hospitalized pediatric patients. Isr J Med Sci 20:519–521, 1984.
52. Doern GV, Jorgensen JW, Thornsberry C. Prevalence of antimicrobial resistance among clinical isolates of *H. influenzae:* A collaborative study. Diagn Microbiol Infect Dis 4:95–107, 1986.
53. Campos J, Garcia-Tornel S, Gairi JM, Fabregues I. Multiply resistant *H. influenzae* type b causing meningitis: Comparative clinical and laboratory study. J Pediatr 108:897–902, 1986.
54. Jorgensen JH. Update on mechanisms and prevalence of antimicrobial resistance in *Haemophilus influenzae.* Clin Infect Dis 14:1119–1123, 1992.

55. Smith AL. Antibiotic resistance in *H. influenzae.* Pediatr Infect Dis J 2:352–355, 1983.
56. Roberts MC, Swenson CD, Owens IM, Smith AL. Characterization of chloramphenicol-resistant *H. influenzae.* Antimicrob Agents Chemother 18:610–615, 1980.
57. Mendelman PM, Doroshow CA, Gandy SL. Plasmid-mediated resistance in multiply resistant *H. influenzae* type b causing meningitis: Molecular characterization of one strain and review of the literature. J Infect Dis 150:30–39, 1984.
58. Centers for Disease Control. Ampicillin and chloramphenicol resistance in systemic *H. influenzae* disease. MMWR Morb Mortal Wkly Rep 33:35–37, 1984.
59. Kenney JF, Isburg CD, Michaels RH. Meningitis due to *H. influenzae* type b resistant to both ampicillin and chloramphenicol. J Pediatr 66:14–16, 1980.
60. Uchiyama N, Greene GR, Kitts DR, Thrupp LD. Meningitis due to *H. influenzae* type b resistant to ampicillin and chloramphenicol. J Pediatr 97:421–424, 1980.
61. Simasathien S, Dhangmani C, Echeverria P. *H. influenzae* type b resistant to ampicillin and chloramphenicol in an orphanage in Thailand. Lancet 1:1214–1217, 1980.
62. Feigin RD, McCracken GH Jr, Klein JO. Diagnosis and management of meningitis. Pediatr Infect Dis J 11:785–814, 1992.
63. Moxon ER. The carrier state: *Haemophilus influenzae.* J Antimicrob Chemother 18:17–24, 1986.
64. Michaels RH, Norden CW. Pharyngeal colonization with *H. influenzae* type b: A longitudinal study of families with a child with meningitis or epiglottitis due to *H. influenzae* type b. J Infect Dis 136:222–228, 1977.
65. Murphy TV, Granoff D, Chrane DF. Pharyngeal colonization with *Haemophilus influenzae* type b in children in a day care center without invasive disease. J Pediatr 106:712–716, 1985.
66. Ginsburg CM, McCracken GH Jr, Rae S. *Haemophilus influenzae* type b disease: Incidence in a daycare center. JAMA 238:604–607, 1977.
67. Granoff DM, Gilsdorf J, Gessert C. *Haemophilus influenzae* type b disease in a day care center: Eradication of carrier state by rifampin. Pediatrics 63:397–401, 1979.
68. Barenkamp SJ, Granoff DM, Munson RS Jr. Outer membrane protein subtypes of *Haemophilus influenzae* type b and spread of disease in day care centers. J Infect Dis 144:210–217, 1981.
69. Li KI, Dashefsky B, Wald ER. *Haemophilus influenzae* type b colonization in household contacts of infected and colonized children enrolled in day care. Pediatrics 78:15–20, 1986.
70. Ward JI, Gorman G, Phillips C. *Haemophilus influenzae* type b disease in a day-care center: Report of an outbreak. J Pediatr 92:713–717, 1978.
71. Campbell LR, Zedd AJ, Michaels RH. Household spread of infection due to *H. influenzae* type b. Pediatrics 66:115–117, 1980.
72. Michaels RH, Poziviak CS, Stonebraker FE, Norden CW. Factors affecting pharyngeal *H. influenzae* type b colonization rates in children. J Clin Microbiol 4:413–417, 1976.
73. Masters PL, Brumfitt W, Mendez RL, Likar M. Bacterial flora of the upper respiratory tract in Paddington families. BMJ 1:1200–1205, 1958.
74. Dawson B, Zinnermann K. Incidence and type distribution of capsulated *H. influenzae* strains. BMJ 1:740–742, 1952.
75. Mpairwe Y. Observations on the nasopharyngeal carriage of *H. influenzae* type b in children in Kampala, Uganda. J Hyg 68:337–341, 1970.
76. Turk DC. Naso-pharyngeal carriage of *H. influenzae* type B. J Hyg 61:247–256, 1963.
77. Lerman SJ, Kucera JC, Brunken JM. Nasopharyngeal carriage of antibiotic-resistant *H. influenzae* in healthy children. Pediatrics 64:287–291, 1979.
78. Hall DB, Lum MK, Knutson LR, et al. Pharyngeal carriage and acquisition of anticapsular antibody to *H. influenzae* type b in a high-risk population in southwestern Alaska. Am J Epidemiol 126:1190–1197, 1987.
79. Michaels RH, Stonebraker FE, Robbins JB. Use of antiserum agar for detection of *H. influenzae* type b in the pharynx. Pediatr Res 9:513–516, 1975.
80. Alpert G, Campos JM, Smith DR. Incidence and persistence of *H. influenzae* type b upper airway colonization in patients with meningitis. J Pediatr 107:555–557, 1985.
81. Band JD, Fraser DW, Ajello G. Prevention of *H. influenzae* type b disease. JAMA 251:2381–2386, 1984.
82. Granoff DM, Munson RS Jr. Prospects for prevention of *H. influenzae* type b disease by immunization. J Infect Dis 153:448-461, 1986.
83. Greenfield S, Peter G, Howie VM. Acquisition of type-specific antibodies to *H. influenzae* type b. J Pediatr 80:204–208, 1972.
84. Stephenson WP, Doern G, Grantz N. Pharyngeal carriage rates of *Haemophilus influenzae* type b and non-b, and prevalence of ampicillin-resistant *Haemophilus influenzae* among healthy day-care children in central Massachusetts. Am J Epidemiol 122:868–875, 1985.
85. Shapiro ED, Wald ER. Efficacy of rifampin in eliminating pharyngeal carriage of *H. influenzae* type b. Pediatrics 66:5–8, 1980.
86. Shapiro ED. Persistent pharyngeal colonization with *H. influenzae* type b after intravenous chloramphenicol therapy. Pediatrics 67:435–437, 1981.
87. Stephens DS, Farley MM. Pathogenic events during infections of the human nasopharynx with *Neisseria meningitidis* and *Haemophilus influenzae.* Rev Infect Dis 13:22–33, 1991.
88. Krasinski K, Nelson JD, Butler S, et al. Possible association of mycoplasma and viral respiratory infections with bacterial meningitis. Am J Epidemiol 125:499–508, 1987.
89. Takala AK, Mourman O, Kleemola M, et al. Preceding respiratory infection predisposing for primary and secondary invasive *Haemophilus influenzae* type b disease. Pediatr Infect Dis J 12:189–195, 1993.
90. Smith AL, Daum RS, Scheifele DW. Pathogenesis of *H. influenzae* meningitis. In Sell SH, Wright PE (eds). *Haemophilus influenzae.* New York, Elsevier Science Publishing, 1982, pp 89–109.
91. Moxon ER. Molecular basis of invasive *Haemophilus influenzae* type b disease. J Infect Dis 165(suppl 1):S77–S81, 1992.
92. Moxon ER, Smith AL, Averill DR, Smith DH. *H. influenzae* meningitis in rats following intranasal inoculation. J Infect Dis 129:154–162, 1974.
93. Ostrow PT, Moxon ER, Vernon N, Kapko R. Studies on the route of meningeal invasion following *H. influenzae* inoculation of infant rats. Lab Invest 40:678–685, 1979.
94. Gregorius FK, Johnson BJ, Stern WE, Brown WJ. Pathogenesis of hematogenous bacterial meningitis in rabbits. J Neurosurg 45:561–567, 1976.
95. Weller PF, Smith AL, Smith DH, Anderson P. Role of immunity in the clearance of bacteremia due to *H. influenzae.* J Infect Dis 138:427–436, 1978.
96. Weller PF, Smith AL, Anderson P, Smith DH. The role of encapsulation and host age in the clearance of *H. influenzae* bacteremia. J Infect Dis 135:34–41, 1977.
97. Rubin LG, Moxon ER. Pathogenesis of bloodstream invasion with *H. influenzae* type b. Infect Immun 24:102–105, 1979.
98. Scheld WM, Parks TS, Winn HR, et al. Clearance of bacteria from cerebrospinal fluid to blood in experimental meningitis. Infect Immun 24:102–105, 1979.
99. Feldman WE, Ginsburg CM, McCracken GH. Relation of concentrations of *H. influenzae* type b in cerebrospinal fluid to late sequelae of patients with meningitis. J Pediatr 100:209–212, 1982.
100. Feldman W. Relation of concentration of bacteria and bacterial antigens in cerebrospinal fluid to prognosis in patients with bacterial meningitis. N Engl J Med 296:433–435, 1977.
101. Chapin KC, Doern GV. Selective media for recovery of *Haemophilus influenzae* from specimens contaminated with upper respiratory tract microbial flora. J Clin Microbiol 17:1163–1165, 1983.
102. Marcon MJ, Hamoudoi AC, Cannon HJ. Comparative laboratory evaluation of three antigen detection methods for diagnosis of *H. influenzae* type b disease. J Clin Microbiol 19:333–337, 1984.
103. Kaplan SL. Antigen detection in cerebrospinal fluid: Pros and cons. Am J Med 75(B):109–188, 1983.
104. McGraw TP, Bruckner DA. Sensitivity of commercial agglutination and counterimmunoelectrophoresis methods for the detection of *Haemophilus influenzae* type b capsular polysaccharide. Am J Clin Pathol 80:703–706, 1983.
105. Rothstein EP, Madore DV, Girone JA, et al. Comparison of

antigenuria after immunization with three *Haemophilus influenzae* type b conjugate vaccines. Pediatr Infect Dis J 10:311–314, 1991.
106. Spinola SM, Sheaffer CI, Philbrick KB, Gilligan PH. Antigenuria after *H. influenzae* type b polysaccharide immunization: A prospective study. J Pediatr 109:835–838, 1986.
107. Kleiman MB, Reynolds JK, Watts NH, et al. Superiority of acridine orange stain versus Gram stain in partially treated bacterial meningits. J Pediatr 104:401–404, 1984.
108. Clausen CR. Detection of bacterial pathogens in purulent clinical specimens by immunofluorescence techniques. J Clin Microbiol 13:1119–1121, 1981.
109. Jacobs RF, Wright MW, Deskin RL, et al. Delayed sterilization of *Haemophilus influenzae* type b meningitis with twice-daily ceftriaxone. JAMA 259:392–394, 1988.
110. Sirinavin S, Chiemchanya S, Visudhipan P, et al. Cefuroxime treatment of bacterial meningitis in infants and children. Antimicrob Agents Chemother 25:273–275, 1984.
111. Korones DN, Marshall GS, Shapiro ED. Outcome of children with occult bacteremia caused by *Haemophilus influenzae* type b. Pediatr Infect Dis J 11:516–520, 1992.
112. Cortese MM, Goepp J, Almeido-Hill J, et al. Children with *Haemophilus influenzae* bacteremia initially treated as outpatients: Outcome in 85 American Indian children. Pediatr Infect Dis J 11:521–525, 1992.
113. Prober CJ. The role of steroids in the management of children with bacterial meningitis. Pediatrics 95:29–31, 1995.
114. Institute of Medicine. Prospects for immunizing against *Haemophilus influenzae* type b. In New Vaccine Development: Establishing Priorities. Washington, DC, National Academy Press, 1985, pp 235–251.
115. Cochi SL, Broome CV. Vaccine prevention of *H. influenzae* type b disease: Past, present and future. Pediatr Infect Dis J 5:12–19, 1986.
116. Murphy TV, Clements JF, Petroni M, et al. Survival of *Haemophilus influenzae* type b in respiratory secretions. Pediatr Infect Dis J 8:148–151, 1989.
117. Makela PH, Takala AK, Peltola H, Eskola J. Epidemiology of invasive *Haemophilus influenzae* type b disease. J Infect Dis 165(suppl 1):S2–S6, 1992.
118. Shapiro ED, Ward JI. The epidemiology and prevention of disease caused by *Haemophilus influenzae* type b. Epidemiol Rev 13:113–142, 1991.
119. Cochi SL, Fleming DW, Hightower AW. Primary invasive *H. influenzae* type b disease: A population-based assessment of risk factors. J Pediatr 108:887–896, 1986.
120. Baraff LJ, Wehrle PF. Epidemiology of pediatric meningitis: Los Angeles County, 1975 [abstract]. Pediatr Res 11:434, 1977.
121. Fraser DW, Hencke CE, Feldman RA. Changing patterns of bacterial meningitis in Olmsted County, Minnesota. J Infect Dis 238:300–307, 1973.
122. Fraser DW, Geil CC, Feldman RA. Bacterial meningitis in Bernalillo County, New Mexico: A comparison with three other American populations. Am J Epidemiol 100:29–34, 1974.
123. Fraser DW, Mitchell JE, Silverman LP, Feldman RA. Undiagnosed bacterial meningitis in Vermont children. Am J Epidemiol 102:394–399, 1975.
124. Istre GR, Conner JS, Broome CV. Risk factors for primary invasive *H. influenzae* disease: Increased risk from day care attendance and school age household members. J Pediatr 106:190–195, 1985.
125. Parke JC Jr, Schneerson R, Robbins JB. The attack rate, age incidence, racial distribution, and case fatality rate of *H. influenzae* type b meningitis in Mecklenburg County, North Carolina. J Pediatr 81:765–769, 1972.
126. Murphy TV, Osterholm MT, Pierson LM. Prospective surveillance of *H. influenzae* type b disease in Dallas County, Texas, and in Minnesota. Pediatrics 79:173–180, 1987.
127. Redmond SR, Pichichero ME. *H. influenzae* type b disease: An epidemiologic study with special reference to day care centers. JAMA 252:2581–2584, 1984.
128. Smith EWP Jr, Haynes RE. Changing incidence of *H. influenzae* meningitis. Pediatrics 50:723–727, 1972.
129. Ward JI, Lum MK, Hall DB. Invasive *H. influenzae* type b disease in Alaska: Background epidemiology for a vaccine efficacy trial. J Infect Dis 153:17–26, 1986.
130. Tarr PI, Peter G. Demographic factors in the epidemiology of *H. influenzae* meningitis in young children. J Pediatr 92:884–888, 1978.
131. Floyd RF, Federspiel CF, Schaffner W. Bacterial meningitis in urban and rural Tennessee. Am J Epidemiol 99:395–397, 1974.
132. Fraser DW. *Haemophilus influenzae* in the community and in the home. In Sell SH, Wright PF (eds). *Haemophilus influenzae.* New York, Elsevier Science Publishing, 1982, pp 11–22.
133. Peltola H, Rod TO, Jonsdottir K, et al. Life-threatening *Haemophilus influenzae* infections in Scandinavia: A five-country analysis of the incidence and the main clinical and bacteriologic characteristics. Rev Infect Dis 12:708–715, 1990.
134. Claesson B, Trollfors B, Jodal U. Incidence and prognosis of *Haemophilus influenzae* meningitis in children in a Swedish region. Pediatr Infect Dis J 3:35–39, 1984.
135. Salwen KM, Vikerfors T, Olcen P. Increased incidence of childhood bacterial meningitis: A 25-year study in a defined population in Sweden. Scand J Infect Dis 19:1–11, 1987.
136. Trollfors B, Claesson BA, Strangert K, Taranger J. *Haemophilus influenzae* meningitis in Sweden, 1981–1983. Arch Dis Child 62:1220–1223, 1987.
137. Valmari P, Kataja M, Peltola H. Invasive *Haemophilus influenzae* and meningococcal infections in Finland. A climatic, epidemiologic and clinical approach. Scand J Infect Dis 19:19–27, 1987.
138. Peltola H, Kayhty H, Virtanen M, Makela PH. Prevention of *H. influenzae* type b bacteremic infection with the capsular polysaccharide vaccine. N Engl J Med 310:1566–1569, 1984.
139. Spanjaard L, Bol P, Ekker W, Zanen HC. The incidence of bacterial meningitis in The Netherlands—a comparison of three registration systems, 1977–1982. J Infect 11:259–268, 1985.
140. Hanna JN. The epidemiology of invasive *Haemophilus influenzae* infections in children under five years of age in the Northern Territory: A three-year study. Med J Aust 152:234–240, 1990.
141. Hanna JN, Wild BE. Bacterial meningitis in children under five years of age in Western Australia. Med J Aust 155:160–164, 1991.
142. Halfon-Yaniv I, Dagan R. Epidemiology of invasive *Haemophilus influenzae* type b infections in Bedouins and Jews in southern Israel. Pediatr Infect Dis J 9:321–326, 1990.
143. Dagan R, The Israeli Pediatric Bacteremia Meningitis Group. A two-year prospective, nationwide study to determine the epidemiology and impact of invasive childhood *Haemophilus influenzae* type b infection in Israel. Clin Infect Dis 15:720–725, 1992.
144. Hammond GW, Rutherford BE, Malazdrewicz R, et al. *Haemophilus influenzae* meningitis in Manitoba and the Keewatin District, NWT: Potential for mass vaccination. Can Med Assoc J 139:743–747, 1988.
145. Varaghese P. *Haemophilus influenzae* infection, in Canada, 1969–1985. Can Dis Wkly Rep 12:37–43, 1986.
146. Broughton SJ, Warren RE. A review of *Haemophilus influenzae* infections in Cambridge, 1975–1981. J Infect Dis 9:30–42, 1984.
147. Davey PG, Cruikshank JK, McManus IC, et al. Bacterial meningitis—ten years' experience. J Hyg 88:383–401, 1982.
148. Cadoz M, Prince-David M, Mar ID, Denis F. Epidemiologie et prognostic des meningites à *Haemophilus influenzae* en Afrique (901 cas). Pathol Biol 31:128–133, 1983.
149. Bijlmer HA, van Alphen L, Greenwood BM. The epidemiology of *Haemophilus influenzae* meningitis in children under five years of age in The Gambia, West Africa. J Infect Dis 161:1210–1215, 1990.
150. Wright PF. Approaches to prevent acute bacterial meningitis in developing countries. Bull World Health Organ 67:479–486, 1989.
151. Cadoz M, Denis F, Diop Mar I. Étude epidemiologique de cas de meningites purulentes hospitalises à Dakar pendant la decennie 1970–1979. Bull World Health Organ 59:575–584, 1981.
152. Bijlmer HA. Worldwide epidemiology of *Haemophilus influenzae* meningitis; industrialized versus nonindustrialized countries. Vaccine 9(suppl):S5–S9, 1991.
153. Clements DA, Booy R, Dagan R, et al. Comparison of the epidemiology and cost of *Haemophilus influenzae* type b disease in five western countries. Pediatr Infect Dis J 12:362–367, 1993.
154. Hansman D, Hanna J, Morey F. High prevalence of invasive *Haemophilus influenzae* disease in central Australia, 1986 [letter]. Lancet 2:927, 1986.
155. Losonsky GA, Santosham M, Sehgal VM, et al. *H. influenzae* in

the White Mountain Apaches: Molecular epidemiology of a high risk population. Pediatr Infect Dis J 3:539–547, 1984.
156. Coulehan JL, Michaels RH, Williams KE, et al. Bacterial meningitis in Navajo Indians. Public Health Rep 91:464–468, 1976.
157. Coulehan JL, Michaels RH, Hallowell C, et al. Epidemiology of *H. influenzae* type b disease among Navajo Indians. Public Health Rep 99:404–409, 1984.
158. Ostroy PR. Bacterial meningitis in Washington State. West J Med 131:339–343, 1979.
159. Wotton KA, Stiver HG, Hildes JA. Meningitis in the central Arctic: A 4-year experience. Can Med Assoc J 124:887–890, 1981.
160. Gilsdorf JR. Bacterial meningitis in southwestern Alaska. Am J Epidemiol 106:388–391, 1977.
161. Ward JI, Lum MK, Margolis HS, et al. *H. influenzae* disease in Alaskan Eskimos: Characteristics of a population with an unusual incidence of invasive disease. Lancet 1:1281–1285, 1982.
162. Sato T, Wada Y, Okazaki M, et al. Study on septicaemia in infants and children in the past 20 years. Part 1. An analysis of causal organisms [in Japanese]. Kansenshogaku Zasshi 70:775–783, 1996.
163. Kam K, Luey K, Fun SM, et al. Emergency of multiple-antibiotic-resistant *Streptococcus pneumoniae* in Hong Kong. Antimicrob Agents Chemother 25:184–187, 1995.
164. Sato T, Wada Y, Okazaki M, et al. Study on septicaemia in infants and children in the past 20 years. Part 2. An analysis of factors that prescribe for the prognosis [in Japanese]. Kansenshogaku Zasshi 70:784–791, 1996.
165. Hsueh P, Wu J, Hsieu T. Invasive *Streptococcus pneumoniae* infection associated with rapidly fatal outcome in Taiwan. J Formos Med Assoc 95:364–371, 1996.
166. Broome CV, Schlech WF III. Recent developments in the epidemiology of bacterial meningitis. In Sande MA, Smith A, Root RD (eds). Bacterial Meningitis. Edinburgh, Churchill Livingstone, 1985, pp 1–10.
167. Bijlmer HA, van Alphen L. A prospective, population-based study of *Haemophilus influenzae* type b meningitis in The Gambia and the possible consequences. J Infect Dis 165(suppl 1):S29–32, 1992.
168. Farley MM, Stephens DS, Brachman PS, et al. Invasive *Haemophilus influenzae* disease in adults. A prospective, population-based surveillance. Ann Intern Med 116:806–812, 1992.
169. Takala AK, Eskola J, van Alphen L. Spectrum of invasive *Haemophilus influenzae* type b disease in adults. Arch Intern Med 150:2573–2576, 1990.
170. Santosham M, Kallman CH, Neff JM, Moxon ER. Absence of increasing incidence of meningitis caused by *H. influenzae* type b. J Infect Dis 140:1009–1012, 1979.
171. Vadheim CM, Greenberg DP, Bordenave N, et al. Risk factors for invasive *Haemophilus influenzae* type b in Los Angeles county children 18–60 months of age. Am J Epidemiol 136:221–235, 1992.
172. Yost GC, Kaplan AM, Bustamante R, et al. Bacterial meningitis in Arizona American Indian children. Am J Dis Child 140:943–946, 1986.
173. Granoff DM, Shackelford PG, Pandey JP, Boies EG. Antibody responses to *H. influenzae* type b polysaccharide vaccine in relation to Km(1) and G2m(23) immunoglobulin allotypes. J Infect Dis 154:257–264, 1986.
174. Takala AK, Clements DA. Socioeconomic risk factors for invasive *Haemophilus influenzae* type b disease. J Infect Dis 165(suppl 1):S11–S15, 1992.
175. Ounsted C. *H. influenzae* meningitis: A possible ecological factor. Lancet 1:161–162, 1950.
176. Granoff DM, Boies EG, Squires JE, et al. Histocompatibility leukocyte antigen and erythrocyte MNS specificities in patients with meningitis or epiglottitis due to *H. influenzae* type b. J Infect Dis 149:373–377, 1984.
177. Michaels RH, Schultz WF. The frequency of *H. influenzae* infections: Analysis of racial and environmental factors. In Sell SW, Karzon DT (eds). *Haemophilus influenzae.* Nashville, TN, Vanderbilt University Press, 1973, pp 243–250.
178. Lum MK, Ward JI, Bender TR. Protective influence of breast feeding on the risk of developing invasive *H. influenzae* type b disease [abstract]. Pediatr Res 16(pt 2):436, 1982.
179. Takala AK, Eskola J, Palmgren J. Risk factors of invasive *Haemophilus influenzae* type b disease among children in Finland. J Pediatr 115:694–701, 1989.
180. Petersen GM, Silimperi DR, Chiu CY, Ward JI. Effects of age, breast feeding, and household structure on *Haemophilus influenzae* type b disease risk and antibody acquisition in Alaskan Eskimos. Am J Epidemiol 134:1212–1221, 1991.
181. Silfverdal SA, Bodin L, Hugosson S, et al. Protective effect of breast-feeding on invasive *Haemophilus influenzae* infection: A case-control study in Swedish preschool children. Int J Epidemiol 26:443–450, 1997.
182. Goldman AS. The immune system of human milk: Antimicrobial, antiinflammatory and immunomodulating properties. Pediatr Infect Dis J 12:664–671, 1993.
183. Pichichero ME, Sommerfelt AE, Steinhoff MC, Insel RA. Breast milk antibody to the capsular polysaccharide of *Haemophilus influenzae* type b. J Infect Dis 142:694–698, 1980.
184. Insel RA, Amstey M, Pichichero ME. Postimmunization antibody to the *Haemophilus influenzae* type b capsule in breast milk. J Infect Dis 152:407–408, 1985.
185. Casadevall A, Dobroszycki J, Small C, Pirofski L. *Haemophilus influenzae* type b bacteremia in adults with AIDS and at risk for AIDS. Am J Med 92:587–590, 1992.
186. Schlamm HT, Yancovitz SR. *Haemophilus influenzae* pneumonia in young adults with AIDS, ARC, or risk of AIDS. Am J Med 86:11–14, 1989.
187. Steinhart R, Reingold AL, Taylor F, et al. Invasive *Haemophilus influenzae* infections in men with HIV infection. JAMA 268: 3350–3352, 1992.
188. Ward JI, Smith AL. *H. influenzae* bacteremia in children with sickle cell disease. J Pediatr 88:261–262, 1976.
189. Powars D, Overturf G, Turner E. Is there an increased risk of *H. influenzae* septicemia in children with sickle cell anemia? Pediatrics 71:927–931, 1983.
190. Zarkowsky HS, Gallagher D, Gill FM, et al. Bacteremia in sickle hemoglobinopathies. J Pediatr 109:579–585, 1986.
191. Chilcote R, Baehner R, Hammond D. Septicemia and meningitis in children splenectomized for Hodgkin's disease. N Engl J Med 295:798–801, 1976.
192. Rosen FS, Janeway CA. The gamma globulins: III. The antibody deficiency syndromes. N Engl J Med 275:709–715, 1966.
193. Farrand RJ. Recurrent *Haemophilus* septicemia and immunoglobulin deficiency. Arch Dis Child 45:582–584, 1970.
194. Figueroa JE, Densen P. Infectious diseases associated with complement deficiencies. Clin Microbiol Rev 4:359–395, 1991.
195. Ross SC, Densen P. Complement deficiency states and infection: Epidemiology, pathogenesis, and consequences of neisserial and other infections in an immune deficiency. Medicine (Baltimore) 63:243–273, 1984.
196. Siber GR. Bacteremias due to *H. influenzae* and *Streptococcus pneumoniae:* Their occurrence and course in children with cancer. Am J Dis Child 134:668–672, 1980.
197. Bartlett AV, Zusman J, Daum RS. Unusual presentations of *H. influenzae* infections in immunocompromised patients. J Pediatr 102:55–58, 1983.
198. Weitzman S, Aisenberg AC. Fulminant sepsis after the successful treatment of Hodgkin's disease. Am J Med 62:47–50, 1977.
199. Granoff DM, Suarez BK, Pandey JP, Shackelford PG. Genes associated with the G2m(23) immunoglobulin allotype regulate the IgG subclass responses to *Haemophilus influenzae* type b polysaccharide vaccine. J Infect Dis 157:1142–1149, 1988.
200. Lenoir AA, Pandey JP, Granoff DM. Antibody responses of black children to *Haemophilus influenzae* type b polysaccharide—*Neisseria meningitidis* outer-membrane protein conjugate vaccine in relation to the Km(1) allotype. J Infect Dis 157:1242–1245, 1988.
201. Whisnant JK, Mann DL, Rogentine GN, Robbins JB. Human cell-surface structures related to *H. influenzae* type b disease. Lancet 2:895–898, 1971.
202. Whisnant JK, Rogentine GN, Gralnick MA, et al. Host factors and antibody response in *H. influenzae* type b meningitis and epiglottitis. J Infect Dis 133:448–455, 1976.
203. Tejani A, Mahadevan R, Dobias B, et al. Occurrence of HLA types in *H. influenzae* type b disease. Tissue Antigens 17:205–211, 1981.

204. Petersen GM, Silimperi DR, Rotter JI, et al. Genetic factors in *H. influenzae* type b disease susceptibility and antibody acquisition. J Pediatr 110:229–233, 1987.
205. Granoff DM, Pandley JP, Boies EG, et al. Response to immunization with *H. influenzae* type b polysaccharide-pertussis vaccine and risk of *Haemophilus meningitis* in children with the Km(1) immunoglobulin allotype. J Clin Invest 74:1708–1714, 1984.
206. Ambrosino DM, Schiffman G, Gotschlich EC, et al. Correlation between G2m(n) immunoglobulin allotype and human antibody response and susceptibility to polysaccharide encapsulated bacteria. J Clin Invest 75:1935–1942, 1985.
207. Granoff DM, Boies EG, Squires J, et al. Interactive effect of genes associated with immunoglobulin allotypes and HLA specificities on susceptibility to *H. influenzae* disease. J Immunogenet 11:181–188, 1984.
208. Petersen GM, Silimperi DR, Scott EM, et al. Uridine monophosphate kinase 3: A genetic marker for susceptibility to *H. influenzae* type b disease. Lancet 2:417–419, 1985.
209. Myerowitz RL, Norden CW. Immunology of the infant rat experimental model of *H. influenzae* type b meningitis. Infect Immun 16:218–225, 1977.
210. Michaels RH, Myerowitz RL, Klaw R. Potentiation of experimental meningitis due to *Haemophilus influenzae* by influenza virus. J Infect Dis 135:641–645, 1977.
211. David DJ. Influenzal meningitis. Arch Intern Med 4:323–329, 1909.
212. Prevention of secondary cases of *Haemophilus influenzae* type b disease. MMWR Morb Mortal Wkly Rep 31:672–680, 1982.
213. Update: Prevention of *Haemophilus influenzae* type b disease. MMWR Morb Mortal Wkly Rep 37:13–16, 1988.
214. Glode MP, Daum RS, Halsey NA, et al. Rifampin alone and in combination with trimethoprim in chemoprophylaxis for infections due to *Haemophilus influenzae* type b. Rev Infect Dis 5(suppl):S549–S555, 1983.
215. Ward JI, Fraser DW, Baraff LJ, Plikaytis BD. *H. influenzae* meningitis: A national study of secondary spread in household contacts. N Engl J Med 301:122–126, 1979.
216. Fleming DW, Liebenhaut MH, Albanes D, et al. Secondary *H. influenzae* type b in daycare facilities: Risk factors and prevention. JAMA 254:509–514, 1985.
217. Centers for Disease Control and Prevention. Recommendations for use of *Haemophilus influenzae* conjugate vaccines and a combined diphtheria, tetanus, pertussis, and *Haemophilus* b vaccine. Recommendations of the Advisory Committee on Immunization Practices (ACIP). MMWR Morb Mortal Wkly Rep 42(RR-13):1–15, 1993.
218. Osterholm MT, Pierson LM, White KE. The risk of subsequent transmission of *H. influenzae* type b disease among children in day care. N Engl J Med 316:1–4, 1987.
219. Murphy TV, Clements JF, Breedlove JA. Risk of subsequent disease among daycare contacts of patients with systemic *H. influenzae* type b disease. N Engl J Med 316:5–10, 1987.
220. Makintubee S, Istre GR, Ward JI. Transmission of invasive *H. influenzae* type b (Hib) disease in day care settings. J Pediatr 111:180–186, 1987.
221. Broome CV, Mortimer EA, Katz SL. Use of chemoprophylaxis to prevent the spread of *Haemophilus influenzae* b in day care facilities. N Engl J Med 316:1226–1228, 1987.
222. Dashefsky B, Wald E, Li K. Management of contacts of children in day care with invasive *Haemophilus influenzae* type b disease. Pediatrics 78:939–941, 1986.
223. Marks MI, Dorchester WL. Secondary rates of *Haemophilus influenzae* type b disease among day care contacts. J Pediatr 111:305–306, 1987.
224. Bachrach S. An outbreak of *Haemophilus influenzae* type b bacteraemia in an intermediate care hospital for children. J Hosp Infect 11:121–126, 1988.
225. Smith PF, Stricof RL, Shaylgani M. Cluster of *Haemophilus influenzae* type b infections in adults. JAMA 260:1446–1449, 1988.
226. Barton LL, Granoff DM, Barenkamp SJ. Nosocomial spread of *H. influenzae* type b infection documented by outer membrane protein subtype analysis. J Pediatr 102:820–824, 1983.
227. Devine LF, Johnson LF, Johnson DP, et al. Rifampin: Levels in serum and saliva and effect on the meningococcal carrier state. JAMA 214:1055–1059, 1970.
228. McCracken GH Jr, Ginsburg CM, Zweighaft TC, Clahsen J. Pharmacokinetics of rifampin in infants and children: Relevance to prophylaxis against *Haemophilus influenzae* type b disease. Pediatrics 66:17–21, 1980.
229. Glode MP, Daum RS, Goldmann DA, et al. *H. influenzae* type b meningitis: A contagious disease of children. BMJ 280:899–901, 1980.
230. Campos J, Garcia-Tornel S, Roca J, Iriondo M. Rifampin for eradicating carriage of multiply resistant *Haemophilus influenzae* b. Pediatr Infect Dis J 6:719–721, 1987.
231. Cox F, Trincher R, Rissing JP, et al. Rifampin prophylaxis for contacts of *Haemophilus influenzae* type b disease. JAMA 245:1043–1045, 1981.
232. Gessert C, Granoff DM, Gilsdorf J. Comparison of rifampin and ampicillin in day care center contacts of *Haemophilus influenzae* type b disease. Pediatrics 66:1–4, 1980.
233. Daum RS, Glode MP, Goldmann DA, et al. Rifampin chemoprophylaxis for household contacts of patients with invasive infections due to *Haemophilus influenzae* type b. J Pediatr 98:485–491, 1981.
234. Glode MP, Daum RS, Boies EG, et al. Effect of rifampin chemoprophylaxis on carriage eradication and new acquisition of *Haemophilus influenzae* type b in contacts. Pediatrics 76:537–542, 1985.
235. Yogev R, Lander HB, Davis AT. Effect of rifampin on nasopharyngeal carriage of *Haemophilus influenzae* type b. J Pediatr 94:840–841, 1979.
236. Yogev R, Melick C, Kabat K. Nasopharyngeal carriage of *Haemophilus influenzae* type b: Attempted eradication by cefaclor or rifampin. Pediatrics 67:430–433, 1981.
237. Darouiche R, Perkins B, Musher D, et al. Levels of rifampin and ciprofloxacin in nasal secretions: Correlation with MIC90 and eradication of nasopharyngeal carriage of bacteria. J Infect Dis 162:1124–1127, 1990.
238. Committee on Infectious Diseases, American Academy of Pediatrics. *Haemophilus influenzae* infections. In Peter G (ed). 1997 Red Book: Report of the Committee on Infectious Diseases (24th ed). Elk Grove Village, IL, American Academy of Pediatrics, 1997, pp 220–231.
239. Committee on Infectious Diseases, American Academy of Pediatrics. *Haemophilus influenzae* type b conjugate vaccines: Recommendations for immunization with recently and previously licensed vaccines. Pediatrics 92:480–488, 1993.
240. Hansen EJ, Frisch CF, Johnston KH. Detection of antibody-accessible proteins on the cell surface of *H. influenzae* type b. Infect Immun 32:950–953, 1981.
241. Gotoff SP. On the surface of *H. influenzae*. J Infect Dis 143:747–748, 1981.
242. Loeb MR, Smith DH. Human antibody response to individual outer membrane proteins of *H. influenzae* type b. Infect Immun 37:1032–1036, 1982.
243. Inzana TJ, Anderson P. Serum factor-dependent resistance of *H. influenzae* type b to antibody to lipopolysaccharide. J Infect Dis 151:869–877, 1985.
244. Shenep JL, Munson RS, Granoff DM. Human antibody responses to lipopolysaccharide after meningitis due to *H. influenzae* type b. J Infect Dis 145:181–190, 1982.
245. Anderson P, Flesher A, Shaw S. Phenotypic and genetic variation in the susceptibility of *H. influenzae* type b to antibodies to somatic antigens. J Clin Invest 65:885–891, 1980.
246. Lagergard T, Nylen O, Sandberg T, Trollfors B. Antibody responses to capsular polysaccharide, lipopolysaccharide and outer membrane in adults infected with *H. influenzae* type b. J Clin Microbiol 20:1154–1158, 1984.
247. Robbins JB, Schneerson R, Pittman M. *H. influenzae* type b infections. In Germanier R (ed). Bacterial Vaccines. Orlando, FL, Academic Press, 1984, pp 290–313.
248. Robbins JB, Parke JC Jr, Schneerson R, Whisnant JK. Quantitative measurement of "natural" and immunization-induced *H. influenzae* type b capsular polysaccharide antibodies. Pediatr Res 7:103–110, 1973.
249. Tosi MF, Kaplan SL, Mason EO. Generation of chemotactic activity in serum by *H. influenzae* type b. Infect Immun 43:593–599, 1984.
250. Tarr PI, Hosea SW, Brown EJ. The requirement of specific

anticapsular IgG for killing of *H. influenzae* by the alternative pathway of complement activation. J Immunol 128:1772–1775, 1982.

251. Quinn PH, Crosson FJ Jr, Winkelstein JA, Moxon ER. Activation of the alternative complement pathway by *H. influenzae* type b. Infect Immun 16:400–402, 1977.
252. Crosson FJ Jr, Winkelstein JA, Moxon ER. Participation of complement in the nonimmune host defense against experimental *H. influenzae* type b septicemia and meningitis. Infect Immun 14:882–887, 1976.
253. Steele NP, Munson RS, Granoff DM. Antibody-dependent alternative pathway killing of *H. influenzae* type b. Infect Immun 44:452, 1984.
254. Winkelstein JA, Moxon ER. The role of complement in the host's defense against *Haemophilus influenzae*. J Infect Dis 165(suppl 1):S62–S65, 1992.
255. Newman SL, Waldo B, Johnston RB Jr. Separation of serum bactericidal and opsonizing activities for *H. influenzae* type b. Infect Immun 8:488–490, 1973.
256. Hayashi K, Lee DA, Quie PG. Chemiluminescent response of polymorphonuclear leukocytes to *Streptococcus pneumoniae* and *H. influenzae* in suspension and adhered to glass. Infect Immun 52:397–400, 1986.
257. Norden CW. Prevalence of bactericidal antibodies to *H. influenzae*, type b. J Infect Dis 130:489–494, 1974.
258. Feigin RD, Richmond D, Hisler MW. Reassessment of the role of bactericidal antibody in *H. influenzae* infection. Am J Med Sci 262:338–346, 1971.
259. Dahlberg-Lagergard T. Target antigens for bactericidal and opsonizing antibodies to *H. influenzae*. Acta Pathol Microbiol Scand 90:209–216, 1982.
260. Stull TL, Jacobs RF, Haas JE. Human serum bactericidal activity against *H. influenzae* type b. J Clin Microbiol 130:665–672, 1984.
261. Lee CJ, Malik FG, Robbins JB. The regulation of the immune response of mice to *H. influenzae* type b capsular polysaccharide. Immunology 34:149–156, 1978.
262. Schneerson R, Robbins JB. Age-related susceptibility to *H. influenzae* type b disease in rabbits. Infect Immun 4:397–401, 1971.
263. Santosham M, Reid R, Ambrosino DM. Prevention of *H. influenzae* type b (Hib) infections in high-risk infants treated with bacterial polysaccharide immune globulin. N Engl J Med 317:923–929, 1987.
264. Kayhty H, Karanko V, Peltola H, Makela PH. Serum antibodies after vaccination with *H. influenzae* type b capsular polysaccharide and responses to reimmunization: No evidence of immunologic tolerance or memory. Pediatrics 74:857–865, 1984.
265. Anderson P, Smith DH, Ingram DL. Antibody to polyribophosphate of *H. influenzae* type b in infants and children: Effect of immunization with polyribophosphate. J Infect Dis 136:S57–S62, 1977.
266. Smith DH, Peter G, Ingram DL. Responses of children immunized with the capsular polysaccharide of *H. influenzae* type b. Pediatrics 52:637–644, 1973.
267. Anderson P, Peter G, Johnston RB Jr, et al. Immunization of humans with polyribophosphate, the capsular antigen of *H. influenzae*, type b. J Clin Invest 51:39–44, 1972.
268. Robbins JB, Schneerson R, Glode MP. Cross-reactive antigens and immunity to diseases caused by encapsulated bacteria. J Allergy Clin Immunol 56:141–151, 1975.
269. Schneerson R, Robbins JB. Induction of serum *H. influenzae* type b capsular antibodies in adult volunteers fed cross-reacting *Escherichia coli* O75:K100:H5. N Engl J Med 292:1093–1096, 1975.
270. Schreiber JR, Barrus V, Cates KL, Siber GR. Functional characterization of human IgG, IgM and IgA antibody directed to the capsule of *H. influenzae* type b. J Infect Dis 153:8–16, 1986.
271. Kayhty H, Peltola H, Karanko V, Makela PH. The protective level of serum antibodies to the capsular polysaccharide of *H. influenzae* type b. J Infect Dis 147:1100, 1983.
272. Anderson P. The protective level of serum antibodies to the capsular polysaccharide of *H. influenzae* type b [letter]. J Infect Dis 149:1034, 1984.
273. Smith DH, Hann S, Howie VM. Studies on the prevalence of antibodies to *H. influenzae* type b. In Sell SH, Karzon DT (eds). *Haemophilus influenzae*. Nashville, TN, Vanderbilt University Press, 1973, pp 175–185.
274. Kayhty H, Jousimies-Somer H, Peltola H, Makela PH. Antibody response to capsular polysaccharides of groups A and C *Neisseria meningitidis* and *H. influenzae* type b during bacteremic disease. J Infect Dis 143:32–41, 1981.
275. Kayhty H, Schneerson R, Sutton A. Class-specific antibody response to *H. influenzae* type b capsular polysaccharide vaccine. J Infect Dis 148:767, 1983.
276. Kaplan SL, Mason EO, Johnson G. Enzyme linked immunosorbent assay for detection of capsular antibodies against *H. influenzae* type b: Comparison with radioimmunoassay. J Clin Microbiol 18:1201–1204, 1983.
277. Griffiss JM, Bertram MA. Immunoepidemiology of meningococcal disease in military recruits. II. Blocking of serum bacterial activity by circulating IgA early in the course of invasive disease. J Infect Dis 136:733–739, 1977.
278. Musher DM, Goree A, Baughn RE, Birdsall HH. Immunoglobulin A from bronchopulmonary secretions block bactericidal and opsonizing effects of antibody to nontypable *H. influenzae*. Infect Immun 45:36–40, 1984.
279. Rosales SV, Lascolea LJ Jr, Ogra PL. Development of respiratory mucosal tolerance during *H. influenzae* type b infection in infancy. J Immunol 132:1517–1521, 1984.
280. Beuvery EC, Van Rossum F, Nagel J. Comparison of the induction of immunoglobulin M and O antibodies in mice with purified pneumococcal type 3 and meningococcal group G polysaccharides and their protein conjugates. Infect Immun 37:15–22, 1982.
281. Riesen WF, Skvaril F, Braun DG. Natural infection of man with group A streptococci: Levels, restriction in class, subclass, and type, and clonal appearance of polysaccharide-group specific antibodies. Scand J Immunol 5:383–390, 1976.
282. Barrett DJ. Human immune responses to polysaccharide antigens: An analysis of bacterial polysaccharide vaccines in infants. Adv Pediatr 32:139–158, 1985.
283. Jennings HJ. Capsular polysaccharides as human vaccines. Adv Carbohydr Chem Biochem 41:155–208, 1983.
284. Oxelius VA, Berkel AI, Hanson LA. IgG2 deficiency in ataxia-telangiectasia. N Engl J Med 306:515–517, 1982.
285. Oxelius VA. Quantitative and qualitative investigations of serum IgG subclasses in immunodeficiency diseases. Clin Exp Immunol 36:112–116, 1979.
286. Oxelius VA. Chronic infections in a family with hereditary deficiency of IgG2 and IgG4. Clin Exp Immunol 17:19–27, 1974.
287. Schur PH, Borel H, Gelfand EW. Selective gamma-G globulin deficiencies in patients with recurrent pyogenic infections. N Engl J Med 283:631–634, 1970.
288. Shackelford PG, Granoff DM, Nahm MH. Relation of age, race and allotype to immunoglobulin subclass concentrations. Pediatr Res 19:846–849, 1985.
289. Ramadas K, Petersen GM, Heiner DC, Ward JI. Class and subclass antibodies to *H. influenzae* type b capsule: Comparison of invasive disease and natural exposure. Infect Immun 53:486–490, 1986.
290. Shackelford PG, Granoff DM, Nelson SJ, et al. Subclass distribution of human antibodies to *Haemophilus influenzae* type b capsular polysaccharide. J Immunol 138:587–592, 1987.
291. Ambrosino DM, Sood SK, Lee MC, et al. IgG1, IgG2 and IgM reponses to two *Haemophilus influenzae* type b conjugate vaccines in young infants. Pediatr Infect Dis J 11:855–859, 1992.
292. Insel RA, Anderson P, Pichichero ME. Anticapsular antibody to *H. influenzae* type b. In Sell SH, Wright PF (eds). *Haemophilus influenzae*. New York, Elsevier Science Publishing, 1982, pp 155–168.
293. Siber GR, Ambrosino DM. Heavy and light chain restriction of human antibodies to bacterial polysaccharide antigens. In Morell A, Nydegger UE (eds). Clinical Use of Intravenous Immunoglobulins. Orlando, FL, Academic Press, 1986, pp 47–54.
294. Lucas AH, Granoff DM. A major cross-reactive idiotype associated with human antibodies to the *Haemophilus influenzae* b polysaccharide. Expression in relation to age and immunoglobulin G subclass. J Clin Invest 85:1158–1166, 1990.
295. Lucas AH. Expression of cross-reactive idiotypes by human antibodies specific for the capsular polysaccharide of *Haemophilus influenzae* b. J Clin Invest 81:480–486, 1988.
296. Tarrand JJ, Scott MG, Takes PA, Nahm MH. Clonal character-

ization of the human IgG antibody repertoire to *Haemophilus influenzae* type B polysaccharide. Demonstration of three types of V regions and their association with H and L chain isotypes. J Immunol 142:2519–2526, 1989.

297. Scott MG, Crimmins DL, McCourt DW, et al. Clonal characterization of the human IgG antibody repertoire to *Haemophilus influenzae* type b polysaccharide III. A single VkII gene and one of several JK genes are joined by an invariant arginine to form the most common L chain V region. J Immunol 143:4110–4116, 1989.
298. Chung GH, Kim KH, Daum RS, et al. The V-region repertoire of *Haemophilus influenzae* type b polysaccharide antibodies induced by immunization of infants. Infect Immun 63:4219–4223, 1995.
299. Huber BT. B cell differentiation antigens as probes for functional B cell subsets. Immunol Rev 64:57–79, 1982.
300. Davie JM. Antipolysaccharide immunity in man and animals. In Sell SH, Wright PF (eds). *Haemophilus influenzae.* New York, Elsevier Science Publishing, 1982, pp 129–134.
301. Landsteiner K. The Specificity of Serologic Reactions. Cambridge, Harvard University Press, 1945. Reprinted by Dover Publications, New York, 1962.
302. Pandey JP, Fudenberg HH, Virella G. Association between immunoglobulin allotypes and immune responses to *H. influenzae* and meningococcus polysaccharides. Lancet 1:190–192, 1979.
303. Andersson B, Porras O, Hanson LA. Inhibition of attachment of *Streptococcus pneumoniae* and *H. influenzae* by human milk and receptor oligosaccharides. J Infect Dis 153:232–237, 1986.
304. Pichichero ME, Insel RA. Relationship between naturally occurring human mucosal and serum antibody to the capsular polysaccharide of *H. influenzae* type b. J Infect Dis 146:243–248, 1982.
305. Pichichero ME, Hall CB, Insel RA. A mucosal antibody response following systemic *H. influenzae* type b infection in children. J Clin Invest 67:1482–1489, 1981.
306. Pichichero ME, Insel RA. Mucosal antibody response to parenteral vaccination with *H. influenzae* type b capsule. J Allergy Clin Immunol 72:481–486, 1983.
307. Mulks MH, Kornfeld SJ, Bragione B, Plaut AG. Relationship between the specificity of IgA proteases and serotypes in *H. influenzae.* J Infect Dis 146:266–274, 1982.
308. Takala AK, Eskola J, Leinonen M, et al. Reduction of oropharyngeal carriage of *Haemophilus influenzae* type b (Hib) in children immunized with an Hib conjugate vaccine. J Infect Dis 164:982–986, 1991.
309. Murphy TV, Pastor P, Medley F, et al. Decreased *Haemophilus* colonization in children vaccinated with *Haemophilus influenzae* type b conjugate vaccine. J Pediatr 122:517–523, 1993.
310. Takala AK, Santosham M, Almeido-Hill J, et al. Vaccination with *Haemophilus influenzae* type b meningococcal protein conjugate vaccine reduces oropharyngeal carriage of *Haemophilus influenzae* type b among American Indian children. Pediatr Infect Dis J 12:593–599, 1993.
311. Mohle-Boetani JC, Ajello G, Breneman E, et al. Carriage of *Haemophilus influenzae* type b in children after widespread vaccination with conjugate *Haemophilus influenzae* type b vaccines. Pediatr Infect Dis J 12:589–593, 1993.
312. Kauppi M, Eskola J, Kayhty H. Anti–capsular polysaccharide antibody concentrations in saliva after immunization with *Haemophilus influenzae* type b conjugate vaccines. Pediatr Infect Dis J 14:286–294, 1995.
313. Drexhage HA, Van de Plassche EM, Kokje M, Leezenberg HA. Abnormalities in cell-mediated immune functions to *H. influenzae* in chronic purulent infections of the upper respiratory tract. Clin Immunol Immunopathol 28:218–228, 1983.
314. Siber GR, Ambrosino DM, McIver J. Preparation of human hyperimmune globulin to influenzae b, *Streptococcus pneumoniae,* and *Neisseria meningitidis.* Infect Immun 45:248–254, 1984.
315. Ambrosino DM, Schreiber JR, Daum RS, Siber GR. Efficacy of human hyperimmune globulin in prevention of *H. influenzae* type b disease in infant rats. Infect Immun 39:709–714, 1983.
316. Siber GR, Thompson C, Reid GR, et al. Evaluation of bacterial polysaccharide immune globulin for the treatment or prevention of *Haemophilus influenzae* type b and pneumococcal disease. J Infect Dis 165(suppl 1):S129–S133, 1992.
317. Ambrosino DM, Landesman SH, Gorham CC, Siber GR. Passive immunization against disease due to *H. influenzae* type b: Concentrations of antibody to capsular polysaccharide in high-risk children. J Infect Dis 153:1–7, 1986.
318. Letson GW, Santosham M, Reid R, et al. Comparison of active and combined passive/active immunization of Navajo children against *Haemophilus influenzae* type b. Pediatr Infect Dis J 7:747–752, 1988.
319. Carvalho ADA, Giampaglia CMS, Kimura H. Maternal and infant antibody response to meningococcal vaccination in pregnancy. Lancet 2:809–811, 1977.
320. Amstey MS, Insel R, Munoz J, Pichichero M. Fetal-neonatal passive immunization against *H. influenzae* type b. Am J Obstet Gynecol 153:607–611, 1985.
321. Glezen WP, Englund JA, Siber GR, et al. Maternal immunization with the capsular polysaccharide vaccine for *Haemophilus influenzae* type b. J Infect Dis 165(suppl 1):S134–S136, 1992.
322. Englund JA, Glezen WP, Turner C, et al. Maternal immunization with PRP and PRP-conjugate vaccines for passive protection of infants [abstract 68]. In Program and Abstracts of the 31st Interscience Conference on Antimicrobial Agents and Chemotherapy; Chicago IL; September 29–October 2, 1991.
323. Rodrigues LP, Schneerson R, Robbins JB. Immunity to *H. influenzae* type b. I. The isolation and some physicochemical, serologic and biologic properties of the capsular polysaccharide of *H. influenzae* type b. J Immunol 107:1071–1080, 1971.
324. Argaman M, Lin TY, Robbins JB. Polyribitol-phosphate: An antigen of four gram-positive bacteria cross-reactive with the capsular polysaccharide of *H. influenzae* type b. J Immunol 112:649–655, 1974.
325. Crisel RM, Baker RS, Dorman DE. Capsular polymer of *H. influenzae* type b. I. Structural characterization of the capsular polymer of strain Eagan. J Biol Chem 250:4926–4930, 1975.
326. Anderson P, Pichichero ME, Insel RA. Immunization of 2-month old infants with protein-coupled oligosaccharides derived from the capsule of *H. influenzae* type b. J Pediatr 107:346–351, 1985.
327. Makela PH, Peltola H, Kayhty H. Polysaccharide vaccines of group A *Neisseria meningitidis* and *H. influenzae* type b: A field trial in Finland. J Infect Dis 136:S43–S50, 1977.
328. Daum RS, Granoff DM. A vaccine against *H. influenzae* type b. Pediatr Infect Dis J 4:355–358, 1985.
329. Ward JI. Is *H. influenzae* type b disease preventable? JAMA 253:554–556, 1985.
330. Deveikis A, Ward J, Kim KS. Functional activities of human antibody induced by the capsular polysaccharide or polysaccharide-conjugate vaccines against *Haemophilus influenzae* type b. Vaccine 6:14–18, 1988.
331. Milstien JB, Gross TP, Kuritsky JN. Adverse reactions reported following receipt of *Haemophilus influenzae* type b vaccine: An analysis after 1 year of marketing. Pediatrics 80:270–274, 1987.
332. Shapiro ED, Murphy TV, Wald ER, Brady CA. The protective efficacy of *Haemophilus* b polysaccharide vaccine. JAMA 260:1419–1422, 1988.
333. Harrison LH, Broome CV, Hightower AW, et al. A day care–based study of the efficacy of *Haemophilus* b polysaccharide vaccine. JAMA 260:1413–1418, 1988.
334. Osterholm MT, Rambeck JH, White KE, et al. Lack of efficacy of *Haemophilus* b polysaccharide vaccine in Minnesota. JAMA 260:1423–1428, 1988.
335. Black SB, Shinefield HR, Hiatt RA, Fireman BH. Efficacy of *Haemophilus influenzae* type b capsular polysaccharide vaccine. Pediatr Infect Dis J 7:149–156, 1988.
336. Ward JI, Broome CV, Harrison LH, et al. *Haemophilus influenzae* type b vaccines: Lessons for the future. Pediatrics 81:886–893, 1988.
337. Daum RS, Marcuse EK, Giebink GS, et al. *Haemophilus influenzae* type b vaccines: Lessons from the past. Pediatrics 81:893–897, 1988.
338. Murphy TV. *Haemophilus* b polysaccharide vaccine: Need for continuing assessment. Pediatr Infect Dis J 6:701–703, 1987.
339. Granoff DM, Osterholm MT. Safety and efficacy of *Haemophilus influenzae* type b polysaccharide vaccine. Pediatrics 80:590–592, 1987.
340. Parke JC Jr, Schneerson R, Robbins JB, Schlesselman J. Interim report of a controlled field trial of immunization with capsular

polysaccharides of *H. influenzae* type b and group c *Neisseria meningitidis* in Mecklenburg County, North Carolina. J Infect Dis 136(suppl):S51–S56, 1977.

341. Peltola H, Kayhty H, Sivonen A. *Haemophilus influenzae* type b capsular polysaccharide vaccine in children: A double-blind field study of 100,000 vaccinees 3 months to 5 years of age in Finland. Pediatrics 60:730–737, 1977.
342. Committee on Infectious Diseases. *Haemophilus* b polysaccharide vaccine. Pediatrics 76:322–324, 1985.
343. Immunization Practices Advisory Committee. Polysaccharide vaccine for prevention of *Haemophilus influenzae* type b disease. MMWR Morb Mortal Wkly Rep 34:102–105, 1985.
344. Granoff DM, Shackelford PG, Suarez BK. *H. influenzae* type b disease in children vaccinated with type b polysaccharide vaccine. N Engl J Med 315:1584–1590, 1986.
345. Osterholm MT, Jacobs JL, White KE, et al. Efficacy of *Haemophilus influenzae* b plain polysaccharide (PRP) vaccine and conjugate vaccine (PRP-D) in Minnesota [abstract 449A]. In Program and Abstracts of the 30th Interscience Conference on Antimicrobial Agents and Chemotherapy; Atlanta, GA; October 21–24, 1990.
346. Loughlin AM, Marchant CD, Lett S, Shapiro ED. Efficacy of *Haemophilus influenzae* type b vaccines in Massachusetts children 18–59 months of age. Pediatr Infect Dis J 11:374–379, 1992.
347. Avery OT, Goebel WF. Chemo-immunological studies on conjugated carbohydrate-proteins. II. Immunological specificity of synthetic sugar-protein antigen. J Exp Med 50:533–550, 1929.
348. Goebel WF, Avery OT. Chemo-immunological studies on conjugated and carbohydrate-proteins. I. The synthesis of *p*-aminophenol B-glucoside, *p*-aminophenol B-galactoside, and their coupling with serum globulin. J Exp Med 50:521–531, 1929.
349. Schneerson R, Barrera O, Sutton A, Robbins JB. Preparation, characterization, and immunogenicity of *H. influenzae* type b polysaccharide-protein conjugates. J Exp Med 152:361–376, 1980.
350. Gordon LK. Characterization of a hapten-carrier conjugate vaccine: *H. influenzae*--diphtheria conjugate vaccine. In Chanock RM, Lerner RA (eds). Modern Approaches to Vaccines. Cold Springs Harbor, NY, Cold Springs Harbor Laboratory, 1984, pp 393–396.
351. Anderson P. Antibody responses to *H. influenzae* type b diphtheria toxin induced by conjugates of oligosaccharides of the type b capsule with the nontoxic protein CRM_{197}. Infect Immun 39:233–238, 1983.
352. Tai JY, Vella PP, McLean AA, et al. *Haemophilus influenzae* type b polysaccharide-protein conjugate vaccine. Proc Soc Exp Biol Med 184:154–161, 1987.

352a. Harrison LH, Broome CV, Hightower AW, *Haemophilus* Vaccine Efficacy Study Group. *Haemophilus influenzae* type b polysaccharide vaccine: An efficacy study. Pediatrics 84:255–261, 1989.

353. Chu C, Schneerson R, Robbins JB, Rastogi SC. Further studies on the immunogenicity of *H. influenzae* type b and pneumococcal type 6A polysaccharide-protein conjugates. Infect Immun 40:245–256, 1983.
354. Berkowitz CD, Ward JI, Meier K, et al. Safety and immunogenicity of *Haemophilus influenzae* type b polysaccharide and polysaccharide diphtheria toxoid conjugate vaccines in children 15 to 24 months of age. J Pediatr 110:509–514, 1987.
355. Holmes SJ, Murphy TV, Anderson RS, et al. Immunogenicity of four *Haemophilus influenzae* type b conjugate vaccines in 17- to 19-month-old children. J Pediatr 118:364–371, 1991.
356. Decker MD, Edwards KM, Bradley R, Palmer P. Responses of children to booster immunization with their primary conjugate *Haemophilus influenzae* type b vaccine or with polyribosylribitol phosphate conjugated with diphtheria toxoid. J Pediatr 122:410–413, 1993.
357. Lepow ML, Samuelson JS, Gordon LK. Safety and immunogenicity of *H. influenzae* type b polysaccharide–diphtheria toxoid conjugate vaccine in infants 9 to 15 months of age. J Pediatr 106:185–189, 1985.
358. Lepow M, Randolph M, Cimma R. Persistence of antibody and responses to booster dose of *H. influenzae* type b polysaccharide diphtheria toxoid conjugate vaccine in infants immunized at 9 to 15 months of age. J Pediatr 108:882–886, 1986.
359. Kayhty H, Eskola J, Peltola H, et al. Immunogenicity in infants of a vaccine composed of *Haemophilus influenzae* type b capsular polysaccharide mixed with DPT or conjugated to diphtheria toxoid. J Infect Dis 155:100–106, 1987.
360. Eskola J, Kayhty H, Peltola H. Antibody levels achieved in infants by a course of *H. influenzae* type b polysaccharide/diphtheria toxoid conjugate vaccine. Lancet 1:1184–1186, 1985.
361. Decker MD, Edwards KM, Bradley R, Palmer P. Comparative trial in infants of four conjugate *Haemophilus influenzae* type b vaccines. J Pediatr 120:184–189, 1992.
362. Jakacki R, Luery N, McVerry P, Lange B. *Haemophilus influenzae* diphtheria protein conjugate immunization after therapy in splenectomized patients with Hodgkin disease. Ann Intern Med 112:143–144, 1990.
363. Frank AL, Labotka RJ, Rao S, et al. *Haemophilus influenzae* type b immunization of children with sickle cell diseases. Pediatrics 82:571–575, 1988.
364. Lange B, Jakacki R, Nasab AH, et al. Immunization of leukemic children with *Haemophilus* conjugate vaccine. Pediatr Infect Dis J 8:883–884, 1989.
365. Feldman S, Gigliotti F, Shenep JL, et al. Risk of *Haemophilus influenzae* type b disease in children with cancer and response of immunocompromised leukemic children to a conjugate vaccine. J Infect Dis 161:926–931, 1990.
366. Vadheim CM, Greenberg DP, Marcy SM, et al. Safety evaluation of PRP-D *Haemophilus influenzae* type b conjugate vaccine in children immunized at 18 months of age and older: Follow-up study of 30,000 children. Pediatr Infect Dis J 9:555–561, 1990.
367. D'Cruz OF, Shapiro ED, Spiegelman KN, et al. Acute inflammatory demyelinating polyradiculoneuropathy (Guillain-Barré syndrome) after immunization with *Haemophilus influenzae* type b conjugate vaccine. J Pediatr 115:743–746, 1989.
368. Gross TP, Hayes SW. *Haemophilus* conjugate vaccine and Guillain-Barré syndrome [letter]. J Pediatr 118:161, 1991.
369. Greenberg DP, Vadheim CM, Bordenave N, et al. Protective efficacy of *Haemophilus influenzae* type b polysaccharide and conjugate vaccines in children 18 months of age and older. JAMA 265:987–992, 1991.
370. Frasch CE, Hiner EE, Gross TP. *Haemophilus* b disease after vaccination with *Haemophilus* b polysaccharide or conjugate vaccine. Am J Dis Child 145:1379–1382, 1992.
371. Nelson WL, Granoff DM. Protective efficacy of *Haemophilus influenzae* type b polysaccharide–diphtheria toxoid conjugate vaccine. Am J Dis Child 144:292–295, 1990.
372. Wenger JD, Pierce R, Deaver KA, et al, *Haemophilus influenzae* Vaccine Efficacy Study Group. Efficacy of *Haemophilus influenzae* type b polysaccharide–diphtheria toxoid conjugate vaccine in US children aged 18–59 months. Lancet 338:395–398, 1991.
373. Loughlin AM, Marchant CD, Lett S, Shapiro ED. Efficacy of *Haemophilus influenzae* type b vaccines in Massachusetts children 18 to 59 months of age. Pediatr Infect Dis J 11:374–379, 1992.
374. Eskola J, Kayhty H, Takala AK, et al. A randomized, prospective field trial of a conjugate vaccine in the protection of infants and young children against invasive *Haemophilus influenzae* type b disease. N Engl J Med 323:1381–1387, 1990.
375. Eskola J, Peltola H, Takala AK, et al. Efficacy of *Haemophilus influenzae* type b polysaccharide–diphtheria toxoid conjugate vaccine in infancy. N Engl J Med 317:717–722, 1987.
376. Ward J, Brenneman G, Letson GW, Heyward WL, the Alaska *H. influenzae* Vaccine Study Group. Limited efficacy of a *Haemophilus influenzae* type b conjugate vaccine in Alaska Native infants. N Engl J Med 323:1393–1401, 1990.
377. Eskola J, Peltola H, Kayhty H, et al. Finnish efficacy trials with *Haemophilus influenzae* type b vaccines. J Infect Dis 165(suppl 1):S137–S138, 1992.
378. Jonsdottir KE, Steingrimsson O, Olafsson O. Immunisation of infants in Iceland against *Haemophilus influenzae* type b. Lancet 340:252–253, 1992.
379. Madore DV, Johnson CL, Phipps DC, et al. Safety and immunogenicity of *Haemophilus influenzae* type b oligosaccharide-CRM_{197} conjugate vaccine in infants aged 15 to 23 months. Pediatrics 86:527–534, 1990.
380. Turner RB, Cimino CO, Sullivan BJ. Prospective comparison of the immune response of infants to three *Haemophilus influenzae* type b vaccines. Pediatr Infect Dis J 10:108–112, 1991.

381. Seppala I, Sarvas H, Makela O, et al. Human antibody responses to two conjugate vaccines of *Haemophilus influenzae* type B saccharides and diphtheria toxin. Scand J Immunol 28:471–479, 1988.
382. Rowe JE, Messinger IK, Schwendeman CA, Popejoy LA. Three-dose vaccination of infants under 8 months of age with a conjugate *Haemophilus influenzae* type B vaccine. Milit Med 155:483–486, 1990.
383. Madore DV, Johnson CL, Phipps DC, et al. Safety and immunologic response to *Haemophilus influenzae* type b oligosaccharide-CRM_{197} conjugate vaccine in 1- to 6-month-old infants. Pediatrics 85:331–337, 1990.
384. Kayhty H, Peltola H, Eskola J, et al. Immunogenicity of *Haemophilus influenzae* oligosaccharide-protein and polysaccharide-protein conjugate vaccination of children at 4, 6, and 14 months of age. Pediatrics 84:995–999, 1989.
385. Makela PH, Eskola J, Peltola H, et al. Clinical experience with *Haemophilus influenzae* type b conjugate vaccines. Pediatrics 85:651–653, 1990.
386. Bulkow LR, Wainwright RB, Letson GW, et al. Comparative immunogenicity of four *Haemophilus influenzae* type b conjugate vaccines in Alaska Native infants. Pediatr Infect Dis J 12:484–492, 1993.
387. Ward JI, Chiu CY, Wainwright RB, et al. Lack of suppressive effect of preexisting antibody on immune responses to 5 *H. influenzae* type b conjugate vaccines in young Alaskan infants [abstract 64]. In Program and Abstracts of the 30th Interscience Conference on Antimicrobial Agents and Chemotherapy; Atlanta, GA; October 21–24, 1990.
388. Insel RA, Anderson PW. Response to oligosaccharide-protein conjugate vaccine against *Haemophilus influenzae* type b in two patients with IgG2 deficiency unresponsive to capsular polysaccharide vaccine. N Engl J Med 315:499–503, 1986.
389. Schneider LC, Insel RA, Howie G, et al. Response to a *Haemophilus influenzae* type b diphtheria CRM_{197} conjugate vaccine in children with a defect of antibody production to *Haemophilus influenzae* type b polysaccharide. J Allergy Clin Immunol 85:948–953, 1990.
390. Anderson P, Insel RA. Prospects for overcoming maturational and genetic barriers to the human antibody response to the capsular polysaccharide of *Haemophilus influenzae* type b. Vaccine 6:188–191, 1988.
391. Gigliotti F, Feldman S, Wang WC, et al. Immunization of young infants with sickle cell disease with a *Haemophilus influenzae* type b saccharide-diphtheria CRM_{197} protein conjugate vaccine. J Pediatr 114:1006–1010, 1989.
392. Gigliotti F, Feldman S, Wang WC, et al. Serologic follow-up of children with sickle cell disease immunized with a *Haemophilus influenzae* type b conjugate vaccine during early infancy. J Pediatr 118:917–919, 1991.
393. Rubin LG, Voulalas D, Carmody L. Immunogenicity of *Haemophilus influenzae* type b conjugate vaccine in children with sickle cell disease. Am J Dis Child 146:340–342, 1992.
394. Edwards KM, Decker MD, Porch CR, et al. Immunization after invasive *Haemophilus influenzae* type b disease. Serologic response to a conjugate vaccine. Am J Dis Child 143:31–33, 1989.
395. Steinhoff MC, Auerbach BS, Nelson KE, et al. Antibody responses to *Haemophilus influenzae* type B vaccines in men with human immunodeficiency virus infection. N Engl J Med 325:1837–1842, 1991.
396. Anderson PW, Pichichero ME, Insel RA. Vaccines consisting of periodate-cleaved oligosaccharides from the capsule of *H. influenzae* type b coupled to a protein carrier: Structural and temporal requirements for priming in the human infant. J Immunol 137:1181–1186, 1986.
397. Vella PP, Ellis RW. Immunogenicity of *Haemophilus influenzae* type b conjugate vaccines in infant rhesus monkeys. Pediatr Res 29:10–13, 1991.
398. Granoff DM, Rathore MH, Holmes SJ, et al. Effect of immunity to the carrier protein on antibody responses to *Haemophilus influenzae* type b conjugate vaccines. Vaccine 11(suppl 1):S46–S51, 1993.
399. Tudor-Williams G, Frankland J, Isaacs D, et al. *Haemophilus influenzae* type b conjugate vaccine trial in Oxford: Implications for the United Kingdom. Arch Dis Child 64:520–524, 1989.
400. Black SB, Shinefield HR, Lampert D, et al. Safety and immunogenicity of oligosaccharide conjugate *Haemophilus influenzae* type b (HbOC) vaccine in infancy. Pediatr Infect Dis J 10:92–96, 1991.
401. Paradiso PR, Hogerman DA, Madore DV, et al. Safety and immunogenicity of a combined diphtheria, tetanus, pertussis and *Haemophilus influenzae* type b vaccine in young infants. Pediatrics 92:827–832, 1993.
402. Black S, Shinefield H, Ray P, et al. Safety of combined oligosaccharide conjugate *Haemophilus influenzae* type b (HbOC) and whole cell diphtheria–tetanus toxoids–pertussis vaccine in infancy. Pediatr Infect Dis J 12:981–985, 1993.
403. Black SB, Shinefield HR, Fireman B, et al, the Northern California Kaiser Permanente Vaccine Study Center Pediatrics Group. Efficacy in infancy of oligosaccharide conjugate *Haemophilus influenzae* type b (HbOC) vaccine in a United States population of 61,080 children. Pediatr Infect Dis J 10:97–104, 1991.
404. Black SB, Shinefield HR. Immunization with oligosaccharide conjugate *Haemophilus influenzae* type b (HbOC) vaccine on a large health maintenance organization population: Extended follow-up and impact on *Haemophilus influenzae* disease epidemiology. Pediatr Infect Dis J 11:610–613, 1992.
405. Eskola J, Peltola H, Takala A. Protective efficacy of the *Haemophilus influenzae* type b conjugate vaccine HbOC in Finnish infants [abstract 60]. In Program and Abstracts of the 30th Interscience Conference on Antimicrobial Agents and Chemotherapy; Atlanta, GA; October 21–24, 1990.
406. *Haemophilus* b conjugate vaccines for prevention of *Haemophilus influenzae* type b disease among infants and children two months of age and older. Recommendations of the Advisory Committee On Immunization Practices (ACIP). MMWR Morb Mortal Wkly Rep 40(RR-1):1–7, 1991.
407. Advisory Committee on Immunization Practices. Recommendations for use of *Haemophilus* b conjugate vaccines and a combined diphtheria, tetanus, pertussis, and *Haemophilus* b conjugate vaccine: Recommendations of the Advisory Committee on Immunization Practices (ACIP). MMWR Morb Mortal Wkly Rep 42(RR-13):1–15, 1993.
408. Weinberg GA, Einhorn MS, Lenoir AA, et al. Immunologic priming to capsular polysaccharide in infants immunized with *Haemophilus influenzae* type b polysaccharide–*Neisseria meningitidis* outer membrane protein conjugate vaccine. J Pediatr 111:22–27, 1987.
409. Ahonkhai VI, Lukacs LJ, Jonas LC, Calandra GB. Clinical experience with PedvaxHIB, a conjugate vaccine of *Haemophilus influenzae* type b polysaccharide--*Neisseria meningitidis* outer membrane protein. Vaccine 9(suppl):S38–S41, 1991.
410. Vella PP, Staub JM, Armstrong J, et al. Immunogenicity of a new *Haemophilus influenzae* type b conjugate vaccine (meningococcal protein conjugate) (PedvaxHIB). Pediatrics 85:668–675, 1990.
411. Ahonkhai VI, Lukacs LJ, Jonas LC, et al. *Haemophilus influenzae* type b conjugate vaccine (meningococcal protein conjugate) (PedvaxHIB): Clinical evaluation. Pediatrics 85:676–681, 1990.
412. Shapiro ED, Capobianco LA, Berg AT, Zitt MQ. The immunogenicity of *Haemophilus influenzae* type B polysaccharide--*Neisseria meningitidis* group B outer membrane protein complex vaccine in infants and young children. J Infect Dis 160:1064–1067, 1989.
413. Campbell H, Byass P, Ahonkhai VI, et al. Serologic responses to an *Haemophilus influenzae* type b polysaccharide--*Neisseria meningitidis* outer membrane protein conjugate vaccine in very young Gambian infants. Pediatrics 86:102–107, 1990.
414. Granoff DM, Anderson EL, Osterholm MT, et al. Differences in the immunogenicity of three *Haemophilus influenzae* type b conjugate vaccines in infants. J Pediatr 121:187–194, 1992.
415. Yogev R, Arditi M, Chadwick EG, et al. *Haemophilus influenzae* type b conjugate vaccine (meningococcal protein conjugate): Immunogenicity and safety at various doses. Pediatrics 85:690–693, 1990.
416. Santosham M, Wolff M, Reid R, et al. The efficacy in Navajo infants of a conjugate vaccine consisting of *Haemophilus influenzae* type b polysaccharide and *Neisseria meningitidis* outer-membrane protein complex. N Engl J Med 324:1767–1772, 1991.
417. Sood SK, Ballanco GA, Daum RS. Duration of serum anticapsular antibody after a two-dose regimen of a *Haemophilus influenzae* type b polysaccharide–*Neisseria meningitidis* outer membrane pro-

tein conjugate vaccine and anamnestic response after a third dose. J Pediatr 119:652–654, 1991.
418. Ward JI, Bulkow L, Wainwright R, Chang S. Immune tolerance and lack of booster responses to *Haemophilus influenzae* (Hib) conjugate vaccination in infants immunized beginning at birth [abstract 984]. In Program and Abstracts of the 32nd Interscience Conference on Antimicrobial Agents and Chemotherapy; Anaheim, CA; October 11–14, 1992.
419. Weinberg GA, Granoff DM. Immunogenicity of *Haemophilus influenzae* type b polysaccharide-protein conjugate vaccines in children with conditions associated with impaired antibody responses to type b polysaccharide vaccine. Pediatrics 85:654–661, 1990.
420. Granoff DM, Chacko A, Lottenbach KR, Sheetz KE. Immunogenicity of *Haemophilus influenzae* type b polysaccharide–outer membrane protein conjugate vaccine in patients who acquired *Haemophilus* disease despite previous vaccination with type b polysaccharide vaccine. J Pediatr 114:925–933, 1989.
421. Granoff DM, Weinberg GA, Shackelford PG. IgG subclass response to immunization with *Haemophilus influenzae* type b polysaccharide–outer membrane protein conjugate vaccine. Pediatr Res 24:180–185, 1988.
422. Gray BM. Opsonophagocidal activity in sera from infants and children immunized with *Haemophilus influenzae* type b conjugate vaccine (meningococcal protein conjugate). Pediatrics 85:694–697, 1990.
423. Schlesinger Y, Granoff DM, Vaccine Study Group. Avidity and bactericidal activity of antibody elicited by different *Haemophilus influenzae* type b conjugate vaccines. JAMA 267:1489–1494, 1992.
424. Stein KE. Thymus-independent and thymus-dependent responses to polysaccharide antigens. J Infect Dis 165(suppl 1):S49–S52, 1992.
425. Advisory Committee on Immunization Practices (ACIP). Update: Report of PedvaxHIB lots with questionable immunogenicity. MMWR Morb Mortal Wkly Rep 41:878–879, 1992.
426. Santosham M, Hill J, Wolff M, et al. Safety and immunogenicity of a *Haemophilus influenzae* type b conjugate vaccine in a high risk American Indian population. Pediatr Infect Dis J 10:113–117, 1991.
427. Dashefsky B, Wald E, Guerra N, Byers C. Safety, tolerability, and immunogenicity of concurrent administration of *Haemophilus influenzae* type b conjugate vaccine (meningococcal protein conjugate) with either measles-mumps-rubella vaccine or diphtheria-tetanus-pertussis and oral poliovirus vaccines in 14- to 23-month-old infants. Pediatrics 85:682–689, 1990.
428. Santosham M, Rivin B, Wolff M, et al. Prevention of *Haemophilus influenzae* type b infections in Apache and Navajo children. J Infect Dis 165(suppl 1):S144–S151, 1992.
429. Vadheim CM, Greenberg DP, Eriksen E, et al. Eradication of *Haemophilus influenzae* type b disease in Southern California. Arch Pediatr Adolesc Med 148:51–56, 1994.
430. Schneerson R, Robbins JB, Parke JC Jr. Quantitative and qualitative analyses of serum antibodies elicited in adults by *H. influenzae* type b and pneumococcus type 6A capsular polysaccharide–tetanus toxoid conjugates. Infect Immun 52:519–528, 1986.
431. Claesson BA, Trollfors B, Lagergard T, et al. Clinical and immunologic responses to the capsular polysaccharide of *Haemophilus influenzae* type b alone or conjugated to tetanus toxoid in 18- to 23-month-old children. J Pediatr 112:695–702, 1988.
432. Claesson BA, Schneerson R, Robbins JB, et al. Protective levels of serum antibodies stimulated in infants by two injections of *Haemophilus influenzae* type b capsular polysaccharide–tetanus toxoid conjugate. J Pediatr 114:97–100, 1989.
433. Holmes SJ, Fritzell B, Guito KP, et al. Immunogenicity of *Haemophilus influenzae* type b polysaccharide–tetanus toxoid conjugate vaccine in infants. Am J Dis Child 147:832–836, 1993.
434. Kayhty H, Eskola J, Peltola H, et al. Antibody responses to four *Haemophilus influenzae* type b conjugate vaccines. Am J Dis Child 145:223–227, 1991.
435. Vadheim CM, Greenberg DP, Partridge S, et al. Effectiveness and safety of an *Haemophilus influenzae* type b conjugate vaccine (PRP-T) in young infants. Pediatrics 92:272–279, 1993.
436. Fritzell B, Plotkin SA. Efficacy and safety of a *Haemophilus influenzae* type b capsular polysaccharide–tetanus protein conjugate vaccine. J Pediatr 121:355–362, 1992.
437. Parke JC Jr, Schneerson R, Reimer C, et al. Clinical and immunologic responses to *Haemophilus influenzae* type b–tetanus toxoid conjugate vaccine in infants injected at 3, 5, 7, and 18 months of age. J Pediatr 118:184–190, 1991.
438. Claesson BA, Schneerson R, Lagergard T, et al. Persistence of serum antibodies elicited by *Haemophilus influenzae* type b–tetanus toxoid conjugate vaccine in infants vaccinated at 3, 5 and 12 months of age. Pediatr Infect Dis J 10:560–564, 1991.
439. Barra A, Cordonnier C, Preziosi M, et al. Immunogenicity of *Haemophilus influenzae* type b conjugate vaccine in allogeneic bone marrow recipients. J Infect Dis 166:1021–1028, 1992.
440. Kaplan SL, Duckett T, Mahoney DH Jr, et al. Immunogenicity of *Haemophilus influenzae* type b polysaccharide–tetanus protein conjugate vaccine in children with sickle hemoglobinopathy or malignancies, and after systemic *Haemophilus influenzae* type b infection. J Pediatr 120:367–370, 1992.
441. Gibb D, Spoulou V, Giacomelli A, et al. Antibody responses to *Haemophilus influenzae* type b and *Streptococcus pneumoniae* vaccines in children with human immunodeficiency virus infection. Pediatr Infect Dis J 14:129–135, 1995.
442. Clemens JD, Ferreccio C, Levine MM, et al. Impact of *Haemophilus influenzae* type b polysaccharide–tetanus protein conjugate vaccine on responses to concurrently administered diphtheria-tetanus-pertussis vaccine. JAMA 267:673–678, 1992.
443. Ferreccio C, Clemens J, Avendano A, et al. The clinical and immunologic response of Chilean infants to *Haemophilus influenzae* type b polysaccharide–tetanus protein conjugate vaccine coadministered in the same syringe with diphtheria-tetanus toxoids–pertussis vaccine at two, four and six months of age. Pediatr Infect Dis J 10:764–771, 1991.
444. Mulholland K, Hilton S, Adegbola R, et al. Randomised trial of *Haemophilus influenzae* type-b tetanus protein conjugate for prevention of pneumonia and meningitis in Gambian infants. Lancet 349:1191–1197, 1997.
445. Vadheim CM, Greenberg DP, Partridge S, et al, UCLA Vaccine Study Group. Effectiveness and safety of an *Haemophilus influenzae* type b conjugate vaccine (PRP-T) in young infants. Pediatrics 92:272–279, 1993.
446. Booy R, Moxon ER, MacFarlane JA, et al. Efficacy of *Haemophilus influenzae* type b conjugate vaccine in Oxford region [letter]. Lancet 340:847, 1992.
447. Booy R, Hodgson S, Carpenter L, et al. Efficacy of *Haemophilus influenzae* type b conjugate vaccine PRP-T. Lancet 344:362–366, 1994.
448. Lagos R, Horwitz I, Toro J, et al. Large scale, postlicensure, selective vaccination of Chilean infants with PRP-T conjugate vaccine: Practicality and effectiveness in preventing invasive *Haemophilus influenzae* type b infections. Pediatr Infect Dis J 15:216–222, 1996.
449. Peltola H, Kilpi T, Anttila M. Rapid disappearance of *Haemophilus influenzae* type b meningitis after routine childhood immunisation with conjugate vaccines. Lancet 340:592–594, 1992.
450. Centers for Disease Control and Prevention. Food and Drug Administration approval of use of *Haemophilus influenzae* type b conjugate vaccine reconstituted with diphtheria-tetanus-pertussis vaccine for infants and children. MMWR Morb Mortal Wkly Rep 42:964–965, 1993.
451. Ward JI, Greenberg DP, Anderson PW, et al. Variable quantitation of *Haemophilus influenzae* type b anticapsular antibody by radioantigen binding assay. J Clin Microbiol 26:72–78, 1988.
452. Peltola H, Eskola J, Kayhty H, et al. Clinical efficacy of the PRP-D vs Hboc conjugate vaccines against *Haemophilus influenzae* type b (Hib) [abstract 975]. In Program and Abstracts of the 32nd Interscience Conference on Antimicrobial Agents and Chemotherapy; Anaheim, CA; October 11–14, 1992.
453. Anderson EL, Decker MD, Englund JA, et al. Interchangeability of conjugate *Haemophilus influenzae* type b vaccines in infants. JAMA 273:849–853, 1995.
454. Scheifele D, Law B, Mitch L, Ochnio J. Study of booster doses of two *Haemophilus influenzae* type b conjugate vaccines including their interchangeability. Vaccine 14:1395–1406, 1996.
455. Kovel A, Wald ER, Guerra N, et al. Safety and immunogenicity of acellular diphtheria–tetanus–pertussis and *Haemophilus* conjugate vaccines given in combination or at separate injection sites. J Pediatr 120:84–87, 1992.

455a. Bewley KM, Schwab JG, Ballanco GA, et al. Interchangeability of *Haemophilus influenzae* type b vaccines in the primary series: Evaluation of a two-dose mixed regimen. Pediatrics 98:898–904, 1996.

456. Mulholland EK, Ahonkhai VI, Greenwood AM, et al. Safety and immunogenicity of *Haemophilus influenzae* type b–*Neisseria meningitidis* group B outer membrane protein complex conjugate vaccine mixed in the same syringe with diphtheria-tetanus-pertussis vaccine in young Gambian infants. Pediatr Infect Dis J 12:632–637, 1993.

457. Watemberg N, Dagan R, Arbelli Y, et al. Safety and immunogenicity of *Haemophilus* type b–tetanus protein conjugate vaccine, mixed in the same syringe with diphtheria-tetanus-pertussis vaccine in young infants. Pediatr Infect Dis J 10:758–763, 1991.

458. Avendano A, Ferreccio C, Lagos R, et al. *Haemophilus influenzae* type b polysaccharide–tetanus protein conjugate vaccine does not depress serologic responses to diphtheria, tetanus, or pertussis antigens when coadministered in the same syringe with diphtheria-tetanus-pertussis vaccine at two, four, and six months of age. Pediatr Infect Dis J 12:638–643, 1993.

459. Granoff DM, Holmes SJ, Osterholm MT, et al. Induction of immunologic memory in infants primed with *Haemophilus influenzae* type b conjugate vaccines. J Infect Dis 168:663–671, 1993.

460. Carlsson RM, Claesson BA, Lagergard T, Kayhty H. Serum antibodies against *Haemophilus influenzae* type b and tetanus at 2.5 years of age: A follow-up of 2 different regimens of infant vaccination. Scand J Infect Dis 28:519–523, 1996.

461. Kurikka S, Kayhty H, Saarinen L, et al. Immunologic priming by one dose of *Haemophilus influenzae* type b conjugate vaccine in infancy. J Infect Dis 172:1268–1272, 1995.

462. Rothstein EP, Madore DV, Long SS, et al. Antibody persistence four years after primary immunization of infants and toddlers with *Haemophilus influenzae* type b CRM_{197} conjugate vaccine. J Pediatr 119:655–657, 1991.

463. Calandra GB, Lukacs LJ, Jonas LC, et al. Anti-PRP antibody levels after a primary series of PRP-OMPC and persistence of antibody titres following primary and booster doses. Vaccine 11(suppl 1):S58–S62, 1993.

463a. Heath PT, Bowen-Morris J, Griffiths H, et al. Antibody persistence after infant immunization with PRP-T. Arch Dis Child 77:488–492, 1997.

464. Booy R, Heath PT, Slack M, et al. Vaccine failures after primary immunisation with *Haemophilus influenzae* type-b conjugate vaccine without booster. Lancet 349:1197–1202, 1997.

465. Granoff DM, Holmes SJ, Belshe RB, et al. Effect of carrier protein priming on antibody responses to *Haemophilus influenzae* type b conjugate vaccines in infants. JAMA 272:1116–1121, 1994.

466. Lieberman JM, Greenberg DP, Wong VK, et al. Effect of neonatal immunization with diphtheria and tetanus toxoids on antibody responses to *Haemophilus influenzae* type b conjugate vaccines. J Pediatr 126:198–205, 1995.

467. Nelson MB, Murphy TF, van Keulen H, et al. Studies on P-6, an important outer-membrane protein antigen of *Haemophilus influenzae*. Rev Infect Dis 10(suppl 2):S331–S336, 1988.

468. Murphy TF, Bartos LC, Campagnari AA, et al. Antigenic characterization of the P-6 protein of nontypable *Haemophilus influenzae*. Infect Immun 54:774–779, 1986.

469. Nelson MB, Apicella MA, Murphy TF, et al. Cloning and sequencing of *Haemophilus influenzae* outer membrane protein P-6. Infect Immun 56:128–134, 1988.

470. van Alphen L, Eijk P, Geelen–van den Broek L, Dankert J. Immunochemical characterization of variable epitopes of outer membrane protein P2 of non-typeable *Haemophilus influenzae*. Infect Immun 59:247–252, 1991.

471. Karasic RB, Beste DJ, To SC, et al. Evaluation of pilus vaccines for prevention of experimental otitis media caused by nontypable *Haemophilus influenzae*. Pediatr Infect Dis J 8:S62–S65, 1989.

472. Broadhurst LE, Erickson RL, Kelley PW. Decreases in invasive *Haemophilus influenzae* diseases in US army children, 1984 through 1991. JAMA 269:227–231, 1993.

473. Murphy TV, White KE, Pastor P, et al. Declining incidence of *Haemophilus influenzae* type b disease since introduction of vaccination. JAMA 269:246–248, 1993.

474. Adams WG, Deaver KA, Cochi SL, et al. Decline of childhood *Haemophilus influenzae* type b (Hib) disease in the Hib vaccine era. JAMA 269:221–226, 1993.

475. Scheifele DW. Recent trends in pediatric *Haemophilus influenzae* type B infections in Canada. Immunization Monitoring Program, Active (IMPACT) of the Canadian Paediatric Society and the Laboratory Centre for Disease Control. Can Med Assoc J 154:1041–1047, 1996.

476. Teare EL, Fairley CK, White J, Begg NT. Efficacy of Hib vaccine. Lancet 344:828–829, 1994.

477. Urwin G, Krohn JA, Deaver-Robinson K, et al. Invasive disease due to *Haemophilus influenzae* serotype f: Clinical and epidemiologic characteristics in the *H. influenzae* serotype b vaccine are. Cin Infect Dis 22:1069–1076, 1996.

478. Kurikka S, Kayhty H, Peltola P, et al. Neonatal immunization response to *Haemophlius influenzae* type b–tetanus toxoid conjugate vaccine. Pediatrics 95:815–822, 1995.

479. Englund JA, Glezen WP, Turner C, et al. Transplacental antibody transfer following maternal immunization with polysaccharide and conjugate *Haemophilus influenzae* type b vaccines. J Infect Dis 171:99–105, 1995.

480. Carlsson RM, Claesson BA, Iwarson S, et al. Antibodies against *Haemophilus influenzae* type b and tetanus in infants after subcutaneous vaccination with PRP-T/diphtheria, or PRP-OMP/diphtheria-tetanus vaccines. Pediatr Infect Dis J 13:27–33, 1994.

481. Livatowski A, Boucher J, Guyot C. Epidemiologie des infections non meningitiques a *Haemophilus influenzae* type b dans deux departments francais. Arch Fr Pediatr 46:181–185, 1989.

482. Voss L, Lennon D, Gillies M. *Haemophilus influenzae* type b disease in Auckland children. N Z Med J 102:149–151, 1989.

483. Ferreccio C, Ortiz E, Astroza L. A population based retrospective assessment of the disease burden resulting from invasive *Haemophilus influenzae* in infants and young children in Santiago, Chile. Pediatr Infect Dis J 9:488–494, 1990.

chapter

12 Measles Vaccine

Stephen C. Redd

Lauri E. Markowitz

Samuel L. Katz

The written history of measles is classically traced to the writings of the Persian physician Rhazes, also known as Abu Becr, who lived during the 10th century.[1–4] However, the disease was apparently recognized as early as the 7th century by such ancients as the Hebrew physician Al Yehudi.[2, 3] Rhazes referred to measles as *hasbah*, which means "eruption" in Arabic.[2, 3] *Rubeola* and *morbilli* are descriptive Latin words first used in the Middle Ages. The latter is a diminutive of *morbus*, meaning "disease," which was reserved to refer to the bubonic plague; *morbilli* referred to a minor disease. "Measles" is probably derived from *mesels*, the anglicized form of *misellus*, which in turn is a diminutive of the Latin word *miser*, meaning miserable and referring to the sufferer of various eruptions or sores. The presence of nonspecific leprous sores was incorrectly identified with the disease called *morbilli* in Latin. Thus, *mesels* came to be equated with the disease and not the sufferer of ill-defined skin lesions.[4]

Rhazes appears to have been the first to make the distinction between measles and smallpox.[3, 4] He considered measles to be a severe disease, "more to be dreaded than smallpox."[3] Although Rhazes did distinguish between the two diseases, he and others still probably considered them to be closely related.[4] Furthermore, although he was aware of the seasonal nature of measles, he did not think the disease was infectious.[3]

As noted by Wilson,[4] the distinction between measles and smallpox was becoming clearer by the beginning of the 17th century when annual bills of mortality in London in 1629 listed the two diseases separately. Thomas Sydenham clearly described the clinical characteristics of measles during this period and believed the disease to be infectious.[3–5] It was, however, Francis Home, a Scottish physician who worked in Edinburgh in the mid-18th century, who truly recognized the infectious nature of the illness in his attempts to prevent it.[6] In 1758, he used an approach similar to variolation, the scarification technique used to induce mild smallpox before jennerian vaccination. The absence of vesicular or pustular lesions, such as those seen in smallpox and from which the variolation material was obtained, presented a challenge to Home. Lacking the knowledge that viremia precedes the rash of measles, he chose to use blood from patients at the peak of their fever and the onset of the rash. Following such a technique, he inoculated 12 children with material from the blood of a measles patient. Ten of them developed a rash that was typical of the disease, preceded by symptoms of upper respiratory infection. This technique came to be known as morbillization but was never widely adopted.

Understanding of the epidemiology of measles was greatly enhanced by the classic investigation of a measles epidemic on the Faroe Islands in 1846 by the young Danish physician Peter Panum.[7] He not only confirmed that measles was contagious but also defined the 14-day interval between exposure and appearance of exanthem, recognized the higher mortality at the extremes of age, and observed that infection provided lifelong immunity.

In 1911, using infected material from acute cases, Goldberger and Anderson[8] transmitted human measles infection to monkeys, clearly demonstrating the existence of an infectious agent or substance responsible for measles. This finding antedated the technology to isolate and culture the measles virus. In 1954, Enders and Peebles[9] successfully isolated the measles virus in human and monkey kidney tissue cultures. Adaptation of the virus to chicken embryos[10] and cultivation in chicken embryo tissue culture[11] paved the road to vaccine development and licensure in 1963.[12–22]

Widespread vaccination of children in this country[23–28] and others[29–42] has had a dramatic effect on the incidence of measles and its associated complications. Reductions in morbidity and mortality have been so great that global eradication has been proposed[43–46] and judged feasible.[47] This would be a fitting end to a disease once confused with smallpox, the first infectious disease eradicated from the world.

This chapter is dedicated to the memory of our friend and colleague, Stephen Preblud, who was responsible in great part for the original version of this chapter.

BACKGROUND

Clinical Description

Usual Clinical Course

The first symptoms of measles occur after a 10- to 12-day incubation period that follows airborne or droplet exposure. If infection occurs after parenteral exposure, the incubation period is shortened by 2 to 4 days.[3, 12, 48–50] Immunosuppressed persons may have a prolonged incubation period.[51] The prodromal stage is heralded by the onset of fever, malaise, conjunctivitis, coryza, and tracheobronchitis (manifesting as cough) and lasts 2 to 4 days. This symptom complex is similar to that seen with any upper respiratory infection. The temperature rises during the ensuing 4 days and may reach as high as 40.6°C (105°F). Koplik spots, the enanthema believed to be pathognomonic of measles, appear on the buccal mucosa 1 to 2 days before the onset of rash and may be noted for an additional 1 to 2 days after rash onset.[52] The rash is an erythematous maculopapular eruption that usually appears 14 days after exposure and spreads from the head (face, forehead, hairline, ears, and upper neck) over the trunk to the extremities during a 3- to 4-day period. The exanthem is usually most confluent on the face and upper body and initially blanches on pressure. During the next 3 to 4 days, the rash fades in the order of its appearance and assumes a nonblanching brownish appearance.

Virus can be isolated from both the nasopharynx and blood during the latter part of the incubation period and during the early stages of rash development.[9, 53] Although virus has been isolated from the urine as late as 4 to 7 days after rash onset,[54] viremia generally clears 2 to 3 days after rash onset in parallel with the appearance of antibody.[55] Individuals with measles are generally considered to be infectious 2 to 4 days before through 4 days after rash onset.

Measles virus infection causes simultaneous activation and suppression of the immune system.[56–61] Measurement of cytokines released during measles suggests activation of $CD8^+$ T cells, which are important for viral clearance, and type 2 $CD4^+$ T cells, which provide optimal antibody production.[61] Recovery from infection is associated with the production of serum and secretory antibodies[55, 62–70] as well as the establishment of cellular immunity.[60, 61, 71–77] Although subclinical infection with boosting of antibody may occur with subsequent exposure,[63, 65] immunity after natural infection is believed to be lifelong.[7, 78]

Complications

The complications associated with measles infection have been the subject of much description and review.[2, 25, 48, 50, 79–100] In industrialized countries, the most commonly cited complications associated with measles infection are otitis media (7 to 9%), pneumonia (1 to 6%), diarrhea (6%), postinfectious encephalitis (1 per 1000 to 2000 cases of measles), subacute sclerosing panencephalitis (SSPE) (1 per 100,000 cases), and death (1.0 to 3.0 per 1000 cases). Complications are likely to be present if the fever has not lysed within 1 to 2 days of rash onset. The risk of serious complications and death is increased in infants and adults.[2, 3, 90, 91, 95, 99] Pneumonia, which is responsible for approximately 60% of deaths, is more common in young patients, whereas acute encephalitis occurs more frequently in adults.[90, 99] Pneumonia may occur as a primary viral pneumonia (Hecht pneumonia) or as a bacterial superinfection, most commonly with staphylococcus, pneumococcus, or typable (encapsulated) *Haemophilus influenzae.* Other described complications include thrombocytopenia, laryngotracheobronchitis, stomatitis, hepatitis, appendicitis and ileocolitis, pericarditis and myocarditis, glomerulonephritis, hypocalcemia, and Stevens-Johnson syndrome.[48, 50] Although it has long been assumed that measles infection exacerbates or activates tuberculosis,[101] it is no longer certain that this is the case.[102]

Measles infection runs a devastating course in children in developing countries, where the mortality rates can be as high as 5 to 15%.[3, 48, 50, 103–119] The rash is intense and often hemorrhagic (black measles), and it resolves after marked desquamation. Inflammation of the mucosa leads to stomatitis and diarrhea. Diarrhea is a frequent cause of death because it may persist long after the acute insult and further aggravate a preexisting malnourished state.[100, 120, 121] Mediastinal and subcutaneous emphysema, keratitis, corneal ulceration, and gangrene of the extremities are not uncommon. The combination of vitamin A deficiency and keratitis results in a high incidence of blindness.[115, 122–124] Secondary bacterial infections, often with staphylococci, produce pustules, furuncles, pneumonia, osteomyelitis, and other pyogenic complications.

SSPE is a rare degenerative central nervous system disease caused by a persistent infection with a defective measles virus.[125–129] The agent has been noted in affected brain tissue by use of antigen detection assays, electron microscopy, polymerase chain reaction (PCR), and in situ RNA hybridization (and has been cultured by cocultivation techniques). Signs and symptoms of mental and motor deterioration begin an average of 7 years after measles infection, which frequently has occurred before the age of 2 years. Patients have progressive personality changes, develop myoclonic seizures and motor disability, lapse into a coma, and die. The average age at onset is 9 years. Males outnumber females 2 to 4:1.[92, 93, 97, 114, 130] Patients with SSPE have high titers of measles-specific antibodies in their sera and cerebrospinal fluid. Measles viruses that have been isolated from affected brain tissue have mutations that prevent normal replication and budding from the host membrane; such mutations can occur in M, H, or F genes of the virus.[126, 131] SSPE occurs as a complication of measles infection with a frequency of about 1 per 100,000 measles cases.

A team of investigators in the United Kingdom has recently suggested an association of exposure to measles (or measles vaccine) and subsequent development of Crohn disease or ulcerative colitis.[132–135] These investigators have concluded that infection with measles virus or measles vaccine virus may result in a persistent infection of the gastrointestinal tract leading to Crohn disease later in life. Other researchers have been unable to replicate the laboratory findings using similar as well as more sensitive and specific methods.[136] Using PCR, the U.K. team has been unable to identify measles virus RNA in specimens in which an immunofluorescence assay, a much less sensitive technique than PCR, has been reported to be positive for measles virus nucleoprotein. This result suggests the possibility of a false-positive interpretation of the immunofluorescence assay. In addition, concerns have been raised about the methods used in the epidemiological studies examining risk of Crohn disease after measles vaccination.[137, 138] An epidemiological study did not find an association with measles vaccination and the development of Crohn disease.[139] In summary, current evidence does not support a causal association between measles or measles vaccine and the subsequent development of Crohn disease.

Infection during pregnancy is associated with an increased risk of miscarriage and prematurity,[140–142] although there is no convincing evidence that maternal infection with measles is associated with congenital malformations.[143, 144] Clinical illness in the newborn after intrauterine exposure follows a shortened incubation period and may vary from mild to severe.[144, 145]

Clinical Variants

The typical course of measles described in the preceding section can be modified by the presence of antibody.[2, 3, 48, 50] This situation usually arises in the infant with residual maternal transplacental antibody or in the individual given immune globulin after exposure in an attempt to abort or attenuate disease.[65, 146–152] Although some individuals have subclinical infection,[153] most will have a mild abbreviated illness that confers lasting immunity.[150, 152, 154] A second clinical measles infection may occur, however, if immunity is incomplete.[2, 50, 155] Typical or modified measles illness may also rarely follow reinfection after either natural infection[156–158] or vaccination.[158–168] Schaffner and colleagues[157] reported a case of typical albeit mild measles in a 16-year-old girl who reportedly had measles 8 years previously. She had a hemagglutination-inhibiting antibody titer of 1:200 on the second day of rash and titers of 1:1600 and 1:320 at 23 days and 6 months after rash onset, respectively. The rapidity of antibody appearance, the high titer achieved, and the absence of immunoglobulin (Ig) M antibody in all of the specimens suggested a secondary immune response. Although reports examining immunity after infection rely on antibody determination, immunity relies heavily on T-lymphocyte memory and function.

Measles infection in the immunocompromised host can be prolonged, severe, and frequently fatal.[169–175] Infection in these persons may occur in the absence of rash.[169, 173, 174, 176] The severity of illness is believed to be due primarily to impaired cell-mediated immunity.[177–180] Two especially severe complications are an acute progressive encephalitis (inclusion body encephalitis)[96, 181, 182] and a characteristic giant cell pneumonia (Hecht pneumonia).[169–172, 183] Measles has been found to be more severe in persons with human immunodeficiency virus (HIV) infection. In the United States, the case-fatality rate was been reported to be as high as 50% in HIV-infected children.[184]

An atypical variant of measles occurred in some recipients of killed measles vaccine who were at risk for developing a severe delayed hypersensitivity reaction after exposure to wild virus.[48, 50, 155, 158, 161, 185–197] Patients with atypical measles lacked antibody to the measles virus F protein[125, 197, 198] and had exaggerated cellular responses to measles antigen.[73, 199] Exposure resulted in an unbalanced response between cellular and humoral immunity with production of extremely high levels of measles-specific circulating antibody.[50, 73, 74, 186, 197] After an incubation period of 1 to 2 weeks, a prodrome consisting of high fever, headache, abdominal pain, myalgia, and cough ensued. In the next 2 to 3 days, an unusual rash erupted on the extremities and spread centripetally. Whereas the exanthem could be erythematous and maculopapular, it was frequently petechial or vesicular and accompanied by edema and was occasionally pruritic. Hepatocellular enzymes were sometimes strikingly elevated. The illness was frequently mistaken for Rocky Mountain spotted fever and had to be differentiated from meningococcemia, Henoch-Schönlein purpura, and drug eruptions.[48, 50, 200, 201] A nodular pneumonitis with pleural effusion was common.[194, 202] In spite of the potential for serious illness, there was only one report of a possible atypical measles–related fatality.[203] This syndrome has also been reported rarely after receipt of live measles vaccine exclusively.[159, 204, 205] Individuals with atypical measles are believed to be noncontagious.[50, 186, 187] On the basis of humoral and cellular immunity studies, they are also thought to be protected from subsequent illness after exposure to measles.[73, 74, 197] The syndrome can probably be prevented by appropriate immunization with live vaccine.[73, 74, 206, 207]

Treatment

A number of preparations such as interferon,[208, 209] thymic humoral factor,[210] thymostimulin,[211] levamisole,[212] ribavirin,[213] and immune globulin[146, 214] have been used to treat measles. None of these is commonly used to treat uncomplicated measles, although limited studies with ribavirin have shown reduced duration of illness.[213] Ribavirin and interferon may be effective in treating severe measles in immunocompromised persons.[215]

High doses of vitamin A have been shown to decrease mortality and morbidity in young children hospitalized with measles in developing countries.[216, 217] The World Health Organization currently recommends vitamin A for children with acute measles.[124] In the United States as well as in developing countries, children with measles have been found to have low levels of serum retinol, and those with more severe illness have lower levels.[218–220] The American Academy of Pediatrics has recommended vitamin A therapy for hospitalized children with measles aged 6 months to 2 years.[221] In addition, vitamin A therapy should be administered to children with measles who are immunosuppressed, who have clinical evidence of vitamin A deficiency, or who have recently immigrated from areas with a high mortality rate from measles.[221]

Antibiotics, in the absence of pneumonia, sepsis, or other signs of a secondary bacterial complication, are not recommended.[222]

Various chemotherapeutic agents have also been used in patients with SSPE in an attempt to treat or at least alter the clinical course of the disease.[129, 223–228] Of these, inosiplex (Isoprinosine) and interferon alfa have been the most extensively studied[225–228]; despite anecdotal evidence of their effectiveness, controlled trials are lacking.

Virology

The measles virus is a spherical, nonsegmented, single-stranded, negative-sense RNA virus with a diameter of 120 to 250 nm.[125, 198, 229] It is a member of the genus *Morbillivirus* in the family Paramyxoviridae and is closely related to the canine distemper, rinderpest, *peste des petits ruminants*, and a recently identified phocine distemper virus of seals.[230, 231] There are six structural proteins. Three are complexed with the RNA and form the nucleocapsid: the phosphoprotein (P), the large protein (L), and the nucleoprotein (N). Three are complexed with the envelope: fusion protein (F), hemagglutinin protein (H), and matrix protein (M).[198] The F and H envelope proteins are glycosylated; the innermost of the three envelope proteins, the M protein, is not. The F and H proteins are responsible for fusion of virus and host cell membranes, allowing viral penetration and hemolysis. Virions enter the cell by binding to the recently identified human cellular receptor CD46,[232, 233] fusing with the membrane, and releasing the nucleocapsid into the cytoplasm. Viral replication takes about 24 hours. After synthesis of viral proteins and RNA, infectious viral particles bud from the cell membrane.

The entire genome of the Edmonston strain of measles virus has been sequenced and is about 16,000 nucleotides in length.[234] Although measles virus is considered a stable virus, sequence analysis of the N, H, P, and M genes has identified differences between wild virus strains as well as differences between wild and vaccine viruses.[235–240] Evolutionary drift in measles viruses in the past 40 years has led to the development of an epidemiological tool to trace measles virus transmission by genetic analysis. For example, the nucleotide sequences of H and N genes from wild-type strains isolated in the United States from 1988 to 1992 differed from those isolated since 1993, suggesting the interruption of transmission of the pre-1993 strain (Fig. 12–1). Comparison of genetic sequences from wild-type strains isolated in the United States with those isolated elsewhere in the world has suggested international importations of measles virus as sources of outbreaks.[241] Eight distinct lineages have been identified through 1997, and despite the wide geographical distribution from which wild-type measles viruses have been collected, these strains differ from each other by no more than 0.5 to 0.6%. The biological significance of these differences is not known[242]; the immune response generated through vaccination appears to protect against all strains.

Measles virus is difficult to culture from clinical specimens and is best isolated in the marmoset lymphocyte cell line B95a,[243] although primary human fetal or infant kidney or primary monkey kidney cells may also be used.[125] However, after initial passage in the laboratory, many other primary and continuous cell lines of both human and nonhuman origin are permissive (e.g., human amnion, human embryonic lung, human carcinoma [HeLa, Hep-2, and KB], and chick embryo).[125, 244, 245]

Measles virus is inactivated rapidly in the presence of sunlight, heat, and extremes of pH.[125] It can, however, be safely stored for long periods at −70°C (−94°F).

In cell cultures, the virus causes two distinct cytopathic effects.[20, 125, 246, 247] The first is formation of multinucleated syncytia (giant cells) containing numerous nuclei of fused cells. This corresponds to the predominant pathological process observed in infected tissues, including skin and Koplik spots.[248] When observed in lymphoid tissue, the giant cells are referred to as Warthin-Finkelday cells, otherwise as epithelial giant cells.[125] Both intracytoplasmic and intranuclear inclusions are characteristic. Whereas this cytopathic effect is characteristic of wild virus isolates, the cytopathic effects of passaged virus may additionally include spindle cell transformation. This difference in cytopathic effects as well as other factors, such as ability to grow in chick embryo fibroblasts, plaque morphology, interferon production, and optimal growth temperature, help differentiate wild virus from attenuated vaccine virus strains.[125, 249–251]

Pathogenesis as It Relates to Prevention

The sequence of events between exposure to measles virus and subsequent primary acute illness in the normal host has been extensively studied, described, and reviewed[48, 50, 79, 80] (Fig. 12–2); it is based on information from both monkeys and humans. First there is localized infection of the respiratory epithelium of the nasopharynx, and possibly of the conjunctivae,[252] with spread to regional lymphatics. Further events then occur in a manner similar to those observed in the Fenner ectromelia–mouse experimental model.[253] Specifically, 2 to 3 days after exposure, there is a primary viremia with further replication of virus at the site of inoculation as well as in regional and distant reticuloendothelial tissue. Then, 5 to 7 days after exposure, there is an intense secondary viremia of 4 to 7 days' duration that leads to infection of and further replication in the skin, conjunctivae, respiratory tract, and other distant organs.[254] The amount of virus in blood and infected tissues peaks 11 to 14 days after exposure and then falls rapidly during the next 2 to 3 days. The characteristic rash is probably a manifestation of a hypersensitivity reaction and may not be seen in persons with suppression of the cell-mediated immune system.

The pathogenesis of measles infection indicates that prevention through immunization could be accomplished by inhibiting replication at and dissemination from the nasopharynx or by inhibiting the viremia that occurs during the incubation period. The first approach requires the presence of local secretory IgA antibody

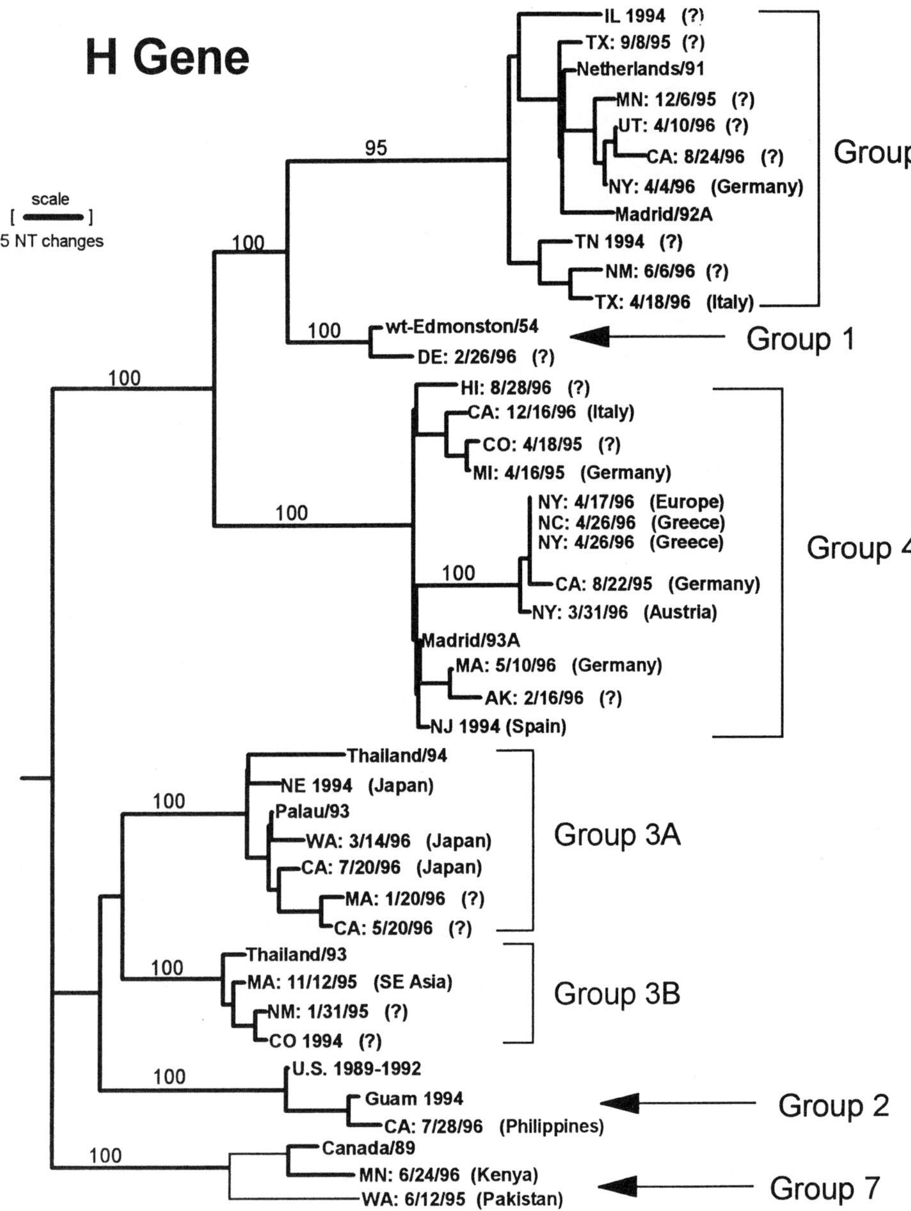

Figure 12–1. Genetic relationship of hemagglutinin gene from measles viruses. Horizontal distance is proportional to genetic relatedness.

or transudated IgG[255, 256]; the second approach requires circulating antibody, either actively or passively acquired, to neutralize the virus. Although infection can be prevented solely after administration of antibody,[146–152] induction of cellular immunity would also seem to be desirable.[3, 251] Children with primary agammaglobulinemia do not have more severe measles infections than do children with normal immune systems, and both develop long-lasting immunity after infection.[178, 179] These observations indicate that the cell-mediated immune system alone is adequate to prevent measles.

On re-exposure, it is uncertain whether prevention of the primary viremia is necessary or even feasible, but it is obvious that the secondary viremia should be prevented. In fact, an initial limited replication and the circulation of a small amount of viral antigen may be necessary to restimulate the immune system and to elicit an anamnestic antibody response.

Diagnosis

Measles should be suspected in children who present with an acute erythematous rash and fever, preceded by a 2- to 4-day prodrome of cough, coryza, conjunctivitis, and photophobia. Recent experience suggests that clinical measles may be difficult to distinguish from other causes of febrile rash illness, particularly in areas where the incidence of measles has been low. Clinical features that support the diagnosis of measles include the following: the presence of Koplik spots, the characteristic 2 to 4 days of intensifying prodromal symptoms, the progression of the rash from the head to the trunk and out to the extremities, and the lysis of fever shortly after the appearance of the rash. Healthcare providers working in measles endemic areas may be more familiar with these clinical findings than are healthcare providers working in areas with a low incidence of measles. A clinical case

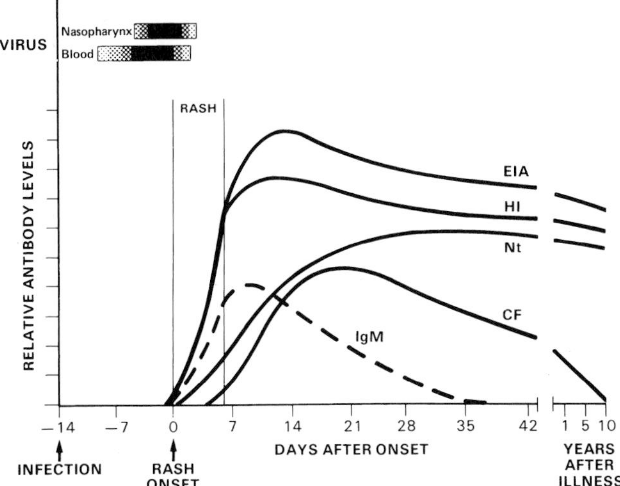

Figure 12–2. Schematic of immune response in acute measles infection. EIA, enzyme immunoassay; HI, hemagglutination; Nt, neutralization; CF, complement fixation; IgM, immunoglobulin M.

definition for epidemiological purposes is the presence of rash lasting 3 or more days; a temperature of 38.4°C (101°F) or higher, if it is measured; and cough, conjunctivitis, or coryza.[257] Its use for clinical diagnosis is limited particularly because of the criterion requiring at least 3 days of rash before the diagnosis is made. Many other illnesses can also meet this clinical definition. In some parts of the world, a less specific clinical definition is being used for epidemiological purposes, not requiring 3 days' duration of rash. Laboratory tests are necessary to confirm the diagnosis, especially when measles is rare. In the United States, it is recommended that clinicians obtain a blood or other suitable specimen for laboratory confirmation from all patients suspected of having measles, unless the patient is part of an already documented measles outbreak.

Although virus isolation, direct cytological examination of clinical material, or demonstration of virus antigen can be used to diagnose measles,[53, 54, 258–263] detection of measles-specific IgM antibody is the most commonly used method. An increase in measles antibodies between acute and convalescent serum specimens is also diagnostic but requires the collection of two blood specimens. PCR can be used to identify measles virus RNA in urine, blood, and nasopharyngeal mucus.[264, 265] Because measles is an RNA virus, RNA must be transcribed to DNA before PCR analysis, resulting in a much reduced sensitivity for diagnosing measles compared with diagnosing DNA viruses.[266]

In primary acute infection, detectable antibodies generally appear in the serum within the first few days of rash onset, peak within about 4 weeks, and subsequently decline somewhat but persist for life[48, 50, 62–65, 267–270] (see Fig. 12–2). Both IgG and IgM antibodies are initially produced.[156, 271–274] However, IgG antibodies are detectable long after infection, whereas IgM antibodies are rarely detected after 6 to 8 weeks. Serum and secretory IgA antibodies are also produced.[68–70, 275, 276] Re-exposure usually induces a characteristic anamnestic response with a rapid boosting of IgG antibody; IgM may not be detected after re-exposure with use of some currently available serological assays.[65, 156, 163, 166, 272, 273] If IgM is detected after re-exposure, it will be at a lower ratio to IgG than the IgM to IgG ratio in a previously unexposed person.[277]

The tests for complement fixation (CF), hemagglutination inhibition (HI), and neutralization (Nt) have been the traditionally employed assays to detect antibody.[156] However, the CF has been shown to be less sensitive,[63–65, 78, 278] and the HI and Nt tests have undergone technical modifications over time.[279, 280] The plaque reduction neutralization (PRN) test is one of the most sensitive assays available at this time, but because it is time and personnel intensive, it is generally limited to research work.[280] Fluorescence tests are available,[281] as are enzyme immunoassays (EIA), also referred to as the enzyme-linked immunosorbent assays (ELISA).[282–291] EIA tests have become popular because they are generally sensitive and convenient. Good correlation between HI and Nt antibody has been shown in many studies[292] as well as between EIA and other serological methods for the diagnosis of acute measles.[275, 283, 284, 293]

Historically, the serological diagnosis of measles required the demonstration of a fourfold or greater rise in antibody titer between acute and convalescent sera.[125] With the advent of the EIA test, the diagnosis is based on significant changes in optical density values, because optical density values cannot be directly translated to antibody concentrations or titers.

A single specimen, however, is adequate to detect the presence of IgM antibody.[276, 288, 290, 291] Indirect EIA tests for IgM, in which measles antigen coats the polystyrene plates before serum is added, require that IgG antibodies be removed before testing for IgM can be done. If IgG is not removed before testing, antimeasles IgG can block antimeasles IgM from binding to the antigen on the plate and can therefore cause a false-negative test result for measles. Reduced sensitivity may also occur if IgM antibodies are inadvertently removed at the same time that IgG antibodies are removed. Rheumatoid factor can also bind IgG and cause false-positive results when that IgG is bound to measles antigen on the plate. IgM capture EIAs have recently been developed that do not require removal of IgG and are not affected by rheumatoid factor.[289]

Correct interpretation of serological data depends on proper timing of specimens with regard to rash onset. This is especially important in interpreting negative IgM results. For example, in one study, only 56% (36 of 64) specimens obtained within 5 days of rash onset had IgM compared with 98% of those obtained 6 to 31 days after rash onset.[291] A higher detection rate early in illness, however, has been found with other IgM assays.[288] In one study, the sensitivity of a capture IgM assay was approximately 80% within the first 72 hours after rash onset and rose to 100% between 3 and 14 days after rash onset.[294] This capture EIA is being used as the reference test for measles in laboratories in the United States and the Western Hemisphere.

In the United Kingdom, a radioimmunoassay has been developed to detect IgM antibodies in saliva or oral secretions.[295] The test was 92% sensitive and 98% specific compared with serum tests to detect IgM and is routinely used to diagnose measles. Immunoglobulin concentrations in oral secretions are approximately 1% of that found in serum, and in the assessment of sensitivity and specificity, 5 of 77 specimens were unsuitable for testing because they contained no immunoglobulin.[295]

EPIDEMIOLOGY

General Epidemiology

In the absence of an immunization program, measles is an ubiquitous, highly contagious, seasonal disease affecting nearly every person in a given population by adolescence.[2, 3, 296–300] An important exception is island populations, which can remain free of infection for variable periods and then, after reintroduction of the virus, experience epidemic disease that involves all those not affected by the last wave of infection.[3, 7, 78, 82, 85, 87, 298] Thus, whereas peak transmission usually occurs among young children, outbreaks in isolated communities involve many older individuals. This is exemplified by Panum's description of measles on the Faroe Islands, in which the disease affected individuals of all ages who were not affected by the last epidemic that had occurred 65 years previously.[7]

Measles is transmitted primarily from person to person by large respiratory droplets but can also be spread by the airborne route as aerosolized droplet nuclei.[2, 3, 301–304] The period of maximal contagion occurs during the prodrome.[8, 48, 50, 88] Secondary attack rates in susceptible household (and institution) contacts are high and can be on the order of 90% or greater.[49, 63, 267, 305–307] Because virus is excreted before and after the appearance of rash, the onset of exanthem in secondary household cases occurs an average of 14 to 15 days (range of 7 to 18 days) after that in the index case.[306] Almost all primary infections (except those modified by maternal antibody or parenteral immune globulin) are thought to be clinically overt.[2, 3] Asymptomatic transmission from exposed immune persons has not been demonstrated.[308] Although susceptible monkeys may contract measles, there is no significant animal reservoir.[3, 48, 125]

Before the introduction of vaccines in most developed countries, school-aged children had the highest risk of infection and accounted for the largest proportion of cases.[2, 3, 25, 296] However, in dense urban areas, transmission among preschoolers took on greater importance.[296, 309] Although serious complications did occur, they were relatively rare compared with the situation in developing countries. In the United States before the introduction of vaccine in 1963, major epidemics occurred approximately every 2 to 3 years.[2, 3, 25, 310–312] Each year, disease peaked in late winter and early spring. The highest occurrence of disease was in children 5 to 9 years of age who accounted for more than 50% of reported cases (Table 12–1). More than 95% of cases had occurred by age 15 years.[2, 3, 296] The highest risk of death was in children younger than 1 year and in adults.[2, 90, 91]

The measles virus is so contagious that it can be expected to circulate wherever a relatively large number of susceptibles congregate, even in the face of a low population susceptibility rate.[3] This explains the outbreaks that were typical among military recruits before the institution of routine measles vaccination.[313] Outbreaks among high-school and college students, most of whom have been vaccinated, demonstrate the virus's capability to seek out the small number of remaining susceptibles.[313–318]

Before widespread vaccination, in many developing countries, the average age at infection was much lower than that observed in developed countries.[3, 103–114] In some areas of Africa, more than 50% of 2-year-old and 100% of 4-year-old children may be expected to have had measles. Poor nutrition and rapid loss of maternal antibody may explain why a greater proportion of these infants are susceptible at an earlier age than are those in developed areas.[292, 319–325] Infection, in turn, results partly from the early age at which infants are exposed to the community at large and prolonged excretion of virus from malnourished children.[107, 109] This is in contrast to developed countries where infants are usually homebound until they enter daycare or school. Although the young age at infection contributes to the high risk of serious complications and death, malnutrition, especially vitamin A deficiency, may also be an important factor leading to the marked severity of measles in the developing world because of defects in cellular (and possibly humoral) immunity.[115, 326] However, there is some evidence that crowding, which leads to an increased dose of virus, may be a more significant determinant of the severity of infection than is malnutrition.[327–330]

Significance as a Public Health Problem

Although remarkable control of measles has been achieved in some areas of the world,[42, 331] measles is

Table 12–1. **AGE DISTRIBUTION AND MEAN ANNUAL INCIDENCE OF REPORTED MEASLES CASES BY AGE GROUP FROM FOUR REPORTING AREAS,* 1960 TO 1964, REPRESENTING PREVACCINE YEARS, AND FROM THE ENTIRE UNITED STATES FOR THREE TIME INTERVALS, 1981 TO 1988, 1989 TO 1991, 1993 TO 1996**

	1960–1964		1981–1988		1989–1991		1993–1996	
AGE (yr)	Total (%)	Cases/100,000	Total (%)	Cases/100,000	Total (%)	Cases/100,000	Total (%)	Cases/100,000
0–4	37.2	766.0	31.9	4.9	43.6	43.7	29.1	0.84
5–9	52.8	1236.9	11.7	1.8	10.4	10.4	9.9	0.28
10–14	6.5	169.1	19.7	3.3	9.2	9.8	12.9	0.36
≥15	3.4	10.0	35.6	0.6	36.9	3.5	48.1	0.12

*New York City, District of Columbia, Illinois, and Massachusetts.

still the leading cause of vaccine-preventable deaths in children. Measles is also responsible for much diarrhea, respiratory disease, and blindness in the developing world.[119, 120, 332] In 1996, approximately 1.67 million measles-associated deaths were prevented because of the impact of vaccination programs. The Global Burden of Disease Study[333] provides data on the public health importance of measles worldwide. In this study, which ranked 107 causes of death among all age groups, measles ranked eighth overall, accounting for 1.1 million deaths worldwide in 1990 and 1 million in 1996.

In the United States in the prevaccine era, approximately 500,000 cases of measles were reported each year, but in reality, an entire birth cohort of approximately 4 million persons was infected annually.[28] Associated with these cases were an estimated 500 deaths; 150,000 cases with respiratory complications; 100,000 cases of otitis media; 48,000 hospitalizations; 7000 seizure episodes; and 4000 cases of encephalitis, which left up to one quarter of patients permanently brain damaged or deaf.[28] On the basis of a 1985 dollar value, the annual cost was in excess of $670 million.[334] Using a 1992 dollar value, the annual estimated costs of measles in 1994 in the absence of vaccination would have been $2.2 billion in direct costs and $1.6 billion in indirect costs.[335]

PREVENTION THROUGH PASSIVE IMMUNIZATION

Immune Globulin

Administration of antibody has the disadvantage that the immunity conferred is only temporary (approximately 3 to 4 weeks, assuming that neither modified nor typical disease occurs).[148, 149, 336] However, there are certain situations in which immediate and relatively reliable prophylaxis against measles is desirable. These situations include exposure of children younger than 1 year, pregnant women, immunocompromised patients, and other susceptible persons with a contraindication to the receipt of live vaccine. Such recommendations are derived from studies indicating that immune globulin administered in doses ranging from 0.05 to 0.5 mL/kg within 6 days after recognized exposure to a case of measles is effective in modifying or preventing subsequent disease.[146–152] Based on data from Janeway, appropriate administration of immune globulin in a dose of 0.22 mL/kg after intimate exposure prevented measles in 80% of cases with less than 5% of cases resembling typical measles.[149]

Current recommendations are to administer immune globulin intramuscularly in a dose of 0.25 mL/kg within 6 days of exposure.[206, 207] The dose should be increased to 0.50 mL/kg for immunocompromised persons. The maximum dose in all cases is 15 mL. In the absence of disease, vaccine should be administered 5 to 6 months later, depending on the dose administered,[337] as long as the patient is at least 12 months of age and there are no contraindications to vaccination.

Intravenous Immune Globulin

Although there are no specific recommendations regarding the use of intravenous immune globulin (IVIG) after measles exposure, information on its potential efficacy is useful for patients who regularly receive this globulin preparation. This may be especially important for persons with the acquired immunodeficiency syndrome (AIDS) who are exposed to measles.[338] Information published by the manufacturers of the various IVIG preparations indicates that they contain varying titers of measles antibodies, but all preparations have a minimum titer based on the same standard that is used for immune globulin (D. Tankersby, personal communication, 1987). Because the standardization process also takes into account the difference in the protein content of IVIG and immune globulin (approximately 5 g/100 mL for IVIG and 16.5 g/100 mL for immune globulin), IVIG can be administered in the same dose as immune globulin expressed as milligrams of protein/per kilogram of body weight (41.25 mg/kg [165 mg/mL × 0.25 mL/kg] for normal individuals and 82.5 mg/kg [165 mg/mL × 0.5 mL/kg] for immunocompromised persons). Thus, the higher doses (e.g., 100 to 400 mg/kg) commonly used for the immunocompromised should be more than sufficient to prevent measles.

PREVENTION THROUGH ACTIVE IMMUNIZATION

Vaccine Strains

Origin and Development

After the isolation and propagation of measles virus in tissue culture by Enders and Peebles[9] in 1954, vaccine development, testing, and licensure quickly followed.[12–22] The Edmonston strain, named after the youth from whom the virus was isolated, was used for many of the vaccines developed worldwide[339–364] (Fig. 12–3). To make the now famous Edmonston B vaccine, Enders and colleagues[13, 20, 251] further passaged the Edmonston strain at 35 to 36°C (95 to 96.8°F) 24 times in primary kidney cells and 28 times in primary human amnion cells, adapted it to chicken embryos (6 passages), and then passaged it in chicken embryo cells. This attenuated Edmonston B vaccine was licensed in the United States in March 1963 along with another Edmonston B virus strain that had been adapted to primary dog kidney cells.[365–368] Although the administration of the Edmonston B vaccine was associated with a high rate of fever (temperature of 39.4°C [103°F] or higher) (20 to 40%) and rash (approximately 50%), the recipients remained remarkably well (Fig. 12–4). However, simultaneous administration of a small dose of immune globulin (eventually set at 0.02 mL/kg) reduced the occurrence of high fever and rash by approximately 50%* (see Fig. 12–4). Approximately 18.9 million doses of Edmonston B vac-

*References 267, 346, 350, 351, 365, 366, 369–377.

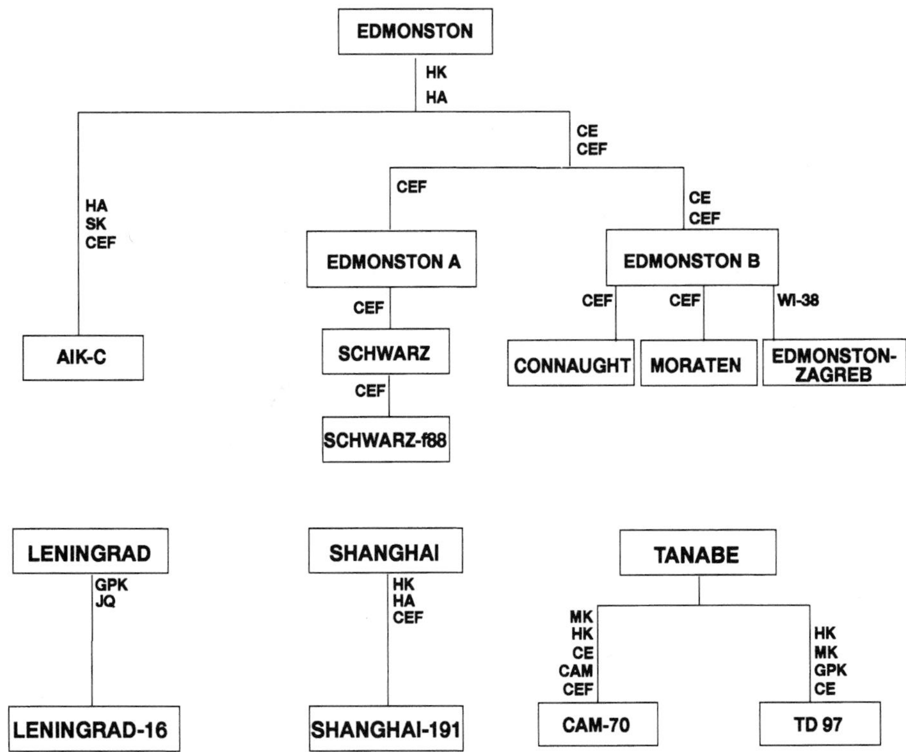

Figure 12–3. Attenuation history of selected measles vaccine strains. Cell cultures in which strains were passed during attenuation: HK, human kidney; HA, human amnion; CE, chick embryo intra-amniotic cavity; CEF, chick embryo fibroblast; WI-38, human diploid cell line; GPK, guinea pig kidney; JQ, Japanese quail; MK, monkey kidney; CAM, chick chorioallantoic membrane; SK, sheep kidney.

cine were administered in the United States between 1963 and 1975 (Table 12–2, Fig. 12–5).

Killed Vaccine

A formalin-inactivated alum-precipitated vaccine derived from the Edmonston strain was also licensed in the United States in 1963 and used until 1967 (see Table 12–2). This vaccine was also used in some provinces in Canada. Usually, three doses of killed vaccine or two doses of killed and one dose of live vaccine were administered at monthly intervals with few side effects.[65, 267, 346, 350, 378–385] Use of killed vaccine was eventually not recommended when it became apparent that this vaccine produced short-lived immunity and placed many recipients at risk for atypical measles infection.[386] It has been estimated that between 600,000 and 900,000 persons in the United States received the 1.8 million doses of killed measles vaccine that were administered[387] (see Table 12–2 and Fig. 12–5).

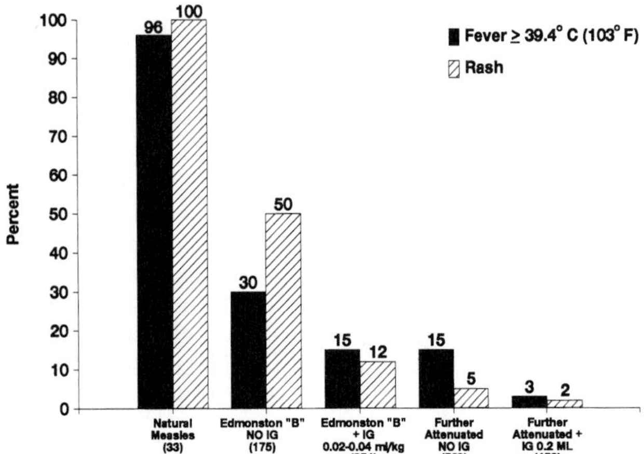

Figure 12–4. Incidence of fever and rash after natural measles infection and vaccination. Number of susceptibles is included in parentheses; IG, immune globulin. (Adapted from Krugman S, Giles JP, Jacobs AM, Friedman H. Studies with a further attenuated live measles-virus vaccine. Pediatrics 31:919–928, 1963. Adapted by permission of Pediatrics.)

Further Attenuated Live Vaccines

Many further attenuated vaccines have been developed and are in active use worldwide (Table 12–3; see also Fig. 12–3). Most were derived from the Edmonston strain. These further attenuated vaccines differ in the viral isolate of origin, the number and temperature of cell culture passages, the type of cell culture used for the passage and production, and whether plaquings were performed during the passages.[13, 20, 354, 359, 360, 364, 388] Although differences in plaque size,[354, 389] subgenomic particles,[390] and temperature sensitivity[391] among the further attenuated vaccine strains have been described, their significance is uncertain. Analysis of the F, H, N, and M genes has found nucleotide sequence differences of no more than 0.6% between the vaccine strains derived from the Edmonston strain.[240] More divergent sequences were found in CAM-70 and S-191, non–Edmonston-derived vaccines. Mori[391] sequenced the entire genome of the AIK-C vaccine and found only 56 nucleotide differences, from a total of 15,894 bases, compared with the Edmonston sequence. Studies have identified nucleotide sequence substitutions in the H gene that appear

Table 12–2. **HISTORY OF MEASLES VACCINE MANUFACTURE AND DISTRIBUTION IN THE UNITED STATES, 1963 TO 1990**

VACCINE	STRAIN	MANUFACTURER	BRAND	YEARS IN USE	DOSES DISTRIBUTED
Inactivated	—	Lilly Pfizer	Generic Pfizer Vax, Measles-K	1963–1967	1.8 million
Live attenuated	Edmonston B	Lederle Lilly Merck Parke Davis Pfizer Philips Roxane	M-Vac Generic Rubeovax Generic Pfizer-vax, Measles-L Generic	1963–1975	18.9 million
Live further attenuated	Schwarz Moraten	Pitman Moore–Dow Merck	Lirugen Attenuvax	1965–1976 1968 to present	>205 million

Adapted from Hayden GF. Measles vaccine failure. A survey of causes and means of prevention. Clin Pediatr 18:155–167, 1979.

to mediate some of the biological characteristics of the Moraten strain of vaccine.[392]

Two further attenuated live measles vaccines derived from the Edmonston strain were licensed in the United States, the Schwarz strain in 1965 and the Moraten strain in 1968 (see Table 12–2 and Fig. 12–3). The Schwarz vaccine was derived from Edmonston virus passaged an additional 85 times at 32°C (89.6°F) in chicken embryo cells.[393–398] The Moraten strain was also passaged at this lower temperature but only an additional 40 times.[399] Compared with the Edmonston B vaccine, the frequency and severity of side effects attributed to these and other further attenuated vaccines were significantly lower[267, 346–352, 393–400] (see Fig. 12–4). A temperature of 39.4°C (103°F) or higher occurred in only 5 to 15% and rash in only 3 to 5% of vaccinees. Simultaneous administration of specially titered immune globulin in a low dose (0.02 mL/kg, 0.1 mL, or 0.2 mL) further reduced the incidence of high fever and rash to approximately 3% each[267] (see Fig. 12–4). These doses of immune globulin did not interfere with seroconversion, but the peak geometric mean antibody titer was lower than that observed without immune globulin administration. The further attenuated vaccines were intended for use without immune globulin.[401]

The Moraten vaccine (Attenuvax, Merck) is now the only measles vaccine used in the United States; the Schwarz vaccine is the predominant product in many other nations.[358] Several different further attenuated measles vaccines, including AIK-C, Schwarz F88, CAM-70, and TD97, have been developed and are being used in Japan.[359, 360, 364, 388] The vaccine developed by Smorodintsev (Leningrad-16) was introduced in Russia in 1967 and was the principal vaccine virus strain in eastern Europe.[356] The CAM-70 and TD97 vaccines were derived from the Tanabe strain.[364, 388] These vaccines, as well as those in use in China since 1965,[361] are the few not derived from the Edmonston virus.

Whereas most measles vaccines were attenuated and are produced in chick embryo fibroblasts, a few currently used vaccines were attenuated in human diploid cells. The Edmonston-Zagreb vaccine, used extensively in Yugoslavia since 1969, was derived from the Edmonston strain and underwent additional passage in WI-38

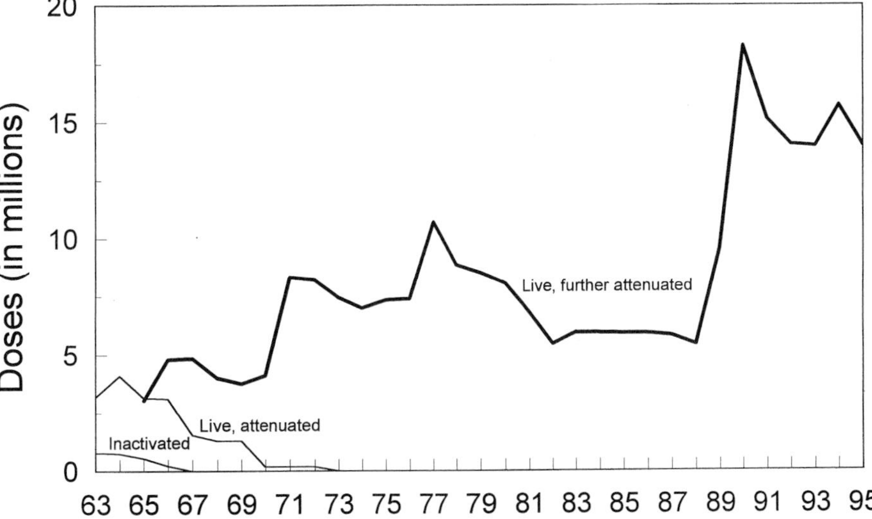

Figure 12–5. Doses of measles virus vaccine distributed, by vaccine type, United States, 1963 to 1995. Live attenuated, Edmonston B; live, further attenuated, Schwarz and Moraten combined.

Table 12–3. **MEASLES VACCINE MANUFACTURERS AND VACCINE STRAINS PRODUCED**

MANUFACTURER	VACCINE STRAIN
Merck, United States	Moraten
RIVM Netherlands	Moraten
Connaught Laboratories, Canada	Connaught
National Institute of Health, Pakistan	Connaught
SmithKline Beecham, Belgium	Schwarz
Pasteur Mérieux–Connaught, France	Schwarz
Evans, United Kingdom	Schwarz
Chiron, Italy	Schwarz
Dong Shin Pharmaceutical, Korea	Schwarz
Institute of Sera and Vaccines, Czechoslovakia	Schwarz
Cantacuzino Institute, Romania	Schwarz
Takeda Chemical Industries, LTD, Japan	Schwarz F88
Swiss Serum and Vaccine Institute, Switzerland	Edmonston-Zagreb
Serum Institute of India, India	Edmonston-Zagreb
Institute of Immunology, Croatia	Edmonston-Zagreb
Gerencia General de Biologicos y Reactivos, Mexico	Edmonston-Zagreb
Research Foundation for Microbial Diseases, Japan	CAM-70
BioManguinhos, Brazil	CAM-70
Perum BioFarma, Indonesia	CAM-70
The Kitasato Institute, Japan	AIK-C
The Razi State Serum Institute, Iran	AIK-HDC*
Chiba-Serum, Japan	TD97
D. Mazay, Russia	Leningrad-16†
Research Institute of Infectious and Parasitic Diseases, Bulgaria	Leningrad-16
National Vaccine and Serum Institute, China	Shanghai-191
Lanzhou Institute of Biological Products, China	Changchun-47
Shanghai Institute of Biological Products, China	
Wuhan Institute of Biological Products, China	
Chengdu Institute of Biological Products, China	

*AIK-C vaccine produced in human diploid cells.
†Not currently in production.

cells.[354] This vaccine is now produced by several other manufacturers (see Table 12–3). Other vaccine strains have been adapted to MRC-5 and R-17 human diploid cells in Iran[357, 362] and in China.[361]

Dosage and Route of Administration

According to current regulations in the United States, measles vaccine must contain at least 1000 median tissue culture infective doses ($TCID_{50}$) at the end of the expiration date of the vaccine.[402] This dose is administered in 0.5 mL. The minimum dose required to immunize a seronegative child has been found to be as low as 20 $TCID_{50}$ in some studies but higher in others.[403–406] The dose in the commercial product is designed to compensate for some of the virus deterioration that may result either from improper storage or reconstitution or from exposure to light or heat before injection.

The recommended route of administration is subcutaneous injection. Although there are only limited data on the intramuscular route, it appears to be as effective as subcutaneous vaccination.[407] Studies with the Edmonston B and further attenuated vaccines have examined the effectiveness of other routes of administration, such as intranasal and conjunctival inoculation.[12, 16, 49, 256, 365, 366, 408–410] Most of the results were not favorable. In contrast, aerosol administration, which was evaluated during the early 1960s and 1970s in Japan, the former Soviet Union, and the United States, showed promising results.[410] More recently, studies have been undertaken to determine whether aerosol administration of measles vaccine could overcome maternal antibody and immunize younger infants.[410–418] Many of these studies have found the Edmonston-Zagreb vaccine strain to be more immunogenic than the Schwarz strain when it is administered by aerosol. However, whereas some investigators reported high seroconversion rates after administration by this route in young infants,[411–414, 416] others found it inferior to subcutaneous administration.[415] The aerosol route is not being used routinely.

Combination with Rubella and Mumps Vaccines

In the United States, vaccination against measles is most often accomplished with combined live vaccines that also contain attenuated rubella and mumps vaccine viruses. Such combined vaccines were licensed in the United States in 1971. They contain at least 1000 $TCID_{50}$ of the measles Moraten strain, at least 5000 $TCID_{50}$ of the mumps Jeryl Lynn strain, and at least 1000 $TCID_{50}$ of the RA27/3 strain of rubella vaccine virus. The RA27/3 strain of rubella virus replaced the HPV-77:DE-5 strain as the rubella component in 1979. Currently, the only licensed measles, mumps, rubella (MMR) vaccine is produced by Merck (MMR II). Measles vaccine is also available in a measles-rubella formulation (M-R-VAX II, Merck). More combination products are being developed as other countries consider vaccinating children against rubella or mumps along with measles.[33–36, 39, 419, 420] For example, SmithKline produces a vaccine that contains Schwarz measles vaccine, RIT 4385 mumps vaccine strain (derived from the Jeryl Lynn strain), and the RA27/3 strain of rubella vaccine. SmithKline also produces a combined vaccine that contains the Schwarz measles vaccine, the Urabe mumps vaccine, and the RA27/3 rubella vaccine. Mérieux produces a combined formulation with Schwarz measles vaccine, Urabe mumps vaccine, and RA27/3 rubella vaccine. In Japan, several formulations of combined vaccines are available, including one containing the AIK-C measles virus, the Hoshino mumps virus, and the Takahashi rubella virus.[421] Two other combined vaccines are also licensed, one containing the CAM-70 measles strain and one the Schwarz F88 strain. A triple vaccine with the Edmonston-Zagreb strain of measles vaccine is being produced by the Institute of Immunology, Zagreb,[422] the Swiss Serum Institute,[424] and the Serum Institute of India.

Safety and immunogenicity data indicate that combining the measles antigen with rubella and mumps antigens is both safe and effective.[419–441]

Production and Constitution of Vaccine

Preparation methods for the Merck vaccine provide generally applicable information regarding the production and constitution of measles vaccines.[442] Although there are minor differences in dose, antibiotic content, and other details among manufacturers, there are no reports of significant differences in side effects or vaccine efficacy.

The vaccine virus is cultured in primary chick embryo cells. After an initial cell growth phase, the cultures are inoculated with the further attenuated Moraten strain of measles virus. After several days' incubation at 32°C (89.6°F), the cells are washed to remove fetal bovine serum and the medium is replaced with one containing 50 μg/mL of neomycin, sucrose, buffered salts, amino acids, and human albumin. Fluids containing virus can be removed from the cultures for a period of time as the cells are maintained at the same temperature. These fluids are frozen until determinations of the virus titer have been performed on retained aliquots. Harvested virus fluids having sufficient virus potency and satisfactorily passing tests are thawed, pooled, sampled for safety testing, clarified, dispensed, and refrozen.

When bulk vaccine has passed all quality control tests, portions of the vaccine are thawed, dispensed into vials, and lyophilized. At the time of use, the vaccine is reconstituted with fluid (sterile distilled water) provided by the manufacturer. The use of a preservative-containing reconstitution fluid is not recommended for general use because it may inactivate the vaccine. Each vaccine dose contains approximately 25 μg of neomycin. Sorbitol and hydrolyzed gelatin are added as stabilizers. When reconstituted with the provided diluent, the vaccine is clear and yellow in color.

In 1996, the existence of reverse transcriptase in several vaccines that were grown in chick embryo fibroblast tissue culture was reported, including measles vaccine,[443] by use of a new and highly sensitive technique to detect the reverse transcriptase activity. With use of similar assays, other laboratories have confirmed the existence of the reverse transcriptase activity.[444] In a subsequent study, evidence was found that this reverse transcriptase activity is associated with the endogenous avian retrovirus EAV-0.[445] Extensive efforts to identify a transmissible virus have failed to link the reverse transcriptase activity with a transmissible virus. Because retroviruses are highly species restricted, these findings represent no apparent risk to vaccine recipients.[446]

Stability of Vaccine

Measles vaccine is extremely stable between −70°C (−94°F) and −20°C (−4°F).[405, 447] Although measles vaccine is affected adversely by higher temperatures, the introduction of more heat stable vaccines in 1979 has led to increased stability under normal working conditions, which is especially important in the developing world.[448] In the United States, manufacturers must demonstrate that a minimum titer of 1000 $TCID_{50}$ is maintained at the end of the dating period when the vaccine is stored at 2 to 8°C. The World Health Organization has a requirement that lyophilized measles vaccine, after exposure to 37°C for at least 1 week, cannot lose more than 1 $\log_{10}$ and must maintain a titer of at least 1000 $TCID_{50}$.[449]

For the currently available vaccine in the United States, when it is stored at 2 to 8°C (35.6 to 46.4°F), a minimum titer of 1000 $TCID_{50}$ can be maintained in unreconstituted vaccine for 2 years or more. This potency can be maintained for 8 months at room temperature and 4 weeks at 37°C (98.6°F). Reconstituted vaccine loses 50% potency in 1 hour at 20 to 25°C (68 to 77°F) and almost all its potency when it is held at 37°C (98.6°F) for 1 hour. Vaccine is also sensitive to sunlight; however, colored glass vials further minimize loss of potency. Notwithstanding its improved thermostability, the vaccine still needs to be handled with care according to the recommendations of the manufacturer.

As stated in the package insert, Merck recommends that its product be shipped at a temperature of 10°C (50°F) or less and stored, before reconstitution, at 2 to 8°C (35.6 to 46.4°F) and protected from sunlight. After reconstitution, the product should be kept in a dark place at 2 to 8°C (35.6 to 46.4°F) and used within 8 hours.

Results of Vaccination

The Immune Response

The immune response after successful vaccination is similar in almost all respects to that noted after natural infection. Although the interval between vaccination and an immune response is a few days shorter than that observed after natural infection,[12, 45, 46, 52] immunization induces both humoral[22, 65, 68, 70, 267] and cellular[73, 74, 76] immunity and the production of interferon.[450–452]

Laboratory evidence of immunity is most conveniently documented by use of antibody assays because tests for cell-mediated immunity are not standardized. However, even with antibody assays, results of studies on vaccine-induced immunity may vary depending on the sensitivity of the antibody assay used.* Although the presence of antibodies detected by HI, ELISA, or CF correlates with immunity, neutralizing antibodies are probably most important in clinical protection.[2, 3, 63, 78, 292]

IgG, IgM, and IgA antibodies can be detected in both serum and nasal secretions.[68, 70, 156, 272, 274, 462] IgM antibody can be detected in the serum between 3 and 4 weeks after vaccination and disappears soon thereafter.[156, 272, 274, 463] Although only small amounts of IgA have been detected in serum, IgA is the predominant antibody found in nasal secretions.[68, 70] Although detectable serum IgA and IgM antibodies are transient, IgG antibodies

*References 63–65, 78, 278, 280–284, 286, 453–461.

Table 12–4. **ANTIBODY RESPONSE 21 TO 28 DAYS AFTER MEASLES VACCINATION WITH OR WITHOUT IMMUNE GLOBULIN***

VACCINATION REGIMEN	TOTAL NUMBER	SEROCONVERSION (%)	GMT†
Edmonston B Vaccine			
Alone	171	96	—
	27	—	1:208
Immune globulin, 0.02 mL/kg	185	99	1:96
Further Attenuated Vaccine‡			
Alone	121	99	1:56
Immune globulin, 0.1 mL total	89	95	1:32
Immune globulin, 0.2 mL total	452	98	1:32
Immune globulin, 0.02 mL/kg	193	95	1:24

*Neutralizing titer of 1:400/0.1 mL.
†Complement fixation assay geometric mean titer.
‡Schwarz strain.
Adapted from Krugman S, Giles JP, Jacobs AM, Friedman H. Studies with live attenuated measles-virus vaccine. Am J Dis Child 103:353–363, 1962; and Krugman S, Giles JP, Jacobs AM, Friedman H. Studies with a further attenuated live measles-virus vaccine. Pediatrics 31:919–928, 1963.

generally persist for many years. The antibody titers elicited by vaccination do decline over time (as do those induced by natural infection) and may become undetectable.* Vaccine-induced antibody titers are typically lower than those induced by natural infection. Vaccine-induced immunity is subject to boosting on challenge, by either vaccine or wild virus; likewise, similar boosting can be observed after natural infection.† Thus, as discussed in more detail later, immunization usually provides immunity as solid as that induced by natural infection.

Although many investigators have described the initial antibody response elicited by live measles vaccination, the studies by Krugman[65, 153, 267–270] serve as an excellent example. Depending on the antibody assay used (CF, HI, or Nt), antibodies first appear between 12 (HI and Nt) and 15 (CF) days and peak 21 to 28 days after vaccination. Although antibodies were detected in 95% or more of susceptible vaccinees, regardless of the vaccine strain, the CF geometric mean titer did vary by strain of vaccine (Table 12–4). The geometric mean titer for children 1 month after receipt of Edmonston B vaccine alone, Edmonston B vaccine plus immune globulin, Schwarz vaccine, and Schwarz vaccine with immune globulin were 1:208,[153] 1:96, 1:56, and 1:24 to 1:32, respectively.[267] The titer observed in 33 children 1 month after natural infection was 1:128.[267] Hilleman and colleagues[399] also noted a difference in the geometric mean titer by vaccine strain using the HI assay (Table 12–5). Although 98% or more of vaccinees seroconverted, the HI geometric mean titer associated with the Edmonston B vaccine was 1:25, whereas that noted after vaccination with either the Schwarz or Moraten further attenuated strains was 1:16. Despite these differences in geometric mean titer, receipt of these vaccines was associated with a markedly reduced risk of infection that did not decrease over time.[65, 268–270]

Measles-specific cell-mediated immunity after live attenuated vaccine has seldom been studied because of the lack of a simple in vitro assay. With the importance that cell-mediated immunity plays in natural infection,[60, 177–180] it would seem that successful vaccination would stimulate such immunity. In studies that have been conducted, cell-mediated immune responses after live attenuated vaccine appear to be similar to but less pronounced than those after natural infection.[177–180, 470] For example, Gallagher and coworkers[76] reported that a positive lymphocyte stimulation index was noted in 9 of 9 subjects with natural immunity and in 10 of 16 vaccinees. More recently, Pabst[471] found good correlation between antibody titers and lymphoproliferative responses in 124 children receiving their first dose of MMR. Ward[472] studied revaccinated children and found good lymphoproliferative responses after revaccination, even among those whose antibody titers dropped to low levels. In vitro cytotoxic T lymphocyte responses have been detected after vaccination but are lower than those after natural infection.[473] It appears that both wild and vaccine infection result in a biphasic immune response beginning with transient production of interleukin-2 and interferon-γ followed by more sustained production of interleukin-4. First, $CD8^+$ T cells are activated, which are important for viral clearance. Later, beginning about the time of rash onset, $CD4^+$ T cells are activated and are involved in antibody production.[61] These responses by the cell-mediated immune system correspond to an initial Th1-type response with a shift to a Th2-type response.

*References 65, 268–270, 440, 454, 460–462, 464–469.
†References 63, 65, 159, 268–270, 397, 462, 467, 468.

Table 12–5. **ANTIBODY RESPONSE 28 DAYS AFTER ATTENUATED AND FURTHER ATTENUATED MEASLES VACCINE**

VACCINE	TOTAL NUMBER	SEROCONVERSION (%)	GMT*
Edmonston B†	258	99	1:25
Schwarz‡	250	98	1:16
Moraten‡	273	98	1:16

*Hemagglutination inhibition assay.
†Attenuated vaccine.
‡Further attenuated vaccine.
Adapted from Hilleman MR, Buynak EB, Weibel RE, et al. Development and evaluation of the Moraten measles virus vaccine. JAMA 206:587–590, 1968.

Vaccination suppresses cell-mediated immune function (as does natural infection).[101, 470, 474–480] This manifests in vitro as suppression of lymphocyte stimulation or in vivo as suppression of cutaneous delayed hypersensitivity to various antigens. Fireman and colleagues[476, 481] noted suppressed cellular immune function up to 4 weeks after administration of live vaccine. Suppression did not occur after receipt of killed vaccine. Recent data suggest that this suppression is due to down-regulation of interleukin-12, which is needed for cell-mediated immunity.[482] Although there was concern initially that this temporary suppression of cellular immunity might be harmful, for example, in patients with unrecognized tuberculosis,[102] it is now clear that there is no such risk.[483–485]

One would assume that the presence of a rash after parenteral injection of vaccine would be associated with viremia. The generalized stimulation of T and B lymphocytes after vaccination also suggests viremia. Few studies documented viremia after vaccination. Early studies with the canine cell vaccine isolated vaccine virus from blood,[365, 367] and more recently, van Binnendijk and colleagues[486] have isolated Schwarz strain vaccine virus from monkeys 7 to 9 days after vaccination. There are no reports of isolation of vaccine virus from blood in normal humans.[12–14, 19, 49] Although Mitus and associates[169] did isolate vaccine virus from the throat and conjunctivae of a susceptible leukemic patient who died of giant cell pneumonia after administration of Edmonston B vaccine, they failed to isolate virus from the blood. The apparent difficulty of isolating vaccine virus may reflect the low level of viremia after vaccination.

Because wild virus is so highly transmissible, both virological and clinical studies with susceptible contacts were conducted in early vaccine investigations.[12, 14–19, 49, 365, 367] These studies showed no evidence of virus excretion by vaccinees. Although sensitivity of methods to isolate virus may have improved since these studies were conducted, person-to-person transmission of vaccine virus has never been documented.

Response to Revaccination

The immune response after revaccination depends on the results of the initial vaccination. Persons who had no response to initial vaccination typically generate a primary immune response to revaccination, with a significant rise in antibody titer and the production of IgM antibody. After revaccination of an individual with some level of immunity, a fourfold or greater rise in antibody may appear sooner than that seen after initial vaccination, but there are no signs of clinical infection.* IgG antibodies are first detected within 5 to 6 days and peak around 12 days. IgM antibodies are not produced. As is the case with immunity after natural infection, these are the characteristics of an anamnestic immune response.[271, 273] Such a boost is more likely to occur in the presence of a low or undetectable preexisting antibody titer, whereas persons with a high level of circulating antibody may not boost.* Krugman and coworkers[65] reported that after revaccination, a significant increase in HI titer occurred in only 1 of 6 children with HI titers of 1:16 or 1:32 but in 25 of 36 children with titers of 1:8 or less. Similar findings were noted in vaccinees exposed to wild virus.

*References 65, 156, 268–270, 272, 274, 460, 461, 469, 487.

*References 65, 159, 268–270, 454, 467–469, 488, 489.

Boosting of antibody titers appears to be transient, with several investigators finding decay of antibody levels to the pre-revaccination level within months to years.[472, 490, 491] In one study in which antibody titers against measles decayed in children with low levels of antibody before revaccination during a 6-month period after revaccination, cellular immunity, measured in a lymphocyte proliferation assay, appeared to persist.[472]

The booster phenomenon is not unique to vaccine-induced immunity. It can also be observed after exposure to measles or after vaccination in persons who have had measles, but it occurs less frequently because antibody titers after natural infection are usually higher than those after vaccination.[63, 65] Stokes and colleagues[63] reported that on re-exposure to wild virus, 6 of 12 naturally immune persons with pre-exposure Nt titers ranging from 1:2 to 1:8 experienced a boost in titer. However, such boosts were not seen in any of 22 individuals with titers between 1:16 and 1:128. These data indicate that subclinical reinfection may occur after both natural infection and successful vaccination.

Studies of the response to revaccination[472, 487, 492–494] have shown that a high proportion of vaccinated persons who lack detectable antibody to measles will respond to the second dose. Among persons initially vaccinated after 12 months of age, at least 90% will respond.

Measures of Protection

The protective effects of measles vaccine have been measured in a variety of ways. Reduction in the occurrence of measles after the introduction of vaccine is one general indicator of vaccine-induced protection. Both Krugman and colleagues[267] and Baba and coworkers[495] noted virtual elimination of measles from a population of institutionalized children after vaccination became routine despite high levels of infection in the surrounding community. Similarly, nationwide surveillance in the United States and other countries with high levels of immunization has documented a significant reduction in reported measles cases since vaccine licensure.[23–41]

Another commonly used method to quantitate the vaccine's protective effect is to compare the risk of infection (i.e., the infection rate or attack rate) in unvaccinated and vaccinated persons and to measure vaccine efficacy.[496, 497] Refer to Chapter 44 for a detailed discussion of vaccine effectiveness.

Calculation of vaccine efficacy can be useful in those situations in which vaccine coverage is high, as it is in the United States. Because the proportion of cases that are vaccinated is also high, it may appear erroneously that vaccine failure is a problem.[498–500] However, approximately 50% of cases can be expected to be vaccinated with vaccine efficacy and vaccine coverage each 90%.[25, 496] This proportion increases to 60% with a 95% coverage rate. The majority of available data indicate vaccine efficacy in the United States of 90 to 95% or greater,[501] consistent with seroconversion data.

Protection can also be documented by examining the immune response and clinical outcome of vaccinees challenged with either wild or vaccine virus.* Such challenges most often result in an anamnestic immune response in the absence of clinical disease.

Despite the fact that any detectable measles antibody has been interpreted as evidence of protection after vaccination, the development of more sensitive antibody tests[280] has raised concerns that low levels of antibody, although indicating previous exposure to wild or vaccine virus,[460] may not be protective. Some persons with low but detectable levels of measles antibody (<1:120) by PRN have been found to be susceptible to clinical measles reinfection.[504] Although it is likely that many persons with low antibody titers will not develop disease after exposure, available data suggest that these low levels of antibody may not be fully protective.

Host Factors Affecting Protection

The quality and durability of measles vaccine–induced immunity is dependent on a number of factors that relate both to the vaccine and to the host.[269, 498] In considering factors affecting protection, it is important to distinguish between primary vaccine failure, that is, a failure to seroconvert after vaccination, and secondary vaccine failure, that is, loss of protection after demonstrated seroconversion.

Maternal Antibody and Age at Vaccination. A number of host factors may be responsible for primary vaccine failure. The most important and well described is maternal antibody. Passively acquired measles antibodies may neutralize vaccine virus before a complete immune response develops. The most common sources of these antibodies are maternal, immune globulin, and other blood products. The presence of maternally derived transplacental antibody is particularly important in evaluating the immunogenicity of live measles vaccine in early childhood.[292, 505]

As noted by Orenstein and colleagues,[505] recommendations for the age at vaccination must balance two factors: (1) the earliest age at which high rates of seroconversion can be obtained and (2) the age group with the greatest risk of severe infection.[505] A balance must be met that optimizes vaccine-induced protection while minimizing the risk of morbidity and mortality that would occur by delaying vaccination.[292, 323] The age at vaccination that achieves this balance is lower in developing countries than in developed nations because of the increased risk of measles exposure and because of earlier loss of maternally derived antibody. The reasons for the variation in duration of passive protection from maternal antibody have been reviewed by Black[292] and include differences in (1) levels of measles antibody in mothers, (2) efficiency of transport of IgG across the placenta, and (3) rate of loss of passively acquired antibody by the infant.

*References 65, 158, 159, 161–164, 270, 460, 461, 467–469, 490, 502, 503.

Early in the clinical investigations of live measles virus vaccine, it was recognized that maternal antibody interfered with seroconversion by in vivo neutralization of vaccine virus before adequate replication had occurred.[498] On the basis of data available at the time, it appeared that maternal antibody rarely persisted beyond 7 months of age and that an adequate immune response could be achieved if vaccination was limited to infants 9 months of age and older.[63, 65, 456, 458, 506, 507] Whereas only 60 to 70% of infants younger than 9 months seroconverted, 95% or more of older infants produced antibodies.[22, 505] Accordingly, when vaccine was licensed in 1963, the recommended age for routine vaccination was 9 months.[508]

In the first few years after licensure, it became apparent, however, that maternal antibodies actually persisted in many infants until 11 months of age.[65, 455, 456, 459] On the basis of these data, vaccination before 1 year would be expected to be associated with a high risk of primary vaccine failure and subsequent infection in exposed vaccinees.* Thus, in 1965, the recommended age for vaccination was raised to 12 months.[401] The importance of this change is illustrated by Krugman's data that only 86% of 123 infants 9 months of age seroconverted after administration of Edmonston B vaccine and immune globulin compared with 97% of 899 vaccinated at 12 months of age or older.[268]

In 1965, it was also recommended that children vaccinated before 1 year of age be revaccinated because a large proportion of these children were susceptible and were expected to respond well to revaccination. A number of studies confirmed these findings,[469, 509, 510, 515, 516] but there are also some data indicating that early vaccination may alter the immune response after revaccination. Wilkins and Wehrle[458] first raised concerns by reporting that 19 (51.4%) of 37 children who did not respond when they were initially vaccinated at 6 to 10 months of age did not have detectable HI antibodies 8 months after revaccination. All 37 did, however, have detectable Nt antibody. Similarly, Linnemann and colleagues[481] reported that 29 (40.3%) of 72 children vaccinated before 10 months of age were HI negative at a mean of 4.8 years after revaccination. In contrast, Lampe and colleagues[503] did not find any difference in seroconversion rates in children vaccinated once at 15 months of age or later compared with children revaccinated after first being vaccinated before 1 year of age. Using an EIA assay, Murphy and colleagues[517] observed high seroprevalence rates at a mean of 6 months after vaccination in 302 children revaccinated after early vaccination and in 300 vaccinated once at 15 months of age or older (98% for both groups). However, they did observe that the titers in the revaccinated group were lower than those in the children vaccinated once. These findings were confirmed by McGraw.[407]

One of the most complete descriptions of an altered

*References 158, 159, 162, 268, 453, 458, 468, 469, 509–514.

immune response is provided by Stetler and colleagues.[461] These authors reported that children revaccinated after an initial vaccination before 1 year had no difficulty seroconverting; post-revaccination HI antibody was detected in 116 (95.9%) of 121 children lacking HI antibody before revaccination. Eight months later, HI antibodies were undetectable in 58 (47.9%); but after retesting with a cytopathic effect neutralization test (CPENt),[248] only 5 (4.2%) of 120 sera were negative. Successful priming in some of the early vaccinees was also suggested by the finding that IgM was detected in the sera of only 22.2% of 63 revaccinated children lacking HI, EIA, and CPENt antibody compared with 74.0% of 50 random control vaccinees. These findings were similar to those noted by Black and coworkers.[502]

Although there may be some alteration of the immune response, the most reliable indicator of the actual effectiveness of revaccination of these children is the evaluation of their risk of infection. Although revaccination may not be 100% effective, available data indicate that revaccination is efficacious.[510, 515, 516, 518] Shasby and colleagues[509] reported that in an outbreak, the attack rate in 73 children vaccinated once before 12 months of age was 35.6%, whereas the attack rate in 55 children revaccinated after 12 months of age was only 1.8%. Davis and coworkers[516] noted that none of 80 students revaccinated after their first vaccination before 12 months of age became infected during an outbreak. For comparison, the attack rate in children vaccinated twice at 12 months of age or older was 1.4% (2 of 138), that in children vaccinated once at 12 months of age or older was 1.8% (21 of 1191), and that in unvaccinated children was 57.1% (4 of 7). Thus, the available data indicate that revaccination of children first vaccinated before 1 year of age will result in good vaccine-induced protection although it may be associated with an altered immune response, manifested as a lower antibody titer. This conclusion is especially important because vaccination of children as young as 6 months with subsequent revaccination is recommended in certain outbreak situations.[206, 207]

The recommended age at vaccination was again changed in 1976 to 15 months from 12 months[519, 520] because newer data indicated that children vaccinated at 15 months of age and older were even more likely to make and maintain antibodies and to be less likely to be infected in outbreak situations than those children vaccinated earlier.[505] Although some studies provide contrary results, examination of data on seroconversion rates and prevalence of antibodies after vaccination indicates that in general, 79 to 89% of children vaccinated at 12 months of age have detectable antibodies compared with 87 to 99% of those vaccinated at 15 months or later.* Similarly, a number of studies measuring the risk of measles in vaccinated and unvaccinated children indicated that measles occurred in children vaccinated at 12 months of age approximately 1.5 to 5.0 times more frequently than in those vaccinated later than 12 months.[505, 509, 514, 525–530]

In 1994, the age of vaccination in the United States was changed again to be between 12 and 15 months.[337] Data on measles antibody titers in umbilical cord blood and in infants suggested that infants may be receiving less maternal antibody than in the prevaccine era because their mothers have lower titers.[471, 512, 524, 531–534] This is because many mothers have either vaccine-induced antibodies or naturally derived antibodies that have not been boosted by repeated exposures. In addition, some mothers may not have had measles or been vaccinated. Because the lower levels of antibody decline earlier, infants are susceptible to disease at a younger age. Higher rates of seroconversion at 12 months have been found in children born to women with vaccine-induced immunity.[531, 534, 535]

Intercurrent Illness and Malnutrition. There is a theoretical concern that interferon produced by an intercurrent infection may interfere with successful vaccination.[468, 536–538] Studies addressing this question, which have been conducted in developing and in developed countries, have produced discordant results. Two studies in developing countries found no differences in seroconversion rates in ill and well children after receipt of measles vaccine.[324, 539] However, a small study in the United States found that 80% of children with rhinorrhea seroconverted, compared with 98% of well children.[540] Subsequent studies conducted in the United States and Canada have found equivalent seroconversion rates among children with upper respiratory infections or mild illness and well children.[541–543] In a study of 128 mildly ill and 258 well children given MMR, seroconversion to measles was 97% in well children compared with 99% in those with mild illnesses, mostly upper respiratory tract infection[543]; no differences were observed in seroconversion to mumps or rubella. A study conducted in Wisconsin found no association of vaccine failure and vaccination during the high-risk season for respiratory infections.[544] One study conducted in Thailand found lower geometric mean titers for children vaccinated at 9 months of age among those who experienced an upper respiratory tract infection in the 2 weeks after vaccination.[545] However, vaccination of mildly ill children and vaccination during the upper respiratory infection season appear to outweigh the theoretical risk of lower seroconversion rates.[546] Several studies have found seroconversion rates in malnourished children similar to those in children who are well nourished.[323, 547, 548]

Immunosuppression. Measles vaccination is not recommended for most immunocompromised patients. However, the increasing number of children with HIV infection, the high risk of severe measles in these children, and few demonstrated side effects to measles vaccine have resulted in recommendations for vaccination. Studies in the United States have found that these children have poor responses to vaccination and lose antibody more quickly after vaccination.[173, 338, 549, 550] Retrospective studies have found that only 12% of 24[173] and 59% of 37[550] vaccinated children had detectable measles antibody. Seroconversion rates in prospective studies range from 33% of 39 children to 60% of 25 children.[184, 549] In the Democratic Republic of Congo, formerly Zaire, seroconversion rates after vaccination at 9 months were 77% in asymptomatic HIV-infected

*References 25, 455–457, 459, 505, 509, 521–524.

children and 36% in symptomatic HIV-infected children (36%).[551] In two other studies in Africa, seroconversion rates after vaccination at 6 months were greater than 75% in HIV-infected children.[552, 553] Children may respond better when they are vaccinated at earlier ages, before they become severely immunocompromised.[550, 554]

Adults who were vaccinated in childhood before becoming infected with HIV appear to retain protective levels of measles antibody. Several studies have documented high seroprevalence of measles antibody in HIV-infected adults in the United States[555, 556] and that antibody levels are maintained, even as immunosuppression progresses.

Other Host Factors. Vitamin A supplementation at the time of measles vaccination has recently been examined. Investigators in Indonesia found a lower rate of seroconversion among children vaccinated at 6 months of age who received supplementary vitamin A compared with children not receiving such a supplement.[557] A subsequent study, conducted in Guinea-Bissau, found similar rates of seroconversion among 9-month-old children receiving and not receiving vitamin A supplements.[558] Although the discordant findings in these two studies remain unexplained, vitamin A supplementation programs should not be modified to separate the timing of measles vaccination and vitamin A supplementation.

Even after receipt of potent vaccine, approximately 2 to 5% of vaccinees will fail to respond for unknown reasons.[22, 65, 267] No genetic factors have been found that predispose a given person to fail repeatedly to respond to the vaccine. However, studies have found an association with one particular HLA type and poor response to measles vaccination.[559] The same investigators also found a similar association with homozygosity for the gene for transport-associated protein 2 and poor response to measles vaccination.[560]

Although there may be some exceptions in the very young,[407, 458, 461, 515, 502] revaccination has been found in both epidemiological and serological studies to induce the same high rate of immune response that follows initial vaccination.*

Vaccine Factors Affecting Protection

Vaccine Antigen and Strain. Although most further attenuated measles vaccines have been found to be equally immunogenic in older children,[399, 411] differences in the ability of vaccine strains to immunize young infants have been reported.[412, 414, 415, 561–566] High measles morbidity and mortality among infants younger than the recommended age for vaccination, 9 months, in developing countries[567–569] has stimulated research on strategies for immunization of younger infants. Sabin and associates[411, 412] in the early 1980s investigated aerosol administration of two measles vaccines, the Edmonston-Zagreb and Schwarz strains.[411, 412] Their finding of higher seroconversion rates after Edmonston-Zagreb than after Schwarz focused attention on this vaccine strain. Several subsequent studies found that the Edmonston-Zagreb strain was more immunogenic than the Schwarz vaccine in this age group. The reasons for these differences are not known.

Vaccine Dose. Small doses of vaccine can effectively immunize older infants and children; however, the dose of vaccine administered has been shown to be important in immunizing young infants.[561, 562, 565] Increasing the Edmonston-Zagreb vaccine dose from 10,000 to 40,000 plaque-forming units in the Gambia resulted in an increase in response rate from 73% to 100% in 4- to 6-month-old infants.[561] In Mexico, serological response to vaccination of 6-month-olds increased for both Schwarz (66 to 91%) and Edmonston-Zagreb vaccines (92 to 98%) with a 100-fold increase in dose[562]; the effect was greater for Schwarz than for Edmonston-Zagreb vaccine. Because of these data and interest in a vaccination strategy for children younger than 1 year in developing countries, in 1990 the World Health Organization recommended that a higher dose (initially defined as >100,000 and later changed to >50,000) Edmonston-Zagreb vaccine be administered at 6 months of age in areas where measles mortality in young infants was a major health problem.[570] However, problems with vaccine availability resulted in little use of the vaccine on a large scale. Questions have been raised regarding the safety of high-dose measles vaccine, with a higher mortality rate in girls in several developing countries who received high-titer vaccines at 5 to 6 months of age compared with those who received standard-titer vaccines at 9 to 10 months.[571–573] Increased mortality rates after vaccination with a high-titer vaccine were not observed in developed countries or in countries with an infant mortality rate below 100 per 1000 births. High-titer measles vaccines are not currently recommended.[574]

Vaccine Handling. Primary vaccine failures with live vaccine have stemmed from improper handling. Loss of potency of live vaccines can result from poor shipping or storage practices.[528, 575, 576] Although administration of impotent vaccine had previously been implicated in outbreaks of measles in vaccinated persons, the likelihood of this occurring now has been greatly reduced by the addition in 1979 of the new stabilizers discussed previously.[405, 447]

Persistence of Immunity

Although vaccine-induced antibody titers are lower than those achieved after natural infection, this difference does not appear to be biologically significant. The majority of data suggest that after seroconversion, a single dose of live vaccine properly administered to an appropriate host will afford lifelong protection.[577] The duration of vaccine-induced immunity has been documented by studying the persistence of measurable antibody, the effects of vaccine challenge, the attack rate in vaccinees as a function of the time since vaccination, and the clinical characteristics and serological response of measles cases in vaccinated persons.

Serological studies limited to children vaccinated at 12 months of age or older indicate that although antibody titers do decline over time, detectable antibodies

*References 460, 469, 478, 481, 492–494, 509, 510.

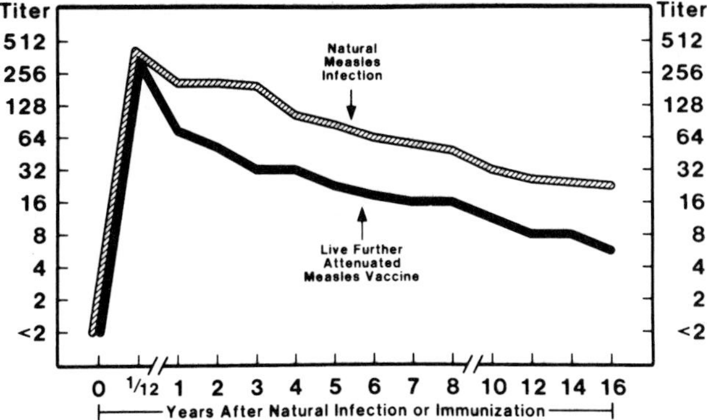

Figure 12–6. Measles geometric mean hemagglutination inhibition antibody titers after natural infection and immunization with live further attenuated vaccine. (Courtesy of S. Krugman.)

are present in most vaccinees.* Because titers can fall to levels undetectable with some assays, the test used is important in the assessment of immune status. Furthermore, many individuals lacking detectable antibody manifest a secondary immune response on revaccination or exposure to wild virus.[277]

The longitudinal observations of greatest duration are provided by Krugman,[65, 269, 270] who observed a population of institutionalized children for 16 years. The HI geometric mean titer in 70 individuals who received further attenuated vaccine was 1:333 at 1 month but in the absence of exposure had fallen to 1:6 after 16 years[270] (Fig. 12–6). Thirteen percent had an HI titer of 1:4, 10% had a titer of 1:2, and 13% had no detectable antibody. In contrast, whereas 47 naturally infected children had a comparable 1-month HI geometric mean titer of 1:410, 16 years after vaccination the geometric mean titer was 1:22 (see Fig. 12–6). Only 4% had an HI titer of 1:2, and none had undetectable antibodies. Sixteen sera with HI titers ranging from below 1:2 to 1:4 obtained from persons vaccinated 6 to 15 years earlier were retested with the more sensitive PRN assay[280]; the PRN titers ranged from 1:4 to 1:46.[270] Typical booster responses after revaccination of some of the HI-negative individuals were also found.

Seroprevalence studies also provide useful information about duration of immunity, but because information on seroconversion is lacking, one cannot be sure whether persons are seronegative because of primary or secondary vaccine failure. In addition, sensitivity of the assay procedure is important. These variables account for some discrepancies in reported findings. For example, Bass and coworkers[454] reported that HI antibodies were detectable in 73% of 40 children more than 8 years after vaccination; however, 98% had Nt antibody. Orenstein and colleagues[440] reported that the seroprevalence among 1871 10th, 11th, and 12th graders, 98.1% of whom had been vaccinated at 14 months of age or older and who had no history of measles, was 86.9% by an HI assay. However, 98.8% were positive with both the HI assay and the same PRN assay used in the Krugman study.[280] Orenstein and colleagues[460] further documented the specificity of the PRN assay by vaccinating HI-negative children. IgM was detected in 14 of 16 students with a PRN titer below 1:4 but in only 1 of 68 who were PRN positive.

Although live virus vaccine–induced immunity is accepted as durable, there have been reports of measles, or modified measles, occurring in some vaccinees who have had laboratory evidence of reinfection without an IgM (i.e., secondary) immune response[158–164, 166] and reports of measles in persons who had a previously documented seroconversion after vaccination.[165, 167, 581] Although reports of measles in persons with unknown initial responses to vaccine are limited by the sensitivity of the assays used to detect IgM antibody,[582] reports of measles in persons with previously documented seroconversions indicate that clinical reinfection can occur. These studies also suggest that the clinical reinfection can be mild and may be more likely to occur in persons vaccinated at younger than 12 months. One study that provides data on the risk of clinical reinfection after vaccination was conducted in Canada; 5% (9 of 175) of persons who initially seroconverted after receipt of measles vaccine developed measles within 10 years of vaccination.[165] In this study, persons who developed measles had lower postvaccination titers than those who did not.

Although some epidemiological studies have shown slight increases in attack rates over time after vaccination with live vaccine at 12 months of age or older, none has yet documented a significant increase[509, 510, 514, 516, 527, 583–586] (Table 12–6). During outbreaks, observed attack rates in persons vaccinated 15 years or more before infection have been on the order of 5% or less, and calculated vaccine efficacies have generally been 90 to 95% or greater. These results are consistent with the expected frequency of primary vaccine failure that occurs in everyday practice. Data from the United Kingdom, the United States, and other countries[577, 580, 587, 588] have not found increases in vaccine failures with time since vaccination. With overall incidence of measles in the

Table 12–6. **EPIDEMIOLOGICAL STUDIES OF THE DURATION OF MEASLES VACCINE–INDUCED IMMUNITY**

STUDY	ATTACK RATE (%) BY YEARS SINCE VACCINATION*			
	0–4	5–9	>10	≥15
[1]Shasby[509]	9.4 (3/32)†	6.9 (7/101)	5.4 (8/52)	—
[2]Nkowane[510]	0 (0/18)	1.1 (1/21)	1.4 (10/158)	—
Davis[516]	1.1 (2/187)	1.7 (11/661)	2.6 (8/308)	0 (0/35)
[3]Marks[514]	4.0/1000	4.2/1000	5.4/1000	11.7/1000
Hutchins[583]	0 (0/33)	0 (0/143)	2.2 (12/549)	3.1 (6/192)
Robertson[584]	0 (0/2)	1.4 (1/74)	3.4 (10/292)	0 (0/3)
Guris[586]	11.8 (2/17)	0 (0/7)		18.2 (2/11)

*Single vaccination at 15 months of age or older except for Shasby, Nkowane, and Davis (12 months of age or older).

†Number ill/total number.

[1]Years since vaccination 5 to 8 and 9 or more.

[2]Projected from a 25% random sample.

[3]Cases per 1000 person-weeks at 0 to 3 (2 of 499), 4 to 6 (6 of 1420), 7 to 9 (5 of 929), and 10 to 12 (4 of 343) years since vaccination.

Adapted from Markowitz LE, Preblud SR, Fine PE, et al. Duration of live measles vaccine–induced immunity. Pediatr Infect Dis J 9:101–109, 1990.

*References 65, 269, 270, 440, 453, 454, 457, 460, 462, 464–467, 578–580.

United States at record low levels and no evidence of increasing incidence among previously vaccinated persons, waning immunity does not appear to constitute a problem. Although secondary vaccine failures have been documented, taken collectively, the serological and epidemiological data during the past 35 years indicate that vaccine provides long-term immunity.

Combined Vaccines and Simultaneous Vaccination

Live measles vaccine has been administered successfully in combination or in conjunction with a variety of immunizing agents, such as yellow fever vaccine, poliovirus vaccine, diphtheria and tetanus toxoids and pertussis vaccine (DTP), meningococcal vaccine, hepatitis B vaccine, and smallpox vaccine.[427, 429, 432, 436, 589–602] There is one report of interference with the measles antibody response after simultaneous administration of meningococcal A and C vaccine,[597] although a different team of investigators did not find interference with simultaneous administration of measles vaccine and meningococcal A vaccine.[595]

Measles vaccine is most commonly administered today along with rubella and mumps vaccines as a combined vaccine (MMR) as part of routine childhood immunization programs.[206, 207] Use of MMR vaccine instead of single-antigen measles vaccine increases the benefit-cost ratio of the measles vaccination program in the United States from 17.2:1 to 21.3:1.[335] Measles vaccine is also frequently administered to susceptible adults, either as MMR or combined with only rubella vaccine.

Studies consistently show that combinations of these three antigens, regardless of the virus strain, elicit the same high rates of seroconversion seen with each component individually and that there is no increased risk of reactions in persons susceptible to all three antigens[404, 420–439, 441] (Tables 12–7 and 12–8). Furthermore, vaccination of persons already immune to one or more of the antigens, from either previous vaccination or infection, is not associated with any increased risk of vaccine-associated adverse events.[599, 603–608] Although there are reports of directly mixing measles vaccine with DTP,[515, 609, 610] this should not be done routinely. Rather, the vaccines should be administered in separate syringes and at separate sites.[611]

Table 12–8. **PROPORTION OF CHILDREN WITH FEVER AND RASH AFTER ADMINISTRATION OF MEASLES VACCINE ALONE AND IN COMBINATION WITH MUMPS AND RUBELLA VACCINES***

VACCINE	TOTAL NUMBER	FEVER (%) (≥39.4°C)	RASH (%)
Measles[1]	43	5	12
Measles,[1] mumps,[2] rubella (RA27/3)	141	11	20
Measles,[1] mumps,[2] rubella (HPV-77 : DE-5)	142	8	17
Placebo	42	0	9

*During the 6 weeks after vaccination.
[1]Moraten strain.
[2]Jeryl Lynn strain.
Adapted from Lerman SJ, Bollinger M, Brunken JM. Clinical and serologic evaluation of measles, mumps and rubella (HPV-77 : DE5 and RA27/3) virus vaccines, singly and in combination. Pediatrics 68:18–22, 1981.

Immunization against varicella along with measles, rubella, and mumps, either as two vaccines (varicella and MMR) or as a quadrivalent vaccine (MMRV), has been studied.[612–615] Seroconversion rates have been reported to be 95% or greater to all antigens, although titers against varicella were lower among persons receiving the quadrivalent vaccine.

Side Effects

Although there are some findings to the contrary, side effects after receipt of live measles vaccine (alone and in combination) are generally mild and limited to susceptible vaccinees.* Peltola and colleagues[420] conducted a study of adverse events in twins, one of whom received MMR vaccine while the other received placebo. This investigation showed that more episodes of fever occurred among children who had received MMR vaccine compared with placebo between 7 and 12 days after vaccination. Fever with temperature greater than 39.5°C attributable to vaccine occurred almost exclusively 9 or 10 days after vaccination. In addition, many adverse events occurring after vaccination were shown to be

*References 267, 313, 346–352, 386, 394–398, 420, 421, 424, 425, 428–436, 438, 454, 599, 612–614, 616–619.

Table 12–7. **ANTIBODY RESPONSE AFTER ADMINISTRATION OF MEASLES VACCINE ALONE AND IN COMBINATION WITH MUMPS AND RUBELLA VACCINES**

VACCINE	TOTAL NUMBER	MEASLES		MUMPS		RUBELLA	
		%	GMT*	%	GMT†	%	GMT*
Measles[1]	23	100	82	—	—	—	—
Measles,[1] mumps,[2] rubella (RA27/3)	91	96	89	90	31	100	301
Measles,[1] mumps,[2] rubella (HPV-77 : DE-5)	85	99	77	89	15	99	144

*Hemagglutination inhibition assay geometric mean titer.
†Indirect immunofluorescent assay geometric mean titer.
[1]Moraten strain.
[2]Jeryl Lynn strain.
Adapted from Lerman SJ, Bollinger M, Brunken JM. Clinical and serologic evaluation of measles, mumps and rubella (HPV-77 : DE5 and RA27/3) virus vaccines, singly and in combination. Pediatrics 68:18–22, 1981.

related only by chance rather than to be caused by vaccine. For example, although fever was reported in vaccine recipients, there were no real differences in rates of fever between vaccinees and placebo recipients in the 1 to 6 days and 13 to 21 days after vaccination. Reactions do follow revaccination of recipients of killed measles vaccine, who are partially immune.[73, 74, 186, 187, 620–624] Anaphylaxis may occur, although since 1990 in the United States, the estimated rate of anaphylaxis is less than 1 per million doses.

Although the incidence of reactions from measles vaccine has been greatly reduced through the use of further attenuated vaccines, fever with a temperature of 39.4°C or higher (≥103°F) occurs in approximately 5 to 15% of vaccinees. The fever usually occurs between the 7th and 12th day after vaccination and lasts approximately 1 to 2 days.[420] In contrast to the fever of natural measles, the fever associated with vaccine is not usually bothersome. However, it may induce a febrile seizure in some vaccinees.[251, 619, 625–628] Rash occurs in approximately 5% of recipients. The rash usually starts 7 to 10 days after vaccination and lasts about 2 days. Serological testing cannot distinguish these vaccine-related events from vaccine-induced modified measles if the vaccine was administered to an individual already incubating natural disease. However, these two situations can be distinguished by isolating virus from a urine or nasopharyngeal mucus specimen, genotyping the virus, and comparing the sequence with known wild-type and vaccine genotypes. Side effects after second doses of measles-containing vaccines are generally less frequent than those after the first dose[618] (C. LeBaron et al., unpublished data), because most children receiving the second dose are already immune from the initial vaccination, thus preventing significant viral replication. A study has found an increased risk of adverse effects after a second dose of MMR when that dose was given to 10- to 12-year-olds compared with 4- to 6-year-olds.[629] Adverse events resulting in medical visits in the 1 month after vaccination of 10- to 12-year-olds were still rare (attributable risk 1.7/1000) and consisted mainly of rashes and joint pain.

There have been a number of reported adverse events involving the nervous system, such as encephalitis, encephalopathy, Guillain-Barré syndrome, Reye syndrome, oculomotor palsy, optic neuritis, retinopathy, hearing loss, and cerebellar ataxia.[630–637] Other reactions such as arthralgia or arthritis, allergic phenomena, and thrombocytopenia have also been reported.[251, 606–608, 638–649] Reactions involving the skin and soft tissues have also been noted.[650–653] It is usually difficult to determine whether these events were truly vaccine related or represent a chance temporal association. An examination of the incidence of Guillain-Barré syndrome after mass vaccination campaigns found no evidence suggesting that measles vaccination was associated with an increased risk.[654]

In 1994, the Institute of Medicine released a report, *Adverse Events Associated with Childhood Vaccine: Evidence Bearing on Causality*, that examined possible adverse events associated with licensed vaccines in the United States.[655, 656] The committee found evidence to establish a causal relationship between measles-containing vaccine and thrombocytopenia, anaphylaxis,[657] and death from measles vaccine strain. The incidence of thrombocytopenic purpura from MMR is estimated to be 1 per 30,000 vaccinated.[658] Several reports have documented death from vaccine strain viral infection in severely immunocompromised patients.[659, 660] The report of progressive vaccine-associated measles pneumonitis in a person with AIDS 1 year after a dose, presumably a second dose, of measles-containing vaccine led to the reevaluation of measles vaccination recommendations for severely immunocompromised persons with HIV infection.[660]

The possible relationship of central nervous system dysfunction, such as encephalitis and encephalopathy, and vaccination has been the subject of considerable interest.[251, 619, 625, 661] The Institute of Medicine report on adverse events caused by measles vaccine has concluded that there are inadequate data to accept or reject a causal relationship between measles vaccination and encephalopathy or encephalitis[656]; these data are summarized here. Using data from 1963 to 1971, Landrigan and Witte[625] estimated that the risk of either encephalitis or encephalopathy occurring within 30 days of vaccination was approximately 1 per 1 million doses of vaccine. During the period 1979 to 1986, nine such cases were reported to the Centers for Disease Control and Prevention (CDC) Monitoring System for Adverse Events Following Immunization after administration of 22.7 million doses of measles antigen–containing vaccine, a rate of 1 per 2.5 million doses (0.4 per 1 million doses).[606–608] This rate is lower than that noted for severe neurological disorders of unknown etiology in unimmunized children of the same age range, suggesting that a chance temporal association rather than cause and effect accounts for some if not most cases.[98] The National Childhood Encephalopathy Study did find an increased risk of encephalopathy or prolonged or complicated convulsions within 7 to 14 days after measles vaccination, but none of the children had any serious permanent sequelae.[661] In a 10-year follow-up of the National Childhood Encephalopathy Study, no increased risk of permanent neurological sequelae was attributable to measles vaccination.[662] To date, there has been only one report of a vaccine isolate recovered from the cerebrospinal fluid of a normal individual; it involved an Edmonston B strain passaged in dog kidney cells.[663]

The association between natural measles infection and SSPE has led to concern that vaccine virus could also cause a persistent central nervous system infection, especially because some patients with SSPE had received vaccine and lacked a history of disease.[92, 97, 128, 130] The virtual disappearance of SSPE, in parallel with the decline in measles cases, suggests that the vaccine protects against SSPE (Fig. 12–7). With immunization levels in the United States exceeding 95%, it is expected that a large proportion of the most recently reported cases of SSPE have a history of vaccination. However, it is not known if such patients had mild measles, perhaps in the first year of life, or if they had failed to seroconvert after vaccination because premorbid sera were unavailable.[98] Epidemiological data have not documented a direct risk from the vaccine.[92, 97, 130] However, if the vaccine is asso-

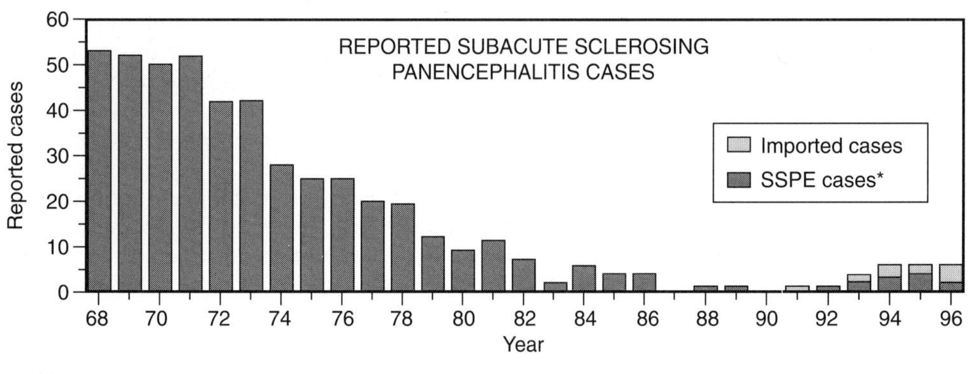

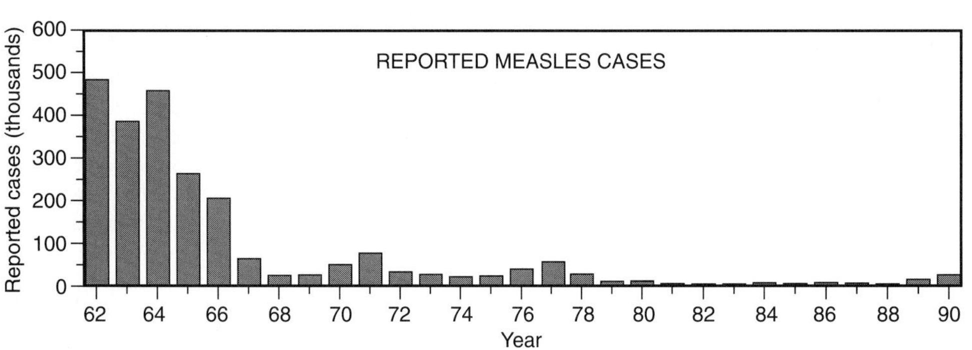

Figure 12–7. Reported measles cases, 1962 to 1990, and subacute sclerosing panencephalitis (SSPE) cases, 1968 to 1996, United States. SSPE data are provisional. *Distinction between imported and nonimported SSPE cases not determined before 1990. (SSPE data courtesy of P. Dyken and S. Cunningham.)

ciated rarely with SSPE, the risk after vaccination is estimated to be approximately one tenth or less that noted after natural infection (approximately 0.7 cases per 1 million doses versus 8.5 cases per 1 million cases of measles).[97]

Measles vaccination has been reported as a possible risk factor for inflammatory bowel disease. One cohort study conducted in England found a relative risk of 3.0 for development of Crohn disease and 2.5 for ulcerative colitis.[135] However, this study has been criticized because of bias due to differential follow-up rates and case ascertainment.[138] Two case-control studies have found no association between measles vaccine and inflammatory bowel disease.[139, 664] Furthermore, researchers have found no evidence of measles virus in small intestine tissue from subjects with Crohn disease using PCR with primers sensitive and specific for the measles virus genome.[136]

Indications

General

The goal of measles vaccination programs is to protect young children from the severe consequences of measles infection, to provide lasting immunity throughout life, and to prevent transmission of this disease. Recommendations for measles vaccination vary by country. The World Health Organization recommends that for most developing countries, measles vaccine be administered at 9 months of age. Many developed and some developing countries now have schedules for two doses. In developed countries, the first dose is usually recommended early in the second year of life; the age for the second dose varies.[32, 34, 35, 207, 665]

Measles vaccine can be given for postexposure prophylaxis, and if it is administered within 3 days of exposure, it may have some effect.[382, 484, 666, 667] However, vaccination should not be deferred until exposure has occurred.

Routine Vaccination Schedule in the United States

All children should receive the first dose of measles-containing vaccine at 12 to 15 months of age (Table 12–9). Children living in high-risk areas should be vaccinated at 12 months of age. A second dose of measles-containing vaccine should be administered at 4 to 6 years of age, usually at the time of school entry. Children who have not received a second dose by 11 to 12 years of age should be vaccinated at that age.

Recommendations for a second dose of measles-containing vaccine, first established in 1989, were made to reduce the number of children experiencing vaccine failure. The Committee on Infectious Diseases of the American Academy of Pediatrics (AAP) and the Advisory Committee on Immunization Practices (ACIP) recommended that both doses be given as combined MMR vaccine. Because of the cost of the additional vaccination, both the ACIP and AAP initially proposed that this recommendation be phased in one birth year or grade cohort per year. In 1989, the ACIP recommended that a second dose be given at school entry (to children 4 to 6 years of age), and the AAP recommended that the second dose be given to middle or junior high-school enterers (to children 11 to 12 years of age).[207, 668] The AAP recommendation was designed to cover children in junior and senior high school, where the majority of measles in school-aged children was occurring,

Table 12–9. **RECOMMENDATIONS FOR MEASLES VACCINATION IN THE UNITED STATES**

Routine childhood schedule	
Most areas	Two doses* First dose: 12–15 mo Second dose: 4–6 yr or 11–12 yr
High-risk areas†	Two doses* First dose: 12 mo Second dose: 4–6 yr or 11–12 yr
Colleges and other educational institutions post high school	Documentation of receipt of two doses of measles vaccine on or after the first birthday‡ or other evidence of measles immunity§
Persons working in healthcare facilities	Documentation of receipt of two doses of measles vaccine on or after the first birthday‡ or other evidence of measles immunity§

*Both doses should preferably be given as a combined measles, mumps, rubella vaccine (MMR). The American Academy of Pediatrics and the Advisory Committee on Immunization Practices recommend the second dose at 4 to 6 years of age or 11 to 12 years of age.

†A county with more than five cases among preschool-aged children during each of the last 5 years; a county with a recent outbreak among unvaccinated preschool-aged children; or a county with a large inner-city urban population. These recommendations may be applied to an entire county or identified risk areas within a county.

‡No less than 1 month apart. If there is no documentation of any dose of vaccine, vaccine should be given at the time of entry or employment and no less than 1 month later.

§Prior physician-diagnosed measles disease, laboratory evidence of measles immunity, or birth before 1957.

more rapidly than the ACIP recommendation. In addition, delaying revaccination until adolescence could boost immunity if waning of vaccine-induced immunity were part of the reason for the increased incidence of vaccine failure among secondary school students. The ACIP recommendation built on the already developed public health infrastructure of primary school entry vaccination requirements. The main drawback to the ACIP recommendation was that vaccinating single cohorts of primary school enterers would take several years before junior and senior high-school–aged children would be covered with second-dose requirements.

Since the initial recommendations for a second measles vaccination were made in 1989, no additional epidemiological evidence has emerged to suggest that waning immunity is a significant problem. Boosting of prevaccination antibody titers, when it occurs, appears to be transient. The major effect of the second dose appears to be in immunizing persons who failed to respond to the initial dose (i.e., persons who experienced primary vaccine failure). On the basis of these considerations, the ACIP recommended, in 1997, that each state ensure that all school-aged children, kindergarten through 12th grade, receive second doses of measles-containing vaccine by 2001. After all schoolchildren are covered by second-dose requirements, routine administration of the second dose should occur at school entry in all states (at age 4 to 6 years).[669] The ACIP, the AAP, and the American Academy of Family Physicians have each endorsed this recommendation.[670]

In addition to routine vaccination, measles vaccine is indicated for all susceptible persons unless there are contraindications to vaccination. Few people in the United States born before 1957 escaped natural infection; therefore, vaccination is not usually recommended for these individuals. In the United States, individuals should be considered susceptible to measles unless they (1) have documentation of adequate vaccination, (2) have laboratory evidence of immunity, (3) were born before 1957, or (4) have documentation of physician-diagnosed measles. Criteria for adequate vaccination will vary by age of the child and recommendations adopted by the local authorities.[207] Because of reduced efficacy of measles vaccine when it is administered to young children, doses of measles vaccine administered to children younger than 12 months are not considered valid doses. Children vaccinated at ages younger than 12 months should be revaccinated at 12 to 15 months of age (provided at least 28 days have elapsed) to be considered to have received a single dose of measles vaccine.

Except in the situations noted in the following, in which the risk of exposure to measles may be increased, evidence of adequate vaccination for most adults consists of at least one dose of vaccine on or after the first birthday.

Recommendations for Other Age Groups

Colleges and universities are the most frequently reported setting of measles transmission for persons 18 years of age and older; outbreaks have occurred most frequently in dormitories.[315] As a result, the ACIP and AAP have recommended that college entrants and students in other post–high school educational institutions be required to provide documentation of measles immunity (i.e., physician-diagnosed measles, serological evidence of immunity, or documentation of two doses of live measles vaccine after the first birthday).

Healthcare workers are at high risk for measles. During 1985 to 1989, physicians had an eightfold increased risk and nurses a twofold increased risk compared with non-healthcare workers of the same age.[671] Even with the low incidence of measles in the United States since 1993, transmission in healthcare settings commonly complicates measles outbreaks (K. Steingart, unpublished data). In the 75 measles outbreaks occurring during 1993 through 1996, transmission of measles in a healthcare facility was documented in 15 (CDC, unpublished data, 1997). The ACIP and AAP have recommended that persons born in or after 1957 working in healthcare facilities be required to provide evidence of two MMR vaccinations, documentation of physician-diagnosed measles, or laboratory evidence of measles immunity.[206, 207] In addition, because measles has occurred in persons born before 1957, healthcare facilities may also consider requiring MMR vaccination for health workers born before 1957 who do not have a history of measles or documentation of immunity to measles. Whereas it may be cost-effective in some situations,[672, 673] serological screening is not routinely recommended because the follow-up vaccination of susceptible persons identified in such screening programs can be difficult to implement.

International Travel

Ensuring immunity for all age groups is important in considering overseas travel.[206, 207] Because of the increased risk of exposure in some areas, special consideration for children younger than 12 months may be necessary. When traveling to areas with endemic or epidemic measles, children 12 months of age should be vaccinated before departure with MMR vaccine; children 6 to 11 months of age should be vaccinated before departure with single measles antigen. Infants younger than 6 months are likely to be protected by maternal antibodies. For infants vaccinated before 12 months of age, revaccination should be at 12 to 15 months of age (12 months of age for those remaining in areas of endemic or epidemic measles). The second revaccination should be administered when the child enters school.

Because the risk of complications from measles is increased in adults, it is also important to protect susceptible young adults. Most persons born in the United States before 1957 are likely to be immune. However, for persons born after 1956 who travel abroad, two doses of measles vaccine should be administered separated by at least 28 days, unless there is documentation of receipt of two doses, other evidence of immunity, or a contraindication.

Outbreak Control

During outbreaks in schools and other institutions, all persons should have documentation of two doses of measles-containing vaccine on or after the first birthday. All persons who do not have such documentation or other evidence of immunity should be revaccinated or excluded from the school. In outbreaks where there is increased risk of exposure for infants younger than 1 year, vaccination with monovalent measles vaccine is recommended for infants as young as 6 months. Children who are vaccinated before their first birthday should be revaccinated when they are 12 months of age (provided at least 28 days have elapsed since the first dose given before age 12 months) and again at school entry. During outbreaks, immune globulin should be administered to immunocompromised persons, susceptible pregnant women, and unvaccinated children younger than 12 months who are exposed to measles. However, immune globulin should not be used to control outbreaks.

Revaccination of Persons Vaccinated According to Earlier Recommendations

Anyone vaccinated at any age with killed vaccine alone or killed vaccine followed by live vaccine within a 3-month period and anyone vaccinated between 1963 and 1967 with a vaccine of unknown type should be revaccinated to ensure protection and to prevent atypical measles illness. Revaccinating persons who received an unknown type of vaccine is recommended because Edmonston B, inactivated, and further attenuated live vaccines were all in use during this interval (see Fig. 12–5). As noted previously, vaccination of an immune individual is not associated with any increased risk of adverse events. However, revaccination of recipients of killed vaccine may be associated with local reactions of pain, swelling, erythema, and regional lymphadenopathy lasting 1 to 2 days.[73, 74, 186, 187, 620–624] These reactions have been reported to occur in 4 to 55% of vaccinees. More severe reactions have been noted but only rarely.[74] Whereas revaccination has not been proved to totally eliminate the risk for atypical measles,[193] available data suggest that the risk is reduced considerably.[73, 74, 197] Thus, the risk of these reactions is outweighed by the risk associated with atypical measles.[674]

A dose of further attenuated live vaccine with immune globulin administered simultaneously should not be considered adequate vaccination. This recommendation is based on the theoretical consideration that passively derived antibody might interfere with seroconversion. Whereas low doses of immune globulin do not appear to interfere with seroconversion,[267] there is no information available about the dose used in general practice shortly after the introduction of further attenuated vaccines in the United States. Furthermore, at least one study has suggested that there is an increased rate of seronegativity when further attenuated vaccine was administered with immune globulin.[509] Finally, and perhaps most important, revaccination is indicated if there is any uncertainty about the vaccination record.[528, 530]

Precautions and Contraindications

In general, vaccination is contraindicated if there is high fever, immunosuppression, pregnancy, a history of an anaphylactic reaction to neomycin, or recent administration of immune globulin or other blood products.

Concurrent Illness

Although vaccine should not be administered in the presence of significant fever because of the likelihood of a concurrent infection that may interfere with seroconversion, vaccination should not be deferred in the presence of mild conditions such as an upper respiratory infection.[536, 537, 543, 546] Furthermore, concern about possible undiagnosed tuberculosis is not a reason to defer vaccination. Whereas vaccination may suppress delayed hypersensitivity for up to 4 to 6 weeks,[474–478] there is no evidence that measles vaccine exacerbates tuberculosis.[483–485] Thus, doing a tuberculin skin test before vaccination is unnecessary; such testing can be undertaken at the same time that vaccine is administered, if testing is indicated. If skin testing is not done at that time, it is advisable to wait 4 to 6 weeks after vaccination before administering a tuberculosis skin test.

Immunosuppression

Because replication of live vaccine virus may be potentiated and prolonged in patients who are immunocompromised,[169, 675] live virus measles vaccine should not be administered to persons who are immunosuppressed because of underlying illness (e.g., congenital illness, leukemia, lymphoma, generalized malignant disease), medication (e.g., high-dose steroids, alkylating agents, and antimetabolites), or therapy such as radiation. This does not include persons receiving topical, localized (e.g., intra-articular, bursal, or tendon injection), or short-term (less than 2 weeks) steroid treatment, unless systemic immunosuppressive levels are achieved.[676]

Although published data are limited,[677] experience indicates that vaccine may be administered to susceptible patients with leukemia who are in remission and who have discontinued all immunosuppressive therapy for at least 3 months. It is not clear whether these patients will all respond to vaccine. The interval between termination of therapy and the ability to respond to vaccine is not known with certainty; however, it probably varies from 3 months to 1 year. Bone marrow transplant recipients have also been vaccinated without problems 2 years after transplantation.[678–680]

Available data indicate that persons with HIV infection who are not severely immunosuppressed may be vaccinated safely.* No adverse events were reported in a survey of 42 HIV-infected children who had received MMR vaccine after infection; 11 had been vaccinated after the onset of symptoms without serious outcome.[681] Prospective studies in the Democratic Republic of Congo, formerly Zaire, and in Rwanda found no difference in adverse reactions to measles vaccine administered at 9 months[551] or 6 months of age[552, 553] between HIV-infected and uninfected children. Small studies of HIV-infected adults who received MMR vaccine also found no increased risk of adverse reactions.[682–684] However, in one study, most subjects had measles antibody at the time of vaccination.[682] A theoretical risk of an increase (probably transient) in HIV viral load after MMR vaccination exists because such an effect has been observed with other vaccines.[685, 686] The clinical significance of such an increase is not known.

Because measles has been documented to be severe in HIV-infected persons in both the United States and developing countries,[173, 207, 338] measles vaccine is recommended routinely for asymptomatic HIV-infected children and adults without evidence of measles immunity and should be considered for those with symptomatic infections who are not severely immunosuppressed. MMR and other measles-containing vaccines are not recommended for HIV-infected persons in the United States with evidence of severe immunosuppression because of the risk of adverse events, the impaired immune response to MMR vaccination, and the current low risk of exposure to measles in the United States.[184, 660] Severe immunosuppression is defined as (1) a $CD4^+$ count of less than 200 cells/mm^3 for persons 6 years of age and older, a $CD4^+$ count of less than 500 cells/mms^3 for children 1 to 5 years old, and a $CD4^+$ count of less than 750 cells/mm^3 for children younger than 12 months of age or (2) $CD4^+$ cells less than 15% of total lymphocytes for children younger than 13 years.[687]

*References 173, 184, 207, 338, 406, 552, 553, 681.

Asymptomatic patients at risk for HIV infection should not be screened before vaccination.

Pregnancy

In contrast to rubella and mumps vaccines, measles vaccine virus has not been shown to cross the placenta and infect the fetus. However, on theoretical grounds, measles vaccine should not be administered to a pregnant woman. Susceptible women of childbearing age may be vaccinated after asking them if they are pregnant (excluding them if they are) and explaining the theoretical risks.

Allergies

Persons with anaphylactic reactions (urticaria, angioneurotic edema, wheezing, hypotension, and shock) after either topical or systemic administration of neomycin should not be vaccinated. Penicillin allergy is not a contraindication because the vaccine does not contain penicillin. In contrast to previous belief,[688, 689] children with anaphylactic reactions after egg ingestion may be vaccinated.[690–693] Recent data suggest that most anaphylactic reactions to measles-containing vaccines are associated with hypersensitivity not to egg but to other components of the vaccine. The risk for anaphylaxis is low and is not predicted by the response to skin tests; therefore, skin testing before vaccination, which had been recommended in the past, is not recommended.[694–696] Allergic reaction to gelatin has recently been recognized as a cause of anaphylaxis after MMR vaccination[697–699]; persons with such allergies should not be vaccinated. Persons with nonanaphylactic reactions to eggs, or allergy to chicken or feathers, may be vaccinated as usual.

Administration of Immune Globulin and Other Blood Products

Because passively derived antibody may interfere with vaccine seroconversion, vaccination should be deferred for 3 to 11 months after receipt of immune globulin and other blood products, depending on the dose of the blood product received.[700] In addition, vaccination should precede receipt of immune globulin by at least 2 weeks whenever possible.

NEW DEVELOPMENTS

Although measles vaccine is one of the most effective vaccines available today, research is being conducted on new vaccines that may be able to (1) overcome maternal antibody and thereby allow immunization of children at younger ages or (2) be administered by routes that allow easy delivery during mass campaigns. Advances have been made in the development of subunit and vectored measles vaccines that could avoid the problems experienced with the previously used formalin-inactivated measles vaccine and may be immunogenic in young infants in the presence of maternal antibody.[701] Current approaches include the development of recombinant vaccines[702, 703] and immune-stimulating complexes.[486] Preliminary work on a DNA measles vaccine is also ongoing.[704] The feasibility and desirability of such vaccines have not been established.

A variety of mucosal routes of administration have been evaluated in the past and continue to be explored. Although aerosol administration of measles is theoretically attractive, the devices available for administration of these preparations are limited. Preclinical studies have been done with an oral measles vaccine preparation that could be administered as a capsule, and there are plans for further evaluation of this concept. The cost and time required for development of any of these new vaccines or routes of administration need to be considered in light of the recent progress in measles control and the future plans for measles elimination.

PUBLIC HEALTH CONSIDERATIONS

Epidemiological Results of Vaccination

The goal of measles vaccination is to prevent illness and death due to measles.[705] Whereas vaccination reduces an individual's risk of measles, as long as measles virus circulates, unvaccinated persons and persons who fail to develop protective immunity after vaccination contract measles. High vaccination coverage with a single dose of measles vaccine will decrease measles incidence and lead to a period referred to as the honeymoon period.[706] During this period, susceptible persons, who either were not vaccinated or failed to develop protective immunity after vaccination, accumulate. Eventually, when the number of susceptible persons surpasses a critical threshold, measles outbreaks occur, mainly among older age groups.[707–709] Many countries introduced measles vaccine as a single-dose schedule and changed to multiple-dose strategies because of continuing outbreaks. Multiple-dose strategies, including strategies relying on periodic mass vaccination campaigns, attempt to prevent outbreaks by preventing this accumulation of susceptible persons. The ultimate aim, and ultimate challenge, of such programs is to prevent all cases of measles.

The feasibility of measles elimination and eradication has been debated for many years.[43, 46, 47, 710–712] Elimination is defined as the interruption of measles virus transmission in a geographically defined area for a sustained period, and eradication is defined as the elimination of the virus reservoir. An area that has achieved measles elimination remains at risk for importations of measles from regions with endemic or epidemic measles. After eradication, there will be no risk of measles importation, and vaccination could be stopped. Hopkins and colleagues[43] have proposed global measles eradication and pointed out both the similarities and differences between measles and smallpox. For a variety of reasons, including the higher contagiousness of measles, younger mean age at infection, and older age at which vaccine is effective, measles would be substantially more difficult to eradicate than was smallpox and would require a different strategy for eradication. Whereas vaccination of a large proportion of a population can strikingly reduce the risk of measles and produce a "herd" effect,[713] protecting even those who are not immune, measles is so contagious that it has the capability to spread in some situations unless virtually every susceptible person has been immunized.[2, 714–717]

Mathematical models have been used to understand measles epidemiology as well as to design vaccination programs and evaluate their impact.[706, 712, 715, 718, 719] Models have suggested that measles will disappear from the United States only if immunity levels are approximately 94%.[717] However, in a measles outbreak in Milwaukee, census tract areas where vaccination coverage in 2-year-old children exceeded 80% were not affected.[720] If an immunity level of more than 94% is required, then vaccine coverage rates of 97 to 98% would be needed with a single dose of vaccine that is 95% efficacious. A two-dose schedule, such as is being implemented in the United States and other countries, would theoretically make measles elimination easier by decreasing vaccine failures.[712] However, even with these schedules, pockets of unimmunized populations can prevent measles elimination, even if high coverage is achieved in the general population.

Measles elimination in developing countries may be more difficult to achieve than in developed countries because of higher contact and reproduction rates and because of less well developed infrastructure for delivering vaccine and conducting surveillance.[119] However, the recent success in controlling measles achieved in Latin America and the Caribbean suggests that measles elimination, following a mass vaccination strategy, although difficult, may be feasible. The success of the global poliomyelitis eradication initiative, also based on mass vaccination campaigns and intensified surveillance, has also contributed to the enthusiasm for measles eradication.[46]

Country Experiences in Measles Control and Elimination

Industrialized Countries

The administration of more than 205 million doses of live measles vaccine between the year of licensure in the United States in 1963 and the end of 1997 has been associated with a dramatic reduction in measles and its associated complications (Fig. 12–8; see also Fig. 12–7) and an estimated savings of billions of dollars.[28, 335] Whereas approximately 4 million cases occurred annually in prevaccine years, on average only 400,000 to 500,000 cases were reported. In 1995, only 309 cases were reported, a reduction of more than 99.9% compared with the years preceding vaccine licensure. The reported occurrence of SSPE has also declined greatly (see Fig. 12–7). Although a small number of cases have been reported each year for most of the past decade,

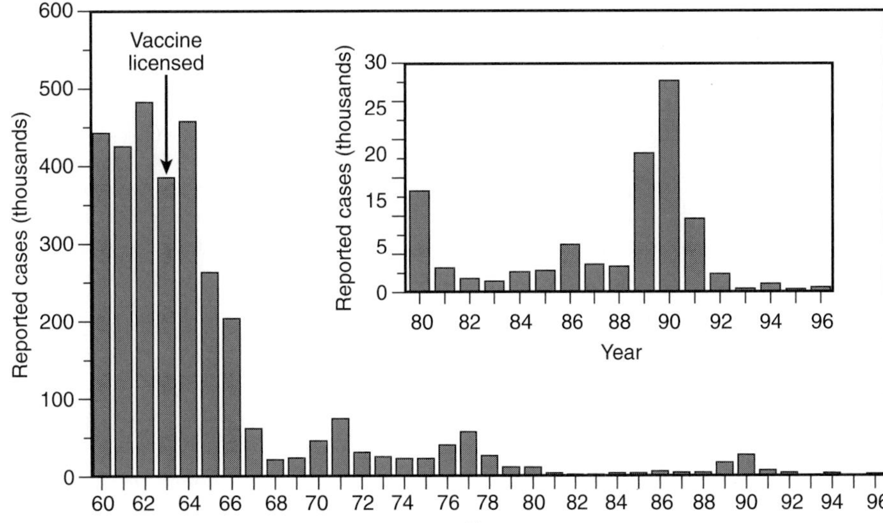

Figure 12–8. Reported measles cases, United States, 1960 to 1996.

numbers are far lower than before the widespread use of measles vaccine, and many cases result from measles acquired outside the United States (P. Dyken, personal communication, 1997) (see Fig. 12–7).

Soon after measles vaccine was licensed for use in the United States, the potential for eliminating this disease from the United States was recognized. In 1966, a program for elimination was announced, and elimination was expected to be achieved by the end of 1967.[721] The program was based on extrapolation of data collected in Baltimore in the mid-1930s showing that biennial measles epidemics occurred when the population susceptibility among schoolchildren was above 47%. It was anticipated that the epidemic cycle could be broken by vaccinating more than 53% of schoolchildren. This program resulted in a decline in measles cases from 204,136 in 1966 to 22,231 in 1968, but not in the interruption of measles virus transmission. After the diversion of federal funds from measles vaccine purchase to rubella vaccine purchase in 1969, measles cases rose to 75,290 in 1971. In assessing the failure of this effort to eliminate measles, Conrad and associates[712] identified no scientific reason to indicate that measles elimination was not feasible. They cited lack of routinely vaccinating a high enough proportion of preschool-aged children as the critical weakness in the program.

In 1978, the United States announced a second goal for eliminating measles, with the target year for elimination of 1982.[23, 24] The elimination strategy had three components: (1) attain a high level of population immunity through vaccination with a single dose of measles vaccine, (2) surveillance, and (3) prompt response to outbreaks.[24] To attain high levels of vaccination coverage, vaccination requirements for school entry were enacted and enforced in every state. These requirements, which mandated not only measles vaccination but also other childhood vaccinations, have become one of the major legacies of this measles elimination initiative. Case definitions for measles and the establishment of a system for timely notification and analysis of measles surveillance data were also established.

These efforts resulted in a drop in measles cases through the 1980s, from an average of 36.7 thousand cases in the 1970s to 5.7 thousand during the 1980s. In 1983, a record low number of reported measles cases, 1497, was reached. Although sustained interruption of indigenous transmission of measles was not achieved, measles was eliminated from most of the country; 54% of counties in the United States were measles free for the entire decade from 1980 to 1989, and only 17 (0.5%) counties reported measles every year during that period.[722]

Two major types of measles outbreaks were recognized in the United States during the 1980s[27]: "preschool outbreaks," in which a large percentage of cases (generally 50 to 75%) occurred in children younger than 5 years, most of whom were unvaccinated; and "school outbreaks," which occurred in highly vaccinated populations. In many large school outbreaks, more than 95% of cases had occurred in school-aged persons with histories of vaccination on or after their first birthday.* However, a few outbreaks occurred in groups with religious exemptions to vaccination in which almost all cases were in unvaccinated persons.[307]

After the relatively low incidence of measles during the 1980s, a 3-year epidemic of measles began in 1989 (see Fig. 12–8); in 1989, 18,193 cases were reported, followed by 27,786 cases in 1990 and 9643 in 1991, the largest number of cases reported for a 3-year period since the late 1970s.[724, 725] The average annual incidence of 7.4 per 100,000 population was a more than fourfold increase above the average incidence for 1981 to 1988 (1.8 per 100,000). During this epidemic, the incidence of measles in all age groups increased. However, the greatest increases were in children younger than 1 year and 1 to 4 years old, resulting in almost half of all cases occurring in children younger than 5 years (see Table 12–1).

The vaccination status of case patients also changed during the 1989 to 1991 epidemic years. Between 1985

*References 315, 316, 510, 516, 530, 583, 584, 723.

and 1988, 47.7% of cases occurred in persons who were vaccinated on or after their first birthday. During the 1989 to 1991 resurgence, this percentage decreased to 29.9%. Whereas most of the cases in school-aged persons occurred in children who were vaccinated, only 11.3% of cases in children younger than 5 years occurred in children who had received vaccine. In 1989 and 1990, 56 and 106 preschool outbreaks occurred. Most of these were in large inner-city areas, and the majority of cases occurred in unvaccinated black and Hispanic children.[724, 725]

The available data indicate that the 1989 to 1991 epidemic was due to widespread measles virus circulation among unvaccinated preschool-aged children.[726, 727] Although measles vaccination levels among school-aged children in the United States have been 97 to 98%, coverage in preschool-aged children has been much lower[728]; during the 1980s, the highest reported coverage among 2-year-old children was 67%. In many of the inner-city areas where the outbreaks occurred, retrospective surveys in children entering school indicated that measles vaccine coverage at 2 years of age in some cities was as low as 50%.[729] There was no evidence of decreased vaccine efficacy during the epidemic; a study conducted in California found measles vaccine 95% effective in preventing measles among preschool-aged children.[501] Large measles outbreaks occurred in Canada, Mexico, and Central America between 1989 and 1991[47]; the epidemic in the United States was part of a hemisphere-wide measles epidemic.[730]

Large outbreaks among preschool-aged children and the persistence of outbreaks in schools with high one-dose vaccination coverage levels led to two specific recommendations for controlling measles: (1) higher coverage in young children was needed to prevent measles outbreaks in preschool-aged children, and (2) a two-dose measles vaccination policy was needed to prevent measles outbreaks in schools.

Higher vaccination coverage levels in preschool-aged children have been achieved. By 1996, the vaccination goal of 90% coverage among 2-year-old children had been exceeded.[731] States are gradually implementing requirements for two doses of measles-containing vaccine, and coverage in school-aged children in 1996 was estimated to be 64% (CDC, unpublished data, 1996).

As a result of these efforts, measles incidence has fallen to record low levels. Between 1993 and 1997, the annual number of reported measles cases in the United States has never exceeded 1000, with the fewest cases (138) reported in 1997. The number of large outbreaks has also declined, with only three outbreaks of greater than 100 cases occurring between 1992 and 1997.[731a, 731b] Beginning in late 1993, surveillance data indicate that indigenous measles virus transmission has been interrupted on several occasions. In late 1996 and early 1997, two 8-week periods without an indigenous case were recorded.[732] Virological surveillance has also indicated interruption of indigenous measles. The genetic structure of circulating wild-type measles viruses isolated between 1988 and 1992 is different from that of the strains isolated since, which are similar to those isolated in other regions of the world, particularly western Europe and east Asia (see Fig. 12–1). These data suggest that the recurrent reintroductions of measles into the United States from other regions are responsible for current measles morbidity in the United States.[241, 733]

Excellent control of measles has also been achieved in other developed countries. A measles vaccination program was begun in Finland in 1975; however, low coverage levels were achieved and measles outbreaks continued to occur. In 1982, Finland initiated a measles elimination program based on a two-dose vaccination strategy. Efforts to improve vaccination coverage included mass media, a registry system to track defaulters, and an intensive outreach program to vaccinate.[36] By 1993, coverage was above 95% for both doses, and measles virus circulation had been interrupted. Only 13 cases were reported in that year.[734] During 1996, no cases of measles were reported.[735] Sweden has reported similar success with a two-dose schedule. The European Region of the World Health Organization is considering a goal for the regional elimination of measles by the year 2007.[736]

The United Kingdom and Canada began their measles immunization programs in the 1960s with single-dose schedules. Both experienced reductions in measles incidence but with persistent measles virus transmission, similar to what had occurred in the United States. Recently, both the United Kingdom and Canada have undertaken mass vaccination campaigns to halt measles virus transmission. In 1994, mathematical models, based on national serosurveillance data in the United Kingdom, predicted a measles epidemic affecting principally secondary school–aged children that might have occurred as early as 1995.[737, 738] Because of the age structure of the predicted epidemic, 150 deaths were forecast. To avert this epidemic, a school-based vaccination campaign, using measles-rubella vaccine, was undertaken in England and Wales during November 1994. During the campaign, 6.2 million doses were administered and a coverage level of 92% was achieved.[739] The number of laboratory-confirmed measles cases dropped sharply after the campaign, and some of these cases were imported from other countries or linked to imported cases.[740]

In Canada, measles vaccination coverage with a single dose exceeded 95% in 2-year-old children throughout the 1980s. Despite this high coverage level, measles outbreaks continued to occur. In 1995, 2362 measles cases were reported in Canada. School outbreaks among children who had received a single dose of measles-containing vaccine accounted for most cases. Despite the formal adoption of a goal for measles elimination and a recommendation for a two-dose policy in 1992, few children in Canada were receiving second doses of vaccine. Mathematical modeling predicted a sizable measles epidemic,[47] and cost-benefit analyses showed that a national vaccination campaign to prevent the predicted epidemic would save $2.50 for every dollar spent.[741] On the basis of these analyses, 11 of the 12 provinces of Canada undertook mass vaccination campaigns targeting school-aged children using measles-rubella vaccine in the spring of 1996. Some provinces also included preschool-aged children in the target group. A coverage level of more than 90% was achieved, and measles cases during 1996 fell to 324 cases.

Developing Countries

In developing countries, two themes in measles control have emerged during the 1990s. First, improving measles vaccination coverage has been recognized as an extremely cost-effective means to prevent deaths in children. Second, efforts in the Western Hemisphere led by the Pan American Health Organization (PAHO) to eliminate measles virus transmission have been highly successful and, along with successes in developed countries, have rekindled interest in the global eradication of measles.

Beginning in the late 1970s, the Expanded Programme on Immunization has fostered remarkable progress in increasing immunization levels in developing countries.[742] Measles vaccination coverage in developing countries rose from 18% in 1981 to 76% in 1990, and an estimated 1.9 million measles deaths were prevented in 1991 alone.[742] Since 1990, overall vaccination coverage levels have plateaued at around 80%. The annual number of deaths in children attributed to measles has also stabilized at around 1 million, as has the annual estimated number of measles cases at between 35 and 40 million.

Although the impact of measles vaccination on overall childhood mortality in developing countries was questioned by one study,[118] several subsequent studies have documented that measles vaccination increases overall child survival.[743–746] In Bangladesh, investigators found that the mortality rate in measles-vaccinated children was 45% lower than in unvaccinated children.[743]

Current measles epidemiology and issues in measles control in Africa, where the highest incidence and death rates occur, have been reviewed.[718] The impact of measles vaccination has varied in urban and rural areas. One of the major factors confronting measles control is the rapid urbanization in Africa and other parts of the world.[747] This has resulted in continued measles transmission despite increasing vaccination levels in some cities.[567–569, 746] In these areas, measles in children younger than 9 months, the recommended age for vaccination in developing countries, is a striking problem. With 62% coverage in 12- to 59-month-olds, measles remained endemic in Kinshasa, the Democratic Republic of Congo, formerly Zaire. A community survey found that 18% of cases were in children younger than 9 months and a total of 37% in children younger than 12 months.[568] In Cape Town, 43% of reported cases were in children younger than 9 months.[746] These data raised concerns that measles cannot be controlled in such settings unless vaccines become available that are effective in children younger than 9 months, the routine age for vaccination. Improving coverage levels can prevent transmission from persons old enough to be vaccinated to those too young to be vaccinated. Because older persons tend to be more mobile and in most areas are likely to be the primary transmitters of measles, achieving high levels of coverage in older children may be sufficient to prevent transmission among children too young for vaccination. The recent experience of interrupting measles virus transmission in São Paulo and Rio de Janeiro, which are densely populated and have large impoverished populations, suggests that immunization of children younger than 9 months may not be necessary, if coverage levels of 90% to 95% can be achieved in older age groups through mass vaccination campaigns. However, in the absence of high coverage, vaccines that could be given to children younger than 9 months would be desirable. The precise vaccination coverage level that must be attained to interrupt virus transmission is unknown. In less densely populated areas where there have been sustained high vaccination levels, outbreaks in older school-aged children have occurred, similar to those in the United States. Many countries have experienced outbreaks after a period of low incidence.[707–709] This pattern that follows introduction of a vaccination program, the honeymoon period, has been well described by mathematical modelers, the length of the interepidemic period being dependent on the vaccination coverage.[719]

The 1990 World Health Assembly and World Summit for Children set global goals for measles control: "Reduction by 95 percent in measles deaths and reduction by 90 percent of measles cases compared to pre-immunization levels by 1995, as a major step to the global eradication of measles in the longer run."[40] Although many developing countries failed to meet these goals, recent success in controlling measles in the Western Hemisphere indicates that new strategies may be effective in controlling measles in developing countries.

The strategy currently being implemented in most countries of the Western Hemisphere to prevent measles was developed in Cuba in the late 1980s.[748] Despite high measles vaccination coverage levels in Cuba during the early and mid-1980s, measles cases continued to occur, mostly in persons who had previously received a single dose of measles-containing vaccine. To prevent measles cases among one-dose recipients as well as to vaccinate any persons not previously vaccinated, the Cuban Ministry of Health executed a mass vaccination campaign, using MMR vaccine, targeting all children 1 through 14 years of age, regardless of history of disease or vaccination. A coverage level of nearly 98% was achieved, and reported measles cases dropped precipitously.[748] A follow-up campaign targeting children 2 through 5 years old, too young to have been reached in the first campaign, was undertaken in 1993. A similarly high level of coverage was achieved, and no laboratory-confirmed cases of measles have been identified between 1993 and 1997.

In 1990, the English-speaking Caribbean countries, supported by the PAHO, adopted a plan for the elimination of indigenous transmission of measles in their region by 1995.[749] In 1991, a mass vaccination campaign targeting all children aged 9 months through 14 years was undertaken in each country. After this campaign in 1991 through 1996, no measles cases have been identified.[750]

In 1994, the members of the Pan American Sanitary Conference, representing PAHO member countries, voted unanimously to approve the goal of measles elimination by the year 2000.[751] To achieve the goal of measles elimination, PAHO has elaborated a three-part strategy.[752] The strategy first calls for each country to undertake a mass vaccination campaign targeting all children aged 9 months through 14 years, regardless of history of disease or vaccination. Second, PAHO recommends changing the age for routine vaccination to 12 months after the campaign. Vaccinating children at 12 months of age instead of 9 months of age results in higher vaccine effectiveness. The risk of exposure to measles is sufficiently low after the mass vaccination campaigns that the danger of contracting measles between 9 and 12 months of age is negligible. Routine one-dose vaccination coverage levels should be maintained at greater than 90%. Third, PAHO recommends that countries undertake additional mass vaccination campaigns when the number of children susceptible to measles, as estimated by vaccination coverage levels and vaccination failure rates, is equivalent to the number of children born in a year. Children aged 12 months through 5 or 6 years should be targeted. In practice, campaigns will be needed every 3 to 5 years, depending primarily on vaccination coverage levels. Through 1995, every country in the Western Hemisphere, except for Canada and the United States, had implemented the first component of the measles elimination strategy, with vaccination coverage levels greater than 85% except for two countries. All countries that have conducted initial mass vaccination campaigns have either implemented or are planning follow-up mass vaccination campaigns to be completed by 1998.

In addition to the vaccination strategy, surveillance has been strengthened throughout the region, with an increased emphasis on laboratory testing. Surveillance indicators have been developed and are being measured in each country to ensure that low numbers of reported cases indicate a decline in the true incidence of measles.

After implementation of the strategy, the decline in measles cases has been remarkable (Fig. 12–9). Reported measles cases in Latin America and the Caribbean fell from 218,000 in 1990 to fewer than 1000 in 1996. Cuba, Chile, and countries in the English-speaking Caribbean have each reported several-year periods without a single indigenous case of measles. Surveillance assessments in Guatemala, Mexico, and Nicaragua in 1995 and 1996 have confirmed the absence of ongoing indigenous transmission. In addition, surveillance of international importations of measles in the United States has provided further evidence of the success of measles control efforts in Latin America. In 1990, more than 200 cases of measles imported from the countries of Latin America were identified; in 1995 and 1996, no imported cases from Latin America were identified.[753] Until measles control in other regions of the world reaches similar levels, imported cases into the countries of the Western Hemisphere will serve as a continual challenge to the ability to sustain these low or absent levels of measles transmission.

Measles Eradication

In July 1996, the World Health Organization, PAHO, and CDC convened a meeting to review progress in measles elimination and to assess the feasibility of global measles eradication.[47] The consultative group concluded that on the basis of the recent successes in both developing and developed countries, measles eradication with use of currently available vaccines was feasible. Although different strategies will be appropriate for different countries, strategies that rely on a single dose of measles vaccine or where extra efforts to reach unvaccinated children are not undertaken will not be successful. The group predicted that a strategy based on periodic mass vaccination campaigns will be needed in most developing countries. Some developed countries have apparently eliminated measles without mass vaccination campaigns, although intensive efforts to locate and vaccinate children who were not vaccinated have been required. Surveillance for measles cases will be needed to guide all control efforts. In elimination programs, laboratory confirmation of every isolated suspected measles case and every measles outbreak will be required. Molecular epidemiological studies will need to become a standard tool in tracing transmission patterns. Understanding measles outbreaks that occur after the initiation of measles elimination efforts will be critical in refining the

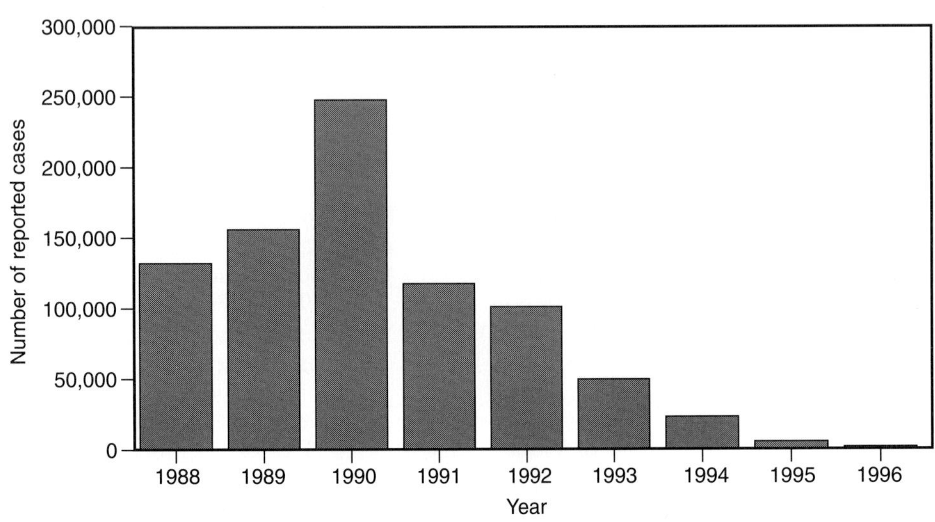

Figure 12–9. Reported measles cases, Latin America and the Caribbean, 1988 to 1996. (Data courtesy of the Special Programme on Vaccines and Immunizations, Pan American Health Organization.)

strategies for measles elimination. The group concluded with defining the major obstacles to measles elimination as perceptual, political, and financial, and not technical.

A follow-up meeting, sponsored by the same organizations, was held in August 1997, and progress toward improved control of measles and measles elimination was discussed. Increased attention to preventing death from measles was agreed on as an urgent priority. Further efforts to better document the financial and health burden of measles and the cost-effectiveness of global measles eradication are under way.

Although no goal for worldwide measles eradication has been established, such a goal, with a subsequent major public health initiative, is likely within the next few years.

REFERENCES

1. Abu Becr M; Mead R (trans). A Discourse on the Smallpox and Measles. London, J Brindley, 1748.
2. Babbott FL Jr, Gordon JE. Modern measles. Am J Med Sci 228:334–361, 1954.
3. Black FL. Measles. In Evans AS (ed). Viral Infections of Humans. Epidemiology and Control (3rd ed). New York, Plenum Publishing, 1989, pp 451–465.
4. Wilson GS. Measles as a universal disease. Am J Dis Child 103:219–223, 1962.
5. Sydenham T. The Works of Thomas Sydenham. Vol. 2. London, Sydenham Society, 1922, pp 250–251.
6. Enders JF. Francis Home and his experimental approach to medicine. Bull Hist Med 38:101–112, 1964.
7. Panum PL. Observation made during the epidemic of measles on the Faroe Islands in the year 1846. Med Classics 3:839–886, 1939.
8. Goldberger J, Anderson JF. An experimental demonstration of the presence of the virus of measles in the mixed buccal and nasal secretions. JAMA 57:476–478, 1911.
9. Enders JF, Peebles TC. Propagation in tissue cultures of cytopathogenic agents from patients with measles. Proc Soc Exp Biol Med 86:277–286, 1954.
10. Milovanovic MV, Enders JF, Mitus A. Cultivation of measles virus in human amnion cells and developing chick embryo. Proc Soc Exp Biol Med 95:120–127, 1957.
11. Katz SL, Milovanovic MV, Enders JF. Propagation of measles virus in cultures of chick embryo cells. Proc Soc Exp Biol Med 97:23–29, 1958.
12. Katz SL, Enders JF. Immunization of children with a live attenuated measles virus. Am J Dis Child 98:605–607, 1959.
13. Enders JF, Katz SL, Milovanovic MV, Holloway A. Studies on an attenuated measles-virus vaccine. I. Development and preparation of the vaccine: Techniques for assay of effects of vaccination. N Engl J Med 263:153–159, 1960.
14. Katz SL, Enders JF, Holloway A. Studies on an attenuated measles-virus vaccine. II. Clinical, virologic and immunologic effects of vaccine in institutionalized children. N Engl J Med 263:159–161, 1960.
15. Kempe CH, Ott EW, St. Vincent L, Maesel JC. Studies on an attenuated measles-virus vaccine. III. Clinical and antigenic effects of vaccine in institutionalized children. N Engl J Med 263:162–165, 1960.
16. Black FL, Sheridan SR. Studies on an attenuated measles-virus vaccine. IV. Administration of vaccine by several routes. N Engl J Med 263:165–169, 1960.
17. Lepow ML, Gray N, Robbins FC. Studies on an attenuated measles-virus vaccine. V. Clinical, antigenic and prophylactic effects of vaccine in institutionalized and home-dwelling children. N Engl J Med 263:170–173, 1960.
18. Krugman SL, Giles JP, Jacobs AM. Studies on an attenuated measles-virus vaccine. VI. Clinical, antigenic and prophylactic effects of vaccine in institutionalized children. N Engl J Med 263:174–177, 1960.
19. Katz SL, Kempe HC, Black FL, et al. Studies on an attenuated measles-virus vaccine. VIII. General summary and evaluation of the results of vaccination. N Engl J Med 263:180–184, 1960.
20. Enders JF. Measles virus: Historical review, isolation and behavior in various systems. Am J Dis Child 103:282–287, 1962.
21. Enders JF, Katz SL, Holloway A. Development of attenuated measles-virus vaccines. A summary of recent investigation. Am J Dis Child 103:335–340, 1962.
22. Seminar on the Epidemiology and Prevention of Measles and Rubella. Arch Virusforsch 16:1–551, 1965.
23. Centers for Disease Control. Goal to eliminate measles from the United States. MMWR Morb Mortal Wkly Rep 41:391, 1978.
24. Hinman AR, Brandling-Bennett AD, Nieberg PI. The opportunity and obligation to eliminate measles from the United States. JAMA 242:1157–1162, 1979.
25. Centers for Disease Control. Measles Surveillance Report No. 11, 1977–1981. US Department of Health and Human Services, Public Health Service. Atlanta, Centers for Disease Control, September 1982.
26. Hinman AR, Orenstein WA, Bloch AB, et al. Impact of measles in the United States. Rev Infect Dis 5:439–444, 1983.
27. Markowitz LE, Preblud SR, Orenstein WA, et al. Patterns of transmission in measles outbreaks in the United States, 1985–1986. N Engl J Med 320:75–81, 1989.
28. Bloch AB, Orenstein WA, Stetler HC, et al. Health impact of measles vaccination in the United States. Pediatrics 76:524–532, 1985.
29. White FMM. Policy for measles elimination in Canada and program implications. Rev Infect Dis 5:577–582, 1983.
30. Ikic DM. Edmonston-Zagreb strain of measles vaccine: Epidemiologic evaluation in Yugoslavia. Rev Infect Dis 5:558–563, 1983.
31. Sejda J. Evaluation of the eight-year period of compulsory measles vaccination in the Czech Socialist Republic (CSR). J Hyg Epidemiol Microbiol Immunol 23:272–283, 1979.
32. Sejda J. Control of measles in Czechoslovakia (CSSR). Rev Infect Dis 5:564–567, 1983.
33. Rabo E, Taranger J. Scandinavian model for eliminating measles, mumps, and rubella. BMJ 289:1402–1404, 1984.
34. Bottiger M, Christenson B, Romanus V, et al. Swedish experience of two dose vaccination programme aiming at eliminating measles, mumps and rubella. BMJ 295:1264–1267, 1987.
35. Peltola H, Kurki T, Virtanen M, et al. Rapid effect on endemic measles, mumps, and rubella of nationwide vaccination programme in Finland. Lancet 1:137–139, 1986.
36. Paunio M, Virtanen M, Peltola H, et al. Increase of vaccination coverage by mass media and individual approach: Intensified measles, mumps, and rubella prevention program in Finland. Am J Epidemiol 133:1152–1160, 1991.
37. Yihao Z, Wannian S. A review of the current impact of measles in the People's Republic of China. Rev Infect Dis 5:411–416, 1983.
38. Yihao Z, Wannian S. Introduction to the control of measles by vaccination in the People's Republic of China. Rev Infect Dis 5:568–573, 1983.
39. van Druten JAM, de Boo T, Plantinga AD. Measles, mumps, and rubella control by vaccination. Dev Biol Stand 65:53–63, 1986.
40. United Nations Children's Fund. State of the World's Children, 1992. New York, Oxford University Press, 1992.
41. Henderson RH, Keja J, Hayden G, et al. Immunizing the children of the world: Progress and prospects. Bull World Health Organ 66:535–543, 1988.
42. Cliff A, Haggett P, Smallman-Raynor M. Measles: An Historical Geography of a Major Human Viral Disease. Cambridge, MA, Blackwell Scientific Publications, 1993.
43. Hopkins DR, Hinman AR, Koplan JP, Lane JM. The case for global measles eradication. Lancet 1:1396–1398, 1982.
44. Hinman AR. Prospects for disease eradication or elimination. N Y State J Med 84:502–506, 1984.
45. Hinman AR, Bart KJ, Hopkins DR. Costs of not eradicating measles. Am J Public Health 75:713–715, 1985.
46. de Quadros CA. Global eradication of poliomyelitis and measles: Another quiet revolution. Ann Intern Med 127:156–158, 1997.
47. Centers for Disease Control and Prevention. Measles eradication: Recommendations from a meeting cosponsored by the World Health Organization, the Pan American Health Organization, and CDC. MMWR Morb Mortal Wkly Rep 46(RR-11):1–20, 1997.

48. Robbins FC. Measles: Clinical features. Pathogenesis, pathology, and complications. Am J Dis Child 103:266–273, 1962.
49. Katz SL, Enders JF, Holloway A. Use of Edmonston attenuated measles strain. A summary of three year's experience. Am J Dis Child 103:340–344, 1962.
50. Kempe CH, Fulginiti VA. The pathogenesis of measles virus infection. Arch Ges Virusforsch 16:103–128, 1965.
51. Case records of the Massachusetts General Hospital: Weekly clinicopathological exercises. Progressive pulmonary consolidations in a 10-year-old boy with Evans' syndrome. N Engl J Med 319:495–509, 1988. Case 34-1988.
52. Koplik H. The diagnosis of the invasion of measles from a study of the exanthema as it appears on the buccal mucous membrane. Arch Pediatr 13:918–922, 1896.
53. Gresser I, Chany C. Isolation of measles virus from the washed leukocyte fraction of blood. Proc Soc Exp Biol Med 113:695–698, 1963.
54. Gresser I, Katz SL. Isolation of measles virus from urine. N Engl J Med 263:452–454, 1960.
55. Ruckle G, Rogers KD. Studies with measles virus. II. Isolation of virus and immunologic studies in persons who have had natural disease. J Immunol 78:341–355, 1957.
56. Griffin DE, Ward BJ, Jauregui E, et al. Immune activation in measles. N Engl J Med 320:1667–1672, 1989.
57. Johnson RT, Griffin DE, Hoench TR. Pathogenesis of measles immunodeficiency and encephalomyelitis: Parallels to AIDS. Microbial Pathol 4:169–174, 1988.
58. Ward BJ, Johnson RT, Vaisberg A, et al. Cytokine production in vitro and the lymphoproliferative defect of natural measles virus infection. Clin Immunol Immunopathol 61:236–248, 1991.
59. McChesney MB, Oldstone BA. Virus-induced immunosuppression: Infections with measles virus and human immunodeficiency virus. Adv Immunol 45:335–380, 1989.
60. Griffin DE. Immune responses during measles virus infection. Curr Top Microbiol Immunol 191:117–134, 1995.
61. Griffin DE, Ward BJ, Esolen LM. Pathogenesis of measles virus infection: An hypothesis for altered immune responses. J Infect Dis 170(suppl 1):S24–S31, 1994.
62. Bech V. Studies on the development of complement fixing antibodies in measles patients. Observations during a measles epidemic in Greenland. J Immunol 83:267–275, 1959.
63. Stokes J Jr, Reilly CM, Buynak EB, Hilleman MR. Immunologic studies of measles. Am J Hyg 74:293–303, 1961.
64. Enders-Ruckle G. Methods of determining immunity, duration and character of immunity resulting from measles. Arch Ges Virusforsch 16:182–207, 1965.
65. Krugman S, Giles JP, Friedman H, Stone S. Studies on immunity to measles. J Pediatr 66:471–488, 1965.
66. Norrby E, Gollmar Y. Appearance and persistence of antibodies against different virus components of regular measles infections. Infect Immun 6:240–247, 1972.
67. Kibler R, ter Meulen V. Antibody-mediated cytotoxicity after measles virus infection. J Immunol 114:93–98, 1975.
68. Bellanti JA, Sanga RL, Klutinis B, et al. Antibody responses in serum and nasal secretions of children immunized with inactivated and attenuated measles-virus vaccines. N Engl J Med 280:628–633, 1969.
69. Polna I, Aleksandrowicz J, Krawczynski K, et al. Measles antibodies in nasal secretions and sera of children with measles. Acta Virol 21:331–337, 1977.
70. Friedman M, Hadari I, Goldstein V, Sarov I. Virus-specific secretory IgA antibodies as a means of rapid diagnosis of measles and mumps infection. Isr J Med Sci 19:881–884, 1983.
71. Ruckdeschel JC, Graziano KD, Mardiney MR Jr. Additional evidence that the cell-associated system is the primary host defense against measles (rubeola). Cell Immunol 17:11–18, 1975.
72. Graziano KD, Ruckdeschel JC, Mardiney MR Jr. Cell-associated immunity to measles (rubeola). The demonstration of in vitro lymphocyte tritiated thymidine incorporation in response to measles complement fixation antigen. Cell Immunol 15:347–359, 1975.
73. Krause PJ, Cherry JD, Naiditch MJ, et al. Revaccination of previous recipients of killed measles vaccine: Clinical and immunologic studies. J Pediatr 93:565–571, 1978.
74. Krause PJ, Cherry JD, Carney JM, et al. Measles-specific lymphocyte reactivity and serum antibody in subjects with different measles histories. Am J Dis Child 134:567–571, 1980.
75. Whittle HC, Werblinska J. Cellular cytotoxicity to measles virus during natural measles infection. Clin Exp Immunol 42:136–143, 1980.
76. Gallagher MR, Welliver R, Yamanaka T, et al. Cell-mediated immune responsiveness to measles. Its occurrence as a result of naturally acquired or vaccine-induced infection and in infants of immune mothers. Am J Dis Child 135:48–51, 1981.
77. Sissons JGP, Colby SD, Harrison WO, Oldstone MBA. Cytotoxic lymphocytes generated in vivo with acute measles virus infection. Clin Immunol Immunopathol 34:60–68, 1985.
78. Black FL, Rosen L. Patterns of measles antibodies in residents of Tahiti and their stability in the absence of re-exposure. J Immunol 88:725–731, 1962.
79. Krugman S, Katz SL, Gershon AA, et al. Measles. In Krugman S (ed). Infectious Diseases of Children (8th ed). St. Louis, CV Mosby, 1985, pp 152–166.
80. Cherry JD. Measles. In Feigen RD, Cherry JD (eds). Textbook of Pediatric Infectious Diseases (2nd ed). Philadelphia, WB Saunders, 1987, pp 1607–1628.
81. Appelbaum E, Dolgopol VB, Dolgin J. Measles encephalitis. Am J Dis Child 77:25–48, 1949.
82. Christensen PE, Schmidt H, Bang HO, et al. An epidemic of measles in southern Greenland, 1951. Measles in virgin soil. II. The epidemic proper. Acta Med Scand 144:430–449, 1953.
83. Peart AFW, Nagler FP. Measles in the Canadian Arctic, 1952. Can J Public Health 45:146–156, 1954.
84. Miller HG, Stanton JB, Gibbons JL. Para-infectious encephalomyelitis and related syndromes: A critical review of the neurologic complications of certain specific fevers. Q J Med 25:247–505, 1956.
85. Bech V. Measles epidemic in Greenland. Am J Dis Child 103:252–253, 1962.
86. Miller DL. Frequency of complication of measles, 1963. Report on a national Inquiry by the Public Health Laboratory Service in Collaboration with the Society of Medical Officer of Health. BMJ 2:75–78, 1964.
87. Bech V. The measles epidemic in Greenland in 1962. Arch Ges Virusforsch 16:53–56, 1965.
88. Littauer J, Sorensen K. The measles epidemic at Umanak in Greenland in 1962. Dan Med J 12:43–50, 1965.
89. McLean DM, Best JM, Smith PA, et al. Viral infections of Toronto children during 1965. II. Measles encephalitis and other complications. Can Med Assoc J 94:906–910, 1966.
90. Barkin RM. Measles mortality: A retrospective look at the vaccine era. Am J Epidemiol 102:341–349, 1975.
91. Barkin RM. Measles mortality. Analysis of the primary cause of death. JAMA 129:307–309, 1975.
92. Modlin JF, Jabbour JT, Witte JJ, Halsey NA. Epidemiologic studies of measles, measles vaccine, and subacute sclerosing panencephalitis. Pediatrics 59:505–512, 1977.
93. Modlin JF, Halsey NA, Eddins DL, et al. Epidemiology of subacute sclerosing panencephalitis. J Pediatr 94:231–236, 1979.
94. Becroft DMO, Osborne DRS. The lungs in fatal measles infection in childhood: Pathological, radiological and immunological correlations. Histopathology 4:401–412, 1980.
95. Englehandt SF, Halsey NA, Eddins DL, Hinman AR. Measles mortality in the United States 1971–1975. Am J Public Health 70:1166–1169, 1980.
96. Johnson RT, Griffin DE, Hirsch RL, et al. Measles encephalomyelitis—clinical and immunologic studies. N Engl J Med 310:137–141, 1984.
97. Centers for Disease Control. Subacute sclerosing panencephalitis surveillance—United States. MMWR Morb Mortal Wkly Rep 31:585–588, 1982.
98. Bloch AB, Orenstein WA, Wassilak SG, et al. Epidemiology of measles and its complications. In Gruenberg EM, Lewis C, Goldston SE (eds). Vaccinating Against Brain Syndromes: The Campaign Against Measles and Rubella. New York, Oxford University Press, 1986, pp 5–20. Monographs in Epidemiology and Biostatistics, Vol. 9.
99. Atkinson WL, Markowitz LE. Measles and measles vaccine. Semin Pediatr Infect Dis 2:100–107, 1991.
100. Greenberg BL, Sack RB, Salazar-Lindo, et al. Measles associated

diarrhea in hospitalized children in Lima, Peru: Pathogenic agents and impact on growth. J Infect Dis 164:495–502, 1991.
101. von Pirquet CE. Das Verhalten der kutanen Tuberkulinreaktion wahrend der Masern. Dtsch Med Wochnschr 34:1297–1300, 1908.
102. Flick JA. Does measles really predispose to tuberculosis? Am Rev Respir Dis 114:257–265, 1976.
103. Morley D, Woodland M, Martin WJ. Measles in Nigerian children. A study of the disease in West Africa, and its manifestations in England and other countries during difficult epochs. J Hyg (Camb) 61:115–134, 1963.
104. Morley D. Severe measles in the tropics. BMJ 1:297–300, 363–365, 1969.
105. O'Donovan C. Measles in Kenyan children. East Afr Med J 48:526–532, 1971.
106. Scheifele DW, Forbes CE. The biology of measles in African children. East Afr Med J 50:169–173, 1973.
107. Morley DC. Measles in the developing world. Proc R Soc Med 67:1112–1115, 1974.
108. Hayden RJ. The epidemiology and nature of measles in Nairobi before the impact of measles immunization. East Afr Med J 51:199–205, 1974.
109. Assaad F. Measles: Summary of worldwide impact. Rev Infect Dis 5:452–459, 1983.
110. Walsh JA. Selective primary health care: Strategies for control of disease in the developing world. IV. Measles. Rev Infect Dis 5:330–340, 1983.
111. Williams PJ, Hull HF. Status of measles in the Gambia, 1981. Rev Infect Dis 5:391–394, 1983.
112. Borgono JM. Current impact of measles in Latin America. Rev Infect Dis 5:417–421, 1983.
113. Hull HF, Williams PJ, Oldfield F. Measles mortality and vaccine efficacy in rural West Africa. Lancet 1:972–975, 1983.
114. Loening UE, Coovadia HM. Age specific occurrence rates of measles in urban, periurban, and rural environments and implication for time of vaccination. Lancet 2:324–326, 1983.
115. Nieberg P, Dibley MJ. Risk factors for fatal measles infections. Int J Epidemiol 15:309–311, 1986.
116. Porter JDH, Gastellu-Etchegorry M, Navarre I, et al. Measles outbreaks in the Mozambican refugee camps in Malawi: The continued need for an effective vaccine. Int J Epidemiol 19:1072–1077, 1989.
117. Narain JP, Khare S, Rana SRS, Banerjee KB. Epidemic measles in an isolated unvaccinated population, India. Int J Epidemiol 18:952–958, 1989.
118. The Kasongo Project Team. Influence of measles vaccination on survival pattern of 7–35 month-old children in Kasongo, Zaire. Lancet 1:764–767, 1981.
119. Foster SO, McFarland DA, John MA. Health sector priorities review, measles. In Jamison DT, Mosley WH (eds). Evolving Health Sector Priorities in Developing Countries. Washington, DC, The World Bank, 1993, pp 161–183.
120. Koster F, Curlin G, Aziz KMA, Haque A. Synergistic impact of measles and diarrheoa in nutrition and mortality in Bangladesh. Bull World Health Organ 59:901–908, 1981.
121. Sarker SA, Wahed MA, Rahaman MM, et al. Persistent protein losing enteropathy in post measles diarrhoea. Arch Dis Child 61:739–743, 1986.
122. Reddy V, Bhaskaram P, Raghuramulu N, et al. Relationship between measles, malnutrition, and blindness: A prospective study in Indian children. Am J Clin Nutr 44:924–930, 1986.
123. Expanded Programme on Immunization: Programme for the prevention of blindness nutrition. Joint WHO/UNICEF statement: Vitamin A for measles. Wkly Epidemiol Rec 62:133–134, 1987.
124. Gilbert CE, Wood M, Waddel K, Foster A. Causes of childhood blindness in east Africa: Results in 491 pupils attending 17 schools for the blind in Malawi, Kenya and Uganda. Ophthalmic Epidemiol 2:77–84, 1995.
125. Gershon AA, Krugman S. Measles virus. In Lennette EH, Schmidt NJ (eds). Diagnostic Procedures for Viral, Rickettsial and Chlamydial Infections (5th ed). Washington, DC, American Public Health Association, 1979, pp 665–693.
126. Sever JL. Persistent measles infection of the central nervous system: Subacute sclerosing panencephalitis. Rev Infect Dis 5:467–473, 1983.
127. Sakaguchi M, Yoshikawa Y, Yamanouchi K, et al. Characteristics of fresh isolates of wild measles virus. Jpn J Exp Med 56:61–67, 1986.
128. Dyken PR. Subsclerosing panencephalitis, current status. Neurol Clin 3:179–196, 1985.
129. Gascon GG. Subacute sclerosing panencephalitis. Semin Pediatr Neurol 3:260–269, 1996.
130. Halsey NA, Modlin JF, Jabbour JT, et al. Risk factors in subacute sclerosing panencephalitis: A case control study. Am J Epidemiol 3:415–420, 1980.
131. Billeter MA, Cattaneo R, Spielhofer P, et al. Generation and properties of measles virus mutations typically associated with subacute sclerosing panencephalitis. Ann N Y Acad Sci 724:367–377, 1994.
132. Ekbom A, Wakefield AJ, Zack M, Adami HO. Perinatal measles infection and subsequent Crohn's disease. Lancet 344:508–510, 1994.
133. Wakefield AJ, Ekbom A, Dhillon AP, et al. Crohn's disease: Pathogenesis and persistent measles virus infection. Gastroenterology 108:991–996, 1995.
134. Ekbom A, Daszak P, Kraaz W, Wakefield AJ. Crohn's disease after in-utero measles virus exposure. Lancet 348:515–517, 1996.
135. Thompson NP, Montgomery SM, Pounder RE, Wakefield AJ. Is measles vaccination a risk factor for inflammatory bowel disease? Lancet 345:1071–1074, 1995.
136. Iizuka M, Nakagomi O, Chiba M, et al. Absence of measles virus in Crohn's disease [letter]. Lancet 345:199, 1995.
137. Patriarca PA, Beeler JA. Measles vaccination and inflammatory bowel disease. Lancet 345:1062–1063, 1995.
138. Farrington P, Miller E. Measles vaccination as a risk factor for inflammatory bowel disease [letter]. Lancet 345:1362, 1995.
139. Feeney M, Clegg A, Winwood P, Snook J. A case-control study of measles vaccination and inflammatory bowel disease. Lancet 350:764–766, 1997.
140. Atmar RL, Englund JA, Hammill H. Complications of measles in pregnancy. Clin Infect Dis 14:217–226, 1992.
141. Eberhart-Phillips JE, Frederick PD, Baron RC, Mascola L. Measles in pregnancy: A descriptive study of 58 cases. Obstet Gynecol 82:797–801, 1993.
142. Young NA, Gershon AA. Chickenpox, measles, and mumps. In Remington JS, Klein JO (eds). Infectious Diseases of the Fetus and Newborn Infant (2nd ed). Philadelphia, WB Saunders, 1983, pp 375–427.
143. Siegel M. Congenital malformations following chickenpox, measles, mumps, and hepatitis. Results of a cohort study. JAMA 226:1521–1524, 1973.
144. Jesperson CS, Littover J, Saglid V. Measles as a cause of fetal defects. A retrospective study of ten measles epidemics in Greenland. Acta Paediatr Scand 66:367–376, 1977.
145. Siegel M, Fuerst HT, Peress NS. Comparative fetal mortality in maternal virus diseases. A prospective study on rubella, measles, mumps, chicken pox, and hepatitis. N Engl J Med 274:768–771, 1966.
146. Stokes J Jr, Maris EP, Gellis SS. Chemical, clinical, and immunologic studies on the products of human plasma fractionation. XI. The use of concentrated normal human serum gamma globulin (human immune serum globulin) in the prevention and attenuation of measles. J Clin Invest 23:531–540, 1944.
147. Ordman CW, Jennings CG Jr, Janeway CA. Chemical, clinical and immunological studies on the products of human plasma fractionation. XII. The use of concentrated normal human serum gamma globulin (human immune serum globulin) in the prevention and attenuation of measles. J Clin Invest 23:541–549, 1944.
148. Janeway CA. Use of concentrated human serum g-globulin in the prevention and attenuation of measles. Bull N Y Acad Med 21:202–222, 1945.
149. Janeway CA. Plasma fractionation. Arch Intern Med 3:295–372, 1949.
150. Black FL, Yannet H. Inapparent measles after gamma globulin administration. JAMA 173:1183–1188, 1960.
151. Brody JA, Bridenbraugh E. Prophylactic g-globulin and live measles vaccine in an island epidemic of measles. Lancet 2:811–813, 1964.
152. Perkins FT. Passive prophylaxis of measles. Arch Ges Virusforsch 16:210–217, 1965.

153. Krugman S, Giles JP, Jacobs AM, Friedman H. Studies with live attenuated measles-virus vaccine. Am J Dis Child 103:353–363, 1962.
154. Karlitz S, Markham FS. Immunity after modified measles. Am J Dis Child 103:682–687, 1962.
155. Linnemann CC Jr. Measles vaccine: Immunity, reinfection and revaccination. Am J Epidemiol 97:365–371, 1973.
156. Schluederberg A. Modification of immune response by previous experience with measles. Arch Virusforsch 16:347–350, 1965.
157. Schaffner W, Schluederberg AES, Byrne EB. Clinical epidemiology of sporadic measles in a highly immunized population. N Engl J Med 279:783–789, 1968.
158. Cherry JD, Feigen RD, Lobes JA Jr, et al. Urban measles in the vaccine era: A clinical, epidemiologic, and serologic study. J Pediatr 81:217–230, 1972.
159. Linneman CC, Rotte TC, Schiff GM, Youtsey JL. A seroepidemiologic study of a measles epidemic in a highly immunized population. Am J Epidemiol 95:238–246, 1972.
160. Linnemann CC, Hegg ME, Rotte TC, et al. Measles IgM response during reinfection of previously vaccinated children. J Pediatr 82:798–801, 1973.
161. Cherry JD, Feigen RD, Shackelford PG, et al. A clinical and serologic study of 103 children with measles vaccine failure. J Pediatr 82:802–808, 1973.
162. Schluederberg A, Lamm SH, Landrigan PJ, Black FL. Measles immunity in children vaccinated before one year of age. Am J Epidemiol 97:402–409, 1973.
163. Smith FR, Curran AS, Raciti A, Black FL. Reported measles in persons immunologically primed by prior vaccination. J Pediatr 101:391–393, 1982.
164. Nagy G, Kosa S, Takatsy, Koller M. The use of IgM tests for analysis of the causes of measles vaccine failures: Experience gained in an epidemic in Hungary in 1980 and 1981. J Med Virol 13:93–103, 1984.
165. Mathias R, Meekison J, Arcand T, et al. The role of secondary vaccine failures in measles outbreaks. Am J Public Health 79:475–478, 1989.
166. Edmonson MB, Addiss DG, McPherson JT, et al. Mild measles and secondary vaccine failure during sustained outbreak in a highly vaccinated population. JAMA 263:2467–2471, 1990.
167. Reyes MA, Franky De Borrero M, Roa J, et al. Measles vaccine failure after documented seroconversion. Pediatr Infect Dis J 6:848–851, 1987.
168. Bin D, Zhihui, Qichang L, et al. Duration of immunity following immunization with live measles vaccine: 15 years of observation in Zhejiang Province, China. Bull World Health Organ 69:415–423, 1991.
169. Mitus A, Enders JF, Craig JM, Holloway A. Persistence of measles virus and depression of antibody formation in patients with giant cell pneumonia after measles. N Engl J Med 261:882–889, 1959.
170. Mitus A, Holloway, Evans AE, Enders JF. Attenuated measles vaccine in children with acute leukemia. Am J Dis Child 103:413–418, 1962.
171. Mitus A, Enders JF, Edsall G, Holloway A. Measles in children with malignancy. Problems and prevention. Arch Ges Virusforsch 16:331–337, 1965.
172. Siegel MM, Walter TK, Ablin AR. Measles pneumonia in childhood leukemia. Pediatrics 60:38–40, 1977.
173. Krasinski K, Borkowsky W. Measles and measles immunity in children infected with human immunodeficiency virus. JAMA 261:2512–2516, 1989.
174. Gray MM, Hann IM, Glass S, et al. Mortality and morbidity caused by measles in children with malignant disease attending four major treatment centres: A retrospective review. BMJ 295:19–22, 1987.
175. Kaplan LJ, Daum RS, Smaron M, McCarthy CA. Severe measles in immunocompromised patients. JAMA 267:1237–1241, 1992.
176. Markowitz LE, Chandler FW, Roldan EO, et al. Fatal measles pneumonia without rash in a child with AIDS. J Infect Dis 158:480–483, 1988.
177. Nahmias AJ, Griffith D, Salsbury C, Yoshida K. Thymic aplasia and lymphopenia, plasma cells and normal immunoglobulins. Relation to measles virus infection. JAMA 201:729–734, 1967.
178. Good RA, Zak SJ. Disturbances in gamma globulin synthesis as "experiments of nature." Pediatrics 18:109–149, 1956.
179. Burnet FM. Measles as an index of immunological function. Lancet 2:610–613, 1968.
180. Coovadia HM, Brain P, Hallett AF, et al. Immunoparesis and outcome in measles. Lancet 1:619–621, 1977.
181. Aicardi J, Goutiere SF, Arsenio-Nunes ML, Lebon P. Acute measles encephalitis in children with immunosuppression. Pediatrics 59:232–239, 1977.
182. Roos RP, Graves MC, Wollmann RL, et al. Immunologic and virologic studies of measles inclusion body encephalitis: The relationship to subacute sclerosing panencephalitis. Neurology 31:1263–1270, 1981.
183. Enders JF, McCarthy K, Mitus A, Cheatham WJ. Isolation of measles virus at autopsy in cases of giant-cell pneumonia without rash. N Engl J Med 261:875–881, 1959.
184. Palumbo P, Hoyt L, Demasio K, et al. Population-based study of measles and measles immunization in human immunodeficiency virus–infected children. Pediatr Infect Dis J 11:1008–1014, 1992.
185. Rauh LW, Schmidt R. Measles immunization with killed virus vaccine. Serum antibody titers and experience with exposure to measles epidemic. Am J Dis Child 109:232–237, 1965.
186. Fulginiti VA, Eller JJ, Downie AW, Kempe CH. Altered reactivity to measles virus. Atypical measles in children previously immunized with inactivated measles virus vaccines. JAMA 202:1075–1080, 1967.
187. Nader PR, Horowitz MS, Rousseau J. Atypical exanthem following exposure to natural measles: Eleven cases in children previously inoculated with killed vaccine. J Pediatr 72:22–28, 1968.
188. Gokiert JG, Beamish WE. Altered reactivity to measles virus in previously vaccinated children. Can Med Assoc J 103:724–727, 1970.
189. Buser F, Montagnon B. Severe illness in children exposed to natural measles after prior vaccination against the disease. Scand J Infect Dis 2:157–160, 1970.
190. O'Neil AE. The measles epidemic in Calgary 1969–70; the protective effect of vaccination for the individual and the community. Can Med Assoc J 105:819–825, 1971.
191. Welliver RC, Cherry JD, Holtzman AE. Typical, modified, and atypical measles: An emerging problem in the adolescent and adult. Arch Intern Med 137:39–41, 1977.
192. Weiner LB, Corwin RM, Nieberg PI, Feldman HA. A measles outbreak among adolescents. J Pediatr 90:17–20, 1977.
193. Chatterji M, Mankad V. Failure of attenuated viral vaccine in prevention of atypical measles. JAMA 238:2635, 1977.
194. Hall WW, Breese Hall C. Atypical measles in adolescents; evaluation of clinical and pulmonary function. Ann Intern Med 90:882–886, 1979.
195. Martin DB, Weiner LB, Nieberg PI, Blair DC. Atypical measles in adolescents and young adults. Ann Intern Med 90:877–881, 1979.
196. Fulginiti VA, Helfer RE. Atypical measles in adolescent siblings 16 years after killed measles virus vaccine. JAMA 244:804–806, 1980.
197. Annuziato D, Kaplan MH, Hull WW, et al. Atypical measles syndrome: Pathologic and serologic findings. Pediatrics 70:203–209, 1982.
198. Norrby E. Measles. In Fields BN (ed). Virology. New York, Raven Press, 1985, pp 1305–1321.
199. Lennon RG, Isacson P, Rosales T, et al. Skin tests with measles and poliomyelitis vaccines in recipients of inactivated measles virus vaccine. JAMA 200:275–280, 1967.
200. Nieberg PI, D'Angelo LJ, Herrmann KL. Measles in patients suspected of having Rocky Mountain spotted fever. JAMA 244:808–809, 1980.
201. Brooks JB, McDade JE, Alley CC. Rapid differentiation of Rocky Mountain spotted fever from chickenpox, measles, and enterovirus infections and bacterial meningitis by frequency-pulsed electron capture gas-liquid chromatography analysis of sera. J Clin Microbiol 14:165–172, 1981.
202. Laptook A, Wind A, Nussbaum M, Shenker IR. Pulmonary lesions in atypical measles. Pediatrics 62:42–26, 1978.
203. Centers for Disease Control. Death from measles, possibly atypical—Michigan. MMWR Morb Mortal Wkly Rep 28:298–299, 1979.
204. Cherry JD, Feigen RD, Lobes LA, Shakelford PG. Atypical measles in children previously immunized with attenuated measles virus vaccines. Pediatrics 50:712–717, 1972.

205. St. Geme JW Jr, Bush BM, George BL. Exaggerated natural measles following attenuated virus immunization: A refraction-toxic shock syndrome [letter]. Pediatrics 67:942, 1981.
206. American Academy of Pediatrics. Measles. In Peter G (ed). 1997 Red Book: Report of the Committee on Infectious Diseases (24th ed). Elk Grove Village, IL, American Academy of Pediatrics, 1997, pp 344–357.
207. Centers for Disease Control. Recommendations of the Immunization Practices Advisory Committee (ACIP). Measles prevention. MMWR Morb Mortal Wkly Rep 38(S-9):1–13, 1989.
208. Olding-Stenkvist E, Forsgren M, Henley D, et al. Measles encephalopathy during immunosuppression: Failure of treatment. Scand J Infect Dis 14:1–4, 1982.
209. Simpson R, Eden OB. Possible interferon response in a child with measles encephalitis during immunosuppression. Scand J Infect Dis 16:315–319, 1984.
210. Beatty DW, Handzel ZT, Pecht M, et al. A controlled trial of treatment of acquired immunodeficiency in severe measles with thymic humoral factor. Clin Exp Immunol 56:479–485, 1984.
211. Tovo PA, Pugliese A, Palomba E, et al. Thymostimulin therapy in patients with measles meningoencephalitis. Thymus 8:91–94, 1986.
212. Wesley AG, Coovadia HM, Kiepiela P. Levamisole therapy in children at risk from severe measles. Ann Trop Paediatr 2:23–29, 1982.
213. Banks G, Fernandez H. Clinical use of ribavirin in measles: A summarized review. In Smith RA, Knight V, Smith JAD (eds). Clinical Applications of Ribavirin. New York, Academic Press, 1984, pp 203–209.
214. Aaby P, Bukh J, Hoff G, et al. Humoral immunity in measles infection: A critical factor? Med Hypotheses 23:278–301, 1987.
215. Ross LA, Kim KS, Mason WH, Gomperts E. Successful treatment of disseminated measles in a patient with acquired immunodeficiency syndrome: Consideration of antiviral and passive immunotherapy. Am J Med 88:313–314, 1990.
216. Hussey GD, Klein M. A randomized, controlled trial of vitamin A in children with severe measles. N Engl J Med 323:160–164, 1990.
217. Barclay AJG, Foster A, Sommer A. Vitamin A supplements and mortality related to measles: A randomized clinical trial. BMJ 294:294–296, 1987.
218. Butler JC, Havens PL, Sowell AL, et al. Measles severity and serum retinol (vitamin A) concentration among children in the United States. Pediatrics 91:1176–1181, 1993.
219. Frieden TR, Sowell AL, Henning KJ, et al. Vitamin A levels and severity of measles. New York City. Am J Dis Child 146:182–186, 1992.
220. Arrieta AC, Zaleska M, Stutman HR, Marks MI. Vitamin A levels in children with measles in Long Beach, California. J Pediatr 121:75–78, 1992.
221. American Academy of Pediatrics, Committee on Infectious Diseases. Vitamin A treatment of measles. Pediatrics 91:1014–1015, 1993.
222. Shann F. Meta-analysis of trials of prophylactic antibiotics for children with measles: Inadequate evidence. BMJ 314:334–336, 1997.
223. Freeman JM. Treatment for subacute sclerosing panencephalitis with 5-bromo-2-deoxyuridine and Pyran copolymer. Neurology 18(pt 2):176–192, 1968.
224. Kackell YM, Grob PJ, Kreth WH, et al. Transfer factor therapy in patients with subacute sclerosing panencephalitis. J Neurol 211:39–49, 1975.
225. Steiner I, Wirguin I, Morag A, Abramsky O. Intraventricular alpha interferon for subacute sclerosing panencephalitis. J Child Neurol 4:20–23, 1989.
226. Gascon GG, Yamani S, Cafege A. Treatment of subacute sclerosing panencephalitis with alpha interferon. Ann Neurol 30:227–228, 1991.
227. Huttenlocher PR, Mattson RH. Isoprinosine in subacute sclerosing panencephalitis. Neurology 29:763–771, 1979.
228. DuRant RH, Dyken PR, Swift AV. The influence of inosiplex treatment on the neurological disability of patients with subacute sclerosing panencephalitis. J Pediatr 101:288–293, 1982.
229. Waterson AP. Measles virus. Arch Ges Virusforsch 16:57–80, 1965.
230. Bostock CJ, Barrett T, Crowther JR. Characterization of the European seal morbillivirus. Vet Microbiol 23:351–360, 1990.
231. Imagawa DT. Relationships among measles, canine distemper and rhinderpest viruses. Prog Med Virol 10:160–193, 1968.
232. Naniche D, Varior-Krishnan G, Cervoni F, et al. Human membrane cofactor protein (CD46) acts as a cellular receptor for measles virus. J Virol 67:6025–6032, 1993.
233. Gerlier D, Varior-Krishnan G, Devaux P. CD46-mediated measles virus entry: A first key to host-range specificity. Trends Microbiol 3:338–345, 1995.
234. Crowley JC, Dowling PC, Menonna J, et al. Sequence variability and function of measles virus 3′ and 5′ ends and intercistronic regions. Virology 164:498–506, 1988.
235. Giraudon P, Jacquier MF, Wild TF. Antigenic analysis of African measles virus field isolates: Identification and localization of one conserved and two variable epitope sites on the NP protein. Virus Res 10:137–152, 1988.
236. Baczko D, Brinckmann U, Padowitz I, et al. Nucleotide sequence of the genes encoding the matrix protein of two wild-type measles virus strains. J Gen Virol 72:2279–2282, 1991.
237. Taylor MJ, Godfrey E, Baczko K, et al. Identification of several different lineages of measles virus. J Gen Virol 72:83–88, 1991.
238. Rota JS, Hummel KB, Rota PA, Bellini WJ. Genetic variability of the glycoprotein genes of current wildtype measles isolates. J Virol 188:135–142, 1992.
239. Rota PA, Bloom AE, Vanchiere JA, Bellini WJ. Evolution of the nucleoprotein and matrix genes of wild-type strains of measles virus isolated from recent epidemics. Virology 198:724–730, 1994.
240. Rota JS, Wang ZD, Rota PA, Bellini WJ. Comparison of sequences of the H, F, and N coding genes of measles virus vaccine strains. Virus Res 31:317–330, 1994.
241. Rota J, Heath JL, Rota PA, et al. Molecular epidemiology of measles virus: Identification of pathways of transmission and implications for measles elimination. J Infect Dis 173:32–37, 1996.
242. Tamin A, Rota PA, Wang ZD, et al. Antigenic analysis of current wild type and vaccine strains of measles virus. J Infect Dis 170:795–801, 1994.
243. Kobune F, Sakata H, Sugiura A. Marmoset lymphoblastoid cells as a sensitive host for isolation of measles virus. J Virol 64:700–705, 1990.
244. Matumoto M. Multiplication of measles virus in cell cultures. Bacteriol Rev 30:152–176, 1966.
245. Forthal DN, Blanding J, Aarnaes S, et al. Comparison of different methods and cell lines for isolating measles virus. J Clin Microbiol 31:695–697, 1993.
246. Enders JF, Katz SL, Grogran E. Markers for Edmonston measles virus. Am J Dis Child 103:473–474, 1962.
247. McCarthy K. Measles in laboratory hosts and tissue cultures systems. Am J Dis Child 103:314–319, 1962.
248. Suringa DWR, Bank LJ, Ackerman AB. Role of measles virus in skin lesions and Koplik's spots. N Engl J Med 283:1139–1142, 1970.
249. Buynak EB, Peck JM, Creamer AA, et al. Differentiation of virulent from avirulent measles strains. Am J Dis Child 103:460–473, 1962.
250. DeMaeyer E, Enders JF. Growth characteristics, interferon production and plaque formation with different lines of Edmonston measles virus. Arch Ges Virusforsch 16:151–160, 1965.
251. Katz SL. Immunization with live attenuated measles virus vaccines: Five years' experience. Arch Virusforsch 16:222–230, 1965.
252. Papp K. Experiences prouvant que la voie d'infection de la rougeole est la contamination de la muqueuse conjunctival. Rev Immunol Ther Antimicrob 20:27–36, 1956.
253. Fenner F. The pathogenesis of the acute exanthems. Lancet 2:915–920, 1948.
254. Moench TR, Griffin DE, Obriecht CR, et al. Acute measles in patients with and without neurological involvement: Distribution of measles virus antigen and RNA. J Infect Dis 158:433–442, 1988.
255. Ogra PL, Morag A. Immunologic and virologic aspects of secretory immune system in human respiratory tract. Dev Biol Stand 28:129–144, 1975.
256. Ogra PL, Fishaut M, Gallagher MR. Viral vaccination via mucosal routes. Rev Infect Dis 2:352–369, 1980.

257. Centers for Disease Control. Classification of measles cases and categorization of measles elimination programs. MMWR Morb Mortal Wkly Rep 31:707–711, 1983.
258. Llanes-Rodas R, Liu C. Rapid diagnosis of measles from urinary sediments stained with fluorescent antibody. N Engl J Med 275:515–523, 1966.
259. Lightwood R, Nolan R, Franco M, White AJS. Epithelial giant cells in measles as an aid in diagnosis. J Pediatr 77:59–64, 1970.
260. Fulton RE, Middleton PJ. Immunofluorescence in diagnosis of measles infection in children. J Pediatr 86:17–22, 1975.
261. Olding-Stenkvist E, Bjorvatn B. Rapid detection of measles virus in skin rashes by immunofluorescence. J Infect Dis 134:463–469, 1976.
262. Nommensen FE, Dekkers NWHM. Detection of measles antigen in conjunctival epithelial lesions staining by Lissamine green during measles virus infection. J Med Virol 7:157–162, 1981.
263. Boyd JF. A fourteen year study to identify measles antigen in urine specimens by fluorescent-antibody methods. J Infect 6:163–170, 1983.
264. Jin L, Richards A, Brown DW. Development of a dual target–PCR for detection and characterization of measles virus in clinical specimens. Mol Cell Probes 10:191–200, 1996.
265. Rota PA, Khan AS, Durigon E, et al. Detection of measles virus RNA in urine specimens from vaccine recipients. J Clin Microbiol 33:2485–2488, 1995.
266. Wassilak SGF, Bernier RH, Herrmann KL, et al. Measles seroconfirmation using dried capillary blood specimens in filter paper. Pediatr Infect Dis 3:117–121, 1984.
267. Krugman S, Giles JP, Jacobs AM, Friedman H. Studies with a further attenuated live measles-virus vaccine. Pediatrics 31:919–928, 1963.
268. Krugman S. Present status of measles and rubella immunization in the United States: A medical progress report. J Pediatr 78:1–16, 1971.
269. Krugman S. Present status of measles and rubella immunization in the United States: A medical progress report. J Pediatr 90:1–12, 1977.
270. Krugman S. Further-attenuated measles vaccine: Characteristics and use. Rev Infect Dis 5:477–481, 1983.
271. Schluederberg A. Immune globulins in human viral infections. Nature 205:1232–1233, 1965.
272. Heffner RR Jr, Schluederberg A. Specificity of the primary and secondary antibody responses to myxoviruses. J Immunol 98:668–672, 1967.
273. Polna I, Aleksandrowicz J, Roszkowska K. Localization of measles antibody and inhibitor activity in fractions of human sera at different stages of the disease, and sera of animals immunized with measles virus. I. Dynamics of increase in measles antibody activity and its localization in children sera after natural infection. Acta Microbiol Pol A 5:131–138, 1973.
274. Aleksandrowicz J, Polna I, Sadowski W. II. Primary and secondary immunological response of experimental animals to attenuated and nonattenuated measles virus. Acta Microbiol Pol A 22:139–145, 1973.
275. Friedman MG, Philip M, Dagan R. Virus-specific IgA in serum, saliva, and tears of children with measles. Clin Exp Immunol 75:58–64, 1989.
276. Erdman DD, Anderson LJ, Adams DR, et al. Evaluation of monoclonal antibody–based capture enzyme immunoassays for detection of specific antibodies to measles virus. J Clin Microbiol 29:1466–1471, 1991.
277. Erdman DD, Heath JL, Watson JC, et al. Immunoglobulin M antibody response to measles virus following primary and secondary vaccination and natural virus infection. J Med Virol 41:44–48, 1993.
278. Cutchins EC. A comparison of the hemagglutination-inhibition, neutralization and complement fixation tests in the assay of antibody to measles. J Immunol 88:788–795, 1962.
279. Norrby E. Hemagglutination by measles virus. IV. A simple procedure for production of high potency antigen for hemagglutination-inhibition (HI) tests. Proc Soc Exp Biol Med 111:814–818, 1962.
280. Albrecht P, Herrmann K, Burns GR. Role of virus strain in conventional and enhanced measles plaque neutralization test. J Virol Methods 3:251–260, 1981.
281. Roesing TG, Meeker J, Garfinkle B, et al. Determination of antibody to measles virus by a fluoroimmunoassay (FIAX). J Biol Stand 9:401–407, 1981.
282. Forghani B, Schmidt NJ. Antigen requirements, sensitivity, and specificity of enzyme immunoassays for measles and rubella viral antibodies. J Clin Microbiol 9:657–664, 1979.
283. Kleiman MB, Blackburn CKL, Zimmerman SE, French ML. Comparison of enzyme-linked immunosorbent assay for acute measles with hemagglutination inhibition, complement fixation, and fluorescent-antibody methods. J Clin Microbiol 14:147–152, 1981.
284. Neumann PW, Weber JM, Jessamine AG, O'Shaughnessy MV. Comparison of measles antihemolysin test, enzyme-linked immunosorbent assay, and hemagglutination inhibition test with neutralization test for determination of immune status. J Clin Microbiol 22:296–298, 1985.
285. Boteler WL, Luiperbeck PM, Fuccillo DA, O'Beirne AJ. Enzyme-linked immunosorbent assay for detection of measles antibody. J Clin Microbiol 17:814–818, 1983.
286. Weigle KA, Murphy MD, Brunell PA. Enzyme-linked immunosorbent assay for evaluation of immunity to measles virus. J Clin Microbiol 19:376–379, 1984.
287. Cremer NE, Cossen CK, Shill G, et al. Enzyme immuno-assay versus plaque neutralization and other methods for determination of immune status to measles and varicella-zoster viruses versus complement fixation for serodiagnosis of infections with those viruses. J Clin Microbiol 21:869–874, 1985.
288. Lievens AW, Brunell PA. Specific immunoglobulin M enzyme-linked immunosorbent assay for confirming the diagnosis of measles. J Clin Microbiol 24:291–394, 1986.
289. Hummel KB, Erdman DD, Heath J, Bellini WJ. Baculovirus expression of the nucleoprotein gene of measles virus and the utility of the recombinant protein in diagnostic enzyme immunoassays. J Clin Microbiol 30:2874–2880, 1992.
290. Rossier E, Miller H, McCulloch B, et al. Comparison of immunofluorescence and enzyme immunoassay for detection of measles-specific immunoglobulin M antibody. J Clin Microbiol 29:1069–1071, 1991.
291. Mayo DR, Brennan T, Cormier DP, et al. Evaluation of a commercial measles virus immunoglobulin M enzyme immunoassay. J Clin Microbiol 29:2865–2867, 1991.
292. Black FL. Measles active and passive immunity in a worldwide perspective. Prog Med Virol 36:1–33, 1989.
293. Ratnam S, Gadag V, West R, et al. Comparison of commercial enzyme immunoassay kits with plaque reduction neutralization test for detection of measles virus antibody. J Clin Microbiol 33:811–815, 1995.
294. Helfand RF, Heath JL, Anderson LJ, et al. Diagnosis of measles with an IgM capture EIA: The optimal timing of specimen collection after rash onset. J Infect Dis 175:195–199, 1997.
295. Brown DW, Ramsay ME, Richards AF, Miller E. Salivary diagnosis of measles: A study of notified cases in the United Kingdom, 1991–1993. BMJ 308:1015–1017, 1994.
296. Langmuir AD. Medical importance of measles. Am J Dis Child 103:224–226, 1962.
297. Black FL. A nationwide screen survey of United States military recruits, 1962. III. Measles and mumps antibodies. Am J Hyg 80:304–307, 1964.
298. Black FL. Measles antibody prevalence in diverse populations. Am J Dis Child 103:242–249, 1962.
299. James JJ, Halvorson GW. Measles-like disease and measles antibody titers in an adult population. Milit Med 144:672–676, 1979.
300. Preblud SR, Gross F, Halsey NA, et al. Assessment of susceptibility to measles and rubella. JAMA 247:1134–1137, 1982.
301. deJong JG. The survival of measles virus in air, in relation to the epidemiology of measles. Arch Ges Virusforsch 16:97–102, 1965.
302. Riley RC, Murphy G, Riley RL. Airborne spread of measles in a suburban elementary school. Am J Epidemiol 107:421–432, 1978.
303. Bloch AB, Orenstein WA, Ewing WM, et al. Measles outbreak in a pediatric practice: Airborne transmission in an office setting. Pediatrics 75:676–683, 1985.
304. Remington PL, Hall WN, Davis IH, et al. Airborne transmission of measles in a physician's office. JAMA 253:1574–1577, 1985.
305. Top FH. Measles in Detroit, 1935. I. Factors influencing the

secondary attack rate among susceptibles at risk. Am J Public Health 28:935–943, 1938.
306. Hope-Simpson RE. Infectiousness of communicable diseases in the household. Lancet 2:549–554, 1952.
307. Sutter RW, Markowitz LE, Bennetch JM, et al. Measles among the Amish: A comparative study of measles severity in primary and secondary cases in households. J Infect Dis 163:12–16, 1991.
308. Brandling-Bennett AD, Landrigan PJ, Baker EL. Failure of vaccinated children to transmit measles. JAMA 224:616–618, 1973.
309. The National Vaccine Advisory Committee. The measles epidemic. The problems, barriers, and recommendations. JAMA 266:1547–1552, 1991.
310. Hedrich AW. The corrected average attack rate from measles among city children. Am J Hyg 11:576–600, 1930.
311. London WP, Yorke JA. Recurrent outbreaks of measles, chickenpox and mumps. I. Seasonal variation in contact rates. Am J Epidemiol 98:453–468, 1973.
312. Yorke JA, London WP. Recurrent outbreaks of measles, chickenpox and mumps. II. Systematic differences in contact rates and stochastic effects. Am J Epidemiol 98:469–482, 1973.
313. Crawford GE, Gremillion DH. Epidemic measles and rubella in Air Force recruits: Impact of immunization. J Infect Dis 144:403–410, 1981.
314. Krause PJ, Cherry JD, Deseda-Tous J, et al. Epidemic measles in young adults: Clinical, epidemiologic, and serologic studies. Ann Intern Med 90:873–876, 1979.
315. Hersh BS, Markowitz LE, Hoffman RE, et al. A measles outbreak at a college with a prematriculation immunization requirement. Am J Public Health 81:360–364, 1991.
316. Chen RT, Goldbaum GM, Wassilak SGF, et al. An explosive point-source outbreak in a highly vaccinated population. Am J Epidemiol 129:173–182, 1989.
317. Centers for Disease Control and Prevention. Measles outbreak among school-aged children—Juneau, Alaska, 1996. MMWR Morb Mortal Wkly Rep 45:777–780, 1996.
318. Centers for Disease Control and Prevention. Measles outbreak—southwestern Utah, 1996. MMWR Morb Mortal Wkly Rep 46:766–769, 1997.
319. Griffith AH. Measles vaccination in tropical countries. Trans R Soc Trop Med Hyg 69:29–30, 1975.
320. Collaborative study by Ministry of Health of Kenya and World Health Organization. Measles immunity in the first year after birth and the optimum age for vaccination in Kenyan children. Bull World Health Organ 55:21–31, 1977.
321. Abdurrahman MB, Taqi AM. Measles immunity and immunization in developing countries of Africa: A review. Afr J Med Sci 10:57–62, 1981.
322. Ministries of Health of Brazil, Chile, Costa Rica, and Ecuador and the Pan American Health Organization. Seroconversion rates and measles antibody titers induced by measles vaccination in Latin American children 6 to 12 months of age. Rev Infect Dis 5:596–605, 1983.
323. Halsey NA. The optimal age for administering measles vaccine in developing countries. In Halsey NA, de Quadros CA (eds). Recent Advances in Immunization. A Bibliographic Review. Publication 451. Washington, DC, Pan American Health Organization, 1983, pp 4–17.
324. Halsey NA, Boulos R, Mode F, et al. Responses to measles vaccine in Haitian infants 6 to 12 months old. Influence of maternal antibodies, malnutrition, and concurrent illnesses. N Engl J Med 313:544–549, 1985.
325. Black FL, Berman LL, Borgono JM, et al. Geographic variation in infant loss of maternal measles antibody and in prevalence of rubella antibody. Am J Epidemiol 124:442–452, 1986.
326. Whittle HC, Mee J, Werblinska J, et al. Immunity to measles in malnourished children. Clin Exp Immunol 42:144–151, 1980.
327. Aaby P, Bukh J, Lisse IM, Smits AJ. Measles mortality, state of nutrition, and family structure: A community study from Guinea-Bissau. J Infect Dis 147:693–701, 1983.
328. Aaby P, Bukh J, Lisse IM, Smits AJ. Overcrowding and intensive exposure as determinants of measles mortality. Am J Epidemiol 120:40–63, 1984.
329. Aaby P, Bukh J, Hoff G, et al. High measles mortality in infancy related to intensity of exposure. J Pediatr 109:40–44, 1986.
330. Morley DC, Aaby P. Managing measles. Size of infecting dose may be important [letter]. Br Med J 314:1692, 1997.
331. Centers for Disease Control and Prevention. Progress toward global measles control and elimination, 1990–1996. MMWR Morb Mortal Wkly Rep 46:893–897, 1997.
332. Markowitz LE, Nieburg P. The burden of acute respiratory infections due to measles in developing countries and the potential impact of measles vaccine. Rev Infect Dis 13(suppl 6):S555–S561, 1991.
333. Murray CJL, Lopez AD. Mortality by cause for eight regions of the world: Global burden of disease study. Lancet 349:1269–1276, 1997.
334. White CC, Koplan JP, Orenstein WA. Benefits, risks, and costs of immunization for measles, mumps, and rubella. Am J Public Health 75:739–744, 1985.
335. Hatziandreu EJ, Brown RE, Halpern MT. A cost benefit analysis of measles-mumps-rubella vaccine. Arlington, VA, Battelle. Final report. 1994, pp 1–66.
336. Stiehm ER. Standard and special human immune serum globulins as therapeutic agents. Pediatrics 63:301–319, 1979.
337. Centers for Disease Control and Prevention. General recommendations on immunization: Recommendations of the Advisory Committee on Immunization Practices (ACIP). MMWR Morb Mortal Wkly Rep 43(RR-1):1–38, 1994.
338. Onorato IM, Markowitz LE, Oxtoby MJ. Childhood immunization, vaccine-preventable diseases and infection with human immunodeficiency virus. Pediatr Infect Dis J 7:588–595, 1988.
339. Okuno Y, Takahashi M, Toyoshima K, et al. Studies on the prophylaxis of measles with attenuated living virus. III. Inoculation tests in man and monkey with chick embryo passage measles virus. Biken J 3:115–122, 1960.
340. Collard P, Hendrickse RG, Montefiore D, et al. Vaccination against measles. Part II. Clinical trial in Nigerian children. Br Med J 2:1246–1250, 1961.
341. Aldous IR, Kirman BH, Butler N, et al. Vaccination against measles. Part III. Clinical trial in British children. Br Med J 2:1250–1253, 1961.
342. Katz SL, Morley DC, Krugman S. Attenuated measles vaccine in Nigerian children. Am J Dis Child 103:402–405, 1962.
343. Halonen P, Forssell P, Halonen H, et al. Clinical and immunological studies on a live attenuated measles virus vaccine in infants and children. Acta Paediatr 51:401–408, 1962.
344. Smorodinstev AA, Boychuk LM, Shikina ES, et al. Further experiences with live measles vaccines in U.S.S.R. Am J Dis Child 103:384–386, 1962.
345. Goffe AP, Woodall JT, Tuckman E, et al. Vaccination against measles in general practice. BMJ 1:26–28, 1963.
346. Report of a WHO Scientific Group. Measles vaccine. World Health Organ Tech Rep Ser 263:5–37, 1963.
347. Hendrickse RG, Montefiore D, Sherman PM, van der Wall HM. Studies on measles vaccination in Nigerian children. BMJ 1:470–474, 1964.
348. Medical Research Council. Vaccination against measles: A study of clinical reactions and serological response of young children. BMJ 1:817–823, 1965.
349. Medical Research Council. Vaccination against measles: A clinical trial of live measles vaccine given alone and live vaccine preceded by killed vaccine. BMJ 1:441–446, 1966.
350. Bolotovskij VM, Nefedova LA, Gelikman BG, et al. Comparative studies of measles vaccine in a controlled trial in the USSR. Bull World Health Organ 34:859–864, 1966.
351. Cockburn WC, Pecenka J, Sundaresan T. WHO supported comparative studies of attenuated live measles vaccines. Bull World Health Organ 34:223–231, 1966.
352. Swartz T, Klingberg W, Nishmi M, et al. A comparative study of four live measles vaccines in Israel. Bull World Health Organ 39:285–292, 1968.
353. Jean-Joseph P, Imperator PH, Sow S, et al. A comparison of Edmonston-B and Schwarz measles vaccine in Malian children. Lancet 1:665–667, 1969.
354. Ikic D, Juzasic M, Beck M, et al. Attenuation and characterization of Edmonston-Zagreb measles virus. Ann Immunol Hung 16:175–181, 1972.
355. Anti-Epidemic Stations of Zhuang Autonomous Region, Qingzhou Prefecture Beihai Municipality and Weizhou People's Commune Hospital, Guangxi and National Vaccine and Serum Institute, Beijing. Clinical reactogenicity and immunogenicity of

five live measles vaccine strains. Chin Med J (Engl) 94:201–206, 1981.
356. Peradze TV, Smorodintsev AA. Epidemiology and specific prophylaxis of measles. Rev Infect Dis 5:487–490, 1983.
357. Mirchamsy H. Measles immunization in Iran. Rev Infect Dis 5:491–494, 1983.
358. Clements CJ, Milstein JB, Grabowsky M, Gibson J. Research into alternative measles vaccines in the 1990's. EPI/Gen/88.11 Rev 1.
359. Hirayama M. Measles vaccine used in Japan. Rev Infect Dis 5:495–503, 1983.
360. Makino S. Development and characteristics of live AIK-C measles virus vaccine: A brief report. Rev Infect Dis 5:504–505, 1983.
361. Jianzhi X, Zhihui C. Measles vaccine in the People's Republic of China. Rev Infect Dis 5:506–510, 1983.
362. Mirchamsy H, Bahrami S, Shafyi A, et al. The isolation and characterization of a human diploid cell strain and its use in production of measles vaccine. J Biol Stand 14:75–79, 1986.
363. Mirchamsy H, Shafyi A, Nazari P, et al. Evaluation of live attenuated measles vaccines prepared in human diploid cells for reimmunization. Epidemiol Infect 101:437–443, 1988.
364. Okuno Y, Ueda S, Kurimura T, et al. Studies on further attenuated live measles vaccine. VII. Development and evaluation of CAM-70 measles virus vaccine. Biken J 14:253–258, 1971.
365. McCrumb FR, Kress S, Saunders E, et al. Studies with live attenuated measles-virus vaccine. I. Clinical and immunologic responses in institutionalized children. Am J Dis Child 101:689–700, 1961.
366. Kress S, Schluederberg AE, Hornick RB, et al. Studies with live attenuated measles-virus vaccine. II. Clinical and immunologic response of children in an open community. Am J Dis Child 101:701–707, 1961.
367. Hornick RB, Schluederberg AE, McCrumb FR Jr. Vaccination with live attenuated measles virus. Am J Dis Child 103:344–347, 1962.
368. Musser SJ, Slater EA. Measles virus growth in canine renal cell cultures. Am J Dis Child 103:476–481, 1962.
369. Stokes J Jr, Hilleman MR, Weibel RE, et al. Efficacy of live attenuated measles-virus vaccine given with human immune globulin. N Engl J Med 265:507–513, 1961.
370. Hilleman MR, Stokes J Jr, Buynak EB, et al. Enders' live measles-virus vaccine with human gamma globulin. II. Evaluation of efficacy. Am J Dis Child 103:272–379, 1962.
371. Stokes J Jr, Hilleman MR, Weibel RE, et al. Persistent immunity following Enders live, attenuated measles-virus vaccine given with human immune globulin. N Engl J Med 267:222–224, 1962.
372. Stokes J Jr, Weibel R, Halenda R, et al. Enders' live measles-virus vaccine with human globulin. I. Clinical reactions. Am J Dis Child 103:366–372, 1962.
373. Weibel R, Halenda R, Stokes J Jr, et al. Administration of Enders' live measles virus vaccine with immune globulin. JAMA 180:1086–1094, 1962.
374. Morley D, Katz SL, Krugman S. The clinical reaction of Nigerian children to measles vaccine with and without gamma globulin. J Hyg (Camb) 61:135–141, 1963.
375. Benson PF, Butler NR, Goeffe AP, et al. Vaccination of infants with living attenuated measles vaccine (Edmonston strain) with and without gamma-globulin. BMJ 2:851–853, 1964.
376. Weibel RE, Stokes J Jr, Halenda R, et al. Durable immunity two years after administration of Enders' live measles-virus vaccine with immune globulin. N Engl J Med 270:172–175, 1964.
377. Warren RJ, Nader PR, Levine RH. Measles immune globulin. Proposed standard dose given with live attenuated measles virus vaccine. JAMA 203:186–188, 1968.
378. Warren J, Gallian MJ. Concentrated inactivated measles-virus vaccine. Preparation and antigenic potency. Am J Dis Child 103:418–423, 1962.
379. Feldman HA. Protective value of inactivated measles vaccine. Am J Dis Child 103:423–424, 1962.
380. Karzon DT, Winkelstein W Jr, Jenss R, et al. Field trial of inactivated measles vaccine. Am J Dis Child 103:425–426, 1962.
381. Karlitz S, Berliner BC, Orange M, et al. Inactivated measles virus vaccine. Subsequent challenge with attenuated live virus vaccine. JAMA 184:673–679, 1963.
382. Fulginiti VA, Kempe CH. Measles exposure among vaccine recipients. Am J Dis Child 106:450–461, 1963.
383. Krugman S, Stone S, Hu R, Friedman H. Measles immunization incorporated in the routine schedule for infants: Efficacy of a combined inactivated-live vaccination regimen. Pediatrics 34:795–797, 1964.
384. Karzon DT, Rush D, Winkelstein W. Immunization with inactivated measles virus vaccine: Effect of booster dose and response to natural challenge. Pediatrics 36:40–50, 1965.
385. Guinee VF, Henderson DA, Casey HL, et al. Cooperative measles vaccine field trial. I. Clinical efficacy. II. Serologic studies. Pediatrics 37:649–657, 657–665, 1966.
386. Centers for Disease Control. Recommendations of the Public Health Service Advisory Committee on Immunization Practice. Measles vaccines. MMWR Morb Mortal Wkly Rep 16:269–271, 1967.
387. Orenstein WA, Halsey NA, Hayden GF, et al. Current status of measles in the United States, 1973–1977. J Infect Dis 137:847–853, 1978.
388. Suzuki K, Morita M, Katoh M, et al. Development and evaluation of the TD97 measles virus vaccine. J Med Virol 32:194–901, 1990.
389. Mann GF, Allison LMC, Copeland JA, et al. A simplified plaque assay system for measles virus. J Biol Stand 8:219–225, 1980.
390. Bellocq C, Roux L. Wide occurrence of measles virus subgenomic RNAs in attenuated live-virus vaccines. Biologicals 18:337–343, 1990.
391. Mori T, Sasaki K, Hashimoto H, Makino S. Molecular cloning and complete sequence of genomic RNA of the AIK-C strain of attenuated measles virus. Virus Genes 7:67–81, 1993.
392. Lecouturier V, Fayolle J, Caballero M, et al. Identification of two amino acids in the hemagglutinin glycoprotein of measles virus (MV) that govern hemadsorption, HeLa cell fusion, and CD46 downregulation: Phenotypic markers that differentiate vaccine and wild-type MV strains. J Virol 70:4200–4204, 1996.
393. Hoekenga MT, Armuelles P, Schwarz AJF, et al. Experimental vaccination against measles. II. Tests of live measles and live distemper vaccine in human volunteers during a measles epidemic in Panama. JAMA 173:868–872, 1960.
394. Schwarz AJF. Preliminary tests of a highly attenuated measles vaccine. Am J Dis Child 103:386–389, 1962.
395. Andelman SL, Schwarz A, Andelman MB, Zackler J. Experimental vaccination against measles. Clinical evaluation of a highly attenuated live measles vaccine. JAMA 184:721–723, 1963.
396. Schwarz AJ. Immunization against measles: Development and evaluation of a highly attenuated live measles vaccine. Ann Paediatr 202:241–252, 1964.
397. Schwarz AJF, Anderson JT. Immunization with a further attenuated live measles vaccine. Arch Virusforsch 16:273–278, 1965.
398. Schwarz AJF, Anderson JT, Ramos-Alvarez M, et al. Extensive clinical evaluations of a highly attenuated live measles vaccine. JAMA 199:84–88, 1967.
399. Hilleman MR, Buynak EB, Weibel RE, et al. Development and evaluation of the Moraten measles virus vaccine. JAMA 206:587–590, 1968.
400. Krugman S, Constantinidis P, Medovy H, Giles JP. Comparison of two further attenuated live measles-virus vaccines. Am J Dis Child 117:137–138, 1969.
401. Centers for Disease Control. Recommendations of the Public Health Service Advisory Committee on Immunization Practice. MMWR Morb Mortal Wkly Rep 14:64–67, 1965.
402. Potency Test. Code of Federal Regulations 21, paragraph 630.34.
403. Sassani A, Mirchamsy H, Shafyi A, et al. Excessive attenuation of measles virus as a possible cause of failure in measles immunization. Ann Inst Pasteur Virol 138:491–501, 1987.
404. Makino S, Sasaki K, Nakayama T, et al. A new combined trivalent live measles (AIK-C strain), mumps (Hoshino strain) and rubella (Takahashi strain) vaccine. Am J Dis Child 144:905–910, 1990.
405. McAleer WJ, Markus HZ, McLeam AA, et al. The stability on storage at various temperatures of the live measles, mumps, and rubella virus vaccines in a new stabilizer. J Biol Stand 8:281–287, 1980.
406. Wallace RB, Landrigan PJ, Smith A, et al. Trial of a reduced dose of measles vaccine in Nigerian children. Bull World Health Organ 53:361–364, 1976.
407. McGraw TT. Reimmunization following early immunization

with measles vaccine: A prospective study. Pediatrics 77:45–48, 1986.
408. Lee GC-Y. Intranasal vaccination with attenuated measles virus. Proc Soc Exp Biol Med 112:656–658, 1963.
409. Kok PW, Kenya PR, Ensering H. Measles immunization with further attenuated heat-stable measles vaccine using five different methods of administration. Trans R Soc Trop Med Hyg 77:171–176, 1983.
410. Sabin AB. Immunization against measles by aerosol. Rev Infect Dis 5:514–523, 1983.
411. Sabin AB, Arechiga AF, Fernandez de Castro J, et al. Successful immunization of infants with and without maternal antibody by aerosolized measles vaccine. I. Different results with undiluted human diploid cell and chick embryo fibroblast vaccines. JAMA 240:2651–2652, 1983.
412. Sabin AB, Arechiga AF, Fernandez de Castro J, et al. Successful immunization of infants with and without maternal antibody by aerosolized measles vaccine. II. Vaccine comparisons and evidence for multiple antibody response. JAMA 251:2363–2371, 1984.
413. Sabin AB, Albrecht P, Takeda AK, et al. High effectiveness of aerosolized chick embryo fibroblast vaccine in seven-month-old and older infants. J Infect Dis 152:1231–1237, 1985.
414. Whittle HC, Rowland MG, Mann GF, et al. Immunization of 4–6 month old Gambian infants with Edmonston-Zagreb measles vaccine. Lancet 2:834–837, 1984.
415. Khanum S, Garelick H, Uddin N, et al. Comparison of Edmonston-Zagreb and Schwarz strains of measles vaccine given by aerosol or subcutaneous injection. Lancet 1:150–153, 1987.
416. Ekunwe EO. Immunization by inhalation of aerosolized measles vaccine. Ann Trop Pediatr 10:145–149, 1990.
417. Torrigoe S, Biritwun RB, Isomura S, Kobune F. Measles in Ghana: A trial of an alternative means of measles vaccine. J Trop Pediatr 32:304–309, 1986.
418. Cutts FT, Clements CJ, Bennett JV. Alternative routes of measles immunization: A review. Biologicals 25:323–338, 1997.
419. Walker D, Carter H, Jones IG. Measles, mumps, and rubella: The need for a change in immunization policy. BMJ 292:1501–1502, 1986.
420. Peltola H, Heinonen OP. Frequency of true adverse reactions to measles-mumps-rubella vaccine. A double-blind placebo-controlled trial in twins. Lancet 1:939–942, 1986.
421. Isozaki M, Kuno-Sakai H, Hoshi N, et al. Effects and side effects of a new trivalent combined measles-mumps-rubella (MMR) vaccine. Tokai J Exp Clin Med 7:547–550, 1982.
422. Beck M, Smerdel S, Dedic I, et al. Immune response to Edmonston-Zagreb measles virus strain in monovalent and combined MMR vaccine. Dev Biol Stand 65:95–100, 1986.
423. Just M, Berger R, Glueck R, Wegmann A. Evaluation of a combined vaccine against measles-mumps-rubella produced on human diploid cells. Dev Biol Stand 65:25–27, 1986.
424. Buynak EB, Weibel RE, Whitman JE Jr, et al. Combined live measles-mumps-rubella virus vaccines. Findings in clinical-laboratory studies. JAMA 207:2259–2262, 1969.
425. Smorodintsev AA, Nasibov MN, Jakovleva NV. Experience with live rubella virus vaccine combined with live vaccines against measles and mumps. Bull World Health Organ 42:283–289, 1970.
426. Krugman S, Muriel G, Fontana VJ. Combined live measles, mumps, rubella vaccine: Immunological response. Am J Dis Child 121:380–381, 1971.
427. Hilleman MR, Weibel RE, Villarejos VM, et al. Combined live virus vaccines. Proceedings of the International Conference on the Application of Vaccines Against Viral, Rickettsial, and Bacterial Diseases of Man. Scientific Publication No. 226. Washington, DC, Pan American Health Organization, 1971, pp 397–400.
428. Stokes J Jr, Weibel RE, Vallarejos VM, et al. Trivalent combined measles-mumps-rubella vaccine. Findings in clinical-laboratory studies. JAMA 218:57–61, 1971.
429. Karchmer AW, Friedman JP, Casey HL, et al. Simultaneous administration of live virus vaccines: Measles, mumps, poliomyelitis, and smallpox. Am J Dis Child 121:382–388, 1971.
430. Landrigan PJ, Murphy KB, Meyer HM Jr, et al. Combined measles-rubella vaccines: Virus dose and serologic response. Am J Dis Child 125:65–67, 1973.
431. Schwarz AJF, Jackson JE, Ehrenkranz NJ, et al. Clinical evaluation of a new measles-mumps-rubella trivalent vaccine. Am J Dis Child 129:1408–1412, 1975.
432. Krugman RD, Witte JJ, Parkman PD, et al. Combined administration of measles, mumps, rubella, and trivalent poliovirus vaccines. Public Health Rep 92:220–222, 1977.
433. Weibel RE, Carlson AJ Jr, Villarejos VM, et al. Clinical and laboratory studies of combined live measles, mumps, and rubella vaccines using the RA 27/3 rubella virus (40979). Proc Soc Exp Biol Med 165:323–326, 1980.
434. Lerman SJ, Bollinger M, Brunken JM. Clinical and serologic evaluation of measles, mumps and rubella (HPV-77:DE5 and RA 27/3) virus vaccines, singly and in combination. Pediatrics 68:18–22, 1981.
435. Sugiura A, Ohtawara M, Hayami M, et al. Field trial of trivalent measles-rubella-mumps vaccine in Japan. J Infect Dis 146:709, 1982.
436. Parkman PD, Hopps HE, Albrecht P, Meyer HM Jr. Simultaneous administration of vaccines. In, Halsey NA, de Quadros CA (eds). Recent Advances in Immunization. A Bibliographic Review. Publication 451. Washington, DC, Pan American Health Organization, 1983, pp 65–80.
437. Brunell PA, Weigle K, Murphy MD. Antibody response following measles-mumps-rubella vaccine under conditions of customary use. JAMA 250:1409–1412, 1983.
438. Vesikari T, Ala-Laurila E-L, Heikkinen A, et al. Clinical trial of a new trivalent measles-mumps-rubella vaccine in young children. Am J Dis Child 138:843–847, 1984.
439. Wegmann A, Gluck R, Just M, et al. Comparative study and evaluation of further attenuated, live measles vaccines alone and in combination with mumps and rubella vaccines. Dev Biol Stand 65:69–74, 1986.
440. Orenstein WA, Herrmann KL, Albrecht P, et al. Immunity against measles and rubella in Massachusetts school children. Dev Biol Stand 65:75–83, 1986.
441. Andre FE, Peetermans J. Effect of simultaneous administration of live measles vaccine on the "take rate" of live mumps vaccine. Dev Biol Stand 65:101–107, 1986.
442. Elliott AY. Manufacture and testing of measles, mumps and rubella vaccine. In 19th Immunization Conference Proceedings; Boston, MA; May 21–24, 1984, pp 79–86.
443. Böni J, Stadler J, Reigel F, Schüpbach J. Detection of reverse transcriptase activity in live attenuated virus vaccines. Clin Diagn Virol 5:43–53, 1996.
444. Mahy BWJ, Hadler SC. Editorial. Clin Diagn Virol 5:1–2, 1996.
445. Weissmahr RN, Schüpbach J, Böni J. Reverse transcriptase activity in chicken embryo fibroblast culture supernatants is associated with particles containing endogenous avian retrovirus EAV-0 RNA. J Virol 71:3005–3012, 1997.
446. Waters TD, Anderson PS, Beebe GW, Miller RW. Yellow fever vaccination, avian leukosis virus, and cancer risk in man. Science 177:76–77, 1972.
447. Peetermans J, Colinet G, Stephenne J, Bouillet A. Stability of freeze-dried and reconstituted measles vaccines. Dev Biol Stand 41:259–264, 1978.
448. Heyman DL, Smith EL, Nakano JH, et al. Further field testing of the more heat-stable measles vaccines in Cameroon. BMJ 285:531–533, 1982.
449. World Health Organization. Requirement for Measles Vaccine (Live) and Measles Vaccine (Inactivated). Geneva, World Health Organization Technical Report Series, 1966, revised 1982, 1988, p 329.
450. Petralli JK, Merigan TC, Wilbur JC. Action of endogenous interferon against vaccinia infection in children. Lancet 2:401–405, 1965.
451. Trubina LM, Yakovenko ZF, Itkis SN, Zakharchenko EM. Interferon formation induced by various viruses in cultures of leukocytes from children vaccinated against measles. Acta Virol 16:446, 1972.
452. Nakayama T, Urano T, Osano M, et al. Long term regulation of interferon production by lymphocytes from children inoculated with live measles virus vaccine. J Infect Dis 158:1386–1390, 1988.
453. Kalis JM, Quie PG, Balfour HH Jr. Measles (rubeola) susceptibility among elementary schoolchildren. Am J Epidemiol 101:527–531, 1975.

454. Bass JW, Halstead SB, Fischer GW, et al. Booster vaccination with further live attenuated measles vaccine. JAMA 235:31–34, 1976.
455. Albrecht P, Ennis FA, Saltzman EJ, Krugman S. Persistence of maternal antibody in infants beyond 12 months: Mechanism of measles vaccine failure. J Pediatr 91:715–718, 1977.
456. Krugman RD, Rosenberg R, McIntosh K, et al. Further attenuated live measles vaccine: The need for revised recommendations. J Pediatr 91:766–767, 1977.
457. Balfour HH, Amren DD. Rubella, measles and mumps antibodies following vaccination of children: A potential rubella problem. Am J Dis Child 132:573–577, 1978.
458. Wilkins J, Wehrle PF. Additional evidence against measles vaccine administration to infants less than 12 months of age: Altered immune response following active/passive immunization. J Pediatr 94:865–869, 1979.
459. Sato H, Albrecht P, Reynolds DW, et al. Transfer of measles mumps and rubella antibodies from mother to infant. Its effect on measles, mumps and rubella immunization. Am J Dis Child 133:1240–1243, 1979.
460. Orenstein WA, Albrecht P, Herrman KL, et al. Evaluation of low levels of measles antibody: The plaque neutralization test as a measure of prior exposure to measles virus. J Infect Dis 155:146–149, 1986.
461. Stetler HC, Orenstein WA, Bernier RH, et al. Impact of revaccinating children who initially received measles vaccine before 10 months of age. Pediatrics 77:471–476, 1986.
462. Pedersen IR, Mordhorst CH, Ewald T, von Magnus H. Long-term antibody response after measles vaccination in an isolated arctic society in Greenland. Vaccine 4:173–178, 1986.
463. Helfand R, Gary HE, Atkinson WL, et al. Decline of measles-specific immunoglobulin M antibodies after primary measles, mumps, and rubella vaccination. Clin Diagn Lab Immunol 5:135–138, 1998.
464. Brown P, Gajdusek C, Tasi T. Persistence of measles antibody in the absence of circulating natural virus five years after immunization of an isolated virgin population with Edmonston B vaccine. Am J Epidemiol 90:514–518, 1969.
465. Weibel RE, Buynak EB, McLean AA, Hilleman MR. Long-term follow-up for immunity after monovalent or combined live measles, mumps, and rubella virus vaccines. Pediatrics 56:380–387, 1975.
466. Weibel RE, Buynak EB, McLean AA, et al. Persistence of antibody in human subjects 7 to 10 years following administration of combined live attenuated measles, mumps, and rubella virus vaccines (40967). Proc Soc Exp Biol Med 165:260–263, 1980.
467. Isomura S, Morishima T, Nishikawa K, et al. A long-term follow-up study on the efficacy of further attenuated live measles vaccine, Biken CAM vaccine. Biken J 29:19–26, 1986.
468. Linnemann CC, Dine MS, Bloom JE, Schiff GM. Measles antibody in previously vaccinated children: The need for revaccination. Am J Dis Child 124:53–57, 1972.
469. Arbeter AM, Arthur JH, Blakeman GJ, McIntosh K. Measles immunity: Reimmunization of children who previously received live measles vaccine and gamma globulin. J Pediatr 81:737–741, 1972.
470. Ward BJ, Griffin DE. Changes in cytokine production after measles virus vaccination: Predominant production of IL-4 suggests induction of a Th2 response. Clin Immunol Immunopathol 67:171–177, 1993.
471. Pabst HF, Spady DW, Marusyk RG, et al. Reduced measles immunity in infants in a well vaccinated population. Pediatr Infect Dis J 11:525–529, 1992.
472. Ward BJ, Boulianne N, Ratnam S, et al. Cellular immunity in measles vaccine failure: Demonstration of measles antigen-specific lymphoproliferative responses despite limited serum antibody production after revaccination. J Infect Dis 172:1591–1595, 1995.
473. Wu VH, McFarland H, Mayo K, et al. Measles virus–specific cellular immunity in patients with vaccine failure. J Clin Microbiol 31:118–122, 1993.
474. Starr S, Berkowitz S. Effects of measles, gamma-globulin modified measles and vaccine measles on the tuberculin test. N Engl J Med 270:386–391, 1964.
475. Brody JA, Overfield T, Hammes LM. Depression of the tuberculin reaction by viral vaccines. N Engl J Med 271:1294–1296, 1964.
476. Fireman P, Friday G, Kumate J. Effect of measles vaccine on immunologic responsiveness. Pediatrics 43:264–272, 1969.
477. Zweiman B, Pappagianis D, Maibach H, Hildreth EA. Effect of measles immunization on tuberculin hypersensitivity and in vitro lymphocyte reactivity. Int Arch Allergy 40:834–841, 1971.
478. Munyer TP, Mangi RJ, Dolan T, Kantor FS. Depressed lymphocyte function after measles-mumps-rubella vaccination. J Infect Dis 132:75–78, 1975.
479. Arneborn P, Biberfeld G. T-lymphocyte subpopulations in relation to immunosuppression in measles and varicella. Infect Immun 39:29–37, 1983.
480. Griffin DE, Moench TR, Johnson RT, et al. Peripheral blood mononuclear cells during natural measles virus infection: Cell surface phenotypes and evidence for activation. Clin Immunol Immunopathol 40:305–312, 1986.
481. Linnemann CC Jr, Dine MS, Rosella GA, Askey MT. Measles immunity after revaccination: Results in children vaccinated before 10 months of age. Pediatrics 69:332–335, 1982.
482. Karp CL, Wysocka M, Wahl LM, et al. Mechanism of suppression of cell-mediated immunity by measles virus. Science 273:228–231, 1996.
483. Kempe CH. Measles vaccine in children with asthma and tuberculosis. Am J Dis Child 103:409, 1962.
484. Berkovich S, Starr S. Use of live-measles-virus vaccine to abort an expected outbreak of measles within a closed population. N Engl J Med 269:75–77, 1963.
485. Bhaskaram P, Madhusudan J, Radhakrishna KV, Raj S. Immunological response to measles vaccination in poor communities. Hum Nutr Clin Nutr 40:197–204, 1986.
486. van Binnendijk RS, Poelen MC, van Amerongen G, et al. Protective immunity in macaques vaccinated with live attenuated, recombinant, and subunit measles vaccines in the presence of passively acquired antibodies. J Infect Dis 175:524–532, 1997.
487. Wittler RR, Veit BC, Mcintyre S, Schydlower M. Measles revaccination response in a school-age population. Pediatrics 88:1024–1030, 1991.
488. Bottiger M. Boosting effect of a second dose of measles vaccine given to 12-year-old children. Scand J Infect Dis 25:239–243, 1993.
489. Christenson B, Bottiger M. Measles antibody: Comparison of long-term vaccination titres, early vaccination titres and naturally acquired immunity to and booster effects on the measles virus. Vaccine 12:129–133, 1994.
490. Deseda-Tous J, Cherry JD, Spencer MJ, et al. Measles revaccination. Persistence and degree of antibody titer by type of immune response. Am J Dis Child 132:287–290, 1978.
491. Markowitz LE, Albrecht P, Orenstein WA, et al. Persistence of measles antibody after revaccination. J Infect Dis 166:205–208, 1992.
492. Watson JC, Pearson JA, Markowitz LE, et al. An evaluation of measles revaccination among school-entry-aged children. Pediatrics 97:613–618, 1996.
493. Poland GA, Jacobson RM, Thampy AM, et al. Measles reimmunization in children seronegative after initial immunization. JAMA 277:1156–1158, 1997.
494. Cote TR, Sivertson D, Horan JM, et al. Evaluation of a two-dose measles, mumps, and rubella vaccination schedule in a cohort of college athletes. Public Health Rep 108:431–435, 1993.
495. Baba R, Yabuuchi H, Takahashi M, et al. Seroepidemiologic behavior of varicella zoster virus infection in a semiclosed community after introduction of VZV vaccine. J Pediatr 105:712–716, 1984.
496. Orenstein WA, Bernier RH, Dondero TJ, et al. Field evaluation of vaccine efficacy. Bull World Health Organ 63:1055–1068, 1985.
497. Marks JS, Hayden GF, Orenstein WA. Methodologic issues in the evaluation of vaccine effectiveness. Measles vaccine at 12 vs. 15 months. Am J Epidemiol 116:510–523, 1982.
498. Hayden GF. Measles vaccine failure. A survey of causes and means of prevention. Clin Pediatr 18:155–167, 1979.
499. Wyll SA, Witte JJ. Measles in previously vaccinated children. An epidemiological study. JAMA 216:1306–1310, 1971.
500. Landrigan PJ. Epidemic measles in a divided city. JAMA 221:567–570, 1972.

501. King GE, Markowitz LE, Patriarca PA, Dales LG. Clinical efficacy of measles vaccine during the 1990 measles epidemic. Pediatr Infect Dis J 10:883–887, 1991.
502. Black FL, Berman LL, Libel M, et al. Inadequate immunity to measles in children vaccinated at an early age: Effect of revaccination. Bull World Health Organ 62:315–319, 1984.
503. Lampe RM, Weir MR, Scott RMC, Weeks JL. Measles reimmunization in children immunized before 1 year of age. Am J Dis Child 139:33–35, 1985.
504. Chen RT, Markowitz LE, Albrecht P, et al. Measles antibody: Reevaluation of protective titers. J Infect Dis 162:1036–1042, 1990.
505. Orenstein WA, Markowitz L, Preblud SR, et al. Appropriate age for measles vaccination in the United States. Dev Biol Stand 65:13–21, 1986.
506. Stokes J Jr, Reilly CM, Hilleman MR, Buynak EB. Use of living attenuated measles-virus vaccine in early infancy. N Engl J Med 263:230–233, 1960.
507. Reilly CM, Stokes J Jr, Buynak EB, et al. Living attenuated measles-virus vaccine in early infancy. Studies of the role of passive antibody in immunization. N Engl J Med 265:165–169, 1961.
508. American Academy of Pediatrics. Report of the Committee on the Control of Infectious Diseases. Evanston, IL, American Academy of Pediatrics, 1964, p 8.
509. Shasby DM, Shope TC, Downs H, et al. Epidemic measles in a highly vaccinated population. N Engl J Med 296:585–589, 1977.
510. Nkowane BM, Bart SW, Orenstein WA, Baltier M. Measles outbreak in a vaccinated school population: Epidemiology, chains of transmission and the role of vaccine failures. Am J Public Health 77:434–438, 1987.
511. Baratta RO, Gitner MC, Price MA, et al. Measles (rubeola) in previously immunized children. Pediatrics 46:397–402, 1970.
512. Wilkins J, Wehrle PF, Portnoy B. Live, further attenuated rubeola vaccine. Serologic responses among term and low birth infants. Am J Dis Child 123:190–192, 1972.
513. Reynolds DW, Start A. Immunity to measles in children vaccinated before and after one year of age. Am J Dis Child 124:848–849, 1972.
514. Marks JS, Halpin TJ, Orenstein WA. Measles vaccine efficacy in children previously vaccinated at 12 months of age. Pediatrics 62:955–960, 1978.
515. McIntyre RC, Preblud SR, Polloi A, Korean M. Measles and measles vaccine efficacy in a remote island population. Bull World Health Organ 60:767–775, 1982.
516. Davis RM, Whitman ED, Orenstein WA, et al. A persistent outbreak of measles despite appropriate prevention and control measures. Am J Epidemiol 126:438–449, 1987.
517. Murphy MD, Brunell PA, Lievens AW, Schehab ZM. Effect of early immunization on antibody response to reimmunization with measles vaccine as demonstrated by enzyme-linked immunosorbent assay (ELISA). Pediatrics 74:90–93, 1984.
518. Vitek CR, Redd SC, Hoffman RE, et al. Effectiveness of preexisting 2 doses of measles containing vaccine in preventing measles during an outbreak. Unpublished data.
519. American Academy of Pediatrics. Measles immunization—new recommendations. News Release. October 21, 1976.
520. Centers for Disease Control. Recommendations of the Public Health Service Advisory Committee on Immunization Practice. Measles vaccine. MMWR Morb Mortal Wkly Rep 25:359–360, 365, 1976.
521. Yeager AS, Davis JH, Ross LA, Harvey B. Measles immunization. Successes and failures. JAMA 237:347–351, 1977.
522. Wilkins J, Wehrle PF. Evidence for reinstatement of infants 12 to 14 months of age into routine measles immunization programs. Am J Dis Child 132:164–166, 1978.
523. Reynolds DW, Stagno S, Herrmann KL, Alford C. Antibody response to live virus vaccines in congenital and neonatal cytomegalovirus infections. J Pediatr 92:738–742, 1978.
524. Yeager AS, Harvey B, Crosson FJ Jr, et al. Need for measles revaccination in adolescents: Correlation with birth date prior to 1972. J Pediatr 102:191–195, 1983.
525. Centers for Disease Control. Measles—Florida. MMWR Morb Mortal Wkly Rep 29:625–628, 1980.
526. Judelsohn RG, Fleissner ML, O'Mara DJ. School-based measles outbreaks: Correlation of age at immunization with risk of disease. Am J Public Health 70:1162–1165, 1980.
527. Faust HS, Thompson FE. Age at and time since vaccination during a measles outbreak in a rural community. Am J Dis Child 137:977–980, 1983.
528. Wassilak SGF, Orenstein WA, Strickland PL, et al. Continuing measles transmission in students despite a school based outbreak control program. Am J Epidemiol 122:208–217, 1985.
529. Shelton JD, Jacobson JE, Orenstein WA, et al. Measles vaccine efficacy: Influence of age at vaccination vs duration of time since vaccination. Pediatrics 62:961–964, 1978.
530. Hull HF, Montes JD, Hays PC, Lucero RL. Risk factors for measles vaccine failure among immunized students. Pediatrics 76:518–523, 1985.
531. Maldonado YA, Lawrence EC, DeHovitz R, et al. Early loss of passive measles antibody in infants of mothers with vaccine-induced immunity. Pediatrics 96:447–450, 1995.
532. Kacica MA, Venezia RA, Miller J, et al. Measles antibodies in women and infants in the vaccine era. J Med Virol 45:227–229, 1995.
533. Lennon JL, Black FL. Maternally derived measles immunity in era of vaccine-protected mothers. J Pediatr 108:671–676, 1986.
534. Markowitz LE, Albrecht P, Rhodes P, et al. Changing levels of measles antibody titers in women and children in the United States: Impact on response to revaccination. Pediatrics 97:53–58, 1996.
535. Redd SC, King GE, Nordin J, et al. Comparison of response to measles-mumps-rubella vaccination at 9, 12, and 15 months of age. Centers for Disease Control and Prevention, unpublished data.
536. Merigan TC, Waddell D, Grossman M, et al. Modified skin lesions during concurrent varicella and measles infections. JAMA 204:123–125, 1968.
537. Tolchin D. Failure of measles vaccination. J Pediatr 83:890–891, 1973.
538. Wheelock EF, Larke RPB, Caroline NL. Interference in human viral infections: Present status and prospects for the future. Prog Med Virol 10:286–347, 1968.
539. Ndikuyeze A, Munoz A, Stewart J, et al. Immunogenicity and safety of measles vaccine in ill African children. Int J Epidemiol 17:448–455, 1988.
540. Krober MS, Stracener CE, Bass JW. Decreased measles antibody response after measles-mumps-rubella vaccine in infants with colds. JAMA 265:2095–2096, 1991.
541. Dennehy PH, Saracen CL, Peter G. Seroconversion rates to combined measles-mumps-rubella-varicella (MMRV) vaccine of children with upper respiratory tract infection. Pediatrics 94:514–516, 1994.
542. Ratman S, West R, Gadag V. Measles and rubella antibody response after measles-mumps-rubella vaccination in children with afebrile upper respiratory tract infection. J Pediatr 127:432–434, 1995.
543. King GE, Markowitz LE, Heath J, et al. Antibody response to measles-mumps-rubella vaccine of children with mild illness at the time of vaccination. JAMA 275:704–707, 1996.
544. Edmonson MB, Davis JP, Hopfensperger DJ, et al. Measles vaccination during the respiratory virus season and risk of vaccine failure. Pediatrics 98:905–910, 1996.
545. Simasathien S, Migasena S, Bellini W, et al. Measles vaccination of Thai infants by intranasal and subcutaneous routes: Possible interference from respiratory infections. Vaccine 15:329–334, 1997.
546. Peter G. Measles immunization: Recommendations, challenges, and more information. JAMA 265:2111–2112, 1991.
547. McMurray DN, Loomis AS, Cassazza LJ, Rey H. Influence of moderate malnutrition on morbidity and antibody response following vaccination with live, further attenuated measles virus vaccine. Bull Pan Am Health Organ 13:52–57, 1979.
548. Ifekwunigwe AE, Grasset N, Glass R, Foster S. Immune response to measles and smallpox vaccinations in malnourished children. Am J Clin Nutr 33:621–624, 1980.
549. Rudy BJ, Rutstein RM, Pinto-Martin JP. Responses to measles immunization in children infected with human immunodeficiency virus. J Pediatr 25:72–74, 1994.
550. al-Attar I, Reisman J, Muehlmann M, McIntosh K. Decline of

measles antibody titers after immunization in human immunodeficiency virus infected children. Pediatr Infect Dis J 14:149–151, 1995.
551. Oxtoby MJ, Ryder R, Mvula M, et al. Patterns of immunity to measles among African children infected with human immunodeficiency virus [abstract]. Presented at the 38th Epidemic Intelligence Service Conference; Atlanta, GA; April 3–7, 1989.
552. Lepage P, Dabis F, Msellati P, et al. Safety and immunogenicity of high dose Edmonston-Zagreb measles vaccine in children with HIV-1 infection. Am J Dis Child 146:550–555, 1992.
553. Cutts FT, Mandala K, St. Louis M, et al. Immunogenicity of high-titer Edmonston-Zagreb measles vaccine in human immunodeficiency virus–infected children in Kinshasa, Zaire. J Infect Dis 167:1418–1421, 1993.
554. Arpadi SM, Markowitz LE, Baughman AL, et al. Measles antibody in vaccinated human immunodeficiency virus type 1–infected children. Pediatrics 97:653–657, 1996.
555. Zolopa AB, Kemper CA, Shiboski S, et al. Progressive immunodeficiency due to infection with human immunodeficiency virus does not lead to waning immunity to measles in a cohort of homosexual men. Clin Infect Dis 18:636–638, 1994.
556. Sha BE, Harris AA, Benson CA, et al. Prevalence of measles antibodies in asymptomatic human immunodeficiency virus–infected adults. J Infect Dis 164:973–975, 1991.
557. Semba RD, Munasir Z, Beeler J, et al. Reduced seroconversion to measles in infants given vitamin A with measles vaccination. Lancet 345:1330–1332, 1995.
558. Benn CS, Aaby P, Balé C, et al. Randomised trial of effect of vitamin A supplementation on antibody response to measles vaccine in Guinea-Bissau, west Africa. Lancet 350:101–105, 1997.
559. Hayney MS, Poland GA, Jacobson RM, et al. The influence of the HLA-DRB1*13 allele on measles vaccine response. J Invest Med 44:261–263, 1996.
560. Hayney MS, Poland GA, Dimanlig P, et al. Polymorphisms of the *TAP2* gene may influence antibody response to live measles vaccine virus. Vaccine 15:3–6, 1997.
561. Whittle HC, Mann G, Eccles M, et al. Effects of dose and strain of vaccine on success of measles vaccination in infants aged 4–5 months. Lancet 1:963–966, 1988.
562. Markowitz LE, Sepulveda J, Diaz-Ortega JL, et al. Immunization of six-month old infants with different doses of Edmonston-Zagreb and Schwarz measles vaccines. N Engl J Med 322:580–587, 1990.
563. Tidjani O, Grunitsky B, Guerin N, et al. Serological effects of Edmonston-Zagreb, Schwarz and AIK-C measles vaccine strains given at ages 4–5 or 8–10 months. Lancet 2:1357–1360, 1989.
564. Whittle HC, Campbell H, Rahman S, Armstrong JR. Antibody persistence in Gambian children after high-dose Edmonston-Zagreb measles vaccine. Lancet 336:1046–1048, 1990.
565. Kiepiela P, Coovadia HM, Loening WEK, et al. Lack of efficacy of the live standard potency Edmonston-Zagreb live, attenuated measles vaccine in African infants. Bull World Health Organ 69:221–227, 1991.
566. Job JS, Halsey NA, Boulos R, et al. Successful immunization of infants at 6 months of age with high dose Edmonston-Zagreb measles vaccine. Pediatr Infect Dis J 10:303–311, 1991.
567. Dabis F, Sow A, Waldman R, et al. The epidemiology of measles in a partially vaccinated African city: Implications for immunization programmes. Am J Epidemiol 127:171–178, 1988.
568. Taylor WR, Mambu RK, Ma-Disu W, Weinman JM. Measles control effort in urban Africa complicated by high incidence of measles in the first year of life. Am J Epidemiol 27:788–794, 1988.
569. Kambarami RA, Nathoo KJ, Nkrumah FK, Pirie DJ. Measles epidemic in Harare, Zimbabwe, despite high measles immunization coverage rates. Bull World Health Organ 69:213–219, 1991.
570. Expanded Programme on Immunization. Measles immunization before 9 months of age. Wkly Epidemiol Rec 2:8, 1990.
571. Expanded Programme on Immunization. Safety and efficacy of high titre measles vaccine at 6 months of age. Wkly Epidemiol Rec 66:249–251, 1991.
572. Garenne M, Leroy O, Beau FP, Sene I. Child mortality after high titer measles vaccines: Prospective study in Senegal. Lancet 338:903–907, 1991.
573. Aaby P, Samb B, Simondon F, et al. Divergent mortality for male and female recipients of low-titre and high-titre measles vaccines in rural Senegal. Am J Epidemiol 138:756–755, 1993.
574. Expanded Programme on Immunization. Safety of high titre measles vaccines. Wkly Epidemiol Rec 67:357–361, 1992.
575. Krugman RD, Meyer BC, Parkman PD, et al. Impotency of vaccines as a result of improper handling in clinical practice. J Pediatr 85:512–514, 1972.
576. Lerman SJ, Gold E. Measles in children previously vaccinated against measles. JAMA 216:1311–1314, 1971.
577. Markowitz LE, Preblud SR, Fine PE, et al. Duration of live measles vaccine–induced immunity. Pediatr Infect Dis J 9:101–109, 1990.
578. Lepow ML, Nankervis GA. Eight-year serologic evaluation of Edmonston live measles vaccine. J Pediatr 75:407–411, 1969.
579. Medical Research Council Committee on Development of Vaccines and Immunization Procedures. Clinical trial of live measles vaccine given alone and live vaccine preceded by killed vaccine. Lancet 2:571–575, 1977.
580. Miller C. Live measles vaccine: A 21 year follow-up. BMJ 295:22–24, 1987.
581. Hirose M, Hidaka Y, Miyazaki C, et al. Five cases of measles secondary vaccine failure with confirmed seroconversion after live measles vaccination. Scand J Infect Dis 29:187–190, 1997.
582. Tischer A, Gerike E. Detection of measles-specific IgM antibodies: Comparison of 2-mercaptoethanol treatment, density gradient centrifugation, protein A–sepharose affinity chromatography, ion-exchange chromatography and haemadsorption techniques. Acta Virol 30:373–380, 1986.
583. Hutchins SS, Markowitz LE, Mead P, et al. School-based measles outbreak: The effect of a selective revaccination policy and risk factors for vaccine failure. Am J Epidemiol 132:157–168, 1990.
584. Robertson SE, Markowitz LE, Berry DA, et al. A million dollar measles outbreak: Epidemiology, risk factors and a selective revaccination strategy. Public Health Rep 107:24–31, 1992.
585. O'Neil AE. The measles epidemic in Calgary, 1974–75: The duration of protection conferred by the vaccine. Can J Public Health 69:325–333, 1978.
586. Guris D, McCready J, Watson JC, et al. Measles vaccine effectiveness and duration of vaccine-induced immunity in the absence of boosting from exposure to measles virus. Pediatr Infect Dis J 15:1082–1086, 1996.
587. Ramsay ME, Moffatt D, O'Connor M. Measles vaccine: A 27-year follow-up. Epidemiol Infect 112:409–412, 1994.
588. Anders JF, Jacobson RM, Poland GA, et al. Secondary failure rates of measles vaccines: A metaanalysis of published studies. Pediatr Infect Dis J 15:62–66, 1996.
589. Meyer HM Jr, Hostetler DD Jr, Bernheim BC, et al. Response of Volta children to jet inoculation of combined live measles, smallpox, and yellow fever vaccines. Bull World Health Organ 30:783–794, 1964.
590. Meyer HM Jr, Bernheim BC, Rogers NG. Titration of live measles and smallpox vaccines by jet inoculation of susceptible children. Proc Soc Exp Biol Med 118:53–57, 1965.
591. Meyer HM Jr. Field experience with combined live measles, smallpox and yellow fever vaccines. Arch Ges Virusforsch 16:366–374, 1965.
592. Sherman RM, Hendrickse RG, Montifiore D. Simultaneous administration of live measles virus vaccine and smallpox vaccine. BMJ 2:672–676, 1967.
593. Weibel RE, Stokes J Jr, Buynak EB, et al. Clinical laboratory experiences with a more attenuated Enders measles virus vaccine (Moraten) combined with smallpox vaccine. Pediatrics 43:567–572, 1969.
594. Ruben FL, Smith EA, Foster SO, et al. Simultaneous administration of smallpox, measles, yellow fever, and diphtheria-pertussis-tetanus antigens to Nigerian children. Bull World Health Organ 48:175–181, 1973.
595. Lapeyssonnie L, Omer IA, Nicolas A, Roumiantzeff M. A study of the serological response of Sudanese children to three associated immunizations (measles, tetanus, meningococcal A meningitis). Med Trop (Mars) 39:71–79, 1979.
596. Marshall R, Habicht J-P, Landrigan PJ, et al. Effectiveness of measles vaccine given simultaneously with DTP. J Trop Pediatr Environ Child Health 20:126–129, 1974.

597. Ajjan N, Fayet MT, Biron G, et al. Combination of attenuated measles vaccine (Schwarz) with meningococcus A and A+C vaccine. Dev Biol Stand 41:209–216, 1978.
598. McBean AM, Gateff C, Manclark CR, Foster SO. Simultaneous administration of live attenuated measles vaccine with DTP vaccine. Pediatrics 62:288–293, 1978.
599. Deforest A, Long SS, Lischner HW, et al. Simultaneous administration of measles-mumps-rubella vaccine with booster doses of diphtheria-tetanus-pertussis and oral poliovirus vaccines. Pediatrics 81:237–246, 1988.
600. Huang L, Lee C, Hsu C, et al. Effect of monovalent measles and trivalent measles-mumps-rubella vaccines at various ages and concurrent administration with hepatitis B vaccine. Pediatr Infect Dis J 9:461–465, 1990.
601. Lhuillier M, Mazzariol MJ, Zadi S, et al. Study of combined vaccination against yellow fever and measles in infants from six to nine months. J Biol Stand 17:9–15, 1989.
602. Adu FD, Omotade OO, Oyedele OI, et al. Field trial of combined yellow fever and measles vaccines among children in Nigeria. East Afr Med J 73:579–582, 1996.
603. Centers for Disease Control. Recommendations of the Immunization Practices Advisory Committee (ACIP). New recommended schedule for active immunization of normal infants and children. MMWR Morb Mortal Wkly Rep 35:577–579, 1986.
604. King GE, Hadler SC. Simultaneous administration of childhood vaccines: An important public health policy that is safe and efficacious. Pediatr Infect Dis J 13:394–407, 1994.
605. Giammanco G, Li Volti S, Salemi I, et al. Immune response to simultaneous administration of a combined measles, mumps and rubella vaccine with booster doses of diphtheria-tetanus and poliovirus vaccine. Eur J Epidemiol 9:199–202, 1993.
606. Centers for Disease Control. Adverse Events Following Immunization Surveillance Report No. 1, 1979–1982. U.S. Department of Health and Human Services, Public Health Service. Atlanta, Centers for Disease Control, August 1984.
607. Centers for Disease Control. Adverse Events Following Immunization Surveillance Report No. 2, 1982–1984. U.S. Department of Health and Human Services, Public Health Service. Atlanta, Centers for Disease Control, December 1986.
608. Centers for Disease Control. Adverse Events Following Immunization Surveillance Report No. 3, 1985–1986. U.S. Department of Health and Human Services, Public Health Service. Atlanta, Centers for Disease Control, February 1989.
609. John TJ, Selvakumar R. Mixing measles vaccine with DTP and DPTP [letter]. Lancet 1:1154, 1985.
610. John TJ, Selvakumar R, Balrai V, Simoes EAF. Antibody response to measles vaccine with DTPP [letter]. Am J Dis Child 141:14, 1987.
611. Chen RT, Haber P, Mullen JR. Surveillance of the safety of simultaneous administration of vaccines. The Centers for Disease Control and Prevention experience. Ann N Y Acad Sci 754:309–320, 1995.
612. Arbeter AM, Baker L, Starr SE, et al. Combination measles, mumps, rubella, and varicella vaccine. Pediatrics 78(suppl):742–747, 1986.
613. Just M, Berger R, Just V. Evaluation of a measles-mumps-rubella-chickenpox vaccine. Dev Biol Stand 65:85–88, 1986.
614. Englund JA, Swarez CS, Kelly J, et al. Placebo-controlled trial of varicella vaccine given with or after measles-mumps-rubella vaccine. J Pediatr 114:37–44, 1989.
615. Watson BM, Laufer DS, Kuter BJ, et al. Safety and immunogenicity of a combined live attenuated measles, mumps, rubella and varicella vaccine ($MMR_{II}V$) in healthy children. J Infect Dis 173:731–734, 1996.
616. Byrne EB, Rosenstein BJ, Jaworski AA, Jaworski RA. A statewide mass measles immunization program. JAMA 199:619–623, 1967.
617. Centers for Disease Control. Measles vaccination reactions among college students—North Carolina, Massachusetts. MMWR Morb Mortal Wkly Rep 29:549–551, 1980.
618. Chen RT, Moses JM, Markowitz LE, Orenstein WA. Adverse events following measles-mumps-rubella and measles vaccinations in college students. Vaccine 9:297–299, 1991.
619. Griffin MR, Ray WA, Mortimer EA, et al. Risk of seizures after measles-mumps-rubella immunization. Pediatrics 88:881–885, 1991.
620. Scott TFM, Bonanno DE. Reactions to live-measles-virus vaccine in children previously vaccinated with killed-virus vaccine. N Engl J Med 277:248–250, 1967.
621. Buser F. Side reaction to measles vaccine suggesting the Arthus phenomenon. N Engl J Med 277:250–251, 1967.
622. Fulginiti VA, Arthur JA, Pearlman DS, Kempe CH. Altered reactivity to measles virus. Local reactions following attenuated measles virus immunization in children who previously received a combination of inactivated and attenuated vaccines. Am J Dis Child 115:671–676, 1968.
623. Harris RW, Isacson P, Karzon DT. Vaccine-induced hypersensitivity: Reactions to live measles and mumps vaccine in prior recipients of inactivated measles vaccine. J Pediatr 74:552–563, 1969.
624. Stetler HC, Gens RD, Seastrom GR. Severe local reactions to live measles virus vaccine following an immunization program. Am J Public Health 73:899–900, 1983.
625. Landrigan PJ, Witte JJ. Neurologic disorders following live measles-virus vaccination. JAMA 223:1459–1462, 1973.
626. Miller CL. Surveillance after measles vaccination in children. Practitioner 226:535–537, 1982.
627. Hirtz DG, Nelson KD, Ellenberg JH. Seizures following childhood immunizations. J Pediatr 102:14–18, 1983.
628. Abe T, Nonaka C, Hiraiwa M, et al. Acute and delayed neurologic reaction to innoculation with attenuated live measles virus. Brain Dev 7:421–423, 1985.
629. Davis RL, Marcuse E, Black S, et al. MMR2 immunization at 4 to 5 years and 10 to 12 years of age: A comparison of adverse clinical events after immunization in the Vaccine Safety Datalink (VSD) project. Pediatrics 100:767–771, 1997.
630. Trump RC, White TR. Cerebellar ataxia presumed due to live, attenuated measles virus vaccine. JAMA 199:165–166, 1967.
631. Grose CG, Spigland I. Guillian-Barré syndrome following administration of live measles vaccine. Am J Med 60:441–443, 1976.
632. Karzarian EL, Gager WE. Optic neuritis complicating measles, mumps, and rubella vaccination. Am J Ophthalmol 86:544–547, 1978.
633. Morens DM, Halsey NA, Schoenberger LB, Baublis JV. Reye syndrome associated with vaccination with live virus vaccines. An exploration of possible etiologic relationships. Clin Pediatr 18:42–44, 1979.
634. Chan CC, Sogg RL, Steinman L. Isolated oculomotor palsy after measles immunization. Am J Ophthalmol 89:446–448, 1980.
635. Halsey NA, Weiner LB, Meyers MG, et al. Clinical evaluation of a new live measles vaccine derived in chick chorioallantoic membranes. J Biol Stand 9:507–511, 1981.
636. Marshall GS, Wright PF, Fenichel GM, Karzon DT. Diffuse retinopathy following measles, mumps, and rubella vaccination. Pediatrics 76:989–991, 1985.
637. Brodsky L, Stanievich J. Sensorineural hearing loss following live measles virus vaccination. Int J Pediatr Otorhinolaryngol 10:159–163, 1985.
638. Oski FA, Naiman JL. Effect of live measles vaccine on the platelet count. N Engl J Med 275:352–356, 1966.
639. Bachand AJ, Rubenstein J, Morrison AN. Thrombocytopenic purpura following live measles vaccine. Am J Dis Child 113:283–285, 1967.
640. Wilhelm DJ, Paegle RD. Thrombocytopenic purpura and pneumonia following measles vaccination. Am J Dis Child 113:534–537, 1967.
641. Alter HJ, Scanlon RT, Schechter GP. Thrombocytopenic purpura following vaccination with attenuated measles virus. Am J Dis Child 115:111–113, 1968.
642. Beeler J, Varricchio F, Wise R. Thrombocytopenia after immunization with measles vaccines: Review of the vaccine adverse events reporting system (1990 to 1994). Pediatr Infect Dis J 15:88–90, 1996.
643. Zwemer R, Hodge S, Owen LG, Fliegelman MT. Persistent toxic erythema and chronic urticaria. Possible association with the use of measles virus vaccine. Arch Dermatol 104:390–392, 1971.
644. Bunch C, Schwartz FC, Bird GW. Paroxysmal cold haemoglobinuria following measles immunization. Arch Dis Child 47:299–300, 1972.
645. Vessal S, Kravis LP. Immunologic mechanisms responsible for

adverse reactions to routine immunizations in children. Clin Pediatr 15:688–696, 1976.
646. Van Aspersen PP, McEniery J, Kemp AS. Immediate reactions following live attenuated measles vaccine. Med J Aust 2:330–331, 1981.
647. McEwen J. Early-onset reaction after measles vaccination: Further Australian reports. Med J Aust 2:503–505, 1983.
648. Neiderud J. Thrombocytopenic purpura after a combined vaccine against morbilli, parotitis, and rubella. Acta Paediatr Scand 72:613–614, 1983.
649. Kalet A, Berger DK, Bateman WB, et al. Allergic reactions to MMR vaccine. Pediatrics 89:168–169, 1992.
650. Glenn MP, McKendrick DW. Varicella bullosa associated with measles vaccine. Br J Dermatol 83:595–596, 1970.
651. Shoss RG, Rayhanzadeh S. Toxic epidermal necrolysis following measles vaccination. Arch Dermatol 110:766–770, 1974.
652. Buntain WL, Missall SR. Local subcutaneous atrophy following measles, mumps, and rubella vaccination [letter]. Am J Dis Child 130:335, 1976.
653. Buck BE, Yang LC, Caleb MH, et al. Measles virus panniculitis subsequent to vaccine administration. J Pediatr 101:366–373, 1982.
654. da Silveira CM, Salisbury DM, de Quadros CA. Measles vaccination and Guillain-Barré syndrome. Lancet 349:14–16, 1997.
655. Stratton K, Howe CJ, Johnston RB Jr. Adverse events associated with childhood vaccines other than pertussis and rubella: Summary of a report from the Institute of Medicine. JAMA 271:1602–1605, 1994.
656. Stratton K, Howe CJ, Johnston RB Jr. Adverse Events Associated with Childhood Vaccinations: Evidence Bearing on Causality. Washington, DC, National Academy Press, 1994.
657. Thurston A. Anaphylactic shock reaction to measles vaccine [letter]. J R Coll Gen Pract 37:41, 1987.
658. Cohn J. Thrombocytopenia in childhood: An evaluation of 433 patients. Scand J Haematol 16:226–240, 1976.
659. Monafo WJ, Haslam DB, Roberts RL, et al. Disseminated measles infection after vaccination in a child with a congenital immunodeficiency. J Pediatr 124:273–276, 1994.
660. Centers for Disease Control and Prevention. Measles pneumonitis following measles-mumps-rubella vaccination of a patient with HIV infection. MMWR Morb Mortal Wkly Rep 45:603–606, 1996.
661. Committee on Safety of Medicines and the Joint Committee on Vaccination and Immunization. Whooping Cough. London, Her Majesty's Stationery Office, 1981, pp 79–169.
662. Miller D, Wadsworth J, Diamond J, Ross E. Measles vaccination and neurological events. Lancet 349:730–731, 1997.
663. Forman ML, Cherry JD. Isolation of measles virus from the cerebrospinal fluid of a child with encephalitis following measles vaccination [abstract 13]. Presented at the 77th Annual Meeting of the American Pediatric Society; April 26–29, 1967.
664. Gilat T, Hacohen D, Lilos P, Langman MJ. Childhood factors in ulcerative colitis and Crohn's disease. An international cooperative study. Scand J Gastroenterol 22:1009–1024, 1987.
665. Rosenthal SR, Clements CJ. Two-dose measles vaccination schedules. Bull World Health Organ 71:421–428, 1993.
666. Fulginiti V. Simultaneous measles exposure and immunization. Arch Ges Virusforsch 16:300–304, 1965.
667. Ruuskanen O, Salmi TT, Halonen P. Measles vaccination after exposure to natural measles. J Pediatr 93:43–46, 1978.
668. American Academy of Pediatrics. Measles: Reassessment of current immunization policy. Pediatrics 84:1110–1113, 1989.
669. Centers for Disease Control and Prevention. Recommended schedule for childhood vaccination, United States, 1998. MMWR Morb Mortal Wkly Rep 47:8–12, 1998.
670. Centers for Disease Control and Prevention. Measles, mumps, and rubella—vaccine use and strategies for measles, rubella, and congenital rubella syndrome elimination and mumps control: Recommendations of the Advisory Committee on Immunization Practices (ACIP). MMWR Morb Mortal Wkly Rep 47(RR-8):1–57, 1998.
671. Atkinson WL, Markowitz LE, Adams NC, Seastrom GR. Transmission of measles in medical settings, 1985–1989. Am J Med 91(suppl 3B):320S–324S, 1991.
672. Subbarao EK, Amin S, Kumar ML. Prevaccination serologic screening for measles in health care workers. J Infect Dis 163:876–878, 1991.
673. Grabowsky M, Markowitz L. Serologic screening, mass immunization and implications for immunization programs. J Infect Dis 164:1237–1238, 1991.
674. Hinman AR, Koplan JP. Public health policy toward atypical measles syndrome in the United States. Med Decis Making 2:71–77, 1982.
675. Bellini WJ, Rota JS, Greer PW, Zaki SR. Measles vaccination death in a child with severe combined immunodeficiency: Report of a case [abstract]. Presented at the Annual Meeting of Laboratory Investigation, 1992.
676. Centers for Disease Control and Prevention. Recommendations of the Advisory Committee on Immunization Practices (ACIP): Use of vaccines and immune globulins in persons with altered immunocompetence. MMWR Morb Mortal Wkly Rep 42(RR-4):1–18, 1993.
677. Torigoe S, Hirai S, Oitani K, et al. Application of live attenuated measles and mumps vaccines in children with acute leukemia. Biken J 24:147–151, 1981.
678. Ljungman P, Fridell E, Lonnqvist B, et al. Efficacy and safety of vaccination of marrow transplant recipients with a live attenuated measles, mumps and rubella vaccine. J Infect Dis 159:610–615, 1989.
679. Ljungman P, Lewensohn-Fuchs I, Hammarstrom V, et al. Long-term immunity to measles, mumps, and rubella after allogeneic bone marrow transplantation. Blood 84:657–663, 1994.
680. Henning KJ, White MH, Sepkowitz KA, Armstrong D. A national survey of immunization practices following allogeneic bone marrow transplantation. JAMA 277:1148–1151, 1997.
681. McLaughlin M, Thomas P, Onorato I, et al. Live viral vaccines in human immunodeficiency virus infected children: A retrospective survey. Pediatrics 82:229–233, 1988.
682. Sprauer MA, Markowitz LE, Nicholson JK, et al. Response of human immunodeficiency virus–infected adults to measles-rubella vaccination. J Acquir Immune Defic Syndr 6:1013–1016, 1993.
683. Rhoads JL, Birx DL, Wright C, et al. Safety and immunogenicity of multiple conventional immunizations administered during early HIV infection. J Acquir Immune Defif Syndr 4:724–731, 1991.
684. Wallace MR, Hooper DG, Graves SJ, Malone JL. Measles seroprevalence and vaccine response in HIV-infected adults. Vaccine 12:1222–1224, 1994.
685. O'Brien WA, Grovit-Ferbas K, Namazi A, et al. Human immunodeficiency virus-type 1 replication can be increased in peripheral blood of seropositive patients after influenza vaccination. Blood 86:1082–1089, 1995.
686. Stanley SK, Ostrowski MA, Justement JS, et al. Effect of immunization with a common recall antigen on viral expression in patients infected with human immunodeficiency virus type 1. N Engl J Med 334:1222–1230, 1996.
687. Centers for Disease Control and Prevention. 1994 Revised classification system for human immunodeficiency virus infection in children less than 13 years of age. Official authorized addenda: Human immunodeficiency virus infection codes and official guidelines for coding and reporting ICD-9-CM. MMWR Morb Mortal Wkly Rep 43(RR-12):1–19, 1994.
688. Kamin PB, Fein BT, Britton HA. Use of live, attenuated measles virus vaccine in children allergic to egg protein. JAMA 193:1125–1126, 1965.
689. Brown FR, Wolfe HI. Chick embryo grown measles vaccine in an egg-sensitive child. J Pediatr 71:868–869, 1967.
690. Herman JJ, Radin R, Schneiderman R. Allergic reactions to measles (rubeola) vaccine in patients hypersensitive to egg protein. J Pediatr 102:196–199, 1983.
691. Greenberg MA, Birx DL. Safe administration of mumps-measles-rubella vaccine in egg-allergic children. J Pediatr 261:2512–2516, 1988.
692. Beck SA, Williams LW, Shirrell A, Wesley B. Egg hypersensitivity and measles-mumps-rubella vaccine administration. Pediatrics 88:913–917, 1991.
693. Stiehm RE. Skin testing prior to measles vaccination for egg-sensitive patients [editorial]. Am J Dis Child 144:320, 1990.
694. Fasano MB, Wood RA, Cooke SK, Sampson HA. Egg hypersen-

sitivity and adverse reactions to measles, mumps, and rubella vaccine. J Pediatr 120:878–881, 1992.
695. Kemp A, Van Asperen P, Mukhi A. Measles immunization in children with clinical reactions to egg protein. Am J Dis Child 144:33–35, 1990.
696. James JM, Burks AW, Roberson PK, Sampson HA. Safe administration of the measles vaccine to children allergic to eggs. N Engl J Med 332:1262–1266, 1995.
697. Kelso JM, Jones RT, Yunginger JW. Anaphylaxis to measles, mumps, and rubella vaccine mediated by IgE to gelatin. J Allergy Clin Immunol 91:867–872, 1993.
698. Sakaguchi M, Ogura H, Inouye S. IgE antibody to gelatin in children with immediate-type reactions to measles and mumps vaccines. J Allergy Clin Immunol 96:563–565, 1995.
699. Sakaguchi M, Nakayama T, Inouye S. Food allergy to gelatin in children with systemic immediate-type reactions, including anaphylaxis, to vaccines. J Allergy Clin Immunol 98:1058–1061, 1996.
700. Siber GR, Werner BG, Halsey NA, et al. Interference of immune globulin with measles and rubella immunization. J Pediatr 122:204–211, 1993.
701. Osterhaus AD, de Vries P, van Binnendijk RS. Measles vaccines: Novel generations and new strategies. J Infect Dis 170(suppl 1):S42–S55, 1994.
702. Taylor J, Weinberg R, Tartaglia J, et al. Nonreplicating viral vectors as potential vaccines: Recombinant canarypox virus expressing measles virus fusion (F) and hemagglutinin (HA) glycoproteins. Virology 187:321–328, 1992.
703. Taylor J, Pincus S, Tartaglia J, et al. Vaccinia virus recombinants expressing either the measles virus fusion or hemagglutinin glycoprotein protect dogs against canine distemper virus challenge. J Virol 65:4263–4274, 1991.
704. Yang K, Mustafa F, Valsamakis A, et al. Early studies on DNA-based immunizations for measles virus. Vaccine 15:888–891, 1997.
705. Cutts FT, Markowitz LE. Successes and failures in measles control. J Infect Dis 170(suppl 1):S32–S41, 1994.
706. Mclean AR, Nokes DJ, Anderson RM. Model-based comparisons of measles immunization strategies using high dose Edmonston-Zagreb type vaccines. Int J Epidemiol 20:1107–1117, 1991.
707. Chen RT, Weierbach R, Bisoffi Z, et al. A "post-honeymoon period" measles outbreak in Muyinga sector, Burundi. Int J Epidemiol 23:185–193, 1994.
708. Agocs MM, Markowitz LE, Straub I, Dômôk I. The 1988–1989 measles epidemic in Hungary: Assessment of vaccine failure. Int J Epidemiol 21:1007–1013, 1992.
709. Kambarami RA, Nathoo KJ, Nkrumah FK, Pirie DJ. Measles epidemic in Harare, Zimbabwe despite high measles immunization coverage rates. Bull World Health Organ 69:213–219, 1991.
710. Henderson DA. Global measles eradication [letter]. Lancet 2:208, 1982.
711. Thacker SB, Millar DJ. Mathematical modeling and attempts to eliminate measles: A tribute to the late professor George Macdonald. Am J Epidemiol 133:517–525, 1991.
712. Conrad JL, Wallace R, Witte JJ. The epidemiologic rationale for the failure to eradicate measles in the United States. Am J Public Health 61:2304–2310, 1971.
713. Fine PEM. Herd immunity: History, theory, practice. Epidemiol Rev 15:265–302, 1993.
714. Fox JP, Elveback L, Scott W, et al. Herd immunity: Basic concept and relevance to public health immunization practices. Am J Epidemiol 94:179–189, 1971.
715. Hethcote HW. Measles and rubella in the United States. Am J Epidemiol 117:2–13, 1983.
716. Levy DL. The future of measles in highly immunized populations. A modeling approach. Am J Epidemiol 120:39–48, 1984.
717. Anderson RM, May RM. Age-related changes in the rate of disease transmission: Implications for the design of vaccination programs. J Hyg 94:365–436, 1985.
718. Cutts FT, Henderson RH, Clements CJ, et al. Principles of measles control. Bull World Health Organ 69:1–7, 1991.
719. McLean AR, Anderson RM. Measles in developing countries. Part II. The predicted impact of mass vaccination. Epidemiol Infect 100:419–442, 1988.
720. Schlenker TL, Bain C, Baughman AL, Hadler SC. Measles herd immunity. The association of attack rates with immunization rates in preschool children. JAMA 267:823–826, 1992.
721. Sencer DJ, Dull HB, Langmuir AD. Epidemiologic basis for eradication of measles in 1967. Public Health Rep 82:253–256, 1967.
722. Hersh BS, Markowitz LE, Maes EF, et al. The geography of measles in the United States, 1980–1989. JAMA 267:1936–1941, 1992.
723. Gustafson TL, Lievens AW, Brunell PA, et al. Measles outbreak in a fully immunized secondary school population. N Engl J Med 316:771–774, 1987.
724. Atkinson WL, Orenstein WA, Krugman S. The resurgence of measles in the United States, 1989–90. Annu Rev Med 43:451–463, 1992.
725. Gindler JS, Atkinson WL, Markowitz LE, Hutchins SS. The epidemiology of measles in the United States in 1989 and 1990. Pediatr Infect Dis J 11:841–846, 1992.
726. National Vaccine Advisory Committee. The measles epidemic: The problems, barriers and recommendations. JAMA 266:1547–1552, 1991.
727. Centers for Disease Control and Prevention. Measles vaccination levels among selected groups of preschool-aged children—United States. MMWR Morb Mortal Wkly Rep 40:36–39, 1990.
728. Centers for Disease Control and Prevention. Vaccination coverage of 2-year-old children—United States, 1991–1992. MMWR Morb Mortal Wkly Rep 42:985–988, 1993.
729. Zell ER, Dietz V, Stevenson J, et al. Low vaccination levels of US preschool and school-age children. Retrospective assessments of vaccination coverage, 1991–1992. JAMA 271:833–839, 1994.
730. Measles in Canada, 1989. Can Dis Wkly Rep 16:213–218, 1990.
731. Centers for Disease Control and Prevention. Status report on the childhood immunization initiative: National, state and urban area vaccination coverage levels among children aged 19–35 months—United States, 1996. MMWR Morb Mortal Wkly Rep 46:657–664, 1997.
731a. Measles—United States, 1994. MMWR Morb Mortal Wkly Rep 44:486–487, 493–494, 1995.
731b. Measles—United States, 1996, and the interruption of indigenous transmission. MMWR Morb Mortal Wkly Rep 46:242–246, 1997.
732. Centers for Disease Control and Prevention. Measles—United States, 1996 and the interruption of indigenous transmission. MMWR Morb Mortal Wkly Rep 46:242–246, 1997.
733. Rota JS, Rota PA, Redd SB, et al. Genetic analysis of measles viruses isolated in the United States, 1995–1996. J Infect Dis 177:204–208, 1998.
734. Peltola H, Heinonen OP, Valle M, et al. The elimination of indigenous measles, mumps, and rubella from Finland by a 12 year, two dose vaccination program. N Engl J Med 331:1397–1402, 1994.
735. Peltola H, Davidkin I, Valle M, et al. No measles in Finland [letter]. Lancet 350:1364–1365, 1997.
736. Communicable Disease Surveillance Centre. World Health Organization aims to eliminate measles in Europe by 2007. Commun Dis Rep CDR Wkly 7:425, 428, 1997.
737. Ramsay ME, Gay NJ, Miller E, et al. The epidemiology of measles in England and Wales: Rationale for the 1994 national vaccination campaign. Commun Dis Rep CDR Rev 4:R141–R146, 1994.
738. Babad HR, Nokes DJ, Gay NJ, et al. Predicting the impact of measles vaccination in England and Wales—model validation and analysis of policy options. Epidemiol Infect 114:319–344, 1995.
739. Salisbury DM, Horsley SD. Measles campaign [letter; comment]. BMJ 310:1334, 1995.
740. Gay N, Ramsay M, Cohen B, et al. The epidemiology of measles in England and Wales since the 1994 vaccination campaign. Commun Dis Rep CDR Rev 7:R17–R21, 1997.
741. Duclos P, Paulsen E. Measles elimination in Canada. Can J Public Health 86:370, 1995.
742. Centers for Disease Control and Prevention. Progress toward global measles control and elimination 1990–1996. MMWR Morb Mortal Wkly Rep 46:893–897, 1997.
743. Clemens JD, Stanton B, Chakraborty J, et al. Measles vaccination and childhood mortality in rural Bangladesh. Am J Epidemiol 128:1330–1339, 1988.

744. Holt EA, Boulos R, Halsey NA, et al. Childhood survival in Haiti: Protective effect of measles vaccination. Pediatrics 85:188–194, 1990.
745. Koenig MA, Khan MA, Wojtyniak B, et al. Impact of measles vaccination on childhood mortality in rural Bangladesh. Bull World Health Organ 68:441–447, 1990.
746. Aaby P, Pedersen IR, Knudsen K, et al. Child mortality related to seroconversion or lack of seroconversion after measles vaccination. Pediatr Infect Dis J 8:197–200, 1989.
747. Yach D. Re: The epidemiology of measles in a partially vaccinated population in an African city: Implications for immunization programs [letter; comment]. Am J Epidemiol 132:193, 1990.
748. Molinert HT, Rodriguez R, Galindo M. Principales Aspectos del Programa Nacional de Immunizacion de la Republica de Cuba. Havana, Cuba, Ministry of Health, 1993.
749. Plan to eliminate indigenous transmission of measles in the English-speaking Caribbean countries. Bull Pan Am Health Organ 24:240–246, 1990.
750. Pan American Health Organization. Record five years measles free! EPI Newsletter 18:1–3, 1996.
751. Pan American Health Organization. Measles elimination by the year 2000. EPI Newsletter 16:1–2, 1994.
752. de Quadros CA, Olivé JM, Hersh BS, et al. Measles elimination in the Americas: Evolving strategies. JAMA 275:224–229, 1996.
753. Vitek CR, Redd SC, Redd SB, Hadler SC. Trends in importation of measles to the United States, 1986–1994. JAMA 277:1952–1956, 1997.

chapter

13 Mumps Vaccine

Stanley A. Plotkin
Melinda Wharton

Hippocrates was the first to describe the clinical picture of mumps in the 5th century BC. His description of an illness characterized by swelling about one or both ears and, in some instances, painful swelling of one or both testes is reported in Book 1 of his *Book of Epidemics*. In 1790, the Royal Society of Edinburgh published a paper by Hamilton titled "An account of a distemper by the common people of England vulgarly called the mumps."[1] Hamilton reported for the first time that some patients with mumps had evidence of involvement of the central nervous system. He also emphasized the importance of orchitis as a manifestation of the disease in adult males. The origin of the word *mumps* is obscure but may be related to the old English verb, which means "grimace, grin or mumble."

Although mumps is generally viewed as an acute communicable disease of childhood, it gained notoriety as an illness that substantially affected armies during times of mobilization. Gordon and Kilham drew attention to this phenomenon in a series of two reviews of the epidemiology of mumps written during the 1940s.[2, 3] They noted that mumps was the leading cause of days lost from active duty in the U.S. Army in France during World War I. The average annual rate of hospitalization due to mumps during World War I was 55.8 per 1000 (a total of 230,356 cases), which was exceeded only by the rates for influenza and gonorrhea.[4, 5] In 1940, the Surgeon General of the United States stated that, next to the venereal diseases, mumps was the most disabling of the acute infections among recruits.[6] Mumps continues to occur in military settings even in the postvaccine era. In the 1980s, mumps was reported frequently among Soviet military recruits,[7] and outbreaks occurred among U.S. military personnel stationed in Korea in 1986[8] and onboard a ship in the western Pacific in 1992.[9]

In 1934, in a landmark study, Johnson and Goodpasture identified the etiological agent of mumps as a virus.[10] They obtained saliva from patients with epidemic parotitis and produced nonsuppurative parotitis in monkeys by inoculating the filtered, bacteria-free infectious material into the Stensen duct. The Koch postulates were fulfilled when filtrate from affected monkey parotid glands caused parotitis in uninfected monkeys and children.[11] Cultivation of the mumps virus in the developing chick embryo was first achieved by Habel[12] and Enders[13] in 1945. Propagation of the mumps virus in chick embryo and tissue culture made it possible to develop inactivated and live virus vaccines. An experimental inactivated vaccine developed in 1946[14] was tested in humans in 1951.[15] The first live attenuated mumps virus vaccines were developed during the 1960s in the former Soviet Union[16] and the United States.[17]

BACKGROUND

Clinical Description

The classic symptom of mumps is parotitis, which may be unilateral or, more commonly, bilateral and develops an average of 16 to 18 days after exposure.[18] Parotitis may be preceded by several days of nonspecific symptoms, including fever, headache, malaise, myalgias, and anorexia. Data from longitudinal studies have suggested that 15 to 20% of mumps virus infections produce typical acute parotitis; as many as 40 to 50% of infections in some studies have been associated with nonspecific or primarily respiratory symptoms.[19, 20] Particularly in children younger than 5 years, mumps may commonly appear as lower respiratory disease.[21] Inapparent infection may be more common in adults than in children,[22] and parotitis may occur more commonly in children aged 2 to 9 years than in other children.[20] Serious complications of mumps virus infection can occur without evidence of parotitis. Fever usually lasts 1 to 6 days, but enlargement of the parotid gland may persist 10 days or longer. An average of 7 days is lost from work or school.[9, 19, 23, 24]

Some complications of mumps are known to occur at higher rates in adults than in children.[19, 25] Orchitis may occur in as many as 38% of postpubertal men who develop mumps.[7, 22, 26] Although testicular involvement can be bilateral in as many as 30% of men with mumps orchitis, sterility is thought to occur only rarely.[27, 28] An increased risk of testicular cancer has been reported after mumps orchitis.[29–31] Pancreatitis, usually mild, may occur in 4% of cases.[19] Although an association with diabetes mellitus has been suggested,[32–35] it remains unproved.

Central nervous system involvement is reported in 4 to 6% of clinical cases in both population-based studies and large outbreaks.[19, 26, 36, 37] Adults are at more risk for mumps meningoencephalitis than are children.[19, 25] Typically, the illness is mild, appearing as aseptic meningitis that is clinically indistinguishable from other forms of aseptic meningitis,[38] and most patients recover fully. Other clinical presentations include encephalitis and rarely cerebellar ataxia.[39, 40] Permanent sequelae may occur, including paralysis, seizures, cranial nerve palsies, aqueductal stenosis, and hydrocephalus.[41–47] As many as half of patients with mumps meningoencephalitis have no evidence of parotid gland involvement.[38, 48] Typical abnormalities of the cerebrospinal fluid in people with mumps virus infection of the central nervous system include mononuclear pleocytosis, elevated protein levels, and normal or low glucose levels. Subclinical involvement of the central nervous system appears to be common, and cerebrospinal fluid pleocytosis is common in people with clinically uncomplicated mumps virus infection.[49] A chronic encephalitis has been reported rarely.[50–52]

Mumps is a major cause of sensorineural deafness among children. Deafness may be sudden in onset, bilateral, and permanent.[53–55] Mumps virus has been isolated from perilymph.[56]

Mastitis has been reported in as many as 31% of female patients older than 15 years who have mumps,[22] and pelvic pain thought to represent oophoritis has also been observed. An association with subsequent infertility has been suggested but remains unconfirmed.[57]

Nephritis is not uncommon but is generally not clinically significant.[58] The pathogenesis of nephritis is uncertain; it may be due to either direct viral infection of the kidney or immune complex glomerulonephritis. Although a limited number of pathological specimens have been examined, there is evidence to suggest that immune complex deposition may play a role in some cases.[59] Autoimmune hemolytic anemia associated with mumps has also been reported.[60]

Mumps arthropathy is a rare complication that reportedly is most common in young adults and more common in men than in women. The arthropathy may be manifested as arthralgias, polyarticular migratory arthritis, or monoarticular arthritis of the knee, hip, or ankle and may have a protracted course.[61, 62] The pathogenesis of mumps arthritis is unknown. Although mumps virus has not been isolated from affected joints, mumps virus can replicate in explants of human joint tissue.[63, 64]

Electrocardiographic abnormalities are sometimes detected in people with mumps virus infection between days 5 and 10 of illness,[65] but clinically apparent myocarditis is rare. The myocarditis is usually self-limited, but fatal cases have been reported.[66, 67] Conduction abnormalities, including complete heart block, may occur.[68]

Endocardial fibroelastosis has long been considered a complication of intrauterine or postnatal mumps infection, based on serological data and positive reactions to mumps skin test antigen.[69] Ni and colleagues reported detecting the mumps virus genome by the polymerase chain reaction (PCR) in cardiac muscle from 21 of 29 (72%) patients with endocardial fibroelastosis.[70] Endocardial fibroelastosis has become less common, perhaps because of the widespread use of mumps vaccine, although mumps does not appear to be a cause of other myopathies.[71–73]

An increase in fetal death has been observed among women who develop mumps during the first trimester of pregnancy.[74] No increased incidence of congenital malformations resulting from maternal mumps infection during pregnancy has been demonstrated,[75] although mumps virus has been shown to cross the placenta and infect the fetus.[76] Virus has been isolated at birth from infants born to women with mumps.[77] Although mumps is generally considered a benign infection among neonates,[78] severe disease may occur.[77, 79–81]

Virology

Mumps virus is a member of the genus *Rubulavirus* in the family Paramyxoviridae, which also includes Newcastle disease virus; human parainfluenza virus types 2, 4a, and 4b; and simian virus 5. It is an enveloped, negative-strand RNA virus consisting of 15,384 nucleotides encoding seven genes.[82] Two surface glycoproteins, the hemagglutinin-neuraminidase (HN) protein and the fusion (F) protein, are responsible for viral adsorption and fusion of the virion membrane with the host cell membrane, respectively; both are required for cell fusion. Antibodies to the HN protein neutralize the infectivity of mumps virus.

The four other structural proteins that have been characterized are located within the virion and are not thought to be important targets of a protective immune response. The nucleocapsid protein confers helical symmetry on the RNA complex. RNA transcriptase activity has been ascribed to both the phospho- (or polymerase) (P) protein and the large (L) protein. The membrane-associated, or matrix (M), protein is thought to play an important role in the assembly of viral proteins and in the budding of virions from the cell surface. Sequencing of the mumps virus genome revealed an additional open reading frame that could encode a small hydrophobic (SH) protein.[83] Although the messenger RNA transcript of the SH gene was found in cells infected with mumps virus,[84] detection of the protein by immunoprecipitation has been reported only more recently. The protein is described as having the characteristics of an integral membrane protein[85]; its function and whether it is a structural protein are both unknown. Two nonstructural proteins, V and I, are encoded by the P gene and are synthesized as a result of cotranscriptional editing of messenger RNA.[86, 87] The V protein is thought to play a role in regulating replication of the genome.

Varying degrees of homology of amino acid sequences have been demonstrated to analogous proteins in related paramyxoviruses. There is moderate homology between the F protein of mumps virus and that of other paramyxoviruses,[88, 89] and similarities also exist between the mumps virus HN protein and that of other paramyxoviruses.[90, 91] These similarities account for the serological cross-reactions that are observed among paramyxoviruses.[92–94] Likewise, homology has been demonstrated for the L,[82] M,[95, 96] NP,[97] and P[98] protein sequences of mumps virus and those of other paramyxoviruses. There is no sequence homology between the SH protein of mumps virus and that in simian virus 5.[96]

In a newborn hamster model, both the HN and F glycoproteins appear to be important in pathogenesis.[99] Wolinsky and colleagues found that monoclonal antibodies to the HN glycoprotein—but not the F glycoprotein—of mumps virus protected newborn hamsters from fatal experimental mumps encephalitis.[100] A monoclonal antibody to F was found by Löve and colleagues to protect newborn hamsters from developing necrotizing mumps encephalitis, but large amounts of viral antigen were present in tissue.[101]

Before monoclonal antibodies were available, no antigenic differences among mumps viruses had been demonstrated.[102, 103] However, by using monoclonal antibodies to distinguish among structural proteins of the mumps virus, researchers have demonstrated a variety of antigenic differences.[104–106] Although strain-specific differences in neutralizing activity have been identified,[104] these differences are thought to be insufficient to result in susceptibility to other strains after infection or vaccination. However, symptomatic mumps virus reinfections have been reported.[107]

Several mumps vaccines have been found to contain more than one strain of mumps virus. The Jeryl Lynn vaccine has been demonstrated to contain two distinct but related viruses in an approximate 1:5 ratio.[108] The Urabe Am9 vaccine from two manufacturers has been demonstrated to contain two viruses in a 1:3 ratio. Although specific differences in the HN gene have been identified, the relatedness of the two strains has not been reported.[109] The Leningrad-3 mumps vaccine has also been reported to contain more than one strain of virus.[110, 111]

Although extensive sequencing data are now available for multiple strains of wild-type mumps virus and vaccine strains, the molecular basis of attenuation is not understood. Differences in the neuroinvasiveness of various strains of mumps virus have been demonstrated in a neonatal hamster model.[112] In a 1993 mumps outbreak in Japan, a high incidence of aseptic meningitis was noted. Subsequent analysis of strains from the outbreak revealed that some circulating strains had lost a restriction endonuclease cleavage site in the P gene, a change previously reported to be specific for the Urabe strain.[113, 114] However, sequencing of one of these strains demonstrated other changes that allowed it to be distinguished from the Urabe vaccine strain.[115] Additional sequencing data may lead to a better understanding of the relationship between these findings and the high rate of aseptic meningitis observed in this outbreak. Brown and colleagues reported that the two virus variants in Urabe vaccine differ in neurovirulence.[109] Sequencing demonstrated a single nucleotide change resulting in an amino acid change at position 335 in the HN glycoprotein, but the contribution of this single change to the differences observed in neurovirulence of the two strains has not been established. The neurovirulent strain has the amino acid lysine at position 335, as do other mumps virus strains (including other vaccine strains).[104] There is evidence based on neutralization studies with monoclonal antibodies that amino acid 335 occupies an important domain, but other amino acid changes have been observed in the variant as well.[116]

Several different methods have been described for differentiating wild-type and vaccine strains of mumps virus. Both strains have been differentiated by amplification and sequencing of segments of the F gene,[117, 118] the HN gene,[119] and the SH gene.[120, 121] Yamada and associates sequenced a 223-nucleotide segment of the P gene from several vaccine strains and wild-type strains and from isolates obtained from patients who developed meningitis or parotitis after vaccination.[113] They found unique nucleotide changes for the Urabe, Hoshino, Miyahara, and Torii vaccine strains, and the postvaccination isolates were identical to the corresponding vaccine strain. They also noted a specific nucleotide change in the Urabe vaccine strain that resulted in the loss of one restriction endonuclease cleavage site. Thus, the Urabe strain could be distinguished from other strains by restriction endonuclease digestion of PCR-amplified P gene segments.[113] The single-strand conformation polymorphism technique has also been used to distinguish among mumps virus strains.[122, 123]

Nucleotide sequence analysis of different segments of the mumps virus genome has allowed mumps vaccine strains and circulating wild-type strains to be grouped on the basis of similarity. Although relationships among mumps virus strains have been inferred from nucleotide sequence analyses of the P,[124] F,[117] and HN[104] genes, the SH gene sequence has been studied the most extensively.[108, 125–129] Based on nucleotide sequence analysis of the SH gene, Yeo and colleagues identified three different groups of mumps virus.[125] Group A included the Jeryl Lynn vaccine strain and the Kilham, Enders, and SBL-1 strains. Group B included the Urabe wild-type and vaccine strains and other isolates from Japan. Group C included isolates from the United Kingdom. Sequence analysis of the SH gene has demonstrated similarity between the two strains that constitute the Jeryl Lynn vaccine.[108] Strains isolated during outbreaks in Switzerland from 1992 to 1993 were later demonstrated to be closely related to isolates from the United Kingdom.[126, 127] In more recent studies, mumps virus strains have been divided into three,[128] five,[129] or six[130] groups based on the similarity of the SH gene sequence. Standardized nomenclature has not yet been adopted.

Pathogenesis as It Relates to Prevention

Mumps can be understood as a respiratory infection that is frequently accompanied by viremia, which leads commonly to organ involvement, particularly of the salivary glands.

Because mumps virus is present in the saliva and urine for long periods, infection is probably transmitted by large droplets that infect the upper respiratory tract. Approximately one third of infected individuals do not manifest salivary gland or other involvement. Because mumps virus has been isolated from patients with undifferentiated respiratory disease, one can infer that many infections do not go beyond the respiratory tract.[21] Mumps virus can be recovered from the saliva approximately 7 days before the onset of symptoms, and it persists for several days thereafter.[131]

Viremia is likely to occur late in the incubation period, which in terms of the interval until parotitis is 12 to 25 days, 16 to 18 days being the usual.[18, 132] In view of the protective effect on the infant exerted by maternal mumps antibodies (see subsequent discussion), it is probable that the viremia is cell free.

Viremia leads to the involvement of many different glandular and other tissues. Parotitis or other salivary gland involvement is certainly the most common, occurring in two thirds of infections. The second most common is meningitis, which may occur in the absence of parotitis. The incidence of central nervous system involvement is difficult to judge. If lumbar punctures are performed routinely, as many as half of the infections show inflammation of the meninges.[49, 133] If the diagnosis is based only on clinical evidence of meningitis, only 0.5 to 15.0% of cases are considered to involve the central nervous system.[134]

In any case, virus isolation from the cerebrospinal fluid confirms that meningitis is a complication of viremia, which also explains mumps nephritis, orchitis, oophoritis, pancreatitis, mastitis, thyroiditis, arthritis, and endolymph infections that lead to deafness.

Viremia during infection in a pregnant woman explains reports of the isolation of mumps virus from the placenta[135] and the fetus.[76] Infection of the kidneys, whether or not accompanied by clinical nephritis, is accompanied by viruria that lasts 10 to 14 days; most patients with mumps show viruria.[13]

The point at which the mumps virus is most susceptible to immune attack is therefore the period of viremia, when antibodies can prevent viral spread. However, it is possible that local antibodies induced by mumps live virus vaccine also act to prevent respiratory infection by the virus. Cellular immunity probably plays a role in protection, as administration of immune globulin has been generally ineffective in preventing mumps after exposure.[136] Nevertheless, the considerable although transient efficacy of an inactivated mumps virus vaccine suggests that antibodies are the most important means of protection.[137]

Although antigenic differences among mumps strains are minor, symptomatic reinfection has been reported.[107] Reinfections may be common, usually resulting in asymptomatic rises in antibody but occasionally accompanied by mild illness.

Diagnosis

The diagnosis of mumps is usually made clinically, based on the presence of parotitis. Although parotitis can result from infection with other viruses, such as the Coxsackie and parainfluenza viruses,[138] these agents do not produce parotitis on an epidemic scale. In the absence of high levels of mumps vaccination, most cases of parotitis that are clinically suspected to be mumps are caused by infection with the mumps virus[131]; nonetheless, before the introduction of mumps vaccination in Alberta, one third of sporadic cases reported by participating family practitioners from 1980 to 1982 could not be confirmed serologically as mumps.[19] The inadequacy of clinical diagnosis is even more apparent when disease incidence is low; as disease incidence declines, laboratory confirmation becomes increasingly important.[139–142] Brunell and colleagues evaluated 20 children with parotitis who had received mumps vaccine 3 to 39 months previously.[143] The diagnosis of mumps could be confirmed in only 8 children, and serological studies and virus isolation failed to identify any infectious cause in the other 12 children. Only 32 of 252 suspected cases reported to the Texas Department of Health in the first 11 months of 1995 could be confirmed, based on documentation of mumps immunoglobulin M (IgM) antibody testing or epidemiological linkage to a laboratory-confirmed case.[144] In England and Wales, only 3% of 1333 reported clinically diagnosed cases that were tested for salivary mumps IgM antibody were confirmed as mumps.[141]

Mumps virus may be readily isolated from swabs of the opening of the Stensen duct, saliva, urine, or cerebrospinal fluid during the first 5 days of illness.

Historically, serological assays, including complement fixation, neutralization, and hemagglutination inhibition, have been employed for the diagnosis of mumps. Paired sera are required for these assays, and the acute serum should be obtained as early as possible in the course of illness. Cross-reactions with other paramyxoviruses may occur. Demonstration of neutralizing antibodies is extremely laborious, and both complement fixation and hemagglutination inhibition assays are relatively insensitive. The hemolysis in gel assay is simple enough to perform to make it feasible for serological screening.[145] However, both false-positive and false-negative results may occur.[146]

At present, enzyme-linked immunosorbent assays (ELISAs) for mumps IgG and IgM antibody are widely available commercially. The use of IgM antibody assays allows for the diagnosis of mumps from the analysis of a single acute serum sample, and cross-reactions with other paramyxoviruses do not occur.[92, 93] Compared with the complement fixation, hemagglutination inhibition, and hemolysis in gel tests, the IgM ELISA is more sensitive.[147] IgM antibodies are detectable within the first few days of illness, reach a maximum level about a week after the onset of symptoms, and remain elevated for several weeks or months.[147, 148] Comparison of antibody levels in serum and cerebrospinal fluid may provide support for local synthesis of antibody in the central nervous system.[149, 150] Maximum antibody titers in cerebrospinal fluid occur 1 to 2 weeks after the onset of meningeal symptoms.

Researchers have described a capture radioimmunoassay for mumps IgM antibody in saliva.[151, 152] The method is highly sensitive compared with serology 1 to 4 weeks after onset, but data are more limited during the first week after onset, and after the fourth week. Based on the measured declines in IgM antibody in saliva in a small number of cases, the test appears to have limited usefulness after 5 to 6 weeks.

Indirect fluorescent antibody assays for mumps IgM antibody testing are offered by some laboratories. False-positive test results for mumps IgM antibody by this technique have been reported.[153]

Direct detection of mumps virus in clinical specimens (oropharyngeal swabs or cerebrospinal fluid) by reverse transcription–PCR (RT-PCR) has been reported.[118] Cusi and colleagues evaluated the use of RT-PCR to detect mumps virus in clinical specimens from children with suspected mumps in Siena, Italy, during the period 1993 to 1995.[118] RT-PCR was more sensitive than mumps IgM ELISA, detecting evidence of mumps infection in 22 of 27 oropharyngeal swabs from children with parotitis, compared with 18 of 27 positive tests for mumps IgM antibody by ELISA. Afzal and colleagues used RT-PCR in evaluation of clinical specimens from patients during the 1996 outbreak in Portugal.[154] In this series, mumps virus was detected more frequently from saliva than from throat swabs by RT-PCR.

Immunity to mumps may be documented by the presence of neutralizing antibodies or by the detection of IgG antibodies by ELISA. In several studies of vaccinated people, seroconversion was demonstrated by ELISA even in the absence of demonstrable neutralizing antibody.[146, 155–157] The reason for this finding is unknown but may be related to antibody directed primarily against the F protein.[156] With the addition of complement, neutralizing antibodies may be detectable.[158] The mumps skin test is not reliable and should not be used for identification of susceptible individuals.[159]

Epidemiology

Prior to the introduction of mumps vaccine in the United States, mumps was a disease of young school-aged children. In the 1920s, mumps incidence was highest among children 6 to 9 years of age.[160] In the years immediately before the introduction of mumps vaccine in the United States, mumps was most commonly reported among young school-aged children, with more than half the reported cases of mumps among children 5 to 9 years of age.[161] There is evidence that preschool-aged children may also have played an important role in the epidemiology of mumps. The longitudinal Seattle Virus Watch Study (1965–1969) found that infants and preschool-aged children (many of whom did not develop typical parotitis) accounted for the majority of probable primary infections in households.[20]

Data on the incidence of mumps in the U.S. military in the 20th century suggest that there have been significant shifts in morbidity from adults to children that are associated with increasing urbanization. During World War I, when mumps was a major cause of days lost from active duty among U.S. troops, cases occurred predominantly among men from rural backgrounds.[162] During World War II, outbreaks did occur among military recruits, but reported rates were less than one tenth of those documented during World War I. Large outbreaks tended to occur only among groups of soldiers from rural areas.[26] Serosurveys of military recruits in 1962 demonstrated little difference in rates of susceptibility to mumps among men from urban, town, and rural backgrounds, although rates remained slightly higher among men from the southern United States. The difference was not statistically significant.[163] A serosurvey of U.S. Army recruits in 1989 found no differences among recruits from urban, suburban, small town, and rural backgrounds, but people from the western United States were more likely to be seronegative than others (relative risk 1.31; 95% confidence interval, 0.94–1.82). Black non-Hispanic recruits were significantly more likely to be seropositive than recruits from other racial or ethnic backgrounds.[164]

Serosurveys from around the world have demonstrated that, in the absence of mumps vaccination, there is substantial variation in the average age at infection with mumps virus. A seroepidemiological study in St. Lucia demonstrated that 70% of children are seropositive for mumps at 4 years of age,[165] whereas studies from the Netherlands,[166] Singapore,[167] and Scotland[168] demonstrated that most children 4 years of age and younger remained susceptible. In the Netherlands, peak acquisition occurred between ages 4 and 6 years; more than 90% of people aged 14 years had mumps-neutralizing antibodies, as did 95% of adults aged 18 to 65 years.[166] Before the initiation of routine mumps vaccination of children in 1988, the average age at infection in the United Kingdom was reported to be 6 to 7 years.[169] Evidence from England indicates that there has been some decrease in the average age at infection, perhaps because of increased contacts among preschool-aged children.[170, 171] Before the introduction of mass vaccination in Spain, two thirds of 3- to 5-year-old children and more than half of 6- to 7-year-old children were susceptible to mumps. The trend within each age group, however, was toward decreased susceptibility with more siblings and years in school.[172]

Hope-Simpson demonstrated in household contact studies that mumps is less infectious than measles or varicella.[18] Secondary attack rates among susceptible household contacts younger than 15 years were 75.6% for measles, 61.0% for varicella, and 31.1% for mumps. Some of the observed differences were undoubtedly due to a higher rate of subclinical infection with mumps, but the higher average age at infection observed for mumps also supports the less efficient transmission of mumps virus.[173]

Most epidemiological reports suggest an interepidemic period for mumps of approximately 3 years.[169, 171] In temperate zones, mumps exhibits seasonality, with peak incidence occurring during the winter and spring and a nadir in the summer.[170] This seasonal pattern was seen in the United States until the mid-1990s but is no longer apparent (Fig. 13–1). Seasonality of mumps has not been noted in tropical areas.

Following licensure of the live virus mumps vaccine in 1967, the number of reported mumps cases in the United States decreased steadily from 152,209 cases in 1968 to 2982 cases in 1985, a record low at the time (Fig. 13–2). However, this downward trend was reversed from 1986 to 1987, when a relative resurgence of mumps occurred in the United States. That resurgence was the result of incomplete vaccination coverage of adolescents and young adults in the years after the introduction of the live virus vaccine (see under *Epidemiological Effects of*

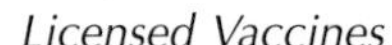

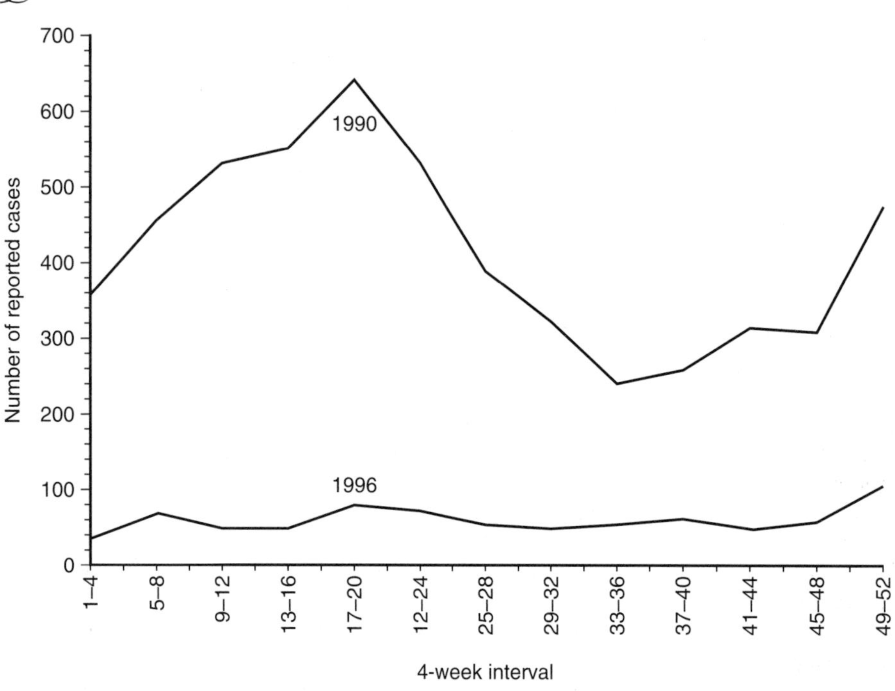

Figure 13–1. Reported mumps cases, by 4-week interval, in the United States, 1990 and 1996. (From National Notifiable Diseases Surveillance System, Centers for Disease Control and Prevention, Atlanta, GA, 1997.)

Vaccination). Since 1989, reported cases of mumps have again decreased: In 1996, only 751 mumps cases were reported in the United States, an all-time low. From 1988 to 1996, reductions were most dramatic among those 5 to 19 years of age (Fig. 13–3). This pattern reflects an increasing implementation of school immunization requirements for two doses of measles-mumps-rubella (MMR) vaccine as well as improved specificity in the reporting of mumps in some states.[144]

Passive Immunization

Immune globulin has not been demonstrated to be effective for postexposure prophylaxis against mumps or for the prevention of complications.[136, 174] Likewise, mumps immune globulin has not been shown to be effective and is no longer available in the United States.[36, 175] In a study that resulted from an outbreak of mumps in Alaska, administration of mumps immune globulin to susceptible people did not appear to decrease attack rates or prevent clinical complications.[36] Maternal antibody is transferred across the placenta and appears to protect infants from developing mumps during the first year of life.[132, 176]

ACTIVE IMMUNIZATION

Vaccine Strains

Origin and Development

Soon after the initial isolation of mumps virus, attempts were made to develop vaccines based on formalin-inactivated virus.[14, 15] Although these vaccines were

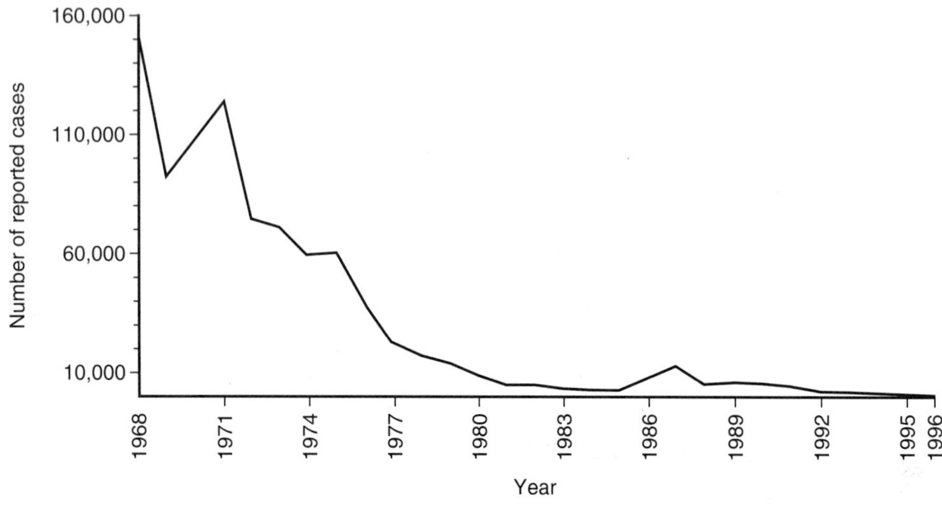

Figure 13–2. Reported mumps cases in the United States, 1968 to 1996. (From National Notifiable Diseases Surveillance System, Centers for Disease Control and Prevention, Atlanta, GA, 1997.)

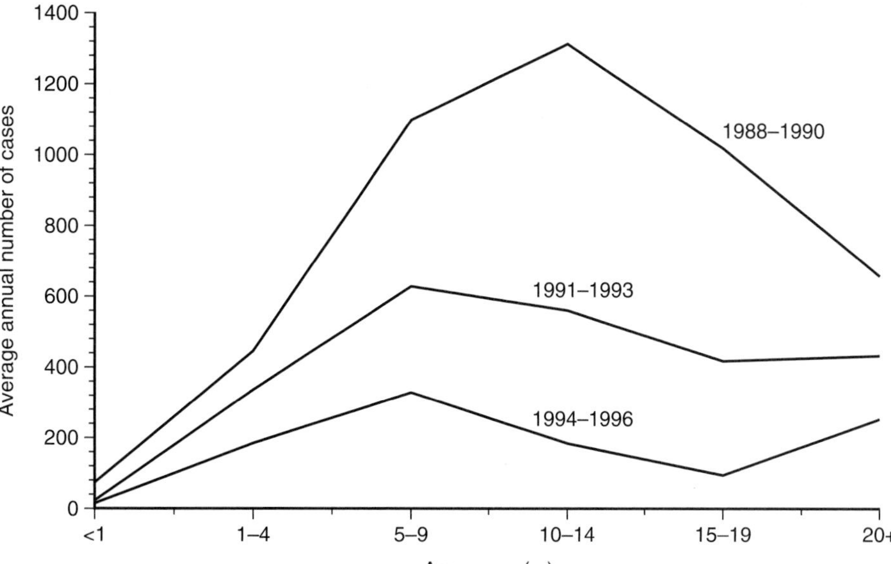

Figure 13–3. Average annual number of reported cases by age group and by 3-year period, 1988 to 1996. (From National Notifiable Diseases Surveillance System, Centers for Disease Control and Prevention, Atlanta, GA, 1997.)

somewhat effective, the duration of immunity was short, and their use was abandoned in the United States in the 1950s.[177, 178]

More than 10 mumps vaccine strains, listed in Table 13–1, are in use throughout the world. Strains have been adapted to the embryonated egg,[179] chick embryo fibroblast cell culture,[179–183] human diploid cell culture,[184, 185] quail embryo fibroblast cell culture,[186] and primary guinea pig kidney cell culture.[187]

Description of Vaccines and Producers: Vaccine Dosage, Route of Administration, and Composition

The live virus mumps vaccine produced in the United States by Merck Sharp & Dohme is derived from the Jeryl Lynn strain of mumps virus isolated from the throat of Jeryl Lynn Hilleman and attenuated by passage in embryonated hens' eggs and chick embryo cell culture.[180] The vaccine is available both as monovalent mumps vaccine and in combination with rubella vaccine (mumps-rubella) or measles and rubella vaccines (MMR).

In its monovalent form, mumps vaccine is supplied as a lyophilized powder containing 20,000 times the median tissue culture infective dose ($TCID_{50}$) of virus, which is reconstituted with sterile, preservative-free water. Sorbitol and hydrolyzed gelatin are used as stabilizers, and 25 μg of neomycin is present in each dose of vaccine. The volume of 0.5 mL is injected subcutaneously above the deltoid area. The vaccine should be kept at 2 to 8°C and should not be exposed to light.

The Urabe Am9 strain was developed by the Biken Institute in Japan from an isolate obtained from the saliva of a mumps patient. The vaccine is produced in Japan by multiple manufacturers and in Europe by SmithKline Beecham and Pasteur Mérieux Connaught. Each dose contains 5000 times the $TCID_{50}$ of lyophilized virus and is administered subcutaneously after rehydration with sterile water in a volume of 0.5 mL. Data concerning vaccine-associated meningitis (see subsequent discussion) have led to the withdrawal of Urabe-containing vaccines from several countries.

Table 13–1. **MUMPS VACCINE STRAINS CURRENTLY IN USE**

STRAIN	MANUFACTURER	CELL SUBSTRATE	MAIN AREA OF DISTRIBUTION
Jeryl Lynn	Merck	CEF	Worldwide
Urabe	SmithKline Beecham	CEF	Worldwide
	Pasteur Mérieux Connaught	CEF	Worldwide
	Biken	CEF	Japan
Hoshino	Kitasato Institute	CEF	Japan
Rubini	Swiss Serum Institute	HEF	Switzerland
Leningrad-3	Bacterial Medicine Institute, Moscow	QEF	Former Soviet Union
L-Zagreb	Institute of Immunology of Zagreb	CEF	Former Yugoslavia
Miyahara	Chem-Sero Therapeutic Research Institute	CEF	Japan
Torii	Takeda Chemicals	CEF	Japan
NK M-46	Chiba	CEF	Japan
S-12	Razi State Serum and Vaccine Institute	HEF	Iran
RIT 4385*	SmithKline Beecham	CEF	Europe

CEF, chick embryo fibroblast; HEF, human embryo fibroblast; QEF, quail embryo fibroblast.
*Derived from the Jeryl Lynn strain.

The Rubini mumps vaccine virus was derived from a mumps isolate obtained from the urine of a child named Carlo Rubini in Switzerland in 1974.[104, 184] Subsequent nucleotide sequence analysis has demonstrated that the strain is closely related to a wild-type strain isolated in Germany from 1987 to 1992[120] as well as to the tissue culture–adapted Enders strain.[104]

The other strains listed in Table 13–1 have had limited usage, often being sold in one country only. Their properties are therefore less well described. Each is characterized by a relatively limited number of passages, during which a level of attenuation was sought that would be sufficient to reduce reactions to an acceptable level without sacrificing immunogenicity.[182] Table 13–2 gives the history of passage during the attenuation of three of the strains listed in Table 13–1 that have gained some prominence.

At least three of the major vaccine strains have been shown to be composed of mixed virus populations. The Jeryl Lynn strain has two distinct viruses, both probably originating from U.S. wild-type isolates and maintained in passage.[108] The Urabe vaccine strain from two manufacturers has also been demonstrated to contain two distinct strains, one of which may be more neurovirulent than the other.[109] The Leningrad-3 strain used in the former Soviet Union is a mixture of large-plaque and small-plaque variants.[110] The significance of these findings is not entirely clear, but findings of the studies of the Urabe strain variants suggest that different populations may have different biological characteristics.

Stability of Vaccine

A study of the stability of the Jeryl Lynn strain of vaccine showed that the lyophilized vaccine could be stored for at least 3 years at −20°C without significant loss of infectivity.[188] A loss of infectivity of 0.5 log $TCID_{50}$ is seen after storage at 4°C after 1 year, at room temperature after 2 months, and at 37°C after 1 week. When reconstituted to a liquid state, the mumps vaccine remains stable at 4°C for about 8 hours.[189]

Combinations Including Mumps Vaccine

Mumps vaccine is available in the United States either as monovalent vaccine or as part of a combined formulation, such as MMR or mumps-rubella vaccines. The administration of MMR vaccine results in immune responses similar to those produced by the administration of individual measles, mumps, and rubella vaccines at different sites or at different times (see later). Combination products including measles, mumps, rubella, and varicella vaccines are currently under development (see Chapter 19).

Table 13–2. **DERIVATION OF THREE ATTENUATED MUMPS STRAINS**

JERYL LYNN	URABE	HOSHINO
7P EHE 10P CEF	2P HEK 4P AGMK 3P EHE 5P QEF 2–5P EHE or CEF	1P EHE 22P CEF

AGMK, African green monkey kidney; CEF, chick embryo fibroblast; EHE, embryonated hen's egg; HEK, human embryo kidney; P, passage; QEF, quail embryo fibroblast.

Results of Vaccination

Immune Responses

In one of the first prelicensure immunogenicity studies of the Jeryl Lynn strain, in Philadelphia in 1965, the seroconversion rate in children who tested initially as seronegative for mumps neutralization antibody was 98.1% (355 of 362 children).[17, 190] Similar results have been reported from other studies.[191–194] The total prelicensure experience in U.S. children showed that 96.9% of 6283 initially seronegative children developed neutralizing antibody after vaccination.[190] One study after licensure suggested that in some recipients of mumps vaccine, the immune response may not be completed by 4 weeks after immunization; seroconversion rates were 86.6% at 4 weeks and 93.3% at 5 weeks after immunization.[195]

In studies of monovalent Urabe vaccine, 94% of recipients seroconverted.[196] In Germany, a total of 94.4% of previously seronegative children developed neutralizing antibody after administration of vaccine from any of four lots of Urabe vaccine. The antibody response was demonstrated to persist for at least 32 months after vaccination.[196] Researchers in Finland compared the immunogenicity of the Urabe vaccine with that of the Jeryl Lynn vaccine in children 14 to 20 months of age. According to the results of the hemolysis in gel and neutralization assays, 55 of 58 (94.8%) of the recipients of the Urabe vaccine experienced seroconversion, as did 58 of 60 children (96.7%) who received the Jeryl Lynn vaccine.[197]

Ninety-three percent of children receiving monovalent Hoshino strain vaccine seroconverted.[198] In another study, 122 previously seronegative children received the Hoshino vaccine, and 95% developed neutralizing antibody to mumps.[182] In a study of preschool-aged children attending daycare, 712 of 775 (92%) who received the Leningrad-3 mumps vaccine seroconverted based on the hemagglutination inhibition assay.[199]

In early field trials of the L-Zagreb vaccine conducted in preschool-aged children, 88 to 94% of children in various districts were demonstrated to have developed mumps antibodies as documented by hemagglutination inhibition. Later trials of the L-Zagreb strain combined with measles and rubella vaccines demonstrated seroconversion rates as high as 98%.[179]

The level of mumps-neutralizing antibody in children 6 to 8 weeks after vaccination is substantially lower than the level after natural mumps. In the Philadelphia prelicensure study, mean neutralization antibody titers were 1:9 after vaccination and 1:6 after natural disease.[17]

The immunogenicity of mumps vaccine has been evaluated as a component of triple MMR vaccines. The Jeryl Lynn strain gave between 90% conversion (geometric mean titer, 31) and 98% conversion in two studies.[200, 201] The Urabe and Jeryl Lynn strains were compared in several studies as part of two different trivalent vaccines.[202–205] Rates of seroconversion based on the presence of neutralizing antibodies in the four studies were 91, 84, 96, and 90% for the Jeryl Lynn strain and 94, 93, 98, and 97% for the Urabe strain, respectively.

Subsequent studies of combined vaccines demonstrated that, in general, the Urabe strain is highly immunogenic when administered in combination with measles and rubella vaccines. In Finland, seroconversion rates of 96 to 98% based on hemagglutination inhibition were demonstrated for MMR preparations containing Urabe or Jeryl Lynn strains in children 14 to 24 months of age.[204] A comparison of Urabe and Jeryl Lynn vaccines administered with measles vaccine in Austria suggested that the Urabe vaccine produced higher antibody responses as determined by ELISA.[205] In the United Kingdom, 88% of 13- to 15-month-old recipients of Urabe-containing MMR were demonstrated to develop neutralizing antibody.[206] However, given the lack of comparable efficacy data, the clinical significance of these observations is unknown.

The immunogenicity of the Rubini mumps vaccine as MMR has been evaluated in several clinical studies. Among children 15 to 24 months of age, 95% of recipients of Rubini mumps vaccine and 100% of recipients of Jeryl Lynn vaccine seroconverted, based on immunofluorescence.[207] In a study comparing the immunogenicity of Jeryl Lynn, Urabe, and Rubini vaccines as MMR among children 15 to 24 months of age, all children who received vaccines containing Jeryl Lynn or Urabe vaccines seroconverted as measured by immunofluorescence. In contrast, the seroconversion rate after use of Rubini vaccine varied among the four lots tested and was as low as 71% for one lot.[208] Another comparative study[208a] showed equal seroconversion with the use of Jeryl Lynn and Rubini vaccines when measured by the indirect immunofluorescence test but not by ELISA. Nevertheless, poor effectiveness of Rubini vaccine has been reported (see later).

Equivalent rates of seroconversion after the administration of monovalent and trivalent vaccines have been demonstrated for the Hoshino vaccine.[182] Similarly, studies with the L-Zagreb vaccine have demonstrated similar rates of seroconversion (approximately 90%) when vaccine is administered to 12- to 14-month-old children as single-antigen mumps vaccine or combined with measles and rubella vaccines.[179]

Researchers have examined several factors that affect vaccine immunogenicity in children. King and colleagues studied serological responses to MMR in children receiving routine vaccination, who frequently have mild illness afterward.[209] Seroconversion to the Jeryl Lynn mumps valence was not influenced by the illnesses, and the children exhibited an overall seroconversion rate of 83% as determined by ELISA. A small study examined the immune responses to the Jeryl Lynn strain among 44 seronegative infants who were identified from 52 infants tested.[189] None of the infants had a documented exposure to mumps virus. The seroprevalence of prevaccination mumps antibody varied by age from 50% (4 of 8) in infants aged 3 to 5 months to 9% (2 of 23) in those aged 6 to 8 months to 10% (2 of 21) in those aged 9 to 11 months. Seroconversion rates among the initially seronegative children also varied among these age groups and were 50%, 95%, and 95%, respectively. The investigators concluded that maternal antibody inhibited response to the vaccine; however, the study was too small to evaluate adequately whether there was an age-related immune responsiveness to the vaccine among seronegative infants.[189] Wagenvoort and associates demonstrated that most infants born to mothers with naturally acquired mumps antibody became seronegative by 4 months of age.[166]

The response to Urabe strain mumps vaccine given as MMR has been evaluated among children younger than 12 months. In a study in India, children 9, 12, and 15 months of age were vaccinated, and their seroresponses as measured by hemagglutination inhibition were reduced from 92% when the vaccine was given at 1 year of age to 75% when vaccine was given at 9 months of age.[210] In contrast in Brazil, 99% of children seroconverted after vaccination at 9 months of age as measured by neutralization, and 100% seroconverted after vaccination at 15 months of age;[211] similar results were reported from South Africa.[212]

Whether immune globulin interferes with the immune response to mumps vaccine has not been well studied. Among 23 children 2 to 13 years of age who were initially seronegative to mumps, coadministration of mumps vaccine and 0.1 to 0.2 mL of immune globulin per lb resulted in 100% seroconversion and no difference in the levels of postvaccination mumps antibody titers compared with those of 11 control children who had received vaccine only.[189]

MMR is now often recommended for older children, and seroconversion rates of mumps-susceptible children vaccinated at 18 months or 12 years of age were compared in Sweden. Whereas 93% of the toddlers converted, only 80% of the 12-year-olds did so.[213]

Seroconversion rates among adults are generally slightly lower than those for children. A prelicensure immunogenicity study demonstrated neutralizing antibody responses after vaccination of 19 of 20 (95%) initially seronegative adults.[214] The total prelicensure experience in adults vaccinated with the Jeryl Lynn strain showed an overall seroconversion rate of 92.6% among 163 initially susceptible adults (132 men and 31 women).[194]

Mumps vaccine administered after exposure to mumps does not provide clinical protection or alter the severity of the disease.[193] However, evidence from an observational study suggests that mass vaccination during a mumps outbreak may help terminate the outbreak.[215]

Persistence of Antibodies

Serological studies have shown that neutralizing antibody titers of 1:2 or higher persisted for at least 12 years after vaccination in a follow-up study of children involved in a clinical efficacy trial.[216–218] Weibel[219] has

Table 13–3. **PERSISTENCE OF MUMPS-NEUTRALIZING ANTIBODY IN SEROPOSITIVE CHILDREN AFTER CLINICAL MUMPS OR VACCINATION WITH JERYL LYNN STRAIN OF MUMPS VACCINE**

	MUMPS-NEUTRALIZING ANTIBODY GEOMETRIC MEAN TITERS	
TIME	Vaccine (34 children)	Clinical Mumps (36 children)
1 mo	10.1	62.8
1 yr	12.8	27.6
2 yr	11.9	42.1
4 yr	11.8	34.5
7 yr	10.3	18.6
9.5 yr	12.5	24.4

From Weibel RE. Mumps vaccine. In Plotkin SA, Mortimer EA (eds). Vaccines. Philadelphia, WB Saunders, 1988, p 231.

summarized data on antibody persistence from this longitudinal study, which demonstrate that, with the passage of time, antibody levels after vaccination remain consistently lower than those after clinical mumps (Table 13–3). In the final report of the mumps data from this longitudinal study,[216] the mumps-neutralizing antibody titers of 22 vaccinated children, all of whom had remained free of clinical mumps disease during the 12 years of follow-up, were compared with those of 24 unvaccinated control children from the original 20-month trial who had developed natural mumps. Antibody measurements had been taken on the two groups of children at intervals of 3 to 4 years, 7 to 8 years, and 11 to 12 years after vaccination and mumps disease, respectively.

Although the initial level of neutralizing antibody reached after vaccination was generally less than that after natural disease, the geometric mean titers after vaccination decreased by 27% in nearly 12 years, whereas those following natural mumps fell 80% during approximately the same time period. Thus, the mean titers after vaccination (mean 9.1) and natural mumps (mean 11.5) were comparable. There was evidence during the follow-up period, however, that suggested asymptomatic boosting of antibody levels due to subclinical natural reinfection, particularly among the vaccinees.[217]

Miller and colleagues followed children given Jeryl Lynn or Urabe vaccine 4 years previously at 12 to 18 months of age.[220] Seronegativity by neutralization assay had developed in 19% of the Jeryl Lynn recipients and 15% of Urabe recipients, a difference that was statistically significant. Among seropositive children, however, geometric mean titers were higher among Jeryl Lynn recipients than among recipients of Urabe vaccine.[220] Canadian children who had received MMR vaccines containing Jeryl Lynn or Urabe strains at 12 to 24 months of age were later evaluated at 6 to 7 years of age. As measured by ELISA, 15% of Jeryl Lynn recipients and 7% of Urabe recipients were seronegative at 6 to 7 years of age.[221] Finnish workers provided data on children vaccinated with Jeryl Lynn vaccine at 14 to 18 months of age and again at 6 years of age. Seroconversion after the first dose was 86%, 76% at 6 years of age, 95% after booster, and 86% 9 years later.[222]

Data are limited on the immunogenicity of mumps vaccine among immunocompromised people. A study in pediatric patients who had received bone marrow transplants revealed that MMR vaccination 2 or more years after transplantation resulted in an increase in seropositivity from 31% to 87%.[223] Among 20 bone marrow transplant patients aged 1 to 29 years who were vaccinated with MMR vaccine 2 to 3 years after transplantation, 11 were seronegative before vaccination and 7 of the 11 seronegative patients seroconverted.[224] In a small study of children with end-stage renal disease undergoing maintenance hemodialysis, only 5 of 10 children seroconverted after receiving mumps vaccine as MMR.[225]

Protective Efficacy in Controlled Clinical Trials

Before the licensure of the Jeryl Lynn strain of mumps vaccine in the United States, two different clinical trials demonstrated that a single dose of live attenuated mumps vaccine was 95 to 96% effective in preventing mumps disease in people who were followed for as many as 20 months after vaccination (Table 13–4).[190, 193, 226] The first clinical trial was conducted in Philadelphia

Table 13–4. **PROTECTIVE EFFICACY OF JERYL LYNN STRAIN OF MUMPS VACCINE AMONG INITIALLY SUSCEPTIBLE CHILDREN, BY MONTHS SINCE VACCINATION, PHILADELPHIA, 1965 TO 1967**

INTERVAL BETWEEN VACCINATION AND MUMPS EXPOSURE (mo)	STUDY GROUP	VACCINATED GROUP			UNVACCINATED GROUP			VACCINE EFFICACY (%)
		No. of Cases	No. at Risk	Attack Rate (%)	No. of Cases	No. at Risk	Attack Rate (%)	
0–10	Household	2*	29	6.9	50	59	84.7	91.7
	Classroom	2*	114	1.8	49	113	43.4	95.9
11–20	Household	1†	14	7.1	22	24	91.7	92.3
	Classroom	1†	28	3.6	24	40	60.0	94.1
Total period	All children‡	5	174	2.9	133	224	59.4	95.2

*Three of these children showed postvaccination neutralizing antibody titers of 1:1; one failed to respond.

†This child, who was in both household and classroom groups, failed to respond serologically to vaccination.

‡Among vaccinated children, 11 counted twice, one of whom contracted mumps; among control children, 12 counted twice, and mumps developed in all 12.

From Hilleman MR, Weibel RE, Buynak EB, et al. Live, attenuated mumps-virus vaccine. 4. Protective efficacy as measured in a field evaluation. N Engl J Med 276:252–258, 1967. Reprinted, by permission, from The New England Journal of Medicine.

from 1965 to 1967 among selected children and their siblings attending nursery school or kindergarten.[190, 226] The children were initially screened serologically, and those lacking mumps antibody were randomized to the vaccinated and control groups (although complete randomization of the siblings was not achieved). Both groups were followed for a total of 20 months for the acquisition of a laboratory-confirmed case of clinical mumps or the documented exposure to a laboratory-confirmed case in a classroom or household setting. Laboratory confirmation was defined as the isolation of mumps virus from mouth or throat specimens or the indication of a fourfold or greater increase in mumps antibody titer by hemagglutination inhibition or neutralization antibody assays. Of the 867 children enrolled, 398 children (174 vaccinees and 224 control subjects) had a documented exposure to mumps during the 20-month follow-up period (see Table 13–4). Five cases of mumps occurred in the vaccinated group, compared with 133 cases among the control children. The overall protective efficacy of the vaccine was 95% (95% confidence interval, 88–98%), and the point estimates of efficacy varied from 92 to 96% by subgroups of exposed individuals (families vs. classrooms) and by interval from vaccination to exposure (0–10 mo vs. 11–20 mo).

The second clinical trial was a double-blind, placebo-controlled study conducted from 1966 to 1967 of first- and second-grade children attending 44 schools in Forsyth County, North Carolina (Table 13–5).[193] Every tenth study child in each school received the placebo vaccine, and no study participants were excluded based on mumps antibody status. After sera were drawn from a sample of children for mumps antibody testing by neutralization, all vaccinations were given during a 2-day period at the onset of the trial, and the children were followed for 6 months. Initial susceptibility to mumps did not differ significantly between the two study groups in the sample of children tested (34.9% among vaccinees vs. 37.1% among control subjects; P = .87). During the follow-up period from 30 to 180 days after vaccination, there were 5 cases of mumps among the 2965 children who received mumps vaccine, compared with 13 cases among the 316 control children, giving a vaccine efficacy of 96% (95% confidence interval, 88–99% [Fisher exact method, two-tailed]).

Smorodintsev and coworkers reported briefly on a small clinical trial of the Leningrad-3 strain among children 3½ to 6 years of age.[16] Two (2.3%) of the 85 vaccinated children developed mumps disease, compared with 42 (38.8%) of the children in the control group, giving a vaccine efficacy of 94% (95% confidence interval, 76–98%).

Effectiveness in Field Use and Duration of Immunity

The two trials just discussed have raised questions about the duration of vaccine-induced immunity.[227] Despite limitations in the design, study size, and duration of follow-up in these two prelicensure clinical trials, vaccine-induced antibody levels in general were found to be substantially lower than levels after naturally acquired mumps infection. Effectiveness of the Jeryl Lynn strain of mumps vaccine in the United States under conditions of routine use has been consistently lower in outbreak-based studies (i.e., 75–91%) than in the original clinical trials (i.e., 95–96%) (Table 13–6).[24, 215, 228–234] Although low calculated vaccine efficacy may be the result of true low efficacy, the methods used in postlicensure field evaluations of vaccine effectiveness have limited our ability to draw firm conclusions about the reasons for the lower estimates for vaccine efficacy compared with the results in controlled clinical trials. Kim-Farley and colleagues have demonstrated that errors such as inaccurate case definition, incomplete surveillance with limited case ascertainment, and inaccurate determination of vaccination status all were factors that potentially contributed to falsely low estimates of vaccine efficacy in observational studies.[230]

The occurrence of serologically or virologically confirmed mumps cases in vaccinated people is also predictable, as with any vaccine of less than 100% efficacy. This problem becomes more prominent as vaccination coverage increases. Although the overall rate of susceptibility decreases, the proportion of remaining susceptible people increases among the vaccinated, and hence cases occur among vaccinated people even when vaccine efficacy is high.[235] Incomplete case ascertainment with selectively better identification of vaccinated than unvaccinated cases may result in low vaccine efficacy estimates. Factors that can confound the analyses include prior mumps disease and subclinical infection occurring before the outbreak and noncomparable levels of exposure of vaccinees and nonvaccinees to mumps virus during the outbreak. Inaccuracies in determining mumps vaccination status from parent histories or school records may also result in misleadingly low estimates of efficacy.[215, 230, 231, 235]

Despite these methodological limitations, the outbreak-based studies taken together suggest that mumps vaccine effectiveness is somewhat lower than the estimates derived from the controlled clinical trials with relatively short follow-up periods. Although earlier studies had not identified the waning of vaccine-induced

Table 13–5. **PROTECTIVE EFFICACY OF JERYL LYNN STRAIN OF MUMPS VACCINE AMONG PRIMARY SCHOOL CHILDREN,* NORTH CAROLINA, 1966 TO 1967**

STUDY GROUP	NO. OF CASES	NO. AT RISK	ATTACK RATE (%)	VACCINE EFFICACY (%)	95% CONFIDENCE INTERVAL†
Vaccines	5	2965	0.17	96	88–99
Control subjects	13	329	3.95		

*Children were enrolled without serological screening to exclude those who were already immune.
†By the Fisher exact text, two-tailed.

Table 13–6. **PUBLISHED CLINICAL STUDIES OF MUMPS VACCINE EFFICACY**

STUDY POPULATION	VACCINE STRAIN	YEAR	VACCINE EFFICACY (%)	95% CONFIDENCE INTERVAL
Clinical trials				
Philadelphia	J	1965–1967	95	88–98
North Carolina	J	1966–1967	96	88–99
Outbreak studies				
New York	J	1973	79	53–91
Canada	J	1977	75	49–87
Ohio	J	1981	81	71–88
Ohio	J	1982	85	39–94
New Jersey	J	1983	91	77–93
Tennessee	J	1986	78	64–87
Spain	J/U	1987	86	65–95
Kansas	J	1988–1989	83	57–94
Spain	J/U	1990	75	53–86
France	U	1995	76	66–83
Switzerland	J	1994	65	11–86
	U	1994	76	36–91
	R	1994	12	−102–62

J, Jeryl Lynn; R, Rubini; U, Urabe.

immunity as an important factor,[215, 232] several more recent outbreaks in highly vaccinated populations have raised the possibility of waning immunity.[24, 236, 237] Two outbreaks occurred in U.S. high schools in which more than 95% of students were vaccinated. In a Tennessee school, serological data suggested that most of the mumps cases resulted from primary failure of the first dose to produce seroconversion; however, students vaccinated more than 3 years earlier had higher attack rates than those vaccinated more recently, suggesting that waning immunity may also have contributed to the outbreak.[236] In a Texas outbreak, 18% of students developed mumps despite prior vaccination. However, there was no evidence for an increase in attack rate with increased time since vaccination.[237] Thus, it appears that failure to seroconvert after a first vaccination, rather than waning immunity, is the major risk factor for mumps among vaccinated people.

The efficacy of the Urabe strain was studied in an outbreak that occurred in a French community. The focus of the epidemic was a primary school in which the calculated efficacy was 76%.[238]

Data have become available from Switzerland concerning the Rubini strain. Analysis of reported mumps cases, supplemented by serological data, suggested that the strain had little or no efficacy.[239] That stark conclusion was supported by a study conducted in five primary schools in Geneva, in which secondary attack rates were calculated in children exposed in school according to the vaccine they had received. The protective efficacy of Jeryl Lynn vaccine was 65%, of Urabe vaccine 76%, and of the Rubini vaccine only 12%.[240]

An outbreak has been described in a Japanese primary school in which some of the students had been vaccinated with two Japanese attenuated strains: the Urabe strain (as MMR) and the Torii strain.[241] Calculations from the reported data suggest a protection level of 61%. The Leningrad-3 strain was reported to have a vaccine effectiveness of 96.4% when given to children attending 19 daycare centers in a program to control an outbreak of mumps.[199]

The relative contributions of primary vaccine failure and secondary vaccine failure (i.e., waning immunity) remain uncertain, but primary vaccine failure seems to be more important. It seems reasonable to assume that a second dose of MMR vaccine given at school entry for the prevention of measles would result in a further decrease in the proportion of children susceptible to mumps on entering school. In one study, U.S. children who had previously received Jeryl Lynn vaccine as MMR were evaluated before receiving a second dose of MMR at either 4 to 6 or 11 to 13 years of age. As determined by ELISA, 97% of 4- to 6-year-old children and 100% of 11- to 13-year-old children were seropositive for mumps antigen, and 100% of both age groups were seropositive after revaccination.[242]

In the United States, the Advisory Committee on Immunization Practices and the American Academy of Pediatrics have recommended since 1989 that all children receive two doses of measles vaccine.[243] Because measles vaccine is generally given to children in the United States as MMR vaccine, the effect of implementation of this recommendation has been that most children have received two doses of mumps vaccine. Although there is limited information on the effectiveness of a second dose of mumps vaccine, a two-dose schedule of MMR vaccine should protect most people who do not respond to initial vaccination. As this recommendation has been implemented in the United States, reported cases of mumps have decreased dramatically.

Risk Factors for Vaccine Failure

Epidemiological studies of mumps outbreaks have examined potential risk factors for mumps vaccine failure by comparing the characteristics of vaccinated cases and vaccinated control subjects. Several studies demonstrated that use of the measles vaccine before 15 months of age was associated with vaccine failure during the 1980s, when most mothers had immunity resulting from prior infection with measles rather than vaccination.[244]

In contrast, mumps vaccination at 12 to 14 months of age has not been associated with mumps vaccine failure.[24, 215, 232, 236, 237, 245] One study conducted in 9-month-old children showed a decreased rate of seroconversion.[210] Two studies have shown a trend toward a lower attack rates among children who have received two doses of mumps vaccine as opposed to those who have received one dose, but in both instances the findings did not reach statistical significance.[24, 237] The type of mumps vaccine preparation (i.e., monovalent vs. MMR) has not been found to affect the risk of vaccine failure.[215, 232, 236, 237, 245] Studies have not shown clear evidence of increased risk with increasing number of years since vaccination (i.e., waning immunity), but such studies have been hampered by an inability to measure the independent effect of this potential risk factor. Reinfection likely resulted in boosting of immunity in vaccinees when mumps incidence was high. With near elimination of mumps in several countries that have achieved high levels of vaccination coverage with two doses of MMR, boosting probably no longer plays a role in maintaining immunity. Further surveillance for mumps in highly vaccinated populations will be required to determine the importance (if any) of boosting in maintaining mumps immunity.

Transmission of Vaccine Virus

In the Philadelphia prelicensure immunogenicity study, none of the 365 children who were classroom or household contacts of the vaccinated children developed mumps vaccine virus infection.[17] This conclusion was based on an analysis of paired serum specimens that documented the absence of contact transmission of the virus. Other studies have shown that recipients of the Jeryl Lynn strain of mumps virus vaccine do not spread this virus to susceptible contacts and that the vaccine virus cannot be isolated from blood, urine, or saliva.[135, 192] However, dissemination of vaccine virus within the body must occur in at least some vaccine recipients. Yamauchi and colleagues isolated mumps virus from placental tissues of two of three seronegative women who were administered the vaccine 7 to 10 days before planned abortions.[135] One study demonstrated transmission of the Urabe strain to a sibling from a child who developed parotitis after vaccination.[246]

Possibility of Herd Immunity

Mathematical models of the potential impact of mass vaccination on the incidence of mumps disease predict that an 85 to 90% level of vaccination coverage by 2 years of age would be required to eliminate the transmission of the mumps virus in western Europe or the United States.[169] High levels of vaccine coverage with two doses of MMR in Sweden and Finland have resulted in dramatic reductions in disease incidence (see later). By 1996, 91% of 19- to 35-month-old children in the United States had received at least one dose of measles-containing vaccine (almost all of which is administered as MMR), and many children had received two doses of MMR. The number of mumps cases was at an all-time low, with only 751 cases reported.[247, 248]

Simultaneous Administration with Other Vaccines

Simultaneous administration of mumps vaccine as MMR with diphtheria and tetanus toxoids and whole-cell pertussis vaccine, with diphtheria and tetanus toxoids and acellular pertussis vaccine, or with oral poliovirus vaccine, *Haemophilus influenzae* type b conjugate vaccine, or hepatitis B vaccine does not impair antibody responses or increase rates of serious adverse events.[249–253] Simultaneous administration of varicella vaccine either in combination with separate measles, mumps, and rubella vaccines or with MMR vaccine but in separate sites has been shown to be safe and immunogenic.[254–257]

Adverse Events

The most common adverse reactions to mumps vaccination are parotitis and low-grade fever. Vaccine-associated parotitis occurs most commonly 10 to 14 days after vaccination.[258] Rash, pruritus, and purpura have been reported after mumps vaccination but are uncommon and usually mild and transient. In one study of Jeryl Lynn and Urabe strains, parotid and/or submaxillary swelling was noted in 1.6% of children who received Jeryl Lynn vaccine and in 1 to 2% of children who received Urabe vaccine[205]; in a large study of Urabe vaccine, there was a 0.7% incidence of parotitis.[259] The Hoshino strain vaccine virus has been isolated from vaccine recipients who developed parotitis 14 to 24 days after vaccination.[260]

Assessing complications after mumps vaccination is exacerbated by the fact that most mumps vaccine is given in combination with measles and rubella vaccines. Based on biological plausibility, however, orchitis,[261] arthritis,[262, 263] sensorineural deafness,[264, 265] and acute myositis[266] may rarely follow vaccination. The role of mumps vaccine in reports of diffuse retinopathy,[267] gait disturbances,[268] and thrombocytopenic purpura[269–271] after MMR vaccination is difficult to evaluate.

A search for mumps virus replication in children with symptomatic human immunodeficiency virus (HIV) infection gave negative results.[272] Encephalitis within 30 days after mumps vaccination does not occur more frequently than the background rate of central nervous system dysfunction in the normal population; 0.4 case of encephalitis has been reported in the United States per million doses of live virus mumps vaccine distributed.[175] Febrile seizures following mumps vaccination have rarely been reported.[273]

Aseptic Meningitis

As noted previously, one of the most frequent complications of natural mumps infection is meningitis.[22, 36]

Mumps strains used as attenuated vaccines have lost most of their potential for viremia and therefore for meningitis as a complication of viremia, but this potential has not been lost entirely. The rate of aseptic meningitis that occurs after vaccination ranges widely from approximately 1 in 800,000 for the Jeryl Lynn strain[274] to as high as 1 in 1000 for the Leningrad-3 strain.[275] The incubation period of the illness has generally been between 2 and 3 weeks after vaccination, and the clinical symptoms and signs, including lymphocytic pleocytosis in the cerebrospinal fluid, have been similar to those of the natural disease.[276]

Of course, coincidental meningitis after vaccination may occur due to other viruses and even due to wild mumps virus,[120] and confirmation of the causative role of vaccine virus requires definitive identification of the mumps virus isolate as vaccine strain (see earlier discussion under *Virology*). Because viruses similar or identical in sequence to the vaccine virus previously administered have been isolated from people with postvaccination meningitis,[113, 117, 119] there is no doubt that some vaccine strains can cause meningitis.

Data bearing on meningitis after vaccination are available from six countries: the United States, the United Kingdom, Canada, Germany, Japan, and France. In the United States, meningitis after vaccination with the Jeryl Lynn strain has been a rare event that is perhaps coincidental with vaccination, occurring after only 1 in 1.8 million doses administered, according to passive surveillance.[277] In a large cohort of children 12 to 23 months of age for whom vaccination and hospitalization records were available, for every 100,000 doses administered, 1 child was hospitalized within 30 days of receiving MMR. In a nested case-control study, receipt of MMR within 8 to 14, 14, or 30 days was not demonstrated to be a risk factor for hospitalization for aseptic meningitis, but the number of cases was very small; odds ratios were 1.00 (95% confidence interval, 0.1–9.2), 0.50 (0.1–4.5), and 0.84 (0.2–3.5), respectively.[278] In Germany, the Jeryl Lynn strain was associated with a meningitis rate of 1 in 1 million doses,[258] and isolation of a Jeryl Lynn–like strain was reported from one patient who developed aseptic meningitis after vaccination.[279] Reported rates of postvaccine meningitis for strains used in Japan have been 1 in 120,000, 30,000, 20,000, and 5000 for the Hoshino, Torii, Miyahara, and Chiba strains, respectively (S. Makino, personal communication), but these rates are based on passive surveillance.

The Urabe strain has been linked with aseptic meningtitis wherever adverse reactions have been studied. In Japan, for reasons that are unclear, the rate of meningitis after vaccination with the Urabe strain was reported to be 1 in 2000 doses, and the rate of meningitis with Urabe strain isolated from cerebrospinal fluid was 1 in 9000.[280, 281] In one prefecture, the rate of proven Urabe meningitis was as high as 1 in 900.[281] Data from Japan suggest that all strains labeled Urabe Am9 may not be the same. A prospective study of meningitis after vaccination with Urabe-containing MMR produced by four different manufacturers revealed no cases after administration of one of the vaccines but similar incidence after administration of any of three others.[282] Retrospective data collected by the Ministry of Health also suggested variation between 1 case in 933 vaccinations to 1 case in 18,686 vaccinations. A follow-up study further confused the picture. Urabe vaccine manufactured by Biken gave an incidence of 25 per 10,000 doses administered in one formulation but 0 per 10,000 doses in another formulation. The rates for Urabe vaccines made by Takeda and Kitasato were 14 and 7.4 per 10,000 doses administered, respectively.[283]

In Canada, the observed rate of meningitis after vaccination with Urabe strain was calculated to be 1 in 62,000 doses of the vaccine manufactured by SmithKline Beecham.[284] In Europe, Urabe strain mumps vaccine manufactured by either SmithKline Beecham or Pasteur Mérieux Connaught was used. Estimates by the capture-recapture method[285] and by retrospective passive surveillance[286] of the rate of meningitis in France after administration of the Urabe strain produced by Pasteur Mérieux Connaught elicited a rate of 1 case of meningitis per 28,400 vaccinations; for SmithKline Beecham, the estimated rate was 1 case per 120,000 vaccinations.

In the United Kingdom, a cluster of cases in the Nottingham area prompted an investigation disclosing that the incidence of vaccine-associated mumps meningitis after vaccination with the Urabe strain was higher than had been previously thought.[287] By linking virology laboratory and hospital discharge records with vaccination histories, 1 case of postvaccination meningitis was found per 3800 doses of MMR administered in the Nottingham health district. During this period, 80% of the MMR used in the district contained the Urabe strain, and all cases of meningitis identified followed inoculation with vaccines that contained the Urabe strain.[288] Data for the entire United Kingdom, based on Public Health Laboratory Service surveillance from all sources, suggested a rate of aseptic meningitis estimated at 1 in 11,000 doses of Urabe-containing vaccine (23 cases), compared with no cases after vaccination with Jeryl Lynn–containing vaccine.[289] Convulsions occurred 15 to 35 days after vaccination with Urabe strain vaccine in 1 of 2600 doses.[290] Urabe-containing mumps vaccine accounted for approximately 85% of the total doses of mumps vaccine distributed during the study period, and Jeryl Lynn–containing doses of mumps vaccine accounted for 15%. As a result of these findings, vaccines containing the Urabe strain have been withdrawn from use in several countries.

Brown and coworkers demonstrated that the strain isolated from cases of aseptic meningitis was one of two variants present in the Urabe vaccine.[109] The meningitis-associated variant had a mutation from guanine to adenine at base 1081, which resulted in a glutamine to lysine change in amino acid 335 of the HN protein.

Fortunately, sequelae to postvaccine meningitis have been rare or absent. Unpublished follow-up data from France, Canada, and the United Kingdom have not revealed sequelae clearly attributable to the illness, although possible sequelae have been noted in about 3 to 5% of cases.

In conclusion, it appears that many attenuated mumps vaccine strains cause aseptic meningitis, although the rates of this complication vary according to the vaccine strain, the manufacturer, the index of clinical suspicion, and the intensity of surveillance. For Urabe strain vaccine, the variation lies between 1 per 1000 and 1 per 20,000 vaccinations. However, in evaluating the importance of this complication, one has to consider the incidence of meningitis that would occur in natural mumps (variously reported as between 1 and 50%, but a conservative estimate would be 1 in 400 cases)[291] and the possible differences in immunogenicity between strains. Nokes and Anderson have argued that if the Urabe strain is more immunogenic than the Jeryl Lynn strain, the risk-benefit ratio would be in favor of the former strain when vaccination coverage is low and mumps virus continues to circulate in the population.[292] Different countries have made different judgments regarding the use of Jeryl Lynn or Urabe strain vaccines for the prevention of mumps.[293]

Indications for Vaccination

In the United States, the Advisory Committee on Immunization Practices has recommended two doses of MMR vaccine for all children and certain high-risk groups of adolescents and adults. The first dose of MMR vaccine should be administered to all children at age 12 to 15 months, and the second dose administered routinely at age 4 to 6 years. Certain adults who may be at increased risk for exposure to and transmission of mumps should receive special consideration for vaccination. These people include international travelers, people attending colleges and other higher educational institutions, and people who work at healthcare facilities.[294]

In general, people can be considered immune to mumps who (1) have documentation of vaccination with live mumps virus vaccine on or after their first birthday, (2) have laboratory evidence of mumps immunity, (3) have documentation of physician-diagnosed mumps, or (4) were born before 1957. People born before 1957 in the United States are likely to have been infected naturally between 1957 and 1977 and may be presumed immune even if they have not had clinically recognizable mumps disease. However, birth before 1957 does not guarantee mumps immunity. Therefore, during mumps outbreaks, vaccination with MMR should be considered for people born before 1957 who may be exposed to mumps and who may be susceptible. Laboratory testing for mumps susceptibility before vaccination is not necessary.[294] There is no increased risk of adverse reactions to vaccination of people who are already immune.

Precautions and Contraindications

Because mumps vaccine produced in chick embryo cell culture contains small quantities of ovalbumin, there have been concerns about the risk for serious allergic reactions in people with egg allergy. However, studies have demonstrated that the risk for serious allergic reactions such as anaphylaxis after the administration of mumps vaccine in people allergic to eggs is extremely low and that skin testing with vaccine is not predictive of allergic reaction to vaccination.[295–299] Therefore, skin testing is not required before administering mumps vaccine to these individuals. Similarly, the administration of gradually increasing doses of vaccine is not required.[294]

Data suggest that most anaphylactic reactions to mumps-containing vaccines are associated not with hypersensitivity to egg antigens but to other components of the vaccines. There are several case reports of people with an anaphylactic sensitivity to gelatin who had anaphylactic reactions after receiving MMR vaccine.[300–302] MMR and its component vaccines contain hydrolyzed gelatin as a stabilizer. Therefore, extreme caution should be exercised when administering MMR or its component vaccines to people who have a history of an anaphylactic reaction to gelatin or gelatin-containing products. Skin testing for sensitivity to gelatin could be considered, but no specific protocols for this purpose have been published.[294] Likewise, people who have a history of anaphylactic reactions to neomycin should not receive the vaccine; a history of contact dermatitis to neomycin is not a contraindication to vaccination. Mumps vaccine does not contain penicillin.

Mumps vaccine should be given at least 2 weeks before the administation of immune globulin or deferred until 3 months after such administration, because passively acquired antibody can interfere with response to the vaccine.

The live virus mumps vaccine should not be given to pregnant women because of the theoretical risk of fetal damage; there is no evidence, however, that the vaccine can cause congenital malformations in humans. Vaccinated women should avoid pregnancy for 3 months after vaccination.

People with severe febrile illnesses should in general not be vaccinated until they have recovered. Vaccination should not be postponed because of minor illness.

Live virus mumps vaccine should not be given to people with acquired immunodeficiency disease or suppressed immunity due to other causes (e.g., leukemia, lymphoma, generalized malignancy, or therapy with corticosteroids, alkylating drugs, antimetabolites, or radiation). An exception is children infected with HIV. MMR vaccination is recommended for all asymptomatic HIV-infected people who do not have evidence of severe immunosuppression and for whom measles vaccination would otherwise be indicated. MMR vaccination should also be considered for all asymptomatic HIV-infected people who do not have evidence of severe immunosuppression. Because the immunological response to vaccines may decrease as HIV disease progresses, HIV-infected infants without severe immunosuppression should routinely receive MMR at age 12 months. Consideration should be given to administering the second dose of MMR vaccine as soon as 1 month after the first dose.[294] Patients with leukemia in remission who have not received chemotherapy in at least 3 months may receive live virus mumps vaccine, as may people who have received short-term (i.e., less than 2 weeks' duration) steroid therapy.[294]

PUBLIC HEALTH CONSIDERATIONS

Epidemiological Effects of Vaccination—United States

Live attenuated mumps vaccine was licensed in the United States in 1967. Since that time, the incidence of mumps in this country has decreased dramatically. However, outbreaks of mumps in the 1980s raised new questions about vaccine efficacy and the duration of immunity (see under *Effectiveness in Field Use and Duration of Immunity*).

Following the licensure of the live virus mumps vaccine in 1967, reported cases of mumps decreased from more than 185,000 in 1967 to 2982 by 1985, a decrease of more than 98% (see Fig. 13–2). In 1986 and 1987, however, a relative resurgence of mumps occurred, with 7790 cases reported in 1986 and 12,848 in 1987. Outbreaks were reported in high schools,[215] in colleges,[24, 303] and in the workplace among young adults.[304] After 1989, the number of reported cases began to decrease again and by 1996 reached a new low of 751 (see Fig. 13–2).

During the prevaccine era, mumps was classically a disease of children 5 to 9 years of age. From 1986 to 1991, however, the highest age-specific incidence was reported for children 10 to 14 years of age.[305–307] From the beginning of the vaccine era, the average age of people with mumps infection gradually increased, resulting in an increasing proportion of cases reported among people 15 years and older. From 1967 to 1971, only 8% of reported cases were among this age group, compared with more than one third from 1987 to 1992 (Fig. 13–4).[306, 307] This shift in reported cases of mumps from school-aged children to adolescents and young adults was an expected result of the implementation of immunization programs, which historically were directed at preschool-aged children and led to widespread interruption of mumps virus transmission; a similar shift was previously observed for measles and rubella.

Several lines of evidence suggest that the increase in reported mumps was primarily the result of failure to vaccinate susceptible people and only secondarily the result of vaccine failures.[308] National immunization policy in the United States historically was slow to endorse mumps vaccine as a routine immunization of childhood. Thus, a decade elapsed between licensure of the vaccine in 1967 and the recommendation at the end of 1977 that it be given routinely to all children. The sluggish pattern of distribution of mumps vaccine during this decade documented that the vaccine only gradually came into widespread use. However, during the decade after licensure of mumps vaccine, the incidence of reported mumps declined markedly. Presumably, this decline was a result of the incremental uptake of sufficient mumps vaccine in the U.S. population to interrupt substantially the transmission of the mumps virus. Data from secondary attack rate studies and mathematical models show that clinical mumps is substantially less communicable than measles, leading to reductions in the transmission of mumps at immunization levels that would have only a minimal impact on measles transmission.[18, 309] Consequently, a cohort of children born between about 1967 and 1977 (i.e., people between 10 and 20 years of age in 1987) grew up when the chance of exposure to wild mumps virus for a preschool-aged or young school-aged child was markedly declining while the opportunity to receive mumps vaccine was uncertain.

In short, the gradual adoption of mumps vaccination during the decade after its licensure resulted in a relatively underimmunized cohort of children born between 1967 and 1977, a period when the risk of exposure to mumps was rapidly declining. The greater mobility of older chldren and adolescents increased the potential for contact among susceptible people in these age groups, which led to mumps outbreaks when mumps disease was introduced into these populations.

At the same time, there was a gradual movement toward the routine use of mumps vaccine in children born since 1977. Although the increasing use of MMR vaccine and the enactment of mumps immunization school laws by 26 states between 1977 and 1986 led to higher levels of mumps immunization in U.S. children, the timing of these events varied among state immuniza-

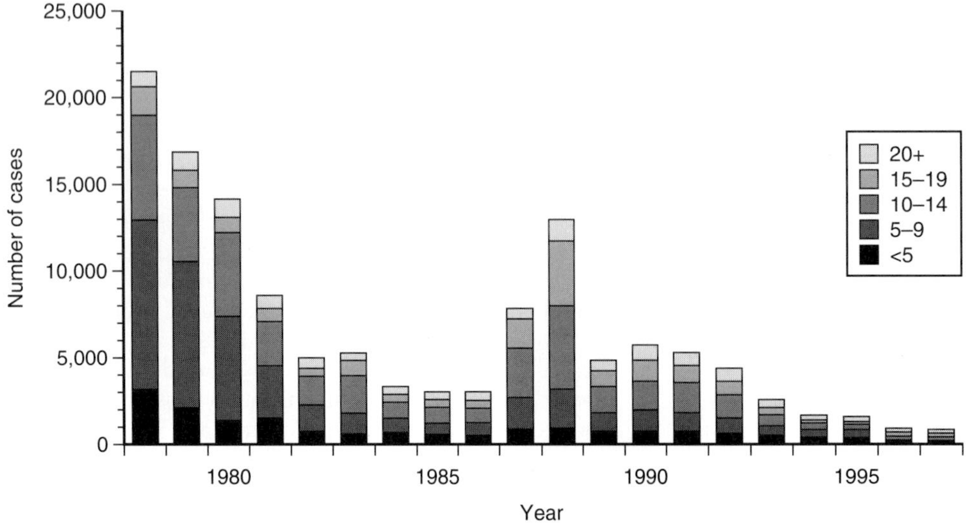

Figure 13–4. Reported cases of mumps by age group, United States, 1977 to 1996. In each year, the age distribution of cases of known age has been applied to the cases of unknown age. (From National Notifiable Diseases Surveillance System, Centers for Disease Control and Prevention, Atlanta, GA, 1997.)

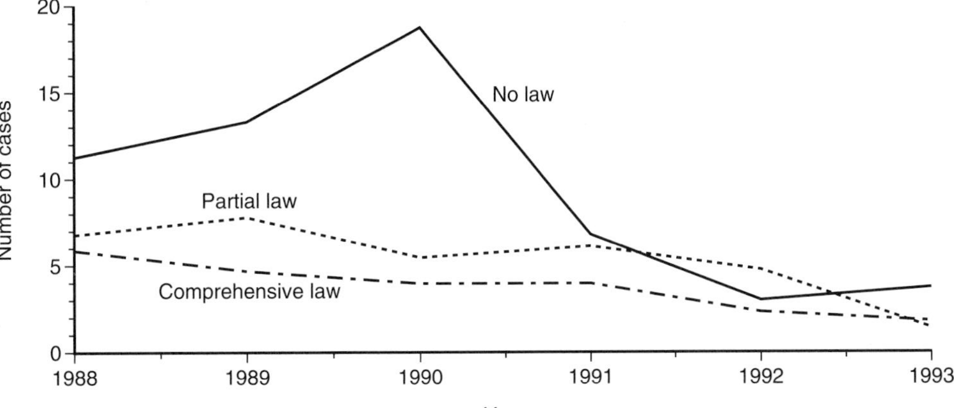

Figure 13–5. Reported incidence of mumps for people 5 to 19 years of age by type of state immunization requirement, United States, 1988 to 1993. (From van Loon FPL, Holmes SJ, Sirotkin BI, et al. Mumps surveillance—United States, 1988–1993. MMWR CDC Surveill Summ 44:1–14, 1995.)

tion programs and the many private providers of vaccine. The gradual implementation of these changes likely resulted in isolated pockets of susceptible, unvaccinated children.

Immunization policy influenced not only the age groups affected but also the areas where outbreaks have occurred. During the relative resurgence of mumps that began in 1986, large outbreaks were generally confined to states that did not have comprehensive (i.e., kindergarten through grade 12) requirements for mumps vaccination for school attendance. In 1986, the reported incidence of mumps in 15 states without any requirement for mumps vaccination was 14-fold higher than that observed in states that had a comprehensive requirement. The incidence in states with requirements that affected only some students (e.g., a requirement that applied only to children first entering school) was more than twice as high as that observed in states with comprehensive laws.[308] More recent data demonstrate that as mumps incidence has decreased nationally, differences in incidences between states with and without comprehensive school vaccination laws have been less striking (Fig. 13–5).[307]

School laws regarding mumps vaccination have consistently been shown to be effective in decreasing the incidence of mumps.[25, 229, 308] The occurrence of a cluster of outbreaks of mumps on university campuses from 1986 to 1987 underscored the need for preadmission immunization requirements that include inoculation with mumps vaccine.[23]

The dramatic reduction in reported cases of mumps in the United States since 1991 reflects increasing implementation of school immunization laws requiring two doses of MMR. In 1998, the Advisory Committee on Immunization Practices recommended that all states take immediate steps to implement the two-dose MMR schedule so that by the year 2001 all children in kindergarten through grade 12 will have received two doses of MMR.[294] This protocol should result in further decreases in mumps among school-aged children. However, with disease now at an all-time record low in the United States, national surveillance data will be inadequate for documenting further decreases without improved case investigation and increased use of laboratory testing for confirmation of mumps.

From 1975 to 1984, there was approximately 1 death from mumps per 5000 reported cases and 1 case of mumps encephalitis per 500 reported cases (Fig. 13–6). Since 1984, these proportions have been more variable owing to smaller numbers of reported events, and since 1995, mumps encephalitis has not been a reportable disease in the United States.[310] Because of underre-

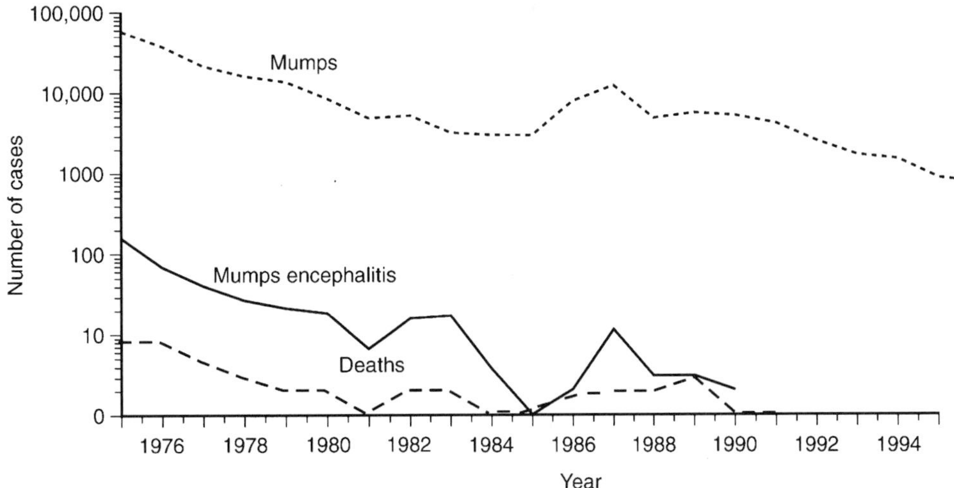

Figure 13–6. Reported cases of mumps and mumps encephalitis and deaths from mumps, United States, 1975 to 1995. There were no deaths due to mumps from 1985 to 1986 and from 1992 to 1995; mortality data for 1996 are not yet available. No cases of mumps encephalitis were reported in 1991 and 1993; beginning in 1995, mumps encephalitis was no longer nationally notifiable.

porting of both mumps and mumps encephalitis, these figures probably overestimate the risk of mortality and underestimate the rate of mumps encephalitis. Indeed, before the introduction of mumps vaccination, mumps was the most commonly diagnosed cause of encephalitis in childhood; introduction of routine vaccination has resulted in the virtual elimination of mumps encephalitis in some areas.[311, 312]

Previous cost-benefit analyses have shown that $7 to 14 are saved for every dollar spent on a program of vaccination with either mumps or MMR vaccine.[313, 314] A more recent analysis found cost-benefit ratios of 6.1 (direct costs only) and 13.0 (direct and indirect costs) for use of monovalent mumps vaccine and 16.3 (direct costs only) and 21.3 (direct and indirect costs) for MMR vaccine (Centers for Disease Control and Prevention, unpublished data).

Epidemiological Effects of Vaccination—Countries Other Than the United States

Compulsory immunization with mumps vaccine was introduced in Croatia in 1976, and a greater than 90% reduction in morbidity was reported by 1978.[179]

In Finland, a two-dose schedule of vaccination with MMR was introduced in November 1982, with a first dose occurring at 14 to 18 months of age and the second at 6 years of age. During the first 2½ years of the vaccination program, 81% of targeted children had been vaccinated, with a resulting 87% decrease in the incidence of mumps.[315] By 1986, more than 95% of eligible children had been vaccinated.[316] In 1989, Koskiniemi and Vaheri reported that no cases of mumps encephalitis had been seen at Helsinki Children's Hospital, the pediatric referral hospital for southern Finland, since the introduction of the vaccination program.[312]

The Finnish program has had spectacular success. By 1994, Peltola and colleagues noted that there were fewer than 30 cases of laboratory-confirmed mumps reported each year and that these were probably imported.[317] The incidence of new cases of type 1 (insulin-dependent) diabetes, which had been rising in Finland, has plateaued since 1990 and has been accompanied by a decrease in mumps antibodies in diabetic children.[318] Whether the relationship is causal remains to be seen, but in any case the overall success of the Finnish program, achieved by the routine two-dose schedule of MMR vaccination, serves as a model for other countries that wish to eradicate measles, rubella, and mumps.[319]

In Sweden, a two-dose vaccination schedule with MMR at 18 months and 12 years of age was introduced in 1982, with approximately 90% coverage for each of the two doses. Before the second dose, according to one study, 27% of prior vaccinees had lost mumps antibodies, but the booster seroconverted all but 7%.[320] Although mumps vaccine was licensed in Sweden in the 1970s, the vaccine was not widely used until 1982. Subsequently, dramatic decreases in reported morbidity for all three diseases were observed.[321] Serological screening demonstrated an increase in the proportion of 12-year-old children who tested seronegative to mumps virus, from 13% in 1985 to 39% in 1989. This trend suggests a decrease in naturally acquired immunity after the introduction of widespread vaccination, thus providing another reason for a two-dose schedule.[322]

Routine vaccination with MMR at 12 to 15 months of age was introduced in England and Wales in 1988. Preschool-aged children were also offered MMR in a 3-year catch-up program, and in some districts, catch-up vaccination was extended to children up to 10 years of age. Vaccination coverage reached 91% of 24-month-old children by 1996.[323] The impact of vaccination on disease incidence was prompt, as reflected in notified cases, which decreased 79% from 1989 to 1990.[324] Based on reports from sentinel surveillance, the annual incidence decreased from 160 per 100,000 population in 1989 to 17 per 100,000 in 1995, with the most dramatic decrease occurring among children 0 to 14 years of age. Since November 1994, salivary mumps IgM antibody testing has been offered for confirmation of clinically diagnosed mumps cases, and 46% of 2868 notified people have been tested. Mumps IgM antibody was detected in only 40 (3%) of these specimens, one of which was obtained from a person who had been recently vaccinated. Serological surveillance demonstrated an increase in seronegativity among people 9 to 20 years of age, reflecting a decreased circulation of mumps virus. With the introduction of a routine second dose of MMR at 4 years of age, further reductions in incidence of mumps are expected.[141]

In January 1989, Israel incorporated mumps and rubella vaccine with measles vaccine into the routine immunization schedule at 15 months of age. The incidence of mumps dropped from 11.6 to 0.6 per 10,000 between the prevaccine era and 1991.[325] A cost-benefit analysis suggested that such a vaccination program was cost saving.[326]

Mumps has been nearly eradicated from Cuba since 1988, when that country embarked on an accelerated MMR vaccination program of preschool-aged children and achieved coverage levels greater than 95%.[327]

A contrasting experience has been reported from Switzerland. The Jeryl Lynn strain mumps vaccine (as MMR) first became available in Switzerland in 1971, and MMR vaccine including Urabe strain was introduced in 1983. Routine vaccination of children at 15 to 24 months of age was recommended by Swiss public health authorities in 1985. MMR containing the Rubini mumps vaccine became available in 1986 and subsequently accounted for more than half the doses of MMR vaccine used in the country. Reports from a sentinel network of physicians demonstrated an increase in reported cases of mumps beginning in 1991. Increases in mumps cases were seen among all age groups but were most striking among children 5 to 9 years of age. Based on information from the sentinel network and manufacturer-specific coverage estimates, the effectiveness of the Rubini vaccine among children 1 to 19 years of age from 1991 to 1993 was estimated at 13 to 73%, compared with 69 to 92% for Jeryl Lynn and Urabe vaccines.[328] By 1993 to 1994, 59% of reported cases were noted to occur in children previously vaccinated, compared with only 9% from 1986 to 1987.[329] A 1991 to 1992 seroprevalence survey suggested that mumps immunity in young children was lagging behind that for measles and rubella, perhaps reflecting the relatively poor immunogenicity of the Rubini strain vaccine.[330]

In Portugal, routine vaccination with MMR at 15 months of age was begun in 1987. In 1990, a second dose of MMR was recommended at 11 to 13 years of age. Reported cases of mumps decreased from 2197 in 1987 to 627 in 1993. In 1994, however, reported cases increased to 1445 and continued to increase from 1995 to 1996. The outbreak accelerated dramatically in early 1996; during the first 8 months of 1996, 7620 cases were reported. Although incidence increased among all age groups, incidence rates were highest among children 1 to 4 years of age. This finding was unexpected because reported MMR vaccination coverage among children 12 to 23 months of age had exceeded 90% since 1991. In 1987, three different mumps vaccines—Urabe, Rubini, and Jeryl Lynn strains—were initially available in Portugal as MMR. Following recognition of aseptic meningitis after vaccination with Urabe mumps vaccine, the sale of Urabe-containing vaccine was suspended in Portugal in October 1992, and subsequently only Rubini-containing MMR was used.[331] Substitution of Rubini for Urabe vaccine was followed by a mumps epidemic.[331]

Disease Control Strategies and Possible Eradication

One issue worthy of note is the experience with aseptic meningitis after vaccination with several strains of mumps vaccine. This event underscores the importance of careful postlicensure monitoring of vaccine safety to detect other uncommon events that may be causally related to vaccination with any new mumps vaccines that are distributed on a wide scale.

A second critical issue for further study concerns the extent and duration of protection conferred by a single dose of mumps vaccine. Widespread use of the live virus mumps vaccine since its licensure in 1967 has resulted in a marked decrease in the incidence of mumps in the United States. However, the outbreaks reported from 1986 to 1991 illustrate both the potential for continued epidemics in susceptible unvaccinated populations and the importance of vaccine failure. The question of whether vaccine failure is due to low seroconversion or to waning immunity remains unresolved, but both elements appear to play a role.

A two-dose MMR vaccination schedule was adopted in Sweden[332] and and Finland[312] in 1982 with the aim of eradicating measles, mumps, and rubella within a decade. Likewise, the two-dose schedule in the United States has reduced reported cases of mumps to a record low. These programs have had a marked impact on the incidence of all three diseases, suggesting that the goal of eradication may be feasible if high immunization coverage levels with two doses of MMR can be achieved.

In 1991, the International Task Force for Disease Eradication concluded that mumps is potentially eradicable through the use of MMR vaccine but that more data are needed to document the impact of mumps and the use of the vaccine in developing countries.[333] With national and regional measles elimination efforts now under way in the Americas and Europe,[334] programs may be established that could lead to elimination and ultimately eradication of measles, mumps, and rubella if MMR vaccine is used. In the absence of such an effort, it remains to be seen whether the benefits of mumps vaccination are of sufficient value globally to incorporate mumps vaccine into the routine childhood vaccination schedule of the Expanded Program of Immunization of the World Health Organization.

REFERENCES

1. Hamilton R. An account of a distemper by the common people of England vulgarly called the mumps. London Med J 11:190–211, 1790.
2. Gordon JE. The epidemiology of mumps. Am J Med Sci 200:412–428, 1940.
3. Gordon JE, Kilham L. Ten years in the epidemiology of mumps. Am J Med Sci 218:338–359, 1949.
4. Stokes J. Mumps. In Preventive Medicine in World War II. Vol. IV. Communicable Diseases Transmitted Chiefly Through Respiratory and Alimentary Tracts. Prepared by the Historical Unit, US Army Medical Service. Washington, DC, US Government Printing Office, 1958, pp 135–140.
5. Feldman HA. Mumps. In Evans AS (ed). Viral Infections of Humans: Epidemiology and Control (3rd ed). New York, Plenum Medical Books, 1990, pp 471–491.
6. Parran T. Health and medical preparedness. JAMA 115:49–51, 1940.
7. Postovit VA. Epidemic parotitis in adults. Voen Med Zh 3:38–41, 1983.
8. Arday DR, Kanjarpane DD, Kelley PW. Mumps in the U.S. Army, 1980–86: Should recruits be immunized? Am J Public Health 79:471–474, 1989.
9. Kuhlman JC. Mumps outbreak aboard the USS Reuben James. Mil Med 3:255–257, 1994.
10. Johnson CD, Goodpasture EW. An investigation of the etiology of mumps. J Exp Med 59:1–19, 1934.
11. Johnson CD, Goodpasture EW. The etiology of mumps. Am J Hyg 21:46–57, 1935.
12. Habel K. Cultivation of mumps virus in the developing chick embryo and its application to studies of immunity to mumps in man. Public Health Rep 60:201–212, 1945.
13. Enders JF. Mumps: Techniques of laboratory diagnosis, tests for susceptibility, and experiments on specific prophylaxis. J Pediatr 29:129–142, 1946.
14. Habel K. Preparation of mumps vaccine and immunization of monkeys against experimental mumps infection. Public Health Rep 61:1655–1664, 1946.
15. Habel K. Vaccination of human beings against mumps; vaccine administered at the start of an epidemic. I. Incidence and severity of mumps in vaccinated and control groups. Am J Hyg 54:295–311, 1951.
16. Smorodintsev AA, Luzianina TY, Mikutskaya BA. Data on the efficiency of live mumps vaccine from chick embryo cell cultures. Acta Virol 9:240–247, 1965.
17. Weibel RE, Stokes J, Buynak EB, et al. Live attenuated mumps virus vaccine. 3. Clinical and serologic aspects in a field evaluation. N Engl J Med 276:245–251, 1967.
18. Hope-Simpson RE. Infectiousness of communicable diseases in the household (measles, chickenpox, and mumps). Lancet 2:549–554, 1952.
19. Falk WA, Buchan K, Dow M, et al. The epidemiology of mumps in southern Alberta, 1980–1982. Am J Epidemiol 130:736–749, 1989.
20. Cooney MK, Fox JP, Hall CE. The Seattle Virus Watch. VI. Observations of infections with and illness due to parainfluenza,

mumps and respiratory syncytial viruses and *Mycoplasma pneumoniae*. Am J Epidemiol 101:532–551, 1975.
21. Foy HM, Cooney KM, Hall CE, et al. Isolation of mumps virus from children with acute lower respiratory tract disease. Am J Epidemiol 94:467–472, 1971.
22. Philip RN, Reinhard KR, Lackman DB. Observations on a mumps epidemic in a virgin population. Am J Hyg 69:91–111, 1959.
23. Mumps outbreaks on university campuses—Illinois, Wisconsin, South Dakota. MMWR Morb Mortal Wkly Rep 36:496–498, 503–505, 1987.
24. Hersh BS, Fine PEM, Kent WK, et al. Mumps outbreak in a highly vaccinated population. J Pediatr 119:187–193, 1991.
25. Mumps Surveillance, January 1977–December 1982. Atlanta, GA, US Department of Health and Human Services, US Public Health Service, 1984.
26. McGuinness AC, Gall EA. Mumps at army camps in 1943. War Med 5:95–104, 1944.
27. Werner CA. Mumps orchitis and testicular atrophy. I. Occurrence. Ann Intern Med 32:1066–1074, 1950.
28. Werner CA. Mumps orchitis and testicular atrophy. II. A factor in male sterility. Ann Intern Med 32:1075–1086, 1950.
29. Beard CM, Benson RC, Kelalis PP, et al. The incidence and outcome of mumps orchitis in Rochester, Minnesota, 1935 to 1974. Mayo Clin Proc 52:3–7, 1977.
30. Swerdlow AJ, Huttly SRA, Smith PG. Testicular cancer and antecedent diseases. Br J Cancer 55:97–103, 1987.
31. Brown LM, Pottern LM, Hoover RN. Testicular cancer in young men: The search for causes of the epidemic increase in the United States. J Epidemiol Community Health 41:349–354, 1987.
32. Dacou-Voutekis C, Constantinidis M, Moschos A, et al. Diabetes mellitus following mumps. Am J Dis Child 127:890–891, 1974.
33. Sultz HA, Hart BA, Zielezny M. Is mumps virus an etiologic factor in juvenile diabetes mellitus? J Pediatr 86:654–656, 1975.
34. Otten A, Helmke K, Stieff T, et al. Mumps, mumps vaccination, islet cell antibodies and the first manifestation of diabetes mellitus type I. Behring Inst Mitt 75:83–88, 1984.
35. Hyöty H, Leinikki P, Reunanen A, et al. Mumps infections in the etiology of type 1 (insulin-dependent) diabetes. Diabetes Res 9:111–116, 1988.
36. Reed D, Brown G, Merrick R, et al. A mumps epidemic on St. George Island, Alaska. JAMA 199:113–117, 1967.
37. Russell RR, Donald JC. The neurological complications of mumps. BMJ 2:27–30, 1958.
38. Levitt LP, Rich TA, Kinde SW, et al. Central nervous system mumps: A review of 64 cases. Neurology 20:829–834, 1970.
39. Miller HG, Stanton JB, Gibbons JL. Para-infectious encephalomyelitis and related syndromes. Q J Med 25:427–505, 1956.
40. Cohen HA, Ashkenazi A, Nussinovitch M, et al. Mumps-associated acute cerebellar ataxia. Am J Dis Child 146:930–931, 1992.
41. Miller HG, Stanton JB, Gibbons JL. Para-infectious encephalomyelitis and related syndromes. Q J Med 25:427–505, 1956.
42. Timmons GD, Johnson KP. Aqueductal stenosis and hydrocephalus after mumps encephalitis. N Engl J Med 283:1505–1507, 1970.
43. Bray PF. Mumps—a cause of hydrocephalus? Pediatrics 49:446–449, 1972.
44. Challapalli M, Varnado SC, Cunningham DG. Fever, abdominal pain and an intracranial mass. Pediatr Infect Dis J 14:725–726, 1995.
45. Lahat E, Aladjem M, Schiffer J, Starinsky R. Hydrocephalus due to bilateral obstruction of the foramen of Monro: A possible late complication of mumps encephalitis. Clin Neurol Neurosurg 95:151–154, 1993.
46. Oldfelt V. Sequelae of mumps-meningoencephalitis. Acta Med Scand 134:405–414, 1949.
47. Oran B, Çeri A, Yilmaz H, et al. Hydrocephalus in mumps meningoencephalitis: Case report. Pediatr Infect Dis J 14:724–725, 1995.
48. Azimi PH, Cramblett HG, Haynes RE. Mumps meningoencephalitis in children. JAMA 207:509–512, 1969.
49. Bang HO, Bang J. Involvement of the central nervous system in mumps. Acta Med Scand 113:487–505, 1943.
50. Julkunen I, Lehtokoski-Lehtiniemi E, Koshiniemi M, Vaheri A. Elevated mumps antibody titers in the cerebrospinal fluid suggesting chronic mumps virus infection in the central nervous system. Pediatr Infect Dis J 4:99, 1985.
51. Ito M, Go T, Okuno T, Mikawa H. Chronic mumps virus encephalitis. Pediatr Neurol 7:467–470, 1991.
52. Julkunen I, Koskiniemi M, Lehtokoski-Lehtiniemi E, et al. Chronic mumps virus encephalitis: Mumps antibody levels in cerebrospinal fluid. J Neuroimmunol 8:167–175, 1985.
53. Hall R, Richards H. Hearing loss due to mumps. Arch Dis Child 62:189–191, 1987.
54. Vuori M, Lahikainen EA, Peltonen T. Perceptive deafness in connection with mumps: A study of 298 servicemen suffering with mumps. Acta Otolaryngol 55:213–236, 1962.
55. Okamoto M, Shitara T, Nakayama M, et al. Sudden deafness accompanied by asymptomatic mumps. Acta Otolaryngol (Stockh) 514(suppl):45–48, 1994.
56. Westmore GA, Pickard BH, Stern H. Isolation of mumps virus from the inner ear after sudden deafness. BMJ 1:14–15, 1979.
57. Prinz W, Taubert HD. Mumps in pubescent females and its effect on later reproductive function. Gynaecologia 167:23–27, 1968.
58. Utz JP, Houk VN, Alling DW. Clinical and laboratory studies of mumps. IV. Viruria and abnormal renal function. N Engl J Med 270:1283–1286, 1964.
59. Lin CY, Chen WP, Chiang H. Mumps associated with nephritis. Child Nephrol Urol 10:68–71, 1990.
60. Ozen S, Damarguc I, Besbas N, et al. A case of mumps associated with acute hemolytic crisis resulting in hemoglobinuria and acute renal failure. J Med 25:255–259, 1994.
61. Gordon SC, Lauter CB. Mumps arthritis: A review of the literature. Rev Infect Dis 6:338–344, 1984.
62. Harel L, Amir J, Reish O, et al. Mumps arthritis in children. Pediatr Infect Dis J 9:928–929, 1990.
63. Huppertz HI, Chantler JK. Restricted mumps virus infection of cells derived from normal human joint tissue. J Gen Virol 72:339–347, 1991.
64. Huppertz HI, Niki NPH, Chantler JK. Susceptibility of normal human joint tissue to viruses. J Rheumatol 18:699–704, 1991.
65. Rosenberg DH. Electrocardiographic changes in epidemic parotitis (mumps). Proc Soc Exp Biol Med 58:9–11, 1945.
66. Roberts WC, Fox SM. Mumps of the heart: Clinical and pathologic features. Circulation 32:342–345, 1965.
67. Chaudary S, Jaski BE. Fulminant mumps myocarditis. Ann Intern Med 110:569–570, 1989.
68. Arita M, Ueno Y, Masuyama Y. Complete heart block in mumps myocarditis. Br Heart J 46:342–344, 1981.
69. Noren GR, Adams P, Anderson RC. Positive skin test reactivity to mumps virus antigen in endocardial fibroelastosis. J Pediatr 62:604–606, 1963.
70. Ni J, Bowles NE, Young-Hwue K, et al. Viral infection of the myocardium in endocardial fibroelastosis. Molecular evidence for the role of mumps virus as an etiologic agent. Circulation 95:133–139, 1997.
71. Leff RL, Love LA, Miller FW, et al. Viruses in idiopathic inflammatory myopathies: Absence of candidate viral genomes in muscle. Lancet 339:1192–1195, 1992.
72. Nishino H, Engel AG, Rima BK. Inclusion body myositis: The mumps virus hypothesis. Ann Neurol 25:260–264, 1989.
73. Fox SA, Ward BK, Robbins PD, et al. Inclusion body myositis: investigation of the mumps virus hypothesis by polymerase chain reaction. Muscle Nerve 19:23–28, 1996.
74. Siegel MS, Fuerst HT, Peress NS. Comparative fetal mortality in maternal virus diseases: A prospective study on rubella, measles, mumps, chicken pox, and hepatitis. N Engl J Med 274:768–771, 1966.
75. Siegel MS. Congenital malformations following chickenpox, measles, mumps and hepatitis: Results of a cohort study. JAMA 226:1521–1524, 1973.
76. Kurtz JB, Tomlinson AH, Pearson J. Mumps virus isolated from a fetus. BMJ 284:471, 1982.
77. Jones JF, Ray CG, Fulginiti VA. Perinatal mumps infection. J Pediatr 96:912–914, 1980.
78. Sterner G, Grandien M. Mumps in pregnancy at term. Scand J Infect Dis 71(suppl):36–38, 1990.
79. Groenendall F, Rothbarth PH, van den Anker JN, Spritzer R. Congenital mumps pneumonia: A rare cause of neonatal respiratory distress. Acta Pediatr Scand 79:1252–1254, 1990.

80. Lacour M, Maherzi M, Vienny H, Suter S. Thrombocytopenia in a case of neonatal mumps infection: Evidence for further clinical presentations. Eur J Pediatr 152:739–741, 1993.
81. Reman O, Freymuth F, Laloum D, Bonte JF. Neonatal respiratory distress due to mumps. Arch Dis Child 61:80–81, 1986.
82. Okazaki K, Tanabayashi K, Takeuchi K, et al. Molecular coding and sequence analysis of the mumps virus gene encoding the L protein and the trailer sequence. Virology 188:926–930, 1992.
83. Elango N, Varsanyi TM, Kövamees J, Norrby E. Molecular cloning and characterization of six genes, determination of gene order and intergenic sequences and leader sequence of mumps virus. J Gen Virol 69:2893–2900, 1988.
84. Elango N, Kövamees J, Varsanyi TM, Norrby E. mRNA sequence and deduced amino acid sequence of the mumps virus small hydrophobic protein gene. J Virol 63:1413–1415, 1989.
85. Takeuchi K, Tanabayashi K, Hishiyama M, Yamada A. The mumps virus SH protein is a membrane protein and not essential for virus growth. Virology 225:156–162, 1996.
86. Elliott GD, Yeo RP, Afzal MA, et al. Strain-variable editing during transcription of the P gene of mumps virus may lead to the generation of non-structural proteins NS1 (V) and NS2. J Gen Virol 71:1555–1560, 1990.
87. Paterson RG, Lamb RA. RNA editing by G-nucleotide insertion in mumps virus P-gene mRNA transcripts. J Virol 64:4137–4145, 1990.
88. Waxham MN, Server AC, Goodman HM, Wolinsky JS. Cloning and sequencing of the mumps virus fusion protein gene. Virology 159:381–388, 1987.
89. Elango N, Varsanyi TM, Kövamees J, Norrby E. The mumps fusion protein mRNA sequence and homology among the Paramyxoviridae proteins. J Gen Virol 70:801–807, 1989.
90. Waxham MN, Aronowski J, Server AC, et al. Sequence determination of the mumps virus HN gene. Virology 164:318–325, 1988.
91. Kövamees J, Norrby E, Elango N. Complete nucleotide sequence of the hemagglutinin-neuraminidase (HN) mRNA of mumps virus and comparison of paramyxovirus HN proteins. Virus Res 12:87–96, 1989.
92. Ukkonen P, Väisänen O, Penttinen K. Enzyme-linked immunosorbent assay for mumps and parainfluenza type 1, immunoglobulin G, and immunoglobulin M antibodies. J Clin Microbiol 11:319–323, 1980.
93. Meurman O, Hänninen P, Krishna RV, Ziegler T. Determination of IgG- and IgM-class antibodies to mumps virus by solid-phase enzyme immunoassay. J Virol Methods 4:249–257, 1982.
94. Örvell C, Rydbeck R, Löve A. Immunological relationships between mumps virus and parainfluenza viruses studied with monoclonal antibodies. J Gen Virol 67:1929–1939, 1986.
95. Elango N. Complete nucleotide sequence of the matrix protein mRNA of mumps virus. Virology 168:426–428, 1989.
96. Elliott GD, Afzal MA, Martin SJ, Rima BK. Nucleotide sequence of the matrix, fusion, and putative SH protein genes of mumps virus and their deduced amino acid sequences. Virus Res 12:61–75, 1989.
97. Elango N. The mumps virus nucleocapsid mRNA sequence and homology among the Paramyxoviridae proteins. Virus Res 12:77–86, 1989.
98. Elango N, Kövamees J, Norrby E. Sequence analysis of the mumps virus mRNA encoding the P protein. Virology 169:62–67, 1989.
99. Merz DC, Wolinsky JS. Biochemical features of mumps virus neuraminidases and their relationship with pathogenicity. Virology 114:218–227, 1981.
100. Wolinsky JS, Waxham MN, Server AC. Protective effects of glycoprotein-specific monoclonal antibodies on the course of experimental mumps virus meningoencephalitis. J Virol 53:727–734, 1985.
101. Löve A, Rydbeck R, Utter G, et al. Monoclonal antibodies against the fusion protein are protective in necrotizing mumps meningoencephalitis. J Virol 58:220–222, 1986.
102. Beveridge WIB, Lind PE. Virus haemagglutination and serological reactions. Aust J Exp Biol Med Sci 24:127–132, 1946.
103. Leprat R, Aymard M. Selective inactivation of hemagglutinin and neuraminidase on mumps virus. Arch Virol 61:273–281, 1979.
104. Yates PJ, Afzal MA, Minor PD. Antigenic and genetic variation of the HN protein of mumps virus strains. J Gen Virol 77:2491–2497, 1996.
105. Server AC, Merz DC, Waxham MN, Wolinsky JS. Differentiation of mumps virus strains with monoclonal antibody to the HN glycoprotein. Infect Immun 35:179–186, 1982.
106. Örvell C. The reactions of monoclonal antibodies with structural proteins of mumps virus. J Immunol 132:2622–2629, 1984.
107. Gut JP, Lablache C, Berh S, Kirn A. Symptomatic mumps virus reinfections. J Med Virol 45:17–23, 1995.
108. Afzal MA, Pickford AR, Forsey T, et al. The Jeryl Lynn vaccine strain of mumps virus is a mixture of two distinct isolates. J Gen Virol 74:917–920, 1993.
109. Brown EB, Dimock K, Wright KE. The Urabe AM9 mumps vaccine is a mixture of viruses differing at amino acid 335 of the hemagglutinin-neuraminidase gene with one form associated with disease. J Infect Dis 174:619–622, 1996.
110. Boriskin YS, Yamada A, Kaptsova TI, et al. Genetic evidence for variant selection in the course of dilute passaging of mumps vaccine virus. Res Virol 143:279–283, 1992.
111. Boriskin YS, Kaptsova TI, Booth JC. Mumps virus variants in heterogeneous mumps vaccine. Lancet 341:318–319, 1993.
112. McCarthy M, Jubelt B, Fay DB, Johnson RT. Comparative studies of five strains of mumps virus in vitro and in neonatal hamsters: Evaluation of growth, cytopathogenicity, and neurovirulence. J Med Virol 5:1–15, 1980.
113. Yamada A, Takeuchi K, Tanabayashi K, et al. Differentiation of the mumps vaccine strains from the wild viruses by the nucleotide sequences of the P gene. Vaccine 8:553–557, 1990.
114. Forsey T, Bentley ML, Minor PD, Begg N. Mumps vaccines and meningitis [letter]. Lancet 340:980, 1992.
115. Saito H, Takahashi Y, Harata S, et al. Isolation and characterization of mumps virus strains in a mumps outbreak with a high incidence of aseptic meningitis. Microbiol Immunol 40:271–275, 1996.
116. Afzal MA, Yates PJ, Minor PD. Nucleotide sequence at position 1081 of the hemagglutinin-neuraminidase gene in the mumps Urabe vaccine strain. J Infect Dis 177:265–266, 1998.
117. Forsey T, Mawn JA, Yates PJ, et al. Differentiation of vaccine and wild mumps viruses using the polymerase chain reaction and dideoxynucleotide sequencing. J Gen Virol 71:987–990, 1990.
118. Cusi MG, Bianchi S, Valassina M, et al. Rapid detection and typing of circulating mumps virus by reverse transcription/polymerase chain reaction. Res Virol 147:227–232, 1996.
119. Brown EG, Furesz J, Dimock K, et al. Nucleotide sequence analysis of Urabe mumps vaccine strain that caused meningitis in vaccine recipients. Vaccine 9:840–842, 1991.
120. Künkel U, Driesel G, Henning U, et al. Differentiation of vaccine and wild mumps viruses by polymerase chain reaction and nucleotide sequencing of the SH gene: Brief report. J Med Virol 45:121–126, 1995.
121. Turner PC, Forsey T, Minor PD. Comparison of the nucleotide sequence of the SH gene and flanking regions of mumps vaccine virus (Urabe strain) grown on different substrates and isolated from vaccinees. J Gen Virol 72:435–437, 1991.
122. Afzal MA, Yates PJ, Forsey T, Minor PD. Use of single-strand conformation polymorphism technique for the initial characterization of virus isolates [letter]. Vaccine 11:1169, 1993.
123. Katayama K, Oya A, Tanabayashi K, et al. Differentiation of mumps vaccine strains from wild viruses by single-strand conformation polymorphism of the P gene. Vaccine 11:621–623, 1993.
124. Yamada A, Takeuchi K, Tanabayashi K, et al. Sequence variation of the P gene among mumps virus strains. Virology 172:374–376, 1989.
125. Yeo RP, Afzal MA, Forsey T, Rima BK. Identification of a new mumps virus lineage by nucleotide sequence analysis of the SH gene of ten different strains. Arch Virol 128:371–377, 1993.
126. Künkel U, Schreier E, Siegl G, Schultz D. Molecular characterization of mumps virus strains circulating during an epidemic in eastern Switzerland 1992/93. Arch Virol 136:433–438, 1994.
127. Ströhle A, Bernasconi C, Germann D. A new mumps virus lineage found in the 1995 mumps outbreak in western Switzerland identified by nucleotide sequence analysis of the SH gene. Arch Virol 141:733–741, 1996.
128. Afzal MA, Buchanan J, Heath AB, Minor PD. Clustering of mumps virus isolates by SH gene sequence only partially reflects geographical origin. Arch Virol 142:227–238, 1997.

129. Örvell C, Kalantari M, Johansson B. Characterization of five conserved genotypes of the mumps virus small hydrophobic (SH) protein gene. J Gen Virol 78:91–95, 1997.
130. Wu L, Bai Z, Rima BK, Afzal MA. Wild type mumps viruses circulating in China establish a new genotype. Vaccine 16:281–285, 1998.
131. Ennis FA, Jackson D. Isolation of virus during the incubation period of mumps infection. J Pediatr 72:536–537, 1968.
132. Meyer MB. An epidemiologic study of mumps: Its spread in schools and families. Am J Hyg 75:259–281, 1962.
133. Brown JW, Kirkland HB, Hein GE. Central nervous system involvement during mumps. Am J Med Sci 215:434–441, 1948.
134. Immunization Practices Advisory Committee. Mumps prevention. MMWR Morb Mortal Wkly Rep 38:392, 397–400, 1989.
135. Yamauchi T, Wilson C, St Geme JW. Transmission of live, attenuated mumps virus to the human placenta. N Engl J Med 290:710–712, 1974.
136. Utz JP. Viruria in man, an update. Prog Med Virol 17:77–90, 1974.
137. Meyer MB, Stifler WC, Joseph JM. Evaluation of mumps vaccine given after exposure to mumps, with special reference to exposed adults. Pediatrics 37:304–315, 1966.
138. Meurman O, Vainionpää, Rossi T, Hänninen P. Viral etiology of parotitis. Scand J Infect Dis 15:145–148, 1983.
139. Gaulin C, DeSerres G. Need for a specific definition of mumps in a highly immunized population. Can Commun Dis Rep 23:14–16, 1997.
140. Manual for the Surveillance of Vaccine-Preventable Diseases. Atlanta, GA, Centers for Disease Control and Prevention, 1997.
141. Gay N, Miller E, Hesketh L, et al. Mumps surveillance in England and Wales supports introduction of two dose vaccination schedule. Commun Dis Rep CDR Rev 7:R21–R26, 1997.
142. Lennette EH, Jensen FW, Guenther RW, Magoffin RL. Serologic responses to para-influenza viruses in patients with mumps virus infection. J Lab Clin Med 61:780–788, 1963.
143. Brunell PA, Brickman A, Steinberg S, Allen E. Parotitis in children who had previously received mumps vaccine. Pediatrics 50:441–444, 1972.
144. Pelosi JW, Besselink LC. Reducing mumps morbidity in Texas. Abstracts of the 30th National Immunization Conference; Washington, DC; April 9–12, 1996.
145. Grillner L, Blomberg J. Hemolysis-in-gel and neutralization tests for determination of antibodies to mumps virus. J Clin Microbiol 4:11–15, 1976.
146. Christenson B, Böttiger M. Methods for screening the naturally acquired and vaccine-induced immunity to the mumps virus. Biologicals 18:213–219, 1990.
147. Ukkonen P, Granström M, Penttinen K. Mumps-specific immunoglobulin M and G antibodies in natural mumps infection as measured by enzyme-linked immunosorbent assay. J Med Virol 8:131–142, 1981.
148. Benito RJ, Larrad L, Lasierra MP, et al. Persistence of specific IgM antibodies after natural mumps infection. J Infect Dis 155:156–157, 1987.
149. Ukkonen P, Granström ML, Räsänen J, et al. Local production of mumps IgG and IgM antibodies in the cerebrospinal fluid of meningitis patients. J Med Virol 8:257–265, 1981.
150. Vandvik B, Nilsen RE, Vartdal F, Norrby E. Mumps meningitis: Specific and nonspecific antibody responses in the central nervous system. Acta Neurol Scand 65:468–487, 1982.
151. Ramsey MEB, Brown DW, Eastcott HR, Begg NT. Saliva antibody testing and vaccination in a mumps outbreak. Commun Dis Rep CDR Review 1:R96–R98, 1991.
152. Perry KR, Brown DWG, Parry JV, et al. Detection of measles, mumps, and rubella antibodies in saliva using antibody capture radioimmunoassay. J Med Virol 40:235–240, 1993.
153. Schluter WW, Reef SE, Dykewicz CA, Jennings CE. Pseudo-outbreak of mumps—Illinois, 1995 [abstract 338]. Abstracts of the 30th National Immunization Conference; Washington, DC; April 9–12, 1996.
154. Afzal MA, Buchanan J, Dias JA, et al. RT-PCR based diagnosis and molecular characterisation of mumps viruses derived from clinical specimens collected during the 1996 mumps outbreak in Portugal. J Med Virol 52:349–353, 1997.
155. Leinikki PO, Shekarchi I, Tzan N, et al. Evaluation of enzyme-linked immunosorbent assay (ELISA) for mumps virus antibodies. Proc Soc Exp Biol Med 160:363–367, 1979.
156. Sakata H, Hishiyama M, Sugiura A. Enzyme-linked immunosorbent assay compared with neutralization test for evaluation of live mumps vaccines. J Clin Microbiol 19:21–25, 1984.
157. Fedová D, Brucková N, Plesnik V, et al. Detection of postvaccination mumps virus antibody by neutralization test, enzyme-linked immunosorbent assay and sensitive hemagglutination inhibition test. J Hyg Epidemiol Microbiol Immunol 31:409–422, 1987.
158. Hishiyama M, Tsurudome M, Ito Y, et al. Complement-mediated neutralization test for determination of mumps vaccine-induced antibody. Vaccine 6:423–427, 1988.
159. Brickman A, Brunell PA. Susceptibility of medical students to mumps: Comparison of serum neutralizing antibody and skin text. Pediatrics 48:447–450, 1972.
160. Collins SD. Age incidence of the common communicable diseases of children. Public Health Rep 44:763–826, 1929.
161. Mumps Surveillance. Report No. 1. Atlanta, GA, US Department of Health, Education, and Welfare, January 1968.
162. Brooks H. Epidemic parotitis as a military disease. Med Clin North Am 2:493–505, 1918.
163. Black FL. A nationwide serum survey of United States military recruits, 1962. III. Measles and mumps antibodies. Am J Hyg 80:304–307, 1964.
164. Kelley PW, Petruccelli BP, Stehr-Green P, et al. The susceptibility of young adult Americans to vaccine-preventable infections: A national serosurvey of U.S. Army recruits. JAMA 266:2724–2729, 1991.
165. Cox MJ, Anderson RM, Bundy DAP, Nokes DJ. Seroepidemiological study of the transmission of the mumps virus in St. Lucia, West Indies. Epidemiol Infect 102:147–160, 1989.
166. Wagenvoort JHT, Harmsen M, Boutahar-Trouw BJK, et al. Epidemiology of mumps in the Netherlands. J Hyg 85:313–326, 1980.
167. Seroepidemiology of measles, mumps and rubella. Wkly Epidemiol Rec 67:231–233, 1992.
168. Narayan KMV, Moffat MA. Measles, mumps, rubella antibody surveillance: Pilot study in Grampian, Scotland. Health Bull (Edinb) 50:47–53, 1992.
169. Anderson RM, Crombie JA, Grenfell BT. The epidemiology of mumps in the U.K.: A preliminary study of virus transmission, herd immunity and the potential impact of immunization. Epidemiol Infect 99:65–84, 1987.
170. Galbraith NS, Young SEJ, Pusey JJ, et al. Mumps surveillance in England and Wales 1962–81. Lancet 1:91–94, 1984.
171. Nokes DJ, Wright J, Morgan-Capner P, Anderson RM. Serological study of the epidemiology of mumps virus infection in north-west England. Epidemiol Infect 105:175–195, 1990.
172. Arroyo M, Alia JM, Mateos ML, et al. Natural immunity to measles, rubella and mumps among Spanish children in the pre-vaccination era. Int J Epidemiol 15:95–100, 1985.
173. Anderson RM, May RM. Vaccination and herd immunity to infectious disease. Nature 318:323–329, 1985.
174. Gellis SS, McGuinness AC, Peters M. A study on the prevention of mumps orchitis by gamma globulin. Am J Med Sci 210:661–664, 1945.
175. Mumps prevention. MMWR Morb Mortal Wkly Rep 38:388–392, 397–400, 1989.
176. Hodes D, Brunell PA. Mumps antibody: Placental transfer and disappearance during the first year of life. Pediatrics 45:99–101, 1970.
177. Hilleman MR. The development of live attenuated mumps virus vaccine in historic perspective and its role in the evolution of combined measles-mumps-rubella. In Plotkin S, Fantini B (eds). Vaccinia, Vaccination, Vaccinology: Jenner, Pasteur, and Their Successors. Paris, Elsevier, 1996, pp 283–292.
178. Hilleman MR. Past, present, and future of measles, mumps, and rubella virus vaccines. Pediatrics 90:149–153, 1992.
179. Beck M, Weisz-Malecek R, Mesko-Prejac M, et al. Mumps vaccine L-Zagreb, prepared in chick fibroblasts. I. Production and field trials. J Biol Stand 17:85–90, 1989.
180. Buynak EB, Hilleman MR. Live attenuated mumps virus vaccine. 1. Vaccine development. Proc Soc Exp Biol Med 123:768–775, 1966.

181. Sasaki K, Hagashihara M, Inoue K, et al. Studies on the development of a live attenuated mumps vaccine. I. Attenuation of the Hoshino wild strain of mumps vaccine. Kitasato Arch Exp Med 49:43–52, 1976.
182. Makino S, Sasaki K, Nakayama T, et al. A new combined trivalent live measles (AIK-C strain), mumps (Hoshino strain), and rubella (Takahashi strain) vaccine. Findings in clinical and laboratory studies. Am J Dis Child 144:905–910, 1990.
183. Yamanishi K, Takahashi M, Ueda S, et al. Studies on live mumps virus vaccine. V. Development of a new mumps vaccine "AM 9" by plaque cloning. Biken J 16:161–166, 1973.
184. Glück R, Hoskins JM, Wegmann A, et al. Rubini, a new live attenuated mumps vaccine virus strain for human diploid cells. Dev Biol Stand 65:29–35, 1986.
185. Sassani A, Mirchamasy H, Shafyi A, et al. Development of a new live attenuated mumps virus vaccine in human diploid cells. Biologicals 19:203–211, 1991.
186. Smorodintsev AA, Kiyachko NS, Nasibov NM, Schickina ES. Experience with live mumps virus vaccine in the USSR. First International Conference of Vaccines Against Viral and Rickettsial Diseases of Man, Pan American Health Organization; Washington, DC; 1967.
187. Odisseev H, Gacheva N. Vaccinoprophylaxis of mumps using mumps vaccine, strain Sofia 6, in Bulgaria. Vaccine 12:1251–1254, 1994.
188. McAleer WJ, Markus HZ, McLean AA, et al. Stability on storage at various temperatures of live measles, mumps and rubella virus vaccines in new stabilizer. J Biol Stand 8:281–287, 1980.
189. Buynak EB, Hilleman MR, Leagus MB, et al. Jeryl Lynn strain live attenuated mumps virus vaccine: Influence of age, virus dose, lot, and gamma-globulin administration on response. JAMA 203:9–13, 1968.
190. Hilleman MR, Buynak EB, Weibel RE, Stokes J Jr. Live attenuated mumps-virus vaccine. N Engl J Med 278:227–232, 1968.
191. Roth A. Immunization with live attenuated mumps virus vaccine in Honolulu. Am J Dis Child 115:459–460, 1968.
192. Stokes J Jr, Weibel RE, Buynak EB, Hilleman MR. Live attenuated mumps virus vaccine: II. Early clinical studies. Pediatrics 39:363–371, 1967.
193. Sugg WC, Finger JA, Levine RH, Pagano JS. Field evaluation of live virus mumps vaccine. J Pediatr 72:461–466, 1968.
194. Young ML, Dickstein B, Weibel RE, et al. Experiences with Jeryl Lynn strain live attenuated mumps virus vaccine in a pediatric outpatient clinic. Pediatrics 40:798–803, 1967.
195. Brunell PA, Brickman A, Steinberg S. Evaluation of a live attenuated mumps vaccine (Jeryl Lynn): With observation on the optimal time for testing serological response. Am J Dis Child 118:435–440, 1969.
196. Ehrengut W, Georges AM, André FE. The reactogenicity and immunogenicity of the Urabe Am 9 live mumps vaccine and persistence of vaccine induced antibodies in healthy young children. J Biol Stand 11:105–113, 1983.
197. Vesikari T, André RE, Simoen E, et al. Evaluation in young children of the Urabe Am 9 strain of live attenuated mumps vaccine in comparison with the Jeryl Lynn strain. Acta Paediatr Scand 72:37–40, 1983.
198. Nakayama T, Urano T, Osano M, et al. Evaluation of live trivalent vaccine of measles AIK-C strain, mumps Hoshino strain and rubella Takahashi strain, by virus specific interferon-γ production and antibody response. Microbiol Immunol 34:497–508, 1990.
199. Garaseferian MG, Bolotovskii VM, Shatova LP, Tetova NS. Prevention of mumps in preschool institutions using a live mumps vaccine made from strain L-3. Zh Mikrobiol Epidemiol Immunobiol 4:39–42, 1988.
200. Lerman SJ, Bollinger M, Brunken JM. Clinical and serological evaluation of measles, mumps, and rubella (HPV-77:DE-5 and RA 27/3) virus vaccines, singly and in combination. Pediatrics 68:18–22, 1981.
201. Brunell PA, Weigle K, Murphy D, et al. Antibody response following measles-mumps-rubella vaccine under conditions of customary use. JAMA 250:1409–1412, 1983.
202. Christenson B, Heller L, Böttiger M. The immunizing effect and reactogenicity of two live attenuated mumps virus vaccines in Swedish schoolchildren. J Biol Stand 11:323–331, 1983.
203. Vesikari T, André FE, Simoen E, et al. Comparison of the Urabe AM 9–Schwarz and Jeryl Lynn–Moraten combinations of mumps-measles vaccines in young children. Acta Paediatr Scand 72:41–46, 1983.
204. Vesikari T, Ala-Laurila EL, Heikkinen A, et al. Clinical trial of a new trivalent measles-mumps-rubella vaccine in young children. Am J Dis Child 138:843–847, 1984.
205. Popow-Kraupp T, Kundi M, Ambrosch F, et al. A controlled trial for evaluating two live attenuated mumps-measles vaccines (Urabe Am 9–Schwarz and Jeryl Lynn–Moraten) in young children. J Med Virol 18:69–79, 1986.
206. Edees S, Pullan CR, Hull D. A randomized single blind trial of a combined measles rubella vaccine to evaluate serological response and reactions in the UK population. Public Health 105:91–97, 1991.
207. Just M, Berger R, Glück R, Wegmann A. Evaluation of a combined vaccine against measles-mumps-rubella produced on human diploid cells. Dev Biol Stand 65:25–27, 1986.
208. Berger M, Just M, Glück R. Interference between strains in live virus vaccines I: Combined vaccination with measles, mumps and rubella vaccine. J Biol Stand 16:269–273, 1988.
208a. Schwarzer S, Reibel S, Lang A, et al. Safety and characterization of the immune response engendered by two combined measles, mumps and rubella vaccines. Vaccine 16:298–304, 1998.
209. King GE, Markowitz LE, Heath J, et al. Antibody response to measles-mumps-rubella vaccine of children with mild illness at the time of vaccination. JAMA 275:704–707, 1996.
210. Singh R, John TJ, Cherian T, Raghupathy P. Immune response to measles, mumps & rubella vaccine at 9, 12, & 15 months of age. Indian J Med Res 100:155–159, 1994.
211. Forleo-Neto E, Carvalho ES, Fuentes ICP, et al. Seroconversion of a trivalent measles, mumps, and rubella vaccine in children aged 9 and 15 months. Vaccine 15:1898–1901, 1997.
212. Schoub BD, Johnson S, McAnerney JM, et al. Measles, mumps and rubella immunization at nine months in a developing country. Pediatr Infect Dis J 9:263–267, 1990.
213. Christenson B, Böttiger M. Vaccination against measles, mumps and rubella (MMR): A comparison between the antibody responses at the ages of 18 months and 12 years and between different methods of antibody titration. J Biol Stand 13:167–172, 1985.
214. Davidson WL, Buynak EB, Leagus MB, et al. Vaccination of adults with live attenuated mumps virus vaccine. JAMA 201:995–998, 1967.
215. Wharton M, Cochi SL, Hutcheson RH, et al. A large outbreak of mumps in the postvaccine era. J Infect Dis 158:1253–1260, 1988.
216. Weibel RE, Buynak EB, McLean AA, Hilleman MR. Followup surveillance for antibody in human subjects following live attenuated measles, mumps and rubella virus vaccines. Proc Soc Exp Biol Med 162:328–332, 1979.
217. Weibel RE, Buynak EB, McLean AA, Hilleman MR. Persistence of antibody after administration of monovalent and combined live attenuated measles, mumps, and rubella virus vaccines. Pediatrics 61:5–11, 1978.
218. Weibel RE, Buynak EB, McLean AA, et al. Persistence of antibody in human subjects for 7 to 10 years following administration of combined live attenuated measles, mumps, and rubella virus vaccines. Proc Soc Exp Biol Med 165:260–263, 1980.
219. Weibel RE. Mumps vaccine. In Plotkin SA, Mortimer EA (eds). Vaccines. Philadelphia, WB Saunders, 1988 p 231.
220. Miller E, Hill A, Morgan-Capner P, et al. Antibodies to measles, mumps and rubella in UK children 4 years after vaccination with different MMR vaccines. Vaccine 13:799–802, 1995.
221. Boulianne N, De Serres G, Ratman S, et al. Measles, mumps, and rubella antibodies in children 5–6 years after immunization: Effect of vaccine type and age at vaccination. Vaccine 13:1611–1616, 1995.
222. Davidkin I, Valle M, Julkunen I. Persistence of anti-mumps virus antibodies after a two-dose MMR vaccination. A nine-year follow-up. Vaccine 13:1617–1622, 1995.
223. King SM, Saunders EF, Petric M, Gold R. Response to measles, mumps and rubella vaccine in paediatric bone marrow transplant recipients. Bone Marrow Transplant 17:633–636, 1996.
224. Ljungman P, Fridell E, Lönnqvist B, et al. Efficacy and safety of vaccination of marrow transplant recipients with a live attenuated

measles, mumps, and rubella vaccine. J Infect Dis 159:610–615, 1989.
225. Schulman SL, Deforest A, Kaiser BA, et al. Response to measles-mumps-rubella vaccine in children on dialysis. Pediatr Nephrol 6:187–189, 1992.
226. Hilleman MR, Weibel RE, Buynak EB, et al. Live, attenuated mumps-virus vaccine. 4. Protective efficacy as measured in a field evaluation. N Engl J Med 276:252–258, 1967.
227. Mumps vaccine: More information needed. N Engl J Med 278:275–276, 1968.
228. Mumps in an elementary school—New York. MMWR Morb Mortal Wkly Rep 22:185–186, 1973.
229. Chaiken BP, Williams NM, Preblud SR, et al. The effect of a school entry law on mumps activity in a school district. JAMA 257:2455–2458, 1987.
230. Kim-Farley R, Bart S, Stetler H, et al. Clinical mumps vaccine efficacy. Am J Epidemiol 121:593–597, 1985.
231. Lewis JE, Chernesky MA, Rawls ML, Rawls WE. Epidemic of mumps in a partially immune population. Can Med Assoc J 121:751–754, 1979.
232. Sullivan KM, Halpin TJ, Marks JS, Kim-Farley R. Effectiveness of mumps vaccine in a school outbreak. Am J Dis Child 139:909–912, 1985.
233. Pena AA, Pitarch SM, Adsuara LS. Epidemia de parotiditis en una población escolar y eficacia de la vacunación antiparotiditis. Med Clin (Barc) 93:607–610, 1989.
234. Guimbao J, Moreno MP, Gutiérrez V, Pac MR, Arribas F. La parotiditis en época posvacunal. Patrón epidemiológico y efectividad vacunal en un brote epidémico. Med Clin (Barc) 99:281–285, 1992.
235. Orenstein WA, Bernier RH, Dondero TJ, et al. Field evaluation of vaccine efficacy. Bull World Health Organ 63:1055–1068, 1985.
236. Briss PA, Fehrs LJ, Parker RA, et al. Sustained transmission of mumps in a highly vaccinated population: Assessment of primary vaccine failure and waning immunity. J Infect Dis 169:77–82, 1994.
237. Cheek JE, Baron R, Atlas H, et al. Mumps outbreak in a highly vaccinated school population. Evidence for large-scale vaccination failure. Arch Pediatr Adolesc Med 149:774–778, 1995.
238. Baron S, Lorente C. Investigation d'une épidémie d'orcillons dans la commune de Millau (Aveyron), janvier–août 1995. Réseau National de Santé Publique Français, 1995, pp 1–22.
239. Germann D, Ströhle A, Eggengerger K, et al. An outbreak of mumps in a population partially vaccinated with the Rubini strain. Scand J Infect Dis 28:235–238, 1996.
240. Toscani L, Batou M, Bouvier P, Schlaepfer A. Comparaison de l'efficacité de différentes souches de vaccin ourlien: Une enquête en milieu scolaire. Soz Praeventivmed 41:341–347, 1996.
241. Oda K, Kato H, Konishi A. The outbreak of mumps in a small island in Japan. Acta Paediatr Jpn 38:224–228, 1996.
242. Johnson CE, Kumar ML, Whitwell JK, et al. Antibody persistence after primary measles-mumps-rubella vaccine and response to a second dose given at four to six vs. eleven to thirteen years. Pediatr Infect Dis J 15:687–692, 1996.
243. Measles prevention. MMWR Morb Mortal Wkly Rep 38(suppl 9):1–18, 1989.
244. Orenstein WA, Markowitz LE, Preblud SR, et al. Appropriate age for measles vaccination in the United States. Dev Biol Stand 65:13–21, 1986.
245. Efficacy of mumps vaccine—Ohio. MMWR Morb Mortal Wkly Rep 32:391–398, 1983.
246. Sawada H, Yano S, Oka Y, Togashi T. Transmission of Urabe Am 9 mumps vaccine between siblings [letter]. Lancet 342:371, 1993.
247. Status report on the Childhood Immunization Initiative: National, state, and urban area vaccination coverage levels among children aged 19–35 months—United States, 1996. MMWR Morb Mortal Wkly Rep 46:657–664, 1997.
248. Status report on the Childhood Immunization Initiative: Reported cases of selected vaccine-preventable diseases—United States, 1996. MMWR Morb Mortal Wkly Rep 46:665–671, 1997.
249. Deforest A, Long SS, Lischner HW, et al. Simultaneous administration of measles-mumps-rubella vaccine with booster doses of diphtheria-tetanus-pertussis and poliovirus vaccines. Pediatrics 81:237–246, 1988.
250. Rothstein E, Bernstein H, Glode M, et al. Simultaneous administration of an acellular pertussis-DT vaccine (APDT) with MMR and OPV vaccines [abstract]. Program and Abstracts of the 32nd Interscience Conference on Antimicrobial Agents and Chemotherapy; Anaheim, CA; October 11–14, 1992.
251. Dashefsky B, Wald E, Guerra N, Byers C. Safety, tolerability, and immunogenicity of concurrent administration of *Haemophilus influenzae* type b conjugate vaccine (meningococcal protein conjugate) with either measles-mumps-rubella vaccine or diphtheria-tetanus-pertussis and oral poliovirus vaccines in 14- to 23-month-old infants. Pediatrics 85(suppl):682–689, 1990.
252. Huang LM, Lee CY, Hsu CY, et al. Effect of monovalent measles and trivalent measles-mumps-rubella vaccines at various ages and concurrent administration with hepatitis B vaccine. Pediatr Infect Dis J 9:461–465, 1990.
253. King GE, Hadler SC. Simultaneous administration of childhood vaccines: An important public health policy that is safe and efficacious. Pediatr Infect Dis J 13:394–407, 1994.
254. Arbeter AM, Baker L, Starr SE, et al. Combination measles, mumps, rubella, and varicella vaccine. Pediatrics 76(suppl):742–747, 1986.
255. Arbeter AM, Baker L, Starr SE, Plotkin SA. The combination measles, mumps, rubella and varicella vaccine in healthy children. Dev Biol Stand 65:89–93, 1986.
256. Englund JA, Suarez CS, Kelly J, et al. Placebo-controlled trial of varicella vaccine given with or after measles-mumps-rubella vaccine. J Pediatr 114:37–44, 1989.
257. Just M, Berger R, Just V. Evaluation of a combined measles-mumps-rubella-chickenpox vaccine. Dev Biol Stand 65:85–88, 1986.
258. Fescharek R, Quast U, Maass G, et al. Measles-mumps vaccination in the FRG: An empirical analysis after 14 years of use. II. Tolerability and analysis of spontaneously reported side effects. Vaccine 8:446–456, 1990.
259. Miller C, Miller E, Rowe K, et al. Surveillance of symptoms following MMR vaccine in children. Practitioner 233:69–73, 1989.
260. Nakayama T, Oka S, Komase K, et al. The relationship between the mumps vaccine strain and parotitis after vaccination. J Infect Dis 165:186–187, 1992.
261. Kuczyk MA, Denil J, Thon WF, et al. Orchitis following mumps vaccination in an adult. Urol Int 53:179–180, 1994.
262. Nakayama T, Urano T, Osano M, et al. Evaluation of live trivalent vaccine of measles AIK-C strain, mumps Hoshino strain and rubella Takahashi strain, by virus-specific interferon-gamma production and antibody response. Microbiol Immunol 34:497–508, 1990.
263. Nussinovitch M, Harel L, Varsano I. Arthritis after mumps and measles vaccination. Arch Dis Child 72:348–349, 1995.
264. Stewart BJA, Prabhu PU. Reports of sensorineural deafness after measles, mumps and rubella immunisation. Arch Dis Child 69:153–154, 1993.
265. Nabe-Nielsen J, Walter B. Unilateral total deafness as a complication of the measles-mumps-rubella vaccination. Scand Audiol Suppl 30:69–70, 1988.
266. Rose C, Viget N, Copin MC, et al. Myosite aiquë sévère et transitoire après vaccination ourlienne (Imovax-Oreillion (R)). Therapie 51:87–89, 1996.
267. Marshall GS, Wright PF, Fenichel GM, Karzon DT. Diffuse retinopathy following measles, mumps, and rubella vaccination. Pediatrics 76:989–991, 1985.
268. Plesner AM. Gait disturbances after measles, mumps, and rubella vaccine [letter]. Lancet 345:316, 1995.
269. Drachtman RA, Murphy S, Ettinger LJ. Exacerbation of chronic idiopathic thromocytopenic purpura following measles-mumps-rubella immunization. Arch Pediatr Adolesc Med 148:326–327, 1994.
270. Jonville-Béra AP, Autret E, Galy-Eyraud C, Hessel L. Thrombocytopenic purpura after measles, mumps and rubella vaccination: A retrospective survey by the French Regional Pharmacovigilance Centres and Pasteur-Mérieux Sérums et Vaccins. Pediatr Infect Dis J 15:44–48, 1996.
271. Nieminen U, Peltola H, Syrjälä MT, et al. Acute thrombocytopenic purpura following measles, mumps and rubella vaccination. A report on 23 patients. Acta Paediatr 82:267–270, 1993.

272. Frenkel LM, Nielsen K, Garakian A, Cherry JD. A search for persistent measles, mumps, rubella vaccine virus in children with human immunodeficiency virus type 1 infection. Arch Pediatr Adolesc Med 148:57–90, 1994.
273. Griffin MR, Ray WA, Mortimer EA, et al. Risk of seizures after measles-mumps-rubella immunization. Pediatrics 88:881–885, 1991.
274. Nalin D. Mumps vaccine complications: Which strain? [letter: comment]. Lancet 2:1396, 1989.
275. Cizman M, Mozetic M, Radescek-Raker R, et al. Aseptic meningitis after vaccination against measles and mumps. Pediatr Infect Dis J 8:302–308, 1989.
276. McDonald JC, Moore DL, Quennec P. Clinical and epidemiological features of mumps meningoencephalitis and possible vaccine-related disease. Pediatr Infect Dis J 8:751–755, 1989.
277. Nalin D. Evaluating mumps vaccines [letter: comment]. Lancet 339:305, 1992.
278. Black S, Shinefield H, Ray P, et al. Risk of hospitalization because of aseptic meningitis after measles-mumps-rubella vaccination in one- to two-year-old children: An analysis of the Vaccine Safety Datalink (VSD) Project. Pediatr Infect Dis J 16:500–503, 1997.
279. Ehrengut W, Zastrow K. Komplikationen nach Mumpsschutzimpfungen in der Bundesrepublik Deutschland (einschließlich Mehrfachschutzimpfungen). Monatsschr Kinderheilkd 137:398–402, 1989.
280. Sugiura A, Yamada A. Aseptic meningitis as a complication of mumps vaccination. Pediatr Infect Dis J 10:209–213, 1991.
281. Fujinaga T, Youichi M, Hiroshi T, Takayoshi K. A prefecture-wide survey of mumps meningitis associated with measles, mumps and rubella vaccine. Pediatr Infect Dis J 10:204–209, 1991.
282. Ueda K, Miyazaki C, Hidaka Y, et al. Aseptic meningitis caused by measles-mumps-rubella vaccine in Japan. Lancet 346:701–702, 1995.
283. Kimura M, Kuno-Sakai H, Yamakazi S, et al. Adverse events associated with MMR vaccines in Japan. Acta Paediatr Jpn 38:205–211, 1996.
284. Furesz J, Contreras G. Vaccine-related mumps meningitis—Canada. Can Dis Wkly Rep 16:253–254, 1990.
285. Rebiere I, Galy-Eyraud C. Estimation of the risk of aseptic meningitis associated with mumps vaccination, France, 1991–1993. Int J Epidemiol 24:1223–1227, 1995.
286. Jonville-Béra AP, Autret E, Galy-Eyraud C, Hessel L. Aseptic meningitis following mumps vaccine. A retrospective survey by the French Regional Pharmacovigilence Centres and by Pasteur-Mérieux Sérums & Vaccins. Pharmacoepidemiol Drug Safety 5:33–37, 1996.
287. Balraj V, Miller E. Complications of mumps vaccines. Rev Med Virol 5:219–227, 1995.
288. Colville A, Pugh S. Mumps meningitis and measles, mumps, and rubella vaccine [letter]. Lancet 340:786, 1992.
289. Miller E, Goldacre M, Pugh S, et al. Risk of aseptic meningitis after measles, mumps, and rubella vaccine in U.K. children. Lancet 341:979–982, 1993.
290. Farrington P, Pugh S, Colville A, et al. A new method for active surveillance for adverse events from diphtheria/tetanus/pertussis and measles/mumps/rubella vaccines. Lancet 345:567–569, 1995.
291. Mumps Surveillance. Report No. 2. Atlanta, GA, US Department of Health, Education, and Welfare, September 1972.
292. Nokes DJ, Anderson RM. Vaccine safety versus vaccine efficacy in mass immunisation programmes. Lancet 338:1309–1312, 1991.
293. Peltola H. Mumps vaccination and meningitis. Lancet 341:994–995, 1993.
294. Measles, mumps, and rubella—vaccine use and strategies for measles, rubella, and congenital rubella syndrome elimination and mumps control: Recommendations of the Advisory Committee on Immunization Practices (ACIP). MMWR Morb Mortal Wkly Rep 47(RR-8):1–57, 1998.
295. Fasano MB, Wood RA, Cooke SK, Sampson HA. Egg hypersensitivity and adverse reactions to measles, mumps, and rubella vaccine. J Pediatr 120:878–881, 1992.
296. Kemp A, Van Asperen P, Mukhi A. Measles immunization in children with clinical reactions to egg protein. Am J Dis Child 144:33–35, 1990.
297. James JM, Burks AW, Roberson PK, Sampson HA. Safe administration of measles vaccine to children allergic to eggs. N Engl J Med 332:1262–1266, 1995.
298. Lavi S, Zimmerman B, Koren G, et al. Administration of measles, mumps, and rubella virus vaccine (live) to egg-allergic children. JAMA 263:269–271, 1990.
299. Beck SA, Williams LW, Shirrell MA, Burks AW. Egg hypersensitivity and measles-mumps-rubella vaccine administration. Pediatrics 88:913–917, 1991.
300. Kelso JM, Jones RT, Yunginger JW. Anaphylaxis to measles, mumps, and rubella vaccine mediated by IgE to gelatin. J Allergy Infect Dis 91:867–872.
301. Sakaguchi M, Ogura H, Inouye S. IgE antibody to gelatin in children with measles and mumps vaccines. J Allergy Infect Dis 96:563–565, 1995.
302. Sakaguchi M, Nakayama T, Inouye S. Food allergy to gelatin in children with immediate-type reactions to measles and mumps vaccines. J Allergy Infect Dis 98:1058–1061, 1996.
303. Sosin DM, Cochi SL, Gunn RA, et al. Changing epidemiology of mumps and its impact on university campuses. Pediatrics 84:779–784, 1989.
304. Kaplan KM, Marder DC, Cochi SL, Preblud SR. Mumps in the workplace: Further evidence of the changing epidemiology of a childhood vaccine-preventable disease. JAMA 260:1434–1438, 1988.
305. Summary of notifiable diseases, United States, 1986. MMWR Morb Mortal Wkly Rep 35:10–11, 1987.
306. Summary of notifiable diseases, United States, 1987. MMWR Morb Mortal Wkly Rep 36:10–11, 1988.
307. van Loon FPL, Holmes SJ, Sirotkin BI, et al. Mumps surveillance—United States, 1988–1993. MMWR CDC Surveill Summ 44:1–14, 1995.
308. Cochi SL, Preblud SR, Orenstein WA. Perspectives on the relative resurgence of mumps in the United States. Am J Dis Child 142:499–507, 1988.
309. Anderson RM, May RM. Directly transmitted infectious diseases: Control by vaccination. Science 215:1053–1060, 1982.
310. Summary of notifiable diseases, United States, 1994. MMWR Morb Mortal Wkly Rep 43:iv, 1994.
311. Rantala H, Uhari M. Occurrence of childhood encephalitis: A population-based study. Pediatr Infect Dis J 8:426–430, 1989.
312. Koskiniemi M, Vaheri A. Effect of measles, mumps, rubella vaccination on pattern of encephalitis in children. Lancet 1:31–34, 1989.
313. Koplan JP, Preblud SR. A benefit-cost analysis of mumps vaccine. Am J Dis Child 136:362–364, 1982.
314. White CC, Koplan JP, Orenstein WA. Benefits, risks and costs of immunization for measles, mumps and rubella. Am J Public Health 75:739–744, 1985.
315. Peltola H, Karanko V, Kurki T, et al. Rapid effect on endemic measles, mumps, and rubella of nationwide vaccination programme in Finland. Lancet 1:137–139, 1986.
316. Paunio M, Virtanen M, Peltola H, et al. Increase of vaccination coverage by mass media and individual approach: Intensified measles, mumps, and rubella prevention program in Finland. Am J Epidemiol 133:1152–1160, 1991.
317. Peltola H, Heinonen OP, Valle M, et al. The elimination of indigenous measles, mumps, and rubella from Finland by a 12-year, two-dose vaccination program. N Engl J Med 331:1397–1402, 1994.
318. Hyöty H, Hiltunen M, Reunanen A, et al. Decline of mumps antibodies in type 1 (insulin-dependent) diabetic children and a plateau in the rising incidence of type 1 diabetes after introduction of the mumps-measles-rubella vaccine in Finland. Diabetologia 36:1303–1308, 1993.
319. Heisler MB, Richmond JB. Lessons from Finland's successful immunization program. N Engl J Med 331:1446–1447, 1994.
320. Broliden K, Rubilar Abreu E, Arneborn M, Bottiger M. Immunity to mumps before and after MMR vaccination at 12 years of age in the first generation offered the two-dose immunization programme. Vaccine 16:323–327, 1998.
321. Böttiger M, Christenson B, Romanus V, et al. Swedish experience of two-dose vaccination programme aiming at eliminating measles, mumps, and rubella. BMJ 295:1264–1267, 1987.

322. Christenson B, Böttiger M. Changes of the immunological patterns against measles, mumps and rubella. A vaccination programme studied 3 to 7 years after the introduction of a two-dose schedule. Vaccine 9:326–329, 1991.
323. Vaccination coverage statistics for children up to two years of age in the United Kingdom. Commun Dis Rep CDR Wkly 6:262, 1996.
324. Jones AGH, White JM, Begg NT. The impact of MMR vaccine on mumps infection in England and Wales. Commun Dis Rep CDR Rev 1:R93–R96, 1991.
325. Slater PE, Roitman M, Costin C. Mumps incidence in Israel—impact of MMR vaccine. Public Health Rev 91:88–93, 1990.
326. Berger SA, Ginsberg GM, Slater PE. Cost-benefit analysis of routine mumps and rubella vaccination for Israeli infants. Isr J Med Sci 26:74–80, 1990.
327. Krugman S, de Quadros C. Eradication of measles, rubella and mumps in Cuba: Report of a technical advisory group. Washington, DC, Pan American Health Organization, May 1989.
328. Zimmermann H, Matter HC, Kiener T, die Sentinella-Arbeitsgemeinschaft. Mumps—Epidemiologie in der Schweiz: Ergebnisse der Sentinella—Überwachung 1986–1993. Soz Praventivmed 40:80–92, 1995.
329. Matter HC, Cloetta J, Zimmermann H, and the Sentinella Arbeitsgemeinschaft. Measles, mumps, and rubella monitoring in Switzerland through a sentinel network, 1986–94. J Epidemiol Community Health 49(suppl 1):4–8, 1995.
330. Matter L, Germann D, Bally F, Schopfer K. Age-stratified seroprevalence of measles, mumps and rubella (MMR) virus infections in Switzerland after the introduction of MMR mass vaccination. Eur J Epidemiol 13:61–66, 1997.
331. Dias JA, Cordiero M, Afzal MA, et al. Mumps epidemic in Portugal despite high vaccine coverage—preliminary report. Eurosurveillance 1:25–28, 1996.
332. Fahlgren K. Two doses of MMR vaccine—sufficient to eradicate measles, mumps and rubella? Scand J Soc Med 16:129–135, 1988.
333. Recommendations of the International Task Force for Disease Eradication. MMWR Morb Mortal Wkly Rep 42(RR-16):11, 1993.
334. Measles eradication: Recommendations from a meeting cosponsored by the World Health Organization, the Pan American Health Organization, and CDC. MMWR Morb Mortal Wkly Rep 46 (RR-11):1–20, 1997.

chapter

14 Pertussis Vaccine

Kathryn M. Edwards
Michael D. Decker
Edward A. Mortimer Jr.

History

Pertussis (whooping cough) is a bacterial respiratory infection caused by *Bordetella pertussis*, a gram-negative bacillus. Its major manifestation is a protracted cough illness that lasts many weeks. The disease is most severe in infants and young children, many of whom suffer the intense paroxysmal coughing that terminates in an inspiratory "whoop."

The first known description of an outbreak of pertussis is that of Guillaume De Baillou, who described an epidemic that occurred in Paris in the summer of 1578.[1] The epidemic primarily affected infants and young children and resulted in high mortality. Apparently, the disease had been known previously in France, because De Baillou referred to its common name of *quinte*, which he hypothesized might have reflected the characteristic sound of the cough or the 5-hour periodicity of the paroxysms.

A disease known in Britain from the early 16th century as *chyne-cough* probably was pertussis, and the terms *whooping cough* and *chincough* appeared in the London Bills of Mortality in 1701.[2] The causative organism was grown by Jules Bordet and Octave Gengou in 1906, and the first crude vaccines appeared soon thereafter.[3]

Importance

Prior to widespread use of whole-cell pertussis vaccine, there were as many as 270,000 cases of pertussis reported each year in the United States (indeed, the true case count likely approximated the annual birth cohort), with 10,000 deaths.[4] The occurrence of pertussis declined markedly after the introduction of whole-cell vaccine, to a nadir of 1010 cases reported in 1976.[5] The occurrence of pertussis has since progressively increased, with 7796 cases reported for 1996, the highest total since 1964. The increase in pertussis has been greatest among older children and adults, probably reflecting waning vaccine-induced immunity. Because pertussis often goes undiagnosed in adolescents and adults, it is likely that the actual number of cases greatly exceeds the number reported.

Worldwide, pertussis remains an important killer of children. In 1994, there were an estimated 40 million cases that resulted in 5 million episodes of pneumonia, 360,000 deaths, and 50,000 patients with long-term neurological complications (including permanent brain damage).[6]

Common Questions Concerning Pertussis Vaccines

The last section of this chapter provides brief answers to some of the most common questions concerning pertussis vaccines.

BACKGROUND

Clinical Description

Infants and Young Children

The incubation period of pertussis averages 9 or 10 days (range, 6–20 d). The onset is insidious, and symptoms are indistinguishable from those of a minor upper respiratory infection. Fever is usually minimal throughout the course of infection. Cough, initially intermittent, progresses within 1 or 2 weeks to become paroxysmal. The paroxysms increase in both frequency and severity and then gradually subside, rarely lasting longer than 2 to 6 weeks. In the absence of immunization, most children experience the full-blown disease; however, some children appear to develop either clinical immunity, serological evidence of prior infection without a history of clinical pertussis, or both of these, suggesting that mild atypical cases occur.[7]

It is during the paroxysmal stage, when the cough is most severe, that the characteristic whoop occurs. The whoop is caused by forced inspiration through a narrowed glottis immediately after a paroxysm of a dozen or more rapid, short coughs without intervening inspiration. The paroxysms apparently result from difficulty in expelling thick mucus from the tracheobronchial tree. During a paroxysm, cyanosis may occur and vomiting may ensue. The clinical picture of a young infant in a severe paroxysm is distressing indeed. After the episode, the child is often exhausted; unfortunately, several paroxysms may occur successively within a few minutes. Between paroxysms, the child may be playful and appear quite normal. Paroxysms may be induced by eating, laughing, crying, and a variety of other stimuli and are usually worse at night.

Recovery is gradual. The paroxysms become less frequent and milder, and the whoop disappears. Nonparoxysmal cough may persist for many weeks. During the convalescent phase, intercurrent respiratory infections may trigger a recurrence of the paroxysmal cough.

Complications and Sequelae. Minor complications of pertussis include subconjunctival hemorrhages and epistaxis secondary to the paroxysms. Edema of the face may occur. An ulcer of the lingual frenulum is frequently seen, owing to protrusion of the tongue during paroxysms. Suppurative otitis media frequently occurs (due to the usual bacteria, such as *Streptococcus pneumoniae* or *Haemophilus influenzae*, not *B. pertussis*).

Major complications, which are sometimes fatal, are of three types: pulmonary, encephalitic, and nutritional. Of these, pulmonary complications are the most frequent. The vast majority of full-blown pertussis cases likely exhibit some degree of atelectasis or bronchopneumonia. Pathologically, the pneumonia is both interstitial and alveolar, and the exudate usually is primarily mononuclear.[8] Pneumonic involvement may be sufficiently severe to compromise respiratory function and cause death. Indeed, 54% of the deaths associated with pertussis are attributed to pneumonia. However, in those children who survive pneumonia, permanent lung damage usually does not occur.[9]

Acute encephalopathy associated with pertussis, usually occurring during the paroxysmal stage, has been recognized for many years. There may be a wide variety of manifestations, the most common of which are convulsions and altered consciousness. Only limited data on the incidence of encephalopathy are available; estimates from population-based studies have ranged from 0.08 to 0.8 per 1000 cases.[10, 11] Of those cases reported to the Centers for Disease Control and Prevention (CDC) between 1992 and 1994, 17 (0.1%) were complicated by encephalopathy.[12] Approximately one third of children with pertussis encephalopathy succumb to the acute illness, one third survive with permanent brain damage, and one third recover without obvious neurological sequelae (D. Annunziato, personal communication, 1985).[13]

Nutritional problems due to repeated vomiting during an episode of pertussis were of major importance in developed countries in the past and remain so in developing nations today. The inability to maintain adequate caloric intake is a severe problem in previously malnourished children who develop pertussis.

Adolescents and Adults

It is becoming clear that pertussis plays an important role in the etiology of cough illness in older children and adults, particularly among populations with high rates of childhood immunization with whole-cell pertussis vaccine (see under *Epidemiology*). Furthermore, older children and adults have been demonstrated to be a reservoir for pertussis infection.[14]

German household contact studies have provided comprehensive descriptions of the signs and symptoms of adult pertussis.[15, 16] Of 79 adults with symptomatic pertussis, 34% had been diagnosed with pertussis as children; 72 (91%) had cough with their present illness, 63 (80%) had cough lasting longer than 21 days, and 1 had a cough for 8 months.[16] Prolonged paroxysmal cough was experienced by 50 patients (63%); cough resulting in sleep disturbance was reported in 41 (52%); cough followed by vomiting occurred in 33 (42%); and whoops occurred in 6 (8%). The adults usually expectorated "a glassy, viscous mucus." Malaise was reported in 24 patients and arthralgia in 12. Eleven patients reported attacks involving flushing and sweating. These episodes lasted 1 to 2 minutes, occurred several times a day, and continued for 2 to 8 weeks.

Family studies of children with culture-confirmed pertussis disease and seroprevalence studies have both shown that asymptomatic infections are common in older children and adults.[17–19] Frequently, these asymptomatic adults have been implicated in the spread of infection to susceptible children.

Complications and Sequelae. Complications of pertussis were seen in 18 (23%) of the 79 adult patients in the German study.[16] These included otitis media (4 patients), pneumonia (2), urinary incontinence (3), rib fracture (1), and severe weight loss (1). Other known complications of pertussis in adults include cough syncope, in which a prolonged coughing attack is followed by unconsciousness; seizures; loss of concentration; and loss of memory.[20–22]

Bacteriology

Overview

The causative agent of pertussis is *Bordetella pertussis*, a small, gram-negative, pleomorphic bacillus. Although the organism was identified before the turn of the century in stained preparations of respiratory secretions from children with pertussis and from pathological specimens,[23] the organism was not recovered in culture until 1906 by Bordet and Gengou.[3] The culture medium originally employed, now called Bordet-Gengou medium, is still used in clinical laboratories, although more complex synthetic media have been devised and are employed in some laboratories to grow this relatively fastidious organism.

Two closely related organisms in the genus *Bordetella* are *B. parapertussis* and *B. bronchiseptica*. The former is responsible for a pertussis-like syndrome in humans, which is usually less severe than pertussis. The latter produces respiratory illnesses in domestic animals.[23] Because the DNA structure of these two organisms is essentially identical to that of *B. pertussis*, it may be that the three organisms are actually subspecies of the same bacterium.[24] Indeed, some have suggested that the curious absence of descriptions of pertussis before the 16th century may represent the adaptation of an animal organism to humans as recently as 5 centuries ago.[24] Others, however, see evidence of pertussis in the ancient folklore of southern India and Malabar.[2]

Although many of the biological activities of *B. pertussis* have been recognized for some time, attempts to determine the components responsible for these various activities were unsuccessful for many years. However, newer techniques have facilitated the identification of several components that apparently contribute to disease manifestations and immunity. This increased understanding of the organism's biology has led to an enhanced understanding of the pathogenesis of the disease and has spurred development of purified component vaccines.

B. pertussis has a marked tropism for and attaches strongly to ciliated respiratory tract epithelial cells.[25, 26] The bacteria may be internalized by epithelial cells but do not penetrate submucosal cells or invade the blood stream. Toxins produced by the organism can enter the blood stream and produce systemic effects, however. *B. pertussis* antigens that have been incorporated in acellular vaccines, as well as other known components of the pertussis organism, are listed in Table 14–1.

Key Components

Pertussis Toxin. Pertussis toxin (PT), previously termed lymphocytosis-promoting factor, or LPF, is a major contributor to the pathogenesis of pertussis and is generally believed to play an important role in the induction of clinical immunity. PT is located on the cell wall of *B. pertussis* and may be recovered from liquid cultures of the organism.

Figure 14–1 is a diagram of PT. The S1 component (A protomer) appears to be largely responsible for the recognized biological activities of PT, including the promotion of lymphocytosis, the stimulation of islet cells,[27] the sensitization to histamines, the clustering of the ovary cells of Chinese hamsters, and the adjuvant properties. The B oligomer comprises five monomers, one of which (S5) serves to link the two dimers, S2-S4 and S3-S4. The primary function of the B oligomer is to facilitate the attachment of PT to the ciliated cells of the respiratory tract.[28, 29] However, the B oligomer does have some enzymatic activities, including hemagglutina-

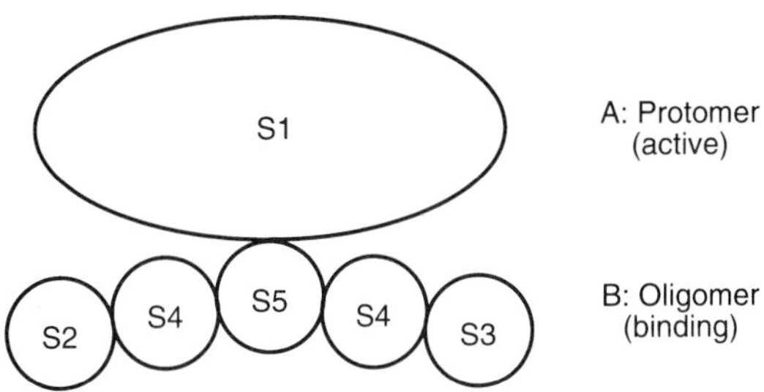

Figure 14–1. Diagrammatic representation of the pertussis toxin (see text).

tion and T-cell mitogenicity. The entire PT molecule is required for the majority of the enzymatic activities of the A protomer (the A protomer does not function in the absence of the B oligomer).[27, 30] PTs produced by different agglutinogen-type strains of *B. pertussis* appear to have a single biological and serological identity.[31] PT is not produced by *B. parapertussis*.

PT appears to play two major roles in the pathogenesis of pertussis, although the precise mechanisms are not entirely clear. First, it facilitates the attachment of *B. pertussis* to ciliated respiratory cells. Second, it appears to be of major importance in cell toxicity. PT is a strong immunogen. Antibodies to PT are associated with clinical immunity to pertussis, and many researchers believe these antibodies to be the most important or even the sole mediators of clinical protection.[32] In the laboratory, antibodies to PT protect mice that undergo intracerebral challenge with live *B. pertussis* (the mouse protection test). These antibodies are similarly protective of mice after aerosol challenge.[27, 33] Studies employing intracerebral or aerosol challenge of mice that have been actively immunized with subunits of PT or passively immunized with monoclonal antibodies to various subunits have suggested that the entire molecule is required for optimum protection.[27, 29, 30, 34] PT is chemically or genetically inactivated (toxoided) for incorporation into a vaccine. Interestingly, however, intravenous injection of substantial quantities of active PT into adult human volunteers caused no adverse effects.[35]

Filamentous Hemagglutinin. Filamentous hemagglutinin (FHA) is a large, rod-like surface protein that has been identified and purified from broth cultures of the organism. The major role of FHA in the pathogenesis of pertussis appears to be the attachment of the

Table 14–1. **KEY COMPONENTS OF THE *Bordetella pertussis* ORGANISM**

COMPONENT	BIOLOGICAL ACTIVITY
Pertussis toxin	Secreted exotoxin that induces lymphocytosis, sensitivity to histamine, pancreatic islet cell activation, and immune enhancement
Filamentous hemagglutinin	Involved in attachment to ciliated respiratory epithelium
Fimbriae (fimbrial agglutinogens)	Involved in attachment to ciliated respiratory epithelium
Pertactin	Outer membrane protein that promotes adhesion to ciliated respiratory epithelium
Adenylate cyclase	Inhibits phagocytic function
Tracheal cytotoxin	Causes ciliary stasis and cytopathic effects on tracheal mucosa
Dermonecrotic or heat-labile toxin	Causes dermal necrosis and vasoconstriction in animals
BrkA	Outer membrane protein that mediates adherence and resists complement
Endotoxin	Contributes to fever and local reactions in animals and probably humans

BrkA, *Bordetella* resistance to killing genetic locus, frame A.

organism to ciliated respiratory epithelial cells. FHA promotes attachment to human ciliated cells in vitro and to ciliated cells in animals. Mutant organisms deficient in FHA adhere poorly to cells in vitro.[25, 36, 37] Mice immunized with FHA are protected against lethal respiratory challenge with pertussis but not against intracerebral challenge.[33, 38] FHA is a strong immunogen, and serum antibodies to FHA are found after natural infection and after immunization with vaccines containing this protein. The results of one epidemiological study in Finland suggested that antibodies to FHA in immunized schoolchildren correlated with protection against pertussis disease.[39]

Fimbrial Agglutinogens. More than a dozen agglutinogens are present on the cell envelope of the three species of the genus *Bordetella*; most, if not all, of these agglutinogens are fimbrial. The terms *fimbriae* and *agglutinogens*, although not synonymous, are used somewhat interchangeably. Agglutinogen patterns differ among the three species. As many as eight are found in *B. pertussis*, six of which are unique to that species, but only agglutinogens 1, 2, and 3 are considered to be of importance in disease pathogenesis and immunity. Antibodies to these agglutinogens have been useful in seroepidemiological studies.

The fimbrial agglutinogens (FIMs) appear to participate in the attachment of *B. pertussis* to respiratory cilia, although their role probably is less than that of FHA or PT. The agglutinogens are also immunogenic. Serum antibodies to the fimbrial agglutinogens are found almost universally after natural disease or after immunization with vaccines containing these proteins.

Evidence is conflicting regarding the role of antibodies to these agglutinogens in clinical immunity. The major evidence for such a role is that the efficacy of whole-cell pertussis vaccines appears to be compromised in the absence of a "match" between the agglutinogens in the vaccine and those of prevalent *B. pertussis* strains. There is some in vitro evidence of shifts in serotypes of *B. pertussis* on serial culture.[40] There is also evidence that a change in serotype occurs during the course of clinical pertussis in some instances.[41] Seroepidemiological data from the United Kingdom indicate that between 1941 and 1953 the circulating strains of *B. pertussis* contained FIM 1, 2, and 3. By 1968, however, 75% of isolated strains contained FIM 1 and 3.[42] There is suggestive evidence (but no proof) that this change resulted from the use of vaccines that contained relatively little FIM 3.[41, 43, 44] The one product that contained considerable FIM 3 was far more effective than the others in preventing pertussis during this time. Subsequent manufacturing changes that incorporated more FIM 3 resulted in higher efficacy.[41] It is, of course, possible that serotype differences are markers for some other antigenic differences in strains of *B. pertussis*; however, the biological activities of PT from different serotypes of *B. pertussis* do not appear to differ.[31] Because of the evidence that the agglutinogens play some role in the induction of clinical immunity to pertussis, the World Health Organization (WHO) has recommended that whole-cell pertussis vaccines contain agglutinogens 1, 2, and 3.[45]

Pertactin. Pertactin (PRN), originally known as the 69-kDa protein, is an agglutinogen of *B. pertussis* that is nonfimbrial instead being located on the outer cell membrane.[46] Somewhat similar proteins are produced by *B. parapertussis* and *B. bronchiseptica*.[47] It seems clear that PRN participates in the mechanism of adherence to human cells, along with PT and FHA,[47, 48] and it has been shown to play a role in cell invasion in vitro.[49]

PRN is highly immunogenic. Antibodies to PRN are found after natural disease or immunization with vaccines containing this protein.[50] Curiously, however, serum antibodies to PRN have consistently been found in unimmunized children without detectable antibodies to PT or FHA or a history of pertussis,[51] although in those with a prior history of pertussis, antibody levels to PRN were higher. This suggests immunological cross-reactivity with other organisms, some but not all of which might have been *B. parapertussis* or *B. bronchiseptica*. Mice that have been protected passively with antibodies to PRN are highly resistant to an otherwise fatal aerosol challenge with virulent *B. pertussis*.[52] However, in the intracerebral mouse protection test, mice that have been actively immunized with PRN are protected only when also immunized with FHA.[47]

More recently, evidence has appeared suggesting the existence of genetic variation in PRN (and PT) molecules, with a shift over time among circulating strains toward variants not represented in the pertussis vaccine(s) in use in the community.[53] If confirmed, such a shift could reduce vaccine efficacy and thus might have implications for vaccine design.

Adenylate Cyclase. Adenylate cyclase is an enzyme that is released into culture medium, is present in all virulent strains of *B. pertussis*, and is noncytoplasmic, apparently being located on the cell membrane. In pertussis, adenylate cyclase compromises phagocytic cell functions (including chemotaxis, phagocytosis, and bacterial killing)[54] by augmenting production within the phagocyte of cyclic adenosine monophosphate from adenosine triphosphate, resulting in an excessive accumulation of cyclic adenosine monophosphate and paralysis of the various phagocytic functions. Adenylate cyclase may contribute to the excessive production of bronchial secretions during pertussis. In the mouse model of aerosol infection, PT and adenylate cyclase appear to be the two most important virulence factors.[55] Adenylate cyclase is immunogenic[56]; in the mouse models of intracerebral and aerosol challenge, prior active immunization with adenylate cyclase was shown to be similar in protective efficacy to whole-cell vaccine.[57] In addition, it has been shown that adenylate cyclase antibodies interfere with the multiplication of organisms in these models.[57]

Tracheal Cytotoxin. Tracheal cytotoxin appears to be a fragment released from the peptidoglycan of the *B. pertussis* cell wall.[58–60] It can be recovered from culture supernatant, is a very small molecule, and is nonimmunogenic. In vitro models suggest that it has a single major function: the paralysis and destruction of respiratory ciliated cells. Tracheal cytotoxin appears to be the only component of *B. pertussis* to exhibit this function.

Heat-Labile Toxin. Heat-labile toxin, so called because it is inactivated at 56°C, is also known as the dermonecrotic or mouse-lethal toxin because of its effects in experimental animals.[61] It is produced by all virulent *Bordetella* species. Located intracellularly, it can be recovered by disruption of *B. pertussis* cells. The mechanism of production of cutaneous lesions after injection of the toxin in animals appears to be vasoconstriction.[62] The role, if any, of heat-labile toxin in the pathogenesis of pertussis is unknown. No consistent effects on cells have been recognized in vitro. It is a weak immunogen, antibodies to it are nonprotective in animal challenge tests, and its absence does not diminish the lethality of experimental pertussis infection in mice.[55]

BrkA. BrkA (*Bordetella* resistance to killing genetic locus, frame A), another outer membrane protein of *B. pertussis* similar in structure to PRN, mediates adherence to respiratory cells and protects the bacterium against complement.[63]

Endotoxin. The endotoxin or lipopolysaccharide of *B. pertussis* exhibits many of the in vivo activities of endotoxins produced by other gram-negative organisms, but its role in the disease process or in recovery is unclear.[64] The endotoxin content of whole-cell vaccine may contribute to immediate adverse reactions in vaccinees.

Pathogenesis

Current knowledge of the components of *B. pertussis* and their actions permits construction of a reasonable hypothesis regarding the pathogenesis of whooping cough in humans.[65, 66] Transmission occurs when airborne bacteria from symptomatic patients reach the ciliated respiratory epithelium of a susceptible host. *B. pertussis* overcomes the mucosal immune defenses of the upper respiratory tract and causes disease in healthy individuals. The organisms attach strongly to the ciliated cells through several adhesins. Although PT and FHA are important attachment proteins, fimbriae, PRN, and BrkA participate in this process as well.[26, 36, 46, 66, 67] The bacteria do not invade beyond the epithelial layers of the respiratory tract, but PT enters the blood stream and exerts its biological effects on systemic sites. PT, adenylate cyclase, and BrkA have marked effects on host immune function.[26, 54, 63, 68] Adenylate cyclase induces production of high levels of cyclic adenosine monophosphate, disrupting the functions of several cell types of the immune system; PT inhibits chemotaxis of phagocytic cells into the site of inflammation; and BrkA protects the bacteria against complement attack.[63] Tracheal cytotoxin and dermonecrotic toxin are likely involved in the damage to the tracheobronchial epithelium that is so characteristic of the disease.[59–61]

Although this sequence may explain the respiratory manifestations of pertussis, the pathogenesis of the encephalopathy that can complicate clinical disease remains unclear.[69] Suggested pathogenetic mechanisms have included anoxia secondary to severe paroxysms, metabolic disturbances, hypoglycemia, or minute hemorrhages[69]; a direct toxic effect on the brain seems unlikely, given the fact that intravenous injection of substantial quantities of active PT into adult human volunteers caused no adverse effects.[35]

Diagnosis

The etiological agent responsible for an infectious disease is generally determined by culture of the organism, detection of antigens produced by the organism, or measurement of the immune response in serological studies. Even when using all these criteria, the confirmation of *B. pertussis* infection is still one of the most difficult diagnostic challenges facing the clinician, particularly in adolescents and adults. Pertussis organisms can be detected in the nasopharynx of patients with pertussis only early in the illness, when the symptoms are similar to those of the common cold. By the time severe cough appears, the organism has typically decreased in number or disappeared from the nasopharynx, making culture or antigen detection difficult.

Bacteriological Diagnosis

Culture. Culture of *B. pertussis* from the nasopharynx of symptomatic patients is compelling evidence of the disease. The optimum likelihood of isolating the organism is achieved by immediate inoculation onto fresh media early in the illness in a laboratory experienced with handling *B. pertussis*. At best, these conditions are difficult to meet, but even under optimum circumstances, the organism is frequently not recovered due to its fastidious nature and its disappearance later in the disease process.[70] Cultures obtained after 21 days of cough are significantly less likely to yield organisms.[71–74] Because the human nasopharynx is colonized with many respiratory bacteria, the use of selective media containing antibiotics such as cloxacillin and cephalexin may increase the yield of positive pertussis cultures by suppressing normal flora and allowing *Bordetella* to grow.[72] Two media are specialized for pertussis cultures: Bordet-Gengou medium, containing defibrinated horse blood and cloxacillin, and Regan-Lowe medium, containing charcoal agar, defibrinated horse blood, and cephalexin. Although Granstrom and colleagues have shown that the two media detect comparable numbers of positive cultures in symptomatic unimmunized children with pertussis,[75] others have reported better yield with Regan-Lowe medium.[72] Direct plating of the specimen at the bedside or clinic has also been shown to increase the yield of positive cultures, whereas prior therapy with erythromycin or sulfamethoxazole reduces the likelihood of positive cultures. Data from pertussis vaccine efficacy studies suggest that immunized individuals with pertussis have lower rates of positive cultures than unimmunized control subjects,[76] which further complicates the diagnosis of pertussis in partially or fully immunized children or adults.

Antigen Detection: Direct Fluorescent Antibody Test and Polymerase Chain Reaction. Antigen detection tests offer the important advantage that organisms do not have to be viable for detection and can therefore be detected later in the disease and in the presence of antibiotics. The first such test, the direct fluorescent antibody test (DFA), can achieve a specificity of 95% and a sensitivity of 61% (compared with culture) in experienced laboratories.[72, 73, 77] When properly performed, the DFA can provide a useful addition to culture and serology, particularly for the confirmation of clinically suspected cases. However, as with any test of less than perfect specificity, the positive predictive value of the test can be quite low when the true prevalence is low in the tested population.

More recently, polymerase chain reaction (PCR) assays have been developed for the identification of unique gene sequences of *B. pertussis* in respiratory secretions.[72, 78–83] Although bacteria can no longer be cultured after 5 days of therapy, the PCR can remain positive for an additional week.[84] Although used primarily for research at present, this rapid, highly sensitive and specific diagnostic method will likely become more widely available. Improved techniques, such as immunomagnetic and solid-phase detection methods, offer the promise that a single organism might be detected with this improved technology.

Two types of clinical samples have been tested: nasopharyngeal aspirates and nasopharyngeal swab specimens. During the investigation of pertussis epidemics, most studies have demonstrated that the PCR assay is more sensitive than culture in the diagnosis of pertussis and that nasopharyngeal swabs provide adequate samples for analysis. Several PCR assays have been developed, the majority of which target one of four chromosomal regions of the organism for PCR amplification: (1) the PT promoter region, (2) repeated insertion sequences, (3) a region upstream from the porin gene, and (4) the adenylate cyclase toxin gene. A more recent study examined the nationwide use of a PCR assay in Finland and Switzerland from nearly 4000 clinical samples and found that the sensitivity of the PT promoter–based PCR was higher than that of the insertion sequence–based PCR.[85] The PCR remained positive longer than culture and offered results more rapidly. *B. pertussis* cultures typically take 3 to 7 days to become positive, whereas PCR can be completed in 1 to 2 days.[85]

Serological Diagnosis

Although they are not available for routine clinical use, serological tests for antibodies to various components of *B. pertussis* have been used extensively for a variety of investigational purposes.[72, 86] Serological testing avoids the lack of sensitivity and other known limitations of culture methods and has also improved our understanding of the clinical spectrum of pertussis, particularly by demonstrating asymptomatic, mild, or atypical infections in partially immune individuals.[19, 87–89] Serological studies have been used to examine the natural history of pertussis in unimmunized populations by determining the prevalence of antibodies at various ages,[90, 91] and they have been shown to be useful in monitoring the incidence of pertussis during regional outbreaks.[92] Serological studies have been of considerable value in monitoring clinical outcomes in trials of newer pertussis vaccines, because partially immune individuals may incur pertussis infection but display few or no symptoms.[76]

Tests used to measure serum antibodies to *B. pertussis* include complement fixation, agglutination tests, toxin neutralization, and enzyme-linked immunosorbent assays (ELISAs).[72] Of these tests, ELISAs are used most frequently because they are the easiest to perform and can detect specific immunoglobulin (Ig) classes. Another advantage of the ELISA method is that serum antibodies against specific antigens of *B. pertussis* can be readily measured; for example, IgG and IgA antibodies to PT and FHA are among those commonly assayed.

The most conclusive serological evidence of an infection is the demonstration of a significant rise in specific antibodies as a consequence of the infection. Pertussis presents a considerable problem in this regard, because the frequently subtle early course of the disease does not excite suspicion of the diagnosis for several weeks. By this time, a substantial rise in serum antibodies has already occurred, thus compromising the likelihood of a significant increase between the initial and follow-up serum specimens. An approach that avoids this problem has been taken in studies of people with respiratory illnesses who are suspected of having pertussis.[87–90] In these studies, the range of antibody levels is determined in a comparable, control population of people who are not suspected to have pertussis. The distribution of antibody levels in single specimens from the population under investigation is determined and compared with that of the normal population. Those subjects whose antibody levels, singly or in various combinations, exceed the mean of the control population by a selected factor (typically, two or three standard deviations) are assumed to have experienced recent infection.

A somewhat different problem is presented by the use of serological testing to detect pertussis in field trials of pertussis vaccine. It is possible to obtain serum specimens from study subjects in advance of infection, thereby enabling one to detect a rise in antibodies if a suspicious illness occurs. Although this approach is valid for nonimmunized control subjects, detection of antibody increases may be compromised in those who were immunized, because immunization itself leads to increases in antibody titer. In this situation, the development of antibodies against an antigen of *B. pertussis* that was not included in the vaccine can be useful. The fact that IgA responses to PT and FHA occur in about half of all infections but rarely after immunization may have useful application to vaccine trials.

Treatment and Prevention with Antibiotics

All patients with suspected pertussis should receive erythromycin therapy. Treatment can be expected to ameliorate the patient's symptoms only if it is begun early in the catarrhal phase. Treatment can still be beneficial, however, even if it is begun after symptoms have become established, since antibiotics may hasten clearance of the organism and limit spread to other susceptible contacts.[4, 93, 94]

Erythromycin, especially the estolate form, has been considered the most active drug against pertussis.[93, 94] The dosage of erythromycin is 40 to 50 mg per kg per day, with a maximum of 2 g per day, given every 6 hours. Because bacterial relapses have been reported with shorter courses of therapy, it has traditionally been recommended that treatment continue for 14 days. A recent trial comparing therapy with erythromycin estolate for 7 days (74 patients) and 14 days (94 patients) found overall failure rates of 2.70 and 1.06%, respectively.[95] Although these rates did not differ significantly and both failure rates are quite low, the point estimates nonetheless indicate a more than twofold higher failure rate with 7-day therapy. Another study has suggested that the necessary duration of therapy is related to the age of the patient, with very young patients requiring longer therapy than older patients.[96]

The newer macrolides azithromycin and clarithromycin have good penetration into relevant tissues, are effective in vitro, and offer reduced adverse effects and a simplified dosing regimen. A small Japanese study compared once-daily azithromycin for 5 days (8 patients) and twice-daily clarithromycin for 7 days (9 patients) with matched historical control subjects given erythromycin for 14 days.[97] Eradication rates after azithromycin and clarithromycin were both 100%, compared with 13 of 16 and 16 of 18 among the respective matched controls; no bacterial relapses were detected.

In situations in which macrolides are not tolerated, trimethoprim-sulfamethoxazole (8 mg of trimethoprim/kg/d in two divided doses) has been recommended, although few data exist to confirm its efficacy.[98]

Bronchodilators have not been shown to be beneficial, and cough suppressants and antihistamines may be counterproductive. Corticosteroids may be considered in seriously ill infants.[94]

A 14-day course of erythromycin is recommended for antibiotic prophylaxis of household and other close contacts, regardless of vaccination status, and for health-care workers with a high risk of or known exposure.[99–101] The newer macrolides presumably might be substituted, but no data are available. Prophylaxis reduces, but does not eliminate, the risk of pertussis.[102, 103] Prophylaxis within a household is substantially more effective if given before the appearance of the first secondary case.[103] Cases and inadequately vaccinated contacts younger than 7 years should be excluded from school, daycare, and similar settings until they have received at least 5 days of prophylaxis or therapy.[99]

EPIDEMIOLOGY

Overview

Pertussis is an endemic disease with epidemic peaks occurring every 2 to 5 years (most commonly, every 3 to 4 years).[104] Widespread vaccination of children and the consequent reduction in the incidence of disease do not appear to have altered these intervals,[104–106] suggesting that there continues to be ongoing endemic circulation of the organism in the community.[107, 108] There is no consistent seasonal pattern. Some studies have reported a summertime peak; others have failed to demonstrate seasonal peaks or have indicated that peaks are more apt to occur during the winter months.[106, 109, 110] From 1980 to 1989, the peak incidence in the United States occurred during the early summer in the warmer states and between June and October in the northern states.[111] Reported morbidity and mortality rates are higher in females than in males. There is no evidence that females are more susceptible to infection than males; furthermore, before the development of pertussis vaccine, it was expected that every child would have whooping cough sooner or later. It is therefore likely that the disease is more severe in female patients, which results in more ready recognition and higher mortality than in male patients. One explanation for this phenomenon is that for the first 6 months of life male infants have considerably higher levels of testosterone than do female infants, which perhaps results in a larger laryngeal airway and thus less likelihood of obstruction (J. Germak, personal communication, 1986).[112] Another explanation might be that the sexes differ in their immune responses to pertussis infection.

Pertussis is acquired through direct transmission from close respiratory contact. Transmission by the indirect route from airborne droplet nuclei or organisms on fomites or in dust occurs extremely rarely, if ever. Whooping cough is highly contagious: As many as 90% of susceptible household contacts acquire the disease. Rates of transmission in school settings range from 50 to 80%.[113]

Pertussis may occur at any age. Infants are susceptible to pertussis within the first few weeks or months of life, when mortality from whooping cough is highest. For many years, it was assumed that one attack of pertussis provided lifelong immunity. Before widespread vaccination, this belief was reflected by the age distribution of pertussis: approximately 20% of all whooping cough cases occurred in infants younger than 1 year, and as much as 60%, among children aged 1 to 4 years.[109] Anecdotal information indicated that second attacks of pertussis did occur in the prevaccine era, such as in older persons exposed to grandchildren with the disease, although these instances were rarely described and incompletely documented.[114] A chronic carrier state has not been demonstrated,[115] but evidence for such a state may be compromised by the insensitivity of culture methods.[116]

More recently, in countries such as the United States in which pertussis vaccination is common, the age distribution of pertussis has changed markedly. Between 1992 and 1994, 28% of reported pertussis cases occurred in individuals 10 years and older,[12] in contrast to less than 3% of patients being older than 15 years before the advent of widespread vaccination[109]; 41% of cases providing age data occurred in infants younger than 1 year, compared with 45% in the prior 3-year period.[117]

Pertussis is seen increasingly in adolescents. In 1965, Lambert reported an outbreak in Michigan, in which the highest attack rates were seen in individuals older than 10 years, and concluded that "the direct relationship of increased pertussis incidence in vaccinated people to increased interval since the last injection of pertussis-containing vaccine was the most significant study finding."[114] During an outbreak in an immunized population in Finland, the attack rate (per 100,000) of laboratory-confirmed pertussis was 317 in children younger than 4 years, 1838 in children 4 to 6 years of age, and 2535 in children 7 to 15 years of age.[118] In a Wisconsin outbreak, adolescents were at a higher risk than any other age group for the acquisition of pertussis.[119] Reports of pertussis outbreaks have appeared in middle-school and high-school populations, and statewide surveillance in Massachusetts has shown that the incidence of confirmed pertussis in people 11 to 19 years of age has increased.[111, 120, 121]

Pertussis occurs in adults of all ages, most of whom were vaccinated or experienced the disease in the past. Of 218 Australian adults referred for investigation of chronic cough, 56 (26%) had pertussis IgA antibody levels more than three standard deviations higher than normal.[122] Similarly, Mink and colleagues found that 26% of students presenting to a university student health service with cough of at least 6 days' duration had serological evidence of pertussis.[88] During the 1993 pertussis epidemic in Chicago, 10 (26%) of 38 adults presenting to a clinic with unexplained cough had serological evidence of pertussis.[123] Of adults presenting to an emergency department with cough persisting 2 weeks or longer, 21% had serological evidence of pertussis.[124] Of adult patients in a large California healthcare plan who were referred for chronic cough, 12.4% had evidence of recent pertussis,[125] representing an incidence of 176 per 100,000 person-years—a rate greater than the annual incidence of reported pertussis (157/100,000) in the United States in the prevaccine era. These reports have shown clearly that chronic cough may be the sole manifestation of pertussis among adolescents and adults and that adults with pertussis cannot be differentiated on clinical grounds from other adult patients with cough.[124]

Further insight into the epidemiology of pertussis in a highly vaccinated population comes from a serosurvey of 600 normal healthy individuals aged 1 to 65 years (Fig. 14–2).[90] The results demonstrated not only the expected peak in PT and FHA titers in the 4- to 6-year-old group, reflecting the administration of booster doses of pertussis vaccine, but also a second, larger peak in the 13- to 17-year-old group, suggesting that natural acquisition of pertussis is frequent during the adolescent years.

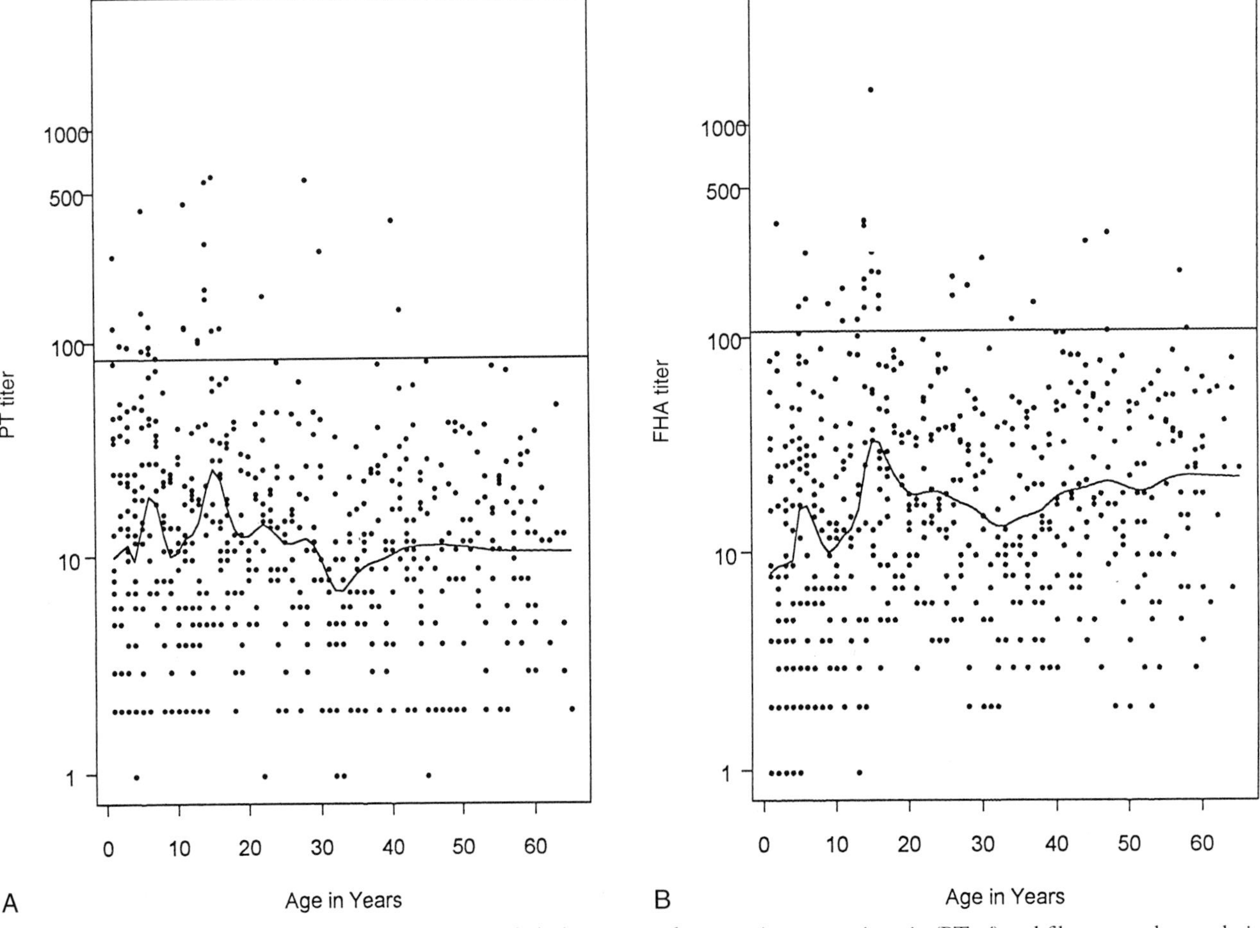

Figure 14–2. Serological responses (as measured by enzyme-linked immunosorbent assay) to pertussis toxin (PT; *A*) and filamentous hemagglutinin (FHA; *B*) of 600 normal healthy individuals aged 1 to 65 years. Solid lines show geometric mean titers by age; each dot represents one subject. (Adapted from Cattaneo LA, Reed G, Haase DH, et al. The seroepidemiology of *Bordetella pertussis* infections: A study of persons aged 1–65 years. J Infect Dis 173:1256–1259, 1996.)

In many adolescent and adult infections, symptoms are mild or even absent, and cases are recognized only because of the presence of an outbreak. Serological studies during outbreaks have demonstrated the occurrence of frequent asymptomatic infections or illnesses, indistinguishable from mild viral upper respiratory disorders, among previously vaccinated people or among those with a past history of pertussis.[19, 87–89] How contagious these infections are is unknown, but it is clear that infected adults have been responsible for the transmission of disease to young infants and children.[14, 19] In the Chicago outbreak, for example, young mothers were an important source of pertussis for their infants.[123]

In part, the increase in recognized cases of pertussis in older individuals may represent enhanced suspicion and recognition, improved reporting of adult pertussis, or better diagnostic methods. However, the most important factor has probably been waning vaccine-induced immunity, coupled with the infrequency of pertussis in well-immunized populations and thus fewer opportunities for the reinforcement of immunity by casual exposure. Immunity after vaccination was previously thought to be of shorter duration than that after natural disease, but this concept has been challenged recently by the frequent diagnosis of pertussis in German adults who had experienced previous natural infection.[16] It is also possible that vaccine-induced immunity is less vigorous or that it provides more protection against disease manifestations than against infection.[19] Whatever the reasons, the increased recognition of pertussis in older individuals has stimulated interest in booster immunization of adolescents and adults.

Incidence of Pertussis in the United States

Disease caused by *B. pertussis* was once a major cause of morbidity and mortality among infants and children. From the 1920s (when pertussis was first a reportable disease) until the early 1940s, there were 115,000 to 270,000 cases of pertussis reported, with 5000 to 10,000 deaths each year, representing approximately 150 cases and 6 deaths per 100,000 population, respectively.[4] As pertussis vaccine came to be used commonly in infants and children, the incidence of pertussis markedly decreased (Fig. 14–3).[111] By the 1970s, the annual incidence of reported disease had been reduced by 99%, and the lowest annual number of cases of pertussis—1010—was reported in 1976. Reported cases began to increase in the 1980s: From 1980 to 1989, 27,826 cases of pertussis were reported to the CDC, for a crude incidence of 1.2 cases per 100,000 population. The U.S. pertussis case-fatality rate during the 1980s was estimated to be 0.6%.[111] Cyclical peaks in pertussis incidence were noted in 1983, 1986, 1990, 1993, and 1996, with each peak surpassing the last. The highest number of cases since 1964 (7796 cases) was reported in 1996. From January 1992 to June 1995, the majority (63%) of reported cases occurred among persons who had received fewer than three doses of pertussis vaccine[12]; however, many of these persons were younger than 6 months and had thus not received three doses. Among reported pertussis patients aged 7 months to 4 years, 23% had received no doses; 22%, one or two doses; and 55%, three or more doses.[12]

Several large pertussis outbreaks have been reported in recent years.[78, 92, 123, 126–128] In the 1993 outbreak, the median age of patients in Chicago was 8 months, and many children had received fewer than three vaccine doses.[123] In Cincinnati, the median age was 17 months, and most of the children had received at least three doses of vaccine.[126] A statewide outbreak of pertussis in 1996 in Vermont, a highly vaccinated population, affected primarily school-aged children and adults.[128] Multiple outbreaks of disease have also been reported from Canada.[78, 92] Many researchers have speculated about the reasons for this increase in pertussis disease. Some have noted that the two commercial whole-cell vaccines used most recently in the United States produce substantially different antibody responses, with one generating little

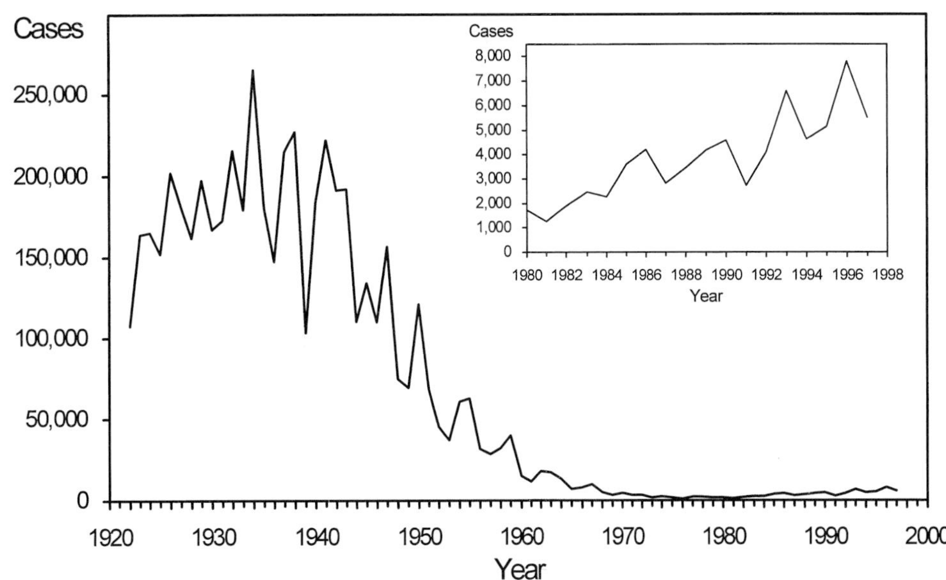

Figure 14–3. Number of reported pertussis cases, by year, in the United States from 1922 to 1997. Data for 1997 are provisional. (Data for 1922–1996 from W. Orenstein, personal communication, Centers for Disease Control and Prevention; data for 1997 from Provisional cases of selected notifiable diseases preventable by vaccination, United States, weeks ending December 27, 1997, and December 28, 1996 [52nd week]. MMWR Morb Mortal Wkly Rep 46:1263, 1996.)

antibody to PT and the other little antibody to FHA. These researchers have suggested that the increase in pertussis disease may be a result of vaccines that are less immunogenic than previously believed.[129, 130] Evidence for this concern has been provided by the pertussis vaccine efficacy trials conducted in Europe in the early 1990s, which found adequate efficacy after three doses for one U.S. whole-cell vaccine[131] but quite low efficacy for the other.[132, 133] Most cases of pertussis among recipients of the latter vaccine occurred after the age at which a fourth dose of vaccine is recommended in the United States.[132, 133] These results are completely consistent with U.S. surveillance data from 1992 to 1994 that found an overall whole-cell pertussis vaccine efficacy of 64% after three doses and of 82% after four or more doses.[12]

Significance of Pertussis as a Global Public Health Problem

During the 1990s in the United States, an average of fewer than 10 deaths from pertussis has been recorded annually. The remarkable decline in mortality from the disease since the 1950s is clearly attributable to widespread use of whole-cell vaccine.[134] Nonetheless, as noted, the occurrence of pertussis appears to be increasing in the United States, particularly among adolescents and adults, and continues to pose a substantial burden.

In the developing world, the situation is very different and is reminiscent of that existing in the United States earlier in the century. Data collected by the Expanded Programme on Immunization (EPI) of the WHO in 1992 indicated that 850,000 of the approximately 110 million children born annually in the developing world a decade earlier succumbed to pertussis before their fifth birthdays. Obviously, complicating factors such as low birth weight, malnutrition, and other infections, particularly intestinal and respiratory, contribute to mortality from pertussis in these population groups. A more recent WHO estimate illustrates both the success of the Expanded Programme on Immunization and the substantial work yet to be done: In 1994, 40 million pertussis infections resulted in 5 million episodes of pneumonia, 360,000 deaths (a nearly 60% reduction), and 50,000 patients with long-term neurological complications (including permanent brain damage).[6]

PASSIVE IMMUNIZATION

Transplacental

Antibodies to PT and FHA readily cross the placenta and are found in infant sera in concentrations comparable to those in maternal sera. The half-life of these transplacental antibodies appears to be about 6 weeks, and they usually disappear by 4 months of age.[135] However, these antibodies appear to offer little or no clinical protection, because infants of mothers who are presumed to be immune to pertussis, whether because of immunization or disease, are susceptible to pertussis on exposure. Indeed, from 1980 to 1989, 31% of the cases of pertussis reported to the CDC were in children younger than 6 months, and the highest average annual age-specific incidence rate during those years was among infants 1 to 2 months of age.[111]

Therapeutic

Before the widespread use of pertussis vaccine and the availability of antibiotics, passive immunization using whole sera was employed in an effort to prevent the spread of disease to exposed susceptible people and to modify the course of the illness in those who had already acquired whooping cough.[136] Most of the studies of preventive efficacy in exposed individuals were not controlled; a few studies that did include control subjects suggested that as many as 40% of recipients were protected.[8, 32, 136]

The subsequent development of methods for purification of serum immune globulins led to the commercial production of pertussis hyperimmune globulin, composed largely of IgG.[137] Although this preparation was widely used for prophylaxis and treatment, controlled studies indicated that it had no effect, and production was discontinued.[138, 139]

More recently, new preparations of pertussis immune globulin have been prepared and evaluated in animal models and humans. Sato and Sato demonstrated that both monoclonal and polyclonal antibodies to PT improved survival of suckling mice after aerosol challenge with live pertussis organisms.[33] The ability to generate high-titer immune globulin by immunizing adults with safe acellular pertussis vaccines led to a reassessment of the use of immune globulin as therapy for pertussis. In 1991, Granstrom and colleagues conducted a double-blind, randomized, placebo-controlled trial of a pertussis immune globulin prepared from adults immunized with an acellular vaccine containing either PT or PT plus FHA.[140] A significant reduction in the duration of whoops was demonstrated in the recipients of the pertussis immune globulin compared with placebo recipients (8.7 vs. 20.6 d; $P = .0041$). A pertussis immune globulin has been prepared by the Massachusetts Biologic Laboratories using serum from adults immunized with monovalent pertussis toxoid vaccine. This product has been evaluated in the mouse aerosol model of pertussis and in phase 1 trials in infants.[141] Preliminary studies have demonstrated clinical improvement, and further studies are under way.

ACTIVE IMMUNIZATION: WHOLE-CELL VACCINES

History

The isolation and propagation of *B. pertussis* on artificial media in 1906 offered hope for the prevention of whooping cough, a disease that at the turn of the century killed more than 5 of every 1000 children born in the United States. Initial steps to develop a vaccine were empirical, given the lack of understanding of the biological anatomy of the organism and its relationship to the pathogenesis of the disease. An improved understanding of the different phases of the organism led to refinement in the methods of production and resulted in a whole-cell vaccine prepared in a standardized and reproducible fashion. During the 1980s and 1990s, knowledge of the components of the pertussis organism and their biological roles has led to the development of the acellular pertussis vaccines.

Whole-cell pertussis vaccine was first licensed in the United States in 1914 and became available combined with diphtheria and tetanus toxoids (DTP) in 1948. Since its introduction, DTP has been recommended and widely used for the routine vaccination of children in the United States. Because of state laws mandating vaccination for school entry, almost all U.S. children are vaccinated.

Development

Whole-cell pertussis vaccines are suspensions of killed *B. pertussis* organisms. Early vaccines were remarkably crude and of uncertain content; they sometimes included mixed respiratory flora along with *B. pertussis* and were used for treatment as well as prophylaxis.[142] One of the first clinical trials of a whole-cell vaccine was conducted during an epidemic of pertussis in the Faroe Islands and provided evidence of efficacy.[143] Subsequent trials of similarly constituted vaccines yielded varying results, and some showed no apparent effect.[8] In the 1930s, steps taken to improve vaccines included increasing the number of bacteria in the vaccine; using standardized culture media; inactivating the organisms by "gentler" methods; and using fresh, rapidly growing (phase 1) organisms.[23, 32]

A major stumbling block in the development and assessment of pertussis vaccines was the lack of a suitable means other than clinical trials for assessing the immunizing capability of a vaccine. Serological tests did not correlate satisfactorily with clinical protection, and attempts to produce disease in mice by respiratory or intraperitoneal inoculation were not useful. Indeed, it was not until after World War II that a laboratory test that reproducibly measured vaccine potency was devised. In this mouse protection test, mice are immunized with pertussis vaccine and then challenged by intracerebral inoculation of living *B. pertussis* organisms.[144] Although several antigens of *B. pertussis* affect the results of the mouse protection test and it is not clear that the mouse-protective and human-protective antigens are identical, the results of the mouse protection test were shown to correlate well with protective efficacy in humans.[145, 146] The mouse protection test enabled standardized whole-cell vaccines to be produced. Although the test has remained the measure of potency for more than 40 years, recent efficacy trials, discussed later, have made it clear that whole-cell vaccines that are of low efficacy (36–48% when given at 2, 4, and 6 months of age without a booster at 12–18 months of age) may nonetheless pass the mouse potency test.

Whole-cell pertussis vaccines have been produced in the United States by methods that vary somewhat among manufacturers.[23] The organism may be grown in liquid or solid media, and, after harvesting, the bacteria are inactivated by any of several methods (usually by formalin). In the United States, pertussis vaccine is almost always administered to children in combination with diphtheria and tetanus toxoids. This combination is adsorbed onto an aluminum salt, which results in greater immunogenicity and less reactivity.

Early attempts to extract *B. pertussis* cells and produce an effective subcellular vaccine resulted in Trisolgen, a product distributed by Eli Lilly and Company from 1962 to 1977.[23] In comparison to whole-cell vaccines, this more purified preparation produced less local reactivity and less fever, probably at least in part because of the removal of some cellular debris and endotoxin[147]; it is not clear what antigens the vaccine contained. Although this vaccine passed the mouse protection test and produced agglutinating antibody, clinical field trials for the determination of protection against disease were never conducted, and it is not known whether this vaccine produced fewer (or more) reactions considered to be worrisome or severe, compared with whole-cell vaccines. This product became unavailable when the manufacturer withdrew from the vaccine market.

Available Preparations

Constituents and Stability

In the early 1970s, DTP vaccine was distributed in the United States by seven commercial manufacturers and three state laboratories. Two non-U.S. manufacturers subsequently received licensure for the distribution of DTP in the United States. In more recent years, however, only four U.S. manufacturers have produced whole-cell DTP vaccine: Connaught Laboratories and Wyeth-Lederle Vaccines and Pediatrics, for commercial distribution; Massachusetts Public Health Biologic Laboratories; and the Michigan Department of Public Health. The Michigan Department of Public Health has also produced a monocomponent pertussis vaccine. Wyeth-Lederle also produces a combination vaccine that incorporates their DTP with their conjugate *H. influenzae* type b (Hib) vaccine; the Connaught DTP can be used to reconstitute their Hib vaccine, thereby permitting both products to be delivered with a single injection.

In the United States, each manufacturer's methods of production must be approved by the Food and Drug Administration (FDA), and each lot of vaccine must be submitted to certain test procedures by the FDA and the manufacturer. For whole-cell vaccines, these procedures include the assessment of potency by the mouse protection test and the assessment of toxicity by the mouse weight-gain (toxicity) test. The opacity of the vaccine is determined to ensure that it does not contain excessive numbers of bacteria. Other standard tests, such as those for sterility, are also employed.

The available DTP vaccines differ slightly in their content of diphtheria and tetanus toxoids (6.5–12.5 limit of flocculation units [Lf] of diphtheria toxoid, and 5–5.5 Lf of tetanus toxoid). All vaccines nominally contain 4 units of pertussis content, as measured by the opacity test, and achieve 12 mouse protection test potency units per total human immunizing dose (normally, three 0.5-mL doses). All contain an aluminum salt as adjuvant; concentrations range from 0.25 to 0.8 mg of aluminum per 0.5 mL. All contain 0.01% thimerosal as preservative. All are to be stored at 2 to 8°C and should not be frozen; all expire within 18 months.

It is likely that all the whole-cell pertussis vaccines will disappear from the U.S. marketplace within the next few years. Acellular vaccines are likely to represent the majority of pertussis vaccines used in a number of other countries as well, particularly in Europe and the Americas, but whole-cell vaccine will remain the most widely used globally for some time to come. Whole-cell vaccines are produced locally in many regions of the world, are efficacious, and are inexpensive to produce. Each country will have to evaluate, based on its own circumstances, the relative virtues of the cost, efficacy, and adverse reactions of available whole-cell and acellular vaccines.

There are far too many whole-cell vaccines produced globally to permit a complete listing here. Prominent commercial vaccines include those produced by Behringwerke Aktiengesellischaft, Pasteur Mérieux Connaught, SmithKline Beecham, and Wellcome Foundation (Evans Medical). Some of these vaccines are available in combination with Hib, enhanced inactivated polio vaccine (IPV), or hepatitis B vaccine (see Chapter 20).

Dosage and Route

All the U.S. whole-cell pertussis vaccines are available in multidose vials except for the Wyeth-Lederle DTP/Hib combination vaccine, which is supplied in single-dose vials. For all vaccines, the standard dose is 0.5 mL given intramuscularly in the anterolateral thigh or, if necessary, the deltoid. It is inappropriate to give a partial dose in the hope of reducing adverse effects.

Indications for Vaccine

With licensure of the combination diphtheria and tetanus toxoids and acellular pertussis vaccine (DTaP) for primary vaccination of infants, recommendations for the use of whole-cell DTP in the United States have been modified extensively. Both the Advisory Committee on Immunization Practices (ACIP) of the CDC and the Committee on Infectious Diseases of the American Academy of Pediatrics (the Red Book Committee) have recommended that the acellular vaccine be preferred for all doses in the vaccination schedule, although DTP remains an acceptable alternative for any of the five doses. A more complete discussion of the recommendations for acellular pertussis vaccine is given later in this chapter.

Immunization of Infants and Children

Unless specifically contraindicated (see later), every infant should receive pertussis vaccine (normally as DTaP or DTP) at ages 2, 4, and 6 months and 15 to 18 months; a booster is indicated at 4 to 6 years of age. The timing of infant vaccination is determined by birth age, without regard to prematurity.[98, 148] Children whose vaccination series has been interrupted need not have prior doses repeated but should have their series resumed at the earliest opportunity.

Immunization of Adolescents and Adults

With the availability of acellular vaccines that are safe and immunogenic (although as yet not licensed) for use in adults (see later in this chapter), it is difficult to conceive of a situation in which one would use whole-cell vaccine to protect adults from pertussis.

Use of Vaccine in Outbreaks

Immunization initiated after an exposure does not protect from that exposure; in an outbreak, however, exposure opportunities are ongoing, and the existence of an outbreak should reinvigorate efforts to properly immunize those who have not completed a full vaccination schedule. An accelerated infant vaccination schedule (e.g., 4, 8, and 12 weeks of age) may be indicated.[99]

Numerous nosocomial pertussis outbreaks involving healthcare workers have been reported.[101] In 1974, whole-cell vaccine was administered to 286 healthcare workers during a hospital outbreak[149]; 77% of vaccinees had a fourfold increase in pertussis agglutinins. Injection-site redness or swelling of 6 cm or more in diameter was seen in 45% of vaccinees; 97% noted pain at the injection site; 27% noted limitation of motion of the inoculated arm; and 10% had oral temperature 100°F (37.8°C) or greater. Two subjects had generalized rash, and one required steroid therapy. The only central nervous system symptoms were headaches, lethargy, and dizziness. Later that year, 449 more hospital staff members were vaccinated. Local reactions were reported to be less severe than in the earlier study; the whole-cell vaccine was generally perceived much as a "tetanus shot." However, one medical student had a transient episode of memory difficulty 1 day after the vaccine.[149]

Contraindications and Precautions

Normal Infants and Children

Older recommendations regarding contraindications and precautions reflected concerns that are not supported by more recent data. At present, there are but two true contraindications to the use of pertussis vaccine: anaphylaxis or encephalopathy following prior administration of a vaccine containing a pertussis component.[98, 148]

An anaphylactic reaction occurring immediately after administration of DTaP or whole-cell DTP is a contraindication to further vaccination with separate diphtheria, tetanus, or pertussis (acellular or whole-cell) components, absent proof as to which of these three components was responsible. Given the importance of tetanus vaccination, referral to an allergist for tetanus toxoid desensitization may be indicated. Acute encephalopathy occurring within 7 days after administration of DTP or DTaP, not attributable to another identifiable cause, is a contraindication to further pertussis immunization. DT vaccine should be administered for the remaining doses in the vaccination schedule, although it may be appropriate to delay vaccination until the patient's neurological status is clear.[98, 148]

The following are now considered precautions, not contraindications, to pertussis vaccine: temperature 40.5°C or greater (105°F) within 48 hours of pertussis vaccination, not due to another identified cause; collapse or shock-like state (termed a *hypotonic-hyporesponsive episode*) within 48 hours; persistent, inconsolable crying lasting 3 or more hours, occurring within 48 hours; and convulsions occurring within 3 days, with or without fever. Decisions regarding the further administration of pertussis vaccine should be guided by an individualized evaluation of benefits and risks.[98, 148] Those risks are likely to be substantially lower if acellular, rather than whole-cell, pertussis vaccine is used (see later).

A family history of seizures, adverse reactions to vaccine, or allergy to vaccine is not a contraindication to the receipt of DTaP. Administration of pertussis vaccine should be deferred briefly for children with moderate or severe acute illnesses, with or without fever; they may be vaccinated as soon as they recover. Children who are immunocompromised or are receiving immunosuppressive therapy may be vaccinated with DTP. If immunosuppressive therapy will be discontinued soon, deferral of vaccination until 1 month after therapy may permit better immune responses.

Children with Neurological Disorders

As is discussed under *Adverse Events*, pertussis vaccine may precipitate febrile convulsions and may unmask neurological disorders that would soon have become evident anyway, but it does not appear to cause or worsen chronic neurological disorders. Because children with neurological impairments are as needful—indeed, perhaps more needful—of protection from pertussis disease as are normal children, any decision to decline pertussis vaccination should reflect a careful consideration of risks and benefits, particularly in light of the increasing incidence of pertussis.[98, 148] It may be appropriate to delay pertussis vaccination of infants with neurological disorders until their status is clarified, but again careful consideration is required. The highest risk of pertussis is in the first 6 months of life, whereas the risk of febrile convulsions is higher thereafter; both factors therefore argue for adherence to the standard schedule.

Children with prior convulsions should probably have pertussis vaccine deferred until the cause of the convulsions is assessed and any necessary treatment is established. Febrile seizures unrelated to pertussis vaccine are not a contraindication to pertussis vaccine, nor is a family history of seizures.[148] Administration of acetaminophen at a dose of 15 mg per kg should also be considered at the time of vaccination and every 4 hours for the ensuing 24 hours.[148]

False Contraindications

A number of situations have incorrectly been considered to be contraindications, and deferral of pertussis vaccination on these bases is inappropriate: redness, swelling, or pain at the injection site; temperature less than 40.5°C (105°F); mild acute illness, even involving diarrhea or low-grade fever; current antibiotic therapy; recent exposure to an infectious disease; prematurity; personal or family history of allergies; and family history of sudden infant death syndrome (SIDS), convulsions, or adverse event after pertussis vaccination.[148] Prior pertussis infection is not a contraindication to vaccination; although a previously infected child may not require vaccination for immunity, proceeding with vaccination obviates the risk that the prior illness was not in fact pertussis.

Simultaneous Administration with Other Vaccines

Whole-cell pertussis vaccine is commonly administered simultaneously not only with diphtheria and tetanus toxoids but also with oral polio vaccine or IPV, conjugate Hib vaccine, hepatitis B vaccine, measles-mumps-rubella vaccine, and varicella vaccine (see Chapter 20). A few studies have found reduced immunogenicity of whole-cell pertussis vaccine when given in combination or association with one or more of these other vaccines, but there are no data to suggest that any of these other vaccines decreases the efficacy of whole-cell pertussis vaccine.[150, 151]

RESULTS OF VACCINATION: WHOLE-CELL VACCINES

Overview

Although some observers have challenged whole-cell pertussis vaccine as being ineffective, dangerous, or superfluous,[152, 153] most authorities agree that the widespread use of the vaccine has had enormous benefits.[134, 154, 155] Observations that have led to this conclusion include the results of clinical trials, including the rapid decline in morbidity and mortality from pertussis concomitant with the implementation of vaccine programs; the recurrence of disease in countries in which immunization has been discontinued, rates of acceptance have declined markedly, or vaccines have become ineffective; the inverse correlation of the pertussis attack rate with the proportion of immunized children in communities in which pertussis becomes epidemic; and the lower attack rates in previously immunized children than in unimmunized children under both endemic and epidemic conditions.

Immune Responses

Several studies have demonstrated substantial differences in the immune responses stimulated by the various whole-cell vaccines in recent use in the United States.[129, 156] One study compared the Wyeth-Lederle and Massachusetts whole-cell vaccines.[156] The Wyeth-Lederle vaccine stimulated substantial levels of antibody to all measured components except FHA, to which it produced a minimal response. In comparison, the Massachusetts vaccine produced higher levels of antibody to FHA (51 vs. 3 ELISA units) and PRN (99 vs. 63) and lower levels of antibody to PT (20 vs. 67) and FIM (70 vs. 191); all differences were significant.[156] Another report comparing the Wyeth-Lederle and Connaught whole-cell vaccines found that the Connaught vaccine produced only minimal responses to PT (5 ELISA units vs. 66 for the Wyeth-Lederle vaccine in one series; 1 vs. 26 in another series) but higher levels of agglutinating antibodies (15 vs. 4 dilutions). These results differed significantly, whereas FHA responses did not.[129] Another study found that the whole-cell DTP produced by Connaught Canada for use in that country stimulated even lower levels of antibody to PT than did either the Wyeth-Lederle or Connaught USA DTPs.[157]

It has been demonstrated that the antibody response to primary immunization of infants with whole-cell vaccine depends on the preimmunization (transplacental) levels of antibody to PT. Higher circulating levels of maternally derived antibody were associated with significantly lower levels of postimmunization antibody.[135] In contrast, PT antibody responses to an acellular vaccine containing 12.5 μg each of PT and FHA were superior to those of the whole-cell vaccine and were not affected by prevaccination antibody levels.[135]

Controlled Clinical Trials

It is well documented by controlled clinical trials that pertussis vaccine provides protection against clinical whooping cough after exposure in the majority of immunized people. The first convincing evidence was provided by studies in the Faroe Islands during two epidemics.[143] These studies showed that pertussis vaccine not only protected against disease but also ameliorated the severity of disease in immunized individuals who contracted the illness. Although studies with early vaccines produced inconsistent results,[8, 134, 155, 158] clinical trials subsequent to standardization of the vaccines by the mouse protection test[154] demonstrated clear-cut, consistent efficacy.[154, 159, 160]

In more recent years, a number of field trials of acellular pertussis vaccines (see under *Efficacy Trials, 1992 to 1997*) have incorporated whole-cell pertussis vaccines as controls and have provided some of the best data ever obtained about the efficacy of the conventional whole-cell vaccines. These studies suggest that whole-cell vaccines vary substantially in efficacy (the following estimates reflect efficacy after three doses and, to the extent possible, consistent case definitions; however, none of these studies was fully blinded and randomized, and these estimates may be generous). The Mainz[161] and Munich[162] studies produced efficacy estimates of 98% and 96% respectively for the German-produced Behringwerke vaccine; the U.S.-made Wyeth-Lederle whole-cell vaccine was reported to be 83% efficacious in the Erlangen trial[131, 163]; and the Senegal trial reported the French-made Pasteur Mérieux whole-cell vaccine to be 96% efficacious.[164] In each of these trials, the whole-cell vaccine was more efficacious than the acellular product.

In marked contrast, the U.S.-made Connaught whole-cell vaccine had very low rates of efficacy after three doses: 48% in Sweden and 36% in Italy.[132, 133] Vaccine efficacy of the Connaught whole-cell vaccine was nearly 74% for the first 6 months after the third dose of vaccine but declined rapidly after that time.[132]

A British national survey of reported whooping cough from 1989 to 1990 determined that the efficacy of the Wellcome whole-cell vaccine, administered at 3, 5, and 10 months of age, was 87 and 93% during epidemic and nonepidemic periods, respectively.[165] Efficacy declined with age but remained high until the age of 8 years. A repeat survey was conducted in 1994 to determine whether efficacy had been altered by the change to an accelerated schedule of immunization at 2, 3, and 4 months of age (with no subsequent booster). Efficacy was not altered and was 94% overall for those subjects between 6 months and 5 years of age.[166] This accelerated schedule was also associated with a reduced rate of adverse reactions compared with the prior schedule.[167]

Other Evidence of Effectiveness

Secular Changes in Morbidity and Mortality

There is no question that the widespread use of pertussis vaccine has been associated with a remarkable decline in reported pertussis in developed countries.[105, 106, 134, 168] However, it is also clear that mortality rates from pertussis were declining in at least some of these countries even before the advent of the vaccine.[105, 134, 154, 169, 170] The latter reductions likely reflect a decrease in case-fatality rates due to such factors as improved social and economic conditions, better nutrition, and declines in concomitant infections that may have enhanced pertussis mortality.

Effects of the Withdrawal of Pertussis Immunization

Strong evidence of the benefits of pertussis vaccine was provided by unintended experiments that occurred in three developed countries when vaccine use was curtailed or abandoned. Japan initiated widespread immunization against pertussis in 1950, and over the ensuing years the numbers of reported cases and the numbers of deaths declined remarkably (Fig. 14–4).[106, 170a] Beginning in 1975, a near boycott of the vaccine occurred and epidemic pertussis recurred, with hundreds of deaths.[106] A similar experience occurred in England and Wales; because of negative publicity concerning pertussis vaccine, rates of acceptance of the vaccine fell from approximately 75% to about 25% during the mid-1970s, and major epidemics of pertussis ensued, with numerous deaths.[105, 171] In Sweden, the administration of pertussis vaccine was suspended in 1979 because recent pertussis outbreaks, despite high vaccination coverage, suggested poor efficacy of the vaccine then in use. The incidence of whooping cough then increased more than fourfold from 1980 to 1985, with several major outbreaks in subsequent years.[172, 173]

Pertussis Rates in Vaccinated and Unvaccinated Communities

Further evidence of the efficacy of whole-cell pertussis vaccine is that during outbreaks of pertussis, the reported incidence of the disease varies inversely with vaccine acceptance rates from community to community. A study in England and Wales found that communities with low pertussis vaccine acceptance rates (<30%) had a 59% higher reported incidence of pertussis among children than did areas with high (>50%) acceptance rates; areas with intermediate acceptance rates had intermediate pertussis rates.[174] These findings were not explained by differences among the communities such as crowding and social class; indeed, after adjustment for these two social indicators, the inverse correlation with immunization status was, if anything, stronger.

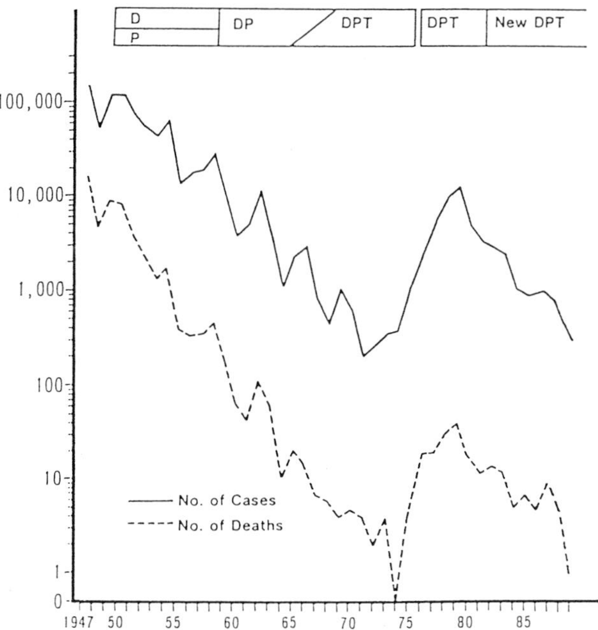

Figure 14–4. Number of reported pertussis cases and deaths, by year, in Japan from 1947 to 1990. "New DPT" refers to the Biken- and Takeda-type acellular vaccines (see text). (From Kimura M. Japanese clinical experiences with acellular pertussis vaccines. Dev Biol Stand 73:5–9, 1991.)

Pertussis Attack Rates in Immunized and Unimmunized Children During Outbreaks

Additional evidence for the efficacy of whole-cell pertussis vaccine is provided by community outbreaks of pertussis in which the attack rates of the disease in immunized children were compared with the rates in those who were incompletely or never immunized. Such studies have been conducted in both Britain and the United States and have been reviewed in detail by Cherry.[105] A more recent study has been conducted in the United States.[175] Although methods of ascertainment and analysis vary, most of these studies indicate that the efficacy of three or more doses of pertussis vaccine in protecting children against clinical disease during outbreaks is 80 to 90%, with incomplete immunization offering partial protection.[175] In children who contracted pertussis in spite of immunization, the disease was milder and complications were far less frequent, despite the fact that younger infants and children are more likely to have received inadequate or no immunization.[176, 177]

Herd Immunity After Immunization

In view of the fact that whole-cell pertussis vaccine is not 100% effective, it could be considered curious that morbidity and mortality from clinical pertussis have been negligible in countries with widespread immunization programs. This is a particularly interesting finding because *B. pertussis* appears to remain ubiquitous in such countries, as indicated by surveillance statistics and studies demonstrating pertussis to be a common cause of protracted cough illness in adolescents and adults.[88, 90, 121–125] Attempts to model mathematically the decline in pertussis incidence attributable to widespread immunization with vaccines of 85% efficacy have underestimated the rates of decline of the disease.[178] Although other factors, such as social and economic changes, may play a role, the probable explanation is herd immunity, a complex phenomenon that varies among different infectious diseases and is difficult to measure with precision.[179] Herd immunity undoubtedly explains the cycles of outbreaks of pertussis every 3 or 4 years; after an outbreak, several years are required for the proportion of susceptible individuals to increase to a level that facilitates a new wave of rapid spread within a population.

Duration of Immunity

A number of studies have evaluated the duration of protection after immunization with whole-cell vaccine, with general agreement. Studies that provide the longest period of evaluation indicate that protection declines by 50% over a period of 6 to 12 years.[180–182] These data are consistent with the incidence and serosurvey data cited previously that suggest an increase in rates of pertussis among 13- to 17-year-olds, representing an interval of 7 to 12 years since last vaccination.[90] It is likely that the duration of protection is influenced by the vaccine used, the number of doses given, and the vaccination schedule.

Adverse Events

Overview

Despite their clear benefits in reducing—nearly to the point of elimination—the substantial mortality and morbidity of pertussis, the whole-cell vaccines have long been recognized as our least satisfactory vaccines with respect to adverse reactions. They commonly cause reactions that are minor but burdensome, occasionally cause reactions that are transient but frightening, and uncommonly cause more serious (but generally self-limited) adverse effects. For some time, there was substantial suspicion that whole-cell vaccines might be causally related to devastating outcomes such as encephalopathy or SIDS, but several careful studies have largely laid these issues to rest.

Untoward events after pertussis immunization began to be of increasing concern to the public and to physicians in the early 1970s, particularly in societies that, because of widespread use of the vaccine, had been spared the ravages of pertussis for a generation or more. Vaccine-associated adverse events loomed large in the eyes of young parents and physicians who had never witnessed the morbidity and mortality of whooping cough. Widespread publicity about the alleged dangers of pertussis vaccine, combined with the infrequency of the disease in some societies and doubts about vaccine efficacy in others, resulted in near boycotts or abandonment of pertussis vaccine in several countries, with consequent recrudescence of disease.[105, 106, 172] In the United States, strong school entry immunization laws enabled vaccination rates to be preserved despite widespread publicity about these concerns, but extensive litigation over alleged personal injuries cost millions of dollars and contributed to the cessation of pertussis vaccine production by several manufacturers.

Establishing or disproving cause and effect, particularly for events of major consequence, proved difficult. The original allegations of causation were largely anecdotal and based on the fallacious assumption that subsequences and consequences were synonymous. The relationships, if any, between whole-cell pertussis vaccine and fatal or disabling events are difficult to study for four reasons including, first, the rarity of such events. Second, DTP is administered to infants at an age when disorders such as encephalopathy, infantile spasms, preexisting neurological conditions, and SIDS are most likely to occur or to be first recognized. Third, all of these disorders can arise from other causes. Fourth, an absolute negative can never be proved, yet some critics would be satisfied by nothing less.

Many earlier estimates of the rates of adverse events proved unsatisfactory owing to the lack of consideration of background rates, ill-defined criteria, and uncertainty of denominators. Since the 1980s, more rigorous epidemiological or interventional studies have improved our understanding of the incidence and spectrum of adverse events after whole-cell pertussis vaccine. Many of these studies, particularly those related to serious untoward events, have been evaluated by a special committee of the Institute of Medicine (IOM) of the U.S. National Academy of Sciences.[183–185]

We expect that the availability of less reactogenic acellular pertussis vaccines will largely put an end to the long debate over the merits of whole-cell vaccines. Therefore, we restrict the following to a summary of the key studies and conclusions regarding adverse events after whole-cell vaccines; readers interested in a more thorough review of these data are referred to the second edition of this text.

Nonfatal, Nondisabling Reactions to Whole-Cell Pertussis Vaccine

Common Reactions. Minor local reactions, consisting of redness, swelling, and pain at the site of injection, occur in about half of DTP recipients. In a study in which 15,752 children received DTP and 784 were randomly assigned to receive DT for one of the first three doses, Cody and colleagues found the rate of minor local reactions to be approximately five times higher after DTP than DT.[186] Similarly, minor systemic reactions such as fever, irritability, and drowsiness are significantly more common after DTP than DT.[186] About half of the children who receive whole-cell pertussis vaccine (usually as DTP) experience some fever, usually minor; less than 1% exhibit an elevation in temperature to 40.5°C (105°F).[186, 187]

Some infants and children may be excessively sleepy during the 12 to 24 hours after vaccination. Participants in the Multicenter Acellular Pertussis Trial (MAPT) experienced somnolence at rates of 62% for whole-cell recipients and 43% for acellular vaccine recipients,[187] suggesting that the somnolence is, at least in part, an effect of the vaccine. Some children are reported to have an unusual high-pitched cry. Somewhat more remarkable is a period of excessive crying, which may last several hours or longer after an injection. This incessant, inconsolable crying usually begins within 12 hours. Persistent crying of 1 hour or more occurred in both the DTP and DT groups in the Cody study but was at least four times as frequent after DTP. Among those with persistent crying, the cry was described as high-pitched or unusual in 3.5% of the children.[186] This reaction appears to be a unique response to inoculation with DTP.

These common reactions vary somewhat in frequency and severity among lots[188] and manufacturers.[155] The vaccine schedule followed may also affect the incidence and severity of adverse reactions. In 1990, the schedule for DTP vaccination in the United Kingdom was changed from 3, 5, and 10 months of age to 2, 3, and 4 months of age. The new schedule was associated with a substantial reduction in postvaccination fever and redness in the injection site after vaccination with the Wellcome whole-cell vaccine.[167] With the accelerated vaccination schedule, reaction rates for the whole-cell vaccine did not differ significantly from those of several acellular vaccines.[167]

Reaction rates also vary with the number of prior DTP injections. In the Cody study, local reactions increased in frequency with successive doses, including the preschool booster.[186] The incidence of fever also increased with successive doses through the 18-month booster but was lower with the preschool booster. Conversely, persistent, inconsolable crying occurred most frequently with the initial dose and less often thereafter. Even in this large study, however, seizures and shock-like episodes were too infrequent to permit differentiation by series number. In the MAPT, the incidence and severity of fever increased substantially with successive primary doses of the reference whole-cell vaccine.[187, 189] Redness increased modestly; the frequency of pain, fussiness, anorexia, vomiting, and the use of antipyretics did not materially increase or decrease with successive doses; and drowsiness decreased.[187] In general, children who have experienced local or systemic reactions after pertussis vaccine have an enhanced likelihood of experiencing the same reaction with a subsequent dose.[190]

Uncommon Reactions. There is no question that DTP is associated with febrile seizures.[186, 191–196] Among the 15,752 children in the Cody study who received DTP, 9 (0.06%) experienced a convulsion, usually associated with fever.[186] In addition, it has been shown that seizures occur at increased rates after DTP in children with personal or family histories of convulsions.[186, 191, 195–197] One study found that children who had a convulsion after immunization were more than seven times as likely as control children to have had a prior seizure and more than four times as likely to have a family history of seizures.[195] Simple convulsions, although distressing, are considered to be benign.[191, 198] Data do not support the concern that seizures after the receipt of DTP might induce epilepsy in some children.[199]

Another worrisome but uncommon reaction to DTP is that of a strange shock-like state, termed a hypotonic-hyporesponsive episode, which usually has its onset within 12 hours of inoculation and may last for several hours but always resolves. Neither death nor adverse sequelae have been observed. The Cody study detected nine hypotonic-hyporesponsive episodes, for an incidence of 0.06%.[186] The mechanism of this phenomenon is unknown.

Serious Reactions Allegedly Due to Pertussis Vaccine

Encephalopathy. The most serious reaction that has been attributed to whole-cell pertussis vaccine is acute encephalopathy, the first anecdotal report of which was made in 1933.[143] Subsequently, numerous anecdotal reports[200] and several series of cases appeared.[201–205] However, in none of these could the risk of the reactions be calculated, because denominators of children receiving pertussis vaccine were not available.

Considerable circumstantial evidence casts doubt on the concept of pertussis vaccine encephalopathy: No plausible mechanism for vaccine-induced encephalopathy has been uncovered, there is no characteristic syndrome that has been ascribed to pertussis vaccine, and there is no characteristic pathological picture.[206] No analogy can be drawn between vaccine-induced encephalopathy and disease-related encephalopathy. There is no basis for believing that vaccine can trigger any of the pathogenetic mechanisms that have been suggested as explanations for whooping cough–associated encephalopathy (most prominently including anoxia, cerebral hemorrhages, and edema).

Early epidemiological studies produced a variety of estimates of the incidence of encephalopathy associated with DTP; however, these studies failed to consider such confounding factors as the background rates of serious neurological disease and of other conditions that occur in this age group and are associated with severe neurological damage. DTP is customarily administered at a time in life when a variety of neurological disorders occur or become manifest; moreover, fever and other responses to the vaccine may unmask preexisting but previously unrecognized neurological and developmental disorders. These issues are complex, and their clarification presents an enormous problem. A useful prospective study would require not only administering pertussis vaccine to millions of subjects but also withholding pertussis vaccine from a randomized control group, which would be ethically unacceptable. However, the decline in DPT use in the United Kingdom in the mid-1970s and the consequent epidemic of pertussis provided an opportunity to clarify the risks of whole-cell pertussis vaccine.

The National Childhood Encephalopathy Study, conducted from 1976 to 1979, examined whether the frequency of vaccination in children with encephalopathy was greater than expected. It compared children aged 2 months to 3 years admitted to a hospital for serious acute neurological disease with a control group of normal children. Based on 11 subjects who appeared to have residua 18 months later, it was estimated that acute encephalopathy with permanent brain damage occurred at the widely quoted rate of 1 per 310,000 doses, with a 95% confidence interval (CI) of 1 in 54,000 to 5,310,000 doses. However, 4 among the 11 with apparent residua had infantile spasms[207] and were subsequently eliminated from consideration when this condition was shown to be unrelated to DTP.[208] Based on the data for the remaining 7 subjects, the relative risk for permanent impairment was 4.7 (95% CI, 1.1–28.0), with an attributable risk of 1 per 330,000 doses (95% CI, 1 case/ 50,000–18,000,000 doses). However, of these seven children, two had disseminated viral infections and one had Reye syndrome,[13] conditions that are unlikely to be related to inoculation with DTP. In addition, three of the remaining four did not appear to be neurologically impaired on subsequent examination.[209]

A 10-year follow-up evaluation was conducted of all

the children included in the original study and their age-matched control subjects. More than 80% of these individuals were traced. Case children who had received DTP vaccine within 7 days before the onset of their original illness were significantly more likely than control subjects to have died or to have some form of neurological dysfunction, with a relative risk of 5.5 (95% CI, 1.6–23.7). However, the prevalence rates for death or other sequelae were similar regardless of whether or not the onset of acute neurological illness was temporally associated with DTP vaccination. The investigators concluded that whole-cell pertussis immunization "may on rare occasions be associated with the development of severe acute neurologic illness that can have serious sequelae."[210]

The results of the National Childhood Encephalopathy Study have been subjected to extensive analysis, reanalysis, challenge, and debate,[209–215] none of which has overturned the investigators' initial cautious interpretation that the data suggested but did not prove a causal relationship between pertussis vaccine and permanent neurological damage. Several U.S. studies also failed to show a relationship between vaccine and acute encephalopathy leading to brain damage.[192–194] However, only the National Childhood Encephalopathy Study was large enough to identify events that occurred a few times per million exposures.

In 1992, the IOM committee examined the evidence for the various alleged reactions to pertussis vaccine and determined that the evidence was consistent with a causal relationship of pertussis vaccine and acute encephalopathy.[184, 185] However, the data were insufficient to conclude that pertussis vaccine caused permanent brain damage, a position with which many other authorities agreed.[98, 216–225] In 1994, after reanalysis of the 10-year follow-up data, the IOM concluded that the "balance of evidence is consistent with a causal relation between DTP and chronic nervous system dysfunction in children whose serious acute neurologic illness occurred within 7 days of DTP vaccination."[226] However, the IOM was not able to determine whether the pertussis vaccine increased the number of children with chronic neurological illness or was simply a precipitating event in children who would have nonetheless developed chronic neurological dysfunction as a result of underlying brain or metabolic abnormalities.

Infantile Spasms. Infantile spasms, which occur in about 40 per 100,000 infants,[227] have been reported in temporal association with pertussis vaccination.[228] Because infantile spasms typically present between 2 and 8 months of age, it is obvious that an association is occasionally seen by chance alone. Four studies have demonstrated no foundation for concern that DTP causes infantile spasms.[208, 229–231] The National Childhood Encephalopathy Study detected an increased risk of infantile spasms during the week after DT or DTP administration,[208] but this was balanced by a decreased risk in the three succeeding weeks, suggesting that the vaccines may unmask infantile spasms that would have become manifest soon even without vaccination.

Sudden Infant Death Syndrome. In the United States in 1996, 2906 infants succumbed to SIDS.[232] Because this calamity occurs most often in the first 6 months of life, it is to be expected by chance alone that some instances would be observed within a day or two of receipt of DTP. Several early reports suggested clustering of SIDS cases within a few days after the administration of DTP,[233–237] but subsequent studies found no evidence of a causal relationship between SIDS and receipt of DTP.[238–245] The IOM panel, after a careful review of all studies, also concluded that no causal relationship existed.[183–185]

Other Serious Conditions. A 5-year study of 13,135 infants born during a single week in the United Kingdom found deficits in speech, intellectual performance, and growth and an excess of convulsive disorders in the unimmunized cohort, compared with immunized children; this difference was due at least in part to an unusual excess of these problems in unimmunized children who had been hospitalized for pertussis.[246] The IOM panel examined the evidence concerning an association between DTP and a variety of syndromes; their conclusions are summarized in Table 14–2.[183–185]

U.S. National Childhood Vaccine Injury Act

Increasing litigation over alleged vaccine injuries and withdrawal from the marketplace of vaccines by several DTP manufacturers prompted the U.S. Congress in 1986 to pass the National Childhood Vaccine Injury Act, which provides compensation for certain untoward events that occur within specified time periods after vaccination. In 1995, program rules were revised in light of the report of the IOM committee.[183–185]

Table 14–2. **INSTITUTE OF MEDICINE CONCLUSIONS REGARDING THE CAUSATION OF SERIOUS ADVERSE EVENTS BY DTP**

CONCLUSION	EVENT
Evidence indicates causation	Anaphylaxis Prolonged or inconsolable crying Febrile seizures
Evidence consistent with causation	Acute encephalopathy Hypotonic-hyporesponsive episodes
Evidence does not indicate causation	Afebrile seizures Hypsarrhythmia Infantile spasms Reye syndrome Sudden infant death syndrome
Insufficient evidence to draw a conclusion	Aseptic meningitis Chronic neurological damage Epilepsy Erythema multiforme or other rashes Guillain-Barré syndrome Hemolytic anemia Juvenile diabetes Learning or attention disorders Peripheral mononeuropathy Thrombocytopenia
No evidence available either way	Autism

DTP, diphtheria and tetanus toxoids and whole-cell pertussis vaccine.
Data from references 183 to 185.

The replacement of whole-cell with acellular pertussis vaccines does not eliminate the need for the compensation program. Coincidental events causally unrelated to DTP will continue to occur and, without the compensation program, would once again lead to the lawsuits that were a major reason for establishing the program.

ACTIVE IMMUNIZATION: ACELLULAR VACCINES

History

Although whole-cell pertussis vaccines have in general been highly effective, they clearly have varied in efficacy. Moreover, the common occurrence of minor but burdensome adverse reactions, the rare occurrence of more severe adverse reactions, and, in particular, public anxiety over allegations of possible devastating complications have stimulated the search for effective, less reactogenic pertussis vaccines. Better understanding of the biology of *B. pertussis* and the isolation of components that appear to be important in disease pathogenesis and induction of clinical immunity led to the development in Japan of purified component (acellular) vaccines that contain FHA plus varying amounts of inactivated PT and, in some cases, agglutinogens and PRN. These vaccines have been used extensively in Japan since 1981 and have clearly been effective.[247–251] This Japanese experience has stimulated the development of additional, more highly purified acellular pertussis vaccines, which are now coming into widespread use.

Japanese Vaccines

With extensive use of the whole-cell vaccine, the reported annual incidence of pertussis in Japan declined more than 99% by the early 1970s.[249, 251] However, pertussis vaccine acceptance decreased from 85 to 15% of eligible children after widely publicized reports in 1975 of two deaths in temporal proximity to pertussis immunization, and reported pertussis cases and deaths increased approximately 20-fold in the next 5 years (see Fig. 14–4).[106, 249, 251]

In late 1981, six acellular pertussis vaccines combined with diphtheria and tetanus toxoids and adsorbed onto an aluminum salt were licensed in Japan and replaced the whole-cell preparations that had been in use.[252] These vaccines, produced by six different manufacturers, varied in composition.[253–256] The vaccines have in general been considered to be of two types, designated *B* and *T* for the two major sources: the Research Foundation for Microbial Diseases of Osaka University (Biken) and Takeda Chemical Industries, Ltd. The B-type vaccine contains approximately equal amounts of PT and FHA, whereas the five T-type vaccines contain more FHA and substantially less PT than the B-type vaccine. The T-type vaccines usually contain agglutinogens, and at least one T-type vaccine (the Takeda product) includes PRN. The acellular pertussis components were recovered and semipurified by sucrose density gradient centrifugation of antigens from supernatants of *B. pertussis* cultures.[247] Approximately 90% of endotoxin is removed in processing. PT is detoxified by formalin, resulting in marked reductions in histamine sensitization and lymphocytosis promotion in laboratory animals.[247, 257] Other acellular vaccines developed subsequently in other countries have used other approaches to detoxification, including glutaraldehyde, hydrogen peroxide, and genetic engineering.[258]

Acceptable criteria for the licensure of these vaccines in Japan included low toxicity in the mouse; documentation of mouse potency, using a somewhat modified test; diminished systemic and local reactivity in children; and antibody production in children similar to or exceeding that of the whole-cell vaccine. Demonstration of clinical protection by field trials was not required, but household-contact studies and pertussis surveillance after implementation of the acellular vaccines gave clear evidence of their effectiveness. By 1989, reported pertussis was again near an all-time low, with approximately 300 cases and 1 death.[259]

Further Development of Acellular Pertussis Vaccines

The encouraging results of the Japanese experience stimulated vigorous efforts in other industrialized nations to evaluate further the Japanese acellular vaccines and to develop other acellular preparations. To date, nearly two dozen acellular pertussis vaccines have been developed; many have been evaluated in immunogenicity and reactogenicity trials, and the efficacy and safety of some have been demonstrated in field trials.

These vaccines vary from one another with respect to their source, number of components, quantity of each component, method of purification, method of toxin inactivation, incorporated adjuvants, and excipients (Tables 14–3 and 14–4). Unfortunately, identifying the optimum formulation for an acellular vaccine has proved difficult, because no simple method exists to determine the protective capability of a pertussis vaccine. The results of the mouse intracerebral protection test correlate reasonably well with the clinical protection afforded by whole-cell vaccine, but the test appears to be unreliable in assessing acellular pertussis vaccines.[260] Antibody studies, although useful, have not been shown to correlate with protection against disease and infection (although analysis of the completed efficacy trials continues, in the hope of establishing such correlations). Thus, each vaccine's utility must be determined in cumbersome and expensive field trials designed to measure the prevention of disease. The lack of animal models or serological correlates of protection largely prevents the stepwise evaluation of alternative formulations that would be desired to ensure optimum vaccine design.

Also unknown are the roles, if any, of cellular immunity and secretory mucosal antibodies in clinical protection.[261] It is possible that the lack of transplacental cellular or secretory immunity contributes to the poor protection of infants of immune mothers. Furthermore, the fact that mucosal IgA is not produced by immuniza-

Table 14–3. **KEY CHARACTERISTICS OF SELECTED ACELLULAR PERTUSSIS VACCINES***

MANUFACTURER OR DISTRIBUTOR	VACCINE†	EVALUATED IN MAPT	PERTUSSIS ANTIGEN (µg/DOSE)				DIPHTHERIA TOXOID (Lf/dose)	TETANUS TOXOID (Lf/dose)
			PT	FHA	PRN	FIM		
Chiron Vaccines (previously Biocine Sclavo)	Acelluvax	Yes	5	2.5	2.5	—	25	10
	BSc-1	Yes	10	—	—	—	15	10
Japan National Institutes of Health	JNIH-6‡	No	23.4	23.4	—	—	—	—
	JNIH-7	No	37.7	—	—	—	—	—
Massachusetts Public Health Biologic Laboratories	SSVI-1	Yes	50	—	—	—	10	5
	SSVI-2	No	25	3	—	—	10	5
Michigan Department of Public Health	Mich-2	Yes	25	25	—	—	15	15
North American Vaccine	Certiva	No	40	—	—	—	15	6
Pasteur Mérieux Connaught (Canada)§	HCP4DT	No	20	20	3	5	15	5
	CLL-4F_2	Yes	10	5	3	5	15	5
	CLL-3F_2	Yes	10	5	—	5	15	5
Pasteur Mérieux Connaught (France)	Triavax‖	Yes	25	25	—	—	15	5
Pasteur Mérieux Connaught (USA)	Tripedia	Yes	23.4	23.4	—	—	6.7	5
SmithKline Beecham Biologicals	Infanrix	Yes	25	25	8	—	25	10
	SKB-2	Yes	25	25	—	—	25	10
Speywood Pharmaceuticals Ltd¶	Por-3F_2	Yes	10	10	—	10	29	6
Wyeth-Lederle Vaccines and Pediatrics	ACEL-IMUNE**	Yes	3.5	35	2	0.8	9	5
	LPB-3P	Yes	10	20	5	—	10	5

*Compositions may differ in various markets; local suppliers should be consulted as necessary.

†For those vaccines without known trade names, designation reflects source and composition of vaccine.[5, 266] Letters before hyphen indicate source; characters after hyphen indicate number and type of components. All monocomponent vaccines contain PT; two-component vaccines contain PT and FHA; three-component vaccines contain PT, FHA, and either PRN or FIM (as indicated by the letter P or F, respectively); four-component vaccines contain PT, FHA, PRN, and FIM. "F_2" signifies that two fimbrial proteins are included.

‡A Biken vaccine, similar to Tripedia.

§FIM component is a mixture of FIM-2 and FIM-3. The CLL-4F_2 ("classic") formulation was used in the MAPT and in the 1992–1993 Swedish trial. Both formulations have been marketed in Canada (as Tripacel, Quadracel, and Pentacel). Products outside of Canada might be based on either formulation; consult local suppliers.

‖Marketed as Triavax in Europe, Triaxim elsewhere. Referred to as Triavax in this chapter.

¶Previously Porton Products Ltd. FIM component is mixture of FIM-2 and FIM-3.

**Contains approximately 40 µg (but not >60 µg) of pertussis antigen proteins in the following approximate proportions: 86% FHA, 8% PT, 4% PRN, and 2% FIM-2.

FHA, filamentous hemagglutinin; FIM, fimbrial proteins; Lf, limit of flocculation; MAPT, Multicenter Acellular Pertussis Trial; PRN, pertactin; PT, pertussis toxin.

tion might explain the disproportionately higher rates of infection than disease in previously immunized adults.[261]

The Vaccines

Constituents and Stability, Storage and Handling, Dosage and Route

Details of the composition and other key characteristics of the acellular pertussis vaccines are listed later and are shown in Tables 14–3 and 14–4. Unless otherwise noted, all vaccines listed should be stored refrigerated at 2 to 8°C (36–46°F; do not freeze) and given as a 0.5-mL intramuscular dose in the anterolateral thigh or, if necessary, in the deltoid muscle.

Preparations Submitted for U.S. Licensure

The following vaccines are licensed, or have been submitted for licensure, in the United States as of summer 1998. They may also be licensed, or under application for licensure, in other jurisdictions. In these jurisdictions, their composition and trade name may vary from the U.S. formulations described here; local suppliers should be consulted as necessary.

Because the intracerebral mouse protection test does not provide a valid measure of the protective capability of the acellular pertussis vaccines, the potency of individual lots of these vaccines produced for the U.S. marketplace is evaluated by measurement of the antibody response to PT (plus FHA, PRN, and FIM, as applicable) in immunized mice, using an ELISA.

Wyeth-Lederle Vaccines and Pediatrics (ACEL-IMUNE). The Lederle-Takeda DTaP, marketed as ACEL-IMUNE, was licensed in the United States on December 17, 1991, for use as the fourth and fifth (booster) doses in the pertussis series. A reformulation of the Lederle-Takeda vaccine was licensed for use in the infant primary series on December 30, 1996. ACEL-IMUNE is produced by Wyeth-Lederle Vaccines and Pediatrics and combines the acellular pertussis vaccine manufactured by Takeda Chemical Industries, Ltd. (Osaka, Japan), with diphtheria and tetanus toxoids manufactured by Lederle Laboratories (Pearl River, New York). All components are detoxified with formaldehyde.

Pasteur Mérieux Connaught, United States (Tripedia). The Connaught-Biken DTaP, marketed as Tripedia, was licensed August 21, 1992, for use as the fourth and fifth (booster) doses in the pertussis series and was licensed for use in the infant primary series on July 31, 1996. Tripedia is produced by Pasteur Mérieux Connaught (United States) and combines the acellular

Table 14–4. **ADDITIONAL CHARACTERISTICS OF SELECTED ACELLULAR PERTUSSIS VACCINES***

MANUFACTURER OR DISTRIBUTOR	VACCINE†	HOW TOXOIDED	ALUMINUM (mg/dose)	DILUENT	PRESERVATIVE	TRACE CONSTITUENTS
Chiron Vaccines (previously Biocine Sclavo)‡	Acelluvax	Genetic	1.0§	NA	Thimerosal	NA
	BSc-1	Genetic	1.0§	NA	Thimerosal	NA
Japan National Institutes of Health	JNIH-6	Formaldehyde	0.08	PBS	Thimerosal	Formaldehyde
	JNIH-7	Formaldehyde	0.075	PBS	Thimerosal	Formaldehyde
Massachusetts Public Health Biologic Labs	SSVI-1	TNM	0.49‖	NA	Thimerosal	NA
	SSVI-2	TNM	0.49‖	NA	Thimerosal	NA
Michigan Department of Public Health	Mich-2	Formaldehyde	0.50‖	NA	Thimerosal	NA
North American Vaccine	Certiva	H_2O_2	0.50§	PBS	Thimerosal	None
Pasteur Mérieux Connaught (Canada)	HCP4DT	Glutaraldehyde	0.33‖	PBS	Phenoxyethanol	Glutaraldehyde, PS
	CLL-4F_2	Glutaraldehyde	0.33‖	PBS	Phenoxyethanol	Glutaraldehyde, PS
	CLL-3F_2	Glutaraldehyde	0.33‖	PBS	Phenoxyethanol	Glutaraldehyde, PS
Pasteur Mérieux Connaught (France)	Triavax	Glutaraldehyde	0.30§	NA	Thimerosal	NA
Pasteur Mérieux Connaught (USA)	Tripedia	Formaldehyde	0.17¶	PBS	Thimerosal	Formaldehyde, gelatin, PS
SmithKline Beecham Biologicals	Infanrix	Formaldehyde**	0.50§**	Saline	Phenoxyethanol	Formaldehyde, PS
	SKB-2	Formaldehyde	0.50§	Saline	Phenoxyethanol	Formaldehyde, PS
Speywood Pharmaceuticals	Por-3F_2	Formaldehyde	0.75§	NA	Thimerosal	NA
Wyeth-Lederle Vaccines and Pediatrics	ACEL-IMUNE	Formaldehyde	0.23††	PBS	Thimerosal	Formaldehyde, gelatin, PS
	LPB-3P	Formaldehyde	0.23††	NA	Thimerosal	NA

*Compositions may differ in various markets; local suppliers should be consulted as necessary.
†For those vaccines without known trade names, designation reflects source and composition of vaccine.[5, 266] See Table 14–3 for details.
‡Pertussis components are formaldehyde stabilized. Aluminum content was 0.35 mg in the MAPT.
§As aluminum hydroxide.
‖As aluminum phosphate.
¶As aluminum potassium sulfate.
**PT component detoxified with both formaldehyde and glutaraldehyde.
††A mixture of aluminum hydroxide and aluminum phosphate.
NA, information not available; MAPT, Multicenter Acellular Pertussis Trial; PBS, phosphate-buffered saline; PS, polysorbate-80; TNM, tetranitromethane.

pertussis vaccine manufactured by Biken and Tanabe Corporation (Osaka, Japan) with diphtheria and tetanus toxoids manufactured by Connaught Laboratories. The vaccine is supplied in 5.0-mL multidose vials.

Owing to the lack of sufficient data, the vaccine is not presently licensed for the fifth dose in children who have received four prior doses of DTaP. However, it is expected that licensure will be received for this indication before such children reach the age at which the fifth dose is given. For the fourth dose (usually given at 15–18 mo), Tripedia may be used to reconstitute Connaught's conjugate Hib vaccine, ActHIB, so that both vaccines may be given via a single injection. The two vaccines are marketed together for this purpose under the trade name TriHIBit. Although licensure is being sought for use of TriHIBit in the infant primary series, the FDA has requested additional data to confirm that the combination produces adequate Hib antibody levels in infants (see Chapters 11 and 20).

SmithKline Beecham (Infanrix). On January 29, 1997, the FDA licensed for use in infants and children a three-component acellular pertussis vaccine distributed by SmithKline Beecham Pharmaceuticals. The SmithKline Beecham DTaP, marketed as Infanrix, consists of acellular pertussis components manufactured by SmithKline Beecham Biologicals (Rixensart, Belgium) plus diphtheria and tetanus toxoids manufactured by Chiron Behring GmbH & Co. (Marburg, Germany). The vaccine is supplied as a turbid white suspension in packages of 10 single-dose vials.

Owing to the lack of sufficient data, the vaccine is not presently licensed for the fifth dose in children who have received four prior doses of DTaP. However, it is expected that licensure will be received for this indication before such children reach the age at which the fifth dose is given.

North American Vaccine (Certiva). The North American Vaccine DTaP, marketed as Certiva, was licensed for use in infants and children on July 29, 1998. It is a monovalent pertussis vaccine (i.e., the pertussis component consists of inactivated PT alone). The vaccine was developed by the National Institute of Child Health and Human Development and is manufactured by North American Vaccine (Beltsville, Maryland; previously known as AMVAX). The vaccine is unique in that the pertussis component is detoxified with hydrogen peroxide.

Chiron Vaccine (Acelluvax). The Chiron Vaccine DTaP, which is expected to be marketed as Acelluvax if approved by the FDA, is a three-component vaccine manufactured by Chiron Vaccines (previously Biocine Sclavo) SpA, Siena, Italy, and distributed in the United States by Chiron Vaccines. The vaccine is unique in that the pertussis toxoid component consists of a recombinant PT that is genetically detoxified using molecular techniques to alter two amino acids for the S1 subunit of *B. pertussis* toxin,[262] resulting in the lack of PT enzymatic activity.

Preparations Licensed Only in Countries Other than the United States

As of spring 1998, two acellular pertussis vaccines have been licensed in other countries but have not (as yet) been offered for licensure in the United States. The characteristics and trade names of these vaccines may vary in some jurisdictions from those given here; local suppliers should be consulted as necessary.

Pasteur Mérieux Connaught, Canada (Tripacel). Connaught Laboratories, Ltd. (Willowdale, Ontario, Canada) produces a four-component acellular pertussis vaccine that is available combined with DT, marketed as Tripacel; combined with DT and conjugate Hib vaccine (ActHIB), marketed as Quadracel; combined with DT, conjugate Hib vaccine, and IPV (IPOL), marketed as Pentacel; or packaged with ActHIB for reconstitution at the time of administration, marketed outside of Canada as Actacel. Tripacel has been produced and marketed in two different formulations, referred to within the company as the "classic" and "hybrid" formulations (shown in Table 14–3 as CLL-4F_2 and HCP4DT, respectively). At present, only the higher-concentration hybrid formulation is marketed in Canada; for the formulation of products marketed outside Canada, consult local suppliers. Because these vaccines contain both FIM-2 and FIM-3, they are often referred to as five-component vaccines.

Pasteur Mérieux Connaught, France (Triavax in Europe, Triaxim elsewhere). The Pasteur Mérieux DTaP is a two-component acellular pertussis vaccine developed by Pasteur Mérieux Connaught (Lyon, France) and, combined with DT, marketed in France by Pasteur Mérieux MSD as Triavax; combined with DT and conjugate Hib vaccine (ActHIB) and marketed as Tetravac; or combined with DT, conjugate Hib vaccine, and IPV (Imovax Polio) and marketed as Pentavac. Triavax is marketed as Triaxim outside Europe.

Preparations Not Submitted for Licensure

A number of acellular pertussis vaccines have been developed but, as of summer 1998, are not yet ready for licensure application or have been abandoned. Those known to us include the following.

Chiron Vaccines. Chiron Vaccines produced a monocomponent vaccine. Subsequent developmental efforts have focused on Chiron Vaccines's previously described three-component vaccine, Acelluvax.

Massachusetts Public Health Biologic Laboratories. A monocomponent vaccine was produced by the Swiss Serum and Vaccine Institute (Berne, Switzerland) using technology and methods developed by the Massachusetts Public Health Biologic Laboratories (Boston). A similar two-component vaccine is undergoing further development at the Massachusetts Public Health Biologic Laboratories.

Michigan Department of Public Health. A two-component vaccine was produced by the Michigan Department of Public Health; we are not aware of further plans to develop this vaccine.

SmithKline Beecham. A two-component vaccine produced by SmithKline Beecham Biologicals, similar to Infanrix minus the PRN component, performed poorly in an efficacy trial (see later) and is not being pursued.

Pasteur Mérieux Connaught, Canada. Connaught Laboratories Ltd. produced a three-component acellular vaccine similar to Connaught Canada's licensed product Tripacel minus the PRN component; we are not aware of further plans to develop this vaccine.

Wyeth-Lederle Vaccines and Pediatrics. Lederle-Praxis Biologics produced a three-component vaccine; we are not aware of further plans to develop this vaccine.

Speywood Pharmaceuticals. Speywood Pharmaceuticals Ltd. (Porton Down, Salisbury, UK; previously Porton Products Limited) produced a three-component vaccine; we are not aware of further plans to develop this vaccine.

Vaccine Schedule Deviations

A failure to adhere to the recommended schedule, causing a delay between doses, should not interfere with the final immunity achieved by any of the DTaP vaccines. There is no need to start the series over again, regardless of the time between doses. Partial doses should not be given; there is no evidence that doing so reduces the frequency of serious adverse events, and there is the risk that efficacy might be impaired.

Interchangeability of Vaccines

No studies are available demonstrating the effects of a change during the scheduled immunization series from one brand of DTaP to another. It is therefore preferred to use the same brand of DTaP vaccine for all doses of the vaccination series for a given child. However, if the vaccine provider does not know, or does not have available, the brand of DTaP previously administered to a child, any of the licensed DTaP vaccines may be used to complete the vaccination series.

Indications for Vaccine—Infants and Children

DTaP is indicated for the primary or booster immunization of infants and children and may be used instead of whole-cell DTP for any scheduled immunization. In the United States, DTaP is preferred to DTP, and administration is recommended at ages 2, 4, and 6 months; 15 to 18 months; and 4 to 6 years, before entering school (this last dose is not necessary if the fourth dose was delayed and was not administered until after the fourth birthday). For children who have started the vaccination series with DTP, DTaP may be used for all remaining doses in the schedule. Although DTaP is preferred, DTP is an acceptable alternative for any of the five doses.

For the first four doses, whole-cell DTP combined with Hib vaccine (DTP/Hib vaccine) is an acceptable alternative to DTaP and Hib vaccine administered at separate sites. At present, no formulation of DTaP combined with Hib vaccine is licensed in the United States for primary immunization of infants; one such formulation (TriHIBit) is approved for the fourth (booster) dose, after primary immunization with any Hib and pertussis vaccines. Combination vaccines containing DTaP and Hib are likely to become available in the United States for use in infants, and some such combinations already are licensed elsewhere (e.g., Quadracel and Pentacel in Canada, Tetravac and Pentavac in France; see Chapter 20).

Contraindications and Precautions

The contraindications and precautions for DTaP are identical to those for DTP, as detailed earlier in this chapter.

Simultaneous Administration with Other Vaccines

Although complete data do not yet exist regarding all possible interactions for the licensed DTaP vaccines, it is nonetheless recommended that oral polio vaccine or IPV, Hib vaccine, measles-mumps-rubella vaccine, varicella vaccine, and hepatitis B vaccine, as appropriate to the age and previous vaccination status of the child, may be given concomitantly with DTaP at the same visit, using separate syringes for injections at separate sites. Most studies have found that the adverse reactions after multiple simultaneous vaccinations are only slightly greater than would be expected from the most reactogenic vaccine alone. However, many of those studies incorporated DTP; one study found a material increase in reactions among infants given DTaP in one thigh and a combination prepared by using a Swedish IPV to reconstitute a French Hib conjugate vaccine in the other thigh, as compared with DTaP alone or DTaP plus IPV.[263, 263a] Presumably, in earlier studies the adverse reactions of DTP were so prominent that the other effects were lost in the background. Once DTaP is used instead, the overall rate of adverse reactions is reduced, and these additive effects can be seen. Further reductions in adverse reactions can often be obtained by using combination vaccines (see Chapter 20), thereby reducing the number of injections given.

Use of Vaccine in Outbreaks—Infants and Children

There is no evidence that supplemental doses of pertussis vaccine are required during an outbreak for the protection of normal children who have received pertussis immunization in accord with the recommended schedule. Of course, children whose immunizations are tardy should be brought into compliance as quickly as possible, and those who have not completed their immunization series and are eligible for their next vaccination should be immunized. Supplemental immunization of children who have immunological or cardiopulmonary compromise may be considered if the benefits of vaccination are believed to outweigh the risks of adverse reactions (a consideration that favors the use of acellular vaccine).

Future Developments

The Children's Vaccine Initiative has proposed that the ideal vaccine would provide all required antigens in a single dose (preferably oral) and would be heat stable, effective when administered soon after birth, and affordable to families of all economic levels. Although this goal may not be reached, present efforts to develop multivalent combination vaccines move us in the right direction (see Chapter 20). It is likely that vaccines combining DTaP, conjugate Hib, hepatitis B, and inactivated poliomyelitis components will soon become available.

Future acellular pertussis vaccines may benefit from an increased use of genetic engineering techniques. Two major advantages of this production method are antigen purity and the possibility of inserting multiple antigens into a single carrier organism that might be administered parenterally (such as vaccinia) or given orally. Another exciting area of research is that of naked DNA vaccines, in which DNA coding for the production of a particular antigen is injected into somatic muscle. Studies have shown that the muscle cells subsequently produce the antigen in question, which escapes the cell and serves as an immunogen. Antigen production typically continues for several months, providing an ongoing antigenic challenge that can serve to boost the initial immune response.[264, 265]

RESULTS OF VACCINATION: ACELLULAR VACCINES

Immune Responses

Humoral Immunity

Numerous immunogenicity and reactogenicity studies have been published, each evaluating one of the various acellular pertussis vaccines. Making comparisons across such studies, however, is an uncertain process, given the variations in study design, study populations, serological assays, and reaction endpoints. To provide such comparisons and facilitate selection of candidate vaccines for anticipated efficacy trials, the U.S. National Institute of Allergy and Infectious Diseases (NIAID) sponsored the MAPT in six of its Vaccine Treatment and Evaluation Units from 1991 to 1992. Thirteen acellular and two whole-cell vaccines were evaluated in the MAPT, including all but one of the acellular vaccines subsequently evaluated in efficacy trials. Although this last vaccine was not made available for the MAPT, it was evaluated thereafter at one of the Vaccine Treatment and Evaluation Units using the MAPT protocol, procedures, and data forms; sera were evaluated in one of the MAPT reference laboratories. Immunogenicity and reactogenicity results from that study are presented here, along with the MAPT results, to provide the most complete available comparison of these vaccines.

Healthy infants enrolled in the MAPT were randomized to receive one of the study vaccines (see Table 14–3) at 2, 4, and 6 months of age. Whole-cell vaccines made by Lederle Laboratories (the reference or control vaccine) and the Massachusetts Public Health Biologic Laboratories were also evaluated. Sera were obtained before the first immunization and 1 month after the third immunization. Serological assays included ELISA of antibody to PT, FHA, PRN, and FIM; Chinese hamster ovary cell and agglutination assays; and assays of diphtheria and tetanus antitoxin.[266]

Each vaccine produced significant increases in antibodies directed against its included antigens, which most often equaled or exceeded those produced by the reference whole-cell vaccine (Table 14–5).[266] Nonetheless, postimmunization antibody titers differed substantially among the acellular vaccines. For PRN and FIM, and to some extent for FHA, antibody levels tended to correlate with the quantity of antigen included in the vaccine. For PT in particular, postimmunization antibody levels did not correlate well with the quantity of antigen in the vaccine, suggesting that manufacturing techniques were important in determining the immunogenicity of the particular PT component of each vaccine. No acellular vaccine was most or least immunogenic with respect to all included antigens.

Cell-Mediated Immunity

Animal studies[267–270] and persistent pertussis infection in human immunodeficiency virus–infected patients[271, 272] have suggested an important role for cell-mediated immunity (CMI) in the host defense against pertussis. Initial studies in adults[273–277] and more recent studies in infants[278] have characterized pertussis-specific CMI after the administration of acellular pertussis vaccine. In infants, acellular pertussis vaccine induced specific T-cell responses for PT, FHA, and PRN that increased progressively over the course of vaccination.[278] Interleukin-2 and γ-interferon were induced preferentially, and T-helper 1 (Th1) cells appeared to be involved in the immune response.[278] CMI responses were more durable than humoral responses. Studies of CMI may prove to be an important tool for assessing protective potency in future vaccine studies.

Controlled Clinical Trials of Vaccine Efficacy

Results are available from nine large efficacy trials of acellular pertussis vaccine that were initiated between 1985 and 1993 in Europe or Africa. The efficacy trials differed by many characteristics: type of study, study population, prevalence of pertussis and other diseases in the community, number of immunizations, timing of immunizations, choice of comparison or control vaccines, methods of surveillance, case definitions, and details of the laboratory support used to evaluate fulfillment of the case definition. These differences confound interpretation of the trials and prevent a simple, direct comparison of their primary efficacy results.

In evaluating these efficacy trials, we have several independent goals: to determine whether the candidate vaccine performs well enough to warrant licensure; to position correctly the evaluated vaccine within the spectrum of available vaccines; to draw inferences concern-

Table 14–5. **ANTIBODY LEVELS 1 MONTH AFTER THE THIRD DOSE OF VACCINE: RESULTS FROM THE MULTICENTER ACELLULAR PERTUSSIS TRIAL AND A FOLLOW-UP TRIAL***

MANUFACTURER OR DISTRIBUTOR	VACCINE†	GEOMETRIC MEAN ANTIBODY LEVEL (95% CI) AFTER IMMUNIZATION AT 2, 4, AND 6 MONTHS OF AGE			
		PT	FHA	PRN	FIM
Chiron Vaccines (previously Biocine Sclavo)	Acelluvax	99 (87–113)	21 (18–25)	65 (53–79)	1.9 (1.7–2.1)
	BSc-1	180 (163–200)	1.2 (1.1–1.4)	3.4 (3.1–3.7)	1.8 (1.7–2.0)
Massachusetts Public Health Biologic Laboratories	SSVI-1	99 (87–111)	1.2 (1.1–1.3)	3.4 (3.1–3.6)	2.1 (1.8–2.4)
Michigan Department of Public Health	Mich-2	66 (59–75)	237 (213–265)	3.2 (3.0–3.4)	2.0 (1.8–2.3)
North American Vaccine	Certiva	55 (42–71)	1.1 (1.0–1.2)	NA	NA
Pasteur Mérieux Connaught (Canada)	CLL-4F_2	36 (32–41)	37 (32–42)	114 (93–139)	240 (204–282)
	CLL-3F_2	38 (33–44)	36 (31–41)	3.4 (3.1–3.6)	230 (182–290)
Pasteur Mérieux Connaught (France)	Triavax	68 (60–76)	143 (126–161)	3.3 (3.1–3.6)	1.9 (1.6–2.1)
Pasteur Mérieux Connaught (USA)	Tripedia	127 (111–144)	84 (73–95)	3.5 (3.2–3.9)	2.0 (1.7–2.3)
SmithKline Beecham Biologicals	Infanrix	54 (46–64)	103 (88–120)	185 (148–231)	1.9 (1.7–2.2)
	SKB-2	104 (94–116)	110 (99–122)	3.3 (3.1–3.5)	1.9 (1.7–2.1)
Speywood Pharmaceuticals	Por-3F_2	29 (25–33)	20 (17–23)	3.0 (3.0–3.1)	361 (303–430)
Wyeth-Lederle Vaccines and Pediatrics	ACEL-IMUNE	14 (12–17)	49 (45–54)	54 (47–62)	51 (41–63)
	LPB-3P	39 (32–48)	144 (127–163)	128 (109–150)	19 (13–27)
	Whole-cell	67 (54–83)	3.0 (2.7–3.4)	63 (54–74)	191 (161–227)

*Results for Certiva are from a separate study conducted at an MAPT study center after completion of the MAPT, using the MAPT protocol, procedures, and data forms; sera were assayed at one of the MAPT reference laboratories.

†For those vaccines without known trade names, designation reflects source and composition of vaccine.[5, 266] For branded products, note that the licensed vaccine's formulation may differ from that of the vaccine evaluated in MAPT. See Table 14–3 for details.

CI, confidence interval; FHA, filamentous hemagglutinin; FIM, fimbrial proteins; NA, not available; PRN, pertactin; PT, pertussis toxin.

Adapted from Edwards KM, Meade BD, Decker MD, et al. Comparison of 13 acellular pertussis vaccines: Overview and serologic response. Pediatrics 96:548–557, 1995.

Table 14–6. **CHARACTERISTICS OF THE IDEAL PERTUSSIS VACCINE EFFICACY TRIAL**

CHARACTERISTIC	COMMENT
Prospective	Avoids recall and other biases.
Randomized	Minimizes risk of unbalanced allocation of confounders.
Fully blinded	Minimizes risk of selection, response, detection, diagnostic, and other biases. Using an unblinded, unimmunized control group is likely to bias efficacy estimates upward, because parents who know their coughing children are unprotected are more likely to suspect pertussis and seek care.
Employs a commonly used immunization schedule	Permits comparison of results to largest possible number of other studies.
Uses a whole-cell control group (ideally, one used in other efficacy trials)	Provides direct comparison with presumed gold standard; improves ability to link results of one study to another.
Uses a placebo control group, if ethically permissible	Allows calculation of absolute efficacy, which is the most useful result. Relative risk (RR), which is the only measure available without a placebo group, can be misleading. For example, if DTaP #1 and DTP #1 have efficacies of 80 and 90%, respectively, then RR = 2 (100–80%) ÷ (100–90%). If DTaP #2 and DTP #2 have efficacies of 92 and 98%, respectively, then RR = 4. Thus, DTaP #2, which is better than DTaP #1, appears to be less effective.
Conducts active surveillance for pertussis and obtains diagnostic specimens in accord with a protocol designed to detect mild as well as severe disease	Minimizes detection bias; improves efficiency, power. Especially in cohort studies, poor surveillance biases toward the null hypothesis (i.e., hides differences between vaccines). In addition, obtaining diagnostic specimens only in more severe cases can bias efficacy estimates upward.[302]
Employs the World Health Organization criteria (at least 21 days of paroxysmal cough plus bacteriological, serological, or epidemiological confirmation) as the primary case definition	Permits comparison of results to largest possible number of other studies.
Obtains specimens for culture from all suspected cases	Cornerstone of bacteriological confirmation. Improves specificity, compared with clinical criteria alone.
Obtains specimens for antigen detection from all suspected cases	May be positive after culture turns negative; improves sensitivity, compared with culture alone.
Obtains specimens for serology (acute and convalescent) from all suspected cases	Improves sensitivity and reduces diagnostic bias, compared with bacteriological confirmation alone (culture is less likely to be positive in immunized than unimmunized cases).
Uses serological definitions appropriate to the vaccines being evaluated (e.g., looks for rises to antigens not included in the vaccine itself)	Immunized subjects who acquire pertussis are less likely than unimmunized subjects to manifest a diagnostic rise in an antibody that has already risen substantially in response to vaccine.
Close contacts of pertussis cases evaluated for pertussis infection	Permits epidemiological confirmation of clinical cases, thereby improving sensitivity and reducing impact of diagnostic biases of culture and serology.
If booster given, separately analyzes the time at risk before and after booster	Necessary for valid comparison with results of other studies.
Provides alternate analyses that differ in case definition or diagnostic tools employed	Permits evaluation of (1) vaccine's ability to protect against mild disease, (2) effect of variations in case definition, and (3) contribution of various confirmatory criteria.

ing the influence on efficacy of various vaccine characteristics; and to draw inferences concerning the effect on vaccine evaluation of various study design characteristics. Various deviations from the ideal study design (Table 14–6) are likely to affect these goals differentially; that is, a study that poses difficulties in accomplishing one goal may nonetheless be useful for accomplishing other goals.

The objectives of pertussis vaccination also play a role in evaluating measurements of efficacy. If the societal goal is focused on the prevention of severe disease, then an inability to detect mild illness (or determine efficacy against that endpoint) may not be important. However, if the goal is to prevent pertussis infection, then mild illnesses must be detected, even though such illnesses may be more difficult to ascertain than classic whooping cough. To the extent that vaccines modify but do not prevent illness, the case definition chosen could have a major impact on interpretation of the efficacy, and hence the benefits, of the vaccine.

Although frustration with the limitations of these trials has led to calls for "definitive studies" that would resolve remaining questions,[279] it is doubtful that any sponsor, public or private, would find the enormous expense of such a study to be both in their interest and of sufficient priority to compete successfully for funds. Thus, these trials will likely remain our only sources of efficacy data, and we must make use of them as best we can.

1986 Swedish Efficacy Trial

The first large-scale efficacy trial of acellular vaccine was conducted in 1986 in Sweden, where routine pertussis immunization had been discontinued in 1979 and pertussis had since become endemic.[172] The randomized, double-blind, placebo-controlled trial (Table 14–7) evaluated a Biken vaccine containing 23.4 μg each of PT and FHA (denoted JNIH-6; see Tables 14–3 and 14–4),[280] a monocomponent vaccine prepared for the purposes of this study and containing 37.7 μg of PT (denoted JNIH-7),[280] and vaccine diluent given as a placebo.[76] There was no whole-cell control group. A two-dose schedule was used: Infants were enrolled and immunized at 5 to 11 months of age, with the second dose given 8 to 12 weeks later.

Antibody responses to PT were dose dependent, being higher in the children who received the monovalent vaccine; FHA antibody rose only in the bivalent vaccine

Table 14–7. OVERVIEW OF NINE ACELLULAR PERTUSSIS VACCINE EFFICACY TRIALS

LOCATION AND YEAR BEGUN	STUDY GROUPS AND VACCINES EVALUATED			AGES AT VACCINATION	TYPE OF SURVEILLANCE			COMMENTS ON STUDY DESIGN
	Acellular*	Whole-Cell	Placebo		Duration†	Active	Passive	
Randomized, Fully Blinded, Controlled Comparative Studies								
Stockholm 1986	JNIH-6 JNIH-7	None	Diluent	5–11 mo, then 8–12 wk later	15 mo‡	Telephone every mo	Parents instructed to report	Lack of whole-cell control hampered interpretation. Schedule (two doses, relatively late in infancy) makes comparisons with other trials difficult. Later analyses revealed differential sensitivity of culture and of serology in vaccine versus placebo groups.
Stockholm 1992	SKB-2 CLL-4F$_2$§	Connaught‖	DT	2, 4, and 6 mo	23.3 mo 23.8 mo	Telephone every 6–8 wk	Parents instructed to report	Stockholm 1992 and Italy are the benchmark studies: prospective, fully randomized and blinded, with both whole-cell and placebo (DT) control groups. Each study evaluated two candidate acellular vaccines head to head, using the same immunization schedules and similar case definitions and diagnostic procedures. (Serological case detection appears to have been less sensitive in Italy.)
Italy 1992	Infanrix Acelluvax	Connaught‖	DT	2, 4, and 6 mo	17 mo	Telephone every mo	Parents instructed to report	
Stockholm 1993	SKB-2 Acelluvax HCP4DT§	Wellcome	None	88% at 3, 5, and 12 mo; 12% at 2, 4, and 6 mo	7.2 mo 21.5 mo 21.5 mo	Clinic visits at 5, 12, and 18 mo	Daily check of culture reports	No placebo control group, thus no absolute efficacy estimates, hampering comparisons with other studies. Formulation of Connaught Canada five-component vaccine changed since Stockholm 1992, further hampering comparisons; however, Acelluvax arm presumably comparable with that of Italy study.
Randomized, Fully Blinded, Controlled Studies								
Göteborg (Sweden) 1991	Certiva	None	DT	3, 5, and 12 mo	17.5 mo	Telephone every mo	Parents instructed to report	Vaccination schedule and lack of whole-cell control group hamper comparisons with other studies.
Other Studies								
Senegal 1990	Triavax	Pasteur Mérieux	DT	2, 4, and 6 mo	21 mo	Field worker visit every week	None	Prospective, double-blind, randomized for relative risk of DTaP versus DTP. Absolute efficacy based on case-contact study using nonrandomized DT/no vaccine group that was unblinded to parents and probably to field workers performing initial case detection. Investigating physicians were said to be blinded.
Erlangen (Germany) 1991	ACEL-IMUNE	Wyeth-Lederle‖	DT	3, 5, 7, and 17 mo	25.6 mo	Telephone every 2 wk	Parents instructed to report to physician	Prospective, double-blind, randomized for relative risk of DTaP versus DTP. Absolute efficacy based on comparison to a nonrandomized DT group that was unblinded to parents and occasionally to investigators.
Mainz (Germany) 1992	Infanrix	Behringwerke or SmithKline Beecham	DT	2, 3, and 4 mo	23 mo	None	Physician report of contact by parent	Household contact study. Vaccine assignment not randomized; parents and physicians responsible for initial case detection not blinded. Central case investigators were said to be blinded.
Munich 1993	Tripedia	Behringwerke	DT	3, 5, and 7 mo	NA	None	Physician report of contact by parent	Nonrandomized (vaccine chosen by parents) and unblinded (parents and investigators knew vaccine status) case-control study.

*Descriptive name given for those without trade name. Letters before hyphen indicate source; characters after hyphen indicate number and type of components. See Tables 14–3 and 14–4 for further details.

†Mean duration of surveillance. Subjects were eligible for inclusion as cases from time of last dose (Stockholm 1992, Stockholm 1993), from 28 to 30 days after last dose (Stockholm 1986, Italy, Göteborg, Senegal, Mainz), or from 14 days after last dose (Erlangen) of DTaP.

‡Passive unblinded surveillance, augmented with inquiries mailed to parents every 6 months and follow-up of positive cultures reported to the National Bacteriology Laboratory, continued for an additional 3 years.

§CLL-4F$_2$ and HCP4DT are the "classic" and "hybrid" (higher-concentration) formulations of Tripacel. CLL-4F$_2$ has 10 μg PT and 5 μg FHA, as compared with 20 μg of each in HCP4DT.

‖U.S.-licensed whole-cell vaccine.

DT, diphtheria and tetanus toxoids vaccine; DTaP, DT plus acellular pertussis vaccine; DTP, DT plus whole-cell pertussis vaccine; NA, not available or not applicable.

group. Efficacy for both vaccines was less than anticipated (Tables 14–8 and 14–9); for culture-confirmed cough of any duration, efficacy was 69% for the two-component vaccine and 54% for the monocomponent vaccine.[76]

During the surveillance period, four vaccinees (one JNIH-7 and three JNIH-6 recipients) died of bacterial infections.[281] Review of hospitalizations for infection found no differences among the three study groups. Analyses of immunoglobulins from prevaccination and postvaccination sera showed no abnormalities, nor did leukocyte counts obtained in a subsample of subjects 2 to 4 months after the second dose.

In January 1989, the Swedish National Bacteriology Laboratory withdrew the acellular vaccine licensure application, citing both the impression that efficacy was lower than that of whole-cell vaccines and the possible association with deaths due to serious bacterial infections. The laboratory called for studies that would directly compare acellular and whole-cell vaccines.[282]

In light of these safety concerns and of animal data suggesting that PT might enhance the susceptibility of animals to bacterial infection,[283] several studies were conducted that demonstrated, if anything, a decreased risk of severe invasive bacterial disease after DTP immunization[284–286] and no increased risk of minor infections.[285] Data from Japan indicated that there was no enhanced risk from the acellular vaccines.[287] Thus, it appears that the four deaths were chance events, with no causal relationship to vaccination.

Subsequent Follow-Up and Analyses. Later evaluations of various case definitions and confirmatory criteria showed that the two-component and monocomponent vaccines were 81% and 75% effective, respectively, in preventing culture-confirmed disease with at least 21 days of coughing spasms.[288] Estimates of efficacy were profoundly influenced by case definition, ranging (using the monocomponent vaccine as an example) from 5% efficacy in preventing spasmodic cough lasting 1 day or longer to 100% efficacy in preventing culture-confirmed pertussis with spasmodic cough lasting 28 days or longer, with whoops on at least 1 day.[288]

It was also found that prior receipt of pertussis vaccine reduced the likelihood of finding positive pertussis cultures or significant antibody rises in patients with cough.[289] Thus, pertussis infection could be confirmed more readily in placebo recipients than in vaccinees, which would tend to bias efficacy estimates upward.

Although the initial results from the 1986 Swedish trial had suggested that the efficacies of the monocomponent and two-component vaccines did not differ, long-term follow-up showed the two-component vaccine to be significantly more efficacious (Fig. 14–5).[173] Following unblinding of the study after 15 months of active observation, passive surveillance continued for 3 additional years, during which vaccine efficacy ranged from 77 to 92% for the bivalent vaccine and from 65 to 82% for the monovalent vaccine, depending on the case definition (see Table 14–9).[173] Clinical immunity after immunization with acellular pertussis vaccine was maintained for at least 4 years.[173]

The monocomponent vaccine, with 50% more PT, appeared to be more effective than the two-component vaccine in preventing the most severe manifestations of disease. Its efficacy exceeded that of the two-component vaccine for every case definition involving whoops (see Table 14–9), a difference that was statistically significant for 28 or more days of cough with whoops.[288] On the other hand, the two-component vaccine appeared to be more effective in preventing mild or moderate disease (e.g., shorter durations of cough or cough without whoops).[173, 288, 289] Thus, efficacy was influenced by both the number of antigens and the quantity of antigen included.

The initial efficacy results[76] gave the impression that these acellular vaccines were substantially less efficacious than whole-cell vaccine.[76, 173, 290] As a result, Japan remained the only country in which they were licensed. However, results of later studies suggest that efficacy would have been higher had a standard three-dose schedule been used. Most important, inclusion of a whole-cell control group might have led to markedly different conclusions regarding the relative efficacy of these vaccines.

World Health Organization Case Definition of Pertussis

In response to the demonstration in the 1986 Swedish trial of the strong influence of pertussis case definition on estimates of vaccine efficacy, and in expectation of the efficacy trials that would be conducted to evaluate the new vaccines being developed, the World Health Organization convened a group of pertussis experts in January 1991 to develop a consensus pertussis case definition for use in clinical trials. The resulting WHO case definition requires the presence of paroxysmal cough for at least 21 days plus confirmation that the cough illness

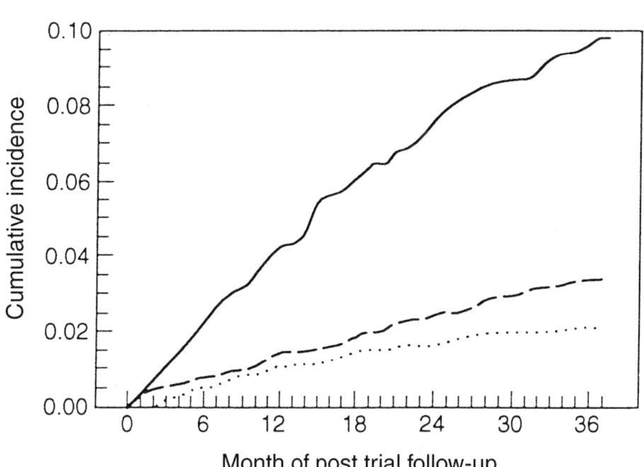

Figure 14–5. Cumulative incidence curves for culture-confirmed pertussis during unblinded posttrial follow-up, in the placebo group (solid line), in the monocomponent (JNIH-7) vaccine group (dashed line), and in the two-component (JNIH-6) vaccine group (dotted line). Unblinded follow-up started August 27, 1987, and ended September 9, 1990. (From Storsaeter J, Olin P. Relative efficacy of two acellular pertussis vaccines during three years of passive surveillance. Vaccine 10:142–144, 1992.)

Table 14–8. RESULTS OF NINE ACELLULAR PERTUSSIS VACCINE EFFICACY TRIALS*

STUDY	CASE DEFINITION‡	VACCINE† (NO. OF COMPONENTS)	EFFICACY (95% CI) No. of Cases	Absolute %	Relative Risk	COMMENT
Randomized, Fully Blinded, Controlled Comparative Studies						
Stockholm 1986[290]	≥21 d cough plus ≥9 coughing spasms on at least 1 d plus positive culture	JNIH-6 (2)	10	81 (61–90)		Differential sensitivity of culture, lack of serological or epi-link criteria may bias estimates upward
		JNIH-7 (1)	12	75 (53–87)		
Stockholm 1992[132]	≥21 d paroxysmal cough plus either positive culture (confirmed by SA or PCR), twofold rise in PT or FHA IgG, or epi link to culture-positive case	SKB-2 (2)	159	59 (51–66)	0.83 (0.66–1.1) vs. DTP	Because of unusually low DTP efficacy, relative risks difficult to compare with other studies
		CLL-4F$_2$§ (4)	59	85 (81–89)	0.29 (0.21–0.40) vs. DTP	
		Connaught DTP	148	48 (37–58)		
Italy 1992[133]	≥21 d paroxysmal cough plus either positive culture (confirmed by SA or PCR), fourfold CHO rise or twofold PT or FHA IgG or IgA rise; no epi-link criterion	Infanrix (3)	37	84 (76–89)	0.25 (0.17–0.36) vs. DTP	Because of unusually low DTP efficacy, relative risks difficult to compare with other studies
		Acelluvax (3)	36	84 (76–90)	0.25 (0.17–0.36) vs. DTP	
		Connaught DTP	141	36 (14–52)		
Stockholm 1993[298]	≥21 d paroxysmal cough plus positive culture (no information on confirmation); no serological or epi-link criteria	HCP4DT§ (4)	13		0.85 (0.41–1.79) vs. DTP	Comparison is to the Wellcome DTP used in this study (see Table 14–7)
		Acelluvax (3)	21		1.38 (0.71–2.69) vs. DTP	
		SKB-2 (2)	99		2.3 (1.5–3.5) vs. DTP‖	Acelluvax, unchanged from the Italy study, provides a link to the Italy study (and thus to Stockholm 1992)
		HCP4DT§(4)	38		0.62 (0.31–1.2) vs. Acelluvax‖	
		SKB-2 (2)	99		2.0 (1.4–2.8) vs. Acelluvax‖	
Randomized, Fully Blinded, Controlled Studies						
Göteborg 1991[299]	≥21 d paroxysmal cough plus either positive culture confirmed by SA or PCR, threefold PT or FHA IgG rise, or epi link	Certiva (1)	72	71 (63–78)		Lack of FHA in vaccine enhanced sensitivity of serological criteria, thereby improving accuracy of estimate
Other Studies						
Senegal 1990[164]	≥21 d paroxysmal cough plus either positive culture confirmed by DIF, twofold PT or FHA IgG rise, or epi link	Triavax (2)	24	74 (51–86)	2.42 (1.4–4.3) vs. DTP	Few cases, thus broad CIs; open DT group may bias absolute efficacy estimates upward
		PMC-Fr DTP	7	92 (81–97)		
Erlangen 1991[131]	≥21 d cough with paroxysms, whoop, or vomiting, plus confirmation¶	ACEL-IMUNE (4)	45	78 (60–88)	1.5 (0.7–3.4) vs. DTP[163]	Open DT group, incomplete case ascertainment may bias absolute efficacy estimates upward
		Wyeth-Lederle DTP	18	93 (83–97)		
Mainz 1992[161]	21 d paroxysmal cough plus either positive culture confirmed by DIF or SA, twofold rise in PT or FHA IgG or IgA	Infanrix (3)	7	89 (77–95)	4.7 (0.6–37.3) vs. DTP	Few cases, thus broad CIs; note how misleading relative risk is if DTP result is close to 100%
		Behring, SKB DTP	1	98 (83–100)		
Munich 1993[162, 348]	21 d paroxysmal cough plus either positive culture confirmed by SA or epi link; no serological criteria	Tripedia (2)	4	93 (63–99)**	2.0 (NA) vs. DTP	Few cases, thus broad CIs; lack of serological criteria, blinding, or randomization may bias efficacy estimates upward
		Behring DTP	1	96 (71–100)		

*Results are based on the case definition most similar to that of the WHO (≥21 d paroxysmal cough plus bacteriological, serological, or epidemiological confirmation that cough is due to *Bordetella pertussis*. Results shown are for complete primary infant immunization series (3 doses, except 2 doses for Stockholm 1986); effects of any booster dose are not included. Some results were obtained by recalculation from data provided in the referenced source and may represent crude, rather than adjusted, efficacies. Blank cells: not applicable or no data.

†Descriptive name given for those without trade name. Letters before hyphen indicate source; characters after hyphen indicate number and type of components. See Tables 14–3 and 14–4 for further details.

‡Unless otherwise noted, all cultures were nasopharyngeal, FHA rises were considered diagnostic only if culture (and PCR, if done) was negative for *Bordetella parapertussis*, and "epi link" means documented contact with a culture-confirmed (PCR-confirmed, for Senegal) case within 28 days before/after illness onset in the subject (for Erlangen or Munich, no time limit was specified). Criteria shown are for the case definition most similar to that of the WHO; different criteria may have been used for alternative case definitions.

§CLL-4F$_2$ and HCP4DT are the "classic" and "hybrid" (higher-concentration) formulations, respectively, of Tripacel.

‖Calculated for time from first dose to soon after the third dose, when SKB-2 recipients were unblinded and given a booster with another vaccine.

¶Confirmation criteria: Positive culture (confirmed by PCR in the last year of study); "significant" PT IgG or IgA result; or household contact to a culture-confirmed case. "Significant" serological result defined as the ratio of convalescent to acute antibody levels that exceeded the 95th, 99th, or 99.9th percentile of a distribution of similar ratios determined among randomly selected subjects at roughly the same time after immunization. Selection of the percentile limit was determined by the number and type of elevated antibody ratios. Efficacy rates reflect adjustment for single adult households and households in which all siblings were unimmunized. Other published efficacy estimates[131] may have also used FHA, PRN, or FIM IgG or IgA values or fourfold agglutinin rises and may not have reflected such adjustment.

**Differs from efficacy reported in patient package insert approved by the Food and Drug Administration, which is based on the primary case definition (≥21 d of any cough) rather than the WHO definition.

CHO, Chinese hamster ovary cell assay; CI, confidence interval; DIF, direct immunofluorescence; DTP, diphtheria and tetanus toxoids and whole-cell pertussis vaccine; FHA, filamentous hemagglutinin; FIM, fimbrial protein; IgA, immunoglobulin A; IgG, immunoglobulin G; NA, not available or not applicable; PCR, polymerase chain reaction; PMC-Fr, Pasteur Mérieux Connaught–France; PRN, pertactin; PT, pertussis toxin; SA, slide agglutination; SKB, SmithKline Beecham; WHO, World Health Organization.

Table 14–9. **RESULTS OF NINE ACELLULAR PERTUSSIS VACCINE EFFICACY TRIALS FOR VARIOUS CASE DEFINITIONS OR SURVEILLANCE PERIODS***

STUDY	VACCINE†	CASE DEFINITION‡	EFFICACY (95% CI) Absolute (%)	EFFICACY (95% CI) Relative Risk
		Randomized, Fully Blinded, Controlled Comparative Studies		
Stockholm 1986	JNIH-6, JNIH-7	≥1 d of any cough + positive culture[76]	69 (47–82), 54 (26–72)	
		Same but including cases from date of first dose[76]	65 (44–78), 53 (28–69)	
		Same but for first 60 d after first dose only[290]	41 (0–79), 42 (0–79)	
		≥1 d cough with spasms (defined in Table 14–8)[290]	16 (3–27), 5 (−10, 17)	
		≥1 d cough with spasms + ≥1 d whoops[288]	39 (16–56), 51 (30–65)	
		≥1 d cough with spasms + culture[288]	75 (54–86), 60 (33–76)	
		≥1 d cough with spasms + whoops + culture[288]	85 (67–94), 89 (72–96)	
		≥21 d cough with spasms[288]	41 (23–55), 27 (6–43)	
		≥21 d cough with spasms + whoops[288]	60 (37–75), 62 (39–76)	
		≥21 d cough with spasms + culture[288]	81 (61–90), 75 (53–87)	
		≥21 d cough with spasms + whoops + culture[288]	84 (63–93), 90 (73–97)	
		3 additional yr of passive surveillance: positive culture[173]	77 (65–85), 65 (50–75)	
		3 additional yr: ≥30 d cough + positive culture[173]	92 (84–96), 79 (67–87)	
		3 additional yr: ≥9 cough spasms/d + positive culture[173]	89 (76–97), 82 (67–90)	
Stockholm 1992	SKB-2, Tripacel (classic or CLL-4F$_2$ formulation)	**≥21 d paroxysmal cough, confirmed as in Table 14–8[132]**	59 (51–66), 85 (81–89)	0.83 (0.66–1.1), 0.29 (0.21–0.40) vs. DTP
		Same but including cases from date of first dose[132]	59 (51–66), 84 (80–88)	0.83 (0.66–1.1), 0.30 (0.22–0.42) vs. DTP
		≥1 d any cough, confirmed as in Table 14–8[132]	42 (33–51), 78 (73–82)	
		≥21 d any cough, confirmed as in Table 14–8[294]	54 (46–62), 81 (76–85)	
Italy	Infanrix, Acelluvax	≥21 d paroxysmal cough + positive culture[133]	85 (NA), 87 (NA)	
		≥21 d paroxysmal cough, confirmed as in Table 14–8[133]	84 (76–89), 84 (76–90)	0.25 (0.17–0.36), 0.25 (0.17–0.36) vs. DTP
		Same but including cases from date of first dose[133]	82 (73–87), 84 (76–89)	0.28 (0.20–0.39), 0.25 (0.17–0.36) vs. DTP
		Same but from 30 d after first dose to 29 d after third[133]	19 (0–84), 83 (0–98)	0.49 (0.17–1.44), 0.10 (0.01–0.79) vs. DTP
		≥7 d any cough, confirmation as before[133]	71 (60–78), 71 (61–79)	0.38 (0.30–0.49), 0.38 (0.29–0.48) vs. DTP
		≥21 d any cough, confirmation as before[133]	79 (70–85), 77 (68–84)	0.29 (0.21–0.39), 0.31 (0.24–0.42) vs. DTP
Stockholm 1993	Acelluvax, Tripacel (hybrid or HCP4DT formulation)	Positive culture, with or without (±) cough[298]		1.40 (0.78–2.52), 2.55 (1.50–4.33) vs. DTP
		≥21 d paroxysmal cough + positive culture[298]		0.85 (0.41–1.79), 1.38 (0.71–2.69) vs. DTP
		Positive culture, ± cough; from date of first dose[298]		1.25 (0.90–1.75), 1.84 (1.36–2.51) vs. DTP
		≥21 d paroxysmal cough + positive culture; from first dose[298]		1.25 (0.82–1.89), 1.65 (1.12–2.45) vs. DTP
		Same but from date of first dose to date of second dose[298a]		1.49 (0.80–2.77), 1.42 (0.76–2.65) vs. DTP
		Same but from date of second dose to date of third dose[298]		1.42 (0.54–3.74), 3.14 (1.34–7.34) vs. DTP

Table continued on following page

Table 14–9. **RESULTS OF NINE ACELLULAR PERTUSSIS VACCINE EFFICACY TRIALS FOR VARIOUS CASE DEFINITIONS OR SURVEILLANCE PERIODS*** *Continued*

STUDY	VACCINE†	CASE DEFINITION‡	EFFICACY (95% CI) Absolute (%)	EFFICACY (95% CI) Relative Risk
		Randomized, Fully Blinded, Controlled Studies		
Göteborg	Certiva	≥7 d any cough, confirmed as in Table 14–8[299]	54 (43–63)	
		≥7 d any cough, confirmed by Göteborg criteria[299]	62 (51–70)	
		≥21 d any cough, confirmed as in Table 14–8[299]	63 (52–71)	
		≥21 d any cough, confirmed by Göteborg criteria[299]	69 (60–77)	
		≥21 d paroxysmal cough, confirmed by Göteborg criteria[299]	77 (69–83)	
		Same; from 30 d after second dose to 29 d after third dose[349]	39 (0–66)	
		≥21 d paroxysmal cough, confirmed as in Table 14–8[299]	71 (63–78)	
		Same; from first dose to 29 d after second dose[299]	≤16 (0–≤64)	
		Same; from 30 d after second dose to 29 d after third dose[299]	55 (12–78)	
		Same; from 18.5 to 24.5 mo after third dose[292]	77 (65–85)	
		Other Studies		
Senegal	Triavax	≥21 d any cough, confirmed as in Table 14–8[164]	31 (7–49)	1.54 (1.23–1.94) vs. DTP
		As above, plus epi-link cases confirmed by PCR[164]	53 (23–71)	1.87 (1.38–2.52) vs. DTP
		≥8 d paroxysmal cough, confirmed as in Table 14–8[350]		3.26 (2.08–5.10) vs. DTP
		≥21 d paroxysmal cough, confirmed as in Table 14–8[164]	74 (51–86)	2.42 (1.35–4.34) vs. DTP
		As above, plus epi-link cases confirmed by PCR[164]	85 (66–93)	2.80 (1.36–5.74) vs. DTP
Erlangen	ACEL-IMUNE	≥7 d any cough, confirmed as in Table 14–8[131]	62 (38–77)§	3.1 (NA) vs. DTP
		≥21 d paroxysmal cough, confirmed as in Table 14–8[131]	78 (60–88)	1.5 (0.7–3.4) vs. DTP
Mainz	Infanrix	≥1 d paroxysmal cough[161]	64 (51–73)	
		≥7 d paroxysmal cough, confirmed as in Table 14–8[161]	81 (68–89)	
		≥21 d paroxysmal cough, with or without confirmation[161]	83 (71–90)	
		≥21 d paroxysmal cough, confirmed as in Table 14–8[161]	89 (77–95)	4.7 (0.6–37.3) vs. DTP
Munich	Tripedia	≥21 d any cough, confirmed as in Table 14–8[162]	80 (63–89)‖	4.0 (NA) vs. DTP
		≥21 d paroxysmal cough, confirmed as in Table 14–8[162]	93 (63–99)	2.0 (NA) vs. DTP

*Results shown are for complete primary infant immunization series (3 doses, except 2 doses for Stockholm 1986); effects of any booster dose are not included. Some results were obtained by recalculation from data provided in the referenced source and may represent crude, rather than adjusted, efficacies. Confidence limits less than zero are shown as zero. Blank cells: not applicable or no data. WHO case definition: ≥21 days paroxysmal cough plus bacteriological, serological, or epidemiological confirmation that cough is due to *Bordetella pertussis*. See Tables 14–7 and 14–8 for additional details, including confirmation methods used by each study.

†Descriptive name given for those without trade name. Letters before hyphen indicate source; characters after hyphen indicate number and type of components. See Tables 14–3 and 14–4 for further details.

‡Definition most similar to that of the WHO is shown in boldface; see Table 14–8 for details. Göteborg criteria: Positive culture; or IgG against both PT and FHA 6000 or greater in a single convalescent specimen; or two major criteria; or one major and one minor criterion. Major criteria: threefold rise in PT or FHA IgG; household contact with confirmed pertussis. Minor criteria: threefold change in PT or FHA IgA or IgM; positive PCR. Unless otherwise specified, subjects were eligible for inclusion as cases from time of last dose (Stockholm 1992; Stockholm 1993), from 28 to 30 days after the last dose (Stockholm 1986, Italy, Göteborg, Senegal, Mainz), or from 14 days after last dose (Erlangen) of DTaP (see Table 14–7 for vaccination schedule).

§Not adjusted for single adult households and households in which all siblings were unimmunized (see Table 14–8).

‖This result, which is based on the primary case definition rather than the WHO definition, is the one reported in the patient package insert approved by the Food and Drug Administration.

See abbreviations in Table 14–8.

actually is due to pertussis. This confirmation can be based on laboratory results (a positive culture for *B. pertussis* or a significant rise in specific antibody, such as IgG or IgA against PT, FHA, or agglutinogens 2 or 3) or on an epidemiological link (e.g., a household contact with a bacteriologically confirmed case within 28 days before or after the onset of illness in the subject).[291] The consensus statement recognized that future laboratory developments might add to the tools available for bacteriological or serological confirmation (e.g., DFA, PCR, assay of antibody to PRN).

Although the WHO case definition has played an essential role in improving comparability of subsequent field trials, its limitations should be recognized. First, it improves but does not eliminate the problem of differential sensitivity of the case definition with respect to detecting pertussis in the various arms of a comparative trial. The yield of cultures is lower in immunized than in unimmunized pertussis patients and varies inversely with the efficacy of the vaccine.[132, 289, 292–294] Thus, a cough illness that is really pertussis is more likely to be confirmed by culture as being pertussis in the unvaccinated group than in the vaccinated group. This disparity leads to a disproportionate discarding of true pertussis cases in the vaccinated group, which can result in falsely elevated estimates of vaccine efficacy. Similarly, the differences between a less effective and a more effective vaccine are likely to be exaggerated because more cases will be confirmed by culture in the group that received the less effective vaccine. Those subjects who have already had a substantial increase in the level of a pertussis antibody, due to the receipt of a highly immunogenic vaccine, will be less likely to show a fourfold (or other diagnostic) rise in the level of that antibody after infection than those subjects who did not receive a vaccine containing that antigen (or a vaccine substantially less immunogenic with respect to that antigen).[289, 292] When comparing two vaccines, one of which stimulates the antibody being tested for and one of which does not, there will be a diagnostic bias favoring the vaccine that stimulates the antibody. If both vaccines contain the antigen in question, the bias will favor the more immunogenic vaccine.

Second, setting the clinical cutoff at "paroxysmal cough of 21 days or more" has been shown to result in the removal from efficacy calculations of a substantial number of laboratory-confirmed pertussis cases.[173, 288, 295] Because these mild cases are more common in vaccinees than in control subjects, the effect is to inflate efficacy estimates, reducing the ability to discriminate among vaccines.

Third, the case definition permits the use of a variety of serological assays for confirmation as well as the future use of additional serological assays or other bacteriological techniques to detect *B. pertussis* organisms. Although commendable, this flexibility means that studies that differ in the laboratory tools employed for case confirmation, and thus in the sensitivity and specificity of case confirmation, nonetheless may characterize themselves as complying with the WHO case definition. Thus, as always, the burden is on the reader to consider carefully the methods employed in each trial.

Efficacy Trials, 1992 to 1997

After the 1986 Swedish clinical trial, worldwide efforts to develop additional acellular pertussis vaccines continued, culminating in eight additional efficacy trials initiated between 1990 and 1993 (see Table 14–7). Four of the trials were randomized, prospective, and fully blinded; of these, three incorporated a whole-cell control arm and evaluated several candidate acellular vaccines head to head. The four remaining trials each evaluated only a single vaccine, using a variety of study designs; all made use of placebo (DT or no vaccine) groups that were neither randomized nor fully blinded.

Key characteristics of all nine efficacy studies are summarized in Tables 14–7 and 14–8. For each trial, Table 14–8 presents results for the case definition that we consider most similar to the WHO standard case definition, and Table 14–9 presents selected results reflecting a variety of alternative case definitions or surveillance intervals. For studies not incorporating a placebo control group (e.g., DT), only relative risks (usually, relative to a DTP used in the same trial) are available. For those trials in which the control groups were not blinded or randomized, relative risks for DTaP compared with DTP (if available) may be less susceptible to bias than the estimates of absolute efficacy. However, relative risks must be interpreted with great caution. As in Table 14–6 (e.g., "Uses a placebo control group") and Table 14–8 (e.g., see comment under Mainz 1992), a DTaP that truly is more efficacious may appear to have a worse relative risk (compared with DTP) than that for another DTaP that was evaluated in a different trial, depending on the relative performance of the DTP vaccines in the two trials.

Sweden and Italy, 1992 to 1993. Of the 13 acellular vaccines evaluated in the MAPT, four were selected, based on evaluations of their safety, immunogenicity, and purity, for evaluation in two NIAID-funded efficacy trials conducted in Sweden and Italy.[132, 133] These two NIAID-sponsored studies were of rigorous design and serve as the benchmarks against which others must be compared. The studies were double blinded, randomized, and used closely coordinated protocols, serological assays, and case definitions. (However, the Italian case definition did not include epidemiologically linked cases, and preexposure sera were not collected routinely in Italy as they were in Sweden.) Infants were immunized at 2, 4, and 6 months of age, and no booster was given. Each study compared two candidate acellular vaccines head to head and incorporated both a placebo control group and a whole-cell control group. The whole-cell vaccine was produced by Connaught Laboratories (Swiftwater, PA) and was licensed for use in the United States.

During the main follow-up period of the Swedish study (hereafter referred to as Stockholm 1992), 737 cases of pertussis were diagnosed that met the primary case definition. Efficacy was 59% for the SmithKline Beecham bivalent vaccine, 85% for the Connaught Canada four-component vaccine, and 48% for the whole-cell vaccine (see Table 14–8).[132] The efficacy of the four-component vaccine was sustained during the 2 years of follow-up, whereas the efficacy of the whole-cell vaccine declined substantially.

The performance of the two-component vaccine was much lower than had been anticipated. (JNIH-6, a similar vaccine, was 81% effective in the 1986 trial, using the most similar case definition.) It was noted that the SmithKline Beecham two-component vaccine produced significantly less antibody to PT in Sweden than it had in the MAPT,[296] prompting both the investigators[132] and other reviewers[296] to speculate that the vaccine's performance in Stockholm 1992 may have in part reflected characteristics unique to the batch of vaccine used in that trial.

The four-component vaccine was 78% effective against laboratory-confirmed pertussis with at least 1 day of cough, suggesting substantial protection against mild or atypical pertussis. In contrast, the two-component and Connaught whole-cell vaccines were 42 and 41% effective, respectively.[132]

During the main follow-up period of the Italian trial, 288 cases of pertussis met the primary case definition. The SmithKline Beecham (Infanrix) and Chiron Vaccines (Acelluvax) three-component acellular vaccines were both 84% effective; efficacy for the Connaught whole-cell vaccine was 36%.[133] Since completion of the main follow-up period, unblinded surveillance of the study cohort has continued. During the first 9 months of extended follow-up, efficacy of the two vaccines differed significantly: 36 cases were detected among recipients of the SmithKline Beecham vaccine, as compared with 18 among recipients of the Chiron vaccine (efficacies, 78% and 89%, respectively).[297] However, a more complete analysis that incorporated results through April 1997 found no material differences in long-term efficacy. For the SmithKline Beecham and Chiron vaccines, respectively, efficacies by year of observation were: 1994, 82.7% and 82.1%; 1995, 81.5% and 85.9%; 1996, 87.6% and 87.7%.[297a]

The similarity in efficacy of the three multicomponent vaccines is noteworthy, particularly given their substantially different compositions (see Tables 14–3 and 14–4). Acelluvax has only one fifth the PT, one tenth the FHA, and one third the PRN content of Infanrix (but the PT is genetically inactivated, rather than being a toxoided natural protein). The Connaught Canada four-component vaccine had far less than half the PT, FHA, and PRN as Infanrix but contained FIM-2 and FIM-3. These facts strongly suggest that the efficacy of an acellular pertussis vaccine is influenced by both the quantity and the particular characteristics of its components.

Sweden, 1993 to 1996. After completion of the immunization phase of Stockholm 1992 (but before completion of the surveillance phase), the Swedish investigators launched another NIAID-supported prospective, randomized, double-blind trial (henceforth referred to as Stockholm 1993) that compared four vaccines: (1) the two-component SmithKline Beecham vaccine evaluated in Stockholm 1992; (2) a four-component Connaught Canada vaccine (HCP4DT) similar to the one evaluated in Stockholm 1992 but reformulated to contain more PT and FHA; (3) the three-component Chiron acellular vaccine (Acelluvax) evaluated in Italy; and (4) a different whole-cell vaccine, the Wellcome whole-cell vaccine (now produced by Evans Medical) used in the United Kingdom.[298] Because of the safety and efficacy of acellular pertussis vaccine demonstrated in Stockholm 1992, Stockholm 1993 did not incorporate a placebo group. Conducted in 22 of 25 Swedish counties, the trial randomized 82,892 children to be immunized at 3, 5, and 12 months of age (the Swedish schedule for DT). Surveillance was predominantly passive; detected rates of pertussis were markedly lower than in Stockholm 1992. Surveillance was terminated early for the group receiving the two-component SmithKline Beecham vaccine, and the subjects were given a booster with another acellular vaccine when results from the Stockholm 1992 study showed this vaccine to be of substantially lower efficacy than the others.

The relative performances of the evaluated vaccines are shown in Tables 14–8 and 14–9. (The absence of a DT or placebo control group precludes calculation of absolute vaccine efficacies.) Relative risks of culture-confirmed *B. pertussis* infection with at least 21 days of paroxysmal cough were 0.85 and 1.38 for the four-component and three-component vaccines, respectively, as compared with whole-cell vaccine. The relative risk of pertussis occurring between administration of the second dose (5 months of age) and third dose (12 months of age) of vaccine was 1.42 for the four-component vaccine, 3.13 for the three-component vaccine, and 7.81 for the two-component vaccine (as compared with whole-cell vaccine). Efficacy of the two-component vaccine differed significantly from that of the other three.

The Stockholm 1993 study provides important new data, but several factors complicate the direct comparison of its results to those of other trials. As noted, there was no placebo control group, precluding calculations of absolute efficacy. The Wellcome whole-cell vaccine was not used in any other efficacy trial. The four-component Connaught Canada vaccine was reformulated after Stockholm 1992 to include twice the PT and four times the FHA as in the original formulation. The SmithKline Beecham two-component vaccine was used in Stockholm 1992, but surveillance of this group was terminated early in the second Stockholm study. Thus, the Chiron three-component vaccine represents the only secure link to the prior trials.

Based on the Stockholm 1992 and Italy 1992 trials (Table 14–8), Infanrix, Acelluvax, and the classic (CLL-4F_2) formulation of Tripacel appear to be of equal efficacy. In Stockholm 1993, however, the relative risk of typical pertussis with the reformulated (hybrid or HCP4DT) version of Tripacel was 0.62 (95% CI, 0.28–1.29) compared to Acelluvax. For combined mild and severe pertussis the hybrid vaccine was equal to the whole cell vaccine, but significantly better than Acelluvax.[298a] Although not conclusive, these results suggest to us that the hybrid formulation of Tripacel may be more efficacious than the classic formulation. The hybrid formulation of Tripacel contains twice the PT and four times the FHA of the classic formulation.

Both the classic and hybrid formulations of Tripacel contain fimbrial agglutinogens, whereas Acelluvax and Infanrix do not. Interestingly, recent analyses of a household contact study nested within the Stockholm 1992 trial have indicated that, among those subjects, high levels of pre-exposure antibody to FIM and PRN were most predictive of efficacy; antibody to PT was of lesser importance, and antibody to FHA appeared to play no role in protection.[298b]

If the hybrid formulation of Tripacel truly is more efficacious than Acelluvax (and by implication, than Infanrix or the classic formulation of Tripacel), this would reinforce the conclusion that efficacy is influenced by both the choice (or number) of components and by the quantity of each component included in the vaccine, and would suggest that fimbrial agglutinogens can contribute to vaccine efficacy.

Serological studies performed on small subsets of subjects in the 1992[294] and 1993[349] Stockholm trials found significantly higher FHA responses with the 1993 Connaught Canada vaccine compared with the 1992 formulation. There were no differences in antibody responses to the SmithKline Beecham bivalent vaccine lots used in the 1992 and 1993 trials.

Göteborg, Sweden. A randomized, double-blind, placebo-controlled trial sponsored by the U.S. National Institute of Child Health and Human Development was conducted in Göteborg, Sweden, from September 1991 to July 1994. This trial evaluated the monocomponent (PT toxoid only) acellular vaccine developed by the National Institute of Child Health and Human Development and manufactured by North American Vaccine (Certiva).[299] Children were immunized with DTaP or DT at 3, 5, and 12 months of age; there was no whole-cell control group.

During the period from 30 days after the third vaccination (at the age of 1 year) to the end of the study, 72 DTaP and 240 DT recipients met the WHO case definition, for an efficacy of 71%. Other case definitions produced efficacy estimates ranging from 54 to 77%, depending on the stringency of the definition. A nested analysis of subjects with household exposure to pertussis found 66% efficacy after two doses and 75% efficacy after three doses.[300] During an additional 6 months of surveillance after unblinding of the study (representing a period averaging 18.5–24.5 mo after the third injection), efficacy was 77% for the full cohort and 76% in a nested household-contact study.[292]

Because this vaccine included only PT toxoid, serological rises to FHA were an unbiased indicator of possible pertussis. Thus, pertussis could be identified more readily among vaccine recipients than if the vaccine had contained FHA. Other vaccines to which this vaccine is compared may have benefited from a lower case ascertainment rate in the vaccine groups, biasing their efficacy estimates upward.

The only other efficacy trial that immunized subjects at 3, 5, and 12 months of age was Stockholm 1993. However, comparing results with that study cannot readily be done; the two studies evaluated no acellular vaccines in common, and there was no DT arm in Stockholm 1993 or a whole-cell arm in Göteborg.

Munich, Germany. An unblinded, nonrandomized case-control study, sponsored by Pasteur Mérieux Connaught, was conducted in 63 pediatric practices from February 1993 to May 1995.[162] A cohort of children was enrolled prospectively to receive, according to parental choice, either the Connaught-Biken two-component DTaP (Tripedia), the Behringwerke DTP, a DT vaccine, or no vaccine at 3, 5, and 7 months of age.

All infants 2 to 24 months of age who presented to their pediatrician with cough for 7 days or more, or with suspected exposure to pertussis, had nasopharyngeal specimens obtained for culture (whether the children were part of the above cohort or not). There were 11,237 such children, including 3245 who were part of the prospective cohort. Children whose cultures were positive and whose cough persisted for 21 days or more were each matched with four control patients from the same practice who were born within 30 days of the subject. Pertinent clinical, demographic, and immunization data were entered into a conditional logistic regression analysis to calculate the relative odds of pertussis while controlling for confounding factors.

Eighty-seven subjects met the case definition of 21 or more days of paroxysmal cough plus either positive culture or household contact with a laboratory-confirmed case. These individuals were matched to 344 control subjects. Eighty-one of the case subjects and 186 of the control subjects had received no pertussis vaccine; 4 and 55, respectively, had received three doses of DTaP; and 1 and 61, respectively, had received three doses of DTP. Adjusted estimates of efficacy were 96% for the DTP and 93% for the DTaP.[162]

This study raises issues that may be applicable to any study that is not completely blinded and randomized. Although these efficacy estimates reflect adjustment for risk factors that differed between cases and controls, such as the number of siblings in daycare, it is not possible to adjust for, or even confirm the existence or magnitude of, any bias that might have arisen because the study was not blinded or randomized. The analysis rested on comparing the proportions of vaccinated patients in two groups: those patients who were brought in because of possible pertussis, and control subjects who were selected in a systematic manner. If unvaccinated children were more likely than vaccinated children to be brought to the pediatrician with suspicious cough, they would be overrepresented in the case (but not control) groups, biasing upward the estimates of efficacy for DTaP and DTP.

Could this bias have happened? Parents knew what vaccine their child received; those whose child received no pertussis vaccine might have been more likely to seek care when their child had a cough illness. (On the other hand, parents who selected a pertussis-containing vaccine may have been more health conscious and more likely to seek medical attention than other parents. Lack of blinding can bias in either direction.)

Even if the parents did not differ in their response to cough illness, we know that vaccinated children who develop pertussis have a milder illness. Such children are less likely to have been brought to the pediatrician and are thus less likely to have been included in the case group. Because the case definition did not allow for serological confirmation of possible cases, confirmation depended on obtaining a positive culture, thus increasing the risk of diagnostic bias (as described after the 1986 Swedish trial).

The effect of each of these factors would be to produce an erroneously high estimate of vaccine efficacy.

The magnitude of the effect and the relative impact on efficacy estimates for the German whole-cell and the Connaught Biken two-component acellular vaccine are impossible to estimate. Given this potential for bias and the small number of cases detected, the efficacy estimates presented should be interpreted with great caution.

Erlangen, Germany. A prospective, randomized, double-blind clinical trial conducted from May 1991 to December 1994 in Erlangen, Germany, compared two U.S.-licensed vaccines produced by study sponsor Wyeth-Lederle: the Lederle-Takeda four-component DTaP (ACEL-IMUNE) and the U.S. DTP that served as the control vaccine in the MAPT.[131, 163] Participants were immunized at approximately 3, 5, 7, and 17 months of age. Infants whose parents declined pertussis immunization received a German DT vaccine at approximately 3, 5, and 17 months of age and served as the control group for estimates of absolute efficacy.

Based on a case definition of 21 or more days of cough with paroxysms, whoop, or posttussive vomiting plus either positive culture, positive serology, or household contact with a culture-proven case, efficacies after three doses of vaccine were 78% for DTaP and 93% for DTP.[131] (The abstract of this trial's published report cites an efficacy of 83% for the DTaP, but that figure reflects the benefit of a fourth, booster dose of vaccine and thus is not comparable to the data presented for any other trial.) As reported in the FDA-approved labeling for ACEL-IMUNE, the relative risk of pertussis was 1.5 for DTaP compared with DTP.[163] A household-contact study nested within the overall trial found efficacy rates similar to those reported from the cohort study.[301]

Although this study also used an unblinded, nonrandomized placebo control group for estimates of absolute efficacy, the potential for ascertainment bias may have been reduced by the use of active surveillance (telephone calls every 2 wk) to detect possible cases. Nonetheless, the relative risk may represent a more reliable estimate than the absolute efficacies.

In a follow-up analysis that has implications for all of the efficacy studies, the local physicians who served as study investigators were stratified into three groups based on the proportion of their patients who underwent investigation for pertussis.[302] For subjects attended by physicians who sought pertussis diligently, efficacy of the DTaP in preventing laboratory-confirmed pertussis with 7 or more days of cough was only 40%, whereas efficacy was 78 and 75% in the physician groups of moderate and low diligence, respectively. These results are not surprising, in that the less diligent physicians detected only the more obvious (i.e., more severe) cases, and it has long been known that the efficacy of pertussis vaccine appears higher when one uses case definitions that focus on more severe disease. Nonetheless, this analysis has illuminated the extent to which fairly subtle differences in diagnostic diligence can alter estimates of efficacy, and it alerts us to another factor that might confound efforts to compare the results of different studies.

The Lederle-Takeda is a four-component vaccine, but it predominantly consists of FHA (86%; about 35 μg), with very little PT, FIM, or PRN, as reflected by both its formulation (see Table 14–3) and its immunogenicity (see Table 14–5). It appears to be of somewhat lower efficacy than the three-component vaccines evaluated in Italy (although the 95% CIs do overlap). If so, this represents further evidence that the quantity and nature of the individual components can be as important as the number of components in determining the efficacy of the vaccine.

Niakhar, Senegal. A prospective, randomized, double-blind study conducted in Senegal from 1990 to 1994 compared a two-component DTaP produced by study sponsor Pasteur Mérieux Connaught (Triavax) with that company's European DTP in children immunized at 2, 4, and 6 months of age.[164] Estimates of absolute efficacy were derived from a nested case-contact study that compared rates of pertussis (after exposure to an index case) among study subjects and nonstudy children (who thus had received either DT or no vaccine) living in the same villages and housing compounds. Thus, the study design was analogous to that of a household-contact study.

Surveillance detected 197 DTaP and 123 DTP recipients who met the primary case definition of confirmed pertussis (see Table 14–8) with cough for 21 or more days, yielding a relative risk of pertussis 1.54 times higher in the DTaP than the DTP group. Requiring the cough to be paroxysmal (the WHO definition) reduced the case counts to 41 and 16, respectively, for a relative risk of 2.42 compared with DTP.

When cases were stratified by age, the relative risk of meeting the primary case definition was 1.16 for children younger than 18 months versus 1.76 for older children, suggesting that protection waned more quickly among DTaP than DTP recipients.

The case-contact study included 197 DTaP recipients, 190 DTP recipients, and 17 unvaccinated children exposed to pertussis, of whom 24, 7, and 8, respectively, met the WHO case definition; the absolute efficacy estimates were 74% for DTaP and 92% for DTP. Owing to the small number of cases, confidence limits for these estimates are wide (95% CIs, 51–86% and 81–97% for DTaP and DTP, respectively). In addition, although field surveillance workers and physician evaluators were blinded to the vaccination status of the randomized children, it is obvious that parents knew whether their children had been vaccinated, a situation that may have increased case detection among unimmunized children. For both reasons, the relative rates are likely to be more reliable than the absolute efficacy estimates.

Initial reports from the investigators cited efficacies of 85 to 86% for DTaP and 95 to 96% for DTP,[303] and some early reviews echo those figures.[304, 305] However, these higher efficacies are based on a requirement that epidemiologically linked cases be confirmed by PCR, a case definition more strict than that of the WHO.

Compared with whole-cell vaccine, relative risks of WHO-defined pertussis were 0.85 and 1.38 in Stockholm 1993 for the four-component Connaught Canada and three-component Chiron vaccines, respectively, as compared with 2.42 for the two-component DTaP evaluated in Senegal. Unless the Pasteur Mérieux whole-cell vaccine is substantially more effective than the Wellcome whole-cell vaccine used in Stockholm 1993, it would appear that this two-component vaccine is less efficacious than the three- and four-component vaccines evaluated in Sweden and Italy. (The data do not permit a direct comparison with the two-component vaccine evaluated in Sweden.)

Mainz, Germany. A prospective household-contact study was conducted from October 1992 to September 1994 in six areas of Germany, in which 22,505 children had been immunized with study sponsor SmithKline Beecham's three-component acellular pertussis vaccine (Infanrix) in a prior safety and immunogenicity trial. Other children in these regions were unimmunized against pertussis or had been immunized with the Behringwerke whole-cell vaccine, because immunizations had been given at 3, 4, and 5 months of age, in accord with the standard German schedule. Passive surveillance for pertussis identified households that contained both an index case of pertussis and at least one contact aged 6 to 47 months who could be evaluated. Prospective surveillance of the 360 eligible contacts identified 104 secondary cases of pertussis (defined as 21 or more days of spasmodic cough plus either culture or serological confirmation of *B. pertussis* infection): 96 of the 173 unvaccinated children, 7 of the 112 DTaP recipients, and 1 of the 75 DTP recipients. The corresponding estimates of vaccine efficacy were 89% for the DTaP and 98% for the Behringwerke DTP.[161]

The use of a household-contact study design largely eliminated the potential for ascertainment bias that would otherwise arise from the fact that study groups were not blinded or randomized, because family members were intensely surveyed by blinded field supervisors for pertussis in households with an index case. However, the authors noted that the efficacy of the Behringwerke whole-cell vaccine may have been overestimated owing to more frequent erythromycin use among contacts who had received the whole-cell vaccine.[161] The simplest explanation for the higher efficacy estimate for Infanrix in this study (89%) than the more-rigorous Italian trial (84%) is that the small number of cases in this study reduced the precision of the estimate, as reflected by the wide confidence limits (95% CI, 77–95%).

Conclusions from the Efficacy Trials

Our conclusions from the efficacy trials are summarized in the last section of this chapter, which presents brief answers to some of the most common questions concerning pertussis vaccines.

Other Evidence of Effectiveness

Both the whole-cell and acellular pertussis vaccines have been highly effective in controlling pertussis in Japan. From 1948 to 1975, pertussis was well controlled by a program that initiated immunization at the age of 3 months (see Fig. 14–4).[249] In response to concerns regarding adverse reactions, in 1975 the age of immunization was raised to 24 months, effectively suspending immunization for 2 years. During this period, reported pertussis cases in Japan rose dramatically, with more than 40,000 cases and nearly 200 deaths for the 8 years 1976 to 1983.[106, 249] By 1980, vaccine acceptance rates were again above 70%, and pertussis cases began to decline.[249] In 1981, whole-cell vaccine was replaced by the new acellular vaccines, and the decline in cases and deaths continued[249]; by 1988, reported pertussis cases were approximately 400, with 5 deaths.[253]

It was hoped that a program that vaccinated children beginning at 2 years of age would prevent transmission of disease to younger children,[249] and national surveillance data indeed revealed that pertussis rates declined sixfold to ninefold among unimmunized children younger than 2 years.[306] Unfortunately, even with this decline, 1984 pertussis rates still remained sixfold higher among these unimmunized children than they had been in 1974, prior to the suspension of whole-cell immunization. For children 3 years and older, however, the incidence of pertussis was essentially the same in 1984 as it had been in 1974.[249] Consequently, the national immunization policy was changed once again, and beginning in 1989, it was recommended that pertussis immunizations once again commence at age 3 months.

A later study provided data showing that the incidence of pertussis among children 2 years and younger continued to decline between 1987 and 1989.[251] Thus, it would appear that use of the acellular pertussis vaccines among older children was capable of protecting younger, unimmunized children but that the full effect did not appear until vaccination had continued long enough, and widely enough, to substantially reduce overall pertussis rates.

Household-contact studies in Japan found that the efficacy of the acellular vaccines ranged from 78 to 94%.[249, 250, 255–258] Studies of the Lederle-Takeda[187, 266, 307–315] and Connaught-Biken[187, 266, 316–318] vaccines found that their immunogenicities were comparable to that of whole-cell vaccine and were similar in Japanese and U.S. infants. In addition, these vaccines caused fewer adverse reactions than the whole-cell vaccine. These data justified licensure of these vaccines in the United States for the fourth and fifth doses.[319, 320]

Duration of Immunity

Few data are available defining the duration of immunity afforded by acellular pertussis vaccines. Long-term follow-up of subjects in the 1986 Swedish efficacy trial did not demonstrate any decline in efficacy of the JNIH-6 or JNIH-7 vaccines through the end of the fourth year after immunization (although it did make clear the higher efficacy of the JNIH-6 vaccine).[173] In the Stockholm 1992 trial, efficacy of the Connaught Canada four-component vaccine was sustained above 80% during 2 years of follow-up, whereas that of the control whole-cell vaccine declined sharply.[132] During extended follow-up in the Italian trial (mean total follow-up, 45 mo; mean time from 6-mo immunization to end of follow-up, 41 mo), efficacies of both the Chiron and the SmithKline Beecham three-component vaccines were fully maintained.[133, 297a] Follow-up of subjects given Certiva in the Göteborg trial showed that protection remained unchanged for at least 2 years after the third dose.

A British study of children immunized at ages 3, 5,

and 9 months with acellular or Wellcome whole-cell vaccine found significantly better PT antibody persistence at age 4 to 5 years among recipients of the Pasteur Mérieux two-component acellular vaccine compared with the whole-cell or Lederle-Takeda vaccines.[167] In contrast, the efficacy trial in Senegal found that the protective efficacy of the same Pasteur Mérieux vaccine, given at ages 2, 4, and 6 months, declined after 18 months of age, as compared with the Pasteur Mérieux whole-cell vaccine.[164]

The duration of immunity will likely depend on the vaccine used, the schedule followed, and the number of doses administered. Although further long-term data are needed, the available results offer hope of improved duration of immunity with at least some acellular vaccines.

Efficacy Against Mild Disease

People with mild disease may play an important role in the spread of pertussis, and vaccines may differ in their effectiveness against mild disease. If so, those vaccines that are more effective against mild disease may be more effective at interrupting the transmission of pertussis, resulting in a greater herd immunity effect.

It has been suggested that vaccines containing attachment proteins (e.g., FHA, PRN, and perhaps FIM) may have a relative advantage in preventing mild disease and may therefore better curtail the spread of pertussis. Figure 14–6 shows the efficacy of various vaccines in preventing culture-confirmed pertussis associated with cough of selected durations. The slope of each line reflects the change in efficacy from mild to severe disease (a horizontal line means that efficacies or relative risks are the same for mild and severe disease). None of the lines is perfectly horizontal; every vaccine was more efficacious against severe than against mild illness (see also Table 14–9). The acellular vaccine with the lowest overall efficacy (the SmithKline Beecham two-component acellular vaccine) has a line that is noticeably steeper than most, and the line for the Connaught Canada four-component vaccine (Tripacel, classic formulation) appears more horizontal than most. Many lines have surprisingly similar slopes, despite representing quite dissimilar vaccines (e.g., slopes are virtually identical for the monocomponent vaccine Certiva and the three-component vaccine Infanrix). Thus, it does not appear that the number of components in the vaccine necessarily affects efficacy against mild disease separately from efficacy against severe disease.

Adverse Events

Numerous safety and immunogenicity studies of the acellular vaccines have been conducted in infants and children[316, 321–326] and have invariably found the acellular vaccines to be associated with lower rates of adverse reactions than whole-cell vaccine. Although most trials have not compared one acellular vaccine with another to detect differences in the rates of adverse reactions, the MAPT evaluated 13 acellular and 2 whole-cell vaccines and thus offers the best comparison of common reactions with these vaccines.[187] The various efficacy trials maintained surveillance for more severe reactions among much larger numbers of infants and thus supplement the MAPT data by providing more precise estimates of rates for these less common events.

Common Adverse Events: Comparative Rates

The MAPT included all acellular vaccines studied in the efficacy trials except one, a monovalent PT vaccine produced by North American Vaccine (similar to Certiva). Fortunately, this vaccine was evaluated using the MAPT protocol in a subsequent trial at one of the MAPT study sites, which allows it to be directly compared with the other vaccines (Table 14–10).

Among the acellular vaccines, there were significant differences with respect to redness, swelling, pain, and vomiting but not fussiness, drowsiness, anorexia, or antipyretic use.[187] No acellular vaccine was consistently the most or least reactogenic. Compared with the reference whole-cell vaccine, all the acellular vaccines were associated with significantly lower rates and severity of every reaction except vomiting.

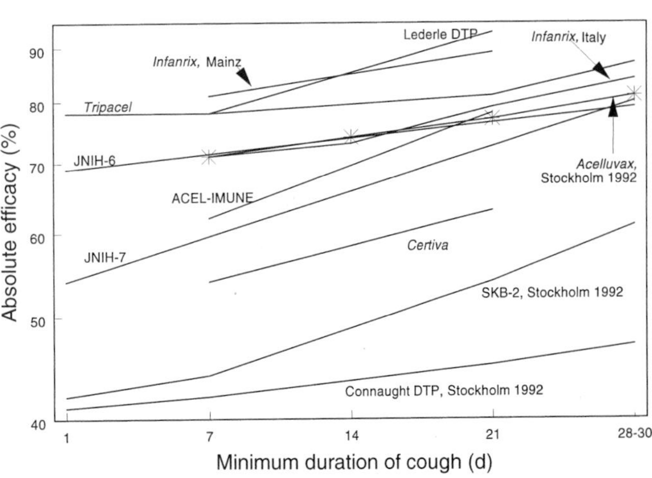

Figure 14–6. Efficacy of pertussis vaccines (names defined in Table 14–3) for preventing various durations of any cough (except Infanrix Mainz and Lederle DTP, paroxysmal cough) associated with culture-confirmed pertussis, based on data from trials providing absolute efficacies (the higher the line, the better the efficacy). A slope of zero (horizontal line) would indicate that the vaccine provides equal absolute or relative protection from mild disease and from severe disease; the steeper the slope, the less the protection from mild disease compared with severe disease. Because estimates were obtained in separate studies, only the slopes, and not the actual values, should be compared. The logarithmic Y-axis scale was chosen to properly display ratios. The Tripacel shown here was the classic (CLL-4F_2) formulation used in the Stockholm 1992 trial.

Table 14–10. **ADVERSE REACTION RESULTS FROM THE MULTICENTER ACELLULAR PERTUSSIS TRIAL AND A FOLLOW-UP TRIAL***

MANUFACTURER OR DISTRIBUTOR	VACCINE†	REPORTED INCIDENCE (%) OF REACTION BY THE THIRD EVENING AFTER VACCINATION AT 2, 4, OR 6 MONTHS OF AGE: Fever (°F)		Redness (mm)		Swelling (mm)							CRUDE OVERALL AVERAGE (%)‖	NO. OF VALUES EXCEEDING MAPT AVERAGE FOR DTaP¶
		100.1–101	*>101.1*	*1–20*	*>20*	*1–20*	*>20*	Pain‡	Fussiness§	Drowsiness	Anorexia	Vomiting		
Chiron Vaccines (previously Biocine Sclavo)	Acelluvax	19.0	1.6	29.4	1.6	17.5	2.4	1.6	16.7	41.3	19.0	9.5	14.5	0
	Monocomponent	18.6	3.6	28.3	5.3	24.8	3.5	3.6	20.4	52.2	25.7	17.7	18.5	6
Massachusetts Public Health Biologic Labs	Monocomponent	21.2	4.1	36.3	1.4	21.9	6.2	8.2	16.4	48.6	22.6	14.4	18.3	8
Michigan Department of Public Health	Two-component	22.1	2.2	30.1	5.9	19.1	3.7	13.2	16.2	46.3	23.5	14.0	17.8	5
North American Vaccine	Certiva	20.0	2.5	20.0	2.5	7.5	2.5	7.5	22.5	30.0	20.0	2.5	12.5	2
Pasteur Mérieux Connaught (Canada)	CLL-4F_2	29.2	3.6	32.8	3.6	21.9	4.4	5.1	18.2	42.3	19.0	12.4	17.5	6
	Three-component	22.4	3.2	44.0	2.4	22.4	8.0	12.0	21.6	45.6	27.2	21.6	20.9	8
Pasteur Mérieux Connaught (France)	Triavax	24.1	4.6	42.9	4.5	28.6	5.3	8.3	12.0	42.1	20.3	7.5	18.2	7
Pasteur Mérieux Connaught (USA)	Tripedia	19.3	5.2	27.4	5.2	16.3	3.7	9.6	19.3	41.5	22.2	7.4	16.1	5
SmithKline Beecham Biologicals	Infanrix	28.3	3.3	35.0	4.2	24.2	5.8	10.8	15.0	46.7	19.2	12.5	18.6	7
	Two-component	18.8	3.1	31.3	2.1	23.4	4.2	6.2	17.2	37.0	17.7	10.9	15.6	2
Speywood Pharmaceuticals	Three-component	17.6	5.0	36.1	2.5	21.0	4.2	4.2	24.4	45.4	18.5	10.9	17.3	5
Wyeth-Lederle Vaccines and Pediatrics	ACEL-IMUNE	16.6	3.2	23.5	2.8	12.4	3.2	3.7	14.3	40.6	24.9	13.4	14.4	2
	Three-component	16.0	5.9	15.1	2.5	10.9	0.8	5.9	12.6	29.4	22.7	12.6	12.2	2
Average for all DTaPs in MAPT	—	**20.8**	**3.7**	**31.4**	**3.3**	**20.1**	**4.2**	**6.9**	**17.1**	**42.7**	**21.7**	**12.6**	**16.8**	**5**
Wyeth-Lederle Vaccines and Pediatrics	Whole-cell	44.5	15.9	56.3	16.4	38.5	22.4	40.2	41.5	62.0	35.0	13.7	—	—

*Results for Certiva are from a separate study conducted at an MAPT study center after completion of the MAPT, using the MAPT protocol, procedures, and data forms.

†Number of pertussis components is shown for those vaccines without known trade names. For branded products, note that the licensed vaccine's formulation may differ from that of the vaccine evaluated in the MAPT. See Table 14–3 for details.

‡Moderate (cried or protested when touched) or severe (cried when leg was moved).

§Moderate (prolonged crying and refused to play) or severe (persistent crying and could not be comforted).

‖Unweighted average of the 11 specific rates shown to the left of this value, which has the effect of giving more weight to less serious reactions but provides a crude overall comparison that may be useful.

¶Of the 11 specific rates, values given indicate the number of times this vaccine's reaction rate exceeded the average for all DTaPs evaluated in the MAPT (see the next-to-last row of the table). This statistic treats small differences and large differences as though they were the same but provides a crude overall comparison that may be useful.

DTaP, diphtheria and tetanus toxoids and acellular pertussis vaccine; MAPT, Multicenter Acellular Pertussis Trial.

Adapted with permission from Decker MD, Edwards KM, Steinhoff MC, et al. Comparison of 13 acellular pertussis vaccines: Adverse reactions. Pediatrics 96:557–566, 1995.

Common and Severe Adverse Events: Data from the Efficacy Trials

Adverse reaction data from the efficacy trials, organized by vaccine, are summarized here and in Table 14–11. Definitions and methods may have differed from study to study, and thus caution should be taken in comparing rates between trials. Note also that Table 14–11 presents per-dose rates whereas the following rates are per subject (these two approaches will produce different rates unless every child with a reaction has the same reaction with every dose).

ACEL-IMUNE (Lederle-Takeda). In the Erlangen trial, minor local and systemic reactions and antipyretic use occurred at nearly identical rates among DTaP and DT recipients but were significantly more common after DTP.[327] Persistent inconsolable crying was experienced by 3.3% of recipients of DTP and 0.7% of recipients of DTaP or DT; convulsions within 72 hours of vaccination occurred in 4, 1, and 0 recipients, respectively.[328] One hypotonic-hyporesponsive episode occurred, in a DTP recipient.

Acelluvax (Chiron) and Infanrix (SmithKline Beecham). In the Italian trial, adverse events were significantly more common among recipients of DTP than DTaP or DT. Temperature of 40.5°C or greater was seen in 6.8% of recipients of DTP, 0.8% of Infanrix, 1.1% of Acelluvax, and 1.3% of DT; crying 3 or more hours in 11.5, 1.9, 1.3, and 0%, respectively; and hypotonic-hyporesponsive episodes in 1.7, 0.2, 0, and 1.3%, respectively.[329] Seizures within 48 hours of vaccination occurred in one Infanrix recipient and in three DTP recipients.[133] The Stockholm 1993 trial also found significantly fewer of these adverse reactions with Acelluvax than whole-cell vaccine.[297]

Certiva (North American Vaccines). Of 1724 children given Certiva in the Göteborg trial, there were no episodes of persistent crying, hypotonic-hyporesponsiveness, afebrile seizures, or withdrawal from the study because of an adverse reaction.[299] Two acellular vaccine recipients (0.1%) developed febrile convulsions within 48 hours after vaccination. Invasive bacterial infections occurred at a lower rate among Certiva than DT recipients.

Triavax (Pasteur Mérieux Connaught, France). In the Senegal efficacy study, Triavax and whole-cell vaccine were each given to approximately 2200 children. Persistent crying was significantly more common among whole-cell recipients (eight vs. zero episodes). Two subjects in each group experienced febrile seizures within 48 hours of vaccine administration. No episodes of hypotonic-hyporesponsive or anaphylactic reactions were seen. In the pilot study preceding this trial, fever, crying, and local reactions were significantly more common with whole-cell than acellular vaccine.[330]

Tripacel (Connaught Laboratories Ltd., Canada). Of 17,686 children given HCP4DT in Stockholm 1993, 0.2% had hypotonic-hyporesponsive episodes, 0.04% had fever 40°C or greater, and 0.02% had convulsions within 48 hours of vaccine administration.[298] Of the 2552 children given the classic (CLL-4F_2) formulation of Tripacel in Stockholm 1992, 1 (0.04%) had a hypotonic-hyporesponsive episode and another was withdrawn due to pronounced local reactions.[132] There were seven episodes of convulsions, but none occurred within 48 hours of vaccination, making a causal association unlikely. Minor local and systemic reactions were sig-

Table 14–11. **INCIDENCE (PER 1000 DOSES) OF MAJOR ADVERSE REACTIONS AFTER PRIMARY IMMUNIZATION: DATA FROM EFFICACY TRIALS, 1992 TO 1997***

PRODUCT	TRIAL	VACCINE	NO. OF DOSES	HIGH FEVER†	HHE	PERSISTENT CRYING‡	SEIZURES§
ACEL-IMUNE	Erlangen[131]	DTaP	16,644	0.06	0	2.0‡	0.06
		DTP	16,424	0.19	0.06	8.8‡	0.18
Tripedia	Munich[162]	DTaP	41,615	NA†	0.05	0.12	0.02
Infanrix	Italy[133]	DTaP	13,761	0.36	0	0.44	0.07
		DTP	13,520	2.4	0.67	4.0	0.22
		DT	4,540	0.44	0.44	0	0
Acelluvax	Italy[133]	DTaP	13,713	0.29	0.07	0.66	0
		DTP	13,520	2.4	0.67	4.0	0.22
		DT	4,540	0.44	0.44	0	0
	Stockholm 1993[298]	DTaP	61,219	0.24	0.26	NA	0.03
		DTP	60,792	0.61	0.56	NA	0.21
Certiva	Göteborg[299]	DTaP	5,124	2.6	0	0‡	0.4
		DT	5,130	1.9	0	0‡	0
Tripacel (classic)	Stockholm 1992[132, 294]	DTaP	7,699	0.26	0.13	0.9	0
		DTP	6,143	4.4	0.81	4.8	0.16
		DT	7,667	0.39	0	0.52	0.26
Tripacel (hybrid)	Stockholm 1993[298]	DTaP	61,220	0.11	0.47	NA	0.06
		DTP	60,792	0.61	0.55	NA	0.21
Triavax	Senegal[164]	DTaP	6,881	NA	0	0	0.29
		DTP	6,595	NA	0	1.2	0.39

*The duration of surveillance or definitions of adverse reactions may have varied from trial to trial. Thus, comparisons within trials are more valid than comparisons across trials.

†Fever 40°C or greater except 40.5°C or greater for Erlangen; for Munich, the rate of "fever" was 2.8 per 1000, but "fever" was not defined.

‡Crying persisting 3 hours or more, except that duration not specified for Erlangen and Göteborg.

§Within 48 hours of vaccination.

HHE, hypotonic-hyporesponsive episode; NA, data not available.

nificantly less common with HCP4DT than with whole-cell vaccine.

Tripedia (Pasteur Mérieux Connaught, USA). Of 12,514 children given Tripedia in the Munich trial, 2.2% experienced the following adverse events related to vaccination: fever, 0.9%; local reactions, 0.4%; unusual crying, 0.3%; irritability, 0.3%; somnolence, 0.2%; crying more than 3 hours, 0.04%; hypotonic-hyporesponsive episodes, 0.02%; and febrile seizure, 0.01%.[162] Ten children given Tripedia had culture-confirmed invasive bacterial disease, a rate not significantly higher than that seen in the control group.

Severe Adverse Events: National Surveillance Data

The claims paid by the Japanese Vaccine Compensation System provide a comparison of severe neurological reactions and deaths with whole-cell versus acellular vaccine and with immunization beginning at 3 months versus 2 years.[249, 251, 331] As shown in Table 14–12, changing the age of administration of whole-cell vaccine from 3 months to 2 years was associated with a dramatic reduction in compensable adverse neurological events and deaths; a further reduction occurred with the change from whole-cell to acellular vaccine. The data strongly suggest that this low rate of serious adverse events was maintained after the initiation in 1989 of immunization with acellular vaccine at the age of 3 months. Severe neurological events and deaths were both reduced more than eightfold during 13 years of acellular vaccine use, as compared with the preceding 11 years of whole-cell vaccine use (see Table 14–12).

Similar data, albeit less dramatic, are available from the U.S. Vaccine Adverse Event Reporting System, maintained by the CDC and the FDA.[332] From 1991 to 1993, rates of reported adverse events after the fourth and fifth doses in the pertussis immunization series were significantly lower for DTaP than DTP. These events included fever (1.9 vs. 7.5 events per 100,000 vaccinations, respectively), seizures (0.5 vs. 1.7), and hospitalization (0.2 vs. 0.9), for a total of 2.9 versus 9.8 cases per 100,000, respectively.[333] There were three reports of encephalopathy after DTP, but none after DTaP.

Results of Booster Doses Given to Children Previously Primed with Acellular Vaccine

A follow-up study to the MAPT evaluated the safety and immunogenicity of a fourth (booster) dose of acellular vaccine given to children primed with acellular or whole-cell vaccine at 2, 4, and 6 months of age.[334] For children primed and given a booster with acellular vaccine, fever and injection site redness, swelling, and pain were seen more frequently with the booster than with the primary series. Of children given a booster with acellular vaccine, those who had been primed with acellular vaccine had local redness and swelling significantly more frequently than did those who had been primed with whole-cell vaccine. However, children who had been both primed and given a booster with whole-cell vaccine had significantly higher rates of irritability, redness, swelling, and pain after the booster than did either of the groups that were given a booster with acellular vaccine. None of 1293 evaluated children experienced seizures, hypotonic-hyporesponsive episodes, or fever greater than 105°F.

A further follow-up study has provided preliminary data that suggests a similar pattern after administration of the fifth dose of pertussis vaccine.[335] Local reactions after a fifth dose of acellular vaccine are more prominent than after the fourth dose but are still less frequent and less severe than those seen after a fifth dose of whole-cell vaccine.

Summary of Adverse Events

Almost every study has found minor local and systemic adverse reactions to be less common with acellular than whole-cell vaccine. Although hypotonic-hyporesponsive episodes and seizures are seen after acellular vaccine, they occur less frequently than with whole-cell vaccine.

Table 14–12. **JAPANESE VACCINE INJURY COMPENSATION SYSTEM CLAIMS, 1970 TO 1993**

REPORTING PERIOD	VACCINES IN USE	MILLIONS OF DOSES	AGE AT FIRST VACCINATION	NO. OF CLAIMS		CLAIMS PER 10^6 DOSES	
				Neurological Events*	Total Deaths†	Neurological Events‡	Total Deaths‡
January 1970–January 1975	Whole-cell		3 mo	86	37		
February 1975–August 1981	Whole-cell		2 yr	23	3		
September 1981–December 1984	Acellular		2 yr	11	2		
1970–1980, overall	Whole-cell	44.9	3 mo, 1970–1975; 2 yr, 1975–1980			18.5	7.4
1981–1993, overall	Acellular	62.6	2 yr, 1981–1988; 3 mo thereafter			2.4	0.9

*Claims approved for neurological illnesses within 7 days after DTP immunization. Data from Kimura M, Kuno-Sakai H. Current epidemiology of pertussis in Japan. Pediatr Infect Dis J 9:705–709, 1990.

†Number of deaths included among claims paid. Data from Nobel GR, Bernier RH, Esber EC, et al. Acellular and whole-cell pertussis vaccine in Japan: Report of a visit by U.S. scientists. JAMA 257:1351–1356, 1987.

‡Rate per 10 million doses of cases applied to the compensation system. Data from Kuno-Sakai H, Kimura M. Epidemiology of pertussis and use of acellular pertussis vaccines in Japan. Dev Biol Stand 89:331–332, 1997.

Rates of rare adverse effects cannot be determined reliably even with large efficacy trials, and they require postmarketing surveillance for their determination. Of course, adverse events temporally but not causally associated with vaccination will continue to occur at their background rates regardless of the vaccine used. Among children primed and boosted with acellular vaccine, reaction rates increase successively with each booster dose but remain lower than seen among children primed and boosted with whole-cell vaccine.

VACCINATION OF ADOLESCENTS AND ADULTS

Numerous acellular pertussis vaccines have been evaluated in adults.[336–342] All appear highly immunogenic, with few adverse reactions.

Adverse Reactions

In a Swedish study of the Biken vaccine in adults, local reactions were common (85%) but described by most subjects as insignificant. One of 20 placebo recipients and 2 of 47 vaccine recipients reported substantial discomfort.[343] In the vaccine group, two distinct patterns of local swelling and redness were noted: an early-onset reaction at 2 to 3 days and a late-onset reaction at 7 to 14 days. Fever 38°C or greater was seen in one placebo and two vaccine recipients. A study of the Pasteur Mérieux two-component acellular vaccine noted fever 37.8°C or greater in 9 of 164 adults.[339] Local redness or swelling was present in one third of subjects, with a maximum diameter of 8 cm. Early and late reactions were seen. In another trial, redness was noted at the injection site in 4 of 76 volunteers given a monovalent PT vaccine similar to Certiva; no fever or late local reactions were seen.[340] In a Tennessee study that randomized 120 adults to receive standard diphtheria and tetanus toxoid (Td) or full-, half-, or quarter-strength Lederle-Takeda acellular vaccine combined with Td, local and systemic adverse reactions were rare and did not differ significantly among the study groups.[338] A series of studies in adolescents and adults of the Chiron Biocine three-component acellular pertussis vaccine demonstrated no serious adverse reactions; rates of minor reactions generally did not differ between the vaccine and placebo groups.[337]

A National Institutes of Health (NIH)-sponsored multicenter trial evaluated the immunogenicity and reactogenicity in adults of varying strengths of five acellular pertussis vaccines (variants of Certiva, Acelluvax, Infanrix, ACEL-IMUNE, and a PT-FHA vaccine supplied by the Massachusetts Public Health Biologic Laboratories).[336, 342] All vaccine dose strengths were well tolerated, although dose-related increases in the rates of injection-site symptoms and the duration of injection-site discomfort were seen in some subjects. Late-onset or biphasic reactions, generally minor, were also noted in this study. The frequency of these late reactions seemed to be greater for the higher strength doses and for vaccines with more antigens.

Immunogenicity

All the studies just mentioned demonstrated excellent immunogenicity of the acellular vaccines in adults, even with doses substantially lower than the standard pediatric dose. In the Tennessee study of the Lederle-Takeda vaccine, antibody responses to PT, FHA, agglutinogens, and PRN, even at the lowest dose, exceeded those seen in infants after complete primary immunization with the same vaccine.[338] No interference was noted with diphtheria or tetanus antibody responses in any of the groups. Similar findings were reported with the same vaccine when studied in German adults.[341] In the NIH dose-ranging study, dose-related increases in serum antibody levels against known vaccine antigens were seen in all vaccine groups.[336, 342] For several vaccines, significant antibody responses were seen against antigens not known to be present in the vaccines, suggesting that the vaccines contained those antigens in trace quantities and were stimulating an anamnestic response in these adults, who had been immunized in childhood with whole-cell vaccine.

Efficacy

An NIH-sponsored study is currently under way to evaluate the efficacy of an acellular pertussis vaccine in adolescents and adults. This trial, being conducted at eight centers across the United States, will randomize 2750 healthy subjects aged 15 to 65 years to receive either an acellular pertussis vaccine similar to Infanrix (at one third the strength and minus the DT components) or hepatitis A vaccine. Subjects will be followed for pertussis illness for at least 1 year; results are expected in 1999. This trial should add substantial data regarding the reactogenicity and immunogenicity (humoral and cell mediated) of this acellular pertussis vaccine. The study's ability to provide definitive conclusions regarding efficacy will depend, of course, on the prevalence of pertussis during the study period.

It can be argued that such an efficacy trial is unnecessary and that licensure of acellular pertussis vaccine for adult use is warranted based on immunogenicity and safety data in adults coupled with efficacy data from studies conducted in children. Certainly, if efficacy of any acellular vaccine is demonstrated in adults, routine use of these vaccines to boost immunity in adolescents and adults should be considered. Healthcare workers, childcare workers, and adults in households containing children are among the likely high-priority target groups for immunization.[344]

Use of Vaccine in Outbreaks—Adolescents and Adults

Although the acellular vaccines are not yet licensed for adult use, at least two reports of their use among healthcare workers in outbreak situations have appeared.[345,346] Pending licensure of acellular pertussis vaccines for adult use, the available data suggest that booster immunization of previously immunized healthcare workers, using one third to one half of the standard pediatric dose of a licensed acellular pertussis vaccine, is safe and immunogenic. Although DTaP was used in the cited outbreaks, if acellular pertussis vaccine were available, its use would be preferred to avoid possible Arthus reactions among people who recently received a booster with Td. The efficacy of such immunization is as yet unproved; pertussis attack rates already were declining in both outbreaks when vaccination was implemented. Clearly, however, vaccination is most likely to be beneficial if it is begun as early as possible in the epidemic. During an outbreak, such booster immunization may also be appropriate for other adolescents and adults at high risk of complications from acute pertussis, but data are lacking.

PUBLIC HEALTH CONSIDERATIONS

Disease Control Strategies

There is but one disease control strategy for pertussis: vaccination. But with which vaccine? Numerous whole-cell and acellular pertussis vaccines have been evaluated in efficacy trials. Which should be licensed, and which should be recommended for use?

In the United States, the answers are relatively simple. All the acellular vaccines evaluated in efficacy trials have superior efficacy and fewer adverse effects than a whole-cell vaccine widely used in the United States, and all therefore merit licensure (assuming other standard requirements are met).[130] The efficacies of the licensed acellular vaccines appear to be sufficiently similar that all are recommended equally over whole-cell vaccine by the advisory bodies. Purchase prices of the whole-cell and acellular vaccines differ little, and all the licensed products are made available to the states by the Federal Vaccines for Children program (see Chapter 42). Given the long-standing public concern regarding the adverse effects of whole-cell vaccine, it is likely that whole-cell vaccine will disappear from the U.S. market within the next few years.

Other countries will have to apply their own relative weights when evaluating the comparative cost, efficacy, and adverse effects of the acellular and whole-cell vaccines.[347] Many countries may decide that their present whole-cell vaccine offers unsurpassed efficacy at low cost; if the vaccine is well accepted by the public, no change would be indicated.

Among the acellular vaccines, there will likely be tradeoffs between efficacy and cost: Multicomponent vaccines may offer the highest efficacy, but they may be the most costly to produce. Most countries electing to use acellular vaccine will likely choose among those that they perceive as the most efficacious. However, because the effectiveness of a pertussis immunization program depends not only on the efficacy of the vaccine but also on the coverage achieved by the program, countries with comprehensive programs that wish to use an acellular vaccine might elect to use a vaccine that is somewhat less efficacious but materially less expensive.

As combination vaccines become available, these decisions will have to be revisited and are likely to become even more complex (see Chapter 20).

Eradication or Elimination

Humans are the only reservoir for pertussis, and chronic carriage is not known to occur. In principle, then, pertussis can be eradicated. Acellular vaccines, as discussed previously, appear suitable for use among all age groups, but it remains to be seen whether their widespread use can interrupt transmission of pertussis within a region. Global eradication, although perhaps possible, clearly must be many years away.

BRIEF ANSWERS TO COMMON QUESTIONS CONCERNING PERTUSSIS VACCINES

Although the efficacy trials and other studies have greatly enriched our understanding of pertussis vaccines, they have left many important questions unresolved. Despite attempts to standardize key variables, no two studies are perfectly comparable. No study has evaluated a multicomponent vaccine directly against versions of itself that contain alternate components or different quantities of each component, and there is no reasonable expectation of such a study. Although the comparative merits of the various acellular vaccines will remain a subject of debate, decisions must nonetheless be made.

The following questions are among those that have been posed to us by physicians or other healthcare professionals after presentations on the acellular pertussis vaccines. The answers, kept as brief as possible, reflect our opinion of the relevant data, as presented in the text and tables elsewhere in this chapter.

The Broad Issues

Do the acellular vaccines really differ?

Very much so. They differ in source, number of components, amount of each component, and method of manufacture, resulting in differences in efficacy and in the frequency of minor adverse effects.

Are acellular vaccines really safer than whole-cell vaccines?

Definitely. Common adverse reactions and serious adverse reactions both are reduced by about two thirds.

Are acellular vaccines as effective as whole-cell vaccines?

Acellular and whole-cell vaccines overlap in their ranges of efficacies. If we could match all the vaccines head to head in a blinded, randomized trial, we would probably find that whole-cell efficacies range from 85 to 95%, with one or two much lower. We would probably find that acellular efficacies range from 75 to 90%, with one or two much lower.

Is vaccine efficacy the most important determinant of the effectiveness of an immunization program?
No, clearly not. Consider how well pediatric pertussis has been controlled in the United States, using one whole-cell vaccine of moderate efficacy and another whose efficacy (without a booster dose) was startlingly low (see Table 14–8). Other important program factors include the immunization schedule (especially the timing and number of boosters) and comprehensiveness of coverage.

If acellular vaccines are better for some countries, are they better for all countries?
No. Most whole-cell vaccines are very effective and, in many countries, inexpensive. The choice of vaccine depends on balancing considerations of relative efficacy, adverse effects, and cost; such decisions would be expected to differ among countries.

Efficacy

Do study designs affect efficacy estimates? If so, how?
Yes, profoundly.[351–353] The choice of overall design affects the confidence we can have that the results are accurate (i.e., that the results would be found again in another study that used the same case definitions). The choice of details such as case definition strongly influences the actual calculated results.

If studies used different designs, how do we compare them?
With great difficulty. Our best efforts are reflected in Table 14–8, but it is impossible to remove all the uncertainties.

Which studies inspire the highest confidence in their results?
The four double-blind, randomized, prospective trials have the best chance of being accurate, all else (such as case definitions) being equal. Of these, the three that incorporated a whole-cell control and compared acellular vaccines head to head are the most useful.

Are the vaccines that were not studied in double-blind, randomized trials inferior?
The quality of the study should not be confused with the quality of the vaccine being studied. The weakest study designs leave us the most uncertain as to the truth, but that uncertainty reflects on the study, not the vaccine.

Are some acellular vaccines more effective than others? If so, which ones?
Yes. It is virtually certain that there are real differences in efficacy among the acellular vaccines. However, vaccine efficacy is only one—and probably not the most important—factor in determining the effectiveness of a vaccine program, and it is only one of the qualities that should be considered in choosing a vaccine (as is discussed further in the final question). Of the evaluated acellular pertussis vaccines, all except SKB-2 appear to have demonstrated sufficient efficacy in the prevention of whooping cough (and all are sufficiently safe, as is discussed later) to warrant their licensure. Licensed vaccines are generally considered equally acceptable; in the United States, for example, recommending bodies (such as the Advisory Committee on Immunization Practices or the Red Book Committee) had expressed no preference for one licensed acellular vaccine over another as of June 1998. Thus, you should not accord undue importance to the following ranking (even if you agree with it).

When we consider the results of the efficacy studies as well as the confidence the design of each study permits us to have in its results, we conclude that the three- and five-component vaccines evaluated in Stockholm 1992, Stockholm 1993, and Italy (Acelluvax, Infanrix, and the two formulations [classic and hybrid] of Tripacel) are probably the most efficacious. The vaccines evaluated in Munich and Senegal (Tripedia and Triavax) may be in an intermediate tier, and the remaining vaccines are less efficacious. Owing to study design limitations, however, we cannot exclude the possibility that the middle and lower tiers are equivalent (or even that the middle and upper tiers are equivalent), let alone try to place those vaccines in order.

We just categorized the Biken and Takeda vaccines as middle or lower tier. Those are the acellular vaccines used in Japan, where national surveillance statistics have shown them to control pertussis exceedingly well (at least as well as whole-cell vaccine; see Fig. 14–4). Note also that widespread use of Certiva in the Göteborg area since mid-1995 has been associated with the near-eradication of pertussis disease. Either we have incorrectly categorized these vaccines, or "middle or lower tier" is more than good enough (we believe the latter is the case).

Is it the choice of components, the number of components, or the amount of each component that matters most?

The number of components, the quantity of each component, and the methods of producing the components (particularly the PT) all influence the efficacy of an acellular vaccine; no one of these factors is determinative irrespective of the others. For example, a vaccine with few components might be more effective than another vaccine that has more components but has them in lesser quantity or of lesser immunogenicity.

Everyone seems to agree that PT is the essential component; most seem to think that adding other components is helpful. The three vaccines previously mentioned as appearing to be the most effective all contain PRN. However, that does not prove that PRN is more important than FHA or FIM; no study has made the necessary comparisons (e.g., PT/FHA plus FIM versus the same PT/FHA plus PRN).

Can efficacy be predicted from immunological results?

Alas, no—at least not yet. Efforts continue to explore correlations between efficacy and both humoral and cell-mediated immunity.

How soon after beginning immunization is protection seen?

Data on this are sparse. It appears that some protection (perhaps 20–40%) accrues with the first dose, and substantially more with the second dose (see Table 14–9). The acellular vaccines likely differ, perhaps markedly, in the degree of protection afforded by the initial doses, but for most of the studies, the data necessary for a proper analysis of this question have not been published.

How many doses are needed, and how is efficacy affected by the choice of schedule?

In general, three doses appear to be necessary for acceptable protection, and, for most of the vaccines and schedules, a booster dose at around 15 months of age will provide substantial additional benefit. There is probably little difference between schedules that immunize at ages 2, 4, and 6 months; 3, 5, and 7 months; or even 2, 3, and 4 months. Immunizing at 3, 5, and 12 months of age gives a little less protection in the second half-year of life and better protection thereafter, as one would intuitively expect.

What is the duration of immunity? Does it vary among the vaccines?

Yes, it does vary. Most of the studies that looked at the question found that the duration of protection with acellular vaccine equaled or exceeded that of the whole-cell vaccine. Some studies have found no apparent decline in efficacy for 2 to 4 years after a three-dose primary infant immunization series; there are few data covering longer periods.

Can the acellular vaccines provide herd immunity or decrease the spread of pertussis?

There is good evidence from Japan that acellular vaccines can induce substantial herd immunity. During a period when only children 2 years or older were being immunized, pertussis rates fell dramatically not only in that group but also among all younger age groups. The experience in Göteborg, Sweden, in household studies and after implementation in 1995 of mass vaccination with Certiva provides further evidence of herd immunity. Whether the acellular vaccines differ in their ability to decrease spread of pertussis, independent of any differences in efficacy, is unclear.

Safety and Adverse Events

Do acellular vaccines reduce adverse reactions compared with whole-cell vaccines?

Absolutely. As noted before, both the common adverse events (e.g., fever, pain, irritability) and uncommon adverse events (e.g., seizures, shock-like episodes) appear to be reduced by about two thirds as compared with whole-cell vaccine.

Will the acellular vaccines also reduce the risk of rare, severe neurological reactions?

We will not know the answer for certain until the vaccines have been widely used for a number of years. However, the data suggest that all adverse reactions that truly are due to pertussis vaccine are reduced with acellular vaccine. Of course, using acellular vaccine will not reduce the risk of events, such as SIDS that are not caused by pertussis vaccine.

Are some acellular vaccines safer or less reactogenic than others?

The MAPT study allows us to directly compare rates of common adverse reactions. As shown in Table 14–10, when we look across all the reactions, no one vaccine is the best or worst, but there are some trends. Of the seven vaccines presently licensed in one or more countries, the fewest reactions are seen with Acelluvax and Certiva (which have unique PT components) and ACEL-IMUNE (perhaps because of its low content of antigens other than FHA). Vaccines more reactogenic than average for all DTaPs evaluated in the MAPT include Infanrix and Tripacel (classic formulation), two of the highest efficacy vaccines, as well as Triavax. The seventh vaccine, Tripedia, had average reactogenicity. With respect to the less common, more severe adverse effects, one presumes that the acellular vaccines must differ from one another at least somewhat, but the safety data from the efficacy trials (see Table 14–11) cannot be compared across studies.

Once again, we must caution against according too much importance to these rankings, even if you agree with them. The reduction in reactogenicity of every acellular vaccine, compared with whole-cell vaccine, is far more substantial than any differences among the acellular vaccines.

Is it true that you get progressively more reactions with later doses of the acellular vaccines?

Yes, but keep in mind that the rate of reactions still remains less than that seen with the use of whole-cell vaccine.

Practical Issues

Of the four acellular vaccines currently licensed in the United States, why is only one licensed for the fifth dose in subjects who received acellular vaccine for the four prior doses?

All four acellular vaccines licensed in the United States are approved for use as the fifth (5-year booster) dose in children who previously received one or more doses of whole-cell vaccine. However, for three of the four vaccines, studies have not yet accrued sufficient subjects who have received acellular vaccine for every injection in the vaccination series, from 2 months to 5 years of age. We would expect all the vaccines to have the fifth-dose indication in plenty of time to boost patients who started out with acellular vaccine.

Can different acellular vaccines be used for different doses in the primary series?

We do not have data yet concerning the effect of such switches, and so as a matter of principle it is preferred to stay with the vaccine that was used previously. However, keeping immunizations on schedule is a far more important principle, and there is no reason to expect that a switch would cause problems. Thus, pending definitive data, do not hesitate to use what you have.

What about combination vaccines?

Combining DTaP with Hib for infant use has been harder than expected, but such combinations (and combinations with IPV or hepatitis B) are on the market already in some countries and should become available everywhere over the next few years (see Chapter 20).

Will we use acellular pertussis vaccine in adults?

Almost certainly. Acellular pertussis vaccines are highly immunogenic and have a reaction profile that appears similar to that of the Td vaccine. Their use in adults may be an essential tool for the control of pertussis. An efficacy trial is under way.

Can we eradicate pertussis?

In principle, yes; in practice, probably not. It is likely, however, that we will be able to control it much better.

How do I choose which acellular pertussis vaccine to use?

Consider five factors (some may not apply in your situation): efficacy, rate of adverse effects, cost, convenience (e.g., how is the vaccine supplied?), and service (e.g., what will the vendor do to make your practice run better?). Make your choice based on the relative weights you assign to each of those factors. As noted, the major immunization advisory committees in the United States have not indicated a preference among the licensed acellular pertussis vaccines; all are considered acceptable and are preferred to whole-cell vaccines.

REFERENCES

1. Holmes WH. Bacillary and Rickettsial Infections. New York, Macmillan, 1940, pp 395–398.
2. Hardy A. Whooping cough. In Kiple KF (ed). The Cambridge World History of Human Disease. New York, Cambridge University Press, 1993, pp 1094–1096.
3. Bordet J, Gengou O. Le microbe de la coqueluche. Ann Inst Pasteur 20:731–741, 1906.
4. Cherry JD, Brunell PA, Golden GS, Karzon DT. Report of the task force on pertussis and pertussis immunization—1988. Pediatrics 81(suppl):933–984, 1988.
5. Pertussis vaccination: Use of acellular pertussis vaccines among infants and young children—recommendations of the Advisory Committee on Immunization Practices (ACIP). MMWR Morb Mortal Wkly Rep 46(RR-7):1–25, 1997.
6. Global Programme on Vaccines. State of the World's Vaccines and Immunization. Geneva, World Health Organization; and New York, UNICEF, 1996.
7. Zackrisson G, Taranger J, Trollfors B. History of whooping cough in nonvaccinated Swedish children, related to serum antibodies to pertussis toxin and filamentous hemagglutinin. J Pediatr 116:190–194, 1990.
8. Lapin LH. Whooping Cough. Springfield, IL, CC Thomas, 1943.
9. Johnston IDA, Bland JM, Ingram D, et al. Effect of whooping cough in infancy on subsequent lung functions and bronchial reactivity. Am Rev Respir Dis 134:270–275, 1986.
10. Department of Health and Social Security, Committee on Safety of Medicines and Joint Committee on Vaccination and Immunisation. Whooping cough. London, Her Majesty's Stationery Office, 1981, pp 1–184.

11. Litvak AM, Gibel H, Rosenthal SE, et al. Cerebral complications in pertussis. J Pediatr 32:357–379, 1948.
12. Pertussis United States, January 1992–June 1995. MMWR Morb Mortal Wkly Rep 44:525–529, 1995.
13. Miller DL, Ross EM, Alderslade R, et al. Pertussis immunisation and serious acute neurological illness in children. BMJ 282:1595–1599, 1981.
14. Nelson JD. The changing epidemiology of pertussis in young infants. The role of adults as reservoirs of infection. Am J Dis Child 132:371–373, 1978.
15. Schmitt-Grohe S, Cherry JD, Heininger U, et al. Pertussis in German adults. Clin Infect Dis 21:860–866, 1995.
16. Postels-Multani S, Schmitt HJ, Wirsing von Konig CH, et al. Symptoms and complications of pertussis in adults. Infection 23:139–142, 1995.
17. Long SS, Lischner HW, Deforest A, et al. Serologic evidence of subclinical pertussis in immunized children. Pediatr Infect Dis J 9:700–705, 1990.
18. Cromer BA, Goydos J, Hackell J, et al. Unrecognized pertussis infection in adolescents. Am J Dis Child 147:575–577, 1993.
19. Long SS, Welkon CJ, Clark JL. Widespread silent transmission of pertussis in families: Antibody correlates of infection and symptomatology. J Infect Dis 161:480–486, 1990.
20. Jenkins P, Clarke SW. Cough syncope: A complication of adult whooping cough. Br J Dis Chest 75:311–313, 1981.
21. Halperin SA, Marrie TJ. Pertussis encephalopathy in an adult: Case report and review. Rev Infect Dis 13:1043–1047, 1991.
22. MacLean DW. Adults with pertussis. J R Coll Gen Pract 32:298–300, 1982.
23. Manclark CR, Cowell JL. Pertussis. In Germanier R (ed). Bacterial Vaccines. New York, Academic Press, 1984, pp 69–106.
24. Kloos WE, Mohapatra N, Dobrogosz WJ, et al. Deoxyribonucleotide sequence relationships among *Bordetella* species. Int J Syst Bacteriol 31:173–176, 1981.
25. Tuomanen E. *Bordetella pertussis* adhesins. In Wardlaw AC, Parton R (eds). Pathogenesis and Immunity in Pertussis. Chichester, John Wiley & Sons Ltd, 1988, pp 75–94.
26. Weiss A. Mucosal immune defenses and the response of *Bordetella pertussis*. ASM News 63:22–28, 1997.
27. Sato H, Sato Y. Relationship between structure and biological and protective activities of pertussis toxin. Dev Biol Stand 73:121–132, 1991.
28. Tamura M, Nogimori K, Murai S, et al. Subunit structure of islet-activating protein, pertussis toxin, in conformity with the A-B model. Biochem 21:5516–5522, 1982.
29. Halperin SA, Issekutz TB, Kasina A. Modulation of *Bordetella pertussis* infection with monoclonal antibodies to pertussis toxin. J Infect Dis 163:355–361, 1991.
30. Nencioni L, Pizza MG, Volpini G, et al. Properties of the B oligomer of pertussis toxin. Infect Immun 59:4732–4734, 1991.
31. Watanabe M. Biological activities of pertussigen from *Bordetella pertussis* of various agglutinogen types. Microbiol Immunol 28:509–515, 1984.
32. Pittman M. The concept of pertussis as a toxin-mediated disease. Pediatr Infect Dis J 3:467–486, 1984.
33. Sato H, Sato Y. *Bordetella pertussis* infection in mice: Correlation of specific antibodies against two antigens, pertussis toxin, and filamentous hemagglutinin with mouse protectivity in an intracerebral or aerosol challenge system. Infect Immun 46:415–421, 1984.
34. Arciniega JL, Shahin RD, Burnette WN, et al. Contribution of the B oligomer to the protective activity of genetically attenuated pertussis toxin. Infect Immun 59:3407–3410, 1991.
35. Griffith AH. Permanent brain damage and pertussis vaccination: Is the end of the saga in sight? Vaccine 7:199–210, 1989.
36. Tuomanen E, Weiss A, Rich R, et al. Filamentous hemagglutinin and pertussis toxin promote adherence of *Bordetella pertussis* to cilia. Develop Biol Stand 61:197–204, 1985.
37. Tuomanen E, Weiss A. Characterization of two adhesions of *Bordetella pertussis* for human ciliated respiratory-epithelial cells. J Infect Dis 152:118–125, 1985.
38. Oda M, Cowell JL, Burstyn DG, Manclark CR. Protective activities of the filamentous hemagglutinin and the lymphocytosis-promoting factor of *Bordetella pertussis* in mice. J Infect Dis 150:823–833, 1984.
39. He Q, Viljanen MK, Olander RM, et al. Antibodies to filamentous hemagglutinin of *Bordetella pertussis* and protection against whooping cough in schoolchildren. J Infect Dis 170:705–708, 1994.
40. Stanbridge TN, Preston NW. Variation of serotype in strains of *Bordetella pertussis*. J Hyg Camb 73:305–310, 1974.
41. Preston NW, Stanbridge TN. Efficacy of pertussis vaccines: A brighter horizon. BMJ 3:448–451, 1972.
42. Bronne-Shanbury CJ, Miller D, Standfast AFB. The serotypes of *Bordetella pertussis* isolated in Great Britain between 1941 and 1948 and a comparison with the serotypes observed in other countries over this period. J Hyg Camb 76:265–275, 1976.
43. Public Health Laboratory Service. Efficacy of whooping-cough vaccines used in the United Kingdom before 1968. BMJ 1:259–262, 1973.
44. Preston NW. Prevalent serotypes of *Bordetella pertussis* in non-vaccinated communities. J Hyg Camb 77:85–91, 1976.
45. WHO Expert Committee on Biological Standardization. Requirements for Diphtheria, Pertussis, Tetanus and Combined Vaccines. WHO Technical Report Series 800. 40th report. Geneva, World Health Organization, 1990, pp 87–179.
46. Brennan MJ, Li Z-M, Cowell JL, et al. Identification of a 69-kilodalton nonfimbrial protein as an agglutinogen of *Bordetella pertussis*. Infect Immun 56:3189–3195, 1988.
47. Novotny P, Chubb AP, Cownley K, et al. Biologic and protective properties of the 69-kDa outer membrane protein of *Bordetella pertussis*: A novel formation for an acellular pertussis vaccine. J Infect Dis 164:114–122, 1991.
48. Leininger E, Kenimer JG, Brennan MJ. Surface proteins of *Bordetella pertussis*: Role in adherence. 1990 Proceedings of the 6th International Symposium on Pertussis. DHHS Publication No. FDA 90–1164. Bethesda, MD, Department of Health and Human Services, United States Public Health Service, pp 100–104.
49. Ewanowich CA, Leininger E, Kenimer JG, et al. Mechanisms of *Bordetella pertussis* invasion of HeLa 229 cells. 1990 Proceedings of the 6th International Symposium on Pertussis. DHHS Publication No. FDA 90–1164. Bethesda, MD, Department of Health and Human Services, United States Public Health Service, pp 106–113.
50. Thomas MG, Redhead K, Lambert HP. Human serum antibody responses to *Bordetella pertussis* infection and pertussis vaccination. J Infect Dis 159:211–218, 1989.
51. Trollfors B, Zackrisson G, Taranger J, et al. Serum antibodies against a 69-kilodalton outer-membrane protein, pertactin, from *Bordetella pertussis* in nonvaccinated children with and without a history of clinical pertussis. J Pediatr 120:924–926, 1992.
52. Shahin RD, Brennan MJ, Li ZM, et al. Characterization of the protective capacity and immunogenicity of the 69-kD outer membrane protein of *Bordetella pertussis*. J Exp Med 171:63–73, 1990.
53. Mooi FR, van Oirschot H, Heuvelman K, et al. Polymorphism in the *Bordetella pertussis* virulence factor P.69/pertactin and pertussis toxin in The Netherlands: Temporal trends and evidence for vaccine-driven evolution. Infect Immun 66:670–675, 1998.
54. Hewlett EL, Gordon VM. Adenylate cyclase toxin of *Bordetella pertussis*. In Wardlaw AC, Parton R (eds). Pathogenesis and Immunity in Pertussis. New York, John Wiley and Sons, 1988, pp 193–209.
55. Weiss AA, Goodwin M St. M, Allison N. Investigation of the role of *Bordetella pertussis* virulence factors in disease. 1990 Proceedings of the 6th International Symposium on Pertussis. DHHS Publication No. FDA 90–1164. Bethesda, MD, Department of Health and Human Services, United States Public Health Service, pp 202–205.
56. Arciniega JL, Hewlett EL, Johnson FD, et al. Human serologic response to envelope-associated proteins and adenylate cyclase toxin of *Bordetella pertussis*. J Infect Dis 163:135–142, 1991.
57. Guiso N, Szatanik M, Rocancourt M. *Bordetella pertussis* adenylate cyclase: A protective antigen against lethality and bacterial colonization in murine respiratory and intracerebral models. 1990 Proceedings of the 6th International Symposium on Pertussis. DHHS Publication No. FDA 90–1164. Bethesda, MD, Department of Health and Human Services, United States Public Health Service, pp 207–231.

58. Cookson BT, Cho HL, Herwaldt LA, et al. Biological activities and chemical composition of purified tracheal cytotoxin of *Bordetella pertussis*. Infect Immun 57:2223–2229, 1989.
59. Goldman WE. Tracheal cytotoxin of *Bordetella pertussis*. In Wardlaw AC, Parton R (eds). Pathogenesis and Immunity in Pertussis. New York, John Wiley and Sons, 1988, pp 231–246.
60. Goldman WE, Collier JL, Cookson BL, et al. Tracheal cytotoxin of *Bordetella pertussis*: Biosynthesis, structure, and specificity. 1990 Proceedings of the 6th International Symposium on Pertussis. DHHS Publication No. FDA 90-1164. Bethesda, MD, Department of Health and Human Services, United States Public Health Service, pp 5–10.
61. Nakase Y, Endoh M. Heat-labile toxin of *Bordetella pertussis*. In Wardlaw AC, Parton R (eds). Pathogenesis and Immunity in Pertussis. New York, John Wiley and Sons, 1988, pp 211–229.
62. Endoh M, Nagai M, Burns DL, et al. Effects of exogenous agents on the action of *Bordetella parapertussis* in heat-labile toxin on guinea pig skin. Infect Immun 58:1456–1460, 1990.
63. Fernandez RC, Weiss A. Cloning and sequencing of a *Bordetella pertussis* serum resistance locus. Infect Immun 62:4727–4738, 1994.
64. Chaby R, Caroff M. Lipopolysaccharides of *Bordetella pertussis* endotoxin. In Wardlaw AC, Parton R (eds). Pathogenesis and Immunity in Pertussis. Chichester, John Wiley & Sons Ltd, 1988, pp 247–271.
65. Weiss A, Hewlett EL. Virulence factors of *Bordetella pertussis*. Ann Rev Microbiol 40:661–686, 1986.
66. Hewlett EL. Pertussis: Current concepts of pathogenesis and prevention. Pediatr Infect Dis J 16:578–584, 1997.
67. Zhang JM, Cowell JL, Steven AC, et al. Purification of serotype 2 fimbriae of *Bordetella pertussis* and their identification as a mouse protective antigen. Devel Biol Stand 61:173–185, 1985.
68. Confer DL, Eaton JW. Phagocyte impotence caused by an invasive bacterial adenylate cyclase. Science 217:948, 1982.
69. Olson LC. Pertussis. Medicine 54:427–469, 1975.
70. Broome CV, Fraser DW, English WJ II. Pertussis—diagnostic methods and surveillance. In Manclark CR, Hill JC (eds). International Symposium on Pertussis. Washington, DC, US Government Printing Office, 1979, pp 19–22.
71. Strebel PM, Cochi SL, Farizo KM, et al. Pertussis in Missouri: Evaluation of nasopharyngeal culture, direct fluorescent antibody testing, and clinical case definitions in the diagnosis of pertussis. Clin Infect Dis 16:276–285, 1993.
72. Onorato IM, Wassilak SGF. Laboratory diagnosis of pertussis: The state of the art. Pediatr Infect Dis J 6:145–152, 1987.
73. Halperin SA, Bortolussi R, Wort AJ. Evaluation of culture, immunofluorescence, and serology for the diagnosis of pertussis. J Clin Microbiol 27:752–757, 1989.
74. Hallander HO, Reizenstein E, Renemar B, et al. Comparison of nasopharyngeal aspirates with swabs for culture of *Bordetella pertussis*. J Clin Microbiol 31:50–52, 1993.
75. Granstrom G, Wretlind B, Granstrom M. Diagnostic value of clinical and bacteriological findings in pertussis. J Infect 22:17–26, 1991.
76. Ad hoc group for the study of pertussis vaccines: Placebo-controlled trial of two acellular pertussis vaccines in Sweden—protective efficacy and adverse events: Lancet 1:955–960, 1988.
77. Donaldson P, Whitaker JA. Diagnosis of pertussis by fluorescent antibody staining of nasopharyngeal smears. Am J Dis Child 99:423–427, 1960.
78. Ewanowich CA, Chui LW-L, Paranchych MG, et al. Major outbreak of pertussis in northern Alberta, Canada: Analysis of discrepant direct fluorescent-antibody and culture results by using polymerase chain reaction methodology. J Clin Microbiol 31:1715–1725, 1993.
79. He Q, Mertsola J, Soini H, Vijanen MK. Sensitive and specific polymerase chain reaction assays for detection of *Bordetella pertussis* in nasopharyngeal specimens. J Pediatr 124:421–426, 1994.
80. Schlapfer G, Cherry JD, Heininger V, et al. Polymerase chain reaction identification of *Bordetella pertussis* infections in vaccinees and family members in a pertussis vaccine efficacy trial in Germany. Pediatr Infect Dis J 14:209–214, 1995.
81. Olcen P, Backman A, Johansson B, et al. Amplification of DNA by the polymerase chain reaction for the efficient diagnosis of pertussis. Scand J Infect Dis 24:339–345, 1992.
82. Reizenstein E, Lofdahl S, Granstrom M, et al. Evaluation of an improved DNA probe for diagnosis of pertussis. Diagn Microbiol Infect Dis 5:569–573, 1992.
83. Glare EM, Paton JC, Premier RR, et al. Analysis of a repetitive DNA sequence from *Bordetella pertussis* and its application to the diagnosis of pertussis using the polymerase chain reaction. J Clin Microbiol 28:1982–1987, 1990.
84. Edelman K, Nikkari S, Ruuskanen O, et al. Detection of *Bordetella pertussis* by polymerase chain reaction and culture in the nasopharynx of erythromycin-treated infants with pertussis. Pediatr Infect Dis J 15:54–57, 1996.
85. He Q, Schmidt-Schlapfer G, Just M, et al. Impact of polymerase chain reaction on clinical pertussis research: Finnish and Swiss experiences. J Infect Dis 174:1288–1295, 1996.
86. Meade BD, Mink CM, Manclark CR. Serodiagnosis of pertussis. 1990 Proceedings of the 6th International Symposium on Pertussis. DHHS Publication No. FDA 90-1164. Bethesda, MD, Department of Health and Human Services, United States Public Health Service, pp 322–329.
87. Steketee RW, Burstyn DG, Wassilak SGF, et al. A comparison of laboratory and clinical methods for diagnosing pertussis in an outbreak in a facility for the developmentally disabled. J Infect Dis 157:441–449, 1988.
88. Mink CAM, Cherry JD, Christenson P, et al. A search for *Bordetella pertussis* infection in university students. Clin Infect Dis 14:464–471, 1992.
89. Addiss DG, Davis JP, Meade BD, et al. A pertussis outbreak in a Wisconsin nursing home. J Infect Dis 164:704–710, 1991.
90. Cattaneo LA, Reed G, Haase DH, et al. The seroepidemiology of *Bordetella pertussis* infections: A study of persons age 1–65 years. J Infect Dis 173:1256–1259, 1996.
91. Giammanco A, Chiarini A, Stroffolini T, et al. Seroepidemiology of pertussis in Italy. Rev Infect Dis 13:1216–1220, 1991.
92. Halperin SA, Bortolussi R, MacLean D, et al. Persistence of pertussis in an immunized population: Results of the Nova Scotia enhanced pertussis surveillance program. J Pediatr 115:686–693, 1989.
93. Bass JW, Klenk EL, Kotherine JB, et al. Antimicrobial treatment of pertussis. J Pediatr 75:768–781, 1969.
94. Hewlett EL. *Bordetella* species. In Mandell GL, Bennett JE, Dolin R (eds). Mandell, Douglas and Bennett's Principles and Practice of Infectious Diseases (4th ed). New York, Churchill Livingstone, 1995, pp 2078–2083.
95. Halperin SA, Bortolussi R, Langley JM, et al. Seven days of erythromycin estolate is as effective as fourteen days for the treatment of *Bordetella pertussis* infections. Pediatrics 100:65–71, 1997.
96. Kawai H, Aoyama T, Goto A, et al. Evaluation of pertussis treatment with erythromycin ethylsuccinate and stearate according to age. Kansenshogaku Zasshi 68:1324–1329, 1994.
97. Aoyama T, Sunakawa K, Iwata S, et al. Efficacy of short-term treatment of pertussis with clarithromycin and azithromycin. J Pediatr 129:761–764, 1996.
98. Committee on Infectious Diseases, American Academy of Pediatrics; Peter G, Hall CB, Halsey NA, et al. (eds). 1997 Red Book: Report of the Committee on Infectious Diseases (24th ed). Elk Grove Village, IL, American Academy of Pediatrics, 1997.
99. Pertussis. In Benenson AS (ed). Control of Communicable Disease Manual (16th ed). Washington, DC, American Public Health Association, 1995.
100. Weber DJ, Rutala WA. Management of healthcare workers exposed to pertussis. Infect Control Hosp Epidemiol 15:411–415, 1994.
101. Decker MD, Schaffner W. Nosocomial diseases of health care workers spread by the airborne or contact route (other than tuberculosis). In Mayhall CG (ed). Hospital Epidemiology and Infection Control. Baltimore, Williams & Wilkins, 1996, pp 871–872.
102. Wirsing von Konig CH, Schmitt HJ, Bogaerts H, et al. Factors influencing the analysis of secondary prevention of pertussis. Dev Biol Stand 89:175–179, 1997.
103. De Serres G, Boulianne N, Duval B. Field effectiveness of erythromycin prophylaxis to prevent pertussis within families. Pediatr Infect Dis J 14:969–975, 1995.
104. Fine PEM, Clarkson JA. The recurrence of whooping cough:

Possible implications for assessment of vaccine efficacy. Lancet 1:666–669, 1982.

105. Cherry JD. The epidemiology of pertussis and pertussis vaccine in the United Kingdom and the United States: A comparative study. Curr Probl Pediatr 14:1–78, 1984.
106. Kanai K. Japan's experience in pertussis epidemiology and vaccination in the past thirty years. Jpn J Sci Biol 33:107–143, 1980.
107. Cherry JD, Baraff LJ, Hewlett E. The past, present, and future of pertussis: The role of adults in epidemiology and future control. West J Med 150:319–328, 1989.
108. Cherry JD. Pertussis in adults. Ann Intern Med 128:64–66, 1998.
109. Luttinger P. The epidemiology of pertussis. Am J Dis Child 12:290–315, 1916.
110. Friedlander A. Whooping cough. In Abt IA (ed). Pediatrics. Vol. 11. Philadelphia, WB Saunders, 1925, pp 128–147.
111. Farizo KM, Cochi SL, Zell ER, et al. Epidemiological features of pertussis in the United States, 1980–1989. Clin Infect Dis 14:708–719, 1992.
112. Forest MG, Cathiard AM, Bertrand JA. Evidence of testicular activity in early infancy. J Clin Endocrinol Metab 37:148–151, 1973.
113. Clark AC, Bradford WL, Berry GP. An epidemiological study of an outbreak of pertussis in a public school. Am J Public Health 36:1156–1162, 1946.
114. Lambert HS. Epidemiology of a small pertussis outbreak in Kent County, Michigan. Public Health Rep 80:365–369, 1965.
115. Linneman CC, Bass JW, Smith MHD. The carrier state of pertussis. Am J Epidemiol 88:422–427, 1968.
116. Lambert HP. The carrier state: *Bordetella pertussis*. J Antimicrob Chemother 18(suppl A):13–16, 1986.
117. Pertussis surveillance—United States 1989–1991. MMWR CDC Surveill Summ 41(SS-8):11–19, 1992.
118. He Q, Viljanen MK, Nikkari S, et al. Outcomes of *Bordetella pertussis* infection in different age groups of an immunized population. J Infect Dis 170:873–877, 1994.
119. Biellik RJ, Patriarca PA, Mullen JR, et al. Risk factors for community- and household-acquired pertussis during a large-scale outbreak in central Wisconsin. J Infect Dis 157:1134–1141, 1988.
120. Mink CM, Sirota NM, Nguent S. Outbreak of pertussis in a fully immunized adolescent and adult population. Arch Pediatr Adolesc Med 148:153–157, 1994.
121. Marchant CD, Loughlin AM, Lett SM, et al. Pertussis in Massachusetts, 1981–1991: Incidence, serologic diagnosis, and vaccine effectiveness. J Infect Dis 169:1297–1305, 1994.
122. Robertson PW, Goldberg H, Jarvie BAH, et al. *Bordetella pertussis* infection: A cause of persistent cough in adults. Med J Aust 146:522–525, 1987.
123. Rosenthal S, Strebel P, Cassiday P, et al. Pertussis infection among adults during the 1993 outbreak in Chicago. J Infect Dis 171:1650–1652, 1995.
124. Wright SW, Edwards KM, Decker MD, Zeldin MH. Pertussis infection in adults with persistent cough. JAMA 273:1044–1046, 1995.
125. Nennig ME, Shinefield HR, Edwards KM, et al. Prevalence and incidence of adult pertussis in an urban population. JAMA 275:1672–1674, 1996.
126. Christie CDC, Marx ML, Marchant CD, et al. The 1993 epidemic of pertussis in Cincinnati: Resurgence of disease in a highly immunized population of children. N Engl J Med 331:16–21, 1994.
127. Resurgence of pertussis—United States, 1993. MMWR Morb Mortal Wkly Rep 42:952–953, 959–960, 1993.
128. Pertussis outbreak—Vermont, 1996. MMWR Morb Mortal Wkly Rep 46:822–826, 1997.
129. Edwards KM, Decker MD, Halsey NA, et al. Differences in antibody response to whole-cell pertussis vaccines. Pediatrics 88:1019–1023, 1991.
130. Edwards KM, Decker MD. Acellular pertussis vaccines for infants. N Engl J Med 334:391–392, 1996.
131. Stehr K, Cherry JD, Heininger U, et al. A comparative efficacy trial in Germany in infants who received either the Lederle/Takeda acellular pertussis component DTP (DTaP) vaccine, the Lederle whole-cell component DTP (DTP) vaccine or DT vaccine. Pediatrics 101:1–11, 1998.
132. Gustafsson L, Hallander HO, Olin P, et al. A controlled trial of a two-component acellular, a five-component acellular, and a whole-cell pertussis vaccine. N Engl J Med 334:349–355, 1996.
133. Greco D, Salmaso S, Mastrantonio P, et al. A controlled trial of two acellular vaccines and one whole-cell vaccine against pertussis. N Engl J Med 334:341–348, 1996.
134. Mortimer EA Jr, Jones PK. An evaluation of pertussis vaccine. Rev Infect Dis 1:927–932, 1979.
135. Van Savage J, Decker MD, Edwards KM, et al. Natural history of pertussis antibody in the infant and effect on vaccine response. J Infect Dis 161:487–492, 1990.
136. Bradford WL. Use of convalescent blood in whooping cough. Am J Dis Child 50:918–928, 1935.
137. Department of Health and Human Services, Food and Drug Administration. Biological products; bacterial vaccines and toxoids; implementation of efficacy review; proposed rule. Fed Register 50:51002–51117, 1985.
138. Balagtas RC, Nelson KE, Levin S, et al. Treatment of pertussis with pertussis immune globulin. J Pediatr 79:203–208, 1971.
139. Morris D, McDonald JC. Failure of hyperimmune gamma globulin to prevent whooping cough. Arch Dis Child 32:236–239, 1957.
140. Granstrom M, Olinder-Nielsen AM, Holmblad P, et al. Specific immunoglobulin for treatment of whooping cough. Lancet 338:1230–1233, 1991.
141. Bruss JB, Malley R, Parker JC, et al. Treatment of severe pertussis with intravenous pertussis immune globulin. Presented at the 33rd Interscience Conference on Antimicrobial Agents and Chemotherapy (ICAAC); New Orleans, LA; October 1993.
142. Luttinger P. Pertussis vaccine: Its value as a curative and prophylactic agent in whooping cough. JAMA 68:1461–1464, 1917.
143. Madsen T. Vaccination against whooping cough. JAMA 101:187–188, 1933.
144. Kendrick PL, Eldering G, Dixon MK, et al. Mouse protection tests in the study of pertussis vaccine: A comparative series using intracerebral route for challenge. Am J Public Health 37:803–810, 1947.
145. Eldering G. Symposium on pertussis immunization, in honor of Dr. Pearl L. Kendrick in her eightieth year: Historical notes on pertussis immunization. Health Lab Sci 8:200–205, 1971.
146. Medical Research Council. Vaccination against whooping-cough: Relation between protection in children and results of laboratory tests. BMJ 2:454–462, 1956.
147. Weihl C, Riley HD, Lapin JH. Extracted pertussis antigen. A clinical appraisal. Am J Dis Child 106:210–215, 1963.
148. Diphtheria, tetanus and pertussis: Recommendations for vaccine use and other preventive measures: Recommendations of the Advisory Committee on Immunization Practices (ACIP). MMWR Morb Mortal Wkly Rep 40(RR-10):1–28, 1991.
149. Linnemann CC Jr, Ramundo N, Perlstein PH, et al. Use of pertussis vaccine in an epidemic involving hospital staff. Lancet 2:540–543, 1975.
150. Edwards KM, Decker MD. Combination vaccines consisting of acellular pertussis vaccines. Pediatr Infect Dis J 16:S97–S102, 1997.
151. Gold R, Scheifele D, Barreto L, et al. Safety and immunogenicity of *Haemophilus influenzae* vaccine (tetanus toxoid conjugate) administered concurrently or combined with diphtheria and tetanus toxoids, pertussis vaccine and inactivated poliomyelitis vaccine to healthy infants at two, four and six months of age. Pediatr Infect Dis 13:348–355, 1994.
152. Hinman AR, Koplan JP. Pertussis and pertussis vaccine. Reanalysis of benefits, risks and costs. JAMA 251:3109–3113, 1984.
153. Miller DL, Alderslade R, Ross EM. Whooping cough and whooping cough vaccine: The risks and benefits debate. Epidemiol Rev 4:1–24, 1982.
154. Kendrick P, Eldering G. Progress report on pertussis immunization. Am J Public Health 26:8–12, 1936.
155. Sauer LW. Whooping cough. New phases of the work of immunization and prophylaxis. JAMA 112:305–308, 1939.
156. Steinhoff MC, Reed GF, Decker MD, et al. A randomized comparison of reactogenicity and immunogenicity of two whole-cell pertussis vaccines. Pediatrics 96:567–570, 1995.
157. Baker JD, Halperin SA, Edwards KM, et al. Antibody response to *Bordetella pertussis* antigens after immunization with American and Canadian whole-cell vaccines. J Pediatr 121:523–527, 1992.

158. Doull JA, Shibley GS, McClelland JS. Active immunization against whooping cough. Interim report of the Cleveland experience. Am J Public Health 26:1097–1105, 1936.
159. Sako W. Studies on pertussis immunization. J Pediatr 30:29–40, 1947.
160. Medical Research Council. Vaccination against whooping-cough. The final report to the Immunization Committee of the Medical Research Council and to the medical officers of health for Battersea and Wandsworth, Bradford, Liverpool and Newcastle. BMJ 1:994–1000, 1959.
161. Schmitt H-J, Wirsing von Konig CH, Neiss A, et al. Efficacy of acellular pertussis vaccine in early childhood after household exposure. JAMA 275:37–41, 1996.
162. Liese JG, Meschievitz CK, Harzer E, et al. Efficacy of a two-component acellular pertussis vaccine in infants. Pediatr Infect Dis J 16:1038–1044, 1997.
163. Wyeth-Ayerst Laboratories. ACEL-IMUNE (Lederle Laboratories) Product Labelling. In Physician's Desk Reference. Montvale, NJ, Medical Economics Company, 1997.
164. Simondon F, Preziosi MP, Yam A, et al. A randomized double-blind trial comparing a two-component acellular to a whole-cell pertussis vaccine in Senegal. Vaccine 15:1606–1612, 1997.
165. Ramsay ME, Farrington CP, Miller E. Age-specific efficacy of pertussis vaccine during epidemic and non-epidemic periods. Epidemiol Infect 111:41–48, 1993.
166. White JM, Fairley CK, Owen D, et al. The effect of an accelerated immunization schedule on pertussis in England and Wales. Commun Dis Rep CDR Rev 6:R86–R91, 1996.
167. Miller E, Ashworth LAE, Redhead K, et al. Effect of schedule on reactogenicity and antibody persistence of acellular and whole-cell pertussis vaccines: Value of laboratory tests as predictors of clinical performance. Vaccine 15:51–60, 1997.
168. Lautrop H, Mikkelson OS. The effect of prophylactic whooping-cough vaccination. An attempt at an evaluation based on experiences in Denmark. Ugeskr Laeger 131:735–741, 1969.
169. Sutter RW, Cochi SL. Pertussis hospitalizations and mortality, 1985–1988. Evaluation of the completeness of national reporting. JAMA 267:386–391, 1992.
170. Dauer CC. Reported whooping cough morbidity and mortality in the United States. Public Health Rep 58:661–676, 1943.
170a. Kimura M, Kuno-Sakai H. Immunization system in Japan: Its history and present situation. Acta Paediatr Jpn 30:109–126, 1988.
171. Stuart-Harris CH. Experiences of pertussis in the United Kingdom. In Manclark CR, Hill JC (eds). International Symposium on Pertussis. Washington, DC, US Government Printing Office, 1979, pp 256–261.
172. Romanus V, Jonsell R, Bergquist S-O. Pertussis in Sweden after the cessation of general immunization in 1979. Pediatr Infect Dis 6:664–671, 1987.
173. Storsaeter J, Olin P. Relative efficacy of two acellular pertussis vaccines during three years of passive surveillance. Vaccine 10:142–144, 1992.
174. Pollard R. Relation between vaccination and notification rates for whooping cough in England and Wales. Lancet 1:1180–1182, 1980.
175. Onorato IM, Wassilak SG, Meade B. Efficacy of whole-cell pertussis vaccine in preschool children in the United States. JAMA 267:2745–2749, 1992.
176. Vesselinova-Jenkins CK, Newcombe RG, Gray OP, et al. The effects of immunisation upon the natural history of pertussis: A family study in the Cardiff area. J Epidemiol Commun Health 32:194–199, 1978.
177. Grob PR, Crowder MH, Robbins JF. Effect of vaccination on the severity and dissemination of whooping cough. BMJ 2:1925–1928, 1981.
178. Cvjetanovic B, Grab B, Uemura K. Diphtheria and whooping cough. Diseases affecting a particular age group. Bull World Health Organ 56(suppl 1):103–133, 1978.
179. Fox JP, Elveback L, Scott W, et al. Commentary. Herd immunity: Basic concept and relevance to public health immunization practices. Am J Epidemiol 94:179–189, 1971.
180. Jenkinson D. Duration of effectiveness of pertussis vaccine: Evidence from a 10 year community study. BMJ 296:612–614, 1988.
181. Fine PE, Clarkson JA. Reflections on the efficacy of pertussis vaccines. Rev Infect Dis 9:866–883, 1987.
182. Weiss ES, Kendrick PL. The effectiveness of pertussis vaccine: An application of Sargent and Merrell's method of measurement. Am J Hyg 38:306–309, 1943.
183. CP Howson, CJ Howe, HV Fineberg (eds). Adverse effects of pertussis and rubella vaccines. Report of the Committee to Review the Adverse Consequences of Pertussis and Rubella Vaccines. Washington, DC, National Academy Press, 1991.
184. Howson CP, Fineberg HV. Adverse events following pertussis and rubella vaccines: Summary of a report of the Institute of Medicine. JAMA 267:392–396, 1992.
185. Howson CP, Fineberg HV. The ricochet of magic bullets: Summary of the Institute of Medicine report: Adverse effects of pertussis and rubella vaccines. Pediatrics 89:318–324, 1992.
186. Cody CL, Baraff LJ, Cherry JD, et al. Nature and rates of adverse reactions associated with DTP and DT immunizations in infants and children. Pediatrics 68:650–660, 1981.
187. Decker MD, Edwards KM, Steinhoff MC, et al. Comparison of 13 acellular pertussis vaccines: Adverse reactions. Pediatrics 96:557–566, 1995.
188. Baraff LJ, Cody CL, Cherry JD. DTP-associated reactions: An analysis by injection site, manufacturer, prior reactions, and dose. Pediatrics 73:31–36, 1984.
189. Pichichero ME, Christy C, Decker MD, et al. Defining the key parameters for comparing reactions among acellular and whole-cell pertussis vaccines. Pediatrics 96:588–593, 1995.
190. Deloria MA, Blackwelder WC, Decker MD, et al. Association of reactions after consecutive acellular or whole-cell pertussis vaccine immunizations. Pediatrics 96:592–594, 1995.
191. Hirtz DG, Nelson KB, Ellenberg JH. Seizures following childhood immunizations. J Pediatr 102:14–18, 1983.
192. Walker AM, Jick H, Perera DR, et al. Neurologic events following diphtheria-tetanus-pertussis immunization. Pediatrics 81: 345–349, 1988.
193. Griffin MR, Ray WA, Mortimer EA Jr, et al. Risk of seizures and encephalopathy after immunization with the diphtheria-tetanus-pertussis vaccine. JAMA 263:1641–1645, 1990.
194. Gale JL, Thapa PB, Bobo JK, et al. Acute neurological illness and DTP: Report of a case-control study in Washington and Oregon. Abstracts of the 6th International Symposium on Pertussis. DHHS Publ. No. 90–1162. Bethesda, MD, Public Health Service, US Department of Health and Human Services.
195. Stetler HC, Orenstein WA, Bart KJ, et al. History of convulsions and use of pertussis vaccine. J Pediatr 107:175–179, 1985.
196. Bellman MH, Ross EM. Pertussis immunization and fits. In Ross E, Reynolds E (eds). Paediatric Perspectives on Epilepsy. New York, John Wiley & Sons, 1985.
197. Livengood JR, Mullen JR, White JW, et al. Family history of convulsions and use of pertussis vaccine. J Pediatr 115:527–531, 1989.
198. Ellenberg JH, Hirtz DG, Nelson KB. Do seizures in children cause intellectual deterioration? N Engl J Med 314:1085–1088, 1986.
199. Shields WD, Nielsen C, Buch D, et al. Relationship of pertussis immunization to the onset of neurologic disorders: A retrospective epidemiologic study. J Pediatr 113:801–805, 1988.
200. Berg JM. Neurological complications of pertussis immunization. BMJ 2:24–27, 1958.
201. Byers RK, Moll FC. Encephalopathies following prophylactic pertussis vaccine. Pediatrics 1:437–456, 1948.
202. Toomey JA. Reactions to pertussis vaccine. JAMA 139:448–450, 1949.
203. Halpern SR, Halpern D. Reactions from DTP administration and its relationship to allergic children. J Pediatr 47:60–67, 1955.
204. Kulenkampf M, Schwartzman JS, Wilson J. Neurological complications of pertussis inoculation. Arch Dis Child 49:46–49, 1974.
205. Murphy JV, Sarff LD, Marquardt KM. Recurrent seizures after diphtheria, tetanus and pertussis vaccine immunization. Am J Dis Child 138:908–911, 1984.
206. Corsellis JAN, Janota J, Marshall AK. Immunization against whooping cough: A neuropathological review. Neuropathol Appl Neurobiol 9:261–270, 1983.
207. Miller DL, Wadsworth MJH, Ross EM. Pertussis vaccine and severe acute neurological illnesses. Response to a recent review by members of the NCES team. Vaccine 7:487–489, 1989.

208. Bellman MH, Ross EM, Miller DL. Infantile spasms and pertussis immunisation. Lancet 1:1031–1034, 1983.
209. Miller D, Wadsworth J, Ross E. Safety of pertussis vaccine [letter]. Lancet 335:655–656, 1990.
210. Miller D, Madge N, Diamond J, et al. Pertussis immunization and serious acute neurological illnesses in children. BMJ 307:1171–1176, 1993.
211. Griffith AH. Pertussis vaccines and permanent brain damage [letter]. Vaccine 7:489–490, 1989.
212. Bowie C. Viewpoint. Lessons from the pertussis vaccine court trial. Lancet 335:397–399, 1990.
213. Stephenson JBP. A neurologist looks at neurological disease temporally related to DTP immunization. Tokai J Exp Clin Med 13:157–164, 1988.
214. Leviton A. Commentary. Neurologic sequelae of pertussis immunization—1989. J Child Neurol 4:311–314, 1989.
215. MacRae KD. Epidemiology, encephalopathy, and pertussis vaccine. FEMS—Symposium Pertussis: Proceedings of the Conference Organized by the Society for Microbiology and Epidemiology of the GDR; Berlin; April 20–22, 1988; pp 302–311.
216. Fulginiti VA. A pertussis vaccine myth dies. Am J Dis Child 144:860–861, 1990.
217. Golden GS. Pertussis vaccine and injury to the brain. J Pediatr 116:854–861, 1990.
218. Wentz KE, Marcuse EK. Diphtheria-tetanus-pertussis vaccine and serious neurological illness: An updated review of the epidemiologic evidence. Pediatrics 87:287–297, 1991.
219. American Academy of Pediatrics, Committee on Infectious Diseases. The relationship between pertussis vaccine and central nervous system sequelae: Continuing assessments. Pediatrics 97:279–281, 1996.
220. Child Neurology Society. Ad hoc committee for the Child Neurology Society consensus statement on pertussis immunization and the central nervous system. Ann Neurol 29:458–460, 1991.
221. American Academy of Neurology. Report of the Therapeutics and Technology Assessment Subcommittee. Assessment: DTP vaccination. Neurology 42:471–472, 1992.
222. British Paediatric Association. Pertussis immunization. In Nicoll A, Rudd P (eds). Manual on Infections and Immunizations in Children. Oxford, England, Oxford University Press, 1989, pp 207–210.
223. Brahams D. Medicine and the law. Pertussis vaccine litigation. Lancet 335:905–906, 1990.
224. National Advisory Committee on Immunization. Statement on pertussis immunization. Can Commun Dis Ref 19:41–45, 1993.
225. Update: Vaccine side effects, adverse reactions, contraindications, and precautions. Recommendations of the Advisory Committee on Immunization Practices (ACIP). MMWR Morb Mortal Wkly Rep 45(RR-12):1–35, 1996.
226. Stratton KR, Howe CJ, Johnston RB (eds). DPT Vaccine and Chronic Nervous System Dysfunction. A New Analysis. Washington, DC, National Academy Press, 1994.
227. Riikonen R, Donner M. Incidence and aetiology of infantile spasms from 1960 to 1976: A population study in Finland. Dev Med Child Neurol 21:333–343, 1979.
228. Millichap JG. Etiology and treatment of infantile spasms: Current concepts, including the role of DPT immunization. Acta Paediatr Jpn 29:54–60, 1987.
229. Melchior JC. Infantile spasms and early immunization against whooping cough. Danish survey from 1970 to 1975. Arch Dis Child 52:134–137, 1977.
230. Fukuyama Y, Tomori N, Sugitate M. Critical evaluation of the role of immunization as an etiological factor of infantile spasms. Neuropaediatrie 8:224–237, 1977.
231. Lombroso CR. A prospective study of infantile spasms: Clinical and therapeutic correlations. Epilepsia 24:135–158, 1983.
232. Guyer B, Martin JA, MacDorman MF, et al. Annual summary of vital statistics 1996. Pediatrics 100:905–918, 1997.
233. Bernier RH, Frank JA Jr, Dondero TJ Jr, et al. Diphtheria-tetanus toxoids-pertussis vaccination and sudden infant deaths in Tennessee. J Pediatr 101:419–421, 1982.
234. Baraff LJ, Ablon WJ, Weiss RC. Possible temporal association between diphtheria-tetanus toxoid-pertussis vaccination and sudden infant death syndrome. Pediatr Infect Dis 2:7–11, 1983.
235. Torch WC. Diphtheria-pertussis-tetanus (DPT) immunization: A potential cause of the sudden infant death syndrome (SIDS). J Pediatr 101:169–170, 1982.
236. Torch WC. Characteristics of diphtheria-pertussis-tetanus (DPT) postvaccinal deaths and DPT-caused sudden infant death syndrome (SIDS): A review. Neurology 36(suppl 1):148, 1986.
237. Nickerson BG, Robison BK. How many sudden infant death syndrome victims were recently immunized? Western Soc Pediatr Res Clin Res 33:121A, 1985.
238. Taylor EM, Emery JL. Immunisation and cot deaths. Lancet 2:721, 1982.
239. Hoffman HS, Hunter JC, Damus K, et al. Diphtheria-tetanus-pertussis immunization and sudden infant death: Results of the National Institute of Child Health and Human Development Cooperative Epidemiological Study of Sudden Infant Death Syndrome Risk Factors. Pediatrics 79:698–711, 1987.
240. Bouvier-Colle MH, Flahaut A, Messiah A, et al. Sudden infant death and immunization. An extensive epidemiological approach to the problem in France—winter 1986. Int J Epidemiol 18:121–126, 1989.
241. Griffin MR, Ray WA, Livengood JR, et al. Risk of sudden infant death syndrome (SIDS) after immunization with the diphtheria-tetanus-pertussis vaccine. N Engl J Med 319:618–623, 1988.
242. Geraghty KC. Presentation to the Immunization Practices Advisory Committee, Centers for Disease Control; Atlanta, GA; October 25, 1985.
243. Walker AM, Jick H, Perera DR, et al. Diphtheria-tetanus-pertussis immunization and sudden infant death syndrome. Am J Public Health 77:945–951, 1987.
244. Solberg LK. DTP immunization, visit to child health center and sudden infant death syndrome (SIDS). Report to the Oslo Health Council, Norway, 1985, 131 pp.
245. Wennergren G, Milerad J, Lagercrantz H, et al. The epidemiology of sudden infant death syndrome and attacks of lifelessness in Sweden. Acta Paediatr Scand 76:898–906, 1987.
246. Butler NR, Haslum M, Golding J, et al. Recent findings from the 1970 child health and education study: Preliminary communication. J Roy Soc Med 75:781–784, 1982.
247. Sato Y, Kimura M, Fukumi H. Development of a pertussis component vaccine in Japan. Lancet 1:122–126, 1984.
248. Kimura M, Hikino N. Results with a new DTP vaccine in Japan. Dev Biol Stand 61:545–561, 1985.
249. Noble GR, Bernier RH, Esber EC, et al. Acellular and whole-cell pertussis vaccine in Japan: Report of a visit by U.S. scientists. JAMA 257:1351–1356, 1987.
250. Aoyama T, Murase Y, Gonda T, et al. Type-specific efficacy of acellular pertussis vaccine. Am J Dis Child 142:40–42, 1988.
251. Kimura M, Kuno-Sakai H. Current epidemiology of pertussis in Japan. Pediatr Infect Dis J 9:705–709, 1990.
252. Kato T, Goshima T, Nakajima N, et al. Protection against pertussis by acellular vaccines. (Takeda, Japan): Household contact studies in Kawasaki City, Japan. Acta Paediatr Jpn 31:698–701, 1989.
253. Kimura M, Kuno-Sakai H. Pertussis vaccines in Japan. Acta Paediatr Jpn 30:143–153, 1988.
254. Kamiya H, Nii R. Overview of currently available Japanese acellular pertussis vaccines and future problems. Tokai J Exp Clin Med 13(suppl):45–49, 1988.
255. Sato Y, Sato H. Further characterization of Japanese acellular pertussis vaccine prepared in 1988 by six Japanese manufacturers. Tokai J Exp Clin Med 13(suppl):79–88, 1988.
256. Ginnaga A, Morokuma K, Aihara K, et al. Characterization and clinical study on the acellular pertussis vaccine produced by a combination of column purified pertussis toxin and filamentous hemagglutinin. Tokai J Exp Clin Med 13(suppl):59–69, 1988.
257. Kimura M, Kuno-Sakai H. Developments in pertussis immunisation in Japan. Lancet 336:30–32, 1990.
258. Pittman M. History of the development of pertussis vaccine. Dev Biol Stand 73:19–29, 1991.
259. Kimura M. Japanese clinical experiences with acellular pertussis vaccines. Dev Biol Stand 73:5–9, 1991.
260. Robinson A, Funnell SGP. Potency testing of acellular pertussis vaccines. Vaccine 10:139–141, 1992.
261. Winsnes R, Lonnes T, Mogster, et al. Antibody responses after vaccination and disease against leukocytosis promoting factor, filamentous hemagglutinin, lipopolysaccharide and a protein

binding to complement-fixing antibodies induced during whooping cough. Proceedings of the Fourth International Symposium on Pertussis. Dev Biol Stand 61:353–365, 1985.
262. Pizza M, Covacci A, Bartoloni A, et al. Mutants of pertussis toxin suitable for vaccine development. Science 246:497–500, 1989.
263. Olin P, Rasmussen F, Gottfarb P. Schedules and protection, simultaneous vaccination and safety: Experiences from recent controlled trials. Int J Infect Dis 1:143–147, 1997.
263a. Olin P. Vaccination and safety: A clarification. Int J Infect Dis 1:235, 1997.
264. Robinson HL, Torres CA. DNA vaccines. Semin Immunol 9:271–283, 1997.
265. Siegrist CA. Potential advantages and risks of nucleic acid vaccines for infant immunization. Vaccine 15:798–800, 1997.
266. Edwards KM, Meade BD, Decker MD, et al. Comparison of 13 acellular pertussis vaccines: Overview and serologic response. Pediatrics 96:548–557, 1995.
267. Mills KHG, Barnard A, Watkins A, Redhead K. Cell-mediated immunity to *Bordetella pertussis*: Role of Th1 cells in bacterial clearance in a murine respiratory infection model. Infect Immun 61:399–410, 1993.
268. Petersen JW, Anderson P, Ibsen PH, et al. Proliferative responses to purified and fractionated *Bordetella pertussis* antigens in mice immunized with whole-cell pertussis vaccine. Vaccine 11:463–472, 1993.
269. Peterson JW, Ibsen PH, Haslov K, Heron I. Proliferative responses and gamma interferon and tumor necrosis factor production by lymphocytes isolated from tracheobroncheal lymph nodes and spleens of mice aerosol infected with *Bordetella pertussis.* Infect Immun 60:4563–4570, 1992.
270. Redhead K, Watkins J, Barnard A, Mills KHG. Effective immunization against *Bordetella pertussis* respiratory infection in mice is dependent on induction of cell-mediated immunity. Infect Immun 61:3190–3198, 1993.
271. Adamson PC, Wu TC, Meade BD, et al. Pertussis in a previously immunized child with human immunodeficiency virus infection. J Pediatr 115:589–592, 1989.
272. Bromberg K, Tannis G, Steiner P. Detection of *Bordetella pertussis* associated with the alveolar macrophages of children with immunodeficiency virus infection. Infect Immun 59:4715–4719, 1991.
273. De Magistris MT, Romano R, Nuti S, et al. Dissecting human T cell responses against *Bordetella* species. J Exp Med 168:1351–1362, 1988.
274. Gearing AJH, Bird CR, Redhead K, Thomas M. Human cellular immune responses to *Bordetella pertussis* infection. FEMS Microbiol Immunol 47:205–212, 1989.
275. Peppoloni S, Nencioni L, Di Tommaso A, et al. Lymphokine secretion and cytotoxic activity of human CD4+ T cell clones against *Bordetella pertussis.* Infect Immun 59:3768–3773, 1991.
276. Petersen JW, Ibsen PH, Bentzon MW, et al. The cell-mediated and humoral immune response to vaccination with acellular and whole-cell pertussis vaccine in adult humans. FEMS Microbiol Immunol 3:279–287, 1991.
277. Podda A, Nencioni L, De Magistris MT, et al. Metabolic, humoral, and cellular responses in adult volunteers immunized with the genetically inactivated pertussis toxin mutant PT-9K/129G. J Exp Med 172:861–868, 1990.
278. Zepp F, Knuf M, Habermehl P, et al. Pertussis-specific cell-mediated immunity in infants after vaccination with a tricomponent acellular pertussis vaccine. Infect Immun 64:4078–4084, 1996.
279. Poland GA. Still more questions on pertussis vaccines. Lancet 350:1564–1565, 1997.
280. Pertussis vaccination: Acellular pertussis vaccine for reinforcing and booster use—supplementary ACIP statement. Recommendations of the Immunization Practices Advisory Committee (ACIP). MMWR Morb Mortal Wkly Rep 41(RR-1):1–10, 1992.
281. Storsaeter J, Olin P, Renemar B, et al. Mortality and morbidity from invasive bacterial infections during a clinical trial of acellular pertussis vaccines in Sweden. Pediatr Infect Dis J 7:637–645, 1988.
282. Anonymous. License application for pertussis vaccine withdrawn in Sweden. Lancet 1:114, 1989.
283. Samore MH, Siber GR. Effect of pertussis toxin on susceptibility of infant rats to *Haemophilus influenzae* type b. J Infect Dis 165:945–948, 1992.
284. Black SB, Cherry JD, Shinefield HR, et al. Apparent decreased risk of invasive bacterial disease after heterologous childhood immunization. Am J Dis Child 145:746–749, 1991.
285. Davidson M, Letson GW, Ward JI, et al. DTP immunization and susceptibility to infectious diseases. Is there a relationship? Am J Dis Child 145:750–754, 1991.
286. Joffe LS, Glode MP, Gutierrez MK, et al. Diphtheria-tetanus toxoids-pertussis vaccination does not increase the risk of pertussis hospitalization with an infectious illness. Pediatr Infect Dis J 11:730–735, 1992.
287. Kimura M, Kuno-Sakai H. Acellular pertussis vaccines and fatal infections [letter]. Lancet 1:881–882, 1988.
288. Blackwelder WC, Storsaeter J, Olin P, Hallander HO. Acellular pertussis vaccines: Efficacy and evaluation of clinical case definitions. Am J Dis Child 145:1285–1289, 1991.
289. Storsaeter J, Hallander H, Farrington CP, et al. Secondary analyses of the efficacy of two acellular pertussis vaccines evaluated in a Swedish phase III trial. Vaccine 8:457–461, 1990.
290. Olin P, Storsaeter J. Vaccine efficacy. In A Clinical Trial of Acellular Pertussis Vaccines in Sweden: Technical Report. Stockholm, National Bacteriological Laboratory, 1988, pp 1–28.
291. WHO meeting on case definition of pertussis: Geneva, 10–11 January 1991. General document MIM/EPI/PERT/91.01 (1245). Geneva, World Health Organization, 1991, pp 4–5.
292. Taranger J, Trollfors B, Lagergård T, et al. Unchanged efficacy of a pertussis toxoid vaccine throughout the two years after the third vaccination of infants. Pediatr Infect Dis J 16:180–184, 1997.
293. Hallander HO, Storsaeter J, Mollby R. Evaluation of serology and nasopharyngeal cultures for diagnosis of pertussis in a vaccine efficacy trial. J Infect Dis 163:1046–1054, 1991.
294. Gustafsson L, Hallander HO, Olin P, et al. Efficacy trial of acellular pertussis vaccines: Technical report, trial 1, with results of preplanned analysis of safety, efficacy and immunogenicity. Stockholm, Swedish Institute for Infectious Disease Control, 1995.
295. Heininger U, Cherry JD, Eckhardt T, et al. Clinical and laboratory diagnosis of pertussis in the regions of a large vaccine efficacy trial in Germany. Pediatr Infect Dis J 12:504–509, 1993.
296. Edwards K, Decker MD. Comparison of serologic results in the NIAID multicenter acellular pertussis trial with recent efficacy trials. Dev Biol Stand 89:265–273, 1997.
297. Greco D, Salmaso S, Mastrantonio P, et al. A difference in relative efficacy of two DTaP vaccines in continued blinded observation of children following a clinical trial [abstract 1021]. Pediatr Res 39:173A, 1996.
297a. Salmaso S, Anemona A, Mastrantonio P, et al. Long-term efficacy of pertussis vaccines in Italy. Proceedings: Preclinical and Clinical Development of New Vaccines. Paris, Institute Pasteur, May 28–30, 1997.
298. Olin P, Rasmussen F, Gustafsson L, et al. Randomised controlled trial of two-component, three-component, and five-component acellular pertussis vaccines compared with whole-cell pertussis vaccine. Lancet 350:1569–1577, 1997.
298a. Plotkin SA, Cadoz M. Acellular vaccine efficacy trials. Pediatr Infect Dis J 16:913–914, 1997.
298b. Storsaeter J, Hallander HO, Gustafsson L, et al. Levels of antipertussis antibodies over time related to protection after household exposure to *Bordetella pertussis.* Vaccine: in press.
298c. Olin P, Gustafsson L, Rasmussen F, et al. Efficacy trial of acellular pertussis vaccines: Technical report, trial 2, with results of preplanned analysis of efficacy, immunogenicity and safety. Stockholm, Swedish Institute for Infectious Disease Control, 1997.
299. Trollfors B, Taranger J, Lagergård T, et al. A placebo-controlled trial of a pertussis-toxoid vaccine. N Engl J Med 333:1045–1050, 1995.
300. Trollfors B, Taranger J, Lagergård T, et al. Efficacy of a monocomponent pertussis toxoid vaccine after household exposure to pertussis. J Pediatr 130:532–536, 1997.
301. Heininger U, Cherry JD, Stehr K, et al. The comparative efficacy of the Lederle/Takeda acellular pertussis component DTP (DTaP) vaccine and Lederle whole-cell component DTP vaccine in German children following household exposure. Pediatrics 102:546–553, 1998.

302. Cherry JD, Heininger U, Stehr K, et al. The effect of investigator compliance (observer bias) on calculated efficacy in a pertussis vaccine trial. Pediatrics:in press.
303. Simondon F. Senegal pertussis trial. Dev Biol Stand 89:63–66, 1997.
304. Plotkin SA, Cadoz M. The acellular pertussis vaccine trials: An interpretation. Pediatr Infect Dis J 16:508–517, 1997.
305. Cherry JD. Comparative efficacy of acellular pertussis vaccines: An analysis of recent trials. Pediatr Infect Dis J 16:S90–S96, 1997.
306. Kumira M, Kuno-Sakai H. Epidemiology of pertussis in Japan. Tokai J Exp Clin Med 13(suppl):1–7, 1988.
307. Aoyama T, Murase Y, Kato M, et al. Efficacy and immunogenicity of acellular pertussis vaccine by manufacturer and patient age. Am J Dis Child 143:655–659, 1989.
308. Isomura S, Suzuki S, Sato Y. Clinical efficacy of the Japanese acellular pertussis vaccine after intrafamilial exposure to pertussis patients. Dev Biol Stand 61:531–537, 1985.
309. Mortimer EA Jr, Kimura M, Cherry JD, et al. Protective efficacy of the Takeda acellular pertussis vaccine combined with diphtheria and tetanus toxoids following household exposure of Japanese children. Am J Dis Child 144:899–904, 1990.
310. Kimura M, Kuno-Sakai H. Pertussis vaccines in Japan. Acta Paediatr Jpn 30:143–153, 1988.
311. Cherry JD, Mortimer EA Jr, Hackell JG, et al. Clinical trials in the United States and Japan with the Lederle-Takeda and Takeda acellular pertussis-diphtheria-tetanus (APDT) vaccines. Dev Biol Stand 73:51–58, 1991.
312. Kuno-Sakai H, Kimura M, Ozaki H, et al. Japanese clinical trials with Takeda acellular pertussis vaccine. Tokai J Exp Clin Med 13(suppl):15–19, 1988.
313. Morgan CM, Blumberg DA, Cherry JD, et al. Comparison of acellular and whole-cell pertussis component DTP vaccines: A multicenter double-blind study in 4- to 6-year-old children. Am J Dis Child 144:41–45, 1990.
314. Glode M, Joffe L, Reisinger K, et al. Safety and immunogenicity of acellular pertussis vaccine combined with diphtheria and tetanus toxoids in 17- to 24-month-old children. Pediatr Infect Dis J 11:530–535, 1992.
315. Blumberg D, Mink CM, Cherry JD, et al. Comparison of an acellular pertussis-component diphtheria-tetanus-pertussis (DTP) vaccine with a whole-cell pertussis-component DTP vaccine in 17- to 24-month-old children, with measurement of 69-kilodalton outer membrane protein antibody. J Pediatr 117:46–51, 1990.
316. Blumberg DA, Mink CM, Cherry JD, et al. Comparison of acellular and whole-cell pertussis-component diphtheria-tetanus-pertussis vaccines in infants. J Pediatr 119:194–204, 1991.
317. Watson B, Cawein A, McKee BL, et al. Safety and immunogenicity of acellular pertussis vaccine, combined with diphtheria and tetanus as the Japanese commercial Takeda vaccine, compared with the Takeda acellular pertussis component combined with Lederle's diphtheria and tetanus toxoids in two-, four- and six-month-old infants. Pediatr Infect Dis J 11:930–935, 1992.
318. Kamiya H, Nii R, Matsuda T, et al. Immunogenicity and reactogenicity of Takeda acellular pertussis-component diphtheria-tetanus-pertussis vaccine in 2- and 3-month-old children in Japan. Am J Dis Child 146:1141–1147, 1992.
319. Pertussis vaccination: Acellular pertussis vaccine for reinforcing and booster use-supplementary ACIP statement. Recommendations of the Immunization Practices Advisory Committee (ACIP). MMWR Morb Mortal Wkly Rep 41(RR-1):1–10, 1992.
320. Pertussis vaccination: Acellular pertussis vaccine for the fourth and fifth doses of the DTP series; update to supplementary ACIP statement. Recommendations of the Advisory Committee on Immunization Practices (ACIP). MMWR Morb Mortal Wkly Rep 41(RR-16):1–5, 1992.
321. Edwards KM, Karzon DT. Pertussis vaccines. In Bellanti JA (ed). Pediatr Clin North Am 37:549–566, 1990.
322. Lewis K, Cherry JD, Holroyd J, et al. A double-blind study comparing an acellular pertussis-component DTP vaccine with a whole-cell pertussis component DTP vaccine in 18-month-old children. Am J Dis Child 140:872–876, 1986.
323. Edwards KM, Lawrence E, Wright PF. Diphtheria, tetanus, and pertussis vaccine. A comparison of the immune response and adverse reactions to conventional and acellular pertussis components. Am J Dis Child 140:867–871, 1986.
324. Edwards KM, Bradley RB, Decker MD, et al. Evaluation of a new highly purified pertussis vaccine in infants and children. J Infect Dis 160:832–837, 1989.
325. Pichichero ME, Badgett JT, Rodgers GC, et al. Acellular pertussis vaccine: Immunogenicity and safety of an acellular pertussis vs. a whole cell pertussis vaccine combined with diphtheria and tetanus toxoids as a booster in 18–24 month old children. Pediatr Infect Dis J 6:352–363, 1987.
326. Anderson EL, Belshe RB, Bartram J. Differences in reactogenicity and antigenicity of acellular and standard pertussis vaccines combined with diphtheria and tetanus in infants. J Infect Dis 157:731–736, 1988.
327. Schmitt-Grohe S, Stehr K, Cherry JD, et al. Minor adverse events in a comparative efficacy trial in Germany in infants receiving either the Lederle/Takeda acellular pertussis component DTP (DTaP) vaccine, the Lederle whole-cell component DTP (DTP) or DT vaccine. The Pertussis Vaccine Study Group. Dev Biol Stand 89:113–118, 1997.
328. Uberall MA, Stehr K, Cherry JD, et al. Severe adverse events in a comparative efficacy trial in Germany in infants receiving either the Lederle/Takeda acellular pertussis component DTP (DTaP) vaccine, the Lederle whole-cell component DTP (DTP) or DT vaccine. The Pertussis Vaccine Study Group. Dev Biol Stand 89:83–89, 1997.
329. Ciofi degli Atti ML, Olin P. Severe adverse events in the Italian and Stockholm I pertussis vaccine clinical trials. Dev Biol Stand 89:77–81, 1997.
330. Simondon F, Yam A, Gagnepain JY, et al. Comparative safety and immunogenicity of an acellular versus whole-cell pertussis component of diphtheria-tetanus-pertussis vaccines in Senegalese infants. Eur J Clin Microbiol Infect Dis 15:927–932, 1996.
331. Kuno-Sakai H, Kimura M. Epidemiology of pertussis and use of acellular pertussis vaccines in Japan. Dev Biol Stand 89:331–332, 1997.
332. Chen RT, Rastogi SC, Mullen JR, et al. The Vaccine Adverse Event Reporting System (VAERS). Vaccine 12:542–550, 1994.
333. Rosenthal S, Chen R, Hadler S. The safety of acellular pertussis vaccine vs whole-cell pertussis vaccine. A postmarketing assessment. Arch Pediatr Adolesc Med 150:457–460, 1996.
334. Pichichero ME, Deloria MA, Rennels MB, et al. A safety and immunogenicity comparison of 12 acellular pertussis vaccines and one whole-cell pertussis vaccine given as a fourth dose in 15 to 20 month old children. Pediatrics 100:772–788, 1997.
335. Pichichero ME, Edwards KM, Anderson EL, et al. The National Institutes of Health (NIH) Vaccine and Treatment Evaluation Units (VTEUs) collaborative study of a fifth sequential dose of 6 DT-acellular pertussis (DTaP) vaccines compared with one whole cell pertussis (DTwP) vaccine in 4- to 6-year-old children. Pediatr Res 43:154A, 1998.
336. Keitel W, Edwards K, Englund J, et al. Dose-response comparisons of 5 acellular pertussis vaccines in healthy adults [abstract 286]. Abstracts of the 34th Annual Meeting of the Infectious Diseases Society of America; New Orleans, LA; September 1996.
337. Decker MD, Cates KL, Maida A, et al. Safety and immunogenicity in adults and adolescents of Biocine acellular pertussis (aP) vaccine [abstract 123.002]. 7th International Congress for Infectious Diseases; Hong Kong; June 1996.
338. Edwards KM, Decker MD, Graham BS, et al. Adult immunization with acellular pertussis vaccine. JAMA 269:53–56, 1993.
339. Cadoz M, Arminjon F, Quentin-Millet MJ, et al. Safety and immunogenicity of Mérieux acellular pertussis in adult volunteers. Transcript of the workshop on Acellular Pertussis Vaccines. Washington, DC, US Department of Health and Human Services, 1986, pp 131–134.
340. Sekura RD, Zhang YL, Robertson R, et al. Clinical, metabolic and antibody responses of adult volunteers to an investigational vaccine composed of pertussis toxin inactivated by hydrogen peroxide. J Pediatr 113:806–813, 1988.
341. Stehr K, Lugauer S, Heninger U, et al. Immunogenicity and reactogenicity of Lederle/Takeda acellular pertussis vaccine in 185 German adults. Pediatr Res 37:189A, 1995.
342. Keitel W. Adult pertussis study results using five acellular vaccines. Acellular pertussis vaccine trials: Results and impact on

US public health. National Institutes of Health Pertussis Conference; Washington, DC; June 3–5, 1996.

343. Sato Y. Acellular pertussis vaccine in adults: Adverse reactions and immune response. Eur J Clin Microbiol 6:18–21, 1987.
344. Wright SW, Edwards KM, Decker MD, et al. Pertussis seroprevalence in emergency department staff. Ann Emerg Med 24:413–417, 1994.
345. Shefer A, Dales L, Nelson M, et al. Use and safety of acellular pertussis vaccine among adult hospital staff during an outbreak of pertussis. J Infect Dis 171:1053–1056, 1995.
346. Christie C, Garrison K, Kiely L, et al. Acellular pertussis vs. meningococcal vaccine trial in hospital workers during the Cincinnati pertussis epidemic [abstract 616]. Abstracts of the 35th Annual Meeting of the Infectious Diseases Society of America; San Francisco; September 1997.
347. Decker MD, Edwards KM. Acellular pertussis vaccines: The authors reply. N Engl J Med 334:1547–1548, 1996.
348. Tripedia (Connaught Laboratories, Swiftwater, PA) Product Labeling. In Physician's Desk Reference. Montvale, NJ, Medical Economics Company, 1997, pp 908–911.
349. Taranger J, Trollfors B, Lagergård T. Clinical Trials of a Monocomponent Pertussis Toxoid Vaccine (NICHD Ptxd)—A Technical Report. Göteborg, Sweden, Göteborg University, 1995.
350. Knudsen KM. Statistical Report on Vaccine Efficacy, Senegal Pertussis Study. Report 3 (May 13, 1996). Copenhagen, Denmark, Statens Seruminstitut, 1996.
351. Fine PEM. Implications of different study designs for the evaluation of acellular pertussis vaccines. In Brown F, Greco D, Mastrantonio P, et al (eds). Pertussis Vaccine Trials. Basel, Dev Biol Stand 123–133, 1997.
352. Hewlett EL, Cherry JD. New and improved vaccines against pertussis. In Levine MM, Woodrow GC, Kaper JB, Cobon GS (eds). New Generation Vaccines (2nd ed). New York, Marcel Dekker, 1997, pp 387–416.
353. Olin P. The best acellular vaccines are multi-component. Pediatr Infect Dis J 16:517–519, 1997.
354. Trollfors B, Taranger J, Langergård T, et al. Immunization of children with pertussis toxoid decreases spread of pertussis within families. Pediatr Infect Dis J 17:196–199, 1998.

chapter

15 Inactivated Polio Vaccine

Stanley A. Plotkin
Andrew Murdin
Emmanuel Vidor

HISTORICAL INTRODUCTION

Not since Louis Pasteur and the introduction of rabies vaccine was public interest in vaccines stirred as much as by the development and testing of inactivated polio vaccine (IPV); and not since Einstein did a scientist receive as much public adulation as Jonas Salk, the vaccine's inventor. The circumstances that contributed to this phenomenon included the rise of poliomyelitis as an epidemic disease, its notoriety with the public (augmented by the paralysis suffered by President Franklin Roosevelt), the publicity diffused by the March of Dimes Foundation in its efforts to raise money for research, and the involvement of hundreds of thousands of U.S. children in the field trial that demonstrated the efficacy of IPV.

Nevertheless, in the early 1960s, IPV was eclipsed by oral polio vaccine (OPV), except in some northern European countries. More recent changes in public health conditions, the accelerating disappearance of poliomyelitis as an epidemic disease, and rare but persistent cases of paralysis caused by the attenuated OPV have restored interest in IPV. An increasing number of countries have adopted its use, and more are likely to do so.

The disease itself is ancient. A famous Egyptian stele dating from 1580 to 1350 BC shows a man with flaccid paralysis of a leg. However, presumably owing to almost universal infection under the protection of maternal antibodies, only sporadic cases were described (perhaps including that of Sir Walter Scott) until the 19th century. Early in that century, small outbreaks were noted, usually among infants living in rural areas. In 1870, Jean-Martin Charcot described the pathological lesions in the gray matter of the spinal cord, and in 1890 Oscar Medin described a major outbreak in Sweden, where epidemics subsequently continued to occur. Epidemics were reported in the United States at the end of the century, and in 1916 thousands of children were paralyzed during an epidemic in the northeastern United States. Fortunately, in 1908 Karl Landsteiner and Eric Popper isolated the virus of poliomyelitis in monkeys, and scientific study of the agent began.[1]

The key scientific discoveries that led to IPV were as follows:

1. Definition of the three serotypes of poliovirus by David Bodian and colleagues[2]
2. Determination that polio viremia precedes paralysis[3]
3. Confirmation that neutralizing antibodies protect against disease[4]
4. Demonstration by John Enders and colleagues that the virus could be grown in cell culture[5]

These discoveries permitted Salk, fresh from his success in developing an inactivated influenza vaccine and also experienced in working with poliovirus, to start efforts at vaccine development. Large quantities of virus were grown in monkey kidney cell culture, and the kinetics of inactivation by formalin were studied. Salk concluded that poliovirus was inactivated at a constant first-order rate, permitting complete killing if the process was of sufficient duration. Pools of trivalent vaccine were prepared at Connaught Laboratories in Toronto for use in a field trial of efficacy, which was conducted by Thomas Francis and his associates in 1954. The trial decisively demonstrated that IPV was protective, and in 1955 IPV was licensed in the United States.[6]

Years later, two major developments improved the quality of IPV. The first was the invention by Anton Van Wezel in Holland of techniques to select the best sources of monkey kidney cells, grow the cells to high density on microbeads, and concentrate the virus produced.[7] The second development was the adaptation of the Vero continuous African green monkey kidney cell line to the production of poliovirus by Montagnon at the Institut Mérieux of Lyon, France.[8] The result of these improvements was the enhanced-potency IPV, which is the subject of this chapter.

Licensure of IPV was the first result of the cell culture revolution that permitted the development of many other vaccines. At the time of licensure, more than 20,000 cases of polio were reported annually in the United States. Polio was a worldwide disease with an incidence in the tropics that was as great as in the developed world but was unrecognized owing to the concentration of cases in infants younger than 2 years.[9, 10]

The description of poliomyelitis as a disease, in addition to its virology, pathogenesis, and epidemiology, is covered in Chapter 16 (Live Attenuated Poliovirus Vaccines).

PASSIVE IMMUNIZATION

A field trial using human γ-globulin proved the efficacy of IPV against poliomyelitis, verified the importance of viremia in the pathogenesis of the disease, and proved the concept that antibodies were protective. This field experience, conducted in 1952 by Hammon and colleagues,[4] involved more than 54,000 children, half of whom received γ-globulin and half of whom received injections of gelatin. From the second to the eighth week after injection, paralytic poliomyelitis was reduced about 80%. Unfortunately, the dose used in the study was large (0.3 mL/kg) and the protection temporary (8 wk), rendering γ-globulin administration impractical as a public health strategy.

Maternally produced antibodies transmitted via the placenta are also protective, but their half-life is only 21 days. By 6 months of age, then, few unvaccinated infants are protected.[11]

ACTIVE IMMUNIZATION

Prior Approaches to Inactivated Polio Vaccines

Before the work of Salk, two attempts were made to inactivate poliovirus in monkey spinal cord for the purposes of vaccination. Formalin was used by Brodie and Park,[12] whereas Kolmer[13] used ricinoleate. Both attempts failed because of inadequate inactivation and probably also inadequate immunogenicity. The occurrence of polio cases possibly caused by the vaccine terminated the development of these vaccines.

Description of Inactivated Polio Vaccine

IPV is a mixture of the three polioviruses made by harvesting cell culture supernatants and submitting them to inactivation by formalin. The first version of IPV was produced in primary monkey kidney cell culture, with all the problems of finding healthy monkeys and of excluding simian viruses that might be latent or replicating actively in cultured cells. The poliovirus strains used by Salk and still used by most manufacturers are Mahoney type 1 (Brunenders in Sweden), MEF1 type 2, and Saukett type 3. The final vaccine is a mixture of three parts type 1 to one part type 2 and one part type 3.

Although the results of the field trial of efficacy were dramatically positive (described under *Efficacy of Inactivated Polio Vaccine*), the Cutter incident (described under *Adverse Events*) led to a change in manufacturing processes that lowered the immunogenicity of the vaccine.[14] The occurrence of paralytic polio in vaccinated children weakened confidence in IPV.[15]

The current enhanced-potency IPV, although based on similar principles to the first-generation vaccine, differs in important aspects, as follows:

1. The cell substrate on which the virulent seed viruses are inoculated is either secondary or tertiary subcultures of kidneys from pathogen-free monkeys, human diploid cell strains, or the Vero African green monkey kidney cell line, rather than primary cultures from newly captured monkeys.

Expansion of cell culture seeds by passage on microbeads to reach density of 10^{12} cells per 1000-L fermenter
↓
Inoculation of seed virus (types 1, 2, or 3)
↓
Incubation at 37°C for 3 to 4 days
↓
Harvest 1000 L supernatant
↓
Filter for clarification
↓
Concentrate to 2 L by ultrafiltration
↓
Purify by column chromatography to volume of 15 L
↓
Filter for sterility
↓
Dilution in medium 199 and new filtration
↓
Inactivate with 1/4000 formalin for 6 days at 37°C
↓
Filter again for elimination of clumps
↓
On days 9 and 12, sample for control*
↓
Combine with other serotypes for trivalent vaccine; adjust antigen concentration*

Figure 15–1. Production of enhanced-potency inactivated polio vaccine. *Sampling of an equivalent of at least 1500 human doses for control of effective inactivation.

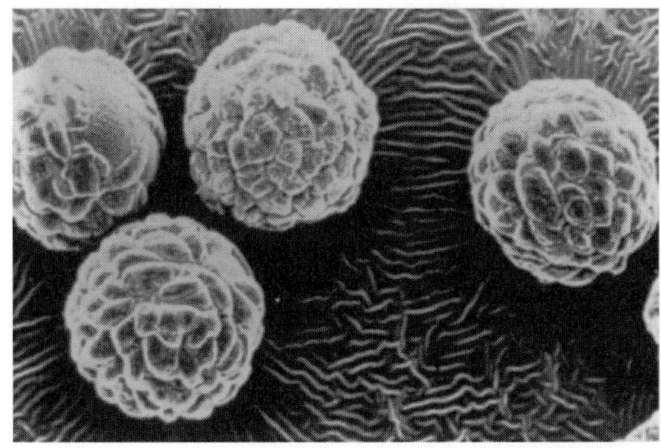

Figure 15–2. Kidney cells from monkeys (Vero) growing on microcarrier beads in cultivation. (Courtesy of Dr. B. Montagnon, Institut Mérieux, Lyon.)

2. To increase density, cells are grown on microbeads in large fermenters.
3. The virus harvest is concentrated before inactivation to increase the final antigen content.

The production of enhanced-potency IPV is outlined in Figure 15–1.[16, 17] The substrate cell culture is expanded by cell division of the working cell bank grown on microcarrier beads (Fig. 15–2) in large vessels until a density of about 1.5×10^{12} cells is reached in each 1000-L fermenter (Fig. 15–3). Growth medium is then removed, the cells are washed, and one of the three types of poliovirus is inoculated. By 72 to 96 hours of incubation at 37°C, the cells have been lysed by viral replication, and the supernatant fluids are collected. After clarification through a 0.2-μm filter, the virus is concentrated 500 fold by ultrafiltration. To remove cellular proteins and DNA, the concentrated virus is passed through column chromatography to yield 15 L of purified material. At this point, there is less than 10 pg of DNA in the material, a level considered to pose no hazard to recipients.[18]

The concentrated, purified virus is inactivated by the addition of formalin to a final concentration of 1 to 4000, followed by incubation at 37°C for 12 days. By 4 days, however, viral inactivation should be almost complete, as confirmed by sampling for residual live virus. During inactivation of the virus, it is important to avoid viral clumping and to maintain a neutral pH. An extra filtration is included during inactivation to remove viral clumps.[19]

The final monovalent material is subjected to tests for residual infectivity, which of course must be negative. The three monovalent lots are then mixed to form the trivalent enhanced-potency IPV. Concentrations of the three vaccine types are adjusted by determination of the poliovirus D antigen (which is expressed only on intact poliovirus particles) by gel diffusion or enzyme-linked immunosorbent assay. The final formula in D units is 40 of type 1, 8 of type 2, and 32 of type 3.

Formalin inactivation does modify some of the epitopes of the virus, particularly antigenic site 1 of viral types 2 and 3.[20] Although this modification has little effect on the overall neutralizing antibody response, it does alter the specificity of that response, which may have some epidemiological effect (see section on Finland under *Public Health Considerations*).

Producers

Table 15–1 lists the manufacturers of enhanced-potency IPV, which are principally based in Europe. The enhanced-potency IPV currently used in the United States is produced by Pasteur Mérieux Connaught in France. As all IPV now in use is of enhanced potency, the chapter hereafter uses the designation IPV to refer to enhanced-potency IPV vaccines.

Dosage and Route

Salk established that the immune response to polio vaccine was directly related to the dose of viral antigen (Table 15–2).[21] Recommended dosage for IPV given as a primary vaccination in adults is three doses (0.5 mL/

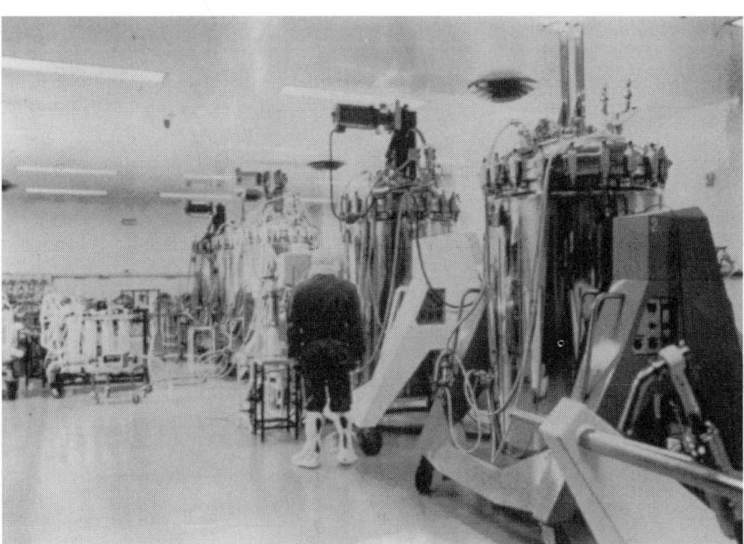

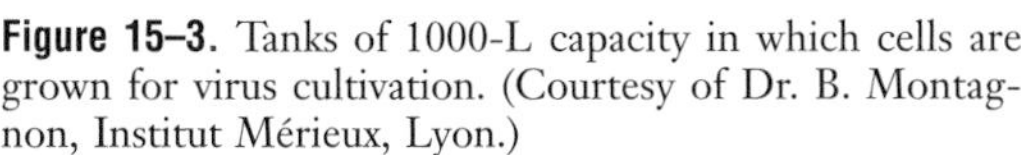

Figure 15–3. Tanks of 1000-L capacity in which cells are grown for virus cultivation. (Courtesy of Dr. B. Montagnon, Institut Mérieux, Lyon.)

Table 15–1. **MANUFACTURERS OF INACTIVATED POLIOVIRUS VACCINE**

MANUFACTURER	LOCATION	CELL SUBSTRATE
National Biological Laboratory (S.B.L.)	Sweden	Vero
Pasteur Mérieux Connaught*	France, Canada	Vero, MRC-5
Rijks Institute	The Netherlands	Vero
SmithKline Beecham	Belgium	Vero
Statens Seruminstitut	Denmark	(Confidential)

*Current U.S. manufacturer.

dose). The first two doses can be given 1 or preferably 2 months apart, with the third dose given 6 to 12 months later. If there is urgency, the third dose can be given earlier, but the immune response will not be as good. IPV can be inoculated either subcutaneously or intramuscularly; however, when given in combination with other antigens such as diphtheria, tetanus, and pertussis (DTP) or hepatitis B, the vaccine should be administered by the intramuscular route only.

When IPV is used for primary vaccination of infants, the schedule is two or three doses during the first 6 months of life, followed by a booster during the second year of life and another booster before school entry (Table 15–3). Two doses are sufficient as priming for the booster in the second year, but when IPV is included in combination vaccines with DTP, convenience may dictate using three doses. In any case, the first two doses should be followed by a third dose at some point.[22] In the United States, infants immunized with IPV alone receive doses at ages 2 months, 4 months, 6 to 18 months, and 4 to 6 years. Infants receiving the U.S. mixed schedule are given IPV at ages 2 and 4 months, followed by OPV at ages 12 to 18 months and 4 to 6 years. The schedules used in the United States and other countries are shown in Table 15–4.

Table 15–2. **COMPARATIVE ESTIMATION OF TYPE 1 IMMUNE STATUS: DETECTABLE SERUM ANTIBODY VERSUS SECONDARY-TYPE RESPONSIVENESS**

NO. OF SUBJECTS*	PRIMARY DOSE†	% OF GROUP WITH DETECTABLE ANTIBODY (≥1:4): 2 Weeks After One Dose	% OF GROUP WITH DETECTABLE ANTIBODY (≥1:4): 1 Year After Two Doses	% OF GROUP WITH SECONDARY-TYPE ANTIBODY RESPONSE (≥1:32)‡ 2 WEEKS AFTER BOOSTER DOSES§
33	None	—	—	6
24	2	100	92	100
21	1	100	85	100
26	½	96	60	96
27	¼	93	73	100
30	⅛	87	45	93
26	1/16	77	35	96

*In the group evaluated 2 wk after booster dose.
†mL of reference vaccine A given in each of two doses 2 wk apart.
‡Antibody titer of 1:32 arbitrarily chosen as criterion for hyperreactive secondary-type antibody response.
§1 mL of vaccine J.
From Salk J, Salk D. Vaccination against poliomyelitis. In Voller A, Friedman H (eds). New Trends and Developments in Vaccines. Lancashire, England, MTP Press, 1978, pp 117–154.

Table 15–3. **RECOMMENDED POLIOVIRUS VACCINATION SCHEDULES FOR U.S. CHILDREN**

VACCINATION SCHEDULE	VACCINE USED FOR GIVEN CHILD'S AGE: 2 Months	4 Months	12–18 Months	4–6 Years
Sequential IPV/OPV	IPV	IPV	OPV	OPV
OPV	OPV	OPV	OPV*	OPV
IPV	IPV	IPV	IPV	IPV

*For children who receive only OPV, the third dose of OPV may be administered as early as 6 months of age.
IPV, inactivated polio vaccine; OPV, live oral polio vaccine.

The issue of additional boosters after the preschool dose is considered later (see under *Duration of Immunity*).

Few data are available on the primary immunization of seronegative adults. However, indications are that three doses should be given on a schedule of 0, 1, and 6 months of age. Adults who are already seropositive need only one booster dose to develop high titers (Pasteur Mérieux Connaught Laboratories, unpublished data).

Available Preparations

Two IPVs are currently licensed in the United States: one produced in France and the second in Canada. The French vaccine is produced in Vero cell culture, whereas the Canadian vaccine is produced in MRC-5 human diploid cell culture.

At present, IPV is available in the United States only as a single entity. However, in Canada and elsewhere, combinations of DTP and IPV are frequently used, and pentavalent vaccines that include *Haemophilus influenzae* type b (Hib) have started to appear in some countries. Other combinations are just coming to the market, including those based on acellular pertussis vaccine to

Table 15–4. **ADMINISTRATION SCHEDULES OF ENHANCED-POTENCY INACTIVATED POLIO VACCINE**

VACCINES	SCHEDULES
Children	
United States	2 mo, 4 mo, 12–18 mo, 4–6 yr
	2 mo, 4 mo, 6 mo, 12–18 mo*
	2 mo, 4 mo, switch to OPV†
Canada	2 mo, 4 mo, 6 mo, 12–18 mo, 4–6 yr
France	2 mo, 3 mo, 4 mo, 12–18 mo, 6 yr, 11 yr, 16 yr
Sweden	3 mo, 5 mo, 12 mo, 6 yr
Netherlands	3 mo, 4 mo, 5 mo, 12 mo, 4 yr, 9 yr
Adults in all countries	0, 1–2, and 6–12 mo

*Permissible with combination vaccines and may be recommended for enhanced-potency inactivated polio vaccine alone in the future.
†Alternative mixed schedule.

which IPV and Hib vaccines have been added.[23] By the end of the 1990s, there will be hexavalent combinations also containing hepatitis B vaccine.

Worldwide, the market for vaccines containing IPV is dominated by Pasteur Mérieux Connaught products, but the situation is likely to change with the expansion of IPV production by SmithKline Beecham and North American Vaccine (see Table 15–1).

A new IPV is under development in Finland because that country experienced an epidemic due to a type 3 antigenic variant (see under *Public Health Considerations*). The new vaccine, produced by Rijksinstituut Voor Volksgezondheid en Milien (RIVM) in Holland, differs from the current IPV in that the Saukett type 3 strain has been treated with trypsin to uncover three neutralizing epitopes additional to antigenic site 1. When wild type 3 virus infects the intestine, antigenic site 1 is destroyed by intestinal trypsin, and thus the virus may not be neutralized by antibodies raised against that particular neutralizing epitope. The new IPV has undergone satisfactory phase 1 and 2 trials.[24]

Vaccine Constituents Other Than Immunizing Antigens

With regard to the vaccine produced in Vero cell culture, streptomycin, neomycin, and polymyxin B are used during the manufacturing process to control bacterial contamination but are largely eliminated during production. Test results for these antibiotics in the final product are negative, but trace amounts (<200 ng of streptomycin, <5 ng of neomycin, and <25 ng of polymyxin B) may still be present. Preservation is conferred by residual formalin (0.02%) and 2-phenoxyethanol (0.5%), which are sufficient to maintain sterility.

The MRC-5–produced vaccine contains trace amounts of streptomycin and neomycin as well as formalin (27 ppm), 2-phenoxyethanol (0.5%), human albumin (0.5%), and Tween 80 (20 ppm).

Stability

In contrast to OPV, IPV is relatively heat stable. The vaccine is stable for 4 years at 4°C and for 1 month at 25°C. At 37°C, there is significant loss of potency of the type 1 component after 1 to 2 days, and of types 2 and 3 after 2 weeks.[25] Freezing diminishes the in vitro potency of IPV and should be avoided.[26]

Results of Vaccination

Immune Responses

Although it is possible to measure serum antibodies to poliovirus by a variety of methods, neutralizing antibodies are considered to be the protective response, and only these are considered here.

The accumulated data were reviewed concerning antibody responses to IPV and to the DTP-IPV combination that is in wide use in Europe.[26–28] Two doses of IPV induced low-titer responses in nearly all recipients in most studies, but in some studies as many as 20% of vaccinees did not seroconvert. After three doses, however, virtually all recipients became seropositive, and the geometric mean titers were elevated. Antibody levels fell subsequently, although the vaccinees usually retained a positive titer and a fourth injection gave a marked anamnestic response.

Figure 15–4 and Table 15–5 present data on the neutralizing antibody responses after two doses of Vero cell–produced IPV.[29–34] The 18 studies represented in Figure 15–4 were conducted in a wide range of geographical locations, including tropical countries, with a range of schedules starting at 2 to 5 months of age. More than 85% of infants responded to all three serotypes, and in many cases the percent seroconversion was close to 100. Five more recent studies conducted in the United States are presented in Table 15–5, along with titer values and percent seropositivity. In the U.S. studies, nearly all infants were seropositive after the second dose, although their titers were generally below 1:100.

The data in Figure 15–4 also show that in terms of immunogenicity, an interval of 2 months between the first two doses is preferable to an interval of 1 month, as is the case for other vaccine antigens in infants.

In Figure 15–5 are represented 22 studies in which titers were measured after three doses of IPV. Virtually all infants are seropositive to the three polioviruses. The U.S. data in Table 15–5 confirm this point and show that the geometric mean titers after three doses are well over 1:100. In the U.S. trials, the third dose of IPV was given either at 6 months of age or in the second year of life. In the former case, titers were between 1:100 and 1:1000, whereas when the third dose was administered after a longer interval, titers rose to more than 1:1000.

Swartz and colleagues[35] showed that a single dose of IPV at birth primed infants to a uniform response to a

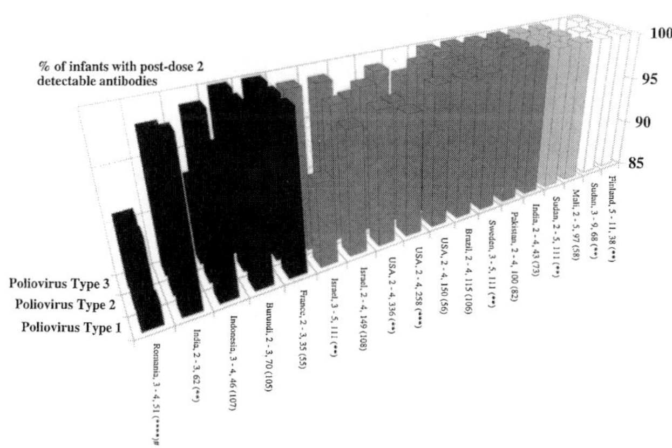

Figure 15–4. Immunogenicity of Vero cell–produced vaccines containing enhanced-potency inactivated polio vaccine administered in two doses during the first year of life. The country, age at vaccination, and number of infants enrolled at the beginning of the study are shown; reference numbers in parentheses refer to the original publication. (From Vidor E, Meschievitz C, Plotkin S. Fifteen years of experience with Vero-produced enhanced potency inactivated poliovirus vaccine. Pediatr Infect Dis J 16:312–322, 1997.)

Table 15–5. **U.S. STUDIES WITH THE VERO CELL–PRODUCED eIPV GIVEN ALONE OR IN MIXED IPV/OPV SEQUENTIAL SCHEDULES**

INVESTIGATORS AND REFERENCE	NO.*	VACCINE ADMINISTERED AT GIVEN AGE				% OF NEUTRALIZING ANTIBODY TO INDICATED STRAIN ≥1/8 (GEOMETRIC MEAN TITER)											
						After Second Dose			After Third Dose†			Before Booster			After Booster‡		
		2 Months	*4 Months*	*6 Months*	*Booster 12–18 Months*	*Type 1*	*Type 2*	*Type 3*	*Type 1*	*Type 2*	*Type 3*	*Type 1*	*Type 2*	*Type 3*	*Type 1*	*Type 2*	*Type 3*
Faden et al.[29]	116	IPV	IPV		IPV	96 (184)	100 (631)	96 (634)				90 (61)	96 (135)	92 (102)	96 (1954)	100 (5835)	100 (5187)
	34	IPV	IPV		OPV	100 (283)	100 (481)	100 (1132)				100 (128)	100 (334)	93 (151)	100 (3044)	100 (10,693)	100 (2347)
	94	IPV	IPV		IPV	97 (44)	96 (105)	95 (83)				92 (22)	65 (42)	87 (23)	100 (2070)	100 (3419)	100 (1968)
Blatter and Starr[34]	68	IPV	IPV		IPV	98 (88)	100 (256)	98 (162)				100 (41)	100 (71)	93 (35)	100 (2029)	100 (4388)	100 (2580)
	75	IPV	IPV		OPV	94 (28)	98 (91)	96 (63)				85 (18)	96 (47)	81 (20)	100 (1568)	100 (7199)	96 (297)
	99	IPV	IPV		OPV	99 (90)	99 (120)	95 (126)				98 (47)	96 (61)	88 (29)	100 (1765)	100 (7516)	99 (709)
Halsey et al.[33]	87	IPV	IPV	IPV	OPV	97 (74)	98 (82)	100 (110)	100 (463)	100 (652)	100 (605)	100 (72)	100 (98)	100 (91)	100 (2141)	100 (7169)	100 (1824)
McBean et al.[30]	331	IPV	IPV		IPV	99	99	99							99	100	100
	332	IPV	IPV		IPV	99	100	100							100	100	100
Modlin et al.[31]	101	IPV	IPV		IPV	97	92	78							100	100	100

*Number of enrolled subjects at beginning of study.
†In infancy.
‡Booster is third or fourth dose, depending on the schedule.
eIPV, enhanced-potency inactivated polio vaccine; OPV, live oral polio vaccine.

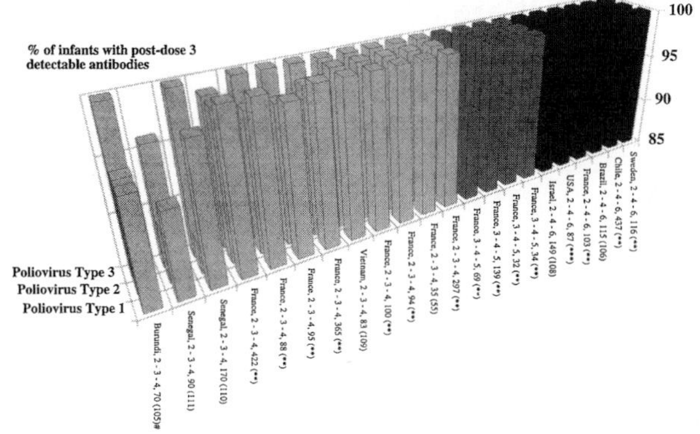

Figure 15–5. Immunogenicity of Vero cell–produced vaccines containing enhanced-potency inactivated polio vaccine administered in three doses during the first year of life. The country, age at vaccination, and number of infants enrolled at the beginning of the study are shown; reference numbers in parentheses refer to the original publication. (From Vidor E, Meschievitz C, Plotkin S. Fifteen years of experience with Vero-produced enhanced potency inactivated poliovirus vaccine. Pediatr Infect Dis J 16:312–322, 1997.)

second dose given at age 6 months. This abbreviated schedule has never been tried in public health practice, however.

As stated previously, IPV has been combined with DTP, acellular DTP, and Hib vaccines without evident effect on its immunogenicity,[26, 36–39] although none of these combinations is yet available in the United States (see Chapter 20).

In a study sponsored by the World Health Organization (WHO),[40] three doses of IPV were given to infants in Oman and Thailand. Whereas 90 to 96% of the Omani infants responded to the three serotypes, the Thai infants showed seroconversion rates of only 67% and 65% to types 1 and 2, respectively. The low responses in Thailand were attributed to high maternal antibody titers, the onset of vaccination at 6 weeks of age, and an interval of 1 rather than 2 months between doses.[41, 42] The results were considered disappointing, however.[40] Comparative serological data after OPV or IPV vaccination are given in Table 15–6.

Table 15–7 and Figure 15–6 present data obtained with IPV produced in MRC-5 cells in the course of studies of combination vaccines. After three doses at 2, 4, and 6 months of age, excellent responses were seen, which were markedly augmented after a booster dose at 18 months. Additional data on the MRC-5–produced IPV are provided in Table 15–8, which also contains information on IPV produced in primary monkey kidney cells.

Immunogenicity of Sequential Schedule of Inactivated and Oral Polio Vaccines

The Centers for Disease Control and Prevention has adopted a recommendation for mixed IPV/OPV vaccination, in which two doses of IPV are administered at 2 and 4 months of age, followed by two doses of OPV administered at 6 to 18 months of age and again at school entry. Table 15–5 provides data on the excellent immunogenicity of this schedule, which is considered in detail in the chapter on OPV (see Chapter 16). Israel, Denmark, and Prince Edward Island in Canada also use a mixed schedule, with successful induction of immune responses and protection. A study in the United Kingdom showed the advantages of a mixed schedule in terms of immunogenicity.[43]

A particular use of mixed schedules was undertaken in Romania, because of an unusually high rate of vaccine-associated paralytic poliomyelitis (VAPP) owing to concurrent intramuscular injections.[44] Infants in one province of Romania received IPV at 2, 3, and 4 months of age, together with OPV at 4 and 9 months of age.[45] The schedule was well tolerated and highly immunogenic. No cases of polio occurred subsequently in this region, but too few children were involved to draw conclusions about the prevention of VAPP.

The WHO study mentioned previously[40] compared four doses of OPV, three doses of IPV, and a mixed schedule consisting of four doses of OPV and three doses of IPV. The vaccines were administered to infants in Oman, the Gambia, and Thailand. Seroconversion rates and geometric mean titers were highest in the mixed OPV/IPV group. In addition, when children of the three groups were challenged with another dose of OPV, virus excretion was as low in the mixed vaccine group as in the OPV group, confirming the presence of mucosal immunity.

Another mixed schedule was tested in the Ivory Coast,

Table 15–6. **STUDIES COMPARING IMMUNOGENICITY AFTER PRIMARY IMMUNIZATION WITH eIPV (OR DPT/eIPV) VERSUS OPV**

STUDY	TYPE OF VACCINE AND NO. OF DOSES	NO. OF SUBJECTS	GMT TO INDICATED STRAIN AFTER VACCINATION			TYPE OF VACCINE	NO. OF SUBJECTS	GMT TO INDICATED STRAIN AFTER VACCINATION		
			Type 1	Type 2	Type 3			Type 1	Type 2	Type 3
United States	eIPV × 2	91	208	552	605	OPV × 2	22	273	2726	351
India	eIPV × 2	62	257	264	479	OPV × 5	64	295	814	102
Mali	eIPV × 2	37	839	944	1054	OPV × 3	31	23	89	122
Mali	DPT/eIPV × 2	60	228	664	638	OPV × 3	31	23	89	122
Pakistan	DPT/eIPV × 2	101	345	368	519	OPV × 3	104	267	409	316
Ivory Coast	eIPV × 3	186	1204	1195	1591	OPV × 3	182	924	1602	609
Ivory Coast	eIPV × 3	177	1954	1593	1977	OPV × 3	169	1589	1736	779

DPT, diphtheria, pertussis, and tetanus; eIPV, enhanced-potency inactivated polio vaccine; GMT, geometric mean titer.

Table 15–7. **POLIOVIRUS-NEUTRALIZING ANTIBODY RESPONSES IN INFANTS TO MRC-5 CELL–PRODUCED eIPV***

TIME OF ADMINISTRATION (mo)	TYPE OF VACCINE	NO. OF SUBJECTS	POLIOVIRUS TYPE 1		POLIOVIRUS TYPE 2		POLIOVIRUS TYPE 3	
			% Antibody ≥4†	GMT‡	% Antibody ≥4	GMT	% Antibody ≥4	GMT
7	Combined	211	100	252	99.5	222	100	919
	Separate	211	100	282	99.5	209	100	1024
18	Combined	188	94	47	88	34.2	98	109
	Separate	188	95	44	90	35.7	98	121
19	Combined	189	100	4961	100.0	4289	100	5180
	Separate	187	100	4686	100.0	4907	100	4572

*Vaccine given at 7, 18, and 19 months of age after a 3-dose primary series at 2, 4, and 6 months of age and a booster at 18 months of age with DPT/IPV and PRP-T given combined or simultaneously at separate sites.

†Percentage of children with a poliovirus-neutralizing antibody titer of ≥4.

‡Geometric mean titer of poliovirus-neutralizing antibodies.

DPT, diphtheria, pertussis, and tetanus; eIPV, enhanced-potency inactivated polio vaccine; GMT, geometric mean titer; PRP-T, Hib vaccine.

From Murdin A, Barreto L, Plotkin S. Inactivated poliovirus vaccine: Past and present experience. Vaccine 14:735–746, 1996.

with the objective of correcting deficiencies in response to OPV in tropical settings.[46] A single dose of IPV or OPV was given after three doses of OPV. Of those 9-month-old children who remained seronegative after the third dose of OPV, 81, 100, and 67% seroconverted to types 1, 2, and 3 polio, respectively, after the IPV booster. The corresponding percentages for an OPV booster were 14, 27, and 5.

Immunogenicity in the Immunocompromised Patient

Because IPV is indicated for immunocompromised people even in countries that recommend OPV, the immunogenicity of IPV in these patients is an important issue.

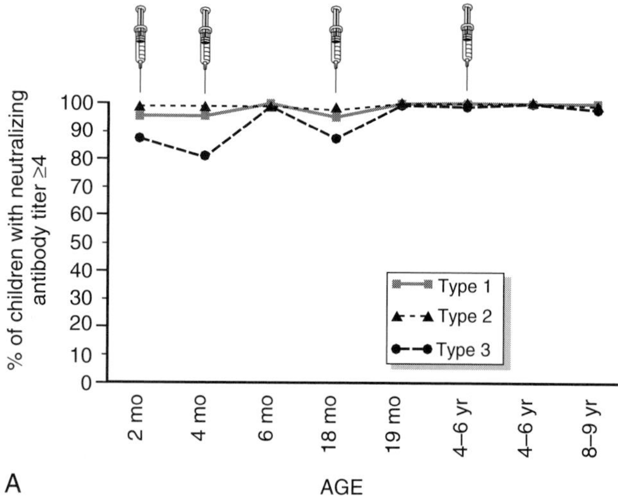

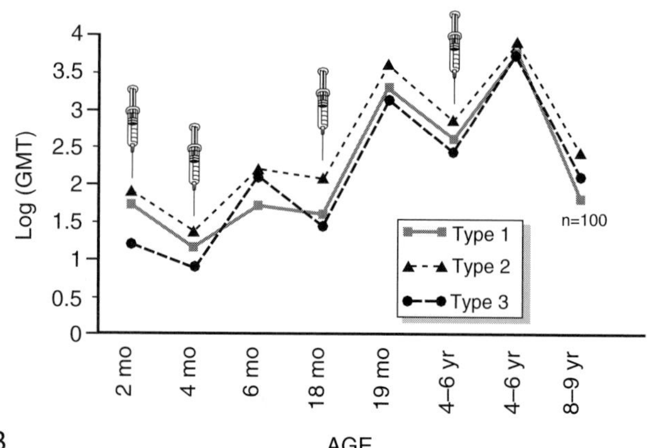

Figure 15–6. Eight- to 9-year follow-up study of poliovirus-neutralizing antibodies in children immunized with MRC-5–produced inactivated polio vaccine. Vaccinees received a two-dose primary series at 2 and 4 months of age and booster vaccinations at 18 months and 4 to 6 years of age (indicated by the syringe symbol). *A*, Percentage of children with a neutralizing antibody titer of 4 or greater. *B*, Natural logarithm of the geometric mean antibody titer (GMT). The number of sera (*n*) tested at each time is shown. (From Murdin A, Barreto L, Plotkin S. Inactivated poliovirus vaccine: Past and present experience. Vaccine 14:735–746, 1996.)

Table 15–8. **NEUTRALIZATION ANTIBODY RESPONSES TO NON–VERO CELL–PRODUCED eIPVs***

				% POSITIVE FOR NEUTRALIZING ANTIBODIES TO INDICATED STRAIN								
				After Second Dose			After Third Dose			Before Fourth Dose		
eIPV USED†	AGE AT VACCINATION (mo)	COUNTRY	NO. OF SUBJECTS‡	Type 1	Type 2	Type 3	Type 1	Type 2	Type 3	Type 1	Type 2	Type 3
PMKC 40/8/32	1.5, 10 or 2.5, 5, 11	India	114	97	88	97						
PMKC 40/8/32	3, 8–9, 14	Burkina Faso	179	94	99	78						
PMKC 40/8/32	2, 4, 6	Kenya	84	94	88	97	100	98	100			
PMKC 40/8/32	2, 4, 6	Thailand	94	100	99	97	100	100	100			
MRC-5 40/8/32	2, 4, 6	Canada	120	90	99	97	99	100	100			
MRC-5 40/8/32	2.4, 15	United States	279	92	94	74	81	92	53	99	100	100
PMKC 40/4/16	2, 3.5, 10	Israel	115	100	97	100	97	95	96	100	100	100
MRC-5 40/8/32	2.4, 18	United States	377	99	100	99	98	99	99	100	100	100
PMKC 40/4/16	2, 4, 18	United States	371	99	99	99	99	99	98	99	100	100
MRC-5 40/8/32	2, 4, 18	Canada	329	99	99	99	98	95	97	87	99	100
MRC-5 40/8/32	2, 4, 6, 18	Canada	443	94	97	96	99	99	99	100	100	100
MRC-5 40/8/32	2, 4, 6, 18	Canada	211	NA	NA	NA	NA	100	99	100	94	88
MRC-5 40/8/32	2, 4, 6, 18	Canada	211	NA	NA	NA	100	99	100	95	90	98
PMKC 40/4/8	3, 4, 5, 18	Netherlands	118	NA	NA	NA	97	95	94	100	99	96

*Two or three doses of eIPV were administered during the first year of life, with or without a booster dose during the second year of life.
†Cell substrate and poliovirus D antigen formulation of the used vaccine.
‡Number of subjects enrolled at beginning of study.
NA, data not available or analysis not performed; PMKC, primary monkey kidney culture; MRC-5, Medical Research Council strain 5 of human diploid fibroblasts.
From Vidor E, Meschiewitz C, Plotkin S. Fifteen years of experience with vero-produced enhanced potency inactivated poliovirus vaccine. Pediatr Infect Dis J 16:312–322, 1997.

Prematurity does not appear to reduce the response to IPV when the vaccine is given at the usual postnatal age[47, 48] unless the infants are chronically ill.[49] However, vaccination of full-term infants at birth results in lower immune responses than does vaccination later in life, presumably because maternal antibody levels are higher in newborns.[48, 50]

Children infected with human immunodeficiency virus (HIV) who were given two doses of IPV in early infancy responded reasonably well, probably because their immune systems were largely intact.[51] In hemophilic adults, however, HIV seropositivity had a negative effect on titer levels after IPV, although all adults responded to some degree.[52] Chronic renal dialysis patients also seroconverted in 90% or more of cases.[53] In patients who had undergone a bone marrow transplantation and were reimmunized after transplantation, vaccination was usually successful in inducing antibodies, although at least two and often three doses were needed.[54, 55]

Secretory Immunoglobulin A Responses and Local Immunity

In general, the secretory immunoglobulin A (IgA) response to IPV is not as high as is the response to OPV. Many of the data come from the laboratory of Ogra, who found that about 90% of IPV recipients showed poliovirus-specific secretory IgA, compared with 100% of OPV recipients.[38, 56–58] Moreover, titers were on average three to four times higher in the OPV vaccinees than in the IPV recipients. Local and systemic antibody responses after three doses of IPV, OPV, or a mixed schedule are shown in Table 15–9.[38] One study

Table 15–9. **LEVELS OF SERUM NEUTRALIZING OR NASOPHARYNGEAL IMMUNOGLOBULIN A ANTIBODIES IN CHILDREN AFTER THREE DOSES OF eIPV, OPV, OR A COMBINED SCHEDULE**

	OPV-OPV-OPV			eIPV-eIPV-eIPV			eIPV-eIPV-OPV		
	Type 1	Type 2	Type 3	Type 1	Type 2	Type 3	Type 1	Type 2	Type 3
Serum neutralizing antibodies									
% Positive	100	100	100	96	100	100	100	100	100
GMT	1470	3578	1522	1954	5835	5187	3044	10,693	2348
Nasopharyngeal secretory immunoglobulin A antibodies									
% Positive	100	100	100	89	91	89	75	81	81
GMT	69	97	128	24	25	31	19	22	23

eIPV, enhanced-potency inactivated polio vaccine; GMT, geometric mean titer; OPV, oral polio vaccine.
From Faden H, Modlin J, Thoms M, et al. Comparative evaluation of immunization with live attenuated and enhanced-potency inactivated trivalent poliovirus vaccines in childhood: Systemic and local immune responses. J Infect Dis 162:1291–1297, 1990.

conducted in another laboratory showed equal secretory IgA levels in pharyngeal and stool samples of prior IPV and OPV vaccinees, suggesting that the titers equalize after a time.[59]

Significant secretory IgA responses to IPV were shown in the breast milk of Pakistani mothers.[60] Both premature and full-term infants developed nasopharyngeal IgA antipolio antibody after immunization in about 90% of cases.

Effect of Inactivated Polio Vaccine on Poliovirus Excretion

Early in the history of IPV, it was shown that IPV vaccinees could excrete poliovirus after challenge,[61–64] which was considered an important disadvantage in relation to OPV. Time has shown that the difference is not between black and white but between two shades of gray. Studies in monkeys demonstrated that pharyngeal excretion of poliovirus was inhibited in IPV vaccinees.[65–67] Marine and colleagues followed families exposed to a natural type 1 outbreak and found that pharyngeal infection was prevented by low levels of neutralizing antibodies, whereas higher levels dampened intestinal infection (Table 15–10).[68] In a more recent study by Onorato and colleagues, children who had received three doses of IPV or OPV were challenged with two different doses of type 1 OPV.[59] The results (summarized in Table 15–11) reveal that whereas few subjects in either group excreted virus from the pharynx, intestinal infection occurred in both groups but was lower in the OPV group. The persistence of local immunity has not been well studied, but there is evidence that resistance to reinfection wanes and that protection ultimately depends on the level of serum antibodies.[69, 70] The issue of gastrointestinal immunity after IPV is discussed in more detail elsewhere.[26, 69]

Studies have examined the effect of IPV on the mutation of OPV strains in the intestinal tract.[71–73] This phenomenon, referred to as *reversion to virulence*, is a regular feature of the replication of attenuated strains, whereby the mutations in those strains responsible for attenuation in humans revert to the virulent genotype. Although the suggestion has been made that prior IPV immunization potentiates that reversion,[74, 75] a relatively large study failed to show a significant difference in the mutation of excreted virus between the IPV and OPV groups.[27]

Table 15–10. **PERCENT EXCRETION OF WILD POLIOVIRUS TYPE 1 IN CHILDREN ACCORDING TO LEVEL OF VACCINE-INDUCED SERUM NEUTRALIZING ANTIBODY**

ANTIBODY TITER	% EXCRETION AT GIVEN TIME AFTER INFECTION			
	1–2 Weeks		3–4 Weeks, S	5–6 Weeks, S
	P	*S*		
<8	75	93	82	60
8–64	38	97	81	54
>64	25	88	59	28

P, pharynx sample; S, stool sample.
Data from Vidor et al.[26] and Marine et al.[68]

Table 15–11. **ISOLATION OF POLIOVIRUS FROM STOOL OR PHARYNX OF PRIOR RECIPIENTS OF eIPV OR OPV AFTER CHALLENGE WITH TYPE 1 OPV**

CHALLENGE DOSE	NO. OF PHARYNGEAL ISOLATIONS (%)		NO. OF STOOL ISOLATIONS (%)	
	eIPV	OPV	eIPV	OPV
High (5,000,000 $TCID_{50}$)	1/45 (2)	3/45 (7)	37/45 (82)	14/45 (31)
Low (500 $TCID_{50}$)	0/48 (0)	0/34 (0)	22/48 (46)	6/34 (18)
Total	1/93 (1)	3/79 (4)	59/93 (63)	20/79 (25)

eIPV, enhanced-potency inactivated polio vaccine; OPV, oral polio vaccine; $TCID_{50}$, median tissue culture infective dose.
From Onorato I, Modlin J, McBean A, et al. Mucosal immunity induced by enhanced-potency inactivated and oral polio vaccines. J Infect Dis 163:1–6, 1991.

Efficacy of Inactivated Polio Vaccine

The efficacy of IPV in its original version was proved beyond a doubt in the original field trial conducted by Thomas Francis.[76] In that trial, approximately 400,000 children randomly received vaccine or placebo, and another 200,000 were vaccinated and observed together with unvaccinated children. There were 71 cases of paralytic polio in vaccinees against 445 in control subjects. In the placebo-controlled part of the study, 70 cases occurred in the placebo arm against 11 in the vaccinated arm.[76] The calculated efficacy of the vaccine was 80 to 90% against paralytic polio and 60 to 70% against all forms of polio.

The efficacy of the IPV was later confirmed in several settings. Melnick and colleagues calculated an efficacy of 96% through two polio seasons in Houston.[77] In Senegal, two doses of DTP/IPV were given in the Kolda area, which subsequently suffered an epidemic of type 1 polio. According to case-control analysis, the efficacy of one dose was 36% and of two doses was 89% (95% confidence limits, 62–97%).[78–80] In another study conducted in the North Arcot region of India, John compared OPV in one district with IPV vaccination in two other districts.[81] Vaccination coverage with three doses rose to 85 to 90% in the OPV districts and 75 to 80% in the IPV districts. Case-control analysis revealed an efficacy of 92% for IPV and 66% for OPV. During the introduction of IPV into Canada, efficacy of the vaccine was calculated at more than 90%.[82]

Herd Immunity

Perhaps the best evidence for a herd immunity effect of IPV is the experience in the United States. IPV was introduced into routine use in 1955 and was replaced by OPV in 1962. A sharp drop in the numbers of cases of

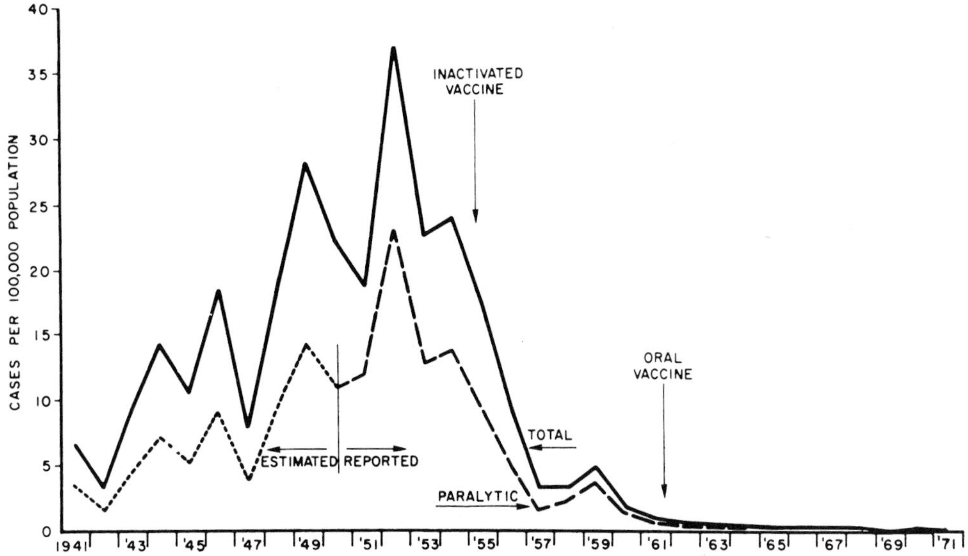

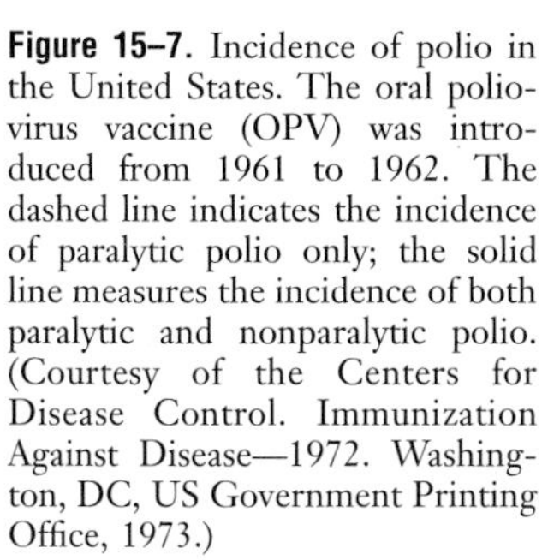

Figure 15–7. Incidence of polio in the United States. The oral poliovirus vaccine (OPV) was introduced from 1961 to 1962. The dashed line indicates the incidence of paralytic polio only; the solid line measures the incidence of both paralytic and nonparalytic polio. (Courtesy of the Centers for Disease Control. Immunization Against Disease—1972. Washington, DC, US Government Printing Office, 1973.)

paralytic and nonparalytic polio is evident during the years 1955 to 1962 (Fig. 15–7). The apparent reduction in the total number of cases observed exceeded the expectation based on the percentage of children vaccinated (Fig. 15–8). More specific regional data were also published that suggested a greater than expected reduction in polio cases.[83] An important point to consider is that studies conducted in families, in which contact is intimate, may show less blockage of transmission than community-based studies. The fecal-oral route may be more important to transmission in families, whereas contact with pharyngeal secretions may be more important to community spread.

The second example of herd immunity is furnished by the example of the Netherlands. Vaccination is refused by a particular religious community of 200,000 individuals who are well dispersed throughout this country, although IPV is routinely administered to the rest of the population. Two outbreaks of polio have occurred in this religious group, one caused by type 1 virus in 1978 (110 cases) and the second by type 3 virus in 1992 (71 cases). Despite the wide circulation of virus in the sect members, there was only a single case of polio in other Dutch people and no laboratory evidence of virus dissemination. Approximately 400,000 unvaccinated individuals not belonging to the sect also remained unaffected.[84–89] The virulent viruses were passed to religious groups in North America in both epidemic years, but cases resulted from only the 1978 outbreak.[90–92]

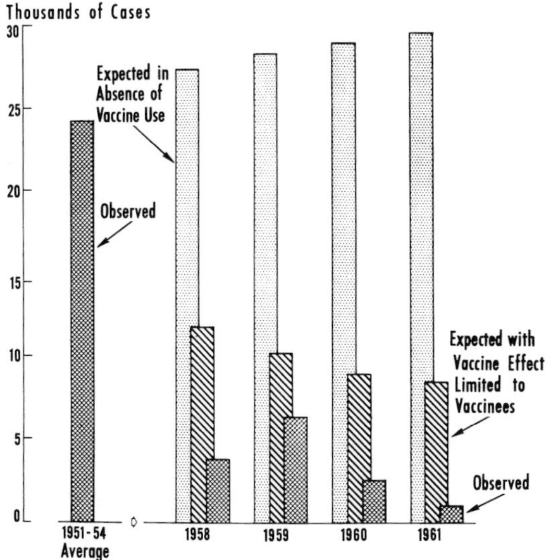

Figure 15–8. Herd effect induced by inactivated poliovirus vaccine in the United States, 1958 to 1961. The number of observed cases of paralytic poliomyelitis was consistently lower than the number expected if vaccination had benefited only vaccinated individuals. (From Stickle G. Observed and expected poliomyelitis in the United States, 1958–1961. Am J Public Health 54:222–229, 1964.)

Duration of Immunity

The importance of an interval between the second and third doses in persistence of the immune response was demonstrated by comparing infants given doses at 2, 4, and 6 months of age with those given doses at 2, 4, and 12 months of age.[93] The latter group maintained higher titers at 4 years of age. French children who were studied after a booster dose at age 18 months had antibodies to the three types of polio in 94% of cases; after an additional booster, 95% were positive at 12 years of age.[28] A group of more than 500 French young adults were 100% seropositive after their childhood vaccinations.[28] Faden and colleagues showed that IPV induced better persistence of antibodies in comparison to OPV.[93] Bottiger has followed Swedish children given four doses of first-generation IPV.[94] After 18 years, all of them had neutralizing antibodies. Persistence data have also been obtained in Israel,[95] the Netherlands,[96] and Canada,[27] showing close to 100% seropositivity 4 years after the administration of three or four doses of IPV. Additional data from a study in Israel are included in Table 15–12.

Both the need for booster vaccination with IPV and the precise schedule to be used remain controversial.

Table 15–12. **PERSISTENCE OF ANTIBODIES AFTER BOOSTER DOSE IN THE SECOND YEAR OF LIFE**

STUDY	VACCINE (MANUFACTURER)	NO. OF SUBJECTS	TIME OF PRIMARY DOSE (mo)	TIME OF BOOSTER DOSE (yr)	TIME AFTER PRIMARY DOSE (yr)	% TESTING POSITIVE FOR ANTIBODIES (GMT)		
						Type 1	Type 2	Type 3
Bottiger[94]	IPV (NBL)	250	9, 10	2, 10	18	100 (217)	100 (247)	100 (181)
Faden et al.[93]	eIPV (PMC-CA)	27	2, 4, 12		4	100 (230)	100 (260)	100 (240)
Guerin*	eIPV (PMC-FR)	39	3, 4, 5	1½, 5	5	94 (62)	100 (81)	95 (40)
Stehlin†	IPV (PMC-FR)	23	3, 4, 5	1½, 5	8	95 (30)	100 (82)	95 (42)
Swartz‡	eIPV (RIVM)	83	2, 4, 10		7	98 (131)	100 (116)	95 (62)

*Unpublished data. Swiftwater, PA, Pasteur Mérieux Laboratories, 1989.
†Unpublished data. Swiftwater, PA, Pasteur Mérieux Laboratories, 1983.
‡Personal communication, 1997.
eIPV, enhanced-potency inactivated polio vaccine; GMT, geometric mean titer; NBL, National Biological Laboratories, Sweden; PMC-CA, Pasteur Mérieux Connaught (Canada); PMC-FR, Pasteur Mérieux Connaught (France); RIVM, Rijksinstituut Voor Volksgezondheid en Milien.

Salk has argued that immunological memory is established by primary vaccination with IPV and that no further immunizations are necessary.[97–99] He showed that whereas unprimed individuals reacted with only low responses to a single dose of IPV, previously vaccinated individuals, even those originally given fractional doses, developed anamnestic responses (see Table 15–2). In his opinion, the vaccinees would respond similarly to an infection, thus preventing viremia and disease. Nevertheless, the fact that in Senegal a single dose of IPV protected only 36% of vaccinees[79] gives no support to the idea; it could be argued, however, that to induce immunological memory, both T- and B-cell responses are required, which a single dose may not induce. Swartz and colleagues showed that newborns could be sensitized to develop an anamnestic response to IPV at age 6 months if they were given a dose at birth.[35]

Whatever the theoretical arguments may be, a moderate position would be to recommend four doses of IPV, as for example in the current U.S. schedule, which is ages 2, 4, and 18 months and 4 to 6 years. We consider that the need for subsequent boosters has not been established.

Adverse Events

IPV is in general a well-tolerated vaccine.[26–28] When the vaccine is injected intramuscularly to infants as IPV alone, injection site erythema is seen in 0.5 to 1.5% of infants, induration in 3 to 11%, and tenderness in 14 to 29%.[24, 47, 100] The combination of IPV with other vaccines, such as DTP or Hib, does not seem to add to the reactions expected with those vaccines alone (Pasteur Mérieux Connaught Laboratories, unpublished data).[26, 27]

IPV-containing vaccines are licensed in more than 40 countries, and at least 125 million people have received them. Overall, the numbers of adverse events reported to the manufacturers have been low, and the types of reactions reported have been banal and without concentration in a single category. In particular, neurological events such as Guillain-Barré syndrome have not exceeded the background incidence. In France, the rate of reported reactions has been consistently on the order of 3 per 100,000 doses (Pasteur Mérieux Connaught Laboratories, unpublished data).

With regard to major events, the Cutter incident is the major blot on the record of IPV. Between April and June 1955, shortly after licensure in the United States, 204 cases of type 1 polio developed in association with use of the vaccine manufactured by Cutter Laboratories.[101–103] After epidemiological analysis, 60 cases in vaccinees and 89 in family contacts were judged to be caused by two lots of vaccine in which infectious virus had not been completely inactivated. Cases in vaccinees peaked about 14 days after inoculation, whereas cases in family contacts peaked at 28 days. About 70,000 children received the two lots, of whom half were probably seronegative to type 1. Virological studies revealed infection in 10 to 25% of vaccinated children and found an incidence of 1 paralytic case in every 100 to 600 infections.

The incriminated lots all had passed safety tests, including monkey neurovirulence and tissue culture infectivity. Studies conducted in retrospect showed that only monkeys immunosuppressed with cortisone and x-irradiation showed paralysis after inoculation of the incriminated lots.[19]

Extensive studies of production techniques attributed the disaster to two causes: failure to remove viral clumps that could hide infectious particles, and a "tailing-off" of viral inactivation at low concentrations of infectious virus, which meant that the inactivation was no longer linear. Addition of a filtration through a Seitz filter midway during formalin inactivation was the major new step taken, the result being increased safety but unfortunately also diminished antigenicity.[19] Other steps taken were to increase the volume of doses tested for residual infectivity after inactivation and to extend the inactivation period.

Since the Cutter incident and the safety measures instituted as a result of that experience, there has been no evidence for defective manufacture of IPV. More than 90 million doses of IPV produced by the major manufacturers have been used without association with subsequent polio, Guillain-Barré syndrome, anaphylaxis, or other serious reaction.[26–28, 104] Augmented use of IPV in routine vaccination in the United States has permitted additional accumulation of data by the Vaccine Adverse Events Reporting System, again without indication of a causal relationship to serious disease. Accumulated data from Canada and France are likewise reassuring. In France, between 1990 and 1994, more than 56 million doses of IPV vaccines were used, with no evidence for a relationship between vaccine and serious reactions. Postmarketing surveillance, conducted principally in France but also more recently in the United States, largely reveals complaints of local reactions and fever. Hypotonic hyporesponsiveness has been reported rarely, but because IPV was given most often as part of combined vaccines containing a whole-cell pertussis component, the relationship to IPV is uncertain. The other serious reactions reported did not cluster in any organ system or show any pattern indicating vaccine causation (Pasteur Mérieux Connaught Laboratories, unpublished data).

Flare-ups of systemic lupus erythematosus were reported in approximately 6% of IPV-vaccinated patients. However, about the same rate was seen in OPV recipients, and no control group was studied.[105]

There is a theoretical risk of hypersensitivity reactions to the streptomycin, polymyxin B, and neomycin present in IPVs, but no confirmation of such reactions has been found in postmarketing surveillance.

Indications for Inactivated Polio Vaccine[32, 106]

Infants. IPV is now an accepted product to vaccinate American children against poliomyelitis, with OPV alone or in a schedule that begins with two doses of IPV and is completed with two doses of OPV. The Advisory Committee on Immunization Practices accepts all three options but has expressed a preference for the mixed schedule.[32] In Canada and a number of other countries principally in Europe, IPV is the routine vaccine against polio (see Table 15–4).[107]

Children. For children who need rapid vaccination because they are traveling to a zone of endemic polio, or for those who have not previously been vaccinated, the recommended schedule is two doses 1 month apart followed by a booster 6 months later (or, if pressed for time, at least 1 month later).

All children should receive a booster dose of IPV at school entry (age 4–6 yr) if they have received this vaccine previously. The recommendation of the Advisory Committee on Immunization Practices is to give OPV if the child has previously received OPV or a mixed schedule.

Adults, Including Travelers.[32] Routine vaccination of adults is not recommended in the United States, but it is recommended in many European countries. If adults need primary polio vaccination, they should always receive IPV, as VAPP after OPV appears to be more common after the age of 18 years. However, adults who have previously received OPV may receive it as a booster.

In principle, vaccination of previously unvaccinated adults, to protect them from VAPP, is recommended when they are in contact with children excreting OPV. How often this recommendation is followed is uncertain.

Those adults traveling to polio epidemic or polio endemic areas should receive IPV as a booster before their first trip. Laboratory personnel working with wild polioviruses should have previously completed vaccination. Healthcare workers should also be vaccinated, as they may come into contact with wild poliovirus or reverted attenuated viruses being excreted by vaccinees.

Immunocompromised People. IPV is universally recommended for patients with congenital or acquired immunodeficiency, including HIV infection, in view of the VAPP risk in those patients after OPV.[108] Those receiving systemic steroid therapy or chemotherapy are included in this indication. In developing countries, OPV is recommended for asymptomatic HIV seropositive people, as the risk of polio is considered larger than the risk of VAPP.

To protect immunosuppressed people from mutant strains of OPV, family contacts should also receive IPV.

Contraindications to Inactivated Polio Vaccine[32, 106]

Formal contraindications to IPV consist of previous severe reaction to IPV or to streptomycin, neomycin, or polymyxin B. Neither pregnancy nor breast-feeding is a contraindication.

Simultaneous Use with Other Vaccines. No significant interference effects have been described when IPV was used in association with DTP, Hib, or hepatitis B vaccines. The largest experiences with IPV combinations have been with DTP-IPV and DTP-IPV-Hib in France, Canada, and elsewhere (see Chapter 20 [Combination Vaccines]).[26–28] In combination vaccines, IPV is compatible with DTP; diphtheria, acellular pertussis, and tetanus; Hib; and hepatitis B, although generalization is difficult owing to the many combinations and the rapidly changing picture of the availability of these vaccines. Spontaneous mixtures should not be made by the physician, as IPV is destroyed by certain substances, such as thimerosal, which is used as a preservative. Bypass syringes have been used to prevent inactivation of IPV by DTP before injection.

PUBLIC HEALTH CONSIDERATIONS

Results of Vaccination with Inactivated Polio Vaccine

Experience with IPV in national programs is greatest in Europe and in Canada. Some countries have used IPV exclusively, and some as part of a mixed schedule with OPV, as reviewed by Murdin and colleagues[27] and Plotkin.[107]

Sweden. Sweden has used IPV since 1957. In 1989, IPV replaced the original vaccine. Indigenous circulation of wild poliovirus was stopped by 1962,[109] although a subsequent case occurred in an unvaccinated religious sect without spread to the larger population.[110] Data showing the persistence of antibodies in Swedish children despite the absence of circulating virus were discussed earlier under *Duration of Immunity.*

Finland. IPV has been used in Finland for many years, starting with first-generation vaccine and changing to enhanced-potency IPV in 1985. The only outbreak of polio since the introduction of vaccine involved 10 cases in 1984 under the following circumstances[111, 112]:

1. The type 3 component of the first-generation IPV being used in Finland was of low potency, with the minority of vaccinees responding with antibodies.[113]
2. Vaccination coverage had slipped to 80%.
3. A type 3 wild virus was introduced probably from Turkey that was genetically distinct from the Saukett virus in the vaccine,[84] so that antibodies against the latter did not always neutralize the wild virus.[113]
4. The mutation in the wild type 3 virus occurred at neutralization antigenic site 1. This site is present on inactivated polioviruses and induces neutralizing antibodies. However, the three other sites present on the virus are destroyed by inactivation, and thus protection depends on the presence of antibody to site 1. If the circulating virus has mutated at this site, it can escape neutralization.

OPV was used to stop the outbreak, after which the Finns returned to the use of IPV, but in the form of the enhanced-potency vaccine that was also used in Sweden. The new IPV did induce antibodies neutralizing to the Finnish isolate. No spread of polio to Sweden occurred during the epidemic.[109]

The Netherlands. The enhanced-potency IPV was developed in the Netherlands in the late 1970s and reached its current form by 1982.[114] Polio has been prevented ever since in the general population. As recounted earlier, however, two outbreaks have occurred in Protestant sects refusing vaccination, without spread to others (see under *Herd Immunity*).

Iceland. Polio disappeared from Iceland in 1960 after the introduction of IPV vaccination in 1956.[109]

Norway. The history of polio vaccination in Norway provides evidence that IPV prevents VAPP. Norway started vaccination with IPV in the late 1950s but switched to OPV in 1965. After that switch, there were six cases of VAPP, of which five were in unvaccinated people and the sixth in an individual given IPV 10 years earlier (L. Flagstrud and H. Nokleby, personal communication, 1996). In view of the fact that most of the susceptible population had received IPV previously but VAPP was concentrated in the remaining unvaccinated, it appeared that VAPP had been almost completely prevented by prior IPV vaccination.

Norway switched back to IPV in 1979, and since then the only reported poliomyelitis has been imported from abroad.[109]

France. France is perhaps the best example of a sizable country exposed to immigration from polio endemic areas in Africa that has kept the disease at bay with IPV vaccination only. France started vaccination with an IPV in 1956, but in 1965 OPV became the recommended vaccine. Both OPV and IPV were in use until 1983, when the Vero cell IPV received official recommendation. Doses are recommended at ages 2, 3, 4, and 15 to 18 months; 5 to 6 years; and 11 years. VAPP occurred sporadically during the use of OPV but in 1986 ceased to be seen.[115–117] The last wild polio case was reported in 1989, and attempts to find virus in sewage have not been successful since 1988.[115–118] The occurrence of polio in France from 1977 to 1992 is shown in Figure 15–9.[115]

Canada. Canadian provinces have used IPV, OPV, or a mixed schedule since the inception of vaccination in 1955. At present, nearly all provinces are using IPV, and the experience has been particularly large in Ontario, Canada's most populous province. Since 1988, the vaccine has been an IPV produced in human diploid cells.

The last indigenous case of polio occurred in 1988, related to importation of the virus. Introductions of poliovirus from the Netherlands in 1979 and 1992 and from the Indian subcontinent in 1996 failed to result in spread to the general population.[26, 82, 119]

The province of Prince Edward Island uses a mixed schedule consisting of IPV at 2, 4, and 6 months of age, followed by OPV at 18 months, 4 to 6 years, and 14 to 16 years of age. No polio has occurred in many years,

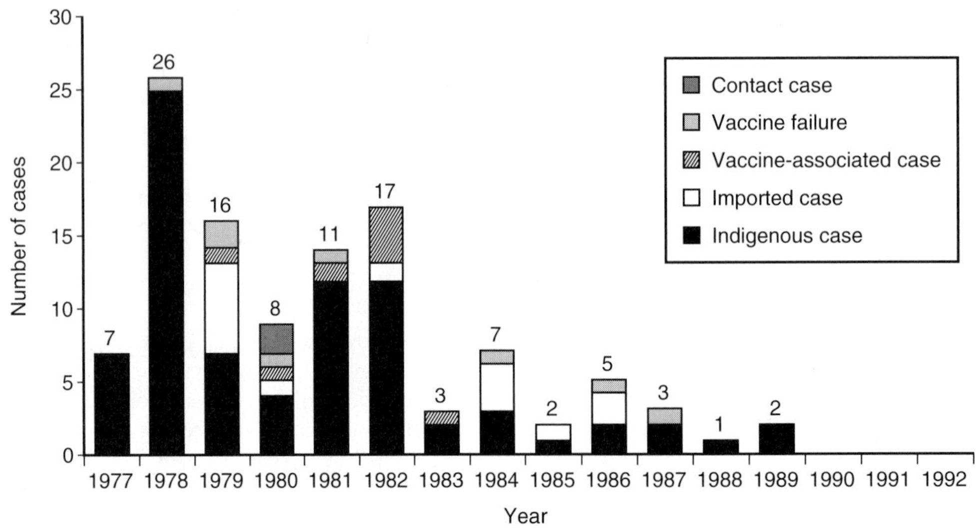

Figure 15–9. Sources of poliomyelitis in France, 1977 to 1992.

but the size of the population (137,000) precludes conclusions.

Israel. Israel has used both polio vaccines in an attempt to solve their particular epidemiological situation, in which two communities that live close together have different hygienic conditions and levels of vaccination coverage. After brief experience with IPV, Israel started routine OPV vaccination in 1960. Vaccination coverage reached high levels among both Jewish and Arab children. Nevertheless, sporadic poliomyelitis continued among Jews, and small epidemics continued to occur in the West Bank and Gaza.[120–124]

In view of the failure of OPV to control polio, in 1978 the Israelis introduced a combined schedule: OPV was administered at 1, 2½, 4, 5½, and 12 months of age, and IPV (as DTP-IPV) was given at 2½ and 4 months of age. For a time in the 1980s, there were no cases in Israel proper and only sporadic cases in the Palestinian areas.[120, 121]

All was more or less well until 1988, when an epidemic of 15 cases of type 1 polio occurred in Israel,[123, 124] localized in one of two districts that had adopted IPV vaccination of infants. Although the analysis of this epidemic is controversial, it is clear that antibody responses to OPV were suboptimal, resulting in a low level of resistance among Israeli young adults. Conversely, the wild virus may have circulated among infants immunized with IPV only, allowing spread to their parents.[124]

The response to the epidemic included mass vaccination with OPV and the institution of three doses of DTP-IPV in the routine vaccination scheme, together with four doses of OPV. Since 1988, no cases of polio have been reported in Israel or its territories, despite an outbreak in neighboring Jordan from 1991 to 1992 that caused wild virus circulation in Gaza.[123]

Denmark. Denmark chose a mixed schedule in 1968. Since 1970, Danish children have received IPV at 5, 6, and 15 months of age, followed by OPV at 2, 3, and 4 years of age. Single polio cases were diagnosed in 1969, 1976, 1980, and 1986, the last two being imported. No wild virus has been identified in sewage samples since 1968. Not surprisingly, seroimmunity has been virtually 100% at all age levels of the Danish population.[27, 125] No VAPP has occurred among 1.5 million Danes who have received two or more doses of IPV.

United States. Early use of first-generation IPV in the United States was discussed previously (see under *Herd Immunity*). Despite incomplete application of the vaccine, polio incidence fell 95% between the introduction of the vaccine in 1955 and its abandonment in 1961 (see Fig. 15–7). The remaining cases, however, many of them in IPV vaccinees, sapped confidence in the vaccine and caused its replacement by OPV.[27, 107]

IPV has been reintroduced into routine use in the United States in its enhanced-potency form and primarily as part of a mixed schedule, although complete vaccination with four doses of IPV is an accepted regimen.[32, 106] The Advisory Committee on Immunization Practices gives preference to a regimen of two doses of IPV at 2 and 4 months of age, followed by two doses of OPV at 18 months and 4 to 6 years of age.[32] Recommendations may change to an abbreviated schedule, with the first dose of OPV being given at 6 months of age and the second at 18 months of age.

The primary reason for the reintroduction of IPV was the perception that polio is vanishing from the world, whereas VAPP exacts a yearly toll of 8 to 10 cases.[107, 108, 126]

Developing Countries. Although not routinely recommended in developing countries, IPV has been studied in those areas (Pasteur Mérieux Connaught Laboratories, unpublished data).[26, 40, 41, 79, 127] The viewpoint of the WHO and other authorities is that only OPV should be used as the principal tool for eradicating polio in developing countries.[128]

Recommendations for the Use of Inactivated Polio Vaccine

IPV is the polio vaccine of choice for immunosuppressed individuals and in most circumstances is the vaccine of choice for adults.

Since the 1960s, the controversy that has consumed much ink is the choice of IPV or OPV for routine vaccination in infancy. Table 15–13 summarizes the advantages and disadvantages of IPV, OPV, or mixed IPV/OPV schedules.[107] In essence, the arguments for IPV are safety, predictable immunogenicity, and the possibility of its inclusion in combination vaccines. The arguments for OPV are induction of mucosal immunity, ease of administration to large populations, and low cost. The argument for a mixed schedule is to fuse the immunogenicity advantages of each vaccine, with less risk of VAPP.

VAPP, which is discussed in detail in the chapter on OPV (Chapter 16), is an inescapable phenomenon that has been consistently observed after OPV.[32, 105, 129, 130] In our view, the following circumstances should lead to the choice of IPV for routine vaccination of infants at the end of the 20th century in a particular country:

1. Absence of paralytic polio and the likelihood that wild polioviruses are not circulating. This criterion applies to countries where eradication of polio has been certified, even if importation is possible through carriage by immigrants. As stated previously, the WHO still recommends OPV in this circumstance.
2. High prior vaccine coverage with either IPV or OPV, equivalent to 80% or better of infants and children, so that introduction of wild virus is unlikely to result in spread.
3. Ability of the medical system or of individual families to afford the higher costs of IPV, although the cost issue may be exaggerated. Reduced wastage and lower needs for a cold chain compensate to some degree for the difference in price, and the price differential between IPV and OPV varies from country to country. In the United States, for example, because of liability tax and other factors, the difference in price is not so evident. In developing countries, however, the relative cost of IPV to OPV is high, but the absolute price of IPV is lower because of the system of two-tiered pricing. The costs of National Vaccination Days with OPV, in which

Table 15–13. **ADVANTAGES AND DISADVANTAGES OF ALL OPV, ALL IPV, OR MIXED VACCINATION SCHEDULES**

FEATURE	ALL OPV	ALL IPV	IPV/OPV
VAPP	1 case per 790,000 first vaccinations	No cases	Estimated 50–75% reduction in VAPP cases
Safety (other than VAPP)	Excellent	Excellent	Presumably excellent
Systemic immunity	Good	Good	Good
Mucosal immunity	Excellent	Slight to moderate in intestine Marked in pharynx Overall less than OPV	Excellent
Transmission to contacts and secondary vaccination	Yes	No	Some
Extra injections	No	Yes if monovalent No if part of combination vaccine	Same as for all IPV
Reduced compliance	No	Possible if monovalent vaccine	Possible if monovalent vaccine
Likelihood of future combinations	Uncertain	High	High
Cost	Low	Higher, although price difference depends on volume, combinations, and so forth	Intermediate

IPV, inactivated polio vaccine; OPV, live oral polio vaccine; VAPP, vaccine-associated paralytic poliomyelitis.
From Plotkin S. Developed countries should use inactivated polio vaccine for the prevention of poliomyelitis. Rev Med Virol 7:75–81, 1997.

large populations are mobilized, must also be taken into account.

The criteria for a mixed schedule are the same, but with the addition of a public health policy factor: the desire to prevent polio by all possible means, taking advantage of both vaccines but also maximizing safety.[131, 132] Although this point refers to schedules beginning with IPV and ending with OPV, in view of the sometimes low rates of seroconversion after the primary vaccination, IPV might be considered in a single booster dose for children living in tropical areas who have been previously vaccinated with OPV.[46]

Role of Inactivated Polio Vaccine in Polio Eradication

Campaigns with OPV have already resulted in the eradication of polio from the Western Hemisphere and are having a marked impact on the incidence of polio in traditionally endemic areas, such as India, Africa, and China.[133] At some point, there will be no clinical evidence of paralytic polio in the world, and thus the question of how to certify eradication is under discussion. One means of verifying eradication would be to stop all vaccination and observe for wild virus circulation and cases of poliovirus-induced paralysis. A second strategy would be to continue OPV vaccination while attempting to detect circulating wild poliovirus. The difficulty here would be in detecting the virus in a sea of excreted attenuated viruses, some mutated toward virulence and some recombinants with other polioviruses.[134, 135] Moreover, a report of an immunosuppressed individual who appears to have excreted poliovirus for 7 years[136] raises the specter that attenuated strains will continue to circulate in a mutated virulent form that pose a danger for an unvaccinated population.

A third strategy could be proposed, consisting of a gradual switch from OPV to combined pediatric vaccines containing IPV (e.g., DTP-Hib-hepatitis B-IPV) as wild poliovirus disappears from more and more countries. Vaccination with IPV would prevent the search for polioviruses in the environment from being hampered by OPV vaccine strains and yet would maintain protection against polio. Such a strategy may be all the more valuable, as it has been calculated that even after a 5-year period without polio cases, there may still be a 0.1 to 1.0% probability of silent transmission.[137] There are obviously many practical difficulties in implementing such a plan, but it is likely that developed countries and the more affluent developing countries will avail themselves of this strategy.

A fourth strategy, a variant of the second, is to switch to an oral vaccine containing only type 1 and type 3 viruses and to search for wild type 2 virus. As type 2 virus may well disappear before the others and this approach would require the development of a new vaccine, this strategy has little to recommend it.

CONCLUSION

More than 40 years after its invention, IPV is renascent, owing to improvements in its manufacture and its outstanding safety record. In the immediate future, this vaccine is certain to have more widespread use, as the world moves toward the eradication of poliovirus with the use of two potent vaccines that can be synergistic for public health programs in terms of safety, immunogenicity, and other attributes.[138]

REFERENCES

1. Gear J. The History of the Poliomyelitis Research Foundation. Rivonia, South Africa, Poliomyelitis Research Foundation, 1996, pp 4–13.
2. Bodian D, Morgan I, Howe H. Differentiation of types of poliomyelitis viruses; the grouping of fourteen strains into three basic immunologic types. Am J Hyg 49:234–245, 1949.

3. Horstmann D, McCollum R, Mascola A. Viremia in human poliomyelitis. J Exp Med 99:355–369, 1954.
4. Hammon WM, Coriell L, Wehrle P, et al. Evaluation of Red Cross gamma globulin as a prophylactic agent for poliomyelitis. 4. Final report of results based on clinical diagnoses. JAMA 151:1272–1285, 1953.
5. Enders J, Weller T, Robbins F. Cultivation of the Lansing strain of poliomyelitis virus in cultures of various human embryonic tissues. Science 109:85–87, 1949.
6. Beale A. The development of IPV. In Plotkin S, Fantini B (eds). Vaccinia, Vaccination, Vaccinology: Jenner, Pasteur, and Their Successors. Paris, Elsevier, 1996, pp 221–227.
7. Van Wezel A. Growth of cell strains and primary cells on micro carriers in homogenous culture. Nature 216:64–65, 1967.
8. Montagnon B. Polio and rabies vaccines produced in continuous cell lines: A reality for Vero cell line. Dev Biol Stand 70:27–47, 1988.
9. Paul J, Melnick J, Barnett V, Goldblum N. A survey of neutralizing antibodies to poliomyelitis in Cairo, Egypt. Am J Hyg 55:402–413, 1952.
10. Lebrun A, Cerf J, Gelfand H, et al. Vaccination with the CHAT strain of type I attenuated poliomyelitis virus in Leopoldville, Belfian Congo. I. Description of the city, its history of poliomyelitis, and the plan of vaccination campaign. Bull World Health Organ 22:203–213, 1960.
11. Plotkin S, Koprowski H, Stokes J Jr. Clinical trials in infants of orally administered attenuated poliomyelitis viruses. Pediatrics 23:1041–1062, 1959.
12. Brodie M, Park W. Active immunization against poliomyelitis. Am J Public Health 26:119–125, 1936.
13. Kolmer J. Vaccination against acute anterior poliomyelitis. Am J Public Health 26:126–135, 1936.
14. Murray R. Standardization licensing and availability of live polio virus vaccine. JAMA 175:843–846, 1961.
15. Berkovich S, Pickering J, Kibrick S. Paralytic poliomyelitis in Massachusetts, 1959: A study of the disease in a well vaccinated population. N Engl J Med 264:1325–1329, 1961.
16. Montagnon B, Fanget B, Vincent-Falquet J. Industrial-scale production of inactivated poliovirus vaccine prepared by culture of Vero cells on microcarrier. Rev Infect Dis 6 (suppl 2):S341–S344, 1984.
17. Duchene M, Peetermans J, D'Hondt E, et al. Production of poliovirus vaccines: Past, present, and future. Viral Immunol 3:243–272, 1990.
18. Horaud F. Viral vaccines and residual cellular DNA. Biologicals 23:225–228, 1995.
19. Melnick J. Virus inactivation: Lessons from the past. Dev Biol Stand 75:29–36, 1991.
20. Ferguson M, Wood D, Minor P. Antigenic structure of poliovirus in inactivated vaccines. J Gen Virol 74:685–690, 1993.
21. Salk J. One-dose immunization against paralytic poliomyelitis using a noninfectious vaccine. Rev Infect Dis 6(suppl 2):S444–S450, 1984.
22. Mellander L, Bottiger M, Hanson L, et al. Avidity and titres of the antibody response to two inactivated poliovirus vaccines with different antigen content. Acta Paediatr 82:552–556, 1993.
23. Halperin S, Davies H, Barreto L, et al. Safety and immunogenicity of two inactivated poliovirus vaccines in combination with an acellular pertussis vaccine and diphtheria and tetanus toxoids in seventeen- to nineteen-month-old infants. J Pediatr 130:525–531, 1997.
24. Piirainen L, Roivainen M, Litmanen L, et al. Immunogenicity of a pilot inactivated poliovirus vaccine with trypsin-treated type 3 component. Vaccine 15:237–243, 1997.
25. Sawyer L, McInnis J, Patel A, et al. Deleterious effect of thimerosal on the potency of inactivated poliovirus vaccine. Vaccine 12:851–856, 1994.
26. Vidor E, Caudrelier P, Plotkin S. The place of DPT/eIPV vaccine in routine paediatric vaccination. Rev Med Virol 4:261–277, 1994.
27. Murdin A, Barreto L, Plotkin S. Inactivated poliovirus vaccine: Past and present experience. Vaccine 14:735–746, 1996.
28. Vidor E, Meschievitz C, Plotkin S. Fifteen years of experience with Vero-produced enhanced potency inactivated poliovirus vaccine. Pediatr Infect Dis J 16:312–322, 1997.
29. Faden H, Modlin J, Thoms M, et al. Comparative evaluation of immunization with live attenuated and enhanced-potency inactivated trivalent poliovirus vaccines in childhood: Systemic and local immune responses. J Infect Dis 162:1291–1297, 1990.
30. McBean A, Thoms M, Albrecht P, et al. Serologic response to oral polio vaccines and enhanced-potency inactivated polio vaccines. Am J Epidemiol 128:615–628, 1988.
31. Modlin J, Halsey N, Thoms M, et al. Humoral and mucosal immunity in infants induced by three sequential inactivated poliovirus vaccine–live attenuated poliovirus vaccine immunization schedules. J Infect Dis 175(suppl 1):S228–S234, 1997.
32. Poliomyelitis prevention in the United States: Introduction of a sequential vaccination schedule of inactivated poliovirus vaccine followed by oral poliovirus vaccine. MMWR Morb Mortal Wkly Rep 46(RR-3):1–25, 1997.
33. Halsey N, Blatter M, Bader G. Safety and Immunogenicity of a Combination DPT/IPV Vaccine Administered to Infants in a Dual-Chamber Syringe. Final Report. Swiftwater, PA, Connaught Laboratories, 1993.
34. Blatter M, Starr S. Safety and Immunogenicity of a Combination DPT/eIPV Vaccine Presented in a Dual-Chamber Syringe, in 2-Month-Old Infants. Swiftwater, PA, Connaught Laboratories, 1994.
35. Swartz T, Handsher R, Stoeckel P, et al. Immunologic memory induced at birth by immunization with inactivated polio vaccine in a reduced schedule. Eur J Epidemiol 5:143–145, 1989.
36. Baker J, Halperin S, Edwards K, et al. Antibody response to *Bordetella pertussis* antigens after immunization with American and Canadian whole-cell vaccines. J Pediatr 121:523–527, 1992.
37. Halperin S, Langley J, Eastwood B. Effect of inactivated poliovirus vaccine on the antibody response to *Bordetella pertussis* antigen when combined with diphtheria-pertussis-tetanus vaccine. Clin Infect Dis 22:59–62, 1996.
38. Halperin S, Eastwood B, Langley J. Immune response to pertussis vaccines concurrently administered with viral vaccines. Ann N Y Acad Sci 754:89–96, 1995.
39. Kurkka S, Kayhty H, Saarinen L, et al. Comparison of five different vaccination schedules with *Haemophilus influenzae* type b–tetanus toxoid conjugate vaccine. J Pediatr 4:524–530, 1996.
40. WHO Collaborative Study Group. Combined immunization of infants with oral and inactivated poliovirus vaccines: Results of a randomized trial in The Gambia, Oman, and Thailand. J Infect Dis 175(suppl 1):S215–S227, 1997.
41. Krishnan R, Jadhav M, John T. Efficacy of inactivated poliovirus vaccine in India. Bull World Health Organ 61:689–692, 1983.
42. Simoes EA, Padmini B, Steinhoff MC, et al. Antibody response of infants to two doses of inactivated poliovirus vaccine of enhanced potency. Am J Dis Child 139:977–980, 1985.
43. Ramsey M, Begg N, Gandhi J, et al. Antibody response and viral excretion after live polio vaccine or a combined schedule of live and inactivated polio vaccines. Pediatr Infect Dis J 13:1117–1121, 1994.
44. Strebel P, Ion-Nedelcu N, Baughman A, et al. Intramuscular injections within 30 days of immunization with oral poliovirus vaccine—a risk factor for vaccine-associated paralytic poliomyelitis. N Engl J Med 332:500–506, 1995.
45. Ion-Nedelcu N, Strebel P, Toma F, et al. Sequential and combined use of inactivated and oral poliovirus vaccines: Dolj District, Romania, 1992–1994. J Infect Dis 175(suppl 1):S241–S246, 1997.
46. Moriniere B, Van Loon F, Rhodes P, et al. Immunogenicity of a supplemental dose of oral versus inactivated poliovirus vaccine. Lancet 341:1545–1550, 1993.
47. Adenyi-Jones S, Faden H, Ferdon M, Kwong M. Systemic and local immune responses to enhance potency inactivated poliovirus vaccine in premature term infants. J Pediatr 120:686–689, 1992.
48. Linder N, Yaron M, Handsher R, et al. Early immunization with inactivated poliovirus vaccine in premature infants. J Pediatr 127:128–130, 1995.
49. O'Shea TM, Dillard RG, Gillis DC, Abramson JS. Low rate of response to enhanced inactivated polio vaccine in preterm infants with chronic illness. Clin Res Reg Affairs 10:49–57, 1993.
50. Weckx L, Schmidt BJ, Herrmann AA, et al. Early immunization of neonates with trivalent oral polivirus vaccine. Bull World Health Organ 70:85–91, 1992.

51. Barbi M, Bardare M, Luraschi C, et al. Antibody response to inactivated polio vaccine (e-IPV) in children born to HIV-positive mothers. Eur J Epidemiol 8:211–216, 1992.
52. Varon D, Handsher R, Dardik R, et al. Response of hemophilic patients to poliovirus vaccination: Correlation with HIV serology and with immunological parameters. J Med Virol 40:91–95, 1993.
53. Sipila R, Hortling L, Hovi T. Good seroresponse to enhanced-potency inactivated poliovirus vaccine in patients on chronic dialysis. Bone Marrow Transplant 8:295–300, 1991.
54. Engelhard D, Handsher R, Naparstek E, et al. Immune response to polio vaccination in bone marrow transplant recipients. Bone Marrow Transplant 8:295–300, 1991.
55. Ljungman P, Duraj V, Magnius L. Response to immunization against polio after allogeneic marrow transplantation. Bone Marrow Transplant 7:89–93, 1991.
56. Ogra P, Karzon D, Righthand F, et al. Immunoglobulin response in serum and secretions after immunization with live and inactivated poliovaccine and natural infection. N Engl J Med 279:893–900, 1968.
57. Zhaori G, Sun M, Faden H, Ogra P. Nasopharyngeal secretory antibody response to poliovirus type 3 virion proteins exhibit different specificities after immunization with live or inactivated poliovirus vaccines. J Infect Dis 159:1018–1024, 1989.
58. Faden H, Duffy L. Effect of concurrent viral infection on systemic and local antibody responses to live attenuated and enhanced-potency inactivated poliovirus vaccines. Am J Dis Child 146:1320–1323, 1992.
59. Onorato I, Modlin J, McBean A, et al. Mucosal immunity induced by enhanced-potency inactivated and oral polio vaccines. J Infect Dis 163:1–6, 1991.
60. Hanson L, Carlsson B, Jalil F, et al. Different secretory IgA antibody responses after immunization with inactivated and live poliovirus vaccines. Rev Infect Dis 6(suppl 2):S356–S360, 1984.
61. Fox J. The influence of natural and artificially induced immunity on alimentary infections with polioviruses. Am J Public Health 48:1181–1192, 1958.
62. Horstmann D, Paul J, Melnick J, Deustch J. Infection induced by oral administration of attenuated poliovirus to persons possessing homotypic antibody. J Exp Med 106:159–177, 1997.
63. David D, Lipson M, Carver D, et al. The degree and duration of poliomyelitis virus excretion among vaccinated household contacts of clinical cases of poliomyelitis. Pediatrics 22:33–40, 1958.
64. Gelfand H, LeBlanc D, Potash L, Fox J. Studies on the development of natural immunity to poliomyelitis in Louisiana: IV. Natural infections with polioviruses following immunization with a formalin-inactivated vaccine. Am J Hyg 70:312–327, 1959.
65. Howe H, O'Leary W, Bender W, et al. Day-by-day response of vaccinated chimpanzees to poliomyelitic infection. Am J Public Health 47:871–875, 1957.
66. Craig D, Brown G. The relationship between poliomyelitis antibody and virus excretion from the pharynx and anus of orally infected monkeys. Am J Hyg 69:4–12, 1959.
67. Selvakumar R, John T. Intestinal immunity induced by inactivated poliovirus vaccine. Vaccine 5:141–144, 1987.
68. Marine W, Chin T, Gravelle C. Limitation of fecal and pharyngeal poliovirus excretion in Salk-vaccinated children. Am J Hyg 76:173–195, 1962.
69. Ghendon Y, Robertson S. Interrupting the transmission of wild polioviruses with vaccines: Immunological considerations. Bull World Health Organ 72:973–983, 1994.
70. Nishio O, Ishihara Y, Sakae K, et al. The trend of acquired immunity with live poliovirus vaccine and the effect of revaccination: Follow-up of vaccinees for ten years. J Biol Stand 12:1–10, 1984.
71. Minor P. The molecular biology of poliovaccines. J Gen Virol 73:3065–3077, 1997.
72. Macadam A, Arnold C, Howlett J, et al. Reversion of the attenuated and temperature-sensitive phenotypes of the Sabin type 3 strain of poliovirus in vaccines. Virology 172:408–414, 1989.
73. Chumakov K, Powers L, Noonan K, et al. Correlation between amount of virus with altered nucleotide sequence and the monkey test for acceptability of oral poliovirus vaccine. Proc Natl Acad Sci U S A 88:548–550, 1991.
74. Abraham R, Minor P, Dunn G, et al. Shedding of virulent poliovirus revertants during immunization with oral poliovirus vaccine after prior immunization with inactivated polio vaccine. J Infect Dis 168:1105–1109, 1993.
75. Ogra P, Faden H, Abraham R, et al. Effect of prior immunity on the shedding of virulent revertant virus in feces after oral immunization with live attenuated poliovirus vaccines. J Infect Dis 164:191–194, 1991.
76. Francis T, Korns R, Voight R, et al. An Evaluation of the 1954 Poliomyelitis Vaccine Trials. Ann Arbor, University of Michigan, 1955.
77. Melnick J, Benyesh-Melnick M, Pena R, Yow M. Effectiveness of Salk vaccine. JAMA 175:1159–1162, 1961.
78. Stoeckel P, Schlumberger M, Parent G, et al. Use of killed poliovirus vaccine in a routine immunization program in West Africa. Rev Infect Dis 6(suppl 2):S463–S466, 1984.
79. Robertson S, Traverso H, Drucker J, et al. Clinical efficacy of a new enhanced-potency, inactivated poliovirus vaccine. Lancet 1:897–899, 1988.
80. Paralytic poliomyelitis—Senegal. MMWR Morb Mortal Wkly Rep 37:257–259, 1988.
81. John T. Poliovirus vaccine and poliomyelitis control in India [abstract]. World Conference on Poliomyelitis and Measles, 1992.
82. Varughese P, Carter A, Acres S, Furesz J. Eradication of indigenous poliomyelitis in Canada: Impact of immunization strategies. Can J Public Health 80:363–368, 1989.
83. Chin TDY. Immunity induced by inactivated poliovirus vaccine and excretion of virus. Rev Infect Dis 6(suppl 2):S369–S370, 1984.
84. Hofman B. Poliomyelitis in the Netherlands before and after vaccination with inactivated poliovaccine. J Hyg 65:547–557, 1967.
85. van Wijngaarden J, van Loon A. The polio epidemic in the Netherlands. Public Health Rev 21:107–116, 1992.
86. Bijkerk H. Poliomyelitis in the Netherlands. Dev Biol Stand 47:233–240, 1981.
87. Bijkerk H. Poliomyelitis epidemic in the Netherlands. Dev Biol Stand 43:195–206, 1997.
88. Oostvogel R, Van Wijngaarden J, Avoort H, et al. Poliomyelitis outbreak in an unvaccinated community in the Netherlands. Lancet 344:665–670, 1994.
89. Schaap G, Bijkerk H, Coutinho R, et al. The spread of wild poliovirus in the well-vaccinated Netherlands in connection with the 1978 epidemic. Prog Med Virol 29:124–140, 1984.
90. Epidemiological notes and reports: Follow-up on poliomyelitis—United States, Canada, Netherlands, 1979. MMWR Morb Mortal Wkly Rep 28:345, 1979.
91. Lack of Evidence for Wild Poliovirus Circulation—United States, 1993. MMWR Morb Mortal Wkly Rep 43:957–959, 1995.
92. Rumke H. Vaccination against polio; inactivated polio vaccine used in the Netherlands and Burkina Faso. Trop Geogr Med 45:202–205, 1993.
93. Faden H, Duffy L, Sun M, Shuff C. Long-term immunity to poliovirus in children immunized with live attenuated and enhanced-potency inactivated trivalent poliovirus vaccines. J Infect Dis 168:452–454, 1993.
94. Bottiger M. Polio immunity to killed vaccine: An 18-year follow-up. Vaccine 8:443–445, 1997.
95. Swartz T, Roumiantzeff M, Peyron L, et al. Use of a combined DTP-polio vaccine in a reduced schedule. Dev Biol Stand 65:159–166, 1986.
96. Salk J, Drucker J, Malvy D. Noninfectious poliovirus vaccine. In Plotkin S, Mortimer E Jr (eds). Vaccines (2nd ed). Philadelphia, WB Saunders, 1994, pp 205–227.
97. Salk J. Persistence of immunity after administration of formalin-treated poliovirus vaccine. Lancet 2:715–723, 1960.
98. Salk J. Are booster doses of poliovirus vaccine necessary? Vaccine 8:419–420, 1990.
99. Salk D. Induction of long-term immunity to paralytic poliomyelitis by use of non-infectious vaccine. Lancet 2:1317–1321, 1984.
100. Poliovirus Vaccine Inactivated (IPOL) package insert. Swiftwater, PA, Mérieux Connaught Laboratories, 1997.
101. Nathanson N, Langmuir A. The Cutter Incident: Poliomyelitis following formaldehyde-inactivated poliovirus vaccination in the United States during the spring of 1955. III. Comparison of the

clinical character of vaccinated and contact cases occurring after use of high rate lots of Cutter vaccine. Am J Hyg 78:61–81, 1963.
102. Nathanson N, Langmuir A. The Cutter Incident: Poliomyelitis following formaldehyde-inactivated poliovirus vaccination in the United States during the spring of 1955. I. Background. Am J Hyg 78:16–28, 1963.
103. Nathanson N, Langmuir A. The Cutter Incident: Poliomyelitis following formaldehyde-inactivated poliovirus vaccination in the United States during the spring of 1955. II. Relationship of poliomyelitis to Cutter vaccine. Am J Hyg 78:29–60, 1963.
104. Plotkin S. Inactivated polio vaccine for the United States: A missed vaccination opportunity. Pediatr Infect Dis J 14:835–839, 1997.
105. Schattner A, Ben-Chetrit E, Schmilovitz H. Poliovaccines and the course of systemic lupus erythematosus—a retrospective study of 73 patients. Vaccine 10:98–100, 1992.
106. Poliovirus infections. In Peter G, Hall C, Halsey N, et al. Red Book: Report of the Committee on Infectious Diseases. Red Book Report (24th ed). Elk Grove Village, IL, American Academy of Pediatrics, 1997, pp 424–433.
107. Plotkin S. Developed countries should use inactivated polio vaccine for the prevention of poliomyelitis. Rev Med Virol 7:75–81, 1997.
108. Sutter R, Prevots D. Vaccine-associated paralytic poliomyelitis among immunodeficient persons. Infect Med 11:426–438, 1994.
109. Bottiger M. The elimination of polio in the Scandinavian countries. Public Health Rev 21:27–33, 1993.
110. Bottiger M, Mellin P, Romanus V, et al. Epidemiological events surrounding a paralytic case of poliomyelitis in Sweden. Bull World Health Organ 57:99–103, 1979.
111. Hovi T, Cantell K, Huovilainen A, et al. Outbreak of paralytic poliomyelitis in Finland: Widespread circulation of antigenically altered poliomyelitis type 3 in a vaccinated population. Lancet 1:1427–1432, 1986.
112. Lapinleimu K. Elimination of poliomyelitis in Finland. Rev Infect Dis 6(suppl 2):S457–S460, 1984.
113. Magrath D, Evans D, Ferguson M, et al. Antigenic and molecular properties of type 3 poliomyelitis responsible for an outbreak of poliomyelitis in a vaccinated population. J Gen Virol 67:899–905, 1986.
114. van Wezel AL, van Steenis P, van deer Marel P, et al. Inactivated poliovirus vaccine: Current production methods and new developments. Rev Infect Dis 6(suppl 2):S335–S340, 1984.
115. Malvy D, Drucker J. Elimination of poliomyelitis in France: Epidemiology and vaccine status. Public Health Rev 21:41–49, 1993.
116. Roure C, Rebiere I, Aymard M, Dubrou S. Surveillance de la poliomyelite en France. Bull Epidemiol Hebd 15:59–61, 1993.
117. Guerin N, Lequellec-Nathan M, Rebiere I, et al. Surveillance de la poliomyelite et des poliovirus en France. Bull Epidemiol Hebd 12:51–53, 1997.
118. Drucker J. Poliomyelitis in France: Epidemiology and vaccination status. Pediatr Infect Dis J 10:967–969, 1991.
119. Ministry of Health Ontario. Wild-type poliovirus isolated in Hamilton. Public Health Epidemiol Rep 7:51–52, 1996.
120. Tulchinsky T, Abed Y, Shaheen S, et al. A ten-year experience in control of poliomyelitis through a combination of live and killed vaccines in two developing areas. Am J Public Health 79:1648–1652, 1989.
121. Lasch E, Abde Y, Abdulla K, et al. Successful results of a program combining live and inactivated poliovirus vaccines to control poliomyelitis in Gaza. Rev Infect Dis 6(suppl 2):S467–S470, 1984.
122. Swartz TA, Ben-Porath E, Kanaaneh H, et al. Comparison of inactivated poliovirus vaccine and oral poliovirus vaccine program in Israel. Rev Infect Dis 6(suppl 2):S556–S561, 1984.
123. Tulchinsky T. Combined OPV and IPV program in control of poliomyelitis in two endemic areas—a potential tool in the struggle to eradicate poliomyelitis. Public Health Rev 21:153–156, 1997.
124. Slater P, Orenstein W, Morag A, et al. Poliomyelitis oubreak in Israel in 1988: A report with two commentaries. Lancet 335:1192–1198, 1990.
125. von Magnus H, Peterson I. Vaccination with inactivated poliovirus vaccine and oral poliovirus in Denmark. Rev Infect Dis 6(suppl 2):S471–S474, 1984.
126. Strebel P, Sutter R, Cochi S, et al. Epidemiology of poliomyelitis in the United States one decade after the last reported case of indigenous wild virus–associated disease. Clin Infect Dis 14:681–682, 1992.
127. John T. Immunisation Against Polioviruses in Developing Countries. Rev Med Virol 3:149–160, 1993.
128. Hull HF, Aylward RB. Ending polio immunization. Science 277:780, 1997.
129. Esteves K. Safety of oral poliomyelitis vaccine: Results of a WHO enquiry. Bull World Health Organ 66:739–746, 1988.
130. Andrus J, Strebel P, deQuadros C, Olive J. Risk of vaccine-associated paralytic poliomyelitis in Latin America, 1989–91. Bull World Health Organ 73:33–40, 1995.
131. McBean A, Modlin J. Rationale for the sequential use of inactivated poliovirus vaccine and live attenuated poliovirus vaccine for routine immunization in the United States. Pediatr Infect Dis J 6:881–887, 1987.
132. Faden H. Poliovirus vaccination: A trilogy. J Infect Dis 168:25–28, 1993.
133. Hull H, Birmingham M, Melgaard B, Lee J. Progress toward global polio eradication. J Infect Dis 175(suppl 1):S4–S9, 1997.
134. Georgescu M, Delpeyroux F, Tardy-Panit M, et al. High diversity of poliovirus strains isolated from the central nervous system from patients with vaccine-associated paralytic poliomyelitis. J Virol 68:8089–9101, 1994.
135. Dove A, Racaniello V. The polio eradication effort: Should vaccine eradication be next? Science 277:779–780, 1997.
136. Prolonged poliovirus excretion in an immunodeficient person with vaccine-associated paralytic poliomyelitis. MMWR Morb Mortal Wkly Rep 46:641–643, 1997.
137. Eichner M, Dietz K. Eradication of poliomyelitis: When can one be sure that polio virus transmission has been terminated? Am J Epidemiol 143:816–822, 1996.
138. Plotkin S. An end to Manicheism. Public Health Rev 21:135–138, 1993.

chapter

16 Live Attenuated Poliovirus Vaccines

Roland W. Sutter
Stephen L. Cochi
Joseph L. Melnick

HISTORY

The written history of poliomyelitis can be traced to the first description of the disease as a separate clinical entity by Michael Underwood in 1789, more than 200 years ago.[1] Since then, many important scientific discoveries and public health milestones have been associated with poliomyelitis. Undoubtedly, the most consequential of these were the development of effective poliovirus vaccines,[2] which paved the way for the implementation of control programs, and a resolution by the World Health Assembly that established the goal of global eradication of poliomyelitis by the year 2000.[3] The polio eradication initiative is operational in all polio endemic countries and within a few years is expected to relegate poliomyelitis to a disease that future generations will know only by history.

Although the written history of poliomyelitis is relatively succinct, an Egyptian stele from the 18th dynasty (1580 to 1350 BC) depicts a "crippled young man, apparently a priest, with a withered and shortened left leg, and with his foot held in a typical equinus position characteristic of flaccid paralysis."[4] This inscription demonstrates that poliomyelitis has probably affected mankind since ancient times. Underwood[1] introduced the term *debility of the lower extremities* in 1789; other researchers suggested a series of alternative terms, including *Lähmungszustände der unteren Extremitäten* in 1840,[5] *morning paralysis* in 1843,[6] *paralysie esséntielle chez les énfants* in 1851,[7] *paralysie atrophiques graisseues de l'énfance* in 1855,[8] *spinale Kinderlähmung* in 1860,[9] *tephromyelitis anterior acuta parenchymatose* in 1872,[10] and *poliomyelitis anterior acuta* in 1874.[11] The last term is based on anatomical location of lesions within the spinal cord—which was discovered in the early 1870s—and constructed from the Greek words *polios* (i.e., gray) and *myelos* (i.e., marrow, the gray matter of the spinal cord) with the ending -itis to imply inflammation. Although the terms Heine-Medin disease in 1907,[12] infantile paralysis, and polio were proposed subsequently, poliomyelitis prevailed and became the standard designation for the disease.

In the late 19th century and early 20th century, a change in the epidemiology of poliomyelitis from a predominantly endemic to an epidemic form was observed in Sweden and Norway,[12–14] heralding similar changes in other industrialized countries. Our understanding of these changes in the epidemiology was greatly aided by groundbreaking investigations of the three largest poliomyelitis outbreaks of the time: (1) 132 cases in Rutland County, Vermont, in 1894 by Charles Caverly,[15] (2) 1031 cases in Sweden in 1905 by Ivar Wickman,[12, 14] and (3) more than 9000 cases in New York in 1916.[16] Wickman was the first to recognize that abortive cases might equal or outnumber cases with paralytic manifestations and that these cases may be significant in the propagation of the infection.[14] These outbreaks were due to an accumulation of a sufficient number of susceptible children to sustain epidemic transmission of poliovirus, presumably because improvements in hygiene and sanitation had delayed poliovirus exposure from infancy to later in life.

Landsteiner and Popper[17] reported in 1908 that a "filtrable agent" (i.e., virus) was the cause of poliomyelitis on the basis of microscopic examination of spinal cords from two monkeys that had been injected intraperitoneally with a suspension of ground up cord from a fatal human case. Burnet and Macnamara[18] determined in 1931 that more than one strain of virus could cause poliomyelitis and that immunity to one strain did not confer immunity to another strain. These investigators based their findings on cross-immunity and serological tests and most importantly showed that three monkeys who had recovered from one strain (and should have been immune) developed paralytic disease after injection of another strain. This report had profound implications, although not immediately appreciated at the time, both in terms of redefining the epidemiology of the disease and with respect to directing the subsequent development of vaccines. In 1948, an effort was launched to determine the number of distinct poliovirus strains. This effort was coordinated by the Committee on Typing of the National Foundation for Infantile Paralysis, which reported in 1951 that three and only three types of poliovirus designated types I, II, and III were the cause of poliomyelitis.[19] Enders, Weller, and Robbins[20] in *Science* demonstrated in 1949 that poliovirus could be grown in nonnervous, human embryonic tissue, work that was later honored with the Nobel Prize. Thus, the determination of the number of poliovirus strains, the ability for large-scale growth of the virus, and the finding that circulating antibody had a protective effect against poliomyelitis[21–26] all were essential preconditions for the development of effective poliovirus vaccines.

Two different approaches for vaccine development pursued at the time were successful: inactivation of poliovirus by formalin pioneered by Dr. Jonas Salk, licensed as inactivated poliovirus vaccine (IPV) in 1955 after the largest controlled field trials ever conducted[2]; and the attenuation of the three serotypes of poliovirus by Dr. Albert Sabin, licensed in 1961 as monovalent oral poliovirus vaccine and in 1963 as trivalent oral poliovirus vaccine (OPV).[27] The widespread use of IPV and OPV rapidly controlled poliomyelitis.

The construction of the Drinker respirator (i.e., "iron lung") beginning in 1928 and its widespread use in the 1930s and 1940s rapidly decreased the case-fatality ratio of bulbar forms of poliomyelitis.[28] Epidemic poliomyelitis in the early part of the 20th century was associated with a high case-fatality rate (27.1% during the New York epidemic of 1916).[16, 29, 30] Further improvements in hygiene and sanitation delayed the median age of poliovirus infection from younger than 5 years in the 1910s to 5 to 9 years in the 1940s[31, 32] and allowed the accumulation of large numbers of people susceptible to poliomyelitis. Epidemics of ever increasing magnitude began to occur in the United States and Europe until the mid to late 1950s when vaccines became available. Because increasing age appeared to be the primary risk factor for bulbar paralysis—the basis for the "central dogma" of the epidemiology of poliomyelitis[33]—an increasing proportion of cases required respiratory support, and whole wards of iron lungs were devoted to caring for poliomyelitis victims in the 1940s and 1950s.

Poliomyelitis is intimately linked with some of the greatest triumphs in medicine, including scientific breakthroughs, public health achievements, and advancements in social justice. Social justice, the indiscriminate benefit of scientific discoveries or access to care and rehabilitation, was pioneered by the National Foundation for Infantile Paralysis, which raised funds through annual March of Dimes campaigns that covered treatment and rehabilitation costs of poliomyelitis victims.[34] The Vaccines for Children Act (1993) ensures that poliovirus vaccines are available for poor children in the United States. Ultimately, the successful conclusion of the poliomyelitis eradication initiative will benefit all children equally, whether rich or poor, whether white or black, and whether living in industrialized or developing countries.

The history of poliomyelitis has been reviewed in detail by Paul[4] and in Chapter 2 of this edition of *Vaccines*.

Why Is the Disease Important?

Poliomyelitis was the leading cause of permanent disability in the prevaccine era.[31] Besides the considerable disease burden, poliomyelitis was much feared in the prevaccine era because it could strike anybody, no means existed of protecting oneself or one's children, and unlike with other diseases such as measles, from which most children either recover or die rapidly, society was reminded every day of the devastating effects of this crippling disease.

Disease control programs using poliovirus vaccines have prevented and continue to prevent millions of children from becoming paralyzed. In 1988, when the global eradication target was adopted, the World Health Organization (WHO) estimated that approximately 350,000 cases of paralytic poliomyelitis were occurring annually.[35] Poliomyelitis has gained renewed attention in recent years because the feasibility of its eradication has been demonstrated[35, 36] and because of the visibility of the ongoing global effort to eradicate poliovirus by the year 2000.[37–39]

BACKGROUND

Clinical Description

Poliomyelitis is an acute infection caused by any of three serotypes of poliovirus that replicate initially in the gastrointestinal tract and rarely in the motor neurons of the anterior horn cells in the spinal cord where the replication of virus results in cell destruction and flaccid paralysis of the muscles the cells innervate (i.e., spinal poliomyelitis). On occasion, brain stem cells innervating respiratory muscles can be affected, resulting in difficulties in breathing (i.e., bulbar paralysis). In addition to the acute paralysis, late manifestations with exacerbation of weakness or new paralysis (i.e., postpolio syndrome) can be observed in a significant proportion of patients decades after the acute paralytic episode.

Poliovirus exposure in a person susceptible to poliomyelitis results in one of the following consequences: (1) inapparent infection without symptoms, (2) minor illness, (3) nonparalytic poliomyelitis (aseptic meningitis), or (4) paralytic poliomyelitis.[31, 40–42] Inapparent infection without symptoms is the most frequent outcome (72%) after poliovirus exposure in susceptible people.[43] Minor illness is the most frequent form (24%) of the disease, characterized by transient illness associated with a few days of fever, malaise, drowsiness, headache, nausea, vomiting, constipation, or sore throat, in various combinations.[43] Nonparalytic poliomyelitis (aseptic meningitis) is a relatively rare outcome (4%) of poliovirus infection. It begins usually as a minor illness characterized by fever, sore throat, vomiting, and malaise. One to 2 days later, signs of meningeal irritation become apparent, including stiffness of the neck or back; vomiting; severe headache; and pain in limbs, back, and neck.[40] This form of the disease lasts 2 to 10 days, and recovery is usually rapid and complete. In a small proportion of these cases, the disease advances to transient mild muscle weakness or paralysis.

Paralytic poliomyelitis is a rare outcome (<1%) of poliovirus infections among susceptible people. Its clinical course is characterized by a minor illness of several days, a symptom-free period of 1 to 3 days, followed by rapid onset of flaccid paralysis with fever and progression to the maximum extent of paralysis within a few days. This characteristic clinical course of a minor illness followed by the major illness with paralysis has been related to the two humps of the dromedary.[44] In actuality, this is a misnomer, because the dromedary is a one-humped camel. Among adolescent and adult cases of poliomyelitis, the minor illness is often absent, and these groups also appear to experience more severe pain in the affected extremities. After temperature returns to normal, there is usually no further progression of paralysis. If paralysis of an extremity is not complete, it is more pronounced proximally. Paralysis is usually asymmetric, associated with diminished or complete loss of deep tendon reflexes and an intact sensory system. Paralytic manifestations in extremities begin proximally and progress to involve distal muscle groups (i.e., descending paralysis). Depending on the anatomical location of motor neuron damage in the spinal cord or in the brain stem, spinal, mixed spinal-bulbar, or bulbar paralysis involving primarily respiratory muscles may be observed. The anterior horn cells (and brain stem cells), just like other nerve cells of the central nervous system (CNS), cannot be regenerated or replaced, and paralysis is permanent. Nevertheless, because of compensation of other, still functioning muscles, partial or total recovery can be achieved, usually within the first 6 months after onset of disease. Detailed clinical descriptions may be found in a number of reviews and books.[45–48]

Postpolio syndrome, a term invented in the early 1980s, refers to a disease entity that encompasses the late manifestations of acute paralytic poliomyelitis.[49] Aside from previously published case reports and case series, the first systematic investigation of postpolio syndrome was published in 1984.[50] After an interval of 15 to 40 years, many people (25 to 40%) who contracted paralytic poliomyelitis in their childhood may experience muscle pain and exacerbation of existing weakness or may develop new weakness or paralysis. Factors that enhance the risk of postpolio syndrome include (1) increasing length of time since acute poliovirus infection, (2) presence of permanent residual impairment after recovery from the acute illness, and (3) female gender. The exact cause of these late effects is currently unknown, although it is not a consequence of persistent infection. The pathogenesis of postpolio syndrome is thought to involve late attrition of oversized motor units that developed during the recovery process of paralytic poliomyelitis.[49] Postpolio syndrome has been described in people infected during the era of wild poliovirus circulation. An excellent summary of the current scientific knowledge of postpolio syndrome has been published recently.[51]

Virology

Polioviruses are part of the *Enterovirus* genus and belong to the family *Picornaviridae* (pico, implying small, and RNA, the nucleic acid component). Polioviruses are small icosahedral viruses (27 to 30 nm in diameter), are nonenveloped, and contain a genome of RNA of molecular weight 2.5×10^6 daltons. The poliovirus genome is a single-stranded messenger molecule, containing about 7500 nucleotides, that is covalently linked to a small protein. Single-stranded RNA constitutes approximately 30% of the virion, and the remainder consists of four major proteins (VP1–4) and one minor protein (VPg). Each surface unit of the capsid is composed of the three proteins (VP1–3); VP4 is associated with the inner surface of the capsid and the viral RNA. There are three antigenic types (serotypes 1, 2, and 3)[52–55] (Table 16–1), whose physical properties are nearly identical. Polioviruses are stable at acid pH (3.0 to 5.0) for 1 to 3 hours. They have a buoyant density in cesium chloride of about 1.34 g/mL. They are inactivated when heated at 55°C for 30 minutes, but $MgCl_2$ prevents this inactivation.[56] The different serotypes share between 36 and 52% of their nucleotide sequences. Neutralizing antibody is directed toward VP1, VP2, and VP3 (present in copies of 60 each of VP1 and VP3 and 58 to 59 copies of VP2 and VP4) containing at least four epitopes located on the surface of the virion. VP1 is the immunodominant antigen. The entire genome of all three serotypes of polioviruses has been sequenced,[57] and the three-dimensional structure of poliovirus type 1 has been revealed by x-ray crystallography.[58]

Polioviruses require a receptor to attach and enter cells.[59] On infection of a susceptible cell, the RNA is translated to yield a large polyprotein that is cleaved after translation into the virus-specific proteins, and the viral RNA becomes susceptible to RNase within 30 to 60 minutes after infection. Progeny viral RNA appears in cells approximately 3 hours after infection.[60] Once virion assembly has started, production of capsid protein and replication of RNA are closely linked, and integration of viral RNA into the virion follows within several minutes. Morphogenesis appears to involve the combination of viral RNA with a shell of viral proteins (VP0, VP1, VP3) during which the VP0 procapsid protein is cleaved to yield VP2 and VP4. After final assembly,

Table 16–1. **POLIOVIRUSES**

POLIOVIRUS SEROTYPE	PROTOTYPE* STRAIN DESIGNATION	GEOGRAPHICAL ORIGIN	ILLNESS IN PERSON YIELDING VIRUS	INVESTIGATORS
1	Brunhilde	Maryland	Paralytic poliomyelitis†	Bodian et al[53]
2	Lansing	Michigan	Fatal paralytic poliomyelitis‡	Armstrong[52]
3	Leon	California	Fatal paralytic poliomyelitis‡	Kessel and Pait[54]

*Prototype strains for serotypes.
†Virus recovered from feces.
‡Virus recovered from spinal cord.

virions are released initially through vacuoles but after several hours escape by cell lysis and death. Thus, the interval from cell entry to release of virions in vitro may require approximately 4 to 5 hours.

Most strains of polioviruses can be grown in primary or continuous cell lines derived from monkey kidney, testis, or muscle but not in cells from lower animals. Poliovirus requires a membrane receptor for infection, and the absence of this receptor on the membrane of nonprimate cells renders them resistant to the virus. This restriction can be overcome by transfection with poliovirus RNA or by introduction of the whole virion into resistant cells by means of synthetic liposomes.

The gene for the human cell receptor for poliovirus has been cloned.[59] On introduction into resistant cells, the human gene coverts them into susceptible cells. The gene for the human poliovirus receptor (PVR) has been introduced into a germ line of mice. The resulting transgenic animals become susceptible to polioviruses, demonstrating that the primary block to infection of normal mice by such strains is at the level of cell entry.[61] Antibodies to the cell receptor protect susceptible cells from infection by polioviruses.

Transgenic mice carrying the human poliovirus receptor gene can be infected and paralyzed by wild poliovirus but do not develop disease on inoculation with the attenuated strain.[61] Such transgenic mice may prove useful for testing neurovirulence of strains during manufacture and field use.

Pathogenesis as It Relates to Prevention

The pathogenesis of poliovirus infection indicates that prevention through immunization can be accomplished by inhibiting replication at and dissemination from the gastrointestinal tract, by inhibiting the viremia that follows, or by doing both. After exposure to poliovirus by way of the oral cavity, the virus attaches and enters specific cells that express the poliovirus receptor.[59] The virus replicates locally at the sites of virus implantation (e.g., tonsils, intestinal M cells, and Peyer patches of the ileum) or at the lymph nodes that drain these tissues. The first approach requires the presence of local secretory immunoglobulin (Ig) A antibody. The second approach—because spread occurs primarily by way of the blood stream to other susceptible tissues, namely, other lymph nodes, brown fat, and the CNS, or by way of retrograde axonal transport to the CNS—requires the presence of neutralizing antibody.

The host range of poliovirus and tissue tropism is determined by the expression of the poliovirus receptor, which belongs to the immunoglobulin superfamily.[59] Tissue tropism refers to the ability of poliovirus to replicate in specific cells.[62] In situ hybridization with nucleic acid probes of PVR in transgenic mice suggested a limited expression of the PVR to the CNS, thymus, lung, kidney, and adrenal glands and more recently in monocytes (mononuclear phagocytes).[63] Even within the CNS, the PVR expression is restricted to neurons.[62] Replication of poliovirus in motor neurons results in cell destruction and paralysis.

Poliovirus may be found in the blood of patients with the abortive form ("minor illness"), and it can be detected several days before onset of clinical signs of CNS involvement in patients who develop nonparalytic or paralytic poliomyelitis.[24, 64] The virus is regularly present in the throat and in the stools before the onset of illness. In individuals who have either clinical or subclinical infection, virus is excreted in the feces for several weeks[43] and in saliva for 1 to 2 weeks. The mean duration of wild poliovirus type 1 excretion in fecal specimens is 24 days (median, 20 to 29 days), with a range of 1 to 114 days.[43]

For further details of pathogenesis and pathology, see Bodian,[45] Bodian and Horstmann,[46] and Sabin.[48]

Diagnosis

Paralytic poliomyelitis due to imported wild poliovirus or due to vaccine-related poliovirus has become a rare disease in the United States and other industrialized countries. Therefore, physicians may not be familiar with the disease or consider the diagnosis of poliomyelitis until other more frequent causes of acute flaccid paralysis have been ruled out. The diagnosis of paralytic poliomyelitis is dependent on (1) clinical course, (2) virological testing, (3) special studies, and (4) residual neurological deficit 60 days after onset of symptoms. For surveillance purposes, any case with physician-diagnosed suspected poliomyelitis is investigated in the United States, and a case is confirmed if a panel of independent experts determines that the case definition* for paralytic poliomyelitis has been met. The WHO has been and is continuing to use similar screening and confirmatory clinical case definitions; however, in countries that have "adequate" surveillance for poliomyelitis (see under *Disease Control Strategies*), any case from which wild poliovirus is isolated is considered confirmed poliomyelitis. This definition is referred to as the virological case definition.

Clinical Course. The clinical course (see *Clinical Description)* is helpful in ruling in or ruling out paralytic poliomyelitis. Several studies in the developing world have attempted to assess the sensitivity and specificity of different clinical case definitions for paralytic poliomyelitis and compared these with the "gold standard" of virologically confirmed poliomyelitis based on poliovirus isolation from stool specimens. These studies reported similar findings.[65–67] The largest study reported a sensitivity of 64% and a specificity of 82% for a case definition that included age younger than 6 years, fever at onset, and rapid progress to maximum extent of paralysis (≤4 days).[65] The addition of a specific pattern of paralysis (proximal, unilateral, or absence of paralysis in all four extremities) increased the specificity with varying degrees of loss in sensitivity. The case definitions and case classification schemes have been reviewed.[68]

*"A patient must have had paralysis clinically and epidemiologically compatible with poliomyelitis and, at 60 days after onset of symptoms, had residual neurologic deficit, had died, or had no information available on neurologic residua." This case definition was formerly known as the Best Available Paralytic Poliomyelitis Case Count (BAPPCC).

Virological Testing. Because other enteroviruses and other diseases may cause acute flaccid paralysis (see *Differential Diagnosis)*, laboratory confirmation is critical to establishing the diagnosis of poliomyelitis. The most important is the recovery of poliovirus and the characterization of virus isolates as wild type or vaccine related. Detailed descriptions of standard laboratory principles and procedures for investigation of enterovirus infections are available,[69] and standard typing antisera for identifying enteroviral isolates are available through the WHO.[70] WHO has published a manual for the virological investigation of poliomyelitis cases that includes protocols for the isolation of poliovirus.[71] This manual has become the standard for conducting virus isolation in the laboratories participating in the WHO's Global Laboratory Network to support polio eradication and is widely used in nonnetwork laboratories.[72]

WHO recommends that stool specimens be inoculated into two cell lines—RD cells, derived from human rhabdomyosarcoma, and Hep2 (Cincinnati) cells, derived from a human epidermoid sarcoma. RD cells have the added advantage that they can support the growth of other nonpolio enteroviruses. Mouse cells (L20b) that have been genetically altered to express the poliovirus receptor have recently been introduced in network laboratories.[61, 72] These cells offer the advantage of being relatively resistant to infection with nonpolio enteroviruses. Poliovirus may be recovered from stool, throat swabs, or cerebrospinal fluid taken soon after the onset of illness and from stool specimens collected over longer periods of time. Isolation of poliovirus from cerebrospinal fluid suggests a causal relationship between a poliovirus serotype and paralytic disease. After treatment with antibiotics, cell cultures are inoculated, incubated, and observed for cytopathogenic effects, which appear typically within 3 to 6 days. A virus isolate is identified and typed by neutralization with specific antiserum. WHO recommends that two stool samples be collected at least 24 hours apart to confirm the diagnosis, because excretion of virus can be intermittent and the sensitivity of isolation is less than 100%.* Wild poliovirus has been found in stool samples of 63 to 93% of patients during the first 2 weeks of illness, in 35 to 75% during the third and fourth weeks, and in less than 50% during the fifth and sixth weeks.[73] The duration of viral shedding was reduced among children who were previously vaccinated, had preexisting homologous antibody, or had a previous intestinal infection with homologous poliovirus.[73]

After determination of serotype is accomplished, intratypic differentiation of poliovirus isolates as vaccine related or wild type should be considered. Five rapid methods are in use: (1) enzyme-linked immunosorbent assay with polyclonal cross-absorbed antisera (PAB-E)[74, 75]; (2) a neutralization assay with type-specific monoclonal antibody (MAB-N)[76]; (3) a restriction fragment length polymorphism (RFLP) assay[77]; (4) a Sabin vaccine virus strain-specific polymerase chain reaction (PCR) assay[78]; and (5) a Sabin vaccine strain-specific cRNA probe hybridization (ProbHyb) assay.[79] In a comparative study, each of these methods performed well (between 91.9 and 97.4% correct results per number of tests performed).[80] However, because misclassification of a vaccine-related virus as wild poliovirus (in an era with a global effort to eradicate poliomyelitis) has wide-ranging programmatic implications, WHO proposes that at least two methods be used for the intratypic differentiation of poliovirus isolates and that each method be based on a different principle (i.e., antigenic properties [PAB-E, MAB-N] or nucleotide sequence composition [RFLP, PCR, ProbHyb]). If the two assays yield discrepant findings, partial nucleotide sequencing—the gold standard assay—should be used for the correct identification of poliovirus.[80–83] The use of genomic sequencing, pioneered with polioviruses,[84] has given rise to a new discipline, molecular epidemiology of viruses, a hybrid discipline that combines the tools and concepts of classical epidemiology with those of microbiology, biochemistry, genetics, and evolutionary biology (see *Molecular Epidemiology of Poliovirus)*.[85]

Serological testing may be helpful in establishing the diagnosis but often does not contribute and sometimes may cause confusion because (1) antibody rises have already occurred by the time the first specimen has been collected, (2) antibody may be present to one or more serotypes because of previous or recent vaccination, and (3) heterotypic responses may be observed to one serotype after exposure to another serotype. There are no reliable means of distinguishing antibody induced by vaccine-related or wild-type poliovirus. Standard protocols for neutralization assays to determine levels of antibody to poliovirus are available.[86–88] Paired serum specimens are required to demonstrate a fourfold or greater rise in antibody titer between acute and convalescent sera. The first serum specimen should be collected as soon as possible after onset of paralytic manifestations, and the second specimen should be collected 2 to 3 weeks later. Neutralizing antibodies appear early and are usually already detectable at the time of onset of paralysis. However, if the first specimen is taken early enough, a rise in titer may be demonstrated during the course of the disease. In a study from Louisiana, specimens were collected as soon as possible after hospital admission from poliomyelitis patients and about 6 weeks later; in 36% of patients, a fourfold rise in poliovirus antibody titer could be demonstrated; in 61%, reciprocal titers were above 320 and did not change; and in 3%, reciprocal titers were below 320 and remained unchanged.[89]

Other assays have been proposed, including indirect immunofluorescence,[90] paper-radioactive virus method,[91] enzyme-linked immunosorbent assay,[92] and microindirect hemagglutination and hemagglutination inhibition.[93] Complement fixation should not be used because of problems in both sensitivity and specificity. Intrathecal immune responses can be measured and offer the advantage of attributing a causal relationship between a poliovirus serotype and paralytic disease.[94]

Neutralization assays continue to be the gold standard

---

*Extensive evaluations of the laboratory network in the Americas have demonstrated that with a well-functioning transport system for specimens and high-quality laboratories that pass proficiency tests, one stool sample is adequate. This is the only region in which there is a recommendation that one stool specimen be collected from acute flaccid paralysis cases.

method for the detection of type-specific antibody in sera.[22] Neutralization antibody induced by a single serotype may not be completely serotype specific. In practical terms, this seldom constitutes a problem because the heterotypic response results in low levels of neutralizing antibody. Because of the limitations described before, serology may be more important in excluding (e.g., no detectable antibody) the diagnosis of poliomyelitis than in confirming it.

Special Studies. Nerve conduction and electromyography studies can point to the anatomical location of the paralysis[95]—destruction of anterior horn cells in the spinal cord versus a demyelinating process in the peripheral nerves—helping to exclude the most frequent cause of acute flaccid paralysis, Guillain-Barré syndrome. Magnetic resonance imaging has been used infrequently; but in at least one patient with poliomyelitis, magnetic resonance imaging has highlighted the anterior column of the spinal cord.[96] Analysis of spinal fluid may be helpful in ruling out other causes. In paralytic poliomyelitis, the cerebrospinal fluid contains an increased number of leukocytes—usually 10 to 200/mL, and seldom more than 500/mL.[97, 98] At the onset of signs of CNS involvement, the ratio of polymorphonuclear cells to lymphocytes is high, but within a few days the ratio is reversed. The total white blood cell count slowly subsides to normal levels. The protein content of the cerebrospinal fluid initially is elevated only slightly (average, about 46 mg/100 mL [range, 15 to 165] in nonparalytic cases and 68 mg/100 mL [range, 25 to 250] among paralytic cases), but it rises gradually in paralytic cases until the third week, generally returning to normal by the sixth week.[97] Glucose levels are usually within the normal range. In fatal cases, spinal cord and brain stem tissue samples should be examined for the typical lesions caused by viral replication and destruction of the motor neuron cells.

Residual Neurological Deficit. The clinical case definition for paralytic poliomyelitis requires a residual neurological deficit at 60 days after onset of paralysis. Such a neurological deficit may be apparent as complete flaccid paralysis of one or more extremities or partial paralysis or weakness of muscles or muscle groups. In the latter instance, because of functional recovery (intact muscles may compensate for muscles that are not innervated), it may be more difficult to establish a neurological deficit. The most severe cases of poliomyelitis in terms of complications and fatal outcomes occur in people with underlying immunodeficiency disorders.

Differential Diagnosis

The list of underlying causes of acute flaccid paralysis is extensive (Table 16–2). The distinguishing features of poliomyelitis, Guillain-Barré syndrome, transverse myelitis, and traumatic neuritis, neuritis secondary to the trauma of injections, are contained in Table 16–3.

In general, Guillain-Barré syndrome accounts for 50% or more of the cases of acute flaccid paralysis,

Table 16–2. **CAUSES AND DIFFERENTIAL DIAGNOSIS OF ACUTE FLACCID PARALYSIS**

Infectious	Viral	Enteroviruses: Poliomyelitis; coxsackievirus A (A7, A9; A4, A5, A10); coxsackievirus B (B1–B5); echoviruses (6, 9; 1–4, 7, 11, 14, 16–18, 30); enterovirus 70; enterovirus 71
		Myxoviruses (mumps virus); togaviruses and arboviruses; Epstein-Barr virus; human immunodeficiency virus
	Bacterial	*Campylobacter jejuni* (leading cause of Guillain-Barré syndrome)
Metabolic	Transient and periodic paralyses	Hypokalemic: familial; Sjögren syndrome; hyperthyroidism; gossypol-induced (toxic phenolic pigment in cottonseed); associated with barium poisoning; associated with hyperaldosteronism
		Normokalemic or hyperkalemic: familial, adynamia episodica hereditaria of Gamstorp
		Hypophosphatemia
Drug-induced	Heroin	
	Antibiotics: aminoglycosides; polymyxin B; tetracyclines	
Organics	Volatile hydrocarbons: hexane; methyl butyl ketone; carbon disulfide	
	Trecresyl phosphate: an ingredient of Jamaican ginger tonic and a potential contaminant of cooking oil, mustard oil, or flour	
	Cantharidin	
	Deet	
	Dithiobiuret (rat)	
	Triethyldodecyl-ammonium bromide (mouse)	
Toxins	Bacterial	Botulinum; diphtheria; tetanus (cephalic form); *Moraxella*
Fungal—mycotoxins	*Penicillium citrea-viride; Penicillium islandicum; Penicillium citrinum*	
Insect	Tick paralysis; spider venom—cockroach, beetle; wasp venom—Lepidoptera larvae	
Parasite/protozoa/dinoflagellates	Paralytic shellfish poisoning—saxitoxin; ichthyotoxism (sardines)	
Reptiles—snake venom	Cobra; Australian elapid; krait; mamba; sea snake	
Plants and plant toxin	*Gloriosa superba* (root); *Lathyrus* species (sweet pea); monkshood; hemlock (parsley); *Karwinskia humboldtiana*—coyotillo; buckthorn; *Callilepsis* species (daisy); *Cassia* (bean); *Cycas* (evergreens, seeds); *Gelsemium* (blossoms); *Heliotropium* (bush tea shrub); *Melochia* species (stems); *Oenanthe* species (parsnips)	
Metals	Organic tin compounds, lead	
Pesticides	EPN, trichlorfon (Dipterex), dichlorvos (DDVP), DEF, isofenphos (Oftanol), leptophos (Phosvel)	
Inherited/congenital/acquired	Werdnig-Hoffmann; Wohlfart-Kugelberg-Welander; porphyric polyneuropathy	
Unknown/multiple causes	Guillain-Barré syndrome; China paralytic syndrome; Bell palsy; transverse myelitis	
Asthma	Polio-like Hopkins syndrome	

Table 16–3. **DISTINGUISHING FEATURES OF FOUR COMMON DIAGNOSES OF ACUTE FLACCID PARALYSIS (POLIOMYELITIS, GUILLAIN-BARRÉ SYNDROME, TRAUMATIC NEURITIS, AND TRANSVERSE MYELITIS)**

FEATURE	POLIOMYELITIS	GUILLAIN-BARRÉ SYNDROME	TRAUMATIC NEURITIS (AFTER INJECTION)	TRANSVERSE MYELITIS
Development of paralysis	24–48 hr onset to full paralysis	From hours to 10 d	From hours to 4 d	From hours to 4 d
Fever at onset	High, always present at onset of flaccid paralysis, gone when progression of paralysis stops	Not common	Commonly present before, during, and after flaccid paralysis	Rarely present
Flaccid paralysis	Acute, usually asymmetrical, principally proximal	Generally acute, symmetrical, and distal	Asymmetrical, acute, and affecting only one limb	Acute, lower limbs, symmetrical
Progression of paralysis	"Descending"	"Ascending"		
Muscle tone	Reduced or absent in affected limb	Global hypotonia	Reduced or absent in affected limb	Hypotonia in affected limbs
Deep tendon reflexes	Decreased or absent	Globally absent	Decreased or absent	Absent in lower limbs early, hyperreflexia late
Sensation	Severe myalgia, backache, no sensory changes	Cramps, tingling, hypoanesthesia of palms and soles	Pain in gluteus, hypothermia	Anesthesia of lower limbs with sensory level
Cranial nerve involvement	Only when bulbar involvement is present	Often present, affecting nerves VII, IX, X, XI, XII	Absent	Absent
Respiratory insufficiency	Only when bulbar involvement is present	In severe cases, enhanced by bacterial pneumonia	Absent	Sometimes
Autonomic signs and symptoms	Rare	Frequent blood pressure alterations, sweating, blushing, and body temperature fluctuations	Hypothermia in affected limb	Present
Cerebrospinal fluid	Inflammatory	Albumin-cytologic dissociation	Normal	Normal or mild in cells
Bladder dysfunction	Rare	Transient	Never	Present
Nerve conduction velocity: third week	Abnormal: anterior horn cell disease (normal during first 2 wk)	Abnormal: slowed conduction, decreased motor amplitudes	Abnormal: axonal damage	Normal or abnormal, no diagnostic value
Electromyography at 3 wk	Abnormal	Normal	Normal	Normal
Sequelae at 3 mo and up to a year	Severe, asymmetrical atrophy, skeletal deformities developing later	Symmetrical atrophy of distal muscles	Moderate atrophy, only in affected limbs	Flaccid diplegia atrophy after years

Adapted from Global Program for Vaccines and Immunization. Field Guide for Supplementary Activities Aimed at Achieving Polio Eradication. Geneva, World Health Organization, 1996.

in the absence of wild virus–induced poliomyelitis, in industrialized countries such as the United Kingdom and Australia as well as in developing countries in Latin America.[99–101] At times, nonpolio enteroviruses have been associated with cases of polio-like paralytic disease, but this has been uncommon. Coxsackievirus A7 has been associated with outbreaks of paralytic disease,[102, 103] and enterovirus 71 has been involved in several outbreaks of CNS disease, including polio-like paralysis, with some fatal cases.[104] Two motor neuron diseases in childhood are Werdnig-Hoffmann disease, a rapidly progressing, often fatal disorder of early childhood, and Wohlfart-Kugelberg-Welander disease, a more benign disorder with a generally later onset.[105] Electromyographic findings are useful in establishing the diagnosis of these disorders.[106] China paralytic syndrome, a distinct disease entity that appears different from Guillain-Barré syndrome and poliomyelitis, has been described among children and adults in northern China.[107] Early symptoms of this disease include leg weakness and resistance to neck flexion. The weakness ascends rapidly, affects symmetrically the arms and respiratory muscles, and progresses to maximum extent of weakness within 6 days on average. Electromyography indicates denervation potentials in weak muscles and suggests that this entity may be a reversible distal motor nerve terminal or anterior horn lesion. Tick bite paralysis occurs infrequently and is manifested by flaccid ascending paralysis that usually resolves rapidly after tick removal. Botulism toxins can also cause descending paralysis—characterized by symmetrical impairment of cranial nerves, followed by a descending pattern of weakness or paralysis of the extremities and trunk.[108] A relatively frequent complication among approximately 10 to 15% of diphtheria patients is the paralysis of the soft palate and peripheral nerves due to diphtheria toxin[109]; tetanus toxin can cause a flaccid paralysis of the muscles innervated by the affected cranial nerves (i.e., cephalic tetanus).[110]

The following signs and symptoms help in distinguishing poliomyelitis from other causes of acute flaccid paralysis: (1) fever is present at onset; (2) there is rapid progression to maximum paralysis; (3) paralysis is usually asymmetric; and (4) paralysis is more pronounced proximally than distally (i.e., descending paralysis) (see Table 16–3).

EPIDEMIOLOGY

General Epidemiology

Poliomyelitis is an ubiquitous, highly contagious, seasonal viral disease (more pronounced in moderate climate countries) caused by three serotypes of poliovirus (types 1, 2, and 3) that infect nearly every person in a given population in the absence of vaccination.[31] Paralytic manifestations are a rare outcome (less than 1%) of poliovirus infections. Important exceptions are island or isolated populations (e.g., Eskimo), which can remain unaffected by the virus for varying periods and after reintroduction can experience outbreaks of poliomyelitis that affect all age groups that were not affected by the previous wave of infection.[111] Poliovirus type 1 appears to be the most neurovirulent of the three serotypes.[112] Most epidemic and endemic cases of poliomyelitis are caused by poliovirus type 1 followed by type 3 and type 2. Peak transmission occurs among infants and young children (tropical areas) and school-aged children (temperate zones). However, outbreaks in isolated communities can give rise to paralytic cases in many older individuals.[31, 111]

Poliomyelitis is transmitted by person-to-person spread through fecal-oral and oral-oral routes or less frequently by a common vehicle (e.g., water, milk).[113, 114] People remain most infectious immediately before and 1 to 2 weeks after onset of paralytic disease, although poliovirus replicates for substantially longer periods and is excreted for 3 to 6 weeks in feces and approximately 2 weeks in saliva.[43] Thus, the period of communicability may be 4 to 8 weeks. Secondary infection rates of susceptible household or institutional contacts, probably mediated by fecal-oral spread, are high, more than 90%.[43] The incubation period between infection and first symptoms (minor illness) is 3 to 6 days and from infection to onset of paralytic disease usually 7 to 21 days, with a range of 3 to 35 days.[115] Most exposures to polioviruses result in inapparent infections.[31, 40, 41] On the basis of serological surveys in the prevaccine era[116, 117] and lameness surveys in developing countries, it appears that in the absence of a control program with vaccines, approximately 1 of 200 (0.5%) children will develop paralytic disease after exposure to polioviruses.[118]

Between 1976 and 1995, 48 outbreaks involving approximately 17,000 cases of paralytic poliomyelitis were reported in the literature.[119] These outbreaks involved primarily unvaccinated or inadequately vaccinated subgroups and were caused predominantly by poliovirus type 1 (74%). On the basis of this review, cases in developing countries occurred mostly among children younger than 2 years, whereas cases in industrialized countries tended to occur in older people who had remained susceptible to poliomyelitis.

Besides age and being unvaccinated or inadequately vaccinated, several factors have been shown to increase the risk of acquiring paralytic manifestations, including intramuscular injections with diphtheria-tetanus toxoids and pertussis vaccine (DTP)[120, 121] or antibiotics,[122, 123] strenuous exercise,[124–126] injury such as fractures, and pregnancy.[127] Provocation poliomyelitis describes the enhanced risk of paralytic manifestations that follows injection in the 30 days preceding paralysis onset. Aggravation poliomyelitis describes the elevated risk of paralytic disease that follows strenuous exercise shortly (preceding 24 to 48 hours) before paralysis onset.

Removal of tonsils and adenoids predisposes to bulbar poliomyelitis.[128] Clinical observations on this fact were reported in the early part of the 20th century.[128, 129] Rhesus monkeys, when inoculated with poliovirus in the tonsillopharyngeal region, developed poliomyelitis with greater frequency than when they were inoculated by other routes.[4] Later, von Magnus and Melnick[130] demonstrated that if cynomolgus monkeys were given poliovirus by the oral route, their susceptibility was greatly enhanced in animals that had their tonsils recently removed. Ogra and Karzon[131, 132] studied 40 children before and after removal of tonsils and adenoids. The children ranged from 3 to 11 years of age and had been immunized with live attenuated poliovirus vaccine 6 months to 6 years previously. Before tonsillectomy, IgA poliovirus antibody was present in appreciable titers in the nasopharynx of all children, but no IgM or IgG antibody was detectable. Significantly, however, after tonsillectomy, the preexisting IgA poliovirus antibody level in the nasopharynx sharply declined in all children studied. Mean antibody titers decreased threefold to fourfold. Thus, removal of tonsils may eliminate a valuable source of immunocompetent tissue particularly important in conferring resistance to poliovirus.

Lower socioeconomic status has been shown to be a risk for paralytic poliomyelitis in developing countries,[133] probably because children belonging to the lower socioeconomic group experience more intense exposure to poliovirus (i.e., a higher virus inoculum, which has been shown in experimental studies to be a risk factor for paralytic disease[29]), and these children are also at higher risk for primary vaccine failure after OPV because of more frequent concurrent enterovirus infections.[133–136]

In a study of twins, concordance with regard to paralytic poliomyelitis was found in 36% of monozygous pairs compared with 6% among dizygous pairs.[137] The authors concluded that the data were consistent with "the theory that susceptibility may be conditioned by the homozygous state of a recessive gene." A histocompatibility leukocyte antigen (HLA) complex study suggested that HLA-encoded genetic factors control resistance to the paralytic form of poliomyelitis.[138] Data on genetic susceptibility to poliomyelitis were reviewed by Wyatt,[139] who proposed that multiple linked genes determine whether an infection with poliovirus results in paralytic disease.

The case-fatality rate is variable and depends primarily on the age groups affected. The highest case-fatality rates have been reported from epidemic cases in the early 20th century[16, 29, 30] and among older people but are commonly between 5 and 10%.[29, 31] Even in the 1990s, the case-fatality rate can be high as occurred in a large outbreak of poliomyelitis in Albania in 1996, which had a case-fatality rate of 10%.[140]

Apes, such as chimpanzees, gorillas, and orangutans, are susceptible to poliovirus and can experience paralytic disease after poliovirus infection; outbreaks of poliomyelitis have been reported both in captivity and in the wild.[141–143] It is unlikely that they play any role in the sustained transmission of this virus.[144] Most monkeys cannot be infected by oral administration of poliovirus and would not be expected to participate in the chain of transmission. In short, there is no significant animal reservoir for poliovirus.[144]

Results from mathematical modeling suggest that the force of poliovirus infection, measured primarily by the average age at infection among populations in the prevaccine era, is substantially higher in developing countries compared with industrialized countries. For example, the basic reproductive rate in the United States is 5, which means that, on average, an infected person would transmit infection to 5 other people if *all* contacts of that infected person were susceptible. In contrast, the average infected person in French Morocco in 1953 would have transmitted infection to 25 people if all contacts had been susceptible. As population immunity increases, and many of the contacts of an infected person are no longer susceptible, the number of transmissions decreases. When the reproductive rate is less than 1 because of high population immunity, transmission ceases. The immunity level at which the reproductive number becomes 1 is known as the herd immunity threshold.

Whereas poliomyelitis outbreaks in industrialized countries can be prevented with overall population immunity levels of approximately 80%, outbreaks in developing countries with poor sanitation and hygiene could still occur with immunity levels as high as 97% (Fig. 16–1). These findings may be helpful in explaining why there was no spread to the general population after the outbreaks in the Netherlands, Canada, and the United States[145, 146] and why there was widespread transmission among fully vaccinated children in many outbreaks in developing countries.[147, 148]

Epidemiological Patterns and Incidence of Poliomyelitis

The epidemiology of poliomyelitis changed substantially during the last century. Three epidemiological patterns have been observed: (1) *endemic*, (2) *epidemic* (prevaccine), and (3) *vaccine era*. Polioviruses probably circulated in an uninterrupted *endemic* fashion for many centuries, infecting new cohorts of susceptible infants continuously, almost all early in life, when maternally derived antibody transferred from mother to the newborn still provided some protection.

A change from endemic transmission to periodic epidemics was first observed in some temperate climate countries (e.g., Norway, Sweden, United States) late in the 19th century and at the beginning of the 20th century.[12–15] The delay in median age of poliovirus exposure permitted the accumulation of sufficient children susceptible to poliomyelitis to permit periodic outbreaks. In the United States, the median age of poliovirus infection increased from younger than 5 years at the beginning of the century to 5 to 9 years in the 1940s, before poliovirus vaccine licensure.[31] In contrast, approximately 80% of the cases were in children younger than 5 years during the large epidemic in New York in 1916.[16] The generally accepted explanation, supported by numerous studies, is that—in a temperate zone climate with increased economic development and correspondingly improved resources for community sanitation and household hygiene—exposure to polioviruses was postponed to later in life. Epidemic transmission became the primary epidemiological pattern in temperate climate

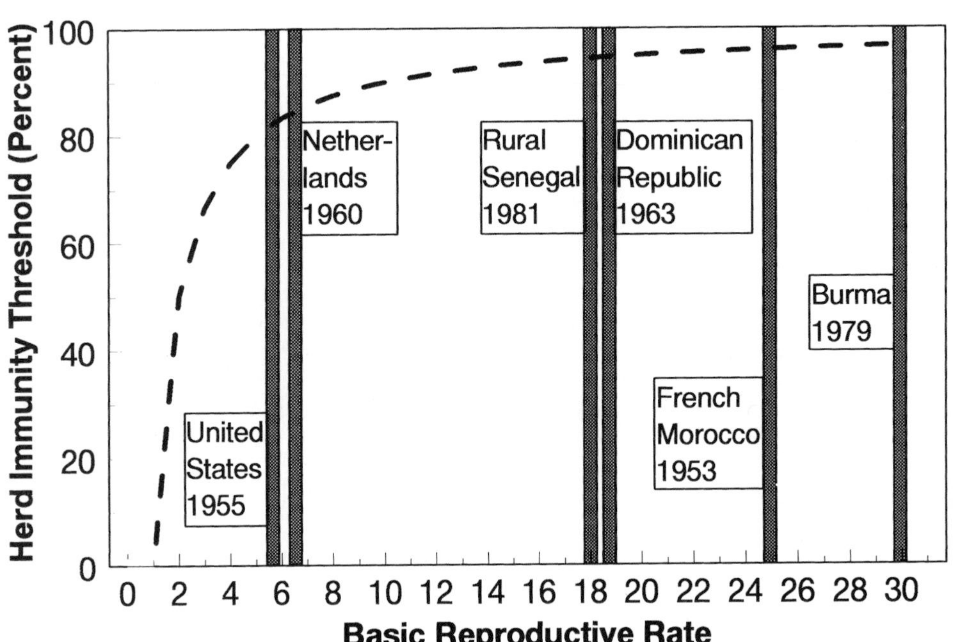

Figure 16–1. Herd immunity threshold levels for selected industrialized and developing countries, based on basic reproductive rate, or R_0. Threshold values for herd immunity were calculated using 1 − (1/R_0), where R_0 is 1 + (life expectancy/average age at infection with poliovirus). Herd immunity threshold values are shown by the dashed line. The solid bars are the basic reproductive rate in a given population. (From Patriarca PA, Sutter RW, Oostvogel PM. Outbreaks of poliomyelitis, 1976–1995. J Infect Dis 175[suppl 1]:S165–S172, 1997.)

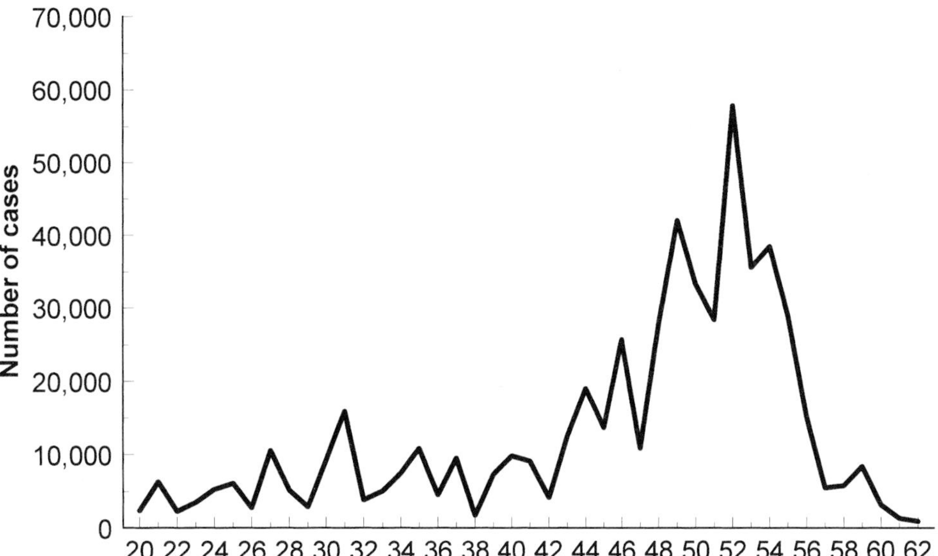

Figure 16–2. Reported cases of poliomyelitis, United States, 1920-1962.

countries, such as the industrialized countries in Europe and North America, until poliomyelitis was brought under control after introduction of effective vaccines (Fig. 16–2).

In developing countries, particularly tropical areas, an endemic epidemiological pattern predominated until recently. Poliovirus exposure occurred early in life. Although earlier theories suggested that paralytic poliomyelitis was not a health burden in tropical countries because of early exposure of infants to virus at a time when levels of maternally derived antibodies protected them from paralytic disease, more recent studies have disproved these theories. The history and scientific evidence for this misconception—that poliomyelitis was not a significant public health problem in developing countries—has been reviewed in detail in the corresponding chapter of the second edition of *Vaccines.*[149] In the last three decades, a series of lameness surveys were conducted in many developing countries that reported between 5 and 10 lameness cases per 1000 children in the age group studied,[118] suggesting that approximately 1:100 to 1:200 children acquire paralytic disease attributable to poliovirus. WHO estimates that in the absence of vaccination, there would be 550,000 cases of paralytic disease annually, the great majority of which would occur in children from developing countries. With improving vaccination coverage, a shift from an endemic to an epidemic pattern of poliovirus transmission has been observed in some developing countries that experienced large epidemics.[119, 148, 150–152]

The vaccine era began in the United States and in many European countries, Canada, Australia, New Zealand, and Japan after introduction of IPV in 1955.[2] The incidence of paralytic poliomyelitis decreased rapidly from 18,308 reported cases in the United States in 1954, the year immediately preceding IPV licensure, to 2499 cases in 1957, a decline of 86% only 3 years after the availability and widespread use of IPV. The relative upswing in reported cases in 1959 (6289 cases) with many cases having a history of receiving several prior doses of IPV raised concerns regarding the clinical efficacy of IPV in preventing paralytic disease, although the concerns were probably unfounded.[153] Nevertheless, continued and accelerated IPV use decreased the incidence of paralytic poliomyelitis to nearly record low levels (2525 cases) in the United States by 1960. Widespread use of IPV in other countries was followed by substantial decreases in the incidence of poliomyelitis and in some European countries, including Finland, Netherlands, and Sweden, resulted in the apparent elimination of indigenous wild poliovirus transmission.[154, 155]

The OPV era started in the United States with licensure of monovalent OPV in 1961, followed by licensure of trivalent OPV in 1963.[27] Although live attenuated oral poliovirus vaccine was developed in the United States, the first large-scale production, as well as the large field trials that proved the safety and efficacy of the vaccine, took place in the Soviet Union. A mass immunization program was initiated in the Soviet Union in 1959 and completed in 1960, covering 77.5 million people or 36.7% of the entire population. The immunization campaign was followed by a sharp decrease in the incidence of poliomyelitis: from 10.6 per 100,000 population in 1958 to 0.43 per 100,000 population in 1963. Since 1964, the incidence has remained at a level of 0.01 to 0.1 per 100,000 population.[156] Similar declines in the incidence of poliomyelitis were observed in other European countries, Australia, New Zealand, Canada, and the United States after the introduction of OPV. In the United States, monovalent OPV was administered initially in mass vaccination campaigns in 1962—called Sabin Oral Saturdays/Sundays (SOS)—followed by a routine vaccination program that administered vaccine to infants year-round.[27, 157, 158] The impact of administering OPV to a population that already had high immunity levels generated by previous natural infection or vaccination with IPV was impressive. Substantial reductions in the reported number of poliomyelitis cases were observed from 988 cases in 1961 to 61 cases in 1965. In 1973, only 7 cases of poliomyelitis were reported. Epidemic poliomyelitis also was brought under control, with the last outbreak in the general population occurring in Texas along the United States–Mexico border in 1970, followed by small outbreaks occurring in 1972 and 1979 among religious groups whose members object to vaccination.[146] The last indigenously acquired case of poliomyelitis due to the wild poliovirus was detected in 1979. Since 1980, aside from less than one imported case of poliomyelitis per year, all cases have been vaccine associated.[159] Rarely has a serious disease been controlled as rapidly and dramatically as has poliomyelitis in the United States and other industrialized countries of the world.

The history of controlling poliomyelitis in many developing, particularly tropical countries has been more recent. There is a notable exception. Cuba appears to have interrupted wild poliovirus after two rounds of mass vaccination campaigns in 1962.[160] In many other developing countries, however, national vaccination programs were not operational until the late 1970s and early 1980s, and global OPV coverage with three doses among children age 1 year only reached 80% by 1990.[161] Wherever moderately high levels of OPV coverage were achieved, the incidence of poliomyelitis decreased by more than would be expected,[162] but endemic transmission of polioviruses continued, and cases of poliomyelitis continued to be reported. In addition to achieving high routine coverage with three doses of OPV, control of poliomyelitis required additional supplemental doses of OPV that were incorporated into the routine schedule in some countries; other countries needed to administer supplemental doses of OPV in mass campaigns. For example, in Brazil, control of poliomyelitis could not be accomplished until mass vaccination campaigns were initiated in 1980 (Fig. 16–3). The impact of these mass campaigns on poliomyelitis incidence was dramatic; the number of reported cases decreased from 1290 in 1980 to 122 cases in 1981, a decrease of more than 90%.[163]

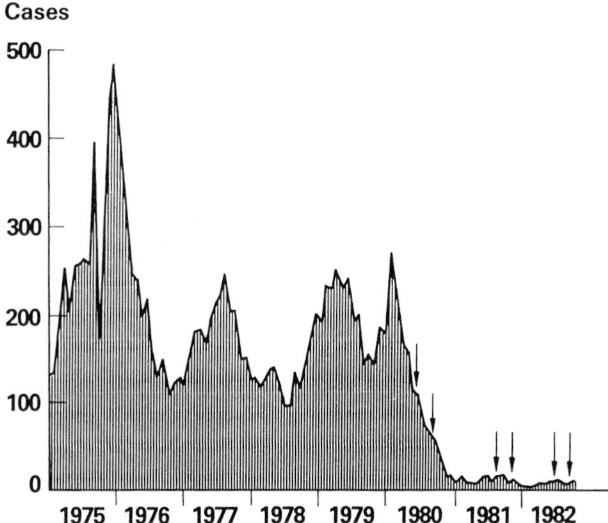

Figure 16–3. Cases of poliomyelitis by 4-week periods in Brazil, 1975 to 1982. Arrows indicate national immunization days. (From Risi JB. The control of poliomyelitis in Brazil. Rev Infect Dis 6[suppl 2]:S400–S403, 1984.)

Significance as a Public Health Problem

In the absence of effective control programs with poliovirus vaccine, approximately 1 of every 200 children (see *Epidemiology*) develops paralysis after exposure to polioviruses,[118] followed in most instances by permanent disability; 5 to 10% of patients with paralytic disease have a fatal outcome.[29, 31] Thus, with a worldwide birth cohort of approximately 129 million in 1997, approximately 645,000 people would be expected to acquire paralytic poliomyelitis resulting in permanent disability each year, and more than 32,000 of the cases would result in poliomyelitis-associated deaths. In the United States, a report estimated that in the absence of a control program, more than $3 billion ($926 million in direct costs and $2.1 billion in indirect costs) would be required each year to cover the treatment and other related costs of patients with poliomyelitis.[164] In addition to the acute manifestations of poliomyelitis, patients may experience postpolio syndrome decades after the acute episode; postpolio syndrome is associated with new muscle pain, exacerbation of existing muscle weakness, or the development of new weakness or paralysis[49] that may require additional therapy, rehabilitation, and respiratory support.

In spite of the availability of two highly effective vaccines, poliomyelitis still exerts a significant public health impact in the world. In the United States in the prevaccine era, the peak incidence year of poliomyelitis was in 1952 when 57,879 cases of poliomyelitis were reported (including 21,269 cases of paralytic disease).[165] After the availability and widespread use of poliovirus vaccines beginning in 1955, poliomyelitis was rapidly controlled in industrialized countries and in other areas where vaccines were used effectively. Globally, the Expanded Programme on Immunization, a program of the WHO established in 1974, provided leadership to national programs in virtually all developing countries to improve vaccination coverage. Coverage levels reached 80% with three doses of OPV among children 1 year of age for the first time in 1990,[161] resulting in substantial decreases in the global morbidity and mortality burden of poliomyelitis. Despite this success, WHO estimates that approximately 350,000 cases of paralytic poliomyelitis associated with permanent disability occurred in 1988, the year the global polio eradication target was adopted.[35] Because of rapid progress toward polio eradication, the worldwide reported incidence of poliomyelitis was 3997 cases in 1996[37]; and since reporting completeness is estimated by WHO to be approximately 10%,[37, 166] an estimated 40,000 cases of paralytic poliomyelitis occurred in 1996.

Paralytic poliomyelitis continues to be a serious threat, albeit a declining threat, to children in polio endemic countries and occasionally to people residing in industrialized countries that have achieved good control of poliomyelitis for many years.[167, 168] Even in countries with well-vaccinated populations that have eliminated indigenous wild poliovirus circulation for decades, gaps in population immunity may persist, particularly in groups objecting to vaccination (e.g., religious groups, Amish in the United States, and the Netherlands Reformatory Church in the Netherlands and related groups in Canada) or groups that are not reached effectively by national vaccination programs (e.g., gypsies).[145, 169–171] In the United States, the last two outbreaks of poliomyelitis occurred in 1972 and 1979 among members of religious groups objecting to vaccination.[146] The 1979 outbreak was an extension of an outbreak affecting first the Netherlands in 1978 and then Canada.[145, 170] An outbreak of poliomyelitis affecting the same religious group in the Netherlands also occurred in 1992 to 1993.[168] On the basis of genomic sequence,[83, 84] the poliovirus type 1 strain causing the epidemic in the Netherlands in 1978 had its origin in Turkey. The recent outbreak was due to poliovirus type 3, which was most likely imported from the Indian subcontinent.[172] In Spain, the last cases of poliomyelitis in 1980 to 1981 were detected among gypsy children,[169] and in both the Bulgarian outbreak in 1990 to 1991[173] and the Romanian outbreak in 1991 to 1992,[174] gypsy children either were exclusively affected or constituted a substantial proportion of poliomyelitis cases. Although no cases of paralytic poliomyelitis were detected in the outbreaks in the United States (1979), Canada (1978), and the Netherlands (1978 and 1992 to 1993) beyond the affected unvaccinated or inadequately vaccinated subpopulations, wild poliovirus exposure of people in the general population and the establishment of subsequent endemic and epidemic transmission remain a concern.

Molecular Epidemiology of Poliovirus

The application of molecular tools, such as genomic sequencing of poliovirus, has added a new dimension and resolution power to our understanding of the epidemiology of poliomyelitis.[85, 175] Because the poliovirus genome evolves rapidly (1–2% nucleotide substitutions per site per year) (Fig. 16–4), links between poliomyelitis cases can now be determined and importations from the remaining poliovirus reservoirs can be established. These molecular methods offer an additional tool to monitor the progress of the global polio eradication initiative and suggest that lineages of poliovirus genotypes (differing by less than 15% in their nucleotide sequences) disappear sequentially through intensive immunization efforts.[84, 85] The experience in the Americas suggests that if a genotype is not detected for a year or more despite adequate surveillance, it probably has become extinct.[81] These methods have established the existence of numerous poliovirus genotypes endemic to different regions of the world,[85] the former Soviet Union,[176] Europe, the Middle East, and the Indian subcontinent[82] and demonstrated that poliovirus type 2 is usually the first serotype to be eliminated, that poliovirus type 3 appears to circulate more locally than other serotypes, and that poliovirus type 1 appears to be most commonly associated with importations from neighboring countries and with intercontinental or global

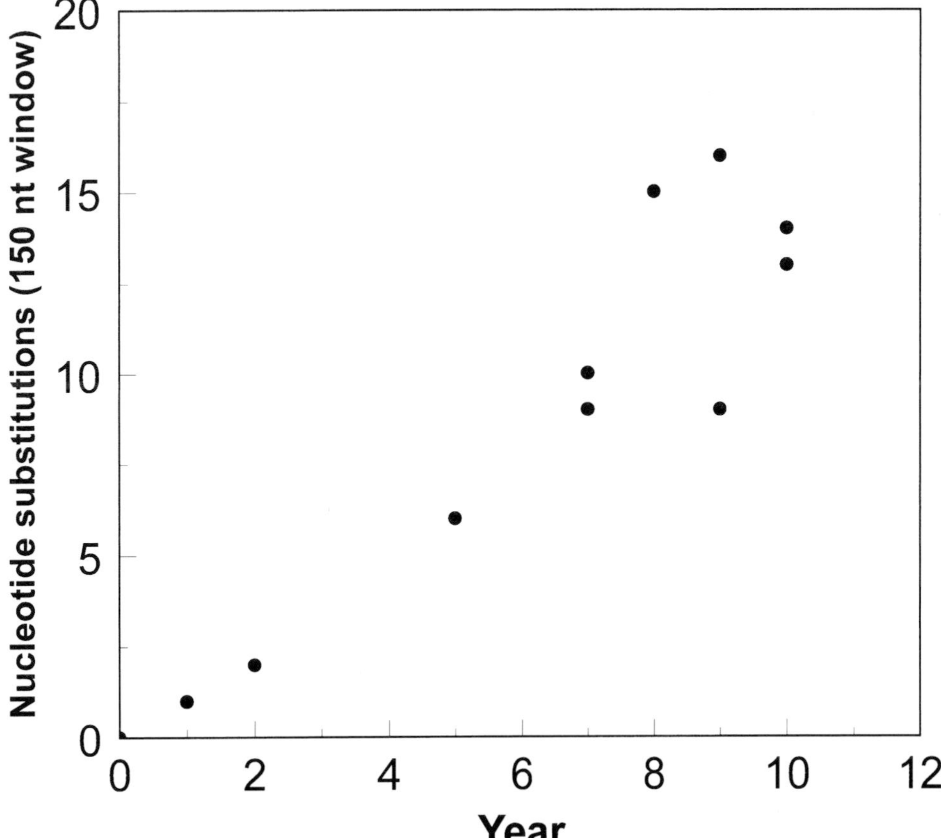

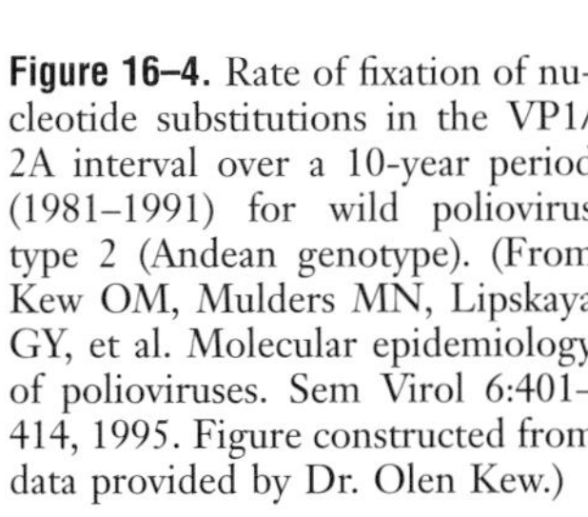
Figure 16–4. Rate of fixation of nucleotide substitutions in the VP1/2A interval over a 10-year period (1981–1991) for wild poliovirus type 2 (Andean genotype). (From Kew OM, Mulders MN, Lipskaya GY, et al. Molecular epidemiology of polioviruses. Sem Virol 6:401–414, 1995. Figure constructed from data provided by Dr. Olen Kew.)

spread of the virus.[81, 84] Genomic sequencing of polioviruses suggested that the viruses responsible for the epidemic in the Netherlands in 1992 to 1993 (type 3) and Albania in 1996 (type 1) were probably imported from reservoirs in the Indian subcontinent.[82] These molecular methods have shown that in some instances, different genotypes of poliovirus can circulate concomitantly and cause poliomyelitis cases in a geographically limited area.[81, 151] Finally, these methods have been critical for determining laboratory contamination. If the nucleotide sequence of a virus has not evolved to the predicted extent over time compared with previous isolates, it is likely that the virus isolated constitutes a laboratory contamination either with virus isolated by that laboratory in previous years or from wild poliovirus used as reference strains in the laboratory.[81, 177]

PASSIVE IMMUNIZATION

Therapeutic use of convalescent serum for poliomyelitis was first recommended as early as 1915.[178] Several trials using convalescent serum, administered by a single intrathecal injection, intraspinally, intravenously, or subcutaneously, reported conflicting results.[179] However, convalescent serum use was advocated by some until a well-controlled trial during a poliomyelitis outbreak in 1931 provided no statistical evidence that the therapy was of value.[180]

Administration of antibody was pursued again in the late 1940s and early 1950s as a means of preventing poliomyelitis by passive immunization. It had been demonstrated previously that low levels of circulating neutralizing antibody were protective against the paralytic manifestations of poliomyelitis both in experimental animal models and in humans.[180] In addition, infants in the first few months of life rarely acquired paralytic poliomyelitis, presumably because maternally derived type-specific poliovirus antibodies provided some protection. However, this protective effect is relatively short-lived. Maternally derived antibody declines with a half-life of approximately 28 days and can rarely be detected in infants older than 6 months.[181]

A large field trial funded by the National Foundation for Infantile Paralysis demonstrated in 1952 that immune globulin (i.e., gamma globulin) was effective in preventing paralytic disease if it was administered before the presumed exposure to poliovirus but that the protective effect was relatively short-lived, about 5 to 8 weeks.[182] In this study, a single dose of 0.14 mL/kg body weight was administered intramuscularly.[182] However, evaluation of large-scale use of gamma globulin in 1953 by the National Advisory Committee for the Evaluation of Gamma Globulin in the Prophylaxis of Poliomyelitis concluded, ". . . Its preventive effect in community prophylaxis during 1953 has not been demonstrated. Also, no modification of the severity of paralysis was shown. Nevertheless, the committee cannot say that the use of gamma globulin by mass inoculation produced no effect."[183] Although these conclusions were modified somewhat by Hammon—who pointed out that this evaluation had serious, perhaps fatal flaws, including (1) the gamma globulin was given far too late to be expected to have much or any effect and (2) this was not a controlled experiment with appropriate controls—the committee report nevertheless dampened enthusiasm for this approach. In addition, in view of the progress toward the subsequent development of effective poliovirus vaccines that induced active immunity, presumably for life, gamma globulin as a tool to prevent poliomyelitis was not further pursued.

Passive immunity to poliomyelitis (and other diseases) among immunodeficient people, particularly those with agammaglobulinemia or hypogammaglobulinemia, is achieved through substitution therapy, namely, the regular administration (monthly) of immune globulin to those individuals. Monthly doses of 100 to 400 mg/kg body weight given intravenously are used.[184] Intramuscular immune globulin may also be used. Immune globulin, whether it is formulated to be administered intramuscularly or intravenously, must pass the requirements of the Food and Drug Administration in the United States, which include minimum titers for antibody to polioviruses. In addition, immune globulin or hyperimmune sera may be used to eliminate chronic enterovirus infections,[185] including chronic infections with poliovirus,[186] and the oral route of administration sometimes has been used.[185]

ACTIVE IMMUNITY

Early Approaches

Research on inducing active immunity in monkeys by administering ground up spinal cord and observing whether the animals succumbed to poliomyelitis began as early as 1910.[187] Inactivation of poliovirus by formalin was first reported in 1911.[188] Brodie[189, 190] first used subinfective doses of live poliovirus and later mixed live poliovirus with hyperimmune serum before using phenol and formalin as inactivating substances. After further small-scale experiments to optimize formalin inactivation and administration of the inactivated vaccine to small numbers of rhesus monkeys, adult volunteers, and children, the vaccine was administered to approximately 3000 children.[191, 192] However, this approach was controversial and not pursued further because of concerns about the efficacy and safety of this vaccine. Kolmer in 1935 pioneered the use of attenuated live poliovirus that had been passaged continually in monkeys and prepared a suspension of monkey spinal cord in 1% sodium ricineolate. The vaccine was administered to approximately 10,000 children, at least 10 of whom acquired paralytic poliomyelitis shortly after vaccination, for a rate of approximately 1 case per 1000 children vaccinated.[193, 194] In short, both approaches—inactivation by formalin and attenuation of live poliovirus—that were successfully used later by Salk and Sabin had been employed during these trials. In retrospect, it is clear that without knowledge of the number of poliovirus serotypes, these early vaccine development efforts were doomed to failure.

Advances in tissue culture growth of poliovirus in the late 1940s[20] renewed interest in poliovirus vaccines, and some of the first reports on attenuation of wild poliovirus for vaccine purposes were published in the early 1950s.[195–198] Essentially, attenuated strains were developed by several passages of virus at high concentration in cell cultures of rodent CNS tissue or nonnervous system tissue from monkeys, followed by selection of attenuated variants at limiting dilutions or from single plaques.

Description of Vaccine: How Strains Were Developed

The history of early developments of oral vaccines can be reviewed in detail in reports of meetings published between 1958 and 1961[199–202] and in the corresponding chapter of the second edition of *Vaccines*.[149] As with most major scientific achievements, crucial contributions came from a number of different investigative teams.[27, 203–205] Hilary Koprowski and colleagues[195] reported the successful immunization of humans against poliomyelitis with a live poliovirus vaccine as early as 1950. Although these attenuated strains were not selected for licensing, this work meant that by 1960, when not only his strains but also several other candidate vaccines were well into their testing and field trial use, a 10-year record of evidence was available on patterns of response in humans who had received the type 2 strain in 1950.[206]

Continued development and testing of candidate strains were conducted in three institutions: the Children's Hospital Research Foundation, Cincinnati (A. B. Sabin); Lederle Laboratories, Wayne, NJ (V. J. Cabasso et al.); and the Wistar Institute, Philadelphia (H. Koprowski et al.).[201, 202] The work with attenuated polioviruses was advanced toward practical usefulness, particularly by Sabin, who meticulously studied a number of progeny of single virus particles for neurotropism in monkeys and finally selected three for small experimental trials in humans.[207] Much of the early efforts in the development of candidate strains were devoted to[147] (1) maintaining high degrees of infectivity in cell culture and the human intestinal tract, (2) inducing detectable levels of neutralizing antibody in a high proportion of susceptible (seronegative) recipients, (3) displaying low neurovirulence in monkeys, (4) demonstrating a lack of association with paralytic disease in humans, and (5) maintaining genetic stability after replication in the human host. The efforts of a number of investigators to develop and test suitable attenuated poliovirus strains came to fruition during 1955 to 1959, and large-scale field trials were held in many countries under a variety of conditions. Many of these trials in humans involved the sequential administration of monovalent formulations of poliovirus types 1, 2, and 3. A number of investigators around the world participated in studies in which these candidate strains were fed to millions of people. At the two conferences held by the Pan American Health Organization (1959 and 1960), these investigators joined in assessing the results.[201, 202]

The field trials[201, 202] and subsequent studies focused not only on the human populations fed candidate virus but also on the virus populations recovered from stool samples of vaccinees. Because the attenuated polioviruses are living organisms that must multiply to immunize, it was essential to know as much as possible about the progeny viruses let loose in nature—agents that still retain their property of infecting humans. All poliovirus strains, regardless of how highly attenuated, retain the property of multiplying and destroying cells in the monkey spinal cord. The degree to which this property is retained, however, varies over an enormous range as one progresses from the virulent strains to the highly attenuated ones suitable for vaccine use. The laboratory techniques are such that different degrees of neurotropism, even among attenuated strains, can be detected.

In 1958, a detailed comparison of candidate strains was conducted.[208, 209] The attenuated strains that had been developed at the Yale Poliomyelitis Study Unit had already been shown to have too high a degree of reversion in chimpanzees and were dropped from consideration.[197, 210] At Baylor College of Medicine in Houston, extensive comparison was made of the Sabin strains and the Lederle-Cox strains for neurovirulence in hundreds of monkeys inoculated by the intracerebral and intraspinal routes.[208–211] At the Division of Biologics Standards of the National Institutes of Health, Murray and colleagues[212] compared three sets of candidate strains as follows: Lederle-Cox, Sabin, and Koprowski-Wistar. In spite of the studies being done in two different laboratories and with some variations in methodology, the overall findings were essentially in agreement. It was clear that the Lederle and Wistar strains were more neurotropic for monkeys than the Sabin strains. Because the results favored the Sabin strains, these strains are the ones that have been licensed, manufactured, and used almost universally since then.

The passage histories of the three Sabin vaccine seeds now in use are shown in Tables 16–4 to 16–7.[213] For example, the type 1 strain was derived from the Mahoney strain, initially isolated by Francis and Mack in

Table 16–4. **POLIOVIRUS TYPE 1, SABIN STRAIN, PASSAGE HISTORY**

YEAR	MANIPULATION	DESIGNATION
1941	*Francis and Mack:* Isolation of Mahoney strain *Salk:* 14 MKTC and 2 monkey testicular cell passages	Mahoney strain
1953	*Li and Schaeffer:* 11 MKTC passages	LS strain
	Additional tissue culture passages in monkey kidney and skin	LS-a LS-b LS-c
1954	*Sabin:* 5 passages in cynomolgus MKTC (3 terminal dilutions) 3 single-plaque passages Selection by neurovirulence testing	 LS-c, 2ab
1956	*Sabin:* 2 passages in cynomolgus MKTC	LS-c, $2ab/KP_2$ = SO
1956	*MSD:* 1 passage in rhesus MKTC	LS-c, $2ab/KP_3$ SO + 1 = SOM

MKTC, monkey kidney tissue culture; MSD, Merck Sharp & Dohme.
From WHO Consultative Group on Poliomyelitis Vaccines, 1985.

Table 16–5. **POLIOVIRUS TYPE 2, SABIN STRAIN, PASSAGE HISTORY**

YEAR	MANIPULATION	DESIGNATION
—	*Fox and Gelfand:* P 712 strain isolated	P 712
1954	*Sabin:* 4 passages (3 terminal dilutions) in cynomolgus MKTC 3 serial passages of plaque isolates	
	Selection by neurovirulence testing	
	Fed to chimpanzees	P 712, Ch
	3 single-plaque passages	P 712, Ch, 2ab
1956	*Sabin:* 2 passages in cynomolgus MKTC	P 712, Ch, 2ab/KP_2 = SO
1956	*MSD:* 1 passage in rhesus MKTC	P 712, Ch, 2ab/KP_3 SO + 1 = SOM

MKTC, monkey kidney tissue culture; MSD, Merck Sharp & Dohme.
From WHO Consultative Group on Poliomyelitis Vaccines, 1985.

1941. Salk made additional monkey kidney and monkey testicular passages. In 1953, Li and Schaeffer made 11 monkey kidney tissue culture passages, yielding the partially attenuated LS strain, and additional passages in monkey kidney and skin to yield the further attenuated strain LS-c. Then, Sabin, in 1954, carried the LS-c strain through terminal dilutions and single-plaque passages, carefully selecting by neurovirulence testing, finally obtaining strain LS-c, 2ab. Two further passes, in cynomolgus kidney, yielded LS-c, 2ab/KP_2, designated SO (Sabin original). Dr. Bettylee Hampil at Merck Sharp & Dohme made one additional passage in rhesus monkey kidney tissue culture to derive LS-c, 2ab/KP_3, designated SO + 1 or SOM. The current vaccine is SO + 4, four tissue culture passages beyond the SO. A maximum of five passages are permitted, after which earlier (grandmother) seeds must be thawed and used to prepare new mother seeds. Because of inherent difficulties in maintaining the genetic stability of the Sabin

Table 16–6. **POLIOVIRUS TYPE 3, SABIN STRAIN, PASSAGE HISTORY**

YEAR	MANIPULATION	DESIGNATION
1937	*Kessel and Stimpert:* Leon strain isolated 20 intracerebral passages in rhesus monkeys	Leon strain
1952	*Melnick:* 8 passages in rhesus testicular tissue culture	
1953	*Sabin:* 3 passages in cynomolgus MKTC	
	30 rapid passages at low dilution in cynomolgus MKTC	
	3 terminal dilution passages	
	1 low-dilution pass	
	9 plaques isolated, single-plaques passed 3 times	
	Selection by neurovirulence testing	Leon 12a,b
1956	*Sabin:* 3 passages in cynomolgus MKTC	Leon 12a,b/KP_3 = SO
1956	*MSD:* 1 passage in rhesus MKTC	Leon 12a,b/KP_4 SO + 1 = SOM

MKTC, monkey kidney tissue culture; MSD, Merck Sharp & Dohme.
From WHO Consultative Group on Poliomyelitis Vaccines, 1985.

Table 16–7. **POLIOVIRUS TYPE 3, SABIN STRAIN, RNA-DERIVED, PASSAGE HISTORY**

YEAR	MANIPULATION	DESIGNATION
1959	*Pfizer:* 1 passage of SOM in cercopithecoid MKTC with SV40 antiserum	SO + 2 = 127-B-111
1962	*Pfizer:* RNA extraction and plaque cloning, selection by rct40° marker test	SO + 3 = 457-111
	2 plaque purifications	SO + 5 = SOR
1978	Seed stocks acquired by Institute Mérieux and distributed to others when Pfizer ceased operations	

MKTC, monkey kidney tissue culture; SV40, simian virus 40.
From WHO Consultative Group on Poliomyelitis Vaccines, 1985.

type 3 seed stock, manufacturers have turned to an RNA-derived passage and clone of the strain, labeled SOR. This seed has yielded a vaccine of greater consistency and stability than the original Sabin seed. Adequate grandmother seeds are available through the WHO Consultative Group to last for centuries.

Molecular biology has provided methods for analyzing the genetic basis of virus attenuation.[214] The molecular differences between the parent and vaccine viruses have been determined. For poliovirus type 1, 56 (0.8%) mutations scattered throughout the 7441 nucleotides in the genome of the virus account for 21 amino acid differences. Reversion to neurovirulence requires several back mutations. This is an unlikely occurrence as the virus replicates in the vaccinated person and accounts for the greater safety of the type 1 component of OPV. For poliovirus type 3, only 10 (0.1%) of the 7429 nucleotides in the genome in the vaccine virus are different from those in the parent strain, and only two or three seem to be important for attenuation. The most essential is a C-to-U point mutation at base 472 in the 5′ noncoding part of the genome and another C-to-U mutation of nucleotide 2034.[213] The point mutation at position 2493 from C to U appears to increase the neurovirulence of type 3 virus independently of other point mutations at position 472 and 2034.[215] For type 2, the situation in regard to frequency of base changes is intermediate, with 23 point mutations in the vaccine virus with the nucleotide at position 481 in the 5′ noncoding region essential for achieving attenuation.[216, 217] For the three types, the most crucial mutations for attenuation seem to be at nucleotide 480 for type 1, at 481 for type 2, and at 472 for type 3.

How Trivalent Vaccine Was Developed

Viral replication in the gastrointestinal tract and seroconversion were usually demonstrated in 80 to 100% of seronegative recipients with a single dose of monovalent vaccines at dosage levels of 10^5 median tissue culture infective doses ($TCID_{50}$).[218–221] However, when doses of 10^5 $TCID_{50}$ of each poliovirus serotype were mixed and administered as trivalent preparations, the replication and antibody production were consistently lower for some types compared with the sequential administration of monovalent vaccines.[222–228] This effect could be modified somewhat by increasing the doses of each type ($\geq 10^7$ $TCID_{50}$).[229, 230] In addition, these studies showed that trivalent OPV of similar potency for each serotype was associated with a predominance of poliovirus type 2 excretion, and significantly higher type 2 antibody titers, than for poliovirus types 1 and 3. These early trials did not evaluate the impact of increasing the quantity of one serotype or reducing the quantity of another on seroconversion to all three serotypes because the interference effect of type 2 could often be overcome by administering three or more doses of the trivalent vaccine.

In 1961, a large study in Canada tested a "balanced" formulation of trivalent OPV (10^6 $TCID_{50}$ for Sabin type 1, 10^5 $TCID_{50}$ for Sabin type 2, and $10^{5.5}$ $TCID_{50}$ for Sabin type 3).[231] A single dose of this balanced (10:1:3) vaccine was administered to nearly 24,000 people, including 106 previously seronegative subjects, 103 (97%) of whom seroconverted to all three serotypes. Although one could conclude from this study that a single dose of OPV may be sufficiently immunogenic for a routine program, only triple seronegative infants were included in this analysis of the Canadian trial, so the results represent the best possible scenario for inducing optimal levels of seroconversion because the infants lacked maternally derived antibody that can interfere with seroconversion. On the basis of these findings and an unpublished study from Guam, the balanced formulation of OPV was licensed in Canada in 1962 and in the United States in 1963.

Dosage and Route

According to current regulations in the United States, trivalent live attenuated oral poliovirus vaccine (OPV) must contain at least $10^{5.5}$ $TCID_{50}$ for poliovirus type 1, $10^{4.5}$ $TCID_{50}$ for type 2, and $10^{5.2}$ $TCID_{50}$ for type 3.[232, 233] However, the U.S. manufacturer routinely exceeds these minimum requirements, and an evaluation by a WHO reference laboratory found potency levels of $10^{6.5}$, $10^{5.4}$, and $10^{6.3}$ $TCID_{50}$ per dose of types 1, 2, and 3, respectively (WHO unpublished data). WHO requires the following minimum $TCID_{50}$ for each vaccine poliovirus serotype: $10^{5.9 \pm 0.5}$ $TCID_{50}$ for type 1, $10^{5.0 \pm 0.5}$ $TCID_{50}$ for type 2, and $10^{5.7 \pm 0.5}$ $TCID_{50}$ for type 3. However, because of evidence from an evaluation in Brazil that poliovirus type 3 immunogenicity is not satisfactory with $10^{5.5}$ (300,000), particularly in tropical countries,[234] the WHO's Global Advisory Group recommended in 1990 that the type 3 component of OPV should be increased to $10^{5.8}$ (600,000) $TCID_{50}$.[235] OPV purchased by the United Nation's Children Fund (UNICEF) beginning with the 1992 to 1993 tender period complied with this recommendation.

The recommended route of administration of OPV is the oral route by releasing the vaccine volume (0.5 mL) contained in single-dose droppers into the oral cavity[236] for vaccine manufactured in the United States or providing 2 drops (~0.1 mL) of OPV contained in multidose vials produced by many non-U.S. manufacturers.[237] Although in the early 1960s some manufacturers put OPV into dragées, at present only OPV produced in China is in dragée form; before administration, the dragée must be ground up and mixed with water.

Producers

At least 18 manufacturers around the world are producing OPV using the Sabin vaccine seeds (now under the control of WHO) (Table 16–8). This includes producers in Belgium, Canada, China, France, Germany, India, Indonesia, Iran, Italy, Mexico, Pakistan, Russia, United Kingdom, United States,* Vietnam, and Yugoslavia. In addition, manufacturers in Egypt, Pakistan, Brazil, India, and Korea are filling and finishing bulk OPV produced by one of these manufacturers.

*Initially, several U.S. companies produced OPV: Merck Sharp & Dohme, Wyeth, Pfizer, and Lederle; but as of this writing, only Wyeth-Lederle Vaccines and Pediatrics continues to produce OPV in the United States.

Table 16–8. **MANUFACTURERS OF ORAL POLIOVIRUS VACCINE (1997)**

MANUFACTURER	CITY	COUNTRY
SmithKline Beecham Biologicals	Rixenart	Belgium
Pasteur Mérieux Connaught	Willowdale	Canada
National Vaccine and Serum Institute	Beijing	China
Polio Institute	Kunming	China
Pasteur Mérieux Connaught	Lyon	France
Chiron Behringwerke	Marburg	Germany
Haffkine Bio-Pharmaceutical Corp., Ltd.	Bombay	India
Persero BioFarma	Bandung	Indonesia
Razi State Serum Institute	Teheran	Iran
Chiron Vaccines	Siena	Italy
Japan Poliomyelitis Research Institute	Tokyo	Japan
Gerencia General de Biologicos y Reactivos, Instituto National de Virologia	Mexico City	Mexico
National Institute of Health	Islamabad	Pakistan
Institute of Poliomyelitis and Viral Encephalitides	Moscow	Russian Federation
Evans Medical Ltd.	Medeva-Speke, Liverpool	United Kingdom
Wyeth-Lederle Vaccines and Pediatrics	Pearl River	United States
Poliomyelitis Vaccine Research Centre (POLIOVAC)	Hanoi	Vietnam
Institute of Immunology and Virology (TORLAK)	Belgrade	Yugoslavia

Most of these manufacturers use seed strains of types 1 and 2 no more than two passages away from the WHO master seed (SO + 1, i.e., Sabin final plus one passage). There is more variation in the type 3 seed used; most manufacturers are now using the Pfizer RNA-derived seed (SOR + 1). The type 3 seed used by China, the CHUNG-3 strain, has been shown by oligonucleotide mapping to be similar to Sabin type 3. Vero cells and human diploid cells are employed by at least one manufacturer each for growing their vaccine viruses; the others continue to employ primary monkey kidney cells. It is recommended that the cells for cultivation be taken from monkeys bred in captivity. Like the cell cultures used, the monkey colony should be shown to be free of extraneous viruses and other pathogens.

Preparations Available (Including Combinations)

Although monovalent OPV formulations of the three poliovirus serotypes were used widely in the early 1960s, they were replaced by trivalent OPV starting in 1963 in the United States and other countries. Exceptions include Hungary, which used all three types of monovalent OPV sequentially until the early 1990s,[238] and South Africa, which routinely used monovalent type 1 OPV in the routine immunization program until the early 1990s.[239] Although monovalent vaccines are still licensed in many countries, they are not used in routine vaccination programs. Thus, trivalent OPV is the only preparation available, either in single-, 10-, or 20-dose vials. No combination products with OPV as one of the components have been licensed.

Constituents Including Antibiotics and Preservatives

The growth medium for the cells consists of Eagle basal medium, the components of which include Earle balanced salt solution, amino acids, antibiotics, and calf serum. After the cells have grown out, the medium is removed and replaced with fresh medium that contains the inoculating virus but no calf serum. The final vaccine is diluted with a modified cell culture maintenance medium that usually contains stabilizer. Each dose (0.5 mL) of vaccine contains less than 25 μg of each of the antibiotics streptomycin and neomycin as well as sorbitol (United States) or $MgCl_2$ (most non-U.S. producers) as a stabilizer. The vaccine contains phenol red as an indicator of pH.

Vaccine Stability

Before any vaccine lot can be released, it must be tested and meet the requirements of the national control authorities. If the vaccine is purchased by UNICEF, the vaccine must also meet the WHO requirements for manufacture, safety, and potency. Because OPV is a live viral vaccine, it is unstable unless it is stored at low temperatures (frozen). Thermostability requirements were defined by WHO as OPV that loses less than 0.5 $\log_{10}$ of titer of each of the three vaccine strains after exposure to 37°C for 2 days.[240] In addition, current regulations require that for maintenance of potency, the vaccine must be stored and shipped frozen and that after thawing, it must be held in the refrigerator at no more than 10°C for a period not to exceed 30 days, after which time it must be discarded.

In the early 1960s, it was found that the infectivity of the enteroviruses could be preserved even when they were heated at 50°C if molar $MgCl_2$ was added,[241] a property that is still used in their identification and characterization. This discovery was applied rapidly to live vaccines[56] not only in the laboratory[242] but also in the field, where stabilized vaccines were used effectively to halt type 1 and type 3 outbreaks.[243] In laboratory studies with OPV containing $MgCl_2$ as a stabilizer,[244] the vaccine showed so little loss in virus titer after long-term storage at −20°C that the predicted half-life was calculated as 92 years. It was also noted that vaccine stabilized with $MgCl_2$ suffered no significant loss of potency after as many as nine cycles of alternate warm and cold conditions. In the United States, the sole producer uses sorbitol,[236] a less effective stabilizer, so this vaccine does not meet the WHO requirements for thermostability. Both sucrose and sorbitol have been used as stabilizers, but they have been less effective, particularly at high temperatures. One manufacturer has introduced concentrated phosphate buffer–lactalbumin hydrolysate as a stabilizer; it works well at 4°C, but more data are needed to learn how effective it would be in the field at higher temperatures. It has recently been shown that D_2O (deuterium oxide) with $MgCl_2$ improves the thermal stability[245]; however, no OPV vaccines in use today contain D_2O.

Individual vaccine vial monitors (VVMs) were introduced in 1996 for all OPV procured by UNICEF.[246] VVMs respond to heat exposure with a change in color. The potential benefits of VVMs include (1) ability to keep opened vials without having to discard partially used vials at the end of the day, (2) decrease of at least 30% in vaccine wastage rates, (3) flexibility to take the vaccine beyond the cold chain to reach remote locations, and most important (4) reassurance for the vaccinator at peripheral vaccination sites that the vaccine is potent.[246]

Regulatory Requirements for OPV Licensure

National control or regulatory agencies, such as the Food and Drug Administration in the United States or the National Institute for Biological Standards and Control in the United Kingdom, provide guidance to manufacturers for the production and licensing of OPV.[232] In addition, WHO provides regulations that manufacturers must follow to be eligible to sell vaccine through the UNICEF tender. The WHO regulations contain three sections: (1) manufacturing requirements, (2) national control requirements, and (3) requirements for poliomyelitis vaccine (oral) prepared in primary cultures of monkey kidney cells. In addition, a summary protocol for poliomyelitis vaccine (oral) production is provided in appendix 7 of that document.[240]

WHO recommends that all candidate vaccine strains be evaluated in large-scale field trials before licensure because of the potential that neurovirulence testing in monkeys may not always predict the actual behavior of vaccine strains (i.e., reversion to neurovirulence and potential for epidemic spread) in humans under field conditions.[247] USOL-D bac, a new poliovirus type 3 vaccine strain, was developed by the Institute of Sera and Vaccines, Prague, Czechoslovakia, in 1962.[248] Virus isolated in stool after administration of Sabin type 3 possessed a higher degree of neurovirulence than the corresponding mutants of USOL-D bac. In addition, this vaccine strain had passed all neurovirulence tests as determined in monkeys and appeared to be safer than the Sabin type 3 strain. In 1968, an extensive outbreak of poliomyelitis caused by poliovirus type 3 occurred in Poland 4 months after a small vaccine trial with Sabin type 3 and USOL-D bac vaccine strains had been carried out.[249] Subsequent molecular investigations indicated that USOL-D bac had been responsible for the epidemic.[250, 251] This experience in humans indicates that monkey neurovirulence testing alone is insufficient to ensure vaccine safety. This conclusion is supported by data from the United States. Neurovirulence information, based on monkey neurovirulence tests, from more than 80 individual vaccine lots of Sabin type 3 virus produced between 1964 and 1983 was reviewed.[252] The authors of this study concluded that "type 3 OPV is, if anything, less neurovirulent than is type 1 OPV. However, in field use type 3 OPV has been associated with vaccine-related poliomyelitis more frequently than has type 1 OPV." The molecular mechanisms for poliovirus attenuation and experiences with neurovirulence testing during the last 40 years were reviewed in a meeting in 1991.[253]

Genetic Stability of Vaccine Seed Strains

To enhance the genetic constancy of the present seed viruses of the Sabin strains, infectious complementary DNA (cDNA) clones of the vaccine viral RNA have been developed and are used by some vaccine manufacturers. cDNA clones are attractive because mutations (see *Molecular Epidemiology of Poliovirus)* during replication of the single-stranded RNA genome of polioviruses occur frequently[85, 175, 254] and because RNA seed viruses are not completely homogeneous. Initiation of replication with cDNA ensures that pure populations of attenuated viral genomes are produced, which reduces the potential for mutations.

cDNA of the poliovirus genome can be cloned into bacterial plasmids, and with propagation large amounts of homogeneous vaccine polioviruses can be produced. To that end, cDNA copies of RNA from all three serotypes of poliovirus have been sequenced and cloned in *Escherichia coli.* Racaniello and Baltimore[255] assembled a full-length clone of the genome of the virulent Mahoney strain of type 1 poliovirus from subgenomic cDNA clones and showed that transfection of plasmid DNA from this clone would produce infectious poliovirus in cultured primate cells. Subsequently, an infectious cDNA clone of the genome of the Sabin 1 strain of poliovirus was isolated. Virus recovered from HeLa S3 cells transfected with the infectious Sabin 1 clone was shown by physical methods and in vitro marker tests to be indistinguishable from the Sabin 1 reference virus. In 1986, Kohara and colleagues[254] described the biological properties of the Sabin 1 viruses recovered from different mammalian cells transfected with the infectious cDNA clone. They also presented satisfactory neurovirulence tests for attenuation in monkeys that were injected intraspinally with these same viruses. Their results suggest that infectious cDNA clones may be used to preserve the vaccine quality of the Sabin 1 viruses and to provide a potentially unlimited supply of constant seed virus for future poliovirus vaccine production.

RESULTS OF VACCINATION

Viral Excretion and Immune Response

OPV administration, similar to natural exposure to polioviruses, initiates a complex process that eventually results in both humoral (systemic) and mucosal (local) immunity. The kinetics of this immune response have been reviewed in detail by Ogra and Karzon.[132] Production of IgM antibody predominates initially, can be detected as early as 1 to 3 days after infection, and disappears after 2 to 3 months. IgG antibody increases during this same period, eventually constitutes the predominant class of persistent antibody, and may last for life.[256] The development of both serum and secretory antibody responses to OPV compared with IPV is shown in Figure 16–5.[132] The broader response of nasal and duodenal IgA associated with OPV administration is apparent. The humoral immune response is not completely serotype specific,[112, 257] and some degree of cross-protection

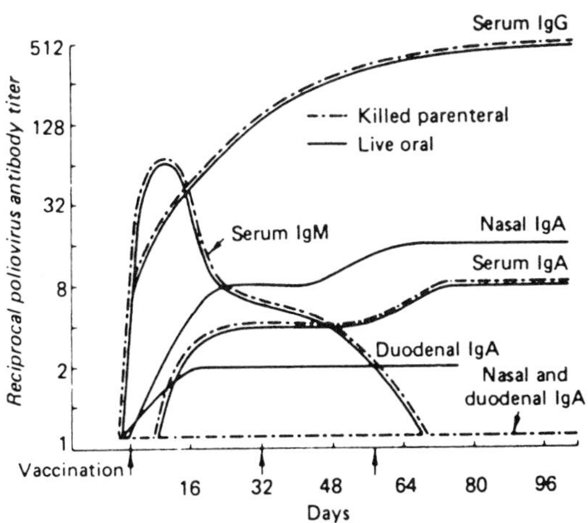

Figure 16–5. Serum and secretary antibody responses to orally administered, live attenuated poliovirus vaccine (OPV) and to intramuscularly administered inactivated poliovirus vaccine (IPV). (From Ogra PL, Fishaut M, Gallagher MR. Viral vaccination via the mucosal routes. Rev Infect Dis 2:352–369, 1980.)

(heterotypic cross-reaction) has been observed. Preexisting antibody to poliovirus type 2 may modify the risk of paralytic poliomyelitis after exposure to poliovirus type 1.[258] The significance of cell-mediated immunity to poliovirus exposure remains to be shown,[259] although cytotoxic T-cell responses may contribute to inflammation and cell necrosis that characterize poliovirus infections of the CNS.

Viremia has been demonstrated commonly after ingestion of type 2 OPV. Free virus is present in serum between days 2 and 5 after vaccination, and virus, bound to antibody, can be detected for an additional few days.[260, 261] Bound virus in serum is detected by acid treatment, which inactivates the antibody and liberates active virus.

The majority of infants (70 to 90%) susceptible to poliomyelitis excrete poliovirus after administration of OPV. A study conducted during the winter of 1960 in Houston reported that 72%, 88%, and 75% of infants 0 to 6 months of age excreted homologous poliovirus types 1, 2, and 3, respectively, after vaccination with monovalent poliovirus vaccines[262] (Fig. 16–6). The same study showed that familial and extrafamilial contacts of vaccinated children get exposed secondarily to excreted poliovirus and in turn also excrete poliovirus in feces. The highest proportion of type 2 monovalent OPV–vaccinated infants excreted homologous virus in the first week after vaccination, the highest proportion of familial contacts excreted virus during the second week, and the highest proportion of nonfamilial contacts excreted virus during the fourth week (Fig. 16–7).

In industrialized countries, after complete primary vaccination with three doses of OPV, 95% or more of recipients seroconvert and develop long-lasting immunity to all three poliovirus serotypes. In a recent trial in

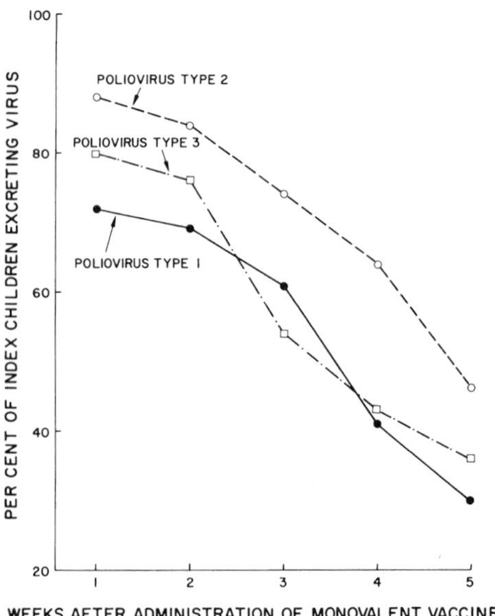

Figure 16–6. Weekly excretion rates of homotypic virus by index children after administration of monovalent poliovaccines. (From Benyesh-Melnick M, Melnick JL, Rawls WE, et al. Studies on the immunogenicity, communicability and genetic stability of oral poliovaccine administered during the winter. Am J Epidemiol 86:112–136, 1967.)

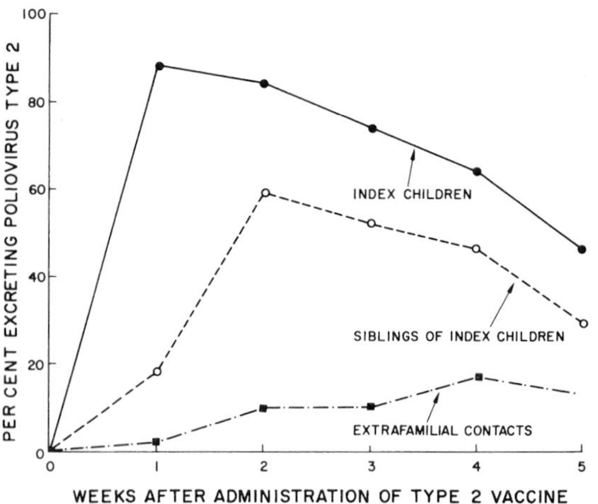

Figure 16–7. Weekly excretion rates of homotypic virus following administration of type 2 monovalent vaccine, for index children, their siblings younger than 5 years, and extrafamilial contacts. (From Benyesh-Melnick M, Melnick JL, Rawls WE, et al. Studies on the immunogenicity, communicability and genetic stability of oral poliovaccine administered during the winter. Am J Epidemiol 86:112–136, 1967.)

the United States, 39% of vaccinees seroconverted to poliovirus type 1, 84% to poliovirus type 2, and 71% to poliovirus type 3 after a single dose of OPV.[263] After receipt of two doses of OPV, seroprevalence was 92% to poliovirus type 1, 100% to poliovirus type 2, and 96% to poliovirus type 3; and after three doses of OPV, 97% had antibodies to poliovirus type 1, 100% to poliovirus type 2, and 100% to poliovirus type 3.[263] This study using the currently formulated trivalent vaccine confirmed earlier studies conducted between 1959 and 1962, which administered OPV to infants and children who were initially seronegative. These earlier studies reported that after two doses, the proportion of recipients seroconverting was 90 to 93% for type 1, 99 to 100% for type 2, and 76 to 98% for type 3; after a third dose, all converted to types 1 and 2, and 87 to 100% seroconverted to type 3.[92, 181, 200–202]

However, OPV appears to be considerably less immunogenic in developing countries. A careful review of the immunogenicity of OPV in developing countries reported that only 73% (range, 36 to 99%), 90% (77 to 100%), and 70% (range, 40 to 99%) of children have detectable antibody to poliovirus types 1, 2, and 3, respectively, after three OPV doses[147] (Table 16–9). Results of controlled trials conducted after the review[147] have confirmed the lower immunogenicity of OPV, particularly to poliovirus type 3, in developing countries.[264–266] A number of hypotheses attempt to explain the differences in OPV performance between industrialized and developing countries. These include interference from concurrent infections with other enteroviruses or diarrhea, both of which are more prevalent in developing countries.[264–267] In addition, there may be nonspecific factors not yet known; and colostrum contains secretory IgA that can influence seroconversion.[268–270] Children with higher levels of maternal antibody have lower seroconversion rates. Maternally derived antibodies are higher in newborns in developing countries compared with newborns in the industrialized world[263, 264]; and

Table 16–9. **SEROCONVERSION/SEROPREVALENCE AFTER RECEIPT OF THREE DOSES OF ORAL POLIOVIRUS VACCINE (OPV) IN THE DEVELOPING WORLD**

COUNTRY	PERCENTAGE WITH NEUTRALIZING ANTIBODY TO INDICATED SEROTYPE			AGE AT FIRST OPV DOSE (mo)	INTERVAL BETWEEN DOSES (mo)	NO. STUDIED	LOWEST DILUTION TESTED*	VACCINE FORMULATION†
	Type 1	Type 2	Type 3					
Thailand	69	95	69	3	1.5	92	1:4	2:2:2
Thailand	90	100	100	3	1.5	82	1:4	5:1:2
Mexico	75	93	59	6	1	75	NA	3:3:3
India	61	77	40	3	1	74	1:10	4:4:4
South Africa	85	96	90	2	1.5	956	1:10	4:2:2
Iran	77	77	60	2	1	354	1:10	5:1:3
Iran	91	92	77	2	1	595	1:10	5:1:3
South Africa	86	96	75	0	1.5	176	1:8	6:2:3
China	99	98	99	0	3	100	1:4	10:1:3
Sri Lanka	97	98	98	3	2	65	1:8	10:1:3
Israel	95	98	93	2	1.5	121	1:10	10:1:3
Kenya	92	98	90	2	2	45	1:8	10:1:3
Brazil	91	98	94	2	2	75	1:5	10:1:3
South Africa	87	95	90	3	1	77	1:10	10:1:3
India	86	84	62	3	1.5	158	1:4	10:1:3
Mali	82	90	76	2	2	118	1:8	10:1:3
Gambia	81	95	56	2	1	182	1:10	10:1:3
Brazil	80	95	56	2	>2	161	1:8	10:1:3
India	73	87	63	0	1	139	1:8	10:1:3
India	72	88	79	1.5	1	86	1:8	10:1:3
Sri Lanka	69	91	78	2	2	68	1:4	10:1:3
India	66	95	72	1.5	1	61	1:8	10:1:3
Kenya	63	92	60	6	2	65	1:8	10:1:3
India	63	75	68	2	1	71	1:10	10:1:3
India	58	92	83	3	1	78	1:10	10:1:3
Brazil	55	71	65	3	1.5	30	1:8	10:1:3
Nigeria	48	92	52	2	1.5	56	1:8	10:1:3
India	47	75	59	3	1.5	50	1:16	10:1:3
Kenya	44	77	60	6	2	31	1:8	10:1:3
India	40	75	51	2	2	87	1:8	10:1:3
Ghana	36	73	61	3	6	75	1:8	10:1:3
Morocco	89	95	74	2	1	122	1:10	20:2:13

*Lowest antibody dilution tested.
†The ratio of potencies to type 1 to type 2 to type 3.
Adapted from Patriarca PA, Wright PF, John TF. Factors affecting the immunogenicity of oral poliovirus vaccine in developing countries: Review. Rev Infect Dis 13:926–939, 1991.

OPV is administered at an earlier age (birth, 6, 10, 14 weeks), an age when the influence of maternally derived antibody on seroconversion is more distinct.[147] Increasing the potency of OPV can correct some of these limitations of the currently formulated OPV[266, 271]; this can also be achieved by administering additional doses of OPV in the routine program or through mass campaigns.[68]

Mucosal immunity is measured primarily by resistance to poliovirus replication and excretion in the pharynx and intestine after challenge with monovalent or trivalent OPV.[201, 202] After challenge, lower titers of virus are excreted for significantly shorter periods among vaccinees compared with unvaccinated children[272] (Table 16–10). Secretory IgA can be measured directly in stool, saliva, and breast milk to assess the degree of mucosal immunity. These methods are difficult to perform, require tedious standardization, and are rarely used. Mucosal immunity may exist even when levels of serum antibody are negligible,[203, 273] although the degree of mucosal immunity appears most closely correlated with the titer of homologous humoral antibody[274]—the lower the titer, the more likely excretion of challenge virus can be demonstrated. One study reported that mucosal immunity may be strain specific, and mucosal immunity induced by one vaccine poliovirus strain may not induce mucosal immunity against another strain.[275] Intestinal mucosal immunity induced by IPV is less effective against infection than that induced by OPV, as measured by the proportion of vaccinees excreting virus or the duration of excretion. However, the clinical importance of these differences in reducing wild virus spread in highly immunized populations in industrialized countries is not clear because (1) IPV does reduce shedding compared with no vaccine and (2) pharyngeal spread may be important in industrialized countries, and IPV induces pharyngeal immunity.[276, 277] IPV and OPV induce equivalent pharyngeal mucosal immunity.[278] On the other hand, in developing countries with poor hygiene and great potential for fecal-oral spread of enteric viruses, the clear increase in mucosal (intestinal) immunity induced by OPV over IPV would appear to offer a major advantage to OPV in reducing the circulation of polioviruses. Secretory IgA has an important role in defense against poliovirus infections,[132, 278, 279] and all available evidence indicates that the immune response

Table 16–10. **INTESTINAL IMMUNITY IN VACCINATED (OPV OR IPV) AND NATURALLY IMMUNE AND SUSCEPTIBLE CHILDREN**

STUDY GROUP	PROPORTION EXCRETING	MEAN DURATION OF EXCRETION (d)	MEAN TITER OF VIRUS EXCRETED (log TCD_{50})	EXCRETION INDEX (million)*	REDUCTION IN VIRAL EXCRETION (%)
Susceptible control subjects	0.80	20.4	5.15	2.305	Reference
IPV vaccinated	0.74	12.3	4.11	0.1173	95
OPV vaccinated	0.37	4.6	2.18	0.00026	99
Naturally immune	0.37	5.4	2.03	0.00022	99

*Excretion index: proportion children excreting challenge type 1 virus × mean duration of excretion days × titer of virus excreted.
IPV, inactivated poliovirus vaccine; OPV, oral poliovirus vaccine.
Table constructed from data in references 372, 378, and 383.

after vaccination with OPV is similar to that after infection with wild poliovirus.

Few studies have provided data on the persistence of mucosal immunity. No data are currently available from developing countries regarding the duration of mucosal immunity for polioviruses. Several studies have assessed resistance to oral challenge by vaccine viruses years after the initial administration of OPV. One study reported that children were completely resistant to intestinal infection 10 years after vaccination, unless prechallenge serum antibodies were 1:8 or lower.[274] Another study reported similar findings on the relationship of humoral antibody and resistance to excretion.[280] No data are available on the long-term persistence of secretary IgA for polioviruses. However, looking at the mucosal immunity induced by another enterovirus, echovirus type 6, might provide some insights. A study assessing the fall-off in secretory IgA titer to echovirus type 6 in the pharynx and intestine reported no declines during a 4-year follow-up period,[281] although the possibility of boosting with echovirus 6 or other enteroviruses in the follow-up period cannot be excluded.

When poliovirus is ingested, the virus has contact with proteolytic enzymes such as trypsin, which may alter viral antigens.[279] Secretory and humoral antibody responses after OPV include those against the new antigens associated with trypsin-cleaved virus. Such antigens are not accessible in IPV, and consequently the immune response after IPV is more limited.[282]

Evidence of OPV Effectiveness

A large body of empirical and scientific evidence has accumulated since the late 1950s that demonstrates the effectiveness of OPV in preventing paralytic disease. OPV use was pioneered in the Soviet Union,[283–285] and the approaches developed in the Soviet Union led to rapid control or elimination of poliomyelitis in many countries. The most prominent example of the effectiveness of OPV is the success of the global polio eradication program,[37] including the Western Hemisphere, which was certified free of wild poliovirus by an International Certification Commission in 1994.[286] OPV has curtailed epidemics and has greatly reduced the incidence of poliomyelitis, often eliminating the pattern of expected seasonal increase in poliomyelitis cases.[46, 158, 162, 243, 285, 287–295] Two vaccine effectiveness studies have been conducted in recent years.[148, 296] The study in Oman estimated that the effectiveness of three doses of OPV in preventing paralytic disease was approximately 90%.[148] Much of the earlier evidence of both small and large trials is contained in meeting reports.[201, 202]

The ability of OPV to infect contacts of vaccine recipients (i.e., "contact spread") and "indirectly vaccinate" these contacts against poliomyelitis is considered by many to be another advantage of OPV compared with IPV. OPV vaccine virus spread has been demonstrated by prospective virological studies and by serological studies in both industrialized and developing countries.[262, 265, 297–300] Serological surveys have shown that the proportion of people who possess antibodies is considerably greater than would be expected either by vaccination or by the circulation of wild polioviruses. After OPV introduction in Yaoundé, Cameroon, the incidence of paralytic poliomyelitis decreased by 85%, although only 35% of children 12 to 13 months of age received three doses of OPV.[162] Among infants who received IPV in Oman, the seroconversion rates were significantly higher among those whose study period coincided with a mass OPV campaign that was conducted elsewhere in the country[265] (Fig. 16–8). A serological survey among unvaccinated inner-city children in the United States demonstrated also that a substantial proportion of these children are exposed secondarily to vaccine viruses[299] (Fig. 16–9). In a study conducted in the United Kingdom, infants received a dose of IPV at 2 months of age. In the ensuing 1-month period and before any OPV was administered, 11% of infants excreted poliovirus type 1 and 4% excreted poliovirus type 2 in stool specimens.[300] These data indicate that vaccine virus spreads easily from OPV recipients to contacts both in industrialized and in developing countries.

Duration of Immunity

Because attenuated viruses contained in OPV are live viruses that induce the same types of antibody as wild poliovirus does, and because wild virus infection is believed to induce lifelong immunity, it has been reasoned by analogy that immunity induced by OPV is also lifelong. In an isolated Eskimo population, antibodies induced by wild poliovirus were shown to have persisted for at least 40 years in the absence of any further exposure during the intervening period.[256] The best evidence

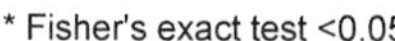

Figure 16–8. Seroconversion to poliovirus types 1, 2, and 3 between birth and 10 weeks of age among children not exposed compared with children exposed secondarily to OPV mass campaigns, by vaccine group, Oman. *P < .05. (From World Health Organization Collaborative Study Group on Oral and Inactivated Poliovirus Vaccines. Combined immunization of infants with oral and inactivated poliovirus vaccines: Results of a randomized trial in The Gambia, Oman, and Thailand. J Infect Dis 175[suppl 1]:S215–S227, 1997.)

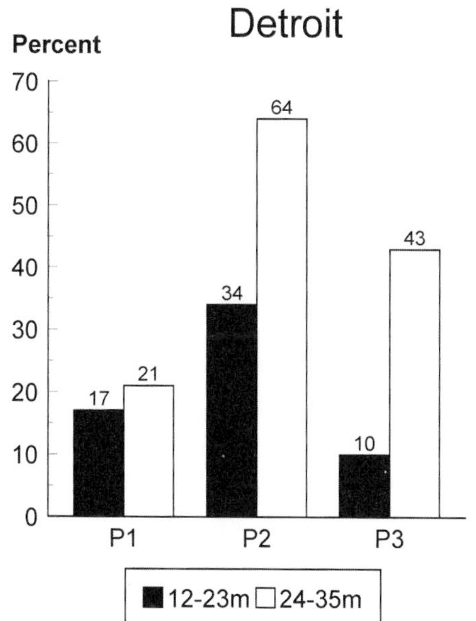

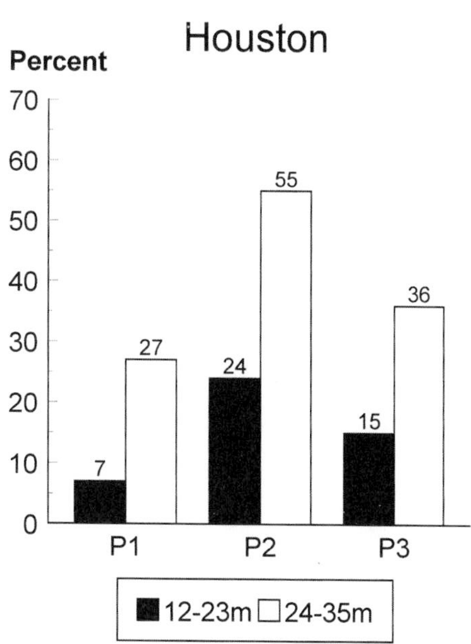

Figure 16–9. Poliovirus antibody seroprevalence among unvaccinated inner-city preschool children, by age groups, Detroit and Houston, 1990 to 1991. Figure constructed from data in reference.[299]

of the persistence of vaccine-induced immunity is the absence of disease in adolescents and adults who had been vaccinated previously with OPV and the persistence of type-specific antibody assessed in population-based surveys.[301, 302] However, interpretation of these data is difficult because of potential repeated exposures to shed virus. In prospective studies in which the same vaccinees were observed for several years, antibodies to types 1 and 2 were found in more than 90% of children and to type 3 in 83 to 95%.[27, 302a–302f] Data from population-based studies of antibody seroprevalence (>95% to poliovirus types 1 and 2, and >85% to poliovirus type 3) conducted among Army recruits in the United States in 1989 and school-aged children in Massachusetts in 1981 (>99% to poliovirus type 1, >99% to poliovirus type 2, and >99% to poliovirus type 3) and in The Gambia (88.1% to poliovirus type 1 and 89.3% to poliovirus type 3 among 3- to 4-year-old children[303]) have demonstrated that poliovirus antibodies induced by OPV persist for many years.[301, 302]

Adverse Events

In the early 1990s, the Institute of Medicine reviewed adverse events associated with childhood vaccines, including poliovirus vaccines.[304] The major adverse event associated with OPV is vaccine-associated paralytic poliomyelitis (VAPP). Shortly after licensure and widespread use of monovalent OPV, cases with paralytic manifestations followed vaccination with monovalent type 3 vaccines. These cases were considered clinically consistent with poliomyelitis and were supported by laboratory findings that did not exclude a possible causal relationship to the administration of oral vaccine. This report by the Surgeon General describes the earliest cases of VAPP.[305]

In 1969, the WHO coordinated a collaborative study to obtain data on the potential risks associated with OPV use. The findings of the first 5- and 10-year follow-up studies were published.[306, 307] During the 5-year period from 1980 to 1984, 395 cases of acute persisting spinal paralysis were reported from 13 countries with a total population of 547 million.[308] The risk of VAPP (either recipients or contacts of recipients) was less than 0.3 per million doses of OPV distributed (or less than 1 case per 3.3 million doses), and the average annual incidence of VAPP was 0.14 per million people (range, 0.0 to 0.33), excluding Romania. Romania reported an average annual incidence of 2.7 per million people. Although some have challenged the existence of VAPP,[27, 309, 310] believing that the cases of paralysis have different etiological factors, the following evidence supports vaccine viruses as causative:

1. Clinical syndromes are typical of poliomyelitis.
2. Vaccine virus is frequently isolated from cases.
3. History of exposure to vaccine is often obtained.
4. Both recipient and contact cases cluster after receipt of the first dose of OPV (one would expect virtually equal numbers of cases after each dose if there were other etiological agents causing the illnesses).
5. Shed viruses have been shown to have mutated toward neurovirulence.
6. The incidence of VAPP is highest in immunodeficient people with B-cell deficiencies, a group also at higher risk of poliomyelitis from wild poliovirus.[311] The completeness of reporting of VAPP cases to the Centers for Disease Control and Prevention (CDC) was estimated to be 81%.[312]

Between 1980 and 1994, a total of 125 cases (94% of all reported cases) classified as VAPP were reported in the United States, including 49 (39%) among immunologically normal vaccine recipients, 46 (37%) among immunologically normal contacts of vaccine recipients, and 30 (24%) among immunologically compromised OPV recipients or contacts of OPV recipients[312] (Fig. 16–10). Six of 46 contact VAPP cases were not epidemi-

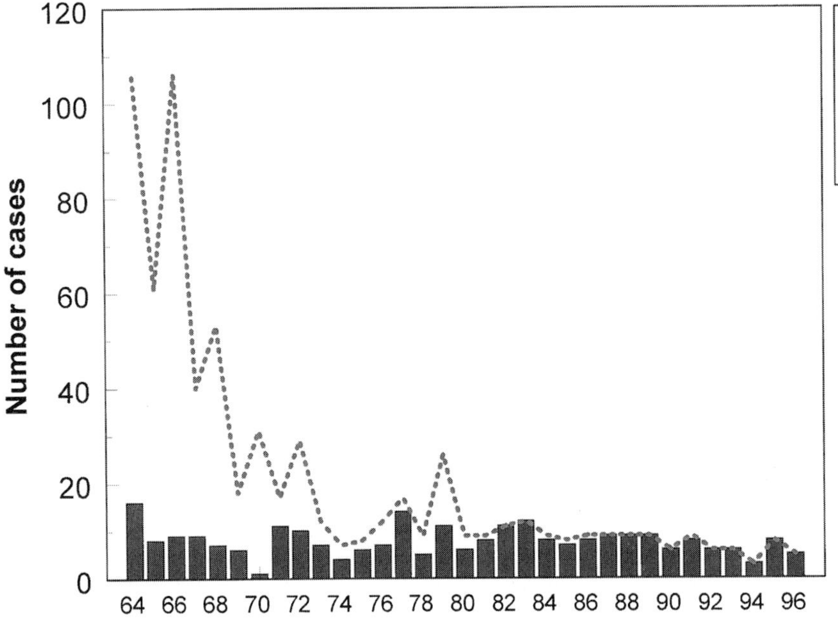

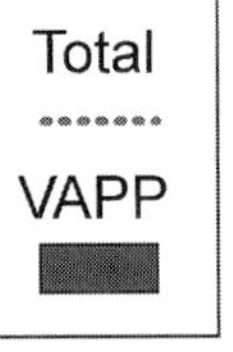

Figure 16–10. Total reported paralytic poliomyelitis cases and vaccine-associated paralytic poliomyelitis (VAPP), United States, 1964 to 1996.

ologically associated with vaccine; however, all had virus isolates characterized as vaccine related. Most contact cases were either unvaccinated or inadequately vaccinated. Therefore, if contacts had been concomitantly vaccinated and immunized, the risk of contact cases would have been smaller or nonexistent.

For the period 1980 to 1994, the risk of VAPP in the United States was estimated as 1 case per 2.4 million doses of OPV distributed; and for children receiving the first doses of OPV, the risk was estimated as 1 case per 750,000 children vaccinated[313] (Table 16–11). The risk of VAPP is highest after the first dose of OPV. Recipients of a first dose and their contacts had a 6.8-fold higher risk of VAPP than did recipients of subsequent doses and their contacts. People with immunodeficiency disorders are at highest risk for VAPP. The risk of VAPP among immunocompromised people is elevated more than 3200 times the risk of immunocompetent people.[314] Almost all cases occurred in people with congenital or acquired immunodeficiency. Immune deficient people with VAPP primarily had abnormalities affecting the B-cell system (humoral immunity), with agammaglobulinemia or hypogammaglobulinemia most frequently associated with VAPP.[314] With the exception of one VAPP case with immunodeficiency disorder, in all other cases, the precipitating event for the diagnosis of immunodeficiency was the onset of paralytic disease. Poliovirus type 3 is the most frequently isolated virus from immunocompetent people with VAPP. In contrast, poliovirus type 2 is the most common virus detected in immunodeficient cases with VAPP. Poliovirus type 1 is rarely isolated from cases with VAPP.[159]

Romania and Hungary have consistently reported higher rates of VAPP than other countries with well-developed surveillance systems. Until recently, both Romania and Hungary used trivalent OPV and monovalent OPV, respectively, solely in campaigns.[174, 238] The high risk of VAPP in Hungary was associated primarily with the administration of monovalent type 3 OPV.[238] The high risk of VAPP in Romania can be attributed to provocation poliomyelitis (i.e., multiple intramuscular injections in the 30 days before paralytic manifestations).[315] VAPP cases in Romania had received, on average, 16.8 intramuscular injections, primarily for antibiotics, in the 30 days before onset of paralysis. Analysis of VAPP cases in the United States between 1980 and 1993 suggested that cases with a history of intramuscular injections received an average of only 1.5 intramuscular injections in the 45 days before onset of paralysis; no clustering of injections during the 45-day period was observed.[316] In contrast, in Romania, most injections were received in the periods 0 to 7 days and 8 to 14 days before onset. It appears unlikely that intramuscular injections contribute substantially to the VAPP burden in the United States. The risk of VAPP in the Americas, where Latin America administered large quantities of OPV in mass campaigns (national immunization days) to eradicate poliomyelitis, was similar to VAPP risk reported in the United States and other countries.[317] Thus, mass campaigns of OPV are unlikely to independently increase the risk of VAPP.

Immunodeficient children are subject to infection, frequently fatal, by a wide variety of normally benign or avirulent agents. Nonpolio enteroviruses may cause serious or fatal illnesses in immunocompromised people.[318, 319] A prominent feature of such infections is the patient's inability to eradicate the virus from the CNS; some patients continue to yield virus from cerebrospinal fluid for up to 3 years,[320] and there is evidence that an immunodeficient patient with VAPP may have excreted vaccine-related poliovirus in stool specimens for up to 7 years.[321] In such people, poliovirus infection, either by a wild virus or by a vaccine strain, may develop in an atypical manner, with an incubation period longer than 28 days, a high mortality rate after a long chronic illness, and unusual lesions in the CNS.[22, 186, 314]

Table 16–11. **RATIO OF NUMBER OF CASES OF VACCINE-ASSOCIATED PARALYTIC POLIOMYELITIS TO NUMBER OF DOSES OF ORAL POLIOVIRUS VACCINE DISTRIBUTED, UNITED STATES, 1980 TO 1994**

	RATIO OF NUMBER OF CASES PER MILLION DOSES OF OPV DISTRIBUTED			
CASE CATEGORY	Overall	First Dose	Subsequent Doses	RELATIVE RISK*
Recipient	1:6.2	1:1.4	1:27.2	19.4
Contact	1:7.6	1:2.2	1:17.5	8.0
Community-acquired	1:50.5	NA	NA	NA
Immunologically abnormal	1:10.1	1:5.8	1:12.9	2.2
Total†	1:2.4	1:0.75	1:5.1	6.8

*First dose ratio to subsequent dose ratio. NA, Not available.

†Includes normal as well as immunologically abnormal cases.

Adapted from Centers for Disease Control and Prevention. Poliomyelitis prevention in the United States: Introduction of a sequential vaccination schedule of inactivated poliovirus vaccine followed by oral poliovirus vaccine. Recommendations of the Advisory Committee on Immunization Practices. MMWR Morb Mortal Wkly Rep 46(RR3):1–25, 1997.

Simian Virus 40

During the early years of OPV production, some cell cultures were contaminated with simian virus 40 (SV40), a virus that causes cancer in rodents.[322] Although concerns were raised about the carcinogenic potential of the SV40 in vaccinees and their offspring, long-term follow-up studies do not support such an association.[323, 324] A meeting convened at the National Institutes of Health in 1997 re-examined the available evidence and concluded that "no measurable increase in neoplastic diseases has occurred in humans exposed to SV40 contaminated polio vaccines."[325] Subsequently, a report evaluated the cancer risks of birth cohorts potentially exposed to SV40 and concluded that these cohorts did not experience a significantly increased risk for the cancer outcomes studied.[326] Cell lines currently used for OPV production come from monkeys raised in colonies free of SV40 or from well-characterized continuous cell lines (Vero cells). In addition, OPV must be screened for known viruses; thus, SV40 is not present in current lots of OPV vaccine.

Guillain-Barré Syndrome

A review by the Institute of Medicine in 1992 suggested that "the evidence favors acceptance of a causal relationship between OPV and Guillain-Barré syndrome."[304] This conclusion was based primarily on data from Finland, where an OPV mass campaign was conducted to control an outbreak of poliomyelitis and 27 patients developed Guillain-Barré syndrome within 10 weeks after initiation of the campaign.[327, 328] However, after the Institute of Medicine review was completed, the Finnish data were reanalyzed and an observational study was completed in the United States.[329, 330] The observational study in the United States showed that rates of Guillain-Barré syndrome after OPV were similar to rates that would have been expected in the absence of vaccination; and the reanalysis in Finland suggested that the increase in Guillain-Barré syndrome risk began before the mass vaccination campaign had been initiated and noted that an influenza epidemic occurred concurrently with the mass campaign. Thus, the available data do not support a causal relationship between OPV and Guillain-Barré syndrome.

Contraindications and Precautions

Contraindications for OPV administration differ somewhat depending on whether the vaccine recipient resides in the industrialized or the developing world (Table 16–12). The risk-benefit ratio of OPV versus no vaccine among children residing in countries with endemic poliomyelitis or recent endemic poliomyelitis favors OPV administration in almost all circumstances. Because of the availability of IPV in a number of industrialized countries and because the need for mucosal (intestinal) immunity is not as great, industrialized countries may have more contraindications than developing countries. In general, OPV is contraindicated in people with known immunodeficiency disorders and those receiving cancer chemotherapy. Age older than 18 years and pregnancy are precautions in the United States, and OPV doses should be repeated in children who vomit within 30 minutes of OPV receipt. In developing countries, OPV doses administered to children with diarrhea should also be repeated. More details on contraindications and precautions are discussed later.

Altered Immune States

In the United States, people with known or suspected immunodeficiency disorders, such as severe combined immunodeficiency syndrome, common variable immunodeficiency disorder, agammaglobulinemia, and hypogammaglobulinemia, should not receive OPV.[313, 314, 331] Similarly, in people with altered immune states due to diseases such as leukemia, lymphoma, or generalized malignant disease or with immune systems compromised by therapy with corticosteroids, alkylating drugs, antimetabolites, or radiation, OPV is contraindicated. Because of the potential for vaccine spread, OPV should not be given to a child who is a member of a family in which there are immunocompromised people. Also, where there has been a family member with immunodeficiency in the past, OPV should not be given to another child unless that child is known to be immunocompetent.

Human Immunodeficiency Virus Infection

In the United States, OPV is contraindicated in people infected with human immunodeficiency virus (HIV), and OPV also should not be used for immunizing household contacts of patients with the immunodeficiency disorder; instead, IPV is recommended.

In developing countries, the HIV status of infants is often not known. IPV is not available as an alternative vaccine. In these settings, OPV is administered early in life (i.e., 6, 10, and 14 weeks of age) on the basis of WHO recommendations; this is at an age when HIV infection would not be expected to have caused immunodeficiency. Several studies showed that OPV induces

Table 16–12. **CONTRAINDICATIONS AND PRECAUTIONS FOR USE OF ORAL POLIOVIRUS VACCINE IN UNITED STATES AND IN DEVELOPING COUNTRIES**

	TYPE	UNITED STATES[313, 331]	DEVELOPING COUNTRY (WHO)[379]
Contraindication	Known or suspected immunodeficiency disorder or immunocompromised	Yes	Yes*
	Family member known to have or suspected of having immunodeficiency disorder or being immunocompromised	Yes	NA
	HIV infection	Yes	No†
	Age ≥18 yr	Yes (use IPV)	NA
	Allergic reaction to a previous dose of OPV or one of its components	Yes	NA
Precaution	Pregnancy	Yes‡	NA
	Diarrhea	No	Yes (repeat dose)

*If immunodeficiency is known.
†Yes, if clinical disease.
‡If immediate protection against poliomyelitis is necessary, IPV or OPV can be used.
HIV, human immunodeficiency virus; IPV, inactivated poliovirus vaccine; OPV, oral poliovirus vaccine; NA, not applicable.

antibody to polioviruses in a similar proportion of HIV-infected infants compared with the response in non–HIV-infected infants.[331a, 331b] HIV infection does not appear to be a risk factor for paralytic poliomyelitis caused by wild poliovirus[332] or for VAPP. There is only a single case report in the literature that links HIV infection and VAPP.[333]

Previous Allergic Reaction

OPV contains trace amounts of neomycin and streptomycin, and a previous allergic reaction to OPV or a similar reaction to these antibiotics constitutes a contraindication to further OPV receipt.[313]

Adult Use

Unvaccinated adults 18 years of age and older in the United States in need of immunization should not receive OPV, because of concerns about a slightly elevated risk of VAPP in adults.[305] Adults at risk may receive OPV if they had been primed by OPV previously.[313]

Pregnancy

In the United States, pregnancy is a precaution to OPV receipt. Two recent evaluations have found no link between adverse outcomes and administration of OPV to pregnant women.[334, 335] Nevertheless, most immunization authorities recommend that immunization during pregnancy generally should be avoided for reasons of theoretical risk. However, if immediate protection against poliomyelitis is needed, IPV or OPV can be used.[313, 331]

Diarrhea

In the United States, OPV may be administered to children with mild diarrhea. In developing countries, OPV may be given to a child with diarrhea; however, because of the lower immunogenicity of OPV in these countries, the dose should not be counted as a valid dose toward completing the routine schedule and should be repeated 4 weeks later.[264, 265, 313, 331, 336]

Simultaneous Administration with Other Vaccines

In industrialized countries as well as in developing countries, OPV is usually administered with other vaccines, including (where appropriate) bacille Calmette-Guérin (BCG), DTP, hepatitis B, measles, *Haemophilus influenzae* type b, and other vaccines used routinely,[313, 337] since no interference between these vaccines and OPV has been observed.

SEQUENTIAL AND COMBINED SCHEDULES

In the United States, there are three acceptable schedules for vaccination against poliomyelitis: an IPV only, an OPV only, or a sequential schedule of IPV followed by OPV. The Advisory Committee on Immunization Practices prefers the sequential schedule of IPV followed by OPV for these scientific and programmatic reasons:

1. The schedule should reduce the number of VAPP cases among recipients by 95% and to some degree among contacts because the mucosal immunity induced by two doses of IPV should reduce spread of vaccine virus.
2. Continued use of OPV will induce effective intestinal immunity,[338] thereby enhancing community resistance to transmission of imported wild poliovirus.
3. There is opportunity for spread of vaccine virus, thus immunizing people missed by routine immunization.
4. The number of injections in the second year of life is reduced from what would be required with use of an IPV only schedule, making compliance with the overall schedule easier.
5. The schedule will lead to stocking of both poliovirus vaccines by healthcare providers, facilitating choice by both parents and providers. In addition to the United States, sequential schedules of IPV followed by OPV have been recommended in several other industrialized countries, including Denmark, Lithuania, Hungary, and Israel.[339] The immunogenicity of sequential schedules depends on the vaccines used, the age at administration, the number of doses, and the interval between doses. In addition to the results of the immunogenicity studies, there is a growing body of evidence suggesting the effectiveness of this approach in controlling poliomyelitis.[340]

In the United States, a small trial first demonstrated the immunogenicity of two sequential schedules of IPV and OPV in inducing antibody.[341] Subsequently, a series of studies were conducted in the United States to assess the immunogenicity of sequential schedules of IPV followed by OPV (Table 16–13). In general, these studies showed that a series of at least three doses of either vaccine—IPV or OPV or with sequential or combined use—was necessary to induce antibody to all three poliovirus serotypes in more than 90% of vaccinees.

To assess effectiveness of three sequential schedules in inducing mucosal immunity in the United States, vaccinees received a dose of OPV at age 18 months (3 months after the last dose of poliovirus vaccine), and stool specimens were obtained before challenge (day 0) and 3, 7, and 21 days thereafter (Table 16–14). One dose of OPV after IPV reduced shedding of poliovirus types 2 and 3 (after challenge with OPV) but did not decrease poliovirus type 1 shedding. Two doses of OPV after IPV decreased shedding of poliovirus type 1 and further decreased shedding of poliovirus type 3. The differences in proportion excreting among groups B (two IPV, two OPV), C (two IPV, three OPV), and E (three OPV)

Table 16–13. **SEROPREVALENCE AFTER VACCINATION WITH INACTIVATED POLIOVIRUS VACCINE (IPV), ORAL POLIOVIRUS VACCINE (OPV), OR IPV FOLLOWED BY OPV IN THE UNITED STATES**

STUDY	VACCINE SCHEDULE AND TYPE OF VACCINE ADMINISTERED: 2 mo	4 mo	6 mo	12–18 mo	NUMBER STUDIED	SEROPREVALENCE (%) AFTER TWO DOSES: Type 1	Type 2	Type 3	SEROPREVALENCE (%) AFTER THREE DOSES: Type 1	Type 2	Type 3
McBean et al[263]	IPV*	IPV		IPV	331	99	99	99	99	100	100
	IPV†	IPV		IPV	332	99	100	100	100	100	100
	OPV	OPV		OPV	337	92	100	96	97	100	100
Faden et al[341]	IPV*	IPV		IPV	91	96	100	100	96	100	100
	OPV	OPV		OPV	22	100	100	100	100	100	100
	IPV*	OPV		OPV	29	94	100	94	100	100	100
	IPV*	IPV		IPV	29	100	100	100	100	100	100
Modlin et al[338]	IPV†	IPV		IPV	101	97	92	78	100	100	100
	OPV	OPV		OPV	98	95	100	90	95	100	100
	IPV†	IPV		OPV	98	90	93	74	97	100	85
	IPV†	OPV	OPV	OPV	106	89	96	71	94	100	81
	IPV†	IPV/OPV	OPV	OPV	101	96	100	85	93	99	97
Blatter and Starr[380]§	IPV*	IPV		IPV	94	97	96	95	100	100	100
	IPV‡	IPV		IPV	68	98	100	98	100	100	100
	IPV*	IPV		OPV	75	94	98	96	100	100	100
	IPV‡	IPV		OPV	99	99	99	95	100	100	100
Halsey et al[381]§	IPV‡	IPV	IPV	OPV	97	98	98	100	100	100	100
	IPV‡	IPV	OPV	OPV	96	100	97	99	100	100	100
	IPV‡	IPV	IPV/OPV	OPV	91	95	96	100	100	100	100

*IPV grown on Vero cells.
†IPV grown on MRC-5 cells.
‡IPV grown in Vero cells and administered through double-barreled syringe with DTP vaccine.
§See reference 382 for additional details.
Adapted from Centers for Disease Control and Prevention. Poliomyelitis prevention in the United States: Introduction of a sequential vaccination schedule of inactivated poliovirus vaccine followed by oral poliovirus vaccine. Recommendations of the Advisory Committee on Immunization Practices. MMWR Morb Mortal Wkly Rep 46(RR3):1–25, 1997.

were statistically not different. The study conducted by Johns Hopkins demonstrated that at least two doses of OPV were needed to induce mucosal immunity sufficient to significantly decrease the proportion of vaccinees excreting poliovirus[338] (Fig. 16–11). The proportion of study subjects who had received prior IPV and excreted type 1 (18%) was much lower than expected based on other challenge studies with OPV. The reasons for this discrepancy are not known, since other challenge studies of IPV vaccinees with trivalent OPV led to 80% shedding of poliovirus type 1[342] and with monovalent

Table 16–14. **PREVALENCE OF OPV VIRUS EXCRETION, BY TYPE, AMONG INFANTS CHALLENGED WITH TRIVALENT ORAL POLIOVIRUS VACCINE AT 18 MONTHS OF AGE (AFTER THREE SEQUENTIAL SCHEDULES OF IPV AND OPV, IPV ALONE, OR OPV ALONE)**

GROUP (N)	VACCINE DOSES	PROPORTION EXCRETING (%)*: Poliovirus Type 1	Poliovirus Type 2	Poliovirus Type 3
A (79)	2 IPV, 1 OPV	27	11	54
B (80)†	2 IPV, 2 OPV	14	4	20
C (70)†	2 IPV, 3 OPV	14	3	17
D (74)	3 IPV	18	39	78
E (73)†	3 OPV	4	3	10

*Alone or in combination with other serotypes.
†Groups B, C, and E are not statistically different.
IPV, inactivated poliovirus vaccine; OPV, oral poliovirus vaccine.
Table constructed from data in reference 338.

OPV led to 70% excretion.[278] We believe the most likely explanation is that the study duration (16 mo) may have allowed participants (including those receiving only IPV) to be exposed to vaccine virus excreted from other OPV-vaccinated infants, masking differences that may have existed shortly after the completion of the primary series.

No combined schedules of IPV and OPV have been evaluated in the United States, except for one study arm, which was part of a larger study of sequential schedules, that used one dose of OPV and IPV simultaneously at 4 months of age (IPV at 2 months, IPV/OPV at 4 months, OPV at 6 and 15 months).[338] In this trial, two doses of IPV and three doses of OPV resulted in seroprevalence levels of 99 to 100% against poliovirus types 1, 2, and 3 compared with 99 to 100% after three doses of IPV and 96 to 100% after three doses of OPV.

In developing countries, the major issue is how to improve the immunogenicity of OPV. In these settings, schedules using OPV followed by IPV were evaluated. These studies demonstrated that IPV after a primary series of OPV can correct the low immunogenicity of OPV alone that was commonly reported from tropical developing countries. In the Ivory Coast, schedules that added a dose of IPV administered simultaneously with measles vaccine, after a course of three doses of OPV administered by the routine program, resulted in a significantly higher proportion of children with antibodies against poliovirus types 1 and 3 compared with a control group that received an additional dose of OPV. Administration of a dose of IPV increased seroprevalence from 85 to 97% for poliovirus type 1 and from 76 to 92% for poliovirus type 3.[343] The experiences in the Gaza Strip

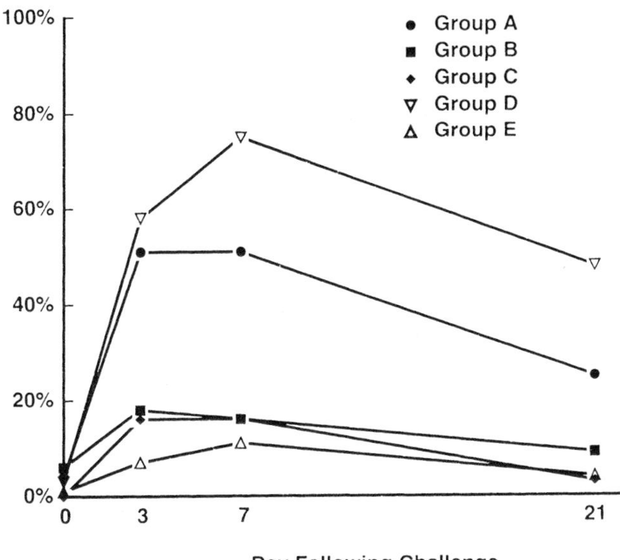

Figure 16–11. Proportion of subjects who shed polioviruses (any type) on day of challenge and 3, 7, and 21 days after challenge, by study group. Group A, 2 IPV doses, 1 OPV dose; Group B, 2 IPV doses, 2 OPV doses; Group C, 2 IPV doses, 3 OPV doses; Group D, 3 IPV doses; Group E, 3 OPV doses. See Table 16–14 for additional information. Groups B, C, and E are statistically not different. (From Modlin JF, Halsey NA, Thoms ML, et al. Humoral and mucosal immunity in infants induced by three sequential inactivated poliovirus vaccine–live attenuated oral poliovirus vaccine immunization schedules. J Infect Dis 175[suppl 1]:S228–S234, 1997.)

are of particular interest. In this area, a new combined and sequential schedule of OPV and IPV (monovalent type 1 OPV during the first month; simultaneous administration of OPV and IPV at 2 to 3 and 3 to 4 months; and OPV at 5 to 6 and 12 to 14 months) reduced the incidence of poliomyelitis during the first 3 years after the change in vaccination schedule from an annual incidence of 10 to 2.2 per 100,000 population.[340, 344, 345] In Israel after the outbreak in 1988,[346] a sequential schedule of IPV and OPV has been adopted for routine use.[347]

In the developing world, however, a large randomized trial in The Gambia, Oman, and Thailand compared the immunogenicity of (1) a combined schedule of four doses of OPV administered at birth, 6, 10, and 14 weeks and IPV administered simultaneously with OPV at 6, 10, and 14 weeks; (2) four doses of OPV administered at birth, 6, 10, and 14 weeks; and (3) three doses of IPV administered at 6, 10, and 14 weeks. The combined schedule with seven doses of poliovirus vaccines performed significantly better (95 to 99% for poliovirus type 1, 99 to 100% for poliovirus type 2, and 97 to 100% for poliovirus type 3) compared with four doses of OPV or three doses of IPV[265] (Table 16–15). In addition, the combined schedule was not affected by socioeconomic status or level of maternal antibody, in contrast to the comparison groups that received OPV or IPV, respectively. This study demonstrated that a combined schedule could correct the lower immunogenicity of OPV in developing countries, but additional doses of vaccine are required.[147] Mucosal immunity induced by the combined schedule in the IPV/OPV group was similar to that of the OPV group and significantly better than that of the IPV group.[265]

One study reported no benefit of one dose of OPV after three doses of IPV in terms of type 3 seroprevalence and mean geometric antibody titer (GMT)[348]; however, a larger study in Oman demonstrated that additional doses of OPV significantly increased seroprevalence and GMT to polioviruses types 1 and 3.[349] This study confirmed earlier observations about the incremental benefit of adding additional doses of OPV in terms of seroconversion and GMT.[68, 147, 271, 349]

Limited data are available on the persistence of poliovirus antibody induced by combined or sequential schedules of poliovirus vaccines. A single study in the United States evaluated the persistence of antibody 4 years after a primary series of sequential schedules.[350] Antibody persistence was excellent but titers decreased by 10- to 100-fold during the first 2 years of follow-up, and thereafter the titers remained relatively stable.

Despite the high immunogenicity of combined schedules in the developing world, there appears to be little need for IPV, particularly considering the success to date

Table 16–15. **PROPORTION SEROPOSITIVE FOR NEUTRALIZING ANTIBODY TO POLIOVIRUS TYPES 1, 2, AND 3 IN INFANTS IMMUNIZED WITH OPV ALONE, IPV ALONE, OR OPV AND IPV SIMULTANEOUSLY, THE GAMBIA, OMAN, AND THAILAND**

AGE AND TYPE OF VACCINES ADMINISTERED					PROPORTION SEROPOSITIVE (%)		
Birth	6 wk	10 wk	14 wk	TYPE	The Gambia (N = 118)	Oman (N = 183)	Thailand (N = 145)
OPV	OPV	OPV	OPV	1	88	90	98
				2	97	98	100
				3	72	73	100
	IPV	IPV	IPV	1	81	88	66
				2	82	92	63
				3	98	91	92
OPV	OPV/IPV	OPV/IPV	OPV/IPV	1	97	95	99
				2	100	99	100
				3	99	97	100

IPV, inactivated poliovirus vaccine; OPV, oral poliovirus vaccine.
Table constructed from data in reference 264.

in eliminating poliomyelitis from much of the developing world with use of OPV alone. Successful use of OPV alone both for routine immunization and in mass campaigns obviates the need for more costly IPV and the injections and more complex logistics required for IPV administration. Accumulating evidence demonstrates that OPV alone will continue to be the vaccine of choice for the global poliomyelitis eradication initiative.

Results of Controlled Trials of Protection Against Disease

There are no data from controlled trials of sequential schedules that used as the outcome measure the prevention of paralytic disease. Because detectable antibody to polioviruses provides an excellent correlate for protection, results of controlled trials are redundant and would be unethical to conduct.[22]

Potential Adverse Reactions With Sequential Schedules

Genetic sequencing studies suggest that reversion of Sabin strains to potentially more neurovirulent phenotypes occurs commonly after OPV administration.[351–358] Two relatively small studies[359, 360] indicated that the use of a sequential schedule may not reduce the frequency of such mutations. However, one larger study suggests that the use of a dose of IPV before two or more doses of OPV may reduce the amount of type 3 virus shed, the most common cause of VAPP, but will probably not influence the shedding of type 1 or type 2 viruses or the extent of reversion.[361]

RECOMMENDATIONS FOR VACCINE USE

Two major objectives of vaccination, protection at the youngest possible age and minimum rates of attrition (i.e., dropout) between OPV doses, govern the development of routine vaccination schedules in industrialized and developing countries. In each of these settings, an optimal balance must be found between these objectives.[68]

Industrialized Countries

Most industrialized countries, including many western European countries, Japan, Australia, and New Zealand, recommend schedules that rely exclusively on OPV for the prevention of poliomyelitis; some countries use only IPV (e.g., Finland, France, Norway, Netherlands), whereas other countries use sequential schedules of both IPV and OPV (e.g., Denmark, Lithuania, Hungary, Israel, and the United States). The major differences in the recommended schedules between industrialized and developing countries include (1) age at first dose, (2) vaccines used for each dose, (3) interval between doses, and (4) dosage volume of OPV in the United States.

The recommendations for poliomyelitis prevention in the United States were revised in 1997.[313] A sequential schedule of IPV followed by OPV is now recommended by the CDC for primary poliovirus vaccination of children in the United States. However, schedules relying only on IPV or OPV remain acceptable alternatives. The American Academy of Pediatrics recommends, with no particular preference, any of the following schedules: (1) two doses of IPV followed by two doses of OPV; (2) four doses of IPV; or (3) four doses of OPV.[331] The current vaccination schedules for the United States are outlined in Table 16–16, and the major advantages and disadvantages of the three poliovirus vaccination schedules are shown in Table 16–17.

The sequential use of IPV and OPV is recommended for infants, children, and adolescents through secondary school age (generally up to age 18 years) in the United States. The schedule consists of four doses administered at age 2 months (IPV), 4 months (IPV), 12 to 18 months (OPV), and 4 to 6 years (OPV). For people of any age, the first three doses should be separated by an interval of at least 4 weeks between doses, although a minimum interval of 6 to 8 weeks is preferred. Both IPV and OPV can be administered simultaneously with DTP or DTaP (diphtheria and tetanus toxoids and pertussis vaccine), *H. influenzae* type b vaccines, hepatitis B vaccine, varicella vaccine, and measles-mumps-rubella vaccines.

The primary series of IPV consists of three doses. In infancy, the primary schedule is usually integrated with the administration of other routine vaccines. Two doses are recommended at 2 and 4 months of age; the third dose customarily should be given 6 to 12 months after the second; however, in circumstances in which acceler-

Table 16–16. **CURRENT POLIOVIRUS VACCINE SCHEDULES IN THE UNITED STATES, 1998**

	MONTH/YEAR OF AGE				
SCHEDULE	2 mo	4 mo	6–18 mo	12–18 mo	4–6 yr
Sequential IPV/OPV*	IPV	IPV		OPV†	OPV
OPV only	OPV	OPV	OPV		OPV
IPV only	IPV	IPV	IPV		IPV

*Recommended schedule by ACIP.[313]
†OPV should be administered between 12 and 18 months.
IPV, inactivated poliovirus vaccine; OPV, oral poliovirus vaccine.
From Centers for Disease Control and Prevention. Poliomyelitis prevention in the United States: Introduction of a sequential vaccination schedule of inactivated poliovirus vaccine followed by oral poliovirus vaccine. Recommendations of the Advisory Committee on Immunization Practices. MMWR Morb Mortal Wkly Rep 46(RR3):1–25, 1997; and American Academy of Pediatrics. Poliovirus infections. In Peter G (ed). 1997 Red Book: Report of the Committee on Infectious Diseases. Elk Grove Village, IL, American Academy of Pediatrics, 1997, pp 424–433.

Table 16–17. **ADVANTAGES AND DISADVANTAGES OF THE THREE POLIOVIRUS VACCINATION SCHEDULES**

	VACCINATION SCHEDULE		
ATTRIBUTE	OPV Only	IPV Only	IPV/OPV Sequential
VAPP	8–9 cases/yr	None	Estimated 2–5 cases/yr
Other serious adverse events	None known	None known	None known
Systemic immunity	High	High	High
Mucosal immunity	High	Lower	High
Secondary transmission of vaccine virus	Yes	No	Some
Extra injections or visits needed	No	Yes	Yes
Compliance with the immunization schedule	High	Possibly reduced	Possibly reduced
Future combination vaccines	Unlikely	Likely	Likely (IPV)
Current cost	Low	Higher	Intermediate

IPV, inactivated poliovirus vaccine; OPV, oral poliovirus vaccine; VAPP, vaccine-associated paralytic poliomyelitis.
Adapted from Centers for Disease Control and Prevention. Poliomyelitis prevention in the United States: Introduction of a sequential vaccination schedule of inactivated poliovirus vaccine followed by oral poliovirus vaccine. Recommendations of the Advisory Committee on Immunization Practices. MMWR Morb Mortal Wkly Rep 46(RR3):1–25, 1997.

ated protection is needed, the minimum interval between doses of IPV is 4 weeks. All children should receive a dose of IPV (fourth dose) before or at school entry, if the third dose of IPV had been given before the fourth birthday. The fourth dose is not needed if the third dose is given on or after the fourth birthday.

The primary series with OPV alone consists of three doses. In infancy, the primary series is usually integrated with the administration of other routine vaccines. Three doses can be given at ages 2, 4, and 6 to 18 months. The minimum recommended interval between doses of OPV for routine vaccination is 6 to 8 weeks. A supplementary dose of OPV should be provided before school entry at 4 to 6 years of age, if the third dose of OPV had been administered before the fourth birthday. The fourth dose is not needed if the third dose is given on or after the fourth birthday. OPV should not be used for the primary immunization of people 18 years of age and older.

The third dose of the sequential schedule is given at 12 to 18 months of age, whereas for OPV only or IPV only, the third dose may be administered at 6 to 18 months of age. The lower limit of 12 months of age for the sequential schedule exists primarily to allow more time to diagnose immunodeficiency disorders before the first dose of OPV is administered, so that VAPP can be reduced further.

Routine immunization for adults residing in the continental United States and other industrialized countries is not believed to be necessary because of the small risk of exposure to wild poliovirus.[313, 331] However, adults who are at increased risk because of contact with a patient infected with wild poliovirus or who are working with polioviruses and those who are planning travel to an epidemic or endemic area should be immunized. Parents and other household members who do not have definite evidence of having been completely immunized should receive IPV at the time the child is vaccinated.[313, 331]

Developing Countries

The WHO-recommended schedule that calls for the administration of four doses of OPV at birth, 6, 10, and 14 weeks of age should be used for polio endemic or recently polio endemic countries. This is particularly important in areas in which frequent importation or endemic circulation of wild polioviruses takes place and in which a majority of infants are exposed to all three poliovirus types early in life.[119, 147, 340, 344] For these areas, the primary immunization schedules not only should begin early, with the first dose being given to newborns, but also—and most important—should be completed as early as possible. Many countries also recommend a dose of OPV in the second year of life, usually at age 18 months given simultaneously with DTP.

This four-dose WHO-recommended schedule is supported by data from China,[362] where a schedule that included a birth dose of OPV performed considerably better than a schedule without a birth dose, particularly for type 3 (97% versus 74% seroprevalence). These recommendations have been further supported and extended by a review of the available literature on the efficacy of early immunization with DTP and OPV.[135, 363–365]

PUBLIC HEALTH CONSIDERATIONS

Epidemiological Results of Vaccination

Surveillance data since 1980 suggest that continuing transmission of indigenous wild poliovirus has been interrupted in the United States, during a period when the country relied on OPV for immunization.[159, 312] As part of the certification of the Western Hemisphere as polio free, all countries in the Americas, including the United States, were certified free of indigenous wild poliovirus in 1994 by an International Commission convened by the Pan American Health Organization on the basis of a detailed review of available data by national committees.[286] Data on poliomyelitis incidence and OPV vaccination coverage during 1988 to 1996 by WHO region can be found in Figure 16–12.

Disease Control Strategies

In 1988, the World Health Assembly, the governing body of the WHO, resolved to eradicate polio globally

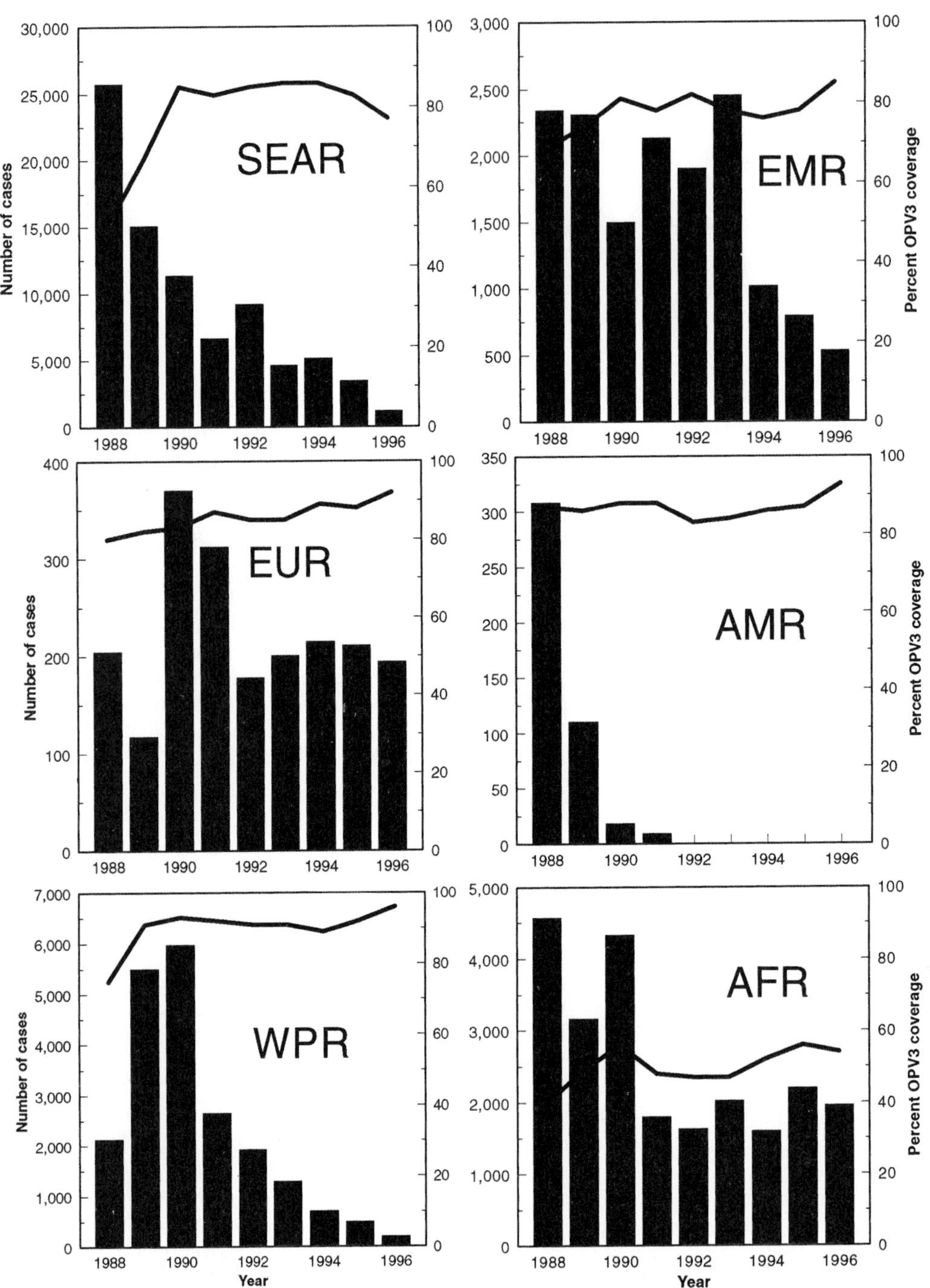

Figure 16–12. Number of reported poliomyelitis cases (bars) and coverage (lines) with three doses of oral poliovirus vaccine (OPV), by region of the World Health Organization, 1988 to 1996. AFR, African Region; AMR, American Region; EMR, Eastern Mediterranean Region; EUR, European Region; SEAR, South-East Asia Region; WPR, Western Pacific Region. (From Expanded Programme on Immunization. EPI Information System. Global Summary, August 1997. Geneva, World Health Organization, 1997.)

by the year 2000.[3] The global resolution followed the 1990 regional elimination goal established in 1985 by the countries of the Western Hemisphere. The last case of poliomyelitis associated with wild poliovirus isolation in the Americas was reported from Peru in 1991, and the entire hemisphere was certified free of indigenous wild poliovirus by an International Certification Commission in 1994.[286]

The following strategies to achieve polio eradication developed in the Western Hemisphere were adopted by WHO for worldwide implementation in all polio endemic countries[35]:

1. achieving and maintaining high routine coverage in infants younger than 1 year with at least three doses of oral poliovirus vaccine (OPV3);
2. administering supplemental doses of OPV to all young children (usually those younger than 5 years) during national immunization days to rapidly interrupt poliovirus transmission;
3. conducting "mopping up" vaccination campaigns—localized campaigns targeting high-risk areas where poliovirus transmission is most likely to persist at low levels; and
4. developing sensitive systems of epidemiological and laboratory surveillance, including establishing surveillance of cases of acute flaccid paralysis.*

Routine Immunization

Control of poliomyelitis and the global eradication initiative are greatly aided by well-functioning routine immunization programs that deliver potent OPV to a high proportion of infants in the first year of life. Global coverage with three doses of OPV among infants younger than 1 year was 81% in 1996. All WHO Regions reported a coverage of more than 80% except for the African Region, where coverage improved from 40% in 1988 to 54% in 1996 but continues to be below the coverage achieved in the other WHO Regions.[161] However, these global and regional figures may mask substantial variation in coverage reported from and within individual countries.

National Immunization Days

Mass campaigns with OPV—administered during national immunization days—are the only proven strategy to reduce widespread transmission of wild poliovirus in endemic countries.[366] National immunization days are conducted twice annually for a short period (1 to 3 days) in which one dose of OPV is administered to all children in the target age group, usually children younger than 5 years, regardless of prior vaccination history. A second dose is administered in the same way after an interval of 4 to 6 weeks. National immunization days usually take place during the low transmission season when conditions are optimal to interrupt the few remaining chains of poliovirus transmission. Most countries provide OPV during national immunization days, relying primarily on fixed sites, including vaccination clinics supplemented by a large number of temporary vaccination sites.

National immunization days are necessary in developing countries to rapidly increase immunity levels in the population to achieve and surpass herd immunity threshold levels for poliomyelitis and, hence, rapidly interrupt the transmission of poliovirus. OPV administered in campaigns also appears to be more immunogenic compared with OPV administered in the routine program,[367, 368] probably because (1) national immunization days are conducted during the low poliovirus transmission season because this is the period when the fewest chains of poliovirus transmission are maintained, (2) national immunization days are conducted during the low transmission season for other enteroviruses that may interfere with poliovirus seroconversion,[369] (3) the cold chain can be better maintained for these short campaigns, and (4) massive use of OPV probably also results in intensive secondary spread of shed virus.[265] Children residing in polio endemic countries using national immunization days may receive 13 to 14 doses of OPV by the time they reach their fifth birthday.[68, 271] These OPV doses are administered both by the routine program (three or four doses) and through national immunization days (two doses annually during the first 5 years of life). These additional doses of OPV, administered during national immunization days, should correct the lower immunogenicity of OPV commonly observed in tropical areas.

During 1985 to 1996, a total of 92 polio endemic countries conducted national immunization days (Fig. 16–13). In 1996 alone, 82 countries conducted national immunization days, providing supplemental doses of OPV to approximately 419 million children younger than 5 years (approximately two thirds of all children younger than 5 years). In 1996, national immunization days were conducted for the first time in 27 sub-Saharan countries of the African Region of WHO. These national immunization days in the African Region targeted approximately 74 million children younger than 5 years. Synchronized national immunization days were conducted in December 1996 and January 1997 in 18 contiguous countries of the European and the Eastern Mediterranean Regions of WHO, vaccinating 58 million children younger than 5 years. Synchronized national immunization days were also implemented among contiguous countries of the Eastern Mediterranean Region (Pakistan), the South Asia Region (Bangladesh, Bhutan, India, Myanmar, Nepal, Thailand), and the Western Pacific Region (China, Vietnam), vaccinating 257 million children younger than 5 years in each of two rounds. The two rounds of national immunization days in India—vaccinating 117 and 127 million children, respectively—represent the largest mass campaigns ever conducted. Even more impressive is that each round of these national immunization days was conducted in a single day.

*A confirmed case of polio is defined as acute flaccid paralysis and at least one of the following: (1) laboratory-confirmed wild poliovirus infection, (2) residual paralysis at 60 days, (3) death, or (4) no follow-up investigation at 60 days.

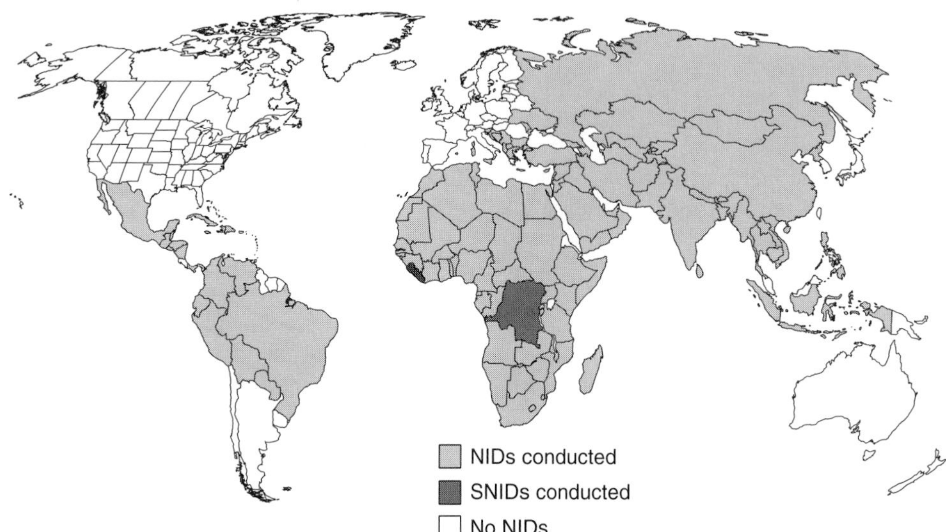

Figure 16–13. Countries that have conducted subnational immunization days (SNIDs) and national immunization days (NIDs), 1985 to 1997. NIDs needed in Sierra Leone, Liberia, and Democratic Republic of Congo.

"Mopping up" Campaigns

To eliminate the last potential or known reservoirs of wild poliovirus circulation, "mopping up" vaccination campaigns are conducted. These mopping up campaigns usually target children younger than 5 years with two doses of OPV separated by an interval of 4 to 6 weeks. In contrast to national immunization days, these campaigns include house-to-house administration of OPV to reach any children who may have been missed by national immunization days. Mopping up is a critical component to achieve interruption of the final chains of poliovirus transmission in all polio endemic countries. Risk areas, usually defined at county or district levels, to be included in mopping up include those with recent circulation of wild poliovirus (usually within the last 3 years), low vaccination coverage, suboptimal surveillance, large migrant or refugee populations, and common borders with known poliovirus endemic areas.

These supplemental immunization activities have been successful in decreasing the number of reported poliomyelitis cases globally from 35,251 in 1988 (when the polio eradication target was adopted) to 5139 in 1997, a decrease of approximately 85%[37] (Fig. 16–14). A detailed review of the current status of the polio eradication initiative was published in 1997.[370]

Surveillance

Surveillance for cases of acute flaccid paralysis and for wild poliovirus is critical for guiding programmatic activities as well as for contributing to the eventual certification of polio-free status. Systems for acute flaccid paralysis surveillance have been established in virtually all polio endemic or recently endemic countries. The major reason for using a symptom (e.g., acute flaccid paralysis) rather than a diagnosis (e.g., poliomyelitis) is to ensure that the sensitivity of the surveillance system can be maximized; all possible cases of poliomyelitis, including those with atypical presentations, will be included in the surveillance system. In addition, acute flaccid paralysis surveillance helps to monitor the quality of surveillance even in the absence of cases of poliomyelitis. In the last stages of the eradication program, no cases of poliomyelitis (except for rare cases of VAPP) would be expected to be detected. Thus, it would be impossible to determine whether the absence of poliomyelitis cases represents "true" absence or deficiencies in surveillance. On the basis of the experience in the Americas, in each population a rate of 1 case of nonpolio acute flaccid paralysis per 100,000 population younger than 15 years would be expected annually, and achievement of such a rate would indicate adequate surveillance, defined as the ability of the surveillance system to detect wild poliovirus circulation due to indigenous transmission or virus importation, should it occur.

Two regions of WHO, the Americas and the Western Pacific Regions, have achieved a rate of more than 1 nonpolio acute flaccid paralysis case per 100,000 population younger than 15 years of age; two other regions, the European and the Eastern Mediterranean Regions, are close to 1 per 100,000. Table 16–18 contains the acute flaccid paralysis rates for the different WHO Regions in 1996.[37] A number of other performance indicators are also used to monitor the quality of acute flaccid paralysis surveillance; the most important are the proportion of people with acute flaccid paralysis from whom two stool specimens were collected within 14 days after onset of paralysis and the proportion of health centers and hospitals reporting the presence or absence (i.e., "zero-case" reporting) of acute flaccid paralysis cases during the previous week. A comprehensive list of performance indicators used to monitor the quality of acute flaccid paralysis surveillance can be found in Table 16–19.

Certification of Polio Eradication

A process that started with the constitution of an International Commission for the Certification of Polio

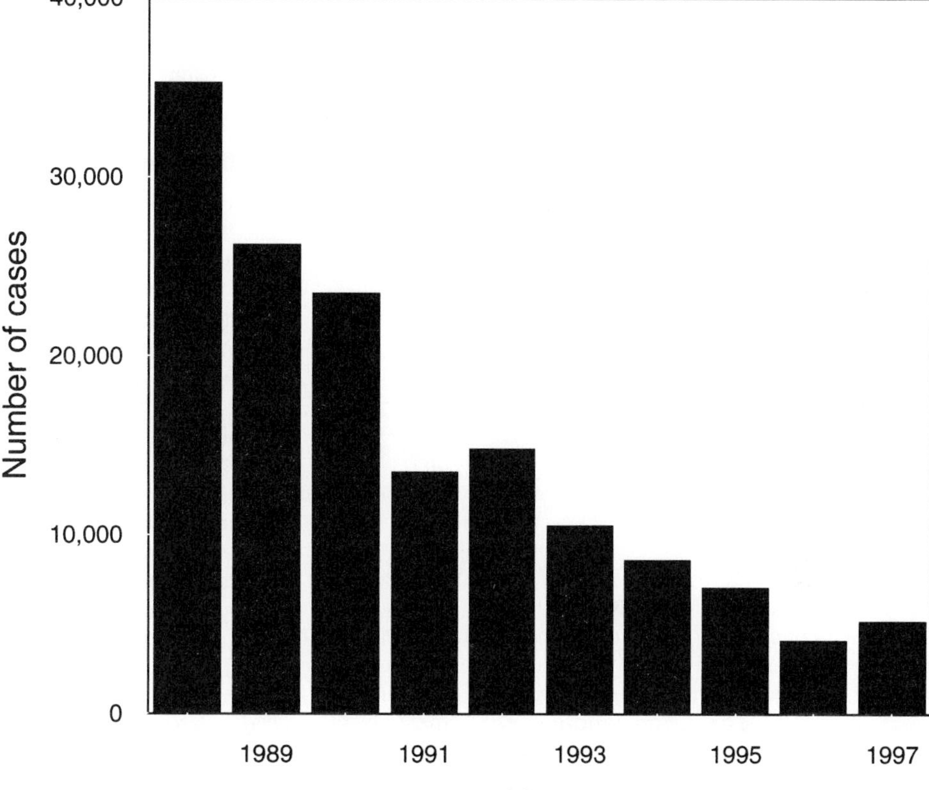

Figure 16–14. Number of reported poliomyelitis cases globally, 1988 to 1997.

Table 16–18. **CONFIRMED POLIOMYELITIS CASES AND ACUTE FLACCID PARALYSIS SURVEILLANCE INDICATORS, BY WORLD HEALTH ORGANIZATION REGION, 1995 AND 1996**

REGION	POLIO ENDEMIC OR RECENTLY ENDEMIC COUNTRIES: Number	POLIO ENDEMIC OR RECENTLY ENDEMIC COUNTRIES: Established AFP Surveillance	NONPOLIO AFP RATE: 1995	NONPOLIO AFP RATE: 1996	AFP CASES WITH TWO STOOL SPECIMENS IN 1996 (%)	NUMBER OF CONFIRMED CASES: 1995	NUMBER OF CONFIRMED CASES: 1996	REDUCTION IN CONFIRMED CASES FROM 1995 TO 1996 (%)
Africa	42	27	<0.1	<0.1	NA	2192	1949	11
America	45*	45	1.2	1.2	76	0	0	—
Eastern Mediterranean	23	20	0.5	0.7	65	789	532	33
Europe	18	16†	0.2	0.7	63	210	193	8
South-East Asia	8	8	<0.1	<0.1	39‡	3349	1203	64
Western Pacific	10	10	1.2	1.2	80	492	197	60
Total	146	137	0.4	0.6	—	7032	4074	42

*The last case of poliomyelitis attributed to indigenous wild poliovirus was detected in 1991.
†In addition, 11 countries in which poliomyelitis is not endemic conduct AFP surveillance in the European Region of WHO.
‡Percentage excludes India, for which these data are not available.
AFP, acute flaccid paralysis; NA, not available.
Data from Centers for Disease Control and Prevention (CDC). Progress toward global eradication of poliomyelitis, 1996. MMWR Morb Mortal Wkly Rep 46:579–584, 1997; and CDC. Progress toward global eradication of poliomyelitis, 1997. MMWR Morb Mortal Wkly Rep 47:414–419, 1998.

Table 16–19. **INDICATORS OF ACUTE FLACCID PARALYSIS DISEASE SURVEILLANCE AND LABORATORY PERFORMANCE**

INDICATOR	TARGET
Nonpolio AFP rate in children <15 yr	≥1/100,000
Completeness of monthly reporting	≥90%
Timeliness of monthly reporting	≥80%
Reported AFP cases investigated ≤48 hr after report	≥80%
Reported AFP cases with 2 stool specimens collected ≤14 d since onset	≥80%
Reported AFP cases with a follow-up examination at least 60 d after paralysis onset to verify the presence or absence of residual paralysis	≥80%
Specimens arriving at national laboratory <3 d of being sent	≥80%
Specimens arriving at laboratory in good condition*	>80%
Specimens with a turnaround time ≤28 d between receipt and reporting of results	≥80%
Stool specimens from which nonpolio enterovirus was isolated	≥10%

*Good condition means that on arrival, (1) there is ice or frozen icepacks or a temperature indicator (showing <8°C) in the container, (2) the specimen volume is adequate (>5 g), (3) there is no evidence of leakage or desiccation, and (4) appropriate documentation (laboratory request/reporting form) is completed.
AFP, acute flaccid paralysis.

Eradication in the WHO Region of the Americas in 1990 (which certified the entire Western Hemisphere free of polio in 1994[286]) is being replicated in each of six WHO regions, guided by the Global Certification Commission.[371] The Commission in the Americas defined four criteria on the basis of which possible poliovirus eradication could be assessed: (1) the absence of virologically confirmed cases for a period of 3 years in the presence of adequate surveillance; (2) the absence of detected wild poliovirus in tests of stools from healthy children (e.g., from the contacts of cases of acute flaccid paralysis being investigated and, when indicated, from waste water); (3) evaluation by a national certification committee convened for that purpose in the country, eventually reporting to the regional commission; and (4) establishment of appropriate measures to deal with importations.

REMAINING ISSUES

A number of issues remain unresolved despite more than 50 years of intensive study of poliomyelitis. These include

1. determination of host factors for paralytic disease;
2. pathogenesis of provocation poliomyelitis;
3. determination of molecular factors (specific mutations) that determine neurovirulence;
4. evaluation of the transgenic mice model for neurovirulence testing of OPV (preliminary results suggest that the neurovirulence test using TgPVR21 mice is excellent and at least as sensitive as the monkey test for the type 3 component of OPV; currently this testing is being expanded to the type 2 component of OPV[372]);
5. evaluation of L20b cells that express the poliovirus receptor for diagnostic purposes;
6. determination of optimal tests to process environmental samples for poliovirus; and
7. pathogenesis of postpolio syndrome.

In addition, there are a number of remaining issues that have gained prominence because of the progress achieved toward global polio eradication. Some of these issues are discussed.

Stopping Polio Vaccination After Eradication Has Been Achieved

Certification of global poliomyelitis eradication will enable discontinuation of poliovirus vaccination, eliminating the risk of VAPP and accruing savings in vaccination program costs in perpetuity. Once poliomyelitis eradication is achieved, for some period of time thereafter (before vaccination is stopped altogether), the only poliovirus administered to the population and detectable in the environment will be derived from the vaccine. Because these circumstances will be unprecedented (administration of a live virus vaccine that can be transmitted easily), it is imperative that a safe and effective strategy be developed regarding how to stop all poliovirus vaccination based on the best available scientific data. Our understanding could benefit from efforts to address a number of gaps in current knowledge: (1) Will vaccine viruses continue to circulate and cause VAPP if vaccination is stopped? (2) Will vaccine virus continue to circulate and mutate toward greater neurovirulence, increasing the risk of VAPP? and (3) Will there be carriers of wild virus (or vaccine virus) among immunodeficient people that can reseed the population at large? Whereas more knowledge is desired, the available information supports the goal of stopping vaccination once wild virus is eradicated. Billions of doses of OPV have been administered during more than 35 years of worldwide use. During these more than three decades of OPV use, there have been only rare documented instances of human carriage of vaccine virus for 1 to 2 years and in one instance for up to 7 years.[321] It remains unclear whether these rare carriers have the potential to reseed the population at large once poliovirus has been eradicated. Arguing against this possibility is the experience of countries relying exclusively on IPV, which have not detected persistent circulation of either wild or vaccine-related polioviruses, even among unvaccinated subgroups that on rare occasions have experienced wild poliovirus outbreaks. These outbreaks occurred at a time when there was much more poliovirus in the world than would be expected at the time of eradication and cessation of vaccination. Nevertheless, more data should be collected to ensure that any decision to stop vaccination has as firm a scientific basis as possible.

A series of studies are now under way in the United States and the United Kingdom to assess what proportion of immunodeficient people with or without VAPP excrete poliovirus chronically and to characterize the findings by type of immunodeficiency disorder (i.e., agammaglobulinemia, common variable immunodeficiency disorder, or selective IgA deficiency). In developing countries, children with HIV infection will be evaluated for persistence of poliovirus excretion. Another study will assess the potential contribution of immunodeficient people in developing countries to the propagation of poliovirus. Mathematical modeling and a detailed review of the available scientific data are necessary to further define parameters that may be important for the development of a strategy to stop poliovirus vaccination.

Although a number of uncertainties continue to exist, several options currently are being considered for stopping poliovirus vaccination. These options include

1. immediate discontinuation of poliovirus vaccination once the world has been certified free of wild poliovirus;
2. selective use of monovalent OPV for types 1 and 3 (because type 2 poliovirus is likely to be eradicated first, one would not need vaccination against this type, and the circulation of poliovirus type 2 could be studied in the population and the environment after discontinuation of this serotype);
3. an intermediate phase of global use of IPV;
4. region by region discontinuation of vaccination; and
5. a global immunization day with OPV followed by the immediate discontinuation of OPV.

Poliovirus Containment

In contrast to the smallpox eradication program in which the virus was restricted to a selected group of laboratories, poliovirus is used in many laboratories conducting serology, research, or vaccine production. Many laboratories store potentially infectious materials (e.g., stool, saliva specimens) that may contain polioviruses. These specimens could have been collected for studies unrelated to poliomyelitis, including studies of other enteric pathogens. In addition, the manufacturing process for IPV relies on wild polioviruses. Thus, polioviruses, either vaccine derived or wild type, may be found in many laboratories and freezers, known or unknown to the laboratory personnel.[373, 374] To recommend measures to prevent the inadvertent reintroduction of virus from the laboratory, a WHO working group developed the following three-phase plan of action in 1997:

1. Laboratories that handle wild poliovirus or potentially infectious materials should immediately institute enhanced biosafety level 2 procedures[375] and develop action plans to implement maximum level containment when required.
2. One year after the last isolation of wild poliovirus, laboratories that have wild poliovirus or potentially infectious material should implement maximum containment (biosafety level 4).
3. After OPV immunization stops, laboratories should place under high containment (biosafety level 4) all polioviruses, including OPV vaccine and vaccine-derived strains.[376]

Vaccine Stock and Destruction of Poliovirus

After achievement of polio eradication, or preferably before, decisions about the stocking of vaccine (whether OPV or IPV), the retention of seed virus for OPV or IPV production, and the destruction of poliovirus will need to be made. IPV vaccine production relies on wild-type poliovirus, and it is likely that IPV production will need to continue several years after achievement of polio eradication. There is a potential danger that wild poliovirus could escape from production facilities. A construct of other viruses expressing the surface protein of poliovirus offers the prospects of producing vaccine without reliance on infectious poliovirus. Finally, a process will need to be developed that will lead to the eventual complete destruction of all poliovirus, avoiding, it is hoped, the controversy that is still associated with the final destruction (extinction) of smallpox virus.

Certification of Polio Eradication

In recently polio endemic countries, the certification process will rely primarily on data from acute flaccid paralysis surveillance; and in countries that have been free of poliovirus for many years (and that have not implemented acute flaccid paralysis surveillance), the process will evaluate data from all relevant sources (i.e., VAPP surveillance, virological surveillance, adverse events reporting systems). Whether environmental surveillance has a role in this process remains to be determined. In the past, the usefulness of environmental surveillance has been limited in countries that routinely use OPV, because large amounts of vaccine-derived virus would be expected to be found in sewage samples, and PCR would need to be employed to amplify wild poliovirus. The use of PCR, however, is somewhat of a problem for the following two reasons: (1) sewage is "toxic" for PCR (thus, it needs to be extensively purified), and (2) to design PCR probes, one must know the RNA of the virus one is looking for (thus, only viruses that have been sequenced already can be detected with PCR). In addition, the sensitivity of environmental surveillance is unknown and needs to be evaluated, using acute flaccid paralysis reporting as the reference point.

CONCLUSION

Poliomyelitis has probably affected mankind since ancient times. It appeared as an epidemic disease in industrialized countries in the last century and the beginning of this one. Development and widespread use of poliovirus vaccines have effectively controlled poliomyelitis in industrialized countries. The global poliomyelitis eradication initiative, adopted in 1988, has led to dramatic decreases in the incidence of poliomyelitis in developing countries. Although some issues remain in regard to defining a strategy to stop vaccination after poliomyelitis eradication has been achieved, it appears likely that the eradication target will be accomplished by the year 2000 or shortly thereafter, thus relegating this once much feared crippling disease to one that future generations will know only by history.[39]

REFERENCES

1. Underwood M. A Treatise of Children with General Directions for Management of Infants from Birth (2nd ed). London, Matthews, 1789.
2. Poliomyelitis Vaccine Evaluation Center. Evaluation of the 1954 Field Trial of Poliomyelitis Vaccine. Ann Arbor, MI, Edwards Brothers, 1957.
3. World Health Assembly. Global Eradication of Poliomyelitis by the Year 2000. Geneva, World Health Organization, 1988.
4. Paul JR. A History of Poliomyelitis. New Haven, Yale University Press, 1971.
5. Heine J. Beobachtungen über Lähmungszustände der unteren Extremitäten und deren Behandlung. Stuttgart, Köhler, 1840.
6. West C. On some forms of paralysis incidental to infancy and childhood. London Med Gaz 32:829, 1843, pp 829–836.
7. Rilliet F. De la paralysie éssentielle chez les énfants. Gaz Med Paris 6:681–704, 1851.
8. de Boulogne D. De l'Electrisation Localisee et de son Application a la Physiologie, a la Pathologie et a la Therapeutique. Paris, Baillière, 1855.
9. von Heine J. Spinale Kinderlähmung. Stuttgart, Cotta, 1860.
10. Charcot JM. Groupe des myopathies de cause spinal: Paralysie infantile. Rev Phot Hop 4:1–36, 1872.
11. Frey A. Ein Fall von subakuter Lähmung Erwachsener, wahrscheinlich Poliomyelitis. Berl Klin Wochenschr 11:549–566, 1874.
12. Wickman I. Beitrage zur Kentniss der Heine-Medinschen Krankheit (Poliomyelitis acuta und verwandte Erkrankungen). Berlin, Karger, 1907.
13. Leegaard C. Die akute Poliomyelitis in Norwegen. Dtsch Z Nervenheilk 53:145–262, 1890.
14. Wickman I. Studien über Poliomyelitis acuta: Zugleich ein Beitrag zur Kentniss der Myelitis acuta. Arb Path Inst Univ Helsingfors. Vol. 1. Berlin, Karger, 1905.
15. Caverly CS. Preliminary report of an epidemic of paralytic disease, occurring in Vermont, in the summer of 1894. Yale Med J i:1–5, 1894–1895.
16. Lavinder CH, Freeman AW, Frost WH. Epidemiologic studies of poliomyelitis in New York City and the northeastern United States during the year 1916. Public Health Bull (Wash) 91, 1918.
17. Landsteiner K, Popper E. Mikroskopische Praparate von einem menschlichen und zwei Affenruckenmarken. Wien Klin Wochenschr 21:1830, 1908.
18. Burnet FM, Macnamara J. Immunological differences between strains of poliomyelitis virus. Br J Exp Pathol 12:57–61, 1931.
19. Committee on Typing of the National Foundation for Infantile Paralysis. Immunologic classification of poliomyelitis viruses: A cooperative program for the typing of one hundred strains. Am J Hyg 54:191–274, 1951.
20. Enders JF, Weller TH, Robbins FC. Cultivation of the Lansing strain of poliomyelitis virus in cultures of various human embryonic tissue. Science 109:85–87, 1949.
21. Hammon WM, Coriell LI, Stokes J. Evaluation of Red Cross gamma globulin as a prophylactic agent for poliomyelitis. I. Plan of controlled field tests and results of 1951 pilot study in Utah. JAMA 150:739–749, 1952.
22. Sutter RW, Pallansch MA, Sawyer LA, et al. Defining surrogate serologic tests with respect to predicting protective vaccine efficacy: Poliovirus vaccination. Ann N Y Acad Sci 754:289–299, 1995.
23. Brown GC, Rabson AS, Schieble JH. The effect of gamma globulin on subclinical infection in familial associates of poliomyelitis cases: II. Serological studies and virus isolations from pharyngeal secretions. J Immunol 74:71–80, 1955.
24. Horstmann DM, McCollum RW, Mascola AD. Viremia in human poliomyelitis. J Exp Med 99:355–369, 1954.
25. McKay HW, Fodor AR, Kokko UP. Viremia following administration of live poliovirus vaccines. Am J Public Health 53:274–285, 1963.
26. Nathanson N, Bodian D. Experimental poliomyelitis following intramuscular virus injection. III. The effect of passive antibody on paralysis and viremia. Bull Johns Hopkins Hosp 111:198–220, 1962.
27. Sabin AB. Oral poliovirus vaccine: History of its development and use and current challenge to eliminate poliomyelitis from the world. J Infect Dis 151:420–436, 1985.
28. Drinker P, Shaw LA. Apparatus for prolonged administration of artificial respiration: I. A design for adults and children. J Clin Invest 7:229–247, 1929.
29. Sabin AB. Paralytic consequences of poliomyelitis infection in different parts of the world and in different population groups. Am J Public Health 41:1215–1230, 1951.
30. Greenberg M, Siegel M, Magee MC. Poliomyelitis in New York City, 1949. N Y State Med J 50:1119–1123, 1950.
31. Sabin AB. Epidemiologic patterns of poliomyelitis in different parts of the world. Poliomyelitis. Papers and discussions presented at the First International Poliomyelitis Conference. Philadelpia, JB Lippincott, 1949, pp 3–33.
32. Das AN. A Study of the Trend of the Age Selection of Poliomyelitis in the United States Since 1910. Baltimore, Johns Hopkins University, 1932.
33. Olin G. The epidemiologic pattern of poliomyelitis in Sweden from 1905 to 1950. Poliomyelitis. Papers and discussions presented at the Second International Poliomyelitis Conference. Philadelpia, JB Lippincott, 1951, pp 367–375.
34. Paul JR. The National Foundation for Infantile Paralysis. A History of Poliomyelitis. New Haven, Yale University Press, 1971, pp 308–323.
35. Hull HF, Ward NA, Hull BP, et al. Paralytic poliomyelitis: Seasoned strategies, disappearing disease. Lancet 343:1331–1337, 1994.
36. de Quadros CA, Hersh BS, Olive JM, et al. Eradication of wild poliovirus from the Americas: Acute flaccid paralysis surveillance, 1988–1995. J Infect Dis 175(suppl 1):S37–S42, 1997.
37. Centers for Disease Control and Prevention. Progress toward global eradication of poliomyelitis, 1996. MMWR Morb Mortal Wkly Rep 46:579–584, 1997.
38. de Quadros CA. Global eradication of poliomyelitis and measles: Another quiet revolution. Ann Intern Med 127:156–158, 1997.
39. Foege WH. A world without polio. 'Future generations will know by history only . . . .' JAMA 270:1859–1860, 1993.
40. Horstmann DM. Clinical aspects of acute poliomyelitis. Am J Med 6:592–605, 1949.
41. Horstmann DM. Poliomyelitis: Severity and type of disease in different age groups. Ann N Y Acad Sci 61:956–967, 1955.
42. Paul JR. Clinical epidemiology of poliomyelitis. Medicine (Baltimore) 20:495–520, 1941.
43. Gelfand HM, LeBlanc DR, Fox JP, Conwell DP. Studies on the development of natural immunity to poliomyelitis in Louisiana. II. Description and analysis of episodes of infection observed in study households. Am J Hyg 65:367–385, 1957.
44. Draper G. Acute Poliomyelitis. Philadelphia, Blakiston's, 1917.
45. Bodian D. Poliomyelitis: Pathogenesis and histopathology. In Rivers TM, Horsfall FL (eds). Viral and Rickettsial Infections of Man. Philadelphia, JB Lippincott, 1959, pp 479–498.
46. Bodian D, Horstmann DM. Polioviruses. In Horsfall FL, Tamm I (eds). Viral and Rickettsial Infections of Man (4th ed). Philadelphia, JB Lippincott, 1965, pp 430–473.
47. Morens DM, Pallansch MA, Moore M. Polioviruses and other enteroviruses. In Belshe RB (ed). Textbook of Human Virology (2nd ed). St. Louis, Mosby, 1991, pp 427–497.
48. Sabin AB. Poliomyelitis. In Braude AI, Davis CE, Fierer J (eds). International Textbook of Medicine. Vol. II. Infectious Diseases and Medical Microbiology (2nd ed). Philadelphia, WB Saunders, 1986, pp 1147–1161.
49. Ramlow J, Alexander M, LaPorte R, et al. Epidemiology of postpolio syndrome. Am J Epidemiol 136:769–786, 1992.
50. Dalakas MC, Sever JL, Madden DL, et al. Late post-poliomyelitis muscular atrophy: Clinical, virological and immunological studies. Rev Infect Dis 6(suppl 2):S562–S567, 1984.
51. Dalakas MC, Bartfeld H, Kurland LT. The postpolio syndrome. Advances in the pathogenesis and treatment. Ann N Y Acad Sci 753:1–412, 1995.
52. Armstrong C. The experimental transmission of poliomyelitis to

the Eastern cotton rat, *Sigmodon hispidus hispidus*. Public Health Rep 54:1719–1721, 1939.
53. Bodian D, Morgan IM, Howe HA. Differentiation of types of poliomyelitis viruses. III. The grouping of fourteen strains into three basic immunologic types. Am J Hyg 49:234–245, 1949.
54. Kessel JF, Pait CF. Differentiation of three groups of poliomyelitis virus. Proc Soc Exp Biol Med 70:315–316, 1949.
55. Murdin AD, Lu HH, Murray MG, Wimmer E. Poliovirus antigenic hybrids simultaneously expressing antigenic determinants from all three serotypes. J Gen Virol 73:607–611, 1992.
56. Melnick JL, Ashkenazi A, Midulla VC, et al. Immunogenic potency of $MgCl_2$-stabilized oral poliovaccine. JAMA 185:406–408, 1963.
57. Toyoda H, Kohara M, Kataoka Y, et al. Complete nucleotide sequences of all three poliovirus serotype genomes: Implications of genetic relationship, gene function and antigenic determinants. J Mol Biol 174:561–585, 1984.
58. Hogle JM, Chow M, Filman DJ. Three-dimensional structure of poliovirus at 2.9 A resolution. Science 229:1358–1365, 1985.
59. Mendelsohn CL, Wimmer E, Racaniello VR. Cellular receptor for poliovirus: Molecular cloning, nucleotide sequence, and expression of a new member of the immunoglobulin superfamily. Cell 56:855–865, 1989.
60. Scharff MD, Levintow L. Quantitative study of the formation of poliovirus antigens in infected HeLa cells. Virology 19:491–500, 1963.
61. Ren R, Constanini F, Gorgacz EJ, et al. Transgenic mice expressing a human poliovirus receptor: A new model for poliomyelitis. Cell 63:353–362, 1990.
62. Freistadt MS, Stoltz DA, Eberle KE. Role of poliovirus receptors in the spread of infection. Ann N Y Acad Sci 753:37–47, 1995.
63. Freistadt MS, Fleit HB, Wimmer E. Poliovirus receptor on human blood cells: A possible extraneural site of poliovirus replication. Virology 195:798–803, 1993.
64. Bodian D, Paffenbarger RS. Poliomyelitis infection in households: Frequency of viremia and specific antibody response. Am J Hyg 60:83–98, 1954.
65. Andrus JK, de Quadros CA, Olive JM, et al. Screening of cases of acute flaccid paralysis for poliomyelitis eradication: Ways to improve specificity. Bull World Health Organ 70:591–596, 1992.
66. Dietz V, Lezana M, Garcia Sancho C, Montesano R. Predictors of poliomyelitis case confirmation at initial clinical evaluation: Implications for poliomyelitis eradication in the Americas. Int J Epidemiol 21:800–806, 1992.
67. Biellik RJ, Bueno H, Olive JM, de Quadros C. Poliomyelitis case confirmation: Characteristics for use by national eradication programmes. Bull World Health Organ 70:79–84, 1992.
68. Patriarca PA, Linkins RW, Sutter RW, Orenstein WA. Optimal schedule for the administration of oral poliovirus vaccine. In Kurstak E (ed). Measles and Poliomyelitis. Vaccine, Immunization, and Control. Wien, Springer-Verlag, 1993, pp 303–313.
69. Melnick JL. Enteroviruses: Polioviruses, coxsackieviruses, echoviruses, and newer enteroviruses. In Fields BN, Knipe DM, Chanock RM, et al (eds). Fields Virology (2nd ed). New York, Raven Press, 1990, pp 549–605.
70. Melnick JL, Mordhorst CH, Pervikov Y. Worldwide use of LBM combination pools for typing enteroviruses. Bull World Health Organ 67:327–332, 1989.
71. Expanded Programme on Immunization. Manual for the Virological Investigation of Poliomyelitis. Geneva, World Health Organization, 1990.
72. Centers for Disease Control and Prevention. Status of the global laboratory network for poliomyelitis eradication. MMWR Morb Mortal Wkly Rep 46:692–694, 1997.
73. Alexander JP, Gary HE, Pallansch MA. Duration of poliovirus excretion and its implications for acute flaccid paralysis surveillance: A review of the literature. J Infect Dis 175(suppl 1):S176–S182, 1997.
74. van Wezel AL, Hazendonk AG. Intratypic differentiation of poliomyelitis virus strains by strain-specific antisera. Intervirology 11:2–8, 1979.
75. Osterhaus ADME, van Wezel AL, Hazendonk T, et al. Monoclonal antibodies to polioviruses. Comparison of intratypic strain differentiation of poliovirus type 1 using monoclonal antibodies versus cross-absorbed antisera. Intervirology 20:129–136, 1983.
76. Jarzabek Z, Jabicka J, John A, et al. Application of monoclonal antibody panels in the virological and epidemiological review of poliomyelitis in Poland, 1981–1990. Bull World Health Organ 70:327–333, 1992.
77. Balanant J, Guillot S, Candrea A, et al. The natural genomic variability of poliovirus analysed by restriction fragment length polymorphism assay. Virology 184:645–654, 1991.
78. Yang CF, De L, Yang SJ, et al. Genotype-specific in vitro amplification of sequences of the wild type 3 polioviruses from Mexico and Guatemala. Virus Res 24:277–296, 1992.
79. De L, Nottay B, Yang CF, et al. Identification of vaccine-related polioviruses by hybridization with specific RNA probes. J Clin Microbiol 33:562–571, 1995.
80. van der Avoort HGAM, Hull BP, Hovi T, et al. Comparative study of five methods for intratypic differentiation of polioviruses. J Clin Microbiol 33:2562–2566, 1995.
81. Kew OM, Nottay BK, Rico-Hesse R, Pallansch M. Molecular epidemiology of wild poliovirus transmission. In Kurstak E, Marusyk RG, Murphy FA, van Regenmortel MHV (eds). Virus Variability, Epidemiology and Control. Applied Virology Research. Vol. 2. New York, Plenum Publishing, 1990, pp 199–221.
82. Mulders MN, Lipskaya GY, van der Avoort HGAM, et al. Molecular epidemiology of wild poliovirus type 1 in Europe, the Middle East, and the Indian subcontinent. J Infect Dis 171:1399–1405, 1995.
83. Poyry T, Kinnunen L, Kapsenberg J, et al. The type 3 poliovirus strain responsible for the outbreak in Finland in 1984–1985 is genetically related to common Mediterranean strains. J Gen Virol 71:2535–2541, 1990.
84. Rico-Hesse R, Pallansch MA, Nottay BK, Kew OM. Geographic distribution of wild poliovirus type 1 genotypes. Virology 160:311–322, 1987.
85. Kew OM, Mulders MN, Lipskaya GY, et al. Molecular epidemiology of polioviruses. Semin Virol 6:401–414, 1995.
86. Albrecht P, Enterline JC, Boone EJ, Klutch MJ. Poliovirus and polio-antibody assay in Hep-2 and Vero cell cultures. J Biol Stand 11:91–97, 1983.
87. Expanded Programme on Immunization. Report of a WHO Consultation on Polio Neutralization Antibody Assays; Nashville, TN, USA; 5–6 December 1991. Geneva, World Health Organization, 1990.
88. Expanded Programme on Immunization and Division of Communicable Diseases. Manual for the Virological Investigation of Poliomyelitis. Geneva, World Health Organization, 1990.
89. Bhatt PN, Brooks M, Fox JP. Extent of infection with poliomyelitis virus in household associates of clinical cases as determined serologically and by virus isolation using tissue culture methods. Am J Hyg 61:287–301, 1955.
90. Pettit C, Minnich LL, Shehab ZM, Ray GC. Comparison between indirect immunofluorescence and microneutralization for detection of antibodies to polioviruses. J Clin Microbiol 25:1325–1326, 1987.
91. Hodes HL, Berger R, Ainbender E, et al. Study of viral antibodies by the paper-reactive virus method. Pediatrics 37:7–18, 1966.
92. Hagenaars AM, van Delft RW, Nagel J, et al. A modified ELISA technique for the titration of antibodies to polio virus as an alternative to a virus neutralization test. J Virol Methods 6:233–239, 1983.
93. Esposito JJ. Detection of poliovirus antigens and antibodies: Microindirect haemagglutination and haemagglutination inhibition tests for poliovirus types I, II, and III. Microbios 16:29–36, 1976.
94. Rovainen M, Agboatwalla M, Stenvik M, et al. Intrathecal immune reponse and virus-specific immunoglobulin M antibodies in laboratory diagnosis of acute poliomyelitis. J Clin Microbiol 31:2427–2432, 1993.
95. Wiechers D. Electrophysiology of acute polio revisited. Utilizing newer EMG techniques in vaccine-associated disease. Ann N Y Acad Sci 753:111–119, 1995.
96. Malzberg MS, Rogg JM, Tate CA, et al. Poliomyelitis hyperintensity of the anterior horn cells on MR images of the spinal cord. AJR Am J Roentgenol 161:863–865, 1993.
97. Bernstein HGG, Clark JMP, Tunbridge RE. Acute anterior poliomyelitis among service personnel in Malta: Account of epidemic. Br Med J i:763–767, 1945.

98. Fraser FR. A study of the cerebrospinal fluid in acute poliomyelitis. J Exp Med 18:242–251, 1913.
99. Salisbury DM, Ramsay ME, White JM, Brown DW. Polio eradication: Surveillance implications for the United Kingdom. J Infect Dis 175(suppl 1):S156–S159, 1997.
100. Olive JM, Castillo C, Castro RG, de Quadros CA. Epidemiologic study of Guillain-Barré syndrome in children <15 years of age in Latin America. J Infect Dis 175(suppl 1):S160–S164, 1997.
101. Herceg A, Kennett M, Antony J, Longbottom H. Acute flaccid paralysis surveillance in Australia: The first year. Commun Dis Intell 20:403–405, 1996.
102. Grist NR, Bell EG. Enteroviral etiology of the paralytic poliomyelitis syndrome. Arch Environ Health 21:382–387, 1970.
103. Voroshilova MK, Chumakov MP. Poliomyelitis-like properties of AB-IV-Coxsackie A7 group of viruses. Prog Med Virol 2:106–170, 1959.
104. Melnick JL. Enterovirus type 71 infections: A varied clinical pattern sometimes mimicking paralytic poliomyelitis. Rev Infect Dis 6(suppl 2):S387–S390, 1984.
105. Dyken P, Krawiecki N. Neurodegenerative diseases in infancy and childhood. Ann Neurol 13:351–364, 1983.
106. Daube JR. Electrophysiologic studies in the diagnosis and prognosis of motor neuron diseases. Neurol Clin 3:473–493, 1985.
107. McKhann GM, Cornbluth DR, Ho T, et al. Clinical and electrophysiological aspects of acute paralytic diseases of children and young adults in northern China. Lancet 338:593–597, 1991.
108. Weber JT, Hatheway CL, St. Louis ME. Botulism. In Hoeprich PD, Colin Jordan M, Ronald AR (eds). Infectious Diseases. A Treatise of the Infectious Process (5th ed). Philadelphia, JB Lippincott, 1994, pp 1185–1194.
109. Hoeprich PD. Diphtheria. In Hoeprich PD, Colin Jordan M, Ronald AR (eds). Infectious Diseases (5th ed). Philadelphia, JB Lippincott, 1994, pp 373–380.
110. Sutter RW, Orenstein WA, Wassilak SG. Tetanus. In Hoeprich PD, Colin Jordan M, Ronald AR (eds). Infectious Diseases (5th ed). Philadelphia, JB Lippincott, 1994, pp 1175–1185.
111. Paul JR, Riordan JT, Melnick JL. Antibodies to three different antigenic types of poliomyelitis virus in sera of North Alaskan Eskimos. Am J Hyg 54:275–285, 1951.
112. Salk J. Requirements for persisting immunity to poliomyelitis. Trans Assoc Am Physicians 69:105–114, 1956.
113. Aycock WL. A milk-borne epidemic of poliomyelitis. Am J Hyg 7:791–803, 1927.
114. Bancroft PM, Engelhard WE, Evans C. Poliomyelitis in Huskerville (Lincoln) Nebraska. Studies indicating a relationship between clinically severe infection and proximate fecal pollution of water. JAMA 164:836–847, 1957.
115. Horstmann DM, Paul JR. The incubation period in human poliomyelitis and its implications. JAMA 135:11–14, 1947.
116. Melnick JL, Ledinko N. Development of neutralizing antibodies against the three types of poliomyelitis virus during an epidemic period. The ratio of inapparent infection to clinical poliomyelitis. Am J Hyg 58:207–222, 1953.
117. Penttinen K, Patiala R, Bremer D. The paralytic/infected ratio in a susceptible population during a polio type 1 epidemic. Ann Med Exp Fenn 39:195–202, 1961.
118. Bernier RH. Some observations on poliomyelitis lameness surveys. Rev Infect Dis 6(suppl 2):S371–S375, 1984.
119. Patriarca PA, Sutter RW, Oostvogel PM. Outbreaks of poliomyelitis, 1976–1995. J Infect Dis 175(suppl 1):S165–S172, 1997.
120. Bradford Hill AB, Knowelden J. Inoculation and poliomyelitis. A statistical investigation in England and Wales in 1949. Br Med J 2:1–6, 1950.
121. Sutter RW, Patriarca PA, Suleiman AJM, et al. Attributable risk of DTP (diphtheria-tetanus toxoids and pertussis vaccine) injection in provoking paralytic poliomyelitis during a large outbreak in Oman. J Infect Dis 165:444–449, 1992.
122. Lambert SM. A yaws campaign and an epidemic of poliomyelitis in Western Samoa. J Trop Med Hyg 39:41–46, 1936.
123. Korns RF, Albrecht RM, Locke FB. The association of parenteral injections with poliomyelitis. Am J Public Health 42:153–169, 1952.
124. Trueta J, Hodes R. Provoking and localising factors in poliomyelitis. An experimental study. Lancet 1:998–1001, 1954.
125. Horstmann DM. Acute poliomyelitis: Relation of physical activity at the time of onset to the course of the disease. JAMA 142:236–241, 1950.
126. Talmey M. Predisposing factors in infantile paralysis. N Y Med J 104:202–204, 1916.
127. Aycock WL. Frequency of poliomyelitis in pregnancy. N Engl J Med 225:405–408, 1941.
128. Aycock WL. Tonsillectomy and poliomyelitis. I. Epidemiological considerations. Medicine (Baltimore) 21:65–94, 1942.
129. Sabin AB. Experimental poliomyelitis by the tonsillopharyngeal route with special reference to the influence of tonsillectomy on the development of bulbar paralysis. JAMA 111:605–610, 1938.
130. von Magnus H, Melnick JL. Tonsillectomy in experimental poliomyelitis. Am J Hyg 48:113–125, 1948.
131. Ogra PL. Effect of tonsillectomy and adnoidectomy on nasopharyngeal antibody response to polivirus. N Engl J Med 284:59–64, 1971.
132. Ogra PL, Karzon DT. Formation and function of poliovirus antibody in different tissues. Prog Med Virol 13:156–193, 1971.
133. Bernkopf H, Medalie J, Yekutiel M. Antibodies to poliomyelitis virus and socioeconomic factors influencing their frequency in children in Israel. Am J Trop Med 1957:697–703, 1957.
134. Pal SR, Banerjee G, Aikat BK. Serological investigation on endemicity of poliomyelitis in Calcutta and in a neighboring rural area. Indian J Med Res 54:507–511, 1966.
135. Sutter RW, Patriarca PA, Suleiman AJM, et al. Paralytic poliomyelitis in Oman: Association between regional differences in attack rate and variations in antibody responses to oral poliovirus vaccine. Int J Epidemiol 22:936–944, 1993.
136. Swartz TA, Skalska P, Gerichter CG, Cockburn WC. Routine administration of oral polio vaccine in a subtropical area. Factors possibly affecting sero-conversion. J Hyg (Camb) 70:719–726, 1972.
137. Herndon CN, Jennings RG. A twin-family study of susceptibility to poliomyelitis. Am J Hum Genet 3:17–46, 1951.
138. van Eden W, Persijn GG, Bijerk H, et al. Differential resistance to paralytic poliomyelitis controlled by histocompatibility leukocyte antigens. J Infect Dis 147:422–426, 1983.
139. Wyatt HV. Is poliomyelitis a genetically-determined disease? I. A genetic model. Med Hyotheses 1:35–42, 1975.
140. Prevots DR, Ciofi M, Sallabanda A, et al. Outbreak of paralytic poliomyelitis in Albania, 1996: High attack rate among adults and apparent interruption of transmission following nationwide mass vaccination. Clin Infect Dis 26:419–425, 1998.
141. Allmond W, Froeschle JE, Gilloud NB. Paralytic poliomyelitis in large laboratory primates. Am J Epidemiol 85:229–239, 1967.
142. Goodall J. The Chimpanzees of Gombe. Boston, Belkap Press of Harvard University, 1986, pp 92–94.
143. Ruch TC. Diseases of Laboratory Primates. London, WB Saunders, 1967, pp 408–410.
144. Dowdle WR, Birmingham ME. The biologic principles of poliovirus eradication. J Infect Dis 175(suppl 1):S286–S292, 1997.
145. Furesz J, Armstrong RE, Contreras G. Viral and epidemiological links between poliomyelitis outbreaks in unprotected communities in Canada and the Netherlands [letter]. Lancet 2:1248, 1978.
146. Schonberger LR, Kaplan J, Kim-Farley R, et al. Control of paralytic poliomyelitis in the United States. Rev Infect Dis 6(suppl 2):S424–S426, 1984.
147. Patriarca PA, Wright PF, John TJ. Factors affecting the immunogenicity of oral poliovirus vaccine in developing countries: Review. Rev Infect Dis 13:926–939, 1991.
148. Sutter RW, Patriarca PA, Brogan S, et al. Outbreak of paralytic poliomyelitis in Oman: Evidence for widespread transmission among fully vaccinated children. Lancet 338:715–720, 1991.
149. Melnick JL. Live attenuated poliovirus vaccines. In Plotkin SA, Mortimer EA (eds). Vaccines. Philadelphia, WB Saunders, 1994, pp 155–204.
150. Otten MW, Deming MS, Jaiteh KO, et al. Epidemic poliomyelitis in The Gambia following the control of poliomyelitis as an endemic disease. I. Descriptive findings. Am J Epidemiol 135:381–392, 1992.
151. Afif H, Sutter RW, Kew OM, et al. Outbreak of poliomyelitis in Gizan, Saudi Arabia: Cocirculation of wild type 1 polioviruses from three separate origins. J Infect Dis 175(suppl 1):S71–S75, 1997.
152. Reichler MR, Abbas A, Kharabsheh S, et al. Outbreak of paralytic

poliomyelitis in a highly immunized population in Jordan. J Infect Dis 175(suppl 1):S62–S70, 1997.
153. Melnick JL, Benyesh-Melnik M, Pena R, Yow M. Effectiveness of Salk vaccine. Analysis of virologically confirmed cases of paralytic and nonparalytic poliomyelitis. JAMA 175:1159–1162, 1961.
154. Bottiger M. Long-term immunity following vaccination with killed poliovirus vaccine in Sweden, a country with no circulating poliovirus. Rev Infect Dis 6(suppl 2):S548–S551, 1984.
155. Lapinleimu K. Elimination of poliomyelitis in Finland. Rev Infect Dis 6(suppl 2):S456–S460, 1984.
156. Grachev VP. Long-term use of oral poliovirus vaccine from Sabin strains in the Soviet Union. Rev Infect Dis 6(suppl 2):S321–S322, 1984.
157. Nathanson N. Epidemiologic aspects of poliomyelitis eradication. Rev Infect Dis 6(suppl 2):S308–S312, 1984.
158. Sabin AB. Oral poliovirus vaccine—recent results and recommendations for optimum use. R Soc Health J 82:51–59, 1962.
159. Strebel PM, Sutter RW, Cochi SL, et al. Epidemiology of poliomyelitis in the United States one decade after the last reported case of indigenous wild virus–associated disease. Clin Infect Dis 14:568–579, 1992.
160. Cruz RR. Cuba: Mass polio vaccination program. Rev Infect Dis 6(suppl 2):S408–S412, 1984.
161. Expanded Programme on Immunization. EPI Information System. Global Summary, August 1997. Geneva, World Health Organization, 1997.
162. Heymann DL, Murphy K, Brigaud M, et al. Oral poliovirus vaccine in tropical Africa: Greater impact on incidence of paralytic disease than expected from coverage surveys and seroconversion rates. Bull World Health Organ 65:495–501, 1987.
163. Risi JB. The control of poliomyelitis in Brazil. Rev Infect Dis 6(suppl 2):S400–S403, 1984.
164. Hatziandreu EJ, Palmer CS, Halpern MT, Brown RE. A Cost Benefit Analysis of OPV. Final Report. Arlington, Batelle, 1994.
165. Centers for Disease Control. Summary of Notifiable Diseases, United States, 1990. MMWR Morb Mortal Wkly Rep 39:1–61, 1991.
166. World Health Organization. Poliomyelitis in 1980. Parts 1 and 2. Wkly Epidemiol Rec 56:329–332, 337–341, 1981.
167. Kubli D, Steffen R, Schar M. Importation of poliomyelitis in industrialised nations between 1975 and 1984: Evaluation and conclusions for vaccination recommendations. Br Med J 295:169–171, 1987.
168. Oostvogel PM, van Wijngaarden JK, van der Avoort HGAM, et al. Poliomyelitis in an unvaccinated community in the Netherlands, 1992–1993. Lancet 344:665–670, 1994.
169. Bernal A, Garcia-Saiz A, Liacer A, et al. Poliomyelitis in Spain, 1982–1984: Virologic and epidemiologic studies. Am J Epidemiol 126:69–76, 1987.
170. Centers for Disease Control. Poliomyelitis—Pennsylvania, Maryland. MMWR Morb Mortal Wkly Rep 28:49–50, 1979.
171. Aylward RB, Porta D, Fiore L, et al. Unimmunized gypsy populations and implications for the eradication of poliomyelitis in Europe. J Infect Dis 175(suppl 1):S86–S88, 1997.
172. Mulders NM, van Loon AM, van der Avoort HGAM, et al. Molecular characterization of a wild poliovirus type 3 epidemic in the Netherlands (1992 and 1993). J Clin Microbiol 33:3252–3256, 1995.
173. World Health Organization. Poliomyelitis outbreak, Bulgaria. Wkly Epidemiol Rec 67:336–337, 1992.
174. Strebel PM, Aubert-Cambiescu A, Ion-Nedelcu N, et al. Paralytic poliomyelitis in Romania, 1984–1992: Evidence for a high risk of vaccine-associated disease and reintroduction of wild-virus infection. Am J Epidemiol 140:1111–1124, 1994.
175. Kew OM, Nathanson N. Molecular epidemiology of viruses. Semin Virol 6:357–358, 1995.
176. Lipskaya GY, Chervonskaya EA, Belova GI, et al. Geographical genotypes (geotypes) of poliovirus case isolates from the former Soviet Union: Relatedness to other known poliovirus genotypes. J Gen Virol 76:1687–1699, 1995.
177. Pinheiro FP, Kew OM, Hatch MH, da Silveira CM. Eradication of wild poliovirus from the Americas: Wild poliovirus surveillance—laboratory issues. J Infect Dis 175(suppl 1):S43–S49, 1997.
178. Netter A. Serotherapie de la poliomyélite. Nos resultats chez 30 malades: Indications, techniques, incidents possible. Bull Acad Med Paris 74:403–423, 1915.
179. Paul JR. Convalescent Serum Therapy. A History of Poliomyelitis. New Haven, Yale University Press, 1971, pp 190–199.
180. Flexner S, Lewis PA. Experimental poliomyelitis in monkeys: Active immunization and passive protection. JAMA 54:1780–1782, 1910.
181. Gelfand HM, Fox JP, LeBlanc DR, Elveback L. Studies on the development of natural immunity to poliomyelitis in Louisiana: V. Passive transfer of polio antibody from mother to fetus, and natural decline and disappearance of antibody in the infant. J Immunol 85:46–55, 1960.
182. Hammon WM, Coriell LL, Wehrle PF. Evaluation of Red Cross gamma globulin as a prophylactic agent for poliomyelitis. IV. Final report of results based on clinical diagnosis. JAMA 151:1272–1285, 1953.
183. National Advisory Committee for the Evaluation of Gamma Globulin in the Prophylaxis of Poliomyelitis. An Evaluation of the Efficacy of Gamma Globulin in the Prophylaxis of Paralytic Poliomyelitis as Used in the United States 1953. Publication No. 358. Washington, DC, US Public Health Service, 1954.
184. Department of Drugs. Drug Evaluations. Annual 1991. Milwaukee, American Medical Association, 1991.
185. O'Neal KM, Pallansch MA, Winkelstein JA, et al. Chronic group A coxsackievirus infection in agammglobulinemia: Demonstration of genomic variation of serotypically identical isolates persistently excreted by the same patient. J Infect Dis 157:183–186, 1988.
186. Davis LE, Bodian D, Price D, et al. Chronic progressive poliomyelitis secondary to vaccination of an immunodeficient child. N Engl J Med 297:214–245, 1977.
187. Flexner S, Lewis PA. Experimental poliomyelitis in monkeys. Seventh and eighth notes. JAMA 54:1789, 1910.
188. Romer PH. Die epidemische Kinderlähmung (Heine-Medinsche Krankheit). Berlin, Springer, 1911.
189. Brodie M, Goldblum A. Active immunization against poliomyelitis in monkeys. J Exp Med 53:885–893, 1931.
190. Brodie M. Active immunization against poliomyelitis. J Exp Med 56:493–505, 1932.
191. Brodie M, Park WH. Active immunization against poliomyelitis. N Y State J Med 35:815–818, 1935.
192. Brodie M, Park WH. Active immunization against poliomyelitis. JAMA 105:1089–1093, 1935.
193. Kolmer JA. Susceptibility and immunity in relation to vaccination in acute anterior poliomyelitis. JAMA 105:1956–1963, 1935.
194. Leake JP. Poliomyelitis following vaccination against this disease. JAMA 105:2152, 1936.
195. Koprowski H, Jervis GA, Norton TW. Immune responses in human volunteers upon oral administration of a rodent-adapted strain of poliomyelitis virus. Am J Hyg 55:108–126, 1952.
196. Li CP, Schaeffer M, Nelson DB. Experimentally produced variants of poliomyelitis virus combining in vivo and in vitro techniques. Ann N Y Acad Sci 61:902–910, 1955.
197. Melnick JL. Variation in poliomyelitis virus on serial passage through tissue culture. Cold Spring Harb Symp Quant Biol 18:178–179, 1953.
198. Sabin AB, Hennessen WA, Winsser J. Studies on variants of poliomyelitis virus. I. Experimental segregation and properties of avirulent variants of three immunologic types. J Exp Med 99:551–576, 1954.
199. Poliomyelitis. Papers and discussions presented at the 4th International Poliomyelitis Conference. Philadelphia, JB Lippincott, 1958.
200. Poliomyelitis. Papers and discussions presented at the 5th International Poliomyelitis Conference. Philadelphia, JB Lippincott, 1961.
201. Pan American Health Organization. Live Poliovirus Vaccines. Washington, DC, Pan American Health Organization, 1960.
202. Pan American Sanitary Bureau. Live Poliovirus Vaccines. Washington, DC, Pan American Sanitary Bureau, 1959.
203. Sabin AB. Present position of immunization against poliomyelitis with live virus vaccines. Br Med J 1:663–680, 1959.
204. Koprowski H. Live poliomyelitis virus vaccines. JAMA 178:1151–1155, 1961.
205. Paul JR. Status of vaccination against poliomyelitis, with particu-

lar reference to oral vaccination. N Engl J Med 264:651–658, 1961.
206. Koprowski H. The 10th Anniversary of the Development of Live Poliovirus Vaccine. In Second International Conference on Live Poliovirus Vaccines. Wahington, DC, Pan American Health Organization, 1960.
207. Sabin AB. Properties and behaviour of orally administered attenuated poliovirus vaccine. JAMA 164:1216–1223, 1957.
208. Melnick JL. Problems associated with the use of live poliovirus vaccine. Am J Public Health 50:1013–1031, 1960.
209. Melnick JL. Tests for safety of live poliovirus vaccine. Acad Med N J Bull 6:146–167, 1960.
210. Melnick JL, Benyesh-Melnick M, Brennan JC. Studies on live poliovirus vaccine. Its neurotropic activity in monkeys and its increased neurovirulence after multiplication in vaccinated children. JAMA 171:1165–1172, 1959.
211. Melnick JL. Attenuation of poliomyelitis viruses on passage through tissue culture. Fed Proc 13:505, 1954.
212. Murray R, Kirschstein R, van Hoosier G, Baron S. Comparative virulence for rhesus monkeys of poliovirus strains used for oral administration. In 1st International Conference on Live Poliovirus Vaccines. Washington, DC, Pan American Sanitary Bureau, 1959, pp 39–64.
213. Westrop GD, Wareham KA, Evans DMA, et al. Genetic basis of attenuation of the Sabin type 3 oral poliovirus vaccine. J Virol 63:1338–1344, 1989.
214. Racaniello VR. Poliovirus neurovirulence. Adv Virus Res 35:217–246, 1988.
215. Mento SJ, Weeks-Levy C, Tatem JM, et al. Significance of a newly identified attenuating mutation in Sabin 3 oral poliovirus vaccine. Dev Biol Stand 78:93–100, 1993.
216. Ren R, Moss EG, Racaniello VR. Identification of two determinants that attenuate vaccine-related type 2 poliovirus. J Virol 65:1377–1382, 1991.
217. Macadam AJ, Pollard SR, Gerguson G, et al. The 5′ noncoding region of the type 2 poliovirus vaccine strain contains determinants of attenuation and temperature sensitivity. Virology 181:451–458, 1991.
218. Horwitz A, Martins da Silva M, Bica AN. Large-scale field studies with live attenuated polioviruses in the Americas. In 5th International Poliomyelitis Conference. Philadelphia, JB Lippincott, 1961, pp 221–227.
219. Cox HR, Cabasso VJ, Markham FS, et al. Immunologic response to trivalent oral poliomyelitis vaccine. In 1st International Conference on Live Poliovirus Vaccines. Washington, DC, Pan American Sanitary Bureau, 1959, pp 229–248.
220. Voroshilova MK. Influence of dose and schedule of oral immunization of people with live poliovirus vaccine on antibody response. In 5th International Poliomyelitis Conference. Philadelphia, JB Lippincott, 1961, pp 296–303.
221. Verlinde JD, Wilterdink JB. A small-scale trial on vaccination and revaccination with live attenuated polioviruses in the Netherlands. In 1st International Conference on Live Poliovirus Vaccines. Washington, DC, Pan American Sanitary Bureau, 1959, pp 355–366.
222. Embil J, Gervais L, Hermandez Miyares C, Cardelle G. Use of attenuated live poliovirus vaccine in Cuban children. In Second International Conference on Live Poliovirus Vaccines. Washington, DC, Pan American Health Organization, 1960, pp 365–370.
223. Kimball AC, Barr RN, Bauer H, et al. Minnesota studies with oral poliomyelitis vaccine. Community spread of orally administered attenuated poliovirus vaccine strains. In Second International Conference on Live Poliovirus Vaccines. Washington, DC, Pan American Health Organization, 1960, pp 161–173.
224. Krugman S, Warren J, Eiger MS, et al. Immunization of newborn infants with live attenuated poliovirus vaccine. In Second International Conference on Live Poliovirus Vaccines. Washington, DC, Pan American Health Organization, 1960, pp 315–321.
225. Paul JR, Horstmann DM, Riordan JT, et al. The capacity of live attenuated polioviruses to cause human infection and to spread within families. In Second International Conference on Live Poliovirus Vaccines. Washington, DC, Pan American Health Organization, 1960, pp 174–184.
226. Tomlinson AJH, Davies J. Trial of live attenuated poliovirus vaccine: A report to the Public Health Laboratory Service from the Poliomyelitis Vaccines Committee of the Medical Research Council. Br Med J 2:1037–1044, 1961.
227. Voroshilova MK, Zhevandrova VI, Tolskaya EA, et al. Virologic and serologic investigations of children immunized with trivalent live vaccine from A. B. Sabin's strains. In Second International Conference on Live Poliovirus Vaccines. Washington, DC, Pan American Health Organization, 1960, pp 240–265.
228. Zhdanov VM, Chumakov MP, Smorodintsev AA. Large-scale practical trials and use of live poliovirus vaccine in the USSR. In Second International Conference on Live Poliovirus Vaccines. Washington, DC, Pan American Health Organization, 1960, pp 576–588.
229. Ramos Alvarez M, Gomez Santos F, Rivera LR, Mayes O. Viral and serological studies in children immunized with live poliovirus vaccine—preliminary report of a large trial conducted in Mexico. In 1st International Conference on Live Poliovirus Vaccines. Washington, DC, Pan American Sanitary Bureau, 1959, pp 483–494.
230. Ramos Alvarez M, Bustamante ME, Alvarez Alba R. Use of Sabin's live poliovirus vaccine in Mexico. Results of a large-scale trial. In Second International Conference on Live Poliovirus Vaccines. Washington, DC, Pan American Health Organization, 1960, pp 386–409.
231. Robertson HE, Acker MS, Dillenberg HO, et al. Community-wide use of a "balanced" trivalent oral poliovirus vaccine (Sabin): A report of the 1961 trial at Prince Albert, Saskatchewan. Can J Public Health 53:179–191, 1962.
232. Food and Drug Administration. Additional standards for viral vaccines; poliovirus vaccine live oral; final rule (21 CFR Part 630). Federal Register 56:21418–21438, 1991.
233. Public Health Service. Public Health Service Regulations. Biological Products. Title 42, Part 73. Washington, DC, US Department of Health, Education and Welfare, 1967.
234. Patriarca PA, Laender F, Palmeira G, et al. Randomised trial of alternative formulations of oral poliovaccine in Brazil. Lancet 1:429–433, 1988.
235. World Health Organization. Report of the 13th Global Advisory Group Meeting; Cairo, Egypt; 14–18 October, 1990. Geneva, World Health Organization, 1991.
236. Lederle Laboratories. Poliovirus Vaccine Live Oral Trivalent [package insert]. Pearl River, NY, Lederle Laboratories, 1993.
237. Global Programme for Vaccines and Immunization. International List of Availability of Vaccines and Sera. Geneva, World Health Organization, 1995.
238. Domok I. Experiences associated with the use of live poliovirus vaccine in Hungary, 1959–1982. Rev Infect Dis 6(suppl 2):S413–S418, 1984.
239. Schoub BD, Johnson S, McAnererney J, et al. Monovalent neonatal polio immunization—a strategy for the developing world. J Infect Dis 157:836–839, 1988.
240. World Health Organization. Requirements for Poliomyelitis Vaccine (Oral). Requirements for Biological Substances No. 7 (Revised 1989). Geneva, World Health Organization, 1990.
241. Wallis C, Melnick JL. Stabilization of poliovirus by cations. Tex Rep Biol Med 19:683–700, 1961.
242. Petersen I, von Magnus H. Polio neutralization tests with $MgCl_2$-stabilized virus. Acta Pathol Microbiol Scand 61:652–653, 1964.
243. Yofe J, Goldblum N, Eylan E, Melnick JL. An outbreak of poliomyelitis in Israel in 1961 and the use of attenuated type 1 vaccine in its control. Am J Hyg 76:225–238, 1962.
244. Mirchamsy H, Shafyi A, Mahinpour M, Nazari P. Stabilizing effect of magnesium chloride and sucrose on Sabin live polio vaccine. Dev Biol Stand 41:255–257, 1978.
245. Milstien JB, Lemon SM, Wright PF. Development of a more thermostable poliovirus vaccine. J Infect Dis 175(suppl 1):S247–S253, 1997.
246. Expanded Programme on Immunization. The Vaccine Vial Monitor. Geneva, World Health Organization, 1994.
247. Ghendon Y. WHO recommendations on potential use of a new poliomyelits vaccine. Dev Biol Stand 78:133–139, 1993.
248. Vonka V, Janda Z, Simon J, et al. A new type 3 attenuated poliovirus for possible use in oral poliovirus vaccine. Prog Med Virol 9:204–255, 1967.
249. Melnick JL, Berencsi G, Biberi-Moroeanu S, et al. WHO collab-

orative studies on poliovirus type 3 strains isolated during the 1968 poliomyelitis epidemic in Poland. Bull World Health Organ 47:287–294, 1972.
250. Kew OM, Nottay BK. Molecular epidemiology of polioviruses. Rev Infect Dis 6(suppl 2):S499–S504, 1984.
251. Kew OM, De L, Yang CF, et al. The role of virologic surveillance in the global initiative to eradicate poliomyelitis. In Kurstak E (ed). Control of Virus Diseases. New York, Marcel Dekker, 1993, pp 215–246.
252. Nathanson N, Horn SD. Neurovirulence tests of type 3 poliovirus vaccine manufactured by Lederle Laboratories, 1964–1988. Vaccine 10:469–474, 1992.
253. Brown F, Lewis BP. Poliovirus Attenuation: Molecular Mechanisms and Practical Aspects. Developments in Biological Standardization. Vol. 78. Basel, S Karger, 1993.
254. Kohara M, Abe S, Kuge S, et al. An infectious cDNA clone of the poliovirus Sabin strain could be used as a stable repository and inoculum for the oral live vaccine. Virology 151:21–30, 1986.
255. Racaniello VR, Baltimore D. Cloned poliovirus complementary DNA is infectious in mammalian cells. Science 214:915–919, 1981.
256. Paul JR, Riordan JT, Melnick JL. Antibodies to three different antigenic types of poliomyelitis virus in sera from North American Eskimos. Am J Hyg 54:275–285, 1951.
257. Sabin AB. Transitory appearance of type 2 neutralizing antibody in patients infected with type 1 poliomyelitis virus. J Exp Med 96:99–106, 1956.
258. Hammon WM, Ludwig EH. Possible protective effect of previous type 2 infection against paralytic poliomyelitis due to type 1 virus. Am J Hyg 66:274–280, 1957.
259. Bogger-Goren S, Baba K, Hurly P, et al. Antibody response to varizella-zoster virus after natural and vaccine-induced infection. J Infect Dis 146:260–265, 1982.
260. Horstmann DM, Opton EM, Klemperer R, et al. Viremia in infants vaccinated with oral poliovirus vaccine (Sabin). Am J Hyg 79:47–63, 1964.
261. Melnick JL, Proctor RO, Ocampo AR, et al. Free and bound virus in serum after administration of oral poliovirus vaccine. Am J Epidemiol 84:329–342, 1966.
262. Benyesh-Melnick M, Melnick JL, Rawls WE, et al. Studies on the immunogenicity, communicability and genetic stability of oral poliovaccine administered during the winter. Am J Epidemiol 86:112–136, 1967.
263. McBean AM, Thoms ML, Albrecht P, et al. Serologic response to oral polio vaccine and enhanced-potency inactivated polio vaccines. Am J Epidemiol 128:615–628, 1988.
264. WHO Collaborative Study Group on Oral and Inactivated Poliovirus Vaccines. Response to an Infant Immunization Schedule Combining Oral and Inactivated Poliovirus Vaccines. Compared With Either Vaccine Alone. Results of a Randomized Trial in The Gambia, Oman, and Thailand. Final Report. Geneva, World Health Organization, 1995.
265. WHO Collaborative Study Group on Oral and Inactivated Poliovirus Vaccines. Combined immunization of infants with oral and inactivated poliovirus vaccines: Results of a randomized trial in The Gambia, Oman, and Thailand. J Infect Dis 175(suppl 1):S215–S227, 1997.
266. World Health Organization Collaborative Study Group on Oral Poliovirus Vaccine. Factors affecting the immunogenicity of oral poliovirus vaccine: A prospective evaluation in Brazil and The Gambia. J Infect Dis 171:1097–1106, 1995.
267. Posey DL, Linkins RW, Oliveria MJ, et al. The effect of diarrhea on oral poliovirus vaccine failure in Brazil. J Infect Dis 175(suppl 1):S258–S263, 1997.
268. Zaman S, Carlsson B, Morikawa A, et al. Poliovirus antibody titres, relative affinity, and neutralizing capacity in maternal milk. Arch Dis Child 68:198–201, 1993.
269. Ogra SS, Weintraub DI, Ogra PL. Immunologic aspects of human colostrum and milk: Interaction with the intestinal immunity of the neonate. Adv Exp Med Biol 107:95–107, 1978.
270. Palmer EL, Gary GW, Black R, Martin ML. Antiviral activity of colostrum and serum immunoglobulins A and G. J Med Virol 5:123–129, 1980.
271. Patriarca PA, Linkins RW, Sutter RW. Poliovirus vaccine formulations. In Kurstak E (ed). Measles and Poliomyelitis. Vaccine, Immunization, and Control. Wien, Springer-Verlag, 1993, pp 265–277.
272. Sutter RW, Patriarca PA. Inactivated and live, attenuated poliovirus vaccines: Mucosal immunity. In Kurstak E (ed). Measles and Poliomyelitis. Vaccines, Immunization and Control. Wien, Springer-Verlag, 1993, pp 279–294.
273. Smorodintsev AA, Davidenkova EF, Drobyshevskaya AI, et al. Results of a study of the reactogenic and immunogenic properties of live antipoliomyelitis vaccine. Bull World Health Organ 20:1053–1074, 1959.
274. Nishio O, Ishihara Y, Sakae K, et al. The trend of acquired immunity with live poliovirus vaccine and the effect of revaccination: Follow-up of vaccinees for ten years. J Biol Stand 12:1–10, 1984.
275. Janda Z, Adam E, Vonka V. Properties of a new type 3 attenuated poliovirus. VI. Alimentary tract resistance in children fed previously with type 3 Sabin vaccine to reinfection with homologous and heterologous type 3 attenuated poliovirus. Arch Virusforsch 20:87–98, 1967.
276. Soloviev VD. Problems connected with live polio vaccine. In 5th International Poliomyelitis Conference. Philadelphia, JB Lippincott, 1961, pp 403–410.
277. Rossen RD, Kasel JA, Couch RB. The secretory immune system: Its relation to respiratory viral infections. Prog Med Virol 13:194–238, 1971.
278. Onorato IM, Modlin JF, McBean AM, et al. Mucosal immunity induced by enhance-potency inactivated and oral polio vaccines. J Infect Dis 163:1–6, 1991.
279. Ogra PL, Fishaut M, Gallagher MR. Viral vaccination via the mucosal routes. Rev Infect Dis 2:352–369, 1980.
280. Smith JWG, Lee JA, Fletcher WB, et al. The response of oral poliovaccine in persons aged 16–18 years. J Hyg (Camb) 76:235–247, 1976.
281. Ogra PL. Distribution of echovirus antibody in serum, nasopharynx, rectum and spinal fluid after natural infection with echovirus type 6. Infect Immun 2:150–155, 1970.
282. Rovainen M, Hovi T. Cleavage of VP1 and modification of antigenic site 1 of type 2 polioviruses by intestinal trypsin. J Virol 62:3536–3539, 1988.
283. Agol VI, Drozdov SG. Russian contribution to OPV. Biologicals 21:321–325, 1993.
284. Sabin AB. Role of my cooperation with Soviet scientists in the elimination of polio. Perspect Biol Med 31:57–64, 1987.
285. Chumakov MP, Voroshilova MK, Drozdov SG, et al. Some results of the work on mass immunization in the Soviet Union with live poliovirus vaccine prepared from Sabin strains. Bull World Health Organ 25:79–91, 1961.
286. Centers for Disease Control and Prevention. Certification of poliomyelitis eradication—the Americas, 1994. MMWR Morb Mortal Wkly Rep 43:720–722, 1994.
287. Hale JH, Doraisingham M, Kanagaratnam K, et al. Large-scale use of Sabin type 2 attenuated poliovirus vaccine in Singapore during a type 1 poliomyelitis epidemic. Br Med J 1:1537–1549, 1959.
288. Knowelden J, Hale JH, Gardner PS, Lee JH. Measurement of the protective effect of attenuated poliovirus vaccine. Br Med J 1:1418–1420, 1961.
289. Fox JP, Gelfand HM, LeBlanc DR, Rowan DF. The influence of natural and artificially induced immunity on alimentary infections with polioviruses. Am J Public Health 48:1181–1192, 1958.
290. Koprowski H, Norton TW, Jervis GA, et al. Clinical investigations of attenuated strains of poliomyelitis virus. Use as a method of immunization of children with living virus. JAMA 160:954–966, 1956.
291. Paul JR, Horstmann DM, Niederman JC. Immunity in poliomyelitis infection: Observations in experimental epidemiology. In Najjar VA (ed). Immunity and Virus Infection. New York, John Wiley & Sons, 1959, pp 233–245.
292. Skovranek V, Zacek K. Oral poliovirus vaccine (Sabin) in Czechoslovakia. Effectiveness of nationwide use in 1960. JAMA 176:524–526, 1961.
293. Plotkin SA, Koprowski H. Epidemiological studies on the safety and efficacy of vaccination with the CHAT strain of attenuated poliovirus in Leopoldville, Belgian Congo. Live Poliovirus Vaccines: Papers and discussions held at the First International Con-

ference on Live Poliovirus Vaccines. Washington, DC, Pan American Sanitary Bureau, 1959, pp 419–436.
294. Rangelova SM. Control of poliomyelitis in Bulgaria: Experiences of two decades. Prog Med Virol 31:183–211, 1984.
295. Dong DX. Immunization with oral poliovirus vaccine in China. Prog Med Virol 31:168–182, 1984.
296. Deming MS, Jaiteh KO, Otten MW, et al. Epidemic poliomyelitis in The Gambia following the control of poliomyelitis as an endemic disease. II. Clinical efficacy of trivalent oral polio vaccine. Am J Epidemiol 135:393–408, 1992.
297. Horstmann DM, Emmons J, Gimpel L, et al. Enterovirus surveillance following a community-wide oral poliovirus vaccination program: A seven-year study. Am J Epidemiol 97:173–186, 1973.
298. Sabin AB, Ramos-Alvarez M, Alvarez-Amezquita J, et al. Live, orally given poliovirus vaccine—effect of rapid mass immunization on population under conditions of massive enteric infections with other viruses. JAMA 173:1521–1526, 1960.
299. Chen RT, Hausinger S, Dajani AS, et al. Seroprevalence of antibody against poliovirus in inner-city preschool children. Implications for vaccination policy in the United States. JAMA 275:1639–1645, 1996.
300. Ramsay ME, Begg NT, Ghandi J, Brown D. Antibody response and viral excretion after live polio vaccine or a combined schedule of live and inactivated polio vaccines. Pediatr Infect Dis J 13:1117–1121, 1994.
301. Orenstein WA, Wassilak SGF, DeForest A, et al. Seroprevalence of poliovirus antibodies among Massachusetts schoolchildren [abstract 512]. In 28th Interscience Conference on Antimicrobial Agents and Chemotherapy. Washington, DC, American Society for Microbiology, 1988, p 198.
302. Kelley PW, Petruccelli BP, Stehr-Green P, et al. The susceptibility of young adult Americans to vaccine-preventable infections: A national serosurvey of US army recruits. JAMA 266:2724–2729, 1991.
302a. WHO Consultative Group. Evidence on the safety and efficacy of live poliomyelitis vaccines currently in use, with special reference to type 3 poliovirus. Bull World Health Organ 40:925–945, 1969.
302b. Oberhofer TR, Brown GC, Monto AS. Seroimmunity to poliomyelitis in an American community. Am J Epidemiol 101:333–339, 1975.
302c. Horstmann DM. Maxwell Finland lecture: Viral vaccines and their ways. Rev Infect Dis 1:502–516, 1979.
302d. Cabasso VJ, Nozell H, Rueggsegger JM, Cox HR. Poliovirus antibody three years after oral trivalent vaccine (Sabin strains). J Pediatr 68:199–203, 1966.
302e. Krugman RD, Hardy GE, Sellers C, et al. Antibody persistence after primary immunization with trivalent oral poliovirus vaccine. Pediatrics 60:80–82, 1977.
302f. Rousseau WE, Noble GR, Tegtmeier GE, et al. Persistence of poliovirus neutralizing antibodies eight years after immunization with live attenuated virus vaccine. N Engl J Med 289:1357–1359, 1973.
303. Fortuin M, Maine N, Mendy M, et al. Measles, polio and tetanus toxoid antibody levels in Gambian children aged 3 to 4 years following routine vaccination. Trans R Soc Trop Med Hyg 89:326–329, 1995.
304. Stratton KR, Howe CJ, Johnston RB. Adverse Events Associated with Childhood Vaccines. Evidence Bearing on Causality. Washington, DC, National Academy Press, 1994.
305. Terry L. The Association of Cases of Poliomyelitis with the Use of Type 3 Oral Poliomyelitis Vaccines. Washington, DC, US Department of Health, Education and Welfare, 1962.
306. WHO Collaborative Study Group. The relationship between persisting spinal paralysis and poliomyelitis vaccine—results of a ten-year enquiry. Bull World Health Organ 60:231–242, 1982.
307. WHO Collaborative Study Group. The relationship between acute and persisting spinal paralysis and poliomyelitis vaccine (oral): Results of a WHO enquiry. Bull World Health Organ 53:319–331, 1976.
308. Esteves K. Safety of oral poliomyelitis vaccine: Results of a WHO enquiry. Bull World Health Organ 66:739–746, 1988.
309. Sabin AB. Commentary on report on oral poliomyelitis vaccine. JAMA 190:52–55, 1964.
310. Sabin AB. Paralytic poliomyelitis: Old dogmas and new perspectives. Rev Infect Dis 3:543–564, 1981.
311. Wyatt HV. Poliomyelitis in hypogammaglobulinemics. J Infect Dis 128:802–806, 1973.
312. Prevots DR, Sutter RW, Strebel PM, et al. Completeness of reporting for paralytic poliomyelitis, United States, 1980 through 1991. Arch Pediatr Adolesc Med 148:479–485, 1994.
313. Centers for Disease Control and Prevention. Poliomyelitis prevention in the United States: Introduction of a sequential vaccination schedule of inactivated poliovirus vaccine followed by oral poliovirus vaccine. Recommendations of the Advisory Committee on Immunization Practices. MMWR Morb Mortal Wkly Rep 46(RR3):1–25, 1997.
314. Sutter RW, Prevots DR. Vaccine-associated paralytic poliomyelitis among immunodeficient persons. Infect Med 11:426, 429–430, 435–438, 1994.
315. Strebel PM, Ion-Nedelcu N, Baughman AL, et al. Intramuscular injections within 30 days of immunization with oral poliovirus vaccine—a risk factor for vaccine-associated paralytic poliomyelitis. N Engl J Med 332:500–506, 1995.
316. Izurieta HS, Sutter RW, Baughman AL, et al. Vaccine-associated paralytic poliomyelitis in the United States: No evidence of elevated risk after simultaneous intramuscular injections with vaccine. Pediatr Infect Dis J 14:840–846, 1995.
317. Andrus JK, Strebel PM, de Quadros CA, Olive JM. Risk of vaccine-associated paralytic poliomyelitis in Latin America, 1989–91. Bull World Health Organ 73:33–40, 1995.
318. Wilfert CM, Buckley RH, Mohanakumar T, et al. Persistent and fatal central-nervous-system echovirus infections in patients with agammaglobulinemia. N Engl J Med 296:1485–1489, 1977.
319. Ziegler JB, Penny R. Fatal echo 30 virus infection and amyloidosis in X-linked hypogammaglobulinemia. Clin Immunol Immunopathol 3:347–352, 1975.
320. Hodes DS, Espinoza DV. Temperature sensitivity of isolates of echovirus type 11 causing chronic meningoencephalitis in an agammaglobulinemic patient. J Infect Dis 144:377, 1981.
321. Centers for Disease Control and Prevention. Prolonged poliovirus excretion in an immunodeficient person with vaccine-associated paralytic poliomyelitis. MMWR Morb Mortal Wkly Rep 46:641–643, 1997.
322. Eddy BE, Borman GS, Berkeley WH, Young RD. Tumors induced in hamsters by injection of rhesus monkey kidney cell extracts. Proc Soc Exp Biol Med 107:191–197, 1961.
323. Mortimer EA, Lepow ML, Gold E, et al. Long-term follow up of persons inadvertently inoculated with SV40 as neonates. N Engl J Med 305:1517–1518, 1981.
324. Shah K, Nathanson N. Human exposure to SV40: Review and comment. Am J Epidemiol 103:1–12, 1976.
325. Lewis AM, Egan W. Meeting report. Workshop on simian virus 40 (SV40): A possible human polyomavirus. Biologicals 25:355–358, 1997.
326. Strickler HD, Rosenberg PS, Devesa SS, et al. Contamination of poliovirus vaccines with simian virus 40 (1955–1963) and subsequent cancer rates. JAMA 279:292–295, 1998.
327. Uhari M, Rantala M, Niemela M. Cluster of childhood Guillain-Barré cases after an oral polio vaccine campaign. Lancet 2:440–441, 1989.
328. Kinnunen E, Farkkila M, Hovi T, et al. Incidence of Guillain-Barré syndrome during a nationwide oral poliovirus campaign. Neurology 39:1034–1036, 1989.
329. Rantala H, Cherry JD, Shields WD, Uhari M. Epidemiology of Guillain-Barré syndrome in children: Relationship of oral polio vaccine administration to occurrence. J Pediatr 124:220–223, 1994.
330. Kinnunen E, Junttila O, Haukka J, Hovi T. Nationwide oral poliovirus vaccination campaign and the incidence of Guillain-Barré syndrome. Am J Epidemiol 147:69–73, 1998.
331. American Academy of Pediatrics. Poliovirus infections. In Peter G (ed). 1997 Red Book: Report of the Committee on Infectious Diseases. Elk Grove Village, IL, American Academy of Pediatrics, 1997, pp 424–433.
331a. Onorato IM, Strebel PM, Sutter RW. Immunizations, vaccine-preventable diseases, and HIV infection. In Wormser GP (ed). AIDS and Other Manifestations of HIV Infection (3rd ed). Philadelphia, Lippincott-Raven, 1998, pp 745–758.
331b. Ryder RW, Oxtoby MJ, Mvula M, et al. Safety and immunogenicity of bacille Calmette-Guérin, diphtheria-tetanus-pertussis,

and oral polio vaccines in newborn children in Zaire infected with human immunodeficiency virus type 1. J Pediatr 122:697–702, 1993.

332. Vernon A, Okwo B, Lubamba N, Miaka MB. Paralytic poliomyelitis and HIV infection in Kinshasa, Zaire. In Sixth International Conference on AIDS; June 20–24, 1990; San Francisco, CA.
333. Ion-Nedelcu N, Dobrescu A, Strebel PM, Sutter RW. Vaccine-associated paralytic poliomyelitis and HIV infection [letter]. Lancet 343:51–52, 1994.
334. Harjulehto-Mervaala T, Aro T, Hiilesmaa VK, et al. Oral polio vaccination during pregnancy: No increase in the occurrence of malformations. Am J Epidemiol 138:407–414, 1993.
335. Harjulehto-Mervaala T, Aro T, Hiilesmaa VK, et al. Oral polio vaccination during pregnancy: Lack of impact on fetal development and perinatal outcome. Clin Infect Dis 18:414–420, 1994.
336. Myaux JA, Unicomb L, Besser RE, et al. Effect of diarrhea on the humoral response to oral polio vaccination. Pediatr Infect Dis J 15:204–209, 1996.
337. American Academy of Pediatrics. 1997 Red Book: Report of the Committee on Infectious Diseases. Elk Grove Village, IL, American Academy of Pediatrics, 1997.
338. Modlin JF, Halsey NA, Thoms ML, et al. Humoral and mucosal immunity in infants induced by three sequential inactivated poliovirus vaccine–live attenuated oral poliovirus vaccine immunization schedules. J Infect Dis 175(suppl 1):S228–S234, 1997.
339. World Health Organization. Overview of Immunization Programmes in the European Region. Copenhagen, World Health Organization, Regional Office for Europe, 1995.
340. Lasch EE, Abed Y, Marcus O, et al. Combined live and inactivated poliovirus vaccine to control poliomyelitis in a developing country—five years after. Dev Biol Stand 65:137–143, 1985.
341. Faden H, Modlin JF, Thoms ML, et al. Comparative evaluation of immunization with live attenuated and enhanced-potency poliovirus vaccines in childhood: Systemic and local immune response. J Infect Dis 162:1291–1297, 1990.
342. Ion-Nedelcu N, Strebel PM, Toma F, et al. Sequential use of inactivated and oral poliovirus vaccines: Dolj district, Romania, 1992–1994. J Infect Dis 175(suppl 1):S241–S246, 1997.
343. Moriniere BJ, van Loon FPL, Rhodes PH, et al. Immunogenicity of a supplemental dose of oral versus inactivated poliovirus vaccine. Lancet 341:1545–1550, 1993.
344. Tulchinsky T, Abed Y, Handsher R, et al. Successful control of poliomyelitis by a combined OPV/IPV polio vaccine program in the West Bank and Gaza, 1978–1993. Isr J Med Sci 30:489–494, 1994.
345. Goldblum N, Gerichter CB, Tulchinsky TH, Melnick JL. Poliomyelitis control in Israel, the West Bank and Gaza Strip: Changing strategies with the goal of eradication in an endemic area. Bull World Health Organ 72:783–796, 1994.
346. Slater PE, Orenstein WA, Morag A, et al. Poliomyelitis outbreak in Israel in 1988: A report with two commentaries. Lancet 335:1192–1198, 1990.
347. Swartz TA, Handsher R. Israel in the elimination phase of poliomyelitis—achievements and remaining problems. Public Health Rev 21:99–106, 1993–1994.
348. Hanlon P, Hanlon L, Marsh V, et al. Serological comparisons of approaches to polio vaccination in The Gambia. Lancet 1:800–801, 1987.
349. Sutter RW, Suleiman AJM, Malankar PG, et al. Sequential use of inactivated poliovirus vaccine followed by oral poliovirus vaccine in Oman. J Infect Dis 175(suppl 1):S235–S240, 1997.
350. Faden H, Duffy L, Sun M, Shuff C. Long-term immunity to poliovirus in children immunized with live attenuated and enhanced-potency inactivated trivalent poliovirus vaccines. J Infect Dis 168:452–454, 1993.
351. Kew OM, Nottay BK, Hatch MH, et al. Multiple genetic changes can occur in the oral poliovaccines upon replication in humans. J Gen Virol 56(pt 2):337–347, 1981.
352. Cann AJ, Stanway G, Hughes PJ, et al. Reversion to virulence of the live attenuated Sabin type 3 oral poliovirus vaccine. Nucleic Acids Res 12:7787–7792, 1984.
353. Cammack NJ, Philipps A, Dunn G, et al. Intertypic genomic rearrangements of poliovirus strains in vaccinees. Virology 167:507–514, 1989.
354. Pollard SR, Dunn G, Cammack N, et al. Nucleotide sequence of a neurovirulent variant of the type 2 oral poliovirus vaccine. J Virol 63:4949–4951, 1989.
355. Evans DMA, Dunn G, Minor PD, et al. Increased neurovirulence associated with a single nucleotide change in a noncoding region of Sabin type 3 poliovaccine genome. Nature 314:548–550, 1985.
356. Dunn G, Begg NT, Cammack N, Minor PD. Virus excretion and mutation by infants following primary vaccination with live oral poliovaccine from two sources. J Med Virol 32:92–95, 1990.
357. Minor PD, Dunn G. The effect of sequences in the 5′ noncoding region on the replication of polioviruses in the human gut. J Gen Virol 69:1091–1096, 1988.
358. Tatem JM, Weeks-Levy C, Mento SJ, et al. Oral poliovirus vaccine in the United States: Molecular characterization of Sabin type 3 after replication in the gut of vaccinees. J Med Virol 35:101–109, 1991.
359. Ogra PL, Faden HS, Abraham R, et al. Effect of prior immunity on the shedding of virulent revertant virus in feces after oral immunization with live attenuated poliovirus vaccines. J Infect Dis 161:191–194, 1991.
360. Abraham R, Minor P, Dunn G, et al. Shedding of virulent poliovirus revertants during immunization with oral poliovirus vaccine after prior immunization with inactivated polio vaccine. J Infect Dis 168:1105–1109, 1993.
361. Murdin AD, Barreto L, Plotkin S. Inactivated poliovirus vaccine: Past and present experience. Vaccine 14:735–746, 1996.
362. De-Xiang D, Xi-Min H, Wan-Jun L, et al. Immunisation of neonates with trivalent oral poliomyelitis vaccine (Sabin). Bull World Health Organ 64:853–860, 1986.
363. Halsey N, Galazka A. The efficacy of DTP and oral poliomyelitis immunization schedules initiated from birth to 12 weeks of age. Bull World Health Organ 63:1151–1169, 1985.
364. Galazka AM, Lauer BA, Henderson RH, Keja J. Indications and contraindications for vaccines used in the Expanded Programme on Immunization. Bull World Health Organ 62:357–366, 1984.
365. Weckx LY, Schmidt BJ, Hermann AA, et al. Early immunization of neonates with trivalent oral poliovirus vaccine. Bull World Health Organ 70:85–91, 1992.
366. Birmingham ME, Aylward RB, Cochi SL, Hull HF. National Immunization Days: State of the art. J Infect Dis 175(suppl 1):S183–S188, 1997.
367. Reichler MR, Kharabsheh S, Rhodes P, et al. Increased immunogenicity of oral poliovirus vaccine administered in mass vaccination campaigns compared with the routine vaccination program in Jordan. J Infect Dis 175(suppl 1):S198–S204, 1997.
368. Richardson G, Linkins RW, Eames M, et al. Immunogenicity of oral poliovirus vaccine administered in mass campaigns versus routine immunization programs. Bull World Health Organ 73:769–777, 1995.
369. Deming MS, Linkins RW, Jaiteh KO, Hull HF. The clinical efficacy of trivalent oral polio vaccine in The Gambia by season of vaccine administration. J Infect Dis 175(suppl 1):S254–S257, 1997.
370. Cochi SL, Hull HF, Sutter RW, et al. Global poliomyelitis eradication initiative: Status report. J Infect Dis 175(suppl 1):1–292, 1997.
371. Global Program for Vaccines and Immunization. Report of the 1st Meeting of the Global Commission for the Certification of Poliomyelitis. Geneva, World Health Organization, 1995.
372. Global Program for Vaccines and Immunization. Vaccine Research and Development: Report of the Technical Review Group Meeting, 9–10 June 1997. Achievements and Plan of Activities, July 1997–June 1998. Geneva, World Health Organization, 1997.
373. Dove AW, Racaniello VR. The polio eradication effort: Should vaccine eradication be next? Science 277:779–780, 1997.
374. Hull HF, Aylward RB. Ending polio immunization. Science 277:780, 1997.
375. Kiley MP, Lloyd G. Safety in the virologic laboratory. In Mahy BWJ, Collier L (eds). Topley & Wilson's Microbiology and Microbial Infections (9th ed). Vol. 1. New York, Oxford University Press, 1998, pp 933–945.
376. World Health Organization. Network labs to provide lead in safe handling and containment of wild polioviruses. Polio Lab Network Quarterly Update 4:1–3, 1998.
377. Global Program for Vaccines and Immunization. Field Guide for

Supplementary Activities Aimed at Achieving Polio Eradication. Geneva, World Health Organization, 1996.

378. Ghendon YUZ, Sanakoyeva II. Comparison of the resistance of the intestinal tract to poliomyelitis vaccine (Sabin strains) in persons after naturally and experimentally acquired immunity. Acta Virol 5:265–273, 1961.
379. Expanded Programme on Immunization. Field Guide for Supplementary Activities Aimed at Achieving Polio Eradication. Geneva, World Health Organization, 1997.
380. Blatter MM, Starr S. Safety and Immunogenicity of a Combination DTP/eIPV Vaccine Presented in a Dual Chamber Syringe, in 2-Month-Old Infants. Swiftwater, PA, Connaught Laboratories, 1993.
381. Halsey NA, Blatter MM, Bader G. Safety and Immunogenicity of a Combination DTP/IPV Vaccine Administered to Infants in a Dual Chamber Syringe. Swiftwater, PA, Connaught Laboratories, 1994.
382. Halsey N, Blatter M, Bader G, et al. Inactivated poliovirus vaccine alone or sequential inactivated and oral poliovirus vaccine in two-, four- and six-month-old infants with combination *Haemophilus influenzae* type b/hepatitis B vaccine. Pediatr Infect Dis J 16:675–679, 1997.
383. Fine PEM, Carneiro IAM. Transmissibility and persistence of oral polio vaccine viruses: Implications for the global poliomyelitis eradication initiative. Meeting on the Scientific Basis for Stopping Immunization Against Poliomyelitis. Geneva; World Health Organization; 23–25 March 1998 (WHO/EPI/POLIO/SIM.98.WP5.3).

chapter

17 Rubella Vaccine

Stanley A. Plotkin

rubella

just
a dead comma of flesh where
the ear should hang, a poxed hole
mottled in bone, and she holds you, as you shiver
curled against the muffled songs we sing as we pass by
in our doctor's clothes and then leave you alone
again, to redefine
the white surgery waiting-room with glazed dum-dum eyes,
not even warming
the living gel of your pulped brain.

Michael O'Reilly. Falling on deaf ears.
Perspect Biol Med 39:204, 1992.

Discovered in the late 18th century, suddenly prominent since 1941, and controlled in the 1980s and 1990s, rubella is an interesting case history in relation to vaccine development and application. Although only a mild exanthematous viral infection of children and young adults, rubella assumes greater importance in pregnant women, from whom the causative virus can be transmitted to the fetus, with disastrous effects.

The first researchers to distinguish the disease from other exanthemas were German physicians; hence, the common English language eponym is German measles.[1] In 1841, a British physician reported an outbreak in a boys' school in India and used the term rubella, a Latin diminutive meaning "little red."[2]

For the next hundred years, rubella received scant attention, but in 1941, Norman McAlister Gregg,[3] an Australian ophthalmologist, published a report relating congenital cataracts to maternal rubella. Gregg noticed that an unusual number of infants with cataracts had been brought to him, and he was curious enough to investigate and determine that their mothers gave histories of rubella infections in pregnancy during the Australian outbreak of 1940.

Gregg's original report was soon followed with reports by Australian,[4] Swedish,[5] American,[6] and British[7] epidemiologists and teratologists, who confirmed the role of rubella in congenital cataracts and also noticed the simultaneous presence of heart disease and deafness in the infants. Thus, the characteristic congenital rubella triad was established.

The next 20 years were spent in trying to isolate the agent and in obtaining statistics on the risk of fetal abnormality after maternal rubella. Various estimates of the incidence of fetal disease were made, ranging from very high to very low. The disparity in estimates stemmed from the absence of a definitive diagnostic test and consequent misdiagnosis of rubella in the mother.

In late 1962, a breakthrough came in the form of the first isolations of rubella virus by Weller and Neva[8] in Boston and by Parkman, Beuscher, and Artenstein[9] in Washington, D.C. To detect the presence of rubella virus, Parkman and coworkers developed the technique of interference with the growth of enteroviruses in African green monkey kidney cell culture, which soon became the standard method for virus isolation.

Meanwhile, a virtual pandemic of rubella started in Europe in the 1962 to 1963 season, with spread to the United States in 1964 to 1965. As a result, from 1964 to 1966, thousands of pregnancies were affected, leaving behind a wake of abnormal infants and induced abortions.[10, 11]

The pandemic had two major effects on biomedicine. First, an expanded congenital rubella syndrome (CRS) was recognized, adding hepatitis, splenomegaly, thrombocytopenia, encephalitis, mental retardation, and numerous other anomalies to the already described deafness, cataracts, and heart disease.[12, 13] Second, it became obvious that a vaccine was needed, and many groups set to work.

Between 1965 and 1967, several attenuated rubella strains were developed and reached clinical trials.[14–16] In 1969 to 1970, rubella vaccine entered into commercial use; and since the late 1970s, vaccines have had a major impact on the epidemiology of rubella and CRS.

BACKGROUND

Clinical Description

Acquired Rubella

The incubation period of rubella is 14 to 21 days, with most patients developing a rash 14 to 17 days after exposure.[17] During the first week after exposure, there are no symptoms. In the second week, lymphadenopathy may be noted, particularly occipital and postauricular,

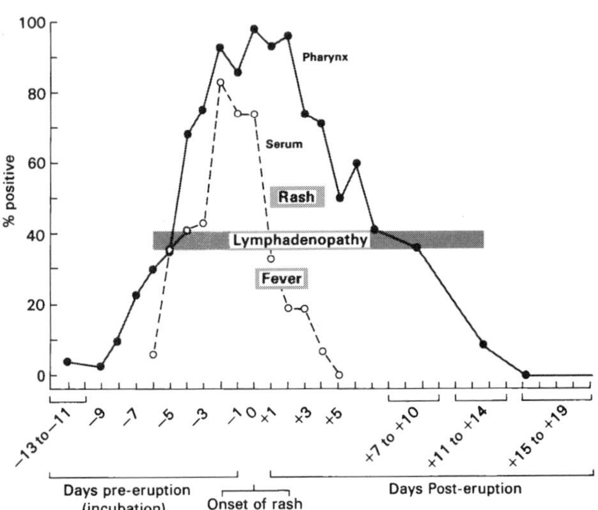

Figure 17–1. The sequence of events in acquired rubella infections, showing the relationship between onset of rash and other clinical symptoms to recovery of rubella virus from diagnostic specimens.

and virus cultures done at this time reveal rubella virus in the nasopharynx. Later in the second week, virus appears in the blood. At about this time, there may be a prodromal illness consisting of low-grade fever (<39.0°C), malaise, and mild conjunctivitis. If not already present, the aforementioned lymphadenopathy is likely to develop.

At the end of the incubation period, a maculopapular erythematous rash appears on the face and neck. The rash may be difficult to detect and is more prominent after hot showers or baths. During a course of 1 to 3 days, the rash spreads downward and begins to fade. Virus excretion in pharynx and urine may continue for another 1 to 2 weeks, but viremia ends with the onset of the rash.[18] The evolution of acquired rubella is illustrated in Figure 17–1.

Although acquired rubella is thought of as a benign disease, arthralgia and arthritis are commonly observed in adults, and chronic arthritis has been reported after rubella infection.[19, 20] Other less common complications are thrombocytopenia[21] and encephalitis, which may be fatal.[22, 23] Encephalitis, which occurs in approximately 1 of 6000 cases, is of the postinfectious type, but the limited available pathological data show little evidence of demyelination.[24] In a Japanese outbreak, the incidence of encephalitis was 1 in 1600 cases of rubella.[25] In addition, there is a rare late syndrome of progressive rubella panencephalitis.[26, 27] Guillain-Barré syndrome after rubella has also been reported.[28] Antibodies to rubella and measles structural proteins are elevated in autoimmune chronic active hepatitis, but whether this is related to viral persistence is unknown.[29]

Congenital Rubella

Rubella is the archetypical fetal infectious pathogen (see *Pathogenesis as It Relates to Prevention*). Because all organs of the fetus are affected, it is not surprising that the CRS comprises a lengthy list of abnormalities, both teratological, resulting from interference with organogenesis, and inflammatory, involving organs such as the liver and spleen[30] (Table 17–1).

Table 17–1. **PROMINENT CLINICAL FINDINGS IN CONGENITAL RUBELLA SYNDROME**

Cataracts Retinitis Microphthalmia Glaucoma	Intrauterine growth retardation Metaphyseal rarefactions Hepatosplenomegaly Thrombocytopenic purpura
Cochlear deafness Central auditory imperception	Interstitial pneumonitis
Patent ductus arteriosus Peripheral pulmonic artery stenosis	Diabetes Hypothyroidism
Encephalitis Microcephaly Mental retardation Autism	

Modified from Cooper LZ, Preblud SR, Alford CA. Rubella. In Remington JS, Klein JO (eds). Infectious Diseases of the Fetus and Newborn Infant (4th ed). Philadelphia, WB Saunders, 1995, p 288.

The time of infection during gestation is important in relation to the fetal outcome; early infection tends to result in serious ocular disease, whereas infection late in the first half of pregnancy is likely to result in deafness. However, the relationship between gestational age and abnormality can be overemphasized, because fetal infection, once established, spreads to all organs, and damage may be cumulative. Table 17–2 demonstrates that organ specificity is only generally related to the stage of gestational infection with rubella virus. The most common congenital defects are sensorineural deafness, cataracts, pigmentary retinopathy, and patent ductus arteriosus; but a myriad of other defects occur, including glaucoma, peripheral pulmonic stenosis, endocrinopathies including diabetes, hyperimmunoglobulinemia M,[31] microcephaly, and mental retardation.

Various estimates have been made of the incidence of

Table 17–2. **AGE OF GESTATION AT TIME OF RUBELLA IN RELATION TO ABNORMALITIES OBSERVED**

	MONTH OF GESTATION MEASURED FROM LAST MENSTRUAL PERIOD				
	0*	**1**	**2**	**3**	**4**
Birth weight <2500 g	0/1†	9/21	9/21	10/18	0/2
<38 weeks' gestation	0/1	5/21	2/21	4/18	0/2
Growth retardation	0/1	7/21	5/20	7/17	0/2
Ocular defects	0/1	14/21	9/21	9/18	0/2
Cardiac defects	0/1	17/21	13/21	6/18	0/2
Deafness	0/1	8/18	10/18	11/17	2/2
Mental retardation	1/1	7/20	7/20	8/16	0/2
Microcephaly	1/1	3/18	2/19	4/17	0/2

*Before conception.
†Ratio of number of patients with condition to total number for whom information is available.
From Plotkin SA, Cochran W, Lindquist J, et al. Congenital rubella syndrome in late infancy. JAMA 200:435–441, 1967. Copyright 1967, American Medical Association.

Table 17–3. **FETAL ABNORMALITY INDUCED BY CONFIRMED RUBELLA AT VARIOUS STAGES OF PREGNANCY**

STAGE OF PREGNANCY (wk)	UNITED KINGDOM STUDY (% DEFECTIVE)*	UNITED STATES STUDY (% DEFECTIVE)†
≤4		70
5–8		40
≤10	90	
11–12	33	
9–12		25
13–14	11	
15–16	24	
13–16		40
≥17	0	8

*Data from Miller E, Cradock-Watson JE, Pollock TM. Consequences of confirmed maternal rubella at successive stages of pregnancy. Lancet 2:781–784, 1982. © The Lancet Ltd., 1982.

†Data from South MA, Sever JL. Teratogen update: The congenital rubella syndrome. Teratology 31:297–307, 1985.

fetal abnormalities after internal infection.[6, 32–37] The two most reliable, one from United States data[34] and the other from United Kingdom data,[33] are tabulated in Table 17–3. The first 12 weeks of pregnancy are clearly the most dangerous time for rubella infection in the mother. The incidence of fetal disease declines during the next 4 weeks, and in the 16th to the 20th weeks only deafness has been reported as a complication. Preconceptional rubella rarely results in fetal infection, but rashes that occur within 12 days of the last menstrual period carry proven risk.[38] Swedish and Australian data appear similar. In contrast, some Japanese workers[39] have claimed that rubella virus is less teratogenic in their country, but these claims have not been supported.[25]

Most prospective studies of the incidence of fetal rubella have accepted clinical diagnosis of rubella in the mother. If only virologically confirmed maternal rubella is considered, the rate of transmission to the fetus during the first trimester of pregnancy is higher than 80%.[33, 40–42] In addition, a variety of autoimmune syndromes, including diabetes mellitus and thyroiditis, have been seen as late complications of congenital rubella infection.[43]

Virology

The agent of rubella is a cubical, medium-sized (70 nm), lipid-enveloped virus with an RNA genome belonging to the togavirus family. Although the other togaviruses are arthropod borne, there is no evidence for such transmission of rubella. Frey[44] has reviewed the virology of rubella. Apart from the complex lipid envelope, rubella virus is composed of three proteins, two in the envelope (E1 and E2) and one in the core. One of the two envelope proteins (E1) is a glycoprotein with neutralizing and hemagglutinating epitopes.[45] The three proteins, which have molecular masses of 60,000 kDa (E1), 42,000 to 47,000 kDa (E2), and 30,000 kDa (C), are derived from a polypeptide of 110 kDa that is translated from a 245-kDa messenger RNA.[46–48]

The RNA genome of rubella virus is infectious,[49, 50] and complementary DNA copies facilitate study of its transcripts.[51] The replication strategy of rubella virus is similar to that of the alphaviruses in that both full-length and subgenomic RNAs are produced, and it is from the subgenomic RNA that viral structural proteins are translated. Three other proteins are produced by the virus in infected cells but are not incorporated into the virion.[52]

There is only one serotype of rubella virus, and analyses of sequence variation among occidental isolates show high conservation of amino acid structure (0 to 3.3% differences), with less conservation of isolates from Asia (up to 7%).[53, 54] An international collaborative group[55] confirmed that the isolates from the occidental pandemic of the 1960s were related to each other, that there is an Asian genotype, and that no antigenic drift has occurred in recent years.

Rubella virus grows in many different primary, semicontinuous, and continuous cells of mammalian origin. In human amnion cells, it produces a subtle cytopathic effect. More pronounced cytopathic effects, sufficient to allow plaque formation, are produced in continuous cell lines, such as rabbit kidney and baby hamster kidney.[18] Even in those cell lines, fresh isolates frequently are not highly cytopathogenic and require adaptation by serial passage. High passage generates defective-interfering RNA and particles.[56]

Virus isolation is generally performed in primary African green monkey kidney cell culture, in which virus growth is detected by “challenging” the cultures with a cytopathogenic agent such as ECHO 11. If rubella virus has infected the cultures, the action of ECHO 11 is blocked; the presence of rubella virus is inferred by this interference. Confirmation is performed by another technique, such as neutralization or fluorescence with specific antirubella serum.[57]

The fact that rubella virus hemagglutinates red blood cells, particularly of avian origin, has been highly important for diagnosis.[58] The viral hemagglutinin is used as an antigen for measurement of antibodies by hemagglutination inhibition. Other serological examinations that are amenable to mass testing have come into use, such as latex agglutination, indirect hemagglutination, enzyme-linked immunosorbent assay (ELISA), and fluorescence inhibition.[42, 59] Detection of antibodies in saliva has simplified testing in developing countries.[60]

Pathogenesis as It Relates to Prevention

The pathogenesis of rubella provides two points at which immune intervention could have an effect. The first point is in the nasopharynx, where the virus first replicates and from which it spreads to local lymph nodes. Secretory immunoglobulin (Ig) A antibody in the nasopharynx, induced by prior disease or vaccination, can block mucosal replication. The second point begins about a week into the incubation period, at which time the viremia can be blocked by the presence of antibody, either passively or actively acquired.

During viremia in a pregnant woman, the virus may

infect the placenta. Placental replication appears to precede fetal infections, leading to entrance of virus into the fetal circulation, from which it infects fetal organs.[61] In vitro experiments show that human embryonic cells of many different lineages are susceptible to the virus and develop chronic infection.[62] The same phenomenon occurs in vivo.[63] If the infected cells are stimulated to divide, either artificially in vitro or in the course of embryological development in vivo, there is an inhibition of mitosis[62, 64] that may be mediated in part by a soluble protein inhibitor[65] or by the induction of apoptosis.[66] Organogenesis is thus disrupted. In a few organs, including the lens, cochlea, and brain, the damage caused by the virus is more destructive.[67] This damage may be related as much to vasculitis and ischemia as to cytopathology, but the question is still open.

Diagnosis

Methods for the diagnosis of acquired rubella are summarized in Table 17–4. Clinical diagnosis is so inaccurate as to be useless without laboratory support. Isolation of virus can be accomplished from the blood and nasopharynx during the prodromal period and from the nasopharynx for as long as 2 weeks after eruption, although the likelihood of virus recovery is sharply reduced by 3 days after the rash. African green monkey kidney cells or the RK_{13} cell line are generally used for virus isolation. Owing to the slow growth of the virus in tissue culture, virus isolation is often bypassed in favor of serological diagnosis.

The polymerase chain reaction has been adapted to the detection of rubella RNA by reverse transcription and amplification.[68] The method appears to be sensitive and specific[69, 70] and is particularly useful for prenatal detection of rubella infection of the fetus.[71]

Serological diagnosis depends on the demonstration of a fourfold rise in titer between acute and convalescent specimens or a demonstration of IgM antibody in the acute specimen.[59] The standard serological test is the hemagglutination inhibition test, based on the property of rubella antigens to agglutinate certain red blood cells. Other tests that are easier to perform and are more sensitive have come into use, including indirect hemagglutination, latex agglutination, hemolysis in gel, and ELISA. For IgM testing, ELISA is the predominant assay in use, and results may be positive for up to 6 weeks after the acute infection.

Susceptibility has been defined as a hemagglutination-inhibiting antibody titer of less than 1:8, a hemolysis in gel result of less than 10 IU, or an optical density by ELISA below the limit set by the manufacturer. Although titers at the borderline level are difficult to evaluate, the consensus is that in the majority of cases they correlate with immunity.[71a] Assays for antibodies to specific peptides have shown promise in distinguishing between congenital and acquired infection.[72]

The recognition of the combination of cataracts, heart disease, and deafness provides a clinical means of diagnosis of CRS that is reasonably accurate. However, laboratory confirmation is always desirable both because isolated abnormalities may occur and for public health reasons.

Congenital rubella infection can be diagnosed in the infant by the isolation of virus, by the demonstration of IgM antibodies, or by the detection of antibodies persisting beyond the predicted decay of passively transmitted maternal antibodies. Virus can often be isolated from tissues obtained at biopsy, autopsy, or surgical procedures such as cataract extraction,[73] but more often, nasopharyngeal swabs, urine specimens, or cerebrospinal fluid serve as the sources. Almost always one or more of these sources are positive for virus at birth, gradually becoming negative during the first year of life.[74] In severe cases, virus excretion may persist for several years.[75] IgM antibodies are present for as long as a year after birth. Persistence of IgG antibodies beyond 6 months of age can be detected in 95% of infants with CRS.[76] An infant with seropositive results for rubella after 6 months of age who has not received rubella vaccine is likely to have been congenitally infected.

Table 17–4. **DIAGNOSIS OF ACQUIRED AND CONGENITAL RUBELLA**

	VIRUS ISOLATION	ANTIBODY TESTS	
		IgG	IgM
Acquired			
Active exanthem	+	Fourfold rise in HI or other tests	+
Recent rash	−	Fourfold rise in CF test	±
Congenital			
<6 mo	+	+	+
6–12 mo	±	+	−

+, Likely to be positive; −, likely to be negative; ±, uncertain; HI, hemagglutination inhibition; CF, complement fixation.

EPIDEMIOLOGY

Acquired Infection

Rubella is a worldwide infection, as may be inferred from serological surveys conducted in many different countries.[77, 78] The age at infection varies from area to area. Although much childhood infection is asymptomatic and therefore unrecognized, infection tends to take place at a young age in countries in which living conditions are crowded. Daycare centers also promote early infection with rubella. In island countries and in countries that are less crowded, the average age at rubella infection is later, and many children reach puberty still in a seronegative state.[79] Under these circumstances, introduction of the virus into places where young people congregate results in epidemic spread.[80] Thus, schools, colleges, and military camps are all places where rubella is likely to become epidemic. Outbreaks at the stock exchange on Wall Street illustrate the potential effect of bringing seronegative individuals together in close quarters. In fact, rubella is highly efficient at infecting susceptible persons in certain epidemiological situations.[81–83]

Transmission of rubella seems to be primarily respiratory, with implantation of virus in the nasopharynx. As is true of other diseases, some individual rubella patients excrete large amounts of virus in respiratory secretions and are highly infectious "spreaders."[80]

In the United States, the epidemiology of rubella before vaccination was both endemic and epidemic.[10] Each spring, rubella tended to occur, primarily in schoolchildren 6 to 10 years of age but also in older individuals. Superimposed on this occurrence was a cycle of major epidemics at 7-year intervals (Fig. 17–2). Susceptibility in young adults varied from 10 to 20%, with the lower figure being found after an epidemic. Similarly, in Israel, approximately 9% of women were infected during a 1972 rubella outbreak[84]; however, even after the epidemic, a significant pool of susceptible individuals remained.

The epidemiology of rubella in developing countries can be deduced from the seroprevalence of rubella antibodies. The large variation seen in seroprevalence suggests that rubella occurs in sporadic epidemics except where population density is high. In the metropolis of S̃ao Paulo, Brazil, nearly everyone is seropositive by 20 years of age,[85] whereas in rural Mexico, seropositivity varies from 29 to 76%.[86] Cutts and colleagues[87] reviewed rubella susceptibility data from 45 developing countries and found remarkable differences among them not correlated with geography. For example, Malaysia, Peru, and Nigeria were among the countries where more than 25% of women were found to be seronegative.

Congenital Infection

Most information on the epidemiology of CRS is available from the United Kingdom and the United States. Table 17–5 presents the tally of fetal damage caused by rubella during the 1963 to 1964 outbreak.[11] A minimum of 30,000 infants were damaged by intrauterine rubella, for an incidence rate of 100 per 10,000 pregnancies. In Philadelphia, the rate was also as high as 1% of pregnancies.[88] After that outbreak, CRS rates fell to 4 to 8 per 10,000 pregnancies until 1970, when the first vaccines were licensed. Since then, the rate has declined further to a vanishingly low incidence of less than 0.01 per 10,000 pregnancies.[89]

The epidemiology of CRS in the United Kingdom has been similar to that in the United States, with rates of approximately 4.6 per 10,000 births in the prevaccine era.[90]

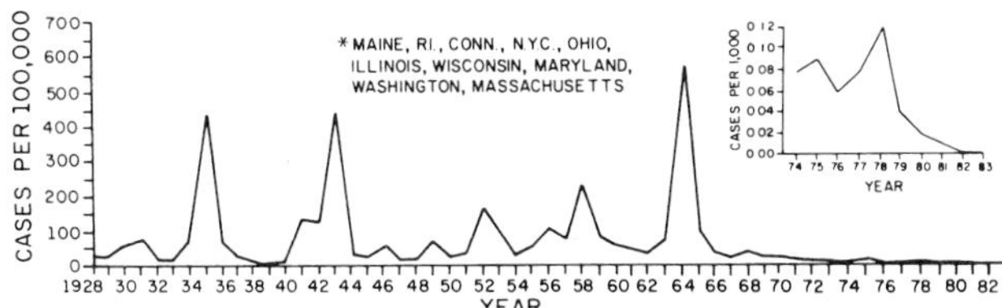

Figure 17–2. Rubella incidence in 10 selected areas* of the United States, 1928 to 1983. (From Williams NM, Preblud SR. Rubella and congenital rubella surveillance, 1983. MMWR CDC Surveill Summ 33:1SS–10SS, 1984.)

Table 17–5. **ESTIMATED MORBIDITY ASSOCIATED WITH THE 1964 TO 1965 RUBELLA EPIDEMIC**

CLINICAL EVENTS	
Rubella cases	12,500,000
Arthritis-arthralgia	159,375
Encephalitis	2084
Deaths	
Excess neonatal deaths	2100
Other deaths	60
Total deaths	2160
Excess fetal wastage	6250
Congenital rubella syndrome	
Deaf children	8055
Deaf-blind children	3580
Mentally retarded children	1790
Other congenital rubella syndrome	6575
Total congenital rubella syndrome	20,000
Therapeutic abortions	5000

From Rubella Surveillance. National Communicable Disease Center, United States Department of Health, Education, and Welfare (No. 1), June 1969.

The epidemiology of CRS is really known only for a few countries of the world. Little information is available for the countries in South America, Africa, and most of Asia, although such data suggest that CRS is common even in the developing world.[91, 92] For example, in India, 26% of 90 infants investigated for congenital malformations had serological evidence of CRS.[93]

Two other Indian studies[94, 95] showed that 15% of children with nontraumatic cataracts and 15% of infants suspected of having congenital infection were rubella positive. Rubella was also frequently the cause of sensorineural hearing loss in Saudi Arabian children.[96] A review of worldwide data concerning CRS revealed rates in developing countries varying between 0.6 and 2.2 per 1000 live births, similar to rates seen in developed countries before universal vaccination.[87]

A virulence factor has been postulated for rubella strains, and it has been argued from laboratory and clinical data that rubella virus is not teratogenic in Japan. Kono and colleagues[39] reported that Japanese strains had no effect on pregnant rabbits, whereas American strains were transmitted across the placenta from dams to fetal rabbits. In addition, they reported that on the main island of Honshu, no CRS was reported even though rubella outbreaks were evident.[97] However, after careful analysis of rubella on the southern Japanese island of Kyushu, Ueda and associates[98] showed that the rates of both rubella and CRS were high. They concluded that the apparently low rate of CRS on Honshu is due to a high seropositivity rate in adult women and a low clinical reporting rate of CRS.

CRS shows a predisposition to affect infants of young mothers, presumably because they are more likely to enter pregnancy in a seronegative state. Women in contact with populations in which rubella outbreaks occur frequently, such as military recruits and school-aged children, are more likely to be exposed. Military dependents and school teachers are thus at increased risk.

Pregnant women with older children are also at greater risk.

Although rubella outbreaks may be explosive, they frequently do not exhaust all susceptible persons in large populations, and thus a history of having been exposed to a rubella outbreak does not necessarily indicate immunity to rubella. Even more important is the fact that 10 to 85% of infections in various outbreaks have been inapparent or at least have been without evidence of eruption.[82] Infection without rash in pregnancy can still lead to fetal disease, although the risk may be lower than that after symptomatic infection with rash.[99]

Significance as a Public Health Problem

The seriousness of congenital rubella as a public health problem can be gauged by the results of the last major American epidemic in 1964 to 1965 (see Table 17–5). An estimated 12.5 million rubella cases occurred, including approximately 2000 cases of encephalitis. There were also many cases in pregnant women, about 5000 of whom had surgical abortions and about 6250 of whom lost fetuses to spontaneous abortions. Another 2100 infants were stillborn or died soon after birth.[11]

CRS occurred in 20,000 infants who survived pregnancy. Of these, 11,600 were deaf, 3580 blind, and about 1800 mentally retarded. The human misery imposed by such severe damage can well be imagined. The economic burden has been estimated to be $221,660 per CRS child, and the total cost of the epidemic may have been $1.5 billion.[11]

Before the use of vaccine, rubella epidemics involved about 5% of the population, although only approximately 10% of these cases were reported to public health authorities.[100] In the years between epidemics, rates were about one tenth of the epidemic peaks, but CRS continued at a low endemic rate even in those years.

Analysis of the age distribution of acquired rubella in the prevaccine era showed 60% of cases in children younger than 10 years and 23% in those older than 15 years.[101] As discussed subsequently, application of vaccine in children did not reduce by much the incidence in adolescents and adults, and CRS continued to occur for some years after the introduction of vaccination.

Lest it be thought that rubella infection in pregnancy has lost its danger, a recent outbreak among unvaccinated Amish people living in Pennsylvania serves as a corrective.[102] Young Amish women were 20% seronegative at the beginning of the outbreak, and infections in pregnancy were common. More than 8% of Amish infants gave laboratory evidence of infection, and more than 2% had CRS. Of infants born after first-trimester infection, 90% had confirmed or possible CRS.

Data on CRS for other countries in the world are few. In the United Kingdom, CRS estimates before the use of vaccine were only about 200 to 300 cases per year, but that figure was from a passive ascertainment system.[90] In Australia, about one CRS baby per 2000 births was recorded before vaccine.[103] During an outbreak of rubella in Israel, there were 1441 confirmed infections in pregnant women, most of whom had abortions.[104] Projection of the experience to the United States would be equivalent to 75,000 pregnancies complicated by rubella. In France, 16% of congenital cataract cases were attributable to CRS.[105] A follow-up study of an epidemic in Poland showed that 15% of pregnant women had been infected. The rate of CRS after first-, second-, or third-trimester infection was 78%, 33%, and 0%, respectively.[106] The picture of rubella in the developing world is complex.[87, 107] Although a frequent seroepidemiological finding has been a high rate of infection early in life,[83] there are many exceptions, including island populations,[108] several West African countries, the city of Calcutta, and Morocco.[109] Thus, the pattern is that of a disease that comes in epidemic waves, sometimes being absent from an area for some time.

Clusters of CRS have been reported in developing countries,[110, 111] and there is little doubt that wherever seronegative pregnant women are exposed to a rubella outbreak, CRS cases will follow.

PASSIVE IMMUNIZATION

Ordinary Immune Serum Globulin

Because most adults have had rubella, ordinary immune serum globulin (ISG) contains rubella antibody.[112] By the hemagglutination inhibition test, rubella antibody titers of about 1:16 are found in immune globulins.[113] Before the development of vaccine, ISG was frequently offered to pregnant women who had been exposed to rubella in the hope that it would prevent fetal infection. The results were equivocal, but if large doses (20 to 30 mL) of material with high titer were given, frank symptoms and viremia could be prevented.[114–117] Experimental studies confirmed the efficacy of passive antibody in preventing clinical rubella,[118, 119] but there were numerous failures of gamma globulin to prevent congenital fetal abnormality in actual practice.[116, 119] In one study of CRS patients, 6% of mothers gave histories of receipt of gamma globulin after exposure.[76] Thus, whatever the real efficacy of ISG, it is unlikely to be complete.

The sole current indication for ISG is the exposure to rubella of a pregnant seronegative woman who will not accept abortion if infection is proved. If 1 week or less has elapsed since exposure and a serum specimen is taken first to confirm susceptibility, ISG in large amounts (20 mL) can be given intramuscularly. Convalescent specimens should be obtained 3 and 4 weeks later to search for IgM antibody and a rise in IgG titer. The absence of a rash in the exposed woman does not mean that viremia and fetal infection have been prevented. The newer intravenous gamma globulins do not have high concentrations of rubella antibodies.[113]

Hyperimmune Rubella Globulin

To overcome the deficiencies of ISG, a hyperimmune globulin was prepared by Cutter Laboratories from the sera of normal individuals who had high rubella antibody titers. The titer of this preparation was 1:8000 by hemagglutination inhibition. A controlled clinical trial of the preparation was performed in volunteers who were inoculated first with live unattenuated rubella virus and then given hyperimmune rubella globulin 24 to 96 hours later. With a challenge given intranasally, viremia was detected in two of five control subjects and in one of 10 subjects given gamma globulin. Pharyngeal excretion was similar in the two groups.[120] Although a previous experimental study with high-titered globulin had given better results,[118] the production of hyperimmune globulin was stopped and it is not now commercially available.

ACTIVE IMMUNIZATION

Killed Virus Vaccine

Advances in molecular biology have allowed consideration of a subunit-inactivated vaccine against rubella. The genome of the virus has been sequenced, in particular the genetic code for the E1 protein[121, 122] that carries multiple neutralizing epitopes located between amino acids 214 and 285 of the 481 amino acids contained in the polypeptide.[123–125] T-cell epitopes were also defined on the E1 protein, although no single epitope was recognized by a majority of individuals.[126–130] The E1 protein has been produced in quantity in baculovirus vectors by truncating the C terminus to allow secretion.[131–134] So far, the immunogenicity of bioengineered E1 has been moderate,[133] but strong adjuvants have produced good responses in animals.[135] Synthetic peptides have also generated neutralizing antibodies,[136] and virus-like particles containing the three main viral proteins have been produced from transfected cell lines, with retention of immunogenicity.[137, 138] Although it is doubtful that an inactivated vaccine could provide protection from infancy throughout the childbearing period, such a vaccine might be useful for immunizing adult women.

Live Virus Vaccine

Vaccine Strains

Origin and Development[139]

Several vaccine strains were developed soon after the isolation of rubella virus in tissue culture. Three vaccines were licensed in the United States in 1969 to 1970 as follows: HPV-77 (duck embryo),[140] HPV-77 (dog kidney),[14] and Cendehill (rabbit kidney).[15] Soon thereafter, the RA27/3 human diploid fibroblast vaccine was licensed in Europe.[16] During the succeeding years, both HPV-77 (dog kidney) and Cendehill were withdrawn from American licensure. Finally, in 1979, RA27/3 was licensed in the United States, and HPV-77 (duck embryo) was withdrawn, leaving RA27/3 as the only American rubella vaccine. The RA27/3 strain is also the most widely used throughout the world with the exception of Japan[141] (Table 17–6). This strain was adopted because of its consistent immunogenicity, induction of resistance to reinfection, and low rate of side effects.[142] Accordingly, most of the information presented hereafter concerns the RA27/3 strain, with the addition of data on the other strains that can be extrapolated to the currently used vaccine.

Table 17–6. **CURRENT MANUFACTURE OF RUBELLA VACCINES**

MANUFACTURER	VIRUS STRAIN	CELL SUBSTRATE
Merck Sharp & Dohme, United States	RA27/3	HDCS
SmithKline-RIT,	RA27/3	HDCS
Belgium	RA27/3	HDCS
Swiss Serum and Vaccine Institute, Switzerland	RA27/3	HDCS
Pasteur Mérieux–Connaught, France	RA27/3	HDCS
Sclavo, Italy	RA27/3	HDCS
Institute of Immunology, Yugoslavia	RA27/3	HDCS
Chemo-sero-therapeutic Research Institute, Japan	Matsuba	Rabbit kidney
Chiba Serum Institute, Japan	DCRB 19	Rabbit kidney
Kitasato Institute, Japan	Takahashi	Rabbit kidney
Osaka University, Japan	Matsuura	Quail embryo fibroblast
Takeda Chemical Industries, Japan	TO-336	Rabbit kidney

HDCS, human diploid cell strain.

Published with permission of the University of Chicago Press from Perkins FT. Licensed vaccines. Rev Infect Dis 7:573–576, 1985.

RA27/3 was isolated from a fetus infected with rubella in early 1965.[139, 143] Culture fluid from a tissue explant was passaged directly into WI-38 cells, and eight serial passages were made in WI-38 cultures incubated at 37°C. Additional passages were then done in cultures incubated at 30°C. After seven passages at 30°C, studies using human volunteers showed that the strain was attenuated. To reduce the pathogenicity even further, 10 additional passages were made.[144] The RA27/3 strain is produced as a vaccine strain between the 25th and 30th passages in human diploid cells (WI-38 or MRC-5).[142] The relatively rapid attenuation by passage may be attributable to the use of cold adaptation, whereas the retention of high immunogenicity may be attributable to the low number of passages required to attenuate.[145] The nucleotide sequence of the envelope genes of RA27/3 has been sequenced, revealing 31 amino acid changes in the vaccine compared with the sequence in the wild strain.[146] In comparison, only five changes were noted in the HPV-77 strain.[147]

Strain-specific nucleotide sequences have been demonstrated in the RA27/3 strain, permitting specific identification.[148] Although some antigenic variations have been discerned with rabbit antibodies against *Escherichia coli*–expressed proteins,[149] monoclonal antibody studies employing a panel of monoclonal antibodies showed no significant differences[151] (see *Virology*).

Dosage and Route of Administration

The vaccine dose of RA27/3 is required to be at least 1000 plaque-forming units (PFU) of virus delivered subcutaneously. However, titration studies in humans showed that in keeping with its being a live vaccine, even small subcutaneous doses (<3 PFU) of RA27/3 are immunogenic.[151]

A peculiar attribute of RA27/3, not so far demonstrated with any other rubella vaccine strain, is its immunogenicity when it is administered intranasally.[152–158] Some studies suggested that intranasal administration might confer an advantage on the vaccinees in terms of quality of the immune response.[159] However, the subcutaneous administration of vaccine gave similar humoral antibody with only slightly less secretory antibody.[143, 159] Moreover, the intranasal dose of RA27/3 required for consistent immunization is high: 10,000 PFU.[154] Lower doses result in frequent failures,[160] particularly in children, possibly owing to the mechanics of administration. Nevertheless, under careful conditions, some workers have been able to achieve 95% seroconversion rates, only slightly inferior to those rates achieved with subcutaneous injection of RA27/3.[157]

Combination with Measles and Mumps

In the United States and increasingly elsewhere, most pediatric rubella vaccination is accomplished with a triple vaccine that also contains measles and mumps vaccine viruses (MMR). The American triple formulation (MMR II, Merck Sharp & Dohme) contains the Moraten attenuated measles virus (1000 $TCID_{50}$), the Jeryl Lynn mumps virus (5000 $TCID_{50}$), and the RA27/3 rubella virus (1000 $TCID_{50}$). A rubella and measles combined vaccine (M-R-Vax II, Merck Sharp & Dohme) is available for those who do not wish to use mumps vaccine. A combined rubella and mumps vaccine (Biavax II, Merck Sharp & Dohme) can be given to older children who have had measles vaccine previously. Two formulations available in Europe and elsewhere (Pluserix, SmithKline-RIT, Belgium; and Trimovax, Pasteur Mérieux) contain the Schwarz measles virus (1000 $TCID_{50}$), the Urabe mumps virus (20,000 $TCID_{50}$), and the RA27/3 rubella virus (1000 $TCID_{50}$). A triple vaccine made in Japan contains the AIK-C measles virus (30,000 $TCID_{50}$), the Urabe mumps virus (10,000 $TCID_{50}$), and the TO-336 rubella virus (10,000 $TCID_{50}$).[161]

Responses to rubella as part of the triple vaccine are equal to those seen after rubella vaccination as a single antigen. Table 17–7 is taken from a study by Weibel and colleagues[162] that compared MMR formulated with RA27/3 with RA27/3 alone. The excellent responses in both groups of vaccinees have been confirmed by other investigators,[163, 164] who also found RA27/3 to be superior to the earlier HPV-77 component.[163] The bivalent measles-rubella and mumps-rubella vaccines also produced rubella antibody levels that were equivalent to those of the monovalent vaccine.[163] A triple vaccine that contained Cendehill virus gave a 96% seroconversion rate to the rubella component.[165]

Production and Constituents of Vaccine

RA27/3 is manufactured on a human diploid cell substrate, either WI-38 or MRC-5 fetal lung fibroblasts. Cell cultures inoculated with the seed virus are incubated at 30°C. After 4 to 7 days of initial incubation, there is sufficient virus in the supernatant medium to harvest. Fresh medium is added, and subsequent harvests can be made every 2 to 3 days for several weeks. Stabilizer is added to the harvest fluids, which are frozen for later safety testing and pooling before eventual lyophilization.[166, 167] The final RA27/3 vaccine is essentially free of animal serum but does contain 0.4% human albumin, 25 to 50 μg/mL neomycin, and, in one case (Sclavo), 50 μg/mL of kanamycin. The lyophilization medium varies according to the manufacturer; however, it generally contains sucrose or sorbitol, glutamic acid and other amino acids, and buffering salts. When lyophilized, the vaccine is hypertonic. Reconstitution is accomplished with sterile distilled water (0.5 to 1.0 mL) according to the manufacturer's directions, which restores the vaccine to a normal or slightly hypertonic state. The water added for reconstitution should not include a preservative, because it would kill the live vaccine virus. All manufacturers provide water for reconstitution with the vaccine.

RA27/3 is produced in the United States, the United Kingdom, France, Belgium, Italy, Switzerland, and Yugoslavia by the manufacturers listed in Table 17–6. Despite minor differences in dose, antibiotic content, and other details among manufacturers, differences in vaccine efficacy or in the nature or severity of side effects have not been reported.

Stability of Vaccine

Rubella vaccine is highly stable in the frozen state at −70°C or −20°C. At 4°C, the viability of the virus and

Table 17–7. **ANTIBODY RESPONSES IN INITIALLY SERONEGATIVE CHILDREN WHO RECEIVED COMBINED MEASLES (MORATEN)–MUMPS (JERYL LYNN)–RUBELLA (RA27/3) OR MONOVALENT RA27/3 RUBELLA VACCINE**

	ANTIBODY RESPONSES VERSUS								
	Measles (HI) Conversion			Mumps (Neutralizing) Conversion			Rubella (HI) Conversion		
VACCINE	*N/ Total*	*%*	*Geometric Mean*	*N/ Total*	*%*	*Geometric Mean*	*N/ Total*	*%*	*Geometric Mean*
Combined	64/68	94	57	65/68	96	8	68/68	100	136
Monovalent	—	—	—	—	—	—	67/67	100	159

HI, hemagglutination inhibition.

From Weibel RE, Carlson AJ, Villarejos VM, et al. Clinical and laboratory studies of combined live measles, mumps, and rubella vaccines using the RA27/3 rubella virus. Proc Soc Exp Biol Med 165:323–326, 1980.

Table 17–8. **COMPARISON OF HEMAGGLUTINATION-INHIBITING ANTIBODY RESPONSE AMONG INITIALLY SERONEGATIVE CHILDREN AND ADULTS WHO RECEIVED RA27/3 or HPV-77 DUCK EMBRYO RUBELLA VIRUS VACCINES**

	CHILDREN			ADULTS		
VACCINE	**Seroconverting/Total (N)**	**HI Titer Range**	**Mean**	**Seroconverting/Total (N)**	**HI Titer Range**	**Mean**
RA27/3	153/153 (100%)	8–1024	153*	98/99 (99)	<8–512	84*
HPV-77:DE	152/156 (97%)	<8–512	81	85/94 (90)	<8–512	35

*Significantly greater than geometric mean titer for HPV-77:DE group (P < .001).
HI, hemagglutination inhibition.
Modified from Weibel RE, Villarejos VM, Klein EB, et al. Clinical laboratory studies of live attenuated RA27/3 and HPV-77 DE rubella virus vaccines. Proc Soc Exp Biol Med 165:44–49, 1980. Copyright 1980. Society for Experimental Biology and Medicine.

the potency of the vaccine are also maintained for at least 5 years. At room temperature, there is significant loss after 3 months; at 37°C, a 3-week period is sufficient to damage vaccine potency.[168] The vaccine should be stored at 2 to 8°C and protected from light. The virus is labile after reconstitution and should be used within 8 hours.

Results of Vaccination

Immune Responses

Vaccination induces antibodies of both IgM and IgG classes and cellular immune responses. The induction of secretory IgA responses depends on the type of immunization, as subsequently described.

Most studies of immunogenicity have been done by measuring hemagglutination inhibition responses, although the neutralizing responses may be more important biologically. By the hemagglutination inhibition technique, 95 to 100% of RA27/3 vaccinees experience seroconversion by 21 to 28 days after vaccination, with geometric mean titers ranging from 1:30 to 1:300, depending on the method of titration[16, 144, 169, 170] (Table 17–8). Some of the apparent failures, at least in young adults, may be explained by preexisting low levels of antibody that neutralize the vaccine virus but that are detectable only by sensitive tests.[171]

Several direct comparative immunogenicity studies have been done with different strains. A trial comparing the administration of the RA27/3 and Cendehill strains to Scottish schoolgirls resulted in a 98% seroconversion for the former and 90% for the latter.[172] In Sweden, Böttiger and Heller[173] found a 98% response after inoculation with RA27/3 and 96% after inoculation with Cendehill. In another Swedish trial, Grillner[174] tested neutralizing titers after vaccination, and 95% of RA27/3 vaccinees were seropositive compared with 56% of Cendehill vaccinees. Menser and colleagues[175] tested RA27/3 and Cendehill in Australian schoolgirls and adults; they found no differences in seroconversion but better boosting of seropositive individuals by RA27/3. Weibel and associates[176] conducted large comparative studies of RA27/3 and HPV-77, obtaining results that are summarized in Table 17–8. The Japanese TO-336 and the Chinese BRD-2 strains compared favorably with RA27/3 in parallel studies.[177, 178]

RA27/3 elicits complement-fixing and precipitating antibody titers in nearly all vaccinees.[143] In a precipitin test system, RA27/3 was the only vaccine strain that evoked antibodies to the iota internal antigen of rubella virus.[179]

The induction of neutralizing antibody is particularly significant and is seen regularly and promptly after the administration of RA27/3. Figure 17–3 and Table 17–9 present comparative data obtained in New Haven, Connecticut,[101] and in Sweden.[173] Immunoblot analysis confirmed the persistence of antibodies for at least 3 years to the E1 protein that bears neutralizing epitopes. Antibodies to the C protein also persisted, but antibodies to E2 disappeared in some cases.[180]

A crucial property of RA27/3 is its ability to induce secretory IgA antibody in the nasopharynx, which, as discussed subsequently, may prevent reinfection with wild virus. This property makes RA27/3 similar to natu-

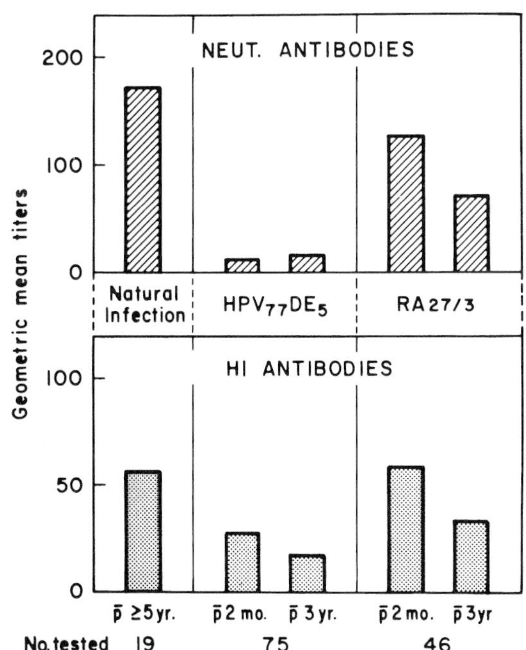

Figure 17–3. Comparison of neutralizing antibodies and hemagglutination-inhibiting (HI) antibodies in three groups of individuals: naturally infected children, children given HPV-77 duck embryo vaccine, and children given RA27/3 vaccine. (From Horstmann DM. Viral vaccines and their ways. Rev Infect Dis 1:502–516, 1979.)

Table 17–9. **NEUTRALIZING ANTIBODY RESPONSE IN 114 RUBELLA-VACCINATED WOMEN WHO DEMONSTRATED SEROCONVERSION WITH HEMAGGLUTINATION-INHIBITING ANTIBODIES**

VACCINE	BEFORE VACCINATION*	AFTER VACCINATION	
		8 Weeks	2 Years
Cendehill	1/45	24/43 (56%)	27/33 (82%)
HPV-77 duck	2/29	23/29 (79%)	16/17 (94%)
RA27/3	1/40	37/39 (95%)	20/20 (100%)

*Number positive/number tested.

From Grillner L. Neutralizing antibodies after rubella vaccination of newly delivered women. A comparison between three vaccines. Scand J Infect Dis 7:169–172, 1975.

ral infection, which also induces local immunity. Although secretory IgA responses are higher after intranasal vaccination, they are also induced by subcutaneous vaccination with RA27/3.[181, 182] Whereas some workers believe that secretory antibodies are important in protection against rubella, Cradock-Watson and colleagues[183] published evidence that nasal antibodies were transient in appearance, and they doubted their ability to prevent reinfection.

Not surprisingly, vaccination, like disease, is followed by the early production of IgM class antibodies. These antibodies reach a peak at 1 month after vaccination[183] and last approximately 1 month more.[184, 185]

Cellular immune responses have been studied, although their significance is unclear. A proliferation of lymphoblasts in response to rubella antigen appears 2 weeks after vaccination, without suppression of tuberculin hypersensitivity.[186] Honeyman and coworkers[187] found sensitization of lymphocytes from Cendehill vaccinees to rubella antigen, which disappeared 1 year later. Relatively short-lived cellular responses were also seen in other studies.[188, 189] Human leukocyte antigen–restricted T-cell cytotoxicity was shown to increase after immunization.[190] Morag and coworkers[191] showed that cytotoxic T-lymphocyte activity was high in tonsillar lymphocytes after intranasal vaccination (with RA27/3) but was low after subcutaneous vaccination (with HPV-77). Unfortunately, subcutaneous administration of RA27/3 was not evaluated.

Although early studies done with relatively insensitive detection systems suggested that rubella vaccines did not cause viremia, viremia has been documented between 7 and 11 days after inoculation.[192] However, the viremia is low and inconstant. Pharyngeal excretion of virus is more frequent, occurring from about 7 to 21 days after vaccination, in low titer of usually less than 10 PFU per swab. Excretion peaks on approximately the 11th day after vaccination; if properly tested, essentially all vaccinees will be shown to excrete virus from the nasopharynx.[193, 194]

In view of the excretion of rubella virus by vaccinees, considerable effort has been made to detect the spread of vaccine virus to susceptible contacts. Initially, contact studies were focused on children in institutions and on families, and no evidence for spread of vaccine virus was found.[15, 16, 141] For example, none of 393 seronegative family members was infected by contact with RA27/3 vaccinees.[16] Veronelli[195] studied 347 familial contacts of HPV-77 vaccinees and also found no evidence of spread.

Subsequently, experience in studies of contact spread produced largely negative results, with the rare asymptomatic seroconversion that could not be fully explained.[196, 197] Scott and Byrne[198] observed 121 seronegative pregnant women exposed to HPV-77 vaccines during a vaccination campaign in Rhode Island; only one experienced seroconversion. Fifteen seronegative husbands who had been exposed to wives vaccinated with Cendehill did not acquire infection.[199] Negative results were also obtained in 67 elementary school teachers exposed to vaccinated pupils.[200] Fleet and colleagues[201] performed a large population surveillance study in Nashville, Tennessee, where 24,000 children were vaccinated. More than 11,000 pregnancies were assessed by virological studies of newborns and abortuses and by serological study of the mothers, without a demonstrated effect of vaccine virus.[201] A possible case of symptomatic reinfection by contact has been reported, but the evidence was unconvincing.[202] Low percentages of seroconversion among contacts were found in large studies of HPV-77 and Cendehill vaccinees.[203, 204] The general lack of evidence for spread by vaccine virus may reflect the maintenance of attenuated markers by excreted virus, as demonstrated for RA27/3.[205]

In summary, rubella vaccine induces immune responses that are similar in quality but lesser in quantity than those after natural disease.[206] The live virus produces viremia and pharyngeal excretion, but both are of low magnitude and are noncommunicable. IgG and IgM antibody responses follow vaccination. Natural infection elicits nasal secretory antibody that may be useful in the prevention of reinfection, and RA27/3 vaccine also has the same property.

Protective Effects

The protective efficacy of rubella vaccination has been assessed (1) by observation of vaccinees and control subjects during natural epidemics and (2) by intranasal challenge of vaccinated volunteers with unattenuated or attenuated viruses.

During an institutional outbreak of rubella, Davis and colleagues[207] were able to evaluate the effect of natural rubella exposure on persons who had been vaccinated with HPV-77. Clinical rubella occurred in 22 of 33 unvaccinated seronegative individuals but in none of 22 vaccinees and 66 naturally immune individuals. Asymptomatic reinfection without viremia was noted in five vaccinees (23.0%) and in one naturally immune subject (1.5%). Grayston and associates[208] compared the effect of HPV-77 vaccine with placebo during an epidemic on Taiwan. Rubella incidence began to drop in the vaccinated group within 2 to 3 weeks, and vaccine efficacy was estimated at 94%. In a separate study undertaken during the same outbreak, RA27/3 vaccine gave a 97% protection rate. A group of children in daycare was observed by Chang and colleagues[209] after some had been vaccinated with Cendehill. The vaccine afforded

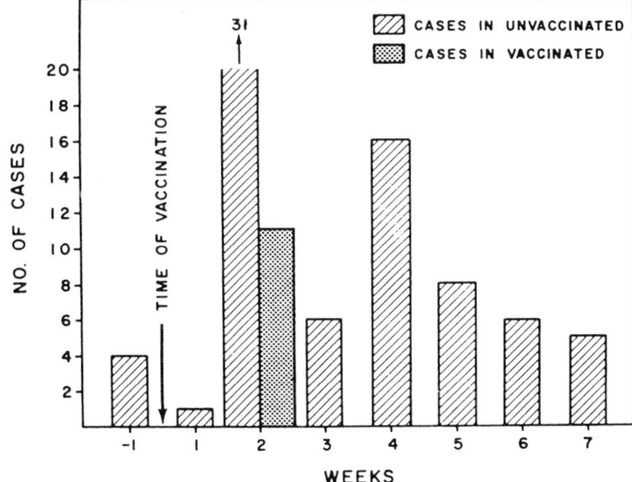

Figure 17–4. Demonstration of protection against rubella during an epidemic in a boys' school at the Toyota car factory near Nagoya, Japan. Boys were selected at random to receive RA27/3 vaccine at the time indicated, and about one third received the vaccine. (From Furukawa T, Miyata T, Kondo K, et al. Rubella vaccination during an epidemic. JAMA 213:987–990, 1970. Copyright 1970, American Medical Association.)

complete protection against disease, but 50% of the vaccinees were reinfected.

A dramatic example of protection by vaccine was reported from Japan.[210] An outbreak started in a school for apprentices at the Toyota automobile factory. RA27/3 vaccine was given randomly to a third of the boys. As shown in Figure 17–4, the epidemic continued for 7 weeks, but rubella ceased to occur in vaccinees 2 weeks after they were vaccinated.

An outbreak of rubella in a primary school in France during 1997 permitted a calculation of efficacy, because only about 75% of children had been vaccinated. Vaccine efficacy was 95% (85 to 99% confidence interval).[211]

In Olmstead County, Minnesota, adolescent girls were vaccinated with Cendehill; unvaccinated boys were used as control subjects, which permitted a calculation of efficacy at 94% during a 1972 outbreak.[212] The introduction of rubella vaccination of recruits at Lackland Air Force Base resulted in a 95% reduction in rubella by 1979.[213] A more recent outbreak in Sanford, Maine, during 1980 to 1981 allowed an assessment of vaccine efficacy 8 years after vaccination; it was 90%.[214]

In Finland, five cases of rubella encephalitis were seen at Helsinki Children's Hospital during a 15-year period starting in the late 1960s, whereas none has been seen since the advent of MMR vaccination in 1982.[215]

Reinfection and Herd Immunity

Early in rubella vaccine studies, it became evident that under conditions of exposure to wild virus, reinfection of persons vaccinated with HPV-77 and Cendehill could occur with a frequency of 50% or greater.[216–220]

Herd immunity was shown to be ineffective when rubella broke out in a company of military recruits who were studied by Horstmann and coworkers.[221] Although most recruits had antibodies due to vaccination or prior infection at the start of the epidemic, 100% of the remaining susceptible individuals were infected. Moreover, 80% of the recruits vaccinated with HPV-77 were reinfected. The same conclusion was reached in another study of recruits, in which rubella singled out the susceptible individuals despite high levels of immunity in the group.[222]

Bermuda experienced a rubella outbreak in 1971. A vaccination campaign with Cendehill resulted in prompt termination of the epidemic; vaccine efficacy was estimated to be 94%.[223] However, a rubella epidemic in Casper, Wyoming, in the same year showed that although the vaccine (HPV-77) prevented rubella in immunized elementary schoolchildren, unimmunized adolescents and adults still suffered an attack rate that was 50% of that expected without vaccination.[224, 225] Fogel and colleagues[216] used intranasal RA27/3 as a challenge to RA27/3, Cendehill, and HPV-77 vaccinees. Their results showed a higher rate of reinfection in the last two groups compared with that in RA27/3 vaccinees (Table 17–10). Harcourt and associates[217] concluded that reinfection is dependent on a number of immunological factors, including but not restricted to the presence of nasopharyngeal IgA rubella antibody. When the RA27/3 virus itself was given intranasally as a challenge virus, O'Shea and coworkers[226] found that reinfection was infrequent in those who had natural immunity or significant titers (>15 IU) of rubella antibody from previous vaccination but was frequent in vaccinees who had low titers (<15 IU), although viremia as part of the reinfection was rare. Among RA27/3 vaccinees, approximately 5% had low titers 6 to 16 years after vaccination.[227] A 9.8% incidence of asymptomatic reinfection was reported 5 years after vaccination.[228]

The significance of reinfection is hotly debated. In some studies, reinfection leads only to an IgG booster response, without IgM,[229] whereas in others the appearance of IgM antibody suggested significant viral replication.[230, 231] Nevertheless, clinical rubella has been documented during reinfection of vaccinees[232] and naturally immune individuals.[233, 234] Moreover, maternal reinfection during pregnancy has resulted in congenital rubella,[235–249] although reinfection is a relatively infrequent event. In a prospective study, Morgan-Capner and associates[250] found definite evidence of passage of virus from reinfected mothers to their fetuses in two of three cases

Table 17–10. **REINFECTION* OF VACCINEES AFTER VIRUS CHALLENGE**

PREVIOUS VACCINE GIVEN	TOTAL VACCINEES	VACCINEES SHOWING REINFECTION	
		N	Percentage
Cendehill	27	18	66.7
HPV-77	30	14	45.7
RA27/3	28	2	7.1

*As revealed by a positive booster in at least one of four serological tests.

From Fogel A, Gerichter CB, Barena B, et al. Response to experimental challenges in persons immunized with different rubella vaccines. J Pediatr 92:26–29, 1978.

in which exposure had occurred in the first trimester and fetal tissue was available. However, follow-up of seven liveborn infants did not reveal CRS. O'Shea and colleagues[251] measured rubella immunity in reinfected women and reinfected seropositive volunteers undergoing a challenge with rubella virus. The presence or absence of neutralizing antibodies or cellular immunity did not correlate with the likelihood of reinfection. However, Matter and coworkers[252] suggested that reinfection may be more likely at low levels of antibody measured by hemolysis in gel (10 to 15 IU), and Mitchell and colleagues[253] reported that reinfection was correlated with lack of prior antibodies to a peptide of the E1 protein.

It is not always easy to distinguish between primary and secondary responses in a person with prior low or nondetectable antibodies who has been exposed to natural infection or been revaccinated. If that distinction is important for clinical care or research, detection of IgM antibodies or low avidity IgG antibodies may be helpful.[230, 252] The best conclusion at this time is that reinfection with fetal transmission of wild rubella virus is a fact, in the presence of both natural and vaccine-induced immunity, but that the risk is probably less than 5% in the first trimester of pregnancy compared with at least 80% in primary infection. The danger of reinfection is another reason for immunizing contacts of pregnant women.

Persistence of Immunity and Revaccination

There are numerous data on persistence of antibody after vaccination. Liebhaber and colleagues[254] found antibodies in all 18 vaccinees 2 years after vaccination with RA27/3. In response to a challenge with unattenuated rubella virus, 16 of the 18 vaccinees showed resistance to reinfection. Amazonian Indians given RA27/3 by Black and coworkers[255] had persistent antibodies in the absence of any possible re-exposure to the virus, although there was a twofold drop during 2.5 years. A 98 to 99% persistence of antibody was noted in schoolchildren 4 years after vaccination.[256] Zealley and Edmond[257] reported on a long-term study of Edinburgh schoolgirls, of whom 97% retained antibodies 6 to 7 years after vaccination with RA27/3. The longest observation periods after vaccination with RA27/3 thus far have been 12 to 17 years,[145] 15 years,[258] and 10 to 21 years.[259] In one long-term study, 75 of 78 (96%) vaccinees retained measurable antibody (Fig. 17–5). In a follow-up of Baltimore schoolchildren, there was a decline of less than fourfold in titer during a 15-year postvaccination period, and 97% remained seropositive.[260]

Miller and colleagues[261] studied 475 children 4 years after MMR and found 97% positive for rubella antibodies. A Canadian study of a similar number of children tested 5 to 6 years after MMR gave identical results.[262] Böttiger[263] observed 220 Swedish children given MMR at 18 months of age. At 12 years of age, 97% had rubella antibodies, although not at the same levels seen immediately after vaccination. A second dose given at 12 years of age raised the titer levels to those seen after primary vaccination. Christenson and Böttiger[264] also observed a cohort of almost 500 girls vaccinated at age

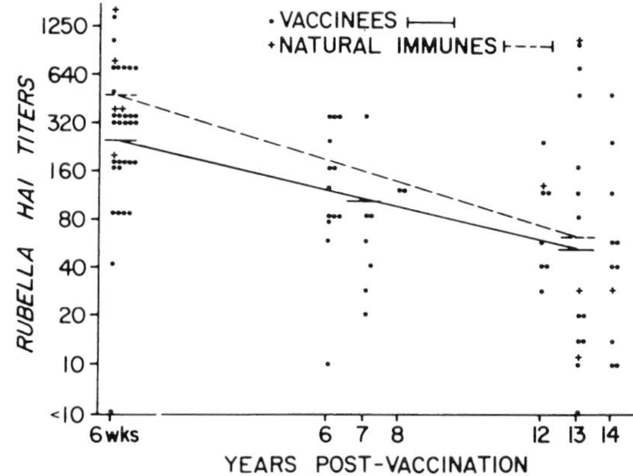

Figure 17–5. Persistence of hemagglutination-inhibiting antibody (HAI) to rubella after natural infection or the administration of RA27/3 vaccine. (From Plotkin SA, Buser F. History of RA27/3 rubella vaccine. Rev Infect Dis 7[suppl]:S77–S78, 1985.)

12 years. After 8 years, 96% were still seropositive, and 94% were still so at 16 years after vaccination, although the mean titers had dropped from 1:110 to 1:18 (Table 17–11).

Different results were reported by Johnson and coworkers,[265] who studied 95 children given MMR at 15 months of age. Children studied at age 4 to 6 years were 100% positive for rubella-neutralizing antibodies, but only 63% of children aged 11 to 13 years were positive. They suggested that immunity had waned. After a second dose of MMR, 100% of children became seropositive with almost a threefold rise in the geometric mean titer of rubella antibodies. In Newfoundland, Ratnam and associates[266] found that 16.5% of children 8 to 17 years of age were seronegative after prior vaccination at 1 year of age.

Reports of persistence of antibody to Cendehill vaccine from Australia, Switzerland, the United States, and the United Kingdom gave, in order, 95% persistence at 5 years,[267] 96% at 15 years,[268] 98% at 10 years,[269] and 100% at 8 to 18 years after vaccination.[257, 270]

Persistence of antibodies after vaccination with the HPV-77 vaccines used earlier has been variable. Whereas some reports were favorable,[259, 270–272] other reports indicated that antibody was less persistent.[273, 274] Follow-up of those vaccinated with Cendehill or HPV-77:DE 20 years previously in Hawaii showed persistent antibody in 92.8%.[275] A study in Milwaukee revealed

Table 17–11. **PERSISTENCE OF RUBELLA ANTIBODIES AFTER VACCINATION OF SERONEGATIVE SCHOOLGIRLS**

TIME AFTER VACCINATION	N	% HI TITERS ≥1:8	GMT (HI)
8 wk	486	100	110
2 yr	346	99	80
4 yr	136	99	53
8 yr	486	96	34
16 yr	190	94	18

HI, hemagglutination inhibition; GMT, geometric mean titer.
Data from reference 264.

13% seronegativity 12 years after vaccination.[276] Best[277] summarized published studies of antibody persistence 9 to 21 years after vaccination and found a seronegativity rate of 1% for RA27/3 vaccinees, 2.7% for Cendehill vaccinees, and 7.3% for HPV-77 vaccinees.

An epidemic of rubella occurred during 1981 to 1982 among students at the University of California at Los Angeles. Strassburg and colleagues[278] performed a case-control study and found that prior immunization with unspecified rubella vaccines conferred a 97% protection, even though some students had been immunized 10 years previously. Natural immunity to rubella lasts at least 26 years.[279]

One study reported good persistence of antibody 10 years after inoculation with the Japanese TO-336 virus.[280] Persistent antibody and protection also followed the use of the Matsuba strain.[281]

Rossier and associates[282] studied persistence of cellular immunity to rubella and found that in contrast to naturally infected individuals, most HPV-77 vaccinees lacked cellular immunity 5 years after vaccination. A similar difference was noted between Cendehill vaccinees and naturally infected adults.[187] In a small group of vaccinees followed 23 years after receipt of the Matsuba strain, 15% were negative by HI, but reimmunization nevertheless induced secondary responses.[282a]

It thus appears that rubella immunity wanes after vaccination, but most vaccinees remain seropositive. Reimmunization has been advocated by some of those who have studied the persistence of immunity to HPV-77:DEV and Cendehill,[283, 284] and subcutaneous RA27/3 could be given as a booster vaccine for those previously immunized.[285, 286] However, ostensibly seronegative individuals usually show secondary immunological responses after boosters, indicating that they had been immune.[287, 288] In any case, the question has now been rendered in part moot by the adoption in many countries of a routine second dose of measles, usually as a triple vaccine containing rubella. Revaccination is a suggested strategy to augment rubella immunity before the age of reproduction. Individuals who fail to seroconvert after rubella vaccination should be given a single repeated dose. Failure to respond to the second dose may be evidence for tolerance to rubella virus antigens,[289] which is definitely seen in survivors of CRS.[290]

Combined Vaccination

As mentioned previously, when rubella vaccine is given to preschool-aged children, it is almost always given in combination with measles and mumps vaccines as MMR vaccine. Excellent results have been reported for both RA27/3 and Cendehill as components of triple vaccines.[162, 291] There is no contraindication to giving MMR even in the presence of immunity to one or two of its components, and some authorities prefer to use MMR exclusively in vaccination programs.

Rubella or MMR vaccine can be given simultaneously (but separately) with diphtheria and tetanus toxoids and pertussis vaccine, *Haemophilus influenzae* vaccine, inactivated poliovirus vaccine, hepatitis B vaccine, oral poliovirus vaccine,[292] and varicella vaccine.[293]

Side Effects

In 1991, the Institute of Medicine of the National Academy of Sciences published a committee report on four possible adverse effects of rubella vaccine: acute arthritis, chronic arthritis, neuropathies, and thrombocytopenia.[294] The committee concluded that RA27/3 causes acute arthritis. With regard to chronic arthritis, the committee stated, "The evidence is consistent with a causal relation between the currently used rubella vaccine strain (RA27/3) and chronic arthritis in adult women, although the evidence is limited in scope and confined to reports from one institution." However, the committee found insufficient evidence to indicate a causal relationship between use of the vaccine and incidence of radiculoneuritis, other neuropathies, and thrombocytopenia. We shall see that many of these conclusions remain controversial or dubious.

Arthritis and Arthralgia. A review of adverse events in Canada gave a reaction rate for rubella vaccine of 28.7 per 100,000 doses distributed, of which 0.3 per 100,000 was arthritis or arthralgia.[295] Arthritis is part of the disease caused by rubella virus, at least in adults, and is also the most important side effect of vaccination.[296] Although the HPV-77 strain is no longer in use, much information on joint reactions was obtained by studying reactions to vaccination with this strain. The HPV-77 dog kidney vaccine was particularly likely to cause reactions in joints, even in children.[297, 298] At times, the reactions included neuropathies, such as the "catcher's crouch" syndrome.[297–302] The HPV-77 duck embryo vaccine produced reactions that were age related; for example, in one study, 0% of girls younger than 13 years, 2% of those 13 to 16 years old, 6% of those 17 to 19 years old, 25% of women 20 to 24 years old, and 50% of women older than 25 years developed reactions in the joints.[303, 304] Symptoms could be prolonged.[305] In two different studies, Cendehill vaccine was reported to cause these reactions in 23% and 16% of women.[306, 307] RA27/3 produced infrequent reactions in children,[308] but approximately 25% of adults had temporary joint symptoms.[309]

Polk and associates[310] performed a comparative trial of rubella vaccines in adult women. Some of their comparative data are represented in Table 17–12. In addition, they reviewed other reports and concluded that the incidence of transient arthralgia or arthritis was 35 to 63% with the use of HPV-77 dog kidney, 27 to 33% with HPV-77 duck embryo, 8 to 10% with Cendehill, and 13 to 15% with RA27/3. Although many different joints can be involved in the reaction to rubella vaccines, knees and fingers are the most common, whereas the hips are seldom involved. Conflicting evidence has been reported regarding the influence of the stage of the menstrual cycle on joint symptoms.[177, 303, 305]

The mechanism of joint inflammation appears to be direct infection of the synovial tissue by the virus, if one extrapolates from recoveries of the virus from joints of patients with arthritis after occurrence of natural rubella[311] and after inoculation with HPV-77 vaccine.[312] Laboratory studies suggesting that rubella RNA and rubella peptides might induce autoimmunity have also

Table 17–12. **SIDE EFFECTS AMONG SERONEGATIVE ADULT FEMALE VACCINEES RECEIVING MEASLES-MUMPS-RUBELLA (MMR) OR MEASLES-MUMPS-RUBELLA II (MMR II) AND AMONG SEROPOSITIVE CONTROL SUBJECTS**

	MMR (HPV-77:DE-5)	MMR II (RA27/3)	CONTROL SUBJECTS
N	59	53	60
Age (yr)			
X ± SD	29.29 ± 9.09	30.00 ± 9.81	30.70 ± 10.36
Median	26	27	27
Range	19–58	19–58	20–58
Any joint manifestation	17 (28.8%)	14 (26.4%)	2 (3.3%)
Arthritis only	9 (15.3%)	6 (11.3%)	0 (0)
Paresthesias	2	0	0
Fever	5	1	4
Rash	4	4	2
Days of work missed because of joint pains	8 (4)*	3 (1)*	0

*Number of vaccinees who missed work in parentheses.
From Polk BF, Modlin JF, White JA, DeGirolami PC. A controlled comparison of joint reactions among women receiving one of two rubella vaccines. Am J Epidemiol 115:19–25, 1982.

been published.[313, 314] Human joint tissue infected in vitro by Miki and Chantler[315] supported high-titer replication of wild viruses and of HPV-77 but relatively restricted replication of RA27/3 and particularly Cendehill. Although RA27/3 has not been recovered from joints, Tingle and associates[316] reported isolating vaccine virus from the peripheral blood mononuclear cells of two women who had prolonged arthritis after administration of the vaccine. Joint reactions were not associated with elevated IgG or prolonged IgM responses.[317] Tingle and coworkers[318] reported a prospective study conducted in British Columbia of arthritis after RA27/3 vaccination or natural disease. The incidence of acute arthritis was 52% in the disease group and 14% in the vaccinees. Recurrent arthropathy developed in 30% of women who had the disease and 5% of women who had been vaccinated. Symptoms were not associated with circulating immune complexes.[319] The occurrence of chronic viremia and the determination of an etiological relationship between rubella vaccination and chronic arthritis await confirmation. The Institute of Medicine committee suggested the need for prospective, double-blind, controlled trials of rubella vaccine in adult women, associated with attempts to isolate rubella virus, to resolve the controversy.[320]

Six studies touching on this issue have since been reported. Phillips and colleagues[321] and subsequently Frenkel[322] and Nielsen[323] and their coworkers were unable to confirm the presence of viremia in vaccinees complaining of chronic arthritis. Rubella genomic RNA was not demonstrated by Zhang and associates[324] in blood and synovial fluid from cases of rheumatoid arthritis. Slater and colleagues[325] observed two cohorts of Israeli women, one of which had received rubella vaccine. Five to 10 years later, the incidence of arthritis in vaccinees and control subjects was 3.9% and 3.2%, respectively, an insignificant difference. At the Kaiser Permanente Northern California Health Maintenance Organization, Ray and colleagues[326] linked rubella vaccination records with cases of chronic arthritis and found no association between the two. Finally, the British Columbia group performed a placebo-controlled prospective study of approximately 500 women, half of whom were vaccinated and observed for 1 year.[327] Their results are summarized in Table 17–13. Not surprisingly, acute arthralgia and arthritis were more common in vaccinees, although the excess attributable to vaccine was only 5%. Chronic arthritis or arthralgia was seen in no less than 15% of placebo recipients but was increased to 22% in vaccinees. However, the difference had only marginal statistical significance (P = .04).

Thus, taking the evidence as a whole, one is left with the conclusion that chronic arthropathy due to RA27/3 is plausible biologically, but unconfirmed by virology or epidemiology, and is rare if it occurs at all. Nevertheless, on the basis of the Institute of Medicine report, the National Vaccine Injury Compensation Program has

Table 17–13. **FREQUENCIES OF ACUTE AND CHRONIC REACTIONS TO RUBELLA VACCINE OR PLACEBO IN ADULT WOMEN**

	GROUP (%)		
	Placebo (N = 275)	Vaccine (N = 268)	ODDS RATIO (95% confidence interval)
Acute Reactions			
Sore throat	32	34	1.09 (0.75–1.59)
Cervical Lymphadenopathy	10	19	2.21 (1.31–3.76)
Rash	11	25	2.57 (1.58–4.21)
Myalgia	16	21	1.36 (0.88–2.10)
Paresthesias	7	7	1.09 (0.57–2.09)
Arthralgia	16	21	1.42 (0.92–2.19)
Arthritis	4	9	2.36 (1.13–4.92)
Arthralgia or arthritis	20	30	1.73 (1.17–2.57)
Chronic Reactions			
Myalgia	9	15	1.68 (0.99–2.84)
Paresthesias	4	5	1.12 (0.50–2.50)
Arthralgia or arthritis	15	22	1.58 (1.01–2.45)

Adapted from Tingle A, Mitchell L, Grace M, et al. Randomised double-blind placebo-controlled study on adverse effects of rubella immunisation in seronegative women. Lancet 349:1277–1281, 1996.

been accepting claims of chronic arthropathy due to rubella vaccination, and compensation has been awarded to 23 of 56 completed cases.[328]

Chiba and colleagues[329] reported a depression of rubella-specific cellular immune responses in children with arthritis. Circulating immune complexes containing rubella antigen were found in 11 of 33 vaccinees who developed arthralgia after vaccination but in only 3 of 19 who did not.[330]

Other Side Effects. Vaccinees sometimes develop mild rubella, including rash, lymphadenopathy, fever, sore throat, and headache. The incidence of each of these side effects varies directly with age, being almost absent in infants but present in up to 50% of women. As stated previously, the severity of reactions is greatest in older women. Fortunately, the minor side effects are seldom severe enough to cause days to be lost from school or work.[173, 175, 309, 331]

A double-blind study of vaccination with MMR in children gave a 1% incidence of arthropathy and little evidence of other reactions.[332] Another controlled study revealed no significant differences in reactions of children receiving either MMR or measles vaccines.[333]

Complications

Although few serious events after vaccination with RA27/3 have been reported, it is useful to review this type of information for all vaccine strains.[334] Polyneuropathy is part of natural rubella and is among the most frequent of the unusual complications of rubella vaccination. Schaffner and associates,[335] who reviewed the problem in 1974, found 299 reports of polyneuropathy after vaccination. The cases they reviewed followed immunization with HPV-77:DEV, HPV-77:DK, and, less frequently, Cendehill vaccines. The symptoms began about 40 days after vaccination, appearing in the form of two syndromes, one consisting of paresthesias and pain in the arms and the other involving pain in the knee and preference for a crouching position. The second syndrome tended to recur. Carpal tunnel syndrome and Horner syndrome were also seen. Children with polyneuropathy showed impairment of motor and sensory nerve conduction.

Two cases of optic neuritis after vaccination for rubella have been reported, the vaccine being HPV-77 in one instance[336] and an unstated vaccine in the other.[337] Transverse myelitis has been reported on two occasions[338] and diffuse myelitis on three occasions after inoculation with RA27/3, Cendehill, and an unstated vaccine.[339, 340] Four cases of transverse myelitis have been reported after vaccination with MMR containing RA27/3.[341] Facial paresthesias were reported after vaccination with RA27/3.[342] Two cases of Guillain-Barré syndrome have been noted after the use of HPV-77:DEV, but an etiological association could not be confirmed.[338, 343]

There are rare reports of Guillain-Barré syndrome after rubella vaccination in combined vaccines,[344] but an epidemiological study in the United Kingdom after a measles-rubella vaccination campaign revealed rates of Guillain-Barré less than that expected by the background rate (1 per 100,000 children).[345] Chantler and associates[346] showed that rubella viruses grow in human astrocytes but poorly in oligodendrocytes, suggesting that demyelinating disease is not likely to be associated with rubella virus replication.

A case of "bone changes" after rubella vaccination was reported,[347] but the negative virus isolation, absence of IgM antibodies, and lack of detail make the association dubious. One case of mild orchitis after the administration of rubella vaccine was reported.[348]

Thrombocytopenia has followed vaccination for rubella on several occasions[349, 350] and has been reported frequently after the administration of triple vaccine.[351, 352] A decrease in platelets may be seen in some asymptomatic vaccinees after vaccination, and symptomatic thrombocytopenia has been reported after natural rubella. A rate of 1 in 3000 is accepted for thrombocytopenia after wild rubella,[353] whereas rates 10 times lower have been reported after rubella vaccination.[351] It appears that either measles or rubella vaccines may be responsible for thrombocytopenia after MMR.[354] In addition, exacerbation of chronic thrombocytopenia has been reported after MMR,[355] as has recurrent thrombocytopenia after repeated administration.[356] Revaccination is not recommended by the Advisory Committee on Immunization Practices for children who suffered thrombocytopenic purpura after MMR,[357] but the balance of risk and benefit should be weighed.[358]

Rubella vaccines have been noted to depress nonspecific cellular immunity transiently,[359] including the tuberculin reaction, cell-mediated immunity to *Candida*, phytohemagglutinin responses, and delayed-type hypersensitivity to recall antigens, and to increase suppressor T cells.[360–362] Follow-up study of RA27/3 vaccinees has shown no increase in cancer incidence.[363]

A double-blind study of vaccination with MMR in children gave a 1% incidence of arthropathy and little evidence of other reactions.[331] Another controlled study revealed no significant differences in reactions of children receiving either MMR or measles vaccines.[333]

In contrast to the Institute of Medicine, I conclude that acute arthritis and thrombocytopenia are caused by RA27/3 vaccination, whereas the relationship to chronic arthritis and neuropathy is unsubstantiated.

Indications for Rubella Vaccine

The targets of rubella vaccination are listed in Table 17–14.

Table 17–14. **TARGET GROUPS FOR RUBELLA VACCINATION**

Infants ≥12 mo
Older unvaccinated children and adolescents
College students
Childcare personnel
Healthcare workers
Military personnel
Adult women before pregnancy
Adult seronegative women post partum
Adult men in contact with pregnant women
All of the above as part of a two-dose elimination strategy

Infants

Rubella vaccine is given to preschool-aged children in the United States and many other developed countries in an effort to immunize them for the future and to protect their mothers through reduction of rubella virus circulation.

Rubella vaccine is usually given at 12 to 15 months of age as part of the MMR vaccine. Children who miss the vaccine at that time can receive it at any later age and in most states must receive it at the time of school entry. The age at first vaccination does not seem to be as critical for rubella as for measles vaccine. From 9 months of age on, successful vaccination is likely,[364–369] but there is little need to prevent rubella in those younger than 1 year.[370] A study done in Brazil showed reliable seroconversion after rubella vaccine from about 6 months of age.[85] The presence of acute respiratory infection at the time of vaccination of infants 12 to 18 months of age was shown in three separate studies to have no influence on seroconversion.[371–373]

In view of the lack of evidence of contagiousness of vaccinees, infants whose mothers are pregnant may be vaccinated.

Adolescents

Vaccination is recommended for all adolescents, male and female, who have not been previously vaccinated. In addition, as described later, revaccination with rubella vaccine as part of MMR is recommended in many countries, either at entry to primary school or at 11 to 13 years. The justification for this practice lies mainly in the prevention of measles outbreaks caused by accumulation of susceptibles resulting from primary vaccine failure. However, it has been argued that revaccination will also boost waning immunity to rubella and mumps. Although the evidence for the need to revaccinate against rubella is slim, two-dose regimens are now standard in the United States and other countries (see *Public Health Considerations*).

In the United Kingdom, public health policy formerly emphasized vaccination of 11- to 14-year-old girls, with the idea that by doing this, a cohort of immune women could be created during a period of 10 to 20 years. The success of this policy is considered subsequently; in brief, its advantage was narrowing the target group to potential mothers, and its disadvantages were a high refusal rate and the lack of effect on the circulation of virus. However, Schiff and colleagues[374] succeeded in vaccinating 97% of the high-school girls in a rural town in Wisconsin, with excellent results.

Immunization of adolescent girls has been done with and without the addition of contraception, depending on the known sexual activity in the particular population.[375, 376]

Adults

The most directed vaccination program, in the sense of having the most immediate impact on CRS, is vaccination of women. The principal problem with this approach is the possibility of unsuspected pregnancy, although, as described subsequently, the actual risk to the fetus may be nonexistent.

Identification of seronegative women cannot be done accurately on the basis of history because clinical diagnosis of rubella is unreliable.[377] Vaccination of women who give negative histories of prior vaccinations is advocated without prior serological testing.[370] A frequent practice has been to test women for immune status and then to vaccinate them while oral contraceptives or other forms of pregnancy precaution are taken.[378–381] Vaccination can be practiced as part of routine gynecological care, premarital screening, and occupational health care or at other medical opportunities, as long as contraception can be ensured for 3 months. A frequently expressed concern is whether to vaccinate women with low positive titers, such as those with ELISA values just beyond the cutoff value with hemolysis in gel values of 10 to 15 IU or with hemagglutination inhibition titers of 1:8. Current evidence suggests that those women are usually immune but may be at higher risk of reinfection,[382] and thus one dose of vaccine should be offered (see *Reinfection)*. There is no evidence that vaccination of seropositive women is attended by increased risk of untoward reactions.

The use of rubella vaccine during the puerperium (postpartum vaccination) has been widely advocated.[306, 383–389] Because 56% of CRS children in the United Kingdom were born to multiparae,[390] this practice should prevent a significant portion of CRS. Indeed, Edmond and Zealley[391] observed that CRS was prevented in Edinburgh by vaccination of girls and postpartum vaccination of women, with most of the failures occurring in women who had been screened but not vaccinated. However, pregnancy can occur even in the immediate postpartum period,[392] and contraceptive measures such as the use of depot progestogen should be undertaken.[393] Administration of blood or blood products such as Rh_O globulin to a vaccinee should be associated with postvaccination tests for seroconversion.

Although the postpartum genital tract is not susceptible to rubella vaccine virus,[394] vaccinated parturient women do excrete vaccine virus in their breast milk.[395] The vaccine virus may then be transmitted to their newborns, but they usually remain asymptomatic and do not develop tolerance to subsequent vaccination.[396–398] Thus, breast-feeding is not a contraindication to vaccination.

Adult men not in high-risk groups are not generally targeted for vaccination, although they are also a reservoir of susceptibles and may serve as the source of infection of pregnant women.[399] An outbreak in Croatia showed that infection can propagate among men even if they do not live in a collectivity, despite routine vaccination of infants and women.[400]

Military Recruits and College Students

Vaccination is routinely practiced in the armed forces of the United States, with the consequence being the virtual eradication of rubella.[401] Rubella was also eradicated in the armed forces of Singapore several years after commencement of routine vaccination.[402] The consequences of failure to vaccinate were recently illustrated by an epidemic in British troops in Bosnia.[403] The French army, which until recently has not practiced routine rubella vaccination of its recruits, has had perennial epidemics.[404] In view of the congregation of large numbers of susceptible young adults in colleges and universities, routine vaccination with MMR at matriculation is also advocated.[370, 405] In principle, these vaccinations will be second doses, but they are considered important to prevent outbreaks of measles and perhaps rubella on college campuses.

Hospital Employees

Outbreaks of rubella in hospitals,[406–409] with the resultant exposure of pregnant women, has led to the recommendation of compulsory rubella vaccination for both male and female hospital employees.[410] In one hospital outbreak,[411] those departments that had a compulsory vaccination policy escaped unscathed, whereas those departments that had a voluntary vaccination policy suffered numerous cases including infections of pregnant women. A recent evaluation reconfirmed the recommendation for vaccination of hospital personnel.[412]

International Travelers

Unimmunized women of childbearing age who travel overseas should be vaccinated to protect against the greater likelihood of exposure to the disease in countries that do not use rubella vaccine.

Contraindications

General Contraindications[370]

Rubella vaccine can be given to patients with minor respiratory illnesses, febrile or afebrile (see *Indications*). Those with congenital immune deficiencies should never receive a live virus vaccine, although in the case of rubella, measles, and mumps, family members should be vaccinated to protect the patients. It would also be prudent to wait until systemic immunosuppressant drug therapy has been terminated for 3 months before vaccinating patients receiving such regimens. A 16-year-old boy with acute lymphoblastic leukemia who received RA27/3 rubella vaccine developed chronic infection of leukocytes and high antibody titers. Symptoms of arthritis required temporary interruption of immunosuppression, but fortunately the patient recovered spontaneously.[413] Short-term (less than 2 weeks) corticosteroid therapy is not a contraindication to the administration of rubella vaccine. Patients whose immunity had been ablated during bone marrow transplantation were given rubella vaccine as part of MMR 2 years later by Ljungman and associates.[414] They observed a 75% seroconversion to the rubella component with no safety problems. King and colleagues[415] performed a similar study and found 91% seroconversion.

Asymptomatic children who are infected with the human immunodeficiency virus (HIV) should receive rubella vaccine as part of MMR. Virological study of 10 HIV-infected patients who received MMR failed to detect rubella virus.[416] MMR should also be considered for symptomatic children who are not severely immunosuppressed.

Persons who have had anaphylactic reactions to neomycin should not receive rubella vaccines containing that antibiotic.[417] Whereas monovalent RA27/3 vaccine is grown in human diploid cells, MMR does contain other viruses grown in avian tissue, but reactions in egg-sensitive individuals are very rare.

Concurrent IgG

Vaccination within 2 weeks before receipt of IgG or 3 months after receipt of IgG is inadvisable.[113, 370] However, anti-Rh(D) globulin did not interfere with vaccination of postpartum women.[389] Women who are vaccinated after receiving anti-Rh(D) globulin should be tested 6 weeks later for rubella antibodies.

Pregnancy

Pregnancy remains a contraindication to rubella vaccination, and women should take precautions against pregnancy for 3 months after vaccination on the basis of a case of wild virus transmission to a fetus conceived 7 weeks after vaccination.[418] However, evidence for damage to the fetus by rubella vaccine strains is nonexistent. Several summaries of the accumulated American, British, and German data have been published[419–421] (Table 17–15). Transplacental passage of vaccine virus is evidently a rare event, having occurred 4 times in 708 pregnancies complicated by RA27/3 vaccination. More important, there was no CRS case demonstrated in more than 1000 pregnancies during which rubella vaccines were given. On the basis of data in Table 17–15, the theoretical maximum risk for CRS after the administration of vaccine is 1.6%, considerably lower than the risk due to wild rubella virus or indeed the risk of non–CRS-induced congenital defects in pregnancy. If only the American women known to be seronegative who received RA27/3 are considered in the calculation, the theoretical risk to the fetus still does not rise above 2.1%. For these reasons, and because the observed risk has been zero, rubella vaccination during pregnancy is no longer considered an indication for abortion.[422, 423]

Children with Congenital Rubella Syndrome

Children with CRS will probably not respond to parenteral rubella vaccine, even when they are seronegative.[424] They can be immunized with RA27/3 intrana-

Table 17–15. **SUMMARY OF DATA ON ACCIDENTAL VACCINATION BEFORE PREGNANCY AND DURING EARLY PREGNANCY OF WOMEN IN THE UNITED STATES AND GERMANY**

STUDY LOCATION AND VACCINE	VACCINATED WOMEN (N)	MOTHER'S IMMUNE STATUS BEFORE VACCINATION			OUTCOME FOR LIVE BIRTHS				PRODUCTS OF CONCEPTION POSITIVE WHEN TESTED FOR RUBELLA	THEORETICAL RISK OF CRS DEFECT (%)
		Susceptible	Immune	Unknown	Total Liveborn	Liveborn to Susceptible Mothers	Asymptomatic Infection	CRS Defect		
United States										
Cendehill and HPV-77	538	149	25	364	290	94	8	0	17/85	0–3.8
RA27/3	683	272	32	379	562	226	3	0	1/35	0–1.6
Germany										
Cendehill	340	130	61	149	177	107	2	0	1/34	
RA27/3	25	16	4	5	17	12	0	0		

CRS, congenital rubella syndrome.

Data from Centers for Disease Control and Prevention. Rubella prevention: Recommendation of the Immunization Practices Advisory Committee. MMWR Morb Mortal Wkly Rep 39(RR-15):1–18, 1990; Rubella vaccination during pregnancy—United States, 1971–1988. MMWR Morb Mortal Wkly Rep 38:289–293, 1989; and Enders G. Rubella antibody titers in vaccinated and nonvaccinated women and results of vaccination during pregnancy. Rev Infect Dis 7(suppl):S103–S107, 1985.

sally,[425] but there is no official recommendation to vaccinate these children.

PUBLIC HEALTH CONSIDERATIONS

Epidemiological Results of Vaccination

United States

Rubella vaccine has had spectacular success in the United States, in terms of the number of people vaccinated and the declining numbers of rubella cases reported. Figure 17–2 shows that since the licensing of the vaccine in 1969, no major epidemic of rubella has occurred, despite the previously observed 6- to 9-year cycle.[426]

These impressive results were obtained initially by the vaccination of children, with a dependence on herd immunity to protect pregnant women. However, assessment in 1977 to 1978 revealed that although the program was having a major impact on rubella in children, rubella rates in those older than 15 years were not substantially different from prevaccination rates.[427] Specific experiences in institutional or city-wide outbreaks showed that the concept of herd immunity had only limited validity, giving a protection of perhaps 50%.[224, 428, 429] Moreover, some doubted that children were often the source of infection for their mothers.[430] Serological surveys showed a persistence of 12 to 24% seronegativity in adolescent and adult populations. As a consequence, programs to expand vaccination of adolescents and adults were increased. Since then, the disease rate in age groups old enough to bear children has dropped markedly, as have the numbers of CRS cases. From an average of 106 cases a year during the 1970s, the number fell to 20 per year, and the prospect of elimination of CRS was discussed.[431, 432] As shown in Figure 17–6, the incidence of rubella has dropped to less than 1 per 100,000 population, and the incidence of CRS has dropped to less than 0.1 per 100,000 births.[426] In fact,

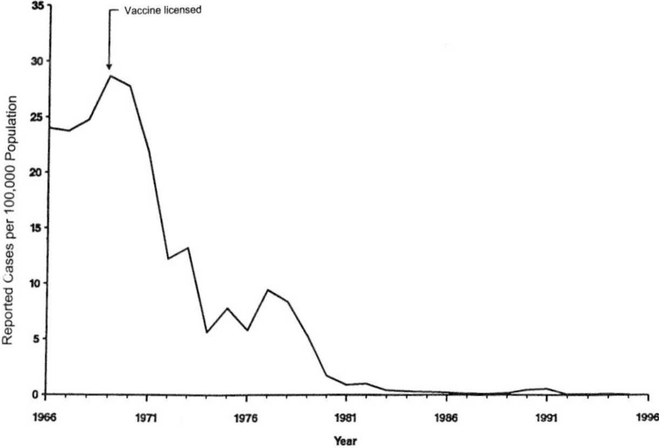

Figure 17–6. Rubella (German measles), by year, United States, 1966 to 1995. In 1995, 128 cases of rubella were reported in the United States, which is the lowest number ever reported. (From Summary of Notifiable Diseases, United States, 1995. MMWR Morb Mortal Wkly Rep 44:1–87, 1996.)

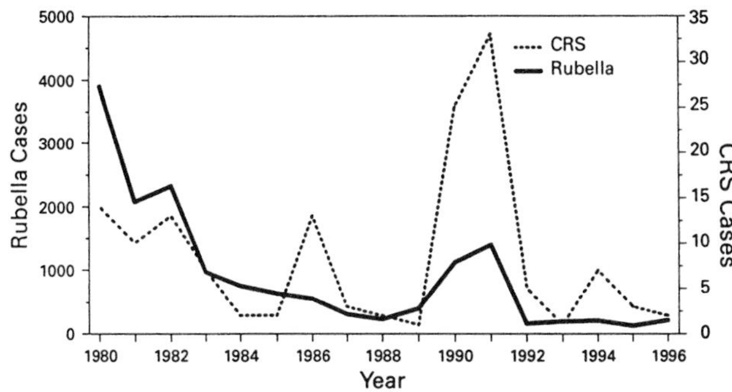

Figure 17–7. Number of reported rubella and congenital rubella syndrome (CRS) cases by year, United States, 1980 to 1996. (From Rubella and congenital rubella syndrome—United States, 1994–1997. MMWR Morb Mortal Wkly Rep 46:350–354, 1997.)

only seven cases of CRS were reported in 1983 in the United States, two in 1984, and two in 1985.[426, 427, 431–433]

In 1988, a nadir was reached in reported postnatal rubella, and only one case of CRS was registered in 1989. A large outbreak of rubella occurred in unimmunized immigrants to California and was followed by the expected cluster of CRS cases.[434]

There was a slight recrudescence in 1990 to 1991, with 10 cases being reported in 1991; but between 1994 and 1996, there was an average of three CRS cases per year, of which about one third were imported[435] (Fig. 17–7).

During recent years, rubella outbreaks have been sporadic and relatively small. Nevertheless, it is troubling that 85% of cases have been in adults. Interestingly, more than half the cases were in patients of Latino origin, implying that unvaccinated immigrants are an important reservoir of rubella susceptibility. Mexico has not conducted routine MMR vaccination, but is scheduled to start in 1998.

In the debate over vaccine policy, cost-benefit analyses were made to assess the various strategies. For every dollar spent on childhood rubella vaccination in the United States, $7.70 was saved.[436] An analysis made in Israel also reached the same favorable conclusion.[437] However, Schoenbaum and colleagues[438] argued that vaccination of schoolgirls would be economically preferable to vaccination of infants.

Meanwhile, the growing resurgence of measles resulted in a recommendation for a routine second dose of measles vaccine, usually in the form of MMR.[439, 440] Thus, revaccination with rubella became standard, practiced at either entrance to primary school (4 to 6 years) or entrance to secondary school (11 to 12 years of age). Although there are theoretical arguments in favor of revaccinating older children,[441] the United States is moving toward uniform revaccination at 4 to 6 years.

Europe in General

Table 17–16 summarizes the vaccine schedules currently in use in various countries.

Every country in western Europe has introduced rubella vaccination into routine childhood vaccination, as

Table 17–16. **SCHEDULES FOR RUBELLA VACCINATION CURRENTLY USED IN SOME NORTH AMERICAN AND EUROPEAN COUNTRIES***

COUNTRY	FIRST DOSE FOR CHILDREN OF BOTH SEXES		SECOND DOSE FOR CHILDREN OF BOTH SEXES		ONLY GIRLS	
	Antigens	Age	Antigens	Age	Antigens	Age
Austria	MMR	13 mo	MMR	6yr	R	10–14 yr
Belgium	MMR	15 mo	MMR	11yr		
Bulgaria	MMR	13 mo			MR	12–15 yr
Canada	MMR	12–15 mo				
Czech	MMR	15 mo	MMR	21–25 mo	R	12 yr
Denmark	MMR	15 mo	MMR	11–12 yr		
Finland	MMR	14–18 mo	MMR	6 yr		
France	MMR	12 mo	MMR	11–13 yr		
Germany	MMR	12–15 mo	MMR	6 yr	R	11–15 yr
Greece	MMR	15 mo	MMR	10 yr		
Hungary	MMR	15 mo			R or MR	11–12 yr
Iceland	MMR	18 mo	MMR	9 yr	R	12 yr
Ireland	MMR	15 mo	MMR	12 yr		
Israel	MMR	15 mo			R	12 yr
Italy	MMR	15 mo			R	11 yr
Netherlands	MMR	14 mo	MMR	9 yr		
Norway	MMR	15 mo	MMR	12 yr		
Poland					R	13 yr
Portugal	MMR	15 mo	MMR	11 yr		
Spain	MMR	15 mo	MMR	11 yr		
Sweden	MMR	18 mo	MMR	12 yr		
Switzerland	MMR	15 mo	MMR	4–7 yr or 12–15 yr		
United Kingdom	MMR	13 mo	MMR	4 yr		
United States	MMR	12–15 mo	MMR	6–12 yr		

*Prepared prior to licensure of Rotavirus vaccine on Aug 31, 1998, for use as three doses at 2, 4, and 6 months of age.
MMR, measles, mumps, and rubella combined vaccine; MR, measles and rubella combined vaccine; R, monovalent rubella vaccine.

part of MMR, with the exception of Italy and Austria, which limit vaccination to adolescent girls. The Scandinavian countries and the Netherlands have adopted a policy of two doses of MMR, and the other countries give a second dose of rubella vaccine to adolescent girls.[442]

United Kingdom

The policy of vaccinating schoolgirls was adopted by the British in 1970.[427, 443] During the subsequent years, the number of reported rubella cases decreased only slightly, but the reported cases of CRS decreased approximately 75%.[444] About 15% of schoolgirls did not accept the vaccine,[445, 446] which explained why 88% of women reporting for assessment for rash disease had not been immunized.[447] Nevertheless, serological studies showed that vaccination had reduced seronegativity of young women,[447–450] although many susceptible persons still remained.[450, 451] Fortunately, acceptance of rubella vaccine among schoolgirls is increasing, and a national program to promote vaccination was started.[443] Nevertheless, after original hesitation, opinion in Britain changed to favor the inclusion of young children in rubella vaccination practice, as is now done in the United States.[452–455] Since October 1988, rubella vaccine has been recommended to all infants as part of MMR,[456] and in 1994 a large-scale vaccination campaign was conducted with measles-rubella combined vaccine. Congenital rubella and terminations of pregnancy for rubella have decreased markedly in England and Wales,[457] with only one CRS case reported in 1995.[458, 459] In 1996, however, the United Kingdom experienced a resurgence of rubella, primarily in adult and adolescent males who were unvaccinated.[459] As might be predicted, cases of CRS followed the outbreak.

Scandinavia

In 1982, Sweden adopted a two-stage vaccination scheme, involving the use of MMR at two ages: 18 months and 12 years.[460] The rationale for this scheme was as follows[461]:

1. Vaccination at 18 months will reduce the incidence of rubella among schoolchildren and, ultimately, among childbearing women when these same children reach maturity.
2. A more immediate effect on rubella in pregnancy is obtained by vaccinating young girls.
3. The second dose also reinforces immunity and replaces the boosters that natural infection formerly provided.

An acceptance rate of 88% was achieved among Swedish schoolgirls and an even higher rate among other children. Some problems with seroconversion for mumps and measles among the 12-year-old girls were reported, but rubella vaccine gave good results in both age groups.[462] Christenson and Böttiger[463] studied the rubella serology of 1343 susceptible 12-year-olds in the Swedish program and found that 100% seroconverted after vaccination. Before 1974, a yearly average of 14

CRS cases were recorded in Sweden, 2 cases per year between 1975 and 1985, and no cases since 1985.[463a]

The Finns vaccinate with MMR at 14 to 18 months and at 6 years. The peak incidence has shifted to adults, whereas children appear to be protected.[464] The success of the MMR two-dose vaccination policy in Finland has been spectacular. Peltola and colleagues[465] summarized the results of the program that succeeded in eliminating indigenous cases of rubella, measles, and mumps. This program was supported by improved surveillance of disease and by ancillary studies demonstrating lack of significant reactions to vaccine and persistence of antibodies. Ukkonen[466] provided data on the disappearance of rubella and the state of rubella immunity in the Finnish population. As shown in Figure 17–8, the two-dose policy has erased seronegativity in adolescents and caused rubella to disappear. Since 1986, no case of CRS has been reported.

Other European Countries

Coverage with MMR in France is only about 60% in adolescent girls and considerably less in adult women. Although vaccination with MMR is increasing in infants, seven French cases of CRS were reported in 1994.[467]

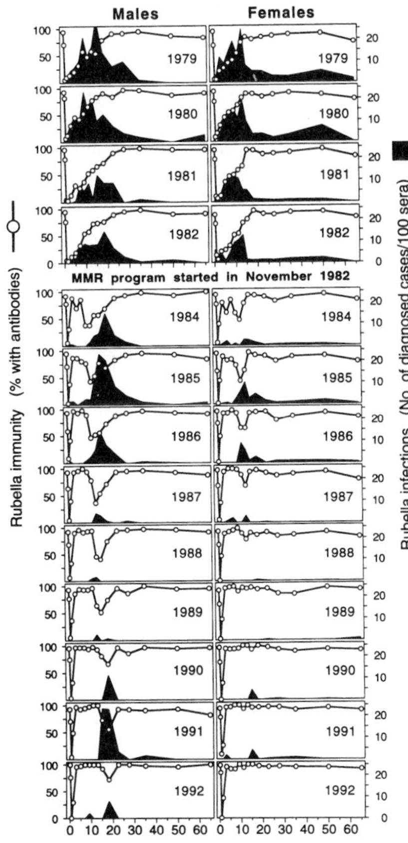

Figure 17–8. Gradual increase in rubella immunity and disappearance of rubella infections as a consequence of measles, mumps, and rubella (MMR) vaccination. *Top*, Before the MMR program (1979 to 1982). *Bottom*, During the MMR program (1984 to 1992). (From Ukkonen P. Rubella immunity and morbidity: Impact of different vaccination programs in Finland 1979–1992. Scand J Infect Dis 28:31–35, 1996.)

Coverage rates in Switzerland are also uncertain, and Matter and colleagues[468] reported the persistence of rubella and CRS cases.

Canada

The provinces of Canada adopted a policy either of mass vaccination of infants or of selective vaccination of preschool-aged girls.[427, 469] Total rubella incidence dropped in the provinces that adopted mass vaccination of infants but was not much changed in those adopting vaccination of preschool-aged girls. However, reported CRS decreased throughout Canada. As of 1983, all provinces give vaccine to infants and also to 12-year-old girls who have not been immunized previously.[469]

Israel

Israel at first adopted the British policy of vaccination of schoolgirls. Subsequent observations showed that whereas the youngest girls were being protected, epidemics could still infect large numbers of pregnant women. Accordingly, family health clinics, which most Israeli women attend, started to screen for rubella antibodies and to vaccinate seronegative women. Universal vaccination of children with MMR was started.[104]

The problem of eliminating rubella in Israel has been exacerbated by the early emphasis on vaccination of women only, by immigration of unvaccinated populations, and by the existence of religious communities that do not accept vaccination. Thus, progress has been slow, and in 1992 five cases of CRS were reported.[470, 471]

Australia

Australia also adopted the policy of vaccinating schoolgirls. By 1983, 12 years after the program had started, 96% of pregnant women were seropositive. Cases of reported CRS have fallen from approximately 120 per year (prevaccine) to 20 per year, despite continued circulation of virus among children.[103] Vaccine efficacy is high,[472] and in west Australia the CRS incidence is below 2 cases per 10,000 births.[473]

Developing Countries

The facts concerning rubella and CRS described earlier under *Epidemiology* suggest that developing countries could also benefit from rubella vaccination. In South Africa, the rubella component of an MMR vaccine elicited seroconversion in 94% of black African infants.[474] A model immunization program for rubella was conducted in São Paolo, Brazil, by Massad and coworkers.[475, 476] A mass campaign was conducted to vaccinate all children 1 to 10 years old with MMR, accompanied by routine MMR vaccination of infants at 15 months of age. Immunity to rubella in the population jumped from 40 to 97%, and more important, the number of CRS cases dropped from 29 confirmed and suspected in 1992 to none in 1994.

Robertson and colleagues[477] have reviewed the use of rubella vaccine in developing countries. They documented use of rubella vaccine in about 30% of nonindustrialized countries but with varied strategies. Although combined childhood and adult female vaccination was used by the majority of countries, 40% did not do so, and the authors expressed concern that selective vaccination of infants might increase the risk of infection in pregnant women by reducing the now prevalent exposure in childhood.[478] Certainly the picture described by Robertson and colleagues[477] is chiaroscuro: Cuba has succeeded in eliminating rubella, but most developing countries, notably Malaysia, Hong Kong, Caribbean islands, and Middle Eastern states, are still working out their strategies. Another example is Korea, where only vaccination of female infants has been practiced.[479]

The Technical Advisory Group of the Pan American Health Organization has recently recommended routine rubella immunization throughout the Americas, after concluding that 20,000 infants with CRS are born each year to that region in the absence of an epidemic.[480] The English-speaking Caribbean countries have added rubella to their measles vaccination campaigns.

Rubella vaccine as part of combination vaccines should be applied in more developing countries.[480a]

Recommended Use

The choice of a strategy for vaccination for rubella should be based on local circumstances. Vaccination of all infants will probably eradicate CRS in 30 to 40 years; vaccination of all schoolgirls will presumably eradicate CRS in 10 to 20 years; and vaccination of adult women will eradicate CRS immediately, but only if 100% are immunized. Because 100% acceptance of vaccine is unlikely and one does not wish to wait for the eradication of CRS, some combination of the aforementioned strategies is necessary. Knox[481] and Anderson and May[482] have argued that where vaccine acceptance rates are less than 84%, the adult vaccination policy is best; where acceptance rates are higher, the childhood vaccination policy is best.[483]

Rubella vaccination of infants should be practiced if the two following conditions are fulfilled: (1) rubella is given as part of MMR or MR, and (2) vaccine acceptance rates are high.

Schoolgirl vaccination is an alternative strategy only if high acceptance rates cannot be guaranteed. Vaccination of seronegative women is now feasible because of the availability of simple serological methods and the evidence described previously that rubella vaccine is not teratogenic. Vaccination of this group has the advantage of a direct effect on the group at highest risk.

The adoption of a two-dose strategy by many developed countries has been highly successful in eliminating pockets of susceptibility, and this policy is likely to be extended as part of efforts to maintain control of infectious diseases in adolescents and adults.

In the United States, a decision has been made to eliminate rubella and CRS,[432] and the goal has been set by the year 2000.[484] The strategy for elimination is essentially childhood vaccinations supplemented by vaccination of women as outlined in Table 17–14. The implementation of universal immunization could mean the end of CRS within 50 years of its discovery.[485, 486] This goal is also feasible in many other parts of the world and should be adopted.

REFERENCES

1. Smith JL. Rotheln (epidemic roseola–German measles–hybrid measles, etc.). Arch Dermatol 1:1–13, 1875.
2. Veale H. History of an epidemic of rotheln, with observation on its pathology. Edinb Med J 12:404–414, 1866.
3. Gregg NM. Congenital cataract following German measles in the mother. Trans Ophthalmol Soc Aust 3:35–46, 1941.
4. Pitt D, Keir EH. Results of rubella in pregnancy. Med J Aust 2:647–651, 1965.
5. Lundstrom R. Rubella during pregnancy: A follow-up study of children born after an epidemic of rubella in Sweden, 1951, with additional investigations on prophylaxis and treatment of maternal rubella. Acta Paediatr Scand 133(suppl):1–110, 1962.
6. Greenberg M, Pellitteri O, Barton J. Frequency of defects in infants whose mothers had rubella during pregnancy. JAMA 165:675–678, 1957.
7. Manson MM, Logan WPD, Loy RM. Rubella and Other Virus Infections During Pregnancy. Ministry of Health, Report on Public Health and Mechanical Subjects, No. 101. London, Her Majesty's Stationery Office, 1960.
8. Weller TH, Neva FA. Propagation in tissue culture of cytopathic agents from patients with rubella-like illness. Proc Soc Exp Biol Med 111:215–225, 1962.
9. Parkman PD, Beuscher EL, Artenstein MS. Recovery of rubella virus from army recruits. Proc Soc Exp Biol Med 111:225–230, 1962.
10. Witte JJ, Karchmer AW, Case G, et al. Epidemiology of rubella. Am J Dis Child 118:107–112, 1969.
11. Rubella surveillance. National Communicable Disease Center, United States Department of Health, Education and Welfare (No. 1), June 1969.
12. Cooper LZ, Ziring PR, Ockerse AB, et al. Rubella: Clinical manifestations and management. Am J Dis Child 118:18–29, 1969.
13. Plotkin SA, Oski FA, Hartnett EM, et al. Some recently recognized manifestations of the rubella syndrome. J Pediatr 67:182–191, 1965.
14. Meyer HM, Parkman PD, Hobbins TE, et al. Attenuated rubella viruses: Laboratory and clinical characteristics. Am J Dis Child 118:155–165, 1969.
15. Prinzie A, Huygelen C, Gold J, et al. Experimental live attenuated rubella virus vaccine: Clinical evaluation of Cendehill strain. Am J Dis Child 118:172–177, 1969.
16. Plotkin SA, Farquhar JD, Katz M, Buser F. Attenuation of RA27/3 rubella virus in WI-38 human diploid cells. Am J Dis Child 118:178–185, 1969.
17. Heggie AD, Robbins FC. Natural rubella acquired after birth. Am J Dis Child 118:12–17, 1969.
18. Plotkin SA. Rubella viruses. In Lennette EH, Schmidt NJ (eds). Diagnostic Procedures for Viral and Rickettsial Infections (4th ed). Washington, DC, American Public Health Association, 1969, pp 364–413.
19. Kantor TG, Tanner M. Rubella arthritis and rheumatoid arthritis. Arthritis Rheum 5:378–383, 1962.
20. Fraser FRE, Cunningham AL, Hayes K, et al. Rubella arthritis in adults. Isolation of virus, cytology and other aspects of infection. Clin Exp Rheumatol 1:287–293, 1983.
21. Morse EE, Zinkham WH, Jackson DP. Thrombocytopenic purpura following rubella infection in children and adults. Arch Intern Med 117:573–579, 1966.
22. Sherman EF, Michaels RH, Kenny FM. Acute encephalopathy (encephalitis) complicating rubella: Reports of cases with viro-

logic studies, cortisol-production determinations and observations at autopsy. JAMA 192:675–681, 1965.
23. Pisternick D, Hoppe J, Dannecker G, et al. Fulminant verlaufende Rotelnenzephalitis mit letalem Ausgang. Monatsschr Kinderheilkd 145:105–108, 1997.
24. Katz M, Plotkin SA. Parainfectious encephalopathies associated with measles, mumps, chickenpox, and German measles. In Goldensohn ES, Appel SH (eds). Scientific Approaches to Clinical Neurology. Vol. 1. Philadelphia, Lea & Febiger, 1977, pp 405–425.
25. Moriuchi H, Yamasaki S, Mori K, et al. A rubella epidemic in Sasebo, Japan in 1987, with various complications. Acta Paediatr Jpn 32:67–75, 1990.
26. Townsend JJ, Baringer JR, Wolinsky JS, et al. Progressive rubella panencephalitis: Late onset after congenital rubella. N Engl J Med 292:990–993, 1975.
27. Weil ML, Itabashi HH, Cremer NE, et al. Chronic progressive panencephalitis due to rubella virus simulating SSPE. N Engl J Med 292:994–998, 1975.
28. Yaginuma Y, Kawamura M, Ishikawa M. Landry–Guillain-Barré–Strohl syndrome in pregnancy. J Obstet Gynaecol 22:47–49, 1996.
29. Kalvenes M, Kalland K, Haukenes G. Radioimmunoprecipitation and immunoblot studies of antibodies to rubella virus in patients with chronic liver disease. Arch Virol 136:73–85, 1994.
30. Cooper LZ, Preblud SR, Alford CA. Rubella. In Remington JS, Klein JO (eds). Infectious Diseases of the Fetus and Newborn Infant (4th ed). Philadelphia, WB Saunders, 1995, pp 268–311.
31. Cosachov J, Frieri M. Hyper-IgM syndrome with congenital rubella. Pediatr Asthma Allergy Immunol 9:79–85, 1995.
32. Siegal M, Fuerst HT, Peress NS. Fetal mortality in maternal rubella: Results of a prospective study from 1957–1964. Am J Obstet Gynecol 96:247–253, 1966.
33. Miller E, Cradock-Watson JE, Pollock TM. Consequences of confirmed maternal rubella at successive stages of pregnancy. Lancet 2:781–784, 1982.
34. South MA, Sever JL. Teratogen update: The congenital rubella syndrome. Teratology 31:297–307, 1985.
35. Ingalls TH. German measles and German measles in pregnancy. Am J Dis Child 93:555–558, 1957.
36. Grillner L, Forsgren M, Barr B, et al. Outcome of rubella during pregnancy with special reference to the 17th to 24th weeks of gestation. Scand J Infect Dis 15:321–325, 1983.
37. Sheridan MD. Final report of a prospective study of children whose mothers had rubella in early pregnancy. BMJ 2:536–539, 1964.
38. Enders G, Nickerl-Pacher U, Miller E, Cradock-Watson JE. Outcome of confirmed periconceptional maternal rubella. Lancet 1:1445–1447, 1988.
39. Kono R, Hibi M, Hayakawa Y. Experimental vertical transmission of rubella virus in rabbits. Lancet 1:343–347, 1969.
40. Rawls WE, Desmyter J, Melnick JL. Serologic diagnosis and fetal involvement in maternal rubella. JAMA 203:627–631, 1968.
41. Thompson KM, Tobin JOH. Isolation of rubella virus from abortion material. BMJ 2:264–266, 1970.
42. Cradock-Watson JE, Bourne MS, Vandervelde EM. IgG, IgA, and IgM responses in acute rubella determined by the immunofluorescent technique. J Hyg (Camb) 70:473–485, 1972.
43. Tomer Y, Davies TF. Infection, thyroid disease, and autoimmunity. Endocr Rev 14:107–120, 1993.
44. Frey T. Molecular biology of rubella virus. Adv Virus Res 44:69–160, 1994.
45. Pettersson RF, Oker-Blom C, Kalkkinen N, et al. Molecular and antigenic characteristics and synthesis of rubella virus structural proteins. Rev Infect Dis 7:S140–S149, 1985.
46. Oker-Blom C, Ulmanen I, Kaanianen L, Pettersson RF. Rubella virus 40S genome RNA specifies a 24S subgenomic mRNA that codes for a precursor to structural proteins. J Virol 49:403–408, 1984.
47. Oker-Blom C, Kalkkinen N, Kaanianen L, Pettersson RF. Rubella virus contains one capsid protein and three envelope proteins, E1, E2a, E2b. J Virol 46:964–973, 1983.
48. Waxham NM, Wolinsky JS. A model of the structural organization of rubella virions. Rev Infect Dis 7(suppl):S133–S139, 1985.
49. Hovi T, Vaheri A. Infectivity and some physicochemical characteristics of rubella virus ribonucleic acid. Virology 42:1–8, 1970.
50. Sedwick W, Sokol F. Nucleic acid of rubella virus and its replication in hamster kidney cells. J Virol 5:478–489, 1970.
51. Wang C, Dominguez G, Frey T. Construction of rubella virus genome-length cDNA clones and synthesis of infectious RNA transcripts. J Virol 68:3550–3557, 1994.
52. Forng R, Frey T. Identification of the rubella virus nonstructural proteins. Virology 206:843–853, 1995.
53. Lonesborough P, Ho-Terry L, Terry G. Sequence variation and biological activity of rubella virus isolates. Arch Virol 140:563–570, 1995.
54. Bosma T, Best J, Corbett K, et al. Nucleotide sequence analysis of a major antigenic domain of the E1 glycoprotein of 22 rubella virus isolates. J Gen Virol 77:2523–2540, 1996.
55. Frey T, Abernathy E, Weaver S, et al. Molecular epidemiology of rubella virus [abstract]. 16th Annual Meeting of the American Society for Virology; Bozeman, MT, July 19–23, 1997, p 158.
56. Derdeyn C, Frey T. Characterization of defective-interfering RNAs of rubella virus generated during serial undiluted passage. Virology 206:215–226, 1995.
57. Herrmann KL. Rubella virus. In Lennette EH, Schmidt NJ (eds). Diagnostic Procedures for Viral, Rickettsial and Chlamydial Infections (5th ed). Washington, DC, American Public Health Association, 1979, pp 725–766.
58. Stewart GL, Parkman PD, Hopps HE, et al. Rubella-virus hemagglutination-inhibition test. N Engl J Med 276:554–557, 1967.
59. Hermann KL. Available rubella serologic tests. Rev Infect Dis 7:S108–S112, 1985.
60. Perry K, Brown D, Parry J, et al. Detection of measles, mumps, and rubella antibodies in saliva using antibody capture radioimmunoassay. J Med Virol 40:235–240, 1993.
61. Alford CA, Neva FA, Weller TH. Virologic and serologic studies on human products of conception after maternal rubella. N Engl J Med 271:1275–1281, 1964.
62. Plotkin SA, Boue A, Boue JG. The in vitro growth of rubella virus in human embryo cells. Am J Epidemiol 81:71–85, 1965.
63. Rawls WE, Melnick JL. Rubella virus carrier cultures derived from congenitally infected infants. J Exp Med 123:795–816, 1966.
64. Naeye RL, Blanc W. Pathogenesis of congenital rubella. JAMA 194:1277–1283, 1965.
65. Plotkin SA, Vaheri A. Human fibroblasts infected with rubella virus produce a growth inhibitor. Science 156:659–661, 1967.
66. Duncan R, Lee N, Atreya C, et al. Variation in rubella virus induced apoptosis corresponds to constitutive differences in levels of regulatory factors [abstract]. 16th Annual Meeting of the American Society for Virology; Bozeman, MT, July 19–23, 1997, p 113.
67. Tondury G, Smith DW. Fetal rubella pathology. J Pediatr 68:867–879, 1965.
68. Ho-Terry L, Lonesborough P. Diagnosis of foetal rubella virus infection by polymerase chain reaction. J Gen Virol 71:1607–1611, 1990.
69. Bosma T, Corbett K, O'Shea S, et al. PCR for detection of rubella virus RNA in clinical samples. J Clin Microbiol 33:1075–1079, 1995.
70. Tanemura M, Suzumori K, Yoshiaki Y. Diagnosis of fetal rubella infection with reverse transcription and nested polymerase chain reaction: A study of 34 cases diagnosed in fetuses. Am J Obstet Gynecol 174:578–582, 1996.
71. Bosma TJ, Corbet KM, Eckstein MB, et al. Use of PCR for prenatal and postnatal diagnosis of congenital rubella. J Clin Microbiol 33:2881–2887, 1995.
71a. Skendzel LP. Rubella immunity. Am J Clin Pathol 106:170–174, 1996.
72. Meitsh K, Enders G, Wolinsky J, et al. The role of rubella-immunoblot and rubella-peptide-EIA for the diagnosis of the congenital rubella syndrome during the prenatal and newborn periods. J Med Virol 51:280–283, 1997.
73. Menser MA, Harley JD, Hertzberg R, et al. Persistence of virus in lens for three years after prenatal rubella. Lancet 2:387–388, 1967.
74. Cooper LZ, Green RH, Krugman S, et al. Neonatal thrombocytopenic purpura and other manifestations of rubella contracted in utero. Am J Dis Child 110:416–428, 1965.
75. Scheie HG, Schaffer DB, Plotkin SA, Kertesz ED. Congenital rubella cataracts. Arch Ophthalmol 77:440–444, 1967.

76. Plotkin SA, Cochran W, Lindquist J, et al. Congenital rubella syndrome in late infancy. JAMA 200:435–441, 1967.
77. Cockburn WC. World aspects of the epidemiology of rubella. Am J Dis Child 118:112–122, 1969.
78. Assaad F, Ljungars-Esteves K. Rubella—world impact. Rev Infect Dis 7:S29–S36, 1985.
79. Ingalls TH. Rubella—epidemiology, virology and immunology. The epidemiology of rubella. Am J Med Sci 253:349–356, 1967.
80. Halstead SB, Diwan AR, Oda AI. Susceptibility to rubella among adolescents and adults in Hawaii. JAMA 210:1881–1883, 1969.
81. Bisno AL, Spence LP, Stewart JA, Casey HL. Rubella in Trinidad: Sero-epidemiologic studies of an institutional outbreak. Am J Epidemiol 89:74–81, 1969.
82. Brody JA. The infectiousness of rubella and the possibility of reinfection. Am J Public Health 56:1082–1087, 1966.
83. Grayston JT, Gale JL, Watten RH. The epidemiology of rubella on Taiwan: Introduction and description of the 1957–1958 epidemic. Int J Epidemiol 1:245–265, 1972.
84. Fogel A, Gerichter CB, Rannon L, et al. Serologic studies in 11,460 pregnant women during the 1972 rubella epidemic in Israel. Am J Epidemiol 103:51–59, 1976.
85. De Azevedo Neto R, Silveira A, Nokes D, et al. Rubella seroepidemiology in a non-immunized population of Šao Paulo State, Brazil. Epidemiol Infect 113:161–173, 1994.
86. Yamamoto L, Mejfa E, Lopez R, et al. Susceptibility to rubella infection in females at high risk. Trop Geogr Med 47:235–238, 1995.
87. Cutts F, Robertson S, Diaz-Ortega J, Samual R. Control of rubella and congenital rubella syndrome (CRS) in developing countries, part 1: Burden of disease from CRS. Bull World Health Organ 75:55–68, 1997.
88. Lindquist J, Plotkin SA, Shaw L, et al. Congenital rubella as a systemic infection. BMJ 2:1401–1406, 1965.
89. Centers for Disease Control. Rubella and congenital rubella surveillance, 1983. MMWR CDC Surveill Summ 33:4SS, 1984.
90. Peckham C. Congenital rubella in the United Kingdom before 1970: The prevaccine era. Rev Infect Dis 7:S11–S16, 1985.
91. Seth P, Manjunath N, Balaya S. Rubella infection: The Indian scene. Rev Infect Dis 7:S64–S67, 1985.
92. Mingle JAA. Frequency of rubella antibodies in the population of some tropical African countries. Rev Infect Dis 7:S68–S71, 1985.
93. Broor S, Kapil A, Kishore J, Seth P. Prevalence of rubella virus and cytomegalovirus infections in suspected cases of congenital infections. Indian J Pediatr 58:75–78, 1991.
94. Eckstein M, Vijayalakshmi P, Killedar M, et al. Aetiology of childhood cataract in south India. Br J Ophthalmol 80:628–632, 1996.
95. Ballal M, Shivananda P. Prevalence of rubella virus in suspected cases of congenital infections. Indian J Pediatr 64:231–235, 1997.
96. Zakzouk S, Al-Muhaimeed H. Prevalence of sensorineural hearing loss due to rubella in Saudi children. ORL J Otorhinolaryngol Relat Spec 58:74–77, 1996.
97. Kono R, Hirayama M, Sugishita C, Miyamura K. Epidemiology of rubella and congenital rubella infection in Japan. Rev Infect Dis 7:S56–S63, 1985.
98. Ueda K, Nishida Y, Oshima K, et al. An explanation for the high incidence of congenital rubella syndrome in Ryukyu. Am J Epidemiol 107:344–351, 1978.
99. Cooper LZ. Birth defects. Original article series: Rubella, a preventable cause of birth defects. Nat Found March of Dimes 4:23–35, 1968.
100. Horstmann DM. Rubella. The challenge of its control. J Infect Dis 123:640–654, 1971.
101. Horstmann DM. Viral vaccines and their ways. Rev Infect Dis 1:502–516, 1979.
102. Mellinger A, Cragan J, Atkinson W, et al. High incidence of congenital rubella syndrome after a rubella outbreak. Pediatr Infect Dis J 14:573–578, 1995.
103. Menser MA, Hudson JR, Murphy AM, Upfold LJ. Epidemiology of congenital rubella and results of rubella vaccination in Australia. Rev Infect Dis 7:S37–S41, 1985.
104. Swartz TA, Hornstein L, Epstein I. Epidemiology of rubella and congenital rubella infection in Israel: A country with a selective immunization program. Rev Infect Dis 7:S42–S46, 1985.
105. Celers J, Aymard M, Feingold J, Godde-Jolly D. Rubeole et cataractes congénitales. Arch Fr Pediatr 40:391–395, 1983.
106. Zgorniak-Nowosielska I, Zawilinska B, Szostek S. Rubella infection during pregnancy in the 1985–86 epidemic: Follow-up after seven years. Eur J Epidemiol 12:303–308, 1996.
107. Miller CL. Rubella in the developing world. Epidemiol Infect 107:63–68, 1991.
108. Gale JL, Detels R, Kim KSW, et al. Epidemiology of rubella on Taiwan. Am J Dis Child 118:143–145, 1969.
109. Gomwalk NE, Ahmad AA. Prevalence of rubella antibodies on the African continent. Rev Infect Dis 11:116–121, 1989.
110. Owens CS, Espino RT. Rubella in Panama: Still a problem. Pediatr Infect Dis J 8:110–115, 1989.
111. Kishore J, Broor S, Seth P. Acute rubella infection in pregnant women in Delhi. Indian J Med Res 91: 245–246, 1990.
112. Millian SJ, Kogon A, Klein S. Rubella antibody levels in commercial gamma globulin preparations. Am J Public Health 61:353–358, 1971.
113. Siber GR, Werner BG, Halsey NA, et al. Interference of immune globulin with measles and rubella immunization. J Pediatr 122:204–211, 1993.
114. Brody J, Sever JL, Schiff GM. Prevention of rubella by gammaglobulin during an epidemic in Barrow, Alaska, in 1964. N Engl J Med 272:127–129, 1965.
115. McDonald JC, Peckham C. Gamma globulin in prevention of rubella and congenital defects: A study of 30,000 pregnancies. BMJ 3:633–637, 1967.
116. Public Health Laboratory Service Working Party on Rubella. Studies of the effect of immunoglobulin on rubella in pregnancy. BMJ 2:497–500, 1970.
117. Martin du Pan R, Koechli B, Douath A. Protection of nonimmune volunteers against rubella by intravenous administration of normal human gamma globulin. J Infect Dis 126:341–344, 1972.
118. Schiff GM. Titered lots of immune globulin (Ig). Am J Dis Child 118:322–327, 1969.
119. Doege TC, Kim KSW. Studies of rubella and its prevention with immune globulin. JAMA 200:104–110, 1967.
120. Cooper L, Giles J, Florman A, et al. Protective effect of antirubella human immunoglobulin [abstract]. Soc Pediatr Res April 30, 1971.
121. Clarke DM, Loo TW, McDonald H, Gillam S. Expression of rubella virus cDNA coding for the structural proteins. Gene 65:23–30, 1988.
122. Frey T, Marr L, Hemphill M, Dominguez G. Molecular cloning and sequencing of the region of the rubella virus genome coding for glycoprotein E1. Virology 154:228–232, 1986.
123. Terry G, Ho L, Londesborough P, Rees K. Localization of the rubella E1 epitopes. Arch Virol 98:189–197, 1988.
124. Chaye HH, Chong P, Tripet B, et al. Localization of the virus neutralizing and hemagglutinin epitopes of E1 glycoprotein of rubella virus. Virology 189:483–492, 1992.
125. Hobman TC, Qiu ZY, Chaye H, Gillam S. Analysis of rubella virus E1 glycosylation mutants expressed in COS cells. Virology 181:768–772, 1991.
126. Wolinsky JS, McCarthy M, Allen CO, et al. Monoclonal antibody–defined epitope map of expressed rubella virus protein domains. J Virol 65:3986–3994, 1991.
127. Ilonen J, Seppänen H, Närvänen A, et al. Recognition of synthetic peptides with sequences of rubella virus E1 polypeptide by antibodies and T lymphocytes. Viral Immunol 5:221–228, 1992.
128. Lovett AE, McCarthy M, Wolinsky JS. Mapping cell-mediated immunodominant domains of the rubella virus structural proteins using recombinant proteins and synthetic peptides. J Gen Virol 74:445–452, 1993.
129. Marttila J, Lehtinen M, Parkkonen P, Salmi A. Definition of three minimal T helper cell epitopes of rubella virus E1 glycoprotein. Clin Exp Immunol 104:394–397, 1996.
130. Mitchell L, Decarie D, Tingle A, et al. Use of synthetic peptides to map regions of rubella virus capsid protein recognized by human T lymphocytes. Vaccine 12:639–645, 1994.
131. Seto N, Gillam S. Expression and characterization of a soluble rubella virus E1 envelope protein. J Med Virol 44:192–199, 1994.
132. Johansson T, Enestam A, Kronqvist R, et al. Synthesis of soluble rubella virus spike proteins in two lepidopteran insect cell lines: Large scale production of the E1 protein. J Biotechnol 50:171–180, 1996.
133. Terry GM, Ho TL, Londesborough P, Rees KR. A bio-engineered rubella E1 antigen. Arch Virol 104:63–75, 1989.

134. Seppanen H, Huhtala ML, Vaheri A, et al. Diagnostic potential of baculovirus-expressed rubella virus envelope proteins. J Clin Microbiol 29:1877–1882, 1991.
135. Trudel M, Nadon F, Seguin C, Payment P. Neutralizing response of rabbits to an experimental rubella subunit vaccine made from immunostimulating complexes. Can J Microbiol 34:1351–1354, 1988.
136. Robinson K, Mostratos A, Grencis R. Generation of rubella virus–neutralising antibodies by vaccination with synthetic peptides. FEMS Immunol Med Microbiol 10:191–198, 1995.
137. Qui Z, Ou D, Wu H, et al. Expression and characterization of virus-like particles containing rubella virus structural proteins. J Virol 68:4086–4091, 1994.
138. Hobman T, Lundstrom M, Mauracher C, et al. Assembly of rubella virus structural proteins into virus-like particles in transfected cells. Virology 202:574–585, 1994.
139. Plotkin SA. History of rubella and the recent history of cell culture. In Plotkin S, Fantini B (eds). Vaccinia, Vaccination, Vaccinology: Jenner, Pasteur, and Their Successors. Paris, Elsevier, 1996, pp 271–282.
140. Hilleman MR, Buynak EV, Whitman JE, et al. Live attenuated rubella virus vaccines: Experiences with duck embryo cell preparations. Am J Dis Child 118:166–171, 1969.
141. Perkins FT. Licensed vaccines. Rev Infect Dis 7:S73–S76, 1985.
142. Plotkin SA, Farquhar JD, Ogra PL. Immunologic properties of RA27/3 rubella virus vaccine. JAMA 225:585–590, 1973.
143. Plotkin SA, Cornfeld D, Ingalls TH. Studies of immunization with living rubella virus: Trials in children with a strain cultured from an aborted fetus. Am J Dis Child 110:381–389, 1965.
144. Plotkin SA, Farquhar J, Katz M, Ingalls TH. A new attenuated rubella virus growth in human fibroblasts: Evidence for reduced nasopharyngeal excretion. Am J Epidemiol 86:468–477, 1967.
145. Plotkin SA, Buser F. History of RA27/3 rubella vaccine. Rev Infect Dis 7:S77–S78, 1985.
146. Nakhasi H, Thomas D, Zheng D, Liu TY. Nucleotide sequence of capsid, E2 and E1 protein genes of rubella virus vaccine strain RA27/3. Nucleic Acids Res 17:4393–4394, 1989.
147. Zheng DX, Dickens L, Liu TY, Nakhasi HL. Nucleotide sequence of the 24S subgenomic messenger RNA of a vaccine strain (HPV-77) of rubella virus: Comparison with a wild-type strain (M33). Gene 82:343–349, 1989.
148. Frey TK, Abernathy ES. Identification of strain-specific nucleotide sequences in the RA27/3 rubella virus vaccine. J Infect Dis 168:854–864, 1993.
149. Londesborough P, Terry G, Ho-Terry L. Reactivity of a recombinant rubella E1 antigen expressed in *E. coli.* Arch Virol 122:391–397, 1992.
150. Best JM, Thomson A, Nores JR, et al. Rubella virus strains show no major antigenic differences. Intervirology 34:164–168, 1992.
151. Zealley H, Morrison AM, Freestone DS. Dose response studies with Wistar RA27/3 strain live attenuated rubella vaccine. J Biol Stand 2:111–119, 1974.
152. Plotkin SA, Ingalls TH, Farquhar JS, Katz M. Intranasally administered rubella vaccine. Lancet 2:9–34, 1968.
153. Puschak R, Young M, McKee TV, Plotkin SA. Intranasal vaccination with RA27/3 attenuated rubella virus. J Pediatr 79:55–70, 1971.
154. Ingalls TH, Horne HW. Immunization of women with rubella (RA27/3) vaccine administered intranasally. Lancet 1:830–832, 1971.
155. Hillary IB. Trials of intranasally administered rubella vaccine. J Hyg (Camb) 69:547–552, 1971.
156. Ganguly R, Durrer B, Waldman RH. Rubella virus immunization of preschool children via the respiratory tract. Am J Dis Child 128:821–823, 1974.
157. Midulla M, Assensio AM, Balducci L, et al. Intranasal versus subcutaneous rubella vaccination in schoolgirls. Dev Biol Stand 33:241–248, 1976.
158. Freestone DS. Clinical trials carried out to assess non-parenteral routes for administration of Wistar RA27/3 strain live attenuated rubella vaccine. Dev Biol Stand 33:237–240, 1976.
159. Ganguly R, Ogra PL, Regas J, Waldman RH. Rubella immunization of volunteers via the respiratory tract. Infect Immun 8:497–502, 1973.
160. Paradise JE, Nemorofsky DT, Huggins GR, et al. Intranasal administration of RA27/3 rubella virus vaccine: A clinical trial in young adults. J Adolesc Health Care 5:75–78, 1984.
161. Isozaki M, Kuno-Sakai H, Hoshi N, et al. Effects and side effects of a new trivalent combined measles-mumps-rubella (MMR) vaccine. Tokai J Exp Clin Med 7:547–550, 1982.
162. Weibel RE, Carlson AJ, Villarejos VM, et al. Clinical and laboratory studies of combined live measles, mumps, and rubella vaccines using the RA27/3 rubella virus. Proc Soc Exp Biol Med 165:323–326, 1980.
163. Lerman SJ, Bollinger M, Brunken JM. Clinical and serologic evaluation of measles, mumps, and rubella (HPV-77:DE-5 and RA27/3) virus vaccines, singly and in combination. Pediatrics 68:18–22, 1981.
164. Brunell PA, Weigle K, Murphy D, et al. Antibody response following measles-mumps-rubella vaccine under conditions of customary use. JAMA 250:1409–1412, 1983.
165. Schwartz AJF, Jackson JE, Ehrenkranz J, et al. Clinical evaluation of a new measles-mumps-rubella trivalent vaccine. Am J Dis Child 129:1408–1412, 1975.
166. Plotkin SA, Beale AJ. Production of RA27/3 rubella vaccine and clinical results with the vaccine. Dev Biol Stand 37:291–296, 1976.
167. Elliott AY. Manufacture and testing of measles, mumps, and rubella vaccine. 19th Immunization Conference Proceedings. US Department of Health and Human Services, Public Health Service. Atlanta, Centers for Disease Control, 1984, pp 79–83.
168. McAleer WJ, Markus HZ, McLean AA, et al. Stability on storage at various temperatures of live measles, mumps, and rubella virus vaccines in new stabilizer. J Biol Stand 8:281–287, 1980.
169. Hillary IB, Meenan PN, Griffiths AH, et al. Rubella vaccine trial in children. BMJ 2:531–532, 1969.
170. Berger R, Just M, Glück R. Interference between strains in live virus vaccines I: Combined vaccination with measles, mumps and rubella vaccine. J Biol Stand 16:269–273, 1988.
171. Vaananen P, Makela P, Vaheri A. Effect of low level immunity on response to live rubella virus vaccine. Vaccine 4:5–8, 1986.
172. Freestone DS, Reynolds GM, McKinnin JA, Prydie J. Vaccination of schoolgirls against rubella: Assessment of serological status and a comparative trial of Wistar RA 27/3 and Cendehill strain live attenuated rubella vaccines in 13-year-old schoolgirls in Dudley. Br J Prev Soc Med 29:258–261, 1975.
173. Böttiger M, Heller L. Experiences from vaccination and revaccination of teenage girls with three different rubella vaccines. J Biol Stand 4:107–114, 1976.
174. Grillner L. Neutralizing antibodies after rubella vaccination of newly delivered women. A comparison between three vaccines. Scand J Infect Dis 7:169–172, 1975.
175. Menser MA, Forrest JM, Bransby RD, Collins E. Rubella vaccination in Australia: Experience with the RA27/3 rubella vaccine and results of a double-blind trial in schoolgirls. Med J Aust 2:85–88, 1978.
176. Weibel RE, Villarejos VM, Klein EB, et al. Clinical and laboratory studies of live attenuated RA27/3 and HPV-77DE rubella virus vaccines. Proc Soc Exp Biol Med 165:44–49, 1980.
177. Best JM, Banatvala JE, Bowen JM. New Japanese rubella vaccine: Comparative trials. BMJ 3:221–224, 1974.
178. Wang S, Han Y, Su W, et al. Studies on the reactogenicity and immunogenicity of the BRD-2 and RA27/3 live attenuated rubella vaccines. Vaccine 2:227–280, 1984.
179. LeBouvier GL, Plotkin SA. Precipitin responses to rubella vaccine RA27/3. J Infect Dis 123:220–223, 1971.
180. Cusi M, Metelli R, Valensin P. Immune responses to wild and vaccine rubella viruses after rubella vaccination. Arch Virol 106:63–72, 1989.
181. Ogra PL, Kerr-Grant D, Umana G, et al. Antibody response in serum and nasopharynx after naturally acquired and vaccine-induced infection with rubella virus. N Engl J Med 285:1333–1339, 1971.
182. Cradock-Watson JE, MacDonald J, Ridehalgh MKS, et al. Nasal immunoglobulin responses in acute rubella determined by the immunofluorescent technique. J Hyg (Camb) 71:603–616, 1973.
183. Cradock-Watson JE, MacDonald J, Ridehalgh MKS, et al. Specific immunoglobulin responses in serum and nasal secretions after the administration of attenuated rubella vaccine. J Hyg (Camb) 73:127–141, 1974.

184. Banatvala JE, Druce A, Best JM, Al-Nakib W. Specific IgM responses after rubella vaccination; potential application following inadvertent vaccination during pregnancy. BMJ 2:1263–1264, 1977.
185. Meegan JM, Evans BK, Horstmann DM. Use of enzyme immunoassays and the latex agglutination test to measure the temporary appearance of immunoglobulin G and M antibodies after natural infection or immunization with rubella virus. J Clin Microbiol 18:745–748, 1983.
186. Lalla M, Vesikari T, Virolainen M. Lymphoblast proliferation and humoral antibody response after rubella vaccination. Clin Exp Immunol 15:192–202, 1973.
187. Honeyman MC, Forrest JA, Dorman DC. Cell-mediated immune response following natural rubella and rubella vaccination. Clin Exp Immunol 17:665–671, 1974.
188. Vesikari T, Buimovici-Klein E. Lymphocyte responses to rubella antigen and phytohemagglutinin after administration of the RA27/3 strain of live attenuated rubella vaccine. Infect Immun 11:748–753, 1975.
189. Heigl Z, Wasserman J, Forsgren M. In vitro lymphocyte reactivity to rubella antigen following vaccination. Scand J Infect Dis 12:13–20, 1980.
190. Steele RW, Hensen SA, Vincent MM, et al. Development of specific cellular and humoral immune responses in children immunized with live rubella virus vaccine. J Infect Dis 130:449–453, 1974.
191. Morag A, Morag B, Bernstein JM, et al. In vitro correlates of cell-mediated immunity in human tonsils after natural or induced rubella virus infection. J Infect Dis 131:4–16, 1975.
192. Balfour HH, Groth KE, Edelman CK, et al. Rubella viremia and antibody responses after rubella vaccination and reimmunization. Lancet 1:1078–1080, 1981.
193. Detels R, Kim KSW, Gale JL, Grayston JT. Viral shedding in Chinese children following vaccination with HPV-77 and Cendehill-51 live attenuated rubella vaccines. Am J Epidemiol 94:473–478, 1971.
194. Marshall WC, Peckham CS, Darby CP, et al. Further studies with rubella vaccines in adults and children. Practitioner 207:632–638, 1971.
195. Veronelli JA. An open community trial of live rubella vaccines: Study of vaccine virus transmissibility and antigenic efficacy of three HPV-77 derivatives. JAMA 213:1829–1836, 1970.
196. Meyer HM, Parkman PD. Rubella vaccination: A review of practical experience. JAMA 215:613–619, 1971.
197. Mogabgab WJ, Stowe FR. Evaluation of attenuated rubella virus vaccine in families. Am J Dis Child 122:122–128, 1971.
198. Scott HD, Byrne EB. Exposure of susceptible pregnant women to rubella vaccinees: Serologic findings during the Rhode Island immunization campaign. JAMA 215:609–612, 1971.
199. Halstead SB, Diwan AR. Failure to transmit rubella virus vaccine: A close-contact study in adults. JAMA 215:634–636, 1971.
200. Fleet WF, Schaffner W, Lefkowitz LB, et al. Exposure of susceptible teachers to rubella vaccines. Am J Dis Child 123:28–30, 1972.
201. Fleet WF, Vaughn WM, Lefkowitz LB, et al. Gestational exposure to rubella vaccinees: A population surveillance study. Am J Epidemiol 101:220–230, 1975.
202. Wolf J, Eisen JE, Fraimow HS. Symptomatic rubella reinfection in an immune contact of a rubella vaccine recipient. South Med J 86:91–93, 1993.
203. Schiff GM, Bloom JE. Evaluation of rubella vaccination in a large school system. J Pediatr 78:211–219, 1971.
204. Lipman RP, Bethel MB, Wooten JH, et al. Attenuated rubella vaccine (HPV-77): Evaluation in a large controlled trial. Am J Public Health 61:1392–1402, 1971.
205. Linnemann CC, Hutchinson L, Rotte TC, et al. Stability of the rabbit immunogenic marker of RA27/3 rubella vaccine virus after human passage. Infect Immun 9:547–549, 1974.
206. Furesz J. Antibody response of school children to live attenuated rubella virus vaccines as measured with various serologic methods. Am J Epidemiol 95:536–541, 1972.
207. Davis WJ, Larson HE, Simsarian JP, et al. A study of rubella immunity and resistance to infection. JAMA 215:600–608, 1971.
208. Grayston JT, Detels R, Chen KP, et al. Field trial of live attenuated rubella virus vaccine during an epidemic on Taiwan. JAMA 207:1107–1110, 1969.
209. Chang TW, Desrosiers S, Weinstein L. Clinical and serologic studies of an outbreak of rubella in a vaccinated population. N Engl J Med 283:246–248, 1970.
210. Furukawa T, Miyata T, Konda K, et al. Rubella vaccination during an epidemic. JAMA 213:987–990, 1970.
211. deValk HM, Garde X, Cohen B, et al. Clinical efficacy of rubella vaccine determined during an outbreak of rubella in a primary school, France, 1997 [abstract]. JET 11:146, 1997.
212. Landrigan PL, Stoffels MA, Anderson E, Witte JJ. Epidemic rubella in adolescent boys: Clinical features and results of vaccination. JAMA 227:1283–1287, 1974.
213. Crawford GE, Gremillion DH. Epidemic measles and rubella in Air Force recruits: Impact of immunization. J Infect Dis 144:403–410, 1981.
214. Greaves WL, Orenstein WA, Hinman AR, Nersesian WS. Clinical efficacy of rubella vaccine. Pediatr Infect Dis 2:284–286, 1983.
215. Koskiniemi M, Vaheri A. Effect of measles, mumps, rubella vaccination on pattern of encephalitis in children. Lancet 1:31–34, 1989.
216. Fogel A, Gerichter CB, Barena B, et al. Response to experimental challenge in persons immunized with different rubella vaccines. J Pediatr 92:26–29, 1978.
217. Harcourt GC, Best JM, Banatvala JE. Rubella-specific serum and nasopharyngeal antibodies in volunteers with naturally acquired and vaccine-induced immunity after intranasal challenge. J Infect Dis 142:145–155, 1980.
218. Schiff GM, Donath R, Rotte T. Experimental rubella studies: Clinical and laboratory features of infection caused by the Brown rubella virus. Artificial challenge studies of adult rubella vaccinees. Am J Dis Child 118:269–276, 1969.
219. Wilkins J, Leedom JM, Portnoy B, Salvatore MA. Reinfection with rubella virus despite live vaccine induced immunity. Am J Dis Child 118:275–294, 1969.
220. Nacify K, Nategh R, Ahangary S, Mohsenin H. Artificial challenge studies in rubella. Am J Dis Child 120:520–523, 1970.
221. Horstmann DM, Leibhaber H, Le Bouvier GL, et al. Rubella reinfection of vaccinated and naturally immune persons exposed in an epidemic. N Engl J Med 283:771–778, 1970.
222. Lehane DE, Newberg NR, Beam WE. Evaluation of rubella herd immunity during an epidemic. JAMA 213:2236–2239, 1970.
223. Judelsohn RG, Wyll SA. Rubella in Bermuda: Termination of an epidemic by mass vaccination. JAMA 223:401–406, 1973.
224. Klock LE, Rachelefsky GS. Failure of rubella herd immunity during an epidemic. N Engl J Med 288:69–72, 1973.
225. Rachelefsky GS, Herrmann KL. Congenital rubella surveillance following epidemic rubella in a partially vaccinated community. J Pediatr 84:474–478, 1974.
226. O'Shea S, Best JM, Banatvala JE. Viremia, virus excretion and antibody responses after challenge to volunteers with low levels of antibody to rubella virus. J Infect Dis 148:639–647, 1983.
227. Banatvala JE, Best JM, O'Shea S, Dudgeon JA. Persistence of rubella antibodies after vaccination: Detection after experimental challenge. Rev Infect Dis 7:S86–S90, 1985.
228. Cusi MG, Rossolini GM, Valensin PE, et al. Serological evidence of reinfection among vaccinees during rubella outbreak. Lancet 336:10–71, 1990.
229. Butler AB, Scott RM, Schydlower M, et al. The immunoglobulin response to reimmunization with rubella vaccine. J Pediatr 99:531–534, 1981.
230. Morgan-Capner P, Hodgson J, Hambling MH, et al. Detection of rubella-specific IgM in subclinical rubella reinfection in pregnancy. Lancet 1:244–246, 1985.
231. Forsgren M, Soren L. Subclinical rubella reinfection in vaccinated women with rubella-specific IgM response during pregnancy and transmission of virus to the fetus. Scand J Infect Dis 17:337–341, 1985.
232. Forrest JM, Menser MA, Honeyman MC, et al. Clinical rubella eleven months after vaccination. Lancet 2:399–400, 1972.
233. Northrop RL, Gardner WM, Geittmann WF. Rubella reinfection during early pregnancy: A case report. Obstet Gynecol 39:524–526, 1972.
234. Morgan-Capner P, Burgess C, Ireland RM, Sharp JC. Clinically apparent rubella reinfection with a detectable rubella specific IgM response. BMJ 286:1616, 1983.

235. Eilard T, Strannegard O. Rubella reinfection in pregnancy followed by transmission to the fetus. J Infect Dis 129:594–596, 1974.
236. Das BD, Lakhani P, Kurtz JB, et al. Congenital rubella after previous maternal immunity. Arch Dis Child 65:545–546, 1990.
237. Keith CG. Congenital rubella infection from reinfection of previously immunised mothers. Aust N Z J Ophthalmol 19:291–293, 1991.
238. Weber B, Enders G, Schlösser R, et al. Congenital rubella syndrome after maternal reinfection. Infection 21:118–121, 1993.
239. Robinson J, LeMay M, Vaudry W. Congenital rubella after anticipated maternal immunity: Two cases and a review of the literature. Pediatr Infect Dis J 13:812–815, 1994.
240. Paludetto R, van den Heuvel J, Stagni A, et al. Rubella embryopathy after maternal infection. Biol Neonate 65:340–341, 1994.
241. Braun C, Kampa D, Fressle R, et al. Congenital rubella syndrome despite repeated vaccination of the mother: A coincidence of vaccine failure with failure to vaccinate. Acta Paediatr 83:674–677, 1994.
242. Fogel A, Handsher R, Barnea B. Subclinical rubella in pregnancy—occurrence and outcome. Isr J Med Sci 21:133–138, 1985.
243. Bott LM, Eisenberg DH. Congenital rubella after successful vaccination. Med J Aust 1:514–515, 1982.
244. Enders G, Calm A, Schaub J. Rubella embryopathy after previous maternal rubella vaccination. Infection 12:96–98, 1984.
245. Connolly JH, Nevin NC, Simpson DM, O'Neill HJ. Outcome of pregnancy in rubella outbreak in Northern Ireland, 1978–1979. Ulster Med J 53:65–73, 1984.
246. Forsgren M, Carlstrom G, Strangert K. Congenital rubella after maternal reinfection. Scand J Infect Dis 11:81–83, 1979.
247. Levine JB, Berkowitz CD, St. Geme JW. Rubella virus reinfection during pregnancy leading to late onset congenital rubella syndrome. J Pediatr 100:589–591, 1982.
248. Schoub BD, Blackburn NK, O'Connell K, et al. Symptomatic rubella re-infection in early pregnancy and subsequent delivery of an infected but minimally involved infant. S Afr Med J 78:484–485, 1990.
249. Gilbert J, Kudesia G. Fetal infection after maternal reinfection with rubella. BMJ 299:12–17, 1989.
250. Morgan-Capner P, Miller E, Vurdien J, Ramsay M. Outcome of pregnancy after maternal reinfection with rubella. Commun Dis Rep 1:R57–R59, 1991.
251. O'Shea S, Corbett K, Barrow S, et al. Rubella reinfection; role of neutralising antibodies and cell-mediated immunity. Clin Diagn Virol 2:349–358, 1994.
252. Matter L, Kogelschatz K, Germann D. Serum levels of rubella virus antibodies indicating immunity: Response to vaccination of subjects with low or undetectable antibody concentrations. J Infect Dis 175:749–755, 1997.
253. Mitchell L, Ho M, Rogers J, et al. Rubella reimmunization: Comparative analysis of the immunoglobulin G response to rubella virus vaccine in previously seronegative and seropositive individuals. J Clin Microbiol 34:2210–2218, 1996.
254. Liebhaber H, Ingalls TH, Le Bouvier GL, Horstmann DM. Vaccination with RA27/3 rubella vaccine. Am J Dis Child 123:133–136, 1972.
255. Black FL, Lamm SH, Emmons JE, Pinheiro FP. Reactions to rubella vaccine and persistence of antibody in virgin-soil populations after vaccination and wild virus–induced immunization. J Infect Dis 133:393–398, 1976.
256. Balfour HH, Groth KE, Edelman CK. RA27/3 rubella vaccine. Am J Dis Child 134:350–353, 1980.
257. Zealley H, Edmond E. Rubella screening and immunization of school girls: Results six to seven years after vaccination. BMJ 284:382–384, 1982.
258. Hillary IB, Griffith AH. Persistence of rubella antibodies 15 years after subcutaneous administration of Wistar 27/3 strain live attenuated rubella virus vaccine. Vaccine 2:274–276, 1984.
259. O'Shea S, Best JM, Banatvala JE, et al. Rubella vaccination: Persistence of antibodies for 10–21 years [letter]. Lancet 2:909, 1988.
260. King JC, Lichenstein R, Feigelman S, et al. Measles, mumps, and rubella antibodies in vaccinated Baltimore children. Am J Dis Child 147:558–550, 1993.
261. Miller E, Hill A, Morgan-Capner P, et al. Antibodies to measles, mumps, and rubella in UK children 4 years after vaccination with different MMR vaccines. Vaccine 13:799–802, 1995.
262. Boulianne N, DeSerres G, Ratnam S, et al. Measles, mumps, and rubella antibodies in children 5–6 years after immunization: Effect of vaccine type and age at vaccination. Vaccine 13:1611–1616, 1995.
263. Böttiger M. Immunity to rubella before and after vaccination against measles, mumps and rubella (MMR) at 12 years of age of the first generation offered MMR vaccination in Sweden at 18 months. Vaccine 13:1759–1762, 1995.
264. Christenson B, Böttiger M. Long-term follow-up study of rubella antibodies in naturally immune and vaccinated young adults. Vaccine 12:41–45, 1994.
265. Johnson C, Kumar M, Whitwell J, et al. Antibody persistence after Primary measles-mumps-rubella vaccine and response to a second dose given at four to six vs. eleven to thirteen years. Pediatr Infect Dis J 15:687–692, 1996.
266. Ratnam S, West R, Gadag V, et al. Rubella antibody levels in school aged children in Newfoundland: Implications for a two-dose rubella vaccination strategy. Can J Infect Dis 8:85–88, 1997.
267. Menser MA, Forrest JM, Bransby RD. Rubella vaccination in Australia. Med J Aust 2:83–85, 1978.
268. Just M, Just V, Berger R, et al. Duration of immunity after rubella vaccination: A long term study in Switzerland. Rev Infect Dis 7(suppl):S91–S94, 1985.
269. Chu SY, Bernier RH, Stewart JA, et al. Rubella antibody persistence after immunization: Sixteen-year follow-up in the Hawaiian Islands. JAMA 259:3133–3136, 1988.
270. Schiff GM, Rauh JL, Young B, et al. Rubella-vaccinated students: Follow-up in a public school system. JAMA 240:2635–2637, 1978.
271. Weibel RE, Buynak EB, McLean AA, Hilleman MR. Follow-up surveillance for antibody in human subjects following live attenuated measles, mumps, and rubella virus vaccines. Proc Soc Exp Biol Med 162:328–332, 1979.
272. Weibel RE, Buynak EB, McLean AA, et al. Persistence of antibody in human subjects for 7 to 10 years following administration of combined live attenuated measles, mumps, and rubella virus vaccines. Proc Soc Exp Biol Med 165:260–263, 1980.
273. Balfour HH, Amren DP. Rubella, measles and mumps antibodies following vaccination of children. Am J Dis Child 132:573–577, 1978.
274. Horstmann DM, Schluederberg A, Emmons JE, et al. Persistence of vaccine-induced immune responses to rubella: Comparison with natural infection. Rev Infect Dis 7(suppl):S80–S85, 1985.
275. Maes EF, Gillan A, Stehr-Green PA, et al. Rubella antibody persistence 20 years after immunization. Abstracts of the 31st Interscience Conference on Antimicrobial Agents and Chemotherapy; Chicago, IL; September 29–October 2, 1991, p 285.
276. Schum T, Nelson D, Duma M, Sedmak G. Increasing rubella seronegativity despite a compulsory school law. Am J Public Health 80:66–69, 1990.
277. Best JM. Rubella vaccines: Past, present and future. Epidemiol Infect 107:17–30, 1991.
278. Strassburg MA, Greenland S, Stephenson TG, et al. Clinical effectiveness of rubella vaccine in a college population. Vaccine 3:109–112, 1985.
279. Forrest JM, Slinn RF, Nowak MJ, Menser MA. Duration of immunity to rubella. Lancet 1:10–13, 1971.
280. Hoshino M, Oka Y, Deguchi M, et al. The ten-year follow-up of the persistence of humoral antibody to rubella virus acquired by vaccination with the Japanese To336 vaccine. J Biol Stand 10:213–219, 1982.
281. Ueda K, Yoshikawa, H, Ohashi K, et al. Clinical experience with a live attenuated rubella virus vaccine, Matsuba strain GMK3SK6ORK6, in special reference to 6-year follow-up of rubella antibodies to prevention of rubella infection during an epidemic. J Pediatr 20:8–14, 1978.
282. Rossier E, Phipps PH, Polley JR, Webb T. Absence of cell-mediated immunity to rubella virus 5 years after rubella vaccination. Can Med Assoc J 116:481–484, 1977.
282a. Asahi T, Ueda K, Hidaka Y, et al. Twenty-three-year follow-up study of rubella antibodies after immunization in a closed population, and serological response to revaccination. Vaccine 15:1791–1795, 1997.

283. Balfour HH. Rubella reimmunization now. Am J Dis Child 133:1231–1233, 1979.
284. Lawless MR, Abramson JS, Harlan JE, Kelsey DS. Rubella susceptibility in sixth graders: Effectiveness of current immunization practice. Pediatrics 65:1086–1089, 1990.
285. Brandling-Bennet AD, Jackson RS, Halstead SB, et al. Serologic response to revaccination with two rubella vaccines. Am J Dis Child 130:1081–1089, 1976.
286. Serdula MK, Halstead SB, Wiebenga NH, Herrmann KL. Serological response to rubella revaccination. JAMA 251:1974–1977, 1984.
287. Robinson RG, Dudenhoeffer FE, Holroyd HJ, et al. Rubella immunity in older children, teenagers, and young adults: A comparison of immunity in those previously immunized with those unimmunized. J Pediatr 101:188–191, 1982.
288. Fitzpatrick SB, Anthony R, Heald F. Serological response to rubella revaccination in adolescent females. J Adolesc Health Care 4:168–170, 1983.
289. Mauracher C, Mitchell L, Tingle A. Selective tolerance to the E1-protein of rubella virus in congenital rubella syndrome. J Immunol 151:2041–2049, 1993.
290. Forrest J, Honeyman M, Menser M. Immunity after congenital rubella. Lancet 1:1075–1076, 1972.
291. Schell K, Kenny MT, Jackson JE. Serological evaluation of measles virus (Schwarz strain), mumps virus (Jeryl Lynn strain) and rubella (Cendehill strain) combination vaccines. J Biol Stand 3:231–239, 1975.
292. Deforrest A, Long SS, Lischner HW, et al. Simultaneous administration of measles-mumps-rubella vaccine with booster dose of diphtheria-tetanus-pertussis and poliovirus vaccines. Pediatrics 81:237–246, 1988.
293. Watson B, Laufer D, Kuter B, et al. Safety and immunogenicity of combined live attenuated measles, mumps, rubella, and varicella vaccine ($MMR_{II}V$) in healthy children. J Infect Dis 173:731–734, 1996.
294. Howson CP, Howe CJ, Fineberg HV. Chronic Arthritis in Adverse Effects of Pertussis and Rubella Vaccines. Washington, DC, Institute of Medicine, National Academy Press, 1991, p 196.
295. Epidemiologic report. Adverse events temporally associated with immunizing agents: 1989 report. Can Med Assoc J 145:1269–1275, 1991.
296. Dudgeon JA, Marshall WC, Peckham CS, Hawkins GT. Clinical and laboratory studies with rubella vaccines in adults. BMJ 1:271–276, 1969.
297. Barnes EK, Altman R, Austin SM, Dougherty WJ. Joint reactions in children vaccinated against rubella. Comparison of three vaccines. Am J Epidemiol 95:59–66, 1972.
298. Spruance SL, Smith CB. Joint complications associated with derivatives of HPV-77 rubella virus vaccine. Am J Epidemiol 122:105–111, 1971.
299. Kilroy AW, Schaffner W, Fleet FW, et al. Two syndromes following rubella immunization: Clinical observations and epidemiologic studies. JAMA 214:2287–2292, 1970.
300. Thompson GR, Weiss JJ, Schills JC, et al. Intermittent arthritis following rubella vaccination: A three-year follow-up. Am J Epidemiol 125:526–530, 1973.
301. Spruance SL, Klock LE, Bailey A, et al. Recurrent joint symptoms in children vaccinated with HPV-77DK12 rubella vaccine. J Pediatr 80:413–417, 1972.
302. Gilmartin RC, Jabbour JT, Duenas DA. Rubella vaccine myeloradiculoneuritis. J Pediatr 80:406–412, 1972.
303. Swartz TA, Klingberg W, Goldwasser RA, et al. Clinical manifestations, according to age, among females given HPV-77 duck rubella vaccine. Am J Epidemiol 94:246–251, 1971.
304. Weibel RE, Stokes J, Buynak EB, Hilleman MR. Influence of age on clinical response to HPV-77 duck rubella vaccine. JAMA 202:805–807, 1972.
305. Lerman SJ, Nankervis GA, Heggie AJ, Gold E. Immunologic response, virus excretion and joint reactions with rubella vaccine. Ann Intern Med 74:67–73, 1971.
306. Horstmann DM, Liebhaber H, Kohorn EI. Postpartum vaccination of rubella-susceptible women. Lancet 2:1003–1006, 1970.
307. Fox JP, Rainey HS, Hall CE, et al. Rubella vaccine in postpubertal women: Experience in western Washington state. JAMA 236:837–843, 1976.
308. Rowlands DF, Freestone DS. Vaccination against rubella of susceptible schoolgirls in Reading. J Hyg (Camb) 69:579-586, 1971.
309. Freestone DS, Prydie J, Hamilton-Smith SG, Laurence G. Vaccination of adults with Wistar RA27/3 rubella vaccine. J Hyg (Camb) 69:471–477, 1971.
310. Polk BF, White JA, DeGirolami PC. A controlled comparison of joint reactions among women receiving one of two rubella vaccines. Am J Epidemiol 115:19–25, 1982.
311. Ogra PL, Chiba Y, Ogra SS, et al. Rubella-virus infection in juvenile rheumatoid arthritis. Lancet 1:1157–1161, 1975.
312. Ogra PL, Herd JK. Arthritis associated with induced rubella infection. J Immunol 107:810–813, 1971.
313. Nepon G, Ou D, Lybrand T, et al. Recognition of altered self major histocompatibility complex molecules modulated by specific peptide interactions. Eur J Immunol 26:949–952, 1996.
314. Pogue G, Hofmann J, Duncan R, et al. Autoantigens interact with *cis*-acting elements of rubella virus RNA. J Virol 70:6269–6277, 1996.
315. Miki NPH, Chantler JK. Differential ability of wild-type and vaccine strains of rubella virus to replicate and persist in human joint tissue. Clin Exp Rheumatol 10:3–12, 1992.
316. Tingle AJ, Chantler JK, Pot KH, et al. Postpartum rubella immunization: Association with development of prolonged arthritis, neurological sequelae and chronic rubella viremia. J Infect Dis 152:606–612, 1985.
317. Tingle AJ, Kettyls GDM, Ford DK. Studies on vaccine induced rubella arthritis. Serologic findings before and after immunization. Arthritis Rheum 22:400–402, 1979.
318. Tingle AJ, Allen M, Petty RE, et al. Rubella-associated arthritis. I. Comparative study of joint manifestations associated with natural rubella infection and RA27/3 rubella immunization. Ann Rheum Dis 45:110–114, 1986.
319. Singh VK, Tingle AJ, Schulzer M. Rubella-associated arthritis. II. Relationship between circulating immune complex levels and joint manifestations. Ann Rheum Dis 45:115–119, 1986.
320. Howson CP, Katz M, Johnston RBJ, Fineberg HV. Chronic arthritis after rubella vaccination. Clin Infect Dis 15:307–312, 1992.
321. Phillips P, Dougherty R, Mican J. Failure to isolate rubella virus (RV) from blood of adults after vaccination. Arthritis Rheum 32:113, 1989.
322. Frenkel L, Garakian A, Cherry J. Rubella virus (RV): No evidence of persistent infection following immunization with RA 27/3 or wild type infection. In Program and Abstracts of the 31st Interscience Conference on Antimicrobial Agents and Chemotherapy; Chicago, IL; September 29–October 2, 1991, p 1294.
323. Nielsen K, Garakian A, Frenkel L, Cherry J. The in vitro growth and serial passage of RA 27/3 rubella vaccine in cord blood mononuclear leukocytes from normal babies. Pediatr Res 37:623–625, 1995.
324. Zhang D, Nikkari S, Vainionpaa R, et al. Detection of rubella, mumps, and measles virus genomic RNA in cells from synovial fluid and peripheral blood in early rheumatoid arthritis. J Rheumatol 24:1260–1265, 1997.
325. Slater P, Ben-Zvi T, Fogel A, et al. Absence of an association between rubella vaccination and arthritis in underimmune postpartum women. Vaccine 13:1529–1532, 1995.
326. Ray P, Black S, Shinefield H, et al. Risk of chronic arthropathy among women after rubella vaccination. JAMA 278:551–556, 1997.
327. Tingle A, Mitchell L, Grace M, et al. Randomised double-blind placebo-controlled study on adverse effects of rubella immunisation in seronegative women. Lancet 349:1277–1281, 1996.
328. Weibel R, Benor D. Chronic arthropathy and musculoskeletal symptoms associated with rubella vaccines. Arthritis Rheum 39:1529–1534, 1996.
329. Chiba Y, Sadeghi E, Ogra PL. Abnormalities of cellular immune response in arthritis induced by rubella vaccination. J Immunol 117:1684–1687, 1976.
330. Coyle PK, Wolinsky JS, Buimovici-Klein E, et al. Rubella-specific immune complexes after congenital infection and vaccination. Infect Immun 36:498–503, 1982.
331. Fogel A, Moshkowitz A, Rannon L, Gerichter CB. Comparative trials of RA27/3 and Cendehill rubella vaccines in adult and adolescent females. Am J Epidemiol 93:392–398, 1971.

332. Peltola H, Heinonen OP. Frequency of true adverse reactions to measles-mumps-rubella vaccine. A double-blind placebo-controlled trial in twins. Lancet 1:939–942, 1986.
333. Edees S, Pullan CR, Hull D. A randomised single blind trial of a combined mumps-measles-rubella vaccine to evaluate serological response and reactions in the UK population. Public Health 105:91–97, 1991.
334. Centers for Disease Control. Adverse Events Following Immunization. Surveillance Report No. 1, 1979–1982. US Department of Health and Human Services, Public Health Service. Atlanta, Centers for Disease Control, August 1984.
335. Schaffner W, Fleet WF, Kilroy AW, et al. Polyneuropathy following rubella immunization: A follow-up study and review of the problem. Am J Dis Child 127:684–688, 1974.
336. Kazarian EL, Gager WE. Optic neuritis complicating measles, mumps and rubella vaccination. Am J Ophthalmol 86:544–547, 1978.
337. Kline LB, Margulies SL, Oh SJ. Optic neuritis and myelitis following rubella vaccination. Arch Neurol 39:443–444, 1982.
338. Centers for Disease Control. Rubella Surveillance No. 2. US Department of Health and Human Services, Public Health Service. Atlanta, Centers for Disease Control, August 1970.
339. Hold S, Hudgins D, Krishnan KR, Critchley EMR. Diffuse myelitis associated with rubella vaccination. BMJ 2:1037–1038, 1976.
340. Behan PO. Diffuse myelitis associated with rubella vaccination [letter]. Br Med J 1:166, 1977.
341. Morton-Kute L. Rubella vaccine and facial paresthesias [letter]. Ann Intern Med 102:563, 1985.
342. Joyce K, Rees J. Transverse myelitis after measles, mumps, and rubella vaccine. BMJ 311:422, 1995.
343. Gunderman JR. Guillain-Barré syndrome: Occurrence following combined mumps-rubella vaccine. Am J Dis Child 125:834–835, 1973.
344. Rees J, Hughes R. Guillain-Barré syndrome after measles, mumps, and rubella vaccine [letter; comment]. Lancet 343:733, 1994.
345. Hughes R, Rees J, Smeeton N, Winer J. Vaccines and Guillain-Barré syndrome. Bull Epidemiol Hebdomadaire 312:1475–1476, 1996.
346. Chantler J, Smyrnis L, Tai G. Selective infection of astrocytes in human glial cell cultures by rubella virus. Lab Invest 72:334–340, 1995.
347. Peters ME, Horowitz S. Bone changes after rubella vaccination. Am J Radiol 143:27–28, 1984.
348. Zeffer K, Sauer M. Orchitis after a rubella vaccination. A case report. J Reprod Med 33:80–81, 1988.
349. Sharma ON. Thrombocytopenia following measles-mumps-rubella vaccination in a 1-year-old infant. Clin Pediatr 12:315–316, 1973.
350. Neiderund J. Thrombocytopenia purpura after a combined vaccine against morbilli, parotitis and rubella. Acta Paediatr Scand 72:613–614, 1983.
351. Nieminen U, Peltola H, Syrjälä MT, et al. Acute thrombocytopenic purpura following measles, mumps and rubella vaccination. A report on 23 patients. Acta Paediatr 82:267–270, 1993.
352. Chang Y, Farrell D, Dougan K, Kobayashi B. Acute idiopathic thrombocytopenic purpura following combined vaccination against measles, mumps, and rubella. J Am Board Fam Pract 9:53–55, 1996.
353. Bayer W, Sherman F, Michaels R, et al. Purpura in congenital and acquired rubella. N Engl J Med 273:1362–1366, 1965.
354. Autret E, Jonville-Béra A, Galy-Eyraud C, Hessel L. Purpura throbopénique après vaccination isolée ou associeé contre la rougeole, la rubéole et les oreillons. Therapie 51:677–680, 1996.
355. Drachtman R, Murphy S, Ettinger L. Exacerbation of chronic idiopathic thrombocytopenic purpura following measles-mumps-rubella immunization. Arch Pediatr Adolesc 148:326–327, 1994.
356. Vlacha V, Forman E, Miron D, Peter G. Recurrent thrombocytopenic purpura after repeated measles-mumps-rubella vaccination. Pediatrics 97:738–739, 1996.
357. Advisory Committee on Immunization Practices. Update: Vaccine side effects, adverse reactions, contraindications and precautions. MMWR Morb Mortal Wkly Rep 45(RR-12):1–35, 1996.
358. Pool V, Chen R, Rhodes P. Indications for measles-mumps-rubella vaccination in a child with prior thrombocytopenia purpura. Pediatr Infect Dis J 15:423–424, 1997.
359. Midulla M, Businco L, Moschini L. Some effects of rubella vaccination on immunologic responsiveness. Acta Paediatr Scand 61:609–611, 1972.
360. Munyer TP, Mangi RJ, Dolan T, Kantor FS. Depressed lymphocyte function after measles-mumps-rubella vaccination. J Infect Dis 132:75–78, 1975.
361. Ganguly R, Cusumano CL, Waldman RH. Suppression of cell-mediated immunity after infection with attenuated rubella virus. Infect Immun 13:464–469, 1976.
362. Arneborn P, Biberfeld G, Wasserman J. Immunosuppression and alterations of T-lymphocyte subpopulations after rubella vaccination. Infect Immun 29:36–41, 1980.
363. Mellor JA, Langford DT, Zealley H, et al. A survey of cancer morbidity and mortality in vaccinees 7 to 12 years after the administration of live vaccine propagated in human diploid cells. J Biol Stand 11:221–225, 1983.
364. Herrmann KL, Wende RD, Witte JJ. Rubella immunization with HPV-77 DE vaccine during infancy. Am J Dis Child 121:474–476, 1971.
365. Wilkins J, Wehrle PF. Further evaluation of the optimum age for rubella vaccine administration. Am J Dis Child 133:1237–1239, 1979.
366. Schoub B, Johnson S, McAnerney J, et al. Measles, mumps, and rubella immunization at nine months in a developing country. Pediatr Infect Dis J 9:263–267, 1990.
367. Volti S, Giammanco-Bilancia G, Grassi M, et al. Duration of the immune response to MMR vaccine in children of two age-different groups. Eur J Epidemiol 9:311–314, 1993.
368. Singh R, John T, Cherian T, Raghupathy P. Immune response to measles, mumps, and rubella vaccine at 9, 12 and 15 months of age. Indian J Med Res 100:155–159, 1994.
369. Ratnam S, Chandra R, Gadag V. Maternal measles and rubella antibody levels and serologic response in infants immunized with MMRII vaccine at 12 months of age. J Infect Dis 168:1596–1598, 1993.
370. Centers for Disease Control and Prevention. Rubella prevention: Recommendation of the Immunization Practices Advisory Committee. MMWR Morb Mortal Wkly Rep 39(RR-15):1–18, 1990.
371. Dennehy P, Saracen C, Peter G. Seroversion rates to combined measles-mumps-rubella-varicella vaccine of children with upper respiratory tract infection. Pediatrics 94:514–516, 1994.
372. Ratnam S, West R, Gadag V. Measles and rubella antibody response after measles-mumps-rubella vaccination in children with afebrile upper respiratory tract infection. J Pediatr 12:432–434, 1995.
373. Cilla G, Pena B, Marimon J, Perez-Trallero E. Serologic response to measles-mumps-rubella vaccine among children with upper respiratory tract infection. Vaccine 14:492–494, 1996.
374. Schiff GM, Linnemann CC, Rotte T, Ashe HS. Rubella surveillance and immunization. Susceptibility in nonurban adolescents. JAMA 226:554–556, 1973.
375. Raugh JL, Schiff GM, Johnson LB. Rubella surveillance and immunization among adolescent girls in Cincinnati. Am J Dis Child 124:71–75, 1972.
376. Mann JM, Montes JM, Hull HF, et al. Risk of pregnancy among adolescent schoolgirls participating in a measles mass immunization program. Am J Public Health 73:527–529, 1983.
377. Lerman SJ, Lerman LM, Nankervis GA, Gold E. Accuracy of rubella history. Ann Intern Med 74:97–98, 1971.
378. Tattersall JM, Freestone DS. Rubella vaccination in young women attending a family planning clinic. Practitioner 221:769–772, 1973.
379. Halstead E, Halstead SB, Jackson RS, et al. Rubella vaccination: Fertility control in a large-scale vaccination program for postpubertal women. Am J Obstet Gynecol 121:1089–1094, 1975.
380. Gringras M, Reisler R, Caisley J, et al. Vaccination of rubella-susceptible women during oral contraceptive care in general practice. Br Med J 2:245–246, 1977.
381. Rowlands S, Bethel RGH. Contraceptive cover for rubella vaccination. Practitioner 226:1155–1156, 1982.
382. Schiff GM, Young BC, Stefanovic GM, et al. Challenge with rubella virus after loss of detectable vaccine-induced antibody. Rev Infect Dis 7(suppl):S157–S163, 1985.

383. Kelly CS, Gibson JL, Williams CS, Leibovitz A. Postpartum rubella immunization. Obstet Gynecol 37:338–342, 1971.
384. Tobin JO. Rubella vaccination of postpartum women and of adolescents in the Northwest of England. Can J Public Health 62:634–667, 1971.
385. Beazley JM, Hurley R, Middlebrook C, Rumpus MF. Rubella vaccination in the puerperium. Br J Prev Soc Med 25:140–143, 1971.
386. Grillner L, Hedstrosom CE, Bergstrom H, et al. Vaccination against rubella of newly delivered women. Scand J Infect Dis 5:237–241, 1973.
387. Cheldelin LV, Francis DP, Tilson H. Postpartum rubella vaccination: A survey of private physicians in Oregon. JAMA 225:158–159, 1973.
388. Griffiths PD, Baboonian C. Is post-partum rubella vaccination worthwhile? J Clin Pathol 35:1340–1344, 1982.
389. Black NA, Parsons A, Kurtz JB, et al. Postpartum rubella immunization: A controlled trial of two vaccines. Lancet 2:990–992, 1983.
390. Marshall WC, Peckham CS, Dudgeon JA, et al. Parity of women contracting rubella in pregnancy: Implications with respect to rubella vaccination. Lancet 1:1231–1233, 1976.
391. Edmond E, Zeally H. The impact of a rubella prevention policy on the outcome of rubella in pregnancy. Br J Obstet Gynecol 93:563–567, 1986.
392. Baldwin JA, Freestone DA. Risk of early post-partum pregnancy in the context of postpartum vaccination against rubella. Lancet 2:366–367, 1971.
393. Sharp DS, MacDonald H. Use of medroxyprogesterone acetate as a contraceptive in conjunction with early postpartum rubella vaccination. BMJ 4:443–446, 1973.
394. Bolognese RJ, Corson SL, Fucillo DA, Traub R. The susceptibility of the postpartum and postabortal cervix and uterine cavity to infection with attenuated rubella virus. Am J Obstet Gynecol 125:525–527, 1976.
395. Buimovici-Klein E, Hite RL, Byrne T, Cooper LZ. Isolation of rubella virus in milk after postpartum immunization. J Pediatr 91:939–943, 1977.
396. Landes RD, Bass JW, Millunchick EW, Oetgen WJ. Neonatal rubella following postpartum maternal immunization. J Pediatr 97:465–467, 1980.
397. Losonsky GA, Fishaut JM, Strussenberg J, Ogra PL. Effect of immunization against rubella on lactation products. 1. Development and characterization of specific immunological reactivity in breast-milk. J Infect Dis 145:654–660, 1982.
398. Losonsky GA, Fishaut JM, Strussenberg J, Ogra PL. Effect of immunization against rubella on lactation products. 2. Maternal-neonatal interactions. J Infect Dis 145:661–666, 1982.
399. Perez-Trallero E, Cilla G, Urbieta M. Rubella immunisation of men: Advantages of herd immunity [letter; comment]. Lancet 348:413, 1996.
400. Bakasun V, Suzanic-Karnincic J. A rubella outbreak in the region of Rijeka, Croatia. Int J Epidemiol 24:453–456, 1995.
401. Crawford GE, Gremillion DH. Epidemic measles and rubella in Air Force recruits: Impact of immunization. J Infect Dis 144:403–410, 1981.
402. Lim MK, Fong YF, Soh CS. Rubella seroprevalence in the Singapore Armed Forces (SAF) and the changing need of the SAF rubella immunisation programme. Ann Acad Med Singapore 26:37–39, 1997.
403. Adams MS, Croft AMJ, Winfield DA, Richards PR. An outbreak of rubella in British troops in Bosnia. Epidemiol Infect 118:253–257, 1997.
404. Migiani R, Renaudat-Olivaud A, Barneche J, et al. Epidémie de rubéole en 1996 dans un centre d'instruction militaire dans le centre de la France. Bull Epidemiol Hebdomadaire 28:124–125, 1996.
405. Centers for Disease Control. Rubella Surveillance Report. US Department of Health and Human Services, Public Health Service. Atlanta, Centers for Disease Control, May 1980.
406. Weiss KE, Falvo CE, Buimovici-Klein E, et al. Evaluation of an employee health service as a setting for a rubella screening and immunization program. Am J Public Health 69:281–283, 1979.
407. Polk BF, White JA, DeGirolami PC, Modlin JF. An outbreak of rubella among hospital personnel. N Engl J Med 303:541–545, 1980.
408. Nosocomial rubella infection—North Dakota, Alabama, Ohio. MMWR Morb Mortal Wkly Rep 29:629–631, 1981.
409. Rubella in hospitals—California. MMWR Morb Mortal Wkly Rep 32:37–39, 1983.
410. Greaves WL, Orenstein WA, Stetler HC, et al. Prevention of rubella transmission in medical facilities. JAMA 242:861–864, 1982.
411. Heseltine PN, Ripper M, Wohlford P. Nosocomial rubella—consequences of an outbreak and efficacy of a mandatory immunization program. Infect Control 6:371–374, 1985.
412. Weber D, Rutala W, Orenstein WA. Prevention of mumps, measles and rubella among hospital personnel. J Pediatr 119:322–326, 1991.
413. Geiger R, Fink F, Solder B, et al. Persistent rubella infection after erroneous vaccination in an immunocompromised patient with acute lymphoblastic leukemia in remission. J Med Virol 47:442–444, 1995.
414. Ljungman P, Fridell E, Lonqvist B, et al. Efficacy and safety of vaccination of marrow transplant recipients with a live attenuated measles, mumps and rubella vaccine. J Infect Dis 159:610–615, 1989.
415. King S, Saunders E, Gold R. Response to measles, mumps, rubella vaccine in paediatric bone marrow transplant recipients. Bone Marrow Transplant 148:57–60, 1994.
416. Frenkel L, Nielsen K, Garakian A, Cherry J. A search for persistent measles, mumps, and rubella vaccine virus in children with human immunodeficiency virus type 1 infection. Arch Pediatr Adolesc Med 148:57–60, 1994.
417. Kwittken PL, Rosen S, Sweinberg SK. MMR vaccine and neomycin allergy. Pediatr Forum 147:128–129, 1993.
418. Fleet WF, Benz EW, Karzon DT, et al. Fetal consequences of maternal rubella immunization. JAMA 227:621–626, 1974.
419. Rubella vaccination during pregnancy—United States, 1973–1983. MMWR Morb Mortal Wkly Rep 33:365–373, 1984.
420. Bart SW, Stetler HC, Preblud SR, et al. Fetal risk associated with rubella vaccine: An update. Rev Infect Dis 7(suppl):S95–S102, 1985.
421. Enders G. Rubella antibody titers in vaccinated and nonvaccinated women and results of vaccination during pregnancy. Rev Infect Dis 7(suppl):S103–S107, 1985.
422. Centers for Disease Control. Rubella vaccination during pregnancy— United States, 1971–1986. MMWR Morb Mortal Wkly Rep 36:457–461, 1987.
423. Sheppard S, Smithells RW, Dickson A, Holsel H. Rubella vaccination and pregnancy: Preliminary report of a national survey. BMJ 292:727, 1986.
424. Cooper LZ, Florman AL, Ziring PR, Krugman S. Loss of rubella hemagglutination inhibition antibody in congenital rubella. Am J Dis Child 122:397–403, 1971.
425. Ingalls TH, Plotkin SA, Philbrook FR, et al. Immunization of school children with rubella (RA27/3) vaccine. Lancet 1:99–101, 1970.
426. Williams NM, Preblud SR. Rubella and congenital rubella surveillance, 1983. MMWR CDC Surveill Summ 33:1SS–10SS, 1984.
427. Preblud SR, Serdula MK, Frank JA, et al. Rubella vaccination in the United States: A 10 year review. Epidemiol Rev 2:171–194, 1980.
428. Weinstein L, Chang TW. Rubella immunization. N Engl J Med 288:100–101, 1973.
429. Farquhar JD. Experience with rubella and rubella immunization in institutional children. J Pediatr 83:51–56, 1973.
430. Schoenbaum SC, Biano S, Mack T. Epidemiology of congenital rubella syndrome. JAMA 233:151–155, 1975.
431. Cochi S, Edmonds L, Dyer K, et al. Congenital rubella syndrome in the United States, 1970–1985. On the verge of elimination. Am J Epidemiol 129:349–361, 1989.
432. Bart KJ, Orenstein WA, Preblud SR, Hinman AR. Universal immunization to interrupt rubella. Rev Infect Dis 7(suppl):S177–S184, 1985.
433. Centers for Disease Control. Rubella and congenital rubella syndrome—United States, 1984–1985. MMWR 35:129–135, 1986.
434. Increase in rubella and congenital rubella syndrome—United States, 1988–1990. MMWR Morb Mortal Wkly Rep 40:93–99, 1991.
435. Rubella and congenital rubella syndrome—United States, 1994–1997. MMWR Morb Mortal Wkly Rep 46:350–354, 1997.

436. White CC, Koplan JP, Orenstein WA. Benefits, risks and costs of immunization for measles, mumps, and rubella. Am J Public Health 75:739–744, 1985.
437. Berger S, Ginsberg G, Slater P. Cost-benefit analysis of routine mumps and rubella vaccination for Israeli infants. Isr J Med Sci 26:74–80, 1990.
438. Schoenbaum SC, Hyde JN, Bartoshesky L, Crampton K. Benefit-cost analysis of rubella vaccination policy. N Engl J Med 294:306–310, 1976.
439. Centers for Disease Control. Measles prevention. MMWR Morb Mortal Wkly Rep 38:1–18, 1989.
440. Committee on Infectious Diseases, American Academy of Pediatrics. Measles: Reassessment of the current immunization policy. Pediatrics 84:110–112, 1989.
441. Beckler N, Rouderfer V. Simultaneous control of measles and rubella by multidose vaccination schedules. Math Biosci 131:81–102, 1996.
442. Galazka A. Rubella in Europe. Epidemiol Infect 107:43–54, 1991.
443. Dudgeon JA. Selective immunization: Protection of the individual. Rev Infect Dis 7(suppl):S185–S190, 1985.
444. Smithells RW, Sheppard S, Marshall WC, Milton A. National congenital rubella surveillance programme—1971–1981. BMJ 285:13–63, 1982.
445. Peckham CS, Marshall WC, Dudgeon JA. Rubella vaccination of schoolgirls: Factors affecting vaccine uptake. Br Med J 1:760–761, 1977.
446. Noah N, Fowle S. Immunity to rubella in women of childbearing age in the United Kingdom. Br Med J 297:1301–1304, 1988.
447. Goldwater PN, Quiney JR, Banatvala JE. Maternal rubella at St. Thomas' Hospital: Is there need to change British vaccination policy? Lancet 2:1298–1300, 1978.
448. Freestone D. Vaccination against rubella in Britain. Benefits and risks. International symposium on immunization, Brussels, 1978. Dev Biol Stand 43:339–348, 1979.
449. Hambling MH. Changes in the distribution of rubella antibodies in women of childbearing age during the first eight years of rubella vaccination programme. J Infect 2:341–346, 1980.
450. Clarke M, Seagroatt V, Schild GC, et al. Surveys of rubella antibodies in young adults and children. Lancet 1:667–668, 1983.
451. Gilmore D, Robinson ET, Gilmour WH, Urquhart GD. Effect of rubella immunity in a general practice population. Br Med J 284:628–630, 1982.
452. Miller CL, Miller E, Sequeira PJL, et al. Effect of selective vaccination on rubella susceptibility and infection in pregnancy. Br Med J 291:1398–1401, 1985.
453. Anderson RM, Grenfell BT. Control of congenital rubella syndrome by mass vaccination. Lancet 2:827–828, 1985.
454. Anderson RM, Grenfell BT. Quantitative investigations of different vaccination policies for the control of congenital rubella syndrome (CRS) in the United Kingdom. J Hyg (Camb) 96:305–333, 1986.
455. Walker D, Carter H, Jones IG. Measles, mumps and rubella: The need for a change in immunization policy. Br Med J 292:1501–1502, 1986.
456. Hutchinson A. Rubella prevention—a new era. J R Coll Gen Pract 38:193–194, 1988.
457. Miller E. Rubella in the United Kingdom. Epidemiol Infect 107:31–42, 1991.
458. Miller E, Tookey P, Morgan-Capner P, et al. Rubella surveillance to June 1994: Third joint report from the PHLS and the National Congenital Rubella Surveillance Programme. Commun Dis Rep 4:R146–R152, 1994.
459. Miller E, Waight P, Gay N, et al. The epidemiology of rubella in England and Wales before and after the 1994 measles and rubella vaccination campaign: Fourth joint report from the PHLS and the National Congenital Rubella Surveillance Programme. Commun Dis Rep 7:R26–R32, 1997.
460. Christenson B, Böttiger M, Heller L. Mass vaccination programme aimed at eradicating measles, mumps, and rubella in Sweden: First experience. Br Med J 287:389–391, 1983.
461. Rabo E, Taranger J. Scandinavian model for eliminating measles, mumps, and rubella. Br Med J 289:1402–1404, 1984.
462. Böttiger M, Christenson B, Taranger J, Bergman M. Mass vaccination programme aimed at eradicating measles, mumps and rubella in Sweden: Vaccination of schoolchildren. Vaccine 3:113–116, 1985.
463. Christenson B, Böttiger M. Changes of the immunological patterns against measles, mumps and rubella. A vaccination programme studied 3 to 7 years after the introduction of a two-dose schedule. Vaccine 9:326–329, 1991.
463a. Böttiger M, Forsgren M. Twenty years' experience of rubella vaccination in Sweden: 10 years of selective vaccination (of 12-year-old girls and of women postpartum) and 13 years of a general two-dose vaccination. Vaccine 15:1538–1544, 1997.
464. Peltola H, Kurki T, Virtanen M, et al. Rapid effect on endemic measles, mumps, and rubella of nationwide vaccination programme in Finland. Lancet 1:137–139, 1986.
465. Peltola H, Heinonen O, Paunio M, et al. The elimination of indigenous measles, mumps, and rubella from Finland by a 12-year, two-dose vaccination program. N Engl J Med 331:1397–4102, 1994.
466. Ukkonen P. Rubella immunity and morbidity: Impact of different vaccination programs in Finland 1979–1992. Scand J Infect Dis 28:31–35, 1996.
467. Fouquet F, Rebière I. Infectious rubéoleuses confirmées au laboratore chez la femme enceinte et le nouveau-né en France—année 1994. Bull Epidemiol Hebdomadaire 43:187–189, 1996.
468. Matter L, Bally F, Germann D, Schopfer K. The incidence of rubella virus infections in Switzerland after the introduction of the MMR mass vaccination programme. Eur J Epidemiol 11:305–310, 1995.
469. Furesz J, Varughese P, Acres SE, Davies JW. Rubella immunization strategies in Canada. Rev Infect Dis 7(suppl):S191–S197, 1985.
470. Fogel A, Barnea B, Aboudy Y, Mendelson E. Rubella in pregnancy in Israel: 15 years of follow-up and remaining problems. Isr J Med Sci 32:300–305, 1996.
471. Slater P, Roitman M, Leventhal A, Anis E. Control of rubella in Israel: Progress and challenge. Public Health Rev 24:183–192, 1996.
472. Cheah D, Hall R, Mead C, Passaris I. The effectiveness of rubella vaccine. Med J Aust 158:434–435, 1993.
473. Condon RJ, Bower C. Rubella vaccination and congenital rubella syndrome in Western Australia. Med J Aust 158:379–382, 1993.
474. Schoub BD, Johnson S, McAnerney JM, et al. Measles, mumps and rubella immunization at nine months in a developing country. Pediatr Infect Dis J 9:263–267, 1990.
475. Massad E, Nascimento Burattini M, De Azevedo Neto R, et al. A model-based design of a vaccination strategy against rubella in a non-immunized community of S̃ao Paulo State, Brazil. Epidemiol Infect 112:579–594, 1994.
476. Massad E, Azevedo-Neto R, Burattini M, et al. Assessing the efficacy of a mixed vaccination strategy against rubella in S̃ao Paulo, Brazil. Int J Epidemiol 24:842–850, 1995.
477. Robertson S, Cutts F, Samuel R, Diaz-Ortega J. Control of rubella and congenital rubella syndrome (CRS) in developing countries, part 2: Vaccination against rubella. Bull World Health Organ 75:69–80, 1997.
478. Gomwalk NE, Ahmad AA. Prevalence of rubella antibodies on the African continent. Rev Infect Dis 11:116–121, 1989.
479. Park K, Kim H. Seroprevalence of rubella antibodies and effects of vaccination among healthy university women students in Korea. Yonsei Med J 37:420–426, 1996.
480. SVI Technical Advisory Group Meets. EPI Newsletter 19(7):1–4, 1997.
480a. Banatvala JE. Rubella—could do better. Lancet 21:849–850, 1998.
481. Knox EG. Epidemiology of prenatal infections: An extension of the congenital rubella model. Stat Med 2:1–12, 1983.
482. Anderson RM, May R. Vaccination against rubella and measles: Quantitative investigations of different policies. J Hyg (Camb) 90:259–325, 1983.
483. Forster J. Rubella vaccination. Eur J Pediatr 147:570–573, 1988.
484. Public Health Service. Healthy People 2000: National Health Promotion and Disease Prevention Objectives—full Report, with Commentary. PHS Publication 91-50212. Washington, DC, US Department of Health and Human Services, 1991.
485. Plotkin SA. Birth and death of congenital rubella syndrome. JAMA 251:2003–2004, 1984.
486. Orenstein WA, Bart KJ, Hinman AR, et al. The opportunity and obligation to eliminate rubella from the United States. JAMA 251:1988–1994, 1984.

chapter

18 Tetanus Toxoid

Steven G. F. Wassilak
Walter A. Orenstein
Roland W. Sutter

Tetanus is unique among the vaccine-preventable diseases in that it is not communicable. Instead, tetanus is acquired through environmental exposure. Many animals in addition to humans can harbor and excrete the organisms. Spores introduced under the proper (anaerobic) conditions germinate to vegetative bacilli, which elaborate toxin. The clinical presentation results from the actions of this toxin on the central nervous system (CNS). Many animal species besides humans are susceptible to the disease. Prevention of tetanus can be achieved by use of a chemically inactivated toxin ("toxoid") that induces production of neutralizing antibodies (antitoxin). It can also be prevented by the introduction of exogenous antibody. The toxoid is highly immunogenic, safe, and protective after a primary series.

The clinical characteristics of tetanus were probably recognized as distinct early in human history because of the constancy of symptom presentation in animals and humans. The first medical description appears in the writings of Hippocrates, but the etiology of tetanus was unknown until 1884. Carle and Rattone[1] demonstrated that the contents of a pustule from a fatal human case led to typical symptoms in rabbits on injection into the sciatic nerve; the disease could subsequently be passed to other rabbits from infected nervous tissue. Inoculation of soil samples into animals also resulted in tetanus. Gram-positive bacilli were often noted in the exudate at the inoculation site but generally not in nervous tissue, leading Nicolaier[2] to hypothesize that a poison produced at the site of inoculation led to the nervous system symptoms. In 1886, spore-forming bacilli were observed in the exudate obtained from a human case.[3] In 1889, the spores of the causative organism, *Clostridium tetani*, in contrast to the vegetative organisms, were shown to survive heating and to germinate under anaerobic conditions; injection of pure cultures caused reproducible disease in animals.[4] After identification and purification of the toxin in 1890, it was shown that repeated inoculation of animals with minute quantities of toxin led to the production of antibodies in survivors that neutralized the effects of the toxin.[5] Preparations of these antibodies derived from animal sera, particularly horses, became the first means of preventing and treating the cause of tetanus. Further research culminated in the preparation of "anatoxin"—chemically inactivated toxin, now termed toxoid—in 1924.[6] These preparations induced active immunity against the disease before exposure.

BACKGROUND

Clinical Description

Although the incubation period has been reported to vary from 1 day to several months, the majority of cases occur within 3 days to 3 weeks after inoculation of spores. In the United States during 1991 to 1994, the median incubation period between identified acute injury and reported onset was 7 days (range of 0 to more than 60 days). For 15% of injury-associated wounds, the interval between wound and onset was reported to be 3 days or less. There appears to be a direct relationship between site of inoculation and incubation period, the longest intervals occurring after injuries farthest away from the CNS; injuries of the head and trunk are likely to be associated with the shortest incubation periods.[7, 8] Historically, the incubation period has been inversely related to severity of illness.[9–14] Incubation periods of 10 days or more tend to result in mild cases, whereas people developing illness within 7 days of injury tend to have more severe disease.

Three clinical syndromes are associated with tetanus: (1) localized, (2) generalized, and (3) cephalic.[7] Local tetanus consists of spasm of muscles in a confined area close to the site of the original injury.[15, 16] These painful contractions may persist for several weeks to months before gradually subsiding. It is thought to occur when toxin produced at the site of the injury is transported solely through the local nerves.[8] In general, localized tetanus is unusual in humans, probably because toxin rapidly disseminates in the blood stream and is taken up by nerve endings closer to the CNS than those at the site of the original injury. Localized tetanus can be produced experimentally by simultaneously injecting toxin into a muscle and antitoxin in blood to prevent hematogenous dissemination.[8] Localized tetanus per se is generally mild with death-to-case ratios of less than 1%.[15] However, it may presage the development of generalized tetanus with more serious outcomes.

More than 80% of cases of tetanus are of the generalized variety; this proportion may be influenced by vaccine status of the population. The most common initial sign is spasm of the muscles of mastication—trismus or lockjaw—occurring in more than 50% of the cases.[7, 17] Trismus associated with spasm of the facial muscles results in a characteristic facial expression—risus sardonicus—consisting of raised eyebrows, tight closure of the eyelids, wrinkling of the forehead, and extension of the corners of the mouth laterally. Trismus may be followed by involvement of other muscles in the neck, thorax and back, abdomen, and extremities. Generalized hyperreflexia is elicited. Persistent and sustained spasm of back muscles can give rise to opisthotonos. Generalized tonic tetanic seizure–like activity (tetanospasms), often triggered by mild external stimuli such as sudden noises, consists of sudden painful contraction of all muscle groups resulting in opisthotonos, abduction at the shoulders, flexion of the elbows and wrists, and extension of the legs. Spasm of the glottis can result in immediate death. Temperature elevations of 2 to 4°C are often associated with severe spasms. Cognitive functions are not overtly affected.

Tetanus may be accompanied by severe autonomic nervous system abnormalities, particularly among the elderly and narcotic addicts, consisting of systemic arterial hypertension or hypotension, flushing, diaphoresis, tachycardia, and arrhythmias.[18–22] Tetanus is also associated with a variety of spasm-related complications including fractures of the long bones and vertebrae, asphyxia from glottic obstruction, and traumatic glossitis. Toxin can also induce urinary retention and dysphagia. In addition, complications can be due to chronic debility: pulmonary embolism, decubitus ulcers, pneumonia, catheter-associated infections, and contractures. Long-term consequences—including prolonged muscle fatigue, hyperostoses and osteoarthritis, and difficulties with speech, memory, and mental capacity—have been documented.[23–25]

Tetanus neonatorum, the most common form of the disease in developing countries, is a form of generalized tetanus occurring in newborn infants often as a result of an infected umbilical cord stump.[7] It usually begins 3 to 14 days after birth in an infant with normal ability to suck in the first 2 days of life. The illness begins with poor sucking and excessive crying.[7, 26] This is followed by variable degrees of trismus, difficulty swallowing, opisthotonos, and other tetanic spasms.

The clinical course of generalized tetanus is highly variable. The disease frequently remains intense for 1 to 4 weeks and then gradually subsides. Death-to-case ratios for reported cases of generalized tetanus vary from about 25 to 70% overall, with the risk of fatality in the past approaching 100% at the extremes of age.[13, 14] With good intensive care, mortality can be reduced to 10 to 20%.[27–32] In the United States during 1972 to 1994, overall reported death-to-case ratios have declined from approximately 50 to 11% overall but nonetheless are influenced by age[33, 33a] (Fig. 18–1) and immunization status.[34] A higher death-to-case ratio has been reported with tetanus after intramuscular injections and particularly with intramuscular injection of quinine.[35]

Cephalic tetanus is a rare manifestation of the disease generally associated with lesions of the head or face, especially in the distribution of the facial nerve and the orbits.[7, 26] The incubation period is usually on the order of 1 to 2 days. It has also been associated with chronic otitis media.[36] On occasion, a portal of injury cannot be identified. In contrast to generalized tetanus, which is associated with generalized spasms, cephalic tetanus is associated with atonic cranial nerve palsies involving nerves III, IV, VII, IX, X, and XII, singly or in combination. Nonetheless, trismus can be present. The disease may progress to generalized tetanus and has a similar prognosis.[7, 37]

Bacteriology

Clostridium tetani is a gram-positive, spore-forming, motile, anaerobic bacillus.[38–40] Typically measuring 0.3 to 0.5 μm in width and 2 to 2.5 μm in length, the vegetative form often develops long filament-like cells in culture. Flagella are attached bilaterally on non–spore-forming bacteria. With sporulation, *C. tetani* takes on the more characteristic drumstick-like appearance. Spores usually form in the terminal position. *Clostridium tetani* is considered a strict anaerobe that grows optimally at 33 to 37°C; however, depending on the strain, growth can occur at 14 to 43°C. *Clostridium tetani* can be cultured in a variety of media used in growing anaerobes such as thioglycolate, casein hydrolysate, and cooked meat. Growth is enhanced in media supplemented with reducing substances at a neutral to alkaline pH. On blood agar, the organism produces characteristic compact colonies extending in a meshwork of fine filaments. Growth is usually accompanied by the production of gas and is associated with a fetid odor.

Sporulation is dependent on a variety of factors including pH, temperature, and media composition. Sporulation can be promoted at 37°C and in the presence of oleic acid, phosphates, 1 to 2% sodium chloride or protein, and magnesium.[38, 39] Aging also promotes sporulation. In contrast, acidification, high (>41°C) or low (<25°C) temperatures, glucose, assorted saturated fatty acids, antibiotics, and potassium can inhibit spore formation. The germination of spores requires anaerobic conditions and is enhanced by the presence of lactic acid and chemicals toxic to cells.[41]

If not exposed to sunlight, the spores may persist in soil for months to years.[7, 38, 39] The spores are resistant to boiling and a variety of disinfectants. Solutions of phenol (5%), formalin (3%), chloramine (1%), and hydrogen hyperoxidates (6%) require 15 to 24 hours to inactivate spores. The spores are more easily destroyed by heating to 120°C for 15 to 20 minutes. Use of aqueous iodine or 2% glutaraldehyde at pH 7.5 to 8.5 kills spores within 3 hours.

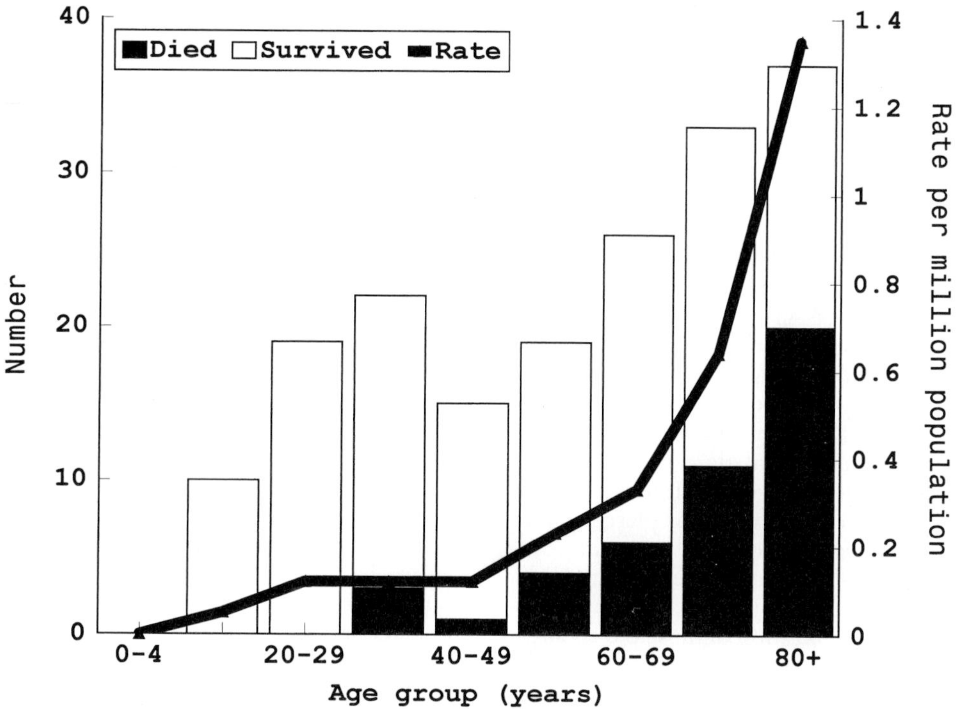

Figure 18–1. Reported number of tetanus cases, average annual incidence rates, and survival status of patients, by age group, United States, 1991 to 1994.

The most common source of environmental exposure to *C. tetani* bacilli and spores is the soil, where the organism is widely but variably distributed. It is difficult to compare different studies of how widespread the organism is in nature, in part because of differences in methodology. For example, the higher the temperatures applied in processing the specimens before culture, the lower the frequency of *C. tetani* isolation and the more likely it is that nontoxigenic strains are isolated.[42] A method of quantifying spores described in 1984 may provide a standard method for future studies.[43] Most studies suggest that viable spores are more commonly present in soils with an alkaline pH and in nutrient-rich soils in warm, moist climates that support multiplication of the bacillus.[44, 45] Within the contiguous United States, however, a limited study in 1975 found spores in 30% of the samples without any apparent geographical or chemical influence on the distribution.[46]

Soil is not the only reservoir of the organism. Animals, both herbivores and omnivores, can carry *C. tetani* bacilli and spores in their intestines and readily disseminate the organism in their feces. In the literature, fecal carriage has been reported in 10 to 20% of horses and 25 to 30% of dogs and guinea pigs; fecal specimens from several other animals, including sheep, cattle, and small animals, may also contain *C. tetani*.[47, 48] Attempts to quantify the frequency of human intestinal colonization have produced varied results from 0 to 40%.[41, 49–55] Rural residents tend to have higher rates of intestinal carriage than city dwellers. *Clostridium tetani* spores have also been detected in street dust[55, 56] and the dust and air of surgical operating theaters.[55]

Pathogenesis

Clostridium tetani produces two exotoxins, tetanolysin and tetanospasmin.[7] Tetanolysin is an oxygen-sensitive hemolysin related to streptolysin and the θ-toxin of *Clostridium perfringens*, and it may play a role in establishing infection at the site of inoculation but is not otherwise involved in pathogenesis of the disease.[57] Tetanospasmin, a neurotoxin and the cause of the manifestations of tetanus, is a highly toxic protein that accumulates intracellularly during the logarithmic phase of growth and is released into the medium on autolysis. The toxin has an approximate molecular weight of 150,000 and is synthesized as a single polypeptide chain. When released in culture medium, the toxin is cleaved by proteases into light (toxic moiety) and heavy (binding) chains with molecular weights of 50,000 and 100,000, respectively, containing two disulfide bonds—one between chains and one internal to the heavy chain.[58–61] Whereas the heavy chain may mediate pore formation after binding, the C-terminal end of the heavy chain (fragment C) is the moiety that binds to gangliosides and is otherwise totally inactive.[62, 63] The light chain is an endopeptidase that cleaves a membrane protein of synaptic vesicles. Toxin production appears to be under the control of a plasmid.[64, 65]

The toxin is one of the most potent known poisons on a weight basis. As little as 1 ng/kg may kill a mouse, and 0.3 ng/kg will kill a guinea pig.[66] The estimated minimum human lethal dose is less than 2.5 ng/kg. Various species have different levels of responsiveness to the toxin. For example, cats, dogs, and particularly birds and poikilotherms appear to be relatively resistant to its effects; guinea pigs, monkeys, sheep, goats, and particularly horses are sensitive to the toxin.[67] As reviewed by Smith,[47] the existence of preexisting antitoxin does not generally account for the differences in animal susceptibility to tetanus toxin.

Infection usually begins with the inoculation of spores through the epithelium. Wounds accompanied by tissue injury and necrosis (with or without the presence of aerobic organisms) leading to anaerobic or hypoaerobic conditions are generally necessary for the spores to germinate and bacilli to replicate. Ionic calcium appears to increase local necrosis and increase the likelihood of *C. tetani* infection, and it may be a factor in soil contamination that particularly enhances germination.[68] The umbilical stump serves as a nontraumatic site where spore contamination can easily lead to germination and bacterial replication, but traditional surgeries or piercings can also be associated with neonatal tetanus.[32, 69]

Transport of toxin from the injured site into the CNS is complex. Toxin injected under the skin appears to enter underlying muscle; infiltration of muscle with antitoxin before subcutaneous toxin injection can block the development of tetanus.[8] Once in the muscle, some toxin makes its way to the CNS directly by intra-axonal transport; other toxin is transported by the lymphatics and then disseminated hematogenously.

Evidence for hematogenous transport came from a variety of studies that showed rapid absorption of toxin into the lymphatics and from there into the blood stream to a variety of tissues.[8, 70] Although most of the toxin is disseminated through the blood stream, toxin does not cross the blood-brain barrier.[70] Neuronal transport is the means by which the toxin enters the CNS with or without hematogenous dissemination.[8, 71–74] The toxin can be demonstrated in motor end plates of muscle nerves. After toxin gains entry at neuromuscular junctions by binding to gangliosides,[63, 75] it proceeds up the nerve to the ventral horns of the spinal cord or motor nuclei of the cranial nerves by intra-axonal transport; this is supported by radiolabeled toxin studies and histological studies of binding to fragment C.[76–78] The disease can progress clinically despite use of parenteral antitoxin. The neuronal binding is not evidently reversible[79]; intracranial injection studies in animals suggest that recovery may depend on new functional connections, whereas spinal cord culture studies suggest that recovery depends on toxin degradation.[80, 81]

Tetanospasmin can act at the peripheral motor end plates, the spinal cord, the brain, and the sympathetic nervous system.[8, 18–22, 82, 83] The toxic moiety cleaves the synaptic vesicle membrane protein synaptobrevin and causes disinhibition of spinal cord reflex arcs by interfering with release of the neurotransmitters glycine and γ-aminobutyric acid (GABA) from presynaptic inhibitory fibers.[8, 82–88] Once inhibition is blocked, excitatory reflexes multiply unchecked, causing the tetanic spasms. The clinical syndrome appears almost identical to strychnine poisoning, which acts by competitively binding to postsynaptic glycine receptors at the motor neurons.[89] Tetanospasmin has also been shown to interfere with release of a variety of other neurotransmitters including acetylcholine in peripheral somatic and autonomic nerves.[90] More detailed information on the nature of the toxin and its effects can be found in reviews by van Heyningen[91] and Bizzini.[59]

Diagnosis

The diagnosis of tetanus is established primarily on clinical and secondarily on epidemiological grounds. A history of a wound contaminated by soil or other material and the presence of a local skin infection are helpful in the diagnosis, although these criteria are not always present. Laboratory investigations are frequently negative. Characteristic-appearing gram-positive bacilli, some with terminal or subterminal spores, may occasionally be seen in aspirates from the affected area. Anaerobic cultures of tissues or aspirates are usually not positive.[29, 92] Low or undetectable levels of circulating antitoxin at the time of onset of symptoms are compatible with the diagnosis; however, there are a number of case reports in which moderately high levels of antitoxin were noted at the time of presentation.[93–99] Changes in antitoxin levels in convalescence are not reliably seen.[100] Given the mild nature of some presentations, electromyography has been suggested to aid in the diagnosis,[101] and elicitation of trismus by posterior pharynx stimulation has been reported to help in differentiation.[102]

The differential diagnosis depends on the clinical form of tetanus and the presenting symptoms. Cephalic tetanus may be confused with Bell palsy and trigeminal neuritis. However, cephalic tetanus is often accompanied by other cranial nerve symptoms, including dysphagia, and signs of trismus and nuchal rigidity.[7, 26] Trismus has a variety of causes including caries, tonsillitis, peritonsillar abscess, temporomandibular joint dysfunction, parotitis, and CNS disturbances other than tetanus. Rabies patients can also present with hyperreflexia; however, rabies is more likely to be associated with hallucinations, hydrophobia, mania, stupor, and a history of animal bites and is unlikely to be accompanied by trismus. In addition, seizures with rabies are usually clonic, whereas tetanospasms are prolonged and tonic. Encephalitis is rarely associated with trismus and is much more likely to be accompanied by disturbances of consciousness than is tetanus. Because of nuchal rigidity, bacterial meningitis could be confused with tetanus.

A variety of metabolic conditions and poisonings can resemble tetanus. Although muscle spasm may be seen with hypocalcemic tetany, it is not generally associated with trismus.[103] A determination of low serum calcium can confirm tetany. Strychnine poisoning can mimic generalized tetanus.[89] However, such poisoning is characterized by (1) rare association with persistent trismus, (2) greater muscle relaxation between spasms, (3) normal body temperature, and (4) presence of detectable strychnine in gastric contents or in urine. Phenothiazine toxicity may be associated with a variety of dystonias including trismus. Detection of phenothiazines in the blood or amelioration by treatment with diphenhydramine confirms the diagnosis. Hysteria can mimic tetanus.[104] However, hysterical patients usually relax during prolonged observation or when they are distracted and are more likely to display clonic rather than tonic spasms.

Because of the unique presentation of neonatal tetanus, postmortem history (even taken by nonclinical personnel) can permit accurate classification of the illness as the cause of death with a high degree of probability, simply by determining the timing of symptoms and verifying that the child was normal after birth. The World Health Organization (WHO) defines neonatal tetanus as an illness occurring in a child who has the normal ability to suck and cry in the first 2 days of life, loses this ability between 3 and 28 days of life, and becomes rigid or has convulsions (see Table 44–6).

Treatment

At the time a patient presents with manifestations of tetanus, some toxin has entered the nervous system (some of it bound to its target site and some in transit), some toxin is circulating in the lymphatics and the blood stream, and some toxin is present within the organisms at the site of infection. Therefore, the purpose of therapy is to (1) give supportive care for the illness caused by toxin that has already reached the CNS (including nutritional support and prevention of thromboemboli),[87, 105] (2) prevent any additional circulating toxin from reaching the CNS, and (3) prevent further toxin production by eliminating the organism. General principles of pharmacotherapy are indicated here; more detailed information and a protocol on treatment can be obtained from review articles or chapters by Bleck.[87, 88, 106]

Good nursing care is critical in the management of patients with tetanus.[29, 30, 107] The patient should be kept in a quiet, dimly lit room, and sudden environmental stimuli such as loud noises should be avoided. Pharmacological treatment of hypertonicity and spasms depends on the severity and frequency of the conditions. The major purpose is to control spasms and tone without impairing, if possible, voluntary movement, consciousness, and most importantly respiration. Because tetanospasmin blocks inhibitory neurons in the CNS, the ideal therapeutic agent would reverse this inhibition.[87, 88, 106] Experimental work with benzodiazepines such as diazepam has demonstrated that these agents enhance inhibition induced by GABA at presynaptic reflexes.[88, 108–110] Intravenous diazepam has proved useful generally in doses of 0.5 to 15 mg/kg/day.[92, 111–114] Some clinicians use standard doses administered every 2 to 8 hours; others give doses at the time of spasms, generally of 5 to 10 mg, as often as three times per hour or more.[7, 30] Higher doses may be used if the lower doses fail. Some adults will tolerate doses of more than 600 mg in 24 hours. Other muscle relaxants that have been used include lorazepam, dantrolene, and intrathecal baclofen.[41, 106, 115] Midazolam by continuous infusion has also been effective and does not contain propylene glycol, a preservative included in diazepam and lorazepam that may produce lactic acidosis.[106] Propofol by continuous infusion has been used as an adjunct sedative with benzodiazepine therapy.[116]

Other drugs used to treat tetanus in the past include the short-acting barbiturates, particularly secobarbital sodium and pentobarbital.[7, 92] However, in contrast to diazepam, barbiturates are more likely to result in respiratory depression and coma. Chlorpromazine intramuscularly in doses of 50 to 150 mg in adults and 4 to 12 mg in infants every 4 to 8 hours has been used with barbiturate therapy.[7] Other sedative drugs used in the past include paraldehyde and meprobamate.[7]

Some studies suggest that pyridoxine may be a useful adjunct to the treatment of neonatal tetanus.[117, 118] Likewise, a study suggesting improvement of the outcome of tetanus in adults with corticosteroid therapy implies that further improvements in therapy may be possible.[119]

Although effective in controlling spasms, these drugs may not decrease sympathetic overactivity. These complications are now the most frequently associated complications in people who go on to die from tetanus. Autonomic dysfunction has been successfully treated with labetalol or morphine.[22, 87, 88, 106, 120–122] Isolated treatment with β-blockers should not be undertaken to avoid potentiation of increased α activity, which could result in severe hypertension. Other agents that have been used include continuous intravenous magnesium sulfate, clonidine, and fentanyl.[123, 124] Spinal anesthesia, given with catecholamine infusion, has been reported to be useful in extreme instances of hemodynamic instability.[125, 126]

If conservative therapy fails or if the patient presents in extreme spasm, neuromuscular block must be considered. Vecuronium is now the agent of choice for this because its use results in minimal autonomic instability; an alternative is atracurium.[87, 106] Older agents can be used in their absence.[7, 88, 92] Of course, whenever neuromuscular blocking agents are used, assisted ventilation is necessary.

Even with neuromuscular blockade, short-term assisted ventilation may be possible and endotracheal intubation may be adequate. However, the severity of tetanospasms before neuromuscular blockade may suggest a prolonged need for mechanical ventilation and the possible need for tracheotomy. Tracheotomy should also be considered in cases in which generalized spasms occur despite pharmacotherapy and when there is respiratory muscle or laryngeal spasm that could potentially compromise ventilation or oxygenation. Inability to cough, difficulty in swallowing, and coma are also indications because of the risk of aspiration.[7, 29, 127] Patients with mild illness such as localized tetanus generally do not require tracheotomy.

Some researchers have suggested that certain biochemical alterations (e.g., elevations in blood urea nitrogen, serum aspartate transaminases, or cerebrospinal fluid protein) may herald more severe disease and, therefore, such alterations indicate early intensive intervention.[128, 129] A protein-catabolic state occurs in severely affected patients, requiring therapy with intravenous alimentation.[126]

Human tetanus immune globulin (TIG) should be given at the time of diagnosis to prevent further intoxication.[7, 106] The dose is generally 3000 to 6000 units given intramuscularly in a single dose.[7] Analyses of tetanus cases reported in the United States from 1965 to

1971 suggested that doses of 500 units were as effective as higher doses in reducing mortality.[130] However, a more recent analysis of data for reported cases from 1972 to 1986 suggested that doses of 3000 to 6000 units resulted in significantly higher benefit than lower doses.[34] No additional benefit was seen with doses higher than 6000 units; no significant benefit was seen for doses of 1000 units or less compared with no TIG treatment. Peak serum levels are achieved 48 to 72 hours after intramuscular TIG administration (a theoretical disadvantage of TIG, which cannot be given intravenously).[131] Equine antitoxin can be given intravenously but is associated with serious allergic side effects such as anaphylaxis and serum sickness.[132, 133] There is no evidence that outcome is less satisfactory after intramuscular administration of the human TIG.[134] Although equine antitoxin remains available outside the United States, its use is not recommended. Intravenous immune globulin has been proposed as an alternative to TIG when TIG is not available.[135] However, there is wide variation in the content of antitoxin by manufacturer, and the tetanus antitoxin content is not controlled. This product is not licensed for this indication in the United States; if used, doses of 200 to 400 mg/kg have been recommended.[131]

There has been considerable controversy in the medical literature over the use of intrathecal therapy with TIG or equine antitoxin.[107, 136] Because systemically administered antibody does not appreciably cross the blood-brain barrier, intrathecal administration theoretically offers the possibility of neutralizing unbound toxin in the CNS. One controlled trial and several noncontrolled studies have reported decreased mortality with intrathecal administration of equine antitoxin or TIG.[107, 137, 138] However, a variety of other studies, including randomized controlled trials, have failed to show benefits of the intrathecal route of equine antitoxin or TIG, particularly in neonatal tetanus.[139–142] Aburtyn and Berlin[136] concluded, after meta-analysis of English-language reports of trials, that methodological difficulties preclude a convincing argument for intrathecal therapy; they recommend a solid, randomized study with clinical blinding and stratification by severity. Given this information and that TIG available in the United States (which contains thimerosal) is not licensed for intrathecal use, this route of administration cannot currently be recommended.

Further production of toxin should be prevented by appropriate antimicrobial therapy and surgical drainage or débridement when necessary. In the past, penicillin has been the drug of choice. Procaine penicillin, 1.2 million units daily, or aqueous crystalline penicillin G, 4 million units daily divided every 6 hours, is administered for 5 to 10 days to kill the vegetative form of the organism.[7] A controlled study from Indonesia suggests that metronidazole significantly improves prognosis compared with penicillin.[143] Theoretically, penicillin may act as an agonist to tetanospasmin by inhibiting release of GABA. Therefore, at a number of centers, metronidazole has become the first choice for antimicrobial therapy.[106] The dosage used for sepsis is given during 1 hour: 15 mg/kg loading dose, followed by 7.5 mg/kg every 6 to 8 hours (maximum, 2–4 g/day).

Tetanus itself may not induce future immunity to tetanospasmin.[100] Recurrent or relapsing cases have been reported.[36, 144–146] Therefore, all suspected tetanus patients should start or complete a primary series of a toxoid-containing preparation at the time of diagnosis or during convalescence. Patients with tetanus appear to respond to tetanus toxoid less vigorously than other individuals do but nevertheless achieve protective levels of antitoxin.[147, 148]

EPIDEMIOLOGY

Incidence and Descriptive Epidemiology of Nonneonatal Tetanus

In spite of the availability of a highly effective immunizing agent, tetanus exerts a substantial health impact in the world.[149] In 1984, estimates based on mortality surveys suggested that there were approximately 1 million deaths due to neonatal tetanus alone.[150] Nonneonatal tetanus also has a substantial health impact. Estimates from reported data suggested that in the early 1980s, 310,000 to 700,000 nonneonatal cases, resulting in 122,000 to 300,000 deaths, occurred annually in the developing world (excluding China).[151] In contrast, approximately 2000 cases and 1000 deaths were estimated to occur annually in the developed world during that period.

Improved hygiene and childbirth practices, improvements in wound care, reduction in exposure to tetanus spores, and active immunization have led to major declines in reported tetanus incidence since the 1950s in Australia, Cuba, Europe, Japan, New Zealand, North America, and the former USSR.[45, 149, 152, 153] In the United States, death certificate data from 1920 onward indicate a relatively constant decline in annual tetanus death rates, which may have accelerated with the use of equine antitoxin in prophylaxis and treatment in the mid-1920s (Fig. 18–2). Cases of tetanus have been monitored nationally since 1947 when incidence was 0.39 per 100,000 total population. The decrease in tetanus occurrence since that time is a historical tribute to wound management and the use of toxoid in the general population. A continual decline in reported cases occurred until 1976; since then, overall incidence rates have declined more gradually from 0.04 to below 0.02 per 100,000 (see Fig. 18–2).

Tetanus generally follows a distinct seasonal trend with a midsummer or "wet" season peak, which may reflect soil and spore conditions but may also reflect more frequent injury-incurring behavior during the warmer months.[45, 154–156] Geographical distribution across the globe is generally on the basis of moist, warm climate and fertile soil; with incomplete public health programs, those areas that have exhibited high incidence of tetanus in the past consistently continue to do so. The highest rates of tetanus occur in the developing world, particularly in countries near the equator.[149] In the United States, although all states have reported cases, tetanus has been predominantly a disease of the South-

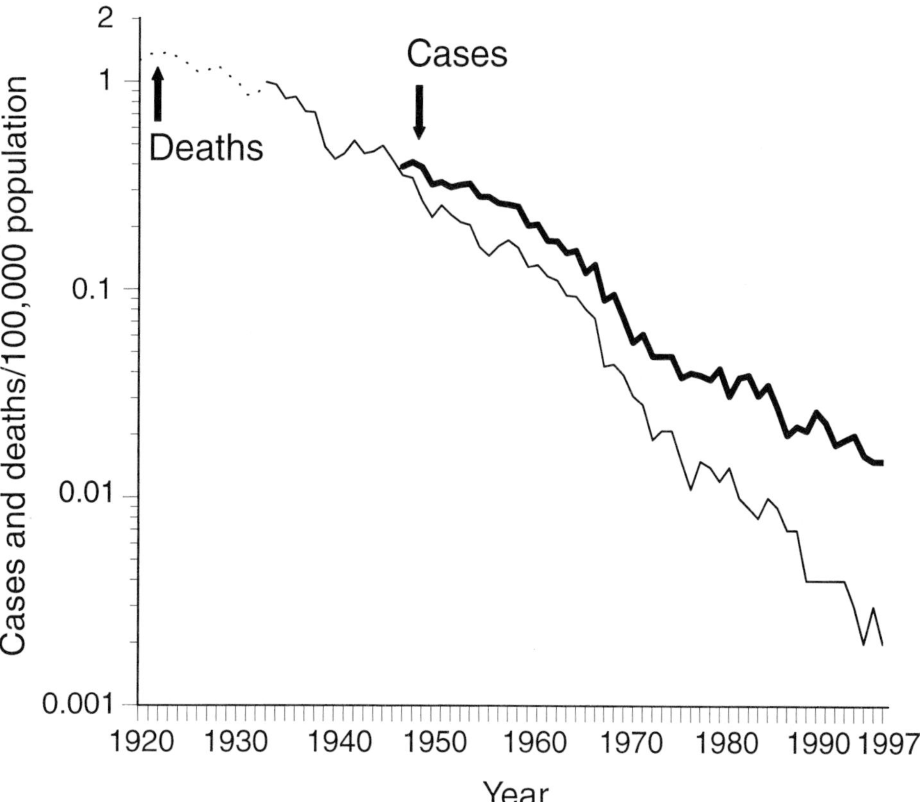

Figure 18–2. Reported tetanus mortality and incidence rates, United States, 1920 to 1997. Reporting of deaths was incomplete from 1920 to 1932; estimates shown are based on the population of reporting areas. National reporting began in 1947, as shown.

east[13, 14, 154–157]; the geographical distribution is currently less distinct with a lower reported incidence.[33a, 158–161]

Aside from neonatal tetanus, the major proportion of victims in underdeveloped nations are male older children and young adults. Wherever immunization programs are in place, tetanus occurrence declines.[45] In the face of immunization programs, sex and age distributions shift to mirror the underimmunized population. The leveling in tetanus incidence in the United States since 1976, in part, reflects this in the shifting age distribution of tetanus cases; even in the years since 1965, average annual age-specific tetanus incidence rates indicate a slightly declining rate in the elderly but drastic declines in the rates for younger age groups[162] (Fig. 18–3). More than one third of tetanus deaths in the 1950s were in children younger than 1 year. In contrast, the elderly during the early to mid-1990s accounted for the majority of cases and virtually all deaths. Also in the 1950s, nonwhite individuals had an incidence more than five times that of whites, and rates of neonatal tetanus were 10-fold higher.[154, 155]

In various case series, even in the early toxoid era, acute wounds were the predominant associated site of infection, including relatively minor wounds; in a small proportion of cases, no history of injury could be elicited.[139, 156, 157, 163–165] Injection drug use is known to place individuals at particular risk.[166–169] Operative procedures, particularly bowel surgery, can infrequently put some individuals at risk.[170, 171]

There has been some debate over whether humans can develop circulating antitoxin against tetanus in the absence of vaccination or disease. Before artificial immunization was possible and the neutralization test was standardized, conflicting results were found on whether the host had detectable antitoxin titer when *C. tetani* was isolated from a human.[50, 51] The majority of studies that purport to show natural immunity did not use toxin neutralization assays in mice, the accepted definitive method of testing that correlates with clinical protection (see *Immune Responses*). Studies in the developing world and some developed nations using other generally acceptable assays (e.g., enzyme-linked immunosorbent assay [ELISA] and passive hemagglutination) have shown substantial proportions of some reportedly unimmunized populations in Brazil, China, Ethiopia, India, Italy, Israel, Spain, and the former USSR with detectable levels of antitoxin.[172–177] Specifically, up to 80% of people in India and up to 95% of people in a group of Ethiopian refugees had levels of antitoxin by these methods exceeding 0.01 IU/mL.[172, 173, 175] This information has led some to suggest that at least in some areas of the developing world, asymptomatic colonization/infection with *C. tetani* occurs—presumably leading to production of antitoxin. Such studies have been criticized because the absence of vaccination cannot be completely ensured and because of the assays used.[47, 178] As discussed later, at low levels of detection, there may be substantial nonspecificity of these testing methods. If seroprevalence were indicative of natural immunity from natural exposure, the rate of seroprevalence should increase with increasing age as a result of increasing cumulative opportunity for exposure; instead, seroprevalence does not appear to appreciably differ throughout multiple age groups, arguing against these levels being indicative of

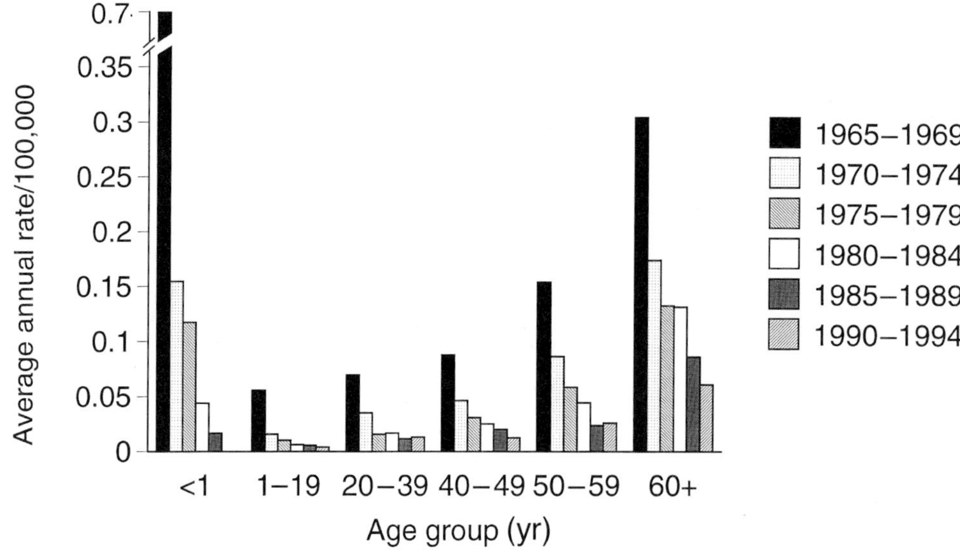

Figure 18–3. Reported age group–specific tetanus incidence rates, by 5-year intervals, United States, 1965 to 1994.

natural immunity.[172, 175] Serosurveys in the United States have found 25% or more of reportedly unimmunized individuals to have circulating antitoxin, although negative immunization histories are perhaps more likely to be unreliable than in undeveloped countries.[179–183] Overall, even if natural immunity occurs in some unimmunized populations, it has no substantial importance in the control of tetanus.

The current epidemiology of tetanus outside of the neonatal period in the United States is here derived from detailed information on 96% (192) of the 201 cases reported from 1991 to 1994.[33] The information is similar to other data collected since 1982.[33a, 158–161] The efficiency of the reporting of tetanus deaths in the United States in the 1979 to 1984 period has been estimated at 40%[184]; continual underreporting of cases overall is therefore also likely. Of the 150 cases with reported clinical presentation, 81% were generalized, 13% were localized, and 6% were cephalic. Of these cases, 121 (64%) were in people 50 years of age or older, including 74 (34%) in people 70 years of age or older. The gender distribution of recent cases is age dependent: below 50 years of age, 67% of the case patients were male; for people 50 years of age and older, 37% of the cases were in men. The decrease in the proportion of men with cases in the elderly probably reflects the systematic immunization of men in military service during World War II and the Korean conflict.

In the United States, past serosurveys using various in vitro antibody assays have indicated that levels of antibody below those considered protective are found in 38 to 59% of men and 53 to 71% of women 60 years of age or older.[179–183] Seroprevalence in younger individuals is substantially higher.[185] A population-based serosurvey of people older than 5 years in the United States during 1988 to 1991 reaffirmed the heightened susceptibility in older age groups; by use of an ELISA with a protective level defined as greater than 0.15 IU/mL (see *Immune Responses*), 70% of the population was protected, falling from 88% in children 6 to 11 years of age to 29% in people 70 years of age or older.[183]

Current tetanus cases continue, for the most part, to be associated with acute trauma of diverse severity in underimmunized individuals. Tetanus occurred after an identified acute injury in 77% (148) of the 192 cases. The most frequently reported injuries were puncture wounds (49%), lacerations (20%), and abrasions (12%). Injuries incurred in outdoor settings accounted for 51% of wound-associated cases. Animal-related wounds (bites and scratches) accounted for 3% (5) of wound-associated tetanus; surgical wounds, some of which were known to have been contaminated (e.g., bowel procedures), were associated with 4% (7). Twelve percent of the 192 cases (23) were associated with chronic wounds (e.g., skin ulcers, gangrene, abscesses) or diabetes. A history of illegal injection drug use was the only associated medical condition for 4% of cases (7), consistent with reports in prior years.[158–161] For 7% of patients (14), no known acute injury, chronic wound, or medical condition was reported. Cases associated with minor or chronic wounds as well as the substantial proportion without a recent history of a wound have been described during many decades, as pointed out in the review article by Bytchenko.[45]

Twenty-three (12%) of the 192 patients, or 26% of the patients with known immunization status, were reported to have received at least a primary series (i.e., three or more doses) of tetanus toxoid before onset of illness (Table 18–1). Of these patients, 13 were reported to have received the last booster 10 years or more before onset of illness; for two patients, this information was verified by healthcare provider records. These and prior cases in immunized individuals supported the observations that cases occurring in previously immunized individuals may exhibit a milder clinical course.[34, 186–188] No deaths were observed among the 23 patients with three or more prior doses of toxoid, as opposed to a case-fatality of 25% in those with zero or one dose and 31%

Table 18–1. **IMMUNIZATION STATUS OF INDIVIDUALS WITH REPORTED TETANUS CASES* FOR WHOM SUPPLEMENTARY INFORMATION IS AVAILABLE, UNITED STATES, 1991–1994**

IMMUNIZATION STATUS	NUMBER (%)	% OF THOSE WITH KNOWN STATUS
No dose	49 (25.5)	55.1
1 dose	17 (8.9)	19.1
2 doses	0 (0.0)	0.0
3 doses	5 (2.6)	5.6
≥4 doses	18 (9.4)	20.2
Unknown	103 (53.6)	
Total	192 (100)	100

*Nonneonatal tetanus only.

in those with unknown immunization status. Multiple regression analysis of cases reported from 1972 to 1986 has shown that people who had received three or more doses previously were 5.2 times more likely to survive compared with people who had no prior doses (95% confidence interval, 1.2 to 22.3).[34]

Of the 148 patients with acute wounds, tetanus toxoid was given as prophylaxis in wound management to 15% (22 cases, 43% of the 51 who had sought medical care); of these, 77% had received toxoid within 3 days of injury. Most of these individuals were also potential candidates for, but did not receive, TIG. Nine percent (13) of the 148 patients with acute wounds underwent prophylactic débridement after injury. Of these 13 patients, 10 did not receive the recommended tetanus and diphtheria toxoids (Td) with or without TIG on the basis of their individual immunization histories.

Incidence of Neonatal Tetanus and Its Public Health Significance

Tetanus occurring within the first month of life results from *C. tetani* infection (most commonly at the umbilical cord stump) of a child born to a mother who did not possess sufficient circulating antitoxin to passively protect the infant by transplacental transfer. The epidemiology of neonatal tetanus is distinct from that of tetanus outside the neonatal period. Neonatal tetanus symptoms occur 3 to 14 days after birth in approximately 90% of cases but can occur from 1 up to 28 days of age.[155, 189–192] This predictable incubation period has led several cultures to apply time-related names to the condition, for example, "three-six disease" in China and "eight day disease" in the Pacific Islands and other locations.[192, 193] Cases are often associated with unsterile conditions of childbirth, with delivery personnel untrained in sterile care of the umbilical cord and stump or not adequately washing their hands,[194–196] and particularly with births followed by unhygienic cultural rituals involving the umbilical stump—such as application of herbs, clarified butter, or animal dung.[190, 194–202] Unless their mothers have received two or more doses of tetanus toxoid, newborns are susceptible.[203] The magnitude of the occurrence of neonatal tetanus is particularly important given a death rate of more than 95% without specific therapy and 10 to 90% with therapy, depending on the intensity of supportive care.[32, 189–192, 197–200, 204–207] Long-term residual effects on neurological and growth status can be seen.[208, 209]

The incidence of tetanus neonatorum in developing nations in the 1960s had been estimated to be approximately 0.1 per 1000 live births on the basis of reported disease.[45] Using hospital-based reporting, Bytchenko and coworkers[149] made an estimate in 1981 of 600,000 neonatal tetanus deaths worldwide, corresponding to approximately 5 neonatal tetanus cases per 1000 live births. A better assessment of the occurrence of neonatal tetanus throughout the globe was only possible with the use of community-based, house-to-house surveys of neonatal deaths.[189, 192] Stanfield and Galazka[192] reviewed these surveys, which documented that the actual incidence of neonatal tetanus was more than 50 per 1000 live births in some areas and above 5 per 1000 in most; overall, there was an estimated annual rate of 10 cases per 1000 live births in the early 1980s, resulting in approximately 1.2 million deaths per year. Among the possible reasons that the full impact of neonatal tetanus had not previously been evident is that the populations at highest risk of neonatal tetanus live in rural areas, meaning more likely exposure to contaminated soil and at the same time with the poorest access to healthcare services and to birth registration.[192]

There is some indication that the risk of neonatal tetanus is lower at higher altitudes.[210] For reasons that are not clear, there is a striking male predominance (2:1 or greater) of tetanus neonatorum as detected by surveillance or by population-based surveys in many areas; in other areas, this predominance is less striking or nonexistent.[152, 155, 160, 164] It has been suggested that separation of the cord stump occurs later in boys[211] and that this may account in part for a male predominance.[212]

In the United States, the occurrence of neonatal tetanus was falling before widespread tetanus toxoid use in women, presumably because of improvements in puerperal hygiene. As followed from the beginning of the 20th century, deaths due to neonatal tetanus have become progressively less common in the United States.[193] Because tetanus occurring under a year of age was and is almost exclusively in the neonatal period, tetanus occurring in this age group can be used as a surrogate measure of neonatal disease. Deaths due to tetanus in those younger than 1 year declined from 0.64 per 1000 live births in 1900 to 0.07 in 1930 to 0.01 by the 1960s.[193] The overall gradual decline in tetanus mortality in part reflects maternal immunity due to the initiation of routine infant and child tetanus toxoid inoculation in the late 1940s as well as hospital delivery and other birth practices. From 1961, tetanus occurrence could be accurately monitored in those younger than 1 year, and trends in occurrence paralleled those in mortality. In the 1-year period from 1967 to 1968, there was a precipitous decrease in the incidence of reported cases and in the incidence of reported tetanus deaths in those younger than 1 year, corresponding to a sharp decline in reported cases from Texas after a rigorous campaign of vaccination of high-risk mothers. After 1968, the annual rate has continued to decline more gradually (see Fig. 18–3). Other developed nations have witnessed similar declines.[149]

Of the 30 cases reported in U.S. infants during the first 4 weeks of life from 1972 to 1995, 27 were in infants born outside of a hospital. Nineteen of the cases (63%) occurred in Texas, which had only 6% of U.S. births. Only five mothers had a history of ever having received tetanus toxoid, and only one was known to have received more than one dose. Twenty (74%) of 27 with known outcome survived. Only two cases of neonatal tetanus have been reported in the United States after 1984, in 1989 and 1995.[213, 214] The case in 1995 followed birth in a hospital after routine prenatal care; the history of only one prior tetanus toxoid dose was never elicited from the foreign-born mother before the birth and subsequent onset of illness in the child.[214]

Given its substantial impact in the developing world, the elimination of neonatal tetanus as a significant public health illness is a current goal of the Expanded Programme on Immunization (EPI) of the WHO (see *Neonatal Tetanus Elimination*).[215, 216]

PASSIVE IMMUNIZATION

Early researchers were able to prevent, modify, or treat tetanus in animal models using antitoxin prepared from large animals. The therapeutic doses required were much larger than the prophylactic ones.[47] Passive immunization for treatment and for prophylaxis after wounds became common practice in World War I, and there was some evidence of prophylactic efficacy.[9] As a means of lessening the antigenicity of equine antitoxin for human use, proteolytic treatment to obtain cleaved Fab fragments (with the binding sites) was introduced.[217] Passive immunity conferred by equine antitoxin is of limited duration. The half-life of refined equine antitoxin in humans is less than 2 weeks and may be eliminated more rapidly by the immunological response in some individuals.[218, 219]

TIG was introduced early in the 1960s and was found to have a fairly constant half-life of 28 days in humans.[220, 221] The frequency of allergic and serum sickness reactions to equine antitoxin,[132, 133] along with its shorter half-life, made TIG more attractive for passive immunization. TIG is derived by cold-ethanol fractionation of the plasma of hyperimmunized adults. This preparation has been shown not to pose a risk of hepatitis transmission. It is distributed in 1-mL vials with 250 IU/mL (see Appendix 2 for U.S. producers). Even in the developing world, TIG is beginning to supplant equine antitoxin as it becomes more widely available. Recommendations for the use of TIG in disease prevention are given in the section *Tetanus Prophylaxis in Wound Management.* Tetanus toxoid is always given with TIG to induce persistence of immunity beyond 28 days in those with any past exposure to toxoid and to initiate active immunization in those without any prior exposure.[222–225]

Quantitation of the potency of antitoxin of animal or human origin has been standardized by comparison with an international standard antitoxin using fixed doses of toxin. Although the international unit defined in 1928 was half of the unit of the U.S. National Institutes of Health (NIH), the WHO reset the international standard unitage in 1950 to be in agreement with that of the NIH. Assay results before that time were generally reported in antitoxin units (or American units) per milliliter (AU/mL) using the NIH reference. Results using the current standard are reported as international units per milliliter (IU/mL).

The level of antitoxin needed to protect has been examined in a number of ways, and it is generally accepted that 0.01 IU/mL of tetanus antitoxin is the minimum level needed to ensure protection against tetanus in humans.[221, 226–228] This is based primarily on animal experiments after passive and active immunization. Early work based on experiments involving passive immunization in animals with heterologous antitoxin led investigators to conclude that levels of 0.1 to 0.25 AU/mL were needed to protect against tetanus. A review of data on the reduction of tetanus in horses following homologous passive immunization by McComb[221] in 1964 found an absence of clinical tetanus in horses following injection of 1500 IU of antitoxin after acute injury (approximately 2.5 IU/kg), similar to earlier data with 2.5 IU/kg in guinea pigs. This corresponded to a level of 0.01 IU/mL. The only experimental studies in humans follow active immunization.

Several papers have appeared suggesting that a level of 0.01 IU/mL may not protect in all cases. Dozens of patients, including many neonates, have been described with pretreatment antitoxin levels greater than 0.01 IU/mL.[94–99] The highest reported titer on presentation was 25 IU/mL. The assessment of serum antitoxin in these reports used in vitro methods, results that sometimes could be questioned regarding relevance to clinical protection—indeed, in one study, a discrepancy was noted between in vitro and neutralization techniques. In addition, it is possible that in previously vaccinated individuals, an intoxicating dose of tetanus toxin could lead to an anamnestic response before the testing of serum antitoxin. Nonetheless, these data strongly suggest that the 0.01 IU/mL level is not absolute. Variations in toxin production are not unexpected, and greater toxin production may overcome a fixed level of antitoxin. Alternatively, toxin may be rapidly transported to the CNS in some patients even in the presence of circulating antitoxin. Nonetheless, given the rarity of tetanus in patients with prior adequate immunization history and given most of the animal data reviewed, it seems reasonable to conclude that the 0.01 IU/mL level by neutralization assays is indicative of protection in most situations.

ACTIVE IMMUNIZATION: TOXOID

Prior Approaches

The purification of tetanus toxoid led to efforts to inactivate it chemically without eliminating its immunogenicity. Early researchers used iodine trichloride. An early human challenge study and seroconversion studies supported the applied use of tetanus toxoid. Later, formaldehyde emerged as the most convenient and efficient means of inactivation. Ramon and Zoeller[229] early on suggested the combination with diphtheria toxoid and demonstrated that there was no antigenic competition for immune responses; he also recognized neonatal tetanus as a disease to be prevented by immunization of pregnant women. Tetanus toxoid became commercially available in the United States in 1938 but was not widely used until the military began routine pre-wound prophylactic inoculation in 1941.

Toxoid Description

To produce toxoid, *C. tetani* is cultured in liquid medium in large-capacity fermenters (up to 1000 liters). The medium, modified by Latham from that of Mueller and Miller, consists of a tryptic digest of casein, free of Berna and Witte peptones and other allergenic substances.[229a] In the United States, media containing human blood group–specific substances, such as beef heart infusion broth, are specifically avoided. Data suggest that tetanus toxin production can be enhanced by bubbling nitrogen through the liquid media.[230] Extracellular toxin is harvested by filtration, purified, and detoxified with 40% formaldehyde at 37°C.

In 1979, WHO attempted to standardize the content of tetanus toxoid preparations. By use of bioassays in mice, comparison with a standard preparation allowed the establishment of international units for toxoid content. However, guinea pig immune responses to tetanus toxoid apparently correspond more closely to human responses than do responses in mice; more importantly, the immune response in mice varies greatly depending on the mouse strain used. Even with a toxoid assessed in one strain of mice, the immune response in humans can vary greatly. For these reasons, the international standard has not been adopted in the United States.[231] WHO derived methods for testing tetanus toxoid potency based on International Immunizing Units (IIU or IU) by challenging mice immunized with the tested toxoid in comparison to mice immunized with standard vaccines. Until 1982, 30 IU was required per human dose; this was changed in 1982 to 40 IU (60 IU in preparations of diphtheria and tetanus toxoids and pertussis vaccine).[232]

Some people have used the results of the limits of flocculation (Lf) test as a surrogate measure of potency. However, this assay measures antigen content, which may not perfectly correlate with antibody production. U.S. requirements for antigen content and potency for commercial tetanus toxoid products are discussed later in *Dosage and Route.*

WHO standards apply as recommendations for commercial and governmental producers and also serve as a requirement for supply to United Nations agencies including WHO and the United Nations Children's Fund (UNICEF).

Producers

In the United States, several manufacturers distribute tetanus toxoid (TT) singly or in combination with diphtheria toxoid with or without whole-cell or acellular pertussis vaccine (DT, Td, DTP, DTaP; see later and see Appendix 2 for U.S. producers). In Canada and some European nations, inactivated poliomyelitis vaccine may be combined with DTP. More recent combinations have been introduced outside the United States for use in childhood, including whole-cell DTP combinations with hepatitis B vaccine or *Haemophilus influenzae* type b (Hib) conjugate vaccines.

Producers who are eligible to supply TT–containing products to UN agencies and meet WHO requirements ("prequalified") as of January 1998 include Chiron Behring, Germany (DTP, DT, TT, Td); Chiron Vaccines, Italy (DT, TT, Td); CSL, Ltd., Australia (DTP, DT, TT, Td); HUMAN, Ltd., Hungary (DT, TT, Td); Pasteur Mérieux–Connaught, Canada (DTP, DT, TT, Td); Pasteur Mérieux–Connaught, France (DTP, DT, TT, Td); Serum Institute of India (DTP, DT, TT, Td); and Swiss Serum and Vaccine Institute, Switzerland (DTP, DT, TT, Td). Tetanus toxoid–containing products are widely made by local manufacturers. The majority of countries with reported neonatal tetanus produce their own vaccines. Despite the promulgation of WHO standards, many local producers as of January 1998 either have no effective quality control mechanism or have not fully adopted WHO standards. In response to problems evident with tetanus toxoid potency in many developing countries, the World Health Assembly in 1992 discussed working toward the exclusive use of vaccines that meet WHO requirements.[233]

Dosage and Route

As with other inactivated vaccines and toxoids, the immunological response to tetanus toxoid requires more than one dose to confer protection and persisting immunity. There is no need to repeat doses if scheduled doses are delayed. Even with long intervals between doses, the immune response to subsequent doses appears similar to or better than that with shorter intervals.[234, 235]

In North America, the preparations available are given as 0.5-mL doses. The adsorbed toxoid is administered intramuscularly; fluid preparations can be given subcutaneously. Either can be given by jet injector. The toxoid content of commercial products is assessed by flocculation with standard antitoxin and measured in Lf. This measure of toxoid protein content does not necessarily correspond directly with immunogenicity as measured by potency in guinea pigs. Adsorbed products available in the United States have a content of 5 to 20 Lf per dose; fluid products contain 10 to 40 Lf. Potency is determined by animal bioassays: for the fluid preparation, immunized guinea pigs are tested for survival after a toxin challenge; for precipitated toxoid, a serum pool from immunized guinea pigs must exceed 2 IU/mL.

Available Preparations

Diphtheria and tetanus toxoids and pertussis vaccine adsorbed (whole-cell DTP), diphtheria and tetanus toxoids and acellular pertussis vaccine adsorbed (DTaP), and diphtheria and tetanus toxoids adsorbed (for pediatric use) (DT) are combinations used in infants and children younger than 7 years. Recent combinations available in the United States include DTP with Hib conjugate vaccines, which can be used for doses one to four of the five-dose DTP series, and DTaP with Hib conjugate vaccines, which as of January 1998 was available only for dose four.

Universal use of DTP/DTaP in infancy and childhood is recommended unless there are contraindications to pertussis vaccine[135, 236]; tetanus and diphtheria toxoids (Td) adsorbed (for adult use) is for use in people 7 years of age and older because it contains less diphtheria toxoid (2 Lf or less) than the pediatric preparation (more than 10 Lf). Single-antigen tetanus toxoid (fluid) and tetanus toxoid adsorbed are also available in the United States for use in people 7 years of age and older. Td is the preferred preparation for tetanus prophylaxis in adults under all circumstances because most adults in need of tetanus toxoid are likely to be susceptible to diphtheria; Td is the recommended formulation for routine boosting of older children, adolescents, and adults. Clinically significant reactions are not substantially more frequent after receipt of Td than single-antigen tetanus toxoid. Although in the 1960s more than 70% of adult tetanus toxoid preparations distributed were single-antigen tetanus toxoid, only 11% of the 13 million doses of tetanus toxoid distributed for adult use in 1996 (i.e., other than DTP and DT) was as single-antigen tetanus toxoid.

Both fluid preparations of tetanus toxoid alone and preparations adsorbed with various precipitating salt adjuvants are available. In the United States, aluminum hydroxide or aluminum phosphate is used as the adjuvant. These salts allow an adequate immune response after fewer doses of toxoid than with the fluid preparation.[237] The primary immunization schedule for fluid toxoids requires four doses, whereas the adsorbed toxoid requires three. In neonatal tetanus prevention trials, three doses of fluid toxoid for pregnant women were necessary to achieve protective levels of antitoxin as opposed to two doses of adsorbed toxoid.[228] At constant levels of antigen content, geometric mean antibody responses are higher after adsorbed toxoid,[228] and the higher the antitoxin response, the slower the absolute rate of decline of antibody.[238, 239] Because fluid and adsorbed preparations are essentially equivalent with regard to adverse events, adsorbed toxoid is preferred because it confers protective levels of antitoxin for a longer time. Response to either form of toxoid as a booster dose is equally brisk. In combined active-passive immunization, TIG does not substantially alter the response to adsorbed toxoid as it does with fluid toxoid.[221, 225, 240] In the United States, therefore, adsorbed products are recommended over fluid. Td preparations are available only as adsorbed products. Outside the United States, a calcium phosphate–adsorbed product is also available.[241] Interest has focused on the theoretical but unproved possibility that calcium-adsorbed preparations may be associated with fewer reactions than the aluminum products.[242, 243]

Constituents

According to WHO, the final product should contain 0.5% formaldehyde or less. In the United States, minimum requirements stipulate a residual formaldehyde content of 0.02% or less. When given as an adsorbed suspension, precipitating calcium or aluminum salt adjuvants are available. A single human dose must contain less than 1.25 mg of aluminum. Preparations outside the United States may contain larger amounts of aluminum. All toxoid preparations in the United States have thimerosal added to a final concentration of up to 0.1% to prevent bacterial contaminant overgrowth; the final concentration is typically 0.01%.

Stability

Preparations should be stored at 2 to 8°C and generally have a 2-year expiration date. Higher ambient temperatures for short periods, generally 7 days or less, do not reduce the potency of the toxoid except at temperatures of 45°C or greater.[244] This indicates that use of this preparation in the developing world is not as dependent on the "cold chain" as are other immunobiologicals. Freezing, particularly repeated freezing, can reduce potency, particularly when the toxoid is a component of DTP.[7, 245, 246] The effect of freezing on different samples of DT or DTP alone is variable. The effect of repeated freezing on adsorbed and fluid single-antigen tetanus toxoids has been shown to reduce the mean antitoxin response time.[247] The available data on temperature stability have recently been reviewed.[248]

ACTIVE IMMUNIZATION: ADMINISTRATION

Immune Responses

The standard for measuring an immune response to tetanus toxoid is the serum toxin neutralization test.[235, 249, 250] Such tests are performed in mice injected with preincubated mixtures of various dilutions of serum and a lethal dose of tetanus toxin and standardized to a reference serum specimen. Toxin neutralization tests allow antitoxin titers as low as 0.001 IU/mL to be detected. These assays are believed to be most reliable because they assess actual neutralization in a living host. However, because in vivo neutralization tests are time-consuming and expensive, a variety of other serological tests have been developed. Among these are passive hemagglutination, enzyme immunoassays (EIA) or ELISA, radioimmunoassays, immunofluorescent assays (IFA), latex agglutination, and a variety of methods using agar gel precipitation.[251–273] All tests can be specific (depending on detection of immunoglobulin [Ig] M or low-avidity antibodies; see later), but sensitivity varies widely by assay. IFA, agar gel diffusion, and latex agglutination are the least sensitive.[178, 256] In general, any of the techniques is useful provided that correlation with toxin neutralization has been performed. The advantages and disadvantages of each technique have been reviewed.[178, 252]

The evaluation of alternatives to toxin neutralization tests has most often involved passive hemagglutination techniques.[252–260, 263–265] Whereas results vary from technique to technique, in general there is a good correlation with toxin neutralization, particularly at high titers. Consistency in testing among laboratories has been aided by the use of turkey erythrocytes in the assay.[252, 263] However, a passive hemagglutination test measures both IgG and IgM, perhaps preferentially IgM.[254, 265] Studies indicate that IgG is a better neutralizer of tetanospasmin than is IgM.[226, 274] Hence, titers detected early in an immunization series by passive hemagglutination, particularly after the first dose, may not represent neutralizing antitoxin. EIA, radioimmunoassays, and IFA can measure specific immunoglobulins and avoid this problem. However, at low levels of antitoxin, EIA may read higher levels than indicated by neutralization assays in mice. This has been in part attributed to more ready detection by EIA of low-affinity IgG, which may not be neutralizing.[266, 267] There is good evidence that with levels below 0.16 IU/mL detected by solid-phase EIA, neutralization tests should be performed to substantiate the antitoxin content.[266] These problems in specificity are apparently due to differences in antibody binding because of conformational changes in tetanus toxoid in solid-phase EIA[269]; this can be alleviated by use of an antigen-competition method. Mixing of antibody in the serum dilution with antigen in solution leads to results that are more comparable with neutralization assays at low antitoxin levels.[269, 270] Another modification of EIA that increases specificity at low antitoxin titers is toxin-binding inhibition in which toxin preincubated with serum dilutions is exposed to antitoxin-coated plates to detect unbound toxin.[271–273]

In reporting results, it is clear that the best approach is always to state the assay method and to indicate the correlation with neutralization. Serosurveys have recently reported solid-phase EIA results with a protective level reported as greater than 0.15 IU/mL.[183, 275] This will underestimate the level of protection in a population because some people with levels less than 0.16 IU/mL may be protected; the reporting of seroprevalence using solid-phase EIA including those results below 0.16 will clearly overestimate the level of protection in a population. The use of antigen-competition EIA and toxin-binding inhibition may allow future serosurveys to indicate levels of protection more accurately.[270, 273]

Cellular immunity (type IV hypersensitivity) to tetanus toxoid is frequently induced by routine immunization (74 to 90%); intradermal skin testing with tetanus toxoid has been used as a screen for anergy,[276–278] although there can be false-positive reactions.[279]

Results of Controlled Studies of Protection Against Disease

A double-blind, randomized, controlled clinical trial in rural Colombia showed that two or three doses of tetanus toxoid administered to women of childbearing age protected their babies.[235, 280] Control infants had a neonatal tetanus mortality rate of 78 per 1000 live births, whereas no neonatal tetanus cases occurred in the children of women who received at least two doses. A mean antitoxin level of 0.01 AU/mL in pregnant women has been associated with protection of infants from neonatal tetanus.[228]

Other Evidence of Effectiveness in Protection

Early data suggesting the efficacy of active immunization with tetanus toxoid come from Wolters and Dehmel,[281] who immunized themselves with toxoid and achieved serum levels of 0.007 to 0.01 AU/mL. This allowed them to resist challenge with “two or three fatal doses” of tetanus toxin, but the actual challenge dose is unknown.[281]

The reduction in neonatal tetanus where tetanus toxoid is used in pregnant women supports the preceding findings. Field assessment of the efficacy of two or more tetanus toxoid doses has been made in neonatal tetanus mortality surveys, reporting 70 to 100% effectiveness.[178, 282–286] Formal assessments of the efficacy of tetanus toxoid against disease in ages outside the neonatal period have not been made because of the rarity of the disease. Nonetheless, the efficacy of a standard preexposure immunization regimen plus postwound booster doses was demonstrated in the application of tetanus toxoid use in the military: only 12 cases of tetanus occurred among 2.73 million wounded U.S. Army personnel on all fronts in World War II (0.44 per 100,000) versus 70 of 520,000 wounded in World War I (13.4 per 100,000); only 4 of the 12 had completed primary immunization.[287] A similar experience occurred in British personnel.[288]

Because of the initial studies in neonatal tetanus prevention and the effect that programs of prenatal immunization to prevent neonatal tetanus have had, and the correlation of immunogenicity with protection, routine use of toxoid has been assumed also to be highly effective.[228, 235] As indicated next, primary immunization of infants and children leads to antitoxin responses well above protective levels in virtually all recipients.

Indications for Use

Because of the success of active immunization in the military, wide spore distribution, the high death-to-case ratio of tetanus, and the frequent reactions with and incomplete efficacy of equine antitoxin,[289] routine inoculation in childhood was recommended in 1944 by the American Academy of Pediatrics (AAP). In the mid-1940s, tetanus toxoid was combined with diphtheria toxoid and pertussis vaccine (DTP), which permitted administration of all three antigens with a single injection. In 1951, the AAP recommended routine use of DTP in infancy, and generalized use by practitioners became more common. Since that time, advisory groups in the United States, including the Advisory Committee on Immunization Practices (ACIP), have recommended that all people receive three or more doses of tetanus toxoid in the appropriate combination based on age followed by routine booster doses every 10 years.

Administration to Infants and Children. The recommended schedule for routine tetanus immunization in the United States is given in Table 18–2.[135, 236, 290, 291] The EPI-recommended schedule for the developing world of DTP at 6, 10, and 14 weeks of age is also being used in many countries in Europe and elsewhere and is discussed further later.[292]

Tetanus toxoid is one of the most potent immunizing agents used routinely in children. Protective levels can be obtained with schedules starting in the newborn period.[231, 292–298] Premature infants have immune responses at a given chronological age comparable to that of term infants.[296, 299]

In contrast to the immunological response to diphtheria toxoid, which may be impeded in the presence of passively transferred maternal antitoxin, the immune response to tetanus toxoid has been considered to be minimally inhibited by maternal antitoxin.[294, 295, 300–302] Many of the studies examining inhibition of response to tetanus toxoid were performed at a time before mothers were likely to be immune.[303] The majority of women of childbearing age in the United States have previously been immunized and have received a booster dose in adolescence; increasing numbers of adult women in the developing world also have been previously immunized. Studies in the United States have shown that term infants have high geometric mean titers (GMTs) of circulating tetanus antitoxin at 2 months of age, before immunization, implying that most term infants currently have levels of antitoxin well above protective levels before beginning immunization.[304–306] Edwards and colleagues[306] evaluated 13 candidate acellular pertussis (DTaP) vaccines (with a U.S. schedule of doses at 2, 4, and 6 months of age) and compared the serological responses with a whole-cell DTP vaccine licensed in the United States. Before the first dose at 2 months of age, GMTs varied from 1.115 to 7.43 IU/mL measured by modified passive hemagglutination. After the third dose at 6 months of age, all infants had levels of antibody of 0.01 IU/mL or higher, and GMTs ranged from 3.094 to 22.513 IU/mL. The whole-cell DTP vaccine induced the highest levels of antitoxin, with GMT at least 10 IU/mL higher than with any DTaP vaccine. Nevertheless, GMTs for the acellular vaccines were all at least 300-fold greater than 0.01 IU/mL. Such high preimmunization antitoxin titers do not inhibit the full induction of active immunity, including in children of mothers vaccinated in pregnancy.[307, 308] With an accelerated scheduled (e.g., 2, 3, 4 months), the tetanus toxoid response may be lower in infants with higher preexisting maternal antitoxin.[309] However, infants are protected after immunization, and by 6 months after completing an accelerated schedule, mean titers are still well above protective levels.[310]

Table 18–2. **RECOMMENDATIONS FOR PRIMARY IMMUNIZATION WITH TETANUS TOXOID BY AGE AT BEGINNING IMMUNIZATION**

	AGE GROUP			
	<1 yr	1–6 yr		≥7 yr
Vaccine	*DTaP* or DT†,‡*	*DTaP**	*DT†,§*	*Td‖*
Interval before				
Dose 1	First visit	First visit	First visit	First visit
Dose 2	1–2 mo	1–2 mo	1–2 mo	1–2 mo
Dose 3	1–2 mo	1–2 mo	6–12 mo	6–12 mo
Dose 4	Approximately 1 yr¶	Approximately 1 yr¶	—	—

*DTaP is the preferred pertussis vaccine preparation for all doses in the series. Whole-cell DTP is an acceptable alternative.

†DT for those with contraindications to pertussis vaccine.

‡Boosters with DT or DTaP (dose five) indicated at 4 to 6 years of age. Boosters with Td indicated at 11 to 12 years of age and every 10 years thereafter. First visit generally at 2 months of age.

§Dose 4 of DT indicated at 4 to 6 years of age unless dose 3 administered at 4 years of age or older. In this instance, dose 4 is not needed. Boosters with Td indicated at 11 to 12 years of age and every 10 years thereafter.

‖Boosters with Td indicated every 10 years.

¶Dose 5 of DTaP/DTP indicated at 4 to 6 years of age unless dose 4 administered at 4 years of age or older. In this instance, dose 5 is not needed. Boosters with Td indicated at 11 to 12 years of age and every 10 years thereafter.

DT, diphtheria and tetanus toxoids for pediatric use; DTaP, diphtheria and tetanus toxoids and acellular pertussis vaccine; DTP, diphtheria and tetanus toxoids and pertussis vaccine; Td, tetanus and diphtheria toxoids for adult use.

During the first year of life, the older a child is at the time of receipt of the third dose of tetanus toxoid, the higher the level of antitoxin produced. Brown and coworkers[311] studied infants beginning immunization at 3 to 7 months of age with three doses of DTP inoculated at 1- or 2-month intervals. In general, regardless of interval, GMTs were higher in infants completing the schedule at older ages versus younger ages (Table 18–3). However, these differences are probably of no clinical significance: all infants, regardless of schedule, had antitoxin titers higher than 0.01 AU/mL for at least 12 to 18 months after completing the initial three-dose series, and both groups had comparable GMTs. Response to boosters was similar under all schedules tested, confirming that immunization against tetanus can begin at an early age with good results. More recent studies support the results of Brown and coworkers. In the United Kingdom, the routine schedule for DTP was changed in 1992 from three doses at 3, 4½ to 5, and 8½ to 11 months to 2, 3, and 4 months.[292, 310] Children vaccinated with the accelerated schedule, completed at 4 months, had only about one sixth the GMT of tetanus antitoxin, approximately 8 weeks after the third dose, compared with children who completed immunization at the older age (0.522 versus 3.43 IU/mL, assessed by radioimmunoassay). By 1 year after the third dose, the differences had narrowed (0.197 IU/mL for the early schedule versus 0.341 IU/mL). No child with either schedule had levels less than 0.01 IU/mL.

Single doses of standard- or high-potency tetanus toxoids have induced protective levels in some studies.[238, 243, 312–314] However, in general, these levels do not greatly exceed 0.01 IU/mL, and long-term follow-up has been lacking. Therefore, a minimum of two doses of standard-potency tetanus toxoids are considered necessary to reach protective levels of circulating antitoxin in infants during the first year of life.[231, 315–320] Data do not support sufficient protection from neonatal tetanus when only one dose of standard potency is administered in pregnancy.[178, 282] Recent data collected in trials of DTP vac-

Table 18–3. **EFFECT OF INTERVAL BETWEEN DOSES ON THE ANTITOXIN RESPONSE TO THREE DOSES OF TETANUS TOXOID**

AGE AT TIME OF FIRST DOSE (mo)	INTERVAL BETWEEN DOSES (mo)	ANTITOXIN TITERS 2 WEEKS AFTER PRIMARY SERIES*			ANTITOXIN TITERS 1 YEAR AFTER PRIMARY SERIES†		
		Number of Participants	GMT‡	% Protected§	Number of Participants	GMT‡	% Protected§
3	1	61	13.5	100	44	1.8	100
3	2	31	24.0	100	24	1.2	100
4	1	86	13.6	100	59	2.0	100
4	2	50	22.6	100	32	1.8	100
5	1	54	21.3	100	35	2.2	100
5	2	28	29.2	100	21	2.4	100
6	1	25	21.2	100	15	2.0	100
7	1	10	29.1	100	6	2.9	100

*Lowest postprimary titer in age group was 0.6 AU/mL (antitoxin units/mL).
†Lowest prebooster titer was 0.125 AU/mL.
‡Geometric mean antitoxin titer in AU/mL.
§≥0.01 AU/mL.
Adapted from Brown GC, Volk VK, Gottshall RY, et al. Responses of infants to DTP-P vaccine used in nine injection schedules. Public Health Rep 79:585–602, 1964.

cines in the United States imply that three doses may be needed in infants before significant production of antitoxin takes place.[304–306]

Most primary immunization schedules used in the developed world consist of two or three doses in the first year of life followed by a reinforcing dose approximately 6 months to 1 year afterward.[135, 236, 290, 321] When combined DTP is used, the schedule for tetanus immunization is often tied to the scheduling requirements of immunization with diphtheria toxoid and pertussis vaccines. Immunization against pertussis requires three doses in the first year of life. The EPI of the WHO, with its emphasis on protection in early infancy, recommends a total of three doses of DTP early in the first year, starting as early as 6 weeks of age with a minimum of 4 weeks between doses.[216, 322]

Intervals for the first two or three doses are generally 1 to 2 months, and there appears to be little reason to prefer one interval over another with regard to tetanus antitoxin production. Data from Brown and colleagues[311] indicate that whereas infants vaccinated at 2-month intervals make higher levels of antitoxin than infants vaccinated at 1-month intervals, all groups of infants had similar GMTs at the time of reinforcing doses.

After two- or three-dose primary schedules during infancy, antibody levels tend to wane.[301, 310, 311, 322–325] Although children who receive two or three doses of vaccine at 1- or 2-month intervals rarely have lost protective levels of antibody 1 year after the last dose, reinforcing doses at this time lead to high levels of antitoxin production and long-term immunity, generally exceeding 10 years.[239, 301, 304, 305, 307–311, 320, 324–328]

In children older than 1 year, two doses at intervals of 1 to 2 months appear to induce protective levels of antitoxin that persist at least 6 to 12 months.[323] A reinforcing dose at this time is associated with a marked booster response and persistent high levels of antitoxin. Therefore, most immunization schedules for children older than 1 year call for three doses: the first two separated by 1 to 2 months and the third dose 6 to 12 months after the second. However, when combined with pertussis vaccine, which requires a minimum of three doses, a schedule similar to that for infants is often used, with three doses 1 to 2 months apart followed by a fourth dose 6 to 12 months later.

Administration to Adults. The immune response to tetanus toxoid appears to decrease with increasing age. In comparative studies, children will generally develop higher levels of antitoxin than adults.[329] Despite the decrease in immunogenicity, the majority of adult vaccinees achieve and maintain protective levels of antitoxin for many years.[234, 239] Most schedules in use in the world today call for two doses 1 to 2 months apart followed by a third dose 6 to 12 months later.

After two doses 4 weeks or more apart, almost all adults produce antitoxin levels higher than 0.01 IU/mL.[329] GMTs vary according to type of vaccine and schedule but in general are below 1.0 IU/mL. In one large-scale field trial in New Guinea, titers persisted at protective levels for 40 months in as many as 78% of adult women given two doses of aluminum phosphate–adsorbed vaccine and for 54 months in 33%.[330] Other studies, particularly in older adults, have confirmed that persistence of protective levels of antitoxin without a reinforcing dose is short-lived.[331, 332]

A reinforcing dose 6 to 12 months after the first two doses is associated with production of high levels of antitoxin (>5 IU/mL) that have long-term duration.[329] Immune response in the elderly may be somewhat impaired. Only 77% of elderly subjects in one study had protective levels of antitoxin 8 years after a three-dose primary series.[331] Other workers have also indicated a weaker immune response in elderly individuals.[333–337] Nevertheless, in most adults, routine boosters every 10 years should be sufficient to maintain immunity.[234, 239, 328, 334]

Administration to Women of Childbearing Age for Prevention of Neonatal Tetanus. A minimum of two doses of tetanus toxoid at least 1 month apart with the last dose at least 2 weeks before the estimated date of delivery appears to provide protective levels of antibody for well above 80% of newborns (see earlier, *Active Immunization: Administration*).[215] However, higher efficacy and long-term protection is desired, so WHO has adopted a schedule of five tetanus toxoid doses adminis-

Table 18–4. **RECOMMENDATIONS OF THE EXPANDED PROGRAMME ON IMMUNIZATION FOR IMMUNIZATION OF WOMEN OF CHILDBEARING AGE FOR PREVENTION OF NEONATAL TETANUS**

NOT PREVIOUSLY IMMUNIZED

Dose	When Given
1	First contact or as early in pregnancy as possible
2	At least 4 wk after dose 1
3	6–12 mo after dose 2 or during subsequent pregnancy
4	1–5 yr after dose 3 or during subsequent pregnancy
5	1–10 yr after dose 4 or during subsequent pregnancy; no further doses indicated

PREVIOUSLY IMMUNIZED

Age at Last Immunization	Previous Immunization	Recommended Immunizations: *At Present Contact/Pregnancy*	Recommended Immunizations: *Later (At Interval of at Least 1 Yr)*
Infancy	3 doses of DTP	2 doses of TT (at least 4 wk apart)	1 dose of TT
Childhood	4 doses of DTP	1 dose of TT	1 dose of TT
School age	3 doses of DTP	1 dose of TT	1 dose of TT
School age	4 doses of DTP + 1 dose of DT/Td	1 dose of TT	None
Adolescence	4 doses of DTP + 1 dose of DT/Td at 4–6 yr + 1 dose of TT/Td at 14–16 yr	None	None

DT, diphtheria and tetanus toxoids; DTP, diphtheria and tetanus toxoids and pertussis; Td, tetanus and diphtheria toxoids; TT, tetanus toxoid.
Adapted from Expanded Programme on Immunization: Issues in Neonatal Tetanus Control. Geneva, World Health Organization, 1987. EPI/GAG/87/WP.11; and Galazka AM. The immunologic basis for immunization: Module 3: Tetanus. Geneva, World Health Organization, 1993, WHO/EPI/GEN/93.14.

tered during a minimum of 2.6 years and preferably more than 10 years to induce sustained levels of circulating antitoxin in all vaccinated women for the duration of their reproductive years[215] (Table 18–4).

In addition, the schedule of recommended immunization must now take into account that the EPI has been in effect since 1974, and many expectant mothers and women of childbearing age also have history of childhood immunization. An immunization schedule has been recommended that considers the woman's prior history of vaccination in infancy, childhood, or adolescence so that an excessive number of doses are not given—a maximum of six doses is administered from infancy through the reproductive years to prevent neonatal tetanus[178] (see Table 18–4).

Some researchers have suggested that active immunization of fetuses can occur as a consequence of vaccination of mothers during pregnancy and that these effects can persist[337]; this work has been disputed.[178, 338]

Duration of Immunity and Booster Immunization

After each subsequent injection, antitoxin levels peak within 2 weeks, fall rapidly during 2 months, and then fall more gradually in the years following.[339] A constant log-linear decline in antitoxin level has been described.[239, 327, 328, 340] Long-term protection has been reviewed by Simonsen.[341] These data, in general, support a need for booster doses after a primary series and repeated boosters throughout life. The best information on long-term duration of protective levels of tetanus antitoxin comes from studies in Denmark. These studies are conducted following the consistent use of three doses of single-source 12-Lf adsorbed tetanus toxoid from 1950 through 1960 and four doses of a 7-Lf toxoid since 1961 in this homogeneous population. These data indicate that after a three-dose primary series consisting of two doses 1 month apart followed by a third dose 9 months to 1 year later, protective levels of antitoxin persist in 96% of recipients for 13 to 14 years and in 72% of recipients for more than 25 years.[326, 340, 341] A study in Sweden indicated that after a series of three doses 4 to 6 weeks apart, protective levels of antibody were retained by more than 94% after 10 years.[342] Information from an American study showed persistence in 91% of recipients for 7 to 13 years after a three-dose primary series 1 month apart without a reinforcing dose.[343] In U.S. children who received four or more doses of tetanus toxoid, none was found to have an antitoxin level below 0.08 IU/mL in the 90 months of follow-up.[328] On the basis of this information and other studies, immunization advisory bodies in the United States have recommended that boosters for preexposure prophylaxis are needed no more frequently than every 10 years.[135, 344] The EPI/WHO recommendation for women of childbearing age for the prevention of neonatal tetanus differs, however[345] (see Table 18–4). With particular emphasis on eliciting high antitoxin titers during pregnancy, this schedule recommends boosting at each subsequent pregnancy.

Recent analyses of data collected over 13 years on women in Bangladesh vaccinated with none, one, or two doses of tetanus toxoid have shown a substantial reduction in overall neonatal mortality in the 4- to 14-day interval after birth for the offspring of vaccinated mothers.[345a] The duration of immunity was up to 10 years for women who received two doses and up to 4 years after one dose. These data not only show the high efficacy of tetanus toxoid and long duration of immunity but also confirm the major contribution neonatal tetanus immunization makes to overall mortality 4 to 14 days after birth.

An acceptable immune response is achieved after boosters even when intervals of longer than 20 years have elapsed since the last dose.[327] If fluid toxoid had been used for primary immunization, booster immunization within 3 years has been recommended, preferably with adsorbed tetanus toxoid.[346]

In the developed world, infants beginning immunization with DTP or DT in the first year of life should receive a booster dose at 4 to 6 years of age and at least one booster of adult type Td; in general, this is given every 10 years thereafter, regardless of the initial schedule used.[135, 236, 344]

The need for booster doses every 10 years has recently been questioned by some experts because few cases of tetanus are reported among people who received a primary series (three or more doses), regardless of whether they have received booster doses.[33, 158–161, 341, 347–350] Furthermore, this low morbidity in vaccinated populations has occurred despite the recommendation for boosters not being widely implemented. In particular, arguments against routine boosting every 10 years have been based on the lack of substantial mortality in immunized people; it has been suggested that as an alternative to decennial boosting after a booster in adolescence, no further assessment of tetanus immunization status is necessary until age 50 years.[351] One prominent reason in the past for the decennial boosting recommendations was the possibility that fluid tetanus toxoid could have been used in prior doses and that dose potencies of preparations may have been highly variable; studies of duration in Scandinavia in which toxoid of constant antigen content and potency was used may not be representative of the situation for other countries. The current predominant reason for adult boosters is to maintain serum antitoxin well above protective levels for nearly all members of the population. Although immunization status has an effect on disease severity, occasional reports of severe tetanus cases and deaths continue to occur despite receipt of prior immunizations.[34, 99] The rationale for boosters of Td every 10 years includes the following: (1) seronegativity increases with increasing age (see under *Epidemiology*), and the elderly may be most in need—that is, a single booster dose at 50 years of age may not protect them; (2) although susceptibility is lower in adults younger than 50 years, because they account for a much greater proportion of the population than the elderly, immunization of younger individuals would have a greater impact on total numbers of susceptible people; and (3) boosting against diphtheria toxin is recommended every 10 years.[236, 352] A cost-effectiveness analysis of this issue by Balestra and Littenberg[350] revealed that decennial boosting prevented four times as many cases as a single booster at 65 years of age even though it was substantially less cost-effective—$143,138 in 1993 dollars for every year of life saved with decennial booster versus $4527 for every year of life saved with a single booster at age 65 years. Because of the greater health impact of decennial boosters, the ACIP continues to recommend boosters every 10 years.[79, 344]

Adverse Events After Immunization

The incidence and severity of adverse events, particularly local reactions, after administration of tetanus toxoid may potentially be influenced by the number of prior doses, the toxoid dosage, the presence of adjuvant (and perhaps quantity), the route and method of injection, and the presence of other antigens in the preparation used. The most common adverse event is a local reaction (defined differently in different studies) reported in 0 to 95% of recipients. The frequency of the reaction after any given dose in the series is uncertain. Most, but not all, studies support an increasing incidence of local reactions with an increasing number of doses.[329, 353–355] In general, 50 to 85% of recipients of booster doses of adsorbed toxoid experience some pain or tenderness at the injection site; 25 to 30% may experience edema and erythema.[356–360] Local reactions characterized by marked swelling occur in less than 2%.[276, 353, 361] Whereas some investigators have claimed that increasing antigen content (Lf) increases local reactions, there is no clear evidence of this.[353, 354, 362]

There have been conflicting reports as to whether aluminum adjuvants increase the incidence of local reactions compared with fluid toxoids.[237, 356, 357, 363, 364] This apparent controversy may be a function of (1) potential differences in the manufacturing of adsorbed toxoids, which can lead to variation in the degree of adsorption and therefore adjuvant activity,[365] and (2) potential differences within the study groups in toxoid potency (with or without equivalent Lf content), which is a problem in all comparisons of adverse events after tetanus toxoid. Aluminum adjuvant in adsorbed products can theoretically invoke local inflammatory responses more frequently than fluid toxoid because of adjuvant-induced activation of complement and stimulation of macrophages.[365]

The frequency of local reactions may be increased when toxoid is administered subcutaneously rather than intramuscularly.[353] This is particularly true for adsorbed toxoid[366]; in subcutaneous injection, aluminum adjuvant can lead to sterile abscesses.[365] Use of jet injectors, which deposit some toxoid in the subcutaneous tissue, has been associated with a twofold higher frequency of site edema than intramuscular injection by needle.[367]

In the United States, it is recommended that tetanus toxoid be given with diphtheria toxoid and, depending on age, with or without pertussis vaccine.[135, 236, 344] Adverse effects of pertussis vaccination and diphtheria toxoid inoculation are addressed in their respective chapters. Some controlled studies, although not with tetanus toxoid of the same lot, have suggested that minor adverse events, such as swelling or pain, may occur more frequently in individuals receiving Td than among those receiving tetanus toxoid, whereas other studies have not[355, 358–360, 368, 369] (Table 18–5). Passive surveillance of adverse events after immunization with privately funded vaccine from 1991 to 1995 has suggested that there may also be a significantly higher frequency of some systemic events, such as myalgia and syncope, after Td compared with TT.[369] However, the overall frequency of all reported events after each toxoid preparation, although

Table 18–5. **REPORTED FREQUENCIES OF ADVERSE EVENTS AFTER TETANUS TOXOID (TT) COMPARED WITH TETANUS AND DIPHTHERIA TOXOIDS FOR ADULT USE (Td)**

STUDY	PREPARATION	DOSE NUMBER	NUMBER OF DOSES IN STUDY*	FEVER (%)	LOCAL REACTIONS (%)		
					Pain	Edema	Massive
Williams and Ellingson	Adsorbed Td	1	1081	1		5	0
	Adsorbed TT	1	1087	1		5	<1
	Adsorbed Td	2	1013	3		19†	0
	Adsorbed TT	2	1012	1		8†	<1
	Adsorbed Td	3	284	7		62	1
Macko	Adsorbed Td	1	100	7	75†	30	
	Adsorbed TT	1	93	2	48†	26	
Ullberg-Olsson	Fluid Td	1	187		63		
	Fluid TT	1	197		74		
Deacon et al.	Adsorbed Td	1	29		21	66	
	Adsorbed TT	1	31		42	61	
Zurrer and Steffan	Adsorbed Td	1	653	6	63	32†	
	Adsorbed TT	1	773	5	58	63†	

*Prior vaccination status variable.

†For the parametric test of the difference between vaccine groups, $P < .05$.

Based on Williams JJ, Ellingson HV. Field trial of commercially-prepared diphtheria-tetanus toxoid: Immunization reactions among recruits. Unpublished report to the Armed Forces Epidemiologic Board, 1954; and Macko MB. Comparison of the morbidity of tetanus toxoid boosters with tetanus-diphtheria toxoid boosters. Ann Emerg Med 14:33–35, 1985.

Ullberg-Olsson K. Vaccinationsreaktioner efter injektion: Av tetanustoxoid med och utan tillsats av difteritoxoid. Lakartidningen 76:2976, 1979.

Deacon SP, Langford DT, Shepard WM, Knight PA. A comparative clinical study of adsorbed tetanus vaccine and adult-type tetanus-diphtheria vaccine. J Hyg (Camb) 89:513–519, 1982.

Zurrer G, Steffen R. Side effects in tetanus vs. diphtheria tetanus vaccination in travellers [abstract WPO3.3]. Proceedings of the First Conference on International Travel Medicine; Zurich, Switzerland; April 5–8, 1988.

differing significantly, was rare—36 events per million doses of Td and 23 per million doses of TT. Further, there were no significant differences in the frequencies of severe adverse events (i.e., associated with death, life-threatening illness, hospitalization, or disability)—2.1 events per million doses of Td and 1.5 per million doses of TT. Therefore, any differences in reported reactions may not be clinically important.

Several studies have found an association between the circulating tetanus antitoxin level and the degree of local reactions,[353, 354, 356, 357, 362, 370, 371] that is, the greater the preexisting level, the higher the incidence of local reactions, although not consistently.[346, 363] Similar trends are seen in comparing people who make a rapid immunological response (e.g., within 4 days), implying that they were primed by prior doses, with those who do not. There have been several reports of massive local reactions (i.e., associated with swelling from elbow to shoulder after deltoid inoculation), particularly in people with a history of multiple booster doses of toxoid. In general, these reactions begin within 2 to 8 hours after an injection. Such people are typically found to have serum antitoxin levels many-fold higher on average (at 2 to 160 IU/mL) than those of people without reactions or with only systemic adverse events.[362, 372–375] Preformed antibody apparently forms complexes with the deposited toxoid to induce an inflammatory response (Arthus reaction, type II hypersensitivity), and this is one of the reasons that frequent boosters of tetanus toxoid in wound management are discouraged. Other undefined associated host factors are involved because the range of antitoxin levels in individuals who exhibit this response is wide and includes levels seen in individuals without such a response. In those with a history of massive local reactions, boosting with lower than standard doses of tetanus toxoid (1 Lf) has been proposed by some researchers and appears successful.[354, 362, 376] This approach should be considered only if patients' antitoxin levels are monitored.

The preservative used in the U.S. preparations of tetanus toxoid is thimerosal, a mercurial known to lead to delayed-type hypersensitivity.[376, 377] It is uncertain to what degree hypersensitivity to either component influences local reactions when it is given intramuscularly. Reports have rarely linked reactions with an exaggerated delayed hypersensitivity response to tetanus toxoid.[372, 378–380]

Lymphadenopathy can occur after toxoid inoculation.[357, 372] Fever can accompany a local response, particularly when there is a marked local reaction or antitoxin levels are high.[358, 361, 375] Overall, booster doses of Td are associated with fever in 0.5 to 7% of recipients, with temperature above 39°C being rare.[355, 358, 361] Other systemic symptoms—headache or malaise—are reported less frequently.[354, 355, 361, 369] There are rare individuals with high antitoxin levels who, when receiving booster doses of toxoid, experience high fever and malaise without experiencing substantial local reactions.[375] Serum sickness–like illnesses (type III hypersensitivity) appear to be rarely associated with tetanus toxoid.[381, 382]

There have been several reports of peripheral neuropathy, particularly brachial plexus neuropathy, hours to weeks after tetanus toxoid.[382–390] These reports and laboratory findings have recently been reviewed.[382, 390, 391] Although anecdotal, the reports could be considered consistent with neuropathy as a manifestation of immune complex disease similar to that occurring after equine tetanus antitoxin.[392] The Vaccine Safety Committee of the National Academy of Sciences concluded in 1994 that there is evidence to support a causal association between tetanus toxoid and brachial plexus neuropathy.[382] The evidence was considered inadequate to accept or reject a causal relationship of tetanus toxoid with mononeuropathy. On the basis of case reports of brachial plexus neuropathy with history of tetanus toxoid exposure,[388, 389] the Institute of Medicine committee estimated that 0.5 to 1 case of brachial neuropathy per 100,000 recipients was attributable to tetanus toxoid within 1 month of immunization.[382] There have been reports of 25 cases of Guillain-Barré syndrome (GBS) after tetanus toxoid[382–386]; one patient had relapsing signs and symptoms after each of three injections of toxoid.[384] One estimated incidence was 0.4 per million doses of toxoid.[385] Although there may be a causal relationship between tetanus toxoid and GBS, the occurrence is rare. Population studies do not support a role for tetanus toxoid–containing preparations in causing GBS. A study of 700,000 children who received DTP revealed an incidence of GBS after immunization similar to background expected rates.[393] Similar results have been reported after administration of tetanus toxoid–containing vaccines to an estimated 1.2 million adults.[394] Other neurological events, including seizures and acute encephalopathy, have been reported after tetanus toxoid or DT.[375, 382, 395, 396] There are insufficient data to support a causal relationship with any of these other illnesses.[382] As is true with other immunizations, the occurrence of systemic symptoms soon after inoculation does not in itself indicate causation but rather may represent an unrelated chance occurrence.

Tetanus toxoid occasionally induces an IgE response, particularly with aluminum salt–adsorbed toxoid.[242, 397–399] Nonetheless, true anaphylactic (type I hypersensitivity) reactions to purified tetanus toxoid appear to be rare.[382, 400–402] When contaminating peptones from the culture media and silk fibers from the filtering process were present in toxoid preparations (before 1942 in the United States), two cases of anaphylaxis were reported after administration of 61,000 doses (0.003%).[403–406] In a large series using Air Force recruits, serious allergic reactions attributable to toxoid occurred in 0.001%.[407] In the United States, passive surveillance for the years 1991 to 1995 revealed 1.6 serious allergic reactions (equivalent of laryngospasm, bronchospasm, or anaphylaxis) reported per million doses of publicly distributed Td.

Although true acute sensitivity resulting in anaphylaxis is apparently rare, skin testing has been urged in management of patients with a history suggestive of such a reaction.[376, 408] In a study of Air Force recruits with a history of an anaphylactic-type adverse event after a prior tetanus toxoid dose, skin testing revealed negative responses to an intradermal skin test in 94 of 95. All recruits tolerated full-dose challenges of toxoid, suggesting lack of IgE-mediated hypersensitivity in the prior reported reaction. Positive test responses were found in people who subsequently tolerated full-dose challenges.[376] Because of the nonspecificity of skin test reactions, undue weight should not be put on skin test results alone.[409] However, caution is indicated because anaphylaxis while undergoing skin testing was reported in 3 of 200 people with a history of sensitivity[408] and has been seen by others.[402]

In eliciting a history of allergic reactions to tetanus toxoid, attention should be paid to details of the injection and of the reaction. One potential problem with purported reaction histories in older subjects may be confusion by the recipient of equine antitoxin or other immunizations with tetanus toxoid. An adverse event after a "tetanus shot" received before tetanus toxoid became available in 1938 would suggest that equine antitoxin or some other product was received. If a patient in need of tetanus toxoid presents with a history of severe local reactions consistent with an Arthus response, no toxoid booster should be given unless 10 years or more have elapsed since the last dose. When the event history is consistent with an immediate hypersensitivity reaction, testing for serum antitoxin level would be helpful to evaluate the need for a booster of toxoid, but such results are unlikely to be rapidly available in an emergency wound care setting. Skin testing before challenge (in the presence of resuscitation medication and equipment) could be attempted if time is available (Table 18–6). If not, or if there is a substantial response on skin testing such that a challenge is not considered prudent or if there is a strongly suggestive history of acute sensitivity, use of TIG should be considered. In an individual presenting for a routine booster dose with such a history, antitoxin determination and skin testing, preferably followed by monitored challenge, would be helpful in management of the patient.

Immunization in pregnancy has rarely been related to mild hemolytic disease of the newborn when toxoid is used that is produced with use of media containing human blood group–related antigens (such as beef heart infusion).[410, 411] Because of the exclusion of these substances in growth media for U.S. manufacturers, this has not been a relevant issue in the United States and can be similarly avoided elsewhere if producers adhere to WHO standards.

Simultaneous Administration with Other Vaccines

Tetanus toxoid has been combined with diphtheria toxoid, pertussis vaccines (both whole-cell and acellular),

Table 18–6. **PROTOCOL FOR SKIN TESTING FOR ACUTE HYPERSENSITIVITY AND CHALLENGE TO TETANUS TOXOID***

STEP	PREPARATION	VOLUME (mL)	CONCENTRATION	ROUTE
1	TT, fluid	—	1:10	Prick
2	TT, fluid	0.02	1:100,000	ID
3	TT, fluid	0.02	1:10,000	ID
4	TT, fluid	0.02	1:1000	ID
5	TT, fluid	0.02	1:100	ID
6	Td, adsorbed	0.02	1:10	SC
7	Td, adsorbed	0.1	1:10	SC
8	Td, adsorbed	0.1	Full strength	SC
9	Td, adsorbed	0.4	Full strength	SC

*Wait 15 minutes between steps for observation of reaction.

ID, intradermal injection; SC, subcutaneous; Td, tetanus and diphtheria toxoids; TT, tetanus toxoid.

Modified from Jacobs RL, Lowe RS, Lanier BQ. Adverse reactions to tetanus toxoid. JAMA 247:40–42, 1982; and Mansfield LE, Ting S, Rawls DO, Frederick R. Systemic reactions during cutaneous testing for tetanus toxoid hypersensitivity. Ann Allergy 57:135–137, 1986.

and Hib conjugate vaccines without compromising the immune response or substantially enhancing adverse events associated with the tetanus component (see under Available Preparations). Combination with whole-cell pertussis vaccines enhances the serological response to diphtheria and tetanus toxoids because of the adjuvant properties of whole-cell vaccines.

With the use of *H. influenzae* type b polysaccharide conjugate vaccine covalently linked to tetanus toxoid (PRP-T), theoretical concerns were raised whether tetanus toxoid in the conjugate vaccine could inhibit or enhance a response to tetanus toxoid. These concerns have not been shown to be clinically relevant. Initial antitoxin responses are slightly higher after simultaneous administration of DTP vaccines with PRP-T compared with DTP alone, but overall antitoxin levels are well above protective levels regardless of whether or not DTP is administered with PRP-T. Maternally acquired tetanus antitoxin does not interfere with the immune response to PRP-T.[412] PRP-T alone induces a substantial tetanus antitoxin response but lower than the response to tetanus toxoid[413]; thus, PRP-T vaccines cannot substitute for tetanus toxoid. Use of simultaneous PRP-T with DTP does not appear to increase the frequency of common adverse events and does not appear to differ in this respect from other Hib conjugate vaccines.[414] DTP combined with PRP-T vaccine in the same syringe is equivalent in immunogenicity and safety to DTP with PRP-T vaccine administered separately.[415, 416]

Contraindications and Precautions

A careful history of possible adverse events is necessary because many patients may have confused equine antitoxin with toxoid. Conditions recognized by the ACIP and the Committee on Infectious Diseases of the AAP as contraindications to the use of tetanus toxoid include a history of severe hypersensitivity or a neurological event after a prior dose.[135, 344] The evaluation should distinguish between a neurologic illness in which further doses are contraindicated and other syndromes, such as syncope, in which they are not. When toxoid is contraindicated, TIG should be given if immune status is unknown and a wound occurs that is not clean and minor. TIG is not necessary for clean and minor wounds. Delayed-type hypersensitivity to thimerosal is not a contraindication.

Although studies have failed to suggest that tetanus toxoid with or without diphtheria toxoid is teratogenic or has any other harmful effect when it is given in pregnancy,[417, 418] in industrialized nations, when providers believe that the woman will return for visits later in pregnancy, it may be prudent to delay immunization to the second trimester to minimize any concern about a theoretical possibility of a relationship with any observed birth defect.

Future Vaccines

Although previous work with high-potency tetanus toxoid has yielded small hope for widescale use,[243, 312–314] high-dose toxoid (250 Lf) has been under investigation to reduce the number of doses needed for primary immunization.[419] Another potential means of reducing the number of tetanus toxoid doses needed is through microencapsulation in a time-release combination of small and large microparticles.[420–422] Microencapsulation allows gradual or pulsed antigen release in parenteral vaccination and also permits the eventual possibility of vaccination by the oral route.[423] In one study, rats that received a single dose of encapsulated toxoid attained equivalent protection against a lethal challenge and equivalent serological responses to those of rats that received three doses of adsorbed toxoid.[422]

Future tetanus toxoid–containing vaccines may be made more simply from genetically altered *C. tetani*, which produces inactive toxin, simplifying production of an effective immunobiological, or by similar molecular technology. Some research has begun into expression of a cloned nontoxic fragment C of tetanus toxin[424–426]; other means of producing nontoxic subunit tetanus vaccines are possible. Researchers have successfully vaccinated mice against lethal challenges of tetanus toxin using carrier bacteria containing the gene segment coding for tetanus toxin fragment C by oral or intravenous vaccination with live attenuated *Salmonella* or intranasal vaccination with *Lactobacillus*.[427, 428]

TETANUS PROPHYLAXIS IN WOUND MANAGEMENT

Although some acute injuries result in wounds that are more likely than others to be contaminated with tetanus spores (e.g., contaminated by soil or feces), an individual who presents for medical care with any type of wound should be evaluated for tetanus prophylaxis. Removal of foreign bodies and débridement of devitalized tissue in a timely fashion have been routinely recommended to prevent reduction of the partial pressure of oxygen as well as co-contamination with other bacterial species.[429–432] Drainage and irrigation should be performed if necessary.

The patient's immunization status requires careful evaluation, including the number of prior doses as well as the time interval since the last dose of toxoid. In the 1950s, it was recommended and common practice to provide a booster dose of toxoid for every wound if more than a year had elapsed since the last dose. The frequency of Arthus-type reactions and examination of antitoxin level kinetics led to a reappraisal of this practice and yielded the current schedule.[239, 324, 328, 343, 374] Recommendations for the use of tetanus toxoid and TIG in the United States for tetanus prophylaxis in the management of wounds have been made by the ACIP and agree with those of the AAP and the Committee on Trauma of the American College of Surgeons.[135, 344, 432] The recommendations of the ACIP are given in Table 18–7.

Although any wound can potentially give rise to tetanus infection, clean wounds are considered to have a low likelihood both of contamination by tetanus spores and of leading to an environment that would support

Table 18–7. **SUMMARY GUIDE TO TETANUS PROPHYLAXIS IN ROUTINE WOUND MANAGEMENT**

HISTORY OF ADSORBED TETANUS TOXOID (DOSES)	CLEAN, MINOR WOUNDS		ALL OTHER WOUNDS*	
	Td†	TIG	Td†	TIG
Unknown or <3	Yes	No	Yes	Yes
≥3‡	No§	No	No‖	No

*Such as, but not limited to, wounds contaminated with dirt, feces, soil, saliva; puncture wounds; avulsions; and wounds resulting from missiles, crushing, burns, and frostbite.

†For children younger than 7 years, DTaP (DT, if pertussis vaccine is contraindicated) is preferred to tetanus toxoid alone. For people 7 years of age and older, Td is preferred to tetanus toxoid alone. Diphtheria and tetanus toxoids and whole-cell pertussis vaccine (DTP) may be used instead of DTaP.

‡If only three doses of *fluid* toxoid have been received, then a fourth dose of toxoid, preferably an adsorbed toxoid, should be given.

§Yes, if more than 10 years since last dose.

‖Yes, if more than 5 years since last dose. (More frequent boosters are not needed and can accentuate side effects.)

From ACIP. Diphtheria, tetanus and pertussis: Guidelines for vaccine prophylaxis and other preventive measures. Recommendations of the Advisory Committee on Immunization Practices (ACIP). MMWR Morb Mortal Wkly Rep 40(RR-10):1–28, 1991.

germination of spores. For people with this category of wounds, Td is recommended if the patient has received fewer than three doses of adsorbed toxoid in the past or it has been more than 10 years since the previous toxoid dose; TIG administration is not necessary. Most individuals will have protective antitoxin levels before exposure, and individuals with three or more prior doses of toxoid respond within 7 days or less to subsequent doses.[433–435] There is experimental evidence suggesting that protection begins before a detectable rise in antitoxin level.[436] Because tetanus is unusual after complete primary immunization, an anamnestic response has been proposed to occur in those with lower antibody levels,[349] but other mechanisms could also be important.

Most patients who had received fluid toxoid in the past and less commonly individuals who received adsorbed toxoid may have circulating antitoxin levels below 0.01 IU/mL after 5 years.[328, 343, 346] Therefore, it is recommended that people with wounds that are at higher risk of contamination receive a dose of toxoid if more than 5 years has elapsed since the last dose. Individuals with such wounds are also potential candidates for TIG if the immunization history indicates fewer than three prior toxoid doses. When administered at a separate site, TIG does not interfere with the immune response to adsorbed tetanus toxoid.[221, 225, 240] A dot-EIA has recently been proposed as a means of rapidly assessing the status of a person presenting for wound management.[437]

In individuals with human immunodeficiency virus (HIV) infection or with significant immunoglobulinopathy, an immune response to tetanus toxoid may not be optimal; therefore, although toxoid is not contraindicated, TIG should be given with toxoid to such an individual if a wound occurs that is not clean and minor.[431, 438] TIG is not needed in HIV patients with clean and minor wounds. Antibody responses of children with acquired immunodeficiency syndrome (AIDS) to tetanus toxoid are lower than in age-matched control subjects. Most children perinatally infected with HIV respond appropriately to infant immunization with tetanus toxoid–containing vaccines. The immune response in symptomatic HIV-infected adults is decreased.[439]

The dose of TIG necessary for adequate passive immunity is somewhat controversial.[440] In the United States, an intramuscular dose of 250 units (1 mL) is recommended by the ACIP and 250 to 500 IU by the American College of Surgeons. A dose of 250 to 400 IU will induce levels above 0.01 IU/mL for 4 weeks in almost all individuals.[225, 441–445] However, there have been reported tetanus cases in individuals with circulating levels of antitoxin above 0.01 IU/mL at the time of diagnosis.[93–99] In addition, fatal tetanus has been reported despite prophylactic receipt of 250 IU of TIG.[446] Doses of 400 IU may induce protective levels earlier than 250 IU.[447] However, by 3 days, virtually all people who received 250 IU will have protective levels of antitoxin (0.01 IU/mL). Therefore, whereas 250 IU seems to be a reasonable prophylactic dose in general, when it is indicated in wound management, use of 400 to 500 IU can be supported.

Before the wide availability of TIG, antibiotics were used for tetanus prophylaxis in wound management as a substitute for or adjunct to equine antitoxin.[448] Smith[449] and earlier researchers demonstrated the efficacy of prophylactic antibiotics in animal models. However, although the prevention of tetanus may be aided, efficacy superior or equal to that of antitoxin was not proved.[450, 451] Antimicrobials may sensitize patients and are not currently recommended for tetanus prophylaxis per se.[429, 450] Instead, careful observation of the wound by the patient or physician and early treatment of infection, if it occurs, is indicated.

On the basis of the analyses of U.S. cases reported in 1982 to 1994, many individuals who subsequently developed tetanus received less than the recommended prophylactic care when medical treatment was sought for wounds.[33, 158–161] Two studies suggest that when patients with wounds do seek care in the United States, 1 to 6% receive fewer prophylactic measures than recommended and 12 to 17% receive more than recommended, that is, Td with or without TIG when not indicated.[452, 453] This problem has been described outside the United States also.[454] Education of physicians regarding the recommendations should decrease the level of inappropriate prophylactic care.

PUBLIC HEALTH PERSPECTIVE

Epidemiological Results of Vaccination

The health burden of tetanus is totally preventable through immunization. Tetanus toxoid is one of the most effective biologicals available; with few doses, the toxoid produces long-term immunity and causes few significant adverse reactions. Elimination of environmental exposure to the causative agent is not feasible; however, total prevention of disease is essentially possible with universal immunization of target populations.

The current epidemiology of tetanus reflects the immunization programs in place. In developed countries, cases of tetanus are now considered rare.[31, 33, 33a, 151–153] The situation in the United States indicates that overall declines in tetanus incidence and mortality (see Fig. 18–2) were accelerated with the onset of routine immunization. In particular, the decline in age group–specific incidence rates is more evident in the younger populations that were vaccinated (see Fig. 18–3). In 1996, the United States was able to declare the absence of reported cases in people younger than 15 years.[455]

The majority of European countries have a reported annual incidence below 0.10 per 100,000 population. The current age distribution of tetanus in developed nations reflects incomplete toxoid coverage, as discussed earlier regarding the United States, with the predominance of cases occurring in the elderly.[31, 151–153] Those European countries with crude incidence rates higher than 0.10 are in southern, central, and eastern Europe, for which differences in soil exposure or bacterial concentration of *C. tetani* could also play a role. Selected countries within Europe continue to report incidence rates in excess of 0.20 per 100,000, including some European developing nations where childhood immunization services have not been completely implemented. Neonatal tetanus continues to be reported from four to six European countries per year, although underreporting is likely; Albania and Turkey report the highest incidence rates of neonatal tetanus at 0.05 to 0.10 per 1000 live births.[456]

WHO has used reported coverage in pregnant women to project the proportion of infants protected at birth, together with background estimates of incidence in the absence of immunization, to estimate the number of cases and deaths due to neonatal tetanus prevented. As toxoid coverage in pregnant women and women of childbearing age has increased, the number of cases of tetanus prevented has increased. In 1997, an estimated 867,000 deaths due to neonatal tetanus were prevented by immunization; an estimated 255,000 deaths occurred.

Disease Control Strategies

The majority of tetanus cases occur in individuals who are not adequately immunized. For further progress in tetanus prevention in the United States, the top priority is completion of routine Td immunization of adult populations, particularly the elderly who have never previously received three doses of toxoid. Scrupulous attention to appropriate wound prophylaxis will also aid in further reductions. Although a higher proportion of tetanus cases occurring in developed nations is associated with minor acute wounds and with nonacute wounds than in the past, most cases continue to be associated with acute trauma.[31, 33] If care for wounds has been sought, tetanus can occur in those individuals who have not received the recommended tetanus prophylaxis in wound management.

Serosurveys for the prevalence of tetanus antitoxin show a direct relationship between absence of protective levels, lack of prior immunization (which is age related), and the distribution of tetanus cases.[176, 177, 179–182, 185, 457–461] In the developed world, the lowest seroprevalence rates and highest incidence rates occur in elderly individuals. Although elderly individuals may have a lessened immune response to antigenic stimulation, primary immunization and booster schedules confer adequate protection against tetanus.[179, 333, 334, 339–341, 460, 461] The ACIP and the American College of Physicians now make specific recommendations for routine primary tetanus and diphtheria immunization of susceptible adults; adult immunization against several diseases has received more emphasis than in the past.[351, 462]

A comprehensive approach to vaccinations has also been recommended for younger people corresponding to recommended ages for physician visits.[135, 290, 291, 462] All people should complete primary immunization against tetanus and diphtheria; after childhood immunization with four or five doses of tetanus toxoid–containing vaccines, a booster dose of Td is currently recommended at the adolescent healthcare visit at 11 to 12 years of age.[290] This is opportune, because the 1988 to 1991 serosurvey indicated that 20% of children 10 to 16 years of age did not have a protective level of antibody as defined.[183] All people providing healthcare to older adolescents and adults should review the immunization status of patients and provide Td as well as measles, rubella, influenza, pneumococcal, and hepatitis B antigens, when indicated.

The most important issue in tetanus control globally is the prevention of neonatal tetanus by vaccination of pregnant women and women of childbearing age (see following section, *Neonatal Tetanus Elimination*). However, nonneonatal tetanus will continue to occur unless susceptible individuals of all ages are inoculated. Remedial mass immunization campaigns have been shown to be cost-beneficial in some nations.[463, 464] Routine vaccination with three doses of DTP in the first year of life under the EPI should ensure immune childhood populations. Indeed, global coverage of children with DTP has increased and has been estimated to exceed 80%.[456] Given the long duration of immunity even in the absence of reinforcing or booster doses, many of the infants immunized should retain protection into the teenage years and, in some, longer. Appropriate surveillance can determine the extent of the tetanus problem in adults and the need to implement programs for appropriate wound prophylaxis and routine immunization of adults other than women of childbearing age.

Use of tetanus toxoid is highly cost-effective. Routine toxoid use in pregnant women costs $2 to $82 (in circa 1972 dollars) to prevent a case of neonatal tetanus in the developing world; combination of this approach with mass inoculation campaigns of women of childbearing age increases costs—approximately twice as much per case averted—but may be more effective in reducing morbidity and mortality by increasing overall immunity.[465–467] Even under the best circumstances of treatment, tetanus remains associated with a significant case-fatality rate. The cost of care for patients can exceed $150,000.[468]

Neonatal Tetanus Elimination

The current global health burden of tetanus exists primarily in the developing world, manifested predominantly as neonatal tetanus. The EPI was launched in 1974 to improve child health by increasing global immunization levels. The WHO included prevention of neonatal tetanus as one of the objectives of the EPI, recommending administration of at least two doses of tetanus toxoid at least 4 weeks apart to pregnant women and advocating training of traditional birth attendants.[215] In 1980, global tetanus toxoid use in pregnant women (two or more doses) was reported to be 4%; by 1988, use had increased to 20%; despite declines in reported neonatal tetanus in many areas, an estimated 787,000 neonatal tetanus deaths (about 6.5 cases per 1000 live births) occurred globally in that year.[469, 470] This improvement in status, however, encouraged the World Health Assembly in 1989 to formulate a goal to eliminate neonatal tetanus worldwide by 1995.[471, 472] In 1993, the elimination of neonatal tetanus as a significant public health problem was defined as less than 1 case of neonatal tetanus for every 1000 live births per year in each administrative district throughout the world.[473]

In addition to expanding vaccination of women to other routine healthcare encounters besides pregnancy, this current WHO initiative emphasizes attention to hygienic delivery practices ("clean" hands, "clean" delivery surface, "clean" cord-cutting and care, which includes the use of local antibiotics) and improved surveillance to identify "high-risk" areas and take appropriate action. The estimated proportion of pregnant women who have access to "clean" deliveries has not increased greatly since 1989 and remains well below 50% globally.[469, 474] Although immunization is more effective per se than the presence of trained attendants, training of traditional birth attendants lowers overall neonatal mortality due to tetanus and also other infections.[280, 475–477] Topical antibiotics have been shown to be an additional protective factor in neonatal tetanus prevention. Two case-control studies have suggested that the use of antiseptics or topical antibiotics at the time of delivery and in postnatal care decreased the risk of neonatal tetanus by up to two thirds; dry cord care in itself did not appear to be a protective factor.[478, 479] On the basis of these findings, a comprehensive approach using immunization of women of childbearing age, attended birth, clean delivery practices, improved cord care by the avoidance of contaminated substances, and topical antimicrobials can provide optimal protection against neonatal tetanus.

Since the elimination goal was set, the reported coverage of pregnant women with two or more doses of tetanus toxoid has not exceeded 50% in the developing world.[456, 469] However, coverage among pregnant women may underestimate the true protection of infants because many women may have received toxoid during childhood or in other health encounters or in mass campaigns. Such women, if they were not immunized during pregnancy, would be considered unimmunized in these coverage reports.[475, 480, 481] WHO currently recommends assessing progress in neonatal tetanus elimination programs by the use of the mother's cumulative immunization history to determine the proportion of children protected at birth. This can be done at the same time as EPI immunization coverage is measured in the childhood population (at 12 to 23 months of age) by using cluster surveys that include a sample of children younger than 12 months and determining the immunization status of their mothers at the time the children were born.[482] Serosurveys allow an immunological assessment of the true protection of mothers and presumably infants without the difficulties in obtaining and interpreting immunization histories of mothers.[270, 481, 483, 484] A study recently performed in Burundi confirmed the correlation of serological protection with the child's estimated "protection at birth" based on cumulative maternal immunization history by maternal recall.[481] WHO also encourages the routine monitoring of the immune status of individual women by eliciting their lifetime history of tetanus toxoid at the time when a child presents for the first dose of DTP[473]; inadequately immunized women who do not have contraindications should be immunized at that health encounter.

The immunization of all women of childbearing age regardless of whether they are pregnant can be more effective than limiting vaccination to pregnant women.[475] Such a strategy circumvents poor access to health services and decreases missed opportunities.[485] Many countries demonstrated substantial progress in controlling neonatal tetanus when they began immunizing all women of childbearing age whenever possible, whether or not they were pregnant, with booster inoculation offered during pregnancy.[215, 282, 474–476] The approach of focusing on "high-risk" districts (see later) and the use of mass vaccination campaigns for women of childbearing age have greatly helped in making substantial progress.[480, 486–492] Immunization schedules have been developed to take account of the mother's prior immunization status[178] (see Table 18–4). In addition, vaccination of women of childbearing age will address tetanus after wounds occurring in women and tetanus related to induced or spontaneous septic abortions or puerperal infection.[493] It has been estimated that there are 15,000 to 30,000 cases of maternal tetanus each year; a review of the published reports of cases indicated that 27% occurred after abortion and 67% occurred in the postpartum period.[494]

The major current strategy for neonatal tetanus elimination (the high-risk approach) is to focus available public health resources on districts with a reported incidence of disease of more than 1 case per 1000 births.[480, 486–492] Because deficient surveillance may fail to identify many high-risk districts, since 1994, districts have been targeted with other indicators suggesting that there probably is a substantial disease burden. These other indicators include rural setting or underserved periurban area, poor sanitation, low tetanus toxoid coverage among pregnant women, and low rate of deliveries attended by a trained birth attendant.[480, 488–492] Once identified, all women of childbearing age are immunized through focal mass campaigns. Ideally, three rounds of immunization are performed, appropriately spaced to provide effective and long-term protection. Since 1994, more countries have taken this approach; for example, China has immunized 10 million women of childbearing age with such campaigns in 560 high-risk districts.[486] The WHO Region of the Americas (Pan American Health Organization) systematically targeted neonatal tetanus using the high-risk approach in 16 countries of the region.[490] From 1992 to 1996, a decrease occurred in the proportion of districts with an incidence of neonatal tetanus of 1 case or more per 1000 live births from 2.5% to 1.0%. Maintenance of this control and elimination are the important next steps and will require further efforts to focus on specific high-risk subgroups within urban areas as well as ensuring that all women who have routine contact with the healthcare system are immunized.

Improved detection of neonatal tetanus cases after implementing the high-risk approach helps to focus intervention activities to the areas and populations of greatest need.[286] Case investigations allow determination of whether the case occurred as a result of failure to access the healthcare system by the mother or failure of the health services to provide toxoid during visits by the mother (missed opportunities).[270, 286, 485]

Although the global elimination goal was not met by the target date, more than 110 developing and developed countries and territories (Fig. 18–4) have succeeded in reaching the WHO definition of elimination—less than 1 case per 1000 live births for all districts—and more than 50 other countries are approaching the target.[469] Nevertheless, 255,000 deaths from neonatal tetanus are estimated to have occurred in 1997. Sixty-five countries and territories do not claim to approach elimination of neonatal tetanus; 26 of these account for 90% of all estimated cases, and 16 of these 26 are in the African continent. In the coming years, WHO emphasis will be placed on seeking partners to support the national programs in these 26 countries.

Two doses of tetanus toxoid, optimally given 4 weeks or more apart with the second at least 2 weeks before delivery, significantly reduce mortality due to neonatal tetanus and confer an appropriate immune response for several years.[280, 330–332, 345a, 495–497] Nonetheless, cases of neonatal tetanus have been reported in children of vaccinated women.[96, 98, 195, 498–502] A case-control study in Bangladesh in 1990, conducted to evaluate risk factors for neonatal tetanus, estimated the efficacy of two doses of tetanus toxoid to be below 50%; a small serosurvey of vaccinated women was consistent with these findings.[195] Subsequent testing at a WHO reference laboratory of samples from three consecutive lots indicated no detectable toxoid potency; toxoid produced within Bangladesh was not subject to independent quality control review. Concerns about potential potency problems with production of tetanus toxoid in countries other than Bangladesh triggered a review by WHO of the quality control procedures in 22 countries with reported neonatal tetanus that produced tetanus toxoid; only four of these countries had a functioning national control authority. Eighty lots of toxoid from 21 manufacturers in 14 of those countries were tested for potency; 15 of the 80 failed to meet WHO minimum potency standards.[503] Efforts have been made to initiate and strengthen the biologicals control authorities in these countries. Unfortunately, problems with potency of tetanus toxoid continue to be reported because of the use of standards that do not comply with WHO requirements or because adequate testing of vaccines has not been done.

Other potential reasons for apparent toxoid failure include poor toxoid handling (particularly repeated freezing),[7, 245–248] use of inadequate immunization sched-

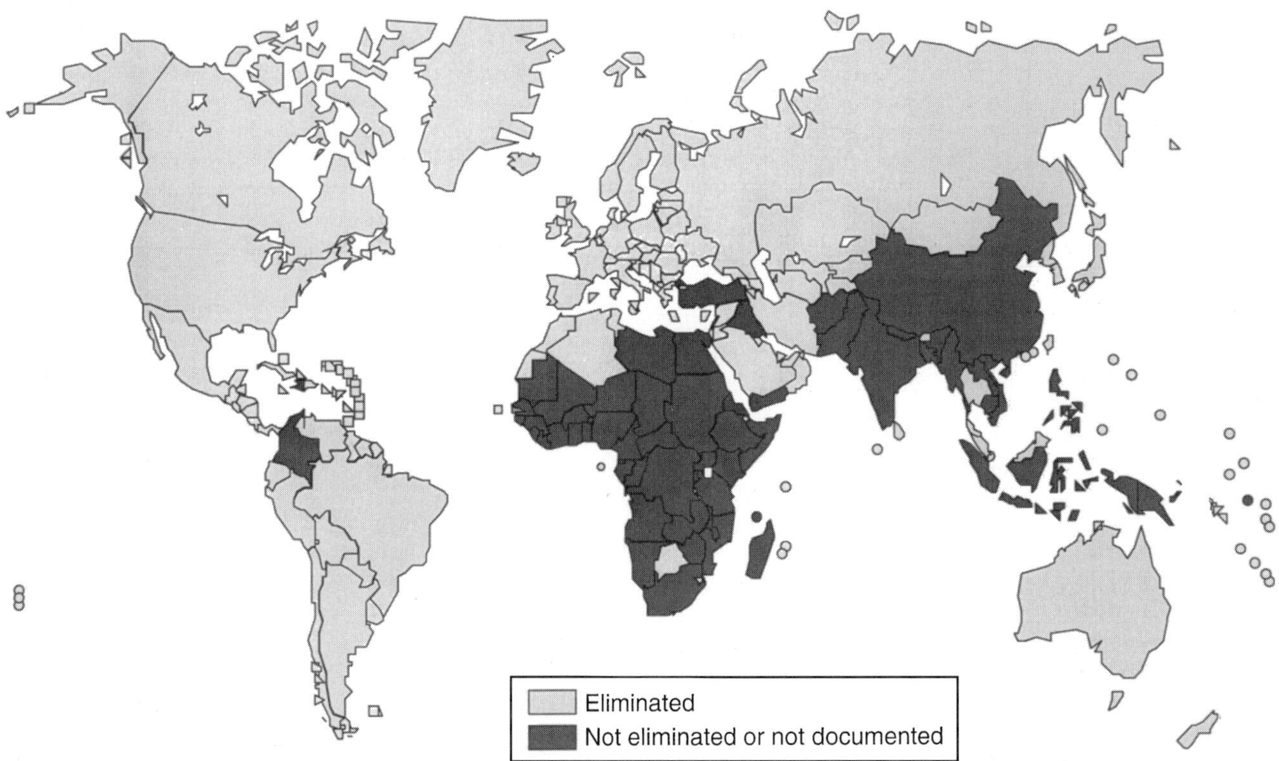

Figure 18–4. Global neonatal tetanus elimination status, by country, 1997. *Elimination* is defined as less than 1 case per 1000 live births in each district of the country.

ules with inappropriately short intervals between doses,[248] and inaccurate histories of prior vaccination. Decreased transport of antitoxin across the placenta in some populations[504, 505] or unusually high toxin challenges that overcome maternal antitoxin may play some role in a small proportion of apparent failures of toxoid to prevent neonatal tetanus. A review by Dietz and colleagues[248] of other factors that may affect the response to tetanus toxoid indicated that malarial infection may decrease, malarial chemoprophylaxis may enhance, and malnutrition may not substantially affect an immune response. Case investigations and the use of other indicators are critical to determine whether the predominant cause of neonatal tetanus in a given area is vaccine failure or failure to vaccinate. Available data suggest that lack of adequate vaccination is a far bigger cause of neonatal tetanus than is vaccine failure.

The four major constraints to reaching the objective of the elimination of neonatal tetanus as a significant health problem in some high-risk countries are (1) limited national funds to acquire potent tetanus toxoid and autodestruct syringes to perform repeated rounds of immunization, (2) lack of adequate healthcare infrastructure, (3) civil unrest, and (4) lack of political commitment due to underreporting from weak surveillance and competing health priorities.[470]

REFERENCES

1. Carle A, Rattone G. Studio sperimentale sull'etiologia del tetano. G Accad Med Torrino 32:174, 1884.
2. Nicolaier A. Über infectiösen Tetanus. Dtsch Med Wochenschr 10:842–844, 1884.
3. Rosenbach. Zur Aetiologie des Wundstarrkrampfes beim Menschen. Arch Klin Chir 34:306–317, 1886.
4. Kitasato S. Über den Tetanusbacillus. Z Hyg 7:225–234, 1889.
5. von Behring E, Kitasato S. Über das Zustandekommen der Diphtherie-Immunität bei Thieren. Dtsch Med Wochenschr 16:1113–1114, 1890.
6. Descombey P. L'anatoxine tetanique. Can R Soc Biol 91:239–241, 1924.
7. Weinstein L. Tetanus. N Engl J Med 289:1293–1296, 1973.
8. Kryzhanovsky GN. Pathophysiology. In Veronesi R (ed). Tetanus, Important New Concepts. Amsterdam, Excerpta Medica, 1981, pp 109–182.
9. Bruce D. Tetanus. J Hyg (Camb) 19:1–32, 1920.
10. Garcia-Palmieri MR, Ramirez R. Generalized tetanus: Analysis of 202 cases. Ann Intern Med 47:721–730, 1957.
11. Adams EB. The prognosis and prevention of tetanus. S Afr Med J 42:739–743, 1968.
12. Patel JC, Mehta BC, Modi KN. Prognosis in tetanus. In Patel JC (ed). Proceedings of the International Conference on Tetanus, 1963. Bombay, PH Ramans Printers, 1965, p 181.
13. Buchanan TM, Brooks GF, Martin S, Bennett JV. Tetanus in the United States, 1968 and 1969. J Infect Dis 122:564–567, 1970.
14. Blake PA, Feldman RA. Tetanus in the United States 1970–1971. J Infect Dis 131:745–748, 1975.
15. Millard AH. Local tetanus. Lancet 2:844–846, 1954.
16. Roistacher K, Griffin JW. Local tetanus. Johns Hopkins Med J 149:84–88, 1981.
17. Pratt EL. Clinical tetanus: A study of fifty-six cases with special reference to methods of prevention and a plan for evaluating treatment. JAMA 129:1243–1247, 1945.
18. Kerr JH, Corbett JL, Prys-Roberts C, et al. Involvement of the sympathetic nervous system in tetanus: Studies on 82 cases. Lancet 2:236–241, 1968.
19. Zacks SI, Shef MF. Tetanus toxin: Fine structure, localization of binding sites in striated muscle. Science 159:643–644, 1968.
20. Kanarek DJ, Kaufman B, Zwi S. Severe sympathetic hyperactivity associated with tetanus. Arch Intern Med 132:602–604, 1973.
21. Hollow VM, Clarke GM. Autonomic manifestations of tetanus. Anaesth Intensive Care 3:142–147, 1975.
22. Buchanan N, Cane GW, DeAndrade M. Autonomic dsyfunction in tetanus: The effects of a variety of therapeutic agents, with special reference to morphine. Intensive Care Med 5:65–68, 1979.
23. Luisto M. Outcome and neurological sequelae of patients after tetanus. Acta Neurol Scand 80:504–511, 1989.
24. Luisto M, Seppalainen AM. Electroencephalopathy in tetanus. Acta Neurol Scand 80:157–161, 1989.
25. Luisto M, Zitting A, Tallroth K. Hyperostosis and osteoarthritis in patients surviving after tetanus. Skeletal Radiol 23:31–35, 1994.
26. Veronesi R, Focaccia R. The clinical picture. In Veronesi R (ed). Tetanus, Important New Concepts. Amsterdam, Excerpta Medica, 1981, pp 459–463.
27. Trujillo MJ, Castillo A, Espana JV, et al. Tetanus in the adult: Intensive care and management experience with 233 cases. Crit Care Med 8:419–423, 1980.
28. Garnier MJ. Tetanus in patients 3 years of age and up. Am J Surg 129:459–463, 1975.
29. Edmondson RS, Flowers MW. Intensive care in tetanus: Management, complications and mortality in 100 cases. Br Med J 1:1401–1404, 1979.
30. Humbert G, Fillastre JP, Dordain M, et al. One hundred cases of tetanus. Scand J Infect Dis 4:129–131, 1972.
31. Peetermans WE, Schepens D. Tetanus—still a topic of present interest: A report of 27 cases from a Belgian referral hospital. J Intern Med 239:249–252, 1996.
32. Sow PS, Diop BM, Barry HL, et al. Tetanos et pratiques traditionnelles a Dakar (a propos de 141 cas). Dakar Med 38:55–59, 1993.
33. Izurieta HS, Sutter RW, Strebel PM, et al. Tetanus surveillance—United States, 1991–1994. MMWR CDC Surveill Summ 46(SS-2):16–24, 1996.
33a. Bardenheier B, Prevots DR, Khetsuriani N, Wharton M. Tetanus surveillance—United States, 1995–1997. MMWR Morb Mortal Wkly Rep 47(SS-2):1–13, 1998.
34. Sutter RU, Cochi SL, Wassilak SG, et al. Epidemiology and therapy of tetanus in the United States, 1972–1986 [abstract 1382]. In Program and Abstracts of the 28th Interscience Conference on Antimicrobial Agents and Chemotherapy; Los Angeles, CA; October 23–26, 1988.
35. Yen LM, Dao LM, Day NPJ, et al. Role of quinine in the high mortality of intramuscular injection tetanus. Lancet 344:786–787, 1994.
36. Oyelami OA, Aladekomo TA, Ononye FO. A 10 year retrospective evaluation of cases of post neonatal tetanus seen in a paediatric unit of a university teaching hospital in southwestern Nigeria (1985 to 1994). Cent Afr J Med 42:73–75, 1996.
37. Jagoda A, Riggio S, Burguieres T. Cephalic tetanus: A case report and review of the literature. Am J Emerg Med 6:128–130, 1988.
38. Bizzini B. Tetanus. In Germanier R (ed). Bacterial Vaccines. Orlando, FL, Academic Press, 1984, pp 38–68.
39. Bytchenko B. Microbiology of tetanus. In Veronesi R (ed). Tetanus, Important New Concepts. Amsterdam, Excerpta Medica, 1981, pp 28–39.
40. Willis AT. *Clostridium:* The spore-bearing anaerobes. In Wilson G, Miles A, Parker MT (eds). Topley and Wilson's Principles of Bacteriology, Virology and Immunity. Vol. 2. Baltimore, Williams & Wilkins, 1983, pp 442–475.
41. Tulloch WJ. Report of bacteriological investigation of tetanus carried out on behalf of the war office committee for the study of tetanus. J Hyg (Camb) 18:103–202, 1919.
42. Sanada I, Nishida S. Isolation of *Clostridium tetani* from soil. J Bacteriol 89:626–629, 1965.
43. Ebisawa I, Kurata M. A quantitative study of *C. tetani* in the earth. In Nistico G, Mastroeni P, Pitzurra M (eds). Seventh International Conference on Tetanus; Copanello, Italy; September 10–15, 1984. Rome, Gangeni Publishing Company, 1985, pp 7–10.
44. Dubovsky J, Meyer K. The occurrence of *B. tetani* in soil and in vegetables. J Infect Dis 31:614–616, 1922.

45. Bytchenko B. Geographical distribution of tetanus in the world, 1951–60. Bull World Health Organ 34:71–104, 1966.
46. Smith LD. The occurrence of *Clostridium botulinum* and *Clostridium tetani* in the soil of the United States. Health Lab Sci 15:74–80, 1978.
47. Smith JWG. Tetanus. In Wilson G, Miles A, Parker MT (eds). Topley and Wilson's Principles of Bacteriology, Virology and Immunity. Vol. 3. Baltimore, Williams & Wilkins, 1984, pp 345–368.
48. Kerrin JC. The distribution of *B. tetani* in the intestines of animals. Br J Pathol 10:370–373, 1929.
49. TenBroeck C, Bauer JH. The tetanus bacillus as an intestinal saprophyte in man. J Exp Med 36:261–271, 1922.
50. TenBroeck C, Bauer JH. Studies on the relation of tetanus bacilli in the digestive tract to tetanus antitoxin in the blood. J Exp Med 37:479–489, 1923.
51. Coleman GE, Meyer KF. Study of tetanus agglutinins and antitoxin in human serums. J Infect Dis 39:332–336, 1926.
52. Bauer JH, Meyer KF. Human intestinal carriers of tetanus spores in California. J Infect Dis 38:295–305, 1926.
53. Kerrin JC. The incidence of *B. tetani* in human feces. Br J Pathol 9:69–71, 1928.
54. Bandmann F. Zum Nachweis von Tetanusbacillen im Darm von Ulcus- und Carcinomträgern. Z Hyg 136:559–567, 1953.
55. Lowbury EJL, Lilly HA. Contamination of operating-theatre air with *Cl. tetani.* Br Med J 2:1334–1336, 1958.
56. Gilles EC. The isolation of tetanus bacilli from street dust. JAMA 109:484–486, 1937.
57. Smith JWG. Tetanus and its prevention. Prog Drug Res 19:391–401, 1975.
58. Matsuda M, Yoneda M. Isolation and purification of two antigenically active, "complementary" polypeptide fragments of tetanus neurotoxin. Infect Immun 12:1147–1153, 1975.
59. Bizzini B. The chemistry of tetanus toxin as a basis for understanding its immunological and biological activities. In Nistico G, Mastroeni P, Pitzurra M (eds). Seventh International Conference on Tetanus; Copanello, Italy; September 10–15, 1984. Rome, Gangeni Publishing Company, 1985, pp 11–28.
60. Robinson JP, Hash JH. A review of the molecular structure of tetanus toxin. Mol Cell Biochem 48:33–44, 1982.
61. Schiavo G, Papini E, Genna G, Montecucco C. An intact interchain disulfide bond is required for the neurotoxicity of tetanus toxin. Infect Immun 58:4136–4141, 1990.
62. Ahnert-Hilger G, Dauzenroth MW, Habermann E, et al. Chains and fragments of tetanus toxin, and their contribution to toxicity. J Physiol 84:229–236, 1990.
63. Parton RG, Critchley DR, Ockleford CD. Tetanus toxin binding to mouse spinal cord cells. An evaluation of the role of gangliosides in toxin internalization. Brain Res 475:118–127, 1988.
64. Laird WJ, Aaronson W, Silver RP, et al. Plasmid-associated toxigenicity in *Clostridium tetani.* J Infect Dis 142:623, 1980.
65. Finn LW Jr, Silver RP, Habig HW, et al. The structural gene for tetanus neurotoxin is on a plasmid. Science 224:881–884, 1984.
66. Gill DM. Bacterial toxins: A table of lethal amount. Microbiol Rev 46:86–94, 1982.
67. Wright GP. The neurotoxins of *Clostridium botulinum* and *Clostridium tetani.* Pharmacol Rev 7:413–456, 1955.
68. Bulloch WE, Cramer W. On a new factor in the mechanism of bacterial infection. Proc R Soc B 90:513–528, 1919.
69. Eregie CO. Uvulectomy as an epidemiological factor in neonatal tetanus mortality: Observations from a cluster survey. West Afr J Med 13:56–58, 1994.
70. Abel JJ, Firor WM, Chalain W. Researches on tetanus. IX. Further evidence to show that tetanus toxin is not carried to central nervous by way of the axis cylinders of motor nerves. Bull Johns Hopkins Hosp 63:373–403, 1938.
71. Friedemann U, Zuger B, Hollander A. Investigations on the pathogenesis of tetanus. J Immunol 36:473–488, 1939.
72. Bizzini B. Tetanus toxin. Microbiol Rev 43:224–240, 1979.
73. Green J, Erdmann JG, Wellhoner HH. Is there retrograde axonal transport of tetanus toxin in both alpha and beta fibres? Nature 265:370, 1977.
74. Schwab ME, Thoenen H. Selective binding, uptake and retrograde transport of tetanus toxin by nerve terminals in the rat iris. J Cell Biol 77:1–13, 1978.
75. Fedinec AA. Current studies on pathogenesis of tetanus. In Nistico G, Mastroeni P, Pitzurra M (eds). Seventh International Conference on Tetanus; Copanello, Italy; September 10–15, 1984. Rome, Gangeni Publishing Company, 1985, pp 61–68.
76. Price DL, Griffin JW, Young A, et al. Tetanus toxin: Direct evidence for retrograde axonal transport. Science 188:945–957, 1975.
77. Manning KA, Erichsen JT, Evinger C. Retrograde transneuronal transport properties of fragment C of tetanus toxin. Neuroscience 34:251–263, 1990.
78. Parton RG, Critchley DR, Ockleford CD. A study of the mechanism of internalisation of tetanus toxin by primary mouse spinal cord cultures. J Neurochem 49:1057–1068, 1987.
79. Sanford JP. Tetanus—forgotten but not gone [editorial]. N Engl J Med 332:812–813, 1995.
80. Habig WH, Nelson PG, Hardegree MC, et al. Tetanus toxin in dissociated spinal cord cultures: Long-term characterization of form and action. J Neurochem 47:930–937, 1986.
81. Empson RM, Gutnick MJ, Jefferys JG, Amitai Y. Injection of tetanus toxin into the neocortex elicits persistent epileptiform activity but only transient impairment of GABA release. Neuroscience 57:235–239, 1993.
82. Brooks VB, Curtis DR, Eccles JC. Mode of action of tetanus toxin. Nature 175:120–121, 1955.
83. Brooks VB, Asanuma H. Action of tetanus toxin in the cerebral cortex. Science 137:674–676, 1962.
84. Bergey GK, Nelson PG, Bigalke H. Differential effects of tetanus toxin on inhibitory and excitatory synaptic transmission in mammalian spinal cord neurons in culture: A presynaptic locus of action for tetanus toxin. J Neurophysiol 57:121–131, 1987.
85. Schiavo G, Benfenati R, Poulain B, et al. Tetanus and botulism-B neurotoxins block neurotransmitter release by proteolytic cleavage of synaptobrevin. Nature 359:832–835, 1992.
86. Cornille F, Fournie-Zaluski MC, Roques BP, et al. Cooperative exosite-dependent cleavage of synaptobrevin by tetanus toxin light chain. J Biol Chem 272:3459–3464, 1997.
87. Bleck TP. Tetanus: Pathophysiology, management, and prophylaxis. Dis Mon 37:545–603, 1991.
88. Bleck TP. Pharmacology of tetanus. Clin Neuropharmacol 9:103–120, 1986.
89. Boyd RE, Brennan PT, Denj J-F, et al. Strychnine poisoning. Am J Med 74:507–512, 1983.
90. Wellhoner JJ. Tetanus neurotoxin. Rev Physiol Biochem Pharmacol 93:1–68, 1982.
91. van Heyningen S. Tetanus toxin. Pharmacol Ther 11:141–157, 1980.
92. Alfery DD, Rauscher LA. Tetanus: A review. Crit Care Med 7:176–181, 1979.
93. Goulon M, Girard O, Grosbuis S, et al. Les anticorps antitetaniques. Nouv Presse Med 1:3049–3050, 1972.
94. Berger SA, Cherubin LE, Nelson S, et al. Tetanus despite preexisting antitetanus antibody. JAMA 240:769–770, 1978.
95. Passen EL, Andersen BR. Clinical tetanus despite a 'protective' level of toxin-neutralizing antibody. JAMA 255:1171–1173, 1986.
96. Masellle SY, Matre R, Mbise R, Hofstad T. Neonatal tetanus despite protective serum antitoxin concentration. FEMS Microbiol Immunol 3:171–175, 1991.
97. Crone NE, Reder AT. Severe tetanus in immunized patients with high anti-tetanus titers. Neurology 42:761–764, 1992.
98. de Moraes-Pinto MI. Neonatal tetanus despite immunization and protective antitoxin antibody. J Infect Dis 171:1076–1077, 1995.
99. Pryor T, Onarecker C, Coniglione T. Elevated antitoxin titers in a man with generalized tetanus. J Fam Pract 44:299–303, 1997.
100. Turner TB, Velasco-Joven EA, Prudovsky S. Studies on the prophylaxis and treatment of tetanus. II. Studies pertaining to treatment. Bull Johns Hopkins Hosp 102:71–84, 1958.
101. Steinegger T, Wiederkehr M, Ludin HP, Roth F. Elektromyogramm als diagnostische Hilfe beim Tetanus. Schweiz Med Wochenschr 126:379–385, 1996.
102. Apte NM, Karnad DR. Short report: The spatula test: A simple bedside test to diagnose tetanus. Am J Trop Med Hyg 53:386–387, 1995.
103. Smith WD, Tobias MA. Tetany, tetanus or drug reaction? Br J Anaesth 48:703–705, 1976.
104. Barnes V, Ware MR. Tetanus, pseudotetanus, or conversion disorder: A diagnostic dilemma? South Med J 86:591–592, 1993.

105. O'Keefe SJD, Wesley A, Jialal I, Epstein S. The metabolic response and problems with nutritional support in acute tetanus. Metabolism 33:482–487, 1984.
106. Bleck TP. *Clostridium tetani.* In Mandell GL, Bennett JE, Dolin R (eds). Principles and Practice of Infectious Diseases (4th ed). New York, Churchill Livingstone, 1995, pp 2173–2178.
107. Rey M, Diop-Mar I, Robert D. Treatment of tetanus. In Veronesi R (ed). Tetanus, Important New Concepts. Amsterdam, Excerpta Medica, 1981, pp 207–237.
108. Tallman JF, Gallager DW. The GABA-ergic system: A locus of benzodiazepine action. Annu Rev Neurosci 8:21–44, 1985.
109. Davidoff RA. Antispasticity drugs: Mechanisms of action. Ann Neurol 17:107–116, 1985.
110. Curtis DR, Lodge D, Bornstein JL, et al. Selective effects of (−)-baclofen on spinal synaptic transmission in the cat. Exp Brain Res 42:158–170, 1981.
111. Joseph A, Pulimood BM. Use of diazepam in tetanus—a comparative study. Indian J Med Res 68:489–491, 1978.
112. Dasta JF, Brier KL, Kidwell GA, et al. Diazepam infusion in tetanus: Correlation of drug levels with effect. South Med J 74:278–280, 1981.
113. Tekur U, Gupta A, Tayal G, et al. Blood concentrations of diazepam and its metabolites in children and neonates with tetanus. J Pediatr 102:145–147, 1983.
114. Vassa T, Yajnik VH, Joshi KR, et al. Comparative clinical trial of diazepam with other conventional drugs in tetanus. Postgrad Med J 50:755–758, 1974.
115. Checketts MR, White RJ. Avoidance of intermittent positive pressure ventilation in tetanus with dantrolene therapy. Anaesthesia 48:969–971, 1993.
116. Borgeat A, Popovic V, Schwander D. Efficiency of a continuous infusion of propofol in a patient with tetanus. Crit Care Med 19:295–297, 1991.
117. Dianto, Mustadjab I. The influence of pyridoxin in the treatment of tetanus neonatorum. Paediatr Indones 31:165–169, 1991.
118. Caglar MK. Pyridoxine in the treatment of tetanus neonatorum. Paediatr Indones 29:233–236, 1989.
119. Paydas S, Akoglu TF, Akkiz H, et al. Mortality-lowering effect of systemic corticosteroid therapy in severe tetanus. Clin Ther 10:276–280, 1988.
120. Domenighetti GM, Savary G, Stricker H. Hyperadrenergic syndrome in severe tetanus: Extreme rise in catecholamines responsive to labetolol. Br Med J 288:1483–1484, 1984.
121. Rie M, Wilson RS. Morphine therapy controls autonomic hyperactivity in tetanus. Ann Intern Med 88:653–654, 1978.
122. Wright DK, Lalloo UG, Nayiager S, Govender P. Autonomic nervous system dysfunction in severe tetanus: Current perspectives. Crit Care Med 17:371–375, 1989.
123. Sutton DN, Tremlett MR, Woodcock TE, Nielsen MS. Management of autonomic dysfunction in severe tetanus: The use of magnesium sulfate and clonidine. Intensive Care Med 16:75–80, 1990.
124. Moughabghab AV, Prevost G, Socolovsky C. Fentanyl therapy controls autonomic hyperactivity in tetanus. Br J Clin Pract 50:477–478, 1996.
125. Shibuya M, Sugimoto H, Sugimoto T, et al. The use of continuous spinal anesthesia in severe tetanus with autonomic disturbance. J Trauma 29:1423–1429, 1989.
126. Hiraide A, Katayama M, Sugimoto H, et al. Metabolic changes in patients severely affected by tetanus. Ann Surg 213:66–69, 1991.
127. Mukherjee DR. Tetanus and tracheostomy. Ann Otol Rhinol Laryngol 86:67–72, 1977.
128. Bademosi O. The prognostic features of biochemical investigations in tetanus. Am J Med Sci 278:167–172, 1979.
129. Idoko JA, Amiobonomo AE, Anjorin FI, et al. Cerebrospinal fluid changes in tetanus: Raised proteins and immunoglobulins in patients with severe disease. Trans R Soc Trop Med Hyg 84:593–594, 1990.
130. Blake PA, Feldman RA, Buchanan TM, et al. Serologic therapy of tetanus in the United States, 1965–1971. JAMA 235:42–44, 1976.
131. Lee DC, Lederman HM. Anti-tetanus toxoid antibodies in intravenous gamma globulin: An alternative to tetanus immune globulin. J Infect Dis 166:642–645, 1992.
132. Moynihan NH. Serum-sickness and local reactions in tetanus prophylaxis. Lancet 2:264–266, 1955.
133. Merson MH, Hughs JM, Dowell VR, et al. Current trends in botulism in the United States. JAMA 229:1305–1308, 1974.
134. McCracken GH Jr, Dowell DL, Marschall FN. Double-blind trial of equine antitoxin and human immune globulin in tetanus neonatorum. Lancet 1:1146–1149, 1971.
135. Committee on Infectious Diseases, American Academy of Pediatrics. Peter G, Lepow ML, McCracken GH, Phillips CF (eds). Report of the Committee on Infectious Diseases (24th ed). Elk Grove Village, IL, American Academy of Pediatrics, 1997.
136. Aburtyn E, Berlin JA. Intrathecal therapy in tetanus: A meta-analysis. JAMA 266:2262–2267, 1991.
137. Gupta PS, Kapoor R, Goyal S, et al. Intrathecal human tetanus immunoglobulin in early tetanus. Lancet 2:439–440, 1980.
138. Sun KO, Li PC, Yu YL, et al. Management of tetanus: A review of 18 cases. J R Soc Med 87:135–137, 1994.
139. Vakil BJ, Armitage P. Therapeutic trial of intracisternal human tetanus immunoglobulin in clinical tetanus. Trans R Soc Trop Med Hyg 73:579–583, 1979.
140. Sedaghatian MR. Intrathecal serotherapy in neonatal tetanus: A controlled trial. Arch Dis Child 54:623–625, 1979.
141. Neequaye J, Nkrumah FR. Failure of intrathecal antitetanus serum to improve survival in neonatal tetanus. Arch Dis Child 58:276–278, 1983.
142. Beague RE, Lindo-Soriano I. Failure of intrathecal tetanus antitoxin in the treatment of tetanus neonatorum. J Infect Dis 164:419–420, 1991.
143. Ahmadsyah I, Salim A. Treatment of tetanus: An open study to compare the efficacy of procaine penicillin and metronidazole. Br Med J 291:648–650, 1985.
144. Cain HD, Falco FG. Recurrent tetanus. Calif Med 97:31–33, 1962.
145. Spenney JG, Lamb RN, Cobbs CG. Recurrent tetanus. South Med J 64:859–862, 1971.
146. Bhatt AD, Dastur FD. Relapsing tetanus: A case report. J Postgrad Med 27:184–186, 1981.
147. Naranyanan K, Gupta PS, Kumar N, Aggarwal SK. Antitoxin response in tetanus. Indian J Med Res 74:482–485, 1981.
148. Yeni P, Carbon C, Tremolieres F, Gibert C. Serum levels of antibody to toxoid during tetanus and after specific immunization of patients with tetanus. J Infect Dis 145:278, 1982.
149. Bytchenko BD, Causse G, Grab B, Kereselidze TS. Tetanus: Recent trends of world distribution. In Mérieux C (ed). Sixth International Conference on Tetanus; Lyon, France; December 3–5, 1981. Lyon, Collection Foundation Mérieux, 1981, pp 97–111.
150. Galazka A, Cook R. Neonatal tetanus today and tomorrow. In Nistico G, Mastroeni P, Pitzurra M (eds). Seventh International Conference on Tetanus; Copanello, Italy; September 10–15, 1984. Rome, Gangeni Publishing Company, 1985, pp 350–363.
151. Rey M, Tikhomirov E. Non neonatal tetanus over the world. In Nistico G, Bizzini B, Bytchenko M, Triau R (eds). Eighth International Conference on Tetanus; Leningrad, USSR; August 25–28, 1987. Rome, Pythagora Press, 1989, pp 506–518.
152. Luisto M. Epidemiology of tetanus in Finland from 1969 to 1985. Scand J Infect Dis 21:655–663, 1989.
153. Galazka A, Kardymowicz B. Tetanus incidence and immunity in Poland. Eur J Epidemiol 5:474–480, 1989.
154. Axnick NW, Alexander ER. Tetanus in the United States: A review of the problem. Am J Public Health 47:1493–1501, 1957.
155. Heath CW, Zusman J, Sherman IL. Tetanus in the United States, 1950–1960. Am J Public Health 54:769–779, 1964.
156. LaForce FM, Young LS, Bennett JV. Tetanus in the United States (1965–1966). N Engl J Med 280:569–574, 1969.
157. Moore RM, Singleton AO. Tetanus at the John Sealy Hospital. Surg Gynecol Obstet 69:146–154, 1939.
158. Centers for Disease Control. Tetanus—United States, 1982–1984. MMWR Morb Mortal Wkly Rep 34:602, 607–611, 1985.
159. Centers for Disease Control. Tetanus—United States, 1985–1986. MMWR Morb Mortal Wkly Rep 36:477–481, 1987.
160. Centers for Disease Control. Tetanus—United States, 1987 and 1988. MMWR Morb Mortal Wkly Rep 39:37–41, 1990.
161. Prevots R, Sutter RW, Strebel PM, et al. Tetanus surveillance–United States, 1989–1990. MMWR CDC Surveill Summ 41(SS-8):1–9, 1992.
162. Frazer DW. Tetanus in the United States, 1900–1969: Analysis by cohorts. Am J Epidemiol 96:306–312, 1972.

163. Christensen NA, Thurber DL. Clinical experience with tetanus: 91 cases. Proc Mayo Clin 32:146–158, 1957.
164. Faust RA, Vickers OR, Cohn I. Tetanus: 2,449 cases in 68 years at Charity Hospital. J Trauma 16:704–712, 1976.
165. Bowen V, Johnson J, Boyle J, Snelling CF. Tetanus—a continuing problem in minor injuries. Can J Surg 31:7–9, 1988.
166. Levinson AK, Marske RL, Shein MK. Tetanus in heroin addicts. JAMA 157:658–660, 1955.
167. Cherubin CE. Urban tetanus: The epidemiologic aspects of tetanus in narcotic addicts in New York City. Arch Environ Health 14:802–808, 1967.
168. Cherubin CE. Epidemiology of tetanus in narcotic addicts. N Y State J Med 70:267–271, 1970.
169. Sangalli M, Chierchini P, Aylward RB, Forastiere F. Tetanus: A rare but preventable cause of mortality among drug users and the elderly. Eur J Epidemiol 12:539–540, 1996.
170. Postoperative tetanus [editorial]. Lancet 2:964–965, 1984.
171. Federmann M, Kotzerke M. Postoperativ tetanus. Dtsch Med Wochenschr 114:1833–1836, 1989.
172. Ray SN, Ray K, Grover SS. Sero-survey of diphtheria and tetanus antitoxin. Indian J Med Res 68:901–904, 1978.
173. Dastur FD, Awatramani VP, Dixit SK. Response to single dose of tetanus vaccine in subjects with naturally acquired tetanus antitoxin. Lancet 2:219–222, 1981.
174. Veronesi R, Bizzini B, Focaccia R, et al. Naturally acquired antibodies to tetanus toxin in humans and animals from the Galapagos Islands. J Infect Dis 147:308–311, 1983.
175. Matzkin H, Regev S. Naturally acquired immunity to tetanus toxin in an isolated community. Infect Immun 48:267–268, 1985.
176. Veronesi R. Naturally acquired tetanus immunity: Still a controversial theme? In Nistico G, Mastroeni P, Pitzurra M (eds). Seventh International Conference on Tetanus; Copanello, Italy; September 10–15, 1984. Rome, Gangeni Publishing Company, 1985, pp 365–372.
177. Leshem Y, Herman J. Tetanus immunity in kibbutz women. Isr J Med Sci 25:127–130, 1989.
178. Galazka AM. The immunologic basis for immunization: Tetanus. Geneva, World Health Organization. WHO/EPI/GEN/91.13.
179. Ruben FL, Nagel J, Fireman P. Antitoxin responses in the elderly to tetanus-diphtheria (Td) immunization. Am J Epidemiol 108:145–149, 1978.
180. Crossley K, Irvine P, Warren B, et al. Tetanus and diphtheria immunity in urban Minnesota adults. JAMA 242:2298–2300, 1979.
181. Weiss BP, Strassburg MA, Feeley JC. Tetanus and diphtheria immunity in an elderly population in Los Angeles County. Am J Public Health 73:802–804, 1983.
182. Stair TO, Lippe MA, Russell H, Feeley JC. Tetanus immunity in emergency department patients. Am J Emerg Med 7:563–566, 1989.
183. Gergen PJ, McQuillan GM, Kiely M, et al. A population-based serologic survey of immunity to tetanus in the United States. N Engl J Med 332:761–766, 1995.
184. Sutter RW, Cochi SL, Brink EW, Sirotkin BI. Assessment of vital statistics and surveillance data for monitoring tetanus mortality, 1979–1984. Am J Epidemiol 131:132–142, 1990.
185. Koblin BA, Townsend TR. Immunity to diphtheria and tetanus in inner-city women of childbearing age. Am J Public Health 79:1297–1298, 1989.
186. Can modified tetanus occur? [editorial]. N Engl J Med 266:1117–1118, 1962.
187. McComb JA. Tetanus in a previously immunized person [letter]. N Engl J Med 273:452–453, 1965.
188. Luisto M, Iivananinen M. Tetanus in immunized children. Dev Med Child Neurol 35:351–355, 1993.
189. Suleman O. Mortality from tetanus neonatorum in Punjab (Pakistan). Pakistan Pediatr J 6:152–183, 1982.
190. Marshall FN. Tetanus of the newborn: With special reference to experiences in Haiti, W. I. Adv Pediatr 15:65–110, 1968.
191. Adams JM, Kenny JD, Rudolph AJ. Modern management of tetanus neonatorum. Pediatrics 64:472–477, 1979.
192. Stanfield JP, Galazka A. Neonatal tetanus in the world today. Bull World Health Organ 62:647–669, 1984.
193. Hinman AR, Foster SO, Wassilak SGF. Neonatal tetanus: Potential for elimination in the USA and the world. Pediatr Infect Dis 6:813–816, 1987.
194. Leroy O, Garenne M. Risk factors of neonatal tetanus in Senegal. Int J Epidemiol 20:521–526, 1991.
195. Hlady WG, Bennett JV, Samadi AR, et al. Neonatal tetanus in rural Bangladesh: Risk factors and toxoid efficacy. Am J Public Health 82:1365–1369, 1992.
196. Bennett J, Schooley M, Traverso H, et al. Bundling, a newly identified risk factor for neonatal tetanus: Implications for global control. Int J Epidemiol 25:879–884, 1996.
197. Jagetiya P, Bhandari B. Analysis of tetanus neonatorum cases admitted in a hospital during 1976–1977. Indian J Public Health 23:103–105, 1979.
198. Hamid ED, Daulay AP, Lubis CP, et al. Tetanus neonatorum in babies delivered by traditional birth attendants in Medan, Indonesia. Paediatr Indones 25:167–174, 1985.
199. Cliff J. Neonatal tetanus in Maputo, Mozambique. Part I: Hospital incidence and childbirth practices. Cent Afr J Med 31:9–12, 1985.
200. Traverso HD, Bennett JV, Kahn AJ, et al. Ghee application to the umbilical cord: A risk factor for tetanus. Lancet 1:486–488, 1989.
201. Bennett J, Azhar, Rahim F, et al. Further observations on ghee as a risk factor for tetanus. Int J Epidemiol 24:643–647, 1995.
202. Roison AJ, Prazuch T, Tall F, et al. Risk factor for neonatal tetanus in west Burkina Faso: A case-control study. Eur J Epidemiol 12:535–537, 1996.
203. Baltazar JC, Sarol JN. Prenatal tetanus immunization and other practices associated with neonatal tetanus. Southeast Asian J Trop Med Public Health 25:132–138, 1994.
204. Salimpour R. Cause of death in tetanus neonatorum: Study of 233 cases with 54 necropsies. Arch Dis Child 52:587–594, 1977.
205. Bhat GJ, Joshi MK, Kandoth PW. Neonatal tetanus: A clinical study of 100 cases. Indian Pediatr 16:159–166, 1979.
206. Gupta SM, Takkar VP, Verma AK. A retrospective study of tetanus neonatorum and comparative assessment of diazepam in its treatment. Indian Pediatr 16:343–346, 1979.
207. Paul SS, Utal DS, Gupta GS. Tetanus neonatorum. Indian Pediatr 21:683–687, 1984.
208. Teknetzi P, Manios S, Katsouyanopoulos V. Neonatal tetanus—long term residual handicaps. Arch Dis Child 58:68–69, 1983.
209. Anlar B, Yalaz K, Dizmen R. Long-term prognosis after neonatal tetanus. Dev Med Child Neurol 31:76–80, 1989.
210. Ball K, Norboo T, Gupta U, et al. Is tetanus rare at high altitudes? [letter]. Trop Doct 24:78–80, 1994.
211. Oudesluys-Murphy AM, Eilers GA, de Groot CJ. The time of separation of the umbilical cord. Eur J Pediatr 146:387–389, 1987.
212. Oudesluys-Murphy AM. Umbilical cord care and neonatal tetanus [letter]. Lancet 1:843, 1989.
213. Kumar S, Malecki JM. A case of neonatal tetanus. South Med J 84:396–398, 1991.
214. Craig AS, Reed GW, Mohon RT, et al. Neonatal tetanus in the United States: A sentinel event in the foreign-born. Pediatr Infect Dis J 16:955–959, 1997.
215. Expanded Programme on Immunization. Issues in Neonatal Tetanus Control. Geneva, World Health Organization, 1987. WHO/EPI/GAG/87/WP.11.
216. Expanded Programme on Immunization. Report of the 14th Global Advisory Group; Antalya, Turkey; October 14–18, 1991. Geneva, World Health Organization, 1992. WHO/EPI/GEN/92.1.
217. Pope CG. Development of knowledge of antitoxins. Br Med Bull 19:230–234, 1963.
218. Reisman RE, Rose NR, Witebsky E, Arbesman CE. Serum sickness: II. Demonstration and characteristics of antibodies. J Allergy 32:531–543, 1961.
219. Suri JC, Rubbo SD. Immunization against tetanus. J Hyg (Camb) 59:29–48, 1961.
220. Rubbo SD, Suri JC. Passive immunization against tetanus with human immune globulin. Br Med J 2:79–81, 1962.
221. McComb JA. The prophylactic dose of homologous tetanus antitoxin. N Engl J Med 270:175–178, 1964.
222. Smith JWG, Evans DG, Jones DA, et al. Simultaneous active and passive immunization against tetanus. Br Med J 1:237–238, 1963.
223. Eckmann L. Active and passive immunization. N Engl J Med 271:1087–1091, 1964.

224. Smith JWG. Simultaneous active and passive immunization of guinea-pigs against tetanus. J Hyg (Camb) 62:379–388, 1964.
225. Levine L, McComb JA, Dwyer RC, Latham WC. Active-passive tetanus immunization. N Engl J Med 274:186–190, 1966.
226. Edsall G. Problems in the immunology and control of tetanus. Med J Aust 2:216–220, 1976.
227. Smith JWG. Diphtheria and tetanus toxoids. Br Med Bull 25:177–182, 1969.
228. MacLennan R, Schofield FD, Pittman M, et al. Immunization against neonatal tetanus in New Guinea: Antitoxin response of pregnant women to adjuvant and plain toxoids. Bull World Health Organ 32:683–697, 1965.
229. Ramon G, Zoeller C. L'anatoxine tetaniqui et l'immunisation active de l'homme vis-à-vis du tetanos. Ann Inn Pasteur 41:808–825, 1927.
229a. Bizzini B. Tetanus. In Germanier R (ed). Bacterial Vaccines. Orlando, Academic Press, 1984, pp 37–68.
230. De Luca MM, Basualdo JA, Bernagozzi JA, Abeiro HD. Nitrogen-gas bubbling during the cultivation of *Clostridium tetani* produces a higher yield of tetanus toxin for the preparation of its toxoid. Microbiol Immunol 41:161–163, 1997.
231. Hardegree MC, Fornwald RE, Farber J, et al. Titration of tetanus toxoids in international units: Relationship to antitoxin responses of Rhesus monkeys. In Mérieux C (ed). Sixth International Conference on Tetanus; Lyon, France; December 3–5, 1981. Lyon, Collection Foundation Mérieux, 1981, pp 409–424.
232. Manahilov R, Solomonova K. Evaluation of the quality of tetanus toxoid preparations. In Nistico G, Bizzini B, Bytchenko M, Triau R (eds). Eighth International Conference on Tetanus; Leningrad, USSR; August 25–28, 1987. Rome, Pythagora Press, 1989, pp 235–237.
233. World Health Assembly. Resolution 42.32, 1992. In Handbook of Resolutions and Decisions of the World Health Assembly and the Executive Board (1985–1992). Vol. 3 (3rd ed). Geneva, World Health Organization, 1993.
234. McCarroll JR, Abrahams I, Skudder PA. Antibody response to tetanus toxoid 15 years after initial immunization. Am J Public Health 52:1669–1675, 1962.
235. Newell KW, LeBlank DR, Edsall G, et al. The serological assessment of a tetanus toxoid field trial. Bull World Health Organ 45:773–785, 1971.
236. Pertussis vaccination: Use of acellular pertussis vaccines among infants and young children—recommendations of the Advisory Committee on Immunization Practices (ACIP). MMWR Morb Mortal Wkly Rep 46(RR-7):1–25, 1997.
237. Jones FG, Moss JM. Studies on tetanus toxoid. I: The antitoxic titer of human subject following immunization with tetanus toxoid and tetanus alum precipitated toxoid. J Immunol 30:115–125, 1936.
238. Maclennan R, Levine L, Newell KW, Edsall G. The early primary immune response to absorbed tetanus toxoid in man: A study of the influence of antigen concentration, carrier concentration, and sequence of dosage on the rate, extent, and persistence of the immune response to one and to two doses of toxoid. Bull World Health Organ 49:615–626, 1973.
239. Gottlieb S, McLaughlin FX, Levine L, et al. Long-term immunity to tetanus: A statistical evaluation and its clinical implications. Am J Public Health 54:961–971, 1964.
240. Mahoney LJ, Aprile MA, Moloney PJ. Combined active-passive immunization against tetanus in man. Can Med Assoc J 96:1401–1404, 1967.
241. Relyveld E, Bengounia A, Huet M, Kreeftenberg JG. Antibody response of pregnant women to two different adsorbed tetanus toxoids. Vaccine 9:369–372, 1991.
242. Vassilev TL. Aluminum phosphate but not calcium phosphate stimulates the specific IgE response in guinea-pigs to tetanus toxoid. Allergy 33:155–159, 1978.
243. Kielmam AA, Vohra SR. Control of tetanus neonatorum in rural communities—immunization effects of high-dose calcium phosphate–adsorbed tetanus toxoid. Indian J Med Res 66:906–916, 1977.
244. Kumar V, Sahai G, Kumar A. Studies on the stability of tetanus and pertussis components of DTP vaccine on exposure to different temperatures. Indian J Pathol Microbiol 23:50–54, 1982.
245. World Health Organization, Expanded Programme on Immunization. The effects of freezing on the appearance, potency and toxicity of adsorbed and unadsorbed DPT vaccines. Wkly Epidemiol Rec 55:385–390, 1980.
246. World Health Organization, Expanded Programme on Immunization. The effects of freezing on the appearance, potency and toxicity of adsorbed and unadsorbed DPT vaccines. Wkly Epidemiol Rec 55:396–398, 1980.
247. Menon PS, Sahai G, Joshi VB, et al. Field trial on frozen and thawed tetanus toxoid. Indian J Med Res 64:25–32, 1976.
248. Dietz V, Galazka A, van Loon F, Cochi S. Factors affecting the immunogenicity and potency of tetanus toxoid: Implications for the elimination of neonatal and non-neonatal tetanus as public health problems. Bull World Health Organ 5:81–93, 1997.
249. Barile MF, Hardegree MC, Pittman M. Immunization against neonatal tetanus in New Guinea. 3. The toxin-neutralization test and the response of guinea-pigs to the toxoids as used in the immunization schedules in New Guinea. Bull World Health Organ 43:453–459, 1970.
250. Christiansen G. Quantification of tetanus antitoxin by toxin neutralization test in mice. A comparison between lethal and paralytic techniques. J Biol Stand 9:453–460, 1981.
251. Melville-Smith ME, Seagroatt VA, Watkins JT. A comparison of enzyme-linked immunosorbent assay (ELISA) with the toxin neutralization test in mice as a method for the estimation of tetanus antitoxin in human sera. J Biol Stand 11:137–144, 1983.
252. Marconi P, Pitzurra M, Bistoni F. Passive hemagglutination as the reference method for evaluation of tetanus immunity. In Nistico G, Mastroeni P, Pitzurra M (eds). Seventh International Conference on Tetanus; Copanello, Italy; September 10–15, 1984. Rome, Gangeni Publishing Company, 1985, pp 259–273.
253. Hardegree MC, Barile MF, Pittman M, et al. Immunization against neonatal tetanus in New Guinea. 4. Comparison of tetanus antitoxin titers obtained by haemagglutination and toxin neutralization in mice. Bull World Health Organ 43:461–468, 1970.
254. Hernandez R, Just M, Burgin-Wolf A. Immunoglobulin classes of human antitoxin after tetanus vaccination studies by immunofluorescence with agarose bound tetanus toxoid. Z Immunol Forsch 145:376–384, 1973.
255. Bernath S, Habermann E. Solid-phase radioimmunoassay in antibody coated tubes for the quantitive determination of tetanus antibodies. Med Microbiol Immunol 160:47–51, 1974.
256. Ourth DD, Murray ES, MacDonald AB, et al. An indirect immunofluorescent test for human antibodies to tetanus toxoid using an insoluble toxoid as antigen. J Clin Exp Immunol 19:571–577, 1975.
257. Winsnes R, Christiansen G. Quantification of tetanus antitoxin in human sera. II. Comparison of counter-immunoelectrophoresis and passive haemagglutination with toxin neutralisation in mice. Acta Pathol Microbiol Scand B 87:197–200, 1979.
258. Peel MM. Measurement of tetanus antitoxin I. Indirect haemagglutination. J Biol Stand 8:177–189, 1980.
259. Layton GT. A micro-enzyme–linked immunosorbent assay (ELISA) and radioimmunosorbent technique (RIST) for the detection of immunity to clinical tetanus. Med Lab Sci 37:323–329, 1980.
260. Wang AS, Burns GF, Kronborg IJ, et al. Detection of antibodies to tetanus toxoid: Comparison of a direct haemagglutination method with a radioimmunoassay. J Clin Pathol 35:1138–1141, 1982.
261. Cox JC, Permier RR, Finger W, et al. A comparison of enzyme immunoassay and bioassay for the quantitative determination of antibodies to tetanus toxin. J Biol Stand 11:123–128, 1983.
262. Sedgwick AK, Ballow M, Sparks K, et al. Rapid quantitative micro-enzyme–linked immunosorbent assay for tetanus antibodies. J Clin Microbiol 18:104–109, 1983.
263. Pitzurra LF, Bistoni M, Pitzurra L, et al. Comparison of passive haemagglutination with turkey erythrocyte assay, enzyme-linked immunosorbent assay and counter immunoelectrophoresis assay for serological evaluation of tetanus immunity. J Clin Microbiol 17:432–435, 1983.
264. Gupta RK, Maheshwari SC, Singh H. The titration of tetanus antitoxin. I. Factors affecting the sensitivity of the indirect haemagglutination test. J Biol Stand 12:11–17, 1984.
265. Gupta RK, Maheshwari SC, Singh H. The titration of tetanus

antitoxin. II. A comparative evaluation of the indirect haemagglutination and toxin neutralization tests. J Biol Stand 12:137–143, 1984.
266. Simonsen O, Bentzon MW, Heron I. ELISA for the routine determination of antitoxic immunity to tetanus. J Biol Stand 14:231–239, 1986.
267. Hagenaars AM, van Delft RW, Nagel J. Comparison of ELISA and toxin neutralization for the determination of tetanus antibodies. J Immunoassay 5:1–11, 1984.
268. Virella G, Hyman B. Quantitation of anti-tetanus and anti-diphtheria antibodies by enzymoimmunoassay: Methodology and applications. J Clin Lab Anal 5:43–48, 1991.
269. Simonsen O, Schou C, Heron I. Modification of the ELISA for the estimation of tetanus antitoxin in human sera. J Biol Stand 15:143–157, 1987.
270. Vernacchio L, Madico G, Verastegui M, et al. Neonatal tetanus in Peru: Risk assessment with modified enzyme-linked immunosorbent assay and toxoid skin test. Am J Public Health 83:1754–1756, 1993.
271. Hendriksen CFM, van der Gun JW, Kreeftenberg JG. The toxin-binding inhibition test as a reliable in vitro alternative to the toxin neutralization test in mice for the estimation of tetanus antitoxin in human sera. J Biol Stand 16:287–297, 1988.
272. Hendriksen CFM, van der Gun JW, Kreeftenberg JG. Combined estimation of tetanus and diphtheria antitoxin in human sera by the in vitro toxin-binding inhibition (ToBi) test. J Biol Stand 17:191–200, 1989.
273. Hong HA, Ke NT, Nhon TN, et al. Validation of the combined toxin-binding inhibition test for determination of neutralizing antibodies against tetanus and diphtheria toxins in a vaccine field study in Vietnam. Bull World Health Organ 74:275–282, 1996.
274. Ourth PP, MacDonald AB. Neutralization of tetanus toxin by human and rabbit immunoglobulin classes and subunits. Immunology 3:807–815, 1977.
275. Yuan L, Lau W, Thipphawong J, et al. Diphtheria and tetanus immunity among blood donors in Toronto. Can Med Assoc J 156:985–990, 1997.
276. Borut TC, Ank BJ, Gard SE, Stiehm ER. Tetanus toxoid skin test in children: Correlation with in vitro lymphocyte stimulation and monocyte chemotaxis. J Pediatr 97:567–573, 1980.
277. Johnson C, Walls RS, Ruwoldt A. Delayed hypersensitivity to tetanus toxoid in man: In vivo and in vitro studies. Pathology 15:369–372, 1983.
278. Delafuente JC, Eisenberg JD, Hoelzer DR, Slavine RG. Tetanus toxoid as an antigen for delayed cutaneous hypersensitivity. JAMA 249:3209–3211, 1983.
279. Kaufman DB, deMendonca WC, Newton J. Diphtheria-tetanus skin testing. Am J Dis Child 134:479–483, 1980.
280. Newell KW, Duenas Lehman A, LeBlanc DR, Garces Osorio N. The use of toxoid for the prevention of tetanus neonatorum. Final report of a double-blind controlled field trial. Bull World Health Organ 35:863–871, 1966.
281. Wolters KL, Dehmel H. Abschliessende Untersuchungen über die Tetanusprophylaxe durch aktive Immunisierung. Z Hyg 124:326–332, 1942.
282. Rahman M, Chen LC, Chakraborty J, et al. Use of tetanus toxoid for the prevention of neonatal tetanus. 1. Reduction of neonatal mortality by immunization of non-pregnant and pregnant women in rural Bangladesh. Bull World Health Organ 60:261–267, 1982.
283. Kumar V, Kumar R, Mathur VN, et al. Neonatal tetanus mortality in a rural community of Haryana. Indian Pediatr 25:167–169, 1986.
284. Maru M, Geahun A, Hosana S. A house-to-house survey on neonatal tetanus in urban and rural areas in the Gondar region, Ethiopia. Trop Geogr Med 40:233–236, 1986.
285. Expanded Programme on Immunization. Neonatal tetanus mortality surveys, Egypt. Wkly Epidemiol Rec 62:332–335, 1987.
286. Cardenas Ayala VM, Nunez Urquiza RM, Brogan DR, et al. Neonatal tetanus mortality in Veracruz, Mexico, 1989. Bull Pan Am Health Organ 29:116–128, 1995.
287. Long AP, Sartwell PE. Tetanus in the U.S. Army in World War II. Bull US Army Med Dept 7:371–385, 1947.
288. Boyd JSK. Tetanus in the African and European theaters of war, 1939–1945. Lancet 1:113–119, 1946.
289. Press E. Desirability of the routine use of tetanus toxoid. N Engl J Med 239:50–56, 1948.
290. General recommendations on immunization: Recommendations of the Advisory Committee on Immunization Practices (ACIP). MMWR Morb Mortal Wkly Rep 43(RR-1):1–38, 1994.
291. Adkins SB. Immunizations: Current recommendations. Am Fam Physician 56:865–874, 1997.
292. Ramsay ME, Corbel MJ, Redhead K, et al. Persistence of antibody after accelerated immunisation with diphtheria/tetanus/pertussis vaccine. BMJ 302:1489–1491, 1991.
293. Cooke JV, Holowach J, Atkins JE, et al. Antibody formation in early infancy against diphtheria and tetanus toxoids. J Pediatr 33:141–146, 1948.
294. Barrett CD, McLeon IW, Molner JG, et al. Multiple antigen immunization of infants against poliomyelitis, diphtheria, pertussis and tetanus. An evaluation of antibody responses of infants one day old to seven months of age at start of inoculations. Pediatrics 30:720–736, 1962.
295. Di Sant'Agnese PA. Combined immunization against diphtheria, tetanus, and pertussis in newborn infants I. Production of antibodies in early infancy. Pediatrics 3:20–33, 1949.
296. Di Sant'Agnese PA. Combined immunization against diphtheria, tetanus, and pertussis in newborn infants III. Relationship of age to antibody production. Pediatrics 3:333–344, 1949.
297. Di Sant'Agnese PA. Simultaneous immunization of newborn infants against diphtheria, tetanus, and pertussis. Production of antibodies and duration of antibody levels in an Eastern Metropolitan area. Am J Public Health 40:674–680, 1950.
298. Gaisford W, Feldman GV, Perkins FT. Current immunization problems. J Pediatr 56:319–330, 1960.
299. Bernbaum JC, Daft A, Anolik R, et al. Response of preterm infants to diphtheria-tetanus-pertussis immunizations. J Pediatr 107:184–188, 1985.
300. Barr M, Glenny AT, Butler NR. Immunization of babies with diphtheria-tetanus-pertussis prophylactic. Br Med J 2:635–639, 1955.
301. Di Sant'Agnese PA. Combined immunization against diphtheria, tetanus, and pertussis in newborn infants II. Duration of antibody levels. Antibody titers after booster dose. Effect of passive immunity to diphtheria on active immunization with diphtheria toxoid. Pediatrics 13:181–194, 1949.
302. Peterson JC, Christie A. Immunization in the young infant: Response to combined vaccines. VI. Tetanus. Am J Dis Child 81:518–529, 1951.
303. Halsey NA, Galazka A. The efficacy of DPT and oral poliomyelitis immunization schedules initiated from birth to 12 weeks of age. Bull World Health Organ 63:1151–1169, 1985.
304. Barkin RM, Samuelson JS, Gotlin LP. DTP reactions and serologic response with a reduced dose schedule. J Pediatr 105:189–194, 1984.
305. Barkin RM, Pichichero ME, Samuelson JS, et al. Pediatric diphtheria and tetanus toxoids vaccine: Clinical and immunologic response when administered as the primary series. J Pediatr 106:779–781, 1985.
306. Edwards KM, Meade BD, Decker MD, et al. Comparison of 13 acellular pertussis vaccines: Overview and serologic response. Pediatrics 96:548–557, 1995.
307. Kutukculer N, Kurugol Z, Egemen A, et al. The effect of immunization against tetanus during pregnancy for protective antibody titres and specific antibody responses of infants. J Trop Pediatr 42:308–309, 1996.
308. Habig WH, Tankersley DL. Tetanus. In Cryz SJ (ed). Vaccines and Immunotherapy. New York, Pergamon Press, 1991, pp 13–19.
309. Booy R, Aitken SJM, Taylor S, et al. Immunogenicity of combined diphtheria, tetanus, pertussis vaccine given at 2, 3, and 4 months versus 3, 5, and 9 months of age. Lancet 339:505–510, 1992.
310. Ramsay MEB, Rao M, Begg NT, et al. Antibody response to accelerated immunisation with diphtheria, tetanus, pertussis vaccine. Lancet 342:203–205, 1993.
311. Brown GC, Volk VK, Gottshall RY, et al. Responses of infants to DTP-P vaccine used in nine injection schedules. Public Health Rep 79:585–602, 1964.
312. Breman JG, Wright GG, Levine L, et al. The primary serologic

response to a single dose of adsorbed tetanus toxoid, high concentration type. Bull World Health Organ 59:745–752, 1981.
313. Stanfield JP, Gall D, Bracken PM. Single-dose antinatal tetanus immunisation. Lancet 1:215–219, 1973.
314. Agrawal K, Pandit K, Kannan AT. Single dose tetanus toxoid—a review of trials in India with special reference to control of tetanus neonatorum. Indian J Pediatr 81:283–285, 1984.
315. Dick G. Combined vaccines. Can J Public Health 57:435–446, 1966.
316. Someya S, Mizuhara H, Murata R, et al. Studies on the adequate composition of diphtheria and tetanus toxoids with reference to the amounts of toxoids and aluminum adjuvant. Jpn J Med Sci Biol 34:21–35, 1981.
317. Ruben FL, Smith EA, Foster SO, et al. Simultaneous administration of smallpox, measles, yellow fever, and diphtheria-pertussis-tetanus antigens to Nigerian children. Bull World Health Organ 48:175–181, 1973.
318. Griffith AH. The role of immunization in the control of diphtheria. Dev Biol Stand 43:3–13, 1979.
319. Miller JJ, Saito TM. Concurrent immunization against tetanus, diphtheria and pertussis. A comparison of fluid and alum-precipitated toxoids. J Pediatr 21:31–44, 1942.
320. Orenstein WA, Weisfeld JS, Halsey NA. Diphtheria and tetanus toxoids and pertussis vaccine, combined. In Recent Advances in Immunization. A Bibliographic Review. PAHO Scientific Publication No. 451. Washington, DC, Pan American Health Organization, 1983, pp 30–51.
321. World Health Organization. Immunization Policies in Europe. Report on a WHO meeting; Karlovy Vary, Czechoslovakia; December 10–12, 1984. Geneva, World Health Organization ICP/EPI 001 m01, 1430G, 1986 PS4.
322. Expanded Programme on Immunization. Global Advisory Group. Wkly Epidemiol Rec 60:13–16, 1985.
323. Volk VK. Safety and effectiveness of multiple antigen preparations in a group of free-living children. Am J Public Health 39:1299–1313, 1949.
324. Barrett CD, Timm EA, Molner JG, et al. Multiple antigen immunization of infants against poliomyelitis, diphtheria, pertussis and tetanus. II. Response of infants and young children to primary immunization and eighteen-month booster. Am J Public Health 49:644–655, 1959.
325. Pichichero ME, Barkin RM, Samuelson JS. Pediatric diphtheria and tetanus toxoids–adsorbed vaccine: Immune response to the first booster following the diphtheria and tetanus toxoids primary series. Pediatr Infect Dis 5:428–430, 1986.
326. Scheibel I, Bentzon MW, Christensen PE, et al. Duration of immunity to diphtheria and tetanus after active immunization. Acta Pathol Microbiol Scand 67:380–392, 1966.
327. Simonsen O, Kjeldsen K, Heron I. Immunity against tetanus and effect of revaccination 25–30 years after primary vaccination. Lancet 2:1240–1242, 1984.
328. Peebles TC, Levine L, Eldred ML, et al. Tetanus-toxoid emergency boosters: A reappraisal. N Engl J Med 280:575–581, 1969.
329. Myers MG, Beckman CW, Vosdingh RA, et al. Primary immunization with tetanus and diphtheria toxoids. Reaction rate and immunogenicity in older children and adults. JAMA 248:2478–2480, 1982.
330. Hardegree ML, Barile MF, Pittman M, et al. Immunization against neonatal tetanus in New Guinea. 2. Duration of primary antitoxin responses to adjuvant tetanus toxoids and comparison of booster responses to adjuvant and plain toxoids. Bull World Health Organ 43:439–451, 1970.
331. Ruben FL, Fireman P. Follow-up study: Protective immunization in the elderly [letter]. Am J Public Health 73:1330, 1983.
332. Solomonova K, Vizev S. Secondary response to boostering by purified aluminum-hydroxide–adsorbed tetanus antitoxin in aging and in aged adults. Immunobiology 158:312–319, 1981.
333. Kishimoto S, Tomino S, Mitsuya H, et al. Age-related decline in the in vitro and in vivo syntheses of anti-tetanus toxoid antibody in humans. J Immunol 125:2347–2352, 1980.
334. Simonsen O, Bloch AV, Klaerke A, et al. I. Immunity against tetanus and response to revaccination in surgical patients more that 50 years of age. Surg Gynecol Obstet 164:329–334, 1987.
335. Murphy SM, Hegarty DM, Feighery CS, et al. Tetanus immunity in elderly people. Age Ageing 24:99–102, 1995.
336. Masar I, Kamienicka L, Novakova I. Immune response of elderly to booster of tetanus. In Nistico G, Bizzini B, Bytchenko M, Triau R (eds). Eighth International Conference on Tetanus; Leningrad, USSR; August 25–28, 1987. Rome, Pythagora Press, 1989, pp 251–253.
337. Gill TJ, Karasic RB, Antoncic J, Rabin BS. Long-term follow-up of children born to women immunized with tetanus toxoid during pregnancy. Am J Reprod Immunol 25:69–71, 1991.
338. Englund JA, Mbawuike IN, Hammill H, et al. Maternal immunization with influenza or tetanus toxoid vaccine for passive antibody protection in young infants. J Infect Dis 168:647–656, 1993.
339. Evans DG. Persistence of antitoxin in man following active immunisation. Lancet 2:316–317, 1943.
340. Simonsen O, Badsberg JH, Kjeldsen K, et al. The fall-off in serum concentration of tetanus antitoxin after primary and booster vaccination. Acta Pathol Microbiol Scand C 94:77–82, 1986.
341. Simonsen O. Vaccination against tetanus and diphtheria. Danish Med Bull 36:24–47, 1989.
342. Christenson B, Böttiger M. Immunity and immunization of children against tetanus in Sweden. Scand J Infect Dis 23:643–647, 1991.
343. Volk VK, Gottshall RY, Anderson HD, et al. Antigenic response to booster dose of diphtheria and tetanus toxoids, seven to thirteen years after primary inoculation of noninstitutionalized children. Public Health Rep 77:185–194, 1962.
344. Centers for Disease Control. Diphtheria, tetanus and pertussis: Guidelines for vaccine prophylaxis and other preventive measures. Recommendations of the Immunization Practices Advisory Committee (ACIP). MMWR Morb Mortal Wkly Rep 40(RR-10):1–28, 1991.
345. Expanded Programme on Immunization. Prevention of neonatal tetanus through immunization. Geneva, World Health Organization, WHO/EPI/GEN/86/9.
345a. Koenig MA, Roy NC, McElrath T, et al. Duration of protective immunity conferred by maternal tetanus toxoid immunization: Further evidence from Matlab, Bangladesh. Am J Public Health 88:903–907, 1998.
346. White WG, Gall D, Barnes GM, et al. Duration of immunity after active immunisation against tetanus. Lancet 2:95–96, 1969.
347. Mathias RG, Schechter MT. Booster immunization for diphtheria and tetanus: No evidence for need in adults. Lancet 1:1089–1091, 1985.
348. Gardner P, LaForce FM. Protection against tetanus [letter]. N Engl J Med 333:599, 1995.
349. Bowie C. Tetanus toxoid for adults—too much of a good thing [editorial]. Lancet 348:1185–1186, 1996.
350. Balestra DJ, Littenberg B. Should adult tetanus immunization be given as a single vaccination at age 65? J Gen Intern Med 8:405–412, 1993.
351. Task Force on Immunization of the American College of Physicians. Guide for Adult Immunization (4th ed). Philadelphia, American College of Physicians, 1997.
352. Sutter RW, Hadler SC, McQuilllan G, Gergen PJ. Protection against tetanus [letter reply]. N Engl J Med 333:600, 1995.
353. Relihan M. Reactions to tetanus toxoid. J Irish Med Assoc 62:430–434, 1969.
354. White WG, Barnes GM, Barker E, et al. Reactions to tetanus toxoid. J Hyg (Camb) 71:283–297, 1973.
355. Williams JJ, Ellingson HV. Field trial of commercially-prepared diphtheria-tetanus toxoid: Immunization reactions among recruits. Unpublished report to the Armed Forces Epidemiologic Board, 1954.
356. Collier LH, Polakoff S, Mortimer J. Reactions and antibody responses to reinforcing doses of adsorbed and plain tetanus vaccines. Lancet 1:1364–1368, 1979.
357. Jones AE, Melville-Smith M, Watkins J, et al. Adverse reactions in adolescents to reinforcing doses of plain and adsorbed tetanus vaccines. Community Med 7:99–106, 1985.
358. Macko MB. Comparison of the morbidity of tetanus toxoid boosters with tetanus-diphtheria toxoid boosters. Ann Emerg Med 14:33–35, 1985.
359. Deacon SP, Langford DT, Shepard WM, Knight PA. A comparative clinical study of adsorbed tetanus vaccine and adult-type tetanus-diphtheria vaccine. J Hyg (Camb) 89:513–519, 1982.

360. Zurrer G, Steffen R. Side effects in tetanus vs. diphtheria tetanus vaccination in travellers [abstract WPO3.3]. Proceedings of the First Conference on International Travel Medicine; Zurich, Switzerland; April 5–8, 1988.
361. Sisk CW, Lewis CE. Reactions to tetanus-diphtheria toxoid (adult). Arch Environ Health 11:34–36, 1965.
362. McComb JA, Levine L. Adult immunization II. Dosage reduction as a solution to increasing reactions to tetanus toxoid. N Engl J Med 265:1152–1153, 1961.
363. Holden JM, Strang DU. Reactions to tetanus toxoid: Comparison of fluid and adsorbed toxoids. N Z Med J 64:574–577, 1965.
364. Griffith AH. Clinical reactions to tetanus toxoid. In Eckmann L (ed). Principles on Tetanus. Bern, Hans Huber, 1967, p 299.
365. Edelman R. Vaccine adjuvants. Rev Infect Dis 2:370–383, 1980.
366. Expanded Programme on Immunization. Reactions to tetanus toxoid. Wkly Epidemiol Rec 57:193–194, 1982.
367. Middaugh JP. Side effects of diphtheria-tetanus toxoid in adults. Am J Public Health 69:246–249, 1979.
368. Ullberg-Olsson K. Vaccinationsreaktioner efter injektion: Av tetanustoxoid med och utan tillsats av difteritoxoid. Lakartidningen 76:2976, 1979.
369. Lloyd JC, Haber P, Chen RT, et al. Adverse events following tetanus-diphtheria and tetanus toxoid vaccinations: Data from the Vaccine Adverse Event Reporting System (VAERS), 1991–1995. Unpublished data.
370. Levine L, Ipsen J, McComb JA. Adult immunization: Preparation and evaluation of combined fluid tetanus and diphtheria toxoids for adult use. Am J Hyg 73:20–35, 1961.
371. Ipsen J. Immunization of adults against diphtheria and tetanus. N Engl J Med 251:459–466, 1954.
372. Eisen AH, Cohen JJ, Rose B. Reaction to tetanus toxoid: Report of a case with immunologic studies. N Engl J Med 269:1408–1411, 1963.
373. Schneider CH. Reactions to tetanus toxoid: A report of five cases. Med J Aust 1:303–305, 1964.
374. Edsall G, Elliot MW, Peebles TC, et al. Excessive use of tetanus toxoid boosters. JAMA 202:17–19, 1967.
375. Levine L, Edsall G. Tetanus toxoid: What determines reaction proneness? J Infect Dis 144:376, 1981.
376. Jacobs RL, Lowe RS, Lanier BQ. Adverse reactions to tetanus toxoid. JAMA 247:40–42, 1982.
377. Reisman RE. Delayed hypersensitivity to merthiolate preservative. J Allergy 43:245–248, 1969.
378. Gold H. Sensitization induced by tetanus toxoid, alum precipitated. J Lab Clin Med 27:26–36, 1941.
379. Church JA, Richards W. Recurrent abscess formation following DTP immunizations: Association with hypersensitivity to tetanus toxoid. Pediatrics 75:899–900, 1985.
380. Osawa J, Kitamura K, Ikezawa Z, Nakejima H. A probable role for vaccines containing thimerosal in thimerosal hypersensitivity. Contact Dermatitis 24:178–182, 1991.
381. Diete GF. Serum sickness after tetanus toxoid injection [question and answer]. JAMA 220:137, 1972.
382. Vaccine Safety Committee. Diphtheria and tetanus toxoids. Adverse events associated with childhood vaccines: Evidence bearing on causality. In Stratton KR, Howe CJ, Johnston RB (eds). Research Strategies for Assessing Adverse Effects Associated with Vaccines. Washington, DC, National Academy Press, 1994, pp 67–117.
383. Quast U, Hennessen W, Widmark RM. Mono- and polyneuritis after tetanus vaccination (1970–1977). Dev Biol Stand 43:25–32, 1979.
384. Pollard JD, Selby G. Relapsing neuropathy due to tetanus toxoid: Report of a case. J Neurol Sci 37:113–125, 1978.
385. Holliday PL, Bauer RB. Polyradiculoneuritis secondary to immunization with tetanus and diphtheria toxoids. Arch Neurol 40:56–57, 1983.
386. Newton N, Janati A. Guillain-Barré syndrome after vaccination with purified tetanus toxoid. South Med J 80:1053–1054, 1987.
387. Kiwit JCW. Neuralgic amyotrophy after administration of tetanus toxoid [letter]. J Neurol Neurosurg Psychiatry 47:320, 1984.
388. Tsairis P, Dyck PJ, Mulder DW. Natural history of brachial plexus neuropathy: Report on 99 patients. Arch Neurol 2:116–120, 1965.
389. Beghi E, Kurland LT, Mulder DW, Nicolosi A. Brachial plexus neuropathy in the population of Rochester, Minnesota, 1970–1981. Ann Neurol 18:320–323, 1985.
390. Dittman S. Tetanusschutzimpfung. Beitr Hyg Epidemiol 25:239–240, 1981.
391. Rutledge SL, Snead OC. Neurologic complications of immunizations. J Pediatr 109:917–923, 1986.
392. Garvey JL. Serum neuritis: 20 cases following use of antitetanic serum. Postgrad Med 13:210–213, 1953.
393. Rantala J, Cherry JD, Shields WD, et al. Epidemiology of Guillain-Barré syndrome in children: Relationship of oral polio vaccine occurrence. J Pediatr 124:220–223, 1994.
394. Update: Vaccine side effects, adverse reactions, contraindications, and precautions—recommendations of the Advisory Committee on Immunization Practices (ACIP). MMWR Morb Mortal Wkly Rep 45(RR-12):1–35, 1996.
395. Schlenska GK. Unusual neurologic complications following tetanus toxoid administration. J Neurol 215:299–302, 1977.
396. Schwarz G, Lanzer G, List WF. Acute midbrain syndrome as an adverse reaction to tetanus toxoid. Intensive Care Med 15:53–54, 1988.
397. Nagel J, Svec D, Waters T, Fireman P. IgE synthesis in man. I. Development of specific IgE antibodies after immunization with tetanus-diphtheria (Td) toxoids. J Immunol 118:334–341, 1977.
398. Matuhasi T, Ikegami H. Elevation of levels of IgE antibody to tetanus toxin in individuals vaccinated with diphtheria-pertussis-tetanus vaccine. J Infect Dis 146:290, 1982.
399. Cogne M, Ballet JJ, Schmitt C, Bizzini B. Total and IgE antibody levels following booster immunization with aluminum adsorbed and nonadsorbed tetanus toxoid in humans. Ann Allergy 54:148–151, 1985.
400. Zalogna GP, Chernow B. Life-threatening anaphylactic reactions to tetanus toxoid. Ann Allergy 49:107–108, 1982.
401. Ratliff DA, Burns-Cox CJ. Anaphylaxis to tetanus toxoid (unreviewed reports). Br Med J 288:114, 1983.
402. Engler RJM, Zalogna G. Anaphylaxis to tetanus toxoid: IgE mediated disease [abstract 422]. Program and abstracts of the 41st annual meeting of the American Academy of Allergy and Immunology; New York, NY; March 16–20, 1985. J Allergy Clin Immunol 75(pt 2), 1985.
403. Cooke RA, Hampton S, Sherman WB, Stull A. Allergy induced by immunization with tetanus toxoid. JAMA 114:1854–1858, 1940.
404. Whittingham HE. Anaphylaxis following administration of tetanus toxoid. Br Med J 1:292–293, 1940.
405. Parrish HJ, Oakley CL. Anaphylaxis after injection of tetanus toxoid: Report of a case. Br Med J 1:294–295, 1940.
406. Miller HG, Stanton JB. Neurologic sequelae of prophylactic inoculation. Q J Med 23:1–27, 1954.
407. Smith RE, Wolnisty C. Allergic reactions to tetanus, diphtheria, influenza and poliomyelitis immunization. Ann Allergy 20:809–813, 1962.
408. Mansfield LE, Ting S, Rawls DO, Frederick R. Systemic reactions during cutaneous testing for tetanus toxoid hypersensitivity. Ann Allergy 57:135–137, 1986.
409. Facktor MA, Bernstein RA, Fireman P. Hypersensitivity to tetanus toxoid. J Allergy Clin Immunol 52:1–12, 1973.
410. Gupte SC, Bhatia HM. Anti-A and anti-B titre response after tetanus toxoid injections in normal adults and pregnant women. Indian J Med Res 70:221–228, 1979.
411. Gupte SC, Bhatia HM. Increased incidence of haemolytic disease of the newborn caused by ABO-incompatibility when tetanus toxoid is given during prenancy. Vox Sang 38:22–28, 1980.
412. Kurikka S, Olander RM, Eskola J, Kayhty H. Passively acquired anti-tetanus and anti-*Haemophilus* antibodies and the response to *Haemophilus influenzae* type b–tetanus toxoid conjugate vaccine in infancy. Pediatr Infect Dis J 15:530–535, 1996.
413. Carlsson RM, Claesson BA, Iwarson S, et al. Antibodies against *Haemophilus influenzae* type b and tetanus in infants after subcutaneous vaccination with PRP-T/diphtheria, or PRP-OMP/diphtheria-tetanus vaccines. Pediatr Infect Dis J 13:27–33, 1994.
414. Holmes SJ, Fritzell B, Guito KP, et al. Immunogenicity of *Haemophilus influenzae* type b polysaccharide–tetanus toxoid conjugate vaccine in infants. Am J Dis Child 147:832–836, 1993.
415. Avendano A, Ferreccio C, Lagos R, et al. *Haemophilus influenzae* type b polysaccharide–tetanus protein conjugate vaccine does not

depress serologic responses to diphtheria, tetanus or pertussis antigens when coadministered in the same syringe with diphtheria-tetanus-pertussis vaccine at two, four and six months of age. Pediatr Infect Dis J 12:638–643, 1993.
416. Kaplan SL, Lauer BA, Ward MA, et al. Immunogenicity and safety of *Haemophilus influenzae* type b–tetanus protein conjugate vaccine alone or mixed with diphtheria-tetanus-pertussis vaccine in infants. J Pediatr 124:323–327, 1994.
417. Silveira CM, Caceres VM, Dutra MG, et al. Safety of tetanus toxoid in pregnant women: A hospital-based case-control study of congenital anomalies. Bull World Health Organ 73:605–608, 1995.
418. Catindig N, Abad-Viola G, Magboo F. Tetanus toxoid and spontaneous abortions: Is there epidemiological evidence of an association? [letter] Lancet 348:1098–1099, 1996.
419. Sethi N, Srivastava RK, Singh RK, Srivastava S. Safety evaluation of a potent tetanus vaccine (250 Lf) in guinea pigs *(Cavia procellus).* Biomed Environ Sci 3:364–367, 1990.
420. Wise DL, Trantolo J, Marino RT, Kitchell JP. Opportunities and challenges in the design of implantable biodegradable polymeric systems for the delivery of antimicrobial agents and vaccines. Adv Drug Delivery Rev 1:19–30, 1987.
421. Davis D, Gregoriadis G. Primary immune response to liposomal tetanus toxoid in mice: The effect of mediators. Immunology 68:277–282, 1989.
422. Singh M, Li XM, Wang H, et al. Immunogenicity and protection in small-animal models with controlled-release tetanus toxoid microparticles as a single-dose vaccine. Infect Immun 65:1716–1721, 1997.
423. Hiraga C, Ishii F, Ichikawa Y. Oral immunization against tetanus using liposome-trapped tetanus toxoid. Kansenshogaku Zasshi 63:1308–1312, 1989.
424. Fairweather NF, Lyness VA, Pickard DJ, et al. Cloning, nucleotide sequencing and expression of tetanus toxin fragment C in *Escherichia coli.* J Bacteriol 165:21–27, 1986.
425. Halpern JL, Habig WH, Neale EA, Stibitz S. Cloning and expression of functional fragment C of tetanus toxin. Infect Immun 58:1004–1009, 1990.
426. Romanos MA, Makoff AJ, Fairweather NF, et al. Expression of tetanus toxin fragment C in yeast: Gene synthesis is required to eliminate fortuitous polyadenylation sites in AT-rich DNA. Nucleic Acids Res 19:1461–1467, 1991.
427. Fairweather NF, Chatfield SN, Makoff AJ, et al. Oral vaccination of mice against tetanus by use of a live attenuated *Salmonella* carrier. Infect Immun 58:1323–1326, 1990.
428. Norton PM, Le Page RW, Macpherson AM, et al. Protection against tetanus toxin in mice nasally immunized with recombinant *Lactococcus lactis* expressing tetanus toxin fragment C. Vaccine 15:616–619, 1997.
429. Smith JWG, Laurence DR, Evans DG. Prevention of tetanus in the wounded. Br Med J 3:453–455, 1975.
430. Percy AS, Kukora JS. The continuing problem of tetanus. Surg Gynecol Obstet 160:307–312, 1985.
431. Furste W. Four keys to 100 per cent success in tetanus prophylaxis. Am J Surg 128:616–623, 1974.
432. Committee on Trauma, American College of Surgeons. Prophylaxis against tetanus in wound management. Am Coll Surg Bull 69:22–23, 1984. Revised.
433. Banton HJ, Miller PA. An observation of antitoxin titers after booster doses of tetanus toxoid. N Engl J Med 240:13–14, 1949.
434. Trinca JC. Active immunization against tetanus: The need for a single all-purpose toxoid. Med J Aust 2:116–120, 1945.
435. Kaiser GC, King RD, Lempe RE, Ruster MH. Delayed recall of active tetanus immunization. JAMA 178:914–916, 1961.
436. Ipsen J. Changes in immunity and antitoxin level immediately after secondary stimulus with tetanus toxoid in rabbits. J Immunol 86:50–55, 1961.
437. Mastroeni P, Leonardi MS, Gazzara D, Bizzini B. Rapid assessment of the antitetanus immune status of a subject using Dot-ELISA. Eur Epidemiol 5:97–100, 1989.
438. Chen RT, Spira TJ. Tetanus prophylaxis in AIDS patients [question and answer]. JAMA 255:1061, 1986.
439. Expanded Programme on Immunization. Global Advisory Group—Part II. Wkly Epidemiol Rec 68:11–16, 1993.
440. Lindsey D. Tetanus prophylaxis—do our guidelines assure protection? [editorial] J Trauma 24:1063–1064, 1984.
441. Rubenstein HM. Studies on human tetanus antitoxin. Am J Hyg 76:276–292, 1962.
442. McComb JA, Dwyer RC. Passive-active immunization with tetanus immune globulin. N Engl J Med 268:857–862, 1963.
443. Moloney PJ. Active-passive immunization against tetanus. In Eckmann L (ed). Principles on Tetanus. Bern, Hans Huber, 1967, pp 393–396.
444. Rubbo SD, Suri JC. Active-passive immunization against tetanus with human immune globulin. Med J Aust 2:109–113, 1965.
445. Cohen H, Leussink AB. Passive-active immunization with human tetanus immunoglobulin and adsorbed toxoid. J Biol Stand 1:313–320, 1973.
446. Johnson DM. Fatal tetanus after prophylaxis with human tetanus immune globulin [letter]. JAMA 207:1519, 1969.
447. Pontecorvo M. The prophylactic dose of TIG. In Nistico G, Mastroeni P, Pitzurra M (eds). Seventh International Conference on Tetanus; Copanello, Italy; September 10–15, 1984. Rome, Gangeni Publishing Company, 1985, pp 375–379.
448. Smith JWG, MacIver AG. Studies in experimental tetanus infection. J Med Microbiol 2:385–393, 1969.
449. Smith JWG. Penicillin in prevention of tetanus. Br Med J 2:1293–1296, 1964.
450. Lucas AO, Willis AJP. Prevention of tetanus. Br Med J 2:1333–1336, 1965.
451. Lowbury EJL, Kidson A, Lilly HA, et al. Prophylaxis against tetanus in non-immune patients with wounds: The role of antibiotics and of human antitetanus globulin. J Hyg (Camb) 80:267–274, 1978.
452. Brand DA, Acampora D, Gottlieg L, et al. Adequacy of antitetanus prophylaxis in six hospital emergency rooms. N Engl J Med 309:636–640, 1983.
453. Giangrosso J, Smith RK. Misuse of tetanus immunoprophylaxis in wound care. Ann Emerg Med 14:573–579, 1985.
454. Ribero ML, Gastaldi G, Fara GM. Ongoing tetanus prophylaxis of injured patients in five hospital emergency rooms. Boll Ist Sieroter Milan 64:70–76, 1985.
455. Centers for Disease Control and Prevention. Status report on the childhood immunization initiative: Reported cases of selected vaccine-preventable diseases—United States. MMWR Morb Mortal Wkly Rep 46:665–671, 1997.
456. World Health Organization. EPI Information System, Global Summary, August 1997. Geneva, World Health Organization, WHO/EPI/GEN/97.02.
457. Galazka A, Sporzynska Z. Immunity to tetanus and diphtheria in various age groups of the Polish population. Arch Immunol Ther Exp 27:715–726, 1979.
458. Matzkin H, Regev S, Kedem R, Nili E. A study of factors influencing tetanus immunity in Israeli male adults. J Infect 11:71–78, 1985.
459. Bouleaud J, Huet M. Contribution in the study of tetanus in France. In Nistico G, Mastroeni P, Pitzurra M (eds). Seventh International Conference on Tetanus; Copanello, Italy; September 10–15, 1984. Rome, Gangeni Publishing Company, 1985, pp 495–497.
460. Murphy SM, Hegarty DM, Feighery CS, et al. Tetanus immunity in elderly people. Age Ageing 24:99–102, 1995.
461. Gareau AB, Eby RJ, McLellan BA, Williams DR. Tetanus immunization status and immunologic response to a booster in an emergency department geriatric population. Ann Emerg Med 19:1377–1382, 1990.
462. Update on adult immunization recommendations of the Advisory Committee on Immunization Practices (ACIP). MMWR Morb Mortal Wkly Rep 40(RR-12):1–52, 1991.
463. Rey M, Guillaumont P, Majnoni d'Intignano B. Benefits of immunization versus risk factors in tetanus. Dev Biol Stand 43:15–23, 1979.
464. Carducci A, Avio CM, Bendinelli M. Cost-benefit analysis of tetanus prophylaxis by a mathematical model. Epidemiol Infect 102:473–483, 1989.
465. Cvjetanovic B, Grab B, Uemura K, Bytchenko B. Epidemiologic model of tetanus and its use in the planning of immunization programmes. Int J Epidemiol 1:125–137, 1972.
466. Smucker CM, Swint JM, Simmons GB. Prevention of neonatal tetanus in India: A prospective cost-effectiveness analysis. J Trop Pediatr 30:227–236, 1984.

467. Berman P, Quinley J, Yusef B, et al. Maternal immunization in Aceh Province, Sumatra: The cost effectiveness of alternative stategies. Soc Sci Med 33:185–192, 1991.
468. Tetanus—Kansas, 1993. MMWR Morb Mortal Wkly Rep 43:309–311, 1994.
469. Expanded Programme on Immunization. Eliminating neonatal tetanus: How near, how far? Geneva, World Health Organization, WHO/EPI/GEN/96.01.
470. Expanded Programme on Immunization. Progress towards the global elimination of neonatal tetanus, 1989–1993. Wkly Epidemiol Rec 70:81–84, 1995.
471. Expanded Programme on Immunization. Global Advisory Group—Part I. Wkly Epidemiol Rec 65:5–11, 1990.
472. World Health Assembly Resolution 42.32, 1989. In Handbook of Resolutions and Decisions of the World Health Assembly and the Executive Board (1985–1992). Vol. 3 (3rd ed). Geneva, World Health Organization, 1993.
473. Expanded Programme on Immunization. Global Advisory Group—Part II. Wkly Epidemiol Rec 69:29–31, 34–35, 1994.
474. Berggren GG, Verly A, Garnier N, et al. Traditional midwives, tetanus immunization, and infant mortality in rural Haiti. Trop Doct 13:79–87, 1983.
475. Expanded Programme on Immunization. Global Advisory Group—Part II. Wkly Epidemiol Rec 68:11–16, 1993.
476. Kessel E. Strategies for the control of neonatal tetanus. J Trop Pediatr 30:145–149, 1984.
477. Hamid ED, Daulay AP, Lubis CP, et al. Tetanus neonatorum in babies delivered by traditional birth attendants in Medan, Indonesia. Paediatr Indones 25:167–174, 1985.
478. Traverso H, Kamil S, Rahim H, et al. A reassessment of risk factors for neonatal tetanus. Bull World Health Organ 69:573–579, 1991.
479. Bennett J, Macia J, Traverso H, et al. Protective effects of topical antimicrobials against neonatal tetanus. Int J Epidemiol 26:897–903, 1997.
480. Aylward RB, Mansour E, Cummings F. Surveillance for neonatal tetanus in high-risk areas [letter]. Lancet 347:690–691, 1996.
481. Expanded Programme on Immunization. Estimating tetanus protection of women by serosurvey, Burundi. Wkly Epidemiol Rec 71:117–124, 1997.
482. Expanded Programme on Immunization. Training for mid-level managers. EPI coverage survey. Geneva, World Health Organization, WHO/EPI/MLM/91.10.
483. Perez-Trallero E, Urbieta M, Diaz-de-Tuesta JL, et al. Antitetanus toxin titers in sera of the women who gave births in 1985 and 1989 in Gipuzkoa (Basque Country, Spain). Eur J Epidemiol 11:231–234, 1995.
484. De Francisco A, Chakraborty J. Maternal recall of tetanus toxoid vaccination. Ann Trop Paediatr 16:49–54, 1996.
485. Ekanem EE, Asindi AA, Antia-Obong OE. Factors influencing tetanus toxoid immunization among pregnant women in Cross Rivers State, Nigeria. Nigerian Med Pract 27:3–5, 1994.
486. Expanded Programme on Immunization. Reassessment of the neonatal tetanus problem, China. Wkly Epidemiol Rec 68:201–204, 1993.
487. Expanded Programme on Immunization. Elimination of neonatal tetanus, Thailand. Wkly Epidemiol Rec 68:337–341, 1993.
488. Expanded Programme on Immunization. Global Advisory Group—Part II. Wkly Epidemiol Rec 69:29–35, 1994.
489. Expanded Programme on Immunization. Progress towards neonatal tetanus elimination, 1988–1994. Wkly Epidemiol Rec 71:33–36, 1996.
490. da Silveira CM, de Quadros CA. Neonatal tetanus: April 1996. Pan American Health Organization, unpublished data.
491. Bennett J, Seward J, Sakai S, Wang LD. Identifying areas at high-risk for neonatal tetanus [letter]. Lancet 346:1628–1629, 1995.
492. Aylward RB, Mansour E, Aly Oon ES, et al. The role of surveillance in 'high risk' approach to the elimination of neonatal tetanus in Egypt. Int J Epidemiol 25:1286–1291, 1996.
493. Brabin L, Kemp J, Maxwell S, et al. Protecting adolescent girls against tetanus. Br Med J 311:73–74, 1995.
494. Farveau V, Mamdani M, Steinglass R, Koblinsky M. Maternal tetanus: Magnitude, epidemiology and potential control measures. Int J Gynecol Obstet 40:3–12, 1993.
495. Dhillon H, Menon PS. Active immunization of women in pregnancy with two injections of absorbed tetanus toxoid for prevention of tetanus neonatorum in Punjab, India. Indian J Med Res 63:583–589, 1975.
496. Chen ST, Edsall G, Peel MM, Sinnathuray TA. Timing of antenatal tetanus immunization for effective protection of the neonate. Bull World Health Organ 61:159–163, 1983.
497. Kutukculer N, Kurugol Z, Egemen A, et al. The effect of immunization against tetanus during pregnancy for protective antibody titres and specific antibody responses of infants. J Trop Pediatr 42:308–309, 1996.
498. Owa JA, Makinde OO. Neonatal tetanus in babies of women immunized with tetanus toxoid during pregnancy. Trop Doct 20:156–157, 1990.
499. Ghosh JB. Prevention of tetanus neonatorum [letter]. Indian Pediatr 27:210, 1990.
500. Deivanayagam N, Nedunchelian K, Kamala KG. Neonatal tetanus: Observations on antenatal immunization, natal and immediate post-natal factors. Indian J Pediatr 58:119–122, 1991.
501. Task Force for Child Survival and Development. Global 2000 Child Survival Project on Neonatal Tetanus in Rural Pakistan, 1988–1991. Carter Center, Atlanta, Georgia, April 1992.
502. Bjerregaard P, Steinglass R, Mutie DM, et al. Neonatal tetanus mortality in coastal Kenya: A community survey. Int J Epidemiol 22:163–169, 1993.
503. Dietz V, Milstien JB, van Loon F, et al. Performance and potency of tetanus toxoid: Implications for eliminating neonatal tetanus. Bull World Health Organ 74:619–628, 1996.
504. Gendrel D, Richard-Lenoble D, Massamba MB, et al. Placental transfer of tetanus antibodies and protection of the newborn. J Trop Pediatr 36:279–282, 1990.
505. Madico G, Salazar G, McDonald J, et al. Rates of tetanus protection and transplacental tetanus antibody transfer in pregnant women from different socioeconomic groups in Peru. Clin Diagn Lab Immunol 3:753–755, 1996.

chapter

19 Varicella Vaccine

Anne A. Gershon
Michiaki Takahashi
C. Jo White

The varicella-zoster virus (VZV) causes two distinct diseases, varicella (chickenpox) and herpes zoster (HZ, shingles). Infection with VZV in temperate climates approaches 100% by the second decade of life. Whereas the disease may be mild in some individuals, more recent epidemiological studies indicate that there is significant morbidity and some mortality with primary infection in previously healthy individuals. A live attenuated VZV (Oka strain) vaccine has been in use for several years in immunocompromised individuals and high-risk adults in Europe and in healthy children in Korea and Japan. Recent efforts have resulted in licensure of the Oka strain vaccine in several countries for the prevention of primary infection in all healthy children and adults. Progress has also been made in the understanding of the pathogenesis of HZ, and there are plans for vaccination of the elderly in hopes of preventing or ameliorating this disease.

HISTORICAL ASPECTS OF VARICELLA-ZOSTER VIRUS

In the early medical literature, varicella and smallpox were often confused. The clinical differentiation was made by Heberden in 1767. Varicella was first proved to be an infectious disease in 1875 when Steiner transmitted the virus by inoculating volunteers with vesicular fluid from patients with varicella.[1] In 1892, Bokay[2] reported that varicella occurred in individuals who were in close contact with people with HZ, suggesting for the first time that the two diseases were caused by the same agent. It was not until the early part of the 20th century that this hypothesis was proved by inducing varicella in children who were inoculated with vesicular fluid from patients with HZ.[3, 4] Garland,[5] in 1943, suggested that HZ might be due to reactivation of VZV acquired earlier in life. The causative virus was first isolated in cell culture by Weller and Stoddard[6] in 1952 from samples of vesicular fluid from patients with varicella. Later studies by Weller and colleagues[7–9] indicated that the viruses isolated from subjects with varicella and HZ were morphologically and serologically identical, and the name VZV was given to the agent. In 1974, Takahashi and colleagues at Osaka University produced a live VZV vaccine by attenuation of a wild-type strain by passage through various diploid cultures. This attenuated VZV vaccine, the Oka strain, was suitable for human use and has subsequently been administered to several million individuals for prevention of varicella. Molecular studies have shown the restriction endonuclease patterns of viral genomes of isolates from subjects with varicella and subsequent HZ,[10] as well as those from vaccine recipients with subsequent HZ,[11, 12] to be identical, proving that HZ is due to reactivation of latent VZV. Therefore, clinical trials are now in progress to determine whether immunization of individuals with a prior history of varicella can prevent or modify HZ.

VIROLOGY

VZV is a herpesvirus, a member of the subfamily *Alphaherpesvirinae.*[13] The virion is composed of approximately 125,000 base pairs, making it one of the smaller agents in the group. The entire genome has been sequenced.[14] The virus is characterized by (1) a linear genome of $80 \pm 3 \times 10^6$ Da with inverted terminal sequences present internally that result in two isomeric DNA molecules,[15–17] (2) a relatively short replication cycle, (3) a host range limited to humans and some higher primates, and (4) frequent latent infection of sensory ganglia. The virions are round or polygonal with a central DNA core. The nucleocapsid is approximately 100 nm in diameter and consists of 162 hexagonal capsomers organized as an icosahedron (20 sides) with a central axial hollow with 5:3:2 axial symmetry.[14] The capsid is surrounded by a tegument and an envelope derived in part from cellular membranes. The entire VZV particle is 180 to 200 nm in diameter. There are 70 open reading frames (ORFs) that encode at least 68 viral gene products. VZV DNA is synthesized in a cascade of expression of immediate early (IE) or α regulatory genes, followed by expression of early (E) or β genes that encode regulatory and structural proteins, followed by expression of late (L) or γ genes that encode structural proteins. Interruption of the cascade, particularly at the IE stage, results in failure to synthesize infectious virus.[18]

At least 30 polypeptides, which are L gene products

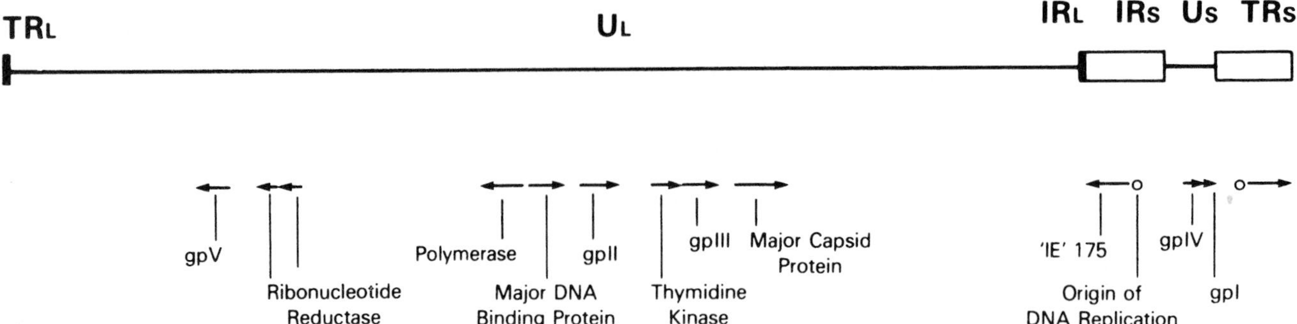

Figure 19–1. The structure of the varicella-zoster virus genome and organization of some genes that have counterparts in herpes simplex virus type I. The horizontal line indicates the long and short unique regions (UL and Us). The two large open rectangles represent the terminal and internal inverted repeats flanking Us (TRs and IRs), and the two small dark rectangles represent the repeats flanking UL (TRL and IRL). The origin of DNA replication within IRs is shown (small open circles). The open reading frame and direction of transcription (shown by arrows) of some important viral genes are indicated below the map. (Adapted from Ostrove JM, Inchauspé G. The biology of varicella-zoster virus. Ann Intern Med 56:600–606, 1988.)

with different molecular weights, have been detected in VZV; at least six of these are glycosylated.[19, 20] The known glycoproteins (g) are termed B, C, E, H, I, and L (Fig. 19–1), corresponding to those of herpes simplex virus (HSV). VZV gB is probably essential to infectivity and is the target of neutralizing antibodies.[19–21] The gE is the most abundantly expressed glycoprotein and is highly immunogenic. It is linked to gI and is an Fc receptor on infected cells.[22] It also binds to mannose 6-phosphate receptors, which may be critical to VZV infection, and it provides signal sequences that mediate assembly of viral proteins in the *trans*-Golgi network.[23, 24] VZV gH is involved in cell-to-cell spread by inducing membrane fusion, and it is a target of neutralizing antibodies. It is complexed with gL.[24–26] Studies in the SCID-hu mouse suggest that gC is essential to replication in skin and to virulence.[205] In addition to glycosylated proteins, some IE gene products of VZV are also immunogenic.[27] The immunogenic protein (p) 170 or IE62 protein is encoded by VZV ORF 62; this protein is closely related to the regulatory polypeptide Vmw175 (or ICP4) of HSV-1.[28] This protein was at one time thought to be purely nonstructural; in contrast to ICP4 for HSV, however, IE62 protein has been identified as a major component of the VZV tegument[29] that is also highly immunogenic.[30] With regard to gene expression and regulation, IE62 protein is the initial *trans*-activating protein of VZV. Other regulatory proteins of VZV are encoded by ORFs 4, 10, 61, and 63.[31–35]

During latent infection, several VZV genes are expressed in sensory ganglia; these are mostly IE genes (ORFs 4, 10, 62, and 63). Although there is also some E gene expression (ORFs 21, 29), L genes are not known to be expressed.[18, 36] Several IE gene products are also expressed during latent infection, including those of ORFs 4, 21, 29, 62, and 63.[37, 38] This degree of gene expression during latency is considerably more extensive than that seen in latent infection with HSV and suggests that there is a certain degree of viral replication even during latent infection. Although some investigators have localized latent VZV infection to either satellite cells[39] or neurons,[40] others have demonstrated latent VZV in both neurons and satellite cells of sensory human ganglia.[41] Reactivation of VZV with production of infectious virions in human neurons in dorsal root ganglia has been visualized with use of in situ hybridization to identify VZV DNA in autopsy specimens.[41] Patients with impaired cell-mediated immunity (CMI) have an increased incidence of HZ, which is consistent with the hypothesis that at least some aspects of suppression of VZV reactivation are under immunological control.[42–44] An animal model of latent VZV infection in the rat has been developed, which may help to clarify how latent infection with VZV is maintained.[45–47]

Varicella is a highly contagious disease due to airborne spread of infectious virions released from skin or the respiratory mucosa of patients with the disease. In contrast, growth of VZV in cell monolayer cultures is slow, with poor infectious yields and the absence of infectious virions in supernatant media. This phenomenon has tended to impede research on VZV and undoubtedly had an influence on vaccine development as well. To obtain cell-free VZV, infectious virions must be released artificially by disruption of cells by methods such as sonication or freeze-thawing.[43]

CLINICAL SYNDROMES AND EPIDEMIOLOGY OF VARICELLA-ZOSTER VIRUS INFECTIONS

The pathogenesis of varicella was conceptualized by Grose[48] in 1981 on the basis of the pathogenesis of mousepox originally outlined by Fenner[49] in 1948 (Fig. 19–2). VZV infects the host by airborne droplets through the conjunctivae or mucosa of the upper respiratory tract. Although less easily transmitted than measles, it is highly contagious, with secondary attack rates in susceptible household contacts of greater than 85%.[50, 51] Varicella can also be transmitted to susceptible individuals from patients with HZ, although analysis of household contacts suggests the risk of viral transmission is less than that from varicella.

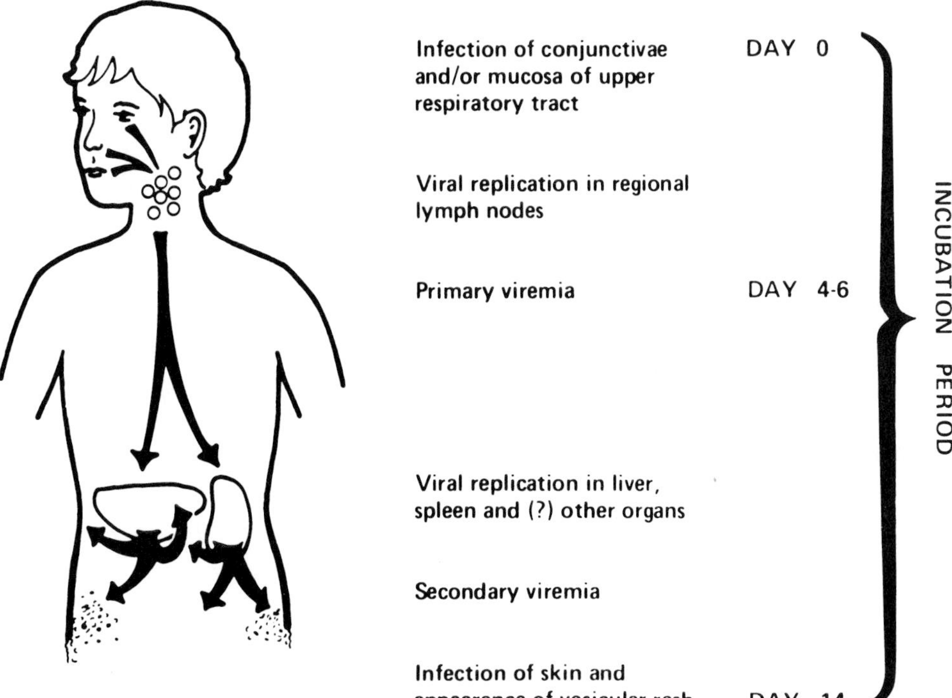

Figure 19–2. Possible pathogenesis of chickenpox. (Adapted from Grose C. Variation on a theme by Fenner: The pathogenesis of chickenpox. Pediatrics 68:735, 1981. Reproduced by permission of Pediatrics.)

Immunocompetent Children and Adults

In the exposed, susceptible immunocompetent individual, the virus replicates during the next 2 to 3 days in regional lymph nodes, followed by a primary viremia on days 4 to 6 after infection. The virus is thought to replicate in the liver and spleen and possibly other organs, and a secondary viremia occurs about 10 to 14 days after infection. This secondary viremia is coincident with the appearance of a vesicular rash characteristic of varicella. In the infected host, there is either a short or absent prodromal period of malaise and fever for 1 or 2 days before the appearance of the characteristic rash. The rash appears in crops and usually progresses rapidly from macules to papules, vesicles, pustules, and finally crusts. New lesions occur in crops during the next 5 to 6 days with various stages of healing noted on the patient in the course of the illness. The lesions are pruritic and can scar if they become secondarily infected. In several published studies, the average number of vesicles ranges from 250 to 500.[51, 52] The height of the fever usually parallels the extent of the rash, and the subject is usually ill for 5 to 7 days. The rash has a central distribution, with a concentration of lesions on the trunk, scalp, and face. Second cases of varicella have been reported in immunocompetent people but are unusual.[53–55] There is evidence that subclinical reinfection with VZV is common.[56–58] Varicella in otherwise healthy children has few extracutaneous manifestations. These include pneumonia, encephalitis, cerebellar ataxia, arthritis, appendicitis, hepatitis, glomerulonephritis, pericarditis, and orchitis.[59–62]

Adults with varicella have a significantly higher per case morbidity with primary VZV infection than healthy children do on the basis of experience by many clinicians as well as retrospective surveys of national healthcare statistics.[62, 63] The height and duration of the febrile response are greater, and rash is frequently more severe with a greater number of lesions and increased time for clearing in comparison to children.[64, 65] Constitutional symptoms such as malaise, myalgias, anorexia, and dehydration are of greater intensity in adults. Complications of varicella in the adult include encephalitis, which is seven times more common than in healthy children. Hospitalizations occur nine times more frequently than in children, and the case-fatality rate is estimated to be 25 times more frequent than for children.[59, 66] With the exception of varicella in the child younger than 1 year, varicella in the adult is the peak age-specific period for morbidity.

It is estimated that there are approximately 4 million cases each year of varicella in the United States. In temperate climates such as the United States, most cases are reported during the winter and early spring (Fig. 19–3), and almost all individuals are infected by the time they reach adulthood, most acquiring the disease between 5 and 14 years of age.[67] The highest incidence rates in a population-based telephone survey conducted in Kentucky were in children 3 to 6 years of age.[68] It may be that the average age of varicella acquisition has fallen because of the increasing number of preschool-aged children participating in daycare.

Seroprevalence studies done as a part of the third National Health and Nutrition Examination Survey (1988 to 1994) demonstrated that 34% of 4- to 5-year-olds, 18% of 6- to 10-year-olds, 6% of 11- to 19-year-olds, and only 4% of 20- to 29-year-olds were susceptible to varicella.[69] The epidemiology is somewhat different in tropical climates, where as many as 30% of 15- to 30-year-olds may be seronegative[70] and where it

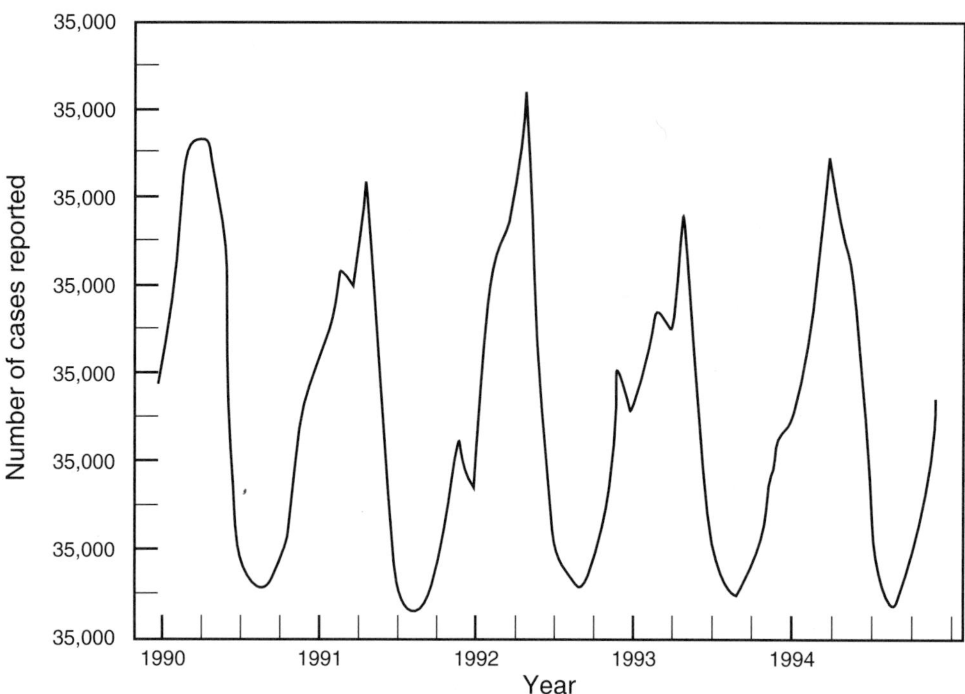

Figure 19–3. Number of cases of varicella reported by month to the National Notifiable Diseases Surveillance Systems, Centers for Disease Control and Prevention, 1990 to 1994. Note peaks in the winter and spring of each year. (From Wharton M. The epidemiology of varicella-zoster virus infection. Infect Dis Clin North Am 10:571–581, 1996.)

has been reported that the peak incidence of disease is in adolescents and young adults.[71]

Although varicella infection in most immunocompetent individuals is not associated with secondary complications, otherwise healthy children and adolescents who contract varicella comprise the largest proportion (80%) of an estimated 9300 annual varicella-related hospitalizations. The rate of complications is substantially higher for people older than 15 years and for infants younger than 1 year.[72] The most common complication in children is secondary bacterial infection of the skin.[59] Staphylococci or group A β-hemolytic streptococci are the usual causative pathogens.[73, 74] The incidence of extracutaneous complications of varicella is low. The most common complication is acute cerebellar ataxia, which develops about 5 to 10 days after the rash, with truncal ataxia often the only neurological sign. Cerebellar ataxia in association with varicella is estimated to occur in 1 in 4000 cases among children younger than 15 years and can result in hospitalization.[75] Varicella encephalitis is a more serious and less common complication than cerebellar ataxia and carries a more guarded prognosis. Other complications include pneumonia and hepatitis. Approximately 60 to 100 previously healthy individuals die of complications of varicella each year in the United States.[72]

Pregnant Women and Newborns

There is increased morbidity of varicella in a varicella-susceptible woman and her fetus.[76] Varicella in the first trimester may cause damage to the fetal central nervous system resulting in mental retardation, permanent scarring of the skin, shortening of the extremities, chorioretinitis, microphthalmia, optic atrophy, cataract, Horner syndrome, blindness, and fetal demise. There appears to be a high correlation between the presence of limb abnormalities and serious central nervous system damage.[76] Although similar fetal abnormalities have been reported after maternal HZ infection, the congenital syndrome due to HZ is exceedingly rare.[76] Patuszak and colleagues[77] conducted a prospective case-controlled study of 106 pregnant women with varicella and performed a meta-analysis combining their study with other published prospective studies. They estimated a 2% risk of varicella embryopathy if infection occurred during the first 20 weeks of gestation.

Infection at any time during fetal life may result in latent infection that subsequently reactivates as childhood or teen HZ.[76, 78–81] Third-trimester infection may cause severe maternal infection, including pneumonia, as well as a life-threatening spread to the newborn. When maternal varicella infection occurs within 5 days before delivery or 2 days after delivery, a severe or fatal infection may develop if the newborn infant contracts varicella.[76] In the days immediately preceding delivery, protective maternal antibodies to VZV would not yet have been formed and crossed the placenta, and after delivery, presumably because of the immaturity of CMI, the baby is at risk for development of an illness resembling varicella in a leukemic child. The infected infant may develop hemorrhagic skin lesions and primary varicella pneumonia, which can be avoided in many cases with prompt administration of VZV immune globulin (VZIG) and judicious use of acyclovir.[76, 78, 79]

Immunocompromised Individuals

Varicella in an immunodeficient individual may lead to a more serious form of illness referred to as progressive varicella.[61] Individuals with malignant disease who are receiving chemotherapy, radiotherapy, or both—especially those with leukemia, those receiving high doses of steroids for any reason (i.e., organ transplantation, severe asthma), and those with congenital deficits in CMI—appear to be at greatest risk of severe varicella with complications. The association of decreased CMI and severe varicella was first noted in the early 1950s.[82] Complications from varicella have become more common as greater numbers of children are treated successfully for malignant disease,[83] are surviving transplantation,[84] and are receiving high-dose steroids for asthma.[85, 86] In addition, cases of severe and fatal varicella have been described in children with human immunodeficiency virus (HIV) infection.[87]

HERPES ZOSTER (SHINGLES)

During the primary infection with VZV, the virus migrates to the dorsal root and trigeminal ganglia where it usually remains latent for the lifetime of the individual. It is hypothesized that the waning of CMI to VZV later in life or during immunosuppression from a variety of causes activates the virus, and a unilateral, dermatomal, usually painful vesicular rash ensues. The rash may remain localized to one to three dermatomes, but in a minority of patients it disseminates outside the dermatomal area and causes widespread lesions that resemble varicella. The rash begins as erythematous, maculopapular lesions that rapidly evolve into a vesicular rash. The vesicles may coalesce to form bullous lesions. In the immunocompetent host, these lesions continue to form for a period of 3 to 5 days with the total duration of disease being 10 to 15 days. It may take as long as 1 month before the skin returns to normal. Occasional patients will develop dermatomal pain without cutaneous lesions *(zoster sine herpete)*, which can be confirmed serologically to be HZ.

HZ may involve the eyelids when the first or second branch of the fifth cranial nerve is affected, but keratitis heralds a sight-threatening condition, herpes zoster ophthalmicus. Keratitis may be followed by severe iridocyclitis, secondary glaucoma, or neuroparalytic keratitis. When the geniculate ganglion is involved, the Ramsay Hunt syndrome may occur, with pain and vesicles in the external auditory meatus, loss of taste in the anterior two thirds of the tongue, and ipsilateral facial palsy. However, thoracic and lumbar dermatomes are most commonly involved. Motor paralysis can occur as a consequence of the involvement of the anterior horn cells in a manner similar to that encountered with poliomyelitis. Neuromuscular disorders associated with HZ include Guillain-Barré syndrome, transverse myelitis, and myositis.[88–90]

The major risk factors for development of HZ are increasing age (older than 50 years), immunosuppression, and VZV infection acquired in utero or during the first year of life (because of a poor CMI response to the virus at young ages).[91–93] In 1965, Hope-Simpson published estimates of incidence rates of 74 per 100,000 people per year among children younger than 10 years increasing to 1010 per 100,000 people per year among those 80 to 89 years of age.[94] Looking at it in a different way, if all people were to live to the ninth decade, approximately 15% would develop HZ in their lifetime, with a sharp increase in the incidence of disease beginning at about age 50 years. In a more recent study by Schmader and colleagues,[95] the lifetime incidence of HZ among African Americans was half that reported by whites in a study of community-dwelling elderly residents of North Carolina. After adjusting for age, cancer history, gender, education, and urban or rural residence, race remained a significant protective factor.

HZ is more common and more severe in immunocompromised than in immunologically normal individuals. Lesion formation continues for up to 2 weeks, and scabbing may not occur until 3 to 4 weeks into the disease course.[96] Immunosuppressed subjects are at risk for cutaneous dissemination and visceral involvement, including varicella pneumonitis, hepatitis, and meningoencephalitis. In leukemic children who have experienced varicella, a rate of HZ of about 15% has been observed.[97, 98] As many as 30% of patients may develop HZ after bone marrow transplantation.[99] A similar percentage of adults with HIV infection may develop HZ.[100] Children who develop varicella after HIV infection has occurred are at even higher risk to develop HZ, especially if varicella occurs in the setting of a low $CD4^+$ level, in which it approaches 70%.[101] Chronic HZ is often reported in HIV-infected patients with HZ. In these individuals, there is sustained new lesion formation with an absence of healing of the existing lesions. Many of these chronic syndromes have been associated with the isolation of VZV isolates resistant to acyclovir.[102]

The most debilitating complication of HZ is postherpetic neuralgia. Postherpetic neuralgia is uncommon in young individuals but may occur in as many as 25 to 50% of patients older than 50 years.[103–107] Among patients older than 60 years, 20 to 40% may experience postherpetic neuralgia of 3 months or longer. The case-incidence of this complication is not precisely known because the definition of postherpetic neuralgia (including measures of severity and effect on quality of life) varies between studies.[108–113] Postherpetic neuralgia may cause constant pain or intermittent stabbing pain in the involved dermatome. Pain is often reported to be worse at night or on exposure to temperature changes. In some, the pain is incapacitating.

PATHOGENESIS AS IT RELATES TO PREVENTION

VZV spreads by the airborne route.[114, 115] Infectivity is maximal in the early stages of the illness.[116] Although the issue is somewhat controversial, the source of infectious virus is probably from both the skin and respiratory secretions.[116–119] Studies of transmission of vaccine-type VZV have implicated skin lesions as a source of infectious virus.[119] Virus from skin is commonly isolated in cell culture, but it is extremely unusual to isolate VZV from respiratory secretions.[120] Limited epidemiological data, however, suggest that respiratory spread can occur.[121] Data from polymerase chain reaction (PCR) studies of respiratory secretions have yielded differing results and have not clarified the issue of whether respiratory spread of VZV occurs. In one study, only 1 of 30 (3.3%) oropharyngeal samples were positive for VZV DNA during the first day of the rash of chickenpox,[118] but in another study, 26% and 90% were positive during the incubation period and after clinical onset, respectively.[117] In yet another study, VZV DNA was detected in the respiratory tract of patients with varicella in 28 of 45 (62%) on day 1, in 50% on day 6, and in 22% after day 6.[122] The different rates of positivity obtained in various studies may reflect differences in primers used as well as differences in techniques for collection of respiratory secretions. The demonstration of VZV DNA, however, does not necessarily indicate the presence of infectious virus in respiratory secretions.

In infection, the site of host invasion of VZV appears to be the conjunctivae or the mucosa of the upper respiratory tract or both. On the basis of the mousepox model of Fenner,[48] it is hypothesized that in primary infection, VZV replicates locally in the lymph nodes for several days, causing a primary viremia of low magnitude, which delivers the virus to the viscera where further multiplication occurs. A demonstrable secondary viremia of greater magnitude subsequently results (see Fig. 19–2). Culture of mononuclear cells from 5 days before to 2 days after appearance of rash in patients with natural varicella (Table 19–1) yielded VZV,[123–128] as has PCR.[122, 129] The presence of VZV in CD4+ and CD8+ T lymphocytes has also been demonstrated by in situ hybridization during early varicella.[118] In a model of varicella in the SCID-hu mouse, not only was VZV found to be present in human T lymphocytes, but infectious VZV was also released from these cells.[130] Viremia has also been demonstrated in patients with disseminated HZ by use of either virus isolation or PCR.[131–133]

DIAGNOSIS

The diagnosis of varicella can usually be made clinically by the characteristic rash and epidemiological factors such as age of the patient, lack of history of the illness, and exposure to individuals with varicella or HZ in the previous 2 to 3 weeks. HZ, however, may be confused with recurrent HSV infection, especially if the face or trunk is involved and there is no previous history of a similar rash.[134] When it is deemed necessary, laboratory diagnosis is best made either by demonstration of viral antigens in scrapings from skin vesicles or by isolation of VZV from these lesions. Rapid diagnosis can be accomplished by scraping a suspicious skin lesion, making a smear on a microscope slide, fixing with ethanol, and staining with commercially available fluorescein-tagged monoclonal antibody to VZV gE.[120, 135]

The virus may be isolated in human embryonic lung fibroblasts (HELF), with the appearance of cytopathic effect within 2 days to several weeks after inoculation. PCR has recently been employed successfully for diagnosis of VZV infection, using vesicular fluid, respiratory secretions, and cerebrospinal fluid.[117, 118, 136–138] Whereas PCR is still a research tool, it is likely to become clinically available and useful in the future. It appears to be more sensitive than either immunofluorescence or virus isolation for diagnosis of infection with this labile agent.[136, 137, 139]

Serological tests for VZV-specific antibody permit documentation of immunity to varicella and also diagnosis of varicella by a fourfold or greater rise in antibody titer after the illness. Serological tests are of limited value for the diagnosis of HZ, however, because heterologous rises in VZV antibody titer may occur when HSV reactivates in an individual immune to varicella.[120] It is possible to make the diagnosis of active VZV infection on a single serum specimen by demonstration of specific antibody to VZV immunoglobulin (Ig) M; VZV IgM may be detected in HZ as well as in varicella.[120] The complement fixation (CF) test has largely been replaced by enzyme-linked immunosorbent assay (ELISA) for measurement of antibodies to VZV. ELISA assays are highly specific and cause few false-positive reactions. Commercially available ELISA tests are less sensitive than the fluorescent antibody to membrane antigen (FAMA) test,[120, 140, 141] but ELISA tests have the advantage of being more adaptable to large-scale testing than the sensitive but cumbersome FAMA test. An ELISA that uses glycoprotein of VZV for antigen has been reported to be highly sensitive,[142] but it is not commercially available. Moreover, positive antibody titers detected by this method in some 2-year-old children (and older children as well) before development of varicella suggest that the assay may be overly sensitive.[143] On the other hand, this assay has shown reproducibility when different batches of vaccine were used for immunization, and there was an excellent linear concordance when neutralizing antibody levels and glycoprotein-based ELISA (gpELISA) titers were compared.[144] An immune adherence assay (IAHA) has been described that has been used to analyze seroconversions to VZV particularly in studies in Japan.[145, 146] A latex agglutination (LA) assay based on the clumping of latex particles coated with VZV glycoprotein, observed in the presence of VZV antibody, combines the sensitivity of FAMA with the ease of performance of ELISA.[147, 148] In addition, this

Table 19–1. **ISOLATION OF VARICELLA-ZOSTER VIRUS FROM MONONUCLEOCYTES OF CHILDREN WITH TYPICAL COURSES OF VARICELLA**

	DAY	VZV ISOLATION	CONTACT
	11	0/1	Family
	7	0/1	School
	6	0/1	Family
Before rash (total 15	5	1/2	Family
cases)	4	1/2	Family
	2	4/4	Family
	1	4/4	Family
Rash	0	1/2	
	1	3/4	
After rash (total 9	2	0/2	
cases)	3	0/1	

Adapted from Ozaki T, Ichikawa T, Matsui Y, et al. Viremic phase in nonimmunocompromised children with varicella. J Pediatr 104:85–87, 1984; and Asano Y, Itakura N, Hiroishi Y, et al. Viremia is present in the incubation period in nonimmunocompromised children with varicella. J Pediatr 106:69–71, 1985.

assay can be performed within 15 minutes and requires no complicated equipment. There is a high degree of correlation between the presence of antibodies to VZV measured by FAMA and LA and protection from varicella after natural infection as well as after immunization.[147, 148] However, as with many serological tests, occasional false-positive and false-negative reactions have been reported.[149] A reliable, sensitive, rapid means of identifying individuals who have immunity to VZV, particularly after immunization, is sorely needed.

IMMUNE RESPONSE TO VARICELLA-ZOSTER VIRUS

Cell-Mediated Immunity. The precise roles of humoral immunity and CMI in protection against VZV infection are not entirely understood but are summarized as follows (reviewed in reference 43). Both structural and regulatory proteins of VZV are recognized during varicella by T lymphocytes, which induce protection from further VZV infection. Immunity is usually maintained for decades and is mediated by both $CD4^+$ and $CD8^+$ T lymphocytes, which can be demonstrated by cell proliferation and cytokine production in vitro after antigenic stimulation. Memory T lymphocyte responses may be maintained in part because of periodic exogenous reexposure to others with either varicella or HZ as well as by endogenous reexposure to the virus during subclinical reactivation of VZV. T lymphocytes from varicella-immune individuals produce cytokines of the Th1 type, such as interleukin-2 and interferon-γ, which potentiate clonal expansion of virus-specific T cells on exposure to VZV antigens.[43] $CD4^+$ lymphocytes provide help so that humoral responses to VZV antigens develop and are maintained after varicella.

CMI to VZV is important in recovery from VZV infections and also in prevention of development of clinical HZ. That CMI is required to maintain the balance between the host and latent VZV is demonstrated by the correlation between diminished CMI and an increased risk of HZ. Susceptibility of individuals to VZV reactivation is related not to diminished levels of VZV antibodies but rather to loss of CMI, which appears to be the response of major importance in control of VZV by the host. This is most clearly seen from clinical observations that patients with isolated agammaglobulinemia have normal courses of varicella and are not subject to an increased incidence of HZ, whereas those with defects in CMI are at risk for development of disseminated and possibly fatal varicella.

CMI to VZV after immunization has been determined mainly by lymphocyte transformation to VZV antigen, measured by a stimulation index, and by an intradermal skin test. CMI responses measured by lymphocyte transformation and skin test are promptly detected after natural infection; peak activity occurs within 1 to 2 weeks and then gradually decreases to lower levels.[150–156] In vitro, CMI to VZV can be detected by stimulation of lymphocytes with VZV antigens[42, 98, 157–160] and by specific lysis of histocompatible target cells by cytotoxic T cells stimulated with VZV antigen.[42, 98, 157–160] Natural killer cell and antibody-dependent cellular toxicity to VZV have also been reported.[161–163]

CMI responses develop within days after onset of clinical varicella and remain positive for many years; however, declining CMI is noted with advancing age, beginning at about age 50 years.[159, 164, 165] Decreased CMI to VZV is a necessary but not sufficient requirement for development of HZ.[43] Patients with poor CMI responses during varicella are also at risk for development of severe or fatal varicella.[43]

CMI responses of normal subjects with remote clinical evidence of varicella are characterized by occasional high activity in the absence of symptoms, suggesting either exposure to VZV with boosting of immunity or possibly subclinical reactivation of VZV.[166] Increases in CMI usually occur after HZ, even in immunocompromised patients, which probably accounts for the observation that second attacks of HZ are uncommon.[167] Subclinical viremia has been demonstrated in immunocompromised individuals after bone marrow transplantation.[168]

Class I–restricted lysis of VZV-infected target cells has been described after immunization of elderly seropositive individuals. This CMI response was more prominent in subjects who were immunized with live varicella vaccine compared with those who were given a similar dose of inactivated vaccine.[169]

Serum IgG Antibody Response. After natural infection, VZV-specific IgG antibody, measured by FAMA, is detected in most patients within the first 4 days after the onset of rash and other symptoms.[151] Peak IgG levels are attained at 4 to 8 weeks, and levels usually remain high for up to 6 to 8 months, after which titers decline twofold to threefold. Positive VZV FAMA titers have been detected in 100% of healthy adults for years to decades after clinical varicella.[58, 141, 147, 170] The kinetics of humoral, nasopharyngeal, and cellular immunity in patients with clinical varicella are shown in Figure 19–4.

Serum IgA Antibody Responses. Serum IgA antibody responses to natural infection are detectable early in the course of varicella, in most cases within the first 3 to 4 days after the onset of symptoms.[151] Serum IgA antibody responses attain peak levels by the fourth week of illness. Although levels subsequently decline, serum IgA antibody was detected in 44% of subjects up to 14 months after varicella.[151]

Nasopharyngeal Humoral Immune Response. Nasopharyngeal VZV-specific IgA antibody responses are detectable at the onset of clinical symptoms in patients with natural infections.[171] Nearly all patients exhibit IgA antibody responses within the first week. Maximum titers are attained at the third week of illness, and the IgA antibody activity declines subsequently.

SIGNIFICANCE AS A PUBLIC HEALTH PROBLEM

Because VZV is a highly contagious virus spread by respiratory droplets or airborne transmission, in temperate climates more than 90% of individuals have been infected by the second decade of life. It is now estimated that there are approximately 4 million cases of varicella

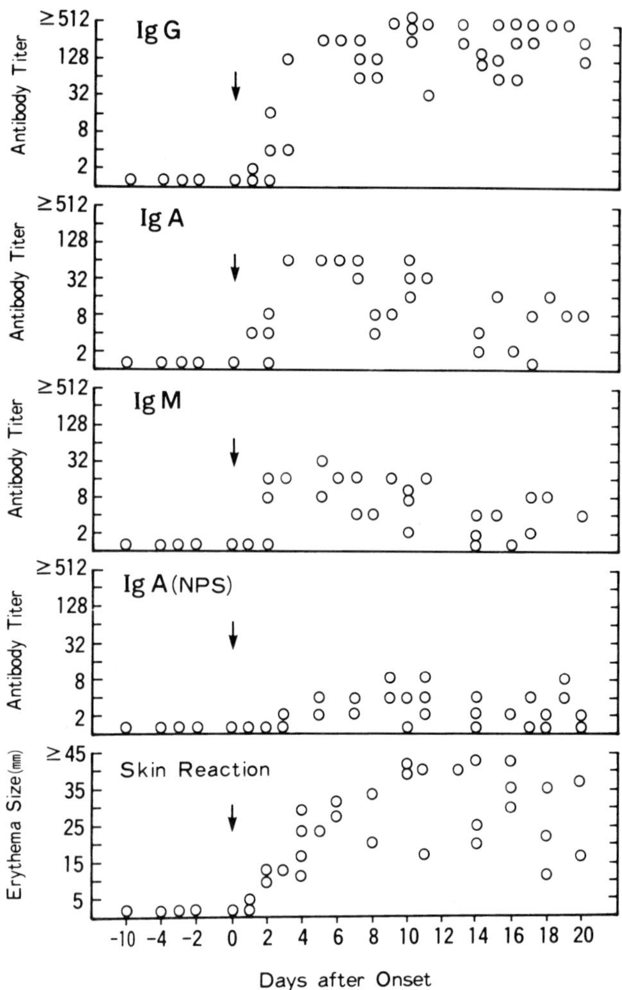

Figure 19–4. The kinetics of appearance of humoral (blood), nasopharyngeal (NPS, secretory), and cellular (skin reactive) immunity in patients with clinical varicella. The antibody titer was measured by fluorescent antibody to membrane antibody. Arrows at day 0 indicate the onset of varicella infection. (From Baba K, Yabuuchi H, Takahashi M, et al. Seroepidemiologic behavior of varicella-zoster virus infection in semiclosed community after introduction of VZV vaccine. J Pediatr 105:712–716, 1984.)

each year in the United States alone. If one accepts a conservative yearly birth rate of 1.5%, assumes that everyone in the cohort will eventually contract varicella, and estimates the world population at 4 billion, an estimated 60 million cases of varicella will occur annually.[172] There will also be an expected 5,200,000 cases of HZ per year, using the rate of 1.3 cases per 1000 derived from the population-based study in Minnesota.[173]

Several studies have been published indicating the significance of varicella as a public health problem. The first studies were done by Preblud and associates[174] in 1985, from the Centers for Disease Control and Prevention (CDC) in the United States.[174] They estimated that without a vaccination program, 3,291,750 cases of varicella would be expected during a 1-year period in normal individuals in the United States. With a vaccine program, the incidence would be reduced by 78%. A similar reduction would occur in the 329,262 physician visits and the 4653 hospitalizations attributable to varicella each year. Deaths and other disease-related events, including medication use, would also be reduced considerably. On the basis of these 1985 assumptions, there would be a savings of $7 for every dollar spent on a vaccination program.

In a study published by Huse and colleagues,[175] the authors estimated that there would be 32 physician visits per 100 cases of varicella among people aged 1 to 15 years and 95 visits per 100 cases among people aged 16 to 25 years in the United States. Their estimates were based on the average annual number of physician visits for varicella reported in the National Health Interview Survey divided by the corresponding average annual numbers of cases. The cost per outpatient visit for treatment of varicella was estimated to be $43.80 on the basis of reports in the National Medical Expenditure Survey. These surveys indicated that there would be 11 prescriptions for anti-infective and antipruritic medications per 100 cases of varicella in people aged 1 to 25 years with the cost per prescription estimated to be $15.50. Review of the National Hospital Discharge Survey indicated that the rates of hospitalizations were 16 and 60 per 10,000 cases of varicella, respectively, for people aged 1 to 15 years and 16 to 25 years. Estimates of costs of work loss assumed the average number of days of home care per case of varicella to be 3.7 days with a value of $103 per day for cases in children aged 5 to 12 years. No work loss was assumed for cases occurring in individuals 13 to 17 years of age. For individuals aged 18 to 25 years, average number of days lost was 5.5 days at $78 per day. With use of these assumptions, the expected costs of varicella to age 25 years among 100,000 children aged 15 months with and without vaccination in the United States are shown in Table 19–2. For the analysis of benefits and costs, the cost of vaccine was estimated to be $35 per dose with an additional charge of $13 by physicians for handling and administration. By use of these assumptions, there would be a net savings of $6,647,000 for universal use of the varicella vaccine.

Lieu and coworkers[176] also evaluated the cost-effectiveness of a routine varicella vaccination program using costs and medical intervention statistics from the Kaiser Permanente Medical Care Program and the California Hospital Discharge Database and several published studies. The cost of the vaccine in their analysis was estimated to be $35 with a $5 to $10 administration fee (Table 19–3). The authors concluded that the program would save more than $5 for every dollar invested in vaccination if one included work loss costs as well as medical costs. However, from the healthcare payer's perspective (medical costs only), the program would cost approximately $2 per varicella case prevented or $2500 per life-year saved.[176]

In a study conducted in Germany, the authors concluded that from a purely economic viewpoint, vaccination of susceptible adolescents was the optimal approach.[177] With use of assumptions collected from physicians and hospitals in Germany, for every Deutsche Mark (DM) spent for a vaccination program, DM 0.82 in medical costs would be recovered by vaccinating children compared with DM 1.94 for vaccinating only susceptible 12-year-olds. However, if indirect costs such as

Table 19–2. **EXPECTED COSTS OF CHICKENPOX TO AGE 25 YEARS* AMONG 100,000 CHILDREN AGED 15 MONTHS, WITH AND WITHOUT VACCINATION**

COSTS	NOT VACCINATED (A)	VACCINATED (B)	NET COST OF VACCINATION (B MINUS A)
Medical care			
Vaccination	—	$4,800,000	$4,800,000
Treatment of side effects	—	12,000	12,000
Treatment of chickenpox	$ 1,766,000	88,000	(1,678,000)
Total medical care costs	$ 1,766,000	4,900,000	3,134,000
Work loss	10,296,000	515,000	(9,781,000)
Total costs	$12,062,000	$5,415,000	(6,647,000)

*Discounted at 5% annually.
From Huse DM, Meissner HC, Lacey MJ, Oster G. Childhood vaccination against chickenpox: An analysis of benefits and costs. J Pediatr 124:869–874, 1994.

wages lost were included, the return on investment was DM 4.60 and 6.02, respectively.

In a study of healthcare workers in a United States hospital, the costs associated with VZV control during 1986 totaled $55,934: $39,658 for work furloughs, $9800 for serologies, $4293 for isolation of patients, $155 for VZIG, and $2028 for infection control personnel time.[178] Studies have not been reported to date analyzing the impact of vaccination on prevention or amelioration of HZ.

The importance of immunization was painfully demonstrated in 1997 in the United States when, in the first 4 months of that year, three young adult women were reported to have died of complications of varicella.[179] In each case, the source of infection was an unvaccinated child. These three deaths were considered vaccine-preventable by the CDC. Two of the women were healthy mothers before developing varicella and were only in their early 20s when they contracted fatal chickenpox.

PREVENTION AND TREATMENT BY ANTIVIRALS

Antiviral therapy for varicella and HZ first became available in the early 1970s. Antiviral therapy is useful to speed recovery from varicella and HZ especially in elderly and immunocompromised patients, but it does not decrease virus shedding or prevent latent infection. Vidarabine was the first successful antiviral drug to be used, but it was supplanted by acyclovir, a DNA chain terminator and an inhibitor of DNA polymerase that is less toxic than vidarabine.[180, 181] Intravenous acyclovir speeds healing of varicella and HZ in immunocompro-

Table 19–3. **AVERAGE ANNUAL VARICELLA-RELATED HEALTH OUTCOMES AND COSTS WITH AND WITHOUT A PROJECTED U.S. VACCINATION PROGRAM***

HEALTH OUTCOMES	NO VACCINATION	VACCINATION	DISEASE CASES PREVENTED BY VACCINATION
Chickenpox cases	3,953,000	240,000	3,713,000
Major sequelae	9,930	610	9,320
Pneumonia	1,000	62	938
Encephalitis	650	40	610
Cases of long-term disability from encephalitis	20	1	18
Deaths	56	4	52
DISCOUNTED COSTS ($ IN MILLIONS)	**NO VACCINATION**	**VACCINATION**	**NET COST (SAVINGS) OF VACCINATION VERSUS NO VACCINATION**
Medical costs†			
Vaccine and administration	0	88	88
Varicella disease costs	90	10	(80)
Total medical costs	90	98	8
Work loss costs (savings)	439	48	(392)
Total medical + work loss varicella-related costs (savings)	529	146	(384)

*Figures are averages for the first 30 years of a vaccination program. Costs are determined at 5% per year; health outcomes are undiscounted.
†Healthcare payer's perspective includes medical costs only. Ratio is the reduction in medical costs divided by the cost of the vaccination program. Societal perspective includes medical and work loss costs. Ratio is the reduction in medical and work loss costs divided by the costs of the vaccination program.
From Lieu TA, Cochi SL, Black SB, et al. Cost-effectiveness of a routine varicella vaccination program for US children. JAMA 271:375–381, 1994. Copyright 1994, American Medical Association.

mised patients, and orally administered acyclovir, at high doses, is useful to treat elderly patients with HZ.[180–182] Orally administered acyclovir may be used to treat otherwise healthy children with varicella, but owing in part to the poor absorption of the drug when it is given orally, the antiviral effect is minimal. A double-blind placebo-controlled study in which 102 healthy children were given acyclovir 40 or 80 mg per kg (or placebo) daily for 5 days, beginning within 24 hours of rash onset, revealed that the mean number of skin lesions was significantly reduced from more than 500 to 336.[52] On average, there was 1 day less of fever, but children who were treated with acyclovir did not return to school any more rapidly than those who received placebo. A multicenter collaborative study involving 815 similarly treated children given 80 mg/kg of acyclovir daily yielded similar results.[183] The benefit to secondary household cases was not increased beyond that of primary cases. The modest benefit conferred by acyclovir therapy is not surprising in view of the self-limited nature of chickenpox in children. Studies in adults have not indicated more striking antiviral effects.[64] The newer oral antiviral drug valacyclovir, which is well absorbed from the gastrointestinal tract and is rapidly converted to acyclovir in the liver, results in blood levels of acyclovir that are significantly higher than those achieved by administering acyclovir orally. Whereas valacyclovir has efficacy for treatment of HZ,[184] no studies of varicella have been performed, nor have children participated in any clinical trials of this drug. Famciclovir, which is also administered orally, is rapidly converted to penciclovir in the body; penciclovir has an action similar to that of acyclovir. Like valacyclovir, famciclovir is useful for treatment of HZ but has not been studied for treatment of varicella.[185] The antiviral drug sorivudine[186] was not approved by the Food and Drug Administration (FDA) in the United States because of the lack of significant benefit over acyclovir and the potential for toxicity in patients being treated for cancer. Antiviral therapy continues to be an important aspect of therapy for VZV in immunocompromised patients. However, for control of varicella, and possibly even for HZ, prevention of chickenpox would seem to offer greater benefit.

PASSIVE IMMUNIZATION

Ordinary Immune Globulin

The first studies indicating that varicella could be modified by administration of human immune globulin after exposure to VZV were reported by Ross.[51] He and his coworkers demonstrated that varicella could be attenuated by giving immune globulin to varicella-susceptible children within 72 hours after household exposure. Larger doses of immune globulin produced decreasing numbers of skin lesions. However, no completely preventive effect of immune globulin was noted at any dosage level.

Varicella-Zoster Immune Globulin

When globulin prepared from serum of patients recovering from HZ with high VZV antibody titers was given to children who had been exposed to varicella, chickenpox was prevented.[187] This material, termed zoster immune globulin (ZIG), was first tested in a double-blind controlled fashion in healthy children, for whom a dose of 2 mL, administered within 72 hours of exposure, prevented varicella. Subsequently, a larger dose, 5 mL of ZIG, was found to modify but not necessarily prevent varicella in leukemic children.[102, 103] In an efficacy study, 15 children who were undergoing therapy for leukemia or other malignant disease who had household exposures to varicella were given ZIG within 72 hours of exposure. Varicella was severe in one child, mild in nine, and subclinical in five. All children had persistence of antibodies to VZV for at least 2 years, suggesting that ZIG modified but did not prevent infection by VZV.[188]

It was subsequently determined that a high-potency globulin with titers equal to those in ZIG could be prepared by using outdated units of plasma with high VZV antibody titers.[189] This material was termed VZIG, and it was licensed for use in the United States in the early 1980s.[72] It is estimated that VZIG contains more than 10 times the amount of antibody to VZV as does ordinary immune globulin.

Zoster immune plasma has efficacy in preventing or modifying varicella in immunocompromised patients,[190, 191] but treatment of immunocompromised patients with disseminated HZ with zoster immune plasma is not effective.[192] This is not surprising because HZ may occur in the face of high antibody titers to VZV.

Passive immunization is thus known to be effective against chickenpox. On occasion, however, varicella may be severe in passively immunized immunocompromised children, including newborns, despite use of the correct dose at the proper time.[188, 192–194] Passive immunization, moreover, is of limited use because an exposure to VZV must be recognized for it to be given.

ACTIVE IMMUNIZATION

The KMcC Candidate Vaccine Strain

The Oka strain of VZV is the only vaccine strain that is currently available for use. Before clinical trials with this vaccine in the 1970s, however, another candidate vaccine strain (KMcC) was developed by serial passage of VZV in human diploid cells and underwent clinical trials.[195, 196] It was tested at the 40th and 50th passage levels in healthy children; 26 children were given the 40th passage vaccine, and 17 were given the 50th passage. The seroconversion rate for children in both groups was 100%. Papular skin lesions occurred in 31% of the passage-40 vaccinees but in only 6% of the passage-50 vaccinees.

A series of 10 clinical trials were performed in which either the Oka or one of the two passages of the KMcC strain of varicella vaccine was administered to 369 children.[152] Postimmunization clinical reactivity, mainly in the form of rash, was minimal with the Oka and the KMcC passage-50 vaccine but was unacceptably high (32%) after the KMcC passage-40 vaccine. Immunogenicity of both KMcC strains was high: 93 to 100% of vaccinees seroconverted by the FAMA assay or developed positive in vitro lymphocyte proliferation responses to VZV antigen. There were at least 281 known varicella exposures in vaccinees. A high degree of protection from or modification of varicella was observed 9 to 48 months after immunization with each strain. Five episodes of mild varicella, however, occurred in children who experienced a seroconversion after immunization. The KMcC passage-50 vaccine was judged unacceptable because all these episodes occurred in children who received it, and thus it seemed insufficiently protective. Comparatively better immunogenicity of the Oka strain to the KMcC strain was also noted in rhesus monkeys.[197] The passage-40 KMcC vaccine was also judged unacceptable because of its high rate of vaccine-associated rash. In summary, it did not seem possible to obtain a passage of the KMcC candidate vaccine strain with an acceptably low degree of reactogenicity that was sufficiently effective; the passage that was highly immunogenic was unacceptably reactogenic, whereas one that was not reactogenic was poorly immunogenic.

The Oka Vaccine Strain: Description and Development

The Oka strain of varicella vaccine was developed as follows[198, 199]: (1) fluid was taken from the vesicles of a 3-year-old boy (with the family name of Oka) who had typical chickenpox but who was otherwise healthy, and (2) VZV was isolated in primary HELF cell cultures. Attempts to obtain an attenuated strain of virus were made by serial cultivation 11 times at 34°C in HELF and 12 passages in guinea pig fibroblast cells (GPFC). Because GPFC are nonprimate cells in which VZV replicates, these cells were hypothesized to be suitable for obtaining a VZV variant that might become attenuated for the human host. The master seed virus was prepared by two passages in WI-38 human diploid cells, followed by three passages in MRC-5 human diploid cells to prepare the seed virus. Vaccine pools are usually made after two to three additional passages in MRC-5 cells.

For the original preparation of Oka vaccine, infected tissue cultures were washed with phosphate-buffered saline, and infected cells were harvested in the presence of ethylenediaminetetraacetic acid (EDTA). The cell suspension in vaccine medium was then sonicated to obtain cell-free virus; a titer of 1500 to 5000 plaque-forming units (PFU) per milliliter of VZV was usually obtained. Initial safety testing of the vaccine included demonstration of lack of pathogenicity after parenteral and intracerebral inoculation of small animals and monkeys. The absence of C-type particles and latent viruses was confirmed morphologically and biochemically.

The vaccine virus was found to have various biological and biophysical attributes that can be used to distinguish it from wild-type viruses.[12, 158, 200–205] Attenuation for humans is correlated with poor growth in skin explants cultivated in SCID-hu mice and may be related to deficient synthesis of gC.[205] Other attributes of attenuation include the following.

Temperature Sensitivities of the Vaccine and Wild-Type Strains. The vaccine strain was found to be slightly temperature sensitive at 39°C, in comparison to wild-type strains. The plaque foci of the vaccine strain in cell culture are also smaller than those of wild-type strains at high temperatures but similar in size to the wild-type strains at lower temperatures.[12]

Difference in Infectivity in Guinea Pig Embryo Fibroblasts (GPEF) and HELF of the Vaccine and Wild-Type Strains. The infectivities of the vaccine strain and wild-type strains were demonstrated to be different by plaque titration assay on GPEF and HELF. The vaccine strain exhibited a ratio of infectivity in GPEF compared with HELF ranging from 10 to 50 times higher than that demonstrated with 12 wild-type strains, including the Oka parental wild-type strain. Presumably, this increased infectivity of the vaccine strain in guinea pig cell cultures is due to its prior adaptation in these cells during attenuation.[12, 201] The immunogenicity of the vaccine virus was also far better than that of other wild viruses in guinea pigs,[201, 206] which is also probably related to the difference in the capacity of the vaccine virus to replicate in cultured guinea pig cells.

DNA Cleavage Profile. Differences in the migration patterns of DNA fragments of the vaccine-type virus and other wild-type strains were found after cleavage of purified DNA obtained from viruses propagated in cell cultures, with restriction endonucleases. In a comparison of DNA from the vaccine-type virus and wild-type viruses, significantly different cleavage patterns were seen with use of *Hpa*I, *Bam*HI, *Bgl*I, and *Pst*I enzymes.[200, 201, 204] In studies from Japan using *Hpa*I, a DNA fragment unique to vaccine-type virus (K) was identified[12, 207] (Fig. 19–5). When clinical isolates were tested with this method, the results were in accordance with those of the infectivity ratio (GPEF-HELF) and also consistent with the clinical picture of the origin of the VZV isolates.[12] In early studies in the United States employing *Bgl*I, it was noted that a novel restriction site in vaccine-type virus resulted in a different pattern of migration of fragments A to C in comparison with wild-type VZV[200] (Fig. 19–6). This distinction was attributed to differences between most but not all American and Japanese circulating wild-type viruses rather than a marker of attenuation.[202] With *Pst*I, an additional cleavage site is present in wild-type virus (between O and L fragments) that is not found in vaccine-type virus.[203, 204] It subsequently became possible to distinguish between vaccine-type and wild-type VZV by use of PCR and restriction endonuclease digestion of the resulting DNA fragments.[203] This approach was based on the differences noted before between wild-type VZV and the Oka strain. Two primer pairs are used, one that generates a 220 base pair fragment flanking a novel *Bgl*I restriction site in vaccine-type virus and another that generates a 350 base pair fragment that is cleaved in all wild-type VZVs. The resulting amplification products are subjected to digestion with *Bgl*I and *Pst*I restriction enzymes, and the fragments are separated by electrophore-

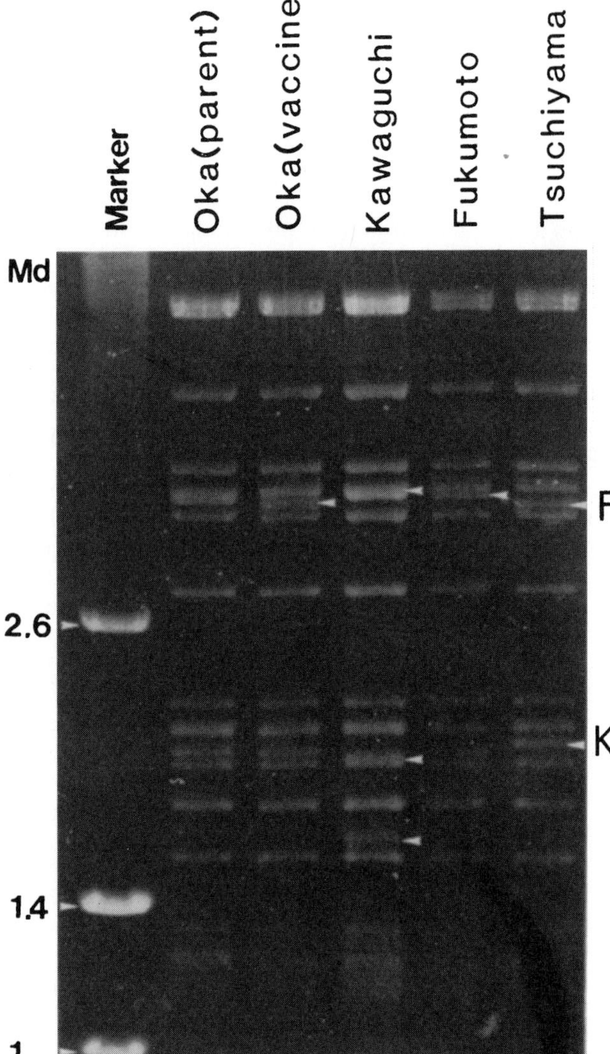

Figure 19–5. Profile of DNA cleavage by endonuclease *Hpa*I as follows: the Oka parent strain, the Oka vaccine strain, two wild-type strains (Kawaguchi and Tsuchiyama), and the Fukumoto strain recovered from a vaccine recipient. The mobility of the K fragment of the Oka strain is unique, whereas that of the F strain varies. (From Hayakawa Y, Torigoe S, Shiraki K, et al. Biologic and biophysical markers of a live varicella vaccine strain [Oka]: Identification of clinical isolates from vaccine recipients. J Infect Dis 149:956–963, 1984, and the University of Chicago Press.)

sis in a 4% agarose gel. By examining the number and sizes of the DNA fragments, wild and vaccine-type viruses can be distinguished (Fig. 19–7). In a series of 19 VZV isolates, there was 100% correlation between standard analysis of VZV isolates by culture, purification of DNA, and restriction endonuclease digestion and the PCR method.[203] All Oka strains lack a *Pst*I restriction site and have a *Bgl*I restriction site. All wild-type VZVs in the United States have a *Pst*I restriction site and most lack a *Bgl*I restriction site.

Studies using the described amplification by PCR and treatment of the amplification products with restriction enzymes have confirmed and extended a number of the analyses described. It is now recognized from studies of 92 clinical isolates from the United States that approximately 20% of circulating American wild-type VZVs have a *Bgl*I cleavage site.[208] All of these circulating wild-type viruses had a *Pst*I restriction site. Studies of viruses obtained from New York, California, and Australia (113 specimens) have indicated that there are no circulating viruses that have the DNA profile of the Oka strain (i.e., that lack a *Pst*I restriction site).[208] One of nine wild-type VZVs studied from Japan, however, had a *Pst*I restriction site as well as a *Bgl*I restriction site.[208] Thus, in countries other than Japan, the best marker for the vaccine strain is the absence of a *Pst*I restriction site. In Japan, the combination of single-stranded conformational polymorphism profile after PCR amplification of the R2 terminal repeat (within *Hpa*I-K fragment, ORF 14) and analysis of the *Pst*I site is useful for distinguishing between Oka and other clinical isolates.[209]

Clinical Evidence of Attenuation

In contrast to natural infection, the Oka strain appears to be less likely to induce a demonstrable viremia after immunization. Viremia was not detected in 18 healthy or 10 immunocompromised vaccine recipients who had no clinical symptoms.[139] Viremia due to vaccine virus, however, was found in a leukemic child in remission for only 6 months when immunized, who had vesicles and fever to 104°F 20 days after vaccination.[210] These observations suggest that vaccine virus is attenuated, because in contrast to natural varicella, development of viremia in healthy hosts has not been demonstrated. The Oka strain does, however, retain the ability to multiply in animal model systems of VZV such as the guinea pig[43] and possibly in the rat model of VZV latency.[45]

The incidence of rash after subcutaneous injection of varicella vaccine is far lower than the incidence of rash in natural infection. This is also suggestive of attenuation, although not conclusive, because the virus is delivered by an unnatural route (i.e., by injection rather than inhalation). There are, however, further indications of attenuation in human studies. When the vaccine (800 to 2500 PFU) was administered to 19 healthy children by inhalation, the incidence of rash remained low.[171] Although the inoculating dose of virus under natural circumstances cannot be known and therefore cannot be compared with the dose of vaccine virus, these observations are highly suggestive of attenuation.

Transmissibility of Vaccine Virus

When rare transmission of vaccine virus to a healthy susceptible inadvertently occurs, the disease is invariably mild or subclinical.[119, 211, 212] Moreover, the rate of transmissibility of the Oka strain in a household setting is four to five times lower than that of wild-type VZV.[119]

A pregnant woman was infected by her healthy 12-month-old child, who had developed approximately 30 vesicular lesions after vaccination.[212a] A vaccinated adult woman developed a similar number of lesions and transmitted mild varicella to two of her children.[212b]

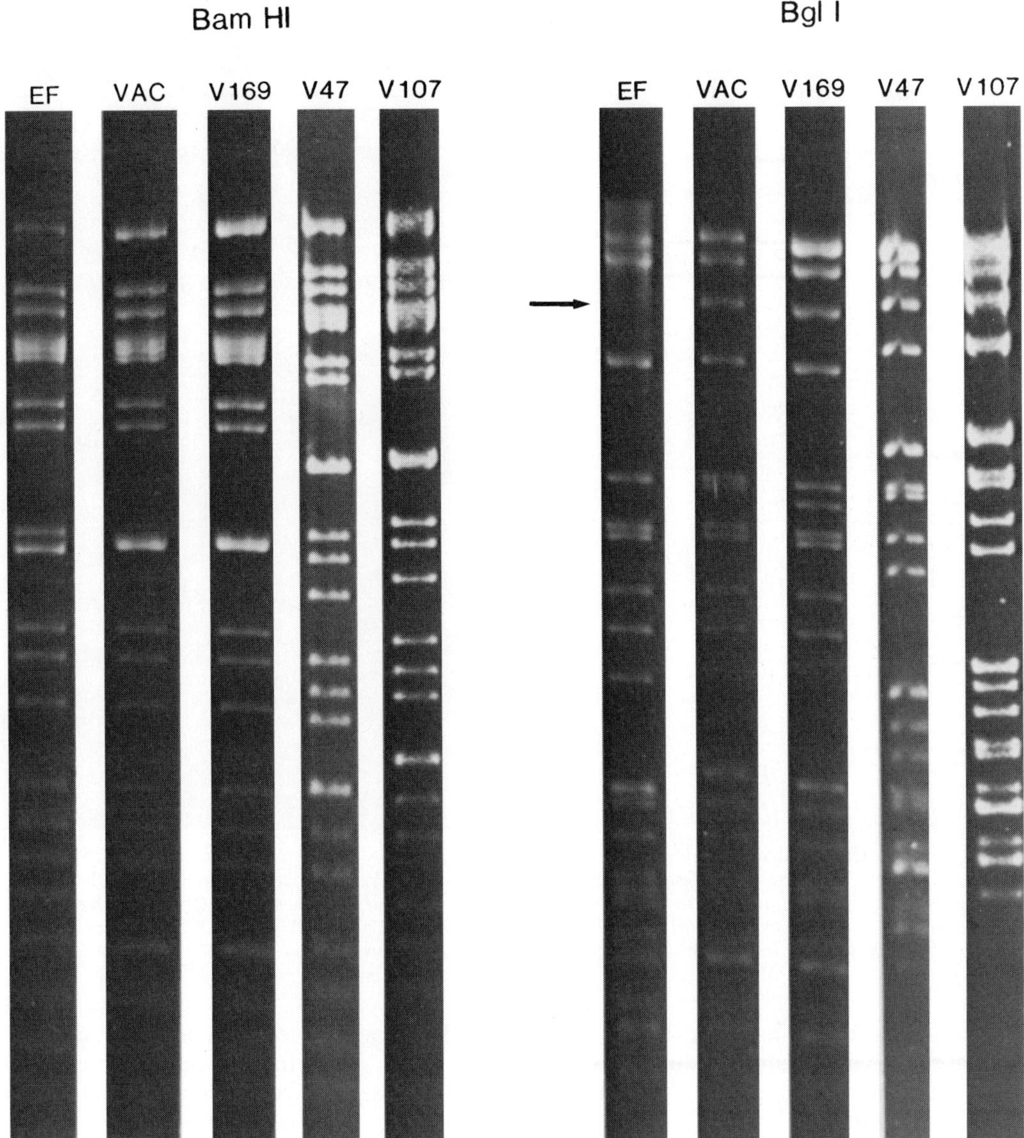

Figure 19–6. Restriction endonuclease analysis of varicella-zoster virus isolates obtained from vaccinees with a rash after immunization (V47 and V107) and from a varicella-susceptible sibling (V169) exposed to a leukemic vaccinee with mild vaccine-associated rash. Strains studied here are all vaccine type. Viral DNA was digested with *Bam*HI or *Bgl*I, processed by electrophoresis through 0.8% agarose, and stained with ethidium bromide. EF is wild-type virus control, and VAC is Oka vaccine control. The illustration is a composite of several gels, causing apparent minor differences between isolates. The arrow points to *Bgl*I A, B, C fragment migration characteristic of Oka vaccine strain. (From Gershon AA, Gelb L, LaRussa P. Live attenuated varicella vaccine: Efficacy for children with leukemia in remission. JAMA 252:355–362, 1984. Copyright 1984, American Medical Association.)

Transmission of vaccine-type virus from leukemic vaccinees has been observed, but only when the leukemic child had a vaccine-associated rash. The likelihood of spread has been reported to be directly proportional to the number of skin lesions in the vaccinee.[119] The likelihood of spread of vaccine virus in a household setting is reported to be about 25%, in contrast to the usual rate of transmission of about 90% for the wild-type virus under similar circumstances.[119] In combined clinical and serological studies of siblings of leukemic vaccinees, there was no transmission to 112 susceptible siblings exposed in a household to a leukemic vaccinee who had no rash. In contrast, of 93 siblings exposed to a leukemic vaccinee with a vaccine-associated rash, 21 (23%) seroconverted. Of these children, 5 of 21 (24%) never developed a rash. In comparison, the normal expected subclinical attack rate of wild-type varicella is about 5%.[51] In siblings who developed a rash, the average number of skin lesions was 38 (median, 12; range, 1 to 200).[211] In comparison, children with wild-type varicella have on average 300 skin lesions.[51] There was only one report of tertiary spread in the collaborative study, suggesting that the vaccine virus has limited ability for transmission.[119] These results are important for two reasons. First, the low transmission rate and the mild rash in contacts infected by a natural route (airborne spread) of vaccine-type virus provide evidence of the attenuation of the Oka strain.[213] Second, these results have potential implications concerning the spread of vaccine-type VZV from healthy vaccinees, such as healthcare workers to other

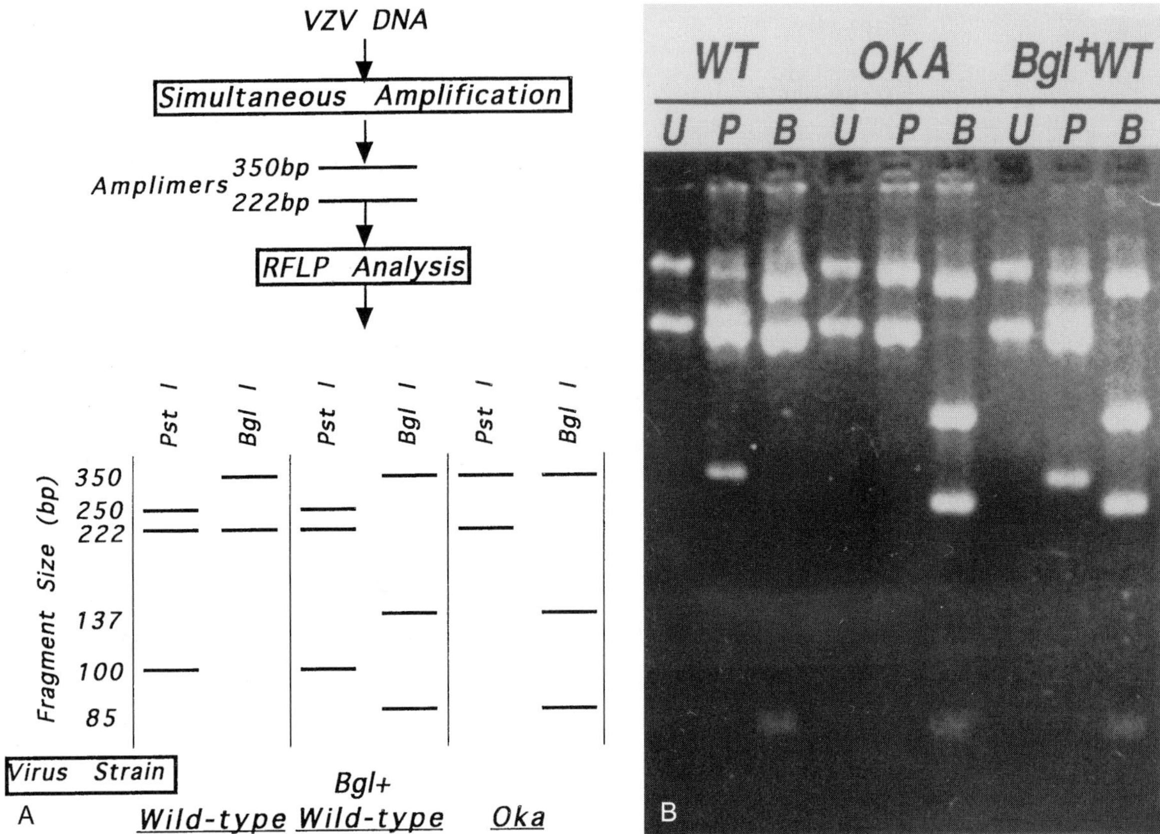

Figure 19–7. Restriction fragment length polymorphism analysis of VZV DNA amplified by polymerase chain reaction. *A*, Schematic representation of the predicted digestion patterns. The virus strain designated Bgl⁻, Pst⁻ is a theoretical recombinant that we have not detected in these analyses. *B*, Representative examples of amplification products from wild-type (lanes 1 through 3), Oka (lanes 4 through 6), and Bgl⁺WT (lanes 7 through 9) strains that were undigested (U) or digested with *Pst*I (P) or *Bgl*I (B). (*A* and *B* from LaRussa P, Lungu O, Hardy I, et al. Restriction fragment length polymorphisms of polymerase chain reaction products from vaccine and wild-type varicella-zoster isolates. J Virol 66:1016-1020, 1992.)

susceptibles. If a healthy vaccinee has no rash, the opportunity for spread of the virus seems vanishingly small.

The mildness of the clinical illness in children infected by the respiratory route with the Oka strain, the high rate of subclinical infection, and the low rate of transmissibility all provide evidence that the Oka strain is attenuated and not simply a geographical variant. Clinical evidence of reversion of the Oka strain to virulence has not been observed.

Constituents of Vaccine

For vaccine preparation, infected cells are harvested, suspended in the vaccine medium, and sonicated or exposed to a high-speed jet stream that shears the cells to obtain cell-free virus. Clinical studies indicate that the ratio of total viral antigen to total infectious viral particles is important in eliciting the appropriate immune response to vaccination.[214] Vaccine medium may vary according to the manufacturer; however, it generally contains sucrose and buffering salts. The vaccine is marketed in a lyophilized form to improve stability during prolonged storage. Reconstitution is accomplished with sterile distilled water (0.5 mL) according to the manufacturer's directions. All manufacturers provide reconstitution fluid with the vaccine.

Oka varicella vaccine is produced in the United States (Merck & Co., Inc.), Belgium (SmithKline Beecham Biologicals), France (Pasteur Mérieux–Connaught), and Japan (Biken). The vaccines vary in (1) passage number in human diploid cells, (2) virus dose (1000 to 10,000 PFU), (3) trace antibiotics added to ensure sterility during preparation, and (4) stabilizers and other minor constituents.

Seed lots of Oka vaccine have been prepared from virus passaged 11 times in HELF, 12 times in GPFC, and 5 times in human diploid cells. Manufacturers add three to nine additional passages in human diploid cells to prepare enough vaccine to meet marketing needs. Varicella vaccine is stable when it is frozen at −70°C for many years and for at least 3 years at −20°C. SmithKline Beecham Biologicals and Pasteur Mérieux–Connaught vaccines have improved stabilizers that allow storage at refrigerator temperatures (4 to 8°C) for up to 2 years. Although there is appreciable decrease in the titer of VZV during this time, enough remains at the end of the dating period to induce protective immunity (see later).

Clinical Development of the Oka Vaccine

Clinical trials with the Oka vaccine were initiated in Japan by Takahashi[198] in 1974. The vaccine was first given to 70 normal children at doses ranging from 100 to 2000 PFU. The Oka strain was immunogenic at doses greater than 200 PFU, and no significant reactions were noted in the children. Initial protective efficacy was demonstrated by giving the vaccine to susceptible household contacts within 3 days of exposure.[215] All of the 19 unvaccinated contacts, but none of the vaccinated contacts, developed typical varicella. The Oka strain was licensed to several other pharmaceutical companies (Merck & Co., Pasteur Mérieux–Connaught, SmithKline Beecham Biologicals) that later conducted clinical trials in Europe, the United States, and Canada.

Immunocompromised Children

Safety and Immunogenicity

Studies continued in Japan to include vaccination of children with malignant diseases for which the severity of varicella was the greatest. In the mid-1970s, a group of 39 children with underlying diseases such as nephrosis, nephritis, asthma, and hepatitis, about one third of whom were receiving steroids, were immunized. They were given a dose of 1000 to 2000 PFU of Oka/Biken vaccine. All of these children developed VZV antibodies as determined by CF.[198, 199]

A major departure in immunization with live virus vaccines occurred when children with leukemia and other malignant diseases were vaccinated.[216] Before this time, live vaccines were considered to be contraindicated for use in immunocompromised children. Given the high risk from natural varicella, however, 11 children with leukemia and 6 with solid tumors who were in remission from their malignant disease were immunized in Japan. Their chemotherapy, 6-mercaptopurine and methotrexate, was empirically withheld for 1 week before and 1 week after immunization.[216–220] In these studies, the seroconversion rate for antibodies against VZV, measured by CF or IAHA, approached 100%. Subsequently, the same workers reported on 326 Japanese leukemic children who were immunized, confirming and extending these data.[221] Most of these children seroconverted to VZV after immunization as determined by FAMA or IAHA.

In the late 1970s in the United States, in children with leukemia and varicella, a dissemination rate of 30% with 7% mortality of chickenpox had been reported.[83] On the basis of the successful studies of immunization of leukemic children in Japan, open label clinical trials in children with acute lymphoblastic leukemia in remission were begun in the United States and Canada in 1979. These studies first introduced varicella vaccine to the United States.

The largest clinical trial in leukemic children was conducted by the Varicella Vaccine Collaborative Study Group, which was organized to conduct these trials under sponsorship of the National Institute of Allergy and Infectious Diseases (NIAID).[44, 210, 219–223] At the time of immunization, children had to meet the following criteria: be in continuous remission from leukemia for at least 1 year, have no detectable antibodies to VZV by FAMA, have a positive response to mitogens in vitro, and have more than 700/mm^3 circulating lymphocytes. Within a decade, 64 children whose chemotherapy for leukemia had been completed and 511 children whose chemotherapy was suspended for 2 weeks were immunized.[213, 227] Chemotherapy for most of these children was daily 6-mercaptopurine, weekly methotrexate, and monthly pulses of prednisone and vincristine, regimens that were more intense than those given to Japanese children in earlier studies. By the late 1980s, in the United States, higher doses of methotrexate, prednisone, and cyclophosphamide were being administered. Although it was initially planned to administer one dose of vaccine, because of a failure of seroconversion after one dose in about 15% and loss of detectable VZV antibody after a year in about 5% of leukemic vaccinees, two doses of vaccine 3 months apart were recommended. In this study, a seroconversion to VZV occurred in 82% of leukemic children after one dose of vaccine and in 95% after two doses of vaccine.[158, 213, 224, 225] In general, about 80% of vaccinees tested developed positive CMI responses after one dose of vaccine and 90% after two doses, mirroring the experience with humoral immune responses.

Rash developed within 1 month after the first dose of vaccine[213] in 5% of leukemic children no longer receiving chemotherapy and in about 50% still receiving maintenance chemotherapy. Rashes were less common after the second dose of vaccine, occurring in only 10% still receiving maintenance chemotherapy. The rash after vaccination in children with acute lymphoblastic leukemia was usually maculopapular and vesicular and resembled a mild form of varicella. About 40% of children receiving chemotherapy who developed rash were treated with high oral doses (900 mg/m^2 four times a day) of acyclovir.[213] Some with more severe rashes (usually those with more than 200 lesions) were treated with intravenous acyclovir at a standard dosage. Oka VZV is sensitive to acyclovir, and acyclovir therapy did not appear to interfere with the development of the immune response.[213] The standard practice after observations of rashes in these children was to administer acyclovir in children with more than 50 lesions or who had rashes lasting more than 7 days.

A retrospective analysis of rash after immunization led to the recommendation that children not be given steroids for at least 2 weeks after immunization.[228] There has been no increase in relapse rate of leukemia in vaccinated leukemic children compared with children who had natural varicella either in the United States or in Japan.[225, 228, 229]

In two other smaller studies conducted in the United States in immunocompromised patients, 84 leukemic children were immunized.[230, 231] The seroconversion rates were similar to those observed in the collaborative study. Twenty-two children with solid tumors (Wilms tumor and rhabdomyosarcoma) were also immunized in the collaborative study (Gershon et al., unpublished data). After two doses of vaccine, 77% seroconverted by the FAMA assay. Thirty-two percent of these children had minor vaccine-associated rashes.

In a study of 23 uremic children, vaccine was given at least 2 months before renal transplantation. The vaccine was well tolerated with an 87% seroconversion rate after one dose of vaccine.[232] In another study in Spain, 34 children, half on dialysis and half after transplantation, were immunized. Their seroconversion rate measured by ELISA was 85% after one dose; 10% had a mild vaccine-associated rash.[233] Nephrotic children have also been vaccinated: There were no significant reactions, but two doses of vaccine were necessary for seroconversion.[233a]

There has been one large study of immunization of children with renal failure. A group of 212 French children were immunized before renal transplantation and observed between 1980 and 1994. They were compared with a group of 49 similar children with no history of vaccination or chickenpox and 415 similar children who had previous varicella. Antibodies to VZV were measured by FAMA and by ELISA. One year after immunization, 62% were VZV antibody positive.[234]

Studies are ongoing to evaluate the immunization of children with HIV infection whose CD4+ lymphocyte levels are relatively normal.

Vaccination of immunocompromised individuals proved to be useful for evaluating the relationship between immunization and development of HZ, because immunocompromised individuals are at high risk for development of HZ if they have had previous varicella infection.[97] A lower incidence of HZ in vaccinees was noted in uncontrolled studies[12, 207, 235] and in controlled trials[98, 226] (see later, *Herpes Zoster in Vaccinated Individuals*). This lower incidence again suggests the attenuation of the Oka strain. In these studies, there was a direct correlation between the risk of HZ and prior presence of VZV on the skin. It is hypothesized that VZV reaches nerve ganglia from skin infection and then becomes latent.[98] One could extrapolate that because vaccinees have a lower incidence of VZV rash, they may be at a lower risk to develop HZ later in life. Definitive information, however, will take another three to four decades of observations.

Efficacy

There is significant efficacy information on immunocompromised leukemic children in the United States and Canada from the collaborative NIAID study. In this group, there were 123 household exposures to varicella in a decade, with 17 cases of breakthrough chickenpox, a rate of protection of 86%.[98, 213, 224, 225] Varicella occurred in a total of 39 vaccinated children, most of whom did not have household exposures to chickenpox; this was generally a modified illness, with an average of 96 skin lesions (range, 1 to 640). None of these leukemic children with breakthrough varicella required treatment with antiviral drugs.

Efficacy of vaccine was also examined in the 212 French children who were immunized before renal transplantation. They were compared with a group of 49 similar children with no history of vaccination or chickenpox and 415 similar children who had previous varicella. The incidence of varicella, 26 of 212 (12%), was significantly lower in vaccinees than in those who were not vaccinated, 22 of 49 (45%). The disease was also less severe in the vaccinated, with no deaths; there were three deaths from varicella in the unvaccinated group. Varicella occurred only in vaccinees who lost detectable VZV antibodies after vaccination; no cases of varicella were observed in those who remained antibody positive. Four of the 415 (10%) patients with a history of past varicella developed a second attack, which was similar to the attack rate in vaccinees.[234]

Healthy Children

Dose and Route Selection

Clinical studies began in Japan in healthy adults and children before they progressed to the immunosuppressed population. After initial safety studies in healthy adults, children in Japan were given varying doses of the Oka strain to determine the minimum effective dose.[221, 236–238] Seroconversion rates of more than 95% were obtained in normal children with 300 to 500 PFU administered by subcutaneous injection. In another dose-response study using the Oka strain vaccine manufactured by SmithKline Beecham, seroconversion rates of 95.5% were induced with approximately 600 PFU.[239]

The Oka strain vaccine manufactured by Merck has been tested in various dose titration studies during the development of the vaccine. Each time there was a change in the manufacturing process, dose titration studies were performed. The first study was conducted in 137 healthy children who were randomized to receive approximately 43, 435, 970, and 4350 PFU.[240] Of the 99 initially seronegative children who received doses of 435 PFU or greater, 94% of those assayed at 2 weeks and 100% of those assayed at 4 or 6 weeks seroconverted. Children who received only 43 PFU seroconverted more slowly than those who received higher doses. The geometric mean titers (GMTs) at 6 weeks were similar for all vaccine doses. All vaccine dose levels were well tolerated with no significant differences in the rate of clinical reactions by dose. The frequency of varicella-like rash was 3%, and all rashes were mild. Two additional studies were performed with later formulations of the vaccine.[241, 242] In these studies, the vaccine was not diluted to obtain the lower dose levels of plaque-forming units but was exposed to slightly elevated temperatures to accelerate the decay of infectious particles. This process mimics what would actually happen during prolonged storage of the vaccine (i.e., constant antigen with decreasing plaque-forming units in the injected dose). Doses lower than 500 PFU resulted in seroconversion rates greater than 90%; moreover, dose levels of 80 to 160 PFU and 439 PFU elicited significantly lower antibody titers compared with dose levels of 1125, 1770, and 3625 PFU.

Administration of the vaccine using an inhalation method was tested in a small study in an institution in Osaka, Japan.[243] Oka strain virus at doses of 800 to 2500 PFU was well tolerated by the 23 children older than 1 year enrolled in the study. All of the children seroconverted. During an outbreak of varicella in the institution 1.5 years after immunization, none of the vaccinees developed clinical varicella. In contrast, all 110 susceptible unvaccinated control children contracted clinical varicella. Unlike in subcutaneous injection, however, the dose of vaccine virus is difficult to control by the inhalation method, and the method itself is somewhat cumbersome.

Efficacy

In the first published study of varicella vaccine, immunization was used to terminate an outbreak of nosocomial chickenpox.[198] All of the healthy children who were immunized developed specific antibodies, and that particular outbreak of varicella was terminated. The vaccinated children were subsequently protected after four subsequent hospital exposures to varicella.[244] Although this was not a classic efficacy study, these data strongly suggested that live attenuated varicella vaccine would be effective in preventing disease.

There have been two published double-blind, placebo-controlled efficacy studies, both performed in children. The first was conducted in the early 1980s using Merck's Oka vaccine in the suburbs of Philadelphia.[245] In this study, 468 children were immunized with one dose of varicella vaccine containing approximately 17,000 PFU (the original report of 8700 PFU was erroneous) and 446 were given placebo. During the following 9 months, there were 39 cases of varicella, all in the placebo recipients, resulting in a vaccine efficacy of 100%. During the second year of follow-up, one vaccinated child developed modified varicella consisting of 17 lesions after exposure to wild-type varicella, resulting in an efficacy rate of 98%. During a 7-year follow-up, 95% of these vaccinees were estimated to have remained free of varicella.[246] These data are somewhat difficult to compare with those of subsequent studies in the United States, however, because these children received the highest dose of vaccine ever used in the United States, and this dose is not currently available or under consideration for future use.[247]

A second controlled study was performed in Finland using vaccine produced by SmithKline Beecham. This study included 513 healthy children aged 10 to 30 months. They were divided into three groups: those who were given a high dose of vaccine (10,000 or 15,850 PFU), those who were given a low dose (1260 or 630 PFU), and those who were given placebo. There was a seroconversion rate approaching 100% in vaccinees, as determined by FAMA. Children were observed for 29 months on average. During this time, there were 65 serologically confirmed cases of varicella, 5 in the high-dose group (3% attack rate), 19 in the low-dose group (11.4% attack rate), and 41 (25.5% attack rate) in the placebo group. The differences in protection were significant for each group, compared with each other and with control subjects. The breakthrough varicella in vaccinees was a minor illness with on average fewer than 30 skin lesions.[248]

Open Label Efficacy Studies

In other efficacy studies, involving either populations at high risk for development of severe varicella or healthy children, advantage was taken of the high degree of communicability of varicella in households and the high clinical attack rate of chickenpox. After household exposure to varicella, 80 to 90% of exposed susceptible children develop clinical disease.[51] In addition, secondary cases in the household are usually more severe. Studies of vaccinated children over time have indicated that the Oka vaccine is approximately 77 to 86% effective in preventing clinical varicella after household exposure, the most intense challenge for vaccine efficacy.[246, 249] The protective efficacy in children who received Oka vaccine manufactured by Merck and who were observed for up to 6 years after vaccination was 77%. In those who developed varicella after household exposure, the disease was usually mild (fewer than 50 lesions) (Table 19–4).

During the late 1980s, 3303 children in the United States were immunized in clinical trials with one of five production lots of Merck's Oka vaccine at a dose of 1000 to 1625 PFU.[249] There were 82 subsequent household exposures to varicella, and the attack rate of breakthrough disease was 12%. Breakthrough infections were mild, with about one tenth the number of expected skin lesions. This observation was consistent with those of many other investigators who also reported cases of mild breakthrough varicella in vaccinated healthy children.[152, 250–256]

Prospective experience from Japan in 2454 healthy children vaccinated between 1991 and 1993 indicated breakthrough varicella in 151 (6.2%) during the first year after vaccination when breakthrough varicella was most frequent. Most cases were clearly attenuated. Earlier, retrospective data in Japanese children immunized between 1987 and 1990 indicated an attack rate of about 12% in the 6 to 36 months after vaccination, again with generally mild breakthrough infections.[257] Another follow-up study reported that over 7 years the attack rate in vaccinated children was 34%; however, all cases were mild.[257a] With a vaccine uptake rate in Japanese children of approximately 20%, there has been no clear decrease in the incidence of clinical disease in Japan.[257]

Most published long-term follow-up studies of vaccinated children report that 1 to 3% annually have developed breakthrough varicella after significant exposure to wild-type varicella.[143, 246, 248, 249, 253, 255] Most cases of breakthrough varicella consist of a rash of fewer than 50 lesions, unaccompanied by fever. The rates and severity of breakthrough varicella do not appear to increase over time after vaccination. Johnson and colleagues reported a 28% yearly rate of varicella in children vaccinated six years previously with production lots.[257a] Only one seri-

Table 19–4. **PROTECTION IN CHILDREN VACCINATED WITH OKA/MERCK FROM NATURAL VARICELLA AFTER HOUSEHOLD EXPOSURE***

ATTACK RATE	PROTECTION FROM		MEDIAN NUMBER OF LESIONS
	Any Disease	Severe Disease	
20%†	80%	~98%	42

*Up to 6 years of follow-up results.
†77% reduction in cases compared with historical attack rate of 87%.

ous complication has been reported in a previously vaccinated child in association with breakthrough varicella.[258] The child had received the Oka strain vaccine manufactured in Japan at the age of 24 months. The child had a documented seroconversion to VZV determined by IAHA 4 weeks after vaccination. At 45 months of age, he developed aseptic meningitis along with an episode of wild-type varicella. Varicella infection was confirmed by the presence of viral DNA in cerebrospinal fluid by PCR with Southern blot hybridization. The child recovered without sequelae.

In an interesting report of an outbreak in a daycare center in which approximately 45% of children had been vaccinated, Izurieta and colleagues reported an efficacy of 86% against all disease and 100% against moderate or severe varicella.[258a]

Overall it appears that varicella vaccine is highly protective, although perhaps not as protective as other live viral vaccines such as measles and poliovirus vaccines. On the other hand, even in the minority of vaccinees who develop a breakthrough infection, there is evidence of partial immunity. Moreover, immunity resulting from natural varicella is not complete, with resultant second cases of varicella in some individuals and development of HZ in others. Overall, imperfect immunity against VZV may be not only reality but also an advantage, because it allows an opportunity for boosting of the immune responses due to exposure to VZV.

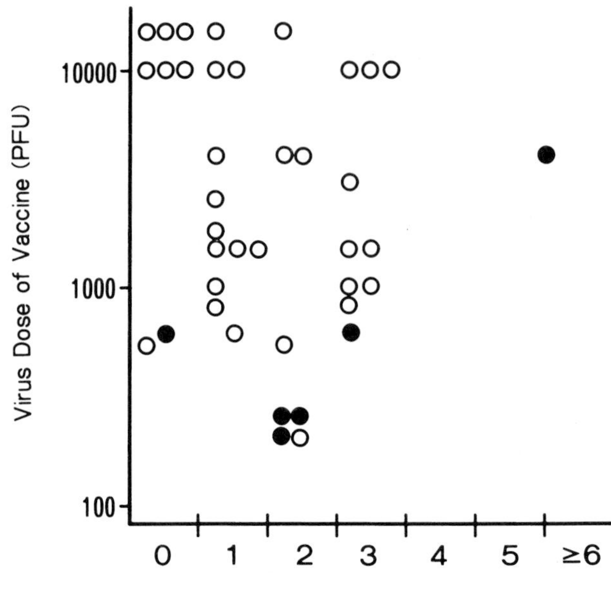

Figure 19–8. The protective effect of inoculation with live varicella vaccine in household contacts with regard to the dose of virus and the time between exposure and vaccination. (Adapted from Asano Y, Hirose S, Iwayama S, et al. Protective effect of immediate inoculation of a live varicella vaccine in household contacts in relation to the viral dose and interval between exposure and vaccination. Biken J 25:43–45, 1982.)

Efficacy of Postexposure Prophylaxis

Varicella vaccine has been useful to prevent chickenpox after an exposure to the virus has already occurred.[215] In one study, 26 contacts in 21 families were vaccinated, mostly within 3 days after exposure to the index case. None of the vaccinated children became ill, but 19 unvaccinated control subjects developed chickenpox.

The relationship between viral dose, interval between exposure and vaccination, and protective effect was examined in household contacts in a study of postexposure prophylaxis.[259] When approximately 1000 PFU of Oka/Biken vaccine was administered within 3 days after exposure, protection against varicella was observed (Fig. 19–8). In a similar study performed in the United States, using a larger dose of virus for immunization, there was also a protective effect.[172] These results are in accordance with the hypothesized pathogenesis of varicella, with initial mucosal replication 4 to 6 days before the virus spreads to visceral sites.[48] Although this method of immunization may be successful, it is not necessarily reliable; therefore, immunization before exposure is recommended.

Safety

The most common adverse events reported after varicella vaccine are mild tenderness and redness at the injection site (~15 to 20% of vaccinees), fever (~14% of vaccinees), and mild rash (~4% of vaccinees). In one double-blind, placebo-controlled clinical trial, the only complaint that occurred more often in vaccinated children than in placebo recipients was pain and redness at the injection site ($P < .05$).[245] The rash usually consists of 10 or fewer lesions occurring 7 to 21 days after vaccination. A similar percentage of children report a rash at the injection site, usually consisting of two to four lesions. It is difficult to culture vaccine-type virus from a child with a vaccine-associated rash, but it has been reported once.[260] Development of more than 30 lesions after vaccination in healthy children would be suggestive of intercurrent infection with wild-type strain.

Transmission of the Oka strain was addressed in two clinical studies in healthy children using the Merck vaccine.[245, 261] (Also, see earlier section, *Transmissibility of Vaccine Virus*.) In one study, children in a household were randomized to receive either vaccine or placebo.[245] In that study, there were no reports of transmission of clinical disease (e.g., rash). However, 3 of the 439 initially seronegative placebo recipients exposed to vaccinees seroconverted to VZV. No rash was reported in either the placebo recipients who seroconverted or the vaccine recipient to whom they were exposed. In the second study, siblings of susceptible immunocompromised children (most with a diagnosis of leukemia) were vaccinated.[261] There was no evidence of clinical or serological transmission of the Oka virus after vaccination in the approximately 30 families studied.

There is one report of spread of vaccine-type VZV from a healthy child vaccinee to a pregnant adult, his varicella-susceptible mother.[262] In view of the distribution of more than 4 million doses of varicella vaccine in the United States at the time of this occurrence, such an event must be considered exceedingly rare. On the basis of the estimated annual childhood risk of developing varicella of 9% and the high degree of transmissibility of the wild-type virus, the risk from natural disease to a susceptible pregnant woman with young children is calculated to be greater than the potential risk due to vaccination of the child.[263]

There have been eight reported cases of HZ in healthy children who previously received the vaccine as discussed later in *Herpes Zoster in Vaccinated Individuals*. The HZ was mild in all individuals.

Immune Responses After Vaccination in Healthy Children

After immunization with at least 500 PFU of the Oka strain, serum IgG antibody responses are easily detected within 1 month after vaccination, and antibody can be detected for months to years in most individuals. However, the individual and mean IgG antibody titers may be 10 to 30 times lower after vaccination than after natural infection, depending on the dose of vaccine virus administered and the age at immunization.[58, 214, 215, 244] Titers of antibodies to VZV have been observed to increase with time, however, so that presumably because of exposure to the wild-type virus, subclinical boosting of the immune response occurs, eventually resulting in IgG titers that are similar to those after natural infection.[247, 251] Serum IgA antibody is detectable only occasionally and at low levels in vaccinees immunized by inhalation, and VZV serum IgA is virtually undetectable in subjects immunized subcutaneously.[171] In contradistinction to the response after varicella, secretory IgA antibody responses to VZV have not been demonstrated after immunization, regardless of the route or dose of administration of vaccine.[171] However, as for many vaccines, immune correlates of protection against VZV infection are not entirely delineated. It is not known what level of IgG is protective or whether IgA at mucosal sites offers protection against infection.

In the 3303 children immunized in the United States in clinical trials during the late 1980s, VZV antibody titers were determined with the VZV gpELISA assay 6 weeks after immunization.[249] Their seroconversion rate was 96% with a GMT of about 1:12. It was noted, however, that the seroconversion rate in adolescents aged 13 to 17 years was only 79%; moreover, their GMT was 1:6, half the levels seen in healthy children.

During vaccine manufacturing campaigns conducted by Merck from 1982 to 1991 in the United States, a clear relationship between the dose of vaccine administered and the antibody titer measured by gpELISA was observed.[247] These data are presented in Table 19–5.

An update concerning 8429 healthy children from Japan, where 1.39 million healthy children were vaccinated between 1987 and 1993, indicates the highly immunogenic behavior of the vaccine. A seroconversion to VZV, using IAHA, was found in 2347 of 2565 (91.5%), with a GMT of 1:12.[257]

There are no published data on the use of commercially available VZV antibody tests to determine seroconversion rates in healthy children. Presumably, how-

Table 19–5. **LONG-TERM CLINICAL FOLLOW-UP OF VARIVAX RECIPIENTS: BREAKTHROUGH INCIDENCE (%) AND NUMBER OF VACCINEES (IN PARENTHESES) STUDIED PER YEAR**[247]

	VACCINE MANUFACTURING CAMPAIGN				
INTERVAL AFTER IMMUNIZATION	**1982 Lot (17,430 PFU)**	**1982 Lot (950 PFU)**	**1984 Lot (2460–14,000 PFU)**	**1987 Lot (1000–1625 PFU)**	**1991 Lot (2900–9000 PFU)**
Active and passive follow-up combined					
1†	0.2% (487)	0.4% (908)	0.3% (1154)	2.1% (3537)	0.2% (1011)
2	0.0% (543)	1.2% (1021)	0.9% (1294)	2.9% (3842)	0.8% (1134)
3	0.6% (534)	2.1% (1004)	0.6% (1279)	3.3% (3713)	1.0% (682)
4	1.3% (528)	1.2% (989)	0.7% (1271)	3.6% (3563)	
5	1.9% (518)	2.1% (971)	0.8% (1261)	3.3% (3371)	
6	1.0% (513)	0.9% (956)	0.9% (1247)	3.0% (2831)	
7	0.6% (508)	0.3% (951)	0.9% (1076)		
8	0.0% (506)	0.4% (943)			
9	0.2% (505)	0.5% (938)			
10	0.0% (504)	0.0% (917)			
Active follow-up alone					
1	0.2% (401)	0.8% (615)		3.0% (2994)	0.6% (955)
2	*	1.2% (417)		3.3% (2415)	0.8% (717)
3	*	2.4% (123)		4.4% (911)	*
4	*	1.8% (111)		4.3% (538)	
5	*	1.9% (108)		4.5% (376)	

For each follow-up interval, the annual incidence (%) of breakthrough varicella and the number of children (in parentheses) included in the study population are shown. When *active and passive follow-up periods* were combined, calculations assumed that all breakthrough cases that occurred in vaccinated individuals were reported. The 12-month follow-up intervals started 6 weeks after initial vaccination in this population. In *active follow-up alone*, only those subjects contacted for information on breakthrough disease within the previous interval were included. Individuals reimmunized with vaccine were excluded from further analysis.

*Fewer than 100 subjects actively observed during preceding 12-month interval.

†Excludes infections occurring within 6 weeks of vaccination.

From Krause P, Klinman DM. Efficacy, immunogenicity, safety, and use of live attenuated chickenpox vaccine. J Pediatr 127:518–529, 1995.

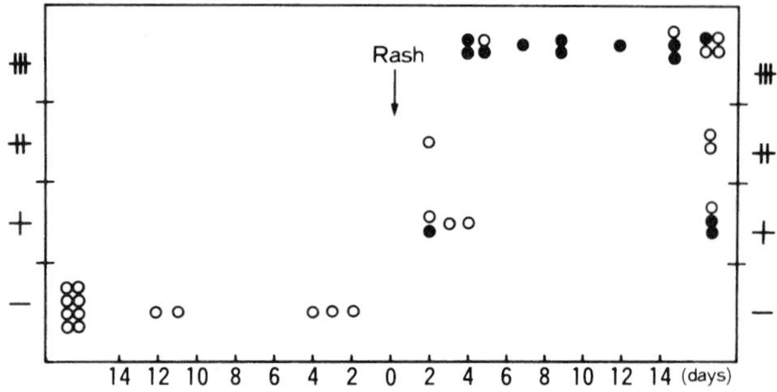

Skin test was done on 22 children

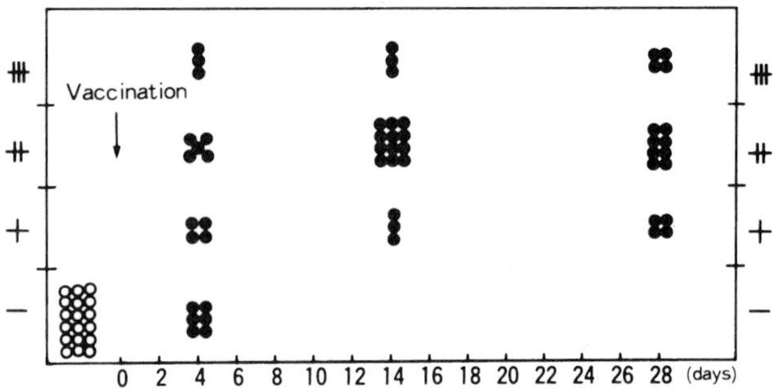

Skin test was done 4 times in all the 18 vaccinated children

o indicates the first skin test

• indicates the 2nd. 3rd. 4th skin tests

Figure 19–9. Comparison of the time of conversion of the varicella skin reaction in children after natural varicella or vaccination. (From Takahashi M, Baba K. A live varicella vaccine. In de la Maza LM, Peterson EM [eds]. Medical Virology. III. New York, Elsevier, 1984, p 255.)

ever, because these tests are less sensitive than the gpELISA assay, many children will have undetectable antibodies when commercial tests are used, despite successful immunization.

In vaccinated healthy children, the skin test response became positive as early as 4 days after immunization in about half the children (Fig. 19–9), 7 to 9 days before detection of neutralizing antibodies.[153] Similarly, in another study, lymphocyte proliferation became positive about 1 week before neutralizing antibodies were detected.[264] The stimulation index against VZV antigen in 74 healthy American children 6 weeks after immunization was 58.6 (±6.5).[265]

Adolescents and Adults

Safety and Immunogenicity

Adults who have been immunized have lower seroconversion rates than healthy children do. Small early studies suggested that the vaccine was more immunogenic in adults than it is now recognized to be. In 1985, in Switzerland, 32 healthy seronegative adults, mainly medical personnel, were given Oka/RIT vaccine, with a 90% seroconversion rate.[266] At a similar time, in the United Kingdom, 34 seronegative nurses were immunized with Oka/RIT, and 94% seroconverted as determined by several serological tests including ELISA and immunofluorescence.[267] After 3 years, however, only 66% remained seropositive. In studies of Alter[268] and Arbeter,[250] 89 to 94% of 53 adults seroconverted after one dose of vaccine as determined by FAMA.

In the NIAID collaborative study, during roughly 1980 to 1990, 268 healthy adults whose average age was 27 years were immunized.[58, 213, 269] Most were given two doses of vaccine 3 months apart; their seroconversion rate was 82% after one dose and 90% after two doses, as determined by FAMA. This experience is also consistent with the experience with rates of seroconversion in 79 vaccinated adolescents after one dose of vaccine.[249] The rate of mild vaccine-associated rash (average of nine skin lesions) was 10%, and although it was possible to isolate vaccine-type VZV from a few vaccinated individuals, there was no recognition of spread to others.

There has been one report of transmission of wild-type varicella from a vaccinated adult with breakthrough varicella to a varicella susceptible.[270] In addition, in studies from Cincinnati, Ohio, a vaccinated adult developed breakthrough varicella and transmitted what was presumably wild-type infection to another adult.[271] The rarity of such reports suggests that spread of vaccine-type or wild-type VZV from healthy vaccinees to others is possible but extremely rare.

Larger studies in adults using vaccine produced by Merck have indicated that adults require two doses of vaccine to achieve a seroconversion rate greater than 90%.[272] As for children, there are no data on seroconversions in healthy adults with use of commercially available tests. However, it would not be surprising, given the insensitivity of commercial tests, to find that many seroconversions in vaccinated adults cannot be detected by this method. In one comparative study of LA, FAMA, and a commercial ELISA, positive VZV antibody levels in 48 adults 1 to 3 years after immunization were detected in 52%, 69%, and 36%, respectively.[273]

Positive VZV CMI responses, including cytotoxic T lymphocytes, have also been observed in vaccinated adults in studies in the United States.[274] A cytotoxic T-cell response in 23 adult vaccinees was found to be similar to that observed in adults with past natural varicella.[274] The CMI responses of adults to varicella vaccine are, however, lower than those observed in children.[275]

Efficacy

In the NIAID collaborative study, 57 adults experienced household exposures to varicella, with 15 resultant breakthrough cases of chickenpox, an attack rate of 26%. From these data, an efficacy of 70% can be inferred against varicella of any type. In addition, the severity of the breakthrough cases was mild in most instances, even when antibodies were no longer present at the time of exposure. This attack rate appears to be higher than that seen in children who have been given similar lots and dosages of vaccine. Although the adults who developed breakthrough varicella had all previously lost detectable VZV antibodies by FAMA or LA, of these adults who had undetectable antibodies within the previous year, only 50% developed clinical varicella after a household exposure.[58, 213, 276] Most experienced a modified form of varicella. In summary, both the seroconversion rate and rate of protection of adults after exposure to VZV are lower than those seen after immunization of children. Nevertheless, vaccination of varicella-susceptible adults offers obvious protection from severe varicella.

PERSISTENCE OF IMMUNITY AFTER VACCINATION

Immunocompromised Patients

There has been a high degree of persistence of antibodies to VZV in vaccinated leukemics, although the rate of persistence is lower than that in healthy children. During an 11-year interval, 13% of vaccinees who originally seroconverted become seronegative by FAMA or LA.[213] Many of these children were exposed to varicella but did not become ill. After a re-seroconversion, titers in leukemic children usually remain detectable, and in a number of patients who re-seroconverted without symptoms, the Western blot antibody pattern was characteristic of an anamnestic response.[224, 277] The attack rate of clinical varicella among leukemic vaccinees who had again become seronegative and who had household exposures, furthermore, was only 30%, not the 80 to 90% that would be expected in varicella-susceptible individuals.[224] Neither the incidence nor the severity of breakthrough varicella in leukemic vaccinees has increased with time, and many of these vaccinees are now young adults.[213] The meaning of loss of a detectable antibody titer years after immunization is difficult to interpret but may represent some waning of immunity. At present, however, no booster immunizations are recommended.

The only other immunocompromised patients for whom there is long-term follow-up are those who received renal transplants. Antibody persistence was determined in French children who had been immunized before renal transplantation. After 10 years, 42% were seropositive by ELISA.[234]

Healthy Children

Several studies indicate that humoral, cellular, and protective immunity last for many years after immunization in healthy children. There has been no concrete evidence of waning of immunity. In Japan, a 5-year follow-up study of 26 healthy immunized children revealed that 100% had detectable neutralizing antibodies and 96% had positive FAMA titers.[251] None of these children developed breakthrough chickenpox, although many had been exposed to VZV. In a subsequent study of 106 Japanese children, 14 of whom had been receiving steroid therapy when they were immunized, there were 5 cases of breakthrough chickenpox.[252] Four of the cases developed in the first year after immunization. There were 147 recognized occasions when these children were exposed to VZV. Serum specimens were available from 38 children; FAMA antibody titers were 1:4 or higher in 37 (97%), with a GMT of 1:9. In 29 control children who had experienced natural varicella, FAMA titers were 1:4 or higher in 100%, with a GMT of 1:10. The VZV skin test response was positive in 97% of each group. Because the average VZV antibody titer after immunization is significantly lower than that after natural varicella, these results indicate that a boost in antibody titer had occurred in vaccinees, probably because of subclinical reinfection after exposure to exogenous virus.

A major question exists as to whether vaccine-induced immunity to VZV will remain positive when exposures to VZV become unusual in the postvaccine era. It was possible to assess whether exposure and consequent boosting are required to maintain positive VZV antibody titers after vaccination in a small group of handicapped institutionalized children who had no exposures to VZV for 5 years after being immunized.[278] The 16 vaccinated children as well as 7 children who had experienced natural varicella maintained positive VZV antibody titers for 5 years. Skin test reactions also remained positive in 14 of 16 vaccinees. Six VZV seronegative children remained seronegative during this 5-year period, indicating that no VZV was circulating in this isolated population during this interval. Thus, humoral and cellular immunity conferred by vaccine lasted at least 5 years, without boosting by natural infection. It is possible that subclinical reactivation of latent VZV may serve to stimulate immunity so that exogenous exposure to VZV may not be required to preserve immunological memory.

A 10-year follow-up as well as a subsequent 20-year follow-up after immunization in Japan has revealed that 25 of 25 young adults remained seropositive and 26 of 26 retained positive CMI responses as indicated by positive skin test reactions.[252, 257, 279]

In studies performed in the United States, persistence of antibodies for 2 years after vaccination was 94% in one study of 36 immunized toddlers.[254] Of more than 200 healthy children who were immunized in various studies in the United States, for whom there is a follow-up of 4 to 6 years, more than 95% remain seropositive.[246, 255, 280] Humoral immune responses against VZV appear to be more durable in healthy children than in immunized adults or leukemic children.[213] A follow-up of 85 vaccinees who were given 17,000 PFU of vaccine revealed that 97% retained positive CMI responses to VZV 5 to 6 years after immunization.[280] It is of the utmost importance to continue to observe healthy children who were immunized for persistence of immunity, particularly after the time when there is widespread use of varicella vaccine and little opportunity for boosting of immunity due to exposure to natural infection. Toward this goal, the FDA has mandated that long-term studies of immunity after varicella vaccination be carried out.[247]

A correlation between protection from varicella and the height of the gpELISA titer 6 weeks after immunization has been observed. Optical density values of more than 10 units at 6 weeks are associated with a lower chance of development of future breakthrough varicella.[143, 255] To achieve high levels of VZV antibodies after immunization that might be associated with better overall protection, several studies using two doses of varicella vaccine 4 to 8 weeks apart have been conducted

Table 19–6. **VARICELLA VACCINE IN HEALTHY ADULTS***

YEAR	NUMBER	NUMBER WITH VARICELLA (%)	PERCENTAGE SERONEGATIVE
1	343	8 (2)	34
2	234	8 (3)	33
3	174	2 (1)	40
4	115	5 (4)	10
5	68	4 (6)	30
6	45	2 (4)	10
7–13	40	2 (5)	18

*Long-term follow-up with regard to breakthrough illness and antibody loss with time. During the past 13 years, breakthrough varicella has developed in 9%.
From Gershon A. Varicella-zoster virus: prospects for control. Adv Pediatr Infect Dis 101:93–104, 1995.

in healthy children. These studies have indicated that this approach is safe, but whether two doses will offer greater protection than one dose for healthy children is not known.[265, 281] Studies of the rate of breakthrough varicella in vaccinated American children for as long as 10 years after vaccination have indicated a rate ranging from 0 to 4% per year, lower rates of breakthrough illness being associated with higher doses of vaccine[247] (see Table 19–5).

Healthy Adults

Studies of American adults vaccinated in the NIAID collaborative study have indicated that about 60 to 90% are seropositive by FAMA or LA antibody tests as long as 13 years after vaccination[213, 282] (Table 19–6). The incidence and severity of varicella have not increased with time in these vaccinated adults[213] (Fig. 19–10).

In summary, all data thus far support long-term persistence of humoral and cellular immunity in healthy vaccinees. Even in immunocompromised patients, although loss of detectable antibodies may occur, excellent immunity to VZV appears to persist. Boosting due to exposure to VZV occurs, but whether it is required for long-term persistence of immunity is not yet known.

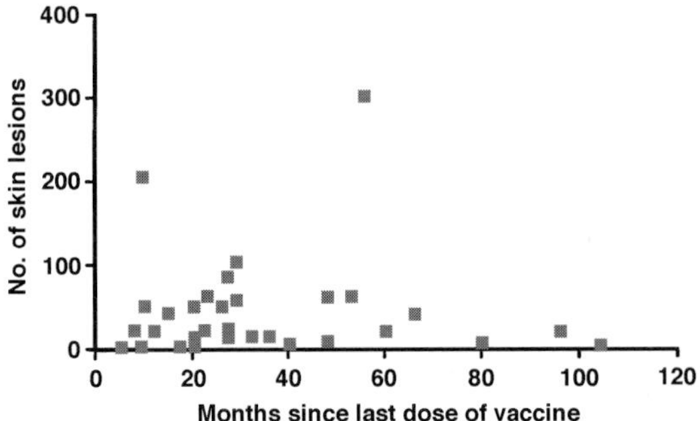

Figure 19–10. Number of skin lesions in 31 vaccinated adults with breakthrough varicella months to years later with respect to the time since the last dose of varicella vaccine was given. Note that the severity of illness did not increase with an increasing interval (in months) since immunization. The average number of skin lesions was 43. (From Gershon A. Varicella-zoster virus: Prospects for control. Adv Pediatr Infect Dis 10:93–124, 1995.)

HERPES ZOSTER IN VACCINATED INDIVIDUALS

A major question concerning the varicella vaccine has been whether the vaccine virus can establish latency, potentially resulting in later development of HZ. A long-term follow-up of vaccinated, healthy children will be required to answer this question definitively, but whether such a study, spanning more than 5 decades, can ever be practically performed is open to question. Nevertheless, it is possible to obtain some significant information on the issue. In U.S. studies, the incidence of HZ has not been increased in healthy immunized children.[283, 284] Table 19–7 outlines the cases of HZ reported in clinical trials.

The reported incidence of HZ in healthy vaccinated children is 13 cases per 100,000 person-years of observation.[285] In children aged 5 to 9 years who experienced natural varicella, it was 30 cases per 100,000 person-years of observation.[92] A few cases of HZ caused by vaccine-type VZV have been recognized since licensure of the vaccine, after which time more than 4 million doses of vaccine have been distributed in the United States (Sharrar et al., personal communication). It is not possible to calculate the incidence of HZ from this information, but it is clear that HZ remains a rare occurrence in healthy vaccinated children.

Comparative information on the frequency of development of HZ in immunized immunocompromised children and those who had natural varicella is available. This is because children with leukemia who have had natural chickenpox develop HZ at a much higher rate than healthy children do.[97] Vaccinated leukemic children have therefore been observed closely for development of HZ and compared with leukemic children who have had natural varicella. In Japan, one study found HZ in 8 of 52 (15%) vaccinated children and in 11 of 63 (18%) control children.[286] In another, 4 of 44 (9%) vaccinees and 8 of 37 (22%) control children developed HZ. In the United States, none of 34 vaccinated leukemics but 15 of 73 (21%) unmatched control subjects developed HZ ($P = .017$),[235] also suggesting that HZ would be less common after immunization than natural infection. In the NIAID collaborative study, the rate of HZ was 2% in vaccinees and 15% in control subjects. A subset of these vaccinees was prospectively matched, according to chemotherapeutic protocol, with 96 leukemic children who had experienced natural varicella. A life-table analysis revealed that the incidence of HZ was significantly lower in vaccinees than in the matched leukemics who had experienced natural varicella[44, 226] (Fig. 19–11).

Similar results were found in vaccinated children who had renal transplantation. In the study of vaccination of French children before renal transplantation, during 10 years, the rate of HZ was 7% in vaccinees, 13% in those with varicella before transplantation, and 38% in those who developed varicella after grafting.[234]

There are several possibilities that are not mutually exclusive as to why HZ may be less common after vaccination than after natural infection. One is that the virus is attenuated and less able to reactivate than the

Table 19–7. **CASES OF HERPES ZOSTER REPORTED AFTER VACCINATION WITH OKA/MERCK**

AGE (yr)	INTERVAL SINCE VACCINATION (yr)	VACCINE DOSE (PFU)	VZV-LIKE RASH AFTER VACCINATION	CULTURE RESULTS	SEROLOGY RESULTS*	DESCRIPTION OF CASES
8	4.2	87	No	Negative	Acute = 1448	10 papular and 25 vesicular lesions on back over right scapula and right arm; no other complaints
6	3.6	872	No	None	Acute = 2750	~9 erythematous patches, ranging in size from 2 × 2 mm to 15 × 9 mm, each composed of clusters of papulovesicular lesions; lesions were located along the right T6 dermatome; some upper airway congestion, itching
7	5.8	950	Chickenpox 1.5 yr before onset of HZ	Negative	Acute = 34.4 Conv = 2155	Vesicular rash on chest, arms (73 vesicles along C8, T1, T2 dermatomes); minimal itching, painful and burning sensation 1 week before onset
4	2.4	1460	Yes—injection site rash	None	Conv = 247.2	"Few" papular lesions in sacral area; no complaints
12	1.8	1460	No	Negative	Acute = 20	22 zoster-like lesions, papules and vesicles with surrounding erythema on left arm–hand; pruritus, local irritation: stinging before onset of lesion
2	1.8	3010	No	Positive; wild type	Acute = 112.2 Conv = 1551.9	Zoster-like lesions in the path of right ulnar nerve, right buttocks, right shoulder; restless; lesions painful to touch
6	3.3	5880	Non–injection site rash	None	Acute = 115 Conv = 2025	1 vesicular chain from upper chest to upper left arm; itching
2	1.2	5850	No	Negative	No sample	5 papular, 6 vesicular, 5 macular lesions on left upper arm and fourth and fifth digit of left hand; minor discomfort on lesions

*Glycoprotein-based enzyme-linked immunosorbent assay; HZ, herpes zoster; conv, convalescent.
From White CJ. Clinical trials of varicella vaccine in healthy children. Infect Dis Clin North Am 10:595–608, 1996.

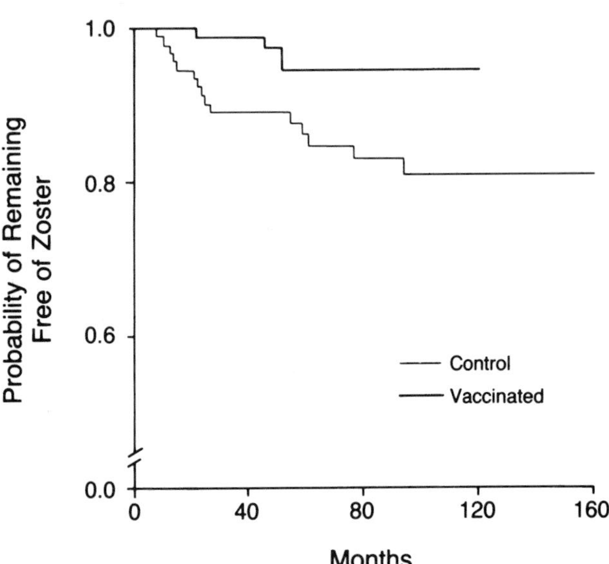

Figure 19–11. Kaplan-Meier product-limit analysis of the probability of remaining free of zoster in 96 children with leukemia who received varicella vaccine and 96 children with leukemia who had naturally acquired chickenpox before or after the diagnosis of leukemia. (From Hardy IB, Gershon A, Steinberg S, et al. The incidence of zoster after immunization with live attenuated varicella vaccine. A study in children with leukemia. N Engl J Med 325:1545–1550, 1991. Reproduced by permission of the New England Journal of Medicine.)

wild-type virus. Another is that the vaccine strain may have less frequent access to sensory nerves because of a lower incidence of viremia and infection of the skin.

It was first observed in Japan that HZ occurred far more frequently in children who had a vaccine-associated rash (16% of 83) than in those with no rash after immunization (2% of 249) (Collaborative Study Group of Varicella Vaccine, Ministry of Health and Welfare, Japan, 1974 to 1983). This observation was confirmed and extended in the NIAID collaborative study.[44, 226] Of 13 vaccinated leukemic children who developed HZ, 11 (85%) had a prior history of a VZV-related rash, either vaccine-associated (8 children) or breakthrough varicella (3 children). Both children with no history of rash developed HZ at the injection site of the vaccine. In the 268 vaccinees who had any type of previous VZV-related rash, the chance of subsequent development of HZ was more than six times greater than in the 280 vaccinees who had no VZV-associated rash. In the NIAID collaborative study, it was possible to type four of the viruses causing HZ. Two were due to vaccine-type virus, and two were caused by wild-type VZV.[213] Because a vaccine-associated rash is unusual in healthy vaccinated children or adults and breakthrough varicella is also unusual, it is expected that the incidence of HZ will be lower in healthy vaccinees than in those who have had the natural infection.[98]

In the NIAID collaborative study, only one adult (of 268) has developed HZ. This physician vaccinee had seroconverted after vaccination, but she lost detectable VZV antibodies after 1 year. She was exposed to a patient with varicella, after which she again seroconverted without any symptoms. About 1 year later, she developed thoracic HZ from which wild-type VZV was cultured.[287] Although the CMI response to VZV has been found to be low in vaccinated adults and this is known to predispose to HZ, the incidence of HZ appears to be low in adult vaccinees, as suggested by this single report of HZ in an adult vaccinee, which was not even caused by the vaccine-type virus.

STUDIES OF SIMULTANEOUS ADMINISTRATION OF VARICELLA VACCINE WITH OTHER VACCINES

Studies have been performed in children to evaluate the safety and immunogenicity of varicella given with measles-mumps-rubella (MMR) vaccine at the same time at different sites using two syringes.[288, 289] In the study reported by Englund and colleagues,[289] seroconversion rates were greater than 95% for all four viral components whether they were given concomitantly at separate anatomical sites or separated by 6 weeks. The varicella vaccine used in that study contained approximately 3450 PFU. All vaccines were well tolerated whether they were given concomitantly or 6 weeks apart. In the study reported by Just and coworkers,[288] there were no statistical differences in seroconversion rates to varicella in children who received the varicella vaccine alone (either ~6000 or ~12,000 PFU) or simultaneously with MMR vaccine. If the two vaccines were mixed together in the same syringe, however, approximately 20% of the children did not seroconvert to varicella.

More recent studies using the Oka vaccine manufactured by Merck containing approximately 3000 PFU given concomitantly at separate sites with MMR vaccine indicated no significant interactions[284] (Table 19–8). Children 12 to 23 months of age were randomized to receive either MMR followed by the varicella vaccine 6 weeks later (group B) or the two vaccines concomitantly (group A). Seroconversion rates were more than 98% to all four components in both groups, and the GMTs were similar.

Clinical studies evaluating the safety and immunogenicity when varicella vaccine manufactured by Merck is administered concomitantly with oral poliovirus vaccine (OPV), *Haemophilus influenzae* type b vaccine (Hib), MMR vaccine, and diphtheria and tetanus toxoids and acellular or whole-cell pertussis vaccine (DTaP, DTwP) have been completed. All vaccines were well tolerated whether they were given concomitantly with or separately from varicella vaccine. In one study, children 12 to 23 months of age were randomized to receive OPV, DTwP-Hib, MMR, and varicella vaccine concomitantly or varicella vaccine given 6 weeks later.[290] Titers to VZV were significantly lower ($P \leq .001$) in the group that received all vaccines concomitantly (11.2 versus 15.2 by gpELISA), but seroconversion rates to VZV were greater than 95% in both groups. At 1 year after vaccination, the GMTs to VZV were similar between the groups (28.2 versus 27.3). In another study, varicella vaccine was given concomitantly with or 6 weeks after DTaP, Hib, and OPV. Results showed similar safety and immunogenicity for all antigens tested (Dr. Joel Ward, personal communication, UCLA).

Table 19–8. **CONCOMITANT USE STUDY: MMR II AND OKA/MERCK VARICELLA VACCINE SEROCONVERSION RATES AND GEOMETRIC MEAN TITERS***

	GROUP A	GROUP B	GEOMETRIC MEAN FOLD DIFFERENCE GROUP A/GROUP B (95% CI)
Viral component	MMR II and Varivax given concomitantly	MMR II and Varivax given 6 wk apart	
Measles			
Seroconversion rate	98% (247/252)	98.2% (224/228)	0.98 (0.85, 1.13)
GMTs	131.0	133.3	
Mumps			
Seroconversion rate	99.6% (239/240)	99.1% (216/218)	1.03 (0.85, 1.25)
GMTs	82.5	80.0	
Rubella			
Seroconversion rate	98.4% (247/251)	100% (225/225)	1.02 (0.88, 1.18)
GMTs	154.8	151.8	
Varicella			
Seroconversion rate	99.5% (199/200)	100% (174/174)	0.74 (0.63, 0.87)
GMTs	13.2	17.9	

*6 weeks after vaccination.

CI, confidence interval; GMTs, geometric mean titers.

From White CJ. Clinical trials of varicella vaccine in healthy children. Infect Dis Clin North Am 10:595–608, 1996.

A combination MMR-varicella vaccine has been tested in children.[291–293] Although earlier studies showed no interference in immune responses when all four viruses were combined, the later studies indicate that the immune response to VZV is significantly lower with the combination vaccine. More studies are needed before a combination vaccine is licensed for general use (see also Chapter 20).

INDICATIONS FOR VACCINATION

Healthy Children

The Oka vaccine was licensed in the late 1980s for use in healthy children in Japan and Korea. The Oka vaccine manufactured by Merck was licensed in the United States in 1995. After licensure, the vaccine was recommended for universal use by the American Academy of Pediatrics[294] and the Advisory Committee for Immunization Practices[72] for healthy, varicella-susceptible children 12 months to 12 years of age. Only one dose (administered subcutaneously) is recommended at present, but it is expected that a booster dose may be recommended in the future, similar to the practice used with MMR vaccines. Oka vaccines manufactured by SmithKline Beecham and Merck were later licensed for use in healthy children in several European countries, such as Germany, and in several countries in the Far East, including the Philippines, Hong Kong, Singapore, Thailand, and Indonesia. It is expected that many of the other developed countries worldwide will license the vaccine for use in healthy children during the next few years.

Immunocompromised Children

The vaccine is licensed for use in immunocompromised children in Japan, Korea, and some European countries. In the United States, the FDA allows the vaccine to be used in leukemic children in remission for at least 1 year on an individual, compassionate use basis. Vaccination can be arranged for this purpose by contacting Varivax Coordinating Center, Bio-Pharm Clinical Services, Inc., 4 Valley Square, Blue Bell, PA 19422 (telephone 215-283-0897). The following guidelines are suggested for vaccination of leukemic children in the United States:

1. The child must be in full remission from leukemia for at least 1 year.
2. The child must have a total peripheral lymphocyte count of 700 cells per mm^3 or more on the day the vaccine is administered.
3. Tests for CMI such as stimulation of peripheral blood lymphocytes with mitogens or antigens before immunization are optional.
4. Antileukemic chemotherapy should be withheld for 1 week before immunization and 1 week afterward. In addition, steroid therapy should not be given for a total of 2 weeks after vaccination.[228] It is only necessary to withhold chemotherapy for the first dose of vaccine.
5. Two doses of vaccine are given 3 months apart. It is desirable to document a seroconversion to VZV by a sensitive, reliable test such as FAMA or LA in leukemic vaccinees. Most commercially available ELISA tests are not sensitive enough for this purpose, and experience with other ELISA tests may be too limited to be used to indicate immunity in these high-risk children.[295] The sensitive LA antibody assay is currently the best test for this purpose.
6. Close follow-up after vaccination is recommended for possible adverse effects. Children who develop more than 50 skin lesions should be given acyclovir. Usually this can be given orally, at a dose of 900 mg per m^2 per dose four times a day. Children who appear ill or toxic or who have extensive rashes (more than 200 lesions) should receive acyclovir intravenously at the usual dosage for varicella (1500 mg/m^2/day).

Children who are somewhat immunocompromised, such as those with asthma or nephrosis who are receiving low doses of steroids, have been safely immunized in Japan[221] and in the United States.[223a] On the basis of these studies, the vaccine is recommended for use in nephrotic children.[72, 294] The American Academy of Pediatrics recommends that children receiving more than 2 mg/kg/day of prednisone (or its equivalent) not be immunized until they have not taken steroids for at least 3 months.

Seronegative Adults

Because healthy adults are at increased risk for development of severe varicella in comparison to children, it is highly desirable that they be immunized if they are susceptible to chickenpox. It is particularly important to immunize those who are likely to be exposed to VZV, such as hospital personnel, teachers, and parents of young children. In the United States, vaccine is recommended for healthy varicella-susceptible adults as two doses of vaccine 4 to 8 weeks apart. It is desirable to perform serological testing for susceptibility to varicella by ELISA or LA before and after vaccination, particularly for women of childbearing age and hospital personnel. A history of prior varicella given by adults is often erroneous.[294a]

Seropositive Adults

Approximately 20% of healthy adults aged 55 to 65 years with a past history of varicella and detectable humoral immunity to VZV have negative CMI to VZV.[164, 165] Because it is now apparent that low CMI to VZV predisposes to development of HZ, there is interest in immunizing elderly individuals with varicella vaccine. In one open label study, 33 healthy individuals in this age group were immunized with live attenuated vaccine, and in 28 (85%), vaccination induced a change from negative to positive VZV CMI measured by lymphocyte transformation.[296] An increase in antibody titer was also observed in more than 75% of the vaccinees. Retesting of a few of the vaccinees showed that the increase in CMI persisted for at least 1 year. In another study, 11 of 11 elderly adults manifested a CMI response, including increased responder cell frequency levels, to VZV vaccine that was similar to that seen in elderly adults after HZ, indicating that immunization can elicit a T-cell response in this group.[167] The incidence of HZ was significantly lower in children who received two doses of vaccine than in those who received one dose in leukemic children vaccinated in the collaborative study, strongly suggesting that immunization of individuals who already have latent infection can prevent HZ.[227] In an uncontrolled study of 202 individuals aged 55 to older than 87 years, there was an increase in CMI to VZV as determined by an increase in responder cell frequency in a lymphocyte transformation assay with VZV as the antigen. The increase lasted as long as 4 years, and although the incidence of HZ was not clearly decreased, all presumed cases were exceedingly mild with little pain and of extremely short duration.[297] A double-blind placebo-controlled efficacy study involving several thousand individuals older than 50 years is planned to determine whether immunization will prevent or modify HZ.

CONTRAINDICATIONS

Severe Immunosuppression

In Japan, five cases of severe reactions to varicella vaccine, consisting of extensive rash and high fever, have been reported.[221] All of these children were receiving high doses of immunosuppressive medications that were not withheld before immunization. None of these children suffered permanent sequelae, and all recovered. In the United States, a few severe reactions to vaccine have been reported in leukemic children who received a lot of vaccine, which is no longer being used, that had a significantly lower antigen-to-infectivity ratio than other varicella vaccines.[224, 298]

Live attenuated varicella vaccine is licensed for use in certain immunosuppressed populations in Europe and the Far East if chemotherapy is suspended around vaccination. The vaccine is available, as described, through a compassionate use program with Merck for children with leukemia in remission for at least 1 year. Individuals with lymphoma, monocytic leukemia, and HIV infection and patients after transplantation may be more immunosuppressed than children with leukemia, and there is little experience with vaccination of such children. Therefore, such children should not be immunized with live attenuated varicella vaccine except on a research basis.

Concurrent Immune Globulin

Because the vaccine is a live attenuated virus, it should not be given concurrently with immune globulin. If immune globulin must be given for other reasons, vaccination should be delayed for 3 to 6 months and titers should be evaluated after vaccination to ensure adequate seroresponse.

Seropositive People

Individuals with preexisting anti-VZV titers have received vaccine in clinical trials and responded with a boost in antibody and CMI. Although it is preferable to immunize seronegative individuals, a positive antibody titer is not a true contraindication to vaccination.

Pregnancy

Although no infants with the congenital varicella syndrome secondary to vaccine-type virus have been reported, vaccination in pregnancy is contraindicated. If a woman inadvertently receives varicella vaccination 3 months before or at any time during pregnancy, it should be reported to the VARIVAX (pregnancy registry to monitor the maternal-fetal outcomes [1-800-986-8999]).

PUBLIC HEALTH IMPACT

As the use of varicella vaccine increases worldwide, the epidemiological features of the disease are expected to change. In studies reported by Halloran,[299] theoretical mathematical modeling was used to examine the morbidity effects of routine varicella immunization of preschool children in the United States. An age-structured theoretical transmission model was used with values for vaccine efficacy based on a review of the literature by an expert panel. According to the author's conclusions, implementation of a vaccination program would result in a shift in the age distribution of remaining varicella cases toward older ages with higher complication rates. However, the overall reduction in cases would result in decreased morbidity as measured by overall number of hospitalizations and number of primary cases. These changes would depend on the level of coverage achieved by the vaccination program. At 97% coverage, endogenous transmission is virtually eliminated. A catch-up program in older children who had not yet had varicella would be important to decrease the shift in age distribution of cases and increased morbidity over time. Surveillance for varicella is essential for monitoring the effectiveness of current immunization strategies and timing of booster doses. Cost-benefit studies of varicella vaccination are discussed earlier under *Significance as a Public Health Problem.*

More information is also needed to determine the impact of routine immunization on the incidence of HZ. Garnett and Grenfell[300] used mathematical modeling techniques to evaluate this issue. Their analysis suggested that if exposure to varicella plays a role in maintenance of immunity and prevention of reactivation, the widespread use of varicella vaccine in children could result in an increased incidence of HZ. However, administration of varicella vaccine has been shown to boost CMI to VZV in the elderly.[296] Ongoing surveillance for changes in the epidemiology of both varicella and HZ are under way in the United States. Because VZV is able to establish latency, it is not expected that a universal immunization program with a live attenuated VZV vaccine will completely eliminate circulation of the virus. Nevertheless, the widespread use of varicella vaccine will improve the health of many children, adolescents, and adults who will no longer have to suffer with varicella and perhaps HZ in the future.

Acknowledgment

Work on this chapter was supported in part by Grant AI24021 of the National Institutes of Health and by Merck & Co., Inc.

REFERENCES

1. Takahashi M. Chickenpox virus. Adv Virus Res 29:285–356, 1983.
2. von Bokay J. Über den aetiologischen Zusammenhang der Varizellen mit Gewissen Fallen von Herpes Zoster. Wien Klin Wochenschr 22:1323–1326, 1909.
3. Bruusgaard E. The mutual relation between zoster and varicella. Br J Dermatol Syph 44:1–24, 1932.
4. Kundratitz K. Experimentelle Übertragung von Herpes Zoster auf den Menschen und die Beziehungen von Herpes Zoster zu Varicellen. Monatss Kinder 29:516–523, 1925.
5. Garland J. Varicella following exposure to herpes zoster. N Engl J Med 228:336–337, 1943.
6. Weller T, Stoddard MB. Intranuclear inclusion bodies in cultures of human tissue inoculated with varicella vesicle fluid. J Immunol 68:311–319, 1952.
7. Weller TH. Serial propagation in vitro of agents producing inclusion bodies derived from varicella and herpes zoster. Proc Soc Exp Biol Med 83:340–346, 1953.
8. Weller TH, Coons AH. Fluorescent antibody studies with agents of varicella and herpes zoster propagated in vitro. Proc Soc Exp Biol Med 86:789, 1954.
9. Weller TH, Witton HM. The etiologic agents of varicella and herpes zoster. Serological studies with the viruses as propagated in vitro. J Exp Med 108:869–890, 1958.
10. Straus SE, Reinhold W, Smith HA, et al. Endonuclease analysis of viral DNA from varicella and subsequent zoster infections in the same patient. N Engl J Med 311:1362–1364, 1984.
11. Williams DL, Gershon A, Gelb LD, et al. Herpes zoster following varicella vaccine in a child with acute lymphocytic leukemia. J Pediatr 106:259–261, 1985.
12. Hayakawa Y, Torigoe S, Shiraki K, et al. Biologic and biophysical markers of a live varicella vaccine strain (Oka): Identification of clinical isolates from vaccine recipients. J Infect Dis 149:956–963, 1984.
13. Roizman B, Carmichael LE, Deinhardt W, et al. Herpesviridae: Definition, provisional nomenclature and taxonomy. Intervirology 16:201–217, 1981.
14. Davison AJ, Scott JE. The complete DNA sequence of varicella-zoster virus. J Gen Virol 67:1759–1816, 1986.
15. Dumas AH, Geelen JLMC, Weststrate MW, et al. *Xba*I, *Pst*I, and *Bgl*II restriction enzyme maps of the two orientations of the varicella-zoster virus genome. J Virol 39:390–400, 1981.
16. Ecker JR, Hyman RW. Varicella zoster virus DNA exists as two isomers. Proc Natl Acad Sci USA 79:156–160, 1982.
17. Straus SE, Aulakh HS, Ruyechan WT, et al. Structure of varicella-zoster virus DNA. J Virol 40:516–526, 1981.
18. Hay J, Ruyechan WT. Varicella-zoster virus: A different kind of herpesvirus latency? Semin Virol 5:241–248, 1994.
19. Grose C. Glycoproteins encoded by varicella-zoster virus: Biosynthesis, phosphorylation, and intracellular trafficking. Annu Rev Microbiol 44:59–80, 1990.
20. Grose C. Glycoproteins of varicella-zoster virus and their herpes simplex virus homologs. Rev Infect Dis 13:S960–S963, 1991.
21. Keller PM, Neff B, Ellis RW. Three major glycoprotein genes of varicella-zoster virus whose products have neutralization epitopes. J Virol 52:293–297, 1984.
22. Yao Z, Grose C. Unusual phosphorylation sequence in the gpIV (gI) component of the varicella-zoster virus gpI-gpIV glycoprotein complex (VZV gE-gI complex). J Virol 68:4204–4211, 1994.
23. Zhu Z, Gershon MD, Gabel C, et al. Entry and egress of VZV: Role of mannose 6-phosphate, heparan sulfate proteoglycan, and signal sequences in targeting virions and viral glycoproteins. Neurology 45:S15–S17, 1995.
24. Zhu Z, Hao Y, Gershon MD, et al. Targetting of glycoprotein I (gE) of varicella-zoster virus to the *trans*-Golgi network by a signal sequence (AYRV) and patch in the cytosolic domain of the molecule. J Virol 70:6563–6575, 1996.
25. Rodriquez JE, Monninger T, Grose C. Entry and egress of varicella virus blocked by same anti-gH monoclonal antibody. Virology 196:840–844, 1993.
26. Forghani B, Grose C. Neutralization epitope of the varicella-zoster virus gH:gL glycoprotein complex. Virology 199:458–462, 1994.

27. Bergen RE, Sharp M, Sanchez A, et al. Human T cells recognize multiple epitopes of an immediate early/tegument protein (IE 62) and glycoprotein I of varicella-zoster virus. Viral Immunol 4:151–166, 1991.
28. Disney GH, Everett RD. A herpes simplex virus type 1 recombinant with both copies of the Vmw175 coding sequences replaced by the homologous varicella-zoster open reading frame. J Gen Virol 71:2681–2689, 1990.
29. Kinchington PR, Hougland J, Arvin A, et al. The varicella-zoster virus immediate-early protein IE62 is a major component of virus particles. J Virol 66:359–366, 1992.
30. Sabella C, Lowry P, Abbruzzi G, et al. Immunization with immediate-early tegument protein (open reading frame 62) of varicella-zoster virus protects guinea pigs against virus challenge. J Virol 67:7673–7676, 1993.
31. Cohen J, Seidel KE. Varicella-zoster virus (VZV) open reading frame (ORF) 10 protein, the homologue of the essential herpes simplex virus protein VP16, is dispensible for VZV replication in vitro. J Virol 68:7850–7858, 1994.
32. Debrus S, Sadzot-Delvaux C, Nikkels AF, et al. Varicella-zoster virus gene 63 encodes an immediate-early protein that is abundantly expressed during latency. J Virol 69:3240–3245, 1995.
33. Moriuchi H, Moriuchi M, Smith HA, Cohen JI. Varicella-zoster virus open reading frame 4 is functionally distinct from and does not complement its herpes simplex virus type 1 homolog, ICP27. J Virol 68:1987–1992, 1994.
34. Perera LP, Kaushal S, Kinchington PR, et al. Varicella-zoster virus open reading frame 4 encodes a transcriptional activator that is functionally distinct from that of herpes simplex virus homology ICP27. J Virol 68:2468–2477, 1994.
35. Moriuchi H, Moriuchi M, Cohen JI. The RING finger domain of the varicella-zoster virus open reading frame 61 protein is required for its transregulatory functions. Virology 205:238–246, 1994.
36. Cohrs RJ, Barbour M, Gilden DH. Varicella-zoster virus (VZV) transcription during latency in human ganglia: Detection of transcripts to genes 21, 29, 62, and 63 in a cDNA library enriched for VZV RNA. J Virol 70:2789–2796, 1996.
37. Mahalingham R, Wellish M, Cohrs R, et al. Expression of protein encoded by varicella-zoster virus open reading frame 63 in latently infected human ganglionic neurons. Proc Natl Acad Sci USA 93:2122–2124, 1996.
38. Lungu O, Panagiotidis C, Annunziato P, et al. VZV gene expression in latency and reactivation. 3rd International Conference on VZV; Palm Beach, FL; March 9–11, 1997.
39. Croen KD, Ostrove JM, Dragovic LY, Straus SE. Patterns of gene expression and sites of latency in human ganglia are different for varicella-zoster and herpes simplex viruses. Proc Natl Acad Sci USA 85:9773–9777, 1988.
40. Mahalingham R, Wellish M, Dueland AN, et al. Localization of herpes simplex virus and varicella zoster virus DNA in human ganglia. Ann Neurol 31:444–448, 1992.
41. Lungu O, Annunziato P, Gershon A, et al. Reactivated and latent varicella-zoster virus in human dorsal root ganglia. Proc Natl Acad Sci USA 92:10980–10984, 1995.
42. Arvin AM, Pollard RB, Rasmussen L, Merigan T. Selective impairment in lymphocyte reactivity to varicella-zoster antigen among untreated lymphoma patients. J Infect Dis 137:531–540, 1978.
43. Arvin A, Gershon A. Live attenuated varicella vaccine. Annu Rev Microbiol 50:59–100, 1996.
44. Hardy IB, Gershon A, Steinberg S, et al. The incidence of zoster after immunization with live attenuated varicella vaccine. A study in children with leukemia. N Engl J Med 325:1545–1550, 1991.
45. Annunziato P, LaRussa P, Lee P, et al. Latent VZV infection in the rat model. 3rd International Conference on VZV; Palm Beach, FL; March 9–11, 1997.
46. Rentier B, Debrus S, Sadzot-Delvaux C, et al. Varicella-zoster virus latency in the nervous system of rats and humans is accompanied by the abundant expression of an immediate-early protein that is also present in acute infection. Keystone Symposium on Virus Entry, Replication, and Pathogenesis; Santa Fe, NM; February 10–16, 1996.
47. Merville-Louis M-P, Sadzot-Delvaux C, Delree P, et al. Varicella-zoster virus infection of adult rat sensory neurons in vitro. J Virol 63:3155–3160, 1989.
48. Grose CH. Variation on a theme by Fenner. Pediatrics 68:735–737, 1981.
49. Fenner F. The pathogenesis of the acute exanthems: An interpretation based on experimental investigations with mousepox (infectious ectromelia of mice). Lancet 2:915–920, 1948.
50. Hope-Simpson RE. Infectiousness of communicable diseases in the household (measles, mumps, and chickenpox). Lancet 2:549, 1952.
51. Ross AH, Lencher E, Reitman G. Modification of chickenpox in family contacts by administration of gamma globulin. N Engl J Med 267:369–376, 1962.
52. Balfour HH, Kelly JM, Suarez CS, et al. Acyclovir treatment of varicella in otherwise healthy children. J Pediatr 116:633–639, 1990.
53. Gershon AA, Steinberg S, Gelb L, NIAID Collaborative Varicella Vaccine Study Group. Clinical reinfection with varicella-zoster virus. J Infect Dis 149:137–142, 1984.
54. Junker AK, Angus E, Thomas E. Recurrent varicella-zoster virus infections in apparently immunocompetent children. Pediatr Infect Dis J 10:569–575, 1991.
55. Terada K, Kawano S, Shimada Y, et al. Recurrent chickenpox after natural infection. Pediatr Infect Dis J 15:179–181, 1996.
56. Arvin A, Koropchak CM, Wittek AE. Immunologic evidence of reinfection with varicella-zoster virus. J Infect Dis 148:200–205, 1983.
57. Gershon A, Steinberg S, Borkowsky W, et al. IgM to varicella-zoster virus: Demonstration in patients with and without clinical zoster. Pediatr Infect Dis 1:164–167, 1982.
58. Gershon AA, Steinberg S, NIAID Collaborative Varicella Vaccine Study Group. Live attenuated varicella vaccine: Protection in healthy adults in comparison to leukemic children. J Infect Dis 161:661–666, 1990.
59. Preblud SR. Varicella: Complications and costs. Pediatrics 76(suppl):728–735, 1986.
60. Quintero-del-Rio AI, Fink CW. Varicella arthritis in childhood. Pediatr Infect Dis J 16:241–243, 1997.
61. Krugman S, Katz S, Gershon A, Wilfert C. Infectious Diseases of Children. St. Louis, Mosby, 1992.
62. Choo PW, Donahue JG, Manson JE, Platt R. The epidemiology of varicella and its complications. J Infect Dis 172:706–712, 1995.
63. Gogos CA, Bassaris HP, Vagenakis AG. Varicella pneumonia in adults. A review of pulmonary manifestations, risk factors, and treatment. Respiration 59:339–343, 1992.
64. Wallace MR, Bowler WA, Murray NB, et al. Treatment of adult varicella with oral acyclovir. A randomized, placebo-controlled trial. Ann Intern Med 117:358–363, 1992.
65. Wallace MR, Bowler WA, Oldfield EC. Treatment of varicella in the immunocompetent adult. J Med Virol Suppl 1:90–92, 1993.
66. Preblud S, Orenstein W, Bart K. Varicella: Clinical manifestations, epidemiology, and health impact on children. Pediatr Infect Dis 3:505–509, 1984.
67. Wharton M, Fehrs LJ, Cochi SL, et al. Health impact of varicella in the 1980s. 30th Interscience Conference on Antimicrobial Agents and Chemotherapy; Atlanta, GA; October 21–24, 1990.
68. Halloran E, Cochi S, Lieu T, et al. Theoretical epidemiologic and morbidity effects of routine immunization of preschool children with varicella vaccine in the United States. Am J Epidemiol 140:81–104, 1994.
69. Van Loon F, Markowitz L, McQuillan G, et al. Varicella seroprevalence in U.S. population. 33rd Interscience Conference on Antimicrobial Agents and Chemotherapy; New Orleans, LA; October 17–20, 1993.
70. Migasena S, Simasathien S, Desakorn V, et al. Seroprevalence of varicella-zoster virus antibody in Thailand. Int J Infect Dis 2:26–30, 1997.
71. Ooi PL, Goh KT, Doraisingham S, Ling AE. Prevalence of varicella-zoster virus infection in Singapore. Southeast Asian J Trop Med Public Health 23:22–25, 1992.
72. Centers for Disease Control. Prevention of varicella: Recommendations of the Advisory Committee on Immunization Practices (ACIP). MMWR Morb Mortal Wkly Rep 45:1–36, 1996.
73. Davies HD, McGeer A, Schwarts B, et al. Invasive group A streptococcal infections in Ontario, Canada. N Engl J Med 335:547–553, 1996.
74. Frenkel LD, Banaji M, Oldenburg N, et al. So you really don't

want to use varicella vaccine? [abstract 612]. 35th Annual Meeting, Infectious Diseases Society of America; San Francisco, CA; September 13–16, 1997.

75. Guess HA, Broughton DD, Melton LJ, Kurland L. Population-based studies of varicella complications. Pediatrics 78(suppl):723–727, 1986.
76. Gershon A. Chickenpox, measles, and mumps. In Remington J, Klein J (eds). Infections of the Fetus and Newborn Infant (4th ed). Philadelphia, WB Saunders, 1994, pp 565–618.
77. Pastuszak AL, Levy M, Schick B, et al. Varicella infection pregnancy. N Engl J Med 330:901–905, 1994.
78. Hanngren K, Grandien M, Granstrom G. Effect of zoster immunoglobulin for varicella prophylaxis in the newborn. Scand J Infect Dis 17:343–347, 1985.
79. Meyers J. Congenital varicella in term infants: Risk reconsidered. J Infect Dis 129:215–217, 1974.
80. Brunell PA, Kotchmar GSJ. Zoster in infancy: Failure to maintain virus latency following intrauterine infection. J Pediatr 98:71–73, 1981.
81. Dworsky M, Whitely R, Alford C. Herpes zoster in early infancy. Am J Dis Child 134:618–619, 1980.
82. Cheatham WJ, Weller TH, Dolan TF, Dower JC. Varicella: Report of two fatal cases with necropsy, virus isolation, and serologic studies. Am J Pathol 32:1015–1035, 1956.
83. Feldman S, Hughes W, Daniel C. Varicella in children with cancer: 77 cases. Pediatrics 80:388–397, 1975.
84. Lynfield R, Herrin JT, Rubin RH. Varicella in pediatric renal transplant patients. Pediatrics 90:216–220, 1992.
85. Lanter R, Rockoff JB, DeMasi J, et al. Fatal varicella in a corticosteroid-dependent asthmatic receiving troleandomycin. Allergy Proc 11:83–87, 1990.
86. Silk H, Guay-Woodford L, Perez-Atayde A, et al. Fatal varicella in steroid-dependent asthma. J Allergy Clin Immunol 81:47–51, 1988.
87. Jura E, Chadwick E, Josephs SH, et al. Varicella-zoster virus infections in children infected with human immunodeficiency virus. Pediatr Infect Dis J 8:586–590, 1989.
88. Hogan EL, Krigman MR. Herpes zoster myelitis. Arch Neurol 29:309–313, 1973.
89. Norris FH, Dramov B, Calder CD, et al. Virus-like particles in myositis accompanying herpes zoster. Arch Neurol 21:25–31, 1969.
90. Rubin D, Fusfeld RD. Muscle paralysis in herpes zoster. Calif Med 103:261–266, 1965.
91. Baba K, Yabuuchi H, Takahashi M, Ogra P. Increased incidence of herpes zoster in normal children infected with varicella-zoster virus during infancy: Community-based follow up study. J Pediatr 108:372–377, 1986.
92. Guess H, Broughton DD, Melton LJ, Kurland L. Epidemiology of herpes zoster in children and adolescents: A population-based study. Pediatrics 76:512–517, 1985.
93. Terada K, Kawano S, Yoshihiro K, Morita T. Varicella-zoster virus (VZV) reactivation is related to the low response of VZV-specific immunity after chickenpox in infancy. J Infect Dis 169:650–652, 1994.
94. Hope-Simpson RE. The nature of herpes zoster: A long term study and a new hypothesis. Proc R Soc Med 58:9–20, 1965.
95. Schmader K, George LK, Burchett GM, et al. Racial differences in the occurrence of herpes zoster. J Infect Dis 171:701–704, 1995.
96. Whitley RJ. Varicella-zoster infections. In Galasso G, Merigan T, Buchanan R (eds). Antiviral Agents and Viral Infections of Man. New York, Raven Press, 1984, pp 517–541.
97. Feldman S, Hughes WT, Kim HY. Herpes zoster in children with cancer. Am J Dis Child 126:178–184, 1973.
98. Hardy IB, Gershon A, Steinberg S, et al. Incidence of zoster after live attenuated varicella vaccine. 31st Interscience Conference on Antimicrobial Agents and Chemotherapy; Chicago, IL; September 29–October 2, 1991.
99. Locksley RM, Flournoy N, Sullivan KM, Meyers J. Infection with varicella-zoster virus after marrow transplantation. J Infect Dis 152:1172–1181, 1985.
100. Veenstra J, Krol A, van Praag R, et al. Herpes zoster, immunological deterioration and disease progression in HIV-1 infection. AIDS 9:1153–1158, 1995.
101. Gershon A, Mervish N, LaRussa P, et al. Varicella-zoster virus infection in children with underlying human immunodeficiency virus infection. J Infect Dis 176:1496–1500, 1997.
102. Jacobson MA, Berger TG, Fikrig S. Acyclovir-resistant varicella-zoster virus infection after chronic oral acyclovir therapy in patients with the acquired immunodeficiency syndrome. Ann Intern Med 112:187–191, 1990.
103. Esmann V, Kroon S, Peterslund NA, et al. Prednisolone does not prevent post-herpetic neuralgia. Lancet 2:126–129, 1987.
104. Gilden DH, Dueland AN, Cohrs R, et al. Postherpetic neuralgia. Neurology 41:1215–1218, 1991.
105. Gilden D. Herpes zoster with postherpetic neuralgia—persisting pain and frustration. N Engl J Med 330:932–934, 1994.
106. Watson PN, Evans RJ, Watt VR, Birkett N. Postherpetic neuralgia: 208 cases. Pain 35:289–297, 1988.
107. Portenoy RK, Duma C, Foley KM. Acute herpetic and postherpetic neuralgia: Clinical review and current management. Ann Neurol 20:651–664, 1986.
108. Hope-Simpson RE. Postherpetic neuralgia. J R Coll Gen Pract 25:571–575, 1975.
109. Lydick E, Epstein RS, Himmelberger D, White CJ. Area under the curve: A metric for patient subjective responses in episodic diseases. Qual Life Res 4:41–45, 1995.
110. McKendrick MW, McGill JI, Wood MJ, et al. Lack of effect of acyclovir on postherpetic neuralgia. Br Med J 298:431, 1989.
111. Rogers RS. Geriatric herpes zoster. J Am Geriatr Soc 19:495–503, 1971.
112. Watson CPN. Postherpetic neuralgia. Neurol Clin 7:231–248, 1989.
113. Wood MJ. Herpes zoster and pain. Scand J Infect Dis 78:53–61, 1991.
114. Gustafson TL, Lavely GB, Brauner ER, et al. An outbreak of nosocomial varicella. Pediatrics 70:550–556, 1982.
115. Leclair JM, Zaia J, Levin MJ, et al. Airborne transmission of chickenpox in a hospital. N Engl J Med 302:450–453, 1980.
116. Moore DA, Hopkins RS. Assessment of a school exclusion policy during a chickenpox outbreak. Am J Epidemiol 133:1161–1167, 1991.
117. Kido S, Ozaki T, Asada H, et al. Detection of varicella-zoster virus (VZV) DNA in clinical samples from patients with VZV by the polymerase chain reaction. J Clin Microbiol 29:76–79, 1991.
118. Koropchak C, Graham G, Palmer J, et al. Investigation of varicella-zoster virus infection by polymerase chain reaction in the immunocompetent host with acute varicella. J Infect Dis 163:1016–1022, 1991.
119. Tsolia M, Gershon A, Steinberg S, Gelb L. Live attenuated varicella vaccine: Evidence that the virus is attenuated and the importance of skin lesions in transmission of varicella-zoster virus. J Pediatr 116:184–189, 1990.
120. Gershon A, Forghani B. Varicella-zoster virus. In Lennette E (ed). Diagnostic Procedures for Viral, Rickettsial, and Chlamydial Infections. Washington, DC, American Public Health Association, 1995, pp 601–613.
121. Brunell PA. Transmission of chickenpox in a school setting prior to the observed exanthem. Am J Dis Child 143:1451–1452, 1989.
122. Sawyer MH, Wu YN, Chamberlin CJ, et al. Detection of varicella-zoster virus DNA in the oropharynx and blood of patients with varicella. J Infect Dis 166:885–888, 1992.
123. Feldman S, Epp E. Isolation of varicella-zoster virus from blood. J Pediatr 88:265–267, 1976.
124. Feldman S, Epp E. Detection of viremia during incubation period of varicella. J Pediatr 94:746–748, 1979.
125. Asano Y, Itakura N, Kajita Y, et al. Severity of viremia and clinical findings in children with varicella. J Infect Dis 161:1095–1098, 1990.
126. Asano Y, Itakura N, Hiroishi Y, et al. Viremia is present in incubation period in nonimmunocompromised children with varicella. J Pediatr 106:69–71, 1985.
127. Myers MG. Viremia caused by varicella-zoster virus: Association with malignant progressive varicella. J Infect Dis 140:229–233, 1979.
128. Ozaki T, Ichikawa T, Matsui Y, et al. Viremic phase in nonimmunocompromised children with varicella. J Pediatr 104:85–87, 1984.
129. Ozaki T, Kajita Y, Asano Y, et al. Detection of varicella-zoster

virus DNA in blood of children with varicella. J Med Virol 44:263–265, 1994.
130. Moffat JF, Stein MD, Kaneshima H, Arvin AM. Tropism of varicella-zoster virus for human CD4+ and CD8+ T lymphocytes and epidermal cells in SCID-hu mice. J Virol 69:5236–5242, 1995.
131. Ito M, Nishihara H, Mizutani K, et al. Detection of varicella zoster virus (VZV) DNA in throat swabs and peripheral blood mononuclear cells of immunocompromised patients with herpes zoster by polymerase chain reaction. Clin Diagn Virol 4:105–112, 1995.
132. Gershon A, Steinberg S, Silber R. Varicella-zoster viremia. J Pediatr 92:1033–1034, 1978.
133. Feldman S, Chaudhary S, Ossi M, Epp E. A viremic phase for herpes zoster in children with cancer. J Pediatr 91:597–600, 1977.
134. Kalman CM, Laskin OL. Herpes zoster and zosteriform herpes simplex virus infections in immunocompetent adults. Am J Med 81:775–778, 1986.
135. Coffin SE, Hodinka RL. Utility of direct immunofluorescence and virus culture for detection of varicella-zoster virus in skin lesions. J Clin Microbiol 33:2792–2795, 1995.
136. LaRussa P, Hughes P, Pearch J, et al. Use of polymerase chain reaction (PCR) assay to identify and type varicella-zoster virus (VZV). 62nd Annual Meeting of the Society for Pediatric Research; Washington, DC; May 6, 1993.
137. LaRussa P, Steinberg S, Gershon A. Diagnosis and typing of varicella-zoster virus (VZV) in clinical specimens by polymerase chain reaction (PCR). 34th Interscience Conference on Antimicrobial Agents and Chemotherapy; Orlando, FL; October 4–7, 1994.
138. Puchhammer-Stockl E, Popow-Kraupp T, Heinz F, et al. Detection of varicella-zoster virus DNA by polymerase chain reaction in the cerebrospinal fluid of patients suffering from neurological complications associated with chicken pox or herpes zoster. J Clin Microbiol 29:1513–1516, 1991.
139. Asano Y, Itakura N, Hiroishi Y, et al. Viral replication and immunologic responses in children naturally infected with varicella-zoster virus and in varicella vaccine. J Infect Dis 152:863–868, 1985.
140. Demmler G, Steinberg S, Blum G, Gershon A. Rapid enzyme-linked immunosorbent assay for detecting antibody to varicella-zoster virus. J Infect Dis 157:211–212, 1988.
141. Williams V, Gershon A, Brunell P. Serologic response to varicella-zoster membrane antigens measured by indirect immunofluorescence. J Infect Dis 130:669–672, 1974.
142. Wasmuth EH, Miller WJ. Sensitive enzyme-linked immunosorbent assay for antibody to varicella-zoster virus using purified VZV glycoprotein antigen. J Med Virol 32:189–193, 1990.
143. White CJ, Kuter BJ, Ngai A, et al. Modified cases of chickenpox after varicella vaccination: Correlation of protection with antibody response. Pediatr Infect Dis J 11:19–22, 1992.
144. Krah DL, Cho I, Schofield T, Ellis RW. Comparison of gpELISA and neutralizing antibody responses to Oka/Merck live varicella vaccine (Varivax) in children and adults. Vaccine 15:61–64, 1997.
145. Forghani B, Schmidt N, Dennis J. Antibody assays for varicella-zoster virus: Comparison of enzyme immunoassay with neutralization, immune adherence hemagglutination, and complement fixation. J Clin Microbiol 8:545–552, 1978.
146. Gershon A, Kalter Z, Steinberg S. Detection of antibody to varicella-zoster virus by immune adherence hemagglutination. Proc Soc Exp Biol Med 151:762–765, 1976.
147. Steinberg S, Gershon A. Measurement of antibodies to varicella-zoster virus by using a latex agglutination test. J Clin Microbiol 29:1527–1529, 1991.
148. Gershon A, Steinberg S, LaRussa P. Detection of antibodies to varicella-zoster virus by latex agglutination. Clin Diagn Virol 2:271–277, 1994.
149. Landry ML, Ferguson D. Comparison of latex agglutination test with enzyme-linked immunosorbent assay for detection of antibody to varicella-zoster virus. J Clin Microbiol 31:3031–3033, 1993.
150. Kumagai T, Chiba Y, Wataya Y, et al. Development and characteristics of the cellular immune response to infection with varicella-zoster virus after natural or vaccine-induced infection. J Infect Dis 141:1–13, 1980.
151. Baba K, Yabuuchi H, Takahashi M, et al. Seroepidemiologic behavior of varicella zoster virus infection in a semiclosed community after introduction of VZV vaccine. J Pediatr 105:712–716, 1984.
152. Arbeter AM, Starr SE, Preblud S, et al. Varicella vaccine trials in healthy children: A summary of comparative follow-up studies. Am J Dis Child 138:434–438, 1984.
153. Baba K, Yabuuchi H, Okuni H, Takahashi M. Studies with live varicella vaccine and inactivated skin test antigen: Protective effect of the vaccine and clinical application of the skin test. Pediatrics 61:550–555, 1978.
154. Kamiya H, Ihara T, Hattori A, et al. Diagnostic skin test reactions with varicella virus antigen and clinical application of the test. J Infect Dis 136:784–788, 1977.
155. LaRussa P, Steinberg S, Seeman MD, Gershon AA. Determination of immunity to varicella by means of an intradermal skin test. J Infect Dis 152:869–875, 1985.
156. Shiraki K, Yamanishi K, Takahashi M. Biological and immunological characterization of the soluble skin test antigen of varicella-zoster virus. J Infect Dis 149:501–504, 1983.
157. Arvin AM. Varicella-zoster virus. In Fields BN (ed). Virology. New York, Raven Press, 1995, pp 2547–2586.
158. Gershon AA, Steinberg S, Gelb L, NIAID Collaborative Varicella Vaccine Study Group. Live attenuated varicella vaccine: Efficacy for children with leukemia in remission. JAMA 252:355–362, 1984.
159. Hayward A, Herberger M. Lymphocyte responses to varicella-zoster virus in the elderly. J Clin Immunol 7:174–178, 1987.
160. Zaia JA, Leary PL, Levin MJ. Specificity of the blastogenic response of human mononuclear cells to herpes antigens. Infect Immun 20:646–651, 1978.
161. Ihara T, Ito M, Starr SE. Human lymphocyte, monocyte and polymorphonuclear leucocyte mediated antibody-dependent cellular cytotoxicity against varicella-zoster virus-infected targets. Clin Exp Immunol 63:179–187, 1986.
162. Ihara T, Starr S, Ito M, Douglas S, Arbeter A. Human polymorphonuclear leukocyte-mediated cytotoxicity against varicella-zoster virus–infected fibroblasts. J Virol 51:110–116, 1984.
163. Kamiya H, Starr S, Arbeter A, Plotkin S. Antibody dependent cell-mediated cytotoxicity against varicella-zoster virus infected targets. Infect Immun 38:554–557, 1982.
164. Berger R, Florent G, Just M. Decrease of the lymphoproliferative response to varicella-zoster virus antigen in the aged. Infect Immun 32:24–27, 1981.
165. Burke BL, Steele RW, Beard OW, et al. Immune responses to varicella-zoster in the aged. Arch Intern Med 142:291–293, 1982.
166. Luby J, Ramirez-Ronda C, Rinner S, et al. A longitudinal study of varicella zoster virus infections in renal transplant recipients. J Infect Dis 135:659–663, 1977.
167. Hayward A, Levin M, Wolf W, et al. Varicella-zoster virus–specific immunity after herpes zoster. J Infect Dis 163:873–875, 1991.
168. Wilson A, Sharp M, Koropchak C, et al. Subclinical varicella-zoster virus viremia, herpes zoster, and T lymphocyte immunity to varicella-zoster viral antigens after bone marrow transplantation. J Infect Dis 165:119–126, 1992.
169. Hayward A, Buda K, Jones M, et al. Varicella-zoster virus–specific cytotoxicity following secondary immunization with live or killed vaccine. Viral Immunol 9:241–245, 1996.
170. Gershon A, Frey H, Steinberg S, et al. Enzyme-linked immunosorbent assay for measurement of antibody to varicella-zoster virus. Arch Virol 70:169–172, 1981.
171. Bogger-Goren S, Baba K, Hurley P, et al. Antibody response to varicella-zoster virus after natural or vaccine-induced infection. J Infect Dis 146:260–265, 1982.
172. Plotkin SA, Arbeter AA, Starr SE. The future of varicella vaccine. Postgrad Med 61:155–162, 1985.
173. Ragozzino ME, Melton LF, Kurland L, et al. Population-based study of herpes zoster and its sequelae. Medicine (Baltimore) 61:310–316, 1982.
174. Preblud SR, Orenstein WA, Koplan JP, et al. A benefit-cost analysis of a childhood vaccination programme. Postgrad Med J 61:17–22, 1985.
175. Huse DM, Meissner C, Lacey MJ, Oster G. Childhood vaccination against chickenpox: An analysis of benefits and costs. J Pediatr 124:869–874, 1994.

176. Lieu T, Cochi S, Black S, et al. Cost-effectiveness of a routine varicella vaccination program for U.S. children. JAMA 271:375–381, 1994.
177. Beutels P, Clara R, Tormans G, et al. Costs and benefits of routine varicella vaccination in German children. J Infect Dis 174:S335–S341, 1996.
178. Weber DJ, Rotala WA, Parham C. Impact and costs of varicella prevention in a university hospital. Am J Public Health 78:19–23, 1988.
179. Centers for Disease Control. Varicella-related deaths among adults—United States, 1997. MMWR Morb Mortal Wkly Rep 46:409–412, 1997.
180. Whitley R. Therapeutic approaches to varicella-zoster virus infections. J Infect Dis 166:S51–S57, 1992.
181. Whitley RJ, Gnann JW. Acyclovir: A decade later. N Engl J Med 327:782–789, 1992.
182. Wood MF, Johnson RW, McKendrick MW, et al. A randomized trial of acyclovir for 7 days or 21 days with and without prednisolone for treatment of acute herpes zoster. N Engl J Med 330:896–900, 1994.
183. Dunkel L, Arvin A, Whitley R, et al. A controlled trial of oral acyclovir for chickenpox in normal children. N Engl J Med 325:1539–1544, 1991.
184. Beutner KR, Friedman DJ, Forszpaniak C, et al. Valaciclovir compared with acyclovir for improved therapy for herpes zoster in immunocompetent adults. Antimicrob Agents Chemother 39:1546–1553, 1995.
185. Tyring S, Barbarash RA, Nahlik JE, et al. Famciclovir for the treatment of acute herpes zoster: Effects on acute disease and post herpetic neuralgia. Ann Intern Med 123:89–96, 1995.
186. Wallace MR, Chamberlin CJ, Sawyer MH, et al. Treatment of adult varicella with sorivudine: A randomized, placebo controlled trial. J Infect Dis 174:249–255, 1996.
187. Brunell P, Ross A, Miller L, Kuo B. Prevention of varicella by zoster immune globulin. N Engl J Med 280:1191–1194, 1969.
188. Gershon A, Steinberg S, Brunell P. Zoster immune globulin: A further assessment. N Engl J Med 290:243–245, 1974.
189. Zaia J, Levin M, Preblud S, et al. Evaluation of varicella-zoster immune globulin: Protection of immunosuppressed children after household exposure to varicella. J Infect Dis 147:737–743, 1983.
190. Balfour HH, Groth KE, McCullough J, et al. Prevention or modification of varicella using zoster immune plasma. Am J Dis Child 131:693–696, 1977.
191. Balfour HH, Groth KE. Zoster immune plasma prophylaxis of varicella: A follow up report. J Pediatr 94:743–746, 1979.
192. Groth KE, McCullough J, Marker S, et al. Evaluation of zoster immune plasma: Treatment of herpes zoster in patients with cancer. JAMA 239:1877–1879, 1978.
193. Bakshi S, Miller TC, Kaplan M, et al. Failure of VZIG in modification of severe congenital varicella. Pediatr Infect Dis 5:699–702, 1986.
194. Feldman S, Lott L. Varicella in children with cancer: Impact of antiviral therapy and prophylaxis. Pediatrics 80:465–472, 1987.
195. Arbeter AM, Starr SE, Weibel RE, et al. Live attenuated varicella vaccine: The KMcC strain in healthy children. Pediatrics 71:307–312, 1983.
196. Neff BJ, Weibel RE, Villerajos VM, et al. Clinical and laboratory studies of KMcC strain of live attenuated varicella virus. Proc Soc Exp Biol Med 166:339–347, 1981.
197. Asano Y, Albrecht P, Behr DE, et al. Immunogenicity of wild and attenuated varicella zoster virus strains in rhesus monkeys. J Med Virol 14:305–312, 1984.
198. Takahashi M, Otsuka T, Okuno Y, et al. Live vaccine used to prevent the spread of varicella in children in hospital. Lancet 2:1288–1290, 1974.
199. Takahashi M, Okuno Y, Otsuka T, et al. Development of a live attenuated varicella vaccine. Biken J 18:25–33, 1975.
200. Martin JH, Dohner D, Wellinghoff WJ, Gelb LD. Restriction endonuclease analysis of varicella-zoster vaccine virus and wild type DNAs. J Med Virol 9:69–76, 1982.
201. Takahashi M, Hayakawa Y, Shiraki K, et al. Attenuation and laboratory markers of the Oka-strain varicella-zoster virus. Postgrad Med 61:37–46, 1985.
202. Gelb LD, Dohner DE, Gershon AA, et al. Molecular epidemiology of live, attenuated varicella virus vaccine in children and in normal adults. J Infect Dis 155:633–640, 1987.
203. LaRussa P, Lungu O, Hardy I, et al. Restriction fragment length polymorphism of polymerase chain reaction products from vaccine and wild-type varicella-zoster virus isolates. J Virol 66:1016–1020, 1992.
204. Brunell P, Geiser C, Novelli V, et al. Varicella-like illness caused by live varicella vaccine in children with acute lymphocytic leukemia. Pediatrics 79:922–927, 1987.
205. Moffat J, Zerboni L, Kinchington P, et al. Virologic basis for the attenuation of the vaccine, Oka strain of varicella-zoster virus [abstract 590]. 35th Annual Meeting, Infectious Diseases Society of America; San Francisco, CA; September 13–16, 1997.
206. Myers M, Duer HL, Haulser CK. Experimental infection of guinea pigs with varicella-zoster virus. J Infect Dis 142:414–420, 1980.
207. Hayakawa Y, Yamamoto T, Yamanishi K, Takahashi M. Analysis of varicella zoster virus (VZV) DNAs of clinical isolates by endonuclease *HpaI*. J Gen Virol 67:1817–1829, 1986.
208. LaRussa P, Steinberg S, Arvin A, et al. PCR and RFLP analysis of VZV isolates from the USA and other parts of the world. 3rd International Conference on VZV; Palm Beach, FL; March 9–11, 1997.
209. Mori C, Takahara R, Toriyama T, et al. Identification of the Oka strain of the live attenuated varicella vaccine from other clinical isolates by molecular epidemiological analysis. J Infect Dis 178:35–38, 1998.
210. Ihara T, Kamiya H, Torigoe S, et al. Viremic phase in a leukemic child after live varicella vaccination. Pediatrics 89:147–149, 1992.
211. Gershon A, LaRussa P, Steinberg S. Varicella vaccine: Clinical trials in immunocompromised patients. Infect Dis Clin North Am 10:583–594, 1996.
212. Hughes P, LaRussa PS, Pearce JM, et al. Transmission of varicella-zoster virus from a vaccinee with underlying leukemia, demonstrated by polymerase chain reaction. J Pediatr 124:932–935, 1994.
212a. Salzman MB, Sharrar RG, Steinberg S, LaRussa P. Transmission of varicella-vaccine virus from a healthy 12-month-old child to his pregnant mother. J Pediatr 131:151–154, 1997.
212b. LaRussa P, Steinberg S, Meurice F, Gershon A. Transmission of vaccine strain varicella-zoster virus from a healthy adult with vaccine-associated rash to susceptible household contacts. J Infect Dis 176:1072–1075, 1997.
213. Gershon A. Varicella-zoster virus: Prospects for control. Adv Pediatr Infect Dis 10:93–124, 1995.
214. Bergen RE, Diaz P, Arvin A. The immunogenicity of Oka/Merck varicella vaccine in relation to infectious varicella-zoster virus and relative viral antigen content. J Infect Dis 162:1049–1054, 1990.
215. Asano Y, Nakayama H, Yazaki T, et al. Protection against varicella in family contacts by immediate inoculation with live varicella vaccine. Pediatrics 59:3–7, 1977.
216. Izawa T, Ihara T, Hattori A, et al. Application of a live varicella vaccine in children with acute leukemia or other malignant diseases. Pediatrics 60:805–809, 1977.
217. Sato Y, Miyano T, Kawauchi K, Yokoyama M. Use of live varicella vaccine in acute leukemia and malignant lymphoma. Biken J 27:111–113, 1984.
218. Ha K, Baba K, Ikeda T, et al. Application of a live varicella vaccine in children with acute leukemia or other malignancies without suspension of anticancer therapy. Pediatrics 65:346–350, 1980.
219. Konno T, Yamaguchi Y, Minegishi M, et al. A clinical trial of live attenuated varicella vaccine (Biken) in children with malignant diseases. Biken J 27:73–75, 1984.
220. Nunoue T. Clinical observations on varicella-zoster virus vaccinees treated with immunosuppressants for a malignancy. Biken J 27:115–118, 1984.
221. Takahashi M, Kamiya H, Baba K, et al. Clinical experience with Oka live varicella vaccine in Japan. Postgrad Med 61:61–67, 1985.
222. Gershon A. Immunoprophylaxis of varicella-zoster infections. Am J Med 76:672–677, 1984.
223. Gershon A, Steinberg S, Gelb L, NIAID Collaborative Varicella Vaccine Study Group. Live attenuated varicella vaccine: Use in immunocompromised children and adults. Pediatrics 78(suppl):757–762, 1986.

224. Gershon AA, Steinberg S, NIAID Collaborative Varicella Vaccine Study Group. Persistence of immunity to varicella in children with leukemia immunized with live attenuated varicella vaccine. N Engl J Med 320:892–897, 1989.
225. Gershon AA, LaRussa P, Steinberg S. Live attenuated varicella vaccine: Current status and future uses. Semin Pediatr Infect Dis 2:171–178, 1991.
226. Lawrence R, Gershon A, Holzman R, Steinberg S, NIAID Varicella Vaccine Collaborative Study Group. The risk of zoster after varicella vaccination in children with leukemia. N Engl J Med 318:543–548, 1988.
227. Gershon A, LaRussa P, Steinberg S, et al. The protective effect of immunologic boosting against zoster: An analysis in leukemic children who were vaccinated against chickenpox. J Infect Dis 173:450–453, 1996.
228. Lydick E, Kuter BJ, Zajac B, Guess H, NIAID Collaborative Varicella Vaccine Study Group. Association of steroid therapy with vaccine-associated rashes in children with acute lymphocytic leukaemia who received Oka/Merck varicella vaccine. Vaccine 7:549–553, 1989.
229. Takahashi M, Gershon A. Varicella vaccines. In Levine M, Woodrow GC, Kaper JB, Cobon GS (eds). New Generation Vaccines. New York, Marcel Dekker, 1997, pp 647–658.
230. Arbeter A, Granowetter L, Starr S, et al. Immunization of children with acute lymphoblastic leukemia with live attenuated varicella vaccine without complete suspension of chemotherapy. Pediatrics 85:338–344, 1990.
231. Brunell PA, Shehab Z, Geiser C, Waugh JE. Administration of live varicella vaccine to children with leukemia. Lancet 2:1069–1073, 1982.
232. Broyer M, Boudailliez B. Prevention of varicella infection in renal transplanted children by previous immunization with a live attenuated varicella vaccine. Transplant Proc 17:151–152, 1985.
233. Zamora I, Simon JM, Da Silva ME, Piqueras AI. Attenuated varicella vaccine in children with renal transplants. Pediatr Nephrol 8:190–192, 1994.
233a. Quien RM, Kaiser BA, Deforest A, et al. Response to the varicella vaccine in children with nephrotic syndrome. J Pediatr 131:688–690, 1997.
234. Broyer M, Tete MT, Guest G, et al. Varicella and zoster in children after kidney transplantation: Long term results of vaccination. Pediatrics 99:35–39, 1997.
235. Brunell PA, Taylor-Wiedeman J, Geiser CF, et al. Risk of herpes zoster in children with leukemia: Varicella vaccine compared with history of chickenpox. Pediatrics 77:53–56, 1986.
236. Horiuchi K. Chickenpox vaccination of healthy children: Immunological and clinical responses and protective effect in 1978–1982. Biken J 27:37–38, 1984.
237. Naganuma Y, Osawa S, Takahashi M. Clinical application of live attenuated varicella vaccine (Oka strain) in a hospital. Biken J 27:59–61, 1984.
238. Ozaki T, Ichikawa T, Asano Y, et al. Clinical trial of the Oka strain of live attenuated varicella vaccine on healthy children. Biken J 27:39–42, 1984.
239. Andre F. Summary of clinical studies with the Oka live varicella vaccine produced by Smith Kline-RIT. Biken J 27:89–98, 1984.
240. Weibel R, Kuter B, Neff B, et al. Live Oka/Merck varicella vaccine in healthy children: Further clinical and laboratory assessment. JAMA 245:2435–2439, 1985.
241. Watson B, Piercy S, Soppas D, et al. The effect of decreasing amounts of live virus, while antigen content remains constant, on immunogenicity of Oka/Merck varicella vaccine. J Infect Dis 168:1356–1360, 1993.
242. Rothstein EP, Bernstein H, Penridge P, et al. Dose titration study of live attenuated varicella vaccine in healthy children. J Infect Dis 175:444–447, 1997.
243. Baba K, Yabuuchi H, Takahashi M, Ogra P. Live attenuated varicella vaccine: Efficacy trial in an institution. 18th International Congress of Pediatrics; Honolulu, HI; July 7–12, 1986.
244. Asano Y, Nakayama H, Yazaki T, et al. Protective efficacy of vaccination in children in four episodes of natural varicella and zoster in the ward. Pediatrics 59:8–12, 1977.
245. Weibel R, Neff BJ, Kuter BJ, et al. Live attenuated varicella virus vaccine: Efficacy trial in healthy children. N Engl J Med 310:1409–1415, 1984.
246. Kuter BJ, Weibel RE, Guess HA, et al. Oka/Merck varicella vaccine in healthy children: Final report of a 2-year efficacy study and 7-year follow-up studies. Vaccine 9:643–647, 1991.
247. Krause P, Klinman DM. Efficacy, immunogenicity, safety, and use of live attenuated chickenpox vaccine. J Pediatr 127:518–525, 1995.
248. Varis T, Vesikari T. Efficacy of high titer live attenuated varicella vaccine in healthy young children. J Infect Dis 174:S330–S334, 1996.
249. White CJ, Kuter BJ, Hildebrand CS, et al. Varicella vaccine (VARIVAX) in healthy children and adolescents: Results from clinical trials, 1987 to 1989. Pediatrics 87:604–610, 1991.
250. Arbeter A, Starr SE, Plotkin SA. Varicella vaccine studies in healthy children and adults. Pediatrics 78(suppl):748–756, 1986.
251. Asano Y, Albrecht P, Vujcic LK, et al. Five-year follow-up study of recipients of live varicella vaccine using enhanced neutralization and fluorescent antibody membrane antigen assays. Pediatrics 72:291–294, 1983.
252. Asano Y, Nagai T, Miyata T, et al. Long-term protective immunity of recipients of the Oka strain of live varicella vaccine. Pediatrics 75:667–671, 1985.
253. Bernstein HH, Rothstein EP, Watson BM, et al. Clinical survey of natural varicella compared with breakthrough varicella after immunization with live attenuated Oka/Merck varicella vaccine. Pediatrics 92:833–837, 1993.
254. Johnson C, Rome L, Stancin T, Kumar M. Humoral immunity and clinical reinfections following varicella vaccine in healthy children. Pediatrics 84:418–421, 1989.
255. Clements DA, Armstrong CB, Ursano AM, et al. Over five-year follow-up of Oka/Merck varicella vaccine recipients in 465 infants and adolescents. Pediatr Infect Dis J 14:874–879, 1995.
256. Watson BM, Piercy SA, Plotkin SA, Starr SE. Modified chickenpox in children immunized with the Oka/Merck varicella vaccine. Pediatrics 91:17–22, 1993.
257. Asano Y. Varicella vaccine: The Japanese experience. J Infect Dis 174:S310–S313, 1996.
257a. Takayama N, Minamitani M, Takayama M. High incidence of breakthrough varicella in healthy Japanese children immunized with live attenuated varicella vaccine (Oka strain). Acta Pediatr Jpn 39:663–669, 1997.
257b. Johnson CE, Stancin T, Fattlar D, et al. A long-term prospective study of varicella vaccine in healthy children. Pediatrics 100:761–766, 1997.
258. Naruse H, Minwata H, Ozaki T, et al. Varicella infection complicated with meningitis after immunization: Case report. Acta Pediatr Jpn 35:345–347, 1993.
258a. Izurieta HS, Strebel PM, Blake PA. Postlicensure effectiveness of varicella vaccine during an outbreak in a child care center. JAMA 278:1495–1499, 1997.
259. Asano Y, Hirose S, Iwayama S, et al. Protective effect of immediate inoculation of a live varicella vaccine in household contacts in relation to the viral dose and interval between exposure and vaccination. Biken J 25:43–45, 1982.
260. Chartrand S, Madison BG, Steinberg S, Gershon A. Varicella vaccine in day care centers. 25th Interscience Conference on Antimicrobial Agents and Chemotherapy; Minneapolis, MN; September 29–October 2, 1985.
261. Diaz PS, Au D, Smith S, et al. Lack of transmission of the live attenuated varicella vaccine virus to immunocompromised children after immunization of their siblings. Pediatrics 87:166–170, 1991.
262. Salzman MB, Sharrar R, Steinberg S, LaRussa P. Transmission of varicella-vaccine virus from a healthy 12 month old child to his pregnant mother. J Pediatr 131:151–154, 1997.
263. Long S. Toddler-to-mother transmission of varicella-vaccine virus: How bad is that? J Pediatr 131:10–12, 1997.
264. Kumagai T, Chiba Y, Fujiyama M, et al. Humoral and cellular immune response to varicella-zoster virus in children inoculated with live attenuated varicella vaccine. Biken J 23:135–141, 1980.
265. Watson B, Boardman C, Laufer D, et al. Humoral and cell-mediated immune responses in healthy children after one or two doses of varicella vaccine. Clin Infect Dis 20:316–319, 1995.
266. Just M, Borger R, Leuscher D. Live varicella vaccine in healthy individuals. Postgrad Med 61:129–132, 1985.
267. Ndumbe PM, Cradock-Watson JE, MacQueen S, et al. Immuni-

sation of nurses with a live varicella vaccine. Lancet 1:1144–1147, 1985.

268. Alter SJ, McVey CJ, Jenski L, Myers M. Varicella live virus vaccine in normal susceptible adults at high risk for exposure. 25th Interscience Conference on Antimicrobial Agents and Chemotherapy; Minneapolis, MN; September 29–October 2, 1985.
269. Gershon A, Steinberg S, Schmidt N. Varicella-zoster virus. In Ballows A (ed). Manual of Clinical Microbiology. Washington, DC, American Society for Microbiology, 1991, pp 838–846.
270. LaRussa P, Steinberg S, Meurice F, Gershon A. Transmission of vaccine strain varicella-zoster virus from a healthy adult with vaccine-associated rash to susceptible household contacts. J Infect Dis 176:1072–1075, 1997.
271. Kacica MA, Connelly BL, Myers MG. Communicable varicella in a health care worker 21 months following successful vaccination with live attenuated varicella vaccine. 28th Interscience Conference on Antimicrobial Agents and Chemotherapy; Los Angeles, CA; October 23–26, 1988.
272. Kuter BJ, Ngai A, Patterson CM, et al. Safety, tolerability, and immunogenicity of two regimens of Oka/Merck varicella vaccine (Varivax) in healthy adolescents and adults. Vaccine 13:967–972, 1995.
273. Gershon A, Steinberg S, LaRussa P. Measurement of antibodies to VZV by latex agglutination. Society for Pediatric Research; Anaheim, CA; May 1992.
274. Sharp M, Terada K, Wilson A, et al. Kinetics and viral protein specificity of the cytotoxic T lymphocyte response in healthy adults immunized with live attenuated varicella vaccine. J Infect Dis 165:852–858, 1992.
275. Nader S, Bergen R, Sharp M, Arvin A. Comparison of cell-mediated immunity (CMI) to varicella-zoster virus (VZV) in children and adults immunized with live attenuated varicella vaccine. J Infect Dis 171:13–17, 1995.
276. Gershon AA, Steinberg S, LaRussa P, et al, NIAID Collaborative Varicella Vaccine Study Group. Immunization of healthy adults with live attenuated varicella vaccine. J Infect Dis 158:132–137, 1988.
277. Dubey L, Steinberg S, LaRussa P, et al. Western blot analysis of antibody to varicella-zoster virus. J Infect Dis 157:882–888, 1988.
278. Ueda K, Tokugawa K, Nakashima F, Takahashi M. A five-year immunological follow-up study of the institutionalized handicapped children vacinated with live varicella vaccine or infected with natural varicella. Biken J 27:119–122, 1984.
279. Asano Y, Suga S, Yoshikawa T, et al. Experience and reason: Twenty year follow up of protective immunity of the Oka live varicella vaccine. Pediatrics 94:524–526, 1994.
280. Watson B, Gupta R, Randall T, Starr S. Persistence of cell-mediated and humoral immune responses in healthy children immunized with live attenuated varicella vaccine. J Infect Dis 169:197–199, 1994.
281. Ngai A, Stahele BO, Kuter BJ, et al. Safety and immunogenicity of one vs. two injections of Oka/Merck varicella vaccine in healthy chidren. Pediatr Infect Dis J 15:49–54, 1996.
282. Hardy I, Gershon A. Prospects for use of a varicella vaccine in adults. Infect Dis Clin North Am 4:160–173, 1990.
283. Plotkin SA, Starr S, Connor K, Morton D. Zoster in normal children after varicella vaccine. J Infect Dis 159:1000–1001, 1989.
284. White CJ. Clinical trials of varicella vaccine in healthy children. Infect Dis Clin North Am 10:595–608, 1996.
285. White CJ. Letter to the editor. Pediatrics 89:354, 1992.
286. Kamiya H, Kato T, Isaji M, et al. Immunization of acute leukemic children with a live varicella vaccine (Oka strain). Biken J 27:99–102, 1984.
287. Hammerschlag MR, Gershon A, Steinberg S, et al. Herpes zoster in an adult recipient of live attenuated varicella vaccine. J Infect Dis 160:535–537, 1989.
288. Just M, Berger R, Just V. Evaluation of a combined measles-mumps-rubella-chickenpox vaccine. Dev Biol Stand 65:85–88, 1986.
289. Englund JA, Suarez CS, Kelly J, et al. Placebo-controlled trial of varicella vaccine given with or after measles-mumps-rubella vaccine. J Pediatr 114:37–44, 1989.
290. Shinefield HR, Black S, Morozumi P, et al. Safety and immunogenicity of concomitant separate administration of MMRII, Tetramune (Wyeth Lederle DPT & HbOC) and Varivax (Oka/Merck Varicella Vaccine) vs concomitant injections of MMRII, and Tetramune with Varivax given six weeks later. Society for Pediatric Research; Washington, DC; May 1996.
291. Arbeter AM, Baker L, Starr SE, et al. Combination measles, mumps, rubella, and varicella vaccine. Pediatrics 78:S742–S747, 1988.
292. Brunell PA, Novelli VM, Lipton SV, Pollock B. Combined vaccine against measles, mumps, rubella, and varicella. Pediatrics 81:779–784, 1988.
293. White CJ, Stinson D, Staehle B, et al. Measles, mumps, rubella, and varicella combination vaccine: Safety and immunogenicity alone and in combination with other vaccines given to children. Clin Infect Dis 24:925–931, 1997.
294. Committee on Infectious Diseases. Live attenuated varicella vaccine. Pediatrics 95:791–796, 1995.

294a. Wallace MR, Chamberlin CJ, Zerboni L, et al. Reliability of a history of previous varicella infection in adults. JAMA 278:1520–1522, 1997.

295. Provost PJ, Krah DL, Kuter BJ, et al. Antibody assays suitable for assessing immune responses to live varicella vaccine. Vaccine 9:111–116, 1991.
296. Berger R, Luescher D, Just M. Enhancement of varicella-zoster-specific immune responses in the elderly by boosting with varicella vaccine. J Infect Dis 149:647, 1984.
297. Levin M, Murray M, Zerbe G, et al. Immune responses of elderly persons 4 years after receiving a live attenuated varicella vaccine. J Infect Dis 170:522–526, 1994.
298. Marwick C. Lengthy tale of varicella vaccine development finally nears a clinically useful conclusion. JAMA 273:833–835, 1995.
299. Halloran ME. Epidemiologic effects of varicella vaccination. Infect Dis Clin North Am 10:631–656, 1996.
300. Garnett GP, Grenfell BT. The epidemiology of varicella-zoster infections: A mathematical model. Epidemiol Infect 108:495–511, 1992.

chapter

20 Combination Vaccines

Michael D. Decker
Kathryn M. Edwards

A combination vaccine consists of two or more separate immunogens that have been physically combined in a single preparation. This concept differs from that of simultaneous vaccines, which, although administered concurrently, are physically separate (i.e., injected at separate sites or delivered by separate routes). In this chapter, the use of a virgule to coordinate the names of two vaccines (e.g., DTP/IPV) indicates a combination of those two vaccines; a plus sign (e.g., DTP + IPV) indicates their concurrent but separate administration.

Rapid growth in the number of effective and important vaccines provides a continuing need to both expand and simplify vaccine administration programs, a need being addressed by ongoing research into new combination vaccines. However, the development, evaluation, and implementation of combination vaccines can pose complex issues, many of which were reviewed by scientists from academia, government, and industry at a 1993 workshop convened by the U.S. Food and Drug Administration (FDA) in Bethesda, Maryland. The proceedings of that workshop provide a useful reference on these topics.[1]

In this chapter, we review the history and importance of combination vaccines, outline study design issues pertinent to the evaluation of combination vaccines, examine relevant immunological principles, and review other impediments to combination vaccines. Most of the vaccine components included in these combinations are discussed in their own chapters elsewhere in this text, and readers are referred to those chapters for additional information.

Simultaneous Vaccines

Although some studies have shown altered immune responses to various vaccines when they are given concurrently with other vaccines, there is no evidence that the efficacy of any vaccine recommended for routine use in childhood is materially altered by concurrent administration with any other vaccines recommended for administration at the same age.[2] Similarly, adverse events after concurrent administration of multiple vaccines generally are increased only modestly, if at all, compared with events after the administration of the most reactogenic vaccine alone. Thus, we do not review the many studies that have evaluated simultaneous administration, except to the extent that they provide reference data against which results from combined vaccines can be compared.

History

The combining of multiple related or unrelated antigens into a single vaccine is not a new concept; combination vaccines have long been a bedrock of our pediatric and adult immunization programs. Those combination vaccines in common use include diphtheria and tetanus toxoids, available alone (DT or Td) or with pertussis vaccine (DTP); inactivated (IPV) or live oral (OPV) trivalent polio vaccine; and measles and rubella vaccine, available alone (MR) or with mumps vaccine (MMR).

The first combination vaccine licensed in the United States was trivalent influenza vaccine, approved in November 1945, and the second was a hexavalent pneumococcal vaccine, licensed in 1947.[3] DTP, although developed in 1943, was not licensed until March 1948. IPV was licensed in 1955, and the individual OPV serotypes were licensed from 1961 to 1962. Efforts to overcome the interference seen with simultaneous administration of three live vaccines delayed the licensure of trivalent OPV until June 1963. MMR and MR were licensed in April 1971, and quadrivalent meningococcal vaccine in 1978. More recently licensed combination vaccines incorporate newer components such as conjugate *Haemophilus influenzae* type b (Hib), acellular pertussis (aP), and hepatitis B (HB) antigens.

Current developmental efforts seek combination vaccines that protect against many more pathogens, in keeping with the ultimate goal of combining all the antigens recommended for routine immunization into a single multivalent product. Table 20–1 outlines the current status of the newer combination vaccines, and Table 20–2 provides further details concerning those that are licensed.

Table 20–1. **COMBINATION VACCINES FOR USE IN INFANCY AND CHILDHOOD, PRESENTLY LICENSED OR UNDER DEVELOPMENT***

VACCINES COMBINED†	MANUFACTURERS HOLDING LICENSE FOR COMBINATION VACCINE			CLINICAL TRIALS CONDUCTED	DEVELOPMENT PLANS ACCOUNTED‡
	Europe or Canada	United States	Other Countries		
Td/IPV	PMC-Fr, PMC-Ca				
DT/IPV	PMC-Ca				
DT/HB	PMC-Fr				
DTP/IPV	PMC-Ca, PMC-Fr		PMC-Fr		
DTP/Hib	PMC-Ca, PMC-Fr, SB, WL	PMC-US, WL	PMC-Fr, PMC-Ca		
DTP/Hib/IPV	PMC-Ca, PMC-Fr		PMC-Fr, PMC-Ca		
DTP/HB	SB		SB		
DTP/Hib/HB	SB		SB	Merck	
DTaP/IPV	NAVA, PMC-Ca, PMC-Fr, SB		PMC-Ca		
DTaP/Hib	SB	PMC-US§	SB	WL	NAVA
DTaP/IPV/Hib	PMC-Ca, PMC-Fr, SB		PMC-Ca	NAVA	WL
DTaP/HB	SB				
DTaP/IPV/HB				SB	
DTaP/Hib/HB				SB	
DTaP/Hib/IPV/HB				PMC-Fr, PMC-US, SB	
DTaP/Hib/IPV/HB/HA					SB
HB/Hib		Merck			
HB/HA	SB		SB		
MMRV				Merck, SB	
PnC/MnC				WL	
PnC/MnC/Hib				WL	

*Products combining only multiple serotypes of a single pathogen are excluded, as are DT, DTP, DTaP, OPV, IPV, and MMR. Only those manufacturers that distribute their products globally are listed; other manufacturers may produce some products (e.g., DTP/IPV) for local or regional use. Some products represent components derived from, or joint efforts of, more than one manufacturer; in such cases, their principal distributor is shown.

†No discrimination is made between products distributed in combined form and those distributed in separate containers, for combination at the time of use.

‡Information based on written communications from manufacturers, January 1998.

§Licensed for the fourth (booster) dose only as of January 1998.

DT, diphtheria and tetanus toxoids vaccine; DTaP, diphtheria, tetanus, and acellular pertussis vaccine; DTP, diphtheria, tetanus, and whole-cell pertussis vaccine; HA, hepatitis A vaccine; HB, hepatitis B vaccine; Hib, conjugate *Haemophilus influenzae* type b vaccine; IPV, enhanced-potency inactivated trivalent polio vaccine; MMRV, measles, mumps, rubella, and varicella vaccine; MnC, meningococcal conjugate vaccine; NAVA, North American Vaccine; PMC, Pasteur Mérieux Connaught (Ca, Canada; Fr, France; US, United States); PnC, pneumococcal conjugate vaccine; SB, SmithKline Beecham; Td, tetanus and diphtheria toxoids vaccine; WL, Wyeth Lederle Vaccines and Pediatrics.

Importance

Growth in the number of effective vaccines suitable for use in infancy and early childhood has posed substantial economic and logistical difficulties. Providing these vaccines as separate injections not only is expensive but also requires a great number of injections, which quickly becomes intolerable for the patient, parent, and provider alike. Scheduling additional vaccination visits to keep the number of injections per visit to a reasonable number increases costs, burdens staff, and jeopardizes the entire immunization program by increasing the likelihood of missed vaccinations. The shipping, handling, and storage of a plethora of vaccines are burdensome and expensive and increase the likelihood of error. These issues are of such intense international interest for the global birth cohort of 125 million children that in 1990 the Children's Vaccine Initiative (CVI) was launched at the World Summit for Children in New York City.[4] Endorsed by multiple governmental and policymaking bodies, the CVI proposed that the ideal vaccine would provide all indicated antigens in a single dose (preferably oral) and would be heat stable, effective when administered soon after birth, and affordable to families of all economic levels. The Institute of Medicine supported the full participation of the United States in the CVI in 1993.[5]

PRINCIPLES OF COMBINED VACCINES

Basic Design Concepts for Combination Vaccine Trials

The Challenges

Combining multiple antigens into one injection requires demonstration in clinical trials that the combination will not materially reduce the safety or immunogenicity of the component vaccines and, in some instances, that efficacy is retained.[6–8]

Combination vaccine trials should be prospective, randomized, and double-blinded and should have appropriate comparison (control) groups. Defining the comparison groups can be problematic when evaluating a multicomponent vaccine. If no pertinent data are available and if one wishes to be able to detect reduced immunogenicity of any component in the combination vaccine, the number of study arms required for the complete evaluation of an n-component vaccine is 2^n, based on the possible combinations alone. Other factors may further increase the number of study arms needed. For example, the sequence of administration of certain antigens may play an important role in immunogenicity. As is discussed later, it has been shown that the response to some Hib vaccines may depend on previous or con-

Table 20–2. **COMBINATION VACCINES PRESENTLY AVAILABLE IN THE UNITED STATES**

CLASS	VACCINE NAME	MANUFACTURER	FORMULATION OF EACH 0.5-mL DOSE
DT	DT vaccine	Wyeth Lederle	12.5 Lf of diphtheria toxoid and 5 Lf of tetanus toxoid. The aluminum content does not exceed 0.80 mg. The final concentration of thimerosal is 0.01%.
		Pasteur Mérieux Connaught	6.6 Lf of diphtheria toxoid and 5 Lf of tetanus toxoid. The aluminum content does not exceed 0.25 mg, and the thimerosal is 0.01%.
		Massachusetts Department of Public Health	7.5 Lf of diphtheria toxoid, 7.5 Lf of tetanus toxoid, and 0.01% of thimerosal.
		Medeva	10 Lf of diphtheria toxoid and 5 Lf of tetanus toxoid. The aluminum content should not exceed 0.85 mg, and the thimerosal is 0.01%.
Td	Td vaccine	Pasteur Mérieux Connaught	2 Lf of diphtheria toxoid and 5 Lf of tetanus toxoid. The aluminum content should not exceed 0.25 mg, and the thimerosal is 0.01%.
		Wyeth Lederle	2 Lf of diphtheria toxoid and 5 Lf of tetanus toxoid. The aluminum content should not exceed 0.80 mg, and the thimerosal is 0.01% thimerosal.
		Massachusetts Department of Public Health	2 Lf of diphtheria toxoid and 2 Lf of tetanus toxoid. The aluminum content should not exceed 0.45 mg, and the thimerosal is 0.0033%.
		Medeva	2 Lf of diphtheria toxoid and 5 Lf of tetanus toxoid. The aluminum content should not exceed 0.85 mg, and the thimerosal is 0.01%.
DTP	DTP vaccine	Pasteur Mérieux Connaught	6.5 Lf of diphtheria toxoid, 5 Lf of tetanus toxoid, 4 units of pertussis vaccine, aluminum not to exceed 0.25 mg, and 0.01% thimerosal as a preservative.
		Massachusetts Department of Public Health	10 Lf of diphtheria toxoid, 5.5 Lf of tetanus toxoid, 4 units of pertussis vaccine, 0.11–0.19 mg of aluminum, and 0.01% thimerosal.
		Michigan Department of Public Health/SKB	10 Lf of diphtheria toxoid, 5.5 Lf of tetanus toxoid, 4 units of pertussis vaccine, 0.2–0.6 mg of aluminum, and 0.01% thimerosal.
	Tri-Immunol	Wyeth Lederle	12.5 Lf of diphtheria toxoid, 5 Lf of tetanus toxoid, 4 units of pertussis vaccine, aluminum not to exceed 0.80 mg, and 0.01% thimerosal as a preservative.
DTP/Hib	Tetramune	Wyeth Lederle	12.5 Lf of diphtheria toxoid, 5 Lf of tetanus toxoid, 10 μg of purified Hib, approximately 25 μg of CRM_{197} protein, and 4 units of pertussis vaccine.
	DTP/ActHib	Pasteur Mérieux Connaught	6.7 Lf of diphtheria toxoid, 5 Lf of tetanus toxoid, and 4 units of pertussis vaccine as DTP to reconstitute lyophilized ActHib (10 μg of Hib polysaccharide).
DTaP	Acel-Immune	Wyeth Lederle	9 Lf of diphtheria toxoid, 5 Lf of tetanus toxoid, 40 μg (but not more than 60 μg) of pertussis antigen protein (representing approximately 86% FHA, 8% inactivated pertussis toxoid, 4% pertactin, and 2% type 2 fimbriae), 0.23 mg of aluminum as aluminum hydroxide and aluminum phosphate, 0.01% thimerosal, and trace amounts of formaldehyde, gelatin, and polysorbate 80.
	Infanrix	SmithKline Beecham	25 Lf of diphtheria toxoid, 10 Lf of tetanus toxoid, 25 μg of pertussis toxoid, 25 μg FHA, 8 μg of pertactin, and not more than 0.625 mg of aluminum.
	Tripedia	Pasteur Mérieux Connaught	6.7 Lf of diphtheria toxoid, 5 Lf of tetanus toxoid, 46.8 μg of pertussis antigens (approximately 23.4 μg of inactivated PT and 23.4 μg of FHA), not more than 0.170 mg of aluminum, 0.01% thimerosal, not more than 100 μg (0.02%) of residual formaldehyde, and trace amounts of formaldehyde, gelatin, and polysorbate 80.
DTaP/Hib	TriHIBit	Pasteur Mérieux Connaught	Tripedia, packaged with and used to reconstitute ActHIB.
Hib/HB	Comvax	Merck	7.5 μg of Hib PRP, 125 μg of *Neisseria meningitidis* OMPC, 5 μg of HBsAg, approximately 225 μg of aluminum hydroxide, 35 μg sodium borate (decahydrate) as a pH stabilizer, and 0.9% sodium chloride. The product contains no preservative.
Measles-containing	M-M-R II	Merck	Not less than 1000 $TCID_{50}$ measles vaccine, 20,000 $TCID_{50}$ of mumps virus, and 1000 $TCID_{50}$ rubella virus; and approximately 25 μg of neomycin.
	M-RVAX II	Merck	Not less than 1000 $TCID_{50}$ measles virus and 1000 $TCID_{50}$ rubella virus; and approximately 25 μg of neomycin. The product contains no preservative.
Streptococcus pneumoniae polysaccharide	Pneumovax 23	Merck	25 μg of each polysaccharide type dissolved in isotonic saline solution containing 0.25% phenol as preservative.
	Pnu-Imune 23	Wyeth Lederle	25 μg of each polysaccharide types. Thimerosal 0.01% is added as a preservative.
Neisseria meningitidis	Menomune-A/C/Y/W-135	Pasteur Mérieux Connaught	50 μg each of "isolated product" from *N. meningitidis* group A, group C, group Y, and group W-135; saline; thimerosal; and 2.5–5 mg of lactose added as a stabilizer.

CRM, cross-reactive mutant No. 197; FHA, filamentous hemagglutinin; Hib, *Haemophilus influenzae* type b; HBsAg, hepatitis B surface antigen; Lf, limit of flocculation; OMPC, outer membrane protein conjugate; PRP, polyribosylribitol phosphate; $TCID_{50}$, median tissue culture infective dose. See also abbreviations in Table 20–1.

current administration of DTP. Evaluation of such interactions may require study arms that receive the implicated antigens in different sequences.

Another complicating factor is that reduced antibody responses to one component of a combination could be due to immunological interference that would occur even if the antigens were injected at different sites during the same visit, or alternatively, to chemical or physical inactivation that occurs only when the antigens are combined in a single injection. The need to differentiate these two possibilities would require additional study arms. Ethical concerns also complicate study design, because vaccines that are recommended for routine use in the study population cannot be withheld in order to study vaccine interactions (although they can be administered at intercalated visits).

The complexity of these studies is increased by the availability of multiple vaccine preparations designed for protection against the same pathogen. Although this consideration does not increase the number of arms required for study of a given combination vaccine, it dramatically increases the number of potential combination vaccines to be studied. If one considers only the three Hib conjugate vaccines, two HB vaccines, and seven aP vaccines presently licensed (anywhere) for use in infancy, there could be as many as 42 DTaP/Hib/HB combination vaccines. Each combination would be unique, and thus demonstration that one combination performed as well as its component antigens given singly would be no assurance that any other combination would also be satisfactory.

Some Solutions

With all these factors serving to increase the number of study arms in combination vaccine trials, what tactics could be used to simplify these design problems and allow for studies of reasonable size? Multicenter studies allow larger enrollments—and thus more arms—than are possible at a single institution. A multicenter trial that is well designed with standardized protocols can be an effective means of evaluating multiple vaccines or multicomponent products, as is shown by the Multicenter Acellular Pertussis Trial.[9] The Swedish and Italian DTaP efficacy trials, with their coordinated protocols and control vaccines, are other pertinent examples.[10, 11]

A straightforward and attractive solution exists to the dilemma of designing combination vaccine studies. If earlier studies have laid an appropriate foundation for the study of a multicomponent vaccine (i.e., if they have evaluated predecessor vaccines that differ from the new combination by lacking only a single component), a study can then compare the new combination to its predecessor plus the new component, given separately. Another solution is to compare the new combination against each of its components given alone, deferring study of the subcombinations in the hope that no interference will be observed.

It may be possible to simplify study of a combination vaccine by administering to one of the comparison arms a similar, previously studied vaccine, thereby allowing comparison of the current results to those obtained in other arms of the prior study. This *bridging technique* has been employed in the Swedish acellular pertussis efficacy trials to compare the results from each trial.[10, 12, 13] The methodological risks of this approach can be reduced through coordinated efforts to enhance the comparability of serological and reaction data gathered for similar vaccines in independent studies. With adequate standardization, incorporation of a prior study arm as a comparison arm in the current study could allow comparison with the results obtained in the other arms of the prior study.

Correlates of Protection

For some antigens, studies of vaccine efficacy and immunogenicity have established correlations between levels of antibody and protection from disease. Such *correlates of protection* have been identified for several common vaccine antigens, including diphtheria toxoid, HB virus, Hib, measles virus, poliovirus, and tetanus toxoid. Studies of some other vaccines, such as pertussis vaccines, have not identified a correlation between humoral antibody levels and vaccine efficacy.

Identifying such correlates provides important benefits. For example, these correlates enable attention to be focused on clinically pertinent performance rather than on numerical differences that may be statistically significant but clinically irrelevant. If a combination vaccine produced serological results for a particular antigen that were significantly lower than those seen in the comparison arm but were nonetheless greater than the level known to provide clinical protection throughout the period of risk, then the diminished immunogenicity would not alter the acceptability of the combination vaccine. Furthermore, such correlates permit the licensure of new vaccines based on immunogenicity studies that compare the performance of these vaccines to that of prior vaccines of proven efficacy. The identification of correlates is of sufficient importance that it should be an explicit objective of any efficacy study of an antigen for which such correlates are not yet determined with confidence. The lack of such correlates poses problems for the licensure of new vaccines containing those antigens[14, 15] and has stimulated the pursuit of more sophisticated analyses in the hopes of identifying useful correlations.[16]

Combination Vaccines and the Immune System

Immune responses to vaccines are in general assessed by measuring humoral antibodies to the vaccine antigens. Although cell-mediated immune responses to included immunogens have not been evaluated for most vaccines, there is little evidence to demonstrate that vaccine efficacy correlates with cell-mediated immunity in humans. Therefore, the following discussion focuses primarily on factors influencing the generation of humoral antibody responses to vaccine.

Antibodies recognize conformationally determined epitopes on protein or polysaccharide antigens. Modification of an antigen's B-cell epitopes during vaccine preparation may reduce the ability of vaccine-induced antibody to bind to the pathogen. Consequently, the techniques used to produce an antigen may have important implications for the immunogenicity (and, presumably, the efficacy) of a vaccine containing that antigen.[17] Results from the Multicenter Acellular Pertussis Trial, which compared 13 acellular pertussis vaccines, showed that levels of antibody to pertussis toxin correlated poorly with the quantity of toxoided pertussis toxin present in the vaccines.[9] For example, one of the acellular vaccines contained a genetically inactivated pertussis toxin produced by recombinant technology. This vaccine produced markedly higher antibody responses per unit antigen than did the remainder of the evaluated vaccines, whose pertussis toxin components were chemically inactivated (e.g., with formaldehyde or glutaraldehyde).[9]

Many bacterial pathogens are protected by a polysaccharide capsule that is antiphagocytic. Generation of antibody to the capsular polysaccharide is needed for optimal opsonization, and levels of anticapsular antibody are correlated with protection against disease.[18] However, most capsular polysaccharides are poor immunogens, especially in young infants, and they do not prime for a memory response.[19, 20] As early as 1929, Avery and Goebel demonstrated the beneficial effect on immunogenicity of coupling carbohydrates to carrier proteins.[21] Such treatment can overcome the poor immunogenicity of polysaccharide in infants, increase the immune response in adults, and prime for a memory response.[22–24]

A review of the mechanism of antibody production by B lymphocytes illustrates how conjugation of the polysaccharide to a protein enhances B-cell responses.[25, 26] B cells have immunoglobulins on their surface that serve as antigen receptors. When polysaccharide antigens are presented to B cells, the antigens are ingested and processed; however, because the antigens do not contain peptides, they cannot associate with major histocompatibility complex molecules and cannot move to the surface of the B cell to stimulate T-cell responses.[27–29] Polysaccharide antigens are thus termed *T cell–independent antigens* and stimulate more restricted primary and memory responses.[30] In contrast, when polysaccharide-protein conjugates are presented to B cells, the antigens are endocytosed and degraded into peptide epitopes that associate with major histocompatibility complex molecules and return to the B-cell surface to be recognized by helper T cells.[31] T cells bind to the B cells, triggering the B cells to proliferate and differentiate into antibody-secreting cells, leading to increased antibody production.[32] Other antigen-presenting cells (e.g., macrophages and dendritic cells) also efficiently stimulate T cells through costimulatory molecules such as CD28 and B7.[33, 34] Once primed, memory T cells can be restimulated by antigen that is presented by a broad range of antigen-presenting cells, including B cells.[32] B cells can also be selected to become memory cells by interactions with T cells and thereby become capable of activation with subsequent exposure to the antigen.[25]

The remarkable success of the polysaccharide-protein conjugate Hib vaccines in eliminating Hib disease is testimony to the utility and effectiveness of the conjugate vaccine approach. However, some bacterial pathogens, such as *Streptococcus pneumoniae*, have many serotypes that cause disease, requiring that numerous conjugates be combined into one vaccine. Theories regarding the human immune response and vaccine studies in animals and humans suggest that simultaneous exposure to multiple conjugate antigens (as with a polyvalent conjugate vaccine) could result in either enhanced or diminished immune responses.[35–39]

The phenomenon of carrier-induced epitope-specific suppression is one in which antibody responses to haptens presented on a carrier are inhibited by prior immunization with the specific carrier. Studies in animals have shown that the dose, route, choice of carrier protein, and presence of adjuvant contribute to determining whether epitopic suppression or enhancement of the immune response occurs. Suppression more frequently occurs when large amounts of carrier protein are used for priming and high anticarrier antibody titers are achieved.[26] Concurrent administration of two conjugate vaccines employing the same carrier may also lead to interference. For example, a study among infants given a combination vaccine containing Hib capsular polysaccharide conjugated to tetanus toxoid (PRP-T) plus a quadrivalent pneumococcal vaccine conjugated to either tetanus or diphtheria toxoid found reduced Hib antibodies among those infants whose pneumococcal vaccine was conjugated to tetanus toxoid rather than diphtheria toxoid.[40]

These data make it clear that the effect of prior or concomitant administration of proteins used in conjugate vaccines is unpredictable and must be evaluated for each vaccine combination.

Other Impediments to the Development of Combination Vaccines

Chemical or physical interactions among the vaccine components being combined can result in an alteration of the immune response to vaccine.[26] Adjuvants such as aluminum hydroxide and aluminum phosphate bind to inactivated vaccines by noncovalent ionic binding. The combination of one vaccine that is generally administered with adjuvant with another vaccine that is not administered with adjuvant may lead to displacement of the adjuvant and reduced immunogenicity of the first vaccine. Furthermore, the adjuvant might combine with the second antigen and thereby alter the immune response to the second vaccine as well.

Buffers, stabilizers, excipients, and similar components included in one vaccine may interfere with the components of another vaccine. For example, some DTP and Hib vaccines contain thimerosal, which can destroy the potency of inactivated polio vaccine. Although such vaccines cannot be mixed in the vial, distribution of the two vaccines in a dual-chambered syringe can circumvent this problem.

Live vaccines can interfere immunologically with each

other. For example, one vaccine might stimulate immune responses, such as interferon production, that inhibit replication of another virus.

Patent and other proprietary issues also complicate the generation of combination vaccines. Vaccine manufacturers cannot market vaccines that contain antigens they do not own or license. The best possible combination vaccine might be one that incorporated components from two or more manufacturers, but absent agreement between the companies, this combination will not become available. Although the dramatic consolidation in recent years among vaccine manufacturers has eased this problem, as have cross-licensing agreements, it has not disappeared.

TRADITIONAL COMBINED VACCINES: DTP, IPV, OPV, ENHANCED-POTENCY IPV, AND MMR

As noted earlier, DTP was developed in 1943 and licensed in the United States in 1948. Its component antigens had long been available separately: The first pertussis vaccine (see Chapter 14) was licensed to the Massachusetts Public Health Biological Laboratories in 1914; mixtures of diphtheria toxin and antitoxin came into use the same year; alum-precipitated diphtheria toxoid (see Chapter 9) was licensed in 1926; and adsorbed tetanus toxoid (see Chapter 18) was licensed in 1937.[3] Pertussis vaccine is a potent adjuvant, and the combining of the three antigens in DTP actually improved the immunogenicity of the toxoids as compared with that of the component products given alone.[41, 42] Adsorption of the vaccines with aluminum further improved immunogenicity while decreasing the severity of adverse reactions associated with pertussis vaccine.[43]

MMR vaccines are produced in many countries (see Chapters 12, 13, and 17, respectively). Multiple strains of each vaccine have been used, although three MMR formulations currently predominate. Rates of adverse reactions after the administration of MMR are only modestly higher than those seen with the individual component products, and seroconversion rates are essentially unchanged.[44–48] The various MMR vaccines all appear to be highly immunogenic.[49, 50]

Advances in tissue culture techniques permitted the development of trivalent IPV (see Chapter 15), which underwent extensive field trials in 1954. These trials found 90% efficacy against poliovirus types 2 and 3 but only about 70% efficacy against type 1.[51] Investigation revealed that thimerosal, used as a preservative, inactivated the vaccine virus and had a relatively greater effect on type 1 poliovirus than on types 2 and 3; other preservatives were substituted. Further improvements in production techniques in the late 1970s allowed the introduction of enhanced-potency IPV, which provides substantially higher immunogenicity.[52–54] There is no evidence of interference between the inactivated vaccine strains themselves, unlike the situation with the trivalent OPV (see Chapter 16). Because enteroviruses can compete with each other in the gut, concerns about such interference initially prompted immunization at three separate visits with the monovalent Sabin OPVs. However, it was soon found that adequate immunogenicity could be obtained by adjusting the relative concentrations of the three strains in the trivalent vaccine and by giving three doses.

EXTENDING THE TRADITIONAL COMBINATIONS

Adding New Valences to DTP

DTP/IPV

Interest in a vaccine combining DTP and IPV first arose before the licensure of OPV. In 1960, Bordt and colleagues compared IPV, DTP, and DTP/IPV among 192 previously unimmunized children ranging in age from 1 month to 6 years.[55] Results were analyzed separately for infants (1–5 mo), toddlers (6 mo–2 yr), and older children; all age groups showed better neutralizing antibody responses to poliovirus, diphtheria, and tetanus, and agglutinating antibodies to pertussis with the combined vaccine than with the separate vaccines.

DTP/Enhanced-Potency IPV

Soon after Bordt and colleagues' study,[55] OPV was licensed in the United States, where interest in DTP/IPV combination vaccines subsequently waned. However, widespread use of these combinations continued in several countries, mostly European. When enhanced-potency IPV became available, its high immunogenicity broadened interest in DTP/IPV combinations, which could simplify vaccination programs and eliminate the necessity for frozen shipment and storage of OPV.[42] Such vaccines would also obviate concerns regarding reduced immunogenicity of OPV in tropical countries due to competition in the gut from other circulating enteroviruses,[56] and they would eliminate the risk of vaccine-associated paralytic poliomyelitis.[57]

In 1980, a noncomparative study in Senegal found good poliovirus immunogenicity and efficacy for a combination DTP/IPV vaccine prepared by Institut Mérieux.[56] However, a comparative study from the same centers comparing responses in infants to a dose of IPV, IPV/pertussis, IPV/DT, or IPV/DTP, followed by IPV/DTP a month later for all groups, found reduced poliovirus antibody responses in the combination vaccine groups.[58] In a third study, 320 Mali infants were given two doses of either the same DTP/IPV used in the other studies, DTP + IPV, or DTP + OPV.[59] Although poliovirus seroconversion rates were 100% for all three serotypes with DTP/IPV and with DTP + IPV, mean antibody levels were markedly higher for the separate than the combined group. When given a booster dose a year later, both groups had excellent poliovirus antibody responses, although mean titers again were about twice as high in the separate-vaccine group. Investigators in

Pakistan compared DTP/IPV with DTP + OPV and found good poliovirus immunogenicity in both groups.[60]

None of these studies found material reductions in responses to the DTP components. A comparison of DTP and DTP/IPV in Scandinavian children found enhanced DTP antibody responses in the group given the combination vaccine,[61] and a noncomparative study in Burkina Faso found that two doses of a DTP/IPV vaccine produced good poliovirus and tetanus antibody responses.[62] Levels of antibodies to diphtheria were lower than those for poliovirus and tetanus, although 98% of children were primed.

The first report clearly documenting reduced antibody responses to the pertussis component of a DTP/IPV vaccine was that of Baker and colleagues,[63] who compared serological responses to DTP and IPV (both produced by Connaught Laboratories Ltd., Ontario, Canada), given combined or separately, versus DTP + OPV (Table 20–3). Unexpectedly, whether the products were administered separately or combined into a single injection, IPV recipients demonstrated significantly lower pertussis antibody responses, for both pertussis toxin and filamentous hemagglutinin, than did OPV recipients.[63] Halperin and colleagues more recently conducted a follow-up study comparing DTP + IPV with DTP/IPV and found significantly lower pertussis antibody responses with the combined than with the separate vaccines (see Table 20–3).[64] Neither of these reports included data concerning the immunogenicity of the IPV component, but another study comparing DTP/IPV versus DTP + IPV reported that 96 to 100% of recipients in both groups had neutralizing antibody to all three poliovirus serotypes at 6 months of age.[65]

Summary of DTP/IPV. It appears that antibody responses to pertussis toxoid and poliovirus components may be substantially reduced with the combined DTP/IPV compared with DTP + IPV. However, poliovirus seroconversion rates and absolute antibody levels remained high even with combined vaccine, and the clinical import of any reduction in mean antibody levels, for either polio or pertussis, is unknown. Antibody responses to diphtheria and tetanus appear to be somewhat lower with DTP/IPV than with the component vaccines alone, but these effects appear minor, with good seroconversion rates. The nature and magnitude of any interactions likely depend on the particular vaccine formulations involved. No study found a material increase in adverse reactions with combined versus separate injections.

Table 20–3. **ANTIBODY RESPONSES TO PERTUSSIS ANTIGENS IN CANADIAN CHILDREN GIVEN DTP/IPV, DTP + IPV, OR DTP + OPV**

	ANTIBODY RESPONSES (EU)			
STUDY AND VACCINE	**Pertussis Toxin**	**Filamentous Hemagglutinin**	**Pertactin**	**Fimbrial Proteins**
Baker et al. (1992)[63]				
DTP + OPV	30.8	69.7	11,092	2,931
DTP + IPV at separate sites	5.4*	30.6*	6,209*	542*
DTP combined with IPV in a single injection	5.6*	14.3*	4,688*	653*
Halperin et al. (1996)[64]				
DTP + IPV at separate sites	35.5	63.9	5,127	2,272
DTP combined with IPV in a single injection	10.0†	24.8†	1,980†	1,276†

*Compared with DTP + OPV, difference significant at $P \leq .05$.
†Compared with DTP + IPV, difference significant at $P \leq .05$.
DTP, diphtheria and tetanus toxoids and whole-cell pertussis vaccine; EU, ELISA (enzyme-linked immunosorbent assay) units; IPV, inactivated polio vaccine; OPV, live oral polio vaccine.
Adapted from Edwards KM, Decker MD. Combination vaccines consisting of acellular pertussis vaccines. Pediatr Infect Dis J 16(suppl 4):S97–S102, 1997.

DTP/Conjugate Hib

During the late 1980s and early 1990s, a number of studies were launched to evaluate vaccines that combined DTP with conjugate Hib vaccine (and, in some instances, also with IPV). The first such studies compared the separate or combined administration of Pasteur Mérieux's PRP-T (ActHIB) and DTP in Israeli infants.[66] No increase in adverse events or interference with DTP antibody responses was detected. The study contained no comparison group given PRP-T alone, but PRP antibody responses appeared consistent with those seen in prior studies. A Canadian study comparing DTP/PRP-D with DTP + PRP-D as boosters at 18 months of age found no differences in antibody responses to the PRP, tetanus, or diphtheria components and found a slight reduction in pertussis agglutinins in the combined group.[67]

Concern was soon raised by a series of studies conducted in Chile and Canada (Vancouver) that evaluated the performance of DTP, PRP-T, and OPV or IPV, with the parenteral vaccines administered combined or concurrently at separate sites.[68–72] Table 20–4 shows the ratio of antibody response after administration of the combination vaccine to antibody response after separate injections. For every antigen except diphtheria, the combined vaccine produced substantially lower antibody levels in at least one study.[68–72]

Not surprisingly, these findings sparked additional studies of DTP/PRP-T combination vaccines with or without IPV.[73–80a] As is shown in Table 20–5, differences in antibody responses between the combined and separately administered vaccines were inconsistent, with few achieving statistical significance. For most antigens, absolute antibody levels, even if somewhat reduced, were still well above levels considered protective. The clinical implications of any reduction in pertussis antibody levels were unclear, given the lack of known correlation between such levels and protection from disease. It is uncertain what role is played by the choice of DTP, or the characteristics of the DTP chosen, in determining the nature of any interactions with a combined Hib vaccine.

The studies shown in Table 20–5 involved lyophilized PRP-T reconstituted with DTP. More recently, a fluid

Table 20–4. **RATIO OF MEAN POSTVACCINATION ANTIBODY LEVELS FOR COMBINED OR SEPARATE ADMINISTRATION OF DTP (OR DTP/IPV) AND PRP-T AMONG INFANTS IN CHILE AND CANADA**

LOCATION	AGE AT VACCINATION (mo)	VACCINES	RATIO OF ANTIBODY LEVELS WITH COMBINED VACCINE TO LEVELS WITH SEPARATE VACCINES*					
			PRP	D	T	PT	FHA	AGG
Chile[68,69]	2, 4, 6	DTP/PRP-T + OPV, DTP + PRP-T + OPV	0.43†	1.00	0.85	0.97	1.07	0.62‡
Chile[70]	2, 4, 6	DTP/PRP-T + OPV, DTP + PRP-T + OPV	0.70	1.32†	0.78	1.10	0.86	1.41
Vancouver[71]	2, 4, 6	DTP/PRP-T (lot 1) + OPV, DTP + PRP-T + OPV	1.16	1.33	1.00	0.80	1.00	0.88
Vancouver[71]	2, 4, 6	DTP/PRP-T (lot 2) + OPV, DTP + PRP-T + OPV	1.03	1.33	0.78	0.80	0.75	0.68†
Vancouver[72]	2, 4, 6	DTP/PRP-T/IPV, DTP/IPV + PRP-T	0.75	1.02	0.66	0.78	0.9	0.79

*A ratio less than 1 indicates that mean antibody levels were lower with the combined vaccine than with separate injections; a ratio higher than 1 indicates that mean antibody levels were higher with combined than with separate injections.

†Difference significant at $P \le .05$.

‡P-value not available. However, the rate of seroconversion (AGG ≥ 320) was significantly lower ($P < .05$) in the combined group (79% vs. 92%).

AGG, pertussis agglutinins; D, diphtheria toxin; DTP, diphtheria and tetanus toxoids and whole-cell pertussis vaccine; FHA, filamentous hemagglutinin; IPV, inactivated polio vaccine; OPV, live oral polio vaccine; PRP, polyribosylribitol phosphate; PRP-T, PRP-tetanus toxoid protein conjugate vaccine (Pasteur Mérieux Connaught); PT, pertussis toxin; T, tetanus toxin.

Adapted from Edwards KM, Decker MD. Combination vaccines consisting of acellular pertussis vaccines. Pediatr Infect Dis J 16(4 suppl):S97–S102, 1997.

preparation of PRP-T combined with DTP has been prepared. A comparative trial found no difference in the immunogenicity and reactogenicity of the two preparations.[81]

Surveillance data provide reassurance that use of the combined DTP/PRP-T does not reduce efficacy in comparison to DTP and PRP-T administered separately. In Chile, surveillance for pertussis in matched areas that used either DPT alone or DTP/PRP-T found no significant difference in the rates of pertussis in the two areas.[81] In the area using DTP/PRP-T, efficacy against invasive Hib disease was more than 90%.[82] Surveillance in Canada found a continued low rate of invasive Hib disease after the licensure and widespread use of DTP/PRP-T in that country, with no change in the extremely low rates of vaccine failure.[83, 84] Similarly, there was no increase in invasive Hib disease in the United States after the 1993 licensure of DTP/PRP-T and a similar product, DTP/PRP-HbOC (Tetramune, Wyeth Lederle Vaccines & Pediatrics; see Chapter 11).[85]

Several studies have compared DTP combinations with unconjugated PRP or with the conjugate Hib vaccines PRP-OMP (PedvaxHIB, Merck & Co.), or PRP-HbOC (HibTITER, Wyeth Lederle Vaccines & Pediatrics).[86–94] As is shown in Table 20–6, the data do not suggest that combining these vaccines materially interferes with the immunogenicity of any components; indeed, improved immunogenicity was seen more often than interference.

None of the combinations that include DTP and any conjugate Hib vaccine have been shown to be associated with materially increased adverse reactions. Typically, adverse reactions were slightly greater with the combinations than with the DTP alone; however, they were less than the aggregate of local reactions seen when separate vaccines were given at separate injection sites.

Table 20–5. **ADDITIONAL STUDIES COMPARING COMBINED OR SIMULTANEOUS ADMINISTRATION OF DTP AND PRP-T VACCINES FOR PRIMARY IMMUNIZATION OF INFANTS**

LOCATION	AGE AT VACCINATION (mo)	VACCINES	RATIO OF ANTIBODY LEVELS WITH COMBINED VACCINE TO LEVELS WITH SEPARATE VACCINES*								
									Poliovirus Serotypes		
			PRP	D	T	PT	FHA	AGG	*1*	*2*	*3*
United States[73]	2, 4, 6	DTP/PRP-T, DTP + PRP-T	0.88	1.09	0.94	1.01	1.00				
Israel[74]	2, 4, 6	DTP/IPV/PRP-T, DTP/IPV		0.86	0.65†			0.70†	1.01	0.78	1.29
United Kingdom[75]	2, 3, 4	DTP/PRP-T, DTP + PRP-T	0.75	1.01	1.83†	1.68	1.11	1.12			
Chile[76]	2, 4, 6	DTP/PRP-T, DTP				1.12	0.94	0.96			
United States[77]	2, 4, 6	DTP/PRP-T, DTP + PRP-T	1.60	1.14	0.96	1.44	0.69		1.55	1.38	0.79
Gambia[78]	2, 3, 4	DTP/PRP-T, DTP + PRP-T	0.96	1.11	1.16	0.91	0.77	‡			
United Kingdom[79]	2, 3, 4	DTP/PRP-T, DTP + PRP-T§	0.73								
Sweden[80]	3, 5, 12	DT/IPV/PRP-T, DT/PRP-T + IPV	‖	‖	‖				‖	‖	‖

*A ratio less than 1 indicates that mean antibody levels were lower with the combined vaccine than with separate injections; a ratio higher than 1 indicates that levels were higher with combined than with separate injections. A blank cell indicates that the comparison was not possible or is not available.

†Difference significant at $P \le .05$.

‡Agglutinin titers were not determined. However, ratios for antibody to pertactin and fimbrial antigens were 0.55 ($P < .05$) and 0.74, respectively.

§Combined vaccine group was compared with historical control subjects in the United Kingdom, who received the same PRP-T on the same schedule but a different DTP.

‖Reported as "not significantly different" or "comparable."

DT, diphtheria and tetanus toxoids vaccine. See also abbreviations in Table 20–4.

Table 20–6. **STUDIES COMPARING COMBINED OR SIMULTANEOUS ADMINISTRATION OF DTP AND Hib VACCINES OTHER THAN PRP-T FOR PRIMARY IMMUNIZATION OF INFANTS**

LOCATION	AGE AT VACCINATION (mo)	VACCINES	RATIO OF ANTIBODY LEVELS WITH COMBINED VACCINE TO LEVELS WITH SEPARATE VACCINES*					
			PRP	D	T	PT	FHA	AGG
United States[86]	2, 4, 6	DTP/PRP (unconjugated), DTP						1.41
Finland[87]	3, 4, 6	DTP/PRP-D, DTP		1.17	0.99			
The Gambia[88]	2, 3, 4	DTP/PRP-OMP, DTP + PRP-OMP	1.03	0.80	0.71			0.88
United States[89, 90]	2, 4, 6	DTP/PRP-HbOC, DTP + PRP-HbOC	1.51†	1.78†	1.82†			2.22†
United States[91]	2, 4, 6	DTP/PRP-HbOC, DTP + PRP-HbOC	‡	‡	‡			‡
United Kingdom[75]	2, 3, 4	DTP/PRP-HbOC, DTP + PRP-HbOC	1.30	0.93	1.48†	1.06	1.39	1.10

*A ratio less than 1 indicates that mean antibody levels were lower with the combined vaccine than with separate injections; a ratio higher than 1 indicates that levels were higher with combined than with separate injections. A blank cell indicates that the comparison was not possible or is not available.

†Difference significant at $P \leq .05$.

‡Serological assays were performed only for the DTP/PRP-HbOC group (PRP, 8.20 μg/mL; D, 0.92 IU/mL; T, 7.52 IU/mL; AGG, 110.1/dilution) and were said to be comparable to values reported in other series.

Hib, *Haemophilus influenzae* type b; PRP-D, PRP-diphtheria toxoid conjugate vaccine; PRP-HbOC, PRP-diphtheria CRM197 protein conjugate vaccine; PRP-OMP, PRP-meningococcal outer membrane protein conjugate vaccine. See also abbreviations in Table 20–4.

DTP/Hepatitis B

A number of studies have evaluated combination vaccines from SmithKline Beecham (SB) that incorporate DTP, HB, and, more recently, Hib components (Table 20–7).[92–98] For one study,[92] the Hib component was a PRP-T (ActHIB) manufactured by Pasteur Mérieux Connaught (PMC); for all others, the PRP-T manufactured by SB (Hiberix) was used. Several additional studies have evaluated DTP/HB versus DTP/HB/PRP-T but have not yet been published.

Results of these studies were variable. The combined vaccines were as likely to show higher as lower antibody responses compared with the separate vaccines for the various antigens. In general, the groups with the lowest antibody responses still attained levels considered protective (where applicable). One study, not yet published, evaluated the effect of a booster dose of DTP/HB/Hib given at 18 months of age to subjects who received DTP/HB + Hib or DTP/HB/Hib for the primary series. Both groups had high antibody responses to the booster; mean levels tended to be higher in the group primed with DTP/HB/Hib and were significantly so for antibody to PRP. Another study evaluated an Australian DTP (Commonwealth Serum Laboratories) with Merck's Hib and HB vaccines and found good antibody responses after booster administration.[99]

DTP/Measles

In 1973, Mérieux and colleagues administered lyophilized measles vaccine reconstituted with DPT/IPV to 20 seronegative children and found good responses to the measles and polio components.[100] From 1970 to 1978, public health nurses working in the Marshall Islands routinely drew up DTP and measles vaccine in the same syringe. Surveillance during a measles epidemic in 1978 revealed no significant difference in protection between those immunized with the combined vaccines (measles attack rate, 16.1%) or with the measles vaccine alone (attack rate, 17.9%).[101] Encouraged by these reports, John and colleagues conducted a series of experiments[102–104] involving the administration of DTP or DTP/IPV combined in the same syringe with measles vaccine. They found no significant difference in adverse reactions, measles antibody titers, or measles seroconversion rates.[104]

Table 20–7. **STUDIES COMPARING COMBINED OR SIMULTANEOUS ADMINISTRATION OF VACCINES CONTAINING DTP AND HB COMPONENTS, WITH OR WITHOUT Hib COMPONENTS, FOR PRIMARY IMMUNIZATION OF INFANTS**

LOCATION	AGE AT VACCINATION (mo)	VACCINES	RATIO OF ANTIBODY LEVELS WITH COMBINED VACCINE TO LEVELS WITH SEPARATE VACCINES*				
			PRP	D	T	WBP	HBs
Spain[98]	3, 5, 7	DTP/HB, DTP		0.79	0.70	0.79	
United States[92]	2, 4, 6	DTP/HB/PRP-T, DTP/HB + PRP-T†		1.63‡	1.08‡	1.47‡	2.02
Chile[93]	2, 4, 6	DTP/HB/PRP-T, DTP/HB + PRP-T§	0.70	0.95	0.98	0.86	0.94
Myanmar[94]	1½, 3, 5	DTP/HB/PRP-T, DTP/HB + PRP-T§	1.07	0.74‡	2.23‡	0.95	1.00‖

*A ratio less than 1 indicates that mean antibody levels were lower with the combined vaccine than with separate injections; a ratio higher than 1 indicates that levels were higher with combined than with separate injections. A blank cell indicates that the comparison was not possible or is not available.

†OmniHIB, SmithKline Beecham (produced by Pasteur Mérieux Connaught and identical to ActHIB).

‡Difference significant at $P \leq .05$.

§Hiberix, SmithKline Beecham.

‖Including only those subjects seronegative at birth.

HB, hepatitis B vaccine (SmithKline Beecham); HBs, hepatitis B surface antigen; Hib, *Haemophilus influenzae* type b; WBP, whole *Bordetella pertussis* (a mixture of serotypes 1, 2, and 3 used in a solid-phase immunoassay). See also abbreviations in Table 20–4.

Adding New Valences to Measles or MMR

Measles Combined with Yellow Fever and/or Smallpox

With the licensure of measles vaccines in the early 1960s, interest arose in administering this vaccine in combination with other antigens. In the West, combination with mumps and rubella antigens became the focus of interest; in Africa, however, smallpox and yellow fever were diseases of greater concern.

The use of combination smallpox/yellow fever vaccines began in 1939, when investigators at the Pasteur Institute of Dakar began to study coadministration of these vaccines through a single scarification site.[105] After successful animal and human studies, mass vaccination campaigns were conducted in French West Africa, with more than 14 million people receiving the combined vaccine between 1939 and 1945 alone.[106] A study among 600 French soldiers in 1945 found that the combined vaccine produced seroconversion to yellow fever in 98% of the participants, compared with 99% in those given the yellow fever vaccine alone.[106]

The yellow fever vaccine used by the French was a neurotropic strain maintained in mouse brains.[106, 107] In 1952, the Rockefeller Foundation supported efforts to develop a combination vaccine using the safer, although less immunogenic, 17D chick-embryo strain.[107] The resulting smallpox/yellow fever combination vaccine appeared to be safe and highly immunogenic in pilot studies and was readily manufactured and stored.[107] However, subsequent studies of this or similar vaccines in British East Africa found only about 70% seroconversion to yellow fever under field conditions, leading those investigators to recommend simultaneous rather than combined immunization.[108–110]

Soon after measles vaccine became available, researchers from the U.S. National Institutes of Health studied its use in combination with smallpox and yellow fever vaccines in Burkina Faso (previously Upper Volta).[111–116] Neutralizing antibody responses to measles, vaccinia, and yellow fever vaccines were materially lower in the combined-vaccine groups. The investigators noted that the ability of measles and yellow fever vaccines, but not vaccinia vaccine, to induce circulating interferon might explain the apparent interference found in the groups receiving combinations containing measles and yellow fever vaccines.[113]

A subsequent study in the United States evaluated a measles/smallpox vaccine in which the components were combined before lyophilization.[114] All subjects developed good responses to the vaccinia virus, and all but two subjects (who were injected intradermally) developed good response to the measles vaccine. A French study evaluated a combination vaccine created by the physician using a high-dose tetanus toxoid vaccine to draw up measles vaccine and found equal rates of seroconversion in the recipients of separate or combined vaccines (bacille Calmette-Guérin, yellow fever, and smallpox vaccines were administered simultaneously).[115]

More recently, investigators in at least four countries of Africa have evaluated the use of a combined measles/yellow fever vaccine.[116–118] In a randomized study in Cote d'Ivoire, infants (aged 6–9 mo) had comparable seroresponse rates to measles vaccine, yellow fever vaccine, or the combined vaccine.[116] Similar results were obtained in Mali for both infants (aged 4–8 mo) and toddlers (aged 12–24 mo).[117] Investigators in Cameroon found higher seroconversion rates with the combined than with the separate vaccines as well as significantly higher yellow fever antibody levels in the group given combined vaccine 30 days after immunization.[118] A trial in Nigeria similarly found that antibody levels and seroconversion rates were higher with combined than separate vaccines.[119]

MMR Combined with Varicella Vaccine

Among the combination vaccines incorporating MMR, the one that is receiving the greatest attention in developed countries results from the addition of varicella vaccine, yielding MMRV. Clinical investigations have evaluated products based on component vaccines from SB and from Merck. Each MMRV incorporates different measles and mumps strains but the same rubella strain (see Chapters 12, 13, and 17) and each company's derivative of the Oka varicella strain (see Chapter 19).

MMRVs Derived from SmithKline Beecham-Components. The first comparative trial of MMRV produced from SB components evaluated combinations of a then-available MMR with varicella vaccine of high potency (4300 plaque-forming units [PFU]) or low potency (1100 PFU), also produced by SB.[120] The combination of MMR plus the low-potency varicella vaccine yielded a varicella seroconversion rate 36% lower with the combined than the separate vaccines (78% vs. 42%). The high-potency varicella vaccine yielded substantially better seroconversion rates alone (98%) or combined with MMR (79%). A follow-up study evaluated the use of a low-potency MMR (measles and mumps virus contents reduced by 80% and 88%, respectively) combined with commercial varicella vaccine (both produced by SmithKline); the new combination yielded seroconversion rates of 98% for measles, 100% for mumps, 99% for rubella, and 98% for varicella.[121]

Finnish investigators subsequently evaluated MMRV vaccines composed of standard or low-potency MMR that was combined, respectively, with high-potency (5300 PFU) or low-potency (2000 PFU) varicella vaccine.[122] Varicella seroconversion rates were reduced substantially by combination with MMR, although less so for high-potency varicella combined with standard MMR (97% vs. 85%) than when both low-potency forms were combined (92% vs. 72%). Combination with high-potency varicella vaccine had little effect on seroconversion rates to standard MMR; seroconversion rates with low-potency MMR were somewhat reduced for mumps, but the difference was not significant. The authors concluded that neither of the evaluated MMRV formulations produced adequate varicella responses but that high-potency varicella plus low-potency MMR might prove suitable.

MMRVs Derived from Merck Components. MMRV formulations derived from Merck components have been evaluated in a number of studies.[123–127] The first report compared standard MMR versus MMR combined with a varicella vaccine containing 2300 peripheral resistance units (PFU) per dose; 6 weeks later, both groups received a varicella vaccine containing 1900 PFU per dose.[123] Mean titers, seroconversion rates, and adverse reactions were very similar between the two groups.[124] A study reported in 1988 compared MMRV vaccine versus varicella vaccine alone. The varicella component contained 2300 PFU per dose; the pure varicella vaccine contained 950 PFU per dose. Varicella conversion rates were higher in the group receiving the MMRV vaccine than in the group receiving only varicella vaccine (90% vs. 74%).

Subsequent studies gave results less favorable to the combination. Watson and colleagues[126] evaluated an MMRV similar to Merck's commercially distributed MMR, which is combined with 3785 PFU of varicella per dose, in comparison to MMR + varicella (3625 PFU/dose) and found 100% seroconversion to all antigens in both groups. Mean antibody titers were essentially identical in both groups for all antigens except varicella, for which titers were more than twice as high in the separate group (15.3 vs. 7.0 ELISA [enzyme-linked immunosorbent assay] units [EU]). Cell-mediated immune (lymphoproliferative) responses to varicella were also somewhat lower in the combined group. Merck researchers evaluated MMRV versus MMR + varicella (study 1) among 494 children and evaluated commercially available MMR + varicella vaccine (3500 PFU/dose, given 6 weeks later) + DTaP (Acel-Imune) + OPV versus MMRV (4000 PFU/dose) + DTaP + OPV (study 2) among 318 children.[127] Seroconversion rates were high for all viral antigens, although they were slightly lower with the combined vaccine in both studies. Mean antibody levels were high and similar between groups for the MMR antigens, but varicella titers were again about twice as high in the separate as in the combined groups (6.8 vs. 12.4 EU for study 1; 6.9 vs. 11.9 EU for study 2). Among study 2 subjects, poliovirus responses were virtually identical for the combined and separate vaccines; responses to the DTaP components were slightly lower in the combined group. Rates and severity of varicella infection did not significantly differ by group during 1 year of follow-up.

A recent study randomized 294 children aged 12 to 18 months to receive MMRV + Hib (PRP-OMP) or MMR + Hib, with varicella vaccine given 6 weeks later.[128] Although seroconversion rates did not differ significantly by group mean postimmunization antibody levels differed significantly for measles (combined, 126.5 EU; separate, 90.9 EU) and varicella (combined, 8.3 EU; separate, 11.7 EU). One year after vaccination, however, mean antibody levels no longer differed.

Summary of MMR Combined with Varicella Vaccine. Based on the foregoing results, it would appear that the more recent formulations of MMRV stimulate uniformly high rates of seroconversion, with no material reduction in postimmunization antibody titers (compared with separate vaccines) except for the varicella component. Some of the studies have evaluated antibody levels 1 year after immunization and have found that varicella antibody levels converge for the combined and separate vaccine groups. The lower peak antibody levels may therefore have little import for duration of protection. Adverse reactions in all the studies were typical of prior experience with the vaccines, except that morbilliform rash tended to be more common among MMRV recipients; the rate of varicelliform rashes generally did not differ.

COMBINATIONS BASED ON ACELLULAR PERTUSSIS OR HEPATITIS B

Combinations Based on DTaP

The development of numerous effective acellular pertussis vaccines (see Chapter 14) and their licensure in combination with diphtheria and tetanus toxoids (DTaP) represented an important advance that quickly stimulated efforts to combine DTaP with other routine vaccines of infancy, such as Hib, IPV, and HB. Efforts turned first to evaluating combinations of DTaP and conjugate Hib vaccines, probably because of their similar schedule, universal use in developed countries, and lack of orally administered alternatives. (Because the compositions of the acellular pertussis vaccines are complex and differ markedly from one product to another, and because simple, unambiguous generic names do not exist for the various products, DTaP products are here referred to by trade names, if available.)

Studies of DTaP/Hib Combinations. A combination consisting of a Biken-type DTaP plus PRP-D (PRP-diphtheria toxoid conjugate vaccine; see Chapter 11) was used as a booster dose in toddlers primed with DTP. Pertussis antibody responses were comparable after combined or separate vaccines. PRP antibody responses were low, as expected with PRP-D, but were materially lower in the combined vaccine group.[129] However, when used to immunize infants at 2, 3, and 4 months of age, the combined vaccine produced somewhat better PRP responses than did PRP-D given separately.[130]

A combination consisting of Acel-Imune/PRP-HbOC was evaluated first as a booster for toddlers primed with HbOC plus DTP or DTaP and then as a three-dose primary series.[131–134] Adverse reactions were mild[131, 134] although somewhat more common after boosting with the combined product.[132] Antibody responses after booster immunization at 12 to 21 months of age did not differ significantly between the combined and separate vaccines (Table 20–8).[132–133] In contrast, there was a markedly reduced antibody response to PRP after primary immunization with the combined product.[134] Similar results became available for other DTaP/Hib combinations, raising concerns that combining Hib with DTaP might prove even more problematic than combining with DTP.

TriHIBit, the combination of Tripedia and PRP-T (ActHIB), is licensed in the United States for use as a

Table 20–8. **STUDIES EVALUATING COMBINED OR SIMULTANEOUS ADMINISTRATION OF DTaP AND Hib VACCINES**

LOCATION	AGE AT VACCINATION (mo)	VACCINES†	PRP ANTIBODY LEVELS (μg/mL)		RATIO OF ANTIBODY LEVELS WITH COMBINED VACCINE TO LEVELS WITH SEPARATE VACCINES*						
			% >1.0	GMC	PRP	D	T	PT	FHA	PRN	FIM
United States[129]	18	DTaP2/PRP-D, DTaP2 + PRP-D	53, 76								
Germany[130]	2, 3, 4	DTaP2/PRP-D, DTaP2 + PRP-D		0.58, 0.44	1.34						
United States[132]	15–21	DTaP4/HbOC, DTaP4 + HbOC		26.9, 32.4	0.83						
United States[133]	12–15	DTaP4/HbOC, DTaP4 + HbOC						0.55‡	0.93	0.96	1.00
United States[133]	15–18	DTaP4/HbOC, DTaP4 + HbOC						0.79	1.32	1.04	1.00
United States[134]	2, 4, 6	DTaP4/HbOC, DTaP4 +HbOC	55, 94‡	1.15, 16.4	0.07‡						
United States[135]	15–20	DTaP2/PRP-T_1, DTaP2 + PRP-T_1	100, 100								
United States[136]	2, 4, 6	DTaP2/PRP-T_1, DTaP2 + PRP-T_1	85, 100‡	4.29, 7.0	0.61‡	1.67‡	0.79‡	1.00	1.29‡		
Germany[137]	2, 3, 4	DTaP2/PRP-T_1, DTaP2 + PRP-T_1	91, 99	2.83, 4.3	0.66‡						
England[138]	2, 3, 4	DTaP2/PRP-T_1	27	0.48							
Belgium[139]	3, 4, 5	DTaP2/PRP-T_1, DTaP2 + PRP-T_1		1.78, 6.19	0.29‡						
Turkey[139]	3, 4, 5	DTaP2/PRP-T_1, DTaP2 + PRP-T_1		5.02, 11.7	0.43‡						
Germany[146, 147]	3, 4, 5	DTaP3/PRP-T_2, DTaP3 + PRP-T_2	72, 88	2.02, 7.20	0.28‡	0.92	0.85‡	0.89‡	0.77‡	0.81‡	
Germany[146, 147]	3, 4, 5	DTaP3/PRP-T_1, DTaP3 + PRP-T_1	N/A, 88	2.75, 5.44	0.51‡						
Taiwan[149]	2, 4, 6	DTaP5/PRP-T_1, DTaP5 + PRP-T_1	95, 99	11.8, 13.0	0.91			1.25	1.00	1.31	1.30

*A ratio less than 1 indicates that mean antibody levels were lower with the combined vaccine than with separate injections; a ratio higher than 1 indicates that levels were higher with combined than with separate injections. A blank cell indicates that the comparison was not possible or is not available.

†aP2 = Tripedia, Triavac, or similar Biken-type aP vaccine; aP3 = Infanrix or similar 3-component aP vaccine; aP4 = Acel-Imune or similar Takeda-type aP vaccine; aP5 = Tripacel or similar 5-component aP vaccine (see Chapter 14 for details of vaccines). PRP-T_1 = ActHib (Pasteur Mérieux Connaught); PRP-T_2 = Hiberix (SmithKline Beecham).

‡Difference significant at $P \leq .05$.

DTaP, diphtheria and tetanus toxoids and acellular pertussis vaccine; FIM, fimbrae; GMC, geometric mean concentration; HbOC, PRP-diphtheria CRM197 protein conjugate vaccine; Hib, *Haemophilus influenzae* type b; N/A, not available; PRN, pertactin; PRP-D, PRP-diphtheria toxoid conjugate vaccine. See also abbreviations in Table 20–4.

booster in children 15 to 18 months of age, in whom it produces PRP antibody levels comparable to those seen with the separate vaccines.[135] When used for primary immunization of infants, TriHIBit produced responses to the DTaP components that equaled or exceeded those of Tripedia; mean PRP antibody levels were high (4.3 μg/mL) with the combined vaccine but were significantly higher (7.0 μg/mL) with the separate vaccines (see Table 20–8).[136, 137]

Another two-component acellular pertussis vaccine (Triavac, PMC) has been evaluated in combination with ActHIB in British,[138] Belgian,[139] and Turkish[139] infants. The British infants developed low levels of antibody to PRP (mean, 0.48 μg/mL) after primary immunization at 2, 3, and 4 months of age,[138] but they developed high levels (mean, 36.8 μg/mL) after a booster dose of PRP-T at 13 months of age.[140] Although the Belgian and Turkish infants, immunized at 3, 4, and 5 months of age, had markedly better mean PRP antibody levels than the British infants after primary immunization with combined vaccine, their responses were substantially higher with separate vaccines (see Table 20–8).[139]

The first published study of a combination vaccine incorporating SB's DTaP (Infanrix) and PRP-T (Hiberix) reported markedly lower antibody responses to PRP among Finnish infants receiving the combination, compared with separate injection of the Hib component (Table 20–9); responses to the DTaP components did not significantly differ by group.[141] The study used the Finnish vaccination schedule, however, in which infants received PRP-T only at ages 4 and 6 months and not at 2 months, even though studies in other populations have suggested that a three-dose series of PRP-T is required to develop optimal antibody levels early in life.[142–144] In a follow-up study, available participants were given a booster with DTaP and PRP-T at 24 months of age. Vaccines were given separately to those who had been primed with separate vaccines; those who had been primed with combination vaccines were randomized to be given a booster with separate or combined vaccines.[145] Despite the large difference in PRP antibody levels at 7 months of age, there was little difference in levels at 24 months of age. After receiving a booster dose, all groups showed strong responses, which were about twice as high among those primed with separate vaccines. The groups primed with combined vaccine had roughly equal

Table 20–9. **ANTIBODY TO PRP AMONG 120 INFANTS GIVEN DTaP AT 2 MO; THEN DTaP, IPV, AND CONJUGATE Hib VACCINE, SEPARATELY OR TOGETHER, AT 4 AND 6 MO; AND THEN DTaP AND PRP-T, SEPARATELY OR TOGETHER, AT 24 MO**

	PRIMARY SERIES		BOOSTER IMMUNIZATION AT 24 MONTHS				
	GMC (μ/mL)		Vaccines Given*		GMC (μg/mL)		
Vaccines Given at 4 and 6 Months	6 Months (No.)†	7 Months (No.)†	4 and 6 Months	24 Months	7 Months (No.)†	24 Months (No.)†	25 Months (No.)*
DTaP3, IPV, and PRP-T_2, all separate[141, 145]	0.19 (30)	3.94 (30)	Separate	Separate	3.49 (60)	0.35 (39)	54.46 (38)
DTaP3 and IPV mixed; PRP-T_2 separate	0.18 (28)	3.10 (30)	Mixed	Separate	0.38 (26)	0.24 (18)	27.99 (17)
DTaP3 and PRP-T_2 mixed; IPV separate	0.10 (29)	0.38 (30)	Mixed	Mixed	0.56 (29)	0.36 (16)	20.76 (17)
DTaP3, IPV, and PRP-T_2 all mixed	0.09 (27)	0.56 (30)					

*Vaccines were given separately to those who were primed with separate vaccines; those who were primed with combination vaccines were randomized to be given a booster dose with separate or combined vaccines.

†Number of subjects providing serum samples for assay.

DTaP3, diphtheria and tetanus toxoids and acellular pertussis vaccine (Infanrix, SmithKline Beecham); GMC, geometric mean concentration; Hib, *Haemophilus influenzae* type b; IPV, inactivated polio vaccine; PRP-T_2, polyribosylribitol phosphate–tetanus toxoid protein conjugate vaccine (SmithKline Beecham).

Data from Eskola J, Olander RM, Hovi T, et al. Randomised trial of the effect of co-administration with acellular pertussis DTP vaccine on immunogenicity of *Haemophilus influenzae* type b conjugate vaccine. Lancet 348:1688–1692, 1996; and Eskola J, Litmanen L, Saarinen L, Kayhty H. Responses at 24 months to a combined DTaP-Hib conjugate vaccine in children vaccinated with the same vaccines at 4 and 6 months. Abstracts of the 36th Interscience Conference on Antimicrobial Agents and Chemotherapy [abstract G060]. Washington, DC, American Society for Microbiology, 1996.

responses to the booster dose, whether they were given combined or separate vaccines as booster doses (see Table 20–9).

When administered to German infants in a conventional three-dose series, the same DTaP/PRP-T combination produced substantially higher PRP antibody levels and seroconversion rates than those seen in the Finnish study. Again, levels were higher with separate than combined vaccine.[146, 147] ActHIB, PMC's PRP-T vaccine, was evaluated in the same study, alone or combined with Infanrix. It produced PRP antibody responses similar to those obtained with Hiberix (see Table 20–9). Both the combined and separate vaccines produced high levels of antibody to the DTaP components; all antibody levels were slightly lower with the combined vaccine.[146, 147] Available subjects were given a booster at 18 to 19 months of age with Hiberix, ActHIB, or either Hib vaccine mixed with Infanrix. PRP antibody levels after the booster dose were high: 24 to 40 μg per mL for those boosted with Hiberix/Infanrix or ActHIB/Infanrix and 85 to 137 μg per mL for those primed and boosted with the separately administered Hib vaccine.[147] Assessment of T-lymphocyte proliferative responses and cytokine production before and after the booster dose found no difference between combined and separate vaccines.[148]

A five-component acellular pertussis vaccine licensed in Canada and elsewhere as Tripacel (PMC) has been evaluated in combination with ActHIB in Canada and in Taiwan.[149, 149a] Antibody responses to the pertussis and Hib components were excellent and did not differ between combined and separate administration (see Table 20–8).

Summary of DTaP/Hib Combinations. Numerous studies have evaluated a variety of DTaP/Hib combinations and have produced remarkably consistent results. All combinations are highly immunogenic when used to boost previously primed children. When used for primary immunization, these vaccines have in general stimulated similar antibody responses to their DTaP components, whether given separately or in combination with Hib. The combination vaccines (other than those containing the relatively poor immunogen PRP-D) have stimulated good Hib responses, but these responses have in general been substantially lower than the high responses obtained with present formulations of PRP-T or HbOC when given separately.[142–144] Several of these DTaP/Hib combinations are licensed in countries other than the United States for primary immunization of infants (e.g., Tripacel/ActHIB, with or without IPV, in Canada; Infanrix + Hiberix in Germany). As of mid-1998, the FDA had not approved any combination DTaP/Hib vaccines for infant immunization in the United States (TriHIBit is approved for use as the fourth dose). Published reports of recent FDA meetings indicate that the FDA remains concerned about the lower PRP antibody levels after combination compared with separate injections. As shown in Tables 20–7 and 20–8, however, the combination vaccines licensed elsewhere have stimulated PRP responses that equal or exceed those reported for some U.S.-licensed monocomponent Hib vaccines.[142–144] Thus, it is hoped that these combinations will soon become available in the United States as well.

Studies of DTaP/IPV Combinations, with or Without Hib. Reports are available concerning DTaP/IPV or DTaP/IPV/Hib combinations from three manufacturers: North American Vaccine (NAVA), SB, and PMC. NAVA's Certiva (a monocomponent acellular pertussis vaccine + DT; see Chapter 14) has been combined with an IPV from the Statens Seruminstitut in Denmark.[150, 151] Workers from NAVA and Statens Seruminstitut reported that (1) the combination achieved protective antibody levels for diphtheria, tetanus, and the polio serotypes; (2) strong cell-mediated immunity was demonstrated for the pertussis component; and (3) 98% of children retained protective levels of antibody to PRP 1 year later.[152] (Unfortunately, none of these abstracts contained sufficient details of the immunogenicity studies to permit inclusion in our tables.)

Combined or separate administration of SB's DTaP/IPV and PMC's PRP-T was evaluated among children aged 15 to 24 months; combining the PRP-T with the DTaP/IPV did not materially alter antibody responses (Table 20–10).[153] Finnish infants given IPV separately or combined with DTaP/PRP-T at 4 and 6 months of age in general had comparable antibody responses.[141] Combined administration resulted in significantly lower antibody to poliovirus type 1 and significantly higher proportions of children achieving PRP antibody levels greater than 1.0 μg per mL. Dagan and colleagues compared DTaP/IPV/PRP-T (SB) with DTP/IPV/PRP-T (Pentacoq, PMC) given at 2, 4, 6, and 12 months of age and found strong antibody responses to all components after both the primary series and the booster dose.[154, 155] Polio antibody levels after primary immunization and PRP antibody levels after the booster dose were significantly higher with the DTaP than the DTP combination. Another study (not yet published) comparing SB's DTaP/IPV and PRP-T, given combined or separately at 2, 3, and 4 months of age, found good responses to all components in both groups.[156] Antibody levels tended to be higher with the combined vaccine than with separate administration for tetanus toxoid, filamentous hemagglutinin, and poliovirus type 3, but they were higher with separate administration for the other components.

A number of studies have evaluated DTaP/IPV or DTaP/IPV/PRP-T vaccines produced by PMC using their French two-component acellular pertussis vaccine (see Chapter 14). French infants immunized at 3, 4, and 5 months of age had better responses to DTaP/IPV than to DTP/IPV (Table 20–10).[157] Lagos and colleagues compared DTaP/IPV, DTaP + IPV, and DTaP + OPV given at 2, 4, and 6 months of age, all groups receiving PRP-T at 3, 5, and 7 months of age, with DTaP/IPV/PRP-T and DTaP/IPV + PRP-T given at 2, 4, and 6 months of age.[158, 159] All groups had poliovirus seroconversion rates of 99% or 100%, with higher antibody levels among the groups receiving IPV in combination than in the groups receiving separate IPV or OPV. Responses to pertussis toxin, filamentous hemagglutinin, and PRP were good in all groups but were superior in those receiving separate injections (see Table 20–10). Whether PRP-T was given combined or separately, PRP antibody levels were markedly higher in study subjects receiving PRP-T at 3, 5, and 7 months of age than in those receiving all antigens at 2, 4, and 6 months of age, despite the fact that levels were determined at 7 months of age (and thus did not reflect the effect of the third injection in the former groups). It is not known whether this effect is caused by age or immunological interference, although the latter seems more likely. When a booster dose of DTaP/PRP-T was given at 12 months, all groups had strong PRP antibody responses (mean levels, 48.6–95.2 μg/mL), but there were significantly higher levels for the groups primed at 3, 5, and 7 months of age.[158, 159]

Other studies also suggest that earlier immunization might worsen the problem of reduced antibody responses to PRP when given in combination with DTaP. In a French study in which PRP-T was administered at 2, 3, and 4 months of age, combined with or separately from DTaP/IPV, PRP antibody levels were 1.95 μg per mL with the combined vaccine and 5.18 μg per mL with separate vaccines (see Table 20–10).[160, 161] Another French study compared administration of DTaP/IPV/PRP-T at ages 2, 3, and 4 months or 2, 4, and 6 months and found higher mean antibody levels for all antigens in the group immunized later.[161–163] Responses to PRP differed significantly for the proportion exceeding 1 μg per mL (70% vs. 89%) and for mean antibody levels (1.7 vs. 4.7 μg/mL).[161] However, when given a booster at 15 months of age, both groups responded equally strongly to all antigens (PRP antibody levels were 36.8 and 31.8 μg/mL for 2-3-4 and 2-4-6, respectively).[161, 163] Similar results have been obtained among Swedish children immunized at ages 3, 5, and 12 months or 2, 4, 6, and 13 months. Not surprisingly, antibody levels were higher after primary immunization with the 2-4-6 schedule, although there was no significant difference in the proportion that achieved defined protective levels or had fourfold rises.[164] Following booster immunization at 12 or 13 months of age, antibody levels were virtually identical in the two groups.

DTaP/IPV and DTaP/IPV/PRP-T combination vaccines based on the five-component acellular pertussis vaccine used in Canada and elsewhere have been evaluated in several studies. A comparison of two different IPVs, given separately or combined with DTaP, showed that the combined vaccines generally produced higher poliovirus and pertussis antibody levels than did vaccination with DTaP plus separate IPV or OPV (see Table 20–10).[165] A comparative trial examined vaccination at 2, 4, 6, and 18 months of age with (1) DTaP/IPV used to reconstitute lyophilized PRP-T, (2) a fully liquid DTaP/IPV/PRP-T, or (3) DTaP/IPV and PRP-T given separately.[166–167a] All three groups responded well after primary and booster immunization. The liquid and lyophilized combinations performed similarly.[166] Antibody responses with the liquid combination did not differ significantly from those of the separate vaccines for any antigen (see Table 20–10).[166–167a]

Summary of DTaP/IPV Combinations, with or Without Hib. Taken together, these studies indicate that combining IPV with DTaP has no consistent effect on antibody responses to those components. Including PRP-T in the combination does not alter that conclusion. On the other hand, studies comparing PRP-T given separately or combined with DTaP/IPV provide further support for the observation that, when used for primary immunization, most DTaP/Hib combinations (whether incorporating IPV or not) stimulate lower PRP antibody responses than does PRP-T given separately. Nonetheless, the conjugate Hib vaccines are so immunogenic that primary immunization with such combinations typically induces PRP antibody levels greater than 1.0 μg per mL in 90% of recipients. The deserved relative reduction in antibody responses may therefore have no material effect on protection of the individual or community.

DTaP/HB Combinations. SB has obtained licensure in Europe of a DTaP/HB combination vaccine. Table 20–11 summarizes studies comparing the performance of this vaccine with the separately administered components and also comparing various administration schedules.[168–172] The combination vaccine retains the immuno-

Table 20–10. **STUDIES EVALUATING COMBINED OR SIMULTANEOUS ADMINISTRATION OF DTaP (OR DTaP/PRP) AND IPV VACCINES**

LOCATION	AGE AT VACCINATION (mo)	VACCINES*	PRP ANTIBODY LEVELS (μg/mL)		RATIO OF ANTIBODY LEVELS WITH COMBINED VACCINE TO LEVELS WITH SEPARATE VACCINES†									
						Poliovirus Serotypes								
			% >1.0	GMC	PRP	*1*	*2*	*3*	D	T	PT	FHA	PRN	FIM
France[153]	15–24	DTaP3/IPV/PRP-T_2, DTaP3/IPV + PRP-T_2	100, 97	60.4, 60.0	1.01	0.89	0.74	1.05	1.19	0.84	1.15	1.11	1.03	
Finland[141]	(2),‡ 4, 6	DTaP3/PRP-T_2/IPV, DTaP3/PRP-T_2 + IPV	48, 19§	0.56, 0.38	1.47	0.34§	0.49	0.61	1.09	1.44	1.02	1.09	1.13	
Israel[154, 155]	2, 4, 6	DTaP3/IPV/PRP-T_1, DTP/IPV/PRP-T_1	89, 96	5.06, 6.66	0.76	2.92§	2.49§	2.44§	1.05	0.70§				
Israel[155]	12	DTaP3/IPV/PRP-T_1, DTP/IPV/PRP-T_1	100, 99	23.1, 13.6	1.70§									
France[157]	3, 4, 5	DTaP2/IPV, DTP/IPV				1.79§	1.24	1.43	2.47§	1.14§				
Chile[158, 159]	3, 5, 7‖	DTaP2/IPV + PRP-T_1, DTaP2 + IPV + PRP-T_1	98, 95	19.0, 21.7	0.88	1.6§	0.5§	0.4§			0.72	0.74§		
Chile[158, 159]	2, 4, 6	DTaP2/IPV + PRP-T_1, DTaP2 + IPV + PRP-T_1	97, 96	7.46, 14.1	0.53§	1.1	1.2	1.0			0.89	0.87		
France[160, 161]	2, 3, 4	DTaP2/IPV/PRP-T_1, DTaP2/IPV + PRP-T_1	71, 88§	1.9, 5.2	0.36§	0.73	0.76	0.58	1.03	0.81	0.98	0.84		
Canada[165]	17–19	DTaP5/IPV, DTaP5 + IPV (MRC-5)¶				1.17	1.61§	0.80	1.28	0.98	1.23	0.96	2.05§	1.61
Canada[165]	17–19	DTaP5/IPV, DTaP5 + IPV (Vero)**				1.17	1.30	0.74	0.90	1.01	1.08	0.96	1.41§	1.14
Canada[166, 167]	2, 4, 6	DTaP5/IPV/PRP-T_1, DTaP5/IPV + PRP-T_1††	85, 89	5.04, 3.83	1.32	0.90	0.85	1.17	0.67§	0.61§	1.20	1.06	1.16	0.83
Canada[166, 167]	2, 4, 6	DTaP5/IPV/PRP-T_1, DTaP5/IPV + PRP-T_1‡‡	89, 89	4.86, 3.83	1.27	0.88	0.92	0.69	0.81	0.68	0.84	0.94	1.37	0.83
Canada[166, 167]	17–19	DTaP5/IPV/PRP-T_1, DTaP5/IPV + PRP-T_1‡‡	99, 100	32.5, 26.9	1.21									

*aP2 = Tripedia, Triavac, or similar Biken-type aP vaccine; aP3 = Infanrix or similar 3-component aP vaccine; aP4 = Acel-Imune or similar Takeda-type aP vaccine; aP5 = Tripacel or similar 5-component aP vaccine (see Chapter 14 for details of vaccines). PRP-T_1 = ActHIB (Pasteur Mérieux Connaught); PRP-T_2 = Hiberix (SmithKline Beecham).

†A ratio less than 1 indicates that mean antibody levels were lower with the combined vaccine than with separate injections; a ratio higher than 1 indicates that levels were higher with combined than with separate injections. A blank cell indicates that the comparison was not possible or is not available.

‡Only DTaP given at 2 months, without IPV or PRP-T.

§Difference significant at $P \leq .05$.

‖DTaP and IPV were given at 2, 4, and 6 months of age; PRP-T was given at 3, 5, and 7 months of age. Polio antibody levels estimated from figures.

¶IPV produced on MRC-5 cells by Connaught Laboratories Ltd. (North York, Canada) division of Pasteur Mérieux Connaught.

**IPV produced on Vero cells by Pasteur Mérieux Serums et Vaccines (Lyon, France) division of Pasteur Mérieux Connaught.

††DTaP5/IPV used to reconstitute lyophilized PRP-T.

‡‡DTaP5/IPV/PRP-T combined, fully liquid, in vial.

DTaP, diphtheria and tetanus toxoids and acellular pertussis vaccine; FIM, fimbrae; GMC, geometric mean concentration; IPV, inactivated poliovirus vaccine; PRN, pertactin. See also abbreviations in Table 20–4.

Table 20–11. **STUDIES EVALUATING COMBINED OR SIMULTANEOUS ADMINISTRATION OF DTaP AND HB VACCINES**

LOCATION	AGE AT VACCINATION (mo)	VACCINES†	COMMENT	MEAN ANTIBODY LEVELS 1 MONTH AFTER LAST INJECTION*					
				HB (mIU/mL)	D (IU)	T (IU)	PT (EU)	FHA (EU)	PRN (EU)
Turkey[168]	3, 4, 5	DTaP/HB	Group 1	343	2.05	4.35	56	89	129
	3, 4, 5	DTaP + HB	Group 2	275	1.88	4.38	52	114	159
	3, 4, 5	DTaP	Group 3	6	1.59	4.03	47	89	125
Lithuania[169]	3, 4½, 6	DTaP/HB	Mixed in vial	667	1.40	2.21	47.9	184	170
	3, 4½, 6	DTaP/HB	Mixed at time of injection	518	1.06	2.00	46.7	131	124
	3, 4½, 6	DTaP + HB	Separate administration	438	1.10	1.76	46.7	158	148
Italy[170]	2, 4, 6	DTaP/HB	Group 1	949			56.1	153	240
	3, 5	DTaP/HB	Group 2, after first 2 injections	572			31.8	86	113
	3, 5, 11	DTaP/HB	Group 2, after third injection	5554			65.3	232	372
United States[171]	2, 4, 6	DTaP/HB	Combined vaccine	1280	1.93	3.82	72.3	459	195
	2, 4, 6	DTaP + HB	HB given at birth, 1, and 6 mo	4620‡	1.00	2.11	52.2	334	138
Not stated[172]	2, 4, 6	DTaP/HB		929	1.96	3.08	66.5	285	233
	2, 4, 6	DTaP			1.88	2.22	60.0	220	170
	2, 4, 6	HB		1895					

*A blank cell indicates that data are not available.
†All vaccines produced by SmithKline Beecham.
‡Difference significant at $P \leq .05$.
DTaP, diphtheria and tetanus toxoids and acellular pertussis vaccine; EU, ELISA (enzyme-linked immunosorbent assay) units; FHA, filamentous hemagglutinin; HB, hepatitis B; PRN, pertactin. See also abbreviations in Table 20–4.

genicity and safety profiles of the separate components and delivers good antibody concentrations at a variety of schedules. A comparison of combined vaccine at ages 2, 4, and 6 months versus a currently recommended schedule in the United States—HB at birth and 1 and 6 months of age and DTaP at 2, 4, and 6 months of age—found significantly higher antibody responses for combined vaccine for every component except HB, which was significantly lower.[171] However, the mean HB antibody with combined vaccine was nonetheless high (1280 mIU/mL), and 98% of subjects had levels greater than 10 mIU per mL, the level considered protective.

DTaP/HB/PRP-T Combinations. A number of studies have been published evaluating SB's DTaP/HB/PRP-T combination vaccine. Not surprisingly, these vaccines tend to produce lower PRP antibody levels than are obtained with separate administration of PRP-T, as seen with the DTaP/Hib and DTaP/IPV/Hib combinations previously described. For example, among children randomized at 2, 4, and 6 months of age to receive (1) DTaP/HB/PRP-T, (2) DTaP/HB + PRP-T, or (3) DTaP + HB + PRP-T, mean PRP antibody levels at 7 months of age were 1.5, 6.9, and 6.4 μg per mL, respectively; proportions achieving 1 μg per mL were 68, 91, and 90%, respectively.[173, 174] No interference was seen in the antibody responses to the other components. Children whose 7-month PRP antibody levels were below 1.0 μg per mL were administered a booster dose at 11 to 15 months of age, resulting in mean PRP antibody levels of 5.1 μg per mL for the combined group and 3.0 μg per mL for the other two groups.[174] A different study also found comparable responses with combined and separate administration for all antigens except PRP-T. PRP antibody levels were 1.2 and 5.5 μg per mL, and proportions achieving 1 μg per mL were 58 and 88% for the combined and separate groups, respectively.[175] Children with low responses to primary immunization again had excellent responses when given booster doses. The same PRP results were found in a German study in which infants were immunized at 3, 4, and 5 months of age; mean PRP antibody levels were 1.2 and 5.5 μg per mL, respectively, for DTaP/HB/PRP-T and DTaP/HB + PRP-T.[176] Zepp and colleagues gave unconjugated PRP to children at 12 months of age who had been immunized at 3, 4, and 5 months of age with DTaP/HB/PRP-T. The children developed good antibody responses to PRP promptly after the booster immunization, demonstrating that the combination vaccine had successfully primed the immune system.[176a]

DTaP/Hib/IPV/HB Combinations. Only preliminary results are available from studies of vaccines that combine DTaP, Hib, IPV, and HB. As might be expected from the preceding data, good antibody responses are seen for all components, although PRP responses are substantially lower with the combination vaccine than with separate administration.[177, 178]

Combinations Based on Hepatitis B Vaccine, Without DTaP

HB/Hib Combinations. Comvax (Merck & Co) is a licensed combination of HB vaccine (5 μg) and PRP-OMP conjugate Hib vaccine (7.5 μg). A study comparing Comvax and its constituent components given at 2, 4, and 12 to 15 months of age found no material difference in antibody responses.[179] Mean PRP antibody levels for the combined and separate products (2.5 and 2.8 μg/mL, respectively) and proportions exceeding 1.0 μg per mL at 6 months of age (72 and 76%, respectively) were in the usual range for PedvaxHIB. When infants were given a booster dose at 12 to 15 months of age, these values rose to 9.5 and 10.2 μg per mL and 92 and 93%, respectively. Responses to the HB component were also as expected, with 92 and 98% of subjects in the respective groups achieving protective levels of antibody (≥10 mIU/mL) at 6 months of age, and with 98 and 100%, respectively, achieving these levels after boosting.

HB/Hepatitis A Combinations. Vaccines combining hepatitis A and HB antigens are under development by several manufacturers, although there are few published reports. One study of adults evaluated administration at 0, 1, and 6 months of combined Havrix (720 EU) and Engerix (20 μg; both from SB) versus the same vaccines given separately or mixed at the time of injection.[180] Antibody responses were excellent, with 100% of combined-vaccine recipients achieving protective levels of both antibodies before the 6-month injection. Another study in adults has found similar responses to a combined HB/hepatitis A vaccine.[181]

OTHER COMBINATIONS

Although we have discussed certain obsolete combination vaccines of historical relevance, such as those containing vaccinia virus, there are many others that we have not mentioned. Some of these, such as the combined tetanus/rabies vaccine,[182] performed well in trials or even in field use but were abandoned as newer products or approaches arrived. The future of others is uncertain, one example of which is the combination of yellow fever and Vi polysaccharide typhoid fever vaccine that was found to be well tolerated and to induce higher yellow fever antibody levels than those seen with separate injection.[183]

Wyeth Lederle is conducting clinical trials of pneumococcal conjugate/meningococcal conjugate and pneumococcal conjugate/meningococcal conjugate/Hib combinations. There are also a host of other new combination vaccines, many of which are (or likely will be) of great importance. These vaccines are well described in other chapters. Among these combination vaccines are trivalent influenza vaccines, including those of novel modes of delivery (Chapters 21 and 37); polyvalent pneumococcal vaccine (Chapter 22) and meningococcal vaccine (Chapter 28), especially the conjugate products presently under development; and polyvalent rotavirus vaccine (Chapter 41). Other targets for combination vaccines include tick-borne infections, arboviruses, and additional diarrheal agents.

PRACTICAL ISSUES IN THE USE OF COMBINATION VACCINES

Interchangeability

When multiple combination vaccines are available from several different manufacturers, practitioners will question whether the vaccines can be used interchangeably. This question can be difficult to answer even for monocomponent vaccines, and there is little hope of definitive answers for multicomponent vaccines. For example, we performed a study to evaluate the interchangeability of the three conjugate Hib vaccines indicated for the infant primary series.[184] Of the 27 theoretically possible permutations of 3 vaccines and 3 injections, we evaluated 5. One alternative we did not evaluate has become pertinent: PRP-OMP has been selected as the predominant Hib vaccine provided through the Vaccines for Children program in 1998, making it more likely that some children will receive PRP-OMP only for their third dose. Despite the lack of data regarding the immunogenicity of this specific regimen, we have little doubt of its acceptability; however, this circumstance does illustrate the limitations of our abilities to rigorously investigate such questions of interchangeability. Once we are faced with multiple, distinct DTaP, DTaP/Hib, DTaP/Hib/IPV (and so on) vaccines, the likelihood shrinks that any particular substitution will have been explicitly studied.

In this day of bulk vaccine purchase through competitive bidding by large health maintenance organizations and the government, it is unrealistic to presume that the same vaccine will always be available for each child at the time of each vaccination. The situation is further complicated by the fact that 25% of children see at least two different healthcare providers for their vaccination series and that the average time for a child to remain in a publicly funded healthcare plan is 10 months. Different practitioners are likely to stock different combination vaccines.

The Advisory Committee on Immunization Practices has recognized certain vaccines as interchangeable: DTP (and its individual components), IPV, OPV, Hib (as long as three doses are given), and HB.[2] For those vaccines for which there are no data on the interchangeability of licensed products from various manufacturers (e.g., DTaP[185] and the newer combination vaccines[186]), the Advisory Committee on Immunization Practices has recommended that the same product be used throughout the primary series. However, if the identity of the product previously used is not known or if the product is not available at the time of the child's visit, then any licensed product appropriate to the child's immunization status and requirements may be used.

Ad Hoc Combinations

Providers should not create their own ad hoc combinations by mixing separate vaccines in the same syringe unless there is published evidence establishing the stability, safety, and immunogenicity of the resultant combination. (If there were such evidence, one would expect it to be reflected in the package inserts.)

Administration of Superfluous Antigens

As a variety of vaccines become available that combine different antigens, physicians will increasingly find that the most simple (and even, perhaps, the least expensive) alternative will be use of a vaccine that will deliver an antigen that the patient does not need, having already received that antigen in the recommended quantity and timing. Some antigens are known to be associated with increased adverse effects when administered too frequently (e.g., tetanus toxoid), but these are few. Fortunately, it has been shown for many vaccine antigens that an extra dose may be given without adverse consequence. In particular, the low reactogenicity of Hib, IPV, and HB vaccines makes it unlikely that an extra dose of any of these antigens would cause a problem.

PUBLIC HEALTH CONSIDERATIONS

Cost Issues

Many of the newer vaccines, such as DTaP and conjugate Hib, are expensive to produce as compared with DTP, OPV, and other traditional combination vaccines. Certainly, cost considerations will constrain the use of some of these vaccines in parts of the world. DTP, for example, is produced locally at low cost in many countries, and its replacement with DTaP would not be a sensible use of healthcare resources. On the other hand, some other relatively expensive vaccines, such as HB or Hib, offer such clear benefits that they are being used in many developing countries. Once a country has committed to using conjugate Hib vaccine, for example, it is likely to find that a combination that also provides other relatively inexpensive antigens (e.g., DTP/IPV/Hib) can be purchased for less than the cost of separately purchasing the component vaccines. The use of such a combination vaccine should offer additional savings in program costs by reducing the number of vaccines that must be stored, shipped, tracked, and injected.

Tracking of Vaccinations

The increasing variety of alternative vaccines, including those with multiple valences, that might be used to satisfy childhood vaccination requirements renders it unlikely that a practitioner will be able to deduce the precise vaccination history of a new patient. Although legislation has mandated since March 1988 that medical records of vaccination should contain the identity of the vaccine manufacturer, the date of administration, and the lot number of the vaccine given, the completeness and accuracy of these data still remain a problem. The optimal solution would be a national vaccination history database, which would not only provide practitioners with individual vaccination histories and health planners with a comprehensive measure of the vaccination status of the community but also greatly facilitate postmarketing surveillance of vaccine efficacy and safety.

Pending the availability of such a database, postmarketing surveillance can be facilitated by the use of large linked databases of pharmacies, healthcare providers, and hospitals that are maintained by some commercial healthcare organizations. The integrated data information systems maintained by some state governments for their Medicaid programs can also be used.

Methods are also needed to improve the accuracy and convenience of recording and transferring vaccine information from the vaccine vial to the medical record. One attractive alternative would be to include machine-readable bar codes or stickers with vaccines to facilitate the electronic transfer of information.

REFERENCES

1. Williams JC, Goldenthal KL, Burns DL, Lewis BP Jr (eds). Combined vaccines and simultaneous administration: Current issues and perspectives. Ann N Y Acad Sci 754:xi–404, 1995.
2. General recommendations on immunization. Recommendations of the Advisory Committee on Immunization Practices (ACIP). MMWR Morb Mortal Wkly Rep 43(RR-1):1–38, 1994.
3. Grabenstein JD. Immunofacts: Vaccines and Immunologic Drugs. St Louis: Facts and Comparisons, 1995.
4. Children's vaccine initiative [news]. World Health Forum 13:93, 1992.
5. Mitchell VS, Philipose NM, Sanford JS. The Children's Vaccine Initiative: Achieving the Vision. Washington, DC, National Academy Press, 1993.
6. Edwards KM, Decker MD. Combination vaccines: Hopes and challenges. Pediatr Infect Dis J 13:345–347, 1994.
7. Decker MD, Edwards KM. Issues in design of clinical trials of combination vaccines. In Williams JC, Goldenthal KL, Burns DL, Lewis BP Jr (eds). Combined Vaccines and Simultaneous Administration: Current Issues and Perspectives. Ann N Y Acad Sci 754:234–240, 1995.
8. Edwards KM, Decker MD. Combination vaccines consisting of acellular pertussis vaccines. Pediatr Infect Dis J 16(suppl 4):S97–S102, 1997.
9. Edwards KM, Meade BD, Decker MD, et al. Comparison of 13 acellular pertussis vaccines: Overview and serologic response. Pediatrics 96:548–557, 1995.
10. Gustafsson L, Hallander HO, Olin P, et al. A controlled trial of a two-component acellular, a five-component acellular, and a whole-cell pertussis vaccine. N Engl J Med 334:349–355, 1996.
11. Greco D, Salmaso S, Mastrantonio P, et al. A controlled trial of two acellular vaccines and one whole-cell vaccine against pertussis. N Engl J Med 334:341–348, 1996.
12. Ad hoc group for the study of pertussis vaccines: Placebo-controlled trial of two acellular pertussis vaccines in Sweden—protective efficacy and adverse events. Lancet 1:955–960, 1988.
13. Olin P, Rasmussen F, Gustafsson L, et al. Randomised controlled trial of two-component, three-component, and five-component acellular pertussis vaccines compared with whole-cell pertussis vaccine. Lancet 350:1569–1577, 1997.
14. Granoff DM, Rappuoli R. Are serological responses to acellular pertussis antigens sufficient criteria to ensure that new combination vaccines are effective for prevention of disease? Dev Biol Stand 89:379–389, 1997.
15. Granoff DM. Challenges for licensure of new diphtheria, tetanus, acellular pertussis (DTaP) combination vaccines: Point. Pediatr Infect Dis J 15:1069–1070, 1996.
16. Edwards KM, Decker MD. Challenges for licensure of new diphtheria, tetanus toxoid, acellular pertussis (DTaP) combination vaccines: Counterpoint. Pediatr Infect Dis J 15:1070–1073, 1996.
17. Arnon R, Van Regenmortel MHV. Structural basis of antigenic specficity and design of new vaccines. FASEB J 6:3265–3274, 1992.
18. Fothergill LD, Wright J. Influenzal meningitis: The relation of age incidence to the bactericidal power of blood against the causal organism. J Immunol 24:273–284, 1933.
19. Moskela M, Leinonen M, Häivä VM, et al. First and second dose antibody responses to pneumococcal polysaccharide vaccine in infants. Pediatr Infect Dis J 5:45–50, 1986.
20. Peltola H, Käyhty H, Sivonen A, Mäkelä PH. *Haemophilus influenzae* type b capsular polysaccharide vaccine in children: A double-blind field study of 100,000 vaccinees 3 months to 5 years of age in Finland. Pediatrics 60:730–737, 1977.
21. Avery OT, Goebel WF. Chemo-immunological studies on conjugated carbohydrate-proteins. II. Immunological specificity of synthetic sugar-protein antigens. J Exp Med 50:522–550, 1929.
22. Berkowitz CD, Ward JI, Meier K, et al. Safety and immunoge-

nicity of *Haemophilus influenzae* type b polysaccharide and polysaccharide diphtheria toxoid conjugate vaccines in children 15 to 24 months of age. J Pediatr 110:509–514, 1987.
23. Granoff DM, Boies HG, Munson RS Jr. Immunogenicity of *Haemophilus influenzae* type b polysaccharide-diphtheria toxoid conjugate vaccine in adults. J Pediatr 105:22–27, 1984.
24. Schneerson R, Robbins JB, Szu SC, Yang Y. Vaccines composed of polysaccharide-protein conjugates: Current status, unanswered questions, and prospects for the future. In Bell R, Torrigiani G (eds). Towards Better Carbohydrate Vaccines. Chichester, England, John Wiley & Sons, 1987, pp 307–332.
25. Janeway CA, Travers P. Immunobiology: The Immune System in Health and Disease (2nd ed). New York, Garland Publishing Inc., 1996, pp 8:1–8:23.
26. Insel RA. Potential alterations in immunogenicity by combining or simultaneously administering vaccine components. Ann N Y Acad Sci 754:35–47, 1995.
27. Ronchese F, Hausmann B. B lymphocytes in vivo fail to prime naive T cells but can stimulate antigen-experienced T lymphocytes. J Exp Med 177:679–690, 1993.
28. Germain RN, Margulies DH. The biochemistry and cell biology of antigen processing and presentation. Annu Rev Immunol 11:403–450, 1993.
29. Lanzavecchia A. Receptor-mediated antigen uptake and its effect on antigen presentation to class II-restricted T lymphocytes. Annu Rev Immunol 8:773–793, 1990.
30. Mosier DE, Subbarao B. Thymus-independent antigens: Complexity of B-lymphocyte activation revealed. Immunol Today 3:217–222, 1982.
31. Moss PAH, Rosenberg WNC, Bell JI. The human T cell receptor in health and disease. Annu Rev Immunol 10:71–96, 1992.
32. Bradley LM, Croft M, Swain SL. T-cell memory: New perspectives. Immunol Today 14:197–199, 1993.
33. Steinman RM. The dendritic cell system and its role in immunogenicity. Annu Rev Immunol 9:271–296, 1991.
34. Linsley PS, Ledbetter JA. The role of the CD28 receptor during T cell responses to inactivation. Annu Rev Immunol 11:191–211, 1993.
35. Chu C, Schneerson R, Robbins JB, Rastogi SC. Further studies on the immunogenicity of *Haemophilus influenzae* type b and pneumococcal type 6A polysaccharide-protein conjugates. Infect Immun 40:245–256, 1983.
36. Castillo de Febres O, Decker MD, Estopinan M, et al. Enhanced antibody response in Venezuelan infants immunized with *Haemophilus influenzae* type b–tetanus toxoid conjugate vaccine. Pediatr Infect Dis J 13:635–639, 1994.
37. Schneerson R, Robbins JB, Chu C, et al. Serum antibody responses of juvenile and infant rhesus monkeys injected with *Haemophilus influenzae* type b and pneumococcus type 6A capsular polysaccharide-protein conjugates. Infect Immun 45:582–591, 1984.
38. Anderson P, Pichichero M, Edwards K. Priming and induction of *Haemophilus influenzae* type b capsular antibodies in early infancy by Dpo20, an oligosaccharide-protein conjugate vaccine. J Pediatr 111:644–650, 1987.
39. Barington T, Skettrup M, Juul L, Heilman C. Non-specific suppression of the antibody response to *Haemophilus influenzae* type b conjugate vaccines by preimmunization with vaccine components. Infect Immun 61:432–438, 1993.
40. Dagan R, Eskola J, Leclerc C, Leroy O. Reduced response to multiple vaccines sharing common protein epitopes that are administered simultaneously to infants. Infect Immun 66:2093–2098, 1998.
41. Greenberg L, Fleming DS. The immunizing efficacy of diphtheria toxoid when combined with various antigens. Can J Public Health 39:131–135, 1948.
42. Spiller V, Barnes JM, Holt LB, Cullington DE. Immunization against diphtheria and whooping-cough: Combined v. separate inoculations. BMJ 2:639–642, 1955.
43. Aprile MA, Wardlaw AC. Aluminium compounds as adjuvants for vaccines and toxoids in man: A review. Can J Public Health 57:343–354, 1966.
44. Lerman SJ, Bollinger M, Brunken JM. Clinical and serologic evaluation of measles, mumps, and rubella (HPV-77:DE5 and RA 27/3) virus vaccines, singly and in combination. Pediatrics 68:18–22, 1981.
45. Berger R, Just M, Gluck R. Interference between strains in live virus vaccines, I: Combined vaccination with measles, mumps and rubella vaccine. J Biol Stand 16:269–273, 1988.
46. Weibel RE, Carlson AJ Jr, Villarejos VM, et al. Clinical and laboratory studies of combined live measles, mumps, and rubella vaccines using the RA 27/3 rubella virus. Proc Soc Exp Biol Med 165:323–326, 1980.
47. Beck M, Smerdel S, Dedic I, et al. Immune response to Edmonston-Zagreb measles virus strain in monovalent and combined MMR vaccine. Dev Biol Stand 65:95–100, 1986.
48. Buynak EB, Weibel RE, Whitman JE Jr, et al. Combined live measles, mumps, and rubella virus vaccines. JAMA 207:2259–2262, 1969.
49. Schwarz AJ, Jackson JE, Ehrenkranz NJ, et al. Clinical evaluation of a new measles-mumps-rubella vaccine. Am J Dis Child 129:1408–1412, 1975.
50. Just M, Berger R, Gluck R, Wegmann A. Evaluation of a combined vaccine against measles-mumps-rubella produced on human diploid cells. Dev Biol Stand 65:25–27, 1986.
51. Francis TM Jr, Napier JA, Voight RB, et al. Evaluation of the 1954 Field Trial of Poliomyelitis Vaccine (Final Report). Ann Arbor, University of Michigan, 1957.
52. Cohen H, Nagel J. Two injections of diphtheria-tetanus-pertussis-polio vaccine as the backbone of a simplified immunization schedule in developing countries. Rev Infect Dis 6:S350–S351, 1984.
53. van Wezel AL, van Steenis G, van der Marel P, Osterhaus AD. Inactivated poliovirus vaccine: Current production methods and new developments. Rev Infect Dis 6:S335–S340, 1984.
54. Salk J. One-dose immunization against paralytic poliomyelitis using a noninfectious vaccine. Rev Infect Dis 6:S444–S450, 1984.
55. Bordt DE, Whalen JW, Boyer PA, et al. Poliomyelitis component in quadruple antigen. JAMA 174:1166–1169, 1960.
56. Stoeckel P, Schlumberger M, Parent G, et al. Use of killed poliovirus vaccine in a routine immunization program in West Africa. Rev Infect Dis 6:S463–S466, 1984.
57. Henderson DA, Witte JJ, Morris L, Langmuir AD. Paralytic disease associated with oral polio vaccines. JAMA 190:41–48, 1964.
58. Cadoz M, Montagnon B, Yvonnet B, et al. Lack of adjuvant effect of the pertussis component on IPV DTP-polio vaccine in children. Dev Biol Stand 65:153–158, 1986.
59. Drucker J, Soula G, Diallo O, Fabre P. Evaluation of a new combined inactivated DPT-polio vaccine. Dev Biol Stand 65:145–151, 1986.
60. Qureshi AW, Zulfiqar I, Raza A, Siddiqi N. Comparison of immunogenicity of combined DPT-inactivated injectable polio vaccine (DPT-IPV) and association of DPT and attenuated oral polio vaccine (DPT + OPV) in Pakistani children. J Pak Med Assoc 39:31–35, 1989.
61. Ruuskanen O, Viljanen MK, Salmi TT, et al. DTP and DTP-inactivated polio vaccines: Comparison of adverse reactions and IgG, IgM and IgG antibody responses to DTP. Acta Paediatr Scand 69:177–182, 1980.
62. Rumke HC, Schlumberger M, Floury B, et al. Serological evaluation of a simplified immunization schedule using quadruple DPT-polio vaccine in Burkina Faso. Vaccine 11:1113–1118, 1993.
63. Baker JD, Halperin SA, Edwards K, et al. Antibody response to *Bordetella pertussis* antigens after immunization with American and Canadian whole-cell vaccines. J Pediatr 121:523–527, 1992.
64. Halperin SA, Langley JM, Eastwood BJ. Effect of inactivated poliovirus vaccine on the antibody response to *Bordetella pertussis* antigens when combined with diphtheria-pertussis-tetanus vaccine. Clin Infect Dis 22:59–62, 1996.
65. Meschievitz C, Blatter M, Starr S, Fritzell B. Safety and immunogenicity of IPV only or a sequential schedule of IPV (given separately or in combination with DTP) followed by OPV [abstract H089]. Abstracts of the 36th Interscience Conference on Antimicrobial Agents and Chemotherapy, American Society for Microbiology; Washington, DC; 1996.
66. Watemberg N, Dagan R, Arbelli Y, et al. Safety and immunogenicity of *Haemophilus* type b-tetanus protein conjugate vaccine, mixed in the same syringe with diphtheria-tetanus-pertussis vaccine in young infants. Pediatr Infect Dis J 10:758–763, 1991.

67. Scheifele D, Bjornson G, Barreto L, et al. Controlled trial of *Haemophilus influenzae* type b diphtheria toxoid conjugate combined with diphtheria, tetanus and pertussis vaccines, in 18-month-old children, including comparison of arm versus thigh injection. Vaccine 10:455–460, 1992.
68. Ferreccio C, Clemens J, Avendano A, et al. The clinical and immunologic response of Chilean infants to *Haemophilus influenzae* type b polysaccharide-tetanus protein conjugate vaccine coadministered in the same syringe with diphtheria-tetanus toxoids-pertussis vaccine at two, four and six months of age. Pediatr Infect Dis J 10:764–771, 1991.
69. Clemens JD, Ferrecio C, Levine M, et al. Impact of *Haemophilus influenzae* type b polysaccharide-tetanus conjugate vaccine on responses to concurrently administered diphtheria-tetanus-pertussis vaccine. JAMA 267:673–678, 1992.
70. Avendano A, Ferrecio C, Lagos R, et al. *Haemophilus influenzae* type b polysaccharide-tetanus protein conjugate vaccine does not depress serologic responses to diphtheria, tetanus, or pertussis antigens when coadministered in the same syringe with diphtheria-tetanus-pertussis vaccine at two, four and six months of age. Pediatr Infect Dis J 12:638–643, 1993.
71. Scheifele D, Barreto L, Meekison W, et al. Can *Haemophilus influenzae* type b–tetanus toxoid conjugate vaccine be combined with diphtheria toxoid–pertussis vaccine–tetanus toxoid? Can Med Assoc J 149:1105–1112, 1993.
72. Gold R, Scheifele D, Barreto L, et al. Safety and immunogenicity of *Haemophilus influenzae* vaccine (tetanus toxoid conjugate) administered concurrently or combined with diphtheria and tetanus toxoids, pertussis vaccine and inactivated poliomyelitis vaccine to healthy infants at two, four and six months of age. Pediatr Infect Dis J 13:348–355, 1994.
73. Kaplan SL, Lauer BA, Ward MA, et al. Immunogenicity and safety of *Haemophilus influenzae* type b–tetanus protein conjugate vaccine alone or mixed with diphtheria-tetanus-pertussis vaccine in infants. J Pediatr 124:323–327, 1994.
74. Dagan R, Botujansky C, Watemberg N, et al. Safety and immunogenicity in young infants of *Haemophilus* b–tetanus protein conjugate vaccine, mixed in the same syringe with diphtheria-tetanus-pertussis–enhanced inactivated poliovirus vaccine. Pediatr Infect Dis J 13:356–362, 1994.
75. Begg NT, Miller E, Fairley CK, et al. Antibody responses and symptoms after DTP and either tetanus or diphtheria *Haemophilus influenzae* type b conjugate vaccines given for primary immunisation by separate or mixed injection. Vaccine 13:1547–1550, 1995.
76. Levine OS, Lagos R, Losonsky GA, et al. No adverse impact on protection against pertussis from combined administration of *Haemophilus influenzae* type b conjugate and diphtheria–tetanus toxoid–pertussis vaccines in the same syringe. J Infect Dis 174:1341–1344, 1996.
77. Miller MA, Meschievitz CK, Ballanco GA, Daum RS. Safety and immunogenicity of PRP-T combined with DTP: Excretion of capsular polysaccharide and antibody response in the immediate post-vaccination period. Pediatrics 95:522–527, 1995.
78. Mulholland EK, Hoestermann A, Ward JI, et al. The use of *Haemophilus influenzae* type b–tetanus toxoid conjugate vaccine mixed with diphtheria-tetanus-pertussis vaccine in Gambian infants. Vaccine 14:905–909, 1996.
79. Bell F, Martin A, Blondeau C, et al. Combined diphtheria, tetanus, pertussis, and *Haemophilus influenzae* type b vaccines for primary immunisation. Arch Dis Child 75:298–303, 1996.
80. Carlsson RM, Claesson BA, Iwarson S, Selstam U. Studies on a Hib conjugate vaccine (PRP-T): The effects of coadministered tetanus toxoid vaccine, combined administration with injectable polio vaccine, and administration route [abstract G74]. Abstracts of the 35th Interscience Conference on Antimicrobial Agents and Chemotherapy, American Society for Microbiology; Washington, DC; 1995.
80a. Mills E, Gold R, Thipphawong J, Barreto L, et al. Safety and immunogenicity of a combined five-component pertussis-diphtheria-tetanus-inactivated poliomyelitis-*Haemophilus* b conjugate vaccine administered to infants at two, four and six months of age. Vaccine 16:576–585, 1998.
81. Amir J, Melamed R, Bader J, et al. Immunogenicity and safety of a liquid combination of DT-PRP-T vs lyophilized PRP-T reconstituted with DTP. Vaccine 15:149–154, 1997.
82. Lagos R, Horwitz I, Toro J, et al. Large scale, postlicensure, selective vaccination of Chilean infants with PRP-T conjugate vaccine: Practicality and effectiveness in preventing invasive *Haemophilus influenzae* type b infections. Pediatr Infect Dis J 15:216–222, 1996.
83. Scheifele DW. Recent trends in pediatric *Haemophilus influenzae* type b infections in Canada. Immunization Monitoring Program, Active (IMPACT) of the Canadian Paediatric Society and the Laboratory Centre for Disease Control. Can Med Assoc J 154:1041–1047, 1996.
84. Scheifele D, Gold R, Marchessault V, Duclos P. Failures after immunization with *Haemophilus influenzae* type b vaccines—1991–1995. Can Commun Dis Rep 22(3):17–20, 1996.
85. Summary of notifiable diseases, United States, 1996. MMWR Morb Mortal Wkly Rep 45:73, 1996.
86. Coulehan JL, Hallowell C, Michaels RH, et al. Immunogenicity of a *Haemophilus influenzae* type b vaccine in combination with diphtheria-pertussis-tetanus vaccine in infants. J Infect Dis 148:530–534, 1983.
87. Eskola J, Kayhty H, Gordon LK, et al. Simultaneous administration of *Haemophilus influenzae* type b capsular polysaccharide-diphtheria toxoid conjugate vaccine with routine diphtheria-tetanus-pertussis and inactivated poliovirus vaccinations of childhood. Pediatr Infect Dis J 7:480–484, 1988.
88. Mulholland EK, Ahonkhai VI, Greenwood AM, et al. Safety and immunogenicity of *Haemophilus influenzae* type b–*Neisseria meningitidis* group B outer membrane protein complex conjugate vaccine mixed in the syringe with diphtheria-tetanus-pertussis vaccine in young Gambian infants. Pediatr Infect Dis J 12:632–637, 1993.
89. Paradiso PR, Hogerman DA, Madore DV, et al. Safety and immunogenicity of a combined diphtheria, tetanus, pertussis and *Haemophilus influenzae* type b vaccine in young infants. Pediatrics 92:827–832, 1993.
90. Paradiso PR. Combination vaccines for diphtheria, tetanus, pertussis, and *Haemophilus influenzae* type b. Ann N Y Acad Sci 754:108–113, 1995.
91. Black SB, Shinefield HR, Ray P, et al. Safety of combined oligosaccharide conjugate *Haemophilus influenzae* type b (HbOC) and whole cell diphtheria-tetanus toxoids-pertussis vaccine in infancy. Pediatr Infect Dis J 12:981–985, 1993.
92. Black S, Shinefield H, Ray P, et al. Safety and immunogenicity of combined DTP-hepatitis B-PRP-T vaccine (DTPHH) (SmithKline Beecham) in infants [abstract G73]. Abstracts of the 35th Interscience Conference on Antimicrobial Agents and Chemotherapy, American Society for Microbiology; Washington, DC; 1995.
93. Win KM, Aye M, Htay-Htay H, et al. Comparison of separate and mixed administration of DTPw-HBV and Hib vaccines: Immunogenicity and reactogenicity profiles. Int J Infect Dis 2:79–84, 1997.
94. Riedmann S, Reinhardt G, Jara J, et al. Reactogenicity and immunogenicity of a diphtheria-tetanus-pertussis-hepatitis B and *Haemophilus influenzae* type B vaccine (DTPw-HBV-Hib) vs. separately administered DTPw-HBV and Hib vaccines in infants [abstract]. J Paediatr Child Health 33(suppl 1):S121, 1997.
94a. Ramkissoon A, Coovadia HM, Jugnundan P, et al. Antibody responses and safety following a pentavalent vaccine: Combined DTP-hepatitis B-*Haemophilus influenzae* type B (Hib) at 2, 4, and 6 months of age [abstract]. 7th International Congress for Infectious Diseases; Hong Kong; June 10–13, 1996; p 72.
95. Papaevangelou G, Karvelis E, Alexiou D, et al. Evaluation of a combined tetravalent diphtheria, tetanus, whole-cell pertussis and hepatitis B candidate vaccine administered to healthy infants according to a three-dose vaccination schedule. Vaccine 13:175–178, 1995.
96. Usonis V, Bakasenas V, Taylor D, Vandepapeliere P. Immunogenicity and reactogenicity of a combined DTPw-hepatitis B vaccine in Lithuanian infants. Eur J Pediatr 155:189–193, 1996.
97. Aristegui J, Garrote E, Gonzalez A, et al. Immune response to a combined hepatitis B, diphtheria, tetanus and whole-cell pertussis vaccine administered to infants at 2, 4 and 6 months of age. Vaccine 15:7–9, 1997.
98. Diez-Delgado J, Dal-Re R, Llorente M, et al. Hepatitis B component does not interfere with the immune response to diphthe-

ria, tetanus and whole-cell *Bordetella pertussis* components of a quadrivalent (DTPw-HB) vaccine: A controlled trial in healthy infants. Vaccine 15:1418–1422, 1997.

99. Nolan T, Hogg G, Darcy M-A, Skeljo M. 18m booster immunogenicity and reactogenicity in infants immunised with a combination DTPw-Hib-hepatitis B vaccine [abstract 751]. Abstracts of the 1997 Pediatric Academic Societies' Annual Meeting; Washington, DC; May 1997.
100. Mérieux C, Triau R, Ajjan N, Eyraud C. Vaccination quintuple: Association du vaccin rougeole hyperattenue (Schwarz) avec le vaccin anti-diphtherique, antitetanique, anticoquelucheux adsorbe et antipoliomyelitique inactive. Rev Pediatr 9:79–84, 1973.
101. McIntyre RC, Preblud SR, Polloi A, Korean M. Measles and measles vaccine efficacy in a remote island population. Bull World Health Organ 60:767–775, 1982.
102. John TJ, Selvakumar R. Mixing measles vaccine with DPT and DPTP. Lancet 1:1154, 1985.
103. John TJ, Selvakumar R, Balrai V, Simoes EAF. Antibody response to measles vaccine with DTPP. Am J Dis Child 141:14, 1987.
104. Simoes EAF, Balraj V, Selvakumar R, John TJ. Antibody response of children to measles vaccine mixed with diphtheria-pertussis-tetanus or diphtheria-pertussis-tetanus-poliomyelitis vaccine. Am J Dis Child 142:309–311, 1988.
105. Peltier M, Durieux C, Jonchere H, Arquie E. Pénétration du virus amaril neurotrope par voie cutanée. Vaccination mixte contre la fièvre jaune et la variole [note préliminaire]. Bull Acad Natl Med (Paris) 17:657, 1939.
106. Peltier M. Yellow fever vaccination, simple or associated with vaccination against smallpox, of the populations of French West Africa by the method of the Pasteur Institute of Dakar. Am J Public Health 37:1026–1032, 1947.
107. Hahn RG. A combined yellow fever–smallpox vaccine for cutaneous application. Am J Hyg 54:50–70, 1951.
108. Dick GWA, Horgan ES. Vaccination by scarification with a combined 17D yellow fever and vaccinia vaccine. J Hyg (Camb) 50:376–383, 1952.
109. Meers PD. Combined smallpox–17D yellow fever vaccine for scratch vaccination. Trans R Soc Trop Med Hyg 53:196–201, 1959.
110. Meers PD. Further observations on 17D–yellow fever vaccination by scarification, with and without simultaneous smallpox vaccination. Trans R Soc Trop Med Hyg 54:493–501, 1960.
111. Meyer HM, Hostetler DD Jr, Bernheim BC, et al. Response of Volta children to jet inoculation of combined live measles, smallpox and yellow fever vaccines. Bull World Health Organ 30:783–794, 1964.
112. Meyer HM Jr. Field experience with combined live measles, smallpox and yellow fever vaccines. Arch Ges Virusforsch 16:365–366, 1965.
113. Meyer HM, Hopps HE, Bernheim BC, Douglas RD. Combined measles-smallpox and other vaccines. First International Conference on Vaccines Against Viral and Rickettsial Diseases in Man. Pan American Health Organization Scientific Publ. No. 147. Washington, DC, Pan American Health Organization, 1967, pp 336–342.
114. Weibel RE, Stokes J Jr, Buynak EB, et al. Clinical-laboratory experiences with combined dried live measles-smallpox vaccine. Pediatrics 37:913–920, 1966.
115. Gateff C, Relyveld EH, Le Gonidec G, et al. Etude d'une nouvelle association vaccinal quintuple. Ann Microbiol (Paris) 124:387–409, 1973.
116. Lhuillier M, Mazzariol MJ, Zadi S, et al. Study of combined vaccination against yellow fever and measles in infants from six to nine months. J Biol Stand 17:9–15, 1989.
117. Mouchon D, Pignon D, Vicens R, et al. The combined measles–yellow fever vaccination in African infants aged 6 to 10 months. Bull Soc Pathol Exot 83:537–551, 1990.
118. Soula G, Sylla A, Pichard E, et al. A new combined vaccine against yellow fever and measles in infants aged 6 to 24 months in Mali. Bull Soc Pathol Exot 84(5 Pt 5):885–897, 1991.
119. Adu FD, Omotade OO, Oyedele OI, et al. Field trial of combined yellow fever and measles vaccines among children in Nigeria. East Afr Med J 73:579–582, 1996.
120. Just M, Berger R, Just V. Evaluation of a combined measles-mumps-rubella-chickenpox vaccine. Dev Biol Stand 65:85–88, 1986.
121. Berger R, Just M. Interference between strains in live virus vaccines. II: Combined vaccination with varicella and measles-mumps-rubella vaccine. J Biol Stand 16:275–279, 1988.
122. Vesikari T, Ohrling A, Baer M, et al. Evaluation of live attenuated varicella vaccine (Oka-RIT strain) and combined varicella and MMR vaccination in 13–17-month-old children. Acta Paediatr Scand 80:1051–1057, 1991.
123. Arbeter AM, Baker L, Starr SE, Plotkin SA. The combination measles, mumps, rubella and varicella vaccine in healthy children. Dev Biol Stand 65:89–93, 1986.
124. Arbeter AM, Baker L, Starr SE, et al. Combination measles, mumps, rubella and varicella vaccine. Pediatrics 78(4 Pt 2):742–747, 1986.
125. Brunell PA, Novelli VM, Lipton SV, Pollock B. Combined vaccine against measles, mumps, rubella, and varicella. Pediatrics 81:779–784, 1988.
126. Watson BM, Laufer DS, Kuter BJ, et al. Safety and immunogenicity of a combined live attenuated measles, mumps, rubella, and varicella vaccine ($MMR_{II}V$) in healthy children. J Infect Dis 173:731–734, 1996.
127. White CJ, Stinson D, Staehle B, et al. Measles, mumps, rubella, and varicella combination vaccine: Safety and immunogenicity alone and in combination with other vaccines given to children. Clin Infect Dis 24:925–931, 1997.
128. Reuman PD, Sawyer MH, Kuter BJ, Matthews H. Safety and immunogenicity of concurrent administration of measles-mumps-rubella-varicella vaccine and PedvaxHIB vaccines to healthy children twelve to eighteen months old. The MMRV Study Group. Pediatr Infect Dis J 16:662–667, 1997.
129. Kovel A, Wald ER, Guerra N, et al. Safety and immunogenicity of acellular diphtheria-tetanus-pertussis and *Haemophilus* conjugate vaccines given in combination or at separate injection sites. J Pediatr 120:84–87, 1992.
130. Liese JG, Harzer E, Hosbach P, et al. Immunogenicity of a combined DTaP-PRP-D conjugate vaccine compared to separate injections in infants [abstract G106]. Abstracts of the 36th Interscience Conference on Antimicrobial Agents and Chemotherapy, American Society for Microbiology; Washington, DC; 1996.
131. Hogerman D, Malinoski FJ, Madore DV, Paradiso PR. Safety and immunogenicity of DTaP-HbOC in toddlers primed by DTP and HbOC as separate injections or DTP-HbOC combination vaccine [abstract 1006]. Pediatr Res 33:171A, 1993.
132. Shinefield H, Black S, Adelman T, et al. Safety and immunogenicity of DTaP-HbOC—a combined oligosaccharide conjugate (HbOC, HibTITER) *Haemophilus influenzae* type b and acellular DTP vaccine (DTaP) in toddlers [abstract 306]. Abstracts of the 32nd Interscience Conference on Antimicrobial Agents and Chemotherapy, American Society for Microbiology; Washington, DC; 1992.
133. Rennels M, Hohenboken M, Clements D, et al. Antibodies to pertussis induced by DTaP and HbOC administered simultaneously versus combined in children <15 months versus ≥15 months [abstract G101]. Abstracts of the 36th Interscience Conference on Antimicrobial Agents and Chemotherapy, American Society for Microbiology; Washington, DC; 1996.
134. Shinefield H, Black S, Ray P, et al. Safety of combined acellular pertussis DTaP-HbOC vaccine (Lederle-Praxis) in infants [abstract G72]. Abstracts of the 36th Interscience Conference on Antimicrobial Agents and Chemotherapy, American Society for Microbiology; Washington, DC; 1996.
135. *TriHIBit* monograph. In Physician's Desk Reference. Montvale, NJ, Medical Economics, 1998, pp 2138–2142.
136. Pichichero ME, Latiolais T, Bernstein DI, et al. Vaccine antigen interactions after a combination diphtheria–tetanus toxoid–acellular pertussis/purified capsular polysaccharide of *Haemophilus influenzae* type b–tetanus toxoid vaccine in two-, four- and six-month-old infants. Pediatr Infect Dis J 16:863–870, 1997.
137. Liese JG, Harzer E, Hosbach P, et al. Hib antibody response of a combined DTaP-PRP-T conjugate vaccine compared to separate injections in infants [abstract G105]. Abstracts of the 36th Interscience Conference on Antimicrobial Agents and Chemotherapy, American Society for Microbiology; Washington, DC; 1996.
138. Bell F, Heath P, Shackley F, et al. Effect of reconstitution with an acellular pertussis, diphtheria, tetanus vaccine on antibody response to Hib vaccine (PRP-T) [abstract 69]. Meeting of the

European Society for Paediatric Infectious Diseases; Paris; May 1997.

139. Hoppenbrouwers K, Kanra G, Silier T, et al. Priming effect of the combined DTaP/Act-HIB vaccine [abstract 73]. Meeting of the European Society for Paediatric Infectious Diseases; Paris; May 1997.

140. Bell F, Heath P, Shackley F, et al. Immunological memory to Hib following combined acellular pertussis, diphtheria, tetanus/ Hib vaccine. Presented at the Paediatric Research Society Meeting; Sheffield, England; September 12–13, 1997.

141. Eskola J, Olander RM, Hovi T, et al. Randomised trial of the effect of co-administration with acellular pertussis DTP vaccine on immunogenicity of *Haemophilus influenzae* type b conjugate vaccine. Lancet 348:1688–1692, 1996.

142. Decker MD, Edwards KM, Bradley R, Palmer P. Comparative trial in infants of four conjugate *Haemophilus influenzae* type b vaccines. J Pediatr 120:184–189, 1992.

143. Greenberg DP, Lieberman JM, Marcy SM, et al. Enhanced antibody responses in infants given different sequences of heterogeneous *Haemophilus influenzae* type b conjugate vaccines. J Pediatr 126:206–211, 1995.

144. Capeding MR, Nohynek H, Pascual LG, et al. The immunogenicity of three *Haemophilus influenzae* type b conjugate vaccines after a primary vaccination series in Philippine infants. Am J Trop Med Hyg 55:516–520, 1996.

145. Eskola J, Litmanen L, Saarinen L, Kayhty H. Responses at 24 months to a combined DTaP-Hib conjugate vaccine in children vaccinated with the same vaccines at 4 and 6 months [abstract G060]. Abstracts of the 36th Interscience Conference on Antimicrobial Agents and Chemotherapy, American Society for Microbiology; Washington, DC; 1996.

146. Schmitt HJ. Immunogenicity and reactogenicity of 2 Hib tetanus conjugate vaccines administered by reconstituting with DTaP or given as separate injections [abstract G63]. Abstracts of the 35th Interscience Conference on Antimicrobial Agents and Chemotherapy, American Society for Microbiology; Washington, DC; 1995.

147. Schmitt HJ, Zepp F, Muschenborn S, et al. Immunogenicity and reactogenicity of a *Haemophilus influenzae* type b tetanus conjugate vaccine when administered separately or mixed with concomitant DTPa primary and booster immunizations. Eur J Pediatr:in press.

148. Meyer CU, Schmidtke P, Habermehl P, et al. Mixed administration of DTaP/Hib Vaccine has no impact on the generation of pertussis-specific cell-mediated immune (CMI) responses [abstract 585]. Abstracts of the 35th Annual Meeting of the Infectious Diseases Society of America; Alexandria, VA; 1997.

149. Lee C-Y, Huang L-M, Lee P-I, et al. An acellular pertussis DTacP combined with a lyophilized *Haemophilus influenzae* type b (PRP-T) vaccine is safe and immunogenic in Taiwanese infants [abstract G93]. Abstracts of the 37th Interscience Conference on Antimicrobial Agents and Chemotherapy, American Society for Microbiology; Washington, DC; 1997.

149a. Mills EL, Russell M, Cuinning L, et al. A fully liquid acellular pertussis vaccine combined with IPV and Hib vaccines (DTaP-IPV-PRP-T) is safe and immunogenic without significant interaction [abstract G95]. Abstracts of the 37th Interscience Congress on Antimicrobial Agents and Chemotherapy; Toronto; September 28–October 1, 1997.

150. Hronowski L, Rohrbaugh J, Prebula R, et al. Immunogenicity of a new *Haemophilus influenzae* type b polysaccharide–tetanus toxoid (Hib-TT) conjugate vaccine and the immunogenicities of the individual components in the pentavalent Hib-TT + DTaP + IPV vaccine [abstract E78]. Abstracts of the 93rd General Meeting of the American Society for Microbiology; Washington, DC; 1993.

151. Gyhrs AG, Olsen A, Petersen JV, et al. T-cell immunity in children vaccinated with hydrogen peroxide detoxified PT in a DTaP-IPV combination vaccine [abstract E92]. Abstracts of the 95th General Meeting of the American Society for Microbiology; Washington, DC; 1995.

152. Heron I, Gyhrs AF, Kristiansen M, Aggerbeck H. Safety and immunogenicity of a DTaP-IPV combination vaccine in infants for the primary immunization series [abstract 543]. Abstracts of the 1997 Pediatric Academic Societies' Annual Meeting; Washington, DC; May 1997.

153. Begue P, Stagnara J, Vie-Le-Sage F, et al. Immunogenicity and reactogenicity of a booster dose of diphtheria, tetanus, acellular pertussis and inactivated poliomyelitis vaccines given concurrently with *Haemophilus* type b conjugate vaccine or as pentavalent vaccine. Pediatr Infect Dis J 16:787–794, 1997.

154. Dagan R, Agbaria K, Piglansky L, et al. Immunogenicity of a combined diphtheria, tetanus, acellular pertussis, inactivated poliovirus and *H. influenzae* type b–tetanus conjugate vaccine (DTPa-IPV-Hib) in infants [abstract G59]. Abstracts of the 36th Interscience Conference on Antimicrobial Agents and Chemotherapy, American Society for Microbiology; Washington, DC; 1996.

155. Dagan R, Igbaria K, Piglansky L, et al. Safety and immunogenicity of a combined pentavalent diphtheria, tetanus, acellular pertussis, inactivated poliovirus and *Haemophilus influenzae* type b–tetanus conjugate vaccine in infants, compared with a whole cell pertussis pentavalent vaccine. Pediatr Infect Dis J 16:1113–1121, 1997.

156. Synopsis of Clinical Trial 213503-003 (DTPa-IPV-003) (Pilot Phase). Risenxart, Belgium; SmithKline Beecham Biologicals; May 29, 1996.

157. David T, Cadoz M, Gobert P, Danve B. Acellular pertussis vaccine combined with diphtheria and tetanus toxoids and inactivated polio vaccine (AcPDT IPV): Comparison to a DTP-IPV with a whole cell pertussis component (WcPDT IPV) in infants [abstract 60]. Abstracts of the 31st Interscience Conference on Antimicrobial Agents and Chemotherapy, American Society for Microbiology; Washington, DC; 1991.

158. Lagos R, Kotloff K, Hoffenbach A, et al. Clinical response to pentavalent parenteral diphtheria, tetanus, acellular pertussis (DTaP), inactivated polio (eIPV) and *Haemophilus influenzae* b (Hib) conjugate vaccine in 2, 4 & 6 mo old Chilean infants [abstract 609]. Abstracts of the 35th Annual Meeting of the Infectious Diseases Society of America; Alexandria, VA; 1997.

159. Lagos R, Kotloff K, Hoffenbach A, et al. Clinical acceptability and immunogenicity of a pentavalent parenteral combination vaccine containing diphtheria, tetanus, acellular pertussis, inactivated poliomyelitis, and *Haemophilus influenzae* type b conjugate antigens in two-, four- and six-month-old Chilean infants. Pediatr Infect Dis J 17:294–304, 1998.

160. Langue J, David T, Roussel F, et al. Safety and immunogenicity of DTaP-IPV and Act-HIB vaccines administered either combined or separately to infants at 2, 3, and 4 months of age [abstract 79]. Abstracts of the 15th Annual Meeting of the European Society for Paediatric Infectious Diseases; Paris; 1997.

161. Hoffenbach A, Langue J, Mallet E, et al. Influence of combining DTaP-IPV and Act-HIB vaccines and of changing the primary immunization schedule on the antibody response to *Haemophilus influenzae* type b [abstract 80]. Abstracts of the 15th Annual Meeting of the European Society for Paediatric Infectious Diseases; Paris; 1997.

162. Mallet E, Hoffenbach A, Salomon H, et al. Primary immunization with combined, acellular DTaP-IPV-Act-HIB vaccine given at 2-3-4 or 2-4-6 months of age [abstract 19]. Abstracts of the 14th Annual Meeting of the European Society for Paediatric Infectious Diseases; Elsinore, Denmark; 1996.

163. Mallet E, Hoffenbach A, Pines E, Salomon H. Immunogenicity of the fourth dose of a combined DTaP-IPV/Act-HIB vaccine administered at 15 months of age to children primed either at 2, 3, and 4 or at 2, 4, and 6 months of age [abstract 81]. Abstracts of the 15th Annual Meeting of the European Society for Paediatric Infectious Diseases; Paris; 1997.

164. Carlsson RM, Claesson B, Selstam U, et al. Safety and immunogenicity of a combined DTaP-IPV/PRP-T vaccine, administered either at 3, 5, and 12 months or at 2, 4, 6 and 13 months [abstract 78]. Abstracts of the 15th Annnual Meeting of the European Society for Paediatric Infectious Diseases; Paris; 1997.

165. Halperin SA, Davies HD, Barreto L, et al. Safety and immunogenicity of two inactivated poliovirus vaccines in combination with an acellular pertussis vaccine and diphtheria and tetanus toxoids in seventeen- to nineteen-month-old infants. J Pediatr 130:525–531, 1997.

166. Thipphawong J, Baretto L, Mills E, et al. A fully-liquid, acellular pertussis vaccine combined with IPV and Hib vaccines (DTaP-IPV-PRP-T) is safe and immunogenic without significant inter-

actions [workshop W3E]. Abstracts of the International Conference on Acute Respiratory Infections; Canberra, Australia; July 7–10, 1997.
167. Mills E, Russell M, Cunning L, et al. A fully liquid acellular pertussis vaccine combined with IPV and Hib vaccines (DTaP-IPV-PRP-T) is safe and immunogenic without significant interaction [abstract G95]. Abstracts of the 37th Interscience Conference on Antimicrobial Agents and Chemotherapy, American Society for Microbiology; Washington, DC; 1997.
167a. Mills E, Gold R, Thipphawong J, et al. Safety and immunogenicity of a combined five-component pertussis-diphtheria-tetanus-inactivated poliomyelitis-*Haemophilus* b conjugate vaccine administered to infants at two, four, and six months of age. Vaccine 16:576–585, 1998.
168. Kanra G, Ceyhan M, Ecevit Z, et al. Primary vaccination of infants with a combined diphtheria-tetanus-acellular pertussis-hepatitis B vaccine. Pediatr Infect Dis J 14:998–1000, 1995.
169. Usonis V, Bakasenas V, Willems P, Clemens R. Feasibility study of a combined diphtheria-tetanus-acellular pertussis-hepatitis B (DTPa-HBV) vaccine, and comparison of clinical reactions and immune responses with diphtheria-tetanus-acellular pertussis (DTPa) and hepatitis B vaccines applied as mixed or injected into separate limbs. Vaccine 15:1680–1686, 1997.
170. Giammanco G, Moiraghi A, Zotti C, et al. Safety and immnogenicity of a combined diphtheria-tetanus-acellular pertussis-hepatitis B vaccine administered according to two different primary vaccination schedules. Vaccine 16:722–726, 1998.
171. Greenberg DP, Wong VK, Partridge S, et al. Safety and immunogenicity of a combination DTPa-hepatitis B vaccine (DTPa-Hep B) administered to infants at 2, 4 and 6 months of age [abstract 602]. Abstracts of the 35th Annual Meeting of the Infectious Diseases Society of America; Arlington, Virginia; 1997.
172. Andre F. The way forward—combined vaccines [abstract SD5]. Extended Abstracts from the 9th Triennial International Symposium on Viral Hepatitis and Liver Disease; Rome; 1996.
173. Greenberg DP, Wong VK, Partridge S, et al. Evaluation of a new combination vaccine that incorporates diphtheria-tetanus-acellular pertussis (DTaP), hepatitis B (HB) and *Haemophilus influenzae* type b (Hib) conjugate (PRP-T) vaccines [abstract G70]. Abstracts of the 35th Interscience Conference on Antimicrobial Agents and Chemotherapy, American Society for Microbiology; Washington, DC; 1995.
174. Greenberg DP, Wong VK, Partridge S, et al. Immunogenicity of a booster dose of Hib conjugate vaccine in children with impaired immune responses following primary vaccination with DTaP-Hep B-PRP-T vaccine [abstract G061]. Abstracts of the 36th Interscience Conference on Antimicrobial Agents and Chemotherapy, American Society for Microbiology; Washington, DC; 1996.
175. Pichichero ME, Passador S. Administration of combined diphtheria and tetanus toxoids and pertussis vaccine, hepatitis B vaccine, and *Haemophilus influenzae* type b (Hib) vaccine to infants and response to a booster dose of Hib conjugate vaccine. Clin Infect Dis 25:1378–1384, 1997.
176. Schmitt HJ, Bock H, Bogaerts H, Clemens R. Single injection of a combined DTPa-Hep B and Hib tetanus conjugate vaccine; a feasibility study [abstract G64]. Abstracts of the 35th Interscience Conference on Antimicrobial Agents and Chemotherapy, American Society for Microbiology; Washington, DC; 1995.
176a. Zepp F, Schmitt HJ, Kaufhold A, et al. Evidence for induction of polysaccharide specific B-cell-memory in the 1st year of life: Plain *Haemophilus influenzae* type b-PRP (Hib) boosters children primed with a tetanus-conjugate Hib-DTPa-HBV combined vaccine. Eur J Pediatr 156:18–24, 1997.
177. Fabre P, Mallet E. Safety and immunogenicity of a fully liquid combination vaccine, with acellular pertussis, diphtheria, tetanus, inactivated poliovirus, *Haemophilus influenzae* serotype b, and hepatitis B when given in infants at 2, 3 and 4 months of age [abstract LB31]. Abstracts of the 36th Interscience Conference on Antimicrobial Agents and Chemotherapy, American Society for Microbiology; Washington, DC; 1996.
178. Final Report 217744/007 (DTaP-HBV-IPV-007). Risenxart, Belgium, SmithKline Beecham Biologicals, April 14, 1997.
179. West DJ, Hesley TM, Jonas LC, et al. Safety and immunogenicity of a bivalent *Haemophilus influenzae* type b/hepatitis B vaccine in healthy infants. Pediatr Infect Dis J 16:593–599, 1997.
180. Ambrosch F, Wiedermann G, Andre FE, et al. Clinical and immunological investigation of a new combined hepatitis A and hepatitis B vaccine. J Med Virol 44:452–456, 1994.
181. Leroux-Roels G, Moreau W, Desombere I, Safary A. Safety and immunogenicity of a combined hepatitis A and hepatitis B vaccine in young healthy adults. Scand J Gastroenterol 31:1027–1031, 1996.
182. Lery L, Rotivel Y, Trabaud MA, et al. Combined tetanus-rabies vaccination. Dev Biol Stand 65:209–220, 1986.
183. Ambrosch F, Fritzell B, Gregor J, et al. Combined vaccination against yellow fever and typhoid fever: A comparative trial. Vaccine 12:625–628, 1994.
184. Anderson EL, Decker MD, Englund JA, et al. Interchangeability of conjugated *Haemophilus influenzae* type b vaccines in infants. JAMA 273:849–853, 1995.
185. Pertussis vaccination: Use of acellular pertussis vaccines among infants and young children—recommendations of the Advisory Committee on Immunization Practices (ACIP). MMWR Morb Mortal Wkly Rep 46:19, 1997.
186. Combination Vaccines for Childhood Immunization. Recommendations of the Advisory Committee on Immunization Practices (ACIP), the American Academy of Pediatrics (AAP), and the American Academy of Family Physicians (AAFP). MMWR Morb Mortal Wkly Rep: in press.

chapter 21

Inactivated Influenza Vaccines

Edwin D. Kilbourne
Nancy H. Arden

Influenza is an "unvarying disease caused by a varying virus."[1] Although lacking the pathognomonic stigmata of poliomyelitis or smallpox, influenza has a clinical and epidemiological picture sufficiently characteristic to support reasonable speculation about the antiquity of the disease. No other acute febrile disease attended by respiratory symptoms is capable of such rapid involvement of such large numbers of the population. It is this *epidemicity* of influenza that is its hallmark. On the basis of compilations by Thompson[2] and Creighton,[3] influenza epidemics have been credibly reported since at least 1510, with probable pandemics occurring at least four times in the previous century (1833, 1836, 1847, and 1849).

Modern knowledge of influenza begins with the first isolation of the virus from humans in 1933, which provided a probe for serological studies.[4] Analysis of serum antibody and immune responses in the elderly has provided evidence of prior circulation of 20th-century viruses in the 19th century.

Study of the pandemic of 1957, the first within the period of modern virology, established that the virus of pandemic influenza differed in no significant way from the viruses of epidemic influenza of the 1930s and 1940s, except in degree of antigenic difference. By retrospective extrapolation, it can be inferred that the notorious agent of the 1918 pandemic was closely related to contemporary viruses. Indeed, serological studies strongly indicate its antigenic similarity to the virus isolated from swine in 1931.[1]

BACKGROUND

Clinical Description

Influenza is an acute, febrile, prostrating infection of sudden onset associated with systemic symptoms of myalgia and headache disproportionate in severity to coincident signs and symptoms referable to the respiratory tract. Cough, usually nonproductive, is almost invariable and derives from destruction of tracheal epithelium that also may produce substernal burning in a few patients. Complaints referable to rhinitis and pharyngitis are less frequent. Gastrointestinal symptoms are uncommon in adults but are progressively more frequent in children, in inverse relationship to age.

Fever in adults usually lasts for about 3 days and rarely beyond 5. Recovery is usually rapid, but some patients may sustain lingering sequelae of depression and asthenia for several weeks.

Rarely in healthy adults, and more commonly in those with preexisting cardiopulmonary disease, primary influenza virus pneumonia may occur; its outcome is usually fatal. Most fatalities from influenza, however, are the result of secondary bacterial pneumonia.

The Viruses

The basic virology of the influenza viruses has been well described in this book (see Chapter 37). A guide to the somewhat confusing taxonomy of the viruses is provided in Table 21–1, in which common vernacular as well as formal designations are given. Note that only influenza A viruses have antigenic subtypes. Not shown are such common names as *Sydney* or *Beijing* "flu" that define, respectively, the current strains of the H3N2 and H1N1 influenza A virus subtypes.

Pathogenesis as It Relates to Prevention

Infection with influenza viruses involves primarily the respiratory tract. Common symptoms of the disease,

Table 21–1. **CLASSIFICATION OF HUMAN INFLUENZA VIRUSES**

TYPE	SUBTYPES	EXAMPLES OF STRAIN DESIGNATION
A	H1N1	A/England/1/51/ (H1N1)*
	H2N2	A/Japan/305/57 (H2N2)
	H3N2	A/Hong Kong/8/68 (H3N2)
B	None	B/Great Lakes/1/54
C	None	C/Paris/1/67

*Type/place of isolation/isolate number/date of isolation (subtype).
H, hemagglutinin; N, neuraminidase.
Data from A revision of the system of nomenclature for influenza viruses: A WHO memorandum. Bull World Health Organ 58:585–591, 1980.

such as cough, nasal discharge, and substernal burning, reflect a complete destruction of respiratory epithelium, especially in the trachea and upper bronchi. In most cases, viremia is not demonstrable, and the systemic symptoms of myalgia, prostration, and fever remain unexplained. In the absence of viremia, prevention or modification of the disease by passive immunization would not be expected to work, and injected immune globulins have had no role in disease prophylaxis. However, studies in animal models have demonstrated that experimental disease can be prevented by administration of preformed antibody.[5] Furthermore, as discussed subsequently, parenteral administration of vaccine can produce immunoglobulin (Ig) G that is detectable in upper respiratory tract secretions.

Diagnosis

The definitive diagnosis of influenza is made in the laboratory by isolation and characterization of the causative virus, by demonstration of viral antigen in exfoliated cells or in respiratory secretions, or by demonstration of an increase in a specific antibody in the serum.

Virus can be found in throat washings or nasal secretions during the first 3 to 4 days of infection. Recovery of virus depends on inoculation of the amniotic or allantoic sac of 10- to 11-day-old chick embryos or certain cell cultures that support viral replication. In recent years, the Madin-Darby canine kidney (MDCK) cell line has proved equal and often superior in efficiency to the chick embryo in laboratory cultivation of virus.[6, 7] Demonstration of hemagglutinating or hemadsorbing virus by either chick embryo or cell culture techniques requires a minimum of 48 hours, and identification of virus types requires 1 to 2 additional days. Therefore, this information cannot assist in the management of the typical short-lived case of influenza but can aid in defining the etiology of a local epidemic.

Direct demonstration of viral antigens in clinical specimens by immunofluorescence microscopy has been used with limited success in the past. More promising results have been obtained with selected monoclonal antibodies specific for the nucleoprotein antigen of the virus.[8] A commercially available enzyme immunoassay membrane test with high sensitivity and specificity for detection of influenza A virus can be completed in 15 minutes. This test can provide rapid diagnosis in clinical and institutional settings, which can be helpful in guiding decisions about the use of antiviral agents.[9]

Specific antibody response in influenza can be shown as early as 10 days after infection, but convalescent blood samples are best obtained at 21 days or later. Serodiagnosis is usually made by the hemagglutinin inhibition (HI) test, which depends on the capacity of influenza virus to agglutinate human or chicken erythrocytes and its inhibition by specific antibody.

Treatment and Prevention with Antiviral Agents

Amantadine and Rimantadine

Although vaccination is the primary method for control of influenza, the antiviral agents amantadine hydrochloride and rimantadine hydrochloride have a role in the treatment and prophylaxis of influenza type A infection. These chemically related drugs interfere with the replication of influenza type A viruses but not of type B. Both drugs have high oral bioavailability and are equally effective. However, the two drugs differ considerably in pharmacokinetics, and amantadine is associated with a higher incidence of side effects.[10, 11]

Amantadine and rimantadine inhibit influenza A viruses by the same mechanism, and virus strains can be cross-sensitive and cross-resistant. Resistance is associated with point mutations in the RNA sequence coding for the M2 protein resulting in amino acid substitutions in one of four sites in the membrane-spanning portion of the protein, which is believed to act as an ion channel. Amantadine and rimantadine inhibit virus replication by blocking this ion channel, and certain amino acid substitutions cause a loss of this specific anti–influenza A activity.[12]

Many studies have shown amantadine and rimantadine to be approximately 70 to 90% effective in preventing illness caused by naturally occurring strains of type A influenza viruses. Efficacy against infection is generally lower as evidenced by the occurrence of subclinical infection during the period of prophylaxis. This offers the advantage of protection from future infection with antigenically similar virus strains. Efficacy against illness and infection may be lower in people with no preexisting antibody compared with those who have even low levels of antibody. This is consistent with the observation that the combination of vaccination and chemoprophylaxis has been shown in some studies to be more effective than either measure alone.[13–18]

Chemoprophylaxis can be used as an adjunct to vaccination in other ways. When influenza vaccine is administered after an outbreak has begun, amantadine or rimantadine can be used to provide protection during the approximately 2-week period required for development of antibody after vaccination. These drugs do not interfere with the immunological response to vaccination. Amantadine or rimantadine can also be used during influenza A epidemics to protect people who are likely to have a poor immunological response to vaccination because of immunosuppression or those for whom influenza vaccine is contraindicated.[19]

Chemoprophylaxis is also effective in stopping outbreaks in closed settings such as nursing homes and boarding schools.[20–22] Using amantadine or rimantadine for outbreak control is most effective when the drug is administered to all residents of the institution early in the course of an outbreak. Use of rapid diagnostic testing will greatly facilitate early detection and confirmation.[23]

When an institutional outbreak of influenza A is recognized, residents who have already become ill may benefit from antiviral treatment. However, because those who are given amantadine or rimantadine for treatment of infection may shed resistant virus during the course of therapy, efforts should be made to isolate residents who are being treated from those who are taking the drug for prophylaxis. This principle also applies to staff members, who may also be offered chemoprophylaxis or therapy.[19] Most studies of the therapeutic efficacy of amantadine and rimantadine have been conducted in previously healthy young adults and children. In these populations, the drugs have been shown to reduce the severity and duration of signs and symptoms of influenza A illness when they are administered within 48 hours of illness onset. Controlled studies have not been conducted to determine whether antiviral therapy can prevent or treat complications in people at high risk for complications after influenza infection.[24–26]

Drug-resistant virus can emerge during treatment with amantadine or rimantadine. Although emergence of resistance during treatment has not been shown to reduce therapeutic efficacy in people shedding resistant virus, resistant viruses can be transmitted to contacts, whether or not they are undergoing chemoprophylaxis. Apparent transmission of resistant virus has been described in nursing homes and within households.[27–29]

The extent of transmission of resistant viruses is unknown. Most amantadine- and rimantadine-resistant viruses have been isolated from people undergoing drug treatment or, less often, from their contacts.[30] International surveillance for drug-resistant influenza A viruses has shown that few isolates obtained from patients with no known history of antiviral treatment are resistant.[31] In most circumstances, the benefits of these drugs outweigh the problems of resistance, at present, but clinical practices that discourage the spread of resistance as well as continued surveillance for resistant stains are recommended.[32, 33]

A new antiviral agent currently under study, GG167, interferes with the replication of both influenza type A and type B viruses by inhibiting enzymatic activity of the viral neuraminidase (NA). Twice-daily intranasal administration has been effective for prophylaxis and treatment. Initial studies suggest that resistant virus does not readily emerge during treatment with GG167, although naturally occurring strains of influenza virus have shown nearly 1000-fold differences in in vitro susceptibility to the drug. The clinical significance of these differences requires further study.[34]

EPIDEMIOLOGY

Antigenic Variation as a Key Epidemiological Determinant

Influenza is a disease of global importance and spares no human population. It is a seasonal disease, which in the northern temperate zones occurs during winter and in the tropics occurs during the rainy season. Transmission of the virus is apparently facilitated by the indoor crowding that takes place in both circumstances. Pandemic infection is less seasonally restricted but can occur at any time of year.

To understand the epidemiology of influenza, one must understand the unique antigenic variability of its virus. The surface antigens, hemagglutinin (HA) and NA, are subject to continuous and apparently sequential evolution within immune or partially immune populations, as depicted schematically in Figure 21–1. Antigenic mutants emerge and are selected as predominant virus to the extent that they differ from antecedent virus, which is suppressed by specific antibody arising in the population. The cycle is repeated when increasing antibody to the mutant forces the selection of yet another variant. Such mutants in the interpandemic period arise by cumulative point mutations in the RNA coding for the hemagglutinin. At irregular intervals of 10 to 40 years, viruses showing major antigenic differences from prevalent subtypes enter the community and, because they are antigenically novel, are rapidly dispersed to cause widespread (pandemic) disease, affecting people of all ages. In this century, this probably occurred in 1957 and 1968 and by presumption in 1918. Except in 1918, when the virus appears to have been intrinsically more virulent than ordinary strains, pandemic influenza is no more severe in the individual case, but because large numbers of people are infected, the number if not the proportion of severe and fatal cases will be large.

Significance of Influenza as a Public Health Problem

Although influenza epidemics vary in size and frequency in any one region, active surveillance reveals infection to be present virtually every winter. In epidemic years, the presence of virus is often reflected by an increase in mortality. This effect is so characteristic of influenza that it has been used for years by epidemiologists as an indication of the presence of influenza in the community.[35] William Farr[36] was the first to assess the number of deaths attributable to influenza by calculating the numbers of deaths during epidemic periods above those recorded during otherwise comparable nonepidemic periods. This concept of "excess mortality" is still used, and during the years a number of statistical methods have been developed to calculate expected and excess mortality.[37, 38]

The most dramatic illustration of the impact of influenza on mortality occurred during the 1918 to 1919 pandemic. This pandemic is estimated to have caused at

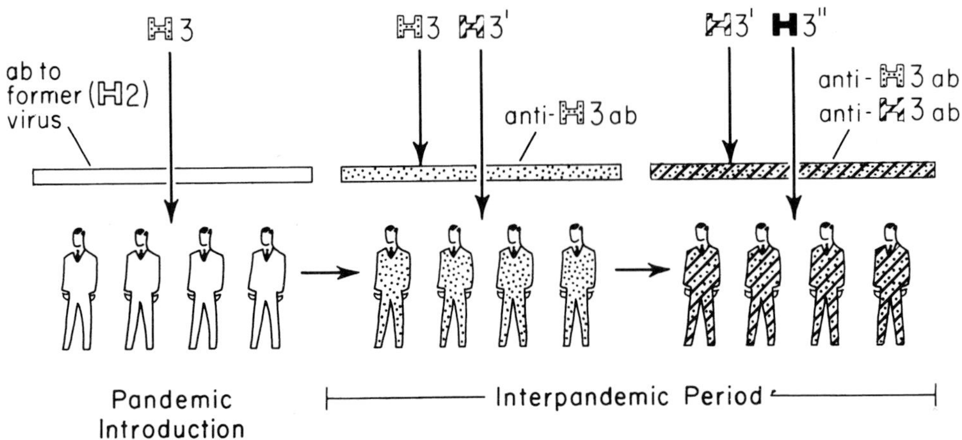

Figure 21–1. Selection of antigenic mutants as a function of population antibody (ab). A new pandemic viral subtype H3 transcends the barrier of antibody to unrelated, previously prevalent, virus H2 and readily infects the population. When a critical percentage of the population has been infected with H3, the survival of H3 is impeded, and antigenically changed mutants H3′, and later H3″, have survival advantage (i.e., minor antigenic variation or antigenic "drift"). (From Kilbourne ED [ed]. The Influenza Viruses and Influenza. New York, Academic Press, 1975, p 522.)

least 20 million deaths worldwide and at least 500,000 in the United States alone. Furthermore, the age-specific mortality was unlike that known to be associated with any other influenza pandemic or epidemic, with the highest mortality among young adults. The impact on mortality was so severe as to decrease the average life expectancy by 10 years.[39]

During interpandemic periods, the age-specific mortality associated with influenza shows a pattern of highest mortality among the age group 65 years and older, with increasingly higher death rates in each age group beyond 65 years. For the years 1972 to 1992, excess mortality attributed to pneumonia and influenza was 69 times higher among people age 65 years and older than among those younger than 65 years.[40] However, of the approximately 60,000 deaths that occurred in the United States as a result of the 1957 to 1958 pandemic, almost 40% occurred among those younger than 65 years.[38]

The risk of death from influenza is also associated with underlying health status. Analyses of United States vital statistics data during the 1957 to 1958 pandemic and the subsequent epidemic during 1960 showed that people with certain chronic diseases were at higher risk for influenza-associated death. Pregnant women, especially those in the later stages of pregnancy, were also shown to be at higher risk during this period, although increased risk of death among pregnant women has not been conclusively demonstrated since that time.[38, 41, 42]

During the present era of cocirculation of influenza A/H1N1, A/H3N2, and type B, excess mortality is most often associated with epidemics in which H3N2 viruses predominate and occasionally during influenza type B epidemics. Excess mortality has not been associated with H1N1 epidemics since this subtype reemerged in 1977 after a 20-year absence, although H1N1 viruses did increase mortality during the previous period of circulation before the mid-1950s. It is estimated that more than 10,000 influenza-related deaths have occurred during each of 21 different epidemics or pandemics occurring from 1957 to 1992 in the United States; more than 40,000 excess deaths occurred in each of six of these epidemics. An average of more than 20,000 influenza-related deaths per season have occurred during the 20 influenza seasons between 1972 to 1973 and 1991 to 1992.[37, 43, 44]

In fact, the cumulative death toll in the United States from influenza epidemics that have occurred since the last pandemic of 1968 to 1969 is greater than that of the 1918 to 1919 pandemic.

In spite of the substantial mortality associated with influenza, the overall case-fatality ratio is small. This is a reflection of the high rates of influenza illness that occur during epidemics.[45] In a study of H3N2 virus infection in Houston, Texas, in 1976, almost half the families had at least one infected member.[46] In Port Chalmers, New Zealand, 46% of selected families had evidence of infection with the 1973 H3N2 variant.[47]

Attack rates vary from one season to another but are highest among school-aged children and lowest among older adults. In fact, influenza in children causes considerable morbidity, and children may be an effective reservoir for disease.[46a] Glezen and colleagues showed that one third of infants in Houston were infected with influenza during the first year of life, mostly between 7 and 12 months of age.[46b] Table 21–2 shows the estimated average annual age-specific rates of influenza illness in the United States based on prospective surveillance among household members during influenza epidemics occurring between 1976 and 1981.

Although most cases of influenza are treated at home, excess rates of hospitalization of adults with respiratory disease ranging from 79 to 270 per 100,000[48, 49] have been found during influenza epidemics. Increased rates

Table 21–2. **ESTIMATED AVERAGE ANNUAL RATE OF INFLUENZA ILLNESS IN THE UNITED STATES DURING INFLUENZA EPIDEMICS FROM 1976 TO 1981**

AGE (yr)	RATE PER 100 PERSON-YEARS
<1	26.4
1–4	37.1
5–14	37.5
15–24	21.8
25–59	15.3
≥60	10.0

Data from Committee on Issues and Priorities for New Vaccine Development, Institute of Medicine. New Vaccine Development: Establishing Priorities. Vol. 1. Diseases of Importance in the United States. Washington, DC, National Academy Press, 1985, pp 342–364.

of hospitalization for acute respiratory disease among infants and young children have also been observed.[50, 51]

School and industrial absenteeism and increase in clinic visits are other measures of the community-wide impact of influenza. A household survey in a community that had experienced an outbreak of influenza B found that 30% of those who became ill sought medical care.[52] Work loss related to medically attended influenza illness has been estimated at 15 million lost work days per year.[53]

The economic impact of influenza reflects not only the cost of medical care but also the loss of human productivity. Of the $1.7 to $3.9 billion cost of epidemics in the 1960s, medically related costs were only 20% of this amount.[54] More recent calculations have estimated that the annual economic cost of influenza in the United States is on the order of $3 to $5 billion per year, with direct medical costs accounting for about 20 to 30% of the total cost.[55] It must be obvious that despite the imperfections of present vaccines, an increase in their use could significantly improve public health.

PASSIVE IMMUNIZATION

Administration of immune globulins has no place in the prophylaxis of influenza. Influenza does not have a viremic stage in pathogenesis, and pooled human antibodies would be lacking in appropriate specificity.

ACTIVE IMMUNIZATION

Vaccines

History of Influenza Vaccine

One of us has reviewed elsewhere the history of influenza vaccines in detail.[56] The basic principles governing influenza vaccination have changed little in the 60 years since the first clearly effective vaccine was administered by Chenoweth, Stokes, and colleagues to institutionalized male subjects in Pennsylvania.[57] Although that vaccine contained live virus in mouse lung suspension, it was effectively inactive because influenza virus does not replicate in humans when it is introduced by the parenteral route. The study by Chenoweth and colleagues was actually preceded by the use of "formol vaccine" in ferret studies by Wilson Smith,[58] a codiscoverer of human influenza virus. Taylor and Dreguss[59] later first demonstrated vaccine failure related to antigenic change in the virus.

In the 1940s, growth of virus in the chick embryo allantoic sac was found to yield an abundant supply of virus, which after inactivation by any of various procedures was a potent immunogen when administered parenterally. The local and systemic reactions associated with these early vaccines were attributable in part to contamination with bacterial endotoxins and in part to the inherent toxicity of the intact, undisrupted virus used in their preparation. These problems have been largely solved by viral purification by zonal centrifugation and chromatography[60, 61] and by splitting the viral lipid membrane with ether or detergents.[62, 63] The early development of live virus vaccines is considered elsewhere in this book.

A major step in influenza vaccine development was the genetic manipulation of potential vaccine strains to effect instant adaptation of poorly growing viruses newly isolated from humans to high-yield growth in the chick embryo host used in production.[64] Such recombinant (reassortant) vaccines have been in use since 1971 and represent the first genetically engineered vaccines of any kind.[65] They have particular value because of the unique requirement for annual vaccine revision that is peculiar to influenza.

Currently Available and Licensed Vaccines

The World Health Organization (WHO) makes recommendations concerning the antigenic properties of influenza virus strains to be used in influenza vaccines for each season. These recommendations are made each February and are based on analyses of data gathered by more than 100 laboratories throughout the world that participate in WHO's global influenza surveillance system. Throughout the year, influenza viruses representative of those in circulation are screened, and selected influenza virus isolates are forwarded to one of three WHO centers in the United States, England, and Australia. In this way, antigenic and genetic changes in the circulating influenza virus strains are monitored continuously. Recommended changes in influenza vaccine composition are based on virological and epidemiological data as well as assessment of the ability of current vaccine strains to produce immunity against newly detected variants.[66]

Current influenza vaccines contain three virus strains representing the strains currently in worldwide circulation: A/H1N1, A/H3N2, and type B. Influenza vaccines manufactured for the Northern Hemisphere are all made with antigenically equivalent virus strains; the same three strains recommended by WHO in February are usually included in vaccines made for the Southern Hemisphere, although more recently detected variants are occasionally used.

All types of inactivated influenza vaccine are prepared from virus grown in embryonated hens' eggs and purified by zonal centrifugation or chromatography. Whole-virus particles are inactivated with formalin or β-propiolactone. Treatment of whole-virus preparations with organic solvents or detergents results in disruption of the lipid-containing viral envelope to release and solubilize the surface glycoproteins. Ether-split preparations contain essentially all the viral structural proteins and portions of the viral membrane and, in this respect, differ from preparations more effectively solubilized with detergents, such as sodium dodecyl sulfate. Detergent-prepared vaccines consist of stellate aggregated HA monomers and are called *subunit* or *purified surface antigen vaccines*. Although they are enriched for HA and NA, they contain residual, internal viral structural proteins—principally NP.[67–69] Split and subunit vaccines are similar in immunogenicity and reactogenicity.[70,71] Split and subunit vaccines are less toxic than whole-virus vaccines. The reason for their lessened reactogenicity is not known but may reflect disturbance of the spatial arrangement of viral lipids during virus disruption.[72,73] Disrupted virus has been most useful in immunization of children, in whom the whole-virus vaccines have prohibitive reactogenic effects. However, split and subunit vaccines are commonly used for vaccination of adults. Some studies have suggested that split and subunit vaccines may be less immunogenic than whole-virus vaccine, but other studies have shown no difference in immunogenicity.[74]

Use of Reassortant Viruses. Viruses newly isolated in the chick embryo—the standard host system for influenza vaccine production—do not usually replicate to high titer and, in the past, were multiply passaged for the empirical selection of a higher yielding virus. Since 1971, on the basis of evidence presented a decade earlier,[64] genetic reassortment of new strains with a high-yield donor virus has been employed to produce virus of the desired antigenic and high-yield phenotype. Reassortants are produced by simultaneous infection of the chick embryo allantoic sac with antigenically dissimilar parental viruses, then selected by passage of post-reassortment virus with antibody suppressive to the antigens of the high-yield donor (Fig. 21–2). The donor viruses employed have been the A/PR/8/34 (H1N1) virus or its H3N2 derivative, X-31,[75] which contains all but the HA and NA proteins of A/PR/8/34. These viruses are standard laboratory strains. The PR8 virus has had many passages in the chick embryo and is maximally adapted to replication in that host. High yield is associated primarily with the M gene (RNA 7) of the virus,[76,77] but other genes,[78] including that coding for the HA,[79] can influence virus yield in the chick embryo.

Reassortant viruses may show slight antigenic differences from wild-type viruses.[80,81] However, these differences are no greater than those encountered among clones of wild-type isolates and have no practical significance. High-yielding influenza B reassortants have not yet been produced.[82]

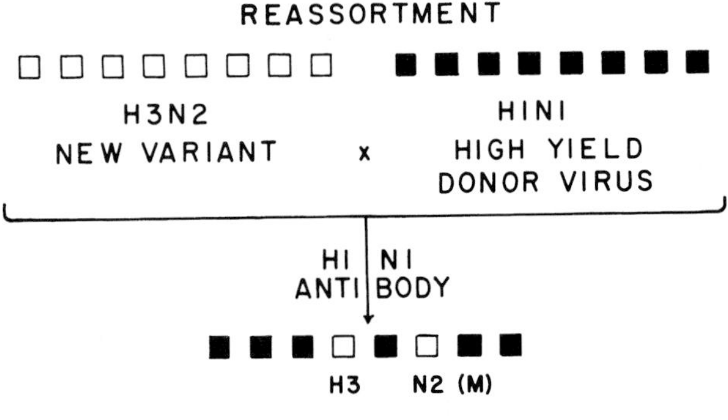

Figure 21–2. Genetic reassortment of a high-yield donor virus and a new antigenic variant to produce a high-yield reassortant vaccine virus. The reassortant contains H3- and N2-coding RNAs from the new variant and high-yield–determining M gene and other genes from the high-yield H1N1 donor virus. (From Kilbourne ED. Influenza. New York, Plenum Publishing, 1987, p 302.)

As the first genetically engineered vaccine viruses, influenza virus high-yield reassortants address three critical problems in influenza vaccine production as follows:

1. need for rapid change in vaccine formulation;
2. limited availability of fertile hens' eggs; and
3. cost of production.

Reassortants can be produced and characterized within a few weeks and, because they usually exceed yields of wild-type virus by 8-fold to 32-fold, require fewer eggs for vaccine production. Reassortants have also proved valuable as experimental live virus vaccines (see Chapter 37).

Vaccine Products (United States). Inactivated influenza vaccines currently available in the United States are prepared by three different manufacturers (Table 21–3) but are similar in composition and method of preparation. All are trivalent and contain antigens representative of the influenza B strain and the two influenza A subtype viruses now circulating. They are standardized to contain 15 μg each of viral hemagglutinin antigen per 0.5 mL dose. All three manufacturers make split-virus or subunit preparations disrupted by ethyl ether or detergents (see Table 21–3), and one manufacturer (Connaught) makes a whole-virus vaccine preparation.

Some manufacturers use antibiotics such as neomycin or gentamicin during virus propagation, and sodium bisulfite may also be used in the manufacturing process. However, except for the preservative thimerosal, pharmacologically active additives or contaminants are not detectable in the final product by current assay procedures. Contamination with egg proteins must be assumed in assessing vaccine use in allergic subjects (see further on).

Inactivated influenza vaccine is stable for at least 1 year when it is stored between 2 and 8°C. Potency is destroyed by freezing. At least one new strain is incorporated into the vaccine almost every year, and vaccines formulated for a previous season should not be used.

Dose and Route of Administration. Currently recommended doses of influenza vaccines (Table 21–4) reflect present interpandemic use of vaccine in populations immunologically primed by infection with H3N2 and H1N1 influenza A viruses. Immunization of immunologically naive young children requires the use of a divided dose schedule, both to provide opportunity for a booster (anamnestic) response and to permit reduction of the amount of antigen in individual doses to lessen reactogenicity.

The required dose of vaccine in nonimmune subjects at the time of pandemic introduction of antigenically novel viruses cannot be predicted accurately. Past experience is not helpful because of different methods of measurement of vaccine HA concentration employed before 1978. However, even small doses of vaccine had demonstrable efficacy in a hospital setting during the pandemic of 1957 to 1958.[83] In 1976, adequate antibody response to a single dose of H1N1 (swine) vaccine occurred only in subjects older than 24 years who were presumably primed by prior exposure to other H1N1 viruses.

Table 21–3. **INFLUENZA VACCINES* LICENSED AND AVAILABLE IN THE UNITED STATES (1997–1998)**

MANUFACTURER	PRODUCT	INACTIVATION	PREPARATION AND DILUENTS
Connaught	Fluzone (whole or split virus)	Formalin Split with Triton X-100	Antigens in 0.01 M phosphate-buffered saline Thimerosal 1:10,000 Gelatin 0.05% in split-virus vaccine
Evans	Fluvirin (subunit/purified surface antigen)	β-Propiolactone Split with Triton N-101	Purified antigens in 0.01 M phosphate-buffered saline Thimerosal 1:10,000
Wyeth-Ayerst	FluShield (split virus)	Formalin Split with tri-*n*-butyl phosphate	Antigens in 0.01 M phosphate-buffered saline Thimerosal 1:10,000

*All influenza vaccines produced for the 1997 to 1998 influenza season contain 15 μg each of A/Bayern/07/95-like (H1N1), A/Wuhan/359/95-like (H3N2), and B/Beijing/184/93-like hemagglutinin antigens in each 0.5 mL. For the A/Bayern/07/95-like, A/Wuhan/359/95-like, and B/Beijing/184/93-like antigens, U.S. manufacturers used the antigenically equivalent strains A/Johannesburg/82/96 (H1N1), A/Nanchang/933/95 (H3N2), and B/Harbin/07/94 because of their growth properties. In addition, manufacturers use high-yield reassortants of the A/Johannesburg/82/96 (H1N1) and A/Nanchang/933/95 (H3N2) viruses.

Dose response to vaccine is linear. A 10-fold increase in vaccine virus concentration induces a two- to threefold increase in geometric mean antibody titer.[84, 85] Antibody responses in primed subjects as measured by fold increase in HI titrations may reach a plateau.[84, 86] Repeated administration of vaccine at 6-month intervals did not increase the number of subjects with protective levels of antibody after initial response had occurred.[87] However, an apparent plateau in response may reflect only the increasing difficulty in demonstrating a significant (i.e., fourfold) response on a geometric dilution scale when initial levels of antibody are high.

It is recommended that inactivated influenza virus vaccines be given by intramuscular injection, but they are also immunogenic by subcutaneous, intradermal, respiratory tract, and oral routes of administration. The intradermal route has been used with the rationale of reducing toxic effects and conserving vaccine during times of vaccine shortage. Evidence from published studies is mixed concerning the frequently alleged superiority of the intradermal route. Few studies have examined the effect in unprimed subjects of equal doses of vaccine by intradermal and subcutaneous injection. A consensus suggests that the limited amount of vaccine that can be given by intradermal administration is equal in efficacy to larger amounts given by parenteral routes only when it is administered to elicit a secondary response in immunologically primed subjects. Topical or aerosol application of vaccine to the upper respiratory tract has proved immunogenic also in primed subjects[88] but may be inferior to parenteral routes in the induction of either serum or nasal antibody.[89]

Few studies have directly compared the immunogenicity and reactogenicity of influenza vaccine administered by the subcutaneous and intramuscular routes. However, there is evidence to suggest that subcutaneous administration is associated with a higher incidence of local reactions.[90, 91]

Contraindications. Influenza vaccines are contraindicated in infants younger than 6 months because of the high incidence of febrile reactions in this age group. In children younger than 13 years, only split-virus vaccines should be used. People with acute febrile diseases should not be vaccinated. Vaccination of a person with a definite history of allergic reactions to eggs should be approached with caution. However, the majority of "egg-allergic" subjects can be safely immunized.[92, 93] Even children with positive skin test reactions to vaccine can be immunized by a rapid, divided dose schedule.[94] Because asthmatic children are more vulnerable to influenza, every effort should be made to immunize them.

Experimental (Nonreplicating Antigen) Vaccines

Research into purified antigen or submolecular vaccines has intensified with the development of cloning and sequencing technology, identification of important epitopes with monoclonal antibody, and increased capability for peptide synthesis. Most efforts have focused on the viral HA as a major antigen of the virus through which viral neutralization is mediated. These approaches include viral gene cloning, synthesis of oligopeptide (submolecular) antigens, and anti-idiotype antibodies.

Purified and Tailored Antigens from Cloned Viral Genes. All influenza A viral genes have now been cloned and sequenced, and the immunogenically important HA and NA genes have been expressed with resultant production of viral antigens. Expression of these proteins in

Table 21–4. **INFLUENZA VACCINE DOSAGE BY PATIENT'S AGE IN THE UNITED STATES (1997–1998)**

AGE GROUP	PRODUCT	DOSAGE	NUMBER OF DOSES	ROUTE
6–35 mo	Split virus only	0.25 mL	1 or 2	IM
3–8 yr	Split virus only	0.50 mL	1 or 2	IM
9–12 yr	Split virus only	0.50 mL	1	IM
>12 yr	Whole or split virus	0.50 mL	1	IM

IM, intramuscular.

From Centers for Disease Control and Prevention. Prevention and control of influenza: Recommendations of the Advisory Committee on Immunization Practices (ACIP). MMWR Morb Mortal Wkly Rep 46(RR-9):1–25, 1997.

mammalian yeast and insect cells results in a glycosylated protein *antigenically* indistinguishable from that produced in natural infection.[95–101] Baculovirus-expressed recombinant HA induced HA-specific antibody response in adult volunteers.[102]

Although this new technology should facilitate the production of isolated viral proteins, it will not necessarily aid in chemical purification of vaccine antigens, nor does it address the primary problem of antigenic variation. However, it is conceivable that site-specific mutagenesis of cloned cDNA might ultimately lead to tailoring of less reactogenic or more immunogenic antigens when cross-reactive epitopes or residues associated with virulence have been identified. More recently, vaccine development has focused on the importance of T-cell recognition of epitopes of internal viral proteins (M1 and NP) in immunity. This approach offers the prospect of broader immunity that is less compromised by antigenic variation. On the other hand, the antiviral protection mediated by memory cytotoxic T lymphocytes (CTL) appears to be short-lived.[103] It remains to be seen if protection induced by NP DNA[104] may be more lasting (see later).

Submolecular (Oligopeptide) Antigens. Definition of major antigenic sites on the HA molecule has led to investigation of oligopeptides corresponding to these sites as possible immunogens. Although synthetic oligopeptides, including epitopic sequences, have proved valuable in confirmation of suspected antigenic sites or demonstration of new ones,[105] they have thus far shown only limited immunogenicity and marginal protection in animal experiments.[106] A variety of recent approaches have included (1) the use of an HA 18mer loaded in intralamellar liposomes[107] in heterovariant (intrasubtypic) protection of mice and (2) the use of a lipid-peptide conjugate[108] and intranasal immunization of mice with synthetic peptides anchored to proteosomes.[109] However, the probable requirement of small peptides for carriers or adjuvants may continue to confound their use as a practical approach to immunization. Again, appropriate tailoring of the HA molecule or combinations of two or more peptides may provide an answer, as has apparently been the case with a synthetic vaccine for foot-and-mouth disease.[110] Such tailoring may also simulate a cryptic or novel antigen that might fortuitously possess enhanced immunogenicity. Still another approach has been to use chimeric proteins derived from relatively invariant antigens of the virus (e.g., NS1/HA2).[111]

Neuraminidase-Specific (Infection-Permissive) Vaccine. A diphasic approach to immunization against influenza entails (1) the administration of influenza viral NA, the minor surface glycoprotein, as a principal antigen, followed by (2) the definitive immunization to all viral proteins by exposure to natural infection or administration of live virus vaccine. The partial immunity induced by NA is infection permissive (i.e., allows infection) but modulates such infection by reduction of virus replication below the threshold required to induce disease (Fig. 21–3). This approach assumes the superiority of infection in inducing effective immunity but achieves its end through the capacity of the NA antigen to induce

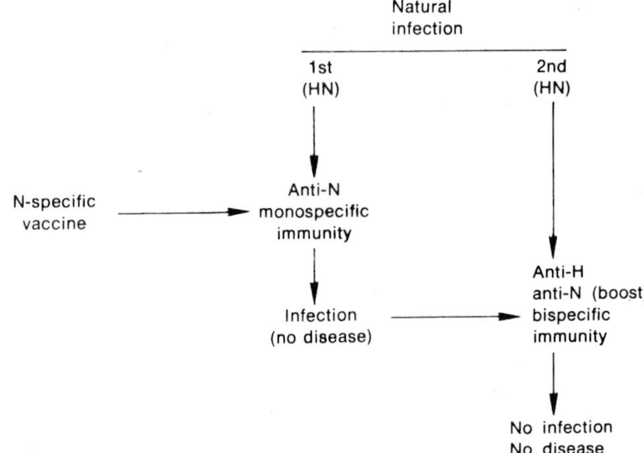

Figure 21–3. The concept of infection-permissive immunization with NA-specific (N) vaccine (see text). (From Couch RB, Kasel JA, Gerin JL, et al. Induction of partial immunity to influenza by a neuraminidase-specific vaccine. J Infect Dis 129:411–420, 1974.)

antibody that is not neutralizing and hence allows antibody-stimulating infection. Clearly, NA antibody is protective, both in animals[112] and in humans.[113, 114] It remains to be determined whether the added immunity induced by the first challenge infection after NA vaccine is lasting and superior to that which may occur after ineffective or partially immunogenic conventional (HA) vaccines. If so, and if this approach does more than merely postpone infection as is the case with conventional inactivated vaccines,[115] it can be equated with live virus vaccination in its durability and efficacy. An immediate role for NA vaccine is as a prelude to live virus vaccine of unknown attenuation. It may also prove useful in supplementing HA oligopeptide vaccines to provide immunity to both viral glycoproteins.

Adjuvants. Adjuvants were used for many years in experimental influenza vaccines and proved effective in enhancing the magnitude and duration of the immune response. Alum has been employed as an immunopotentiator but is inferior to oil adjuvants.[116] Both mineral and vegetable oils have been used as adjuvants but have not received licensure because of (1) the occurrence of local reactions, some even leading to abscess formation, and (2) their potential for carcinogenicity—especially the mineral oil formulations.

If new vaccines consist of only oligopeptide portions of the immunizing viral proteins, adjuvants, carrier proteins, or both may be essential to their immunogenicity (see earlier). Whether the peptidoglycan and other immunopotentiators[117] now under study will prove acceptable remains to be seen.

DNA Vaccines. DNA or nucleotide vaccines represent an exciting but essentially untested prospect for human immunization, in general.

Work to date with influenza virus genome–derived nucleotides appears to offer the stimulation of both B- and T-cell–mediated immunity without the need to actually infect to accomplish this end. In mice, DNA immunization has been shown to elicit protective cellular immunity against both immunodominant and immunorecessive CTL epitopes.[118] An early finding of particular interest was the induction of heterosubtypic immunity in mice by injection of plasmid DNA encoding influenza A virus NP.[104] The method and route of immunization may be of importance, as was shown in studies of ferrets immunized intradermally with DNA-coated gold beads injected with a "gene gun."[119]

Before this approach is used in humans, important safety questions must be answered, including the possibility of nucleic acid–mediated transformation or tumorigenic events, the potential for forming DNA antibodies, and the dangers of long-term expression of a foreign antigen.[120]

Live Attenuated Vaccines. These are discussed in Chapter 37.

Results of Vaccination

Nature of the Immune Response to Inactivated Viral Vaccines

Humoral Antibody Response

Kinetics and Duration of Response. Within 7 days after injection of inactivated whole-virus influenza vaccine, there is an increase in circulating antibody to the viral HA, and peripheral blood lymphocytes are primed to respond to in vitro stimulation by vaccine antigens.[121] However, most adults, even if devoid of demonstrable antibodies to the test virus, have had experience with epitopes shared by influenza strains, even of different subtypes. Therefore, response may be less brisk in truly inexperienced subjects such as children.

The duration of immune response to vaccines as measured by the persistence of humoral antibody will reflect not only prior immunizing experience with the vaccine antigens but possible antigenic stimulation by cryptic infections subsequent to vaccination. A valid indication of the half-life of vaccine-induced antibody was provided in 1976 in children vaccinated with swine influenza virus, to which antigen they had had no previous exposure or subsequent stimulation. Only 58% of the 100% in whom response had been demonstrated had detectable antibody 10 to 15 months later, compared with 91% of young adults and middle-aged adults.[122]

Assessment of actual immunity to influenza on the basis of humoral antibody levels is difficult because the presence or absence of other determinants of immunity (i.e., cell-mediated immunity) must be taken into consideration. In other words, how the antibody was acquired—whether by natural infection or by vaccination—may be important. However, Clark and colleagues[123] found that the incidence of induced infection by a challenge virus, 8 months after immunization with either live virus vaccine or inactivated virus vaccines, was *inversely* related to the titer of serum antibodies 1 month after vaccination.

For practical purposes, it is a fair assumption that immunity after inactivated influenza vaccine rarely exceeds 1 year.

Specificity of the Humoral Antibody Response to Vaccination—The Role of "Original Antigenic Sin." Antibody-mediated immunity to influenza varies in specificity in relation to the challenge virus, as shown in Table 21–5. Vaccine-induced immunity probably is never exclusively variant specific because of shared HA epitopes common to other strains within a subtype (homosubtypic or heterovariant immunity) or even between subtypes (homotypic). Heterovariant immunity has been well documented (Table 21–6), reminding us that in an emergency, "outdated" vaccine could be used, although with less than optimal effect.

Cross-reactive anamnestic response to influenza viruses has been called *original antigenic sin.*[124] In this phenomenon, an HA or NA antigen heterovariant to the one originally administered will evoke (1) the formation of antibodies specific to itself and (2) the accelerated production of antibodies to the original antigen. Thus, the primary homologous response to the new antigen may be impaired at the expense of enhanced response through recognition of shared epitopes.[125]

This response to the second (new) antigen, although partially relevant to the problem of immunizing against a new virus, is not necessarily in the best interests of the host if formation of a less relevant (i.e., heterovariant) antibody is preferentially stimulated. However, heterovariant antibody as produced in a secondary response may be sufficient in quantity and high enough in affinity[126] to provide cross-protection among intrasubtype variants. The need for change in vaccine formula may depend on the duration of subtype prevalence.[127] With progressive increase in population experience with mutants of the prevalent subtype, extensive priming occurs to create a population more responsive to heterovariant immunization.

Although heterosubtypic antibody response among HA subtypes is not uncommonly demonstrated in HI tests and has been found by enzyme-linked immunosorbent assay in infected children,[128] intersubtypic immunity is insignificant as, indeed, is attested to by the occurrence of pandemics with the introduction of new antigen subtypes.

Some studies suggest that influenza virus grown in mammalian (MDCK) cells may more closely match the antigenicity of native human virus and therefore offers advantages in greater specificity.[129–131] Evidence on this point is not yet sufficiently strong to favor the abandonment of present production of vaccine in chick embryos. Furthermore, egg-grown viral isolates, which like those in MDCK cells contain an Ile-186 amino acid substitution in the HA, should be equally effective.[129]

Local Antibody Response. Topical administration of inactivated vaccine induces the formation of secretory IgA antibody, and its administration by aerosol inhala-

Table 21–5. **CROSS-REACTIVE IMMUNITY IN INFLUENZA (A GLOSSARY)**

PRIMARY IMMUNITY	VIRUS CHALLENGE	IMMUNITY REQUIRED
A/H1N1	A/H1N1	Homologous (variant-specific)
A/H1N1	A/H1N1	Homosubtypic (heterovariant)
A/H1N1	A/H3N2	Homotypic (heterosubtypic)
A/H1N1	B	Heterotypic

From Kilbourne ED. Influenza. New York, Plenum Publishing, 1987, p 185.

Table 21–6. **EXAMPLES OF HETEROVARIANT IMMUNITY INDUCED WITH INFLUENZA A VIRUS VACCINES**

VACCINE STRAIN	VACCINE TYPE	CHALLENGE VIRUS	ANTIGENIC SIMILARITY‡	RESULT	REFERENCE
A/Hong Kong/68	I*	A/England/42/72	50%	"Marginal"	Dunn and Wormald,[207] 1973
A/Aichi/68	I	A/England/42/72	50%	60% reduction of influenza frequency	Stiver et al,[208] 1973
A/Hong Kong/68	I	A/England/42/72	50%	69% reduction of influenza frequency	Hoskins et al,[209] 1973
A/Scotland/74	L†	A/Victoria/3/75	—	Reduced frequency and severity of illness	Betts et al,[210] 1977
A/Victoria/3/75	I	A/Texas/1/77	13%	80% reduction of influenza frequency	Meiklejohn et al,[127] 1978
A/Chile/1/83	I	A/Taiwan/86	9%	38% reduction of infection	Clover et al,[211] 1991

*Inactivated whole-virus vaccine.
†Live attenuated vaccine.
‡Defined by hemagglutination inhibition tests.
Modified from Kilbourne ED. Influenza. New York, Plenum Publishing, 1987, p 296.

tion stimulates both nasal IgA and serum IgG neutralizing antibody.[132] Intramuscular injection of inactivated vaccine does not induce secretory IgA in the respiratory tract but does lead to the presence of local IgG antibody in the upper and lower respiratory tract.[133] Although the presence of IgG in the respiratory tract cannot necessarily be equated with the local induction of secretory IgA by live virus, it appears that any inadequacy of inactivated vaccine in comparison to live virus vaccines cannot be attributed categorically to the absence of local antibody response with inactivated virus vaccines.

Cellular Immunological Response to Vaccination. A cytotoxic T lymphocyte (CTL), or cytotoxic T (Tc) cell, response occurs after administration of either killed or live virus vaccines and is detectable in the absence of demonstrable antibody response.[134] Whole-virus vaccine is superior to subunit vaccines in the induction of Tc cell response. High CTL response is inversely correlated with virus shedding in experimental challenge infections in humans.[135] Induction of CTL in mice has been potentiated by a recombinant influenza vaccine in an aluminum hydroxide adjuvant[136] or by inactivated whole-virus vaccine administered with the cholera toxin β-subunit.[137]

Host Differences in Immune Response to Influenza Vaccines. Differences in immunological response to influenza vaccines are principally determined by differences in individual exposure to influenza viruses in nature. The cumulative priming induced by natural infection probably accounts for most age-related differences in host response. However, the proliferative response to influenza vaccines of both T and B lymphocytes is reduced in old age.[138] Although most studies have shown influenza vaccines to be effective in the elderly,[139, 140] some failures have been reported in carefully studied populations. In one such study, 85% of the population consisted of women,[141] and the failure might be explained by a transient T-cell defect in interleukin 2 secretion in healthy elderly women.[142] When differences in sex and nursing care are considered, reduction in mortality of about 60% can be demonstrated.[143, 144] One critical review of the subject of immunological response to influenza vaccines in the elderly concludes that (1) many studies have suffered from poor methodological design and (2) an association between advanced age per se and response to influenza vaccines has not been established.[145] A study in healthy old people also showed a lower response to H1N1 and B antigens, although not to H3N2. Interestingly, whole-virus vaccine was more immunogenic than split-product vaccine.[146] Surely, present evidence does not justify exclusion of these high-risk patients from vaccination target groups.

Curtailment of immunological response to influenza vaccines may be found in patients with neoplastic disease—particularly those receiving immunosuppressive therapy. A substantial proportion of symptomatic human immunodeficiency virus–infected patients have a suboptimal response to vaccine even after a two-dose regimen.[147] Normal response has been reported in patients 30 days or more after cessation of cancer chemotherapy.[148] There is certainly no contraindication to providing inactivated influenza virus vaccine to cancer patients or to others (e.g., those with renal disease) who have suspected immunological impairment.[149–152] Both adults and children with asthma (prime targets for influenza vaccine) tolerate vaccine well and demonstrate unimpaired immunological response.[153, 154] Vaccine response is also normal in children with cystic fibrosis.[155]

Administration with Other Vaccines

There is no contraindication to administration of inactivated influenza vaccine with other vaccines. Simultaneous administration of pneumococcal and influenza vaccines at different sites did not decrease antibody response to either vaccine, nor were reaction rates increased.[156] However, response to pneumococcal antigens was reduced with administration of a combined influenza-pneumococcal vaccine.[157] Children can receive influenza vaccine at the same time they receive other routine vaccinations, including combination diphtheria, tetanus, and pertussis vaccines (DTaP or DTP). Because influenza vaccine can cause fever when it is administered to young children, DTaP (which is less frequently associated with fever and other adverse events) is preferable.[19]

Vaccine Efficacy

Variable estimates of the efficacy and effectiveness of inactivated influenza vaccine reflect the following:

- Differences in study design and surveillance and laboratory methods
- Differences in age and health status among study populations
- Differences in the extent of circulation of influenza and other respiratory viruses
- Differences in vaccine dose
- Differences in interval between vaccine and challenge
- Variability in the antigenic match-up of vaccine and challenge viruses
- Mistaken inclusion of noninfluenza respiratory disease as a criterion for vaccine efficacy

The efficacy or effectiveness of influenza vaccines has been evaluated since the 1940s. Controlled clinical trials yield the most precise determinations of vaccine efficacy, whereas observational studies offer the advantage of studying larger populations but often underestimate the true clinical efficacy of the vaccine in preventing illness, complications, and death. In recent years, the term *efficacy* has been used to describe the findings of controlled trials, whereas the term *effectiveness* refers to the observed effect of an intervention as it is commonly used. Thus, observational studies determine vaccine effectiveness.[158] Observational studies examine relevant outcomes such as hospitalization and death due to pneumonia among nonrandomized vaccinated and unvaccinated groups during periods of known influenza activity. However, not all relevant outcomes are caused by influenza, resulting in an underestimation of vaccine efficacy. For example, if 50% of hospital admissions for pneumonia among a study population were actually caused by influenza infection, an estimated vaccine effectiveness of 30% would indicate true vaccine efficacy of 60%.[159] An example of an effectiveness study, conducted in Manitoba, Canada, is presented in Table 21–7.[158]

Controlled trials among children and young adults have shown influenza vaccine to be approximately 70 to 90% effective in preventing influenza illness when there has been a good match between the vaccine and circulating strains.[160–163] Efficacy may be somewhat lower among older and middle-aged adults but is approximately 70% when there is a good antigenic match and 40 to 60% when there are antigenic differences between the vaccine and circulating strains.[164]

Because influenza vaccination is recommended for people 65 years and older in most countries, studies assessing the benefit of vaccination in this population have usually been observational. However, in the Netherlands, influenza vaccination was not recommended on the basis of age during the 1991 to 1992 influenza season, when a double-blinded, placebo-controlled trial was conducted among people 60 years of age and older. This study showed vaccine to be 58% effective in preventing laboratory-proven influenza illness.[165] Vaccine efficacy in preventing complications or death was not examined, presumably because of the low incidence of these events among the study population.

A meta-analysis of observational studies of the effectiveness of influenza vaccine in preventing respiratory illness and hospitalization or death due to pneumonia among the elderly reported the following pooled estimates from 20 cohort studies: 56% for preventing respiratory illness, 50% for preventing pneumonia hospitalization, and 68% for preventing death. Pooled vaccine effectiveness estimates from case-control studies ranged from 32 to 45% for preventing hospitalization for pneumonia and 31 to 65% for preventing death from pneumonia or influenza.[166] Large population-based studies have shown reductions in hospitalization for pneumonia and influenza among vaccinated elderly people ranging from 31 to 72%.[167–170]

In elderly nursing home residents, although reduction of illness is relatively low (about 30%), vaccine effectiveness in reducing disease severity, hospitalization, pneumonia, and death is much higher (47 to 95%).[171, 172] Studies among nursing home populations have also shown that homes with high rates of vaccination among residents are less likely to experience influenza out-

Table 21–7. **EFFECTIVENESS OF INFLUENZA VACCINE IN PREVENTING PNEUMONIA AND INFLUENZA AND ALL RESPIRATORY CONDITIONS (FIRST POSITION IN ICD-9), MANITOBA, CANADA**

RESPIRATORY ILLNESS	OUTBREAK PERIOD	AGE GROUP (yr)	NUMBER OF MATCHED SETS	EFFECTIVENESS (%)	95% CONFIDENCE INTERVAL
Pneumonia and influenza	1982–1983	All ages	609	33	6–53
		>64	415	38	11–57
	1985–1986	All ages	530	32	6–50
		>64	412	35	8–54
All respiratory conditions	1962–1963	All ages	1447	26	7–42
		>64	984	27	7–43
	1985–1986	All ages	1361	32	15–45
		>64	1015	64	17–48

ICD-9, International Classification of Diseases, ninth revision.

From Monto AS, Ohmit SE. Effectiveness evaluation of inactivated influenza vaccines: Methods and results. In Brown LE, Hampson AW, Webster RG (eds). Options for the Control of Influenza III. Amsterdam, Elsevier Science BV, 1996, pp 93–96.

breaks, suggesting indirect protection by herd immunity.[140, 173, 174]

Complications of Vaccination

The early, relatively crude preparations of influenza virus first used in vaccines were sometimes contaminated with bacterial endotoxins and sometimes provoked severe local and systemic reactions. Present highly purified vaccines (see Table 21–3) are much less reactogenic. The rare febrile and local reactions to these endotoxin-free vaccines are related in part to the intrinsic cytotoxicity of inactivated influenza virus. Other reactions represent host variability in response related to host hypersensitivity or idiosyncrasy. When placebo-controlled and blinded studies are performed (Table 21–8), symptoms attributable to vaccination are surprisingly few.[175]

Acute Side Effects Related to Intrinsic Viral Cytotoxicity

Inactivated influenza virus can injure cells, impair cell function, or induce fever in rabbits. The nature of the toxic factor is unknown, but toxicity is reduced by solubilization of the viral lipid bilayer—the basis for the reduced toxicity of split-virus vaccine preparations. The incidence and severity of the vaccine reactions are proportional to dose.[176] Systemic reactions are less frequent in subjects who have preexisting HI antibodies. Therefore, viral surface components may participate in toxicity.[177]

Local Reactions. Erythema, pain, tenderness, and itching may develop at the site of injection 12 to 24 hours after administration of the vaccine. Rarely, reactions may proceed to induration but are infrequently incapacitating. Local reactions are more frequent in adults[178] and may have an immunological or hypersensitivity basis, in part.

Systemic Reactions. In less than 1% of adults, moderate, briefly sustained fever may appear within 48 hours of vaccination.[85] Other systemic symptoms include myalgia, arthralgia, headache, and malaise—a symptom complex that simulates influenza without the respiratory symptoms.

The frequency of febrile reactions to whole-virus vaccine in infants and children, which ranges from 8 to 50%, is prohibitive and necessitates the use of a two-dose immunization schedule and administration of split-virus vaccine.[71]

Hypersensitivity Reactions. Although the vaccine carries warnings about its use in those with allergy to egg protein (the vaccine is made in chick embryos), the majority of egg-allergic subjects can safely be immunized,[92] although IgE-specific antibody to egg white allergen may increase after vaccination.[93] Influenza vaccine should not be withheld from allergic children. Even those with positive skin test reactions to vaccine can be immunized by a rapid, divided dose schedule.[94]

Pulmonary Function. A well-controlled trial of pulmonary function in vaccinated patients with asthma showed a decrease in function in less than 5%.[94a] However, function returned to normal within 2 days, and the authors considered that the benefits of vaccination outweighed the risk.

Although influenza vaccines contain thimerosal as a preservative, most patients do not develop reactions to thimerosal when it is administered as a component of a vaccine, even when patch or intradermal tests indicate hypersensitivity. When reported, hypersensitivity to thimerosal has usually consisted of local, delayed-type hypersensitivity reactions.[19]

Neurological Complications of Vaccination

A variety of neurological syndromes have been temporally associated with influenza vaccination. These neurological manifestations include rare instances of optic neuritis, brachial neuritis, and cranial palsies. Only in the case of Guillain-Barré syndrome has a statistically significant association with influenza vaccine been established, and that was only with the swine influenza vaccine of 1976.

The Guillain-Barré syndrome is a subacute, usually symmetrical ascending paralysis reflecting segmental demyelination and polyneuronitis with associated sensory disturbances that are associated with lymphocytic infiltration of peripheral nerves. It appears as a sequel to a variety of infections or immunizations after an interval of 1 to 6 weeks and has been reported to occur sporadically also in temporal association with a number of vaccines. National surveillance for Guillain-Barré syndrome was established in 1976 in association with the National Immunization Program against the threat of swine influenza. A definitive study of approximately 1300 cases reported by state health departments to the

Table 21–8. **SIDE EFFECTS* ASSOCIATED WITH VACCINATION**

SYMPTOM	PLACEBO GROUP (%) N = 425	VACCINE GROUP (%) N = 424	P VALUE
Fever	6.1	6.2	.96
Tiredness	19.4	18.9	.93
Feeling "under the weather"	17.5	16.0	.63
Muscle aches	5.7	6.2	.84
Headaches	14.4	10.8	.14
Arm soreness	24.1	63.8	<.001

*The data represent the proportions of subjects who reported having the symptoms during the 7 days after the study injection.
From Nichol KL, Lind A, Margolis KL, et al. The effectiveness of vaccination against influenza in healthy, working adults. N Engl J Med 333:891, 1995.

Centers for Disease Control and Prevention (CDC) defined the vaccine-associated risk as 4.9 to 5.9 per million up to 8 weeks after vaccination.[179]

Subsequent surveillance between 1977 and 1981 did not show a similar increased risk after vaccination.[180, 181] However, investigations after the 1992 to 1993 and the 1993 to 1994 seasons found a relative risk for Guillain-Barré syndrome in vaccinees of 1.8.[181a] As the background incidence of the syndrome is 1 to 2 per 100,000 adults, the excess due to vaccination may be 1 to 1.6 cases per 100,000 adults. It is possible that widescale immunization with any foreign antigen might evoke the same increased incidence of disease in those individuals predisposed to this complication. Swine influenza virus is not uniquely neurotropic, nor can the vaccine alone elicit experimental Guillain-Barré syndrome in animal models.

Contraindications

Influenza vaccines are contraindicated in infants younger than 6 months because of the high incidence of febrile reactions in this age group. In children younger than 12 years, only split-virus vaccines should be used. Adults with acute febrile illnesses usually should not be vaccinated until their symptoms have abated. However, minor illnesses with or without fever should not contraindicate the use of vaccine, particularly among children with mild upper respiratory tract infection or allergic rhinitis.[19]

Vaccination of a person with a definite history of allergic reactions to eggs should be approached with caution. However, the majority of egg-allergic subjects can be safely immunized.[92] Even children with positive skin test reactions to vaccine can be immunized by a rapid, divided dose schedule.[94] Because asthmatic children are more vulnerable to influenza, every effort should be made to immunize them.

Effects of Influenza Vaccination on Drug Metabolism

Some studies have reported a depressive effect of influenza vaccines on the metabolism by the liver of certain drugs, including theophylline, aminopyrine, and phenytoin.[182–184] Other studies indicate that clinical reactions to warfarin and theophylline are rare after influenza vaccination.[185, 186] Current evidence is insufficient to interdict the use of influenza vaccines in a high-risk population because of concern about vaccine-induced impairment of drug metabolism.

Indications for Influenza Vaccine

Prevention of Mortality

Although influenza is a disease with a low case-fatality rate (less than 0.1%), it has a substantial impact on mortality because epidemics involve large numbers of people. Death from influenza usually results from secondary bacterial pneumonia but can also result from primary viral pneumonia in the absence of bacterial invasion.[187] Pneumonia and mortality are clustered in high-risk segments of the population, including the elderly and those with chronic disease or disabilities, notably cardiovascular or pulmonary types. In a study comparing rates of hospitalization during epidemic and nonepidemic seasons among people age 15 years and older, excess rates of hospitalization for pneumonia and influenza were higher among people with high-risk conditions compared with those without high-risk conditions in every age group studied.[188]

Children with deficient pulmonary function associated with cystic fibrosis, chronic asthma, and bronchopulmonary dysplasia are also vulnerable to severe manifestations of influenza and are included among the high-risk groups that have traditionally been given priority in immunization programs.

Pregnancy may also increase the risk of hospitalization during influenza epidemics. A retrospective study of hospitalizations among women of childbearing age during 17 influenza epidemics between 1974 and 1993 demonstrated that the relative risk of hospitalization for selected cardiac or respiratory conditions increased from 1.4 during the first 6 weeks of the second trimester of pregnancy to 4.7 during the last 6 weeks of the third trimester compared with rates of hospitalization among women 1 to 6 months post partum. The study also showed that the rate of hospitalization among women in the third trimester of pregnancy was comparable to that of nonpregnant women with high-risk medical conditions.[19, 189]

Specific recommendations providing rationales for vaccination have been made by the Immunization Practices Advisory Committee of the CDC.[19] These recommendations are summarized in Table 21–9. Traditionally, emphasis has been placed on the prevention of serious complications and death from influenza in subjects in the high-risk categories. However, there is increasing recognition of the enormous impact of even regional interpandemic epidemics caused by morbidity in previously healthy people.

Potency of present vaccines is such that nearly all vaccinated young adults develop antibody titers that are likely to protect them against infection by strains similar to those in the vaccine and, often, by related variants that emerge. The elderly, the very young, and patients with certain chronic diseases may develop lower postvaccination antibody titers than young adults do. Under these circumstances, however, influenza vaccine may be more effective in preventing lower respiratory tract involvement or other complications of influenza than in preventing infection and involvement of the upper respiratory tract. Influenza vaccine will not prevent primary illnesses caused by other respiratory pathogens.

Annual vaccination against influenza has been recommended since 1963 for individuals at high risk of complications and death after influenza infection (e.g., for the elderly; for patients with chronic disorders of the cardiovascular, pulmonary, and renal systems; and for people

Table 21–9. **INFLUENZA VACCINATION STRATEGIES**

Prevent influenza in patients at increased risk of complications and mortality
People 65 years of age and older
Patients with chronic diseases, especially cardiopulmonary
Immunosuppressed patients, including those with human immunodeficiency virus infection
Children and adolescents receiving long-term aspirin therapy (risk of Reye syndrome with influenza)
Women who will be beyond the first trimester of pregnancy during the influenza season
Immunize potential transmitters of infection to those at high risk for complications
Medical and paramedical personnel
Household contacts of high-risk people
Prevent morbidity
Community workers (e.g., firefighters and police officers)
People subject to high exposure to the virus (e.g., those in boarding schools, colleges, and nursing homes as well as medical personnel)
People considering foreign or frequent domestic travel (increased risk of infection)
Any people who wish to reduce their risk of acquiring influenza

with metabolic diseases, severe anemia, and compromised immune function). These groups have been identified primarily by reviews of death certificate data, supported by hospital-based or population-based studies.[38] Each group encompasses patients along a continuum of underlying general health. Within each broadly defined high-risk category, some people may be more likely than others to develop severe complications from influenza infection.

Investigations of influenza outbreaks in nursing homes, for example, have demonstrated attack rates as high as 60%, with case-fatality ratios of 30% or more.[161] Chronic diseases and other debilitating conditions are common among nursing home residents, and spread of infection can often be explosive in such relatively crowded and closed environments. Retrospective studies of noninstitutionalized patients also suggest that chronic underlying diseases, particularly those that affect the cardiovascular and pulmonary systems, may contribute more than age alone to the severity of illness. Since influenza infections are also known to invoke abnormalities in gas exchange and peripheral airways dysfunction in adults, children with compromised pulmonary function, including those with cystic fibrosis, chronic asthma, and bronchopulmonary dysplasia, as well as neonates in intensive care units, may also be at higher risk of severe illness, although firm evidence is lacking. Children with congenital heart disease may also be considered at high risk, because respiratory viruses in general often produce severe infections in this population.

Target Groups for Vaccination

On the basis of the aforementioned observations, groups for which active, targeted vaccination efforts are most necessary are as follows:

- People 65 years of age or older
- Residents of nursing homes and other chronic care facilities that house people of any age who have chronic medical conditions
- Adults and children who have chronic disorders of the pulmonary or cardiovascular systems, including children with asthma
- Adults and children who have required regular medical follow-up or hospitalization during the preceding year because of chronic metabolic diseases (including diabetes mellitus), renal dysfunction, hemoglobinopathies, or immunosuppression
- Children and teenagers (aged 6 months to 18 years) who are receiving long-term aspirin therapy and therefore might be at risk for developing Reye syndrome after influenza
- Women who will be in the second or third trimester of pregnancy during the influenza season

Some of those at high risk for influenza-related complications may have a poor immunological response to influenza vaccine. Protection of such people might be improved by reducing the chances of exposure from their caregivers. There is evidence to suggest that medical personnel can transmit influenza infections to their high-risk patients while they are themselves incubating infections, undergoing subclinical infections, or working, despite the existence of mild symptoms.[190, 191] In many winters, nosocomial outbreaks of influenza are reported. People who have contact with high-risk patients, including providers of home care, should receive influenza vaccinations annually. For the same reasons, household members (including children) of those in high-risk groups should also be vaccinated every year.

Prevention of Morbidity

Even in the absence of lower respiratory tract complications, influenza is not a trivial disease. Therefore, it may seem surprising that except in the military, prevention of morbidity has received only secondary consideration as an objective of influenza vaccination. But general immunization of the population is neither advisable nor feasible given (1) the continuous antigenic variation of the virus and (2) the impermanence of immunity from inactivated virus vaccine. Furthermore, there is evidence in boarding school populations that annual vaccination may simply postpone ultimate infection.[115] However, in another study of sequential vaccination in a free-living population, vaccine efficacy appeared to be somewhat greater after repeated annual vaccination than after first administration.[192] Nevertheless, influenza vaccine has an important role in the prevention of disease in certain categories of healthy people as follows:

- Hospital and other medical personnel in contact with patients. Immunization of this group has two purposes: reduction of virus transmission from infected workers to vulnerable patients and prevention of absenteeism, especially during epidemics when sharp increases in hospitalization rates can occur.

- Personnel indispensable to military or community service, such as police and firefighters
- Any people, such as travelers, and others who may not have good access to medical care and in whom influenza would constitute an intolerable burden or inconvenience

PUBLIC HEALTH CONSIDERATIONS

Epidemiological Results of Vaccination

Unlike the situation with some other vaccine-preventable diseases, changing rates of morbidity and mortality among the general population cannot be used as reliable measures of the effectiveness of influenza vaccine. The most important reason for this is that the impact of influenza varies greatly from one season to another, depending on the intensity of virus circulation and the susceptibility of the general population and specific age groups to the influenza strain or strains that circulate during a given season. If age-specific vaccination rates and vaccine efficacy were the same each year, rates of influenza-associated morbidity and mortality would still vary widely from one year to another.

This is most easily illustrated by examining influenza-associated mortality in the United States, because unlike the case with influenza-associated morbidity, methods have been established to provide reliable national estimates on an ongoing basis. During the present interpandemic period since 1968–1969, excess mortality attributed to a single influenza season in the United States has ranged from more than 47,000 deaths to no detectable excess.[37] During this period, the highest death rates have occurred during epidemics when type A/H3N2 viruses have predominated, but there is also wide variability in death rates from one H3N2 season to another, depending in large part on the extent to which the epidemic strain has drifted from those that circulated during previous seasons. Furthermore, the number of deaths caused by pneumonia and influenza in the United States has been increasing since the 1980s after declining during the 1960s and 1970s. From 1979 to 1992, pneumonia and influenza death rates among people 65 years and older increased 44%, from 146 to 209 per 100,000 population; the majority of these deaths were not associated with influenza epidemics.[193] Thus, although rates of influenza vaccination among the age group 65 years and older in the United States have increased from 23% in 1885 to 55% in 1994,[19] it has not been possible to demonstrate a corresponding decrease in mortality using vital statistics data. Instead, the epidemiological impact of vaccination must be assessed by indirect methods for individual seasons, extrapolating from the types of vaccine efficacy studies described earlier.

A mathematical model developed by Carrat and Valleron[194] was used to estimate the number of influenza-related deaths among the elderly in France that were prevented by vaccination during the period 1980 to 1990. After the number of influenza-associated deaths during each influenza season was estimated by the use of vital statistics data, formulas were developed to estimate deaths avoided on the basis of varying rates of vaccination and vaccine efficacy. Estimates of influenza-associated death rates per season ranged from 28 per 100,000 to 482 per 100,000 during the 10-year period. For the same time period, it was estimated that influenza vaccination prevented between 7 deaths per 100,000 in 1981 to 1982 and 697 deaths per 100,000 during the severe epidemic of 1989 to 1990. The range of estimated deaths prevented varied depending on the intensity of the epidemic, the rates of vaccine coverage in the elderly population, and the estimated vaccine efficacy each year.

Although the epidemiological result of influenza vaccination cannot be directly assessed with use of national vital statistics data, it has been assessed at the community level during prospective studies. Although routine vaccination of school-aged children has not been practiced in most countries, studies have shown that vaccination of schoolchildren can decrease rates of influenza infection not only among the children themselves but also among their teachers and household members.[195, 196] In Japan, an aggressive policy of immunization of schoolchildren was pursued beginning in the mid-1970s. Detailed, controlled studies of efficacy were not done, but it was shown that when vaccination rates exceeded 50 to 70%, closing of classes on the basis of 33% absenteeism was reduced.[197] Although findings have not been consistent, an organized approach to vaccination among adults in the workplace has also shown a significant reduction in morbidity among vaccinated personnel.[175, 198, 199] Table 21–10 gives data on a study of the benefits of influenza vaccination in healthy working adults.[175]

Cost-Benefit Studies

Cost-benefit studies and other economic evaluations of influenza vaccination have produced different conclusions depending on different estimations of and assumptions about relevant factors, such as (1) the population of interest, (2) influenza attack rates, (3) the cost of vaccine and its administration, (4) vaccine efficacy, (5) direct costs of medical care, and (6) indirect costs of illness. One of the most rigorous economic analyses of the value of influenza vaccination was conducted by the Office of Technology Assessment of the United States Congress.[53] This study, published in 1981 and using 1978 economic data, concluded that influenza vaccination was cost-saving for people 65 years and older and would cost $10 per vaccination per year of healthy life gained for people of any age with high-risk medical conditions. Estimates of the cost of vaccination per year of healthy life for the general population ranged from $23 to $258, with the cost increasing with decreasing age.

A more recent study that did not take indirect costs of influenza into account concluded that influenza vaccination provided to members of a health maintenance organization (HMO) saved the HMO $6.11 for each high-risk elderly member vaccinated. The HMO incurred a net cost of $4.82 per vaccination of non–high-risk elderly but a net savings of $1.10 for all elderly people.[200]

Table 21–10. **HEALTH-RELATED BENEFITS ASSOCIATED WITH VACCINATION IN HEALTHY WORKING ADULTS**

STUDY OUTCOME	RATE PER 100 SUBJECTS* Placebo Group	Vaccine Group	DIFFERENCE (95% CI)	VACCINE EFFECTIVENESS (%)†	P VALUE
Primary					
Episodes of upper respiratory illness	140	105	35 (17–53)	25	<.001
Days of sick leave due to upper respiratory illness	122	70	52 (21–84)	43	.001
Visits to physicians' offices for upper respiratory illness	55	31	24 (8–40)	44	.004
Secondary					
Days of upper respiratory illness	974	780	194 (15–373)	20	.034
Days of sick leave due to all illnesses	203	129	74 (23–125)	36	.004

*The values mean cumulative totals for the 4-month period from December 1, 1994, through March 31, 1995 (the influenza season).
†Vaccine effectiveness was calculated as the difference in the rates of outcome variables (placebo group − vaccine group) divided by the rate in the placebo group, multiplied by 100.
CI, confidence interval.
From Nichol KL, Lind A, Margolis KL, et al. The effectiveness of vaccination against influenza in healthy, working adults. N Engl J Med 333:892, 1995.

In a Canadian study to estimate the cost-benefit of vaccinating the elderly, the net benefit per person vaccinated was calculated by use of best estimates (base case), and a sensitivity analysis was performed in which a range of values for key variables such as attack rate, vaccine efficacy, and healthcare costs were used. The base case estimated a net benefit of $3.86 (1982 Canadian dollars) per vaccination; the best case yielded an estimated benefit of $53.52 per vaccination. Not surprisingly, vaccination was not cost-saving under the worst case explored, with a net cost of $6.82.[201]

Although most economic evaluations of the costs and benefits of influenza vaccination have focused on the elderly and other high-risk populations, in recent years there has been increasing interest in the economic benefits of vaccinating other age groups, particularly working-age adults. An analysis of the expected benefits of influenza vaccination of the employed adult population of France concluded that vaccination would be cost-saving from a societal and personal perspective under most scenarios explored. As with other similar analyses, indirect costs of influenza contributed greatly to the overall cost-benefit estimates.[202] Another type of economic evaluation of the benefits of vaccinating healthy, working adults in the United States estimated the cost savings to be $46.85 per person vaccinated.

Whereas numerous studies and economic analyses have concluded that influenza vaccination can be cost-saving for a variety of populations under different sets of circumstances, Nicholson[203] has pointed out that results of such analyses from one country may not be generalizable to other countries. Although there is no reason to believe that overall attack rates differ from one country to another, other factors that influence costs and benefits may vary, and Nicholson has expressed the opinion that influenza vaccine cost-effectiveness needs to be assessed country by country.

Universal (Mass) Vaccination for the Prevention of Pandemic Morbidity

Present policy for vaccination addresses only the problems of interpandemic influenza, as it occurs in a partially immune population in focal epidemics. The irregular appearance of major antigenic variants confronts the entire population, few of whom will now have specific immunity to the new virus, irrespective of age, with the risk of disease and the prospect of attack rates of 30 to 50%.

In this situation, the potential impact on the community is staggering. In 1976, when swine influenza threatened, it was estimated in economic terms at $6 billion.[204] Past efforts to modify pandemics in 1957 and 1968 were essentially unavailing,[205] and organized efforts such as the one mounted in 1976 with the National Immunization Program for swine influenza will be necessary to ensure production of an adequate supply of vaccines, effect their proper distribution, and carry out the vaccination procedure. It is clear from the 1976 experience that optimal immunization may require more than a single dose of vaccine, but earlier experience in 1957 indicates that even a single dose of suboptimal vaccine will have some protective effect.[83] The choice (i.e., the artificial induction of primary immunization for the new virus through vaccination or through uncontrolled natural infection) is a simple one on medical grounds. The implementation of mass vaccination calls for a solution to the complex sociological and political problems that plagued the "swine flu" program.[206]

SUMMARY

Inactivated influenza vaccines are safe and usually effective in the prevention of influenza and its complications. Because they are narrowly immunogenic, they soon become obsolete as the nature of the circulating virus changes. Irrespective of such changes, inactivated influenza vaccines do not induce durable immunity, so repeated vaccination is obligatory in those people unusually susceptible to the life-threatening effects of the disease. Future vaccines must meet the need for broader and more sustained immunity.

REFERENCES

1. Kilbourne ED. The influenza viruses and influenza—an introduction. In Kilbourne ED (ed). The Influenza Virus and Influenza. New York, Academic Press, 1975, p 1.

2. Thompson T. Annals of Influenza or Epidemic Catarrhal Fever in Great Britain from 1510 to 1837. London, Sydenham Society, 1852.
3. Creighton C. A History of Epidemics in Britain, AD 664–1666. New York, Cambridge University Press, 1891.
4. Smith W, Andrewes CH, Laidlaw PP. A virus obtained from influenza patients. Lancet 2:66–68, 1933.
5. Schulman JL, Khakpour M, Kilbourne ED. Protective effects of specific immunity to viral neuraminidase on influenza virus infection of mice. J Virol 2:778–786, 1968.
6. Davies HW, Appleyard G, Cunningham P, Pereira MS. The use of a continuous cell line for the isolation of influenza viruses. Bull World Health Organ 56:991–993, 1978.
7. Tobita K, Sugiura A, Enomoto C, Furuyama M. Plaque assay and primary isolation of influenza A viruses in an established line of canine kidney cells (MDCK) in the presence of trypsin. Med Microbiol Immunol 162:9–14, 1975.
8. McQuillin J, Madeley CR, Kendal AP. Monoclonal antibodies for the rapid diagnosis of influenza A and B virus infections by immunofluorescence. Lancet 2:911–914, 1985.
9. Waner JL, Todd SJ, Shalaby H, et al. Comparison of Directigen FLU-A with viral isolation and direct immunofluorescence for the rapid detection and identification of influenza A virus. J Clin Microbiol 29:479–482, 1991.
10. Douglas RG. Drug therapy: Prophylaxis and treatment of influenza. N Engl J Med 322:443–450, 1990.
11. Tominack RL, Hayden FG. Rimantadine hydrochloride and amantadine hydrochloride use in influenza A virus infections. Infect Dis Clin North Am 1:459–478, 1987.
12. Hay AJ. The action of adamantanamines against influenza A viruses: Inhibition of the M2 ion channel protein. Semin Virol 3:21–30, 1992.
13. Clover RD, Crawford SA, Abell TD, et al. Effectiveness of rimantadine prophylaxis of children within families. Am J Dis Child 140:706–709, 1986.
14. Dolin R, Reichman RC, Madore HP, et al. A controlled trial of amantadine and rimantadine in the prophylaxis of influenza A infection. N Engl J Med 307:580–584, 1982.
15. Galbraith AW, Oxford JS, Schild GC, et al. Study of 1-adamantanamine hydrochloride used prophylactically during the Hong Kong influenza epidemic in the family environment. Bull World Health Organ 41:677–682, 1969.
16. Monto AS, Gunn RA, Bandyk MG, et al. Prevention of Russian influenza by amantadine. JAMA 241:1003–1007, 1979.
17. Pettersson RF, Hellstrom PE, Penttinen K, et al. Evaluation of amantadine in the prophylaxis of influenza A (H1N1) virus infection: A controlled field trial among young adults and high-risk patients. J Infect Dis 142:377–383, 1980.
18. Van Voris LP, Newell PM. Antivirals for the chemoprophylaxis and treatment of influenza. Semin Respir Infect 7:61–70, 1992.
19. Centers for Disease Control and Prevention. Prevention and control of influenza: Recommendations of the Advisory Committee on Immunization Practices (ACIP). MMWR Morb Mortal Weekly Rep 46(RR-9):1–25, 1997.
20. Arden NH, Patriarca PA, Fasano MB, et al. The roles of vaccination and amantadine in controlling an outbreak of influenza A(H3N2) in a nursing home. Arch Intern Med 148:865–868, 1988.
21. O'Donoghue JM, Ray CG, Terry DW Jr, et al. Prevention of nosocomial influenza infection with amantadine. Am J Epidemiol 97:276–282, 1973.
22. Payler DK, Purdham PA. Influenza A prophylaxis with amantadine in a boarding school. Lancet 1:502–504, 1984.
23. Gomolin IH, Leib HB, Arden NH, Sherman FT. Control of influenza outbreaks in the nursing home: Guidelines for diagnosis and management. J Am Geriatr Soc 43:71–74, 1995.
24. Van Voris LP, Betts RF, Hayden FG, et al. Successful treatment of naturally occurring influenza A/USSR/77 H1N1. JAMA 245:1128–1131, 1981.
25. Wingfield WL, Pollack D, Grunert RR. Therapeutic efficacy of amantadine HCl and rimantadine HCl in naturally occurring influenza A2 respiratory illness in man. N Engl J Med 281:579–584, 1969.
26. Younkin SW, Betts RF, Roth FK, et al. Reduction in fever and symptoms in young adults with influenza A/Brazil/78 H1N1 infection after treatment with aspirin or amantadine. Antimicrob Agents Chemother 23:577–582, 1983.
27. Hayden FG, Belshe RB, Clover RD, et al. Emergence and apparent transmission of rimantadine-resistant influenza A virus in families. N Engl J Med 321:1696–1702, 1989.
28. Hayden FG, Hay AJ. Emergence and transmission of influenza A viruses resistant to amantadine and rimantadine. Curr Top Microbiol Immunol 176:120–130, 1992.
29. Mast EE, Harmon MW, Gravenstein S, et al. Emergence and possible transmission of amantadine-resistant viruses during nursing home outbreaks of influenza A(H3N2). Am J Epidemiol 13:988–997, 1991.
30. Belshe RB, Burk B, Newman F, et al. Resistance of influenza A virus to amantadine and rimantadine: Results of one decade of surveillance. J Infect Dis 159:430–435, 1989.
31. Ziegler T, Hemphill M, Zeigler ML, et al. Rimantadine resistance of influenza A viruses: An international surveillance. Presented at the 7th Conference of the International Society for Antiviral Research; Charleston, SC; March 1994.
32. Monto AS, Arden NH. Implications of viral resistance to amantadine in control of influenza A. Clin Infect Dis 15:362–367, 1992.
33. Hayden FG. Amantadine and rimantadine: Clinical aspects. In Richman D (ed). Antiviral Drug Resistance. New York, John Wiley & Sons, 1996, pp 59–77.
34. Hayden FG, Loba M, Jussey EK, Eason CU. Efficacy of intranasal GG167 in experimental human influenza A and B virus infection. In Brown LE, Hampston AW, Webster RG (eds). Options for the Control of Influenza III. Amsterdam, Elsevier Science BV 1996, pp 718–725.
35. Collins SD, Frost WH, Gover M, Sydenstricker E. Mortality from influenza and pneumonia in 50 large cities of the United States, 1910–1929. Public Health Rep 45:2277–2329, 1930.
36. Farr W. Vital Statistics. London, Office of the Sanitary Institute, 1885.
37. Simonsen L, Clarke MJ, Williamson GD, et al. The impact of influenza epidemics on mortality: Introducing a severity index. Am J Public Health 87:1944–1950, 1997.
38. Eickhoff TC, Sherman IL, Serfling RE. Observations on excess mortality associated with epidemic influenza. JAMA 176:776–782, 1961.
39. Crosby AW. America's Forgotten Pandemic: The Influenza of 1919. Cambridge, Cambridge University Press, 1989.
40. Simonsen L, Schonberger LB, Stroup DF, et al. The impact of influenza on mortality in the USA. In Brown LE, Hampson AW, Webster RG (eds). Options for the Control of Influenza III. Amsterdam, Elsevier Science BV, 1996, pp 26–33.
41. Freeman DW, Barno A. Deaths from Asian influenza associated with pregnancy. Am J Obstet Gynecol 78:1172–1175, 1959.
42. Schoenbaum SC, Weinstein L. Respiratory infection in pregnancy. Clin Obstet Gynecol 22:293–300, 1979.
43. Lui KJ, Kendal AP. Impact of influenza epidemics on mortality in the United States from October 1972 to May 1985. Am J Public Health 77:712–716, 1987.
44. Noble GR. Epidemiological and clinical aspects of influenza. In Beare AS (ed). Basic and Applied Influenza Research. Boca Raton, FL, CRC Press, 1982, pp 11–50.
45. Perrotta DM, Decker M, Glezen WP. Acute respiratory disease hospitalizations as a measure of impact of epidemic influenza. Am J Epidemiol 122:468–476, 1985.
46. Taber LH, Paredes A, Glezen WP, Couch RB. Infection with influenza A/Victoria virus in Houston families, 1976. J Hyg (Lond) 86:303–313, 1981.
46a. Glezen WP. Emerging infections: Pandemic influenza. Epidemiol Rev 18:64–76, 1996.
46b. Glezen WP, Taber LH, Frank AL, et al. Influenza virus infections in infants. Pediatr Infect Dis J 16:1065–1068, 1997.
47. Jennings LC, Miles JAR. A study of acute respiratory disease in the community of Port Chalmers. II. Influenza A/Port Chalmers/1/73: Intrafamilial spread and the effect of antibodies to the surface antigens. J Hyg (Lond) 81:67–75, 1978.
48. Barker WH, Mullooly JP. Impact of epidemic type A influenza in a defined adult population. Am J Epidemiol 112:798–813, 1980.
49. Glezen WP, Couch RB, Six HR. The influenza herald wave. Am J Epidemiol 116:589–598, 1982.

50. Couch RB, Kasel WP, Glezen TR, et al. Influenza: Its control in persons and populations. J Infect Dis 153:431–440, 1986.
51. Glezen WP. Serious morbidity and mortality associated with influenza epidemics. Epidemiol Rev 4:25–44, 1982.
52. Retailliau HF, Storch GA, Curtis AC, et al. The epidemiology of influenza B in a rural setting in 1977. Am J Epidemiol 109:639–649, 1979.
53. Office of Technology Assessment, US Congress. Cost-Effectiveness of Influenza Vaccination. Washington, DC, US Government Printing Office, 1982.
54. Kavet J. Vaccine utilization: Trends in the implementation of public policy in the U.S.A. In Selby P (ed). Virus Vaccines Strategy. New York, Academic Press, 1976, pp 297–308.
55. Schoenbaum SC. Economic impact of influenza: The individual's perspective. Am J Med 82(suppl 6A):26–30, 1987.
56. Kilbourne ED. A race with evolution—a history of influenza vaccines. In Plotkin S, Fantini B (eds). Vaccinia, Vaccination and Vaccinology: Jenner, Pasteur and Their Successors. Paris, Elsevier, 1996, pp 183–188.
57. Chenoweth A, Waltz AD, Stokes J Jr, et al. Active immunization with the viruses of human and swine influenza. Am J Dis Child 52:757, 1936.
58. Smith W. The influenza problem. St. Mary's Hsp Gazette 43:112–120, 1937.
59. Taylor RM, Dreguss M. An experiment in immunization against influenza with a formaldehyde-inactivated virus. Am J Hyg 31:31–35, 1940.
60. Williams MS, Wood JM. A brief history of inactivated influenza virus vaccines. In Hannoun C (ed). Options for the Control of Influenza II. Amsterdam, Elsevier Science Publishers, 1993, pp 169–170.
61. Reimer CB, Maker RS, van Frank RM, et al. Purification of large quantities of influenza virus by density gradient centrifugation. J Virol 1:1207–1216, 1967.
62. Hoyle L. Structure of the influenza virus. J Hyg 50:229–245, 1952.
63. Kilbourne ED. Influenza 1970: Unquestioned answers and unanswered questions. Arch Environ Health 21:284–292, 1970.
64. Kilbourne ED, Murphy JS. Genetic studies of influenza viruses. I. Viral morphology and growth capacity as exchangeable genetic traits. Rapid in ovo adaptation of early passage Asian strain isolates by combination with PR8. J Exp Med 11:387–406, 1960.
65. Kilbourne ED. Future influenza vaccines and the use of genetic recombinants. Bull World Health Organ 41:643–645, 1969.
66. Ghendon Y. Influenza surveillance. Bull World Health Organ 69:509–515, 1991.
67. Crawford CR, Faiza Mukhlis FA, Jennings R, et al. Use of zwitterionic detergent for the preparation of an influenza virus vaccine. 1. Preparation and characterization of disrupted virions. Vaccine 2:193–198, 1984.
68. Jennings R, Smith TL, Spencer RC, et al. Inactivated influenza virus vaccines in man: A comparative study of subunit and split vaccines using two methods for assessment of antibody responses. Vaccine 2:75–80, 1984.
69. Webster RG, Kasel JA, Couch RB, Laver WG. Influenza virus subunit vaccines. II. Immunogenicity and original sin in humans. J Infect Dis 134:48–58, 1976.
70. Bernstein DI, Cherry JD. Clinical reactions and antibody responses to influenza vaccines. Am J Dis Child 137:622–626, 1983.
71. Gross PA, Ennis FA, Gaerlan PF, et al. A controlled double-blind comparison of reactogenicity, immunogenicity, and protective efficacy of whole virus and split-product influenza vaccines in children. J Infect Dis 136:623–632, 1977.
72. Grossebauer K, Langmaack H, Schmidt B, Kucchler R. Enhancement and neutralisation of pyrogenicity of influenza viruses by biologically active substances. Arch Ges Virusforsch 28:151–164, 1969.
73. Siegert R, Braune P. The pyrogens of myxoviruses. II. Resistance of influenza A pyrogens to heat, ultraviolet and chemical treatment. Virology 24:218–224, 1964.
74. Potter CW. Inactivated virus vaccine. In Beare AS (ed). Basic and Applied Influenza Research. Boca Raton, FL, CRC Press, 1982, pp 119–158.
75. Kilbourne ED, Schulman JL, Schild GC, et al. Correlated studies of a recombinant influenza-virus vaccine. I. Derivation and characterization of virus and vaccine. J Infect Dis 124:449–462, 1971.
76. Baez M, Palese P, Kilbourne ED. Gene composition of high-yielding influenza vaccine strains obtained by recombination. J Infect Dis 141:362–365, 1980.
77. Klimov A, Ghendon Y, Zavadova H, et al. High reproduction capacity of recombinants between H3N2 human influenza and fowl plague viruses is due to the gene coding for M proteins. Acta Virol 27:434–438, 1983.
78. Schulman JL, Palese P. Biological properties of recombinants of A/Hong Kong and A/PR8 viruses: Effects of genes for matrix protein and nucleoprotein in virus yield in embryonated eggs. In Mahy BWJ, Barry RD (eds). Negative Strand Viruses and the Host Cell. New York, Academic Press, 1978, pp 663–674.
79. Kilbourne ED. Genetic dimorphism in influenza viruses: Characterization of stably associated hemagglutinin mutants differing in antigenicity and biological properties. Proc Natl Acad Sci USA 75:6258–6262, 1978.
80. Downie JC. A genetic and monoclonal analysis of high-yielding reassortants of influenza A virus used for human vaccines. J Biol Stand 12:101–110, 1984.
81. Pemberton RM, Jennings R, Smith TL. Morphology and antigenicity studies on reassortant influenza (H3N2) viruses for use in inactivated vaccines. J Hyg (Lond) 94:229–239, 1985.
82. Goodeve AC, Jennings R, Potter CW. Reassortants of influenza B viruses for use in vaccines: An evaluation. Arch Virol 83:169–179, 1985.
83. Blumenfeld HL, Kilbourne ED, Louria DB, Rogers DE. Studies on influenza in the pandemic of 1957–58. I. An epidemiologic, clinical and serologic investigation of an intrahospital epidemic, with a note on vaccination efficacy. J Clin Invest 38:199–212, 1959.
84. Hirst GK, Rickard ER, Whitman L, Horsfall FL Jr. Antibody response of human beings following vaccination with influenza viruses. J Exp Med 75:495–511, 1942.
85. Mostow SR, Schoenbaum SC, Dowdle WR, et al. Studies on inactivated influenza vaccines. II. Effect of increasing dosage on antibody response and adverse reactions in man. Am J Epidemiol 92:248–256, 1970.
86. Salk JE. Reactions to concentrated influenza vaccines. J Immunol 58:369–395, 1948.
87. Powers RD, Hayden FG, Samuelson J, Gwaltney JM. Immune response of adults to sequential influenza vaccination. J Med Virol 14:169–175, 1984.
88. Waldman RH, Mann JJ, Small PA. Immunization against influenza. JAMA 207:520–524, 1969.
89. Shore SL, Potter CW, Stuart-Harris CH. Antibody response to inactivated influenza vaccine given by different routes in patients with chronic bronchopulmonary disease. Thorax 28:721–728, 1973.
90. Rubin FL, Jackson GG. A new subunit influenza vaccine: Acceptability compared with standard vaccines and effect of dose on antigenicity. J Infect Dis 125:656–664, 1972.
91. Khan AS, Polezhaev F, Vasiljeva R, et al. Comparison of US inactivated split-virus and Russian live attenuated, cold-adapted trivalent influenza vaccines in Russian schoolchildren. J Infect Dis 173:453–456, 1996.
92. Bierman CW, Shapiro GG, Pierson WE, et al. Safety of influenza vaccination in allergic children. J Infect Dis 136:S652–S655, 1977.
93. Yamane N, Uemura H. Serological examination of IgE- and IgG-specific antibodies to egg protein during influenza virus immunization. Epidemiol Infect 100:291–299, 1988.
94. Murphy KR, Strunk RC. Safe administration of influenza vaccine in asthmatic children sensitive to egg proteins. J Pediatr 106:931–933, 1985.
94a. Nicholson KG, Nguyen-Van-Tam S, Ala'eldin HA, et al. Randomised placebo-controlled crossover trial on effect of inactivated influenza vaccine on pulmonary function in asthma. Lancet 351:326–331, 1998.
95. Gething MJ, Sambrook J. Cell surface expression of influenza haemagglutinin from a cloned DNA copy of the RNA gene. Nature 293:620–625, 1981.
96. Gething MJ, Sambrook J. Construction of influenza haemagglutinin genes that code for intracellular and secreted forms of the protein. Nature 300:598–603, 1982.

97. Hartman JR, Nayak DP, Fareed GC. Human influenza virus hemagglutinin is expressed in monkey cells using simian virus 40 vectors. Proc Natl Acad Sci USA 79:233–237, 1982.
98. Jabbar MA, Sivasubramanian N, Nayak DP. Influenza viral (A/WSN/33) hemagglutinin is expressed and glycosylated in yeast, *Saccharomyces cerevisiae*. Proc Natl Acad Sci USA 82:2019–2023, 1985.
99. Sveda MM, Lai CJ. Functional expression in primate cells of cloned DNA coding for the hemagglutinin surface glycoprotein of influenza virus. Proc Natl Acad Sci USA 78:5488–5492, 1981.
100. Kuroda K, Groener A, Frese K, et al. Synthesis of biologically active influenza virus hemagglutinin in insect larvae. J Virol 63:1677–1685, 1989.
101. Price PM, Reichelderfer CF, Johansson BE, Kilbourne ED. Complementation of recombinant baculoviruses by coinfection with wild-type virus facilitates production in insect larvae of antigenic proteins of hepatitis B virus and influenza virus. Proc Natl Acad Sci USA 86:1453–1456, 1989.
102. Lakey DL, Treanor JJ, Betts RF, et al. Recombinant baculovirus influenza A hemagglutinin vaccines are well tolerated and immunogenic in healthy adults. J Infect Dis 174:838–841, 1996.
103. Rimmelzwaan GF, Osterhaus ADME. Cytotoxic T lymphocyte memory: Role in cross-protective immunity against influenza? Vaccine 13:703–705, 1995.
104. Ulmer JB, Donnelly JJ, Parker SE, et al. Heterologous protection against influenza by injection of DNA encoding a viral protein. Science 259:1745–1749, 1993.
105. Wilson IA, Niman HL, Houghten RA, et al. The structure of an antigenic determinant in a protein. Cell 37:767–778, 1984.
106. Shapira M, Jibson M, Muller G, Arnon R. Immunity and protection against influenza virus by synthetic peptide corresponding to antigenic sites of hemagglutinin. Proc Natl Acad Sci USA 81:2461–2465, 1984.
107. Naruse H, Ogasawara K, Kaneda R, et al. A potential peptide vaccine against two different strains of influenza virus isolated at intervals of about 10 years. Proc Natl Acad Sci USA 92:9588–9592, 1994.
108. Friede M, Muller S, Briand JP, et al. Selective induction of protection against influenza virus infection in mice by a lipid-peptide conjugate delivered in liposomes. Vaccine 12:791–797, 1994.
109. Levi R, About-Pirak E, Leclerc C, et al. Intranasal inmmunization of mice against influenza with synthetic peptides anchored to proteosomes. Vaccine 13:1353–1359, 1995.
110. DiMarchi R, Brooke G, Gale C, et al. Protection of cattle against foot-and-mouth disease by a synthetic peptide. Science 232:639–641, 1986.
111. Mbawuike IN, Dillon SB, Demuth SG, et al. Influenza A subtype cross-protection after immunization of outbred mice with a purified chimeric NS_1HA_2 influenza virus protein. Vaccine 12:1340–1348, 1994.
112. Allan WH, Madeley CR, Kendal AP. Studies with avian influenza A viruses: Cross protection experiments in chickens. J Gen Virol 12:79–84, 1971.
113. Beutner KR, Chow T, Rubi E, et al. Evaluation of a neuraminidase specific influenza A virus vaccine in children: Antibody responses and effects on two successive outbreaks of natural infection. J Infect Dis 140:844–850, 1979.
114. Couch RB, Kasel JA, Gerin JL, et al. Induction of partial immunity to influenza by a neuraminidase-specific vaccine. J Infect Dis 129:411–420, 1974.
115. Hoskins TW, Davies JR, Smith AJ, et al. Assessment of inactivated influenza A vaccine after three outbreaks of influenza A at Christ's Hospital. Lancet 1:33–35, 1979.
116. Woodhour AF, Friedman A, Tytell AA, Hilleman MR. Hyperpotentiation by synthetic double-stranded RNA of antibody responses to influenza virus vaccine in adjuvant 65 (33983). Proc Soc Exp Biol 131:809–817, 1969.
117. Stewart-Tull DES. Immunopotentiating conjugates. Vaccine 3:40–44, 1985.
118. Fu T-M, Friedman A, Ulmer JB, et al. Protective cellular immunity: Cytotoxic T-lymphocyte responses against dominant and recessive epitopes of influenza virus nucleoprotein induced by DNA immunization. J Virol 71:2715–2721, 1997.
119. Webster RG, Fynan EF, Santoro JC, et al. Protection of ferrets against influenza challenge with a DNA vaccine to the haemagglutinin. Vaccine 12:1495–1498, 1994.
120. Robertson JS. Safety considerations for nucleic acid vaccines. Vaccine 12:1526–1528, 1994.
121. Mitchell DM, Fitzharris P, Knight RA, Schild GC. Kinetics of specific in vitro antibody production following influenza immunization. Clin Exp Immunol 48:491–498, 1982.
122. Lerman SJ, Wright PF, Patil KD. Antibody decline in children following A/New Jersey/76 influenza virus immunization. J Pediatr 96:271–274, 1980.
123. Clark A, Potter CW, Jennings R, et al. A comparison of live and inactivated influenza A (H1N1) virus vaccines. J Hyg (Lond) 90:361–370, 1983.
124. Francis T, Davenport FM, Hennessy AV. A serological recapitulation of human infection with different strains of influenza virus. Trans Assoc Am Physicians 66:231–239, 1953.
125. Masurel N, Ophof P, de Jong P. Antibody response to immunization with influenza A/USSR/77 (H1N1) virus in young individuals primed or unprimed for A/New Jersey/76 (H1/N1) virus. J Hyg (Lond) 87:201–209, 1981.
126. Webster RG. Original antigenic sin in ferrets: The response to sequential infections with influenza viruses. J Immunol 97:177–183, 1966.
127. Meiklejohn G, Eickhoff TC, Graves P, Josephine I. Antigenic drift and efficacy of influenza virus vaccines, 1976–1977. J Infect Dis 138:618–624, 1978.
128. Burlington DB, Wright PF, van Wyke KL, et al. Development of subtype-specific and heterosubtypic antibodies to the influenza A virus hemagglutinin after primary infection in children. J Clin Microbiol 21:847–849, 1985.
129. Kodiahalli S, Justewicz DM, Gubareva LV, et al. Selection of a single amino acid substitution in the hemagglutinin molecule by chicken eggs can render influenza A virus (H3) candidate vaccine ineffective. J Virol 69:4888–4897, 1995.
130. Katz JM, Wang M, Webster RG. Direct sequencing of the HA gene of influenza (H3N2) virus in original clinical samples reveals sequence identity with mammalian cell-grown virus. J Virol 64:1808–1811, 1990.
131. Robertson JS, Nicolson C, Bootman JS, et al. Sequence analysis of the haemagglutinin (HA) of influenza A (H1N1) viruses present in clinical material and comparison with the HA of laboratory-derived virus. J Gen Virol 72:2671–2677, 1991.
132. Waldman RH, Wood SH, Torres EJ, Small PA. Influenza antibody response following aerosol administration of inactivated virus. Am J Epidemiol 91:575–584, 1970.
133. Zahradnik JM, Kasel JA, Martin RR, et al. Immune response in serum and respiratory secretions following vaccination with a live cold-recombinant (CR35) and inactivated A/USSR/77 (H1N1) influenza virus vaccine. J Med Virol 11:277–285, 1983.
134. Ennis FA, Yi-Hua Q, Schild GC. Antibody and cytotoxic T lymphocyte responses of humans to live and inactivated influenza vaccines. J Gen Virol 58:273–281, 1982.
135. McMichael AJ, Askonas BA, Webster RG, Laver WG. B-cell or T-cell immunity? Immunol Today 3:255–260, 1982.
136. Dillon SB, Demuth SG, Schneider MA, et al. Induction of protective class I MHC-restricted CTL in mice by a recombinant influenza vaccine in aluminium hydroxide adjuvant. Vaccine 10:309–318, 1992.
137. Mbawuike IN, Wyde PR. Induction of $CD8^+$ cytotoxic T cells by immunization with killed influenza virus and effect of cholera toxin B subunit. Vaccine 11:1205–1213, 1993.
138. Biro J, Beregi E. The influence of influenza vaccinations on human peripheral lymphocytes relating to aging. Aktuelle Gerontol 10:319–322, 1980.
139. Barker WH, Mullooly JP. Influenza vaccination of elderly persons. JAMA 244:2547–2549, 1980.
140. Serie C, Barme M, Honnoun C, et al. Effects of vaccination on an influenza epidemic in a geriatric hospital. Dev Biol Stand 39:317–321, 1977.
141. Currier M, Coffman T, Boyd P, et al. Influenza vaccine efficacy in a Maryland nursing home. Md Med J 37:781–783, 1988.
142. Huang Y-P, Pechere J-C, Michel M, et al. In vivo T cell activation, in vitro defective IL-2 secretion, and response to influenza vaccination in elderly women. J Immunol 148:715–722, 1992.
143. Gross PA, Quinnan GV, Rodstein M, et al. Association of influ-

enza immunization with reduction in mortality in an elderly population. Arch Intern Med 148:562–565, 1988.
144. Gross PA, Quinnan GV Jr, Weksler ME, et al. Immunization of elderly people with high doses of influenza vaccine. J Am Geriatr Soc 36:209–212, 1988.
145. Beyer WEP, Palache AM, Baljet M, Masurel N. Antibody induction by influenza vaccine in the elderly: A review of the literature. Vaccine 7:385–394, 1989.
146. McElhaney JE, Graydon SM, Lechelt KE, et al. Antibody response to whole-virus and split-virus influenza vaccines in successful aging. Vaccine 11:1055–1060, 1993.
147. Miotti PG, Nelson KE, Dallabetta GA, Farzadegan H. The influence of HIV infection on antibody responses to a two-dose regimen of influenza vaccine. JAMA 262:779–783, 1989.
148. Steinberg E, Overturf GD, Portnoy B, et al. Serologic and clinical response of children with sickle cell disease to bivalent influenza A split virus vaccine. J Pediatr 92:823–825, 1978.
149. Ganz PA, Shanley JD, Cherry JD. Responses of patients with neoplastic diseases to influenza virus vaccine. Cancer 42:2244–2247, 1978.
150. Lange B, Shapiro SA, Waldman MTG, et al. Antibody responses to influenza immunization of children with acute lymphoblastic leukemia. J Infect Dis 140:402–406, 1979.
151. Ortbals DW, Marks ES, Liebhaber H. Influenza immunization in patients with chronic renal disease. JAMA 239:2562–2563, 1978.
152. Sheth KJ, Freeman ME, Eisenberg C, Sedmak GV. Influenza virus immunization: Antibody response and adverse effects in children with renal disease. JAMA 239:2559–2561, 1978.
153. Kava T, Lindqvist A, Karjalainen J, Laitinen LA. Unchanged bronchial reactivity after killed influenza virus vaccine in adult asthmatics. Respiration 51:98–104, 1987.
154. Ghirga G, Ghirga P, Rodino P, Presti A. Safety of the subunit influenza vaccine in asthmatic children. Vaccine 9:913–914, 1991.
155. Adlard P, Bryett K. Influenza immunization in children with cystic fibrosis. J Int Med Res 15:344–351, 1987.
156. Carlson AJ, Davidson WL, McLean AA, et al. Pneumococcal vaccine: Dose, revaccination, and coadministration with influenza vaccine (40596). Proc Soc Exp Biol Med 161:558–563, 1979.
157. Mufson MA, Krause HE, Tarrant CJ, et al. Polyvalent pneumococcal vaccine given alone and in combination with bivalent influenza virus vaccine (40804). Proc Soc Exp Biol Med 163:498–503, 1980.
158. Monto AS, Ohmit SE. Effectiveness evaluation of inactivated influenza vaccines: Methods and results. In Brown LE, Hampson AW, Webster RG (eds). Options for the Control of Influenza III. Amsterdam, Elsevier Science BV, 1996, pp 93–96.
159. Fedson DS. Influenza and pneumococcal vaccination of the elderly: Newer vaccines and prospects for clinical benefits at the margin. Prev Med 23:751–755, 1994.
160. Davenport FM. Inactivated influenza virus vaccines: Past, present, and future. Am Rev Respir Dis 83(suppl):146–150, 1961.
161. Dowdle WR. Influenza immunoprophylaxis after 30 years' experience. In Nayak DP (ed). Genetic Variation Among Influenza Viruses. New York, Academic Press, 1981, pp 525–534.
162. Meiklejohn G. Viral respiratory disease at Lowry Air Force Base in Denver, 1952–82. J Infect Dis 148:775–784, 1983.
163. Migiliani R, Dart T, Spiegel A, et al. Évaluation de l'efficacité du vaccin grippal 1995 dans une unité militare de la région Île-de-France. Bul Epidem Hebdomadaire 35:157–158, 1997.
164. Couch RB, Keitel WA, Cate TR, et al. Prevention of influenza virus infections by current inactivated influenza vaccines. In Brown LE, Hampson AW, Webster RG (eds). Options for the Control of Influenza III. Amsterdam, Elsevier Science BV, 1996, pp 97–106.
165. Govaert ThME, Thijs CTMCN, Masurel N, et al. The efficacy of influenza vaccination in elderly individuals: A randomized double-blind placebo-controlled trial. JAMA 272:1661–1665, 1994.
166. Gross PA, Hermogenes AW, Sacks HS, et al. The efficacy of influenza vaccine in elderly persons: A meta-analysis and review of the literature. Ann Intern Med 123:518–527, 1995.
167. Barker WH, Mullooly JP. Effectiveness of inactivated influenza vaccine among non-institutionalized elderly persons. In Kendal AP, Patriarca PA (eds). Options for the Control of Influenza. New York, Alan R Liss, 1986, pp 169–182.
168. Fedson DS, Wajda A, Nichol JP, et al. Clinical effectiveness of influenza vaccination in Manitoba. JAMA 270:1956–1961, 1993.
169. Foster DA, Talsma AN, Furumoto-Dawson A, et al. Influenza vaccine effectiveness in preventing hospitalization for pneumonia in the elderly. Am J Epidemiol 136:296–307, 1992.
170. Nichol KL, Margolis KL, Wuorenema J, Sternberg T. The efficacy and cost effectiveness of vaccination against influenza among elderly persons living in the community. N Engl J Med 331:778–784, 1994.
171. Arden NH, Patriarca PA, Kendal AP. Experience in the use and efficacy of inactivated influenza vaccine in nursing homes. In Kendal AP, Patriarca PA (eds). Options for the Control of Influenza. New York, Alan R Liss, 1986, pp 155–165.
172. Patriarca PA, Weber JA, Parker RA, et al. Efficacy of influenza vaccine in nursing homes: Reduction in illness and complications during an influenza A(H3N2) epidemic. JAMA 253:1136–1139, 1985.
173. Arden N, Monto AS, Ohmit SE. Vaccine use and the risk of outbreaks in a sample of nursing homes during an influenza epidemic. Am J Public Health 85:399–401, 1995.
174. Patriarca PA, Weber JA, Parker RA, et al. Risk factors for outbreaks of influenza in nursing homes: A case-control study. Am J Epidemiol 124:114–119, 1986.
175. Nichol KL, Lind A, Margolis KL, et al. The effectiveness of vaccination against influenza in healthy, working adults. N Engl J Med 333:889–893, 1995.
176. Goodeve A, Potter CW, Clark A, et al. A graded-dose study of inactivated, surface antigen influenza B vaccine in volunteers: Reactogenicity, antibody response and protection to challenge virus infection. J Hyg (Lond) 90:107–115, 1983.
177. Dolin R, Wise TG, Mazur MH, et al. Immunogenicity and reactogenicity of influenza A/New Jersey/76 virus vaccines in normal adults. J Infect Dis 136(suppl):435–442, 1977.
178. Barry DW, Mayner RE, Staton E, et al. Comparative trial of influenza vaccines. I. Immunogenicity of whole virus and split product vaccines in man. Am J Epidemiol 104:34–46, 1976.
179. Langmuir AD, Bregman DJ, Kurland LT, et al. An epidemiologic and clinical evaluation of Guillain-Barré syndrome reported in association with the administration of swine influenza vaccines. J Epidemiol 119:841–879, 1984.
180. Hurwitz ES, Schonberger LB, Nelson DB, Holman RC. Guillain-Barré syndrome and the 1978–1979 influenza vaccine. N Engl J Med 304:1557–1561, 1981.
181. Kaplan JE, Katona P, Hurwitz ES, Schonberger LB. Guillain-Barré syndrome in the United States, 1979–1980 and 1980–81. JAMA 248:698–700, 1982.
181a. Prevention and control of influenza: Recommendations of the Advisory Committee on Immunization Practices (ACIP). MMWR 47(RR-6):1–26, 1998.
182. Kramer P, McClain CJ. Depression of aminopyrine metabolism by influenza vaccination. N Engl J Med 305:1262–1264, 1981.
183. Levine M, Jones MW, Gribble M. Increased serum phenytoin concentration following influenza vaccination. Clin Pharmacokinet 3:505–509, 1984.
184. Renton KW, Gray JD, Hall RI. Decreased elimination of theophylline after influenza vaccination. Can Med Assoc J 123:288–290, 1980.
185. Bukowskyz M, Munt PW, Wigle R, Nakatsu K. Theophylline clearance. Am Rev Respir Dis 129:672–675, 1984.
186. Patriarca PA, Kendal AP, Stricof RL, et al. Influenza vaccination and warfarin or theophylline toxicity in nursing-home residents. N Engl J Med 308:1601–1602, 1983.
187. Louria DB, Blumenfeld HL, Ellis JT, et al. Studies on influenza in the pandemic of 1957–58. II. Pulmonary complications of influenza. J Clin Invest 38:213–265, 1959.
188. Barker WH, Mullooly JP. Impact of epidemic type A influenza in a defined adult population. Am J Epidemiol 112:798–813, 1980.
189. Neuzil KM, Reed GW, Mitchel EF, Simonsen L. The impact of influenza on acute cardiopulmonary hospitalizations in pregnant women. Am J Epidemiol 1998, in press.
190. Pachucki CT, Walsh Pappas SA, Fuller GF, et al. Influenza A among hospital personnel and patients: Implications for recognition, prevention, and control. Arch Intern Med 149:77–80, 1989.
191. Potter J, Stott DJ, Roberts MA, et al. Influenza vaccination of health care workers in long-term-care hospitals reduces the mortality of elderly patients. J Infect Dis 175:1–6, 1997.

192. Keitel WA, Cate TR, Couch RB. Efficacy of sequential annual vaccination with inactivated influenza virus vaccine. Am J Epidemiol 127:353–364, 1988.
193. Centers for Disease Control and Prevention. Pneumonia and influenza death rates—United States, 1979–94. MMWR Morb Mortal Weekly Rep 44:535–536, 1995.
194. Carrat F, Valleron AJ. Influenza mortality among the elderly in France, 1980–90: How many deaths may have been avoided through vaccination? J Epidemiol Community Health 49:419–425, 1995.
195. Monto AS, Davenport FM, Napier JA, Francis T. Modification of an outbreak of influenza in Tecumseh, Michigan by vaccination of schoolchildren. J Infect Dis 122:16–25, 1970.
196. Rudenko LG, Slepshukin AN, Monto AS, et al. Efficacy of live attenuated and inactivated influenza vaccines in schoolchildren and their unvaccinated contacts in Novgorod, Russia. J Infect Dis 168:881–887, 1993.
197. Oya A, Nerome N. Experience with mass vaccination of young age groups with inactivated vaccines. In Kendal AP, Patriarca PA (eds). Options for the Control of Influenza. New York, Alan R Liss, 1986, pp 183–192.
198. Heller L, Bottiger M. Attempt to estimate the protective efficacy of routinely performed mass-vaccination against Hong Kong influenza in some industrial populations in Sweden. In Proceedings of the International Symposium on Influenza Vaccines for Men and Horses, London, 1972. Symposium Series on Immunobiological Standards Vol. 20. Basel, S Karger, 1973, pp 258–264.
199. Wesselius-de Casparis A, Hogerzeil HHW, van Beek A. Eleven years of experience in industry with vaccination against influenza: Reduction in absenteeism. In Proceedings of the International Symposium on Influenza Vaccines for Men and Horses, London, 1972. Symposium Series on Immunobiological Standards Vol. 20. Basel, S Karger, 1973, pp 268–274.
200. Mullooly JP, Bennett MD, Hornbrook MC, et al. Influenza vaccination programs for elderly persons: Cost-effectiveness in a health maintenance organization. Ann Intern Med 121:947–952, 1994.
201. Helliwell BE, Drummond MF. The costs and benefits of preventing influenza in Ontario's elderly. Can J Public Health 79:175–180, 1988.
202. Levy E. French economic evaluations of influenza and influenza vaccination. Pharmacoeconomics 9(suppl 3):62–66, 1996.
203. Nicholson K. Socioeconomics of influenza vaccination in Europe. Pharmacoeconomics 9(suppl 3):75–78, 1996.
204. Schoenbaum SC, McNeil BJ, Kavet J. The swine-influenza decision. N Engl J Med 295:759–765, 1976.
205. Kilbourne ED. Influenza. New York, Plenum Publishing, 1987.
206. Kilbourne ED. Influenza pandemics in perspective. JAMA 237:1225–1228, 1977.
207. Dunn GFN, Wormald PJ. Influenza-A Hong Kong vaccine and the new variant A/ENG/42/72. Lancet 1:95, 1973.
208. Stiver HG, Graves P, Eickhoff TC, Meiklejohn G. Efficacy of "Hong Kong" vaccine in preventing "England" variant influenza A in 1972. N Engl J Med 289:1267–1271, 1973.
209. Hoskins TW, Davies JR, Allchin A, et al. Controlled trial of inactivated influenza vaccine containing the A/Hong Kong strain during an outbreak of influenza due to the A/England/42/72 strain. Lancet 2:116–120, 1973.
210. Betts RF, Douglas RG Jr, Roth FK, Little JW II. Efficacy of live attenuated influenza A/Scotland/74 (H3N2) virus vaccine against challenge with influenza A/Victoria/3/75 (H3N2) virus. J Infect Dis 136:746–753, 1977.
211. Clover RD, Crawford S, Glezen WP, et al. Comparison of heterotypic protection against influenza A/Taiwan/86 (H1N1) by attenuated and inactivated vaccines to A/Chile/83-like viruses. J Infect Dis 163:300–304, 1991.

chapter

22 Pneumococcal Vaccine

David S. Fedson
Daniel M. Musher
Juhani Eskola

The modern development of pneumococcal polysaccharide vaccine exemplifies the full cycle of scientific discovery regarding the pathogenesis, treatment, and eventual prevention of a major infectious disease. At each stage, new knowledge has brought forth questions not only about the basic biology of pneumococcal infections and the immune response to pneumococcal vaccination but also about the epidemiological importance of pneumococcal infections and the benefits that might be realized if pneumococcal vaccine were widely used.

In recent years, several critical reviews have added to classic older works,[1–3] providing comprehensive summaries of all aspects of pneumococcal infections[4–15] and pneumococcal vaccine.[4, 7, 11, 12, 16–19] The chapters on pneumococcal vaccine in the first[20] and second editions[21] of this book reviewed studies reported up to 1992. This chapter covers reports published since then and retains essential information from earlier studies. The two earlier chapters can be consulted for additional information and pertinent references on many aspects of pneumococcal infections and pneumococcal vaccine.

For more than 100 years the study of *Streptococcus pneumoniae* and pneumococcal infections has occupied a central position in the development of a scientific basis for the control of infectious diseases.[3, 10] The organism was first isolated and grown in the laboratory almost simultaneously by Sternberg and Pasteur in 1880 (Table 22–1). During the same decade the pneumococcus was shown to be the chief cause of lobar pneumonia. By the first part of the 20th century, the principles of humoral immunity had been elucidated, in great part because of studies of *S. pneumoniae*, and the potential protective effects of antiserum and whole-cell vaccine were beginning to be understood.

The first large-scale clinical trial of a crude whole-cell pneumococcal vaccine was conducted in 1911 at a time when the importance of type-specific immunity was not fully recognized. During the next two decades the experimental foundation was laid for understanding the importance of antibody to pneumococcal capsular polysaccharide and for developing an effective polyvalent, type-specific pneumococcal vaccine. The first clinical trial of a tetravalent pneumococcal polysaccharide vaccine was reported at the close of World War II. Two hexavalent vaccines were marketed in 1946, only to be withdrawn within a few years, primarily because of the apparent success and ease of treating pneumococcal infections with penicillin.

It remained for Austrian and Gold to demonstrate in the early 1960s the continued severe morbidity and mortality of pneumococcal infections in spite of appropriate antimicrobial therapy.[22] Led by Austrian, efforts to develop a modern pneumococcal capsular polysaccharide vaccine were begun once again. Within a decade, pneumococcal vaccination was shown to be effective in clinical trials conducted among gold miners in South Africa.[23, 24] This finding was soon followed by licensure in the United States of a 14-valent capsular polysaccharide vaccine and 6 years later by a 23-valent vaccine.

BACKGROUND

Clinical Pneumococcal Infections

The major clinical syndromes caused by *S. pneumoniae* are widely recognized and discussed in all standard medical textbooks.[25] Infections of the middle ear (otitis media), paranasal sinuses, tracheobronchial tree, and lung are the result of direct spread of the organism from the nasopharynx. Invasive pneumococcal disease is the result of hematogenous spread to the central nervous system (meningitis), heart valves (endocarditis) and, less commonly, other sites such as joints, peritoneal cavity, and fallopian tubes. Primary (occult) bacteremia usually affects children and is much less common in adults. The organism may also spread directly to adjacent sites: from the lung to the pleural space (pleuritis) or from the paranasal sinuses to the central nervous system. Recurrent meningitis suggests a defect in the dura (cerebrospinal fluid [CSF] leak). Pneumococcal infections occur throughout the year, although the number of cases is

Table 22–1. **HISTORICAL MILESTONES IN THE STUDY OF PNEUMOCCAL DISEASE AND PNEUMOCOCCAL VACCINE**

1881	Pasteur, Sternberg—Pneumococcus first isolated and grown in vitro
1880s	Pneumococcus shown to be a major cause of lobar pneumonia
1884	Gram's stain developed
1891	Klemperer, Klemperer—Protective effect of antiserum demonstrated
1897	Bezancon, Griffin—Distinct pneumococcal serotypes demonstrated
1902	Neufeld—Capsular swelling (quellung) with specific antiserum shown
1904	Neufeld, Rimpau—Opsonization by immune serum demonstrated
1910	Neufeld, Handel—Type-specific immunity discovered
1911	Wright—Clinical trials of whole-cell pneumococcal vaccine conducted in South Africa
1913	Lister—Type-specific antibodies found to develop after infection or injection of heat-killed organisms
1917–1927	Avery, Dochez, Heidelberger, Goebel—Capsular antigens shown to be complex polysaccharides that are antigenic and determine serological reactivity
1928	Griffith—Capsular transformation demonstrated
1930	Francis, Tillett—Purified capsular polysaccharides shown to be immunogenic in humans
1931	Dubos, Avery—Capsular polysaccharide found to determine pneumococcal virulence
1931	Finland, Sutliff—Serum therapy for lobar pneumonia shown to be effective
1933	Etinger, Tulezynska—Pneumococcal typing based on quellung reaction developed
1938	Felton—Clinical protection against type-specific disease shown in people injected with purified capsular polysaccharides
	Ekwursel—Clinical trial of capsular polysaccharides shown to reduce incidence of pneumonia and its mortality
1941	Abraham, Chain, and coworkers—Penicillin successful in treating infections with Gram-positive bacterial infections
1944	Avery, MacLeod, McCarty—Capsular transformation by DNA demonstrates that DNA is the bearer of genetic information
1945	MacLeod, Heidelberger, and coworkers—Successful clinical trial of tetravalent pneumococcal vaccine conducted in military recruits
1947	Kaufman—Trivalent vaccine shown to produce type-specific protection in elderly patients
1946–1948	Hexavalent pneumococcal vaccines introduced but soon withdrawn
1964	Austrian, Gold—Pneumococcal infections shown to be a continuing problem in patients treated with antibiotics
1967	Hansman, Bullen—Penicillin-resistant pneumococcus reported
1968	Program to develop polyvalent pneumococcal vaccine begun
1977	14-valent pneumococcal vaccine licensed
1983	23-valent pneumococcal vaccine licensed
1980s	Pneumococcal conjugate vaccine development begun

usually higher during mid-winter periods when outbreaks of viral diseases and increases in air pollution occur.[26]

For this review of pneumococcal vaccine, the clinical features of each of these conditions are less relevant than is their epidemiology. Also relevant to vaccination are the characteristics of the organism itself, certain aspects of the pathogenesis of disease and host defense, problems encountered in establishing a valid diagnosis in each clinical syndrome, and difficulties encountered in treatment because of antibiotic resistance.

Streptococcus pneumoniae

The organism was initially called *Pneumococcus* by Fraenkel in 1886.[10] It was classified in the United States as *Diplococcus pneumoniae* in 1920 because of its distinctive morphology. The name was changed to *Streptococcus pneumoniae* in the United States in 1974 because of the organism's many similarities to other streptococci. Historically, the demonstration in 1944 by Avery, MacLeod, and McCarty that DNA is the active substance responsible for the genetic transformation from rough (noncapsulated) to smooth (capsulated) cells is one of the cornerstones of modern molecular biology.[27–29] Since then, other biological markers, including type specificity and antibiotic resistance, have also been shown to be genetically transferable.

Pneumococci are relatively fastidious, facultative organisms that grow in short chains in broth culture and appear frequently as gram-positive diplococci when examined microscopically. *S. pneumoniae* capsular types 3 and 37 grow as large mucoid colonies; other serotypes produce colonies that are not obviously mucoid. Hydrogen peroxide is one of the end-products of bacterial metabolism. Because pneumococci lack catalase or peroxidase, the addition of red blood cells to the growth medium as a source of catalase serves to inactivate hydrogen peroxide and thus enhance bacterial viability. Under aerobic conditions, colonies of pneumococci alter hemoglobin, producing a greenish discoloration of the surrounding blood-containing medium, incorrectly called α-hemolysis. A similar discoloration is visible around colonies grown on chocolate agar. The sensitivity of pneumococci but not of most other streptococci to growth inhibition by ethylhydrocupreine (Optochin) is widely used as a criterion for laboratory identification. However, because some pneumococcal isolates are resistant to ethylhydrocupreine,[30] the unique property of solubility in bile is still useful for presumptively identifying *S. pneumoniae*.

The cell wall consists of a peptidoglycan backbone and teichoic acid.[25, 31–33] Unique to *S. pneumoniae*, and present in all isolates, is a specific cell wall polysaccharide (C-polysaccharide), a teichoic acid constituent that is covalently linked to peptidoglycan on the outer surface of the cell wall. C-polysaccharide is responsible for serological cross-reactivity between *S. pneumoniae* and other streptococci, reacts with a specific β-globulin in human serum (C-reactive protein) in the early stages of the inflammatory response, and can activate the alternative complement pathway. Antibody to C-polysaccharide appears early in life and can be found in virtually all children and adults, but does not appear to protect against pneumococcal infection.[34] Peptidoglycan plays the major role in stimulating the intense inflammation associated with pneumococcal infection.[14, 35]

The capsular polysaccharide on the cell surface is the primary factor responsible for the virulence of *S. pneumoniae* in the normal host.[7, 25, 31–33] Invasiveness depends more on the composition than on the amount of capsular polysaccharide produced—for example, types 3 and 37 are both heavily encapsulated, but type 3 is highly invasive, whereas type 37 seldom causes disease.[8] Within a single serotype, however, the size of the capsule may correlate directly with the ability to cause disease. Capsular polysaccharide inhibits phagocytosis, presumably by preventing recognition of antibody or complement adherent to bacterial cell wall by polymorphonuclear leukocytes. In addition, capsular polysaccharide may interfere with intracellular killing of phagocytized pneumococci by activating a mechanism that is not dependent on immune globulin or complement.[36]

Several *S. pneumoniae* protein antigens and toxins have been identified.[31, 32, 37, 38] Pneumolysin is a cytolytic toxin that may assist the organism in evading host defenses.[31, 37–40] This toxin damages the alveolar capillary barrier[41, 42] and inhibits the respiratory burst, chemotaxis, and the antimicrobial activities of polymorphonuclear leukocytes and macrophages.[40, 43] It also inhibits the proliferative response of lymphocytes to mitogens and can activate the classic complement pathway. A pneumolysin-negative mutant of *S. pneumoniae* has reduced virulence in experimental infection in mice,[44–46] and inactivated pneumolysin has been studied as a possible vaccine.[39, 40, 47] Pneumococcal surface protein A (PspA) is an antigenically variable surface protein that appears to be essential for full virulence[31, 37, 38]; an antiphagocytic effect may be responsible.[48, 49] Antibody to this substance partially protects mice against pneumococcal challenge,[50, 51] and its potential as a vaccine is being actively explored. Immunoglobulin A1 (IgA) protease is an enzyme that cleaves IgA1 and thus may help pneumococci evade local mucosal defenses,[31, 52] although its precise role in pathogenesis is uncertain.[38] Lysis of pneumococci by autolysin may contribute to bacterial virulence by releasing several potentially damaging or inflammatory cell wall components and pneumolysin.[31, 32, 38, 53] The contributions of pneumococcal neuraminidase,[54] hyaluronidase, surface adhesin A (PsaA), and other pneumococcal adhesins and permeases to the virulence of *S. pneumoniae* are poorly understood.[7, 31–33, 37, 38]

Since the early 1980s, the Danish system for classifying *S. pneumoniae* has been used worldwide. Differences in the chemical structures of pneumococcal capsular polysaccharides provide the basis for classifying them into serotypes. Currently, 90 different serotypes have been described.[55] Some of the serogroups include several serotypes that are serologically related. For example, in serogroup 7, the original type 7 was called 7F (for "first") and related serotypes identified later were named 7A, 7B, etc. Within each capsular serotype, further differences among strains can be demonstrated by DNA fingerprinting,[56] multilocus enzyme electrophoresis and ribotyping,[57] and polymerase chain reaction (PCR) techniques.[58]

The lower-numbered serotypes are generally responsible for causing invasive disease in humans, but shifts in the prevalence of individual serotypes have occurred in a given area over time. Thus, type 1, the first to be recognized, now causes no more than 1 to 2% of pneumococcal disease in the United States, and type 2 is almost never seen, whereas type 3 remains a frequently isolated serotype from patients with invasive disease. Differences in the epidemiology of individual serogroups have also been demonstrated among different age groups in different regions during the same time period,[59] although the clinical syndromes caused by all pneumococcal serotypes are essentially the same.[60]

Each serotype can be identified by its chemical structure and its reaction with type-specific antisera. Perhaps the most widely known serotyping test is the quellung reaction. When bacteria in suspension are mixed with homologous antiserum, a distinct capsular immunoprecipitation reaction can be observed under the microscope, either using phase contrast or after adding methylene blue.

Serotyping of *S. pneumoniae* is usually accomplished using antisera provided by the Statens Seruminstitut in Copenhagen, Denmark.[61] The antisera are available commercially as (1) Omni-serum, which reacts with all 90 types, (2) 14 pooled antisera, each of which reacts with 7 to 12 types, and (3) 46 antisera, each specific for a single type or group. A special set of twelve pooled antisera (A-F, H, P-T; PNEUMOTEST) provides a simple typing system that can be used for surveillance in other than specialized laboratories.[62] These twelve antisera cover 23 different vaccine-related types and 25 other cross-reacting types that together account for 90 to 95% of pneumococcal blood and CSF isolates.

Coagglutination and latex agglutination (LA) tests have been used for serotyping with results that have been equivalent to those obtained with the classic quellung test.[63] The simplicity and low cost of these agglutination tests may permit wider use of serotyping in epidemiological studies, especially those conducted in developing countries.

Pathogenesis and Host Defense as They Relate to Prevention

Many factors, both nonimmunological and immunological, act together to defend the host against pneumococcal infection.[4, 5, 8, 9, 14, 25, 31, 32, 37] Nonimmunological mechanisms include normal function of the gag and cough reflexes and intact clearance mechanisms in the bronchial tree. Immunological mechanisms include the presence of a sufficient number of normally functioning phagocytic cells and sufficient concentrations of antibody and complement.

In most cases of pneumococcal infection, one or more nonimmunological or immunological deficiencies in the mechanisms of host defense can be implicated.[25, 32] Suppression of the cough reflex by alcohol, opiates, or aging, and damage to clearance mechanisms by exposure to cigarette smoke or other air pollutants, are the most commonly identified nonimmunological problems. Exposure to alcohol, renal or hepatic insufficiency, glucocorticoid treatment, and diabetes mellitus adversely affect migration of and bacterial killing by polymorphonuclear leukocytes. People who undergo splenectomy lose the benefit of blood clearance mechanisms that function in the absence of anticapsular antibody and are at risk of overwhelming pneumococcalinfection. Immunoglobulin production is deficient in human immunodeficiency virus (HIV) infection, multiple myeloma, and lymphoma and may be altogether absent in congenital or acquired hypogammaglobulinemia. The extremes of age are associated with the highest incidence of pneumococcal infection. The higher frequency among infants and young children probably reflects the initial exposure of an immature immune system to new antigens. In contrast, the susceptibility of the elderly is probably multifactorial, with a major role being played by nonimmunological mechanisms. Malnutrition and recent hospitalization[64] are important risk factors for pneumococcal infection, the latter probably as a direct reflection of underlying medical conditions on susceptibility.

A clearer understanding of the relationships among the various constituents of *S. pneumoniae* and the molecular events that define pneumococcal infections has emerged.[14, 33, 65] Successful nasopharyngeal colonization occurs with organisms that exhibit transparent, not opaque, colonial morphology. Once aspirated into the lung, pneumococci preferentially activate type II pneumocytes, which increase their expression of platelet activating factor (PAF) receptor. Transparent but not opaque phase variants of *S. pneumoniae* adhere to the PAF receptor in an interaction that involves the phosphorylcholine component of pneumococcal cell-wall teichoic acid. Adherence to type II pneumocytes and endothelial cells occurs in a two-stage process: an initial rapid phase stimulated by a thrombin-dependent mechanism and a later more prolonged phase stimulated by the cytokines tumor necrosis factor-α (TNF-α) and interleukin-1α (IL-1α). Entry of pneumococci into activated cells appears to involve internalization and recycling of PAF receptors. The intense inflammatory response to pneumococcal infection is mediated by cell wall components, not capsular polysaccharide; the latter by itself provides little stimulus to inflammation.

The two most potent inflammatory components of the cell wall are the phosphorylcholine-containing C-polysaccharide and teichoic acid. The precise role of other proteins as determinants of virulence is uncertain. Mixtures of cell wall components alone can recreate all of the characteristic pathological findings that accompany pneumococcal infections, including the intense edema and the deposition of fibrin. Left unchecked, this process inevitably leads to death. It can be interrupted by leukocytes that are recruited to the site of infection by adhesin molecules (integrin CD18) and a non–CD18-dependent process. This inflammatory process is mediated by several cytokines and is distinct from that induced by the endotoxins of gram-negative bacteria.

The molecular events thought to occur during pneumococcal infection explain several of the clinical features of disease. The classic pneumococcal crisis followed by lysis of fever, which occurs in untreated disease or in modified form after antiserum or antibiotic treatment, can be understood as the consequence of the sudden release of inflammatory cell wall components. Once bacterial replication is controlled, the inflammatory process and fever decline. In overwhelming infection, however, antibiotic treatment can release massive amounts of cell wall components that might exacerbate the inflammatory response. Until treatments are developed that down-regulate or interrupt this process,[66] the host's ability to respond effectively to vaccination by producing antibody to capsular polysaccharide remains the best single mechanism of protection against pneumococcal infection.

Experimental studies in mice have helped to define the regulation of the antibody response to pneumococcal vaccine.[8, 67–69] The response to capsular polysaccharide antigens is largely independent of control by the thymus,[69] whereas the response to protein antigens is thymus-dependent, requiring T cells for both its induction and regulation. Although pneumococcal antigens can activate B cells in the absence of T cells, T cells can influence the immunoglobulin class and the magnitude of the antibody response (i.e., pneumococcal capsular polysaccharide functions as a thymus-independent type 2 [TI-2] antigen).[67–69] The antibody response is regulated by T cells that have amplifier (as distinct from helper) and suppressor functions. Both amplifier and helper T cells are $CD4^+$, $CD8^-$, and both positively influence the antibody response, which in mice is largely IgG3. Amplifier T cells do not become active until 2 days after immunization, and their activity peaks around day 4 or 5. Thus, amplifier T cells expand an already ongoing antibody response.[67, 68] Suppressor T cells are $CD8^+$, $CD4^-$, and their activity can be demonstrated as early as 18 to 24 hours after immunization.[68] Suppressor T cells limit the extent to which B cells proliferate after antigenic stimulation. The activity of suppressor T cells may be influenced for a short period (from 4 to 8 days after immunization) by contrasuppressor T cells, although the overall importance of this process in regulating the antibody response to pneumococcal capsular polysaccharide antigens is controversial.[68]

Amplifier and suppressor T cells are not activated directly by antigen. Instead, they respond to idiotypic determinants of cell-associated, type-specific antibody on the surface of immune B cells. Activated but not resting suppressor T cells are influenced by lymphokines produced by helper T cells. Recombinant IL-2, recombinant IL-4, recombinant IL-5, and interferon-γ all appear to be required for the activation or clonal expansion of suppressor T cells.[70] Antigen-antibody complexes may also have a role in immunoregulation: When formed in the presence of antibody excess, they can suppress the antibody response to pneumococcal polysaccharide antigens in mice.[71]

In newborn mice, suppressor T-cell activity develops within 2 weeks, whereas amplifier T cells are not fully mature until 8 to 10 weeks.[68] The early dominance of suppressor T cells helps to explain the poor response of newborn mice to TI-2 antigens such as pneumococcal capsular polysaccharides. Efforts to improve the antibody response of newborns could involve enhancing the functioning of amplifier T cells or eliminating the inhibitory effects of suppressor T cells.

The characteristic features of the human immune response to pneumococcal capsular polysaccharides are similar to some of those found in the murine system. Human B cells from people sensitized in vivo to pneumococcal antigens spontaneously secrete type-specific IgM antibodies in vitro in the absence of T cells. This response lasts no longer than 2 weeks, although it can be reactivated by stimulation with pokeweed mitogen but not by exposure to specific antigen. These findings point to its relative but not absolute independence from regulation by T cells; an amplifier role for $CD4^+$ but not $CD8^+$ T cells has been shown to enhance B cell responses to pneumococcal polysaccharide antigens.[72] Pneumococcal vaccination also increases the expression of IL-2 receptors on peripheral blood lymphocytes, especially $CD8^+$ T cells.[73] In addition, spleen cells isolated from people recently immunized with pneumococcal vaccine can be stimulated to produce specific antibody by pokeweed mitogen.[74] Other studies of B-cell activation by pneumococcal polysaccharides also suggest a role for T cells, as yet not fully defined.[67, 75]

The poor response of human infants to pneumococcal vaccination also parallels that in mice. Children younger than 2 years of age show little antibody response to vaccination with pneumococcal capsular polysaccharide; delayed maturation of specific subsets of B cells is the most likely explanation.[76, 77]

The antibody response to pneumococcal and other bacterial polysaccharides is subject to genetic modification. Adults who possess the G2m(23) allele, an antigenic marker on the heavy chain of the IgG2 idiotype, may have higher postvaccination antibody levels to capsular polysaccharides of types 4 and 18C as well as to the capsular polysaccharide of *Haemophilus influenzae* type b (Hib) than those who lack this gene.[78, 79] Other studies have shown interaction between the G2m(23) and Km(1) allotypes. How allotype-linked hyporesponsiveness to pneumococcal antigens relates to the switching from B-cell production of IgM to that of IgG or to the regulating of T-cell interactions with B cells is not well understood.

Antibodies to pneumococcal capsular polysaccharides can activate and fix complement through the classic pathway.[8] The Fc receptor of attached immunoglobulin and the presence of complement play critical roles in mediating the protective effect of type-specific antibody. The third component of complement (C3) is the site of convergence of the classic and alternative complement pathways and the source of the opsonically active fragments C3b and iC3b. Polymorphonuclear leukocytes possess receptors for each of these fragments, and phagocytosis is initiated through their interaction. In the absence of antibody, complement can be activated via the alternative pathway. Peptidoglycan is largely responsible, although cell wall and even capsular polysaccharides may contribute to this reaction. Complement components are not fixed to the bacterial surface but generate C5a, thereby causing inflammation. This process does not lead to successful opsonization because Fc components are found at the cell wall and are not recognized by phagocytic cells.

Attempts to explain differences in the virulence of pneumococcal serotypes according to differences in their abilities to fix complement by the alternative pathway have not provided consistent results.[80] Experimental studies have shown that pneumococcal serotypes differ in the amount and site of covalently bound C3b and iC3b. Highly immunogenic and virulent serotypes such as type 3 do not inhibit C3b deposition; instead, they increase its proteolytic degradation to fragments, some of which do not function as ligands for phagocytic cell receptors.[81] Some of these fragments (e.g., C3d) appear to interact with receptors on B cells to promote antibody synthesis. Thus, complement also plays a role in regulating antibody production. C3d, which is generated in the process of iC3b degradation, can bind to pneumococcal capsular polysaccharide and be recognized by complement receptor type 2 on type-specific B cells. This complex is more immunogenic than capsular polysaccharide alone. These and other observations indicate that, in addition to its role in opsonophagocytosis, complement participates in the activation and proliferation of B cells and in the production of antibodies.

The spleen is of critical importance in host defense against pneumococcal bacteremia. In the absence of opsonizing antibody, virulent organisms are cleared from the blood stream during their slow passage through the sinusoids of Billroth. Experimental studies have shown that pneumococcal vaccination protects against pneumococcal bacteremia after splenectomy.[82, 83] The spleen is also involved to a varying degree, depending on the structure of the antigen, in regulating the antibody response to pneumococcal capsular polysaccharides.[84] In mice, the antibody response to some antigens (e.g., type 3) may be reduced after splenectomy, but other antibody-producing tissues can compensate.

For other antigens (e.g., type 14), there is no compensatory extrasplenic synthesis of antibody. This important difference may be due to the tendency of neutral polysaccharide antigens such as type 14 to localize to the marginal zone of the spleen, whereas highly acidic antigens such as type 3 localize to the red pulp.[84] Marginal zone macrophages may have unique functions in the transport of antigen-antibody complexes or in the presentation of TI-2 antigens. Pneumococcal capsular polysaccharides that are bound to C3d preferentially localize to the marginal zone and can be found at the surface of $CD21^+$ B cells, the C3d receptors, leading to a rapid immune response.[85] Immaturity of the marginal zone in infancy may contribute to the failure of the antibody response to some pneumococcal polysaccharides (e.g., type 14) but not to others (e.g., type 3).[86] The role of the human spleen in regulating antibody responses to pneumococcal vaccine has not been well studied, although the responses to vaccination after splenectomy appear to be normal.

Diagnosis of Pneumococcal Infections

Pneumococcal infection is diagnosed with certainty when the organism is cultured from blood or from extrapulmonary sites (e.g., cerebrospinal, pleural, or synovial fluid) that are normally sterile. When cultures are negative, establishing a diagnosis becomes problematic.[87, 88]

The question of whether microscopic examination or culture of sputum is reliable in diagnosing nonbacteremic pneumococcal pneumonia has been discussed extensively. The diagnosis is seldom in question when an individual patient with clinical pneumonia coughs up sputum that, under 100× magnification, contains many polymorphonuclear leukocytes and very few epithelial cells and under 1000× magnification shows greater than or equal to 10 elongated, gram-positive cocci for each white blood cell.[89] Studies have reaffirmed the value of microscopic examination of a gram-stained sputum specimen in providing useful information about the cause of community-acquired pneumonia and in guiding the initial choice of antimicrobial therapy.[90] Unfortunately, many patients with pneumonia do not provide adequate sputum specimens, and routine processing of sputum specimens for Gram stain and culture is variable and often imprecise.[91]

These factors cause difficulty in interpreting individual laboratory reports and confound the interpretation of many case series reported in the literature.[89] The American Thoracic Society has recommended "empiric" antibiotic therapy for the initial management of patients with community-acquired pneumonia, meaning that therapy should be given without regard to microscopic examination of the sputum.[92] This recommendation is based on the view that interpretation of the Gram-stained sputum is unreliable in up to one half of cases. It should be emphasized, however, that the accuracy of the sputum examination can be maximized by excluding poor specimens and those obtained from people previously treated with antibiotics.

Considerable attention has been given to improving the accuracy of diagnosing pneumococcal infections by detecting pneumococcal antigen in sputum, blood, CSF, and urine specimens.[93–100] Four methods have been used in most studies: LA, enzyme-linked immunosorbent assay (ELISA),[101–103] counterimmuno-electrophoresis, and staphylococcal coagglutination. The antigens usually sought in these tests are pneumococcal capsular polysaccharide and/or C-polysaccharide. In general, these newer techniques have not added substantially to the diagnostic utility of classic bacteriological methods alone. Reports of quantitative enzyme immunoassay and ELISA tests for C-polysaccharide in sputum have shown positive predictive values of 86%[104] and 93%.[101] Unless sputum specimens are of high quality, however, these and other antigen detection tests can be confounded by cross-reactions with the antigens of viridans streptococci.[105, 106] Adding these tests to routine laboratory procedures may somewhat increase the proportion of patients in whom pneumococcal pneumonia is diagnosed, especially those who have been treated previously with antibiotics and have negative sputum cultures. They may also increase the diagnostic yield of bronchoalveolar lavage[107] and transthoracic needle[96] or pleural fluid[97] aspirates. In patients with pneumococcal bacteremia, detection of C-polysaccharide in blood by latex-agglutination and ELISA has given mixed results.[98, 102, 108]

Pneumococcal antigen has also been sought in the CSF of patients with meningitis.[99, 100] In spite of enthusiasm for these tests, especially in developing countries where reliable bacteriological cultures may be unavailable, they add little to what can be learned from a properly prepared Gram stain and culture of CSF.[99, 109] In one teaching hospital, only 2 of 438 CSF specimens yielded true-positive results for *S. pneumoniae* capsular polysaccharide antigens.[110] Nonselective overuse of these tests[110] as well as technical factors such as pH changes in CSF specimens[111] reduce their usefulness. Likewise, routine detection of pneumococcal antigen in urine has proven to be disappointing for both technical reasons[112] and lack of clinical utility.[110, 113]

Several attempts have been made to develop diagnostic tests based on antibodies to either the capsular or C-polysaccharide or to pneumolysin.[114–118] Tests for circulating immune complexes that contain pneumolysin antigens and antipneumolysin antibodies[119] or IgG antibodies and capsular polysaccharide antigens[120] have also been developed. In the largest experience, Finnish investigators have used antibody tests to study children with lower respiratory tract infections. They have shown that each of the three antibody tests by itself is insensitive[116] and that more than 90% of serological diagnoses that are made require either an antigen or an antibody test, but not both.[117] Thus, establishing a pneumococcal etiology for all of these infections requires a battery of antigen and antibody tests. Furthermore, no commercial bacterial antibody assays are available for routine clinical use.[121] Although these assays have been helpful in studies of the etiology of lower respiratory tract infections,[118] their use is likely to be limited to epidemiological surveys and perhaps to clinical trials of pneumococcal vaccines.[121]

The newest approach to the diagnosis of pneumococcal infections has been the use of PCR techniques. Using primers derived from the genes for pneumolysin,[122, 123] autolysin (PytA),[122, 124] DNA polymerase I (pol I)[125] and penicillin-binding protein (PBP) 2B,[126, 127] blood specimens from patients with culture-proven pneumococcal bacteremia have been tested by using PCR. In three of these studies, all culture-proven cases of pneumococcal infection were also identified by PCR.[123–125] When only one of two blood culture specimens was positive, both were positive by PCR.[124] In another study, however, not all patient specimens positive by culture were positive by PCR.[122] Similarly promising results have also been obtained in PCR studies of CSF specimens taken from patients with meningitis.[127–129]

Sputum specimens from patients with pneumonia[130] and middle ear fluid from those with otitis media have also been studied.[131–133] In each instance, PCR assays were positive in virtually all patients with culture-proven disease. In addition, PCR assays were often positive in patients with negative cultures. In one study of an autolysin-based PCR assay of sputum specimens, the predictive values of positive and negative results were 100% and 95%, respectively.[130] Using a pneumolysin PCR assay, Finnish investigators have shown that positive diagnoses were increased from 18% (culture-positive only) to 28% for acute otitis media[133] and from 11% to 46% for otitis media with effusion.[132] In these studies, the PCR assays have been shown to be exquisitely sensitive and specific for *S. pneumoniae*.

PCR methods have also been used to distinguish between upper respiratory tract isolates of pneumococci and other streptococci when conventional biochemical tests have given equivocal results.[134] Nonetheless, whether a person in whom a PCR assay is positive truly has pneumococcal disease rather than colonization is something that must be determined primarily by clinical criteria. Furthermore, PCR assays are expensive and labor-intensive[125]; whether they can be modified for routine diagnostic use is uncertain. If this proves feasible, PCR-based diagnostic assays could eventually supplant antigen and antibody techniques for diagnosing pneumococcal infections.

Treatment and Antimicrobial Resistance

Until recently there were well-established principles for treating pneumococcal infections.[25] When *S. pneumoniae* was known or expected to be sensitive to penicillin, adults with uncomplicated pneumococcal pneumonia could be adequately treated with 600,000 units of procaine penicillin G intramuscularly twice daily or with 500,000 to 1 million units of aqueous penicillin G intravenously every 4 hours. An acceptable alternative for parenteral therapy was a first-generation cephalosporin. Because of its more reliable absorption and longer half-life than penicillin G, oral amoxicillin could often be used to complete a 5- to 10-day course of treatment. More serious invasive infections, such as meningitis or endocarditis, could initially be treated parenterally with 12 to 24 million doses of penicillin daily. Most children with acute otitis media caused by penicillin-sensitive pneumococci could be successfully treated with oral amoxicillin.

In spite of the clarity and established effectiveness of these general principles, they are becoming increasingly difficult to apply in clinical practice. In most patients infected with *S. pneumoniae*, the causative organism is not known at the time treatment is begun, and in many cases it is never established with certainty. Of necessity, broad-spectrum treatment to cover other potential pathogens is required. Unfortunately, treatment decisions are becoming more problematic because of the increasing occurrence of pneumococcal infections caused by organisms that are resistant to penicillin and to other commonly used antimicrobial agents.

In the late 1960s, isolates of *S. pneumoniae* emerged in Papua New Guinea[135] and elsewhere that were moderately resistant to penicillin (minimum inhibitory concentration [MIC] > 0.1–1.0 μg/mL). A decade later, isolates with greater resistance to penicillin, resistance to several other antibiotics, or both were reported.[136] Since then, antibiotic-resistant pneumococci have been isolated from patients with increasing frequency throughout the world, and these infections are now regarded as among the most important of the newly emerging infectious diseases in humans.[137] The published literature on antimicrobial resistance among *S. pneumoniae* is now extensive. A number of excellent general reviews[138–140] and commentaries[141–143] have been published, along with summaries of issues related to the molecular mechanisms involved in the development of antibiotic resistance,[144–146] laboratory diagnosis,[147, 148] epidemiology[149, 150] and the clinical features[151] and treatment[152–158] of these infections.

The resistance of *S. pneumoniae* to penicillin and to other β-lactam antibiotics is due to alterations in one or more of the organism's PBPs (1a, 1b, 2x, 2a, 2b and 3). In highly resistant strains, as many as four PBPs have been shown to have reduced capacities to bind penicillin.[143, 146] The genes encoding for each of these PBPs have been modified by acquiring new DNA sequences from heterologous DNA donors, many of which appear to be viridans streptococci such as *S. mitis*. Because each of these changes initially occurs as an independent event, the resultant PBP patterns vary widely and each resistant isolate, with its "mosaic" of altered PBP genes, represents a distinct clone.[146, 159] This mosaic of penicillin-resistant PBP genes can then spread "horizontally" to other pneumococcal strains.[143] Furthermore, individual penicillin-resistant strains characterized by a unique PBP pattern may also share other characteristics, such as resistance to other antibiotics, capsular type, and rate of autolysis. Clonal expansion allows these resistant strains to become established in populations and to spread to distant geographic sites.[160, 161]

Once penicillin resistance is acquired, it can increase, perhaps by point mutation. External pressure from antibiotic overuse and the unique resistance-selecting capacity of different β-lactam antibiotics[162] may account for some of these changes. Penicillin-resistant pneumococci can also acquire new and different capsular serotypes, again through genetic transformation, as shown by the appearance of a penicillin-resistant serotype 14 isolate in a day care center.[163] This isolate had the specific PBP mosaic pattern of a previously circulating serotype 23F resistant isolate. It is not known how frequently capsular transformation occurs. Although possible, capsular transformation involving highly invasive serotypes (e.g., type 3) has thus far not been observed clinically.

The increased resistance of pneumococci to other β-lactam antibiotics, including third-generation cephalosporins, can be acquired more rapidly than penicillin resistance, most likely because no more than two genetic determinants are involved.[146] Resistance to other antimicrobial agents is not due to changes in PBPs, although genetic determinants associated with resistance may be acquired from other, unrelated bacteria.

The most reliable tests for antibiotic susceptibility of pneumococci include determination of MIC in broth dilution, disk diffusion, and the more recently developed E-test.[147] The E-test is relatively rapid and reliable and has been adopted in many clinical laboratories. Broth dilution techniques are more commonly employed in epidemiological studies. Current terminology classifies pneumococci with MIC values of 0.1 to 1.0 μg/mL as being of intermediate susceptibility and those with MIC values of greater than or equal to 2.0 μg/mL as being highly resistant. The terms penicillin-nonsusceptible *S. pneumoniae* (PNSP; MIC ≥ 0.1 μg/mL) and penicillin-resistant pneumococci (PRP; MIC ≥ 2.0 μg/mL) have been proposed as more appropriate, following the convention used to describe antibiotic resistance of other bacteria.[164] These new terms have not yet been adopted for routine use.

In the United States, data from the ongoing Pneumococcal Sentinel Surveillance System of the Centers for Disease Control and Prevention (CDC) showed that from 1993 to 1994, 14.1% of 740 invasive isolates were of intermediate susceptibility and 3.2% were highly resistant.[164] These rates were considerably higher than those reported 2 years earlier.[165] Resistance to at least one antibiotic had also increased over this period to 25.5% of all isolates. Isolates that were of intermediate susceptibility were more commonly found in children than in adults, and resistance to at least one other antibiotic was found in almost two thirds of these strains. In another report of 1527 clinically significant isolates obtained from 30 outpatient units, 12.6% of isolates from children 5 years or younger were highly resistant, whereas rates for older people were 7.5 to 8.1%.[166] Another survey of 33 clinical laboratories reported that 5.7% of 1627 isolates were highly resistant.[167] In child day care centers, nasopharyngeal carriage rates for pneumococci that are of intermediate susceptibility can be particularly high,[150, 168] and in acute otitis media almost one third of middle ear isolates can be resistant to penicillin.[169] In the 1993 to 1994 CDC study, 89% of all intermediately susceptible invasive isolates and 100% of all highly resistant isolates were serotypes included in the 23-valent pneumococcal vaccine.[164]

Reports from other countries indicate that, in many, the incidence of antibiotic-resistant pneumococci continues to increase,[138, 149, 170] with highest rates being reported in Southwest Europe, Israel, South Africa, the southern region of South America, Central and Eastern Europe, Korea, and New Guinea.[149, 170, 171] Studies conducted in the 1990s in western Europe[172–182] confirm the growing importance of this problem. Reported rates from individual countries cannot be compared directly because of differences in the completeness of the bacteriological diagnosis in suspected cases, differences in the laboratory methods for demonstrating resistance, and differences in the populations studied.

One effort to overcome some of these limitations has been the Alexander Project.[183] This international collaborative study has involved 10 centers in Europe and five in the United States. Using standardized methods and only one laboratory, workers have compared the antimicrobial susceptibilities of bacterial isolates from patients with community-acquired lower respiratory tract infections. The results for *S. pneumoniae* are shown in Table 22–2. Rates for intermediately susceptible isolates varied substantially among these countries; the high rate in Munich probably reflected antimicrobial treatment of the cystic fibrosis patients who were studied. In 6 of the 14 centers, very resistant isolates were not found, but especially high rates of high-level resistance were observed in France and Spain. Resistance rates to almost all of the other antibiotics tested were higher in penicillin-resistant compared with penicillin-susceptible strains. Although many factors account for these differences, higher rates of penicillin resistance in certain European countries are associated with high rates of antibiotic consumption and low rates of completing full courses of prescribed oral antimicrobial treatment.[184]

Table 22–2. **PENICILLIN RESISTANCE OF *Streptococcus pneumoniae*, 1992 TO 1993***

LOCATION	TOTAL NO. OF ISOLATES	PENICILLIN NONSUSCEPTIBLE STRAINS (MIC 0.12–1 μg/mL)		PENICILLIN-RESISTANT STRAINS (MIC ≥2 μg/mL)	
		No.	%	No.	%
United Kingdom					
London	233	4	1.7	1	0.4
Belfast	83	5	6.0	—	—
France					
Toulouse	241	40	16.6	45	18.7
Paris	153	11	7.2	17	11.1
Spain					
Barcelona	495	85	17.2	122	24.6
Madrid	54	8	14.8	21	38.9
Germany					
Weingarten	110	4	3.6	—	—
Munich	46	23	50.0	—	—
Italy					
Genoa	128	10	7.8	—	—
United States					
Portland, OR	33	2	6.1	—	—
Johnson City, TN	20	3	15.0	—	—
Worcester, MA	57	9	15.8	1	1.8
New York, NY	125	11	8.8	9	7.2
Cleveland, OH	75	13	17.3	6	8.3

*Isolates were obtained from patients with community-acquired lower respiratory infections and were tested in one laboratory.
MIC, minimal inhibitory concentration.
Data from reference 183.

The treatment of infections caused by antimicrobial-resistant pneumococci has been widely discussed.[152–154, 156–158] There appears to be no difference in the treatment response of adults with severe pneumococcal pneumonia caused by penicillin- and cephalosporin-resistant compared with that caused by penicillin- and cephalosporin-sensitive strains.[185] Similar findings have been reported in children with pneumococcal bacteremia, excluding cases of meningitis.[154] Furthermore, analysis of published reports of apparent failures of penicillin treatment of adults with penicillin-resistant pneumococcal pneumonia[152] indicates that few if any of these reports withstand careful scrutiny.[153, 156]

The one clinical situation in which infection with resistant pneumococci poses a serious therapeutic challenge is meningitis. Even with high doses, penicillin and other β-lactam antibiotics may not adequately penetrate into the CSF and treatment failures occur.[152, 158, 186–188] Because the causative organisms may also be resistant to other antimicrobial agents, combination therapy with ceftriaxone and vancomycin is becoming more widely used in the treatment of pneumococcal meningitis.[152, 158] In addition, strains that are highly resistant to penicillin are being increasingly isolated from children with otitis media who have not responded to oral antibiotic treatment, although most of them are sensitive to clindamycin and vancomycin.[169] The widespread problem of vancomycin resistance among enterococci[189] and its recent emergence in *Staphylococcus aureus*[190] has increased concern that pneumococci too might develop resistance to this agent.

Antibiotic resistance among pneumococci, especially in children younger than 2 years, has added to the urgency of developing more effective pneumococcal vaccines for this age group.[191] Resistant strains also account for an increasing proportion of pneumococcal infections in older people, however, and the burden of disease caused by these strains in older people may be greater than it is in young children. Few would doubt that concern about antibiotic-resistant pneumococci is one of the major factors underlying the recent upsurge in interest in pneumococcal polysaccharide vaccine.

EPIDEMIOLOGY OF PNEUMOCOCCAL INFECTIONS

The Carrier State

Pneumococcal infections almost always occur in people who are asymptomatic nasopharyngeal carriers of the organism. Thus, it is not surprising that the greater incidence of pneumococcal infections in young children, compared with that in adults, is paralleled by higher carrier rates. Studies conducted in the 1970s showed carrier rates of 38 to 60% in preschool children, 29 to 35% in grammar school children, and 9 to 25% in junior high school students.[192] Carrier rates among adults were lower: 18 to 29% in those with children at home but only 6% in those without children at home.

Adults often have measurable levels of serum antibody against a number of pneumococcal serotypes. These antibodies may reduce the likelihood of acquisition of nasopharyngeal carriage or its duration. Studies in military recruits have provided insight into the serological response of adults after exposure to a new pneumococcal serotype.[193] In one unusual outbreak of serotype 1 pneumonia, serum antibody was detected in 3.6% of unexposed controls and 27.8% of the asymptomatic contacts of those infected. In a second outbreak of pneumonia due to serotypes 7F and 8, paired sera from those who were colonized but asymptomatic showed that 12 (48%) of 25 who were initially seronegative developed antibodies within the next month. Similarly, among those who initially were both asymptomatic and culture-negative, 25 (52%) of 48 who were also seronegative experienced antibody development 1 month later. These findings demonstrate that serum antibody develops in a substantial proportion of adults after nasopharyngeal colonization in the absence of recognized local or invasive disease.

Children younger than 2 years of age seldom have type-specific serum antibody before being colonized, and virtually all eventually become nasopharyngeal carriers at one time or another. In one study of 1273 Australian children 6 to 54 months of age, 368 (29%) were found to be nasal carriers.[194, 195] Serotypes 6, 9, 14, 18, 19, and 23 accounted for 74% of all organisms carried. Carriage was associated with a significant elevation in serum antibody for some types (e.g., 18C, 19F, and 23F) but not for others (e.g., 6A and 14). Monthly samples taken over a 5-month period showed that 91% of all children became nasal carriers at least once, 18% became carriers on four or five occasions, and 36% of carriers harbored two or more serotypes simultaneously on at least one occasion.

Another large study in Sweden focused on nasopharyngeal colonization in the first year of life.[196] At 2 months of age, 12% of children were colonized by *S. pneumoniae* and 30 to 32% were colonized at 6 and 10 months of age. More recent data from Sweden on the nasopharyngeal carriage of penicillin resistant strains have shown that the duration of carriage is longest in children less than 1 year of age (median 30 days) compared with older children and adults, and that after 3 months, 17% of these infants are still carrying the organism.[197] In most children, nasopharyngeal carriage is followed by the appearance of type-specific antibody.[198, 199] Such antibody decreases the likelihood of recolonization with the same serotype, although in young children recolonization may occur with certain serotypes because of a poor antibody response following the first episode of colonization.

The relationship between the acquisition of nasopharyngeal carriage of individual serotypes and their likelihood of causing invasive disease is not well understood.[200] Some serotypes (e.g., 6, 14, 19, 23) are acquired frequently and carried for extended periods; others (e.g., type 12) are acquired infrequently and are rapidly eliminated, whereas others have intermediate patterns of acquisition and invasiveness. A longitudinal study of the acquisition and duration of nasopharyngeal carriage among children in Papua New Guinea has shown that serotypes regarded as more immunogenic (e.g., 3, 7, 9) were less frequently acquired than were less-immunogenic (e.g., 6, 19, 23) serotypes, and they were carried for shorter periods of time.[200] No relationship was found between the immunogenicity of individual serotypes and their invasiveness, however. Whether the same pattern would be found in developed countries is uncertain; in children in Papua New Guinea, the more highly immunogenic "adult" serotypes are more frequent causes of invasive disease, unlike what occurs in developed countries.

Age and season of the year can have modest effects on acquisition and carrier rates, but living circumstances are usually more important. In families, the spread of *S. pneumoniae* carriage is often associated with symptoms of viral upper respiratory tract infection.

Pneumococcal Infections in Adults

Pneumococcal Pneumonia

Pneumococcal infections continue to be the major cause of adult community-acquired pneumonia requiring hospital admission. The annual incidence of pneumococcal pneumonia, however, has not been well defined. Most studies are case series that have focused on community-acquired pneumonia in general, and several excellent reviews have been published.[201–206] In the United States, much of the clinical research in this area has focused on defining risk factors that are useful in establishing prognosis.[207–213] Similar reports have appeared from other countries.[214–216] The goal in most of these studies has been to establish criteria for intensive care unit admission or for outpatient rather than inpatient treatment.[217] Less attention has been given to estimating the population-based incidence of community-acquired pneumonia or to determining the proportion of cases caused by various microbial agents, including *S. pneumoniae*.

A study of trends in infectious diseases in the United States noted a 20% increase in mortality due to respiratory tract infections during the period 1980 to 1992.[218] In 1992, there were 77,336 deaths in which the underlying cause was listed as respiratory tract infection (30 per 100,000 population). Based on multiple cause-of-death analysis, the overall number of such deaths was considerably higher. Approximately 85% of these deaths that occurred in elderly people (≥65 years) were recorded as being due to pneumonia of unspecified etiology. The reasons for the increase in respiratory infection mortality over this period are unclear and may reflect changes in the way death certificate data are recorded. Nonetheless, pneumonia and influenza are still the sixth leading cause of death in the United States.[219]

Only a few population-based studies of the incidence of community-acquired pneumonia have ever been published. One report described a study conducted in Finland from 1981 to 1982.[220] In an area with a population of almost 50,000 residents, there were 546 cases of pneumonia, giving an overall rate of 11.6 cases per 1000 people per year. In people 60 to 74 years old and 75 or more years of age, the rates were 15.4 and 34.7 cases per 1000 people per year, respectively. Men had higher incidence and higher mortality rates than women. Among all patients, 31% were at least 60 years of age, and 67% of these patients were admitted to hospital. The mortality rate in this elderly group was 11%. Overall, 54% of elderly patients were free of major underlying medical conditions that are associated with an increased risk for pneumonia. The results of this Finnish study are similar to those obtained in four other studies conducted in the United States in the 1970s and 1980s.[220] Another study of community-acquired lower respiratory tract infection has been reported from a single general practice in the United Kingdom.[221] The overall incidence of disease was 44 cases per 1000 people per year. Findings on physical examination were abnormal in only 47% of patients, however, and only 10% of those with chest radiographs had evidence of acute pulmonary infiltrates. Thus, the rate for community-acquired pneumonia was probably not much different from that reported from Finland.

The incidence of community-acquired pneumonia requiring hospitalization was reexamined in the United States in 1991.[221a] The study included adults 18 years and older who lived in an area of Ohio with a total population of 1.1 million people. Based on 2776 patients, the annual incidence among adults was 2.7 cases per 1000 population. In people aged 18 to 44 years, 45 to 64 years, and 65 or more years, the incidence was 0.9, 2.8, and 10.1 cases per 1000 population, respectively. (The hospitalization rate for elderly pneumonia patients in Ohio was somewhat lower than that for similar patients in Finland who were studied 10 years eariler.[220] Moreover, by 1993 the pneumonia hospitalization rate for elderly people in Finland had risen to 24 cases per 1000 population.[221b]) In Ohio, pneumonia hospitalization rates (cases/1000 population) were higher in men (2.9) than in women (2.5) and in African Americans (3.4) than in whites (2.6). The overall mortality rate was 8.8%, but in the elderly it was 12.5%.

Determining the microbial cause of community-acquired pneumonia continues to be a challenging task. The clinical and laboratory features and the prognoses for the pneumonias caused by specific microorganism show considerable overlap and, in spite of careful analysis, the causative agent cannot be reliably predicted in more than half of cases.[222] As a result, it has been difficult to know with certainty the proportion of all adult community-acquired pneumonias requiring hospitalization that is caused by *S. pneumoniae*.

A review of 29 studies of community-acquired pneumonia conducted during the 1980s indicated that approximately 30 to 50% of all cases requiring hospitalization were caused by *S. pneumoniae*.[21] This finding was consistent with the conclusions of several,[204–206] although not all,[201–203] authors who have reviewed smaller numbers of reports. In all but 3 of the 29 studies reviewed, *S. pneumoniae* ranked first among all known causes of pneumonia. The 29 reports could not be compared with each other for several reasons. Individual studies often excluded one or more groups of patients (e.g., those with terminal illness, cancer, immunosuppression, HIV infection, intravenous drug abuse, nosocomial infection, previous antimicrobial treatment, or nursing home residence). Different diagnostic tests were used in different studies to diagnose pneumococcal pneumonia, and it was seldom stated what proportion of patients received each test. Special tests for other microbial agents were used in some but not all studies.

Since the earlier review, at least 30 additional reports of adult community-acquired pneumonia have been published from the United States,[223–226] western Europe[227–246] and other countries (Table 22–3).[216, 247–250] Like the earlier reports,[21] these reports vary considerably in quality; some describe clinical experience in community hospitals in which routine diagnostic tests such as blood cultures were seldom performed,[246] whereas others exclude from consideration sputum Gram's stain and culture results.[224] Several studies not only include blood and sputum culture results but also use special diagnostic tests for pneumococcal capsular antigen, pneumolysin, or pneumolysin antigen-antibody complexes (i.e., so-called "enhanced" diagnostic studies).[229, 230, 235, 246, 250]

In spite of the variability among these studies, several conclusions can be drawn from these reports. First, although *S. pneumoniae* was reported to cause 6 to 55% of all cases of community-acquired pneumonia, in 26 of 30 studies it was the first-ranked cause of infection among all microbial agents that could be identified. Second, if a study reported a low proportion of pneumococcal infections, it usually reported a high proportion of cases for which no causative agent was identified. For example, among 12 studies in which 6 to 18% of all cases were caused by *S. pneumoniae*, 8 reported that 54% or more cases had no identified microbial cause (see Table 22–3). Likewise, if there was a high proportion of cases of pneumococcal pneumonia, there was usually a low proportion with no known cause. For example, among five reports in which 41 to 55% of cases were thought due to pneumococcal infection, three reported that no microbial cause was identified in 19% or fewer cases. Finally, *S. pneumoniae* was the most common cause of severe community-acquired pneumonia requiring intensive care unit admission. The 30 studies summarized in Table 22–3 reaffirm earlier findings[21] that pneumococcal pneumonia is the most common cause of adult community-acquired pneumonia requiring hospitalization.

Pneumococcal infections are an underappreciated cause of nosocomial pneumonia on general medical units,[251, 252] in intensive care units,[253] and in long-term care facilities,[252, 254] accounting for as many as 20 to 25% of cases in each setting. Although nursing home residents who develop pneumonia often do not have adequate studies to establish an etiological diagnosis,[255] distinct outbreaks of pneumococcal pneumonia have been described in several chronic care facilities,[256] and *S. pneumoniae* is probably the most common cause of bacterial pneumonia acquired in nursing homes. Focal outbreaks of pneumococcal pneumonia continue to occur in settings with severe crowding and poor ventilation.[257] At the other end of the spectrum, pneumococcal infection is the commonest bacterial cause of all community-acquired lower respiratory tract infections, most cases of which are not pneumonia. In one study that used "enhanced" diagnostic methods, pneumococcal infection was diagnosed in almost 40% of patients who were 60 to 79 years of age (the upper age limit for the study) or who had underlying medical conditions.[221]

The generally accepted mortality rate for community-acquired pneumonia is 5 to 10% in people of all ages and 10 to 30% in people at least 65 years of age.[258] The mortality rate for community-acquired pneumococcal pneumonias is not well known, however, largely because accurate diagnosis of all cases that are not bacteremic remains elusive. Surprisingly, none of the studies of community-acquired pneumonia reported earlier[21] or in Table 22–3 provides separate mortality rates for patients with bacteremic and nonbacteremic pneumococcal disease. In all likelihood, most fatal cases of pneumococcal pneumonia are associated with bacteremia. Thus, a better estimate of the mortality for pneumococcal pneumonia can probably be obtained from an analysis of bacteremic or invasive pneumococcal disease.

Invasive Pneumococcal Disease

Invasive pneumococcal disease is defined as any infection in which *S. pneumoniae* is isolated from the blood or another normally sterile site. Most recently published case series have included all cases of pneumococcal bacteremia,[259–270] although a few reports have focused on only bacteremic pneumococcal pneumonia[271, 272] or pneumococcal meningitis.[273–276] Among all cases of pneumococcal bacteremia, approximately 70 to 90% are associated with pneumococcal pneumonia,[259, 263, 265, 268–270] and 5 to 10% with pneumococcal meningitis.[259, 269] Splenectomy patients have accounted for as many as 2 to 7% of all bacteremic patients in a few reported series,[266, 268, 269] and nosocomial infection has characterized 4 to 23% of cases in other reports.[264–268, 272] Surprisingly, 8 to 16% of adults with pneumococcal bacteremia have had no identified source of infection.[265, 266, 268, 270] Moreover, 17 to 34% of patients with pneumococcal bacteremia have had no identifiable underlying high-risk medical condition.[259–261, 264, 266, 270] This last finding is not widely appreciated.

The mortality rates for pneumococcal bacteremia in recent case series have been 16 to 36% among all adults[259, 262–269, 271, 272] and 28 to 51% in people at least 65 years of age.[260, 262, 263, 265, 268–270] In some reports, recurrent[277] or relapsing[278] pneumococcal bacteremia or pneumonia has been a sign of underlying immunocompromise or complement deficiency,[279] and mortality rates in these patients have been high.[277] The low mortality rates in bacteremic pneumococcal pneumonia (5% in all people and 3% in those 65 years and older) reported from Stockholm during the period 1977 to 1984[280] have not been characteristic of any of the more recent studies. In pneumococcal meningitis, case-fatality rates have been 23% overall[275] and 33[274] and 48%[276] in the elderly. In the few case series of invasive pneumococcal disease in which serotype data have been reported, 90% or more of the isolates have been vaccine-type organisms.[269, 274, 276]

Population-based studies rather than case series provide a better indication of the burden of invasive pneu-

Table 22–3. ADULT COMMUNITY-ACQUIRED PNEUMOCOCCAL PNEUMONIA

LOCATION	YEAR(S) OF STUDY	PROSPECTIVE STUDY	MEAN/MEDIAN AGE (yr)	TOTAL NO. OF CASES	CASES OF PNEUMOCOCCAL PNEUMONIA				UNKNOWN CAUSE NO. (%)	REFERENCE
					Definite* (No.)	Presumptive† (No.)	Total (%)	Rank‡		
United States										
Little Rock, AR	1985	Yes	64	154	8	1	9 (6)	2	75 (49)	224
Dallas, TX	1985–1986	No	NS	222	39	NS	39 (18)	1	175 (79)	223
Yountville, CA	1989–1991	Yes	80	104	1	30	31 (30)	1	30 (29)	225
Baltimore, MD	1990–1991	Yes	≈44	385	31	38	69 (18)	1	156 (41)†	226
Ohio—15 hospitals	1991	Yes	NS	2776	154	197	351 (13)	2	1545 (56)	221a
United Kingdom										
20 hospitals	1987	No	54	60 ICU	4	7	11 (18)	1	25 (42)	230
France										
Tourcoing	1987–1991	No	64	299 ICU	25	55	80 (27)	1	102 (34)	237
Paris	1987–1989	Yes	58	132 ICU	22	21	43 (33)§	1	37 (28)	235
Montpellier	1989–1994	NS	46	55	NS	NS	26 (47)	1	9 (16)	238
Clermont-Ferrand	NS	Yes	NS	117	NS	NS	29 (25)	1	73 (62)	241
17 centers	1990–1991	Yes	63	117	NS	NS	35 (30)	1	63 (54)	236
Tours	1992–1993	Yes	62	115	NS	NS	12 (10)	1	86 (75)	242
Spain										
Barcelona	1988–1990	Yes	45	58 ICU	7	6	13 (22)	1	23 (40)	243
Barcelona	1990–1991	Yes	48	105	7	6	13 (12)	2	59 (56)	232
Barcelona	1991–1992	Yes	72	95 ICU	18	10	28 (29)	1	45 (47)	231
Murcia	1991–1994	Yes	58	342	11	32	43 (13)	1	242 (71)	244
Germany										
Berlin	1984–1985	Yes	NS	442	NS	NS	68 (15)	1	238 (54)	227
Bonn	1985–1993	No	51	93	6	NS	6 (17)		74 (80)	228
Berlin	1991–1992	Yes	57	237	16	14	30 (13)	1	77 (32)	245
Italy										
Milan	1991–1992	Yes	51	108	NS	NS	10 (9)	3	50 (46)	233
Denmark										
Aarhus	NS	NS	NS	254	11	24	35 (14)	1	161 (63)	234
Finland										
Varkaus	1982–1985	Yes	NS	64	0	33	33 (52)§	1	NS	246
Oulu	1986–1987	Yes	67	125	28	41	69 (55)§	1	15 (12)	239
The Netherlands										
Leiden	1991–1993	Yes	65	334	44	46	90 (27)	1	151 (45)	240
Ireland										
Dublin	1986–1987	Yes	77	127*	NS	NS	47 (37)§	1	53 (42)	229
Israel										
Beersheba	1991–1992	Yes	49	346	NS	NS	148 (43)§	1	67 (19)	247
New Zealand										
Christchurch	1992–1993	Yes	58	255	NS	NS	100 (39)	1	74 (29)	249
South Africa										
Johannesburg	1982–1992	No	44	259 ICU	≥57	≤19	76 (29)	1	100 (39)	216
	1990–1991	Yes	32	102	13	29	42 (41)	1	36 (35)	248
Cameroon										
3 centers	1991–1992	Yes	39	110	10	21	31 (28)§	1	53 (48)	250

*A definite diagnosis of pneumococcal pneumonia was based on isolation of *Streptococcus pneumoniae* from a normally sterile site.
†The clinical and laboratory criteria for diagnosing probable pneumococcal pneumonia varied from study to study.
‡Rank order of pneumococcal pneumonia among all known causes of pneumonia reported in each study.
§Diagnostic studies were "enhanced," usually with tests for pneumococcal capsular polysaccharide antigen.
ICU, intensive care unit; NS, not stated.

mococcal disease. Studies conducted in several areas of the United States in the 1980s suggested that the annual incidence of pneumococcal bacteremia or invasive pneumococcal disease was approximately 16 to 19 cases per 100,000 population (Table 22–4).[281–284] In these studies, the incidence in people at least 65 years of age was 42 to 57 cases per 100,000 population. More recently, population-based data from Atlanta,[285] Franklin County, Ohio,[286] and Dallas[287] have given rates of 19 to 30 cases per 100,000 total population and 80 to 85 cases per 100,000 elderly people. Lower rates have been observed in Hawaii;[288] Southern California;[289] Huntington, West Virginia (M. A. Mufson, personal communication, 1997); and San Francisco[290] (J. P. Nuorti, personal communication, 1997). The 1991 study of community-acquired pneumonia in Ohio, in which 76% of patients had blood cultures, reported that the incidence of bacteremic pneumococcal pneumonia in adults 18 years and older was 14.2 cases per 100,000 population.[221a]

Several epidemiological reports have also provided estimates of the incidence of invasive pneumococcal disease in countries other than the United States (see Table 22–4). Studies from Canada (D. Kertesz, personal communication, 1997),[291] Sweden (A. Ortqvist, personal communication, 1997), Norway (V. Hasseltvedt, personal communication, 1997),[292] Denmark,[293, 294] and Israel[295] have shown rates of disease similar to the higher rates observed in many areas in the United States. In these countries, the incidence of invasive pneumococcal disease in the elderly has ranged from 47 to 80 cases per 100,000 population. Much lower rates, however, have been observed in Finland,[296] Australia (G. Hogg, personal communication, 1997), and England and Wales (R. C. George and E. Miller, personal communication, 1997). Low rates have also been reported from Belgium, where isolates from middle ear aspirates have been included along with invasive isolates.[175]

The substantial differences in the observed rates of invasive pneumococcal disease among different countries are disturbing. Variation in the frequency with which blood cultures are obtained in patients with pneumonia probably explains some of these differences. In Finland, for example, blood cultures are seldom obtained in patients with community-acquired pneumonia.[246] Furthermore, rates of disease can vary substantially in different regions of the same country in the same year. For example, in the 19 counties of Norway, the incidence of invasive pneumococcal disease in 1996 ranged from 5 to 33 cases per 100,000 total population,[292] and the incidence of disease in Oslo that year exceeded the incidence observed in Atlanta 2 years earlier (see Table 22–4).[285, 292]

More accurate blood culturing techniques may also be responsible for some these increases.[297] Nonetheless, some investigators believe that the increasing rates of disease observed in Sweden,[298–300] Norway,[292] Finland,[301] Denmark,[293, 294, 302] and the United Kingdom[303] during the 1990s represent a true increase in the occurrence of disease rather than improved ascertainment of all cases. In Sweden and Denmark, the increases have occurred among elderly people, not children. Moreover, in Sweden the increase has coincided with a substantial increase in the number of serotype 14 isolates.[300] For the time being, no single explanation seems to account for the rising incidence of invasive pneumococcal disease observed in these countries.

Several studies in the United States have documented substantially higher rates of invasive pneumococcal disease in African Americans compared with those in whites and Hispanics.[281, 283–286, 290] This finding applies to both elderly people and younger adults, regardless of whether they have HIV infection.[290] Far higher rates of invasive disease have been reported among the White Mountain Apaches in Arizona,[304] the Native population in Alaska,[305] and the Aboriginal population in central Australia.[306, 306a] In these three areas, the rates for invasive disease in people of all ages have been 156, 74, and 297 cases per 100,000 population, respectively.

The data on mortality from invasive pneumococcal disease obtained in population-based studies (see Table 22–4) confirm those reported in case series; mortality rates have ranged from 8 to 22% in people of all ages and from 16 to 44% in the elderly. Likewise, virtually all studies with serogroup/serotype data report that greater than or equal to 90% of the isolates belong to the serogroups or serotypes included in 23-valent pneumococcal vaccine (see Table 22–4).

Pneumococcal Infections in Children

Otitis Media

Nearly all children experience one or more episodes of otitis media during the first years of life. Several biological factors may increase the susceptibility of young children to otitis media, including eustachian tube abnormalities, early cessation of breast-feeding,[307] increased attachment of pathogens to nasopharyngeal epithelial cells[308] with resultant earlier nasopharyngeal colonization,[309] lower rates of nasopharyngeal colonization with α-streptococci that have inhibitory activity against bacterial pathogens,[310] and decreased ability of the middle ear cavity to coat organisms with secretory IgA, IgM, or IgG during the early stages of infection.[311]

Epidemiological studies from United States have shown that 10% of children have at least one attack of otitis media by 3 months of age, approximately 60% by 1 year of age, and more than 80% by 3 years of age.[312, 313] More recent data suggest that these figures might be too conservative; in a close follow-up of 2253 infants in the Pittsburgh area, 48% had at least one episode of otitis media between the ages of 2 and 6 months, 79% between 2 and 12 months of age, and 91% by 24 months of age.[314] In Finnish studies in the 1980s, the annual incidence rates varied from 0.47 to 1.05 episodes per child among infants aged 0 to 12 months and from 0.51 to 1.42 in children aged 13 to 24 months.[315–317] The prevalence of chronic otitis media with effusion in young children varies from 5% to 25%.[318, 319] Otitis media and its sequelae also are common in developing countries: community studies have shown that perforation of the tympanic membrane is found in 0.4 to 33.3%, otorrhea in 0.4 to 6.1%, and mastoiditis in 0.19 to 0.74% of children.[320]

Table 22–4. **INCIDENCE OF INVASIVE PNEUMOCOCCAL DISEASE IN DEVELOPED COUNTRIES**

COUNTRY	YEAR(S)	NO. OF CASES	ANNUAL INCIDENCE PER 100,000 PEOPLE		MORTALITY (%)		SEROGROUP/SEROTYPE COVERAGE BY 23-VALENT VACCINE (%)	REFERENCE
			All Ages	Older Than 65 Years	All Ages	Older Than 65 Years		
United States								
Hawaii	1986–1987	220*	9†	22	16	35	—‡	288
Oklahoma City, OK	1984	139	16	55	—	—	—	281
	1990	144	17	42	15	—	86	282
Charleston, SC	1986–1987	110*	19	53	18	44	—	283
Monroe County, NY	1985–1989	671*	19	57	15	29	—	284
Southern California	1992–1995	814	13	32	8	16	—	289
Franklin County, OH	1991–1993	419*	19§	83	19	26	92	286
Atlanta, GA	1994	712	30	85	—	—	—	285
Dallas County, TX	1995	432	22	80	16	30	—	287
Huntington, WV	1990–1996	194	17	45	11	21		‖
San Francisco, CA	1994–1996	500	34	48	12	24	—	290
Canada								
Toronto	1995	470	15	63	19	28	94	291
9 sites	1996	431	15	45	11	20	94	‖
Finland	1983–1992	1045	9¶	27	—	—	95	296
Sweden	1996	1336	15	47	—	—	—	‖
Norway	1996	885	21	62	—	—	90	292, ‖
Denmark	1993	962	19	55	—	—	≥90	293
	1996	1417	27	80**	—	—	≥90	294
Israel	1994–1996	603*	15¶	55	28	36	94	295
Australia—Victoria	1994–1996	1043	8	25	—	—	99	‖
England and Wales	1996	4802	9	31	22††	28††	98	‖

*Pneumococcal bacteremia only.
†Reported rates have been rounded to the nearest whole number.
‡Dash indicates no data available.
§People older than 18 years.
‖Data for Huntington, WV, from M. A. Mufson, personal communication, 1997; for Canada, 9 sites, from D. Kertesz, personal communication, 1997; for Sweden, from A. Örtqvist, personal communication, 1997; for Norway, from V. Hasseltvedt, personal communication, 1997; for Australia, G. Hogg, personal communication, 1997; for England and Wales, from R. C. George and E. Miller, personal communication, 1997.
¶People older than 16 years.
**People older than 60 years.
††Mortality based on 32% of all cases.

The hearing impairment that often follows otitis media can directly affect language development and cognitive abilities.[321, 322] In addition to the consequences for the individual child, otitis media also has a major impact on the health care system. Almost half of all antimicrobial agents prescribed for children younger than 10 years of age are used for the treatment of otitis media.[313] In the mid-1980s, otitis media was the reason for almost one of every four physician contacts for respiratory disease in the United States,[323] and its annual direct and indirect costs were then estimated to be $3.5 billion. Antibiotics constitute only a small portion of the total treatment costs, which in one study averaged $116 per episode.[324] Treatment of recurrent otitis media was significantly more costly than treatment of the initial episode.

S. pneumoniae is the major bacterial cause of otitis media in children, accounting for 30 to 60% of middle ear fluid culture-positive episodes.[20, 325–327] The true proportion of cases of pneumococcal otitis may be larger if one accepts cases diagnosed by antigen detection[325, 328] or PCR[131–133] methods. Children with acute otitis media are more likely than healthy control subjects to be nasopharyngeal carriers of pneumococci[329] and to have nasopharyngeal antibodies to capsular polysaccharide[330] and pneumolysin.[331, 332] Because many healthy children are carriers of *S. pneumoniae*, a positive nasopharyngeal culture is not a good predictor of the cause of acute otitis media. A negative culture, however, makes a pneumococcal etiology unlikely. In children with negative cultures of middle ear fluid, *S. pneumoniae* might still be important in the pathogenesis of more prolonged disease. Experimental[333, 334] and clinical[335] data suggest that pneumococcal C-polysaccharide alone can initiate chronic middle ear inflammation. Thus, the effects of pneumococcal infection may persist long after the acute attack.

The treatment of otitis media has been extensively studied. A detailed review of several meta-analyses concluded that the long-term natural history of otitis media is favorable, although important complications such as hearing loss were not considered in these studies.[336] Modern antimicrobial treatment has virtually eliminated mastoiditis as a complication of otitis media, but the treatment of both simple acute otitis media and otitis media with effusion has had only a modest impact on other outcomes; it has been estimated that seven children must be treated to cure one child.[336] Moreover, host and environmental factors and copathogens also affect outcome. The increasing prevalence of antibiotic-resistant organisms, especially multidrug-resistant *S. pneumoniae*, has made evaluation of treatment more complex and problematic.[337] Increasing proportions of highly penicillin-resistant isolates obtained from children with otitis media are also resistant to the oral antibiotics usually used in its treatment.[169]

Antibiotic treatment does not increase the risk of nasopharyngeal carriage of penicillin-resistant pneumococci after treatment is completed, but there is an increase in the ratio of resistant to sensitive organisms as a result of the reduction in carriage of susceptible strains.[338] In one case series in which treatment was considered to have failed, however, *S. pneumoniae* was isolated from middle ear fluid in 28% of children, and 86% of these isolates were penicillin-resistant.[339] An earlier study of otitis-prone children younger than 2 years showed that recurrent attacks of otitis media could be reduced by intermittent penicillin prophylaxis,[307] but this approach is unlikely to be effective in an era of increasing antimicrobial resistance. Intravenous immune globulin (IVIG) prophylaxis has been tried in these patients, but the results have been mixed.[340, 341]

Pneumococcal Pneumonia

In children with pneumonia, establishing a bacterial diagnosis is difficult; nasopharyngeal carriage of potential pathogens is more common and sputum production less common than in older patients. In addition, the clinical and radiographic presentations of viral and bacterial pneumonia rarely help in the differential diagnosis.[342, 343] A positive bacterial culture from blood or a needle aspirate from the lung confirms a specific diagnosis, but in children both techniques are insensitive.[344] Rapid diagnostic tests based on antigen detection in serum[115, 345] or urine[346] may sometimes be helpful, but other methods are often needed, including antigen-antibody complex measurements,[119] pneumolysin antibody assays, and PCR techniques.[123]

In children 6 months of age or younger who live in developed countries, pneumococcal infection rarely causes serious lower respiratory tract disease requiring hospitalization.[347] In older children who are hospitalized for community-acquired pneumonia, however, *S. pneumoniae* is usually the most common bacterial cause of infection.[348–350] In Scandinavian countries, *S. pneumoniae* has been involved in up to 41% of cases of childhood pneumonia.[115, 345, 348, 351] A recent study from the United Kingdom[350] reported 251 children who were 5 years or younger who had been discharged from hospital with the diagnoses of lobar pneumonia, bronchopneumonia, and pneumonia, organism unspecified (ICD-9-CM 481, 485, 486). Although only 3 (1.2%) of these children had positive blood cultures for *S. pneumoniae*, an additional 184 (73%) had clinical and laboratory findings or positive sputum and nasopharyngeal cultures consistent with pneumococcal pneumonia. In developing countries, the percentage of childhood pneumonias attributable to the pneumococcus is also high, and rates for positive sputum cultures of as many as 88% have been reported.[352] In addition to infections in which *S. pneumoniae* is the only pathogen identified, it is often associated with other bacteria or viruses. In children hospitalized with pneumonia due to respiratory syncytial virus, *S. pneumoniae* is often the most common coinfecting bacterial pathogen.[353–356]

Invasive Pneumococcal Disease

Invasive pneumococcal infections are far less common than pneumococcal otitis media or pneumonia. Nonetheless, *S. pneumoniae* is one of the leading causes of invasive bacterial infections in children. In a prospective, 5-year nationwide study in Finland, *S. pneumoniae* caused

15% of all blood culture–positive infections.[357] The epidemiological features of 452 of these infections were analyzed in depth.[358] The annual incidence rate was 8.9 per 100,000 children younger than 16 years, 24.2 per 100,000 among those younger than 5 years, and 45.3 per 100,000 among those younger than 2 years. The most common clinical entities among the blood culture–positive cases were bacteremia without an apparent source (69%), pneumonia (15%), and meningitis (11%). Close contact with other children, especially in day care centers, was a major risk factor for invasive disease.[359]

Studies from other countries have usually reported higher rates of invasive pneumococcal disease than those reported in Finland. Annual incidence rates per 100,000 children 5 years or younger have been 42 in Israel,[360] 56 in New Zealand,[361] 72 in Southern California,[289] 161 in Alaska,[305] and 240 in The Gambia.[362] In Massachusetts, the age-adjusted rate for invasive pneumococcal disease in 1991 was 53.1 cases per 100,000 children, far higher than the rates for invasive disease caused by *Neisseria meningitidis* (10.2 per 100,000) or *H. influenzae* type b (2.9 per 100,000).[363]

In most studies, bacteremia from an occult focus has accounted for 30 to 40% of all cases of invasive pneumococcal disease.[360, 364, 365] Almost all children with occult pneumococcal bacteremia recover uneventfully if they are treated with parenteral antibiotics when first seen, but if they are not so treated, meningitis may occur in 6 to 10% and bacteremia may persist in 20 to 30%.[366, 367] A meta-analysis of oral antibiotic treatment of occult pneumococcal bacteremia has given lower figures: persistent bacteremia in 4.5% and meningitis in 2.7% of untreated patients.[368] It is unclear whether decisions not to treat less ill-appearing children accounted for these lower rates. In case series of pneumococcal bacteremia, pneumonia has been reported in 17 to 34% and meningitis in 14 to 34% of all cases.[360, 364, 365] The long-term sequelae of childhood pneumococcal meningitis are both frequent and severe. A meta-analysis of 9 studies involving 122 children showed that the acute illness was followed by mental retardation in 17%, spasticity or paresis in 12%, and seizure disorder in 14%.[369] Deafness was found in 28% of children and was severe in 16%. In other reports, serious neurological sequelae have affected 25 to 30% of children who survive pneumococcal meningitis.[370, 371] Repeated episodes of invasive pneumococcal infection can occur in a small proportion of young children, but they usually do not signal the presence of an underlying immunodeficiency.[372]

For all cases of invasive pneumococcal disease, mortality rates have varied from 1.3% in Finland[358] to as high as 6.6% in other settings.[360, 364, 365] The incidence of invasive pneumococcal disease observed in some centers has increased dramatically.[301, 373] Whether this reflects a true increase in disease incidence or simply greater efforts to establish a bacteriological diagnosis in suspected cases is uncertain; other centers have observed no such increase.[374]

Most episodes of invasive pneumococcal disease in children are caused by a limited number of pneumococcal capsular types. Data from 16 countries on six continents were reviewed to determine the geographic and temporal distribution of sterile site isolates and to estimate coverage of several possible pneumococcal vaccine formulas.[375] The most common pneumococcal serotypes or groups from developed countries were, in descending order, 14, 6, 19, 18, 9, 23, 7, 4, 1, and 15. In developing countries the order was 6, 14, 8, 5, 1, 19, 9, 23, 18, 15, and 7. These serotypes are also among the leading serotypes isolated from children with pneumococcal otitis media or pneumonia.[376, 377] For example, in United States, a study of 1837 children with pneumococcal isolates from middle ear fluid showed that the rank order of pneumococcal serotypes/groups isolated was 19, 23, 6, 14, 3, and 18.[378] Similar distributions have been demonstrated in Finnish[316] and Belgian[175, 316] children.

Pneumococcal Infections in Developing Countries

In 1990, there were approximately 12.5 million deaths among children younger than 5 years in developing countries.[379] Of these deaths, approximately 21% were attributable to lower respiratory tract infections. In addition, complications of otitis media are estimated to cause 51,000 childhood deaths in these countries each year.[320] Because acute respiratory tract infection (ARI) is the major cause of preventable death in developing countries, several international collaborative research programs have been initiated to study its etiology, epidemiology, and treatment.[379–381] (ARI includes both upper and lower respiratory tract infections.) As a result, many new studies of ARI have been reported from Africa,[382–387] South and Southeast Asia,[388–390] and Latin America.[391–394] The results of many of these studies are summarized in several comprehensive reviews.[320, 381, 395–397]

Community-based studies have shown that young children in developing countries experience 12 to 17 episodes of ARI and 0.2 to 3.4 episodes of acute lower respiratory tract illness per 100 child-weeks of exposure. Risk factors for developing ARI and for ARI mortality are those usually associated with poverty: low birth weight, malnutrition, lack of breast-feeding, vitamin A deficiency, crowding, parental smoking, and indoor and outdoor air pollution.[387, 394, 396] The incidence of disease is greatest in the first year of life. ARI occurs with different patterns of seasonality in different countries.[395, 398]

Microbiological studies to determine the etiology of cases of ARI, pneumonia, and meningitis have been conducted in several settings. In earlier studies, bacterial agents were usually cultured from only 10 to 30% children with ARI, including those who were hospitalized.[395] More recently, newer methods of antigen detection and serological tests for antipneumococcal antibody have been used. Using these methods, studies of acute lower respiratory tract infection in The Gambia have shown that in both infants and young children seen in hospitals and in children younger than 5 years living in rural communities, infection with *S. pneumoniae* occurred in 20, 61, and 90% of cases, respectively.[382–384] Although the specificities of these indirect tests are less than perfect, these reports indicate that *S. pneumoniae* is responsible for a greater proportion of serious respiratory illnesses than can be confirmed by conventional laboratory criteria.

Reports of childhood bacterial meningitis from several African countries have shown that *S. pneumoniae* accounts for 20 to 50% of all cases[399–403] and can have a mortality rate of 35%.[399, 403] Other studies have reported on the annual incidence of invasive pneumococcal disease. In The Gambia, the annual rates in children younger than 1 year and younger than 5 years were estimated to be 554 and 240 cases per 100,000 people, respectively,[362] rates far higher than those reported from developed countries. Subsequent observations in The Gambia from 1993 to 1995 documented annual rates of invasive pneumococcal disease of 224, 139 and 82 cases per 100,000 children aged 2 to 11, 12 to 23, and 24 to 35 months, respectively.[403a]

There is far less information on the occurrence of serious pneumococcal infections in adults in developing countries. In Kenya, however, the incidence of invasive disease in HIV-positive sex workers was 42.5 cases per 1000 patient-years (1 in 24), and for recurrent disease it was 264 cases per 1000 patient-years (1 in 4).[404]

Current efforts to reduce childhood mortality from ARI have concentrated on training indigenous community health workers to diagnose and treat pneumonia according to explicit case-management protocols.[381] Using this approach, health workers in developing countries have achieved a 25 to 30% reduction in mortality from all causes for children younger than 5 years.[405] Even greater success might be expected with a strategy that includes pneumococcal vaccination as well as treatment.

In developing countries, approximately 75 to 90% of clinically significant pneumococcal isolates obtained from children and, less commonly, from adults represent serotypes included in the current 23-valent vaccine.[406–412] Nonetheless, compared with developed countries, there is much less information on the serotype distribution of pneumococcal isolates obtained in developing countries, especially those taken from children 6 months or younger. Such information will be essential for determining the serotype composition of future vaccines: A recent analysis of available data has shown that nine serotypes account for 87% of invasive cases in developed countries but for only 71% in developing countries.[375] Moreover, in one study conducted in Kenya, 31% of nasopharyngeal isolates obtained from HIV-infected and uninfected children (younger than 1 year) were serotype 13, a serotype not included in the 23-valent vaccine.[413]

PASSIVE IMMUNIZATION

People at greatest risk for serious pneumococcal infections are often unable to respond to pneumococcal vaccine. In the preantibiotic era, type-specific antisera prepared in animals were used successfully to treat patients with pneumococcal infections.[414] Human immune globulin has been used successfully for both prophylaxis and treatment of experimental pneumococcal bacteremia in mice[415, 416] and otitis media in chinchillas.[416a] The problems of increasing antimicrobial resistance, the poor response to active immunization among immunocompromised patients, and technological progress in producing safer, more specific human immunoglobulins[414] have led to renewed interest in these preparations for preventing pneumococcal infections.

Several clinical trials have evaluated the efficacy of BPIG, a hyperimmune preparation obtained from adults immunized with 14-valent pneumococcal, meningococcal AC, and Hib polysaccharide vaccines. In one study, 76 children 24 months or younger with a history of one to three previous episodes of acute otitis media were given two doses of either BPIG or placebo at 30-day intervals.[341] During a 3-month follow-up period, those who had received BPIG experienced significantly fewer episodes of pneumococcal otitis media and more time spent free from illness due to otitis media. In another large study of 2515 Apache children, there was a 75% reduction (95% CI, 22–95%) in bacteremic pneumococcal infections that occurred within 90 days of injection of BPIG (16 cases) compared with placebo (4 cases).[417] More prolonged protection was not observed.

The six preparations of IVIG commercially available in the United States contain varying amounts of antibody to pneumococcal capsular polysaccharides.[418, 419] Each is safe to administer and none has been shown to transmit hepatitis B or HIV infections. IVIG should not be given to patients with selective IgA deficiency, however, because approximately 40% of these patients produce antibodies to IgA and these antibodies have been implicated in IVIG-associated anaphylactic reactions.[420] For long-term prophylaxis in patients with immunodeficiency disorders, the usual dose of IVIG is 400 mg per kg every 28 days.

Clinical trials have shown that monthly infusions of IVIG significantly reduce the occurrence of pneumococcal infections in adults with multiple myeloma[421] and lymphoma.[420] When given to children with HIV infections, IVIG has had no effect on overall mortality, and it has not been effective in those with $CD4^+$ counts that are lower than 200 cells per mL.[422] In addition, continuous IVIG prophylaxis is expensive: The annual cost of treating a 10-kg infant is approximately $5000 to 8000 and for a 70-kg adult it is $25,000 to 45,000.[420] Furthermore, the cost-effectiveness of IVIG prophylaxis for HIV-infected and other immunodeficient patients at risk of pneumococcal infections is not well established.[423]

ACTIVE IMMUNIZATION: PNEUMOCOCCAL POLYSACCHARIDE VACCINE

The first pneumococcal polysaccharide vaccines to appear in the United States were two hexavalent preparations. They were licensed in the late 1940s but were soon withdrawn from the market. The first 14-valent vaccine was licensed in the United States in 1977. Each 0.5-mL dose contained 50 μg of each purified capsular polysaccharide. The amount of each antigen was reduced to 25 μg per dose in the 23-valent vaccine that was introduced in 1983.[219, 424]

Current pneumococcal vaccines contain capsular polysaccharides of serotypes 1, 2, 3, 4, 5, 6B, 7F, 8, 9N, 9V, 10A, 11A, 12F, 14, 15B, 17F, 18C, 19A, 19F, 20, 22F, 23F, and 33F. The polysaccharides are dissolved in isotonic saline, and either phenol (0.25%) or thimerosal (0.01%) is added as a preservative. The vaccines contain no adjuvant. They should be stored at 2 to 8°C and should not be frozen; under these conditions, they are stable for 24 months. Two preparations are marketed in the United States: Pneumovax 23 by Merck Sharp & Dohme and Pnu-Imune 23 by Wyeth-Lederle Pediatrics and Vaccines. In Canada, Pneumo 23 is marketed by Pasteur Mérieux-Connaught, along with Pneumovax 23. One or more of these three vaccines is marketed in many Western European countries and elsewhere throughout the world.

The composition of pneumococcal vaccine has been determined by the relative distribution of the individual serotypes that cause invasive disease. These serotypes account for approximately 90% or more of the types responsible for invasive pneumococcal infections in developed countries (see Table 22–4). There are fewer data on the distribution of invasive serotypes from developing countries, although several studies indicate that it is similar to the distribution in developed countries.

The serotypes included in 23-valent pneumococcal vaccine reflect more than their observed frequencies as causes of invasive disease.[424] Although most serotypes within serogroups (e.g., 7F, 10A, 11A, 22F, and 33F) were chosen solely because of their epidemiological occurrence, both serotypes 9N and 9V and 19F and 19A are included because heterologous antibody responses to the individual capsular polysaccharides are poor. The polysaccharides of serotypes 15B and 15C are nearly identical and their antibodies are highly cross-reactive, however; hence only serotype 15B is included. Serotypes 6A and 6B are both frequent causes of invasive disease, and antibodies to the two polysaccharides are highly cross-reactive. Serotype 6B is included in the vaccine instead of 6A because it is a more stable antigen. Serotype 5 is included because it is a frequent cause of infection in Africa and other developing areas.

Vaccine Administration

Pneumococcal vaccine should be administered as a single 0.5-mL dose intramuscularly or subcutaneously, although the intramuscular route is generally preferred.[219] Intradermal vaccination can cause severe local reactions and should not be used. The vaccine can be administered simultaneously with influenza and other vaccines, including those used for routine childhood immunization. When given with influenza vaccine, but at a separate site, there is no decrease in the individual antibody responses to the two vaccines.[425] In addition, malaria prophylaxis with chloroquine and proguanil does not affect the antibody responses to pneumococcal vaccination.[426]

Adverse Reactions and Contraindications

There are no contraindications to pneumococcal vaccination other than a severe reaction to a previous dose of the vaccine.

Local side effects such as erythema, induration, and pain occur in approximately 30 to 50% of all recipients of pneumococcal vaccine. These reactions last 1 to 3 days and are well-tolerated.[219, 427] They may be more prominent in young and middle-aged adults, but their severity diminishes with advancing age, such that elderly people often have little or no local discomfort after vaccination. When intramuscular and subcutaneous injections are compared, local soreness lasts longer after the former, but erythema is more common after the latter. In general, local and febrile reactions following vaccination are more likely to occur in people with higher concentrations of antibodies to pneumococcal polysaccharides, and these reactions probably reflect an Arthus-like phenomenon.[428] More severe systemic reactions are infrequent, and severe febrile reactions (>103°F) are decidedly rare.

Primary pneumococcal vaccination of healthy children is well tolerated,[429, 430] and no marked local reactions have been reported following revaccination in infants.[431] Although a relationship between preexisting antibody levels and local or systemic reactions has been detected in adults, no such correlation has been observed in children,[432] perhaps because they generally have lower antibody concentrations than adults. Local reactions and fever but not other systemic reactions are more frequent in children who have been given *H. influenzae* type b and meningococcal vaccines at the same time as pneumococcal vaccine.[433] The antibody responses to each of the individual vaccines are not compromised by giving them simultaneously.

Although pneumococcal vaccination of HIV-infected people may be followed by a transient increase in viral load,[434] this phenomenon has also been observed following vaccination with other inactivated vaccines (e.g., influenza, tetanus toxoid)[435] and its clinical significance is unknown. A few patients with underlying immunological disorders have been observed to have more serious reactions following pneumococcal vaccination, but these events are likely to have been chance associations rather than causally related. Neurological disorders such as Guillain-Barré syndrome have not been reported following pneumococcal vaccination.

When pneumococcal vaccine is given simultaneously with influenza vaccine, there is no increase in the rate of systemic reactions compared with influenza vaccine alone and little or no increase in the rate of local reactions, although two injections are given.[425, 436]

RESULTS OF VACCINATION

Methods of Assessing Antibody Response

In the 1970s and 1980s, the method most widely used for measuring antibody responses to pneumococcal vaccine was the radioimmunoassay (RIA).[436a, 437] The RIA technique was sensitive and reproducible, but it had several disadvantages, including expense, the need to use radiolabeled type-specific polysaccharides, and the inability to distinguish among the different antibody classes that constitute the response to vaccination. Also, because of the prevalence of measurable antibody before vaccination, antibody responses after vaccination were often reported as n-fold increases, and such derivative data made it difficult to appreciate which levels might be associated with protection. In addition, the RIA-determined antibody levels did not always accurately reflect the levels of functional antibodies specific for each pneumococcal capsular polysaccharide type. This characteristic was due to the use in the assay of antigens that contained both capsular and C-polysaccharides and the ability of the RIA method to detect low- as well as high-avidity antibodies.[335, 438–442] Consequently, the contributions of anti–C-polysaccharide and low-avidity anticapsular polysaccharide antibodies to the overall results determined by the RIA method varied greatly, depending on the type of sera (prevaccination or postvaccination, adult or pediatric) and the individual capsular type being tested. Moreover, the poor correlation often observed between RIA antibody levels and opsonophagocytosis in vitro[443, 444] or protection in vivo may have reflected the ability of the RIA method to detect low-avidity antibodies as well as the high-avidity anticapsular polysaccharide antibodies thought to be responsible for these activities.

Several ELISA[335, 438, 439, 445] and other enzyme immunoassays[446–448] have been developed for measuring antibodies to pneumococcal polysaccharides. The advantages of the ELISA method over RIA include its simplicity, lower cost, lack of need for radiolabeled reagents, and ability to distinguish IgM, IgG, and IgA antibodies. The ELISA method also permits gravimetric conversion of the results so that they can be reported in micrograms per milliliter. Because the capsular polysaccharide antigens used in earlier ELISA assays also contained C-polysaccharide,[440, 449] an adsorption step that removes antibody to C-polysaccharide is required. Noncapsulated mutants of *S. pneumoniae* have been used for this purpose,[450] and a relatively purified preparation of C-polysaccharide is now supplied by the Statens Seruminstitut in Copenhagen.

Modifications in ELISA methods have included the use of phenylated capsular polysaccharides as antigens[451] and the use of secondary anion groups bound to the surface of microtiter plates that, in the presence of a coupling agent, facilitate the direct binding of capsular polysaccharides.[452] It has also been suggested that a modified RIA method is more specific than ELISA for measuring antibody to capsular polysaccharide.[453] However, this difference applies only to ELISA results obtained before adsorption to remove antibodies to C-polysaccharide; the results obtained by the modified RIA method (using unadsorbed serum) and ELISA after adsorption are similar. In addition, a nitrocellulose-based solid-phase multiantigen immunoassay is more specific than ELISA for measuring antibody to capsular polysaccharide.[454]

Measurement of anticapsular polysaccharide antibody after adsorption of serum by any of these methods has shown that most normal subjects lack anticapsular polysaccharide antibody to most pneumococcal serotypes.[455] Antibodies to the majority of capsular polysaccharide antigens appear after pneumococcal vaccine is administered to healthy people, and both IgM and IgG antibodies can be detected within 5 to 8 days of vaccination. Circulating antibody-secreting cells that produce IgA and IgG also appear during this period, indicating a secretory IgA response in saliva.[456] IgM antibody declines rapidly and is no longer detectable after a few months, whereas IgG antibody usually persists, albeit at declining levels, for 5 or more years.

Clinical and experimental observations have firmly established the association between the presence of type-specific anticapsular polysaccharide antibody and protection against homologous serotype pneumococcal infections. Using ELISA to measure the IgG that reacts specifically with capsular polysaccharide, IgG doses can be titrated to determine the levels that protect mice against different multiples of the median lethal dose of *S. pneumoniae*.[449] For serotypes 3, 4, and 8, similar doses of specific IgG have been shown to protect against infection with each serotype. Data in humans on what constitutes a minimally protective level of antibody for each pneumococcal serotype are unavailable, however. Such studies need to be undertaken. Eventual standardization of the methods for quantitating antibodies to pneumococcal capsular polysaccharides should permit meaningful comparison of results obtained in different laboratories.[457, 458]

Antibodies that develop after pneumococcal vaccination enhance bacterial opsonization and phagocytosis by both polymorphonuclear leukocytes and alveolar macrophages.[459] Opsonic activity to most serotypes appears to be proportional to the concentration of serum antibody measured by ELISA after removal of antibody to C-polysaccharide,[459–464] although in some cases discrepancies, especially with cross-reactive serotypes,[464] have been observed. Studies are underway to determine the clinical relevance of this finding, and whether IgG of low avidity is responsible. Some older people produce antibody that has reduced avidity for capsular polysaccharide antigens.

Immunogenicity in Normal Adults

Healthy young adults develop good antibody responses following vaccination with 23-valent pneumococcal vaccine. In earlier studies, antibody levels measured by RIA were found to be similar following vaccination with 25 or 50 μg of each polysaccharide.[424] These comparisons have not been repeated using newer antibody assays.

The antibody responses of small groups of healthy adults vaccinated with 23-valent vaccine have been assayed by an ELISA method before and after adsorption of C-polysaccharide.[439, 449] After adsorption, fully one third of the apparent antibody responses detected in preadsorbed sera were no longer present.[439] Among subjects who responded with increases in type-specific antibody, approximately 75% yielded positive results at levels of 1 μg per mL or greater of IgG. In a more recent study, 72 healthy Caucasian adults were vaccinated with 23-valent pneumococcal vaccine and, 1 month later, IgG antibody responses to 10 representative serotypes were measured (Table 22–5).[465] Altogether, 621 (86%) of 720 possible responses were positive. Only 75% of people had a measurable antibody response to type 12F polysaccharide (mean IgG level, 4.16 μg/mL), whereas 99% responded to type 18C (mean IgG level 20.2 μg/mL). The capacity to generate detectable antibody was not randomly distributed in the study group; 53% of subjects had IgG responses to all 10 polysaccharides, whereas 36% responded to six to nine polysaccharides and 11% to five or fewer polysaccharides. People who responded to a larger number of type-specific polysaccharides also had higher mean IgG levels than did those who responded to fewer antigens.

Several other investigators have also reported increases in total IgG and in IgG subclasses following pneumococcal vaccination of healthy adults.[446, 460, 466, 467] In general, IgG2 subclass antibodies have shown the greatest increase. Among the IgG responses, small amounts of IgG1 are detected in some people, and barely measurable levels of IgG3 or IgG4 can be found occasionally.[465] The failure of healthy adults to make IgG antibody after vaccination is not associated with abnormal levels of total serum IgG, IgM, or IgA, nor does it not reflect a failure to switch from IgM to IgG production; assays for IgM antibody are also negative in IgG nonresponders.[465] Failure to respond to vaccination also does not indicate a global defect in production of IgG2; in the previously cited study,[465] every subject was shown to generate an IgG2 response to at least one type-specific polysaccharide, and responses to a protein antigen (tetanus toxoid) were entirely normal.

Patients who have recovered from community-acquired pneumonia of bacterial or unknown cause may have lower levels of IgG subclass antibody than normal controls, but they respond as well as controls to pneumococcal vaccine.[468] In addition, healthy adults respond well to pneumococcal, meningococcal, and *H. influenzae* type b vaccines when they are given simultaneously.[469]

Pneumococcal vaccination also induces IgM and IgA antibodies. The brisk polymeric serum IgA2 subclass antibody response that often occurs may reflect previous contact with pneumococcal antigens at mucosal surfaces.[470, 471] This polymeric response persists much longer than the initially polymeric but later monomeric response to pneumococcal infection, perhaps reflecting the limited maturation of the immune response following the smaller antigenic stimulus of vaccination.[472]

Several studies have shown that some people respond vigorously to all or nearly all of the components of pneumococcal vaccine, whereas others respond to fewer components and with lower levels of IgG antibody. This variability in the antibody response to vaccination may be reflected in the IgG and IgG2 deficiency that sometimes occurs in people who have had bacteremic pneumococcal infections.[473] Genes that govern Gm and Km allotypes of IgG have been thought to influence the human antibody response to capsular polysaccharides of *S. pneumoniae*, *H. influenzae* type b, *N. meningitidis*, and other streptococci,[78, 79, 474–476] although no such correlation has been detected in mice.[68] In general, Caucasians who have the G2m(23) allotype (an antigenic marker on the heavy chain of the IgG2 idiotype) or who lack the Km(1) allotype experience increased responses to polysaccharide antigens.[78, 79, 474]

Two studies have shown a significant association between G2m(23)$^+$ and the response to pneumococcal capsular polysaccharides.[465, 477] In one, an association with Km(1)$^-$ was also observed,[477] whereas in the other it was not detected.[465] Interestingly, in one Ashkenazic family that was studied, no clear association of responses with G2m(23) was found,[465] a finding consistent with other observations on variations in antibody responses within ethnic or racial groups. Other studies have dem-

Table 22–5. **ANTIBODY RESPONSE TO PNEUMOCOCCAL POLYSACCHARIDE VACCINE IN HEALTHY ADULTS***

	BEFORE VACCINATION			AFTER VACCINATION			
	Detectable Antibody†			Detectable Antibody			
SEROTYPE	*No.*	*%*	**Mean IgG (μg/mL)**	*No.*	*%*	**Mean IgG (μg/mL)**	**95% CI**
1	20	28	.03	59	82	6.97	5.32–8.32
3	35	49	.08	62	86	7.00	6.19–7.91
4	18	25	.03	61	85	3.89	3.41–4.43
6B	24	33	.04	56	78	4.92	4.21–5.74
8	23	32	.04	68	94	5.55	4.81–6.40
12F	14	19	.02	54	75	4.16	3.58–4.84
14	15	21	.02	64	89	10.90	9.16–12.97
18C	42	58	.13	71	99	20.20	17.46–23.22
19F	19	26	.03	62	86	5.75	5.08–6.55
23F	33	46	.07	64	89	12.50	10.74–14.45

*Subjects were 72 unrelated healthy adults who were given one dose of 23-valent pneumococcal polysaccharide vaccine. Serum obtained before and 4 to 6 weeks after vaccination was assayed for serotype-specific IgG antibody by ELISA after cross-reacting antibody to cell-wall polysaccharide was removed by adsorption.

†Detectable antibody indicates the presence of serotype-specific antibody measured by ELISA when compared with negative control sera.

CI, confidence interval; ELISA, enzyme-linked immunosorbent assay; IgG, immunoglobulin G.

Data from reference 465.

onstrated that, in spite of the closer correlation in mean IgG and IgG2 antibody levels after vaccination in monozygotic compared with dizygotic twins,[478, 479] there are differences even within pairs of monozygotic twins[480] as well as with other subjects,[481] suggesting individual variability in V region genes, the genes that determine the final specificity of B cells.

Not surprisingly, HLA type is not related to the capacity to make antibody following pneumococcal vaccination. Polysaccharides interact directly with surface receptors of B1 cells to stimulate the generation of a clone of antibody producing cells,[482] whereas protein antigens are broken down into relatively small sequences of amino acids for surface presentation, a process that requires major histocompatibility complex (MHC) participation.

Immunogenicity in Normal Children

Earlier studies of the antibody responses of young children to pneumococcal vaccine were based on data obtained from sera tested by RIA without adsorption to remove antibody to C-polysaccharide. More recent studies using ELISA assays have greatly expanded our understanding of the specific antibody responses of infants and children to both pneumococcal infections and pneumococcal vaccination.

Preimmunization antibody levels to pneumococcal capsular polysaccharides are low in young infants. Mean IgG titers in 2-month-old infants, however, are higher than those found in older infants for each polysaccharide, reflecting transplacental transfer of maternal IgG1 antibodies.[483, 484] Nasopharyngeal colonization and infection induce variable antibody responses to capsular polysaccharides, depending on the age of the child and the capsular type.[485, 486]

Following one dose of pneumococcal vaccine, good antibody responses have been seen in Finnish and Australian infants to types 3, 4, 8, and 9N; intermediate responses to types 1, 2, 7F, 18C, 19F, and 25; and poor responses to types 12, 14, 23F, and especially to type 6A or 6B.[432, 487, 488] These responses have included all immunoglobulin classes, although IgG2 and IgG4 have been the predominant subclasses affected.[489] A second dose of the vaccine did not, as a rule, improve the response. In contrast, poor immunogens elicited a weak response after the first dose and an even weaker response after the second.

Similar findings concerning the relative immunogenicity of different serotypes have been reported in studies from other countries.[430, 483, 485] In Papua New Guinea, good responses occurred to types 2, 3, 5, 7F, and 23F and poor responses to types 6B and 19F.[485, 490] In The Gambia, vaccine was given to groups of children starting at 2 or 9 months of age and modest IgG responses to types 1, 3, and 5 occurred in children of both age groups.[483] Only children in the older age group developed antibodies to types 19F and 23F, however, and few children in any group responded to type 6A. IgA responses showed patterns similar to those seen for IgG, although they were generally lower.

The local immune response on mucosal membranes may help to protect children from acute and recurrent pneumococcal otitis media.[491] IgM and IgG antibodies to pneumococcal polysaccharides and to pneumolysin are rarely detected in the nasopharynx of children with acute otitis media.[491] IgA antibodies are frequently detected, however. Their appearance occurs independently of serum IgA and correlates with the presence of secretory component in the same antibodies, indicating local production.[330, 331] In addition, a considerable amount of specific anticapsular polysaccharide antibody, both IgA and IgG, is transferred from serum into the middle ear cavity during the acute phase of disease.[492] Pneumococcal vaccination has been shown to elicit an antibody response in both the middle ear and the serum.[493]

The practical implications of these immunogenicity data are clear. Because bacterial capsular polysaccharides induce antibodies primarily by T-cell–independent mechanisms, they are poor immunogens in children whose immune systems are still under development.[463] Although the most immunogenic serotypes, notably serotype 3, can induce antibodies in infants as young as 3 months of age, the antibody responses to most other pneumococcal capsular types are generally poor in children younger than 2 years. For this reason, pneumococcal polysaccharide vaccine is not recommended for these children.[219]

Immunogenicity in People with High-Risk Conditions

Immunocompetent People

The Elderly. Among unvaccinated elderly people, estimates of the prevalence of IgG antibodies to individual pneumococcal serotypes range from 30 to 90%,[455, 494] a pattern similar to that seen in younger adults. Furthermore, most healthy older people respond well to pneumococcal vaccine. In one earlier study, older subjects who had been vaccinated when they were approximately 65 years of age had antibody levels (measured by RIA) 6 years later that were half those detected 1 month after vaccination.[495] Revaccination was followed by an increase in antibody, although not to earlier peak levels. In studies that have used ELISA methods, antibody levels[496–499] and 5-year antibody persistence[497] in elderly people have been generally similar to what has been observed in younger people. Studies of antibody avidity in the elderly have shown conflicting results.[497, 499a]

In one report of 350 subjects, antibody levels to certain serotypes were higher in elderly men than in women, both before and after vaccination.[499] Furthermore, unlike antibody levels in women, those in men showed little decline with increasing age. Several other studies, however, suggest that antibody levels decline substantially after vaccination. In one report of 15 people who were 60 to 67 years of age when vaccinated, the decline in antibody levels was such that 60% were considered candidates for revaccination after 5 years.[497] In another report of 62 people (mean age 72.3 years; 19 men and 43 women), geometric mean antibody levels (serotypes 4, 6B, 9V, 19F, and 23F) observed 3 years after vaccination declined to levels close to or similar to those seen before vaccination.[500] The most important factor predicting sustained antibody levels was the magnitude of the initial antibody response to vaccination.

Chronic Cardiovascular and Pulmonary Diseases. Following pneumococcal vaccination, antibody levels to capsular polysaccharides in older patients with chronic obstructive pulmonary disease (COPD) are often similar to those of older people who are healthy or have cardiovascular disease and to those of younger people who are healthy or who have asthma.[501] One study of 14 asthmatic subjects treated with alternate-day corticosteroids (10–35 mg) showed that mean pre- and post-vaccination antibody levels to the four serotypes tested were similar to those of age-matched normal control subjects.[502] Other studies of COPD patients, however, showed significant reductions in both the mean levels of antibody attained and the number of antigens to which antibody responses were observed when compared with controls.[439, 501]

Several reports have described children who experience recurrent episodes of respiratory tract infection (otitis media, sinusitis, bronchitis, and pneumonia) and who have low or nondetectable levels of antipneumococcal antibodies.[503–508] When those with normal levels of IgG were immunized with pneumococcal vaccine, 4 to 14% were complete nonresponders[505–508] and 40 to 50% showed no specific IgG2 antibody responses,[507] despite often normal IgG2 levels.[506] The exact nature of this apparent isolated defect in antipneumococcal antibody production is not known. Not surprisingly, most children in whom a humoral immunodeficiency is already evident respond poorly to pneumococcal vaccine.[505, 507] Adults with IgA deficiency have also been studied.[509] Recurrent lower respiratory tract infections affect only those who also have low levels of IgG4 and IgG2. Again, the specific nature of this defect is not known.

Diabetes Mellitus. Diabetes mellitus is a frequent underlying condition in patients with pneumococcal bacteremia, although one or more comorbid conditions are usually present. Earlier RIA studies showed that diabetic adults and children who require insulin respond as well as normal subjects to pneumococcal vaccine.[20] No reports of antibody responses using modern ELISA methods have been published.

Chronic Alcoholism and Cirrhosis. The immunogenicity of pneumococcal vaccine has been studied in 41 chronic alcoholics in Alaska, of whom 21 were Alaska natives.[510] Age- and sex-matched native and non-native nonalchoholics served as controls. In general, the antibody responses of both groups were adequate, although occasionally there were significant differences between groups for some of the 12 serotypes tested. Whether vaccination is clinically protective in alcoholics with cirrhosis is not yet known; in one experimental study, vaccine-induced protection was less in cirrhotic animals than in noncirrhotic controls.[511]

Immunocompromised People

Human Immunodeficiency Virus Infection. The increase in the number of patients with HIV infections has brought with it a remarkable increase in the number of pneumococcal infections in both young adults[271, 512–517] and children.[518–520] Nasopharyngeal carriage rates for *S. pneumoniae* are similar in HIV-positive and HIV-negative people,[413, 521] perhaps because there is no decrease in mucosal IgA2 levels.[522] Carriage rates can increase in HIV-infected children and those born of HIV-infected mothers, but only in association with concomitant respiratory illness.[413] Once established, nasopharyngeal carriage may persist for prolonged periods in some patients, increasing the possibility that the organism will develop antimicrobial resistance, especially in people receiving prophylaxis with trimethoprim-sulfamethoxazole (TMP-SMX).[523] One report has documented capsular transformation occurring in a patient with HIV infection: Two sequential isolates of different serotypes were shown to be otherwise the same by ribotyping and PCR techniques.[524]

Population-based studies have shown that hospital admissions for community-acquired pneumonia have risen rapidly in people 25 to 50 or 60 years of age, largely as a result of HIV infection.[525, 526] In the United States, a large multicenter study of 1130 patients documented a hospitalization rate for bacterial pneumonia of 5.5 per 1000 person-years,[515] and rates were considerably higher among those who also had a history of intravenous drug abuse.[515, 527] Community-acquired pneumonia has often been the first manifestation of HIV infection.[513, 528, 529]

Pneumococcal infection is the leading cause of bacterial pneumonia in HIV-infected people.[226, 515, 527, 530] Furthermore, the proportion of all pneumonia cases that become bacteremic appears to be higher in HIV-infected than in non–HIV-infected people.[513, 515] In one area of the United States, the rate for pneumococcal bacteremia in patients with acquired immunodeficiency syndrome (AIDS) was 1 case per 100 patient-years, a rate approximately 100-fold greater than that reported in the same age group in the pre-AIDS era.[531] Experience in several centers in the United States indicates that HIV-infected people account for 40% or more of all cases of invasive pneumococcal disease in adults up to 55 or 60 years of age.[514, 516, 517] An earlier study suggested that surveillance for invasive pneumococcal disease in younger adults might be a useful epidemiological marker to estimate the size of the HIV-infected population.[532] Given wider use of TMP-SMX prophylaxis[533] and multidrug treatment for HIV infection itself, this may no longer be the case.

The clinical features of pneumococcal pneumonia and invasive pneumococcal disease in HIV-infected adults[513, 527, 534–536] and children[518, 519] are generally similar to those in people without HIV infection. Mortality rates in the two groups are also probably similar,[226, 516] although some studies suggest that death rates in HIV-infected patients may be lower[513, 531] or higher.[271, 517] A few patients may present with manifestations of disease not commonly seen since the preantibiotic era,[536] and those with other underlying medical conditions such as sickle cell disease have an especially severe course.[537] Once infected with *S. pneumoniae*, HIV-infected people may experience as much as a 15-fold increase in their risk for a second episode of pneumococcal disease.[516] Thus far, antibiotic-resistant pneumococci have not posed particular problems for managing HIV-infected patients: Rates for colonization,[514, 523] invasive disease,[516] and death[538] do not appear to be increased. Finally, vaccine serogroup/serotype organisms account for approximately 90% of invasive pneumococcal infections in HIV-infected people.[516, 517] HIV-infected adults with invasive pneumococcal disease, however, are more likely than HIV-negative adults to be infected with serotypes that are more common in children and are more frequently associated with antimicrobial resistance.[539]

Several studies have reported the responses of HIV-infected adults[540–550] and children[551–553] to pneumococcal vaccination. Before vaccination, many HIV-seropositive adults have higher total IgG levels than non–HIV-infected control subjects, but antipneumococcal antibody levels in the HIV-infected patients vary considerably.[540, 541, 549] Following vaccination, many respond with increases in total IgG and IgG2 antibody levels, although these responses may be less than those in normal controls. Responses also tend to be lower in those with more clinically advanced HIV disease. In several reports, antibody responses to pneumococcal vaccination have been reasonably good in patients with low CD4 counts.[544, 545, 547] The overall conclusion from these studies, however, is that many HIV-infected people will show no response to vaccination,[549, 550] and even in those with normal responses, antibody levels often decline rapidly.[547] In addition, compared with IgG antibody responses of HIV-infected adults to vaccination, IgM and IgA antibody responses are more frequently suboptimal.[547, 549]

In HIV-infected children, antibody response to pneumococcal vaccination range from poor to near normal.[551–553] Children born of HIV-infected mothers also have low levels of maternally transferred antipneumococcal antibodies.[554]

HIV-infected patients who are treated with zidovudine have better antibody responses after pneumococcal vaccination than do comparable patients who are not being treated.[555] Vaccination with pneumococcal[434] and other[435] vaccines may be followed by a transient increase in HIV viral load as measured in blood, but there is no indication that this has any effect on the overall course of the clinical disease.[434, 556] There are as yet no data on the response to pneumococcal vaccination in HIV-infected patients on multidrug therapy who are in clinical remission and have low or undetectable levels of HIV in their blood.

The epidemiological and clinical evidence to date document the greatly increased risk of pneumococcal infections in people with HIV infection. The antibody response to vaccination is better in the earlier stages of infection when patients are asymptomatic and CD4 counts are high. Once the diagnosis of HIV infection is made, pneumococcal vaccine should be given without delay.[219]

Splenectomy. In both children and adults, the increased risk of overwhelming postsplenectomy infection (OWPI) is greater for those with immunological or hematological disorders than it is for those whose spleens have been removed because of trauma. In one study from Australia, the incidence of OWPI due to any cause was approximately four cases per 1000 patient-years for all patients, a 12.6-fold increase in risk compared with that for the general population.[557] Other studies have estimated the incidence of OWPI to be 3.3 cases per 1000 patient-years for patients with Hodgkin disease, 1.7 for those with idiopathic thrombocytopenia, 0.7 for those with hereditary spherocytosis, and 0.3 for those with trauma.[558] Almost half of these episodes occurred more than 5 years after splenectomy.

In all reported series, *S. pneumoniae* has been the most common cause of OWPI, accounting for 30 to 60% of cases. A 1992–1993 study from Norway showed that among patients who had undergone splenectomy, the rate for pneumococcal sepsis alone was 2.7 cases per 1000 patient-years, a rate 25 times greater than that for the population who had not undergone splenectomy.[559] These cases accounted for 1.7% of all cases of pneumococcal bacteremia reported in Norway during the same period. None had received pneumococcal vaccine, and their mortality rate was 50%.

Studies of antibody responses to pneumococcal vaccination following splenectomy have given variable results, often because these patients have had conditions or treatments associated with immunocompromise. Some splenectomized patients without underlying immunological diseases may also have moderately reduced antibody responses,[560, 561] although the IgG subclass distribution in these patients is similar to that of normal subjects.[560]

Pneumococcal vaccine is strongly recommended for all patients who have undergone splenectomy.[219, 562] In all likelihood, the great majority of physicians know that patients who have undergone splenectomy are at increased risk for pneumococcal infections,[563] but patients themselves are far less likely to be aware of their risk[564] or, if taught, have difficulty remembering information on the disease and the need for vaccination.[565] Comprehensive programs for identifying patients who have undergone splenectomy, however, have been successful in vaccinating most of them.[566–569] Routine measurement of specific antibody levels after vaccination has been recommended by some investigators,[570, 571] but this is unlikely to be undertaken except for research purposes.

Because patients who have undergone splenectomy remain at increased risk indefinitely, the need for revaccination at least every 5 years is generally accepted, and revaccination is well tolerated.[565] Long-term antimicrobial prophylaxis is also recommended, but this does not necessarily mean lifelong treatment.[572] A large proportion of pneumococcal infections occur more than 5 years after splenectomy, and compliance with long-term continuous prophylaxis is often difficult. A more promising approach would be to instruct all vaccinated patients who have undergone splenectomy to begin self-treatment with an oral antimicrobial agent at the first sign of an infection that might be caused by encapsulated bacteria. In Denmark this strategy has been highly effective in preventing OWPI in children.[566]

Sickle Cell Disease. Children with homozygous sickle cell disease (hemoglobin SS) have a greatly increased risk of pneumococcal infections: They may be 600 times more likely to develop pneumococcal meningitis than normal children and are more likely to experience fulminant pneumococcal sepsis. The most significant period of risk begins approximately 4 months after birth and continues until at least 4 to 5 years of age. An epidemiological study has shown that during the period 1957–1989 the annual incidence of bacterial septicemia due to either *S. pneumoniae* or *H. influenzae* varied from 64 to 420 per 1000 patient-years for children younger than 2 years of age but was never more than 10.2 per 1000 patient-years for those 4 years of age or older.[573, 574]

In a more recent report, infants enrolled in the Cooperative Study of Sickle Cell Disease in the United States were followed for a mean of 1.2 years.[575] Among those with homozygous (SS) sickle cell disease, those 6 to 12 months of age had an incidence of 9.9 episodes of pneumococcal bacteremia per 100 patient-years, whereas the rates in those 1, 2, and 3 years of age were 6.5, 8.7, and 4.7 cases per 100 patient-years, respectively. During the first 2 years of life, rates for children with hemoglobin SC disease (32% of all subjects) were only slightly lower. Among all children enrolled in the study, the mortality rate from pneumococcal bacteremia was 14.5%, similar to what has been reported in smaller case series.[576, 577] In some reports an increasing proportion of serious pneumococcal infections in children with sickle cell disease has been caused by organisms that are antibiotic-resistant.[576, 577]

The most common pathophysiological defect that predisposes patients with sickle cell disease to pneumococcal infection is functional asplenia. Reduced serum opsonic activity caused by defects in the classic and alternative complement pathways that are associated with deficiencies in type-specific antibody can also be present.[578] This deficiency may reflect a defect in B-cell maturation that is related to low IL-4 levels.[579] It has also been suggested that the susceptibility of some children to systemic pneumococcal infection may also be due to persistence of *S. pneumoniae* in infected tonsils,[580] although this is not widely accepted. Other research suggests that susceptibility is not due to genotypic variation in the binding of IgG2 and altered clearance of capsulated organisms.[581]

Children with sickle cell disease who are 2 years or older may initially respond to pneumococcal vaccination, but their responses are usually short-lived.[582] Revaccination at 5 years of age is followed by poor serotype-specific antibody responses in most children, and in those who do respond, almost half show a decline in antibodies greater than or equal to twofold 10 to 15 months later. Older children (13–17 years of age) may respond better than younger children to revaccination.[583]

Because of the greatly increased susceptibility of younger children with sickle cell disease to pneumococcal infection, several studies have examined the efficacy of prophylactic penicillin in these patients. A multicenter clinical trial completed in the 1980s demonstrated that penicillin prophylaxis dramatically reduced the incidence of pneumococcal bacteremia, whether or not the children had received pneumococcal vaccine.[584] Moreover, discontinuing penicillin prophylaxis at 5 years of age was not followed by an increased rate of bacteremic disease.[585] Penicillin prophylaxis may reduce the overall rate of nasopharyngeal colonization with *S. pneumoniae*,[586] but it may also increase the proportion of colonizing organisms that are antibiotic-resistant.[586, 587]

The management of children with sickle cell disease has improved dramatically since the 1970s.[588] Hospitalization and death from pneumococcal infection have been largely eliminated by meticulous adherence to penicillin prophylaxis during the first 5 years of life. It is unclear whether pneumococcal vaccination has contributed significantly to the improved outcomes of these children.

Hematological Neoplasms. Patients with Hodgkin disease, multiple myeloma, and chronic lymphocytic leukemia are at increased risk for severe pneumococcal infections. In one report, patients with these disorders had an overall annual incidence of invasive pneumococcal disease of 2.6%.[589] In patients with chronic lymphocytic leukemia, low levels of anticapsular polysaccharide antibodies have been associated with frequent or severe pneumococcal infections.[590]

Several factors influence the antibody response to pneumococcal vaccine in these patients, including the stage of the disease, whether or not splenectomy has been performed, the extent of previous radiation therapy or chemotherapy, and the time between completion of treatment and vaccination. Before radiation therapy or chemotherapy, patients with Hodgkin disease respond to vaccination as well as normal people do.[591, 592] This is true regardless of splenectomy, and the response is independent of the stage of disease. In patients with non-Hodgkin lymphoma, antibody levels before vaccination tend to be lower than those of normal subjects or patients with Hodgkin disease.[591, 592] Once radiation therapy or chemotherapy has begun, the antibody response in these patients is reduced. In some, the antibody levels fall below what they were before vaccination, whereas in others the response is delayed for several months. After completion of treatment, antibody levels may not return to pretreatment levels, and patients seldom respond to revaccination. These studies indicate that patients with Hodgkin disease and non-Hodgkin lymphoma should be vaccinated as soon as possible after the diagnosis is established, before treatment is begun.

Patients with multiple myeloma are also at increased risk for severe pneumococcal infections. Antibody levels before vaccination are generally much lower in these patients than they are in normal subjects. Following vaccination, the antibody response is poor, although some patients may show a response to at least some capsular polysaccharide antigens.[421] The response does not correlate with the severity of the disease or the timing of chemotherapy, and when it occurs it is usually not sustained. A rapid decline in antibody levels also occurs after passive immunization with IVIG.[593] Nonetheless, a randomized controlled trial has shown that prophylactic IVIG (0.4 g/kg body weight monthly) given to stable multiple myeloma patients is significantly protective against pneumonia and septicemia.[421]

Patients with chronic lymphocytic leukemia do not respond to pneumococcal vaccine, even when they are not receiving chemotherapy.[594] In children with acute leukemia who are on maintenance chemotherapy, antibody responses are lower than those of age-matched normal controls, but postvaccination levels achieved in some may be protective.[595] Most children whose disease has been in remission for at least 2 years respond well to pneumococcal vaccination.[596]

Other Neoplasms. The antibody responses to pneumococcal vaccination in patients with nonhematological neoplasms have not been studied extensively. In general, patients with solid tumors have slightly lower pre- and post-vaccination antibody levels when compared with those of healthy controls, but their levels are considerably higher than those of patients with hematological neoplasms. Prior radiation therapy or chemotherapy also has less effect on their responses to vaccination.

Renal Diseases. Children with nephrotic syndrome are at increased risk for serious pneumococcal infections, as are renal transplant and hemodialysis patients. Both transplant and hemodialysis patients usually respond to an initial dose of pneumococcal vaccine, although antibody levels may be lower than those seen in normal subjects.[597] Antibody levels decline substantially 2 years after vaccination. Revaccination leads to a modest antibody increase, and there have been no serious adverse reactions.[598] In children with nephrotic syndrome[599] and other chronic renal diseases,[600, 601] the initial response to vaccination is usually adequate. Except in children with minimal change nephrotic syndrome, there may be a rapid falloff in antibody levels.[599] In one study of 22 children and young adults who were revaccinated 1 year after their initial vaccination, significant immune responses occurred in 50%, but antibody levels declined rapidly over the next 6 months.[600]

Hematopoietic Cell, Cardiac, and Liver Transplantation. Recipients of allogenic hematopoietic (bone marrow) transplants are at considerable risk of pneumococcal infections. These infections usually do not occur in the first 6 months after transplantation, probably because of antimicrobial chemoprophylaxis given to prevent *Pneumocystis carinii* infections. In patients who experience pneumococcal infections, decreased IgG, IgG subclass, IgM, and type-specific antibody levels and serum opsonic activity have been found.[602–604] Patients who do not experience pneumococcal infections after allogenic transplantation have higher levels of IgG2 and IgG4.[603] Pneumococcal vaccination of matched sibling donors before transplantation does not lead to improvement in the antibody levels of transplant recipients.[604]

When pneumococcal vaccine is given 6 months after transplantation or during corticosteroid treatment of graft-versus-host disease, the antibody response in most patients is limited, especially for IgG2 antibodies.[604–607a] When vaccination is delayed until 12 months after transplantation or if two doses are given at 12 and 24 months after transplantation, antibody responses are still poor.[607a, 608] Antibody levels do not return to pretransplantation levels until 1 to 2 years after transplantation. The slow return of IgG2 levels and the poor response to pneumococcal polysaccharide antigens in these patients are similar to what is seen during the immunological maturation of young children.[605, 607] Prevention of pneumococcal infection during this interval depends on other measures such as antimicrobial prophylaxis.

In contrast with recipients of allogenic hematopoietic cell transplants, those who receive autologous transplants generally have normal levels of IgG2 antibodies after pneumococcal vaccination and maintain these levels 1 year after transplantation.[606] A survey of European transplant centers, however, showed that most centers relied on antimicrobial prophylaxis to prevent pneumococcal and other bacterial infections.[609]

Cardiac and liver transplantation have been observed to increase the risk of pneumococcal infection.[610, 611] One study of 31 heart or liver transplant patients who were given pneumococcal vaccine 4 to 85 months after transplantation showed that their antibody responses overall and to most of the 9 individual vaccine serotypes tested were similar to those of healthy controls.[612] However, another report of 34 heart transplant patients vaccinated at least 5 years after transplantation showed that geometric mean levels of postvaccination antibody were significantly reduced when compared with those of healthy, age-matched control subjects.[613] Vaccination has been well-tolerated by these patients.[612, 613]

Other Disorders. Clinical observations suggest that some patients with systemic lupus erythematosus,[614] Felty's syndrome,[615] and celiac sprue[616] may be at increased risk for pneumococcal infections because they have functional asplenia. Earlier studies of the antibody responses of patients with systemic lupus erythematosus to pneumococcal vaccine showed them to be either normal or somewhat lower than those in normal subjects.[20] They were not correlated with drug therapy, renal function, immunoglobulin levels, or disease activity. Patients with celiac sprue respond normally to pneumococcal vaccination.[616]

Although inherited deficiencies of the complement system are known to predispose to pneumococcal infections, one report has noted that three of four patients with C3 deficiency were also almost totally deficient in antipneumococcal capsular polysaccharide antibodies.[617] Only a few patients with other complement deficiencies had such deficits. Whether C3-deficient patients respond to pneumococcal vaccine is not known.

A study of 15 elderly patients with low serum vitamin B_{12} levels showed that their antibody responses to pneumococcal vaccination were significantly lower than those of age-matched control subjects with normal B_{12} levels.[618] As yet, no clinical or epidemiological data suggest an increased risk of pneumococcal infection in B_{12}-deficient patients.

Vaccination in Pregnancy

The safety of pneumococcal vaccine for pregnant women has not been determined, but there is no reason to expect that vaccination in the first trimester should have any adverse effect on fetal development. Whenever possible, however, the vaccine should be given to high-risk women before rather than during pregnancy.

Vaccinating pregnant women might also prevent pneumococcal infections in newborns and infants up to 6 months of age. In developed countries, primary pneumococcal colonization of the female genital tract and maternal pneumococcal sepsis are rare.[619] Pneumococcal bacteremia in newborns is also rare but has a mortality rate approaching 50%.[619–622] The incidence of maternal pneumococcal bacteremia is approximately 4 cases per 100,000 subjects,[623] and in neonates it is 4 to 6 cases per 100,000.[623, 624] In several instances, concomitant infections of mother and newborn infant with the same serotype organism have been demonstrated. During the first 6 months of life, otitis media is common and may be associated with low cord blood levels of maternally derived antibodies to at least some pneumococcal capsular types.[624a] Pneumococcal meningitis occurring during this period has a high mortality rate. Hearing loss and neurological and developmental disabilities are common in those who survive.

Transplacental transfer of IgG antibodies, especially IgG1, has been documented.[625–627] Administration of pneumococcal polysaccharide vaccine to pregnant women in the third trimester elicits levels of type-specific anticapsular antibodies in the cord blood of newborn infants that are higher than the levels in infants whose mothers have not been vaccinated.[628, 629] Neonatal cord blood levels of IgG antibody, however, are approximately 25 to 50% of maternal levels, depending on serotype. Similar findings have been observed after maternal vaccination with other polysaccharide vaccines, suggesting a more general problem with transplacental transfer of maternal antibodies to polysaccharide antigens. This is unlike the efficient transfer of maternal antibodies to protein antigens, wherein cord blood/maternal blood antibody ratios are often greater than or equal to 1.0.[629] Moreover, the half-life of maternally transferred antipneumococcal antibodies is little more than 1 month, and by 3 months of age serum antibody levels in children born of vaccinated and unvaccinated mothers are similar.[628, 629]

Maternal vaccination has been suggested as a way to stimulate protection in newborns via breast milk. In the postpartum period, unvaccinated women usually have measurable breast milk antibodies to some pneumococcal serotypes, and these antibodies can be detected for as long as 5 months after delivery.[628] The antibody levels, however, may be low and do not correlate with rates of nasopharyngeal colonization or otitis media in their breast-fed infants.[630]

Whether maternal immunization with pneumococcal polysaccharide vaccine is safe for infants or will modify their antibody response to pneumococcal conjugate vaccine is not known. Moreover, whether maternal immunization with pneumococcal conjugate vaccine or other polysaccharide-conjugate vaccines[631] will protect infants against infection during the first 6 months of life will require careful study.

Revaccination

Initial recommendations for 14-valent pneumococcal vaccine stated that it should be given only once, and revaccination was not recommended.[632] These recommendations were based on reports of local Arthus-like reactions and systemic reactions after early revaccination. With 23-valent vaccine, the frequency and severity of local and systemic adverse reactions following revaccination of adults (especially ≤4 years after the initial dose) may be similar to[633, 634] or greater than[635] what occurs after primary vaccination. Local adverse reactions tend to be more common among those with higher levels of serum antibody before revaccination.[635] Reactions serious enough to require hospitalization, however, have not been observed.[636] In children, revaccination is also well-tolerated.[583, 637]

After revaccination, the overall increase in antibody levels in most people is lower than[495] or similar to[455, 638] the increase observed after primary vaccination. Although antibody levels increase, no anamnestic response occurs because of the absence of immunological memory. Thus, revaccination should not be considered to be a booster dose of vaccine.

People with surgical or functional asplenia constitute the group for whom revaccination is most strongly recommended. In those who have undergone splenectomy, at least one third to one half or more experience a decline in antibody levels after 5 to 10 years and require revaccination.[639, 640] In patients with renal disease, the decline in antibody levels can be rapid,[598, 600] especially in those who have also undergone splenectomy. Revaccination every 2 years has been successful in preventing recurrent pneumococcal infections in splenectomized patients.

Little is known about the long-term antibody response following pneumococcal revaccination. In one study of children and adolescents with sickle cell disease, antibody levels measured 3 to 7 years after revaccination were substantially lower than levels observed shortly after revaccination.[583] Except for patients who have undergone splenectomy,[639] the clinical effectiveness of revaccination is largely unknown.

PNEUMOCOCCAL VACCINE EFFICACY AND VACCINATION EFFECTIVENESS

Pneumococcal vaccine is not a single vaccine; it is 23 individual vaccines. Any statement about its efficacy (or effectiveness), therefore, must be understood to indicate the aggregate efficacy of its 23 component antigens. Most monovalent vaccines in general use have an efficacy of 90 to 95% or greater. This level of protection cannot be achieved with a 23-valent pneumococcal vaccine. Ideally, the aggregate efficacy of pneumococcal vaccine could be calculated by multiplying the point estimates of efficacy of all 23 antigens, adjusting for the relative frequencies of infection caused by each individual capsular type. In practice, this would be extremely difficult to do, and it is never done. Although the concept of aggregate efficacy is of fundamental importance to understanding the benefits to be expected from pneumococcal vaccine, unfortunately, it is often misunderstood or simply not recognized.

The Carrier State

Some of the beneficial effects of pneumococcal polysaccharide vaccine could be the result of reduced nasopharyngeal carriage of vaccine-type organisms and hence reduced rates of disease. Studies conducted in the setting of outbreaks of pneumococcal disease in military camps during the Second World War showed a 50% reduction in the acquisition of nasopharyngeal carriage of pneumococci in subjects given an experimental pneumococcal vaccine.[641] Several long-term studies in nonoutbreak settings, however, have compared patterns of pneumococcal carriage before and after vaccination with 14-valent vaccine.[194, 642–644] None showed a significant reduction in pneumococcal carrier rates among vaccinees, nor was there a shift among carriers in the distribution of vaccine-type and nonvaccine-type organisms. It is difficult to compare directly the results of studies conducted in the 1940s with those conducted in recent decades, in part because only the earlier studies used mouse inoculation to isolate pneumococci from nasopharyngeal carriers.

The effect of vaccination with pneumococcal conjugate vaccines on nasopharyngeal carriage may be different; recent studies in children at least 2 years of age show a reduction in nasopharyngeal carriage of vaccine-type organisms,[645, 646] but there may be replacement colonization with nonvaccine-type organisms.[646] The clinical and epidemiological importance of these changes remains to be defined.

Vaccine Efficacy and Vaccination Effectiveness in Children

Several randomized controlled trials in the 1980s assessed the efficacy of 14-valent pneumococcal vaccine in preventing otitis media. In Australia, a study of 1158 healthy children showed no consistent differences between vaccinees and controls in the mean number of episodes of otitis media per child or in rates for a variety of clinical signs and symptoms, restricted activity, physician visits, and hospital admissions.[647] These findings were observed in children at least 2 years of age as well as in younger children. Other studies of vaccine efficacy in otitis-prone children younger than 2 years of age have given mixed results; an early study of 320 children in Finland reported a 51% reduction in recurrent pneumococcal otitis media,[648] but later studies showed negligible effects.[316, 649] Another report indicated that African American but not white children 6 to 11 months of age had significantly fewer recurrences of otitis media in both the first and second years after vaccination.[650] The reason for the apparent effect of race on outcome in this study is not known. Considered together, these studies document the limited efficacy of pneumococcal vaccine in preventing otitis media in young children.

In contrast with its equivocal protection against otitis media, pneumococcal vaccine may reduce mortality from acute lower respiratory tract infections that commonly affect children in developing countries.[644, 651, 652] In a clinical trial conducted on more than 7000 children in Papua New Guinea, half of whom were immunized at 6 months to 5 years of age, pneumococcal vaccine reduced pneumonia mortality by 59% in children of all ages (P = .008; 95% CI = 19–79%) and by 50% in children vaccinated when 2 years of age or younger (P = .043; 95% CI = 1–75%). The vaccine was only marginally protective against moderate to severe disease, however, and did not protect against mild illness.[652] More recently, CDC investigators have used the indirect cohort method (see later) to show that pneumococcal vaccination of children 2 to 5 years of age was 62% effective (95% CI = 35–78%) in preventing invasive pneumococcal disease due to vaccine serotypes.[653] Vaccination effectiveness was lower in children with sickle cell disease (perhaps because of antimicrobial prophylaxis of those who were not vaccinated) than it was in children without sickle cell disease.

Vaccine Efficacy and Vaccination Effectiveness in Adults

In the 1940s, clinical trials of trivalent and tetravalent pneumococcal polysaccharide vaccines established their efficacy in preventing pneumococcal pneumonia and bacteremia in military recruits and residents of a long-term care facility.[641, 654] Evidence of the efficacy of modern pneumococcal vaccines emerged in the early 1970s from prospective randomized controlled trials conducted among novice gold miners in South Africa.[23, 24] These young men experienced very high rates of pneumococcal disease, ensuring that clinical trials with several thousand subjects would yield definitive results. In one of these studies, a 13-valent pneumococcal vaccine was shown to be 82% effective against vaccine-type pneumococcal bacteremia, 78.5% effective against vaccine-type bacteremia and pneumonia combined, and approximately 53% effective against pneumonia detected by radiography, irrespective of microbial cause.[23]

In contrast with those in South Africa, attack rates for pneumococcal infections in the United States and other developed countries are much lower. Consequently, clinical trials in older, high-risk people have been difficult to conduct. These difficulties are illustrated by the Veterans Administration Cooperative Study that was undertaken in the early 1980s.[655] In this 3-year study, 36 (3.1%) of 1145 vaccine recipients and 27 (2.3%) of 1150 placebo controls experienced proven or probable pneumococcal pneumonia or bronchitis. Vaccine-type organisms were recovered in 14 episodes of infection in vaccinees and in 11 episodes in controls. The investigators concluded they were unable to demonstrate the efficacy of pneumococcal vaccine in preventing pneumococcal pneumonia or bronchitis in their study population.

Several questions have been raised about the methods used in the Veterans Administration Cooperative Study.[219, 656, 657] First, the success of the randomization process itself has been questioned; compared with control subjects, significantly more vaccinated subjects had a previous history of pneumococcal pneumonia and significantly more died of all causes during the follow-up period.[656] Second, pneumococcal bronchitis was included as an outcome event and accounted for 48% of all pneumococcal infections that were considered in the analysis of the results. This end-point had not been included in any previous clinical trial of pneumococcal vaccine, and it is still not known whether pneumococcal vaccination can be expected to protect against this condition. Third, if only well-accepted outcome measures were considered in the analysis (i.e., vaccine-type pneumococcal bacteremia or pneumonia), the size of the study population was too small to have given a statistically meaningful result.[219, 656, 658] For these and other reasons,[656] the Veterans Administration Cooperative Study should be regarded as an inconclusive rather than a "negative" clinical trial.

Two prospective clinical trials of 14-valent pneumococcal vaccine have provided evidence that it may be efficacious in preventing pneumococcal pneumonia in older people. One was an open, randomized, controlled trial conducted in France in the 1980s.[659] In this study, 1686 people living in geriatric hospitals or homes for the aged were observed for 2 years. In the vaccinated group there was a significant reduction in the occurrence of radiographically confirmed pneumonia ($P < .01$) and in all pneumonias, whether diagnosed clinically, radiographically, or by laboratory studies ($P < .0001$). By these measures, vaccine efficacy was estimated to be 77%. In addition to the French study, a report from Finland has described a clinical trial that was conducted during the period 1982–1985.[246] In elderly people (≥60 years old) with underlying medical risk factors (34% of all elderly people in the study), pneumococcal vaccine was 59% protective (95% CI = 6–82%) against pneumococcal pneumonia. Vaccination was not protective in people without medical risk factors, although the small study population and the use of influenza vaccine in both pneumococcal vaccinated and control subjects may have contributed to this inconclusive result.

One additional prospective trial has been reported from Sweden.[659a] In this study, 691 patients (mean age, 69 years) discharged from hospital after treatment for pneumonia were randomized to receive either 23-valent pneumococcal vaccine or placebo. During the follow-up period (mean, 2.3 years), 63 (19%) of 339 vaccinated patients and 57 (16%) of 352 placebo patients developed recurrent pneumonia. Pneumococcal pneumonia was diagnosed in 19 (5.6%) vaccine and 16 (4.5%) placebo recipients; 60% of these diagnoses were made serologically. The authors concluded that pneumococcal vaccine did not prevent pneumonia overall or pneumococcal pneumonia in middle-aged or elderly individuals. This conclusion must be interpreted with caution: The study lacked adequate statistical power and was conducted among an unrepresentative group of subjects who were at extremely high risk of pneumococcal infection. Interestingly, bacteremic pneumococcal infection was observed in only one vaccine recipient but in five who received placebo. The difference between the two groups, however, was not statistically significant.

Because randomized controlled trials of pneumococcal vaccine in older high-risk adults have been difficult to conduct, investigators have turned to retrospective methods to evaluate the clinical effectiveness of pneumococcal vaccination.[660] Five case-control studies have been reported (Table 22–6).[661–665] In each, pneumococcal bacteremia, not pneumococcal pneumonia, has been the outcome evaluated. The Philadelphia[662] and Charlottesville[665] studies have shown vaccination effectiveness rates of 70% and 81%, respectively. A full report on the Alaska case-control study has not been published.[664] The failure to demonstrate clinical effectiveness in the Denver study[661] is thought to be due to incomplete ascertainment of the vaccination status of study subjects and possible bias in the selection of controls.[657]

The most convincing case-control study has been reported from Connecticut.[663] In this study, the aggregate effectiveness of pneumococcal vaccination in preventing pneumococcal bacteremia caused by vaccine and vaccine-related type organisms was 56%, and it was 47% effective in preventing all pneumococcal bacteremias, regardless of capsular type (see Table 22–6). In a subset of 175 immunocompromised patients, clinical effectiveness against vaccine and vaccine-related serotype infection was only 21% (95% CI = −55–60%). In the remaining 808 immunocompetent patients (82% of all patients studied), however, vaccination was 61% protective (95% CI = 47–72%). The effectiveness of vaccination declined with increasing patient age and time since

Table 22–6. **CLINICAL EFFECTIVENESS OF PNEUMOCOCCAL VACCINATION IN PREVENTING INVASIVE PNEUMOCOCCAL DISEASE***

TYPE OF INFECTION	LOCATION (NO. OF CASES/CONTROL SUBJECTS)	% VACCINATION EFFECTIVENESS (95% CI)	REFERENCE
All serotypes	Connecticut (1054/1054)	47 (30 to 59)	663
	Philadelphia, PA (122/244)	70 (37 to 86)	662
	Charlottesville, VA (85/152)	81 (34 to 94)	665
	Alaska (159/159)	64 (32 to 81)	664
Vaccine type ± VT related	Connecticut (983/983)	56 (42 to 67)	663
	Denver, CO (89/89)	−21 (−221 to 92)	661
	Alaska (87/87)	79 (49 to 92)	664
	CDC†	57 (45 to 66)	666
Nonvaccine type ± non–VT related	Connecticut (983/983)	−73 (−263 to 18)	663

*Only patients with pneumococcal isolates from normally sterile body sites were included. CI indicates confidence interval; VT, vaccine-type pneumococcal infection.
†Centers for Disease Control and Prevention indirect cohort study: 515 vaccinated and 2322 unvaccinated subjects.

vaccination. Nonetheless, in immunocompetent patients aged 65 to 74 years, vaccination effectiveness over a 5-year period was at least 71% (95% CI = 30–88%), and for those 75 to 84 years of age its effectiveness over 3 years was 67% (95% CI = 20–87%). Not surprising, vaccination was not effective in preventing bacteremia due to nonvaccine-type organisms (see Table 22–6).

Another approach to assessing the effectiveness of pneumococcal vaccination has used an indirect cohort method.[666] This method is based on the assumption that if pneumococcal vaccination is effective, fewer illnesses caused by vaccine-type organisms will occur in vaccinated compared with unvaccinated people, whereas infections caused by nonvaccine-type organisms will occur with equal frequency in both groups. Using 14 years of data from a nationwide pneumococcal surveillance program, CDC investigators showed that pneumococcal vaccine was 57% effective in preventing bacteremia due to vaccine-type organisms (see Table 22–6). Moreover, vaccination was effective in preventing pneumococcal bacteremia in people with diabetes mellitus (effectiveness 84%; 95% CI = 50–95%), coronary vascular disease (73%; 95% CI = 23–90%), congestive heart failure (69%; 95% CI = 17–88%), and chronic pulmonary disease (65%; 95% CI = 14–95%). In all immunocompetent people at least 65 years of age, it was 75% protective (95% CI = 57–85%). For other high-risk conditions, the numbers of people available for study were too small to provide conclusive results. The CDC's epidemiological method has been validated by using data from the Connecticut case-control study.[663] For immunocompetent people, the 62% effectiveness (95% CI = 24–81%) determined by the CDC's method was virtually the same as the 61% effectiveness demonstrated by the case-control method.

In one small nested case-control study, the effectiveness of pneumococcal vaccination was assessed in people with HIV infection.[666a] Among the 85 cases, 36 (42%) had invasive pneumococcal disease, whereas the others had clinical pneumonia and sputum cultures positive for *S. pneumoniae*. There were fewer pneumococcal infections in people with a history of pneumococcal vaccination and an equal or greater number of $CD4^+$ cells per mm^3 (adjusted odds ratio, 0.22; 95% CI, 0.05–0.98). Similar studies in larger groups of patients are urgently needed.

The evidence from these retrospective studies supports the conclusion that pneumococcal vaccination is effective in preventing invasive pneumococcal disease in immunocompetent older people, many of whom have high-risk conditions. The earlier clinical trial from France and the more recent report from Finland suggest that the vaccine may also be efficacious in preventing pneumococcal pneumonia in some groups of older people. This conclusion is supported by evidence from a large retrospective cohort study (K. L. Nichol, personal communication, 1997) using methods similar to those that have successfully demonstrated the clinical effectiveness of influenza vaccination.[667]

Although several observers have commented on the failure of some prospective clinical trials to show vaccine efficacy in older people,[668–671] the absence of such proof is not proof of its absence, and the methodological problems of these clinical trials are self-evident. Furthermore, in spite of the difficulty in demonstrating that pneumococcal vaccination prevents nonbacteremic pneumococcal pneumonia,[656, 668] the public health importance of vaccination in preventing invasive pneumococcal disease alone is firmly established.[656]

Cost-Effectiveness of Pneumococcal Vaccination

The cost-effectiveness of pneumococcal vaccination for preventing pneumococcal pneumonia in elderly people has been evaluated by the U.S. Congress's Office of Technology Assessment (OTA). Following the introduction of the 23-valent vaccine, the OTA reevaluated an earlier study of the 14-valent vaccine, incorporating newer information on the disease and the effectiveness of vaccination.[672] Assuming a duration of protection of 3 years and excluding the costs of future medical care, pneumococcal vaccination was estimated to cost \$2286 (1983 dollars) to achieve 1 quality-adjusted life-year (QALY). With a duration of protection of 8 years, vaccination would be cost-saving. These estimates compared favorably with those for other preventive, screening, and treatment interventions for elderly people (Table 22–7).[673, 674]

Since publication of the OTA study, other investigators have examined the cost-effectiveness of pneumococcal vaccination for the United States,[19, 675] the Netherlands,[676] and Spain.[677, 678] Each study has concluded that vaccination of all elderly people to prevent pneumococcal pneumonia would be similarly cost-effective. Nonetheless, acceptance of these results has been limited by the lack of definitive evidence that pneumococcal vaccination prevents nonbacteremic as well as bacteremic pneumococcal pneumonia in this age group.[668–670] For this reason, it was suggested that the cost-effectiveness of vaccination to prevent pneumococcal bacteremia alone should be evaluated.[656] Such a study has been reported for the United States.[679] The investigators followed the guidelines of the Panel on Cost-Effectiveness in Health and Medicine[680–682] and used the most recent data on the incidence of invasive pneumococcal disease in the elderly[284–286] and the clinical effectiveness of vaccination.[663] The analysis showed that pneumococcal vaccination of all elderly people to prevent pneumococcal bacteremia alone would be cost-saving.

Studies of the cost-effectiveness of pneumococcal vaccination in preventing bacteremic or invasive disease need to be repeated for other countries. These studies may be difficult to conduct because some of these countries lack epidemiological data on the incidence of invasive disease. Nonetheless, the finding that pneumococcal vaccination was cost-saving in the United States when the incidence of pneumococcal bacteremia was 57 cases per 100,000 people 65 years of age and older,[284] and observations that similar or greater rates of invasive disease have been observed in Canada, Denmark, Norway, Sweden, and Israel (see Table 22–4) suggest that pneumococcal vaccination of elderly people is probably

Table 22–7. **COST-EFFECTIVENESS OF PNEUMOCOCCAL VACCINATION COMPARED WITH OTHER INTERVENTIONS USED IN THE CARE OF OLDER PEOPLE IN THE UNITED STATES**

INTERVENTION	COST PER LIFE-YEAR GAINED ($U.S.)*
Pneumococcal vaccination, age ≥65 yr, once†	1,300
Influenza vaccination, age ≥65 yr, annually	1,800
Cancer screening	
Hemoccult once, age 55 yr, asymptomatic	1,300
Mammogram, age 50–65 yr, every 3 yr	2,700
Papanicolaou test, age ≥65 yr, every 3 yr	2,800
Blood donors to detect human immunodeficiency virus	14,000
Heart disease	
β-blocker treatment for high-risk survivor of myocardial infarction	3,000
Heart transplant, age ≥55 yr, good prognosis	3,600
Coronary angioplasty, men age 55 yr, severe angina	5,300
Bypass surgery, men age 55 yr, left main disease	5,600
Hypertension screening, age 60 yr, asymptomatic	11,000
Cholesterol 180 mg/dL, men age ≥60 yr, diet only	12,000
Cholesterol 300 mg/dL, men age ≥60 yr, lovastatin and diet	26,000
Other interventions	
Nicotine gum and smoking cessation advice, men age 65–69 yr	9,100
Estrogen-progestin, women age ≥50 yr, symptomatic	15,000
Home dialysis for end-stage renal disease	20,000–46,000
Cadaver kidney transplant and cyclosporine	29,000

*All costs estimated in 1993 U.S. dollars.

†Prevention of pneumococcal pneumonia. For this and other reasons, the cost per life-year gained with pneumococcal vaccination differs from the cost mentioned in the text.

Data from reference 674.

highly cost-effective in most if not all developed countries.

Vaccine Failure

Not everyone who receives pneumococcal vaccine is protected against serious pneumococcal infection; the 23-valent vaccine covers approximately 90% of the serotypes responsible for invasive disease, and people at greatest risk are usually those with the poorest antibody response to vaccination. Published reports often describe immunocompromised patients who would be expected to experience vaccine failure. Many of their infections have been caused by one of the serotypes that are weak vaccine antigens (e.g., types 6A, 19F, and 23F). Even among fully immunocompetent people, studies of antibody responses to individual serotypes usually reveal several serotypes to which there has been little or no antibody increase.[465] In the absence of knowledge about what antibody levels ensure protection against infection caused by each serotype, it is difficult to draw meaningful conclusions about relationships between serological responses to vaccination and vaccine failure. Given these limitations, it is encouraging that the aggregate effectiveness of 23-valent pneumococcal vaccine is as high as it is.

IMMUNIZATION POLICIES AND VACCINE USE

Recommendations for Pneumococcal Vaccination

United States

The Advisory Committee on Immunization Practices (ACIP) issued its fifth set of recommendations on pneumococcal vaccination in 1997 (Table 22–8).[219] The ACIP strongly recommends vaccination for all people 65 years of age and older and for those between 2 and 65 years of age who are at increased risk for serious pneumococcal infection. All people with functional or anatomic asplenia (e.g., sickle cell disease, splenectomy) should be

Table 22–8. **RECOMMENDATIONS FOR PNEUMOCOCCAL VACCINATION AND REVACCINATION IN THE UNITED STATES**

VACCINATION*	REVACCINATION
Immunocompetent People 2 Years and Older	
Age ≥65 yr	Once if vaccinated before age 65 yr and vaccine was given >5 yr previously
Age <65 yr	
With functional or anatomic asplenia	Once after 5 yr if age >10 yr; if age ≤10 yr, consider revaccination after 3 yr
With chronic cardiovascular or pulmonary disease	Not recommended
With diabetes mellitus	Not recommended
With alcoholism and chronic liver disease	Not recommended
With cerebrospinal fluid leak	Not recommended
Inhabiting special environments or social settings (e.g., Native Alaskan, Native American)	Not recommended
Immunocompromised People 2 Years and Older	
With human immunodeficiency virus	Once after 5 yr
With congenital immunodeficiency	Once after 5 yr
With leukemia, lymphoma, Hodgkin disease, multiple myeloma	Once after 5 yr
With generalized malignancy	Once after 5 yr
With immunosuppressive or corticosteroid therapy	Once after 5 yr
With chronic renal failure	Once after 5 yr
With nephrotic syndrome	If age ≤10 yr, consider revaccination after 3 yr
After organ or hematopoietic cell transplantation	Once after 5 yr

*If previous vaccination status is unknown, pneumococcal vaccine should be given.

Data from reference 219.

informed that fulminant pneumococcal disease has a high mortality rate and be vaccinated. Whenever possible, pneumococcal vaccine should be given 2 weeks before elective splenectomy. Vaccination does not ensure complete protection, and for this reason any unexplained fever or septic illness requires prompt medical evaluation and treatment if pneumococcal bacteremia is suspected. Chemoprophylaxis may be considered for many of these patients, and it is prudent for all to carry a 12- to 24-hour supply of an oral antibiotic active against *S. pneumoniae* and to begin treatment if prompt access to medical care is unavailable.

For people younger than 65 years, it is recommended that at 50 years of age their overall vaccination status be reviewed to determine whether high-risk conditions are present; among those in the 50- to 64-year age group, at least 36% have cardiovascular conditions and 12% have pulmonary conditions that are indications for pneumococcal vaccination.[683] The recommendation for people living in special environments includes residents of nursing homes and chronic care facilities and those who live in homeless shelter because outbreaks of pneumococcal disease have occurred in these settings.[256, 684] There is no evidence to support a recommendation that pneumococcal vaccine be given to children in day care centers, however, or to those with recurrent upper respiratory tract disease, otitis media, and sinusitis.

Among immunocompromised people, in whom pneumococcal vaccination is less effective,[219] vaccination is still recommended because of the increased risk of disease and the potential benefits, safety, and low cost of vaccination. People with HIV infection should be vaccinated as soon as the diagnosis is confirmed. Those being considered for immunosuppressive therapy should be vaccinated at least 2 weeks before treatment begins or, if this is not possible, 3 months after treatment stops because the response to vaccination during or shortly after chemotherapy or radiation therapy is poor.

Routine revaccination with 23-valent pneumococcal vaccine is not recommended in the United States (see Table 22–8). Revaccination is contraindicated for anyone who has experienced a severe reaction to a first dose of pneumococcal vaccine. Revaccination once is recommended for people at least 65 years of age who were vaccinated more than 5 years before reaching the age of 65. It is also recommended for those with functional or anatomic asplenia and those who are immunocompromised. For children 10 years and younger with asplenia or conditions associated with a rapid decline in antibody levels, revaccination after 3 years can be considered. The clinical effectiveness of a single revaccination and the need for additional doses are unknown. Although many patients have probably received three or more doses of pneumococcal vaccine, there are no data on the safety of repeated vaccination. In the United States, a second revaccination is not routinely recommended.

Other Developed Countries

Current (1997) recommendations for pneumococcal vaccination vary among developed countries (Table 22–9).[685] All countries with national recommendations include functional or anatomic asplenia and almost all include chronic cardiopulmonary diseases, diabetes mellitus, and conditions associated with immunocompromise. Several countries, however, do not recommend pneumococcal vaccination for all elderly people. Table 22–9 shows the recommendations for pneumococcal vaccination of elderly people in 20 developed countries.[685] Also shown are the year in which 23-valent pneumococcal vaccine was registered and whether vaccination is reimbursed by national or social health insurance. For comparison, the table includes recommendations and reimbursement for influenza vaccination.[686]

Several major differences among developed countries are evident. During the period 1983 to 1986, only 11 of the 20 countries registered 23-valent pneumococcal vaccine. Excluding Iceland, of the eight remaining countries, four did not register the vaccine until 1995 or 1996, and it is still not registered in Spain and Portugal. Although three countries have never issued national recommendations for pneumococcal vaccination, almost all of the others issued their first recommendations or updated previous recommendations in the 1990s. In 1997, seven countries with recommendations did not include all elderly people, although six of the seven (Ireland, the Netherlands, France, Germany, Switzerland, and Australia) recommended influenza vaccination for this age group. In contrast, in Sweden, Denmark, and Finland, pneumococcal but not influenza vaccination is recommended for all elderly people. Eleven of the 20 countries did not provide public reimbursement for pneumococcal vaccination, although four of these 11 provided public reimbursement for influenza vaccination. Many of the inconsistencies within individual countries regarding policies for pneumococcal and influenza vaccination reflect different interpretations of the clinical effectiveness of the two vaccines. Most of these differences are likely to disappear within the next few years.

Use of Pneumococcal Vaccine

United States

As many as 40 to 50 million people in the United States are candidates for pneumococcal vaccination, including 33 million who are 65 years of age or older. During the 14-year period from 1978 through 1991, approximately 23 million doses of pneumococcal vaccine were distributed in the United States.[21] During the 5-year period from 1992 through 1996, an additional 23 million doses were distributed nationwide.[685] Nonetheless, data from the National Health Interview Survey for 1993 suggested that no more than 30% of elderly people had ever been vaccinated.[687] The 1995 Behavioral Risk Factor Surveillance Study indicated that only 35.6% of the elderly population reported they had received a "pneumonia vaccination."[688]

In the late 1980s, a CDC study showed that, regardless of whether elderly people had negative or positive attitudes toward pneumococcal vaccination, the recommendation of a health care provider determined whether

Table 22–9. **REGISTRATION, RECOMMENDATIONS, AND REIMBURSEMENT FOR PNEUMOCOCCAL AND INFLUENZA VACCINATION IN 20 DEVELOPED COUNTRIES**

COUNTRY	23-VALENT PNEUMOCOCCAL VACCINE		VACCINATION RECOMMENDATION FOR ALL ELDERLY PEOPLE (≥65 YR)		VACCINATION REIMBURSED BY NATIONAL OR SOCIAL HEALTH INSURANCE	
	Year Registered	Year of Most Recent Recommendation	Pneumococcal	Influenza	Pneumococcal	Influenza
United States	1983	1997	Yes	Yes	Yes	Yes
Canada	1983	1993	Yes	Yes	Yes	Yes
Sweden	1984	1994	Yes	—*	—	—
Denmark	1996	1996	Yes	—	—	—
Norway	1996	1996	Yes†	Yes	—	Yes
Finland	1984	1996	Yes†	—	—	Yes
Iceland	—‡	1991	Yes§	Yes§	—	—
United Kingdom	1989	1996	—	—	Yes	Yes
Ireland	1985	1996	—	Yes	—	—
Netherlands	1984	1993	—	Yes	Yes	Yes
Belgium	1995	1993	Yes§	Yes§	—	Yes‖
France	1983	1995	—	Yes¶	—	Yes
Germany	1984	1995	—	Yes	Yes	Yes
Switzerland	1983	1996	—	Yes	—	—
Austria	1995	1997	Yes	Yes	—	—
Italy	1992	—	—	Yes	Yes	Yes
Spain	—	—	—	Yes	Yes	Yes
Portugal	—	—	—	Yes	Yes	Yes
Australia	1986	1986	—	Yes	Yes	Yes
New Zealand	1984	1986	Yes	Yes	—	—

*Dash indicates no registration, recommendation, or reimbursement.
†In Finland, national guidelines for physicians issued in 1996 included a recommendation to vaccinate all elderly people. Pneumococcal vaccination, however, is not included in the publicly reimbursed program that covers influenza vaccination.
‡Vaccine registration is not required in Iceland.
§60 years and older.
‖40% of the cost of influenza vaccination is reimbursed.
¶70 years and older.
Adapted from references 685 and 686. The information in this table was current as of October 1, 1997.

an individual was vaccinated: If vaccination was not recommended, only 5 to 7% were immunized, whereas if it was recommended, 63 to 84% were immunized.[689] A similar study conducted almost a decade later showed that without a physician's recommendation, only 16% (negative patient attitude) to 46% (positive patient attitude) were vaccinated, whereas with a recommendation, 85 to 86% were vaccinated.[690] These results show the primary importance of a physician's recommendation, although they also suggest that in the intervening decade, positive patient attitudes had become an important contributing factor to being vaccinated.

Several studies have shown that most physicians in the United States recognize which patients are at risk for pneumococcal infections and understand the benefits of pneumococcal vaccination.[691] Yet little is known about their vaccination practices, especially the practices of office-based physicians who are probably responsible for vaccinating most of those who are vaccinated. Nonetheless, a number of programs to enhance the delivery of pneumococcal vaccine in the outpatient clinics of teaching hospitals have been reported.[692] In these settings, medical house officers almost always have correct knowledge about the vaccine, but many fail to translate this knowledge into clinical practice, often because more urgent clinical issues demand attention.[693] Substantial improvements in vaccination rates have followed the introduction of administrative and organizational changes in the way vaccination is offered.[692, 694] Nurses, pharmacists, and other health care providers have been important contributors to these efforts.[695] As a result, immunization rates for high-risk patients in many of these programs have reached 50 to 80% or higher.[690, 692, 694] Other hospital units such as the emergency department have also been identified as appropriate sites for pneumococcal vaccination.[696, 697]

One often overlooked setting for pneumococcal vaccination is the hospital inpatient unit. Previous hospital care is a useful marker for identifying high-risk people; approximately two thirds of patients hospitalized with pneumococcal bacteremia or pneumonia (all causes) have been discharged from a hospital at least once within the previous 5 years.[64] Efforts to vaccinate inpatients have met with mixed results, however. One program that provided daily computer-generated reminders to medical housestaff had no effect,[698] but systems-oriented approaches have been considerably more effective in increasing inpatient vaccination.[699–701] Other hospital-based programs have specifically targeted surgeons who perform splenectomies.[702]

Several population-based programs to improve pneumococcal vaccine delivery have been organized by large health care organizations[703] and by state[704, 705] and local[706] public health agencies. One noteworthy program has targeted a remote population of high-risk Alaskan Natives, increasing vaccination rates from 30% to 84%

within 3 years.[707] At the national level, the National Coalition for Adult Immunization has regularly sponsored National Adult Immunization Awareness Week each October to emphasize the importance of vaccinating adults against several diseases, including pneumococcal disease.[687]

At the federal level, several initiatives have been undertaken to improve levels of pneumococcal vaccination. In the early 1980s the Surgeon General established the goal of vaccinating 60% of the elderly by 1990. When this goal was not met, it was reset for the year 2000.[708] In 1981, Congress authorized the Health Care Financing Administration (HCFA) to reimburse physicians for the cost of pneumococcal vaccine and its administration, but until 1993 the HCFA's payments covered only the cost of the vaccine, not its administration.[708] Perhaps as a result, claims for Medicare reimbursement in the late 1980s accounted for only 25% of the doses of pneumococcal vaccine distributed nationwide.[708, 709] In 1993, when the HCFA finally authorized Medicare reimbursement for influenza vaccine, it also established a separate billing code for vaccine administration. This has improved the level of physician reimbursement for pneumococcal vaccination. Finally, in 1994 the National Vaccine Advisory Committee presented its report on adult immunization to the Assistant Secretary for Health recommending several initiatives to improve pneumococcal vaccination.[710]

In spite of shortcomings in federal activities identified by the General Accounting Office,[711] the 1990s have seen greatly enhanced federal efforts and expenditures to improve pneumococcal vaccination levels nationwide.[712] These efforts are reflected in changes in pneumococcal vaccine use (Fig. 22–1).[685] From 1991 to 1996, annual vaccine distribution increased from 108 to 267 doses per 10,000 population. The increase was especially noticeable in 1993, when influenza vaccine also became covered benefit under Medicare. Pneumococcal vaccine use fell the following year because of manufacturers' production problems, but it rebounded in 1995 and 1996. If this trend continues, the Surgeon General's goal of vaccinating 60% of the elderly may soon be achieved.

Other Developed Countries

In 1988, the World Health Organization (WHO) convened a group of technical advisers to consider the status of pneumococcal immunization in developed countries, especially those in Western Europe.[713] One of the group's main conclusions was to recommend vaccination for all elderly people and for people of any age who are at increased risk of pneumococcal infection. The response to this recommendation was slow in coming, but by the mid-1990s change was clearly evident.

Figure 22–1 shows the annual use of pneumococcal vaccine in the United States and 13 of the 19 other developed countries shown in Table 22–9. None of these other countries used appreciable amounts of vaccine until 1991. In that year, Iceland and later the United Kingdom (1994), Sweden (1995), and Norway, Belgium, and Canada (1996) increased their use of pneumococcal vaccine dramatically.[685] In five of these six countries, change followed new vaccine registrations, new or expanded national recommendations for pneumococcal vaccination, or both.

The change in Canada occurred for different reasons. As in the United States, pneumococcal vaccine was licensed in Canada in the late 1970s and national recommendations for its use were similar to those issued by the ACIP.[714] What was missing was the willingness of provincial health departments to purchase vaccine and distribute it free-of-charge to practitioners. (Provincial health departments purchase ≥90% of the influenza vaccine used in Canada, and as a result its rate of use has been similar to that in the United States.[714]) The 1996 increase in pneumococcal vaccination in Canada was due entirely to the decision of the provincial health department in Ontario to vaccinate all people at least 65 years of age over a 3-year period. As a result of provincial vaccine purchase and a public and professional education program, the 1996 rate of vaccine use in Ontario (426 doses/10,000 population) was almost 1.5 times greater than that in the United States (see Fig. 22–1). Ontario accounted for 91% of the pneumococcal vaccine used throughout Canada. In the rest of the country, the rate of vaccine use was similar to that in France.[685]

For countries that have not begun using pneumococcal vaccine, the lessons to be learned from these six countries are clear. The vaccine must be registered, broad recommendations for its use must be issued, and vaccination must be promoted by public health officials and professional groups. Given the experience of these six countries, it is likely that within the next few years several other countries will begin to use large amounts of pneumococcal vaccine.

NEWER PNEUMOCOCCAL VACCINES

The limitations of 23-valent pneumococcal polysaccharide vaccine are widely recognized: Some capsular type polysaccharides are weak antigens and probably not very efficacious, the level of clinical protection appears to decline within a few years of vaccination, and revaccination does not elicit a booster antibody response. Newer pneumococcal conjugate[715] and protein vaccines may overcome these limitations.

Pneumococcal Conjugate Vaccines

Several bacterial polysaccharides have been conjugated covalently to carrier proteins, improving their immunogenicity and resulting in antigens with novel characteristics.[716–720] Antigen-presenting cells take up the conjugated polysaccharide-protein molecules and present the peptides in association with MHC class II molecules on their surface. This induces helper T cells to stimulate polysaccharide-specific B cells that have also taken up the conjugate molecules. These B cells then produce antibody and mature into memory cells. A polysaccharide covalently linked to a protein carrier thus becomes recognized by the immune system as a T cell–

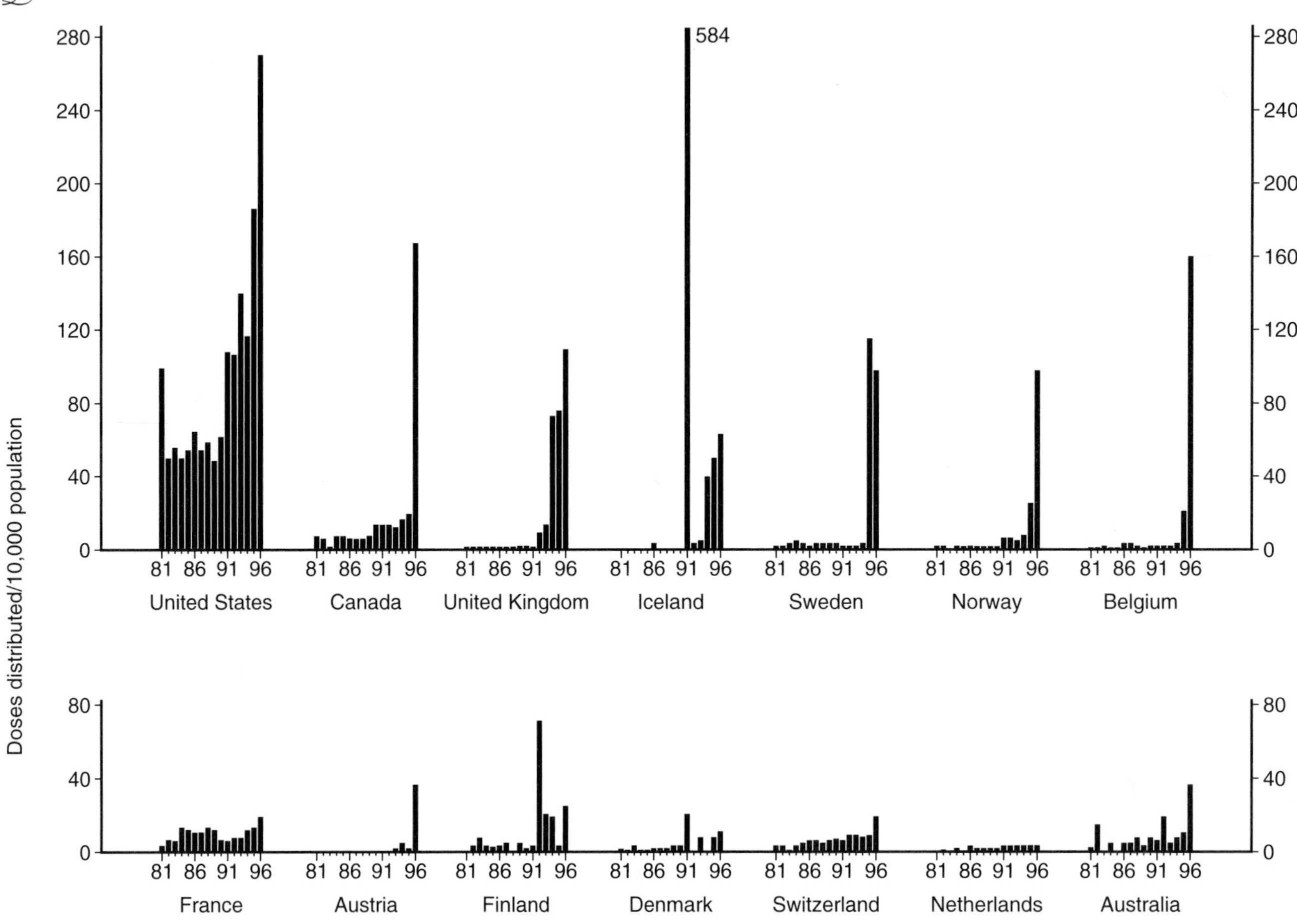

Figure 22–1. Pneumococcal vaccine distribution in 14 developed countries, 1981 to 1996. Data from Fedson DS. Clin Infect Dis 26:1117–1123, 1998.

dependent antigen.[721, 722] Immunological properties of such antigens include increased production of antibodies, development of immunological memory, and maturation of the antibody response so that the majority of the antibodies produced are of high avidity and of the IgG class. These immunological responses can be seen when conjugated polysaccharides are given during the first months of life, in contrast with the poor antibody response when only polysaccharide antigens are given.

For pneumococcal conjugate vaccines, each candidate capsular polysaccharide, either in its native form or as an oligosaccharide, is coupled individually to a carrier protein. The final vaccines are mixtures of these polysaccharide- or oligosaccharide-protein conjugates. Several different chemical methods have been tested for conjugation in order to obtain optimal cross-linking of the polysaccharide to the carrier proteins and to ensure that conformational epitopes are maintained. Although it would be preferable to include a large number of different polysaccharides in a conjugate vaccine, the total amount of carrier protein in the final vaccine must be limited. It must be sufficient to induce T-cell memory for each polysaccharide, yet small enough to minimize the induction of antibodies to the carrier protein. Furthermore, too much carrier protein may impair the antibody response to the polysaccharide antigen through antigenic competition or carrier-mediated epitope suppression.

The carrier proteins used in pneumococcal conjugate vaccines are the same as those present in Hib conjugate vaccines: tetanus (T) and diphtheria (D) toxoids, a nontoxic mutant of diphtheria toxin (CRM 197 protein), and the outer membrane protein complex (OMPC) of *N. meningitidis* group B. Other potential carrier proteins that have been tested in experimental animal studies include bovine serum albumin, human IgG, keyhole limpet hemocyanin,[723] flagellar protein of *Salmonella*, pertussis toxoid,[724] and pneumolysin toxoid.[725–727] Synthetic peptides have also been used as carriers in experimental pneumococcal conjugate vaccines.

Initial studies were conducted with monovalent and later with multivalent conjugate vaccines. In clinical studies, all of these preparations have been well tolerated. The antibody responses in adults have generally been modest,[728, 729] perhaps because the dose of each polysaccharide in the conjugate vaccines has been low, preimmunization antibody concentrations of study subjects have been high, or vaccinees have been given only one dose. In toddlers, the primary response to Pnc-OMPC vaccine has been only slightly higher than the response to the polysaccharide vaccine alone, although after the second dose a booster-type response has occurred in most vaccinees.[730] The Pnc-CRM, Pnc-D, and Pnc-T vaccines have also been shown to be immunogenic and to induce immunological memory.[731, 732] Compared with polysaccharide vaccine, one dose of any of these three conjugate vaccines greatly increases the serotype-specific opsonophagocytic activity of postvaccination serum.[733] Furthermore, individuals who do not respond to the polysaccharide vaccine may show vigorous IgG responses to conjugate vaccine.[733a]

In addition to immunologically normal subjects, patients with impaired natural immunity to pneumococcal infections have been vaccinated with pneumococcal conjugate vaccines. Adults with treated Hodgkin disease who were vaccinated with one dose of a Pnc-OMPC vaccine had lower mean antibody responses than similar patients given one dose of polysaccharide vaccine.[734] After a booster dose of polysaccharide vaccine, however, antibody levels were significantly higher in the group that had been primed with the conjugate vaccine.[735] A monovalent Pnc-T vaccine was shown to be immunogenic in children with sickle cell anemia,[736] as was a pentavalent Pnc-CRM vaccine in HIV-infected adults.[729] HIV-infected children with relatively mild disease were more likely to have moderate or high antibody levels after the first and second doses of conjugate vaccine than were HIV-infected children with more advanced disease. These differences disappeared after the third dose of conjugate vaccine, however.[737] In HIV-infected children at least 2 years of age, one dose of pneumococcal conjugate vaccine is substantially more immunogenic than one dose of the polysaccharide vaccine.[738]

Infants are currently considered the main target group for pneumococcal conjugate vaccines. Most studies have therefore concentrated on safety and immunogenicity in young infants, starting at the age of 2 months. All pneumococcal conjugates tested thus far have been well tolerated, as could be expected from the extensive experience with Hib conjugate vaccines. No immediate serious, vaccine-related adverse events have been reported. Local reactions after pneumococcal conjugate vaccination have been similar in frequency and severity to those reported with Hib conjugate vaccines and have usually been less marked than those seen with whole-cell pertussis-containing vaccines. Reaction rates have been lower and their intensity less marked in young infants than in adults.

In general, all pneumococcal conjugates tested have been immunogenic in infants. Depending on the serotype,[730] three doses of a tetravalent Pnc-OMPC vaccine given between the ages of 2 to 6 months induced 1.4- to 14.1-fold increases in anticapsular polysaccharide antibody levels. When only two doses were given at 4 and 6 months, the antibody increases were lower, but secondary responses occurred following a third dose given at 14 months of age.[730] Polysaccharide-based Pnc-CRM vaccines (bivalent, pentavalent, or heptavalent) have been shown to be immunogenic in infants, whereas antibody responses to the corresponding oligosaccharide formulations have remained relatively modest.[731, 739–741] Tetravalent and octavalent Pnc-T and Pnc-D conjugates have also been shown to be immunogenic. All of these pneumococcal conjugates seem able to induce immunological memory; a secondary type antibody response has occurred after a booster dose of either conjugate or polysaccharide vaccine.[742] In addition, experimental studies in mice suggest that the immune response of infants to pneumococcal conjugate vaccination might be enhanced by maternal immunization with the same vaccine.[743] Important for the future development of multivalent pneumococcal conjugate vaccines is the observation that inclusion of additional serotypes does not seem to significantly affect the immunogenicity of each individual conjugated polysaccharide.[744]

Clear-cut differences exist in the antibody responses to different capsular type polysaccharides in the conjugate vaccines. Serotypes 6B and 23F appear to be poor immunogens in spite of conjugation. A study of a serotype 6B Pnc-T conjugate given to children at either 3, 4, and 6 months or at 7 and 9 months, however, showed that in spite of low antibody responses at 7 or 10 months, respectively, another dose at 18 months elicited a solid booster response in 62% and 79% of the children.[745] For conjugates of other serotypes, such as 3 and 18C, antibody responses are usually satisfactory, even after the first dose. The immunogenic properties of other serotype conjugates tested fall between these two extremes. These differences seem to reflect inherent properties of the individual polysaccharides rather than the specific conjugation procedure.

The immune response needed to prevent mucosal infection may be different from what is needed to protect against invasive disease. For example, acute otitis media is an infection largely restricted to the mucosal surfaces. Pneumococcal conjugate vaccines induce immune responses that protect against experimental pneumococcal otitis media in chinchillas.[746, 747] Preliminary studies suggest that similar protection may be expected in humans; pneumococcal conjugate vaccines induce specific IgA antibody-secreting cells in the peripheral blood of immunized subjects,[748, 749] and these cells are thought to reflect the induction of mucosal immunity. Nonetheless, whether secretory IgA antibodies make an essential contribution to mucosal defense in pneumococcal otitis media is unknown.

Encouraging data on the immunogenicity of pneumococcal conjugate vaccines have been supplemented by clinical experience. In one study from Israel, 12- to 18-month-old children received one or two doses of the Pnc-OMPC vaccine or pneumococcal polysaccharide vaccine.[645] During a 1-year follow-up, there was a significant reduction in carriage of vaccine-type pneumococci in the conjugate vaccine groups but no such reduction in those who received the polysaccharide vaccine. A subsequent study by the same investigators showed that infants given tetravalent Pnc-T or Pnc-D vaccines at 2, 4, and 6 months of age followed by a booster dose of 23-valent polysaccharide at 12 months had markedly reduced carriage rates compared with unvaccinated control subjects.[750] Other reports from The Gambia,[646] Iceland,[751] and South Africa[752] also suggest that conjugate vaccination is associated with a reduction in nasopharyngeal carriage of vaccine-type organisms. If followed by reduced transmission to others, this could be important for preventing the spread of antimicrobial resistant *S. pneumoniae* in the community. Replacement colonization with nonvaccine serotypes has been reported after vaccination with pneumococcal conjugates,[646, 753] but it is unclear whether this will become an important clinical problem.

The pneumococcal conjugate vaccines currently being developed contain 11 serotypes; types 1, 3, 4, 5, 6B, 7F, 9V, 14, 18C, 19F, and 23F. Epidemiological studies indicate that these serotypes account for approximately 75 to 90% of all cases of invasive pneumococcal disease and pneumococcal otitis media in children (Table 22–10).[289, 293, 306, 358, 361, 377, 754–758b] The first results of a large-scale trial of the Pnc-CRM vaccine have just been reported.[757b] Heptavalent vaccine or placebo was administered to 36,000 children, divided randomly into two equal groups. In the placebo groups, 31 cases of pneumococcal bacteremia were reported, of which 22 were caused by serotypes in the vaccine. All 22 infections occurred in the placebo group, 17 in those who had received three doses, 5 in those who had received one or two doses. There were also 8 isolations of pneumococcal serotypes not in the vaccine, about equally divided between vaccinees and placebo recipients. Thus, efficacy of the vaccine was 100%(CI, 81–100%) against serotypes in the vaccine, and 89% against all pneumococci. Data concerning prevention of acute otitis media and pneumonia are forthcoming, but these initial results raise hopes that pneumococcal conjugate vaccines will soon be licensed. Because pneumonia is a major cause of childhood mortality in developing countries, demonstration of the efficacy of pneumococcal conjugate vaccines against pneumococcal pneumonia and meningitis will be important.

To avoid repeating time-consuming and expensive efficacy trials, it would be of great importance to be able to predict clinical protection by means of one or more clearly defined laboratory tests. Unfortunately, even the simplest measure of protection—the serum antibody level—is not known for any pneumococcal serotype. Experience with Hib conjugate vaccines has shown that the development of immunological memory might be decisive for clinical protection.[759–761] No consensus has yet been reached on laboratory correlates of clinical protection for either Hib or pneumococcal conjugate vaccines, however.

Thus far, the magnitude of the antibody response, induction of immunological memory, persistence of antibodies, isotype and subclass distribution of antibodies, and avidity and functional capacity of antibodies have all been proposed as potential surrogates for clinical protection.[761, 762] New methods to measure the avidity[763] or opsonophagocytic activity[733] of vaccine-induced pneumococcal antibodies of different isotypes and subclasses have been developed. These methods should be used in the analysis of sera and other samples from future efficacy trials. Correlates of protection should be sought on the individual level by investigating longitudinal follow-up data on children who contract pneumococcal infection in spite of vaccination. They should also be sought in populations by comparing cross-sectional information on antibody concentrations and estimates of protection in the same group of subjects.

Pneumococcal Protein Vaccines

Although conjugated pneumococcal polysaccharide vaccines have demonstrated enhanced immunogenicity

Table 22–10. **SEROTYPE COVERAGE IN CHILDREN BY THE PROPOSED 11-VALENT PNEUMOCOCCAL CONJUGATE VACCINE**

LOCATION	YEARS	AGE GROUP (YR)	SOURCE OF ISOLATES	TOTAL NUMBER	11 CONJUGATE VACCINE SEROTYPES* No.	%	REFERENCE
United States							
CDC	1978–1994	≤2	Blood, CSF, middle ear	3007	2574	86†	377
		≤6		3884	2964	76	
Connecticut	1984–1993	≤2	Invasive	502	458	91	755
		≤15		722	654	91	
Alabama	1985–1989	Pediatric	Blood, CSF	303	271‡	89	754
			Middle ear	228	198‡	87	
Alaska	1986–1990	<2, Native	Invasive	103	78	76	756
		<2, Non-native		107	92	86	
Southern California	1992–1995	≤2	Invasive	61	52	85	289
		≤10		79	71	90	
Finland§	1985–1992	≤15	Invasive	365	336‡	92	358
Israel§	1988–1996	≤13	Invasive	718	619‡	86	‖
New Zealand	1989–1992	≤14	Blood, CSF	129	104‡	81	361
Denmark	1989–1994	≤14	Blood, CSF	482	416	86	293
Germany	1992–1996	<14	Blood, CSF	121	92	76	757
Central Australia	1992–1993	≤15	Invasive	41	30	73	306a
Uruguay	1994–1996	≤2	Invasive	121	105	87	758
Brazil	1993–1996	≤6	Invasive	360	295	82	758a

*Serotypes 1, 3, 4, 5, 6B/6A, 7, 9V, 14F, 18C, 19F, 23F
†Rates have been rounded to the nearest whole number.
‡Serogroup data only.
§Population-based study.
‖R. Dagan, personal communication, 1997.
CDC, Centers for Disease Control and Prevention; CSF, cerebrospinal fluid; Invasive, isolation of *S. pneumoniae* from a normally sterile site.

to the serotypes included in the vaccines, they cannot provide protection against infection by nonvaccine serotypes. For this reason investigators have looked for other potentially protective antigens. Ideally, these antigens would be one or more common proteins that would not exhibit serotype variation and would provide protection against infection by a broad range of pneumococcal capsular serotypes. As proteins they would also be thymus-dependent antigens and thus be capable of stimulating durable immunological memory in early infancy. It is still uncertain, however, whether the critical epitopes of the pneumococcal proteins that have been proposed as vaccine candidates are sufficiently exposed on the bacterial cell surface to induce antibodies that are protective in vivo.

Several pneumococcal proteins, including pneumolysin, PspA, pneumococcal surface adhesin A (PsaA), neuraminidase, and autolysin, are considered essential for bacterial virulence.[31, 32] Specific inactivation of their respective genes in the pneumococcal chromosome significantly reduces the virulence of these bacteria for mice.[38] Immunization with pneumolysin, PspA, and PsaA have been shown in mice to be capable of eliciting partial protection against challenge infection with virulent *S. pneumoniae*. Each of these proteins has been suggested as a potentially broadly protective protein-based vaccine. Alternatively, it has been suggested they be used as carrier proteins for pneumococcal conjugate vaccines.

Pneumolysin is a cytolytic toxin produced by all pneumococci, regardless of serotype.[38] Genetically engineered pneumolysin-negative mutants of *S. pneumoniae* have significantly reduced virulence for mice.[764] Mice injected with inactivated pneumolysin or recombinant pneumolysin toxoid exhibit enhanced survival when challenged with at least nine different pneumococcal serotypes.[38, 47] Pneumolysin toxoids have also been conjugated to pneumococcal capsular polysaccharides.[725–727] These conjugates elicit antipolysaccharide antibodies in mice, and subsequent injections elicit a clear booster response.[726, 727]

PspA is a surface protein present in all clinically relevant strains of *S. pneumoniae*.[765] Although PspAs from different pneumococcal strains are serologically variable, some elicit antibodies that are cross-reactive with PspAs from unrelated strains. Active immunization of mice with PspA or with truncated PspAs generates antibodies that protect against subsequent challenge with several strains of pneumococci.[50, 51, 766] Moreover, orally administered PspA given with the mucosal adjuvant cholera toxin induces significant levels of serum IgG and IgA antibodies and protects mice against challenge infection.[767]

PsaA is a putative adhesin that may be important for pneumococcal virulence.[768] PsaA is immunogenic and protective in mice,[766] but it is unclear whether its variability in different pneumococcal serotypes will compromise its ability to induce sufficient cross-protection and thus diminish its usefulness as a vaccine antigen.

Although one or more of these pneumococcal proteins offers several theoretical advantages over capsular polysaccharide-based vaccines, no experimental studies have been published that directly compare the protection induced by these two types of vaccines. Such studies are needed.

CONSIDERATIONS FOR THE FUTURE

Since pneumococcal polysaccharide vaccine was first licensed in 1977, much has been learned about the burden of pneumococcal disease (see Tables 22–3 and 22–4), the effectiveness of pneumococcal vaccination (see Table 22–6), the value of pneumococcal vaccination to society (see Table 22–7), and patterns of vaccine use (see Table 22–9 and Fig. 22–1).[769] Nonetheless, important questions persist and must be answered before the full potential of pneumococcal vaccination can be realized.

In most developed countries, population-based estimates of the occurrence of invasive pneumococcal disease have yet to be obtained and are needed. Additional retrospective studies to assess the effectiveness of pneumococcal vaccination in preventing pneumococcal pneumonia and in reducing the burden of community-acquired pneumonias requiring hospital care are also required. Equally important is the need to accurately assess the duration of protection afforded by pneumococcal vaccine, for in spite of its being licensed for 20 years, little is known about the persistence of antibody and long-term protection following a single dose. Comparative studies also need to be undertaken simultaneously in several countries to determine the cost-effectiveness of pneumococcal vaccination in preventing invasive pneumococcal disease alone as well as pneumococcal pneumonia. Finally, much more needs to learned about the microepidemiology of pneumococcal vaccination practices by individual physicians and the rapidly changing macroepidemiology of vaccine use among different countries.

Pediatricians are eagerly awaiting the arrival of pneumococcal conjugate vaccines, although these vaccines are unlikely to become available for several years. In developed countries their greatest impact will likely be on the occurrence of otitis media, and if they are free of serious adverse effects, conjugate vaccines of even low efficacy might be acceptable to parents.[770] As with *H. influenzae* type b conjugate vaccines,[771] however, the public health importance of pneumococcal conjugate vaccines may be better measured by their impact on nasopharyngeal carriage of *S. pneumoniae* and the corresponding reduction in the occurrence of not only otitis media but also invasive pneumococcal disease, including meningitis and other invasive infections caused by antibiotic-resistant pneumococci. Epidemiological studies are needed in many countries to monitor the changing rates and serotype distribution of *S. pneumoniae* nasopharyngeal carriage and antimicrobial resistance over time in order to assess the changes that are expected to occur once pneumococcal conjugate vaccines come into use. At the same time, ongoing clinical surveillance is needed to determine whether antimicrobial resistance will become associated with a broader pattern of treatment failures and involve a larger number of serotypes.

The potential contributions of pneumococcal polysaccharide and conjugate vaccines to the control of acute respiratory infections in developing countries has received little attention. Until now, the WHO Program for Acute Respiratory Infections has focused only on children younger than 5 years.[379] The remarkable effects of Hib conjugate vaccination in The Gambia in not only controlling Hib meningitis but also reducing deaths from childhood pneumonia[758] has heightened expectations of what might be accomplished with pneumococcal conjugate vaccines, and clinical trials in developing countries are expected to begin soon. Whether it will be feasible for pneumococcal conjugate vaccines to actually be used in developing countries is only beginning to receive attention. Several major obstacles need to be overcome, not the least of which are competing demands to introduce other new vaccines (e.g., hepatitis B, Hib conjugate, and meningococcal conjugate) into the same countries. Although vaccine cost is not the only factor that must be considered,[772, 773] cost will inevitably be a central issue, especially for poorer countries.[774] A preliminary study to evaluate some of these issues has been reported.[775]

The contribution that pneumococcal vaccination might make in controlling the morbidity and mortality of respiratory infections among adults in developing countries has received practically no attention. The WHO-sponsored Global Burden of Disease Study has shown that in developing countries, increased mortality rates for respiratory tract infections, although greatest in very young children, extend across the life span and, in virtually all age groups, greatly exceed those in developed countries.[637, 776] Children in developing countries who survive to adulthood, often as a result of successful childhood immunization programs, continue to show high mortality rates throughout their adult years.[777] An appreciable proportion of this mortality is undoubtedly due to pneumococcal infection.

The potential utility of 23-valent pneumococcal polysaccharide vaccine for adults in developing countries has been largely ignored, except for the possibility of maternal immunization to protect young infants. It is conceivable that pneumococcal conjugate vaccines could have a major impact on pneumococcal disease among adults as well as children in both developing and developed countries: Conjugate priming followed by natural or polysaccharide vaccine boosting might provide a foundation of life-long protection against pneumococcal disease. Moreover, the development of pneumococcal conjugate vaccines for adults in developed countries might lead the vaccine manufacturers to greatly expand capacity for their production and distribution, thus facilitating tiered pricing and speeding the availability of conjugate vaccines for children in developing countries.[772, 773]

To date, however, published studies of pneumococcal conjugate vaccines in adults have been few and limited to a single dose of conjugate vaccine, sometimes followed by a booster dose of polysaccharide vaccine. Whether the use of a three-dose prime and boost schedule, similar to what is used for primary immunization of adults with other vaccines (e.g., tetanus and diphtheria toxoids and inactivated polio and hepatitis B vaccines), would be immunogenic and safe[778] is not known because it has not been studied. Yet, if such a schedule were found to more immunogenic and as safe as pneumococcal polysaccharide vaccine alone, pneumococcal conjugate vaccines would likely be licensed as replacement vaccines for people 2 years and older. There would be no requirement for a clinical efficacy trial, just as there was no such requirement when Hib conjugate vaccines were licensed as replacements for Hib polysaccharide vaccines in older children.

The potential of pneumococcal conjugate vaccines for immunizing people of all ages can be achieved only if clinical development is undertaken with this goal in mind. The promise of these new vaccines to bring enormous improvements in public health deserves the broadest possible discussion worldwide.

Acknowledgments

The authors thank C. Eyraud, M. Trellu, K. Farkh, M.-C. Tardy, and E. Montgour for their assistance in preparing the manuscript and R. Austrian, J. C. Butler, D. Goldblatt, and J. Henrichsen for their comments and criticism.

REFERENCES

1. Heffron R. Pneumonia with Special Reference to Pneumococcus Lobar Pneumonia. Harvard University Press. A Commonwealth Fund book. Cambridge, Harvard University Press, 1979.
2. White B. The Biology of Pneumococcus: The Bacteriologic, Biochemical and Immunological Characters and Activities of *Diplococcus pneumoniae*. Harvard University Press. A Commonwealth Fund book. Cambridge, Harvard University Press, 1979.
3. Austrian R. Pneumococcus: The first one hundred years. Rev Infect Dis 3:183–189, 1981.
4. Austrian R. Pneumococcal pneumonia: Diagnostic, epidemiologic, therapeutic and prophylactic considerations. Chest 90:738–743, 1986.
5. Musher DM. Pneumococcal pneumonia including diagnosis and therapy of infection caused by penicillin-resistant strains. Infect Dis Clin North Am 5:509–521, 1991.
6. Johnston RB Jr. Pathogenesis of pneumococcal pneumonia. Rev Infect Dis 13(suppl 6):S509–S517, 1991.
7. Lee CJ, Banks SD, Li JP. Virulence, immunity, and vaccine related to *Streptococcus pneumoniae*. Crit Rev Microbiol 18:89–114, 1991.
8. Bruyn GA, Zegers BJ, van Furth R. Mechanisms of host defense against infection with *Streptococcus pneumoniae*. Clin Infect Dis 14:251–262, 1992.
9. Musher DM. Infections caused by *Streptococcus pneumoniae*: Clinical spectrum, pathogenesis, immunity, and treatment. Clin Infect Dis 14:801–807, 1992.
10. Watson DA, Musher DM, Jacobson JW, Verhoef J. A brief history of the pneumococcus in biomedical research: A panoply of scientific discovery. Clin Infect Dis 17:913–924, 1993.
11. Lee CJ, Wang TR. Pneumococcal infection and immunization in children. Crit Rev Microbiol 20:1–12, 1994.
12. Austrian R. Preventing pneumococcal infection in modern approaches to new vaccines, including prevention of AIDS. In Norby E, Brown F, Chanock RM, Ginsburg HS (eds). Vaccines 94. New York, Cold Spring Harbor Laboratory Press, 1994, pp 91–98.
13. Mufson MA. Pneumococcal infection. Curr Opin Infect Dis 7:178–183, 1994.
14. Tuomanen EI, Austrian R, Masur HR. Pathogenesis of pneumococcal infections. N Engl J Med 332:1280–1284, 1995.
15. Obaro SK, Monteil MA, Henderson DC. Fortnightly review: The pneumococcal problem. BMJ 312:1521–1525, 1996.
16. Makela PH, Jokinen C, Pyhala R, et al. Use of vaccines for respiratory infections: Strategies for influenza and pneumococcal vaccines. Scand J Infect Dis Suppl 70:141–148, 1990.

17. Torzillo PJ. Pneumococcal vaccine: Current status. Aust N Z J Med 23:285–290, 1993.
18. Monto AS, Terpenning MS. The value of influenza and pneumococcal vaccines in the elderly. Drugs Aging 8:445–451, 1996.
19. Gable CB, Botteman M, Savage G, Joy K. The cost effectiveness of pneumococcal vaccination strategies. Pharmacoeconomics 12:161–174, 1997.
20. Fedson DS. Pneumococcal vaccine. In Plotkin SA, Mortimer EA Jr (eds). Vaccines. Philadelphia, WB Saunders, 1988, pp 271–299.
21. Fedson DS, Musher DM. Pneumococcal vaccine. In Plotkin SA, Mortimer EA Jr (eds). Vaccines (2nd ed). Philadelphia, WB Saunders, 1994, pp 517–564.
22. Austrian R, Gold J. Pneumococcal bacteremia with special reference to bacteremic pneumococcal pneumonia. Ann Intern Med 60:759–776, 1964.
23. Austrian R, Douglas RM, Schiffman G, et al. Prevention of pneumococcal pneumonia by vaccination. Trans Assoc Am Physicians 89:184–194, 1976.
24. Smit P, Oberholzer D, Hayden-Smith S, et al. Protective efficacy of pneumococcal polysaccharide vaccines. JAMA 238:2613–2616, 1977.
25. Musher DM. *Streptococcus pneumoniae*. In Mandel GL, Bennett JE, Dolin R (eds). Principles and Practices of Infectious Diseases (4th ed). New York, Churchill Livingstone, 1995, pp 1811–1826.
26. Kim PE, Musher DM, Glezen WP, et al. Association of invasive pneumococcal disease with season, atmospheric conditions, air pollution, and the isolation of respiratory viruses. Clin Infect Dis 22:100–106, 1996.
27. McCarty M. A retrospective look: How we identified the pneumococcal transforming substance as DNA. J Exp Med 179:385–394, 1994.
28. Lederberg J. The transformation of genetics by DNA: An anniversary celebration of Avery, MacLeod and McCarty (1944). Genetics 136:423–426, 1994.
29. Avery OT, MacLeod CM, McCarty M. Studies on the chemical nature of the substance inducing transformation of pneumococcal types: Induction of transformation by a desoxyribonucleic acid fraction isolated from pneumococcus type III [republication of a 1944 paper]. Mol Med 1:344–365, 1995.
30. Munoz R, Fenoll A, Vicioso D, Casal J. Optochin-resistant variants of *Streptococcus pneumoniae*. Diagn Microbiol Infect Dis 13:63–66, 1990.
31. Alonso De Velasco E, Verheul AF, Verhoef J, Snippe H. *Streptococcus pneumoniae*: Virulence factors, pathogenesis, and vaccines. Microbiol Rev 59:591–603, 1995.
32. Watson DA, Musher DM, Verhoef J. Pneumococcal virulence factors and host immune responses to them. Eur J Clin Microbiol Infect Dis 14:479–490, 1995.
33. Cundell D, Masure HR, Tuomanen EI. The molecular basis of pneumococcal infection: A hypothesis. Clin Infect Dis 21:s204–s212, 1995.
34. Musher DM, Watson DA, Baughn RE. Does naturally acquired IgG antibody to cell wall polysaccharide protect human subjects against pneumococcal infection? J Infect Dis 161:736–740, 1990.
35. Tuomanen E, Tomasz A, Heugstler B, Zak O. The relative role of bacterial cell wall and capsule in the induction of inflammation in pneumococcal meningitis. J Infect Dis 151:535–540, 1985.
36. Schweinle JE. Pneumococcal intracellular killing is abolished by polysaccharide despite serum complement activity. Infect Immun 54:876–881, 1986.
37. Boulnois GJ. Pneumococcal proteins and the pathogenesis of disease caused by *Streptococcus pneumoniae*. J Gen Microbiol 138:249–259, 1992.
38. Paton JC, Andrew PW, Boulnois GJ, Mitchell TJ. Molecular analysis of the pathogenicity of *Streptococcus pneumoniae*: The role of pneumococcal proteins. Annu Rev Microbiol 47:89–115, 1993.
39. Gillespie SH. Aspects of pneumococcal infection including bacterial virulence, host response and vaccination [review]. J Med Microbiol 28:237–248, 1989.
40. Paton JC. The contribution of pneumolysin to the pathogenicity of *Streptococcus pneumoniae*. Trends Microbiol 4:103–106, 1996.
41. Rayner CF, Jackson AD, Rutman A, et al. Interaction of pneumolysin-sufficient and -deficient isogenic variants of *Streptococcus pneumoniae* with human respiratory mucosa. Infect Immun 63:442–447, 1995.
42. Rubins JB, Charboneau D, Paton JC, et al. Dual function of pneumolysin in the early pathogenesis of murine pneumococcal pneumonia. J Clin Invest 95:142–150, 1995.
43. Nandoskar M, Ferrante A, Bates EJ, et al. Inhibition of human monocyte respiratory burst, degranulation, phospholipid methylation and bactericidal activity by pneumolysin. Immunology 59:515–520, 1986.
44. Berry AM, Yother J, Briles DE, et al. Reduced virulence of a defined pneumolysin-negative mutant of *Streptococcus pneumoniae*. Infect Immun 57:2037–2042, 1989.
45. Benton KA, Everson MP, Briles DE. A pneumolysin-negative mutant of *Streptococcus pneumoniae* causes chronic bacteremia rather than acute sepsis in mice. Infect Immun 63:448–455, 1995.
46. Berry AM, Alexander JE, Mitchell TJ, et al. Effect of defined point mutations in the pneumolysin gene on the virulence of *Streptococcus pneumoniae*. Infect Immun 63:1969–1974, 1995.
47. Alexander JE, Lock RA, Peeters CC, et al. Immunization of mice with pneumolysin toxoid confers a significant degree of protection against at least nine serotypes of *Streptococcus pneumoniae*. Infect Immun 62:5683–5688, 1994.
48. McDaniel LS, Yother J, Vijayakumar M, et al. Use of insertional inactivation to facilitate studies of biological properties of pneumococcal surface protein A (PspA). J Exp Med 165:381–394, 1987.
49. Briles DE, Yother J, McDaniel LS. Role of pneumococcal surface protein A in the virulence of *Streptococcus pneumoniae*. Rev Infect Dis 10(suppl)2:s372–s374, 1988.
50. McDaniel LS, Sheffield JS, Delucchi P, Briles DE. PspA, a surface protein of *Streptococcus pneumoniae*, is capable of eliciting protection against pneumococci of more than one capsular type. Infect Immun 59:222–228, 1991.
51. Briles DE, King JD, Gray MA, et al. PspA, a protection-eliciting pneumococcal protein: Immunogenicity of isolated native PspA in mice. Vaccine 14:858–867, 1996.
52. Lomholt H. Evidence of recombination and an antigenically diverse immunoglobulin A1 protease among strains of *Streptococcus pneumoniae*. Infect Immun 63:4238–4243, 1995.
53. Berry AM, Lock RA, Hansman D, Paton JC. Contribution of autolysin to virulence of *Streptococcus pneumoniae*. Infect Immun 57:2324–2330, 1989.
54. Lock RA, Paton JC, Hansman D. Purification and immunological characterization of neuraminidase produced by *Streptococcus pneumoniae*. Microb Pathog 4:33–43, 1988.
55. Henrichsen J. Six newly recognized types of *Streptococcus pneumoniae*. J Clin Microbiol 33:2759–2762, 1995.
56. Lefevre JC, Faucon G, Sicard AM, Gasc AM. DNA fingerprinting of *Streptococcus pneumoniae* strains by pulsed-field gel electrophoresis. J Clin Microbiol 31:2724–2728, 1993.
57. Takala AK, Vuopio-Varkila J, Tarkka E, et al. Subtyping of common pediatric pneumococcal serotypes from invasive disease and pharyngeal carriage in Finland. J Infect Dis 173:128–135, 1996.
58. van Belkum A, Sluijuter M, de Groot R, et al. Novel BOX repeat PCR assay for high-resolution typing of *Streptococcus pneumoniae* strains. J Clin Microbiol 34:1176–1179, 1996.
59. Scott JAG, Hall AJ, Dagan R, et al. Serogroup-specific epidemiology of *Streptococcus pneumoniae*: Associations with age, sex, and geography in 7,000 episodes of invasive disease. Clin Infect Dis 22:973–981, 1996.
60. Hedlund J. Should pneumococcal infections continue to be classified as a single disease? Lancet 349:371–372, 1997.
61. Sorensen UB. Typing of pneumococci by using 12 pooled antisera. J Clin Microbiol 31:2097–2100, 1993.
62. Henrichsen J, Robbins JB. Production of monovalent antisera by induction of immunological tolerance for capsular typing of *Streptococcus pneumoniae*. FEMS Microbiol Lett 73:89–93, 1992.
63. Lalitha MK, Pai R, John TJ, et al. Serotyping of *Streptococcus pneumoniae* by agglutination assays: A cost-effective technique for developing countries. Bull World Health Organ 74:387–390, 1996.
64. Fedson DS, Harward MP, Reid RA, Kaiser DL. Hospital-based pneumococcal immunization: Epidemiologic rationale from the Shenandoah study. JAMA 264:1117–1122, 1990.
65. Spellerberg B, Tuomanen EI. The pathophysiology of pneumococcal meningitis. Ann Med 26:411–418, 1994.

66. Idanpaan-Heikkilä I, Simon PM, Zopf D, et al. Oligosaccharides interfere with the establishment and progression of experimental pneumococcal pneumonia. J Infect Dis 176:704–712, 1997.
67. Heilmann C. Human B and T lymphocyte responses to vaccination with pneumococcal polysaccharides. APMIS 15(suppl):1–23, 1990.
68. Baker PJ. Regulation of magnitude of antibody response to bacterial polysaccharide antigens by thymus-derived lymphocytes. Infect Immun 58:3465–3468, 1990.
69. Mond JJ, Vos Q, Lees A, Snapper CM. T cell independent antigens. Curr Opin Immunol 7:349–354, 1995.
70. Taylor CE, Fauntleroy MB, Stashak PW, Baker PJ. Antigen-specific suppressor T cells respond to recombinant interleukin-2 and other lymphokines. Infect Immun 59:575–579, 1991.
71. Caulfield MJ, Shaffer D. Immunoregulation by antigen/antibody complexes: I. Specific immunosuppression induced in vivo with immune complexes formed in antibody excess. J Immunol 138:3680–3683, 1987.
72. Griffioen AW, Toebes EA, Rijkers GT, et al. The amplifier role of T cells in the human in vitro B cell response to type 4 pneumococcal polysaccharide. Immunol Lett 32:265–272, 1992.
73. Tvede N, Heilmann C, Christensen LD. Interleukin 2 receptor expression by human blood lymphocytes after vaccination with pneumococcal polysaccharides. Clin Exp Immunol 76:404–411, 1989.
74. Ambrosino DM, Delaney NR, Shamberger RC. Human polysaccharide-specific B cells are responsive to pokeweed mitogen and IL-6. J Immunol 144:1221–1226, 1990.
75. Griffioen AW, Rijkers GT, Toebes EA, Zegers BJ. The human in vitro anti-type 4 pneumococcal polysaccharide antibody response is regulated by suppressor T cells. Scand J Immunol 34:229–236, 1991.
76. Rijkers GT, Dollekamp EG, Zegers BJ. The in vitro B-cell response to pneumococcal polysaccharides in adults and neonates. Scand J Immunol 25:447–452, 1987.
77. Barrett DJ, Sleasman JW, Schatz DA, Steinitz M. Human anti-pneumococcal polysaccharide antibodies are secreted by the CD5-B cell lineage. Cell Immunol 143:66–79, 1992.
78. Granoff DM, Suarez BK, Pandey JP, Shackelford PG. Genes associated with the G2m(23) immunoglobulin allotype regulate the IgG subclass responses to *Haemophilus influenzae* type b polysaccharide vaccine. J Infect Dis 157:1142–1149, 1988.
79. Winkelstein JA, Childs B. Genetically determined variation in the immune system: implications for host defense. Pediatr Infect Dis J 8:s31–s34, 1989.
80. Hostetter MK. Serotypic variations among virulent pneumococci in deposition and degradation of covalently bound C3b: Implications for phagocytosis and antibody production. J Infect Dis 153:682–693, 1986.
81. Angel CS, Ruzek M, Hostetter MK. Degradation of C3 by *Streptococcus pneumoniae*. J Infect Dis 170:600–608, 1994.
82. Hebert JC. Pneumococcal vaccine improves pulmonary clearance of live pneumococci after splenectomy. J Surg Res 47:283–287, 1989.
83. Iinuma H, Okinaga K. Prevention of pneumococcal bacteremia by immunization with type 6 pneumococcal capsular polysaccharide vaccine in splenectomized rats. J Infect Dis 160:66–75, 1989.
84. Cohn DA, Schiffman G. Immunoregulatory role of the spleen in antibody responses to pneumococcal polysaccharide antigens. Infect Immun 55:1375–1380, 1987.
85. Peset Llopis MJ, Harms G, Hardonk MJ, Timens W. Human immune response to pneumococcal polysaccharides: Complement-mediated localization preferentially on CD21-positive splenic marginal zone B cells and follicular dendritic cells. J Allergy Clin Immunol 97:1015–1024, 1996.
86. Timens W, Boes A, Rozeboom-Uiterwijk T, Poppema S. Immaturity of the human splenic marginal zone in infancy: Possible contribution to the deficient infant immune response. J Immunol 143:3200–3206, 1989.
87. Perlino CA. Laboratory diagnosis of pneumonia due to *Streptococcus pneumoniae*. J Infect Dis 150:139–144, 1984.
88. Roback MG, Tsai AK, Hanson KL. Delayed incubation of blood culture bottles: Effect on recovery rate of *Streptococcus pneumoniae* and *Haemophilus influenzae* type B. Pediatr Emerg Care 10:268–272, 1994.
89. Musher DM. Gram stain and culture of sputum to diagnose bacterial pneumonia [letter]. J Infect Dis 152:1096, 1985.
90. Gleckman R, DeVita J, Hibert D, et al. Sputum gram stain assessment in community-acquired bacteremic pneumonia. J Clin Microbiol 26:846–849, 1988.
91. Fine MJ, Orloff JJ, Rihs JD, et al. Evaluation of housestaff physicians' preparation and interpretation of sputum Gram stains for community-acquired pneumonia. J Gen Intern Med 6:189–198, 1991.
92. Anonymous. Guidelines for the initial management of adults with community-acquired pneumonia: Diagnosis, assessment of severity, and initial antimicrobial therapy. Am Rev Respir Dis 198:1418–1426, 1993.
93. Farrington M, Rubenstein D. Antigen detection in pneumococcal pneumonia. J Infect 23:109–116, 1991.
94. Wellstood S. Evaluation of a latex test for rapid detection of pneumococcal antigens in sputum. Eur J Clin Microbiol Infect Dis 11:448–451, 1992.
95. Boersma WG, Lowenberg A, Holloway Y, et al. Pneumococcal antigen persistence in sputum from patients with community-acquired pneumonia. Chest 102:422–427, 1992.
96. Bella F, Tort J, Morera MA, et al. Value of bacterial antigen detection in the diagnostic yield of transthoracic needle aspiration in severe community acquired pneumonia. Thorax 48:1227–1229, 1993.
97. Boersma WG, Lowenberg A, Holloway Y, et al. Rapid detection of pneumococcal antigen in pleural fluid of patients with community acquired pneumonia. Thorax 48:160–162, 1993.
98. Jesudason MV, Sridharan G, Arulselvan K, et al. C substance—specific latex agglutination for early and rapid detection of *Streptococcus pneumoniae* in blood cultures. Indian J Med Res 102:258–260, 1995.
99. Finlay FO, Witherow H, Rudd PT. Latex agglutination testing in bacterial meningitis. Arch Dis Child 73:160–161, 1995.
100. Camargos PA, Almeida MS, Cardoso I, et al. Latex particle agglutination test in the diagnosis of *Haemophilus influenzae* type B, *Streptococcus pneumoniae* and *Neisseria meningitidis* A and C meningitis in infants and children. J Clin Epidemiol 48:1245–1250, 1995.
101. Gillespie SH, Smith MD, Dickens A, et al. Diagnosis of *Streptococcus pneumoniae* pneumonia by quantitative enzyme linked immunosorbent assay of C-polysaccharide antigen. J Clin Pathol 47:749–751, 1994.
102. Gillespie SH, Smith MD, Dickens A, et al. Detection of C-polysaccharide in serum of patients with *Streptococcus pneumoniae* bacteraemia. J Clin Pathol 48:803–806, 1995.
103. Salih MA, Ahmed AA, Sid Ahmed H, Olcen P. An ELISA assay for the rapid diagnosis of acute bacterial meningitis. Ann Trop Paediatr 15:273–278, 1995.
104. Parkinson AJ, Rabiego ME, Sepulveda C, et al. Quantitation of pneumococcal C polysaccharide in sputum samples from patients with presumptive pneumococcal pneumonia by enzyme immunoassay. J Clin Microbiol 30:318–322, 1992.
105. Ballard TL, Roe MH, Wheeler RC, et al. Comparison of three latex agglutination kits and counterimmunoelectrophoresis for the detection of bacterial antigens in a pediatric population. Pediatr Infect Dis J 6:630–634, 1987.
106. Boersma WG, Lowenberg A, Holloway Y, et al. The role of antigen detection in pneumococcal carriers: A comparison between cultures and capsular antigen detection in upper respiratory tract secretions. Scand J Infect Dis 25:51–56, 1993.
107. Jimenez P, Meneses M, Saldias F, Velasquez M. Pneumococcal antigen detection in bronchoalveolar lavage fluid from patients with pneumonia. Thorax 49:872–874, 1994.
108. Schaffner A, Michel Harder C, Yeginsoy S. Detection of capsular polysaccharide in serum for the diagnosis of pneumococcal pneumonia: Clinical and experimental evaluation. J Infect Dis 163:1094–1102, 1991.
109. Maxson S, Lewno MJ, Schutze GE. Clinical usefulness of cerebrospinal fluid bacterial antigen studies. J Pediatr 125:235–238, 1994.
110. Perkins MD, Mirrett S, Reller LB. Rapid bacterial antigen detection is not clinically useful. J Clin Microbiol 33:1486–1491, 1995.
111. Cunniffe JG, Whitby Strevens S, Wilcox MH. Effect of pH changes in cerebrospinal fluid specimens on bacterial survival and antigen test results. J Clin Pathol 49:249–253, 1996.

112. Boersma WG, Holloway Y. Clinical relevance of pneumococcal antigen detection in urine [letter]. Infection 20:240–241, 1992.
113. Adcock PM, Paul RI, Marshall GS. Effect of urine latex agglutination tests on the treatment of children at risk for invasive bacterial infection. Pediatrics 96:951–954, 1995.
114. Jalonen E, Paton JC, Koskela M, et al. Measurement of antibody responses to pneumolysin—a promising method for the presumptive aetiological diagnosis of pneumococcal pneumonia. J Infect 19:127–134, 1989.
115. Nohynek H, Eskola J, Laine E, et al. The causes of hospital-treated acute lower respiratory tract infection in children. Am J Dis Child 145:618–622, 1991.
116. Korppi M, Koskela M, Jalonen E, Leinonen M. Serologically indicated pneumococcal respiratory infection in children. Scand J Infect Dis 24:437–443, 1992.
117. Korppi M, Heiskanen-Kosma T, Leinonen M, Halonen P. Antigen and antibody assays in the aetiological diagnosis of respiratory infection in children. Acta Paediatr 82:137–141, 1993.
118. Nohynek H, Eskola J, Kleemola M, et al. Bacterial antibody assays in the diagnosis of acute lower respiratory tract infection in children. Pediatr Infect Dis J 14:478–484, 1995.
119. Leinonen M, Syrjala H, Jalonen E, et al. Demonstration of pneumolysin antibodies in dissociated immune complexes—a new method for etiological diagnosis of pneumococcal pneumonia: Serodiag Immunother Infectious Dis 4:451–458, 1990.
120. Holloway Y, Snijder JA, Boersma WG. Demonstration of circulating pneumococcal immunoglobulin G immune complexes in patients with community-acquired pneumonia by means of an enzyme-linked immunosorbent assay. J Clin Microbiol 31:3247–3254, 1993.
121. Leinonen M. Serological diagnosis of pneumococcal pneumonia—will it ever become a clinical reality. Semin Respir Infect 9:189–191, 1994.
122. Rudolph KM, Parkinson AJ, Black CM, Mayer LW. Evaluation of polymerase chain reaction for diagnosis of pneumococcal pneumonia. J Clin Microbiol 31:2661–2666, 1993.
123. Salo P, Ortqvist A, Leinonen M. Diagnosis of bacteremic pneumococcal pneumonia by amplification of pneumolysin gene fragment in serum. J Infect Dis 171:479–482, 1995.
124. Hassanking M, Baldeh I, Secka O, et al. Detection of *Streptococcus pneumoniae* DNA in blood cultures by PCR. J Clin Microbiol 32:1721–1724, 1994.
125. Friedland LR, Menon AG, Reising SF, et al. Development of a polymerase chain reaction assay to detect the presence of *Streptococcus pneumoniae* DNA. Diagn Microbiol Infect Dis 20:187–193, 1994.
126. Zhang Y, Isaacman DJ, Wadowsky RM, et al. Detection of *Streptococcus pneumoniae* in whole blood by PCR. J Clin Microbiol 33:596–601, 1995.
127. Isaacman DJ, Zhang Y, Rydquist White J, et al. Identification of a patient with *Streptococcus pneumoniae* bacteremia and meningitis by the polymerase chain reaction (PCR). Mol Cell Probes 9:157–160, 1995.
128. Olcen P, Lantz PG, Backman A, Radstrom P. Rapid diagnosis of bacterial meningitis by a seminested PCR strategy. Scand J Infect Dis 27:537–539, 1995.
129. Hall LM, Duke B, Urwin G. An approach to the identification of the pathogens of bacterial meningitis by the polymerase chain reaction. Eur J Clin Microbiol Infect Dis 14:1090–1094, 1995.
130. Gillespie SH, Ullman C, Smith MD, Emery V. Detection of *Streptococcus pneumoniae* in sputum samples by PCR. J Clin Microbiol 32:1308–1311, 1994.
131. Post JC, Preston RA, Aul JJ, et al. Molecular analysis of bacterial pathogens in otitis media with effusion. JAMA 273:1598–1604, 1995.
132. Jero J, Virolainen A, Salo P, et al. PCR assay for detecting *Streptococcus pneumoniae* in the middle ear of children with otitis media with effusion. Acta Otolaryngol (Stockh) 116:288–292, 1996.
133. Virolainen A, Salo P, Jero J, et al. Comparison of PCR assay with bacterial culture for detecting *Streptococcus pneumoniae* in middle ear fluid of children with acute otitis media. J Clin Microbiol 32:2667–2670, 1994.
134. Messmer TO, Black CM, Facklam RR. Discrimination of *Streptococcus pneumoniae* from other upper respiratory tract streptococci by arbitrarily primed PCR. Clin Biochem 28:567–572, 1995.
135. Hansman D, Bullen MM. A resistant pneumococcus. Lancet 2:264–265, 1967.
136. Jacobs MR, Koornhof HJ, Robins-Browne RM, et al. Emergence of multiply resistant pneumococci. N Engl J Med 299:735–740, 1978.
137. Hughes JM, LaMontagne JR. Emerging infectious diseases. J Infect Dis 170:263–264, 1994.
138. Klugman KP. Pneumococcal resistance to antibiotics. Clin Microbiol Rev 3:171–196, 1990.
139. Lonks JR, Medeiros AA. The growing threat of antibiotic-resistant *Streptococcus pneumoniae*. Med Clin North Am 79:523–535, 1995.
140. Schreiber JR, Jacobs MR. Antibiotic-resistant pneumococci. Pediatr Clin North Am 42:519–537, 1995.
141. Austrian R. Confronting drug-resistant pneumococci. Ann Intern Med 121:807, 1994.
142. Schutze GE, Kaplan SL, Jacobs RF. Resistant pneumococcus: A worldwide problem. Infection 22:233–237, 1994.
143. Tomasz A. The pneumococcus at the gates. N Engl J Med 333:514–515, 1995.
144. Dowson CG, Coffey TJ, Spratt BG. Origin and molecular epidemiology of penicillin-binding-protein-mediated resistance to beta-lactam antibiotics. Trends Microbiol 2:361–366, 1994.
145. Hakenbeck R. Target-mediated resistance to beta-lactam antibiotics. Biochem Pharmacol 50:1121–1127, 1995.
146. Tomasz A. Antibiotic resistance in *Streptococcus pneumoniae*. Clin Infect Dis 24:s85–s88, 1997.
147. Appelbaum PC. Antibiotic-resistant pneumococci—facts and fiction. J Chemother 6(suppl 4):7–15; discussion 23–24, 1994.
148. McGowan JE Jr, Metchock BG. Penicillin-resistant pneumococci—an emerging threat to successful therapy. J Hosp Infect 30(suppl):472–482, 1995.
149. Baquero F. Pneumococcal resistance to beta-lactam antibiotics: A global geographic overview. Microb Drug Resist 1:115–120, 1995.
150. Appelbaum PC. Epidemiology and in vitro susceptibility of drug-resistant *Streptococcus pneumoniae*. Pediatr Infect Dis J 15:932–934, 1996.
151. Caputo GM, Appelbaum PC, Liu HH. Infections due to penicillin-resistant pneumococci: Clinical, epidemiologic, and microbiologic features. Arch Intern Med 153:1301–1310, 1993.
152. Friedland IR, Mccracken GH. Drug therapy—management of infections caused by antibiotic-resistant *Streptococcus pneumoniae*. N Engl J Med 331:377–382, 1994.
153. Klugman KP. Management of antibiotic-resistant pneumococcal infections. J Antimicrob Chemother 34:191–193, 1994.
154. Friedland IR. Comparison of the response to antimicrobial therapy of penicillin-resistant and penicillin-susceptible pneumococcal disease. Pediatr Infect Dis J 14:885–890, 1995.
155. Bradley JS, Kaplan SL, Klugman KP, Leggiadro RJ. Consensus: Management of infections in children caused by *Streptococcus pneumoniae* with decreased susceptibility to penicillin. Pediatr Infect Dis J 14:1037–1041, 1995.
156. Feldman C, Klugman K. Antibiotic-resistant pneumococcal pneumonia. S Afr Med J 86:28–30, 1996.
157. Goldstein FW, Garau J. 30 years of penicillin-resistant *S. pneumoniae*: Myth or reality? Lancet 350:233–234, 1997.
158. Bradley JS, Scheld WM. The challenge of penicilin-resistant *Streptococcus pneumoniae* meningitis: Current antibiotic therapy in the 1990s. Clin Infect Dis 25:213–221, 1997.
159. Munoz R, Musser JM, Crain M, et al. Geographic distribution of penicillin-resistant clones of *Streptococcus pneumoniae*: Characterization by penicillin-binding protein profile, surface protein A typing, and multilocus enzyme analysis. Clin Infect Dis 15:112–118, 1992.
160. Munoz R, Coffey TJ, Daniels M, et al. Intercontinental spread of a multiresistant clone of serotype 23F *Streptococcus pneumoniae*. J Infect Dis 164:302–306, 1991.
161. Soares S, Kristinsson KG, Musser JM, Tomasz A. Evidence for the introduction of a multiresistant clone of serotype 6B *Streptococcus pneumoniae* from Spain to Iceland in the late 1980s. J Infect Dis 168:158–163, 1993.
162. Negri MC, Morosini MI, Loza E, Baquero F. In vitro selective antibiotic concentrations of beta-lactams for penicillin-resistant *Streptococcus pneumoniae* populations. Antimicrob Agents Chemother 38:122–125, 1994.

163. Barnes DM, Whittier S, Gilligan PH, et al. Transmission of multidrug-resistant serotype 23F *Streptococcus pneumoniae* in group day care: Evidence suggesting capsular transformation of the resistant strain in vivo. J Infect Dis 171:890–896, 1995.
164. Butler JC, Hofmann J, Cetron MS, et al. The continued emergence of drug-resistant *Streptococcus pneumoniae* in the United States: An update from the Centers for Disease Control and Prevention's Pneumococcal Sentinel Surveillance System. J Infect Dis 174:986–993, 1996.
165. Breiman RF, Butler JC, Tenover FC, et al. Emergence of drug-resistant pneumococcal infections in the United States. JAMA 271:1831–1835, 1994.
166. Doern GV, Brueggemann A, Holley HP Jr, Rauch AM. Antimicrobial resistance of *Streptococcus pneumoniae* recovered from outpatients in the United States during the winter months of 1994 to 1995: Results of a 30-center national surveillance study. Antimicrob Agents Chemother 40:1208–1213, 1996.
167. Mason EO, Lamberth L, Lichenstein R, Kaplan SL. Distribution of *Streptococcus pneumoniae* resistant to penicillin in the USA and in vitro susceptibility to selected oral antibiotics. J Antimicrob Chemother 36:1043–1048, 1995.
168. Boken DJ, Chartrand SA, Goering RV, et al. Colonization with penicillin-resistant *Streptococcus pneumoniae* in a child-care center. Pediatr Infect Dis J 14:879–884, 1995.
169. Block SL, Harrison CJ, Hedrick JA, et al. Penicillin-resistant *Streptococcus pneumoniae* in acute otitis media: Risk factors, susceptibility patterns and antimicrobial management. Pediatr Infect Dis J 14:751–759, 1995.
170. Appelbaum PC. Antimicrobial resistance in *Streptococcus pneumoniae*: An overview. Clin Infect Dis 15:77–83, 1992.
171. Lehmann D, Gratten M, Montgomery J. Susceptibility of pneumococcal carriage isolates to penicilin provides a conservative estimate of susceptibility of invasive pneumococci. Pediatr Infect Dis J 16:297–305, 1997.
172. Kristinsson KG, Hjalmarsdottir MA, Steingrimsson O. Increasing penicillin resistance in pneumococci in Iceland [letter]. Lancet 339:1606–1607, 1992.
173. Reichmann P, Varon E, Gunther E, et al. Penicillin-resistant *Streptococcus pneumoniae* in Germany: Genetic relationship to clones from other European countries. J Med Microbiol 43:377–385, 1995.
174. Wust J, Huf E, Kayser FH. Antimicrobial susceptibilities and serotypes of invasive *Streptococcus pneumoniae* strains in Switzerland. J Clin Microbiol 33:3159–3163, 1995.
175. Verhaegen J, Glupczynski Y, Verbist L, et al. Capsular types and antibiotic susceptibility of pneumococci isolated from patients in Belgium with serious infections, 1980–1993. Clin Infect Dis 20:1339–1345, 1995.
176. Arason VA, Kristinsson KG, Sigurdsson JA, et al. Do antimicrobials increase the carriage rate of penicillin resistant pneumococci in children? Cross sectional prevalence study. BMJ 313:387–391, 1996.
177. Doit C, Denamur E, Picard B, et al. Mechanisms of the spread of penicillin resistance in *Streptococcus pneumoniae* strains causing meningitis in children in France. J Infect Dis 174:520–528, 1996.
178. Bedos JP, Chevret S, Chastang C, et al. Epidemiological features of and risk factors for infection by *Streptococcus pneumoniae* strains with diminished susceptibility to penicillin: Findings of a French survey. Clin Infect Dis 22:63–72, 1996.
179. Johnson AP, Speller DC, George RC, et al. Prevalence of antibiotic resistance and serotypes in pneumococci in England and Wales: Results of observational surveys in 1990 and 1995. BMJ 312:1454–1456, 1996.
180. Syrogiannopoulos GA, Grivea IN, Beratis NG, et al. Resistance patterns of *Streptococcus pneumoniae* from carriers attending day care centers in Southwestern Greece. Clin Infect Dis 25:188–194, 1997.
181. Hermans PWM, Sluijtzer M, Elzenaar K. Penicillin-resistant *Streptococcus pneumoniae* in the Netherlands: Results of a 1-year molecular epidemiologic survey. J Infect Dis 175:1413–1422, 1997.
182. Weber M, Roussel-Delvallez M, Laurans G, et al. Enquêtes épidemiologiques régionales sur la résistance aux antibiotiques de *S. pneumoniae*: Résultats préliminaires de 6 Observatoires Régionaux. Méd Mal Infect 27(spécial):7–15, 1997.
183. Felmingham D, Gruneberg RN. A multicentre collaborative study of the antimicrobial susceptibility of community-acquired, lower respiratory tract pathogens 1992–1993: The Alexander project. J Antimicrob Chemother 38:1–57, 1996.
184. Pradier C, Dunais B, Carsenti-Etesse H, Dellamonica P. Pneumococcal resistance patterns in Europe. Eur J Clin Microbiol Infect Dis 16:644–647, 1997.
185. Pallares R, Linares J, Vadillo M, et al. Resistance to penicillin and cephalosporin and mortality from severe pneumococcal pneumonia in Barcelona, Spain. N Engl J Med 333:474–480, 1995.
186. Friedland IR, Istre GR. Management of penicillin-resistant pneumococcal infections. Pediatr Infect Dis J 11:433–435, 1992.
187. Sloas MM, Barrett FF, Chesney PJ, et al. Cephalosporin treatment failure in penicillin- and cephalosporin-resistant *Streptococcus pneumoniae* meningitis. Pediatr Infect Dis J 11:662–666, 1992.
188. Friedland IR, Shelton S, Paris M, et al. Dilemmas in diagnosis and management of cephalosporin-resistant *Streptococcus pneumoniae* meningitis. Pediatr Infect Dis J 12:196–200, 1993.
189. Boyce JM. Vancomycin-resistant enterococcus: Detection, epidemiology, and control measures. Infect Dis Clin North Am 11:367–384, 1997.
190. Reduced susceptibility of *Staphylococcus aureus* to vancomycin—Japan. MMWR Morb Mortal Wkly Rep 46:624–626, 1997.
191. Dagan R, Melamed R, Muallem M, et al. Nasopharyngeal colonization in southern Israel with antibiotic-resistant pneumococci during the first 2 years of life: Relation to serotypes likely to be included in pneumococcal conjugate vaccines. J Infect Dis 174:1352–1355, 1996.
192. Hendley JO, Sande MA, Stewart PM, Gwaltney JMJ. Spread of *Streptococcus pneumoniae* in families: I. Carriage rates and distribution of types. J Infect Dis 132:55–61, 1975.
193. Musher DM, Groover JE, Reichler MR, et al. Emergence of antibody to capsular polysaccharides of *Streptococcus pneumoniae* during outbreaks of pneumonia: Association with nasopharyngeal colonization. Clin Infect Dis 24:441–446, 1997.
194. Douglas RM, Hansman D, Miles HB, Paton JC. Pneumococcal carriage and type-specific antibody: Failure of a 14-valent vaccine to reduce carriage in healthy children. Am J Dis Child 140:1183–1185, 1986.
195. Hansman D, Morris S. Pneumococcal carriage amongst children in Adelaide, South Australia. Epidemiol Infect 101:411–417, 1988.
196. Aniansson G, Alm B, Andersson B, et al. Nasopharyngeal colonization during the first year of life. J Infect Dis 165(suppl)1:s38–s42, 1992.
197. Ekdahl K, Ahlinder I, Hansson HB, et al. Duration of nasopharyngeal carriage of penicillin-resistant *Streptococcus pneumoniae:* Experiences from the South Swedish pneumococcal intervention project. Clin Infect Dis 25:1113–1117, 1997.
198. Gray BM, Dillon HC Jr. Epidemiological studies of *Streptococcus pneumoniae* in infants: Antibody to types 3, 6, 14, and 23 in the first two years of life. J Infect Dis 158:948–955, 1988.
199. Gray BM, Dillon HC Jr. Natural history of pneumococcal infections. Pediatr Infect Dis J 8:s23–s25, 1989.
200. Smith T, Lehmann D, Montgomery J, et al. Acquisition and invasiveness of different serotypes of *Streptococcus pneumoniae* in young children. Epidemiol Infect 111:27–39, 1993.
201. Granton JT, Grossman RF. Community-acquired pneumonia in the elderly patient: Clinical features, epidemiology, and treatment. Clin Chest Med 14:537–553, 1993.
202. Marrie TJ. New aspects of old pathogens of pneumonia. Med Clin North Am 78:987–995, 1994.
203. Marrie TJ. Community-acquired pneumonia. Clin Infect Dis 18:501–515, 1994.
204. Macfarlane J. An overview of community acquired pneumonia with lessons learned from the British Thoracic Society Study. Semin Respir Infect 9:153–165, 1994.
205. Bartlett JG, Mundy LM. Community-acquired pneumonia. N Engl J Med 333:1618–1624, 1995.
206. Marston BJ. Epidemiology of community-acquired pneumonia. Infect Dis Clin Pract 4:s232–s239, 1995.
207. Farr BM, Sloman AJ, Fisch MJ. Predicting death in patients hospitalized for community-acquired pneumonia. Ann Intern Med 115:428–436, 1991.

208. Gilbert K, Fine MJ. Assessing prognosis and predicting patient outcomes in community-acquired pneumonia. Semin Respir Infect 9:140–152, 1994.
209. Carson CA, Fine MJ, Smith MA, et al. Quality of published reports of the prognosis of community-acquired pneumonia. J Gen Intern Med 9:13–19, 1994.
210. Localio AR, Hamory BH, Sharp TJ, et al. Comparing hospital mortality in adult patients with pneumonia: A case study of statistical methods in a managed care program. Ann Intern Med 122:125–132, 1995.
211. Coley CM, Li YH, Medsger AR, et al. Preferences for home vs hospital care among low-risk patients with community-acquired pneumonia. Arch Intern Med 156:1565–1571, 1996.
212. Fine MJ, Smith MA, Carson CA, et al. Prognosis and outcomes of patients with community-acquired pneumonia: A meta-analysis. JAMA 275:134–141, 1996.
213. Fine MJ, Auble TE, Yealy DM, et al. A prediction rule to identify low-risk patients with community-acquired pneumonia. N Engl J Med 336:243–250, 1997.
214. Hedlund JU, Ortqvist AB, Kalin M, et al. Risk of pneumonia in patients previously treated in hospital for pneumonia. Lancet 340:396–397, 1992.
215. Hedlund J, Hansson LO, Ortqvist A. Short- and long-term prognosis for middle-aged and elderly patients hospitalized with community-acquired pneumonia: Impact of nutritional and inflammatory factors. Scand J Infect Dis 27:32–37, 1995.
216. Feldman C, Ross S, Mahomed AG, et al. The aetiology of severe community-acquired pneumonia and its impact on initial, empiric, antimicrobial chemotherapy. Respir Med 89:187–192, 1995.
217. Farr BM. Prognosis and decisions in pneumonia. N Engl J Med 336:288–289, 1997.
218. Pinner RW, Teutsch SM, Simonsen L, et al. Trends in infectious diseases mortality in the United States. JAMA 275:189–193, 1996.
219. Prevention of pneumococcal disease: Recommendations of the Advisory Committee on Immunization Practices (ACIP). MMWR Morb Mortal Wkly Rep 46(RR-8):1–24, 1997.
220. Jokinen C, Heiskanen L, Juvonen H, et al. Incidence of community-acquired pneumonia in the population of four municipalities in eastern Finland. Am J Epidemiol 137:977–988, 1993.
221. Macfarlane JT, Colville A, Guion A, et al. Prospective study of aetiology and outcome of adult lower-respiratory-tract infections in the community. Lancet 341:511–514, 1993.
221a. Marston BJ, Plouffe JF, File TM Jr, et al. Incidence of community-acquired pneumonia requiring hospitalization. Arch Intern Med 157:1709–1718, 1997.
221b. Säynäjäkangas P, Keistinen T, Honkanen PO, Kivelä S-L. Hospital discharge for pneumonia in Finland between 1972 and 1993 in the population aged 65 years or over. Age Ageing 26:269–273, 1997.
222. Farr BM, Kaiser DL, Harrison BD, Connolly CK. Prediction of microbial aetiology at admission to hospital for pneumonia from the presenting clinical features: British Thoracic Society Pneumonia Research Subcommittee. Thorax 44:1031–1035, 1989.
223. Carpenter JL, Huang DY. Community-acquired pulmonary infections in a public municipal hospital in the 1980s. South Med J 84:299–306, 1991.
224. Bates JH, Campbell GD, Barron AL, et al. Microbial etiology of acute pneumonia in hospitalized patients. Chest 101:1005–1012, 1992.
225. Phillips SL, Branaman-Phillips J. The use of intramuscular cefoperazone versus intramuscular ceftriaxone in patients with nursing home-acquired pneumonia. J Am Geriatr Soc 41:1071–1074, 1993.
226. Mundy LM, Auwaerter PG, Oldach D, et al. Community-acquired pneumonia: Impact of immune status. Am J Respir Crit Care Med 152:1309–1315, 1995.
227. Ruf B, Schürmann D, Horbach I, et al. Incidence and clinical features of community-acquired legionellosis in hospitalized patients. Eur Respir J 2:257–262, 1989.
228. Ewig S, Bauer T, Hasper L, et al. Prognostic analysis and predictive rule for outcome of hospital-treated community-acquired pneumonia. Eur Respir J 8:392–397, 1995.
229. Carr B, Walsh JB, Coakley D, et al. Prospective hospital study of community acquired lower respiratory tract infection in the elderly. Respir Med 85:185–187, 1991.
230. Anonymous. The aetiology, management and outcome of severe community-acquired pneumonia on the intensive care unit: The British Thoracic Society Research Committee and The Public Health Laboratory Service. Respir Med 86:7–13, 1992.
231. Rello J, Quintana E, Ausina V, et al. A three-year study of severe community-acquired pneumonia with emphasis on outcome. Chest 103:232–235, 1993.
232. Almirall J, Morato I, Riera F, et al. Incidence of community-acquired pneumonia and *Chlamydia pneumoniae* infection: A prospective multicentre study. Eur Respir J 6:14–18, 1993.
233. Blasi F, Cosentini R, Legnani D, et al. Incidence of community-acquired pneumonia caused by *Chlamydia pneumoniae* in Italian patients. Eur J Clin Microbiol Infect Dis 12:696–699, 1993.
234. Ostergaard L, Andersen PL. Etiology of community-acquired pneumonia: Evaluation by transtracheal aspiration, blood culture, or serology. Chest 104:1400–1407, 1993.
235. Moine P, Vercken JB, Chastang C, and the French Study Group of community-acquired pneumonia in ICU. Severe community-acquired pneumonia: Etiology, epidemiology, and prognosis factors. Chest 105:1487–1495, 1994.
236. Gaillat J, Bru JP, Sedallian A. Penicillin G/ofloxacin versus erythromycin/amoxicillin-clavulanate in the treatment of severe community-acquired pneumonia. Eur J Clin Microbiol Infect Dis 13:639–644, 1994.
237. Leroy O, Santré C, Beuscart C, et al. A five-year study of severe community-acquired pneumonia with emphasis on prognosis in patients admitted to an intensive care unit. Intensive Care Med 21:24–31, 1995.
238. Paganin F, Chanez P, Brousse C, et al. Community acquired pneumonias in the region of Montpellier: Increase of pneumococci with reduced sensitivity to penicillins [French]. Presse Med 24:1341–1344, 1995.
239. Kauppinen MT, Herva E, Kujala P, et al. The etiology of community-acquired pneumonia among hospitalized patients during a *Chlamydia pneumoniae* epidemic in Finland. J Infect Dis 172:1330–1335, 1995.
240. Bohte R, van Furth R, van den Broek PJ. Aetiology of community-acquired pneumonia: A prospective study among adults requiring admission to hospital. Thorax 50:543–547, 1995.
241. Cluzel R, Portier H, Modai J. Treatment of bacterial pneumonias with cefuroxime-axetil: Predictive value of measurement of the in vitro susceptibility. Pathol Biol [French] 44:217–223, 1996.
242. Sow O, Frechet M, Diallo AA, et al. Community acquired pneumonia in adults: A study comparing clinical features and outcome in Africa (Republic of Guinea) and Europe (France). Thorax 51:385–388, 1996.
243. Rello J, Rodriguez R, Jubert P, Alvarez B. Severe community-acquired pneumonia in the elderly: Epidemiology and prognosis: Study Group for Severe Community-Acquired Pneumonia. Clin Infect Dis 23:723–728, 1996.
244. Gomez J, Banos V, Ruiz Gomez J, et al. Prospective study of epidemiology and prognostic factors in community-acquired pneumonia. Eur J Clin Microbiol Infect Dis 15:556–560, 1996.
245. Steinhoff D, Lode H, Ruckdeschel G, et al. *Chlamydia pneumoniae* as a cause of community-acquired pneumonia in hospitalized patients in Berlin. Clin Infect Dis 22:958–964, 1996.
246. Koivula I, Stén M, Leinonen M, Mäkelä PH. Clinical efficacy of pneumococcal vaccine in the elderly: A randomized, single-blind population-based trial. Am J Med 103:281–290, 1997.
247. Lieberman D, Schlaeffer F, Boldur I, et al. Multiple pathogens in adult patients admitted with community-acquired pneumonia: A one year prospective study of 346 consecutive patients. Thorax 51:179–184, 1996.
248. Seedat MA, Feldman C, Skoularigis J, et al. A study of acute community-acquired pneumonia, including details of cardiac changes. Q J Med 86:669–675, 1993.
249. Neill AM, Martin IR, Weir R, et al. Community acquired pneumonia: Aetiology and usefulness of severity criteria on admission. Thorax 51:1010–1016, 1996.
250. Koulla-Shiro S, Kuaban C, Belec L. Acute community-acquired bacterial pneumonia in Human Immunodeficiency Virus (HIV) infected and non-HIV-infected adult patients in Cameroon: Aetiology and outcome. Tuber Lung Dis 77:47–51, 1996.

251. Louie M, Dyck B, Parker S, et al. Nosocomial pneumonia in a Canadian tertiary care center: A prospective surveillance study. Infect Control Hosp Epidemiol 12:356–363, 1991.
252. Schleupner CJ, Cobb DK. A study of the etiologies and treatment of nosocomial pneumonia in a community-based teaching hospital. Infect Control Hosp Epidemiol 13:515–525, 1992.
253. Nielsen SL, Roder B, Magnussen P, et al. Nosocomial pneumonia in an intensive care unit in a Danish university hospital: Incidence, mortality and etiology. Scand J Infect Dis 24:65–70, 1992.
254. Alvarez S, Shell CG, Woolley TW, et al. Nosocomial infections in long-term facilities. J Gerontol 43:m9–m17, 1988.
255. Marrie TJ, Blanchard W. A comparison of nursing home-acquired pneumonia patients with patients with community-acquired pneumonia and nursing home patients without pneumonia. J Am Geriatr Soc 45:50–55, 1997.
256. Outbreaks of pneumococcal pneumonia among unvaccinated residents of chronic-care facilities—Massachusetts, October 1995, Oklahoma, February, 1996, and Maryland, May–June 1996. MMWR Morb Mortal Wkly Rep 46:60–62, 1997.
257. Hoge CW, Reichler MR, Dominguez EA, et al. An epidemic of pneumococcal disease in an overcrowded, inadequately ventilated jail. N Engl J Med 331:643–648, 1994.
258. Markowitz JS, Pashko S, Gutterman EM, et al. Death rates among patients hospitalized with community-acquired pneumonia: A reexamination with data from three states. Am J Public Health 86:1152–1154, 1996.
259. Singh KP, Voolmann T, Lang SD. Pneumococcal bacteraemia in south Auckland: A five year review with emphasis on prescribing practices. N Z Med J 105:394–395, 1992.
260. Teira R, Munoz J, Zubero Z, et al. Epidemiologic characteristics of pneumococcal bacteremia in the era of AIDS [Spanish]. Enferm Infecc Microbiol Clin 10:138–142, 1992.
261. Roca V, Perez Cecilia E, Santillana T, et al. Comparative study of pneumococcal bacteremia in patients with and without HIV infection [Spanish]. Rev Clin Esp 192:21–24, 1993.
262. Watanakunakorn C, Greifenstein A, Stroh K, et al. Pneumococcal bacteremia in three community teaching hospitals from 1980 to 1989. Chest 103:1152–1156, 1993.
263. Jensen C, Nielsen CM, Kolmos HJ. Pneumococcal bacteremia in Hvidovre Hospital 1986–1990 [Danish]. Ugeskr Laeger 155:3665–3670, 1993.
264. Noriega LM, Gonzalez P, Canals C, Michaud P. Sepsis due to *Streptococcus pneumoniae*: Report of 40 cases. Rev Med Chile 122:1385–1392, 1994.
265. Afessa B, Greaves WL, Frederick WR. Pneumococcal bacteremia in adults: A 14-year experience in an inner-city university hospital. Clin Infect Dis 21:345–351, 1995.
266. Carey I, Glauser MP, Bille J. Pneumococcal bacteremia: What is new? [German]. Schweiz Med Wochenschr 125:952–958, 1995.
267. Gomez J, Banos V, Gomez JR, et al. Clinical significance of pneumococcal bacteraemias in a general hospital: A prospective study 1989–1993. J Antimicrob Chemother 36:1021–1030, 1995.
268. Laaveri T, Nikoskelainen J, Meurman O, et al. Bacteraemic pneumococcal disease in a teaching hospital in Finland. Scand J Infect Dis 28:41–46, 1996.
269. Mirzanejad Y, Roman S, Talbot J, et al. Pneumococcal bacteremia in two tertiary care hospitals in Winnipeg, Canada. Chest 109:173–178, 1996.
270. Holm A, Berild D, Ringertz S, Hoiby EA. Incidence and characteristics of invasive pneumococcal infections 1993–1996 in Aker University Hospital, Oslo. Abstracts of the 37th Interscience Conference on Antimicrobial Agents and Chemotherapy; Toronto; 1997; p 343.
271. Pesola GR, Charles A. Pneumococcal bacteremia with pneumonia. Mortality in acquired immunodeficiency syndrome. Chest 101:150–155, 1992.
272. Marfin AA, Sporrer J, Moore PS, Siefkin AD. Risk factors for adverse outcome in persons with pneumococcal pneumonia. Chest 107:457–462, 1995.
273. Hoen B, Viel JF, Gerard A, et al. Mortality in pneumococcal meningitis: A multivariate analysis of prognostic factors. Eur J Med 2:28–32, 1993.
274. Kragsbjerg P, Kallman J, Olcen P. Pneumococcal meningitis in adults. Scand J Infect Dis 26:659–666, 1994.
275. Almirante B, Cortes E, Pigrau C, et al. Therapy and outcome of pneumococcal meningitis in adults: A recent series of 70 episodes [Spanish]. Med Clin 105:681–686, 1995.
276. Urwin G, Yuan MF, Hall LM, et al. Pneumococcal meningitis in the North East Thames Region UK: Epidemiology and molecular analysis of isolates. Epidemiol Infect 117:95–102, 1996.
277. Rodriguez-Creixems M, Munoz P, Miranda E, et al. Recurrent pneumococcal bacteremia: A warning of immunodeficiency. Arch Intern Med 156:1429–1434, 1996.
278. Kuhls TL, Viering TP, Leach CT, et al. Relapsing pneumococcal bacteremia in immunocompromised patients. Clin Infect Dis 14:1050–1054, 1992.
279. Ekdahl K, Truedsson L, Sjoholm AG, Braconier JH. Complement analysis in adult patients with a history of bacteremic pneumococcal infections or recurrent pneumonia. Scand J Infect Dis 27:111–117, 1995.
280. Ortqvist A, Kalin M, Julander I, Mufson MA. Deaths in bacteremic pneumococcal pneumonia: A comparison of two populations—Huntington, W Va, and Stockholm, Sweden. Chest 103:710–716, 1993.
281. Istre GR, Tarpay M, Anderson M, et al. Invasive disease due to *Streptococcus pneumoniae* in an area with a high rate of relative penicillin resistance. J Infect Dis 156:732–735, 1987.
282. Haglund LA, Istre GR, Pickett DA, et al. Invasive pneumococcal disease in central Oklahoma: Emergence of high-level penicillin resistance and multiple antibiotic resistance. J Infect Dis 168:1532–1536, 1993.
283. Breiman RF, Spika JS, Navarro VJ, et al. Pneumococcal bacteremia in Charleston County, South Carolina: A decade later. Arch Intern Med 150:1401–1405, 1990.
284. Bennett NM, Buffington J, LaForce FM. Pneumococcal bacteremia in Monroe County, New York. Am J Public Health 82:1513–1516, 1992.
285. Hofmann J, Cetron MS, Farley MM, et al. The prevalence of drug-resistant *Streptococcus pneumoniae* in Atlanta. N Engl J Med 333:481–486, 1995.
286. Plouffe JF, Breiman RF, Facklam RR. Bacteremia with *Streptococcus pneumoniae*: Implications for therapy and prevention. JAMA 275:194–198, 1996.
287. Pastor P, Medley F, Murphy TV. Invasive pneumococcal disease in Dallas County, Texas: Results from population-based surveillance in 1995. Clin Infect Dis 26:590–595, 1998.
288. Campbell JF, Donohue MA, Mochizuki RB, et al. Pneumococcal bacteremia in Hawaii: Initial findings of a pneumococcal disease prevention project. Hawaii Med J 48:513–514, 1989.
289. Zangwill KM, Vadheim CM, Vannier AM, et al. Epidemiology of invasive pneumococcal disease in southern California: Implications for the design and conduct of a pneumococcal conjugate vaccine efficacy trial. J Infect Dis 174:752–759, 1996.
290. Nuorti P, Vugia D, Butler J, et al. Invasive pneumococcal disease among HIV-infected and uninfected residents of San Francisco, California. Abstracts of the 35th Annual Meeting of the Infectious Diseases Society of America; San Francisco, CA; 1997; p 172.
291. McGeer A, Landry L, Goldenberg E, Green K. Population-based surveillance for invasive pneumococcal infections in Toronto, Canada: Implications for prevention. Abstracts of the 36th Interscience Conference on Antimicrobial Agents and Chemotherapy; Atlanta, GA; 1996; p 251.
292. Hasseltvedt V, Hoiby EA, Iversen BG, Nokelby H. Systemisk pneumokokksydom 1996. MSIS-Rapport 25:8, 1997.
293. Nielsen SV, Henrichsen J. Incidence of invasive pneumococcal disease and distribution of capsular types of pneumococci in Denmark, 1989–94. Epidemiol Infect 117:411–416, 1996.
294. Henrichsen J, Nielsen SV. Incidence of invasive pneumococcal disease in Denmark. Microb Drug Resist 1998: in press.
295. Raz R, Elhanan G, Shimoni Z. Pneumococcal bacteremia in hospitalized Israeli adults: Epidemiology and resistance to penicillin. Clin Infect Dis 24:1164–1168, 1997.
296. Sankilampi U, Herva E, Haikala R, et al. Epidemiology of invasive *Streptococcus pneumoniae* infections in adults in Finland. Epidemiol Infect 118:7–15, 1997.
297. Schonheyder HC, Sorensen HT. Reasons for increase in pneumococcal bacteremia [letter]. Lancet 349:1554, 1997.
298. Hedlund J, Svenson SB, Kalin M, et al. Incidence, capsular types,

and antibiotic susceptibility of invasive *Streptococcus pneumoniae* in Sweden. Clin Infect Dis 21:948–953, 1995.

299. Giesecke J, Fredlund H. Increase in pneumococcal bacteraemia in Sweden [letter]. Lancet 349:699–700, 1997.
300. Kallenius G, Hedlund J, Swenson SB, et al. Pneumococcal bacteremia in Sweden [letter]. Lancet 349:1910, 1997.
301. Baer M, Vuento R, Vesikari T. Increase in bacteraemic pneumococcal infections in children [letter]. Lancet 345:661, 1995.
302. Nielsen SV, Henrichsen J. Capsular types of *Streptococcus pneumoniae* isolated from blood and CSF during 1982–1987. Clin Infect Dis 15:794–798, 1992.
303. Aszkenasy OM, George RC, Begg NT. Pneumococcal bacteraemia and meningitis in England and Wales 1982 to 1992. Commun Dis Rep CDR Wkly 5:r45–50, 1995.
304. Cortese MM, Wolff M, Almeido-Hill J, et al. High incidence rates of invasive pneumococcal disease in the White Mountain Apache population. Arch Intern Med 152:2277–2282, 1992.
305. Davidson M, Parkinson AJ, Bulkow LR, et al. The epidemiology of invasive pneumococcal disease in Alaska, 1986–1990—ethnic differences and opportunities for prevention. J Infect Dis 170:368–376, 1994.
306. Torzillo PJ, Hanna J, Morey F, et al. Invasive pneumococcal disease in central Australia. Med J Aust 162:182–186, 1995.
306a. Trotman J, Hughes B, Mollison L. Invasive pneumococcal disease in central Australia. Clin Infect Dis 20:1553–1556, 1995.
307. Prellner K, Fogle-Hansson M, Jorgensen F, et al. Prevention of recurrent acute otitis media in otitis-prone children by intermittent prophylaxis with penicillin. Acta Otolaryngol (Stockh) 114:182–187, 1994.
308. Stenfors LE, Raisanen S. Abundant attachment of bacteria to nasopharyngeal epithelium in otitis-prone children. J Infect Dis 165:1148–1150, 1992.
309. Faden H, Duffy L, Wasielewski R. Relationship between nasopharyngeal colonization and the development of otitis media in children. J Infect Dis 175:1440–1445, 1997.
310. Fujimori I, Hisamatsu K, Kikushima K, et al. The nasopharyngeal bacterial flora in children with otitis media with effusion. Eur Arch Otorhinolaryngol 253:260–263, 1996.
311. Stenfors LE, Raisanen S. Immunoglobulin- and complement-coated bacteria in middle ear effusions during the early course of acute otitis media. Scand J Infect Dis 24:759–763, 1992.
312. Klein JO. Epidemiology of otitis media. Pediatr Infect Dis J 8:S91, 1989.
313. Teele DW, Klein JO, Rosner B. Epidemiology of otitis media during the first seven years of life in children in greater Boston: A prospective, cohort study. J Infect Dis 160:83–94, 1989.
314. Paradise JL, Rockette HE, Colborn K. Otitis media in 2253 Pittsburg-area infants: Prevalence and risk factors during the first two years of life. Pediatrics 99:318–333, 1997.
315. Pukander J, Karma P, Sipila M. Occurence and recurrence of acute otitis media among children. Acta Otolaryngol (Stockh) 94:479–486, 1982.
316. Karma P, Pukander J, Sipila M. Prevention of otitis media in children by pneumococcal vaccination. Am J Otolaryngol 6:173–184, 1985.
317. Sipila M, Pukander J, Karma P. Incidence of acute otitis media up to the age of 1 1/2 years in urban infants. Acta Otolaryngol (Stockh) 104:138–145, 1987.
318. Henderson FW, Giebink GS. Otitis media among children in day care: Epidemiology and pathogenesis. Rev Infect Dis 8:533–538, 1986.
319. Wald ER, Guerra N, Byers C. Frequency and severity of infections in day care: Three-year follow-up. J Pediatr 118:509–514, 1991.
320. Berman S. Otitis media in developing countries. Pediatrics 96:126–131, 1995.
321. Teele DW. Long term sequelae of otitis media: Fact or fantasy? Pediatr Infect Dis J 13:1069–1073, 1994.
322. Gravel JS, Wallace IF, Ruben RJ. Early otitis media and later educational risk. Acta Otolaryngol (Stockh) 115:279–281, 1995.
323. Stool SE, Field MJ. The impact of otitis media. Pediatr Infect Dis J 8:s11–s14, 1989.
324. Kaplan B, Wandstrat TL, Cunningham JR. Overall cost in the treatment of otitis media. Pediatr Infect Dis J 16:s9–s11, 1997.
325. Luotonen J, Herva E, Karma P. The bacteriology of acute otitis media in children with special reference to *Streptococcus pneumoniae* as studied by bacteriological and antigen detection methods. Scand J Infect Dis 13:177–183, 1981.
326. Giebink GS. The microbiology of otitis media. Pediatr Infect Dis J 8:s18–s20, 1989.
327. Bluestone CD, Stephenson JS, Martin LM. Ten-year review of otitis media pathogens. Pediatr Infect Dis J 11:s7–s11, 1992.
328. Leinonen M. Detection of pneumococcal capsular polysaccharide antigens by latex agglutination, counterimmunoelectrophoresis, and radioimmunoassay in middle ear exudates in acute otitis media. J Clin Microbiol 11:135–140, 1980.
329. Faden H, Stanievich J, Brodsky L, et al. Changes in nasopharyngeal flora during otitis media of childhood. Pediatr Infect Dis J 9:623–626, 1990.
330. Virolainen A, Vero J, Kayhty H, et al. Nasopharyngeal antibodies to pneumococcal capsular polysaccharides in children with acute otitis media. J Infect Dis 172:1115–1118, 1995.
331. Virolainen A, Jero J, Kayhty H, et al. Nasopharyngeal antibodies to pneumococcal pneumolysin in children with acute otitis media. Clin Diagn Lab Immunol 2:704–707, 1995.
332. Virolainen A, Jero J, Chattopadhyay P, et al. Comparison of serum antibodies to pneumolysin with those to pneumococcal capsular polysaccharides in children with acute otitis media. Pediatr Infect Dis J 15:128–133, 1996.
333. Ripley-Petzoldt ML, Giebink GS, Juhn SK, et al. The contribution of pneumococcal cell wall to the pathogenesis of experimental otitis media. J Infect Dis 157:245–255, 1988.
334. Carlsen BD, Kawana M, Kawana C, et al. Role of the bacterial cell wall in middle ear inflammation caused by *Streptococcus pneumoniae*. Infect Immun 60:2850–2854, 1992.
335. Koskela M. Serum antibodies to pneumococcal C polysaccharide in children: Response to acute pneumococcal otitis media or to vaccination. Pediatr Infect Dis J 6:519–526, 1987.
336. Rosenfeld RM. What to expect from medical treatment of otitis media. Pediatr Infect Dis J 14:731–737, 1995.
337. McCracken GHJ. Emergence of resistant *Streptococcus pneumoniae*: A problem in pediatrics. Pediatr Infect Dis J 14:424–428, 1995.
338. Cohen R, Bingen E, Varon E, et al. Change in nasopharyngeal carriage of *Streptococcus pneumoniae* resulting from antibiotic therapy for acute otitis media in children. Pediatr Infect Dis J 16:555–560, 1997.
339. Cohen R, de La Rocque F, Boucherat M, et al. Treatment failure in otitis media: An analysis. J Chemother 6(suppl)4:17–22; discussion 23–24, 1994.
340. Jorgensen F, Andersson B, Larsson S, Nylen O. Nasopharyngeal bacterial flora in otitis prone children treated with immunoglobulin. Acta Otolaryngol 112:530–538, 1992.
341. Shurin PA, Rehmus JM, Johnson CE, et al. Bacterial polysaccharide immune globulin for prophylaxis of acute otitis media in high-risk children. J Pediatr 123:801–810, 1993.
342. Turner RB, Lande AE, Chase P, et al. Pneumonia in pediatric outpatients: Cause and clinical manifestations. J Pediatr 111:194–200, 1987.
343. Isaacs D. Problems in determining the etiology of community-acquired childhood pneumonia. Pediatr Infect Dis J 8:143–148, 1989.
344. Hickey RW, Bowman MJ, Smith GA. Utility of blood cultures in pediatric patients found to have pneumonia in the emergency department. Ann Emerg Med 27:721–725, 1996.
345. Claesson BA, Trollfors B, Brolin I, et al. Etiology of community-acquired pneumonia in children based on antibody responses to bacterial and viral antigens. Pediatr Infect Dis J 8:856–862, 1989.
346. Ramsey BW, Marcuse EK, Foy HM, et al. Use of bacterial antigen detection in the diagnosis of pediatric lower respiratory tract infections. Pediatrics 78:1–9, 1986.
347. Davies HD, Matlow A, Petric M, et al. Prospective comparative study of viral, bacterial and atypical organisms identified in pneumonia and bronchiolitis in hospitalized Canadian infants. Pediatr Infect Dis J 15:371–375, 1996.
348. Ruuskanen O, Nohynek H, Ziegler T, et al. Pneumonia in childhood: etiology and response to antimicrobial therapy. Eur J Clin Microbiol Infect Dis 11:217–223, 1992.
349. Gendrel D, Raymond J, Moulin F. Etiology and response to antibiotic therapy of community-acquired pneumonia in French children. Eur J Clin Microbiol Infect Dis 16:388–391, 1997.

350. Djuretic T, Ryan MJ, Miller E, et al. Hospital admissions in children due to pneumococcal pneumonia in England. J Infect 1998: in press.
351. Korppi M, Heiskanen-Kosma T, Jalonen E. Aetiology of community-acquired pneumonia in children treated in hospital. Eur J Pediatr 152:24–30, 1993.
352. Berman S, Mcintosh K. Selective primary health care: Strategies for control of disease in developing world. Acute respiratory infections. Rev Infect Dis 7:674–691, 1985.
353. Timmons OD, Yamauchi T, Collins SR, et al. Association of respiratory syncytial virus and *Streptococcus pneumoniae* infection in young infants. Pediatr Infect Dis J 6:1134–1135, 1987.
354. Hall CB, Powell KR, Schnabel KC, et al. Risk of secondary bacterial infection in infants hospitalized with respiratory syncytial viral infection. J Pediatr 113:266–271, 1988.
355. Tristram DA, Miller RW, McMillan JA, Weiner LB. Simultaneous infection with respiratory syncytial virus and other respiratory pathogens. Am J Dis Child 142:834–836, 1988.
356. Korppi M, Leinonen M, Koskela M, et al. Bacterial coinfection in children hospitalized with respiratory syncytial virus infections. Pediatr Infect Dis J 8:687–692, 1989.
357. Saarinen M, Takala AK, Koskenniemi E. Spectrum of 2,836 cases of pediatric invasive infections: Results of a prospective nationwide 5-year surveillance in Finland. Clin Infect Dis 21:1134–1144, 1995.
358. Eskola J, Takala AK, Kela E, et al. Epidemiology of invasive pneumococcal infections in children in Finland. JAMA 268:3323–3327, 1992.
359. Takala AK, Jero J, Kela E, et al. Risk factors for primary invasive pneumococcal disease among children in Finland. JAMA 273:859–864, 1995.
360. Dagan R, Engelhard D, Piccard E, Englehard DC. Epidemiology of invasive childhood pneumococcal infections in Israel. JAMA 268:3328–3332, 1992.
361. Voss L, Lennon D, Okesene Gafa K, et al. Invasive pneumococcal disease in a pediatric population, Auckland, New Zealand. Pediatr Infect Dis J 13:873–878, 1994.
362. O'Dempsey TJ, McArdle TF, Lloyd-Evans N, et al. Pneumococcal disease among children in a rural area of west Africa. Pediatr Infect Dis J 15:431–437, 1996.
363. Loughlin AM, Marchant CD, Lett SM. The changing epidemiology of invasive bacterial infections in Massachusetts children, 1984 through 1991. Am J Public Health 85:392–394, 1995.
364. Davis CW, McIntyre PB. Invasive pneumococcal infection in children, 1981–92: A hospital-based study. J Paediatr Child Health 31:317–322, 1995.
365. Grimprel E, Floret D. Pneumococcal bacteremia and sepsis in children: A multi-center study in France [French]. Mod Mal Infect 24:975–981, 1994.
366. Jaffe DM. Occult bacteremia in children. Adv Pediatr Infect Dis 9:237–260, 1994.
367. Harper MB, Bachur R, Fleisher GR. Effect of antibiotic therapy on the outcome of outpatients with unsuspected bacteremia. Pediatr Infect Dis J 14:760–767, 1995.
368. Rothrock SG, Harper MB, Green SM, et al. Do oral antibiotics prevent meningitis and serious bacterial infections in children with *Streptococcus pneumoniae* occult bacteremia? A meta-analysis. Pediatrics 99:438–444, 1997.
369. Baraff LJ, Lee SI, Schriger DL. Outcomes of bacterial meningitis in children: A meta-analysis. Pediatr Infect Dis J 12:389–394, 1993.
370. Kornelisse RF, Westerfeek CML, Spoor AB, et al. Pneumococcal meningitis in children: Prognostic indicators and outcome. Clin Infect Dis 21:1390–1397, 1995.
371. Pikis A, Kavaliotis J, Tsikoulas J, et al. Long-term sequelae of pneumococcal meningitis in children. Clin Pediatr 35:72–78, 1996.
372. Orlicek SL, Herrod HG, Leggiadro RJ, et al. Repeated invasive pneumococcal infections in young children without apparent underlying immunodeficiency. J Pediatr 130:284–288, 1997.
373. Foster JA, Mcgowan KL. Rising rate of pneumococcal, bacteremia at the Childrens Hospital of Philadelphia. Pediatr Infect Dis J 13:1143–1144, 1994.
374. Booy R, Heath P, Willocks L, et al. Invasive pneumococcal infections in children [letter]. Lancet 345:1245–1246, 1995.
375. Sniadack DH, Schwartz B, Lipman H, et al. Potential interventions for the prevention of childhood pneumonia: Geographic and temporal differences in serotype and serogroup distribution of sterile site pneumococcal isolates from children—implications for vaccine strategies. Pediatr Infect Dis J 14:503–510, 1995.
376. Gray BM, Dillon HC. Clinical and epidemiologic studies of pneumococcal infection in children. Pediatr Infect Dis 5:201–207, 1986.
377. Butler JC, Breiman RF, Lipman HB, et al. Serotype distribution of *Streptococcus pneumoniae* infections among preschool children in the United States, 1978–1994: Implications for development of a conjugate vaccine. J Infect Dis 171:885–889, 1995.
378. Klein JO. The epidemiology of pneumococcal disease in infants and children. Rev Infect Dis 3:246, 1981.
379. Kirkwood BR, Gove S, Rogers S, et al. Potential interventions for the prevention of childhood pneumonia in developing countries: A systematic review. Bull World Health Organ 73:793–798, 1995.
380. Bale JR. Creation of a research program to determine the etiology and epidemiology of acute respiratory tract infection among children in developing countries. Rev Infect Dis 12(suppl)8:s861–s866, 1990.
381. Douglas RM. Acute respiratory infections in children in the developing world. Semin Respir Infect 6:217–224, 1991.
382. Forgie IM, O'Neill KP, Lloyd-Evans N, et al. Etiology of acute lower respiratory tract infections in Gambian children: I. Acute lower respiratory tract infections in infants presenting at the hospital. Pediatr Infect Dis J 10:33–41, 1991.
383. Forgie IM, O'Neill KP, Lloyd-Evans N, et al. Etiology of acute lower respiratory tract infections in Gambian children: II. Acute lower respiratory tract infection in children ages one to nine years presenting at the hospital. Pediatr Infect Dis J 10:42–47, 1991.
384. Forgie IM, Campbell H, Lloyd-Evans N, et al. Etiology of acute lower respiratory tract infections in children in a rural community in The Gambia. Pediatr Infect Dis J 11:466–473, 1992.
385. von Schirnding YE, Yach D, Klein M. Acute respiratory infections as an important cause of childhood deaths in South Africa. S Afr Med J 80:79–82, 1991.
386. Adegbola RA, Falade AG, Sam BE, et al. The etiology of pneumonia in malnourished and well-nourished Gambian children. Pediatr Infect Dis J 13:975–982, 1994.
387. de Francisco A, Morris J, Hall AJ, et al. Risk factors for mortality from acute lower respiratory tract infections in young Gambian children. Int J Epidemiol 22:1174–1182, 1993.
388. Ghafoor A, Nomani NK, Ishaq Z, et al. Diagnosis of acute lower respiratory tract infections in children in Rawalpindi and Islamabad, Pakistan. Rev Infect Dis 12(suppl 8):s907–s914, 1990.
389. Jayanetra P, Vorachit M, Rittaporn A, et al. *Haemophilus influenzae* and *Streptococcus pneumoniae* in children with acute respiratory infection. Southeast Asian J Trop Med Public Health 21:195–202, 1990.
390. John TJ, Cherian T, Steinhoff MC, et al. Etiology of acute respiratory infections in children in tropical southern India. Rev Infect Dis 13(suppl 6):s463–s469, 1991.
391. Hortal M, Benitez A, Contera M, et al. A community-based study of acute respiratory tract infections in children in Uruguay. Rev Infect Dis 12(suppl 8):s966–s973, 1990.
392. Weissenbacher M, Carballal G, Avila M, et al. Etiologic and clinical evaluation of acute lower respiratory tract infections in young Argentinian children: An overview. Rev Infect Dis 12(suppl 8):s889–s898, 1990.
393. Carballal G, Siminovich M, Murtagh P, et al. Etiologic, clinical, and pathologic analysis of 31 fatal cases of acute respiratory tract infection in Argentinian children under 5 years of age. Rev Infect Dis 12(suppl 8):s1074–s1080, 1990.
394. Fonseca W, Kirkwood BR, Victora CG, Fuchs SR. Risk factors for childhood pneumonia among the urban poor in Fortaleza, Brazil: A case-control study. Bull World Health Organ 74:199–208, 1996.
395. Selwyn BJ. The epidemiology of acute respiratory tract infection in young children: Comparison of findings from several developing countries: Coordinated Data Group of BOSTID Researchers. Rev Infect Dis 12(suppl 8):s870–s888, 1990.

396. Graham NMH. The epidemiology of acute respiratory infections in children and adults: A global perspective. Epidemiol Rev 12:149–178, 1990.
397. Rogers ZR, Buchanan GR. Risk of infection in children with hemoglobin S-beta-thalassemia [letter; comment]. J Pediatr 127:672–3476. 1995.
398. Mogdasy MC, Camou T, Fajardo C, Hortal M. Colonizing and invasive strains of *Streptococcus pneumoniae* in Uruguayan children: Type distribution and patterns of antibiotic resistance. Pediatr Infect Dis J 11:648–652, 1992.
399. Mackie EJ, Shears P, Frimpong E, Mustafa-Kutana SN. A study of bacterial meningitis in Kumasi, Ghana. Ann Trop Paediatr 12:143–148, 1992.
400. al-Jurayyan NA, al Mazyad AS, al-Nasser MN, et al. Childhood bacterial meningitis in Al-Baha province, Saudi Arabia. J Trop Med Hyg 95:180–185, 1992.
401. Commey JO, Rodrigues OP, Akita FA, Newman M. Bacterial meningitis in children in southern Ghana. East Afr Med J 71:113–117, 1994.
402. Akpede O, Abiodun PO, Sykes M, Salami CE. Childhood bacterial meningitis beyond the neonatal period in southern Nigeria: Changes in organisms/antibiotic susceptibility. East Afr Med J 71:14–20, 1994.
403. Gedlu E, Rahlenbeck SI. Pyogenic meningitis in children in north-western Ethiopia. Ann Trop Paediatr 15:243–247, 1995.
403a. Usen S, Adegbola R, Mulholland K, et al. Epidemiology of invasive pneumococcal disease in the Western Region, The Gambia. Pediatr Infect Dis J 17:23–28, 1998.
404. Gilks CF, Ojoo SA, Ojoo JC, et al. Invasive pneumococcal disease in a cohort of predominantly HIV-1 infected female sex-workers in Nairobi, Kenya. Lancet 347:718–723, 1996.
405. Sazawal S, Black ER. Meta-analysis of intervention trials on case-management of pneumonia in community setting. Lancet 340:528–533, 1992.
406. Bogaerts J, Lepage P, Taelman H, et al. Antimicrobial susceptibility and serotype distribution of *Streptococcus pneumoniae* from Rwanda, 1984–1990. J Infect 27:157–168, 1993.
407. Capeding MR, Sombrero LT, Lucero MG, Saniel MC. Serotype distribution and antimicrobial resistance of invasive *Streptococcus pneumoniae* isolates in Filipino children [letter]. J Infect Dis 169:479–480, 1994.
408. Sessegolo JF, Levin AS, Levy CE, et al. Distribution of serotypes and antimicrobial resistance of *Streptococcus pneumoniae* strains isolated in Brazil from 1988 to 1992. J Clin Microbiol 32:906–911, 1994.
409. Hein N, Ejzenberg B, Lotufo JP, et al. Serotypes of pneumococci isolated from children with pneumonia: Implication of pneumococcal specific immunization [Portuguese]. Rev Hosp Clin Fac Med Sao Paulo 50:280–283, 1995.
410. Brandileone MC, Vieira VS, Zanella RC, et al. Distribution of serotypes of *Streptococcus pneumoniae* isolated from invasive infections over a 16-year period in the greater Sao Paulo area, Brazil. J Clin Microbiol 33:2789–2791, 1995.
411. Echaniz Aviles G, Carnalla Barajas N, Velazquez Meza ME, et al. Capsular types of *Streptococcus pneumoniae* causing disease in children from Mexico City. Pediatr Infect Dis J 14:907–909, 1995.
412. Hsueh PR, Wu JJ, Hsiue TR. Invasive *Streptococcus pneumoniae* infection associated with rapidly fatal outcome in Taiwan. J Formos Med Assoc 95:364–371, 1996.
413. Rusen IA, Fraser-Roberts L. Nasopharyngeal pneumococcal colonization among Kenyan children: Antibiotic resistance, strain types and associations with human immunodeficiency virus type 1 infection. Pediatr Infect Dis J 16:656–662, 1997.
414. Casadevall A, Scharff MD. Serum therapy revisited: Animal models of infection and development of passive antibody therapy. Antimicrob Agents Chemother 38:1695–1702, 1994.
415. Rubin LG, Mardy GV, Pais L, Carlone G. Human anti-capsular concentration required for protection against experimental pneumococcal bacteremia. Abstracts of the 35th Interscience Conference on Antimicrobial Agents and Chemotherapy; 1995; p 166.
416. Chudwin DS. Prophylaxis and treatment of pneumococcal bacteremia by immune globulin intravenous in a mouse model. Clin Immunol Immunopathol 50:62–71, 1989.
416a. Shurin PA, Giebink GS, Wegman DL, et al. Prevention of pneumococcal otitis media in chinchillas with human bacterial polysaccharide immune globulin. J Clin Microbiol 26:755–759, 1988.
417. Santosham M, Reid G, Almeido-Hill J. Efficacy of bacterial polysaccharide immune globulin for prevention of bacteremia pneumococcal infections in Apache children. Pediatr Res 1:178A, 1992.
418. Hamill RJ, Musher DM, Groover JE, et al. IgG antibody reactive with five serotypes of *Streptococcus pneumoniae* in commercial intravenous immunoglobulin preparations. J Infect Dis 166:38–42, 1992.
419. Weisman LE, Cruess DF, Fischer GW. Opsonic activity of commercially available standard intravenous immunoglobulin preparations. Pediatr Infect Dis J 13:1122–1125, 1994.
420. Buckley RH, Schift RI. The use of intravenous immune globulin in immunodeficiency diseases. N Engl J Med 325:110–117, 1991.
421. Chapel HM, Lee M, Hargreaves R, et al. Randomised trial of intravenous immunoglobulin as prophylaxis against infection in plateau-phase multiple myeloma: The UK Group for Immunoglobulin Replacement Therapy in Multiple Myeloma. Lancet 343:1059–1063, 1994.
422. Anonymous. Intravenous immune globulin for the prevention of bacterial infections in children with symptomatic human immunodeficiency virus infection. N Engl J Med 325:73–80, 1991.
423. Weeks JC, Tierney MR, Weinstein MC. Cost effectiveness of prophylactic immune globulin in chronic lymphocytic leukemia. N Engl J Med 325:81–86, 1991.
424. Robbins JB, Austrian R, Lee CJ, et al. Considerations for formulating the second-generation pneumococcal capsular polysaccharide vaccine with emphasis on the cross-reactive types within groups. J Infect Dis 148:1136–1159, 1983.
425. Fletcher TJ, Tunnicliffe WS, Hammond K. Simutaneous immunisation with influenza vaccine and pneumococcal polysaccharide vaccine in patients with chronic respiratory disease. BMJ 314:1663–1665, 1997.
426. Gyhrs A, Pedersen BK, Bygbjerg I, et al. The effect of prophylaxis with chloroquine and proguanil on delayed-type hypersensitivity and antibody production following vaccination with diphtheria, tetanus, polio, and pneumococcal vaccines. Am J Trop Med Hyg 45:613–618, 1991.
427. Nichol KL, MacDonald RM, Hauge M. Side effects associated with pneumococcal vaccination. Am J Infect Control 25:223–228, 1997.
428. Sankilampi U, Honkanen PO, Pyhala R, Leinonen M. Associations of prevaccination antibody levels with adverse reactions to pneumococcal and influenza vaccines administered simultaneously in the elderly. Vaccine 15:1133–1137, 1997.
429. Sell SH, Wright PF, Vaughn WK. Clinical studies of pneumococcal vaccines in infants: I. Reactogenicity and immunogenicity of two polyvalent polysaccharide vaccines. Rev Infect Dis 3:s97–s107, 1981.
430. Lee HJ, Kang JH, Henrichsen J, et al. Immunogenicity and safety of a 23-valent pneumococcal polysaccharide vaccine in healthy children and in children at increased risk of pneumococcal infection. Vaccine 13:1533–1538, 1995.
431. Borgono JM, Mclean AA, Vella PP. Vaccination and revaccination with polyvalent pneumococcal polysaccharide vaccines in adults and infants. Proc Soc Exp Biol Med 157:148–154, 1978.
432. Koskela M, Leinonen M, Haiva VM. First and second dose antibody responses to pneumococcal polysaccharide vaccine in infants. Pediatr Infect Dis 5:45–50, 1986.
433. Eskola J, Kayhty H, Takala A, et al. Reactogenicity and immunogenicity of combined vaccines for bacteraemic diseases caused by *Haemophilus influenzae* type b, meningococci and pneumococci in 24-month-old children. Vaccine 8:107–110, 1990.
434. Brichacek B, Swindells S, Janoff EN, et al. Increased plasma human immunodeficiency virus type 1 burden following antigenic challenge with pneumococcal vaccine. J Infect Dis 174:1191–1199, 1996.
435. Stanley SK, Ostrowski MA, Justement JS, et al. Effect of immunization with a common recall antigen on viral expression in patients infected with human immunodeficiency virus type 1. N Engl J Med 334:1222–1230, 1996.
436. Honkanen PO, Keistinen T, Kivela SL. Reactions following administration of influenza vaccine alone or with pneumococcal vaccine to the elderly. Arch Intern Med 156:205–208, 1996.

436a. Schiffman G, Douglas RM, Bonner MJ, et al. A radioimmunoassay for immunologic phenomena in pneumococcal disease and for the antibody response to pneumococcal vaccines. I. Method for the radioimmunoassay of anticapsular antibodies and comparison with other techniques. J Immunol Meth 33:133–144, 1980.
437. Musher DM, Watson DA, Dominguez EA. Pneumococcal vaccination: Work to date and future prospects. Am J Med Sci 300:45–52, 1990.
438. Siber GR, Priehs C, Madore DV. Standardization of antibody assays for measuring the response to pneumococcal infection and immunization. Pediatr Infect Dis J 8:s84–s91, 1989.
439. Musher DM, Luchi MJ, Watson DA, et al. Pneumococcal polysaccharide vaccine in young adults and older bronchitics: Determination of IgG responses by ELISA and the effect of adsorption of serum with non-type-specific cell wall polysaccharide. J Infect Dis 161:728–735, 1990.
440. Goldblatt D, Levinsky RJ, Turner MW. Role of cell wall polysaccharide in the assessment of IgG antibodies to the capsular polysaccharides of *Streptococcus pneumoniae* in childhood. J Infect Dis 166:632–634, 1992.
441. Goldblatt D, Jadresic LP, Levinsky RJ, Turner MW. Antibody responses to pneumococcal capsular polysaccharide: What is being measured? Immunodeficiency 4:47–50, 1993.
442. Sorensen UB. Pneumococcal polysaccharide antigens: Capsules and C-polysaccharide. An immunochemical study. Dan Med Bull 42:47–53, 1995.
443. Musher DM, Chapman AJ, Goree A, et al. Natural and vaccine-related immunity to *Streptococcus pneumoniae*. J Infect Dis 154:245–256, 1986.
444. Fine DP, Kirk JL, Schiffman G, et al. Analysis of humoral and phagocytic defenses against *Streptococcus pneumoniae* serotypes 1 and 3. J Lab Clin Med 112:487–497, 1988.
445. Nieuwhof WN, Hodgen AN. An enzyme-linked immunosorbent assay suitable for the routine estimation of specific immunoglobulin G responses to polyvalent pneumococcal polysaccharide vaccine in humans. J Immunol Methods 84:197–202, 1985.
446. Shyamala GN, Roberton DM, Hosking CS. Human-isotype-specific enzyme immunoassay for antibodies to pneumococcal polysaccharides. J Clin Microbiol 26:1575–1579, 1988.
447. Zigterman GJ, Verheul AF, Ernste EB, et al. Measurement of the humoral immune response against *Streptococcus pneumoniae* type 3 capsular polysaccharide and oligosaccharide containing antigens by ELISA and ELISPOT techniques. J Immunol Methods 106:101–107, 1988.
448. Verheul AF, Versteeg AA, Westerdaal NA, et al. Measurement of the humoral immune response against *Streptococcus pneumoniae* type 14-derived antigens by an ELISA and ELISPOT assay based on biotin-avidin technology. J Immunol Methods 126:79–87, 1990.
449. Musher DM, Johnson B Jr, Watson DA. Quantitative relationship between anticapsular antibody measured by enzyme-linked immunosorbent assay or radioimmunoassay and protection of mice against challenge with *Streptococcus pneumoniae* serotype 4. Infect Immun 58:3871–3876, 1990.
450. Watson DA, Musher DM. Interruption of capsule production in *Streptococcus pneumoniae* serotype 3 by insertion of transposon Tn916. Infect Immun 58:3135–3138, 1990.
451. Konradsen HB, Sorensen UB, Henrichsen J. A modified enzyme-linked immunosorbent assay for measuring type-specific anti-pneumococcal capsular polysaccharide antibodies. J Immunol Methods 164:13–20, 1993.
452. Zielen S, Broker M, Strnad N, et al. Simple determination of polysaccharide specific antibodies by means of chemically modified ELISA plates. J Immunol Methods 193:1–7, 1996.
453. Nahm MH, Siber GR, Olander JV. A modified Farr assay is more specific than ELISA for measuring antibodies to *Streptococcus pneumoniae* capsular polysaccharides. J Infect Dis 173:113–118, 1996.
454. Roth F, Burkart T, Mühlemann K. A new multiantigen immunoassay for the quantification of IgG antibodies to capsular polysaccharides of *Streptococcus pneumoniae*. J Infect Dis 176:526–529, 1997.
455. Musher DM, Groover JE, Rowland JM, et al. Antibody to capsular polysaccharides of *Streptococcus pneumoniae*: Prevalence, persistence, and response to revaccination. Clin Infect Dis 17:66–73, 1993.
456. Nieminen T, Käyhty H, Virolainen A, Eskola J. Circulating antibody secreting cell response to parenteral pneumococcal vaccines as an indicator of a salivary IgA antibody response. Vaccine 16:313–319, 1998.
457. Rudolph KM, Parkinson AJ. Measurement of pneumococcal capsular polysaccharide serotype-specific immunoglobulin G in human serum, a method for assigning weight-based units to proposed reference sera. Clin Diagn Lab Immunol 1:526–530, 1994.
458. Quataert SA, Kirch CS, Wiedl LJ, et al. Assignment of weight-based antibody units to a human antipneumococcal standard reference serum, lot 89-S. Clin Diagn Lab Immunol 2:590–597, 1995.
459. Vioarsson G, Jonsdottir I, Jonsson S, Valdimarsson H. Opsonization and antibodies to capsular and cell wall polysaccharides of *Streptococcus pneumoniae*. J Infect Dis 170:592–599, 1994.
460. Bardardottir E, Jonsson S, Jonsdottir I, et al. IgG subclass response and opsonization of *Streptococcus pneumoniae* after vaccination of healthy adults. J Infect Dis 162:482–488, 1990.
461. Kaniuk AS, Lortan JE, Monteil MA. Specific IgG subclass antibody levels and phagocytosis of serotype 14 pneumococcus following immunization. Scand J Immunol Suppl 11:96–98, 1992.
462. Vitharsson G, Jonsdottir I, Jonsson S, Valdimarsson H. Opsonization and antibodies to capsular and cell wall polysaccharides of *Streptococcus pneumoniae*. J Infect Dis 170:592–599, 1994.
463. Rijkers GT, Sanders EAM, Breukels MA, Zegers BJM. Responsiveness of infants to capsular polysaccharides: Implications for vaccine development. Rev Med Microbiol 7:3–12, 1996.
464. Nahm MH, Olander JV, Magyarlaki M. Identification of cross-reactive antibodies with low opsonophagocytic activity for *Streptococcus pneumoniae*. J Infect Dis 176:698–703, 1997.
465. Musher DM, Groover JE, Watson DA, Pandey JP. Genetic regulation of the capacity to make immunoglobulin G to pneumococcal capsular polysaccharides. J Invest Med 45:57–68, 1997.
466. Barrett DJ, Ayoub EM. IgG2 subclass restriction of antibody to pneumococcal polysaccharides. Clin Exp Immunol 63:127–134, 1986.
467. Chudwin DS, Artrip SG, Schiffman G. Immunoglobulin G class and subclass antibodies to pneumococcal capsular polysaccharides. Clin Immunol Immunopathol 44:114–121, 1987.
468. Herer B, Labrousse F, Mordelet-Dambrine M, et al. Selective IgG subclass deficiencies and antibody responses to pneumococcal capsular polysaccharide antigen in adult community-acquired pneumonia. Am Rev Respir Dis 142:854–857, 1990.
469. Ambrosino DM, Siber GR. Simultaneous administration of vaccines for *Haemophilus influenzae* type b, pneumococci, and meningococci. J Infect Dis 154:893–896, 1986.
470. Lue C, Tarkowski A, Mestecky J. Systemic immunization with pneumococcal polysaccharide vaccine induces a predominant IgA2 response of peripheral blood lymphocytes and increases of both serum and secretory anti-pneumococcal antibodies. J Immunol 140:3793–3800, 1988.
471. Tarkowski A, Lue C, Moldoveanu Z, et al. Immunization of humans with polysaccharide vaccines induces systemic, predominantly polymeric IgA2-subclass antibody responses. J Immunol 144:3770–3778, 1990.
472. Johnson S, Opstad NL, Douglas JM Jr, Janoff EN. Prolonged and preferential production of polymeric immunoglobulin A in response to *Streptococcus pneumoniae* capsular polysaccharides. Infect Immun 64:4339–4344, 1996.
473. Ekdahl K, Braconier JH, Svanborg C. Impaired antibody response to pneumococcal capsular polysaccharides and phosphorylcholine in adult patients with a history of bacteremic pneumococcal infection. Clin Infect Dis 25:654–660, 1997.
474. Sarvas H, Rautonen N, Sipinen S, Makela O. IgG subclasses of pneumococcal antibodies—effect of allotype G2m(n). Scand J Immunol 29:229–237, 1989.
475. Ambrosino DM, Schiffman G, Gotschlich EC, et al. Correlation between G2m(n) immunoglobulin allotype and human antibody response and susceptibility to polysaccharide encapsulated bacteria. J Clin Invest 75:1935–1942, 1985.
476. Ambrosino DM, Schiffman G, Gotschlich EC, et al. Correlations of G2m(n) and Km(1) allotypes with subclass and light-chain specific antibody. Monographs Allergy 23:244–255, 1988.
477. Ambrosino DM, Barrus VA, DeLange GG, Siber GR. Correlation of the Km(1) immunoglobulin allotype with anti-polysaccha-

ride antibodies in Caucasian adults. J Clin Invest 78:361–365, 1986.
478. Konradsen HB, Henrichsen J, Wachmann H, Holm N. The influence of genetic factors on the immune response as judged by pneumococcal vaccination of mono- and dizygotic Caucasian twins. Clin Exp Immunol 92:532–536, 1993.
479. Konradsen HB, Oxelius VA, Hahn Zoric M, Hanson LA. The importance of G1m and 2 allotypes for the IgG2 antibody levels and avidity against pneumococcal polysaccharide type 1 within mono- and dizygotic twin-pairs. Scand J Immunol 40:251–256, 1994.
480. Konradsen HB, Hahn Zoric M, Nagao AT, Hanson LA. Differences within mono- and dizygotic twin-pairs in spectrotypes and clones of IgG2 antibodies to pneumococcal polysaccharide type 1 and C-polysaccharide after vaccination. Scand J Immunol 40:423–428, 1994.
481. Park MK, Sun Y, Olander JV, et al. The repertoire of human antibodies to the carbohydrate capsule of *Streptococcus pneumoniae* 6B. J Infect Dis 174:75–82, 1996.
482. Kantor AB, Leonore AH. Origin of murine B cells lineages. Annu Rev Immunol 11:501–538, 1993.
483. Temple K, Greenwood B, Inskip H, et al. Antibody response to pneumococcal capsular polysaccharide vaccine in African children. Pediatr Infect Dis J 10:386–390, 1991.
484. Hazlewood M, Nusrat R, Kumararatne DS, et al. The acquisition of anti-pneumococcal capsular polysaccharide *Haemophilus influenzae* type b and tetanus toxoid antibodies, with age, in the UK. Clin Exp Immunol 93:157–164, 1993.
485. Witt CS, Pomat W, Lehmann D, Alpers MP. Antibodies to pneumococcal polysaccharides in pneumonia and response to pneumococcal vaccination in young children in Papua New Guinea. Clin Exp Immunol 83:219–224, 1991.
486. Brussow H, Baensch M, Sidoti J. Seroprevalence of immunoglobulin M (IgM) and IgG antibodies to polysaccharides of *Streptococcus pneumoniae* in different age groups of Ecuadorian and German children. J Clin Microbiol 30:2765–2771, 1992.
487. Douglas RM, Paton JC, Duncan SJ. Antibody response to pneumococcal vaccination in children younger than five years of age. J Infect Dis 148:131–137, 1983.
488. Leinonen M, Sakkinen A, Kalliokoski R. Antibody response to 14-valent pneumococcal capsular polysaccharide vaccine in preschool age children. Pediatr Infect Dis 5:39–44, 1986.
489. Lim PL, Lau YL. Occurrence of IgG subclass antibodies to ovalbumin, avidin, and pneumococcal polysaccharide in children. Int Arch Allergy Immunol 104:137–143, 1994.
490. Pomat WS, Lehmann D, Sanders RC, et al. Immunoglobulin G antibody responses to polyvalent pneumococcal vaccine in children in the highlands of Papua New Guinea. Infect Immun 62:1848–1853, 1994.
491. van den Dobbelsteen GP, van Rees EP. Mucosal immune responses to pneumococcal polysaccharides: Implications for vaccination. Trends Microbiol 3:155–159, 1995.
492. Virolainen A, Jero J, Kayhty H. Antibodies to pneumolysin and pneumococcal capsular polysaccharides in middle ear fluid of children with acute otitis media. Acta Otolaryngol 115:796–803, 1995.
493. Koskela M. Antibody response of young children to parenteral vaccination with pneumococcal capsular polysaccharides: A comparison between antibody levels in serum and middle ear effusion. Pediatr Infect Dis J 5:431–434, 1986.
494. Sankilampi U, Isoaho R, Bloigu A, et al. Effect of age, sex and smoking habits on pneumococcal antibodies in an elderly population. Int J Epidemiol 26:420–427, 1997.
495. Mufson MA, Hughey DF, Turner CE, Schiffman G. Revaccination with pneumococcal vaccine of elderly persons 6 years after primary vaccination. Vaccine 9:403–407, 1991.
496. Hedlund JU, Kalin ME, Ortqvist AB, Henrichsen J. Antibody response to pneumococcal vaccine in middle-aged and elderly patients recently treated for pneumonia. Arch Intern Med 154:1961–1965, 1994.
497. Konradsen HB. Quantity and avidity of pneumococcal antibodies before and up to five years after pneumococcal vaccination of elderly persons. Clin Infect Dis 21:616–620, 1995.
498. Musher DM, Groover JE, Graviss EA, Baughn RE. The lack of association between aging and postvaccination levels of IgG antibody to capsular polysaccharides of *Streptococcus pneumoniae*. Clin Infect Dis 22:165–167, 1996.
499. Sankilampi U, Honkanen PO, Bloigu A, et al. Antibody response to pneumococcal capsular polysaccharide vaccine in the elderly. J Infect Dis 173:387–393, 1996.
499a. Rubins JB, Puri AKG, Loch J, et al. Magnitude, duration, quality, and function of pneumococcal vaccine responses in elderly adults. J Infect Dis 179:431–440, 1998.
500. Sankilampi U, Honkanen PO, Bloigu A, Leinonen M. Persistence of antibodies to pneumococcal capsular polysaccharide vaccine in the elderly. J Infect Dis 176:1100–1104, 1997.
501. Bruyn GA, Hiemstra PS, Matze-van der Lans A, van Furth R. Pneumococcal anticapsular antibodies in patients with chronic cardiovascular and obstructive lung disease in The Netherlands. J Infect Dis 162:1192–1194, 1990.
502. Lahood N, Emerson SS, Kumar P, Sorensen RU. Antibody levels and response to pneumococcal vaccine in steroid-dependent asthma. Ann Allergy 70:289–294, 1993.
503. Shapiro GG, Virant FS, Furukawa CT, et al. Immunologic defects in patients with refractory sinusitis. Pediatrics 87:311–316, 1991.
504. Zora JA, Silk HJ, Tinkelman DG. Evaluation of postimmunization pneumococcal titers in children with recurrent infections and normal levels of immunoglobulin. Ann Allergy 70:283–288, 1993.
505. Sanders LA, Rijkers GT, Kuis W, et al. Defective antipneumococcal polysaccharide antibody response in children with recurrent respiratory tract infections. J Allergy Clin Immunol 91:110–119, 1993.
506. Epstein MM, Gruskay F. Selective deficiency in pneumococcal antibody response in children with recurrent infections. Ann Allergy Asthma Immunol 75:125–131, 1995.
507. Sanders LA, Rijkers GT, Tenbergen Meekes AM, et al. Immunoglobulin isotype-specific antibody responses to pneumococcal polysaccharide vaccine in patients with recurrent bacterial respiratory tract infections. Pediatr Res 37:812–819, 1995.
508. Hidalgo H, Moore C, Leiva LE, Sorensen RU. Preimmunization and postimmunization pneumococcal antibody titers in children with recurrent infections. Ann Allergy Asthma Immunol 76:341–346, 1996.
509. French MA, Denis KA, Dawkins R, Peter JB. Severity of infections in IgA deficiency: Correlation with decreased serum antibodies to pneumococcal polysaccharides and decreased serum IgG2 and/or IgG4. Clin Exp Immunol 100:47–53, 1995.
510. McMahon BJ, Parkinson AJ, Bulkow L, et al. Immunogenicity of the 23-valent pneumococcal polysaccharide vaccine in Alaska Native chronic alcoholics compared with nonalcoholic Native and non-Native controls. Am J Med 95:589–594, 1993.
511. Preheim LC, Mellencamp MA, Snitily MU, Gentry MJ. Effect of cirrhosis on the production and efficacy of pneumococcal capsular antibody in a rat model. Am Rev Respir Dis 146:1054–1058, 1992.
512. Janoff EN, Breiman RF, Daley CL, Hopewell PC. Pneumococcal disease during HIV infection: Epidemiologic, clinical, and immunologic perspectives. Ann Intern Med 117:314–324, 1992.
513. Garcia-Leoni ME, Moreno S, Rodeno P. Pneumococcal pneumonia in adult hospitalized patients infected with the human immunodeficiency virus. Arch Intern Med 152:1808–1812, 1992.
514. Janoff EN, O Brien J, Thompson P, et al. *Streptococcus pneumoniae* colonization, bacteremia, and immune response among persons with human immunodeficiency virus infection. J Infect Dis 167:49–56, 1993.
515. Hirschtick RE, Glassroth J, Jordan MC, et al. Bacterial pneumonia in persons infected with the human immunodeficiency virus. Pulmonary complications of HIV infection study group. N Engl J Med 333:845–851, 1995.
516. Frankel RE, Virata M, Hardalo C, et al. Invasive pneumococcal disease: Clinical features, serotypes, and antimicrobial resistance patterns in cases involving patients with and without human immunodeficiency virus infection. Clin Infect Dis 23:577–584, 1996.
517. Hibbs JR, Douglas RMJ, Judson FN, et al. Prevalence of human immunodeficiency virus infection, mortality rate, and serogroup distribution among patients with pneumococcal bacteremia at Denver General Hospital, 1984–94. Clin Infect Dis 25:195–199, 1997.

518. Gesner M, Desiderio D, Kim M, et al. *Streptococcus pneumoniae* in human immunodeficiency virus type 1-infected children. Pediatr Infect Dis J 13:697–703, 1994.
519. Farley JJ, King JC, Nair P, et al. Invasive pneumococcal disease among infected and uninfected children of mothers with human immunodeficiency virus infection. J Pediatr 124:853–858, 1994.
520. Mao C, Harper M, Mcintosh K, et al. Invasive pneumococcal infections in human immunodeficiency virus-infected children. J Infect Dis 173:870–876, 1996.
521. Falguera M, Perez-Mur J, Galindo C, Garcia M. Prevalence and outcome of pneumococcal carrier human immunodeficiency virus-infected patients [letter]. J Infect Dis 168:511, 1993.
522. Opstad NL, Daley CL, Thurn JR, et al. Impact of *Streptococcus pneumoniae* bacteremia and human immunodeficiency virus type 1 on oral mucosal immunity. J Infect Dis 172:566–570, 1995.
523. Rodriguez-Barradas MC, Tharapel RA, Groover JE, et al. Colonization by *Streptococcus pneumoniae* among human immunodeficiency virus-infected adults: Prevalence of antibiotic resistance, impact of immunization, and characterization by polymerase chain reaction with BOX primers of isolates from persistent S. pneumoniae carriers. J Infect Dis 175:590–597, 1997.
524. Jordens JZ, Paul J, Bates J, et al. Characterization of *Streptococcus pneumoniae* from human immunodeficiency virus–seropositive patients with acute and recurrent pneumonia. J Infect Dis 172:983–987, 1995.
525. Increase in pneumonia mortality among young adults and the HIV epidemic—New York City, United States. MMWR Morb Mortal Wkly Rep 37:593–596, 1988.
526. Drucker E, Webber MP, McMaster P, Vermund SH. Increasing rate of pneumonia hospitalizations in the Bronx: A sentinel indicator for human immunodeficiency virus. Int J Epidemiol 18:926–933, 1989.
527. Boschini A, Smacchia C, Di Fine M, et al. Community-acquired pneumonia in a cohort of former injection drug users with and without human immunodeficiency virus infection: Incidence, etiologies, and clinical aspects. Clin Infect Dis 23:107–113, 1996.
528. Selwyn PA, Feingold AR, Hartel D, et al. Increased risk of bacterial pneumonia in HIV-infected intravenous drug users without AIDS. AIDS 2:267–272, 1988.
529. Manos GE, van Deutekom H, Peerbooms PG, et al. Community-acquired pneumonia in drug abusers in Amsterdam [letter]. Lancet 336:939–940, 1990.
530. Miller RF, Foley NM, Kessel D, Jeffrey AA. Community acquired lobar pneumonia in patients with HIV infection and AIDS. Thorax 49:367–368, 1994.
531. Redd SC, Rutherford GW III, Sande MA, et al. The role of human immunodeficiency virus infection in pneumococcal bacteremia in San Francisco residents. J Infect Dis 162:1012–1017, 1990.
532. Schuchat A, Broome CV, Hightower A, et al. Use of surveillance for invasive pneumococcal disease to estimate the size of the immunosuppressed HIV-infected population. JAMA 265:3275–3279, 1991.
533. Earhart KC, Wallace MR. The changing epidemiology of pneumococcal bacteremia in human immunodeficiency virus infection. J Infect Dis 174:242–243, 1996.
534. Krumholz HM, Sande MA, Lo B. Community-acquired bacteremia in patients with acquired immunodeficiency syndrome: Clinical presentation, bacteriology, and outcome. Am J Med 86:776–779, 1989.
535. Magnenat JL, Nicod LP, Auckenthaler R, Junod AF. Mode of presentation and diagnosis of bacterial pneumonia in human immunodeficiency virus-infected patients. Am Rev Respir Dis 144:917–922, 1991.
536. Rodriguez-Barradas MC, Musher DM, et al. Unusual manifestations of pneumococcal infection in human immunodeficiency virus-infected individuals: The past revisited. Clin Infect Dis 14:192–199, 1992.
537. Godeau B, Bachir D, Schaeffer A, et al. Severe pneumococcal sepsis and meningitis in human immunodeficiency virus–infected adults with sickle cell disease. Clin Infect Dis 15:327–329, 1992.
538. Meynard JL, Barbut F, Blum L, et al. Risk factors for isolation of *Streptococcus pneumoniae* with decreased susceptibility to penicillin G from patients infected with human immunodeficiency virus. Clin Infect Dis 22:437–440, 1996.
539. Crewe-Brown HH, Karstaedt AS, Saunders GL, et al. *Streptococcus pneumoniae* blood culture isolates from patients with and without human immunodeficiency virus infection: Alterations in penicillin susceptibilities and in serogroups or serotypes. Clin Infect Dis 25:1165–1172, 1997.
540. Ballet JJ, Sulcebe G, Couderc LJ, et al. Impaired anti-pneumococcal antibody response in patients with AIDS-related persistent generalized lymphadenopathy. Clin Exp Immunol 68:479–487, 1987.
541. Janoff EN, Douglas JM Jr, Gabriel M, et al. Class-specific antibody response to pneumococcal capsular polysaccharides in men infected with human immunodeficiency virus type 1. J Infect Dis 158:983–990, 1988.
542. Rodriguez-Barradas MC, Musher DM, Lahart C. Antibody to capsular polysaccharides of *Streptococcus pneumoniae* after vaccination of human immunodeficiency virus-infected subjects with 23-valent pneumococcal vaccine. J Infect Dis 165:533–536, 1992.
543. Unsworth DJ, Rowen D, Carne C, et al. Defective IgG2 response to Pneumovax in HIV seropositive patients. Genitourin Med 69:373–376, 1993.
544. Kroon FP, van Dissel JT, de Jong JC, van Furth R. Antibody response to influenza, tetanus and pneumococcal vaccines in HIV-seropositive individuals in relation to the number of CD4+ lymphocytes. AIDS 8:469–476, 1994.
545. Weiss PJ, Wallace MR, Oldfield EC 3rd, et al. Response of recent human immunodeficiency virus seroconverters to the pneumococcal polysaccharide vaccine and *Haemophilus influenzae* type b conjugate vaccine. J Infect Dis 171:1217–1222, 1995.
546. Loeliger AE, Rijkers GT, Aerts P, et al. Deficient antipneumococcal polysaccharide responses in HIV-seropositive patients. FEMS Immunol Med Microbiol 12:33–41, 1995.
547. Mascartlemone F, Gerard M, Libin M, et al. Differential effect of human immunodeficiency virus infection on the IgA and IgG antibody responses to pneumococcal vaccine. J Infect Dis 172:1253–1260, 1995.
548. Vandenbruaene M, Colebunders R, Mascart Lemone F, et al. Equal IgG antibody response to pneumococcal vaccination in all stages of human immunodeficiency virus disease. J Infect Dis 172:551–553, 1995.
549. Carson PJ, Schut RL, Simpson ML, et al. Antibody class and subclass responses to pneumococcal polysaccharides following immunization of human immunodeficiency virus–infected patients. J Infect Dis 172:340–345, 1995.
550. Rodriguez-Barradas MC, Groover JE, Lacke CE, et al. IgG antibody to pneumococcal capsular polysaccharide in human immunodeficiency virus-infected subjects: Persistence of antibody in responders, revaccination in nonresponders, and relationship of immunoglobulin allotype to response. J Infect Dis 173:1347–1353, 1996.
551. Arpadi SM, Back S, O Brien J, Janoff EN. Antibodies to pneumococcal capsular polysaccharides in children with human immunodeficiency virus infection given polyvalent pneumococcal vaccine. J Pediatr 125:77–79, 1994.
552. Peters VB, Diamant EP, Hodes DS, Cimino CO. Impaired immunity to pneumococcal polysaccharide antigens in children with human immunodeficiency virus infection immunized with pneumococcal vaccine. Pediatr Infect Dis J 13:933–934, 1994.
553. Gibb D, Spoulou V, Giacomelli A, et al. Antibody responses to *Haemophilus influenzae* type b and *Streptococcus pneumoniae* vaccines in children with human immunodeficiency virus infection. Pediatr Infect Dis J 14:129–135, 1995.
554. de Moraes Pinto MI, Almeida AC, Kenj G, et al. Placental transfer and maternally acquired neonatal IgG immunity in human immunodeficiency virus infection. J Infect Dis 173:1077–1084, 1996.
555. Glaser JB, Volpe S, Aguirre A, et al. Zidovudine improves response to pneumococcal vaccine among persons with AIDS and AIDS-related complex. J Infect Dis 164:761–764, 1991.
556. Farber CM, Barath AA, Dieye T. The effects of immunization in human immunodeficiency virus type 1 infection [letter]. N Engl J Med 335:817, 1996.
557. Cullingford GL, Watkins DN, Watts AD, Mallon DF. Severe late postsplenectomy infection. Br J Surg 78:716–721, 1991.
558. Styrt BA. Risks of infection and protective strategies for the asplenic patient. Infect Dis Clin Pract 5:94–100, 1996.

559. Aavitsland P, Froholm LO, Hoiby EA, Lystad A. Risk of pneumococcal disease in individuals without a spleen [letter]. Lancet 344:1504, 1994.
560. Aaberge IS, Michaelsen TE, Heier HE. IgG subclass antibody responses to pneumococcal polysaccharide vaccine in splenectomized, otherwise normal, individuals. Scand J Immunol 31:711–716, 1990.
561. Reinert RR, Kaufhold A, Kuhnemund O, Lutticken R. Serum antibody responses to vaccination with 23-valent pneumococcal vaccine in splenectomized patients. Int J Med Microbiol Virol Parasitol Infect Dis 281:481–490, 1994.
562. Cavill I, Baddeley PG, Barnes RA, et al. Guidelines for the prevention and treatment of infection in patients with an absent or dysfunctional spleen. BMJ 312:430–434, 1996.
563. Palejwala AA, Hong LY, King D. Managing patients with an absent or dysfunctional spleen: Under half of doctors know that antibiotic prophylaxis should be life long. BMJ 312:1360, 1996.
564. White KS, Covington D, Churchill P, et al. Patient awareness of health precautions after splenectomy. Am J Infect Control 19:36–41, 1991.
565. Rutherford EJ, Livengood J, Higginbotham M, et al. Efficacy and safety of pneumococcal revaccination after splenectomy for trauma. J Trauma 39:448–452, 1995.
566. Konradsen HB, Henrichsen J. Pneumococcal infections in splenectomized children are preventable. Acta Paediatr Scand 80:423–427, 1991.
567. Kinnersley P, Wilkinson CE, Srinivasan J. Pneumococcal vaccination after splenectomy: Survey of hospital and primary care records. BMJ 307:1398–1399, 1993.
568. Baddeley P, Boyer P, Mayon-White D. Fact sheets, posters and protocol cards available [letter]. BMJ 308:132, 1994.
569. Glass JM, Gilbert JM. Splenectomy in a general hospital. J R Soc Med 89:199–201, 1996.
570. Aaberge IS, Nokleby H, Froholm LO. All persons without spleen should be given pneumococcal vaccine [Norwegian]. Tidsskr Nor Laegeforen 114:2732–2733, 1994.
571. Obaro S, Henderson DC, Monteil M. Long term management after splenectomy. Monitor antibody levels after vaccination [letter]. BMJ 308:338–339, 1994.
572. McMullin MF, Johnston G. Long term management of patients after splenectomy. BMJ 307:1372–1373, 1993.
573. Wong WY, Overturf GD, Powars DR. Infection caused by *Streptococcus pneumoniae* in children with sickle cell disease: Epidemiology, immunologic mechanisms, prophylaxis, and vaccination. Clin Infect Dis 14:1124–1136, 1992.
574. Wong WY, Powars DR, Chan L, et al. Polysaccharide encapsulated bacterial infection in sickle cell anemia: A thirty year epidemiologic experience. Am J Hematol 39:176–182, 1992.
575. Gill FM, Sleeper LA, Weiner SJ, et al. Clinical events in the first decade in a cohort of infants with sickle cell disease. Blood 86:776–783, 1995.
576. Chesney PJ, Wilimas JA, Presbury G, et al. Penicillin- and cephalosporin-resistant strains of *Streptococcus pneumoniae* causing sepsis and meningitis in children with sickle cell disease. J Pediatr 127:526–532, 1995.
577. Wang WC, Wong WY, Rogers ZR, et al. Antibiotic-resistant pneumococcal infection in children with sickle cell disease in the United States. J Pediatr Hematol Oncol 18:140–144, 1996.
578. Bjornson AB, Lobel JS. Direct evidence that decreased opsonization of *Streptococcus pneumoniae* via the alternative complement pathway in sickle cell disease is related to antibody deficiency. J Clin Invest 79:388–398, 1987.
579. Rautonen N, Martin NL, Rautonen J, et al. Low number of antibody producing cells in patients with sickle cell anemia. Immunol Lett 34:207–211, 1992.
580. Ajulo SO. The significance of recurrent tonsillitis in sickle cell disease. Clin Otolaryngol 19:230–233, 1994.
581. Norris CF, Surrey S, Bunin GR, et al. Relationship between Fc receptor IIA polymorphism and infection in children with sickle cell disease. J Pediatr 128:813–819, 1996.
582. Bjornson AB, Falletta JM, Verter JI, et al. Serotype-specific immunoglobulin G antibody responses to pneumococcal polysaccharide vaccine in children with sickle cell anemia: Effects of continued penicillin prophylaxis. J Pediatr 129:828–835, 1996.
583. Rao SP, Rajkumar K, Schiffman G, et al. Anti-pneumococcal antibody levels three to seven years after first booster immunization in children with sickle cell disease, and after a second booster. J Pediatr 127:590–592, 1995.
584. Gaston MH, Verter JI, Woods G, et al. Prophylaxis with oral penicillin in children with sickle cell anemia. A randomized trial. N Engl J Med 314:1593–1599, 1986.
585. Falletta JM, Woods GM, Verter JI, et al. Discontinuing penicillin prophylaxis in children with sickle cell anemia: Prophylactic Penicillin Study II. J Pediatr 127:685–690, 1995.
586. Steele RW, Warrier R, Unkel PJ, et al. Colonization with antibiotic-resistant *Streptococcus pneumoniae* in children with sickle cell disease. J Pediatr 128:531–535, 1996.
587. Norris CF, Mahannah SR, Smith-Whitley K, et al. Pneumococcal colonization in children with sickle cell disease. J Pediatr 129:821–827, 1996.
588. Pearson HA. Prevention of pneumococcal disease in sickle cell anemia [editorial]. J Pediatr 129:788–789, 1996.
589. Gowda R, Razvi FM, Summerfield GP. Risk of pneumococcal septicaemia in patients with chronic lymphoproliferative malignancies. BMJ 311:26–27, 1995.
590. Griffiths H, Lea J, Bunch C, et al. Predictors of infection in chronic lymphocytic leukaemia (CLL). Clin Exp Immunol 89:374–377, 1992.
591. Grimfors G, Bjorkholm M, Hammarstrom L, et al. Type-specific anti-pneumococcal antibody subclass response to vaccination after splenectomy with special reference to lymphoma patients. Eur J Haematol 43:404–410, 1989.
592. Grimfors G, Soderqvist M, Holm G, et al. A longitudinal study of class and subclass antibody response to pneumococcal vaccination in splenectomized individuals with special reference to patients with Hodgkin's disease. Eur J Haematol 45:101–108, 1990.
593. Sklenar I, Schiffman G, Jonsson V, et al. Effect of various doses of intravenous polyclonal IgG on in vivo levels of 12 pneumococcal antibodies in patients with chronic lymphocytic leukaemia and multiple myeloma. Oncology (Huntingt) 50:466–477, 1993.
594. Mellemgaard A, Brown P, Heron I. Ranitidine improves the vaccination response in patients with chronic lymphocytic leukemia—a randomized, controlled study. Immunol Infect Dis 3:109–111, 1993.
595. Rautonen J, Siimes MA, Lundstrom U, et al. Vaccination of children during treatment for leukemia. Acta Paediatr Scand 75:579–585, 1986.
596. Smith S, Schiffman G, Karayalcin G, Bonagura V. Immunodeficiency in long-term survivors of acute lymphoblastic leukemia treated with Berlin-Frankfurt-Munster therapy. J Pediatr 127:68–75, 1995.
597. Rytel MW, Dailey MP, Schiffman G, et al. Pneumococcal vaccine immunization of patients with renal impairment. Proc Soc Exp Biol Med 182:468–473, 1986.
598. Linnemann CC, First R, Schiffman G. Revaccination of renal transplant and hemodialysis patients with pneumococcal vaccine. Arch Intern Med 146:1554–1556, 1986.
599. Spika JS, Halsey NA, Le CT, et al. Decline of vaccine-induced antipneumococcal antibody in children with nephrotic syndrome. Am J Kidney Dis 7:466–470, 1986.
600. Fuchshuber A, Kuhnemund O, Keuth B, et al. Pneumococcal vaccine in children and young adults with chronic renal disease. Nephrol Dial Transplant 11:468–473, 1996.
601. Furth SL, Neu AM, Case B, et al. Pneumococcal polysaccharide vaccine in children with chronic renal disease: A prospective study of antibody response and duration. J Pediatr 128:99–101, 1996.
602. Giebink GS, Warkentin PI, Ramsay NK, Kersey JH. Titers of antibody to pneumococci in allogeneic bone marrow transplant recipients before and after vaccination with pneumococcal vaccine. J Infect Dis 154:590–596, 1986.
603. Sheridan JF, Tutschka PJ, Sedmak DD, Copelan EA. Immunoglobulin G subclass deficiency and pneumococcal infection after allogeneic bone marrow transplantation. Blood 75:1583–1586, 1990.
604. Lortan JE, Vellodi A, Jurges ES, Hugh Jones K. Class- and subclass-specific pneumococcal antibody levels and response to immunization after bone marrow transplantation. Clin Exp Immunol 88:512–519, 1992.

605. Ambrosino DM. Impaired polysaccharide responses in immunodeficient patients: Relevance to bone marrow transplant patients. Bone Marrow Transplant 7(suppl 3):48–51, 1991.
606. Hammarstrom V, Pauksen K, Azinge J, et al. Pneumococcal immunity and response to immunization with pneumococcal vaccine in bone marrow transplant patients: The influence of graft versus host reaction. Support Care Cancer 1:195–199, 1993.
607. Avanzini MA, Carra AM, Maccario R, et al. Antibody response to pneumococcal vaccine in children receiving bone marrow transplantation. J Clin Immunol 15:137–144, 1995.
607a. Parkkali T, Kayhty H, Ruutu T, et al. A comparison of early and late vaccination with *Haemophilus influenzae* type b conjugate and pneumococcal polysaccharide vaccines after allogeneic BMT. Bone Marrow Transplant 18:961–967, 1996.
608. Guinan EC, Molrine DC, Antin JH, et al. Polysaccharide conjugate vaccine responses in bone marrow transplant patients. Transplantation 57:677–684, 1994.
609. Ljungman P, Cordonnier C, de Bock R, et al. Immunisations after bone marrow transplantation: Results of a European survey and recommendations from the infectious diseases working party of the European Group for Blood and Marrow Transplantation. Bone Marrow Transplant 15:455–460, 1995.
610. Amber IJ, Gilbert EM, Schiffman G, Jacobson JA. Increased risk of pneumococcal infections in cardiac transplant recipients. Transplantation 49:122–125, 1990.
611. Barkholt LB, Ericson BG, Tollemar J. Infections in human liver recipients: Different patterns early and late after transplantation. Transplant Int 6:77–84, 1993.
612. Dengler TJ, Strnad N, Zimmermann R, et al. Pneumococcal vaccination after heart and liver transplantation: Immune responses in immunosuppressed patients and in healthy controls [German]. Dtsch Med Wochenschr 121:1519–1525, 1996.
613. Blumberg A, Brozena SC, Groover JE, et al. Immunogenicity of pneumococcal vaccine (PV) in heart transplant recipients. Abstracts of the 35th Annual Meeting of the Infectious Diseases Society of America; San Francisco, CA; 1997; p 181.
614. Liote F, Angle J, Gilmore N, Osterland CK. Asplenism and systemic lupus erythematosus. Clin Rheumatol 14:220–223, 1995.
615. Brzeski M, Smart L, Baird D, et al. Pneumococcal septic arthritis after splenectomy in Felty's syndrome. Ann Rheum Dis 50:724–726, 1991.
616. McKinley M, Leibowitz S, Bronzo R, et al. Appropriate response to pneumococcal vaccine in celiac sprue. J Clin Gastroenterol 20:113–116, 1995.
617. Hazlewood MA, Kumararatne DS, Webster AD, et al. An association between homozygous C3 deficiency and low levels of anti-pneumococcal capsular polysaccharide antibodies. Clin Exp Immunol 87:404–409, 1992.
618. Fata FT, Herzlich BC, Schiffman G, Ast AL. Impaired antibody responses to pneumococcal polysaccharide in elderly patients with low serum vitamin B12 levels. Ann Intern Med 124:299–304, 1996.
619. Westh H, Skibsted L, Korner B. *Streptococcus pneumoniae* infections of the female genital tract and in the newborn child. Rev Infect Dis 12:416–422, 1990.
620. Johnsson H, Bergstrom S, Ewald U, Schwan A. Neonatal septicemia caused by pneumococci. Acta Obstet Gynecol Scand 71:6–11, 1992.
621. Primhak RA, Tanner MS, Spencer RC. Pneumococcal infection in the newborn. Arch Dis Childh 69:317–318, 1993.
622. Simpson JM, Patel JS, Ispahani P. *Streptococcus pneumoniae* invasive disease in the neonatal period: An increasing problem? Eur J Pediatr 154:563–566, 1995.
623. Kaplan M, Rudensky B, Beck A. Perinatal infections with *Streptococcus pneumoniae*. Am J Perinatol 10:1–4, 1993.
624. Johnsson H, Ewald U. The incidence of neonatal pneumococcal septicemia in Sweden 1991–92: The result of a national survey. Ups J Med Sci 99:161–165, 1994.
624a. Salazar JC, Daly KA, Giebink GS, et al. Low cord blood pneumococcal immunoglobulin G (IgG) antibodies predict early onset acute otitis media in infancy. Am J Epidemiol 145:1048–1056, 1997.
625. Chudwin DS, Wara DW, Schiffman G, et al. Maternal-fetal transfer of pneumococcal capsular polysaccharide antibodies. Am J Dis Child 139:378–380, 1985.
626. Lee CJ, Takaoka Y, Saito T. Maternal immunization and the immune reponse of neonates to pneumococcal polysaccharides. Rev Infect Dis 9:494–510, 1987.
627. Anderson P, Porcelli S, Pichichero M. Natural maternal and cord serum antibodies to pneumococcal serotypes 6A, 14, 19F and 23F polysaccharides. Pediatr Infect Dis J 11:677–679, 1992.
628. Shahid NS, Steinhoff MC, Hoque SS, et al. Serum, breast milk, and infant antibody after maternal immunisation with pneumococcal vaccine. Lancet 346:1252–1257, 1995.
629. O'Dempsey TJ, McArdle T, Ceesay SJ, et al. Immunization with a pneumococcal capsular polysaccharide vaccine during pregnancy. Vaccine 14:963–970, 1996.
630. Rosen IAV, Hakansson A, Aniansson G, et al. Antibodies to pneumococcal polysaccharides in human milk: Lack of relationship to colonization and acute otitis media. Pediatr Infect Dis J 15:498–507, 1996.
631. Mulholland K, Suara RO, Siber G, et al. Maternal immunization with *Haemophilus influenzae* type b polysaccharide-tetanus protein conjugate vaccine in The Gambia. JAMA 275:1182–1188, 1996.
632. Pneumococcal polysaccharide vaccine. MMWR Morb Mortal Wkly Rep 38:64–68, 1989.
633. Mufson MA, Krause HE, Schiffman G, Hughey DF. Pneumococcal antibody levels one decade after immunization of healthy adults. Am J Med Sci 293:279–284, 1987.
634. Rodriguez R, Dyer PD. Safety of pneumococcal revaccination. J Gen Intern Med 10:511–512, 1995.
635. Jackson LA, Sneller VP, Kvartskhava T, et al. Safety of revaccination with pneumococcal polysaccharide (PPV). Abstracts of the 35th Annual Meeting of the Infectious Diseases Society of America; San Francisco, CA; 1997; p 181.
636. Snow R, Babish JD, McBean AM. Is there any connection between a second pneumonia shot and hospitalization among Medicare beneficiaries? Public Health Rep 110:720–725, 1995.
637. Kaplan J, Sarnaik S, Schiffman G. Revaccination with polyvalent pneumococcal vaccine in children with sickle cell disease. Am J Pediatr Hematol Oncol 1:80–82, 1986.
638. Davidson M, Bulkow LR, Grabman J, et al. Immunogenicity of pneumococcal revaccination in patients with chronic disease. Arch Intern Med 154:2209–2214, 1994.
639. Konradsen HB, Pedersen FK, Henrichsen J. Pneumococcal revaccination of splenectomized children. Pediatr Infect Dis J 9:258–263, 1990.
640. Konradsen HB, Henrichsen J. The need for revaccination 10 years after primary pneumococcal vaccination in splenectomized adults [letter]. Scand J Infect Dis 23:397, 1991.
641. MacLeod M, Hodges RG, Heidelberger M, Bernhard WG. Prevention of pneumococcal pneumonia by immunization with specific capsular polysaccharides. J Exp Med 82:445–465, 1945.
642. Herva E, Luotonen J, Timonen M. The effect of polyvalent pneumococcal polysaccharide vaccine on nasopharyngeal and nasal carriage of *Streptococcus pneumoniae*. Scand J Infect Dis 12:97–100, 1980.
643. Rosen C, Christensen P, Hovelius B, Prellner K. A longitudinal study of the nasopharyngeal carriage of pneumococci as related to pneumococcal vaccination in children attending day-care centres. Acta Otolaryngol (Stockh) 98:524–532, 1984.
644. Riley ID, Lehmann D, Alpers MP. Pneumococcal vaccine trials in Papua New Guinea: Relationships between epidemiology of pneumococcal infection and efficacy of vaccine. Rev Infect Dis 13(suppl 6):s535–s541, 1991.
645. Dagan R, Melamed R, Muallem M, et al. Reduction of nasopharyngeal carriage of pneumococci during the second year of life by a heptavalent conjugate pneumococcal vaccine. J Infect Dis 174:1271–1278, 1996.
646. Obaro SK, Adegbola RA, Banya WA, Greenwood BM. Carriage of pneumococci after pneumococcal vaccination [letter]. Lancet 348:271–272, 1996.
647. Douglas RM, Miles HB. Vaccination against *Streptococcus pneumoniae* in childhood: Lack of demonstrable benefit in young Australian children. J Infect Dis 149:861–869, 1984.
648. Mäkela PH, Leinonen M, Pukander J, Karma P. A study of the pneumococcal vaccine in prevention of clinically acute attacks of recurrent otitis media. Rev Infect Dis 3:s124–s132, 1981.
649. Teele DW, Klein JO. Use of pneumococcal vaccine for prevention of recurrent acute otitis media in infants in Boston. Rev Infect Dis 3:s113–s118, 1981.

650. Howie VM, Ploussard J, Sloyer JL, Hill JC. Use of pneumococcal polysaccharide vaccine in preventing otitis media in infants: Different results between racial groups. Pediatrics 73:79–81, 1984.
651. Riley ID, Lehmann D, Alpers MP, et al. Pneumococcal vaccine prevents death from acute lower-respiratory-tract infections in Papua New Guinean children. Lancet 2:877–881, 1986.
652. Lehmann D, Marshall TF, Riley ID, Alpers MP. Effect of pneumococcal vaccine on morbidity from acute lower respiratory tract infections in Papua New Guinean children. Ann Trop Paediatr 11:247–257, 1991.
653. Fiore AE, Elliott JA, Franklin AR, et al. Pneumococcal polysaccharide vaccine effectiveness among children of ages 2 through 5. Abstracts of the 35th Annual Meeting of the Infectious Diseases Society of America; San Francisco, CA; 1997; p 186.
654. Kaufman P. Pneumonia in old age active immunization against pneumonia with pneumococcal polysaccharide—results of a six year study. Arch Intern Med 79:518–531, 1947.
655. Simberkoff MS, Cross AP, Al-Ibrahim M, et al. Efficacy of pneumococcal vaccine in high-risk patients: Results of a Veterans Administration Cooperative Study. N Engl J Med 315:1318–1327, 1986.
656. Fedson DS. Pneumococcal vaccination in the prevention of community-acquired pneumonia: An optimistic view of cost-effectiveness. Semin Respir Infect 8:285–293, 1993.
657. Fedson DS, Shapiro ED, LaForce FM, et al. Pneumococcal vaccine after 15 years of use: Another view. Arch Intern Med 154:2531–2535, 1994.
658. Shapiro ED. Pneumococcal vaccine failure [letter]. N Engl J Med 316:1272–1273, 1987.
659. Gaillat J, Zmirou D, Mallaret M, et al. Clinical trial of pneumococcal vaccine among institutionalized elderly [French]. Rev Epidémiol Santé Publ 33:437–444, 1985.
659a. Örtqvist Å, Hedlund J, Burman LA, et al. Randomized trial of 23-valent pneumococcal capsular polysaccharide vaccine in the prevention of pneumonia in middle-aged and elderly people. Lancet 351:399–403, 1998.
660. Clemens JD, Shapiro ED. Resolving the pneumococcal vaccine controversy: Are there alternatives to randomized clinical trials? Rev Infect Dis 6:589–600, 1984.
661. Forrester HL, Jahnigen DW, LaForce FM. Inefficacy of pneumococcal vaccine in a high-risk population. Am J Med 83:425–430, 1987.
662. Sims RV, Steinmann WC, McConville JH, et al. The clinical effectiveness of pneumococcal vaccine in the elderly. Ann Intern Med 108:653–657, 1988.
663. Shapiro ED, Berg AT, Austrian R, et al. The protective efficacy of polyvalent pneumococcal polysaccharide vaccine. N Engl J Med 325:1453–1460, 1991.
664. Davidson M, Parkinson AJ, Bulkow LR, et al. Epidemiology of invasive pneumococcal disease—reply. J Infect Dis 171:1065–1066, 1995.
665. Farr BM, Johnston BL, Cobb DK, et al. Preventing pneumococcal bacteremia in patients at risk: Results of a matched case-control study. Arch Intern Med 155:2336–2340, 1995.
666. Butler JC, Breiman RF, Campbell JF, et al. Pneumococcal polysaccharide vaccine efficacy: An evaluation of current recommendations. JAMA 270:1826–1831, 1993.
666a. Gebo KA, Moore RD, Keruly JC, Chaisson RE. Risk factors for pneumococcal disease in human immunodeficiency virus-infected patients. J Infect Dis 173:857–862, 1996.
667. Nichol KL, Margolis KL, Wuorenma H, Von Sternberg T. The efficacy and cost-effectiveness of vaccination against influenza among elderly persons living in the community. N Engl J Med 331:778–784, 1994.
668. Simberkoff MS. Pneumococcal vaccine in the prevention of community-acquired pneumonia: A skeptical view of cost-effectiveness. Semin Respir Infect 8:294–299, 1993.
669. Hirschmann JV, Lipsky BA. The pneumococcal vaccine after 15 years of use. Arch Intern Med 154:373–377, 1994.
670. Fine MJ, Smith MA, Carson CA, et al. Efficacy of pneumococcal vaccination in adults: A meta-analysis of randomized controlled trials. Arch Intern Med 154:2666–2677, 1994.
671. Hak E, van Essen GA, Grobbee DE, Verheij ThJM. Effectiveness of pneumococcal vaccine [letter]. Lancet 351:1283, 1998.
672. Sisk JE, Riegelman RK. Cost effectiveness of vaccination against pneumococcal pneumonia: An update. Ann Intern Med 104:79–86, 1986.
673. Fedson DS. Influenza and pneumococcal vaccination of the elderly: Newer vaccines and prospects for clinical benefits at the margin. Prev Med 23:751–755, 1994.
674. Tengs TO, Adams ME, Pliskin JS, et al. Five-hundred life-saving interventions and their cost-effectiveness. Risk Anal 15:369–390, 1995.
675. Holzer SS, Gable CB, Friedman RB. Cost-effectiveness of pneumococcal vaccine: Implications for managed care. J Res Pharm Econ 5:79–95, 1993.
676. Baltussen RMPM, Ament AJHA, Leidl RM, van Furth R. Cost-effectiveness of vaccination against pneumococcal pneumonia in The Netherlands. Eur J Public Health 7:153–161, 1997.
677. Plans Rubio P, Garrido Morales P, Salleras Sanmarti L. The cost-effectiveness of pneumococcal vaccination in Catalonia [Spanish]. Rev Esp Salud Publica 69:409–417, 1995.
678. Jimenez FJ, Guallar P. Cost-effectiveness analysis of pneumococcal vaccination in the elderly Spanish population. Br J Med Econ 10:193–202, 1996.
679. Sisk JE, Moskowitz AJ, Whang W, et al. Cost-effectiveness of vaccination against pneumococcal bacteremia among elderly people. JAMA 278:1333–1339, 1997.
680. Russell LB, Gold MR, Siegel JE, et al. The role of cost-effectiveness analysis in health and medicine: Panel on Cost-Effectiveness in Health and Medicine. JAMA 276:1172–1177, 1996.
681. Weinstein MC, Siegel JE, Gold MR, et al. Recommendations of the Panel on Cost-effectiveness in Health and Medicine. JAMA 276:1253–1258, 1996.
682. Siegel JE, Weinstein MC, Russell LB. Recommendations for reporting cost-effectiveness analyses. JAMA 276:1339–1341, 1996.
683. Assessing adult vaccination status at age 50 years. MMWR Morb Mortal Wkly Rep 44:561–563, 1995.
684. Quick RE, Hoge CW, Hamilton DJ, et al. Underutilization of pneumococcal vaccine in nursing home in Washington State: Report of a serotype-specific outbreak and a survey. Am J Med 94:149–152, 1993.
685. Fedson DS. Pneumococcal vaccination in the United States and 20 other developed countries, 1981–1996. Clin Infect Dis 26:1117–1123, 1998.
686. Fedson DS, Hirota Y, Shin HK, et al. Influenza vaccination in 22 developed countries: An update to 1995. Vaccine 15:1506–1511, 1997.
687. Pneumococcal and influenza vaccination levels among adults aged ≥ 65 years—United States, 1993. MMWR Morb Mortal Wkly Rep 45:853–859, 1996.
688. Pneumococcal and influenza vaccination levels among adults aged 65 years—United States, 1995. MMWR Morb Mortal Wkly Rep 46:913–919, 1997.
689. Adult immunization: Knowledge, attitudes and practices—Dekalb and Fulton Counties, Georgia, 1988. MMWR Morb Mortal Wkly Rep 37:657–661, 1988.
690. Nichol KL, MacDonald R, Hauge M. Factors associated with influenza and pneumococcal vaccination behavior among high-risk adults. J Gen Intern Med 11:673–677, 1996.
691. Fedson DS. Influenza and pneumococcal immunization strategies for physicians. Chest 91:436–443, 1987.
692. Gyorkos TW, Tannenbaum TN, Abrahamowicz M, et al. Evaluation of the effectiveness of immunization delivery methods. Can J Public Health 85(suppl 1):s14–s30, 1994.
693. Rushton TC, Ganguly R, Sinnott JT4, Banerji M. Barriers to immunization—an examination of factors that influence the application of pneumococcal vaccine by house staff. Vaccine 12:1173–1179, 1994.
694. Fiebach N, Beckett W. Prevention of respiratory infections in adults: Influenza and pneumococcal vaccines. Arch Intern Med 154:2545–2557, 1994.
695. Herman CJ, Speroff T, Cebul RD. Improving compliance with immunization in the older adult: Results of a randomized cohort study. J Am Geriatr Soc 42:1154–1159, 1994.
696. Rodriguez RM, Baraff LJ. Emergency department immunization of the elderly with pneumococcal and influenza vaccines. Ann Emerg Med 22:1729–1732, 1993.

697. Wrenn K, Zeldin M, Miller O. Influenza and pneumococcal vaccination in the emergency department: Is it feasible? J Gen Intern Med 9:425–429, 1994.
698. Overhage JM, Tierney WM, McDonald CJ. Computer reminders to implement preventive care guidelines for hospitalized patients. Arch Intern Med 156:1551–1556, 1996.
699. Bloom HG, Bloom JS, Krasnoff L, Frank AD. Increased utilization of influenza and pneumococcal vaccines in an elderly hospitalized population. J Am Geriatr Soc 36:897–901, 1988.
700. Clancy CM, Gelfman D, Poses RM. A strategy to improve the utilization of pneumococcal vaccine. J Gen Intern Med 7:14–18, 1992.
701. Landis S, Scarbrough ML. Using a vaccine manager to enhance in-hospital vaccine administration. J Fam Pract 41:364–369, 1995.
702. Silcox MM, Selph AK, Armbruster P, et al. Postsplenectomy sepsis: A case review and one hospital's campaign to prevent other needless tragedies. J Emerg Nurs 17:15–18, 1991.
703. Increasing pneumococcal vaccination rates among patients of a National Health-Care Alliance—United States, 1993. MMWR Morb Mortal Wkly Rep 44:741–744, 1995.
704. Pneumococcal immunization program—California, 1986–1988. MMWR Morb Mortal Wkly Rep 38:517–519, 1989.
705. Campbell JF, Donohue MA, Nevin-Woods C, et al. The Hawaii pneumococcal disease initiative. Am J Public Health 83:1175–1176, 1993.
706. Comprehensive delivery of adult vaccination—Minnesota, 1986–1992. MMWR Morb Mortal Wkly Rep 42:768–770, 1993.
707. Davidson M, Chamblee C, Campbell HG, et al. Pneumococcal vaccination in a remote population of high-risk Alaska Natives. Public Health Rep 108:439–446, 1993.
708. Fedson DS. Clinical practice and public policy for influenza and pneumococcal vaccination of the elderly. Clin Geriatr Med 8:183–199, 1992.
709. McBean AM, Babish JD, Prihoda R. The utilization of pneumococcal polysaccharide vaccine among elderly Medicare beneficiaries, 1985 through 1988. Arch Intern Med 151:2009–2016, 1991.
710. Fedson DS. Adult immunization: Summary of the National Vaccine Advisory Committee report. JAMA 272:1133–1137, 1994.
711. Lee JS. Adult immunization priorities in the United States. Milbank Q 74:285–307, 1996.
712. Orenstein WA, Tilghman J. A closer look at adult immunization in the United States. Milbank Q 74:309–316, 1996.
713. Fedson D, Henrichsen J, Makela PH, Austrian R. Immunization of elderly people with polyvalent pneumococcal vaccine. Infection 17:437–441, 1989.
714. Fedson DS. Influenza and pneumococcal vaccination in Canada and the United States, 1980–1993: What can the two countries learn from each other? Clin Infect Dis 20:1371–1376, 1995.
715. Klein DL, Ellis RW. Conjugate vaccines against *Streptococcus pneumoniae.* In Levine MM, Woodrow GC, Kaper JB, Cobon GS (eds). New Generation Vaccines (2nd ed). New York, Marcel Dekker, 1997, pp 503–526.
716. Avery OT. Chemoimmunological studies on conjugated carbohydrate proteins: II. Immunological specificity of synthetic sugar-protein antigens. J Exp Med 50:533–550, 1929.
717. Robbins JB, Schneerson R. Polysaccharide-protein conjugates: A new generation of vaccines. J Infect Dis 161:821–832, 1990.
718. Siber GR. Pneumococcal disease: Prospects for a new generation of vaccines. Science 265:1385–1387, 1994.
719. Eby R. Pneumococcal conjugate vaccines. Pharm Biotechnol 6:695–718, 1995.
720. Kayhty H, Eskola J. New vaccines for the prevention of pneumococcal infections. Emerg Infect Dis 2:289–298, 1996.
721. van den Dobbelsteen GP, Kroes H, van Rees EP. Characteristics of immune responses to native and protein conjugated pneumococcal polysaccharide type 14. Scand J Immunol 41:273–280, 1995.
722. Alonso de Velasco E, Merkus D, Anderton S, et al. Synthetic peptides representing T-cell epitopes act as carriers in pneumococcal polysaccharide conjugate vaccines. Infect Immun 63:961–968, 1995.
723. Alonso de Velasco E, Verheul AF, van Steijn AM, et al. Epitope specificity of rabbit immunoglobulin G (IgG) elicited by pneumococcal type 23F synthetic oligosaccharide- and native polysaccharide-protein conjugate vaccines: Comparison with human anti-polysaccharide 23F IgG. Infect Immun 62:799–808, 1994.
724. Schneerson R, Levi L, Robbins JB, et al. Synthesis of a conjugate vaccine composed of pneumococcus type 14 capsular polysaccharide bound to pertussis toxin. Infect Immun 60:3528–3532, 1992.
725. Paton JC, Lock RA, Lee CJ, et al. Purification and immunogenicity of genetically obtained pneumolysin toxoids and their conjugation to *Streptococcus pneumoniae* type 19F polysaccharide. Infect Immun 59:2297–2304, 1991.
726. Lee CJ, Lock RA, Andrew PW, et al. Protection of infant mice from challenge with *Streptococcus pneumoniae* type 19F by immunization with a type 19F polysaccharide-pneumolysoid conjugate. Vaccine 12:875–878, 1994.
727. Kuo J, Douglas M, Ree HK, Lindberg AA. Characterization of a recombinant pneumolysin and its use as a protein carrier for pneumococcal type 18C conjugate vaccines. Infect Immun 63:2706–2713, 1995.
728. Powers DC, Anderson EL, Lottenbach K, Mink CM. Reactogenicity and immunogenicity of a protein-conjugated pneumococcal oligosaccharide vaccine in older adults. J Infect Dis 173:1014–1018, 1996.
729. Ahmed F, Steinhoff MC, Rodriguez Barradas MC, et al. Effect of human immunodeficiency virus type 1 infection on the antibody response to a glycoprotein conjugate pneumococcal vaccine: Results from a randomized trial. J Infect Dis 173:83–90, 1996.
730. Kayhty H, Ahman H, Ronnberg PR, et al. Pneumococcal polysaccharide-meningococcal outer membrane protein complex conjugate vaccine is immunogenic in infants and children. J Infect Dis 172:1273–1278, 1995.
731. Steinhoff MC, Edwards K, Keyserling H, et al. A randomized comparison of three bivalent *Streptococcus pneumoniae* glycoprotein conjugate vaccines in young children: Effect of polysaccharide size and linkage characteristics. Pediatr Infect Dis J 13:368–372, 1994.
732. Pichichero ME, Shelly MA, Treanor JJ. Evaluation of a pentavalent conjugated pneumococcal vaccine in toddlers. Pediatr Infect Dis J 16:72–74, 1997.
733. Antilla M, Eskola J, Kayhty H. Opsonic activity and concentration of antibodies to *Streptococcus pneumoniae* type 6B polysaccharide. Abstracts of the 35th Annual Meeting of the Infectious Diseases Society of America; San Francisco, CA; 1997; p 183.
733a. Musher DM, Groover JE, Rodriguez-Barradas MC, Baughn RE. IgG responses to protein-conjugated pneumococcal capsular polysaccharides in persons who are genetically incapable of responding to unconjugated polysaccharides. Clin Infect Dis 111:222–233, 1998.
734. Molrine DC, George S, Tarbell N, et al. Antibody responses to polysaccharide and polysaccharide-conjugate vaccines after treatment of Hodgkin disease. Ann Intern Med 123:828–834, 1995.
735. Chan CY, Molrine DC, George S, et al. Pneumococcal conjugate vaccine primes for antibody responses to polysaccharide pneumococcal vaccine after treatment of Hodgkin's disease. J Infect Dis 173:256–258, 1996.
736. Sarnaik S, Kaplan J, Schiffman G, et al. Studies on pneumococcus vaccine alone or mixed with DTP and a pneumococcus type 6B and *Haemophilus influenzae* type b capsular polysaccharide-tetanus toxoid conjuguates in two- to five-year-old children with sickle cell anemia. Pediatr Infect Dis J 9:181–186, 1990.
737. King JC, Vink PE, Farley JJ, et al. Safety and immunogenicity of three doses of a five-valent pneumococcal conjugate vaccine in children younger than two years with and without human immunodeficiency virus infection. Pediatrics 99:575–580, 1997.
738. King JC, Vink PE, Farley JJ, et al. Comparison of the safety and immunogenicity of a pneumococcal conjugate with a licensed polysaccharide vaccine in human immunodeficiency virus-infected and non-human immunodeficiency virus-infected children. Pediatr Infect Dis J 15:192–196, 1996.
739. Ahman H, Kayhty H, Tamminen P, et al. Pentavalent pneumococcal oligosaccharide conjugate vaccine PncCRM is well-tolerated and able to induce an antibody response in infants. Pediatr Infect Dis J 15:134–139, 1996.
740. Leach A, Ceesay SJ, Banya WAS, Greenwood BM. Pilot trial of a pentavalent pneumococcal polysaccharide/protein conjugate

vaccine in Gambian infants. Pediatr Infect Dis J 15:333–339, 1996.

741. Daum RS, Hogerman D, Rennels MB, Bewley K. Infant immunization with pneumococcal CRM 197 vaccines: Effect of saccharide size on immunogenicity and interactions with simultaneously administered vaccines. J Infect Dis 176:445–455, 1997.
742. O'Brien KL, Steinhoff MC, Edwards K, et al. Immunologic priming of young children by pneumococcal glycoprotein conjugate, but not polysaccharide, vaccines. Pediatr Infect Dis J 15:425–430, 1996.
743. Lu CH, Lee CJ, Kind P. Immune responses of young mice to pneumococcal type 9V polysaccharide-tetanus toxoid conjugate. Infect Immun 62:2754–2760, 1994.
744. Anderson EL, Kennedy DJ, Geldmacher KM, et al. Immunogenicity of heptavalent pneumococcal conjugate vaccine in infants. J Pediatr 128:649–653, 1996.
745. Sigurdardottir ST, Vidarsson G. Immune responses of infants vaccinated with serotype 6B pneumococcal polysaccharide conjugated with tetanus toxoid. Pediatr Infect Dis J 16:667–674, 1997.
746. Giebink GS, Koskela M, Vella PP, et al. Pneumococcal capsular polysaccharide-meningococcal outer membrane protein complex conjugate vaccines: Immunogenicity and efficacy in experimental pneumococcal otitis media. J Infect Dis 167:347–355, 1993.
747. Giebink GS, Meier JD, Quartey MK, et al. Immunogenicity and efficacy of *Streptococcus pneumoniae* polysaccharide-protein conjugate vaccines against homologous and heterologous serotypes in the chinchilla otitis media model. J Infect Dis 173:119–127, 1996.
748. Lue C, Prince SJ, Fattom A. Antibody-secreting peripheral blood lymphocytes induced by immunization with a conjugate consisting of *Streptococcus pneumoniae* type 12F polysaccharide and diphtheria toxoid. Infect Immun 58:2547–2554, 1990.
749. Nieminen T, Virolainen A, Kayhty H, et al. Antibody-secreting cells and their relation to humoral antibodies in serum and in nasopharyngeal aspirates in children with pneumococcal acute otitis media. J Infect Dis 173:136–141, 1996.
750. Dagan R, Muallem M, Melamed R, et al. Reduction of pneumococcal nasopharyngeal carriage in early infancy after immunization with tetravalent pneumococcal vaccines conjugated to either tetanus toxoid of diphtheria toxoid. Pediatr Infect Dis J 16:1060–1064, 1997.
751. Kristinsson KG, Sigurdardottir ST, Gudnason T, et al. Effect of vaccination with octavalent protein conjugated pneumococcal vaccines on pneumococcal carriage in infants. Abstracts of the 37th Interscience Conference on Antimicrobial Agents and Chemotherapy; Toronto; 1997; p 193.
752. Mbelle N, Wasas A, Huebner R, et al. Immunogenicity and impact on carriage of 9-valent pneumococcal conjugate vaccine given to infants in Soweto, South Africa. Abstracts of the 37th Interscience Conference on Antimicrobial Agents and Chemotherapy [program addendum]; Toronto; 1997; p 13.
753. Dagan R, Givon N, Yagupsky P, et al. Effect of a 9-valent pneumococcal vaccine conjugated to CRM<197 (PncCRM9) on nasopharyngeal (NP) carriage of vaccine type and non-vaccine type *S. pneumoniae* (Pnc) strains among day care center (DCC) attendees, abstract G52 of 38th Interscience Conference on Antimicrobial Agents and Chemotherapy. San Diego, Sept 24–27, 1998.
754. Orange M, Gray BM. Pneumococcal serotypes causing disease in children in Alabama. Pediatr Infect Dis J 12:244–246, 1993.
755. Shapiro ED, Austrian R. Serotypes responsible for invasive *Streptococcus pneumoniae* infections among children in Connecticut. J Infect Dis 169:212–214, 1994.
756. Parkinson AJ, Davidson M, Fitzgerald MA, et al. Serotype distribution and antimicrobial resistance patterns of invasive isolates of *Streptococcus pneumoniae*: Alaska 1986–1990. J Infect Dis 170:461–464, 1994.
757. Reinert RR, Kaufhold A, Schlaeger JJ, et al. Serotype distribution and antibiotic susceptibility of *Streptococcus pneumoniae* isolates causing systemic infections among children in Germany, 1992 to 1996. Pediatr Infect Dis J 16:244–245, 1997.
758. Hortal M, Algorta G, Bianchi I. Capsular type distribution and susceptibility to antibiotics of *Streptococcus pneumoniae* clinical strains isolated from Uruguayan children with systemic infections. Microb Drug Resist 3:159–163, 1997.
758a. Brandileone MCdC, Viera VSD, Casagrande ST, et al. Prevalence of serotypes and antimicrobial resistance of *Streptococcus pneumoniae* strains isolated from Brazilian children with invasive infections. Microb Drug Resist 3:141–146, 1997.
758b. Black S, Shinefield H, Ray P, et al. Efficacy of heptavalent conjugate pneumococcal vaccine (Wyeth Lederle) in 37,000 infants and children: Results of the Northern California Kaiser Permanente Efficacy Trial, abstract LB9 of 38th Interscience Conference on Antimicrobial Agents and Chemotherapy, San Diego, Sept. 24–27, 1998.
759. Eskola J, Kayhty H, Takala AK. A randomized prospective field trial of a conjugate vaccine in the protection of infants and young children against invasive *Haemophilus influenzae* type b disease. N Engl J Med 323:1381–1387, 1990.
760. Schlesinger Y, Granoff D. Avidity and bactericidal activity of antibody elicited by different *Haemophilus influenzae* type b conjugates vaccines. JAMA 267:1489–1494, 1992.
761. Kayhty H. Difficulties in establishing a serological correlate of protection after immunization with *Haemophilus influenzae* conjugate vaccines. Biologicals 22:397–402, 1994.
762. Granoff DM, Lucas AH. Laboratory correlates of protection against *Haemophilus influenzae* type b disease: Importance of assessment of antibody avidity and immunologic memory. Ann N Y Acad Sci 754:278–288, 1995.
763. Antilla M, Eskola J, Kayhty H. Avidity of IgG antibodies to capsular polysaccharides of *Streptococcus pneumoniae* elicited by pneumococcal conjugates. Abstracts of the 35th Annual Meeting of the Infectious Diseases Society of America; San Francisco, CA; 1997; p 183.
764. Berry AM, Paton JC, Hansman D. Effect of insertional inactivation of the genes encoding pneumolysin and autolysin on the virulence of *Streptococcus pneumoniae* type 3. Microb Pathog 12:87–93, 1992.
765. Russell H, Tharpe JA. Monoclonal antibody recognizing a species-specific protein from *Streptococcus pneumoniae*. J Clin Microbiol 28:2191–2195, 1990.
766. Tart RC, McDaniel LS, Ralph BA, Briles DE. Truncated *Streptococcus pneumoniae* PspA molecules elicit cross-protective immunity against pneumococcal challenge in mice. J Infect Dis 173:380–386, 1996.
767. Yamamoto M, McDaniel LS, Kawabata K, et al. Oral immunization with PspA elicits protective humoral immunity against *Streptococcus pneumoniae* infection. Infect Immun 65:640–644, 1997.
768. Berry AM, Paton JC. Sequence heterogeneity of PsaA, a 37-kilodalton putative adhesin essential for virulence of *Streptococcus pneumoniae*. Infect Immun 64:5255–5262, 1996.
769. Fedson DS. Pneumococcal vaccination: Four issues for Western Europe. Biologicals 25:215–220, 1997.
770. Wischnack LL, Jacobson RM, Poland GA, et al. The surprisingly high acceptability of low-efficacy vaccines for otitis media: A survey of parents using hypothetical scenarios. Pediatrics 95:350–354, 1995.
771. Robbins JB, Schneerson R, Anderson P, Smith DH. Prevention of systemic infections, especially meningitis, caused by *Haemophilus influenzae* type b: Impact on public health and implications for other polysaccharide-based vaccines. JAMA 276:1181–1185, 1996.
772. Hausdorff WP. Prospects for the use of new vaccines in developing countries: Cost is not the only impediment. Vaccine 14:1179–1186, 1996.
773. Levine MM, Levine OS. Influence of disease burden, public perception, and other factors of new vaccine development, implementation and continued use. Lancet 350:1386–1392, 1997.
774. Ashley RV, Murray CJL. Economic perspectives on vaccine needs. In Kaufman SHE (ed). Concepts in Vaccine Development. Berlin, de Gruyter, 1996, pp 27–69.
775. Miller MA, Schwartz B. Assessment of pneumococcal conjugate vaccine incorporation into the Global Expanded Programme on Immunization. Abstracts of the 37th Interscience Conference on Antimicrobial Agents and Chemotherapy; Toronto; 1997; p 383.
776. Murray CJL, Lopez AD. Mortality by cause for eight regions of the world: Global burden of disease study. Lancet 349:1269–1276, 1997.
777. Kitange HM, Machibya H, Black J. Outlook for survivors of childhood in sub-Saharan Africa: Adult mortality in Tanzania. Br Med J 312:216–220, 1996.
778. Kantor E, Luxenberg JS, Lucas AH. Phase I study of the immunogenicity and safety of conjugated *Hemophilus influenzae* type b vaccines in the elderly. Vaccine 15:129–132, 1997.

VACCINES FOR SPECIAL RISK GROUPS AND SELECTED GEOGRAPHICAL AREAS

chapter

23 Adenovirus Vaccines

Charlotte A. Gaydos
Joel C. Gaydos

Adenoviruses have been associated with many clinical syndromes, particularly with a variety of infections that affect the respiratory tract, the gastrointestinal system, and the eye. The virus, which was recovered from surgically removed human adenoids, was first isolated by Rowe and coworkers as "adenoid degeneration agent" in 1953.[1] Hilleman and Werner independently reported the isolation of "respiratory illness agents" from an acute respiratory disease epidemic at Fort Leonard Wood, Missouri.[2] References to clinical keratoconjunctivitis and "shipyard eye" probably caused by adenoviruses were made as early as 1889 and in the 1940s.[3, 4] These agents comprised a group of related viruses associated with several clinical syndromes such as acute respiratory disease, pharyngitis, conjunctivitis, pneumonitis, and atypical pneumonia.[5] They were named adenoviruses by a committee chaired by Enders.[6] Certain types of adenoviruses soon became identified as causes of severe epidemics of acute respiratory disease in military recruit populations.[7]

Adenovirus infections can be fatal in immunocompromised patients and a cause of serious infection and pneumonia in children, especially infants.[8–13] They have also been associated with infections in acquired immunodeficiency syndrome (AIDS) and bone marrow transplant patients.[14, 15] Acute hemorrhagic cystitis and other infections in patients with immune deficiencies are often fatal.[11, 15] Adenovirus infections are responsible for approximately 10% of pneumonia cases in hospitalized children and cause up to 15% of cases of gastroenteritis in infants and children.[8, 16, 17] Epidemic keratoconjunctivitis, usually caused by adenovirus type 8 or 37, is a severe eye disease that may lead to subepithelial corneal keratitis.[18, 19]

By the 1960s, adenoviruses were recognized as causes of significant respiratory illness in military populations.[7, 20, 21] As many as 80% of recruits developed adenovirus infections, of which 20% required hospitalization.[20] Median attack rates for new recruits ranged from 6 to 16.7 per 100 per month at the most affected military posts in the North and Midwest and from 2.3 to 2.6 per 100 per month for posts in the South and West.[21] The loss of up to 40% of the men in a training unit within a 2-week period, the requirement to restart training for those men who were hospitalized, and the costs associated with excessive hospitalizations, additional medical personnel, and additional training presented serious problems for which an immediate solution was urgently needed.[22] In addition to the severe morbidity suffered by military trainees, at least three pneumonia deaths associated with adenovirus type 7 were recorded for young, otherwise healthy trainees undergoing Army basic training.[23]

BACKGROUND

Clinical Description

A variety of clinical syndromes have been associated with the 47 serotypes of human adenoviruses that have been described (Table 23–1). Two new adenoviruses, which have been isolated mainly from AIDS patients, have been proposed as serotypes 48 and 49.[24] Excellent reviews describing the most common serotypes associated with particular diseases have been published.[25–28]

Endemic Respiratory Adenovirus in Children. Although most children become infected with some of the common adenoviruses early in life, only about 50% of these infections result in disease.[25, 29, 30] Up to 80% of children acquire antibodies to adenovirus types 1, 2, and 5.[30–32] Isolation studies indicate that adenovirus types 1, 2, 5, 3, and 6 are most common, in that order.[25] The syndromes of ill children include pharyngitis, bronchitis, bronchiolitis, croup, and pneumonia.[10, 33] Pneumonia may occasionally be fatal, especially when it is associated with adenovirus type 7.[34–37] The incidence of diseases

Table 23–1. **CLINICAL SYNDROMES ASSOCIATED WITH ADENOVIRUS INFECTIONS**

CLINICAL SYNDROME	SUBGENUS	COMMON SEROTYPES	POPULATION AT RISK
Endemic respiratory	B, C	1, 2, 3, 5, 6, 7	Infants, children
Epidemic respiratory	B, C	5, 7	Children (daycare)
Acute respiratory disease	B, E	3, 4, 7, 14, 21	Military recruits
Pharyngoconjunctival fever	B, C, E	1, 3, 4, 7, 14	School-aged children, young adults
Keratoconjunctivitis	B, D	8, 11, 19, 37	All age groups
Hemorrhagic cystitis	B	11, 21, 34, 35	Immunocompromised patients, children
Infantile gastroenteritis	F, G	40, 41	Children
Other syndromes	B, C, E, D	2, 4, 7, 12, 19, 32, 37	Children, adults
Immune deficiency	B, D	34, 35, 43–49	Transplant patients, AIDS patients, immunocompromised

AIDS, acquired immunodeficiency syndrome.

caused by adenoviruses is higher in late winter, spring, and early summer, and both sexes are equally affected.[29, 38] The mode of transmission in children is thought to be primarily fecal-oral.[30]

Epidemic Respiratory Adenovirus in Children. On occasion, epidemics occur in daycare facilities and orphanages, especially with adenovirus types 5 and 7 but also with other types.[39, 40]

Acute Respiratory Disease of Military Recruits. In young adults who live in closed communities such as boarding schools and military recruit camps, adenoviruses may cause epidemics of illnesses similar to influenza, including tracheobronchitis and pneumonia severe enough to require hospitalization.[2, 7, 41, 42] The incubation period of the disease is 4 to 5 days.[42] Before the use of vaccines in the U.S. military, adenovirus types 4 and 7 accounted for 60% of all respiratory illnesses in recruits who were hospitalized; types 3, 14, and 21 were less frequently observed.[21] At some northern basic training posts, peak rates of 6 to 8 per 100 men per week translated into 600 to 800 acute respiratory disease hospitalized admissions per week.[22]

Typical acute respiratory disease is a febrile disease with symptoms of sore throat, fever, cough, coryza, rhinorrhea, headache, and chest pain.[2, 25, 42] Physical examinations reveal rales and rhonchi with little evidence of consolidation, and chest radiography shows patchy interstitial infiltrates, principally in the lower lung fields.[2, 28, 42] Symptoms last 3 to 10 days.[25] The infection is characteristically self-limited, no specific therapy exists, and superinfection and death are rare but do occur.[2, 23] Transmission is thought to occur primarily through inhalation of aerosolized virus into the lung. The virus is not demonstrable in the respiratory tract after 4 days.[2, 43] Up to 7% of pneumonia cases during an 18-month period in naval military recruits were caused by adenoviruses.[44]

Pharyngoconjunctival Fever. This syndrome is characterized by pharyngitis, conjunctivitis, and spiking fever.[45] First described in the 1920s as associated with swimming, the cause has been subsequently linked to insufficient chlorination.[46–48] Either one or both eyes are affected, and diarrhea, coryza, tonsillar exudate, and lymphadenopathy may be observed. The most frequent association has been with adenovirus types 3 and 7, but other types such as 1, 4, and 14 have been observed.[45] The disease is associated with summer camps, swimming pools, and lakes and occurs in children and young adults, often spreading to other family members.[45, 48, 49] The incubation period is 6 to 9 days, and the virus may be isolated from pool water.[45, 47] There is little bacterial superinfection and no permanent damage to the eye.[28]

Epidemic Keratoconjunctivitis. Epidemics of conjunctivitis in adults caused by adenoviruses were first described by German investigators and later by Jawetz[4] and others[50] as shipyard eye. The disease was observed at industrial settings where shipbuilding took place and was probably transmitted when workers sought care for chemical irritation and minor trauma from paint and rust chips.[4] The disease, with an incubation time of 8 to 10 days, is characterized by conjunctivitis, edema of the eye, pain, photophobia, and lacrimation. Superficial erosions as well as subepithelial infiltrates of the cornea can occur.[25] Preauricular lymph gland swelling and involvement of cervical and submaxillary lymph glands may be observed.[25]

The disease has been associated with adenovirus types 8, 19, and 37 and rarely other types.[51–55] In addition, adenovirus types 19 and 37 have been isolated from the genital tract of young adults with epidemic keratoconjunctivitis, and the possibility of sexual transmission has been considered.[56, 57] Many epidemics of epidemic keratoconjunctivitis have been associated with ophthalmology practices, where spread from contaminated ophthalmic solutions, fingers, and instruments has been implicated.[51, 52, 54, 58, 59]

Hemorrhagic Cystitis. Hemorrhagic cystitis syndrome in children has been shown to be caused by adenovirus infections in 23 to 51% of cases in America and Japan.[60] Although the route of spread is unknown, adenovirus types 11 and 21 (group B adenoviruses), which are uncommon in respiratory infections, were isolated most frequently.[60] Boys were two to three times more commonly affected than girls. Clinical findings included gross hematuria of 3 days' duration. Dysuria, microscopic hematuria, and urinary frequency lasted a few days longer.[60, 61] No viremia or structural abnormalities were found. Adenoviral antigen in exfoliated bladder epithelial cells can be demonstrated by immunofluorescence.[60] Cases of acute hemorrhagic cystitis after renal and bone marrow transplantation have been increasingly reported.[62, 63] Adenovirus types 34 and 35, also group B adenoviruses, were first isolated from renal transplant patients, but neither was associated with symptoms of hemorrhagic cystitis.[64] Tubulointerstitial nephritis due to adenovirus type 11 in adults and children receiving bone marrow transplants has been described.[65]

Infantile Gastroenteritis. Adenoviruses were first visualized by electron microscopy as etiological agents of diarrhea, but they could not be grown on standard tissue culture cells. These adenoviruses are defective and require transformed human embryonic kidney (HEK) cells or Chang's conjunctival cells for isolation. They can be detected by enzyme immunoassay.[66–68] Numerous outbreaks have been described, and adenoviruses may account for up to 12% of all infant diarrhea.[69–71] The diarrhea is watery, is usually associated with fever, and may last 1 to 2 weeks.[28] The etiological serotypes, adenovirus types 40 and 41, are related serologically and belong to subgenus F and subgenus G, respectively.

Other Syndromes Associated with Adenoviral Infections. Encephalitis as well as meningoencephalitis cases associated with adenoviruses have occurred occasionally.[72, 73] Fatal neonatal disseminated infections with adenovirus types 4, 7, 12, and 32 have been reported.[74] A pertussis-like syndrome has also been described, as has a relationship between pertussis and infections with adenoviruses.[64, 75–78] Persistent adenoviral infection has also been associated with chronic airway obstruction in children.[79] Adenovirus types 2, 19, and 37 have been isolated from genital lesions and have been associated with orchitis, urethritis, and cervicitis.[27] Nosocomial transmission to susceptible healthcare workers and other patients has been reported, probably related to the long periods that the virus is secreted in the stool, the possible aerosolization of the virus, and fomite transmission.[27]

Association with Immunocompromised Patients. Adenoviruses have been implicated as opportunistic agents in patients with immune deficiency states, such as those with AIDS, receiving cancer chemotherapy, having bone marrow transplants, or undergoing renal and lung transplantation.[13, 14, 63, 80–84] These patients are prone to pneumonia and disseminated adenoviral infection. Adenovirus type 35 has been associated with urinary tract disease in people with AIDS.[85] Some of the newer types, such as 43 to 47, have been discovered in AIDS patients.[85] Adenoviruses have also been described as a cause of parotitis in patients with AIDS.[86]

A review of 201 bone marrow recipients during 4 years indicated that adenovirus infections occurred in 20.9% of patients, with a higher incidence in pediatric patients than in adult patients (31.3% versus 13.6%, P = .003).[87] Type 35 was the most common serotype identified.[87] Thirty-one percent of patients (13 of 42) with isolates had adenovirus disease, and 7 died.[87] An excellent review of adenoviruses in the immunocompromised host was done by Hierholzer.[88] Adenovirus infections in these patients were associated with case-fatality rates as high as 60% in those with pneumonia, compared with only 15% in immunocompetent hosts with pneumonia. Radiographs often demonstrate patchy interstitial infiltrates usually in the lower lung fields.[89] Figure 23–1 shows the chest radiograph of a 20-year-old recipient of an autologous bone marrow transplant for diffuse large-cell lymphoma (B-cell type) with systemic adenovirus type 11 infection, which was obtained on day 45 after transplantation. He expired on day 80.

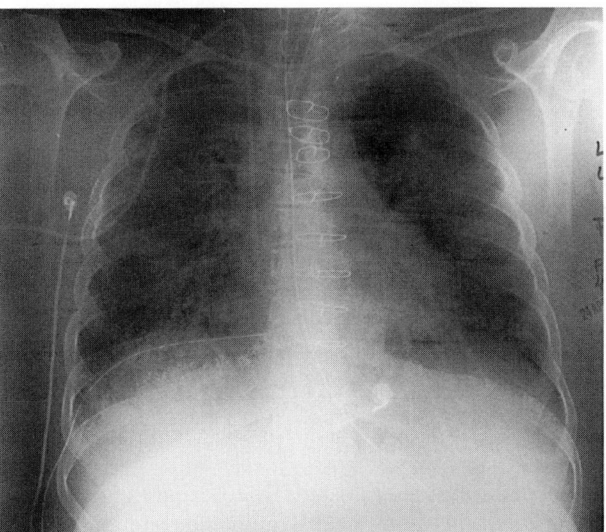

Figure 23–1. Pneumonia caused by adenovirus type 11 in a 20-year-old recipient of an autologous bone marrow transplant. (Courtesy of Stuart Ray, M.D., Johns Hopkins University, Baltimore, MD.)

Adenovirus was recovered from conjunctival, urine, and bronchoalveolar lavage cultures. Similarly, a case-fatality rate of 50% occurred in immunocompromised people with hepatitis and associated adenovirus infections, compared with 10% in similarly infected immunocompetent patients with hepatitis.[88]

Virology

Human adenoviruses are double-stranded, nonenveloped DNA viruses belonging to the genus *Mastadenovirus*, family *Adenoviridae*. The capsid demonstrates icosahedral symmetry and contains 252 capsomers. The capsomers consist of 240 hexons and 12 pentons with a projecting fiber on each of the pentons (Fig. 23–2). The pentons and hexons are each derived from different viral polypeptides. The fibers, which are responsible for type-specific antibodies, vary in length among human strains and are sometimes absent in some animal strains.[90–93] The hexons are group-specific antigens, primarily inducing group-specific complement-fixing antibodies, whereas the pentons are especially active in hemagglutination.[94] The virions are 70 to 90 nm in diameter and composed of 10 structural proteins with molecular weights of 5000 to 120,000.[27] In cesium chloride, they have a buoyant density of 1.33 to 1.34 g/cm^3 and a molecular weight of 170 $\times$ 10^6 to 175 $\times$ 10^6 by sedimentation coefficient.[27] There is a single molecule of linear, double-stranded DNA of 20 $\times$ 10^6 to 24 $\times$ 10^6 molecular weight inside the capsid, and the G + C base compositions of the human virus genomes range from 47 to 60%.[87, 95]

Adenoviruses are unusually stable to physical and chemical agents, as well as adverse pH, and thus survive for long periods outside the host, making them available for transmission to others. They can be destroyed by heat at 56°C for 30 minutes, ultraviolet irradiation, 0.25% sodium dodecyl sulfate, chlorine at 0.5 μg/mL,

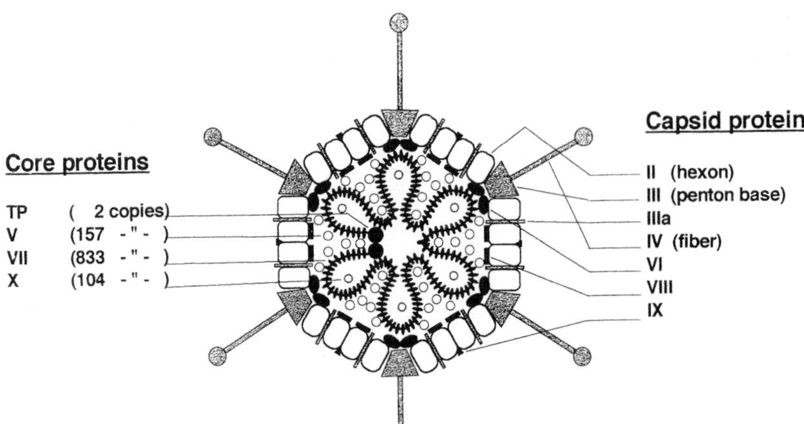

Figure 23–2. Schematic model illustrating the adenovirus particle. The tentative location and copy number of peptides are indicated for the core and capsid proteins. (From Russkanen O, Meurman O, Kusjavi A. Adenoviruses. In Richman DD, Whitley RJ, Hayden FG [eds]. Clinical Virology. New York, Churchill Livingstone, 1997, pp 525–547.)

and formalin but are resistant to ether and chloroform. These viruses replicate in the cell nucleus, tending to be host specific. By determination in reference horse antisera, there are 49 serotypes of human adenoviruses now accepted or proposed, and these have been grouped into subgenera A to G.[96] Historically, hemagglutination properties have also allowed a separation of the human adenoviruses into the subgenera A to G, with the scheme being based primarily on complete agglutination of monkey or rat erythrocytes, partial agglutination of rat erythrocytes, and level of agglutination and secondarily on complete agglutination of human, chicken, and other erythrocytes[27, 28] (Table 23–2).

Some adenovirus serotypes have been determined to be oncogenic in animals and to transform cell lines, but oncogenicity has not been observed in humans. This potential and other viral properties, such as percentage of DNA homology, percentage of G + C content of the DNA, and restriction fragment analysis with *Sma*I endonuclease enzyme, have also been applied to classification schemes and appear to support the existing typing scheme[95–99] (see Table 23–2). Use of restriction endonucleases has also demonstrated that variants of the same serotype can occur.[100] For example, adenovirus type 7 isolates from five continents have been subdivided into 15 different genotypes.[101] Similarly, restriction endonuclease typing has been applied to adenovirus types 3 and 4, as well as types 3 and 7 from pneumonia cases.[102–105] Hybridization or genetic recombination of viruses may occur in vivo, and types 34 and 35 may be recombinants with type 7.[82, 83]

Pathogenesis

Depending on the route of inoculation, the serotype, and the immune state of the host, adenoviruses can cause diseases or asymptomatic infections in the respiratory tract and in other sites. Respiratory infection is presumed to result primarily from inhalation of aerosolized virus; ocular infection, gastroenteritis, and nosocomial infections may arise from fomites, water, or fecal-oral contamination. Reactivation of the latent virus is believed to occur.[42] Some 50% of tonsils removed surgically may have adenoviruses isolated from the tissue, suggesting that these viruses may stay in a latent state for long periods.[106] Virus has also been isolated from lymphocytes, kidney, blood, cerebrospinal fluid, and most body organs.[13, 14, 34, 36, 73, 82, 88, 107–109] In the lungs, extensive pathologic change has been found with microscopic necrosis of the tracheal and bronchial epithelium.[25] Acidophilic intranuclear inclusions are seen in bronchial epithelial cells in addition to basophilic masses of cells surrounded by clear halos, which may indicate aggregations of viral material.[34] A mononuclear infil-

Table 23–2. **CLASSIFICATION SCHEMES FOR ADENOVIRUSES OF HUMANS**

SUBGENUS*	HEMAGGLUTINATION GROUP	SEROTYPES	TUMORS IN ANIMALS	TRANSFORMING POTENTIAL	PERCENTAGE OF G + C in DNA
A	Rat (incomplete)	12, 18, 31	High potential	Moderate	48–49
B	Monkey (complete)	3, 7, 11, 14, 16, 21, 34, 35	Moderate	Moderate	50–52
C	Rat (incomplete)	1, 2, 5, 6	Low or none	Low	57–59
D	Rat (complete)	8, 9, 10, 13, 15, 17, 19, 20, 22–30, 32, 33, 36–39, 42, 43–47	Low or none	Moderate	57–61
E	Rat (incomplete)	4	Low or none	Low	57–59
F	Rat (atypical)	40	None	None	Not done
G	Rat (atypical)	41	None	None	Not done

Adapted from Baum SG. Adenovirus. In Mandell GL, Bennett JE, Dolin R. Principles and Practice of Infectious Diseases. New York, Churchill Livingstone, 1995, pp 1082–1387.

*Subgenus is also referred to as a subgroup.

trate, rosette formation, and focal necrosis of mucous glands are characteristically seen.[25]

Three types of interaction of virus with infected cells may occur. A lytic infection may take place during which the virus completes an entire replicative cycle.[28] From 10^5 to 10^6 progeny viruses per cell may be produced, of which only 1 to 5% are actually infectious.[28] The second type of interaction is the chronic, inapparent, or latent infection; small amounts of virus may be produced, and an inapparent infection results. Viral shedding from the gastrointestinal tract may occur for years.[25] In addition to aerosolization, intestinal shedding of respiratory virus is an important factor to consider in the prevention of nosocomial spread in hospitals and chronic care homes.[25, 110, 111] Persistent infection has been reported in epithelial cells from monkeys.[112] Lymphoid cells are thought to be the reservoir for these persistent infections.[113, 114] The third type of interaction is oncogenic transformation, whereby the viral DNA is integrated into the host genome, where it is replicated with the cellular host DNA; but only the early steps in the viral cycle occur, and no infectious virions are produced.[115]

The genes from adenoviruses are expressed in the cell nucleus in two phases: "early" (E), which precedes viral DNA replication, and "late" (L).[113] Early genes encode proteins that function to counteract immunosurveillance, especially those from the E3 transcription unit.[113] The "late" genes primarily encode viral structural proteins. The function of the E1 proteins includes the induction of DNA synthesis in quiescent cells, immortalization of primary cells in cooperation with activated *ras* or with the E1B proteins, *trans*-activation of delayed early genes, induction or repression or several cellular genes, and induction of apoptosis. These proteins are responsible for inducing sensitivity to tumor necrosis factor (TNF), a key inflammatory cytokine with antiviral properties.[113] None of the E3 genes is required for adenovirus replication in cultured cells, but several of the E3-coded proteins (10.4K, 14.5K, and 14.7K) inhibit TNF cytolysis.[113, 116] Because a major function of TNF may be to prevent viral replication, the inhibition of TNF by these viral proteins could be a significant mechanism of pathogenesis.

Another significant E3-coded protein is glycoprotein 19K. This glycoprotein is located in the endoplasmic reticulum and forms a complex with class I antigens of the major histocompatibility complex (MHC), preventing cells from being killed by cytotoxic T lymphocytes (CTL).[113] A cotton rat animal model was used by Ginsberg and colleagues[116, 117] to study the pathogenesis of adenovirus types 2 and 5, which cause a pneumonia similar to that seen in humans. Two phases of infection were seen, the initial phase, characterized by the infiltration of monocytes and neutrophils, and a later phase associated with the infiltration of lymphocytes. The pathologic process appeared to reflect the response by host immune defenses to viral infection. The glycoprotein 19K markedly reduced the transport of the class I MHC to the surface of the infected cells and therefore the attack of cytotoxic T cells.[117] In support of this mechanism of pathogenesis is the finding that mutants lacking the glycoprotein 19K are more pathogenic than wild-type virus because the mutants do not block the CTL response or the synthesis of cytokines associated with this CTL response.[113, 116] It is now known that only the early genes are required to induce the complete pathogenesis of adenovirus infection in cotton rats.[117] Although several cytokines, such as TNF-α, interleukin-1, and interleukin-6, were elaborated during the first 2 to 3 days of the infection in the cotton rat model, only TNF-α played a major role in pathogenesis.[117] Steroids almost completely eliminated the pneumonic inflammatory response to infection.[117]

Pathologic change caused by latent infection with adenoviruses has been linked to chronic obstructive pulmonary disease (COPD).[114, 118] Some have suggested that childhood viral diseases represent an independent risk factor for COPD.[119] The adenoviral E1A proteins can stimulate the transcription of many heterologous viral and cellular genes. These proteins possess the ability to interact with the DNA binding domains of several cellular transcription factors and activate a wide variety of genes.[120, 121] The adenoviral genome has been found to be present in the lungs of more patients with COPD than in control subjects.[122] E1A proteins are expressed in epithelial cells of human lung tissue, and by increasing the expression of several genes important in controlling the inflammatory process, these may contribute to the pathogenesis of COPD. The events described may amplify the airway inflammation associated with cigarette smoking.[118]

The recent isolation and cloning of a 46-kDa protein adenovirus receptor, which mediates attachment and infection, may facilitate the development of new strategies to limit diseases caused by adenoviruses.[123] This protein has been identified as the receptor for coxsackievirus B and adenovirus types 2 and 5 and has been referred to as coxsackievirus and adenovirus receptor.

Diagnosis

Adenoviral infections cannot be diagnosed on clinical grounds alone because the clinical pictures of these infections resemble those due to other microorganisms and are variable.[79] Laboratory support and qualified personnel are necessary to diagnose adenoviruses in clinical specimens or to perform serological assays. Detailed diagnostic procedures have been outlined.[26, 27, 64] Considerations include specimen type, collection, and storage procedures; types of laboratory tests including serological assays; and availability of newer types of diagnostic assays.

Specimen Types. The optimal specimen depends on the clinical picture as well as the suspected serotype.[79] Adenoviruses can be isolated from a variety of specimens, including throat swabs, nasal washes, conjunctival scrapings and swabs, stool, blood, cerebrospinal fluid, and tissue biopsy specimens. Because they are relatively stable viruses, adenoviruses can be recovered if they are properly transported to the laboratory. Specimens for viral isolation should be collected early in the illness and shipped promptly to the local laboratory at 4°C or frozen at −20°C for shipment to a reference laboratory.

Swab and tissue specimens must be transported in viral transport media containing antibiotics and 0.5% gelatin or bovine serum albumin.[26, 27, 64, 79] Freezing specimens at −70°C is recommended if immediate culture inoculation is not possible.

Fresh urine specimens (20 mL) should be sedimented at 2000 × g for 5 minutes to pellet exfoliated cells, and both the pellet and supernatant should be cultured.[26, 27] Urine, stool, and cerebrospinal fluid should be transported in clean containers but not in transport media. Stool suspensions give better yield than rectal swabs.[25] Blood should be collected in heparin and fractionated on Ficoll Hypaque gradients.[26]

Serological diagnosis requires paired blood samples. The first (acute) specimen should be collected as early as possible in the illness, and the second (convalescent) specimen should be collected 2 to 4 weeks later. Stored sera should be kept at −20°C until testing.

Cell Culture. Because adenoviruses are host specific, isolation is most easily accomplished in human cells.[79] Even though the best isolation sensitivity is achieved in HEK cells, which are difficult to obtain, other continuous cell lines such as A549, HeLa, Hep-2, KB, and MRC-5 are in common use today. All serotypes of adenoviruses grow well and produce typical cytopathic effect, except adenovirus types 40 and 41.[27] Types 40 and 41 require the Graham-293 adenovirus type 5–transformed secondary HEK cell line but may grow in A549 cells or tertiary cynomolgus monkey kidney cells.[26, 27] Specimen preparation before inoculation is extremely important with regard to centrifugation, treatment with antibiotics, and homogenization and is described in detail by Hierholzer.[27] Typical cytopathic effect may be relatively slow and characteristically begins at the periphery on the monolayer. Infected cells become rounded, enlarged, and refractile; they are intranuclear and aggregate into clusters that are irregular.[27] A 4-week incubation with blind passage is recommended.[27] Isolation is the laboratory "gold standard" and the most sensitive (85 to 100%) means for adenovirus diagnosis, except for gastroenteritis cases.[79] An improved culture technique for adenovirus isolation using centrifugation of 24-well plates has been reported to enhance sensitivity of culture.[124]

Identification of Isolated Viruses. Subsequent identification of isolated viruses as adenoviruses can be made by immunofluorescence using monoclonal antibodies, complement fixation (CF), enzyme immunoassay (EIA), time-resolved fluoroimmunoassay (TR-FIA), DNA hybridization assays, counterimmunoelectrophoresis, and latex agglutination.[27, 125–128] In general, IFA, EIA, TR-FIA, and CF are used to classify a viral isolate to genus level as an adenovirus. Agglutination with monkey, human, and rat erythrocytes is employed to assign the virus to a subgroup, and further hemagglutination inhibition and serum neutralization tests are used to serotype the isolate.[27] A rapid diagnostic procedure is the shell vial culture modification, which uses centrifugation and staining with monoclonal antibodies to the hexon protein.[126]

Typing Tests. Serum neutralization assays have been the standard method used to type adenoviruses.[27] Hemagglutination inhibition is convenient but requires fresh rat and monkey erythrocytes. Reference antisera can be obtained from the American Type Culture Collection, Rockville, Maryland. Three types of serum neutralization tests have been described: conventional 7-day assays using Hep-2, A549, HeLa, HEK, or Graham-293 cells; the 3-day test in primary rhesus monkey kidney cells; and microneutralization tests in secondary monkey kidney cells, Vero cells, and Hep-2 cells.[27]

Restriction enzyme analysis can be used for the separation of a serotype into multiple genotypes.[98, 100] The genomic variability of the adenovirus type 3 and type 7 genome types has been investigated extensively with use of a panel of 12 restriction enzymes.[101, 102, 105] In addition, type 4 isolates have been genotyped by use of restriction enzymes.[103, 104] These analyses have been applied mainly for molecular epidemiology studies and may be useful in outbreak investigations. A nomenclature system has been suggested and described in detail, with a recommended protocol for the designation of new genome types.[101, 105]

Direct Detection. Electron microscopy and immunoelectron microscopy have been used in the past as the principal direct detection methods for identifying adenoviruses in clinical material, especially biopsy and autopsy specimens, as well as for the detection of these agents as causes of gastroenteritis.[27, 129–131]

Immunofluorescence can be useful for rapid identification of cells from unfrozen specimens by use of antibodies, which are commercially available, against the group-specific hexon antigen.[125, 132] EIA and TR-FIA as well as latex agglutination can be used to detect antigenic proteins in clinical specimens.[127, 128, 133, 134] The sensitivity of EIA was 84.8% in one large series.[133] A commercial EIA used for the diagnosis of conjunctivitis had a sensitivity of only 62.3% compared with culture, however.[135]

Nucleic Acid Hybridization and Polymerase Chain Reaction. Nucleic acid hybridization using dot blot, sandwich hybridization, and in situ hybridization have also been used for diagnosis but have not been adopted for routine use in clinical laboratories.[136–141]

Polymerase chain reaction (PCR) assays have been developed for the diagnosis of adenoviruses, especially for the types 40 and 41, since they are difficult to grow.[142–147] Allard and colleagues[144, 146] first developed a set of primers with homology to the conserved sequences of the hexon gene, which would amplify adenovirus strains from all six subgenera A to F. Their second pair of primers detected only the enteric types 40 and 41; a third set was specific for type 40, thus differentiating types 40 and 41. PCR with restriction fragment length polymorphism (RFLP) analysis has been used to detect and also differentiate types 40 and 41.[148] The combination of PCR amplification with liquid-phase hybridization quantitated by time-resolved fluorometry has been used by Hierholzer and coworkers[142] to identify adenoviruses from a variety of clinical specimens including urine, stool, and tissue suspensions. Procedures for the performance of PCR assays have been well described.[143, 145, 147] Primers published by Allard and colleagues,[144, 146] useful for some types of adenoviruses, failed to detect the adenovirus type 11 from the patient shown in Figure 23–1. Newly designed primers, HEX3/HEX4, were used successfully to amplify DNA from the specimens from this patient (Marcela Echavarria et al., Johns Hopkins University, personal communication).

PCR has been used with myocardial tissue samples for the diagnosis of adenovirus infection.[149, 150] Ventricular endomyocardial biopsy specimens from pediatric transplant patients were positive for adenoviruses in 14 of 129 (10.8%) samples,[149] and 15 of 38 (39.4%) ventricular biopsy samples were positive from 34 pediatric patients with acute myocarditis.[150]

PCR for adenovirus detection has been used with success on formalin-fixed, paraffin-embedded autopsy specimens from children with viral pneumonitis and disseminated infection.[151, 152] Adenoviral DNA was demonstrated by PCR in 3 of 44 (6.8%) lung specimens from immunocompromised patients with pneumonia.[139]

Adenoviruses from throat, nasopharyngeal, and ocular specimens have also been diagnosed by PCR, offering improved sensitivity and greater speed over culture.[145, 153–155] The combination of PCR with RFLP analysis was used to detect and to type adenoviruses from conjunctival specimens.[156] The PCR was 100% sensitive compared with culture in 127 specimens.[156] PCR with rapid subgenus identification using one-step RFLP with three endonucleases has been described.[157] The use of a multiplex PCR assay for detection of both adenoviruses and herpes simplex viruses in eye swabs has the potential to rapidly detect more than one pathogen with one assay.[158] PCR has additionally been used to detect adenoviruses in polluted waters.[159]

Serology. Acute adenovirus infection can be diagnosed by significant (fourfold) titer rises to the hexon antigen by testing acute and convalescent sera by one of several methods. The CF method, measuring group-specific antibodies, is the most widely used and best standardized.[27] The sensitivity is about 50 to 70%.[79, 160] CF antibody production in infants and young children may be poor and the test can be falsely negative; in adults, CF antibodies from previous infections may cause difficulty in diagnosing a new infection.[25] EIA, also measuring group-specific antibodies, is more sensitive than the CF test and can be automated.[27] Sensitivity of the EIA assay has been reported to be 73 to 87%.[79, 160] Hemagglutination inhibition and serum neutralization assays are more sensitive than CF, but because they measure type-specific antibodies, these are not suitable for routine diagnosis and most reagents are not commercially available.[27] A colorimetric microneutralization assay automates the neutralization test and is useful for testing large numbers of specimens.[161]

Treatment

Topical human fibroblast (β) interferon has been reported to have a beneficial effect on epidemic keratoconjunctivitis.[162] Nucleoside analogues have been demonstrated to have a potent, nontoxic inhibitory effect on replication of adenoviruses in human embryonic fibroblast cultures.[163]

Although ribavirin is active against adenoviruses in vitro, no specific antiviral treatment for adenoviral infections is presently recommended.[79] Nebulized ribavirin was used with some success for two children with pneumonia caused by adenovirus.[164] Intravenous ribavirin has reportedly been used in immunocompromised patients as well as in patients with hemorrhagic cystitis and disseminated disease.[165–169]

The activities of ganciclovir and acyclovir were tested in cell culture and in cotton rat eyes against adenovirus type 5, which is known to cause severe eye disease.[170] The 50% inhibitory dose (ID_{50}) was determined by plaque reduction assays in human cells to be 47 and 604 μM for ganciclovir and acyclovir, respectively. When cottontail rabbits were inoculated with 10^5 plaque-forming units per eye, topical treatment for 21 days with 3%, 1%, or 0.3% demonstrated that only the highest dose of 3% reduced the incidence, duration, and titer of virus shed. The differences were not statistically significant, but the observed trend suggested that the 3% dose had a suppressive effect on some disease parameters.[170]

EPIDEMIOLOGY

Incidence and Prevalence

The epidemic characteristics of the adenoviruses vary somewhat among the subgenera.[25] The reason for the tissue tropism exhibited by various types is unknown.[171] However, there are many similar characteristics among the adenoviruses. They are all transmitted by direct contact, aerosolized virus, the fecal-oral route, or water. Those in subgenus C (types 1, 2, 5, and 6) are usually endemic and acquired in early childhood.[25] Many of the other types occur either sporadically or in epidemics. Many adenovirus infections are subclinical or asymptomatic, especially those in subgenera A and D. Conversely, the types (especially 4, 7, and 21) in subgenera B and E usually cause symptomatic respiratory disease.[25] The enteric adenoviruses (types 40 and 41) of subgenera F and G cause gastroenteritis. The highest incidence of infection for the most common adenoviruses (types 1, 2, 5, and 6) occurs in children younger than 2 years.

Because only about 50% of childhood adenovirus infections result in disease, prevalence as detected by antibody studies is high.[30–32] By school age, most children have been exposed to several types of adenoviruses. Infections caused by adenovirus types 4, 7, 14, and 21 may occur at a later age.

Geographically, most types of adenoviruses have been recovered from all areas of the world.[38] From approximately 25,000 isolation reports to the World Health Organization, a periodicity during 10 years was noted for the incidence of adenovirus types 7, 8, and 19 and less so for types 3 and 4.[38] Age predilections were highly significant for infants for subgenus A (types 12, 18, and 31); for infants and small children for subgenus C (types 1, 2, 5, and 6); for schoolchildren for type 3; for schoolchildren and adults for type 7; and for adults for types 4, 8, and other species of subgenera B and D.[38] A predilection for males was observed for all types in subgenera B and C and with types 4 and 19.[38]

A national surveillance report for 1982 to 1993 from Japan indicated that the most common illnesses associated with adenoviruses were upper respiratory tract infection (51% of 17,265 patients), conjunctivitis (32%), and gastroenteritis (18%).[172] Adenovirus type 3 was the most frequently isolated; yearly fluctuations were observed for types 3 and 4; and few isolates occurred for type 7, which is considered to cause severe pneumonia in many countries.[172]

Significance as a Public Health Problem

The site of transmission for adenoviruses for most endemic infections has been considered to be the home. Transmission rates are higher in children's institutions and daycare centers as well as in lower socioeconomic groups.[39, 40] Enteric adenoviruses may be an important pathogen in the daycare setting.[173] Epidemics associated with type 3 often occur in association with swimming activities.[49] Adenovirus type 8 has been associated with transmission in physicians' offices.[51]

Nosocomial outbreaks of adenovirus keratoconjunctivitis have been reported from the accident and emergency department of a major eye hospital in the United Kingdom.[140, 174, 175] Nosocomial conjunctivitis, pharyngitis, and pneumonia caused by adenoviruses have been noted in hospital intensive care units.[16, 176, 177]

In current hospital practice, there are increasing numbers of immunocompromised patients, and a growing problem with adenoviral disease is that of severe infection among the immunocompromised.[88] The epidemiological concern relates to acquisition from a nosocomial perspective, because these patients may be hospitalized for long periods. In addition, reactivation of a latent infection could possibly initiate a nosocomial outbreak. People with deficient cell-mediated immunity are at greatest risk for adverse outcomes.[25] Bone marrow transplant patients are especially susceptible to adenovirus infections.[63, 87] Immunodeficient patients with pneumonia may experience fatality rates as high as 60%.[88]

Chronic diarrhea in AIDS patients is often a diagnostic problem. A prospective study using extensive diagnostic techniques, such as duodenal, jejunal, and rectal biopsies, found 6.5% of such patients to have adenovirus infections.[178]

Acute Respiratory Disease of Military Recruits

The epidemic nature of certain adenovirus strains in military recruits has been well documented.[7] Before the use of vaccines in the U.S. military, serotypes 4 and 7 accounted for 60% of all acute respiratory disease in recruits who were hospitalized; serotypes 3, 14, and 21 were less frequently observed.[21] Up to 80% of recruits became infected, whereas seasoned military personnel experienced lower rates.[7] Patterns of infections in Dutch military recruits demonstrated that types 4, 7, and 21 were the prevalent types with attack rates of 20 to 60% and with 7 to 14% of recruits requiring hospitalizations.[179]

Extensive studies in unimmunized Marine Corps personnel showed three different patterns of disease.[180] In contrast to Army recruits in whom adenovirus infections were prevalent throughout the year with peaks in fall and winter, Marines experienced sharply demarcated winter epidemics in both advanced recruits and more experienced soldiers. Most of the isolates were type 4, except for a few type 7 isolates. More than 85% of febrile illnesses were associated with adenovirus disease.[181]

Although the civilian experience has not established a requirement for a vaccine, the epidemic nature and extensive morbidity suffered by military recruits during the 1960s demonstrated an overwhelming need for adenovirus vaccines for military use. One well-studied and typical epidemic at Fort Dix, New Jersey, exemplified this requirement.[22] A platoon of 48 men were observed prospectively for their 8 weeks of basic training. Of 92 episodes of respiratory illness, 24 required hospitalization. The documented hospitalization rate for acute respiratory disease due to adenovirus type 4 was 5 per 100 soldiers per week.[22] At large basic training posts, this rate translated to approximately 500 to 800 acute respiratory disease admissions per week, which had a devastating impact on military hospitals.[22, 182] Excess medical costs and the fact that soldiers had to be recycled because of lost training time resulted in significant economic loss to the military. Serious disruptions to training schedules led to administrative attempts to control epidemics, such as sleeping head-to-foot and keeping military units separated (cohorting).[182]

PASSIVE IMMUNIZATION

There have never been attempts to passively immunize people against adenoviruses.

ACTIVE IMMUNIZATION

Prior Approaches That Have Been Abandoned

The first adenovirus vaccine, which was bivalent for types 4 and 7, was grown in monkey kidney cells and formalin inactivated.[182] After safety tests, a small trial in 1957 reduced admissions due to adenoviruses by 98%, and a large trial of 8238 soldiers was 90% effective in reducing hospitalization.[183, 184] A trivalent vaccine, which included type 3, was also tested.[185] Large-scale production of vaccine lots led to variation in antigenicity, resulting in a loss of protection rates, with only a 52% reduction in hospital illnesses due to adenoviruses.[186] Even this low rate of protection was reported in 1965 to have saved the Army about $5 million a year.[186] Adenovirus seed lots were found to be contaminated with SV40, an oncogenic virus, in 1963, and the license for the vaccine was rescinded.[22]

Development of the Current Vaccine

Early Vaccines. Use of a live vaccine for acute respiratory disease caused by adenovirus type 7 was investigated, and oral administration was reported to induce high antibody levels in 1960.[187] Couch and Chanock demonstrated that some adenoviruses infect the gastrointestinal tract but do not produce symptoms in adults. This led to the administration of the virus as a vaccine in an enteric-coated capsule, which produced an asymptomatic, intestinal infection.[188, 189] Many safety studies were performed in human volunteers, including the administration of the adenovirus type 4 and type 7 vaccines separately and the simultaneous administration of both the type 4 and type 7 vaccines.[188] Neutralizing responses were observed, and asymptomatic infections were evidenced by the recovery of virus from rectal specimens. Initial vaccine work using human embryonic kidney cells was later modified to use human diploid fibroblast strains WI-26 and WI-38, because the primary cell line was not suitable for large-scale production and there was fear of contamination of the primary cells with other human pathogens.[189] Because some adenoviruses are oncogenic in animals, much attention was paid to safety studies in hamsters and the transformation of cell lines by adenoviruses.[190, 191]

Additional field trials for adenovirus type 4 vaccine were conducted at Parris Island, South Carolina, and Great Lakes, Illinois, and showed that the vaccine was highly protective, safe, antigenic, and not communicable. Vaccine use led to reductions in acute respiratory disease rates of 50%.[192, 193] Intrinsic vaccine efficacy was as high as 82%, and specific disease reduction was as high as 69%.[193]

Combined Adenovirus Vaccines. Use of the monotypic type 4 vaccine was followed by the appearance of acute respiratory disease due to adenovirus type 7 at Fort Dix, New Jersey.[22] The Army Adenovirus Surveillance Program was initiated to identify the agents of acute respiratory disease and to assess fluctuations in disease patterns.[21]

Before a type 7 vaccine could be developed, numerous studies addressed the oncogenicity potential to humans of the type 7 virus.[194–197] A trial of adenovirus type 7 vaccine demonstrated safety, infectivity, antigenicity, and lack of communicability similar to that observed for the type 4 vaccine.[198] Additional trials indicated that when the types 4 and 7 vaccines were given simultaneously, no decrease in antigenicity occurred, and with mass immunization there was 95% suppression of type 7–associated disease.[198–200] Numerous appearances and outbreaks of adenovirus type 21 in military populations in the United States and in Europe led to the initiation of studies using a type 21 prototype vaccine in safety and immunogenicity trials.[201–205] Because of the absence of prolonged outbreaks associated with adenovirus type 21, the type 21 vaccine was never licensed or tested for efficacy.[182]

Producers

The sole supplier for the adenovirus types 4 and 7 vaccines had been Wyeth Laboratories Incorporated (Marietta, Pennsylvania). However, they ceased production of the vaccine in 1996. The U.S. Department of Defense has been trying to identify a new source for the vaccines.

Dosage, Route, and Preparations

Original trials for adenovirus type 7 vaccine were conducted using 0.05 mL of a 1:10 dilution of the adenovirus type 7 pool (10^6 median tissue culture infective dose [$TCID_{50}$]) within a hard gelatin capsule and given orally.[188] Time of disintegration within the intestine was assayed roentgenographically using a barium sulfate–containing capsule and varied between 1 and 5 hours.[188] Dosage studies using the Wyeth vaccine for type 7 virus in clinical trials used three doses: $10^{6.8}$ $TCID_{50}$, $10^{4.8}$ $TCID_{50}$, and less than 10 $TCID_{50}$.[198, 199] There was 100% antibody response with the highest dose, 95% response with the intermediate dose, and 56% response with the lowest dose. Another study evaluated the response when both vaccines were given individually at doses of $10^{5.4}$ $TCID_{50}$ for type 7 and of 10^4 $TCID_{50}$ for type 4 and simultaneously at the same doses.[198] There was no decrease in the antigenicity of the type 4 vaccine when it was given with the type 7 vaccine.[199]

In 1971, the U.S. military began routinely administering both vaccines to men reporting to recruit training centers, but only during the winter months.[22] The incoming recruits were given the vaccines within hours of arrival at a training center to obtain protection as early as possible in the training program. Initially, women were not given the vaccines because acute respiratory disease outbreaks due to adenoviruses had never been documented among military women, and there was concern about the possibility of administering the vaccines to women who were pregnant.[182]

The program of administering the vaccines only during the high-risk winter months was directed at control rather than eradication of acute respiratory disease due to adenoviruses.[22] With this schedule, late spring and early fall outbreaks occurred. These outbreaks prompted the U.S. Army and the U.S. Navy to adopt a policy of year-round administration of both adenovirus vaccines in 1983.[182] Taking a different course, the U.S. Air Force stopped the administration of adenovirus vaccines at its only recruit training center in Texas in the mid-1980s and adopted a program of surveillance with use of the vaccines only as needed.[182]

When the military started immunizations to protect against acute respiratory disease due to adenoviruses, training programs were segregated by sex. These separate training programs have since been combined, leading to concern that the risk for acute respiratory disease due to adenoviruses may now be the same for both men and women. The current U.S. military regulation for immunizations requires that on the basis of risk, adenovirus types 4 and 7 vaccines be administered simultaneously and only once to Army, Navy, and Marine Corps recruits.[206] In the Air Force and Coast Guard, the vaccines are administered when it is directed by the appropriate authority.[206] The same regulation describes precautions to be taken to avoid unintentional administration of the vaccines during pregnancy and counseling instructions regarding the possibility of pregnancy for 3 months after immunization.[206]

In response to the cessation of adenovirus vaccine production in 1996, the Army, Navy, and Marine Corps modified their policy of year-round vaccine administration to conserve the remaining vaccine for use in higher risk months only. The modified policy directed that the vaccines be given to arriving military recruits only during the period of September 1 through March 31 until all vaccine stocks have been used. The existing vaccine stocks are expected to be exhausted early in 1999.

Preparations

The only adenovirus vaccine stocks currently available are the live, oral, enteric-coated tablets that were produced by Wyeth before production was stopped. These tablets were developed to replace the capsules used earlier. The type 4 vaccine (white tablets) and the type 7 vaccine (yellow tablets) are packaged separately, and each tablet contains approximately 10^5 $TCID_{50}$. Individual tablets consist of three components, an inner core and two outer layers. The core, measuring 6 mm in diameter and 2.5 mm in thickness, contains lyophilized live virus obtained from a stored seed lot system. Each vaccine production lot contained the same virus passage. Compression of the core contents was accomplished without a significant temperature increase. The core was covered by a layer of inert materials, such as starch. This inert layer was applied by use of special equipment and was uniformly 2 mm in thickness. To form the outermost layer, an enteric coating solution was sprayed over the inert layer by use of a pharmaceutical tumbler. This resulted in the uniform fixation of 37 mg per tablet of a dry coat to protect the live vaccine viruses from gastric fluids (Dr. R. Thiboutot, Wyeth-Ayerst Laboratories, personal communication).

The tablets may be administered simultaneously but must be swallowed quickly without chewing. Vomiting and diarrhea may interfere with vaccine effectiveness. These vaccines are indicated in military populations shown to be at risk of acute respiratory disease due to the specific adenovirus serotypes represented in the tablets. Use of the vaccines in pregnant women is not recommended because the possible effects on fetal development have not been studied.

Constituents

The vaccine tablets contain live viruses, materials added for the growth and maintenance of viruses and cells, and other pharmaceutical materials. Human diploid fibroblast cells (strain WI-38) are used for virus preparation, and growth is maintained in minimal essential medium, Eagle's solution, antibiotics (neomycin sulfate, gentamicin sulfate, and amphotericin B), fetal calf serum, and sodium bicarbonate. After harvesting, the viral growth is freed of particulate material by filtration and dried by lyophilization. During drying, additives including human serum albumin, plasdone, sucrose, D-mannose, D-fructose, dextrose, potassium phosphate, and monosodium glutamate are used to preserve viability. Before processing into tablets, the virus preparation is diluted with lactose powder.[207] The vaccine tablets also contain cellulose acetate, phthalate, alcohol, acetone, castor oil, magnesium stearate, and Amberlite. The type 7 vaccine tablets can be distinguished from the type 4 tablets by their yellow color. The color is produced by FD & C Yellow No. 5 (tartrazine), which may cause allergic-type reactions (Dr. Thiboutot, personal communication).

Vaccine Stability

Problems occurred with stability of the vaccines in the early 1970s, with disease control being less than desired. The loss of potency was traced to a several-fold log decrease in the virus titer a few months after manufacture. This was due to contamination of the vaccine viruses in the core by the acetone solvent used in the enteric coating process to inactivate residual live virus that persisted on the surface of the tablets.[22] Live virus outside the protective enteric coating poses a risk to those handling the tablets and could possibly cause an upper respiratory infection in those swallowing the tablets. The problem was resolved by adequate ventilation of the solvent during production.[22] The acetone was sprayed on the tablets' outermost coating in three stages, and between each stage the tablets were dried in a vacuum chamber to rapidly remove the solvent. This prevented the acetone from penetrating the tablet and inactivating the vaccine virus.

The license under which Wyeth produced the vaccines allowed a 12-month cold storage period after packaging of the vaccines. This equated to annual shipments to the military of products that were dated to expire in 18 months. When stored at ordinary refrigeration temperatures (between 2 and 8°C) but not frozen, adenovirus vaccine tablets will remain stable for at least 2 years (Dr. Thiboutot, personal communication).

RESULTS OF VACCINATION

Immune Responses

Oral adenovirus vaccine recipients may shed virus fecally after about 4 days and may continue to do so for an additional 7 to 8 days.[203] Vaccinees develop neutralizing humoral antibody (immunoglobulins G, M, and A).[203] In soldiers who are free of preexisting antibody, an average of 80 to 95% develop a neutralizing antibody level of 1:8, whereas less than 50% demonstrate complement-fixing antibody.[199, 208] Neutralizing antibody responses develop in 2 to 3 weeks. In general, antibody titers are less than those achieved after natural infection.[209, 210] Local secretory immunoglobulin A antibody is not induced by the oral vaccine, and reinfection of

Table 23–3. **SUMMARY OF CLINICAL TRIALS USING ENTERIC-COATED ORAL ADENOVIRUS VACCINES**

STUDY*	TOTAL VACCINATED	REDUCTION IN HOSPITALIZATION (%)	REDUCTION IN ADENOVIRUS ARD (%)
1	125	Not done	100
2	339	Not done	100
3	6,883	Not done	96
4	386	46	69
5	23,015	50	Not done
6	607	69	94
7	10,863	47	95
8	4,364	Not done	98
9	3,867	Not done	95

*Studies 1 to 7, adenovirus type 4 vaccine was administered. Studies 8 and 9, adenovirus types 4 and 7 vaccines were administered.
ARD, acute respiratory disease.
Adapted from Lee SG, Hung PP. Vaccines for control of respiratory disease caused by adenoviruses. Med Virol 209:209–216, 1993.

the respiratory tract is possible but usually mild or asymptomatic.[211] Because viremia and viruria can occur in patients with febrile disease, invasiveness beyond mucosal surfaces may be important in the pathogenesis of the disease and infection.[212] The serum neutralizing antibody produced as a result of vaccination may prevent the typical febrile disease associated with natural infection.[208] Local immunoglobulin A antibody can be produced experimentally in the respiratory tract by the intranasal inoculation of an adenovirus type 4 vaccine in liquid.[211]

Results of Controlled Trials of Protection Against Disease

Military recruits who received adenovirus type 4 vaccine exhibited increased resistance to respiratory disease caused by this virus.[189, 192, 213] A number of major well-controlled studies of military personnel were performed from 1963 to 1966, in which more than 42,000 soldiers were studied.[214] Use of the vaccine reduced acute respiratory disease by 50% on average and adenovirus infection in recruits by more than 90%. Table 23–3 shows the summary results of some of the clinical trials for type 4 vaccine.

Field trials began in 1969 for the adenovirus type 7 vaccine and indicated protection against disease in susceptible individuals.[199, 200, 215] In addition, the two vaccines for type 4 and type 7 could be administered simultaneously without interference or loss of efficacy.[199, 200, 216] As a result of using the vaccines at one large Air Force base during a 9-year period, acute respiratory disease due to adenovirus disappeared.[217] The adenovirus surveillance program demonstrated that the combination of the two adenovirus vaccines was highly effective in controlling epidemic acute respiratory disease.[21] Table 23–3 summarizes some of the clinical trials performed for the type 7 vaccine. Since 1971, the live, enteric-coated adenovirus vaccines for types 4 and 7 have been administered to new military recruits and have successfully controlled acute respiratory disease due to adenoviruses.

Other Evidence of Effectiveness

The successful impact of the adenovirus vaccination program can be seen in Figure 23–3, which demon-

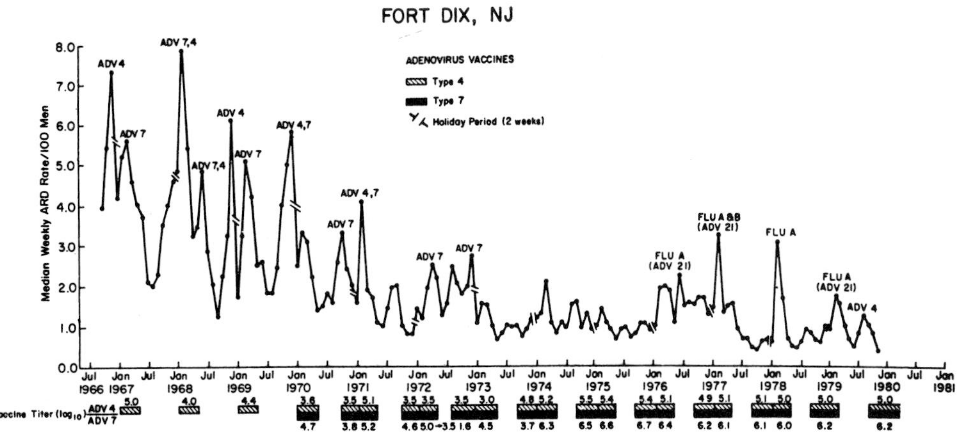

Figure 23–3. The median weekly acute respiratory disease (ARD) rate per 100 men at Fort Dix, New Jersey, during the years 1966 to 1980, demonstrating the impact of adenovirus vaccines type 4 and type 7. The vaccine titer is listed for each year across the bottom of the graph. (Courtesy of Colonel William H. Bancroft, U.S. Army Headquarters Medical Research and Material Command, Fort Detrick, MD.)

Table 23–4. **REDUCTION IN ACUTE RESPIRATORY DISEASE RATES AFTER VACCINATION WITH A SINGLE TABLET EACH OF ADENOVIRUS SEROTYPES 4 AND 7 (10^5 $TCID_{50}$/TABLET)***

		FT. LEWIS		FT. LEONARD WOOD	
WEEK	**PERCENTAGE IMMUNIZED**	**ARD Rate per 100**	**Percentage Rate Reduction Over Peak**	**ARD Rate per 100**	**Percentage Rate Reduction Over Peak**
1	50	6.6		7.8	
2	63	5.4	19	8.4	
3	75	3.7	45	4.8	43
4	88	1.9	72	2.3	74
5	100	2.1	69	1.4	84
6	100	2.1	69	1.6	80

*Reduction of 69 to 80% includes *all* acute respiratory disease (ARD). The adenovirus disease component is reduced by about 95%.
From Dudding BA, Top RH Jr, Winter P. Acute respiratory disease in military trainees. The adenovirus surveillance program 1966–1971. Am J Epidemiol 97:187–198, 1973.

strates the median weekly acute respiratory disease rate per 100 men at one large Army basic training post, Fort Dix, New Jersey. Table 23–4 shows the decline in acute respiratory disease in two military installations after inauguration of vaccination with adenovirus types 4 and 7. No herd immunity can be assumed, because the new recruit cohort changes with every new basic trainee group. Except for the loss of vaccine potency that occurred in the 1970s with solvent contamination,[22] there has never been an outbreak of acute respiratory disease in the U.S. military due to adenovirus type 4 or adenovirus type 7 in groups receiving these vaccines.

The excess morbidity caused by acute respiratory disease and associated costs are of significant concern to the military. A cost-benefit analysis was performed by Collis and associates,[218] which estimated that the use of the vaccines for adenovirus types 4 and 7 in 1970 to 1971 saved \$7.53 million. The costs of the vaccines are expected to increase, but a cost-effectiveness analysis for the continued use of the vaccines indicated that use of these vaccines is still cost-effective, having the potential to save approximately \$15.5 million annually over no vaccination.[218a]

Duration of Immunity

The duration of immunity and persistence of circulating antibody after immunization have never been determined. The adenovirus vaccines were developed to protect new members of the military (recruits) against acute respiratory disease due to adenovirus types 4 and 7 during training required on entry in the services, which consists of elementary military training (basic training) and training to develop special military skills. The adenovirus vaccines have been effective in accomplishing the outcome for which they were intended, and there was never a need to determine the duration of protection against disease or the persistence of circulating antibodies over time.

Adverse Events

Adverse reactions after the oral administration of the types 4 and 7 vaccines have not been reported. Four study groups were observed for inpatient and outpatient episodes of illness during vaccine safety and immunogenicity trials at Lackland Air Force Base, Texas, in 1976. In addition to the placebo group, one group received three vaccines simultaneously (types 4, 7, and 21), another group received two vaccines simultaneously (types 4 and 7), and the last group received the type 21 vaccine only.[205] No appreciable differences were noted in the inpatient or outpatient experiences of the different groups.[205] Of 146 soldiers who received vaccines to adenoviruses 4 and 7, there were 2 (1.4%) hospitalizations for acute respiratory disease, 2 (1.4%) for gastrointestinal disease, and 3 (2%) for other illnesses.[205] Compared with 101 soldiers in the placebo group, who had hospitalizations for 3 (3%), 2 (2.0%), and 1 (1.0%) for the same categories, respectively, the rates were not different.[205] The outpatient episodes recorded for the same categories of illness also did not differ: acute respiratory disease, 14.4% for vaccinees compared with 19.8% for placebo group; gastrointestinal disease, 5.5% compared with 4.0%; and other illnesses, 24% compared with 31.7%.

Spread to sites outside the gastrointestinal tract has not been reported in vaccine recipients.[208] Because the virus is shed fecally for up to 8 days, the virus may be spread to family members or close contacts by fecal-oral transmission.[219]

Indications for Vaccines

Adenovirus vaccines are indicated for the prevention and control of specific adenovirus-associated acute respiratory disease in populations with a high risk of exposure, a high level of susceptibility, and a high risk of subsequent infection and disease. In 1976, 42% of Army recruits tested lacked neutralizing antibody to adenovirus types 4 and 7,[205] and the initial analysis of data from a seroprevalence study of more current recruits supports a continuing high level of susceptibility.[220] In 1995, an outbreak of adenovirus type 4 was reported in Army basic trainees at Fort Jackson, South Carolina, who had not been immunized. The attack rate for the most affected unit at the height of the outbreak was 11.6% per week.[221] Therefore, the vaccines are indicated for use in selected military populations undergoing their initial military training. The vaccine is not recommended for use in other populations.

Contraindications and Precautions

Gentamicin sulfate, neomycin sulfate, and amphotericin B are used in the vaccine manufacturing process, and traces may be found in the final product. People with known sensitivity to any of these antibiotics should not receive the vaccines. The FD & C Yellow No. 5 (tartrazine) in the type 7 tablets may cause bronchial asthma or other allergic-type reactions in susceptible people. Sensitivity to this substance occurs infrequently but is often seen in people with aspirin hypersensitivity.

The live, oral adenovirus vaccines have never been subjected to animal reproduction studies. Therefore, it is not known whether these vaccines have the potential to cause fetal damage if given to a pregnant woman or to affect reproductive capacity. Administration of the vaccines to pregnant women should be avoided.

Adenoviruses have caused severe, overwhelming, and often fatal infections in immunocompromised individuals. Concern about potentially severe adverse effects if an adenovirus vaccine were to be given to such an individual prompted a study of recruits who had early human immunodeficiency virus (HIV) infection and received the standard vaccines required for military induction, including the adenovirus vaccines.[222] Although significantly fewer ($P < .03$) HIV subjects responded to the adenovirus type 4 vaccine than did normal soldiers, no clinically apparent adverse reactions were detected.[222] Response to the type 7 vaccine was difficult to define because many vaccine recipients in both groups had high neutralizing antibody titers at the time of vaccination.[222] More severely immunocompromised individuals, who might inadvertently be infected through fecal shedding from normal vaccine recipients, have not been studied.

Simultaneous Vaccination with Other Vaccines

The adenovirus vaccines are routinely given to military recruits with many other vaccines in the first 8 days after induction into the military. Table 23–5 shows an example of an immunization schedule for military trainees.[222] Type-specific neutralizing antibodies to the adenovirus vaccines are produced in the vaccinated trainees and are associated with protection against acute respiratory disease. Interference with immune responses when the adenovirus vaccines are given with other vaccines has not been identified.[222]

Table 23–5. **EXAMPLE OF AN IMMUNIZATION SCHEDULE FOR MILITARY TRAINEES**

Day 0 (arrival)	Adenovirus, live, oral, types 4 and 7
Day 1	Influenza, zonal purified, formaldehyde inactivated, whole virion for intramuscular injection Meningococcal polysaccharide vaccine, groups A, C, Y, and WI-135 combined for subcutaneous injection
Day 3	Tetanus and diphtheria toxoids adsorbed for intramuscular injection
Day 8	Poliovirus vaccine, live, oral types 1, 2, and 3 Measles virus, live for subcutaneous administration Rubella virus, live for subcutaneous injection, given only if the recruit is not immune by enzyme-linked immunoassay

Adapted from Rhodes JL, Birx DL, Wright C, et al. Safety and immunogenicity of multiple conventional immunizations administered during early HIV infection. J Acquir Immune Defic Syndr 4:724–731, 1991.

Future Vaccines

Subunit Vaccine. In 1963, soluble viral subunit antigens were found to be highly immunogenic on parenteral administration in animals.[208, 223] Crystalline hexon and fiber antigens from adenovirus type 5 have been shown to induce neutralizing antibody and protection in human volunteers who were challenged.[224] There has been no additional development of these antigens as potential vaccines. However, adenovirus vaccines consisting of soluble viral subunit antigens would be free of DNA and could alleviate any fear of the oncogenic potential of adenoviruses.[208]

Recombinant Vaccines. Advances in molecular biology have permitted the in vitro and in vivo gene transfer into mammalian cells. Genetically engineered adenoviruses, which are deficient in genes noted for oncogenicity, have been altered to carry heterologous genes from other pathogens.[225] Use of adenoviruses as multiple carrier vaccines could induce immunity to a number of other pathogens as well as to adenoviruses.[208] Because of their nonpathogenicity compared with adenovirus types 4 and 7, serotypes 2 and 5 have been mostly used for the development of recombinant vaccines.[226] The adenovirus recombinants have been generated by a variety of strategies. The cloning into the E1 region of a transgene uses a bacterial plasmid carrying the foreign DNA flanked by two subsegments of the wild-type viral genome, which provide the nucleotide sequences for the recombination. The chimeric plasmid is cotransfected with the wild-type adenovirus genome into E1 *trans*-complementing 293 cells.[226] The recombinant viruses are produced by in vivo homologous recombination between the two input DNA molecules and are defective for the E1A and E1B genes and require 293 cells for growth.[226] Another strategy uses in vitro ligation between plasmid DNA and viral DNA to make up the complete recombinant DNA before transfection.[226] The expression of the hepatitis B surface antigen in the adenovirus E3 gene region has been reported to induce antibody in animals.[227–229]

Studies have investigated the immunogenicity of recombinant adenovirus vaccines (type 4-, 5- and 7-vectored) carrying the *env* or *gag* protease genes of the HIV virus.[230–232] Chimpanzees responded with type-specific neutralizing anti-HIV antibodies at secretory sites and cell-mediated immune responses to both Gag and Env antigens.[231, 232] Adenoviruses have also been used to express DNA inserts from other viruses, such as human cytomegalovirus, bovine herpesvirus, pseudorabies virus, rabies virus, Epstein-Barr virus, human parainfluenza virus, respiratory syncytial virus, and rotavirus.[226, 233, 234] Some of these have been tested in a variety of animals, including dogs and chimpanzees, as well as in a variety of laboratory animals.[226, 235] Some of the advantages and disadvantages of the potential use of adenovirus-vectored vaccines and the safety issues, as well as foreseen obstacles related to their future use, have been addressed.[226, 236–238] Imler[236] reviewed the desired characteristics of the second-generation adenovirus-vectored vaccines.

Genetically engineered adenoviruses have also been investigated recently as gene transfer vectors for such genes as the cystic fibrosis gene and α_1-antitrypsin in preclinical experiments.[239–241] Early genes that are required for viral replication are deleted, rendering the adenoviruses nonreplicative and potentially efficient agents of gene transfer.[239–241] Inefficient gene transfer has also been reported.[242] Dose-dependent inflammatory lung infiltrates as a result of use of such constructs may prove to be a problem.[241] However, an investigation provided data that do not support a role for the production of cytokines by bronchial epithelial cells in the pathogenesis of such inflammation.[243] Others have reported that a similar E1/E3-deficient vector induced increased interleukin-8 production in A549 alveolar epithelial cells.[242] Future uses of adenovirus vaccines as carriers of genes from other pathogens and as gene transfer agents for genetic diseases await safety and efficacy trials in both animals and human subjects.

PUBLIC HEALTH CONSIDERATIONS

Epidemiological Results of Vaccination

In the prevaccine era, acute respiratory disease due to adenoviruses caused significant morbidity at military training centers. These outbreaks were extremely costly in terms of medical care requirements and time lost from training.[182] The routine administration of the type 4 and type 7 adenovirus vaccines, which began in 1971, resulted in an extremely efficacious, cost-effective, and safe immunization program.[182, 218] Initially, the vaccines were administered only during the high-risk winter months. The occurrence of spring and fall outbreaks prompted a modification of the program to administration of the vaccines year-round.[182] From 1971 to the present, with the exception of a period in the 1970s when defective vaccines contaminated with solvent were used,[22] there has never been an outbreak of acute respiratory disease due to adenovirus type 4 or adenovirus type 7 in U.S. military units that received the vaccines. Outbreaks of acute respiratory disease due to adenovirus type 21 have occurred, but these have been sporadic.[182, 205]

A problem in the administrative system used to procure vaccines for the U.S. military resulted in an adenovirus vaccine production delay that began in the spring of 1994 and lasted until late February 1995.[182] There was only one outbreak of acute respiratory disease due to adenoviruses reported in conjunction with that production delay.[221] When Wyeth Laboratories announced in 1996 that it would no longer produce the adenovirus vaccines, many within the U.S. Department of Defense and the different military services asked if the vaccines were still needed. Some thought that improved military barracks with modern heating, ventilation, and air-conditioning systems may have significantly reduced the risk of transmission of the adenoviruses and subsequent disease in susceptible people. The assessment of current risk was hampered by an absence of data on the prevalence of antibodies to adenoviruses in recruits and an absence of studies to assess carriage, transmission, infection, and disease associated with adenoviruses when the vaccines were not given. Owing to the success of the vaccines in controlling acute respiratory disease, the military lost the capability to do serological studies and had no incentive to study the behavior of adenoviruses in Air Force recruits who had not been routinely receiving the vaccine.

Recently, interest in acute respiratory disease due to adenoviruses in military populations has increased greatly, and several studies have been initiated to develop current data and information. This is because the U.S. Department of Defense may face several winters without the vaccines until a new manufacturer is found and their products are licensed. Because the variables that contributed to the high acute respiratory disease rates observed in the military in the prevaccine era were never defined, the risk of significant outbreaks in contemporary military training populations can only be surmised.[182] The U.S. Department of Defense is attempting to find a new manufacturer for the adenovirus vaccines and to limit the time that the vaccines are not available. This decision was based on a continuing low prevalence of antibodies to types 4 and 7 in people coming into the military,[220] the occurrence of a documented outbreak when the vaccines were not given,[221] and 25 years of experience of not having any acute respiratory disease outbreaks when potent adenovirus vaccines were being administered.[182]

Disease Control Strategies Now and in the Future

Adenovirus vaccines types 4 and 7 are the primary means for controlling acute respiratory disease due to adenoviruses in the U.S. military. Other means consist of administrative measures and adherence to industry-accepted standards for heating, air-conditioning, and ventilation systems. The administrative measures, such as providing each trainee a minimum amount of floor space and enforcing other practices, are aimed at reducing contact and transmission among the trainees (M.R. Howell et al., unpublished data). Cohorting is a practice whereby military training units are formed into cohorts at the beginning of the training period, and contact between people in different cohorts is kept to a minimum during the training period. Within the military barracks, in a line of beds, the recruits can be required to sleep in an alternating head-to-foot pattern, rather than having all heads at the same end of the bed. This is done to increase the distance between breathing zones during the night. In addition, recruits sleeping in an open area may be required to hang sheets from the ceiling to provide physical barriers between beds. Personal hygiene practices, to include use of a handkerchief when sneezing or coughing and hand washing, are supposed to be stressed at all times.

Standards for environmental variables address indoor air temperature, humidity, contaminants, and air exchanges per hour. These standards are intended to define minimum criteria for indoor air quality that will be acceptable to human occupants. Any association between the standards and the risk of acquiring acute respiratory disease due to adenoviruses is weak or empirical. However, these are the only standards available and are recommended for use in military buildings.[244]

Recommended Use

Adenovirus vaccines are recommended for use in military populations at risk of developing acute respiratory disease due to adenoviruses. Use of these vaccines is currently not recommended for other populations.

Acknowledgment

The authors thank Ronald P. Thiboutot, Ph.D., Managing Director, Wyeth-Ayerst Laboratories, Marietta, PA, for his assistance with the sections of this chapter dealing with vaccine preparation, constituents, and stability.

REFERENCES

1. Rowe WP, Huebner RJ, Gilmore LK. Isolation of a cytopathogenic agent from human adenoids undergoing spontaneous degeneration in tissue culture. Proc Soc Exp Biol Med 84:570–573, 1953.
2. Hilleman RM, Werner JH. Recovery of new agent from patients with acute respiratory illness. Proc Soc Exp Biol Med 85:183–188, 1954.
3. Adler H. Keratitis subepithelialis. Sentralbl Prakt Augenheilkd 16:289–294, 1889.
4. Jawetz E. The story of shipyard eye. Br Med J 1:873–878, 1959.
5. Huebner RJ, Rowe WP, Ward TJ. Adenoidal-pharyngeal-conjunctival agents. N Engl J Med 251:1077–1087, 1954.
6. Enders JF, Bell JA, Dingle J. Adenoviruses group name proposed for new respiratory tract viruses. Science 124:119–120, 1956.
7. Dingle JH, Langmuir AD. Epidemiology of acute respiratory disease in military recruits. Am Rev Respir Dis 97:1–65, 1968.
8. Chang C, Lepine P, Lelong M, Le-Tan-Vinn SP. Severe and fatal pneumonia in infants associated with adenovirus infections. Am J Hyg 67:367–378, 1958.
9. Johanson ME, Brown M, Hierholzer JC. Genome analysis of adenovirus type 31 from immunocompromised and immunocompetent patients. J Infect Dis 163:293–299, 1991.
10. Brandt CD, Kim HW, Vargosko AJ, et al. Infections in 18,000 infants and children in a controlled study of respiratory tract disease. I. Adenovirus pathogenicity in relation to serologic type and illness syndrome. Am J Epidemiol 90:484–500, 1969.
11. Hierholzer JC. Adenoviruses in the immunocompromised host. Clin Microbiol Rev 5:262–274, 1992.
12. Pinto A, Beck R, Jadavji T. Fatal neonatal pneumonia caused by adenovirus type 35. Arch Pathol Lab Med 116:95–99, 1992.
13. Stalder H, Hierholzer JC, Oxman MN. New human adenovirus candidate (adenovirus type 35) causing fatal disseminated infection in a renal transplant recipient. J Clin Microbiol 6:257–265, 1977.
14. Hierholzer JC, Wigand R, Anderson IJ, et al. Adenoviruses from patients with AIDS: A plethora of serotypes and a description of five new serotypes of subgenus D types 43–47. J Infect Dis 158:804–813, 1988.
15. Ambinder RF, Burns W, Forman M, et al. Hemorrhagic cystitis associated with adenovirus infection in bone marrow transplantation. Arch Intern Med 146:1400–1401, 1986.
16. Pingleton SK, Pingleton WW, Hill RH, et al. Type 3 adenoviral pneumonia occurring in a respiratory intensive care unit. Chest 73:554–555, 1978.
17. Albert MJ. Enteric adenoviruses. Arch Virol 88:1–17, 1986.
18. Warren D, Nelson KE, Farrar JA, et al. A large outbreak of epidemic keratoconjunctivitis—problems in controlling nosocomial spread. J Infect Dis 160:938–943, 1989.
19. Wishart PK, James C, Wishart MS, Darougar S. Prevalence of acute conjunctivitis caused by chlamydia, adenovirus, and herpes simplex virus in an ophthalmic casualty department. Br J Ophthalmol 68:653–655, 1984.
20. Hilleman MR, Gauld RL, Butler RL. Appraisal of occurrence of adenovirus caused respiratory illness in military populations. Am J Hyg 66:29–51, 1957.
21. Dudding BA, Top FH, Winter P. Acute respiratory disease in military trainees. The adenovirus surveillance program 1966–1971. Am J Epidemiol 97:187–198, 1973.
22. Top JHR. Control of adenovirus acute respiratory disease in U.S. Army trainees. Yale J Biol Med 48:185–195, 1975.
23. Dudding BA, Wagner SC, Zeller JA. Fatal pneumonia associated with adenovirus type 7 in three military recruits. N Engl J Med 286:1289–1292, 1972.
24. Schnurr D, Dondero ME. Two new candidate adenovirus serotypes. Intervirology 36:79–83, 1993.
25. Foy HM. Adenoviruses. In Evans AS (ed). Viral Infections of Humans. New York, Plenum Publishing, 1989, pp 77–89.
26. Rubin BA. Clinical picture and epidemiology of adenovirus infections. Acta Microbiol Hung 40:303–323, 1993.
27. Hierholzer JC. Adenoviruses. In Murray PR, Baron EJ, Pfaller MA, et al (eds). Manual of Clinical Microbiology. Washington, DC, American Society for Microbiology, 1997, pp 947–953.
28. Baum SG. Adenovirus. In Mandell GL, Bennett JE, Dolin R (eds). Principles and Practice of Infectious Diseases. New York, Churchill Livingstone, 1995, pp 1382–1387.
29. Brandt CD, Kim HW, Jeffries BC, et al. Infections in 18,000 infants and children in a controlled study of respiratory tract disease. Variation in adenovirus infections by year and season. Am J Epidemiol 95:218–227, 1972.
30. Fox JP, Brandt CD, Wassermann FE, et al. The virus watch program: A continuing surveillance of viral infections in metropolitan New York families. Observations of adenovirus infections: Virus excretion patterns, antibody response, efficiency of surveillance, patterns of infection and relation to illness. Am J Epidemiol 89:25–50, 1969.
31. Cooney MK, Hall CE, Fox JP. The Seattle virus watch. Evaluation of isolation methods and summary of infections detected by virus isolations. Am J Epidemiol 96:286–305, 1972.
32. Hall CE, Brandt CD, Frothingham TE, et al. The virus watch program. A continuing surveillance of viral infections in metropolitan New York families. A comparison of infections with several respiratory pathogens in New York and New Orleans families. Am J Epidemiol 94:367–385, 1971.
33. Foy HM, Cooney MK, McMahan R, Grayston JT. Viral and mycoplasmal pneumonia in a prepaid medical care group during an eight-year period. Am J Epidemiol 161:123–126, 1973.
34. Benyesh-Melnick M, Rosenberg HS. The isolation of adenovirus type 7 from a fatal case of pneumonia and disseminated disease. J Pediatr Gastroenterol 64:83–87, 1964.
35. Chany C, Lepine P, Lelong M, et al. Severe and fatal pneumonia in infants and young children associated with adenovirus infections. Am J Hyg 67:367–378, 1958.
36. Simla S, Ylikorkala O, Wasz-Hockert O. Type 7 adenovirus vaccine in volunteers: Clinical and immunological responses. J Infect Dis 79:605–611, 1971.

37. Straube RC, Thompson MA, Van Dyke RB, et al. Adenovirus type 7b in a children's hospital. J Infect Dis 147:814–819, 1983.
38. Schmitz H, Wigand R, Heinrich W. Worldwide epidemiology of human adenovirus infections. Am J Epidemiol 117:455–466, 1983.
39. Pacini DL, Collier AM, Henderson FW. Adenovirus infections and respiratory illnesses in children in group day care. J Infect Dis 156:920–927, 1987.
40. Cole RM, Mastrota FM, Floyd TM, Chanock RM. Illness and microbial experiences of nursery children at Junior Village. Am J Hyg 74:267–292, 1961.
41. Commission on Acute Respiratory Disease. Experimental transmission of minor respiratory illness to human volunteers by filter-passing agents. Demonstration of two types of illness characterized by long and short incubation periods and different clinical features. J Clin Invest 26:957–973, 1947.
42. Baum SG. Adenoviruses. In Gorbach SL, Bartlett JB, Blacklow NB (eds). Infectious Diseases. Philadelphia, WB Saunders, 1992, pp 1663–1667.
43. Couch RB, Cate TR, Douglas RG Jr, et al. Effect of route of inoculation on experimental respiratory viral disease in volunteers and evidence for airborne transmission. Bacteriol Rev 30:517–531, 1966.
44. Amundson DE, Weiss PJ. Pneumonia in military recruits. Milit Med 159:629–631, 1994.
45. Bell JA, Rowe WP, Engler JI, et al. Pharyngoconjunctival fever. Epidemiological studies of a recently recognized disease entity. JAMA 157:1083–1092, 1955.
46. Bahn C. Swimming bath conjunctivitis. New Orleans Med Sci J 79:586–590, 1927.
47. D'Angelo LJ, Hierholzer JC, Keenlyside RA, et al. Pharyngoconjunctival fever caused by adenovirus type 4. Report of a swimming pool–related outbreak with recovery of virus from pool water. J Infect Dis 140:42–47, 1979.
48. Parrott RH, Rowe WP, Huebner RJ, et al. Outbreak of febrile pharyngitis and conjunctivitis associated with type 3 adenoidal-phryngeal-conjunctival virus infection. N Engl J Med 251:1087–1090, 1954.
49. Foy HM, Cooney MK, Hatlen JB. Adenovirus type 3 epidemic associated with intermittent chlorination of a swimming pool. Arch Environ Health 17:795–802, 1968.
50. Hogan MJ, Crawford JW. Epidemic keratoconjunctivitis, superficial punctate keratitis, keratitis subepithelialis, keratitis maculosa, keratitis nummularis. Am J Ophthalmol 25:1057–1078, 1942.
51. D'Angelo LJ, Hierholzer JC, Holman RC, Smith JD. Epidemic keratoconjunctivitis caused by adenovirus type 8. Epidemiologic and laboratory aspects of a large outbreak. Am J Epidemiol 113:44–49, 1981.
52. Darougar S, Grey RHB, Thaker U, McSwiggan DA. Clinical and epidemiological features of adenovirus keratoconjunctivitis in London. Br J Ophthalmol 67:1–7, 1983.
53. Guyer B, O'Day DM, Hierholzer JC, Schafner W. Epidemic keratoconjunctivitis. A community outbreak of mixed adenovirus type 8 and type 19 infection. J Infect Dis 132:142–150, 1975.
54. Kemp MC, Hierholzer JC, Cabradilla CP, Obijeski JF. The changing etiology of epidemic keratoconjunctivitis. Antigenic and restriction enzyme analyses of adenovirus type 19 and 37 isolated over a 10-year period. Acta Paediatr Scand 148:24–33, 1983.
55. Darougar S, Walpita P, Thaker U, et al. Adenovirus serotype isolated from ocular infections in London. Br J Ophthalmol 67:111–114, 1983.
56. Muzerie CJ, Wermenbol AG, Schaap GJP. Adenovirus 37. Identification and characterization of a medically important new adenovirus type of subgroup D. J Med Virol 7:105–118, 1981.
57. Harnett GB, Newnham WA. Isolation of adenovirus type 19 from the male and female genital tracts. Br J Vener Dis 57:55–57, 1981.
58. Sprague JB, Hierholzer JC, Currier RW II, et al. Epidemic keratoconjunctivitis. A severe industrial outbreak due to adenovirus type 8. N Engl J Med 289:1341–1346, 1973.
59. Keenlyside RA, Hierholzer JC, D'Angelo LJ. Keratoconjunctivitis associated with adenovirus type 37: An extended outbreak in an ophthalmologist's office. J Infect Dis 147:191–198, 1983.
60. Mufson MA, Belshe RB. A review of adenoviruses in the etiology of acute hemorrhagic cystitis. J Urol 115:191–194, 1976.
61. Numazaki Y, Kimasaka T, Yano N, et al. Further study of acute hemorrhagic cystis due to adenovirus type 11. N Engl J Med 289:344–347, 1973.
62. Koga S, Shindo K, Matsuya F, et al. Acute hemorrhagic cystitis caused by adenovirus following renal transplantation: Review of the literature. J Urol 149:838–839, 1993.
63. Londergan TA, Walzak MP. Hemorrhagic cystitis due to adenovirus infection following bone marrow transplantation. J Urol 151:1013–1014, 1994.
64. Horwitz MS. Adenoviridae and their replication. In Fields BN, Knipe DM, Chanock RM, et al (eds). Virology. New York, Raven Press, 1990, pp 1679–1721.
65. Ito M, Hirabayashi N, Uno Y. Necrotizing tubulointerstitial nephritis associated with adenovirus infection. Hum Pathol 22:1225–1231, 1991.
66. Koc J, Wigand R, Weil M. The efficiency of various laboratory methods for the diagnosis of adenovirus conjunctivitis. Zentralbl Bakteriol Mikrobiol Hyg 263:607–615, 1987.
67. Yolken RH, Lawrence F. Gastroenteritis associated with enteric type adenovirus in hospitalized infants. J Pediatr Gastroenterol 101:21–26, 1982.
68. Brandt CD, Kim HW, Rodriguez WJ, et al. Comparison of direct electron microscopy, immune electron microscopy, and rotavirus enzyme-linked immunosorbent assay for detection of gastroenteritis viruses in children. J Clin Microbiol 13:976–981, 1981.
69. Chiba S, Nakatq S, Nakamuba I, et al. Outbreak of infantile gastroenteritis due to type 40 adenovirus. Lancet 2:954–957, 1983.
70. Rodriguez WJ, Kim HW, Brandt CD, et al. Fecal adenoviruses from a longitudinal study of families in metropolitan Washington, D.C. Laboratory, clinical and epidemiologic observations. J Pediatr Gastroenterol 107:514–520, 1985.
71. Uhnoo I, Wadell G, Svensson L, Johansson ME. Importance of enteric adenoviruses 40 and 41 in acute gastroenteritis in infants and young children. J Clin Microbiol 20:365–372, 1984.
72. Simla S, Jouppila R, Salmi A, Pohjonen R. Encephalomeningitis in children associated with an adenovirus type 7 epidemic. Acta Paediatr Scand 59:310–316, 1970.
73. Kelsey DS. Adenovirus meningoencephalitis. Pediatrics 61:291–293, 1978.
74. Abzug ML, Levine MJ. Neonatal adenovirus infection: Four patients and review of the literature. Pediatrics 87:890–896, 1991.
75. Connor JD. Evidence for an etiologic role of adenoviral infection in pertussis syndrome. N Engl J Med 283:390–394, 1970.
76. Klenk EL, Gwaltney JM, Bass JW. Bacteriologically proved pertussis and adenovirus infection. Am J Dis Child 124:203–207, 1972.
77. Sturdy PM, Court SD, Gardner PS. Viruses and whooping-cough. Lancet 2:978–979, 1971.
78. Nelson KE, Gavitt F, Batt MD, et al. The role of adenoviruses in the pertussis syndrome. J Pediatr Gastroenterol 86:335–341, 1975.
79. Russkanen O, Meurman O, Kusjavi A. Adenoviruses. In Richman DD, Whitley RJ, Hayden FG (eds). Clinical Virology. New York, Churchill Livingstone, 1997, pp 525–547.
80. Shields AF, Hackman RC, Fife KH, et al. Adenovirus infections in patients undergoing bone-marrow transplantation. N Engl J Med 312:529–533, 1985.
81. Carmichael GP Jr, Zahradnick JM, Moyer GH, Porter DD. Adenovirus hepatitis in an immunosuppressed adult patient. Clin Pathol 71:352–355, 1979.
82. de Jong PJ, Valderrama G, Spigland I, Horwitz MS. Adenovirus isolates from urine of patients with acquired immunodeficiency syndrome. Lancet 1:1293–1296, 1983.
83. Horwitz MS, Valderrama G, Korn R, Spigland I. Adenovirus isolates from the urines of AIDS patients: Characterization of group B recombinants in acquired immune deficiency syndrome. In Gottlieb MS, Groopman JE (eds). UCLA Symposia on Molecular and Cellular Biology. New York, Alan R Liss, 1984, pp 187–207.
84. Ohori NP, Michaels MG, Jaffe R, et al. Adenovirus pneumonia in lung transplant recipients. Hum Pathol 26:1073–1079, 1995.

85. Flomenberg PR, Chen M, Munk G. Molecular epidemiology of adenovirus type 35 infections in immunocompromised host. J Infect Dis 155:1127–1134, 1987.
86. Gelfand MS, Cleveland KO, Lancaster D, et al. Adenovirus parotitis in patients with AIDS. Clin Infect Dis 19:1045–1048, 1994.
87. Flomenberg P, Babbitt J, Drobyski WR, et al. Increasing incidence of adenovirus disease in bone marrow transplant recipients. J Infect Dis 169:775–781, 1994.
88. Hierholzer JC. Adenoviruses in the immunocompromised host. Clin Microbiol Rev 5:262–274, 1992.
89. Dolin R. Viral pneumonia. In Gorbach SL, Bartlett JB, Blacklow NB (eds). Infectious Diseases. Philadelphia, WB Saunders, 1992, pp 485–490.
90. Ginsberg HS, Pereira HG, Valentine RC, Wilcox WC. A proposed terminology for the adenovirus antigens and virion morphological subunits. Virology 28:782–783, 1966.
91. Horne RW, Bonner S, Waterson AP. The icosohedral form of an adenovirus. J Mol Biol 1:84–86, 1956.
92. Maizel JV Jr, White DO, Scharff MD. The polypeptides of adenovirus. Evidence for multiple protein components in the virion and a comparison of types 2, 7A and 12. Virology 36:115–125, 1968.
93. Van Oostrum J, Burnett RM. Molecular composition of the adenovirus type 2 viron. J Virol 56:439–488, 1985.
94. Philipson J, Peterson U, Lindberg U. Molecular biology of adenoviruses. Virol Monogr 14:1–115, 1975.
95. Wadell G. Adenoviridae: The adenoviruses. In Lennett EH, Halonen P, Murphy FA (eds). Laboratory Diagnosis of Infectious Disease: Principles and Practice. New York, Springer-Verlag, 1988, pp 284–300.
96. Hierholzer JC, Stone YO, Broderson JR. Antigenic relationships among the 47 human adenoviruses determined in reference horse antisera. Arch Virol 121:179–197, 1991.
97. Hierholzer JC, Wigand R, de Jong JC. Evaluation of human adenoviruses 38, 39, 40 and 41 as new serotypes. Intervirology 29:1–10, 1988.
98. Wadell G. Molecular epidemiology of human adenoviruses. Curr Top Microbiol Immunol 110:191–220, 1984.
99. Adrian T, Wadell G, Hierholzer JC, Wigand R. DNA restriction analysis of adenovirus prototypes 1 to 41. Arch Virol 91:277–290, 1986.
100. Adrian T, Becker M, Hierholzer JC, Wigand R. Molecular epidemiology and restriction site mapping of adenovirus 7 genome types. Arch Virol 106:73–84, 1989.
101. Li Q, Waddell G. Analysis of 15 different genome types of adenovirus type 7 isolated on five continents. J Virol 60:331–335, 1986.
102. Li Q, Wadell G. Comparison of 17 genome types of adenovirus type 3 identified among strains recovered from six continents. J Clin Microbiol 20:1009–1015, 1988.
103. Adrian T. Genome type analysis of adenovirus type 4. Intervirology 34:180–183, 1992.
104. Cooper RJ, Bailey AS, Killough R, Richmond SJ. Genome analysis of adenovirus 4 isolated over a six year period. J Med Virol 39:62–66, 1993.
105. Li Q, Zheng Q, Liu Y, Wadell G. Molecular epidemiology of adenovirus type 3 and 7 isolated from children with pneumonia in Beijing. J Med Virol 49:170–177, 1996.
106. Evans AS. Latent adenovirus infections of the human respiratory tract. Am J Hyg 67:256–266, 1958.
107. Andiman WA, Miller G. Persistent infection with adenovirus type 5 and 6 in lymphoid cells from humans and wooly monkeys. J Infect Dis 145:83–88, 1982.
108. Zahradnik JM, Spencer MJ, Porter DD. Adenovirus infection in the immunocompromised patient. Am J Med 68:725–732, 1980.
109. Yolken RH, Bishop CA, Townsend TR. Infectious gastroenteritis in bone-marrow transplant recipients. N Engl J Med 306:1009–1012, 1982.
110. Brummitt CF, Cherrington JM, Katzenstein DA. Nosocomial adenovirus infections. Molecular epidemiology of an outbreak due to adenovirus. J Infect Dis 158:423–432, 1988.
111. Reid JA, Breckon D, Hunter PR. Infection of staff during an outbreak of viral gastroenteritis in an elderly persons' home. J Hosp Infect 16:81–85, 1990.
112. Baum SG. Persistent adenovirus infections of nonpermissive monkey cells. J Virol 23:412–420, 1977.
113. Wold WSM. Adenovirus genes that modulate the sensitivity of virus-infected cells to lysis by TNF. J Cell Biochem 53:329–335, 1993.
114. Horvath J, Palkonyay L, Weber J. Group C adenovirus DNA sequences in human lymphoid cells. J Virol 59:189–192, 1986.
115. Huebner RJ, Rowe WP, Lane WT. Oncogenic effects in hamsters of human adenoviruses types 12 and 18. Proc Natl Acad Sci USA 48:2051–2058, 1962.
116. Ginsberg HS, Lundholm-Beauchamp U, Horswood RL, et al. Role of early region 3 (E3) in pathogenesis of adenovirus disease. Proc Natl Acad Sci USA 86:3823–3827, 1989.
117. Ginsberg HS, Prince GA: The molecular basis of adenovirus pathogenesis. Infect Agents Dis 3:1–8, 1994.
118. Elliott WM, Hayashi S, Hogg JC. Immunodetection of adenoviral E1A proteins in human lung tissue. Am J Respir Cell Mol Biol 12:642–648, 1995.
119. Gold DR, Tager IB, Weiss ST, et al. Acute lower respiratory illness in childhood as predictor of lung function and chronic respiratory symptoms. Am Rev Respir Dis 140:877–884, 1989.
120. Liu F, Green MR. Promoter targeting by adenovirus E1a through interaction with different cellular DNA binding domains. Nature 368:520–525, 1994.
121. Shenk T, Flint J. Transcriptional and transforming activities of the adenovirus E1a proteins. Adv Cancer Res 57:47–85, 1991.
122. Matsuse T, Hayashi S, Kuwano K, et al. Latent adenoviral infection in the pathogenesis of chronic airways obstruction. Am Rev Respir Dis 146:177–184, 1992.
123. Bergelson JM, Cunningham JA, Droguett G, et al. Isolation of a common receptor for coxsackie b viruses and adenoviruses 2 and 5. Science 275:1320–1323, 1997.
124. Durepaire N, Ranger-Rogez S, Denis F. Evaluation of rapid culture centrifugation method for adenovirus detection in stool. Diagn Microbiol Infect Dis 24:25–29, 1996.
125. Hierholzer J, Schmidt I, Emmons NJ. Diagnostic Procedures for Viral, Rickettsial, and Chlamydial Infections (6th ed). Washington, DC, American Public Health Association, 1989, pp 219–264.
126. Rabalais GP, Stout GG, Ladd KL, Cost KM. Rapid diagnosis of respiratory viral infections by using a shell vial assay and monoclonal antibody pool. J Clin Microbiol 30:1505–1508, 1992.
127. Thomas EE, Roscoe DL. The utility of latex agglutination assays in the diagnosis of pediatric viral gastroenteritis. Am J Clin Pathol 101:742–746, 1994.
128. Hierholzer JC, Johansson KH, Anderson LJ, et al. Comparison of monoclonal time-resolved fluoroimmunoassay with monoclonal capture biotinylated detector enzyme immunoassay for adenovirus antigen detection. J Clin Microbiol 25:1662–1667, 1987.
129. Madeley CR. The emerging role of adenoviruses as inducers of gastroenteritis. Pediatr Infect Dis 5:S63–S74, 1986.
130. Brown M, Petric M, Middleton PJ. Diagnosis of fastidious enteric adenoviruses 40 and 41 in stool specimens. J Clin Microbiol 20:334–338, 1984.
131. Schmidt W, Schneider T, Heise W, et al. Stool viruses, coinfections, and diarrhea in HIV-infected patients. J Acquir Immune Defic Syndr Hum Retrovirol 13:33–38, 1996.
132. Wood DJ, Bijlsma K, de Jong JC, Tonkin C. Evaluation of a commercial monoclonal antibody-based enzyme immunoassay for detection for adenovirus types 40 and 41 in stool specimens. J Clin Microbiol 27:1155–1158, 1989.
133. Kok T, Mickan LD, Burrell CJ. Routine diagnosis of seven respiratory viruses and *Mycoplasma pneumoniae* by enzyme immunoassay. J Virol 50:87–100, 1994.
134. Wood SR, Sharp IR, de Jong JC, Uijterwaal-Verweij MW. Development and preliminary evaluation of an enzyme immunosorbent assay for the detection of adenovirus type 8. J Med Virol 44:348–352, 1994.
135. Bryden AS, Bertrand J. Diagnosis of adenovirus conjunctivitis by enzyme immunoassay. Br J Biomed Sci 53:182–184, 1996.
136. Hyypia T. Detection of adenovirus in nasopharyngeal specimens by radioactive and nonradioactive DNA probes. J Clin Microbiol 21:730–733, 1985.
137. Ranki M, Virtanen M, Palva A. Nucleic acid sandwich hybridization in adenovirus diagnosis. Curr Top Microbiol Immunol 104:307–318, 1983.

138. Bateman ED, Hayashi S, Kuwano K. Latent adenoviral infection in follicular bronchiectasis. Am J Respir Crit Care Med 151:170–176, 1995.
139. Nuovo MA, Nuovo GJ, Becker J, et al. Correlation of viral infection, histology, and mortality in immunocompromised patients with pneumonia. Diagn Mol Pathol 2:200–209, 1993.
140. Ankers HE, Klapper PE, Cleator GM, et al. The role of a rapid diagnostic test adenovirus immune dot blot in the control of an outbreak of adenovirus type 8 keratoconjunctivitis. Eye 7(suppl): 15–17, 1993.
141. Wiley LA, Roba LA, Kowalski RP, et al. A 5 year evaluation of the adenoclone test for the rapid diagnosis of adenovirus from conjunctival swabs. Cornea 15:363–367, 1996.
142. Hierholzer JC, Halonen PE, Dahlen PO, et al. Detection of adenovirus in clinical specimens by polymerase chain reaction and liquid phase hybridization quantitated by time resolved fluorometry. J Clin Microbiol 31:1886–1891, 1993.
143. McDonaugh M, Olen K, Hierholzer J. PCR detection of human adenoviruses. In Persing DH, Smith TF, Tenover FC, White TJ (eds). Diagnostic Molecular Microbiology in Principles and Applications. Washington, DC, American Society for Microbiology, 1993.
144. Allard A, Girones R, Juto P, Waddell G. Polymerase chain reaction for detection of adenoviruses in stool samples. J Clin Microbiol 28:2659–2667, 1990.
145. Hussain MAS, Costelli P, Morris DJ, et al. Comparison of primer sets for detection of fecal and ocular adenovirus infection using the polymerase chain reaction. J Med Virol 49:187–194, 1996.
146. Allard A, Albinsson B, Wadell G. Detection of adenoviruses in stool from healthy persons and patients with diarrhoea by two-step polymerase chain reaction. J Med Virol 37:149–157, 1992.
147. Arthur R. PCR based methods for the detection of adenoviruses. In Ehrlich GD, Greenberg SJ (eds). PCR-Based Diagnostics in Infectious Disease. Boston, Blackwell Scientific Publications, 1994, pp 447–454.
148. Timessen CT, Nell MJ. Detection and typing of subgroup F adenoviruses using the polymerase chain reaction. J Virol 59:73–82, 1996.
149. Schowengerdt KO, Ni J, Denfield SW, et al. Diagnosis, surveillance, and epidemiologic evaluation of viral infections in pediatric cardiac transplant recipients with the use of the polymerase chain reaction. J Heart Lung Transplant 15:111–123, 1996.
150. Martin AB, Webber S, Fricker J, et al. Acute myocarditis. Rapid diagnosis by PCR in children. Circulation 90:330–339, 1994.
151. Akhtar N, Ni J, Langston C, et al. PCR diagnosis of viral pneumonitis from fixed-lung tissue in children. Biochem Mol Med 58:66–76, 1996.
152. Turner PC, Bailey AS, Cooper RJ, Morris DJ. The polymerase chain reaction for detecting adenovirus DNA in formalin fixed paraffin embedded tissue obtained post mortem. J Infect Dis 27:43–48, 1993.
153. Kinchington PR, Turse SE, Kowalski RP, Jerold GY. Use of polymerase chain amplification reaction for the detection of adenoviruses in ocular swab specimens. Invest Ophthalmol Vis Sci 35:4126–4134, 1994.
154. Morris DJ, Cooper RJ, Barr T, Bailey AS. Polymerase chain reaction for rapid diagnosis of respiratory adenovirus infection. J Infect Dis 32:113–117, 1996.
155. Morris DJ, Bailey AS, Cooper RJ, et al. Polymerase chain reaction for rapid detection of ocular adenovirus infection. J Med Virol 46:126–132, 1995.
156. Saitoh-Inagawa W, Oshima A, Aoki K, et al. Rapid diagnosis of adenoviral conjunctivitis by PCR and restriction fragment length polymorphism analysis. J Clin Microbiol 34:2113–2116, 1997.
157. Kidd AH, Jonsson M, Garwicz D, et al. Rapid subgenus identification in human adenovirus isolates by a general PCR. J Clin Microbiol 34:622–627, 1996.
158. Jackson R, Morris DJ, Cooper RJ, et al. Multiplex polymerase chain reaction for adenovirus and herpes simplex virus in eye swabs. J Virol Methods 56:41–49, 1996.
159. Puig M, Jofre J, Lucena F, et al. Detection of adenoviruses and enteroviruses in polluted waters by nested PCR amplification. Appl Environ Microbiol 60:2963–2970, 1994.
160. Meurman O, Ruuskanen O, Sarkkinen H. Immunoassay diagnosis of adenovirus infections in children. J Clin Microbiol 18:1190–1195, 1983.
161. Crawford-Miksza LK, Schnurr DP. Quantitative colorimetric microneutralization assay for characterization of adenoviruses. J Clin Microbiol 32:2331–2334, 1994.
162. Ramano A, Ladizenski E, Guarari-Rotman D, Revel M. Clinical effect of human fibroblast derived interferon in treatment of adenovirus epidemic keratoconjunctivitis and its complications. Tex Rep Biol Med 41:559–565, 1981.
163. Baba M, Mori S, Shigeta S, DeClerco E. Selective inhibitory effects of (s)-9-3(3-hydroxy-2-phosphonylmethoxypropyl)adenine and 2′-nor-cyclic GMP on adenovirus replication in vitro. Antimicrob Agents 31:337–339, 1987.
164. Buchdall RM, Taylor P, Warner JO. Nebulised ribavirin for adenovirus pneumonia. Lancet 2:1070–1071, 1985.
165. Cassano WF. Intravenous ribavirin therapy for adenovirus cystis after allogeneic bone marrow transplantation. Bone Marrow Transplant 7:247–248, 1991.
166. Murphy GF, Wood DP, McRoberts JW, Henslee-Downey PJ. Adenovirus associated hemorrhagic cystitis treated with intravenous ribavirin. J Urol 149:565–566, 1993.
167. McCarthy AJ, Bergin M, DeSilva LM, Stevens M. Intravenous ribavirin therapy for disseminated adenovirus infection. Pediatr Infect Dis 14:1003–1004, 1995.
168. Kapelunshnik J, Delukina M. Intravenous ribavirin therapy for adenovirus gastroenteritis after bone marrow transplantation. J Pediatr Gastroenterol 21:110–112, 1995.
169. Sabroe I, McHale J, Tait DR. Treatment of adenoviral pneumonitis with intravenous ribavirin and immunoglobulin. Thorax 50:1219–1220, 1995.
170. Trousdale MD, Goldschmidt PL, Nobrega R. Activity of ganciclovir against human adenovirus type 5 infection in cell culture and cotton rat eyes. Cornea 13:435–439, 1994.
171. Wright PF. Respiratory disease. In Viral Pathogenesis. New York, Academic Press, 1996, pp 703–711.
172. Yamadera S, Yamashita K, Akatsuka M, et al. Adenovirus surveillance. Jpn J Med Sci Biol 48:199–210, 1995.
173. Prado V, O'Ryan ML. Acute gastroenteritis in Latin America. Dis Latin Am 8:77–106, 1994.
174. Klapper PE, Cleator GM. Adenovirus cross-infection: A continuing problem. J Hosp Infect 30:262–267, 1995.
175. Richmond SJ, Burman R, Crosdale E. A large outbreak of keratoconjunctivitis due to adenovirus type 8. J Hyg 93:285–291, 1984.
176. Holladay RC, Campbell DG. Nosocomial viral pneumonia in the intensive care unit. Clin Chest Med 16:121–133, 1995.
177. Larsen RA, Jacobson JT, Jacobson JA. Hospital associated epidemic of pharyngitis and conjunctivitis caused by adenovirus. J Infect Dis 154:706–709, 1986.
178. Blanshard C, Francis N, Gazzard BG. Investigation of chronic diarrhoea in acquired immunodeficiency syndrome. A prospective study of 155 patients. Gut 39:824–832, 1996.
179. Van der Veen J, Oki KG, Abarbanel MFW. Patterns of infection with adenovirus types 4, 7, and 21 in military recruits during a 9-year survey. J Hyg 67:255–268, 1969.
180. Bloom HH, Forsyth BR, Johnson KM. Patterns of adenovirus infections in Marine Corps personnel. I. A 42-month survey in recruit and nonrecruit populations. Am J Hyg 80:328–342, 1964.
181. Forsyth BR, Bloom HH, Johnson KM, Chanock RM. Patterns of adenovirus infections in Marine Corps personnel. II. Longitudinal study of successive advanced recruit training companies. Am J Hyg 80:343–356, 1964.
182. Gaydos CA, Gaydos JC. Adenovirus vaccines in the U.S. Military. Milit Med 160:300–304, 1995.
183. Stallones RA, Hilleman MR, Gauld RL. Adenovirus vaccine for prevention of acute respiratory illness. JAMA 163:9–15, 1957.
184. Hilleman MR, Greenberg JH, Warfield MS. Second field evaluation of bivalent types 4 and 7 adenovirus vaccine. Arch Intern Med 102:428–436, 1958.
185. Culver JO, Lennetti EH, Flintjer JD. Adenovirus vaccine, a field evaluation of protective capacity against respiratory desease. Am J Hyg 69:120–126, 1959.
186. Sherwood RW, Buescher EL, Nitz RE. Effect of adenovirus vaccine on acute respiratory disease in U.S. Army recruits. JAMA 178:1115–1127, 1961.
187. Hitchcock G, Tyrell DA, Bynol ML. Vaccination of man with attenuated live adenovirus. J Hyg (Camb) 58:288–292, 1960.
188. Couch RB, Chanock RM, Cate TR. Immunization with types 4

and 7 adenovirus by selective infection of the intestinal tract. Am Rev Respir Dis 88:394–403, 1963.
189. Chanock RM, Ludwig W, Huebner RJ, et al. Immunization by selective infection with type 4 adenovirus grown in human diploid tissue culture. I. Safety and lack of oncogenicity and tests for potency in volunteers. JAMA 195:445–452, 1966.
190. Trentin JJ, Van Hoosier JL, Samper L. The oncogenicity of human adenoviruses in hamsters. Proc Soc Biol Med 127:683–689, 1968.
191. McBride WD, Wiener A. In vitro transformation of hamster kidney cells by human adenovirus type 12. Proc Soc Exp Biol Med 115:870–874, 1964.
192. Edmonson WP, Purcell RH, Gundelfinger BF, et al. Immunization by selective infection with type 4 adenovirus grown in human diploid tissue culture. II. Specific protective effect against epidemic desease. JAMA 195:453–459, 1966.
193. Pierce WE, Rosenbaum MJ, Edwards EA. Live and inactivated adenovirus vaccines for the prevention of acute respiratory illness in naval recruits. Am J Epidemiol 87:237–246, 1968.
194. Huebner RJ. The problem of oncogenicity of adenoviruses. In First International Conference on Vaccines Against Viral and Rickettsial Diseases of Man; Washington, DC; November 7–11, 1966. Washington, DC, Pan American Health Organization, 1967.
195. Gilden RV, Kern J, Lee YK. Serologic surveys of human cancer patients for antibody to adenovirus T antigens. Am J Epidemiol 91:500–509, 1970.
196. McAllister RM, Gliden RV, Green M. Adenoviruses in human cancer. Lancet 1:831–833, 1972.
197. National Cancer Institute. The Virus Cancer Program. Bethesda, MD, Viral Oncology Area, Division of Cancer Cause and Prevention, 1974.
198. Top FH, Grossman RA, Bartelloni PJ. Immunization with live types 7 and 4 adenovirus vaccine. Safety, infectivity and potency of adenovirus type 7 vaccine in humans. J Infect Dis 124:148–154, 1971.
199. Top FH, Buescher EL, Bancroft WH. Immunization with live types 7 and 4 adenovirus vaccines. Antibody response and protective effect against acute respiratory disease due to adenovirus type 7. J Infect Dis 124:155–160, 1971.
200. Top FH, Dudding BA, Russell PK. Control of respiratory disease in recruits with types 4 and 7 adenovirus vaccines. Am J Epidemiol 94:142–146, 1971.
201. Van der Veen J, Dykman JH. Association of type 21 adenovirus with acute respiratory illness in military recruits. Am J Hyg 76:149–159, 1962.
202. Dudding BA, Bartelloni PJ, Scott RM. Enteric immunization with live adenovirus type 21 vaccine. Tests for safety, infectivity, immunogenicity, and potency in volunteers. Infect Immun 5:295–299, 1972.
203. Scott RM, Dudding BA, Romano SV. Enteric immunization with live adenovirus type 21 vaccine. Systemic and local immune responses following immunization. Infect Immun 5:300–304, 1972.
204. Top FH, Brandt WE, Russell PK. Adenovirus acute respiratory disease in basic combat trainees. In Research in Biological and Medical Sciences. Annual Progress Report. Washington, DC, Walter Reed Army Institute of Research, 1976, pp 462–465.
205. Takafuji ET, Gaydos JC, Allen RG. Simultaneous administration of live enteric-coated adenoviruses type 4, 7 and 21 vaccines, safety and immunogenicity. J Infect Dis 140:48–53, 1979.
206. Departments of the Army (AR40-562) TN1, The Navy (BUMEDINST 6230.15), The Air Force (Joint Instruction 48-110), and Transportation (CG COMDTINST M623.4E). Immunizations and Chemoprophylaxis. Washington, DC, US Government Printing Office, 1995; 1996-404-611:20059.
207. Tint H, Stone JL, Minecci LC, Rubin BA. Type 4 adenovirus vaccine, live, prepared in human diploid cell for oral administration. Prog Immunobiol Stand 3:113–122, 1969.
208. Lee SG, Hung PP. Vaccines for control of respiratory disease caused by adenoviruses. J Med Virol 3:209–216, 1993.
209. Bellanti JA, Artenstein BC, Brand BS, et al. Immunoglobin responses in serum and nasal secretions after natural adenovirus infections. J Immunol 103:891–898, 1969.
210. Rosenbaum MJ, De Berry P, Sullivan EJ. Characteristics of vaccine-induced and natural infection with adenovirus type 4 in naval recruits. Am J Epidemiol 88:45–54, 1997.
211. McCown WA, McCown JW. Experimental respiratory infection with type 4 adenovirus vaccine in volunteers. Clinical and immunological responses. J Infect Dis 122:239–248, 1970.
212. Gutekunst RR, Heggie AD. Viremia and viruria in adenovirus infection. N Engl J Med 261:374–378, 1961.
213. Van der Veen J, Abarbanel NFW, Oki KG. Vaccination with live type 4 adenoviruses: Evaluation of antibody responses and protective efficacy. J Hyg (Camb) 66:499–511, 1968.
214. Peckinpaugh RO, Pierce WE, Rosenbaum MJ, et al. Mass enteric live adenovirus vaccination during epidemic acute respiratory disease. JAMA 205:75–80, 1968.
215. Rosenbaum MJ, Edwards EA, Hoeffler DF, et al. Recent experiences with live adenovirus vaccines in navy recruits. Milit Med 4:251–257, 1975.
216. Gooch WM, Mogabgab WJ. Simultaneous oral administration of live adenovirus types 4 and 7 vaccine. Arch Environ Health 25:388–394, 1972.
217. Meiklejohn G. Viral respiratory disease at Lowry Air Force Base in Denver 1952–1982. J Infect Dis 148:775–784, 1983.
218. Collis PB, Dudding BA, Winter PE, et al. Adenovirus vaccines in military recruit populations: A cost benefit analysis. J Infect Dis 128:745–752, 1973.
218a. Howell MR, Nang RN, Gaydos CA, Gaydos JC. Prevention of adenoviral acute respiratory disease in army recruits: Cost-effectiveness of a military vaccination policy. Am J Prev Med 14:168–175, 1998.
219. Stanley ED, Jackson GG. Spread of enteric live adenovirus type 4 vaccine in married couples. J Infect Dis 119:51–59, 1969.
220. Towle C, Ludwig SL, Gaydos JC, et al. Seroprevalence survey of antibodies to adenovirus types 4 and 7 among U.S. Army recruits. US Navy Occupational and Preventive Medicine Workshop; Norfolk, VA; February 7–14, 1997.
221. Barraza EM. Adenovirus outbreak—basic trainees, Fort Jackson, SC. Medical Surveillance Monthly Report (US Army Center for Health Promotion and Preventive Medicine, Aberdeen Proving Ground, MD) 1:9–10, 1995.
222. Rhoads JL, Birx DL, Wright DC, et al. Safety and immunogenicity of multiple conventional immunizations administered during early HIV infections. J Acquir Immune Defic Syndr Hum Retrovirol 4:724–731, 1991.
223. Wilcox WC, Ginsberg HS. Production of specific neutralizing antibody with soluble antigens of type 5 adenovirus. Proc Soc Exp Biol Med 114:37–42, 1963.
224. Couch RB, Kasel JA, Pereira HG, et al. Induction of immunity in man by crystalline adenovirus type 5 capsid antigens. Proc Soc Exp Biol Med 143:905–910, 1973.
225. Rubin BA, Rorke LB. Adenovirus vaccines. In Plotkin M, Mortimer EA (eds). Vaccines. Philadelphia, WB Saunders, 1994, pp 475–502.
226. Randrianarison-Jewtoukoff V, Perricaudet M. Recombinant adenoviruses and vaccines. Biologicals 23:145–157, 1995.
227. Chengalvala M, Lubeck MD, Davis AR. Evaluation of adenovirus type 4 and 7 recombinant hepatitis B vaccines in dogs. Vaccine 9:485–490, 1991.
228. Morin JE, Lubeck MD, Barton JE. Recombinant adenovirus induces antibody response to hepatitis B virus surface antigen in hamsters. Proc Natl Acad Sci USA 84:4626–4630, 1987.
229. Morin JE, Lubeck MD, Mason BB. Recombinant adenovirus vaccines for hepatitis B virus. In Woodrow GC, Levine MM (eds). New Generation Vaccines. New York, Marcel Dekker, 1990, pp 448–457.
230. Prevec I, Bhristie BS, Laurie KE. Immune response to HIV-1 gag antigens induced by recombinant adenovirus vectors in mice and rhesus macaque monkeys. J Acquir Immune Defic Syndr Hum Retrovirol 4:568–576, 1991.
231. Natuk RJ, Lubeck MD, Chanda PK, et al. Immunogenicity of recombinant human adenovirus human immunodeficiency virus vaccines in chimpanzees. AIDS Res Hum Retroviruses 9:395–404, 1993.
232. Lubeck MD, Natuk RJ, Chengalvala M, et al. Immunogenicity of recombinant adenovirus human immunodeficiency virus vac-

cines in chimpanzees following intranasal administration. AIDS Res Hum Retroviruses 10:1443–1449, 1994.

233. Lutze-Wallace C, Sapp T, Sidhu M, Wandeler A. In vitro assessments of the genetic stability of a live recombinant human adenovirus vaccine against rabies. Can J Vet Res 59:157–160, 1995.
234. Xiang ZQ, Yang Y, Wilson JM, Ertl HCJ. A replication defective human adenovirus recombinant serves as a highly efficacious vaccine carrier. Virology 219:220–227, 1996.
235. Natuk RJ, Davis AR, Chanda PK, et al. Adenovirus vectored vaccines. Dev Biol Stand 82:71–77, 1994.
236. Imler JL. Adenovirus vectors as recombinant viral vaccines. Vaccine 13:1143–1151, 1995.
237. Ginsberg HS. The ups and downs of adenovirus vectors. Bull N Y Acad Med 1:53–58, 1996.
238. Limbach KJ, Paoletti E. Nonreplicating expression vectors: Application in vaccine development and gene therapy. Epidemiol Infect 116:241–256, 1996.
239. Lemarchand P, Jaffe HA, Daniel C, et al. Adenovirus mediated transfer of a recombinant human cx 1-antitrypsin cDNA to human endothelial cells. Proc Natl Acad Sci USA 89:6482–6486, 1992.
240. Rosenthal W, Dalemans M, Fukayama M, et al. In vivo transfer of the human cystic fibrosis transmembrane conductance regulator gene to the airway epithelium. Cell 68:143–155, 1992.
241. Crystal RG, McElvaney NG, Rosenfeld MA, et al. Administration of an adenovirus containing the human CFTR cDNA to the respiratory tract of individuals with cystic fibrosis. Nat Genet 8:42–51, 1994.
242. Grubb BR, Pickles RJ, Ye H, et al. Inefficient gene transfer by adenovirus vector to cystic fibrosis airway epithelia of mice and humans. Nature 371:802–806, 1994.
243. Noah TL, Wortman IA, Hu PC, et al. Cytokine production by cultured human bronchial epithelial cells infected with a replication-deficient adenoviral gene transfer vector or wild-type adenovirus type 5. Am J Respir Cell Mol Biol 14:417–424, 1996.
244. ASHRAE Standard: Ventilation for Acceptable Indoor Air Quality. Atlanta, GA, American Society of Heating, Refrigerating and Air-Conditioning Engineers (ASHRAE), Standard 62, 1989.

chapter

24 Anthrax

Philip S. Brachman

Arthur M. Friedlander

Anthrax, a zoonotic disease, has three forms—cutaneous, inhalational, and gastrointestinal. Meningitis may be a complication of any of the three forms. The disease is not a major public health problem in the world today, although occasional epidemics do occur. Cases are primarily associated with industrial, agricultural, or laboratory exposure. Mortality is extremely low in cutaneous cases and is less than 5% if antibiotics are given. Inhalational anthrax is almost 100% fatal, and gastrointestinal cases have a mortality rate of 25 to 75%.

Historically, anthrax is reported to have been the fifth plague described in Biblical times (1491 BC). Hippocrates described the disease in approximately 300 BC. Epizootics and epidemics were reported in Europe in the 16th century. Between 1750 and 1850, the disease in humans and animals was described in detail, and the organism was characterized.

In the 1870s, Koch cultured *Bacillus anthracis* on artificial media and used his postulates in the first demonstration of the microbial etiology of an infectious disease. In 1881, Pasteur attenuated the organism and conducted a successful field test of his animal vaccine. In the late 1800s and early 1900s, cases of cutaneous and inhalational industrial anthrax involving rag pickers (Germany) and wool sorters (England)[1] were reported. The term *woolsorters' disease* referred to inhalational anthrax. Because of the large number of reported cases in England, a wool disinfection station was established in Liverpool, England.[2] All incoming wool and other animal fibers were disinfected using formaldehyde baths before being further processed. Subsequently, the number of cases of anthrax among these workers decreased significantly.

Cases of anthrax have been reported from almost every country. However, the actual number of cases in the world is at best an estimate. In 1958, Glassman estimated the annual worldwide incidence at 20,000 to 100,000 cases.[3] In the 1980s and 1990s, the estimate decreased to approximately 2000 cases annually.

Industrial cases occur primarily in European and North American countries and are associated with the processing of animal materials, such as hair, wool, hides, and bones. Agricultural cases occur primarily in Asian and African countries and result from contact with diseased domestic animals or their products, such as hair, wool, hides, bones, and carcasses including meat.

Several unusual epidemics have been reported since the late 1970s. The largest epidemic in modern times occurred in Zimbabwe, where approximately 10,000 human cases were reported between 1979 and 1985, including approximately 7000 cases occurring in 1979 and 1980.[4, 4a, 4b] Most of the affected people had cutaneous lesions, but some gastrointestinal cases were also reported. The source of infections was infected cattle. An unusual epidemic occurred in Sverdlovsk, Russia, in 1979. After an accidental release of spores from a military laboratory, at least 66 human cases of inhalational anthrax occurred among people exposed to an aerosol containing *B. anthracis* organisms.[5, 6] There were also some cases in sheep that were grazing up to 50 km from the laboratory. The revelation that Iraq had produced weapons containing anthrax spores during the 1991 Gulf War confirmed fears of the potential use of anthrax as a biological weapon.

In the United States, the earliest reports of animal anthrax were from Louisiana in the early 1700s. Sporadic animal cases were later reported from almost every state. Areas with more regularly reported cases are now called *anthrax districts* and primarily include the Great Plains states. Human anthrax was first reported from Kentucky in 1824. Human cases were subsequently reported throughout the United States, with the majority from industrialized states in the Northeast. However, as the textile industry moved to other parts of the country, human cases were reported from the new locations.

BACKGROUND

Clinical Description

There are three primary forms of anthrax: cutaneous, inhalational, and gastrointestinal. Secondary meningitis has been reported with all three forms of anthrax. Rarely, a case of anthrax meningitis has been reported in which the primary site was not identified. In the United States, approximately 95% of reported cases have been cutaneous and 5% inhalational; there have been no confirmed gastrointestinal cases.

Cutaneous Anthrax

The incubation period for cutaneous anthrax is 1 to 7 days (usually 2 to 5 days). The lesion is first noted as a small, pruritic papule. Within several days, the papule develops into a vesicle that may be 1 to 2 cm in diameter. Occasionally, the initial papule becomes surrounded by a ring of vesicles, which then coalesce to form a large vesicle. The vesicular fluid is clear or serous colored and contains numerous *B. anthracis* organisms and a paucity of leukocytes. Nonpitting edema and erythema may develop around the lesion. Pain is not present unless there is secondary infection. The vesicle may enlarge to 2 to 3 cm in diameter. Systemic symptoms are usually mild and can include malaise and low-grade fever. There may be regional lymphangitis and lymphadenopathy. Approximately 5 to 7 days after the onset of disease, the vesicle ruptures, revealing a straight-edged, depressed ulcer crater with a black eschar developing at its base. Over a period of 2 to 3 weeks, the eschar loosens and eventually falls off, and a scar may persist.

The lesion usually occurs on an exposed part of the body, such as the face, neck, or arm. Large, irregularly shaped cutaneous lesions similar to those seen in some industrial cases have formed when many organisms were rubbed into the skin. Occasionally, a lesion involving the ocular area is more extensive. The cutaneous lesion may be larger, and the edema may be more extensive, eventually including the entire face and spreading to the cervical area and upper thorax. The orbit may become involved, with subsequent damage to the lids and ductal system.

More severe cutaneous involvement occasionally occurs that is referred to as *malignant edema*, in which multiple bullae surround the site of the initial lesion and extensive local edema, induration, and toxemia are present.

Rarely, multiple cutaneous lesions have occurred that probably represent multiple inoculations of spores through the skin. Reinfections have been reported, but in no instances have both of the lesions been confirmed as anthrax.

Inhalational Anthrax

One to 5 days after inhaling an infectious dose of *B. anthracis* organisms, nonspecific influenza-like symptoms develop that include malaise, fatigue, myalgia, slight temperature elevation, and nonproductive cough. There may be a feeling of precordial oppression. Auscultation of the chest may reveal rhonchi. A slight improvement may occur within 2 to 4 days, but then severe respiratory distress develops suddenly, including dyspnea, cyanosis, stridor, profuse diaphoresis, and possible subcutaneous edema of the neck and chest. Physical examination reveals a patient with toxic symptoms who has an elevated pulse, respiratory rate, and temperature. Auscultation of the lungs reveals moist, crepitant rales and possible minimal pleural effusion. Widening of the mediastinum, as demonstrated on radiographic examination of the chest, is frequently seen. The leukocyte count may be elevated moderately. Shock may develop, and death usually occurs within 24 hours of the onset of the acute phase.

Anthrax meningitis has been reported to occur in approximately 50% of inhalational anthrax cases, but it can develop after bacteremia secondary to the other forms and, very rarely, without an obvious primary source. Clinically, it resembles other meningitides, although it is frequently hemorrhagic.

Gastrointestinal Anthrax

Symptoms of gastrointestinal anthrax develop 2 to 5 days after the ingestion of contaminated meat. The initial symptoms consist of nausea, vomiting, anorexia, and fever followed by abdominal pain and diarrhea, which may be bloody. Hematemesis, possibly severe, may develop. In some cases, the abdominal pain is reported to be as severe as that seen in an acute abdomen and has prompted surgical exploration of the abdomen. Physical examination reveals an elevated temperature, pulse, and respiratory rate. In severe forms, general toxemia with shock, sepsis, and death may develop.

Oral-oropharyngeal anthrax occurs when ingested organisms gain entrance to the subcutaneous tissues through the oral or oropharyngeal tissue. In these cases, local ulcers, fever, anorexia, cervical or submandibular lymphadenopathy, or edema may develop.

Bacteriology

Bacillus anthracis, the causative agent of anthrax, is a large, gram-positive, spore-forming, nonmotile bacillus (1.0–1.5 × 3–10 μm). The organism grows readily on sheep blood agar aerobically and is nonhemolytic under these conditions. The colonies are large, rough, and gray-white, with irregular, tapered, curving outgrowths that cause the typical "Medusa head" appearance. In the presence of high concentrations of carbon dioxide, the organisms form capsules, and colonies are smooth and mucoid. A loop drawn up through a colony makes the disturbed part of the colony stand upright like whipped egg white. In tissue, the bacteria are encapsulated and appear singly or in chains of two or three bacilli. Spores do not occur in living tissue and develop only after the body has been opened. The spores are quite resistant and may survive in the environment for decades in certain soil conditions. Bacterial identification is confirmed by the production of toxin antigen; lysis by a specific bacteriophage; the presence of a capsule, as determined by fluorescent antibody; and virulence for mice and guinea pigs.

Pathogenesis

The known virulence determinants of *B. anthracis* that are important in pathogenesis are the capsule and two protein exotoxins. The importance of the capsule was appreciated early in this century when Bail demonstrated that organisms that lost the ability to produce capsule were avirulent.[7] Extensive studies by Sterne[8] and others in the 1930s expanded this idea and further showed that such unencapsulated strains could induce immunity to anthrax, thus demonstrating that the capsule is not necessary to induce protective immunity. The strains developed by Sterne have proved remarkably effective as live vaccines for domestic animals[9] and are used worldwide. As is true for many bacterial virulence factors, the genes encoding the anthrax capsule are carried on an extrachromosomal plasmid.[10, 11] This discovery allowed more definitive confirmation that the capsule is necessary for virulence. Anthrax strains lacking the capsule plasmid failed to produce capsule and were attenuated.[12] The capsule, a protein composed of poly-D-glutamic acid, enhances virulence by making the organism resistant to phagocytosis and may also protect the bacilli from lysis by cationic proteins in serum.[13] Although the capsule is a necessary virulence factor, it is not an effective immunogen in most experimental animals.

A role for toxins in anthrax pathogenesis was suspected from the earliest studies of Koch[14]; however, it was not firmly established until 1954, when Smith and Keppie demonstrated that sterile plasma from experimentally infected guinea pigs was lethal after being injected into other animals.[15] Much work was done in the 1950s and 1960s to study the role of toxins in disease and immunity.[16, 17] Although since the mid-1980s there have been great advances in our understanding of the molecular biology of the toxins,[18] the exact role of the toxins in pathogenesis remains less well defined. Anthrax has been characterized as being due to a large bacterium that produces a feeble toxin.[19] Although it is clear that anthrax is an invasive disease and that the lethal toxin, when given intravenously, is relatively impotent compared with other bacterial toxins, both the lethal and edema toxins are thought to be important in the establishment of disease by impairing host defenses.

The anthrax toxins, like many bacterial toxins (e.g., diphtheria, tetanus, and botulinum), possess a *binding domain* by which they bind to target cell receptors and an *active domain* that is responsible for the biochemical and usually enzymatic activity of the toxin. The anthrax toxins are unusual in that the binding and active domains are present on two distinct proteins, and the two toxins share the same binding protein. This binding protein, called *protective antigen*, when combined with a second protein, *lethal factor*, constitutes the anthrax lethal toxin, which is lethal when injected into experimental animals.[20, 21] The same protective antigen, together with a third protein, *edema factor*, constitutes the edema toxin, which causes edema when injected into experimental animals.[20, 21] The edema toxin is undoubtedly responsible for the massive edema that may be present in cases of anthrax, especially inhalational anthrax. The edema factor is an adenylate cyclase, which raises intracellular cyclic adenosine monophosphate levels,[22] and the lethal factor has recently been shown to be a metalloprotease.[22a, 22b] Consistent with this model, each of the individual proteins alone lacks biological activity. Recent work has shown that, in vitro, the protective antigen first binds to cellular receptors, after which it is cleaved proteolytically, creating a second binding domain to which either of the active proteins—the lethal or edema factor—binds. The complex then enters the cell and exerts its toxic effect.

The genes for the toxin proteins are carried on a second plasmid.[23] The pathogenic role of the toxins was demonstrated clearly when strains deleted of the plasmid coding for the toxin genes but still encapsulated were shown to be attenuated.[12, 23] Of historical significance, it appears that the veterinary vaccine strains produced by Pasteur by passage at high temperature do not contain the plasmid for the toxin genes.[23] This characteristic explains the lack of virulence of these vaccines. Further work has shown that deleting the protective antigen gene alone eliminates the organism's virulence,[24] thus confirming the central role of the protective antigen in the activity of the two toxins as well as their role in virulence. Early studies showed that crude toxin preparations or combinations of edema and lethal toxins inhibited neutrophil killing,[25] chemotaxis,[26] or phagocytosis.[13] More recent work has shown that the edema toxin inhibits neutrophil phagocytosis[27] and priming of the respiratory burst of neutrophils.[28] At low concentrations, the lethal toxin acts on macrophages to release the cytokines interleukin 1 and tumor necrosis factor[29]; at higher concentrations, it is specifically cytolytic for these cells.[30] In terms of pathogenesis, the greater importance of lethal toxin versus edema toxin was demonstrated with a mouse model, in which an anthrax strain containing the lethal toxin alone retained some virulence, whereas a strain containing only the edema toxin was avirulent when compared with the parent strain containing both toxins.[31]

Infection begins when the spore is introduced through the skin or mucosa. At the local site, the spore germinates into the vegetative bacillus with production of the antiphagocytic capsule. The edema and lethal toxins produced by the organism impair leukocyte function and contribute to the distinctive findings of tissue necrosis, edema, and relative absence of leukocytes. If not contained, the bacilli spread to the draining lymph node, thereby leading to the further production of toxins and the induction of the typical hemorrhagic, edematous, and necrotic lymphadenitis. In inhalational anthrax, spores are ingested by alveolar macrophages and are transported to the tracheobronchial and mediastinal lymph nodes, where they germinate.[32] Local production of toxins by extracellular bacilli leads to the massive hemorrhagic, edematous, and necrotic lymphadenitis and mediastinitis that is so characteristic of this form of the disease. The bacilli then spread through the blood, causing septicemia and, at times, hemorrhagic meningitis. Late in the disease, toxin is present in the blood at high concentrations,[16] with the lethal toxin occurring as a complex of protective antigen and lethal factor.[33] The site of action and the role of lethal toxin in the mechanism of death from infection remain obscure, but the uncontrolled release of cytokines and other possible mediators from macrophages may be involved. Death is due to respiratory failure with overwhelming bacteremia that is often associated with meningitis and subarachnoid hemorrhage.

Diagnosis

A diagnosis of cutaneous anthrax should be considered after the appearance of a painless, pruritic papule that develops into a vesicle, revealing a black eschar at the base of a shallow ulcer. Examination by Gram's stain or culture of the vesicular fluid should confirm the diagnosis. The differential diagnosis should include staphylococcal disease, tularemia, plague, milkers' nodules, and contagious pustular dermatitis. In addition, there should be a history of exposure to materials that have been contaminated by *B. anthracis*.

Diagnosis of inhalational anthrax is difficult, but it should be suspected with a history of exposure to an aerosol that contains *B. anthracis*, followed by a nonspecific initial phase described previously. At this early stage, inhalational anthrax is difficult to distinguish from a mild respiratory infection. Once the acute stage has developed, no specific diagnostic test can distinguish it from a disease in which acute respiratory distress and shock occur; however, a widened mediastinum seen on a chest radiograph should suggest the diagnosis. Because primary pneumonia is not usually a feature of inhalational anthrax, sputum examinations are not of assistance in making the diagnosis.

Gastrointestinal anthrax is difficult to diagnose because of its similarity to other severe gastrointestinal diseases. The incriminating evidence is a history of ingesting contaminated meat, with the development of signs and symptoms as described earlier. Microbiological cultures are not helpful in confirming the diagnosis unless bacteremia is present. The diagnosis of oral-oropharyngeal anthrax can be made from the clinical and physical findings. Adequate data are not available to assess the value of bacteriological cultures in confirming the diagnosis.

TREATMENT AND PREVENTION WITH ANTIBIOTICS

Mild cases of cutaneous anthrax may be effectively treated orally with penicillin or tetracycline. If spreading infection or prominent systemic symptoms are present, then high-dose parenteral therapy should be given as for inhalational anthrax until there is a clinical response. The cutaneous lesion progresses regardless of the timing or amount of antibiotic treatment. Effective therapy reduces the edema and systemic symptoms but does not change the evolution of the skin lesion itself.

Treatment of inhalational or gastrointestinal anthrax requires high-dose intravenous penicillin. Limited animal data suggest that the addition of an aminoglycoside would provide additional benefit. Based on in vitro sensitivities and the treatment of experimental infections in animal models, the fluoroquinolones should be effective, but there is no reported use in humans.

Prophylactic treatment to prevent anthrax after exposure to an infectious spore aerosol should include oral antibiotics for 4 weeks as well as vaccination. Vaccine alone would not be expected to be effective.[34]

EPIDEMIOLOGY

The number of reported human anthrax cases in the United States has declined steadily since adequate surveillance data have been available. Between 1916 and 1925, the annual average number of cases was 127; between 1948 and 1957, 44 cases; between 1978 and 1987, 0.9 case; and between 1988 and 1996, 0.25 case. Of the 234 cases reported from 1955 to 1996, 20 were fatal (Fig. 24–1).[35]

Among the 234 human cases reported from 1955 to 1996, 223 had cutaneous lesions (118 on an arm, 64 on the head and neck, 11 on the trunk, 8 on a leg, and 22 unknown), and 11 were inhalational cases.

The classification of cases is related to the source of infection, that is, whether it is acquired in an industrial, an agricultural, or a laboratory setting. The basic epidemiological principles are the same in developing and developed countries. Agricultural anthrax is a more significant problem in developing countries, and industrial anthrax occurs more commonly in developed countries. Industrial anthrax results from the exposure of susceptible individuals to contaminated animal products that include wool, goat hair, hides, or bones. These materials

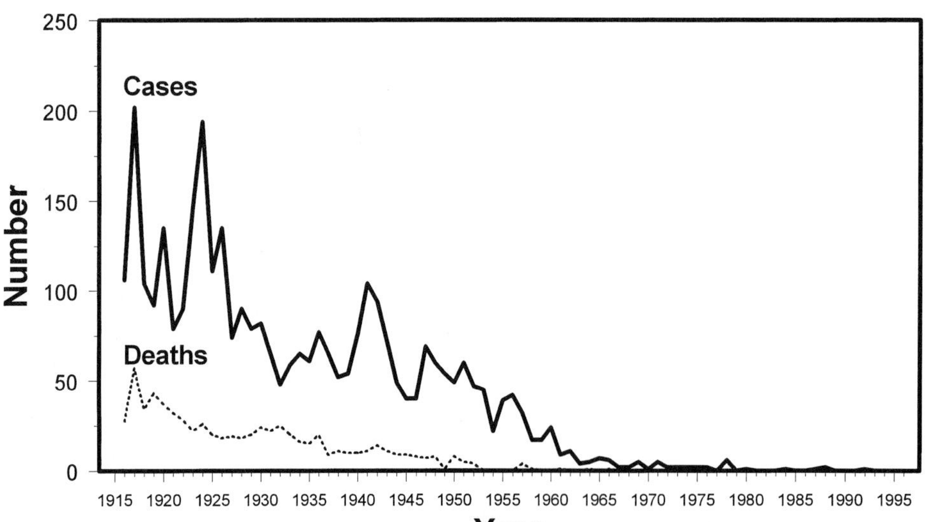

Figure 24–1. Number of cases of anthrax and deaths caused by anthrax in humans, United States, 1916 to 1996. (Data from the National Office of Vital Statistics.)

either come from animals that were infected with *B. anthracis* before death or are contaminated after the death of the animal (e.g., from contaminated soil with which the carcass or animal products came into contact). The wool and hair from infected animals may be clipped from live animals or pulled from carcasses. A hide may be obtained from an animal that has died of anthrax. Bones can be collected from grazing areas on which animals die or from rendering plants that may handle carcasses of animals that have died from anthrax.

Wool and goat hair are processed into yarn that is used in the textile and carpet industries or in the preparation of other cloth-like materials. Hides are processed into leather goods. Bones are used in preparing bone meal, gelatin, or fertilizer.

In industrial cases, cutaneous anthrax results from spores that gain entrance through the skin by entering preexisting wounds or by being rubbed through the skin or on a hair fiber that may penetrate the skin. At times, the processing of goat hair and wool creates infectious aerosols that when inhaled may result in inhalational anthrax. A rendering plant is another source of potential infection.

Cases associated with agricultural settings result from contact with diseased animals or with the products of animals that have died of anthrax. Affected individuals are primarily agricultural workers, veterinarians, or individuals who kill and butcher infected animals or butcher the carcasses of animals that have died of anthrax. This contact results in cutaneous anthrax or, if the infected meat is ingested, gastrointestinal or oral-oropharyngeal anthrax. Veterinarians have developed cutaneous anthrax after contact with infected animals or carcasses or after accidental self-inoculation with the animal anthrax vaccine.

Animal anthrax results from animals ingesting *B. anthracis* spores, either from eating contaminated feed or while grazing on pastures. Soil becomes contaminated from contaminated fertilizer or contaminated feed spread on the ground or from diseased animals that contaminate the soil with their secretions before or after death.

Several theories explain the ecology of soil infected with *B. anthracis*. One theory suggests that the *B. anthracis* spores can persist for many years in some types of soil under certain conditions. These conditions are a soil rich in nitrogen and organic material and with adequate calcium, a pH greater than 6.0, and an ambient temperature greater than 15.5°C. At times of major changes in the microenvironment, such as those produced by drought or heavy rain, spores germinate, and the organism proliferates to maintain the population.[36] An opposing theory is that the spores cannot persist in soil for many years, and thus the persistence of infected soil is the result of repeated reinfection of the soil from infected animals.

Laboratory-associated anthrax cases are rare and occur among people working with the organism. These cases can be either cutaneous or inhalational. Rarely, cases have been reported after contact with contaminated clothing, such as woolen coats or pilots' leather helmets. Table 24–1 presents the sources of infection of the 234 cases reported in the United States from 1955 to 1996. The two vaccine-associated cases of agricultural anthrax resulted from the inadvertent injection of animal vaccine into the hand of the vaccinator.

Table 24–1. **SOURCES OF INFECTION IN 234 CASES OF HUMAN ANTHRAX IN THE UNITED STATES, 1955 TO 1996**

INDUSTRIAL	AGRICULTURAL
Goat hair (113)	Animal (41)
Wool (34)	Vaccine (2)
Goat skin (16)	Unknown (8)
Meat (3)	*Total:* 51
Bone (4)	
Unknown (13)	
Total: 183	

PASSIVE IMMUNIZATION

There is experimental evidence that passive immunization with antibody produced against attenuated Sterne veterinary vaccine strains or against crude toxins protects animals when given before infection.[37] Before the introduction of antibiotics, horse antiserum against Sterne vaccine strains was used to treat anthrax in humans,[38] although no controlled studies were performed to demonstrate efficacy. Although the importance of the toxins in pathogenesis suggests that antiserum may have a role in treating serious infections, no product is available for human use.

ACTIVE IMMUNIZATION

History of Vaccine Development

Although there is great historical interest in Pasteur's development of the first effective live bacterial vaccine, and live attenuated veterinary vaccines are still used, human vaccines against anthrax consist of proteins purified from anthrax cultures, except as indicated in the following discussion.

There has been confusion in the older literature over the use of the term *protective antigen*. Before the identification of the anthrax toxins, this term was applied to uncharacterized material derived from sterile extracts of experimental anthrax lesions[39, 40] or from crude culture supernatants,[41] which were effective immunogens in experimental animals. *Protective antigen* is the term also applied to one of the toxin proteins, which is the plasmid-encoded binding component of the anthrax toxins described previously. It has become clear that these terms apply to the same protein. The major effective immunogen in culture supernatants is the protective antigen component of the toxins, although smaller amounts of lethal and edema factors may be present; their contribution to protective immunity has remained controversial.[42] In older studies, edema factor enhanced the protective efficacy of protective antigen in some experimental animals.[43, 44] The results of these studies are difficult to interpret because the preparations used may not have been pure and free from cross-contamination. Studies using the protective antigen gene cloned into *Bacillus subtilis* demonstrated conclusively that protective antigen alone, in the absence of edema factor, lethal factor, or other *B. anthracis* proteins, protects animals against experimental infection.[45] Although other experiments have shown that purer preparations of protective antigen, free of immunologically detectable lethal or edema factor,[46] or recombinant protective antigen,[46a] can protect experimental animals, it remains unknown whether adding edema or lethal factor enhances the vaccine efficacy of protective antigen.

Description of Vaccine

The human vaccine against anthrax that is licensed in the United States is made by the Michigan Biologic Products Institute, Lansing, Michigan, from sterile filtrates of microaerophilic cultures of an attenuated, unencapsulated, nonproteolytic strain (V770-NP1-R) of *B. anthracis*. The cell-free culture filtrate, thought to contain predominantly protective antigen, is adsorbed to aluminum hydroxide, and the final product contains no more than 2.4 mg of aluminum hydroxide per 0.5-mL dose. Formaldehyde, in a final concentration of no more than 0.02%, and 0.0025% benzethonium chloride are present as preservatives. Some lots appear to contain small amounts of lethal factor and lesser amounts of edema factor as determined by induction of antibody responses in animal recipients,[12, 46, 47] although this has not been reported in the limited observations in human vaccinees.[48] As discussed earlier, although it is clear that protective antigen by itself is an effective immunogen, it remains unresolved whether the small amounts of lethal or edema factor that may be present in some lots of the vaccine contribute to the vaccine's protective efficacy. Potency testing of the vaccine is performed by parenterally challenging guinea pigs. No direct determinations of the content or structure of the protective antigen in the vaccine have been made, and it is unknown whether the protective antigen is biologically active. The vaccine is stored at 2 to 8°C. The recommended schedule for vaccination is 0.5 mL given subcutaneously at 0, 2, and 4 weeks, followed by 0.5-mL boosters at 6, 12, and 18 months. With continued exposure, additional yearly boosters are recommended.

A vaccine licensed in the United Kingdom is made by alum precipitation of the sterile culture filtrate of a derivative of the attenuated Sterne strain.[49] Significant but varying amounts of contaminating lethal factor and edema factor are present in this vaccine at higher levels than those found in the U.S. vaccine.[48, 50] The vaccine is not licensed for use in the United States.

A live spore vaccine, STI, similar to the Sterne strain is used for humans in the former Soviet Union. The vaccine is given by scarification. Its developers claim that it is reasonably well tolerated and shows some degree of protective efficacy.[51]

Results of Vaccination

Immune Responses

The results of two studies indicated that immunization with the licensed U.S. vaccine induced an immune response (as measured by indirect hemagglutination) to protective antigen in 83% of vaccinees 2 weeks after the first three doses[52] and in 91% of those tested after receiving two or more doses.[53] The titers fell over time, but 100% of vaccinees responded with an anamnestic response to the annual booster dose. This hemagglutination assay correlated with results obtained by using an enzyme-linked immunosorbent assay against protective antigen,[54] which is the current test of choice. More recent analysis of the response using a more sensitive enzyme-linked immunosorbent assay against protective antigen demonstrated that seroconversion occurs in 100% of vaccinees after the second dose (P. Pittman et al., personal communication, 1998). In experimental animals, there is generally a correlation between immunity and antibody titer to protective antigen after immunization with the human vaccine (M.L.M. Pitt et al., personal communication, 1998). However, the live veterinary vaccine provides significantly greater protection against anthrax in experimental animals than does the human vaccine, and it often induces lower levels of antibody to protective antigen.[46–48] Thus, the relationship between antibody to protective antigen, as measured in these assays, and immunity remains obscure. Further analysis of the antibody response in terms of epitope specificity for different functional domains of protective antigen may reveal a relationship with a protective immune response.

After a naturally acquired infection, antibody to protective antigen develops in 68 to 93% of cases as reported in different series, depending on the time when samples are drawn.[50, 53–55] Antibody to lethal factor occurs in 42 to 55% of cases, whereas antibody to edema factor is less frequently observed.[50, 54] Antibody to the anthrax capsule occurs in 67 to 94% of cases.[54, 55] This reaction contrasts with that of vaccinees, in which no response to capsule is expected because the vaccine strain is nonencapsulated. In the first such preliminary study reported in the industrialized world, a positive skin test with anthraxin (an undefined skin test antigen developed in Russia from the edematous fluid of infected animals) proved useful in identifying cases of anthrax.[56] This result has not been confirmed by others, however.

Protective Efficacy

The protective efficacy of different experimental protective antigen-based vaccines that were derived from culture filtrates of *B. anthracis* was clearly demonstrated with the use of various animal models and routes of challenge.[42, 49]

A controlled clinical trial was conducted with a vaccine similar to the currently licensed U.S. vaccine.[57] This field-tested vaccine was composed of an alum-precipitated, cell-free culture supernatant from an attenuated, unencapsulated, nonproteolytic strain of *B. anthracis.* This strain differed from that used to produce the licensed vaccine and was grown under aerobic rather than microaerophilic conditions.[58] The study was conducted in a susceptible population working in four mills in the northeastern United States, where raw imported goat hair contaminated with *B. anthracis* was used. The results indicated that vaccination, compared with inoculation with a placebo, provided 92.5% protection against cutaneous anthrax (lower 95% confidence limit, 65%). No assessment of the effectiveness of the vaccine against inhalational anthrax could be made because there were too few cases. This same vaccine was previously shown to protect rhesus monkeys against an aerosol exposure to anthrax spores.[57] A review of the methodology and results of the trial noted above, as well as results of a trial with the live spore vaccine developed in the former Soviet Union, concluded that both products were effective.[57a]

There have been no controlled clinical trials in humans of the efficacy of the currently licensed U.S. vaccine. This vaccine has been extensively tested in animals and has protected guinea pigs against both an intramuscular[47, 48] and an aerosol[46] challenge. More recent experiments show that this vaccine also protected rhesus monkeys against a lethal aerosol challenge with anthrax spores.[47a]

Duration of Immunity

The duration of immunity induced by vaccination has not been clearly established. In field trials that evaluated a vaccine similar to the currently licensed U.S. vaccine, one case of cutaneous anthrax occurred 5 months after the initial three-dose series and just before the scheduled 6-month booster.[57] Although data are insufficient to support any firm conclusions, this observation suggests that the immunity induced by the current vaccine may not be long-lasting and that the recommended schedule of three boosters at 6-month intervals followed by annual boosters is necessary.

Adverse Events

Studies of the protective antigen vaccine used in the human field trial showed that during the initial series of three injections, the incidence of systemic or significant local reactions was 0.7 and 2.4%, respectively.[58] An increase to 1.3 and 2.7%, respectively, was noted with the booster doses. A more detailed study showed that local reactions increased in frequency up to the fifth inoculation and then declined.[57] In this study, there was a 0.2% incidence of systemic reactions and a 2.8% overall incidence of significant local reactions. Systemic reactions consist of mild generalized myalgia, slight headache, and mild to moderate malaise for 1 to 2 days. Most local reactions are mild, consisting of 1 to 2 cm of erythema and slight local tenderness appearing the first day and disappearing within 1 to 2 days. Significant local reactions consist of induration, erythema greater than 5 cm in diameter, edema, pruritus, local warmth, and tenderness. These reactions are maximal at 1 to 2 days after vaccination and usually disappear over 2 to 3 days. Very rarely, the edema may be extensive and extend from the deltoid to the forearm. A small, painless nodule at the injection site, persisting for several weeks, has also been observed, but only rarely. Severe local reactions were observed in individuals with a history of cutaneous anthrax who were inadvertently immunized.[58] All local reactions resolved without complication.

The licensed aluminum hydroxide–adsorbed protective antigen vaccine gave an incidence of local reactions similar to that of the alum-precipitated vaccine, although no detailed observations were reported.[59]

Indications

Routine immunizations are recommended for industrial workers who handle potentially contaminated animal products, including wool, goat hair, hides, and bones imported from countries in which animal anthrax continues to occur. These countries are primarily in Asia and Africa but are occasionally in South America or the Caribbean. A veterinarian or agricultural worker who has contact with potentially infected animals should be immunized, as should laboratory workers who work with *B. anthracis*.

Special circumstances that warrant vaccination with anthrax vaccine include a threat of biological warfare. In addition, if there is a persisting epizootic of anthrax, it may be appropriate to immunize people who have contact with infected animals or with the environmental area.

Contraindications

A contraindication to being vaccinated is a hypersensitive reaction to the vaccine. This is uncommon, but several individuals who have received the initial dose or doses developed moderately severe local reactions with some systemic response. If it is necessary to immunize such individuals, it may be possible to use very small doses of vaccine, although the value of this approach has not been tested scientifically.

PUBLIC HEALTH CONSIDERATIONS

The use of the vaccine in industrialized populations has had a significant impact on the occurrence of anthrax among industrial workers and is one of the main methods by which industrial anthrax has been controlled in the United States and other industrialized countries. Improvement in the industrial environment, with better manufacturing equipment and environmental control, has helped reduce the industrial risks of anthrax. The number of agricultural cases has been reduced by control of the disease in animals through the employment of animal vaccines. The routine immunization of animals in areas with continuing cases of animal anthrax and the immunization of appropriate humans agriculturally and industrially exposed to *B. anthracis* will serve to reduce the number of human cases.

UNRESOLVED PROBLEMS AND FUTURE DEVELOPMENTS

The incidence of human anthrax in the developed world is extremely low. The only impetus for the development of an improved human vaccine is the threat of using anthrax as a biological weapon. There has long been concern about the possible use of anthrax as a military weapon. This horrendous possibility was unfortunately given credence by revelations concerning the 1979 outbreak of inhalational anthrax that occurred after the accidental release of spores from a military microbiology laboratory in Sverdlovsk in the former Soviet Union, as well as by the fact that Iraq weaponized anthrax spores during the Gulf War of 1991. These events have now prompted the Department of Defense to require anthrax vaccination for the Armed Forces. More recent events have also raised the specter of using anthrax as a bioterrorist weapon against civilian populations, with possible catastrophic consequences.[59a] There is evidence in animals of the persistence of spores in host tissues after treatment with antibiotics alone for 30 days.[34] For this reason, the major efforts in public health management of such an event must rely on early diagnosis and include postexposure prophylaxis with both antibiotics and vaccination.

The current vaccine against anthrax is unsatisfactory for several reasons. The vaccine is composed of an undefined crude culture supernatant adsorbed to aluminum hydroxide. There has been no quantification of the protective antigen content of the vaccine or of any of the other constituents, so the degree of purity is unknown. Standardization is determined by an animal potency test. The undefined nature of the vaccine and the presence of constituents that may be undesirable may account for the level of reactogenicity observed. The vaccine is less than optimal, in that six doses are required over 18 months, followed by annual boosters. There is also evidence in rodents that the efficacy of the vaccine may be lower against some strains of anthrax than others,[47, 48, 50] although this has not been observed in rhesus monkeys.[47a] Clearly, a highly desirable anthrax vaccine would be completely defined and less reactogenic and would require one or two doses to produce long-lasting immunity.

Further understanding of the molecular pathogenesis of anthrax and of the structure of the protective antigen and its interaction with lethal and edema factors can be expected to lead to significant progress toward the development of improved vaccines. For example, genetically defined mutations in the cell receptor-binding domain,[60, 61] the protease-sensitive domain,[62] or other parts of the molecule[63] may generate a less toxic protective antigen preparation to be used either alone or as a complex with edema or lethal factor. Similarly, mutations in either the edema or lethal toxin may allow evaluation of nontoxic complexes with protective antigen. Evidence in experimental animals suggests that adjuvants other than aluminum may substantially increase the protective efficacy of protective antigen even after a single dose.[64, 65] Another approach has been to develop live vaccines for human use, because several reports demonstrated that a live vaccine protects experimental animals better than does the licensed human protective antigen vaccine.[46–48, 66] The precedent exists for using such a vaccine in humans in the former Soviet Union. Live vaccines that are known to protect experimental animals against anthrax include aromatic compound–dependent, toxigenic, unencapsulated strains of *B. anthracis*,[65] *B. subtilis*,[66] and vaccinia virus,[67] each constructed to contain the cloned protective antigen gene. Although these efforts are in the experimental stage, they may lead to the production of a vaccine that is less reactogenic, requires fewer doses, and provides more effective and long-lasting immunity.

REFERENCES

1. LaForce FM. Woolsorters' disease, England. Bull N Y Acad Med 54:956–963, 1978.
2. Wool disinfection and anthrax: A year's working of the model station. Lancet 2:1295–1296, 1922.
3. Glassman HN. World incidence of anthrax in man. Public Health Rep 73:22–24, 1958.
4. Davies JCA. A major epidemic of anthrax in Zimbabwe. Part 1. Cent Afr J Med 28:291–298, 1982.

4a. Davies JCA. A major epidemic of anthrax in Zimbabwe. Part 2. Cent Afr J Med 29:8–12, 1983.

4b. Davies JCA. A major epidemic of anthrax in Zimbabwe. Part 3. Cent Afr J Med 31:176–180, 1985.

5. Abramova FA, Grinberg IM, Yampolskaya OV, Walker DH. Pathology of inhalational anthrax in 42 cases from the Svendlovsk outbreak in 1979. Proc Natl Acad Sci U S A 90:2291–2294, 1993.
6. Meselson M, Guillemin J, Hugh-Jones M, et al. The Sverdlovsk anthrax outbreak of 1979. Science 266:1202–1208, 1994.
7. Bail O. In Sterne M. Anthrax. In Stableforth AW, Galloway IA (eds). Infectious Diseases of Animals. Vol. 1. London, Butterworth Scientific Publications, 1959, p 22.
8. Sterne M. Anthrax. In Stableforth AW, Galloway IA (eds). Infectious Diseases of Animals. Vol. 1. London, Butterworth Scientific Publications, 1959, pp 16–52.
9. Sterne M. Distribution and economic importance of anthrax. Fed Proc 26:1493–1495, 1967.
10. Green BD, Battisti L, Koehler TM, Thorne CB. Demonstration of a capsule plasmid in *Bacillus anthracis*. Infect Immun 49:291–297, 1985.
11. Uchida I, Sekizaki T, Hashimoto K, Terkado N. Association of the encapsulation of *Bacillus anthracis* with a 60 megadalton plasmid. J Gen Microbiol 131:363–367, 1985.
12. Ivins BE, Ezzell JW Jr, Jemski J, et al. Immunization studies with attenuated strains of *Bacillus anthracis*. Infect Immun 52:454–458, 1986.
13. Keppie J, Harris-Smith PW, Smith H. The chemical basis of the virulence of *Bacillus anthracis*. IX. Its aggressins and their mode of action. Br J Exp Pathol 44:446–453, 1963.
14. Koch R. Beitrage zur Biologie der Pflanzen. Med Classics 2:787–820, 1938.
15. Smith H, Keppie J. Observations on experimental anthrax: Demonstration of a specific lethal factor produced in vivo by *Bacillus anthracis*. Nature 173:869–870, 1954.
16. Lincoln RE, Fish DC. Anthrax toxin. In Montie TC, Kadis S, Ajl SJ (eds). Microbial Toxins. Vol. 3. New York, Academic Press, 1970, pp 361–414.
17. Stephen J. Anthrax toxin. In Dorner F, Drews J (eds). Pharmacology of Bacterial Toxins. Oxford, Pergamon Press, 1986, pp 381–395.
18. Leppla SH. The anthrax toxin complex. In Alouf JE, Freer JH (eds). Sourcebook of Bacterial Protein Toxins. London, Academic Press, 1991, pp 277–302.
19. Dalldorf FGF, Kaufmann AF, Brachman PS. Woolsorters' disease: An experimental model. Arch Pathol 92:418–426, 1971.
20. Stanley JL, Smith H. Purification of factor I and recognition of a third factor of the anthrax toxin. J Gen Microbiol 26:49–66, 1961.

21. Beall FA, Taylor MJ, Thorne CB. Rapid lethal effects in rats of a third component found upon fractionating the toxin of *Bacillus anthracis*. J Bacteriol 83:1274–1280, 1962.
22. Leppla SH. Anthrax toxin edema factor: A bacterial adenylate cyclase that increases cyclic AMP concentrations of eukaryotic cells. Proc Natl Acad Sci U S A 79:3162–3166, 1982.
22a. Hammond SE, Hanna PC. Lethal factor active-site mutations affect catalytic activity in vitro. Infect Immun 66:2374–2378, 1998.
22b. Duesbury NS, Webb CP, Leppla SH, et al. Proteolytic inactivation of MAP-kinase-kinaso by anthrax lethal factor. Science 280:734–737. 1998.
23. Mikesell P, Ivins BE, Ristroph JD, Dreier TM. Evidence for plasmid-mediated toxin production in *Bacillus anthracis*. Infect Immun 39:371–376, 1983.
24. Cataldi A, Labruyere E, Mock M. Construction and characterization of a protective antigen-deficient *Bacillus anthracis* strain. Mol Microbiol 4:1111–1117, 1990.
25. Bail O, Weil E. Beitrage zum Studium der Milzbrandinfektion. Arch Hyg Bakteriol 73:218–264, 1911.
26. Kashiba S, Morishima T, Kato K, et al. Leucotoxic substance produced by *Bacillus anthracis*. Biken J 2:97–104, 1959.
27. O'Brien J, Friedlander A, Dreier T, et al. Effects of anthrax toxin components on human neutrophils. Infect Immun 47:306–310, 1985.
28. Wright GG, Read PW, Mandell GL. Lipopolysaccharide releases a priming substance from platelets that augments the oxidative response of polymorphonuclear neutrophils to chemotactic peptide. J Infect Dis 157:690–696, 1988.
29. Hanna PC, Acosta D, Collier RJ. On the role of macrophages in anthrax. Proc Natl Acad Sci U S A 90:10198–10201, 1993.
30. Friedlander AM. Macrophages are sensitive to anthrax lethal toxin through an acid-dependent process. J Biol Chem 261:7123–7126, 1986.
31. Pezard C, Berche P, Mock M. Contribution of individual toxin components to virulence of *Bacillus anthracis*. Infect Immun 59:3472–3477, 1991.
32. Ross JM. The pathogenesis of anthrax following the administration of spores by the respiratory route. J Pathol Bacteriol 73:485–494, 1957.
33. Ezzell JW Jr, Abshire TG. Serum protease cleavage of *Bacillus anthracis* protective antigen. J Gen Microbiol 138:543–549, 1992.
34. Friedlander AM, Welkos SL, Pitt MLM, et al. Postexposure prophylaxis against experimental inhalation anthrax. J Infect Dis 167:1239–1243, 1993.
35. Summary of notifiable diseases, United States 1990. MMWR Morb Mortal Wkly Rep 39:55–60, 1991.
36. Kaufmann AF. Observations on the occurrence of anthrax as related to soil type and rainfall. Salisbury Med Bull Suppl 68:16–17, 1990.
37. Belton FC, Strange RE. Studies on a protective antigen produced in vitro from *Bacillus anthracis*: Medium and methods of production. Br J Exp Pathol 37:144–152, 1954.
38. Fleming A, Petrie GF. Recent Advances in Vaccine and Serum Therapy. Philadelphia, P Blakiston's Son & Co, 1934, pp 152–156.
39. Bail O. Untersuchungen über naturliche und kunstliche Milzbrandimmunitat. Zentralbl Bakteriol I Abt Orig 37:270–280, 1904.
40. Cromartie WJ, Watson DW, Bloom WL, Heckly RJ. Studies on infection with *Bacillus anthracis*. II. The immunological and tissue damaging properties of extracts prepared from lesions of *B. anthracis* infection. J Infect Dis 80:14–27, 1947.
41. Gladstone GP. Immunity to anthrax. Protective antigen present in cell-free culture filtrates. Br J Exp Pathol 27:394–418, 1946.
42. Lincoln RE, Fish DC. Anthrax toxin. In Montie TC, Kadis S, Ajl SJ (eds). Microbial Toxins. Vol. 3. New York, Academic Press, 1970, pp 361–414.
43. Stanley JL, Smith H. The three factors of anthrax toxin: Their immunogenicity and lack of demonstrable enzymic activity. J Gen Microbiol 31:329–337, 1963.
44. Mahlandt BG, Klein F, Lincoln RE, et al. Immunologic studies of anthrax. IV. Evaluation of the immunogenicity of three components of anthrax toxin. J Immunol 96:727–733, 1966.
45. Ivins BE, Welkos SL. Cloning and expression of the *Bacillus anthracis* protective antigen gene in *Bacillus subtilis*. Infect Immun 54:537–542, 1986.
46. Ivins BE, Welkos SL. Recent advances in the development of an improved, human anthrax vaccine. Eur J Epidemiol 4:12–19, 1988.
46a. Ivins BE, Pitt MLM, Fellows PF, et al. Comparative efficacy of experimental anthrax vaccine candidates against inhalation anthrax in rhesus macaques. Vaccine: in press.
47. Little SF, Knudson GB. Comparative efficacy of *Bacillus anthracis* live spore vaccine and protective antigen vaccine against anthrax in the guinea pig. Infect Immun 52:509–512, 1986.
47a. Ivins BE, Fellows PF, Pitt MLM, et al. Efficacy of a standard human anthrax vaccine against *Bacillus anthracis* aerosol spore challenge in rhesus monkeys. Salisbury Med Bull 87(suppl):125–126, 1996.
48. Turnbull PCB, Broster MG, Carman JA, et al. Development of antibodies to protective antigen and lethal factor components of anthrax toxin in humans and guinea pigs and their relevance to protective immunity. Infect Immun 52:356–363, 1986.
49. Hambleton P, Carman JA, Melling J. Anthrax: The disease in relation to vaccines. Vaccine 2:125–132, 1984.
50. Turnbull PCB, Leppla SH, Broster MG, et al. Antibodies to anthrax toxin in humans and guinea pigs and their relevance to protective immunity. Med Microbiol Immunol 177:293–303, 1988.
51. Shuylak VP. Epidemiological efficacy of anthrax STI vaccine in Tadjik SSR [in Russian]. Zh Mikrobiol Epidemiol Immunobiol 47:117–120, 1970.
52. Johnson-Winegar A. Comparison of enzyme-linked immunosorbent and hemagglutination assays for determining anthrax antibodies. J Clin Microbiol 20:357–361, 1984.
53. Buchanan TM, Feeley JC, Hayes PS, Brachman PS. Anthrax indirect microhemagglutination test. J Immunol 107:1631–1636, 1971.
54. Sirisanthana T, Nelson KE, Ezzell J, Abshire TG. Serological studies of patients with cutaneous and oral-oropharyngeal anthrax from northern Thailand. Am J Trop Med Hyg 39:575–581, 1988.
55. Harrison LH, Ezzell JW, Veterinary Laboratory Investigation Center, et al. Evaluation of serologic tests for diagnosis of anthrax after an outbreak of cutaneous anthrax in Paraguay. J Infect Dis 160:706–710, 1989.
56. Pfisterer RM. Retrospective verification of the diagnosis of anthrax by means of the intracutaneous skin test with the Russian allergen "anthraxin" in a recent epidemic in Switzerland. Salisbury Med Bull Suppl 68:80, 1990.
57. Brachman PS, Gold H, Plotkin SA, et al. Field evaluation of a human anthrax vaccine. Am J Public Health 52:632–645, 1962.
57a. Demicheli V, Rivetti D, Decks JJ, et al. The effectiveness and safety of vaccines against human anthrax: A systematic review. Vaccine 16:880–884, 1998.
58. Wright GG, Green TW, Kanode RG Jr. Studies on immunity in anthrax. V. Immunizing activity of alum-precipitated protective antigen. J Immunol 73:387–391, 1954.
59. Puziss M, Wright GG. Studies on immunity in anthrax. X. Gel-adsorbed protective antigen for immunization of man. J Bacteriol 85:230–236, 1963.
59a. Kaufman AF, Meltzer MI, Schmid GP. The economic impact of a bioterrorist attack: Are prevention and postattack intervention programs justifiable? Emerg Infect Dis 3:83–94, 1997.
60. Singh Y, Klimpel KR, Quinn CP, et al. The carboxy-terminal end of protective antigen is required for receptor binding and anthrax toxin activity. J Biol Chem 266:15493–15497, 1991.
61. Little SF, Lowe JR. Location of receptor-binding region of protective antigen from *Bacillus anthracis*. Biochem Biophys Res Commun 180:531–537, 1991.
62. Singh Y, Chaudhary VK, Leppla SH. A deleted variant of *Bacillus anthracis* protective antigen is non-toxic and blocks anthrax toxin action in vivo. J Biol Chem 264:19103–19107, 1989.
63. Novak JM, Stein MP, Little SF, et al. Functional characterization of protease-treated *Bacillus anthracis* protective antigen. J Biol Chem 267:17186–17193, 1992.
64. Ivins BE, Welkos SL, Little SF, et al. Immunization against anthrax with *Bacillus anthracis* protective antigen combined with adjuvants. Infect Immun 60:662–668, 1992.
65. Turnbull PCB, Quinn CP, Hewron R, et al. Protection conferred by microbially-supplemented UK and purified PA vaccines. Salisbury Med Bull Suppl 68:89–91, 1990.
66. Ivins BE, Welkos SL, Knudson GB, Little SF. Immunization against anthrax with aromatic compound-dependent (aro-) mutants of *Bacillus anthracis* and with recombinant strains of *Bacillus subtilis* that produce anthrax protective antigen. Infect Immun 58:303–308, 1990.
67. Iacono-Connors LC, Welkos SL, Ivins BE, Dalrymple JM. Protection against anthrax with recombinant virus-expressed protective antigen in experimental animals. Infect Immun 59:1961–1965, 1991.

chapter

25 Cholera Vaccines

David A. Sack
Michel Cadoz

Cholera is an acutely dehydrating, watery diarrheal disease caused by intestinal infection with the bacterium *Vibrio cholerae* serogroup O1. It is one of the dread epidemic and pandemic diseases. Historically, it has had an unusual ability to spread rapidly to large numbers of people, to spread internationally, and to kill a high proportion of those affected. Before the discovery of effective therapy, cholera epidemics were associated with case-fatality rates that exceeded 40% and led to tens of thousands of deaths in single outbreaks. John Snow is credited with understanding the importance of water as a key vehicle for the spread of the disease,[1] but it was not until the early 1880s that Robert Koch recovered the causative agent from the fecal specimen of a patient with the disease.[2]

Preparations of killed parenteral whole-cell cholera vaccine began to be produced shortly after Koch's discovery. Although later controlled studies showed the injectable vaccine to have limited public health usefulness, it did have some short-term efficacy. In Spain in 1884, Ferran produced a killed bacterial vaccine and inoculated thousands of people with it in an area experiencing an epidemic.[2a] Of those inoculated, 1.3% came down with cholera, compared with 7.7% of those who were not vaccinated. This work was not recognized, however, because Ferran refused to provide key information to a commission from the Pasteur Institute, which came to Spain in 1885 to investigate this new vaccine.

Shortly after Ferran, Haffkine began working on a cholera vaccine. His work was stimulated by the cholera epidemics in his native Russia. He was unable to return to his homeland, so he instead went to India, where he began giving vaccine to many people living in the Delhi and Calcutta areas. He became convinced of the success of his vaccine in 1894, when none of the 116 immunized people in a Calcutta slum developed cholera, whereas 9 cases were reported among 84 unimmunized control subjects.[2a]

Popularity of the vaccine grew during the early part of the 1900s, as the cholera problem continued and no effective therapy existed to combat it. Notable during this period is the account of Russell, who carried out large-scale trials of injectable cholera vaccines in the 1920s.[2b, 3] In a vaccine efficacy trial in which more than 8000 people received two doses of the parenteral vaccine, 17,000 received one dose, and 25,000 were not immunized, the vaccines were associated with a protective efficacy of about 80% during a 3-month follow-up period. In further studies involving as many as 3 million people in (uncontrolled) trials in India, the injectable vaccine also appeared to show excellent efficacy.[4]

For the expatriates living in cholera endemic areas, vaccination was especially important. There were numerous anecdotal reports concerning the effectiveness of the parenteral vaccine. For example, 3 cases and 1 death occurred among 8000 European immunized expatriates then living in Java, whereas 32 cases and 15 deaths occurred among 2700 unimmunized Europeans (protective efficacy = 98% for disease).[5]

In the 1920s, Russell tested a killed oral cholera vaccine in India.[2b] This vaccine is especially interesting because of developments in the 1980s with a "new" killed oral cholera vaccine (described later in the chapter). Termed *Bezredka's bilivaccine* because it was developed at the Pasteur Institute by Bezredka and contained bile salts in addition to killed *V. cholerae*, this vaccine was tested in India along with the parenteral vaccine described earlier. The oral vaccine provided protection that was approximately equal (82%) to that of the injectable vaccine, and it appeared to be highly protective against cholera-related deaths. Because of the bile salts, however, the vaccine caused diarrhea in some people and was considered unacceptable by many potential recipients who feared that the vaccine teams were in fact spreading cholera. This apparent success with an oral cholera vaccine was not to be followed up for more than 50 years.

Because of the efficacy of vaccine evident in these early but poorly controlled studies, the panic that accompanied cholera epidemics, and the lack of consistently effective treatment, the parenteral vaccine became widely used. For expatriates such as colonists living in cholera endemic areas, this approach was wise at the time, especially in the absence of safe water and refrigeration. The requirement to receive booster doses every 6 months was not considered a serious constraint because cholera was an ever-present risk, and the vaccine undoubtedly prevented many cases during this early colonial period. With the accompanying panic stimulated by cholera epidemics, many countries began requiring proof of vaccination for travelers who crossed international boundaries. This strategy was based on the (mistaken) belief that vaccination would prevent the international traveler from spreading the bacterium between countries.

After the period of optimism, the vaccine fell from favor for several reasons. During the 1960s, several controlled studies from Bangladesh (formerly East Pakistan), India, the Philippines, and Indonesia showed that the vaccine had only limited (approximately 50%) efficacy and that protection lasted only about 6 months.[6–14] Some vaccine preparations were associated with higher efficacies, but these tended to be associated with a greater occurrence of side effects. More important, each of the injectable vaccines needed to be given frequently (every 6–12 mo) to maintain clinically significant protection. Resources for intensive vaccination programs were not available in areas endemic for cholera and, if mobilized, they would have distracted resources from other more effective interventions.

During this time, the risk of cholera declined substantially for the expatriate upper classes residing in cholera endemic areas and for the military. This decline was due to improved water and food quality associated with the boiling and chlorination of water and the more hygienic preparation of food. Thus, cholera vaccine was no longer needed by groups of people who had previously strongly desired vaccination and had the economic capability to pay for it.

Use of the vaccine was strongly encouraged under the vaccination requirements for international travelers, in an attempt to prevent the spread of the organism between countries. When it was realized that the vaccine did not prevent carriage of the vibrio,[15] these requirements became inappropriate and harmful by placing unnecessary restrictions on travel.

Most important were analyses of the available field trials, which demonstrated that whole-cell parenteral vaccine was not cost-effective in cholera control programs.[8] This poor cost-effectiveness was related to the cost and difficulty of requiring injections every 6 months, the poor acceptability of the relatively reactogenic vaccine, the potential danger from the spread of needle-borne diseases, the vaccine's failure to prevent spread of the vibrio,[16] and the distraction from other potentially more cost-effective interventions. Methods other than parenteral vaccination, such as the provision of safe food and water and effective case management of cholera cases as they occurred, were felt to be more useful in managing cholera epidemics. Also important was the development of effective rehydration fluid therapy, using standardized intravenous and oral solutions, which lowered case-fatality rates to less than 1%, making cholera much less feared than it had been previously.

Cholera vaccination was therefore not needed by the upper classes and expatriates, and it was not cost-effective for the lower socioeconomic groups. Unfortunately, large population groups in Asia, Africa, and South America (including refugees) today remain without safe water or food and may not have access to medical care; thus, a serious cholera risk and a need for an alternative effective cholera vaccine remain for these populations at risk.[17, 18]

BACKGROUND

Clinical Description

Severe cholera (cholera gravis) is characterized by acute diarrhea and usually vomiting, which lead rapidly (within 4–18 hr) to moderate and frequently profound dehydration. Typically, previously healthy individuals are suddenly stricken with watery diarrhea and copious projectile vomiting. Ten and more voluminous stools may be passed within a few hours, at first liquid in consistency and then becoming like rice water. The complications from cholera arise from the loss of fluid volume and electrolytes, especially sodium, potassium, and bicarbonate, in the stool and vomitus. These losses result in hypovolemia, metabolic acidosis, and potassium deficiency.

Secondary complications may arise from the hypovolemia or from inadequate or inappropriate fluid and electrolyte replacement. Complications can include renal failure, hypokalemia, arterial occlusions (especially in the elderly), pulmonary edema, and premature delivery or abortion. Most patients experience a decrease in blood glucose levels during treatment, but some young children experience profound hypoglycemia and seizures. The cause of severe hypoglycemia is not known.

Not all patients with cholera experience the severe cholera gravis syndrome just described. In fact, most infected people have only mild diarrhea or may be asymptomatic. The case-to-infection ratio (number of symptomatic cases per asymptomatic people infected) has ranged from 1:3 to 1:100 depending on the geographical region, biotype, phase of epidemic, and size of inoculum. In general, El Tor strains are associated with a higher proportion of asymptomatic infections than are other strains. The nature of the epidemic also appears to affect the case-to-infection ratio, because explosive epidemics, regardless of biotype, tend to have more severe cases, probably because of higher inoculum sizes.

The Agent. Formerly, it was thought that epidemic cholera could be caused only by toxigenic strains of *V. cholerae* serogroup O1. However, another serogroup, O139, has since caused epidemic cholera in Asia, with a clinical syndrome and epidemiological spread identical to those caused by serogroup O1.[19] Thus, there are now two serogroups of *V. cholerae* that can cause epidemic cholera. However, these serogroups must be distinguished from vibrios that belong to other species, to other serogroups of *V. cholerae*, and even to *V. cholerae* O1 and O139 serogroups that do not produce the toxin. These other bacteria do have pathogenic potential (i.e., they are able to cause diarrhea), but they have not been associated with epidemics. Similarly, some strains of *V. cholerae* of a non-O1, non-O139 serogroup may produce the identical cholera toxin (CT) but not lead to epidemics.

Certain markers of *V. cholerae* are useful for identifying the strains. The serotype (Ogawa or Inaba) arising from different factors in the lipopolysaccharide (LPS) can be determined using agglutination tests with specific antisera. Ogawa strains have factors A and B in their LPS, whereas Inaba strains have factors A and C. (Rarely, strains agglutinate with both monospecific antisera; have factors A, B, and C in their LPS; and are termed serotype Hikojima.) Tests for biotype (classic or El Tor) are determined using agglutination to chicken red blood cells, sensitivity to vibriostatic compounds, and phage-sensitivity patterns. Each strain is thus identified by both its serotype and biotype, resulting in four potential bioserotypes of *V. cholerae* O1. Strains of serogroup O139 need not be further subdivided.

Molecular methods are increasingly being used to identify genetic relatedness between different strains. These molecular epidemiological methods have largely superseded phage typing systems in the evaluation of strains to determine the relatedness between strains.[20–23]

Pathogenesis as It Relates to Prevention

Crucial steps in the pathogenesis of cholera include colonization of the small intestinal mucosa and the elaboration of the enterotoxin, CT, as shown in Figure 25–1. The likelihood of colonization is affected by both host and bacterial factors. People with low levels of gastric acid are more susceptible to colonization and severe disease, because gastric acid normally kills a large proportion of these acid-sensitive bacteria. Lack of gastric acid, on the other hand, allows a higher proportion of the bacteria to survive transit through the stomach to reach the intestine, where colonization can occur.[24, 25] Colonization occurs more readily in people with type O blood, at least for El Tor strains.[26, 27] The mechanism for the increased susceptibility of people with this blood type is not known but may be related to a receptor on the cell surface. Colonization is also inhibited in people with intestinal antibody to the bacteria, which would likely occur from past exposure to the vibrio.

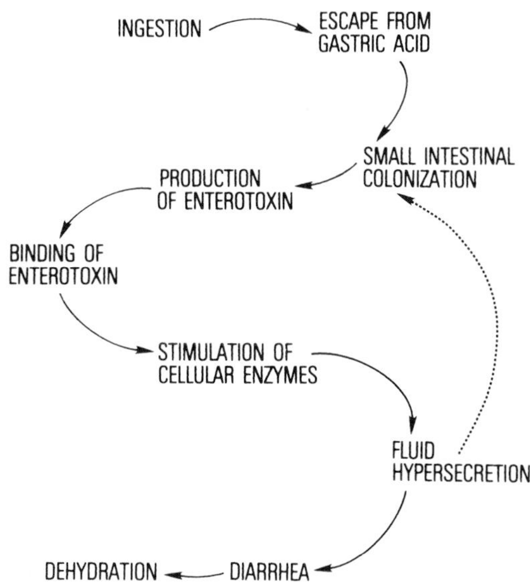

Figure 25–1. Essential steps in the pathophysiology of cholera. After bacteria are ingested, they must escape gastric acid and move into the small intestine. The vibrios then colonize the mucosal cells of the small intestine, using motility (flagella) and colonizing pili, such as toxin coregulated pili. Toxin secreted by the vibrio attaches to the receptor, GM_1 ganglioside, whereupon the A subunit enters the cell and stimulates intracellular enzymes, leading to hypersecretion of water and salts. The fluid secretion exceeds the capacity of the intestinal cells for reabsorption and is passed as watery diarrheal stool, leading to severe and rapid dehydration. The composition of the diarrheal fluid may facilitate further growth of the vibrio.

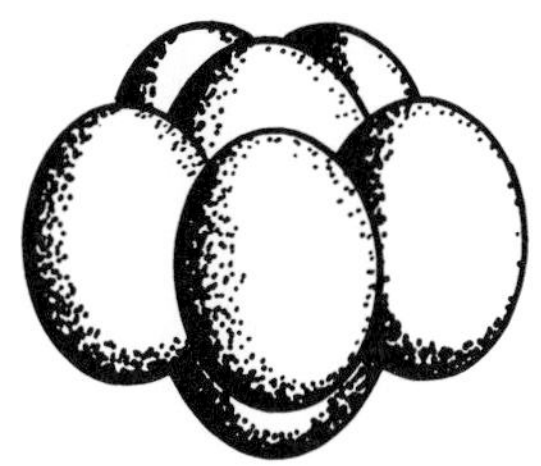

Figure 25–2. Model of the cholera toxin. The cholera toxin is composed of five binding subunits surrounding a central active (A) subunit. The binding (B) subunit binds specifically to GM_1 ganglioside and is the immunodominant portion of the toxin but stimulates no physiological activity. The A subunit is responsible for the toxic activity.

Bacterial factors that facilitate colonization are also important. Bacterial motility allows the bacteria to penetrate the mucous lining of the mucosa and come into close association with the epithelium.[28] Colonization is further facilitated by protein pilus antigens, including the toxin-coregulated pilus or the mannose-sensitive hemagglutinin.[29, 30]

If the bacteria colonize the mucosa in sufficient numbers, they are able to secrete quantities of CT close to the mucosa and thereby cause disease. However, intestinal antitoxin, if present in high concentrations, can block the CT from binding and is therefore protective.[31]

CT, a protein with a molecular weight of 84,000, has a subunit structure consisting of a central active subunit (A subunit) and a surrounding pentomeric binding subunit (B subunit) (Fig. 25–2).[32] The A subunit is responsible for the physiological and toxic activity of the toxin, and the B subunit is responsible for the characteristic tight binding to the GM_1 ganglioside on the cell's surface. After attachment to the surface of the cells, CT stimulates the enzyme adenylate cyclase, which initiates a cascade of biochemical events that lead to hypersecretion of fluid and electrolytes far in excess of the absorptive capacity of the gut. The excess fluid is thus passed out as diarrheal fluid. In cholera, the activity of CT is limited to the intestinal mucosa because CT is not absorbed. If CT were to enter the blood stream, it would have major systemic effects in many tissues of the body, because the receptor (GM_1 ganglioside) and enzyme system (cyclic adenosine monophosphate) are present in all mammalian cells; however, systemic effects from CT are not seen clinically because toxin is not absorbed.

Diagnosis

The diagnosis of cholera can be suspected clinically but is confirmed by culturing the organism from a fecal culture. *V. cholerae* is preserved well in routine fecal transport media, although Cary-Blair medium is preferred. Primary bacteriological plates should include selective media such as thiosulfate citrate bile salts sucrose.[33] Bacteriological confirmation of initial cases in a region is essential because of the epidemic implications, but during major epidemics, laboratory confirmation is not needed except on a sample basis. A rapid diagnostic test based on monoclonal antibody has been developed for both O1 and O139 *V. cholerae* strains and allows for diagnosis within a few minutes of collecting the stool sample.[34, 35] Clinical management of the individual case, however, does not depend on laboratory confirmation, because treatment is aimed at rehydration and only secondarily toward eradicating the bacteria.

Acute and convalescent sera can be tested for vibriocidal or agglutinating antibodies to confirm the diagnosis of cholera due to serogroup O1; a fourfold rise in titer is diagnostic of recent cholera infection. A similar assay is possible for serogroup O139 but is more difficult, because the capsule found on this strain makes it less sensitive to complement-mediated killing and the assay is performed in only a few research laboratories. Antitoxin antibodies can also be measured; however, this procedure is not completely specific, because other vibrios as well as *Escherichia coli* can produce an immunologically similar cholera-like toxin and stimulate antitoxin responses. In general, acute and convalescent sera are not needed to diagnose an individual patient; however, the measurement of serum titers can be helpful during epidemiological evaluations.

Epidemiology: Significance of Cholera as a Public Health Problem

The 1990s have been especially notable for cholera because of the occurrence of two major epidemiological events. In 1991, the El Tor biotype of *V. cholerae* O1, which caused the seventh pandemic of cholera, entered Latin America by way of Peru. It has since spread throughout South and Central America and has thus invaded all regions of the world.[36, 37] Because conditions seemed favorable for cholera to spread to Latin America much sooner, the fact that cholera had not appeared in these countries seemed to provide hope that it would not reach this region. These hopes were unfounded, however, and an explosive epidemic occurred in Peru and other Andean countries, spreading to neighboring countries of South and Central America in a stepwise manner. Since the initial peak, rates have decreased in the region. The decline may be due in part to control measures, but it may also be due to changes in acquired immunity among susceptible people or to ecological changes. Because a high proportion of people in Latin America have type O blood, the epidemic was likely heightened, especially among Native American populations who also had less access to treatment than did other groups.

The second major event of the 1990s was the epidemic due to a new strain of cholera, beginning in India and Bangladesh.[19] All previous epidemics of cholera had been associated with serogroup O1 *V. cholerae*, but this epidemic was caused by the new serogroup O139. Because of its origins in the region around the Bay of Bengal, the new strain has been termed *V. cholerae* Bengal. Although the illness is indistinguishable from cholera due to serogroup O1, the new serogroup is especially important for vaccine development because immunity to serogroup O1 vibrio does not confer immunity to serogroup O139.[38–40] Since its first recognition in Bangladesh and India, *V. cholerae* Bengal has spread to other countries in Asia but not outside this region. Within India and Bangladesh, the strain continues to be isolated, with variations in the proportion of cases due to this strain depending on the season and location. It is not possible to know if this strain represents the next pandemic strain or whether it will remain localized in the area around the Bay of Bengal, but it appears to have established an endemic focus in this region and threatens to spread to other areas. Sporadic cases have appeared in other areas among travelers from Asia to other parts of the world, including the United States, but there have been no secondary cases in these other areas.

The annual number of cholera cases due to serogroups O1 and O139 is not known because of considerable under-reporting, but it probably exceeds 1 million. More than 1 million cases occurred in Latin America during the first 3 years of the current epidemic, causing about 9000 deaths.[36] Although most countries in Asia do not report cholera, rates of illness in the Ganges delta area are approximately 1 to 4 cases per 1000 population.[41] Estimates of cholera-specific mortality are believed to be 100,000 to 130,000 deaths per year, with most of the cholera deaths occurring in Asia and Africa.[17] A recent massive outbreak due to El Tor cholera occurred in 1994 among Rwandan refugees in Zaire, killing about 40,000 people in a few weeks.[42, 43] In addition to the endemic and epidemic cases occurring in developing countries, sporadic cases occur along the U.S. Gulf Coast and are almost always associated with undercooked shellfish, especially crabs.[44]

Most cholera cases occur in older children or adults, although in endemic areas the highest age-specific rates of disease occur between 2 and 5 years of age. An exception is Latin America, where rates have been highest in men, probably as a result of their eating food outside the home. Cholera is unusual in children younger than 2 years and is especially rare in breast-fed children.[45]

Transmission occurs through contaminated water or food and is often the result of combined contamination. Contaminated water, for example, is often used to "wash" fresh food, and thus the food becomes contaminated and can become the vehicle of transmission. Leftover contaminated food, if kept at room temperature, supports the growth of *V. cholerae* and may lead to common source outbreaks.

Although the vibrio is generally thought to be spread by the fecal-oral route, it can also persist in environmental waters without continued contamination with human feces.[46] During epidemics, environmental waters may become heavily contaminated with *V. cholerae* from infected human feces, and this contamination further spreads the epidemic. Once the surface waters become contaminated, an environmental reservoir can maintain the bacterium without further fecal contamination if appropriate conditions of salinity, temperature, and the like exist. As demonstrated in Louisiana, the environmental reservoir can lead to additional sporadic primary cases from contaminated seafood, but if sanitation is adequate, secondary cases do not occur.[44] If sanitation is poor, the sporadic cases may be followed by additional secondary cases and may lead to another epidemic through amplification of the inoculum and further contamination of the waters.

In the environment, the vibrio associates with certain plankton, chitinous shelled animals (e.g., crabs),[47, 48] and vegetation.[49] These associations appear to be crucial for the vibrio's long-term survival. Further, the association with chitinous shells increases the risk of transmission via crabs, shrimp, and other shellfish, many of which are eaten only partially cooked. In some cultures, raw fish may also become a vehicle of transmission. Unfortunately, even if the fish are caught in uncontaminated waters, they may become contaminated when washed in harbor water as the catch is brought to market.

In addition to the consumption of specific high-risk foods, other risk factors for cholera include low socioeconomic status, which correlates with the use of impure water, poor sanitation, and poverty; hypochlorhydria; lack of breast-feeding (in infants); and having type O blood (for El Tor biotype). Among people living in the cholera endemic area of the Ganges delta region, the proportion of people with type O blood is relatively low compared with that of other areas of the world. Some researchers have speculated that this unusual distribution of blood groups is related to cholera-related pressure against people with type O blood.[27] The protection infants receive from breast-feeding may be due to antibodies in the breast milk but may also be due to less exposure to contaminated food and liquids.

IMMUNOLOGY

Passive Immunity

Protection using passive immunization (injected immune globulin) is theoretically possible because very high titers of serum antibody can protect against disease. This passive immunity was demonstrated in the short-lived protection seen after parenteral immunization and also in animal studies in which dogs were protected by injected immune globulin.[31] From a practical standpoint, however, sustaining the high levels of antibody required is not possible with passive immunization.

In contrast, passive immunity for infants through the ingestion of breast milk is feasible and is likely to be critically important. Protection of breast-feeding infants appears to be partially mediated by antibody.[50] Other enteric infections (e.g., with enterotoxigenic *E. coli*) have been prevented in volunteer studies by administering immune milk to the volunteers being challenged with homologous bacteria.[51]

Naturally Acquired Immunity

People who have had cholera develop a protective immune response as demonstrated both by volunteer studies and by epidemiological follow-up of cholera patients.[52, 53] After challenge with classic cholera, and in the absence of further known antigenic challenge, volunteers were solidly protected after a second cholera challenge 3 years later. Protection after El Tor cholera also occurred in volunteers but appeared to be less solid. Epidemiological studies from Bangladesh confirmed the occurrence of naturally acquired immunity after disease, but the differential protection after classic cholera (as opposed to El Tor) was even greater.

The fact that immune protection follows disease provides optimism that effective vaccination is possible. Using naturally occurring immune protection as the gold standard, it is hoped that vaccines can stimulate comparable immune protection. So far, however, there has been no demonstrable way to acquire protection any greater than that experienced after natural infection.

Serological responses after an episode of cholera occur to bacterial LPS and CT, and both of these antibody responses can be protective.[52] The anti-LPS antibodies likely block colonization, whereas antitoxin neutralizes the toxin. Antibodies to toxin-coregulated pilus antigen could also block the colonizing process; however, antibodies to the pilus antigen are not regularly produced after natural infection. Because the B subunit surrounds the A subunit of the toxin, the predominant antitoxic response is to the B subunit, and antibodies to purified B subunit effectively neutralize the toxin in a manner similar to that of antibodies to CT. Although serum titers of antivibrio antibodies are routinely measured using a complement-dependent vibriocidal assay and are useful correlates of bacterial exposure, complement-dependent bacterial killing is not a protective mechanism, because complement-mediated killing does not appear to be an antibacterial mechanism in the gut lumen.

More important from the standpoint of protection is the local intestinal antibody response. Within a few days of infection, peak levels of secretory immunoglobulin A (IgA), anti-LPS, and antitoxin antibodies can be found in intestinal secretions.[54] Although the high titers of IgA antibodies persist for only a few weeks, protection resulting from the immune stimulation appears to last for years.[55, 56] Such protection is likely related to the priming of the intestinal immune system, enabling it to respond quickly when rechallenged with a *V. cholerae* inoculum. Therefore, the protective immune status of an individual cannot be determined simply by measuring antibody titers in intestinal secretions; rather, a measure of the "preparedness" is needed, and there is no standard method for measuring this.

IMMUNIZATION WITH KILLED PARENTERAL VACCINE

Description of Vaccine

Although the killed parenteral vaccine is not recommended, it is available commercially and is the only licensed cholera vaccine in the United States. The vaccine consists of killed *V. cholerae* and contains both Ogawa (usually classic strain NIH 41) and Inaba (usually classic strain NIH 35A3) serotypes. The strains are grown on trypticase soy agar, harvested with isotonic sodium chloride solution, and killed and preserved with 0.5% phenol. Optical density measurements show that the vaccine contains 4 billion organisms of each serotype per mL.

Primary immunization consists of two doses, 1 week to 1 month apart. For adults and children older than 10 years, the dosage is 0.5 mL per dose. For children 6 months to 4 years of age, the dosage is 0.2 mL, and for children 5 to 10 years of age, the dosage is 0.3 mL. Booster doses with the same volume are given at 6-month intervals. The vaccine is not recommended for children younger than 6 months.

Results of Immunization

Approximately 90% of those immunized with the killed whole-cell parenteral vaccine develop a serological response as measured by vibriocidal titer rises.[57] In endemic areas, older children (≥5 yr) and adults usually respond after a single dose, but two doses may be needed for those younger than 5 years. Older individuals (≥5 yr) from endemic areas generally start with a higher titer before immunization because of natural exposure, and the geometrical mean peak titer after immunization is about twice as high as that seen in children younger than 5 years. Titer rises are relatively short lived, with significant decreases in titer occurring within 6 months.

In controlled trials with the commercial vaccine, vaccine efficacy has been approximately 50% for about 6 months. Protection resulting from the vaccine usually correlates with vibriocidal titer.[58] Some studies have suggested that a doubling of titer decreases the risk by approximately 50%; however, there are exceptions to this general finding. Specifically, when a monovalent Ogawa vaccine was given in Bangladesh, the vaccine induced a rise in both Inaba and Ogawa vibriocidal titers but protected only against the homologous serotype, suggesting that the antibody in the serum is not the protective factor.[59] No titer is defined as being highly protective, since a high inoculum can overcome immunity.

See also the introduction to this chapter for historical data on the killed parenteral vaccines.

Side Effects

Side effects from parenteral whole-cell cholera vaccine are similar to those from killed whole-cell typhoid vaccine, although perhaps somewhat less severe.[57] Approximately 50% of vaccinees develop a soreness and inflammation at the site, and 10 to 30% develop generalized symptoms of fever and malaise. Approximately 1 to 5% stay in bed for a day or two. Symptoms usually last 1 to 3 days, although some individuals experience a delayed reaction and develop a sore arm between days 4 and 7. Life-threatening reactions have been extremely rare, but allergic anaphylactic reactions are possible.

Indications

The World Health Organization lists no indications for administering parenteral whole-cell cholera vaccine to a person of any age. However, people who may benefit from the vaccine are those who can receive the vaccine on a regular basis (i.e., boosters at 6-month intervals), who are at very high risk for cholera, and who have no access to medical care should cholera occur. People fitting this description are extremely few and certainly do not include the usual tourists to cholera endemic areas. For people who may fit this description, attempts should be made to use one of the oral vaccines described later.

Contraindications

As with other killed vaccines, there is no specific contraindication for people with immunosuppression. Data on safety during pregnancy are lacking. Simultaneous vaccination for yellow fever is a contraindication because the cholera vaccine may interfere with the immune response to yellow fever vaccine.

IMMUNIZATION WITH KILLED ORAL VACCINES

Description of Vaccines

Killed oral vaccines were designed to stimulate an immune response in the local intestinal mucosa similar to that induced with natural exposure.[60] Animal data showed that oral whole inactivated bacteria induced antibacterial antibodies, that the B subunit of the toxin induced antitoxic antibodies, and that these antibodies protected synergistically.[61] Thus, the vaccine contains both whole bacteria and the B subunit of the toxin. The vaccine is prepared from four strains of killed *V. cholerae*, each in a dose of 2.5×10^{10} organisms, for a total dose of 10^{11} organisms, and 1 mg of B subunit per dose. The *V. cholerae* strains used include a heat-killed classic Inaba, a heat-killed classic Ogawa, a formalin-killed El Tor Inaba, and a formalin-killed classic Ogawa. The rationale for the two methods of killing is the preservation of the protein antigens (by formalin killing) and the LPS antigens (by heat killing). The Inaba and Ogawa strains are included to stimulate immune responses to both LPS antigens.

The B subunit originally used in the Bangladesh field trial[62] was purified chemically from affinity-purified holotoxin. A genetically engineered *V. cholerae* strain was later developed that hyperproduces B subunit but does not produce holotoxin.[63, 64] This recombinant B subunit has been used in subsequent trials and in the commercially available vaccine. The whole-cell/B subunit vaccine is administered with an antacid buffer to neutralize stomach acid, which is known to disaggregate the B subunit.[65]

Another vaccine containing the whole-cell component only (without the B subunit) has been developed and was tested in parallel to the whole-cell/B subunit vaccine to assess the respective value of each component.[62, 66]

Results of Immunization

Volunteers immunized with the killed oral vaccine developed both local intestinal IgA and serum IgG antibody responses.[55, 64, 65, 67–71] Serum titers were lower than those occurring after live challenge, but intestinal responses were similar to those observed in cholera patients. Most important, volunteers were significantly protected after a virulent cholera challenge.[67]

Although the killed oral vaccine is immunogenic, no single assay or titer correlates with protection. Serum *antibacterial* (vibriocidal) responses are seen in approximately 50 to 80% of those immunized, but the geometric mean rises only twofold to fourfold. After administration of the B subunit–containing vaccine, serum *antitoxin* responses are seen in 60 to 80% of recipients, with threefold to fivefold increases on average. The increased titers reach a peak in about 2 weeks and are short lived; titers usually fall to baseline levels within about 3 to 6 months even though protection lasts much longer. The vaccines containing only whole-cell components do not stimulate antitoxin responses.

With the whole-cell/B subunit vaccine, intestinal IgA responses are seen in most vaccinees; however, a rise in antitoxin is generally seen after the first dose, whereas an antibacterial response frequently requires two doses to produce.[68] Because the vaccine stimulates local IgA antibodies and because there is evidence of a common mucosal immune system, titers of antibody in other secretions have been examined after immunization. Titer rises of IgA antitoxin and anti-LPS are frequently seen in saliva, for example, but the correlation between the saliva and intestinal titers is poor.[69] Rises in breast milk antibodies are rarely seen after immunization[70] and do not correlate with intestinal titers.[72]

The immune response has been examined using the enzyme-linked immunosorbent spot (ELISPOT) assay, in which numbers of IgA, IgM, or IgG antibody-secreting cells are determined in peripheral blood specimens.[73] After immunization, increased numbers of IgA and IgG (but not IgM) antitoxin-secreting cells can be seen, with a peak at about 7 days. These numbers fall to baseline levels by 2 or 3 weeks. The IgA lymphocytes detected in the enzyme-linked immunosorbent spot assay are thought to represent cells that have undergone proliferation secondary to the stimulation by intestinal antigen and are passing through the circulation before returning to the intestinal mucosa.

In a field trial in Bangladesh that included more than 60,000 people older than 2 years, the efficacy of the whole-cell/B subunit vaccine was compared with that of an identical whole-cell vaccine without the B subunit and with that of a placebo.[74] The overall 3-year protective efficacy for those older than 5 years was 63%. For those younger than 5 years, protection was similar but only for the first year. Both the whole-cell/B subunit and the whole-cell–only vaccines significantly protected against cholera for 3 years, and the addition of a B subunit appeared to induce a higher level of protection during the first 6 to 8 months but not thereafter (Table 25–1). The whole-cell/B subunit vaccine, but not the whole-cell–only vaccine, protected briefly (a few months) against diarrhea due to enterotoxigenic *E. coli* organisms, which produce heat-labile toxin.[75] There was no evidence of protection against diarrhea due to other Vibrionaceae species with which the vaccine shared certain somatic antigens.[76, 77] The observation related to cross-protection against diarrhea caused by enterotoxigenic *E. coli* was confirmed by studies showing some protection against *E. coli* diarrhea in travelers to Morocco.[78]

In Bangladesh, the level of protection varied significantly with certain risk factors. Age was crucial because protection waned rapidly (within 1 yr) in children younger than 5 years. The vaccine protected against episodes of cholera due to classic strains better than those due to El Tor strains, and it protected vaccinees who did not have type O blood better than it did individuals who had type O blood.

Two efficacy studies in Peru[79, 80] also documented the efficacy of the whole-cell/B subunit vaccine, and a third study from Vietnam confirmed the efficacy of the whole-cell–only vaccine. The second study from Peru used a different dosing regimen in which two doses were followed by a booster dose a year later.[80] Based on this study, it seems that periodic booster doses are needed to maintain high levels of protection. Studies from Vietnam using locally produced, killed, oral whole-cell–only cholera vaccine provided protection similar to that of the whole-cell/B subunit vaccine.[66]

Given the need for an inexpensive vaccine for use in endemic areas, there has been a reevaluation of the need for the B subunit in the vaccine. The inclusion of B subunit induces greater protection during the initial 6 months after vaccination, and it also appears to provide

Table 25–1. **PROTECTIVE EFFICACY OF THREE DOSES OF KILLED ORAL CHOLERA WHOLE-CELL VACCINE WITH AND WITHOUT B SUBUNIT DURING THE FIRST YEAR AND THE FIRST 3 YEARS CUMULATIVELY BY AGE GROUP AT TIME OF IMMUNIZATION**

	PROTECTIVE EFFICACY (%)			
	Whole-Cell Vaccine Only		Whole-Cell Vaccine with B Subunit	
PERIOD AFTER VACCINATION	*Aged 2–5 Years*	*Aged >5 Years*	*Aged 2–5 Years*	*Aged >5 Years*
1 yr	31	67	38	78
3 yr	23	68	26	63

Data from Clemens J, Sack DA, Harris J, et al. Field trial of oral cholera vaccines in Bangladesh: Results from three-year follow-up. Lancet 335:270–273, 1990.

some cross-protection against enterotoxigenic *E. coli* diarrhea due to strains that produce heat-labile toxin. (Heat-labile toxin is similar to CT, and antibodies to one toxin cross-neutralize the other.) However, the long-term (3-yr) efficacy against cholera appears to be the same whether or not the B subunit is included. Furthermore, the whole-cell–only vaccine is simpler to produce and requires neither a cold chain nor the antacid buffer, making it much less expensive and more convenient to distribute.[66]

The whole-cell/B subunit vaccine is licensed in Sweden. Side effects attributable to the vaccine have not been observed.[68] Some individuals have noted abdominal cramps and mild diarrhea, but these complaints have occurred with equal frequency in placebo and vaccine groups, and it is thought that the symptoms have been due to the buffer that is generally given with the vaccine. Data are not available on simultaneous immunization with other vaccines, but no interaction is expected.

Indications

Indications for the use of a killed oral vaccine are the prevention of cholera among those at high risk for the disease. Current studies are attempting to determine the utility of this vaccine for public health for groups such as those living in endemic areas, refugees,[80a] and travelers. Reports from the Centers for Disease Control and Prevention have suggested that rates in travelers are low and do not warrant vaccination in this group[81]; however, the surveillance system used detected cases that occurred in returning travelers but not while traveling abroad, and the rates may be much higher than previously thought.[82] It is not known with certainty whether prevention of diarrhea due to enterotoxigenic *E. coli* will become an indication, but it seems likely that a vaccine that includes the cholera B subunit but also contains whole *E. coli* will be more effective than a vaccine containing the B subunit alone.

Contraindications

At present, there are no specific contraindications for the killed oral vaccines. The safety of the vaccines in pregnant women or immunosuppressed people has not been studied. Because this is a killed oral vaccine, the risk seems minimal. Concurrent administration of IgG has not been studied.

Whole-Cell–Only Vaccine. The whole-cell–only vaccine is being developed in Vietnam for local use. The vaccine is inexpensive (<$0.20/dose) and is easier to produce and more convenient to use and distribute than the whole-cell/B subunit vaccine. There are no known contraindications.

IMMUNIZATION WITH LIVE ORAL VACCINE

Description of Vaccine

A live oral cholera vaccine, CVD103-HgR, has been licensed in Switzerland and is now also available in several other countries (but not in the United States). The vaccine is a genetically engineered mutant derived from a *V. cholerae*, classic Inaba strain that was attenuated by deleting the toxin genes but retaining the genes for B subunit, thus making this a toxin-negative, B subunit–positive strain. A mercury resistance marker was included to assist in differentiating the vaccine strain from wild strains.[83, 84] Earlier vaccine candidate strains either reverted to virulence or were associated with mild but unacceptably frequent side effects—most commonly, diarrhea—which were apparently related to the presence of other virulence factors of *V. cholerae*.

Advantages of this live vaccine include (1) the potential for bacterial replication, resulting in a stronger immune response with fewer organisms administered, and (2) the possibility of immunizing with a single dose. Because the vaccine strain is live, the viability of the bacteria must be preserved while in storage, and the bacteria must be protected from stomach acid by administering the vaccine with a buffer. The vaccine must be kept refrigerated to preserve its viability.

Results of Immunization

Vibriocidal and antitoxic antibodies are stimulated in most vaccinees. Nonimmune individuals respond more consistently than do partially immune individuals, and a dose of 10^9 organisms stimulates a more consistent response than one of 10^8 organisms per dose. People in developing countries appear to require a higher dose of vaccine than do U.S. volunteers. Serum antibodies are similar to those seen after natural infection, and studies found that immunized volunteers were protected against virulent challenge.[83–85] A field trial of the vaccine is underway in Indonesia, where a preliminary analysis found that the vaccine did not confer protection. Reasons why the vaccine was not protective in this endemic area but was protective in volunteers have not been determined, but they may relate to preexisting naturally acquired immunity in the Indonesian population.

Side Effects

Early studies of volunteers in North America suggested that the vaccine might cause mild diarrhea in a small proportion of vaccinees,[83] but side effects have not been seen in subsequent studies in developing countries.

Indications

Indications for the use of this vaccine are the prevention of cholera among travelers at high risk for the disease. Studies are needed to determine the utility of this vaccine for public health use for groups such as those living in endemic areas, refugees, and travelers. In view of the poor results from the field trial in Indonesia, the vaccine will likely not be useful in residents living in cholera endemic areas. There are no data regarding protection against diarrhea due to enterotoxigenic *E. coli.*

Contraindications

There are no known contraindications to the vaccine, but since this is a live attenuated vibrio vaccine, precautions are needed for use in immunocompromised people or people with chronic liver disease. Data are not available regarding safety in pregnancy.

Other Vaccines for Cholera Caused by Serogroup O1 Strains

Other live oral vaccines, including Peru-15[86–88] and CVD-111,[89, 90] have been developed for cholera due to serogroup O1 *V. cholerae* and are being tested. Because the pandemic strain of *V. cholerae* is an El Tor biotype, it was reasoned that a vaccine strain derived from an El Tor strain might provide improved protection against the homologous biotype. Both of these strains, like CVD103-HgR, are genetically engineered strains of *V. cholerae* that produce a B subunit but not an A subunit. However, these strains are genetically more stable because of the deletion of the *recA* gene, without which they are unable to accept foreign genes into their chromosome. Peru-15 is nonmotile and therefore lacks an additional virulence factor. Peru-15 is safe in volunteers at a doses of 10^7 to 10^9 organisms per dose, but about 20% of U.S. volunteers receiving CVD-111 did develop mild diarrhea symptoms after immunization. Peruvian volunteers did not experience side effects.[90]

Like other live oral cholera vaccines, these vaccines are given with a buffer to protect against gastric acid. One study demonstrated that when Peru-15 was given with a rice-based buffer (CeraVacx), the vaccine stimulated higher vibriocidal titers than when given with other buffers, suggesting that the choice of buffer as well as the vaccine strain may be important in maximizing the immune response to the vaccine.[87] Both Peru-15 and CVD-111 demonstrated protection in volunteers, but further studies are needed for both.[88, 89] One concept is to combine CVD103-HgR (derived from a classic strain) with a strain derived from an El Tor strain,[90] in the hopes of stimulating higher protective efficacy. It is not known if this approach will be cost-effective.

Vaccines for Cholera Due to *Vibrio cholerae* O139

Vaccines for serogroup O1 cholera do not protect against cholera due to serogroup O139 strains[8, 39]; thus, another vaccine will be needed for the new group. Based on genetic methods used to develop vaccines for serogroup O1, oral vaccines have been developed for cholera that is due to serogroup O139. These vaccines (Bengal-15 and CVD-112) also produce a B subunit but not an A subunit and lack the *recA* gene. In preliminary volunteer studies, they appear to be safe, immunogenic, and protective,[91, 92] but additional studies are needed to establish the magnitude of their protective efficacy. When Peru-15 (an El Tor strain) was combined with Bengal-15 (the O139 strain) the combination was safe and immunogenic; however, there are no data on the efficacy of the combination. From an epidemiological perspective, it is not possible to know if a vaccine will be needed for serogroup O139 cholera, since the rates of O139 cholera have varied from year to year and from season to season within India and Bangladesh, and the new strain has not yet spread to other regions. If a bivalent O1/O139 vaccine becomes needed, it appears that a combined bivalent vaccine will be feasible to protect against both serogroups.

PUBLIC HEALTH ASPECTS OF CHOLERA VACCINE

The World Health Organization does not currently recommend cholera vaccines. With the availability of the new oral vaccines and the apparent increase in cholera epidemics, however, especially among displaced people, this assessment is undergoing reevaluation in terms of the cost-effectiveness of the vaccines. None of the available oral vaccines is likely to give complete protection, since even natural disease does not protect completely. Primary control measures must continue to be (1) provision of treatment of patients with cholera, (2) prevention of the spread of the bacteria through improvement of water and sanitation facilities, and (3) health education. The new killed oral vaccines may contribute significantly as an additional measure to decrease the rate of cholera in regions with high incidence if they can be made available in a form that is easily distributed and sufficiently inexpensive.[18] The potential usefulness of the oral vaccines will be greatly enhanced if they are able to interrupt transmission of the vibrio sufficiently to provide herd immunity and stop epidemics. This attribute of vaccines has not yet been determined with certainty, although there is some evidence that immunization may at least partially block transmission.[45] Evaluation of the usefulness of oral vaccines in refugee settings in Africa suggests that an inexpensive vaccine will be cost-effective if used before the onset of outbreaks.[80a]

For travelers, military personnel, and expatriates living in endemic areas, the oral vaccine is likely to be welcomed because it is safe; the killed whole-cell/B subunit vaccine will also prevent some episodes of travelers' diarrhea due to enterotoxigenic *E. coli*.

REFERENCES

1. Snow J. Snow on Cholera. New York, Hafner Publications Co, 1962.
2. Koch R. An address on cholera and its bacillus. Br Med J 2:403–407, 453–459, 1884.
2a. Lutzker E, Jochnowitz C. Waldemar Haffkine: Pioneer of cholera vaccine. ASM News 7:366–369, 1987.
2b. Russell AJH. Besredka's cholera bilivaccin versus anti-cholera vaccine: A comparative field test. Trans 7th Congr Far East Assoc Trop Med 1:523–534, 1927.
3. Russell AJH. Cholera in India. Trans 9th Congr Far East Assoc Trop Med 1:389–398, 1934.
4. Chandr Sekar C. Statistical assessment of the efficacy of anti-

cholera inoculation from the data of 63 cheris in south Srcot district. Indian J Med Res 35:153, 1947.
5. Nijland AH. Resultaten met choleravaccinverregen. Geneesk Tijdschr Ned-Indie 53:1, 1913.
6. Benenson AS, Mosley WH, Fahimuddin M, Oseasohn RO. Cholera vaccine field triala in East Pakistan. 2. Effectiveness in the field. Bull World Health Organ 38:359–372, 1968.
7. Mosley WH, McCormack WM, Fahimuddin M, et al. Report of the 1966–67 cholera vaccine field trial in rural East Pakistan. 1. Study design and results of the first year of observation. Bull World Health Organ 40:177–185, 1969.
8. Mosley WH, Aziz KMA, Rahman ASMM, et al. Report of the 1966–67 cholera vaccine trial in rural East Pakistan. 4. Five years of observation with a practical assessment of the role of a cholera vaccine in cholera control programs. Bull World Health Organ 47:229–238, 1972.
9. Mosley WH, Aziz KMA, Rahman ASMM, et al. Field trials of monovalent Ogawa and Inaba cholera vaccines in rural Bangladesh—three years of observation. Bull World Health Organ 49:381–387, 1973.
10. Saroso JS, Bahrawi W, Witjaksono H, et al. A controlled field trial of plain and aluminum hydroxide–adsorbed cholera vaccines in Surabaya, Indonesia, during 1973–75. Bull World Health Organ 56:619–627, 1978.
11. Gupta AD, Sinha R, Shrivastava KL, et al. Controlled field trial of the effectiveness of cholera and cholera El Tor vaccines in Calcutta. Bull World Health Organ 37:371–385, 1967.
12. Pal SC, Deb BC, Sen Gupta PG, et al. A controlled field trial of an aluminum phosphate–adsorbed cholera vaccine in Calcutta. Bull World Health Organ 58:741–745, 1980.
13. Philippines Cholera Committee. A controlled field trial of the effectiveness of various doses of cholera El Tor vaccine in the Philippines. Bull World Health Organ 38:917–23, 1968.
14. Philippines Cholera Committee. A controlled field trial of the effectiveness of the intradermal and subcutaneous administration of cholera vaccine in the Philippines. Bull World Health Organ 49:389–394, 1973.
15. Sommer A, Khan M, Mosley WH. Efficacy of vaccination of family contacts of cholera cases. Lancet 1:1230–1232, 1973.
16. Sommer A, Mosley WH. Ineffectiveness of cholera vaccination as an epidemic control measure. Lancet 1:1232–1235, 1973.
17. Committee on Issues and Priorities for New Vaccine Development. The prospects for immunizing against *V. cholerae*. In New Vaccine Development, Establishing Priorities. Vol 2. Diseases of Importance in Developing Countries. Washington, DC, National Academy of Science, 1986, pp 376–289.
18. Sack DA, Freij L, Holmgren J. Swedish Agency for Research Cooperation with Developing Countries. Prospects for public health benefits in developing countries from new vaccines against enteric infections. J Infect Dis 163:503–506, 1991.
19. Cholera Working Group. Large epidemic of cholera-like disease in Bangladesh caused by *Vibrio cholerae* O139 synonym Bengal. Lancet 342:387–390, 1993.
20. Wachsmuth IK, Evins GM, Fields PI, et al. The molecular epidemiology of cholera in Latin America. J Infect Dis 167:621–626, 1993.
21. Popovic T, Fields PI, Olsvik O, et al. Molecular subtyping of toxigenic *Vibrio cholerae* O139 causing epidemic cholera in India and Bangladesh, 1992–1993. J Infect Dis 171:122–127, 1995.
22. Faruque SM, Abdul Alim AR, Rahman MM, et al. Clonal relationships among classical *Vibrio cholerae* O1 strains isolated between 1961 and 1992 in Bangladesh. J Clin Microbiol 31:2513–2516, 1993.
23. Evins GM, Cameron DN, Wells JG, et al. The emerging diversity of the electrophoretic types of *Vibrio cholerae* in the Western Hemisphere. J Infect Dis 172:173–179, 1995.
24. Sack FH, Pierce NF, Hennessey KN, et al. Gastric acid in cholera and non-cholera diarrhea. Bull World Health Organ 47:31–36, 1972.
25. van Loon FP, Clemens JD, Shahrier M, et al. Low gastric acid as a risk factor for cholera transmission: Application of a new non-invasive gastric acid field test. J Clin Epidemiol 43:1361–1367, 1990.
26. Clemens JD, Sack DA, Harris JR, et al. ABO blood groups and cholera: New observations on specificity of risk and modification of vaccine efficacy. J Infect Dis 159:770–773, 1989.
27. Glass RI, Holmgren J, Haley CE, et al. Predisposition for cholera of individuals with O blood group. Possible evolutionary significance. Am J Epidemiol 121:791–796, 1985.
28. Gardel CL, Mekalanos JJ. Alterations in *Vibrio cholerae* motility phenotypes correlate with changes in virulence factor expression. Infect Immun 64:2246–2255, 1996.
29. Herrington DA, Hall RH, Losonsky G, et al. Toxin, toxin-coregulated pili, and the toxR regulon are essential for *Vibrio cholerae* pathogenesis in humans. J Exp Med 168:1487–1492, 1988.
30. Sun DX, Mekalanos JJ, Taylor RK. Antibodies directed against the toxin-coregulated pilus isolated from *Vibrio cholerae* provide protection in the infant mouse experimental cholera model. J Infect Dis 161:1231–1236, 1990.
31. Pierce NF, Reynolds HY. Immunity to experimental cholera. I. Protective effect of humoral IgG antitoxin demonstrated by passive immunization. J Immunol 113:1017–1023, 1974.
32. Holmgren J, Svennerholm AM, Clemens JD, et al. An oral B subunit–whole cell vaccine against cholera: From concept to successful field trial. Adv Exp Med Biol 216b:1649–1660, 1987.
33. Laboratory Methods for the Diagnosis of *Vibrio cholerae*. Centers for Disease Control and Prevention, Atlanta, GA, 1994.
34. Hasan JA, Huq A, Tamplin ML, et al. A novel kit for rapid detection of *Vibrio cholerae* O1. J Clin Microbiol 32:249–252, 1994.
35. Hasan JA, Huq A, Nair GB, et al. Development and testing of monoclonal antibody–based rapid immunodiagnostic test kits for direct detection of *Vibrio cholerae* O139 synonym Bengal. J Clin Microbiol 33:2935–2939, 1995.
36. Guthmann JP. Epidemic cholera in Latin America: Spread and routes of transmission. J Trop Med Hyg 98:419–427, 1995.
37. Ries AA, Vugia DJ, Beingolea L, et al. Cholera in Piura, Peru: A modern urban epidemic. J Infect Dis 166:1429–1433, 1992.
38. Qadri F, Wenneras C, Albert MJ, et al. Comparison of immune responses in patients infected with *Vibrio cholerae* O139 and O1. Infect Immun 65:3571–3576, 1997.
39. Albert MJ, Alam K, Ansaruzzaman M, et al. Lack of cross-protection against diarrhea due to *Vibrio cholerae* O139 (Bengal strain) after oral immunization of rabbits with *V. cholerae* O1 vaccine strain CVD103-HgR. J Infect Dis 169:230–231, 1994.
40. Qadri F, Mohi G, Hossain J, et al. Comparison of the vibriocidal antibody response in cholera due to *Vibrio cholerae* O139 Bengal with the response in cholera due to *Vibrio cholerae* O1. Clin Diagn Lab Immunol 2:685–688, 1995.
41. Glass RI, Becker S, Huq MI, et al. Endemic cholera in rural Bangladesh, 1966–1980. Am J Epidemiol 116:959–970, 1982.
42. Siddique AK, Salam A, Islam MS, et al. Why treatment centres failed to prevent cholera deaths among Rwandan refugees in Goma, Zaire. Lancet 345:359–361, 1995.
43. Goma Epidemiology Group. Public health impact of Rwandan refugee crisis: What happened in Goma, Zaire, in July, 1994? Lancet 345:339–344, 1995.
44. Blake PA, Allegra DT, Snyder JD, et al. Cholera—a possible endemic focus in the United States. N Engl J Med 302:305–309, 1980.
45. Clemens JD, Sack DA, Harris JR, et al. Breast feeding and the risk of severe cholera in rural Bangladeshi children. Am J Epidemiol 131:400–411, 1990.
46. Colwell RR, Huq A. Environmental reservoir of *Vibrio cholerae*. The causative agent of cholera. Ann N Y Acad Sci 740:44–54, 1994.
47. Huq A, West PA, Small EB, et al. Influence of water temperature, salinity, and pH on survival and growth of toxigenic *Vibrio cholerae* serovar 01 associated with live copepods in laboratory microcosms. Appl Environ Microbiol 48:420–424, 1984.
48. Huq A, Huq SA, Grimes DJ, et al. Colonization of the gut of the blue crab (*Callinectes sapidus*) by *Vibrio cholerae*. Appl Environ Microbiol 52:586–588, 1986.
49. Islam MS, Drasar BS, Sack RB. The aquatic flora and fauna as reservoirs of *Vibrio cholerae*: A review. J Diarrhoeal Dis Res 12:87–96, 1994.
50. Glass RI, Svennerholm AM, Stoll BJ, et al. Protection against cholera in breast-fed children by antibodies in breast milk. N Engl J Med 308:1389–1392, 1983.
51. Levine MM. Vaccines and milk immunoglobulin concentrates for prevention of infectious diarrhea. J Pediatr 118:S129–S136, 1991.
52. Levine MM, Kaper JB, Black RE, Clements ML. New knowledge

on pathogenesis of bacterial enteric infections as applied to vaccine development. Microbiol Rev 47:510–550, 1983.

53. Clemens JD, van Loon F, Sack DA, et al. Biotype as determinant of natural immunising effect of cholera. Lancet 337:883–884, 1991.
54. Svennerholm AM, Jertborn M, Gothefors L, et al. Mucosal antitoxic and antibacterial immunity after cholera disease and after immunization with a combined B subunit–whole cell vaccine. J Infect Dis 149:884–893, 1984.
55. Sack DA, Clemens JD, Huda S, et al. Antibody responses after immunization with killed oral cholera vaccines during the 1985 vaccine field trial in Bangladesh. J Infect Dis 164:407–411, 1991.
56. Clemens JD, Harris JR, Sack DA, et al. Field trial of oral cholera vaccines in Bangladesh: Results of one year of follow-up. J Infect Dis 158:60–69, 1988.
57. Benenson AS, Joseph PR, Oseasohn RO. Cholera vaccine field trials in East Pakistan. 1. Reaction and antigenicity studies. Bull World Health Organ 38:347–357, 1968.
58. Mosley WH, McCormack WM, Ahmed A, et al. Report of the 1966–67 cholera vaccine field test in rural East Pakistan. 2. Results of the serological surveys in the study population—the relationship of case rate to antibody titre and an estimate of the inapparent infection with *Vibrio cholerae*. Bull World Health Organ 40:187–197, 1969.
59. Mosley WH, Woodward WE, Aziz KMA, et al. The 1968–1969 cholera-vaccine field trial in rural East Pakistan. Effectiveness of monovalent Ogawa and Inaba vaccines and a purified Inaba antigen, with comparative results of serological and animal protection tests. J Infect Dis 121(suppl):1–9, 1970.
60. Blake PA. Epidemiology of cholera in the Americas. Gastroenterol Clin North Am 22:639–660, 1993.
61. Svennerholm AM, Holmgren J. Synergistic protective effect in rabbits of immunization with *Vibrio cholerae* lipopolysaccharide and toxin/toxoid. Infect Immun 13:735–740, 1976.
62. Clemens JD, Sack DA, Harris JR, et al. Field trial of oral cholera vaccines in Bangladesh. Lancet 2:124–127, 1986.
63. Jertborn M, Svennerholm AM, Holmgren J. Safety and immunogenicity of an oral recombinant cholera B subunit–whole cell vaccine in Swedish volunteers. Vaccine 10:130–132, 1992.
64. Sanchez J, Holmgren J. Recombinant system for overexpression of cholera toxin B subunit in *Vibrio cholerae* as a basis for vaccine development. Proc Natl Acad Sci U S A 86:481–485, 1989.
65. Clemens JD, Jertborn M, Sack DA, et al. Effect of neutralization of gastric acid on immune responses to an oral B subunit, killed whole cell cholera vaccine. J Infect Dis 154:175–178, 1986.
66. Trach DD, Clemens JD, Ke NT, et al. Field trial of a locally produced, killed, oral cholera vaccine in Vietnam. Lancet 349:231–235, 1997.
67. Black RE, Levine MM, Clements ML, et al. Protective efficacy in humans of killed whole-vibrio oral cholera vaccine with and without the B subunit of cholera toxin. Infect Immun 55:1116–1120, 1987.
68. Clemens JD, Stanton BF, Chakraborty J, et al. B subunit–whole cell and whole cell only oral vaccines against cholera: Studies on reactogenicity and immunogenicity. J Infect Dis 155:79–85, 1987.
69. Jertborn M, Svennerholm AM, Holmgren J. IgG and IgA subclass distribution of antitoxin antibody responses after oral cholera vaccination or cholera disease. Int Arch Allergy Immunol 85:358–363, 1988.
70. Svennerholm AM, Sack DA, Holmgren J, Bardhan PK. Intestinal antibody responses after immunisation with cholera B subunit. Lancet 1:305–308, 1982.
71. Svennerholm AM, Gothefors L, Sack DA, et al. Local and systemic antibody responses and immunological memory in humans after immunization with cholera B subunit by different routes. Bull World Health Organ 62:909–918, 1984.
72. Jertborn M, Svennerholm AM, Holmgren J. Saliva, breast milk, and serum antibody responses as indirect measures of intestinal immunity after oral cholera vaccination or natural disease. J Clin Microbiol 24:203–209, 1986.
73. Lycke N, Hellstrom U, Holmgren J. Circulating cholera antitoxin memory cells in the blood one year after oral cholera vaccination in humans. Scand J Immunol 26:207–211, 1987.
74. Clemens JD, Sack DA, Harris JR, et al. Field trial of oral cholera vaccines in Bangladesh: results from three-year follow-up. Lancet 335:270–273, 1990.
75. Clemens JD, Sack DA, Harris JR, et al. Cross-protection by B subunit–whole cell cholera vaccine against diarrhea associated with heat labile–toxin producing enterotoxigenic *Escherichia coli*: Results of a large-scale field trial. J Infect Dis 158:372–377, 1988.
76. Clemens JD, Harris JR, Kay BA, et al. Oral cholera vaccines containing B-subunit–killed whole cells and killed whole cells only. II. Field evaluation of cross-protection against other members of the Vibrionaceae family. Vaccine 7:117–120, 1989.
77. Ciznar I, Hussain N, Ahsan CR, et al. Oral cholera vaccines containing B-subunit–killed whole cells and killed whole cells only. I. Cross-reacting antigens of members of family Vibrionaceae and the vaccines. Vaccine 7:111–116, 1989.
78. Peltola H, Siitonen A, Kyronseppa H, et al. Prevention of travellers' diarrhoea by oral B-subunit/whole-cell cholera vaccine. Lancet 338:1285–1289, 1991.
79. Sanchez JL, Vasquez B, Begue RE, et al. Protective efficacy of oral whole-cell/recombinant-B-subunit cholera vaccine in Peruvian military recruits. Lancet 344:1273–1276, 1994.
80. Begue RE, Castellares G, Cabezas C, et al. Immunogenicity in Peruvian volunteers of a booster dose of oral cholera vaccine consisting of whole cells plus recombinant B subunit. Infect Immun 63:3726–3728, 1995.
80a. Nafizy A, Rao MR. Paquet C, et al. Treatment and vaccination strategies to control cholera in sub-Saharan refugee settings: A cost-effectiveness analysis. JAMA 279:521–525, 1998.
81. Snyder JD, Blake PA. Is cholera a problem for US travelers? JAMA 247:2268–2269, 1982.
82. Taylor DN, Rizzo J, Meza R, et al. Cholera among Americans living in Peru. Clin Infect Dis 22:1108–1109, 1996.
83. Levine MM, Kaper JB, Herrington DA, et al. Safety, immunogenicity, and efficacy of recombinant live oral cholera vaccines, CVD 103 and CVD 103-HgR. Lancet 2:467–470, 1988.
84. Cryz SJ Jr, Levine MM, Kaper JB, et al. Randomized double-blind placebo controlled trial to evaluate the safety and immunogenicity of the live oral cholera vaccine strain CVD 103-HgR in Swiss adults. Vaccine 8:577–580, 1990.
85. Migasena S, Pitisuttitham P, Prayurahong B, et al. Preliminary assessment of the safety and immunogenicity of live oral cholera vaccine strain CVD 103-HgR in healthy Thai adults. Infect Immun 57:3261–3264, 1989.
86. Sack DA, Sack RB, Shimko J, et al. Evaluation of Peru-15, a new live oral vaccine for cholera in volunteers. J Infect Dis 176:201–205, 1997.
87. Sack DA, Shimko J, Sack RB, et al. Comparison of alternative buffers for use with a new live oral cholera vaccine, Peru-15, in outpatient volunteers. Infect Immun 65:2107–2111, 1997.
88. Kenner JR, Coster TS, Taylor DN, et al. Peru-15, an improved live attenuated oral vaccine candidate for *Vibrio cholerae* O1. J Infect Dis 172:1126–1129, 1995.
89. Tacket CO, Kotloff KL, Losonsky G, et al. Volunteer studies investigating the safety and efficacy of live oral El Tor *Vibrio cholerae* O1 vaccine strain CVD 111. Am J Trop Med Hyg 56:533–537, 1997.
90. Taylor DN, Tacket CO, Losonsky G, et al. Evaluation of a bivalent (CVD 103-HgR/CVD 111) live oral cholera vaccine in adult volunteers from the United States and Peru. Infect Immun 65:3852–3856, 1997.
91. Coster TS, Killeen KP, Waldor MK, et al. Safety, immunogenicity, and efficacy of live attenuated *Vibrio cholerae* O139 vaccine prototype. Lancet 345:949–952, 1995.
92. Tacket CO, Losonsky G, Nataro JP, et al. Initial clinical studies of CVD 112 *Vibrio cholerae* O139 live oral vaccine: Safety and efficacy against experimental challenge. J Infect Dis 172:883–886, 1995.

chapter

26 Hepatitis A Vaccine

Stephen M. Feinstone
Ian D. Gust

HISTORY

Although episodes of jaundice have been known since the time of Hippocrates, the earliest outbreaks that on epidemiological grounds seem likely to have been hepatitis A occurred in Europe in the 17th and 18th centuries.[1, 2] Sporadic cases of jaundice were recognized in the 19th century and became known as catarrhal jaundice, reflecting the view of some pathologists that blockage of the common bile duct by inspissated mucus was the cause of the disease.[3] Early this century, Cockayne concluded that sporadic and epidemic forms of jaundice were probably manifestations of the same disease,[4] and McDonald postulated that a virus might be involved.[5]

The first hard data that hepatitis A was an enterically transmitted viral infection were obtained during World War II from a series of studies among experimentally infected volunteers. Hepatitis has been a military problem for centuries, and major outbreaks occurred among British, French, German, and Romanian troops in World War I and among German, French, American Commonwealth, and Axis troops in World War II.[6]

Epidemic hepatitis, which the British referred to as infective hepatitis, was a serious problem among troops in the Middle East in 1941 and 1942—with at times 8 to 9% of troops and a third of officers out of action through illness.[7] Army physicians formed the opinion that the disease was transmitted from infected feces and that poor sanitation was an important factor in its spread.

In 1943, major government-sanctioned studies were commenced in Britain and the United States; in both countries, research groups of clinicians, virologists, and epidemiologists were established and asked to determine how the disease was being spread and to devise means for its control.[8] It soon became apparent that the disease could not be transmitted to laboratory animals and that the only suitable experimental animal was the human. During the next 2 years, a series of experiments were conducted in human volunteers that provided much basic knowledge on the natural history of the disease and its mode of spread and established reliable methods of interrupting transmission.

Both MacCallum and Bradley[9] in the United Kingdom and Neefe and coworkers[10] in the United States succeeded in transmitting infectious hepatitis to volunteers by feeding them bacteria-free suspensions of feces collected from patients early in the disease or fecally contaminated water that had been collected from a well during an epidemic. Whereas transmission studies also demonstrated that the infectious agent was present in the blood during the late incubation period and early acute phase of the disease, attempts to transmit infection with urine or nasopharyngeal washings were equivocal.[11]

In a classic series of experiments, Havens[12] and Neefe and colleagues[13] were able to show that volunteers who had developed infectious hepatitis were protected from subsequent challenge with the same virus and with infectious material obtained from a separate outbreak. Given this result, attention turned to the potential use of convalescent human serum or normal immune globulin for the prevention of disease. It was soon demonstrated that intramuscular injection of pooled normal human immune globulin could prevent or attenuate the disease.[12, 14] These findings had important applications, and the practice was rapidly adopted. During an epidemic in 1945 in the Mediterranean arena, more than 2700 American soldiers were immunized. The value of this approach was rapidly apparent by an 86% reduction in the incidence of disease among immunized troops.[15]

Subsequently, when it became apparent that infectious hepatitis was clearly distinct from serum hepatitis in both mode of transmission and etiology, MacCallum suggested that the diseases be known as hepatitis A and B. This suggestion was adopted in 1952 by the World Health Organization's First Expert Committee on Viral Hepatitis but not widely accepted by physicians and virologists until the early 1970s, replacing the terms infectious hepatitis (hepatitis A) and homologous serum hepatitis (hepatitis B).

By the end of World War II, volunteer studies had clearly established that infectious hepatitis was enterically transmitted and was caused by a filterable agent—presumably a virus—that was relatively heat stable but could be inactivated by chlorine.[16] The disease appeared to be caused by a single agent, seemed to be associated with lifelong immunity, and was preventable by administration of normal immune globulin.

In the 1950s, these data were expanded and refined by a further series of studies conducted by Krugman and colleagues[17] at the Willowbrook State School in New York and by Boggs and Melnick[18] and their colleagues at the Joliet prison, Illinois. Fecal samples collected from the latter studies were critical in the subse-

Table 26–1. **CLINICAL SPECTRUM OF HEPATITIS A IN 1988 SHANGHAI EPIDEMIC**

310,746 identified cases from January to May 1988
Case-fatality rate: 0.015%: 47 deaths during hepatitis A
25 fulminant hepatitis
15 hepatitis A with underlying chronic liver disease
7 miscellaneous diseases

Clinical manifestations of 8647 hospitalized patients
Age: 12 to 71 yr (90.8% between 20 and 40 yr)
Incubation period: 21.6 d (range, 12 to 36 d)

SYMPTOM	%	CLINICAL FINDING	%	COMPLICATIONS	%
Jaundice	84	Hepatomegaly	87	Cholestasis	1.6–5.3
Weight loss	82	Splenomegaly	9	Upper gastrointestinal bleeding	0.5–1.2
Malaise	80	Rash	3	Thrombocytopenia purpura, Guillain-Barré syndrome, red cell aplasia, autoimmune hemolytic anemia, transverse myelitis, optic neuritis	<0.1 each
Fever	76	Mild edema	2		
Nausea	69	Petechiae	2		
Abdominal pain	37				
Arthralgia	6				

Adapted from Yao G. Clinical spectrum and natural history of viral hepatitis A in a 1988 Shanghai epidemic. In Hollinger FB, Lemon SM, Margolis HS (eds). Viral Hepatitis and Liver Disease. Baltimore, Williams & Wilkins, 1991, pp 76–78.

quent identification of the etiological agent of the disease by electron microscopy.[19] The ability to detect the presence of hepatitis A virus (HAV) in clinical and environmental samples, to grow it in cell culture, and to test for infectivity and virulence in tamarins and chimpanzees has eliminated the need for volunteer studies, other than for evaluation of vaccines.

BACKGROUND

Clinical Description

Before the development of specific diagnostic tests, physicians tended to distinguish between the two classical forms of viral hepatitis on the basis of certain epidemiological features such as incubation period when available, a history of exposure to similar cases in the household or community, or a recent history of blood transfusion or shared needles and syringes.

When specific serological tests for hepatitis A and B were developed, it became apparent that diagnostic decisions based on such epidemiological features were frequently wrong. Although some differences in symptoms are found when large numbers of patients with hepatitis A, B, C, D, and E are studied, there is much overlap; consequently, there is no single clinical feature or group of features that enables a clinician to make a confident etiological diagnosis without recourse to specific laboratory tests. In 1988, an outbreak involving more than 300,000 clinical cases associated with ingestion of clams from contaminated waters occurred in Shanghai, China.[20] Table 26–1 shows an analysis of the clinical picture presented in this outbreak as the most comprehensive description of the clinical spectrum of hepatitis A.

Numerous studies have been conducted to define the incubation period of hepatitis A after natural or experimental infection in children or adults. Although disease has been seen as early as 15 days and as late as 50 days from exposure, the mean incubation period appears to be about 28 days.[13, 20, 21]

Hepatitis A is an acute infection with generalized symptoms often accompanied by jaundice (see Table 26–1). It usually commences with a brief prodromal illness lasting for several days and characterized by increasing fatigue, malaise, loss of appetite, nausea, and vomiting, which although distressing are not severe enough to cause the patient to stop work or see a physician. In most patients, the first objective sign of illness is darkening of their urine, yellowing of the sclera, or the passage of pale-colored stools. One of these signs stimulates the patient to seek medical attention. At this stage, other than jaundice and an enlarged and tender liver, physical examination is often unremarkable. The clinical diagnosis is confirmed by liver function tests and the specific serological assays (Table 26–2).

Table 26–2. **AVAILABLE TESTS FOR HEPATITIS A VIRUS AND ANTIBODY TO HAV**

TEST	UTILITY
Anti-HAV/total antibody (RIA/ELISA) Commercially available	Test for susceptibles before vaccination should *not* be used in postexposure situation to determine use of immune globulin. Epidemiological investigation
Anti-HAV/IgM-specific (RIA/ELISA) Commercially available	Primary test for diagnosis of present or recent infection
Viral culture (cell culture)	Research use only because virus grows slowly on initial isolation
HAV antigen (RIA/ELISA)	Research use for detecting virus in various specimens, i.e., cell culture
HAV RNA (molecular hybridization/PCR)	Research applications Environmental studies
Liver biopsy (light or fluorescent microscopy)	Research with animal inoculations Rare diagnostic dilemma or unusual clinical presentation. Biopsy is not indicated for most hepatitis A cases.

HAV, hepatitis A virus; IgM, immunoglobulin M; RIA, radioimmunoassay; ELISA, enzyme-linked immunosorbent assay; PCR, polymerase chain reaction.

Infection with HAV may produce a wide spectrum of outcomes from silent or subclinical hepatitis at one end, through typical acute hepatitis with jaundice, to fulminant hepatitis at the other. The single most important factor in determining the outcome of HAV infection appears to be age. Whereas greater than 90% of infections acquired before the age of 5 years are silent, the proportion of infected individuals with symptoms increases steadily, reaching approximately 25% by 15 years and 90% or above in adults.[22] The duration of illness varies but most patients feel better, have lost their hepatomegaly, and have nearly normal liver function test results within 3 weeks. In the large 1989 Shanghai outbreak, 90% of a subset of 8647 hospitalized patients observed carefully had completely recovered in 4 months and all had recovered in 1 year.[20, 23] Relapse consisting of renewed symptoms, elevated liver function test results, and possibly detection of virus in stools has been found in up to 10% of cases, but recovery is universal.[24, 25] Hepatitis A never becomes chronic.

A cholestatic form of hepatitis A has been reported in which the patient experiences persistent jaundice usually accompanied by itching. A short course of corticosteroids may reduce these symptoms and hasten recovery, but even without treatment, recovery is universal. Clinical relapses that may include jaundice after initial resolution of illness have also been reported, but again, total recovery is the rule.[26, 27]

Fulminant hepatitis, the most severe form of the disease, is fortunately rare, but special caution should be observed in elderly patients. Case-fatality rates are usually obtained from hospital series that are self-selected for patients with more severe disease. Even so, it is apparent that fulminating hepatitis, liver failure, and death are rare especially among children and young adults but become significant in older adults (Table 26–3). In a large hospital-based series from Fairfield Hospital in Melbourne, only three deaths occurred among more than 2000 patients with serologically confirmed hepatitis A, a case-fatality rate of 0.14%.[28] In the 1988 Shanghai epidemic that involved primarily adolescents and young adults, there were only 47 deaths recorded among the 310,746 diagnosed (0.015%) cases. Twenty-five of the deaths were due to fulminant hepatitis, and 15 were related to exacerbations of underlying chronic hepatitis B infections.[20]

Table 26–3. **AGE-SPECIFIC MORTALITY DUE TO HEPATITIS A**

AGE GROUP (yr)	NO. OF CASES (%)	NO. OF DEATHS (%)	CASE-FATALITY PER 1000
<5	6,165 (5.3)	9 (2.4)	1.5
5–14	22,548 (19.5)	1 (0.3)	0.004
15–29	49,642 (43)	28 (7.3)	0.57
30–49	26,961 (23.3)	67 (17.6)	2.5
>49	10,235 (8.8)	276 (27.4)	27
Total	115,551	381	3.3

From Centers for Disease Control. Viral Hepatitis Surveillance Program, 1983–1989.

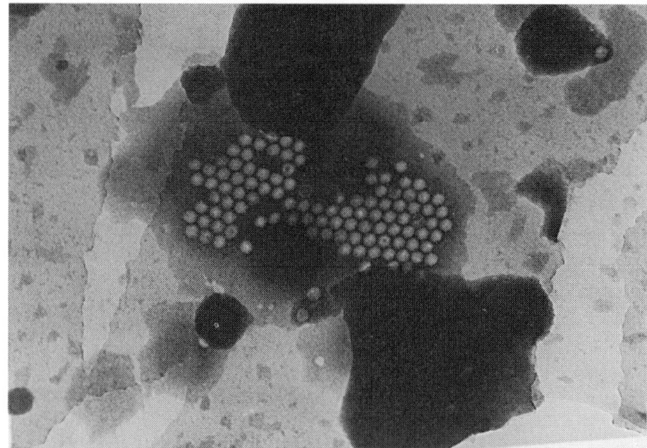

Figure 26–1. Electron micrograph of purified hepatitis A particles. Magnification × 125,000.

Virology

HAV is a member of the *Picornaviridae* family, which includes both the enteroviruses and rhinoviruses of humans. Because of several unique features, HAV has been placed into its own genus, *Hepatavirus*.[29–34] There are four recognized human genotypes of HAV based on primary sequence variability, but there is only one known serotype.[35, 36] Many strains of HAV have been described on the basis of different growth characteristics, nucleotide sequence, or geographical origin.[37–39] Polyclonal and monoclonal antibodies directed against the major antigenic determinant appear to be capable of detecting strains of HAV isolated in different parts of the world, suggesting that there is only one serotype.[40–42]

HAV is a nonenveloped, 27- to 28-nm-diameter spherical virus (Fig. 26–1) with a surface structure that suggests icosahedral symmetry, although fine resolution of the virus structure by x-ray crystallography has not yet been achieved.[19] Mature HAV virions purified from feces collected from infected humans or chimpanzees band at 1.32 to 1.34 g per cm^3 in CsCl and sediment at approximately 160 S.[43–45] A lower density fraction can often be detected that bands at about 1.27 g per cm^3 in CsCl and sediments at 70 to 80 S, which consists primarily of empty capsids. In addition, a high-density fraction (1.4 g/cm^3) that may represent particles with a more open virion structure (allowing increased penetration and binding of CsCl into the viral particle) may also be found. These high-density particles have been shown to contain HAV RNA but tend to be less stable than mature virions.[45–47]

Resistance to Physical and Chemical Agents. HAV is more resistant to heat than other picornaviruses are.[48, 49] Whereas HAV may be incompletely inactivated (depending on the conditions) by exposure to 60°C for 10 to 12 hours,[49] complete inactivation is attained after exposure to 100°C for 5 minutes, after heating for 4 minutes to 70°C, after 5 seconds at 80°C, and virtually instantly at 85°C.[50] HAV may survive for days to weeks in shellfish, water, soil, or marine sediment.[51] Outbreaks of hepatitis A have been reported after ingestion of partially cooked shellfish, suggesting that the usual steaming conditions used to cook shellfish may be insufficient to destroy the virus. HAV can be reliably inactivated by autoclaving (121°C for 30 minutes).[52] The virus is resistant to most organic solvents and detergents as well as pH as low as 3.[46, 52] HAV can be inactivated by many common disinfecting chemicals, including hypochlorite (bleach), and quaternary ammonium formulations containing 23% HCl, found in many toilet bowl cleaners.[52] Currently licensed vaccines are inactivated by 1:4000 formalin at room temperature for at least 15 days to exceed complete inactivation by at least threefold.

Molecular Structure. The HAV genome is composed of single-stranded linear RNA of 7478 nucleotides (strain HM175) and a molecular weight of approximately 2.25×10^6.[32, 53, 54] The genomic RNA has positive polarity, a relatively long 5′ untranslated region of 735 nucleotides typical of picornaviruses followed by a single long open reading frame of approximately 6678 nucleotides coding for a polyprotein of about 2226 amino acids, and a short 3′ untranslated region ending with a virus-coded poly(A) tail. Sequence analysis of the HAV genome reveals that its gene order is also characteristic of picornaviruses with the structural genes coded by the 5′ third of the open reading frame and the nonstructural proteins coded by the remainder. Whereas HAV is similar to the other picornaviruses in physical and molecular structure, it has little similarity to other picornaviruses at the nucleotide or amino acid sequence level.

As with other picornaviruses, the 5′ end of the genome does not have a cap structure but instead has a small, covalently bound, virus-coded protein termed VPg.[55] This 5′ untranslated region has predicted secondary structure similar to other picornavirus untranslated regions and includes an internal ribosomal entry site for cap-independent translation.[56, 57] Translation begins at one of two in-frame AUG codons at nucleotide position 735 or 741, which initiates a single long open reading frame of 6681 nucleotides that encodes a potential polyprotein of 2227 amino acid residues in length.[58, 59] After a translation terminator sequence, the genome ends with a 3′ noncoding region of 63 nucleotides that is followed by a poly(A) tail of varying lengths typical of picornavirus genomes. The polyprotein of picornaviruses has been arbitrarily divided into three parts, termed P1, P2, and P3. The four capsid proteins are coded by the first 2373 nucleotides (P1) and the nonstructural proteins by the remainder (P2 and P3). The gene order and protein function of HAV are similar to those of the other picornaviruses. There are differences in the details of the protein cleavages, and HAV has only one known viral protease, protein 3C, that is responsible for all the cleavages except the final maturation cleavage of the capsid protein VP0 into VP4 and VP2.[60–63]

The predicted VP4 molecule has never been experimentally shown to be a part of the virion particle and at just 23 amino acids is about one third the size of VP4 proteins of other picornaviruses. In addition, VP4 of picornaviruses are myristylated at the N terminus after cleavage of the initial methionine or a leader peptide.[62, 64] Whereas a potential myristylation site could be revealed in the HAV VP4 by cleavage of the first four amino acids, mutations of this myristylation site have no effect on virus replication and it is assumed to be not active.[65]

The 2A protein of poliovirus has proteinase activity and makes the VP1/2A cleavage. However, the 2A of HAV has no known function, and the VP1/2A cleavage seems to be performed by the major viral protease 3C.[60] Mutants in which the central portion of 2A was deleted produced small foci in cell culture but remained virulent in marmosets.[66] The 2B and 2C proteins are believed to be involved in replication. Mutations leading to cell culture adaptation and attenuation in animals have been mapped to these regions.[67, 68] The protein 3AB appears to be the precursor to VPg. Protein 3C is the virion protease that appears to be responsible for all the proteolytic cleavages of the HAV polyprotein except for the VP0 cleavage.[60, 61, 69] Protein 3D is the viral polymerase responsible for the replication of the genomic RNA.

Antigenic Composition. Although a variety of genotypes of HAV have been identified on the basis of genomic sequence analysis, there appears to be only one serotype throughout the world.[35, 36, 40] Individuals who were infected by HAV in one part of the world are not susceptible to reinfection by virus in another part of the world, and immune serum globulin prepared in a variety of developed countries appears to protect travelers from disease irrespective of their destination. Recently, data from newly approved vaccines have shown that vaccines prepared from virus isolates from Australia or Costa Rica induce antibody that protects worldwide.[70, 71] The HAV genotypes I and III are the most genetically diverse viruses identified. A genotype I virus, HM175, and a genotype III virus, PA21, which differed by 16.8% in their nucleotide sequence in the structural protein coding region, were shown to have no significant antigenic differences in a crisscross neutralization assay.[35, 72] In addition, both viruses reacted nearly identically with a panel of 18 monoclonal antibodies.[72]

Stapleton and colleagues[73] have made an extensive analysis of the antigenic composition of the HAV capsid through binding studies of neutralizing monoclonal antibodies analysis of neutralization escape mutants. They have shown that neutralization epitopes of HAV are contained primarily within predicted loop regions on the structural proteins VP1 and VP3. However, neutralizing monoclonal antibodies do not recognize either oligopeptides predicted to contain neutralization epitopes or denatured individual viral capsid proteins, and antibodies raised against synthetic oligopeptides do not neutralize or even bind to whole virus, which suggests that these neutralization epitopes are conformational and not linear. Binding competition assays of neutralizing monoclonal antibodies have indicated that the neutralization epitopes are contained within a closely related antigenic site.[73]

Cellular Replication. Details of HAV replication have been incompletely elucidated because of its relatively inefficient growth in vitro. Like other picornaviruses, HAV is believed to bind to the cell through a specific cellular receptor inserted into the plasma membrane. A previously unidentified receptor molecule from monkey kidney cells termed HAVcr1 appears to be a mucin-like glycoprotein. Binding of HAV to cells that express HAVcr1 is blocked by a specific monoclonal antibody to the receptor, and the cDNA can be transfected into nonpermissive cells, rendering them permissive for virus binding, entry, and translation, although nonpermissive cells transfected with HAVcr1 cDNA have not been found to replicate complete, infectious virus.[74]

Replication of HAV seems to be intimately related to the cytoplasmic membranes. Intracellular virus is only seen within membrane-bound vesicles, whereas enteroviruses can be seen free in the cytoplasm. These vesicles might be released directly from the cell because virus-laden vesicles have been observed both in cell culture supernatants and in intestinal contents.[75–77]

Many HAV strains have been isolated in cell culture directly from clinical material, although the procedure may take several weeks or even months.[38] Until recently, only epithelial or fibroblast cells of primate origin had been conclusively shown to support the growth of HAV.[38, 78–80] However, certain porcine, guinea pig, and dolphin cells can support the replication of HAV.[81] HAV tends to grow more slowly and generate lower yields than other picornaviruses do.[38, 82] In addition, the virus is largely cell associated, does not usually produce cytopathic effect, and readily leads to persistently infected cell lines. Rapidly replicating variants of HAV have been selected that induce cytopathic effects in some cell lines.[83, 84]

Cell culture of HAV has been used to alter the phenotype of the virus primarily for growth characteristics and attenuation of virulence. Attenuated strains of HAV have been selected by multiple tissue culture passages, and cold adaptation has been achieved by passage at reduced temperature.[85–87] Some of the mutations responsible for these altered phenotypes have been determined by molecular cloning and sequencing of the mutant and comparing its sequence with the parental strain. Mutations within the 5′ untranslated region and mutations within the 2B and 2C coding regions of HAV RNA have been shown to enhance virus replication in vitro.[68, 88]

Host Range. HAV is known to infect humans and other great apes and some species of monkeys. The most extensively characterized models are the chimpanzee and two New World monkeys, tamarins and *Aotus* (owl) monkeys.[89–92] The presence of antibodies in some primate species at the time of capture may indicate that there is a reservoir of infection in nature, or these antibodies may represent cross-reactive antibodies with monkey viruses. There are several reports of isolation of human HAV–related viruses from monkeys.[35, 89, 92] Several of these isolates have been shown to have significant sequence variation and minor antigenic differences with human HAV. Although transmission of HAV to primate handlers is well documented, it has not yet been determined whether these monkey isolates are true simian HAVs or human viruses that have infected monkey colonies where they have persisted and adapted. Neither is it known if there is a monkey reservoir of human HAV that can serve as a source of continued human infections.[35, 89, 93]

Pathogenesis as It Relates to Prevention

HAV is generally transmitted by the fecal-oral route, and this acid-resistant virus probably can survive passage through the stomach. Its primary site of replication is somewhere in the intestine, although there are also experimental data in chimpanzees that HAV may replicate in the oropharynx.[94, 95] The virus has been identified by immunofluorescence in the epithelial cells of the intestinal crypts of both the jejunum and ileum of experimentally infected monkeys.[94, 96] A viremic stage has been detected beginning up to 2 weeks before the onset of clinical illness and persisting for a variable period after symptoms begin in both humans and experimentally infected primates.[97–99] Although it is possible that other organs would be seeded by the viremia, HAV, like many other picornaviruses, appears to be organ specific, and the only recognized pathological process in hepatitis A is restricted to the liver. Virus is shed from infected liver cells into the hepatic sinusoids and the bile canaliculi, passes into the intestine, and is excreted in the feces, where it may be found in high titers early in the infection.[100–102]

Because HAV is generally not cytopathic in cell culture and the pathological findings in both experimental animals and humans show little of hepatocyte damage at the peak of viral replication, immune mechanisms, in particular cell-mediated immune responses, have been postulated to explain the hepatic injury.[103, 104] In contrast, circulating antibodies are probably more important in limiting spread of virus to uninfected liver cells, which in combination with interferon is responsible for termination of the infection.[104–106]

Although liver damage occurs at the same time that circulating antibodies become detectable, studies failed to prove that the pathological process is antibody dependent. Whereas circulating immune complexes containing HAV and mostly HAV-specific immunoglobulin M (IgM) antibodies have been found during infection, immunoglobulin and complement deposits were not found at the sites of liver cell damage, and resolution of disease occurred at a time when antibody levels were rising and hepatitis A antigen could still be detected in the liver.[107] Although circulating antibody limits the spread of virus and prevents reinfection, it appears to have no role in liver damage.

Immunity

Because second infections with HAV are unknown, it is assumed that immunity to the disease persists for life. In some endemic areas where exposure to the virus is common, the mean antibody levels in the population decline in older age groups, suggesting that anti-HAV confers complete protection against reinfection.

It is known that passive immunization with immune globulin can provide complete protection against infection, indicating that serum antibody alone is sufficient to prevent infection.[108] It has been difficult to judge the effect of mucosal immunity because antibody in saliva or feces either is not detected or is present at very low levels.[109, 110]

Not all aspects of the pathogenesis of HAV are understood, but it is clear that after ingestion, the virus replicates briefly in the gut without pathological change and then is transported to the liver possibly through the portal circulation. The liver is the major site of replication and is the source of virus that is shed into the bile and excreted in the feces. Liver cell damage is probably mediated by cytotoxic lymphocytes.

Diagnosis

Because hepatitis A is usually indistinguishable from other forms of acute viral hepatitis on clinical grounds, the diagnosis is usually dependent on the results of liver function tests and the detection of specific antibodies (Fig. 26–2). Biochemical evidence of hepatitis consisting of elevated levels of serum bilirubin and elevations in certain liver enzymes, especially alanine aminotransferase and aspartate aminotransferase, combined with the clinical impression of acute viral hepatitis, although not specific, should lead to serological studies for hepatitis A. Biochemical abnormalities generally persist for 3 weeks or more and are often accompanied by elevation of total serum IgM.[111, 112]

Viral detection assays are generally not useful for the diagnosis of hepatitis A infections. Wild-type HAV is extremely difficult to isolate in cell culture, usually requiring weeks or months. Because the virus shedding peaks before the onset of clinical illness, antigen detection systems usually are insufficiently sensitive to detect HAV in stool samples. Newer technologies such as polymerase chain reaction have been used in certain clinical, epidemiological, or environmental studies and could potentially be used on clinical samples, but the difficulty and expense of performing these tests as well as the ease, accuracy, and sensitivity of the serological tests preclude the necessity of these types of specialized assays.[113–115]

The clinical diagnosis of hepatitis A is commonly confirmed by detection of hepatitis A–specific IgM in a single acute-phase serum sample[116–118] (see Table 26–2). HAV-specific IgM antibodies appear early in the course of the illness, are almost invariably present at the time the patient seeks medical attention, and decline to undetectable levels within 6 months. Their presence in the serum is regarded as evidence of current or recent infection.[119] Other tests that measure the total serum antibody to HAV are not helpful for diagnosis of acute illness based on a single serum sample because patients with distant past exposures maintain IgG class antibody against HAV for their lifetime. The total antibody assays are most often used in epidemiological investigations or in determining whether a person is susceptible to HAV infection before use of immune globulin or vaccination.

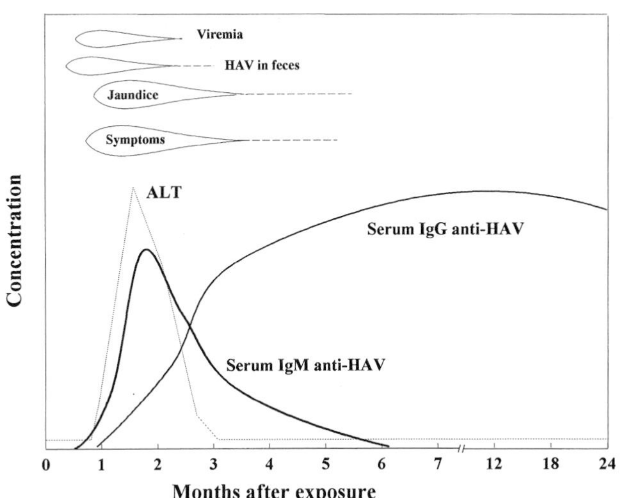

Figure 26–2. The clinical, virological, and serological events after hepatitis A virus (HAV) infection. ALT, alanine aminotransferase.

Treatment

Whereas hepatitis A is preventable by immunization, no specific therapy is available and management is supportive. Bed rest has been the traditional mainstay, although its benefits are difficult to quantitate. Similarly, it is usual to recommend against vigorous exercise and to encourage abstinence from alcohol, although there are few objective data for benefit. Hospital admission is rarely required provided that the patient can be cared for at home.

Hepatitis A is occasionally complicated by cholestasis, which can be treated with a brief course of corticosteroids to shorten the course and reduce symptoms, primarily itching.[27] In the rare occurrence of fulminant hepatitis, the difficult decision of if and when to perform a liver transplantation may be required. Such decisions are always made by teams of physicians with experience in dealing with this problem.[120]

EPIDEMIOLOGY

Prevalence of Infection

Hepatitis A infections occur worldwide, but major geographical differences exist in their prevalence (Fig. 26–3). Like other enteric pathogens, HAV targets primarily children, who then become immune to infection for the remainder of their lives. The analysis of the age-stratified prevalence of antibodies to HAV in a population is an excellent reflection of current and past standards of hygiene and sanitation. Under conditions of overcrowding, especially when there is limited access to clean water and inadequate disposal of human feces, HAV infects most people early in life. These childhood infections are rarely clinically apparent. Where high standards of hygiene and sanitation apply, most children reach adult life without encountering the virus. Currently only 7% of Austrians aged between 18 and 30 years have antibodies to HAV,[121] 12% of U.S. Marines stationed in Okinawa were seropositive, and the prevalence in Scandinavian seamen younger than 40 years was reported to be only 0.3%.[122] Whereas HAV infections are presently uncommon among children and adults in

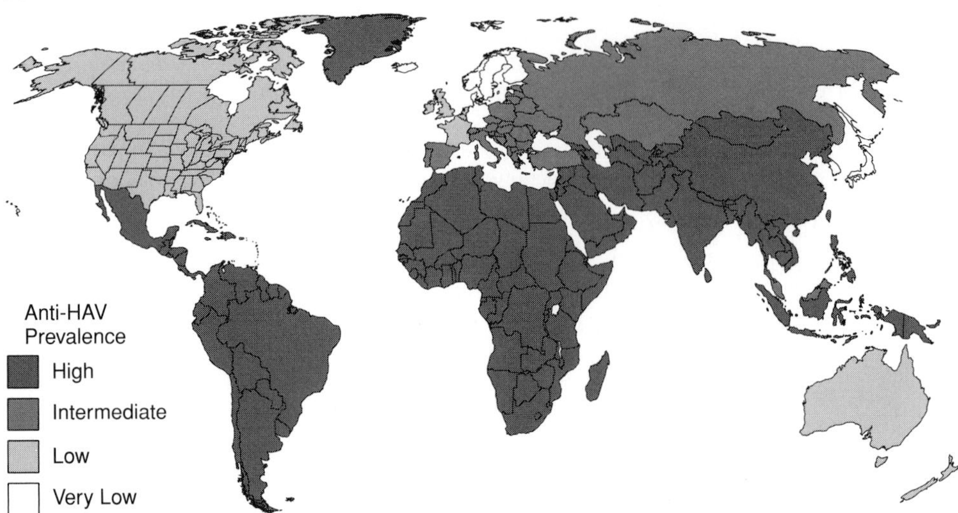

Figure 26–3. World map indicating countries of high, intermediate, low, and very low prevalence of antibody to HAV. Antibody prevalence is an indicator of endemicity of hepatitis A in that particular country (see Table 26–4). (From Centers for Disease Control and Prevention, Atlanta, GA.)

the most developed countries in Scandinavia, parts of western Europe, North America, Japan, Australia, and New Zealand, the majority of people older than 50 years in these countries have detectable levels of anti-HAV, probably reflecting infections acquired in childhood, when living conditions were different.[121] Sequential serological surveys in several developing and rapidly developing countries have demonstrated striking declines in the pattern of infection during just one or two decades.[123] At present in the United States, 26,796 cases of hepatitis A were reported to the Centers for Disease Control and Prevention in 1994, and after accounting for asymptomatic and unreported cases, a total of 134,000 infections were estimated to have occurred.[124]

In areas of high endemicity, infection is nearly universal in childhood but the disease expression in this group is low, resulting in the appearance of a low disease rate (Table 26–4). Seronegative adults in these areas are at high risk of infection and disease, but outbreaks of disease are unusual because of the high prevalence of antibody in the population.[125] High endemicity patterns may also be seen in some ethnic or geographical groups within highly developed countries. For example, the prevalence of anti-HAV was reported to be high among 6- to 10-year-old aboriginal children in the north of Australia (96.6%),[126] in the black population in South Africa,[127] and among recent immigrants from the Asian and Caucasian regions to Israel.[128] In areas of moderate endemicity, the disease rate may be high owing to the delay in the average age at exposure to late childhood and young adults. Food- and water-associated outbreaks are common, although person-to-person spread probably still accounts for most cases.[125] In the United States, for instance, outbreaks accounted for only 4.7% of the reported cases in 1992 (Viral Hepatitis Surveillance Program, Centers for Disease Control and Prevention). Paradoxically, as living standards improve, the incidence of hepatitis A disease may rise because those infections that occur are more frequently associated with jaundice. Brisk epidemics may happen if there is a breakdown in sanitation. The most spectacular outbreak recorded occurred in Shanghai in 1988 when more than 300,000 people, mainly young adults, developed the disease after eating clams harvested from water contaminated with human sewage.[129] In countries of low endemicity, the disease rate also appears low, and although people of all ages are affected, young adults are the most common targets, possibly because of lifestyle. Even in the United States, there are large differences in infection rates in different geographical areas (Fig. 26–4), which reflect local epidemiological conditions.

Some countries have a low incidence of hepatitis A, with most cases occurring in travelers returning from areas of high endemicity. Good sanitation facilities and standards of hygiene in these countries limit the spread of the disease so that outbreaks are also uncommon.

In most developed countries, there is a gradual increase in the prevalence of anti-HAV with increasing age, reflecting the changing childhood infection rates over time. Outbreaks of hepatitis A associated with contaminated food and water continue to be reported throughout the world.[130, 131] Other outbreak situations have been reported in recent years among homosexual men in Australia, Europe, and the United States and among individuals with hemophilia receiving certain batches of factor VIII concentrate.[132, 133] No important gender differences exist in hepatitis A infections except when occupation (e.g., military personnel) or other be-

Table 26–4. **GLOBAL PATTERNS OF HEPATITIS A VIRUS TRANSMISSION**

ENDEMICITY	DISEASE RATE	PEAK AGE AT INFECTION	TRANSMISSION PATTERNS
High	Low to high	Early childhood	Person to person; outbreaks uncommon
Moderate	High	Late childhood/young adults	Person to person; foodborne and waterborne outbreaks
Low	Low	Young adults	Person to person; foodborne and waterborne outbreaks
Very low	Very low	Adults	Travelers; outbreaks uncommon

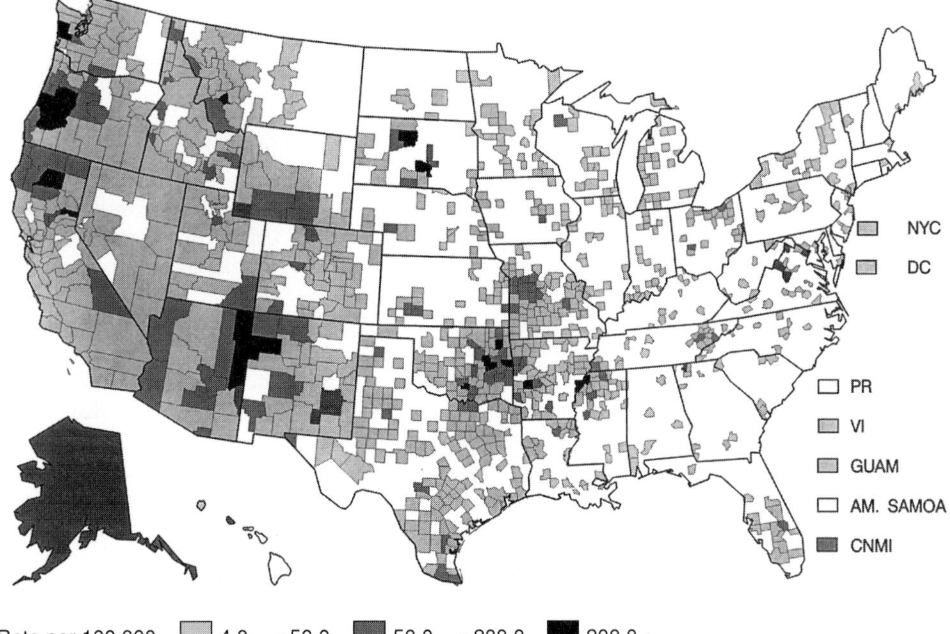

Figure 26–4. Reported cases per 100,000 population in the United States in 1995, by county. (From Centers for Disease Control and Prevention, Atlanta, GA.)

havior (male homosexuality) exposes one gender to a greater risk of infection.

Seasonal Patterns. Seasonal peaks of disease in autumn or early winter have been noted in the past in some temperate countries but are less pronounced in tropical or semitropical countries. Seasonal patterns are no longer observed in the United States or western Europe except as a reflection of travel patterns.

Epidemic Waves. Cyclic patterns of disease prevalence with peaks every 5 to 10 years have been noted in some developed countries with temperate climates. In North America, major waves of disease occurred in 1954, 1961, and the early 1970s (Fig. 26–5); in Australia in 1956 and 1961; in Denmark in the immediate postwar period and again in the mid-1950s; and in the Netherlands in 1954 and 1960. However, declining rates of infection in the last two decades have dampened this periodic wave pattern.[134]

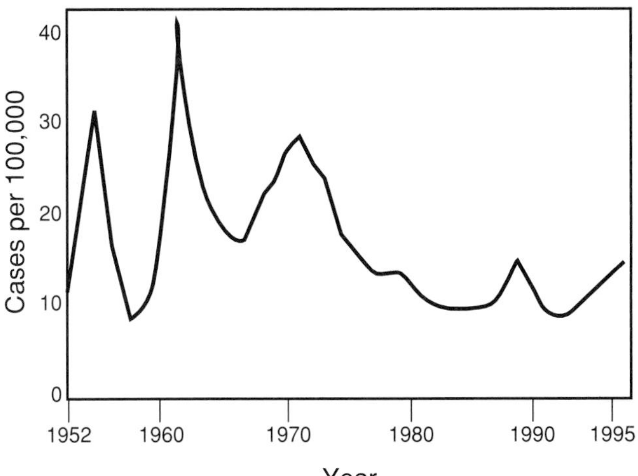

Figure 26–5. Incidence of hepatitis A in the United States between 1952 and 1995. (From Centers for Disease Control and Prevention, National Notifiable Diseases Surveillance System, Atlanta, GA.)

Socioeconomic and Other Factors. In some parts of the world, rural living conditions may be primitive while the urban areas have developed good water supplies and sewage disposal. Inner cities in the United States, on the other hand, may have higher rates than suburban or rural areas for reasons such as crowding and drug abuse rather than sanitation systems.[135]

In developed countries, the risk of becoming infected with HAV is greatest among individuals or groups exposed to poorer conditions of hygiene and sanitation (e.g., some Native American or Australian aboriginal populations and the inner-city poor). Others may be at increased risk because of behavior or occupations. Table 26–5 shows risk factors associated with hepatitis A cases in the United States.[127, 135] Homosexual men who engage in oral-anal contact, intravenous drug users, staff and children of large daycare centers caring for large numbers of children who have not been toilet trained, staff and patients of institutions for the developmentally challenged, and travelers to endemic areas (especially those living under local conditions for extended periods in the developing world) and military personnel posted overseas for prolonged periods all have a demonstrated

Table 26–5. **RISK FACTORS FOR HEPATITIS A IN THE UNITED STATES**

RISK FACTOR	PERCENTAGE OF TOTAL CASES
Personal contact	24.0
Daycare associated	15.1
Foreign travel	5.5
Outbreak associated	4.7
Male homosexual	3.8
Parenteral drug use	2.4
Unknown	44.5

increased risk of hepatitis A. Whereas seroprevalence studies can point out populations at increased risk, the most common risk factors identified by patients with clinical hepatitis are contact with a jaundiced individual, recent travel overseas, and contact with a childcare center. However, about 45% of individuals with sporadic, community-acquired hepatitis A have no known source of infection[134, 135] (see Table 26–5).

Hepatitis A among travelers is an increasingly recognized problem as large numbers of people from low-prevalence countries vacation in regions with high rates of infection.[136–138] Hepatitis A is now the most important vaccine-preventable disease encountered by travelers. It has been estimated that the risk of a susceptible, nonvaccinated traveler acquiring hepatitis A is 100 times greater than for typhoid fever and 1000 times greater than for cholera.[139] In such travelers, hepatitis A has been demonstrated to occur in 3 to 6 susceptible individuals per 1000 per month with sixfold higher rates among backpackers living under completely local conditions. Travelers who acquire hepatitis A during their trip have been a common source of spread to others on their return.[140]

Mode of Transmission

Transmission of HAV depends on how the virus is excreted or in which body fluid it resides. Fecal excretion of HAV is the primary source of virus in person-to-person spread. Infectivity of stools has been demonstrated 14 to 21 days before to 8 days after onset of jaundice.[97] Specimens collected from day 19 after the onset of jaundice have consistently failed to transmit disease.[141] With the use of electron microscopy or radioimmunoassay (RIA), HAV has been detected in the feces commonly for 5 days and occasionally up to 14 days after the onset of jaundice.[142, 143]

Although HAV is present in the blood for a significant period during the incubation period and early acute phase of the disease, blood-transmitted hepatitis A appears to be rare. Volunteer studies conducted in the 1950s and 1960s demonstrated the presence of HAV in blood samples collected as early as 21 days before the onset of jaundice. The chance in a low-incidence country of an individual's donating blood during the viremic phase is low, but the rare incidence of transfusion-associated hepatitis A may also be influenced by the prevalence of antibody in the older age groups that receive most transfusions. Nevertheless, transmission by blood transfusion[144, 145] and transmission by blood derivatives[146, 147] have been reported.

Although HAV may occasionally be detected in saliva, urine, and nasopharyngeal secretions, there is no evidence that any of these fluids is of major epidemiological significance.

Person to Person. The most important means of transmission is undoubtedly from person to person by the fecal-oral route (see Tables 26–4 and 26–5). Transmission is generally limited to close contacts, especially those within families. Young children still have the highest rates of infection and are frequently involved in the spread of infection in households, because infections in this group are often silent and standards of hygiene are generally lower in children than among adults.[135]

Hepatitis A is rarely spread by casual contact, and a study of distribution of cases in school and neighborhood suggested that play contacts are more important than classroom contacts. Contact with feces and personal contact also undoubtedly are important factors in daycare and neonatal care outbreaks.[148–150] Hepatitis A outbreaks have also been reported in neonatal intensive care units.[151, 152] The major features of these outbreaks are a low incidence of clinically apparent disease in the children but a high rate of disease among adult contacts including staff and family members.

Foodborne and Waterborne. Common vehicle epidemics of hepatitis A due to the consumption of contaminated food continue to be reported in the United States but account for less than 5% of reported cases (see Table 26–5). In many countries, an important cause of hepatitis A cases and outbreaks appears to be consumption of raw or partially cooked shellfish (e.g., oysters harvested from waters that have been contaminated with human sewage).[153] Shellfish are particularly likely to transmit hepatitis A because they filter large quantities of water to obtain adequate supplies of food and oxygen and may serve as reservoirs of infection by concentrating virus.[154–156] Shellfish are often eaten raw or after gentle steaming that is sufficient to cause the shell to open but inadequate to inactivate the virus.[157] In an epidemic of hepatitis A in 1988 in Shanghai, the attack rate among individuals eating raw clams was 18% compared with those eating cooked clams, 7%, and those not eating clams, 2%.[158]

Although hepatitis A cases associated with an infected food handler are uncommon, they result in intense public health response.[159, 160] Food may be contaminated during restaurant preparation at the supplier or even at the point of origin, as was the case in a school lunch outbreak caused by contaminated frozen strawberries.[161] Many uncooked foods have been associated with outbreaks, but even cooked foods may transmit hepatitis A if the cooking is inadequate to kill the virus or if the food is contaminated after the cooking. In most outbreaks, transmission of infection can be traced to a food handler who failed to observe hand washing procedures after defecation, but contaminated water that is used for washing or preparation of the food could also be the source.

Waterborne epidemics of hepatitis A have been reported for many years[162, 163] but are uncommon in developed countries and account for less than 1% of all cases seen in the United States. Acquisition of hepatitis A by swimming in a sewage-contaminated water pool has been documented but is rare.[164] Contaminated water can be rendered safe by addition of high levels of chlorine to a total residual of 1 mg per L, and a free chlorine residual of 0.4 ml per L during 30 minutes, or by boiling.

Blood Products. The first recorded outbreak associated with injection of a blood product occurred in 1986 among cancer patients experimentally treated with interleukin-2 and autologous lymphokine-activated killer cells cultured in media containing pooled human serum.[146] Thirty-nine percent of susceptibles developed acute HAV infections. Small outbreaks of hepatitis A have been detected among hemophilia patients receiving prophylactic factor VIII concentrate in Italy, Germany, Belgium, and Ireland.[165] Analysis of the HAV genomic sequences that could be detected in 5 of 12 implicated lots of factor VIII in the Italian outbreak revealed at least three different HAV strains that could be linked to the viruses detected in the recipients, providing strong evidence that the hepatitis A was transmitted by the factor VIII.[114, 166]

Plasma fractionation products treated by solvent/detergent methods have proved free from the risk of transmission of enveloped bloodborne viruses (hepatitis B virus, hepatitis C virus, human immunodeficiency virus), but the process would not be expected to inactivate HAV.[167, 168] Because measures to identify HAV viremic donors are impractical, other methods to inactivate or eliminate HAV from pooled plasma derivatives are under development.[169] It remains difficult to explain why the HAV that may have been in these starting plasma pools was not neutralized by the antibody that must have also been in the pools. Regardless of the effectiveness of viral removal steps, it is recommended that all susceptible chronic recipients of pooled plasma products be immunized against HAV.

Hepatitis A on a worldwide basis is largely an enteric infection of children. The most important aspects of prevention are sanitation rather than medical. Provision of a clean water supply and proper waste management would significantly reduce the rate of HAV infections in most populations. Because these problems are reasonably well solved in the developed world but hepatitis A cases continue to occur, more medically oriented solutions need to be applied, such as vaccination.

PASSIVE IMMUNIZATION

Until recently, immune globulin was the mainstay for prevention of hepatitis A in people who either were likely to be exposed or had recently been exposed. This product has proved useful for prevention of hepatitis A in travelers, Peace Corps volunteers, and military personnel and even for postexposure prophylaxis in common source or family outbreaks. However, immune globulin has never been successful in altering the epidemiology of hepatitis in a high-risk community owing to the transient nature of the protection, low coverage rates, and perhaps lack of herd immunity.

Immune globulin is manufactured from large pools of plasma collected from tens of thousands of donors. Because the prevalence of antibody to HAV in the population has been declining, there is a concern that antibody levels against HAV in immune globulin preparations might drop below effective levels. Whereas in the United States there is no standard for anti-HAV levels in immune globulin preparations even though hepatitis A is the primary use for this product, at this time the anti-HAV levels remain adequate to provide short-term protection.[170] Eventually, consideration may need to be given to the manufacture of immune globulin from selected antibody-positive donors or the development of a hyperimmune globulin for hepatitis A prevention analogous to other agent-specific hyperimmune globulins.[171] With the recent licensure of inactivated hepatitis A vaccines, the use of immune globulin for pre-exposure prophylaxis has been largely eliminated, but immune globulin still has a role in the prevention of hepatitis A after exposure has already occurred, when an exposure is expected before the vaccine would become effective, and in children younger than 2 years for whom the vaccine has not been approved.

The efficacy of immune globulin was first demonstrated in an outbreak at a summer camp in 1944[172] and has been confirmed many times since.[173] Several studies have demonstrated the effectiveness of immune globulin in pre-exposure settings, such as for travelers, military personnel,[174] and Peace Corps workers.[175] The rate of HAV infections among Peace Corps volunteers dropped from 1.6 to 2.1 cases per 100 per year to 0.1 to 0.3 cases per 100 per year after the institution of a mandatory program of immune globulin every 4 months.[175] Active prophylaxis with the recently licensed killed vaccines has largely supplanted the use of immune globulin in this setting. Nevertheless, immune globulin is still recommended for postexposure prophylaxis. If administered within 2 weeks of exposure, immune globulin is effective in eliminating or attenuating the severity of clinical disease while actual infection might still occur. Passive/active immunization often results from the use of immune globulin in the postexposure setting. Immune globulin is useful for limiting the spread of hepatitis in small, defined outbreaks. However, it has not been highly effective in preventing large community-wide persistent epidemics of hepatitis A.[176]

Tables 26–6 and 26–7 outline the recommended use of immune globulin for the prevention of hepatitis A. In general, immune globulin is recommended for postexposure prophylaxis and for those unvaccinated individuals who expect to be in a high-risk situation in less than 2 weeks. Immune globulin is also recommended for pre-exposure prophylaxis for anyone who cannot take the vaccine because of known allergy to one of its components. This category would also include children

Table 26–6. **RECOMMENDATIONS FOR HEPATITIS A PREEXPOSURE IMMUNOPROPHYLAXIS**

AGE (yr)	EXPOSURE DURATION	RECOMMENDED PROPHYLAXIS
<2	Short-term (<3 mo)	IG 0.02 mL/kg
<2	3–5 mo	IG 0.06 mL/kg
<2	>5 mo	IG 0.06 mL/kg repeated every 5 mo
>2	Short- or long-term	HAV vaccine
		HAV vaccine + IG as above if exposure is expected in less than 2 wk
		Substitute IG as above if vaccine is contraindicated or refused

HAV, hepatitis A virus; IG, immune globulin.

Table 26–7. **RECOMMENDATIONS FOR HEPATITIS A POSTEXPOSURE PROPHYLAXIS**

TIME SINCE EXPOSURE	FUTURE EXPOSURE LIKELY	RECOMMENDED PROPHYLAXIS
<2 wk	No	IG 0.02 mL/kg
<2 wk	Yes	IG 0.02 mL/kg + HAV vaccine
>2 wk	No	None
<2 wk	Yes	IG 0.06 mL/kg repeated every 5 mo during exposure (after age 2 yr)
>2 wk	Yes	HAV vaccine

HAV, hepatitis A virus; IG, immune globulin.

younger than 2 years, for whom the vaccine has not yet been approved. Cost analysis studies have also shown that individuals such as travelers who expect to have no more than two short-term exposures to hepatitis A during a 10-year period could be protected by immune globulin at a lower cost than with vaccine. Vaccine becomes more cost-effective for those who expect to travel three or more times in a 10-year period or stay in an endemic area more than 6 months.[177]

Postexposure prophylaxis is recommended for those known to have been exposed less than 2 weeks before immunization. In many postexposure situations, it is often too late for prophylaxis to be effective by the time the index case is discovered. Close personal contacts of those thought to be incubating hepatitis A should be immunized with immune globulin. Casual contacts such as school classmates who have not had physical contact usually do not require immune globulin prophylaxis. The proper use of immune globulin can limit a defined outbreak or a family outbreak of hepatitis A. However, immune globulin has generally not been successful in controlling larger epidemic situations. In these instances, exposure is too broad and the immunity may not last long enough for the virus to be eliminated from the population. Other recommended uses of immune globulin (see Table 26–6) include pre-exposure prophylaxis for children younger than 2 years for whom vaccine has not yet been approved, for individuals who are allergic to the vaccine or components of the vaccine, and in those who expect to be exposed to hepatitis A before the vaccine would become effective in about 2 weeks.

The usual dose of immune globulin is a single intramuscular injection of 0.02 or 0.06 mL per kg. The lower dose is adequate to provide protection for up to 3 months and the higher dose is effective for up to 6 months.[170] Intramuscular preparations of immune globulin should never be given intravenously, and the intravenous preparations of immune globulin are not intended for routine hepatitis A prophylaxis but are used for patients with immune deficiencies and are formulated at a lower globulin concentration.

ACTIVE IMMUNIZATION

Active immunization with hepatitis A vaccines was developed along classic lines similar to the path followed for poliovirus vaccines. As for poliovirus, the initial breakthrough came with the in vitro cultivation of HAV in cell lines suitable for vaccine production.[78] Formalin-inactivated, cell culture–produced whole-virus vaccines have now been approved in much of the world. Live attenuated vaccines based on the CR326 and the HM175 strains have also been tested in primates and to a limited extent in humans, and the H2 strain has been used in extended clinical studies in China.[87, 178–181] Both strains have been evaluated as candidate live vaccines and found to be highly attenuated in humans.[179, 182] For both strains, an inoculum dose of greater than 10^6 tissue culture infective doses was required to induce an antibody response in volunteers. That the vaccines infected volunteers was never proved because the only evidence was seroconversion, which could have been induced by the antigenic mass contained in the inoculum rather than new antigen produced by replication. The entire nucleotide sequences of both the wild type and the vaccine variant of HM175 were determined.[54, 58] A full-length, infectious cDNA clone of the cell culture–adapted virus was made,[183] and the mutations responsible for cell culture adaptation and attenuation were determined by the molecular construction of chimeric viruses.[68, 88, 184] It was found that substitutions and deletions in the 5′ noncoding region and substitutions in the 2B/C coding regions are highly important for cell culture adaptation and attenuation of virulence. However, mutations throughout the genome contributed to improved in vitro replication.[185] It may be difficult to develop a live vaccine that is both adequately immunogenic and attenuated because the properties of replication and pathogenesis may be closely linked.

Vaccine Strains and Producers

Two HAV killed vaccines have been approved for use in the United States and broadly throughout the world. A third vaccine has now been licensed in Europe, and several other similar inactivated vaccines have been developed and registered at least in their country of manufacture.[186, 187] The two broadly licensed products are Havrix (SmithKline Beecham Biologicals) based on strain HM175 and Vaqta (Merck & Co., Inc.) based on strain CR326F. The HM175 strain of HAV was isolated from stool of a patient in a family outbreak in Australia.[188] It was originally adapted to cell culture by a series of 30 passages in primary green monkey kidney cells followed by adaptation to human embryonic lung diploid fibroblasts, MRC-5 cells.[189] The CR326F strain was initially isolated from Costa Rica and was the first strain to be successfully cultivated in vitro.[78] CR326F was initially isolated in a fetal rhesus kidney line, FRhK6. After 15 passages, it was transferred to MRC-5 for an additional 28 passages.[190]

Pasteur Mérieux–Connaught has recently licensed a hepatitis A vaccine in Europe called Avaxim, based on the GBM strain of HAV. This strain was isolated and propagated on primary human kidney cell culture for 10 passages, followed by adaptation to human diploid fibroblast cells during 20 passages.[191–193] Inoculation of chimpanzees showed that the strain had been attenuated by passage.[194] The vaccine is produced in the MRC-5 human diploid fibroblast cell strain. Lysed virus is formalin inactivated (125 μg/mL) and adjuvanted with 0.3 mg of aluminum as the hydroxide.[186]

A vaccine developed at the Swiss Serum Institute uses liposomes as the adjuvant rather than aluminum salts.[187, 195] This vaccine, called Epaxal, is licensed in Switzerland and some other countries. The strain of HAV used in the vaccine is RG-SB, harvested from disrupted MRC-5 cells and inactivated by formalin. The liposome adjuvant is composed of phosphatidylcholine, phosphatidylethanolamine, and hemagglutinin from an H1N1 strain of influenza virus.

Production and Purification

HAV vaccines are produced in similar ways with only details of the manufacturing process differing. Most vaccines are grown in MRC-5 cell culture and harvested by cell lysis. The HAV in Havrix is concentrated and purified by sterile filtration, ultrafiltration, and column chromatography. The virus is then inactivated by 250 μg formaldehyde per mL for 15 days at 37°C. The purified/inactivated virus is adsorbed on aluminum hydroxide (alum) as an adjuvant, and phenoxyethanol at 5 mg per mL is added as a preservative. No antibiotics are present in the vaccine. Havrix is formulated at either 720 or 1440 enzyme-linked immunosorbent assay (ELISA) units per mL (EU/mL) defined by a standard, and each mL contains approximately 0.5 mg of aluminum as aluminum hydroxide.[189]

Vaqta, based on strain CR326F, is grown in MRC-5 cells, extracted by organic solvents, concentrated by precipitation in polyethylene glycol, purified by chromatography, inactivated by 100 μg formaldehyde per mL for 20 days at 37°C, and adsorbed on alum. Vaqta is formulated at 50 units per mL (defined by a standard), contains approximately 0.45 mg per mL of aluminum as aluminum hydroxide, and contains no preservatives or antibiotics.[190]

Formalin inactivation conditions have been set empirically by determining the killing kinetics, extrapolating the curve to the zero intercept where 100% inactivation is theoretically achieved, and exceeding that time by a factor of three. Inactivation is monitored throughout the process, and steps are employed to avoid aggregation of the virus. Because HAV grows slowly in cell culture without cytopathic effect, completeness of inactivation is difficult to prove. Inactivation of these vaccines has been demonstrated by serial blind passages designed to amplify a low level of residual live virus to the point that it would be immunologically detectable. An additional margin of safety is achieved in both Havrix and Vaqta by the use of HAV strains that are highly attenuated in humans. Both vaccines should be stored at 2 to 8°C and can be kept for at least 2 years under those conditions without loss of potency.[189, 196, 197] Freezing destroys the vaccine, causing aggregation of the alum particles. Any vaccine that inadvertently was frozen should be discarded. HAV is a stable virus, and studies are presently under way to determine how long the vaccines retain potency when they are stored without refrigeration.

Dosage and Route

Table 26–8 outlines the recommended dosages and schedules for Havrix, Vaqta, and Avaxim. Havrix has been formulated in two concentrations. The 720 EL per mL is intended as a pediatric vaccine for individuals 2 through 18 years of age to be administered in three 0.5-mL (360 EU) intramuscular injections at time 0, 1 month, and 6 to 12 months. The vaccine formulated at 1440 EU per mL is intended for either pediatric or adult use, with the pediatric dose at 0.5 mL (720 EU) and the adult dose at 1 mL (1440 EU) administered as a single intramuscular injection; a booster 6 to 12 months after the primary dose is recommended for anyone expecting repeated or long-term exposure.[193] Vaqta is formulated at 50 units per mL to be administered as a single dose of 0.5 mL (25 units) for children and adolescents 2 through 17 years of age and 1 mL for adults. A booster dose at 6 months is recommended for long-term protection.[198]

Avaxim is licensed in Europe for individuals older than 15 years. It is administered as a single intramuscular injection of 0.5 mL containing 160 antigen units (defined by a standard) with a booster dose at 6 to 12 months for long-term protection (Avaxim package insert).

Epaxal is given at a dose of 500 RIA units of hepatitis A antigen, associated with 10 μg of influenza hemagglutinin and 300 μg of phospholipids.[199] The recommended schedule is two doses at 0 and 6 to 18 months.

Unfortunately, owing to the different assays used and the lack of an accepted standard, it is not possible to compare the antigen content of the various vaccines. Two doses at least 6 months apart are recommended for all of the vaccines. However, these vaccines are so

Table 26–8. **RECOMMENDED DOSES AND SCHEDULES FOR INACTIVATED HEPATITIS A VIRUS VACCINES**

AGE (yr)	VACCINE	DOSE	VOLUME (mL)	NO. OF DOSES	SCHEDULE
2–18	Havrix	360 EU	0.5	3	0, 1, and 6–12 mo
	Havrix	720 EU	0.5	2	0 and 6–12 mo
	Vaqta	25 units	0.5	2	0 and 6–12 mo
>15	Avaxim	160 antigen units	0.5	2	0 and 6–12 mo
>18	Havrix	1440 EU	1.0	2	0 and 6–12 mo
	Vaqta	50 units	1.0	2	0 and 6–12 mo

EU, enzyme-linked immunosorbent assay (ELISA) units.

immunogenic that shorter schedules will probably work.[200] A study of Avaxim showed that the intramuscular and subcutaneous routes of injection were comparable in immunogenicity.[201]

Hepatitis A particles are concentrated and purified during the manufacture of all of the vaccines. Differences in the content of nonvirion proteins exist between the vaccines, but no correlation between those proteins and reactions has been reported thus far.

Havrix and Avaxim contain polyanethanol as a preservative, whereas Vaqta contains no preservative.

Combined Vaccines

Havrix (720 EU) has been combined with SmithKline Beecham's Engerix hepatitis B vaccine (20 μg) under the trade name Twinrix. This vaccine induces immune responses to both hepatitis A and hepatitis B[202, 203] and is licensed in Europe.

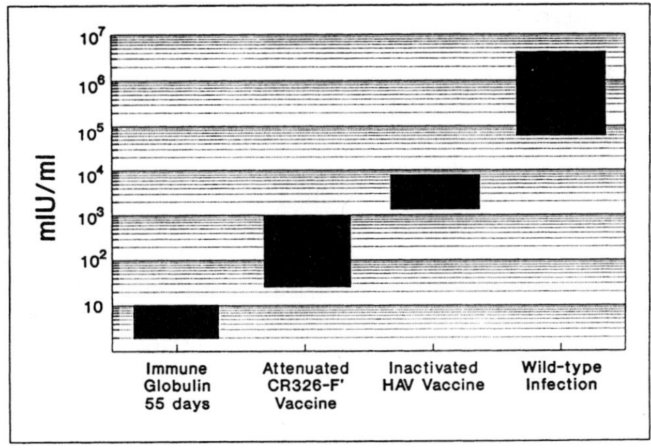

Figure 26–6. Comparative levels of antibody to HAV after administration of immune serum globulin, one dose of an attenuated HAV vaccine, three doses of an inactivated HAV vaccine, and natural infection. The detection limits of the HAVAB assay are approximately 100 mIU per mL. (From Lemon SM. Hepatitis A virus: Current concepts of the molecular virology, immunology and approaches to vaccine development. Rev Med Virol 2:73–87, 1992.)

RESULTS OF VACCINATION

Clinical trials indicate that inactivated hepatitis A vaccines are safe, are highly immunogenic, and provide durable protection against infection expected to last at least 10 years for those receiving the primary vaccine plus the booster.[70, 71, 186, 204] The licensed inactivated hepatitis A vaccines have all been shown to be highly and rapidly immunogenic. They induce seroconversions to protective levels of antibody in as little as 2 weeks after the initial dose.[205, 206] Therefore, travelers, military personnel, or others who had no previous vaccine could be vaccinated as little as 2 weeks before their expected exposure instead of receiving immune globulin.[207] The level of antibody after vaccination varies with the dose and schedule of the vaccine. However, after a single dose of vaccine, antibody titers are higher than titers produced by known protective levels of immune globulin but generally lower than titers measured after natural infection.[123, 205–207]

Seroconversion is defined as a level of antibody equivalent to that induced by immune globulin administration and shown to be protective. This level is defined as 10 to 20 mIU, the titer seen about 2 months after immune globulin administration. Figure 26–6 shows the relationship of titers obtained after immune globulin or after vaccination.

By 4 weeks after the first dose, 95 to 100% of vaccinees are seroconverted. Titers fall subsequently, but a booster injection 6 months after the first dose results in a profound anamnestic response and prolonged seropositivity.

Like hepatitis B vaccine, hepatitis A vaccine is less immunogenic in adults older than 40 years and in the obese, although satisfactory responses are generally obtained after the booster dose.[208]

Immunization of infants younger than 2 years is currently under study. It appears that maternal antibody is inhibitory to antibody response, and further clinical trials are therefore necessary to find the right schedule.[209]

Owing to the interlaboratory variation, no inferences can be drawn as to differences in immunogenicity between vaccines from antibody data obtained in studies of single vaccines.[210–212] One reported comparative study[213] showed a more rapid response to Avaxim than to Havrix, but the significance of this difference with regard to protection is unknown.

In view of the possible application of hepatitis A vaccines to universal vaccination of infants or children (see *Public Health Considerations*), pediatric studies are particularly important. Data obtained with Havrix[214] and Vaqta[215, 216] show excellent immunogenicity in children, who if anything develop higher antibody titers than adults do.

Simultaneous administration of immune globulin with the first dose of Havrix or Avaxim reduced antibody responses by twofold to threefold, an effect that persisted even after booster, although the level of seroconversion remained high in both groups.[217, 218] The reduction of active responses in the presence of passive antibodies is significant with regard to the possibility of immunization of infants. Presumably, infants of mothers immune to hepatitis A will have suppressed antibody formation owing to the presence of transplacental antibodies. Studies are now in progress to evaluate the extent of this suppression.

The quality of the antibody response after vaccination has also been studied. As measured by several different immunoassays, there are distinct differences between the antibody induced by vaccine and the antibody in people who received immune globulin, which should be similar to antibody induced by infection.[219] With similar radioimmunoassay titers (HAVAB), the immune globulin recipients had higher neutralization titers but negligible radioimmunoprecipitation titers compared with the group that was vaccinated. However, it has also been shown that immune globulin prepared from the serum of vaccinees could protect a chimpanzee from HAV challenge when the titer of antibody achieved in the chimpanzee was similar to that found in humans receiving immune globulin prophylaxis.[220]

Efficacy of Protection

All evidence points to the high effectiveness of hepatitis A vaccines. In one study, 1037 healthy seronegative children 2 to 16 years of age in a community experiencing yearly outbreaks of hepatitis A received either a single dose of formalin-inactivated vaccine derived from strain CR326F (Vaqta) or placebo. No cases of hepatitis occurred in the vaccinated group except a few that appeared within 3 weeks of vaccination. These cases represented patients who were already incubating the infection at the time of vaccination. In the placebo group, 34 cases of hepatitis A were observed during the period beginning 3 weeks after vaccination, indicating a 100% vaccine protective efficacy.[204, 221] In a large field trial, inactivated vaccine derived from strain HM175 (Havrix) was evaluated in a study involving more than 40,000 children in Thailand. Under field conditions, the vaccine was found to be at least 80% effective compared with the placebo and was without serious adverse reactions.[70] In a nonrandomized but controlled study in toddlers in a daycare center, Avaxim was completely protective against hepatitis A, which occurred in 5 of 27 control subjects but 0 of 40 vaccinees.[222]

Duration of Immunity

The common recommended schedule of a single dose followed by a booster dose 6 to 12 months later produces high levels of antibody although still below the titers sometimes seen after natural infection.[123, 223–227] On the basis of titers achieved after passive immunization with immune globulin, it appears that only low levels of serum antibody are protective. Antibody data obtained for periods up to 5 years after vaccination for the most part show protective levels.[224–228] After the booster dose, it is estimated from mathematical models that protective levels of antibody will persist for 24 to 47 years.[229] Because the incubation period for hepatitis A is usually 4 weeks and the anamnestic responses observed after the 12-month booster are rapid and robust, it has been suggested that vaccinees who have seroconverted will be protected even if their antibody levels have fallen below protective levels.[71] Long-term follow-up studies will have to be performed to confirm this hypothesis.

Adverse Reactions

Serious adverse reactions clearly associated with hepatitis A vaccines have not been reported. Accumulated experience so far reveals principally nonspecific reactions.[186, 196, 197, 204, 210] Local injection site reactions (pain, tenderness, or erythema) that are mild and transient have been reported in as many as 21% of children and 56% of adults vaccinated. Systemic reactions that include fatigue, fever, diarrhea, and vomiting occur in less than 5% of vaccinees. Headache has been associated with vaccination in up to 16% of adults and 9% of children. Rare adverse events associated with Havrix have been reported in postmarketing surveys including syncope, jaundice, erythema multiforme, convulsions, and others. However, causal relationships have not been established.[195, 196]

A case of leukocytoclastic vasculitis has been described after Havrix vaccination, which resolved without therapy.[230]

Indications

Inactivated hepatitis A vaccine is indicated for anyone 2 years of age or older at increased risk of exposure to hepatitis A who does not have preexisting antibody. It is generally not cost-effective to screen children for anti-HAV before vaccination unless they spent part of their childhood in a high-endemicity area or have a history of exposure. Depending on the local epidemiological situation, prescreening of adults who would be predicted to have greater than a 50% chance of being anti-HAV positive should be considered if time permits. Vaccination of people with preexisting antibody has not been shown to carry any risk. Those considered for pre-exposure prophylaxis include travelers to countries where HAV is endemic, military personnel, certain ethnic or geographical populations that have high rates of hepatitis C virus, homosexual or bisexual men, intravenous drug users, those routinely receiving plasma fractionation products such as factor VIII, and those engaged in high-risk employment such as primate handlers or laboratory personnel who work with HAV. In addition, vaccine may be considered for certain individuals who, although not at higher risk of infection, carry special risks if infected.

Travelers. The risk of hepatitis A among Europeans traveling to Africa, Asia, or South America was 3 per 1000 per month of stay and 20 per 1000 per month for those living under local conditions.[139] Between 1985 and 1990, the number of travel-related cases of hepatitis A in Sweden remained constant at about 140 per year. However, as a proportion of the total cases in Sweden, travel-related cases rose during that period from about 20% to about 55%, and travel became the largest single cause of hepatitis A.[231] Among seronegative American missionaries to sub-Saharan Africa in the prevaccine era, 28% were infected by HAV within 2 years and more than 90% were seropositive after 20 years of service.[232] As of 1992, before the vaccine was licensed, foreign travel accounted for 5.5% of U.S. cases.[233] Protection rates among vaccinated travelers are estimated to exceed 97%.[234]

Military Personnel. Hepatitis A has caused morbidity and affected outcome in wars throughout recorded history. Military personnel deployed in high-risk areas are at special risk because of their field living conditions. The long-term protection afforded by vaccine over immune globulin is a considerable advantage for the armed services, in which the logistics of administration every few months limited the utility of immune globulin.[207]

High-Risk Ethnic or Geographical Populations. Many Native American and Alaskan people have experienced cyclic epidemics of hepatitis A and have a continuing endemic problem. It has been recommended that vaccine programs be established to prevent HAV infections in these groups and to break the cycles of epidemics. The vaccines have been shown to perform well in these high-risk Native American populations.[176, 235, 236]

Tradition-observant Jews also have a high incidence of hepatitis A, and indeed the efficacy study of Vaqta was carried out in that population.[204]

Male Homosexuals. Surveillance data show that male homosexuals account for 3.8% of reported hepatitis A cases in the United States,[233] perhaps because of multiple partners or sexual practices. Vaccination of this group should reduce the rate quickly and could possibly have a herd immunity effect in the homosexual community.

Intravenous Drug Users. Drug users also have a high rate of HAV infections possibly related to sharing needles with an individual who is viremic or to lifestyle factors. Vaccine is indicated for this group, although drug users are notoriously hard to reach for immunizations.

Regular Recipients of Blood or Plasma-Derived Products. The risk of hepatitis A from a blood transfusion or from plasma derivatives is extremely small, but both have been reported.[144, 147] Individuals who receive these products regularly should be immunized against virtually any vaccine-preventable disease. For example, many recipients of factor VIII have been infected by hepatitis C virus or hepatitis B virus, and there is no reason for them to run the risk of another assault to their liver. Presently, these products are treated by a viral inactivation process often based on solvents or heat, but HAV is resistant to organic solvents and is relatively resistant to heat. The cases of hepatitis A associated with factor VIII have caused the manufacturers to begin development of new methods that would eliminate infectious HAV from their products. Nevertheless, vaccination of recipients is prudent.

Chronic Hepatitis C. Individuals chronically infected with hepatitis C have a 40% risk of developing fulminant disease if infected with hepatitis A.[237] Therefore, they should be vaccinated against hepatitis A.[238]

High-risk Employment. Several occupations carry at least a potential for HAV exposure, including employees of institutions for developmentally challenged individuals and staff of daycare centers, especially those who care for children before bowel training. These institutions have been the nidus of outbreaks during recent years. However, it is difficult to show that individual staff members are at higher risk, because these outbreaks remain generally uncommon compared with the total number of such centers. Some studies have shown that sewer workers have a higher rate of HAV infections than the general population, which seems reasonable, but these findings have not been confirmed in every study.[239] Healthcare personnel have not been shown to be at increased risk, and most hepatitis A cases are not admitted to the hospital. If there is a particular problem in a community, it may be prudent to vaccinate healthcare personnel who are expected to be in contact with those infected.

Individuals Who Do Not Have Increased Risk but Should Consider Vaccination. People with chronic liver disease of any etiology should consider vaccination. Whereas the risk for any individual is low, HAV infection superimposed on chronic liver disease can be serious and may result in death. Food handlers are another special category in whom the risk of infection may be no higher than in the general population, but if they become infected, they have the potential to pass the disease to a large number of people. Many food establishments in communities with high rates of hepatitis A have opted to vaccinate their employees because a case of hepatitis A traced back to their establishment can destroy the business. Primate handlers have often been associated with outbreaks of hepatitis A and should be considered for vaccination.

Community Outbreaks. Persistent outbreaks occur from time to time in counties and states. Sporadic vaccination may not control these epidemics, and some experts recommend routine vaccination of preschool children, perhaps as an entry requirement to daycare or to school as a way of controlling the outbreak.

Contraindications and Precautions

The presently licensed inactivated hepatitis A vaccines are not approved for use in children younger than 2 years. The only other contraindication to inactivated hepatitis A vaccines is allergy or hypersensitivity to the vaccine or any of its components.

Simultaneous Vaccination with Other Vaccines

Administration of inactivated hepatitis A vaccine concomitantly with immune globulin to produce both immediate and long-term immunity has been studied several times. The rate of seroconversion in these instances has not been reduced by coadministration of immune globulin. However, the antibody titers elicited were lower than when vaccine alone was given. Because the titers induced by the vaccine far exceed that needed for protection, these reductions are not considered clinically significant.[218, 240, 241] Because hepatitis A vaccine is indicated for travelers to high-incidence countries, the use of HAV vaccine with other common traveler vaccines has been studied. There was no effect on either the immunogenicity or reactogenicity of hepatitis A vaccine administered concurrently with hepatitis B, yellow fever, or typhoid vaccines.[242–244]

Future Vaccines

The ideal HAV vaccine would be cheap and easy to produce, provide lifelong immunity, be orally administered, and have a safety profile enabling universal childhood immunization. Live vaccines have potential to be cheaper because the dose may be much lower, and they should induce long-term immunity after oral administration. However, safety issues of live vaccines may be difficult to overcome. Live attenuated vaccines have been tested in humans and were shown to be safe when given orally or parenterally. Unfortunately, the vaccines studied to date replicate poorly in humans and therefore do not induce a satisfactory immune response.[179, 180] In China, Mao and colleagues[87, 181] have developed a cold-adapted, live attenuated vaccine and reported that this strain is both effective and free of serious adverse reactions. Further studies on this vaccine may show it to be a useful alternative to the inactivated vaccine.

Cohen and colleagues[183] have assembled a full-length infectious cDNA and transcribed from the cDNA a full-length RNA that on transfection into permissive cells results in complete HAV replication. This achievement allows the development of a specifically "engineered" virus that might have the desired growth and attenuation features of an ideal vaccine. Many of the mutations responsible for cell culture adaptation and attenuation have now been identified, although to date the goal of a virus with the ideal characteristics of in vitro growth combined with attenuation and immunogenicity in humans has not been achieved.[68, 88, 184]

The important neutralizing epitopes of HAV appear to be conformational, and immunization with synthetic peptides or expressed capsid proteins has not induced an effective neutralizing antibody response.[245] Stapleton[246–248] has taken the approach of expressing the entire open reading frame of the HAV genome in recombinant vaccinia virus or baculovirus expression systems. Complete or partial capsid assembly seems to occur in cells infected with this recombinant vaccinia, and antibodies raised to these purified HAV synthetic capsids are neutralizing in vitro and protective in animals. Although the immunizing effect of such a vaccine might not be greater than that of inactivated vaccines, the reduced production costs would solve a significant problem.

PUBLIC HEALTH CONSIDERATIONS

Control of community outbreaks of hepatitis A may be one of the most important uses for the vaccine and provides the clearest evidence of its effectiveness. A vaccine program was initiated in schoolchildren in two adjoining villages of 5000 total inhabitants in Slovakia that were experiencing a community-wide outbreak of hepatitis A. There were 8 cases of hepatitis among the 157 susceptible children (5.1%) who were not vaccinated and 1 case among the 404 children (0.25%) who received at least one dose of vaccine. Soon after the vaccine program was initiated in the students, there were no new cases reported in the general population of the villages.[249]

Large outbreaks of hepatitis A have been reported in rural Alaska every 8 to 12 years since the 1960s. McMahon and colleagues[176] have studied these outbreaks and tried to control them in the past with immune globulin. Whereas massive immunization campaigns using immune globulin were able to temporarily reduce the number of cases reported, there was never a lasting effect and the epidemics always recurred and spread. In August 1992, an outbreak of hepatitis A began in the Tok/Glennallen area termed region 1 and another outbreak began in the Kotzebue area (region 2) and began to spread to adjoining areas (region 3). During the next 12 months, despite the liberal administration of immune globulin to household contacts, 529 clinical cases were reported from these regions with a population of 22,629. After a serological survey of a population sample from an affected village in region 1 and analysis of previously collected sera from regions 2 and 3, vaccine was offered to all people 40 years of age and younger and to all seronegative people older than 40 years residing in region 1. In the other regions, all individuals younger than 20 years and all seronegatives between 20 and 34 years of age were offered vaccine. The seroprevalence rate was so high in people older than 34 years that vaccine was not offered to that group. Vaccination began in April 1993 and consisted of a single dose of Havrix, 720 EU for those younger than 20 years and 1440 EU for those 20 years and older. The overall seroconversion rate was about 90%. Region 2 was the most thoroughly analyzed. Of 2826 people eligible, 1829 were vaccinated. The hepatitis A infection rate within 60 weeks of the initiation of the vaccine program was 2.1% in the vaccinees in region 2, 12% in nonvaccinated eligibles, and 0.1% in nonvaccinated ineligibles. Most of the cases among the vaccinees occurred soon after the vaccination. The vaccine program did not completely eliminate hepatitis A in the city of Kotzebue, where only about 50% of the eligibles were vaccinated. However, in the outlying villages where vaccine coverage was about 80% of the eligible, hepatitis was virtually eliminated within 8 weeks of the initiation of the vaccination program.[176]

Disease Control Strategies. Experience gained from vaccination programs intended to interdict ongoing broad-based outbreaks of hepatitis A among some groups of Native Americans, communities of observant Jews living in New York, and other urban areas indicates that these vaccine programs especially targeted at children can dramatically control the outbreaks.[176, 236, 250]

For example, after several outbreaks had occurred in a Jewish religious community in Brooklyn, New York, a program of routine vaccination of children (who had the highest attack rate) was put in place. Subsequently, no case of hepatitis A was observed in vaccinated children, although sporadic cases persisted in the nonvaccinated.[251]

The Advisory Committee for Immunization Practices has recommended that in communities experiencing high rates of hepatitis A, routine vaccination of children begin at age 2 years with an accelerated vaccination program for older unvaccinated children until the vaccine coverage among children exceeds 70% (Table 26–9). In communities with an intermediate rate of hepatitis A, it is recommended that local surveillance and epidemiological data determine the best vaccine strategy. Because these communities are often in large metropolitan areas, the most feasible and cost-effective strategy may

Table 26–9. **FEATURES OF COMMUNITIES THAT HAVE HIGH AND INTERMEDIATE RATES OF HEPATITIS A**

	HIGH-RATE COMMUNITY	INTERMEDIATE-RATE COMMUNITY
Anti-HAV prevalence	<5 yr = 30–40% >15 yr = 70–100%	<5 yr = 10–25% >15 yr = <50%
Age of most patients	5–14 yr	5–20 yr
Reported annual incidence	700–1000/100,000	50–200/100,000
Outbreak periodicity	5–10 yr	May be periodic
Populations	Well-defined geographically or ethnically	Less well defined than high-rate communities
Examples	Alaskan native villages Native American reservations	Zanesville, OH St. Louis, MO Selected religious communities

be to target certain areas or groups that have the highest rates of disease.[250] If such a strategy is contemplated, the sensitivities of the local communities must be considered if such a program is to be accepted. Targeting risk groups such as daycare centers and male homosexuals in these communities may also be beneficial if surveillance data indicate that any one of these groups could be a substantial source of infection.

Previous and ongoing epidemiological studies have identified certain risk groups in developed countries that might benefit from HAV vaccine. Vaccine programs that target these risk groups will undoubtedly benefit individuals in these groups, but such programs are not likely to significantly affect the overall disease rates. Some groups will require vaccination even if cost-benefit analyses are not favorable. For instance, the military clearly sees an importance for use of this vaccine in certain troops although a strict cost analysis might not be favorable.[207, 252] People who are in the high-risk groups mentioned before could individually benefit from vaccination, and cost-effectiveness analyses may be favorable.[177, 253] From a public health point of view, a strategy based only on vaccination of risk groups is unlikely to be useful for controlling hepatitis A in the broad population.[233] Although the aggressive use of vaccine in high-rate and intermediate-rate communities might alter the rates of disease in the country as a whole, if the goal is to substantially reduce the national incidence of hepatitis A, the only strategy that is likely to work would be to include the vaccine in the routine childhood vaccination schedule.[254] Universal immunization of infants should result in a largely immune childhood population in which the HAV would circulate with difficulty, resulting in protection of adults by herd immunity. This strategy will probably have to await the development of combination vaccines including hepatitis A and additional studies of safety and immunogenicity in infants with and without maternal antibodies leading to licensure of HAV vaccine for children younger than 2 years.

At present, there are no plans to begin vaccination programs in developing countries where infection in early childhood is nearly universal but disease is uncommon. As standards of living improve in these areas, greater problems with hepatitis A often arise. Whereas vaccine strategies in parts of these countries such as urban areas that have good water and sanitation facilities could be devised, the cost of such a program today may not make it a high priority compared with other major health problems encountered by those populations. If vaccine could be locally produced at a low cost, some emerging countries in which a significant nonimmune older child and adult population has developed may find it useful to include hepatitis A in their vaccination programs. The duration of immunity to killed vaccines is of some concern and will take some time to evaluate but has been estimated to be at least 10 years and may in fact produce lifelong protection from disease.[71] If children were vaccinated and the duration of immunity were limited to one or two decades, after which natural hepatitis A infection could occur, danger would exist of trading asymptomatic childhood infections leading to permanent immunity for serious clinical disease and possibly epidemics among adults. If long-lasting immunization requires periodic booster inoculations, a killed vaccine would have little practical use in many developing countries. However, if a live attenuated vaccine such as the one being tested in China proves to be highly successful, it could be used in developing and emerging countries.[87]

Finally, hepatitis A will undoubtedly be discussed as a target for eradication. Many problems of epidemiology, virology, and costs would need to be solved before such an undertaking is contemplated. At present, the disease can best be controlled by improving living conditions and wise application of the existing vaccines.

REFERENCES

1. Hirsh A. Handbook of Geographic and Historical Pathology. London, New Sydenham Society, 1886.
2. Bachman L. Infectious hepatitis in Europe. In Rodenwalt E (ed). World Atlas of Epidemic Diseases. Hamburg, Falk-Verlag, 1952.
3. Virchow R. Über das Vorkommen und den Nachweis des Hepatogenen, insbesondere des katarrhalischen Icterus. Virchows Arch Pathol Anat 32:117, 1865.
4. Cockayne EA. Catarrhal jaundice, sporadic and epidemic, and its relation to acute yellow atrophy of the liver. Q J Med 6:1–29, 1912.
5. McDonald S. Acute yellow atrophy of the liver. Edinburgh Med J 1:83, 1908.
6. Paul JR, Gardner HT. Viral hepatitis. In Coates JB, Hoff EC, Hoff PM (eds). Preventive Medicine in World War II. Vol. 4. Washington, DC, US Government Printing Office, 1960.
7. Spooner ETC. The 1942 epidemic of infective hepatitis in the Middle East. Proc R Soc Med 37:171, 1944.
8. MacCallum FO. Early studies on viral hepatitis. Br Med Bull 28:105–108, 1972.
9. MacCallum FO, Bradley WH. Transmission of infective hepatitis to human volunteers. Lancet 2:228, 1944.

10. Neefe JR, Gellis SS, Stokes J Jr. Homologous serum hepatitis and infectious (epidemic) hepatitis; studies in volunteers bearing on immunological and other characteristics of the etiological agents. Am J Med 1:9, 1946.
11. Havens WP Jr. Elimination in human feces of infectious hepatitis virus parenterally introduced. Proc Soc Exp Biol Med 59:148, 1945.
12. Havens WP Jr. Immunity in experimentally induced infectious hepatitis. J Exp Med 84:403, 1946.
13. Neefe JR, Stokes J Jr, Gellis SS. Homologous serum hepatitis and infectious (epidemic) hepatitis: Experimental study of immunity and cross immunity in volunteers; preliminary report. Am J Med Sci 210:561–575, 1945.
14. Havens WP Jr, Paul JR. Prevention of infectious hepatitis with gamma globulin. JAMA 129:270–272, 1997.
15. Gellis SS, Stokes J Jr, Brother GM, et al. The use of immune globulin (gamma globulin) in infectious (epidemic) hepatitis in the Mediterranean theatre of operations. JAMA 128:1062, 1945.
16. Neefe JR, Stokes J Jr, Baty JB, et al. Disinfection of water containing the causative agent of infectious (epidemic) hepatitis. JAMA 128:1076, 1945.
17. Ward R, Krugman S, Giles JP, et al. Infectious hepatitis: Studies of its natural history and prevention. N Engl J Med 258:407, 1958.
18. Melnick JL, Boggs JD. Human volunteer and tissue culture studies of viral hepatitis. Can Med Assoc J 106:461–467, 1972.
19. Feinstone SM, Kapikian AZ, Purcell RH. Hepatitis A: Detection by immune electron microscopy of a viruslike antigen associated with acute illness. Science 182:1026–1028, 1973.
20. Yao G. Clinical spectrum and natural history of viral hepatitis A in a 1988 Shanghai epidemic. In Hollinger FB, Lemon SM, Margolis HS (eds). Viral Hepatitis and Liver Disease. Baltimore, Williams & Wilkins, 1991, pp 76–78.
21. Krugman S, Giles JP, Hammond J. Infectious hepatitis: Evidence for two distinctive clinical, epidemiological and immunological types of infection. JAMA 200:365–373, 1967.
22. Skinhoj P, Gluud C, Ramsoe K. Traveller's hepatitis. Origin and characteristics of cases in Copenhagen 1976–1978. Scand J Infect Dis 13:1–4, 1981.
23. Tong MJ, el-Farra NS, Grew MI. Clinical manifestations of hepatitis A: Recent experience in a community teaching hospital. J Infect Dis 171(suppl 1):S15–S18, 1995.
24. Koff RS. Clinical manifestations and diagnosis of hepatitis A virus infection. Vaccine 10(suppl 1):S15–S17, 1992.
25. Sjogren MH, Tanno H, Fay O, et al. Hepatitis A virus in stool during clinical relapse. Ann Intern Med 106:221–226, 1987.
26. Gordon SC, Reddy KR, Schiff L, et al. Prolonged intrahepatic cholestasis secondary to acute hepatitis A. Ann Intern Med 101:635–637, 1984.
27. Schiff ER. Atypical clinical manifestations of hepatitis A. Vaccine 10(suppl 1):S18–S20, 1992.
28. McNeil M, Hoy JF, Richards MJ, et al. Aetiology of fatal viral hepatitis in Melbourne. A retrospective study. Med J Aust 141:637–640, 1984.
29. Franki RIB, Fauquet CM, Knudson DL, et al. Classification and nomenclature of viruses: The Fifth Report of the International Committee on the Taxonomy of Viruses. Arch Virol Suppl 2, 1993.
30. Melnick JL. Classification of hepatitis A virus as enterovirus type 72 and of hepatitis B virus as hepadnavirus type 1. Intervirology 18:105–106, 1982.
31. Gust ID, Coulepis AG, Feinstone SM, et al. Taxonomic classification of hepatitis A virus. Intervirology 20:1–7, 1983.
32. Ticehurst JR. Hepatitis A virus: Clones, cultures, and vaccines. Semin Liver Dis 6:46–55, 1986.
33. Cohen JI. Hepatitis A virus: Insights from molecular biology. Hepatology 9:889–895, 1989.
34. Melnick JL. Properties and classification of hepatitis A virus. Vaccine 10(suppl 1):S24–S26, 1992.
35. Lemon SM, Jansen RW, Brown EA. Genetic, antigenic and biological differences between strains of hepatitis A virus. Vaccine 10(suppl 1):S40–S44, 1992.
36. Robertson BH, Jansen RW, Khanna B, et al. Genetic relatedness of hepatitis A virus strains recovered from different geographical regions. J Gen Virol 73:1365–1377, 1992.
37. Weitz M, Siegl G. Variation among hepatitis A virus strains. I. Genomic variation detected by T1 oligonucleotide mapping. Virus Res 4:53–67, 1985.
38. Siegl G, de Chastonay J, Kronauer G. Propagation and assay of hepatitis A virus in vitro. J Virol Methods 9:53–67, 1984.
39. Bradley DW, Schable CA, McCaustland KA, et al. Hepatitis A virus: Growth characteristics of in vivo and in vitro propagated wild and attenuated virus strains. J Med Virol 14:373–386, 1984.
40. Lemon SM, Binn LN. Antigenic relatedness of two strains of hepatitis A virus determined by cross-neutralization. Infect Immun 42:418–420, 1983.
41. Lemon SM, Chao SF, Jansen RW, et al. Genomic heterogeneity among human and nonhuman strains of hepatitis A virus. J Virol 61:735–742, 1987.
42. Stapleton JT, Jansen R, Lemon SM. Neutralizing antibody to hepatitis A virus in immune serum globulin and in the sera of human recipients of immune serum globulin. Gastroenterology 89:637–642, 1985.
43. Siegl G, Frosner GG. Characterization and classification of virus particles associated with hepatitis A. I. Size, density, and sedimentation. J Virol 26:40–47, 1978.
44. Siegl G, Frosner GG, Gauss-Muller V, et al. The physicochemical properties of infectious hepatitis A virions. J Gen Virol 57:331–341, 1981.
45. Bradley DW, Fields HA, McCaustland KA, et al. Biochemical and biophysical characterization of light and heavy density hepatitis A virus particles: Evidence HAV is an RNA virus. J Med Virol 2:175–187, 1978.
46. Siegl G, Weitz M, Kronauer G. Stability of hepatitis A virus. Intervirology 22:218–226, 1984.
47. Lemon SM, Jansen RW, Newbold JE. Infectious hepatitis A virus particles produced in cell culture consist of three distinct types with different buoyant densities in CsCl. J Virol 54:78–85, 1985.
48. Nissen E, Konig P, Feinstone SM, et al. Inactivation of hepatitis A and other enteroviruses during heat treatment (pasteurization). Biologicals 24:339–341, 1996.
49. Murphy P, Nowak T, Lemon SM, et al. Inactivation of hepatitis A virus by heat treatment in aqueous solution. J Med Virol 41:61–64, 1993.
50. Parry JV, Mortimer PP. The heat sensitivity of hepatitis A virus determined by a simple tissue culture method. J Med Virol 14:277–283, 1984.
51. Sobsey MD. Survival and persistence of hepatitis A virus in environmental samples. In Zuckerman AJ (ed). Viral Hepatitis and Liver Disease. New York, Alan R Liss, 1988, pp 121–124.
52. Peterson DA, Hurley TR, Hoff JC, et al. Effect of chlorine treatment on infectivity of hepatitis A virus. Appl Environ Microbiol 45:223–227, 1983.
53. Ticehurst JR, Racaniello VR, Baroudy BM, et al. Molecular cloning and characterization of hepatitis A virus cDNA. Proc Natl Acad Sci USA 80:5885–5889, 1983.
54. Cohen JI, Ticehurst JR, Purcell RH, et al. Complete nucleotide sequence of wild-type hepatitis A virus: Comparison with different strains of hepatitis A virus and other picornaviruses. J Virol 61:50–59, 1987.
55. Weitz M, Baroudy BM, Maloy WL, et al. Detection of a genome-linked protein (VPg) of hepatitis A virus and its comparison with other picornaviral VPgs. J Virol 60:124–130, 1986.
56. Brown EA, Zajac AJ, Lemon SM. In vitro characterization of an internal ribosomal entry site (IRES) present within the 5′ nontranslated region of hepatitis A virus RNA: Comparison with the IRES of encephalomyocarditis virus. J Virol 68:1066–1074, 1994.
57. Glass MJ, Jia XY, Summers DF. Identification of the hepatitis A virus internal ribosome entry site: In vivo and in vitro analysis of bicistronic RNAs containing the HAV 5′ noncoding region. Virology 193:842–852, 1993.
58. Cohen JI, Rosenblum B, Ticehurst JR, et al. Complete nucleotide sequence of an attenuated hepatitis A virus: Comparison with wild-type virus. Proc Natl Acad Sci USA 84:2497–2501, 1987.
59. Summers DF, Ehrenfeld E. Host antibody response to viral structural and nonstructural proteins after hepatitis A virus infection. J Infect Dis 165:273–280, 1992.
60. Schultheiss T, Kusov YY, Gauss-Muller V. Proteinase 3C of hepatitis A virus (HAV) cleaves the HAV polyprotein P2–P3 at all sites including VP1/2A and 2A/2B. Virology 198:275–281, 1994.

61. Schultheiss T, Sommergruber W, Kusov Y, et al. Cleavage specificity of purified recombinant hepatitis A virus 3C proteinase on natural substrates. J Virol 69:1727–1733, 1995.
62. Jia XY, Summers DF, Ehrenfeld E. Primary cleavage of the HAV capsid protein precursor in the middle of the proposed 2A coding region. Virology 193:515–519, 1993.
63. Siegl G. Replication of hepatitis A virus and processing of proteins. Vaccine 10(suppl 1):S32–S35, 1992.
64. Kusov YY, Kazachkov YA, Dzagurov GK, et al. Identification of precursors of structural proteins VP1 and VP2 of hepatitis A virus. J Med Virol 37:220–227, 1992.
65. Tesar M, Jia XY, Summers DF, et al. Analysis of a potential myristoylation site in hepatitis A virus capsid protein VP4. Virology 194:616–626, 1993.
66. Harmon SA, Emerson SU, Huang YK, et al. Hepatitis A viruses with deletions in the 2A gene are infectious in cultured cells and marmosets. J Virol 69:5576–5581, 1995.
67. Nigro G, Taliani G, Bartmann U, et al. Hepatitis in children with thalassemia major. Arch Virol Suppl 4:265–267, 1992.
68. Funkhouser AW, Purcell RH, D'Hondt E, et al. Attenuated hepatitis A virus: Genetic determinants of adaptation to growth in MRC-5 cells. J Virol 68:148–157, 1994.
69. Jia XY, Ehrenfeld E, Summers DF. Proteolytic activity of hepatitis A virus 3C protein. J Virol 65:2595–2600, 1991.
70. Innis BL, Snitbhan R, Kunasol P, et al. Protection against hepatitis A by an inactivated vaccine [see comments]. JAMA 271:1328–1334, 1994.
71. Nalin DR, Kuter BJ, Brown L, et al. Worldwide experience with the CR326F-derived inactivated hepatitis A virus vaccine in pediatric and adult populations: An overview. J Hepatol 18(suppl 2):S51–S55, 1993.
72. Brown EA, Jansen RW, Lemon SM. Characterization of a simian hepatitis A virus (HAV): Antigenic and genetic comparison with human HAV. J Virol 63:4932–4937, 1989.
73. Stapleton JT, Lemon SM. Neutralization escape mutants define a dominant immunogenic neutralization site on hepatitis A virus. J Virol 61:491–498, 1987.
74. Kaplan G, Totsuka A, Thompson P, et al. Identification of a surface glycoprotein on African green monkey kidney cells as a receptor for hepatitis A virus. EMBO J 15:4282–4296, 1996.
75. Asher LV, Binn LN, Marchwicki RH. Demonstration of hepatitis A virus in cell culture by electron microscopy with immunoperoxidase staining. J Virol Methods 15:323–328, 1987.
76. Shimizu YK, Mathiesen LR, Lorenz D, et al. Localization of hepatitis A antigen in liver tissue by peroxidase-conjugated antibody method: Light and electron microscopic studies. J Immunol 121:1671–1679, 1978.
77. Shimizu YK, Shikata T, Beninger PR, et al. Detection of hepatitis A antigen in human liver. Infect Immun 36:320–324, 1982.
78. Provost PJ, Hilleman MR. Propagation of human hepatitis A virus in cell culture in vitro. Proc Soc Exp Biol Med 160:213–221, 1979.
79. Daemer RJ, Feinstone SM, Gust ID, et al. Propagation of human hepatitis A virus in African green monkey kidney cell culture: Primary isolation and serial passage. Infect Immun 32:388–393, 1981.
80. Frosner GG, Deinhardt F, Scheid R, et al. Propagation of human hepatitis A virus in a hepatoma cell line. Infection 7:303–305, 1979.
81. Dotzauer A, Feinstone SM, Kaplan G. Susceptibility of nonprimate cell lines to hepatitis A virus infection [published erratum appears in J Virol 68:6829, 1994]. J Virol 68:6064–6068, 1994.
82. Anderson DA, Locarnini SA, Coulepis AG, et al. Restrictive events in the replication of hepatitis A virus in vitro. Intervirology 24:26–32, 1985.
83. Cromeans T, Fields HA, Sobsey MD. Replication kinetics and cytopathic effect of hepatitis A virus. J Gen Virol 70:2051–2062, 1989.
84. Cromeans T, Sobsey MD, Fields HA. Development of a plaque assay for a cytopathic, rapidly replicating isolate of hepatitis A virus. J Med Virol 22:45–56, 1987.
85. Provost PJ, Bishop RP, Gerety RJ, et al. New findings in live, attenuated hepatitis A vaccine development. J Med Virol 20:165–175, 1986.
86. Talukder MA, Waller DK, Nixon P, et al. Prevalence of antibody to hepatitis A virus in a Saudi Arabian hospital population [letter]. J Infect Dis 148:1167, 1983.
87. Mao JS. Development of live, attenuated hepatitis A vaccine (H2-strain). Vaccine 8:523–524, 1990.
88. Cohen JI, Rosenblum B, Feinstone SM, et al. Attenuation and cell culture adaptation of hepatitis A virus (HAV): A genetic analysis with HAV cDNA. J Virol 63:5364–5370, 1989.
89. Balayan MS. Natural hosts of hepatitis A virus. Vaccine 10(suppl 1):S27–S31, 1992.
90. Rakela J, Mosley JW. Fecal excretion of hepatitis A virus in humans. J Infect Dis 135:933–938, 1977.
91. Maynard JE, Lorenz D, Bradley DW, et al. Review of infectivity studies in nonhuman primates with virus-like particles associated with MS-1 hepatitis. Am J Med Sci 270:81–85, 1975.
92. LeDuc JW, Lemon SM, Keenan CM, et al. Experimental infection of the New World owl monkey *(Aotus trivirgatus)* with hepatitis A virus. Infect Immun 40:766–772, 1983.
93. Dienstag JL, Davenport FM, McCollum RW, et al. Nonhuman primate-associated viral hepatitis type A. Serologic evidence of hepatitis A virus infection. JAMA 236:462–464, 1976.
94. Asher LVS, Binn LN, Mensing TL, et al. Pathogenesis of hepatitis A in orally inoculated owl monkeys *(Aotus trivirgatus)*. J Med Virol 47:260–268, 1995.
95. Ruiz-Gomez J, Bustamante-Calvillo ME. Hepatitis A antibodies: Prevalence and persistence in a group of Mexican children. Am J Epidemiol 121:116–119, 1985.
96. Karayiannis P, Jowett T, Enticott M, et al. Hepatitis A virus replication in tamarins and host immune response in relation to pathogenesis of liver cell damage. J Med Virol 18:261–276, 1986.
97. Krugman S, Ward R, Giles JP. Infectious hepatitis: Detection of virus during the incubation period and in clinically inapparent infection. N Engl J Med 261:729–734, 1959.
98. Yotsuyanagi H, Iino S, Koike K, et al. Duration of viremia in human hepatitis A viral infection as determined by polymerase chain reaction. J Med Virol 40:35–38, 1993.
99. Cohen JI, Feinstone S, Purcell RH. Hepatitis A virus infection in a chimpanzee: Duration of viremia and detection of virus in saliva and throat swabs. J Infect Dis 160:887–890, 1989.
100. Schulman AN, Dienstag JL, Jackson DR, et al. Hepatitis A antigen particles in liver, bile, and stool of chimpanzees. J Infect Dis 134:80–84, 1976.
101. Krawczynski KK, Bradley DW, Murphy BL, et al. Pathogenetic aspects of hepatitis A virus infection in enterally inoculated marmosets. Am J Clin Pathol 76:698–706, 1981.
102. Bradley DW, Hollinger FB, Hornbeck CL, et al. Isolation and characterization of hepatitis A virus. Am J Clin Pathol 65:876–889, 1976.
103. Vallbracht A, Fleischer B. Immune pathogenesis of hepatitis A. Arch Virol Suppl 4:3–4, 1992.
104. Kurane I, Binn LN, Bancroft WH, et al. Human lymphocyte responses to hepatitis A virus-infected cells: Interferon production and lysis of infected cells. J Immunol 135:2140–2144, 1985.
105. Davis GL, Hoofnagle JH, Waggoner JG. Acute type A hepatitis during chronic hepatitis B virus infection: Association of depressed hepatitis B virus replication with appearance of endogenous alpha interferon. J Med Virol 14:141–147, 1984.
106. Zachoval R, Abb J, Zachoval V, et al. Circulating interferon in patients with acute hepatitis A. J Infect Dis 153:1174–1175, 1986.
107. Margolis HS, Nainan OV. Identification of virus components in circulating immune complexes isolated during hepatitis A virus infection. Hepatology 11:31–37, 1990.
108. Winokur PL, Stapleton JT. Immunoglobulin prophylaxis for hepatitis A. Clin Infect Dis 14:580–586, 1992.
109. Stapleton JT. Host immune response to hepatitis A virus. J Infect Dis 171(suppl 1):S9–S14, 1995.
110. Stapleton JT, Lange DK, LeDuc JW, et al. The role of secretory immunity in hepatitis A virus infection. J Infect Dis 163:7–11, 1991.
111. Mosley JW, Visona KA, Villarejos VM. Immunoglobulin M level in the diagnosis of type A hepatitis. Am J Clin Pathol 75:86–87, 1981.
112. Norkrans G, Nilsson LA, Frosner G, et al. Serum immunoglobulin levels in hepatitis non-A, non-B: A comparison with hepatitis A and B. Infection 8:98–100, 1980.
113. Jansen RW, Siegl G, Lemon SM. Molecular epidemiology of

human hepatitis A virus defined by an antigen-capture polymerase chain reaction method. Proc Natl Acad Sci USA 87:2867–2871, 1990.
114. Purcell RH, Mannucci PM, Gdovin S, et al. Virology of the hepatitis A epidemic in Italy. Vox Sang 67(suppl 4):2–7; discussion 24–26, 1994.
115. L'Hote P, Alouani S, Marq JB, et al. Concomitant cellular expression of heat shock regulated genes of hepatitis B virus surface antigen and of human growth hormone by a NIH-3T3 cell line. Cell Biol Toxicol 9:319–332, 1993.
116. Locarnini SA, Coulepis AG, Stratton AM, et al. Solid-phase enzyme-linked immunosorbent assay for detection of hepatitis A–specific immunoglobulin M. J Clin Microbiol 9:459–465, 1979.
117. Hansson BG, Calhoun JK, Wong DC, et al. Serodiagnosis of viral hepatitis A by a solid-phase radioimmunoassay specific for IgM antibodies. Scand J Infect Dis 13:5–9, 1981.
118. Duermeyer W, Wielaard F, van der Veen J. A new principle for the detection of specific IgM antibodies applied in an ELISA for hepatitis A. J Med Virol 4:25–32, 1979.
119. Kao HW, Ashcavai M, Redeker AG. The persistence of hepatitis A IgM antibody after acute clinical hepatitis A. Hepatology 4:933–936, 1984.
120. O'Grady J. Management of acute and fulminant hepatitis A. Vaccine 10(suppl 1):S21–S23, 1992.
121. Prodinger WM, Larcher C, Solder BM, et al. Hepatitis A in Western Austria—the epidemiological situation before the introduction of active immunisation. Infection 22:53–55, 1994.
122. Chitambar SD, Murthy-Grewal S, Bokil M, et al. Indigenous anti-hepatitis A virus IgM capture ELISA for the diagnosis of hepatitis A. Indian J Med Res 99:243–251, 1994.
123. Fujiyama S, Odoh K, Kuramoto I, et al. Current seroepidemiological status of hepatitis A with a comparison of antibody titers after infection and vaccination. J Hepatol 21:641–645, 1994.
124. Centers for Disease Control and Prevention. Summary of notifiable diseases, United States. MMWR Morb Mortal Wkly Rep 43:1–80, 1994.
125. Shapiro CN, Margolis HS. Worldwide epidemiology of hepatitis A virus infection. J Hepatol 18(suppl 2):S11–S14, 1993.
126. Bowden FJ, Currie BJ, Miller NC, et al. Should aboriginals in the top end of the Northern Territory be vaccinated against hepatitis A? Med J Aust 161:372–373, 1994.
127. Martin DJ, Blackburn NK, Johnson S, et al. The current epidemiology of hepatitis A infection in South Africa: Implications for vaccination. Trans R Soc Trop Med Hyg 88:288–291, 1994.
128. Karetnyi YV, Mendelson E, Shlyakhov E, et al. Prevalence of antibodies against hepatitis A virus among new immigrants in Israel. J Med Virol 46:61–65, 1995.
129. Halliday ML, Kang LY, Zhou TK, et al. An epidemic of hepatitis A attributable to the ingestion of raw clams in Shanghai, China. J Infect Dis 164:852–859, 1991.
130. Glerup H, Sorensen HT, Flyvbjerg A, et al. A "mini epidemic" of hepatitis A after eating Russian caviar [letter]. J Hepatol 21:479, 1994.
131. Divizia M, Gnesivo C, Amore Bonapasta R, et al. Hepatitis A virus identification in an outbreak by enzymatic amplification. Eur J Epidemiol 9:203–208, 1993.
132. Stewart T, Crofts N. An outbreak of hepatitis A among homosexual men in Melbourne. Med J Aust 158:519–521, 1993.
133. Koziel MJ, Dudley D, Afdhal N, et al. Hepatitis C virus (HCV)–specific cytotoxic T lymphocytes recognize epitopes in the core and envelope proteins of HCV. J Virol 67:7522–7532, 1993.
134. Shapiro CN, Shaw FE, Mandel EJ, et al. Epidemiology of hepatitis A in the United States. In Hollinger FB, Lemon SM, Margolis H (eds). Viral Hepatitis and Liver Disease. Baltimore, Williams & Wilkins, 1991, pp 71–76.
135. Shapiro CN, Coleman PJ, McQuillan GM, et al. Epidemiology of hepatitis A: Seroepidemiology and risk groups in the USA. Vaccine 10(suppl 1):S59–S62, 1992.
136. Schiff E. Viral hepatitis—1993: An update. Proceedings of the Annual Meeting of the Medical Section of the American Council of Life Insurance; Boca Raton, FL; June 13–18, 1993; pp 181–193.
137. Mele A, Sagliocca L, Palumbo F, et al. Travel-associated hepatitis A: Effect of place of residence and country visited [see comments]. J Public Health Med 13:256–259, 1991.
138. Steffen R. Risk of hepatitis A in travellers. Vaccine 10(suppl 1):S69–S72, 1992.
139. Steffen R. Hepatitis A in travelers: The European experience. J Infect Dis 171(suppl 1):S24–S28, 1995.
140. Christenson B. Epidemiological aspects of acute viral hepatitis A in Swedish travellers to endemic areas. Scand J Infect Dis 17:5–10, 1985.
141. Havens WPJ. Period of infectivity of patients with experimentally induced infectious hepatitis. J Exp Med 83:251–258, 1946.
142. Dienstag JL, Feinstone SM, Kapikian AZ, et al. Faecal shedding of hepatitis-A antigen. Lancet 1:765–767, 1975.
143. Dienstag JL, Routenberg JA, Purcell RH, et al. Foodhandler-associated outbreak of hepatitis type A. An immune electron microscopic study. Ann Intern Med 83:647–650, 1975.
144. Hollinger FB, Khan NC, Oefinger PE, et al. Posttransfusion hepatitis type A. JAMA 250:2313–2317, 1983.
145. Barbara JA, Howell DR, Briggs M, et al. Post-transfusion hepatitis A [letter]. Lancet 1:738, 1982.
146. Weisfuse IB, Graham DJ, Will M, et al. An outbreak of hepatitis A among cancer patients treated with interleukin-2 and lymphokine-activated killer cells. J Infect Dis 161:647–652, 1990.
147. Mannucci PM, Gdovin S, Gringeri A, et al. Transmission of hepatitis A to patients with hemophilia by factor VIII concentrates treated with organic solvent and detergent to inactivate viruses. The Italian Collaborative Group [see comments]. Ann Intern Med 120:1–7, 1994.
148. Hadler SC, McFarland L. Hepatitis in day care centers: Epidemiology and prevention. Rev Infect Dis 8:548–557, 1986.
149. Drusin LM, Sohmer M, Groshen SL, et al. Nosocomial hepatitis A infection in a paediatric intensive care unit. Arch Dis Child 62:690–695, 1987.
150. Rosenblum LS, Villarino ME, Nainan OV, et al. Hepatitis A outbreak in a neonatal intensive care unit: Risk factors for transmission and evidence of prolonged viral excretion among preterm infants. J Infect Dis 164:476–482, 1991.
151. Fenton A, Sinclair JA, Entrican G, et al. A monoclonal antibody capture ELISA to detect antibody to border disease virus in sheep serum. Vet Microbiol 28:327–333, 1991.
152. Nagashima H, Imai M, Iwakura Y. Aberrant tissue specific expression of the transgene in transgenic mice that carry the hepatitis B virus genome defective in the X gene. Arch Virol 132:381–397, 1993.
153. Desenclos JC, Klontz KC, Wilder MH, et al. A multistate outbreak of hepatitis A caused by the consumption of raw oysters. Am J Public Health 81:1268–1272, 1991.
154. Zhou YJ, Estes MK, Jiang X, et al. Concentration and detection of hepatitis A virus and rotavirus from shellfish by hybridization tests. Appl Environ Microbiol 57:2963–2968, 1991.
155. Enriquez R, Frosner GG, Hochstein-Mintzel V, et al. Accumulation and persistence of hepatitis A virus in mussels. J Med Virol 37:174–179, 1992.
156. Cromeans TL, Nainan OV, Margolis HS. Detection of hepatitis A virus RNA in oyster meat. Appl Environ Microbiol 63:2460–2463, 1997.
157. Millard J, Appleton H, Parry JV. Studies on heat inactivation of hepatitis A virus with special reference to shellfish. Part 1. Procedures for infection and recovery of virus from laboratory-maintained cockles. Epidemiol Infect 98:397–414, 1987.
158. Wang JY, Hu SL, Liu HY, et al. Risk factor analysis of an epidemic of hepatitis A in a factory in Shanghai. Int J Epidemiol 19:435–438, 1990.
159. Carl M, Francis DP, Maynard JE. Food-borne hepatitis A: Recommendations for control. J Infect Dis 148:1133–1135, 1983.
160. Kosatsky T, Middaugh JP. Linked outbreaks of hepatitis A in homosexual men and in food service patrons and employees. West J Med 144:307–310, 1986.
161. Centers for Disease Control and Prevention. Hepatitis A associated with consumption of frozen strawberries—Michigan, March 1997. JAMA 277:1271, 1997.
162. Bowen GS, McCarthy MA. Hepatitis A associated with a hardware store water fountain and a contaminated well in Lancaster County, Pennsylvania, 1980. Am J Epidemiol 117:695–705, 1983.
163. Bloch AB, Stramer SL, Smith JD, et al. Recovery of hepatitis A virus from a water supply responsible for a common source outbreak of hepatitis A. Am J Public Health 80:428–430, 1990.

164. Mahoney FJ, Farley TA, Kelso KY, et al. An outbreak of hepatitis A associated with swimming in a public pool. J Infect Dis 165:613–618, 1992.
165. Vermylen J, Peerlinck K. Review of the hepatitis A epidemics in hemophiliacs in Europe. Vox Sang 67(suppl 4):8–11; discussion 24–26, 1994.
166. Mannucci PM, Santagostino E, Di Bona E, et al. The outbreak of hepatitis A in Italian patients with hemophilia: Facts and fancies. Vox Sang 67(suppl 1):31–35, 1994.
167. Horowitz B. Specific inactivation of viruses which can potentially contaminate blood products. Dev Biol Stand 75:43–52, 1991.
168. Lemon SM, Murphy PC, Smith A, et al. Removal/neutralization of hepatitis A virus during manufacture of high purity, solvent/detergent factor VIII concentrate. J Med Virol 43:44–49, 1994.
169. Hamman J, Zou J, Horowitz B. Removal and inactivation of hepatitis A virus (HAV) during processing of factor VIII concentrates. Vox Sang 67(suppl 1):72–76; discussion 77, 1994.
170. Lerman Y, Shohat T, Ashkenazi S, et al. Efficacy of different doses of immune serum globulin in the prevention of hepatitis A: A three-year prospective study. Clin Infect Dis 17:411–414, 1993.
171. Smallwood LA, Tabor E, Finlayson JS, et al. Antibodies to hepatitis A virus in immune serum globulin [letter]. Lancet 2:482–483, 1980.
172. Stokes N. The prevention and attenuation of infectious hepatitis by gamma globulin. JAMA 127:144–145, 1945.
173. Stapleton JT. Passive immunization against hepatitis A. Vaccine 10(suppl 1):S45–S47, 1992.
174. Weiland O, Niklasson B, Berg R, et al. Clinical and subclinical hepatitis A occurring after immunoglobulin prophylaxis among Swedish UN soldiers in Sinai. Scand J Gastroenterol 16:967–972, 1981.
175. Pierce PF, Cappello M, Bernard KW. Subclinical infection with hepatitis A in Peace Corps volunteers following immune globulin prophylaxis. Am J Trop Med Hyg 42:465–469, 1990.
176. McMahon BJ, Beller M, Williams J, et al. A program to control an outbreak of hepatitis A in Alaska by using an inactivated hepatitis A vaccine. Arch Pediatr Adolesc Med 150:733–739, 1996.
177. Van Doorslaer E, Tormans G, van Damme P. Cost-effectiveness analysis of vaccination against hepatitis A in travellers. J Med Virol 44:463–469, 1994.
178. Karron RA, Daemer R, Ticehurst J, et al. Studies of prototype live hepatitis A virus vaccines in primate models. J Infect Dis 157:338–345, 1988.
179. Sjogren MH, Purcell RH, McKee K, et al. Clinical and laboratory observations following oral or intramuscular administration of a live attenuated hepatitis A vaccine candidate. Vaccine 10(suppl 1):S135–S137, 1992.
180. Midthun K, Ellerbeck E, Gershman K, et al. Safety and immunogenicity of a live attenuated hepatitis A virus vaccine in seronegative volunteers. J Infect Dis 163:735–739, 1991.
181. Mao JS, Dong DX, Zhang HY, et al. Primary study of attenuated live hepatitis A vaccine (H2 strain) in humans. J Infect Dis 159:621–624, 1989.
182. Cho MW, Ehrenfeld E. Rapid completion of the replication cycle of hepatitis A virus subsequent to reversal of guanidine inhibition. Virology 180:770–780, 1991.
183. Cohen JI, Ticehurst JR, Feinstone SM, et al. Hepatitis A virus cDNA and its RNA transcripts are infectious in cell culture. J Virol 61:3035–3039, 1987.
184. Emerson SU, Huang YK, McRill C, et al. Molecular basis of virulence and growth of hepatitis A virus in cell culture. Vaccine 10(suppl 1):S36–S39, 1992.
185. Emerson SU, Huang YK, Purcell RH. 2B and 2C mutations are essential but mutations throughout the genome of HAV contribute to adaptation to cell culture. Virology 194:475–480, 1993.
186. Vidor E, Fritzell B, Plotkin S. Clinical development of a new inactivated hepatitis A vaccine. Infection 24:447–458, 1996.
187. Gluck R, Mischler R, Brantschen S, et al. Immunopotentiating reconstituted influenza virus virosome vaccine delivery system for immunization against hepatitis A. J Clin Invest 90:2491–2495, 1992.
188. Gust ID, Lehmann NI, Crowe S, et al. The origin of the HM175 strain of hepatitis A virus. J Infect Dis 151:365–367, 1985.
189. Peetermans J. Production, quality control and characterization of an inactivated hepatitis A vaccine. Vaccine 10(suppl 1):S99–S101, 1992.
190. Armstrong ME, Giesa PA, Davide JP, et al. Development of the formalin-inactivated hepatitis A vaccine, VAQTA, from the live attenuated virus strain CR326F. J Hepatol 18(suppl 2):S20–S26, 1993.
191. Flehmig B, Vallbracht A, Wurster G. Hepatitis A in cell culture. 3. Propagation of hepatitis virus in human embryo cells and human embryo fibroblast strains. Med Microbiol Immunol 170:83–89, 1981.
192. Heinricy U, Stierhof YD, Pfisterer M, Flehmig B. Properties of a hepatitis A virus candidate vaccine strain. J Gen Virol 68:2487–2493, 1987.
193. Flehmig B, Heinricy U, Pfisterer M. Prospects for a hepatitis A virus vaccine. Prog Med Virol 37:56–71, 1990.
194. Flehmig B, Mauler RF, Noll G, et al. Viral Hepatitis and Liver Disease. New York, Alan R Liss, 1988, pp 87–90.
195. Ambrosch F, Wiedermann G, Jonas S, et al. Immunogenicity and protectivity of a new liposomal hepatitis A vaccine. Vaccine 15:1209–1213, 1997.
196. Havrix [package insert]. SmithKline Beecham Biologicals, Philadelphia, Pa, 1998.
197. Vaqta [package insert]. Merck & Co., Inc., West Point, PA, 1998.
198. American Academy of Pediatrics. Hepatitis A. In Peter G (ed). 1997 Red Book: Report of the Committee on Infectious Diseases (24th ed). Elk Grove Village, IL, American Academy of Pediatrics, 1997, pp 237–246.
199. Poovorawan Y, Theamboonlers A, Chumderpadetsuk S, et al. Safety, immunogenicity, and kinetics of the immune response to a single dose of virosome-formulated hepatitis A vaccine in Thais. Vaccine 13:891–893, 1995.
200. Westblom TU, Gudipati S, DeRousee C, et al. Safety and immunogenicity of an inactivated hepatitis A vaccine: Effect of dose and vaccination schedule. J Infect Dis 169:996–1001, 1994.
201. Fisch A, Cadilhac P, Vidor E, et al. Immunogenicity and safety of a new inactivated hepatitis A vaccine: A clinical trial with comparison of administration route. Vaccine 14:1132–1136, 1996.
202. Leroux-Roels G, Moreau E, Desombere, et al. Safety and immunogenicity of a combined hepatitis A and hepatitis B vaccine in young healthy adults. Scand J Gastroenterol 31:1027–1031, 1996.
203. Bruguera M, Bayas JM, Vilella A, et al. Immunogenicity and reactogenicity of a combined hepatitis A and B vaccine in young adults. Vaccine 14:1407–1411, 1996.
204. Werzberger A, Mensch B, Kuter B, et al. A controlled trial of a formalin-inactivated hepatitis A vaccine in healthy children [see comments]. N Engl J Med 327:453–457, 1992.
205. Shouval D, Ashur Y, Adler R, et al. Safety, tolerability, and immunogenicity of an inactivated hepatitis A vaccine: Effects of single and booster injections, and comparison to administration of immune globulin. J Hepatol 18(suppl 2):S32–S37, 1993.
206. van Damme P, Mathei C, Thoelen S, et al. Single dose inactivated hepatitis A vaccine: Rationale and clinical assessment of the safety and immunogenicity. J Med Virol 44:435–441, 1994.
207. Hoke CH Jr, Binn LN, Egan JE, et al. Hepatitis A in the US Army: Epidemiology and vaccine development. Vaccine 10(suppl 1):S75–S79, 1992.
208. Reuman PD, Kubilis P, Hurni W, et al. The effect of age and weight on the response to formalin inactivated alum-adjuvanted hepatitis A vaccine in healthy adults. Vaccine 15:1157–1161, 1997.
209. Troisi CL, Holliner FB, Krause DS, et al. Immunization of seronegative infants with hepatitis A vaccine (HAVRIX); SKB: A comparative study of two dosing schedules. Vaccine 15:1613–1617, 1997.
210. Andre FE, D'Hondt E, Eelem A, Safary A. Clinical assessment of the safety and efficacy of an inactivated hepatitis A vaccine: Rationale and summary of findings. Vaccine 10(suppl 1):S160–S168, 1992.
211. Nalin D, Kuter BJ, Brown L, et al. Worldwide experience with the CR326F-derived inactivated hepatitis A virus vaccine in pediatric and adult populations: An overview. J Hepatol 18(suppl 2):S51–S55, 1993.
212. Vidor E, Xueref C, Blondeau C, et al. Analysis of the antibody response in humans with a new inactivated hepatitis A vaccine. Biologicals 24:235–242, 1996.

213. Goilav C, Zuckerman J, Lanfrenz M, et al. Immunogenicity and safety of a new inactivated hepatitis A vaccine in a comparative study. J Med Virol 46:287–292, 1995.
214. Lee SD, Lo KJ, Chan CY, et al. Immunogenicity of inactivated hepatitis A vaccine in children. Gastroenterology 104:1129–1132, 1993.
215. Nalin D, Brown L, Kuter B, et al. Inactivated hepatitis A vaccine in childhood: Implications for disease control. Vaccine 11(suppl 1):S15–S17, 1993.
216. Bock S, Hedrick J, Tyler R, et al. Safety, tolerability and immunogenicity of a formalin-inactivated hepatitis A vaccine (VAQTA) in rural Kentucky children. Pediatr Infect Dis J 12:976–980, 1993.
217. Green MS, Cohen D, Lerman Y, et al. Depression of the immune response to an inactivated hepatitis A vaccine administered concomitantly with immune globulin. J Infect Dis 168:740–743, 1993.
218. Zanetti A, Pregliasco F, Andreassi A, et al. Does immunoglobulin interfere with the immunogenicity to Pasteur Mérieux inactivated hepatitis A vaccine? J Hepatol 26:25–30, 1997.
219. Lemon SM, Murphy PC, Provost PJ, et al. Immunoprecipitation and virus neutralization assays demonstrate qualitative differences between protective antibody responses to inactivated hepatitis A vaccine and passive immunization with immune globulin. J Infect Dis 176:9–19, 1997.
220. Purcell RH, D'Hondt E, Bradbury R, et al. Inactivated hepatitis A vaccine: Active and passive immunoprophylaxis in chimpanzees. Vaccine 10(suppl 1):S148–S151, 1992.
221. Werzberger A, Kuter B, Shouval D, et al. Anatomy of a trial: A historical view of the Monroe inactivated hepatitis A protective efficacy trial. J Hepatol 18(suppl 2):S46–S50, 1993.
222. Richtman R, Chaves R, Mendonca J, et al. Immunogenicity and efficacy of a killed hepatitis A vaccine in day care center children. J Med Virol 48:147–150, 1996.
223. Zaaijer HL, Leentvaar-Kuijpers A, Rotman H, et al. Hepatitis A antibody titres after infection and immunization: Implications for passive and active immunization. J Med Virol 40:22–27, 1993.
224. Fujiyama S, Iino S, Odoh K, et al. Time course of hepatitis A virus antibody titer after active and passive immunization. Hepatology 15:983–988, 1992.
225. Totos G, Papaevagelou G. Persistence of vaccine-induced antibodies for hepatitis A vaccine [letter]. Vaccine 12:475, 1994.
226. Wiens BL, Bohidar NR, Pigeion JG, et al. Duration of protection from clinical hepatitis A disease after vaccination with (VAQTA). J Med Virol 49:235–241, 1996.
227. Maiwald H, Jilg W, Bock HL, et al. Long-term persistence of anti-HAV antibodies following active immunization with hepatitis A vaccine. Vaccine 15:346–348, 1997.
228. Fan PC, Chang MH, Lee PI, et al. Follow-up immunogenicity of an inactivated hepatitis A virus vaccine in healthy children: Results after 5 years. Vaccine 16:232–235, 1998.
229. Wiedermann G, Kundi M, Ambrosch F, et al. Inactivated hepatitis A vaccine: Long term antibody persistence. Vaccine 15:612–615, 1997.
230. Cone L, Sneider R, Nazemi R, Dietrich EJ. Vasculitis related to hepatitis A vaccination. Brief report. Clin Infect Dis 22:596, 1996.
231. Nordenfelt E. Hepatitis A in Swedish travellers. Vaccine 10(suppl 1):S73–S74, 1992.
232. Lange WR, Frame JD. High incidence of viral hepatitis among American missionaries in Africa. Am J Trop Med Hyg 43:527–533, 1990.
233. Lemon SM, Shapiro CN. The value of immunization against hepatitis A. Infect Agents Dis 3:38–49, 1994.
234. Steffen R, Kane MA, Shapiro CN, et al. Epidemiology and prevention of hepatitis A in travelers [see comments]. JAMA 272:885–889, 1994.
235. Newcomer W, Rivin B, Reid R, et al. Immunogenicity, safety and tolerability of varying doses and regimens of inactivated hepatitis A virus vaccine in Navajo children. Pediatr Infect Dis J 13:640–642, 1994.
236. Welty TK, Darling K, Dye S, et al. Guidelines for prevention and control of hepatitis A in American Indian and Alaska Native communities. S D J Med 49:317–322, 1996.
237. Vento S, Garofano T, Renzini C, et al. Fulminant hepatitis associated with hepatitis A virus superinfection in patients with chronic hepatitis C. N Engl J Med 338:286–290, 1998.
238. Berenguer M, Wright TL. Are HCV-infected individuals candidates for hepatitis A vaccine? Lancet 351:924–925, 1998.
239. Maguire H. Hepatitis A virus infection. Risk to sewage workers unproved [letter; comment]. BMJ 307:561, 1993.
240. Wagner G, Lavanchy D, Darioli R, et al. Simultaneous active and passive immunization against hepatitis A studied in a population of travellers. Vaccine 11:1027–1032, 1993.
241. Leentvaar-Kuijpers A, Coutinho RA, Brulein V, et al. Simultaneous passive and active immunization against hepatitis A. Vaccine 10(suppl 1):S138–S141, 1992.
242. Ambrosch F, Andrë FE, Delem A, et al. Simultaneous vaccination against hepatitis A and B: Results of a controlled study. Vaccine 10(suppl 1):S142–S145, 1992.
243. Gil A, Gonzalez A, Dal-Re R, et al. Interference assessment of yellow fever vaccine with the immune response to a single-dose inactivated hepatitis A vaccine (1440 EL.U.). A controlled study in adults. Vaccine 14:1028–1030, 1996.
244. Bienzle U, Bock HL, Kruppenbacher JP, et al. Immunogenicity of an inactivated hepatitis A vaccine administered according to two different schedules and the interference of other "travellers" vaccines with the immune response. Vaccine 14:501–505, 1996.
245. Emini EA, Hughes JV, Perlow DS, et al. Induction of hepatitis A virus-neutralizing antibody by a virus-specific synthetic peptide. J Virol 55:836–839, 1985.
246. Stapleton JT, Raina V, Winokur PL, et al. Antigenic and immunogenic properties of recombinant hepatitis A virus 14S and 70S subviral particles. J Virol 67:1080–1085, 1993.
247. Winokur PL, McLinden JH, Stapleton JT. The hepatitis A virus polyprotein expressed by a recombinant vaccinia virus undergoes proteolytic processing and assembly into viruslike particles. J Virol 65:5029–5036, 1991.
248. Rosen E, Stapleton JT, McLinden J. Synthesis of immunogenic hepatitis A virus particles by recombinant baculoviruses. Vaccine 11:706–712, 1993.
249. Prikazsky V, Olear V, Cernoch A, et al. Interruption of an outbreak of hepatitis A in two villages by vaccination. J Med Virol 44:457–459, 1994.
250. Centers for Disease Control and Prevention. Prevention of hepatitis A through active or passive immunization: Recommendations of the Advisory Committee on Immunization Practices (ACIP). MMWR Morb Mortal Wkly Rep 45:1–31, 1996.
251. Hepatitis A vaccination programs in communities with high rates of hepatitis A. MMWR Morb Mortal Wkly Rep 46:600–603, 1997.
252. Jefferson TO, Behrens RH, Demicheli V. Should British soldiers be vaccinated against hepatitis A? An economic analysis. Vaccine 12:1379–1383, 1994.
253. Behrens RH, Roberts JA. Is travel prophylaxis worth while? Economic appraisal of prophylactic measures against malaria, hepatitis A, and typhoid in travellers [see comments]. BMJ 309:918–922, 1994.
254. Margolis HS, Shapiro CN. Considerations for the development of recommendations for the use of hepatitis A vaccine. J Hepatol 18(suppl 2):S56–S60, 1993.

chapter

27 Japanese Encephalitis Vaccines

Theodore F. Tsai

Gwong-Jen J. Chang

Yong Xin Yu

Japanese encephalitis (JE), a mosquito-borne flaviviral infection, is the leading recognized cause of childhood encephalitis in Asia. Approximately 35,000 cases and 10,000 deaths are reported annually, but in many locations the disease is not under systematic surveillance, and official reports undoubtedly underestimate the true number of cases (Fig. 27–1).[1–3] Although the disease is transmitted only in Asia, because the region contains more than 3 billion people and 60% of the world's population, regional JE-associated morbidity may exceed worldwide morbidity from herpes encephalitis, the latter estimated at 5 per 1 million per year, or approximately 30,000 cases worldwide.[4, 5] With the near eradication of poliomyelitis, JE now is the continent's leading cause of childhood viral neurological infection. By any standard, JE is a major public health problem that potentially can be controlled by proven effective vaccines.

Summer-fall encephalitis outbreaks consistent with JE were recorded in Japan as early as 1871, of which the largest, in 1924, led to more than 6000 cases, 60% of them fatal.[6] A filterable agent from human brain tissue was isolated in rabbits that year, and in 1934, Hayashi transmitted the disease experimentally to monkeys.[7] Soon after, the availability of JE and related St. Louis encephalitis (StLE) viral isolates made possible serological confirmation of encephalitis cases occurring elsewhere in the region, including a cluster of cases occurring in 1934 through 1935 in Beijing.[8] The virus initially was called Japanese B encephalitis (the modifying "B" has since fallen into disuse) in deference to Von Economo's type A encephalitis, which had different clinical and epidemiological characteristics. The mosquito-borne mode of JE transmission was elucidated with the isolation of JE virus from *Culex tritaeniorhynchus* mosquitoes in 1938, and subsequent field studies established the role of aquatic birds and pigs in the viral enzootic cycle. Viruses isolated from human cases in Japan in 1935 and in Beijing in 1949 provided the prototype Nakayama, Beijing, and P3 strains, respectively, that are in principal use in vaccine production today.

During the first half of this century, JE was recognized principally in temperate areas of the continent in the form of perennial outbreaks in Japan, Korea, and China.[1] Annual outbreaks of several thousand cases recurred in Japan until as recently as 1966, with a public impact that was further magnified by the concentration of these outbreaks during the summer season. In Korea, after 5616 cases and 2729 deaths were recorded in 1949, epidemics continued every 2 or 3 years, culminating in an unprecedented 6897 cases in 1958 (Fig. 27–2).[9] However, China has accounted for the majority of cases in the region; between 1965 and 1975, more than 1 million cases were reported, 175,000 in 1971 alone (Fig. 27–3).[10] Public health efforts that placed a great emphasis on vaccination produced a dramatic decline in cases; however, coverage remains low in many provinces, and in recent years incidence in the rural population has remained stable. In Japan, Korea, and Taiwan, the introduction of national immunization programs after 1965

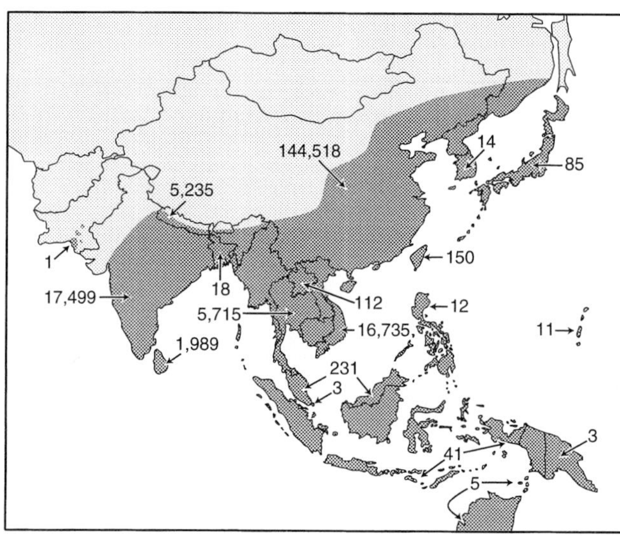

Figure 27–1. Reported cases of Japanese encephalitis, 1986 to 1996, and areas with proven or suspected enzootic viral transmission. Provisional 1997 to 1998 cases from Australia and Papua New Guinea also are included. (From World Health Organization and other reports; see Table 27–20 for updated geographical distribution.)

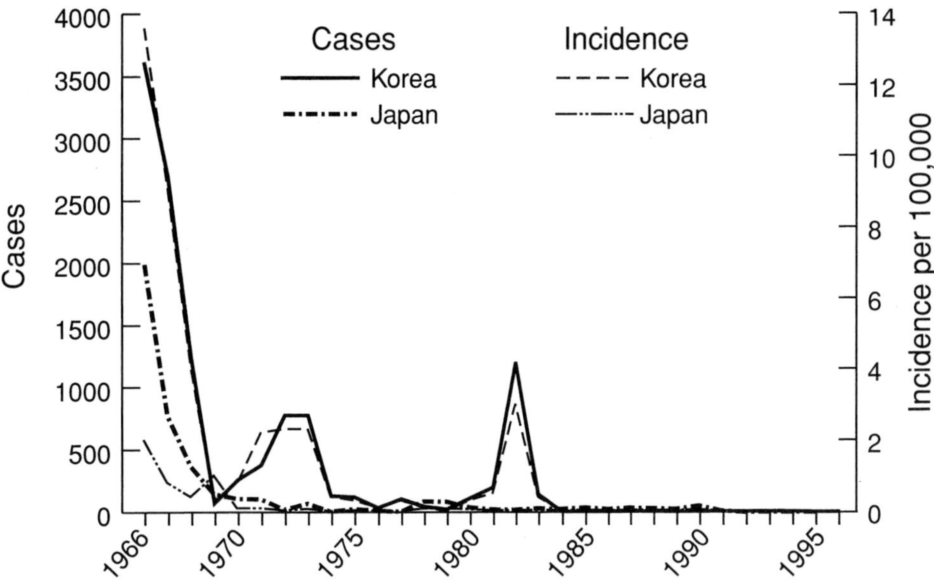

Figure 27–2. Reported Japanese encephalitis cases and incidence, Japan and Korea, 1966 to 1995 (World Health Organization reports).

led to the near elimination of the disease; however, the absence of reported cases is disarming, as enzootic transmission of the virus in its enzootic cycle continues in these locations, and periodic outbreaks have occurred (e.g., in 1982, when 1197 cases were reported in Korea[11]) (Fig. 27–4).

Although sporadic viral encephalitis cases had been noted in northern Thailand, JE was not a recognized public health problem in Southeast Asia until 1969, when an epidemic of 685 cases was reported from the Chiang Mai Valley.[12] Yearly outbreaks producing thousands of cases and hundreds of deaths followed in the northern region, and JE became recognized as a leading cause of childhood mortality and disability (Fig. 27–5).[13] Subsequently, the first of several epidemics was recorded in an adjacent area of the Chiang Mai Valley in Burma in 1974.[14] In Vietnam, since reinstatement of notification in 1979, several thousand JE cases have been reported annually, and the disease has been recognized as a public health threat in the densely populated deltas of the Mekong and Red Rivers.[15] Incidence rates exceeding 20 per 100,000 have been reported from areas of the northern delta near Hanoi. The disease probably occurs with equal frequency in Laos and Cambodia, where clinically and epidemiologically compatible cases have been reported but medical and public health infrastructure are lacking to confirm the etiology. Recent studies in Penang, Malaysia, and Bali, Indonesia, indicate that 40 to 50% of hospitalized encephalitis cases are caused by JE, thereby underscoring the inadequacy of public health surveillance, as few cases previously had been reported from these locations, and even the occurrence of JE had been questioned.[16, 17] The continued public health impact of JE in the region has led to efforts in Thailand and, more recently, in Vietnam to implement programs of childhood immunization and vaccine production.[15, 18]

JE transmission was first recognized in Southwest Asia after an outbreak occurred in 1948 in Sri Lanka. Sporadic cases and later epidemics were recognized on the Indian subcontinent around Vellor.[19, 20] Outbreaks recurred exclusively in southern India until 1973, when JE epidemics were reported in the north for the first time in the Burdwan and Bankura districts of West Bengal and afterward in Bihar and Uttar Pradesh. Apparently novel occurrences of JE subsequently were reported from various states, and the disease is currently recognized to be hyperendemic in northern India and southern Nepal, central India (Andrha Pradesh), and southern India (Goa, Karnataka, and Tamil Nadu) (Fig. 27–6). JE recently has been shown to occur as far west as the Indus valley in Pakistan.[21] The apparent spread to or amplification of JE in new areas has been correlated with agricultural development and intensive rice cultivation supported by irrigation schemes.[22] In Sri Lanka and southern Nepal, hyperendemic transmission of malaria and JE were documented to have followed deforestation and development in the Mahaweli River Valley and Terai, respectively.[23, 24] The potential spread of JE is being watched closely in Irian Jaya, Indonesia, the irrigated Thar desert of Rajasthan, and other places under development where conditions receptive to viral transmission and amplification have recently been created. Recent novel introductions leading to outbreaks on Saipan and the Torres Strait islands between New Guinea and northern Australia, and a sporadic case on the Cape York peninsula of mainland Australia, illustrate the potential for JE virus to be transferred over significant distances, possibly by viremic migratory birds or by windblown mosquitoes.[25, 26] Although development has led to the near elimination of JE in economically advanced Asian countries (Japan, Korea, Taiwan, and Singapore) development in its earlier stages, emphasizing agricultural productivity, seems to have increased JE transmission.

CLINICAL ILLNESS

The great majority of infections are not apparent, and only 1 in 250 infections results in symptomatic

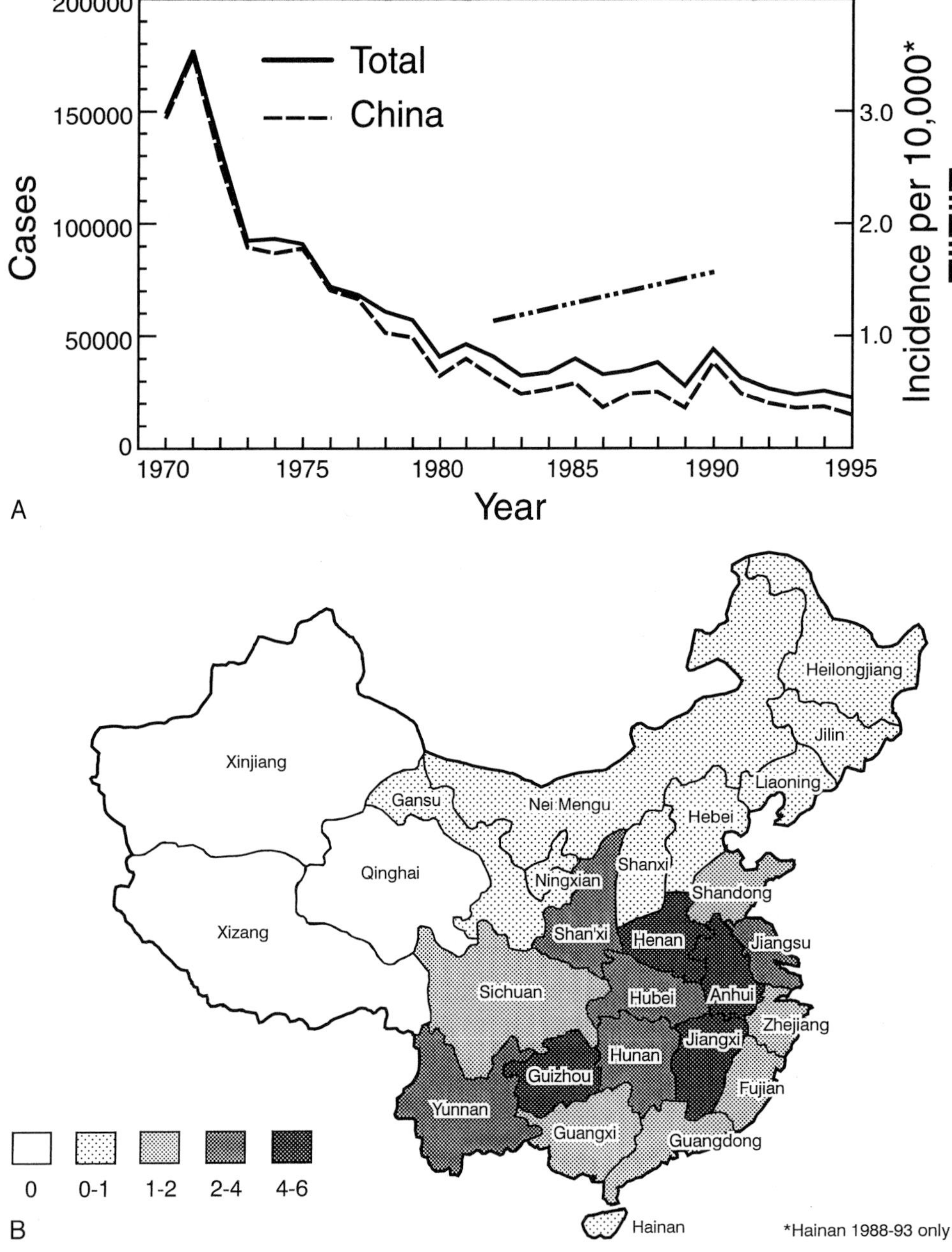

Figure 27–3. *A*, Reported cases of Japanese encephalitis (JE) for Asian and for China only, 1970 to 1995. Incidence rates for China are based on enumerated rural populations of children younger than 15 years in 1982 and 1990. *B*, Incidence of JE per 100,000 by province, China, 1983 to 1993. (From Yu YX. Japanese encephalitis in China. Southeast Asian J Trop Med Public Health 26S3:17–21, 1995.)

illness.[27, 28] The principal clinical manifestation of illness is encephalitis, and milder clinical presentations, such as aseptic meningitis and simple febrile illness with headache, usually escape recognition.[29–38] The incubation period is 5 to 15 days. Illness usually begins with abrupt onset of high fever, change in mental status, gastrointestinal symptoms, and headache, followed gradually by disturbances in speech or gait or other motor dysfunction. Irritability, vomiting, and diarrhea or an acute convulsion may be the earliest signs of illness in an infant or child. Seizures occur in more than 75% of pediatric patients and less frequently in adults. Conversely, a presentation with headache and meningism is more common in adults than in children.

A progressive decline in alertness eventually leads to stupor and coma. A substantial proportion of patients become totally unresponsive and require ventilatory assistance. Generalized weakness and changes in tone, especially hypertonia and hyperreflexia, are common, but focal motor deficits—including paresis, hemiplegia, or tetraplegia; cranial nerve palsies (especially central facial palsy); and abnormal reflexes—also may be present. Sensory disturbances are seen less frequently. Central hyperpnea, hypertension, pulmonary edema, and urinary retention also may complicate the illness. Although symptoms suggest elevated intracranial pressure in many cases, papilledema and other signs of increased intracranial pressure are rarely seen, and in a controlled trial, dexamethasone therapy did not improve outcome.[39, 40] Signs of extrapyramidal involvement, including tremor, mask-like facies, rigidity, and choreoathetoid movements, are characteristic of JE, but these signs may be obscured initially by generalized weakness.

Clinical laboratory examination discloses a moderate

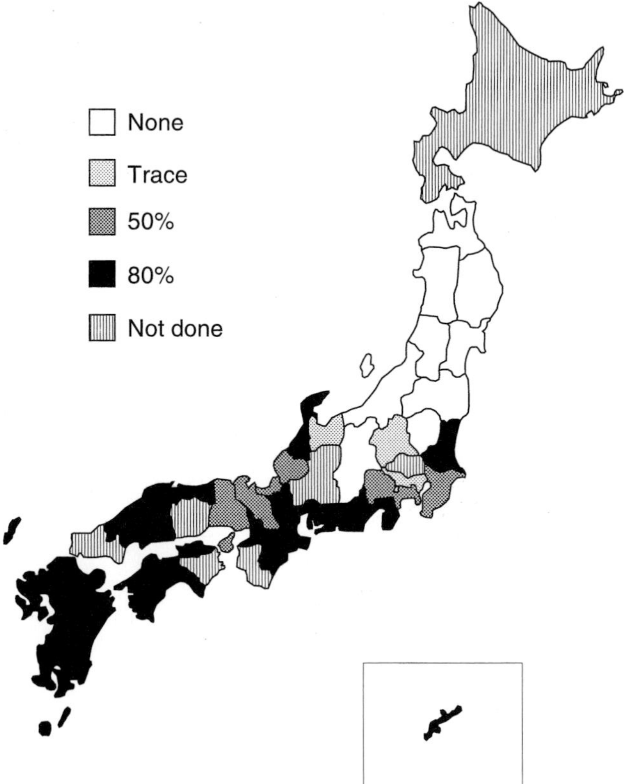

Figure 27–4. Japanese encephalitis seroprevalence in swine by district, Japan, October 1996. The absence of reported human cases belies continued transmission of the virus in its enzootic cycle, as demonstrated by high rates of pig infections. (From Taniguchi K, Matsunaga Y. National epidemiologic surveillance of vaccine-preventable diseases, Japan, October 1995. Available at http://www.nih.go.jp/yoken/idsc/ryukou/japa_Efig1.gif.)

peripheral leukocytosis with neutrophilia and mild anemia. Hyponatremia reflecting inappropriate antidiuretic hormone (ADH) secretion is a frequent complication. Cerebrospinal fluid (CSF) pressure is usually normal. Pleocytosis ranges from a few to several hundred cells per cubic millimeter, with a lymphocytic predominance; neutrophils may prevail in early samples. CSF protein is moderately elevated in about 50% of cases. Reduced levels of CSF monoamine (homovanillic and 5-hydroxyindoleacetic acids) have been found in the acute phase of illness and in recovery, but these reductions have not correlated consistently with clinical parkinsonism.[41]

Computed tomographic (CT) and magnetic resonance imaging (MRI) scans reveal low-density areas and abnormal signal intensities, respectively, in the thalamus, basal ganglia, pons, and putamen.[42–46] Acute changes in the thalamus may be a helpful differentiating feature: When compared with encephalitis cases resulting from other causes, in JE cases, T2-weighted MRI images more frequently disclose bilateral thalamic high-intensity lesions representing hemorrhages, and single photon emission CT more often shows increased activity in the thalami and putamina.[45] MRI abnormalities may be seen in the spinal cord, underscoring that JE is an encephalomyelitis. Electromyographic changes reflecting anterior horn cell degeneration are detected, especially in patients with clinical wasting; however, abnormalities in somatosensory evoked potentials are rare, which is consistent with the infrequency of clinical sensory deficits. Delays in central motor conductance time reflect widespread involvement of white matter, thalamus, brain stem, and spinal cord.[46] Electroencephalography (EEG) tracings typically show diffuse δ wave activity, but α coma also may be seen. Imaging and neurophysiological abnormalities indicative of thalamic damage correlate with several of the clinical manifestations typifying the acute phase of illness.

Five percent to 30% of cases are fatal, with some deaths occurring after a brief prodrome and fulminant course lasting a few days and others occurring after a more protracted course of persistent coma. Young children (<10 years) are more likely to die, and if they survive, they are more likely to have residual neurological deficits. Overall, approximately one third of surviving patients exhibit serious residual neurological disability.[30, 47–52] Principal sequelae include memory loss, impaired cognition, behavioral disturbances, convulsions, motor weakness or paralysis, and abnormalities of tone and coordination. In children, motor abnormalities frequently improve or eventually resolve, but behavioral changes and psychological deficits have been detected 2 to 5 years after recovery in up to 75% of pediatric cases; EEG abnormalities also may persist in the absence of detectable clinical signs.[53] Evidence of previous dengue immunity is associated with better outcome.

Poor prognosis has been associated with a short prodromal interval, clinical presentation in deep obtundation, respiratory dysfunction, prolonged fever, focal presentation, status epilepticus, and the presence of extrapyramidal signs or pathological reflexes.[47, 54–58] In some locations concurrent neurocysticercosis has been reported in more than one third of JE cases, with evidence of increased mortality in coinfected patients (see later discussion).[59]

Anecdotal observations suggest that infection may fail to clear in certain individuals, with the possibility of clinical relapse several months after resolution of the acute illness.[60] In several cases symptoms recurred, and virus was recovered from persistently infected peripheral lymphocytes despite circulating antibody. Other recovered patients who were studied months after recovery had apparently asymptomatic viremias. The possibility of subacute or persisting infection in the central nervous system (CNS) was demonstrated in 5% of patients whose CSF contained virus or viral antigen for 3 weeks or who had intrathecal immunoglobulin M (IgM) antibodies 50 to 180 days after onset.[61] The clinical significance of these observations and conditions under which JE virus persists in humans are unclear.

No specific therapy is available, but supportive treatment can significantly reduce morbidity and mortality. Mannitol and other modalities to control intracerebral pressure often are needed. Trihexyphenidyl hydrochloride and central dopamine agonists have been used to treat acute extrapyramidal symptoms.[62] Neutralizing murine monoclonal antibodies, developed in China, have been reported to improve clinical outcome in small controlled clinical trials, and licensure in that country has been sought.[63] Experimental studies in mice and

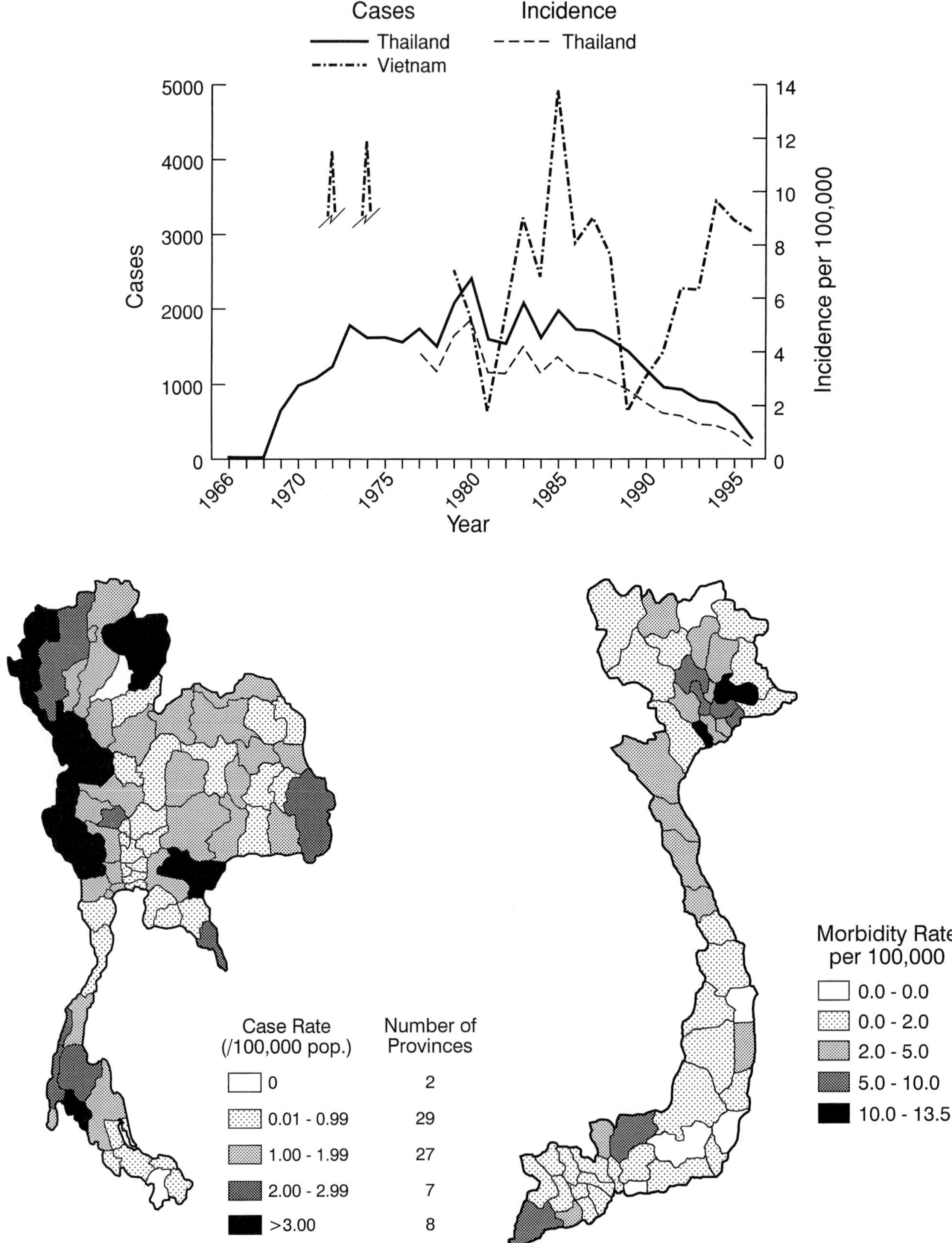

Figure 27–5. *Top*, Reported Japanese encephalitis cases and incidence, Thailand and Vietnam, 1966 to 1995. *Lower left*, Incidence per 100,000 by province, Thailand, 1993. *Lower right*, Incidence per 100,000 by province, Vietnam, 1993. (Thai data from Chunsuttiwat S, Warachit P. Japanese encephalitis in Thailand. Southeast Asian J Trop Med Public Health 26S3:43–46, 1995. Vietnamese data from Nguyen HT, Nguyen TY. Japanese encephalitis in Vietnam 1985–93. Southeast Asian J Trop Med Public Health 26S3:47–50, 1995.)

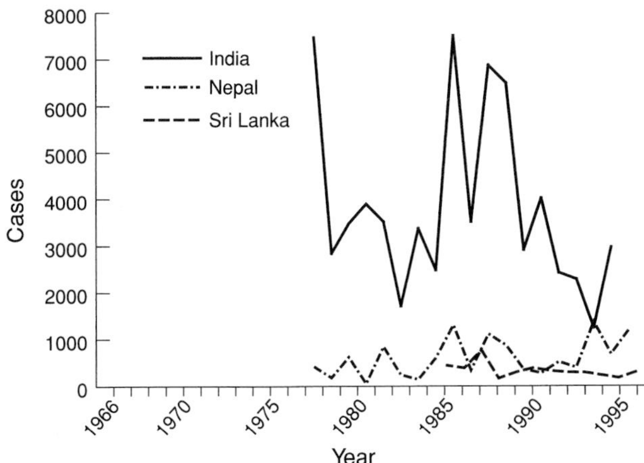

Figure 27–6. Reported Japanese encephalitis cases, India, Nepal, and Sri Lanka, 1977 to 1995 (World Health Organization reports).

monkeys also suggest the potentially beneficial effect of interferon, and in an uncontrolled series of 14 patients treated with recombinant interferon-α, 13 survived; however, further studies have not been undertaken.[64, 65] A number of antiviral compounds, including ribavirin, exhibit activity in vitro but have not been evaluated clinically.

Pathological abnormalities are found chiefly in the CNS; however, inflammatory changes in the myocardium and lung and hyperplasia of reticuloendothelial cells in the spleen, liver, and lymph nodes have been described.[66] Cerebral edema and congested leptomeninges are visible on gross examination of the brain, and "punched-out" necrolytic lesions in the gray matter may be conspicuous.[66–72] Histopathological examination discloses a pattern of diffuse microglial proliferation with nodular formation around dead or degenerating neurons, in which viral antigen can be demonstrated by immunohistochemical staining.[40, 68, 72] Viral antigen is distributed principally in the thalamus, midbrain, hippocampus, and temporal cortex, but also in Purkinje and granular cells of the cerebellum and in the brain stem reticular formation. However, viral antigen also has been demonstrated in well-preserved neurons independent of glial reaction—in some cases, well after the acute phase of illness, suggesting intracellular viral persistence. Gliomesenchymal nodules are seen in a parallel distribution within the brain and anterior horn of the spinal cord. In patients dying with residual neurological impairment several years after resolution of the acute illness, scarred rarified foci are found in a characteristic distribution in the thalamus, substantia nigra, and hippocampus.[73]

Congenital Infection

Relatively little is known of the risks of JE acquired in pregnancy and the consequences of intrauterine infection. In areas where the disease is endemic, children are exposed and become immune at an early age. Consequently, few women of childbearing age are at risk for the disease. Although the virus is an established cause of abortions and abnormal births in pigs, the first associations of JE with adverse events in human pregnancy were not reported until as late as 1980.[74–76] In a series of outbreaks in Uttar Pradesh, India, JE infections were documented in nine pregnant women (Table 27–1). Four who acquired JE in the first or second trimester miscarried, and the virus was recovered from products of conception in two cases. In five women who acquired the illness in the third trimester, no adverse outcomes of pregnancy were observed. However, JE virus–specific IgM was not measured in the infants, and it is unknown whether they were congenitally infected. Experimental data also suggest that risk of congenital infection may be related to gestational age. Human placental organ cultures, obtained from medically terminated pregnancies at 8 to 12 weeks' gestation, supported JE viral replication, but tissues from full-term pregnancies were resistant to infection.[77] Experimental studies have shown that JE viral neurotropism is related to neuronal immaturity.[78, 79]

The spectrum of adverse outcomes associated with congenital JE viral infections is undefined. It is unknown whether congenital infection causes fetal malformation or asymptomatic infection during pregnancy leads to fetal infection or adverse outcome.

VIROLOGY

JE virus is one of 70 viruses in the *Flavivirus* genus of the Flaviviridae family.[80, 81] The complete genomic sequences of JE virus and several other flaviviruses have been determined, including yellow fever (YF) virus, the prototype virus in the family. Morphologically, flaviviruses are spherical, approximately 40 to 50 nm in diameter, with a lipid membrane enclosing an isometric 30-nm-diameter nucleocapsid core comprising a capsid (C) protein and a single-stranded messenger (positive) sense viral RNA.[82] Membrane surface projections are composed of a glycosylated envelope (E) and membrane (M) protein, a mature form of the premembrane (prM) protein. JE viral RNA, 10,976 bases in length, encodes an uninterrupted open reading frame (ORF), flanked by 95 and 585 base untranslated regions at the 5′ and 3′ ends, respectively.[83, 84] Protein translation at the first encountered AUG codon near the 5′ end yields a poly-

Table 27–1. **FETAL OUTCOME AFTER LABORATORY-CONFIRMED JAPANESE ENCEPHALITIS DURING PREGNANCY, UTTAR PRADESH, INDIA, 1978 TO 1980**

WEEKS OF GESTATION	OUTCOME
8	Aborted; Japanese encephalitis (JE) virus isolated from placenta and fetal brain
10	Aborted; no virus isolated from placenta or fetal brain
20	Aborted; cord blood and products of conception not tested
22	Aborted; JE virus isolated from placenta, fetal brain, and liver
28 (2 cases)	Normal full-term delivery; cord blood not tested
30 (2 cases)	Normal full-term delivery; cord blood not tested
36	Normal full-term delivery; cord blood not tested

protein precursor of 3432 amino acids that is co- or post-translationally processed by a virus-specific nonstructural (NS) protease complex, NS2B-NS3, host cell signal peptidase, or unidentified host cell–specific protease into at least 10 mature viral proteins (Fig. 27–7). The order of proteins encoded in the JE virus ORF, as with other flaviviruses, is 5′-C-prM-E-NS1-NS2A-NS2B-NS3-NS4A-NS4B-NS5-3′.

Flaviviruses replicate in a variety of cultured cells of vertebrate and arthropod origin. Viral entry occurs by receptor-mediated endocytosis, with the formation of coated vesicles, or by direct fusion with plasma membranes.[85–87] The nucleocapsid is uncoated by acid-dependent fusion of viral and endosomal membranes, releasing genomic RNA into the cytoplasm, where viral replication continues with immediate translation of the uncoated viral genome.[85] The translated polyprotein then is processed and assembled into a virus-specific replication complex.

Extensive proliferation of membranous organelles in the perinuclear region may be a unique feature of flavivirus-infected cells.[84, 87] Ultrastructural examination discloses convoluted membranes (CM), paracrystalline structures (PC), proliferating endoplasmic reticulum (ER), spherical smooth structures (SMS) of about 100 nm in diameter found adjacent to other induced membranes, and vesicle packets (VP).[88] Membranous structures are partially surrounded by virus particles, many in aggregates within smooth membranes continuous with paired ER membranes.[89] In Kunjin virus–infected cells, RNA synthesis and RNA polymerase activity are not detected until 8 hours after infection, after which smooth membrane associated–VPs are seen. NS3 and NS5 proteins, functioning as a helicase or RNA-dependent RNA polymerase, respectively, are directed to VP membranes through an interaction with NS1 to assemble the flavivirus replication complex. Subsequently, PC and SMS develop, and an interconversion of PC to CM appears.[87, 88] The collection of induced membranes may represent virus factories in which translation, RNA synthesis, and virus assembly occur.

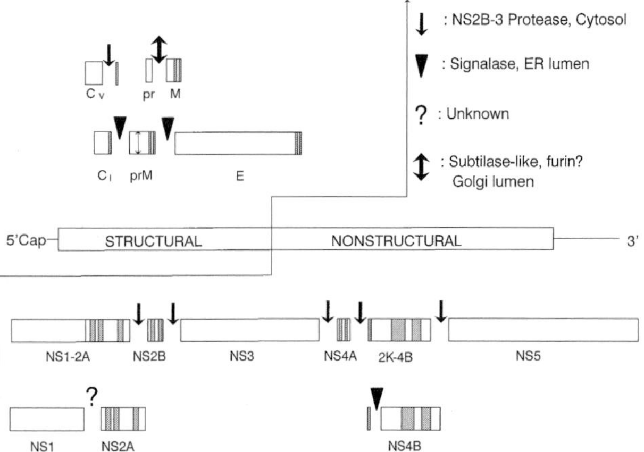

Figure 27–7. Schematic representation of flaviviral polyprotein processing. The middle region outlines the viral genome: line regions, the 5′ and 3′ nontranslated regions; boxed region, open reading frame for structural and nonstructural proteins. Cotranslational cleavage by host cell–encoded signalase separating structural and nonstructural proteins occurs at the E protein C-terminus. A subtilase-like cellular enzyme, furin, may be responsible for prM cleavage. Potential transmembrane regions of the viral polyprotein are indicated by shaded areas.

Of the two viral membrane-associated proteins, the 53-kd surface protein E exhibits the most important biological properties, including viral attachment to cellular receptors, specific membrane fusion, and elicitation of virus-neutralizing, hemagglutination-inhibiting, and anti-fusion antibodies.[81] Immature intracellular virions contain prM, the glycosylated precursor of the 7–8 kd M protein. Cotransport of prM-E protein heterodimers through an exocytic pathway is essential for maturation and biosynthesis of authentic E protein; prM prevents low-pH-induced rearrangements of E, acting as a chaperone for its efficient secretion and proper folding.[90–92] Before release from the cell, the prM protein is cleaved by a putative subtilase-like enzyme associated with the trans-Golgi membrane, leaving only M protein associated with the mature virion.[93]

The hydrophobic carboxyl terminus of the E protein provides a membrane-associated anchor, while an extensive ectodomain, stabilized by disulfide bridging, is folded into three antigenic domains, A, B, and C, which are variably related to (1) determinants representing flaviviral group-, subgroup-, and virus-specific epitopes and (2) biological functions.[94] Crystallographic examination of the tick-borne encephalitis (TBE) viral E protein reveals it to be a homodimer lying parallel to the viral surface. The monomers fold into three distinct structural domains—I, II, and III—corresponding to the antigenic domains, C, A, and B, respectively.[95] Domain III contains an immunoglobulin-like module extending perpendicular to the viral surface that is likely to be involved in receptor binding. Binding of JE virions to certain cells of CNS lineage may be associated with the presence of specific neurotransmitter receptors.[96] Dengue 2 virus selectively binds cellular heparan sulfates of the glycosaminoglycan (GAG) family via E protein GAG-binding motifs within the carboxyl terminal and externally accessible regions of domains I and III.[97–99] Similar mechanisms may apply to JE and other flaviviruses.

Virus-specific and cross-reactive neutralizing epitopes have been mapped to specific regions of the JE E glycoprotein.[94–100] Comprehensive cross-neutralization studies indicate the close antigenic relationship of JE virus to StLE, West Nile, Koutango, and Usutu viruses and several flaviviruses found in Australia (e.g., Murray Valley encephalitis and Kunjin, Alfuy, Stratford, and Kokobera viruses) and their classification into a single antigenic complex.[101, 102] Sequence analysis suggests they are genetically related to members of other flavivirus clades.[80] No serological cross-reactions with hepatitis C virus have been observed.[103]

The biochemical, antigenic, and genetic relationships of JE viruses isolated from different geographic regions and at various times have been compared by using polyclonal and monoclonal antibodies, two-dimensional gel electrophoresis of T1 ribonuclease (RNase)-digested virion RNA, and genomic sequencing.[104–106] The molecular phylogeny of JE viruses, based on the 240 base

Table 27–2. **GEOGRAPHICAL DISTRIBUTION OF JAPANESE ENCEPHALITIS VIRUSES BY GENOTYPE**

GENOTYPE	COUNTRY OR REGION (YEAR OF ISOLATION)
1	Japan (1935, 1955, 1957, 1959, 1979, 1982); China (1949, 1960); Korea (1982, 1987, 1991, 1994); Okinawa (1968–1992); Taiwan (1972, 1987); Philippines (1977, 1984); Vietnam (1964–1988); Nepal (1985); India (1963, 1970, 1972, 1975, 1978–1980, 1982, 1985); Sri Lanka (1969, 1987)
2	Thailand (1979, 1982–1985, 1992, 1993); Cambodia (1969)
3	Indonesia (1970, 1978, 1979, 1981); Thailand (1983); Malaysia (1970); Sarawak (1968); Australia (1995)
4	Indonesia (1981)

Data from Chen et al.,[107, 108] Huong et al.,[109] Ma et al.,[111] Ritchie et al.,[112] and Chung et al.[113]

nucleotide sequence of viral prM, divides JE isolates into four distinct genotypes, with a maximum divergence of 21% among the isolates (Table 27–2).[107–113] The largest genotype consists of viruses from Japan, Okinawa, China, Taiwan, Vietnam, the Philippines, Sri Lanka, India, and Nepal. A second genotype comprises isolates from northern Thailand and Cambodia, and a third comprises isolates from southern Thailand, Malaysia, Sarawak, Australia, and Indonesia. Five Indonesian isolates—two from Java, two from Bali, and one from Flores—similar to each other and distinct from other Indonesian isolates, form the fourth genotype. Cocirculation of multiple genotypes was observed only in Thailand and Indonesia. An antigenic analysis using five virus-specific monoclonal antibodies classified strains into four antigenic types, without correspondence to the genotypes above.

JE virus isolates from the same region but from different years show a high degree of nucleotide similarity. Sixteen Vietnam and 23 Okinawa strains of JE virus isolated between 1964 and 1988 and between 1968 and 1992 differed by only 3.2% and 4%, respectively.[108, 110] However, viruses from the same region were distinguishable chronologically, before and after 1986 in Okinawa and before and after 1975 in Vietnam. Genetic drift appears to be the main mechanism by which JE virus continuously evolves in nature, although novel viral introductions have been documented, indicating the potential for genotypic displacement.[25, 111]

PATHOGENESIS

After an infectious mosquito bite, viral replication occurs locally and in regional lymph nodes. Virions disseminate to secondary sites, where further replication contributes to an augmented viremia. Invasion of the CNS probably occurs from the blood by antipodal transport of virions through vascular endothelial cells.[40, 114–116] Infection in the CNS spreads by viral dissemination through the extracellular space or by direct intercellular spread. Sensitized helper T cells stimulate an inflammatory response by recruiting macrophages and lymphocytes to the perivascular space and parenchyma, where the inflammatory response clears infected neurons, with subsequent formation of glial nodules.[40, 66–68] The predominant cell type in the CSF and in the parenchyma are helper/inducer (CD4+) T cells, with B lymphocytes confined chiefly to the perivascular space.[116, 117]

Why only one in several hundred infections develops into symptomatic neuroinvasive disease is unclear. Factors that contribute to neuroinvasion include age and, potentially, genetic and acquired host factors.[78, 79, 118–120] Genetic resistance to infection and haplotype restriction of the immune response have been described in mice, and some observations suggest epidemiological differences in case-infection ratios in white and indigenous Asian populations.[27] Macrophages are important in the nonspecific clearance of virus, and their depletion leads to extended viremia, CNS invasion, and death in experimentally infected mice.[121] However, circulating antibody plays a critical role in modulating infection by limiting viremia in the preneuroinvasive phase. Both JE virus–specific and heterologous (e.g., dengue) antibodies contribute to protection, and low levels of neutralizing antibody may be sufficient to prevent viremia.[122–125] Guinea pigs or mice that had been previously immunized with attenuated JE vaccine and that no longer had detectable neutralizing antibodies (<1:4) were protected against intraperitoneal challenge infection and, moreover, their serum passively protected mice.[126] Experimentally infected monkeys immunosuppressed with cyclophosphamide have no measurable antibody response and exhibit an increased susceptibility to paralytic encephalitis and a diminished CNS inflammatory reaction.[127] On the other hand, passive transfer of specific monoclonal antibodies can enhance neurovirulence in intracerebrally challenged mice.[128]

Clinically, high CSF interferon alfa levels and low CSF virus-specific IgM and immunoglobulin G (IgG) antibodies have been associated with a fatal outcome, suggesting that delayed or poor local antibody response and uninhibited CNS virus proliferation determines outcome.[129, 130] The reactivities of intrathecal and serum antibodies differ in Western blot analyses, but the relationship of these response patterns to outcome is unknown. Recovered patients develop antibodies to both structural and nonstructural proteins and exhibit CD4+ and CD8+ T-cell proliferative responses to JE viral lysate, in favor of an antigen containing structural E and prM/M proteins only.[131] In the largest clinical study, only 24% of patients developed a proliferative response to whole virus or viral E protein (structural proteins), and response was not correlated with survival.[132]

Other studies have suggested an important role for immunopathological events in JE pathogenesis. Although in these studies intrathecal IgM or neutralizing antibodies did not correlate with outcome, antibodies to neural antigens (neurofilament and myelin basic protein) were associated with death, suggesting that neural damage directed a destructive autoimmune response.[72, 129, 133, 134] CSF viral immune complex formation also was associated with mortality, further implicating the potential for autoimmune injury.

Cell-mediated immune mechanisms have been described in athymic nude mice, which, in contrast to normal adult mice, die or develop an extended illness with secondary viremias after peripheral inoculation.[135, 136] Antibodies did not appear in nude mice, indicating the functional importance of helper T cells. Interestingly, although virus replicated to high titers in brain tissue, histopathological evidence of encephalitis was absent, indicating that T cells are required in mediating pathological changes. Mice immunosuppressed with cyclophosphamide and then immunized with live attenuated vaccine but not inactivated vaccine, are able to resist experimental challenge. Specific JE viral immunity can be transferred passively with spleen cells from immune mice, including animals immunized with live attenuated JE vaccine but not from those immunized with inactivated vaccine.[137–139] Both Lyt2.2$^+$ and L3T4$^+$ cells are needed to protect adult mice against intracerebral challenge, and direct intracerebral introduction of the effector cells is required, suggesting the importance of local T-cell enhancement of antibody production in the CNS.

The role of cytokines in recovery and pathogenesis has not been investigated extensively. Complementing the limited experience with interferon, experimental prophylaxis with a combination of interferon alfa and interleukin-12 (IL-12) protected mice challenged with related StLE virus; however, interferon had no effect after infection was established.[140] Nitric oxide (NO) has been shown to inhibit JE viral replication in vitro. However, in experimental TBE virus infection, NO had no effect on viral replication and exacerbated the infection.[141, 142] A viral-induced macrophage-derived chemotactic factor that modulates neutrophil activity and increases capillary permeability in mice also has been described: Its action to increase blood-brain barrier permeability was implicated in increasing viral neuroinvasion.[143]

Conditions that compromise the integrity of the blood-brain barrier have been suspected to increase risk for neuroinvasion and neurodissemination. Several observations suggest that dual infection with another infectious agent, especially neurocysticercosis, is a risk factor.[59, 69, 144–147] The incidental finding of cysts in a disproportionate number of JE cases at autopsy has indicated their potential contribution to a fatal outcome.[69, 144, 145] In addition, anecdotal observations of dual herpes and JE viral infections in autopsied human JE cases and, in one epidemic, simultaneous CNS infections with mumps and JE have been described.[147] The mechanisms by which dual infections apparently augment the risk of symptomatic illness are unclear, but increased CNS dissemination of JE virus was shown experimentally in mice infected with both JE and herpes.[146] Other physiological or structural conditions that compromise the integrity of the cerebrovasculature or the blood-brain barrier may also contribute to risk. Atherosclerotic and hypertensive cerebrovascular diseases are suspected risk factors for StLE, and foreign bodies (e.g., ventricular shunts) have predisposed patients to poliovirus neuroinvasion. Experimental disruption of the blood-brain barrier by microwave irradiation was shown to predispose mice to JE viral neuroinvasion.[25, 148, 149]

The impact of human immunodeficiency virus (HIV) infection and acquired immunodeficiency syndrome (AIDS) on the outcome of JE has not been reported; however, in several StLE outbreaks, HIV infection appeared to increase the risk for developing overt encephalitis after infection.[150]

DIAGNOSIS

Although a history of exposure to an endemic area and certain clinical features may suggest JE, clinical diagnosis is unreliable, and laboratory confirmation, usually by serological tests, is necessary. JE virus occasionally can be recovered from blood in the preneuroinvasive phase (up to 3 to 7 days after onset), but patients presenting with encephalitis usually are no longer viremic.[7, 29, 55, 151] Virus has been recovered from CSF in 68% of patients when the highly sensitive system of isolation in *Toxorhynchites splendens* mosquitoes was used.[152] Viral antigen often can be demonstrated in brain tissue when no virus can be isolated from the same specimen and when viral antibodies are undetectable. JE virus produces cytopathic effects in Vero, LLCMK$_2$, and PS cells and kills suckling mice inoculated intracerebrally. C6/36 and AP61 mosquito cell lines and *T. splendens*, inoculated intrathoracically, also are sensitive systems for viral isolation. Infection is silent in C6/36 cells, so inoculated cultures must be examined for viral antigen by immunofluorescent (IF) antibody or other techniques. Viral isolates are readily identified by IF techniques using virus-specific monoclonal antibodies or by neutralization.

The most widely used diagnostic method is IgM-capture enzyme-linked immunosorbent assay (ELISA).[57, 153] Specific IgM can be detected in CSF, serum, or both in approximately 75% of patients within the first 4 days after illness onset, and nearly all patients are positive 7 days after onset. Both fluids should be tested to maximize sensitivity. Rapid membrane-based systems for bedside serological diagnosis are in development.

In approximately 30% of cases, antigen-bearing infected cells can be identified in CSF by IF antibody before intrathecal IgM is detected, yielding a specific diagnosis within hours of a lumbar puncture. However, the procedure's sensitivity (58%) was lower than that of combined IgM-capture ELISA testing of acute serum and CSF (84%).[152] In preliminary studies, JE viral genomic sequences have been detected in CSF by polymerase chain reaction; however, detection of CSF IgM by ELISA was more sensitive. Additional comparative evaluations are needed, particularly of acute phase serum samples, which may provide a better yield than CSF.[29, 154]

A specific diagnosis also can be confirmed by demonstrating fourfold or greater changes in antibody titer by conventional serological procedures (e.g., hemagglutination inhibition, complement fixation, IF antibody, ELISA, or neutralization). Heterologous flaviviral antibodies (e.g., to dengue and West Nile viruses) are a potential source of false-positive reactions. These infections can be differentiated by epitope-blocking ELISA or by obtaining ELISA absorbance ratios to the respective antigens.[155] Synthetic antigens, including recombinant virus-like particles expressing the viral E protein, are a potential source of standardized antigen with improved specificity.[156]

EPIDEMIOLOGY

Endemic Areas in Asia

JE is transmitted in epidemics or in an endemic pattern, or both, in virtually every country of Asia (see Fig. 27–1). Officially reported cases significantly underestimate the magnitude and geographic extent of risk because of underreporting and, in some countries, widespread immunization. Transmission is seasonal, occurring approximately from May to September in temperate areas of China, Korea, Japan, and far eastern Russia. Farther south, the transmission season is somewhat longer, extending from March through October (Fig. 27–8). In tropical areas of Southeast Asia and India, seasonal transmission is particular to local patterns of monsoon rains and bird migration, with the possibility of two transmission intervals in a calendar year. The virus is transmitted throughout the year in some sites.

JE is principally a disease of rural areas in which vector mosquitoes proliferate in close association with pigs, wading birds, and ducks, the principal vertebrate amplifying hosts (Fig. 27–9).[1, 2, 29, 157, 158] Humans and horses may become ill after infection, but such illness is incidental to the transmission cycle.[159, 160] Experimental observations and field studies indicate that the virus can overwinter in vertically infected mosquitoes.[157] However, viral persistence in vertebrate hosts, such as bats and reptiles, and annual reintroductions of the virus through migrations of birds or wind-borne mosquitoes also have been hypothesized as mechanisms by which endemic foci are maintained.[157, 161] Self-limited outbreaks on Western Pacific islands, on Guam in 1947, Saipan in 1990, and the Australian Torres Strait islands in 1995 and 1998 were examples of viral introductions possibly by migratory birds or, in the last case, by windblown mosquitoes.[25, 26, 147]

Culex tritaeniorhynchus is the principal JE vector in most areas of Asia, but various principally ground pool– and rice paddy–breeding species, including *Culex vishnui*,

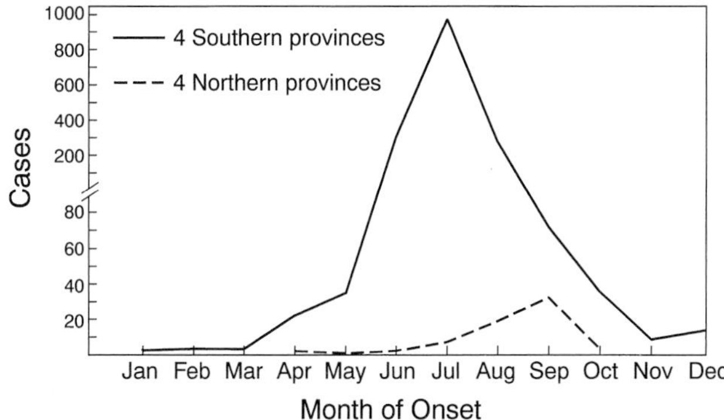

Figure 27–8. Seasonal distribution of Japanese encephalitis cases in four southern and four northern provinces, China, 1993. (From Yu YX. Japanese encephalitis in China. Southeast Asian J Trop Med Public Health 26S3:17–21, 1995.)

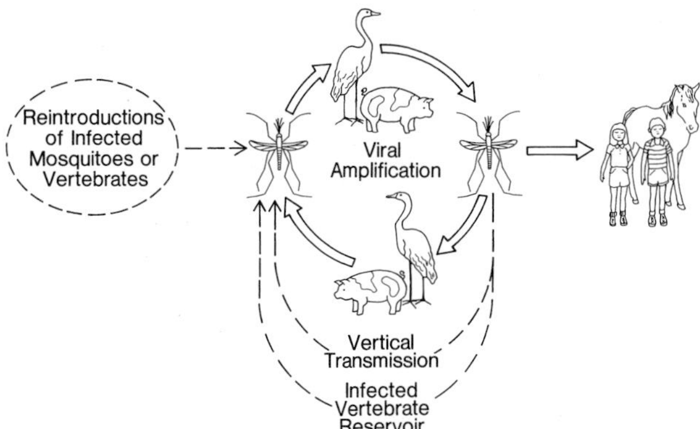

Figure 27–9. Transmission cycle of Japanese encephalitis (JE) virus. The solid arrows indicate known portions of the cycle, and the dashed arrows indicate speculative portions. Infections and clinical illnesses in humans and horses are incidental to the transmission cycle. The overwintering mechanism for JE virus is undefined, but experimental and field observations suggest a role for vertical transmission in vector mosquitoes.

Culex pseudovishnuri, *Culex gelidus*, *Culex fuscocephala*, *Culex bitaeniorhynchus*, *Culex infula*, *Culex whitmorei*, and *Culex annulus*, are also important locally.[157, 158] JE virus has been recovered from *C. pipiens pallens* and *C. quinquefasciatus* in urban locations. In addition, *Culex annulirostris* has been identified as a vector in the Western Pacific, *Aedes togoi* in sylvatic locations in Siberia, and members of the *Anopheles hyrcanus* group in northeastern India.[20, 111] Although vector abundance and risk for human infection are associated with rainfall, with increased implementation of irrigation in rice cultivation, paddy-flooding schedules increasingly influence vector bionomics. Single paddies can produce more than 30,000 adult mosquitoes in a day, so collectively, these artificial breeding sites overpower the impact of natural sources. In these circumstances, mosquito abundance fluctuates with periodic rice field flooding and can peak at any time of the year, including the dry season.[162, 163]

In temperate regions vector mosquitoes emerge in May, and after several initial rounds of viral amplification, high rates of pig seroconversion are detected, followed almost immediately by the onset of human cases, typically in July and August. By virtue of high levels and lengthy periods of viremia after infection and their prevalence as domestic animals, pigs are the key hosts for viral amplification. Infections in adult pigs are asymptomatic, but infection during pregnancy frequently results in abortions and stillbirths, with significant economic losses. In some locations enzootic transmission of the virus is initiated among aquatic birds, and in well-characterized outbreaks in which pigs were absent, such birds have served as epidemic amplifying hosts.[164, 165] Other domesticated animals, such as cattle, dogs, sheep, cows, and chickens, and peridomestic rodents may become infected, but these fail to develop a sufficient viremia to support further viral amplification.[166] JE mosquito vectors are zoophilic; consequently, cows and certain other animals can reduce risk to humans by diverting vector mosquitoes (zooprophylaxis).[167] Immunization of pigs prevents abortion and stillbirths and also may reduce viral transmission by nullifying

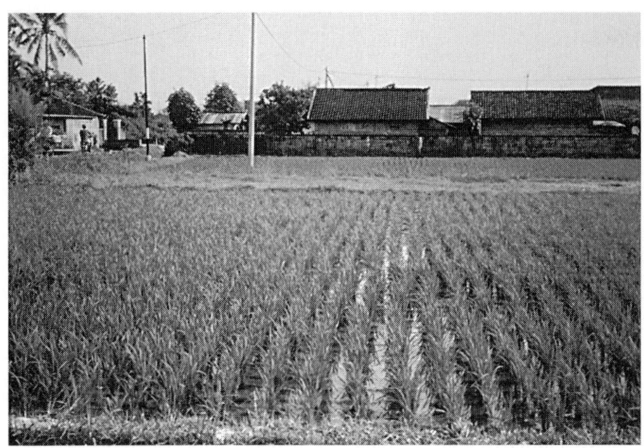

Figure 27–10. Indonesia. Flooded rice paddies are the principal breeding sites for larval stages of Japanese encephalitis virus mosquito vectors. The disease is transmitted chiefly in rural areas, especially in those employing irrigation schemes, where vector mosquitoes and pigs, the principal vertebrate amplifying host, are abundant near human residences.

the role of pigs as viral amplifiers.[167–169] Experimental immunization of nearly the entire pig inventory on one island led to a significant reduction in human cases.[167]

In rural villages all elements of the enzootic transmission cycle are found in proximity to human residences and activities (Fig. 27–10). Consequently, exposure and infection occur at an early age. In areas where transmission is hyperendemic, half of all cases occur in children younger than 4 years of age, and nearly all cases are found in children younger than 10 years (Fig. 27–11). Usually cases in males exceed those in females, possibly reflecting greater outdoor exposure in boys. Typical incidence rates in those younger than 19 years range from 1 to more than 10 per 10,000 per year. For example, in Tamil Nadu (southern India) and in the Changmai Valley (northern Thailand), rates were 6 and 4 per 10,000, respectively. Seroprevalence studies disclose nearly universal infection by early adulthood, and in areas where enzootic viral transmission is particularly intense, seroprevalence rates may increase by 25% per year during childhood. By one estimate, the minimum probability of an infectious mosquito bite in Tamil Nadu was 0.47 to 0.77 per year.[28, 170]

Behavioral and other factors associated with the risk of acquiring JE vary regionally. Household crowding, religion, ethnicity, exposure to domestic animals, and lack of air conditioning were detected as risk factors in some studies.[6, 25, 171] Use of permethrin-impregnated mosquito nets, but not untreated nets, is protective.[172] Although risk for acquiring JE is greatest in rural areas, conditions that permit enzootic viral transmission exist within or at the periphery of many Asian cities. For example, JE cases in Taiwan are reported principally from areas surrounding Taipei; in Vietnam, JE incidence is highest in and near Hanoi; and in India, urban outbreaks have occurred in Lucknow. Cases frequently are reported from suburban areas of major cities such as Bangkok, Beijing, and Shanghai. In a study to determine the causes of childhood encephalitis cases hospitalized in Beijing, JE was the etiology in 5% of cases, herpes virus in 2%, mumps in 7%, and enteroviruses in 15%.[173] The relative frequency of JE cases is notable, since the disease is not considered to be endemic in northern China and immunization coverage in Beijing is high. Sporadic reports of cases from Hong Kong and, previously, Singapore (vide infra) attest to the possibility of enzootic viral transmission near highly developed urban areas.

In developed Asian countries (e.g., Japan and Korea), JE incidence has decreased over several decades to fewer than 5 cases annually (see Fig. 27–2). A number of factors other than immunization have contributed to the decline, including secular trends toward a higher standard of living; a reduction in land under cultivation; and changes in agricultural practices, especially the increased use of pesticides and centralized pig production. The impact of economic development and secular factors has been demonstrated most clearly in Singapore, which has no national immunization program. Although JE previously was endemic on the island, no indigenous cases have been detected since 1992, and serosurveys have shown no antibodies in children younger than 12 years of age, indicating the near elimination of viral transmission through indirect secular changes, mosquito control, and complete prohibition of pig rearing on the island.[174] Although imported pigs are held briefly in quarantine, their segregation from the human population probably has had a major impact on viral amplification.

In countries where childhood cases have been prevented by immunization, the age distribution of cases has shifted toward adults, and particularly to the elderly. In Japan the previous bimodal age distribution of cases, with peaks in young children and in the elderly, has shifted toward a predominance of cases in adults (Fig. 27–12).[11, 175] A similar pattern holds in Korea and has emerged in developed municipalities of China. An analysis of age-specific incidence by decade in an area of Shanghai showed that since 1961, case rates declined most dramatically in children, reflecting the impact of

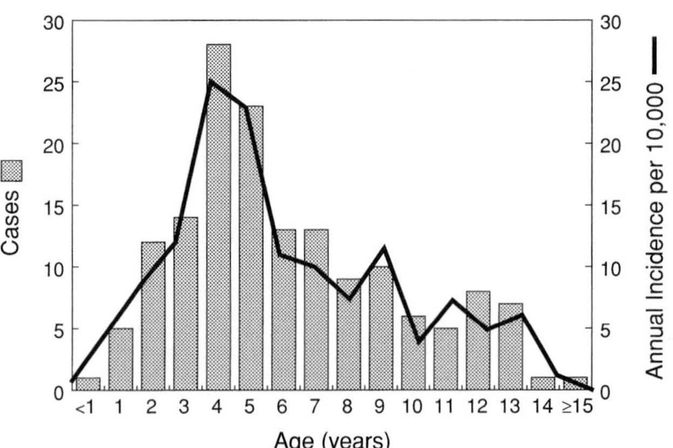

Figure 27–11. Reported Japanese encephalitis cases and age-specific incidence, Nallur Primary Health Centre, South Arcot District, Tamil, Nadu, India, 1986 to 1990. (Adapted with permission from Gajanana A, Thenmozi V, Samuel P, Reuben R. A community-based study of subclinical flavivirus infections in children in an area of Tamil Nadu, India, where Japanese encephalitis is endemic. Bull World Health Organ 73:237–244, 1995.)

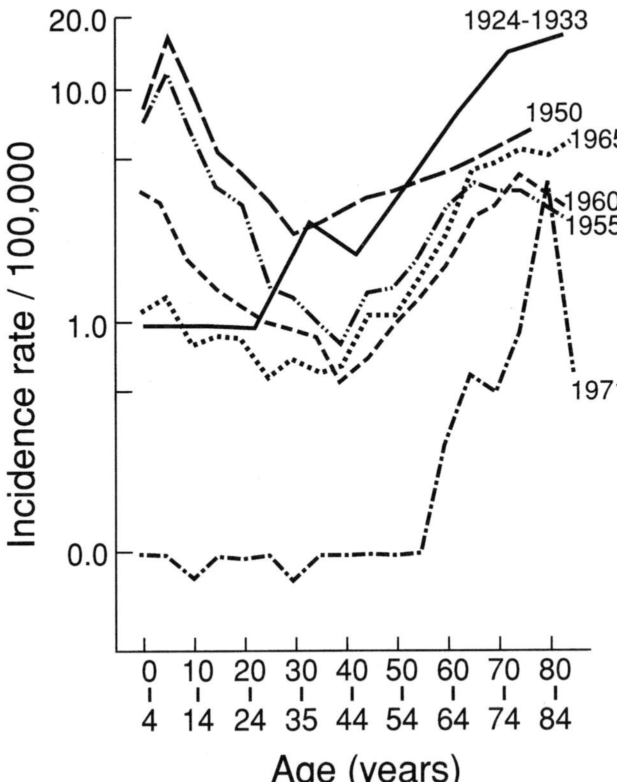

Figure 27–12. Age-specific incidence of Japanese encephalitis in Japan, 1924 to 1971. Although Japanese encephalitis is most visible as a childhood disease, the age-specific incidence is bimodal, with elevated risk in children and the elderly. As a result of universal childhood immunization, sporadic cases now occur almost exclusively in the elderly. The causes of increased risk with advanced age are unknown. (Adapted from Oya A. Epidemiology of Japanese encephalitis, Rinsho to Biseibutsu. Clin Diagn Microbiol 16:5–9, 1989.)

immunization; however, rates also declined in other age groups, reflecting a secular decrease in risk (Fig. 27–13).[176] The result is that incidence rates are similar in both adults and children.

In Taiwan, age-specific incidence is highest in adults 20 to 39 years old, probably because this cohort is too old to have been immunized fully when mass vaccinations began in 1968 and too young to have acquired infections naturally in a developing society. The loss of vaccine-derived immunity can be inferred from declining JE antibody prevalence rates, from 49% in primary school to 38% in junior high school, 34% in junior college, and 29% in university students.[177] A similar trend also has been seen in Japan, where the induction and maintenance of immunity, presumably by immunization, through the first decade of life is followed by a subsequent decline, reflecting loss of vaccine-induced antibodies (Fig. 27–14).[11] The subsequent rise in antibody rates in people older than 35 probably represents naturally acquired immunity in cohorts born before national JE immunization was established in the 1960s.

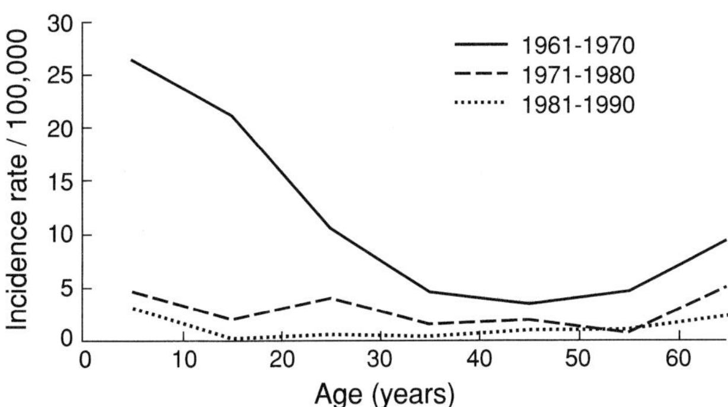

Figure 27–13. Age-specific incidence of Japanese encephalitis, Nanshi District, Shanghai, by decade. (From Xu ZY, personal communication, 1997.)

Waning vaccine-induced immunity, age-related host factors, and reduced opportunities for natural exposure and "boosting" infections in an increasingly urban population undoubtedly will contribute to a rising risk in adults. Although the paradigm that JE is principally a pediatric disease has changed in locations with universal childhood immunization, the relative importance of cases in adults has yet to be addressed as a public health priority. Surveillance to measure JE incidence in adults and to detect cases of secondary vaccine failure should be undertaken to determine the need for booster doses after childhood.

Travelers and Expatriates

Although JE vaccine is used principally in Asia to protect local populations, the vaccine also is marketed in developed countries for travelers to Asia, expatriates, and especially military personnel. (For the purposes of this discussion, *expatriates* are defined as residents through a transmission season.) Sporadic cases have been reported in travelers from North America, Europe, Russia, Israel, and Australia and, paradoxically, in Japanese and Taiwanese tourists to other endemic areas of Asia (see Chapter 24, previous edition).[178–182]

No systematically collected data on cases in travelers are available; however, informal surveillance of diagnos-

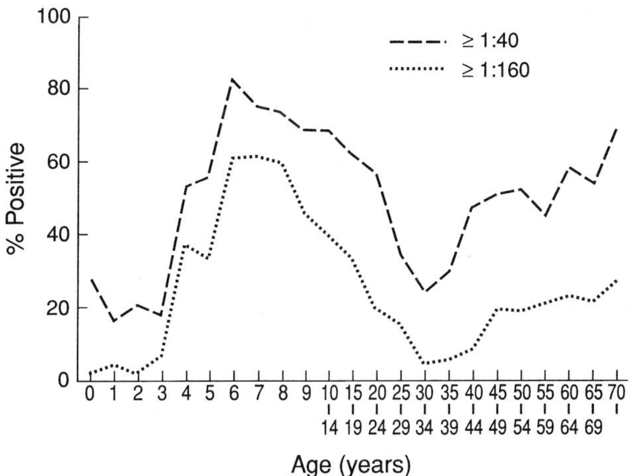

Figure 27–14. Age-specific seroprevalence of Japanese encephalitis neutralizing antibodies, Japan, 1994; age-balanced random sample of 10 prefectures (n = 2027). (From Taniguchi K, Matsunaga Y. National epidemiologic surveillance of vaccine-preventable diseases, Japan. Available at http://www.nih.go.jp/yoken/idsc/ryukou/japa_Efig1.gif. October 1995.)

Table 27–3. **JAPANESE ENCEPHALITIS IN NONIMMUNIZED AMERICAN AND OTHER WESTERN MILITARY PERSONNEL, 1945 TO 1991**

LOCATION	YEAR	NO. OF CASES	APPROXIMATE POPULATION AT RISK	RATE/10,000/WEEK	REFERENCE
Okinawa	1991	3	19,000	0.1*	182
Thailand	1972	9	2,500	2.1†	32
Vietnam‡	1966–1967	2	2,000	0.9§	183
Korea	1958	3	860	1.6§	27
Korea‖	1950	103	114,813	0.4§	187
Korea	1946	3	1,500	0.9§	186
Okinawa	1945	11	77,000¶	0.05*	200

*Rate based on exposure during a 6-month transmission season.
†Rate based on exposure during 4 months.
‡Australian personnel.
§Rate based on exposure during a 5-month transmission season.
‖American and British personnel.
¶Partially immunized population.

tic laboratories suggests that risk is extremely low. Among 24 cases reported to the Centers for Disease Control and Prevention (CDC) from 1978 through 1992, 11 occurred in expatriates, 8 of whom were U.S. military personnel or their dependents. Among other cases in Americans, only one was in a tourist, one was in a summer student, and in one case the exposure history was unknown. U.S. Department of Transportation statistics indicate that 2 to 3 million U.S. citizens travel by air to Asia each year; however, these figures overestimate the population at risk, because most travelers have brief itineraries without exposure to at-risk areas, and others may have been immunized. Annual incidence in American travelers can be estimated roughly at well under 1 per 1 million.

Risk also can be extrapolated from attack rates in unimmunized American, Australian, and British soldiers exposed in Asia. Rates have ranged from 0.05 to 2.1 per 10,000 per week in soldiers who were exposed intensely under field conditions, in some instances during epidemics (Table 27–3).[27, 32, 182–187] These rates are similar to those among children residing in hyperendemic areas, where annual reported incidence rates typically are in the range of 0.1 to 1 per 10,000. Accepting the high estimate and recognizing that transmission is limited to about a 5-month period in most areas, the monthly risk can be estimated as 1 per 50,000 per month, or 1 per 200,000 per week.

The relatively low risk for acquiring JE after a single mosquito bite can be appreciated by considering the following probabilities of infection and illness:

1. Only bites of vector species are potentially infectious.
2. Even in extreme circumstances, viral infection rates in vector mosquitoes rarely exceed 3%.
3. If an individual is infected, infection results in symptomatic neuroinvasive illness in fewer than 1 per 200 cases.

Further reducing the risk of an infectious bite, *C. tritaeniorhynchus* and other JE vectors are chiefly zoophilic and prefer animal rather than human hosts. They feed chiefly in the evening and during the crepuscular (twilight) periods at dawn and dusk, and though they may enter houses to feed, they principally are exophilic and seek hosts outdoors. Travelers can lower risk further by wearing mosquito repellant and long-sleeved shirts and trousers, by avoiding outdoor activities in the evening, and by sleeping under permethrin-impregnated mosquito nets or in screened or air-conditioned rooms.[188, 189]

Risk for acquiring JE during travel is highly variable and depends on the destination and season of travel and the activities of the individual (Table 27–4). Although travelers who remain in rural areas for extended periods are at greatest risk, well-publicized cases have been reported in travelers with brief itineraries in resorts or urban locations.[178–180] For example, in 1996, three cases were reported among travelers to Bali, perhaps a unique situation that may reflect the proximity of local tourist hotels and beaches to areas with intense enzootic viral transmission.

IMMUNIZATION

Passive Immunization

JE immune plasma and immune globulin are not commercially available. Experimental data in mice, goats, and rhesus monkeys indicate a prophylactic and therapeutic potential for polyclonal or a mixture of JE mono-

Table 27–4. **RISK FACTORS FOR ACQUIRING JAPANESE ENCEPHALITIS DURING TRAVEL TO ASIA**

Risk factors
Travel to developing country
Travel during transmission season
Travel to rural areas
Extended period of travel or residence
Outdoor activities, especially in twilight period and evenings
Advanced age
Pregnancy (risk to developing fetus)
Protective factors
Repellents
Protective clothing
Residence in air-conditioned or well-screened areas
Permethrin-treated mosquito nets

clonal antibodies, although combined peripheral and either intraspinal or subdural administration was required for maximum effect with the latter.[63, 190–192] A small controlled trial in humans suggested a potential therapeutic benefit of passive immunization with the antibody combination (see preceding section on clinical illness).[63] However, experience with prophylaxis of TBE using human TBE-specific immune globulin indicates that antibody must be administered within a short period after tick exposure to be effective and that late administration (i.e., after 4 days) may worsen outcome.[193] Although there are few data, early treatment with interferon alfa, perhaps in combination with immune plasma, may be an effective approach to prophylaxis of illness after known exposure, such as in a laboratory accident.[29, 64, 140] Information on availability of immune plasma can be obtained from the U.S. Army Medical Research Institute for Infectious Diseases, Frederick, MD, or the Walter Reed Army Medical Center, Washington, DC.

Active Immunization

Worldwide, three JE vaccines are in widespread production and use (Table 27–5); however, only inactivated JE vaccine produced in mouse brain is distributed commercially and is available internationally.[194, 195] Inactivated JE vaccine and live attenuated JE vaccine, both grown in primary hamster kidney (PHK) cells, are manufactured and distributed exclusively in the People's Republic of China (PRC). Despite an apparently limited pattern of domestic distribution, more than 70 million doses of inactivated PHK vaccine and 30 million doses of live attenuated vaccine are produced and distributed annually in the PRC, whereas all manufacturers in Japan produce approximately 11 million doses of mouse brain–derived vaccine for domestic use in Japan. Biken, the principal Japanese manufacturer of inactivated mouse brain vaccine, distributes about 2 million doses abroad by arrangement through Pasteur Mérieux Connaught. The vaccine is licensed as JE-VAX in the United States, Canada, Israel, and several Asian countries, but is still distributed under special exemptions in most European countries.

Inactivated Mouse Brain–Derived Japanese Encephalitis Vaccine

Inactivated mouse brain–derived JE vaccines were produced in Russia and Japan in the 1930s, and the former was shown to be efficacious against Russian autumnal encephalitis (a synonym for JE).[196] During World War II, a simple uncentrifuged 10% suspension of infected mouse brain, inactivated with formalin, was produced in the United States as a vaccine for the military. The vaccine was variably immunogenic, but efficacy field trials could not be completed.[197–200]

A more stable inactivated chick embryo–derived vaccine, also developed by the U.S. military, had an 80% efficacy in children given a combination of mouse brain– and chick embryo–derived vaccines.[201–205] However, the latter vaccine was less immunogenic in adults, and its efficacy in soldiers never could be evaluated. Although this vaccine was given to all U.S. soldiers assigned to Asia from 1948 to 1951, use was discontinued in 1952 after review of available data failed to produce convincing evidence of immunogenicity and efficacy.[183–187]

Successive refinements of the mouse brain vaccine were introduced by research institutes in Japan, leading to the current purified vaccine (Fig. 27–15).[195, 206, 207] Mouse brain–derived vaccines are produced in Japan and elsewhere using a similar sequence of centrifugation, ultrafiltration, protamine sulfate precipitation, and formalin inactivation in the cold, followed by further purification by ultrafiltration, ammonium sulfate precipitation, and continuous zonal centrifugation on sucrose density gradients. National standards in Japan specify minimal immunogenicity and potency in mice (compared with a vaccine standard) and maximal total protein (80 μg per mL) and myelin basic protein content (2 ng per mL), among other specifications. Bulk vaccine is diluted with medium 199 and phosphate buffer to meet a potency standard.[208, 209] Although the quantity of JE E protein is not controlled, in one study a dose was estimated to contain approximately 50 μg. The vaccine is stabilized with gelatin and sodium glutamate and preserved with thimerosal. In Japan, the vaccine is distributed principally in liquid form; for international distribution, it is lyophilized and reconstituted with sterile water.

Table 27–5. **JAPANESE ENCEPHALITIS VACCINES**

VACCINE TYPE	SUBSTRATE	VIRAL STRAINS	MANUFACTURERS
Inactivated	Mouse brain	Nakayama, Beijing-1 (P1)	*India:* Central Research Institute (currently inactive) *Japan:* Biken (Research Foundation for Microbial Disease of Osaka University), Chiba, Denka-Seiken Co., Ltd., Chemo-Sero Therapeutic Research Institute, Kitasato Institute, Saikin-Kagaku Institute, Takeda *Korea:* Green Cross *Taiwan:* National Institute of Preventive Medicine, Guo-Guang *Thailand:* Government Pharmaceutical Organization *Vietnam:* National Institute of Hygiene
Inactivated	Primary hamster kidney cells	P3	*People's Republic of China:* Beijing, Shanghai, and Changchun Institutes of Biological Products
Live attenuated	Primary hamster kidney cells	SA14-14-2	*People's Republic of China:* Chengdu, Wuhan Institutes of Biological Products

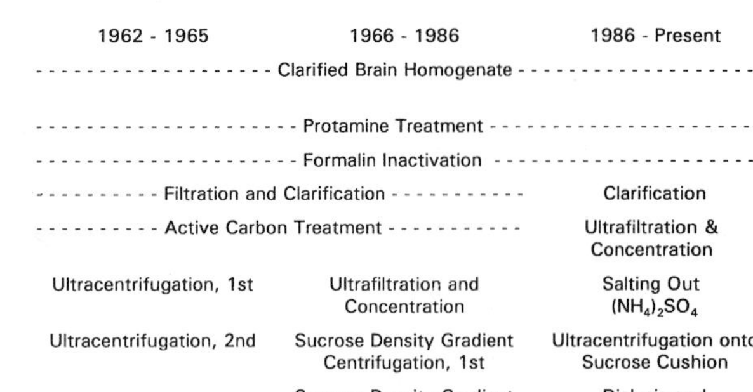

Figure 27–15. Evolution of purification procedure for inactivated Japanese encephalitis vaccine derived from infected mouse brain. (Adapted from Oya A. Japanese encephalitis vaccine. In Fukumi H [ed]. Vaccination Theory and Practice. Tokyo, International Medical Foundation of Japan, 1975, pp 69–82; and Oya A. Japanese encephalitis vaccine. Acta Pediatr Japon 30:175–184, 1988.)

Vaccine Stability and Storage. Lyophilized Biken vaccine is stable at 4°C for at least 1 year and retains more than 90% of its potency after 28 weeks at 22°C. At 37°C, lyophilized vaccine retains 95% of its original potency after 4 weeks. After reconstitution, vaccine is stable at 22°C for at least 2 weeks, but at 37°C, potency declines to 85%.[210]

A field study in Thailand showed that seroconversion rates were higher after immunization with lyophilized vaccine than after immunization with liquid vaccine. A moderate loss of potency was demonstrated after liquid vaccine was exposed to simulated field conditions.[211]

Viral Strains. The Nakayama strain of JE virus, isolated from the CSF of a patient in 1935 and maintained by continuous mouse brain passage, has been the principal strain used in mouse brain–derived vaccines produced throughout Asia.[195] The strain was chosen because of good propagation characteristics and because it provided cross-protection against other JE viral strains in mice. Cross-immunization studies in mice with strains from diverse areas of Asia indicated that strains of the JaGAr01/Beijing type (e.g., Beijing-1, known as P1 in China, and the equivalent P3 strain; see later discussion) confer a broader neutralizing antibody response against various JE viral isolates than does the Nakayama strain (Fig. 27–16).[212–216] The Beijing-1 strain grows to higher titer and the vaccine produces higher heterologous antibody titers in immunized mice than does the Nakayama strain vaccine. Although vaccine produced from either strain meets standardized mouse protection tests for potency, the Beijing-1 vaccine is formulated in half the volume. Biken, the principal Japanese manufacturer of JE vaccine, has used the Beijing-1 strain since 1989 in vaccine produced for domestic consumption, whereas the Nakayama strain is used in vaccines distributed internationally.

A natural diversity of JE viral strains has been demonstrated in minor antigenic differences and in biological characteristics such as growth in cell culture and neuroinvasiveness in experimentally infected mice. However, there is no evidence of corresponding differences in human pathogenicity and no evidence that immunity to one strain would not protect against disease caused by another.[217, 218]

Dosage and Route of Administration. In most areas of Asia, vaccine produced from the Nakayama strain is given subcutaneously in two 0.5-mL doses 1 to 4 weeks apart (1.0 mL for people >3 years of age) usually beginning at the age of 12 to 36 months, with a booster dose at 1 year and additional booster doses thereafter at 1- to 3-year intervals.[195] In practice, immunization schedules are quite variable. The Biken package insert recommends an interval of 1 to 2 weeks for primary immunization; however, many immunogenicity studies have used a 4-week interval. Primary vaccination is recommended at 18 months of age in Thailand, at 15 to 27 months of age in Taiwan, at 3 years of age in Korea, and at 6 to 90 months of age (usually 36 months) in Japan. Boosters are given a year later and, in Taiwan, once again at school entry; in Korea, boosters previously were given annually until 15 years of age, but a revised schedule of triennial boosters recently has been recommended. Boosters are given at 4 years, 9 to 12 years, and 14 to 15 years of age in Japan. Beijing-1 strain–derived vaccine is formulated with a higher antigen concentration, and the recommended dose is 0.5 mL (0.25 mL for children under 3 years of age).[216, 219]

The primary series has been administered to infants (with diphtheria, pertussis, and tetanus vaccine) as early as 2 months of age in clinical trials, but because JE rarely occurs in infants younger than 1 year, there is no need to begin immunization at that age other than to save administration costs.[220]

Immunogenicity studies in subjects from areas with-

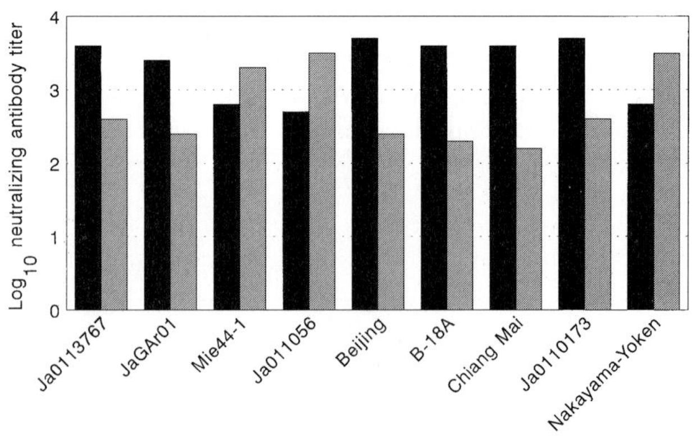

Figure 27–16. Neutralizing antibody response to various Japanese encephalitis (JE) viral strains in mice immunized with inactivated Nakayama or Beijing strains of JE vaccines. The latter conferred a broader heterologous response in immunized mice, but evidence of better protective efficacy in humans is lacking. (Adapted from The Research Foundation for Microbial Diseases of Osaka University. Japanese encephalitis vaccine lyophilized, "Biken." Unpublished report, 1991, pp 1–149.)

Table 27–6. **RECOMMENDED IMMUNIZATION SCHEDULE FOR INACTIVATED JAPANESE ENCEPHALITIS VACCINE**

VACCINEES	PRIMARY*	BOOSTER*
Adults and children ≥3 yr	1.0 mL given on days 0, 7, and 30†	1.0 mL given at 2 yr of age and thereafter at intervals of 3 yr or as determined by serological testing
Children >6 mo and <3 yr	0.5 mL in schedule as above	0.5 mL in schedule as above

*All doses given subcutaneously.
†An abbreviated schedule of immunization on days 0, 7, and 14 should be used only when the recommended schedule cannot be followed.

out endemic transmission (Western countries and areas of India) indicate that three doses are necessary for an adequate antibody response (see later discussion).[181, 221–223] The U.S. Public Health Service (Advisory Committee on Immunization Practices) (ACIP) recommends three doses, on days 0, 7, and 30 (Table 27–6).[224] An abbreviated schedule in which doses are administered on days 0, 7, and 14 also results in uniform seroconversion; however, neutralizing antibody titers are significantly lower. Although approximately 80% of vaccinees respond after two doses, this schedule is not recommended.[181] Recommendations for booster doses are based on limited data. Neutralizing antibody titers were maintained for 3 years in 37 of 39 U.S. Army vaccinees given the Biken vaccine; however, recent field studies indicate greater variability in antibody persistence.[221] Until further data become available, a booster dose is recommended 2 years after the primary series and thereafter as determined by serological monitoring.[224]

In a study of infants less than 1 year of age, simultaneous administration of inactivated JE vaccine with measles, the DPT vaccine and the oral polio vaccine (OPV) did not result in reduced immunogenicity or increased side effects. Under Thailand's Expanded Program of Immunization, JE vaccine is given concurrently with the fourth dose of DPT and OPV at 18 months.[220, 225] A comparison of administration routes in adults showed that a 0.1-mL intradermal dose may be as immunogenic as the standard administration of 1.0 mL subcutaneously, at least when given as a booster.[226] It is unknown whether malaria prophylaxis with chloroquine or mefloquine adversely affects the immune response to JE vaccine in a way similar to the effect on inactivated rabies and live oral cholera vaccines.

Inactivated Primary Hamster Kidney Cell–Derived Japanese Encephalitis Vaccine

Inactivated JE vaccine prepared from the P3 strain in PHK cells is produced exclusively in the PRC and has been that country's principal JE vaccine since 1968.[194] Approximately 70 million doses are distributed annually, making this the most widely used JE vaccine worldwide. The PRC previously had relied on a succession of inactivated mouse brain– and whole chick embryo–derived vaccines, as described earlier. Attempts to produce a cell culture–derived JE vaccine were motivated by concerns about potential contaminating neural antigens and allergic reactions associated with the crude vaccines, and also by the desire to improve immunogenicity and ease of production. Among the numerous primary and continuous cell culture systems that were examined, PHK cells were discovered to produce the highest infectious yield.[227]

Vaccine is prepared in primary cell cultures derived from kidneys of golden Syrian hamsters. Monolayers are washed of growth medium and infected with JE virus. One day later, infected monolayers are washed and refed. The supernatant cell culture fluid is inactivated with 0.05% formalin, stabilized with 0.1% human albumin, and tested for residual infectivity and potency. Liquid vaccine retains potency for more than 2 years at 4 to 8°C.

Viral Strain. The P3 strain of JE virus was recovered in 1949 from the brain of a human patient during the P1 (Beijing-1) strain epidemic. The virus was passaged 70 times in mouse brains and is maintained at the National Institute for Control of Pharmaceutical and Biological Products (NICPBP) in Beijing. Inactivated PHK cell–derived vaccine made from the P3 strain is more immunogenic, produces a better heterologous antibody response (to Nakayama virus), and confers greater cross-protection in mice than the Biken manufactured mouse brain–derived Nakayama strain vaccine. The inclusion of both P3 and Nakayama strains in a bivalent inactivated PHK cell culture vaccine was synergistic in mouse protection tests.[194] This experimental formulation has not been evaluated in humans.

Dosage and Route of Administration. JE vaccine is given seasonally in early spring without concurrent administration of other vaccines. Vaccination schedules vary locally. In the officially recommended schedule, the vaccine is administered subcutaneously in two 0.5-mL doses, 1 week apart, to children 12 months of age. Three booster doses are given 1 year later (0.5 mL) and at 6 years of age and again at 10 years of age (1.0 mL). In some provinces boosters are given annually until age 10. In Hunan province, where JE cases were occurring at a young age, primary immunization with two doses was begun at 6 months, with four subsequent boosters—the so-called "6-6" schedule.[228]

Because vaccination is given only during annual spring campaigns rather than at a specific chronological age in childhood, children who miss the annual opportunity for vaccination remain unprotected through the transmission season.

In one study, concurrent administration with the bacille Calmette-Guérin (BCG), measles, or DPT vaccine at 6 to 10 months of age was not associated with increased adverse events and, compared with JE vaccine administered alone, led to higher JE ELISA antibodies in the first two groups and to no change in the last. Concurrent JE vaccine administration did not lead to significant changes in responses to measles or DPT antibody titers or in the size of BCG reactions.[229]

Enhanced Inactivated Japanese Encephalitis Vaccine Produced in Primary Hamster Kidney Cells.

Experimental inactivated vaccines with higher potencies were formulated by concentrating the standard inactivated PHK cell–derived vaccine through an ultrafilter (10-fold concentrated vaccine), followed by ultracentrifugation (purified virion vaccine). In a field trial, one subcutaneous 1.0-mL dose of enhanced-potency vaccine produced uniform seroconversion to homologous P3 antigen and levels of heterologous antibody to Nakayama virus similar to those obtained with two doses of standard vaccine.[194] Efforts to develop these vaccines further have been discontinued, because the complexity and expense of the purification procedures were thought to be impractical.

Live Attenuated Japanese Encephalitis Vaccine

Attenuated JE viral strains have been sought by passaging wild strains serially in various cell culture systems, including PHK, chick embryo, and embryo mouse skin cells.[230–233] Loss of neurovirulence in mice, hamsters, or pigs, or any combination of the three, initially suggested the possibility of safe use in humans. Attenuation may be correlated with decreased binding to mouse brain cell receptors.[233a] Typical of laboratory attenuated viruses, OCT-541, a temperature-dependent strain obtained by serial PHK cell passage, was overattenuated, with a loss of infectivity in horses and in humans. Workers at the NICPBP in Beijing pursued attenuation of JE virus in PHK cells and derived strain SA14-14-2, which proved to be safe and immunogenic in animals and humans (see Table 27–5).[234–238] The vaccine's efficacy was demonstrated in field trials and was licensed in the PRC in 1988. Currently, 30 million doses are distributed annually in 13 southwestern provinces and in other selected regions, but expanded production and distribution are planned.

Several hundred ampules of seed virus, prepared from the seventh passage level of SA14-14-2 virus, are maintained in lots at the NICPBP in Beijing. Lyophilized seed virus (PHK_6) is provided to the production institute, where it is passaged twice for the production seed (PHK_8). PHK cells are obtained from 10- to 12-day-old golden Syrian hamsters maintained in closed colonies at the Chengdu and Wuhan Production Institutes. Monolayers are inoculated with diluted virus, and cells are fed with minimal essential medium containing 0.25% human albumin, gentamicin, and kanamycin. Infected cell culture fluid with an infectious titer of approximately $10^{7.2}$ pfu per mL is harvested at 78 to 96 hours and coarsely filtered, and the resulting liquid vaccine is lyophilized. Gelatin (1%) and sucrose (5%) are added as stabilizers. Lyophilized vaccine is reconstituted and diluted with sterile phosphate-buffered saline (PBS) (pH 7.4–7.6).[239]

Vaccine must meet standards for freedom from adventitious agents, absence of neurovirulence in adult mice, and stability against reversion to neurovirulence after intracerebral passage in suckling mice. Although examination for contaminating retroviruses has not been required in the PRC, an evaluation in the United States found no evidence of reverse transcriptase activity (dual-template method) in finished or bulk vaccine or in production cell cultures. Potency is confirmed in a mouse assay by measuring protection against P3 viral challenge 14 days after immunization with a single vaccine dose. The vaccine should provide more than 80% protection against challenge with approximately 1000 mouse median lethal dose (LD_{50}) (a 10^{-5} dilution of standard viral challenge dose of approximately 10^8 mouse LD_{50}). Recently potency testing has been required on only 50% of lots. The finished vaccine must have an infectious titer exceeding $10^{5.7}$ pfu per mL.

Vaccine Stability and Storage. The infectious titer of lyophilized vaccine is not appreciably changed after storage at 37°C for 7 to 10 days, at room temperature for 4 months, or at 4 to 8°C for at least 1.5 years. After reconstitution with sterile saline or distilled water and storage at 23°C, the vaccine's infectious titer is stable for 2 to 4 hours or 2 hours, respectively.[239]

Viral Strain. The vaccine parent strain, SA14, was isolated in 1954 from *C. pipiens* larvae collected in Xian (Table 27–7). After isolation and 11 serial passages in weanling mice, the virus was attenuated through 100 passages in PHK cells at 36 to 37°C. Neurovirulence in monkeys had been lost at this passage level. Further plaque selection and cloning in chick embryo cells and subpassages in mice and hamsters by peripheral and oral infection were necessary, however, to obtain a stable aneurovirulent virus. The resulting SA14-5-3 strain no longer reverted to an established criterion of neurovirulence after intracerebral passage in suckling mice while remaining potent in mouse immunization-challenge studies.[234–238, 240–245]

SA14-5-3 virus did not kill 3-week-old mice by either subcutaneous or direct intracerebral inoculation. Direct intrathalamic and intraspinal inoculation of the virus in monkeys resulted in no mortality or morbidity and a minimal degree of CNS inflammation, limited to areas around the injection sites. Histopathological changes were characterized by perivascular lymphocytic cuffs and focal mononuclear cell infiltration, with rare direct neuronal degeneration or necrosis.

SA14-5-3 vaccine was shown to be safe in humans,

Table 27–7. **PASSAGE HISTORY OF JAPANESE ENCEPHALITIS SA14-14-2 VIRUS**

• SA14 virus isolated from pool of *Culex pipiens* larvae	Parent
• One hundred serial passages in primary hamster kidney (PHK) cells; three plaque purifications in primary chick embryo (CE) cells	Clone 12-1-7
• Two× plaque purification in CE cells	Clone 17-4
• One mouse IP passage; spleen harvested for CE cell plaque passage	Clone 2
• Three× plaque purification in CE cells	Clone 9
• One mouse SC passage; skin harvested for one CE cell plaque passage	Clone 9-7
• Six hamster PO passages; spleens harvested for 2× plaque purification in PHK cells	Clone 5-3
• Five suckling mouse SC passages (using skin and peripheral lymph node inocula); 2× PHK cell plaque purifications	Clone 14-2

IP, intraperitoneal; PO, per os; SC, subcutaneous.

Table 27–8. **EFFICACY OF SA14-5-3 ATTENUATED JAPANESE ENCEPHALITIS VACCINE, GUANGTONG, PEOPLE'S REPUBLIC OF CHINA**

YEAR	VACCINATED	JE CASES	UNVACCINATED	JE CASES	EFFICACY (95% CI) (%)
1973	205,359	58	26,180	63	88 (85–92)
1974	205,301	12	26,117	22	93 (90–97)
1975	205,289	8	26,095	7	85 (70–95)
1976	205,281	7	26,088	13	93 (88–97)
1977	205,274	3	26,075	9	96 (92–99)

CI, confidence interval; JE, Japanese encephalitis.

and field trials in endemic areas disclosed seroconversion rates greater than 85%. However, rates of only 61% were obtained in subjects from nonendemic areas.[234] Expanded field trials in southern China involving more than 200,000 immunized children confirmed the vaccine's safety and yielded efficacies ranging from 88 to 96% over 5 years (Table 27–8).[246] However, the vaccine's poor immunogenicity in flavivirus-naive subjects from nonendemic areas suggested that SA14-5-3 virus, like previous live JE virus candidate vaccines, had been overattenuated and did not replicate uniformly in humans. To increase immunogenicity, SA14-5-3 virus was serially passaged five times by subcutaneous inoculation of suckling mice, using skin, subcutaneous tissue, and local peripheral lymph nodes as the passage material.[235] After plaque selection and cloning twice in PHK cells, the SA14-14-2 strain was obtained. SA14-14-2 virus was equally attenuated but more immunogenic in mice, pigs, and humans, producing seroconversion rates greater than 90% in nonimmune subjects.[237, 238]

The reduced neurovirulence of the SA14-14-2 strain was confirmed in 3-week-old mice and monkeys (Table 27–9). Compared with the parent SA14 strain, which killed weanling mice by subcutaneous or intracerebral inoculation with LD_{50}s in the range of $10^{5.5}$ to $10^{8.3}$ LD_{50} per mL, respectively, SA14-14-2 virus produced no mortality and only minor clinical signs in a few intracerebrally inoculated animals. Combined intrathalamic and intraspinal inoculation of rhesus monkeys produced no clinical illness and only minor inflammatory reactions in the substantia nigra and cervical spinal cord. Mice were more sensitive than monkeys to intracerebral infection, with some animals showing mild neuronal lesions in the cerebral cortex, hippocampus, or basal ganglia.[247] Compared with histopathological lesions produced by the parent SA14 virus, the inflammatory reaction to SA14-14-2 virus was greater and neuronal necrosis was significantly less. In 5-week-old mice inoculated intracerebrally with the virus pair, ultrastructural studies showed that the parent virus produced cytopathological changes in the majority of neurons, particularly in the rough endoplasmic reticulum and Golgi apparatus of the neuronal secretory system, while it could not be confirmed that the vaccine strain replicated at all and neurons appeared normal.[243]

Further evidence of the strain's reduced neurotropism comes from experimental studies in athymic nude mice. No deaths or histopathological abnormalities were observed after intraperitoneal or subcutaneous inoculation of a viral dose greater than 10^7 median tissue culture infective dose ($TCID_{50}$), and virus could not be recovered from brain tissue.[137] Although cyclophosphamide increases susceptibility of mice (and also of monkeys, as discussed earlier) to virulent JE virus, immunosuppression with cyclophosphamide did not lead to encephalitis in mice inoculated peripherally with SA14-14-2 virus.[138, 139] The strain also did not kill intracerebrally inoculated weanling hamsters. Phenotypic characteristics of the vaccine strain (PHK_8), such as small plaque size and reduced mouse neurovirulence, were stable

Table 27–9. **COMPARATIVE NEUROVIRULENCE OF ATTENUATED SA14-14-2 AND PARENT SA14 JAPANESE ENCEPHALITIS VIRUSES IN 3-WEEK-OLD MICE AND ADULT RHESUS MONKEYS**

VIRUS STRAIN (VIRUS TITER, pfu/mL)	INOCULATION ROUTE	MICE			RHESUS MONKEYS	
		DILUTION	Died/Tested	Histopathological Score (Neuronal Lesions)*	Died/Tested	Histopathological Score (Neuronal Lesions)*†
SA14 parent (6.15 × 10^8)	IC	10^{-1}	ND	ND	2/2	2–4
		10^{-4}	8/8	2–4	0/1	2–3
		10^{-5}	ND	ND	2/2	2–4
		10^{-6}	8/8	2–3	2/2	2–4
		10^{-7}	8/8	2–4	2/2	2–4
		10^{-8}	8/8	2–4	ND	ND
	SC	10^{-1}	30/30	2–4 (day 5)	ND	ND
SA14-14-2 (8 × 10^6)	IC	1:5	0/30³	0–2	0/4	0–1
	SC	1:5	0/30‡	0(1)§	ND	ND

*0 = No lesion; 1 = ≤5%, 2 = 6–20%, 3 = 21–50%, 4 = >50% of neurons died.
†Inoculation in thalami bilaterally (each 0.5 mL) and lumbar spinal cord (0.2 mL).
‡No clinical illness in mice inoculated subcutaneously; only a few minor clinical signs in intracerebrally inoculated mice.
§One mouse showed a few dead nerve cells.
IC, intracerebral; ND, no data; SC, subcutaneous.

through at least 10 additional PHK cell culture passages.[244]

Compared with two doses of inactivated P3 vaccine, a single dose of live vaccine is more immunogenic and potent in protecting mice and guinea pigs against challenge, as measured by survival after intraperitoneal inoculation and suppression of viremia, respectively. Six months after immunization, when neutralizing antibody titers declined to low levels (1:5), mice receiving attenuated vaccine were protected at higher rates (100%) than mice receiving inactivated vaccine (33%). Adoptive immunity, obtained by transfer of immune spleen cells from immunized mice (50% protection versus 10%), and passive protection from immune serum (80% versus 33%) were better in mice immunized with live vaccine.[248] Induction of cellular immunity also was shown by higher levels of protection in cyclophosphamide-suppressed immunized mice (see earlier discussion). Attenuated vaccine provided more effective protection than inactivated P3 vaccine against a spectrum of JE strains isolated in China.[240]

Attenuation of SA14-14-2 virus was produced empirically by serial cell culture passage, and the underlying molecular basis of its neuroattenuation still is under active investigation. The nucleotide sequence of the neurovirulent parent SA14 virus differs from that of SA14-14-2 and two other attenuated SA14-2–derived vaccine viruses in only seven amino acid substitutions found in all three attenuated strains. Four were in the envelope protein (E138, E176, E315, and E439), one was in nonstructural protein 2B (NS2B63), one was in NS3 (NS3105), and one was in NS4B (NS4B106).[249–251] Studies of other attenuated JE viral strains have shown the spectrum of mutations associated with phenotypical attenuation. ML-17, a pig vaccine strain derived by serial passage in primary monkey kidney cells, contains six amino acid changes in the protein coding region and one nucleotide change within the 3′ noncoding region (nt-10512) (G. J. Chang, unpublished results, 1997). An amino acid change at E-138, also present in SA14-14-2 virus, was shown to be sufficient for mouse neuroattenuation when introduced into a JE complementary DNA (cDNA) infectious clone. The other five changes are unique in ML-17 virus: E-146, NS3-192, NS4A-72, NS4B-274, and NS4B-315. Only six passages of virulent Nakayama and 826309 viruses in HeLa cells (HeLa p6) resulted in significantly reduced neuroinvasiveness and neurovirulence for mice and altered receptor-binding activity.[96] Nucleotide sequences of their structural protein genes revealed that the viruses differed by eight and nine amino acid mutations, respectively. Attenuated viruses also have been obtained by selecting neutralizing-resistant variants. Attenuation was associated with single base changes resulting in single E protein amino acid changes and was linked with altered early virus–cell interactions but not with replication.[252, 253] Manipulations of infectious cDNA will be essential to analyze the contribution of individual mutations in JE viral neuroattenuation.

SA14-14-2 virus also is propagated in BHK-21 cells as a swine vaccine that has been shown to protect against JE virus–associated abortions. SA14-14-2 and the 2-8 strain, obtained from further attenuation of the 12-1-7 strain (see Table 27–7), also are manufactured into effective equine vaccines distributed in China.[254, 255] Other attenuated viruses, such as the "m" and ML-17 strains, are used in swine vaccines in Japan and other Asian countries.

Inferences from several studies indicate a negligible potential for mosquito transmission of attenuated JE viruses from a vaccinated pig or human; however, more definitive experiments are needed. SA14-14-2 virus can be isolated from blood of vaccinees, but it is present at infectious titers below the usual oral infection threshold of mosquitoes. Attenuated JE 2-8 virus, which has a pedigree similar to that of SA14-14-2 virus, replicates in intrathoracically inoculated *C. tritaeniorhyncus* mosquitoes; however, infected mosquitoes failed to transmit the virus, and infection rates after oral feeding were low. The virus did not revert to a neurovirulent phenotype after mosquito passage.[254] Transmission experiments with the SA14-14-2 strain itself are needed.

Dosage and Route of Administration. A 0.5-mL dose is administered subcutaneously to children at 1 year of age and again at 2 years. In some areas, a booster dose is given at 6 years. No other vaccines are given concurrently. Like the inactivated PHK cell–derived vaccine, SA14-14-2 vaccine is distributed in annual spring campaigns rather than according to an age-based schedule. There are no data on combined administration with other vaccines.

A more conventional administration schedule in which the two primary doses were given at intervals of 1 or 2.5 months was shown to produce immunity in 94 to 100% of immunized school-aged children.[256] If similar results can be shown in infants, it may be possible to administer the vaccine with other immunogens, such as measles, according to an age-based immunization schedule.

EXPERIMENTAL VACCINES

Several candidate JE vaccines are in various stages of early clinical and preclinical development or research.[257] The most extensively evaluated candidate vaccines have been a recombinant virus pair engineered by inserting four JE viral genes (prM, E, NS1, and NS2a) into attenuated vaccinia (NYVAC) or canarypox (ALVAC) viruses. Both recombinants expressed the encoded JE structural and nonstructural gene products and stimulated JE protective antibodies in mice; two doses of the former also protected rhesus monkeys against lethal viral challenge. In a phase 1 human trial, the vaccines provoked mild local reactions but were otherwise safe. Two doses of the NYVAC-JE recombinant were nearly as immunogenic as three doses of inactivated mouse brain JE vaccine, but only in vaccinia-naive volunteers. JE neutralizing antibodies were elicited in all non–vaccinia-immune recipients but in none of the vaccinia-immune volunteers and in only 1 of 10 ALVAC-JE vaccinees.[258] Although the NYVAC-JE recombinant virus proved safe and potent, its apparent failure to replicate in vaccinia-immune subjects limits its utility. Further development of vaccines for human use evidently has been halted, but development of animal vaccines still may be pursued.

Several groups have produced experimental inactivated whole-virion vaccines from infected Vero cell cultures. Cell culture medium with high viral infectious titers, harvested continuously from microcarrier cultures, inactivated with formalin, and further concentrated, has yielded candidate vaccine meeting mouse protection potency standards established for the inactivated mouse brain vaccine. Phase 1 clinical trials are scheduled in the near term. Inactivated vaccines produced by similar means for polio and rabies have been safe, highly immunogenic, and compatible with DPT vaccines given to infants. A similarly potent inactivated JE vaccine that could be given in a conventional immunization schedule would lower administration costs and improve JE vaccine coverage in the region.

The potential for adventitious agents in the PHK cell substrate of attenuated SA14-14-2 vaccine has stimulated attempts to adapt the virus to more conventional cell systems. The strain was adapted to primary canine kidney (PCK) cells and, after passing monkey neurovirulence and other safety tests, was produced under Good Manufacturing Practices (GMP) conditions in its ninth PCK cell passage by the Walter Reed Army Institute of Research as a candidate vaccine. The Investigational New Drug (IND) vaccine, containing an infectious titer of more than $10^{5.5}$ pfu per mL, was given safely to adults and children in phase 1 human trials, but neutralizing antibody responses to a single dose were detected in only two of four and 14 of 45 vaccinees (31%), respectively, with geometric mean titers (GMTs) ranging from 7 to 40. In view of the apparently low antibody responses, the PCK-passaged strain was considered further attenuated, and development was discontinued. Subsequently the virus was adapted to Vero cells, and its potential either as a live virus or inactivated whole-virion vaccine is currently under investigation. Adaptation of the SA14-14-2 strain to insect cells has been reported to improve propagation.[259]

The possibility of genetically engineering neuroattenuated JE viruses by introducing defined nucleotide substitutions has been demonstrated conceptually in mouse protection studies.[260] However, technical difficulties have led to further development using a novel JE–YF viral chimera, in which the SA14-14-2 prM and E genes were substituted into a YF 17D viral infectious clone. Comparative neurovirulence properties of the $YF/JE_{SA14-14-2}$ chimera and a "control" chimeric virus constructed with the corresponding genes of the virulent Nakayama JE strain reflected those of the parent JE viruses. Mice immunized with the $YF/JE_{SA14-14-2}$ chimera were protected against lethal challenge, indicating its potential as a candidate vaccine.

JE viral subunit proteins produced in various expression systems, including *Spondoptera frugiperda*, *Escherichia coli*, *Saccharomyces cerevisiae*, and *Drosophila* Schneider 2 cells, have had variable success in eliciting mouse immunogenicity and protective potency, depending on the expressed epitopes and their conformation.[261–265] The identification of peptides mimicking the conformation of viral epitopes may be expedited by screening pentapeptide libraries against monoclonal antibodies with previously defined specificity.[266] The best-characterized candidate subunit vaccine is a vaccinia-JE virus recombinant that releases extracellular particles (EPs) composed of JE, prM, and E proteins in an apparently more authentic configuration than when presented as simple peptides.[267] When given without adjuvant, EP induced long-lasting antibody and memory T cells in immunized mice. Immunogenic subviral particles containing JE E protein also have been produced in other systems, including an alphaviral recombinant virus.[268, 269] Novel delivery systems and adjuvants have been explored as a means to improve immunogenicity, to direct the TH1 or TH2 response, or to improve the convenience of immunization (e.g., the inactivated mouse brain vaccine has been microencapsulated in glycolide and lactide polymer microspheres designed to degrade at specific intervals).[270]

A promising avenue of research is the intramuscular injection of naked DNA plasmids encoding viral prM and E genes under the control of a cytomegalovirus immediate early promotor. For both JE and related StLE-derived plasmids, immunized mice were protected against challenge with the respective viruses. The potential for continued antigen expression and long-term humoral immunity has been illustrated in mice that maintained neutralizing antibodies for more than 18 months after newborn immunization with one or two doses of JE virus–derived DNA. Another important advantage of DNA vaccination is the induction of cellular immunity, which may be significant in protection and viral clearance. Mice immunized with StLE virus–derived DNA were protected independent of their humoral immune response. Continued evaluation of DNA-based vaccine in pigs and monkeys is planned for the near future.

Protective Effects of Immunization

Inactivated Mouse Brain–Derived JE Vaccine

A neutralizing antibody titer of more than 1:10 generally is accepted as evidence of protection and postvaccination seroconversion. Passively immunized mice that acquire this level of neutralizing antibody are protected against challenge from 10^5 LD_{50} of JE virus, a typical dose transmitted by an infectious mosquito bite. Indirect observations from human trials have associated efficacy with this criterion.[175] Although individual laboratories employ test procedures of varying sensitivity to measure neutralizing antibody, results are surprisingly robust. Plaque reduction neutralization tests are used most frequently, and procedural differences, such as choice of challenge virus strain, cell systems, addition of exogenous complement, and choice of end points (ranging from 50 to 90% plaque reduction in serum dilution tests), affect test sensitivity. Some laboratories still employ log neutralization indices (LNIs) in tests using a single serum dilution. However, despite procedural differences, neutralizing antibody titers in three laboratories (the CDC, Japan's National Institutes of Health [NIH], and the Yale Arbovirus Unit) were shown to be highly correlated (R. DeFraites, unpublished observa-

Table 27–10. **HOMOLOGOUS AND HETEROLOGOUS NEUTRALIZING ANTIBODY RESPONSES IN CHILDREN IMMUNIZED WITH INACTIVATED NAKAYAMA OR BEIJING STRAIN JAPANESE ENCEPHALITIS VACCINES**

VACCINE STRAIN	CHALLENGE VIRUS IN NEUTRALIZING ANTIBODY DETERMINATION	AFTER SECOND DOSE		1 YEAR AFTER PRIMARY SERIES		AFTER THIRD DOSE (1 YR BOOSTER)	
		No.	% Response (GMT)	No.	% Response (GMT)	No.	% Response (GMT)
Nakayama	Nakayama[258]	186	99	123	89*	107	100
	Nakayama[259]	93	94* (120)	40	78 (35)	40	100 (562)
	Beijing[259]	93	74* (43)	40	35 (26)	40	95 (190)
	Nakayama[257]	329	97 (63)	311	79 (20)	—	
Beijing	Beijing[258]	196	99	141	100*	114	100
	Nakayama[259]	93	82† (42)	40	52* (34)	40	100 (501)
	Beijing[259]	93	94† (79)	40	88* (66)	40	100 (2754
	Nakayama[257]	59	80† (20)	58	55* (13)	—	
	Beijing[257]	54	94† (79)	51	92* (63)	—	

*P < .001.
†P < .03.
GMT, geometric mean titer.

tions). No international standard for protective antibody units has been established.

Immunogenicity. Among Asian children immunized with two doses of Nakayama or Beijing-1 strain–derived vaccines, neutralizing antibody responses to the respective homologous vaccine strains are in the range of 94 to 100%; responses to strains representing a heterologous antigenic group are lower (selected recent studies are shown in Table 27–10).[271–273] The proportion of vaccinees retaining detectable neutralizing antibodies and their GMTs declined rapidly in the year after the primary two-dose series, so that only 78 to 89% of Nakayama vaccine recipients and 88 to 100% of Beijing-1 vaccine recipients still had protective levels before the scheduled 1-year booster. Antibody persistence was greater among Beijing-1 vaccine recipients. After booster immunization (third vaccine dose), antibody response rates were uniformly high (100%).

Immunogenicity studies in Asian subjects should be interpreted in light of the immunological background of vaccinees. Although some studies have been carried out in nonendemic areas and in subjects without JE viral antibodies, in other studies, undetected exposures to JE, dengue, and other flaviviruses prevalent in Asia may have resulted in an augmented antibody response after immunization and apparently better immune responses. Where the influence of previous flaviviral infections was unlikely, vaccinees receiving two doses produced lower seroconversion rates and lower GMTs (Table 27–11 and Fig. 27–17*A*).[20, 221–223] Moreover, as rapidly as 6 to 12 months after primary immunization with two doses, neutralizing antibody titers declined below 1:8 in 90% of vaccinees (Fig. 17*B*).[181] A three-dose primary schedule was more immunogenic, resulting in seroconversion rates exceeding 90% and significantly higher neutralizing antibody titers.[20, 221–223] A comparison of long (days 0, 7, and 30) and short (days 0, 7, and 14) three-dose schedules disclosed uniform seroconversion in all subjects but significantly higher neutralizing antibody titers in vaccinees immunized over the longer period (30 days).

Vaccine prepared from the Beijing-1 strain appears to be more immunogenic, despite its smaller delivered volume, yielding higher seroconversion rates and higher antibody titers to heterologous Nakayama virus (see Table 27–10).[271–276] Similar but more marked differences were seen in comparative neutralization of field viral strains from Taiwan, paralleling those in experimentally immunized mice (see Figure 27–16).[277] The clinical im-

Table 27–11. **IMMUNOGENICITY OF NAKAYAMA STRAIN INACTIVATED JAPANESE ENCEPHALITIS VIRUS MOUSE BRAIN–DERIVED VACCINE IN SUBJECTS FROM NONENDEMIC AREAS AFTER TWO OR THREE DOSES**

STUDY GROUP	TWO-DOSE SERIES			THREE-DOSE SERIES		
	No.	Seroconversion Rate (%)	GMT	No.	Seroconversion Rate (%)	GMT
United States (1984–1987)[181]	118	77	28	72	98	141
United Kingdom (1983)[222]	27	33	31–61	94	88	146–214
United States (1990)[223]	20	80		25	100*	
United States (1990)[221]				526	100	140/692†
Kolhapur, India (1990)[20]‡	250	50		242	95	
Bagalore, India (1990)[20]‡	184	73		184	98	

*Dose 3 at week 26.
†Day 60 serum; short and long three-dose schedules, P < .0001.
‡Children, 7 to 14 years old.
GMT, geometric mean titer.

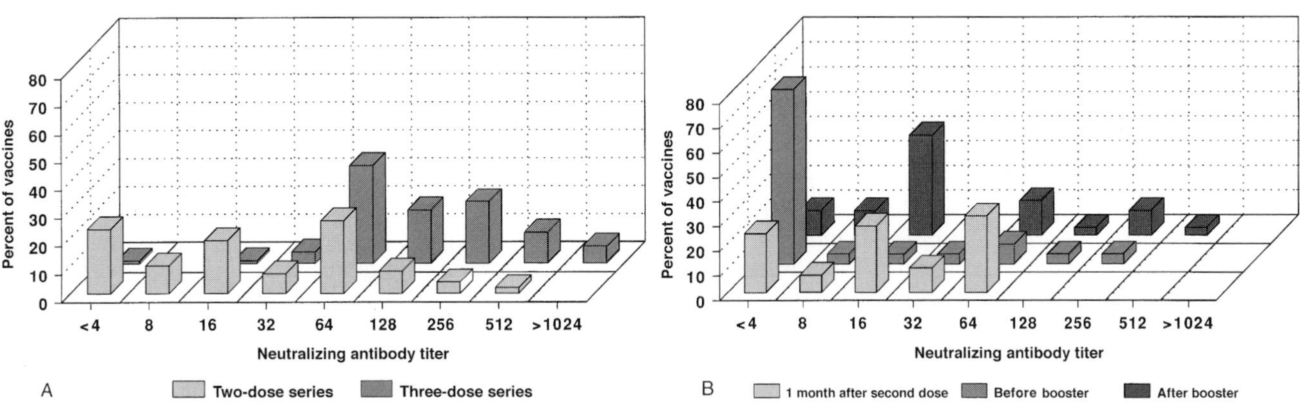

Figure 27–17. *A*, Antibody response to inactivated mouse brain–derived Japanese encephalitis vaccine in a trial among U.S. citizens. Only 77% of vaccinees who received two doses seroconverted, compared with 99% of vaccinees who received three doses. Geometric mean titers also were higher in the latter group (28 vs. 141). (Adapted from Poland JD, Cropp CB, Craven RB, Monath TP. Evaluation of the potency and safety of inactivated Japanese encephalitis vaccine in US inhabitants. J Infect Dis 161:878–882, 1990.) *B*, Six to 12 months after primary immunization, only 10% of vaccinees who were given two doses retained protective levels of neutralizing antibody. Booster immunization led to a greater than 90% response.

portance of these differences in strain reactivity is uncertain. Results of the efficacy trial comparing a monovalent Nakayama strain vaccine with a bivalent vaccine also containing Beijing-1 antigen showed that the two were equally efficacious (see later discussion).[278] JE vaccines produced locally in Thailand, India, Vietnam, and Taiwan all employ the Nakayama strain, and no field observations have suggested a geographic pattern of vaccine failure. Neutralizing activity may be present below the threshold of detection in in vitro assays, and T-cell memory may have been established in vaccinees who appear to be seronegative, providing sufficient help to clear infections upon reexposure.

Although previous exposures to dengue and certain other flaviviruses probably enhance the immune response to JE vaccine, antibody responses did not differ in people with a history of YF vaccination, unlike the accelerated response to inactivated TBE vaccine seen among YF-vaccinated individuals.[279]

Vaccinees are exposed only to viral structural proteins, and in contrast to recovered patients, they do not produce radioprecipitating antibodies to viral nonstructural proteins. Their memory T-cell proliferative responses to a viral-like particle containing only structural proteins also differ from recovered patients, whose $CD4^+$ and $CD8^+$ cell responses also include viral nonstructural proteins.[131] The implications of these immune response differences are uncertain.

Impaired responses to vaccination were observed in infants with vertically acquired HIV infection when compared with control seroreverting infants born to HIV-infected women: five of 14 (36%) HIV-infected children and 18 of 27 (67%) control children developed JE antibodies after immunization (odds ratio 0.3; P = .06); among those with positive titers, the GMT of HIV-infected children also was lower (15.1 vs. 23.8; P = .17).[280] The response to additional doses beyond the primary two doses was not studied. Immune response in other immunocompromised states has not been studied systematically.[281]

Efficacy. Efficacy of the Nakayama vaccine has been evaluated in two masked, randomized, placebo- (tetanus toxoid–) controlled field trials. In the first evaluation, a prototype of the current vaccine was field-tested in 1965 in Taiwan; two doses yielded an 80% efficacy in the first year after immunization (Table 27–12).[282–284] A subsequent masked, randomized, placebo-controlled field trial in Thailand compared the efficacies of the currently produced monovalent Nakayama vaccine with a specially formulated bivalent vaccine also containing Beijing-1

Table 27–12. **EFFICACY OF INACTIVATED MOUSE BRAIN–DERIVED JAPANESE ENCEPHALITIS VACCINE***

COUNTRY	STUDY GROUP	NO. AT RISK	CASE RATE/100,000	EFFICACY (95% CI) (%)
Taiwan, 1965[282, 284]	Total vaccinated	133,943	4.48	76 (63–90)
	1 dose	22,194	9.01	50 (26–88)
	2 doses	111,749	3.58	80 (71–93)
	Placebo	131,865	18.20	—
	Nonvaccinated	140,514	24.91	—
Thailand, 1984–1985[278]	Total vaccinated	43,708	4.60	91 (70–97)
	Monovalent	21,628	4.60	91 (54–98)
	Bivalent	22,080	4.50	91 (54–98)
	Placebo	21,516	51.10	—

*Two doses of Nakayama or bivalent Nakayama/Beijing mouse brain–derived vaccines.
CI, confidence interval.

antigen (see Table 27–12).[278] Two doses of vaccine or placebo were given 1 week apart to children 1 year of age and older. After a 2-year observation period, efficacies of the monovalent and bivalent vaccines were identical, with an overall efficacy of 91%. Lower risks of dengue and dengue hemorrhagic fever also were observed in the JE-vaccinated groups, although the differences were not significant. Experimental studies in monkeys suggest that immunization against JE might provide cross-protection against West Nile virus.[125]

Persistence of Immunity and Protection. Studies in Asia to determine the persistence of vaccine-derived immunity are complicated by natural infections with dengue, West Nile virus, or other flaviviruses and reexposure to JE virus itself, all of which act to reinforce and broaden vaccine-derived immunity to JE virus.[101, 102, 122–124, 153] Even with the potential for these reinforcing infections, several studies in Asian and in Western subjects (see previous discussion) indicate a progressive decline in antibody levels in the first year after primary immunization with two doses (see Fig. 27–17 and Table 27–10).[181, 206] Cross-sectional serosurveys in Japan and Taiwan (see earlier discussion) (see Fig. 27–14) indicate a rapid decline of immunity in childhood. Observations of vaccine efficacy in the Taiwan field trial parallel these results: In the second year after immunization, protective efficacy declined from 80 to 55% (95% confidence interval [CI] = 39–75%).[283] In the Thailand field trial of the current vaccine formulation, efficacy was shown through 2 years of observation. Further follow-up data are not available.

These and other data (see Table 27–11) indicate the need for boosters after a two-dose primary immunization series. A third dose generally has been given at 1 year and subsequently at intervals of 1 to 3 years (Fig. 27–18). Booster doses are followed by significant increases in neutralizing antibody titer and uniform anamnestic responses in subjects who had reverted to seronegative. A small study of vaccinees receiving an Indian-manufactured JE vaccine found that 34 of 35 (97%) retained neutralizing antibodies 3 years after a primary series of three doses, and 31 of 34 (91%) retained antibodies at 4.5 years, with GMTs of 71 and 32, respectively. However, the boosting effect of naturally acquired flaviviral infections in these subjects cannot be ruled out.[285]

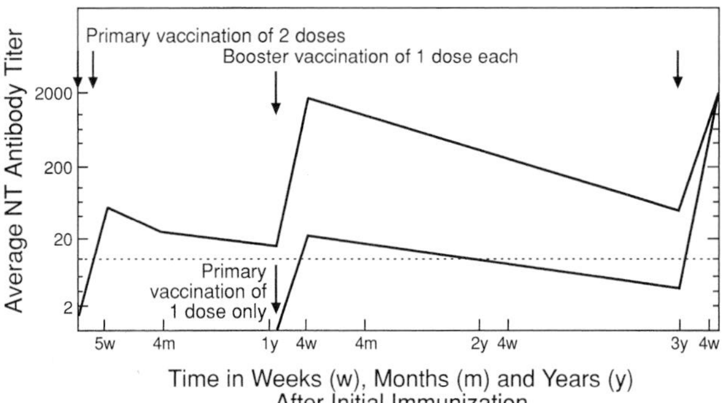

Figure 27–18. A schematic of the antibody response to two doses of inactivated mouse brain–derived Japanese encephalitis (JE) vaccine and of booster doses. Antibody levels declined to subprotective levels within 1 year after primary immunization. Protective levels recovered after booster immunization and declined after 3 to 4 years. Although this study was carried out in an area of Japan where JE transmission is limited, the effects of natural infection on antibody response and persistence of immunity cannot be ruled out. NT, Neutralizing. (Adapted from Kanamitsu M, Hashimoto N, Urasawa S, et al. A field trial with an improved Japanese encephalitis vaccine in a nonendemic area of the disease. Biken J 13:313–328, 1970.)

Flavivirus-naive U.S. Army soldiers who received a three-dose primary immunization series retained protective neutralizing antibody titers for at least 1 year (GMT = 76). Antibody titers at 12 months were unchanged from those observed 3 months after immunization (GMT = 78). A booster dose given at 12 months was followed by a significant anamnestic response (GMT = 1117). In a limited number of subjects studied 3 years after the primary series, 16 of 17 (94%) who had neither traveled to Asia nor received a booster retained neutralizing antibody titers >1:10, and their GMTs at 3 years and at 6 months after primary immunization were unchanged.[221] Although these observations suggest that the first booster immunization is needed no sooner than 2 to 3 years after primary immunization, the interval for subsequent boosters has not been established.

Inactivated Primary Hamster Kidney Cell–Derived Japanese Encephalitis Vaccine

Two doses of inactivated PHK cell–derived vaccine, given 1 week apart, produced an LNI greater than 50 in only 60 to 68% of children who had no prevaccination JE viral antibodies (Table 27–13).[286–289] Immunity wanes rapidly after primary immunization with two doses, and only 10% of vaccinees have an LNI greater than 50 1 year later. The rapid decline in antibody provides some justification for the vaccine's administration in spring campaigns before the onset of the transmission season. A booster dose results in an anamnestic response in 93 to 100% of recipients. After 3 to 4 years, seropositivity is maintained at an LNI of greater than 50 in 64% of vaccinees, and a subsequent booster dose is followed by 100% seroconversion.[194, 290] Extensive randomized field trials among 480,000 children have demonstrated vaccine efficacies in the range of 76 to 95% (Table 27–14).[194, 289]

Table 27–13. **NEUTRALIZING ANTIBODY RESPONSE TO INACTIVATED P3 JAPANESE ENCEPHALITIS VACCINE, YANJI, JILIN, CHINA**

YEAR	VACCINATION	INTERVAL BETWEEN VACCINATION AND BLEEDING	PROPORTION SEROPOSITIVE (%)
1973	Dose 1	1 mo	15/25 (60)
	Dose 2	3 mo	8/28 (29)
		1 yr	3/29 (10)
1974	Booster	1 mo	27/29 (93)
1975		1 yr	50/63 (79)
1976		2 yr	32/47 (68)
1977		3 yr	42/64 (64)
1978		4 yr	40/62 (64)
1978	Booster 2	1 mo	62/62 (100)

Table 27–14. **EFFICACY OF INACTIVATED P3 JAPANESE ENCEPHALITIS VACCINE, PEOPLE'S REPUBLIC OF CHINA**

YEAR	REGION	STUDY GROUP	NO. OF SUBJECTS	CASES OF JAPANESE ENCEPHALITIS	INCIDENCE RATE/100,000	EFFICACY (95% CI) (%)
1967	Wuxi	Vaccinated*	38,482	3	7.8	84 (75–95)
		Nonvaccinated	34,182	17	52.8	
1968	Nanjing	Vaccinated	52,004	3	5.8	87 (73–96)
		Nonvaccinated	18,584	8	43.0	
1968	Hunan	Vaccinated	75,083	7	9.3	76 (63–90)
		Nonvaccinated	48,543	19	39.1	
1969	Beijing	Vaccinated	86,847	3	3.5	87 (81–96)
		Nonvaccinated	76,260	21	27.5	
1973	Guangxi	Vaccinated	58,211	2	3.4	95 (90–100)
		Nonvaccinated	10,165	7	68.9	

*Two doses with an interval of 1 week.
CI, confidence interval.

Although regional trials in Wuxi and Nanjing disclosed partial protection against acquiring JE (efficacies of 85 to 87%), more detailed clinical studies showed that cases in vaccinated children were milder than those in unvaccinated children. None of the six cases in immunized children resulted in death or neurological sequelae, whereas 3 of the 25 cases in unimmunized children were fatal, and 3 led to sequelae. These observations suggest that clinical efficacy is better than the reported protective efficacy.[194] A case-control study measuring vaccine effectiveness in Henan province, China, found that full immunization (two primary doses and annual boosters until age 10) was 78% effective (95% CI = 16–94%) in preventing the disease, and partial immunization was 68% effective (95% CI = 29–92%). The relative risk of acquiring JE was 4.54 in unimmunized children and 3.12 in partially immunized children.[290]

The aggregated data indicate that the inactivated P3 vaccine has some utility in preventing the disease; however, the need for repeated booster doses and its relatively low efficacy limit its use.

Immune responses to single doses of concentrated or purified inactivated PHK cell vaccines (see previous discussion) were similar to those observed after two doses of the standard vaccine. All subjects seroconverted, and respective geometric mean neutralizing antibody titers were 45, 72, and 46.[194] No data on efficacy or persistence of immunity are available, and further work has been discontinued.

Live Attenuated Japanese Encephalitis Vaccine

A comparison of vaccines derived from SA14-5-3 and SA14-14-2 showed that the former was less immunogenic, producing seroconversion in only 61% of 13 vaccinees and having a GMT of 5, compared with a 92.3% seroconversion rate in subjects receiving a similar infectious dose of SA14-14-2 vaccine.[237] Several small immunogenicity studies of the SA14-14-2 vaccine have been reported, with variable results. After a single dose, antibody responses are produced in 85 to 100% of nonimmune 1- to 12-year-old children, with a response gradient that parallels progressive vaccine dilution (Table 27–15).[237, 238, 291, 292] Lower seroconversion rates were obtained with vaccine dilutions that had infectious titers less than $10^{6.7}$ $TCID_{50}$ per mL, which has been established as the minimal standard of vaccine infectivity.

Because of variable immune response rates after one dose, SA14-14-2 vaccine is given in a schedule of two doses separated by a year, according to the custom of administering JE vaccines in annual spring campaigns. The immunogenicity of two doses given at intervals of either 1 or 2.5 months was shown in 12- to 15-year-old children. Response rates were similar: 75 to 100% after one dose and 94 to 100% after two doses (two vaccine lots were compared), but there was a trend toward better seroconversion with the longer interval, and GMTs were approximately two-fold higher (65–89 versus 115–158, respectively). If these results can be confirmed in infants, the SA14-14-2 vaccine could be integrated into a routine childhood immunization schedule, potentially improving vaccine coverage.[256] The effect of maternal immunity on antibody response in infants has not been examined.[292]

Efficacy trials in children 1 to 10 years old have consistently yielded high protection rates above 98% (Table 27–16).[246, 293, 294] In the 1991 Yunnan field study,

Table 27–15. **IMMUNE RESPONSE TO ONE DOSE OF SA14-14-2 ATTENUATED JAPANESE ENCEPHALITIS VACCINE BY VACCINE INFECTIOUS TITER**

YEAR	VACCINE TITER*	SEROCONVERSION RATE (%)†	GMT	REFERENCE
1979	6.7	12/13 (92)	29	237
	5.7	12/17 (71)	10	
	4.7	10/16 (62)	10	
1985	>7.0	23/23 (100)	>32	238
	6.0	10/12 (83)	23	
1987	7.0	33/39 (85)	23	292
1992	6.0–6.5‡	18/19 (95)	25	
1994	6.8‡	29/29 (100)	31	
	6.5‡	24/26 (92)	27	

*Log_{10} median tissue culture infective dose ($TCID_{50}$) per mL.
†>1:10 neutralizing antibody titer.
‡Log (plaque-forming units/mL).
GMT, geometric mean titer.

Table 27–16. **PROTECTIVE EFFICACY OF SA14-14-2 ATTENUATED JAPANESE ENCEPHALITIS VACCINE, CHINA**

PROVINCE	YEAR	STUDY GROUP	NO. OF SUBJECTS	CASES OF JAPANESE ENCEPHALITIS	INCIDENCE/100,000	EFFICACY (95% CI) (%)
Guizhou	1988	Vaccinated*	86,132	1	1.16	98.0 (96–100)
		Nonvaccinated	21,149	12	56.7	
	1989	Vaccinated†	86,933†	0	2.30	100
		Nonvaccinated	16,869	12	71.1	
Jiang-Xi	1989	Vaccinated*	64,027	2	3.12	98.4 (97–100)
		Nonvaccinated	4,546	9	198.0	
	1990	Vaccinated†	63,927	1	1.56	99.8 (98–100)
		Nonvaccinated	5,784	37	639.6	
	1991–1993	Vaccinated†	~65,000	0		100
		Nonvaccinated	~7,000	24 (3 yr)	~109.6	
Yunnan	1991	Vaccinated‡	29,639	2	6.75	95.7 (94–99)
		Nonvaccinated	29,006	46	158.6	
Anhui	1992	Vaccinated	145,758	2	1.37	99.3 (99–100)
		Nonvaccinated	11,264	22	195.3	

*Children 1 to 10 years old immunized with single primary dose.
†Combination of 1- to 10-year-old children immunized in previous year(s), 1-year-old children given primary dose, and 2-year-old children given booster dose.
‡Children 1 to 7 years old immunized with single primary dose only.
CI, confidence interval.

neither of the two cases in vaccinated children produced serious illness, but three deaths occurred in the unvaccinated cohort, and more than 50% of the remaining cases were considered severe. In the Guizhou study, equally good protection was observed through a second year after a booster dose was given. Efficacy was shown with the more attenuated prototype SA14-5-3 vaccine, although protection was lower than that achieved with the SA14-14-2 vaccine (see Table 27–8).[246, 293, 294]

A study measuring the effectiveness of the SA14-14-2 vaccine, using case-control methods, disclosed protection levels similar to those estimated by previous efficacy studies. When immunization histories were compared among 56 hospitalized laboratory-confirmed JE cases and 1299 age-matched village controls, the vaccine's effectiveness was 80% for one dose (95% CI = 44–93%) and 98% for two doses (95% CI = 86–99.6%).[295] Because of uncertainties about the methodological approach of earlier efficacy studies, the consistency of this result with previous estimates was reassuring. Furthermore, effectiveness is a measure of the vaccine's performance under the usual circumstances of health care delivery rather than the artificial conditions of a study, which is additional evidence of the vaccine's robustness.

Interestingly, the vaccine's variable immunogenicity, the relatively low neutralizing antibody titers elicited, and the need for two doses suggest that the strain may be overattenuated. However, vaccination evidently provides sufficient immunological memory, supplemented possibly by natural exposures to the virus, to be highly effective in protecting against clinical illness.

Side Effects of Immunization

Inactivated Mouse Brain–Derived Japanese Encephalitis Vaccine

Local and Nonspecific Adverse Events. Local tenderness, redness, or swelling at the injection site occur in approximately 20% of individuals immunized with inactivated mouse brain–derived vaccines. Mild systemic symptoms, chiefly headache, low-grade fever, myalgias, malaise, and gastrointestinal symptoms, are reported by 10 to 30% of vaccinees (Table 27–17).[181, 222, 223, 271]

Neurological Adverse Events. The vaccine's neural tissue substrate has raised concern about the possibility of postvaccination neurological side effects.[296] The manufacturing process purifies the infected mouse brain suspension extensively, and myelin basic protein (MBP) content is controlled below 2 ng per mL, well below the dose considered to have an encephalitogenic effect in a guinea pig test system. However, measurements of other acute disseminated encephalomyelitis (ADE)–associated neural proteins (e.g., proteolipid protein, myelin-oligodendrocyte glycoprotein) have not been reported. Experimental immunization of guinea pigs and *Cynomolgus* monkeys with adjuvant and 50 times the normal dose of vaccine did not result in clinical or histopathological evidence of encephalomyelitis.[297, 298]

In 1945, in one of the first mass uses of mouse brain–derived JE vaccine, 53,000 American soldiers on Okinawa were immunized with a crude inactivated mouse brain suspension after a JE outbreak occurred on the island.[200] Acute vaccine-associated side effects, including the occurrence of acute neurological events, were monitored. Eight neurological reactions, principally polyneuritis, were observed. However, similar cases were reported concurrently in nonvaccinated individuals, and it is unclear whether the illnesses were vaccine related. One case of Guillain-Barré syndrome, temporally related to JE immunization, was reported among approximately 20,000 American soldiers immunized with the vaccine prior to U.S. licensure.

An early prospective study in Japan to detect vaccine-associated adverse events found no neurological complications occurring within a month after vaccination in 38,384 subjects receiving crude or purified vaccine.[296] A country-wide study to detect neurological complications found 26 temporally related cases (meningitis, convul-

Table 27–17. **REPORTED SIDE EFFECTS OF INACTIVATED MOUSE BRAIN–DERIVED JAPANESE ENCEPHALITIS VACCINE**

COUNTRY	SUBJECTS	LOCAL SIDE EFFECTS (%)*	SYSTEMIC SIDE EFFECTS (%)†	REFERENCE
Thailand	490	<1	1.7–2.9	278
United States	59	18	9	181
United States	1328	12	2	
	526			
	1st dose	20	5	221
	2nd dose	12	2	
	3rd dose	11	1	
United States	3573	23	10–13	223
Thailand	448	2	1.3–1.8	271

*Local tenderness, redness, swelling, itching, and numbness.
†Chiefly fever, headache, malaise, rash; also chills, dizziness, myalgia, nausea, vomiting, abdominal pain, diarrhea, sore throat, blurred vision, increased salivation and taste, difficulty concentrating, and emotional instability.

sions, demyelinating disease, polyneuritis) between 1957 and 1966, but rates and comparisons with nonimmunized controls were not available. Passive surveillance of vaccine-related adverse events (AEs) in Japan is conducted through sentinel hospitals, clinics, and pharmacies and through manufacturers. Surveillance data on JE vaccine AEs come principally from the manufacturer (Biken and others). Few neurological complications temporally related to JE vaccination were reported, but denominators of vaccinees were not available in all years, and the sensitivity of this passive surveillance system is unknown (Table 27–18).[216, 297, 299]

In 1992, two anecdotal cases of temporally related vaccine-associated ADE in Japan prompted a survey of 162 Japanese medical institutions to solicit additional cases.[300] Five more cases spanning 22 years were reported, including two with elevated CSF MBP levels.[301] Neither the numerator of cases nor the denominator of vaccinees was defined rigorously, but the authors estimated that ADE occurred in fewer than 1 in 1 million vaccinees. In an unrelated report, three ADE cases (one fatal) temporally related to vaccination were reported in Korea in 1994; one, also fatal, was reported in 1996. An additional fatal case of acute encephalopathy occurred in a 15-year-old girl who received her ninth dose of JE vaccine and her third dose of hantaviral vaccine (also made in mouse brain) 4 and 2 weeks, respectively, before onset of stupor and seizures (Y. M. Sohn, unpublished observations).

An additional report of vaccination-associated ADE

Table 27–18. **REPORTED NEUROLOGICAL MANIFESTATIONS TEMPORALLY ASSOCIATED WITH JAPANESE ENCEPHALITIS VACCINATION, JAPAN**

YEARS	NO. OF CASES	ESTIMATED RATE
1965–1970	75	$1/10^6$
1971–1978	?	$2.3/10^6$†
1979–1980	6	—
1981–1982	3	—
1983–1986	?	—
1987–1989	2	—

*Inactivated mouse brain–derived vaccine.
†1971 to 1973 data from Tokyo only: two cases per 883,373 vaccinees.

cases in Danish travelers, unprompted by previous reports from Japan and Korea, suggests that the issue of neurological complications should be reinvestigated.[302] After a vaccinee developed ADE in 1995, a review of the national database disclosed two similar temporally related cases in 1983 and 1989, all in adults. Because JE vaccine distribution in Denmark is controlled, the denominator of vaccinees and a rate for AEs could be estimated. The rate of temporally related ADE, 1 in 50,000 to 75,000 vaccinees, is far above previous estimates of all neurological complications and in the same range as JE incidence in countries where the disease is endemic.

The significance of anecdotal reports from Asia is difficult to interpret, as systematic data for children are unavailable. The incidence of serious vaccine-related neurological complications, if any can be shown, probably is low, because no clear association has emerged during the more than three decades the vaccine has been used. Notwithstanding this impression, anecdotal reports and the high rate of serious events in the Danish study suggest the need for a controlled study in routinely vaccinated children. In Korea, where no naturally acquired JE case has occurred in recent years, public objections to the vaccine have cited greater risk from the vaccine than from the disease itself.

Although the bovine spongiform encephalopathy outbreak has raised concern over the potential for contamination of biologicals with prions from animal sources, there has been little discussion about risks of the JE vaccine mouse brain substrate. Factors mitigating against such a risk are (1) the low, if any, natural incidence of a mouse-transmissible spongiform encephalopathy; (2) the vaccine purification process that removes certain proteins from the final product; and (3) the species barrier. In the absence of a naturally occurring murine spongiform encephalopathy, the principal concern is comixing of mice designated for vaccine production with mice infected in a research project. Although this seems unlikely, mice used in vaccine production are supplied by multiple subcontractors whose facilities may be difficult to monitor. The vaccine formalin inactivation process does not inactivate and potentially could stabilize contaminating prions. However, on balance it seems highly unlikely that the vaccine poses a risk for transmission of a spongiform encephalopathy agent.

Hypersensitivity Reactions. Vaccine-related allergic AEs not reported previously from Asia were recognized after 1989 in Australia and several European and North American countries as the vaccine became used widely in travelers.[181, 182, 303–309] Hypersensitivity reactions have consisted principally of generalized urticaria, angioedema, or both, which in a few patients were potentially life threatening. These reactions generally have responded to oral antihistamines or corticosteroids, but recalcitrant cases have required hospitalization and parenteral steroid therapy. A temporally related death was reported in a man with multiple hypersensitivities who also had received plague vaccine.[182] Numerous lots and different manufacturers have been implicated.[307] In retrospect, allergic side effects, including urticaria, angioedema, and moderate dyspnea, were observed in recipients of the crude mouse brain vaccine administered on Okinawa in 1945.[200]

An important feature of the reactions is the potential for delayed onset, particularly after a second dose. In a prospective study of 14,249 U.S. Marines, the median interval between immunization and onset was 18 to 24 hours after the first dose, with 74% of reactions occurring within 48 hours.[181, 182, 304] Among reactors to a second dose, there was a greater delay, with a median interval of 96 hours and a range of 20 to 336 hours. Reactions have developed after a second or third dose when previous doses were given uneventfully. A nested case-control study found an elevated risk with history of various allergic disorders (e.g., urticaria: OR 11.4 [95% CI = 2.4–62.1]; allergic rhinitis: OR 9.2 [95% CI = 2.8–23.1]; asthma, rhinitis, or both: OR 6.5 [95% CI = 2.1–20.8]; and any allergy: OR 5.7 [95% CI = 1.8–18.1]).[182] Another small study also implicated alcohol consumption and receipt of another vaccine 1 to 9 days previously, as opposed to simultaneously, as risk factors.[310]

Reported rates have varied according to the approach to ascertainment (Table 27–19). Recent prospective or retrospective studies have found risk of an allergic AE, usually defined as objective urticaria or angioedema, in the range of 18 to 64 per 10,000 vaccinees.[304, 306, 309–312] A cluster of two deaths owing to anaphylactic shock in children receiving JE vaccine were reported in Korea in 1994. In a follow-up study to measure the incidence of JE vaccine–related AEs, one case of anaphylactic shock with syncope and collapse, three cases of generalized urticaria, and three cases of severe erythema were found in 15,487 Korean children immunized between May 15 and June 30, 1995. The rate of 0.03% was lower than that observed in adult travelers, which could reflect either biological differences in reactivity or the sensitivity of surveillance (Y. M. Sohn, unpublished observations).

Although the pathogenesis of the hypersensitivity reactions is not proven, in three Japanese children experiencing systemic reactions, immunoglobulin E (IgE) antibodies to gelatin were demonstrated, suggesting that gelatin, which is added as a vaccine stabilizer, may be a provoking antigen.[313] Further analysis of reactions showed two patterns: One was a combination of urticarial rash and wheezing, which was associated with the presence of antigelatin IgE in the serum, and the second was a cardiovascular collapse syndrome apparently due to another mechanism.[313a] A similar syndrome has been described in recipients of diploid cell–derived rabies vaccine in whom symptoms developed after a delay of as long as 1 week after booster immunization.[314] Immunological studies demonstrated IgE antibodies to human albumin, which is added to the vaccine as a stabilizer and chemically altered by the inactivating agent β-propionolactone.[315] Allergic reactions in recipients of crude mouse brain vaccine in Okinawa were attributed to formalin-altered proteins.

Inactivated Primary Hamster Kidney Cell–Derived Japanese Encephalitis Vaccine

Few adverse reactions have been reported in connection with the P3 inactivated vaccine. Local reactions, including swelling at the injection site, are observed in about 4% of vaccinees, and mild systemic symptoms, such as headache and dizziness, are reported by fewer than 1% of vaccinees. Fever higher than 38°C previously was a complication in 12% of vaccinees, but after a reduction in bovine serum in the currently formulated vaccine, febrile reactions have been halved. An urticarial allergic reaction was observed in only 1 of nearly 15,000 vaccinees surveyed.[288] Recent clusters of reactions temporally related to vaccination and consisting of acute asthenia, syncope, and disorientation have been reported from disparate areas of the country. Some features of the reactions suggest that they may be outbreaks of

Table 27–19. **HYPERSENSITIVITY REACTIONS* AFTER IMMUNIZATION WITH INACTIVATED MOUSE BRAIN–DERIVED JAPANESE ENCEPHALITIS VIRUS VACCINE**

COUNTRY	CASES/VACCINEES	RATE/10,000 VACCINEES	95% CI (%)	REFERENCE
Denmark	68/≈175,150	1–17†	—	304
United Kingdom	2/314	64	8–200	309
Australia (Torres Strait)	10/3511	28	14–500	312
United States (postmarketing surveillance, travelers)	4/767	52	14–130	311
Active duty military (Okinawa)	26	18	11–25	182

*Generalized urticaria or angioedema.
†Rates varied by vaccine lot.
CI, confidence interval.

hysteria, but their consistency and occurrence in a widespread geographical distribution are difficult to explain.

Live Attenuated Japanese Encephalitis Vaccine

An estimated 100 million children have been immunized with the live attenuated vaccine without apparent complication. Clinical monitoring of experimentally immunized subjects has documented the absence of local or systemic symptoms after immunization; specifically, headache and symptoms that might be associated with neuroinvasive infection as well as fever and signs and symptoms of systemic infection have not been observed after immunization. In a study of 867 children in whom fever was monitored over a 21-day period after immunization, temperatures above 37.6°C were recorded in fewer than 0.5% of vaccinees, and fever-onset days were distributed throughout the observation interval, mitigating against a vaccine-related febrile illness after a specific incubation period. In the same study, symptoms were recorded from 588,512 other vaccinees; fever was reported in 0.046% of subjects, rash in 0.01%, dizziness in 0.0003%, and nausea in 0.0003%, but these rates are difficult to interpret in the absence of similar observations in controls.[238, 316]

A block randomized cohort study of 13,266 vaccinated and 12,951 nonvaccinated 1- to 2-year-old children followed prospectively for 30 days confirmed the vaccine's safety. No cases of encephalitis or meningitis were detected in either group, and rates of hospitalization; new onset of seizures; fever lasting more than 3 days; and allergic, respiratory, and gastrointestinal symptoms were similar in the two groups. The observations excluded a vaccination-related encephalitis risk above 1 in 3400.[317]

The rates of clinical encephalitis among children vaccinated in field trials (see Table 27–16) provide additional reassurance that the SA14-14-2 virus does not itself cause encephalitis at a detectable rate. Rates of clinical encephalitis in children receiving SA14-14-2 vaccine—1.16 to 6.75 per 100,000—are lower than reported population-based incidence rates of childhood encephalitis (15 to 30 per 100,000).

No observations on the vaccine's safety in pregnant women or in immunocompromised individuals, specifically those with HIV infection, have been reported.

Indications for Immunization

Endemic Areas

In rural areas of Asia, intense JE virus transmission in the enzootic cycle leads to a high risk of exposure at an early age. Universal primary immunization is indicated for children between 1 and 2 years of age. The peak risk of infection is in children between 1 and 4 years of age, which may reflect the waning protective effects of maternal immunity and patterns of outdoor activity that place young children at risk. However, cases occur in children through the first decade of life, and in most areas with risk of enzootic transmission, immunity should be maintained by boosters through the age of 10 years.

Although incidence may vary regionally in countries at risk, universal childhood immunization is desirable, because even in economically advanced countries, viral transmission cannot be eliminated, and the cumulative risk of acquiring the illness over a lifetime of exposure probably justifies universal protection. Furthermore, conditions leading to epidemic transmission are unpredictable, and at intervals, outbreaks may lead to large numbers of cases even in urban areas. Hong Kong and Singapore may be special cases in which despite the absence of a national immunization policy, the possibility of enzootic viral transmission is limited by the exclusively urban environment.[174] For the most part, stepwise implementation of national JE vaccination programs, initially in epidemic foci and in areas with hyperendemic transmission, has been necessary because of economic considerations.[18]

Expatriates

JE vaccine is recommended for expatriates whose principal residence is in an area where JE is endemic or epidemic. Risk of acquiring JE among expatriates is variable and depends principally on the specific location of intended residence, housing conditions, nature of activities, and the possibility of unanticipated exposure to high-risk areas (see next section). Risk varies regionally and within specific countries. Viral transmission is seasonal in most areas and can fluctuate from year to year in a given location. Figure 27–1 and Table 27–20 summarize and extrapolate available data on locations and seasonality of risk by country. Patterns of viral transmission may change, and physicians and travelers are cautioned to consult public health officials for current data and trends.

Travelers

JE vaccine is recommended for selected travelers to Asia and should not be considered a routine immunization. Risk of acquiring JE during travel is extremely low (see earlier discussion), and the vast majority of visitors to Asia on business or in tours are at low risk and need not be immunized. In addition, the vaccine is costly; the average wholesale price (AWP) of three doses in the United States is $147. Because JE viral transmission is confined to certain seasons and occurs principally in rural areas, only visitors with such a travel itinerary have a high risk of acquiring the disease. Travelers and their physicians should weigh individual risk factors and disease risk in the area and season of anticipated travel in light of the potential for vaccine side effects (see Fig. 27–1 and Tables 27–4 and 27–20).[188, 189, 306, 318]

Immunization is recommended for visitors to epidemic or endemic areas during the transmission season, especially when there will be an extended period of exposure (more than 30 days) or the individual is at high

Table 27–20. **RISK OF JAPANESE ENCEPHALITIS BY COUNTRY, REGION, AND SEASON**

COUNTRY	AFFECTED AREAS/JURISDICTIONS	TRANSMISSION SEASON	COMMENTS
Bangladesh	Few data, probably widespread	Possibly July–December, as in northern India	Outbreak reported from Tangail district, Dacca division; sporadic cases in Rajshahi division
Bhutan	No data	No data	
Brunei	Presumed to be sporadic-endemic, as in Malaysia	Presumed year-round transmission	
Cambodia	Probably endemic-hyperendemic country-wide	Presumed to be May–October	Cases from Phnom Penh recognized
India	Reported cases from all states except Arunachal, Dadra, Daman, Diu, Gujarat, Himachal, Jammu, Kashmir, Lakshadweep, Meghalaya, Nagar Haveli, Orissa, Punjab, Rajasthan, and Sikkim	*South India:* May–October in Goa; October–January in Tamil Nadu; August–December in Karnataka; second peak, April–June in Mandya district *Andrha Pradesh:* September–December *North India:* July–December	Outbreaks in West Bengal, Bihar, Karnataka, Tamil Nadu, Andrha Pradesh, Assam, Uttar Pradesh, Manipure, Maharashtra, and Goa; urban cases reported (e.g., Lucknow)
Indonesia	Kalimantan, Bali, Nusa Tenggara, Sulawesi, Mollucas, West Irian, Java, Lombok	Probably year-round risk; varies by island; peak risks associated with rainfall, rice cultivation, and presence of pigs; peak period of risk: November–March; June–July in some years	Hyperendemic on Bali; sporadic cases recognized elsewhere; vaccine not recommended if travel is to major cities only
Japan*	Rare-sporadic cases on all islands, except Hokkaido	June–September except Ryukyu Islands (Okinawa), April–October	Vaccine not routinely recommended if travel is to major cities only; enzootic transmission without human cases observed on Hokkaido
Korea*	*North Korea:* no data *South Korea:* rare sporadic cases	July–October	Last major outbreaks in 1982–1983; vaccine not recommended if travel is to major cities only
Laos	Presumed to be endemic-hyperendemic country-wide	Presumed to be May–October	No data
Malaysia	Sporadic-endemic in all states of Peninsula, Sarawak, and probably Sabah	No seasonal pattern; year-round transmission	Vaccine not recommended if travel is to major cities only
Myanmar	Presumed to be endemic-hyperendemic country-wide	Presumed to be May–October	Repeated outbreaks in Shan State in Chiang Mai Valley
Nepal	Hyperendemic in southern lowlands (Terai); sporadic cases now recognized in Kathmandu Valley	July–December	Vaccine recommended for travelers to lowlands
Papua-New Guinea	Sporadic cases (1956 and 1997–1998) reported from Western, Gulf, and South Highland Provinces	Unknown	Vaccine not routinely recommended
People's Republic of China	Cases in all provinces except Xizang (Tibet), Xinjiang, and Qinghai; hyperendemic in southern China; endemic–periodically epidemic in temperate areas; Hong Kong: rare cases in New Territories	*Northern China:* May–September *Southern China:* April–October (Guangshi, Yunnan, Gwangdong, and Southern Fujian, Szechuan, Guizhou, Hunan, and Jiangsi provinces)	Vaccine not routinely recommended for travelers to major cities only (including Hong Kong)
Pakistan	May be transmitted in central deltas	Presumed to be June–January	Cases reported near Karachi; endemic areas overlap those for West Nile virus
Philippines	Presumed to be endemic on all islands	Uncertain; speculations based on locations and agroecosystems *West Luzon, Mindoro, Negro Palowan:* April–November *Elsewhere:* Year-round; greatest risk, April–January	Outbreaks described in Nueva Ecija, Luzon, and Manila
Russia	Far Eastern maritime areas south of Khabarousk	Peak period, July–September	Rare human cases reported
Singapore	Rare cases—last indigenous case in 1992	Year-round transmission not detected recently	Vaccine not routinely recommended
Sri Lanka	Endemic in all but mountainous areas; periodically epidemic in northern and central provinces	October–January; secondary peak of enzootic transmission, May–June	Recent outbreaks in central (Anuradhapura) and northwestern provinces
Taiwan*	Sporadic cases except in central mountains	April–October; June peak	Cases in and around Taipei
Thailand	Hyperendemic in north; sporadic-endemic in south	May–October	Annual outbreaks in Chiang Mai Valley; sporadic cases in Bangkok suburbs
Vietnam	Endemic-hyperendemic in all provinces	May–October	Highest rates in and near Hanoi
Western Pacific and Australia	Discrete epidemics reported on Guam, Saipan (northern Mariana Islands); sporadic cases in Torres Strait and Cape York peninsula, Australia	Uncertain; possibly September–January in the Pacific; February–April in far northern Australia	Enzootic cycle may not be sustainable; epidemics may follow introductions of virus; single case reported on Australian mainland (Cape York peninsula) in 1998

*Reported human cases may not accurately reflect risks to nonimmune visitors because of high immunization rates in local populations. Humans are incidental to the transmission cycle. High levels of viral transmission may occur in the absence of human disease.

Notes:

1. Assessments are based on publications, surveillance reports, and personal correspondence.
2. Extrapolations have been made from available data.
3. Transmission patterns may change.
4. Consult the Centers for Disease Control and Prevention (970-221-6400) or other public health authorities for the latest trends.

risk of exposure to vectors because of the nature of his or her activities or housing. For example, bicyclists on tours and workers on field projects in rural areas may have greater outdoor exposure to vector mosquitoes. In addition, advanced age and pregnancy may affect risk and outcome of JE. Repellents and other protective measures are recommended in any case, because other vector-borne diseases may be transmitted in the same areas. General precautions are especially important to travelers in whom vaccine is contraindicated, who are unable to complete immunization because of departures on short notice, or who do not choose to be immunized because their visits to high-risk areas are brief or carry an equivocal risk.

Because allergic reactions to mouse brain–derived JE vaccine may be delayed for 1 week after immunization, and to allow protective antibody levels to develop, vaccinees ideally should defer travel until 7 days after receiving the last vaccine dose. Travelers should remain in areas accessible to medical care for 7 days after immunization.

Research Laboratory Workers

There have been 22 cases of laboratory-acquired JE virus, principally in research settings where infectious JE virus was used.[319] Infection can be transmitted by percutaneous or mucous membrane exposures and potentially by aerosols, especially from preparations containing high viral concentrations, which occur during viral purification. Immunization presumably protects against percutaneous exposures; however, it is unknown whether vaccine-derived immunity, especially from inactivated vaccine, protects against aerosol infection. Immunization is advised for all research laboratory personnel who potentially may be exposed to field or virulent strains of the virus. Although no formal biosafety recommendations have been issued for work with the attenuated vaccine SA14-14-2 strain, sufficient data are available on its attenuation such that immunized workers should be permitted to handle that virus under Biosafety Level 2 conditions, paralleling recommendations for the attenuated vaccine strains of YF, Junin, Rift Valley fever, chikungunya, and Venezuelan equine encephalitis.[306]

Contraindications to Immunization

Mouse brain–derived JE vaccine is contraindicated in people who have had an allergic reaction to the vaccine, to gelatin, or to other rodent-derived products, including previous doses of JE vaccine. Other biologicals made in rodent tissue include vaccines against rabies, the hantaviral agents of hemorrhagic fever with renal syndrome, Hantaan and Seoul viruses, products derived from Chinese hamster ovary cells, and murine monoclonal antibodies. Hantaan virus vaccine made in mouse brain and purified by methods similar to those used in JE vaccine manufacture is produced in Korea and is under evaluation in China. A hantaviral vaccine produced in primary gerbil (*Meriones unguiculatus*) kidney cells also has limited distribution in China. YF vaccine made from the French neurotropic strain previously was produced in mouse brain, but production was discontinued in 1982.

Anecdotal reports of ADE occurring in temporal relationship to vaccination suggest that the mouse brain–derived vaccine should not be used in individuals who have recovered from ADE or Guillain-Barré syndrome or who have multiple sclerosis or other demyelinating disorders.

Hypersensitivity reactions to mouse brain–derived JE vaccine are more common in individuals with allergic conditions (e.g., asthma; allergic rhinitis; drug or hymenoptera venom sensitivity; and food allergy, especially to gelatin-containing foods [see earlier discussion]). If these individuals are offered JE vaccine, they should be advised of the potential for vaccine-related angioedema and generalized urticaria. Hypersensitivity to a protein found in mouse urine is common in animal caretakers and certain laboratorians. It is unknown whether this sensitivity carries a specific risk in recipients of JE vaccine.

There are no specific contraindications to the use of PHK-derived inactivated JE vaccine except history of allergic reaction to a previous dose.

JE vaccines pose a theoretical risk to the developing fetus. No adverse outcomes of pregnancy have been associated directly with JE vaccine. Travelers and their physicians must balance the theoretical risks of JE vaccine in pregnancy against the potential risks of acquiring JE and the adverse outcome of the disease.

There are few data on the safety and efficacy of inactivated JE vaccines in immunocompromised individuals. A small study of children with various chronic diseases, including some oncology patients, disclosed no difference in immunogenicity or reactogenicity in recipients of mouse brain–derived vaccine.[281] Infants vertically infected with HIV responded less well to the vaccine (see earlier discussion), but no unusual AEs were recorded.[280]

Live attenuated JE vaccine potentially carries an additional risk in pregnant women and immunocompromised patients. Although experimental data suggest that JE SA14-14-2 virus may not be neurotropic in immunosuppressed animals, there are no data on the vaccine's safety in immunocompromised individuals, specifically, HIV-infected patients. When JE vaccine must be given to pregnant women or to immunocompromised patients, available inactivated JE vaccine should be used rather than live vaccine.

PUBLIC HEALTH CONSIDERATIONS

Although a secular trend toward declining JE incidence has been observed with widespread use of JE vaccine, coincident socioeconomic changes also may have contributed to falling disease incidence (Fig. 27–19). In Thailand, for example, encephalitis incidence had begun a steady decline since the mid-1970s, nearly two decades before the national JE immunization program was instituted in 1990 (see Fig. 27–5) and in Singapore, reductions in disease incidence and viral transmission have been attributed solely to factors other

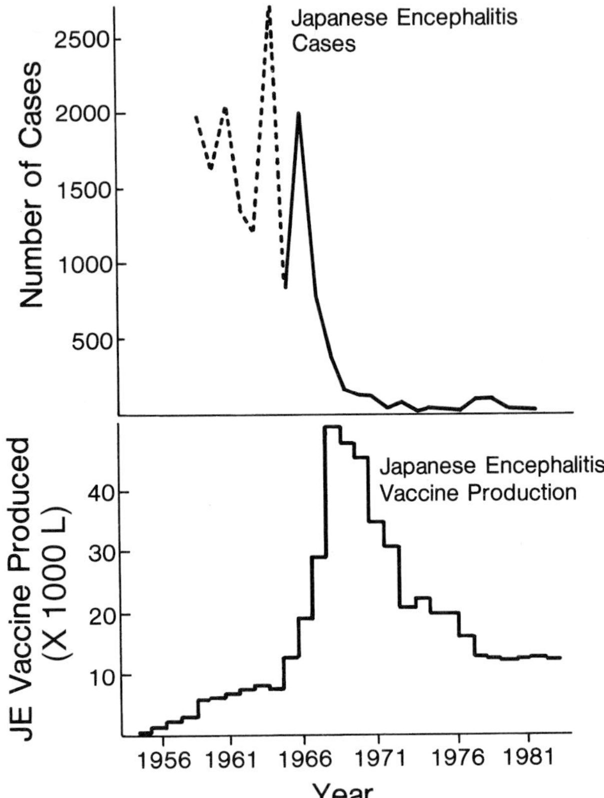

Figure 27–19. Incidence of Japanese encephalitis (JE) in relationship to vaccine distribution in Japan, 1956 to 1981. Dotted line = reported cases; solid line = confirmed cases since 1965. (Adapted from Oya A. Japanese encephalitis vaccine. Acta Pediatr Jpn 30:175–184, 1988.)

than vaccination (see earlier discussion).[13, 174] The most important have been (1) improved agricultural productivity and increasing urbanization, resulting in fewer rural dwellers at risk; (2) a decline in land area under rice cultivation; and (3) increased use of agricultural pesticides, which have reduced numbers of vector mosquitoes (Fig. 27–20).[320] Although pig inventories actually have increased, changes in husbandry practices, especially centralized rearing, probably have resulted in an overall reduction of infected vectors in areas where people are active. Improvements in the general standard of living and, in specific locations, vector control programs have further reduced risk of exposure and infection.

Observations from the PRC, where development has been less extensive, are somewhat clearer in demonstrating the impact of immunization. JE incidence rates in Beijing and in other areas of China where high immunization rates are maintained have declined dramatically and have remained low (Figs. 27–13 and 27–21 and Table 27–21).[10, 194] Although vaccine coverage is high in cities and in prosperous districts, coverage remains low in many rural locations, often in the very places with greatest risk. The principal barriers to immunization include the cost of the vaccine, which must be borne by families, as JE vaccine is not government subsidized as a childhood vaccine, and inaccessibility to the health care system.

As a zoonotic disease with natural viral reservoirs, JE never can be eliminated. Although its transmission can

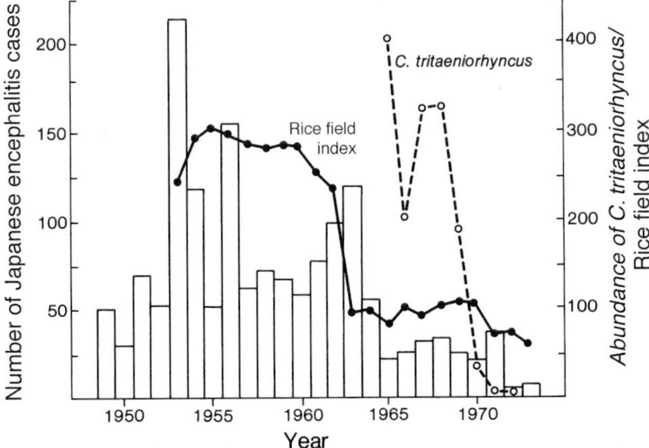

Figure 27–20. The relationship of reduced land area in rice paddies, declining abundance of vector *Culex tritaeniorhyncus* mosquitoes, and reported Japanese encephalitis (JE) cases on Okinawa, 1949 to 1973. JE vaccine was licensed in Japan in 1954, but in addition to immunization, incidental factors associated with development may have contributed to the decline in reported cases. The rice field index is expressed as a percentage of area cultivated in 1964 (100%). (Adapted from T. Fukunaga, personal communication.)

be modulated by factors mentioned earlier, these approaches alone or in combination cannot be relied on to reduce disease incidence as effectively as human vaccination. Successful control of JE by universal immunization in at least three countries in the region suggests that an extension of these efforts throughout the continent could lead to the near elimination of the disease. However, for all of the approved vaccines, unresolved issues potentially limit their acceptability as a solution for region-wide control of the disease.

The inactivated mouse brain–derived vaccine is troubled by safety and other issues. Moreover, the vaccine's 91% efficacy, when extrapolated to the entire cohort of children younger than 15 years in Asia—approximately 1 billion children—yields an absolute number of primary vaccine failures of questionable acceptability. Assuming a JE incidence rate of 1 per 10,000 in children younger than 15 years, approximately 100,000 cases would occur in the absence of any immunization. If every child was immunized but only 91% were protected, 9000 residual

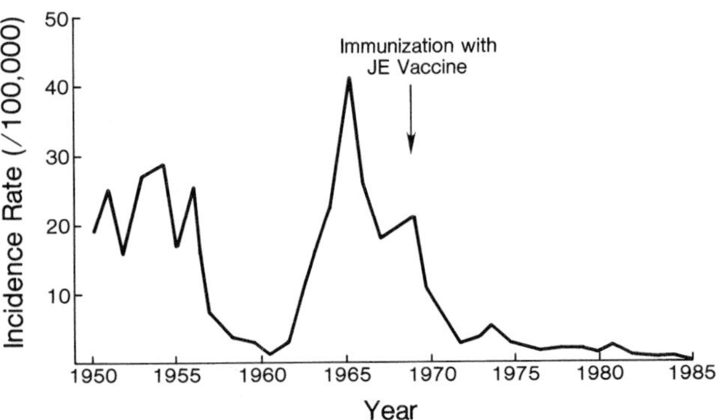

Figure 27–21. Declining incidence of Japanese encephalitis (JE) in Beijing and association with mass immunization, 1950 to 1985. (Adapted from Gu PW, Ding ZF. Inactivated Japanese encephalitis [JE] vaccine made from hamster cell culture [a review]. Jpn Encephalitis Hemorrhagic Fever Renal Synd Bull 2:15–26, 1987.)

Table 27–21. **JAPANESE ENCEPHALITIS IMMUNIZATION COVERAGE AND INCIDENCE, LIAONING**

DISTRICT	POPULATION OF 1- TO 10-YEAR-OLDS	NO. OF CHILDREN IMMUNIZED	% IMMUNIZED	INCIDENCE IN 1- TO 10-YEAR-OLDS
Zhuang Ho	237,457	33,637	14.2	35.0
Fu Hsien	187,414	161,491	86.7	6.5
Xin Chin	135,754	120,839	89.0	3.6

From Zhang Liu Xing Bing Fang Zhi Yan Jin (1978), p 247. Cited in Huang CH. Studies of Japanese encephalitis in China. Adv Virus Res 27:71–101, 1982.

cases would occur annually as a result of primary vaccine failure. Although additional booster doses presumably would improve efficacy, the strategy also would lead to increased costs for a vaccine that already is considered costly and of marginal cost-benefit.

A study of the vaccine's benefits and costs in Thailand showed that a national immunization program of 18-month-old infants had an effectiveness of $15,715 per case prevented and a benefit-cost ratio of 4.6:1 at the current Thai domestic production cost of $2.16 for two 0.5-mL doses.[321] A sensitivity analysis based on varying JE incidence rates showed that the program no longer was economical (where the ratio fell below 1:1) at an incidence rate of 3 per 100,000. In less developed countries where the prevention of lost productivity would yield lower savings, national vaccination programs would be uneconomical at higher incidence rates. Whether vaccine cost could be reduced further by economies of scale is uncertain, because unlike viral vaccines produced in cell cultures, scaling up production involves considerable labor in the rearing, inoculation, and harvesting of mice, as well as an extensive purification process.

The SA14-14-2 vaccine, produced under government subsidy in China, "costs" $0.03 per dose; however, under internationally accepted manufacturing standards, its estimated cost per dose will be in the same range as the inactivated mouse brain vaccine. Fewer doses are required for long-term protection, which reduces the overall costs per child protected. The vaccine is under consideration for licensure in Korea, and if it is approved, it may be manufactured for international distribution in the future. The principal concerns for its broader acceptance are the potential for adventitious agents associated with the PHK cell substrate and its safety in areas of Asian where HIV infections are prevalent.

Acknowledgments

We gratefully acknowledge the support of SB Halstead and the Rockefeller Foundation.

REFERENCES

1. Igarashi A. Epidemiology and control of Japanese encephalitis. World Health Stat Q 45(2–3):299–305, 1992.
2. Burke DS, Leake CJ. Japanese encephalitis. In Monath TP (ed). The Arboviruses: Epidemiology and Ecology. Vol. 3. Boca Raton, FL, CRC Press, 1988, pp 63–92.
3. Umenai T, Krzysko R, Bektimirov TA, Assaad FA. Japanese encephalitis: Current worldwide status. Bull World Health Organ 63:625–631, 1985.
4. Whitley RJ. Herpes simplex virus. In Fields BN, Knipe DM (eds). Virology. New York, Raven Press, 1990, pp 1843–1997.
5. Nicolosi A, Hauser VA, Beghi E, Kurland LT. Epidemiology of central nervous system infection in Olmsted County, Minnesota, 1950–1981. J Infect Dis 154:399–408, 1986.
6. Hiroyama T. Epidemiology of Japanese encephalitis (in Japanese). Saishin-Igaku 17:1272–1280, 1962.
7. Inada R. Compte rendu des recherches sur l'encephalite epidemique au Japon. Off Int d'Hyg Pub Bull Mens 29:1389–1401, 1937.
8. Kuttner AG, T'sun T. Encephalitis in north China. Results obtained with neutralization tests. J Clin Invest 15:525–530, 1936.
9. Sohn YM. Control of Japanese encephalitis through immunization in Korea: Past, present and future. In preparation; Seoul, Korea; 1997.
10. Yu YX. Japanese encephalitis in China. Southeast Asian J Trop Med Public Health 26S3:17–21, 1995.
11. Taniguchi K, Matsunaga Y. National epidemiologic surveillance of vaccine-preventable diseases, Japan. Available at http://www.nih.go.jp/yoken/idsc/ryukou/japa_Efig1.gif. October 1995.
12. Grossman RA, Edelman R, Willhight M, et al. Study of Japanese encephalitis virus in Chiang Mai Valley, Thailand. Am J Epidemiol 98:133–149, 1973.
13. Chunsuttiwat S, Warachit P. Japanese encephalitis in Thailand. Southeast Asian J Trop Med Public Health 26S3:43–46, 1995.
14. Thein S, Aung H, Sebastian AA. Study of vector, amplifier, and human infection with Japanese encephalitis virus in a Rangoon community. Am J Epidemiol 128:1376–1382, 1988.
15. Nguyen HT, Nguyen TY. Japanese encephalitis in Vietnam 1985–93. Southeast Asian J Trop Med Public Health 26S3:47–50, 1995.
16. Kari IK, Suharyono, Jennings GB. Clinical aspects of Japanese encephalitis. Denpasar, Indonesia, unpublished observations, 1990–1995.
17. Cardosa MJ, Hooi TP, Kaur P. Japanese encephalitis virus is an important cause of encephalitis among children in Penang. Southeast Asian J Trop Med Public Health 26:272–275, 1995.
18. Vasakarava S. Japanese encephalitis vaccine implementation in Thailand. Southeast Asian J Trop Med Public Health 26S3:54–56, 1995.
19. Carey DE, Myers RM, Reuben R, Webb JKG. Japanese encephalitis in South India. A summary of recent knowledge. J Indian Med Assoc 52:10–15, 1969.
20. Banerjee K. Japanese encephalitis in India (a country report). Proceedings of a regional workshop on control strategies for Japanese encephalitis; Department of Medical Sciences, Ministry of Public Health, Nonthaburi, Thailand; October 4–6, 1994.
21. Igarashi A, Tanaka M, Morita K, et al. Detection of West Nile and Japanese encephalitis viral genome sequences in cerebrospinal fluid from acute encephalitis cases in Karachi, Pakistan. Microbiol Immunol 38(10):827–830, 1994.
22. Service MW. Agricultural development and arthropod-borne disease—a review. Revista Saudé Publica 25:165–178, 1991.
23. Joshi DD. Current status of Japanese encephalitis in Nepal. Southeast Asian J Trop Med Public Health 26:34–40, 1995.
24. Peiris JSM, Amerasinghe FP, Amerasinghe PH, et al. Japanese encephalitis in Sri Lanka: I. The study of an epidemic-vector incrimination, porcine infection and human disease. Trans R Soc Trop Med Hyg 86:307–323, 1992.
25. Paul WS, Moore PS, Karabatsos N, et al. Outbreak of Japanese encephalitis on the island of Saipan, 1990. J Infect Dis 167:1053–1058, 1993.
26. Hanna JN, Ritchie SA, Phillips DA, et al. An outbreak of Japa-

nese encephalitis in the Torres Strait, Australia, 1995. Med J Aust 165:256–260, 1996.
27. Halstead SB, Grosz CR. Subclinical Japanese encephalitis. I. Infection of Americans with limited residence in Korea. Am J Hyg 75:190–201, 1962.
28. Gajanana A, Thenmozhi V, Samuel P, Reuben R. A community-based study of subclinical flavivirus infections in children in an area of Tamil Nadu, India, where Japanese encephalitis is endemic. Bull World Health Organ 73:237–244, 1995.
29. Innis B. Japanese encephalitis. In Porterfield J (ed). Exotic Viral Infections. Oxford, Chapman & Hall, 1995.
30. Kalayanarooj S. Japanese encephalitis: Clinical manifestations, outcome and management. Southeast Asian J Trop Med Public Health 26S3:9–10, 1995.
31. Lincoln AF, Sivertson SE. Acute phase of Japanese B encephalitis. Two hundred and one cases in American soldiers, Korea, 1950. JAMA 150:268–273, 1952.
32. Benenson MW, Top FH, Gresso W, et al. The virulence of Japanese B encephalitis virus in Thailand. Am J Trop Med Hyg 24:974–980, 1975.
33. Bu'lock FA. Japanese B virus encephalitis in India—a growing problem. Q J Med 233:825–836, 1986.
34. Misra UK, Kalita J. Movement disorders in Japanese encephalitis. J Neurol 244:299–3030, 1997.
35. Kamala CS, Venkatwshwara Rao M, George S, Prasanna NY. Japanese encephalitis in children in Bellary Karnataka. Indian Pediatr 26:445–452, 1989.
36. Rathi AK, Kushwaha KP, Singh YD, et al. JE virus encephalitis: 1988 epidemic at Gorakhpur. Indian Pediatr 30:325–333, 1993.
37. Kumar R, Mathur A, Singh KB, et al. Clinical sequelae of Japanese encephalitis in children. Indian J Med Res 97:9–13, 1993.
38. Kumar R, Mathur A, Kumar A, et al. Clinical features and prognostic indicators of Japanese encephalitis in children in Lucknow (India). Indian J Med Res 91:321–327, 1990.
39. Hoke CH, Vaughn DW, Nisalak A, et al. Effect of high-dose dexamethasone on the outcome of acute encephalitis due to Japanese encephalitis virus. J Infect Dis 165:631–637, 1992.
40. Johnson RT, Burke DS, Elwell M, et al. Japanese encephalitis: Immunocytochemical studies of viral antigen and inflammatory cells in fatal cases. Ann Neurol 18:567–573, 1985.
41. Kusuhara T, Ayabe M, Hino H, et al. Cerebrospinal fluid levels of monoamines in patients with Japanese encephalitis. Eur Neurol 36:236–237, 1996.
42. Misra UK, Kalita J. Encephalopathy with bilateral thalamotegmental lesions? Japanese encephalitis. Am J Neuroradiol 17:192–193, 1996.
43. Koelfen W, Freund M, Guckel F, et al. MRI of encephalitis in children: Comparison of CT and MRI in the acute stage with long-term follow-up. Paediatr Neuroradiol 38:73–79, 1996.
44. Misra UK, Kalita J, Jain SK, Mathur A. Radiological and neurophysiological changes in Japanese encephalitis. J Neurol Neurosurg Psychiatry 57:1484–1487, 1994.
45. Kimura K, Dosaka A, Hashimoto Y, et al. Single-photon emission CT findings in acute Japanese encephalitis. Am J Neuroradiol 18:465–469, 1997.
46. Kumar R, Misra UK, Kalita J, et al. MRI in Japanese encephalitis. Neuroradiology 39:180–184, 1997.
47. Kumar R, Mathur A, Singh KB, et al. Clinical sequelae of Japanese encephalitis in children. Indian J Med Res [A] 97:9–13, 1993.
48. Schneider RJ, Firestone MH, Edelman R, et al. Clinical sequelae after Japanese encephalitis: A one year follow-up study in Thailand. Southeast Asian J Trop Med Public Health 5:560–568, 1974.
49. Huang PJ, Huang YH, Wu PH, et al. A survey of clinical sequelae of Japanese encephalitis. Epidemiol Bull 12:19–26, 1996.
50. Weaver OM. Japanese encephalitis: Clinical features. Neurology 8:887–889, 1958.
51. Pieper SJL, Kurland LT. Sequelae of Japanese B and mumps encephalitis. Recent follow-up of patients affected in 1947–1948 epidemic on Guam. Am J Trop Med Hyg 7:481–490, 1958.
52. Simpson TW, Meiklejohn G. Sequelae of Japanese B encephalitis. Am J Trop Med 27:727–731, 1947.
53. Edelman R, Schneider RJ, Chieowanich P, et al. The effect of dengue virus infection on the clinical sequelae of Japanese encephalitis: A one year follow-up study in Thailand. Southeast Asian J Trop Med Public Health 6:308–315, 1975.
54. Kumar R, Selvan AS, Sharma S, et al. Clinical predictors of Japanese encephalitis. Neuroepidemiology 13:97–102, 1994.
55. Burke DS, Lorsomrudee W, Leake CJ, et al. Fatal outcome in Japanese encephalitis. Am J Trop Med Hyg 34:1203–1210, 1985.
56. Burke DS, Morrill JC. Levels of interferon in the plasma and cerebrospinal fluid of patients with acute Japanese encephalitis. J Infect Dis 155:797–799, 1987.
57. Burke DS, Nisalak A, Ussery MA, et al. Kinetics of IgM and IgG responses to Japanese encephalitis virus in human serum and cerebrospinal fluid. J Infect Dis 151:1093–1099, 1985.
58. Ravi V, Parida S, Desai A, et al. Correlation of tumor necrosis factor levels in the serum and cerebrospinal fluid with clinical outcome in Japanese encephalitis. J Med Virol 51:132–136, 1997.
59. Desai A, Shankar SK, Jayakumar PN, et al. Co-existence of cerebral cysticercosis with Japanese encephalitis: A prognostic indicator. Epidemiol Infect 118:165–171, 1997.
60. Sharma S, Mathur A, Prakash R, et al. Japanese encephalitis virus latency in peripheral blood lymphocytes and recurrence of infection in children. Clin Exp Immunol 85:85–89, 1991.
61. Ravi V, Desai A, Shenoy PK, et al. Persistence of Japanese encephalitis virus in the human nervous system. J Med Virol 40:326–329, 1993.
62. Huy BV, Tu HC, Luan TV, Lindqvist R. Early mental and neurological sequelae after Japanaese B encephalitis. Southeast Asian J Trop Med Public Health 25:549–553, 1994.
63. Ma WY, Jiang SZ, Zhang MJ, et al. Preliminary observations on treatment of patients with Japanese B encephalitis with monoclonal antibody. J Med Coll PLA 7:299–302, 1992.
64. Harinasuta C, Nimmanitya S, Titsyakorn U. The effect of interferon alpha A on two cases of Japanese encephalitis in Thailand. Southeast Asian J Trop Med Public Health 16:332–336, 1985.
65. Harrington DG, Hilmas DE, Elwell MR, Whitmire RE, Stephen EL. Intranasal infection of monkeys with Japanese encephalitis virus: Clinical response and treatment with a nuclease-resistant derivative of poly(I)-poly(C). Am J Trop Med Hyg 26:1191–1198, 1977.
66. Hiyake M. The pathology of Japanese encephalitis. Bull World Health Organ 30:153–160, 1964.
67. Esiri MM, Reading MC, Squier MV, Hughes JT. Immunocytochemical characterization of the macrophage and lymphocyte infiltrate in the brain in six cases of human encephalitis of varied aetiology. Neuropathol Appl Neurobiol 15:289–395, 1989.
68. Li ZS, Hong SF, Gong NL. Immunohistochemical study of Japanese B encephalitis. Chin Med J 101:768–771, 1988.
69. Shankar SK, Rao TV, Mruthyunjayanna BP, et al. Autopsy study of brains during an epidemic of Japanese encephalitis in Karnataka. Indian J Med Res 78:431–440, 1983.
70. Zimmerman HM. The pathology of Japanese B encephalitis. Am J Pathol 22:965–991, 1946.
71. Haymaker W, Sabin AB. Topographic distribution of lesions in central nervous system in Japanese B encephalitis. Arch Neurol Psychiatry 57:673–692, 1947.
72. Desai A, Shankar SK, Ravi V, et al. Japanese encephalitis virus antigen in the human brain and its topographic distribution. Acta Neuropathol 89:368–373, 1995.
73. Ishii T, Matsushita M, Hamada S. Characteristic residual neuropathological features of Japanese B encephalitis. Acta Neuropathol (Berl) 38:181–186, 1977.
74. Burns KF. Congenital Japanese B encephalitis infection of swine. Proc Soc Exp Biol Med 75:621–625, 1950.
75. Chaturvedi UC, Mathur A, Chandra A, et al. Transplacental infection with Japanese encephalitis virus. J Infect Dis 141:712–715, 1980.
76. Mathur A, Tandon HO, Mathur KR, et al. Japanese encephalitis infection during pregnancy. Indian J Med Res 81:9–12, 1985.
77. Bhonde RR, Wagh UV. Susceptibility of human placenta to Japanese encephalitis virus in vitro. Indian J Med Res 82:371–373, 1985.
78. Ogata A, Nagashima K, Hall WW, et al. Japanese encephalitis virus neurotropism is dependent on the degree of neuronal maturity. J Virol 65:880–886, 1991.

79. Kimura-Kuroda J, Ichikawa M, Ogata A, et al. Specific tropism of Japanese encephalitis virus for developing neurons in primary rat brain culture. Arch Virol 130:477–484, 1993.
80. Kuno G, Chang G-JJ, Tsuchiya KR, et al. Phylogeny of the genus *Flavivirus*. J Virol 72:73–83, 1998.
81. Chambers TJ, Hahn CS, Galler R, Rice CM. Flaviviruses genome organization, expression and replication. Annu Rev Microbiol 44:649–688, 1990.
82. Murphy PA. Togavirus morphology and morphogenesis. In Schlesinger RW (ed). The Togaviruses: Biology, Structure and Replication. New York, Academic Press, 1980, pp 241–316.
83. Sumiyoshi H, Mori C, Fuke I, et al. Complete nucleotide sequence of the Japanese encephalitis virus genome RNA. Virology 161:497–510, 1987.
84. Nitayaphan S, Grant JA, Chang GJ, Trent DW. Nucleotide sequence of the virulent SA-14 strain of Japanese encephalitis virus and its attenuated vaccine derivative, SA-14-14-2. Virology 177:541–552, 1990.
85. Gollins SW, Porterfield JS. Flavivirus infection enhancement in macrophages: An electron microscopic study of viral cellular entry. J Gen Virol 66:1969–1982, 1985.
86. Hase T, Summers PL, Dubois DR. Ultrastructural changes of mouse brain neurons infected with Japanese encephalitis virus. Int J Exp Pathol 71:493–505, 1990.
87. Ng ML, Hong SS. Flavivirus infection: Essential ultrastructural changes and association of Kunjin virus NS3 protein with microtubules. Arch Virol 106:103–120, 1989.
88. Westaway EG, Mackenzie JM, Kenney MT, et al. Ultrastructure of Kunjin virus–infected cells: Colocalization of NS1 and NS3 with double-stranded RNA, and of NS2B with NS3, in virus-induced membrane structures. J Virol 71:6650–6661, 1997.
89. Mackenzie JM, Jones MK, Young PR. Immunolocalization of the dengue virus nonstructural glycoprotein NS1 suggests a role in viral RNA replication. Virology 220:232–240, 1996.
90. Konishi E, Mason P. Proper maturation of the Japanese encephalitis virus envelope glycoprotein requires cosynthesis with the premembrane protein. J Virol 67:1672–1675, 1993.
91. Allison SL, Stadler K, Mandl CW, et al. Synthesis and secretion of recombinant tick-borne encephalitis virus protein E in soluble and particulate form. J Virol 69:5816–5820, 1995.
92. Heinz FX, Stadler K, Püschner-Auer G, et al. Structural changes and functional control of the tick-borne encephalitis virus glycoprotein E by the heterodimeric association with protein prM. Virology 198:109–117, 1994.
93. Stadler K, Allison S, Schalich J, Heinz FX. Proteolytic activation of tick-borne encephalitis virus by furin. J Virol 71:8475–8481, 1997.
94. Mandl CW, Guriakhoo FG, Holzmann H, et al. Antigenic structure of the flavivirus envelope protein E at the molecular level, using tick-borne encephalitis virus as a model. J Virol 63:564–571, 1989.
95. Rey FA, Heinz FX, Mandl C, et al. The envelope glycoprotein from tick-borne encephalitis virus at 2 Å resolution. Nature 375:291–298, 1995.
96. Cao JX, Ni H, Wills MR, et al. Passage of Japanese encephalitis virus in HeLa cells results in attenuation of virulence in mice. J Gen Virol 76:757–764, 1995.
97. Chen Y, Maguire T, Marks RM. Demonstration of binding of dengue virus envelope protein to target cells. J Virol 70:8765–8772, 1996.
98. Chen Y, Maguire T, Hileman RE, et al. Dengue virus infectivity depends on envelope protein binding to target cell heparan sulfate. Nat Med 3:866–871, 1997.
99. Kimura T, Kimura-Kuroda J, Nagashina K, Yasui K. Analysis of virus-cell binding characteristics on the determination of Japanese encephalitis virus susceptibility. Arch Virol 139:239–251, 1994.
100. Becker Y. Computer analysis of antigenic domains and RDG-like sequences (RCW6) in the E glycoprotein of flaviviruses: An approach to vaccine development. Virus Genes 4:267–282, 1990.
101. Calisher CH, Karabatsos N, Dalrymple JM, et al. Antigenic relationships among flaviviruses as determined by cross-neutralization tests with polyclonal antisera. J Gen Virol 70:37–43, 1989.
102. Porterfield JS. The flaviviruses (group B arboviruses): A cross-neutralization study. J Gen Virol 23:91–96, 1974.
103. Wu JS, Lu CF, Lin SY. Prevalence of antibody to hepatitis C virus (anti-HVC) in different populations in Taiwan. Chung Hua Min Kuo Weishong Wu Chi Mein J Hsueh Tsa Chih 24:55–60, 1991.
104. Poidinger M, Hall RA, Mackenzie JS. Molecular characterization of the Japanese encephalitis serocomplex of the flavivirus genus. Virology 218:417–421, 1996.
105. Hasegawa T, Yoshida M, Kobayashi Y, Fujita S. Antigenic analysis of Japanese encephalitis viruses in Asian by using monoclonal antibodies. Vaccine 13:1713–1721, 1995.
106. Hasegawa T, Yoshida M, Fujita S, Kobayashi Y. Comparison of structural proteins among antigenically different Japanese encephalitis virus strains. Vaccine 12:841–844, 1994.
107. Chen WR, Tesh RB, Rico-Hesse R. Genetic variation of Japanese encephalitis virus in nature. J Gen Virol 71:2915–2920, 1990.
108. Chen WR, Rico-Hesse R, Tesh RB. A new genotype of Japanese encephalitis virus from Indonesia. Am J Trop Med Hygiene 47:61–69, 1992.
109. Huong VT, Ha QDQ, Deubel V. Genetic study of Japanese encephalitis viruses from Vietnam. Am J Trop Med Hyg 49:538–544, 1993.
110. Tsuchie H, Oda K, Vythilingam I, et al. Genotypes of Japanaese encephalitis virus isolated in three states in Malaysia. Am J Trop Med Hyg 56:153–158, 1997.
111. Ma SP, Arakaki S, Makino Y, Fukunaga T. Molecular epidemiology of Japanese encephalitis virus in Okinawa. Microbiol Immunol 40:847–855, 1996.
112. Ritchie SA, Phillips D, Broom A, et al. Isolation of Japanese encephalitis virus from *Culex annulirostris* in Australia. Am J Trop Med Hyg 56:80–84, 1997.
113. Chung YJ, Nam JH, Ban SJ, Cho HW. Antigenic and genetic analysis of Japanese encephalitis viruses isolated from Korea. Am J Trop Med Hyg 55:91–97, 1996.
114. Hase T, Summers PL, Ray P. Entry and replication of Japanese encephalitis virus in cultured neurogenic cells. J Virol Methods 30:205–214, 1990.
115. Dropulic B, Masters CL. Entry of neurotropic arboviruses into the central nervous system: An in vitro study using mouse brain endothelium. J Infect Dis 161:685–691, 1990.
116. Johnson RT, Intralawan P, Puapanwatton S. Japanese encephalitis: Identification of inflammatory cells in cerebrospinal fluid. Ann Neurol 20:691–695, 1986.
117. Iwasaki Y, Sako K, Tsunoda I, Ohara Y. Phenotypes of mononuclear cell infiltrates in human central nervous system. Acta Neuropathol (Berl) 85:653–657, 1993.
118. Kiura K, Onodera T, Nishida A, et al. A single gene controls resistance to Japanese encephalitis virus in mice. Arch Virol 112:261–270, 1990.
119. Miura K, Goto N, Suzuki H, Fujisaki Y. Strain difference of mouse in susceptibility to Japanese encephalitis virus infection. Exp Anim 37:365–373, 1988.
120. Wills MR, Singh BK, Debnath NC, Barrett AD. Immunogenicity of wild-type and vaccine strains of Japanese encephalitis virus and the effect of haplotype restriction on murine immune responses. Vaccine 11:761–766, 1993.
121. Ben-Nathon D, Huitinga I, Lustig S, et al. West Nile virus neuroinvasion and encephalitis induced by macrophage depletion in mice. Arch Virol 141:459–469, 1996.
122. Sather GE, Hammon WM. Protection against St. Louis encephalitis and West Nile arboviruses by previous dengue virus (types 1–4) infection. Proc Soc Exp Biol Med 135:573–578, 1970.
123. Tarr GC, Hammon WM. Cross-protection between group B arboviruses: Resistance in mice to Japanese B encephalitis and St. Louis encephalitis viruses induced by dengue virus immunization. Infect Immunol 9:909–915, 1974.
124. Edelman R, Nisalak A, Pariyanonda A, et al. Immunoglobulin response and viremia in dengue-vaccinated gibbons repeatedly challenged with Japanese encephalitis virus. Am J Epidemiol 97:208–218, 1973.
125. Goverdhan MK, Kulkarni AB, Gupta AK, et al. Two-way cross protection between West Nile and Japanese encephalitis viruses in bonnet Macaques. Acta Virol 36:277–283, 1992.
126. Jia LL, Zheng Z, Yu YX. Study on the immune mechanism of JE attenuated live vaccine (SA-14-14-2 strain). Chin J Immunol Microbiol 12:366–367, 1992.

127. Nathanson N, Cole GA. Fatal Japanese encephalitis virus infection in immunosuppressed spider monkeys. Clin Exp Immunol 6:161–166, 1970.
128. Gould EA, Buckley A. Antibody-dependent enhancement of yellow fever and Japanese encephalitis virus neurovirulence. J Gen Virol 70:1605–1608, 1989.
129. Ghosh SN, Prasad SR, Thakare JP, et al. Evidence for synthesis of immunoglobulins within central nervous system of Japanese encephalitis cases. Indian J Med Res 86:276–283, 1987.
130. Burke DS, Nisalak A, Lorsomrudee W, et al. Virus-specific antibody-producing cells in blood and cerebrospinal fluid in acute Japanese encephalitis. J Med Virol 17:283–292, 1985.
131. Konishi E, Kurane I, Mason PW, et al. Japanese encephalitis virus-specific proliferative responses of human peripheral blood T lymphocytes. Am J Trop Med Hyg 53:278–283, 1995.
132. Desai A, Ravi V, Chandramuki A, Gourie-Devi M. Proliferative response of human peripheral blood mononuclear cells to Japanese encephalitis virus. Microbiol Immunol 39:269–273, 1995.
133. Desai A, Ravi V, Guru SC, et al. Detection of autoantibodies to neural antigens in the CSF of Japanese encephalitis patients and correlation of findings with the outcome. J Neurol Sci 122:109–116, 1994.
134. Desai A, Ravi V, Chandremuki A, Gourie-Devi M. Detection of immune complexes in the CSF of Japanese encephalitis patients: Correlation of findings with outcome. Intervirology 37:352–355, 1994.
135. Lad VJ, Gupta AK, Goverdhan MK, et al. Susceptibility of BL6 nude (congenitally athymic) mice to Japanese encephalitis virus by the peripheral route. Acta Virol 37:232–240, 1993.
136. Murali-Krishna K, Ravi V, Manjunath R. Protection of adult but not newborn mice against lethal intracerebral challenge with Japanese encephalitis virus by adoptively transferred virus-specific cytotoxic T lymphocytes: Requirement for L3T4$^+$ cells. J Gen Virol 77:705–714, 1996.
137. Yu YX, Wang JF, Zheng GM, Li HM. Response of normal and athymic mice to infection by virulent and attenuated Japanese encephalitis viruses. Chin J Virol 1:203–209, 1985.
138. Jia LL, Zheng Z, Yu YX. Pathogenicity and immunogenicity of attenuated Japanese encephalitis vaccine (SA14-14-2) in immune-inhibited mice. Virol Sinica 8:20–24, 1993.
139. Jia LL, Zheng Z, Yu YX. Study on the immune mechanism of JE attenuated live vaccine (SA14-14-2 strain). Chin J Immunol Microbiol 12:364–366, 1992.
140. Brooks TJ, Lukaszewski, Phillpotts R. Cytokine prophylaxis for St. Louis encephalitis virus infection in mice [abstract G-15]. 37th Interscience Conference on Antimicrobial Agents and Chemotherapy; Toronto; Sept. 28–Oct. 1, 1997.
141. Lin Y, Huang Y, Ma S, et al. Inhibition of Japanese encephalitis virus infection by nitric oxide: Antiviral effect of nitric oxide on RNA virus replication. J Virol 71:5227–5235, 1997.
142. Kreil T, Eibl MM. Nitric oxide and viral infection: No antiviral activity against a flavivirus in vitro, and evidence for contribution to pathogenesis in experimental infection in vivo. Virology 219:304–306, 1996.
143. Khanna N, Mathur A, Chaturvedi UC. Regulation of vascular permeability by macrophage-derived chemotactic factor produced in Japanese encephalitis. Immunol Cell Biol 72:200–204, 1994.
144. Liu YF, Teng CL, Liu K. Cerebral cysticercosis as a factor aggravating Japanese B encephalitis. Chin Med J 75:1010–1017, 1957.
145. Das SK, Nityanand S, Sood K. Japanese B encephalitis with neurocysticercosis. J Assoc Physicians India 39:643–644, 1991.
146. Hayashi K, Arita T. Experimental double infection of Japanese encephalitis virus and herpes simplex virus in mouse brain. Jpn J Exp Med 47:9–13, 1977.
147. Hammon WM, Tigertt WD, Sather GE. Epidemiologic studies of concurrent "virgin" epidemics of Japanese B encephalitis and of mumps on Guam, 1947–1948, with subsequent observations including dengue, through 1957. Am J Trop Med Hyg 7:441–467, 1958.
148. Lange DG, Sedmak J. Japanese encephalitis virus (JEV): Potentiation of lethality in mice by microwave radiation. Bioelectromagnetics 12:335–348, 1991.
149. Gutierrez K, Abzug MJ. Vaccine-associated poliovirus meningitis in children with ventriculoperitoneal shunts. J Pediatr 117:424–427, 1990.
150. Okhuysen PC, Crane JK, Pappas J. St. Louis encephalitis in patients with human immunodeficiency virus infection. Clin Infect Dis 17:140–141, 1993.
151. Kedarnath N, Prasad SR, Dandawate CN, et al. Isolation of Japanese encephalitis and West Nile viruses from peripheral blood of encephalitis patients. Indian J Med Res 79:1–7, 1984.
152. Gajanana A, Samuel PP, Thenmozhi V, Rajendran R. An appraisal of some recent diagnostic assays for Japanese encephalitis. Southeast Asian J Trop Med Public Health 27:673–679, 1996.
153. Innis BL, Nisalak A, Nimmannitya S, et al. An enzyme-linked immunosorbent assay to characterize dengue infections where dengue and Japanese encephalitis cocirculate. Am J Trop Med Hyg 40:418–427, 1989.
154. Meiyu F, Huosheng C, Cuihua C, et al. Detection of flaviviruses by reverse transcriptase-polymerase chain reaction with the universal primer set. Microbiol Immunol 41:209–213, 1997.
155. Burke DS, Nisalak A, Gentry MK. Detection of flavivirus antibodies in human serum by epitope-blocking immunoassay. J Med Virol 23:165–173, 1987.
156. Konishi E, Mason PW, Shope RE. Enzyme-linked immunosorbent assay using recombinant antigens for serodiagnosis of Japanese encephalitis. J Med Virol 48:76–79, 1996.
157. Rosen L. The natural history of Japanese encephalitis virus. Annu Rev Microbiol 40:395–414, 1986.
158. Scherer WF, Buescher EL. Ecologic studies of Japanese encephalitis virus in Japan. I. Introduction. Am J Trop Med Hyg 8:644–650, 1959.
159. Gould DJ, Byrne RJ, Hayes DE. Experimental infection of horses with Japanese encephalitis virus by mosquito bite. Am J Trop Med Hyg 13:742–746, 1964.
160. Wang YJ, Gu PW, Liu PS. Japanese B encephalitis virus infection of horses during the first epidemic season following entry into an infected area. Chin Med J 95:63–66, 1982.
161. Min JG, Xue M. Progress in studies on the overwintering of the mosquito *Culex tritaeniorhynchus*. Southeast Asian J Trop Med Public Health 27:810–817, 1996.
162. Olson JG, Atmosoedjono S, Lee VH, Ksiazek TG. Correlation between population indices of *Culex tritaeniorhynchus* and *Cx. gelidus* (Diptera: Culicidae) and rainfall in Kapuk, Indonesia. J Med Entomol 20:108–109, 1983.
163. Phanthumachinda B. Ecology and biology of Japanese encephalitis. Southeast Asian J Trop Med Public Health 2653:11–16, 1995.
164. Soman RS, Rodrigues FM, Guttikar SN, Guru PY. Experimental viraemia and transmission of Japanese encephalitis virus by mosquitoes in ardeid birds. Indian J Med Res 66:709–718, 1977.
165. Fang R, Hus DR, Lim TW. Investigation of a suspected outbreak of Japanese encephalitis in Pualau Langkawi. Malays J Pathol 3:23–30, 1980.
166. Ilkal MA, Dhanda V, Rao BU, et al. Absence of viraemia in cattle after experimental infection with Japanese encephalitis. Trans R Soc Trop Med Hyg 82:628–631, 1988.
167. Takahashi K, Matsuo R, Kuma M, et al. Use of vaccine in pigs. A. Effect of immunization of swine upon the ecological cycle of Japanese encephalitis virus. In Hammon WM, Kitaoka M, Downs WG (eds). Immunization for Japanese Encephalitis. Amsterdam, Excerpta Medica, 1972, pp. 292–303.
168. Sasaki O, Karoji Y, Kuroda A, et al. Protection of pigs against mosquito-borne Japanese encephalitis virus by immunization with a live attenuated vaccine. Antiviral Res 2:355–360, 1982.
169. Vaughn DW, Hoke CH. The epidemiology of Japanese encephalitis: Prospects for prevention. Epidemiol Rev 14:197–221, 1992.
170. Gajanana A, Rajendran R, Samuel PP, et al. Japanese encephalitis in south Arcot District, Tamil Nadu: A three year longitudinal study of vector density and vector infection frequency. J Med Entomol 34:651–659, 1997.
171. Chaudhuri N, Shaw BP, Mondal KC, Maity CR. Epidemiology of Japanese encephalitis. Indian Pediatr 297:861–865, 1992.
172. Dapeng L, Konghua Z, Jinduo S, et al. The protective effects of bed nets impregnated with pyrethroid insecticide and vaccination against Japanese encephalitis. Trans R Soc Trop Med Hyg 88:632–634, 1994.
173. Xu YH, Zhaori GT, Vene S et al. Viral etiology of acute childhood encephalitis in Beijing diagnosed by analysis of single samples. Pediatr Infect Dis J 15:1018–1024, 1996.

174. Goh KT. Vaccines for Japanese encephalitis. Lancet 348:340, 1996.
175. Oya A. Epidemiology of Japanese encephalitis. Rinsho to Biseibutsu 16:5–9, 1989.
176. Xu ZY, personal communication, 1997.
177. Chang KY, Tseng TC. Seroepidemiological investigation on Japanese encephalitis in Taiwan. Chin J Microbiol Immunol 26:25–37, 1993.
178. Buhl MR, Black FT, Andersen PL, Laursen A. Fatal Japanese encephalitis in a Danish tourist visiting Bali for 12 days. Scand J Infect Dis 28:189, 1996.
179. MacDonald WBG, Tink AR, Ouvrier RA, et al. Japanese encephalitis after a two-week holiday in Bali. Med J Aust 150:334–336, 1989.
180. Rose MR, Hughes SM, Gatus BJ. A case of Japanese B encephalitis imported into the United Kingdom. J Infect 6:261–265, 1983.
181. Poland JD, Cropp CB, Craven RB, Monath TP. Evaluation of the potency and safety of inactivated Japanese encephalitis vaccine in U.S. inhabitants. J Infect Dis 161:878–882, 1990.
182. Berg SW, Mitchell BS, Hanson RK, et al. Systemic reactions in US Marine Corps personnel who received Japanese encephalitis vaccine. J Infect Dis 24:265–266, 1997.
183. Ognibene AJ. Japanese B encephalitis. In Ognibene AJ, Barrett O (eds). Internal Medicine in Vietnam: General Medicine and Infectious Diseases. Washington, DC, U.S. Army Office of Surgeon General and Center for Military History, 1982.
184. Pond WL, Smadel JE. Neurotropic viral diseases in the Far East during the Korean War. Army Medical Science Graduate School Medical Science Publ. No. 4. Recent Adv Med Surg 2:219–233, 1954.
185. Sabin AB. Encephalitis. In Communicable Diseases: Arthropod-Borne Diseases Other than Malaria. Washington, DC, US Army Medical Department. Prevent Med World War II 7:9–21, 1947.
186. Sabin AB, Schlesinger RW, Ginder DR, Matumoto M. Japanese B encephalitis in American Soldiers in Korea. Am J Hyg 46:356–375, 1947.
187. Long AP, Hullinghorst RL, Gauld RL. Japanese B encephalitis—Korea 1950. Army Medical Science Graduate School Medical Science Publ. No. 4. Recent Adv Med Surg 2:317–329. 1954.
188. Tsai TF, Niklasson B, Goujon C. Arboviruses and zoonotic viruses. In Dupont HL, Steffen R (eds). Textbook of Travel Medicine and Health. Hamilton, Ontario, Canada, BC Decker, 1997, pp. 200–214.
189. Centers for Disease Control. CDC Health Information for International Travel, 1996–7. Washington DC, U.S. Government Printing Office, 1996, pp 112–116.
190. Zhang M, Wang M, Jiang S, Ma W. Passive protection of mice, goats, and monkeys against Japanese encephalitis with monoclonal antibodies. J Med Virol 29:133–138, 1989.
191. Ohyama A, Ishiga A, Fujita N, et al. Effect of human gamma globulin upon encephalitis viruses. Jpn J Microbiol 3:159–169, 1959.
192. Lubiniecki AS, Cypess RH, Hammon WM. Passive immunity of arbovirus infection. II. Quantitative aspects of naturally and artificially acquired protection in mice for Japanese (B) encephalitis virus. Am J Trop Med Hyg 22:535–542, 1973.
193. Waldvogel K, Bossart W, Huisman T, et al. Severe tickborne encephalitis following passive immunization. Eur J Pediatr 155:775–779, 1996.
194. Gu PW, Ding ZF. Inactivated Japanese encephalitis (JE) vaccine made from Hamster cell culture (a review). JE HFRS Bull 2:15–26, 1987.
195. Oya A. Japanese encephalitis vaccine. Acta Pediatr Jpn 30:175–184, 1988.
196. Smorodintsev AA, Shubladse AK, Neustroer VD. Etiology of autumn enecephalitis in the Far East of the USSR. Arch Ges Virus Forsch 1:549–559, 1940.
197. Sabin AB, Duffy CE. Antibody response of human beings to centrifuged, lyophilized Japanese B encephalitis vaccine. Proc Soc Exp Med Biol 65:123–126, 1947.
198. Sabin AB. Antibody response of people of different ages to two doses of uncentrifuged, Japanese B encephalitis vaccine. Proc Soc Exp Med Biol 65:127–135, 1947.
199. Sabin AB, Ginder DR, Matumoto M, Schlesinger RW. Serological response of Japanese children and old people to Japanese B encephalitis mouse brain vaccine. Proc Soc Exp Med Biol 65:135–139, 1947.
200. Sabin AB. Epidemic encephalitis in military personnel. Isolation of Japanese B virus on Okinawa in 1945, serologic diagnosis, clinical manifestations, epidemiologic aspects, and use of mouse brain vaccine. JAMA 133:281–293, 1947.
201. Smadel JE, Randall R, Warren J. Preparation of Japanese encephalitis vaccine. US Army Med Dept Bull 7:963–973, 1947.
202. Sabin AB, Tigertt WD. Evaluation of Japanese B encephalitis vaccine. I. General background and methods. Am J Hyg 63:217–227, 1956.
203. Ando K, Satterwhite JP. Evaluation of Japanese B encephalitis vaccine. III. Okayama field trial, 1946–1949. Am J Hyg 63:230–237, 1956.
204. Tigertt WD, Hammon WM, Berge TO, et al. Japanese B encephalitis: A complete review of experience on Okinawa 1945–1949. Am J Trop Med 30:689–722, 1950.
205. Tigertt WD, Berge TO, Burns KF, Satterwhite JP. Evaluation of Japanese B encephalitis vaccine. IV. Pattern of serologic response to vaccination over a five-year period in an endemic area (Okayama, Japan). Am J Hyg 63:238–249, 1956.
206. Kanamitsu M, Hashimoto N, Urasawa S, et al. A field trial with an improved Japanese encephalitis vaccine in a nonendemic area of the disease. Biken J 13:313–328, 1970.
207. Takaku K, Yamashita T, Osanai T, et al. Japanese encephalitis purified vaccine. Biken J 11:25–39, 1968.
208. Shope RE. The potency test for inactivated Japanese encephalitis (JE) vaccines. JE HFRS Bull 2:27–32, 1987.
209. World Health Organization. Requirements for Japanese encephalitis vaccine (inactivated) for human use. WHO Tech Rep Series 77:1133–1156, 1988.
210. Gowal D, Singh G, Rao Bhau LN, Saxena SN. Thermostability of Japanese encephalitis vaccine produced in India. Biologicals 19:37–40, 1990.
211. Fukunaga T, Rojanasuphot S, Wungkorbkiat S, et al. Japanese encephalitis vaccination in Thailand. Biken J 17:21–31, 1974.
212. Kobayashi Y, Hasegawa H, Oyama T, et al. Antigenic analysis of Japanese encephalitis virus by using monoclonal antibodies. Infect Immunol 44:117–123, 1984.
213. Hashimoto H, Nomoto A, Watanabe K, et al. Molecular cloning and complete nucleotide sequence of the genome of Japanese encephalitis virus Beijing-1 strain. Virus Genes 1:305–317, 1988.
214. Kitano T, Yabe S, Kobayashi M, et al. Immunogenicity of JE Nakayama and Beijing-1 vaccines. JE HFRS Bull 1:37–41, 1986.
215. Kitano T. Immunogenicity and field trial of Beijing-1 vaccine. Working group on vaccine development and vaccination strategies for Japanese encephalitis, Osaka. 1–8, 1985.
216. The Research Foundation for Microbial Diseases of Osaka University. Japanese encephalitis vaccine lyophilized, "Biken." Unpublished report, 1991, pp 1–149.
217. Huang CH. Studies of virus factors as causes of inapparent infection in Japanese B encephalitis: Virus strains, viraemia, stability to heat and infective dosage. Acta Virol 1:36–45, 1957.
218. Huang CH. Studies of Japanese encephalitis in China. Adv Virus Res 27:71–101, 1982.
219. Kitano T. Field trial of inactivated JE Beijing vaccine in Japan. Working group on Japanese encephalitis vaccines, Osaka. 1–5, 1987.
220. Rojanasuphot S, Nachiangmai P, Srijaggrawalong A, Nimmannitya S. Implementation of simultaneous Japanese encephalitis vaccine in the expanded program of immunization of infants. Mosq Borne Dis Bull 9:86–92, 1992.
221. Gambel JM, DeFraites R, Hoke C, et al. Japanese encephalitis vaccine: Persistence of antibody up to 3 years after a three-dose primary series. J Infect Dis 171:1074, 1995.
222. Henderson A. Immunization against Japanese encephalitis in Nepal: Experience of 1152 subjects. J R Army Med Corps 130:188–191, 1984.
223. Sanchez JL, Hoke CH, McCowan J, et al. Further experience with Japanese encephalitis vaccine. Lancet 335:972–973, 1990.
224. Immunization Practices Advisory Committee (ACIP). Inactivated Japanese encephalitis virus vaccine: Recommendations of the ACIP. MMWR Morb Mortal Wkly Rep 42(RR1):1–15, 1993.
225. Intralawan P, Puapanwatana S, Hansuttivejakul R, Ratanisirisub

P. Integration of Japanese encephalitis vaccine in EPI. Thai J Pediatr 30:5–10, 1991.

226. Intralawan P, Paupunwatana S. Immunogenicity of low dose Japanese encephalitis vaccine (BIKEN) administered by the intradermal route: Preliminary data. Asian Pacific J Allergy Immunol 11:79–83, 1993.

227. Lee CYG, Grayston JT, Kenny GE. Growth of Japanese encephalitis virus in cell culture. J Infect Dis 115:321–329, 1965.

228. Li GM, Li CG, Bye CR, et al. Efficacy of a newly established Japanese encephalitis vaccination schedule in Hunan. Hunan Med 6:150–152.

229. Zhang XC, Nie SX, Din CS, Wang MJ. Observations on the efficacy of inactivated Japanese encephalitis vaccine in combination with other vaccines. Chin J Pub Health 6:203, 1990.

230. Inoue YK. An attenuated mutant of Japanese encephalitis virus. Bull World Health Organ 30:181–185, 1964.

231. Yoshida I, Takagi M, Inokuma E, et al. Establishment of an attenuated ML-17 strain of Japanese encephalitis virus. Biken J 24:47–67, 1981.

232. Kodama K, Sasaki N, Inoue YK. Studies of live attenuated Japanese encephalitis vaccine in swine. J Immunol 100:194–200, 1968.

233. Hammon WM, Darwish MA, Rhim JS, et al. Studies on Japanese B encephalitis virus vaccines from tissue culture. V. Response of man to live, attenuated strain of OCT541 virus vaccine. J Immunol 96:518–524, 1966.

233a. Ni H, Barrett A. Attenuation of Japanese encephalitis virus by selection of its mouse brain membrane receptor preparation escape variants. Virology 241:30–36, 1998.

234. Yu YX, Ao J, Chu YG, et al. Studies on mutation of JE virus V. Biological characteristics of the attenuated vaccine strain. Acta Microbiol Sinica 13:16–24, 1973.

235. Yu YX, Fang C, Wu PF, Li HM. Studies on the variation of JE virus VI. The changes in virulence and immunity after passaging subcutaneously in suckling mice. Acta Microbiol Sinica 15:133–138, 1975.

236. Yu YX, Wu PF, Ao J, et al. Selection of a better immunogenic and highly attenuated live vaccine virus strain of JE. I. Some biological characteristics of SA14-14-2 mutant. Chin J Microbiol Immunol 1:77–84, 1981.

237. Ao J, Yu Y, Tang YS, et al. Selection of a better immunogenic and highly attenuated live vaccine strain of Japanese encephalitis. II. Safety and immunogenicity of live JBE vaccine SA14-14-2 observed in inoculated children. Chin J Microbiol Immunol 3:245–248, 1983.

238. Yu YX, Ming AG, Pen GY, et al. Safety of a live-attenuated Japanese encephalitis virus vaccine (SA14-14-2) for children. Am J Trop Med Hyg 39:214–217, 1988.

239. Wang SG, Yang HJ, Den YY, et al. Studies on the production of SA14-2 Japanese encephalitis live vaccine. Chin J Virol 6:38–43, 1990.

240. Yu YX, Zhang GM, Zheng Z. Studies on the immunogenicity of live and killed Japanese encephalitis (JE) vaccines to challenge with different Japanese encephalitis virus strains. Chin J Virol 5:106–110, 1989.

241. Wills MR, Sil BK, Cao JX, et al. Antigenic characterization of the live attenuated Japanese encephalitis vaccine virus SA14-14-2: A comparison with isolates of the virus covering a wide geographic area. Vaccine 10:861–872, 1992.

242. Sil BK, Wills MR, Cao JX. Immunogenicity of experimental live attenuated Japanese encephalitis vaccine viruses and comparison with wild-type strains using monoclonal and polyclonal antibodies. Vaccine 10:329–333, 1992.

243. Hase T, Dubois DR, Summers PL, et al. Comparison of replication rates and pathogenicities between the SA14 parent and SA14-14-2 vaccine strains of Japanese encephalitis virus in mouse brain neurons. Arch Virol 130:131–143, 1993.

244. Jia LL, Zhong Z, Yu YX. Study on the stability of viral strains of live-attenuated Japanese encephalitis vaccine. Chin J Biolog 5:174–176, 1992.

245. Eckels KH, Yu XY, Dubois DR, et al. Japanese encephalitis virus live-attenuated vaccine, Chinese strain SA14-14-2; adaptation to primary canine kidney cell cultures and preparation of a vaccine for human use. Vaccine 6:513–518, 1988.

246. Regional Antiepidemic Station, Hueyang, Guangtong: Preliminary observation on epidemiological effectiveness of JE live vaccine. Bull Biol Prod 7:111–114, 1978

247. Ling JP, Zhu YG, Du GZ, et al. Comparative susceptibilities of rhesus monkeys and mice to Japanese encephalitis virus. Beijing, Institute for Control of Pharmaceutical and Biological Products, unpublished report, 1996.

248. Jia LL, Zheng Z, Wang SW, Yu YX. Protective effects and antibody responses in guinea pigs immunized with Japanese encephalitis live-attenuated vaccine SA14-14-2 after challenge with virulent JE virus. Adv Microbiol Immunol (China) 23:73–75, 1995.

249. Ni H, Chang GJ, Xie H, et al. Molecular basis of attenuation of neurovirulence of wild-type Japanese encephalitis virus strain SA14. J Gen Virol 76:409–413, 1995.

250. Ni HL, Barrett ADT. Molecular differences between wild-type Japanese encephalitis virus strains of high and low mouse neurovirulence. J Gen Virol 77:1449–1455, 1996.

251. Aihara S, Rao CM, Yu YX. Identification of mutations that occurred on the genome of Japanese encephalitis virus during the attenuation process. Virus Genes 5:95–109, 1991.

252. Cecilia D, Gould EA. Nucleotide changes responsible for loss of neuroinvasiveness in Japanese encephalitis virus neutralization-resistant mutants. Virology 181:707, 1991.

253. Hasegawa H, Yoshida M, Shiosaka T, et al. Mutations in the envelope protein of Japanese encephalitis virus affect entry into cultured cells and virulence in mice. Virology 191:158–165, 1992.

254. Chen BQ, Beaty BJ. Japanese encephalitis vaccine (28 strain) and parent (SA 14 strain) viruses in *Culex tritaeniorhynchus* mosquitoes. Am J Trop Med Hyg 31:403–407, 1982.

255. Ao J, Yu YX, Wu PF, Zhang GM. Further observations on JBE attenuated live vaccines used for prevention of stillbirths in swine. Acta Microbiol Sinica 21:174–179, 1981.

256. Tsai TF, Yu YX, Jia LL, et al. Immunogenicity of live attenuated SA14-14-2 Japanese encephalitis vaccine—a comparison of 1- and 3-month immunizaton schedules. J Infect Dis 177:221–223, 1998.

257. Chambers TJ, Tsai TF, Pervivkov Y, Monath TP. Vaccine development against dengue and Japanese encephalitis: Report of a World Health Organization meeting. Vaccine 15:1494–1502, 1997.

258. Konishi E, Kurane I, Mason PW, et al. Induction of Japanese encephalitis virus–specific cytotoxic T lymphocytes in humans by poxvirus-based JE vaccine candidates. Vaccine 16:842–849, 1998.

259. Fu DW, Zhand PF. Establishment and characterization of Japanese B encephalitis virus persistent infection in the Sf9 cell line. Biologicals 24:225–233, 1996.

260. Sumiyoshi H, Tignor GH, Shope RE. Characterization of a highly attenuated Japanese encephalitis virus generated from molecularly cloned cDNA. J Infect Dis 171:1144–1151, 1995.

261. Seif SA, Morita K, Igarashi A. A 27 amino coding region of JE virus E protein expressed in *E. coli* as fusion protein with glutathione-S-transferase elicit neutralizing antibody in mice. Virus Res 43:91–96, 1996.

262. Fuijta H, Sumiyoshi H, Mori C, et al. Studies in the development of Japanese encephalitis vaccine: Expression of virus envelope glycoprotein V3 (E) gene in yeast. Bull World Health Organ 65:303–308, 1987.

263. McCown J, Cochran M, Putnak R, et al. Protection of mice against lethal Japanese encephalitis with a recombinant baculovirus vaccine. Am J Trop Med Hyg 42:491–499, 1990.

264. Srivastava AK, Morita K, Igarishi A. Immunogenicity of Japanese encephalitis virus envelope glycoprotein E prepared by four different methods. Trop Med 32:103–113, 1990.

265. Jan LR, Yang CS, Henchal LS, et al. Increased immunogenicity and protective efficacy in outbred and inbred mice by strategic carboxyl-terminal truncation of Japanese encephalitis virus envelope glycoprotein. Am J Trop Med Hyg 48:412–423, 1993.

266. Hirabayashi Y, Fukuda, Kimura J, et al. Identification of peptides mimicking the antigenicity and immunogenicity on Japanese encephalitis virus protein using synthetic peptide libraries. J Virol Methods 61:23–26, 1996.

267. Konishi E, Win KS, Kurane I, et al. Particulate vaccine candidate for Japanese encephalitis induces long-lasting virus-specific memory T lymphocytes in mice. Vaccine 15:281–286, 1997.

268. Pugachev K, Mason PW, Frey TK. Sindbis vectors suppress

secretion of subviral particles of Japanese encephalitis virus from mammalian cells infected with SIN-JEV recombinants. Virology 209:155–166, 1995.

269. Yeolekar LR, Banerjee K. Immunogenicity of immunostimulating complexes of Japanese encephalitis virus in experimental animals. Acta Virol 40:245–250, 1996.
270. Eldridge JH, Hammond CJ, Meulbroek HA, et al. Controlled vaccine release in the gut-associated lymphoid tissues. I. Orally administered biodegradable microspheres target the Peyer's patches. J Controlled Release 11:205–214, 1990.
271. Rojanasuphot S, Charoensook OA, Ungchusak K, et al. A field trial on inactivated mouse brain Japanese encephalitis vaccines produced in Thailand. Mosquito-Borne Dis Bull 8:11–16, 1991.
272. Wu YC. Neutralizing antibody responses to Nakayama and Beijing strain JE vaccine in children of Taipei City, 1993–4. Taipei, National Institute of Preventive Medicine, unpublished report, 1994.
273. Nimmannitya S, Hutami S, Kalayanarooj S, Rojanasuphot S. A field study on Nakayama and Beijing strains of Japanese encephalitis vaccines. Southeast Asian J Trop Med Pub Health 26:689–693, 1995.
274. Susilowati S, Okuno Y, Fukunaga T, et al. Neutralization antibody responses induced by Japanese encephalitis virus vaccine. Biken J 24:137–145, 1981.
275. Okuno Y, Okamoto Y, Yamada A, et al. Effect of current Japanese encephalitis vaccine on different strains of Japanese encephalitis virus. Vaccine 5:128–132, 1987.
276. Juang RF, Okuno Y, Fukunaga T, et al. Neutralizing antibody responses to Japanese encephalitis vaccine in children. Biken J 26:25–34, 1983.
277. Ku CC, King CC, Lin DY, et al. Homologous and heterologous neutralization antibody responses after immunization with Japanese encephalitis vaccine among Taiwan children. Med Virol 44:122–131, 1994.
278. Hoke CH, Nisalak A, Sangawhipa N, et al. Protection against Japanese encephalitis by inactivated vaccines. N Engl J Med 319:608–614, 1988.
279. Kayser M, Klein H, Paasch I, et al. Human antibody response to immunization with 17D yellow fever and inactivated TBE vaccine. J Med Virol 17:35–45, 1985.
280. Rojanasuphot S, Shaffer N, Chotpitayasunondh T, et al. Response to Japanese encephalitis vaccine among HIV-infected children, Bangkok, Thailand. Submitted for publication to Trans Roy Soc Trop Med Hyg.
281. Yamada A, Imanishi J, Juang RF, et al. Trial of inactivated Japanese encephalitis vaccine in children with underlying diseases. Vaccine 4:32–34, 1986.
282. Hsu TC, Chow LP, Wei HY, et al. A controlled field trial for an evaluation of effectiveness of mouse-brain Japanese encephalitis vaccine. J Formosa Med Assoc 70:55–61, 1971.
283. Okuno T, Tseng PT, Hsu ST, et al. Japanese encephalitis surveillance in China (province of Taiwan) during 1958–1971. II. Age-specific incidence in connection with Japanese encephalitis vaccination program. Jpn J Med Sci Biol 28:255–267, 1975.
284. Hsu TC, Chow LP, Wei HY, et al. A completed field trial for an evaluation of the effectiveness of mouse-brain Japanese vaccine. In McDHammon W, Kitaoka M, Downs WG (eds). Immunization for Japanese Encephalitis. Amsterdam, Excerpta Medica, 1972, pp 285–291.
285. Gowal D, Tahlan AK. Evaluation of effectiveness of mouse brain inactivated Japanese encephalitis vaccine produced in India. Indian J Med Res 102:267–271, 1995.
286. National Vaccine and Serum Institute, An Yang Municipal Health Station, Jiangsu Provincial Health Station, et al. Effectiveness of the Japanese B encephalitis inactivated vaccine of hamster kidney cell culture type. Acta Microbiol Sinica 16:48–53, 1976.
287. Wang SG, Yang HJ, Den YY, et al. Improved inactivated Japanese encephalitis vaccine produced in primary hamster kidney cells. National Serum and Biologics Institute, Hebei Health Station, Funien County Health Station. Biol Prod Comm 8:283–285, 1979.
288. National Serum and Biologics Institute, Jiling Yang Gi Health Station. Studies on immunization schedules for Japanese encephalitis vaccine. Chin J Prev Med 6:360–363, 1981.
289. Ren YL, Biol Prod Com (Chinese) 7:111, 1978. Cited in Huang CH. Studies of Japanese encephalitis in China. Adv Virus Res 27:72–101, 1982.
290. Luo DP, Yin HJ, Liu XL, et al. The efficacy of Japanese encephalitis vaccine in Henan, China: A case-control study. Southeast Asian J Trop Med Public Health 25:643–646, 1994.
291. Ao G, Yu YX, Wu PF, et al. Studies on mutation of Japanese B encephalitis virus. VII. An observation of persistence of immunity in children inoculated with JBE attenuated live vaccine (SA-14-5-3 mutant). Acta Microbiol Sinica 21:501–505, 1981.
292. Jia LL, Yu YX, Zheng Z. Neutralizing antibody response of Japanese encephalitis live vaccine in children residing in JE endemic area. Chin J Zoonoses 11:343–344, 1995.
293. Chengdu Biologics Institute. Report on epidemiologic results of lyophilized Japanese encephalitis vaccine. Unpublished report, 1991.
294. Wang JL, Na JC, Zhao SS, et al. An epidemiologic study of the efficacy of live Japanese encephalitis vaccine. Chin J Biolog 6:36–37, 1993.
295. Hennessy S, Liu ZL, Tsai TF, et al. Effectiveness of live-attenuated Japanese encephalitis vaccine (SA14-14-2): a case-control study. Lancet 347:1583–86, 1996.
296. Kitaoka M. Follow-up on use of vaccine in children in Japan. In McDHammon W, Kitaoka M, Downs WG (eds). Immunization for Japanese Encephalitis. Amsterdam, Excerpta Medica, 1972, pp 275–277.
297. Egashira Y, Okawa T, Oya A, et al. Allergic encephalitis in guinea pigs and monkeys with special reference to the relationship between the properties of the antigen and the reaction of the host. Proc Comm Jpn Encephal Vaccine 1:66–70, 1966.
298. Shiraki H. Etiological study of demyelinating disease. Proc Comm Jpn Encephal Vaccine 1:70–71, 1966.
299. Okinaka S, Toyokura Y, Tsukagoshi H, et al. Physical reactions following vaccination against Japanese B encephalitis with special reference to neurological complications. Adv Neurol Sci 11:410–424, 1965.
300. Ohtaki E, Murakami Y, Komori H, et al. Acute disseminated encephalomyelitis after Japanese B encephalitis vaccination. Pediatr Neurol 8:137–139, 1992.
301. Ohtaki E, Matsuishi T, Hirano Y, Maekawa K. Acute disseminated encephalomyelitis after treatment with Japanese B encephalitis vaccine (Nakayama-Yoken and Beijing strains). J Neurol Neurosurg Psychiatry 59:316–317, 1995.
302. Plesner AM, Soborg PA, Herning M. Neurological complications and Japanese encephalitis vaccination. Lancet 348:202–203, 1996.
303. Andersen MM, Ronne T. Side effects with Japanese encephalitis vaccine. Lancet 337:1044, 1991.
304. Plesner AM, Ronne T. Allergic mucocutaneous reactions to Japanese encephalitis vaccine. Vaccine 15:1239–1243, 1997.
305. Ruff TA, Eisen D, Fuller A, Kass R. Adverse reactions to Japanese encephalitis vaccine. Lancet 338:881–882, 1991.
306. Tsai TF. Inactivated Japanese encephalitis virus vaccine—recommendations of the Advisory Committee on Immunization Practices (ACIP). MMWR Morb Mortal Wkly Rep 42:RR-1:1–15, 1993.
307. Beecham HJ III, Pock AR, May LA, Tsai TF. A cluster of severe reactions following improperly administered Takeda Japanese encephalitis vaccine. J Travel Med 4:8–10, 1997.
308. Nothdurft HD, Jelinek T, Marschang A, et al. Adverse reactions to Japanese encephalitis in travellers. J Infect 32:119–122, 1996.
309. Nazareth B, Levin J, Johnson H, Begg N. Systemic allergic reactions to Japanese encephalitis vaccines. Vaccine 12:666, 1994.
310. Robinson P, Ruff T, Kass R. Australian case-control study of adverse reactions to Japanese encephalitis. J Travel Med 2:159–164, 1995.
311. Froeschle J, unpublished report. Swiftwater, PA, Pasteur Mérieux Connaught, 1994.
312. Hanna J, Barnett D, Ewald D. Vaccination against Japanese encephalitis in the Torres Strait. Commun Dis Intell 20:188–190, 1996.
313. Sakaguchi M, Yoshida M, Kuroda W, et al. Systemic immediate-type reactions to gelatin included in Japanese encephalitis vaccines. Vaccine 15:121–122, 1997.

313a. Sakaguchi M, Inouye S. Two patterns of systemic immediate-type reactions to Japanese encephalitis vaccines. Vaccine 16:68–69, 1998.

314. Dressen DW, Bernard KW, Parker RA, et al. Immune complex-

like disease in 23 persons following a booster dose of rabies diploid cell vaccine. Vaccine 4:45–49, 1986.

315. Anderson MC, Baer H, Frazier DJ, Quinnan GV. The role of specific IgE and beta-propiolactone in reactions resulting from booster doses of human diploid cell rabies vaccine. J Allergy Clin Immunol 80:861–868, 1987.
316. Ma X, Yu YX, Wang SG. Observations on safety and serological efficacy from a large-scale field trial of Japanese encephalitis vaccine. Chin J Biolog 6:188–191, 1993.
317. Liu ZL, Hennessy S, Strom BL, et al. Short-term safety of live-attenuated Japanese encephalitis vaccine (SA14-14-2): Results of a 26,239-subject randomized trial. J Infect Dis 176:1366–1369, 1997.
318. Ruff TA. Japanese B encephalitis vaccine—time for a reappraisal? Med J Aust 161:511, 1994.
319. U.S. Public Health Service, Centers for Disease Control and National Institutes of Health. Biosafety in Microbiological and Biomedical Laboratories. Washington, DC, U.S. Government Printing Office, 1988, pp. 82–92.
320. Nakamura H. A consideration of the low incidence of Japanese encephalitis cases during recent years in the southwestern region of Japan. Trop Med 30:191–198, 1988.
321. Siraprapasiri T, Sawaddiwudhipong W, Rojanasuphot S. Cost benefit analysis of Japanese encephalitis vaccination program in Thailand. Southeast Asian J Trop Med Public Health 28:143–148, 1997.

chapter

28 Meningococcal Vaccines

Martha L. Lepow

Bradley A. Perkins

Patricia A. Hughes

Jan T. Poolman

Whether new and virulent strains of meningococcus have been introduced into the population, whether old strains have assumed enhanced virulence or whether individual resistance has been lowered, has not been and probably never will be definitely ascertained.

Norton JF, Gordon JE. Meningococcus meningitis in Detroit in 1928–1929: Epidemiology. J Prevent Med 4:207–214, 1930

History

Neisseria meningitidis is unique among major causes of bacterial meningitis for its ability to cause endemic and epidemic disease. Willis probably reported the first epidemic in 1661,[1] Weiselbaum discovered the meningococcus in 1887,[2] and Vieusseux published the first definitive description of meningococcal meningitis in 1905.[3]

Importance of Meningococcal Disease

Meningococcal disease is a major cause of morbidity and mortality worldwide[4] and the most common cause of bacterial meningitis in persons 2 to 18 years of age in the United States.[5] There are an estimated 2600 cases of systemic meningococcal disease in the United States yearly,[6] of which approximately half are meningitis.

Before the use of serum therapy and the discovery of sulfonamides and antibiotics, meningococcal disease was fatal in about 70% of cases.[7] Today, despite an increased understanding of its pathogenesis and appropriate treatment, the mortality rate is still 7 to 19% for meningococcal disease, and the reported mortality from meningococcemia ranges from 18 to 53%.[8] The potential for increased resistance to current antibiotics makes prevention by vaccination a more urgent task for the future.[9] Much is unknown about meningococcal disease, including why one individual on acquiring the organism develops invasive disease whereas hundreds of others acquiring the same strain do not. Other baffling features include the geographical distribution of serogroup A compared with serogroups B and C as well as the virtual disappearance of serogroup A disease from the United States for almost 50 years.

BACKGROUND

Clinical Description and Presentation

Among the wide range of clinical expressions of the disease, the two most common manifestations are meningitis and meningococcemia.[8] Meningococcemia begins with a sudden onset of fever, malaise, myalgia, and headache, with seizures occurring in 20% of cases. Diarrhea and vomiting are common and the patient may be encephalopathic, although mental status is usually normal when the rash starts. Sixty percent of cases have experienced symptoms for less than 24 hours when they present to the hospital. Receipt of adequate antibiotic therapy before admission to the hospital has been shown to reduce the likelihood of death.[10] A rash, which is present in the majority of cases, starts as a macular eruption on the chest and extremities but rapidly becomes petechial or ecchymotic. Septicemia may be fulminant, with hypotension, extensive purpura due to intravascular coagulation, and dissemination to many organs; death may occur within hours of onset. Such patients are usually not responsive to antimicrobials, steroids, or vasopressor agents. White blood cell counts may be very low or high. Meningitis is usually absent.

More commonly, the course of meningococcal disease is less fulminant, and therapeutic interventions are more likely to be successful. When meningitis follows hematogenous dissemination, vomiting, headache, and photophobia are common. Other manifestations include myocarditis, endocarditis, or pericarditis; arthritis; conjunctivitis; urethritis; pharyngitis; and cervicitis. Arthritis or pericarditis may also occur later in the course as a result of immune complex formation. Chronic meningococcemia, occurring with rash, recurrent low-grade fever, and occasional joint swelling, is rare. Endocarditis has been described in a number of cases.[11]

Complications of Meningococcemia

Kirsch and coworkers reported on 44 patients with severe meningococcemia.[8] Of these, 12 had neurological complications, including 4 with seizures, 4 with infarcts, 2 with atrophy, 1 with a subdural hematoma, and 1 with hearing loss. Six had amputations, and seven required skin grafts.

Complications of Meningitis

Sensorineural deafness (which occurs early in the course of disease)[12] was reported in 9% of survivors in a study of 86 cases of systemic meningococcal disease mainly due to serogroup B. Other complications of meningitis include seizures, cerebral infarctions, and occasionally permanent disabilities. With serogroup A disease, as many as 20% of meningitis survivors may have neurological sequelae including mental retardation and hearing loss.[13]

BACTERIOLOGY

N. meningitidis organisms are gram-negative, spherical or kidney-shaped bacilli commonly seen in pairs intracellularly on Gram's stain. They are aerobic and are best isolated on chocolate agar. The organisms can be found in the nasopharynx in 5 to 11% of the adult population. At least 13 different serogroups exist that are based on the chemical and immunological specificity of the capsular polysaccharides. Most human disease is caused by serogroups A, B, and C, and these strains are responsible for nearly all the outbreaks of disease.[14] Meningococci are serologically classified based on the immunological reactivity of their capsular polysaccharide (serogroup), class 2 or 3 outer membrane protein (serotype), class 1 outer membrane protein subtype and lipopolysaccharide (immunotype). Defining a serotype is most useful for epidemiological purposes; however, certain serotypes may be important in natural immunity to serogroup B disease. The standard nomenclature lists serogroup, serotype,[15] serosubtype, and immunotype, each separated by a colon (e.g., B:4:P1.15:L3,7,9).

Multilocus enzyme electrophoresis has been the gold standard for molecular subtyping of meningococci.[16] Its utility comes from the ability to classify strains belonging to or closely related to genetically similar strains that have increased potential to cause epidemics (e.g., III-1 serogroup A, ET-5 serogroup B, and the serogroup C clones responsible for epidemics). Pulse field gel electrophoresis is often used to rapidly distinguish among similar and dissimilar organisms to assist in identifying clusters from nonrelated groups of endemic cases.[17]

It has been shown that meningococci have the capacity to exchange genetic material responsible for capsule production and thereby switch serogroups B to C or vice versa.[18] Because protection afforded by vaccines is serogroup specific, this phenomenon could have implications for vaccine use and formulation, especially future serogroup C vaccines.

PATHOGENESIS AS IT RELATES TO PREVENTION

N. meningitidis is transmitted from person to person by aerosolization or by contact with respiratory secretions (e.g., kissing or sharing a glass). Nasopharyngeal colonization occurs first, resulting in a carrier state, and is followed by penetration through the mucosa. In a nasopharyngeal organ culture model, an inoculum of more than 10^6 meningococci was necessary for consistent infection. Nasopharyngeal mucous contains components that bind meningococci. Pili are important in attachment to nonciliated epithelial cells.[19] The exact determinants of invasion are unknown, but certain proteins of the outer membrane may insert into host cell membranes. Goldschneider and colleagues showed that the primary host defense is circulating antibody against the capsular polysaccharide.[20, 21] Natural immunity develops as a result of asymptomatic carriage of typable and nontypable meningococci and the antigenically related species *Neisseria lactamica*.[22] Some strains of *Escherichia coli* and other bacteria that constitute normal intestinal flora possess polysaccharide capsules and other cell wall antigens that are immunologically similar or identical to those of meningococci. Robbins and coworkers found that 1% of the 1335 strains of enteric bacteria studied had cross-reacting antigens identical to one or more strains of serogroup A, B, or C meningococci.[23] These strains could enhance natural immunization.

Rates of carriage of typable meningococci range from 5 to 15%. Factors that increase carriage include smoking and passive smoke inhalation[24] and concurrent viral and mycoplasma infections.[25–27] There have been several accounts of outbreaks of meningococcal disease that followed epidemics of influenza A, the most recent occurring in England in 1989.[28] Eight days after a 1996 epidemic of influenza B in a military installation in Greece, seven confirmed and three presumptive cases of serogroup C meningococcal disease occurred during a 4-day period.[29] A case-control study in Oregon and Washington indicated that among the meningococcal cases in people younger than 18 years of age, having a mother who smoked in the house was a substantial risk factor; among those older than 18, smoking was the only identified, potentially modifiable risk factor.[30] Crowded living conditions such as military barracks favor the spread of meningococcal disease.[31]

People with underlying immune deficiencies appear to be at an increased risk of recurrent neisserial disease. Susceptible people include those with C3 and C5-9 deficiencies who are not only at risk for recurrent meningococcal disease but also frequently have disease caused by uncommon serogroups such as X, Y, Z, and W-135.[32, 33] The mechanism is believed to be insufficient killing of primarily intracellular organisms.[34] Asplenia, hypogammaglobulinemia, and agammaglobulinemia are other risk factors.[35] Infection with the human immunodeficiency virus (HIV) poses greater risk for severe meningococcal disease in United States studies.[36] However, an increased risk for disease was not identified for people with HIV infection during an epidemic of serogroup A meningococcal disease in Africa.[37]

DIAGNOSIS

The diagnosis of meningococcal disease can be established by culture of blood, cerebrospinal fluid, skin lesions, and other infected sites. A Gram stain of buffy coat (spun-down blood that is anticoagulated), cerebrospinal fluid, and a smear of "unroofed" petechiae are important diagnostic tools for revealing the characteristic organisms inside polymorphonuclear leukocytes. The cerebrospinal fluid has characteristics of a bacterial infection: a high polymorphonuclear cell count, a depressed sugar content, and elevated protein concentrations. In fulminant meningococcemia, the spinal fluid may be normal but often reveals meningococci in culture. Serological diagnosis and polymerase chain reaction are now being used in some public health laboratories (e.g., in the United Kingdom) to detect meningococcal DNA in the cerebrospinal fluid.[38] Latex particle agglutination tests on cerebrospinal fluid are no longer recommended because of low sensitivity and specificity.

TREATMENT AND PREVENTION

Antibiotics

Aqueous penicillin G is the antibiotic of choice with an intravenous dose of 300,000 U given every 4 hours. Although most meningococci are still susceptible to this antibiotic, resistance has been described.[9, 39–42]

Cefotaxime in four divided intravenous doses of 200 mg per kg per day and ceftriaxone in two divided intravenous or intramuscular doses of 100 mg per kg per day have been shown to be as effective as penicillin in treating meningococcemia and meningitis.[43] Chloramphenicol at 100 mg per kg per day every 6 hours is still recommended if penicillin and cephalosporins cannot be used. Antibiotic treatment for 5 to 7 days is adequate for most systemic meningococcal illnesses.

Other Therapies

Dexamethasone, if given in a dose of 0.15 mg per kg every 6 hours for 4 days with the first dose given before the initiation of antibiotic therapy (when meningitis is present), may decrease deafness and some of the undesirable effects of acute phase reactants in the central nervous system.[8, 9] The high mortality rate with fulminating meningococcemia may be attributed to the release of cytokines such as tumor necrosis factor and interleukin 1 from macrophages, which leads to capillary leakage.[44] Other treatments include airway management, control of shock with fluid resuscitation and intravascular coagulation, and control of increased intracranial pressure. The use of systemic steroids for the treatment of shock still remains controversial. Anti-endotoxic and anticytokine therapies are experimental. Plasmophoresis has been successfully used under some circumstances.[45]

Chemoprophylaxis

Antibiotics are used to eradicate carriage of *N. meningitidis* among people who have had close contact with a person with a confirmed case of meningococcal disease. People likely to have such contact are (1) household members, (2) daycare center contacts, and (3) anyone directly exposed to the patient's oral secretions (e.g., through kissing, mouth-to-mouth resuscitation, endotracheal intubation, or endotracheal tube management).[6] The attack rate for household contacts exposed to patients who have sporadic meningococcal disease has been estimated to be 4 cases per 1000 people exposed, which is 500 to 800 times greater than the rate for the total population.[46] Because the rate of secondary disease for close contacts is highest during the first few days after onset of disease in the index patient, antimicrobial chemoprophylaxis should be administered as soon as possible (ideally within 24 hours of identification of the case). Chemoprophylaxis administered more than 14 days after the onset of illness in the index case is not indicated. Nasopharyngeal cultures are not helpful in determining the need for chemoprophylaxis and may unnecessarily delay institution of this preventive measure. Table 28–1 lists prophylactic drugs and their dosing and administration schedules. Rifampin is the oral drug of choice for children, but there are alternatives for adults.[6]

Administration of prophylactic antibiotics to large populations is not usually effective where community-based or organization-based outbreaks have occurred. However, in outbreaks involving small populations such as a single school, administration of chemoprophylaxis to all people within the population may be considered. If mass chemoprophylaxis is undertaken, the medication should be administered to all members at the same time.[6]

EPIDEMIOLOGY

Incidence and Prevalence

The incidence of meningococcal disease in the United States from 1920 to 1995 is shown in Figure 28–1.[6] Meningococcal disease can be endemic (or sporadic) or epidemic (outbreak or cluster). There is no strict cutoff point between endemic and epidemic rates of the disease. To recognize epidemics, public health officials must usually rely on comparisons of rates of disease with earlier surveillance data from the same population. Other factors such as the clonality of meningococcal strains or changes in the age distribution of cases can be useful in confirming epidemics.[47–49] In a multistate

Table 28–1. **SCHEDULE FOR ADMINISTERING CHEMOPROPHYLAXIS AGAINST MENINGOCOCCAL DISEASE**

DRUG	AGE GROUP	DOSAGE	DURATION OF VACCINE ADMINISTRATION
Rifampin	Children <1 mo	5 mg/kg every 12 hr	2 d
	Children >1 mo–10 yr	10 mg/kg every 12 hr*	2 d
	Adults	600 mg every 12 hr	2 d
Ciprofloxacin	Adults	500 mg	Single dose
Ceftriaxone	Children <15 yr	125 mg	Single intramuscular dose
Ceftriaxone	Adults	250 mg	Single intramuscular dose

*Maximum of 600 mg total.

From Control and prevention of meningococcal disease: Recommendations of the Advisory Committee on Immunization Practices (ACIP). MMWR Morb Mortal Wkly Rep 46(RR-5):1–10, 1997.

surveillance project in 1995, bacterial meningitis was identified in 248 people. Rates per 100,000 people of meningitis due to specific pathogens were 1.14 for *Streptococcus pneumoniae*, 0.60 for *N. meningitidis*, and 0.18 for *Haemophilus influenzae* type b. In infants 1 to 23 months of age, *S. pneumoniae* caused 45% of cases and *N. meningitidis* 31%. Among those 2 to 18 years of age, *N. meningitidis* caused the majority (59%) of cases; in people 19 years and older, however, *S. pneumoniae* caused 62% of meningitis cases. One hundred and thirty cases of invasive disease due to *N. meningitidis* occurred in children and young adults, and 48% of these were meningitis. Serogroups C, Y, B, and W-135 accounted for 39, 32, 24, and 4% of all strains that could be serogrouped, respectively.[5]

The incidence of endemic meningococcal disease generally ranges from 1 to 3 cases per 100,000 population in the United States, England, Wales, and Scandinavia[50, 51] to 10 to 25 cases per 100,000 people in some developing countries.[52] Rates of disease during epidemics may range from 4 to more than 1000 cases per 100,000 people.[52] Overall mortality from meningococcal disease is usually reported as 7 to 14%, although this is likely to be an underestimate in some developing countries.[53] These populations as well as populations that do not have large regular epidemics are generally at some risk for occasional, usually less intense, smaller epidemics.

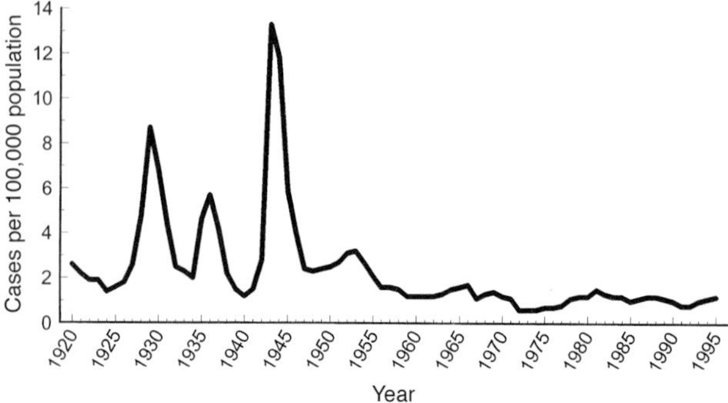

Figure 28–1. Incidence of meningococcal disease in the United States, 1920 to 1995. (From Wenger JD, Perkins BA. Patterns in the emergence of epidemic meningococcal disease. In Scheld WM, Armstrong D, Hughes JM (eds). Emerging Infections 1. Washington, DC, American Society for Microbiology Press, 1998, pp 125–136.)

Meningococcal Disease Due to Serogroup A

Serogroup A meningococci are the most common cause of large epidemics and can also cause endemic disease. In an English study, for example, when epidemics of serogroup A disease occurred in developed countries, cases were more likely than controls to come from lower socioeconomic households.[54] Major epidemics occur most frequently but are not restricted to an area in the African *meningitis belt* that extends across Africa from east to west and includes all or part of 15 countries (Fig. 28–2).[6] Epidemics start in the dry season (December–June) and end promptly when the rainy season begins. They often extend over more than one dry season and are thought to typically recur in 8- to 12-year cycles (this estimate appears to be somewhat more variable than originally believed).[55] Among 125 patient strains isolated in 11 African countries between 1989 to 1994, 92% belonged to a clone-complex of serogroup A meningococcus.[56]

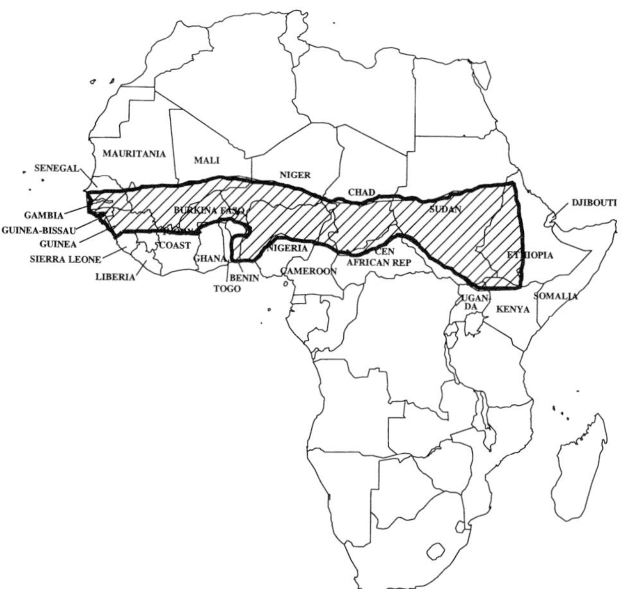

Figure 28–2. The sub-Saharan African meningitis belt. (From Control and prevention of meningococcal disease and control and prevention of serogroup C meningococcal disease: Evaluation and management of suspected outbreaks: Recommendations of the Advisory Committee on Immunization Practices (ACIP). MMWR Morb Mortal Wkly Rep 46[RR-5; suppl]:1–21, 1997.)

In sub-Saharan Africa, attack rates have exceeded 1200 per 100,000 population (1%). Major epidemics have occurred in Ethiopia, Chad, Sudan, and Kenya, in the meningitis belt and beyond. The reasons for the peculiar pattern of disease are not clear. However, it is possible that new clones with increased virulence are introduced to populations who either have not been previously exposed or were exposed years earlier and now have decreased immunity. Such a scenario would lead to higher attack rates in older children and young adults.[56]

During the first 4 months of 1996, the estimated number of cases of meningitis reported in the African region of the World Health Organization was 149,166, with 15,783 deaths. The highest number of cases was reported from Burkina Faso (42,129, with 10% mortality) and Nigeria (75,000 and a similar mortality rate). The peak incidence occurred in the early spring months. The strains isolated were of the III-1 clone.[57]

Meningococcal Disease Due to Serogroup C

Serogroup C meningococci are a leading cause of endemic meningococcal disease in the United States and throughout the world, accounting for a significant proportion of sporadic disease in Europe and Canada and recently in Spain.[58–60] In maritime Canada from 1989 to 1992, the incidence of meningococcal disease was 10 times greater than background levels, with the majority due to group C and affecting an older age group than endemic serogroup C or serogroup B diseases.[61]

In the United States, the majority of cases of meningococcal disease are sporadic. Since 1991, however, an increasing number of localized outbreaks* of serogroup C meningococcal disease have occurred, often associated with the arrival of a new meningococcal strain in the community. A large percentage were related to a specific subtype. Whereas endemic disease continued to occur in infants and young children, there was a shift of the age distribution toward school-aged children and young adults. Associations between cases were typically lacking. In general, outbreaks occurred in small communities or in university populations, with 5 to 15 cases occurring at the same time of year as the peak in endemic disease and without an increase in morbidity or mortality rates. Institutional outbreaks involving primarily children or young adults in single universities or schools were of short duration, with cases occurring within 1 to 2 weeks.[47]

Meningococcal Disease Due to Serogroup B

Worldwide, serogroup B meningococci are probably the most common cause of endemic meningococcal disease. Serogroup B meningococcal organisms have also been responsible for significant outbreaks in Europe, including Scandinavian countries.[62] Although one clonal type (ET-5) has been prevalent, globally, serotypes of serogroup B have been variable.[15] There has also been intercontinental spread, with outbreaks in South America.[63] In Brazil in 1988 to 1990, a new epidemic due to serogroup B occurred in São Paulo, Brazil, and was paralleled by an increased prevalence of a single serogroup B clone, B:4:P1:15, of the ET-5 complex.[64] Epidemics caused by serogroup B meningococci are less intense than those caused by serogroup A meningococci but may extend over a more prolonged period, often for several to many years.[15]

In the early 1990s, an outbreak of serogroup B meningococcal disease was recognized in Oregon and Washington state.[65] The overall rate of disease rose from 1 to 2 cases per 100,000 people to five times that number. Along with this increased incidence, the age distribution of cases changed, with the most dramatic increase occurring in older children and young adults. The enzyme type strain had been rare in the United States previously and belonged to the ET-5 complex reported by Caugant and colleagues, which caused increased rates of serogroup B disease in Europe and Latin America.[16] Non–ET-5 serogroup B outbreaks have been described in Florida, Missouri, and the Los Angeles county jail system.[66]

Serogroup Y Meningococcal Disease in Illinois and Connecticut, 1989 to 1996

During 1992 to 1995 serogroup Y meningococcal (SYM) disease accounted for an increasing proportion of meningococcal disease cases. In Illinois among 589 cases of invasive meningococcal disease, the proportion attributable to SYM disease increased from 6% in 1991 to 29% in 1995, whereas the incidence of diseases from serogroups B and C decreased.

In Connecticut from January 1991 to June 1996, there were 190 culture-proven cases of meningococcal disease. Of the 144 cases that could be serogrouped, nearly half (69) were SYM disease; the remainder were equally divided between serogroups B and C, and two patients had serogroup W-135 disease. Clinically, pneumonia was more common among patients with SYM disease. Nationally, 21% of cases were due to serogroup Y in 1995.[67]

A statewide increase in meningococcal disease due to serogroup Y occurred in Minnesota from April 1995 to April 1997, when 36 cases were identified. These cases accounted for 30% of meningococcal cases in 1995, 51% in 1996, and 25% in the first 4 months of 1997. People with the disease were older than those with diseases due to other serogroups, and 78% of isolates belonged to two clonal groups; however, no epidemiological associations between cases were found.[68]

Significance as a Public Health Problem

In 1996, the global burden of endemic disease due to *N. meningitidis* was 1.3 per 100,000 people, but in some

*An outbreak is defined as the occurrence of 3 or more cases in less than 3 months in people who have a common affiliation or live in the same area but who have no close contact, resulting in a primary disease attack rate of at least 10 cases per 100,000.[6]

areas it reached 1.7 per 100,000 people. The highest age-specific incidence occurred in children 0 to 4 years of age, and disease occurred during the winter months. Meningococcemia without meningitis accounted for an endemic rate of 0.9 per 100,000 people.[4] These data do not include epidemic disease due to serogroup A, which in some years can double the burden. The epidemic potential of *N. meningitidis* increases its importance as a public health problem. Certain clinical features such as the rapidity of illness, which can occur in otherwise healthy young people, increase the importance of the public health problem.

In most developed countries, chemoprophylaxis is given to close contacts of sporadic disease. This approach requires significant public health resources to identify and provide antimicrobials. Although outbreaks or epidemics attract most of the attention to meningococcal disease, it is increasingly clear that to make substantial progress in controlling meningococcal disease, another approach (e.g., routine immunization of infants) is needed to prevent endemic disease in young children.

MECHANISMS OF IMMUNITY TO MENINGOCOCCAL DISEASE

Passive Immunization: The Role of Humoral Immunity in Meningococcal Disease

Landmark observations of Flexner[7] on the efficacy of antimeningococcal serum in reducing mortality during the preantibiotic era provided evidence supporting the importance of humoral immunity in resistance to meningococcal disease.

Natural Acquisition of Humoral Immunity to Serogroup C

Between 2 and 12 years of age, there is a progressive annual increase of approximately 5% in the proportion of children with antibody against meningococcal serogroups A, B, and C and a progressive and marked decrease in the incidence of disease.[20] By 6 to 8 years of age, more than 90% have antibodies to serogroup C. These trends are further evidence of the role of humoral immunity in protection.

Studies of human immunity to meningococcal disease were begun in 1966 by Goldschneider and colleagues at the Walter Reed Army Institute of Research.[21] They were able to demonstrate a direct correlation between the susceptibility to systemic meningococcal disease and the absence of detectable bactericidal antibody. Army recruits who acquired a serogroup C strain and who lacked bactericidal antibody against the strain had a 38% chance of developing disease. Recruits who had detectable antibody frequently became carriers but did not develop disease. Killing of meningococci by antibodies is mediated by terminal complement components (5th–9th) through the assembly of a membrane attack complex on the bacterial surface.[69]

Natural Acquisition of Humoral Immunity to Serogroup A

Natural acquisition of anti-A antibody occurs much earlier than acquisition of anti-C antibody; by 18 months of age, more than 90% of the children in the United States have detectable anti-A antibodies. Because the incidence of disease due to serogroup A meningococcus has been very low in the United States, these natural antibodies must be derived as a result of exposure to other antigens that cross-react with serogroup A organisms.[70]

Griffiss and coworkers compared the immune response of infants and children with that of adults who had disseminated infections with *N. meningitidis* by measurement of antipolysaccharide antibody.[71] Most of the children older than 2 years infected with serogroup C or Y strains developed bactericidal antibody. Response to the serogroup B polysaccharide was poor in younger children, whereas adults developed antipolysaccharide antibody to serogroup B. Bactericidal antibody in the sera of children who did not respond to the serogroup B capsular polysaccharide was often produced against a lipo-oligosaccharide antigen.[71]

Active Immunization

Approaches to Vaccine Development Before the 1960s

Several attempts were made before 1940 to develop a vaccine against meningococcal disease. These early vaccines consisted of either killed whole organisms or crude extracts of broth cultures. During the mid-1940s, several investigators demonstrated that antibodies to the group-specific capsular polysaccharide antigens could passively protect mice against lethal challenge.[72] However, purified preparations of these polysaccharides failed to induce antibody responses in human volunteers.[73] The success of sulfonamides for the treatment and prevention of meningococcal disease at that time made vaccine development less essential.

Development of Polysaccharide Vaccines

In 1963, sulfonamide-resistant strains of serogroup B meningococci became widespread, first among U.S. military personnel[74] and then among civilians. Sulfonamide-resistant serogroup C meningococci became the predominant cause of disease throughout the armed forces, and vaccine development was undertaken to control epidemic disease in recruits.

Description of the Vaccine

After the demonstration that circulating antibody directed toward the group-specific capsular polysaccharide of serogroups A and C confers resistance to meningococcal disease,[20] the stage was set for purification of high–molecular weight polysaccharides of serogroups A and C and subsequently Y and W-135 by Gotschlich and colleagues.[75] The sialic acid found in the serogroup B polysaccharide capsule is identical to that found in association with human neural tissues and is thus unlikely to be effective as an immunogen.[76]

Methods of Determining Immunogenicity of Serogroups A and C Polysaccharides in Humans

The serological response to the serogroups A and C meningococcal polysaccharides depends on many factors, including the age of recipients, the dose of vaccine, the number of exposures to vaccines, prior experience with natural cross-reacting antigens, and the molecular size of vaccines.

A variety of methods have been employed to measure the antibody responses to the meningococcal polysaccharides, such as bactericidal and fluorescent antibody assays; radioactive antigen binding by the Farr technique,[77] later modified by Gotschlich[78]; and solid-phase radioimmunoassay.[79] An enzyme-linked immunosorbent assay (ELISA) test has been developed and is the international standard for antibodies to serogroups A and C. The serum bactericidal test, which is the principal assay for protection afforded by antipolysaccharide antibody to serogroups A, C, Y, and W-135 as well as serogroup B, has not been completely correlated with other antibody assays, nor has the level of antibody required for protection been standardized.[69]

Immunogenicity of Serogroup C Polysaccharide Vaccine

In adult volunteers given a single 50-μg dose of serogroup C vaccine, peak antibody titers were attained by 2 weeks after immunization. Increases in immunoglobulin (Ig) G, IgM, and IgA antimeningococcal antibodies were demonstrated by immunofluorescence.[80]

Among infants, age is the major determinant of the antibody response to the serogroup C polysaccharide vaccine[81] as well as the antibody response after natural disease.[71] The antibody response of infants and children appears to peak at 3 to 4 weeks after immunization. A protective level of antibody has not been identified. Table 28–2 lists the mean anti-C concentrations, as determined by radioactive antigen-binding and seroconversion rates at different ages after a single dose of 25 to 100 μg of serogroup C vaccine.[82] By 3 months of age, most infants have lost detectable maternal antibodies and begin to respond to the vaccine, although the maximum response is only about 2% of that of an adult. By 2 years of age, a child achieves a mean level of antibody that is about 10% of that of an adult. A 50-μg dose is recommended for individuals 2 years of age and older.[83]

No differences have been observed in the immunogenicity of different lots of serogroup C vaccine; moreover, the vaccine appears to be very stable when diluted at 4°C for 2 weeks, at −20°C for 6 months, and up to 5 years at −70°C when stored lyophilized.[84]

The persistence of antibody in adults after a single dose of serogroup C vaccine was reported to be 30% of peak levels 4 years after vaccination.[85] Infants immunized before 1 year of age demonstrated a decline to baseline levels after 3 to 5 months. In slightly older children, the antibody persistence is somewhat more prolonged but declines continuously over 1 to 4 years of observation to less than 25% of the peak level.[83]

Response to Booster Doses of Serogroup C Vaccine. No response was seen to a booster dose of serogroup C vaccine given to adults 10 to 14 days or 8 months after the first dose.[86] Significant responses to booster doses were not observed with serogroup C vaccine administered at 7 and 12 months of age to babies who had initially responded at 3 months of age. Indeed, except for a 10 μg dose, booster injections of 25 or 100 μg of serogroup C vaccine in infants 7 and 12 months of age resulted in lower anti–serogroup C antibody concentrations than did primary immunization at those ages.[83] By 18 months of age, however, there were no differences in the anti–serogroup C antibody responses to primary and booster immunization of serogroup C

Table 28–2. **ANTIBODY RESPONSE 1 MONTH AFTER IMMUNIZATION WITH A SINGLE DOSE OF SEROGROUP C MENINGOCOCCAL POLYSACCHARIDE VACCINE**

AGE AT VACCINATION	NO. VACCINATED	MEAN ANTI–SEROGROUP C CONCENTRATION (mg/mL)*	SEROCONVERSION (%)†
3 mo	76	0.42	90
7 mo	41	1.25	100
12 mo	38	2.10	94
18 mo	24	3.10	96
2–5 yr	33	5.54	100
6–8 yr	49	7.64	94
18–25 yr	22	33.5	100

*Although antibody levels to primary immunization appear high, particularly among children younger than 2 years, type C vaccine was not demonstrated to be effective against disease in such children because antibody levels decline rapidly and a second dose does not result in a booster response. (This response differs from that to serotype A vaccine; see text.)

†Seroconversion indicates either a change from nondetectable preimmunization antibody levels to detectable postimmunization anti–serogroup C antibody concentrations or a twofold increase in anti–serogroup C concentrations by radio immunoassay.

Data from references 82, 83, and 93.

vaccine.[81] Lepow and coworkers found that booster doses of serogroup C vaccine given 3 years after primary immunizations of children 2 to 11 years of age restored the concentrations of anti–serogroup C antibodies to levels similar to those seen after initial doses but that booster responses to higher levels did not occur.[87] Several studies have been carried out comparing the responses to polysaccharide and conjugate vaccines in infants and adults. A comparative study of two doses of Chiron-R conjugate serogroup C vaccine with two doses of polysaccharide vaccine in toddlers 15 to 23 months of age indicated a poor response to the second dose of polysaccharide vaccine as well as to the 1-year booster dose in the polysaccharide-immunized group.[88]

Granoff and coworkers demonstrated that among 34 adults receiving a single 50-μg dose of meningococcal ACY W-135 polysaccharide vaccine, 5 who had received the polysaccharide 4 years earlier had a poorer serogroup C response to the booster than those who were vaccinated for the first time with the polysaccharide vaccine or the 18 adults who had been given a conjugate Chiron-R vaccine.[89]

Immunogenicity of Serogroup A Polysaccharide Vaccine in Infants and Children

In a trial of serogroup A meningococcal vaccine in infants, the geometric mean concentration of anti–serogroup A antibody was 0.36 μg per mL before immunization at 3 months of age, and 60% of infants had concentrations of anti–serogroup A antibodies below 0.13 μg per mL, the lowest detectable level. Primary immunization with one dose at 3 months of age resulted in no detectable increase in antibody.[83] There was an increasing response to primary immunization with age, as indicated in Table 28–3. One-year-old infants achieved mean anti–serogroup A antibody levels that were 4% of those of adults (see Table 28–3),[80] and 6- to 8-year-old children achieved levels that were 25% of the level in adults.[87] A 50-μg dose seemed optimal, but, as with serogroup C vaccine, a protective antibody titer is yet to be determined.

A significant difference in the immunogenicity of different lots of serogroup A vaccine was shown to be related to molecular size.[77] Lots of serogroup A polysaccharide with average molecular weights below 50,000 induced significantly lower anti–serogroup A antibody concentrations than did lots with average molecular weights greater than 80,000.

Storage requirements for the serogroup A polysaccharide vaccine were similar to those defined for the serogroup C vaccine. Failure of serogroup A vaccine to induce significant protection against disease in a field trial in Nigeria was attributed to depolymerization of the serogroup A polysaccharide to a nonimmunogenic, low–molecular weight form, an effect believed to be a result of unavoidable, prolonged exposure to high ambient temperatures.[90]

Several features differ in the persistence of serogroup A antibody after vaccination when compared with serogroup C antibody. The concentration of anti–serogroup A antibody appeared to plateau after an initial decline in infants monitored for a year or longer after immunization, whereas the anti–serogroup C titers continued to decline.[81]

Antibody Response to Booster Doses of Serogroup A Vaccine. The response of infants to boosters of serogroup A vaccine markedly contrasts with that seen to boosters of serogroup C vaccine.[83] Infants who received initial immunizations at 3 months of age show significant anamnestic responses when given a second dose at 7 or 12 months of age. At 7 months of age, an injection of 25 μg of serogroup A vaccine induces a 2.09 μg per mL geometric mean concentration of anti–serogroup A antibody and a seroconversion rate of 88%, compared with 0.37 μg per mL and 60%, respectively, after primary immunization at that age and at 12 months of age (4.0 ug/ml vs. 0.77). Similar responses to the second dose were observed in Finnish children given 2 doses of vaccine between 3 and 18 months of age.[91] Three doses of serogroup A vaccine at 2-month intervals from 2 months of age results in even higher concentrations of anti–serogroup A antibody at 7 months of age

Table 28–3. **ANTIBODY RESPONSE 1 MONTH AFTER PRIMARY IMMUNIZATION WITH GROUP A MENINGOCOCCAL POLYSACCHARIDE VACCINE***

	MEAN ANTI-SEROGROUP A CONCENTRATION (mg/mL)		
AGE AT VACCINATION	Before Vaccination	After Vaccination	SEROCONVERSION (%)*
3 mo	0.37	0.33	9
7 mo	0.19	0.39	68
12 mo	0.19	0.84	85
18 mo	0.23	3.14	91
2–5 yr	0.79	5.23	97
6–8 yr	1.37	7.71	93
15–25 yr	4.70	31.4	100

*In all studies, a second dose results in a booster response for all ages, including young infants (see text).

†Seroconversion indicates either a change from nondetectable preimmunization antibody levels to detectable postimmunization anti–serogroup A concentrations or a twofold increase in anti–serogroup A concentrations by radio immunoassay.

Data from references 82, 83, and 93.

than those observed with two doses at 3 and 7 months of age.[92] Further studies by Gold and Lepow in 282 infants showed no effect of administering a booster dose at 24 months of age in children who had received 1 or 2 doses of serogroup A vaccine at 3, 7, or 12 months of age. Antibody responses were similar to those obtained with a single dose at 24 months of age, implying that natural immunizing infections occurred before this age. Accordingly, the 24-month dose constitutes a reinforcing dose.[93]

In the only such study in African children, Leach and coworkers reported on the antibody response, measured by an ELISA test and by a bactericidal test, to serogroup A polysaccharide vaccine administered at 18 to 24 months of age to Gambian children.[94] The study showed that bactericidal titers in children previously immunized during their first year with serogroup A polysaccharide vaccine and given a booster dose with the same polysaccharide vaccine did not differ from the titers in children immunized for the first time with the same vaccine at 2 years of age, again suggesting that natural immunization occurs during the first 2 years of life.

Thus, the limited studies with serogroup A polysaccharide vaccine demonstrate an age-dependent booster effect only in the first year of life as well as a persistence of antibody concentration of approximately 1 μg per mL at 2 years of age.

The decline in anti–serogroup A antibody levels after a booster dose parallels that seen with primary immunization. After an initial decline in the first year, a plateau is reached during the second year. This trend was also noted in Finnish children.[95] In 1345 U.S. schoolchildren 6 to 8 years of age who were followed for 1 to 3 or 4 years after receiving a single dose of either serogroup A or C vaccine, the mean concentration of anti–serogroup A antibody declined from a peak level of 9.35 μg per mL of antibody protein 1 month after vaccination to 5.54 and 3.62 μg per mL of antibody protein, respectively, 1 and 3 or 4 years after immunization.[87] These results contrast with levels of anti–serogroup C antibodies, which declined much more rapidly: Mean levels of antibody protein were 9.12 μg per mL 1 month after immunization and 2.35 and 1.47 μg per mL, respectively, 1 and 3 or 4 years after immunization. The 4-year group consisted of 90 schoolchildren followed in one private practice.

Efficacy of Serogroup C Vaccine

Two large-scale field trials of the serogroup C vaccine were undertaken in 1969 and 1970 and involved 20,000 troops in the U.S. Army.[96] The results indicated 90% efficacy under the epidemic conditions that existed in basic training centers. Since October 1972, the serogroup C vaccine has been administered to all incoming recruits, and serogroup C meningococcal disease has been eliminated as a health problem in the U.S. Army.[97] The protection induced by the serogroup C vaccine is group specific. The attack rate of serogroup B meningococcal disease was slightly higher in the vaccinated groups compared with that in the control group in the Army trials.

The efficacy of the serogroup C vaccine in infants and young children was evaluated in a placebo-controlled trial during a major epidemic in São Paulo, Brazil, in 1974.[98, 99] Approximately 67,000 children 6 to 35 months of age received a single 50-μg dose of serogroup C vaccine, and a control group of equal size received diphtheria, pertussis, and tetanus vaccine. The meningococcal vaccine was effective in preventing disease in 67% of immunized children aged 24 to 36 months, but no protection was apparent in children 6 to 23 months of age. Although the minimal protective level of anti–serogroup C antibody has not been determined, the Brazilian children older than 2 years responded with approximately 2 μg per mL geometric mean concentrations of anti–serogroup C antibody protein.[100] Similar anti–serogroup C antibody concentrations were achieved by 12 to 18 months of age in U.S. infants.[81] It is clear that the currently available serogroup C polysaccharide vaccines are not likely to consistently protect infants younger than 2 years. In the Brazilian epidemic, administration of the vaccine to pregnant women demonstrated no adverse effects, with good antibody levels noted in maternal and cord bloods. There was no adverse effect on subsequent immunization of infants.[101]

An outbreak of serogroup C meningococcal meningitis occurred in the British Royal Air Force, and serogroup C vaccine was used when chemoprophylaxis failed. With one exception, no further cases of serogroup C disease occurred.[102]

Use of Serogroup C Vaccine for Outbreak Control in Civilian Populations in North America. A mass immunization campaign with Canadian-produced quadravalent vaccine was conducted in Quebec, Canada, during the winter of 1993, after an increase in the incidence of meningococcal disease caused by a virulent clone of *N. meningitidis* serogroup C.[103] Approximately 1.6 million doses of the polysaccharide vaccine were administered to 84% of the target population aged 6 months to 20 years. In the first year after the campaign, the incidence of the disease dropped markedly in vaccinees and in the unvaccinated fraction of the target population, whereas it remained unchanged in people older than 20 years. The overall field efficacy of the vaccine was estimated to be 79%, with efficacies greater in teenagers and less in children younger than 5 years. It was estimated that at least 37 cases were prevented during the first year of the campaign.

During a mass vaccination program, King and coworkers evaluated total and functional antibody responses to the serogroup C polysaccharide component of the Canadian-produced meningococcal polysaccharide vaccine.[104] Immune responses were measured in 345 individuals in seven different age groups selected from more than 2000 participants. One month after vaccination, the geometric mean antibody concentration to serogroup C was 7.56 μg per mL of antibody protein. An overall 113-fold increase over baseline levels was shown in 68.1% of infants 6 to 11 months old, and more than 85% of all other age groups had levels of antibody protein equal to or greater than 2 μg per mL. By 1 year after vaccination, there was a significant decline in titers in children younger than 5 years; revaccination would have to be considered in these individuals if the risk of persistent disease warranted it. Total antibody concentration was a useful surrogate for bactericidal antibody in children older than 18 months.

Jackson and coworkers reported that in the United States in 1992 and in the first half of 1993, 100,000 doses of meningococcal vaccine were administered to contacts of people with meningococcal disease due to serogroup C. Only 34,000 doses were administered from 1980 to 1991. The effectiveness of vaccine for outbreak control in communities or schools is difficult to evaluate. In several schools, additional cases occurred in the same population during the next meningococcal disease season, thus raising questions about the duration of immunity.[47] In Gregg County, Texas, high rates of disease occurred in 3 consecutive years despite large immunization programs. A case-control study showed that the vaccine was 85% effective, but further studies demonstrated that only a small proportion of the population at risk had received vaccine in the mass campaigns, thus leaving a large segment of the population unprotected.[105] Since targeted vaccination programs with the current polysaccharide vaccines do not appear to provide herd immunity, more universal immunization may be required.

Efficacy of Serogroup A Vaccine

Controlled Trials and Case-Control Studies to Estimate Efficacy. Two types of investigations have been reported: controlled trials[91, 106–109] and case-control studies.[37, 110] There are major differences between these types of investigations in study design, number of doses, age groups immunized, and duration of study; however, it is clear that the vaccine has been shown to be effective in a number of settings.

The only controlled trial of serogroup A vaccine in young children was conducted in Finland during an epidemic of meningococcal A disease. Approximately 130,000 children 3 months to 5 years of age were enrolled from 1975 to 1976, of whom 49,925 received serogroup A vaccine (two doses in infants 3–18 mo), 48,977 received *H. influenzae* type b polysaccharide vaccine, and 32,000 served as uninoculated control subjects. After 1 year of observation, no cases of serogroup A disease occurred in those subjects receiving the serogroup A vaccine, but 6 and 13 cases, respectively, were identified in the other two groups.[91]

Although the minimally protective concentration of anti–serogroup A antibody is not known, the response of infants to booster doses of serogroup A vaccine coupled with the promising results of the Finnish field trials suggest that the serogroup A vaccine currently available could be effective in providing short-term protection against serogroup A meningococcal disease at all ages.

In Auckland, New Zealand, where epidemic meningococcal serogroup A disease occurred in the winter seasons of 1985 and 1986, the highest rate of disease was in children younger than 23 months. 130,000 children were immunized. The populations at highest risk were Maori and Pacific Island Polynesian children. There was an estimated 100% efficacy of meningococcal vaccine administered as two doses to children 3 to 23 months of age and as one dose in children older than 2 years. Although persistence of protection is unknown, serogroup A disease had not returned to Auckland as of 1992.[111]

No studies have evaluated the efficacy of disease prevention in Africa of a vaccination regimen of two or more doses given to infants or other age groups. Moreover, in areas where malaria incidence is high, malaria-infected individuals had a depressed immune response, although chloroquine administration before vaccination improved the antibody response.[112] Infant responses were consistent with a low level of vaccine efficacy: Antibody levels declined to 50% of peak levels after 2 years and to less than 10% persistence after 3 years.[110] Long-term protection has not been studied in older children. It is not known when revaccination should be undertaken in children if there is continuing exposure.

Serogroup A vaccine has been used mainly under the emergency conditions of outbreaks. To ensure effective control of outbreaks, an outbreak has to be recognized early, and mobilization for mass immunization must be rapid. An emergency response plan by World Health Organization outlines necessary steps for identifying and responding to outbreaks.[113] It has been proposed by Robbins and others that the entire population of the meningitis belt receive serogroup A vaccine in a mass program.[114] Thereafter, they propose routine immunization with one dose of serogroup A vaccine at 2 years of age and another at 5 years of age. They believe that this will approach will eliminate serogroup A disease in the region.

Control strategies have been evaluated by Miller and colleagues for the World Health Organization Children's Vaccine Initiative in concert with the Centers for Disease Control and Prevention.[115] They formulated models of 1, 2, or 3 doses of the current vaccine for routine immunization in each country and in a campaign response for Burkina Faso, the country with the highest incidence of disease. Immunization for the entire meningitis belt would require 8.2 to 23.8 million doses for each cohort annually at a cost of $20 to 26 million for 1 or 3 doses, respectively. One dose per person would prevent 7800 cases, and three doses per person would prevent 19,000 cases; the cost per death prevented of these two regimens would be $11,000 and $13,000, respectively. Catch-up costs would be considerable. Only one third of cases would be prevented in Burkina Faso with this protocol.

An emergency response strategy on the other hand, would prevent 27% of cases at a cost of $1200 per death prevented. One conclusion, then, is that these countries should improve routine measles elimination programs rather than add meningococcal vaccine to the standard regimen and should instead emphasize a rapid response for outbreak control of meningococcal disease.[115] Even under optimal conditions, it is estimated that only 60% of outbreak-related cases could be prevented; more effective vaccines are sorely needed.

Effect of Meningococcal Vaccination on Carriage

The principal controlled studies of the effect of serogroup C vaccine on the carriage of meningococci were those of Gotschlich and coworkers (1969) in U.S. Army recruits.[116] The researchers found a decreased acquisition (20%) of serogroup C bacteria within 6 weeks of immunization, compared with 47% in unvaccinated recruits.[116]

In the Gambia, carriage of serogroup A meningococci was studied 6 months before and 6 and 18 months after a mass vaccination campaign with serogroup A and C vaccine. Carriage was the same 6 months before and 6 months after widespread vaccination, but it was decreased by 18 months after vaccination. The conclusion is that factors other than vaccine-induced antibody affected carriage.[117]

RECOMMENDATIONS FOR THE USE OF MENINGOCOCCAL A, C, Y, AND W-135 VACCINES IN THE UNITED STATES

The four polysaccharide antigens (A, C, Y, and W-135) have been combined in a tetravalent vaccine.[118] The Advisory Committee on Immunization Practices (ACIP) has made recommendations for the use of meningococcal polysaccharide vaccines. The quadravalent vaccine is administered to all U.S. military recruits. Routine vaccination of civilian populations in industrialized countries is not recommended. In household contacts, routine vaccination may be used as an adjunct to antibiotic chemoprophylaxis. Routine immunization with the quadrivalent vaccine is recommended for asplenic people and those with previously described immunodeficiencies. Vaccination is recommended for outbreak control for diseases caused by the serotypes carried by vaccine and for travelers to hyperendemic or endemic areas such as Nepal, Saudi Arabia, Kenya, and the meningitis belt of sub-Saharan Africa (from Mauritania in the west to Ethiopia in the east). Because epidemics occur in the dry season (December–June), vaccination in Africa is recommended during that time.[6] In general, the use of polysaccharide meningococcal vaccine should be restricted to people older than 2 years; however, short-term protection could result from two doses of serogroup A vaccine in children 3 to 18 months of age, based on a significant booster response when a second dose of vaccine is administered 3 months after the first dose.[91]

Use of Serogroup C in Mass Vaccination Programs to Control Outbreaks. Serogroup C outbreaks have occurred in organizations and communities. An outbreak is defined as the occurrence of three or more cases in less than 3 months in people who have a common affiliation or who live in the same area but have no close contact, resulting in a primary disease attack rate of at least 10 cases per 100,000 persons.[6] The Centers for Disease Control and Prevention have summarized 10 steps to be used in evaluating and managing serogroup C meningococcal disease (Table 28–4).[6]

Table 28–4. **SUMMARY OF 10 STEPS IN THE EVALUATION AND MANAGEMENT OF SUSPECTED OUTBREAKS OF SEROGROUP C MENINGOCOCCAL DISEASE**

1. Establish a diagnosis of serogroup C meningococcal disease.
2. Administer chemoprophylaxis to appropriate contacts.
3. Enhance surveillance, save isolates, and review historical data.
4. Investigate links between cases.
5. Consider subtyping.
6. Exclude secondary and coprimary cases.
7. Determine if the suspected outbreak is organization or community based.
8. Define the population at risk and determine its size.
9. Calculate the attack rate. If it exceeds 10 cases per 100,000 people in a 3-month period, vaccination should be considered.)
10. Select the target group for vaccination (may be limited to a specific age range).

From Control and prevention of meningococcal disease: Recommendations of the Advisory Committee on Immunization Practices (ACIP). MMWR Morb Mortal Wkly Rep 46(RR-5):1–21, 1997.

Use of Serogroup C Vaccination in Colleges. The American College Health Association has recently recommended that college students consider preexposure vaccination against meningococcal meningitis. However, cost-benefit analysis of routine vaccination of college students against serogroup C meningococcal disease documented that such a policy would not be cost-effective unless the incidence rate were at least 6.5 per 100,000 people. The actual rate of disease in this age group is approximately 1.3 per 100,000 people. After reviewing these data as well as the recommendation of the American College Health Association, the ACIP (in October 1997) did not support universal vaccination of college students. However, vaccination could still be indicated for the control of serogroup C disease outbreaks.[119] The ACIP called for more data to better assess the risk among college students.

Specifications of Meningococcal Vaccines. The A, C, Y, and W-135 quadrivalent vaccine is produced and marketed as Menomune A/C/Y/W-135 by Connaught Laboratories in Swiftwater, Pennsylvania. It is available in single-dose and multidose vials distributed as lyophilized powder that contains 50 μg of each component per dose. The vaccine should be stored at −20°C. For both adults and children, vaccine when reconstituted is administered subcutaneously as a 0.5 mL dose. It can be administered simultaneously with other vaccines at different sites. Protective levels of antibody can be expected after 7 to 10 days.[6]

Precautions and Contraindications. Adverse reactions are mild and consist of pain and tenderness at the injection site for 1 to 2 days. Estimates of the incidence of mild to moderate local reactions range from infrequent to more than 40% among vaccine recipients. Fever is rare. No adverse effects have been documented among women vaccinated during pregnancy or their newborns.[120] There are no known contraindications.

Revaccination. Revaccination may be indicated for people at high risk for infection (e.g., people remaining in areas where the disease is epidemic), particularly for children who were first vaccinated when they were younger than 4 years; such children should be considered for revaccination after 2 to 3 years if they remain at high risk. Although the need for revaccination of older children and adults has not been determined, antibody levels decline rapidly over 2 to 3 years, and if indications still exist for immunization, revaccination may be considered within 3 to 5 years.

Vaccination Against Serogroup B Meningococcus. Attempts to develop serogroup B polysaccharide vaccines have been unsuccessful, and antibody response after disease is poor. The capsular polysaccharide is a 2- to 8-linked polysialic acid found in most mammalian tissues during development.[121] The approach to a serogroup B vaccination has been focused on the use of outer membrane proteins to stimulate protective immunity. Two-dose regimens of three outer membrane protein–based serogroup B meningococcal vaccines have been effective in older children and young adults in large clinical trials: Estimated efficacies ranged from 57 to 83%.[15] One commercially available vaccine produced in Cuba (not licensed for use in the United States) was used in São Paulo, Brazil, where approximately 2.4 million children aged 3 months to 6 years were vaccinated from 1989 to 1990. The vaccine was estimated to be 74% effective in children 4 to 6 years of age.[122] A Norwegian outer membrane protein (OMP) vaccine was 57% effective in secondary school children.[123] Because protein serotypes generally have a narrow range of protection, future vaccines would have to include the prevalent serotypes, although some cross-reactive bactericidal antibodies have been identified in postimmunization sera.

NEW DIRECTIONS IN MENINGOCOCCAL A, C, Y, AND W-135 VACCINE DEVELOPMENT

Approach to the Control of Disease with Conjugate Vaccines. Polysaccharides are T cell–independent antigens and are poorly immunogenic in infants and young children; immunity is short lived. It is difficult to demonstrate responses to booster doses. Following the lead provided by *H. influenzae* type b vaccines—in which infant response was enhanced by protein carriers, IgG booster responses were elicited, and nasopharyngeal colonization and transmission were decreased—several meningococcal serotypes A and C vaccines have been developed and conjugated to proteins and are being evaluated in clinical trials.

A vaccine produced by Chiron Biocine (Italy) containing serogroups A and C meningococcal oligosaccharide-protein conjugates has been evaluated in Los Angeles for safety and immunogenicity in toddlers 18 to 24 months of age. A comparable group received 1 or 2 doses of polysaccharide vaccine at the same time. The immune response induced by the conjugate vaccine was qualitatively different from the polysaccharide vaccine, and the antibodies produced by the former had greater bactericidal activity.[124]

In the Gambia, the Chiron Biocine vaccine was evaluated in 304 Gambian infants aged 8 to 10 weeks. Infants were immunized with one, two, or three doses of conjugate vaccine at 2 and 6 months of age; 2, 3, and 4 months of age; or at 6 months of age only. An additional group was immunized with two doses of meningococcal serotypes A and C polysaccharide vaccine at 3 and 6 months of age.[125] Few side effects were noted with either vaccine. Antibodies were measured by ELISA tests. One dose of conjugate vaccine at 6 months of age induced higher antibody levels to serogroup C than did two doses at 2 and 6 months of age. However, mean postvaccination serogroup C antibody titers after three doses were significantly higher than those after two doses at 2 and 6 months of age, suggesting that the first dose induced a short-lived hyporesponsive state, a phenomenon described previously when the serogroup C polysaccharide vaccine was given to young infants in the United States.[82] Nevertheless, levels achieved in all groups were substantially higher than those achieved with the polysaccharides at comparable ages.

The highest levels of preimmunization antibodies to serogroup A were found at 6 months of age, suggesting prior exposure to natural antigens.[125] Postvaccination serogroup A antibody levels increased progressively after the administration of one, two, or three doses. The highest levels of postimmunization IgG anti–serogroup A antibodies were found in infants who received two doses of vaccine at 2 and 6 months of age. Higher levels were achieved to the conjugate vaccine than to the polysaccharides A and C vaccines. Serogroups A and C antibody titers declined after 3 months in both polysaccharide and conjugate vaccine recipients, but it was believed that immunological memory would be established.[125]

In a separate study, 221 subjects were revaccinated at 18 to 24 months of age with one dose of either serogroups A and C polysaccharide vaccine or the conjugate vaccine.[94] A group of previously unvaccinated children of the same age was recruited as control subjects to receive one dose of combined serogroups A and C polysaccharide vaccine. Fourteen children in the prior three-dose conjugate group died, compared with one death in the two-dose group. Causes of death were malnutrition, acute gastroenteritis, and pneumonia; none of the deaths was believed to be vaccine related. No significant differences in deaths were found among the other groups. Children who received conjugate vaccine previously had significantly higher anti–serogroup C antibody responses after revaccination with conjugate vaccine than did the age-matched control subjects who received one dose of polysaccharide vaccine. Among those who received polysaccharide vaccine initially, those who received a booster dose of polysaccharide vaccine had lower serogroup C antibody responses than did those who received a booster dose of conjugate vaccine.[94]

Antibody titers to serogroup A after revaccination with either conjugate or polysaccharide vaccine were not significantly higher in the prior polysaccharide or conjugate recipients than in the control children who received the first dose of polysaccharide at 18 to 24 months of age.[94] Bactericidal titers paralleled the ELISA titers.

Capsular polysaccharides of meningococcal serogroups A, B, and C and oligosaccharides have been covalently joined to tetanus toxoid. Jennings and Lugowski have also prepared an oligosaccharide from the serogroup C polysaccharide that is linked to bovine albumin. These conjugates, except for serogroup B, elicited high antimeningococcal titers in mice.[126]

Wyeth-Lederle has developed oligosaccharides of meningococcal serogroups A and C that are noncovalently complexed to a nontoxigenic diphtheria toxoid (CRM197).[127] The preliminary results of serogroup C trials in the United States have been published. The vaccine was safe and immunogenic: 98% of responses were greater than 1 μg per mL antibody protein after three doses.[128] Follow-up data from this group with a fourth dose of vaccine at 12 to 15 months of age indicated a brisk response with high titers of bactericidal antibody.[129] This combined serogroups A and C vaccine was evaluated in 58 infants in the United Kingdom with three doses at 2, 3, and 4 months of age. Antibody titers to both serogroups A and C were significantly higher than 2 μg at 5 months of age. Although there was a decline at 14 months of age, titers were then higher than 2 μg, suggesting possible longer term protection.[130] A meningococcal serogroups A and C diphtheria toxoid vaccine produced by Pasteur Mérieux Connaught has been evaluated in varying combinations in infants 6, 10, and 14 weeks of age. Compared with pure polysaccharide, the diphtheria toxoid vaccine produced significantly greater functional antibodies to both serogroups A and C. Phase 2 trials are planned.[131] A phase 1 evaluation of a meningococcal serogroup C–tetanus toxoid conjugate has been evaluated in 30 adult volunteers and was shown to be both safe and immunogenic.[132]

In the future, a vaccine that is immunogenic in infants, provides protection through early adulthood, and can be given as a routine infant vaccination will be likely to prevent or dramatically reduce the severity of serogroup A meningococcal disease epidemics.

The phenomenon of hyporesponsiveness to booster doses of serogroup C vaccines in infants and children and some adults has been documented in a number of studies, and the question of safety and efficacy has to be raised if multiple doses of vaccine are required to maintain population immunity. The development of conjugate vaccines appears to be appropriate for long-term protection.[81, 83, 88, 89, 94, 97]

A conjugate vaccine with serogroup C polysaccharide—possibly in combination with diphtheria, tetanus, and pertussis vaccine and *H. influenzae* type b vaccine—that is immunogenic in infants and young children could have a significant impact in the United States and in other developed countries on the control of endemic serogroup C disease and on the severity of epidemics, or outbreaks, caused by this serogroup.

PROSPECTS FOR THE CONTROL OF DISEASE DUE TO MENINGOCOCCAL SEROGROUP B BY VACCINATION

In contrast to the situation with serogroups A and C meningococci, there is no vaccine available for serogroup B meningococci in the United States.

There have been several approaches to enhance the immunogenicity of the polysaccharide. One technique is adsorption on aluminum hydroxide.[133, 134] Another approach by Jennings and colleagues is to chemically alter the polysaccharide by substituting *N*-propionyl for the *N*-acetyl groups and then chemically binding it to tetanus toxoid.[135] The compound has stimulated bactericidal antibodies when tested experimentally.

Poolman has demonstrated that the class 1 outer membrane vesicle (OMV) or PorA (Por from Porin) is a vaccine component recognized in a number of studies to be an important inducer of bactericidal antibodies.[136] Laboratory results of induction of bactericidal antibodies and animal protection in addition to findings from clinical immunization studies led to the development of a hexavalent PorA vaccine using the six most prevalent serosubtypes.[137] Three PorA genes were introduced into one vaccine strain by way of consecutive deletion of the expression of various other surface components. Two such strains were used to produce an OMV vaccine that contained more than 90% PorA protein. Immunization studies of adults gave promising results,[138] and an immunogenicity study in English infants was initiated. It was possible to induce relevant levels of bactericidal antibodies against all six PorA serosubtype-specific target strains with four doses administered at 2, 3, 4, and 12 to 15 months of age. An immunogenicity study in Chilean infants with a Norwegian OMV vaccine demonstrated a PorA specific induction of bactericidal antibodies, with administration of the vaccine at 2 and 4 months of age.[139] These studies support the importance of PorA as well as the conformation of OMPs preserved by the OMP formulation, but further studies are needed to determine the duration of antibody response, booster dose effect, and, ultimately, efficacy in humans.

Another approach with the *N*-proprionylated serogroup B polysaccharide is to conjugate it with a recombinant *N. meningitidis* class 3 porin; this compound has been evaluated in mice and nonhuman primates, and all the antibody production is related to the polysaccharide without contribution from the porin.[140]

Of the many OMPs being expressed by the meningococcus, the OMPs induced by iron limitation and transferrin-binding proteins are being investigated for vaccine potential, although antigenic heterogeneity has been found.[141] Other vaccine candidates include pili[142] and exotoxins. Another experimental approach being evaluated is intranasal administration of OMVs from serogroup B meningococci, a technique that shows promise in adults for the induction of bactericidal antibodies.[143] A new vaccine providing durable protection when given to infants and young children would offer an option to accelerate the control of endemic serogroup B disease and decrease the likelihood of serogroup B disease epidemics.

REFERENCES

1. Willis T. A description of an epidemical fever in 1661. Practice of Physick. Treatise VIII. London, T Dring, 1684, pp 46–54.
2. Weichselbaum A. Über die aetiologie der akuten meningitis cerebro-spinal. Fortschr Med 5:573–583, 620–626, 1887.

3. Vieusseux M. Memoire sur le maladie qui a regne a Geneva au printemps de 1805. J Med Clin Pharm 11:163–182, 1805.
4. Murray JL, Lopez AD (eds). Global health statistics. Global Burden of Disease and Injury Series. Vol 2. Cambridge, MA, Harvard School of Public Health, 1996, p 293.
5. Schuchat A, Deaver-Robinson K, Wenger JD, et al. Bacterial meningitis in the United States in 1995. N Engl J Med 337:970–976, 1997.
6. Control and prevention of meningococcal disease: Recommendations of the Advisory Committee on Immunization Practices (ACIP). MMWR Morb Mortal Wkly Rep 46(RR-5):1–21, 1997.
7. Flexner S. The results of serum treatment in 1300 cases of epidemic meningitis. J Exp Med 17:553–576, 1913.
8. Kirsch EA, Barton RP, Kitchen L, Giroir BP. Pathophysiology, treatment and outcome of meningococcemia: A review and recent experience. Pediatr Infect Dis J 15:967–979, 1996.
9. Quagliarello VJ, Scheld WM. Treatment of bacterial meningitis. N Engl J Med 336:708–716, 1997.
10. Barquet N, Domingo P, Cayla J, Gonzales J. Prognostic factors in meningococcal disease. JAMA 278:491–496, 1997.
11. Benoit FL. Chronic meningococcemia: Case report and review of literature. Am J Med 35:103–112, 1963.
12. Edwards MS, Baker CJ. Complications and sequelae of meningococcal infections in children. J Pediatr 99:540–545, 1981.
13. Baraff LJ, Lee SI, Schriger DL. Outcomes of bacterial meningitis in children: A meta-analysis. Pediatr Infect Dis J 12:389–394, 1993.
14. Apicella MA. *Neisseria meningitidis.* In Mandell GL, Bennett JE, Dolin R (eds). Principles and Practice of Infectious Diseases (4th ed). Vol. 2. New York, Churchill Livingstone Inc, 1995, pp 1896–1909.
15. Fischer M, Perkins BA. *Neisseria meningitidis* is serogroup B: Emergence of the ET-5 complex. Semin Pediatr Infect Dis 8:50–56, 1997.
16. Caugant DA, Froholm LO, Bovre K, et al. Intercontinental spread of a genetically distinctive complex of clones of *Neisseria meningitidis* causing epidemic disease. Proc Natl Acad Sci U S A 83:4927–4931, 1986.
17. Tenover FC, Arbeit RD, Goering RV, et al. Interpreting chromosomal DNA restriction patterns produced by pulsed-field gel electrophoresis: Criteria for bacterial strain typing. J Clin Microbiol 33:2233–2239, 1995.
18. Swartley JS, Marfin AA, Edupuganti S, et al. Capsule switching of *Neisseria meningitidis.* Proc Natl Acad Sci U S A 94:271–276, 1997.
19. Stephens DS, Farley MM. Pathogenic events during infection of the human nasopharynx with *Neisseria meningitidis* and *Haemophilus influenzae.* Rev Infect Dis 13:22–23, 1991.
20. Goldschneider I, Gotschlich EC, Artenstein MS. Human immunity to the meningococcus I. The role of humoral immunity. J Exp Med 129:1307–1326, 1969.
21. Goldschneider I, Gotschlich EC, Artenstein MS. Human immunity to the meningococcus. II. The development of natural immunity. J Exp Med 129:1327–1348, 1969.
22. Gold R, Goldschneider I, Lepow ML, et al. Carriage of *Neisseria meningitidis* and *Neisseria lactamica* in infants and children. J Infect Dis 137:112–121, 1978.
23. Robbins JB, Schneerson R, Glode MP, Wann W, et al. Cross-reactive antigens and immunity to disease caused by encapsulated bacteria. J Allerg Clin Immunol 56:141–151, 1975.
24. Stuart JM, Cartwright KA, Robinson PM, Noah ND. Effect of smoking on meningococcal carriage. Lancet 2:723–725, 1989.
25. Young LS, LaForce FM, Head J, et al. A simultaneous outbreak of meningococcal and influenza infections. N Engl J Med 287:5–9, 1972.
26. Moore PS, Hierholzer J, Dewitt W, et al. Respiratory viruses and mycoplasma as cofactors for epidemic group A meningococcal meningitis. JAMA 264:1271–1275, 1990.
27. Knight V, Kasel JA. Adenoviruses. In Knight V (ed). Viral and Mycoplasmal Infections of the Respiratory Tract. Philadelphia, Lea & Febiger, 1973, pp 65–86.
28. Cartwright KA, Jones DM, Smith AJ, et al. Influenza A and meningococcal disease. Lancet 338:554–557, 1991.
29. Hatzigeorgiou D, Makras P, Alexiou-Daniel S, et al. Outbreak of meningococcal disease following an influenzae B epidemic [abstract K128]. 37th Interscience Conference on Antimicrobial Agents and Chemotherapy; Toronto; September 28–October 1, 1997; p 351.
30. Fischer M, Hedberg K, Cardosi P, et al. Epidemic meningococcal disease and tobacco smoke. Pediatr Infect Dis J 16:979–983, 1997.
31. Gauld JR, Nitz RE, Hurler DH, et al. Epidemiology of meningococcal meningitis at Fort Ord. Am J Epidemiol 82:56–72, 1965.
32. Ross SC, Densen P. Complement deficiency states and infection: Epidemiology, pathogenesis and consequences of neisserial and other infections in an immune deficiency. Medicine 63:243–273, 1984.
33. Fijen CA, Kuijper EJ, Hannema AJ, et al. Complement deficiencies in patients over ten years old with meningococcal disease due to uncommon serogroups. Lancet 2:585–588, 1989.
34. Schlesinger M, Greenberg R, Levy J, et al. Killing of meningococci by neutrophils: Effect of vaccination on patients with complement deficiency. J Infect Dis 170:449–453, 1994.
35. Francke EL, Neu HC. Postsplenectomy infection. Surg Clin North Am 61:135–155, 1981.
36. Stephens DS, Hajjeh RA, Baughman WS, et al. Sporadic meningococcal disease in adults: Results of a 5-year, population-based study. Ann Int Med 123:937–940, 1995.
37. Pinner RW, Onyango F, Perkins BA, et al. Epidemic meningococcal disease in Nairobi, Kenya, 1989. The Kenya Centers for Disease Control (CDC) Meningitis Study Group. J Infect Dis 166:359–364, 1992.
38. Ni H, Knight AI, Cartwright K, et al. Polymerase chain reaction for diagnosis of meningococcal meningitis. Lancet 340:1432–1434, 1992.
39. Riedo FX, Plikaytis BD, Broome CV. Epidemiology and prevention of meningococcal disease. Pediatr Infect Dis J 14:643–657, 1995.
40. Woods CR, Smith AL, Wasilauskas BL, et al. Invasive disease caused by *Neisseria meningitidis* relatively resistant to penicillin in North Carolina. J Infect Dis 170:453–456, 1994.
41. Berron S, Vasquez JA. Increase in moderate penicillin resistance and serogroup C in meningococcal strains isolated in Spain. Is there any relationship? Clin Infect Dis 18:161–165, 1994.
42. Jackson LA, Tenover FC, Baker C, et al. Prevalence of *Neisseria meningitidis* relatively resistant to penicillin in the United States, 1991. Meningococcal Disease Study Group. J Infect Dis 169:438–441, 1994.
43. Grubbauer HM, Dornbusch HF, Dittrich P, et al. Ceftriaxone monotherapy for bacterial meningitis in children. Chemotherapy 36:441–447, 1990.
44. Girardin E, Grau GE, Dayer JM, et al. Tumor necrosis factor and interleukin-1 in the serum of children with severe infectious purpura. N Engl J Med 319:397–400, 1988.
45. Drapkin MS, Wisch JS, Gelfaud JA, et al. Plasmapheresis for fulminant meningococcemia. Pediatr Infect Dis J 8:399–400, 1989.
46. The Meningococcal Disease Surveillance Group. Analysis of endemic meningococal disease by serogroup and evaluation of chemoprophylaxis. J Infect Dis 134:201–204, 1976.
47. Jackson LA, Schuchat A, Reeves MW, Wenger JD. Serogroup C meningococcal outbreaks in the United States. An emerging threat. JAMA 273:383–389, 1995.
48. Peltola H, Kataja JM, Makela PH. Shift in age-distribution of meningococcal disease as predictor of an epidemic? Lancet 2:595–597, 1982.
49. Jackson LA, Wenger JD. Laboratory-based surveillance for meningococcal disease in selected areas, United States, 1989–1991. MMWR CDC Surveill Summ 42(SS-2):21–30, 1993.
50. Jones DM, Abbott JD. Meningococcal disease in England and Wales. In Vedros NA (ed). Evaluation of Meningococcal Disease in England and Wales (1st ed). Vol 1. Boca Raton, FL, CRC Press, 1987, pp 65–90.
51. Peltola H. Meningococcal disease: An old enemy in Scandinavia. In Vedros NA (ed). Evolution of Meningococcal Disease (1st ed). Vol 1. Boca Raton, FL, CRC Press, 1987, pp 91–92.
52. Tikhomirov E. Meningococcal meningitis: Global situation and control measures. World Health Stat Q 40:98–109, 1987.
53. Greenwood BM, Bradley AK, Smith AW, Wall RA. Mortality from meningococcal disease during an epidemic in the Gambia, West Africa. Trans R Soc Trop Med Hyg 81:536–538, 1987.

54. Stuart JM, Cartwright KAV, Dawson JA, et al. Risk factors for meningococcal disease: A case control study in Southwest England. Commun Med 10:139–146, 1988.
55. Greenwood BM, Blakebrough IS, Bradley AK, et al. Meningococcal disease and season in sub-Saharan Africa. Lancet 1:1339–1342, 1984.
56. Guibourdenche M, Hoiby EA, Riou JY, et al. Epidemics of serogroup A *Neisseria meningitidis* of subgroup III in Africa, 1989–1994. Epidemiol Infect 116:115–120, 1996.
57. Cerebrospinal meningitis in Africa. Weekly Epidemiological Record No. 42. Geneva, World Health Organization, October 1996, pp 318–319.
58. Jones DJ. Epidemiology of meningococcal disease in Europe and the USA. In Cartwright K (ed). Meningococcal Disease. Chichester, England, John Wiley & Sons, 1995, pp 147–157.
59. Ashton EA, Ryan JA, Borczyk A, et al. Emergence of a virulent clone of *Neisseria meningitidis* serotype 2a that is associated with meningococcal group C disease in Canada. J Clin Microbiol 29:2489–2493, 1991.
60. Marin M, Diaz S, Rodriguiz-Creixems E, et al. Emergence of severe infections caused by serogroup C *Neisseria meningitidis* [abstract K131]. 37th Interscience Conference on Antimicrobial Agents and Chemotherapy; Toronto; September 28–October 1, 1997; p 351.
61. LeBlanc JC, Marrie TJ, Ashfield R, et al. Meningococcal disease in maritime Canada [abstract K133]. 37th Interscience Conference on Antimicrobial Agents and Chemotherapy; September 28–October 1, 1997; p 351.
62. Poolman JT, Lind I, Jonsdottir K, et al. Meningococcal serotypes and serogroup B disease in northwest Europe. Lancet 2:555–558, 1986.
63. Cruz C, Pavez G, Aquilar E, et al. Serotype-specific outbreak of group B meningococcal disease in Iquique, Chile. Epidemiol Infect 105:119–126, 1990.
64. Sacchi CT, Pessoa LL, Ramos SR, et al. Ongoing group B *Neisseria meningitidis* epidemic in São Paulo, Brazil, due to increased prevalence of a single clone of the ET-5 complex. J Clin Microbiol 30:1734–1738, 1992.
65. Serogroup B meningococcal disease—Oregon, 1994. MMWR Morb Mortal Wkly Rep 44:121–124, 1995.
66. Tappero JW, Reporter R, Wenger JD, et al. Meningococcal disease in Los Angeles County, California, and among men in the county jails. N Engl J Med 335:833–840, 1996.
67. Serogroup Y Meningococcal Disease—Illinois, Connecticut, and selected areas, United States, 1989–1996. MMWR Morb Mortal Wkly Rep 45:1010–1013, 1996.
68. Danila RN, Rainbow J, Lexau CA, et al. Statewide increase in meningococcal disease due to serogroup Y. Epidemiologic and laboratory investigations [abstract K129]. 37th Interscience Conference on Antimicrobial Agents and Chemotherapy; Toronto; September 28–October 1, 1997; p 351.
69. Carlone GM, Wenger JD, Perkins BA, et al. *Haemophilus influenzae* type b, *Neisseria meningitidis*, *Streptococcus pneumoniae*, and *Corynebacterium diphtheriae* vaccines. In Rose NR, deMacario EC, Folds JD, et al. (eds). Manual of Clinical Laboratory Immunology (5th ed). Washington, DC, ASM Press, 1997, pp 460–462.
70. Gold R, Lepow ML. Present status of polysaccharide vaccines in the prevention of meningococcal disease. Adv Pediatr 23:71–87, 1976.
71. Griffiss JM, Brandt BL, Broud DD, et al. Immune response of infants and children to disseminated infections with *Neisseria meningitidis*. J Infect Dis 150:71–79, 1984.
72. Scherp HW, Rake G. Studies on meningococcal infection. XIII. Correlation between antipolysaccharide and the antibody which protects mice against infection with type I meningococci. J Exp Med 8:85–92, 1945.
73. Kabot EA, Kaiser H, Sikarski H. Preparation of the type specific polysaccharide of the type I meningococcus and a study of its effectiveness as an antigen in human beings. J Exp Med 80:229–307, 1944.
74. Miller JW, Siess EE, Feldman HA, et al. In vivo and in vitro resistance to sulfadiazine in strains of *Neisseria meningitidis*. JAMA 186:139–141, 1963.
75. Gotschlich EC, Liu TY, Artenstein MS. Human immunity to the meningococcus. III. Preparation and immunochemical properties of the group A, group B and group C meningococcal polysaccharides. J Exp Med 129:1349–1365, 1969.
76. Finne J, Bitter-Suermann D, Goridis C, Finne U. An IgG monoclonal antibody to group B meningococci cross-reacts with developmentally regulated polysialic acid units of glycoproteins in neural and extraneural tissues. J Immunol 138:4402–4407, 1987.
77. Gotschlich EC, Rey M, Triau R, Sparks KJ. Quantitative determination of the human immune response to immunization with meningococcal vaccines. J Clin Invest 51:89–96, 1972.
78. Gotschlich EC. A simplification of the radioactive antigen binding test by a double label technique. J Immunol 107:910–911, 1971.
79. Ruben FA, Hankins WA, Ziegler Z, et al. Antibody responses to meningococcal polysaccharide vaccine in adults without a spleen. Am J Med 76:115–121, 1984.
80. Gotschlich EC, Goldschneider I, Artenstein MS. Human immunity to the meningococcus. IV. Immunogenicity of group A and group C meningococcus in human volunteers. J Exp Med 129:1367–1384, 1969.
81. Goldschneider I, Lepow ML, Gotschlich EC. Immunogenicity of the group A and group C meningococcal polysaccharides in children. J Infect Dis 125:509–519, 1971.
82. Gold R, Lepow ML, Goldschneider I, et al. Immune response of human infants to polysaccharide vaccines of group A and C *Neisseria meningitidis*. J Infect Dis 136:531–535, 1977.
83. Gold R, Lepow ML, Goldschneider I, et al. Clinical evaluation of group A and group C meningococcal polysaccharide vaccines in infants. J Clin Invest 56:1536–1547, 1975.
84. Artenstein MS. Meningococcal infections. 4. Stability of the group A and group C polysaccharide vaccines. Bull World Health Organ 45:287–290, 1971.
85. Brandt BL, Artenstein MS. Duration of antibody responses after vaccination with group C *Neisseria meningitidis* polysaccharide. J Infect Dis 131:569–575, 1975.
86. Artenstein MS, Brandt BL. Immunologic hyporesponsiveness in man to group C meningococcal polysaccharide. J Immunol 115:5–7, 1975.
87. Lepow ML, Goldschneider I, Gold R, et al. Persistence of antibody following immunization of children with groups A and C meningococcal polysaccharide vaccines. Pediatrics 60:673–680, 1977.
88. MacDonald N, Halperin S, Law B, et al. Immunization of toddlers with Chiron-R conjugated meningococcal C (Men.C) vaccine induces immunologic memory while plain Men. polysaccharide (PS) vaccine induces tolerance [abstract G3]. 37th Interscience Conference on Antimicrobial Agents and Chemotherapy; Toronto; September 28–October 1, 1997; p 192.
89. Granoff DM, Gupta RK, Belshe RB, et al. Induction of immunologic tolerance in adults by meningococcal C (men C) polysaccharide (PS) vaccination [abstract 417]. 35th Annual Meeting of the Infectious Disease Society of America; San Francisco, CA; September 13–16, 1997; p 149.
90. Sanborn WR, Bencic Z, Cvjetanovic B, et al. Trial of a serogroup A meningococcus polysaccharide vaccine in Nigeria. Prog Immunobiol Stand 5:497–505, 1972.
91. Peltola H, Makela PH, Kayhty H, et al. Clinical efficacy of meningococcus group A capsular polysaccharide vaccine in children three months to five years of age. N Engl J Med 297:686–691, 1977.
92. Gold R, Lepow ML, Goldschneider I, et al. Antibody responses of human infants to three doses of group A *Neisseria meningitidis* meningococcal polysaccharide vaccine administered at 2, 4, and 6 months of age. J Infect Dis 138:731–735, 1978.
93. Gold R, Lepow ML. Present status of polysaccharide vaccines in the prevention of meningococcal disease. Adv Pediatr 23:71–93, 1976.
94. Leach A, Twumasi PA, Kumah S, et al. Induction of immunologic memory in Gambian children by vaccination in infancy with a group A plus group C meningococcal polysaccharide-protein conjugate vaccine. J Infect Dis 175:200–204, 1997.
95. Kayhty H, Karanko V, Peltola H, et al. Serum antibodies to capsular polysaccharide vaccine of group A *Neisseria meningitidis* followed for 3 years in infants and children. J Infect Dis 142:861–868, 1980.
96. Gold R, Artenstein MS. Meningococcal infections. 2. Field trial

of group C meningococcal polysaccharide vaccine in 1969–70. Bull World Health Organ 45:279–282, 1971.
97. Artenstein MS, Gold R, Winter PE, Smith CD. Immunoprophylaxis of meningococcal infection. Mil Med 139:91–95, 1974.
98. Taunaey A de E, Galvao PA, deMorais JS, et al. Disease prevention by meningococcal serogroup C polysaccharide vaccine in preschool children [abstract]. Pediatr Res 8:429, 1974.
99. Taunay AE, Feldman RA, Bastos C, et al. Avaliacae do efeito protector de vacina polissacaridica antimeningococica do groupo C, em criancas DE6 A36 meses. Rev Inst Adolfo Lutz 38:77–82, 1978.
100. Amata NV, Finger E, Gotschlich EC, et al. Serologic response to serogroup C meningococcal polysaccharide in Brazilian preschool children. Rev Inst Med Trop Sao Paulo 16:149–153, 1974.
101. McCormick JB, Gusmao HH, Nakamura S, et al. Antibody response to serogroup A and C meningococcal vaccines in infants born to mothers vaccinated during pregnancy. J Clin Invest 65:1141–1144, 1980.
102. Masterton RG, Youngs ER, Wardle JC, et al. Control of an outbreak of group C meningococcal meningitis with a polysaccharide vaccine. J Infect Dis 17:177–182, 1988.
103. DeWals P, Dionne M, Douville-Fradet M, et al. Impact of a mass immunization campaign against serogroup C meningococcus in the province of Quebec, Canada. Bull World Health Organ 74:407–411, 1996.
104. King WJ, MacDonald NE, Wells G, et al. Total and functional antibody response to a quadrivalent meningococcal polysaccharide vaccine among children. J Pediatr 128:196–202, 1996.
105. Rosenstein N, Levine O, Taylor J, et al. Persistant serogroup C meningococcal disease outbreak in a vaccinated population, Gregg County, Texas (ABS). 36th Interscience Conference on Antimicrobial Agents and Chemotherapy; New Orleans, LA; September 15–18, 1996.
106. Wahdan MH, Rizk F, El-Akkad AM, et al. A controlled field trial of serogroup A meningococcal polysaccharide vaccine. Bull World Health Organ 48:667–673, 1973.
107. Erwa HH, Haseeb MA, Idris AA, et al. Studies in the Sudan to combat cerebrospinal meningitis caused by *Neisseria meningitidis* group A: A serogroup A meningococcal polysaccharide. Bull World Health Organ 49:301–305, 1973.
108. Makela PH, Kayhty H, Weckstrom P, et al. Effect of group-A meningococcal vaccine in army recruits in Finland. Lancet 2:883–886, 1975.
109. Wahdan MH, Sallam SA, Hassan MN, et al. A second controlled field trial of a serogroup A meningococcal polysaccharide vaccine in Alexandria. Bull World Health Organ 55:645–651, 1977.
110. Reingold AL, Broome CV, Hightower AW, et al. Age-specific differences in duration of clinical protection after vaccination with meningococcal polysaccharide A vaccine. Lancet 2:114–118, 1985.
111. Lennon D, Gellin B, Hood D, Voss L. Successful intervention in a group A meningococcal outbreak in Auckland, New Zealand. Pediatr Infect Dis J 11:617–623, 1992.
112. Greenwood AM, Greenwood BM, Bradley AK, et al. Enhancement of the immune response to meningococcal polysaccharide vaccine in a malaria endemic area by administration of chloroquine. Ann Trop Med Parasitol 75:261–263, 1981.
113. Moore PS, Plikaytis BD, Bolan GA, et al. Detection of meningitis epidemics in Africa: A population-based analysis. Int J Epidemiol 21:155–162, 1992.
114. Robbins JB, Towne DW, Gotschlich EC, Schneerson R. "Love's labours lost" failure to implement mass vaccination against group A meningococcal meningitis in sub-Sahara Africa. Lancet 350:880–882, 1997.
115. Miller MA, Wenger J, Rosenstien N, et al. Evaluation of meningococcal meningitis control strategies for the meningitis belt in Africa [abstract K127]. 37th Interscience Conference on Antimicrobial Agents and Chemotherapy; Toronto; September 28–October 1, 1997; p 350.
116. Gotschlich EC, Goldschneider I, Artenstein MS. Human immunity to the meningococcus V. The effect of immunization with meningococcal group C polysaccharide on the carrier state. J Exp Med 129:1385–1395, 1969.
117. Hassan King MK, Wall RA, Greenwood BM. Meningococcal carriage, meningococcal disease and vaccination. J Infect Dis 16:55–59, 1988.
118. Armand J, Arminjon F, Mynard MC, Lafaix C. Tetravalent meningococcal polysaccharide vaccine groups A, C, Y, W-135: Clinical and serological evaluation. J Biol Stand 10:335–339, 1982.
119. Jackson LA, Schuchat A, Gorsky RD, Wenger JD. Should college students be vaccinated against meningococcal disease? A cost-benefit analysis. Am J Public Health 85:843–845, 1995.
120. McCormick JB, Gusmao HH, Nakamura S, et al. Antibody response to serogroup A and C meningococcal polysaccharide vaccines in infants born of mothers vaccinated during pregnancy. J Clin Invest 65:1141–1144, 1980.
121. Finne J, Leinonen M, Makela PH. Antigenic similarities between brain components and bacteria causing meningitis. Implications for vaccine development. Lancet 2:355–357, 1983.
122. deMoraes JC, Perkins BA, Camargo MC, et al. Protective efficacy of a serogroup B meningococcal vaccine in Sao Paulo, Brazil. Lancet 340:1074–1078, 1992.
123. Bjune G, Hoiby EA, Gronnesby JK, et al. Effect of outer membrane vesicle vaccine against group B meningococcal disease in Norway. Lancet 338:1093–1096, 1991.
124. Lieberman JM, Chiu SS, Wong VK, et al. Safety and immunogenicity of a serogroups A/C *Neisseria meningitidis* oligosaccharide-protein conjugate vaccine in young children. A randomized controlled study. JAMA 275:1499–1503, 1996.
125. Twumasi PA Jr, Kumah S, Leach A, et al. A trial of group A plus group C meningococcal polysaccharide-protein conjugate vaccine in African infants. J Infect Dis 171:632–638, 1995.
126. Jennings HJ, Lugowski C. Immunochemistry of groups A, B, and C meningococcal polysaccharide-tetanus toxoid conjugates. J Immunol 127:1011–1018, 1981.
127. Constantino P, Viti S, Podda A, et al. Development and phase I clinical testing of a conjugate vaccine against meningococcus of A and C. Vaccine 10:691–698, 1992.
128. Rennels MB, Edwards KM, Keyserling HI, et al. Immunogenicity and safety of conjugate meningococcal vaccine in infants [abstract 1083]. Ped Res 39:183A, 1996.
129. Rennels M, Edwards K, Keyserling H, et al. Immunogenicity and safety of a 4th dose of meningococcal group C oligosaccharide conjugated to CRM 197 (Wyeth-Lederle) vaccine [abstract 601]. 35th Annual Meeting of the Infectious Diseases Society of America; September 12–15, 1997; p 183.
130. Fairley CK, Begg N, Borrow R, et al. Conjugate meningococcal serogroup A and C vaccine: Reactogenicity and immunogenicity in United Kingdom infants. J Infect Dis 174:1360–1363, 1996.
131. Campagne G, Garba A, Fabre P, et al. Safety and immunogenicity of 3 doses of *N. meningitidis* A/C diphtheria conjugate vaccine in infants in Niger [abstract GI]. 37th Interscience Conference on Antimicrobial Agents and Chemotherapy; Toronto; September 28–October 1, 1997; p 192.
132. Richmond P, Goldblatt D, Fusco P. Phase I evaluation of a meningococcal C-tetanus toxoid conjugate vaccine [abstract G111]. 37th Interscience Conference on Antimicrobial Agents and Chemotherapy; Toronto; September 28–October 1, 1997; p 212.
133. Moreno C, Lifely MR, Esdaile J. Effect of aluminum ions on chemical and immunological properties of meningococcal group B polysaccharide. Infect Immun 49:587–592, 1985.
134. Frasch CE, Zahradnik JM, Wang LY, et al. Antibody response of adults to an aluminum hydroxide adsorbed *Neisseria meningitidis* serotype 2b protein group B polysaccharide vaccine. J Infect Dis 158:700–708, 1988.
135. Jennings J, Roy R, Gamian A. Induction of meningococcal group B polysaccharide-specific IgG antibodies in mice using an *N*-propronylated B polysaccharide tetanus toxoid conjugate vaccine. J Immunol 137:1708, 1986.
136. Poolman JT. Development of a meningococcal vaccine. Infect Agents Dis 4:13–28, 1995.
137. van der Ley P, Biezen J, Poolman JT. Construction of *Neisseria meningitidis* strains carrying multiple chromosomal copies of the PorA gene for use in the production of a multivalent outer membrane vesicle vaccine. Vaccine 13:401–407, 1995.
138. Peeters CC, Rumke HC, Sundermann LC, et al. Phase 1 clinical trial with a hexavalent PorA containing meningococcal outer membrane vesicle vaccine. Vaccine 13:1009–1015, 1996.
139. Tappero JW, Lago R, Maldonado A, et al: Serum bactericidal

activity and reactogenicity elicited by two outer membrane protein–based serogroup B meningococcal vaccines among infants, children, and adults in Santiago, Chile. Submitted for publication.

140. Moore S, Farley EK, Hebblewaite DL, et al. Specificity of the immune response to the modified meningococcal B polysaccharide/PorB conjugate vaccine [abstract G2]. 37th Interscience Conference on Antimicrobial Agents and Chemotherapy; Baltimore; September 28–October 1, 1997; p 192.
141. Ala'Aldeen DA. Transferrin receptors of *Neisseria meningitidis*: Promising candidates for a broadly cross-protective vaccine. J Med Microbiol 44:237–243, 1996.
142. Parge HE, Forest KT, Hickey MJ, et al. Structure of the fibre-forming protein pilin at 2.6 Å resolution. Nature 378:32–38, 1995.
143. Maneberg B, Hoiby EA, Wedege E, et al. Nasal immunization with a meningococcal OMV vaccine can induce long-lasting serum antibodies with strong bactericidal activity [abstract G112]. 37th Interscience Conference on Antimicrobial Agents and Chemotherapy; Baltimore; September 28–October 1, 1997; p 213.

chapter

29 Miscellaneous Limited-Use Vaccines

George R. French
Stanley A. Plotkin

Military troops may be exposed to a variety of infectious agents in assignments throughout the world. Because there is limited commercial interest in vaccines against many of these agents, the U.S. Army has developed a number of vaccines intended primarily for the protection of defense personnel from biological warfare and other infectious disease threats potentially facing the U.S. military.

The vaccines presented in Table 29–1 are all Investigational New Drug products developed in U.S. Army medical research laboratories—first at the U.S. Army Medical Unit (a subordinate unit of the Walter Reed Army Institute of Research) at Fort Detrick in Frederick, Maryland, and later the U.S. Army Medical Research Institute of Infectious Diseases at Fort Detrick (better known as USAMRIID), and a subordinate unit of the U.S. Army Medical Research and Development Command. All vaccines discussed here underwent further development, primarily scale-up or stabilization studies at the Salk Institute, Government Services Division (TSI-GSD) (formerly National Drug Laboratories), at Swiftwater, Pennsylvania. Human experience with these products is extensive in some cases and moderate in others. For example, Junin vaccine has been administered to tens of thousands of individuals, successfully fulfilling phase 3 clinical trial requirements, whereas Venezuelan equine encephalitis (VEE) TC-83 vaccine, eastern equine encephalitis (EEE) vaccine, western equine encephalitis (WEE) vaccine, Tularemia LVS vaccine, and one of the two Q fever vaccines have been administered to a thousand or more recipients. The Rift Valley fever Entebbe vaccine has been tested in several hundred people, and the remainder have been administered to fewer than 100 people. To date, the primary use of these vaccines has been for the protection of laboratory personnel in development laboratories. Vaccines have been used in male and female personnel with appropriate precautions to prevent administration to immunocompromised individuals or women who are pregnant.

In the case of live attenuated vaccines, the approach has been to assume they are teratogenic. Efficacy data are lacking or can only be inferred for the majority of these vaccines. This is a result of the absence of a suitable field setting of predictable disease occurrence to test the product. A summary of efficacy testing and an assessment of known safety profiles is shown in Table 29–2.

The military has, in the past, made some of these vaccines available to civilian laboratories and vaccine producers for immunization of at-risk personnel. Distribution is subject to the statutory limitations and requirements of the applicable Code of Federal Regulations and may be subject to reimbursement of the government's cost to produce and monitor the use of the product or products. Inquiries should be addressed to Commander, USAMRMC, attn: MCMR-SGS, Fort Detrick, Frederick, MD 21702-5012. A brief discussion of each vaccine follows.

Table 29–1. **LIMITED-USE VACCINES, CHARACTERISTICS AND ADMINISTRATION**

NAME	TYPE	DOSAGE (mL)	ROUTE
VEE TC-83	Live attenuated	0.5	SC
VEE C-84	Inactivated	0.5	SC
EEE*	Inactivated	0.5	SC
WEE†	Inactivated	0.5	SC
RVF†	Inactivated	1.0	SC
RVF ZH-548	Live attenuated	0.5	SC
Junin	Live attenuated	0.5	SC
Q fever	Inactivated	0.5	SC
Q fever CMR	Inactivated	0.5	SC
Tularemia LVS	Live attenuated	0.06	Scarification
Vaccinia/Hantaan	Live attenuated	0.06/0.5	Scarification/IM

*EEE vaccine normally requires two doses, days 0 and 28, but this may vary depending on plaque reduction neutralization test (PRNT) antibody titer response to the first and second dose. A third dose of EEE vaccine, if required, is administered ID (0.1 mL) when a PRNT antibody titer of less than 1:40 is achieved with the first two doses.

†WEE vaccine and inactivated RVF vaccine are administered in three doses, on days 0, 7, and 28.

VEE, Venezuelan equine encephalitis virus; WEE, western equine encephalitis virus; EEE, eastern equine encephalitis virus; RVF, Rift Valley fever virus; Junin, Junin virus (etiological agent of Argentine hemorrhagic fever); Tularemia, *Francisella tularensis* infection; Q fever, *Coxiella burnetii* infection; Vaccinia/Hantaan, vaccinia virus-vectored Hantaan virus, small and medium-sized segments of RNA.

Table 29–2. **ASSESSMENT OF EFFICACY AND SAFETY OF SELECTED LIMITED-USE VACCINES**

NAME	TESTS OF EFFECTIVENESS	EFFECTIVE	REACTIONS
VEE TC-83, live	Reduction in laboratory-associated infections	Yes	+ +
VEE C-84, inactivated	Unknown	Probably	±
EEE, inactivated	Reduction in laboratory-associated infections	Probably	±
WEE, inactivated	Reduction in laboratory-associated infections	Probably	±
RVF, inactivated	Reduction in laboratory-associated infections	Yes	+
RVF ZH-548, live	In progress	To be determined	?
Junin, live	Formal phase II field trial	Yes	−
Q Fever, inactivated	Reduction in laboratory-associated infections	Probably	+ +
Q Fever CMR, inactivated	In progress	To be determined	+
Tularemia LVS, live	Reduction in laboratory-associated infections	Yes	±
Vaccinia/Hantaan, live	In progress	To be determined	?

+ +, moderate to severe, may be systemic; +, mild to moderate, primarily local erythema; ±, mild local; −, none reported.
See Table 29–1 for abbreviations.

ALPHAVIRUS VACCINES

Venezuelan Equine Encephalitis Virus Vaccines

As shown in Table 29–1, two VEE virus vaccines are in use. The live attenuated vaccine is a freeze-dried product produced in fetal guinea pig heart (FGPH) cell cultures. The seed virus was isolated from donkey brain and subsequently passaged 13 times in embryonated eggs.[1] Attenuation was achieved by successive passage in FGPH cells (78 passages), one plaque-pick passage in chick embryo fibroblasts (CEFs), and finally, four additional passages in FGPH cell cultures.[2] This total of 83 passages in tissue cultures resulted in the designation of the strain as VEE TC-83 virus.

The formalin-inactivated vaccine, known as C-84, utilized TC-83 virus vaccine production seed (TC-82) with one additional passage in CEFs as its production seed. The vaccine was prepared by one additional passage in CEF cells, inactivated with 0.1% formalin, and then freeze-dried.[3] The inactivation procedure is based on the well-known methodology of poliovirus inactivation.[4] The harvested viral fluids, containing 9 to 10 $\log_{10}$ of infectious virus, are filtered through a 0.45 μm pore size membrane filter and warmed to 37°C, and formalin is added to a final concentration of 0.1%. After 24 hours of incubation, with constant stirring at 37°C, the inactivating viral fluids are refiltered and transferred to a fresh container, and incubation is continued for an additional 48 hours at the same temperature. The inactivated virus is then moved to a 4°C refrigeration chamber and safety tested for residual live virus. Residual formaldehyde is neutralized with sodium bisulfite, and the finished vaccine is aliquoted and freeze-dried. Both VEE vaccines contain streptomycin and neomycin (50 μg/mL of each).

The two vaccines are highly effective in inducing long-term neutralizing antibody and, at least in the case of the attenuated product, effective in preventing laboratory-associated disease.[5] In this study of 624 vaccinees, 82% developed satisfactory levels of neutralizing antibody in response to the VEE vaccine. Of the 18% that did not respond, 76% responded satisfactorily to a C-84 vaccine administered booster. Before the deployment of the TC-83 vaccine, virtually all laboratory workers exposed to epizootic strains of VEE became infected and developed clinically apparent disease. The successful administration of TC-83 VEE vaccine essentially eliminates laboratory-associated disease due to epizootic strains of VEE. Use of the live attenuated TC-83 vaccine is not without risk. Experience at TSI-GSD indicates that 10 to 15% of recipients will experience mild febrile reactions. Reports from USAMRIID document the clinical reaction rate to be as high as 23%.[5] A smaller but significant percentage experience fairly serious reactions of severe headache, short-term but significant fever, and sore throats. Further, the original virus isolate from donkey brain and the production seed and vaccine substrate, FGPH cells, were never scrutinized for the presence of adventitious agents peculiar to those species. All of the TC-83 vaccine in inventory was produced before the establishment of procedures for their detection. There is no evidence indicating short- or long-term harm from these vaccines to date, although studies to detect adventitious agents have not been performed. Evidence of their presence may eventually surface.

Because of the reactogenic nature of TC-83 vaccine and the questionable suitability of the substrates for both vaccines, a next-generation product has been developed and should enter into scale-up development shortly. This vaccine will utilize at least two site-directed mutations of a full-length complementary DNA clone of the virulent virus RNA.[6] The mutations include a lethal deletion at the PE2 cleavage signal site combined with a suppressor mutation at site 253 of the E1 glycoprotein. This combination should prevent reversion to wild type; for example, a reversion at site 253 results in nonviable progeny virus because of the deletion mutation in the cleavage signal.

Western Equine Encephalitis Virus Vaccines

WEE virus vaccine is made in the same manner as VEE C-84 except the seed virus was isolated from a mosquito squash.[7,8] Laboratory experience with this vaccine is fairly extensive. It appears to be safe and effective in that recipients experience few problems other than local erythema at the site of inoculation, and most develop suitable levels of neutralizing antibody. There apparently have been no instances of laboratory-associated disease following successful immunization, but no field trial has been performed with the vaccine that could substantiate its effectiveness. The WEE virus vaccine presently in inventory contains 50 μg per mL of neomycin, but like the VEE virus vaccines and in fact all of the products to be described, the WEE virus vaccine is configured in a multiple-dose container without benefit of an additional antibacterial additive.

Eastern Equine Encephalitis Virus Vaccine

The seed for the EEE virus vaccine suffers from the same problem that clouds the use of the VEE products. Its passage history includes two passages in adult mice (not pathogen-free) and two passages in guinea pigs. In addition, there are nine passages in embryonated eggs, six of which are probably not pathogen-free. Nevertheless, the experience with multiple lots of this product has been good in that, like the experience with the VEE C-84 virus vaccine, there have been no problems attributable to the possible presence of adventitious agents. The procedure for propagation of the virus for this vaccine is unique in that it employs three successive undiluted passages of the production seed and the subsequent viral fluid harvests in CEF cells.[9] The inactivation procedure is similar to that of the other vaccines, but 0.05% formalin is used in place of 0.1% formalin. Again, there has been no formal field trial of this vaccine, but it is effective in inducing neutralizing antibody and preventing laboratory-associated disease.

Chikungunya Virus Vaccine

A live attenuated vaccine has been developed for chikungunya virus by passage and plaque selection in fetal rhesus lung (FRhL) cells.[10] It appears to be safe, but very little evaluation of this product has been completed.

RIFT VALLEY FEVER VACCINES

Both inactivated and live attenuated vaccines have been developed for the prevention of disease caused by Rift Valley fever virus. The inactivated vaccine was made with a derivative of the original Entebbe strain of virus.[11] The isolate was obtained from a mosquito pool collected in Bwamba county, Uganda, and passaged 184 times in adult mice and, finally, twice in FRhL cells to form the present production seed. The substrate for the existing vaccine is also FRhL cells, although earlier lots were produced in primary African green monkey kidney cells.[12, 13] Viral fluids are harvested 4 days after infection when the cells demonstrate total destruction. The virus pool is filtered through a prefilter and a 0.45 μm pore size membrane filter and, warmed to 37°C, and formalin is added to a final concentration of 0.05%. After 24 hours at this temperature, the inactivating vaccine is refiltered and transferred to a fresh container. Inactivation at 37°C is continued for an additional 48 hours plus 4 days at 4°C. After verification of viral inactivation, the residual formaldehyde is reduced to less than 0.01% by neutralization with sodium bisulfite. Experience with this vaccine has been good.[12] It is safe and effective in preventing laboratory-associated disease.

The live attenuated vaccine virus is derived from a human isolate obtained at Zagzig hospital in Egypt from a patient hospitalized during the first Egyptian epidemic.[14] This virus, designated ZH-548, underwent two passages in suckling mice, one passage in FRhL cells, and 12 passages in diploid fetal human lung (MRC-5) cells in the presence of 200 μg per mL of 5-fluorouracil.[15] The production seed was made by one additional passage in MRC-5 cells without the drug. The resulting mutant virus selected by this procedure is fully attenuated for laboratory and typical farm animals and stable in terms of not readily reverting to wild type. This vaccine has undergone extensive safety testing in both small and large animals, including pregnant sheep, and has proved to be innocuous to the test animals and highly immunogenic.[16] There have been no reports of transmission of vaccine virus from animal recipients to humans. Phase I trials in human volunteers are presently under way.

JUNIN VIRUS VACCINE

Junin virus, the causative agent of Argentine hemorrhagic fever, is the first arenavirus to be formulated into a vaccine that has been highly successful. The vaccine virus is derived from the XJ-44 clone of Junin virus, which, on a small scale, was used as a prototype vaccine in Argentina. The XJ-44 strain virus was subjected to a highly selective procedure to isolate progeny virus of lesser virulence. A clone was selected, passaged 18 times in FRhL cells, and identified as candidate number 1 virus.[17] The vaccine virus was propagated by an additional passage in FRhL cells, stabilized with a proprietary formula, aliquoted in multidose containers, and freeze-dried. Animal safety tests, including tests in nonhuman primates and human clinical trials, have been extensive.[18] Most of the human clinical trial tests, exclusive of the initial phase 1 safety tests, which were conducted on U.S. Army volunteers, were conducted in Argentina. Formal phase 2 field trials, to reaffirm safety and establish efficacy, were conducted in endemic areas of disease in Argentina and firmly established that the vaccine was safe and effective in reducing disease. A total of 6500 at-risk individuals participated in this double-blind study. One half received vaccine (3255 people), and the remainder (3245 people) received placebo. When the study was terminated and the code broken, it was found that 22 individuals in the placebo group had developed clinically apparent Argentine hemorrhagic fever as opposed to one case of disease in the vaccine group. The authors concluded that the vaccine was 95.5% effective in preventing clinically apparent Junin virus disease.[19] This vaccine appears to be well tolerated. There is no evidence that recipients shed virus in urine or semen. It is clearly indicated for administration to laboratory workers who inadvertently or knowingly are exposed to wild-type Junin virus and to grain harvesters naturally exposed in the endemic areas of disease prevalence.

VACCINES IN USE TO PREVENT Q FEVER DUE TO *Coxiella burnetii* INFECTION

Q fever is a highly infectious zoonotic disease caused by aerosol transmission of *Coxiella burnetii.* Three inactivated vaccines are presently in use or in experimental evaluation. All three are formulated with embryonated chicken egg–produced phase 1 organisms (not to be confused with clinical trial status, but indicating guinea pig virulence). The whole cells are extracted in some fashion in an attempt to remove the offending lipopolysaccharide components to reduce reactogenicity of the vaccine. A second-generation Australian vaccine is prepared by precipitation of the offending substances with high concentrations of NaCl, and the resulting vaccine is licensed in that country.[20] This vaccine is reported to be effective in preventing disease in abattoir workers who are exposed to high concentrations of aerosolized organisms in skins and body organs of infected domestic sheep.[21] In a 5-year retrospective cohort study at three Australian abattoirs, the authors claimed 100% protective efficacy in 2555 vaccinated employees compared with 55 cases among the 1365 unvaccinated employees. Two cases in the vaccinated group apparently involved individuals immunized during the incubation period of the disease. The U.S. Army vaccine, which has been the mainstay of their inventory for a number of years, is also extracted with NaCl, then subjected to ethanol-freon 113 extraction, and finally, purified further on a $CaHPO_4{\cdot}2H_2O$ (brushite) column.[22]

The problem with both these products is that, in spite of enormous effort to remove the toxic components, they produce moderate to severe local reactions in individuals who have experienced prior infections, and they cannot be administered without prior skin testing of the recipient to detect delayed hypersensitivity (DHS) to the product. It is understandable, from a military perspective, that the requirement for skin testing before immunization is not acceptable in a fast-moving military deployment situation. Further, it has been our experience that properly evaluating a Q fever skin test is no easy task. Almost all recipients develop a prominent flare, and without proper training to detect induration, DHS is almost always improperly assessed. The consequence of misreading the skin test as negative is a very sore arm for the recipient and a large area of red hot erythema ($\geq$110 mm in diameter is not uncommon) with induration or the development of a long-term, perhaps permanent, subcutaneous granuloma that is commonly described as the size and consistency of a walnut. An individual whose skin test was misread as positive (and therefore is not immunized) may subsequently develop disease that is complicated as a result of chronic infection.

With these considerations in mind, a third-generation vaccine was placed into development by U.S. Army and Public Health Service scientists. The goal was to develop a product sufficiently reduced in reactogenicity so it could be administered without requirement for prior skin testing or other time-consuming immunologic evaluation. The result was a product developed by J. C. Williams and associates that subjected highly purified whole cells to four cycles of extraction with a chloroform-methanol azeotrope.[23] The residue, designated *CMR* for chloroform-methanol residue, was than utilized to formulate the vaccine. This product is still in phase 1 clinical trial evaluation.[24] The results to date are disappointing and may indicate that the vaccine, formulated with sufficient antigen to induce immunity, will not eliminate the need for prior skin testing.

TULAREMIA VACCINE FOR THE PREVENTION OF DISEASE CAUSED BY *Francisella tularensis*

The tularemia vaccine that presently exists is the direct result of collaborative efforts between Soviet and U.S. medical scientists. The Soviet vaccine was received by U.S. representatives from the Gamaleia Institute in Russia during the 1956 U.S.-USSR Medical Exchange Mission. The account of this transfer, and the Soviet experience in utilizing this vaccine, has been documented by W. D. Tigertt.[25] The seed, as obtained by Eigelsbach and Downs, was a mixture of two colony types, one blue and one gray, as seen on peptone cysteine agar when viewed by obliquely transmitted light.[26] The blue variant was infectious and immunogenic for mice and guinea pigs. It was selected and passaged five times in mice and then utilized as seed for several experimental lots of vaccine. The L3 lot of vaccine was transferred to the National Drug Company laboratories, where it was used as seed for numerous lots of vaccine produced by fermentation in shaker flasks. This vaccine has been administered to more than 1000 volunteers and laboratory workers, and an analysis of the results by Burke show that the vaccine was safe and highly efficacious in preventing laboratory-associated disease, reducing the incidence of typhoidal tularemia from 5.70 cases per 1000 at-risk employee years to 0.27 cases per 1000 risk years.[27] Subsequent lots of this product, made at TSI-GSD, utilized lot 9 of the National Drug Vaccine as seed. These lots were produced in a 50-L glass fermentor and appear similar, if not identical, to the shaker flask vaccine.

ROSS RIVER VIRUS

The Ross River arbovirus, an alphavirus similar to chikungunya virus, is transmitted by mosquitoes to humans in Australia, Fiji, and neighboring islands.[28] The important symptom that accompanies infection is polyarthritis, both acute and chronic.[29] Thousands of cases have occurred in Australia, mainly in adults, and it is therefore a target of vaccine research.

Inactivated whole-virus vaccines have been prepared and shown to be protective in mice,[30] and vaccines for humans are under development.

HANTAVIRUS

First Hantavirus Vaccine

The hantaviruses are transmitted to humans by various rodents. At least 14 distinct viral strains are distributed throughout the world, some causing a pulmonary syndrome but the majority causing hemorrhagic fever with renal syndrome (HFRS).[31] The prototype hantavirus, Hantaan, was first isolated in Korea, and the first vaccine was also developed there to protect against HFRS.[32, 33]

The vaccine is prepared in mouse brain by the Korean Green Cross Corporation, using the ROK84/105 strain isolated locally. The virus is harvested from the mouse brains and concentrated by protamine sulfate precipitation and centrifugation. The concentrate is then exposed to formalin inactivation, following which it is purified by ultrafiltration and sucrose gradient ultracentrifugation. $Al(OH)_3$ is added to the vaccine as adjuvant, thiomerosal as preservative, and gelatin as stabilizer.[34]

The recommended regimen is two doses of 5120 enzyme-linked immunosorbent assay units given 1 month apart by the subcutaneous or intramuscular routes. Little has been published on the vaccine, but the manufacturer reports that tolerance is good, although allergic reactions occur, presumably due to mouse brain antigens. A serological response measurable by indirect fluorescence is seen in nearly all vaccinees. There are no controlled data on the efficacy of the vaccine.

Vaccinia Virus–Vectored Hantaan Virus Vaccine

The production seed for the live attenuated Vaccinia virus–vectored Hantaan virus vaccine is derived from the Connaught vaccinia virus strain 17633 (Connaught Laboratories Inc.) It, in turn, had been derived from the Bureau of Laboratories, Department of Public Health, City of New York strain. In 1980, the U.S. Army purchased the seed and transferred it to the USAMRIID, where it was subjected to three plaque-to-plaque picks in MRC-5 cells. Each pick was sonicated and filtered through a 0.45 μm pore size membrane filter in an attempt to preclude passage of aggregated virus. Through several steps of genetic manipulation, the thymidine kinase gene of the virus was deleted. In its place, the medium-size segment of the Hantaan virus genome, coding for the GP-1 and GP-2 proteins, and the small segment of the Hantaan virus genome, coding for the nucleocapsid protein, were inserted.[35] Vaccine prepared from this seed was propagated in MRC-5 cells and laboriously purified by either layering sonicated virus on a sucrose gradient (early lots) or by pelleting the sonicated virus through a 36% sucrose cushion. The purified vaccine virus was aliquoted to yield a target 2×10^8 plaque-forming units per mL and freeze-dried. The goal of this ambitious project was to formulate a vaccine that could be administered by a peripheral route without scarification (hence, the reason for purification). This was to avoid the potential for generalized vaccinia and to eliminate the risk of human-to-human transmission of the virus. Evaluation of this product and other vaccinia-derived vaccines is ongoing, and a conclusion as to success or failure is premature.[36]

REFERENCES

1. Kubes V, Rios FA. The causative agent of infectious equine encephalitis in Venezuela. Science 90:20–21, 1939.
2. Berge TO, Banks IS, Tigertt WD. Attenuation of Venezuelan encephalomyelitis virus by in vitro cultivation in guinea pig heart cells. Am J Hyg 73:209–218, 1961.
3. Cole FW, May SW, Eddy GA. Inactivated Venezuelan equine encephalomyelitis virus prepared from attenuated (TC-83) virus. Appl Microbiol 27:150–153, 1974.
4. Salk JE, Krech U, Youngner JS, et al. Formaldehyde treatment and safety testing of experimental poliomyelitis vaccines. Am J Public Health 44:563–570, 1954.
5. Pittman PR, Makuch RS, Mangiafico JA, et al. Long-term duration of detectable neutralizing antibodies after administration of live-attenuated VEE vaccine and following booster vaccination with inactivated VEE vaccine. Vaccine 14:337–343, 1996.
6. Davis NL, Brown KW, Greenwald GF, et al. Attenuated mutants of Venezuelan equine encephalitis virus containing lethal mutations in the PE2 cleavage signal combined with a second site suppressor mutation in E1. Virology 212:102–110, 1995.
7. Robinson DM, Berman S, Lowenthal JP, Hetrick FM. Western equine encephalitis vaccine produced in chick embryo cell cultures. Appl Microbiol 14:1011–1014, 1966.
8. Bartelloni PJ, McKinney RW, Calia FM, et al. Inactivated western equine encephalomyelitis vaccine propagated in chick embryo cell culture. Am J Trop Med Hyg 20:146–149, 1971.
9. Maire LF III, McKinney RW, Cole FE Jr. An inactivated eastern equine encephalomyelitis vaccine propagated in chick-embryo cell culture. Am J Trop Med Hyg 19:119–122, 1970.
10. Levitt NH, Ramsburg HH, Hasty SE, et al. Development of an attenuated strain of chikungunya virus for use in vaccine production. Vaccine 4:179–184, 1986.
11. Smithburn KC. Rift Valley fever; the neurotropic adaptation of the virus and the experimental use as a vaccine. Br J Exp Pathol 30:1–16, 1949.
12. Kark JD, Aynor Y, Peters CJ. A Rift Valley fever vaccine trial. I. Side effects and serologic response over a six month follow-up. Am J Epidemiol 116:808–820, 1982.
13. Randall R, Gibbs CJ Jr, Aulisio CG, et al. The development of a formalin-killed Rift Valley fever virus vaccine for use in man. J Immunol 89:660–671, 1962.
14. Meegan JM, Hoogstraal H, Moussa MI. An epizootic of Rift Valley in Egypt in 1977. Vet Rec 105:124–125, 1979.
15. Caplen H, Peters CJ, Bishop DH. Mutagen directed attenuation of Rift Valley fever vaccine. J Gen Virol 66:2271–2277, 1985.
16. Morrill JC, Carpenter L, Taylor D, et al. Further evaluation of a mutagen-attenuated Rift Valley fever vaccine in sheep. Vaccine 9:35–41, 1991.
17. Barrera Oro JG, McKee KT Jr. Toward a vaccine against Argentine hemorrhagic fever. Bull Pan Am Health Organ 25:118–126, 1991.
18. McKee KT Jr, Barrera Oro JG, Kuehne AI, et al. Safety and immunogenicity of a live attenuated Junin (Argentine hemorrhagic fever) vaccine in rhesus macaques. Am J Trop Med Hyg 48:403–411, 1993.
19. Maiztegui JI, McKee KT, Barrera Oro JG, et al., and the AHF Study Group. Protective efficacy of a live attenuated vaccine against Argentine hemorrhagic fever. J Infect Dis 177:277–283, 1998.
20. Ormsbee RA, Marmion BP. Prevention of *Coxiella burnetii* infection: Vaccines and guidelines for those at risk. In Marrie TJ (ed). Q Fever. Vol. I. The Disease. Boca Raton, FL, CRC Press, 1990, pp 225–248.
21. Ackland JR, Worswick DA, Marmion BP. Vaccine prophylaxis of Q fever. A follow-up study of the efficacy of Q-Vax (CSL) 1985–1990. Med J Aust 160:704–708, 1994.

22. Spicer DC, De Sanctis AN. Preparation of phase I Q fever antigen suitable for vaccine use. Appl Environ Microbiol 32:85, 1976.
23. Williams JC, Damrow TA, Waag DM, Amano KI. Characterization of phase I *Coxiella burnetii* chloroform-methanol residue vaccine that induces active immunity against Q fever in c57BL/10ScN mice. Infect Immun 24:935–939, 1986.
24. Fries LF, Waag DM, Williams JC. Safety and immunogenicity in human volunteers of a chloroform-methanol residue vaccine for Q fever. Infect Immun 61:1251–1258, 1993.
25. Tigertt WD. Soviet viable *Pasturella tularensis* vaccines. A review of selected articles. Bacteriol Rev 26:354–373, 1962.
26. Eigelsbach HT, Downs CT. Prophylatic effectiveness of live and killed tularemia vaccines. I. Production of vaccine and evaluation in the white mouse and guinea pig. J Immunol 87:415–425, 1961.
27. Burke DS. Immunization against tularemia: Analysis of effectiveness of live *Francisella tularensis* vaccine in prevention of laboratory-acquired tularemia. J Infect Dis 135:55–60, 1977.
28. Hawkins RA, Boughton CR, Naim HM, Stallman ND. A major outbreak of epidemic polyarthritis in New South Wales during the summer of 1983–84. Med J Aust 143:330–333, 1985.
29. Fraser J. Epidemic polyarthritis and Ross River virus disease. Clin Rheum Dis 12:369–388, 1986.
30. Yu S, Aaskov JG. Development of a candidate vaccine against Ross River virus infection. Vaccine 12:1118–1124, 1994.
31. Schmaljohn C, Hjelle B. Hantaviruses: A global disease problem. Emerg Infect Dis 3:95–104, 1997.
32. Lee HW, Lee PW, Johnson KM. Isolation of the etiologic agent of Korean hemorrhagic fever. J Infect Dis 137:298–308, 1978.
33. Lee HW, Ahn CN. Field trial of an inactivated vaccine against HFRS in humans. Arch Virol (suppl 1):35–47, 1990.
34. A major breakthrough in Preventive Medicine: Hantavax (HFRS Vaccine, KGCC). Seoul, Korea, Korea Green Cross Corporation, 1997.
35. Schmaljohn CS, Hasty SE, Dalrymple JM. Preparation of candidate vaccinia vectored vaccines for haemorrhagic fever with renal syndrome. Vaccine 10:10–13, 1992.
36. McClain DJ, Harrison S, Yeager CL, et al. Immunologic responses to vaccinia vaccines administered by different parenteral routes. J Infect Dis 175:756–763, 1997.

chapter

30 Plague

Richard W. Titball
Stephen Eley
E. Diane Williamson
David T. Dennis

During the last two millennia, the bacterium *Yersinia pestis* has been responsible for social and economic devastation on a scale unmatched by other infectious diseases or armed conflicts. The first reliable reference is to the Justinian plague (AD 542–750), which originated in central Africa and spread throughout the Mediterranean Basin. The second pandemic, the Black Death, which started on the Eurasian border in the mid-14th century, may have caused 25 million deaths in Europe (25–30% of the population), persisted on the continental land mass for several centuries, and culminated in the Great Plague of London in 1665. The third pandemic started in China in the middle of the 19th century, spread east and west, and caused 10 million deaths in India alone. Credible estimates indicate that almost 200 million deaths could be attributed to plague,[1] which swept across Europe in these three major epidemics.[2] The disease occurred in both bubonic and pneumonic ("black death") forms. The bubonic form spreads as a result of transmission of the bacterium from rodents to humans via the bites of infective fleas (usually the rat flea, *Xenopsylla cheopsis*[2]). The close contact of humans with infected rats undoubtedly contributed to the spread of the disease by this route. In some instances, subsequent spread of plague bacilli to the lungs leads to the development of the pneumonic form of the disease; person-to-person transmission by respirable droplets can result in rapid epidemic spread of the disease.[3] It is the pneumonic form of the disease that is most feared and that is associated with a mortality rate approaching 100% when untreated.[4, 5] For reasons that are not fully understood, epidemics of urban plague have dramatically waned, but data from the World Health Organization indicate that plague is still a significant public health problem, especially in Africa, Asia, and South America (Fig. 30–1).[6, 7] In plague endemic areas of the world, vaccines may be useful in preventing plague in people at high risk. Such vaccines are also of use in protecting people who handle *Y. pestis* in research and diagnostic laboratories.

BACKGROUND

Clinical Description

Bubonic Plague. Bubonic plague is the form of disease that typically occurs after a flea that has previously fed on an infected rodent then bites humans. In some circumstances, infection occurs via open wounds that are exposed to infected material.[4] Within 2 to 6 days of infection, the patient develops a fever, headache, and chills.[8] Occasionally, lesions develop at the site of inoculation. The classic feature of bubonic plague is the development of swollen and tender lymph nodes called *buboes*, from the Greek *bubon*, meaning groin. (The buboes are often located in the inguinal and femoral lymph nodes, which drain the original site of infection.[4]) Bacteremia is common in patients with bubonic plague, typically resulting in blood culture counts ranging from fewer than 10 to 4 × 10^7 colony-forming units [cfu] per mL.[4] In many of these cases, there is involvement of the gastrointestinal tract, which can cause vomiting, nausea, and diarrhea.[4] Early intervention during the course of disease with antibiotics such as tetracycline, streptomycin, gentamicin, or chloramphenicol usually leads to rapid recovery.[9]

Septicemic Plague. The demonstration of a bacteremia without evidence of buboes is generally considered to be indicative of primary septicemic plague. Clinically, the disease appears similar to other gram-negative septicemias, with elevated temperature, chills, headache, malaise, and gastrointestinal disturbances. In the absence of aggressive treatment, life-threatening complications of the systemic inflammatory response syndrome occur, such as disseminated intravascular coagulation and bleeding, adult respiratory distress syndrome, shock, and organ failure. Owing to the absence of buboes, a diagnosis of septicemic plague is often delayed, and, even with medical intervention at this stage, 50% of patients die.[8]

Pneumonic Plague. Some colonization of pulmonary tissues occurs in virtually all untreated fatal cases of plague, but most of these patients do not develop a transmissible plague pneumonia.[8] However, when there is colonization of the alveolar spaces after a respiratory exposure, a suppurative pneumonia develops, and during the terminal stages of disease there is coughing and the production of a highly infectious, watery, and bloody sputum. Pneumonic plague is the most widely feared form of the disease because *Y. pestis* can be spread from person to person as respiratory droplets formed during coughing.[10] Inhalation of these airborne droplets by susceptible individuals leads to the rapid (1–3 days) devel-

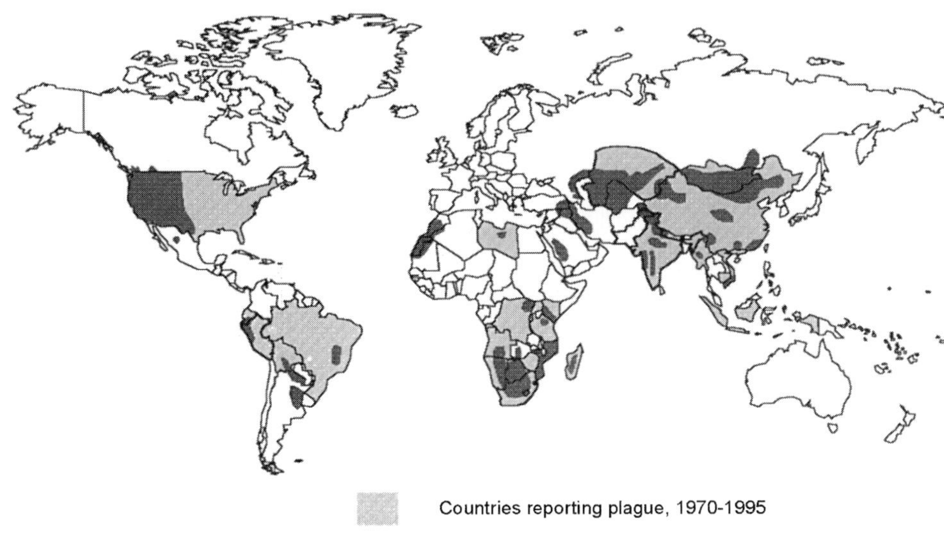

Figure 30–1. Worldwide incidence of plague, 1970 to 1995. (Data from the World Health Organization, the Centers for Disease Control and Prevention, and country sources.)

opment of pneumonic plague.[8] The rapidity with which the infection spreads between individuals, along with the relatively short incubation period, makes control of the disease difficult. Antibiotic therapy may be ineffective after pulmonary symptoms have developed.[4, 8, 9] Pneumonic plague is now rare; in the United States, most cases are acquired by veterinarians and owners of cats that are experiencing a plague pneumonia.[4, 5] Nevertheless, the potential for pneumonic plague to quickly spread in human populations is evident from the reports of the great plagues of the Middle Ages.

Bacteriology

The etiological agent of plague is *Y. pestis*, a gram-negative bacterium that is a member of the family Enterobacteriaceae. The bacterium is able to grow at temperatures between 4 and 40°C and has nutritional requirements for L-isoleucine, L-valine, L-methionine, L-phenylalanine, and glycine. The species has been subdivided into three biovars (*orientalis*, *mediaevalis* and *antigua*) on the basis of their ability to convert nitrate to nitrite and to ferment glycerol; however, all three biovars show similar virulence in animal models.[4] The genus *Yersinia* also includes *Y. enterocolitica* and *Y. pseudotuberculosis* species, both of which are pathogens of humans but rarely cause disease with a fatal outcome.[1, 9] The pathogenic differences among these three organisms have been shown to be related, in the main, to the presence or absence of plasmids that encode virulence determinants. All three species contain a 70-kilobase (kb) low calcium response (Lcr) plasmid that encodes a variety of *Yersinia* outer membrane peptides (Yops[11, 12]). The 9.5-kb pesticin plasmid and the 100-kb Tox plasmids are present only in *Y. pestis*. The *pla* gene on the pesticin plasmid encodes a surface-bound protease (plasminogen activator), which has potent fibrinolytic activity.[1] Post-translational processing of the *pla* gene product results in the formation of a coagulase enzyme. Although it is possible that many virulence determinants are encoded by the Tox plasmid, only the F1 capsular antigen has been studied in detail. The *caf* operon encodes the 17-kd polypeptide F1 antigen (Caf1[13]); the Caf1M chaperone, which allows export from the cell[14]; and the Caf1A polypeptide, which anchors the F1 antigen into the outer membrane.[15] The Caf1R regulatory protein, which is responsible for the induction of F1 capsule production at 37°C, is also encoded by the *caf* operon.[16]

Pathogenesis

Plague is a zoonosis in which *Y. pestis* is transferred most commonly from its animal reservoir (rodents) to humans via fleas (Fig. 30–2). The flea ingests blood-borne bacteria from the infected rodent, and growth of the bacteria leads to blockage of the foregut. The hemin storage system is thought to play an important role in the formation of this blockage.[17] The blockage prevents digestion of the blood meal, and further ingestion of blood leads to regurgitation of bacteria-contaminated material.[18] Movement of the flea to a new rodent host leads to infection of the rodent, and it is thought that the bacterium persists in the environment as the result of a stable rodent-flea infection cycle. However, in situations in which humans and rodents are in close proximity or when the rodent population is reduced, either as a result of the disease or rodent control measures, humans and other warm-blooded mammals serve as alternative hosts. In this respect, *Y. pestis* differs from the other human pathogenic *Yersinia* species in that it is an obligate pathogen. The organism circulates in a "sylvatic" form in wild rodent populations, typically causing a fatal disease in murines and sciurines and a milder, subclinical infection in gerbillines and dipodids.[19]

Infection of humans usually occurs as the result of a bite from an infected flea. It has been suggested that as many as 24,000 bacteria are delivered into the host with a single bite.[4] The expression of many of the virulence

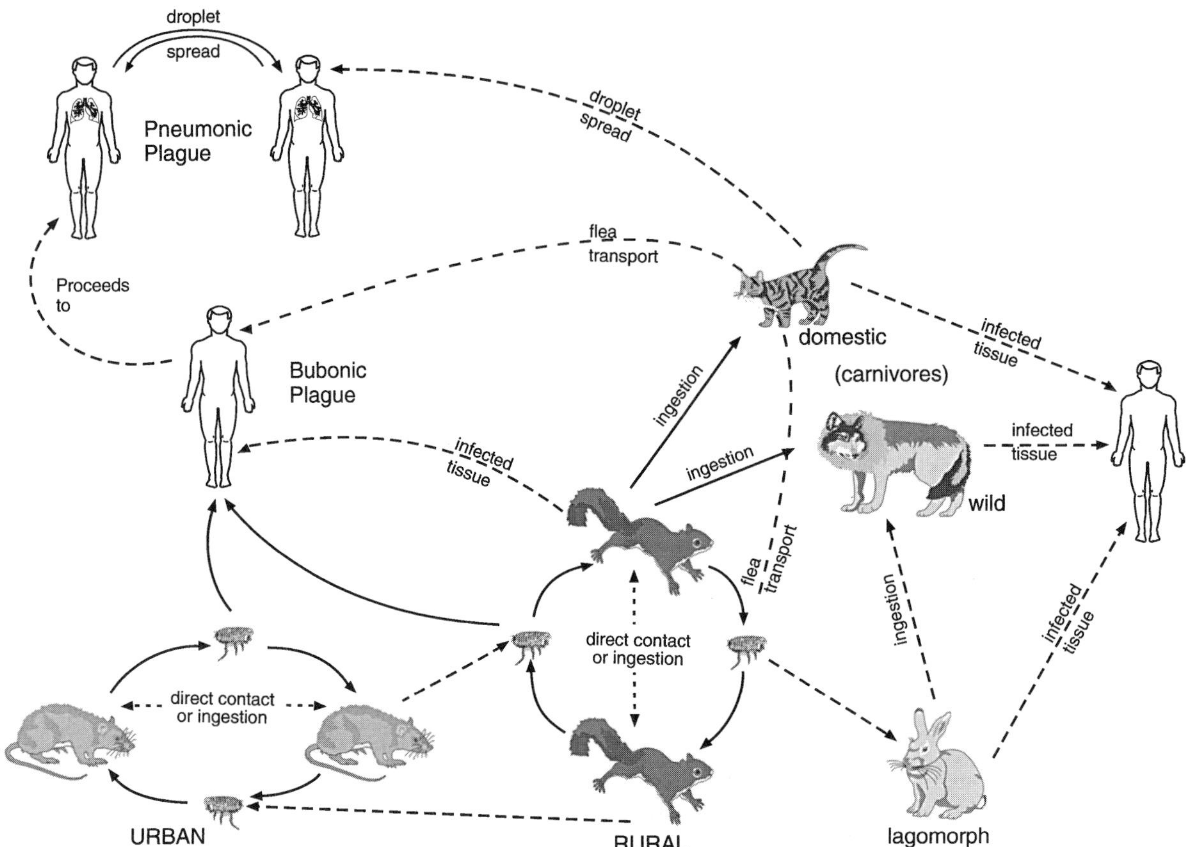

Figure 30–2. Transmission routes of plague. Solid lines indicate the usual routes of transmission, and occasional routes are shown with dashed lines. (From Perry RD, Fetherston JD. *Yersinia pestis*—etiologic agent of plague. Clin Microbiol Rev 10:35–66, 1997.)

genes in *Y. pestis* is upregulated at 37°C, and bacteria delivered by the flea, where they have been growing for several days at ambient temperatures of 28°C or less, do not express the F1 antigen or many of the Lcr plasmid products that are thought to allow the bacteria to resist phagocytosis. Therefore, many of the bacteria that are delivered into the host are easily phagocytosed by polymorphonuclear leucocytes or monocytes. The bacteria within polymorphonuclear leucocytes are destroyed, but those within monocytes survive and express various virulence determinants, thereby allowing growth and eventual release from the monocytes.[20] One such virulence determinant is the pH6 antigen, a fibrillar adhesin induced by low pH conditions such as those encountered in the phagosome, which has a pH of 4.5.[21] The expression of the pH6 antigen may facilitate entry into naive monocytes or participate in the delivery of *Yersinia*-secreted proteins to monocytes and polymorphonuclear leucocytes. Bacteria released from monocytes are resistant to phagocytosis. The F1 capsule might be expected to play a key role in avoiding further phagocytosis.[22] However, mutants of *Y. pestis* that are unable to produce F1 antigen are still able to cause disease in the mouse, albeit in a more protracted form.[23] Other Yops might also play a role in killing phagocytic cells. For example, the YopE protein is a cytotoxin that is transferred into host cells after bacterial contact[12]; the YopH protein is a tyrosine phosphatase that has antiphagocytic cell activity[12]; and the V antigen that is exported from the bacterial cell has been reported to have a profound immunomodulatory effect on cells of the host immune system, by down-regulating the production of γ-interferon and tumor necrosis factor-α.[24, 25] The expression of Yops is further regulated by the environmental calcium concentration, such that maximum expression of these proteins occurs at 37°C when the calcium concentration is below 2.5 mmol (the so-called low calcium response[1]). These are the conditions encountered within the phagosome, and intracellular V antigen is thought to play a key role in the regulation of this response.[26] Under these conditions in vitro, however, growth of the bacterium virtually ceases. Yop production certainly does occur in vivo, but, paradoxically, the bacteria are also able to grow. Either Yop expression in the mammalian host is induced by conditions yet to be identified, or growth in vivo is subject to a different regulatory system than that which occurs in vitro.

An ability to proliferate at the site of infection in host tissues indicates that the bacterium possesses efficient iron acquisition systems. The role of the surface-bound hemin storage proteins in iron acquisition is not proven, but it is known that the bacterium does have an iron scavenging system based on the yersiniabactin siderophore.[4] The bacteria become disseminated from the site of primary infection into regional lymph nodes that drain these tissues. Within the lymph node, further growth of the bacteria, accompanied by a massive inflammatory reaction, leads to lymphadenopathy and the formation of buboes. Eventually, the bacteria can be disseminated by the lymphatic system, gain access to the blood stream, and colonize pulmonary tissues, which may lead to development of the pneumonic form of the disease. Untreated pneumonic plague is almost invariably fatal, but the precise mechanisms that lead to death of the host have not been identified. The bacterium does produce a soluble exotoxin,[4, 27] but this exotoxin is reported to be active only in murines. Because an overwhelming septicemia is a feature of fatal plague infection, it seems likely that lipopolysaccharide is responsible for the systemic inflammatory response syndrome and its sequelae, such as disseminated intravascular coagulation in the terminal stages of the disease.

Models of Disease and Protection

Y. pestis causes disease in a wide variety of laboratory animals,[4, 10] and animal models of the disease in humans have been developed using mice, guinea pigs, and other primates. Most experimental work has been carried out with the mouse model of disease, which has been accepted as a meaningful indicator of the likely responses to infection and protection in humans. However, the disease in the mouse model may not faithfully mimic disease in humans because of the susceptibility of mice to the murine exotoxin.[27] Although this limitation might be resolved by using the guinea pig model of disease, the protracted nature of the disease in this species[4] suggests that this model is a better indicator of the infection that occurs in animal reservoirs. In a comparative study with mice and guinea pigs, it was concluded that mice were more suitable for the evaluation of plague vaccines,[28] and this species is approved by the U.S. Public Health Service for the testing of plague vaccines. Disease arising from the delivery of *Y. pestis* by the subcutaneous route (median lethal dose [MLD], 1–2 cfu[29, 30]) is considered to mimic bubonic plague, whereas the exposure of mice to the bacteria via aerosols inhaled through the nose results in the pneumonic form of the disease (MLD, 2×10^4 cfu[30]). The efficacy of currently licensed plague vaccines is determined by measuring the ability of sera from immunized mice, guinea pigs, monkeys, or humans to protect mice passively against *Y. pestis*. Serum is injected intravenously into groups of 10 mice (0.5 mL serum per mouse), and the mice are then challenged subcutaneously with 100 MLD of *Y. pestis*.[31, 32] The mouse protection index (MPI) is expressed as the percentage mortality of the group of mice (over 14 days) divided by the average time to death. MPI values of 10 or less are considered to be indicative of protection.[33]

EPIDEMIOLOGY

More than 200 mammalian species have been reported to be susceptible to infection with *Y. pestis*,[4] although rodents are considered to be the most important hosts for the bacterium. The observation that distinct geographical foci of infection occur indicates that the bacterium can persist for long periods in some relatively resistant (enzootic) animal hosts and their fleas (see Fig. 30–2).[34] However, the nature of the enzootic host for the bacterium has not been clearly demonstrated and may even vary from location to location. Some types of mice, voles, and gerbils all have been suggested as enzootic hosts.[4, 35] The rapid spread of disease is associated with infection of highly susceptible epizootic hosts such as rats, prairie dogs, squirrels, or mice.[8] In principle, any flea that is capable of feeding on these hosts might transfer the disease to humans,[8] but the usual vector in epidemic plague is the oriental rat flea (*Xenopsylla cheopis*).

Endemic foci of plague occur mainly in semiarid regions of the world (see Fig. 30–1). The main foci have been identified in the southwestern United States, the former Soviet Union, South America, South Africa, and Asia. Not surprisingly, these are the regions of the world that report the highest incidence of human plague. Data from the World Health Organization indicate that the average incidence of plague worldwide was 1666 cases from 1967 to 1993[7, 34]; although the trend was downward until 1981, there has been an apparent increase in the incidence of disease during the 1990s. It is possible that this increase is the result of more efficient diagnosis and reporting of cases. However, the outbreak of disease in Surat, India, during 1994, although overstated by the press, serves as a reminder that the disease can reappear explosively. Serological testing of individuals during this outbreak showed that there were 876 presumptive cases of plague and 54 fatalities.[4] In the United States, a new trend in plague epidemiology appears to be related to the residential encroachment on former rural areas that contain enzootic foci.[4] Inhabiting of such areas can lead to bites of humans by infected fleas or to infection as the result of close contact with infected wild rodents or other animals (e.g., domestic cats) that have become infected.

PASSIVE IMMUNIZATION

Early studies showed that serum from human volunteers immunized with purified F1 antigen or with a killed whole-cell vaccine could be used in the passive protection of mice against a parenteral challenge with 100 MLD of *Y. pestis*.[32] Indeed, this is the basis of the MPI test that is used to evaluate the efficacy of killed vaccines. More recently, there have been several reports that the passive immunization of mice with antiserum against the V antigen provides protection against parenteral challenge with *Y. pestis*.[36–38] However, there is no antiserum that can be used in humans to prevent or treat plague.

ACTIVE IMMUNIZATION

Killed Whole-Cell Vaccines

Killed *Y. pestis* organisms have been used as a vaccine since 1897, when Waldemar Haffkine inoculated himself with an experimental vaccine. The first killed vaccine for human use was the Army Vaccine, which was produced in the United States in 1946. Improvements to this vaccine have led to the plague vaccine, which is produced from the virulent 195/P strain of *Y. pestis*.[39] During the 1990s, there have been several commercial suppliers of killed whole-cell vaccines against plague. Plague vaccine, which contains formaldehyde-killed bacteria, was formerly manufactured by Cutter Laboratories but since 1994 has been manufactured by Greer Laboratories Inc. (P.O. Box 800, Lenoir, North Carolina, 28645-0800).[5] The killed bacteria (strain 195/P) are resuspended in 0.9% saline to a concentration of 1.8×10^9 to 2.2×10^9 cells per mL. The vaccine also contains traces of growth media components and 0.5% weight per volume of phenol as a preservative. The Greer vaccine is given intramuscularly (preferably into the deltoid muscle) as an initial dose of 1.0 mL and is followed 1 to 3 months later with a 0.2-mL dose of vaccine and a third dose of 0.2 mL after 6 months. Booster doses (0.2 mL) may be needed at 6-month intervals[5] (Table 30–1).

An alternative killed vaccine is manufactured by the Commonwealth Serum Laboratories (CSL Ltd., 45 Poplar Road, Parkville, 3052, Australia). This vaccine contains heat-killed bacteria (*Y. pestis* strain 195/P) that are resuspended in saline containing 0.5% weight per volume of phenol to a concentration of 3×10^9 organisms per mL. The vaccine is given subcutaneously, and the initial course in adults is two 0.5-mL doses of vaccine at an interval of 1 to 4 weeks (see Table 30–1). The vaccine can be administered to children using modified immunization schedules. For example, children 6 months to 2 years of age are given three 0.1-mL doses of vaccine at intervals of 1 to 4 weeks (see Table 30–1).

Live Attenuated Vaccines

Vaccination of humans has also been achieved using a live attenuated vaccine strain of *Y. pestis* (strain EV76). This vaccine strain, which was derived from a fully virulent strain by in vitro passage,[40] has been used since 1908, especially in the former Soviet Union and the French colonies. At present, however, the vaccine is not commercially available. The genetic lesion that results in attenuation has not been defined, but the strain is known to be a pigmentation (*pgm*) mutant. This mutation prevents the bacterium from assimilating hemin[4] and may also result in a change in surface properties of the bacterium.[17] The recommended dosing regime for EV76 is to use 5.8×10^6 cfu as a priming dose and to boost with the killed whole-cell vaccine.[40, 41]

Indications for Vaccine Use

The killed whole-cell vaccine is recommended for use in individuals who are working with fully virulent strains of *Y. pestis* (e.g., researchers and laboratory workers). The vaccine is also indicated for use in personnel who are deployed to work in areas where the disease is endemic (e.g., military personnal, field workers, and agricultural consultants), especially if they may be exposed to epizootic plague.[5] The vaccines currently available are not suitable for postexposure use, as several months are required to complete the primary vaccination schedule. In the case of possible exposure to *Y. pestis*, prophylactic use of antibiotics should be considered, even in vaccinees who have completed the full vaccination schedule. Vaccination against plague is not a statutory requirement for travel to any country. The vaccination of populations in plague endemic areas of the world is not routinely indicated, because the incidence of disease is relatively low and most cases of disease are of the bubonic form, which can be treated with antibiotics. Use of the vaccine in the indigenous population might be considered in areas where there is recurrent or intense plague activity that cannot be controlled by other measures. This situation might arise after natural disasters, especially when there is disruption to sanitation systems. Because several months are required to complete the course of vaccination, however, the vaccine has a limited use in controlling sporadic plague epidemics. Use of the vaccine might be indicated in individuals who regularly come into contact with animals where enzootic plague foci are known to be present.[5]

Precautions and Contraindications

The Greer vaccine should not be used in individuals who have a history of hypersensitivity to any of the

Table 30–1. **SCHEDULES AND DOSAGES OF GREER AND COMMONWEALTH SERUM LABORATORIES KILLED WHOLE-CELL VACCINES**

		VOLUME ADMINISTERED			
VACCINE	AGE OF RECIPIENT	First Dose	Second Dose	Third Dose	Booster Dose
Greer	>18 yr	1.0 mL	0.2 mL*	0.2 mL†	0.2 mL‡
Commonwealth Serum Laboratories	6 mo–2 yr	0.1 mL	0.1 mL§	0.1 mL§	0.1 mL‖
	3–6 yr	0.2 mL	0.2 mL§	0.2 mL§	0.2 mL‖
	7–11 yr	0.3 mL	0.3 mL§	0.3 mL§	0.3 mL‖
	>12 yr	0.5 mL	0.5 mL§	—	0.5 mL¶

*One to 3 months after start.
†Six months after start.
‡At 6-month intervals after dose 3, can be extended to 1- to 2-year intervals in the case of individuals who have received three or more booster doses at 6-month intervals.
§One to 4 weeks after previous dose.
‖At 6-month intervals after dose 3.
¶At 6-month intervals after dose 2, dose can be reduced to 0.1 mL intradermally for individuals who have reactions to previous doses of the vaccine.

vaccine components (e.g., beef protein, soy, casein, sulphite, phenol, or formaldehyde). The safety and efficacy of the vaccine in people younger than 18 years or in pregnant women are not known.

RESULTS OF VACCINATION

Immune Responses

Although *Y. pestis* produces a variety of potentially protective antigens (including F1 antigen, V antigen and other Yops, and lipopolysaccharide), most workers consider that antibody against the F1 antigen is the key protective response induced by killed whole-cell vaccines. Although the V antigen is known to also induce a protective response against *Y. pestis*, the level of V antigen is low or undetectable in killed whole-cell vaccines.[42] There is good experimental evidence that the titer of F1 antibody, determined by passive hemagglutination, does correlate with protection against plague in animal models.[41] Ninety percent of animals with anti-F1 passive hemagglutination titers of 128 survived challenge with 1×10^3 to 5×10^5 cfu of *Y. pestis*, whereas the proportions of animals with titers of 32 to 64 or 16 that survived were 46 and 6%, respectively. Passive immunization studies with sera obtained from immunized animals[33] or humans[43] also suggest that anti-F1 passive hemagglutination titers of 1:128 or greater were protective. However, the accepted test for demonstrating the efficacy of vaccines involves passive immunization of mice with sera and the demonstration of an MPI of 10 or less. More recent trials with the Greer Laboratories vaccine suggest that 55 to 58% of individuals develop an antibody response with an MPI of 10 after two vaccinations[5]; however, even after multiple (an average of 5) vaccinations, 8% of individuals fail to develop any antibody response.

Protective Efficacy

None of the plague vaccines available have been subjected to a randomized, clinically controlled study in humans. Although controlled clinical studies are desirable, the sporadic and relatively low incidence of plague means that such studies would be difficult to conduct. Evidence for the efficacy of killed whole-cell vaccines is based mainly on studies in animals, on evidence that they induce antibody in humans that can passively protect animals, and on data obtained from Vietnam. From 1961 to 1971, many thousands of Vietnamese civilians developed plague (333 cases/10^6 person-years of exposure), but the incidence of disease in immunized U.S. troops based in Vietnam during this period was low. (The total of 8 cases represents 1 case per 10^6 person-years of exposure.[5, 44]) Although this difference in the incidence of disease might be attributed to different exposures of these populations to *Y. pestis*, it is worth noting that many military personnel developed murine typhus, which is also transmitted by *X. cheopis*.[5] Furthermore, serological studies indicated that some immunized individuals were exposed to *Y. pestis* and developed subclinical infections.[44] The effectiveness of this vaccine against the pneumonic form of the disease is more questionable, however, and cases of pneumonic plague have been reported in vaccinated individuals.[33, 45] In the murine model of disease, immunization with the killed whole-cell vaccine provided protection against a subcutaneous challenge with *Y. pestis*[29] but not against an inhaled challenge with the bacterium.[46] Although these data alone do not necessarily indicate the effectiveness of the vaccine in humans, when viewed alongside the reports previously cited, the overall evidence is that the vaccine is better able to protect against bubonic plague than against pneumonic plague. Most of these studies, however, have been carried out using $F1^+$ strains of *Y. pestis*, and the ability of the vaccine to provide protection against $F1^-$ strains of *Y. pestis*, which are rarely encountered in natural infections, has not been tested.

Immunization of mice with the EV76 strain does induce protection against both subcutaneous and inhalation challenges with virulent strains of *Y. pestis*,[29] and in this respect the performance of this vaccine is superior to the performance of the killed vaccines. The enhanced protection offered by the live vaccine might be due to three factors. First, it is known that the killed vaccine does not contain immunogenic levels of several outer membrane proteins such as V antigen[42]; second, it has been suggested that the chemical or heat inactivation of the bacterium results in structural changes in other surface components such as the F1 antigen[30]; third, local responses to vaccination with EV76 in mice suggest that a limited local infection is initiated and that the duration of exposure to the antigenic complement is therefore prolonged. The immune response induced by the live attenuated vaccine may be more authentic than that induced by the killed whole-cell preparations.

Persistence of Immunity

There have been few studies to examine the duration of immunity to *Y. pestis* after immunization with killed whole-cell vaccines. However, it is generally considered that immunity is short lived. Booster immunizations may be needed at 6-month intervals to ensure that a protective response is maintained.

Side Effects

The use of killed whole-cell vaccines in humans has highlighted the reactogenicity of the vaccine.[47, 48] The manufacturer of the Cutter vaccine reported that reactions such as malaise, headaches, local erythema and induration, or mild lymphadenopathy occurred in approximately 10% of vaccinees; this frequency of side effects is reported by other workers.[40] Data provided by the manufacturer of the Greer vaccine suggest that more than 10% of vaccinees suffer side effects (Table 30–2). Allergic reactions, evidenced mainly as urticaria, occur infrequently.[47] One study found that the frequency of

Table 30–2. **PERCENTAGE OF INDIVIDUALS REPORTING LOCAL OR SYSTEMIC SIDE EFFECTS WITHIN 48 HOURS OF VACCINATION WITH THE GREER PLAGUE VACCINE***

	% OF RECIPIENTS REPORTING REACTIONS	
REACTION	After First Dose (n = 67)	After Second Dose (n = 59)
Local		
Tenderness	71.6	18.6
Decreased arm motion	11.9	1.7
Erythema	4.5	0
Warmth	3.0	1.7
Edema	1.5	0
Systemic		
Headache	19.4	6.8
Nausea	13.4	3.4
Malaise	10.4	5.1
Dizziness	6.0	0
Chills	4.5	3.4
Joint pain	4.5	0
Muscle pain	4.5	0
Anorexia	1.5	0
Diarrhea	1.5	0
Vomiting	1.5	0

*Vaccinees received the second dose 30 days after the first dose.

side effects was much greater in individuals who had previously been immunized with the live EV vaccine.[40]

The safety of the EV76 vaccine has been questioned by several workers. Russell and colleagues reported that immunization of mice induced severe side effects and occasional (approximately 1%) fatalities.[29]

FUTURE DEVELOPMENTS

Subunit Vaccines

Although the killed or attenuated vaccines just described have several shortcomings, they do indicate that protection against both the bubonic and pneumonic forms of the plague is possible. Work toward the development of a subunit vaccine is supported by two observations. First, the major antibody response to *Y. pestis* (in sera from either vaccinated or convalescent individuals) is known to be directed against the F1 antigen.[49] Second, the V antigen has attracted attention as a component of a vaccine,[50] and the improved performance of live vaccines over killed vaccines might be explained by the ability of only the live vaccines to induce an antibody response to the V antigen.[42]

The F1 antigen can be produced from cultures of *Y. pestis*,[51, 52] but recent studies have used recombinant F1 antigen produced by expressing the *caf* operon in *Escherichia coli* bacteria.[53] Intraperitoneal or intramuscular immunization with native F1 or rF1 antigens adjuvanted with alum induced an immune response that protected mice against a subcutaneous challenge with as many as 10^5 cfu of virulent *Y. pestis*.[30, 42] Although the F1 antigen also induced protection against inhalation challenge with 100 MLD of an $F1^+$ strain of *Y. pestis*,[30] there was concern that a vaccine based solely on the F1 antigen would not provide protection against naturally occurring but virulent $F1^-$ strains of *Y. pestis*. The production of V antigen for vaccine studies has, until recently, been difficult. The V antigen is produced at low levels by *Y. pestis* and readily degrades during purification. As a result, difficulties in preparing the V antigen from this source precluded the evaluation of this antigen in active immunization studies. The fusion of the gene that encodes the V antigen (*lcrV*) with a carrier protein such as protein A or glutathione-s-transferase allows a high level of production of the V antigen in *E. coli* bacteria. The V antigen can be cleaved from the carrier protein using a site-specific protease such as thrombin or factor X_a. Immunization of mice intraperitoneally with either the fusion protein or the V antigen adjuvanted with alum induced protection against a subcutaneous challenge with 4×10^6 cfu of *Y. pestis*.[50] A significant advantage over the F1 antigen is the ability of the V antigen to induce protection against virulent $F1^-$ strains of *Y. pestis* such as the Java 9 strain. Protection against 1000 or more MLD of either virulent $F1^+$ or $F1^-$ strains of *Y. pestis* given by the inhalation route has been reported.[54]

The protection afforded individually by the F1 and V antigens was defeated by subcutaneous challenges of 10^9 cfu of *Y. pestis*.[42] Protection against this challenge was achieved after intraperitoneal immunization with a mixture of the F1 and V antigens.[42] The vaccine also protected mice against 100 MLD of *Y. pestis* given by the inhalation route (Table 30–3), suggesting that the vaccine would provide protection against pneumonic plague in humans.[46] The advantages of such a combined subunit vaccine lie not only with the enhanced level of protection afforded against disease but also with the ability of the vaccine to confer protection against both $F1^+$ and $F1^-$ strains of *Y. pestis*.

The mechanism by which this vaccine induces protective immunity has been the subject of considerable investigation during the past few years. The F1 capsule is thought to inhibit phagocytosis of the bacterium by

Table 30–3. **PROTECTION AFFORDED BY KILLED WHOLE-CELL VACCINE, EV76 VACCINE, OR F1- AND V-ANTIGEN SUBUNIT EXPERIMENTAL VACCINE AGAINST PARENTERAL OR INHALATION CHALLENGE WITH *Yersinia pestis* STRAIN GB**

	PROTECTION (% SURVIVAL) AGAINST CHALLENGE (MLD)	
VACCINE	Subcutaneous Route	Inhalation Route
Control	0 (10^1)*	0 (10^1)†
Killed whole-cell vaccine	60 (2×10^6)*	50 (2×10^3)†
EV76	100 (2×10^9)*	66 (8.5×10^3)‡
F1 + V	100 (2×10^9)*	100 (4×10^4)†

*Tested in Balb/c mice.
†Tested in CBA mice.
‡Tested in Porton strain outbred mice.
EV76, attenuated live vaccine strain of *Y. pestis;* F1 + V, subunit vaccine containing the F1 and V antigens of *Y. pestis.*

preventing complement-mediated opsonization.[22, 55] Therefore, it is possible that induced antibody against the F1 antigen opsonizes the bacterium and promotes antibody-dependent cellular cytotoxicity. Some vaccinated animals do appear to harbor the pathogen even in a mutated F1$^-$ form.[30] The killed whole-cell vaccines are less effective than purified F1 antigen in inducing high titers of antibody to F1.[30, 42] Antibody against the V antigen may also be of overriding importance in protection against plague, and immunization with V antigen has been shown to restore the ability of the host to produce tumor necrosis factor-α and γ-interferon in response to infection.[25] Therefore, immunization with the V antigen would enable the host to mount a normal inflammatory response and thereby enable the host phagocytes to clear bacteria opsonized by antibody against F1 antigen.

The F1/V antigen subunit vaccine shows good promise for development as a replacement for the killed whole-cell vaccines. A further improvement might be achieved by developing an oral or intranasal formulation. Although the oral delivery of purified F1 antigen did not induce an antibody response,[56] microencapsulation of the F1 and V antigens and induction of a protective response have been achieved and will facilitate intranasal or oral delivery.[57] Liposomal encapsulation of the plague subunit vaccine offers an alternative approach to mucosal delivery.[57] Another approach relies on the oral delivery of *Salmonella typhimurium* that expresses the F1 encoding operon, which induced a high level of protection against subcutaneous challenge with *Y. pestis*.[58, 59]

Live Attenuated Vaccines

The finding that the live EV76 vaccine induces protection against plague, although its use is accompanied by unacceptable side effects, has promoted some studies to develop rationally attenuated strains of *Y. pestis* as a vaccine. Work towards this goal has been based on the finding that other Gram-negative pathogens can be attenuated by the introduction of mutations into genes essential for bacterial growth, virulence, or survival in the host. Mutations within genes involved in aromatic amino acid biosynthesis have been shown to attenuate a variety of pathogens, *including Y. enterocolitica*, *S. typhimurium*, and *Salmonella typhi*. An *aroA* mutant of *Y. pestis* was not attenuated in mice but was attenuated in guinea pigs, which subsequently developed antibodies to the F1 and V antigens.[60] Although these guinea pigs were also protected against a subsequent challenge with 10^7 cfu of virulent *Y. pestis*,[60] further work is needed to determine the reason for the species-dependent virulence of the *aroA* mutant before it can be considered for further studies.

REFERENCES

1. Brubaker B. Factors promoting acute and chronic diseases caused by yersiniae. Clin Microbiol Rev 1991;4:309–324.
2. Pollitzer R. Plague. World Health Organ Monogr Ser 22:1–698, 1954.
3. Butler T. Plague and Other *Yersinia* Infections. New York, Plenum Press, 1983.
4. Perry RD, Fetherston JD. *Yersinia pestis*—etiologic agent of plague. Clin Microbiol Rev 10:35–66, 1997.
5. Prevention of plague: Recommendations of the Advisory Committee on Immunization Practices (ACIP). MMWR Morb Mortal Wkly Rep 45(RR-14):1–15, 1996.
6. Vessereau A. Le reglement sanitaire international bilan et perspectives. World Health Stat Q 41:37–45, 1988.
7. Human plague in 1994. Wkly Epidemiol Rec 22:165–168, 1996.
8. Poland JD, Barnes AM. Plague. In Steele JH, Stoenner H, Kaplan W, Torten M (eds). CRC Handbook Series in Zoonoses. Boca Raton, CRC Press, 1979, pp 515–597.
9. Christie AB, Corbel MJ. Plague and other yersinial diseases. In Smith GR, Easmon CSF (eds). Topley and Wilson's Principles of Bacteriology, Virology and Immunity. Vol 3. London, Edward Arnold, 1990, pp 399–410.
10. Meyer KF. Pneumonic plague. Bacteriol Rev 35:249–261, 1961.
11. Cornelis GR, Biot T, Lambert de Rouvroit C, et al. The *Yersinia yop* regulon. Mol Microbiol 3:1455–1459, 1989.
12. Straley SC, Skrzypek E, Plano GV, et al. Yops of *Yersinia* spp. pathogenic for humans. Infect Immun 61:3105–3110, 1993.
13. Galyov EE, Smirnov OY, Karlishev AV, et al. Nucleotide sequence of the *Yersinia pestis* gene encoding F1 antigen and the primary structure of the protein. FEBS Lett 277:230–232, 1990.
14. Galyov EE, Karlishev AV, Chernovskaya TV, et al. Expression of the envelope antigen F1 of *Yersinia pestis* is mediated by the product of *caf1M* gene having homology with the chaperone protein PapD of *Escherichia coli*. FEBS Lett 286:79–82, 1991.
15. Karlyshev AV, Galyov EE, Smirnov OY, et al. A new gene of the *f1* operon of *Y. pestis* involved in the capsule biogenesis. FEBS Lett 297:77–80, 1992.
16. Karylshev AV, Galyov EE, Abramov VM, et al. *Caf1R* gene and its role in the regulation of capsule formation of *Y. pestis*. FEBS Lett 305:37–40, 1992.
17. Hinnesbusch BJ, Perry RD, Schwan TG. Role of the *Yersinia pestis* hemin storage (*hms*) locus in the transmission of plague by fleas. Science 273:367–370, 1996.
18. Cavanaugh DC. Specific effect of temperature upon transmission of the plague bacillus by the oriental rat flea, *Xenopsylla cheopis*. Am J Trop Med Hyg 20:264–272, 1971.
19. Van Zwanenberg D. The last epidemic of plague in England? Suffolk 1906–1918. Med Hist 14:63–74, 1970.
20. Cavanaugh DC, Randall R. The role of multiplication of *Pasteurella pestis* in mononuclear phagocytes in the pathogenesis of flea-borne plague. J Immunol 83:348–363, 1959.
21. Lindler LE, Klemper MS, Straley SC. *Yersinia pestis* pH 6 antigen: Genetic, biochemical and virulence characterisation of a protein involved in the pathogenesis of bubonic plague. Infect Immun 58:2569–2577, 1990.
22. Williams RC, Gewurz H, Quie PG. Effects of fraction 1 from *Yersinia pestis* on phagocytosis in vitro. J Infect Dis 126:235–241, 1972.
23. Friedlander AM, Welkos SL, Worsham PL, et al. Relationship between virulence and immunity as revealed in recent studies of the F1 capsule of *Yersinia pestis*. Clin Infect Dis 21:S178–S181, 1995.
24. Nakajima R, Brubaker RR. Association between virulence of *Yersinia pestis* and supression of gamma interferon and tumor necrosis factor alpha. Infect Immun 61:23–31, 1993.
25. Nakajima R, Motin VL, Brubaker RR. Suppression of cytokines in mice by protein A-V antigen fusion peptide and restoration of synthesis by active immunisation. Infect Immun 63:3021–3029, 1995.
26. Price SB, Cowan C, Perry RD, et al. The *Yersinia pestis* V antigen is a regulatory protein necessary for Ca^{2+}-dependent growth and maximal expression of low-Ca^{2+}-response virulence genes. J Bacteriol 173:2649–2657, 1991.
27. Montie TC, Montie DB. Protein toxins of *Pasturella pestis*. Subunit composition and acid binding. Biochemistry 10:2094–2100, 1971.
28. Von Metz E, Eisler DM, Hottle GA. Immunogenicity of plague vaccines in mice and guinea pigs. Appl Microbiol 22:84–88, 1971.
29. Russell P, Eley SM, Hibbs SE, et al. A comparison of plague vaccine, USP and EV76 vaccine induced protection against *Yersinia pestis* in a murine model. Vaccine 13:1551–1556, 1995.

30. Andrews GP, Heath DG, Anderson GW Jr, et al. Fraction 1 capsular antigen (F1) purification from *Yersinia pestis* CO92 and from an *Escherichia coli* recombinant strain and efficacy against lethal plague challenge. Infect Immun 64:2180–2187, 1996.
31. Bartelloni PJ, Marshall JD, Cavanaugh DC. Clinical and serological responses to plague vaccine. Mil Med 138:720–722, 1973.
32. Meyer KF, Foster LE. Measurement of protective serum antibodies in human volunteers inoculated with plague prophylactics. Stanford Med Bull 6:75–79, 1948.
33. Meyer KF. Effectiveness of live or killed plague vaccines in man. Bull World Health Organ 42:653–666, 1970.
34. WHO report on plague in 1973. World Health Organ Wkly Epidemiol Rec 49:253–254, 1974.
35. Barnes AM. Surveillance and control of bubonic plague in the United States. Symp Zool Soc Lond 50:237–270, 1982.
36. Lawton WD, Erdman RL, Surgalla MJ. Biosynthesis and purification of V and W antigens in *Pasteurella pestis*. J Immunol 91:179–184, 1963.
37. Motin VL, Nakajima R, Smirnov GB, et al. Passive immunity to yersiniae mediated by anti-recombinant V antigen and by protein A-V fusion peptide. Infect Immun 62:4192–4201, 1994.
38. Une T, Nakajima R, Brubaker RR. Roles of V antigen in promoting virulence in *Yersinia*. Contrib Microbiol Immunol 9:179–185, 1986.
39. Williams JE, Altieri PL, Berman S, et al. Potency of killed plague vaccines prepared from avirulent *Yersinia pestis*. Bull World Health Organ 58:753–756, 1980.
40. Meyer KF, Smith G, Foster LE, et al. Plague immunization. IV. Clinical reactions and serologic response to inoculations of Haffkine and freeze-dried plague vaccine. J Infect Dis 129:S30–S36, 1974.
41. Williams JE, Cavanaugh DC. Measuring the efficacy of vaccination in affording protection against plague. Bull World Health Organ 57:309–313, 1979.
42. Williamson ED, Eley SM, Griffin K, et al. A new improved sub-unit vaccine for plague: The basis of protection. FEMS Immunol Med Microbiol 12:223–230, 1995.
43. Marshall JD, Cavanaugh DC, Bartelloni PJ, et al. Plague immunization. III. Serologic response to multiple inoculations of vaccine. J Infect Dis 129:S26–S29, 1974.
44. Cavanaugh DC, Elisberg BL, Llewellyn C, et al. Plague immunization. V. Indirect evidence for the efficacy of plague vaccine. J Infect Dis 129:S37–S40, 1974.
45. Cohen RJ, Stockard JL. Pneumonic plague in an untreated plague vaccinated individual. JAMA 202:365–366, 1967.
46. Williamson ED, Eley SM, Stagg AJ, et al. A sub-unit vaccine elicits IgG in serum, spleen cell cultures and bronchial washings and protects immunized animals against pneumonic plague. Vaccine 15:1079–1084, 1997.
47. Reisman RE. Allergic reactions due to plague vaccine. J Allergy 46:49–56, 1970.
48. Marshall JD, Bartelloni PJ, Cavanaugh DC, et al. Plague immunization. II. Relation of adverse clinical reactions to multiple immunizations with killed vaccine. J Infect Dis 129:S19–S25, 1974.
49. Williams JE, Arntzen L, Tyndal GL, et al. Application of enzyme immunoassays for the confirmation of clinically suspect plague in Nambia, 1982. Bull World Health Organ 64:745–752, 1982.
50. Leary SEC, Williamson ED, Griffin KF, et al. Active immunization with V-antigen from *Yersinia pestis* protects against plague. Infect Immun 63:2854–2858, 1995.
51. Baker EE, Sommer H, Foster LE, et al. Studies on immunization against plague. I. The isolation and characterization of the soluble antigen of *Pasteurella pestis*. J Immunol 68:131–145, 1952.
52. Meyer KF, Hightower JA, McCrumb FR. Plague immunization VI. Vaccination with the fraction 1 antigen of *Yersinia pestis*. J Infect Dis 129:S41–S45, 1974.
53. Simpson WJ, Thomas RE, Schwan TG. Recombinant capsular antigen (fraction 1) from *Yersinia pestis* induces a protective antibody response in BALB/C mice. Am J Trop Med Hyg 43:389–396, 1990.
54. Anderson GW, Leary SEC, Wiliamson ED, et al. Recombinant V antigen protects mice against pneumonic and bubonic plague caused by F1-capsule–positive and –negative strains of *Yersinia pestis*. Infect Immun 64:4580–4585, 1996.
55. Rodrigues CG, Carneiro CMM, Barbosa CFT, et al. Antigen F1 from *Yersinia pestis* forms aqueous channels in lipid bilayer membranes. Braz J Med Biol Res 25:75–79, 1992.
56. Thomas RE, Simpson WJ, Perry LL, et al. Failure of intragastrically administered *Yersinia pestis* capsular antigen to protect mice against challenge with virulent plague: Suppression of fraction 1–specific antibody response. Am J Trop Med Hyg 47:92–97, 1992.
57. Williamson ED, Sharp GJE, Eley SM, et al. Local and systemic immune response to a microencapsulated sub-unit vaccine for plague. Vaccine 14:1613–1619, 1996.
58. Oyston PCF, Williamson ED, Leary SEC, et al. Immunization with live recombinant *Salmonella typhimurium aroA* producing F1 antigen protects against plague. Infect Immun 63:563–568, 1995.
59. Titball RW, Howells AM, Oyston PCF, et al. Expression of the *Yersinia pestis* capsular antigen (F1 antigen) on the surface of an *aroA* mutant *of Salmonella typhimurium* induces high level protection against plague. Infect Immun 65:1926–1930, 1997.
60. Oyston PFC, Russell P, Williamson ED, et al. An *aroA* mutant of *Yersinia pestis* is attenuated in the guinea pig but virulent in mice. Microbiology 142:1847–1853, 1995.

chapter 31

Rabies Vaccine

Stanley A. Plotkin
Charles E. Rupprecht
Hilary Koprowski

I have seen agony in death only once, in a patient with rabies; he remained acutely aware of every stage in the process of his own disintegration over a twenty-four-hour period, right up to his final moment.

Lewis Thomas. *The Lives of a Cell.* New York, Bantam Books, 1974.

BACKGROUND

Historical Perspective

Rabies has been known since before 2300 BC from its description in the Mesopotamian Laws of Eshnunna.[1] Homer, Democritus, and Aristotle referred to *lyssa* (Greek, rabies) in their writings, and in the 1st century AD, the Roman scholar Aulus Cornelius Celsus was perhaps the first to provide an accurate description of the disease and the wide range of species susceptible to infection. In the 15th century AD, the Italian savant Girolamo Fracastoro established the principle of the incurable wound, that is, the disease is always lethal. The Talmud also mentions that one should not believe people who say that they were bitten by a rabid animal and lived.

Shortly after Cortez's exploration of the Americas, the first Bishop of Oceania described "small animals" that bit the toes of Spanish soldiers during the night. The soldiers later died of a disease that could have been rabies, and the small animals may have been vampire bats that even now play a major role in the transmission of rabies in Latin America.

Rabies is defined as an acute viral encephalitis usually transmitted from animal to animal or from animal to human by exposure to saliva. Virus in saliva attaches to peripheral nerve endings and travels to the brain. In nature, rabies is a disease of terrestrial and airborne mammals, involving the Canidae (dogs, wolves, foxes, coyotes, and jackals), Procyonidae (raccoons), Viverridae (mongooses), Mustelidae (skunks, weasels, and martens), and Chiroptera (bats) as reservoirs, although all mammalian species are believed to be susceptible.

Human infection with rabies is nearly always secondary to animal bite, although exposures through the inhalation of virus or through the transplantation of infected cornea also occur. In most of the world, the major reservoir for human rabies is the dog, responsible for an enormous incidence of bites in humans. Although they do not function as reservoirs, cats are important vectors of the disease.

The dramatic symptoms and nearly 100% fatality rate of rabies attracted the curiosity of the first modern microbiologists, and by the end of the 19th century, an effective vaccination procedure was developed.[2, 3] It was recently speculated that Edgar Allan Poe died of rabies in Baltimore.[4]

Experimental transmission of rabies by inoculation of saliva was first demonstrated in 1804 by the German scientist Zinke. In 1879 in Lyon, France, Victor Galtier transmitted rabies from dog to rabbit and from rabbit to rabbit and used intravenous injections of rabid material to immunize sheep and goats. However, Galtier's work was to be overshadowed by that of his famed contemporary, Louis Pasteur. Obviously, much of the credit for rabies research belongs to Pasteur, but one must not overlook the contributions of his collaborators, Roux, Chamberland, and Thuillier. These three investigators carried out most of his laboratory manipulations, because Pasteur, more than 60 years old, was partially disabled by stroke.

The Pasteur group established in 1881 that the central nervous system is the principal site of rabies virus replication. They transmitted the disease by submeningeal inoculation into rabbits and were able to maintain the virus in this host for more than 100 passages. It was Roux who noticed originally that the virulence of rabies-infected spinal cords decreased rapidly when they were suspended in dry air and was extinguished completely in 15 days. From this observation, Pasteur developed a practical method of vaccination. Dogs injected subcutaneously with serial suspensions of fragments of rabies virus–infected spinal cords, beginning with cord dried long enough to be avirulent and using successively less dried cords, resisted rabies when they were injected intracerebrally with a virulent virus.

Fifty dogs were protected this way. Although experiments performed to demonstrate that dogs can be made refractory to rabies by vaccination *after* they have been bitten by "mad" dogs were inconclusive, treatment of a human patient, Joseph Meister, was attempted on July

6, 1885, perhaps subsequent to other nonpublished attempts at human vaccination. Meister, who had been bitten 14 times by a rabid dog 60 hours previously, received a subcutaneous inoculation of spinal cord suspension derived from rabid rabbits and preserved in a flask of dry air for 15 days. Twelve successive inoculations were made with cords of increasing virulence, for a total of 13 inoculations during a 10-day period. The boy not only resisted natural rabies but also escaped large quantities of highly virulent virus that were contained in the last five doses of vaccine.

The Pasteur method of treatment aroused great interest in medical circles and, despite some disagreements, was rapidly accepted. The Pasteur Institute of Paris was founded in 1888, and within a decade, there were Pasteur Institutes throughout the world.

Criticism, however, was forthcoming. The occasional failures raised questions about the safety of the vaccine, especially because virulent material was being inoculated into the patients at the end of the treatment. Also, there were obviously no controls for comparison to confirm the effectiveness of the method. Pasteur thought that vaccine failures could be attributed to prolonged delays in initiating treatment or to excessive bites on the face or head that resulted in a short incubation period.

The original Pasteur vaccination method has not been used in humans since 1953, when it was last employed at the Pasteur Institute in Paris. Only in recent years has an understanding of rabies pathogenesis allowed significant changes in rabies vaccines. Even today, the success of vaccination is only partly explained.

Clinical Description

Reported incubation periods for rabies have been as short as 5 to 6 days and as long as several years, but in the majority of cases, the incubation period is between 20 and 60 days.[5] Although incubation periods of longer than 6 months are reported in less than 1% of cases, identification of strains by monoclonal antibodies and genetic sequencing has permitted positive confirmation of periods as long as 6 years.[6] Incubation periods are usually shorter when the site of the bite is on the head rather than an extremity.[7]

Signs and symptoms of rabies in animals and humans have been well described. After a nonspecific prodromal period, a variable proportion of animals develop aggressive or combative behavior, irritability, viciousness, and hyperreaction to external stimuli. In these cases, the clinical course is described as *furious* rabies. A paralytic phase then develops characterized by weakness of one of more limbs, jaw drop due to paralysis of muscles of head and neck, and difficulty in phonation and respiration, leading ultimately to death. Alternatively, paralysis may predominate with no aggressive signs.

The clinical illness in humans may be divided into the following five stages: incubation period, prodrome, acute neurological phase, coma, and death or rare recovery.[8] Clinical rabies presents either in a furious form (two thirds of the cases) or in a paralytic form. The furious form is characterized by fluctuating consciousness, phobic spasms, and signs of autonomic dysfunction such as dilated pupils and hypersalivation. In the paralytic form, the patient is conscious but appears to have the Guillain-Barré syndrome. In distinction from the latter syndrome, rabies patients usually have fever, intact sensory function, and urinary incontinence.

During the incubation period, there are no symptoms; clinical illness begins with the prodromal complaints of malaise, anorexia, fatigue, headache, and fever. Pain or paresthesia at or close to the site of exposure is reported in 50 to 80% of cases, and apprehension, anxiety, agitation, irritability, nervousness, insomnia, or depression may be prominent during this period. After a prodromal period that lasts 2 to 10 days, objective signs of nervous system involvement develop, including hyperactivity, disorientation, hallucinations, seizures, bizarre behavior, nuchal stiffness, and paralysis. As in animals, a period of hyperactivity lasting hours to days develops in a majority of cases. In humans, this hyperactivity is characteristically intermittent and consists of periods of agitation lasting 1 to 5 minutes. These hyperactive periods may occur spontaneously or may be precipitated by a variety of tactile, auditory, visual, or other stimuli.[9] Between these periods, the patient is usually cooperative and able to communicate. Hydrophobia (the fear of water) appears to develop in most cases of furious human rabies. Attempts to drink or eat may produce severe painful spasms of the pharynx and larynx and precipitate an episode of hyperactivity that is extremely frightening to the patient. Subsequently, simply the sight of liquids may precipitate episodes of pharyngeal spasms.

Other abnormalities during the acute and neurological phase include muscle fasciculation (particularly near the site of the exposure), hyperventilation, hypersalivation, focal or generalized convulsions, and, rarely, priapism or increased libido. Unless the patient dies abruptly, paralysis generally becomes the major problem. Paralysis may be symmetrical; asymmetrical with maximal involvement of the bitten extremity; or ascending, as in the Guillain-Barré syndrome.[10] Paralysis may be the presenting symptom, as seems often to be the case after bat bites.

In the acute neurological phase, the mental status of the patient gradually deteriorates during a period of 2 to 12 days. This phase ends either with abrupt death due to cardiac or respiratory arrest or with onset of coma. Coma may last for hours or months, depending on the intensity of care. Without supportive care, respiratory arrest usually develops shortly after the onset of coma and leads to death. With intensive medical support, respiratory arrest may not occur, and the patient may live with assisted ventilation for up to several months. To date, there are only seven cases of known survival among humans who showed signs of disease, at least four of whom recovered with sequelae and one with severe psychogenic disturbance.[11–15] Despite trials of steroids, interferon, and other antivirals, there is no therapy of proven value.[16]

Virology

Rabies virus belongs to the family *Rhabdoviridae*, genus *Lyssavirus*, consisting of genetically related enveloped viruses with a single, nonsegmented, negative-stranded ribonucleic acid (RNA). The virus contains multiple copies of the following five structural proteins: virion transcriptase (L), glycoprotein (G), nucleoprotein (N), nucleocapsid phosphoprotein (NS), and matrix protein (M). The L, N, and NS proteins are noncovalently bound to the virion RNA, and the resulting ribonucleoprotein complex forms a helically coiled structure within the virion. The nucleocapsid complex is surrounded by a lipoprotein envelope consisting of the M protein, and the surface projection of the G proteins extends to the exterior of the virus.[17]

The rabies virus G protein, which is a trimer of about 67 kDa, is the major antigen responsible for inducing production of virus-neutralizing antibodies (VNA) and for conferring immunity against lethal infection with rabies virus.[18, 19] The G gene was the first rabies virus gene to be cloned and sequenced.[20] From the nucleotide sequence, a polypeptide 524 amino acids long was deduced, which included a signal sequence of 19 amino acids.[17] An arginine at position 333 appears necessary for virulence.[21]

The immunogenic activity of purified native G protein and of smaller fragments of G protein, both naturally occurring and derived by chemical cleavage of the rabies virus G protein, has been compared in a variety of ways to determine the structural basis of VNA production after immunization.[17] Although the protective immune response to rabies is debated,[22–24] evidence for the importance of VNA in prevention of viral infection is convincing both in humans (see later) and in animals. With regard to a cellular response, T helper cells are necessary to antibody induction but are not in themselves protective, whereas cytolytic T cells directed against the nucleocapsid (N) induced by vaccination may be important to destroy already infected cells before entry of virus into the central nervous system. Interestingly, the cytolytic T-cell response may be suppressed in natural infection.

Rabies-Related Viruses

Since the early 1970s, viruses have been isolated from animals and humans that are serologically related to rabies virus. Although members of this group showed some immunological cross-reactivity with the rabies virus, they were sufficiently different to be originally classified as *rabies-related viruses*. The *Lyssavirus* genus is now considered to contain seven viruses.[25] Type 1 is the rabies virus itself as type species; type 2 is the Lagos bat virus, originally isolated from bats in Nigeria[26]; type 3 is the Mokola virus, isolated from a shrew in Nigeria[27]; type 4 is the Duvenhage virus, isolated from a human with a case of rabies-like illness in South Africa[27]; type 5 is European bat lyssavirus 1, isolated from a human case in Russia; type 6 is European bat lyssavirus 2, isolated from a human case in Finland[28]; and type 7 is a new isolate from Australian bats. At present, it is difficult to relate any human disease to either type 2 or type 7 viruses. Mokola virus can cause lethal infection in rabies-vaccinated dogs and cats.[29, 30] European bat lyssavirus 1 has been isolated from bats captured in Poland, Denmark, Finland, and northern provinces of Germany.[27] Strains of lyssavirus types 5 and 6 are apparently widely distributed in European bats.[31] Although tests in mice showed that human diploid cell rabies vaccine could protect against the European bat viruses,[32] and vaccination of exposed humans has so far been successful,[31] only 73% of vaccinated patients developed neutralizing antibodies to these viruses, usually when they had mounted a strong antibody response to the rabies vaccine virus.[33] The larger public health significance of the rabies-related viruses remains to be determined.

Pathogenesis as It Relates to Prevention

When inoculated in a wound, rabies virus may take days or weeks to reach the central nervous system. It is this fact that makes postexposure prophylaxis possible. During this early period, the virus is susceptible to VNA and even to mechanical removal by washing. There is some evidence that initial replication occurs in muscle cells surrounding the wound, providing an amplification of the original inoculum. However, experimental data show that central nervous system entry can occur without any prior replication in the muscle.[34] Another site proposed for possible persistence of rabies virus before entry into the central nervous system is the macrophage, from which the virus could reactivate to cause disease,[35] but the importance of replication in nonnerve cells to the pathogenesis of rabies remains controversial.[36] In any event, at some point in time, the virus attaches to receptors, which may include the acetylcholine receptors of the neuromuscular junction or lipoproteins on the membrane (see later), and begins a passive journey to the cell body, where it replicates and spreads within the central nervous system.[37, 38] Dietzschold and colleagues[39] have demonstrated that the action of rabies VNA is not solely exerted outside of the cell. They showed in an animal model that the effectiveness of antibody was associated with entry into the cell by endocytosis and inhibition of viral transcription.

The rabies virus G protein has sequences similar to certain neurotoxins and binds to the α-subunit of acetylcholine receptor.[40–42] This receptor undoubtedly functions in the entry of virus into muscle, but other lipoprotein receptors function on the nerve cell.[43] Once entered into nerve cells, the virus travels in the nerve at a rate of 12 to 24 mm per day in rodents but perhaps faster in humans. In rodents, virus may reach the central nervous system in 3 to 5 days, where it causes a widespread encephalitis[44] progressing at 20 to 40 mm per day.

Once established in the neurons of the brain, the virus starts to move in the opposite direction, down the axons to replicate in peripheral tissues, most notably the salivary glands, from which excretion in saliva permits transmission by bite to maintain the circuit of infection.[25]

The pathophysiology of the fatal outcome is not completely understood. Although encephalitis is widespread, neuronal destruction is not. Death probably results from the involvement of brain centers controlling the cardiorespiratory system. Although the fatality rate in rabies is extremely elevated, rare documented recovery and even chronic persistent infection have been documented in dogs.[45]

Evidence of a serological response to rabies virus can be demonstrated by a variety of laboratory techniques, including mouse neutralization, fluorescent focus inhibition, indirect fluorescent antibody, plaque neutralization, immunolysis of rabies-infected cells, and binding techniques using the radioimmunoassay or enzyme-linked immunosorbent assay procedures. Serum antibodies develop late after natural infection in humans. In individuals without history of vaccination, serum antibodies are first detected on about the 10th day of illness and thereafter rise rapidly to high levels. Antibodies are also present in cerebrospinal fluid (CSF) late in the clinical course. Antibody titers of CSF are much higher than would be expected from seepage into CSF from circulating blood. Because vaccination does not induce CSF antibodies, the presence of high CSF antibody titers supports the diagnosis of clinical rabies.[11, 12]

The absence of detectable serum antibodies until around the second week of illness (if at all) and of CSF antibodies until approximately the third week of illness (when significant systemic and neurological problems occur) raises the possibility that some of the clinical symptoms result from the interaction of host antibodies with rabies virus–infected cells.[37] In individuals who receive postexposure prophylaxis, antibody titers after the onset of clinical illness rise more rapidly and to higher titers than in individuals who do not receive such immunization.

Diagnosis

Clinical diagnosis of rabies requires differentiation from a wide variety of diseases that can cause neurological symptoms. Because laboratory diagnosis is usually not possible during the first week of illness unless rabies is suspected, presumptive diagnosis based on clinical symptoms is important. As noted previously, the clinical symptoms of rabies encephalitis that may distinguish it from other forms of encephalitis are as follows: pain and paresthesia near the site of exposure, hydrophobia, hypersalivation, hyperventilation, agitated behavior, asymmetrical or ascending paralysis, and aerophobia—all developing during a 2- to 10-day period. These symptoms and a history of exposure to a rabid animal strongly suggest the diagnosis of rabies.

Definitive diagnosis of rabies infection of humans and suspected animal vectors depends on the detection and identification in infected brain tissue of specific rabies antigen, of inclusions (Negri bodies), or of rabies nucleic acid by the polymerase chain reaction[46]; on the presence of antibodies in the CSF; and on the isolation and identification of the virus from brain tissue or saliva. The standard diagnostic technique is to search for rabies antigen by fluorescent antibody staining or by enzyme-linked immunosorbent assay. Identification of rabies nucleic acid by dot blot hybridization or by reverse transcriptase–polymerase chain reaction (RT-PCR) is useful, particularly if specimens are in poor condition. Demonstration of Negri bodies has a variable sensitivity and is of only historical interest, whereas virus isolation is a procedure used for confirmation of other positive test results. Isolation can be accomplished in tissue culture or by intracerebral inoculation of suckling mice.[47] Although diagnostic procedures are generally initiated in tissue specimens collected post mortem, rabies infection can also be identified in vivo during the extended course of the disease. In those cases, the fluorescent antibody staining technique enables detection of rabies antigen in impressions of cornea or in cryoscopic sections of skin biopsy samples from the hairline of the neck, where antigen can be detected in the nerves surrounding the hair follicles.[48] Between 1980 and 1996, 32 cases of rabies were diagnosed in the United States, but only 20 were diagnosed before death, probably because only 7 had a known history of exposure to potentially rabid animals. This problem arose in large part because most of the patients had been infected with rabies strains from bats, presumably as a result of bat bites.[49]

EPIZOOTIOLOGY AND EPIDEMIOLOGY

Animals

Rabies is a disease of both domestic and wild mammals, particularly dogs and related species, raccoons, mongooses, skunks, and bats. In areas in which animal control programs are not extensively developed, dogs and cats account for most of the rabid animals reported and cause the majority (90%) of human rabies exposures and cases. After effective domestic animal rabies control programs in these areas, the numbers of rabid dogs and cats markedly decrease, as illustrated in the United States from the 1940s to the 1960s. Wildlife then becomes the main reservoir of rabies virus. In the United States since 1960, the majority of cases of animal rabies has been in wildlife species, and most of the human rabies cases have been secondary to bites by rabid wildlife, including bats.[10, 50] The situation is similar in western Europe, where foxes account for up to 80% of rabid animals.[51]

Figure 31–1 is a composite map of the United States showing the terrestrial animal reservoirs present in each region.[52] The salient features are that skunks are the important vectors for rabies in the western and central United States, whereas two foci of raccoon rabies exist in the East. The original focus of raccoon rabies was in the Southeast, but a second developed in the Northeast owing to importation of animals, and now raccoon rabies is contiguous from Maine to Florida and is now spreading west to Ohio.[53] Foci of fox rabies are evident in the eastern states bordering Canada and in Alaska. Table 31–1 lists rabies cases by species for the United States in 1995.[52]

Canine rabies is still widespread in Asia, Africa, and parts of Latin America, including Mexico, where control of dogs has proved difficult. However, vaccination of pet dogs can be an effective strategy for protection of humans and has eliminated rabies in Great Britain and

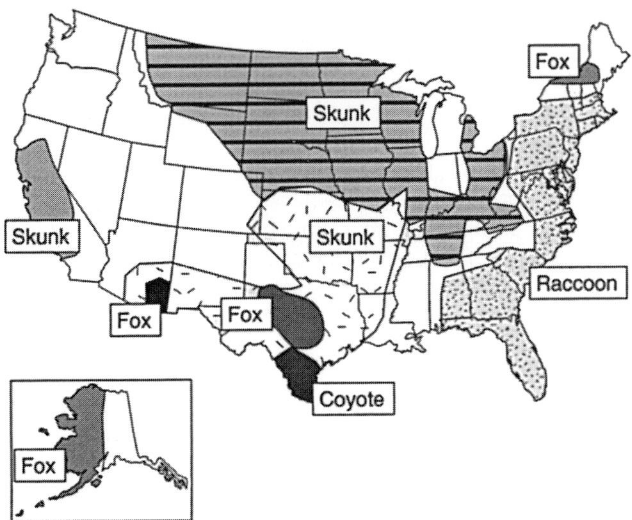

Figure 31–1. Distribution of major terrestrial reservoirs of rabies in the United States.

Japan.[37] An immunization coverage of 70% is estimated to prevent canine rabies outbreaks.[54]

Foxes are important vectors in Europe, Canada, Alaska, and the former USSR. The raccoon dog is now an important rabies vector in eastern Europe. Mongooses imported into the Caribbean Islands now form a reservoir for rabies, and that animal plays the same role in southern Africa. The vampire bat is a major threat to cattle in Latin America and has been involved in many biting incidents in humans. Insectivorous bats in North America are widely infected with rabies. Like all mammals, rodents, squirrels, and voles are susceptible to infection[37] but are infrequently rabid, and human transmission of disease by these animals has not resulted. In Thailand, an Asian country in which rabies has been extensively studied, 95% of the animals involved in biting incidents are dogs, with cats accounting for another 3%. The remaining 2% include monkeys, rats, rabbits, civets, tigers, squirrels, and other animals, which testifies to the high infectiousness of rabies virus. Dogs randomly captured in Thailand developed rabies within 1 month in 3 to 4% of cases, and more interesting, there was

Table 31–1. **CASES OF RABIES IN THE UNITED STATES BY TYPE OF ANIMAL, 1995**

ANIMAL	NO. OF CASES REPORTED	PERCENTAGE OF CASES REPORTED
Wild	7247	92
Domestic	630	8
Raccoons	3964	50
Skunks	1774	23
Bats	787	10
Foxes	513	6.5
Cats	288	3.7
Cows, horses, swine, sheep, goats	193	2.4
Dogs	146	1.9
Humans	4	0.05
Other	212	2.7
Total	7881	100

serological evidence of prior rabies infection in 15 to 20% of dogs.[55]

Widespread infection of insectivorous bats throughout the United States was well documented in the 1950s. However, the importance of bat rabies, particularly from the silver-haired bat *Lasionycteris noctivagans*, to human transmission has become evident recently, as described later. The rabies virus recovered from the silver-haired bat is a variant that appears to be able to replicate better in dermal tissues.[56]

The epidemiology of rabies has been revolutionized by the development of monoclonal antibodies.[57] Panels of these antibodies, directed against epitopes specific to isolates from different animal species and from different geographical locations, are used to identify viruses. Thus, it is now possible to identify an isolate from humans or animals as to the source and to demonstrate that the infection was transmitted far away in time and place. Sequencing of viral genome after RT-PCR has supplemented our knowledge of strain variability.[58] Vaccine strains differ in sequence from wild strains by as much as 10 to 15% of nucleotides. Sequence data suggest that some rabies strains in the Western Hemisphere and in South Africa were imported from Europe.[59, 60]

Human Rabies

The epidemiology of human rabies closely follows the epizootiology of animal rabies. The dog is the major global reservoir of rabies. In the United States alone, a million dog bites occur each year,[61] and the situation is worse in some other parts of the world.[62] Human rabies has been reported from all continents except Australia and Antarctica, but the majority of cases occur in countries where canine rabies is not well controlled. The World Health Organization (WHO) estimate of humans vaccinated for exposure to rabies exceeds 3 million annually. More than 50,000 rabies-related deaths were estimated by the WHO in 1983, and this number certainly represents only a fraction of the actual cases.[63] Human rabies is most common in people younger than 15 years, with about 40% of cases found in children 5 to 14 years, but all age groups are susceptible. The majority of rabies victims are male. In the United States, the highest incidence of human rabies postexposure prophylaxis occurs among rural boys, primarily during the summer months.[64]

Aside from direct animal contact, aerosol and direct implantation of infected tissue may transmit rabies to humans. Infection by aerosol has been suspected in caves heavily contaminated with bat guano and in laboratories.[10, 65] Unwitting corneal transplantation from patients deceased from rabies has also resulted in transmission.[10, 66] Human-to-human transmission by bite is extremely rare.[67, 68]

In the United States, the recent salient fact has been the emergence of bats as the leading transmitter to humans. Between 1980 and 1996, bat-related variants were identified in 15 of 23 diagnosed human rabies cases of domestic origin. No history of contact with bats could be elicited in 8 of the 15 cases, suggesting that unperceived bites in sleeping individuals may have been responsible.[69–71]

IMMUNIZATION

Passive Immunization

Antiserum alone will not prevent rabies and is not recommended except in combination with vaccine (see under *Serum and Vaccine Treatment*).

Active Immunization

Prior Approaches

Table 31–2 summarizes the history of the development of rabies vaccines and lists currently available vaccines. Many different strains have been used for preparation of rabies vaccines. The history of some of these strains is given in Figure 31–2.

For more than 70 years after Pasteur's original work, only vaccines containing nerve tissue were available. Major modifications in nerve tissue vaccine preparation were introduced by Fermi[72] and by Semple,[73] who used phenol to partially or completely inactivate virus. Adverse reactions to rabies vaccines containing brain tissue have been recognized since the time of Pasteur. In addition to neurological complications attributed to the presence of myelinated tissue in the vaccine, fixed virus may be pathogenic for humans, contrary to the "Pasteurian dogma," although it took 75 years before it was proved that some cases of paralysis after vaccination were caused by imperfectly inactivated vaccine virus.

Myelin-free vaccines prepared from neonatal mouse brains were introduced by Fuenzalida and colleagues[74] in 1956 and are still widely used in South America and the former Soviet Union. Introduction of the duck embryo vaccine (DEV) prepared from virus propagated in embryonated duck eggs[75] greatly reduced the number and severity of postvaccinal reactions; however, DEV was less immunogenic than the brain tissue vaccine. Fourteen to 23 daily inoculations were recommended for both these vaccines, but even this "heroic" dosage did not always protect against rabies after severe exposure. Thus, there had long been a pressing need for a highly immunogenic antirabies vaccine that could be used safely and effectively at low doses, both for primary immunization and for treatment after exposure.

Cell Culture Rabies Vaccines

The solution to the problem of safety of rabies vaccines lay in the development of vaccines prepared from rabies virus grown in tissue culture free of neuronal tissue. The first attempts to develop a tissue culture vaccine were made by Kissling[76] in 1958 and by Fenje[77] in 1960. Both investigators used the primary hamster kidney cell for rabies virus production. However, to avoid the injection of foreign proteins, the ideal cell culture substrate for vaccine is of human origin.

Human Diploid Cell Vaccine

In the early 1960s, workers at the Wistar Institute in Philadelphia selected the human diploid cell strain WI-38 for virus propagation to avoid most of the difficulties

Table 31–2. **IMPORTANT PAST AND PRESENT RABIES VACCINES FOR HUMANS**

VACCINE NAME	MANUFACTURER	TYPE	SUBSTRATE	REMARKS	WHERE USED
Nerve Tissue					
Pasteur	None	Inactivated by drying	Rabbit spinal cord	Residual live virus	NLU
Fermi	None	Phenolized live virus	Sheep, goat, or rabbit brains	Contained nerve tissue, residual live virus?	NLU
Semple	Many	Phenol-inactivated	Sheep, goat, or rabbit brains	Contains nerve tissue	Asia, Africa
Fuenzalida	Many	Inactivated	Suckling mouse brain	Decreased myelin content	South America
Avian					
PDEV	Berna	β-Propiolactone–inactivated	Duck embryo	Purified by ultracentrifugation	Europe, ROW
DEV	None	Inactivated	Duck embryo	Allergy to avian antigens	NLU
Cell Culture					
HDCV	PMC, Berna, Chiron Behring	β-Propiolactone–inactivated	Human cultured fibroblasts	Expensive, world standard for rabies vaccine	United States, Europe, ROW
RVA	Michigan	β-Propiolactone–inactivated	Fetal rhesus cell culture	Fewer allergic reactions	United States
PHKCV	Local	Formalin-inactivated	Primary Syrian hamster kidney cell culture	Used in People's Republic of China	China, Russia
PCECV	Chiron Behring	β-Propiolactone–inactivated	Chick embryo cell culture	Purified by ultracentrifugation	Germany, United States, ROW
PVRV	PMC	β-Propiolactone–inactivated	Vero cell line	Purified by ultracentrifugation	France, ROW

Abbreviations for vaccines listed here are those used in the text. NLU, no longer used; ROW, rest of world; PMC, Pasteur Mérieux–Connaught.

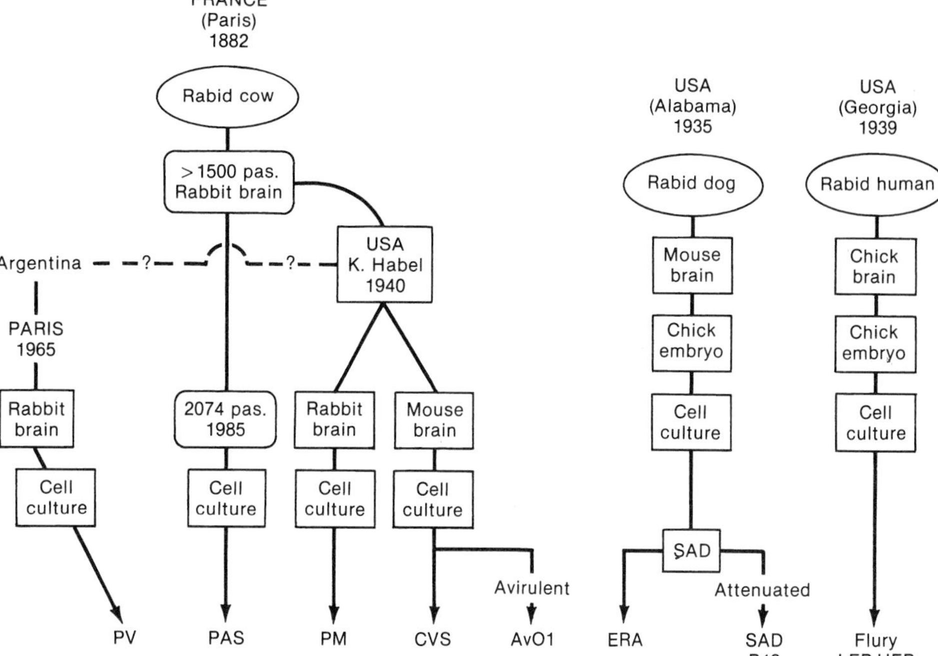

Figure 31–2. History of strains of rabies virus used as vaccine seeds. (From Sacramento D, Badrane H, Bourhy H, Tordo N. Molecular epidemiology of rabies virus in France: Comparison with vaccine strains. J Gen Virol 73:1149–1158, 1992.)

inherent in the use of primary tissue cultures.[78, 79] The vaccine thus developed, the human diploid cell vaccine (HDCV), containing concentrated and purified virus, evoked much better immune responses in experimental animals and in humans than did DEV, suckling brain, or adult brain tissue vaccines.[80, 81] Not only were antibody levels higher after immunization with the cell culture vaccine, but also antibodies appeared earlier. However, the most spectacular result obtained in the course of animal studies was the demonstration, for the first time, that a single injection of a vaccine given several hours after challenge with street virus could protect animals from rabies, although this particular vaccine was of exceptional potency.[82]

The steps leading to the development of the vaccine included the adaptation of the Pitman-Moore strain of virus to WI-38,[83] the inactivation of cell-free virus by β-propiolactone, and the concentration of virus by ultrafiltration.[84]

Currently, HDCV is produced in MRC-5 human fibroblasts, with use of the Pitman-Moore L503 3M strain. Virus-containing supernatants are concentrated 10 to 20 times by ultrafiltration or ultracentrifugation, reaching a titer of about 10^7 median lethal dose per mL before inactivation, which is done with 1:4000 β-propiolactone. Potency is assessed by the National Institutes of Health (NIH) test and is at least 2.5 international units (IU) per dose.

After 4 years of clinical studies in volunteers,[85] the vaccine was used in humans exposed to severe wounds by rabid dogs and wolves in Iran. All vaccinated people developed VNA, survived, and remained free of rabies.[86] Since 1976, HDCV has been recommended for preexposure and postexposure immunization of humans. It is estimated that more than 1,500,000 people have been treated throughout the world.

HDCV was licensed in the United States in June 1980 for preexposure and postexposure rabies immunization. The results of 5 years of clinical experience without failure to prevent rabies were evaluated by Winkler.[87] An estimated 85% of doses are used for preexposure immunization and booster doses for maintenance of antibody; 15% are for postexposure immunization.

Vaccine Constituents. HDCV is basically the supernatant of MRC-5 human embryo fibroblast cell cultures infected with rabies virus. Each dose of the vaccine sold in the United States contains rabies virus inactivated by β-propiolactone, 5% human albumin, phenolsulfonphthalein, and neomycin sulfate (<150 μg) as an antibiotic. The vaccine is lyophilized to a powder form and reconstituted in sterile water. The rabies antigen content is at least 2.5 IU. The vaccine contains no preservative or stabilizer.

Producers. HDCV was formerly produced in the United States by Wyeth Laboratories, with use of *N*-tributyl phosphate as the inactivating agent. As of 1984, all vaccine sold in the United States is manufactured by Pasteur Mérieux–Connaught (Lyon, France). Pasteur Mérieux–Connaught in Canada also produces an HDCV based on the ERA strain of rabies virus. In Europe, Chiron Behring (Marburg, Germany) and Berna (Bern, Switzerland) also produce HDCV. None of the last three HDCVs contain human albumin or phenolsulfonphthalein.

Storage Conditions. Ideal storage conditions are 2 to 8°C, at which temperatures the vaccine is stable for at least 3.5 years.[88] However, vaccine stored for 1 month at 37°C was still potent.[89, 90]

Other Cell Culture Vaccines (CCVs)

There have been intense efforts worldwide to produce vaccines at a low cost that meet or improve on the levels of safety and efficacy achieved with HDCV. These new tissue culture vaccines are listed in Table 31–2. All cell culture vaccines must have a potency of at least 2.5 IU per dose as measured by the NIH test.

A continuous African green monkey kidney cell line, called *Vero*, has come into use as a cell substrate for viral vaccines, and a new cell culture rabies vaccine *(PVRV)* has been developed and licensed by Pasteur Mérieux–Connaught in Europe and in many countries in the developing world.[91] An advantage of the Vero cell is that it can be grown and infected on microcarrier beads and cultivated in fermenters to produce large volumes of tissue culture fluid containing rabies virus.

The rabies virus strain in PVRV is the same as that used for HDCV production. It is inactivated with β-propiolactone and concentrated and purified by zonal centrifugation and ultrafiltration. Clinical studies have shown that the VNA responses after primary and booster injections are equivalent to those seen after preexposure or postexposure treatment with HDCV.[92] Postexposure protection has been demonstrated in Thailand,[93] without unusual adverse reactions.

Purified chick embryo cell culture vaccine (PCECV), prepared by Chiron Behring, has been evaluated together with HDCV in postexposure protection of animals and humans.[94–97] No significant differences between the two vaccines were observed. To prepare PCECV, the Flury LEP-C25 strain is grown in primary chick embryo fibroblasts. The virus is inactivated by β-propiolactone and then concentrated and purified by density gradient centrifugation. The vaccine contains processed gelatin as stabilizer and traces of neomycin, chlortetracycline, and amphotericin B. PCECV is now registered worldwide, including the United States, and about 20 million doses have been used. Sehgal and colleagues[98] reviewed 10 years' experience with PCECV. The vaccine was well tolerated, with only 4% of 1375 people reporting reactions, although some urticarial reactions have been seen.[99] Immunogenicity was also good, with geometric mean titers (GMTs) of neutralizing antibodies after postexposure treatment of about 4 IU and of less than 1 IU in only 0.9% of patients. A similar type of vaccine (Flury HEP strain) is produced in Japan with limited distribution.[100]

Primary hamster kidney cell rabies vaccine (PHKCV) is produced by the Institute of Poliomyelitis and Virus Encephalitides, Moscow, and was approved for use in China in 1980, where it has completely replaced the Semple-type rabies vaccine. The Chinese vaccine contains the Beijing strain, which is inactivated by formalin. The final material contains 0.012% thimerosal and 10 mg human albumin. In addition, a freeze-dried concentrated PHKCV has been developed and is being administered on a five- or six-dose schedule in China.[101]

Swiss Serum and Vaccine Institute, Bern, has introduced a *purified DEV (PDEV)* that contains only about 1% of the protein of the previous DEV with thiomerosal as preservative. This vaccine is also based on the Pitman-Moore strain. Concentration is achieved by density gradient ultracentrifugation and inactivation by β-propiolactone. Potency testing and antibody responses evoked in humans are comparable to those of HDCV. Mild local reactions are noted that occur only slightly more frequently than with HDCV. PDEV differs from other cell culture vaccines in that, after reconstitution, it is a slightly turbid suspension. Its nucleoprotein content is higher than that of other vaccines.[102] If it is used intradermally, the dose must be 0.2 mL.[103, 104]

To provide an alternative to vaccine made in human cells, the Michigan State Health Department prepared a rhesus diploid cell strain vaccine. It adapted the Kissling rabies strain of CVS to DBS-FRHL-2 cell cultures, a fetal *rhesus monkey lung* fibroblast, inactivated it with β-propiolactone, and added alum phosphate.[105, 106] This vaccine *(RVA)* is now licensed in the United States and is available through SmithKline Beecham in liquid form. It is given on the same preexposure schedules as HDCV and is considered to be equally safe and effective,[107] but it is not licensed for intradermal use.

Despite the aforementioned developments, cell culture vaccines are still used far less throughout the world than are nerve tissue vaccines. For development of an even less expensive rabies vaccine, a baby hamster kidney cell line (BHK-21) is under study as vaccine substrate.[108]

Preexposure Immunization

The recommended preexposure immunization regimen in the United States is three doses of HDCV or RVA on days 0, 7, and 21 or 28. The dose is either 1 mL administered intramuscularly or 0.1 mL administered intradermally (see later discussion of intradermal vaccination). An estimated 50,000 people have received rabies preexposure immunization with HDCV in the United States; there have been no rabies cases in any of these individuals.

An attempt was made to use suckling mouse brain vaccine in a preexposure schedule of 0, 2, 4, and 30 days, but the results were unsatisfactory.[109]

Postexposure Prophylaxis

The postexposure regimen recommended in the United States and by WHO is rabies immune globulin (RIG) on day 0 and HDCV on each of days 0, 3, 7, 14, and 28; 1 mL of vaccine is administered intramuscularly in the deltoid area only.[110] In Europe, a sixth dose used to be recommended at 90 days, but the fifth dose may not substantially raise titers beyond those obtained after four doses.[111]

Those who have received prior preexposure or postexposure treatment with a cell culture vaccine, or who have proven VNA to rabies after other vaccines, should receive an intramuscular injection on each of days 0 and 3, without RIG. Anamnestic responses are excellent.[109] Those who have received a non–cell culture vaccine without a documented VNA response must undergo the full postexposure regimen.

Alternative Vaccine Schedules

The application of rabies vaccination faces several practical problems, particularly in developing countries. These include the cost of the vaccine, the cost and the unavailability of antiserum, and the difficulty in getting patients to return a sufficient number of times to complete the series of injections. Therefore, alternatives have been suggested, based on decreasing the number of visits and using the intradermal rather than the intramuscular route of injection.

One such schedule is the 2-1-1 developed in Yugoslavia and also extensively used in France.[113, 114] It consists of two injections of 1.0 mL intramuscularly on day 0 and one each on days 7 and 21. Suckling mouse brain vaccine has also been successfully used according to this schedule.[115] However, if passive immunization is simultaneously used, some reports[116, 117] show that the average antibody response and the persistence of antibody are compromised, whereas other reports[118, 119] show no interference. Immunosuppression by human rabies immune globulin (HRIG) appears to be absent when HDCV is the vaccine used in the 2-1-1 schedule, but in any case, no failures of protection have yet occurred with any vaccine used in this abbreviated schedule.

Intradermal Route of Vaccination

The expense of a full regimen of intramuscular HDCV (about $600 in the United States for a five-dose regimen) has led to attempts to reduce the cost by taking advantage of the intradermal route. Aoki, Turner, Nicholson, and their colleagues demonstrated that rapid antibody responses could be induced by various intradermal regimens, including multisite postexposure inoculations.[120–122] Although injection by the intramuscular and subcutaneous routes results in higher titers, intradermal administration for preexposure or booster vaccinations appears to be adequate.[64, 123] Two intradermal doses of 0.1 mL successfully boosted titers in those previously given DEV.[64, 124]

Intradermal postexposure regimens have now undergone extensive evaluations and are indicated in the circumstances of insufficient vaccine, insufficient funds, and the availability of staff experienced in intradermal injection technique. The vaccines that may be used by this route are HDCV, PVRV, PCECV, and PDEV. The antigenic content of the rehydrated vaccine should always be at least 0.25 IU per 0.1 mL. The injection should be given with use of a 1.0-mL syringe and a 25- or 27-gauge needle, with the needle introduced parallel to the skin into the epidermal layer. A papule should always be produced at the site of the injection.

The manufacturer of HDCV for the United States has developed a prepackaged delivery system for *preexposure* intradermal vaccination. Antibody titers are lower than after intramuscular inoculation but still adequate. Local reactions are annoying but tolerable after preexposure intradermal vaccination, and systemic reactions are virtually absent.[125] Three doses are necessary.[126] The exact number of individuals immunized intradermally is not known, but this route has been widely used to immunize veterinary students and others at high risk of rabies exposure.

However, the death in Kenya in 1983 of a Peace Corps volunteer who had been preimmunized with HDCV by the intradermal regimen raised questions regarding the efficacy of this route.[127] Intensive review of immunization records revealed that people vaccinated overseas, whether intramuscularly or intradermally, often had lower and shorter lived antibody responses than expected from observations made in people immunized in the United States. One factor that has now been shown to be significantly associated with lower immunological responses is the concurrent administration of chloroquine for antimalarial chemoprophylaxis.[128] People receiving concurrent antimalarial chemoprophylaxis or other immunogens are now recommended to receive the intramuscular and not the intradermal regimen for antirabies preexposure immunization. Moreover, those who receive an intradermal preexposure regimen in developing countries should have titers checked after immunization.[129]

Warrell and colleagues[130, 131] developed the concept of multiple intradermal vaccinations to reduce the vaccine dose and the number of visits. HDCV was given intradermally at eight different sites (deltoid, suprascapular, thigh, and abdominal wall on day 0; four 0.1-mL doses over the deltoid and thigh on day 7; and single doses over the deltoid on days 28 and 91).[132] Phanuphak and associates[133] developed another intradermal schedule that is now the standard regimen used in Thailand. PVRV is given over both deltoids in a volume of 0.1 mL on days 0, 3, and 7 followed by single injections on days 30 and 90. This regimen is considerably cheaper than the full intramuscular use of HDCV and has been demonstrated to be protective in Thailand.[55, 134–136]

Intradermal vaccination with HDCV, PVRV, PCECV, and PDEV has been extensively applied in developing countries, particularly Thailand, to make cell culture vaccines available more readily. In the Thai Red Cross schedule, 0.1 or 0.2 mL of PVRV, PCECV, or PDEV is administered at two sites on days 0, 3, and 7, followed by single injections on days 28 and 90. The volume of injection is decided by the volume of reconstitution: 0.1 mL from a 0.5-mL vial and 0.2 mL from a 1.0-mL vial.[137]

Neutralizing responses after intradermal vaccination with HDCV or PVRV were compared in Thailand.[138] All vaccinees in both groups were seropositive at day 14, whereas at day 90, adequate VNA levels were found in 95% of PVRV recipients and 96% of HDCV recipients. In addition, Thai workers simulated two-dose postexposure booster vaccination in subjects previously vaccinated intradermally or intramuscularly with PVRV. The subjects vaccinated and boosted intradermally all developed anamnestic responses, although these were slower and of lower magnitude than in the all intramuscular group.[139]

With use of the same Thai regimen, PDEV was shown to be immunogenic by the intradermal route if the intradermal dose was 0.2 mL, as shown in Table 31–3.[103] PDEV given by either intramuscular or intradermal routes was studied in the Philippines.[139] By day 90, 94% of the intradermal vaccinees and 98% of the intramuscular vaccinees had antibodies above 0.5 IU, and the GMTs were about 3 IU in both groups.

PCECV was also studied in Thailand,[140] both with and without concomitant administration of HRIG. Neutralizing antibodies peaked at a GMT of about 10 IU in

Table 31–3. **GEOMETRIC MEAN TITERS IN INTERNATIONAL UNITS OF NEUTRALIZING ANTIBODIES AFTER VARIOUS INTRADERMAL REGIMENS**

VACCINE	ROUTE	SCHEDULE*	N	DAY 14	DAY 28	N < 0.5 IU
PDEV	IM (for comparison)	A	15	3.1	4.0	0
PVRV	ID	B	9	11.9	5.2	0
PDEV	ID (0.1 mL)	B	11	2.9	1.4	1
PDEV	ID (0.2 mL)	B	12	2.9	1.5	0
PDEV	ID (0.1 mL)	C	16	4.6	3.2	0
PDEV + ERIG	ID (0.2 mL)	B	15	3.0	1.1	0†

*A = One dose on days 0, 3, 7, 14, 28.
B = Two doses on days 0, 3, 7, and one dose on days 28 and 90.
C = Four doses on days 0, 3, 7, and one dose on days 28 and 90.
†One patient was negative at day 90.
ERIG, equine rabies immune globulin; ID, intradermal; IM, intramuscular; PDEV, purified duck embryo vaccine; PVRV, purified Vero cell rabies vaccine.
Adapted from Khawplod P, Glueck R, Wilde H, et al. Immunogenicity of purified duck embryo rabies vaccine "Lyssabvac-N" with use of the WHO-approved intradermal postexposure regimen. Clin Infect Dis 20:646–651, 1995.

both groups, and there were no failures. About 40 patients exposed to rabies were all protected by PCECV.

Currently in India, intradermal vaccination is practiced with the four WHO-approved vaccines, enabling a reduction in cost from $81 for the intramuscular regimen to about $13 for an intradermal regimen.[141]

Serum and Vaccine Treatment

The postexposure protective ability of brain tissue vaccine alone in people bitten by rabid wolves has been frequently questioned. In Iran, Baltazard and Ghodssi[142] observed an overall mortality of 25% in patients bitten by confirmed rabid wolves and treated with nerve tissue vaccine, regardless of the severity and site of the wounds. Among individuals wounded in the head and face, mortality was 42%. When these results were compared with mortality rates observed in individuals exposed to rabid wolves but untreated for various reasons, it appeared that the postexposure treatment of severely exposed individuals with vaccine alone conferred insignificant protection.

The use of antirabies serum in postexposure prophylaxis serum goes back many years; in 1891, Babes and Cerchez[143] treated people severely bitten by rabid wolves with whole blood from vaccinated humans and dogs. Between that year and the 1940s, immune serum was sometimes given in the prevention of experimental rabies in animals or in the postexposure treatment of humans. Results ranged from complete protection to no protection at all.

The efficacy of the combined use of vaccine and rabies serum in postexposure prophylaxis was finally established through studies of the WHO Committee on Rabies. The superior results obtained experimentally by Habel and Koprowski[144] were confirmed in a field study in Iran in 1954.[145] Of 5 patients severely bitten by rabid wolves and treated with vaccine alone, 3 contracted rabies and died, whereas of 13 patients similarly bitten by the same wolf and treated with vaccine and serum, only 1 died. Cho and Lawson[146] performed an experiment on postexposure rabies vaccination. When dogs were inoculated in the masseter muscle with rabies virus, only about 50% of the animals were protected by serum and HDCV. When dogs were inoculated in the femoral muscle, vaccine alone was not protective because of the short incubation period in this experimental system, whereas serum alone protected about 50% and serum together with vaccine protected 100%. Baer and Cleary[147] have shown that HRIG has synergistic activity with HDCV in a mouse challenge model. Thus, these investigators demonstrated again the importance of rapid protection with antibodies and the synergy of serum with postexposure vaccination.

The intended purpose of the RIG is to provide rabies antibody before an active response to the vaccine takes place. Isotyping of antibody after vaccination suggests that immunoglobulin G (IgG) antibody may not appear for 14 days.[148] Evidence that the need for simultaneous RIG and HDCV is not merely theoretical is provided by reports of two cases of rabies that occurred after administration of HDCV without RIG.[149, 150]

HRIG was prepared originally by Cutter and Pasteur Mérieux–Connaught from the plasma of volunteers immunized with HDCV to provide an antibody preparation that would not produce serum sickness. Berna, Bayer, and Centeon (formerly Behringwerke AG) now also produce an HRIG. The products sold in the United States currently are from Pasteur Mérieux–Connaught and Bayer. Administration of RIG has not been associated with reactions other than occasional local pain and low-grade fever.[151] The dose is 20 IU per kg, with as much as possible of the volume instilled at the site of the bite, and the remainder, if any, given into the muscle at a distant site. This recommendation is new, as it has been determined (see later) that VNA after IM administration is low and that local administration of RIG is therefore preferable. That dose should not be exceeded, because too much passive antibody has a dampening effect on the active antibody responses.[152] For the same reason, the dose should not be repeated. However, if the RIG was not given immediately, it should still be given up to the seventh day after exposure. After administration of HRIG, serum neutralizing antibodies can be detected within 24 hours, reach a level of about 0.1 IU at 3 days, and decay with a half-life of about 21 days.[153]

The first commercially available rabies antisera were produced in horses, but because approximately 40% of adult recipients developed serum sickness, they are no longer available in the United States.[154, 155] A purified and pepsin-treated equine rabies immune globulin (ERIG, produced by Swiss Serum Institute and Pasteur Mérieux–Connaught) is available in some countries and is associated with only a 1% rate of serum sickness reactions.[156] The dose is 40 IU per kg.

Wilde and coworkers[156, 157] in Thailand have carefully studied the use of ERIG. In their experience, the risk of anaphylaxis is only 1 in 35,000 people, and only 1 to 1.6% of recipients develop serum sickness. Moreover, although a skin test with 0.02 mL of a 1:100 dilution of ERIG is recommended before use, and the response is positive in 5 to 10% of patients, a positive test response was not predictive of serum sickness. They consider a risk of anaphylaxis to be present only if there is a wheal of 10 mm or greater in diameter or if a wheal of 5 to 10 mm is accompanied by a flare of 20 mm or more.

The Thai group also attempted to answer an often asked question concerning patients who are started on vaccine before coming for RIG treatment. They found that a delay of up to 5 days was acceptable, in that suppression of the active immune response did not occur.[158] Another issue is the importance of local infiltration of antibodies. In fact, serum levels of VNA achieved after intramuscular administration alone may be low or negligible.[159, 160] Local infiltration provides additional VNA at the site of contamination with the virus. To have a sufficient volume for infiltration in the case of multiple bites, particularly in children, the RIG can be diluted in normal saline.[158, 161] Rabies developed in five children in whom local infiltration was not performed as recommended.[162]

American recommendations now call for the local infiltration of the total RIG dose, if feasible. If not, the remainder should be given intramuscularly at a site distant from the vaccine injection.

Results of Immunization

Immune Responses

Extensive studies have been conducted of antibody responses to CCVs.[81, 91–107, 115, 163–173] The essential points discovered during those studies are as follows.

1. The most important immune response to rabies vaccines is antibodies to the G protein of the viral envelope.[18, 163] Antibody is normally measured by neutralization or inhibition of fluorescent foci induced by whole virus.
2. Antibodies appear by 7 to 14 days after the first dose.
3. Vaccine doses given during the first 14 days prime the immune system, but at least one dose at 21 days or later is necessary for high and persistent titers.
4. Three doses of CCV delivered during 21 to 28 days induce antibodies in 100% of individuals and can be used as a preexposure regimen.
5. With this regimen, the GMTs after HDCV were 12.9 IU on day 49 and 5.1 IU on day 90 in one study.[64]
6. With intramuscular vaccination, the primary regimen for postexposure use is four doses given in the first 2 weeks and a fifth dose given as a booster at day 28 or later.
7. Antibody titers after vaccination are usually greater than 10 IU, significantly higher than obtained in control groups given nerve tissue vaccine or DEV.
8. It is not necessary to check rabies antibody titers after preexposure or postexposure immunization with CCV, unless the vaccinee is immunosuppressed, has received chloroquine, or has undergone anesthesia.[174] HIV-infected patients may respond poorly to rabies vaccines[174a] and should be monitored serologically.
9. Subjects older than 50 years respond less well than those younger, but all seroconvert after five doses.[175]
10. The place of cellular immunity in protection remains uncertain. Although cellular responses of both the T helper and the HLA-restricted cytotoxic T-cell types are clearly produced, direct proof of a protective function is lacking, whereas antibodies are demonstrably effective.[21, 176, 177]
11. Vaccinees of HLA group B7 and Dr2 show early and high antibody responses, whereas those of HLA group Dr3 respond late and with low levels.[102]
12. There is molecular mimicry of the nicotine receptor-binding motif between rabies G protein and HIV pg120, which may induce antibodies to HIV in rabies vaccines.[177a]

Protection

The efficacy of Semple-type nerve tissue vaccine has been estimated to be about 84% in India,[178] although protection may be less after severe exposure. For cell culture vaccines, Nicholson[179] estimates a failure rate of 1 in 80,000 in developed countries and between 1 in 12,000 and 1 in 30,000 in developing countries.

During the development of HDCV, efficacy studies were carried out in Iran, Germany, and the United States. In Iran, 45 people exposed in eight different incidents to eight proven rabid wolves or dogs were given six doses of HDCV after exposure. Antirabies serum was also given with the first vaccine doses. The presence of rabies virus in the brain was confirmed for all eight animals. In four animals tested, high virus titers were also found in the salivary glands. All vaccinees developed antibodies (Table 31–4), and none developed rabies.[86] In Germany, 63 individuals bitten by rabid animals were uniformly protected. The accumulated experience of the Centers for Disease Control and Prevention in the United States was summarized in 1980, at which time 90 people exposed to rabid animals had all survived after HDCV vaccination.[180]

The HDCV produced by Berna was subjected to trial in 100 Thai patients exposed to proven rabid animals. All patients were protected by the standard five-dose regimen, although the GMT of rabies neutralizing antibodies at 90 days after the first vaccination was relatively

Table 31–4. **ANTIBODY RESPONSES AFTER ANTISERUM AND HUMAN DIPLOID CELL VACCINE IN IRANIANS EXPOSED TO PROVEN RABID WOLVES AND DOGS**

	DAYS AFTER TREATMENT BEGUN						
TITERS (IU/mL)	0	3	7	14	30	90	100
0	37	1	0	2	0	0	0
<1	0	14	17	4	0	0	0
1–9.9	0	9	8	18	9	7	1
10–99	0	0	0	11	24	27	8
>100	0	0	0	0	5	3	26

From Bahmanyar M, Fayaz A, Nour-Salehi S, et al. Successful protection of humans exposed to rabies infection. Post-exposure treatment with the new human diploid cell rabies vaccine and antirabies serum. JAMA 236:2751–2754, 1976. Copyright 1976, American Medical Association.

low at 2.57 IU.[181] Understandably, there have been no placebo-controlled studies of the efficacy of rabies vaccines. The CCV have been accepted based on the induction of neutralizing antibodies and lack of failures after postexposure vaccination.[93–107]

Protection studies in mice show that antibodies induced by the G protein contained in HDCV neutralized 17 different street rabies viruses.[182]

Persistence of Immunity and Booster Doses. Rabies VNA do not stay at elevated levels for long periods after vaccination with the usual preexposure schedules. By 1 year, VNA fall to levels between 1 and 3.5 IU,[84, 183, 184] and by 2 years, they may fall below the minimum acceptable level of 0.5 IU, which is usually equivalent to a serum dilution of 1:5. Nevertheless, Thraenhart and colleagues[185] reported the presence of VNA in the serum of 18 people vaccinated 2 to 14 years earlier. Antibodies reacting with many virus proteins were still present, in addition to lymphocyte proliferation responses to the same proteins. Booster doses of vaccine were efficient in restoring VNA, with 100% of subjects showing a fivefold rise by day 7.[183] Two booster doses enhance somewhat the speed of the booster response.[186] Therefore, previously immunized individuals who are again exposed to rabies should receive two booster doses 3 days apart, without RIG. Boosters can be given either intramuscularly or intradermally, although a preparation approved for intradermal use is available only in the United States.[187] However, because of allergic reactions to the HDCV used in the United States (see later), routine boosters are not recommended in that country in the absence of definite exposure. Laboratory workers or others who have continuous exposure to rabies should have antibody levels checked every 6 months and should receive a single booster immunization if the titer falls below 0.5 IU.

Briggs and Schwenke[188] compared the persistence of antibodies in civilians and in Peace Corps volunteers who receive chloroquine for prophylaxis of malaria. At 1.5 to 2 years after primary vaccination, adequate titers were found in 99% of civilians and 88% of Peace Corps volunteers who received the vaccine intramuscularly and in 93% of civilians and 64% of Peace Corps volunteers who received the vaccine intradermally, showing that chloroquine was immunosuppressive.

Mechanism of Protection. Preexposure vaccination with potent rabies vaccines leads to the development of VNA. Vaccination also induces production of cytotoxic T cells, which have been shown to protect vaccinated mice in the absence of neutralizing antibodies. A high level of cell-mediated cytotoxic activity can be maintained by repeated inoculations of vaccine, and the presence of VNA does not interfere with the secondary stimulation of sensitized lymphocytes.

The exact mechanism of protection of humans through postexposure vaccination is still unknown, although it is certain that VNA play the major role in this system. The fact that only monoclonal antibodies that interact with macrophages are effective in protection of mice against disease may indicate that a complex mechanism is involved in antibody protection after challenge.

Concentrated and inactivated rabies vaccine of tissue culture origin is able to induce high levels of circulating interferon a few hours after its administration and can protect animals from rabies infection if it is given shortly before or after challenge with virus. This interferon-induced protection, however, is not specific because similar protection can be obtained with concentrated vaccines produced from unrelated viruses, such as influenza and Kern Canyon. However, only the rabies vaccine can protect when it is given several days before challenge with rabies virus. The combined treatment with interferon or interferon inducers in addition to rabies vaccine is more efficacious than vaccine alone in experimental animals when treatment is initiated several hours after challenge.[189] The role of interferon in human prophylaxis is undefined.

Treatment Failures

Thraenhart and colleagues[102] reviewed 28 cases of rabies that developed despite postexposure treatment with modern vaccines. In 90% of cases, RIG had not been administered or had been administered incorrectly. Other errors included passive immunization more than 24 hours before vaccine, incorrect local wound cleansing, injection of vaccine into the buttocks instead of the deltoid, and late initiation of immunization. Only two patients, both of whom had severe facial injuries, could be considered true treatment failures.

A follow-up study of treatment failures after 15 million doses of PCECV reported 47 treatment failures. All had occurred in India and Thailand, and in no case were WHO treatment guidelines completely followed.[190]

Reactions to Rabies Vaccines Containing Animal Brain Tissues[83]

General Systemic Reactions. The various minor disorders that may develop during or after a course of antirabies treatment include fever, headache, insomnia, palpitations, and diarrhea. Sensitization to proteins contained in older vaccines can cause a sudden shock-like collapse, usually toward the end of the course of treatment.

Local Reactions. Erythematous patches may develop approximately 7 to 10 days after the beginning of antirabies treatment. Lesions appear a few hours after vaccine injection and fade in 6 to 8 hours, reappearing after the next vaccine inoculation.

Severe and Fatal Reactions. A patient may suffer from serious and often fatal illness after nerve tissue vaccine. These accidents are of two types: (1) *rage de laboratoire*, a disease induced by the living "fixed virus" present in the old Pasteur vaccine, and (2) *neuroparalytic accidents*, which present the greatest danger from rabies vaccination. All types of vaccine containing adult mammalian nervous tissues exhibit similar capacities for inducing neuroparalytic reactions. The neuroparalytic accident usually develops between the 13th and 15th days of the treatment and may assume one of the following three forms:

1. *Landry type*. In this type of accident, the patient rapidly becomes pyrexial and suffers pain in the back. Flaccid paralysis of the legs begins, and within 1 day, the arms become paralyzed. Later, the paralysis spreads to the face, tongue, and other muscles. The fatality rate is about 30%; in the remaining 70%, recovery usually occurs rapidly.
2. *Dorsolumbar type*. Less severe than the Landry type, this is the most common form of neuroparalytic accident. Clinical features are explicable by the presence of dorsolumbar myelitis. The patient may be febrile and feel weak, with paralysis of the lower limbs, diminished sensation, and sphincter disturbances. The fatality rate does not exceed 5%.
3. *Neuritic type*. In this type of accident, the patient may be pyrexial and usually shows a temporary paralysis of the facial, oculomotor, glossopharyngeal, or vagus nerves.

Neuroparalytic accidents are caused by allergic "encephalomyelitis," attributable specifically to sensitization to adult nerve tissue antigen (myelin basic protein).[191] The incidence of these reactions to nerve tissue vaccine varies widely from 0.017% (1:6000) to 0.44% (1:230) and is definitely lower in people receiving DEV (1:32,000) and in people receiving properly manufactured vaccine of newborn rodent brain (1:8000).

A recently published study observed 1392 Tunisian adults who were given a Semple-type vaccine prepared by phenol inactivation of rabies-infected lamb brains.[192] Seven patients developed neurological complications, including paralysis or paresis in five. Most of the patients had elevated cell counts in their cerebrospinal fluids. A rate of 1 neurological complication in 200 vaccinations is unacceptable and illustrates the desirability of replacing nerve tissue vaccines with cell culture vaccines.

Reactions to Cell Culture Vaccines

General Reactions. CCVs are widely accepted as well-tolerated rabies vaccines, although reported reaction rates to primary immunization have varied with the monitoring system. In a large-scale testing of the safety and immunogenicity of HDCV performed on American veterinary students, adverse reaction rates observed in more than 1770 volunteers were as follows: significantly sore arm (15 to 25%); headache (5 to 8%); malaise, nausea, or both (2 to 5%); and allergic edema (0.1%).[84] In another study of postexposure vaccination, 21% had local reactions, 3.6% had fever, 7% had headache, and 5% had nausea.[180] The most common local reactions are erythema, pain, and induration. When HDCV is administered to children, in whom psychological overlay is presumably less than in adults, there are few complaints.

Allergic Reactions. After licensure of HDCV in the United States and widespread use, allergic reactions began to be reported, principally after booster doses.[193, 194] The overall incidence of reactions was 11 per 10,000 (0.11%) vaccinees, but after boosters, the incidence rose to 6%.[195] Anaphylactic type 1 (IgE) reactions occurred in about 10% of the reported cases, all during the primary series (1 per 10,000 vaccinations), but the majority appeared to be type 3 hypersensitivity (IgG-IgM) reactions occurring 2 to 21 days after booster doses (Table 31–5). These reactions have been attributed to antigenicity conferred on human albumin used as stabilizer in the vaccine by the β-propiolactone used to inactivate the virus, which increases the capacity of the albumin to form immune complexes.[196–198]

Fortunately, respiratory symptoms are mild, and there have been no fatalities. Antihistamines, epinephrine, and occasionally steroids have been used in successful treatment of the reactions, which have resolved in 2 to 3 days.

The Pasteur Mérieux–Connaught Canada, Berna,

Table 31–5. **SIGNS AND SYMPTOMS IN THREE COHORTS CONTAINING 255 SUBJECTS REPORTING PRESUMED IMMUNE COMPLEX–TYPE HYPERSENSITIVITY REACTIONS* AFTER BOOSTER IMMUNIZATION WITH HUMAN DIPLOID CELL RABIES VACCINE (PASTEUR MÉRIEUX–CONNAUGHT) GIVEN INTRADERMALLY OR INTRAMUSCULARLY**

	NUMBER WITH REACTION (%)
Number with any sign or symptom	29 (11.4)
Pruritic rash	17 (59)
Urticaria	24 (90)
Edema	14 (48)
Joint pain	4 (14)
Fever	1 (3)
Difficulty breathing	1 (3)
Mean delay after booster before reaction (range)	9.6 d (3–13 for ID) (8–11 for IM)

* Coombs and Gell type 3.

ID, intradermal; IM, intramuscular.

From Centers for Disease Control. Systemic allergic reactions following immunization with human diploid cell rabies vaccine. MMWR Morb Mortal Wkly Rep 33:185–188, 1984.

and Behring HDCVs are produced by use of additional purification steps to remove human albumin. Systemic reactions to booster doses are uncommon with these vaccines.[199, 199a] The manufacturers of PVRV and PCECV contend that allergic reactions are absent after primary or booster doses with those two CCVs.

Neurological Reactions. Although five cases of central nervous system disease, including transient neuroparalytic illness of the Guillain-Barré type, have been reported among the millions of individuals given HDCV,[200–204] this rate is too low to be certainly related to vaccination, because the background incidence of such diseases is about 1 per 100,000 per year. The low incidence after HDCV compares with a neurological complication rate of 1:1600 people for nerve tissue vaccine, 1:8000 for suckling mouse brain vaccine, and 1:32,000 for DEV.

In Thailand, a switch from Semple-type vaccine to HDCV resulted in a drop in the rate of neurological complications from 1 per 155 to less than 1 per 50,000 treatments. At the same time, the failure rate dropped from 1 per 2000 to 1 per 25,000 treatments without the use of RIG.[205] If reactions occur after one CCV, a switch can be made to another without danger.

Indications for Vaccination

Preexposure Vaccination

All high-risk professionals, such as veterinarians, hunters, trappers, dog catchers, mail carriers, speleologists, and laboratory workers contemplating working with rabies virus, should be prophylactically immunized against rabies. The recommended regimens are given in Table 31–6. After receiving the three-dose preexposure regimen, those who are repeatedly exposed to high concentrations of rabies virus aerosols in the laboratory should have VNA levels checked every 6 months and should be given a booster dose intramuscularly or intradermally if the titer is less than 0.5 IU. Veterinarians and others exposed to rabid animals should be similarly checked every 2 years.

Immunization of travelers against rabies is controversial. Peace Corps workers or others who remain for long periods in rabies enzootic countries certainly deserve preexposure vaccination. A survey of travelers revealed that after an average of 17 days in Thailand, 1.3% and 8.9% had been bitten or licked by a dog, respectively, and 0.5% had required rabies vaccination.[206] Moreover, vaccination in developing countries is often complicated by problems of availability of potent vaccine and RIG.[207] On the other hand, a decision analysis concluded that routine preexposure vaccination would cost $275,000 per case averted and that it should be individualized according to the traveler's situation.[208] Our recommendation would be to vaccinate those who will be staying in remote areas for more than a few days, particularly children.

In countries where rabies is endemic and children are frequently exposed to rabid animals, one might contemplate prophylactic vaccination against rabies as part of pediatric immunization. Dog bites are a considerable problem in many areas of the world and accounted for more than 5% of visits to the emergency department of a Bangkok hospital, of which 55% were by children.[209] So far, prophylaxis has been restricted to the children of Westerners going to live in areas enzootic for rabies,[210] but clinical trials in children have been performed in developing countries.[211] A preliminary study was done with the PVRV vaccine in Thailand, where two doses were given in association with routine pediatric immunizations at 2 and 4 months of age.[212] Seroconversion to rabies occurred in 100% of infants, without significant interference with the other vaccines.

Booster Vaccination

After preexposure vaccination, antibodies decline sharply within the first year of vaccination. If a booster dose is given 1 year later, subjects segregate themselves into two groups: good responders, who develop a titer

Table 31–6. **REGIMENS FOR PREEXPOSURE AND POSTEXPOSURE VACCINATION WITH RABIES VACCINES**

VACCINATION	ROUTE	DAYS ON WHICH DOSES ARE GIVEN	REMARKS
Preexposure	IM†	0, 7, 21 or 28	Standard regimen
	ID‡	0, 7, 21, or 28	Economical, but not to be used in those taking antimalarial medications
Postexposure*	IM†	0, 3, 7, 14, 28	U.S. and WHO recommendation
	IM†	0 (2 doses), 7, 21	Used in some countries when RIG is not indicated
	ID‡	0, 3, 7 (2 doses each), 28, 90	Used in Thailand with PVRV, PCECV, or PDEV
	ID‡	0 (8 doses), 7 (4 doses), 28, 90	Used in developing countries with cell culture vaccine
Booster (for reexposure)	IM†	0, 3	Only after documented vaccination with cell culture vaccine§
	ID‡	0, 3	Only after documented vaccination with cell culture vaccine§

*Together with rabies immune globulin.
†0.5 mL or 1.0 mL, depending on the vaccine, given into the deltoid.
‡0.1 mL or 0.2 mL, depending on the vaccine, given over the deltoid. HDCV is the only vaccine licensed for intradermal use in the United States.
§Or demonstrated presence of virus-neutralizing antibodies after other vaccines.
ID, intradermal; IM, intramuscular; PCECV, purified chick embryo cell culture vaccine; PDEV, purified duck embryo vaccine; PVRV, purified Vero cell rabies vaccine; RIG, rabies immune globulin; WHO, World Health Organization.

greater than 30 IU by 14 days after booster; and poor responders, whose titers are lower. The former, who represent 75% of subjects, may not need further booster vaccination for 10 years, whereas the latter may need more frequent boosters.[213]

Primary vaccination by the intradermal route gives less sustained immunity, but the intradermal route is an effective means of giving a routine booster.[214]

Postexposure Vaccination

The essential triad of postexposure rabies prophylaxis is local treatment, vaccination, and antiserum administration.

Local treatment of bites and scratches consists of vigorous washing with soap and water, followed, if possible, with 70% alcohol, 0.1% quaternary ammonium compound, or povidone-iodine. If possible, surgical suturing should be avoided for 7 days; but in any case, RIG (see later) should always be administered before suturing.[215]

A decision to give postexposure rabies vaccine should be based on consideration of the following issues.[216, 217]

1. Was the patient's skin broken by the bite or scratch, or were mucous membranes contaminated? If not, no real exposure has occurred. The risk of rabies after bite by a rabid animal has been estimated at 5 to 80%, whereas the risk of scratches is much less (0.1 to 1%). The risk after mucous membrane contact is low.[218] However, see number 10 relative to bat exposures.

2. If the bite was by a dog or cat, is domestic animal rabies found in the particular geographical area? Many areas of the world, such as Australia, Antarctica, and the United Kingdom, are free of rabies in mammals. In many cities of the United States, even stray animals are unlikely to be rabid.

3. Was the dog or cat vaccinated against rabies? Vaccination diminishes the risk, but not completely. Proper vaccination of pets should not be accepted at face value. Documentation should be required to show at least two vaccinations with a potent vaccine; one dose of inactivated vaccines is insufficient to guarantee protection.[215, 219]

4. Is the biting animal a domestic dog or cat and available for observation? If yes, vaccination may be postponed. However, in rabies enzootic areas, vaccination may be advisable, even if the domestic animal appears normal, because rabies may be subclinical.[220]

5. If the bite was inflicted by a wild animal, was it a species likely (e.g., skunk and raccoon) or unlikely (e.g., squirrel and rat) to be rabid?

6. Was the bite provoked or unprovoked? This criterion is useful only in areas of low incidence and not where the incidence of rabies in dogs is elevated.[215] In Thailand, even when the animal's behavior appeared normal, an assessment of provocation did not correlate with the presence of rabies at autopsy of the animal.[221] Attempts to play with wild animals should be considered provocative.

7. If exposure was to a rabid human, use the same criteria for vaccination as with a biting animal. Only individuals who were bitten or scratched, who gave mouth-to-mouth respiration, or who were exposed to saliva or nerve tissues need to be vaccinated.[108]

8. RIG should always be given in combination with vaccine according to the Advisory Committee on Immunization Practices, but only for certain categories of exposures according to WHO. (See previous discussion on serum and vaccine treatment.) The dose of HRIG is 20 IU per kg, that of ERIG 40 IU per kg. As much as possible of the RIG should be inoculated locally, diluted if necessary in saline to provide sufficient volume. If necessary, local anesthesia can be provided with procaine-type compounds.[222] The remainder, if any, should be given in the deltoid or gluteus muscles.

9. The dose is the same regardless of age; children tolerate vaccination well and demonstrate excellent antibody response, as has been demonstrated in different ethnic groups.[223–226]

10. Rabies postexposure prophylaxis is recommended for all people with bite, scratch, or mucous membrane exposure to a bat, unless the bat is available for testing and is negative for evidence of rabies. The inability of care providers to elicit information surrounding potential exposures may be influenced by the limited injury inflicted by a bat bite (in comparison to lesions inflicted by terrestrial carnivores) or by circumstances that hinder accurate recall of events. Therefore, postexposure prophylaxis is also appropriate even in the absence of a demonstrable bite or scratch when there is reasonable probability that such contact occurred (e.g., a sleeping individual awakens to find a bat in the room, an adult witnesses a bat in the room with a previously unattended child, mentally deficient person, intoxicated individual).

Fortunately, tests of antigens obtained from humans postvaccination with HDCV or PECECV show good neutralization of rabies virus from bats.[226a]

Useless vaccination can be avoided if circumstances are found that make the chances of rabies exposure remote. Tables 31–7 to 31–9 should be consulted as a guide for the selection of postexposure prophylaxis in the United States and elsewhere in the world.[219, 227] Table 31–6 describes preexposure and postexposure regimens.

If an individual is vaccinated with a cell culture rabies vaccine and later exposed again to rabies, one booster injection of a vaccine may be sufficient for protection. However, *two* doses are recommended. Patients who give a history of vaccination with nerve tissue vaccines responded poorly to boosters in 18% of cases,[228] and they should therefore receive a full primary regimen unless antibodies were previously shown to be present.

Contraindications to Vaccination

Because rabies is a lethal disease, any contraindication to postexposure treatment should be considered carefully before disqualifying an individual for antirabies treatment after high-risk exposure.

Individuals with histories of severe allergies are more prone to develop allergic reactions to rabies vaccine, for

Table 31–7. **RABIES POSTEXPOSURE PROPHYLAXIS GUIDE, UNITED STATES, 1998**

ANIMAL	EVALUATION AND DISPOSITION OF ANIMAL	POSTEXPOSURE PROPHYLAXIS RECOMMENDATIONS
Dogs, cats, and ferrets	Healthy and available for 10 days of observation	Should not begin prophylaxis unless animal develops clinical signs of rabies*
	Rabid or suspected rabid	Immediate vaccination
	Unknown (e.g., escaped)	Consult public health officials
Skunks, raccoons, foxes, and most other carnivores; bats	Regarded as rabid unless animal proven negative by laboratory tests†	Consider immediate vaccination
Livestock, small rodents, lagomorphs (rabbits and hares), large rodents (woodchucks and beavers), and other mammals	Consider individually	Consult public health officials Bites of squirrels, hamsters, guinea pigs, gerbils, chipmunks, rats, mice, other small rodents, rabbits, and hares almost never require antirabies postexposure prophylaxis

*During the 10-day observation period, begin postexposure prophylaxis at the first sign of rabies in a dog, cat, or ferret that has bitten someone. If the animal exhibits clinical signs of rabies, it should be euthanized immediately and tested.

†The animal should be euthanized and tested as soon as possible. Holding for observation is not recommended. Discontinue vaccine if immunofluorescence test results of the animal are negative.

From Centers for Disease Control and Prevention Advisory Committee on Immunization Practices (ACIP). Rabies Prevention—United States, 1998, recommendations of the ACIP. MMWR: in Press, 1998.

Table 31–8. **RABIES POSTEXPOSURE PROPHYLAXIS SCHEDULE, UNITED STATES, 1998**

VACCINATION STATUS	TREATMENT	REGIMEN*
Not previously vaccinated	Local wound cleansing	All postexposure treatment should begin with immediate thorough cleansing of all wounds with soap and water. If available, a virucidal agent such as a povidone-iodine solution should be used to irrigate the wounds.
	HRIG	20 IU/kg body weight. If anatomically feasible, *the full dose* should be infiltrated around the wound(s), and any remaining volume should be administered IM at an anatomic site distant from vaccine administration. Also, HRIG should not be administered in the same syringe as the vaccine. Because HRIG may partially suppress the active production of antibody, no more than the recommended dose should be given.
	Vaccine	HDCV, RVA, or PCECV, 1.0 mL, IM (deltoid area†), one each on days 0, 3, 7, 14, and 28.
Previously vaccinated‡	Local wound cleansing	All postexposure treatment should begin with immediate thorough cleansing of all wounds with soap and water. If available, a virucidal agent such as a povidone-iodine solution should be used to irrigate the wounds.
	HRIG	HRIG should *not* be given.
	Vaccine	HDCV, RVA, or PCECV, 1.0 mL, IM (deltoid area†), one each on days 0 and 3.

*These regimens are applicable for all age groups, including children.

†The deltoid area is the only acceptable site of vaccination for adults and older children. For younger children, the outer aspect of the thigh may be used. Vaccine should never be administered in the gluteal area.

‡Any person with a history of preexposure vaccination with HDCV, RVA, or PCEC; prior postexposure prophylaxis with HDCV, RVA, or PCEC; or previous vaccination with any other type of rabies vaccine and a documented history of antibody response to the prior vaccination.

From Centers for Disease Control and Prevention Advisory Committee on Immunization Practices (ACIP). Rabies Prevention—United States, 1998, recommendations of the ACIP. MMWR: in Press, 1998.

HDCV, human diploid cell vaccine; HRIG, human rabies immune globulin; IM, intramuscularly; PCECV, purified chick embryo cell culture vaccine; RVA, rabies vaccine, adsorbed.

Table 31–9. **WORLD HEALTH ORGANIZATION POSTEXPOSURE PROPHYLAXIS RECOMMENDATIONS**

CATEGORY	TYPE OF CONTACT WITH A SUSPECTED OR CONFIRMED RABID ANIMAL	RECOMMENDED TREATMENT
I	Touching or feeding of animals Licks on intact skin	None, if reliable case history is available. Preexposure treatment may be offered.
II	Nibbling of uncovered skin Minor scratches or abrasions without bleeding Licks on broken skin	Administer vaccine immediately. Stop treatment if animal remains healthy throughout an observation period of 10 days or if animal is killed humanely and found to be negative for rabies by appropriate laboratory techniques.
III	Single or multiple transdermal bites or scratches Contamination of mucous membrane with saliva, i.e., licks	Administer rabies immune globulin and vaccine immediately. Stop treatment if animal remains healthy throughout an observation period of 10 days or if animal is killed humanely and found to be negative for rabies by appropriate laboratory techniques.

From WHO Expert Committee on Rabies. World Health Organ Tech Rep Ser 824:1–84, 1992.

which prophylactic antihistamines may be helpful. When those individuals are vaccinated, epinephrine should be available. If an allergic reaction occurs, one may give an alternative vaccine of different tissue origin, for example, RVA (in the United States), PVRV, or PCECV in the case of a reaction to HDCV. A similar strategy was applied in allergic individuals in whom brain tissue vaccine caused symptoms of central nervous system involvement during the course of injections. Administration of nerve tissue vaccine was immediately interrupted, and the series was completed with vaccine produced in tissue other than brain.

However, only severe reactions not controlled with premedication are grounds for interruption of rabies vaccination. Treatment with steroids may control allergy but may also inhibit VNA responses. Accordingly, antibody titers should be determined after the last dose if steroids have been used. Similarly, patients receiving immunosuppressive medications for other diseases should have VNA levels checked after immunization to verify an adequate response to the vaccine.[229]

Pregnancy is not a contraindication to rabies vaccination.[230, 231] Follow-up of 202 Thai women vaccinated during pregnancy revealed no excess of medical complications or abnormal births.[232]

The "Fourth"-Generation Rabies Vaccines

Excellent results have been obtained with a recombinant vaccine in which the genome for the rabies glycoprotein has been inserted in vaccinia virus,[233] as evidenced by the development of VNA and protection against virus challenge. Recombinant poxvirus vaccines are being used extensively in animals (see under *Rabies Vaccination of Animals*), and both vaccinia and canarypox vectors containing the rabies G protein have been prepared and tested in humans.[234, 235] With both vectors, two injections at 1-month intervals raised protective levels of rabies neutralizing antibodies, although at lower levels than two injections of HDCV given at the same interval. A third dose of the vectors gave striking booster effects, both to those who had received the vectors previously and to those who had received the HDCV previously.

A plasmid containing the cDNA of the gene for the rabies G glycoprotein was constructed and tested in mice.[236] Even one inoculation induced VNA, and three inoculations produced high titers. The mice were protected on challenge with wild virus.

An exciting development is the discovery of the importance of the rabies nucleoprotein (N) in protection.[237, 238] Although the G protein alone is protective in experimental animals, so is the N protein, but without the induction of neutralizing antibodies. After vaccination with cell culture rabies vaccine, antibodies appear to both N and G proteins.[239] The function of N may be to induce protective cellular immune responses, but it also appears to enhance antibody responses to G.[22, 240] The N protein might be used to sensitize hosts to rabies proteins, so that subsequent injection of cell culture vaccine would result in prompt development of high titers of neutralizing antibodies. The N protein can be produced in a baculovirus vector, which is a potential source of antigen for large-scale preexposure immunization of humans and animals.[241] Large amounts of G protein can also be produced by baculovirus vectors.[242]

Although synthetic peptides have been constructed that in laboratory animals produce antibodies binding to the respective peptide and to components of rabies virus, none of the peptides has so far induced either development of VNA or protection against rabies virus challenge. Anti-idiotypic antibodies as vaccines are still experimental.[243]

PUBLIC HEALTH CONSIDERATIONS

Rabies Vaccination of Animals

From the beginning of his involvement with rabies, Pasteur recognized that, for the most part, protection of humans could be effectively achieved through the vaccination of dogs. Although dogs were used to obtain most of the experimental data on protection from 1884 to 1885, it was not until the early 1920s that a practical and successful canine vaccine was developed.

The first vaccine for mass vaccination of dogs was a modified Semple type prepared by Umeno and Doi[244] in Tokyo in 1921. It proved effective in controlling rabies in dogs in Japan and in other countries that produced and used this type of vaccine. The quality of vaccine improved greatly with Habel's introduction of a standard mouse potency test for the Semple-type vaccine, which ensured the potency of the vaccines in mass vaccination programs.[245]

In 1945, Johnson[246] demonstrated that a single dose of a potent, phenol-inactivated vaccine protected dogs against a challenge with street rabies virus for a period of more than 1 year. From 1945 on, this was virtually the only type of vaccine used for control of rabies in dogs, cats, and other domestic animals.

A modified live virus vaccine was introduced by Koprowski and Cox[247] in 1948. Successive passages of a strain of virus of human origin, first in 1-day-old chicks and then in embryonated hens' eggs, resulted in the loss of pathogenicity for dogs, providing an attenuated strain safe for dogs, called Flury low egg passage, or LEP. Further passages of Flury LEP virus in embryonated hens' eggs resulted in a vaccine that was no longer effective for adult laboratory animals yet was lethal for newborn mice, called Flury high egg passage, or HEP. Both Flury LEP and HEP are still given to many types of domestic animals in different parts of the world. However, the live attenuated Flury LEP virus vaccine was discontinued in the late 1970s.

Another attenuated strain of rabies virus, Evelyn-Rokitnicki-Abelseth (ERA), was introduced by Canadian workers in 1964.[248] The ERA vaccine was shown to provide excellent immunity, lasting for at least 3 years. However, several vaccine-induced cases of rabies in cats resulted in the cessation of its use.

Several inactivated rabies vaccines for animals prepared from brains of newborn mice or from virus of tissue culture origin were introduced in the 1980s and are now in general use in Europe and the Americas. However, only inactivated virus vaccines are licensed for domestic animals in the United States.

Oral vaccination of wildlife to prevent the spread of rabies in terrestrial animals such as foxes and raccoons has become possible. The SAD B19 (Street Alabama Dufferin) attenuated strain has been put into fish and bone meal baits for the vaccination of foxes.[249] The virus is grown on a baby hamster kidney cell line and is stable even at high environmental temperatures. A dose of approximately 10^6 infectious units immunizes 100% of foxes, which has allowed its wide application in Germany and elsewhere in central Europe.[250] However, because the SAD B19 strain retains residual pathogenicity for rodents, a more attenuated strain called SAG2 has recently been developed.[251]

Genetic engineering has been applied to rabies immunization by the construction of a vaccinia virus recombinant (V-RG) containing the gene for the G protein.[252] The recombinant is placed in baits, and on ingestion by animals it multiplies only in the tonsils and the buccal area. Extensive tests conducted in many species have confirmed the safety and efficacy of vaccination with this construct, and field tests in France, Belgium, Pennsylvania, and Virginia have confirmed the promising laboratory results.[253–255] Widespread application of V-RG in Belgium starting in 1989 reduced fox rabies from 841 cases in that year to 2 cases in 1993. Concomitantly, a marked drop occurred in human exposures requiring vaccination.[256] The widespread use of these oral vaccines has changed the epizootiology of rabies in Europe, and some vaccination with V-RG has begun in the United States, including New Jersey, New York, Massachusetts, Florida, Texas, Vermont, and Ohio.

Rabies Vaccination of Humans

At least 4 million people are vaccinated each year after presumed exposure to rabies, particularly in Asia.[257] It is difficult to define precisely the effect of rabies vaccination on the incidence of human rabies, because the risk of the disease is variable. Nevertheless, when untreated patients who were bitten by proven rabid animals are followed, disease rates of between 3 and 80% have been observed,[5, 258] depending on the location and severity of bites.[259] In the United States, relatively few of the 30,000 to 40,000 people vaccinated annually are actually at risk of rabies. However, the paucity of cases of rabies in individuals given potent vaccines together with antiserum argues that many cases of rabies are being prevented. In Texas in 1989, 34% of the skunks, 19% of the foxes, and 15% of the bats involved in biting incidents were rabid.[260]

Control of dog rabies is jointly responsible with vaccination of exposed humans for the current rarity of human rabies in the United States and Europe. In developing countries, nerve tissue vaccine reduces the incidence of rabies in vaccinees,[258] but large numbers of exposed individuals never receive vaccine. Thus, need exists for inexpensive cell culture vaccines and for health education to aid in appropriate vaccine use.

The majority of human and animal rabies could be prevented by control of the canine population through responsible pet ownership, contraception, capture of stray dogs, and vaccination. The last is a widely effective technique only in developed countries where the cost is acceptable, where booster vaccination of pets can be required, and where there is an adequate medical and veterinary infrastructure. In other areas, with different social conditions, only the first three methods may be feasible, although often with difficulty. An oral vaccine for dogs would be a great advance in the control of rabies, and as stressed before, oral vaccines for certain wildlife vectors have already had an impact on rabies epizootiology. Control of rabies in other mammals, particularly bats, is not presently possible.

Preexposure vaccination with cell culture vaccines could also reduce human rabies in high-risk areas and professions, as has been achieved among veterinarians and Peace Corps workers. Routine preexposure vaccination of children in areas where animal rabies is prevalent is under consideration. The production of recombinant rabies antigens vaccines produced in transgenic plants may be a future consideration for rabies prevention and control in the next century.

REFERENCES

1. Steele JH. History of rabies. In Baer GM (ed). The Natural History of Rabies. Vol. 1. New York, Academic Press, 1975, pp 1–29.
2. Wiktor T. Historical aspects of rabies treatment. In Koprowski H, Plotkin SA (eds). World's Debt to Pasteur. New York, Alan R Liss, 1985, pp 141–151.
3. Pasteur L. Méthode pour prevenir la rage après morsure. C R Acad Sci 101:765–772, 1885.
4. Benitez RM. A 39-year-old man with mental status change. Md Med J 45:765–769, 1996.
5. Hattwick MAW. Human rabies. Public Health Rev 3:229–274, 1974.
6. Smith JS, Fishbein DB, Rupprecht CE, Clark K. Unexplained rabies in three immigrants in the United States. A virologic investigation. N Engl J Med 324:205–211, 1991.
7. Held JR, Tierkel ES, Steele JH. Rabies in man and animals in the US, 1946–1965. Public Health Rep 82:1009–1011, 1967.
8. Hemachuda T. Human rabies: Clinical aspects, pathogenesis, and potential therapy. Curr Top Microbiol Immunol 187:121–143, 1994.
9. Warrell DA. Clinical picture of rabies in man. Trans R Soc Trop Med Hyg 70:188–195, 1976.
10. Anderson LJ, Nicholson KG, Tauxe RV, Winkler WG. Human rabies in the United States, 1960 to 1979: Epidemiology, diagnosis and prevention. Ann Intern Med 100:728–735, 1984.
11. Hattwick MAE, Weis TT, Stechschulte CJ, et al. Recovery from rabies: A case report. Ann Intern Med 76:931–942, 1972.
12. Porras C, Barboza JJ, Fuenzalida E, et al. Recovery from rabies in man. Ann Intern Med 85:44–48, 1976.
13. Winkler WG, Fashinell TR, Leffingwell L, et al. Airborne rabies transmission in a laboratory worker. JAMA 226:1219–1221, 1973.
14. Gode GR, Saksena R, Batra RK, et al. Treatment of 54 clinically diagnosed rabies patients with two survivals. Indian J Med Res 88:564–566, 1988.
15. Alvarez L, Fajardo R, Lopez E, et al. Partial recovery from rabies in a nine-year-old boy. Pediatr Infect Dis J 13:1154–1155, 1994.
16. Dutta JK, Dutta TK. Treatment of clinical rabies in man: Drug

therapy and other measures. Int J Clin Pharmacol Ther 32:594–597, 1994.

17. Wunner WH, Dietzschold B, Wiktor TJ. Antigenic structure of rhabdoviruses. In Von Regenmortel MHV, Neurath AD (eds). Immunochemistry of Viruses. The Basis for Serodiagnosis and Vaccines. New York, Elsevier Science Publishing, 1985, pp 367–388.
18. Wiktor TJ, Gyorgy E, Schlumberger HD, et al. Antigenic properties of rabies virus components. J Immunol 110:269–276, 1973.
19. Gaudin Y, Ruigrok R, Tuffereau C, et al. Rabies virus glycoprotein is a trimer. Virology 187:627–632, 1992.
20. Anilonis A, Wunner WH, Curtis PJ. Structure of the glycoprotein gene in rabies virus. Nature 294:275–278, 1981.
21. Dietzschold B. Rabies virus infection: Genetic mutations and the impact on viral pathogenicity and immunity. Contrib Microbiol Immunol 8:103–124, 1987.
22. Dietzschold B, Ertl HC. New developments in the pre- and post-exposure treatment of rabies. Crit Rev Immunol 10:427–439, 1991.
23. Nathanson N, Gonzalez-Scarano F. Immune response to rabies virus. In Baer GM (ed). The Natural History of Rabies. Boca Raton, FL, CRC Press, 1991, pp 145–161.
24. Xiang ZQ, Knowles BB, McCarrick JW, Ertl HCJ. Immune effector mechanisms required for protection to rabies virus. Virology 214:398–404, 1995.
25. Smith JS. New aspects of rabies with emphasis on epidemiology, diagnosis, and prevention of the disease in the United States. Clin Microbiol Rev 9:166–176, 1996.
26. Crick J, Tignor GH, Moreno K. A new isolate of Lagos bat virus from the Republic of South Africa. Trans R Soc Trop Med Hyg 76:211–213, 1982.
27. Schneider LG, Barnard BJH, Schneider H. Application of monoclonal antibodies for epidemiological investigations and oral vaccine studies. I. African viruses. Proceedings of an International Conference on Rabies Control in the Tropics; Institut Pasteur, Tunis; October 3–6, 1983.
28. Lumio J, Hillbom M, Roine R, et al. Human rabies of bat origin in Europe [letter]. Lancet 2:378, 1986.
29. Foggin CM, Swanepoel R. Rabies in Africa with emphasis on rabies-related viruses. In Koprowski H, Plotkin SA (eds). World's Debt to Pasteur. New York, Alan R Liss, 1985, pp 219–234.
30. Shope RE. Rabies virus antigenic relationships. In Baer GM (ed). The Natural History of Rabies. Vol. 1. New York, Academic Press, 1975, pp 141–152.
31. Gardner SD. Bat rabies in Europe. J Infect 18:205–208, 1989.
32. Lafon M, Herzog M, Sureau P. Human rabies vaccines inducing neutralising antibodies against the European bat rabies virus (Duvenhage) [letter]. Lancet 2:515, 1986.
33. Herzog M, Fritzell C, Lafage M, et al. T and B cell human responses to European bat *Lyssavirus* after post-exposure rabies vaccination. Clin Exp Immunol 85:224–230, 1991.
34. Shankar V, Dietzschold B, Koprowski H. Direct entry of rabies virus into the central nervous system without prior local replication. J Virol 65:2736–2738, 1991.
35. Ray NB, Ewalt LC, Lodmell DL. Rabies virus replication in primary murine bone marrow macrophages and in human and murine macrophage-like cell lines: Implications for viral persistence. J Virol 69:764–772, 1995.
36. Charlton KM. The pathogenesis of rabies and other lyssaviral infections: Recent studies. Curr Top Microbiol Immunol 187:95–119, 1994.
37. Clark HF, Prabhakar BS. Rabies. In Oslen RG, Krakowa S, Blakeslee JR (eds). Comparative Pathobiology of Viral Diseases. Boca Raton, FL, CRC Press, 1985, pp 165–214.
38. Spriggs DR. Rabies pathogenesis: Fast times at the neuromuscular junction. J Infect Dis 152:1362–1363, 1985.
39. Dietzschold B, Kao M, Zheng YM, et al. Delineation of putative mechanisms involved in antibody-mediated clearance of rabies virus from the central nervous system. Proc Natl Acad Sci USA 89:7252–7256, 1992.
40. Lentz TL, Wilson PT, Hawrot E, Speicher DW. Amino acid sequence similarity between rabies virus glycoprotein and snake venom curaremimetic neurotoxins. Science 226:847–848, 1984.
41. Bracci L, Antoni G, Cusi MG, et al. Antipeptide monoclonal antibodies inhibit the binding of rabies virus glycoprotein and alpha-bungarotoxin to the nicotinic acetylcholine receptor. Mol Immunol 25:881–888, 1988.
42. Gastka M, Horvath J, Lentz TL. Rabies virus binding to the nicotinic acetylcholine receptor alpha subunit demonstrated by virus overlay protein binding assay. J Gen Virol 77:2437–2440, 1996.
43. Tsiang H. An in vitro study of rabies pathogenesis. Bull Inst Pasteur 83:41–56, 1985.
44. Tsiang H. Pathophysiology of rabies virus infection of the nervous system. Adv Virus Res 42:375–412, 1993.
45. Fekadu M. Latency and aborted rabies. In Baer GM (ed). The Natural History of Rabies. Boca Raton, FL, CRC Press, 1991, pp 191–198.
46. Kamolvarin N, Tirawatnpong T, Rattanasiwamoke R, et al. Diagnosis of rabies by polymerase chain reaction with nested primers. J Infect Dis 167:207–210, 1993.
47. King AA, Turner GS. Rabies: A review. J Comp Pathol 108:1–39, 1993.
48. Matsumoto S. Electron microscopy of central nervous system infection. In Baer GM (ed). The Natural History of Rabies. New York, Academic Press, 1975, pp 33–61.
49. Sang E, Farr RW, Fisher MA, Hanna SD. Antemortem diagnosis of human rabies. J Family Pract 43:83–87, 1996.
50. Rabies Surveillance Annual Summary, 1983. Atlanta, GA, Centers for Disease Control, November 1985.
51. Steck F, Wandeler A. The epidemiology of fox rabies in Europe. Epidemiol Rev 2:71–96, 1980.
52. Krebs JW, Strine TW, Smith JS, et al. Rabies surveillance in the United States during 1995. J Am Vet Med Assoc 209:2031–2044, 1996.
53. Update: Raccoon rabies epizootic—United States, 1996. MMWR Morb Mortal Wkly Rep 45:1117–1120, 1997.
54. Coleman PG, Dye C. Immunization coverage required to prevent outbreaks of dog rabies. Vaccine 14:185–186, 1996.
55. Wilde H, Chutivongse S, Tepsumethanon W, et al. Rabies in Thailand: 1990. Rev Infect Dis 13:644–652, 1991.
56. Morimoto K, Patel M, Corisdeo S, et al. Characterization of a unique variant of bat rabies virus responsible for newly emerging human cases in North America. Proc Natl Acad Sci USA 93:5653–5658, 1996.
57. Dietzschold B, Rupprecht CE, Tollis M, et al. Antigenic diversity of the glycoprotein and nucleocapsid proteins of rabies and rabies-related viruses: Implications for epidemiology and control of rabies. Rev Infect Dis 10:S785–S798, 1988.
58. Sacramento D, Badrane H, Bourhy H, Tordo N. Molecular epidemiology of rabies virus in France: Comparison with vaccine strains. J Gen Virol 73:1149–1158, 1992.
59. von Teichman BF, Thomson GR, Meredith CD, Nel LH. Molecular epidemiology of rabies virus in South Africa: Evidence for two distinct virus groups. J Gen Virol 76:73–82, 1995.
60. Smith JS, Orciari LA, Yager PA, et al. Epidemiologic and historical relationships among 87 rabies virus isolates determined by limited sequence analysis. J Infect Dis 166:296–307, 1992.
61. Brogan T, Bratton S, Dowd M, Hegenbarth M. Severe dog bites in children. Pediatrics 96:947–950, 1995.
62. Wilde H. Managing facial dog bites [letter; comment]. J Oral Maxillofac Surg 53:1368, 1995.
63. Bögel K, Motschwiller E. Incidence of rabies and post-exposure treatment in developing countries. Bull World Health Organ 64:883–887, 1986.
64. Bernard KW, Roberts MA, Summer J, et al. Human diploid cell rabies vaccine: Effectiveness of immunization with small intradermal or subcutaneous doses. JAMA 247:1138–1142, 1982.
65. Immunization Practices Advisory Committee (ACIP). Rabies prevention—United States, 1991. MMWR Morb Mortal Wkly Rep 40(RR3):1–19, 1991.
66. World Health Organization. Sixth Report of the Expert Committee on Rabies. Geneva, WHO Technical Report No. 523, 1973.
67. Remington PL, Shope T, Andrews J. A recommended approach to the evaluation of human rabies exposure in an acute-care hospital. JAMA 254:67–69, 1985.
68. Fekadu M, Endeshaw T, Alemu W, et al. Possible human-to-human transmission of rabies in Ethiopia. Ethiop Med J 34:123–127, 1996.

69. Human rabies—California, 1995. MMWR Morb Mortal Wkly Rep 45:353–356, 1996.
70. Krebs JW, Strine TW, Smith JS, et al. Rabies surveillance in the United States during 1995. J Am Vet Med Assoc 209:2031–2044, 1996.
71. Warrell MJ. Human deaths from cryptic bat rabies in the USA. Lancet 346:65–66, 1995.
72. Fermi C. Über die Immunisierung gegen Wutkrankheit. Z Hyg Infectionskrankh 58:233–276, 1908.
73. Semple D. The preparation of a safe and efficient antirabic vaccine. Sci Mem Med Sanit Dep India, No. 44, 1911.
74. Fuenzalida E, Palacios R, Borgono JM. Anti-rabies antibody response in man to vaccine made from infected suckling-mouse brains. Bull World Health Organ 30:431–436, 1964.
75. Peck FB, Powell HM, Culbertson CG. Duck-embryo rabies vaccine: Study of fixed virus vaccine grown in embryonated duck eggs and killed with betapropiolactone. JAMA 162:1373–1376, 1956.
76. Kissling RE. Growth of rabies virus in non-nervous tissue culture. Proc Soc Exp Biol 98:223–225, 1958.
77. Fenje P. A rabies vaccine from hamster kidney tissue cultures: Preparation and evaluation in animals. Can J Microbiol 6:605–610, 1960.
78. Hayflick L, Moorhead PS. The serial cultivation of human diploid cell strains. Exp Cell Res 25:585–621, 1961.
79. Plotkin SA. Vaccine production in human diploid cell strains. Am J Epidemiol 94:303–306, 1971.
80. Wiktor TJ, Sokol F, Kuwert E, Koprowski H. Immunogenicity of concentrated and purified rabies vaccine of tissue culture origin. Proc Soc Exp Biol Med 131:799–805, 1969.
81. Wiktor TJ, Plotkin SA, Grella DW. Human cell culture rabies vaccine. JAMA 224:1170–1171, 1973.
82. Sikes RK, Cleary WF, Koprowski H, et al. Effective protection of monkeys against death by street virus by post-exposure administration of tissue culture rabies vaccine. Bull World Health Organ 45:1–11, 1971.
83. Wiktor TH. Virus vaccines and therapeutic approaches. In Bishop HDL (ed). Rhabdoviruses. Vol. 3. Boca Raton, FL, CRC Press, 1980, pp 99–112.
84. Plotkin SA. Rabies vaccine prepared in human cell cultures: Progress and perspectives. Rev Infect Dis 2:433–447, 1980.
85. Plotkin SA, Wiktor TJ. Rabies vaccination. Annu Rev Med 29:583–591, 1978.
86. Bahmanyar M, Fayaz A, Nour-Salehi S, et al. Successful protection of humans exposed to rabies infection. Post-exposure treatment with the new human diploid cell rabies vaccine and antirabies serum. JAMA 236:2751–2754, 1976.
87. Winkler WG. Current status of use of human diploid cell strain rabies vaccine in the United States, May, 1984. In Vodopija I, Nicholson KG, Smerdel S, Bijok U (eds). Improvements in Rabies Post-Exposure Treatment. Zagreb Institute of Public Health, 1985, pp 3–9.
88. Chippaux A, Chaniot S, Piat A, Netter R. Stability of freeze-dried tissue culture rabies vaccine. In Kuwert EK, Merieux C, Koprowski H, Bogel K (eds). Rabies in the Tropics. Berlin, Springer-Verlag, 1985, pp 322–324.
89. Nicholson KG, Ali S, Burnery MI, Perkins FT. Stability of human diploid-cell strain rabies vaccine at high ambient temperatures. Lancet 1:916–917, 1983.
90. Turner GS, Nicholson KG, Tyrrell DAJ, Aoki FY. Evaluation of a human diploid cell strain rabies vaccine: Final report of a three year study of pre-exposure immunization. J Hyg (Lond) 89:101–110, 1982.
91. Montagnon BJ. Polio and rabies vaccines produced in continuous cell lines: A reality for Vero cell line. Dev Biol Stand 70:27–47, 1989.
92. Ajjan N, Pilet C. Comparative study of the safety and protective value, in pre-exposure use, of rabies vaccine cultivated on human diploid cells (HDCV) and of the new vaccine grown on Vero cells. Vaccine 7:125–128, 1989.
93. Suntharasamai P, Warrell MJ, Warrell DA, et al. New purified Vero-cell vaccine prevents rabies in patients bitten by rabid animals. Lancet 2:129–131, 1986.
94. Bijok U, Vodopija I, Smerdel S, et al. Purified chick embryo cell (PCEC) rabies vaccine for human use: Clinical trials. Behring Inst Mitt 76:155–164, 1984.
95. Scheiermann N, Baer J, Hilfenhaus J, et al. Reactogenicity and immunogenicity of the newly developed purified chick embryo cell (PCEC)–rabies vaccine in man. Zentralbl Bakteriol Hyg A 265:439–450, 1987.
96. Nicholson KG, Farrow PR, Bijok U, Barth R. Pre-exposure studies with purified chick embryo cell culture rabies vaccine and human diploid cell vaccine: Serological and clinical responses in man. Vaccine 5:208–210, 1987.
97. Dreesen DW, Fishbein DB, Kemp DT, Brown J. Two-year comparative trial on the immunogenicity and adverse effects of purified chick embryo cell rabies vaccine for pre-exposure immunization. Vaccine 7:397–400, 1989.
98. Sehgal S, Bhattacharya D, Bhardwaj M. Ten year longitudinal study of efficacy and safety of purified chick embryo cell vaccine for pre- and post-exposure prophylaxis of rabies in Indian population. J Commun Dis 27:36–43, 1995.
99. Dutta JK. Adverse reactions to purified chick embryo cell rabies vaccine [letter]. Vaccine 12:1484, 1994.
100. Arai YT, Ogata T, Oya A. Studies on Japanese-produced chick embryo cell culture rabies vaccines. Am J Trop Med Hyg 44:131–134, 1991.
101. Fangtao L. The protective effect of the large-scale use of PHKC rabies vaccine in humans in China. Bull World Health Organ 68:449–454, 1990.
102. Thraenhart O, Marcus I, Kreuzfelder E. Current and future immunoprophylaxis against human rabies: Reduction of treatment failures and errors. Curr Top Microbiol Immunol 187:173–194, 1994.
103. Khawplod P, Glueck R, Wilde H, et al. Immunogenicity of purified duck embryo rabies vaccine "Lyssabvac-N" with use of the WHO-approved intradermal postexposure regimen. Clin Infect Dis 20:646–651, 1995.
104. Rubin RH, Hattwick MA, Jones S, et al. Adverse reactions to duck embryo rabies vaccine. Range and incidence. Ann Intern Med 78:643–649, 1973.
105. Berlin BS, Mitchell JR, Burgoyne GH, et al. Rhesus diploid rabies vaccine (adsorbed), a new rabies vaccine. Results of clinical studies simulating prophylactic therapy for rabies exposure. JAMA 249:2663–2665, 1983.
106. Burgoyne GH, Kajiya KD, Brown DW, Mitchell JR. Rhesus diploid rabies vaccine (adsorbed): A new rabies vaccine using FRhL-2 cells. J Infect Dis 152:204–210, 1985.
107. Berlin BS. Rabies vaccine adsorbed: Neutralizing antibody titers after three-dose pre-exposure vaccination. Am J Public Health 80:476–477, 1990.
108. Perrin P, Madhusudana S, Gontier-Jallet C, et al. An experimental rabies vaccine produced with a new BHK-21 suspension cell culture process: Use of serum-free medium and perfusion-reactor system. Vaccine 13:1244–1250, 1995.
109. Zanetti CR, Chaves LB, Silva ACR, et al. Studies on human antirabies immunization in Brazil. I—evaluation of the 3 + 1 pre-exposure vaccination schedule under field conditions. Rev Inst Med Trop São Paulo 37:349–352, 1995.
110. Fishbein DB, Sawyer LA, Reid-Sanden FL, et al. Administration of human diploid-cell rabies vaccine in the gluteal area [letter]. N Eng J Med 318:124, 1988.
111. Hasbahceci M, Kiyan M, Eyol E, et al. Human diploid-cell rabies vaccine: Efficacy of four doses. Lancet 347:976–977, 1996.
112. Plotkin SA, Wiktor TJ, Koprowski H, et al. Immunization schedules for the new human diploid cell vaccine against rabies. Am J Epidemiol 103:75–80, 1976.
113. Vodopija I, Sureau P, Lafon M, et al. An evaluation of second generation tissue culture rabies vaccines for use in man: A four-vaccine comparative immunogenicity study using a pre-exposure vaccination schedule and an abbreviated 2-1-1 postexposure treatment. Vaccine 4:245–248, 1986.
114. Vodopija I. Current issues in human rabies immunization. Rev Infect Dis 10:S758–S763, 1988.
115. Zanetti CR, Lee LM, Chaves LB, et al. Studies on human antirabies immunization in Brazil. II—preliminary evaluation of the 2-1-1 schedule for human pre-exposure anti-rabies immunization, employing suckling mouse brain vaccine. Rev Inst Med Trop São Paulo 37:353–356, 1995.
116. Chutivongse S, Wilde H, Fishbein DB, et al. One-year study of the 2-1-1 intramuscular postexposure rabies vaccine regimen in

100 severely exposed Thai patients using rabies immune globulin and Vero cell rabies vaccine. Vaccine 9:573–576, 1991.
117. Vodopija I, Sureau P, Smerdel S, et al. Interaction of rabies vaccine with human rabies immunoglobulin and reliability of a 2-1-1 schedule application for postexposure treatment. Vaccine 6:283–286, 1988.
118. Vodopija L, Sureau P, Smerdel S, et al. Comparative study of two human diploid rabies vaccines administered with antirabies globulin. Vaccine 6:489–490, 1988.
119. Wasi C, Chaiprasithikul P, Auewarakul P, et al. The abbreviated 2-1-1 schedule of purified chick embryo cell rabies vaccination for rabies postexposure treatment. Southeast Asian J Trop Med Public Health 24:461–466, 1993.
120. Aoki FY, Tyrrell DAH, Hill LE. Immunogenicity and acceptability of a human diploid cell culture rabies vaccine in volunteers. Lancet 1:660–662, 1975.
121. Turner GS, Aoki FY, Tyrrell DA, et al. Human diploid cell strain rabies vaccine. Lancet 1:1379–1380, 1976.
122. Nicholson KG, Prestage H, Cole PJ, et al. Multisite intradermal antirabies vaccination: Immune responses in man and protection of rabbits against death from street virus by postexposure administration of human diploid-cell strain rabies vaccine. Lancet 2:915–918, 1981.
123. Ajjan N, Soulebot JP, Triau R, Biron G. Intradermal immunization with rabies vaccine: Inactivated Wistar strain cultivated in human diploid cells. JAMA 244:2528–2531, 1980.
124. Burridge MJ, Baer GM, Sumner JW, Sussman O. Intradermal immunization with human diploid cell rabies vaccine. JAMA 248:1611–1614, 1982.
125. Dreesen DW, Brown WJ, Kemp DT, et al. Pre-exposure rabies prophylaxis: Efficacy of a new packaging and delivery system for intradermal administration of human diploid cell vaccine. Vaccine 2:185–188, 1984.
126. Turner GS, Nicholson KG, Tyrrell DAJ, Aoki FY. Evaluation of a human diploid cell strain rabies vaccine: Final report of a three year study of pre-exposure immunization. J Hyg (Camb) 89:101–110, 1982.
127. Centers for Disease Control. Human rabies—Kenya. MMWR Morb Mortal Wkly Rep 32:494–495, 1983.
128. Pappaioanou M, Fishbein DB, Dreesen DW, et al. Antibody response to reexposure human diploid cell rabies vaccine given concurrently with chloroquine. N Engl J Med 314:280–284, 1986.
129. Bernard KW, Fishbein DB, Miller KD, et al. Pre-exposure rabies immunization with human diploid cell vaccine: Decreased antibody responses in persons immunized in developing countries. Am J Trop Med Hyg 34:633–647, 1985.
130. Warrell JM, Nicholson KG, Chathavanich P, et al. Multi-site intradermal and multi-site subcutaneous rabies vaccination: Improved economical regimens. Lancet 1:874–876, 1984.
131. Warrell JM, Warrell DA, Chathavanich P, et al. Economical multiple-site intradermal immunization with human diploid-cell strain vaccine is effective for post-exposure rabies prophylaxis. Lancet 1:1059–1062, 1985.
132. Warrell MJ, Nicholson KG, Warrel DA, et al. Economical multiple-site intradermal immunisation with human diploid-cell-strain vaccine is effective for post-exposure rabies prophylaxis. Lancet 1:1059–1062, 1985.
133. Phanuphak P, Khawplod P, Sirivichayakul S, et al. Humoral and cell-mediated immune responses to various economical regimens of purified Vero cell rabies vaccine. Asia Pac J Allergy Immunol 5:33–37, 1987.
134. Chutivongse S, Wilde H, Supich C, et al. Post-exposure prophylaxis for rabies with antiserum and intradermal vaccination. Lancet 335:896–898, 1990.
135. Suntharasamai P. Clinical trials of rabies vaccines in Thailand. Southeast Asian J Trop Med Public Health 19:537–547, 1988.
136. Phanuphak P, Khawplod P, Sirivichayakul S, et al. Humoral and cell-mediated immune responses to various economical regimens of purified Vero cell rabies vaccine. Asia Pac J Allergy Immunol 5:33–37, 1987.
137. Report of a WHO Consultation on Intradermal Application of Human Rabies Vaccines [abstract]. Geneva, World Health Organization, 1995, pp 2–19.
138. Chutivongse S, Wilde H, Supich C, et al. Post-exposure prophylaxis for rabies with antiserum and intradermal vaccination. Lancet 335:896–898, 1990.
139. Kositprapa C, Limsuwun K, Wilde H, et al. Immune response to simulated postexposure rabies booster vaccination in volunteers who received preexposure vaccinations. Clin Infect Dis 25:614–616, 1997.
140. Suntharasamai P, Chaiprasithikul P, Wasi C, et al. A simplified and economical intradermal regimen of purified chick embryo cell rabies vaccine for postexposure prophylaxis. Vaccine 12:508–512, 1994.
141. Dutta JK, Warrell MJ, Dutta TK. Intradermal rabies immunization for pre- and post-exposure prophylaxis. Natl Med J India 7:119–122, 1994.
142. Baltazard M, Ghodssi M. Prévention de la rage humaine. Rev Immunol 17:366–375, 1953.
143. Babes V, Cerchez T. Traité de la rage. Ann Inst Pasteur 10:625–702, 1891.
144. Habel K, Koprowski H. Laboratory data supporting the clinical trial of antirabies serum in persons bitten by a rabid wolf. Bull World Health Organ 13:773–779, 1955.
145. Baltazard M, Bahmanyar M. Essai pratique du serum antirabique chez les mordus par loups enragés. Bull World Health Organ 13:747–772, 1955.
146. Cho HC, Lawson KF. Protection of dogs against death from experimental rabies by postexposure administration of rabies vaccine and hyperimmune globulin (human). Can J Vet Res 53:434–437, 1989.
147. Baer GM, Cleary WF. A model in mice for the pathogenesis and treatment of rabies. J Infect Dis 125:520–527, 1972.
148. Gluck R, Wegmann A, Germanier R, et al. Confirmation of need for rabies immunoglobulin as well as post-exposure vaccine. Lancet 2:1216–1217, 1984.
149. Devriendt J, Staroukine M, Costy F, Vanderhaegen JJ. Fatal encephalitis apparently due to rabies: Occurrence after treatment with human diploid cell vaccine but not rabies immune globulin. JAMA 248:2304–2306, 1982.
150. Wattanastri S, Boonthai P, Thongcharoen P. Human rabies after late administration of human diploid cell vaccine without hyperimmune serum. Lancet 2:870–896, 1982.
151. Helmick CG, Johnstone C, Sumner J, et al. A clinical study of Mérieux human rabies immune globulin. J Biol Stand 10:357–367, 1982.
152. Anderson JA, Daly FT, Kidd JC. Human rabies after antiserum and vaccine postexposure treatment. Case report and review. Ann Intern Med 64:1297–1302, 1966.
153. Loofbourow JC, Cabaso VJ, Roby RE, Anuskiewicz W. Rabies immune globulin (human). Clinical trials and dose determination. JAMA 217:1825–1831, 1971.
154. Centers for Disease Control. Rabies prevention—United States. MMWR Morb Mortal Wkly Rep 33:393–408, 1984.
155. Karliner JS. Incidence of reactions following administration of antirabies serum. JAMA 193:359–362, 1965.
156. Wilde H, Chomchey P, Punyaratabandhu P, et al. Purified equine rabies immune globulin: A safe and affordable alternative to human rabies immune globulin. Bull World Health Organ 67:731–736, 1989.
157. Tantawichien T, Benjavongkulchai M, Wilde H, et al. Value of skin testing for predicting reactions to equine rabies immune globulin. Clin Infect Dis 21:660–662, 1995.
158. Khawplod P, Wilde H, Chomchey P, et al. What is an acceptable delay in rabies immune globulin administration when vaccine alone had been given previously? Vaccine 14:389–391, 1996.
159. Lang J, Gravenstein S, Briggs D, et al. Evaluation of the safety and immunogenicity of a new, human rabies immune globulin using a sham, post-exposure prophylaxis or rabies. Biologicals 26:7–15, 1998.
160. Lang J, Attanath P, Quimbao B, et al. Evaluation of the safety, immunogenicity, and pharmacokinetic profile of a new, highly purified, heat-treated equine rabies immunoglobulin, administered either alone or in association with a purified, Vero-cell rabies vaccine. Acta Tropica:in press, 1998.
161. Wilde H, Khawplot P, Benjavongkulchai M, Sitprija V. Method of administration of rabies immune globulin. Vaccine 12:1150–1151, 1994.
162. Wilde H, Sirikawin S, Sabcharoen A, et al. Failure of postexpo-

sure treatment of rabies in children. Clin Infect Dis 22:228–232, 1996.

163. Turner GS. Immunoglobulin (IgG) and (IgM) antibody responses to rabies vaccine. J Gen Virol 40:595–604, 1978.
164. Cabasso VJ, Dobkin MB, Roby RE, Hammar AH. Antibody response to a human diploid cell rabies vaccine. Appl Microbiol 27:553–561, 1974.
165. Soulebot JP. Resultats serologiques d'immunization et de hyperimmunization de l'homme avec un nouveau vaccin antirabique obtenu sur cultures de cellules diploides humaines WI-38. La rage: colloque; Paris; Décembre 7, 1973.
166. Bahmanyar M. Results of antibody profiles in man vaccinated with the HDCS vaccine with various schedules. Symp Series Immunol Stand 21:231–239, 1974.
167. Shah U, Jaswal GS, Mansharamani HJ, et al. Trial of human diploid cell rabies vaccine in human volunteers. Br Med J 1:977, 1976.
168. Kuwert EK, Marcus I, Werner J, et al. Postexposure use of human diploid cell culture rabies vaccine. Dev Biol Stand 37:273–286, 1977.
169. Kuwert EK, Marcus I, Werner J, et al. Some experiences with human diploid cell strain (HDCS) rabies vaccine in pre- and post-exposure vaccinated humans. Dev Biol Stand 40:79–88, 1978.
170. Cox JH, Kleitmann W, Schneider LG. Human rabies immunoprophylaxis using HDC (MRC-5) vaccine. Dev Biol Stand 40:105–108, 1978.
171. Plotkin SA, Wiktor TJ. Vaccination of children with human cell culture rabies vaccine. Pediatrics 63:219–221, 1979.
172. Hafkin B, Hattwick MA, Smith JS, et al. A comparison of a WI-38 vaccine and duck embryo vaccine for pre-exposure rabies prophylaxis. Am J Epidemiol 107:439–443, 1978.
173. Kuwert EK, Marcus I, Hoher PB. Neutralizing and complement-fixing antibody responses in pre- and post-exposure vaccines to a rabies vaccine prepared in human diploid cells. J Biol Stand 4:249–262, 1976.
174. Fescharek R, Franke V, Samuel MR. Do anaesthetics and surgical stress increase the risk of post-exposure rabies treatment failure? Vaccine 12:12–13, 1994.
174a. Thisyakorn U, Pancharoen C, Ruxrungtham K, et al. Safety and immunogenicity of preexposure rabies immunization in HIV-infected children. Abstract (83.001) from papers presented and discussions held at the 8th International Congress on Infectious Diseases; International Society for Infectious Diseases; Boston, MA; May 15–18, 1998; p 236.
175. Mastroeni I, Vescia N, Pompa MG, et al. Immune response of the elderly to rabies vaccines. Vaccine 12:518–520, 1994.
176. Suss J, Sinnecker H. Immune reactions against rabies viruses—infection and vaccination. Exp Pathol 42: 1–9, 1991.
177. Celis E, Wiktor TJ, Dietzschold B, Koprowski H. Amplification of rabies virus induces stimulation of human T-cell lines and clones by antigen-specific antibodies. J Virol 56:426–431, 1985.
177a. Bracci L, Ballas SK, Spreafico A, et al. Molecular mimicry between the rabies virus glycoprotein and human immunodeficiency virus-1 GP120: Cross-reacting antibodies induced by rabies vaccinations. Blood 90:3623–3628, 1997.
178. Veeraraghavan N, Subrahmanyan TP. The value of 5 per cent Semple vaccine prepared in distilled water in human treatment: Comparative mortality among the treated and untreated. Indian J Med Res 46:518–524, 1958.
179. Nicholson KG. Modern vaccines. Rabies. Lancet 335:1201–1205, 1990.
180. Anderson LJ, Sikes RK, Langkop CE, et al. Post-exposure trial of a human diploid cell strain rabies vaccine. J Infect Dis 14:133–138, 1980.
181. Wilde H, Glueck R, Khawplod P, et al. Efficacy study of a new albumin-free human diploid cell rabies vaccine (Lyssavac-HDC, Berna) in 100 severely rabies-exposed Thai patients. Vaccine 13:593–596, 1995.
182. Lodmell DL, Smith JS, Esposito JJ, Ewalt LC. Cross-protection of mice against a global spectrum of rabies virus variants. J Virol 69:4957–4962, 1995.
183. Rosanoff E, Tint H. Responses to human diploid cell rabies vaccine: Neutralizing antibody responses of vaccinees receiving booster doses of human diploid cell rabies vaccine. Am J Epidemiol 110:322–327, 1979.
184. Nicholas KG, Turner GS, Aoki FY. Immunization with a human diploid cell strain of rabies virus vaccine: Two year results. J Infect Dis 17:783–788, 1978.
185. Thraenhart O, Kreuzfelder E, Hillebrandt M, et al. Long-term humoral and cellular immunity after vaccination with cell culture rabies vaccines in man. Clin Immunol Immunopathol 71:287–292, 1994.
186. Fishbein DB, Bernard KW, Miller KD, et al. The early kinetics of the neutralizing antibody response after booster immunization with human diploid cell rabies vaccine. Am J Trop Med Hyg 35:663–670, 1986.
187. Burridge MJ, Sumner JW, Baer GM. Intradermal immunization with human diploid cell rabies vaccine: Serological and clinical responses of immunized persons to intradermal booster vaccination. Am J Public Health 74:503–505, 1984.
188. Briggs DJ, Schwenke JR. Longevity of rabies antibody titre in recipients of human diploid cell rabies vaccine. Vaccine 10:125–129, 1992.
189. Baer GM, Moore SA, Shaddock JH, Levy HB. An effective rabies treatment in exposed monkeys: A single dose of interferon inducer and vaccine. Bull World Health Organ 57:807–813, 1979.
190. Fescharek R. What can be learned from a decade of worldwide postmarketing surveillance? [program/abstract 6.07]. International Rabies Meeting; Institut Pasteur, Paris; March 13–14, 1997.
191. Javier RS, Kunishita T, Koike F, Tabira T. Semple rabies vaccine: Presence of myelin basic protein and proteolipid protein and its activity in experimental allergic encephalomyelitis. J Neurol Sci 93:221–230, 1989.
192. Bahri F, Letaief A, Ernez M, et al. Neurological complications in adults following rabies vaccine prepared from animal brains. Presse Med 25:491–493, 1996.
193. Centers for Disease Control. Systemic allergic reactions following immunization with human diploid cell rabies vaccine. MMWR Morb Mortal Wkly Rep 33:185–188, 1984.
194. Dreesen DW, Bernard KW, Parker RA, et al. Immune complex-like disease in 23 persons following a booster dose of rabies human diploid cell vaccine. Vaccine 4:45–49, 1986.
195. Fishbein DB, Yenne KM, Dreesen DW, et al. Risk factors for systemic hypersensitivity reactions after booster vaccinations with human diploid cell rabies vaccine: A nationwide prospective study. Vaccine 14:1390–1394, 1993.
196. Centers for Disease Control. ACIP Rabies Prevention—United States, 1984. MMWR Morb Mortal Wkly Rep 33:393–407, 1984.
197. Anderson MC, Baer H, Frazier DJ, Quinnan JV. The role of specific IgE and β-propiolactone in reactions resulting from booster doses of human diploid cell rabies vaccine. J Allergy Clin Immunol 80:861–868, 1987.
198. Swanson MC, Rosanoff E, Furwith M, et al. IgE and IgG antibodies to β-propiolactone and human serum albumin associated with urticarial reactions to rabies vaccine. J Infect Dis 155:909–913, 1987.
199. Fishbein B, Dreesen D, Holmes D, et al. Human diploid cell rabies vaccine purified by zonal centrifugation: A controlled study of antibody response and side effects following primary and booster pre-exposure immunizations. Vaccine 7:437–442, 1989.
199a. Briggs DJ, Dreesen DW, Morgan P, et al. Safety and immunogenicity of Lyssavac Berna human diploid cell rabies vaccine in healthy adults. Vaccine 14:1361–1365, 1996.
200. Bernard KW, Smith PW, Kader FJ, Moran MJ. Neuroparalytic illness and human diploid cell rabies vaccine. JAMA 248:3136–3138, 1982.
201. Boe E, Nyland H. Guillain-Barré syndrome after vaccination with human diploid cell rabies vaccine. Scand J Infect Dis 12:231–232, 1980.
202. Knittel T, Ramadori G, Mayet WT, et al. Guillain-Barré syndrome and human diploid cell rabies vaccine. Lancet 1:1334–1335, 1989.
203. Tornatore C, Richert J. CNS demyelination associated with diploid cell rabies vaccine. Lancet 335:1346–1347, 1990.
204. Moulignier A, Richer A, Fritzell C, et al. Meningo-radiculite secondaire à une vaccination antirabique. Presse Med 20:1121–1123, 1991.

205. Thongcharoen P, Wasi C, Chavanich L, Sirikawin S. Rabies in Thailand. In Mackenzie JS (ed). Viral Disease in South-East Asia and Western Pacific. New York, Academic Press, 1982, p 606.
206. Phanuphak P, Ubolyam S, Sirivichayakul S. Should travellers in rabies endemic areas receive pre-exposure rabies immunization? Ann Med Interne (Paris) 145:409–411, 1994.
207. Wilde H. Preexposure rabies vaccination. J Travel Med 1:51–54, 1996.
208. LeGuerrier P, Pilon PA, Deshaies D, Allard R. Pre-exposure rabies prophylaxis for the international traveller: A decision analysis. Vaccine 14:167–176, 1996.
209. Fridell E, Grandien M, Johnasson R. Preexposure prophylaxis against rabies in children by human diploid cell vaccine [letter]. Lancet 1:623, 1984.
210. Lumbiganon P, Chaiprasithikul P, Sookpranee T, et al. Pre-exposure vaccination with purified chick embryo cell rabies vaccines in children. Asia Pac J Allergy Immunol 7:99–101, 1989.
211. Bhanganada K, Wilde H, Sakolsataydorn P, Oonsombat P. Dog-bite injuries at a Bangkok teaching hospital. Acta Trop 55:249–255, 1993.
212. Lang J, Duong QH, Nguyen VG, et al. Randomised feasibility trial of pre-exposure rabies vaccination with DTP-IPV in infants. Lancet 349:1663-1665, 1997.
213. Strady A, Lang J, Lienar M, et al. Antibody persistence using pre-exposure regimens of cell-culture rabies vaccines: A ten-year follow up and proposal for a new booster policy. J Infect Dis 177:1290–1295, 1998.
214. Turner GS, Nicholson KG, Tyrell DAJ, Aoki F. Evaluation of a human diploid strain rabies vaccine: Final report of a three year study of pre-exposure immunization. J Hyg (Camb) 89:101–110, 1982.
215. Wilde H. Rabies, 1996. Int J Infect Dis 1:135–142, 1997.
216. Plotkin SA, Clark HF. Rabies. In Feigin RD, Cherry JD (eds). Textbook of Pediatric Infectious Diseases. Philadelphia, WB Saunders, 1998, pp 2111–2125.
217. Mann JM. Systematic decision-making in rabies prophylaxis. Pediatr Infect Dis 2:162–167, 1983.
218. Fishbein DB, Robinson LE. Rabies. N Engl J Med 329:1632–1638, 1993.
219. Rabies prevention—United States, 1991. Recommendations of the Immunization Practices Advisory Committee (ACIP). MMWR Morb Mortal Wkly Rep 40:1–19, 1991; update in press, 1998.
220. Hemachudha T, Chutivongse S, Wilde H, Phanuphak P. Latent rabies. N Engl J Med 324:1890–1891, 1991.
221. Siwasothiwat D, Lumlertdatcha B, Polsuwan C, et al. Rabies: Is provocation of the biting dog relevant to risk assessment? Trans R Soc Trop Med Hyg 86:443, 1992.
222. Kaplan MM, Cohen D, Koprowski H, et al. Studies on the local treatment of wounds for the prevention of rabies. Bull World Health Organ 26:765–775, 1962.
223. Plotkin SA, Wiktor TJ. Vaccination of children with human cell culture rabies vaccine. Pediatrics 63:219–221, 1979.
224. Ajjan N, Strady A, Roumiantzeff M, Xueref C. Effectiveness and tolerance of rabies post-exposure treatment with human diploid cell rabies vaccine in children. In Kuwert EK, Merieux C, Koprowski H, Bogel K (eds). Rabies in the Tropics. Berlin, Springer-Verlag, 1985, pp 85–90.
225. Thongcharoen PW, Wasi C, Chavanich L. Postexposure prophylaxis against rabies in children by human diploid cell vaccine. Lancet 2:436–437, 1982.
226. Lang J, Plotkin SA. Rabies risk and immunoprophylaxis in children. Adv Ped Infect Dis 13:219–255, 1998.
226a. Dietzchold B, Hooper DC. Efficacy of human rabies vaccines for a newly emerging rabies virus strain in North America. Abstract (53.005) from papers presented and discussions held at the 8th International Congress on Infectious Diseases; International Society for Infectious Diseases; Boston, MA; May 15–18, 1998; p 158.
227. WHO Expert Committee on Rabies. World Health Organ Tech Rep Ser 824:1–84, 1992.
228. Khawplod P, Wilde H, Yenmuang W, et al. Immune response to tissue culture rabies vaccine in subjects who had previous postexposure treatment with Semple or suckling mouse brain vaccine. Vaccine 14:1549–1552, 1996.
229. Thongcharoen PW, Wasi C. Possible factors influencing unsuccessful protection of post-exposure prophylaxis for rabies by human diploid cell vaccine. J Med Assoc Thai 68:386–387, 1985.
230. Chabala S, Williams M, Amenta R, Ognjan AF. Confirmed rabies exposure during pregnancy: Treatment with human rabies immune globulin and human diploid cell vaccine. Am J Med 91:423–424, 1991.
231. Chutivongse S, Wilde H. Post-exposure rabies vaccination during pregnancy: Experience with 21 patients. Vaccine 7:546–548, 1989.
232. Chutivongse S, Wilde H, Benjavongkulchai M, et al. Postexposure rabies vaccination during pregnancy: Effect on 202 women and their infants. Clin Infect Dis 20:818–820, 1995.
233. Wiktor TJ, MacFarlane RI, Reagan KJ, et al. Protection from rabies by vaccinia virus recombinant containing the rabies virus glycoprotein gene. Proc Natl Acad Sci USA 81:7194–7198, 1984.
234. Cadoz M, Strady A, Meignier B, et al. Immunisation with canarypox virus expressing rabies glycoprotein. Lancet 339:1429–1432, 1992.
235. Cadoz M, Strady A, Jaussaud B, et al. Tolérance et immunogénicité de deux vaccins antirabiques recombinants: ALVAC-RG et NYVAC-RG. International Rabies Meeting; Institut Pasteur, Paris; March 13–14, 1997.
236. Xiang ZQ, Spitalnik S, Tran M, et al. Vaccination with a plasmid vector carrying the rabies virus glycoprotein gene induces protective immunity against rabies virus. Virology 199:132–140, 1994.
237. Dietzschold B, Wang H, Rupprecht CE, et al. Induction of protective immunity against rabies by immunization with rabies virus ribonucleoprotein. Proc Natl Acad Sci USA 84:9165–9169, 1987.
238. Fekadu M, Sumner JW, Shaddock JH, et al. Sickness and recovery of dogs challenged with a street rabies virus after vaccination with a vaccinia virus recombinant expressing rabies virus N protein. J Virol 66:2601–2604, 1992.
239. Kasempimolporn S, Hemachudha T, Khawplod P, Manatsathit S. Human immune response to rabies nucleocapsid and glycoprotein antigens. Clin Exp Immunol 84:195–199, 1991.
240. Celis E, Rupprecht C. New and improved vaccines against rabies. In Woodrow GC, Levine M (eds). New Generation Vaccines. New York, Marcel Dekker, 1990, pp 419–438.
241. Fu ZF, Dietzschold B, Schumacher CL, et al. Rabies virus nucleoprotein expressed in and purified from insect cells is efficacious as a vaccine. Proc Natl Acad Sci USA 88:2001–2005, 1991.
242. Prehaud C, Takehara K, Flamand A, Bishop DH. Immunogenic and protective properties of rabies virus glycoprotein expressed by baculovirus vectors. Virology 173:390–399, 1989.
243. Reagan KJ, Wunner WH, Wiktor TH, Koprowski H. Anti-idiotypic antibodies induce neutralizing antibodies to rabies virus glycoprotein. J Virol 48:660–666, 1983.
244. Umeno S, Doi Y. The study on the anti-rabic inoculation of dogs and the results of its practical application. Kitasato Arch Exp Med 4:89, 1921.
245. Habel K. Evaluation of a mouse test for the standardization of the immunizing power of antirabies vaccines. Public Health Rep 55:1473, 1940.
246. Johnson HN. Proceedings of the 49th Annual Meeting: United States Livestock Sanitary Association. Washington, DC, 1945, pp 99–107.
247. Koprowski H, Cox HR. Studies on chick embryo adapted rabies virus. J Immunol 60:533–554, 1948.
248. Abelseth MK. An attenuated rabies vaccine for domestic animals produced in tissue cultures. Can Vet J 5:279–293, 1964.
249. Brochier B, Thomas I, Iokem A, et al. A field trial in Belgium to control fox rabies by oral immunisation. Vet Rec 123:618–621, 1988.
250. Schneider LG. Rabies virus vaccines. Dev Biol Stand 84:49–54, 1995.
251. Lafay F, Benejean J, Tuffereau C, et al. P Vaccination against rabies: Construction and characterization of SAG2, a double avirulent derivative of SAD (Bern). Vaccine 12:317–320, 1994.
252. Wiktor T, MacFarlane RI, Dietzschold B, et al. Immunogenic properties of vaccinia recombinants expressing the rabies glycoprotein. Ann Inst Pasteur 136:405–411, 1985.
253. Koprowski H. Rabies oral immunization. Curr Top Microbiol Immunol 146:137–151, 1989.

254. Desmettre P, Languet B, Chappuis G, et al. Use of vaccinia rabies recombinant for oral vaccination of wildlife. Vet Microbiol 23:227–236, 1990.
255. Brochier B, Kieny MP, Costy F, et al. Large-scale eradication of rabies using recombinant vaccinia-rabies vaccine. Nature 354:520–522, 1991.
256. Brochier B, Boulanger D, Costy F, Pastoret PP. Towards rabies elimination in Belgium by fox vaccination using a vaccinia-rabies glycoprotein recombinant virus. Vaccine 12:1368–1371, 1994.
257. Meslin FX, Fishbein DB, Matter HC. Rationale and prospects for rabies elimination in developing countries. Curr Top Microbiol Immunol 187:1–26, 1994.
258. Veeraraghavan N. Scientific report for 1968 of the Pasteur Institute of Southern India, 36, 1969.
259. Hattwick MA, Gregg MB. The disease in man. In Baer GM (ed). The Natural History of Rabies. New York, Academic Press, 1975, pp 281–304.
260. Fishbein DB. Rabies. Infect Dis Clin North Am 5:53–71, 1991.

chapter

32 Tick-Borne Encephalitis Vaccine

P. Noel Barrett

Friedrich Dorner

Stanley A. Plotkin

Tick-borne encephalitis (TBE) virus is a member of the family *Flaviviridae*,[1] which comprises approximately 70 different viruses that cause many serious diseases in a wide variety of vertebrates, including humans. These viruses all are serologically related as determined by hemagglutination inhibition assays.[2] However, by cross-neutralization tests, flaviviruses can be divided into eight serological subgroups, each containing more closely related viruses.[3, 4] The first subgroup contains TBE virus, which can be further differentiated into a Western and a Far Eastern subtype by agar gel diffusion and antibody absorption tests[5] as well as by peptide mapping and monoclonal antibodies.[6, 7]

TBE virus is one of the major human pathogenic flaviviruses. The Far Eastern subtype established itself in 1930 as a major public health problem in central Russia. The effects of the Western subtype, which is prevalent in western, central, and eastern parts of Europe, were first described as early as 1931 by Schneider,[8] who reported a seasonal outbreak of meningitis cases in the district of Neunkirchen in Lower Austria. This was the first report of TBE in the literature. Shortly afterward, the disease was reported from the Far Eastern part of Russia and from 1939 onward also in its European part. In 1949, the virus was isolated for the first time outside of Russia. In subsequent years, TBE has been identified in the majority of European countries. The name *tick-borne encephalitis* refers to the tick, its chief vector. The disease has also been referred to as *spring-summer meningoencephalitis*, *central European encephalitis*, *Far Eastern encephalitis*, *Taiga encephalitis*, or *Russian spring-summer encephalitis*.

Among the flaviviruses, TBE virus has one of the highest impacts as a human pathogen, as indicated by the disease prevalence in endemic areas (for review, see reference 9). According to a study conducted in 1958, 56% of all viral central nervous system diseases in Austria were caused by TBE virus infection.[10] Thus, before the start of the vaccination program, it was the most important and most frequent disease of this type in adults, with several hundred hospitalization cases reported each year.[11]

BACKGROUND

Clinical Description

The clinical course of the disease is largely determined by the TBE virus subtype. Compared with the virus prevalent in Europe, the eastern variety has proved to be more virulent and to lead to paresis far more often; its associated mortality is also higher.[12, 13] The typical course of TBE is diphasic and can be outlined as follows: the incubation period, which is clinically silent, may last between 2 and 28 days,[14, 15] but in most cases it is between 7 and 14 days. The first stage, which may last 1 to 8 days, corresponds to the viremic phase. It is associated with nonspecific systemic signs and symptoms such as fatigue, headache, aching back and limbs, nausea, and general malaise with temperatures rising to 38°C or higher in most cases. Sometimes exceptionally high initial temperatures may occur, rising as high as 40.9°C.[16]

An afebrile interval follows the first stage of TBE and lasts 1 to 20 days. During this time, patients are usually free of symptoms. Another sudden rise of temperature marks the beginning of the second stage of the disease. Only about one third of those symptomatic with TBE virus infection proceed into the second phase of the disease. The clinical manifestations in this second febrile episode are far more serious. The patients run temperatures that are higher than the average temperatures in other forms of viral meningitis or meningoencephalitis. In the majority of cases, there is central nervous system involvement in the form of meningitis with lymphocytosis and elevated cerebrospinal fluid protein. About a third of cases have more severe disease with signs of encephalitis, including paralysis, stupor, and pyramidal tract signs.[17, 18] In paralytic forms of the disease, paralysis, especially in the region of the shoulder girdle, develops 5 to 10 days after the remission of fever. Paralysis may progress up to 2 weeks, followed by a moderate tendency toward improvement.

Hospitalization varies between 3 and 40 weeks,[19, 20] depending on the severity of the illness. In children and juveniles, meningitis is the predominant form of the disease; this is why the infection usually takes a milder course than that observed in adults. Pareses and lasting sequelae are rare in young patients. However, a few cases of severe TBE have been reported, even in young children.[21–23] After the approximate age of 40 years, patients affected by TBE increasingly develop the encephalitic form of the disease. In older patients, especially those older than 60 years, TBE increasingly takes a severe course, leading to paralysis and sometimes resulting in death.[22]

Not all people infected with TBE run the entire course of the disease. In approximately 65% of cases, the infection remains silent, although viremia can be demonstrated; or the patient shows the clinical picture of the initial phase of TBE, but the symptoms subside without developing into full-blown TBE. Approximately 35% of those infected develop the second phase of TBE, the majority of whom run the typical biphasic course. In the remainder, the infection is inapparent during the first stage and the onset of clinical illness coincides with the beginning of the second phase of the disease.[15, 19]

The course of disease in the Far Eastern variety differs clinically from the European form. The onset of illness is more often gradual than acute with a prodromal phase including fever, headache, anorexia, nausea, vomiting, and photophobia. These symptoms are followed by stiff neck; sensorial changes; visual disturbances; and variable neurological dysfunctions, including paresis, paralysis, sensory loss, and convulsions. In fatal cases, death occurs within the first week after onset. The case-fatality rate is approximately 20% compared with 1 to 2% for the European form,[24] but these figures may be biased by the different standards of medical treatment available in western Europe and eastern regions. In contrast to the European form, the disease caused by the Far Eastern variety is more severe in children than in adults. Neurological sequelae occur in 30 to 80% of survivors, especially residual flaccid paralyses of the shoulder girdle and arms.

Virology

Electron microscopy of negatively stained TBE virus shows it to be spherical, with a diameter of about 50 nm, carrying a fringe of small projections on its surface. The virus particle consists of an electron-dense spherical nucleocapsid of approximately 30 nm in diameter that is surrounded by a lipid bilayer. In sucrose density gradients, purified virus sediments homogeneously at about 200 S and bands after equilibrium centrifugation at a density of about 1.19 g per cm^3 (for review, see reference 9). The virus genome consists of a single, positive-stranded RNA molecule of about 11,000 nucleotides in length. Mature virions are composed of three structural proteins termed envelope (E), core (C), and membrane (M) protein with molecular weights of 55,000, 15,000, and 8000, respectively.[25, 26] The envelope proteins E and M are type 1 membrane proteins embedded in the lipid bilayer by C-terminal hydrophobic anchors. In addition, a precursor of the membrane protein (prM) is present in immature intracellular virus particles. C is the only protein constituent of the isometric nucleocapsid that contains the virion RNA. The virus RNA also codes for seven nonstructural (NS) proteins that can be detected only in infected cells. The coding sequence of the positively stranded RNA is 5′-C-prM-E-NS1-NS2A-NS2B-NS3-NS4A-NS4B-NS5-3′. All viral proteins are encoded within a single open reading frame. The individual proteins are released from a precursor polyprotein by cotranslational and posttranslational cleavage.[27]

Glycoprotein E plays a central role in the biology of flaviviruses. It contains the important antigenic determinants responsible for hemagglutination inhibition and neutralization and is responsible for induction of immunological responses in the infected host. Structural elements of the E protein determinants are known to be involved in the binding of virions to cell receptors and in intraendosomal fusion at low pH.[28]

Because it is the critical structural component of the virus involved in the induction of protective immune responses, the antigenic structure of the glycoprotein has been extremely well characterized. In a number of studies using a panel of monoclonal antibodies, 19 different epitopes have been identified and characterized with respect to serological specificity, functional activity, structural properties, and topological relationships.[29–32] Except for three isolated epitopes, other epitopes cluster to form three nonoverlapping domains termed A, B, and C. The epitopes within each domain vary with respect to their serological specificities and functional activities. Domain A contains not only comprehensive flavivirus cross-reactive epitopes (A1, A2) but also flavivirus subtype-specific epitopes (A3, A4). Most of the epitopes in domain B are specific for the tick-borne group of flaviviruses, whereas those in domain C are predominantly subtype-specific epitopes.

The epitopes within each antigenic domain also characteristically have similar structural properties (e.g., sensitivity to denaturation, low pH, proteolysis, reduction of disulfide bridges).[30] For a precise localization of individual epitopes in the sequence of glycoprotein E, antigenic variants of TBE virus that were selected in the presence of neutralizing antibodies were sequenced. In addition, the locations of several immunoreactive fragments of glycoprotein E were determined by amino-terminal sequence analysis.[33] By combining those data with those on the location of disulfide bridges[34, 35] and the structural characteristics of epitopes, such as dependency on confirmation or on intact disulfide bridges or both, a structural model for protein E was constructed that contains information on the folding of the polypeptide chain into distinct protein domains.[33]

A major advance has recently been made in the understanding of the structure and function of glycoprotein E after analysis of the x-ray structure of the protein at 2 Å resolution.[36] X-ray crystallography was carried out using a soluble fragment of the E protein ectodomain produced by trypsin digestion of intact virions.[37] The glycoprotein E is known to exist as a dimer. The x-ray structure demonstrated that the dimer is a head-to-tail oligomer in the shape of a 170 Å rod and predicts that the dimer is anchored in the bilayer at both distal ends, that is, the glycoprotein does not form spike-like projections, like other lipid enveloped viruses, but is aligned parallel to the viral surface (Fig. 32–1). The curvature of the dimer fits with its location on the surface of the 500 Å virion and confirms that these oligomers do not form long projections or spikes. In each monomer, three structural entities are discernible, two of which are related to the previously defined antigenic domains. The carboxy-terminal 100 amino acids (domain III in Fig. 32–1) correspond to antigenic domain B and form a β-barrel composed of seven antiparallel β-strands resembling an immunoglobulin constant domain. This structure is connected by a flexible region to the central domain I, which is folded as an eight-stranded β-barrel with up-and-down topology. It includes the amino-terminal 50 amino acids as well as a sequence element that carries the single carbohydrate side chain and was previously referred to as antigenic domain C. Two long loops extending from this central part of the protein are primarily involved in dimer contacts (domain II) and correspond to antigenic domain A. The localization of neutralization sites can be inferred from the position of amino acid substitutions on monoclonal antibody escape mutants. Mutations leading to escape from neutralization have been mapped to each of the structural domains shown in Figure 32–1.[33, 38–42] The scattered distribution of these neutralization escape mutations over the entire subunit indicates that antibody binding to any of the structural domains can lead to virus neutralization. The mechanisms of neutralization by these antibodies remain a subject of speculation. The functional sites of protein E have not yet been mapped, although it has been suggested that domain III may be involved in receptor binding[43] and that the highly conserved sequence from residues 98 to 111 at the tip of one of the domain II loops (Fig. 32–1) may be involved in fusion activity.[44] Fusion activity requires conformational changes that affect several neutralization epitopes, primarily within the central domain I and II.[44, 45] These changes are apparently associated with a reorganization of the subunit interaction on the virion surface, with trimer contacts favored in the low pH form, as opposed to dimer contacts in the native form.[46] It can be assumed that the interference with these structural rearrangements by antibody binding represents one mechanism leading to virus neutralization.

At present, in addition to the glycoprotein E, only one other viral protein, the nonstructural protein 1 (NS1), has been associated with a role in protective immunity. This is a glycoprotein with molecular weight of approximately 48,000,[47] which is not present in the virion but is found on the surface of infected cells. It has been demonstrated that protective immunity can be elicited by immunization with NS1 from the flaviviruses yellow fever and dengue 2[48–50] and that monoclonal antibodies directed against the NS1 protein of yellow fever virus can also protect animals against infection with this virus.[48] This protection cannot be due to the neutralization of free virus but may result from antibody-dependent cell-mediated cytotoxicity or complement-fixing activity of the antibodies. However, because the NS1 protein is not a component of the successful inactivated whole-virus TBE vaccines, it is clearly not essential for the induction of protective immune responses in the TBE system.

Pathogenesis

The picture of manifest TBE depends on the virulence of the virus and the individual resistance of the patient.[16, 51] After the bite of an infected tick, the virus usually replicates in the dermal cells at the site of the bite. From there the virus is transferred by afferent

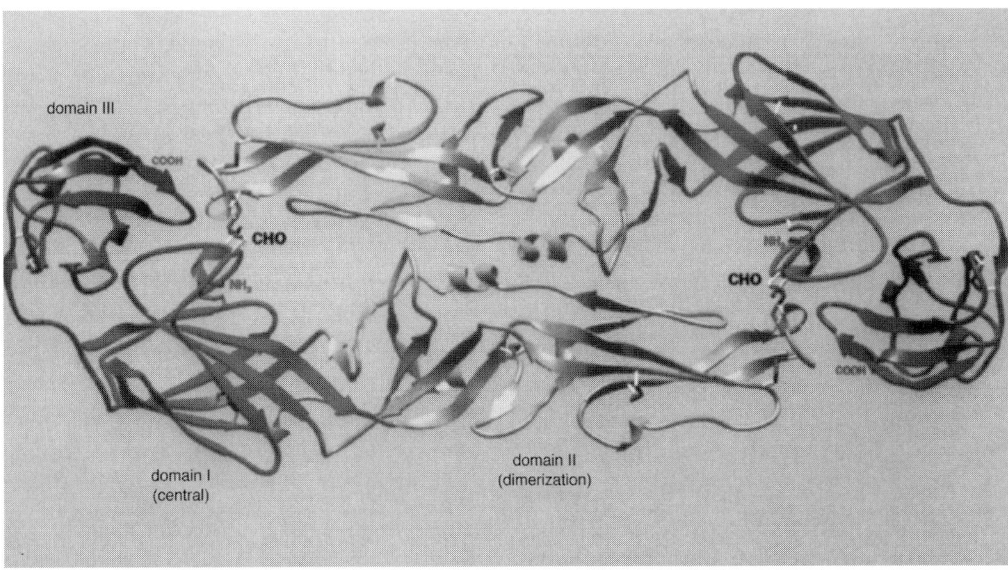

Figure 32–1. Ribbon diagram representing the structure of the membrane anchor-free envelope protein dimer isolated from tick-borne encephalitis virus. The positions of amino acid substitutions in monoclonal antibody escape mutants are indicated by white circles and designated according to Mandl and coworkers.[35] Disulfide bridges and the single carbohydrate side chain (G) attached to domain I are shown as ball and stick representations. (From Rey FA, Heinz FX, Mandl C, et al. The envelope glycoprotein from tick-borne encephalitis virus at 2 Å resolution. Nature 375:291–298, 1995.)

lymphatics to the regional lymph nodes. After further replication in lymphoid tissue, the virus is spread through the lymphatic system and the blood stream, and it invades other susceptible organs or tissues, especially the reticuloendothelial system. Massive virus replication takes place there, and only after this stage is it possible for the virus to reach the central nervous system. High production of virus in the primarily affected organs is a prerequisite for the virus to cross the blood-brain barrier, because the capillary endothelium is not easily infected. Once it has invaded these endothelial cells from the lumen, the virus replicates and enters the central nervous system by seeding through the capillary endothelium into the brain tissue. TBE virus may also spread along nerve fibers. This route may play a role, especially in laboratory infections by aerosols. After infecting the neuroepithelial cells of the nasal mucous membrane, the virus directly enters the brain through the fila olfactoria. Considering the short incubation period and the often extremely severe course of such infections, this route of entry seems likely.[52] However, in arthropod-borne infections, neural spread of the virus is of little importance.

Diagnosis

TBE can be diagnosed definitively only by means of laboratory techniques, because the clinical manifestations of the disease are not specific and are usually not sufficient for diagnosis. However, the laboratory results have no influence on the treatment of TBE and mainly serve for differential diagnosis, because similar symptoms may also be observed in other infections.

In the viremic phase of the initial stage of the disease, the virus can be identified by cultivation in a suitable cell line or in suckling mice.[53] With the onset of the second phase of the disease, the virus can be isolated only from the cerebrospinal fluid.[53, 54]

Because the symptoms that affect the central nervous system are not usually observed until 2 to 4 weeks after the tick bite, antibodies against the virus are nearly always present at the time of admission to hospital and can be detected readily by standard serological tests. Initially a recent infection with TBE virus was established by an increase of the titer in the hemagglutination inhibition test, neutralization test, or complement fixation test or by titer reduction in the hemagglutination inhibition test by 2-mercaptoethanol treatment in one serum sample.[53, 55–57] These tests are now used mainly for confirmatory purposes and are being replaced by rapid, sensitive, and reliable enzyme-linked immunosorbent assay (ELISA) systems based on the detection of immunoglobulin M (IgM) antibodies in the early phase of TBE. A four-layer ELISA system for the detection of TBE virus-specific IgM has been developed that is extremely sensitive and that prevents interference when high-titer virus-specific IgG antibodies for TBE are present.[58] In this system, the solid phase is coated with μ chain–specific antiserum to human IgM. After incubation with the serum sample, purified TBE virus is added, followed by enzyme-labeled anti-TBE virus immunoglobulin. At an early stage after the onset of illness, anti-TBE virus IgM could be detected in serum dilutions up to 10^{-4}. A commercial development of this system (Immunozym FSME, Immuno AG, Austria) allows measurement of both IgM and IgG antibodies.

Treatment

No specific therapy for TBE has been established so far.[16, 51] The treatment of TBE patients with RNAase obtained from bovine pancreas[59] and with emetine[60] has not been generally accepted. Corticosteroids apparently lead to a rapid temperature decrease and an improvement of subjective symptoms[61] but at the same time seem to prolong the period of hospitalization compared with patients receiving only symptomatic treatment. The administration of TBE immune globulin is recommended only within 96 hours after a suspected infection that follows a tick bite (see section on passive immunization).

Because there is no specific treatment targeting the virus itself, symptomatic treatment of patients with TBE is required. The most important measures that can be taken in the clinical management of patients are maintenance of the water and electrolyte balances and of sufficient calorie intake and administration of analgesics, vitamins, and antipyretics.[11, 51, 62, 63] Physiotherapy of paralyzed limbs is essential to prevent muscle atrophy. Because person-to-person transmission of the virus has never been observed, there is no need to isolate TBE patients.[64]

EPIDEMIOLOGY

Incidence and Prevalence

Ticks are the chief vectors and reservoir hosts of TBE virus in nature.[65] In Europe, eight species of ticks have been identified so far that are capable of transmitting TBE virus. *Ixodes ricinus*, the common castor bean tick, is the chief vector and thus is mainly responsible for the spread of the virus in western and central Europe and the European part of Russia, but *Dermacentor* and *Haemaphysalis* species can also transmit the virus.[66] The Far Eastern subtype of the virus is found in the eastern part of Russia, and its vector is primarily *Ixodes persulcatus*.[12, 55] The virus can be transmitted to humans or other hosts by larvae, nymphs, or adult ticks (Fig. 32–2). TBE virus is transferred to the host with the saliva of the infected tick. On humans, ticks attach themselves to the hair-covered portion of the head, the ears, the arm and knee joints, and the hands and feet. The epidermis is punctured with the chelicerae, and the hypostome is inserted. Owing to the anesthetizing effect of the tick's saliva, the bite causes no pain and often passes unnoticed by the host. This may be the main reason that people with manifest TBE sometimes cannot recall having been bitten by a tick.

Ticks parasitize more than 100 different species of mammals, reptiles, and birds. Infection of *I. ricinus* with

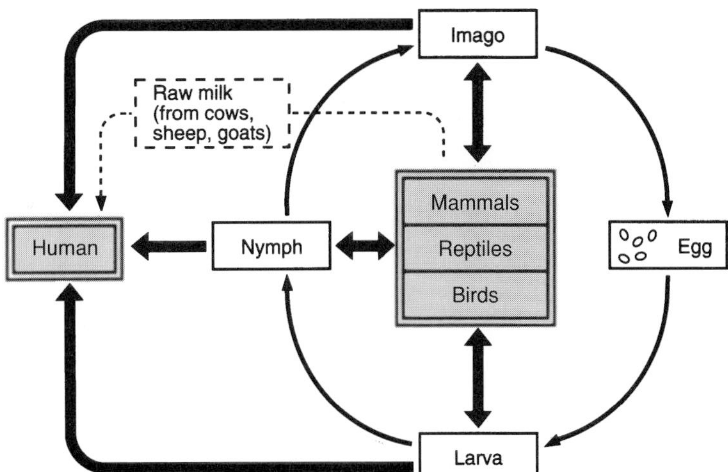

Figure 32–2. Transmission cycle of the tick-borne encephalitis virus in a natural focus.

TBE virus by a host harboring the virus is possible only during the viremic stage in the host, provided the virus titer in its blood is high enough to infect the vector. A long viremic stage, along with a high virus titer, is most likely to be observed in small vertebrates, such as the yellow-necked field mouse, the red-backed vole, the common vole, the dormouse, and the like. In large mammals (e.g., roe, deer, goat), viremia is short-lived, and only low virus titers are reached. During the viremic stage, milk from goats, cows, and sheep may contain the virus and may be a source of infection for humans. Infection by the alimentary route as a result of the ingestion of raw milk has been reported from Poland and the former Yugoslavia,[54, 67] and in 1974, several cases of TBE occurred in Slovakia after the patients had eaten cheese made from raw sheep's milk.[68] However, this route of infection probably does not play any role in western Europe. Laboratory infections have likewise been reported.[69] Although it has not been observed, human-to-human transmission is a theoretical possibility, for example, when blood from a viremic donor is transfused to a patient.

The map presented in Figure 32–3 gives all regions in central and western Europe where TBE infections have so far been recorded. The distribution of the TBE virus covers almost the entire southern part of the non-tropical Eurasian forest belt, from Alsace Lorraine in the West to Vladivostok and northern and eastern regions of China in the East through to Hokkaido in Japan.

Data on TBE prevalence among the inhabitants of endemic areas are presented in Table 32–1. In most endemic areas of Austria and southern Germany, TBE prevalence has been found to be 4 to 8%. In the most severely affected areas in the East and Southeast of Austria, figures up to 14% prevalence may be reached. Prevalence is also extremely high in Russia, followed by the Baltic states, Czech and Slovak republics, eastern Germany, Sweden, and Finland. Little is known about the rate of infection in China.

A much higher percentage of TBE antibody-positive people has been observed among high-risk groups, such as people working in agriculture and forestry, hikers, ramblers, people engaged in outdoor sports, and collectors of mushrooms and berries.

Significance as a Public Health Problem

Table 32–2 lists the number of TBE infections reported in those countries in which the disease is a public health issue or where infections have been reported for a long time. In many of those countries, morbidity has been continually increasing for years. This may partly be due to improved diagnosis of the disease. However, peaks of infection such as that observed in 1994 in Austria may be due to increased activity, after mild winters, in combination with a proliferation of small mammals and as a consequence also of ticks.

PASSIVE IMMUNIZATION

An immunoglobulin concentrate (FSME-Bulin, Immuno AG, Austria) has been developed for the immediate prophylaxis of TBE. This is available as a 16% protein solution and contains specific gamma globulin against TBE virus, with an antibody titer of at least 1:640 as measured in a hemagglutination inhibition test. A similar product (Encegam, Behring, Germany) has recently been licensed in Germany. These can be administered before exposure or up to 96 hours after a tick bite in an endemic area. If more than 4 days have elapsed since an established or assumed tick bite, TBE immune globulin should not be administered for 28 days (the maximum incubation period of TBE) because it may have a negative influence on the course of disease.

Before a possible exposure, a dose of 0.05 mL per kg body weight should be administered intramuscularly. The protection takes effect within 24 hours and lasts approximately 4 weeks. If the risk of exposure continues, the administered dose must be repeated after 4 weeks to maintain the immunological protection. With respect to postexposure prophylaxis, a dose of 0.2 mL per kg body weight should be administered up to 96 hours after the tick bite.

Active immunization with live virus vaccine (e.g., measles, mumps, or rubella) should be postponed until 6 weeks to 3 months after the last administration of the immune globulin, because the efficacy of the live virus vaccine may otherwise be impaired. If the interval be-

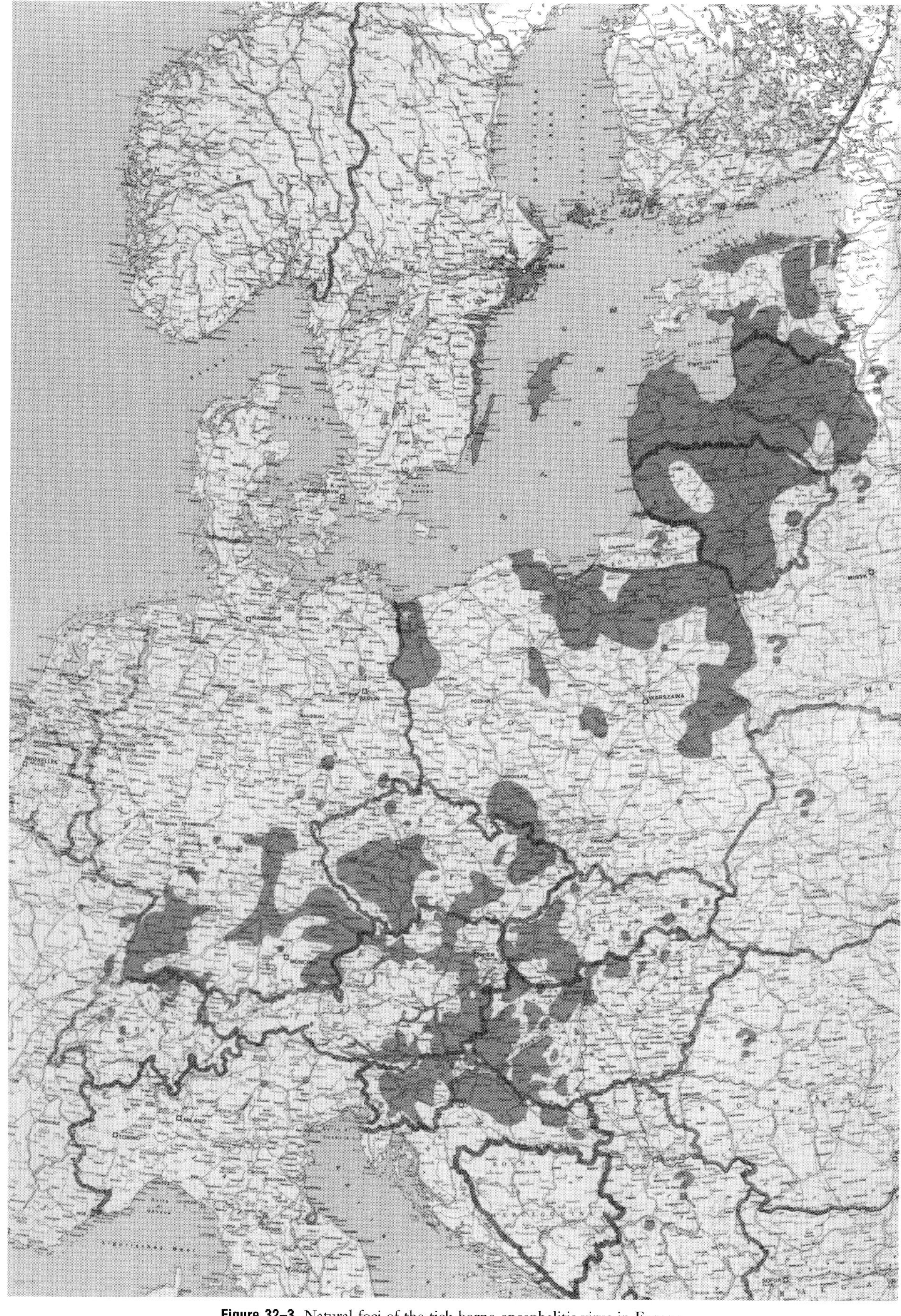

Figure 32–3. Natural foci of the tick-borne encephalitis virus in Europe.

Table 32–1. **PREVALENCE OF ANTIBODY TO TICK-BORNE ENCEPHALITIS VIRUS IN THE POPULATION OF ENDEMIC AREAS**

COUNTRY	PREVALENCE (%)
Austria	4–8
Former Czechoslovakia	2–38
Finland	0.4–39
Former GDR	7–42
Germany	4–8
Hungary	17
Italy	1.5
Sweden	7–29
Switzerland	1.4
Former USSR	30–100

tween the administration of TBE immune globulin and a subsequent injection of TBE vaccine is less than 4 weeks, an impairment of the protective effect of the vaccine may occur.

A number of cases of suspected enhancement of infection have been reported after use of TBE immune globulin in children.[70] For this reason, it has recently been recommended that TBE immune globulin not be used in children younger than 14 years. There is, however, no direct evidence of enhancement of TBE virus infection after correct use of immune globulins in humans, and such enhancement has been demonstrated not to occur in a mouse model.[71]

ACTIVE IMMUNIZATION

Prior Approaches That Have Been Abandoned

In 1937, a few months after identification of the agent responsible for Russian spring-summer encephalitis, the Far Eastern subtype of TBE, vaccinations were carried out in the Russian Army with use of an inactivated suspension from infected mouse brain. This vaccine was the first flavivirus vaccine to be used in humans and was only the third human virus vaccine. Subsequent studies in the former Soviet Union with a similar formalin-inactivated preparation demonstrated the vaccine to be 90% effective in preventing disease.[72] However, the presence of myelin in this crude preparation resulted in an unacceptable level of allergic complications. At that time, attempts to remove the mouse brain component resulted in the loss of most of the viral antigen. Research was then directed toward attempts to produce the vaccine in cell culture, and at the present time two types of formalin-inactivated TBE vaccines derived from chicken embryo cells are in use in the former Soviet Union, both using the Sofjin isolate of TBE virus. The first vaccine is manufactured from nonconcentrated, unpurified virus containing culture fluid.[73] This vaccine, however, contains residual chicken embryo cell impurities and requires a long vaccination schedule. The second vaccine, which is produced only in small quantities, is manufactured by 20- to 30-fold concentration of the initial culture fluid with simultaneous purification of the virus.[74] Although these procedures reduce the reactogenicity of the vaccine, they do not eliminate the problem, because comprehensive data from volunteers still indicate that the vaccine is moderately reactogenic.

First attempts to develop a vaccine against the Western subtype of TBE virus were made in Czechoslovakia in the 1960s.[75, 76] This formalin-inactivated preparation was grown in primary avian fibroblast cultures. The vaccine was shown to be effective in a variety of laboratory animals and also in human volunteers.[77, 78]

Description of Strains and How They Were Developed

In 1971, a cooperative project for the development of an inactivated vaccine that could be produced commercially in large quantities was initiated between Professor Christian Kunz at the Institute of Virology in Vienna, Austria, and the Microbiological Research Establishment in Porton Down, United Kingdom. A vaccine was prepared with use of an Austrian tick virus isolate (Neudörfl), which was cloned in specific pathogen-free chicken embryo cells. The vaccine was prepared by growing virus in suspensions of primary specific pathogen-free chicken embryo cells, clarifying by centrifugation, and purifying by hydroxylapatite chromatography after inactivation with formalin. Aluminum hydroxide was added as an adjuvant. More than 400,000 people were vaccinated in Austria, and serological tests revealed highly satisfactory seroconversion rates of more than 90% after two vaccinations, as measured in the hemagglutination inhibition test.[79] However, because antibodies tended to decline after the second dose, it was necessary to inject a third dose 9 to 12 months later. Despite its efficacy, however, local and systemic side effects, such as headache, malaise, and pyrexia, were common. There were reasons to assume that these side effects were caused by contaminating cellular proteins, and attempts were made to establish a more efficient purification procedure in collaboration with Immuno AG, Austria. This was achieved by the use of continuous-flow zonal centrifugation.[80] Calculated from the potency per microgram of protein, this zonally purified vaccine had a level of purity approximately 90 times higher than that of the previously used vaccine. Subsequent trials in human volunteers showed that the efficacy of this new vaccine was high, and the level of side effects had been reduced drastically.[81]

Producers

This vaccine is now produced commercially by two manufacturers: Immuno AG, Austria, and Chiron Behring, Marburg, Germany. The Austrian manufacturer uses the following manufacturing process for FSME-Immun. A seed virus is prepared from a virus isolated from a pool of five ticks from the area of Neudörfl in Austria. This is passaged once by intracerebral injection of specific pathogen-free (SPF) baby mice, and the virus recovered from the mouse brain suspension is cloned on

Table 32–2. **NUMBER OF ANNUAL DIAGNOSED TICK-BORNE ENCEPHALITIS CASES IN EUROPE AND ASIA**

YEAR	AUSTRIA	FINLAND	FRANCE	GERMANY	ITALY	SWEDEN	SWITZERLAND	CHINA	CROATIA	CZECH R.	ESTONIA	HUNGARY	LATVIA	LITHUANIA	POLAND	SLOVENIA	SLOVAK R.	RUSSIA
1964	101					19			26				6					
1965	129					35			57				6					
1966	136					19			49				9					
1967	60	1				7			36				21					
1968	78		1			13			140				20					
1969	135					16			47				47					
1970	320		1			22	7		107				78		69			
1971	288					22	9		83		9		72		41			
1972	389					33	21		152		10		81		50			
1973	642					18	55		103		12		116		22			
1974	296					29	30		72		13		141		27			
1975	545				3	25	22		86		19		256		26			
1976	346					27	39		84		64		322		40			
1977	318					2	20		34		40		347		54			
1978	351			8		25	31		69		26	287	318		36			
1979	677			11	1	23	41				35	281	220		35			
1980	438	2		32	1	30	13				47	245	184		25			
1981	294	3		30		22	15				43	295	103	13	17			
1982	612	4		97	3	22	57			348	16	351	166	16	9			1365
1983	242	4		29	1	17	10			172	47	207	133	18	20	111		2912
1984	336	11		50		41	32			320	69	406	179	21	25	209		
1985	300	5	1	26		52	15			350	37	226	152	10	14	274	36	
1986	258	5			1	70	27			333	65	372	184	12	10	226	22	
1987	215	6			1	65	34		63	178	91	208	246	9	24	107	24	
1988	201	7	2			43	34		49	191	68	218	119	17	15	114	31	
1989	131	10	3			38	43		62	166		295	117	8	6	65	19	
1990	89	9	2			54	26		23	193	37	222	122	9	8	235	14	5486
1991	128		1	44		75	37		60	356	68	288	227	14	4	245	25	5225
1992	84	14	3	142		83	66		27	337	163	206	287	17	8	210	16	6301
1993	102	25	5	118	3	51	44		76	621	166	329	791	198	249	194	51	7520
1994	178	16	4	306	2	116	97	3500	87	619	177	258	1366	284	181	492	58	5593
1995	109	23	5	220	5	68	60		59	744	175	234	1341	426	270	260	89	5982
1996	128			101	3	40?	62		59	558	177	224	716	309	259		93	9174

primary chicken embryo cells. The cloned virus is then subjected to further passages in SPF baby mice to make a final seed virus that consists of a 2% mouse brain suspension. This material is then passaged once in SPF mouse brain to make the virus suspension used for the inoculation of a primary culture of chicken embryo cells derived from SPF eggs. After inoculation and adsorption of virus, the chicken embryo cells are repeatedly washed to remove mouse brain material. The virus-containing cell supernatant is harvested at the time of maximum virus content and is inactivated by treatment with 0.0185% weight of solute per volume of solvent (w/v) formaldehyde at 37°C. It is then clarified, concentrated, and purified by sucrose density gradient centrifugation. The fraction corresponding to the peak of virus antigen is then diluted, filtered, adsorbed with $Al(OH)_3$, and filled into syringes.

A second European TBE vaccine, similar to FSME-Immun, was licensed in Germany in 1991 (Encepur, Chiron Behring). The K23 virus strain is also grown in primary chicken embryo cells, inactivated by formaldehyde, and purified by continuous-flow density gradient centrifugation.[82] The vaccine is stabilized by processed bovine gelatin and adsorbed onto $Al(OH)_3$.[83, 84] Two concentrations of vaccine were furnished by Chiron Behring, one containing half the dose recommended for children younger than 12 years (Encepur-K).[85] However, the pediatric vaccine has since been withdrawn (see under *Adverse Events*).

Dosage, Route, Preparations, and Constituents

Each FSME-Immun syringe contains 2 to 3.5 μg TBE virus antigen, 1 mg $Al(OH)_3$, less than 0.6 mg human albumin, less than 0.005 mg formaldehyde, and 0.05 mg thimerosal as preservative in a volume of 0.5 mL. The antibiotics gentamicin and neomycin are used in the medium for the production cells but are not detectable in the final product.

An Encepur vaccine dose (0.5 mL) contains 1.5 μg TBE virus antigen, 1 mg $Al(OH)_3$, not more than 0.01 mg formaldehyde, not more than 5 mg polygelin (gelatin) as stabilizer, and trace amounts of the antibiotics neomycin, gentamicin, and chlortetracycline. A pediatric vaccine (Encepur-K) was licensed in 1994 with half the amount of virus antigen (0.75 μg) as in the adult vaccine.

The immunization regimen for FSME-Immun consists of a first dose, followed by a second dose 2 weeks to 3 months later, and a third dose 9 to 12 months after the second dose. According to present experience, the protection achieved by this immunization schedule persists for at least 3 years. A booster injection is recommended 3 years after the last immunization. The vaccine is applied by intramuscular injection, preferably into the upper arm. The immunization schedule for the Chiron Behring vaccine is three injections at 0, 1 to 3 months, and 9 to 12 months after the second dose. A rapid immunization schedule also available for those with immediate risk is three injections on days 0, 7, and 21, followed by a fourth dose 12 to 18 months later.

RESULTS OF VACCINATION

Efficacy and Duration of Immunity

No controlled clinical trials have been carried out to demonstrate the efficacy of vaccination in protecting against disease. However, both commercially available Western vaccines have been demonstrated to be highly effective in inducing seroconversion. A randomized phase II study of the Encepur vaccine reported 100% seroconversion in ELISA after two vaccinations,[86] and a study with the FSME-Immun vaccine reported 98.2% seroconversion in ELISA, also after two vaccinations (unpublished data). The criteria for seroconversion in ELISA were not identical, so it is not possible to directly compare the two vaccines on the basis of these studies. Other studies with FSME-Immun have reported seroconversion rates of 99.5% and 100% after three vaccinations.[81, 87] When blood samples were drawn from different groups of vaccinees 3 to 6 years after the final immunization, a large proportion still had antibodies (Table 32–3). On revaccination, people who had been successfully vaccinated and turned seronegative almost invariably exhibited an IgG response without forming IgM antibodies. Thus, the vaccine appears to establish an immunologic memory that is long lasting. Nevertheless, booster injections are recommended every 3 to 5 years to ensure continuous protection in the vaccinated population.

Seroconversion by ELISA during the basic immunization scheme with the Chiron Behring vaccine is 50%, 98%, and 99% after the first, second, and third doses, respectively. During the rapid immunization schedule, seroconversion occurs in 90% and 99% of subjects after the second and third doses, respectively.[88]

Although it is not widely used in Russia and Asia, cross-protection potency studies in mice showed that the TBE virus vaccine is effective not only against European strains but also against Russian and Asian strains of the virus.[89]

Adverse Events

As with all intramuscularly administered vaccines, occasional local reactions may occur, such as reddening

Table 32–3. **RATE OF SEROCONVERSION AFTER THREE OR MORE TICK-BORNE ENCEPHALITIS VIRUS VACCINATIONS**

TIME AFTER THIRD VACCINATION	HI* N	HI* No. Positive (%)	ELISA* N	ELISA* No. Positive (%)
2 wk	1937	1899 (98)	1723	1714 (99.5)
3 yr	514	384 (74)	490	438 (89)
4 yr	160	126 (79)	145	138 (96)
5 yr	141	126 (88)	144	140 (97)
6 yr	90	73 (82)	88	80 (91)

*Antibody titer measured by hemagglutination inhibition (HI) and enzyme-linked immunosorbent assay (ELISA) tests.

Adapted from Kunz C. Epidemiology of tick-borne encephalitis and the impact of vaccination on the incidence of disease. In Eibl MM, Huber C, Peter HH, Wahn U (eds). Symposium in Immunology V. Berlin, Springer-Verlag, 1996, pp 143–149.

and swelling around the injection site; swelling of the regional lymph nodes; or general reactions, such as fatigue, pain in a limb, nausea, and headache. On rare occasions, temperature higher than 38°C for a short time, vomiting, or temporary rash may occur. In very rare cases, neuritis of a varying degree of severity may be present, although the etiologic relationship to vaccination is uncertain.[89a] After a single dose of vaccine, it was reported that a young woman developed inflammation of the nerves to the gravity muscles in the legs and feet,[90] and neurological complications have also been reported after simultaneous immunization against TBE virus and tetanus.[91] The vaccination is suspected of causing an aggravation of autoimmune diseases such as multiple sclerosis or iridocyclitis in some patients.

Because of the large number of side effects reported with the Encepur vaccine in young children, a pediatric vaccine (Encepur-K) was introduced with a reduced amount of virus antigen (0.75 μg compared with 1.5 μg in the adult vaccine). In a controlled clinical study, it was reported that the frequency of temperature above 38°C was reduced from 30% with the adult formulation to 19% with the pediatric formulation.[85] A survey was carried out among 2800 German pediatricians to determine the rate of side effects associated with this pediatric vaccine in comparison to the standard vaccine FSME-Immun, which is used for both adults and children.[92] The rate of reported side effects was higher for the pediatric vaccine Encepur-K (27%) compared with the FSME-Immun vaccine (3%). All side effects were of a minor nature, consisting of febrile reactions, aching limbs, and headaches.

However, an accumulation of notifications of allergic reactions in children receiving Encepur-K resulted in a withdrawal of that product from the market. The reactions appear to be due to IgE responses to the gelatin stabilizer, reactions also reported after the formulation of other products with gelatin, such as measles-mumps-rubella and Japanese encephalitis vaccines (see relevant chapters).

Indications

Vaccination is warranted for people living in endemic areas (see Fig. 32–3), people working under high-risk conditions (foresters, woodcutters, farmers, military personnel, laboratory workers), and tourists engaged in high-risk activities (e.g., field work, camping, hunting).

Contraindications and Precautions

TBE vaccine should not be given to patients with acute febrile infections. Allergies to components of the vaccines (e.g., thimerosal in FSME-Immun or gelatin in Encepur) or severe reactions to egg ingestion constitute contraindications.

For the Encepur vaccine, it is now recommended that adults with histories of allergies not be vaccinated and that those who have had systemic reactions after vaccination not receive a subsequent dose. All Encepur vaccinees should be kept under observation for a 60-minute period. In the case of a known or suspected autoimmune disease, an unfavorable influence of the vaccination on the autoimmune disease must be weighed against the risk of a TBE virus infection. The safety of both vaccines for use during pregnancy and lactation has not been established in controlled clinical trials, and therefore vaccine should be given only with caution after individual consideration of potential risks and benefits.

Simultaneous Vaccination with Other Vaccines

No time interval is necessary after the administration of other vaccines, either live or inactivated.

Future Vaccines

New formulations of the FSME-Immun vaccine are currently in clinical trials. All are based on a vaccine derived from a modified manufacturing process, which includes two further passages of the mouse brain–derived working virus in chicken embryo cells, before infecting the cells for vaccine production. This development was initiated to eliminate any theoretical possibility that mouse brain material was present in the purified vaccine. Formulations of this vaccine without stabilizers such as human albumin and preservatives such as thimerosal were developed to further reduce the low level of side effects associated with use of this vaccine.

Substrates other than chick embryo cells have also been used for development of experimental TBE vaccines. An experimental Far Eastern Sofjin strain vaccine propagated in primary green monkey kidney cells has been developed in Russia. The use of this substrate provided uniformly higher TBE virus titers than in chick embryo cells, and up to 600,000 doses of TBE vaccine could be produced from every pair of monkey kidneys. Studies on human volunteers also demonstrated this vaccine to be highly immunogenic and have low reactogenicity.[93]

An experimental Neudörfl strain vaccine propagated in a continuous cell line (Vero) has also been developed by Immuno AG.[94] Higher virus titers were achieved in this cell substrate than in chick embryo cells, and the purified vaccine has been demonstrated to be highly immunogenic in mouse protection studies.

A number of recombinant experimental vaccines have been developed in which glycoprotein E was expressed in recombinant vaccinia virus or in mammalian cell lines.[95–99] Whereas soluble envelope glycoproteins were much less immunogenic than inactivated whole-virus particles, micellar aggregates of glycoprotein E or recombinant subviral particles were excellent immunogens and exhibited efficacies similar to those of inactivated virus vaccine with respect to antibody induction and protection against challenge in a mouse model.[98] These studies emphasize that major quantitative and possibly qualitative differences in the immune response are observed when the protein is presented in particulate or soluble form. The best candidate for a recombinant vaccine would thus appear to be particulate subviral particles, which consist of recombinant glycoprotein E in association with prM in dimer form and lipid.

There have been reports of the efficacy of a recombinant NS1 candidate vaccine in protecting mice from challenge with TBE virus.[99, 100] It has also been reported that subneutralizing concentrations of antibodies to glycoprotein E of another flavivirus (i.e., dengue) can mediate antibody-dependent enhancement of infectivity, which has been implicated in the pathogenesis of dengue hemorrhagic fever and dengue shock syndrome.[101] It could therefore be argued that it would be advantageous to use NS1 as the only vaccine component not to incorporate glycoprotein E in a vaccine preparation. However, there is no evidence for TBE vaccine–induced antibody enhancement in humans.

All inactivated and subunit vaccines suffer from the intrinsic disadvantage that booster injections may be required to maintain protective immunity. TBE vaccine booster injections are recommended at 3- to 5-year intervals after an initial immunization schedule of three vaccinations. The development of an attenuated live virus vaccine would provide major advantages with respect to generation of a long-lasting immunity without frequent booster injections. The large amount of information concerning neurovirulence of TBE virus generated by sequencing,[102] monoclonal antibody escape mutant studies,[42] and x-ray crystallography analysis[36] should facilitate the specific generation of stable attenuated live virus vaccines with use of infectious cDNA clone technology.

PUBLIC HEALTH CONSIDERATIONS

Epidemiological Results of Vaccination

The TBE vaccine is widely used in central Europe (approximately 35 million doses have been administered since 1980), and it appears that the vaccine has been a major success in preventing TBE infections in this region. Although the vaccine is not incorporated into routine pediatric immunization, a campaign of voluntary immunization has been instituted since 1980 by the Austrian Health Ministry, so that the majority of children older than 2 years are immunized. This campaign is carried out in early spring of each year, and the vaccine is often given simultaneously with other routine vaccines in children. Figure 32–4 shows that since the beginning of this vaccination campaign in Austria, the number of cases of TBE has been reduced from a high of 677 in 1979 to a low of 84 in 1992. The number of cases increased to 128 in 1996, mainly owing to the climatic conditions of that year. The extensive diagnostic service for TBE in Austria permits calculation of the protection rate of the vaccine using clinical and epidemiological data from the Austrian population.

A calculation of the protection rate of the vaccine for the years 1994 to 1996 in Austria is presented in Table 32–4. Assuming that the total population of Austria (7.8 million) is exposed to the disease, these calculations can be made on the basis of the number of TBE cases occurring in vaccinated and unvaccinated individuals. Protection rates varying from 95.6 to 100% could be calculated after two or three immunizations in these 3 years. These data suggest that TBE virus is one of the most effective viral vaccines.

Disease Control Strategies

Because ticks attach to any spot on the host and from there try to reach an uncovered part of the skin, adequate clothing may help to make access to the skin more difficult for ticks.

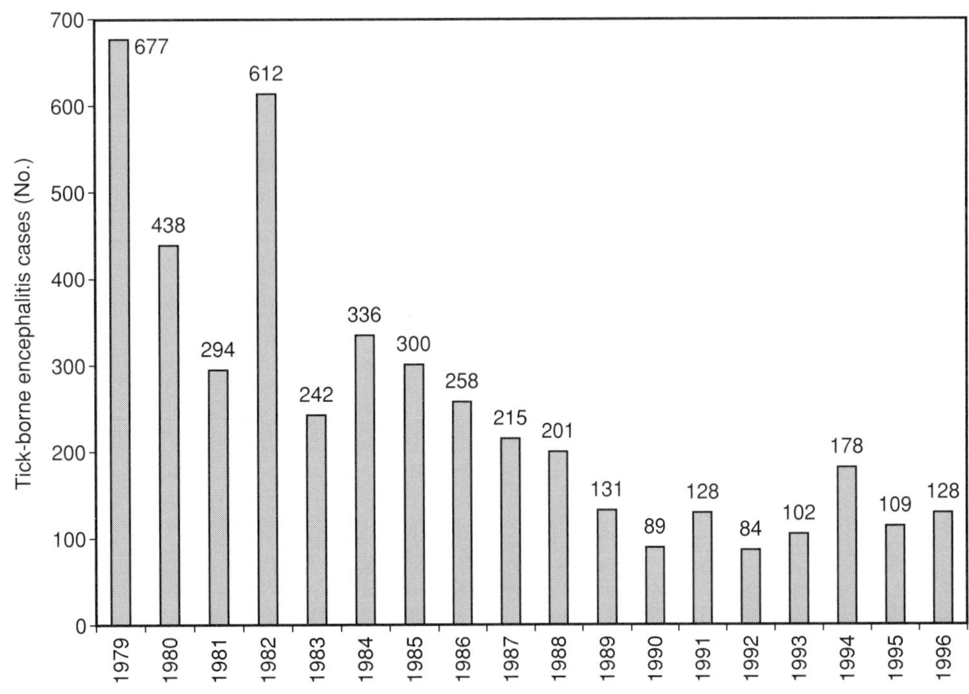

Figure 32–4. Cases of tick-borne encephalitis in Austria (1979–1996).

Table 32–4. **CALCULATION OF THE EFFICACY OF TICK-BORNE ENCEPHALITIS VIRUS VACCINATION IN AUSTRIA AFTER TWO OR THREE VACCINATIONS**

	EXPOSED POPULATION (×1000)/NUMBER OF CASES			PROTECTION RATE (%)	
YEAR	Not Vaccinated	Two Vaccinations	Three or More Vaccinations	Two Vaccinations	Three or More Vaccinations
1994	2340/165	390/1	5070/6	96.4	98.3
1995	2110/104	460/1	5230/4	95.6	98.45
1996	2051/116	328/0	5421/9	100	97

Adapted from Kunz C. Epidemiology of tick-borne encephalitis and the impact of vaccination on the incidence of disease. In Eibl MM, Huber C, Peter HH, Wahn U (eds). Symposium in Immunology V. Berlin, Springer-Verlag, 1996, pp 143–149.

Protective clothes must be completely closed to be really effective, but this may be found intolerable by people spending their leisure time or holidays in endemic areas in the warm season.

In former Czechoslovakia, forestry workers were given protective clothing impregnated with DDT and were regularly disinfested after work.[103] Furthermore, a variety of repellents were used, such as diethyl toluamide, indalone, dimethyl carbate, dimethyl phthalate, and benzyl benzoate. These preparations provided protection for only a few hours, however. Moreover, there have been reports from Russia of ticks becoming resistant to repellents.[104]

Eradication or Elimination

Efforts to eradicate the disease in the past were concentrated on the extermination of the tick population in TBE virus endemic areas. In former Czechoslovakia and USSR, large-scale eradication measures using tetrachlorvinphos, DDT, or hexachlor did not produce the desired effect. Because the virus persists not only in ticks but also in a large number of wild animals, such measures are unlikely to eradicate or even control the disease. The most effective method to prevent infection is vaccination.

Acknowledgments

We thank Ms. Stefanie Fabi for her assistance in preparing the manuscript and Dr. Busch-Petersen for helpful discussions and critical reading of the manuscript.

REFERENCES

1. Westway EG, Brinton MA, Gaidamovitch SY, et al. Flaviviridae. Intervirology 24:183–192, 1985.
2. Casals J. The arthropod-borne group of animal viruses. Trans N Y Acad Sci 19:219–235, 1957.
3. DeMadrid AT, Porterfield JS. The flaviviruses (group B arboviruses): A cross-neutralization study. J Gen Virol 23:91–96, 1974.
4. Calisher CH, Karabatsos N, Dalrymple JM, et al. Antigenic relationships between flaviviruses as determined by cross-neutralization tests with polyclonal antisera. J Gen Virol 70:37–43, 1989.
5. Clarke DH. Further studies on antigenic relationship among the viruses of the group B tick-borne complex. Bull World Health Organ 31:45–56, 1964.
6. Heinz FX, Kunz C. Homogeneity of the structural glycoprotein from European isolates of tick-borne encephalitis virus. Comparison with other flaviviruses. J Gen Virol 57:263–274, 1981.
7. Heinz FX, Berger R, Tuma W, et al. A topological and functional model of epitopes of the structural glycoprotein of tick-borne encephalitis virus defined by monoclonal antibodies. Virology 126:525–537, 1983.
8. Schneider H. Über epidemische akute "Meningitis serosa." Wien Klin Wochenschr 44:350–352, 1931.
9. Monath TP, Heinz FX. Flaviviruses. In Fields BN, Knipe DM, Howley PM (eds). Fields Virology (3rd ed). Philadelphia, Lippincott-Raven, 1996, pp 961–1034.
10. Krausler J, Kraus P, Moritsch H. Klinische und virologisch-serologische Untersuchungsergebnisse bei Frühsommer-Meningoencephalitis und anderen Virusinfektionen des ZNS im Bezirk Neunkirchen. Wien Klin Wochenschr 70:634–637, 1958.
11. Radda A. Die Frühsommer-Meningoenzephalitis in Österreich. In Jusatz H (ed). Beiträge zur Geoökologie der zentraleuropäischen Zecken-Encephalitis. Berlin, Springer-Verlag, 1978, pp 42–47.
12. Blaskovic D. Tick-borne encephalitis in Czechoslovakia. Arch Environ Health 21:453–461, 1970.
13. Grinschgl G, Richling E. Die zentraleuropäische Enzephalomyelitis, eine "Arthropod borne" Erkrankung vom Typ der russischen Frühjahr-Sommer-Enzephalitis. Giorn Mal Infect Paras 9:3–15, 1957.
14. Duniewicz M. Klinisches Bild der zentraleuropäischen Zeckenencephalitis. Munch Med Wochenschr 118:1609–1612, 1976.
15. Reisner H. Clinic and treatment of tick-borne encephalitis (TBE): Introduction. In Kunz C (ed). Tick-Borne Encephalitis. Wien, Facultas Verlag, 1981, pp 1–5.
16. Conrads R, Plassmann E. Frühsommer-Meningoenzephalitis (FSME). Fortschr Med 100:799–801, 1982.
17. Koletzko B, Reinhardt D. Frühsommermeningoenzephalitis (FSME). Monatsschr Kinderheilkd 144:426–434, 1996.
18. Kaiser R, Vollmer H, Schmidtke K, et al. Course and prognosis of tick-borne encephalitis. Nervenarzt 68:324–330, 1997.
19. Ziebart-Schroth A. Frühsommermeningoenzephalitis (FSME). Klinik und besondere Verlaufsformen. Wien Klin Wochenschr 84:778–781, 1972.
20. Bodemann H, Hoppe-Seyler P, Blum H, et al. Schwere und ungünstige Verlaufsformen der Zeckenenzephalitis (FMSE) 1979 in Freiburg. Dtsch Med Wochenschr 105:921–942, 1980.
21. Kunz C. Die Frühsommer-Meningoenzephalitis. Pediatr Prax 14:189–192, 1974.
22. Krausler J. 23 years of TBE in the district of Neunkirchen (Austria). In Kunz C (ed). Tick-Borne Encephalitis. Wien, Facultas Verlag, 1981, pp 6–12.
23. Messner H. Pediatric problems of TBE. In Kunz C (ed). Tick-Borne Encephalitis. Wien, Facultas Verlag, 1981, pp 25–27.
24. Gresikova M, Beran GW. Tick-borne encephalitis. In Beran GW (ed). CRC Handbook Series in Zoonoses. Section B: Viral Zoonoses. Vol. 1. Boca Raton, FL, CRC Press, 1981, pp 201–208.
25. Heinz FX, Kunz C. Characterization of TBE virus and immunogenicity of its surface components in mice. Acta Virol 21:308–316, 1977.
26. Blaskovic DJ, Slavik J. Fine structure of tick-borne encephalitis virus. In Kunz C (ed). Tick-Borne Encephalitis. Wien, Facultas Verlag, 1981, pp 133–141.
27. Rice CM. Flaviviridae: The viruses and their replication. In

Fields BN, Knipe DM, Howley PM (eds). Fields Virology (3rd ed). Philadelphia, Lippincott-Raven, 1996, pp 931–959.

28. Heinz FX. Epitope mapping of flavivirus glycoproteins. In Maramorosh K, Murphy FA (eds). Advances in Virus Research. New York, Academic Press, 1986, pp 103–167.
29. Heinz FX, Berger R, Tuma W, et al. A topological and functional model of epitopes on the structural glycoprotein of tick-borne encephalitis virus defined by monoclonal antibodies. Virology 126:525–537, 1983.
30. Guirakhoo F, Heinz FX, Kunz C. Epitope model of tick-borne encephalitis virus envelope glycoprotein E: Analysis of structural properties, role of carbohydrate side chain, and conformational changes occurring at acidic pH. Virology 169:90–99, 1989.
31. Heinz FX, Mandl CW, Guirakhoo F, et al. The envelope protein E of tick-borne encephalitis virus and other flaviviruses: Structure, functions and evolutionary relationships. Arch Virol Suppl 1:125–135, 1990.
32. Heinz FX, Berger R, Tuma W, et al. Location of immunodominant antigenic determinants on fragments of the tick-borne encephalitis virus glycoprotein: Evidence for two different mechanisms by which antibodies mediate neutralization and hemagglutination inhibition. Virology 130:485–501, 1983.
33. Winkler G, Heinz FX, Kunz C. Characterization of a disulfide bridge–stabilized antigenic domain of tick-borne encephalitis virus structural glycoprotein. J Gen Virol 68:2239–2244, 1987.
34. Nowak T, Wengler G. Analysis of disulfides present in the membrane proteins of the West Nile flavivirus. Virology 156:127–137, 1987.
35. Mandl CW, Guirakhoo F, Holzmann H, et al. Antigenic structure of the flavivirus envelope protein E at the molecular level, using tick-borne encephalitis virus as a model. J Virol 63:564–571, 1989.
36. Rey FA, Heinz FX, Mandl C, et al. The envelope glycoprotein from tick-borne encephalitis virus at 2 Å resolution. Nature 375:291–298, 1995.
37. Heinz FX, Mandl CW, Holzmann H, et al. The flavivirus envelope protein E: Isolation of a soluble form from tick-borne encephalitis virus and its crystallization. J Virol 65:5579–5583, 1991.
38. Cecilia D, Gould EA. Nucleotide changes responsible for loss of neuroinvasiveness in Japanese encephalitis virus neutralization-resistant mutants. Virology 181:70–77, 1991.
39. Gao GF, Hussain MH, Reid HW, et al. Identification of naturally occurring monoclonal antibody escape variants of louping ill virus. J Gen Virol 75:609–614, 1994.
40. Hasegawa H, Yoshida M, Shiosaka T, et al. Mutations in the envelope protein of Japanese encephalitis virus affect entry into cultured cells and virulence in mice. Virology 191:158–165, 1992.
41. Holzmann H, Utter G, Norrby E, et al. Assessment of the antigenic structure of tick-borne encephalitis virus by the use of synthetic peptides. J Gen Virol 74:2031–2035, 1993.
42. Holzmann H, Stiasny K, Ecker M, et al. Characterization of monoclonal antibody–escape mutants of tick-borne encephalitis virus with reduced neuroinvasiveness in mice. J Gen Virol 78:31–37, 1997.
43. Lobigs M, Usha R, Nestorowicz A, et al. Host cell selection of Murray Valley encephalitis virus variants altered at an RGD sequence in the envelope protein and in mouse virulence. Virology 176:587–595, 1990.
44. Roehrig JT, Johnson AJ, Hunt AR, et al. Antibodies to dengue 2 Jamaica E-glycoprotein synthetic peptides identify antigenic conformation. Virology 177:668–675, 1990.
45. Heinz FX, Stiasny K, Püschner-Auer G, et al. Structural changes and functional control of the tick-borne encephalitis virus glycoprotein E by the heterodimeric association with protein prM. Virology 198:109–117, 1994.
46. Allison SL, Schalich J, Stiasny K, et al. Oligomeric rearrangement of tick-borne encephalitis virus envelope proteins induced by an acidic pH. J Virol 69:695–700, 1995.
47. Lee JM, Crooks AJ, Stephenson JR. The synthesis and maturation of a non-structural extracellular antigen from tick-borne encephalitis virus and its relationship to the intracellular NS1 protein. J Gen Virol 70:335–343, 1989.
48. Schlesinger JJ, Brandriss MW, Walsh EE. Protection against 17D yellow fever encephalitis in mice by passive transfer of monoclonal antibodies to the nonstructural glycoprotein gp48 and by active immunization with gp48. J Immunol 135:2805–2809, 1985.
49. Schlesinger JJ, Brandriss MW, Cropp CB, et al. Protection against yellow fever in monkeys by immunization with yellow fever virus nonstructural protein NS1. J Virol 60:1153–1155, 1986.
50. Schlesinger JJ, Brandriss MW, Walsh EE. Protection of mice against dengue 2 virus encephalitis by immunization with the dengue 2 virus nonstructural glycoprotein NS1. J Gen Virol 68:853–857, 1987.
51. Ackermann B, Rehse-Küpper B. Die zentraleuropäische Enzephalitis in der Bundesrepublik Deutschland. Fortschr Neurol Psychiatr 47:103–122, 1979.
52. Hofmann H. Die unspezifische Abwehr bei neurotropen Arbovirusinfektionen. Zentralbl Bakteriol Hyg I Abt Orig A 223:143–163, 1973.
53. Hofmann H. Diagnosis of TBE in the virological routine laboratory. In Kunz C (ed). Tick-Borne Encephalitis. Wien, Facultas Verlag, 1981, pp 129–132.
54. Blessing J. Epidemiologie und Diagnose der Frühsommer-Meningoenzephalitis. Med Welt 32:1345–1347, 1981.
55. Ackermann R, Rehse-Küpper B, Löser R, et al. Neutralisierende Serumantikörper gegen das Virus der Zentraleuropäischen Enzephalitis bei der ländlichen Bevölkerung der Bundesrepublik Deutschland. Dtsch Med Wochenschr 93:1747–1754, 1968.
56. Kunz C, Hofmann H, Dippe H. Die Frühdiagnose der Frühsommer-Meningoenzephalitis (FSME) im Hämagglutinationshemmungstest durch Behandlung des Serums mit 2-Mercaptoäthanol. Zentralbl Bakteriol Hyg I Abt Orig A 218:273–279, 1971.
57. Kunz C, Krausler J. Bildung und Überdauern der komplementbindenden Antikörper nach Infektionen mit Frühsommer-Meningoencephalitis (tick-borne encephalitis). Virus Arch Ges Virusforsch 14:499–507, 1964.
58. Heinz F, Roggendorf M, Hofmann H, et al. Comparison of two different enzyme immunoassays for detection of immunoglobulin M antibodies against tick-borne encephalitis virus in serum and cerebrospinal fluid. J Clin Microbiol 14:141–146, 1981.
59. Glukhov N, Jerusalimsky A, Canter V, et al. Ribonuclease treatment of tick-borne encephalitis. Arch Neurol 33:598–603, 1976.
60. Synek P. Treatment of tick-borne meningoencephalitis with Emetine. Rev Czechosl Med 20:29–33, 1974.
61. Duniewicz M, Kulkova H. Kortikoide in der Behandlung von Zecken und anderen Virus-Meningoenzephalitiden. Munch Med Wochenschr 124:63–64, 1982.
62. Duniewicz M. Klinisches Bild der zentraleuropäischen Zeckenenzephalitis. Munch Med Wochenschr 118:1609–1612, 1976.
63. Kunz C. Die Prophylaxe der Frühsommer-Meningoenzephalitis (FSME) in der dermatologischen Prax. Schrifttum Prax 5:55–58, 1974.
64. Moritsch H, Krausler J. Die Frühsommer-Meningo-Enzephalitis in Niederösterreich 1956–1958. Epidemiologie und Klinik im Seuchengebiet Neunkirchen. Dtsch Med Wochenschr 84:1934–1939, 1959.
65. Jettmar HM. Über die Rolle der Zecken bei der Verbreitung der zweiwelligen Meningoenzephalitis in Österreich. Anzeig Schädlingsk 30:129–132, 1957.
66. Gresikova M, Kozuch O, Nosek J. Die Rolle von *Ixodes ricinus* als Vektor des Zeckenenzephalitisvirus in verschiedenen mitteleuropäischen Naturherden. Zentralbl Bakteriol Parasit 207:423–429, 1968.
67. Blaskovic D. Epidemiologische und immunologische Probleme bei der Zeckenencephalitis. Wien Klin Wochenschr 70:742–749, 1958.
68. Gresikova M, Sekeyova M, Stupalova S, et al. Sheep milk–borne epidemic of tick-borne encephalitis in Slovakia. Intervirology 5:57–61, 1975.
69. Bodemann H, Pausch J, Schmitz H, et al. Die Zeckenenzephalitis (FSME) als Labor-Infektion. Med Welt 28:1779–1781, 1977.
70. Kluger G, Schöttler A, Waldvogel K, et al. Tickborne encephalitis despite specific immunoglobulin prophylaxis [letter]. Lancet 346:1502, 1995.
71. Kreil TR, Eibl MM. Pre- and postexposure protection by passive immunoglobulin but no enhancement of infection with a flavivirus in a mouse model. J Virol 71:2921–2927, 1997.

72. Smorodintsev AA, Ilyenko VI. Results of laboratory and epidemiological study of vaccination against tick-borne encephalitis. In Livikova H (ed). Biology of Viruses of TBE Complex (Symposia of Czechoslovak Academy of Sciences, Vol. 3). New York, Academic Press, 1962, pp 332–343.
73. Lvov DK, Gagarina AV. Immunoprophylaxis of tick-borne encephalitis. In Chumakov MP (ed). Tick-Borne Encephalitis and Other Arboviral Diseases. Viruses and Viral Diseases. Vol. 1 [in Russian]. Moscow, VNIIMI, 1965, pp 97–127.
74. Elbert LB, Krasilnikov IV, Drozdov SG, et al. Concentrated purified vaccine against tick-borne encephalitis produced by ultrafiltration and chromatography [in Russian]. Vopr Virusol 1:90–93, 1985.
75. Danes L, Benda R. Study of the possibility of preparing a vaccine against tick-borne encephalitis using tissue culture methods. I. Propagation of tick-borne encephalitis virus in tissue culture for vaccine preparation. Acta Virol 4:25–31, 1960.
76. Danes L, Benda R. Study of the possibility of preparing a vaccine against tick-borne encephalitis using tissue culture methods. II. The inactivation by formaldehyde of the tick-borne encephalitis virus in liquids prepared from tissue cultures. Immunogenic properties. Acta Virol 4:32–36, 1960.
77. Benda R, Danes L. Study of the possibility of preparing a vaccine against tick-borne encephalitis using tissue culture methods. V. Experimental data for the evaluation of the efficiency of formol treated vaccines in laboratory animals. Acta Virol 5:37–49, 1961.
78. Danes L, Benda R. Study of the possibility of preparing a vaccine against tick-borne encephalitis using tissue culture methods. IV. Immunization of humans with test samples of inactivated vaccine. Acta Virol 4:335–340, 1960.
79. Kunz C, Hofmann H, Stary A. Field studies with a new tick-borne encephalitis (TBE) vaccine. Zentralbl Bakteriol Hyg J Abt Orig A 243:141–144, 1976.
80. Heinz FX, Kunz C, Fauma H. Preparations of a highly purified vaccine against tick-borne encephalitis by continuous flow zonal ultracentrifugation. J Med Virol 6:213–221, 1980.
81. Kunz C, Heinz FX, Hofmann H. Immunogenicity and reactogenicity of a highly purified vaccine against tick-borne encephalitis. J Med Virol 6:103–109, 1980.
82. Klockmann U, Bock HL, Franke V, et al. Preclinical investigations of the safety, immunogenicity and efficacy of a purified, inactivated tick-borne encephalitis vaccine. J Biol Stand 17:331–342, 1989.
83. Kockmann U, Bock HL, Kwasny H, et al. Humoral immunity against tick-borne encephalitis virus following manifest disease and active immunization. Vaccine 9:42–46, 1991.
84. Klockmann U, Krivanec K, Stephenson JR, Hilfenhous J. Protection against European isolates of tick-borne encephalitis virus after vaccination with a new tick-borne encephalitis vaccine. Vaccine 9:210–212, 1991.
85. Girgsdies OE, Rosenkrantz G. Tick-borne encephalitis: Development of a paediatric vaccine. A controlled, randomized, double-blind and multicentre study. Vaccine 15:1421–1428, 1996.
86. Harabacz I, Bock H, Jüngst C, et al. A randomized phase II study of a new tick-borne encephalitis vaccine using three different doses and two immunization regimens. Vaccine 10:145–150, 1992.
87. Kunz C. Epidemiology of tick-borne encephalitis and the impact of vaccination on the incidence of disease. In Eibl MM, Huber C, Peter HH, Wahn U (eds). Symposium in Immunology V. Berlin, Springer-Verlag, 1996, pp 143–149.
88. Data on File, Chiron Behring Laboratories, 1997.
89. Holzmann H, Vorobyova MS, Ladyzhenskaya IP, et al. Molecular epidemiology of tick-borne encephalitis virus: Cross-protection between European and Far Eastern subtypes. Vaccine 10:345–349, 1992.
89a. Kunz C. Tick-borne encephalitis in Europe. Acta Leidensia 60:1–14, 1992.
90. Scholz E, Wiethölter H. Postvakzinale Schwerpunktneuritis nach prophylaktischer FSME-Impfung. Dtsch Med Wochenschr 112:544–546, 1987.
91. Schabet M, Wiethölter H, Grodd W, et al. Neurological complications after simultaneous immunization against tick-borne encephalitis and tetanus. Lancet 2:959–960, 1989.
92. Frühsommer-Meningoenzephalitis: Probleme mit speziellem FSME-Kinderimpfstoff? Fortschr Med 114:9, 1996.
93. Chumakov MP, Rubin SG, Semashko IV, et al. New perspective vaccines from tick-borne encephalitis virus propagated in green monkey kidney cell cultures. Arch Virol Suppl 1:161–168, 1990.
94. Mundt W, Barrett N, Dorner F, Eibl J. Matrix mit daran adhärent gebundenen Zellen, sowie Verfahren zur Produktion von Virus/Virusantigen. EP 0 506 714 B1, 1994.
95. Venugopal K, Gould EA. Towards a new generation of flavivirus vaccines. Vaccine 12:966–975, 1994.
96. Allison SL, Mandl CW, Kunz C, et al. Expression of cloned envelope protein genes from the flavivirus tick-borne encephalitis virus in mammalian cells and random mutagenesis by PCR. Virus Genes 8:187–198, 1994.
97. Allison SL, Stadler K, Mandl C, et al. Synthesis and secretion of recombinant tick-borne encephalitis virus protein E in soluble and particulate form. J Virol 69:5816–5820, 1995.
98. Heinz FX, Allison SL, Stiasny K, et al. Recombinant and virion-derived soluble and particulate immunogens for vaccination against tick-borne encephalitis. Vaccine 13:1636–1642, 1995.
99. Jacobs SC, Stephenson JR, Wilkinson GWG. High-level expression of the tick-borne encephalitis virus NS1 protein by using an adenovirus-based vector: Protection elicited in a murine model. J Virol 66:2086–2095, 1992.
100. Jacobs SC, Stephenson JR, Wilkinson GWG. Protection elicited by a replication-defective adenovirus vector expressing the tick-borne encephalitis virus non-structural glycoprotein NS1. J Gen Virol 75:2399–2402, 1994.
101. Halstead SB. Antibody, macrophages, dengue virus infection, shock and hemorrhage: A pathogenetic cascade. Rev Infect Dis 11(suppl 4):830–839, 1989.
102. Wallner G, Mandl CW, Ecker M, et al. Characterization and complete genome sequences of high- and low-virulence variants of tick-borne encephalitis virus. J Gen Virol 77:1035–1042, 1996.
103. Heinz F, Asmera J, Januska J. Present activity in natural foci of tick-borne encephalitis in the CSSR. In Tick-Borne Encephalitis. International Symposium, Baden/Vienna, 1979. Wien, Facultas Verlag, 1981, pp 279–281.
104. Hoffmann G. Zeckenprophylaxe und bekämpfung. In Probleme der Insekten und Zeckenbekämpfung: Ökologische, medizinische und rechtliche Aspekte. Berlin, Schmidt Verlag, 1978, pp 72–75.

chapter

33 Typhoid Fever Vaccines

Myron M. Levine

History

Typhoid fever is an acute generalized infection of the reticuloendothelial system, intestinal lymphoid tissue, and gallbladder that is caused by *Salmonella typhi*. A broad spectrum of clinical illness can ensue, with more severe forms being characterized by persisting high fever, abdominal discomfort, malaise, and headache. In the preantibiotic era, the disease ran its course over several weeks and was accompanied by a case-fatality rate of 10 to 20%.

Before the first quarter of the 19th century, typhoid fever was not recognized as a distinct clinical entity and was often confused with other prolonged febrile syndromes, particularly typhus fever of rickettsial origin. There is considerable debate over who first clearly differentiated typhus fever from typhoid (i.e., typhus-like) fever. Medical historians have argued over who should receive credit for this clinical clarification, and it has been variously bestowed on Huxham (1782),[1] Louis (1829),[2] Gerhard (1837),[3] and Schoenlein (1839).[4] Gerhard, in Philadelphia, argued that two similar, yet distinct, febrile illnesses existed that were clearly discernible from one another on the basis of pathological findings; one (typhoid) manifested marked intestinal lesions. Schoenlein referred to two distinct forms of typhus: "exanthematicus" and "abdominalis." However, Jenner is responsible for definitively dispelling controversy on the subject.[5, 6] He provided precise clinical descriptions and observations of pathological conditions from postmortem examinations that allowed a clear-cut differentiation between the two illnesses. He also argued that the pathological lesions in Peyer's patches and mesenteric lymph nodes were peculiar to typhoid and were never seen with typhus. In 1847, the term *enteric fever* was introduced in an attempt to replace typhoid fever and avoid confusion with typhus.[7] Although this term is frequently used, it has by no means replaced the appellations *typhoid fever* and *paratyphoid fever* in common usage.

William Budd's book, *Typhoid Fever: Its Nature, Mode of Spreading and Prevention*, published in 1873,[8] is a milestone in epidemiology, because it clearly described the contagious nature of the disease and incriminated transmission via fecally contaminated water sources years before the causative organism was identified. Eberth (1880)[9] visualized the causative bacilli in tissue sections from infected patients, and Gaffky (1884)[10] grew it in pure culture. Known in earlier years as *Bacillus typhosus*, *Eberthella typhosa*, and *Salmonella typhosa*, it is currently referred to as *Salmonella typhi* or *Salmonella enterica* serovar Typhi.[11, 12]

Salmonella paratyphi A and B also cause enteric fever (paratyphoid fever), which in most instances is clinically indistinguishable from typhoid fever. In general, where enteric fever is endemic, typhoid accounts for approximately 90% of the clinical cases and paratyphoid for the rest.

Inactivated (heat-killed, phenol-preserved) *S. typhi* was utilized as a parenteral vaccine as far back as 1896 by Pfeiffer and Kolle[13] in Germany and Wright in England.[14] Wright administered his vaccine (three doses 2 weeks apart) to two medical officers in the Indian Army, one of whom thereafter ingested wild typhoid bacilli without developing illness. Wright then evaluated his vaccine in 2835 volunteers in the Indian Army.[15] Although local and generalized adverse reactions were common, results were considered to be sufficiently encouraging for a decision to be made to vaccinate troops embarking for the Boer War in South Africa. Outcry over the frequency of adverse reactions led to a suspension of vaccination. However, on Wright's insistence, a board of inquiry was established to review data on the reactogenicity and efficacy of the vaccine. The committee concluded that the vaccine was efficacious and that its value in preventing typhoid fever exceeded the price paid in adverse reactions. As a consequence, by World War I typhoid vaccination became virtually routine in the British Army.

Importance of Typhoid Fever

The transmission of typhoid fever is fostered where sanitation is primitive and water supplies are not treated and there exist chronic or short-term carriers of *S. typhi* (who serve as a reservoir of infection). In such situations, human fecal material can contaminate water supplies. In endemic areas, the peak incidence of typhoid fever is typically observed among school-aged children. Typhoid constitutes the main enteric disease threat faced by children in developing countries after they have survived the gauntlet of diarrheal and dysenteric infections encountered during the first 5 years of life.

Because the case-fatality rate in the preantibiotic era was 10 to 20%, typhoid fever was a much-feared disease. After the discovery in 1948 that chloramphenicol (and subsequently certain other antibiotics) can successfully treat typhoid fever, dropping the case-fatality rate to well below 1%, the interest in typhoid vaccines thereafter historically became a weathervane for the prevalence of antibiotic-resistant strains of *S. typhi*. Interest in vaccines waned as long as effective inexpensive oral antibiotics were available, only to resurge when resistant strains appeared and made treatment difficult. Beginning around 1990, strains of *S. typhi* that exhibited plasmid-encoded resistance to all the oral antibiotics that were the mainstays of therapy in the 1970s and 1980s (i.e., chloramphenicol, trimethoprim-sulfamethoxazole, and amoxicillin) began to disseminate throughout Asia and northeast Africa.[16–22] This emergence of multiply antibiotic-resistant typhoid during the last decade of the 20th century has led to an increase in the incidence of severe cases, hospitalizations, and complications as well as an increase in typhoid mortality.[16–19, 22]

BACKGROUND

Clinical Description of Typhoid Fever and Its Most Frequent Complications

Typhoid fever exhibits a wide range of clinical severity. Classic full-blown cases begin with malaise, anorexia, myalgia, fever that increases in stepwise fashion to reach 39 to 40°C, abdominal discomfort, and headaches.[23–25] A bronchitic cough is common in the early stage of illness. The fever often follows three stages. Initially, it rises gradually, in stepwise fashion, with daily increments of 0.5 to 1°C until, after 5 to 7 days, sustained fever of 39 to 41°C is present. Without appropriate antimicrobial therapy, the fever remains at this level for 10 to 14 days. With convalescence, the fever diminishes, also in stepwise fashion, over several days. During the period of sustained fever, approximately 20% of white patients manifest an exanthem (so-called rose spots) consisting of subtle, 2- to 4-mm salmon-colored macules, which blanch with pressure. Rose spots are most often seen on the chest, abdomen, and back; *S. typhi* can be cultured from rose spots.[26] Constipation is typical in older children and adults, whereas diarrhea may occur in young children with typhoid fever.

The peripheral leukocyte count in typhoid fever is often below 4500 per mm³, which helps in the differential diagnosis. Thrombocytopenia is also common, with platelets dropping below 80,000 per mm³. Liver dysfunction, as detected by mildly elevated serum transaminase values, is observed in most patients. Before the availability of fluoroquinolone antibiotics such as ciprofloxacin, approximately 10% of patients treated with earlier antimicrobials of choice such as chloramphenicol, trimethoprim-sulfamethoxazole, or amoxicillin, manifested clinical relapses; notably, the clinical illness in relapse is much milder.

Two of the most feared complications of typhoid fever, intestinal perforation and hemorrhage, are a consequence of the intestinal lesions that are so prominent in the pathology of *S. typhi* infection. These complications occur in 0.5 to 1.0% of cases and are more common in individuals who have been ill for several weeks without proper antibiotic therapy. Other uncommon complications of typhoid fever include typhoid hepatitis, empyema, osteomyelitis, and psychosis. More rarely, arthritis, meningitis, myocarditis, and empyema of the gallbladder can occur. In Indonesia, a particularly severe form of typhoid fever is commonly encountered in which cerebral dysfunction, including obtundation, delirium or coma, and shock are present.[27] Unless corticosteroid therapy accompanies appropriate antimicrobial therapy in patients suffering from this form of the disease, the case-fatality rate exceeds 20%.[27]

Although infants may manifest severe clinical forms of typhoid fever, bacteremic *S. typhi* infection in children younger than 2 years is often remarkably mild and is not recognized clinically as enteric fever.[28, 29]

Two to 5% of patients with typhoid fever, depending on age and sex, become chronic gallbladder carriers of the organism.[30, 31] More rarely, chronic renal carriers occur.

Bacteriology

Taxonomy within the genus *Salmonella* continues to evolve and is a source of considerable confusion. Originally, speciation was based on association with distinct clinical syndromes. With the Kauffman-White serological classification, each distinct O:H serotype was given species status, a situation that rather quickly became ponderous. In 1980, the Approved Lists described five species: *S. enteritidis*, *S. typhi*, *S. typhimurium*, *S. choleraesuis*, and *S. arizonae*.[32] The most recent classification and speciation, based on DNA relatedness and molecular analysis, reduces the genus *Salmonella* to two species, *S. enterica* and *S. bongori*. *S. enterica* is further subdivided into subspecies designated with Roman numerals.[11, 12, 33] Serotypes within *S. enterica* subspecies I are still almost always referred to by their previous genus/species designations. Thus, for example, to avoid confusion, *S. enterica* serovar Typhi continues to be referred to in most international journals of microbiology, infectious diseases, epidemiology, and vaccinology as *Salmonella typhi*. Accordingly, *S. typhi* is the terminology that will be used in this chapter.

Serologically, *S. typhi* falls into group D *Salmonella* on the basis of its O antigens 9 and 12.[34] *S. typhi* is motile, and its peritrichous flagella bear flagellar (H) antigen d, which is also encountered in approximately 80 other bioserotypes of *Salmonella*.[34] Occasional isolates from Indonesia have flagella that bear other antigens (j and z66).[35, 36] Strains freshly isolated from patients express on their surface a polysaccharide capsule, the Vi (for virulence) antigen.[34, 37–40] Vi consists of a homopolymer of *N*-acetyl galacturonic acid[41–43]; the presence of Vi prevents O antibody from binding to the O antigen.[38]

At the level of the clinical microbiology laboratory, *S. typhi* exhibits a remarkable degree of homogeneity, in comparison with the other species of *Salmonella*. *S. typhi* rarely exhibits biochemical or serological variability. One exception is found in Indonesia where a few percent of isolates bear flagellar antigen j or z66 rather than d. Previously, only phage typing using Vi phages was helpful in differentiating strains from different geographical areas. More recently, several molecular epidemiological techniques, including pulsed field gel electrophoresis and ribotyping, have proven their worth in differentiating *S. typhi* strains from diverse sources.[44–49]

S. typhi does not ferment lactose; it produces hydrogen sulfide (H_2S) but does not produce gas. As a consequence, suspicious colonies are evident on usual lactose-containing media such as *Salmonella-Shigella* agar or MacConkey's agar as lactose-negative colonies. The biochemical pattern in triple sugar iron agar is rather characteristic, manifested by an acid butt without gas, an alkaline slant, and obvious H_2S production. Fresh isolates typically agglutinate with Vi but not necessarily with group D antiserum. However, if the bacteria are boiled to remove the Vi capsule, a reaction with group D antiserum is then readily seen.

Pathogenesis

Acute Typhoid Fever

S. typhi and *S. paratyphi* A and B are highly invasive bacteria that pass through the intestinal mucosa of humans rapidly and efficiently to eventually reach the reticuloendothelial system, where, after an 8- to 14-day incubation period, they precipitate a systemic illness.[50] *S. typhi* is a highly host-adapted pathogen; humans comprise the only natural host and reservoir of this infection.

Our comprehension of the steps involved in the pathogenesis of typhoid fever comes from four sources: (1) clinicopathological observations in humans[51, 52]; (2) volunteer studies[53]; (3) studies of a chimpanzee model[54, 55]; and (4) analogies drawn from *S. typhimurium* and *S. enteritidis* infection in mice, the "mouse typhoid" model.[56, 57] The probable steps in the pathogenesis of *S. typhi* infection in humans are summarized in what follows.

Susceptible human hosts ingest the causative organisms in contaminated food and water. The inoculum size and the type of vehicle in which it is ingested greatly influence the attack rate for typhoid fever and also affect the incubation period. Doses of 10^9 and 10^8 pathogenic *S. typhi* ingested by volunteers in 45 mL of skim milk induced clinical illness in 98% and 89% of individuals, respectively; doses of 10^5 organisms caused typhoid fever in 28 to 55% of volunteers, whereas none of 14 subjects who ingested 10^3 organisms developed clinical illness.[53]

When the ingested typhoid bacilli pass through the pylorus and reach the small intestine, they rapidly penetrate the mucosal epithelium by one of two mechanisms to arrive in the lamina propria. One mechanism of invasion involves typhoid bacilli being actively taken up by M cells, the dome-like epithelial cells that cover Peyer's patches and other organized lymphoid tissue of the gut. From here they enter the underlying lymphoid cells. In the second, quite distinct, invasive mechanism, bacilli are internalized by enterocytes where they enter membrane-bound vacuoles that pass through the cell and ultimately release the bacteria at the basal portion of the cell without destroying the enterocyte. Takeuchi provides a highly descriptive electron photomicrographic documentation of the analogous passage of *S. typhimurium* through intestinal mucosa.[58]

On reaching the lamina propria in the nonimmune host, typhoid bacilli elicit an influx of macrophages that ingest the organisms but are generally unable to kill them. Some bacilli apparently remain within macrophages of the small intestinal lymphoid tissue. Other typhoid bacilli are drained into mesenteric lymph nodes, where further multiplication and ingestion by macrophages take place. Shortly after invasion of the intestinal mucosa, a primary bacteremia is believed to take place in which *S. typhi* organisms are filtered from the circulation by fixed phagocytic cells of the reticuloendothelial system. It is believed that the main route by which typhoid bacilli reach the blood stream in this early stage is by lymph that drains from mesenteric nodes to eventually reach the thoracic duct and then the general blood circulation. It is conceivable that ingestion of a massive inoculum followed by widespread invasion of the intestinal mucosa could result in rapid and direct invasion of the blood stream. As a result of this primary bacteremia, the pathogen rapidly attains an intracellular haven throughout the organs of the reticuloendothelial system, where it resides during the incubation period (usually 8–14 days) until the onset of clinical typhoid fever.

Clinical illness is accompanied by a fairly sustained "secondary" bacteremia. In their report of experimental *S. typhi* challenge studies in volunteers, Hornick and colleagues described one volunteer who began a 7-day course of oral chloramphenicol only 1 day after ingesting pathogenic *S. typhi* and who developed clinical typhoid fever 9 days after the antibiotic was discontinued.[53] This report provides evidence that the typhoid bacilli have attained their intracellular haven within 24 hours after ingestion.

The Vi antigen is a virulence property.[37, 40, 59] Felix and Pitt, who originally described the antigen and gave it its name, showed that Vi antigen enhanced the pathogenicity of *S. typhi* for mice.[37, 59] Virtually all strains freshly isolated from patients possess this polysaccharide capsule. Both epidemiological observations and studies in volunteers support the contention that *S. typhi* strains that possess Vi are more virulent than strains lacking this polysaccharide.[53]

Chronic Typhoid Carrier State

During the primary bacteremia that follows ingestion of typhoid bacilli and seeds the reticuloendothelial system, organisms also reach the gallbladder, an organ for which *S. typhi* has a remarkable predilection. After intravenous inoculation, *S. typhi* rapidly appear in the gallbladder of rabbits.[60, 61] *S. typhi* can be readily cultured from bile or from bile-stained duodenal fluid in patients with acute typhoid fever.[62–64] In 2 to 5% of patients, the gallbladder infection becomes chronic.[30, 31] The proclivity to become a chronic carrier is greater in females and increases with age at the time of acute *S. typhi* infection, thereby resembling the epidemiology of gallbladder disease. The infection tends to become chronic in individuals who have a preexisting pathological gallbladder condition at the time of acute *S. typhi* infection.

Diagnosis

Bacteriological Diagnosis

Confirmation of the diagnosis of typhoid fever requires recovery of *S. typhi* from a suitable clinical specimen. Because of practicality and relative ease of access, multiple blood cultures should be obtained from patients in whom the diagnosis is suspected clinically. The rate of recovery of *S. typhi* in blood cultures depends on many factors, including the volume cultured, the ratio of the volume of blood to the volume of culture broth in which it is inoculated (the ratio should be at least 1:8), the inclusion of anticomplementary substances in the medium (such as sodium polyanethol sulfonate or bile), and whether the patient has already received antibiotics to which the *S. typhi* is sensitive. With the use of three 5-mL blood cultures, *S. typhi* can be recovered from the blood in approximately 70% of suspected cases.

The gold standard of bacteriological confirmation of typhoid fever is the bone marrow culture, which is positive in 85 to 96% of cases, even when the patient has received antibiotics.[26, 65] In the 1980s, great interest was shown in the use of duodenal string devices to obtain bile-stained duodenal fluid for culture.[62–64, 66] The combination of a duodenal string and two blood cultures generally provides a sensitivity of bacteriological confirmation equal to that achieved with bone marrow cultures but without the invasiveness of the latter.[62]

Stool cultures lead to recovery of the organism in only 45 to 65% of cases. The yield tends to be somewhat higher in children.[64]

Serodiagnosis of Typhoid Fever

Serodiagnosis of typhoid fever has been attempted since the late 19th century, when Widal and Sicard (1896),[67] among others,[68, 69] showed that the serum of patients with typhoid fever agglutinated typhoid bacilli. The Widal test, which is still practiced today in many areas, involves the search for agglutinins in the patient's serum and may be performed with antigen in tubes or on slides; the former is generally more accurate. By careful choice of antigen, both O and H antibodies can be selectively measured. By use of *S. typhi* strain O901, which lacks flagellar and Vi antigens, *S. typhi* O antibody can be selectively measured. To detect antibodies against the appropriate H antigen (d), a strain such as *S. virginia* is selected that possesses the identical flagellar antigen (d) as *S. typhi* but shares no O somatic antigens with *S. typhi*.[70] Most patients with typhoid fever have elevated levels of O and H antibody at the time of onset of clinical illness.[70] Anderson[71, 72] and Anderson and Gunnell[73] have emphasized the importance and usefulness of H titers in serodiagnosis of typhoid fever. However, in general, the prevalence of H antibodies in adults living in endemic areas is too high for the test to be useful in that age group.[70] Nevertheless, it can be helpful in diagnosing children younger than 10 years of age in endemic areas and people of any age from nonendemic areas. A history of inoculation with parenteral killed whole-cell vaccines invalidates the use of the Widal test. Interest has reappeared in the use of the slide test for O agglutinins of *S. typhi*, even for adults in endemic areas.[74]

Serological tests to measure Vi antibody using highly purified Vi antigen are available.[75–77] Although this serology, including passive hemagglutination,[75] enzyme-linked immunosorbent assay (ELISA),[77] and radioimmunoassay, is practical for the detection of chronic *S. typhi* carriers, most of whom have quite elevated levels of Vi antibody, it is of little help in diagnosing acute typhoid fever because only a minority of patients with acute infection manifest detectable Vi antibody.

Rapid Immunoassays

Over the years many attempts have been made to develop tests that detect *S. typhi* antigens or nucleic acid in blood, urine, or body fluids, thereby providing a rapid diagnostic test for typhoid fever.[78–89] With few exceptions, these tests have been disappointing and have failed to warrant the enthusiasm of the initial reports. The immunoassays are based on the detection of the O or Vi antigens of *S. typhi* in blood or urine using coagglutination, ELISA, or countercurrent immunoelectrophoresis, whereas the polymerase chain reaction and DNA probe methods attempt to amplify *S. typhi* genes and hybridize them with labeled specific gene probes. These assays aim to be more sensitive, practical, economical, and rapid than bacteriological culture, yet comparably specific. Unfortunately, so far no assay has adequately accomplished these objectives and a satisfactory test that might replace bacteriologic culture remains a laudable but elusive goal.

EPIDEMIOLOGY

Basic Epidemiological Features

Humans are the sole reservoir of *S. typhi* infection as well as the only natural host. The infection is transmitted when susceptible hosts ingest food or water that has been contaminated by fecal matter. In contrast, transmission from person to person by direct contact is exceedingly uncommon. As a consequence of these epidemiological features, typhoid fever represents the quintessential infectious disease for which transmission is related to levels of sanitation and quality of water supply. Typhoid fever can abound where sanitation and food hygiene are primitive. The highest incidence usually occurs where water supplies serving large populations are contaminated by fecal matter. This situation existed at the end of the 19th century in most large cities in the United States and western Europe where piped water supplies were available but the water was usually untreated.[90] The water sources (usually rivers) were also the repository for the discharged sewage of the cities. In this manner, the transmission of typhoid fever was amplified, causing the disease to be highly endemic in large cities throughout the United States and Europe. With the introduction of water treatment at the turn of the 20th century, including sand filtration and chlorination, the incidence of typhoid fever plummeted precipitously in the large cities of the United States despite the continued existence within those cities of many chronic carriers of *S. typhi*.[90, 91] Typhoid fever remains endemic in most of the less-developed areas of the world, where fecal contamination of water sources still occurs. This includes many countries in Africa, Asia, and Latin America.

Incidence and Prevalence

In endemic areas, a characteristic age-specific incidence of typhoid fever occurs, with a low incidence in children younger than 2 years of age, a peak incidence in school-aged children (5–19 years), and a low incidence in adults older than 35 years. The apparent low incidence in young children in part relates to decreased exposure to vehicles of transmission. However, other evidence suggests that infection of children younger than 2 years of age may be much more common than previously appreciated but the clinical consequence of *S. typhi* infection in the infant host is often mild or atypical illness, even in the presence of bacteremic infection.[28, 29]

It is presumed that in developing countries, with primitive conditions of human waste disposal and widespread contamination of water supplies, water represents the most common vehicle of transmission, and the number of organisms ingested is usually small. Thus, multiple subclinical and mild infections are believed to occur for each full-blown clinical case. In contrast, in more developed countries, with good sanitation, typhoid is transmitted when chronic carriers contaminate food vehicles through a breakdown in proper practices of personal and food hygiene. In these common-source foodborne outbreaks, the inocula ingested are presumably often relatively large and high attack rates ensue; under these conditions, fewer subclinical cases occur.

It is difficult to quantify the magnitude of the typhoid fever problem worldwide because the clinical picture is confused with that of many other febrile infections and the capacity for routine bacteriological confirmation is absent in most areas of the less-developed world.[92–94] Nevertheless, in the course of several vaccine field trials carried out during the 1980s in Latin America, Asia, and Africa, it was possible to confirm the incidence of typhoid fever that occurred in the unimmunized control subjects during several years of surveillance. In these trials, high annual incidence rates were recorded, including 810 cases per 10^5 population in Indonesia, 653 per 10^5 in Nepal, 442 per 10^5 in South Africa, and 227 cases per 10^5 people in Chile.[95–98]

Seroepidemiological studies that have measured the prevalence of *S. typhi* H antibody have been very useful in quantifying the prevalence of typhoid fever in different geographical areas.[70, 92, 99] However, this seroepidemiological technique has not been widely applied.

Typhoid as a Public Health Problem

It has been estimated that each year more than 33 million cases and more than 500,000 deaths occur worldwide that are due to typhoid fever.[92, 93, 100] Surveillance data generated by quantifying the incidence of typhoid fever in placebo groups participating in large-scale field trials of typhoid vaccines show annual incidence rates from 227 to 810 cases per 10^5 population in typhoid-endemic areas.[95–98] These data suggest that the previous estimates of the annual worldwide burden of typhoid fever grossly underestimate the magnitude of the problem.

Three populations are at particularly high risk of developing typhoid fever and would benefit from immunoprophylaxis with a safe, effective, inexpensive, and practical vaccine. These include children in endemic areas,[28, 70, 101–103] travelers and military personnel from industrialized countries who visit endemic areas in less-developed countries,[104–107] and clinical microbiology technicians.[108–110]

Seroepidemiological studies in Peru and Chile have shown that by 15 to 19 years of age, 50 to 80% of teenagers have serological evidence of past infection with *S. typhi*.[70, 92, 99] In endemic areas, typhoid fever is a major cause of absenteeism from school and from employment. Direct expenditures for hospitalization and medication further raise the public health costs of this disease.[111] For areas in which it is unlikely that improved sanitation and treated water supplies will become a reality in the near future, a safe vaccine that provides long-term protection would be particularly beneficial in relation to its cost, because an initial investment in immunization provides many years of protection. Because typhoid fever exhibits its peak incidence in school-aged children—a "captive" population in many countries—a school immunization program could target the high risk population of schoolchildren.[112–114]

Travelers from industrialized countries who visit less-developed countries in which typhoid fever is endemic are at particular risk of developing the disease.[92, 104–107] Travelers are probably at special risk in endemic areas because they do not have the background immunity that much of the indigenous population has acquired as a consequence of multiple subclinical infections. For U.S. travelers, South America and the Indian subcontinent have been the areas of highest risk.[105] Since 1990, isolates from Asia and northeast Africa have increasingly been resistant to many clinically relevant antibiotics, including chloramphenicol, amoxicillin, and trimethoprim-sulfamethoxazole.[21, 93, 115]

In recent years it has become recognized that microbiology technicians in laboratories, particularly clinical laboratories, constitute a high-risk group for the development of typhoid fever. A review from the Centers for Disease Control and Prevention[110] revealed that 11.2% of the reported sporadic (i.e., not outbreak-associated) cases of typhoid fever in the United States in a 33-month period occurred in laboratory technicians. In the course of their work, these individuals process stool or blood cultures containing *S. typhi* before it is recognized that the pathogen is present. The predilection for laboratory workers to develop typhoid fever suggests that under these special conditions the disease may be spread by aerosol or by direct contact. This observation is in contrast to the lack of contact spread of this infection under more natural conditions and may be related to the organism existing in pure culture in the laboratory.

PASSIVE IMMUNIZATION

Passive protection by means of antiserum or immunoglobulin (Ig) is not used to prevent typhoid or paratyphoid fever.

ACTIVE IMMUNIZATION

For historical as well as practical purposes, we can group the various typhoid vaccines that have been evaluated in clinical trials and the few that have been used as licensed vaccine products into three categories:

1. Early vaccines that are no longer in use or that are no longer under investigation
2. Vaccines that are available in various countries as licensed products
3. Future vaccines that are under active clinical evaluation

The various past, present, and future typhoid vaccines can be considered to fall into five broad groups for review.

1. Inactivated whole-cell parenteral vaccines
2. Subunit parenteral or aerosolized vaccines
3. Inactivated whole-cell oral vaccine
4. Attenuated *S. typhi* strains used as live oral vaccines
5. Parenteral polysaccharide-carrier protein conjugate vaccines

Early Vaccines Not Presently in Use

For a more detailed review of these vaccines readers are referred to the chapters on typhoid vaccine in the first two editions of this book.[116, 117] A few of the vaccines mentioned in this section were licensed products that at one time were in fairly widespread use. Others among the vaccines mentioned did not progress beyond early clinical trials or large-scale field trials because of unsatisfactory safety profiles, poor immunogenicity, disappointing efficacy relative to other typhoid vaccines, or difficulty in manufacture (e.g., loss of potency after lyophilization).

Parenteral Inactivated Whole-Cell Vaccines

Alcohol-Inactivated Vaccine

The prototype alcohol-inactivated vaccine was prepared in the 1940s by Felix, who published experimental evidence contending that alcohol treatment of *S. typhi* was superior in preserving the Vi antigen because it resulted in a vaccine that outperformed the heat-inactivated phenol-preserved vaccine in the mouse-protection assay.[118, 119] For some years this vaccine replaced the heat-inactivated phenol-preserved vaccine in routine use in the British Armed Forces.

Formalin-Inactivated Phenol-Preserved Vaccine

This vaccine, which was evaluated for efficacy in a controlled field trial,[120] was prepared by inactivating *S. typhi* with formalin and then preserving the vaccine in phenol.

Oral Inactivated Whole-Cell Vaccines

As early as the 1920s, Besredka[121, 122] promulgated the use of killed *S. typhi* or attenuated strains as oral vaccines to elicit "local immunity." In the 1960s and 1970s, several large-scale field trials[123–129] and experimental challenge studies in volunteers[130] were carried out to assess the efficacy of oral inactivated whole-cell vaccines, which at that time were widely sold and used in Europe. The oral killed vaccines that were evaluated in field trials or volunteer studies include acetone-inactivated vaccine and formalin-inactivated vaccine.

Parenteral or Aerosolized Subunit Vaccines

Many attempts were made to prepare extracts and sonicates of *S. typhi* and to purify antigens for use as parenteral vaccines. The various subunit immunizing agents (which in the 1960s were referred to as "chemical" vaccines) that have been evaluated for efficacy in controlled field trials (or in volunteer studies) include the following:

1. Freeze and thaw extract vaccines[131]
2. Trypsinized extract vaccines[132]
3. Purified lipopolysaccharide (LPS) vaccines (hot water-phenol extraction method)[133]
4. Purified Vi polysaccharide vaccine prepared by denaturing conditions[134, 135]

One chemical vaccine of the trypsinized extract variety was also evaluated for efficacy in a controlled field trial after administration by the aerosol route.[123]

Freeze and Thaw Extract Vaccines

A parenteral vaccine prepared by the method of Grasset[131] was assessed for efficacy in a controlled field trial in Poland.[136]

Trypsinized Extract Vaccines

Several trypsinized extract vaccines, prepared according to the method of Topley and associates,[132] were subjected to field trials of efficacy in the Soviet Union and Poland.[120, 136, 137]

Purified Lipopolysaccharide Vaccines

Two parenteral vaccines consisting of *S. typhi* LPS O antigen prepared by the hot water/phenol extraction method[133] were evaluated in controlled field trials in Poland[136] and the Soviet Union.[120]

Purified, Denatured Vi Polysaccharide

In the early 1950s, Landy and coworkers[134, 138] isolated Vi antigen from *Citrobacter freundii* (previous designations of this bacterium include *Paracolon ballerup*, *Bethesda ballerup*, and *Escherichia coli* 5396/38) and *S. typhi* for use as a parenteral vaccine. Organisms grown on solid agar were inactivated with acetone, after which the dried acetone-killed bacteria were submitted to multiple extractions with saline, ethanol, and acetic acid to separate Vi from protein, LPS, and nucleic acid. This early method of preparation of purified Vi antigen apparently denatured the polysaccharide, resulting in a complete loss of *O*-acetyl and a diminution of *N*-acetyl moieties.[40, 139, 140] Landy's denatured Vi vaccine was never evaluated for efficacy in field trials. However, in experimental challenge studies in volunteers, a single 25-μg parenteral dose conferred only modest (25% vaccine efficacy), insignificant protection.[53]

Attenuated Strains as Live Oral Vaccines

Attenuated *S. typhi* strains that were evaluated in phase 1 and 2 clinical trials but were abandoned from further development include the following:

1. Streptomycin-dependent strains[141–143]
2. Vi-positive variant of *galE* mutant Ty21a[144]
3. *galE*, via (Vi-negative) recombinant mutant strain EX642 derived from wild-type strain Ty2[145]
4. G 2260 hybrid strain (carrying DNA from *E. coli* K-12 and *Shigella flexneri*)[146]
5. Δ*aroA*, Δ*purA* auxotrophic strain 541Ty derived from wild-type strain CDC1080 (phage type A)[147]
6. 543Ty, Vi-negative derivative of auxotrophic strain 541Ty[147]
7. Δ*aroC*, Δ*aroD* double-mutant recombinant strain CVD 906 (derived from wild-type strain ISP 1896, phage type 46)[148, 149]
8. Δ*cya*, Δ*crp* mutant strain X3927 (derived from wild-type strain Ty2)[150, 151]

Streptomycin-Dependent Mutant Vaccines

The streptomycin-dependent strains of Reitman[141] and Mel and colleagues[142, 143] were developed by repeated cultivation of pathogenic *S. typhi* in the presence of streptomycin. These strains were unable to proliferate in the absence of streptomycin. However, the basis for their attenuation extends beyond dependency on streptomycin to maintain growth because these vaccine strains are innocuous even when administered orally along with streptomycin, which allows the organisms to proliferate.[143, 152, 153] In volunteer challenge studies, freshly harvested organisms of Reitman's streptomycin-dependent oral vaccine proved to be highly protective whereas lyophilized preparations were not.[152, 153]

Vi-Positive Variant of Ty21a

Cryz and associates[144] constructed a Vi-positive variant of strain Ty21a (see later) that was shown to be well tolerated and comparably immunogenic as Ty21a in phase 1 clinical trials.[155] The protective efficacy of this attenuated strain was never evaluated in clinical trials.

ΔgalE, Via-Negative Strain EX642

Using recombinant techniques, Hone and colleagues[145] deleted a 0.4-kilobase (kb) internal portion of *galE* from wild-type strain Ty2. A further mutant that lacked Vi antigen was selected and referred to as strain EX642. When fed to four adult volunteers in a dose of 7×10^8 colony-forming units (CFU) with buffer to neutralize gastric acid, two of the four volunteers developed typhoid fever.[145]

Strain G 2260

G 2260 is a hybrid strain of *S. typhi* that has incorporated into its genome chromosomal segments from both *E. coli* K-12 (the rha$^+$ xyl$^+$ fuc$^+$ region) and *S. flexneri* 2a (the pro$^+$ his$^+$ region).[146] This oral vaccine was well tolerated and modestly immunogenic in a small phase 1 study. Seven vaccinees were challenged with 2×10^5 CFU of a virulent *S. typhi* strain; two subjects shed the challenge strain and none developed illness.[146] Because no unimmunized control volunteers were concomitantly challenged, the stringency of that challenge model and the level of vaccine efficacy cannot be ascertained.

ΔaroA, ΔpurA Mutant 541Ty

Vaccine strain 541Ty was derived from wild *S. typhi* strain CDC10-80 by transducing deletions in two separate genes, each previously characterized in *S. typhimurium* and affecting a different biosynthetic pathway such that the mutations cause requirements for metabolites that are unavailable in adequate concentration in mammalian tissues.[147, 156, 157] The deletion mutation in *aroA* creates a requirement for aromatic compounds, including two (para-aminobenzoic acid and 2,3-dihydroxybenzoic acid) that are not available in adequate concentration in human tissues. The second deletion mutation, in *purA*, causes a specific requirement for adenine (or an assimilable compound such as adenosine).[147, 158] These nutritional requirements rendered *S. typhi* mutant 541Ty unable to sustain growth in mammalian tissues. A third mutation, in *hisG*, leads to a histidine requirement. Although the *hisG* mutation did not affect virulence, it provided an additional biochemical marker to clearly differentiate the vaccine strain from wild *S. typhi*.

In phase 1 clinical trials, Ty541 was well-tolerated but poorly immunogenic in eliciting serologic responses to *S. typhi* antigens.[154]

ΔaroA, ΔpurA *Vi-Negative Strain 543Ty*

Strain 543Ty is a spontaneously derived mutant of 541Ty that lacks the Vi polysaccharide capsular antigen; in all other ways this Vi-negative variant was identical to 541Ty.[147] Like 541Ty, in phase 1 clinical trials, Ty543 was well tolerated but poorly immunogenic in eliciting serologic responses to *S. typhi* antigens.[154] The protective efficacy of 541Ty and 543Ty was never examined in clinical trials.

ΔaroC, ΔaroD *Recombinant Strain CVD 906*

By recombinant techniques, precise deletions of 0.65 and 0.35 kb, respectively, were made in *aroC* and *aroD* of wild-type strain ISP1820 (phage type 46, isolated in 1983 from the blood culture of a Chilean schoolchild with uncomplicated typhoid fever), resulting in vaccine strain CVD 906.[148] In phase 1 clinical trials, CVD 906 given as a single oral dose was found to be highly immunogenic but insufficiently attenuated because several vaccinees developed febrile adverse reactions.[149, 151]

Δcya, Δcrp *Strain X3927*

In *Salmonella*, the products encoded by *cya* (adenylate cyclase) and *crp* (the cyclic adenosine monophosphate receptor protein) comprise a global regulatory system that regulates the transcription of multiple genes and operons.[150] These include genes concerned with the transport and breakdown of catabolites; the expression of fimbriae, flagella, and one outer membrane protein; and the transport systems for carbon sources. Deletion mutations were made in *cya* and *crp* of *S. typhimurium* by illegitimate excision of a transposon that had been inserted into each of these genes.[150] The Δ*cya* and Δ*crp* of *S. typhimurium* were then moved into wild-type *S. typhi* strain Ty2 by transduction with phage P22. The resultant *S. typhi* vaccine strain was designated X3927.[151, 159]

In phase 1 dose-response clinical trials, strain X3927 was moderately immunogenic but caused unacceptable febrile reactions in some subjects, so further clinical trials were discontinued.[151]

Currently Available and Used Vaccines

Currently used and commercially available typhoid vaccines include the following:

1. Heat-inactivated, phenol-preserved whole-cell parenteral vaccine (both liquid and lyophilized formulations and occasionally adsorbed to alum adjuvant)
2. Acetone-inactivated and dried whole-cell parenteral vaccine (lyophilized formulation)
3. Purified (nondenatured) Vi polysaccharide parenteral vaccine
4. Attenuated *galE*, Vi-negative strain Ty21a, used as a live oral vaccine

The results of the various clinical trials and field trials that established the safety, immunogenicity, and efficacy of the currently available typhoid vaccines are described in other sections of this chapter.

Parenteral Inactivated Whole-Cell Vaccines

Parenteral inactivated whole-cell vaccines to prevent typhoid fever have been used since the end of the 19th century. The experience with the early killed *S. typhi* parenteral vaccines has been reviewed.[160] Not until the mid 1950s were randomized, controlled field trials undertaken to assess the absolute and relative efficacy of more modern parenteral killed whole-cell typhoid vaccines.

Heat-Inactivated Phenol-Preserved Vaccine

By far, the most widely available and utilized parenteral killed whole-cell vaccine worldwide is the heat-inactivated phenol-preserved vaccine, which is relatively easy to prepare and standardize and is produced in essentially the same manner as that originally reported by Pfeiffer and Kolle[13] and Wright and co-workers.[14, 15, 161] The heat-killed phenol-preserved vaccine is made by heating agar or broth-grown *S. typhi* (usually to 56°C for 1 hour) and then suspending them in a 0.5% phenol solution, usually to a concentration of 10^9 organisms per milliliter.

Acetone-Inactivated and Dried Vaccine

This type of vaccine was prepared because of evidence showing that acetone-inactivation preserves the Vi antigen (thereby increasing potency in active mouse-protection assays) and improves the stability of the vaccine on long-term storage.[162–164] In preparing acetone-inactivated and dried vaccine, *S. typhi* organisms are precipitated and inactivated with acetone and then air dried or lyophilized.[163] The manufacturing process required to prepare acetone-inactivated, dried vaccine is much more demanding than that for making heat-phenolized vaccine.

Purified Vi Polysaccharide Vaccine

In a modern approach to purify Vi under nondenaturing conditions, Wong and coworkers[165] and Robbins and Robbins[40] treated *S. typhi* with hexadecyltrimethylammonium bromide (Fisher Scientific, Pittsburgh), the detergent that was previously instrumental in the preparation of purified meningococcal polysaccharide vaccines.[166] This extraction method results in purified Vi that is not denatured and that preserves the *O*- and *N*-acetyl moieties, as opposed to the methods used by Landy and coworkers that yielded denatured Vi. The chemical structure of Vi polysaccharide is shown in Figure 33–1.

Scale-up of production of Vi to an industrial manufacturing process was worked out by scientists from the

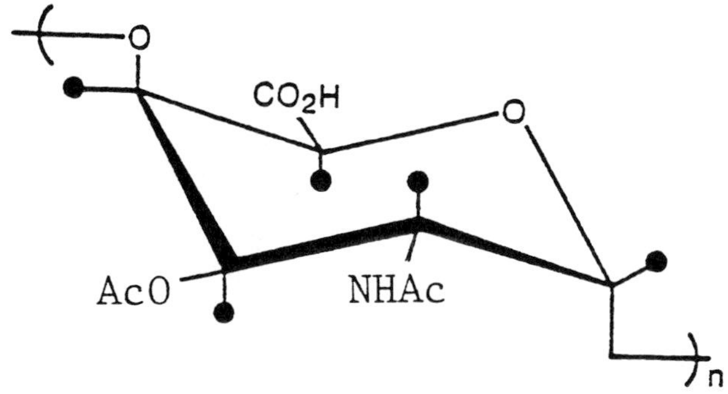

Figure 33–1. Chemical composition of Vi polysaccharide, which is a homopolymer of (1→4)-α-D-GalpANAC that is variably acetylated at carbon 3.

laboratory of John B. Robbins at the National Institute of Child Health and Human Development and Pasteur Mérieux Connaught.[167] The Ty2 strain of *S. typhi* is cultured in 1000-L fermentors, after which the bacteria are fixed with formaldehyde and Vi polysaccharide is extracted from supernatants using cetrimonium bromide. The Vi is further purified, dried, dissolved in a buffer solution, and filter-sterilized. After appropriate controls of this material, it is filled into single-dose syringes.

Attenuated S. typhi *Strain Ty21a as a Live Oral Vaccine*

Ty21a was derived from wild-type strain Ty2 by treatment with the mutagenic agent nitrosoguanidine.[168] A mutant was selected that exhibited a complete absence of activity of the enzyme uridine diphosphate (UDP)-galactose-4-epimerase and a reduction of approximately 80% in the activity of two other Leloir enzymes, galactokinase and galactose-1-phosphate uridyl transferase. A further mutant was then selected that lacked the Vi antigen. This strain was designated Ty21a.[168]

Galactose residues are an important component of the smooth LPS O antigen in wild-type *S. typhi*. The enzyme encoded by the *galE* gene, UDP-galactose-4-epimerase, isomerizes UDP-glucose to UDP-galactose and vice versa (Fig. 33–2). UDP-galactose provides galactose residues that can be incorporated into the smooth LPS O antigen of *S. typhi*. When grown in the absence of galactose, Ty21a does not express smooth O antigen, because it has no source of UDP-galactose; in this state it is not immunogenic.[169] In contrast, when *galE* mutant Ty21a is grown in the presence of exogenous galactose, the two other Leloir pathway enzymes (see Fig. 33–2) allow this monosaccharide to be assimilated to UDP-galactose and utilized to synthesize smooth O antigen. However, because of the lack of epimerase, strain Ty21a (like other *galE* mutants) accumulates galactose-1-phosphate and UDP-galactose when grown in the presence of exogenous galactose (see Fig. 33–2). In vitro, it can be shown that accumulation of these intermediate products leads to bacterial death by lysis.[168]

For many years it was thought that the *galE* and Vi mutations together accounted for the impressive in vivo safety of Ty21a. In the light of more recent data, it is now recognized that the *galE* and Vi mutations in Ty21a do not by themselves explain the attenuation of this strain.[145] Other mutations within strain Ty21a that were also induced by the nonspecific chemical mutagenesis contribute importantly to the safety of this oral vaccine strain. One such mutation may be in *rpoS* (*katF*), which encodes a RNA polymerase sigma factor; this mutation diminishes the ability of the bacteria to survive various stress conditions, including nutrient deprivation.[170]

Producers of Currently Available Vaccines

Killed Whole-Cell Vaccines

At present, the only United States manufacturer of parenteral inactivated whole-cell typhoid vaccine for ci-

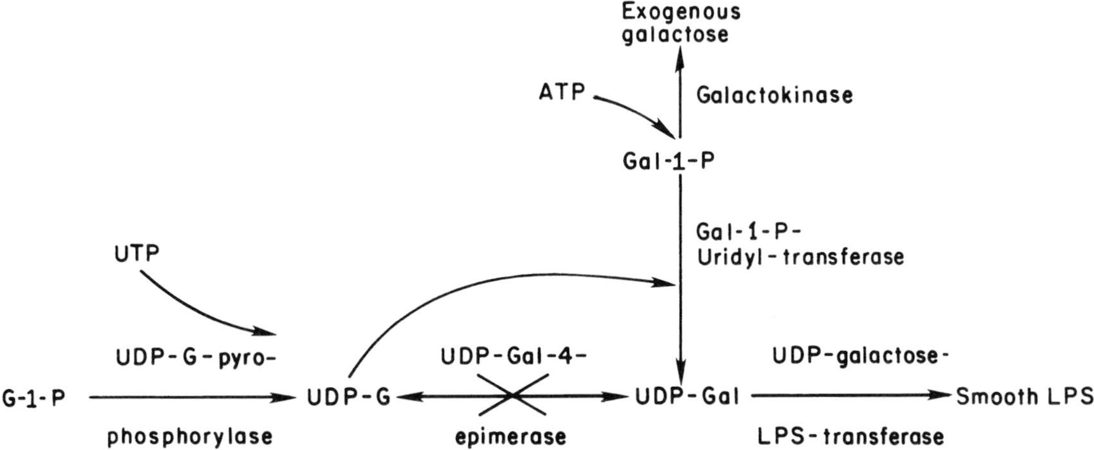

Figure 33–2. Scheme of incorporation of exogenous galactose by galE mutant Ty21a; attenuated *Salmonella typhi* vaccine strain is shown. When grown in the absence of galactose, Ty21a does not produce smooth lipopolysaccharide (LPS) O antigen and is nonimmunogenic. Grown in the presence of exogenous galactose, this hexose is sequentially processed to become galactose-1-phosphate (Gal-1-P) and then uridine diphosphate-galactose (UDP-Gal). Because of the complete lack of UDP-Gal-4-epimerase in Ty21a, UDP-Gal cannot be converted to UDP-glucose (UDP-G), but it can be further incorporated into smooth LPS O antigen. However, the accumulation of UDP-Gal and Gal-1-P consequent to the block of UDP-Gal-4-epimerase activity results in bacteriolysis. (Adapted from Germanier R, Furer E. Isolation and characterization of Gal E mutant Ty21a of *Salmonella typhi:* A candidate strain for a live oral typhoid vaccine. J Infect Dis 141:553–558, 1975.)

vilian use is Wyeth-Lederle, which makes a heat-inactivated phenol-preserved whole-cell liquid product. However, in recent years the supply of this vaccine has been intermittent. Wyeth is also licensed to make a lyophilized acetone-inactivated parenteral vaccine in the United States, on occasion, for the U.S. Armed Forces. However, the U.S. military has since switched to the use of Ty21a or Vi.

Elsewhere throughout the world there are many producers of heat-inactivated phenol-preserved typhoid vaccines and a few manufacturers of acetone-inactivated vaccine for parenteral use. The available products are published in the World Health Organization's *International List of Availability of Vaccines.*[171] In addition to commercial sources, government public health institutes in many countries in Asia, Latin America, and Africa manufacture their own typhoid vaccine.

Purified Vi

At the time of writing this chapter, the only licensed manufacturer of purified Vi was Pasteur-Mérieux-Connaught. However, it is anticipated that in 1998 a purified Vi polysaccharide vaccine manufactured by SmithKline Beecham will become licensed in Europe. A few government vaccine institutes in Asia also already make Vi for local consumption (China) or are considering doing so (Vietnam, India), and the ATV D-Team company manufactures a chromatographically purified Vi polysaccharide vaccine that is licensed in Russia.

Ty21a

Ty21a is manufactured by the Swiss Serum and Vaccine Institute. Under license, it is also distributed by a number of other vaccine distributors such as Medeva in the United Kingdom, Chiron-Biocine in Italy, and Chiron-Behring in Germany.

Dosage and Immunization Schedules

Parenteral Inactivated Whole-Cell Vaccines

The various parenteral killed whole-cell vaccines are usually administered subcutaneously with 0.5-mL injections containing approximately 5×10^8 bacteria; two doses are given 1 month apart. In an effort to diminish both local and systemic adverse reactions associated with these vaccines, some investigators have recommended the administration of 0.1 mL intradermally.[172–181] Although the antigenicity of vaccine given by the intradermal route has been compared with vaccine administered by the subcutaneous route, no controlled field trials of efficacy have been carried out to assess the protective value of intradermal immunization.

Subunit Vaccines

The modern nondenatured Vi vaccine is administered as a single subcutaneous injection containing 25 μg.[96, 97, 167] Single doses that contain 50 μg of purified polysaccharide have also been utilized in phase 2 and 3 clinical trials.[96, 182]

Ty21a Live Oral Vaccine

Irrespective of the formulation or whether a three-dose or four-dose oral immunization schedule is followed, each dose (capsule or sachet of lyophilized vaccine) contains 2 to 6×10^9 CFU of Ty21a.

With the enteric-coated capsule formulation, a four-dose oral immunization schedule is recommended in the United States and Canada, whereas in other countries throughout the world a three-dose regimen is used. Ty21a vaccine is administered with an interval of 1 day between doses. Increasing the interval between doses of enteric-coated vaccine to 21 days does not enhance protection.[113, 183] One of the field trials with the enteric-coated capsule formulation of Ty21a carried out in Santiago, Chile, showed that immunization with four doses within an 8-day period provides significantly greater protection than three doses.[114] Based on results of this field trial, the U.S. Food and Drug Administration and the Canadian Drug Board licensed Ty21a as a four-dose immunization schedule with a dose given every other day.

Two field trials, carried out in Chile[184] and Indonesia,[95] each directly compared the relative efficacy of three doses of Ty21a given in enteric-coated capsules versus vaccine administered as a liquid suspension (that is reconstituted by emptying a sachet containing lyophilized vaccine and a sachet containing buffer into 100 mL of water). The doses of vaccine were given every other day in the trial in Chile, whereas in Indonesia the doses were administered 1 week apart. In each of these trials, three doses of Ty21a in the liquid formulation provided better protection than the enteric-coated capsules. In the Chilean field trial the difference in the level of efficacy conferred by the two formulations was highly significant.[184] Since 1997, the liquid formulation of Ty21a has been licensed by a number of countries with a three-dose immunization regimen that recommends an interval of 1 day between doses.

A practical question arises when a subject fails to complete the full course of immunization with three to four doses of Ty21a. Does one need to simply complete the number of doses or must one reinitiate the full schedule? A definitive answer is not available. However, as a rule of thumb, if less than 3 weeks have passed since the last dose, one may continue to complete the immunization with the missing doses. If more than 3 weeks have passed, the full regimen of this well-tolerated vaccine should be administered de novo.

Formulations Available

Heat-Phenolized Parenteral Vaccine

The heat-inactivated, phenol-preserved vaccine is usually available as a liquid suspension containing 1×10^9 bacilli per milliliter.

Purified Vi Polysaccharide Parenteral Vaccine

Purified Vi is available as a solution containing 25 μg of Vi polysaccharide in 0.5 mL of phenolic isotonic buffer.

Ty21a

There have been three successive commercial formulations of Ty21a, each representing a notable improvement over the earlier versions. The initial commercial formulation of Ty21a (which was available for only a short time) consisted of gelatin-coated capsules containing either $NaHCO_3$ (0.4–0.5 g) or lyophilized vaccine (2 to 6 × 10^9 CFU per dose).[113, 183, 185, 186] Vaccination with this initial formulation involved the ingestion of two gelatin capsules, each containing bicarbonate, followed by a third capsule containing vaccine; doses were ingested every other day for a total of three vaccine doses.

Field trials in Santiago, Chile, compared the efficacy of the gelatin capsule-$NaHCO_3$ formulation with a formulation consisting of lyophilized vaccine in enteric-coated capsules (2 to 6 × 10^9 CFU per capsule) that requires no pretreatment with buffer to neutralize gastric acid.[113, 183] After results of controlled field trials that demonstrated the superiority of the enteric-coated capsule formulation over the gelatin capsule formulation, the latter was withdrawn and replaced with the enteric-coated capsule formulation. Enteric-coated capsules should be ingested on a fasting stomach with a little water.

Since 1997, the liquid suspension formulation of Ty21a has been licensed in several countries with a three-dose immunization regimen that recommends an interval of 1 day between doses. This formulation comes as a double sachet, one sachet containing 2 to 10 × 10^9 CFU of lyophilized vaccine and the other containing buffer. The contents of the two sachets are added to 100 mL of water with stirring, resulting in the vaccine suspension.

Constituents

Heat-Phenolized Parenteral Vaccine

Each vial of heat-inactivated, phenol-preserved vaccine typically contains 1 × 10^9 bacilli per milliliter in 0.5% phenol.

Purified Vi Polysaccharide Parenteral Vaccine

Purified Vi is available as a solution containing 25 μg of Vi polysaccharide in 0.5 mL of phenolic isotonic buffer. Each immunizing dose contains 25 μg of Vi polysaccharide, less than 1.25 mg of phenol, q.s. 0.5 mL of isotonic buffer (4.15 mg sodium chloride; 0.065 mg sodium dibasic phosphate, $2H_2O$; 0.023 mg sodium monobasic phosphate, $2H_2O$; q.s. 0.5 mL water for injection).

Ty21a

Enteric-Coated Capsules

Gelatin capsules are coated with phthalate to render them resistant to acid. Each coated capsule contains 2 to 6 × 10^9 CFU of Ty21a, 5 to 50 × 10^9 nonviable Ty21a, 26 to 130 mg of sucrose, 1 to 5 mg of ascorbic acid, 1.4 to 7.0 mg of an amino acid mixture, 100 to 180 mg of lactose, and 3.6 to 4.4 mg of magnesium stearate.

Liquid Suspension Formulation

The vaccine sachet contains 2 to 10 × 10^9 CFU of Ty21a, 5 to 60 × 10^9 nonviable Ty21a, 15 to 250 mg of sucrose, 0.6 to 10 mg of ascorbic acid, 0.8 to 15 mg of an amino acid mixture, 1.5 g of lactose, and 20 to 30 mg of aspartame. The accompanying sachet of buffer contains 2.4 to 2.9 g of sodium bicarbonate, 1.5 to 1.8 g of ascorbic acid, and 0.18 to 0.22 g of lactose.

Vaccine Stability

Parenteral Inactivated Whole-Cell Vaccines

Driesens has shown that the stability of the pH of liquid formulations of acetone-inactivated vaccine is the major determinant of the vaccine's shelf life and that this stability is related to the type of glass vial.[187] Acetone-inactivated fluid vaccines stored in buffered saline solutions maintained potency for more than 30 months when stored at 4°C. By contrast, the same vaccine in unbuffered saline solution lost potency as the pH increased. Vaccines packaged in U.S. Pharmacopeia borosilicate glass vials retained stable pH and potency, whereas vaccines stored in type III U.S. Pharmacopeia soda-lime glass vials were less stable. If kept refrigerated, heat-inactivated phenol-preserved vaccine has a shelf life of 18 months after leaving the manufacturer's cold storage.

Using the active mouse-protection test as the measure of vaccine potency, Joo and Zsidai[188] systematically investigated the stability of fluid and lyophilized forms of heat-inactivated phenol-preserved and acetone-inactivated vaccines stored at 37°C or 4°C for 12 weeks. Their results showed that fluid vaccines must be maintained in the cold chain to maintain potency; the fluid vaccines lost significant potency within 2 weeks of storage at 37°C. By contrast, the lyophilized vaccine retained potency even after 12 weeks of storage at high temperature. The potency of lyophilized vaccine after long-term storage has been corroborated by Dimache and associates,[174] who showed that lyophilized vaccine was still antigenic and still gave acceptable results in the mouse-protection test after 5 years of storage at 4°C. The shelf life of lyophilized typhoid vaccine is dependent on the residual moisture content of the lyophilate; the lower the residual moisture, the longer the shelf life.[188] Vaccines with moisture contents below 3% have a long shelf life.

Purified Vi Polysaccharide Vaccine

The Vi polysaccharide vaccine, even as a liquid formulation, is fairly stable and retains its physicochemical characteristics 6 months after storage at 37°C and after 2 years at 22°C. Nevertheless, the manufacturer recommends that the vaccine be stored in a refrigerator at 2 to 8°C for up to 18 months.

Ty21a

Long-term storage of Ty21a should be at 4°C. The shelf life of lyophilized Ty21a is dependent on residual moisture content and maintenance of a cold chain.[189, 190]

The potency requirements of Ty21a dictate that the viable counts within each dose (enteric-coated capsule or packet of lyophilized vaccine) exceed 2×10^9 CFU. Prolonged storage for 7 days at room temperature (20–25°C [73–82°F]) resulted in progressively lower viable counts over time. Nevertheless, after a 7-day test period all 10 lots tested still met the minimum potency requirements.[191] Similarly, three separate lots of Ty21a maintained potency when stored at 37°C (98.6°F) for 12 hours.[191]

Laboratory Control of Vaccine Lots (Potency Assays)

Parenteral Inactivated Whole-Cell Vaccines

Many laboratory tests of typhoid vaccine "potency" were carried out in conjunction with the large-scale controlled field trials of vaccine efficacy sponsored by the World Health Organization in an attempt to identify a test, an animal model, or an assay that can predict vaccine potency in humans reliably.[192–208] These tests have consisted mainly of measurement of antibody responses in animals (and humans) and active protection assays in small laboratory animals. Unfortunately, no satisfactory laboratory test has been identified that clearly predicts the potency of all parenteral killed or extract typhoid vaccines or attenuated strains used as live oral vaccines.

The World Health Organization Expert Committee on typhoid vaccines concluded that no single potency test can be used to predict reliably the efficacy of typhoid vaccines in humans.[209] Nevertheless, two assays have shown sufficient correlation with field trial results of parenteral vaccines to have advocates: (1) an elicitation of H antibodies after parenteral immunization of rabbits and (2) an active mouse-protection test.

In conjunction with field trials of the fluid alcohol-inactivated and heat-inactivated phenol-preserved parenteral vaccines in Yugoslavia,[210] investigators in several laboratories found that the more effective heat-inactivated, phenol-preserved vaccine elicited significantly higher levels of H antibody in rabbits.[54, 202, 208] Similarly, in conjunction with the later field trials comparing the lyophilized heat-inactivated, phenol-preserved (L) and acetone-inactivated (K) reference vaccines,[120, 136, 211–214] the more effective K vaccine was again found to stimulate significantly higher H antibody titers in both rabbits and humans (Table 33–1).[194, 195, 201, 203, 211, 215] Debate has raged as to whether this observation implies that protection is directly related to H antigens and mediated by H antibodies or whether the H agglutinins rather serve as a marker to denote that a gentler method of inactivation of *S. typhi* has preserved other highly labile and uncharacterized protective antigens.[216]

S. typhi is an impressively human host–adapted parasite. This fact has greatly impeded the development of a relevant and practical animal model for the testing of typhoid vaccines. Among primates, only chimpanzees develop an experimental infection with *S. typhi* that in its pathogenesis rather closely resembles that found in humans. Furthermore, after inoculation by whatever route, no small laboratory animal species manifests a general infection that resembles human typhoid fever. Several types of active immunization of mice (subcutaneous or intraperitoneal) followed by intraperitoneal challenge with *S. typhi* in saline or mucin have been evaluated in various laboratories.[192, 195–198, 200–206, 208, 214, 215, 217, 218] The different techniques gave varying results; sometimes results from different laboratories were contradictory, despite ostensibly using essentially the same procedure with reference reagents. Nevertheless, several investigators have argued that active intraperitoneal immunization of mice followed 7 to 14 days later by intraperitoneal challenge with pathogenic *S. typhi* in mucin represents the best potency test for typhoid vaccines, among the various alternatives. Results of this assay paralleled the results of the field trials of K and L vaccines (see Table 33–1). Much controversy surrounds the overall usefulness and applicability of this assay be-

Table 33–1. **COMPARISON OF ACETONE-INACTIVATED (K) AND HEAT AND PHENOL–INACTIVATED (L) REFERENCE VACCINES: ABILITY TO STIMULATE ANTIBODY, ACTIVITY IN MOUSE-PROTECTION TESTS, AND EFFICACY IN FIELD TRIALS**

TEST	VACCINE GROUP		TETANUS TOXOID CONTROL
	K	L	
Agglutinins in humans*			
H	1008	720	16
O	13	17	2
Vi†	21	20	4
Agglutinins in rabbits			
H	320	40‡	—
O	320	640	—
Active mouse protection test			
Relative potency	3.6	1.0	—
Efficacy in controlled field trials			
Guyana (7 yr of surveillance)	88%	67%	—
Yugoslavia (2½ yr of surveillance)	79%	51%	—

*Geometric mean titer 2 weeks after second dose of vaccine.
†Measured by passive hemagglutination.
‡Geometric mean titer 7 days after fourth inoculation with vaccine diluted 1:100.

cause it strongly favors vaccines that have a high Vi antigen content; vaccines that are potent in stimulating Vi antibody are highly protective in mice because Vi is a major virulence property in this species.[118, 219–222] Because acetone-inactivation of *S. typhi* enhances the preservation of Vi,[162, 221, 222] the K vaccine performed particularly well in this assay when compared with the L vaccine, which preserves Vi less well.

The field trial in Egypt[223] of an acetone-inactivated typhoid vaccine prepared from a nonflagellated mutant (TNM1) of *S. typhi* strain Ty2[72, 73] provided the opportunity to evaluate which was more important: elicitation of H antibody or potency in the mouse-protection test. This vaccine did not stimulate H antibody because it lacked flagella; however, it was as potent in mouse-protection tests as the acetone-inactivated reference vaccine K. Nevertheless, in the field trial this vaccine was not protective,[223] suggesting that the active mouse-protection test is not an adequate predictor of efficacy of typhoid vaccines in humans.

Despite the controversy that surrounds it, the active mouse-protection test is used in the United States to assay the potency of parenteral killed whole-cell typhoid vaccines.[224]

Purified Vi Polysaccharide Parenteral Vaccine

The active protection test in mice, as used for the inactivated whole-cell parenteral vaccines, can serve as a potency test for the Vi vaccine.

Ty21a and Other Live Oral Vaccines

At present, viable counts of vaccine organisms are used as the measure of potency of live oral vaccines. Until a more relevant potency test is developed, the active protection test in mice can also serve as a potency test for attenuated strain vaccines; here the vaccine is also inoculated intraperitoneally in mice even though it is administered orally in humans.

RESULTS OF VACCINATION

Immune Response

Because of the complex nature of the pathogenesis of *S. typhi* clinical infection, a protective role is probably played by secretory intestinal antibody (in preventing mucosal invasion), circulating antibody (against bacteremic organisms), and cell-mediated immunity (to eliminate intracellular bacilli). With parenteral vaccines, the circulating antibody response is substantial and presumably provides the predominant protective effect. In contrast, with live attenuated oral vaccines, the circulating antibody response may be modest, but vigorous intestinal secretory immunoglobulin A (sIgA) and cell-mediated immune responses occur that are believed to be responsible for the protection conferred by that type of vaccine.

Unfortunately, with *S. typhi* the critical antigens responsible for protection are not agreed on, and data are somewhat contradictory. With parenteral vaccines, elicitation of serum H (flagellar) antibodies in humans correlates with protection, whereas stimulation of O and Vi antibodies does not.[194, 208, 211, 223] In contrast, with live oral vaccines the mucosal IgA and systemic cell-mediated immune responses appear in large part to be directed toward the O and H antigens but not to the Vi antigen.[113, 149, 151, 187, 225–239] In fact, the licensed attenuated strain (Ty21a) lacks Vi antigen[126] yet provides significant protection.[95, 98, 113, 183, 184, 240, 241]

Parenteral Inactivated Whole-Cell Vaccines

Serum Antibody Response

Typically, in assessing the seroconversion after vaccination with a parenteral inactivated whole-cell typhoid vaccine, serum antibodies are measured to the O, H (d), and Vi antigens. O antibodies were formerly assayed by bacterial agglutination (Widal test),[194] but ELISA using purified LPS has become popular in recent years.[149, 151, 225, 226, 228–230, 242] H antibody is measured by agglutination using an appropriate whole-cell antigen such as *Salmonella virginia* (which has the same d flagellar antigen as *S. typhi* but lacks Vi and has distinct O antigens) or by ELISA using purified *S. typhi* flagella.[225, 226, 228, 229] Vi antibody can be measured by passive hemagglutination,[75, 76, 182] radioimmunoassay,[40, 96, 243, 244] or ELISA.[77, 97] It is important to utilize highly purified undenatured Vi antigen to avoid cross reactions. For this reason, only since the 1980s did Vi serology become reliably specific.

The evidence suggesting that anti-H antibodies may play a role in protection has been discussed in part in the section on vaccine potency. In Yugoslavia, Poland, the Soviet Union, and Guyana, field trials of efficacy were carried out with several different well-characterized parenteral killed whole-cell vaccines including alcohol-inactivated, heat-phenolized, and acetone-inactivated vaccines. Measurement of serological responses to these vaccines in groups of vaccinees and in immunized laboratory animals allowed protective efficacy to be correlated with antibody response. Those killed whole-cell parenteral vaccines that were most protective in the field stimulated the highest levels of H antibody. A similar correlation between H titer and protection against typhoid fever was found in healthy young adult volunteers who in the 1960s and 1970s participated in experimental challenge studies to assess the efficacy of typhoid vaccines.[153, 169, 245] Control volunteers who had elevated H titers (presumably derived by natural infection or vaccination many years earlier during military service) were significantly protected against development of typhoid fever.

However, the most convincing evidence that H antibody is important comes from the field trial by Wahdan and colleagues[223] of an acetone-killed and dried vaccine prepared from a strain of *S. typhi* that lacks H antigen. This vaccine, which did not elicit H antibodies, failed to confer significant protection.

In Table 33–1 are shown the serum antibody responses to *S. typhi* O, H, and Vi antigens after vaccination of children with parenteral acetone-inactivated or heat-inactivated, phenol-preserved whole-cell vaccines.[193] These data from children in the Guyana field trial are representative of the serological responses encountered with these types of vaccines.

O antibody that appears after inoculation with parenteral inactivated whole-cell typhoid vaccines is largely IgM, whereas the H antibody response is initially IgM and then becomes IgG.[236, 246–250]

Mucosal Immune Response

Not surprisingly, the few studies that have examined mucosal immunity after administration of parenteral inactivated whole-cell vaccine have reported minimal secretory IgA antibody or gut-derived IgA antibody-secreting cell (ASC) responses.[236, 251–253]

Cell-Mediated Immune Response

Some cell-mediated immune responses have been measured after vaccination with parenteral killed whole-cell vaccines.[231, 237, 254, 255] The assays utilized have included lymphocyte replication or antibody-dependent mononuclear cell migration inhibition in the presence of soluble antigen or inhibition of growth of *S. typhi* by mononuclear cells. The cell-mediated response after administration of these vaccines has not been prominent.

Purified Vi Polysaccharide Parenteral Vaccine

Serum Antibody

Parenteral Vi polysaccharide vaccine elicits serum IgG Vi antibody responses in 85 to 95% of adults or children older than 2 years of age. In Table 33–2 are shown the serum Vi and O antibody responses reported by Tacket and colleagues[243] after vaccination of young adults with one of two purified Vi antigen vaccines prepared from *S. typhi.* The vaccines differed in their degree of purity; one Vi vaccine had 5% residual contamination with LPS, but the other was 99.8% pure. This difference was reflected in the serological response. Although similar Vi antibody seroconversions occurred in approximately 90% of recipients of either preparation, those who received the more purified preparation had only a 26% seroconversion of O antibody versus 83% who seroconverted to O antigen after inoculation with the less purified vaccine.

The serological responses of other groups of adults and children in nonendemic and endemic areas are shown in Table 33–3.[96, 97, 167, 244, 256, 257] In contrast to the strong responses in adults and children older than 2 years of age, the Vi antibody response in toddlers in Indonesia was weak and short lived.[167]

Purified Vi polysaccharide behaves like a T-lymphocyte–independent antigen. The serum antibody response is not boosted by administration of additional doses of Vi vaccine.[244, 256] A second dose of Vi given by Keitel and colleagues[244] 27 to 34 months after a primary inoculation stimulated fourfold rises in serum Vi antibody titer in 33 to 50% of subjects. However, the titers only returned to the levels achieved 1 month after the primary immunization. Titers of Vi antibody progressively fall over time.[244] Klugman[258] has proposed that a serum Vi antibody titer of greater than or equal to 1.0 μg per mL be considered a conservative estimate of the threshold required to confer protection.

As with other T-independent purified polysaccharide vaccines, Vi is not a good immunogen in infants. Most infants do not respond; among those who do, the responses are meager and short lived.

Ty21a

Serum Antibody Response

The serum antibody response has been extensively studied with Ty21a. Gilman and colleagues noted that Ty21a vaccine grown in the presence of galactose (which leads to organisms bearing smooth LPS O antigen) was highly protective, whereas vaccine grown in the absence of galactose (resulting in rough organisms) was not.[169] These investigators reported that recipients of vaccine

Table 33–2. **IMMUNE RESPONSE TO TWO *SALMONELLA TYPHI* Vi POLYSACCHARIDE VACCINE CANDIDATES**

	Vi TITERS*			***S. TYPHI* LIPOPOLYSACCHARIDE TITERS (ELISA)**		
	Geometric Mean Titer			**Geometric Mean Titer**		
	Before	*After*	**Seroconversions (%)†**	*Pre*	*Post*	**Seroconversions (%)‡**
Vi Lot 53226						
Maryland students	0.17	2.57	100	0.11	0.78	83
Chilean recruits				0.15	0.77	83
Vi Lot IMS1569						
French volunteers	0.07	2.73	95	0.12	0.22	26§

*Measured by radioimmunoassay.
†Increase in antibody of 0.15 μg/mL.
‡Increase in net optical density of 0.15.
§X^2 = 28.3; $P < .0001$ versus recipients of lot 53226.
Data from Tacket CO, Ferreccio C, Robbins JB, et al. Safety and characterization of the immune response to two *Salmonella typhi* Vi capsular polysaccharide vaccine candidates. J Infect Dis 154:342–345, 1986.

Table 33–3. **SERUM Vi ANTIBODY RESPONSES MEASURED BY RADIOIMMUNOASSAY IN ADULTS AND CHILDREN IMMUNIZED WITH 25-μg DOSES OF A LIQUID FORMULATION OF PURIFIED Vi POLYSACCHARIDE VACCINE**

			Vi ANTIBODY			
			Geometric Mean Titer (μg/mL)			
STATE	AGE GROUP (yr)	N	*Pre*	*Post**	Rate of Seroconversion (%)†	REFERENCE
United States	18–40	54	0.2	3.2	93	244
Nepal	45–55	8	0.5	4.4	63	96
	15–44	43	0.4	3.7	79	
	5–14	65	0.2	1.9	77	
Indonesia	>22	22	0.8	11.3	68	167
	5–12	80	0.3	5.0	88	
	2–4	54	0.2	5.8	96	
Kenya	5–15	97	0.3	2.0	76	257

*One month after immunization.
†Fourfold or greater rise in titer.

grown in the presence of galactose experienced a significantly greater seroconversion of O antibody.

Using serum IgG O antibody measured by ELISA in Chilean 15-to 19-year olds, Levine and associates showed a correlation between seroconversion to various dosage schedules and formulations and protective efficacy in field trials (Table 33–4).[113] With the currently licensed enteric-coated capsule formulation, there is a stepwise increase in the proportion of vaccinees who manifest significant rises in serum IgG O antibody depending on whether one, two, or three doses of vaccine are administered within 1 week. Although serum O antibody is not believed to be the operative mechanism of immunity elicited by attenuated strains, it clearly correlates with protection. Because measurement of serum IgG ELISA antibody to *S. typhi* O antigen is a simple technique, it provides investigators with a practical tool for comparing immunization schedules and formulations and for evaluating new candidate live oral vaccines.

Mucosal Immune Response

During the past decade, the intestinal mucosal immune response to Ty21a and several new live oral vaccines has been studied rather extensively. Most recipients of the usual three-dose oral regimen of Ty21a develop local antibody responses to O antigen.[232–236, 239, 252, 253, 259–262] Forrest has reported that the propensity to develop a significant rise in intestinal sIgA O antibody after immunization with Ty21a is inversely correlated with the preimmunization baseline level of intestinal antibody.[263] Subjects who have elevated baseline titers of sIgA O antibody mount significantly lowerfold rises than those of vaccinees with absent or low titers. This inverse correlation between baseline titer and propensity to seroconvert has also been reported for the serum vibriocidal antibody response after immunization with live oral cholera vaccines[264] and with Ty21a expressing *Vibrio cholerae* O1 antigen.[265]

After oral administration of antigen, activated lymphocytes in the Peyer's patches and other gut-associated lymphoid tissue migrate to local lymph nodes to mature. After maturation they return to the lamina propria of the intestine as well as to other organs of the mucosal immune system such as the salivary glands, respiratory tract, genitourinary tract, and mammary glands. Kantele and coworkers[232–236, 260, 262] and Forrest[266] have shown that such gut-derived migrating cells can be detected in peripheral blood and that the ability of these cells to secrete specific IgA antibody in the presence of specific antigen can be quantified by means of the ELISA spot[267] or similar techniques.[266] These IgA-producing migrating cells are only detectable during a few days after immunization. The peak detection of gut-derived IgA ASCs in peripheral blood after oral immunization occurs approximately 7 days after vaccination.[151, 226, 228, 229, 232–236, 260]

Table 33–4. **RATES OF SEROCONVERSION OF IgG-ELISA *S. TYPHI* O ANTIBODY AFTER ONE TO THREE ORAL DOSES OF Ty21a LIVE ORAL TYPHOID VACCINE GIVEN WITHIN 1 WEEK**

		SEROCONVERSION		
FORMULATION	NO. DOSES	Rate	%	EFFICACY IN FIELD TRIALS (%)
Enteric-coated capsules	3	61/96	64	67
	2	22/50	44	47
	1	9/50	18	18
Vaccine/$NaHCO_3$ in gelatin capsules	3	99/195	50	21

Serological data from Levine MM, Ferreccio C, Black RE, et al. Progress in vaccines to prevent typhoid fever. Rev Infect Dis 11(suppl 3):S552–S567, 1989. Field trial surveillance data are from the first 36 months of follow-up in field trials in Area Norte (Black RE, Levine MM, Ferreccio C, et al. Efficacy of one or two doses of Ty21a *Salmonella typhi* vaccine in enteric-coated capsules in a controlled field trial. Vaccine 8:81–84, 1990) and Area Occidente, Santiago, Chile (Levine MM, Ferreccio C, Black RE, et al. Large-scale field trial of Ty21a live oral typhoid vaccine in enteric-coated capsule formulation. Lancet 1:1049–1052, 1987.)

Table 33–5. **THE MAGNITUDE OF TRAFFICKING, GUT-DERIVED IgA ANTIBODY-SECRETING CELL RESPONSE TO *S. TYPHI* O ANTIGEN AFTER IMMUNIZATION WITH DIFFERENT FORMULATIONS AND DOSAGE SCHEDULES OF LIVE ORAL TYPHOID VACCINE Ty21a**

VACCINE STRAIN	FORMULATION	NO. OF DOSES	NO. OF VIABLE ORGANISMS/DOSE	IgA ASC RESPONSE	
				% Responders	GMN‡
Ty21a	Gelatin capsule/$NaHCO_3$	3*	2×10^9	7/10†	6
Ty21a	Enteric-coated capsules	3*	2×10^9	18/20	23
Ty21a	Liquid suspension	3*	2×10^9	19/20	63
	Liquid suspension	2*	2×10^9	16/20	12
	Liquid suspension	1	2×10^9	10/20	3

*Every other day schedule.
†Number of responders/number of subjects vaccinated.
‡Geometric mean number of IgA antibody-secreting cells (ASCs) per 10^6 peripheral blood mononuclear cells.

Kantele immunized adult Finnish volunteers with different formulations and immunization schedules of Ty21a, attempting to parallel the different regimens that were used in field trials of the efficacy of Ty21a in Chile and Indonesia.[232] Kantele's results demonstrate that the gut-derived IgA ASC response closely correlates with the efficacy results recorded in field trials (Table 33–5). Thus, three doses (taken every other day) of Ty21a in enteric-coated capsules are markedly more immunogenic than one dose, and Ty21a in a liquid suspension is more immunogenic than vaccine in enteric-coated capsules.

Forrest and associates studied the mucosal immune response when three doses of Ty21a are administered per rectum on days 0, 2, and 5.[268] Each dose of vaccine contained 2×10^{11} CFU, a 100-fold larger dose than is contained in the commercial Ty21a preparation. These vaccinees showed a significant increase in sIgA anti–*S. typhi* O antibody in jejunal fluid, serum, and saliva and in gut-derived IgA ASCs.[268]

Cell-Mediated Immune Response

Cell-mediated immune responses have been measured after vaccination with Ty21a.[231, 237, 238, 253, 269, 270] The assays utilized have included lymphocyte replication in the presence of soluble or particulate antigen[269, 270] or inhibition of growth of *S. typhi* by mononuclear cells in the presence of antibody.[231, 237, 238, 253] Newer live oral vaccines stimulate fairly potent cell-mediated immune responses.[227, 271]

In their studies of the lymphocyte replication response to various *S. typhi* antigens after oral immunization with Ty21a, Murphy and coworkers[269, 270] observed that heat-inactivated phenol-preserved particulate *S. typhi* served as a sensitive and specific antigen. Sztein and associates have found purified flagella from *S. typhi* to be an excellent antigen for stimulation of immune lymphocytes.[227]

Tagliabue and coworkers described a potent anti-*Salmonella* immune response after oral immunization with Ty21a that involves peripheral blood mononuclear cells and immune serum. Mixing peripheral blood mononuclear cells from a neutral donor with postimmunization sera from vaccinees results in marked inhibition of growth of *S. typhi*.[231, 237, 238, 253] Neither mononuclear cells by themselves nor postvaccination serum alone had this effect. These investigators reported that the peripheral blood mononuclear cell that mediates this effect is a $CD4^+$ lymphocyte and that the specific serum antibodies are of the IgA class. This group also showed that intestinal sIgA could substitute for serum IgA.

Comparison with Natural Infection

The circulating, secretory, and cell-mediated immune response is relatively strong after natural infection and includes both prominent serum and cell-mediated components.[53, 70, 272–278] Parenteral killed whole-cell vaccines elicit a serum response equal to that of natural infection but not a comparable cell-mediated response. With live oral vaccines the opposite is true.

Murphy and associates[269, 270] observed that the peripheral blood mononuclear cells from healthy adults living in typhoid-endemic areas who have no known history of acute typhoid fever often specifically proliferate when exposed to *S. typhi* antigens. This corroborates the results of antibody prevalence studies that indicate that in such endemic areas mild or subclinical infections are common.

Results of Controlled Field Trials

Parenteral Inactivated Whole-Cell Vaccines

From the mid-1950s to the early 1970s, the World Health Organization sponsored a series of well-designed, randomized, controlled field trials in countries with endemic typhoid to assess the absolute and relative efficacy of various typhoid vaccines and their duration of protection. In these studies, only culture-confirmed cases were used in calculating incidence rates and vaccine efficacy. In the first trial, in Yugoslavia, the efficacy of two doses of alcohol-killed vaccine was compared with that of heat-inactivated phenol-preserved vaccine, with tetanus toxoid serving as the control vaccine.[208, 210, 279] Both vaccines gave significant protection, but the heat-inactivated phenol-preserved vaccine proved to be superior to the alcohol-killed vaccine (Table 33–6).

In the early 1950s, laboratory studies demonstrated that acetone-inactivated typhoid vaccine resulted in better preservation of the Vi antigen,[162] thus raising the question of whether such a vaccine might be superior to the heat-inactivated phenol-preserved vaccine. The

Table 33–6. **COMPARISON OF HEAT-INACTIVATED, PHENOL-PRESERVED AND ALCOHOL-KILLED, ALCOHOL-PRESERVED FLUID PARENTERAL TYPHOID VACCINES GIVEN AS TWO PRIMARY DOSES WITH OR WITHOUT A REINFORCING DOSE 1 YEAR LATER (YUGOSLAVIA, 1954–1960)**

VACCINE GROUP	NO. VACCINATED	CASES OF TYPHOID PER 10^5	VACCINE EFFICACY (%)	DURATION OF SURVEILLANCE (yr)
Heat inactivated				
Two primary doses	11,503	61[a]	68	1
Two primary and booster doses	8595	81[b]	74	5*
Alcohol inactivated				
Two primary doses	12,017	141[c]	27	1
Two primary and booster doses	8913	157[d]	50	5*
Control (tetanus toxoid)				
Two primary doses	11,988	192[e]	—	5*
Two primary and booster doses	9002	311[f]	—	5*

a versus e; $P = .0086$.
a versus c; $P = .083$.
c versus e; $P = .42$.
b versus f; $P = .0012$.
d versus f; $P = .048$.
b versus d; $P = .22$.
*Period of surveillance after inoculation with booster dose.
Adapted from Yugoslav Typhoid Commission. A controlled field trial of the effectiveness of phenol and alcohol typhoid vaccines. Bull World Health Organ 26:357–369, 1962.

Walter Reed Army Institute of Research prepared for the World Health Organization large reference lots of acetone-inactivated and heat-inactivated phenol-preserved vaccines,[163, 164] designated vaccines K and L, respectively, for large-scale field trials to be carried out in Yugoslavia,[213] Guyana,[211, 212] Poland,[136, 214] and the Soviet Union.[120] The K and L vaccines and the methods for their production also served as international standards to prepare future lots of vaccines of these types for subsequent field trials. For example, in addition to the K and L reference vaccines themselves, two additional K-type vaccines have been tested in controlled field trials and have provided critical information. These include a K-type vaccine used in a randomized, controlled field trial in Tonga to directly compare the efficacy of one versus two doses of vaccine[280]; a K-type vaccine made from a nonflagellated *S. typhi* strain, which was field tested for efficacy in Alexandria, Egypt[223]; and a K-type vaccine evaluated in a single dose against an alum-adsorbed heat-inactivated, phenol-preserved vaccine.[281, 282]

Results of the trials with K, L, and K-type vaccines are summarized in Table 33–7. The major conclusions that can be drawn are the following:

1. Both acetone-inactivated and heat-inactivated, phenol-preserved typhoid vaccines provide significant protection against typhoid fever after two subcutaneous doses, but the acetone-killed vaccine is somewhat superior (79–88% protection for the K vaccine versus 51–66% for the L vaccine).[120, 136, 212, 213]

2. The efficacy of the reference K and L vaccines varied from one geographical site to another.

3. When directly compared in a randomized trial (Tonga), two doses of an acetone-inactivated vaccine gave significantly superior protection to that of a single dose.[280] Previously, in nonrandomized comparisons little difference had been noted between the efficacy conferred by one or two doses.[212]

4. A K-type vaccine prepared from a nonflagellated *S. typhi* strain failed to provide significant protection.[223]

5. A single dose of a K-type vaccine, without adjuvant, provided comparable protection to that of a single dose of an alum-adsorbed heat-inactivated, phenol-preserved vaccine.[281, 282]

The K and L vaccines were also evaluated for efficacy in experimental challenge studies in North American volunteers.[53] Perhaps the most important insight to come from these studies was the observation that protection conferred by the vaccines was relative to the number of pathogenic *S. typhi* used for the experimental challenge (Table 33–8). When 10^5 pathogenic *S. typhi* comprised the challenge inoculum, the K and L vaccines provided approximately 70% protection. However, when the challenge inoculum contained 10^7 bacilli, there was virtually no protection demonstrable (0–14% vaccine efficacy). Differences in inoculum size in nature may be responsible for some of the differences of vaccine efficacy encountered among different field sites and over time.

Vi Polysaccharide Parenteral Vaccine

Two randomized, controlled field trials were carried out in Nepal[96] and South Africa[97] to investigate the efficacy of the nondenatured purified Vi vaccine. A single 25 μg dose conferred 72% protection against typhoid fever in Nepal during 17 months of follow-up and 64% efficacy in South Africa over 21 months of surveillance (Table 33–9). The Nepal trial included all ages from preschool to adults, whereas the South African trial was performed in schoolchildren. A subsequent report from the South African trial showed that over 3 years of follow-up vaccine efficacy was 55% (see Table 33–9).[258]

Ty21a

In early studies in adult volunteers, multiple doses of freshly harvested Ty21a organisms were found to be safe

Table 33–7. **RESULTS OF CONTROLLED FIELD TRIALS OF LYOPHILIZED ACETONE-INACTIVATED AND HEAT AND PHENOL–INACTIVATED REFERENCE VACCINES**

FIELD SITE, DATES	AGE GROUPS	VACCINE (NO. DOSES)	NO. VACCINATED	DURATION OF SURVEILLANCE	INCIDENCE OF TYPHOID PER 10^5	VACCINE EFFICACY (%)	REFERENCE
Yugoslavia 1960–1963	2–50 yr (mostly schoolchildren)	K (2)	5028	2½ yr	318[a]	79	213
		L (2)	5068	2½ yr	727[b]	51	
		Control (2)	5039	2½ yr	1488[c]	—	
Guyana 1960–1967	5–15 yr (schoolchildren)	K (2)	24,046	7 yr	67[d]	89	212
		L (2)	23,431	7 yr	209[e]	65	
		Control (2)	27,241	7 yr	602[f]	—	
Poland 1961–1964	5–14 yr (schoolchildren)	K (2)	81,534	3 yr	7[g]	85	136
		Control (2)	83,734	3 yr	47[h]	—	
Soviet Union 1962–1965	Schoolchildren and young adults (92 age 7–15 yr)	L (2)	36,112	2½ yr	55[i]	66	120
		Control (2)	36,999	2½ yr	162[j]	—	
Tonga 1966–1973	All ages (69 <21 yr)	K-type* (2)	11,128	7 yr	288 (180)†[k]	39 (56)†	280
		K-type* (1)	11,391	7 yr	500 (272)†[l]	0 (34)†	
		Controls (2)	11,129	7 yr	476 (413)†[m]	—	
Egypt 1978–1981	6–7 yr (schoolchildren)	Nonflagellated K-type (2)‡	16,679	11 mo	114[m]	0	223
		Control (2)	16,650	11 mo	84[m]	—	
Soviet Union 1966	7–20 yr	K-type (1)§	52,347	10 mo	21[n]	53	282
		Control (1)	52,816	10 mo	45[o]	—	

*A distinct lot of lyophilized acetone-inactivated vaccine made at the Walter Reed Army Institute of Research in a manner identical to their product of reference vaccine K.

†Numbers in parentheses are results of the first 5 years of surveillance.

‡A lyophilized acetone-inactivated vaccine prepared by the Lister Institute, London, from strain TNM1, a nonflagellated mutant of *S. typhi* Ty2.

§Lyophilized acetone-inactivated vaccine prepared at the Institute of Vaccines and Sera, Zagreb, according to methods for K vaccine Production (Walter Reed Army Institute of Research, 1964[95]).

a versus c; $P = .00001$.
b versus c; $P < .0004$.
a versus b; $P = .0064$.
d versus f; $P < .000001$.
e versus f; $P < .000005$.
d versus e; $P < .000046$.
g versus h; $P = .0000025$.
i versus j; $P = .000021$.
k versus m; $P < .03$.
l versus m; $P = .87$.
k versus l; $P = .015$.
n versus o; $P = .045$.

and to confer significant protection against experimental challenge.[169] Thereafter, a field trial of efficacy was carried out in Alexandria, Egypt, where 16,486 schoolchildren aged 6 and 7 years were given three 10^9 organism doses of vaccine on Monday, Wednesday, and Friday of 1 week.[240, 241] Lyophilized vaccine in glass vials was reconstituted with 30 mL of diluent and ingested by the children 1 to 3 minutes after they chewed a tablet containing 1.0 g of $NaHCO_3$. A similar number (15,902) of other children received placebo in this randomized, double-blind, controlled field trial. During 3 years of epidemiological surveillance, only one culture-confirmed case of typhoid fever occurred among the vaccinees, as opposed to 22 cases among the controls (96% protection) (Table 33–10).

Table 33–8. **EFFICACY OF PARENTERAL ACETONE-INACTIVATED (K) AND HEAT AND PHENOL–INACTIVATED (L) REFERENCE VACCINES AND Vi POLYSACCHARIDE VACCINE IN EXPERIMENTAL CHALLENGE STUDIES IN VOLUNTEERS: EFFECT OF SIZE OF CHALLENGE INOCULUM ON EFFICACY**

VACCINE GROUP	10^5 *S. TYPHI** Attack Rate	Vaccine Efficacy	10^7 *S. TYPHI** Attack Rate	Vaccine Efficacy
K†	4/43 (9%)	63%	12/28 (43%)	14%
L†	3/45 (7%)	71%	13/24 (54%)	0
Vi‡	3/17 (18%)	25%	10/14 (71%)	0
Control	28/104 (24%)	—	15/30 (50%)	—

*Inoculum of pathogenic *S. typhi* ingested by volunteers.

†Three subcutaneous doses were administered.

‡One 50 μg subcutaneous dose of Landy's denatured Vi vaccine was given.

Data from Hornick RB, Greisman SE, Woodward TE, et al. Typhoid fever: Pathogenesis and control. N Engl J Med 283:686–691, 739–746, 1970.

Although this preliminary field trial with Ty21a provided highly encouraging results, considerable work needed to be done to ascertain whether Ty21a could be a practical public health tool. The liquid formulation used in Egypt was not readily amenable to mass production, so alternate formulations had to be prepared and evaluated. It was necessary to determine whether fewer (one or two) doses could protect, to assess the duration of protection, to investigate the effect of increased spacing between vaccine doses, and to ascertain whether infants and young children could be immunized safely and successfully. Many of these questions were answered in a series of five randomized, controlled field trials carried out in Santiago, Chile (four trials), and Indonesia (one trial), under auspices of the World Health Organization and the Pan American Health Organization.[98, 112–114, 183, 184]

The four field trials in Chile involved approximately 550,000 children, aged 6 to 19 years, who were vaccinated in school-based programs after which epidemiological surveillance was maintained through the health centers of the National Health Service. Only culture-confirmed cases were used in the computation of incidence rates and vaccine efficacy.

In the field trial in the Western (Occidente) adminis-

Table 33–9. **RESULTS OF RANDOMIZED, CONTROLLED, DOUBLE-BLIND FIELD TRIALS IN NEPAL AND SOUTH AFRICA ASSESSING THE EFFICACY OF A SINGLE 25-μg DOSE OF NONDENATURED PURIFIED Vi POLYSACCHARIDE SUBUNIT VACCINE IN PREVENTING CULTURE-CONFIRMED TYPHOID FEVER**

	PERIOD OF FOLLOW-UP	Vi VACCINE	CONTROL VACCINE
Nepal Trial*	17 mo		
No. of subjects		3457	3450
Cases		9	32
Incidence/10^5		260	928
Efficacy		72%	—
(95% CI)		(42–86%)	—
South Africa Trial†	21 mo		
No. of subjects		5692	5692
Cases		16	44
Incidence/10^5		281	773
Efficacy		64%	—
(95% CI)		(36–79%)	—
	36 mo		
Cases		30	66
Incidence/10^5		527	1160
Efficacy		55%	—
(95% CI)		(30–71%)	—

*Participants were randomized to receive a 0.5-mL intramuscular inoculation containing either 25 μg of purified Vi or 23-valent pneumococcal polysaccharide. (Data from Acharya VL, Shrestha MB, Cadoz M, et al. Prevention of typhoid fever in Nepal with the Vi polysaccharide of *Salmonella typhi:* A preliminary report. N Engl J Med 317:1101–1104, 1987.)

†Participants were randomized to receive a single 25-μg intramuscular dose of Vi or a 50-μg dose of meningococcal polysaccharide vaccine. (Data from Klugman K, Gilbertson IT, Koornhof HJ, et al: Protective activity of Vi polysaccharide vaccine against typhoid fever. Lancet 2:1165–1169, 1987; and Klugman KP, Koornhof HJ, Robbins JB, et al: Immunogenicity, efficacy and seriological correlate of protection of *Salmonella typhi* Vi capsular polysaccharide vaccine three years after immunization. Vaccine 14:435–438, 1996.)

CI, confidence interval.

trative area of Santiago,[183] the efficacy conferred by three doses of vaccine in enteric-coated capsules was compared with that provided by three doses of vaccine in the gelatin capsule–$NaHCO_3$ formulation. As seen in Table 33–11, over 3 years of surveillance the enteric-coated vaccine provided significantly superior protection. Over 7 years of follow-up, the regimen of three doses of Ty21a in enteric-coated capsules (every other day interval between doses) conferred 62% protection.

A randomized, controlled, double-blind field trial in the Northern (Norte) area of Santiago showed that immunization with only one or two doses of Ty21a in enteric-coated capsules resulted in a moderate level of protection that was short lived (Table 33–12).[98] Although two doses of vaccine conferred 60% protection during the first 2 years of surveillance, efficacy dropped to insignificant levels during the third year and virtually disappeared by the fourth year of surveillance.

A very large trial involving more than 200,000 schoolchildren was carried out in the Southern and Central administrative areas of Santiago to compare directly the protective effects of two, three, or four doses of Ty21a vaccine in enteric-coated capsules and to assess the use of Ty21a as a public health tool.[114] No placebo group was included in this trial. The salient feature of this trial is the observation that four doses of vaccine provided significantly greater protection than three doses (Table 33–13). The results of this trial formed the basis for the recommended four-dose immunization schedule after licensure of Ty21a in the United States and Canada (a three-dose regimen is used elsewhere).

In the mid-1980s the Swiss Serum and Vaccine Institute succeeded in preparing a "liquid suspension" formulation of Ty21a for large-scale field trials that was amenable to large-scale manufacture. The new formulation consists of two packets, one containing a dose of lyophilized vaccine and the other containing buffer. Contents of the two packets are mixed in a cup containing 100 mL of water, and the suspension is then ingested by the subject to be vaccinated. Field trials were initiated in Santiago, Chile,[184] and in Plaju, Indonesia,[95] to directly compare this new liquid formulation of Ty21a (which somewhat resembles what was used in the Alexandria, Egypt, field trial) with the enteric-coated capsule formulation. Results of these trials are summarized in Table 33–14. Vaccine administered as a liquid suspension was superior to vaccine in enteric-coated capsules. In the Santiago trial the difference was highly significant. Ty21a given as a liquid suspension protected young children as well as older children.[184] In previous trials with enteric-coated vaccine, young children were not as well protected as older children.[183]

Table 33–10. **FIELD TRIAL OF EFFICACY OF THREE DOSES OF A LIQUID FORMULATION OF Ty21a VACCINE GIVEN WITH $NaHCO_3$ TO 6- AND 7-YEAR-OLD SCHOOLCHILDREN IN ALEXANDRIA, EGYPT**

PERIOD OF OBSERVATION (1978–1981)	CONFIRMED CASES OF TYPHOID FEVER	INCIDENCE PER 10^5	VACCINE EFFICACY (%)
Vaccinees n = 16,486	1	6.1	96 (77–99)*
Placebo n = 15,902	22	138.3	

*95% confidence interval.

Adapted from Wahdan MH, Serie C, Cerisier Y, et al. A controlled field trial of live *Salmonella typhi* strain Ty21a oral vaccine against typhoid: Three year results. J Infect Dis 145:292–296, 1982.

Duration of Vaccine-Derived Immunity

Parenteral Inactivated Whole-Cell Vaccines

The longest periods of surveillance (7 years) for efficacy of the parenteral killed whole-cell vaccines were carried out in the Guyana and Tonga field trials. In Guyana, two doses of the acetone-killed K vaccine conferred a high level of protection (88%) for 7 years.[212] In contrast, in Tonga, two doses of a K-type vaccine provided moderate protection for a period of only 5 years, after which protection was no longer demonstrable.[280] Two doses of the heat-inactivated, phenol-preserved vaccine (L) tested in Guyana showed moderate (77%) protection during the first 3 years, but this level fell to 47%

Table 33–11. **COMPARISON OF THE EFFICACY OF TWO DIFFERENT FORMULATIONS OF Ty21a LIVE ORAL VACCINE GIVEN BY TWO DIFFERENT IMMUNIZATION SCHEDULES IN AREA OCCIDENTE, SANTIAGO, CHILE: RESULTS OF 36 MONTHS OF FOLLOW-UP (9/1983–8/1986)**

	ENTERIC-COATED CAPSULES		GELATIN CAPSULES WITH $NaHCO_3$		
	Long Interval*	**Short Interval†**	**Long Interval**	**Short Interval**	**PLACEBO**
N	21,598	22,170	21,541	22,379	21,906
Cases	34	23	46	56	68
Incidence	157.4[a]	103.7[b]	213.5[c]	250.3[d]	310.4[e]
Efficacy	49%	67%	31%	19%	—
	(24–66)†	(47–79)	(0–52)	(0–43)	

*Three doses, 21 days between doses.
†Three doses, 1 to 2 days between doses.
a versus e; $P = .0006$. d versus e; $P = .21$.
b versus e; $P < .00001$. a versus c; $P = .23$.
c versus e; $P = .0023$. b versus d; $P = .00052$.
a + b vs c + d; $P = .001$.
Data from Levine MM, Ferreccio C, Black RE, et al. Large-scale field trial of Ty21a live oral typhoid vaccine in enteric-coated capsule formulation. Lancet 1:1049–1052, 1987.

protection during the last 4 years of surveillance. In several other field trials in which the period of surveillance was only 2½ years, the acetone-inactivated and the heat-inactivated, phenol-preserved vaccines conferred significant protection for at least 30 months.[120, 136, 213]

Vi Polysaccharide Vaccine

In the South African field trial, surveillance was maintained for 3 years. During this period the efficacy of the Vi vaccine was 55% (see Table 33–9).[258]

Table 33–12. **COMPARISON OF THE EFFICACY OF ONE VERSUS TWO DOSES OF Ty21a LIVE ORAL TYPHOID VACCINE GIVEN IN ENTERIC-COATED CAPSULE FORMULATION: RESULTS OF A RANDOMIZED, CONTROLLED, DOUBLE-BLIND TRIAL IN AREA NORTE, SANTIAGO, CHILE**

	ONE DOSE (27,618)	TWO DOSES (27,620)	PLACEBO (27,305)
	Year 1 (7/82–6/83)		
No. of cases	47	30	62
Incidence/10^5	170.2[a]	108.6[b]	227.1[c]
Efficacy	25%	52%	—
	Year 2 (7/83–6/84)		
No. of cases	25	11	38
Incidence/10^5	90.5	39.8	139.2
Efficacy	35%	71%	—
	Year 3 (7/84–6/85)		
No. of cases	19	15	19
Incidence/10^5	68.8	54.3	69.6
Efficacy	0%	22%	—
	Year 4 (7/85–6/86)		
No. of cases	30	23	28
Incidence/10^5	108.6	83.3	102.5
Efficacy	−6%	19%	—

a versus c; $P = .42$.
a versus b; $P = .037$.
b versus c; $P = .0032$.
Data from Black RE, Levine MM, Ferreccio C, et al. Efficacy of one or two doses of Ty21a *Salmonella typhi* vaccine in enteric-coated capsules in a controlled field trial. Vaccine 8:81–84, 1990.

Ty21a Live Oral Vaccine

In the field trial in Alexandria, Egypt, three doses of a liquid formulation of vaccine conferred a high level of protection (96%) that persisted for 3 years, the point at which surveillance was discontinued.[240] Three doses of vaccine in enteric-coated capsules given at an interval of every other day conferred 67% protection over 3 years[183] and 62% protection over 7 years of follow-up in a field trial in Santiago, Chile (Levine and coworkers, unpublished data).

Three doses of Ty21a in a liquid formulation provided 78% protection for 3 years[184] and 79% protection during a fourth and fifth year of follow-up in a field trial in Santiago (Levine and colleagues, unpublished data).

Comparison of Vaccine-Derived Immunity with Natural Immunity

Several sources of data suggest that the immunity that follows clinical infection with pathogenic *S. typhi* is relative and can be overcome. Marmion and col-

Table 33–13. **COMPARISON OF THE EFFICACY OF TWO, THREE, AND FOUR DOSES OF Ty21a VACCINE IN ENTERIC-COATED FORMULATION: RESULTS OF A RANDOMIZED FIELD TRIAL IN AREA SUR AND AREA CENTRAL, SANTIAGO, CHILE**

SURVEILLANCE FROM 11/1984 TO 10/1987	TWO DOSES	THREE DOSES	FOUR DOSES
No. of vaccinees	66,615	64,783	58,421
No. of cases	123	104	56
Incidence/10^5	184.6[a]	160.5[b]	95.8[c]
95% confidence interval	152–271	130–191	71–121

a versus c; $P = .0004$.
b versus c; $P = .002$.
a versus b; $P = .32$.
Data from Ferreccio C, Levine MM, Rodriguez H, et al. Comparative efficacy of two, three, or four doses of Ty21a live oral typhoid vaccine in enteric-coated capsules: A field trial in an endemic area. J Infect Dis 159:766–769, 1989.

Table 33–14. **COMPARISON OF THE EFFICACY OF THREE DOSES OF Ty21a ADMINISTERED IN ENTERIC-COATED CAPSULES OR AS A LIQUID SUSPENSION OF VACCINE ORGANISMS: RESULTS OF RANDOMIZED, PLACEBO-CONTROLLED FIELD TRIALS IN SANTIAGO, CHILE, AND PLAJU, INDONESIA**

	SANTIAGO, CHILE			PLAJU, INDONESIA		
	Enteric-Coated Capsules	**Liquid Suspension**	**Placebo**	**Enteric-Coated Capsules**	**Liquid Suspension**	**Placebo**
No. of subjects	34,696	36,623	10,302	5209	5066	10,268
No. of cases of typhoid	63	23	28	61	48	208
Incidence/10^5	182	63	272	468	379	810
Efficacy	33%	77%	—	42%	53%	—
95% confidence interval	0–57%	60–87%	—	23–57%	36–66%	—

Data from Levine M, Ferreccio C, Cryz S, Ortiz E. Comparison of enteric-coated capsules and liquid formulation of Ty21a typhoid vaccine in a randomized controlled field trial. Lancet 336:891–894, 1990; and Simanjuntak C, Paleologo F, Punjabi N, et al. Oral immunisation against typhoid fever in Indonesia with Ty21a vaccine. Lancet 338:1055–1059, 1991.

leagues[283] and others have reported successive outbreaks of typhoid fever in soldiers who, in the space of a few months, experienced two separate bouts of typhoid fever. In the volunteer studies carried out by Hornick and colleagues[53] and DuPont and associates,[130] two relevant observations were reported. The first is that immunity to typhoid fever is relative and can be overcome if a large infecting dose is ingested. Second, the protective effect of a prior clinical typhoid infection was only 28%; that is, 5 of 22 volunteers (23%) who recovered from an induced *S. typhi* infection developed typhoid fever when rechallenged with pathogenic organisms as opposed to 11 of 34 control volunteers ($P > .05$).

Based on these observations, it can be argued that Vi polysaccharide vaccine and Ty21a, as well as the parenteral killed whole-cell vaccines, stimulate rather credible immunity compared with natural immunity elicited by infection with wild type *S. typhi*. Undoubtedly, in endemic areas most individuals experience multiple subclinical *S. typhi* infections, each serving to further boost the state of immunity; individuals who develop overt disease represent a minority of all those infected.

Adverse Events

Parenteral Inactivated Whole-Cell Vaccines

Common

Although the parenteral killed whole-cell vaccines provide moderate to good protection, high rates of systemic and local adverse reactions make them unsatisfactory public health tools.[120, 211, 213, 284–286] Table 33–15 summarizes the adverse reaction rates from several controlled, double-blind evaluations of parenteral killed whole-cell vaccines. The high rates of fever, malaise, local erythema, induration, and pain are obvious. Acetone-inactivated and heat-inactivated, phenol-preserved vaccines administered by jet gun cause higher rates of local adverse reactions than vaccine given by syringe.[287]

Many investigators have compared the reactogenicity and antigenicity of small intradermal doses of parenteral killed whole-cell vaccines with those of full subcutaneous doses. Most of these studies have shown that 0.1-mL intradermal doses elicit significantly fewer adverse reactions than full (0.5 mL) subcutaneous doses of vaccine, and the serological response is only slightly diminished.[172–179] Nevertheless, the protective efficacy of intradermal vaccine has never been assessed in a field trial.

Rare

Rarely, more significant reactions have been attributed to vaccination with parenteral killed whole-cell typhoid vaccines. These include thrombocytopenic purpura,[288, 289] acute renal disease,[290–294] dermatomyositis,[295] appendicitis,[296] erythema nodosum,[297] multiple sclerosis,[298] and a syndrome of high fever, severe malaise, and toxemia,[285, 286] sometimes accompanied by coagulopathy, thrombocytopenia, hepatitis, and renal insufficiency.[299] Rarely, sudden death occurs after parenteral inoculation with inactivated whole-cell typhoid vaccine.[300]

Vi Polysaccharide

Common

When Vi vaccine is highly purified, it is well tolerated.[167, 243, 244] As little as 5% impurity with LPS results in systemic adverse reactions in a proportion of recipients.[243] In controlled phase 2 trials in U.S. adults, local reactions including pain and tenderness were the most common adverse events.[243, 244] Passive surveillance carried out during field trials showed the Vi vaccine to be as well tolerated as the licensed (meningococcal and pneumococcal) polysaccharide vaccines that served as the control preparations in these trials.[96, 97]

Ty21a

Ty21a provides significant protection without causing adverse reactions.[95, 113, 241, 301–303] Results of three double-blind, placebo-controlled studies that utilized active surveillance methods to assess the reactogenicity of Ty21a in adults and children are shown in Table 33–16. The rates of adverse reactions in the vaccine recipients were not significantly higher than those for the placebo group for any symptom or sign. In large-scale field trials with

Table 33–15. **THE FREQUENCY OF FEVER, MALAISE, AND PAIN AT THE INJECTION SITE APPROXIMATELY 24 HOURS AFTER SUBCUTANEOUS INOCULATION WITH HEAT AND PHENOL–INACTIVATED (L) AND ACETONE-INACTIVATED (K) WHOLE CELL TYPHOID VACCINES OR TETANUS TOXOID**

	NO. OF VACCINEES			FEVER AFTER VACCINATION (%)			INABILITY TO WORK (%)	LOCAL PAIN (%)	
VACCINE GROUP	Yugoslavia	Guyana	USSR	Yugoslavia*	Guyana†	USSR‡	Yugoslavia	Yugoslavia	Guyana
Heat and phenol–inactivated	343	86	1656	24	29	6.7	23	35	54
Acetone-inactivated	326	80	—	22	26	—	21	32	45
Tetanus toxoid	328	86	1757	3	7	2.4	5	4	—

*>37°C.
†>37.8°C.
‡37.5°C.
Data from Yugoslav Typhoid Commission. A controlled field trial of the effectiveness of acetone-dried and inactivated and heat-phenol–inactivated typhoid vaccines in Yugoslavia. Bull World Health Organ 30:623–630, 1964; Ashcroft MT, Morrison-Ritchie J, Nicholson CC. Controlled field trial in British Guyana school-children of heat-killed-phenolized and acetone-killed lyophilized typhoid vaccines. Am J Hyg 79:196–206, 1964; and Hejfec LB, Salmin LV, Lejtman MZ, et al. A controlled field trial and laboratory study of five typhoid vaccines in the USSR. Bull World Health Organ 34:321–339, 1966.

Ty21a, involving approximately 550,000 schoolchildren in Chile and 32,000 in Egypt and approximately 20,000 subjects ranging in age from 3 years to adulthood in Indonesia, passive surveillance failed to identify vaccine-related adverse reactions.[95, 98, 183, 184, 241, 304]

Indications

Populations for whom vaccine is indicated include the following:

1. Travelers to less-developed areas where typhoid is known or believed to be endemic
2. Military personnel (who represent a special group of travelers)
3. School-aged children in areas in which typhoid is endemic, particularly where multiply antibiotic-resistant strains are prevalent
4. Microbiology technicians in clinical microbiology laboratories or in research laboratories in which *S. typhi* is handled

Table 33–17 summarizes the immunization schedules and dosages, for different age groups, for the oral Ty21a and the parenteral Vi and heat-phenolized whole-cell vaccines.[112, 305]

Typhoid vaccine is *not* generally indicated after floods, earthquakes, or other natural disasters during which the water supply and sewage systems may suffer structural damage.[306, 307] Resources should rather be directed toward repairing the contaminated water sources, which, it is hoped, could be achieved long before a mass vaccination could be completed and the protective effect of vaccine initiated. Nevertheless, there are situations in which typhoid vaccines may serve as a helpful adjunct to other control measures. For example, if a major upheaval occurs in a region of a country where typhoid is endemic and formidable economic or political obstacles are expected to impede timely improvements in water supply

Table 33–16. **RANDOMIZED, PLACEBO-CONTROLLED, DOUBLE-BLIND CLINICAL TRIALS OF THREE DOSES OF Ty21a IN ENTERIC-COATED CAPSULES, IN MILK WITH $NaHCO_3$ OR IN BUFFER SUSPENSION TO ASSESS REACTOGENICITY OF THE VACCINE IN ADULTS, SCHOOL-AGED CHILDREN, AND PRESCHOOL-AGED CHILDREN**

	ADULTS, CHILE		6- AND 7-YEAR-OLDS		ALL AGES, INDONESIA			
ADVERSE REACTION	Enteric-Coated Vaccine (385)*	Placebo (367)*	Enteric-Coated Vaccine (172)*	Placebo (172)*	Enteric-Coated Vaccine (311)*	Placebo (291)*	Liquid Suspension Vaccine (333)*	Placebo (255)*
Diarrhea	1.8†	1.1	1.2	9.9	3.9	3.1	3.8	5.5
Vomiting	0.5	0.3	2.3	11.0	1.0	1.7	1.5	0.8
Fever	0.3	0.5	0.6	0.6	4.8	1.7	4.8	3.5
Rash	0.5	0.5	ND	ND	1.0	0.3	1.2	0.4

No adverse reactions occurred significantly more frequently in vaccinees than in placebo controls in these clinical trials, all of which utilized active surveillance methods to detect adverse reactions.
*Total number of subjects.
†Percent of total subjects in the group with reactions.
ND, Not determined.
Data from Levine MM, Black RE, Ferreccio C, et al. The efficacy of attenuated *Salmonella typhi* oral vaccine strain Ty21a evaluated in controlled field trials. In Holmgren J, Lindberg A, Molly R (eds). Development of vaccines and drugs against diarrhea. Lund, Sweden, Studentlitteratur, 1986, pp 90–101; Black RE, Levine MM, Young C, et al. Immunogenicity of Ty21a attenuated *Salmonella typhi* given with sodium bicarbonate or in enteric-coated capsules. Dev Biol Stand 53:9–14, 1983. S. Karger, Basel; and Simanjuntak C, Paleologo F, Punjabi N, et al. Oral immunisation against typhoid fever in Indonesia with Ty21a vaccine. Lancet 338:1055–1059, 1991.

Table 33–17. **IMMUNIZATION SCHEDULES FOR Ty21a, Vi, AND HEAT-INACTIVATED, PHENOL-PRESERVED TYPHOID VACCINES**

VACCINE	FORMULATION	ROUTE	AGE	NO. DOSES	INTERVAL BETWEEN DOSES	INTERVAL UNTIL NEXT BOOSTER
Ty21a live strain						
Primary	Enteric-coated capsules	Oral	≥6 yr	3 or 4*	2 d	5 yr
	Reconstituted liquid suspension†	Oral	≥2 yr	3	2 d	5 yr
Booster	Enteric-coated capsules	Oral	≥6 yr	3 or 4	2 d	5 yr
	Reconstituted liquid suspension†	Oral	≥6 yr	3	2 d	5 yr
Vi capsular polysaccharide						
Primary	Liquid	Intramuscular (0.5 mL)	≥2 yr	1	—	3 yr
Booster	Liquid	Intramuscular (0.5 mL)	≥2 yr	1	—	3 yr
Heat-inactivated, phenol-preserved whole cell‡						
Primary	Liquid	Subcutaneous				
		(0.25 mL)	6 mo–10 yr	2	4 wk	3 yr
		(0.50 mL)	>10 yr	2	4 wk	3 yr
Booster	Liquid	Subcutaneous				
		(0.25 mL)	6 mo–10 yr	1	4 wk	3 yr
		(0.50 mL)	>10 yr	1	4 wk	3 yr

*Four doses in the United States and Canada; three doses in all other countries.
†Liquid suspension is currently licensed in only a few countries.
‡Because of frequency of severe adverse reactions associated with this vaccine (e.g., fever, malaise), it is not recommended for routine use. Rather, Ty21a or Vi should be used.

quality and sanitation infrastructure, selective vaccination of high risk groups may be helpful.

It has been suggested by some that a period of increased risk of acquisition of typhoid fever occurs for approximately 10 days after the administration of the first dose of parenteral killed whole-cell vaccine; this has been referred to as the "negative phase" after vaccination.[308–311] Such a phenomenon has not been described for Vi or Ty21a vaccines.

Contraindications

There are no contraindications to immunization with parenteral Vi polysaccharide vaccine. Although there are no definitive contraindications to immunization with killed whole-cell vaccines, in view of the reactogenicity of this vaccine, it should not be given to people who have experienced severe systemic reactions on previous inoculation with this vaccine. Moreover, it would be prudent to avoid giving this vaccine to debilitated or elderly people with chronic health problems such as individuals with cardiac, renal, collagen vascular, or oncologic disease.

As a general rule, Ty21a should not be given to pregnant women, although adverse effects on the pregnant woman or fetus have not been reported. Similarly, caution should be taken before anyone with a known depression of cell-mediated immunity is given Ty21a. On the other hand, there would appear to be no risk for immunocompromised household contacts of Ty21a vaccinees, because excretion of Ty21a has never been detected in any subject given the available formulations that contain 2 to 6 $\times$ 10^9 CFU per dose.

If immunocompromised individuals, including human immunodeficiency virus (HIV)–infected people, must travel to endemic areas, Vi vaccine should be administered. It is important to immunize such travelers because studies of HIV-infected individuals in typhoid-endemic areas have revealed that they are at greatly increased risk of developing typhoid fever.[312]

Ty21a should not be administered to individuals who are taking antibiotics. Certain antimalarials, particularly mefloquine, exhibit activity against Ty21a in vitro.[191, 313, 314] In clinical trials, coadministration of chloroquine, mefloquine, or chloroquine plus pyrimethamine/sulfadoxine did not significantly suppress the serum IgG O antibody response after immunization with Ty21a,[315, 316] whereas coadministration of proguanil did.[315] Based on these data, it has been proposed that Ty21a should not be taken with proguanil; it may be taken with chloroquine, and one should wait 8 to 24 hours after administration of mefloquine before initiating immunization with Ty21a.

Simultaneous Administration of Typhoid Vaccines with Other Vaccines

Parenteral killed whole-cell and subunit typhoid vaccines have been administered concomitantly with *paratyphi* A and B, *Shigella flexneri* or *Shigella sonnei*, or tetanus (toxoid) antigens in field trials[120]; the typhoid components remained immunogenic and protective. Typhoid vaccines have also been administered parenterally in combination with tetanus and diphtheria toxoids and inactivated *Bordetella pertussis* and *V. cholerae*, with serological assessment.[172, 176, 317–319]

Vi Polysaccharide Parenteral Vaccine

Clinical studies have also been carried out in which purified Vi polysaccharide was coadministered along with other parenteral vaccines, including inactivated poliovirus vaccine, yellow fever vaccine,[320] hepatitis B vaccine, hepatitis A vaccine, rabies vaccine,[321] diphtheria and tetanus toxoids, acellular pertussis vaccine, meningococcal vaccine,[322] and measles/mumps/rubella vaccine.

A combination typhoid/hepatitis A vaccine has been developed at SmithKline Beecham for use in travelers. This vaccine, which contains 25 μg of Vi and 1440 units of inactivated hepatitis A virus antigen adsorbed to 0.5 mg of alum, is presently in advanced clinical trials.[323] A similar combination hepatitis A/Vi polysaccharide vaccine is under development by Pasteur Mérieux Connaught.

Ty21a

Ty21a can be coadministered along with oral attenuated poliovirus or with parenteral 17-D-strain yellow fever vaccine.[191, 315] Several large, phase 2 clinical trials have examined the safety and immunogenicity of coadministering the first or the third dose of the liquid suspension formulation of Ty21a in a combination oral vaccine cocktail along with single-dose live oral cholera vaccine CVD 103-HgR (available under the trade name Orochol in Europe, Asia, and Latin America and under the name Mutacol in Canada).[315, 324, 325] These studies have shown that there is no diminution in either the serum IgG *S. typhi* O antibody response or the vibriocidal antibody response when these vaccines are coadministered as a combined oral vaccine cocktail versus when they are administered alone.[324, 326, 327]

Future Vaccines

Vi Conjugates

Because purified Vi polysaccharide acts like a T-lymphocyte–independent antigen, the serum antibody response cannot be readily boosted by administration of additional doses of Vi vaccine. In contrast, when Vi is conjugated to carrier proteins, such as tetanus or diphtheria toxoids, cholera toxin, cholera toxin B subunit, or recombinant exotoxin A of *Pseudomonas aeruginosa*, it behaves as a T-lymphocyte–dependent antigen.[43, 256, 328, 329] In studies in animal models, subsequent inoculations with Vi conjugate vaccine clearly boost the serum Vi antibody titer.[43, 256, 328, 329] The molecular weight of the Vi polysaccharide that is conjugated to the carrier protein influences the magnitude of the serological response. Native Vi was superior to a derivative of lower molecular weight.[328] Early conjugates that Szu and colleagues[256, 329] prepared utilizing tetanus toxoid as the carrier protein met with technical difficulties, apparently because of the large molecular mass of Vi and its rigidity, which led to poor solubility and low yields. One lot of Vi tetanus toxoid conjugate depolymerized during storage and was poorly immunogenic in a safety/immunogenicity trial in North American adults.

Szu and colleagues[256] reported success when 15 μg of Vi was covalently conjugated to *E. coli* LT B subunit or to recombinant exoprotein A of *Pseudomonas aeruginosa*. The conjugates were well tolerated and significantly more immunogenic than unconjugated purified Vi polysaccharide.[256]

Clinical studies in adults, school-aged children, and toddlers in endemic areas in developing countries are underway with Vi conjugates from two different sources. Preliminary results show a high rate of seroconversion in all age groups from toddlers to adults but a gradation in geometric mean titer that decreases progressively from adults to toddlers. These studies are also examining the duration of the serum Vi antibody response.

Pectin, a common polysaccharide of plants, has a homopolymer composition similar to Vi in its backbone. Szu and colleagues have also shown that the treatment of pectin with acetic anhydride results in *O*-acetylation of C-2 and C-3, resulting in a moiety that now reacts with Vi antibody (whereas untreated pectin does not). Szu and colleagues are investigating conjugates in which *O*-acetylated pectin rather than Vi is linked to the protein carrier.[330]

New Recombinant *S. typhi* Strains as Live Oral Vaccines

Various investigators have applied recombinant DNA technology to engineer new candidate vaccine strains of *S. typhi* that will be as well tolerated as Ty21a but much more immunogenic so that protective immunity can be elicited with a single dose. Toward that ambitious goal, putative attenuated vaccine strains have been prepared by inactivating genes encoding various biochemical pathways,[145, 147, 148] global regulatory systems,[150, 159] stress proteins,[331] other regulatory genes,[332, 333] and putative virulence properties.

aro *Mutants Including 541Ty, 543Ty, and CVD 908*

Stocker and coworkers pioneered the use of auxotrophic mutants of *Salmonella* in which the genes encoding enzymes in the aromatic amino acid biosynthesis pathway were inactivated,[147, 156] thereby rendering the *Salmonella* nutritionally dependent on substrates (para-aminobenzoic acid and 2,3-dihydroxybenzoate) that are not available in sufficient quantity in mammalian tissues. As a result, the vaccine strain should be inhibited in its ability to proliferate, although it remains viable.

Edwards and Stocker[147] constructed prototype *aroA* strains 541Ty and 543Ty (a Vi-negative variant of 541Ty) that also harbored deletion mutations in *purA* (which results in a specific requirement for adenine or an assimilable compound such as adenosine).[147] In phase 1 studies, strains 541Ty and 543Ty were quite well tolerated in dosages up to 5×10^{10} CFU but the serologic responses were so feeble that further clinical development of 541Ty and 543Ty was discontinued.[225]

Hone and associates[148] made precise deletion mutations in *aroC* and *aroD* in wild type parent Ty2 (the wild type from which Ty21a was derived), resulting in vaccine strain CVD 908, the first engineered *S. typhi* vaccine candidate that proved to be clinically well tolerated yet highly immunogenic.[151, 226] In phase 1 trials with freshly harvested organisms, a single well-tolerated dose of 5×10^7 CFU elicited IgG O antibody seroconversions in 92% of subjects and 92% had marked rises in gut-derived circulating ASCs that make IgA *S. typhi* O antibody.[226]

The clinical trials with CVD 908 provided an opportunity to perform sophisticated measurements of cell-mediated immunity in recipients of the new generation of attenuated live oral vaccine strains. CVD 908 triggered strong CMI responses to *S. typhi* antigens, including cytokine production (particularly interferon-γ) and proliferative responses to heat-phenolized whole-cell *S. typhi* particles and purified flagella.[227] This type of T lymphocyte response would be expected to help eliminate *S. typhi* in fixed macrophages of the reticuloendothelial system and other cells.

Because *S. typhi* are intracellular pathogens, it has also been assumed that cytotoxic lymphocytes (CTLs) might limit the progression of typhoid infection by destroying host cells harboring *S. typhi*. To address this question, Sztein and associates[271] developed a CTL assay and clearly demonstrated that adult North Americans immunized with attenuated *S. typhi* CVD 908 exhibit CTL effectors in blood capable of killing Epstein-Barr virus–transformed autologous B lymphocytes infected with wild-type *S. typhi*. The CTL effector cell was a classic $CD8^+$, major histocompatibility class I–restricted, cytotoxic T-lymphocyte population.[271] These observations support the contention that CTLs play a role in limiting the progression of human typhoid infection by eliminating host cells harboring bacteria.

The one possible drawback observed in the phase 1 clinical trials with freshly harvested CVD 908 is that 50% of subjects who ingested this vaccine strain at a dose of 5×10^7 CFU and 100% of subjects who received a 5×10^8 CFU dose manifested silent vaccinemias between days 4 and 8 after vaccination detected by systematic daily culturing of blood.[226, 334] No blood cultures from any vaccinee were positive before day 4 nor after day 8. The vaccinemias appeared to have no clinical corollary (e.g., they were not associated with fever); moreover, they were short lived and spontaneously disappeared without the use of antibiotics. There is ample precedent for the licensure by regulatory agencies of live vaccine strains that cause curtailed vaccinemia and the successful use of those vaccines in public health. For example, viremia occurs in many recipients of attenuated rubella vaccine strain RA27/3[335] or attenuated poliomyelitis vaccine (mostly serotype 2 component).[336, 337] However, for a live strain such as CVD 908 that causes vaccinemias to become licensed, convincing data would have to be amassed to document that vaccinemias are indeed not associated with any untoward reactions.

CVD 908-htrA

An additional attenuating mutation was introduced into CVD 908 to yield a derivative that remains well tolerated and immunogenic yet does not cause vaccinemias. Chatfield and coworkers[331] observed that inactivation of *htrA*, a gene encoding a stress protein that functions as a serine protease, attenuates wild type *S. typhimurium* for mice. They further reported that mice immunized orally with *S. typhimurium* harboring a deletion mutation in *htrA* were protected against challenge with a lethal dose of wild type *S. typhimurium*. Based on these observations, a deletion mutation was made into *htrA* of CVD 908, resulting in strain CVD 908-*htrA*.[228, 334] In phase 1 clinical trials, single doses of CVD 908-*htrA* ranging from 5×10^7 to 5×10^9 CFU were as well tolerated as the CVD 908 parent,[228, 334] although 2 of the 22 subjects developed loose stools[228]; mild diarrhea had not been observed in any recipients of CVD 908 during phase 1 studies.[151, 226] CVD 908-*htrA* was highly immunogenic, stimulating significant rises in serum IgG O antibody, gut-derived IgA antibody ASCs and cell-mediated immune responses in 90 to 100% of vaccinees. These immunologic responses are very similar to those observed in recipients of similar doses of CVD 908. The one remarkable difference was in the lack of vaccinemias. No vaccinemias were detected in any of the 22 individuals who ingested well-tolerated, highly immunogenic $5 \times 10^{7-9}$ CFU doses of CVD 908-*htrA* ($P<.001$).[228, 334] CVD 908-*htrA* is being evaluated in phase 2 clinical trials.

Strains with Mutations in cya, crp, cdt

Curtiss and coworkers[150] showed that in *Salmonella* the genes *cya* (encoding adenylate cyclase) and *crp* (cyclic adenosine monophosphate receptor protein) comprise a global regulatory system that affects many genes and operons. They showed that *S. typhimurium* mutants that harbor deletions in *cya* and *crp* are attenuated compared with their wild type parent, and oral immunization protects mice against challenge with virulent *S. typhimurium*.

Curtiss and coworkers[159] constructed vaccine candidate strain χ3927, a *cya*, *crp* double mutant of *S. typhi* strain Ty2. In phase 1 clinical trials, Tacket and associates[151] demonstrated that χ3927 was attenuated from wild type but insufficiently so to serve as a live oral vaccine in humans because occasional subjects developed high temperatures and typhoid-like symptoms. Several subjects also manifested vaccinemias.[151] To achieve a greater degree of attenuation, Curtiss and coworkers[159] introduced into χ3927 a deletion mutation in *cdt*, a gene that affects the dissemination of *Salmonella* from gut-associated lymphoid tissue to deeper organs of the reticuloendothelial system such as the liver, spleen, and bone marrow.[338] The resultant *cya*, *crp*, *cdt* triple mutant strain, χ4073, which was fed to healthy adult North Americans, with buffer, in single doses containing 5×10^5, 5×10^6, 5×10^7, or 5×10^8 CFU,[229] was well tolerated except in one individual who developed diarrhea. No subjects manifested vaccinemia. Four of five subjects who ingested 5×10^8 CFU exhibited significant rises in serum IgG O antibody and had ASCs that made IgA O antibody.

Strains with Mutations in phoP/phoQ

Hohmann and coworkers constructed two candidate *S. typhi* strains harboring deletions in phoP/phoQ.[230, 339] Strain Ty445, which also harbors a deletion in *aroA*, was found to be overly attenuated and only minimally immunogenic.[339] In contrast, strain Ty800, a derivative of Ty2 deleted only in phoP, phoQ, was generally well tolerated and immunogenic when evaluated in dosage levels from 10^7 to 10^{10} CFU in a phase 1 clinical trial involving 11 subjects.[230] At the highest dosage level, 1 of 3 vaccinees developed diarrhea (10 loose stools). Ty800 stimulated vigorous IgA ASCs and serum O antibody responses.

All four of the new attenuated strains, CVD 908, CVD 908-*htrA*, 04073, and Ty800, appear to be markedly more immunogenic than Ty21a.

Attenuated Recombinant *S. typhi* Strains as Live Vector Vaccines

Attenuated *S. typhi* strains can function as so-called live vectors to express critical genes of other organisms and deliver them to the host immune system.[272–274] The appealing features of *Salmonella* strains that make them attractive as live vectors include the following: the vaccines can be given by mucosal (oral or nasal) immunization; *Salmonella* strains elicit a broad immune response that includes serum antibodies, mucosal sIgA antibodies, and different types of cell-mediated immune responses; and considerable experience has been gained in recent years in genetically manipulating *Salmonella*. A few clinical trials with the new generation of attenuated *S. typhi* carrying foreign antigens and serving as live vectors have been published.[229, 340]

PUBLIC HEALTH ASPECTS

Epidemiological Results of Vaccination

Because of their reactogenicity, parenteral killed whole-cell vaccines have rarely been employed in a systematic fashion in public health programs in endemic areas. The one exception is in Thailand, where, in the 1980s, school-based immunization programs utilized parenteral heat-inactivated, phenol-preserved vaccine to control endemic typhoid. A retrospective review suggested that the Thai control program was highly successful.[341]

The lack of adverse reactions associated with live oral vaccine Ty21a or with parenteral Vi polysaccharide vaccine renders them particularly suitable for public health use in school-based immunization programs. In a large effectiveness trial involving immunization of more than 200,000 schoolchildren in Santiago, Chile, with the enteric-coated capsule formulation of Ty21a, the vaccine was found to be quite practical for large-scale use in schools.[114]

There is epidemiological evidence that the large-scale field trials with Ty21a in Santiago, Chile, have produced a "herd immunity" effect.[113] In children within the placebo group in the first field trial of Ty21a in Area Norte, Santiago, the incidence of typhoid progressively fell as each of three field trials was initiated in subsequent years in other administrative areas of the city.[113] The incidence rate in this group has diminished by approximately 70% from the mean incidence in the 3 years before the field trials. These data suggest that systematic application of live oral typhoid vaccine, even with a formulation that provides only 60 to 70% efficacy, can notably diminish the incidence of the disease in endemic areas.

Table 33–18 contains a summary of the salient features of the two typhoid vaccines that have become available in recent years: oral Ty21a and parenteral Vi polysaccharide.

Disease Control Strategies

Because the peak incidence of clinical typhoid fever in most endemic areas occurs in school-aged children of 5 to 19 years, and because this is a "captive" population, in theory, it should be possible to design control programs to incorporate school-based immunization with well-tolerated Ty21a or Vi vaccines. Field trials have clearly demonstrated that both Ty21a and Vi confer a moderate level of protection that endures for several years. Moreover, field experiences with Ty21a support the logistical practicality of such an approach. Ferreccio and associates[114] reported the practicality of school-based immunization in an effectiveness trial in about 200,000 schoolchildren that compared two-dose, three-dose, and four-dose regimens (all within 8 days) of Ty21a. Further encouragement for programmatic use of typhoid vaccines comes from the observation of Levine and associates[113] that a herd immunity effect was evident in geographically separate areas of Santiago after the large-scale use of typhoid vaccine in other areas.

Unfortunately, heretofore, no public health authorities in endemic areas have embraced the use of Ty21a or Vi in school-based immunization programs. The main reason that health authorities have heretofore declined to institute school-based immunization with Ty21a or Vi is the concern that such a program would deflect scarce resources from the Expanded Program on Immunization (EPI), which in most developing countries is restricted to immunization of infants younger than 12 months of age. This is a valid concern because in most developing countries the EPI infrastructure is fragile and personnel resources are meager. For this reason, as an alternative strategy, several national health authorities have expressed interest in the possible inclusion of a typhoid vaccine in the EPI for infants. Such a strategy would allow typhoid fever control to proceed without deflecting resources from the traditional infant-targeted EPI. Unfortunately, heretofore, no data are available to demonstrate that if either Ty21a or Vi is given to infants the immunity elicited would endure and protect years later when the children reach the high-risk school-age years. Although Ty21a has been shown to be immunogenic in toddlers and preschool children 2 to 5 years of age,[302, 303] there have been no published reports of studies

Table 33–18. **A COMPARISON OF THE CHARACTERISTICS OF LIVE ORAL VACCINE Ty21a AND PARENTERAL Vi POLYSACCHARIDE VACCINE**

CHARACTERISTIC	Ty21a	Ty21a	Vi
Formulation	Enteric-coated capsules	"Liquid suspension"*	Liquid
Type of vaccine	Live	Live	Subunit
Route of administration	Oral	Oral	Parenteral
Immunization schedule	3 or 4 doses†	3 doses†	1 dose
Cold chain required by manufacturer	Yes	Yes	Yes
Well tolerated	Yes	Yes	Yes
Range of efficacy	35–67%	55–96%	64–72%
Duration of efficacy	62% for ≥7 yr	78% for ≥5 yr	55% for ≥3 yr
Herd immunity effect	Yes	Yes	?
Can interfere with use of serum Vi antibody as a screening test to detect chronic typhoid carriers	No	No	Yes

*Lyophilized vaccine that is added to 100 mL of water, along with a buffer parameter, resulting in a vaccine suspension.
†Given every other day.

in infants younger than 12 months of age. Vi polysaccharide vaccine has stimulated seroconversions of antibody in the majority of inoculated toddlers, but the titers achieved were notably lower than the titers observed in older children, and they fell after several months.[167] If public health authorities in endemic areas are insistent in their demand for typhoid vaccines that are immunogenic and protective in infants so that they can be added to the EPI, it will be necessary to await the licensure of the new generation of Vi conjugates and the improved attenuated live oral vaccine strains that are presently in clinical trials.

Eradication or Elimination

Whereas chronic carriers constitute the reservoir of *S. typhi*, the maintenance of a high incidence of typhoid fever requires conditions that permit amplified transmission of *S. typhi* to susceptibles. Usually this involves fecal contamination of water sources consumed by large numbers of individuals. In the late 19th and early 20th century it was demonstrated in Europe and the United States that treatment of municipal water supplies caused the incidence of typhoid fever to plummet, despite the continued existence in the population of large numbers of chronic carriers. Over 1 to 2 decades this led to near elimination of typhoid fever from many areas.[90]

It is not known if programmatic use of Ty21a or Vi could accomplish the same near elimination of typhoid fever as a public health problem. However, it is not likely that these vaccines would be the lynch pin of elimination campaigns. On the other hand, future typhoid vaccines currently under development, including several attenuated strains that may function as single-dose oral vaccines and Vi conjugates, may be amenable for this purpose. If these future vaccines are well tolerated and highly immunogenic in infants and confer a high level of long-lasting protection, they could serve as the basis of typhoid fever control programs. Aggressive control programs that achieved a high level of coverage might nearly eliminate typhoid fever in certain populations.

It is epidemiologically feasible that typhoid fever can someday be eradicated from the world. This would require a combination of treatment of water supplies and provision of sanitation to diminish transmission; systematic screening to detect chronic typhoid carriers and treatment of the carriers to diminish the reservoir of infection; and, finally, programmatic use of well-tolerated, highly effective future typhoid vaccines.

REFERENCES

1. Huxham J. To which is now added a dissertation on the malignant, ulcerous sore throat. In An Essay on Fevers. London, SA Cumberledge, 1782, pp 72–125.
2. Louis PCA. Recherches Anatomiques, Pathologiques et Therapeutiques sur la Maladie Connue Sous les Noms de Gastroentérite, Fièvre Putride, Adynamique, Ataxique, Typhoide, etc., Comparée avec les Maladies Aigues les Plus Ordinaires. Paris, Bailliere, 1829.
3. Gerhard WW. On the typhus fever, which occurred at Philadelphia in the spring and summer of 1836. Am J Med Sci 19:289–322, 1837.
4. Schoenlein J. Allgemaine und Specielle Pathologie und Therapie. Freiburg, St. Gallen, 1839.
5. Jenner W. Monthly on typhoid fevers—An attempt to determine the question of their identity or non-identity, by an analysis of the symptoms, and of the appearances found after death in 66 cases observed at the London Fever Hospital from Jan. 1847–Feb. 1849. J Med Sci 9:663–680, 1849.
6. Jenner W. On the identity or non-identity of typhoid and typhus fevers. London, C & J Allard, 1850.
7. Ritchie C. Practical remarks on the continued fevers of Great Britain, and on the generic distinctions between enteric fever and typhus. Monthly J Med Sci 7:347–358, 1846.
8. Budd W. Typhoid Fever: Its Nature, Mode of Spreading and Prevention. London, Longmans, 1873.
9. Eberth C. Organismen in den Organen bei Typhus abdominalis. Virchows Arch Path Anat 81:58–74, 1880.
10. Gaffky G. Zur Aetiologie des Abdominaltyphus: Mittheilungen aus dem kaiserlichen Gesundheitsante. Berlin, Reichsgesundheitsamt, 1884, pp 372–420.
11. Reeves MW, Evins GM, Heiba AA, et al. Clonal nature of *Salmonella typhi* and its genetic relatedness to other salmonellae as shown by multilocus enzyme electrophoresis, and proposal of *Salmonella bongori* comb. nov. J Clin Microbiol 27:313–320, 1989.
12. Le Minor L, Popoff MY. Designation of *Salmonella enterica* sp. nov., nom. rev., as the type and only species of the Genus *Salmonella*. Int J Syst Bacteriol 37:465–468, 1987.
13. Pfeiffer R, Kolle W. Experimentelle Untersuchungen zur Frage der Schutzimpfung des Menschen gegen Typhus abdominalis. Dtsch Med Wochenschr 22:735–737, 1896.
14. Wright A. On the association of serous hemorrhages with conditions and defective blood coagulability. Lancet 2:807–809, 1896.

15. Wright A, Leishman W. Remarks on the results which have been obtained by the antityphoid inoculations and on the methods which have been employed in the preparation of the vaccine. BMJ 1:122–129, 1900.
16. Anand AC, Kataria VK, Singh W, et al. Epidemic multiresistant enteric fever in eastern India [letter]. Lancet 335:352, 1990.
17. Bhutta ZA, Naqvi SH, Razzaq RA, et al. Multidrug-resistant typhoid in children: Presentation and clinical features. Rev Infect Dis 13:832–836, 1991.
18. Bhutta ZA. Impact of age and drug resistance on mortality in typhoid fever. Arch Dis Child 75:214–217, 1996.
19. Gupta A. Multidrug-resistant typhoid fever in children: Epidemiology and therapeutic approach. Pediatr Infect Dis 13:124–140, 1994.
20. Mikhail IA, Haberberger RL, Farid Z, et al. Antibiotic-multiresistant *Salmonella typhi* in Egypt. Trans R Soc Trop Med Hyg 83:120, 1989.
21. Rowe B, Ward LR, Threlfall EJ. Spread of multiresistant *Salmonella typhi*. Lancet 336:1065–1066, 1990.
22. Nguyen TA, Ha Ba K, Nguyen TD. Typhoid fever in South Vietnam, 1990–1993. Bull Soc Pathol Exot 86:476–478, 1993.
23. Osler W. Typhoid fever. In Osler W (ed). The Principles and Practice of Medicine. New York, D Appleton, 1892, pp 2–43.
24. Huckstep R. Typhoid fever and the other *Salmonella* infections. Edinburgh, E & S Livingstone, 1962.
25. Hoffman T, Ruiz C, Counts G, et al. Waterborne typhoid fever in Dade County, Florida. Am J Med 59:481–487, 1975.
26. Gilman R, Terminel M, Levine M, et al. Relative efficacy of blood, urine, rectal swab, bone-marrow, and rose-spot cultures for recovery of *Salmonella typhi* in typhoid fever. Lancet 1:1211–1213, 1975.
27. Hoffman S, Punjabi N, Kumala S, et al. Reduction of mortality in chloramphenicol-treated severe typhoid fever by high-dose dexamethasone. N Engl J Med 310:82–88, 1984.
28. Ferreccio C, Levine MM, Manterola A, et al. Benign bacteremia caused by *Salmonella typhi* and *paratyphi* in children younger than 2 years. J Pediatr 104:899–901, 1984.
29. Mahle WT, Levine MM. *Salmonella typhi* infection in children younger than five years of age. Pediatr Infect Dis J 12:627–631, 1993.
30. Ames W, Robins M. Age and sex as factors in the development of the typhoid carrier state and a method of estimating carrier prevalence. Am J Public Health 33:221–230, 1943.
31. Ledingham J, Arkwright J. The Carrier Problem in Infectious Diseases. London, Arnold, 1912.
32. Skerman VBD, McGowan V, Sneath PHA. Approved lists of bacterial names. Int J Syst Bacteriol 30:225–420, 1980.
33. Baumler AJ, Heffron F, Reissbrodt R. Rapid detection of *Salmonella enterica* with primers specific for *iroB*. J Clin Microbiol 35:1224–1230, 1997.
34. Edwards P, Ewing W. Identification of Enterobacteriaceae. (3rd ed). Minneapolis, Burgess Publishing Co, 1972.
35. Frankel G, Newton S, Schoolnik G, et al. Intragenic recombination in a flagellin gene: Characterization of the H1-j gene of *Salmonella typhi*. EMBO J 8:3149–3152, 1989.
36. Guinée P, Jansen W, Maas W, et al. An unusual H antigen (z66) in strains of *Salmonella typhi*. Ann Microbiol 132:331–334, 1981.
37. Felix A, Pitt R. A new antigen of *B. typhosus*. Lancet 2:186–191, 1934.
38. Felix A, Pitt R. The pathogenic and immunogenic activities of *Salmonella typhi* in relation to its antigenic constituents. J Hyg 49:92–109, 1951.
39. Felix A, Krikorian A, Reitler R. The occurrence of typhoid bacilli containing Vi antigen in cases of typhoid fever and of Vi-antibody in their sera. J Hyg 35:421–427, 1935.
40. Robbins J, Robbins J. Reexamination of the protective role of the capsular polysaccharide Vi antigen of *Salmonella typhi*. J Infect Dis 150:436–449, 1984.
41. Baker EE, Whiteside RE, Basch R, et al. The Vi antigen of the Enterobacteriaceae: I. Purification and chemical properties. J Immunol 83:680–686, 1961.
42. Clark W, McLaughlin J, Webster M. An aminohexuronic acid as the principal hydrolytic component of the Vi antigen. J Biol Chem 230:81–89, 1958.
43. Szu SC, Stone AL, Robbins JD, et al. Vi capsular polysaccharide-protein conjugates for prevention of typhoid fever: Preparation, characterization, and immunogenicity in laboratory animals. J Exp Med 166:1510–1524, 1987.
44. Navarro F, Llovet T, Echeita MA, et al. Molecular typing of *Salmonella enterica* serovar *typhi*. J Clin Microbiol 34:2831–2834, 1996.
45. Thong KL, Passey M, Clegg A, et al. Molecular analysis of isolates of *Salmonella typhi* obtained from patients with fatal and nonfatal typhoid fever. J Clin Microbiol 34:1029–1033, 1996.
46. Thong KL, Cordano AM, Yassin RM, et al. Molecular analysis of environmental and human isolates of *Salmonella typhi*. Appl Environ Microbiol 62:271–274, 1996.
47. Thong KL, Puthucheary S, Yassin RM, et al. Analysis of *Salmonella typhi* isolates from Southeast Asia by pulsed-field gel electrophoresis. J Clin Microbiol 33:1938–1941, 1995.
48. Thong KL, Cheong YM, Puthucheary S, et al. Epidemiologic analysis of sporadic *Salmonella typhi* isolates and those from outbreaks by pulsed-field gel electrophoresis. J Clin Microbiol 32:1135–1141, 1994.
49. Fica AE, Prat-Miranda S, Fernandez-Ricci A, et al. Epidemic typhoid in Chile: Analysis by molecular and conventional methods of *Salmonella typhi* strain diversity in epidemic (1977 and 1981) and nonepidemic (1990) years. J Clin Microbiol 34:1701–1707, 1996.
50. Levine M, Kaper J, Black R, et al. New knowledge on pathogenesis of bacterial enteric infections as applied to vaccine development. Microbiol Rev 47:510–550, 1983.
51. Mallory F. A histological study of typhoid fever. J Exp Med 3:611–638, 1898.
52. Salas M, Angulo O, Villegus J. Patología de la fiebre tifoidea en los niños. Biol Med Hosp Mex 17:63–68, 1960.
53. Hornick RB, Greisman SE, Woodward TE, et al. Typhoid fever: Pathogenesis and immunologic control. N Engl J Med 283:686–691, 739–746, 1970.
54. Edsall G, Gaines S, Landy M, et al. Studies on infection and immunity in experimental typhoid fever. J Exp Med 112:143–166, 1960.
55. Gaines S, Sprinz H, Tully J, et al. Studies on infection and immunity in experimental typhoid fever: VII. The distribution of *Salmonella typhi* in chimpanzee tissue following oral challenge and the relationship between the numbers of bacilli and morphologic lesions. J Infect Dis 118:293–306, 1968.
56. Carter P, Collins R. The route of enteric infection in normal mice. J Exp Med 139:1189–1203, 1974.
57. Collins F. Salmonellosis in orally infected specific pathogen-free C57B1 mice. Infect Immun 6:191–198, 1972.
58. Takeuchi A. Electron microscope studies of experimental *Salmonella* infection: I. Penetrations into the intestinal epithelium by *Salmonella typhimurium*. Am J Pathol 50:109–136, 1967.
59. Felix A, Pitt R. Virulence of *B. typhosus* and resistance to O antibody. J Pathol Bacteriol 38:409–420, 1934.
60. Meyer K, Neilson N, Feusier M. The mechanism of gallbladder infections in laboratory animals: Experimental typhoid-paratyphoid carriers: V. J Infect Dis 28:456–509, 1921.
61. Nichols H. Observations on experimental typhoid infection of the gallbladder in the rabbit. J Exp Med 20:573–581, 1914.
62. Avendãno A, Herrera P, Horwitz, I, et al. Duodenal string cultures: Practicality and sensitivity for diagnosing enteric fever in children. J Infect Dis 53:359–362, 1986.
63. Benavente L, Gotuzzo E, Guerra J, et al. Diagnosis of typhoid fever using a string capsule device. Trans R Soc Trop Med Hyg 78:404–406, 1984.
64. Vallenas C, Hernandez H, Day B, et al. Efficacy of bone marrow, blood, stool, and duodenal contents cultures for bacteriologic confirmation of typhoid fever in children. Pediatr Infect Dis J 4:496–498, 1985.
65. Guerra-Caceres J, Gotuzzo-Herencia E, Crosby-Dagnino E, et al. Diagnostic value of bone marrow culture in typhoid fever. Trans R Soc Trop Med Hyg 73:680–683, 1979.
66. Hoffman S, Punjabi N, Rockhill R, et al. Duodenal string-capsule culture compared with bone-marrow, blood and rectal swab cultures for diagnosing typhoid and paratyphoid fever. J Infect Dis 149:157–161, 1984.
67. Widal G, Sicard A. Recherches de la réaction agglutinante dans le sang et le sérum dessechés des typhiques et dans la serosité des vesications. Bull Soc Med Paris (3rd ser) 13:681–682, 1896.

68. Durham H. Note on the diagnostic value of the serum of typhoid fever patients. Lancet 2:1746–1747, 1896.
69. Grunbaum A. Preliminary note on the use of the agglutinative action of human serum for the diagnosis of enteric fever. Lancet 2:806–807, 1896.
70. Levine MM, Grados O, Gilman RH, et al. Diagnostic value of the Widal test in areas endemic for typhoid fever. Am J Trop Med Hyg 27:795–800, 1978.
71. Anderson ES. Proposed use of a non-motile variant of *Salmonella typhi* for the preparation of vaccine against typhoid fever. Symp Ser Immunobiol Stands 15:79–86, 1971.
72. Anderson ES. Suggested adoption of a non-motile variant of strain Ty2 for vaccination against typhoid fever. Progr Immunobiol Stand 5:373–377, 1972.
73. Anderson ES, Gunnell A. A suggestion for a new antityphoid vaccine. Lancet 2:1196–1200, 1964.
74. Hoffman S, Flanigan TP, Klaucke D, et al. The Widal slide agglutination test, a valuable rapid diagnostic test in typhoid fever patients at the infectious diseases hospital of Jakarta. Am J Epidemiol 123:869–875, 1986.
75. Lanata CF, Levine MM, Ristori C, et al. Vi serology in detection of chronic *Salmonella typhi* carriers in an endemic area. Lancet 2:441–443, 1983.
76. Nolan CM, Feeley JC, White PCJ, et al. Evaluation of a new assay for Vi antibody in chronic carriers of *Salmonella typhi*. J Clin Microbiol 12:22–26, 1980.
77. Losonsky GA, Ferreccio C, Kotloff KL, et al. Development and evaluation of an enzyme-linked immunosorbent assay for serum Vi antibodies for detection of chronic *Salmonella typhi* carriers. J Clin Microbiol 25:2266–2269, 1987.
78. Barrett TJ, Snyder JD, Blake PA, et al. Enzyme-linked immunosorbent assay for detection of *Salmonella typhi* Vi antigen in urine from typhoid patients. J Clin Microbiol 15:235–237, 1982.
79. Gupta AK, Rao KM. Simultaneous detection of *Salmonella typhi* Vi antigen and antibody in serum by counter-immunoelectrophoresis for an early and rapid diagnosis of typhoid fever. J Immunol Methods 30:349–353, 1979.
80. John TJ, Sivasan K, Kurien B. Evaluation of passive bacterial agglutination for the diagnosis of typhoid fever. J Clin Microbiol 20:751–753, 1984.
81. Rockhill RC, Rumans LW, Lesmana M, et al. Detection of *Salmonella typhi* D, VI, and d antigens, by slide coagglutination in urine from patients with typhoid fever. J Clin Microbiol 11:213–216, 1980.
82. Shetty NP, Hiresave S, Bhat P. Coagglutination and counterimmuno-electrophoresis in the rapid diagnosis of typhoid fever. Am J Clin Pathol 84:80–84, 1985.
83. Sivadasan K, Kurien B, John TJ. Rapid diagnosis of typhoid fever by antigen detection. Lancet 1:134–135, 1984.
84. Sundaraj T, Hango B, Subramanian S. A study on the usefulness of counter immunoelectrophoresis for the detection of *Salmonella typhi* antigen in the sera of suspected cases of enteric fever. Trans R Soc Trop Med Hyg 77:194–197, 1983.
85. Taylor DN, Harris JR, Barrett TJ, et al. Detection of urinary Vi antigen as a diagnostic test for typhoid fever. J Clin Microbiol 18:872–876, 1983.
86. Tsang RW, Chau PY. Serological diagnosis of typhoid fever by counter immunoelectrophoresis. BMJ 282:1505–1507, 1981.
87. Rubin FA, Kopecko DJ, Sack RB, et al. Evaluation of a DNA probe for identifying *Salmonella typhi* in Peruvian and Indonesian bacterial isolates. J Infect Dis 157:1051–1053, 1988.
88. Song JH, Cho H, Park MY, et al. Detection of *Salmonella typhi* in the blood of patients with typhoid fever by polymerase chain reaction. J Clin Microbiol 31:1439–1443, 1993.
89. Zhu Q, Lim CK, Chan YN. Detection of *Salmonella typhi* by polymerase chain reaction. J Appl Bacteriol 80:244–251, 1996.
90. Wolman A, Gorman A. The Significance of Waterborne Typhoid Fever Outbreaks. Baltimore, Williams & Wilkins, 1931.
91. JAMA. Typhoid in the large cities of the United States in 1919. JAMA 74:672–675, 1920.
92. Edelman R, Levine MM. Summary of an international workshop on typhoid fever. Rev Infect Dis 8:329–349, 1986.
93. Ivanoff B, Levine MM. Typhoid fever: Continuing challenges from a resilient bacterial foe. Bull Inst Pasteur 95:129–142, 1997.
94. Committee on Issues and Priorities for New Vaccine Development. New Vaccine Development: Establishing Priorities. Volume II. Diseases of Importance in Developing Countries. Washington, DC, National Academy Press, 1985.
95. Simanjuntak C, Paleologo F, Punjabi N, et al. Oral immunisation against typhoid fever in Indonesia with Ty21a vaccine. Lancet 338:1055–1059, 1991.
96. Acharya VI, Lowe CU, Thapa R, et al. Prevention of typhoid fever in Nepal with the Vi capsular polysaccharide of *Salmonella typhi:* A preliminary report. N Engl J Med 317:1101–1104, 1987.
97. Klugman K, Gilbertson IT, Kornhoff HJ, et al. Protective activity of Vi polysaccharide vaccine against typhoid fever. Lancet 2:1165–1169, 1987.
98. Black RE, Levine MM, Ferreccio C, et al. Efficacy of one or two doses of Ty21a *Salmonella typhi* vaccine in enteric-coated capsules in a controlled field trial. Chilean Typhoid Committee. Vaccine 8:81–84, 1990.
99. Levine MM, Black RE, Ferreccio C, et al. Interventions to control endemic typhoid fever: Field studies in Santiago, Chile. In Control and Eradication of Infectious Diseases: An International Symposium. Washington, DC, Pan American Health Organization, PAHO Copublication Series No. 1, pp 37–53, 1986.
100. Committee on Issues and Priorities for New Vaccine Development. The burden of disease resulting from various diarrheal pathogens. In New Vaccine Development: Establishing Priorities. Volume II. Diseases of Importance in Developing Countries. Washington, DC, National Academy Press, 1986.
101. Ashcroft MT. The morbidity and mortality of enteric fever in British Guyana. W Ind Med J 11:62–71, 1962.
102. Ashcroft MT. Typhoid and paratyphoid fever in the tropics. J Trop Med Hyg 67:185–189, 1964.
103. Kligler IJ, Bachi R. An analysis of the endemicity and epidemicity of typhoid fever in Palestine. Acta Med Orient 4:243–261, 1945.
104. Rice PA, Baine WB, Gangarosa EJ. *Salmonella typhi* infections in the United States, 1967–1972: Increasing importance of international travelers. Am J Epidemiol 106:160–166, 1977.
105. Ryan CA, Hargrett-Bean NT, Blake PA. *Salmonella typhi* infections in the United States, 1975–1984: Increasing role of foreign travel. Rev Infect Dis II:1–8, 1989.
106. Ryder RW, Blake PA. Typhoid fever in the United States, 1975 and 1976. J Infect Dis 139:124–126, 1979.
107. Taylor DN, Pollard RA, Blake PA. Typhoid in the United States and risk to the international traveler. J Infect Dis 148:599–602, 1983.
108. Blaser MJ, Feldman RA. Acquisiton of typhoid fever from proficiency-testing specimens. (Correspondence). JAMA 303:1481–1482, 1980.
109. Blaser MJ, Lofgren JP. Fatal salmonellosis originating in a clinical microbiology laboratory. J Clin Microbiol 13:855–858, 1981.
110. Blaser MJ, Hickman FW, Farmer JJ, et al. *Salmonella typhi:* The laboratory as a reservoir of infection. J Infect Dis 142:934–938, 1980.
111. Ferreccio C. Typhoid—Policy quandaries about use of Ty21a in Chile. In Sack DA, Freij L (eds). Prospects for Public Health Benefits in Developing Countries from New Vaccines Against Enteric Infections. Stockholm, Gotab, 1990, pp 67–81.
112. Levine MM, Taylor DN, Ferreccio C. Typhoid vaccines come of age. Pediatr Infect Dis J 8:374–381, 1989.
113. Levine MM, Ferreccio C, Black RE, et al. Progress in vaccines against typhoid fever. Rev Infect Dis 11(suppl 3):S552–S567, 1989.
114. Ferreccio C, Levine MM, Rodriguez H, et al. Comparative efficacy of two, three, or four doses of Ty21a live oral typhoid vaccine in enteric-coated capsules. A field trial in an endemic area. J Infect Dis 159:766–769, 1989.
115. Rowe B, Ward LR, Threlfall EJ. Multidrug-resistant *Salmonella typhi:* A worldwide epidemic. Clin Infect Dis 24(suppl 1):S106–S109, 1997.
116. Levine MM. Typhoid fever vaccines. In Plotkin SA, Mortimer A Jr (eds). Vaccines. Philadelphia, WB Saunders, 1988, pp 333–361.
117. Levine MM. Typhoid fever vaccines. In Plotkin SA, Mortimer E Jr (eds). Vaccines (2nd ed). Philadelphia, WB Saunders, 1994, pp 597–633.
118. Felix A. New type of typhoid and paratyphoid vaccine. BMJ 1:391–395, 1941.
119. Felix A, Rainsford SG, Stokes EJ. Antibody response and sys-

temic reactions after inoculation of a new T.A.B.C. vaccine O. BMJ 1:435–440, 1941.
120. Hejfec LB, Salmin LV, Lejtman MZ, et al. A controlled field trial and laboratory study of five typhoid vaccines in the USSR. Bull World Health Organ 34:321–339, 1966.
121. Besredka A. De la vaccination contre les états typhoides par voie buccale. Ann Inst Pasteur 33:882–890, 1919.
122. Besredka A. Local Immunization. Baltimore, Williams & Wilkins, 1927.
123. Hejfets LB, Levina IA, Salmin LV, et al. Assessment of effectivity of oral killed typhoid and paratyphoid B vaccines and aerosol chemical typhoid vaccine in controlled field trials. J Hyg Epidemiol Microbiol Immunol 20:292–299, 1976.
124. Borgoño JM, Corey G, Engelhardt H. Field trials with killed oral typhoid vaccines. Dev Biol Stand 33:80–84, 1976.
125. Chuttani CS. Controlled field trials of three different oral killed typhoid vaccines in India. Dev Biol Stand 33:98–101, 1976.
126. Chuttani DS, Prakash K, Gupta P, et al. Controlled field trial of a high dose oral killed typhoid vaccine in India. Bull World Health Organ 55:643–644, 1977.
127. Chuttani CS, Prakash K, Vergese A, et al. Ineffectiveness of an oral killed typhoid vaccine in a field trial. Bull World Health Organ 48:756–757, 1973.
128. Chuttani CS, Prakash K, Vergese A, et al. Effectiveness of oral killed typhoid vaccine. Bull World Health Organ 45:445–450, 1971.
129. Hejfec LB, Levina LA, Antanova AA, et al. Controlled field trials of killed oral typhoid and paratyphoid B vaccines and cell-free chemical aerosol tyhoid vaccine. Dev Biol Stand 33:93–97, 1975.
130. DuPont LH, Hornick RB, Snyder MJ, et al. Studies of immunity in typhoid fever: Protection induced by killed oral antigens or by primary infection. Bull World Health Organ 44:667–672, 1971.
131. Grasset E. L'endoanatoxine typho-paratyphique dans la prophylaxie des infections typhoidiques. Rev Immunol (Paris) 15:1–19, 1951.
132. Topley WWC, Raistrick H, Wilson J, et al. Immunising potency of antigenic components isolated from different strains of *Bact. typhosum.* Lancet 1:252–260, 1937.
133. Westphal O, Luderitz O, Bister F. Über die Extraktion von Bakterien mit Phenol/Wasser. Z Naturforsch 7b:148–155, 1952.
134. Landy M. Studies on Vi antigen: VI. Immunization of human beings with purified Vi antigen. Am J Hyg 60:52–62, 1954.
135. Landy M, Gaines S, Seal JP, et al. Antibody responses of man to three types of antityphoid immunizing agents. Am J Public Health 44:1572–1579, 1954.
136. Polish Typhoid Committee. Controlled field trial and laboratory studies on the effectiveness of typhoid vaccines in Poland 1961–64. Bull World Health Organ 34:211–222, 1966.
137. Hejfec LB. Results of the study of typhoid vaccines in four controlled field trials in the USSR. Bull World Health Organ 32:1–14, 1965.
138. Webster ME, Landy M, Freeman ME. Studies on Vi antigen: II. Purification of Vi antigen from *Escherichia coli* 5396/38. J Immunol 69:135–142, 1952.
139. Landy M, Johnson AG, Webster ME. Studies on Vi antigen: VIII. Role of acetyl in antigenic activity. Am J Hyg 73:55–65, 1961.
140. Whiteside RE, Baker EE. The Vi antigens of the Enterobacteriaceae: V. Serologic differences of Vi antigens revealed by deacetylation. J Immunol 86:538–542, 1961.
141. Reitman M. Infectivity and antigenicity of streptomycin-dependent *Salmonella typhosa*. J Infect Dis 117:101–107, 1967.
142. Cvjetanovic B, Mel DM, Felsenfeld O. Study of live typhoid vaccine in chimpanzees. Bull World Health Organ 42:499–507, 1970.
143. Mel DM, Arsic BL, Radovanovic ML, et al. Safety tests in adults and children with live oral typhoid vaccine. Acta Microbiol Acad Sci Hung 21:161–166, 1974.
144. Cryz SJJ, Furer E, Baron LS, et al. Construction and characterization of a Vi-positive variant of the *Salmonella typhi* live oral vaccine strain Ty21a. Infect Immun 57:3863–3868, 1989.
145. Hone DM, Attridge SR, Forrest B, et al. A galE via (Vi antigen-negative) mutant of *Salmonella typhi* Ty2 retains virulence in humans. Infect Immun 56:1326–1333, 1988.
146. Dima VF. Volunteer studies in the development of a live oral typhoid vaccine. Arch Roumaines Pathol Exp Microbiol 42:196–198, 1983.
147. Edwards MF, Stocker BAD. Construction of aroA his pur strains of *Salmonella typhi.* J Bacteriol 170:3991–3995, 1984.
148. Hone DM, Harris AM, Chatfield S, et al. Construction of genetically-defined double *aro* mutants of *Salmonella typhi.* Vaccine 9:810–816, 1991.
149. Hone DM, Tacket C, Harris A, et al. Evaluation in volunteers of a candidate live oral attenuated *S. typhi* vector vaccine. J Clin Invest 90:1–9, 1992.
150. Curtiss R III, Kelly SM. *Salmonella typhimurium* deletion mutants lacking adenylate cyclase and cyclic AMP receptor protein are avirulent and immunogenic. Infect Immun 55:3035–3043, 1987.
151. Tacket CO, Hone DM, Curtiss RI, et al. Comparison of the safety and immunogenicity of *aroC, aroD* and *cya, crp Salmonella typhi* strains in adult volunteers. Infect Immun 60:536–541, 1992.
152. DuPont HL, Hornick RB, Snyder MJ, et al. Immunity in typhoid fever: Evaluation of live streptomycin-dependent vaccine. Antimicrob Agents Chemother 10:236–239, 1970.
153. Levine MM, DuPont LH, Hornick RE, et al. Attenuated streptomycin-dependent *Salmonella typhi* oral vaccine: Potential deleterious effects of lyophilization. J Infect Dis 133:424–429, 1976.
154. Levine MM, Herrington D, Murphy JR, et al. Safety, infectivity, immunogenicity and in vivo stability of two attenuated auxotrophic mutant strains of *Salmonella typhi,* 541Ty and 543Ty, as live oral vaccines in man. J Clin Invest 79:888–902, 1987.
155. Tacket CO, Losonsky G, Taylor DN, et al. Lack of immune response to the Vi component of a Vi-positive variant of the *Salmonella typhi* live oral vaccine strain Ty21a in human studies. J Infect Dis 163:901–904, 1991.
156. Hoiseth S, Stocker BAD. Aromatic-dependent *Salmonella typhimurium* are non-virulent and effective as live vaccines. Nature 292:238–239, 1981.
157. Stocker BAD, Hosieth SK, Smith BP. Aromatic-dependent "*Salmonella* sp" as live vaccine in mice and calves. Dev Biol Stand 53:47–54, 1983.
158. Bacon GA, Burrows TW, Yates M. The effects of biochemical mutation on the virulence of *Bacterium typhosum:* The loss of virulence of certain mutants. Br J Exp Pathol 32:85–96, 1951.
159. Curtiss R III, Kelly SM, Tinge SA, et al. Recombinant *Salmonella* vectors in vaccine development. Dev Biol Standard 82:23–33, 1994.
160. Groschel DHM, Hornick RB. Who introduced typhoid vaccination: Almoth Wright or Richard Pfeiffer? Rev Infect Dis 3:1251–1254, 1981.
161. Wright AE, Semple D. Remarks on vaccination against typhoid fever. BMJ 1:256–258, 1897.
162. Landy M. Enhancement of the immunogenicity of typhoid vaccine by retention of the Vi antigen. Am J Hyg 58:148–164, 1953.
163. Walter Reed Army Institute of Research. Preparation of dried acetone-inactivated and heat-phenol–inactivated typhoid vaccines. Bull World Health Organ 30:635–646, 1964.
164. Walter Reed Army Institute of Research, International Laboratory for Biological Standards SS. Physical and chemical studies on two dried inactivated typhoid vaccines (vaccine K and L). Bull World Health Organ 30:647–652, 1964.
165. Wong KH, Feeley JC, Northrup RS, et al. Vi antigen from *Salmonella typhosa* and immunity against typhoid fever: I. Isolation and immunologic properties in animals. Infect Immun 9:348–353, 1974.
166. Gotschlich EC, Liu TY, Artenstein MS. Human immunity to the meningococcus: III. Preparation and immunochemical properties of the group A, group B and group C meningococcal polysaccharides. Exp Med 129:1349–1365, 1969.
167. Plotkin SA, Bouveret-Le Cam N. A new typhoid vaccine composed of the Vi capsular polysaccharide. Arch Intern Med 155:2293–2299, 1995.
168. Germanier R, Furer E. Isolation and characterization of gal E mutant Ty21a of *Salmonella typhi:* A candidate strain for a live oral typhoid vaccine. J Infect Dis 141:553–558, 1975.
169. Gilman R, Hornick R, Woodward W, et al. Immunity in typhoid fever: Evaluation of Ty21a—An epimeraseless mutant of *S. typhi* as a live oral vaccine. J Infect Dis 136:717–723, 1977.
170. Robbe-Saule V, Coynault C, Norel F. The live oral typhoid vaccine Ty21a is a *rpoS* mutant and is susceptible to various

environmental stresses. FEMS Microbiol Lett 126:171–176, 1995.
171. World Health Organization. International List of Availability of Vaccines. Geneva, 1995.
172. Barr M, Sayers MHP, Stamm WP. Intradermal T.A.B.T. vaccine for immunization against enteric fever. Lancet 1:816–817, 1959.
173. Dimache GL, Dimache V, Ciudin L, et al. Intradermal typhoid vaccination in men by jet-injection. Immunological estimation by laboratory test. Arch Roumaines Pathol Exp Microbiol 36:227–232, 1977.
174. Dimache GL, Dimache V, Croitoru M. The immunization of a five year's old dried typhoid vaccine. Arch Roumaines Pathol Exp Microbiol 40:55–59, 1981.
175. Iwarson S, Larsson P. Intradermal versus subcutaneous immunization with typhoid vaccine. J Hyg 84:11–15, 1980.
176. Keen TEB, Batholomeusz C. Immunization with intradermal T.A.B. tetanus vaccine. Med J Aust 49:591–593, 1962.
177. Perry RM. Comparison of typhoid "O" and "H" agglutinin responses following intracutaneous and subcutaneous inoculation of typhoid, paratyphoid A and B vaccine. Am J Hyg 26:388–393, 1937.
178. Tuft L, Yagle EL, Rogers S. Comparative study of the antibody response after various methods of administration of mixed typhoid vaccine. J Infect Dis 50:98–110, 1932.
179. Van Gelder DW, Fister S. Intradermal immunization: III. Typhoid fever. Am J Dis Child 62:93–98, 1941.
180. Vella W. On vaccines and vaccination: Typhoid-paratyphoid fevers. Postgrad Med J 48:98–100, 1972.
181. Dimache GL, Dimache V, Paxel A, et al. Intradermal various subcutaneous typhoid vaccination. Arch Roumaines Pathol Exp Microbiol 40:143–147, 1965.
182. Tacket CO, Ferreccio C, Robbins JB, et al. Safety and immunogenicity of two *Salmonella typhi* Vi capsular polysaccharide vaccines. J Infect Dis 154:342–345, 1986.
183. Levine MM, Ferreccio C, Black RE, et al. Large-scale field trial of Ty21a live oral typhoid vaccine in enteric-coated capsule formulation. Lancet 1:1049–1052, 1987.
184. Levine MM, Ferreccio C, Cryz S, et al. Comparison of enteric-coated capsules and liquid formulation of Ty21a typhoid vaccine in randomised controlled field trial. Lancet 336:891–894, 1990.
185. Hirschel B, Wuthrich R, Somain B, et al. Inefficacy of the commercial live oral Ty21a vaccine in the prevention of typhoid fever. Eur J Clin Microbiol 4:295–298, 1985.
186. Levine MM, Black RE, Ferreccio C, et al. The efficacy of attenuated *Salmonella typhi* oral vaccine strain Ty21a evaluated in controlled field trials. In Holmgren J, Lindberg A, Molly R (eds). Development of Vaccines and Drugs Against Diarrhea. Lund, Sweden, Studentlitteratur, 1986, pp 90–101.
187. Driesens RJ. Effect of glass on pH-dependent stability of typhoid vaccine. J Clin Microbiol 2:85–88, 1975.
188. Joo I, Zsidai J. Stability of cholera and typhoid vaccines. J Biol Stand 6:341–348, 1977.
189. Cryz SJ Jr, Pasteris O, Varallyay SJ, et al. Factors influencing the stability of live oral attenuated bacterial vaccines. Dev Biol Stand 87:277–281, 1996.
190. Corbel MJ. Reasons for instability of bacterial vaccines. Dev Biol Stand 87:113–124, 1996.
191. Cryz SJ Jr. Post-marketing experience with live oral Ty21a vaccine (Vivotif Berna). Lancet 341:49–50, 1993.
192. Olitzki A. Causing Organisms and Host's Reactions. In Enteric Fevers. Basel, S Karger, 1972, pp 430–486.
193. Ashcroft MT, Morrison-Ritchie J, Nicholson CC, et al. Antibody responses to vaccination of British Guiana school children with heat-killed-phenolized and acetone-killed lyophilized vaccines. Am J Hyg 80:221–228, 1964.
194. Benenson AS. Serological responses of man to typhoid vaccines. Bull World Health Organ 30:653–662, 1964.
195. Cvjetanovic B. Standardization and assay of typhoid reference vaccines K and L. Progr Immunobiol Stand 1:196–203, 1965.
196. Edsall G, Carlson MC, Formal SB, et al. Laboratory tests of typhoid vaccines within a controlled field study. Bull World Health Organ 20:1017–1032, 1959.
197. Ikic D. Ten years of field trials and laboratory examinations of vaccine against typhoid given. Progr Immunobiol Stand 2:175–182, 1965.
198. Joo I, Pusztai ZS, Julasz VP. Mouse protective ability of the international reference preparations of typhoid vaccine. Z Immun-Forsch 135:365–387, 1968.
199. Karolcek JM, Rusinko M, Draskovicova M, et al. Attempts to elaborate a new laboratory test for evaluation of the immunogenic efficiency of typhoid vaccines. J Hyg Epidemiol Microbiol Immunol 10:47–66, 1966.
200. Melikova BN, Lesnjak SV. International reference preparations of typhoid vaccine: Potency by the active mouse protection test with three different routes of immunization. Bull World Health Organ 37:575–579, 1967.
201. Pittman M, Bohner HJ. Laboratory assays of different types of field trial typhoid vaccines and relationships to efficacy in man. J Bacteriol 91:1713–1723, 1966.
202. Standfast AFB. A report on the laboratory assays carried out at the Lister Institute of Preventive Medicine on the typhoid vaccine used in the field study in Yugoslavia. Bull World Health Organ 23:37–45, 1960.
203. Standfast AFB. Some observations on typhoid vaccine assay in 1964. Progr Immunobiol Stand 2:190–195, 1965.
204. Sterne M, Frim G. Assay of typhoid vaccines in man. J Med Microbiol 7:197–203, 1970.
205. Sterne M, Frim G. The significance of protection tests in mice for evaluating typhoid vaccines. Progr Immunobiol Stand 5:382–388, 1972.
206. Ungar J, Addison IE. The comparison of the antigenic assay in mice with that of antibody titration of immune rabbit serum. Progr Immunobiol Stand 2:183–189, 1965.
207. Cvjetanovic B, Uemura K. The present status of field and laboratory studies of typhoid and paratyphoid vaccines: With special reference to studies sponsored by the World Health Organization. Bull World Health Organ 32:29–36, 1965.
208. Yugoslav Typhoid Commission. Field and laboratory studies with typhoid vaccines. Bull World Health Organ 16:897–910, 1957.
209. World Health Organization Expert Committee on Biological Standardization. Typhoid vaccine. World Health Organ Tech Rep Ser 413:19–20, 1969.
210. Yugoslav Typhoid Commission. A controlled field trial of the effectiveness of phenol and alcohol typhoid vaccines. Bull World Health Organ 26:357–369, 1962.
211. Ashcroft MT, Morrison-Ritchie J, Nicholson CC. Controlled field trial in British Guyana schoolchildren of heat-killed-phenolized and acetone-killed lyophilized typhoid vaccines. Am J Hyg 79:196–206, 1964.
212. Ashcroft MT, Nicholson CC, Balwant S, et al. A seven-year field trial of two typhoid vaccines in Guiana. Lancet 2:1056–1060, 1967.
213. Yugoslav Typhoid Commission. A controlled field trial of the effectiveness of acetone-dried and inactivated and heat-phenol-inactivated typhoid vaccines in Yugoslavia. Bull World Health Organ 30:623–630, 1964.
214. Polish Typhoid Committee. Evaluation of typhoid vaccines in the laboratory and in a controlled field trial in Poland. Bull World Health Organ 31:15–27, 1965.
215. Spaun J, Uemura K. International reference preparations of typhoid vaccine. Bull World Health Organ 31:761–791, 1964.
216. Tully JG, Gaines S, Tigertt WD. Studies on infection and immunity in experimental typhoid fever: IV. Role of H antigen in protection. J Infect Dis 112:118–124, 1963.
217. Carter PB, Collins FM. Assessment of typhoid vaccines by using the intraperitoneal route of challenge. Infect Immun 17:555–560, 1977.
218. Spaun J. Studies on the influence of the route of immunization in the active mouse protection test with intraperitoneal challenge for potency of typhoid vaccines. Bull World Health Organ 31:793–798, 1964.
219. Landy M. Studies of Vi antigen: VII. Characteristics of the immune response in the mouse. Am J Hyg 65:81–93, 1957.
220. Landy M, Lamb E. Estimation of Vi antibody employing erythrocytes treated with purified Vi antigen. Proc Soc Exp Bio Med 82:593–598, 1953.
221. Wong KH, Feeley JC, Pittman M. Effect of Vi-degrading enzyme on potency of typhoid vaccines in mice. J Infect Dis 125:360–366, 1972.
222. Wong KH, Feeley JC, Pittman M, et al. Adhesion of Vi antigen

and toxicity in typhoid vaccines inactivated by acetone or by heat and phenol. J Infect Dis 129:501–506, 1974.
223. Wahdan MH, Sippel JE, Mikhail EA. Controlled field trial of a typhoid vaccine prepared with non-motile mutant of *Salmonella typhi* Ty2. Bull World Health Organ 52:69–73, 1975.
224. United States Government Code of Federal Regulations. National Archives and Records Administration. Food and Drugs. Title 21. Point 620. Subpart B. Food and Drugs Title 21 Point 620 Subpart B 620:69–70, 1986.
225. Levine MM, Herrington D, Murphy JR, et al. Safety, infectivity, immunogenicity and *in vivo* stability of two attenuated auxotrophic mutant strains of *Salmonella typhi*, 541Ty and 543Ty, as live oral vaccines in man. J Clin Invest 79:888–902, 1987.
226. Tacket CO, Hone DM, Losonsky GA, et al. Clinical acceptability and immunogenicity of CVD 908 *Salmonella typhi* vaccine strain. Vaccine 10:443–446, 1992.
227. Sztein MB, Wasserman SS, Tacket CO, et al. Cytokine production patterns and lymphoproliferative responses in volunteers orally immunized with attenuated vaccine strains of *Salmonella typhi*. J Infect Dis 170:1508–1517, 1994.
228. Tacket CO, Sztein MB, Losonsky GA, et al. Safety and immune response in humans of live oral *Salmonella typhi* vaccine strains deleted in *htrA* and *aroC, aroD*. Infect Immun 65:452–456, 1997.
229. Tacket CO, Kelly SM, Schodel F, et al. Safety and immunogenicity in humans of an attenuated *Salmonella typhi* vaccine vector strain expressing plasmid-encoded hepatitis B antigens stabilized by the ASD balanced lethal system. Infect Immun 65:3381–3385, 1997.
230. Hohmann EL, Oletta CA, Killeen KP, et al. *phoP/phoQ*-deleted *Salmonella typhi* (Ty800) is a safe and immunogenic single-dose typhoid fever vaccine in volunteers. J Infect Dis 173:1408–1414, 1996.
231. D'Amelio R, Tagliabue A, Nencioni L, et al. Comparative analysis of immunological responses to oral (Ty21a) and parenteral (TAB) typhoid vaccines. Infect Immun 56:2731–2735, 1988.
232. Kantele A. Antibody-secreting cells in the evaluation of the immunogenicity of an oral vaccine. Vaccine 8:321–326, 1990.
233. Kantele A. Immune response to prolonged intestinal exposure to antigen. Scand J Immunol 33:225–229, 1991.
234. Kantele A, Makela PH. Different profiles of the human immune response to primary and secondary immunization with an oral *Salmonella typhi* Ty21a vaccine. Vaccine 9:423–427, 1991.
235. Kantele A, Arvilommi H, Jokinen I. Specific immunoglobulin-secreting human blood cells after peroral vaccination against *Salmonella typhi*. J Infect Dis 153:1126–1131, 1986.
236. Kantele A, Arvilommi H, Kantele JM, et al. Comparison of the human immune response to live oral, killed oral or killed parenteral *Salmonella typhi* Ty21a vaccines. Microb Pathog 10:117–126, 1991.
237. Tagliabue A, Nencioni CA, et al. Cellular immunity against *Salmonella typhi* after live oral vaccines. Clin Exp Immunol 52:242–247, 1985.
238. Tagliabue A, Villa L, De Magistiris MT, et al. IgA-driven T-cell–mediated antibacterial immunity in man after live oral Ty21a vaccine. J Immunol 137:1504–1510, 1986.
239. Panero C, Saletti M, DiTommaso I. The detection of intestinal IgA in children following oral typhoid vaccine. Progr Immunobiol Stand 5:369–372, 1972.
240. Wahdan MH, Serie C, Cerisier Y, et al. A controlled field trial of live *Salmonella typhi* strain Ty21a oral vaccine against typhoid: Three year results. J Infect Dis 145:292–296, 1982.
241. Wahdan MH, Serie C, Germanier R, et al. A controlled field trial of live oral typhoid vaccine Ty21a. Bull World Health Organ 58:469–474, 1980.
242. Ambrosch F, Hirschhl A, Kremsher P, et al. Investigations on the humoral immune response to oral live typhoid vaccination with strain Ty21a. Munchen Med Wochenschr 127:775–778, 1985.
243. Tacket CO, Ferreccio C, Robbins JB, et al. Safety and immunogenicity of two *Salmonella typhi* Vi capsular polysaccharide vaccines. J Infect Dis 154:342–345, 1986.
244. Keitel WA, Bond NL, Zahradnik JM, et al. Clinical and serological responses following primary and booster immunization with *Salmonella typhi* Vi capsular polysaccharide vaccines. Vaccine 12:195–199, 1994.
245. Woodward WE. Volunteer studies of typhoid fever and vaccines. Trans R Soc Trop Med Hyg 74:553–556, 1980.
246. Altemeir WA, Bellanti JA, Buescher EL. The IgM response of children to *Salmonella typhosa* vaccine: II. Comparison of amounts of IgM specific for the somatic, flagellar and Vi antigens. J Immunol 103:924–930, 1969.
247. Chernokhvostova E, Luxemburg KI, Starshinova V, et al. Study on the production of IgG, IgA, and IgM antibodies to somatic antigens of *Salmonella typhi* in humans. Clin Exp Immunol 4:407–421, 1969.
248. Kumar R, Malaviga AN, Murthy RGS, et al. Immunological study of typhoid: Immunoglobulins, C3, antibodies, and leukocyte migration inhibition in patients with typhoid fever and TAB-vaccinated individuals. Infect Immun 10:1219–1225, 1974.
249. Lospallato J, Miller W, Dorward B, et al. The formulation of microglobulin antibodies: I. Studies on adult humans. J Clin Invest 41:1415–1421, 1962.
250. May RP, Barnett JA, Sanford JP. Characterization of the antibody response to acetone-killed typhoid vaccine. Public Health Rec 82:257–259, 1967.
251. Forrest BD, LaBrooy JT, Dearlove CE, et al. The human humoral immune response to *Salmonella typhi* Ty21a. J Infect Dis 163:336–345, 1991.
252. Sarasombath S, Banchuin N, Sukosol T, et al. Systemic and intestinal immunities after different typhoid vaccinations. Asian Pac J Allergy Immunol 5:53–61, 1987.
253. Nisini R, Biselli R, Matricardi PM, et al. Clinical and immunological response to typhoid vaccination with parenteral or oral vaccines in two groups of 30 recruits. Vaccine 11:582–586, 1993.
254. Nath TR, Malaviva AN, Kumar R, et al. A study of the efficacy of typhoid vaccine in inducing humoral and cell-mediated immune responses in human volunteers. Clin Exp Immunol 30:38–43, 1977.
255. Rajagopalan P, Kumar R, Malaviya N. A study of humoral and cell-mediated response following typhoid vaccination in human volunteers. Clin Exp Immunol 47:275–282, 1982.
256. Szu SC, Taylor DN, Trofa AC, et al. Laboratory and preliminary clinical characterization of Vi capsular polysaccharide-protein conjugate vaccines. Infect Immun 62:4440–4444, 1994.
257. Mirza NB, Wamola IA, Estambale BA, et al. Typhim Vi vaccine against typhoid fever: A clinical trial in Kenya. East Afr Med J 72:162–164, 1995.
258. Klugman KP, Koornhof HJ, Robbins JB, et al. Immunogenicity, efficacy and serological correlate of protection of *Salmonella typhi* Vi capsular polysaccharide vaccine three years after immunization. Vaccine 14:435–438, 1996.
259. Bartholomeusz RCA, LaBrooy JT, Johnson M, et al. Gut immunity to typhoid—The immune response to a live oral typhoid vaccine, Ty21a. J Gastroenterol Hepatol 1:61–67, 1986.
260. Kantele A, Kantele JM, Arvilommi H, et al. Active immunity is seen as a reduction in the cell response to oral live vaccine. Vaccine 9:428–431, 1991.
261. Cancellieri V, Fara GM. Demonstration of specific IgA in human feces after immunization with line Ty21a *Salmonella typhi* vaccine. J Infect Dis 151:482–484, 1985.
262. Kantele A, Kantele JM, Savilahti E, et al. Homing potentials of circulating lymphocytes in humans depend on the site of activation: Oral, but not parenteral, typhoid vaccination induces circulating antibody-secreting cells that all bear homing receptors directing them to the gut. J Immunol 158:574–579, 1997.
263. Forrest BD. Impairment of immunogenicity of *Salmonella typhi* Ty21a due to preexisting cross-reacting intestinal antibodies. J Infect Dis 166:210–212, 1992.
264. Su-Arehawaratana P, Singharaj P, Taylor DN, et al. Safety and immunogenicity of different immunization regimens of CVD 103-HgR live oral cholera vaccine in soldiers and civilians in Thailand. J Infect Dis 165:1042–1048, 1992.
265. Attridge S. Oral immmunization with *Salmonella typhi* Ty21a-based clones expressing *Vibrio cholerae* O-antigen: Serum bactericidal antibody responses in man in relation to preimmunization antibody levels. Vaccine 9:877–882, 1991.
266. Forrest BD. Identification of an intestinal immune response using peripheral blood lymphocytes. Lancet 1:81–83, 1988.
267. Czerkinsky CC, Prince SJ, Michalek SM, et al. IgA antibody-producing cells in peripheral blood after ingestion of antigen:

Evidence for a common mucosal immune system in humans. Proc Natl Acad Sci U S A 84:2449–2553, 1987.
268. Forrest BD, Shearman DJC, LaBrooy JT. Specific immune response in humans following rectal delivery of live typhoid vaccine. Vaccine 8:209–211, 1990.
269. Murphy JR, Baqar S, Munoz C, et al. Characteristics of humoral and cellular immunity to *Salmonella typhi* in residents of typhoid-endemic and typhoid-free regions. J Infect Dis 156:1005–1009, 1987.
270. Murphy JR, Wasserman SS, Baqar S, et al. Immunity to *Salmonella typhi:* Considerations relevant to measurement of cellular immunity in typhoid-endemic regions. Clin Exp Immunol 75:228–233, 1989.
271. Sztein M, Tanner MK, Polotsky Y, et al. Cytotoxic T lymphocytes after oral immunization with attenuated vaccine strains of *Salmonella typhi* in humans. J Immunol 155:3987–3993, 1995.
272. Balakrishna-Sarma VN, Malaviva AN, Kumar R, et al. Development of immune response during typhoid fever in man. Clin Exp Immunol 28:35–39, 1977.
273. Mabel TJ, Paniker CKJ. The role of cell-mediated immunity in typhoid. Asian J Infect Dis 3:69–75, 1979.
274. Mogensen HH. *Salmonella typhi*–induced stimulation of blood lymphocytes from persons with previous typhoid fever. Acta Pathol Microbiol Scand [C] 87C:41–45, 1979.
275. Nyerges G, Ferencz A, Funk O. Development of specific cellular immunoreactivity in typhoid fever. Acta Microbiol Acad Sci Hung 26:321–324, 1979.
276. Rajagopalan P, Kumar R, Malaviva N. Immunological studies in typhoid fever: II. Cell-mediated immune responses and lymphocyte subpopulations in patients with typhoid fever. Clin Exp Immunol 47:269–274, 1982.
277. Sarasombath S, Banchuin N, Sukosal T, et al. Systemic and intestinal immunities after natural typhoid infection. J Clin Microbiol 15:1088–1093, 1987.
278. Thevanesam V, Arseculertne SN, Weliange LV, et al. Cell-mediated and humoral immune responses in human typhoid fever. Trop Geogr Med 34:13–17, 1982.
279. Cvjetanovic B. Field trial of typhoid vaccines. Am J Publ Health 47:578–585, 1957.
280. Tapa S, Cvjetanovic B. Controlled field trial on the effectiveness of one and two doses of acetone-inactivated and dried typhoid vaccine. Bull World Health Organ 52:75–80, 1975.
281. Hefjec LB. Duration of postvaccination antityphoid immunity according to the results of strictly controlled field trials. J Hyg Epidemiol Microbiol Immunol 13:154–165, 1969.
282. Hefjec LB, Levina LA, Kuz'minova ML, et al. A controlled field trial to evaluate the protective capacity of a single dose of acetone-killed agar-grown and heat-killed broth-grown typhoid vaccines. Bull World Health Organ 40:903–907, 1969.
283. Marmion DE, Naylor GRE, Stewart IO. Second attacks of typhoid fever. J Hyg 53:260–267, 1953.
284. McAnally TP, Ten Eyck RP. Influenza-like syndrome following typhoid immunization. Milit Med 149:200–201, 1984.
285. Rone JK, Friedstrom S. Severe systemic reactions to typhoid vaccination: Two cases and a review of the literature. Milit Med 155:272–274, 1990.
286. Hoyt RE, Herip DS. Severe systemic reactions attributed to the acetone-inactivated parenteral typhoid vaccine. Milit Med 161:339–341, 1996.
287. Edwards EA, Johnson DP, Pierce WE, et al. Reactions and serologic responses to monovalent acetone-inactivated typhoid vaccine and heat-killed T.A.B. vaccine when given by jet-injection. Bull World Health Organ 541:501–505, 1974.
288. Goel RA. Idiopathic thrombocytopenic purpura: Precipitation relapse with T.A.B. vaccine. Indian Pediatr 18:267, 1981.
289. Tewari SA, Khan CR, Khan AS. Symptomatic thrombocytopenic purpura due to T.A.B. vaccine. J Assoc Physicians India 27:461–462, 1979.
290. Eisinger AJ, Smith JG. Acute renal failure after T.A.B. and cholera vaccination. BMJ 1:381–382, 1979.
291. Joekes AM, Gabriel JRJ, Goggin MJ. Renal disease following prophylactic inoculation. Nephron 9:162–170, 1972.
292. Khan RI. Anaphylactoid reaction to typhoid-paratyphoid A and B vaccine. Trop Geogr Med 23:115–116, 1971.
293. Mittermayer CH. Lethal complications of typhoid-cholera-vaccination (case report and review of the literature. Beitr Path Bd 158:212–224, 1976.
294. Pounder DJ. Sudden, unexpected death following typhoid-cholera vaccination. Forensic Sci Int 24:95–98, 1984.
295. Cotterkill JA, Shapiro H. Dermatomyositis after immunization. Lancet 1:1158–1159, 1978.
296. Bowers WF, Shupe I. Acute appendicitis: Sequela of typhoid inoculation. Milit Surg 90:413, 1942.
297. Thomson BJ, Nuki G. Erythema nodosum following typhoid vaccination. Scott Med J 30:173, 1985.
298. Miller H, Candrowski W, Schapira K. Multiple sclerosis and vaccination. BMJ 2:210–213, 1967.
299. Kelleher PC, Kelley LR, Rickman LS. Anaphylactoid reaction after typhoid vaccination [letter]. Am J Med 89:822–824, 1990.
300. Pounder DJ. Sudden, unexpected death following typhoid-cholera vaccination. Forensic Sci Int 24:95–98, 1984.
301. Black R, Levine MM, Young C, et al. Immunogenicity of Ty21a attenuated "Salmonella typhi" given with sodium bicarbonate or in enteric-coated capsules. Dev Biol Stand 53:9–14, 1983.
302. Cryz SJJ, Vanprapar N, Thisyakorn U, et al. Safety and immunogenicity of *Salmonella typhi* Ty21a vaccine in young Thai children. Infect Immun 61:1149–1151, 1993.
303. Olanratmanee T, Levine MM, Losonsky G, et al. Safety and immunogenicity of *Salmonella typhi* Ty21a liquid formulation vaccine in 4- to 6-year old Thai children. J Infect Dis 166:451–452, 1992.
304. Levine MM. Field trials of efficacy of attenuated *Salmonella typhi* oral vaccine Ty21a. In Robbins J (ed). Bacterial Vaccines. New York, Praeger, 1987.
305. Centers for Disease Control and Prevention. Typhoid Immunization. Recommendations of the Committee on Immunization Practices. MMWR 43:1–7, 1994.
306. Bollag U. Practical evaluation of a pilot immunization campaign against typhoid fever in a Cambodian refugee camp. Int J Epidemiol 9:121–122, 1980.
307. Sunderbruch JH. The case against typhoid immunization during flood periods. J Iowa Med Soc 55:488–489, 1965.
308. Hejfec LB. On the negative phase of postvaccination immunity to typhoid with reference to the results of epidemiological studies. J Hyg Epidemiol Microbiol Immunol 15:393–401, 1971.
309. Joo I. Benefit versus risk factors in cholera and typhoid immunization. Dev Biol Stand 43:47–52, 1979.
310. Topley WCC. The role of active or passive immunization in the control of enteric infection. Lancet 1:181–186, 1938.
311. Wilson GS. The Hazards of Immunization. London, Anthone Press, 1967, p 265.
312. Gotuzzo E, Frisancho O, Sanchez J, et al. Association between the acquired immunodeficiency syndrome and infection with *Salmonella typhi* or *Salmonela paratyphi* in an endemic typhoid area. Arch Intern Med 151:381–382, 1991.
313. Brachman PS Jr, Metchock B, Kozarsky PE. Effects of antimalarial chemoprophylactic agents on the viability of the Ty21a typhoid vaccine strain. Clin Infect Dis 15:1057–1058, 1992.
314. Horowitz H, Carbonaro CA. Inhibition of the *Salmonella typhi* oral vaccine strain, Ty21a, by mefloquine and chloroquine. J Infect Dis 166:1462–1464, 1992.
315. Kollaritsch H, Que JU, Kunz C, et al. Safety and immunogenicity of live oral cholera and typhoid vaccines administered alone or in combination with antimalarial drugs, oral polio vaccine, or yellow fever vaccine. J Infect Dis 175:871–875, 1997.
316. Wolfe MS. Precautions with oral live typhoid (Ty 21a) vaccine [letter]. Lancet 336:631–632, 1990.
317. Clasener HAL. Immunization of man with *Salmonella* vaccine and tetanus-diphtheria vaccine: Dose-response relationship, secondary response and competition of antigens. J Hyg 65:457–466, 1967.
318. Clasener HAL, Beunders BJW. Immunization of man with typhoid and cholera vaccine: Agglutinating antibodies after intracutaneous and subcutaneous injections. J Hyg 65:449–456, 1967.
319. Cvjetanovic B, Ikic D, Lane WR, et al. Studies of combined quadruple vaccines against diphtheria, pertussis, tetanus and typhoid fever: Reactogenicity and antigenicity. Bull World Health Organ 46:47–52, 1972.
320. Ambrosch F, Fritzell B, Gregor J, et al. Combined vaccination against yellow fever and typhoid fever: A comparative trial. Vaccine 12:625–628, 1994.

321. Fritzell C, Rollin PE, Touir M, et al. Safety and immunogenicity of combined rabies and typhoid fever immunization. Vaccine 10:299–300, 1992.
322. Khoo SH, St Clair Roberts J, Mandal BK. Safety and efficacy of combined meningococcal and typhoid vaccine. BMJ 310:908–909, 1995.
323. Van Hoecke C, Lebacq E, Beran J, et al. Concomitant vaccination against hepatitis A and typhoid fever. J Trav Med 5:116–120, 1998.
324. Cryz SJ Jr, Que JU, Levine MM, et al. Safety and immunogenicity of a live oral bivalent typhoid fever (*Salmonella typhi* Ty21a)-cholera (*Vibrio cholerae* CVD 103-HgR) vaccine in healthy adults. Infect Immun 63:1336–1339, 1995.
325. Kollaritsch H, Furer E, Herzog C, et al. Randomized, double-blind placebo-controlled trial to evaluate the safety and immunogenicity of combined *Salmonella typhi* Ty21a and *Vibrio cholerae* CVD 103-HgR live oral vaccines. Infect Immun 64:1454–1457, 1996.
326. McAleer WJ, Buynak EB, Maigetter RZ, et al. Human hepatitis B vaccine from recombinant yeast. Nature 307:178–180, 1984.
327. Hilleman MR, Ellis R. Vaccines made from recombinant yeast cells. Vaccine 4:75–76, 1986.
328. Szu SC, Li X, Schneerson R, et al. Comparative immunogenicities of Vi polysaccharide-protein conjugates composed of cholera toxin or its B subunit as a carrier bound to high- or low-molecular weight-Vi. Infect Immun 57:3823–3827, 1989.
329. Szu SC, Li XR, Stone AL, et al. Relation between structure and immunologic properties of the Vi capsular polysaccharide. Infect Immun 59:4555–4561, 1991.
330. Szu SC, Bystricky S, Hinojosa-Ahumada M, et al. Synthesis and some immunologic properties of an O-acetyl pectin [poly(1->4)-alpha-D-GalpA]-protein conjugate as a vaccine for typhoid fever. Infect Immun 62:5545–5549, 1994.
331. Chatfield SN, Strahan K, Pickard D, et al. Evaluation of *Salmonella typhimurium* strains harbouring defined mutations in *htrA* and *aroA* in the murine salmonellosis model. Microb Pathog 12:145–151, 1992.
332. Pickard D, Li J, Roberts M, et al. Characterization of defined *ompR* mutants of *Salmonella typhi: ompR* is involved in the regulation of Vi polysaccharide expression. Infect Immun 62:3984–3993, 1994.
333. Miller SI, Loomis WP, Alpuche-Aranda C, et al. The PhoP virulence regulon and live oral *Salmonella* vaccines. Vaccine 11:122–125, 1993.
334. Levine MM, Galen J, Barry E, et al. Attenuated *Salmonella* as live oral vaccines against typhoid fever and as live vectors. J Biotechnol 44:193–196, 1995.
335. Balfour HH, Groth KE, Edelman CK, et al. Rubella viremia and antibody responses after rubella vaccination and reimmunization. Lancet 1:1078–1080, 1981.
336. Horstmann DM, Opton EM, Klemperer R, et al. Viremia in infants vaccinated with oral poliovirus vaccine (Sabin). Am J Hyg 79:47–63, 1964.
337. Melnick JL, Proctor RO, Ocampo AR, et al. Free and bound virus in serum after administration of oral poliovirus vaccine. Am J Epidemiol 84:329–342, 1966.
338. Kelly SM, Bosecker BA, Curtiss R III. Characterization and protective properties of attenuated mutants of *Salmonella cholerasuis*. Infect Immun 60:4881–4890, 1992.
339. Hohmann EL, Oletta CA, Miller SL. Evaluation of a *phoP/phoQ*-deleted, *aroA*-deleted live oral *Salmonella typhi* vaccine strain in human volunteers. Vaccine 14:19–24, 1996.
340. Gonzalez C, Hone D, Noriega F, et al. *Salmonella typhi* vaccine strain CVD 908 expressing the circumsporozoite protein of *Plasmodium falciparum:* Strain construction and safety and immunogenicity in humans. J Infect Dis 169:927–931, 1994.
341. Bodhidatta L, Taylor DN, Thisyakorn U, et al. Control of typhoid fever in Bangkok, Thailand, by annual immunization of school children with parenteral typhoid fever. Rev Infect Dis 9:841–845, 1987.

chapter

34 Yellow Fever

Thomas P. Monath

Yellow fever is the prototype member of the *flaviviridae* (*flavus*, L. "yellow"), which includes 68 single-stranded RNA viruses, most of which are transmitted by mosquitoes or ticks. The disease caused by yellow fever virus is the original "viral hemorrhagic fever"—a systemic illness characterized by high viremia; hepatic, renal, and myocardial injury; hemorrhage; and high lethality. Sequence analysis of the envelope gene revealed that yellow fever virus diverged earlier than other mosquito-borne viruses from the ancestral flaviviral lineage, approximately 3000 years ago.[1]

HISTORY

The early history of yellow fever is uncertain, due to the inexactness of clinical and epidemiological descriptions. Carter found the earliest record in a Mayan manuscript describing an epidemic with hematemesis (black vomit, *xekik*) in Yucatan in 1648 and suggested that the virus and mosquito vector were introduced from Africa during the slave trade.[2] The nosological term *yellow fever* was first used in 1750 during an outbreak in Barbados.[3] Yellow fever became a major problem in the 18th century in colonial settlements in the Americas and West Africa. It was introduced repeatedly into seaports in the United States and Europe via sailing vessels infested with *Aedes aegypti* mosquitoes that sustained transmission among the crew. In 1793, for example, yellow fever appeared in Philadelphia, the federal capital of the United States, killing 10% of the population.[4] Similar fates befell other cities throughout the 18th and 19th centuries.[5, 6] In one of the worst medical disasters in the early history of the United States, yellow fever caused over 13,000 deaths in the lower Mississippi Valley in 1878.

Until the 20th century, yellow fever was widely believed to be an airborne "miasma" arising from filth, sewage, and rotting organic matter. Several physicians, most notably Carlos Finlay in Cuba,[7] suggested that yellow fever is transmitted by mosquitoes. Proof was not obtained until 1900, when Walter Reed and colleagues conducted experiments on human volunteers in Cuba demonstrating that the agent is a filterable virus transmitted by *A. aegypti* mosquitoes.[8] This led to successes in disease prevention through mosquito abatement during the first 20 years of the 20th century. The last outbreak in the United States occurred in New Orleans in 1905, with 8399 cases and 908 deaths.

In 1925, the Rockefeller Foundation's West African Yellow Fever Commission laboratory in Yaba (Lagos), Nigeria, set out to determine the etiology of yellow fever, using imported monkeys for isolation of the causative agent. On June 30, 1927, blood of a 28-year-old man, Asibi, a resident of the village of Kpeve, Ghana, obtained 33 hours after the onset of mild yellow fever was inoculated into a rhesus monkey at the field laboratory in Accra. The animal was moribund 4 days later and had hepatic lesions consistent with yellow fever. Blood from this monkey was inoculated intraperitoneally into a second animal, which was transported during the incubation period to Yaba, where it developed clinical yellow fever the day after arrival. Stokes and colleagues established the Asibi strain by continuous direct passage in monkeys and indirect passage through *A. aegypti* mosquitoes.[9] Contemporary efforts at the Institut Pasteur, Dakar, led to isolation of the French strain from a Syrian (François Mayali) with mild yellow fever.[10] Isolation of the Asibi and French strains in 1927 enabled the development of vaccines, and research was initiated immediately in England, the United States, West Africa, and Brazil. Many years later, comparison of the genomes of the Asibi and French viruses confirmed that despite differing passage histories, they were 99.8% identical at the sequence level, divergent at only 23 nucleotides and nine amino acids.[11, 12]

In 1928, Edward Hindle of the Wellcome Research Laboratories, London, described the first attempt to produce an inactivated vaccine.[13] This and subsequent efforts on inactivated yellow fever vaccines were, however, unsuccessful. In 1931, Sawyer and associates at the Rockefeller Institute in New York first vaccinated humans with a live attenuated virus (the neuroadapted French strain) mixed with immune serum.[14] Vaccine development was spurred by a growing number of laboratory infections. In the 5 years following isolation of yellow fever virus, 32 cases (5 fatal) had occurred among laboratory workers.[15]

In 1932, Sellards and Laigret tested the French mouse brain virus without immune serum in humans,[16] and in 1934, Mathis, Laigret, and Durieux described the first field trial of this vaccine.[17] Rejecting mouse brain tissue as a dangerous substrate, Theiler and Smith at the Rockefeller Foundation developed a live vaccine (17D) attenuated by serial passage of the Asibi strain in cell cultures prepared from embryonated chicken eggs.[18, 19] In 1936, the 17D vaccine was tested in a small number of human volunteers in New York,[20] and it entered field trials in Brazil the following year.[21] By 1939, over 1 million Brazilians had received the 17D vaccine,[22] and over 100,000 persons in French West Africa had received the French neurotropic vaccine.[23, 24] During the 1940s, control of yellow fever at a population level was achieved in francophone Africa.[25] Immunization of laboratory workers, travelers, military, and expatriate residents in endemic areas removed the threat of acquiring the disease, and the disease faded from public view, having been transformed from a major human plague to a medical curiosity by the end of World War II.

The availability of 17D—widely regarded as one of the safest and most effective viral vaccines ever developed—has not ensured the adequate control of the disease. This represents a failure of public health policy and implementation of routine vaccination. In the past decade, there has been a resurgence of yellow fever[26, 27] and reappearance of the disease among unvaccinated tourists. Reinvasion of South America by *A. aegypti* (the vector responsible for interhuman transmission), the expansion of human populations in endemic regions, and increasing air travel raise concern about the reappearance of urban epidemics in the Americas and increase the risk of introduction into Asia,[27] where yellow fever has never occurred.

BACKGROUND

Virology

The principal focus here is on the molecular basis for the attenuation of yellow fever 17D vaccine. For comprehensive reviews of flavivirus genome structure and replication, see Chambers and associates[28] and Rice.[29]

Genome Structure and Gene Products

Flaviviruses are small (40–60 nm) positive-sense, single-stranded RNA viruses. The genome of the prototype yellow fever virus contains 10,862 nucleotides, composed of a short 5′ noncoding region, a single open reading frame of 10,233 nucleotides, and a 3′ noncoding region.[28, 29] The 5′ and 3′ noncoding regions have conformational structure and interactive, complementary sequences important in cyclization of the viral genome during encapsidation and replication. The open reading frame encodes three structural proteins at the 5′ end (capsid [C], premembrane [preM], and envelope [E] proteins), followed downstream by eight nonstructural (NS) proteins (Fig. 34–1). The structural proteins are included in the mature virion, whereas the NS proteins are responsible for replication and polypeptide processing. Viral proteins are cleaved after translation of the entire polyprotein at the rough endoplasmic reticulum (ER). Cell-associated virions form within the ER and are morphologically identical to extracellular particles.

The C protein (molecular mass approximately 11 kDa) interacts with RNA to form the virion nucleocapsid. The prM protein (approximately 27 kDa) forms an intracellular heterodimer that stabilizes the E polypeptide during exocytosis. The prM protein is processed by a furin-like cellular protease before viral release from the cell, leaving a small M structural protein (approximately 8 kDa) anchored at the C terminus in the viral envelope. The larger pr segment is released into the extracellular medium, although prM/M cleavage is sometimes incomplete, with incorporation of prM sequences into mature virions. Retention of prM protein may affect conformation and antigenicity of the E protein[30] and may reduce infectivity by inhibiting acid-dependent fusion.

The viral envelope comprises a lipid bilayer derived from the host cell, with dimers of the flavivirus E protein on the surface and anchored at their hydrophobic, basal ends. Like other enveloped viruses, flaviviruses are inactivated by organic solvents and detergents. The E protein is glycosylated and contains distinct determinants with biological function, including hemagglutination and neutralization, attachment to cell receptors, and internalization by membrane fusion. Antibodies to epitopes on the E protein interfere with these functions. The E protein plays a pivotal role in cell tropism, virulence, and immunity, and mutations in the E gene may alter these biological functions.

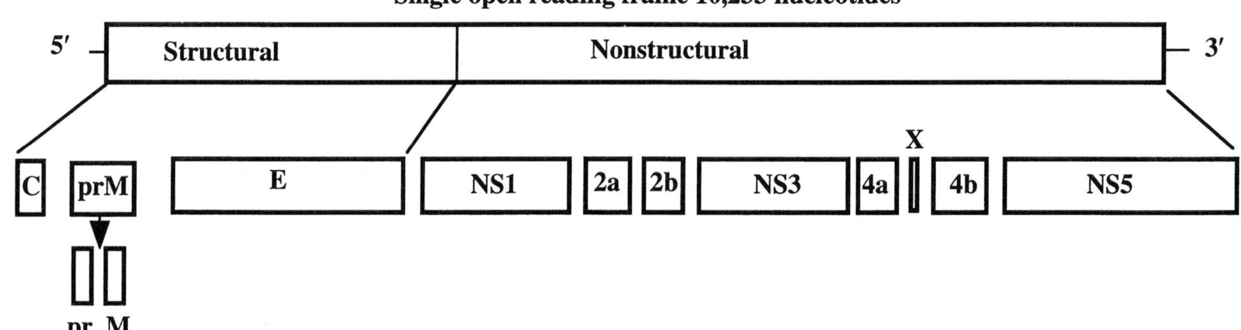

Figure 34–1. Genome organization of flaviviruses, consisting of a single long open reading frame (ORF) of 10,862 nucleotides and flanking short nontranslated regions. The ORF encodes three structural genes at the 5′ end (C-prM-E) and eight nonstructural genes encoding enzymes required for replication and posttranslational processing of viral proteins. (Modified from Chambers TJ, Tsai TF, Pervikov Y, et al. Vaccine development against dengue and Japanese encephalitis: Report of a World Health Organization meeting. Vaccine 15:1494, 1997; and Rice CM.[29])

The crystallographic structure of the E glycoprotein reveals a head-to-tail dimer composed of a 170 Å–long rod anchored to the membrane at its basal end with its long axis parallel to the virion surface (Fig. 34–2).[31] The C terminus resembles an immunoglobulin constant domain and is connected by a flexible region to the central part of the molecule (domain I) with up-and-down topology having eight antiparallel β strands and containing the N terminus. Two long loops (domain II) extending laterally are responsible for dimerization. A conserved stretch of 14 amino acids at the tip of one of the domain II loops constitutes the fusion domain responsible for internalization of nucleocapsids from endosomes into the cytoplasm of the infected cell. Domain III contains ligands involved in binding cell receptors. Neutralization determinants are conformational and are scattered on the outer surface of all three flavivirus structural domains.[32, 33]

Noninfectious subviral structures are released from infected cells. The slowly sedimenting hemagglutinin consists of 14-nm particles containing M and E proteins that are immunogenic and protective in animals. The NS1 protein is both released extracellularly and expressed on the surface of infected cells as a dimeric structure. The secreted form (soluble complement-fixing antigen) contains virus-specific and cross-reactive epi-

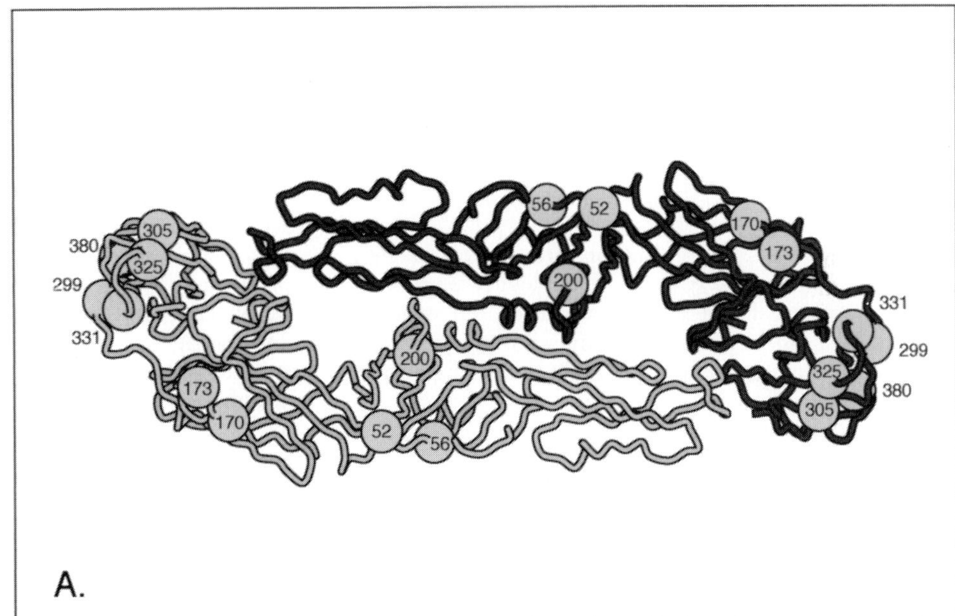

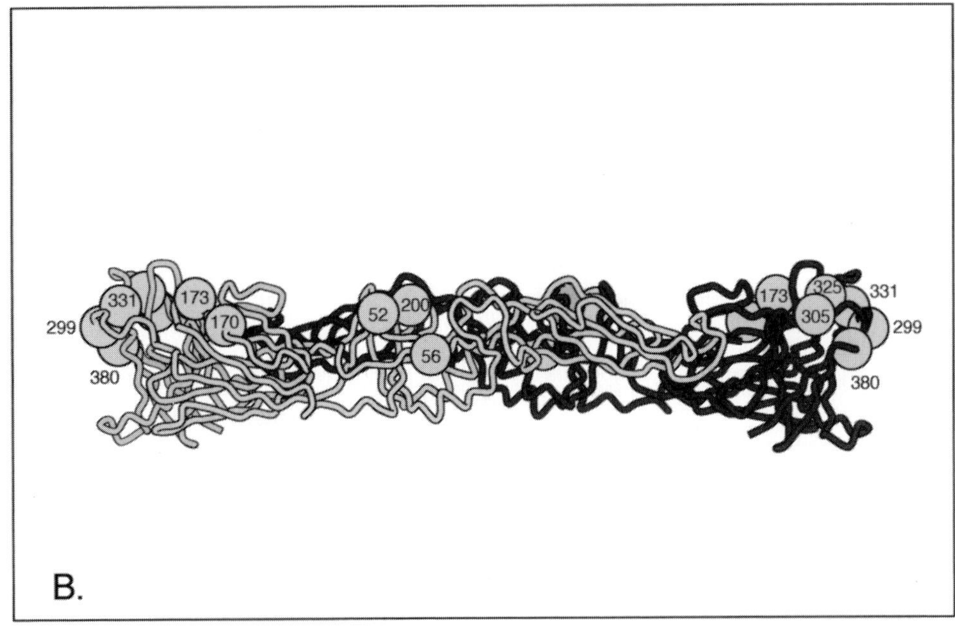

Figure 34–2. Three-dimensional structure of the flavivirus envelope (E) glycoprotein, determined by crystallography.[31] The E protein consists of a flat dimer parallel to the viral membrane, each molecule having three domains. *A*, Top view of the molecule. *B*, Side view. Amino acid determinants that differ between yellow fever 17D vaccine and the parental Asibi virus are shown (circles with amino acid number); their possible functions are described in the text and in Table 34–2. (Figure prepared by Dr. Stanley Watowich, Sealy Center for Structural Biology, based on data provided by Dr. Alan Barrett, both of the University of Texas Medical Branch, Galveston, Texas.)

topes. Antibodies to NS1 do not neutralize viral infectivity but provide protective immunity by complement-mediated lysis of infected cells.[34]

NS3 (molecular mass approximately 70 kDa) and NS2b have serine protease activity in posttranslational cleavage of the viral polyprotein and also have RNA helicase and RNA triphosphatase activities. Because of its critical functions, the NS3 gene sequence is highly conserved at the sequence level. The protein is present in cell membranes, contains virus-specific T-cell epitopes, and is a target for attack by cytotoxic T cells.[35–37] The NS5 protein (molecular mass 103 kDa) is also highly conserved and functions both as the RNA-dependent RNA polymerase in viral replication and as a methyltransferase in 5′ cap methylation. The functions of the other NS proteins are poorly defined. NS2a is localized in cell membranes and may play a role in processing of NS1; NS4a and NS4b may participate in the assembly of virus replication complexes.[38]

Replication

The major steps in replication are shown in Fig. 34–3. Flaviviruses enter cells by attachment to undefined receptors and are taken up in clathrin-coated vesicles. The nucleocapsids are released from endosomes into the cytoplasm by acid-mediated change in the configuration of domain II of the E protein, and fusion with the endosomal membrane. The positive-sense RNA is then translated to synthesize complementary negative RNA strands, which serve in turn as templates for progeny plus-strands. The mRNA encodes polymerase and helicase enzymes (NS5 and NS3) required for continued replication, and structural proteins for virion assembly. Assembly of virus particles occurs in close association with the ER. Virus particles are transported in intracellular vesicles to the plasma membrane, where they are exocytosed.

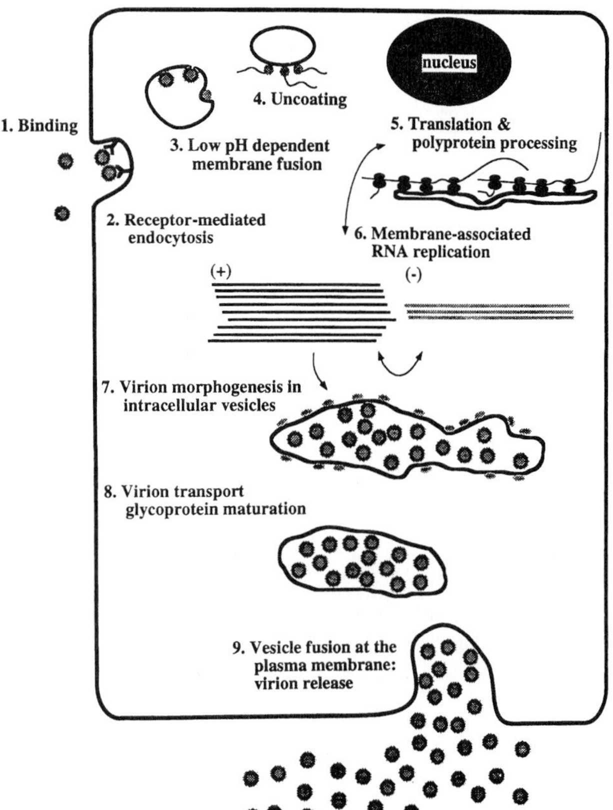

Figure 34–3. Steps in the replication cycle of flaviviruses. (From Rice CM. Flaviviridae; the viruses and their replication. In Fields BN [ed.]. Fields Virology. Vol. 1 (3rd ed). Philadelphia, Lippincott-Raven, 1996, p 931.)

Molecular Distinctions Between Attenuated (Vaccine) and Virulent Yellow Fever Viruses

The entire genomes of the 17D and the French neurotropic vaccines (FNV) and their wild-type progenitors, Asibi and the French viscerotropic virus, have been sequenced.[12, 39–41] Two substrains of 17D (17D-204 and 17DD) used for vaccine production, and variants of 17D-204 virus (ATCC and France), have been fully sequenced, and partial sequences are available for the 17D-204 WHO vaccine strain[12] and for 17DD vaccines produced in Senegal and Brazil.[12, 42] Because a large number of mutations occurred during the more than 230 passages that separate vaccines from their parental strains, it is impossible to define those responsible for attenuation, nor is it clear which determinants encode viscerotropism and neurotropism. Sequence comparison of strains with different biological properties has reduced the number of possibilities and allowed some educated guesses. Although some potentially important mutations have been identified, it is clear that virulence is multigenic.

The first comparison of nucleotide and amino acid differences between 17D-204 (ATCC) and Asibi virus was made by Hahn and coworkers.[40] Of a total of 10,862 nucleotides, 67 changes (0.62%) were found, resulting in mutations in 31 (0.91%) of 3411 amino acids. The changes were not randomly distributed across the genome; the highest rates of change were in genes encoding E, NS2a, and NS2b, and in the 3′ noncoding region. As additional sequences of 17D-204 and 17DD substrain vaccines became available, the number of amino acid differences between parental Asibi virus and attenuated viruses was reduced from 31 to 20, and the number of nucleotide differences in the 3′ noncoding region from 6 to 4 (Table 34–1).[43, 44] Because of the functional importance of the E protein in attachment and entry to cells, one or more of the seven amino acid differences that separate Asibi and the vaccine strains are likely to play a role in attenuation. The role of the E glycoprotein in neurovirulence of flaviviruses has been established by studies in which the E gene of a nonneurovirulent virus has been replaced by the corresponding gene of a virulent virus, resulting in a conversion to neurovirulent phenotype.[45]

The locations of the seven amino acid differences between Asibi and 17D vaccines in the three-dimensional crystallographic structure of the E glycoprotein is shown in Figure 34–2 and Table 34–2. Four are

Table 34–1. **AMINO ACID DIFFERENCES BETWEEN ASIBI VIRUS AND ATTENUATED 17D VACCINES**

NUCLEOTIDE	GENE FOR	AMINO ACID	ASIBI	17D-204 AND 17DD VACCINES
854	M	36	Leu	Phe
1127	E	52	Gly	Arg
1482		170	Ala	Val
1491		173	Thr	Ile
1572		200	Lys	Thr
1870		299	Met	Ile
1887		305	Ser	Phe
2112		380	Thr	Arg
2193		407	Ala	Val
3371	NS1	307	Ile	Val
3860	NS2a	118	Met	Val
4007		167	Thr	Ala
4022		172	Thr	Ala
4056		183	Ser	Phe
4505	NS2b	109	Ile	Leu
6023	NS3	485	Asp	Asn
6876	NS4a	146	Val	Ala
7171	NS4b	95	Ile	Met
10142	NS5	836	Glu	Lys
10338		900	Pro	Leu
10367	(3′ NCR)		U	C
10418			U	C
10800			G	A
10847			A	C

M, membrane; E, envelope; NS, nonstructural; NCR, noncoding region.
From Duarte dos Santos CN, Post PR, Carvalho R, et al: Complete nucleotide sequence of yellow fever virus vaccine strains 17DD and 17D-213. Virus Res 95:35, 1995; and Barrett ADT. Yellow fever vaccine. Biologicals 25:17, 1997.

nonconservative changes ($52^{Gly \to Arg}$; $200^{Lys \to Thr}$; $305^{Ser \to Phe}$; and $380^{Thr \to Arg}$). At least three wild-type yellow fever strains with different passage histories or geographic origins (Asibi,[40] the French viscerotropic virus,[12] and Peruvian strain 1899/81[46]) are identical at these amino acid codons, suggesting that the mutations in 17D play a role in attenuation.[43]

Residues 52 and 200 are located at the base of domain II. Mutations in this region could affect acid-dependent conformational change in the endosome and virion internalization. The conservative change at position $173^{Thr \to Ile}$ corresponds to a site in tick-borne encephalitis (TBE) virus at which a neutralization escape mutant had reduced neuroinvasiveness in mice[47]; mutations in this region may also interfere with acid-dependent fusion events.[48] Further evidence for the importance of residue 173 was obtained by Ryman and colleagues, who showed that it encodes an epitope recognized by wild-type specific monoclonal antibody and that reversion at this site may have contributed to the neurovirulence phenotype of a variant [17D(wt+)] recovered from a 17D-204 vaccine.[49] The nonconservative changes at E-305 and E-380 are located in domain III, which contains the determinants involved in tropism and cell attachment. Residue 305 is located on the outer surface of domain III, and residue 380 is located in a highly conserved region in mosquito-borne flaviviruses implicated in cell receptor interactions.[31] The change at residue E-380 alters the sequence at the putative cell attachment motif from Thr-Gly-Asp in Asibi virus to Arg-Gly-Asp in 17D strains.[42] Mutations in the Arg-Gly-Asp (RGD) sequence of another flavivirus (Murray Valley encephalitis) resulted in attenuation of virulence for mice.[50] Additionally, a mutation at TBE residue E-384 resulted in attenuation.[51] Changes in the cell attachment motif could alter neuro- or viscerotropism of the virus.

The potential importance of residue E-305 in the attenuation phenotype of 17D vaccine was suggested by sequence analysis of virus recovered from the brain of a 3-year-old child in the United States who died of encephalitis after 17D immunization.[52] The brain virus differed from 17D vaccine at a locus in domain III located near the E-305 residue (at $303^{Glu \to Lys}$) and was found to have increased neurovirulence for mice and monkeys.[53] Two other mutations (at E-155 and NS4b-72) were also present in the brain isolate; however, the mutation at 155 is less likely to be responsible since some attenuated vaccine strains have a wild-type residue at this locus.[42, 53]

The complexity of the genetic basis for virulence is underscored by a study of a 17D vaccine strain having increased neurovirulence due to multiple mouse brain passages.[54] It has been repeatedly shown that 17D vaccine is not "fixed" with respect to neurovirulence and that sequential mouse brain passage of the vaccine results in increasing virulence.[55] The neuroadapted 17D

Table 34–2. **LOCATION AND POTENTIAL FUNCTION OF AMINO ACID DIFFERENCES BETWEEN ASIBI AND 17D VACCINE VIRUSES IN THREE-DIMENSIONAL STRUCTURE OF FLAVIVIRUS ENVELOPE (E) GLYCOPROTEIN**

AMINO ACID	ASIBI	17D	DOMAIN	POTENTIAL FUNCTIONAL ROLE IN VIRULENCE OR ATTENUATION
52	Gly	Arg	II	Hinge region between domains I and II; may affect fusion activation (low-pH conformational change)
170	Ala	Val	I	Outer surface of domain I, near known attenuating mutation in TBE virus
173	Thr	Ile	I	Outer surface of domain I, known attenuating mutation in TBE virus
200	Lys	Thr	II	Hinge region between domains I and II; may affect fusion activation (low-pH conformational change)
299	Met	Ile	I/III	
305	Ser	Phe	III	External face of cell attachment domain
380	Thr	Arg	III	Cell attachment motif
407	Ala	Val	III	

TBE, tick-borne encephalitis.
Data from Ray FA, Heinz FX, Mandl C, et al. The envelope glycoprotein from the tick-borne encephalitis virus at 2Å resolution. Nature 375:291, 1995; and Barrett ADT. Yellow fever vaccine. Biologicals 25:17, 1993.

virus reverted to the wild-type (Asibi) sequence at residues 52 and 173 and had other mutations, including one at the putative virulence determinant at residue $305^{Ser \rightarrow Val}$. However, a chimera generated from an infectious clone of 17D virus and containing the E protein of the neuroadapted virus (with the mutations noted previously at residues 52, 173, and 305) did not exhibit increased neurovirulence in the mouse model. This result illustrated the multigenic nature of virulence and suggested that one or more of the mutations in the nonstructural proteins or the 3′ noncoding region of the virus may contribute. Studies with other flaviviruses have demonstrated that mutations in the nonstructural coding region may reduce neurovirulence,[56] presumably by restricting replication efficiency.

There are 11 amino acid changes in the nonstructural proteins of 17D viruses (Table 34–1). One change occurs in the NS1 protein; four in NS2a; and one each in NS2b, NS4a, and NS4b. None of these mutations alter the hydrophobicity profile of the proteins and thus may not affect function.[43] One change occurs in NS3 at position 485, in a region of the protein with RNA helicase and triphosphatase activities, and two mutations occur in the RNA polymerase (NS5). The latter changes may affect replication efficiency and may contribute to attenuation of 17D.

Although none of the specific differences in nonstructural genes of 17D viruses can be precisely implicated, other lines of evidence indicate their potential role in attenuation. Mutations at glycosylation sites in NS1 resulted in reduced neurovirulence of yellow fever 17D virus.[57] A medium-sized plaque variant recovered from 17D-204 vaccine was shown to have reduced neurovirulence for mice.[58] A similar plaque variant purified from 17D-204 vaccine produced in South Africa had reduced mouse neurovirulence and differed from large plaque and uncloned vaccine at a single amino acid in NS5 $137^{Pro \rightarrow Ser}$.[59] This mutation is in a region encoding the methyltransferase activity of NS5.

Little is known about the molecular basis of viscerotropism (the ability of wild-type yellow fever virus to replicate and damage nonneural tissue, particularly the liver), or the mutations responsible for loss of this trait in 17D vaccine. To approach this question, Wang and associates compared the sequence of the French viscerotropic strain with that of the FNV,[41] which was developed by over 100 sequential mouse brain passages. The principal phenotypic change in FNV is loss of viscerotropism for monkeys and humans. Comparison of the parental and vaccine strains revealed 77 (0.7%) nucleotide and 35 (1%) amino acid changes scattered throughout the genome, with the highest frequency of mutations in the C, M, E, NS2a, 2K, and NS4b proteins. The large number of differences and lack of biological data on the role of these mutations preclude speculations on the genetic basis of viscerotropism. Sequence comparison of FNV with 17DD and 17D-204 vaccines (both of which have markedly attenuated viscerotropism) revealed only two shared differences from the parental and other wild-type yellow fever viruses. These common differences, which evolved during the development of vaccine strains by completely distinct processes, were at positions in the M protein ($35^{Leu \rightarrow Phe}$) and NS4b ($95^{Ile \rightarrow Met}$). It is unclear whether these mutations are involved in loss of viscerotropism.

Molecular Identification of Antigenic Determinants in Yellow Fever Virus and Vaccine Strains

Monoclonal antibodies recognize structurally distinct regions in the E protein of yellow fever virus,[60–66] including vaccine strain–specific epitopes, yellow fever virus–specific epitopes, and determinants cross-reactive with specific heterologous flaviviruses and with broad flavivirus group epitopes. Antibodies against vaccine strain–specific, virus-specific, and flavivirus group–reactive epitopes neutralize virus, and many passively protect mice against intracerebral challenge. Interestingly, immunization with 17D virus generated monoclonal antibodies that neutralized wild-type (Asibi) virus but not 17D,[60] and flavivirus group–reactive monoclonals generated after immunization with 17D,[60] Asibi,[64] or heterologous flaviviruses[65] neutralized wild-type virus. This multiplicity of neutralizing determinants helps to explain the broad protective immunity afforded by 17D vaccine against wild yellow fever virus strains, and the partial cross-protection by heterologous flaviviruses against yellow fever. Additional studies have defined epitopes that are substrain specific, differentiating 17D-204 vaccine from other yellow fever viruses, differentiating 17D-204 from 17DD vaccines, and even distinguishing between vaccines of the same substrain from different manufacturers.[65, 67] Plaque-size variants purified from 17D vaccine can also be distinguished in neutralization and hemagglutination inhibition (HI) tests.[66, 68] This antigenic heterogeneity is due to the uncloned nature and different passage histories during manufacture and laboratory manipulation. Some monoclonals are specific for 17D and do not recognize wild-type virus.[60, 69] At present, there is no recognized practical consequence, with respect to protective immunity, of the absence of some wild-type antigenic determinants in 17D vaccines.

Gould and coworkers identified a plaque variant in 17D vaccine that reacted with a monoclonal antibody specific for wild-type viruses and variants recovered from Asibi virus that reacted with a 17D-204 specific monoclonal,[70] suggesting that 17D was derived by a process of selection of subpopulations during serial passage.

Some neutralizing epitopes have been localized by sequencing escape mutants or wild-type antigenic variants recovered from 17D vaccine. An epitope at residue E-173 is the only wild-type antigenic determinant that has been localized[49]; as mentioned previously, this site is a putative neurovirulence factor. Other virus-specific neutralization determinants in the E protein have been identified at residues E-71/72, 155, 158, and 305 or 325[32, 33] and thus occur on the exposed surfaces of all three domains of the glycoprotein (Fig. 34–2). Their location is consonant with the effector roles of antibody in blocking cell attachment and intracellular uncoating events. Neutralization determinants are variable across viral strains, are involved in multiple functional attributes of the E protein, and are structurally diverse, consistent with the broad protective activity of yellow fever vaccine against wild viral strains.

Antigenic determinants involved in cell-mediated immunity have not yet been specifically localized in yellow fever virus. However, epitopes recognized by $CD4^+$ and $CD8^+$ cytotoxic T cells have been identified in dengue[36, 71–75] and Murray Valley encephalitis viruses.[37, 76] These cytotoxic T lymphocyte (CTL) determinants are found in all three structural proteins and in multiple NS proteins, particularly NS3. The location of some epitopes has been fine-mapped to precise locations in these proteins. Dengue and Murray Valley encephalitis have common T-cell determinants in the E protein at residues approximately 225 to 250 and approximately 350 to 370, and it is possible that these domains are functionally similar in yellow fever virus and other flaviviruses.

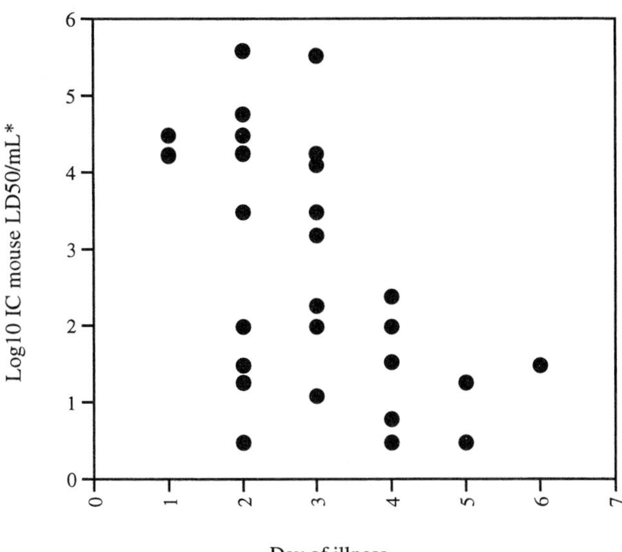

Figure 34–4. Virus titers in blood in yellow fever patients, Nigeria, 1951–1953. Minimal titer endpoint not determined in all cases. (Data from MacNamara FN. Man as the host of the yellow fever virus. MD thesis. Cambridge University, Cambridge, pp 1–140; and MacNamara FN. A clinico-pathological study of yellow fever in Nigeria. West Afr J Med 6:137, 1957.)

Clinical Description

The clinical spectrum of yellow fever is very broad, including truly subclinical infection, abortive infection with nonspecific grippe-like illness, and potentially lethal pansystemic disease with fever, jaundice, renal failure, and hemorrhage. This variability makes the clinical diagnosis of sporadic cases difficult and is responsible for the underestimation of morbidity and inflation of case-fatality rates when only cases of full-blown yellow fever are enumerated. As for many other infections, this variability in response is due to intrinsic and acquired host resistance factors, and probably to differences in the pathogenicity of viral strains.

After an incubation period of 3 to 6 days, the onset is abrupt, with rigors and headache. The classical illness is characterized by three stages.[15, 77–79] During the first *period of infection*, lasting 3 to 4 days, virus is present in blood.[8, 15, 80] Fatal cases appear to have a longer duration of viremia than those of survivors. MacNamara found peak viremias on day 2 to 3 of illness, with titers of up to 5.6 $\log_{10}$ mouse intracerebral median lethal dose ($ICLD_{50}$) per mL (Fig. 34–4).[80] Nassar and associates studied one patient on days 5 and 7 after onset; titers in whole blood were 4.6 and 2.7 $\log_{10}$ $ICLD_{50}$ per mL, respectively.[81]

The frequency of clinical symptoms and signs in yellow fever patients is shown in Fig. 34–5. The period of infection is characterized by fever, malaise, prostration, headache, photophobia, lumbosacral pain, pain in the lower extremities (particularly the knee joints), generalized myalgia, anorexia, nausea, vomiting, restlessness, irritability, and dizziness. On physical examination, the patient appears toxic, with hyperemia of the skin; congestion of the conjunctivae, gums, and face; epigastric tenderness; and tenderness and enlargement of the liver. The tongue is characteristically small, pointed, bright red at the tip and sides, with a white coating in the center. Early clinicians made much of this arcane sign, and it has stood the test of time. Initially the pulse rate is high, but by the second day there is a bradycardia relative to fever (Faget's sign). The average fever is 102 to 103°F and lasts 3.3 days, but the temperature may rise as high as 105°F, a bad prognostic sign. Young children may experience febrile convulsions. Laboratory abnormalities include leukopenia ($1.5–2.5 \times 10^9$/L) with a relative neutropenia. The leukopenia occurs precipitously, in concert with the onset of illness.[15] Between 48 and 72 hours after the onset of illness, an elevation of serum transaminase levels precedes the appearance of jaundice, the levels often predicting the severity of hepatic dysfunction later in the illness.[82]

The period of infection may be followed by a distinct *period of remission* with abatement of fever and symptoms lasting up to 48 hours. The remission is often not obvious or very brief. In cases of abortive infection, the patient simply recovers at this stage. Such cases remain anicteric, and the nonspecificity of the syndrome makes it impossible to diagnose yellow fever clinically except during an epidemic. It is not known what proportion of patients infected with yellow fever virus develop truly subclinical infections versus abortive (anicteric) infections.

Approximately 15% of persons infected with yellow fever virus develop moderate or severe disease characterized by jaundice.[79, 83] These patients enter the third stage of the disease, the *period of intoxication* on the third to sixth day after the onset of illness, with a return of fever, relative bradycardia, nausea, vomiting, epigastric pain, jaundice, oliguria, and a hemorrhagic diathesis. Virus disappears from blood, and antibodies appear. The subsequent course reflects dysfunction of multiple organ systems, including the liver, kidneys, and cardiovascular system. Serum aspartate aminotransferase (AST) and alanine aminotransferase (ALT) levels peak early in the second week of illness and fall rapidly over a few days in patients who recover. AST levels exceed ALT levels,

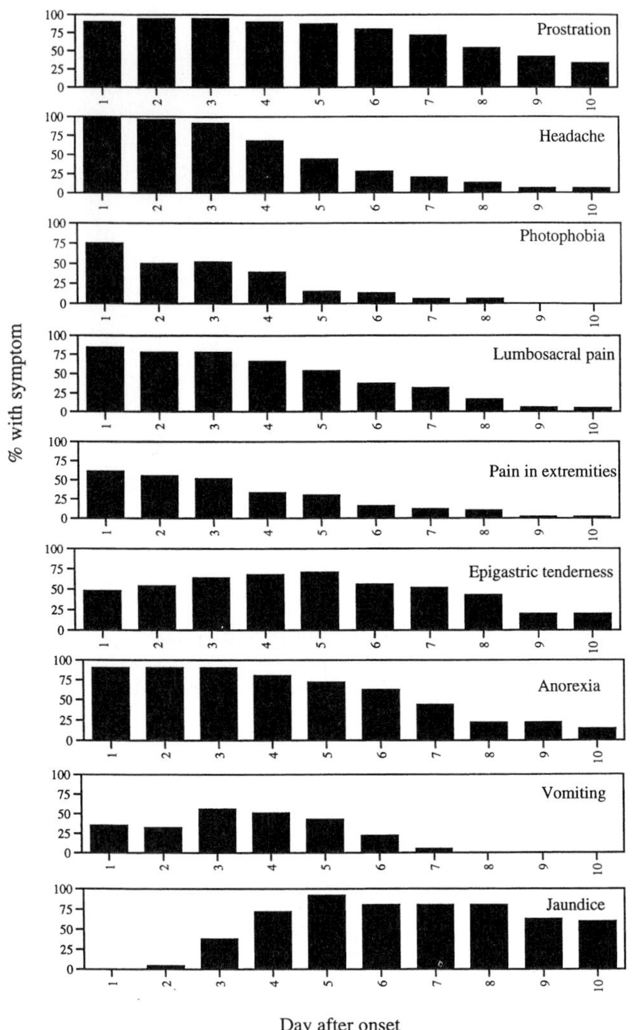

Figure 34–5. Proportion of cases of severe, nonfatal yellow fever with symptoms and signs by day of illness. (After Beeuwkes H. Clinical manifestations of yellow fever in the West African native as observed during four extensive epidemics of the disease in the Gold Coast and Nigeria. Trans R Soc Trop Med Hyg 1:61, 1936.)

probably due to direct viral injury to myocardium and skeletal muscle. This distinguishes yellow fever from viral hepatitis, in which ALT levels typically exceed AST levels. Serum aminotransferase levels are proportional to the severity of the disease. In one study, the mean AST and ALT levels in fatal cases were 2766 and 660 U, respectively, whereas in surviving patients with jaundice the mean levels were 929 and 351 U.[82] Alkaline phosphatase levels are normal or only slightly elevated. Direct bilirubin levels are typically between 5 and 10 mg per dL, with higher levels in fatal than in nonfatal cases.[84]

Renal dysfunction is marked by an increase in albuminuria, a reduction in urine output, and rising azotemia. Albumin levels in the urine typically range between 3 and 5 g per L but may reach 20 g per L. Serum creatinine levels are three to eight times normal. In some patients who survive the hepatitic phase, renal failure predominates.[85] Death is preceded by virtually complete anuria. The hemorrhagic diathesis is manifested as coffee-ground hematemesis, melena, hematuria, metrorrhagia, petechiae, ecchymoses, epistaxis, oozing of blood from the gums, and excessive bleeding at needle puncture sites. Laboratory correlates include thrombocytopenia, prolonged clotting and prothrombin times, and reductions in levels of clotting factors synthesized by the liver (factors II, V, VII, IX, and X). Some patients have clotting abnormalities suggesting disseminated intravascular coagulation, including diminished fibrinogen and factor VIII levels and the presence of fibrin split products.[86, 87]

The clinical significance of myocardial injury remains poorly understood. The electrocardiogram may show sinus bradycardia without conduction defects, and ST-T abnormalities, particularly elevated T waves, and extrasystoles,[15, 88] presumably the result of virus replication and direct viral injury to the myocardium. Bradycardia may contribute to the physiological decompensation associated with hypotension, reduced perfusion, and metabolic acidosis in severe cases. Acute cardiac enlargement may occur during the course of yellow fever infection.[15]

Central nervous system signs include delirium, agitation, convulsions, stupor, and coma. In severe cases, the cerebrospinal fluid is under increased pressure and may have elevated protein levels but no cells. In one case, yellow fever virus was recovered from cerebrospinal fluid after death.[89] In patients dying of yellow fever, central nervous system signs appear to result from cerebral edema or metabolic factors, based on the virtual absence of inflammatory changes in brain tissue. Pathological changes include petechiae (perivascular hemorrhages) and edema.[90] True yellow fever viral encephalitis is exceedingly rare, with few extant clinical case reports of paralysis, optic neuritis, and cranial nerve palsy suggesting neurologic infection, but without substantiating virological evidence to differentiate encephalitis from encephalopathy.[91, 92]

The critical phase of the illness occurs between the fifth and tenth day, at which point the patient either dies or rapidly recovers. Case-fatality rates vary widely, in part because of missed mild cases, but possibly reflect differences in the virulence of viral strains. In recent investigations, the case-fatality rate in West African patients with jaundice approximated 20%.[93, 94] The clinical severity and lethality of yellow fever is highest in older adults.[78, 80, 95–97] Events associated with a poor prognosis or imminent demise include leukocytosis, hypothermia, agitated delirium, intractable hiccups, seizures, hypoglycemia, hyperkalemia, metabolic acidosis, Cheyne-Stokes respirations, stupor, and coma.

In one series of 103 patients in Nigeria, the average hospital stay for surviving patients was 14 days (range 5–42 days) and the average duration of the acute illness was 17.8 days.[96] Although convalescence may be associated with weakness and fatigability lasting several weeks, healing of the liver and kidney is typically complete, without postnecrotic fibrosis. In some cases, jaundice and elevations in serum aminotransferase levels may persist for months after the onset of illness.[82, 84, 98] It is uncertain whether such atypical cases have had other underlying hematological or hepatic diseases. In one study, the outcome of yellow fever in hepatitis B surface antigen–positive and –negative patients was similar.[99] Complications of yellow fever include superimposed bacterial pneumonia, parotitis, and sepsis associated with recovery from renal tubular necrosis. Late deaths during convalescence have been ascribed to myocarditis, arrhythmia, or heart failure,[97] but documentation is poor.

Pathogenesis

Mosquito Vector

Infection of mosquitoes is initiated by the ingestion of a blood meal containing a threshold concentration of virus (approximately 3.5 $\log_{10}$/mL), resulting in infection of the midgut epithelium. The virus is released from the midgut into the hemolymph and spreads to other tissues, notably the reproductive tract and salivary glands. Seven to 10 days elapse between the ingestion of virus and secretion in saliva (the so-called extrinsic incubation period), at which point the vector is capable of transmitting virus when she refeeds on a susceptible host. Infection of reproductive tissues of the mosquito provides a mechanism for vertical transmission of yellow fever virus from the female mosquito to her progeny and from congenitally infected males to females during copulation.[100–102]

Mosquito infection is relevant to the subject of vaccines in the following ways:

1. *Transmission of live vaccine viruses.* The use of a live vaccine might engender a risk of secondary spread by mosquitoes, and passage of vaccine virus could result in a reversion to a more virulent phenotype. This is unlikely for two reasons: (1) viremia following 17D vaccination is very low and below the threshold of oral infection of the vector,[21, 103, 104] (with the proviso that viremia has not been measured in infants, who may sustain more active infections than adults, or in immunosuppressed individuals); and (2) 17D virus is poorly infectious for mosquitoes. Whitman infected *A. aegypti* larvae with 17D virus after immersion in virus, but infected adult progeny were incapable of transmitting the virus.[105] Jennings and associates showed that 45% of adult female *A. aegypti* fed on a high concentration of 17D vaccine in an artificial blood meal developed midgut infections, but no virus was detected in head tissue.[53] In another study, only 1 of 32 *A. aegypti* orally exposed to 17D virus developed infection in head tissue, and none of the mosquitoes transmitted the virus.[106] Thus, yellow fever 17D virus has lost its ability to be transmitted by *A. aegypti*, possibly because of an inability of the virus to cross the "midgut barrier." At the molecular level, it has not been determined which mutations in 17D virus are responsible for restricted transmission by mosquitoes.

2. *Mode of human infection and interaction with the immune system.* Approximately 10^3 virions are inoculated during mosquito feeding.[107] Salivary virus is deposited mainly in the extravascular tissues of the host during probing, as saliva that is injected intravascularly is apparently reingested by the mosquito during blood feeding.[108] Viral replication is initiated at the site of inoculation and spreads through lymphatic channels to regional lymph nodes. In the immunized host, the small inoculum would encounter antibodies in extracellular transudate and lymph. This suggests that a low level of immunity is sufficient to protect the host against disease. It is not known whether immunity is sufficient to sterilize the mosquito inoculum. However, under conditions of artificial inoculation of 17D vaccine to previously vaccinated subjects[104] or coadministration of vaccine viruses and immune serum,[14] sufficient virus replication occurs for a booster or primary immune response, respectively.

The expression of neutralization epitopes (determined with monoclonal antibodies) may differ between yellow fever virus propagated in mosquito and mammalian cells.[65] The evolutionary and functional relevance of this observation are uncertain but may represent a means whereby mosquitoes infected with yellow fever virus would avoid the effects of neutralizing antibodies ingested in a blood meal. In terms of flavivirus vaccine development, host specificity of neutralization determinants suggests that certain arthropod cells may not yield effective inactivated or subunit immunogens for vertebrates.

Vertebrate Hosts

Two biological properties are inherent to all wild-type yellow fever viruses: *viscerotropism*, referring to the ability to cause viremia and to infect and damage liver, spleen, heart, and kidneys, and *neurotropism*, the ability to infect the brain parenchyma and cause encephalitis. Wild-type yellow fever viruses are predominantly viscerotropic in primate hosts.

Wild-type yellow fever virus has a relatively broad host range. In rodents (mice, hamsters, and guinea pigs), the virus is principally neurotropic, and the only extraneural organ showing significant viral replication is the adrenal gland.[109] Rodents develop encephalitis only after IC, intraocular, or intranasal inoculation. The time to death is typically 7 to 10 days, depending on the strain and the passage history (neuroadaptation). Adult mice infected by the peripheral route develop encephalitis if the blood-brain barrier is not completely developed (as in suckling mice up to 5–7 days of age) or is compromised by sham IC inoculation. The human correlate is in very young human infants the increased risk of neuroinvasion after vaccination with 17D vaccine, and in children the increased risk of encephalitis after immunization with the FNV. The basis for age-related resistance is uncertain. Zisman and coworkers suggested that the development of resistance is related to the maturation of macrophages involved in yellow fever virus clearance.[110]

In nature, only nonhuman primates and humans develop viscerotropic infections (hepatitis). Most nonhuman primate species develop viremic infections, and some New World and Asian monkeys develop lethal infections with fulminant hepatitis resembling the human disease.[111, 112] The only nonprimate species that develops viscerotropic infection in response to experimental infection is the European hedgehog.[113]

The pathophysiology of yellow fever in rhesus monkeys and humans is characterized by hepatic dysfunction, renal failure, coagulopathy, and shock[114–116]; monkeys develop a more fulminating illness than humans, lasting only 3 to 4 days. The LD_{50} of the Asibi strain in the monkey is 0.01 mouse $ICLD_{50}$, or approximately 0.2 Vero cell plaque-forming units. Higher viral doses shorten the incubation period but do not alter the duration or outcome of illness (Table 34–3),[117] implying that early, innate host immune responses (e.g., natural killer [NK] cells) are insufficient to clear even a minimal infection. The susceptibility of human peripheral blood mononuclear cells to infection, and evidence from experimental animals, suggest that lymphoid cells are important targets for early replication. After intraperitoneal inoculation of rhesus monkeys, Kupffer cells in the liver were infected first (24 hours after inoculation). Virus was detectable on day 2 in serum and kidney and on day 3 in bone marrow, spleen, and lymph nodes.[115] Early injury to Kupffer cells was also noted after subcutaneous infection of monkeys.[116, 118] Infection and degeneration of hepatocytes is a relatively late event, occurring in the last 24 to 48 hours before death in the monkey[115, 116] and in the last phase of infection in humans. In fatal human cases, 5 to 100% (mean, 80%) of hepatocytes undergo coagulative necrosis.[119] The midzone of the liver lobule is principally affected, with sparing of cells bordering the central vein and portal tracts. The reason for this peculiar distribution of hepatic injury is unknown. Midzonal necrosis has been described in low-flow hypoxia, due to ATP depletion and oxidative stress of marginally oxygenated cells at the border between anoxic and normoxic cells,[120] and a similar mechanism might contribute to injury in yellow fever infection. However, yellow fever viral antigen and RNA have been observed principally in hepatocytes in the midzone,[121] suggesting a predilection of these cells to viral replication. Injury to hepatocytes is characterized by eosinophilic degeneration with condensed nuclear chromatin (Councilman bodies), rather than by ballooning and rarefaction necrosis seen in viral hepatitis.[122] The morphological features suggest that chromatin fragmentation and apoptosis of Kupffer cells and liver cells are induced by yellow fever virus. Apoptosis has been confirmed in liver tissue of a fatal human case (P. Marianneau, M. Huerre, V. Deubel, personal communication, 1997). This mode of cell death may explain the virtual absence of inflammation in tissues affected by yellow fever. Other hepatic changes include microvesicular fat and ceroid or lipofuchsin deposits, and intranuclear (Torres) bodies. Since little inflammation occurs, the reticulin framework is preserved and complete healing occurs without residual fibrosis.

Table 34–3. **EXPERIMENTAL YELLOW FEVER IN RHESUS MONKEY: EFFECT OF VIRAL DOSE ON INCUBATION PERIOD AND DURATION OF ILLNESS**

SUBCUTANEOUS DOSE ($MICLD_{50}$)	MORTALITY (%)	HOURS (MEAN) Incubation Period	Duration of Illness	Time of Death
1000	100	60	40	100
10	100	67	44	111
1	100	90	40	130
0.1	100	186	43	224
0.01	67	182	39.5	222
0.001	0	—	—	—

$MICLD_{50}$, mouse intracerebral LD_{50}.

Data from Spertzl RO, Kosch PC, Gilbertson SH, et al. Annual Progress Report. Ft. Detrick, Frederick, MD, US Army Medical Research Institute of Infectious Diseases, 1972. Similar results were obtained in early studies (see Hindle[299]).

Renal abnormality is characterized by eosinophilic degeneration and fatty changes of renal tubular epithelium without inflammation. These changes may represent late-stage injury following shock. In monkeys, oliguria with maintenance of tubular function indicated prerenal failure associated with hypotension and the hepatorenal syndrome; acute tubular necrosis was a terminal event.[116] Yellow fever antigen was found in renal tubular cells in fatal human cases,[123] suggesting that direct viral injury is responsible. Glomerular lesions (Schiff-positive changes in basement membrane[124] and degeneration of cells lining the Bowman capsule) and yellow fever antigen in glomerulae 2 to 3 days after the infection of monkeys (T. P. Monath, unpublished observations) have been observed, implying that direct viral injury accounts for albuminuria observed in advance of renal failure.

Lymphocytic elements in the germinal centers of spleen, lymph nodes, tonsils, and Peyer patches are depleted, and large mononuclear or histiocytic cells accumulate in the splenic follicles.[116, 125] Necrosis of germinal centers is more striking in monkeys than in humans. It is unknown to what extent the lymphoid injury is the direct result of viral replication.

In addition to hepatic and renal dysfunction, the disease is characterized by hemorrhage and circulatory collapse. Decreased synthesis of vitamin K–dependent coagulation factors by the liver, and disseminated intravascular coagulation, contribute to the bleeding diathesis.[87, 114] Platelet dysfunction, demonstrated by collagen- and ADP-stimulated aggregation, has been demonstrated in the monkey model (S. Fisher-Hoch, J. McCormick, T. P. Monath, unpublished observations).

Direct viral injury to myocardial fibers, which show cloudy swelling and fatty changes[126, 127] and viral antigen,[123] may contribute to shock. It is tempting to speculate that the circulatory shock seen in the terminal stage of yellow fever is mediated by cytokine dysregulation, as in the sepsis syndrome. Tumor necrosis factor-α (TNF-α) produced by infected or activated Kupffer cells and splenic macrophages in response to viral injury might, together with interleukin 1, interferon-γ, platelet-activating factor, and other cytokines, be responsible for cell injury; oxygen free radical formation; endothelial damage and microthrombosis; disseminated intravascular coagulation; tissue anoxia; oliguria; and shock. Patients dying of yellow fever show cerebral edema at autopsy, probably the result of microvascular dysfunction.

Immunopathological Events

Neutralizing antibodies appear within 4 to 5 days after the onset of natural infection with yellow fever virus (i.e., 7–8 days after infection).[15] Antibody and (presumably) cellular responses occur coincident with the clinical crisis (period of intoxication), and both free virions and hemagglutinating, complement-fixing, or immunoprecipitating antigen[115, 128] may be found in blood together with antibody at this time, suggesting that immune clearance of infected cells, associated with release of cytokines, might play a role in the pathogenesis of capillary leak and shock. Although there is no direct evidence to support the notion of an immunopathologic mechanism in acute yellow fever infection, this is an area for future investigation. In an artificial model, the administration of monoclonal antibodies to mice challenged intracerebrally with yellow fever virus caused enhanced perivascular inflammation and accelerated death.[129, 130] There is no known correlate of this phenomenon in humans.

Host Factors Affecting Susceptibility

Young age increases susceptibility to neuroinvasion of yellow fever vaccine strains. In some outbreaks, infection with viscerotropic strains was more lethal in infants than in older children,[95] and in adults older than 50 years than in younger persons.[78, 80, 95–97] Genetic determinants are known to affect the pathogenesis of flavivirus infections, and resistance to yellow fever virus in mice is determined by an autosomal dominant allele (*Flv^r*).[131] Genetic background has been shown also to influence the immune response to flaviviruses in mice.[132] The role of genetic factors in human responses to yellow fever infection is uncertain. The older literature makes repeated reference to racial differences in the lethality of yellow fever, rates being lower in blacks than whites during outbreaks in western Africa,[95] tropical America,[133] and the United States.[134] It is uncertain whether the apparent increased resistance of blacks reflects acquired immunity or is due to genetic factors. Moreover, epidemics of yellow fever in Africa have been associated with high case-fatality rates. The question of racial differences in susceptibility to yellow fever will be resolved only by well-controlled epidemiological and serological studies in the setting of an outbreak affecting both races. In the case of the related flavivirus, dengue, whites had a higher incidence of dengue hemorrhagic fever than persons of the black race during an epidemic in Cuba, a finding that could not be explained on the basis of a racial difference in the background of immunity.[134a] An association between HLA haplotype and disease severity was found in patients with dengue hemorrhagic fever.[135]

Virus-Specified Factors

Wild-type yellow fever viral strains in Africa and South America have been classified into at least three genotypes (representing West Africa, Central-East Africa, and South America) based on sequence analysis (see under *Geographic Distribution*), and there is microheterogeneity at the sequence level among strains within these groupings.[136] Since single mutations can affect the biological behavior of yellow fever virus, it is not surprising that viral strains differ with respect to neurovirulence for mice[137–139] or viscerotropism for monkeys.[140] Variation in virulence may explain differences in mortality rates observed in human epidemics, which have ranged from 3 to 20% in recent outbreaks.[112] Despite the probable importance of virus-specified factors in the pathogenesis of yellow fever, they remain poorly understood. Deubel and coworkers found that South American strains were neuroinvasive for 8-day-old mice, whereas African viruses were not, and suggested that the higher case-fatality rates in South America could be due to strain differences in virulence.[141] On the other hand, it was the impression of early workers that the South American viruses were less often lethal for rhesus monkeys.[109] Miller and colleagues showed that the mosquito responsible for epidemic transmission in Nigeria had a low vector capacity and proposed that the vector served as a genetic bottleneck for the selection of a virulent viral strain able to elicit high viremias in humans.[142]

Nonspecific Resistance Mechanisms and Specific Immune Responses

Nonspecific Responses

NK cells and interferons appear during the early phase of viral replication, before the advent of virus-specific cytotoxic T cells and immunoglobulin. Sabin demonstrated in humans that the inoculation of dengue virus simultaneously with or shortly after the inoculation of yellow fever 17D vaccine delayed the onset of and ameliorated dengue illness.[143] Interference between yellow fever virus and an unrelated orbivirus was demonstrated in a mouse model.[144] Monkeys given yellow fever 17D vaccine and challenged with virulent virus 1 to 3 days later (before the appearance of antibodies) were partially protected.[145] These interference phenomena were not due to specific immunity and may have been mediated by interferon, NK cells, or other host resistance factors.

Peripheral blood mononuclear cells from yellow fever vaccinees demonstrated cytotoxicity against uninfected K562 cell targets, consistent with NK-cell activity.[146] In vitro replication of yellow fever is inhibited by type I interferons but is 250 times less sensitive than vesicular stomatitis virus and more than 500 times less sensitive than alphaviruses (P. Canonico, unpublished data). Nevertheless, monkeys treated with a potent inducer of interferon-α [poly(I)-poly(C)] developed modestly elevated serum interferon levels and were protected against lethal yellow fever infection.[146a] Vaccination of humans with 17D virus results in a serum interferon response (Fig. 34–6). During the early phase of infection with 17D virus, elevated levels of the interferon-dependent enzyme 2′,5′-oligoadenylate synthetase were found in T and B cells.[146b] Since interferon appears shortly after

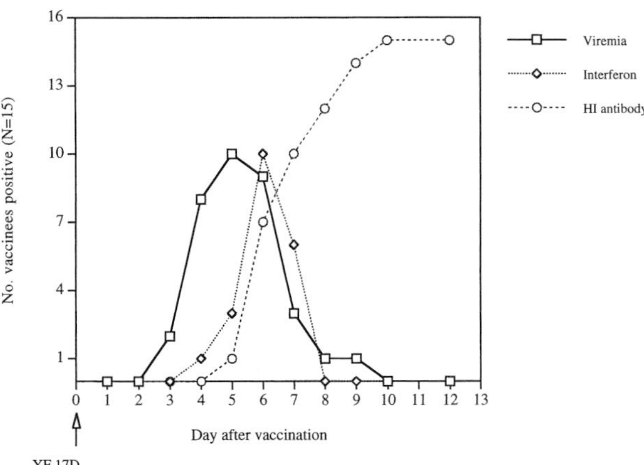

Figure 34–6. Circulating virus, interferon, and hemagglutination-inhibiting (HI) antibodies in adults given yellow fever 17D vaccine. (Modified from Wheelock EF, Sibley WA. Circulating virus, interferon and antibody after vaccination with the 17-D strain of yellow fever virus. N Engl J Med 273:194, 1965.)

viremia and interferon may be effective if given shortly after infection,[147] it could play a role in recovery from natural infection.

Interferon-γ activates nonspecific antiviral host defense mechanisms, including NK cells and macrophages. Interferon-γ enhances antiviral activity of type I interferons, upregulates major histocompatibility complex (MHC) class I and II, helper T cell type 1 (Th1)-dependent immunoglobulin synthesis, and cytotoxic T-cell activity. Dengue infection is characterized by activation of CD4+ T cells that secrete interferon-γ,[148, 149] and it is likely that interferon-γ exerts important immunoregulation in yellow fever. The administration of interferon-γ to monkeys inhibited yellow fever viremia and hepatic necrosis.[150]

Specific Immunity

Infection with yellow fever virus or vaccine is followed by a rapid specific immune response (see under *Immune Responses*). Neutralizing antibodies, cytolytic antibodies against viral proteins on the surface of infected cells, antibody-dependent cellular cytotoxicity (ADCC), and cytotoxic T cells are presumed to mediate the clearance of primary infection. However, there are few data on responses other than humoral immunity in yellow fever.

The humoral response to wild-type fever virus is characterized by the appearance of immunoglobulin M (IgM) antibodies during the first week of illness.[151–153] IgM levels peak during the second week after the onset of illness and decline rapidly over 30 to 60 days. The magnitude of the IgM response in cases of primary yellow fever infection is significantly greater than in patients with prior flavivirus exposure, in whom the ratio of IgM to IgG is low. Antibodies with biological activity (HI and neutralizing) appear rapidly, typically by the fifth day of illness.[15, 154, 155] However, HI and neutralizing antibody responses are not linked in all cases, reflecting different HI and neutralizing antigenic determinants on the viral envelope.[156] HI antibodies peak between 30 and 60 days after infection, and a significant decline in titer occurs during the succeeding 6 months. Neutralizing antibodies persist for many years, if not lifelong after natural yellow fever infection, and provide complete protection against disease on reexposure to the virus. Neutralizing antibodies have been documented as long as 78 years after illness.[157, 158] No documented case of a second clinical yellow fever infection has been reported. Complement-fixing (CF) antibodies appear during the second week after the onset of illness, rise during the convalescent period, and decline between 4 and 12 months after onset.

Antibody responses following primary yellow fever are specific for yellow fever antigen. With affinity maturation, specificity declines, and cross-reactions with related flaviviruses appear during the second week after the onset of illness.[154] Individuals with prior heterologous flavivirus immunity develop broadly cross-reactive antibody responses. The specificity of the immune response differs with the test used, the HI test being least specific, complement fixation being intermediate, and neutralization being most specific. The IgM antibody-capture enzyme-linked immunosorbent assay (ELISA) is specific in cases of primary infection, but cross-reactions develop over time and in cases with prior flavivirus experience. Because of the lower sensitivity of the indirect fluorescent antibody test, IgM antibodies were specific in patients with secondary infections.[153]

Cross-Protection

Previous infection with some flaviviruses may ameliorate the clinical severity of yellow fever. As early as 1923, dengue immunity was suggested as the basis for resistance to yellow fever in long-term residents of endemic areas[159–161] and was later proposed as a barrier to the introduction of yellow fever into Asia.[162–164] Early experiments indicated that the passive transfer of dengue antibodies does not protect monkeys against challenge with yellow fever virus.[159] In contrast, monkeys *actively* immunized with dengue were relatively resistant to challenge with yellow fever virus, suggesting that cellular immunity plays a role in cross-protection.[165] Monkeys actively immunized with two African flaviviruses (Zika and Wesselsbron), but not with West Nile or Banzi viruses, resisted challenge with yellow fever virus.[166] Humans with prior flavivirus immunity had a lower risk of severe disease during an epidemic than individuals with primary yellow fever.[93] Cross-protection is dependent on the virus causing the primary infection, the interval between the primary and the secondary infection, and quantitative and qualitative aspects of the heterologous immune response. The importance of prior flavivirus immunity in vaccination is considered under *Immune Responses.*

Protein and Epitope Specificity and Functionality of Antibody Responses to Yellow Fever

The E protein of yellow fever virus (and other flaviviruses) contains antigenic determinants responsible for neutralization and thus plays the principal role in protective immunity. This was demonstrated by active immunization of mice with recombinant vaccinia virus expressing the E protein[167] and by passive immunization of mice with anti-E monoclonal antibodies.[168, 169] Neutralizing epitopes are conformational (composed of discontinuous peptide sequences).[156] Yellow fever virus contains multiple neutralizing determinants, some of which are highly conserved across strains.[32, 33, 67] The composite polyclonal immune response is therefore capable of protecting against multiple strains of virus that may differ at one (or several) but not all epitopes. This antigenic structure underlies the efficacy of vaccination with a single yellow fever strain (17D) against all wild-type strains of yellow fever virus. Although vaccine and wild strains vary at other epitopes, and neutralizing titers in persons receiving 17D vaccine are higher against the homologous (vaccine virus) strain than against wild strains, antigenic conservation of neutralizing epitopes is sufficient to ensure vaccine efficacy.

Neutralization is presumed to occur both as an extracellular event (in which antibody bound to virus interferes with virion attachment to undefined cell receptors) and intracellularly. Intracellular neutralization is mediated by antibodies inhibiting acid-dependent fusion of virions to the endosomal membrane, thus preventing the release of viral RNA into the cytoplasm.[170] The importance of the Fc domain of neutralizing antibody was demonstrated by comparing the in vitro and in vivo activities of $F(ab')_2$ fragments of monoclonal antibodies.[171] $F(ab')_2$ fragments neutralized strongly in vitro but did not protect against yellow fever virus infection, whereas the full IgG molecule was protective. Presumably, the mediator of protection is complement or Fc-mediated ADCC, but alteration in reactivity of the hypervariable domain with antigenic determinants could also be involved.

Although the immune responses to nonstructural yellow fever proteins have not been elucidated in human infections, their role has been partially explored experimentally. The NS1 protein is present in the cytoplasm and on the surface of infected cells, is secreted from infected cells, and contains determinants that elicit CF antibodies. Monoclonal antibody analysis of NS1 revealed the presence of both type-specific and cross-reactive epitopes, which are principally conformation-dependent.[172] Mice and monkeys actively immunized with native or recombinant NS1 were protected against lethal yellow fever in the absence of neutralizing antibody,[173–175] the principal correlate of protection being complement-mediated cytolytic antibodies. Passive transfer of monoclonal antibodies against NS1 having high CF activity, but not antibodies with low or no CF activity, afforded protection.[176] These studies suggested that antibodies recognizing cell membrane–bound NS1 may promote viral clearance by sensitizing infected cells to complement-mediated cytolysis. An intact Fc portion of the immunoglobulin molecule is required for protection by anti-NS1,[171, 177] and antibody isotype-dependent differences in protective activities have been demonstrated.[34, 176] The mechanism of protection by anti-NS1 and the role of Fc receptor–dependent effector functions, including complement-fixation, remain uncertain. Natural infection with yellow fever virus is associated with the presence of soluble CF antigen (NS1) in blood during the acute phase of infection[115] and is followed by strong CF-antibody responses (presumably directed against NS1). However, because CF-antibody responses occur late after infection, and vaccination with 17D virus does not induce a CF-antibody response,[178, 179] it is uncertain to what extent anti-NS1 plays a role in vivo in recovery or protection. Further studies in humans are needed to define the kinetics of the anti-NS1 response after natural infection and artificial immunization. There are no data on antibody responses to other nonstructural proteins of yellow fever.

Antibody-Dependent Enhancement

Antibody-dependent enhancement of flavivirus replication in monocyte-macrophages has been demonstrated in vitro for a number of flaviviruses, including yellow fever. Schlesinger and Brandriss demonstrated enhanced growth of yellow fever virus in U-937 cells in the presence of serum IgG from human subjects previously immunized with 17D vaccine.[180, 181] Monoclonal antibodies with yellow fever type-specific or flavivirus group reactivity also enhanced yellow fever infection in murine macrophage (P388D1) cells. Enhancement is typically mediated by nonneutralizing antibody-virus complexes that attach to cells via Fcγ type I or II receptors or complement receptors and increase viral internalization.[182–184] However, enhancement in macrophage-like cells occurred in the presence of neutralizing antibody, suggesting that cells bearing Fcγ receptors may facilitate infection after inoculation of yellow fever virus into an immune host, whereas other cells bearing other viral receptors are protected.[181] Active replication of immune complexes may explain the observation that persons re-immunized with 17D vaccine develop increases in levels of serum antibodies.[185]

Immune enhancement is believed to play a role in the pathogenesis of dengue hemorrhagic fever in patients with nonneutralizing antibodies from a previous dengue infection who are infected with a new dengue serotype. The evidence for in vivo enhancement mediated by yellow fever antibodies is mixed. In one study, human volunteers previously immunized with yellow fever 17D had increased immune responses to live dengue-2 vaccine, possibly due to antibody-mediated enhancement of dengue virus replication[186, 187] or to rapid expansion of group-reactive memory T- and B-cell clones. There is no evidence, however, that yellow fever vaccination increases the risk of dengue hemorrhagic fever. Nor does prior heterologous flavivirus infection appear to enhance yellow fever infection, since prior Japanese encephalitis immunity did not increase viremia following yellow fever 17D vaccination.[104]

Cellular Immunity

Little is known about the cellular responses to yellow fever, and inferences are therefore drawn from studies on other flaviviruses, particularly dengue. CTLs mediate killing of flavivirus-infected cells and are the principal effector mechanism of viral clearance during recovery from infection. They may also contribute to protection against subsequent infection or cross-protection against heterologous flaviviruses. Human dengue virus infection is associated with the appearance of activated peripheral blood mononuclear cells that proliferate on stimulation with dengue antigens. MHC class II–restricted $CD4^+CD8^-$ T-cell clones, as well as class I–restricted $CD4^-CD8^+$ T-cell clones from dengue-immune donors lyse infected cells.[75, 188, 189] The majority of the T-cell clones studied target epitopes in nonstructural proteins, particularly NS3, and demonstrate both type specificity and various patterns of cross-reactivity. $CD8^+$ T-cell–reactive epitopes in the prM, E, NS3, and NS1-2A proteins have also been identified.[74, 190] Both MHC class I- and class II–restricted responses have also been described in mice to flaviviruses in the Japanese encephalitis virus complex. In persons with prior flavivirus experience, memory T helper and B cells reactive to specific and cross-reactive antigenic determinants contribute to the rapid anamnestic antibody response.

Diagnosis

The isolated case of yellow fever obviously presents a more difficult diagnostic challenge than a cluster of similar cases. The pathognomonic picture of bi- or triphasic acute illness; conjunctival injection; the characteristic appearance of the tongue; jaundice; relative bradycardia; leukopenia; albuminuria; oliguria; and black vomit in an unvaccinated patient with a history of residence in or recent travel to a yellow fever endemic zone presents little difficulty in clinical differentiation, but in many patients, this full array of clinical signs is not present.

Leptospirosis (Weil disease) and louse-borne relapsing fever (*Borrelia recurrentis*), characterized by jaundice, hemorrhage, disseminated intravascular coagulation, and a high case-fatality rate, closely resemble yellow fever.[97, 191] Other diseases that must be differentiated clinically from yellow fever include viral hepatitis (especially hepatitis E in pregnancy and delta hepatitis), Q fever, West Nile virus hepatitis, Rift Valley fever, typhoid, and malaria. Malaria (blackwater fever) is usually distinguishable by the absence of proteinuria. Dengue hemorrhagic fever; Lassa, Marburg, and Ebola virus diseases; Bolivian and Argentine hemorrhagic fevers; and Congo-Crimean hemorrhagic fever are not usually associated with jaundice but may cause diagnostic confusion. Mild yellow fever may resemble many other arboviral infections and influenza characterized by fever, headache, malaise, and myalgias.

Specific laboratory diagnosis is made by the detection of virus or viral antigen in blood or by serologic examination. Virus is readily isolated from blood during the first 4 days after the onset of illness, but isolations as late as 12 days or longer are recorded.[192] Of 90 cases confirmed during a yellow fever outbreak in Ivory Coast in 1982, 27 (30%) were diagnosed by viral isolation from blood; all but two virus-positive patients were in the preicteric stage.[193] The virus may also be recovered from postmortem liver tissue.

Viral isolation is accomplished by intracerebral inoculation of suckling mice, intrathoracic inoculation of *Toxorhynchites* mosquitoes, or inoculation of cell cultures. Suckling mice develop encephalitis 7 to 14 days after inoculation; a virus-specific diagnosis may be made by immunofluorescence on impression slides of brain tissue or by serologic methods. Viral antigen is detected by immunofluorescence in head-squash preparations of inoculated mosquitoes after an incubation period of 10 to 12 days. *A. pseudoscutellaris* (AP61) cells are more sensitive than other in vitro methods for primary isolation of yellow fever virus[194, 195] and show cytopathic effects within 5 to 7 days after inoculation. Viral antigen is detectable by immunofluorescence in advance of cytopathic effects (e.g., day 3 after inoculation). *A. albopictus* (C6/36) cells, *Toxorhynchites amboinensis* cells, and mammalian cells (e.g., Vero, SW13) may be used, particularly if combined with polymerase chain reaction (PCR) or detection of viral antigen. PCR employing primers spanning a conserved region of the E gene and a digoxigenin-labeled probe detected 10 plaque-forming units (PFU) in cell cultures infected with most, but not all, strains of yellow fever virus.[196] PCR has been used to detect viral genome in clinical samples that were negative by viral isolation.[197] The method requires further field testing but will undoubtedly be useful for the rapid identification of virus in original samples or early after inoculation of AP61 cells.

Rapid, early diagnosis is possible by the measurement of yellow fever antigen in serum by immunoassay.[195, 198, 199] Antigen in serum is captured by a yellow fever type-specific monoclonal antibody affixed to the solid phase and detected by group-reactive monoclonal antibody conjugated to alkaline phosphatase. The sensitivity of the assay for the detection of virus in serum is approximately 3 $\log_{10}$ PFU per 0.1 mL. Under field conditions, antigen detection ELISA had a sensitivity of 69% and a specificity of 100% compared with viral isolation in AP61 cell culture.[195] Samples for PCR and ELISA do not need to be handled in a way that preserves infectivity; specimens may also be intentionally inactivated as a safety precaution when the diagnosis of dangerous pathogens (e.g., other viral hemorrhagic fevers) is considered.

Examination of liver reveals the typical pathoanatomical features of yellow fever, including midzonal necrosis. Liver biopsy during the illness should *never* be performed, as fatal hemorrhage may ensue. Histopathological diagnosis may be difficult in patients who die after the second week of illness. Electron microscopy may reveal typical flavivirus particles in intracellular vacuoles.[200] Definitive postmortem diagnosis may be made by immunocytochemical staining for yellow fever antigen in liver, heart, or kidney even in specimens stored for years at ambient temperature.[121, 123, 201] The distribution of virus in the liver is midzonal, suggesting that hepatocytes bordering the central veins and portal tracts undergo less active viral replication. Viral genome may also be detected by RNA-RNA hybridization,[121] and it may be possible to utilize PCR techniques to obtain yellow fever sequences from historical materials for epidemiological and evolutionary studies.

Although older serological methods for diagnosis (HI, CF, indirect immunofluorescence, and neutralization tests) are useful,[153–155] they have been replaced by the IgM-capture ELISA. The presence of IgM antibodies in a single sample provides a presumptive diagnosis, and confirmation is made by a rise in titer between paired acute and convalescent samples or fall between early and late convalescent samples. The specificity of the IgM ELISA is high in primary infections, and in many cases of secondary infection.[152] However, cross-reactions complicate the diagnosis of yellow fever by all serological methods, particularly in Africa where multiple flaviviruses cocirculate. The phenomenon of "original antigenic sin" complicates flavivirus serological investigations. Individuals with prior heterologous infection who develop yellow fever may have higher responses to the original virus, and those with prior yellow fever infection or vaccination subsequently infected with another flavivirus may have higher responses to yellow fever virus.[202]

Treatment

The management of patients with yellow fever has not been optimized, because the disease occurs in remote areas with rudimentary medical services. An expert panel recommended supportive care including maintenance of nutrition and prevention of hypoglycemia; nasogastric suction to prevent gastric distension and aspiration; treatment of hypotension by fluid replacement and, if necessary, vasoactive drugs; administration of oxygen; correction of metabolic acidosis; treatment of bleeding with fresh-frozen plasma; dialysis if indicated by renal failure; and treatment of secondary infections with antibiotics.[79] The use of heparin to reverse disseminated intravascular coagulation is reserved for cases with documented consumption of clotting factors and activation of fibrinolytic mechanisms.

Antiserum to yellow fever produced in horses, monkeys, or chimpanzees protected rhesus monkeys against lethal yellow fever when given 1 to 3 days after challenge.[203, 204] In contrast, treatment by the administration of immune serum or by cross-circulation from an immune donor animal after the clinical onset of yellow fever had no therapeutic effect.[205] Newer treatments aimed at supporting the patient through the phase of acute liver injury have not been tested clinically or experimentally in yellow fever, for example, inhibitors of mitochondrial membrane permeability transition (L-carnitine), or inhibitors of Ca^{2+}-dependent proteases and phospholipases. Inhibitors or antibodies against TNF-α or other cytokines have not been investigated. A role for endotoxin in shock and liver injury in yellow fever was suggested, based on the global damage to the reticuloendothelial system and the presence of lesions in the Peyer patches of experimentally infected monkeys.[116] Therapeutic interventions based on this hypothesis have not been investigated.

Interferons have been investigated for the prevention and treatment of yellow fever in monkeys. Animals receiving 3.0 mg per kg of the interferon inducer poly(I)-poly(C) intravenously 8 hours before or 8 hours after challenge had low viremias and were significantly protected (71–75% survival) compared with untreated controls (0% survival), but those treated 24 hours after challenge were not protected.[146a] Interferon-γ administered to monkeys 24 hours in advance of challenge and at daily intervals for 4 days reduced yellow fever viremia and significantly delayed hepatic dysfunction and death.[150] The requirement to administer interferons before infection or during the incubation period precludes their clinical use. In an individual with known exposure (for example in the case of an unimmunized laboratory worker with accidental infection), early postexposure prophylaxis with interferon alfa, preferably with immune plasma, would be indicated.

Antiviral activity against yellow fever has been demonstrated in vivo for a number of nucleosides and plant-derived alkaloids.[79, 206, 207] Ribavirin is active against yellow fever virus in vitro, but at concentrations that are too high (9–10 mg/mL) for safe and effective treatment in vivo. Monkeys treated with ribavirin were not significantly protected against yellow fever challenge (G. Tignor, unpublished, 1990), but the dose and formulation may not have been optimized. Synergistic effects of ribavirin and related compounds, such as tiazofurin and selenazole, have been demonstrated in vitro but not investigated in vivo. A number of other nucleosides, including analogues of 6-azauridine, as well as natural plant alkaloids, have shown in vitro activity, but have not been tested in animals.[79]

EPIDEMIOLOGY[1]

Geographic Distribution

Yellow fever occurs in tropical South America and sub-Saharan Africa, where the enzootic transmission cycle involves tree-hole–breeding mosquitoes and nonhuman primates. A detailed comprehension of the geography of yellow fever activity is critical to the proper utilization of yellow fever vaccine, in terms of both public health policy and the protection of persons at risk of exposure during international travel. Yellow fever is one of three quarantinable diseases subject to International Health Regulations (others are plague and cholera).

The first map of endemic regions—based on yellow fever immunity surveys conducted 50 to 60 years ago[208, 209]—was prepared by the International Quarantine Commission and published by the United Nations Relief and Rehabilitation Administration (UNRRA) in 1946. This map has been modified from time to time based on new information[26, 210, 211] (the present version is shown in Fig. 34–7) but is still not an accurate reflection of yellow fever activity. The surveys on which it is based are out of date, and some areas are included based on

[1]More extensive reviews of yellow fever epidemiology and ecology may be found in references 112, 259, and 260 through 263.

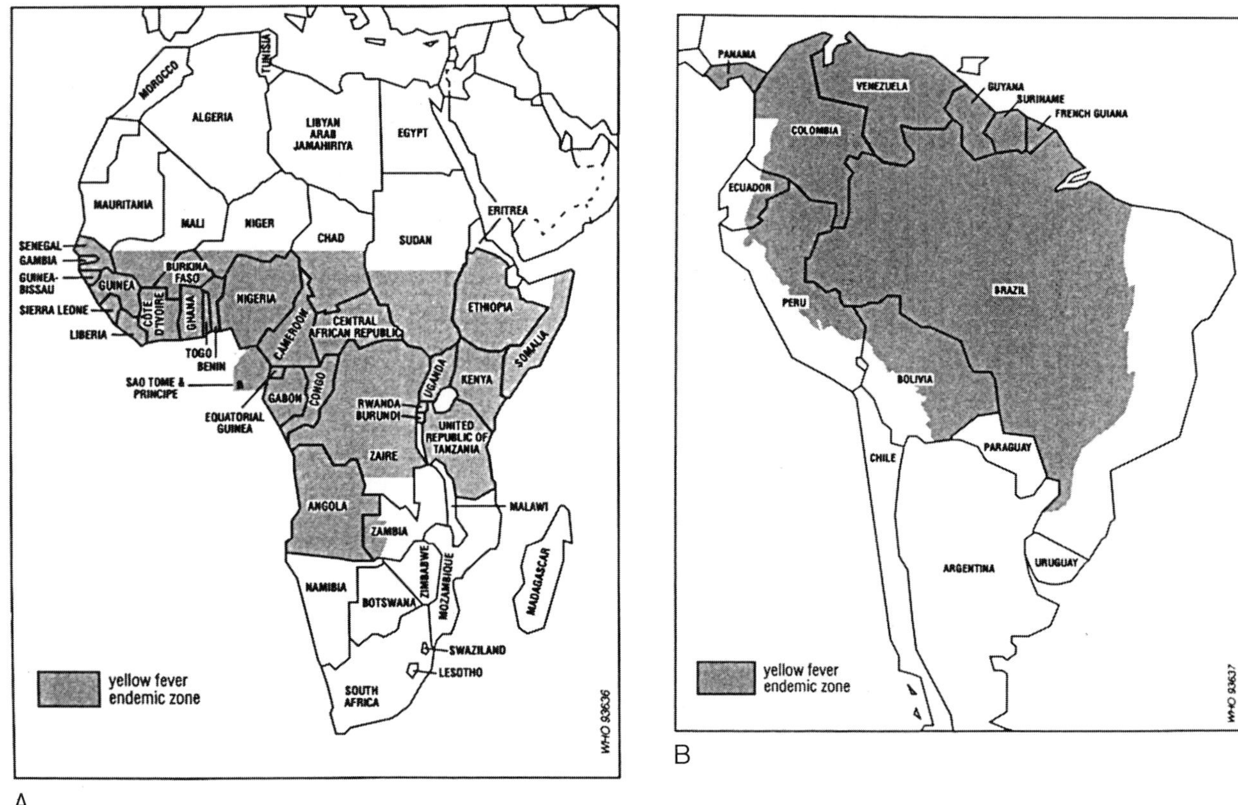

Figure 34–7. Regions (shaded) of Africa *(A)* and South America *(B)* considered endemic for yellow fever. (From World Health Organization. International Travel and Health Vaccination Requirements and Health Advice. Geneva, WHO, 1997.)

scanty serological data without there ever having been a notified human case (e.g., Somalia, Tanzania). The artificial nature of the maps is emphasized by the demarcation along entire national borders and latitude lines.

Current yellow fever activity is published in the World Health Organization (WHO) *Weekly Epidemiological Record (WER)*, and by the Centers for Disease Control and Prevention (CDC), Division of Quarantine. Annual or biannual summaries of morbidity and epidemiological trends are also published in the *WER.*[212–215] Current information can also be found in CDC's home page on the Internet (http://www.cdc.gov/travel/travel.html). Although these materials have limitations, they provide a picture of current "hot spots" of yellow fever activity. The user should keep in mind that endemic (and even epidemic) yellow fever occurs in areas that are silent with respect to official reports.

Most countries in receptive areas (in which yellow fever does not exist but where the presence of the domiciliary vector, *A. aegypti,* would permit its development if introduced) require a valid yellow fever immunization certificate for entry from a yellow fever–endemic region. A 1997 listing of receptive countries that require a valid certificate is provided in references 210 and 211 and Table 34–4.

Areas at highest risk for the introduction and secondary spread by *A. aegypti* are in the Americas and include coastal regions of Brazil, Peru, and Ecuador, western Panama, Central America, the West Indies, Mexico, and the southern United States—areas historically affected by yellow fever in the past. Trinidad, Central America, and Mexico also have the capacity to sustain enzootic and epizootic transmission (jungle yellow fever). Between 1948 and 1954, the virus swept northward from Panama to Mexico in this fashion, causing multiple human outbreaks.[216] Jungle yellow fever has intermittently appeared on the island of Trinidad (e.g., 1954, 1959, 1978) with long-silent interepidemic periods.[217]

A. aegypti–infested regions of southern Europe, the Middle East, Asia, Australia, and Oceania are also at risk of introduction of yellow fever. The virus has never been recorded in India or other parts of Asia. The possible reasons for its absence include both demographic and biological factors.[164] The most likely mode of introduction of yellow fever from endemic areas to Asia is by air travel of viremic humans, and all receptive areas can be reached by air from an endemic region within less than the incubation period of yellow fever.[218] However, yellow fever occurs in remote areas and affects individuals engaged in subsistence farming, who are infrequent international travelers. Biological factors that limit the risk of introduction include cross-protection, principally by dengue, against which nearly all persons residing in Asia are immune (see under *Cross-Protection*). A third hypothesis is that *A. aegypti* strains in Asia have low vector competence for yellow fever virus.[219, 220]

Geographic Variation in Viral Strains

Three (possibly four) distinct genotypes have been found by sequencing wild-type yellow fever virus strains

Table 34–4. **COUNTRIES REQUIRING VALID CERTIFICATE OF YELLOW FEVER VACCINATION (COUNTRIES NOT LISTED HAVE NO REQUIREMENTS FOR IMMUNIZATION)**

COUNTRY	REQUIREMENT	COUNTRY	REQUIREMENT
Afghanistan	A	Malawi	A
Albania	B	Malaysia	B
Algeria	B	Maldives	A
American Samoa	B	Mali	E
Angola	B	Malta	D
Antigua and Barbuda	B	Martinique	B
Australia	C	Mauritania	J
Bahamas	B	Mauritius	B
Bangladesh	A*	Mexico	G
Barbados	B	Mozambique	B
Belize	A	Myanmar	B
Benin	E	Namibia	B*
Bhutan	B	Nauru	B
Bolivia	A, F*	Nepal	A
Brazil	D*	Netherlands Antilles	G
Brunei	C	New Caledonia	B
Burkina Faso	B	Nicaragua	B
Burundi	B	Niger	E
Cambodia	A	Nigeria	B
Cameroon	B	Niue	B
Cape Verde	B*	Oman	A
Chad	E	Pakistan	G*
China	A	Panama	F*
Colombia	F*	Papua New Guinea	B
Congo	E	Paraguay	A*
Djibouti	B	Peru	G, F*
Dominica	B	Philippines	C
Ecuador	B	Pitcairn	B
Egypt	B*	Portugal (Azores and Madeira only)	B
El Salvador	G	Reunion	B
Equatorial Guinea	A	Rwanda	E
Eritrea	A	Saint Helena	B
Ethiopia	B	St. Kitts and Nevis	B
Fiji	B	Saint Lucia	B
French Guiana	E	St. Vincent and the Grenadines	B
French Polynesia	B	Samoa	B
Gabon	E	Sao Tome and Principe	B
Gambia	B	Saudi Arabia	A
Ghana	H	Senegal	A
Greece	G	Seychelles	C
Grenada	B	Sierra Leone	A
Guadeloupe	B	Singapore	C
Guatemala	B	Solomon Islands	A
Guinea	B	Somalia	A
Guinea-Bissau	B*	South Africa	B
Guyana	A*	Sri Lanka	B
Haiti	A	Sudan	B
Honduras	A	Suriname	A
India	I*	Swaziland	A
Indonesia	A	Syrian Arab Republic	A
Iraq	A	Tanzania	B
Ivory Coast	E	Thailand	B
Jamaica	B	Togo	E
Jordan	B	Tonga	B
Kazakhstan	A	Trinidad and Tobago	B
Kenya	B	Tunisia	B
Kiribati	B	Turkmenistan	A
Lao People's Democratic Republic	A	Uganda	B
Lebanon	A	Vietnam	B
Lesotho	A	Yemen	B
Liberia	E	Zaire	B
Libya	B	Zimbabwe	A
Madagascar	I		

*See World Health Organization[211] for additional details regarding requirements from this country.

A, travelers entering country from infected area; B, travelers >1 yr of age entering country from infected area; C, travelers 1 yr of age entering within 6 d of travel (see World Health Organization[211] for details) in infected country; D, travelers >9 mo of age entering country from infected area; E, travelers >1 yr of age entering country; F, travelers going to specified sections of country; G, travelers >6 mo of age entering country from infected area; H, all travelers entering country; I, travelers who have been in or been in transit in infected country; J, as E except travelers arriving from noninfected country and staying <2 wk.

Modified from World Health Organization. International Travel and Health. Vaccination Requirements and Health Advice. Geneva, World Health Organization, 1997.

of different geographic origin. The database includes the entire genome sequences of the Asibi[40] and French viscerotropic[41] viruses (Ghana and Senegal, 1927) and partial sequences of the E gene, the 5′ and 3′ termini, and the NS4a-NS4b region of multiple isolates from South America and Africa isolated over a 60-year period.[46, 136, 221–223] These studies support the concept that yellow fever virus arose in Africa, with divergence of western and eastern African genotypes before the introduction of the virus into the Americas. The yellow fever virus genome has been highly conserved, presumably because of restrictions imposed by the host range. Yellow fever strains in Africa fall into only two genotypes, one represented by western African viruses[223a] and the other by central and eastern African strains. South American viruses fall into one major phylogenetic group with respect to the E gene sequence, but two genotypes are separable when the NS4a-NS4b and 3′ noncoding regions are compared.[222] In contrast to the situation in Africa, the two South American genotypes do not segregate into discrete geographic distributions, but one genotype has not been recovered since 1974, suggesting that this virus may have been lost. The relatively high genetic stability of yellow fever viruses compared with many other RNA viruses is critical to the effectiveness of a single viral strain (17D) as a vaccine.

By cross-absorption with polyclonal antisera, African and New World yellow fever viruses can be serologically distinguished.[224] Slight differences were discerned between eastern and western African strains.[225] Wild-type strains vary with respect to reactivities with monoclonal antibodies[67] but have not been classified to geographic origin or genotype.[141]

Incidence

Endemic or Epidemic Areas

For reviews of yellow fever epidemic activity in the interval from 1950 to 1990 and 1985 to 1994 see Monath[226] and Robertson and colleagues,[26] respectively. During the last decade (1986–1995), 23,543 cases and 6421 deaths were reported to WHO—a dramatic increase compared with previous reporting intervals. In Africa, which accounted for 21,541 cases (91%), the annual incidence varied between approximately 200 and 5000 cases (Figs. 34–8 and 34–9). The case-fatality rate of yellow fever in Africa based on official reports between 1986 and 1995 is 24%. The frequency and intensity of epidemics in Africa are due to interhuman transmission by mosquito vectors present in high-density, high-human populations, and low immunization coverage. In South America, yellow fever occurs in the Amazon region and contiguous areas. Between 1986 and 1995, 2002 cases and 1302 deaths were reported to WHO (mean, 202 cases; range 88–515 cases/year) (Figs. 34–8 and 34–9). The annual incidence varies by country due to fluctuating epizootic activity. The lower incidence of yellow fever in South America than in Africa is due to transmission by enzootic vectors (principally from monkey to human); low densities of vectors, monkeys, and human hosts; and relatively high vaccination coverage. The higher case-fatality rate (65%) in South America probably reflects surveillance based on death reports and the postmortem examination of livers, although it remains possible that the South American genotype(s) are more virulent than those in Africa.[141]

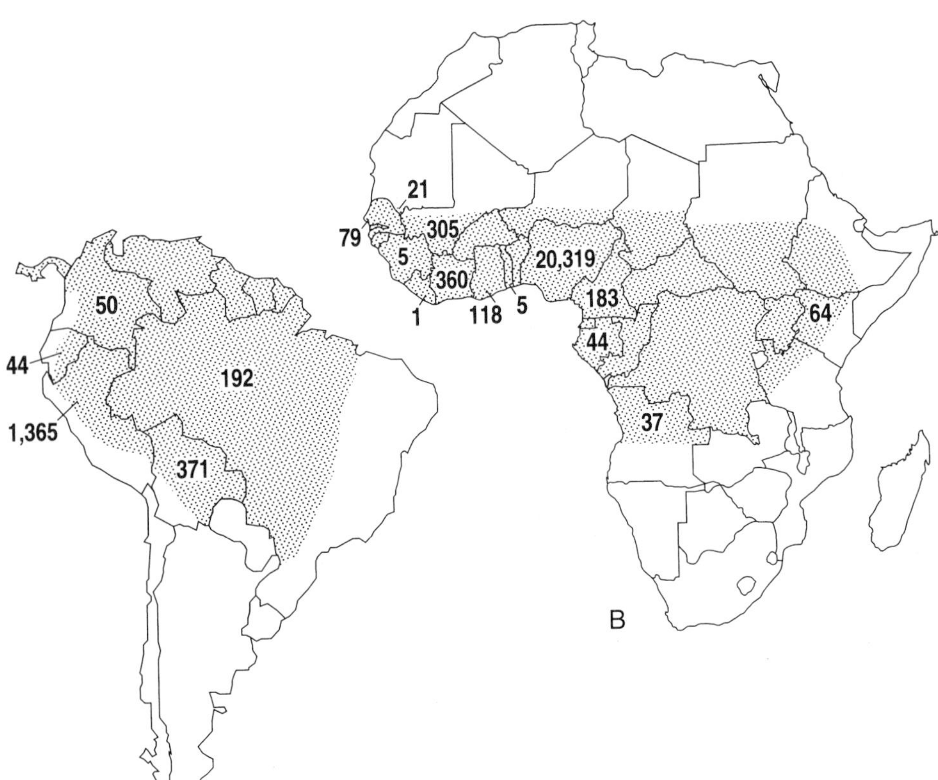

Figure 34–8. Number of yellow fever cases reported to the World Health Organization in South America *(A)* and Africa *(B)*, 1986 to 1995. Regions endemic for yellow fever are shaded. (From Monath TP. Epidemiology of yellow fever: current status and speculations on future trends. In Saluzzo J-F, Dudet B [eds]. Factors in the Emergence of Arbovirus Disease. Paris, Elsevier, 1997, pp 143–156. Data from Robertson SE, Hull BP, Tomori O, et al. Yellow fever. A decade of reemergence. JAMA 276:1157, 1996; and World Health Organization. Yellow fever in 1994 and 1995. Wkly Epidemiol Rec 71:313, 1996.)

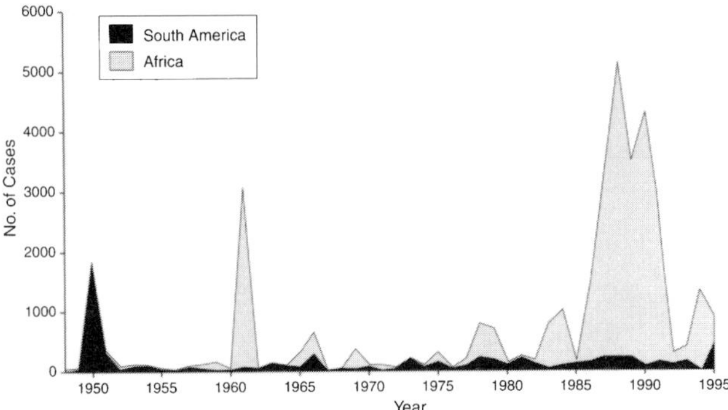

Figure 34–9. Annual incidence of yellow fever cases notified to the World Health Organization, 1950 to 1995. (From Robertson SE, Hull BP, Tomori O, et al. Yellow fever. A decade of reemergence. JAMA 276:1157, 1996.)

The recent resurgence of yellow fever is due to a series of epidemics in western Africa, particularly in Nigeria.[94, 227] Smaller outbreaks have also occurred in Cameroon (1990), Ghana (1993–1994), Liberia (1995), Gabon (1994), Senegal (1995), and Benin (1996). In 1992, an epidemic was recognized in Kenya for the first time in 26 years.[214, 228, 229] In South America, Peru experienced an increased number of cases in the late 1980s and in 1995, reflecting the relatively low vaccine coverage in that country (between 30 and 50% of the at-risk population[230]), and migrations of nonimmunized laborers into forested regions. In 1995, the number of jungle yellow fever cases in Peru (492 cases, 192 deaths[215]) was the highest on record for any country in South America since 1927 (the earliest year for which statistics are available). Closer inspection of the fluctuations of yellow fever activity by country reveals only partial synchrony, indicating that epizootic waves occur as localized events (Fig. 34–10). Increased viral transmission occurs with a periodicity of 7 to 10 years, in part because immunologically susceptible monkey populations are replenished at a slow rate after epizootics.

Only a small proportion of cases are reported, owing to occurrence of the disease in remote areas, late recognition of outbreaks, and lack of diagnostic facilities. Where specific investigations have been undertaken, the ratio of cases to official notifications varies between 3 and 280:1. In recent epidemics, case-finding and census data were used to estimate attack rates (Table 34–5). The incidence of disease in The Gambia (1978–1979) was 44 per 1000 population, the mortality rate 8 per 1000, and the case-fatality rate 19.4%.[93] In Nigeria (1986), the incidence was 49 per 1000, mortality 28 per 1000, and the case-fatality rate 47%; of 200,000 residents in the affected region (Oju Local Government Area), 38,000 persons were infected, 10,000 developed jaundice, and 4700 died.[227] Based on serologic investigations, remarkably similar incidences of yellow fever infection were found in African outbreaks: 35% in Ethiopia (1960–1962),[231] 44% in Senegal (1965),[232] 33% in The Gambia (1978–1979),[93] 29% in Ivory Coast (1982),[233] 31% in Burkina Faso (1983),[234] 19% in Nigeria Oju region, 1986),[227] 21% in Nigeria (Oyo State, 1987),[94] 20% in Cameroon (1990),[235] and 20% in Nigeria (Imo State, 1994).[197]

These serological data provide a basis for estimating the ratio of infection to illness (Table 34–6); in two western African outbreaks, the infection-to-illness ratio was 3.8 to 7.4:1. Since illness was defined by a case definition that included jaundice, the ratio would be lower if mild cases were included. In an epidemic of jungle yellow fever in Brazil, serological evidence for recent infection was found more often in persons with a history of febrile illness than in those without fever (odds ratio 4.5; 95% confidence interval 2.3–8.5).

The evidence that prior heterologous flavivirus infection modified the incidence of yellow fever is conflicting. In The Gambia (1978–1979), the infection-to-illness (jaundice) ratio was higher in persons with prior flavivirus exposure.[93] However, in Nigeria (Oju region, 1986), jaundice rates were not significantly different for patients with primary yellow fever infection (14/84, 17%) and superinfections (13/53, 25%) (odds ratio 0.62, 95% confidence interval 0.24–1.56) (K. M. DeCock, T. P. Monath, unpublished data, 1987). The discrepancy could reflect differences in the specific heterologous flaviviruses responsible for prior immunity.

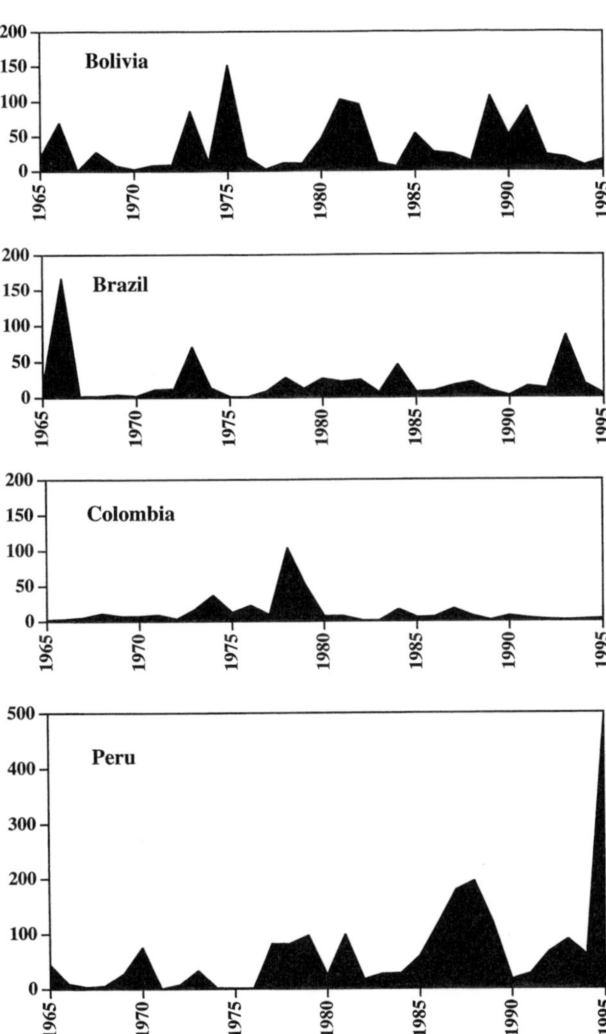

Figure 34–10. Incidence of yellow fever in selected countries in South America, 1965 to 1995. Years of high incidence are not generally synchronous, indicating that epizootic activity occurs in discontinuous regions of the continent.

Table 34–5. **EPIDEMIC YELLOW FEVER IN AFRICA (A PARTIAL LISTING), SHOWING OFFICIALLY NOTIFIED CASES AND ESTIMATED ACTUAL NUMBER OF CASES BASED ON EPIDEMIOLOGICAL INVESTIGATION**

COUNTRY	EPIDEMIC YEAR	OFFICIAL NOTIFICATION	ESTIMATED BY DIRECT INVESTIGATIONS	RATIO ACTUAL:REPORTED	REFERENCE
Ethiopia	1960–1962	3010	100,000	33:1	231
Senegal	1965	243	2000–20,000	8–82:1	232
West Africa	1969	322	>100,000	311:1	473
Nigeria	1970	4	786	197:1	474
Ghana	1977–1978	713	2400	3:1	475
Gambia	1978–1979	30	8400	280:1	93
Mali	1987	305	1500	5:1	476
Nigeria	1986	1289	9100	7:1	227
Nigeria	1987	2676	120,000	45:1	94
Cameroon	1990	173	5000–20,000	29–116:1	212

The burden of yellow fever in Africa has been estimated almost entirely in terms of epidemic disease, and only limited attempts have been made to define the incidence of *endemic* yellow fever infection. In Nigeria (1970–1971), a laboratory diagnosis of yellow fever was made in 2 (1%) of 205 patients hospitalized with jaundice in areas without epidemic activity.[236] With the use of data from serological surveys in Nigeria and an estimated 7:1 infection-to-illness ratio, the annual incidence of overt infection with jaundice was estimated to be between 1.1 and 2.4 per 1000 population and yellow fever deaths between 0.2 and 0.5 per 1000.[237] Although indicating that endemic yellow fever may be a "silent" cause of significant morbidity, the incidence levels are 25- to 50-fold lower than those occurring during epidemics and are thus below the threshold of detection by existing passive surveillance systems. It is likely that endemic yellow fever activity varies considerably from year to year but that it causes thousands of unrecorded deaths annually in western Africa. This provides a strong rationale for preventive immunization.

Expatriate Residents, Travelers, and Military Personnel

In the prevaccine era, yellow fever was a major threat to expatriates living in and travelers to tropical America and Africa, including U.S. military stationed overseas. Fourteen cases occurred in Navy personnel in Honduras and Nicaragua in 1919,[238] and a suspect case was reported in Brazil in 1929.[239] A single case (acquired in Fernando Po in 1938) was found among 2300 seamen of the Polish merchant fleet serving in the tropics.[240] Such cases became rare during World War II, after vaccination came into general use. A few cases among Europeans were reported during[97] and after[241] the 1941 outbreak in the Sudan, and among British forces in western Africa in 1942.[242] In 1952, a fatal case of yellow fever occurred in a previously vaccinated European working in Uganda.[243] In 1979, two fatal cases occurred in unvaccinated French tourists who visited an area of Senegal bordering The Gambia.[244–246] These infections

Table 34–6. **AGE- AND SEX-SPECIFIC ATTACK RATES AND INFECTION-TO-ILLNESS RATIOS IN YELLOW FEVER EPIDEMICS IN THE GAMBIA AND NIGERIA**

LOCATION	AGE (YR)	ATTACK RATE/1000 POPULATION		INFECTION RATE PER 1000 POPULATION		INFECTION-ILLNESS RATIO	
		Males	Females	Males	Females	Males	Females
I. The Gambia (1978–1979)*							
	0–9	70	63	528	333	7.5	5.3
	10–19	56	43	395	387	7.1	9.0
	20–29	39	27	441	238	11.3	8.8
	30–39	49	19	105	394	2.1	20.7
	40+	6	31	231	170	38.5	5.5
	Subtotal	47	41	359	295	7.6	7.2
	All ages, both genders	44		326		7.4	
II. Nigeria (Oju region, 1986)†							
	0–9	62	0	147	238	2.4	—
	10–19	37	93	197	234	5.3	2.5
	20–29	113	44	184	263	1.6	6.0
	30–39	83	19	194	140	2.3	7.4
	40+	33	39	114	156	3.5	4.0
	Subtotal	62	35	166	211	2.7	6.0
	All ages, both genders	49		187		3.8	

*Infection incidence based on complement fixation test.
†Infection incidence based on IgM enzyme-linked immunosorbent assay.
Part I from Monath TP, Craven RB, Adjukiewicz, et al. Yellow fever in The Gambia, 1978–1979: Epidemiologic aspects with observations on the occurrence of Orungo virus infections. Am J Trop Med Hyg 29:912, 1980. Part II from K. M. DeCock, T. P. Monath, unpublished data.

were acquired 1 year after a major outbreak in a region where the resident population had a high background of vaccine immunity. The French tourists returned to France during the early phase of illness and died in a hospital in Paris. In 1979, a nonfatal case also occurred in a European resident of Dakar who visited the Gambian border,[245] and in 1981, an unvaccinated Lebanese resident in Senegal died of yellow fever after visiting a camp near The Gambia.[247] In 1985, a nonfatal case of yellow fever occurred in the Netherlands in a female traveler to The Gambia, Senegal, and Guinea-Bissau.[248] In 1988, a vaccinated Spanish woman acquired yellow fever during travels through Mali, Burkina Faso, Niger, and Mauritania,[249] 1 year after a widespread increase in yellow fever activity in western Africa. In 1996, two fatal cases occurred in unvaccinated American[250] and Swiss[251] tourists who had visited jungle areas near Manaus, Brazil, and returned home during the early phase of illness or during the incubation period, respectively. These cases occurred during a period of increased yellow fever activity in the Amazon basin.

Cases Imported into Receptive Areas

Because the southern United States is infested with *A. aegypti,* importation of yellow fever has long been considered a significant threat.[252, 253] The last outbreak resulting from the introduction of the virus occurred in New Orleans in 1905. Between 1906 and 1996, 27 yellow fever cases (exclusive of laboratory infections) were reported in the United States, 23 of which were intercepted on ships arriving at Public Health Service Quarantine facilities.[253] The last imported case in the prevaccine era occurred in a Mexican immigrant who died in Texas in 1924. In 1996, an unvaccinated American acquired a fatal case of yellow fever during a visit to Brazil.[250]

Within countries affected by yellow fever, the disease may be acquired by unvaccinated residents who travel from an uninfected area to a region of endemic activity.[254] This is a recurring theme in South America, where unvaccinated migrant workers move from a coastal area or the Andean highlands into the Amazon region. In Africa, similar episodes undoubtedly are common but have been recorded infrequently and exclusively in expatriate residents, as noted previously.

The risk of acquiring yellow fever during travel is related to the level of viral transmission at the time and location of the visit. Exposure in an area undergoing an outbreak, even for a short period of time, may be associated with a high risk of infection. In recent outbreaks in western Africa, up to 30% of native populations have acquired the infection during a period of 2 to 3 months. Although nearly all recent episodes of yellow fever among unvaccinated travelers have occurred in conjunction with increases in yellow fever activity, information about increased risk was often not readily available at the time. Increased yellow fever activity in a region often spans 2 or more years and affects contiguous areas in an expanding fashion, but such extensions in time and place may be invisible to passive surveillance systems. Moreover, in areas where vaccination is widely practiced, yellow fever virus may circulate silently between monkeys and mosquitoes, with few human cases in the indigenous population. Season is an important risk factor, and most cases in travelers have occurred during the period of viral amplification (late rainy season to early dry season).

Risk Factors

The age, sex, and occupational distribution of yellow fever victims in Africa and South America differ. In South America, the virus is transmitted by *Haemagogus* mosquitoes in the rain forest canopy, and humans are infected by mosquitoes that previously fed on viremic monkeys (*jungle yellow fever*).[112, 255] Since human infection is linked to occupational activities, such as forest clearing, lumbering, and road construction, most patients are young adults, and 70 to 90% are male (Fig. 34–11).[214, 230, 256] The prevalence of immunity in males exceeds that in females by 2.5- to 7.5-fold.[257] The age and sex distribution of jungle yellow fever patients differs from that observed in South America during *A. aegypti*–borne epidemics in the early 20th century. *A. aegypti* breeds in and around houses and sustains interhuman transmission of virus (*urban* yellow fever), with a high prevalence of infection in children and females.

In Africa, tree-hole–breeding (sylvatic) *Aedes* mosquitoes are responsible for yellow fever transmission between monkeys, from monkeys to humans, and between humans. During the rainy season, these vectors reach high densities in the moist savanna vegetational zone, and some species *(A. furcifer, A. africanus)* enter villages and houses. Yellow fever infection is endemic, and the prevalence of natural immunity accumulates rapidly with age, so that children are at highest risk (Table 34–7). A high attack rate in children (>70% of the total cases) typically reflects an area where older individuals are protected by previous yellow fever vaccination campaigns (e.g., Senegal, 1965; Burkina Faso and Ghana, 1983; Mali, 1987). However, in some epidemics affecting populations without prior vaccination, the attack rate has also been higher in children (see Table 34–6). In The Gambia, the disease incidence in persons aged 0 to 19 years was significantly higher than that in older adults ($P < .01$), possibly due to naturally acquired yellow fever or heterologous flavivirus immunity in adults.[93] There are few data on the relationship between the severity of illness and age. In the 1921 epidemic in Peru, the case-fatality rate was highest in infants and children 0 to 5 years old and in older adults (Fig. 34–12).[95] Other authors noted a higher case-fatality rate among the elderly, but lethality in infants was not assessed in these studies.[78, 80, 96, 97] Increased severity of illness in elderly individuals is known to occur in other flaviviral infections, notably Japanese encephalitis, St. Louis encephalitis, and West Nile encephalitis.

In Africa, a slight excess of cases among males has been observed during epidemics (Table 34–8; see also Table 34–7). This pattern was seen regardless of the role of domiciliary *A. aegypti* or sylvatic vectors and is thus

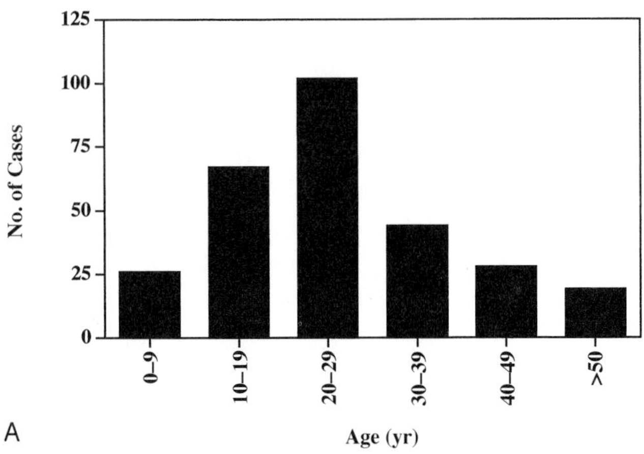

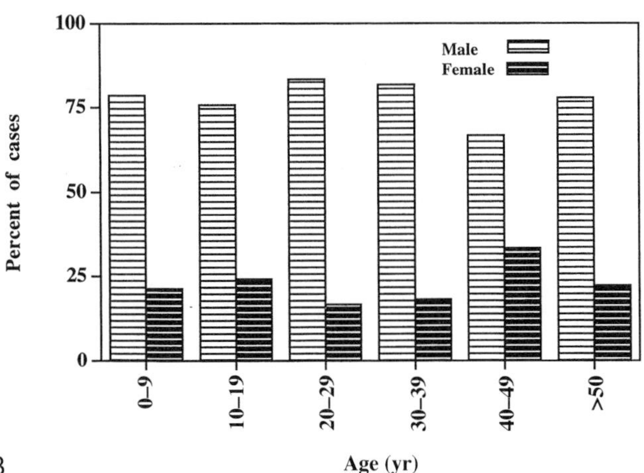

Figure 34–11. Age (*A*) and gender (*B*) distribution of cases of yellow fever, South America, 1992 to 1993. Eight cases during this interval were of undetermined age. (Data from World Health Organization. Yellow fever in 1992 and 1993. Wkly Epidemiol Rec 70:65, 1995.)

difficult to explain on the basis of differences in human behavior or exposure to mosquito bites. The higher proportion of male cases has been observed not only among notified or hospitalized patients, but also in population-based surveys, indicating that it is not due to reluctance of females to seek medical treatment. Serological data have shown neither a consistently higher incidence of infection nor susceptibility to illness among males (see Table 34–6), but a small sample size and sampling biases in these surveys may preclude detection of small differences. Males may be more susceptible to yellow fever, since severe adverse events associated with 17D and French neurotropic vaccines have been more frequent in males (see *Adverse Events*).

Season and Climate

In South America, the incidence of yellow fever is highest during months of high rainfall, humidity, and temperature (January to May, peak incidence February and March), corresponding to the activity of *Haemagogus* mosquitoes, which breed in tree holes and are thus dependent on rainwater. Human exposure during agricultural activities is also increased at this time of the year. In the savanna zone of western Africa, cases appear during the mid–rainy season (August) and peak during the early dry season (October), corresponding to the period of maximal longevity of sylvatic mosquito vectors.[258] The domiciliary vector *A. aegypti* breeds in receptacles used by humans for water storage and is thus less dependent on rainfall. Where this mosquito is involved in viral transmission, yellow fever may occur in the dry season in both rural and heavily settled urban areas. Thus, season is only a partially reliable guide to determining the risk of exposure and to making decisions on the need for immunization of travelers.

Fluctuations in rainfall profoundly affect mosquito vector abundance and the potential for yellow fever epidemics.[218, 259–263] Surveillance of yellow fever in eastern Senegal has been actively maintained for 20 years.[264] Enhanced viral activity in this region, reflected by viral isolations from mosquitoes, coincided with human epidemics over the entire western African region. This correlation may reflect prolonged rainfall or other undefined regional ecological changes. The yellow fever outbreak in The Gambia in 1978 occurred after a period of 2 successive years of excess rainfall.[260] Similarly, excessive rainfall and prolongation of the rainy season reflected by vegetational indices in satellite images preceded the emergence of a sylvatic yellow fever epidemic in Nigeria in 1986.[263]

Temperature influences yellow fever transmission rates.[265] The extrinsic incubation period of yellow fever virus in the mosquito vector is very sensitive to temperature, and an increase of a few degrees may shorten

Table 34–7. **AGE AND SEX DISTRIBUTION, YELLOW FEVER CASES, SELECTED EPIDEMICS IN AFRICA, 1926–1994**

EPIDEMIC	NO. CASES IN CHILDREN/ TOTAL CASES (%)	MALE:FEMALE RATIO	PRESUMED VECTORS	REFERENCE
Ghana, Nigeria, 1926–1928	32‡/122 (26)	2.3:1	? *A. aegypti*	78
Sudan (Nuba Mountains), 1940	110‡/306 (36)	1.7:1	*A. aegypti, A. vittatus,* other Sylvatic vectors	97
Senegal (Diourbel), 1965	86‡/89 (97)	—	*A. aegypti*	232
Nigeria (Jos Plateau area), 1969	38‡/209 (18)	2.5:1	*A. luteocephalus*	P. Brès, unpublished data
Ghana, 1969–1970	99†/164 (60)	—	*A. aegypti*	475
Nigeria (Okwoga District), 1970	35‡/76 (46)	~1:1	*A. africanus*	474
Ivory Coast (Mbahiakro Subprefecture), 1982	43†/90 (48)	—	*A. aegypti*	193
Ghana (Volta and Eastern Regions), 1977–1980	87†/294 (30)	—	*A. aegypti*	475
Burkina Faso (Manga and Fada N'Gourma Regions), 1983	40†/45 (89)	~1:1	*A. furcifer*	477, 478
Ghana (Northern Region), 1983	74†/87 (85)	—	*A. aegypti*	479
Nigeria (Oju LGA), 1986	20‡/39 (51)	2:1	*A. africanus*	227
Nigeria (Oyo State), 1987	72‡/102 (71)	1.4:1	*A. aegypti*	94
Mali (Kati Cercle), 1987	100†/143 (70)	2.1:1	*A. furcifer, A. aegypti*	480
Cameroon (Extreme North Province), 1990	91*/182 (73)	—	*A. aegypti*	235
Nigeria, 1991	1209†/2229 (54)	1.1:1	*A. aegypti*	481
Kenya (Baringo and Elgeyo Marakwet Districts), 1992–1993	18‡/54 (33)	1.8:1	*A. africanus, A. bromeliae*	482
Ghana (Upper Western Region), 1993–1994	47†/69 (68)	2.0:1	?	482a
Nigeria (Imo State), 1994	37†/116 (32)	1.3:1	? *A. africanus*	197

*0–9 years.
†0–15 years.
‡0–19 years.

the extrinsic incubation period by days, resulting in a significantly increased rate of transmission.[266, 267] Even brief exposure to high temperatures (e.g., in a sunlit forest clearing) can have this effect. Warm temperature also increases biting and reproductive rates of *A. aegypti.*[268] Thus, long-term environmental change (global warming) may increase transmission rates of yellow fever.[269]

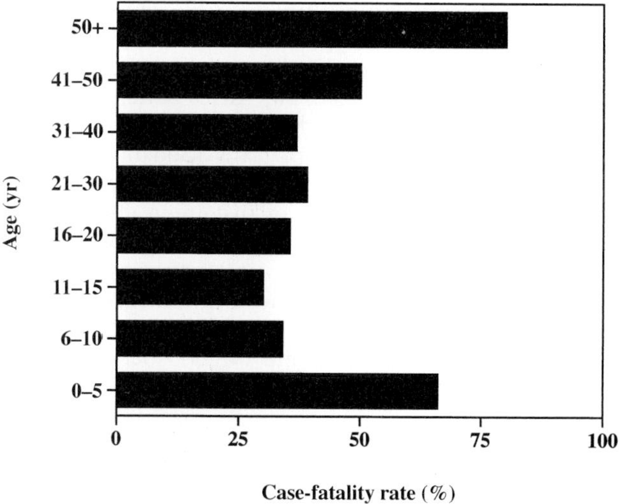

Figure 34–12. Case-fatality rates by age group of 478 cases of yellow fever, Peru, 1921, suggesting a bimodal pattern of increased severity in very young and elderly people. (Data from Hanson H. Observations or the age and sex incidence of deaths and recoveries in the yellow fever epidemic in the department of Lambayeque, Peru, in 1921. Am J Trop Med Hyg 9:233, 1929.)

Transmission Cycles

The enzootic transmission cycle involves monkeys and diurnally active tree-hole–breeding mosquitoes (*Haemagogus* spp. in South America, and *A. africanus* in Africa) (Fig. 34–13). The density of vectors and human disease incidence are low, and human cases occur in a sporadic fashion. This transmission cycle accounts for jungle yellow fever cases in South America and in the rain forest zone of Africa. Many species of nonhuman primates are susceptible to yellow fever infection (reviewed by Bugher[111] and Monath[112]). The majority of African spe-

Table 34–8. **MANUFACTURERS OF YELLOW FEVER 17D VACCINE IN 1997**

COUNTRY	MANUFACTURER
United States	Connaught Laboratories, Swiftwater, PA
Brazil	Bio-Manguinhos, Oswaldo Cruz Foundation, Rio de Janeiro
United Kingdom	Evans Medical, Speke, Liverpool
France	Pasteur Mérieux, Marcy l'Etoile
Russia	Institute of Poliomyelitis and Viral Encephalitides, Moscow
Senegal	Pasteur Institute, Dakar
Germany	Robert Koch Institute, Berlin

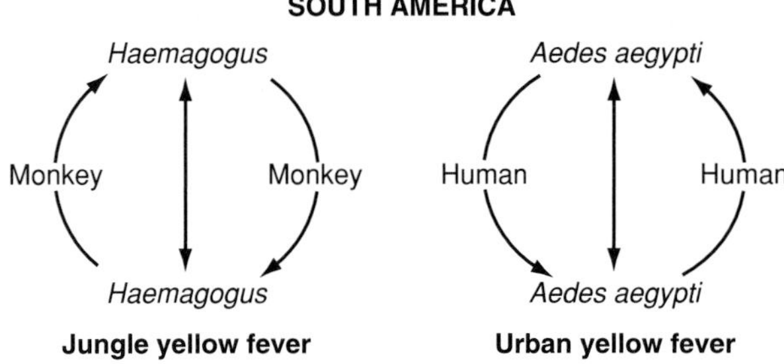

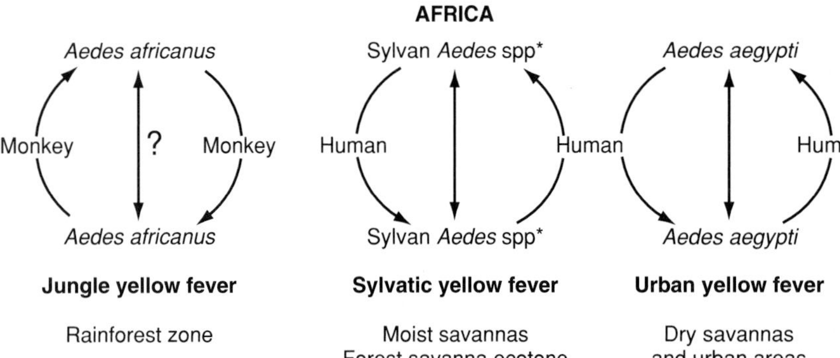

Figure 34–13. Transmission cycles of yellow fever virus in South America *(top)* and in Africa *(bottom)*. In both continents, jungle yellow fever is transmitted through an enzootic cycle, whereas urban and sylvatic yellow fevers are transmitted through epidemic cycles. Transovarial transmission is indicated by vertical arrows showing viral transfer between mosquitoes and may be an important mechanism for viral survival over the long dry season. *West Africa: *A. furcifer, A. taylori, A. luteocephalus, A. africanus, A. opok, A. vittatus,* and *A. metallicus.* East Africa: *A. bromeliae, A. africanus,* and others.

cies have viremic infections sufficient to infect mosquitoes without developing clinical illness, whereas some neotropical species (e.g., howler monkeys) develop lethal infections. Depletion of vertebrate hosts through natural immunization and death during epizootic waves is a factor in the cyclic appearance of yellow fever activity. In many areas, deforestation and hunting pressure have markedly reduced monkey populations, and human beings serve as hosts in the yellow fever transmission cycle.[270] Although still debated, there is little evidence that nonprimate species are involved in enzootic transmission.[111, 112, 259, 271]

The ecology of yellow fever differs in areas bordering the rain forest block in Africa. This transitional vegetational zone is characterized by a mosaic of savanna and forest in galleries along rivers. In this region and surrounding moist (Guinea) savanna, yellow fever transmission is effected by a wide variety of tree-hole–breeding mosquito vectors.[112, 258, 259, 262] In western Africa, the principal vectors responsible for yellow fever transmission in the savanna zone include *A. furcifer, A. vittatus,* and *A. luteocephalus* as well as *A. africanus.* In eastern Africa, *A. africanus* and human-biting populations of *A. bromeliae* (a member of the *A. simpsoni* complex) play a similar role.[272, 273] During the wet and early dry seasons, the vector density reaches high levels. Vectors are active in plantation areas and in proximity to human dwellings and may enter houses.[262] Both humans and nonhuman primates may be involved as hosts in the transmission cycle, and the rate of viral transmission far exceeds that found in the rain forest zone. The savanna-forest ecotone and surrounding Guinea savanna have been described as the *zone of emergence* of yellow fever and represents the region principally affected by epidemics.[259]

An epidemiologically distinct transmission cycle involves *A. aegypti,* which breeds in containers used to store water or in artificial containers that collect rainwater around human habitations. *A. aegypti* transmits yellow fever virus between humans, the sole viremic hosts in the cycle. The vector occurs in dry areas and heavily settled areas but is also widely dispersed in settlements in rural areas. Urban outbreaks have followed introduction of the virus by viremic persons from areas of jungle yellow fever activity.[94, 274] In the Americas, urban yellow fever outbreaks were common before the successful eradication of the vector.[255, 275, 276] The last urban outbreak in continental South America occurred in western Brazil in 1942, and the last episode of *A. aegypti*–transmitted yellow fever in the Americas occurred in Trinidad in 1954.[277] In contrast, Africa suffers many *A. aegypti*–borne epidemics, and the vector is prevalent in urban and rural areas. In dry areas (Sudan and Sahel savanna zones), where domiciliary *A. aegypti* may represent the only species capable of sustaining yellow fever transmission, outbreaks occur after introduction of the virus by viremic person(s). *A. aegypti*–borne epidemics in the past 30 years include those in Senegal in 1965; Angola in 1971; Ghana in 1969, 1977 to 1980, and 1983; Ivory Coast in 1982; and Nigeria between 1987 and 1991.[226]

Maintenance of Yellow Fever in Nature

The means of survival of yellow fever virus across the long dry season, when sylvatic mosquito vectors are virtually absent, remains incompletely understood. *Aedes* and *Haemagogus* eggs survive desiccation in tree holes and hatch with the return of rain. Experimental and field studies indicate that transovarial transmission is an important means of viral survival across the dry season.[101, 102, 278, 279] Low-level horizontal transmission by drought-resistant vectors, and alternative horizontal and vertical transmission cycles involving ticks,[280] have been suggested as ancillary mechanisms. Persistent infection of experimentally infected nonhuman primates has been documented,[59, 281] but such infections are probably not accompanied by viremias sufficient to infect vectors.

Prospects for Future Changes in Yellow Fever Epidemiology

The most alarming prospect for the future involves the reemergence of urban (*A. aegypti*–borne) yellow fever in South America and the spread of yellow fever to heavily populated, *A. aegypti*–infested areas of the world that are currently free from the disease. These regions include both areas historically affected, such as the coastal regions of South America, the Caribbean, and North America, and regions that have not heretofore been reached by the disease but are considered receptive, including the Middle East, coastal eastern Africa, the Indian subcontinent, Asia, and Australia. Alterations in human demography and behavior, in viral activity, and in the distribution of *A. aegypti* underlie the potential for epidemiological change. These alterations include (1) a recent upsurge of yellow fever virus activity and incidence of human infections, which increases the opportunity for geographic spread; (2) the reinvasion of the South American continent by the domestic vector, *A. aegypti* (Fig. 34–14)[263, 282]; (3) changes in human demography, principally the shifting balance of human populations from rural to urban residence, the expansion of internal communications, and the opening of remote rural areas to commerce within countries in the yellow fever endemic zone; (4) economic development and the growth of air travel, which have diminished the barriers to the spread of yellow fever; (5) relaxation of regulations and enforcement of vaccination certification for travelers; and (6) global warming. Spread of yellow fever outside its traditional boundaries and reemergence of the urban disease in the Americas would greatly increase the demand for yellow fever vaccine.

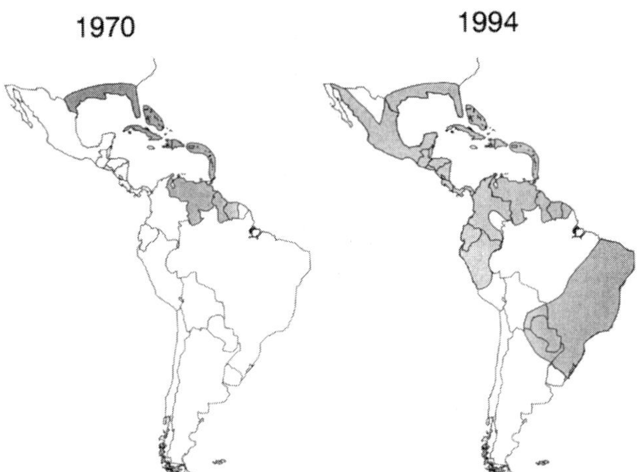

Figure 34–14. Reinvasion of the South American continent by the urban vector of yellow fever, *A. aegypti*, during the period between 1970 and 1994. The vector had been eliminated from many countries during intensive vector control efforts, under the leadership of the Pan American Health Organization. The reinfestation led to the introduction and spread of epidemic dengue and raises the risk of reemergence of urban yellow fever. (From Gubler DJ, Trent DW. Emergence of epidemic dengue/dengue hemorrhagic fever as a public health problem in the Americas. Infect Agents Dis 2:383, 1994.)

Other Modes of Transmission

Laboratory infections with yellow fever were common in the prevaccine era and remain of concern today, particularly where unvaccinated clinical laboratory personnel encounter blood from patients during the early stage of illness. Some laboratory infections were probably acquired by the bite of mosquitoes experimentally infected in the laboratory or of wild mosquitoes infected after feeding on experimental animals; others were the result of direct contact with blood or aerosols of dried virus.[15, 283, 284] The stability of yellow fever virus is sufficient to permit transmission within short periods after the generation of an infectious aerosol in the laboratory.[285] Under experimental conditions, a dose of only 10 mouse LD_{50} (MLD_{50}, i.e., LD_{50} determined by intracerebral inoculation of mice 4 to 6 weeks of age) delivered by aerosol was sufficient to induce lethal infection in rhesus monkeys.[286] The absence of direct interhuman transmission indicates that virus is not shed in secreta or excreta at sufficiently high levels for transfer by contact or aerosols. There is no evidence that black vomit or urine is infectious. However, on multiple occasions, transmission has occurred between separately caged monkeys housed in a single room, possibly by aerosol spread.[109] Findlay and MacCallum infected monkeys by a mucosal (intragastric) route,[287] and Bauer and Hudson transmitted yellow fever to monkeys by rubbing virus on unabraded skin.[288] Some infections in laboratory workers may be explained by contact with viremic blood, but it remains unclear whether infection occurred via intact skin, abrasions, or contact with mucosal surfaces.

PASSIVE IMMUNIZATION AND PASSIVE-ACTIVE IMMUNIZATION

Passive immunization was widely used before the development of vaccines. The concept was established in the 19th century,[289] and convalescent serum was first used in the early 20th century.[290] Experimental validation was after isolation of yellow fever virus. In 1928, Stokes and colleagues reported that pretreatment with a small volume of convalescent serum protected monkeys against a lethal challenge.[9] Because of an increasing number of laboratory infections, standard practice was to administer convalescent serum to at-risk laboratory workers and to inject large amounts after accidental exposures. The potency of passive antibody and the schedule of immunization were not carefully controlled, and laboratory-acquired disease occurred in persons who had been previously immunized[291]; such cases were due to an inadequate dose of antibody and the long interval between the transfer of serum and exposure.[117] In monkey studies, transfer of immune serum before a challenge was protective, whereas immunization 24 hours after an experimental challenge protected 55% of the animals, and transfer at 48 or 72 hours protected only 15 to 20%.[292] Administration of antibody after the clinical onset of disease was ineffective.

Because of the difficulty of obtaining sufficient amounts of potent human serum, hyperimmune antibodies were prepared in nonhuman primates, horses, and goats.[293, 294] Antibodies raised in monkeys and horses were shown to protect susceptible rhesus macaques. Heterologous antisera had limited usefulness for repeated administration to humans but were applied together with partially attenuated virus to achieve active immunization. *Passive-active immunization* using an excess of human or animal serum mixed with partially attenuated virus (French neurotropic strain) elicited active immunity without untoward effects and became standard practice.[14] However, it was a cumbersome method, requiring that the amount of immune serum be sufficient to protect against disease but not completely neutralize the virus and prevent active infection.[295] The use of heterologous serum was problematic, as allergic reactions occurred in 85% of recipients of goat serum, and late reactions similar to abortive yellow fever infection were noted in some cases, possibly due to rapid clearance of the heterologous serum, allowing replication of the underattenuated vaccines used in these studies (e.g., the 17E strain). The use of monkey serum was safer, but frequent failure to seroconvert was attributed to vaccine neutralization by the antiserum. Passive-active immunization was discontinued in 1936 with the advent of vaccines that could be administered safely without serum.[20]

Maternal Antibody

Transplacental transfer of yellow fever neutralizing antibodies has been documented in monkeys[296] and humans,[297] and antibody has also been found in breast milk of immune mothers.[298] Since yellow fever 17D vaccine is not administered to infants younger than 6 months of age for safety reasons, maternal immunity does not pose an obstacle to effective immunization.

ACTIVE IMMUNIZATION

Prior Approaches That Have Been Abandoned

Inactivated Vaccines

After the isolation of the virus in 1927, attempts to develop an inactivated vaccine were made at the Wellcome Bureau of Scientific Research,[13, 299] at the Oswaldo Cruz Institute in Brazil,[300] and at the Pasteur Institute in Paris.[203] The vaccines were prepared by phenol or formaldehyde treatment of infected monkey liver or spleen, or both. Hindle inoculated rhesus monkeys with a single dose of inactivated liver tissue emulsion containing more than 10,000 monkey lethal doses per g and found that 80% of the immunized monkeys were protected against challenge.[299] However, his and others' studies were not controlled for residual live virus, nor were serological studies performed. Subsequent studies in monkeys yielded erratic results,[301, 302] and human trials in Brazil involving 25,000 people were inconclusive.[203] Burke and Davis reported yellow fever in an individual who had received inactivated liver tissue vaccine.[291]

As virological techniques improved, antigens were tested that were more suitable for vaccine production than infected monkey viscera. Gordon and Hughes prepared vaccines from heat- or ultraviolet-inactivated virus tissue cultures (viscerotropic virus) or from mouse brain (neurotropic virus) containing known amounts of virus.[303] Preparations containing residual live virus caused illness in monkeys, and survivors were immune to challenge. However, monkeys given various doses of fully inactivated vaccines did not develop antibodies and were not protected. It appeared that methods that fully inactivated virus also destroyed its antigenic properties. It should be noted, however, that all studies employed a single inoculum of antigen, a procedure that would not be expected to be very effective in the case of an inactivated vaccine. Sellards and Bennett inoculated mice with multiple sequential doses of phenol-inactivated mouse brain and demonstrated protection against challenge,[304] and rabbits immunized sequentially with inactivated virus developed neutralizing antibodies. However, prime-boost vaccination strategies were not used in monkeys or humans.

Methodological problems in antigen production, inactivation, and potency assays; ignorance about immunological principles; and the lack of adjuvants were obstacles to the development of inactivated vaccines. Given the growth characteristics of yellow fever virus, with titers of 10^9 achievable in cell culture, and the success of inactivated vaccines against other flaviviruses, there is little doubt that a satisfactory product could be developed today. The failure of the early efforts to produce inactivated vaccines was certainly auspicious, as success might have sidetracked the development of live vaccines.

Passive-Active Immunization

See *Passive Immunization and Passive-Active Immunization.*

French Neurotropic Vaccine

In 1930, Theiler showed that mice are susceptible to intracerebral inoculation of yellow fever virus.[305] Following the lead of Pasteur, who had attenuated rabies virus by passage in rabbit brains, Theiler made a series of mouse brain passages of the French strain and showed that the adapted virus lost its viscerotropism for monkeys and protected them against challenge. However, in subsequent studies the neuroadapted virus caused fever and viremia in a high proportion of monkeys, and lethal encephalitis after intracerebral or intranasal inoculation, and even, in individual animals, after subcutaneous inoculation.[14, 109, 306–308] The virus was considered too dangerous without the coadministration of immune serum. The first human volunteers, therefore, were given immune human serum and neuroadapted virus (see *Passive Immunization and Passive-Active Immunization*). This regimen resulted in the development of active immunity.[14]

In 1932, Sellards and Laigret reported the first human immunizations with the French strain in the absence of immune serum.[16, 309] Systemic adverse reactions were attributed to underattenuation. To address this problem, a method was devised for "attenuating" the mouse brain virus by aging at room temperature. Subjects received three inoculations at intervals of 20 days with virus that had been aged for decreasing lengths of time.[310] Preliminary studies indicated that the regime was well tolerated and that 90% seroconverted after the second dose. By 1934, 3196 people in French West Africa had received this regime, and 70% of those studied developed antibodies after the first dose.[17] One third of the recipients experienced a febrile reaction after the first dose, and there were two serious adverse events (myelitis, meningitis). In 1935, Nicolle and Laigret simplified the method to a single inoculation of mouse brain virus aged for 24 hours and treated with olive oil or egg yolk to retard diffusion from the inoculation site.[311] By 1939, over 20,000 people in western Africa had recieved the single- or three-dose schedule. Concerns about reactogenicity decreased with vaccine use, despite occasional reports of postvaccinal encephalitis.[312, 313] Careful follow-up studies were not routinely conducted, and the threat of natural infection superseded concerns about vaccine safety.

In 1939, Peltier and coworkers simplified yellow fever immunization by conversion from subcutaneous inoculation to the scarification technique used to deliver smallpox vaccine.[314] In 1939, nearly 100,000 people were given FNV and smallpox vaccines simultaneously, without recognized adverse events. Of 1387 subjects followed up, 96.3% developed neutralizing antibodies 1 month after immunization. By 1941, FNV by scarification had been given to 1.9 million people in francophone Africa, and immunization was then made compulsory in these countries. By 1947, 14 million people had been immunized.[315] In 1946, FNV was approved by the UNRRA Standing Technical Committee on Health, and similar approval was granted in 1948 by the WHO.

FNV was prepared at the Pasteur Institute, Dakar, by the intracerebral inoculation of 2.5- to 3-month-old mice with approximately 20,000 LD_{50} of the French virus.[316] A seed lot system was not used, although the passage level was restricted. Mice showing illness were killed and brains aseptically removed and lyophilized. After sterility tests, brains from a batch were pooled, ground to powdered form, and again tested for sterility. The vaccine powder was filled into ampoules containing one-tenth of a mouse brain (0.4 g), equivalent to 100 doses, and tested for sterility and potency. After reconstitution in 2 mL, the recommended minimum potency was 5000 LD_{50} per dose. The vaccine was quite stable and was stored at 4°C but shipped at ambient temperature. After being reconstituted in a solution of gum arabic, a drop of the solution was placed on the skin, and scarification was performed with a bifurcated needle.

By 1953, 56 million doses had been delivered in francophone Africa (twice the population of the region).[317] As a result, the incidence of yellow fever declined in francophone countries (Fig. 34–15) but not in neighboring Nigeria and Ghana, where immunization was not practiced. Seroconversion rates were shown to exceed 95%,[318] and population surveys in French West Africa showed that the prevalence of immunity rose from approximately 20% before vaccination to 86% in 1952 to 1953.[319]

The safety of FNV was not carefully evaluated during the campaign to achieve full coverage. It was known that FNV caused viremia in two thirds of the subjects, that 10 to 15% experienced a "mild" reaction with fever, headache, and backache on days 4 to 6, and that rare

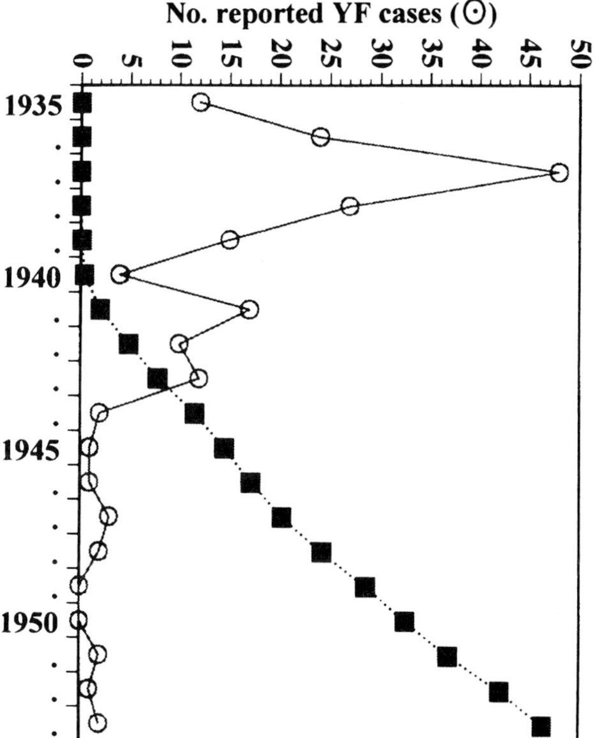

Figure 34–15. Cumulative number of doses of French neurotropic vaccine administered and incidence of yellow fever (YF), French West Africa, 1935 to 1953. Compulsory vaccination of the indigenous population resulted in virtual disappearance of the disease. Neighboring anglophone countries, which did not practice immunization, continued to have epidemic yellow fever. (From Monath TP. Yellow fever vaccines: The success of empiricism, pitfalls of application, and transition to molecular vaccinology. In Plotkin S, Fantini B [eds]. Vaccinia, Vaccination and Vaccinology: Jenner, Pasteur and Their Successors. Paris, Elsevier, 1996, pp 157–182. Data from Durieux C. Mass yellow fever vaccination in French Africa south of the Sahara. Smithburn KC, Durieux C, Koerber R, et al. [eds]. Yellow Fever Vaccination. Geneva, World Health Organization, 1956, pp 51–63.)

cases of meningoencephalitis occurred 10 to 15 days after vaccination.[313, 320–322] The incidence of encephalitis was initially estimated at between 1 in 3000 and 1 in 10,000,[322] but its importance was minimized because full recovery was the rule, and because no serious reactions were noted during campaigns in French West Africa involving over 40 million people.[315, 323] However, contemporary reports described outbreaks of encephalitis and deaths following yellow fever immunization in French Equatorial Africa.[324] English and American workers considered FNV too dangerous for routine use, but when epidemics struck Nigeria (1951–1952) and Central America (1950–1952), the danger of yellow fever exceeded vaccine-associated risks. In Nigeria, the use of FNV was followed by an outbreak of encephalitis principally in children, with an incidence of 3 to 4% and a case-fatality rate of 40%.[325, 326] Autopsies showed lesions of encephalitis consistent with direct viral injury, and yellow fever virus was isolated from brain tissue, confirming that FNV and not an adventitious agent was responsible. In Costa Rica and Honduras, 10 definite and 5 possible cases of postvaccinal encephalitis occurred in children.[327]

The increased recognition of severe reactions in children led to a change in the policy for use of FNV. In 1959 to 1960, vaccination was restricted to people older than 10 years.[328] The distribution of vaccine decreased from approximately 8 million doses to 4 million doses per year. Within 5 years of the cessation of routine immunization of children, epidemic yellow fever reappeared in Senegal for the first time in 28 years.[232] The 1965 epidemic at Diourbel was the largest on record in West Africa, affecting up to 20,000 people. Because of the high incidence of yellow fever in children and limited supplies of the safer 17D vaccine, the age limit for the use of FNV was reduced to the original 2 years. Among 498,887 people vaccinated with FNV vaccine, there were 231 cases of postvaccinal encephalitis.[329] The majority of cases occurred in children aged 2 to 11 years, in whom the incidence of encephalitis was approximately 1.4 per 1000 and the case-fatality rate 9%.[329, 330] The clinical syndromes associated with acute encephalitis and the neuropsychiatric residua were described by Collomb and colleagues.[331] This unfortunate episode confirmed the need both to provide a high rate of coverage of the childhood population in Africa and to utilize a safer method of immunization. In 1966, the Pasteur Institute, with the assistance of the WHO, expanded production of 17D vaccine at Dakar, and by 1970 an official policy was established for the use of 17D people younger than 5 years.[332] Small amounts FNV were used in regions with poor accessibility where the use of the more thermolabile 17D vaccine was problematic, but in 1982 the production of the vaccine was discontinued.

The potential contamination of the FNV with murine viruses (e.g., lymphocytic choriomeningitis) has not been fully clarified. However, the isolation of yellow fever virus from brain tissue in fatal cases[325] and the absence of murine viruses in FNV lots[333] support the hypothesis that the vaccine and not an adventitious agent was responsible for encephalitis.

17D Vaccine Delivered by Scarification

In 1950, a decision was made in Nigeria to prepare 17D vaccine for immunization by scarification, to simplify and reduce the cost of delivery, and to permit the use of formulations with less stringent requirements for sterility.[334] Beginning in 1951, trials were initiated using 17D vaccine alone, combined with smallpox vaccine, or with smallpox vaccine given at different sites.[334–338] The vaccine was prepared in eggs or by passage of the egg vaccine in mouse brain. Clinical trials revealed a lack of seroconversion in up to 15% of those vaccinated with 17D alone and in 35% of those receiving combined yellow fever and smallpox immunization.[339] Revaccination with 17D at an interval of 14 days increased the seroconversion rate.[340] Studies in western Africa and Malaya suggested that vaccine failures may have been due to cross-protective heterologous flavivirus immunity.[341–344] A head-to-head comparison of 17D and FNV delivered by scarification showed a higher seroconversion rate with the French vaccine.[334] The apparent lower seroconversion rate of 17D applied by scarification was probably not due to vaccine titer differences,[340] but rather to the inherently higher capacity of FNV to replicate at the dose delivered by this method. Scarification was not adopted for routine delivery of 17D vaccine in anglophone Africa because of uncertainties about efficacy; the lack of an efficient cold chain, the absence of a public health policy for yellow fever vaccine production and immunization after independence from colonial rule; and the development of improved methods for vaccine delivery (the jet injector).

Yellow Fever 17D Vaccine

17D is the only strain currently used for human immunization against yellow fever.

Development and Early Clinical Testing

The original development of 17D vaccine, described by Lloyd and associates[345] and Theiler and Smith,[18] was achieved by empirical methods of sequential passage of the prototype Asibi virus in a substrate that was restrictive for growth. This process enhanced the selection of variants with altered biological properties, without neuroadaptation by mouse brain passage as in the case of FNV. The first successful in vitro passages of Asibi virus were achieved in cultures of minced mouse embryo tissues. After 18 subcultures, the virus was passed to cultures of minced whole chick embryo. After 58 passages, the virus, now designated as subculture series *17D*, was propagated by subcultures in minced chick embryo cultures from which the brain and spinal cord had been removed. The final passage before human inoculation was in embryonated eggs.

A reduction in monkey neurovirulence and a loss of viscerotropism occurred between the 89th and 114th passages, and reduction in mouse neurovirulence between the 114th and 176th passages. Monkeys inoculated by peripheral routes did not develop encephalitis; those inoculated intracerebrally developed histopathological changes, but only 5 to 10% succumbed to encephalitis. The animals developed antibodies and resisted challenge with Asibi virus.

Preclinical safety and efficacy were deemed sufficient to permit human studies. The initial trials using virus at the 227th and 229th passage levels were conducted in 1936, first in yellow fever immunes and then in nonimmune volunteers.[20, 21] The trials showed acceptable tolerability and the development of neutralizing antibodies. In early 1937, 17D vaccine was taken to Brazil, where it was used in trials of increasing size, leading to the establishment of local manufacturing and the initiation of a mass vaccination campaign in 1938.[21, 22, 346] Between 1938 and 1941, over 2 million people were immunized in Brazil.

Seed Lot System

During the initial phase of yellow fever vaccine production at the Rockefeller Foundation in New York and in Brazil between 1937 and 1941, a number of different substrains were used, representing independent parallel subculture lineages originating at about the 200th passage of the original 17D line (Fig. 34–16). Two main lineages (17D-204 and 17DD) were used for vaccine production (see under *Substrains, Passage Histories, and Molecular Heterogeneity of 17D Vaccines in Current Use*).

Between 1938 and 1941, field trials and experimental studies revealed the importance of controlling the passage level and viral substrain. Substrains 17DD high (305th to 395th passage levels) and $17D_2$ (passage 220) were found to be overattenuated, with poor seroconversion rates in humans and low viremias and poor immunogenicity in monkeys,[347, 348] indicating that a loss of immunogenicity could occur in as few as 20 passages in minced chicken embryo tissue cultures. More important, some substrains were associated with the appearance of encephalitis. In 1941, after an outbreak of postvaccinal encephalitis in Brazil, a survey of 55,073 people who received different lots of the same substrain (17D-NY 104) revealed the occurrence of 273 (0.5%) severe systemic reactions, including 199 (0.36%) with central nervous system signs and 1 fatal case of encephalitis.[349] A controlled study was performed, in which over 19,000 individuals received different vaccine lots (including EP, $17D_3$, 17D-NY 310, and 17D-NY 104; Fig. 34–16) that had been associated with the highest incidence of severe reactions or a control vaccine prepared from uninfected chick embryos. Children 5 to 14 years old sustained the highest incidence of encephalitis, with the onset of central nervous system signs 9 to 12 days after immunization. The highest incidence of encephalitis (13 in 1000) was observed in recipients of the 17D-NY 104 vaccine. This substrain was shown also to produce the highest frequency of encephalitis in monkey neurovirulence tests. Other substrains (17D-NY 310 and $17D_3$) associated with encephalitis in humans, but at a lower incidence than 17D-NY 104, caused early-onset and prolonged fever in monkeys.

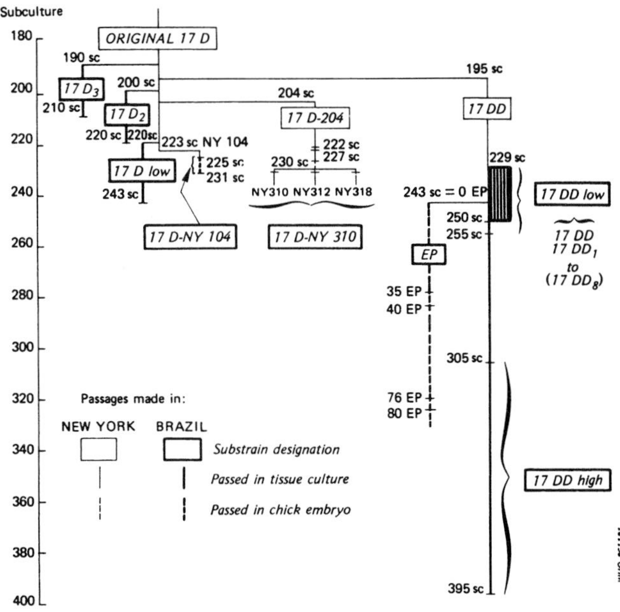

Figure 34–16. Derivation of early vaccine lots from the original 17D virus, before the institution of a seed lot system (see text). (From Fox JP, Penna HA. Behavior of 17D yellow fever virus in rhesus monkeys. Relation to substrain, dose and neural or extraneural inoculation. Am J Hyg 38:152, 1943; and Brès P, Koch M. Production and testing of the WHO yellow fever primary seed lot 213–77 and reference batch 168–73. In WHO Expert Committee on Biological Standardization, 36th Report. Technical Report Series No. 745. Annex 6:113. Geneva, World Health Organization, 1987.)

Recognizing that continued serial passage could lead to unwanted alterations in the biological properties of 17D vaccine, the Rio de Janeiro laboratory instituted a *seed lot* system in 1941, in which primary seed and secondary seed lots were prepared, and the latter was used to prepare multiple vaccine batches. The primary and secondary seeds were extensively characterized, and all vaccine lots were restricted to a single passage from the secondary seed.

This system was used from 1942 onward by many manufacturers and was formally established as a biological standard by UNRRA in 1945.[350] However, appropriate seed lots were not distributed to all manufacturers, and preparation of vaccines by serial passage and without adequate neurovirulence testing continued in some countries in the 1950s. Several cases of encephalitis were reported after the use of such vaccines at the Pasteur Institute during that time.[351] In 1957, publication of WHO Requirements for Yellow Fever Vaccine further standardized the seed lot and manufacturing procedures.[352]

Vaccine Producers

Currently there are seven active manufacturers of yellow fever 17D vaccine (Table 34–8; E. Griffiths, WHO, personal communication, 1997). Three manufacturers in Brazil, France, and Senegal produce large amounts of vaccine for the Expanded Program of Immunization (EPI) and mass vaccination campaigns during routine and emergency operations. Pasteur Mérieux Connaught and Evans Medical export vaccine for the travelers' market. Global vaccine production is currently approximately 60 million doses, with a full capacity of 170 million doses (E. Griffiths, WHO; J.-F. Saluzzo, Pasteur Mérieux, personal communication, 1997). The number of manufacturers has decreased during the last 20 years, with facilities in the Netherlands, India, Australia, South Africa, and Colombia no longer active. Nigeria has completed renovation of its vaccine manufacturing facility to Good Manufacturing Practices (GMP) standards with a potential capacity of producing up to 20 million doses annually but has not implemented production (A. Nasidi, personal communication, 1997). There are concerns about GMP standards at some of the current manufacturers, and it is likely that facility renovations and operational changes will be required to maintain WHO approval for continued production.

All yellow fever vaccines are live attenuated vaccines derived from the 17D strain, are produced in embryonated eggs, and meet WHO standards of safety and potency (see *Method of Manufacture, Control, and Lot Release Tests*). Their biological performance is presumed to be similar or identical with respect to the seroconversion rate; the quality of the immune response; the durability of immunity; safety; and tolerability. Vaccines in current production differ, however, with respect to the 17D substrain; the passage level; the formulation with stabilizers; the thermostability; and the contamination with avian leukosis virus. 17D vaccines are not biologically cloned and are heterogeneous mixtures of multiple virion subpopulations. Not surprisingly, differences have been found in the plaque size,[58] the oligonucleotide fingerprints,[353] and the nucleotide sequences of vaccines in current use.[43, 44, 354] There is no evidence to suggest that such variations affect safety or efficacy.

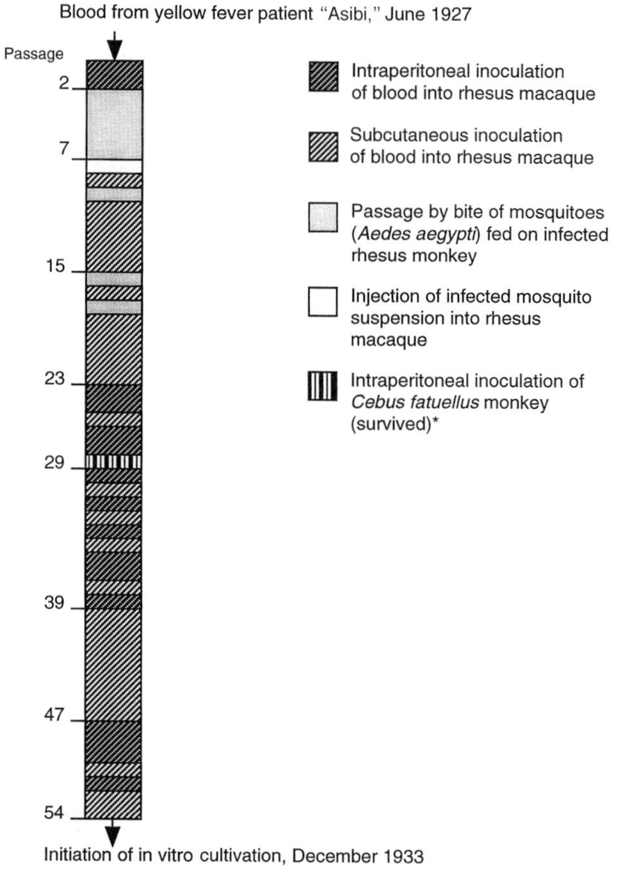

Substrains, Passage Histories, and Molecular Heterogeneity of 17D Vaccines in Current Use

Before initiating the attenuation process, Asibi virus was passaged sequentially 54 times in monkeys, either by the direct injection of blood from the previous animal or with an intervening passage in *A. aegypti* mosquitoes (Fig. 34–17). Throughout this passage history the virus maintained its virulence for rhesus monkeys. Figures 34–16 and 34–18 through 34–20 show the viral passage history during the original development of 17D vaccines. In vitro cultivation began in December, 1933, with the passage of the virulent Asibi strain in mouse embryo tissue culture and subsequently in chick embryo tissue culture to produce attenuated 17D vaccines (Fig. 34–18).[345] Two 17D substrains—17DD and 17D-204—currently used for vaccine manufacture represent independent subcultures performed at the Rockefeller Foundation, New York (see Fig. 34–16). The 17DD and 17D-204 substrains were derived from passage levels 195 and 204, respectively, of the original 17D virus (Figs. 34–16 and 34–18). 17DD virus was sent to Brazil

Figure 34–17. Passage history of Asibi virus from the original isolation to the initiation of in vitro culture for development of the 17D vaccine.*Not counted by authors but represents a passage in the history of Asibi virus before cultivation in vitro.

at passage level 229, whereupon it was passaged 14 times in minced chicken embryo tissue cultures and then, beginning at passage 243, in whole embryonated eggs (the *EP* lineage, Fig. 34–16). Primary and secondary seeds were prepared in Brazil at passages 284 and 285, respectively, and the current vaccine is at passage 286 (Fig. 34–19). One of two 17DD primary seeds was transferred to the Pasteur Institute, Dakar, Senegal, and used to prepare new seed stocks for vaccine manufacture.

The 17D-204 substrain has been used by all other manufacturers. At passage level 222, the virus was propagated in embryonated eggs in order to prepare a vaccine lot (NY 75) (see Fig. 34–18). This vaccine was transferred to the Yellow Fever Laboratory, Bogota, Colombia, where additional egg passages were performed. Colombia No. 88 was returned to the Rockefeller Institute in 1940, whereupon a small number of passages in eggs were made at the Rockefeller Foundation or the Rocky Mountain Laboratory (National Institutes of Health) before the manufacture of primary seed stocks in France, the United States, Australia, the Netherlands, Germany, Colombia, South Africa, England, and India (Fig. 34–20). The Pasteur Institute, Dakar, switched from 17DD to 17D-204 virus for the preparation of secondary seed free from avian leukosis virus. In 1977, the Robert Koch Institute (Berlin) prepared for WHO a primary seed free from avian leukosis virus and maintains this as a

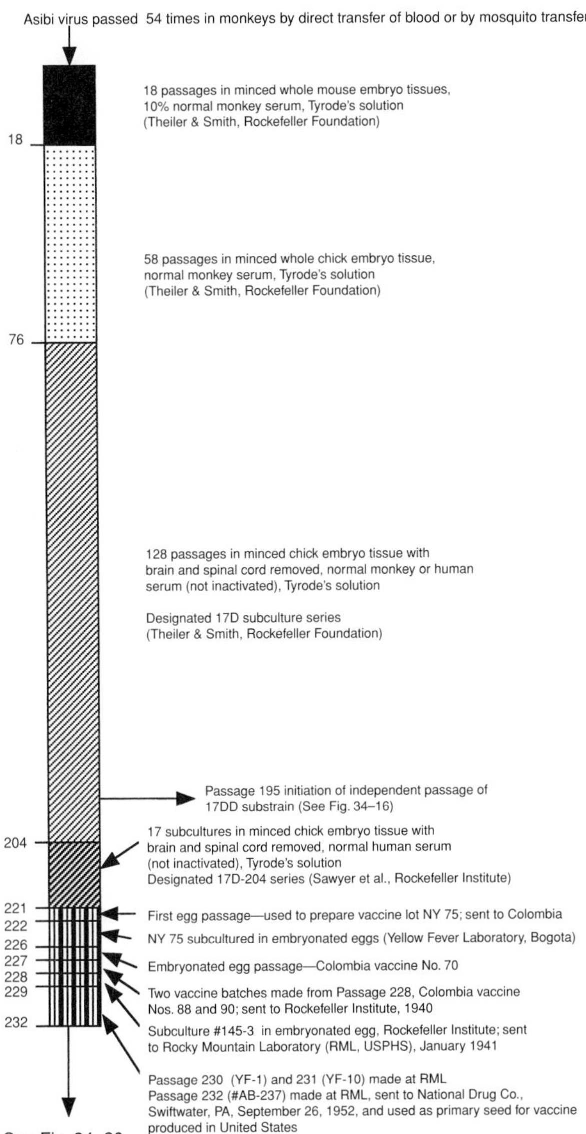

Figure 34–18. Passage history of the seed virus used to prepare yellow fever vaccines. (Modified from Brès P, Koch M. Production and testing of the WHO yellow fever primary seed lot 213–77 and reference batch 168–73. In WHO Expert Committee or Biological Standardization, 36th Report. Technical Report Series No. 745. Annex 6:113. Geneva, World Health Organization, 1987.)

reference stock (designated 17D-213-77[355]) available to new manufacturers and as a source for emergency production. All current 17D-204 vaccines are produced at passage levels between 233 and 239.

The 17DD and 17D-204 substrains are distinguishable by monoclonal antibody analysis, indicating variations in antigenic determinants on the E protein.[60, 68, 69, 353, 356] Antigenic differences between vaccines produced from the 17D-204 substrain by different manufacturers have also been identified.[68] A comparison of the structural proteins of the 17DD substrain vaccine produced in Brazil and Senegal and the WHO reference vaccine (17D-213) at the sequence level revealed that 17DD vaccine had accumulated fewer nucleotide changes per passage than 17D-204.[357] 17DD and 17D-204 (repre-

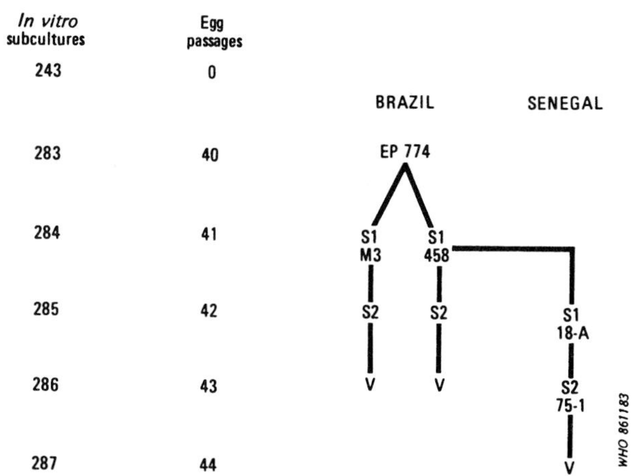

Figure 34–19. Passage history of the 17DD substrain (derivation shown in Fig. 34–16) to prepare seed viruses and vaccines in Brazil and Senegal. (From Brès P, Koch M. Production and testing of the WHO yellow fever primary seed lot 213–77 and reference batch 168–73. In WHO Expert Committee on Biological Standardization, 36th Report. Technical Report Series No. 745. Annex 6:113. Geneva, World Health Organization, 1987.)

sented by the WHO reference seed, 17D-213) differ at five amino acid residues in the E protein (at positions 56, 153, 155, 325, and 416) (Table 34–9).[12, 42] At positions 56, 153, 155, and 325, at least one of the vaccine substrains is identical to the parental Asibi virus, suggesting that these residues are not important in attenuation of virulence.

The neurovirulence phenotypes of 17DD and 17D-204 substrains have been examined in mice[139] and monkeys.[358] Vaccines were compared with respect to the average survival time and mortality after intranasal inoculation of young adult mice. 17DD substrain vaccines were neurovirulent after intranasal inoculation, whereas those derived from 17D-204 were not. In monkeys subjected to the WHO standard intracerebral neurovirulence test, slightly higher histopathologic lesion scores were found in the brains of animals inoculated with

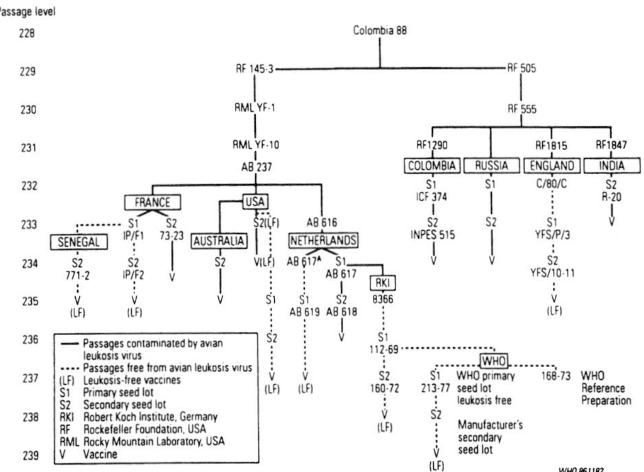

Figure 34–20. Passage history of the 17-204 substrain vaccines (derivation shown in Fig. 34–18) to prepare seed viruses and vaccines in various countries. (From Robertson SE. The Immunological Basis for Immunization. 8. Yellow Fever. Document WHO/EPI/GEN/93.18. Geneva, World Health Organization, 1993.)

Table 34–9. **AMINO ACID DIFFERENCES IN THE STRUCTURAL CODING REGION BETWEEN THE TWO YELLOW FEVER 17D SUBSTRAINS CURRENTLY USED FOR HUMAN IMMUNIZATION (17DD AND 17D-204) AND ASIBI VIRUS (DIFFERENCES BETWEEN 17DD AND 17D-204 ARE IN BOLD)**

AMINO ACID (E PROTEIN)	VIRUS		
	Asibi	17DD*	17D-204†
52	Gly	Arg	Arg
56	**Ala**	**Ala**	**Val**
153	**Asn**	**Asn**	**Thr**
155	**Asp**	**Ser**	**Asp**
170	Ala	Val	Val
173	Thr	Ile	Ile
200	Lys	Thr	Thr
299	Met	Ile	Ile
305	Ser	Phe	Phe
325	**Pro**	**Pro**	**Ser**
331	Lys	Arg	Arg
380	Thr	Arg	Arg
407	Ala	Val	Val
416	**Ala**	**Val**	**Thr**

*17DD vaccine produced in Brazil and Senegal.

†17D-213 World Health Organization vaccine (17D-204 substrain).

Data from Jennings AD, Whitby JE, Minor PD, et al. Comparison of the nucleotide and deduced amino acid sequences of the structural protein genes of the yellow fever 17DD vaccine strain from Senegal with those of other yellow fever vaccine viruses. Vaccine 11:679, 1993; and Post PR, Santos CND, Carvalho R, et al. Heterogeneity in envelope protein sequence and *N*-linked glycosylation among yellow fever virus vaccine strains. Virology 188:160, 1992.

17DD than with 17D-204 vaccines.[358] However, both 17DD and 17D-204 vaccines passed WHO standards and were well within the limits of acceptable safety in the monkey test. Overall, the data suggest that 17DD vaccine may be somewhat more neurovirulent than 17D-204 substrain vaccines as determined in animal models. Since both substrains have a long history of use in many millions of persons, and since all reported cases of postvaccinal encephalitis after stabilization of vaccine passage level have in fact involved 17D-204 substrain vaccines, there is no reason to suspect that the 17DD and 17D-204 substrains differ with respect to safety for humans.

Examination of yellow fever vaccines manufactured in 11 countries by T_1 oligonucleotide fingerprinting revealed a very high degree of genetic similarity.[353] The primary seed and vaccine produced in South Africa (see Fig. 34–20) differed at one and two oligonucleotides, respectively. This difference was confirmed at the sequence level by Xie, who found two changes in the 3′ noncoding region.[59] Minor differences in nucleotide sequences were noted between the 17DD and 17D-204 substrains and between 17D-204 vaccines,[12, 42, 43, 354] but the strains differ by less than 0.2%. Interpretation of the true degree of heterogeneity is clouded somewhat by the fact that 17D vaccines contain heterogeneous mixtures of viral subpopulations, that some of the 17D vaccines studied underwent laboratory passages before sequencing, and that the comparison of strains was by reverse transcription–PCR consensus sequences, which may not elucidate differences in minority virion subpopulations.

Method of Manufacture, Control, and Lot Release Tests

Biological standards for yellow fever vaccines have been established by WHO,[359] and all vaccines must comply with these basic standards and be produced according to GMP. Approval for use is governed by national authorities, for example, the Food and Drug Administration in the United States, and thus biological standards differ somewhat from country to country. All manufacturers currently use seeds free from avian leukosis virus, but testing for other viral adventitious agents varies.

Primary (master) and secondary (manufacturer's working) seeds are tested for bacteria, fungi, mycoplasma, and adventitious viruses and are subjected to a standard safety and immunogenicity test in rhesus or cynomolgus monkeys.[359] A minimum of 10 monkeys is inoculated intracerebrally with 0.25 mL of virus containing 5000 to 50,000 MLD_{50}. Animals are monitored for clinical signs, viremia, antibody responses, and neuropathological lesions (Table 34–10). For comparison, a reference control is inoculated into 10 other animals. Some authorities have advised using a reference vaccine that has failed the safety test, for example, 17D Lot 6766.[358, 360]

Table 34–10. **BIOLOGICAL STANDARDS FOR MONKEY SAFETY TESTS ON 17D VACCINE SEEDS (10 NONIMMUNE RHESUS OR CYNOMOLGUS MONKEYS INOCULATED IN FRONTAL LOBE WITH 5000–50,000 MLD_{50}* AND MONITORED FOR 30 D)**

CRITERION	TEST	RESULT
Viscerotropism	Viremia level on days 2, 4, and 6	Viremia <500 MLD_{50}*/0.03 mL in all samples, and not greater than 100 MLD_{50} in more than one sample
Immunogenicity	Neutralizing antibody	>90% seroconversion on day 30
Neurotropism	Clinical observation daily for 30 days	Frequency of encephalitis and semiquantitative clinical score < reference seed
	Histological evaluation (day 30)	Mean lesion scores < reference seed†

*Or equivalent in plaque-forming units.

†Histological grading performed on five levels of brain and six of cervical and lumbar spinal cord, using semiquantitative grading score of inflammation and neuronal degeneration. Areas of brain studied include "target" areas (areas that show more severe lesions irrespective of degree of neurovirulence of virus tested); "spared" areas; and "discriminator" areas that distinguish between vaccines of low and high neurovirulence. Mean group scores for target + discriminator areas combined and for discriminator areas alone are calculated.

From World Health Organization. Requirements for Yellow Fever Vaccine (Requirements for Biological Substances No. 3). Technical Report Series. Geneva, World Health Organization, 1997.

Vaccine is produced by aseptic inoculation of secondary seed into viable embryonated eggs.[361–363] Most manufacturers use eggs from closed, special pathogen-free flocks. The dose of secondary seed virus inoculated into 7- to 9-day-old embryonated eggs is 2000 to 5000 MLD_{50} (or equivalent in PFU). After incubation for 3 to 4 days, infected embryos are aseptically harvested. Embryos must be 12 days of age or less at the time of harvest. A single harvest is the pool of embryos inoculated together in a single production run. Methods for recovery of virus from infected embryos vary, but all include homogenization to "pulp" and clarification by centrifugation to yield supernatant fluid harvest. Sterility tests are performed at one or more steps before pooling single harvests. The final bulk may contain one or a pool of single harvests. The amount of final bulk prepared is determined principally by the volume capacity of the lyophilizer. The final bulk is diluted based on potency (infectivity titer), filled into glass containers, and lyophilized. The infectivity titer of final bulk varies by manufacturer but is typically in the range of 6 to 7 $\log_{10}$ MLD_{50} per mL. The volume of supernatant recovered from a single chicken embryo is approximately 1.5 mL. Thus, the yield per embryo is in the range of 100 to 300 human doses (1 human dose = 1000 MLD_{50}). If a plaque assay is used for potency, the manufacturer must establish the relationship between MLD_{50} and plaque titer, since the WHO biological standard is tied to MLD_{50}. This relationship has sometimes been difficult to establish, reflecting the variability of plaque titrations.[363] The final bulk is tested for the absence of bacteria, fungi, mycoplasma, and (in some countries) avian leukosis virus. The protein content before the addition of stabilizers may not exceed 0.25 mg per dose. After filling, the final product is tested for identity by neutralization test, potency, thermostability, sterility, general safety in mice and guinea pigs, residual moisture, residual ovalbumin, and endotoxin. As specified by the WHO standards, potency must exceed 1000 MLD_{50} (or equivalent in plaque titer) per dose.[359] Typically, the dose in the final container exceeds the minimal specification by at least fivefold to account for losses during storage.

Cost of Manufacture and Vaccine Price

The cost of manufacture of yellow fever vaccine is modest but highly dependent on local conditions (personnel wages, overhead, and so forth.) Price and sales margins vary by market segment. Current pricing for vaccine supplied to WHO or the United Nations Children's Fund (UNICEF) for use in emergencies or for the EPI is approximately U.S. $0.18 per dose, whereas the price for yellow fever vaccine sold to travelers in developed countries is as high as $50.

Adventitious Viruses

In 1966, Harris and coworkers discovered that yellow fever 17D vaccine was contaminated with avian leukosis virus.[364] All vaccines produced at that time contained the agent, due to the high prevalence of infection of chicken embryos. New seeds free from avian leukosis virus were developed in the 1970s, and all manufacturers now employ leukosis-free seeds as stipulated by WHO standards. One current manufacturer uses embryos contaminated with avian leukosis virus for vaccine production (a practice permitted by WHO).[359] Although the presence of leukosis virus in yellow fever vaccine is certainly undesirable because of the possibility of the insertion of leukosis viral oncogenes, there is no evidence to implicate the virus in human disease. The question was addressed by a retrospective survey of World War II veterans for cancer deaths.[365] The incidence of all cancers, lymphoma, and leukemia was not significantly different (and in fact was lower) in persons vaccinated 5 to 22 years previously with 17D vaccine than in those not vaccinated. Current vaccines, although not contaminated with leukosis virus, contain endogenous sequences encoding leukosis reverse transcriptase (RT) activity, and in some cases RT activity is associated with noninfectious particles. RT activity and particles are not considered to represent a hazard to humans.

During the original formulation and early use of 17D vaccines, pooled human serum was used as a stabilizer. Vaccines were thereby contaminated with hepatitis B virus, resulting in outbreaks of jaundice (see *Adverse Events*). Human serum was eliminated from yellow fever vaccines by 1942.

Dose and Route of Administration

Yellow fever vaccine is given by the subcutaneous route in a volume of 0.5 mL. The usual site of inoculation is the upper arm; there are no data to suggest that the anatomical site of inoculation is relevant to the immune response. Care is taken to avoid exposure of the live vaccine to alcohol or other skin disinfectants. The minimal dose requirement is 1000 MLD_{50}, or the equivalent in PFU. Since commercial vaccines contain an excess of virus to provide for losses during storage, the delivered dose is higher than the minimal standard. The actual dose contained in commercial vaccines varies but at the time of release ranges from 5 to 50 times the minimum.

Preparations Available Including Combinations

All yellow fever vaccines in current use are live attenuated 17DD or 17D-204 substrain viruses, prepared in embryonated chicken eggs and formulated as lyophilized powder. Vaccines vary with respect to stabilizer additives and salt content. Some contain sodium chloride and buffer salts and are reconstituted with sterile water, whereas others are reconstituted with saline solution. Vaccines differ with respect to expiry date, but all require storage at the point of use at 2 to 8°C and must be discarded 1 hour after reconstitution. Vaccines are supplied in single- and multiple-dose containers, the largest of which contains 100 doses for use in jet injectors. Vaccines produced in France (Stamaril, Pasteur Mérieux); England (Arilvax, Evans Medical); and Brazil (Bio-Manguinhos) are exported for international use or supplied to the EPI through the UNICEF bid market. The vaccines produced in the United States (YF-Vax, Connaught Laboratories) and in Russia (Institute of Poliomyelitis and Viral Encephalitides) are used almost exclusively in country for travelers and military personnel, with small amounts exported to foreign distributors. Although certain combination vaccines have been clinically tested (including yellow fever–measles and yellow fever–typhoid), no products are currently commercialized.

Constituents, Including Antibiotics and Preservatives

There are no antibiotics or preservatives in yellow fever vaccines. Salt, buffer, and stabilizers vary by manufacturer.

Vaccine Thermostability

In 1987, WHO published an addendum to the biological standards, with a guideline (not a formal requirement) that vaccines meet a stability standard.[366] The specification included two criteria: the lyophilized vaccine held at 37°C for 14 days must (1) maintain minimal potency (>1000 MLD_{50} per 0.5-mL dose) and (2) show a mean loss of titer less than 1.0 $\log_{10}LD_{50}$. Of the vaccines produced by the 12 approved manufacturers at that time, only five met the stability specifications.[367] Current WHO Requirements for Yellow Fever Vaccine make the stability standard a requirement and also stipulate that the minimal vaccine expiry date shall be not less than 2 years after the last satisfactory potency test.[359]

Without stabilizers, yellow fever vaccine loses 1.5 to 2.5 $\log_{10}$ per dose during 14 days at 37°C. Stabilized vaccines lose only 0.3 to 0.5 $\log_{10}$ per dose during this interval.[368] In one study, a stabilized vaccine met WHO standards after storage at 2 to 8°C and ambient temperature for more than 2 years.[368] Stabilized yellow fever vaccine has a similar or better stability profile than other thermolabile vaccines used in the EPI (including polio, measles, and pertussis vaccines). Thus, although the lyophilized vaccine requires proper storage and handling under cold chain conditions in the field, yellow fever vaccine is not the "weak link" in the EPI system. Stabilizers differ by manufacturer. The vaccines produced in the United States and England use sorbitol and gelatin. The vaccine made in France employs sugars, amino acids, and divalent cations (lactose [4%], sorbitol [2%], histidine [0.01 M], and alanine [0.01 M] in phosphate-buffered saline containing Ca^{2+} and Mg^{2+}).[369, 370] A disadvantage of yellow fever vaccine is its instability after reconstitution. The vaccine must be held on ice after reconstitution and is generally discarded after 1 hour. Unpublished studies indicate that some vaccines may be somewhat more stable and could be held on ice for longer intervals (several hours). This instability leads to wastage under field conditions during mass immunization campaigns and to potential vaccine failures if directions for use are not followed. Lopes and associates found that vaccine maintained potency at 37°C for more than 3 hours in distilled water, whereas vaccine in phosphate buffer or saline with or without stabilizers lost potency.[371] However, the water diluent was found to cause severe pain at the injection site, and its use has been discontinued.

Genetic Stability During Replication in the Host

17D vaccines are not biologically cloned and contain heterogeneous subpopulations of plaque-size variants with differing mouse neurovirulence.[58, 59, 70] One variant recovered from 17D vaccine by plaque purification had a wild-type epitope and amino acid change at position E-173.[33, 49, 70] The relative proportion of plaque-size variants in 17D vaccines changes with passage.[58] However, given the safety record of 17D vaccines since stabilization of the passage level, heterogeneity does not pose a safety problem and in fact has been proposed to be a positive attribute of the vaccine.[44] No individual plaque variant has shown a neurovirulence phenotype that exceeds the vaccine itself, and thus changes in their relative proportions on replication in humans might not alter virulence. Recently, Xie and coworkers sequenced 17D viral strains isolated from the sera of six subjects given the 17D-204 vaccine produced in the United States.[372] No mutations were found in the structural genes, and no more than two nucleotide changes were found in NS5 regions. Similarly, viral strains recovered from sera of monkeys 30 days after intracerebral inoculation of 17D-204 vaccine contained no mutations or a single silent mutation in NS5.[59] These results indicate a high degree of genetic stability of 17D virus during in vivo replication. Mutations tend to accumulate at a significantly lower rate (10^{-5}–10^{-6}) than expected for an RNA virus, and in a nonrandom fashion, principally in the NS5 gene.

On the other hand, rare mutational events in 17D vaccine during replication in the host have been shown to alter pathogenicity. The only recorded fatal case of encephalitis occurred in 1965 in a 3-year-old child who received 17D-204 vaccine.[52] The characteristics of the virus from brain tissue and commercial 17D vaccines at similar laboratory passage level were defined by Jennings and colleagues.[53] Compared with commercial vaccine, the brain isolate had higher neurovirulence for mice, caused severe encephalitis in a cynomolgus monkey, and reacted with a wild-type specific monoclonal antibody. The brain isolate differed from 17D-204 at two residues in the E gene (E-155 and E-303) and one in NS4b. The potential role of these mutations in neurovirulence, particularly the change at position E-303, has been discussed under *Virology*.

RESULTS OF VACCINATION

Viremia Following 17D Vaccination

Whereas wild-type yellow fever virus causes high viremias in monkeys and humans, 17D vaccine induces minimal virus titers in circulating blood. A control test for the reduced viscerotropism of 17D vaccines is the measurement of viremia in monkeys on days 2, 4, and 6 following intracerebral inoculation, which must not exceed 500 MLD_{50} per 0.03 mL on any day and must not exceed 100 MLD_{50} per 0.03 mL on more than 1 day.[359]

Viremia following 17D vaccination has been measured in adult humans. Smith and associates found virus in the serum of 13 (46%) of 28 subjects given 3 to 4 $\log_{10}$ MLD_{50} of 17D vaccine.[21] The earliest onset of viremia occurred on day 4 and the latest on day 10. Of the 13 viremic individuals, 4 were viremic for 1 day, 5 for 2 days, and 4 for 3 days. The quantity of virus in blood was extremely small in all cases (<2 MLD_{50}/0.03 mL). Sweet and coworkers measured viremias in subjects with and without prevaccination neutralizing antibodies to Japanese encephalitis virus.[104] The 17D vaccine (National Drug Company, United States) contained approximately 6.4 $\log_{10}$ *suckling mouse* $ICLD_{50}$ per dose (equivalent to approximately 5.3–5.8 $\log_{10}MLD_{50}$,[373] and thus substantially higher than the dose used by Smith and associates[21]). Viremia was measured by IC inoculation of infant mice with undiluted serum. Of 25 subjects without preexisting flavivirus immunity, 15 (60%) had detectable viremia on 1 or more days during the 6-day sampling period (days 3–8 after vaccination.) The highest incidence of viremia (48%) was on day 5, and the mean duration was 1.9 days. Titers were very low, as none of the sera caused 100% mortality in infant mice. There was no difference in the incidence or duration of viremia in subjects with preexisting immunity to Japanese encephalitis virus.[104]

In a study of 15 young adults, Wheelock and Sibley determined 17D viremia by a more sensitive method (inoculation of 0.1 mL of plasma into tube cultures of BHK-21 cells).[374] Fourteen subjects (93.3%) had detectable viremia. The average time to the onset of viremia was 4.4 days (range 3–6 days), and the mean duration was 2.5 days (range 1–5 days). Viremic days were sequential and continuous in most cases, but one individual had detectable viremia on days 4, 8, and 9. A rough estimation of the level of viremia was possible based on the detection in cell cultures inoculated with differing volumes of plasma. Virus titers were exceedingly low; in only 3 of 14 individuals was virus detected in cultures inoculated with 0.001 mL of plasma.

Actis and Sa Fleitas studied 12 adults who received an unspecified dose of 17DD-EP vaccine produced in Brazil.[375] The duration and level of viremia, detected by IC inoculation of weanling mice, was similar to that of previous studies, but a somewhat higher proportion of subjects were viremic than in other studies using mice for the detection of viremia.

Taken together, these studies confirm that very low levels of virus are present in circulating blood for a brief period following 17D vaccination. The proportion of viremic subjects in published studies is variable (Fig. 34–21) but is less than 100%. Viremia occurs during the latter half of the first week after vaccination, and thus the incubation period and duration of viremia are not dissimilar to natural infection with yellow fever virus. Cessation of viremia corresponds to the time of appearance of neutralizing antibodies around 7 days after immunization (see *Kinetics of the Immune Response*). Titers of virus in blood are far below the infection threshold for mosquito vectors. The low viremia following 17D vaccine administration may also explain the apparently low risk of transmission of the virus to the fetus in women who have been immunized during pregnancy (see under *Pregnancy and Lactation*) and the low incidence of postvaccinal encephalitis. The detection of viremia is influenced by the test methodology. No studies have been published using PCR, which is unlikely to be more sensitive than infectivity assays but might detect viral genome in the absence of infectivity, for example, after the appearance of antibody.

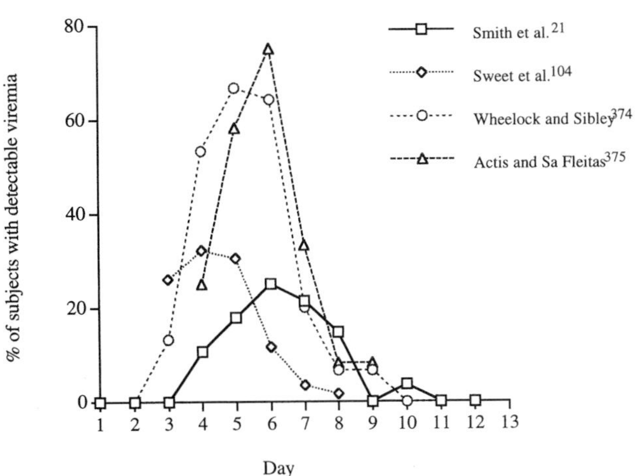

Figure 34–21. Viremic responses in healthy adults inoculated with yellow fever 17D vaccine; results of four published studies.

There are no data on viremia levels in infants or children given 17D vaccine. The higher risk of postvaccinal encephalitis in young infants suggests the possibility that viremia levels may be higher or more prolonged (alternatively, susceptibility could reflect immaturity of the blood-brain barrier). Nor are data available on the height and duration of viremia in people who are immunosuppressed.

Immune Responses

The neutralizing antibody response to 17D vaccine has been evaluated in numerous studies since the development of the vaccine in the late 1930s. Theiler and Smith[20] and Smith and coworkers[21] demonstrated the appearance of neutralizing antibodies within 1 to 2 weeks after immunization. In a field study in Brazil (1937–1938), 94.1% of 882 vaccinees seroconverted after vaccination.[21] Subsequent clinical trials have confirmed the high immunogenicity of yellow fever 17D vaccine, with the development of neutralizing antibodies exceeding 90% in nearly all studies (Table 34–11). Response rates have been similar for vaccines produced from the 17DD and 17D-204 substrains, for vaccines formulated with or without stabilizers, and for vaccines with and without avian leukosis virus. Although some early reports suggested that young children did not re-

Table 34–11. **SEROCONVERSION RATES AND NEUTRALIZING ANTIBODY RESPONSES TO YELLOW FEVER 17D VACCINE IN CLINICAL TRIALS**

STUDY	VACCINE MANUFACTURER	VACCINE SPECIFICATION	DOSE (LOG_{10})	METHOD	INTERVAL*	AGE	STUDY SITE	N	SEROCONVERSION (%)	TITER	TEST USED	REFERENCE
1	National Drug Co. (USA)		6.1–6.4 $SMLD_{50}$	NSI	21 d	Adults	USA, Japan	41†	100	>500	SDNT (IC, mice)‡	394
2	National Drug Co. (USA)		6.8 MLD_{50}	JI	3 wk	5–54 mo	Burkina Faso	72	97	NT	LNI (IC, mice)	456
3	Wellcome (UK)	ALV-contaminated	4.1–4.4 MLD_{50}	NSI	1 mo	Adults	England	38	97.4	1.6	LNI (IC, mice)	483
		ALV-free	4.1–4.4 MLD_{50}	NSI	1 mo	Adults	England	59	98.3	1.7	LNI (IC, mice)	
4	National Drug Co. (USA)	ALV-contaminated	6.2–6.7 MLD_{50}	NSI or JI	28 d	Adults	USA	187	>99	2.2–3.5	LNI (cell culture)	386
		ALV-free	5.6–6.0 MLD_{50}	NSI	28 d	Adults	USA	187	>98	2.2–3.1	LNI (cell culture)	
5	National Drug Co. (USA)	Administered with or without smallpox vaccine at varied intervals	4.3–5.0 MLD_{50}	NSI	28 d	Adults	USA	483	99.8	2.2–2.6	LNI (cell culture)	484
6	Wellcome (UK)	Not stabilized	4.4 MLD_{50}	NSI	28 d	Adults	England	10	100	2.7	LNI (cell culture)	390
		Stabilized	4.2 MLD_{50}	NSI	28 d	Adults	England	20	100	2.9	LNI (cell culture)	
7	Institut Pasteur (Senegal)		ND	JI	25 d	Adults and children	Gambia	41	92.7	≥13.1	PRNT	179
8	Wellcome (UK)	ALV-free, stabilized	>3.0 MLD_{50}	NSI	2–11 wk	Adults	England	600	96.0	2.19	LNI (cell culture)	421
9	Connaught (USA)	ALV-free	3.7 PFU (LLC-MK2)	NSI	1 mo	Adults	USA	28§	100	415	PRNT	485
10	Pasteur Mérieux (France)	Stabilized, ALV-free	5.3–5.4 PFU (PS)	NSI	1 mo	1–5 yr	Central African Republic	209	94	‖	PRNT	486
11	Pasteur Mérieux (France)	Not stabilized	ND	NSI	1 mo +	Adults	France	143	99.3	14	PRNT	487
		Stabilized	ND	NSI	1 mo +	Adults	France	115	100	13	PRNT	
12	Institut Pasteur (Senegal)	Combined with DTP-polio, measles with or without HBV	ND	NSI	60 d	18–26 mo	Senegal	188	91.5–93.6	19.4–31.8	PRNT	457
13	FioCruz (Brazil)	17DD substrain; not stabilized	3.7 MLD_{50}	NSI	28 d	Adults	Brazil	15	100	1656	PRNT	391
		17DD substrain; stabilized	3.8 MLD_{50}	NSI	28 d	Adults	Brazil	31	100	1790	PRNT	
14	Pasteur Mérieux (France)	Stabilized, ALV-free	ND	NSI	45 d	6–7 mo	Ivory Coast	50	91	>1:5	PRNT	488
15	Pasteur Mérieux (France)	Stabilized, ALV-free	3.91 MLD_{50}	NSI	30 d	6–12 mo	Cameroon	68	92.6	22.63	PRNT	455
16	Pasteur Mérieux (France)	Stabilized, ALV-free	ND	NSI	195–240 d	4–8 mo	Mali	52	96.2	19.8	PRNT	489
		Stabilized, ALV-free	ND	NSI	195–240 d	12–24 mo	Mali	19	94.7	29.5		
17	Connaught (USA)		ND	BJS	4–6 wk	Adults	USA	32	81	49.5	PRNT	490
18	Pasteur Mérieux (France)	Stabilized, ALV-free	ND	JI	2–4 wk	Adults	Nigeria	331¶	88.5	NT	PRNT	409
19	Pasteur Mérieux (France)	Stabilized, ALV-free	ND	NSI	45 d	Adults	France	36	100	NT	PRNT	491
20	Pasteur Mérieux (France)	Stabilized, ALV-free	3.9 $TCID_{50}$	NSI	35 d	Adults	Europe	41	100	26.6	PRNT	453
21	Pasteur Mérieux (France)	Combined with measles or HBV + measles	ND	NSI	30 d	9 mo	Senegal	172	96	16.8	PRNT	492
22	FioCruz (Brazil)	17DD substrain; stabilized	ND	JI	6 mo	>6 years	Brazil	161	86.8	NT§	PRNT	493
23	Pasteur Mérieux (France)	Combined with HAV and typhoid	ND	NSI	28 d	Adults	Switzerland	56	100	752	PRNT	494
24	Connaught (USA)	Stabilized, ALV-free	ND	NSI	28–30 d	Adults	USA	Approx. 35	Not specified	226.3	PRNT	454

*Interval between vaccination and serological testing.
†Volunteers in study with no preexisting yellow fever immunity.
‡Serum-dilution constant-virus neutralization test performed in suckling mice inoculated IC.
§17/28 subjects had previously received an experimental vaccine against dengue type 2.
‖78% of vaccinees had high neutralizing antibody titers (≥320).
¶Includes all subjects in study except pregnant women.

ALV, avian leukosis virus; DTP, diphtheria, pertussis, and tetanus; HBV, hepatitis B virus; HAV, hepatitis A virus; LNI, log neutralization index; PRNT, plaque-reduction neutralization test; M, mouse neutralization test; $SMLD_{50}$, suckling mouse LD_{50}; MLD_{50}, mouse LD_{50} performed per World Health Organization (WHO) requirements in 4- to 6-wk-old animals; NSI, needle and syringe injection; BJS, BioJect system; JI, jet injection; NT, not tested; ND, not determined, but vaccine meets WHO standards (>1000 MLD_{50}); PFU, plaque-forming units, titration in cell culture (type specified); $TCID_{50}$, tissue culture median infective dose; IC, intracerebral.

Table 34–12. **NEUTRALIZING ANTIBODY RESPONSE TO YELLOW FEVER 17D VACCINE CORRELATES WITH PROTECTION AGAINST CHALLENGE WITH 5.0 LOG_{10} LD_{50} OF VIRULENT ASIBI VIRUS**

LOG NEUTRALIZATION INDEX (PLAQUE REDUCTION)	PROTECTED	
	Yes	No
≥0.7	51/54 (94%)	1/11 (9%)
<0.7	3/54 (6%)	10/11 (91%)

Chi-square $P < .0001$.
From Mason RA, Tauraso NM, Spertzel RO, et al. Yellow fever vaccine: Direct challenge of monkeys given graded doses of 17D vaccine. Appl Microbiol 25:539, 1973.

spond as well as older persons to 17D vaccine or lost immunity more rapidly,[376, 377] this was not confirmed in other contemporary studies[378, 379] or in recent trials (Table 34–11). Race and gender do not appear to influence response rates, but specific studies are lacking.

Neutralizing antibody levels following the administration of 17D vaccine show individual variability. In the majority of cases, antibody titers are lower and their appearance is delayed compared with natural infection with yellow fever virus,[15, 21, 157] reflecting less viral replication and antigen expression of the attenuated strain. The minimal protective level of neutralizing antibodies induced by 17D vaccine has been estimated by dose-response studies in rhesus monkeys that were challenged after immunization with virulent yellow fever.[347, 373, 380] A $\log_{10}$ neutralization index (LNI, measured by plaque reduction) of 0.7 or more measured before challenge (20 weeks after immunization) was strongly associated with protection (Table 34–12). Of 11 vaccinated monkeys that succumbed to challenge, 10 had a prechallenge LNI of 0.5 or less and 1 had an LNI of 0.9. Clinical trials of 17D vaccine have shown geometric mean LNI values of 2.2 or more measured within a relatively brief interval (usually 1 month) after vaccination (Table 34–11). As pointed out later, antibody titers measured by serum dilution plaque-reduction tests have been much more variable, and no cutoff correlating with protection has been established.

Other experimental evidence supports the concept that minimal immunity is required for protection. Neutralizing antibodies appear in the sera of rhesus monkeys on day 6 to 7 after inoculation of 17D virus. However, some monkeys survive a challenge performed after a shorter interval (1, 3, 5 days) after vaccination, despite the absence of detectable antibodies.[18, 145] Early protection may be mediated by a low-level specific antibody response (see *Kinetics of the Immune Response*), or by nonspecific responses (interferon, NK cells).

Test Methods Affecting Interpretation of Antibody Responses

Various methods have been used to measure neutralizing antibodies, and these methods vary with respect to sensitivity (Table 34–13). Tests in mice were used through the 1950s and in some laboratories thereafter, but these tests were subject to considerable variability (reviewed by Smithburn[381]). The intraperitoneal neutralization test in newborn or 18- to 21-day-old mice was shown to be more sensitive for the detection of neutralizing antibodies than the IC test, because of the higher and more rapid lethality of virus for mice inoculated by the latter route.[145, 382]

Tissue culture neutralization tests have replaced tests in mice. These tests avoid the need for animals, are considerably more convenient and less costly, provide results in a shorter time (5–7 days versus 21 days in mice), and are more reliable and quantitative.[382, 383] A standardized plaque-reduction test has been de-

Table 34–13. **METHODS USED TO MEASURE YELLOW FEVER–NEUTRALIZING ANTIBODY RESPONSES IN ANIMALS AND HUMANS**

HOST (AGE)	DESCRIPTION	ENDPOINT	COMMENT
Monkey (rhesus)	Simultaneous subcutaneous (SC) or intraperitoneal (IP) inoculation of test serum and virus	Death	Used in early studies before development of mouse model
Mouse (adult)	Intracerebral (IC) inoculation of preincubated mixture of serum with constant virus dose (100 LD_{50})	Survival ratio or survival time. Quantitative test (neutralization index*) measures difference in viral titer between test and control sera	In screening test, survival time endpoint more sensitive
Mouse (adult)	IC inoculation of starch followed by IP inoculation of serum-virus mixture	Survival ratio	Extensively employed in early serological surveys
Mouse (18–21 d)	IP inoculation of serum-virus mixture	Survival ratio	More sensitive (higher serum antibody titers) than adult mouse tests
Mouse (newborn)	SC, IP, or IC inoculation of serum-virus mixtures	Survival ratio	More sensitive (higher serum antibody titers) than adult mouse tests
Cell culture	Constant serum–varying virus dilution	Neutralization index* determined by plaque reduction or CPE	Measures quantity of virus neutralized by neat or low dilution of serum
Cell culture	Constant virus–varying serum dilution	Highest serum dilution reducing a defined proportion of plaques	Sensitivity varies with endpoint selected (50, 70, 90% plaque reduction)

*$\log_{10}$ neutralization index.
CPE, cytopathic effect.

scribed.[382, 384] A variety of continuous cell lines, including monkey kidney cells (MA-104, LLC-MK2, Vero), hamster kidney cells (BHK-21), porcine kidney cells (PS), and primary chick or duck embryo cells, may be used, and no clear differences in results have been found among these host cells. A comparative study showed that the intraperitoneal neutralization test performed in newborn mice was somewhat more sensitive for the assay of neutralizing antibodies than the constant serum–varying virus plaque–reduction test in MA-104 cells.[382] The cell culture test was, however, more sensitive than the IC suckling or adult mouse tests. Similarly, Poland and colleagues showed that a constant virus–serum dilution plaque-reduction test in Vero cells was more sensitive than the IC adult mouse neutralization test.[385]

Although differences in test sensitivity account for the variable geometric mean antibody responses noted in clinical trials (Table 34–11), they do not appear to influence seroconversion rates, when seroconversion is measured relatively early (e.g., 1 month or several months) after vaccination. However, the determination of low antibody levels, for example many years after vaccination, may be problematic if an insensitive test is used. In a study of persons vaccinated 30 to 35 years earlier, Poland and coworkers found that the IC adult mouse neutralization test had a 52% false-negative rate compared with plaque reduction, with the false-negative sera having low antibody titers.[385]

As shown in Table 34–11, the serum dilution plaque-neutralization test has been used in recent years as the method of choice in clinical studies of yellow fever vaccines. However, a standardized assay was not used in these clinical trials. The sensitivity (reflected by the geometric mean antibody titer) has varied considerably, presumably due to methodological differences (use of accessory factor [complement]; agar overlay composition; plaque-detection staining methods; and the end-point [proportion of plaques reduced]). These variables make it impossible to compare immunogenicity in terms of antibody titers across different clinical trials. For these reasons, the constant serum–varying virus neutralization test is considered a preferable method for the determination of the antibody response to yellow fever vaccine. This method has been standardized, is reproducible, and has been rigorously compared with the mouse neutralization test.[382] The cutoff for a positive test has been established by experience and convention (log_{10} neutralization index of 0.7), and the level of neutralization (quantity of virus neutralized) in undiluted or minimally diluted serum may be biologically more meaningful than a serum dilution endpoint titer. For the measurement of the immune response in an individual, the difference in titer between pre- and postvaccination sera expressed as the log_{10} neutralization index represents the neutralizing capacity of the serum. Since complement increases the sensitivity of the yellow fever neutralization test, and since complement levels may be unstable in stored sera, it is preferable to heat-inactivate test samples and to add complement (or a standard source of fresh-frozen serum) to the virus-serum mixture.

The HI and CF methods have been used to measure responses to yellow fever vaccine.[343, 379, 382, 386, 387] The HI test is less sensitive than neutralization and is complicated by low specificity in persons with prior flavivirus exposure.[388] The choice of yellow fever antigen may affect results; the use of 17D viral antigen provided a more sensitive assay for detecting vaccine-induced immunity than antigens prepared from the FNV or a wild-type (JSS) strain.[387]

Individuals without prior flavivirus exposure generally do not develop CF antibodies after the administration of 17D vaccine.[178, 179] The CF test has therefore been thought to distinguish recent infection with wild-type virus from vaccine-induced immunity. However, in one study, individuals with prior heterologous flavivirus immunity developed broadly cross-reactive CF antibodies to yellow fever after 17D vaccination.[179] IgG ELISA is unsatisfactory for the detection of seroconversion to 17D vaccine.[146b]

Vaccine Dose

The minimal potency requirement for yellow fever 17D vaccine is 3.0 log_{10} MLD_{50} (or the number of plaque-forming units in cell culture shown to be equivalent to that dose).[359] The vaccine potency of manufactured lots exceeds this minimal limit by at least fivefold to account for losses on storage.

A dose-response relationship was observed in rhesus monkeys inoculated intramuscularly with 17D vaccine (Fig. 34–22).[373, 380] The dose at which 90% of the animals developed a rise in LNI greater than 0.7 was approximately 1000 MLD_{50}, and the 90% protective dose against lethal challenge was approximately 200 adult MLD_{50}. The 50% immunizing dose (ID_{50}) was approximately 2 MLD_{50}.

The dose-response relationship in humans was first determined by Fox and associates in 1943.[389] The mini-

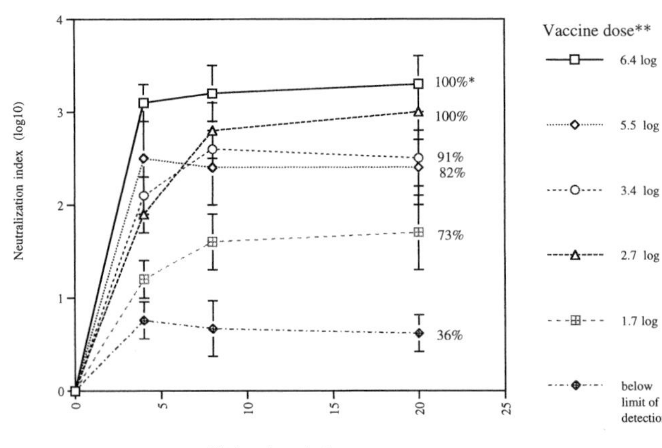

Figure 34–22. Neutralizing antibody responses (mean + SE) in rhesus monkeys immunized with graded doses of yellow fever 17D vaccine. *Percent of monkeys positive (log neutralization index ≥0.7) 20 weeks after immunization. **Suckling mouse median lethal dose of 0.5 mL inoculum. (Data from Mason RA, Tauraso NM, Ginn RK. Yellow fever vaccine. V. Antibody response in monkeys inoculated with graded doses of the 17D vaccine. Appl Microbiol 23:908, 1972.)

mal dose resulting in seroconversion was between 14 and 140 MLD_{50}. At a dose of 14 MLD_{50}, 70% of the volunteers seroconverted. Large-scale field trials of various vaccine lots, some of which were of suboptimal potency, indicated that the administration of doses in the range of 10 to 50 MLD_{50} immunized more than 85% of vaccinees. More recent dose-response measurements (Table 34–14) indicate that doses of 100 to 200 MLD_{50} result in seroconversion of more than 90% of people vaccinated. Thus, the minimal potency requirements set by WHO for yellow fever vaccines exceeds the 90% immunizing dose by fivefold to 50-fold.

Interestingly, an inverse relationship between vaccine dose and antibody titer has been consistently observed.[344, 347, 390, 391] Smith and colleagues found significantly higher responses in subjects given doses of 5 to 50 MLD_{50} than in those given doses of 500 to 5000 MLD_{50}.[344] In monkeys, inoculation of large doses of 17D virus resulted in earlier appearance of viremia, but viremia was inconsistent, lower in magnitude, and briefer in duration than after inoculation of diluted virus.[347] Limited replication of the virus after the inoculation of very large doses may explain the lower magnitude of the immune response. This dose prozone effect is also clearly evident in mice (Fig. 34–23) and may be explained by the presence of interferon (produced in the infected egg), defective interfering particles, or noninfectious antigen competing for cell receptors.

Panthier suggested that a low dose of 17D vaccine may cause a delay in antibody response and an increased risk of encephalitis.[351] This hypothesis was based on a single case of encephalitis in a 4-week-old infant after pricking the skin with a needle dipped in 17D vaccine, and on the work of Fox and Penna in monkeys.[347] A low dose due to loss of vaccine potency was suggested as a factor in encephalitis caused by FNV in some epidemics.[392] It is now known, however, that the vaccination of

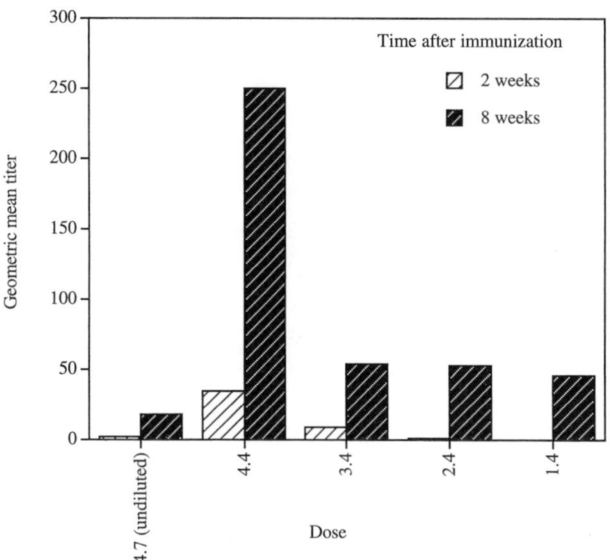

Figure 34–23. Neutralizing antibody response to yellow fever 17D vaccine in mice, showing the geometric mean titer of groups of five Swiss Webster mice inoculated subcutaneously with 0.1 mL of graded doses of commercial yellow fever 17D vaccine and tested 2 and 8 weeks after immunization. The plaque-reduction endpoint was 50%. (From Guirakhoo F, Monath TP, unpublished data, 1997.)

infants younger than 4 months carries a higher risk of encephalitis due to age susceptibility, not vaccine dose (see under *Adverse Events*). Moreover, the application of low doses of 17D vaccine by scarification was not associated with adverse reactions.[334, 335] The administration of small, intradermal doses of 17D vaccine is standard practice in people with a history of egg allergy,[392a, 393] and there are no reports of an increased risk of encephalitis after this procedure. Finally, an epidemic of postvaccinal encephalitis due to FNV occurred in Senegal in 1965, when vaccine potency was not in question.[329]

Table 34–14. **RELATIONSHIP BETWEEN DOSE OF YELLOW FEVER 17D VACCINE AND NEUTRALIZING ANTIBODY RESPONSE**

VACCINE MANUFACTURER	DOSE	NO. SUBJECTS	SEROCONVERSION RATE (%)	MEAN ANTIBODY TITER*	50% IMMUNIZING DOSE†	REFERENCE
South African Institute for Medical Research	5000 MLD_{50}	4	100	1.55	~5 MLD_{50}	344
	500	7	100	1.80		
	50	8	100	3.04		
	5	8	62.5	2.80		
Wellcome (UK)	200,000 PFU	20	100	2.93–2.96	42 PFU (~7 MLD_{50})	390
	200	13	85	2.97		
	50	12	58	3.10		
	10	13	0	—		
BioManguinhos (Brazil)	2000 PFU‡	12	100	—	~20 PFU (~60 MLD_{50})	391
	1000–2000	34	100	—		
	500–1000	10	100	—		
	200–500	34	100	—		
	100–200	32	93.7	—		
	50–100	59	81.3	—		
	20–50	25	84.0	—		
	<20	53	41.5	—		

* Log neutralization index.

† LD_{50}/PFU ratio varies for different vaccines, based on differences between the sensitivity of the assays employed or (possibly) mouse virulence of the vaccines. The Wellcome vaccine (Freestone et al[390]) had an MLD_{50}/PFU ratio of 0.17, whereas the FioCruz vaccine (Lopes et al[391]) had an MLD_{50}/PFU ratio of 2.9.

‡ Range of doses for volunteers receiving different vaccine lots tested in the study.

MLD_{50}, mouse LD_{50}; PFU, plaque-forming units.

Kinetics of the Immune Response

Studies in rhesus monkeys established that neutralizing antibodies were detectable in serum on day 6 or 7 following inoculation of 17D virus, at which time the animals were completely refractory to challenge. Significant protection was present 1 to 2 days before the appearance of detectable neutralizing antibodies,[20, 145, 381] suggesting that very low levels of antibody were protective. Occasional animals survived challenge at even earlier times after 17D immunization, suggesting that interferon or other antiviral mechanisms may also play a role in protection.

Human immunization with 17D virus is also followed by the rapid appearance of neutralizing antibodies, the detection of antibodies being dependent on the sensitivity of the neutralization assay. Early studies using the mouse protection test failed to detect antibodies 7 days after vaccination, but the majority of individuals had seroconverted on day 14.[20, 21] Smithburn and Mahaffy found neutralizing antibodies in 10% of a small group of subjects on day 7 and in 90% on day 10 after immunization.[145] Wisseman and associates found no evidence for immunity on day 6, but all subjects had seroconverted by day 14 after vaccination.[394] Based on human and monkey studies, Courtois concluded that ". . .man seems unable to form antibodies so early as the rhesus but by the 10th day his serum has a very high degree of protectivity. Judging from the studies carried out in monkeys, it seems probable that a protective mechanism begins to operate in man by the 8th or 9th day."[395] This conclusion was incorporated into the International Health regulations, which stipulate that the vaccination certificate for yellow fever is valid 10 days after the administration of 17D vaccine.[396]

Studies employing more sensitive neutralization tests have demonstrated antibodies at earlier times following the administration of 17D vaccine. Monath found the earliest evidence for neutralizing antibodies by a plaque-reduction assay on day 4 in one of four volunteers, with all subjects seroconverting by day 8.[397] The time to appearance of antibodies was not shortened by the use of a kinetic neutralization test. Bonnevie-Nielsen and coworkers found no antibodies by plaque-reduction neutralization test on day 4 after vaccination; 25% were immune on day 7 and 87.5% on day 12.[146b] Thus, it appears that immunity to yellow fever may appear in a minority subset of individuals during the first week after immunization. Neutralizing antibody levels continue to increase during the first month after immunization, with peak titers found at 3 to 4 weeks.[394, 397]

Antibody Subclass Response

The primary immune response is characterized by the appearance of neutralizing antibodies of the IgM class between days 4 and 7, several days before the detection of IgG antibodies.[397] Titers of IgM neutralizing antibodies were 16- to 256-fold higher than IgG antibodies during the first 4 to 6 weeks after immunization, and IgM antibodies were found to persist for at least 18 months (the longest time examined). Prolonged synthesis of IgM antibodies may indicate the persistence of antigen, possibly explaining the durability of yellow fever immunity (see *Duration of Immunity*).

During a field study in Nigeria, 141 (36.6%) of 385 persons vaccinated with 17D seroconverted by IgM antibody–capture ELISA.[94] However, prior flavivirus exposure in this population was high, and this may have reduced IgM responses. In a clinical study in Europe, IgM antibodies measured by capture ELISA appeared in five of six volunteers between the seventh and 12th day after primary immunization.[146b] IgM antibodies were, however, not detected by this method in subjects tested 2 years and 2 months after primary immunization. As expected, the memory B-cell response after yellow fever revaccination was not associated with an IgM response.

Revaccination

According to International Health Regulations,[396] the yellow fever immunization certificate for international travel is valid for 10 years, whereupon revaccination is required. The regulation is conservative, since vaccine immunity appears to last several decades if not for life.[385]

In some studies, prior immunity inhibited the response to revaccination, an expected finding for a live vaccine. In others, revaccination or vaccination of individuals with naturally acquired immunity was followed by a booster response in the majority of subjects, indicating that sufficient virus replication had occurred or that the antigenic mass of neutralized virus in the vaccine dose was sufficient to elicit a memory response. A booster response to revaccination was more likely in individuals with a low neutralizing antibody titer.[398]

Smith and coworkers revaccinated eight subjects who had received 17D vaccine at least once (and up to five times) between 1 and 14 years previously and who had LNIs of 2.1 to 3.6.[344] Only one subject developed a significant rise in neutralizing antibodies. Wisseman and Sweet revaccinated 11 adults 14 months after primary immunization.[185] None had detectable viremia after revaccination, but all responded with a rise in neutralizing antibodies, and 7 (64%) had greater than fourfold increases in titer (Fig. 34–24). The geometric mean titer rose from 121 to 576 after revaccination, but in most subjects the response was lower than to primary immunization. The dose of virus administered by the latter authors was 10- to 30-fold higher that that administered by Smith and coworkers[344]; this plus the lower number of prior immunizations may explain the difference between the studies. Fox and Cabral also concluded that a higher dose of 17D was required to boost individuals with preexisting immunity.[376]

Revaccination of 10 subjects 2 years after primary immunization was characterized by an increase in IgG antibodies detected by ELISA.[146b] This response was greater than that observed in controls undergoing primary immunization, indicating a memory response due to prior sensitization. In another study, two individuals who were revaccinated 3 to 18 months after their last

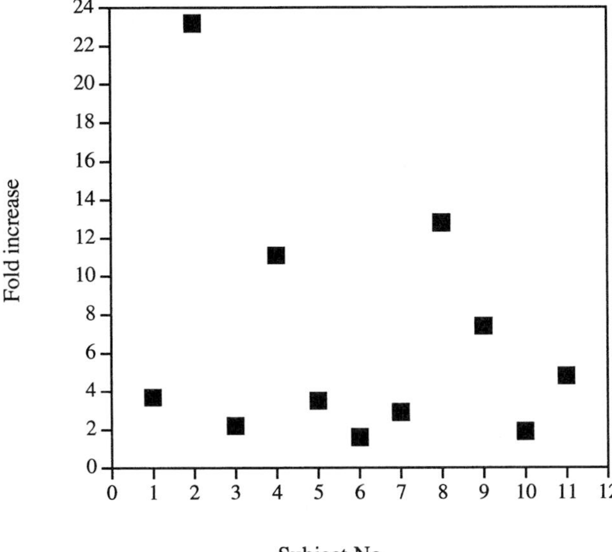

Figure 34–24. Fold increase in neutralizing antibody titer in adults reimmunized with yellow fever 17D vaccine 14 months after primary immunization. Antibodies were measured by a serum dilution constant virus test in weanling mice. (Data from Wisseman CLJ, Sweet B. Immunological studies with group B arthropod-borne viruses. III. Response of human subjects to revaccination with 17D strain yellow fever vaccine. Am J Trop Med Hyg 11:570, 1962.)

immunization had a rise in HI, but not neutralizing antibody titers.[397]

Immunization in Individuals with Prior Flavivirus Immunity

Yellow fever is distinct by neutralization test from other flaviviruses,[383, 399] but it shares antigenic determinants detected by binding assays, hemagglutination inhibition, and complement fixation.[154] Due to these cross-reactive determinants, the immune response to 17D vaccine is qualitatively different in naive individuals and in those with prior heterologous immunity. The principal question is: Does preexisting heterologous immunity reduce (by virtue of cross-protective antigens) or increase (through immune enhancement) the seroconversion rate, antibody titer, or antibody duration following 17D immunization? Conversely, Does prior 17D vaccination modify the response to other flavivirus vaccines or natural infection?

Interference with 17D Vaccine Caused by Heterologous Immunity

Interference by naturally acquired heterologous flavivirus immunity with the response to 17D vaccine is anticipated by experimental and field studies showing that heterologous immunity to dengue, Wesselsbron, and Zika viruses can cross-protect against infection with wild-type yellow fever virus.[93, 165, 166]

The evidence for interference with 17D vaccine in humans is conflicting, and discrepancies across studies may be due to the number of prior flavivirus infections, the breadth of the heterotypic response, or the identity of the viruses responsible for prior infection. Dengue immunity appears to blunt the response to 17D vaccine in some studies, whereas prior infection with members of the Japanese encephalitis complex does not. Pond and associates observed that people with natural immunity to dengue, but not St. Louis encephalitis, had lower seroconversion rates to 17D vaccine.[388] Individuals with monotypic neutralizing antibodies to Japanese encephalitis or with broad flavivirus cross-reactions had equivalent neutralizing antibody responses to 17D as immunological virgins.[394] Moreover, viremic responses to 17D were not significantly different in persons with and without prior Japanese encephalitis immunity, indicating that replication of 17D virus was not reduced.[104] The results of these studies and those of Pond and colleagues are consistent, since St. Louis and Japanese encephalitis viruses are close antigenic relatives.[388]

Naturally acquired yellow fever antibodies, due to infection with heterologous flaviviruses, significantly blunted the magnitude of the neutralizing antibody response to 17D vaccine.[179, 344] Interference was particularly evident when 17D vaccine was given by scarification, presumably due to the lower dose of 17D administered by this route. Low response rates to 17D vaccine administered by scarification were associated with preexisting heterologous flavivirus immunity in multiple studies in Africa.[340–342] In contrast, volunteers who had previously received a live attenuated dengue vaccine and were subsequently given 17D vaccine had similar immune responses to yellow fever as dengue nonimmune controls, suggesting no interference with yellow fever replication.[186] It is possible that the lack of interference was related to the attenuated properties of the dengue infection. In a study conducted in Nigeria, Omilabu and coworkers found no restriction of neutralizing antibody responses to 17D vaccine in people with various patterns of preexisting flavivirus immunity.[400]

There is no evidence that prior flavivirus immunity enhances the replication of yellow fever 17D virus or the immune response to 17D virus.

Heterologous Immunization in People Immune to Yellow Fever 17D

The only live attenuated flavivirus vaccine that has been evaluated in people with prior immunity to 17D vaccine is dengue-2.[187, 401] In yellow fever–immune individuals, the response to dengue vaccine was independent of dose and was of greater magnitude and duration than in nonimmunes.[187] The results suggested that cross-reactive nonneutralizing antibodies may have enhanced dengue virus replication in vivo.

Prior 17D immunization modulates the response to inactivated flavivirus vaccines through memory responses of IgG-producing B cells and restimulation of Th and follicular dendritic cells. In yellow fever–immune subjects receiving inactivated TBE vaccine, anti-TBE antibodies appeared earlier and in higher titers than in nonimmunes.[402] The anamnestic response was also characterized by the appearance of cross-reactive heterologous antibodies.

Serological Specificity

The primary neutralizing antibody response to 17D vaccine is highly specific, characterized by no or very low titer antibodies to other flaviviruses.[394] Neutralizing antibodies in the IgG and IgM fractions of serum display similar specificity in primary vaccinees, whereas IgG (but not IgM) from an individual who had been vaccinated three times and was tested 18 months after the last immunization showed some flavivirus cross-reactivity.[397] The HI antibody response to primary immunization is also monotypic (type specific).[388] In contrast, people with heterologous immunity respond to 17D vaccination with the development of a broadened response and the appearance of both homologous (yellow fever) and heterologous neutralizing, HI, and CF antibodies.[179, 394, 397] Similarly, people with prior 17D immunity respond to natural infection with heterologous flaviviruses with the development of a broadened flavivirus group response.[403]

The phenomenon of "original antigenic sin" has been noted in people previously vaccinated with 17D virus and subsequently infected with another flavivirus. In such cases, an anamnestic response leads to a rapid rise in yellow fever antibodies, whereas the response to the current (heterologous) antigen is delayed. This phenomenon was observed in yellow fever–immune volunteers who were vaccinated with experimental dengue-2 vaccines.[186, 401] Original antigenic sin may lead to diagnostic confusion in patients with clinical syndromes resembling naturally acquired yellow fever.[202]

Genetic Restriction

No studies have been reported on the genetic restriction of immune responses to yellow fever. This is an area deserving study, since studies in mice indicate that haplotype influences the replication of flaviviruses[131] and the immune response to live viruses.[132]

Interferon Response

In a study of adult volunteers given 17D vaccine, circulating interferon was detected in 10 of 15 subjects.[374] Interferon appeared and peaked 24 hours after viremia, in concert with the appearance of HI antibodies (see Fig. 34–6), and levels declined rapidly thereafter. These results are consistent with a subsequent study showing that 2′,5′-oligoadenylate synthetase activity in peripheral blood mononuclear cells increased by day 4 and peaked on day 7 after 17D immunization.[146b] The role of interferon in the clearance of 17D, and the inhibition of replication of or immune response to coadministered vaccines, has not been clarified.

Synthesis of tumor necrosis factor-α and IL-1 receptor antagonist was also elevated after yellow fever vaccination and might account for the fever occasionally seen.[402a]

Evidence That Yellow Fever Vaccine Protects Against Disease

A large body of preclinical data in nonhuman primates has demonstrated the protective activity of yellow fever 17D vaccination against lethal challenge.[380, 381] The development of neutralizing antibodies is strongly correlated with protection. The principal role of humoral antibodies in protection was also shown by transferring serum from immune monkeys before or shortly after challenge with virulent yellow fever.[117, 292]

The effectiveness of 17D vaccine is based on preclinical observations and the demonstration of neutralizing antibodies in more than 95% of people who received the vaccine but has never been tested in controlled clinical trials. However, several observations attest to the effectiveness of the vaccine: (1) laboratory infections with yellow fever were commonplace before routine immunization but disappeared thereafter; (2) observations over 50 years showed that jungle yellow fever in Brazil and other South American countries occurs only in people who have not been immunized with 17D and that immunization during outbreaks results in rapid disappearance of cases[275]; and (3) yellow fever in francophone Africa virtually disappeared after the institution in 1941 of mandatory immunization with FNV (see Fig. 34–15).[317] A high rate of coverage of the population was followed by a marked reduction in the incidence of yellow fever, despite continued human exposure to the enzootic cycle. Yellow fever epidemics were reported during the 1940s and 1950s from neighboring anglophone countries, particularly Nigeria, in which routine vaccination was not practiced.

An assessment of the efficacy of 17D vaccine was made during an epidemic in Nigeria in 1986 (K. M. DeCock, T. P. Monath, unpublished). By a determination of the vaccine coverage and the number of serologically confirmed yellow fever cases among vaccinated and unvaccinated subjects, vaccine efficacy was estimated to be 85%. The assessment was complicated by the simultaneous occurrence of natural infection and immunization in the population, by the potential for natural infection before the onset of vaccine immunity, and by the reliance on historical data about disease and vaccination.

Since yellow fever vaccination is the standard of care, placebo-controlled efficacy trials cannot be performed today. New yellow fever vaccines will be licensed based on immunological surrogates or, perhaps, comparability field trials. Further studies on the effectiveness of yellow fever vaccines, which could be done using case-control methodology, are nevertheless warranted, particularly in populations affected by human immunodeficiency virus (HIV) or malnutrition, where vaccine efficacy may be impaired.

Duration of Immunity

Immunity following 17D vaccination is remarkably durable, and it has been concluded that vaccination "confer(s) an immunity which . . . (is) almost lifelong . . . ."[403] The yellow fever immunization certificate for international travel is valid for 10 years, an interval that was established based on published studies showing that neutralizing antibodies were present in 92 to 97% of people 16 to 19 years after vaccination.[387, 403] The last analysis was performed in 1980, when World War II veterans were tested 30 to 35 years after a single dose of 17D vaccine.[385] Overall, 80.6% of the subjects were seropositive by a plaque-reduction neutralization test. However, the service records used to determine immunization of some veteran groups were undependable; in a subset of 58 Navy and Air Corps veterans, 97% were seropositive.

The basis of durable yellow fever immunity is a matter of speculation. Persistent infection of human cells in culture by yellow fever 17D virus has been described.[404] A human macrophage cell line and human peripheral blood mononuclear cells became persistently infected, with continued production of infectious virus without the appearance of cytopathic effects, in a fluctuating pattern suggesting a role for defective interfering particles.[181] Yellow fever virus was recovered from the brains of rhesus monkeys up to 159 days[281] and from sera 30 days after IC inoculation of monkeys.[59] In addition, a variant virus recovered from a 17D vaccine pool caused persistent infection of mouse brain without overt disease.[70] These observations, as well as the prolonged synthesis of IgM antibodies in persons immunized with 17D virus,[397] suggest that chronic persistent infection or storage of antigen in vivo, possibly in follicular dendritic cells, may explain the durability of the human immune response.

Primary Vaccine Failure

A small minority of healthy individuals inoculated with 17D vaccine do not develop detectable neutralizing antibodies (see Table 34–11). Although there are few reports on this question, it appears that failure to mount a response on primary immunization does not represent an absolute refractoriness, since revaccination may be followed by the development of neutralizing antibodies.[146b]

The development of clinical yellow fever in people with a history of 17D vaccination has been reported on rare occasions. Three cases (two fatal) occurred in British and Allied soldiers serving in western Africa during World War II.[242] In 1952, a fatal case of yellow fever occurred in a previously vaccinated European working in Uganda.[243] In 1988, a previously vaccinated Spanish woman acquired yellow fever during travels in western Africa.[249] It is uncertain whether these individuals had actually received 17D vaccine, had received vaccine that had deteriorated through improper storage or handling after reconstitution, or had simply failed to respond to the vaccine.

Host Factors Responsible for Vaccine Failures

Malnutrition

Protein-calorie malnutrition has been associated with failure to respond immunologically to 17D vaccine. In a study of eight children (mean age 2 years) with kwashiorkor, only one seroconverted after 17D vaccination, compared with five of six controls.[405] Further studies are required to assess the relevance of this finding to the use of 17D vaccine in the EPI in Africa, particularly where covariates such as HIV infection may diminish immunoresponsiveness. Although there were no obvious adverse effects of immunization in the small series of kwashiorkor patients, the safety of yellow fever immunization in infants with malnutrition has not been fully assessed. Gandra and Scrimshaw showed that 17D vaccine administered to children 4 to 11 years old recovering from malnutrition resulted in a significant catabolic effect lasting up to 12 days, in the absence of fever or other signs of increased metabolic rate.[406] This suggests that 17D vaccine could result in a net loss of body nitrogen and aggravate the clinical effects of protein malnutrition. Further studies in fasted adults showed that metabolic changes and mobilization of protein associated with yellow fever immunization were related to dietary factors; a catabolic effect was not observed in subjects consuming a high-protein diet.[407, 408]

Pregnancy

In a field study conducted in Nigeria, the IgM ELISA and neutralizing antibody responses to 17D vaccine were statistically significantly impaired in pregnant women compared with nonpregnant females of child-bearing age, male students, and the general population.[409] Only 38.6% of the pregnant women developed neutralizing antibodies, compared with 81.5 to 93.7% of the other groups. The difference was attributed to the immunosupression associated with pregnancy, emphasizing the need to reimmunize at-risk women who have been inadvertently vaccinated during pregnancy.

Human Immunodeficiency Virus Infection

HIV infection has been shown to reduce immunological responsiveness to a number of nonreplicating and live childhood vaccines. In the case of inactivated flaviviral vaccines, HIV infection reduced the seroconversion rate to Japanese encephalitis[410] and diminished the humoral and T-cell responses to TBE vaccine.[411] Yellow fever 17D vaccine was administered to 33 adult travelers with HIV infection and $CD4^+$ cell counts greater than 200 per mm^3.[412] Only 70% percent responded by 1 month after vaccination, and one individual seroreverted between 1 and 3 months after vaccination. In another study, 10-month-old HIV-infected infants in Ivory Coast were simultaneously immunized with 17D and measles vaccines.[413] Only 3 (17%) of 18 HIV-infected infants developed neutralizing antibodies 2 to 10 months after 17D vaccination, compared with 42 (74%) of 57 HIV-uninfected controls matched for age and nutritional status. These results indicate that HIV infection can impair the immune response to 17D vaccine, but the mechanism is uncertain. Since both HIV and 17D viruses exhibit tropism for human lymphoid cells,[413a] it is possible that HIV infection interferes with replication of 17D vaccine. This question could be addressed by in vitro studies and clinical trials in which 17D viremia is compared across HIV-infected and uninfected subjects.

Adverse Events

Yellow fever 17D is widely acknowledged as one of the safest vaccines in use. Over 300 million people have been immunized, with a remarkable record of tolerability and safety.[392, 414, 415]

Historical Problems: Adverse Events Before Standardization of Vaccine Manufacture

Two significant events in the history of manufacture and use of 17D vaccine are of special interest. The first (described under *Seed Lot System*) was the occurrence of postvaccinal encephalitis associated with the uncontrolled passage of 17D substrains during the early years of vaccine manufacture.[349, 392] The problem was resolved when stabilization of the passage level during vaccine manufacture was instituted in 1941. The second event was the development of acute hepatitis in persons who received 17D vaccine and was recognized as early as 1937 by Findlay and MacCallum.[416] Cases were reported in Brazil during the vaccination campaigns between 1938 and 1940 and, after careful study, were attributed to an adventitious agent in the vaccine rather than to viscerotropism of 17D virus.[417] In 1942, a massive outbreak of hepatitis appeared in U.S. military personnel immunized with 17D vaccine, resulting in approximately 28,000 cases and 62 deaths.[418] These reactions were due to the use of pooled human serum (contaminated with hepatitis virus) as a vaccine stabilizer. This practice was discontinued in Brazil in 1940 and in the United States in 1943,[419] with resolution of the problem. Subsequent retrospective serological studies confirmed that the responsible agent was hepatitis B virus.[420]

Common Adverse Events Following Administration of 17D Vaccines

No placebo-controlled trial has ever been performed to assess adverse reactions associated with 17D vaccine. Fever, headache, and backache, described as mild in severity, were noted since the earliest studies of 17D vaccine.[20] During large-scale field trials in Brazil in 1937 to 1938, Soper and colleagues noted mild systemic reactions in 5 to 8% of vaccinees.[348] Among 2457 people in Brazil from whom "reasonably accurate" clinical follow-up was obtained by Smith and associates, 14.6% complained of headache for 1 to 2 days, 10.2% developed pains in the body (usually accompanied by headache), 1.4% missed time from work (usually only 1 day), and 0.16% spent one or more days in bed.[21] These reactions, which were generally considered mild, occurred on the fifth to seventh day after immunization. Local reactions at the site of inoculation were not observed, and no systemic allergic reactions were noted.

Reactogenicity of 17D vaccine was monitored in 10 clinical trials conducted between 1953 and 1994 (Table 34–15). Self-limited and mild local reactions (erythema and pain at the inoculation site) and systemic reactions (headache, headache and fever, and fever without symptoms), occurred in a minority of subjects 5 to 7 days after immunization. The lack of placebo controls in all published reports makes interpretation of data on adverse events unreliable, although the lower incidence of adverse events in previously vaccinated subjects in one study suggests that these events are real. Reactogenicity in infants is no greater (or perhaps less) than in adults; this conclusion was also made during the early studies in Brazil in 1937 to 1938.[21]

Where subjects were under daily surveillance, a higher frequency of adverse events was detected. Moss-Blundell and coworkers[421] and Freestone and associates[390] determined adverse events in subjects in the United Kingdom who received stabilized 17D vaccine (Table 34–16). Assessment may have been biased by the characteristics of the study populations (military personnel and Wellcome employees, respectively). In Moss-Blundell's study, 514 adult military personnel were questioned for adverse events 2 and 11 weeks after vaccination, and a subset of 90 volunteers filled out a daily diary and took their temperatures for 10 days after vaccination. An interesting aspect of this trial was the determination of adverse events in those with and without preexisting yellow fever immunity, providing a control for reactions due to primary 17D virus replication versus the more limited replication following revaccination. Twenty (3.9%) of 514 seronegative and 1 (1.6%) of 64 seropositive vaccinees reported any adverse event at the routine follow-up visits. Of the 20 reactions in the seronegative group, 17 (85%) were local reactions (erythema or pain at the injection site, or both, noted immediately or within a few days after vaccination). The subset completing a daily diary reported a substantially higher rate of adverse reactions. Thirty-six (42%) of 86 seronegative subjects reported any adverse reaction (there were too few seropositives to draw a valid conclusion). Headache (10%) and local reactions (8%) were most frequently reported. In the study by Freestone and colleagues, subjects completed diary cards for 8 days after vaccination.[390] Mild reactions were noted in 10 (33%) of 30 subjects. A third study of 370 travelers followed by a telephone survey for 1 week provided similar data. Twenty-five percent of those immunized reported one or more reactions, generally mild, characterized by systemic flulike symptoms (22%) or local reactions (5%, typically pain).[422]

Rare Adverse Events Caused by 17D Vaccine

Postvaccinal Encephalitis

The 17D vaccine retains a degree of neurovirulence as demonstrated by intracerebral inoculation of mice and monkeys and by the occurrence of rare cases of postvaccinal encephalitis in humans. These cases have occurred principally, but not exclusively, in very young infants. After the institution of standardized manufacturing procedures in the early 1940s, no cases of meningoencephalitis temporally associated with 17D vaccine were reported for approximately 10 years.[392, 423] In 1952 to 1953, five cases occurred among 1800 children younger than 1 year vaccinated at the Pasteur Institute, Paris.[392] These cases (numbers 1–5 in Table 34–17), constitute the first evidence that 17D vaccine manufactured according to biological standards and with re-

Table 34–15. **ADVERSE EVENTS NOTED IN CLINICAL TRIALS OF 17D VACCINES MANUFACTURED USING STANDARDIZED METHODS, IN WHICH ADVERSE EVENTS WERE SPECIFICALLY MONITORED**

REFERENCE	VACCINE	PLACEBO-CONTROLLED?	SUBJECTS (NO. TESTED)	RESULT
Kouwenaar, 1953[435]	Rocky Mountain Laboratory, USA	No	Adults, Netherlands (1130*)	4.5% with low-grade fever, 7.6% with mild headache, muscle ache, malaise lasting hours to 4 d
Tauraso et al, 1972[386]	National Drug Co., USA	No	Adult prisoners, USA (1676)	"Low reactogenicity, minimal subjective and objective reactions"
Tauraso et al, 1972[484]	National Drug Co., USA	No	Merchant Marine Cadets, USA (181†)	No local or generalized adverse reactions
Freestone et al, 1977[390]	Wellcome, UK	No	Adults, UK (30‡)	33% with various symptoms (headache, fever, pain or redness at injection site [see text])
Moss-Blundell et al, 1981[421]	Wellcome, UK	No	Adult male military, UK	
			514 seronegative§	3.9% reported any reaction; 0.2% headache only; 3.3% local reactions; 0.4% other (see text)
			64 seropositive§	1.6% reported local reaction (see text)
Roche et al, 1986[487]	Pasteur-Mérieux, France	No	Adult male military, France (297)	No adverse events attributable to vaccine
Lhuillier et al, 1989[488]	Pasteur-Mérieux, France	No	6–9 mo infants, Ivory Coast (74‖)	No adverse reactions
Mouchon et al, 1990[455]	Pasteur-Mérieux, France	No	6–12 mo infants, Cameroon (75‖)	No adverse reactions
Soula et al, 1991[489]	Pasteur-Mérieux, France	No	4–24 mo infants, Mali (115‖)	21% with fever >38°C; 2.6% with local induration; 1.7% with rash; 7% with conjunctivitis*
Ambrosch et al, 1994[453]	Pasteur-Mérieux, France	No	Young adults, Austria (41)	2.4% with fever >38°C; 4.8% malaise; short duration

* Including 465 with a history of atopy or other allergic reactions.
† This was a study of sequential or simultaneous inoculation of smallpox and yellow fever 17D vaccines; in the group of 181 subjects included here, the vaccines were separated by 28 days.
‡ Subjects receiving standard dose of 17D vaccine.
§ Yellow fever neutralizing antibody status before 17D vaccination; numbers differ from those of Table 34–11 since not all subjects were interviewed for adverse events.
‖ This was a study of combined or sequential vaccination; only subjects receiving yellow fever 17D vaccine alone are included in the table.

stricted passage may be encephalitogenic in very young infants.* Since 1952, an additional 16 cases have been reported, for a total of 21 cases. Fifteen cases occurred during the 1950s, when there was no age restriction on the use of the vaccine in infants. Of the 15 cases, 13 (87%) occurred in infants younger than 4 months of age, and all were 7 months of age or younger. Recommendations for restriction of the use of 17D vaccine to infants older than 6 months[426] were followed by a reduction in the incidence of encephalitis. Since 1960, only six cases have been reported, one of which occurred in a 1-month-old infant in France, where the age limitation was not universally practiced.[427] Current recommendations for the minimal age for vaccination differ, based on the risk of exposure to natural infection with yellow fever (see *Contraindications and Precautions*), but in no case should the vaccine be administered to infants 4 months old or younger.

The incidence of postvaccinal encephalitis in very young infants may be estimated at 0.5 to 4 per 1000 based on two reports that provide denominator data (Table 34–18). In contrast, the risk of developing encephalitis in people older than 9 months of age (the current minimal age recommended for routine immunization in the United States[392a]) is extremely low. Only

*It is uncertain, however, whether these cases and several others reported subsequently at the Pasteur Institute by Panthier could be due to variations in the substrain and passage level of vaccine,[351] which may not have been adequately controlled at the time. In his review, Stuart states that the vaccine used in case numbers 1–5 were immunized with vaccine prepared by a single passage from seed virus supplied by the Rockefeller Foundation, New York, in 1946.[392]

In addition to those cases described in Table 34–17, two fatal cases of possible encephalitis among 67,325 children between 6 months and 2 years of age who received 17D vaccine were noted during an emergency vaccination campaign in Senegal in 1965, an incidence of 3 per 100,000.[329] The relationship of the reactions to 17D vaccine is in doubt, since both had a very short incubation time (1 and 4 days); one of the cases was ascribed to anaphylaxis.[330] In contrast, there were 231 cases of encephalitis among 498,887 persons given the FNV, for an overall incidence of 46 per 100,000; however, the incidence in children aged 2 to 11 years was 150 per 100,000.

Two other possible cases, not included in the table have been mentioned in the literature. Dick and Horgan make reference to a 6-year-old child in England given 17D vaccine 3 days after smallpox vaccination. The child developed encephalitis 11 days after 17D immunization and made a full recovery. The administration of smallpox vaccine in this case makes the cause uncertain.[424] Thomson cites the case of a 3-month-old child in England inoculated in 1954, in a personal reference from another physician.[425]

Table 34–16. **FREQUENCY OF NONSERIOUS ADVERSE EVENTS AFTER YELLOW FEVER 17D VACCINATION***

REFERENCE	NO. OF SUBJECTS	ADVERSE EVENT	NO. WITH AE	PERCENTAGE WITH AE
Freestone et al, 1977[390]	30 (adult)	Any reaction	10	33
		Headache only	1	3
		Headache and fever	2	7
		Local reaction only†	2	7
		Local reaction and headache	4	13
		Lymphadenopathy	1	3
Moss-Blundell et al, 1981[421]	86 (adult)	Any reaction	36	42
		Headache only	9	10
		Fever only	7	8
		Headache and fever	4	5
		Local reaction only	1	1
		Local reaction and headache	6	7
		Other‡	9	10
Pivetaud et al, 1986[422]	370 (age 1–84 yr; majority 20–39 yr)	Any reaction	94	25
		Grippe-like systemic reaction	42	11
		Fatigue, weakness	28	8
		GI complaints, with or without vomiting	9	2
		Headache only	5	1
		Headache, fever, vomiting	1	0.3
		Headache, dizziness	1	0.3
		Local reaction only†	17	5.0

*Results are from three studies in which subjects without preexisting yellow fever immunity completed a daily diary or were actively followed up after vaccination; trials were not blinded or placebo-controlled.

†Pain and/or redness at site of inoculation.

‡Abdominal pain (1), nausea and vomiting (1), upper respiratory infection (6), rash (1).

AE, adverse event; GI, gastrointestinal.

Table 34–17. **CASES OF MENINGOENCEPHALITIS TEMPORALLY ASSOCIATED WITH OR PROVED TO BE CAUSED BY YELLOW FEVER 17D VACCINE MANUFACTURED ACCORDING TO BIOLOGICAL STANDARDS ESTABLISHED IN 1945***

CASE NO.	YEAR	LOCATION	AGE	SEX	INCUBATION PERIOD (d)	OUTCOME	REFERENCE
1	1952–1953	France	7 mo	F	19	Survived	392
2	1952–1953	France	1.5 mo	M	11	Survived	392
3	1952–1953	France	1 mo	M	12	Survived	392
4	1952–1953	France	6 mo	M	12	Survived	392
5	1952–1953	France	4 mo	F	10	Survived	392
6	1952	So. Africa/England†,‡	5 wk	M	21	Survived	495
7	1953	So. Africa/England†,‡	4 mo	M	8	Survived	496
8	1953	Scotland‡	7 wk	M	17	Survived	425
9	1954	England	5 wk	F	9	Survived	497
10	1954	England	13 wk	?	~9	Survived	498
11	1954	Nigeria/England†	8 wk	M	~14§	Survived	499
12	1954	England	3 mo	M	8	Survived	500
13	1954	France	3 mo	M	8	Survived	501
14	1954	Portugal	6 wk	F	11	Survived	502
15	1959	United States	10 wk	F	12	Survived	503
16	1965	United States	3 yr	F	6	Died	52
17	1979	France	1 mo	M	13	Survived	427
18	1989	South Africa	13 yr	M	7	Survived	504
19	1990		19 yr	M	13	Survived	505
20	1990		59 yr	F	2‖	Survived	505
21	1991	Switzerland	29 yr	M	3 (18)¶	Survived	428

*There are less well substantiated but plausible records of other cases possibly due to 17D vaccine (a 3-mo-old child in England, Parrish, 1954, quoted in Thompson, 1954,[425] and a 6-yr-old child who received 17D vaccine 3 days after smallpox vaccination reported by Dick and Horgan, 1952.[424])

†Country where immunized/where hospitalized, if different.

‡Vaccinated simultaneously or within a few days with smallpox (vaccination unsuccessful).

§Date of onset and hospitalization inaccurate in original publication; see Stuart, 1956.[392]

‖Event occurred 2 days after revaccination with 17D (prior vaccination 10 years in the past).

¶Patient had biphasic illness starting 3 days after immunization, with partial remission and central nervous system signs developing 18 days after immunization.

Table 34–18. **INCIDENCE OF ENCEPHALITIS ASSOCIATED WITH ADMINISTRATION OF 17D VACCINE TO INFANTS**

LOCATION	YEARS	AGE (mo)	NO. VACCINATIONS	NO. ENCEPHALITIS CASES	INCIDENCE/1000	CASE-FATALITY (%)	REFERENCE
France (Paris)	1952–1953	<6	1000	4	4	0	392
		7–12	800	1	1.25	0	
France (Lyon)	1958–1978	<1	1830	1	0.5	0	427

three such cases have been reported among travelers. In the United States, only one case has occurred since 1965, for an approximate incidence of less than 1 in 8 million.

The total number of yellow fever immunizations administered worldwide in the last 50 years approximates 300 million, the majority of which have been performed in developing countries. Surveillance for adverse events has been passive and insensitive to the discovery of rare events. In 1993, an active hospital-based surveillance system for postvaccinal encephalitis was established during a vaccination campaign in response to a yellow fever epidemic in Kenya (D. Heymann, personal communication, 1997). Four encephalitis cases (one child aged 2 years; three adults) were recorded, for an estimated incidence of 5.8 per million vaccinees. Surprisingly, three of the four encephalitis cases had a fatal outcome. Although the population had a high prevalence of HIV infection, the rate of severe reactions to 17D vaccine was not significantly higher in HIV-infected and noninfected people. Further studies in large-scale campaigns, preferably using case-control methodology and the application of laboratory techniques to establish the cause, are needed to clarify the risk of encephalitis following 17D vaccine.

The syndrome associated with 17D encephalitis is characterized by the onset, 7 to 21 days after immunization, of fever and variable neurological signs including meningismus, convulsions, obtundation, and paresis. The cerebrospinal fluid contains 100 to 500 cells (mixed polymorphonuclear and lymphocytic) and an increased protein concentration. The clinical course has typically been brief and recovery generally complete. One patient died[52] and a 29-year-old described by Merlo and associates[428] had residual mild ataxia 11 months after the onset of illness.[428]

The basis for increased risk of encephalitis in young infants is unknown, but it parallels the increased susceptibility of neonatal mice to neuroinvasion and neurovirulence of yellow fever and other flaviviruses. Possibilities include (1) immaturity of the blood-brain barrier; (2) prolonged or higher viremia; and (3) immaturity of the immune system and delayed clearance of the infection. There are no data on 17D viremia levels or on the kinetics of the immune response in infants or children. The incidence of encephalitis following 17D vaccine has been more common in males (13 in 20 cases, 65%) than in females. A slight excess of males (56%) was noted also in the cases of encephalitis following use of the FNV[329] and in epidemics of naturally acquired yellow fever, where no gender difference in exposure to the virus was evident (see *Risk Factors*).

Immediate Allergic Reactions to Egg Proteins

Hypersensitivity reactions to egg proteins in yellow fever vaccine have been extremely infrequent. No such reactions were observed during the initial use of the vaccine in over 2 million people.[429] Guinea pig sensitization tests with 17D vaccine showed that anaphylactic reactions were reduced when the test vaccine was prepared from embryos younger than 13 days. For this reason, the age of embryos at the time of harvest for the production of 17D vaccine is 12 days or younger.[361] Yellow fever vaccine contains multiple proteins derived from egg white and yolk.[430] In one study, 17D vaccine produced in the United States contained 7.8 μg ovalbumin per 0.5 mL dose.[431]

The first report of allergic phenomena associated with use of 17D vaccine was in 1942, during large-scale immunization of military personnel. Sulzberger and Asher described three patients with a serum sickness syndrome (urticaria or erythema multiforme–like rash accompanied by malaise, fever, arthralgia, pruritis, nausea, and vomiting) with an onset between 3 and 7 days after the receipt of different lots of 17D vaccine.[432] In 1943, Swartz described a patient with a strong history of egg and other food allergies who developed anaphylaxis 5 minutes after receiving simultaneous injections of 17D and cholera vaccines.[433] Skin testing revealed marked reactions to egg white and chicken meat, and a moderate reaction to 17D (but not cholera) vaccine. Sprague and Barnard reported a case of severe anaphylaxis occurring within 15 minutes after 17D vaccine in a man with a known egg allergy.[434]

The general consensus based on observations during the first 20 years of use of 17D vaccine was that allergic reactions are extremely rare, occurring at an incidence of less than 1 per million, with reactions occurring principally in persons with known egg sensitivity. Reactions are typically mild and thus may be underreported. Kouwenaar found the frequency of allergic reactions to yellow fever vaccine to be higher than expected, particularly in people with a history of various allergies.[435] He vaccinated 242 people having allergic histories with 0.1 mL of 17D vaccine by the intradermal route; if no reaction occurred within 45 minutes, they received the remaining 0.4 mL subcutaneously. Nine (3.7%) of the subjects experienced allergic reactions, characterized clinically as exacerbations of known but dormant allergy (eczema, asthma, rhinitis) in four patients; urticaria occurring less than 3 days after vaccination in two patients; and "serum sickness–like disease"—urticaria or rash—occurring 6 to 14 days after vaccination in three patients. Of the nine subjects reacting to yellow fever vaccination, two had a known history of egg allergy and the others had various other food allergies, asthma, or hay fever. In a "control" group of 465 persons without a history of allergy, only three patients (0.6%) had a late reaction to yellow fever vaccine (facial erythema [two cases] and urticaria [one case]). In an additional group of 185 nonallergic individuals who were *reimmunized* with 17D vaccine, one (0.5%) experienced generalized urticaria. The skin test had a very low positive predictive value for the development of allergic response to yellow fever vaccine. There were insufficient data on the more important question of the negative predictive value of the skin test.

More recent and definitive data on the incidence of allergic reactions are few, principally because a prior history of intolerance or allergy to eggs or to egg-based vaccines is considered a contraindication to the use of 17D vaccine, and few immunizations are given to such individuals. Guidelines for the use of yellow fever and other egg-based vaccines recommend that egg-sensitive patients undergo scratch, prick, or needle puncture testing with 1:10 diluted vaccine and a negative and positive (histamine) control. If the test is negative, an intradermal test is performed with 0.02 mL of 1:100 vaccine.[393, 436, 437] The application of this skin test procedure in clinical practice was described recently by Mosimann and coworkers.[438] In the case of a positive intradermal test (a wheal 5 mm or larger) and an established need for yellow fever vaccine, the patient may undergo a desensitization procedure consisting of increasing subcutaneous doses at 15- to 20-minute intervals under the supervision of an experienced physician.

In one study, 30,000 Navy and Marine Corps personnel were screened for a history of egg sensitivity and 42 allergic patients underwent scratch and intradermal testing with crude egg white and a variety of egg-based vaccines including yellow fever 17D; most patients also underwent oral egg challenge.[439] The study demonstrated that a history of egg allergy was not a strong contraindication to the administration of egg-based vaccines, since only 16% of the egg-sensitive subjects experienced any reaction, and these were mild in all cases. Skin tests were positive in 31% of the egg-sensitive subjects. Vaccination was performed in 39 subjects (excluding three subjects with strongly positive intradermal tests), using the egg-based vaccines causing the greatest reaginic activity. Intradermal skin testing with vaccine had reasonably high negative predictive value (0.80), but a lower positive predictive value (0.57) for an allergic reaction. However, the strength of positivity of the intradermal test appeared to correlate with the severity of symptoms after vaccination.

Since 1990, the Centers for Disease Control and Prevention has enhanced procedures for reporting adverse events to vaccines.[440] A preliminary assessment of data collected between 1990 and 1995 revealed 31 cases of nonfatal hypersensitivity-type reactions (urticaria, angioedema, bronchospasm, anaphylaxis) temporally associated with yellow fever vaccine; in 14 cases 17D was the only vaccine administered (T. F. Tsai, personal communication, 1997). The incidence of allergic reactions cannot be established with accuracy. However, based on the number of vaccine doses distributed annually in the United States and the assumption that all reported events are caused by 17D vaccine, the incidence of allergic reactions may be estimated at between 5 and 20 per million doses. Although egg protein has been implicated in hypersensitivity reactions to yellow fever vaccine, other components may also play a role, for example, hydrolyzed gelatin incorporated as a stabilizer by some manufacturers.

Other Rare Adverse Events Temporally Related to 17D Vaccine

There are a number of individual case reports of adverse events possibly associated with yellow fever vaccination. Although some are credible, such as the occurrence of ketoacidosis in an insulin-dependent diabetic patient 4 days after vaccination,[441] others (e.g., chronic lymphocytic leukemia,[442] malaria recrudescence,[443] and multiple sclerosis[444]) probably represent chance associations in time. The absence of similar observations over the long history of use of yellow fever vaccine supports this view. Postmarketing surveillance by vaccine manufacturers, as well as the Vaccine Adverse Events Reporting System have accumulated cases of neurological syndromes (Guillain-Barré syndrome, ataxia, Bell's palsy, mononeuritis), jaundice, and bursitis, but the relationship of these events to vaccination is uncertain, since they also occur as independent events in the population.

Mention is made in the literature of a favorable effect of yellow fever vaccine on reducing the incidence of recurrent herpes labialis in 11 patients,[445] but this observation has not been explored in controlled trials.

Reactions Due to Improper Handling and Use of Yellow Fever Vaccine

Since yellow fever vaccine contains no preservative, improper handling of multiple-dose vials can lead to bacterial contamination, sometimes with serious consequences. Repeated use of the same needle and syringe, rubbing dirt or other materials into the inoculation site, and other practices may also contribute to infection. The author has personally observed a number of cases of superficial abscess formation at the site of jet injector immunization in Africa; the common practice of rubbing dirt, bark, balms, and native medicines or other materials onto the inoculation site was probably responsible.

Four known outbreaks of serious illness have been associated with contamination of yellow fever vaccine vials or inoculation equipment in Africa (Table 34–19). The clinical picture in all four episodes was similar, with marked swelling and pain of the vaccinated arm beginning hours after immunization and progressing in the most severe cases to cardiovascular shock and death within hours to several days.[446–448] Some, but not all, patients had signs of necrotizing myositis (gangrene). In all episodes, known or potential problems with use of multiple-dose vaccine containers contaminated after reconstitution, improperly sterilized jet injector equipment, or reuse of syringes and needles was involved. Although no etiologic agent was implicated, *Clostridia* and group A or anaerobic streptococci were suspected.

Table 34–19. **EPISODES INVOLVING MULTIPLE SERIOUS ADVERSE EVENTS CHARACTERIZED BY CELLULITIS OR NECROTIZING MYOSITIS ASSOCIATED WITH PROBABLE BACTERIAL CONTAMINATION OF 17D VACCINE AFTER RECONSTITUTION OR INFECTION OF INOCULATION SITE**

YEAR	LOCATION	NO. CASES	NO. DEATHS (%)	INCIDENCE*	CIRCUMSTANCES	REFERENCE
1974	Ivory Coast	39	8 (20.5)	5.3/100,000 immunizations	Cases occurred at nine designated vaccinating centers; five-dose vials pooled to prepare 50–100 doses for jet injection	446
1982	Ghana	6	2 (33.3)		Cases occurred at single center; possible contaminated 50-dose vial or syringe	446
1984	Benin	31	11 (35.5)	4/10,000	Cases associated with one vaccinating team, six vaccinating sessions using multiple-dose vials, jet injectors	447
1987	Nigeria	25	5 (20)		Illegal clinics, unauthorized inoculators, reuse of syringes, multiple-dose vials	448

* Estimate, since number of persons vaccinated with vaccine vial(s) implicated in the contamination is unknown.

Indications for Yellow Fever Vaccine

All inhabitants of countries, or areas within countries, endemic for yellow fever should be routinely immunized, preferably at 9 months of age. Areas endemic for yellow fever are shown in Figure 34–7. Within these countries, priorities may be established for immunization, related to the risk of exposure to yellow fever virus. For example, residents in rural areas and areas of historical yellow fever epidemic activity are at higher risk than residents of large cities or areas in which yellow fever has not occurred in many years. People migrating from nonendemic to endemic areas are at high risk and should be immunized. Since such movements are difficult to control and the potential exists for the spread of yellow fever from rural to urban areas, a policy of universal immunization in countries within the endemic zone is favored.

During epidemics of yellow fever, mass immunization should be instituted at the earliest possible stage of the outbreak. Priorities for immunizing population subsets according to geography or age group will be determined by local information on the progress of the outbreak and on the history of prior vaccination coverage.

Immigrants, travelers, and military personnel and dependents require immunization at least 10 days before their arrival in endemic areas. As noted under *Incidence*, even a short stay in an area of viral transmission is dangerous. Since native inhabitants may be immune and the virus can circulate in a silent zoonotic cycle, the absence of recent notification of yellow fever in an area is not an indication that it is safe to enter without vaccination. On the other hand, the notification of human cases within the past 1 to 2 years is an indication of high risk. Short-stay travelers to large cities within endemic areas, such as the coastal metropolises of western Africa (Accra, Lagos, Dakar, Abidjan, and so forth) are at very low risk in the absence of a reported outbreak and need not be immunized. Coastal areas of eastern Africa and most of South America are currently outside the area of yellow fever transmission.

Some countries in the endemic zones, and some countries outside the endemic zones but infested with *A. aegypti* and receptive to the introduction of yellow fever require a valid certificate of immunization for travelers from endemic countries (see Table 34–4). A full listing is given in the WHO document International Travel and Health,[211] available from WHO Distribution and Sales, CH-1211 Geneva 27, Switzerland, and in the CDC's Health Information for International Travel,[210] available from the Superintendent of Documents, U.S. Government Printing Office, Washington, D.C. 20402 (phone 202-512-1800). Some countries require a valid certificate even if the traveler has been in transit through an endemic country and even if the disembarking traveler is in transit. Controls at airports and borders are highly variable, but travelers respecting the regulations will avoid unnecessary delays. Persons with a contraindication to immunization (see later) should obtain a letter from their physician stating why immunization could not be performed.

Contraindications and Precautions

Age Restriction

Infants are at higher risk of postvaccinal encephalitis, and this risk is inversely proportional to age. Published guidelines differ somewhat on the minimal age for vaccination.[211, 392a, 393, 446, 449] There is complete agreement, however, that the vaccine should never be administered to infants 4 months of age or younger and that routine immunization may be performed at 9 months of age. Infants between the ages of 5 and 8 months should be immunized if there is a significant risk of natural infection, for example residence in or travel to a rural area in the yellow fever endemic zone or in the context of an ongoing epidemic. Where the risk of exposure to yellow fever is very low (for example in large urban areas in endemic countries, especially in the context of brief visits by tourists), it is advisable to delay immunization until 12 months of age.

Pregnancy and Lactation

Initially, the use of yellow fever vaccine in pregnancy was not constrained, and many women were vaccinated without any reported adverse effects. In Paris, Stefanopoulo and Duvolon immunized over 200 pregnant women between 1936 and 1946,[423] and in Brazil, Smith and colleagues vaccinated ". . . a considerable number of women in all stages of pregnancy . . . with no untoward effects."[21] Spontaneous abortion, stillbirth, and congenital malformation have not been observed in the aftermath of yellow fever epidemics. In one report of yellow fever death of a naturally infected pregnant woman, there was no evidence that the fetus had developed hepatitis.[450] In another report, two women 2 and 5 months pregnant died of yellow fever; in neither case did the fetal livers show necrosis.[450a]

The hypothetical risk of transplacental infection and the recognition that young infants (and thus, potentially, the unborn fetus) were susceptible to neuroinvasion by 17D virus led to the general recommendation that the vaccine not be administered during pregnancy unless clearly required, based on the judgment that a high risk of natural infection exists. Specific recommendations on this issue vary considerably. The position of the WHO is that vaccination is generally contraindicated in pregnancy, but ". . . is permitted after the sixth month of pregnancy when justified epidemiologically."[211] The American Committee on Immunization Practices does not specify a stage of pregnancy but emphasizes the need to establish a clear need for immunization.[392a] Inadvertent immunization of women (generally in the early stages of pregnancy) is definitely not an indication for therapeutic abortion. Women should be cautioned that there is a hypothetical risk but should be reassured that no harm to the fetus has ever been demonstrated. Fear of potential adverse effects may have led to an increase in therapeutic abortions during a vaccination campaign in Trinidad in 1977 to 1978.[451]

Two recent studies have addressed the risk of congenital infection in pregnant women who were inadvertently immunized with 17D vaccine during emergency vaccination campaigns. Nasidi and associates studied 101 women who were immunized in Nigeria in 1986.[409] Four women (4%) were immunized in the first trimester, eight (8%) in the second trimester, and 89 (88%) in the third trimester. There were no adverse effects on fetuses or neonates attributable to vaccination among 40 infants who were carefully followed up. No evidence for transplacental infection was obtained in 40 babies whose cord blood was tested for IgM antibodies. The most important aspect of this study was the finding that women immunized during pregnancy had a significantly lower seroconversion rate (39%) compared with control groups immunized during the campaign. It was concluded that immunization of pregnant women may be justified in epidemic emergencies when there is a high risk of natural infection, but that response rates may be low due to the immunosuppression associated with pregnancy.

A second study was conducted after a vaccination campaign in Trinidad in 1989.[452] Approximately 400,000 people were immunized, and 100 to 200 were estimated to have inadvertently received 17D vaccine during pregnancy. Forty-one cord blood samples were obtained from babies born to mothers who had received 17D vaccine during the first trimester. One infant (normal, full-term) had IgM antibody in the cord blood, suggesting that congenital infection with 17D virus may have occurred.

A recent study of spontaneous abortion after yellow fever vaccination of Brazilian women found an odds ratio of 2.29, but the confidence limits overlapped 1.0, and thus the difference was not significant.[452a]

Thus, although the risk of immunization during pregnancy appears small, both prudence and current vaccine labeling make pregnancy a precaution or contraindication to yellow fever immunization unless clearly indicated by the risk of acquiring natural infection. Further studies are required to determine the frequency and relevance of congenital infection.

Recommendations regarding the use of 17D vaccine in breast-feeding mothers are absent or vary in different documents and are purely hypothetical. A very large number of lactating women have been (appropriately) immunized during emergency vaccination campaigns, but no studies on subsequent effects on or vaccine virus transmission to infants have been conducted. Lactation is not considered a contraindication to 17D vaccination in the United States[393] but is in the United Kingdom[449] because of the theoretical risk of transmission of 17D virus to the breast-fed infant. The theoretical concern is based in part on the knowledge that some tick-borne flaviviruses are secreted in the milk of domesticated livestock.

Concurrent Infections, Medications, and Immunosuppression

Some national authorities recommend that vaccination be delayed in people with acute concurrent infections.[449] Because of the theoretical risk of neuroinvasion and encephalitis, the vaccine is contraindicated in patients with known immunosuppression due to HIV infection or immunological deficiency states (leukemia; lymphoma; generalized malignancy; other conditions affecting humoral and cellular immune responses; or treatment with immunosuppressive drugs, including high-dose corticosteroids). Low-dose corticosteroid treatment or intra-articular injections of corticosteroids do not pose a contraindication to yellow fever vaccination.[392a, 393] Asymptomatic HIV infection is not considered a contraindication in the United States[392a, 393] but is in the United Kingdom.[449] As noted previously, preliminary studies indicate that asymptomatic HIV infection may reduce the immune response to 17D vaccine. Despite an earlier study to the contrary, yellow fever vaccine does not appear to depress tuberculin skin test sensitivity[452b] and is unlikely to adversely affect the course of active tuberculosis.

Bone Marrow and Organ Donation

No formal recommendations have been made on the suitability of people who have received 17D vaccine at a remote point in time as organ or bone marrow donors. This issue has been raised because of the possibility that 17D virus causes a latent, persistent infection (reviewed under *Duration of Immunity*), which is contained and irrelevant in the immune host but might cause systemic infection in an immunosuppressed transplant recipient. The risks to recipients are purely hypothetical. Unless the vaccine changed its tropism and virulence during latency, the risk to the recipient, even if infected, would appear to be small. In a single report, bone marrow from a donor twin immunized 1 month previously with yellow fever 17D was grafted to an identical twin.[452c] The recipient failed to develop yellow fever antibodies, indicating that no yellow fever B-cell clone had been transferred or that immunosuppressive therapy may have masked an immune response by the recipient to transferred virus. There were no untoward events attributable to the potential transfer of 17D virus.

Simultaneous and Combined Vaccination

Yellow fever vaccine has been given simultaneously at different sites or as a mixture, combined with a variety of other vaccines, including vaccinia, diphtheria-pertussis-tetanus, bacille Calmette-Guérin, measles, typhoid, cholera, hepatitis A, hepatitis B, and meningococcal A/C plus typhoid vaccines (Table 34–20). These studies are relevant to the use of 17D vaccine in routine childhood immunization programs, and to the immunization of travelers. In particular, the ability to coadminister or combine yellow fever and measles vaccines could reduce the cost and complexity of childhood immunization.

No increase in reactogenicity has been noted in studies of combined or simultaneous immunization, and with a few exceptions noted later, there have been no alterations in reciprocal immune responses. On theoretical grounds alone, it is recommended that live vaccines (such as measles) be given either concurrently at different sites or the vaccinations separated by 4 weeks; however, where this is impractical, the schedule may be modified. Lipopolysaccharide is known to have adjuvant activity, and coadministration of the typhoid Vi vaccine appeared to enhance antibody titers to yellow fever, especially when the typhoid vaccine was combined with yellow fever.[453] However, in another study, no enhancement was observed when typhoid Vi and meningococcal A/C conjugate vaccines were coadministered with 17D.[454] An enhanced neutralizing antibody response to yellow fever was observed in a study of combined 17D-measles vaccine, perhaps due to cytokine induction by the unrelated virus.[455] Possible interference with yellow fever immune responses was noted when vaccinia and measles vaccine[456] or hepatitis B vaccine[457] was combined with 17D, but these results were not confirmed in other trials (see Table 34–20). An interesting observation, not relevant to current vaccination practices, was the mutual interference due to simultaneous or sequential administration of 17D and inactivated, parenteral whole-cell cholera vaccines.[458, 459] The interference induced by 17D vaccine with vibriocidal responses was not confirmed in another study[460] and may not be real. The basis for interference is obscure, since the interval between cholera and yellow fever immunization was as long as 4 weeks. A trial of combined yellow fever and live oral cholera vaccine (alone or with Ty21a live typhoid vaccine) showed no one-way interference with anticholera immunity,[461] but yellow fever antibody responses have not yet been reported.

Coadministration of Immune Serum Globulin and Yellow Fever Vaccine

Seroconversion rates and neutralizing antibody titers were not affected by the intramuscular administration of 5 mL of commercial pooled immune serum globulin containing high titers of yellow fever neutralizing antibodies zero to 7 days before or at intervals after yellow fever 17D immunization[462]—a finding of practical importance before the advent of vaccines against hepatitis A. The results are not unexpected given the success of passive-active immunization and the observation that revaccination of individuals with neutralizing antibodies results in a booster response.[185]

Yellow Fever Vaccine and Antimalarial Drugs

Chloroquine is known to inhibit the immune response to inactivated rabies vaccine and to interfere with flavivirus replication in vitro. In humans, there was no inhibitory effect of chloroquine at doses used for malaria prophylaxis on the response to yellow fever 17D.[463]

Future Yellow Fever Vaccines

Research sponsored by WHO at the Oswaldo Cruz Foundation, Rio de Janeiro, aims at the development of a novel method for manufacturing 17D vaccine. The approach begins with a full-length cDNA clone of 17D-204 virus,[358] which has been modified by site-directed mutagenesis to substitute a number of 17DD substrain residues. R. Galler (personal communication) and his colleagues[358] have predicted that these changes will further attenuate the marginally acceptable neurovirulence profile of the original infectious clone. The mutated 17DD-like clone has been used to produce a new primary seed virus under GMP, and a full evaluation according to WHO manufacturing standards is under way. Unlike current yellow fever vaccines, which are heterogeneous mixtures of virion subpopulations, the new vaccine is genetically homogeneous. An important aspect of this work is that it sets a precedent for novel, chimeric vaccines in which heterologous flavivirus E genes (e.g., of Japanese encephalitis virus) have been inserted into the yellow fever 17D virus infectious clone.[464] The use of yellow fever 17D as a live vector is a promising

Table 34–20. SIMULTANEOUS AND COMBINED IMMUNIZATION WITH YELLOW FEVER 17D AND OTHER VACCINES IN OPEN-LABEL TRIALS

VACCINE COADMINISTERED WITH 17D	METHOD	YF-ONLY CONTROL GROUP	AGE GROUP	REACTOGENICITY	IMMUNOGENICITY		REFERENCE
					To YF	To Other Vaccine	
Vaccinia	Simultaneous	Yes	Adults	Not altered	Not altered	Not altered	484
Vaccinia + measles	Combined	Yes	Children 5 mo–4.5 yr	Not altered	Possible decrease in seroconversion rate†	Not altered	456
Vaccinia + measles and vaccinia + measles + DPT	Simultaneous	No	Children 6 mo–2 yr	Not altered	Appropriate	Not altered	506
Vaccinia, measles, BCG, tetanus	Simultaneous	No	Children 1–5 yr	Not altered	No different than vaccinia + YF control	No significant decrease	507
Measles	Combined	Yes	Infants	Not altered	Enhanced GMT (P < .05)	Enhanced GMT (not significant)	455
Measles	Combined	Yes	Infants	Not altered	Not altered	Not altered	488
Hepatitis B (plasma derived)	Simultaneous‡	Yes	Infants	Not altered	Seroconversion rate unaffected but GMT lower (P = .02)	Not altered	457
Hepatitis B (plasma derived and recombinant)	Simultaneous§	Yes	Infants	Not altered	Not altered	Not determined	492
Hepatitis A	Simultaneous	No	Adults	Not altered	Not determined	Not altered	508
Hepatitis A	Simultaneous	Yes	Adults	Not altered	Not altered	Not altered	491
Hepatitis A + typhoid Vi	Hepatitis A simultaneous with 17D-typhoid combined	No	Adults	Not altered	Appropriate	Not altered	494
Typhoid Vi	Combined or simultaneous	Yes	Adults	Not altered	Enhanced GMT (P < .05)	Not altered	453
Cholera (whole cell, inactivated)‖	Simultaneous or 1 to >24 wk apart	Yes	Adults	No information provided	Decreased antibody titer when vaccines given 0–3 wk apart	Decreased antibody titer when vaccines given 0–3 wk apart	458
Cholera (whole cell, inactivated)	Simultaneous or 4 wk apart	Yes	Children 2–5 yr	Not determined	Decreased seroconversion rate and titer	Not determined	459
Cholera (whole cell, inactivated)	Simultaneous	Yes	Children (school age)	Not determined	Not determined	Not altered (vibriocidal titers)	460
Cholera (live oral CVD 103 HgR)	Simultaneous	No	Adults	Not altered	Not determined	Not altered	461
Cholera (live oral + live typhoid Ty21a)	Simultaneous	No	Adults	Not altered	Not determined	Not altered	461
Meningococcus A/C + typhoid Vi	Simultaneous	Yes	Adults	Not altered	Not altered	Enhanced meningococcal A and C significant	454

*In addition an unpublished study showed that BCG could be successfully coadministered with 17D by jet injector, with appropriate responses to both vaccines (Chambon L, et al. Unpublished data, 1971).
†Seroconversion rate by survival time method 85% in combined group, 97% in YF 17D–only controls.
‡Subjects also received DTP-polio and measles vaccines at the same time that 17D or 17D and hepatitis B were administered.
§Subjects in all groups also received measles vaccine.
‖Some subjects also received vaccinia.
DPT, diphtheria, pertussis, and tetanus; BCG, bacille Calmette-Guérin; YF, yellow fever; GMT, geometric mean titer.

approach for the development of new vaccines against other flaviviruses. In addition, Galler and coworkers have produced the new seed (and vaccines derived therefrom) in primary chick embryo cell culture, rather than in embryonated eggs (R. Galler, personal communication, 1997). The cell culture–derived vaccine is expected to significantly increase vaccine viral yields, thereby reducing costs. Although modernization of manufacture of 17D vaccine in cell culture has been a goal for many years,[465] previous attempts have failed because of alterations in the virulence phenotype during passage in cell culture (a problem avoided by a genetically uniform infectious clone) or because of poor yields due to in vitro interferon production.

New combination vaccines have been investigated. These include the combination of yellow fever and measles vaccines for the EPI, and combinations of 17D vaccine with inactivated vaccines (e.g., hepatitis A, typhoid) as a means of simplifying immunization regimes for travelers.

PUBLIC HEALTH CONSIDERATIONS

Recommended Usage and Epidemiological Results of Vaccination

South America

Yellow fever immunization has been implemented for decades in all countries with endemic yellow fever in South America, but vaccination coverage and strategies vary by country. Venezuela and Brazil conduct routine immunization using both stationary centers in endemic areas and mobile teams. Vaccination campaigns in endemic areas are also conducted at varied intervals (e.g., every 5 years in Brazil). Since jungle yellow fever affects principally adults, there is less urgency to immunize young children than in Africa. In the mid-1980s, coverage rates in the "at-risk" population (living in the endemic zone; see Fig. 34–7) varied considerably by country, with relatively high coverage (>70%) in Venezuela, Brazil, and Bolivia and low rates in some other countries, notably Ecuador and Peru (approximately 30%).[230, 466] The mass campaigns result in the unnecessary revaccination of large numbers of individuals; in Brazil, for example, 37 million doses were delivered in the endemic population (17 million) between 1980 and 1988.[467] A chronic problem in South America is the movement of unimmunized people from coastal regions, where immunization is not practiced, into the endemic zone. Improvements in roads, increased settlement within the Amazon region, and the fluidity of human population movements hamper vaccination of immigrants and migrant workers.[230] Moreover, the reinvasion of South America by *A. aegypti* has increased the potential for urbanization of the disease and introduction into coastal regions where immunization is not practiced. New recommendations have been made for the integration of yellow fever vaccine into the routine EPI schedule in South America, and implementation has begun in the endemic region of Brazil.

The result of vaccination policies in South America is difficult to assess by historical comparisons with the prevaccine era, since confounding events coincided with the introduction of widescale immunization, including the introduction of active surveillance (using viscerotomy, initiated in 1930) and the expansion of human settlements into endemic areas. Nevertheless, in countries like Brazil that instituted a program of immunization, the incidence of jungle yellow fever declined as vaccination coverage increased (Fig. 34–25),[467] whereas in other countries, where coverage was low (e.g., Peru), large numbers of cases have occurred in recent years.

Africa

The increased incidence of epidemic yellow fever in Africa, beginning in the mid-1980s,[26, 226] and the recognition that the disease predominantly affects children led to a reassessment of vaccination policy for Africa. In 1988, a joint UNICEF/WHO Technical Group on Immunization for the African Region and the EPI Global Advisory Group recommended that countries endemic for yellow fever incorporate 17D vaccine into the routine EPI schedule, either at 6 months of age or at 9 months of age, together with measles vaccine.[212, 468, 469] In 1990, this recommendation was reemphasized, with the additional suggestion that catch-up immuniza-

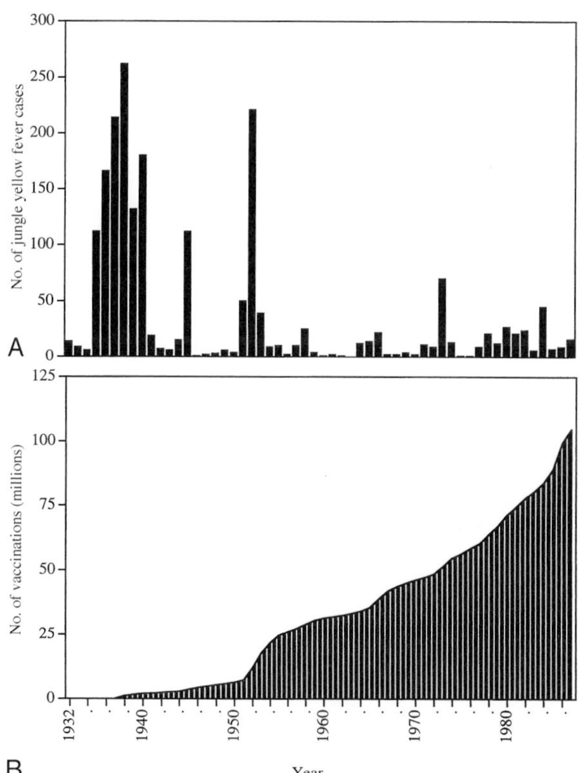

Figure 34–25. Incidence of jungle yellow fever in Brazil (*A*) and the cumulative number of doses of 17D vaccine administered in the endemic area (*B*), 1932 to 1988. (Data from Calheiros LB. A febre amarela no Brasil. Simpósio Internacional sobre Febre Amarela e Dengue. Cingüentenário da Introdução da Cepa 17D no Brasil. Rio de Janeiro, Funação Oswaldo Cruz, 1988, pp 74–85.)

tion of older children is needed in countries at high risk. Surveys conducted between 1987 and 1990 indicated coverage of approximately 80% of infants by 1 year of age in The Gambia, Ivory Coast, and Senegal, but rates of approximately 40% in Burkina Faso, Chad, Mauritania, and the Central African Republic. By 1991, 14 of 33 African countries at risk of yellow fever (Angola, Burkina Faso, Cameroun, Central African Republic, Chad, Ivory Coast, The Gambia, Ghana, Mali, Mauritania, Niger, Nigeria, Senegal, Togo) had officially incorporated 17D vaccine into the EPI, but the uptake of the vaccine was poor in most countries, principally because of a lack of donor funding for the purchase of vaccine. In 1992 (13 countries reporting), the overall coverage was 19%; in 1993 (12 countries reporting), coverage was 14%; and in 1994 (11 countries reporting), coverage was 29%.[470] By 1994, rates were less than 50% in all countries (Fig. 34–26), excepting The Gambia. The Gambia, which suffered a major outbreak in 1978 to 1979 and responded with mass immunization of children and adults, followed by sustained high rates of coverage of infants in the EPI, is the only African country that is fully protected against yellow fever.[93]

Whereas a policy of routine immunization of infants in the EPI is an important goal, it should be emphasized that even assuming the achievement of high coverage rates, it would take at least 15 years to create herd immunity sufficient to prevent epidemic spread without "catch-up" immunization of older children. Since 17D vaccine induces lifelong immunity, as shown by studies of populations that do not have an opportunity for boosting by natural exposure,[385] revaccination is unnecessary.

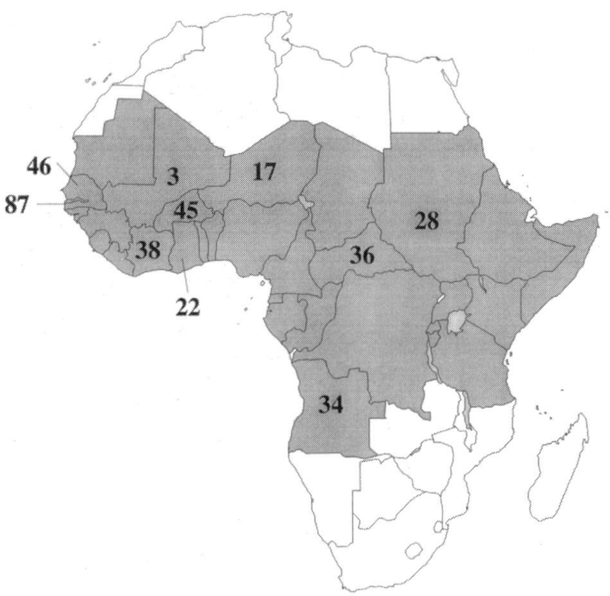

Figure 34–26. Yellow fever vaccine coverage (%) of infants by 1 year of age, 1994; data from WHO Expanded Program of Immunization. Countries shaded are considered at risk of yellow fever. (Data from Meegan JM. Yellow Fever Vaccine. Unofficial Report WHO/EPI/GEN/91.6. Geneva, World Health Organization, 1991.)

Cost-Benefit of Immunization

In an analysis of the benefit of immunization versus the risk of yellow fever, Brès concluded that a "fire-fighting" approach (emergency mass immunization in the face of outbreaks) was less costly than preventive immunization.[415] This question was explored by Monath and Nasidi, using a model in which routine yellow fever vaccination was hypothetically introduced into the EPI in Nigeria.[237] They concluded that 15 to 18 years would be required to achieve an effective immune barrier to epidemic spread, at which time routine immunization would be sevenfold to eightfold more efficient than emergency control in the number of cases and deaths prevented. The cost of routine immunization was estimated at $763 per case and $3817 per death prevented during epidemics, with lower costs if the prevention of endemic disease was taken into account. These cost-effectiveness ratios compared favorably to those for other infections preventable by EPI vaccines in Africa.[471] The authors concluded that "the exceptional ability of a single dose of 17D vaccine to provide lifelong immunity is the keystone of its value in the EPI; an infant vaccinated . . . is fully protected over a 50-year lifetime for an investment of $0.01/year!"

Eradication or Elimination? Level of Herd Immunity Required

Eradication by means of human vaccination is not feasible, since virus circulates independent of humans in nonhuman primates and mosquitoes.

Elimination of the disease is achievable by vaccination, but 100% coverage would be necessary to prevent cases of jungle yellow fever acquired by exposure to enzootic vectors. Prevention of epidemics involving interhuman transmission by *A. aegypti* or sylvatic vectors in Africa would also require a high prevalence of immunity. This was shown in the case of the severe epidemic in Senegal (1965), where the prevalence of immunity before the epidemic in children younger than 10 years (the age group affected during the outbreak) was estimated to have been 57%.[232] Brès concluded that herd immunity must exceed 90% to preclude epidemic yellow fever.[415] Mathematical models have been applied to the calculation of the proportion of human hosts susceptible to infection required to sustain an epidemic (reproductive rate of infection >1), but they require an understanding of the biting rate, probability of feeding on a human host, and transmission efficiency of the vector.[142, 266] The effect of herd immunity on yellow fever transmission under different assumptions of vectorial capacity were explored by Monath and Nasidi.[237] The prevalence of immunity in human population required to preclude an epidemic was estimated to be between 60 and 90% (Fig. 34–27).

Restrictions on Distribution of Yellow Fever Vaccine to at-Risk Travelers

The International Sanitary Regulations specify that yellow fever vaccine be administered only by approved

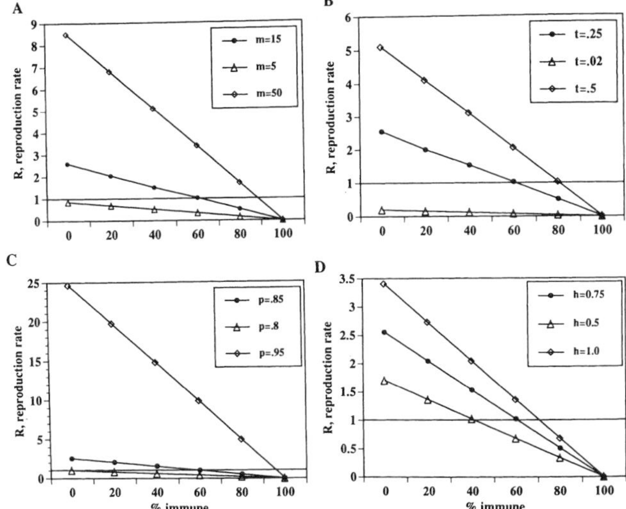

Figure 34–27. Relationship between R, the reproductive rate of an epidemic, and the prevalence of herd immunity in the host population under different assumptions of vectorial capacity. *A*, Effect of varying the number of mosquito bites per day (m). *B*, Effect of varying vector competence (T = proportion of mosquitoes transmitting the virus). *C*, Effect of varying in the average daily survival time of the vector. *D*, Effect of varying the average proportion of vectors feeding on a human host (h). (*A–D* from Monath TP, Nasidi A. Should yellow fever vaccine be included in the Expanded Program of Immunization in Africa? A cost-effectiveness analysis for Nigeria. Am J Trop Med Hyg 48:274, 1993.)

vaccinating centers, which are listed in a 1991 WHO publication[472] and updated in the WHO *WER*. This restriction provides assurances that the vaccine will be properly stored and delivered using aseptic technique within the specified time after reconstitution. A vaccination certificate, specifying the date of immunization and the vaccine lot number and signed by personnel at the vaccinating center, constitutes proof of valid immunization for the purposes of international travel. Although this system has obvious benefits, especially where the medical care system is not highly developed, it also has important drawbacks. It the United States, for example, where there are 800 to 1000 vaccinating centers, the administration of the system by federal and state health departments has become unwieldy and inaccurate. More important, some states are underserved by vaccinating centers, with in excess of 26% of the population residing 25 miles or more from the nearest center (T. P. Monath and colleagues, unpublished data, 1997). This logistic barrier to access to yellow fever vaccine may result in underutilization, as demonstrated by a fatal case in a Tennessee man who was not vaccinated because of the inconvenience of traveling to a distant vaccinating center.[250] The requirements for the proper storage and use of yellow fever vaccine are less stringent than for varicella vaccine, which is available to all physicians through normal distribution channels. A cogent argument can thus be made for open access of yellow fever vaccine to all physicians in countries with well-developed drug distribution systems and large numbers of international travelers. Certification of vaccination would be provided by the vaccinating physician.

REFERENCES

1. Zanotto PM, Gould EA, Gao GF, et al. Population dynamics of flaviviruses revealed by molecular phylogenies. Proc Natl Acad Sci U S A 93:548, 1996.
2. Carter HR. Yellow Fever. An Epidemiological and Historical Study of its Place of Origin. Baltimore, Williams & Wilkins, 1931, pp 1–308.
3. Garrison FH. An Introduction to the History of Medicine with Medical Chronology, Suggestions for Study, and Bibliographical Data. Philadelphia, WB Saunders, 1929, pp 1–996.
4. Powell JH. Bring Out Your Dead. Philadelphia, University of Pennsylvania Press, 1949, pp 1–300.
5. Duffy J. Sword of Pestilence. Baton Rouge, LSU, 1966, pp 1–254.
6. Coleman W. Yellow Fever in the North. Madison, University of Wisconsin Press, 1987, pp 1–260.
7. Finlay C. El mosquito hipoteticamente considerado como agente de transmision de la fiebre amarilla. Anal Real Acad Ciencias Med Fisicas Naturales 18:147, 1881.
8. Yellow Fever. A compilation of various publications. Results of the work of Maj Walter Reed, Medical Corps, United States Army, and the Yellow Fever Commission. 61st Congress Document No. 822, Washington, DC, US Government Printing Office, 1911.
9. Stokes A, Bauer JH, Hudson NP. Experimental transmission of yellow fever to laboratory animals. Am J Trop Med 8:103, 1928.
10. Mathis C, Sellards AW, Laigret J. Sensibilité du *Macacus rhesus* au virus de la fièvre jaune. C R Acad Sci 186:604, 1928.
11. Deubel V, Ekue EK, Diop MM, et al. Introduction à l'analyse de la virulence du virus de la fièvre jaune (*Flaviviridae*): Études génétiques, immunochimiques et biologiques comparatives entre les souches atténuées vaccinales et leurs souches parentales. Ann Inst Pasteur Virol 137E:191, 1986.
12. Jennings AD, Whitby JE, Minor PD, et al. Comparison of the nucleotide and deduced amino acid sequences of the structural protein genes of the yellow fever 17DD vaccine strain from Senegal with those of other yellow fever vaccine viruses. Vaccine 11:679, 1993.
13. Hindle E. A yellow fever vaccine. BMJ 1:976, 1928.
14. Sawyer WA, Kitchen SF, Lloyd W. Vaccination against yellow fever with immune serum and virus fixed for mice. J Exp Med 55:945, 1932.
15. Berry GP, Kitchen SF. Yellow fever accidentally contracted in the laboratory. A study of seven cases. Am J Trop Med Hyg 11:365, 1931.
16. Sellards AW, Laigret J. Vaccination de l'homme contre la fièvre jaune. C R Acad Sci 194:1609, 1932.
17. Mathis C, Laigret J, Durieux C. Trois mille vaccinations contre la fièvre jaune en Afrique Occidentale Française au moyen du virus vivant souris, atténué par le vieillissment. C R Acad Sci 199:742, 1934.
18. Theiler M, Smith HH. The effect of prolonged cultivation in vitro upon the pathogenicity of yellow fever virus. J Exp Med 65:767, 1937.
19. Smith HH, Theiler M. The adaptation of unmodified strains of yellow fever virus to cultivation in vitro. J Exp Med 65:801, 1937.
20. Theiler M, Smith HH. The use of yellow fever virus modified by in vitro cultivation for human immunization. J Exp Med 65:787, 1937.
21. Smith HH. Penna HA, Paoliello A. Yellow fever vaccination with cultured virus (17D) without immune serum. Am J Trop Med Hyg 18:437, 1938.
22. Monath TP. Yellow fever vaccines: The success of empiricism, pitfalls of application, and transition to molecular vaccinology. In Plotkin S, Fantini B (eds). Vaccinia, Vaccination, Vaccinology: Jenner, Pasteur and Their Successors. Paris, Elsevier, 1996, pp 157–182.
23. Sorel F. La vaccination anti-amarile en Afrique Occidentale Française, mise en application du procédé de vaccination Sellards-Laigret. Bull Off Int Hyg Pub 28:1325, 1936.
24. Durieux C. Mass yellow fever vaccination in French Africa south of the Sahara. In Smithburn KC, Durieux C, Koerber R, et al. (eds). Yellow Fever Vaccination. Geneva, World Health Organization, 1956, pp 115–121.

25. Peltier M. Yellow fever vaccination, simple or associated with vaccination against smallpox, of the populations of French West Africa by the method of the Pasteur Institute of Dakar. Am J Public Health 37:1026, 1947.
26. Robertson SE, Hull BP, Tomori O, et al. Yellow Fever. A decade of reemergence. JAMA 276:1157, 1996.
27. Monath TP. Epidemiology of yellow fever: Current status and speculations on future trends. In Saluzzo J-F, Dodet B (eds). Factors in the Emergence of Arbovirus Diseases. Paris, Elsevier 1997, pp 143–156.
28. Chambers TJ, Hahn CS, Galler R, Rice CM. Flavivirus genome organization, expression, and replication. Annu Rev Microbiol 44:649, 1990.
29. Rice CM. Flaviviridae; the viruses and their replication. In Fields BN (ed). Fields Virology. Vol. 1 (3rd ed). Philadelphia, Lippincott-Raven, 1996, p 931.
30. Guirakhoo F, Bolin RA, Roehrig JT. The Murray Valley encephalitis virus prM protein confers acid resistance to virus particles and alters the expression of epitopes within the R2 domain of E glycoprotein. Virology 191:921, 1992.
31. Rey FA, Heinz FX, Mandl C, et al. The envelope glycoprotein from the tick-borne encephalitis virus at 2Å resolution. Nature 375:291, 1995.
32. Lobigs M, Dalgarno L, Schlesinger JJ, et al. Location of a neutralization determinant in the E protein of yellow fever virus (17D vaccine strain). Virology 161:474, 1987.
33. Ryman KD, Ledger TN, Weir RC Jr, et al. Yellow fever virus envelope protein has two discrete type-specific neutralizing epitopes. J Gen Virol 78:1353, 1997.
34. Schlesinger JJ, Brandriss MW, Putnak JR, et al. Cell surface expression of yellow fever virus non-structural glycoprotein NS1: Consequences of interaction with antibody. J Gen Virol 71:593, 1990.
35. Mathews JH, Allan JE, Roehrig JR, et al. T-helper cell and associated antibody response to synthetic peptides of the E glycoprotein of Murray Valley encephalitis virus. J Virol 65:5141, 1991.
36. Rothman AL, Kurane I, Ennis FA. Multiple specificities in the murine $CD4^+$ and $CD8^+$ T-cell response to dengue virus. J Virol 70:6540, 1996.
37. Lobigs M, Arthur CE, Mullbacher A, et al. The flavivirus nonstructural protein NS3 is a dominant source of cytotoxic T cell peptide determinants. Virology 202:196, 1994.
38. Westaway EG, Khromykh AA, Kenney MT, et al. Proteins C and NS4B of the flavivirus Kunjin translocate independently into the nucleus. Virology 234:31, 1997.
39. Rice CM, Lenches EM, Eddy SR, et al. Nucleotide sequence of yellow fever virus: Implications for flavivirus gene expression and evolution. Science 229:726, 1985.
40. Hahn CH, Dalrymple JM, Strauss JH, et al. Comparison of the virulent Asibi strain of yellow fever virus with the 17D vaccine strain derived from it. Proc Natl Acad Sci U S A 84:2019, 1987.
41. Wang E, Ryman KD, Jennings AD, et al. Comparison of the genomes of the wild-type French viscerotropic strain of yellow fever virus with its vaccine derivative French neurotropic vaccine. J Gen Virol 76:2749, 1995.
42. Post PR, Santos CND, Carvalho R, et al. Heterogeneity in envelope protein sequence and *N*-linked glycosylation among yellow fever virus vaccine strains. Virology 188:160, 1992.
43. Duarte dos Santos CN, Post PR, Carvalho R, et al. Complete nucleotide sequence of yellow fever virus vaccine strains 17DD and 17D-213. Virus Res 95:35, 1995.
44. Barrett ADT. Yellow fever vaccine. Biologicals 25:17, 1997.
45. Pletnev AG, Bray M, Lai C-J. Chimeric tick-borne encephalitis and dengue type 4 viruses: Effects of mutations on neurovirulence in mice. J Virol 67:4956, 1993.
46. Ballinger-Crabtree M, Miller BR. Partial nucleotide sequence of South American yellow fever strain 1899/91: Structural proteins and NS1. J Gen Virol 71:2115, 1990.
47. Holzmann H, Stiasny K, Ecker M, et al. Characterization of monoclonal antibody-escape mutants of tick-borne encephalitis virus with reduced neuroinvasiveness in mice. J Gen Virol 78:31, 1997.
48. Guirakhoo F, Heinz FX, Kunz C. Epitope model of tick-borne encephalitis virus envelope glycoprotein E: Analysis of structural properties, role of carbohydrate side-chain, and conformational changes occurring at acidic pH. Virology 169:90, 1989.
49. Ryman KD, Xie H, Ledger TN, et al. Short communication. Antigenic variants of yellow fever virus with an altered neurovirulence phenotype in mice. Virology 230:376, 1997.
50. Lobigs M, Usha R, Nestorowicz A, et al. Host cell selection of Murray Valley encephalitis virus variants altered at the RGD sequence in the envelope protein and in mouse virulence. Virology 176:587, 1990.
51. Holzmann H, Heinz FX, Mandl CW, et al. A single amino acid substitution in envelope protein E of tick-borne encephalitis virus leads to attenuation in the mouse model. J Virol 64:5156, 1990.
52. Fatal viral encephalitis following 17D yellow fever vaccine inoculation. Report of a case in a 3-year-old child. JAMA 198:671, 1966.
53. Jennings AD, Gibson CA, Miller BR. Analysis of a yellow fever virus isolated from a fatal case of vaccine-associated human encephalitis. J Infect Dis 169:512, 1994.
54. Schlesinger JJ, Chapman S, Nestorowicz A, et al. Replication of yellow fever virus in the mouse central nervous system: Comparison of neuroadapted and nonneuroadapted virus and partial sequence analysis of the neuroadapted strain. J Gen Virol 77:1277, 1996.
55. Collier WA, De Roever-Bonnet H, Hoekstra J. A neurotropic variety of the vaccine strain 17D. Trop Geogr Med 11:80, 1959.
56. McMinn PC, Marshall ID, Dalgarno L. Neurovirulence and neuroinvasiveness of Murray Valley encephalitis virus mutants selected by passage in a monkey kidney cell line. J Gen Virol 76:865, 1995.
57. Muylaert IR, Chambers TJ, Galler R, et al. Mutagenesis of the *N*-linked glycosylation sites of the yellow fever virus NS1 protein: Effects on virus replication and mouse neurovirulence. Virology 222:159, 1996.
58. Liprandi F. Isolation of plaque variants differing in virulence from the 17D strain of yellow fever virus. J Gen Virol 56:363, 1981.
59. Xie H. Mutations in the genome of yellow fever 17D-204 vaccine virus accumulate in the non-structural protein genes. PhD dissertation. University of Texas Medical Branch, Galveston, TX, 1997.
60. Schlesinger JJ, Brandriss MW, Monath TP. Monoclonal antibodies distinguish between wild and vaccine strains of yellow fever virus by neutralization, hemagglutination inhibition, and immune precipitation of the virus envelope protein. Virology 125:8, 1983.
61. Schlesinger JJ, Walsh EE, Brandriss MW. Analysis of 17D yellow fever virus envelope protein epitopes using monoclonal antibodies. J Gen Virol 65:1637, 1984.
62. Monath TP, Schlesinger JJ, Brandriss MW, et al. Yellow fever monoclonal antibodies: Type-specific and cross-reactive determinants identified by immunofluorescence. Am J Trop Med Hyg 33:695, 1984.
63. Geske T, Nichtila P, Seethaler H, et al. Establishment of hybridomas producing antibodies to viral surface epitopes related to pathogenic properties of yellow fever virus strains. Immunobiology 165:263, 1983.
64. Cammack N, Gould EA. Antigenic analysis of yellow fever virus glycoproteins: Use of monoclonal antibodies in enzyme-linked immunosorbent assays. J Virol Methods 13:135, 1986.
65. Barrett ADT, Matthews JH, Miller BR, et al. Identification of monoclonal antibodies that distinguish between 17D-204 and other strains of yellow fever virus. J Gen Virol 71:13, 1990.
66. Barrett ADT, Pryde A, Medlen AR, et al. Examination of the envelope glycoprotein of yellow fever vaccine viruses with monoclonal antibodies. Vaccine 7:333, 1989.
67. Buckley A, Gould EA. Neutralization of yellow fever virus studied using monoclonal and polyclonal antibodies. J Gen Virol 66:2523, 1985.
68. Ledger TN, Sil BK, Wills MR. Variation in the biological function of envelope protein epitopes of yellow fever vaccine viruses detected with monoclonal antibodies. Biologicals 20:117, 1992.
69. Sil BK, Dunster LM, Ledger TN, et al. Identification of envelope protein epitopes that are important in the attenuation process of wild-type yellow fever virus. J Virol 66:4265, 1992.
70. Gould EA, Buckley A, Cane PA, et al. Use of a monoclonal

antibody specific for wild-type yellow fever virus to identify a wild-type antigenic variant in 17D vaccine pools. J Gen Virol 70:1889, 1989.
71. Gagnon SJ, Zeng W, Kurane I, et al. Identification of two epitopes on the dengue-4 virus capsid protein recognized by a serotype-specific and a panel of serotype-cross-reactive human $CD4^+$ cytotoxic T-lymphocyte clones. J Virol 70:141, 1996.
72. Roehrig JT, Risi PA, Bribaker JR, et al. T helper cell epitopes on the E glycoprotein of dengue-2 Jamaica virus. Virology 198:31, 1994.
73. Saikh KU, Tammza M, Kuwano K, et al. Protective cross-reactive epitope on the nonstructural protein NS1 of influenza virus. Viral Immunol 6:229, 1993.
74. Mathew A, Kurane I, Rothman A, et al. Dominant recognition by human $CD8^+$ cytoxic T lymphocytes of dengue virus nonstructional proteins NS3 and NS2a. J Clin Invest 98:1684, 1996.
75. Kurane I, Brinton MA, Sampson AL, et al. Dengue virus-specific human $CD4^+CD8^-$ cytotoxic T-cell clones; multiple patterns of virus cross-reactivity by NS3-specific T-cell clones. J Virol 65:1823, 1991.
76. Mathews JH, Allan JE, Roehrig JR, et al. T-helper cell and associated antibody response to synthetic peptides of the E glycoprotein of Murray Valley encephalitis virus. J Virol 65:5141, 1991.
77. Kerr JA. The clinical aspects and diagnosis of yellow fever. In Strode GK (ed). Yellow Fever. New York, McGraw-Hill, 1951, pp 385–426.
78. Beeuwkes H. Clinical manifestations of yellow fever in the West African native as observed during four extensive epidemics of the disease in the Gold Coast and Nigeria. Trans R Soc Trop Med Hyg 1:61, 1936.
79. Monath TP. Yellow fever: A medically neglected disease. Report on a seminar. Rev Infect Dis 9:165, 1987.
80. MacNamara FN. Man as the host of the yellow fever virus. MD thesis. Cambridge University, Cambridge, 1955, pp 1–140.
81. Nassar EdS, Chamelet ELB, Coimbra TLM. Jungle yellow fever: Clinical and laboratorial studies emphasizing viremia on a human case. Rev Inst Med Trop Sao Paulo 37:337, 1995.
82. Oudart J-L, Rey M. Protéinurie, protéinémie et transaminasémies dans 23 cas de fièvre jaune confirmée. Bull World Health Organ 42:95, 1970.
83. MacNamara FN. A clinico-pathological study of yellow fever in Nigeria. W Afr J Med 6:137, 1957.
84. Elton NW, Romero A, Trejos A. Clinical pathology of yellow fever. Am J Clin Pathol 25:135, 1955.
85. Boulos M, Segurado AA, Shirome M. Severe yellow fever with 23-day survival. Trop Geog Med 40:356, 1988.
86. Borges APA, Oliveira GSC, Almeida Netto JC. Estudo da coagulaçao sanguinea na febre amarela. Rev Patologia Trop 2:143, 1973.
87. Santos F, Pereira Lima C, Paiva P, et al. Coagulaçao intravascular disseminada aguda na febre amarela: Dosagem dos factores da coagulaçao. Brasilia Med 9:9, 1973.
88. Chagas E, De Freitas L. Electrocardiogramma na febre amarela. Mem Inst Oswaldo Cruz Suppl 7:72, 1929.
89. Williams MC, Woodall JP, Simpson DIH. Yellow fever in central Uganda, 1964. III. Virus isolation from man and laboratory studies. Trans R Soc Trop Med Hyg 59:444, 1965.
90. Stevanson LD. Pathological changes in the central nervous system in yellow fever. Arch Pathol 27:249, 1939.
91. Stefanopoulo GJ, Mollaret P. Hémiplégie d'origine cérébrale et névrite optique au cours d'un cas de fièvre jaune. Bull Mem Soc Med Hop Paris 50:1463, 1934.
92. Findlay GM, Stern RO. Essential neurotropism of yellow fever virus. J Pathol Bacteriol 41:431, 1935.
93. Monath TP, Craven RB, Adjukiewicz A, et al. Yellow fever in The Gambia, 1978–1979: Epidemiologic aspects with observations on the occurrence of Orungo virus infections. Am J Trop Med Hyg 29:912, 1980.
94. Nasidi A, Monath TP, DeCock K. Urban yellow fever epidemic in western Nigeria, 1987. Trans R Soc Trop Med Hyg 83:401, 1989.
95. Hanson H. Observations on the age and sex incidence of deaths and recoveries in the yellow fever epidemic in the department of Lambayeque, Peru, in 1921. Am J Trop Med Hyg 9:233, 1929.
96. Jones MM, Wilson DC. Clinical features of yellow fever cases at Vom Christian Hospital during the 1969 epidemic on the Jos Plateau, Nigeria. Bull World Health Organ 46:653, 1972.
97. Kirk R. Epidemic of yellow fever in Nuba Mountains, Anglo-Egyptian Sudan. Ann Trop Med Parasitol 35:67, 1941.
98. Klotz O, Simpson W. Jaundice and the liver lesions in West African yellow fever. Am J Trop Med Hyg 7:271, 1927.
99. Monath TP, Hadler SC. Type B hepatitis and yellow fever infections in West Africa. Trans R Soc Trop Med Hyg 81:172, 1987.
100. Cornet M, Robin Y, Héme G, et al. Une pousée épizootique de fièvre jaune selvatique au Sénégal oriental. Isôlement du virus de lots de moustiques adultes et mâles et femelles. Med Malad Infect 9:63, 1979.
101. Beaty BJ, Tesh RB, Aitken THG. Transovarial transmission of yellow fever virus in *Stegomyia* mosquitoes. Am J Trop Med Hyg 29:125, 1980.
102. Aitken THG, Tesh RB, Beaty B, et al. Transovarial transmission of yellow fever virus by mosquitoes (*Aedes aegypti*). Am J Trop Med Hyg 29:125, 1980.
103. Wheelock EF, Edelman R. Specific role of each human leukocyte type in viral infections. III. 17D yellow fever virus replication and interferon production in homogeneous leukocyte cultures treated with phytohemagglutinin. J Immunol 103:429, 1969.
104. Sweet BH, Wisseman CJ Jr, Kitaoka M. Immunological studies with group B arthropod-borne viruses. II. Effect of prior infection with Japanese encephalitis virus on the viremia in human subject following administration of 17D yellow fever vaccine. Am J Trop Med Hyg 11:562, 1962.
105. Whitman L. Failure of *Aedes aegypti* to transmit yellow fever cultured virus (17D). Am J Trop Med 19:19, 1939.
106. Miller BR, Adkins D. Biological characterization of plaque-size variants of yellow fever virus in mosquitos and mice. Acta Virol 32:227, 1988.
107. Turell MJ. Horizontal and vertical transmission of viruses by insect and tick vectors. In Monath TP (ed). The Arboviruses; Epidemiology and Ecology. Vol. I. Boca Raton, CRC, 1988, pp 127–152.
108. Turell MJ, Tammariello RF. Nonvascular delivery of St. Louis encephalitis and Venezuelan equine encephalitis by infected mosquitoes during feeding on a vertebrate host. Am J Trop Med Hyg 49:197, 1993.
109. Theiler M. The virus. In Strode GK (ed). Yellow Fever. New York, McGraw Hill, 1951, pp 46–136.
110. Zisman B, Wheelock EF, Allison AC. Role of macrophages and antibody in resistance of mice against yellow fever virus. J Immunol 107:236, 1971.
111. Bugher JC. The mammalian host in yellow fever. In Strode GK (ed). Yellow Fever. New York, McGraw-Hill, 1951, pp 299–384.
112. Monath TP. Yellow fever. In Monath TP (ed). The Arboviruses: Ecology and Epidemiology. Vol V. Boca Raton, FL, CRC, 1988, pp 139–231.
113. Findlay GM, Clarke LP. Susceptibility of hedgehog to yellow fever: Viscerotropic virus. Trans R Soc Trop Med Hyg 28:193, 1934.
114. Dennis LH, Reisberg BE, Crosbie J, et al. The original haemorrhagic fever: Yellow fever. Br J Haematol 17:455, 1969.
115. Tigertt, WD, Berge TO, Gochenour WS, et al. Experimental yellow fever. Trans N Y Acad Sci 22:323, 1960.
116. Monath TP, Brinker KR, Chandler FW, et al. Pathophysiologic correlations in a rhesus monkey model of yellow fever. Am J Trop Med Hyg 30:431, 1981.
117. Bauer JH. The duration of passive immunity in yellow fever. Am J Trop Med Hyg 11:451, 1931.
118. Bearcroft WGC. The histopathology of the liver of yellow fever infected rhesus monkey. J Pathol Bacteriol 74:295, 1957.
119. Klotz O, Belt TH. Pathology of the liver in yellow fever. Am J Pathol 6:663, 1930.
120. Marotto ME, Thurman RG, Lemasters JJ. Early midzonal cell death during low-flow hypoxia in the isolated, perfused rat liver: Protection by allopurinol. Hepatology 8:585, 1988.
121. Monath TP, Ballinger ME, Miller BR, et al. Detection of yellow fever viral RNA by nucleic acid hybridization and viral antigen by immunocytochemistry in fixed human liver. Am J Trop Med Hyg 40:663, 1989.
122. Vieira WT, Gayotto LC, De Lima CP, et al. Histopathology of

the human liver in yellow fever with special emphasis on the diagnostic role of the Councilman body. Histopathology 7:195, 1983.

123. De Brito T, Siqueira SAC, Santos RTM, et al. Human fatal yellow fever. Immunohistochemical detection of viral antigens in the liver, kidney and heart. Pathol Res Pract 188:177, 1992.
124. Barbareschi G. Glomerulosi tossica in fiebre gialla. Rev Biol Trop 5:201, 1957.
125. Klotz O, Belt TH. Pathology in spleen in yellow fever. Am J Pathol 6:655, 1930.
126. Cannell DE. Myocardial degenerations in yellow fever. Am J Pathol 4:431, 1928.
127. Lloyd W. The myocardium in yellow fever. II. The myocardial lesions in experimental yellow fever. Am Heart J 6:504, 1931.
128. Hughes TP. Precipitin reaction in yellow fever. J Immunol 25:275, 1933.
129. Gould EA, Buckley A, Groeger BK, et al. Immune enhancement of yellow fever virus neurovirulence for mice: Studies of mechanisms involved. J Gen Virol 68:3105, 1987.
130. Barrett ADT, Gould EA. Antibody-mediated early death in vivo after infection with yellow fever virus. J Gen Virol 67:2539, 1986.
131. Sangster MY, Mackenzie JS, Shellam GR, et al. Genetically determined resistance to flavivirus infection in wild *Mus musculus domesticus* and other taxonomic groups in the genus *Mus*. Arch Virol 143:697, 1998.
132. Wills MR, Singh BK, Debnath NC, et al. Immunogenicity of wild-type and vaccine strains of Japanese encephalitis virus and the effect of haplotype restriction murine immune responses. Vaccine 7:761, 1993.
133. Elton NW. Sylvan yellow fever in Central America. Public Health Rep 67:426, 1952.
134. Matas R. Nursing in yellow fever and the duties of trained nurses in epidemics. Trained Nurse Hosp Rev Oct–Dec 3–24, 1905.
134a. Bravo JR, Guzman MG, Kouri GP. Why dengue haemorrhagic fever in Cuba? I. Individual risk factors for dengue haemorrhagic fever/dengue shock syndrome. Trans R Soc Trop Med Hyg. 81:816, 1987.
135. Paradoa Perez ML, Trujillo Y, Basanta P. Association of dengue hemorrhagic fever with the HLA system. Hematologia 20:83, 1987.
136. Chang GJ, Cropp CB, Kinney RM, et al. Nucleotide sequence variation of the envelope protein gene identifies two distinct genotypes of yellow fever virus. J Virol 69:5773, 1995.
137. Fox JP. Non-fatal infection of mice following intracerebral inoculation of yellow fever virus. J Exp Med 77:507, 1943.
138. Fitzgeorge R, Bradish CJ. The in vivo differentiation of strains of yellow fever virus in mice. J Gen Virol 46:1, 1980.
139. Barrett ADT, Gould EA. Comparison of neurovirulence of different strains of yellow fever virus in mice. J Gen Virol 67:631, 1986.
140. Laemmert HW Jr. Susceptibility of marmosets to different strains of yellow fever virus. Am J Trop Med 24:71, 1944.
141. Deubel V, Schlesinger JJ, Digoutte J-P, et al. Comparative immunochemical and biological analysis of African and South American yellow fever viruses. Arch Virol 94:331, 1987.
142. Miller BR, Monath TP, Tabachnick WJ, et al. Epidemic yellow fever caused by an incompetent mosquito vector. Trop Med Parasitol 40:396, 1989.
143. Sabin A. Research on dengue during World War II. Am J Trop Med Hyg 1:30, 1952.
144. David-West TS. Concurrent and consecutive infection and immunization with yellow fever and UGMP-359 virus. Arch Virol 48:21, 1975.
145. Smithburn KC, Mahaffy AF. Immunization against yellow fever. Am J Trop Med 45:217, 1945.
146. Fagaeus A, Ehrnst A, Klein E, et al. Characterization of blood mononuclear cells reacting with K 562 cells after yellow fever vaccination. Cell Immunol 67:37, 1982.
146a. Stephen EL, Sammons ML, Pannier WL, et al. Effect of a nuclease-resistant derivative of polyriboinosinic-polyribocytidylic acid complex on yellow fever in rhesus monkeys (*Macaca mulatta*). J Infect Dis 136:122, 1977.
146b. Bonnevie-Nielsen V, Heron I, Monath TP, et al. Lymphocytic 2′,5′-oligoadenylate synthetase activity increases prior to the appearance of neutralizing antibodies and immunoglobulin M and immunoglobulin G antibodies after primary and secondary immunization with yellow fever vaccine. Clin Diag Lab Immunol 2:302, 1995.
147. Stephen EL, Scott SK, Eddy GA, et al. Effect of interferon on togavirus and arenavirus infections of animals. Tex Rep Biol Med 35:449, 1977.
148. Kurane I, Meager A, Ennis FA. Dengue virus–specific human T-cell clones. Serotype cross-reactive proliferation, interferon-gamma production, cytotoxic activity. J Exp Med 170:763, 1989.
149. Kurane I, Innis BL, Nisalak A, et al. Human T cell responses to dengue antigens: Proliferative responses and interferon-gamma production. J Clin Invest 83:506, 1989.
150. Arroyo JI, Apperson SA, Cropp CB, et al. Effect of human gamma interferon on yellow fever virus infection. Am J Trop Med Hyg 38:647, 1988.
151. Lhuillier M, Sarthou JL, Cordellier R, et al. Émergence endémique de la fièvre jaune en Côte d'Ivoire: Place de la détection des IgM antiamariles dans la stratégie de surveillance. Bull World Health Organ 64:415, 1986.
152. Lhuillier M, Sarthou JL. Intérêt des IgM antiamariles dans le diagnostic et la surveillance épidémiologique de la fièvre jaune. Ann Inst Pasteur Virol 134E:349, 1983.
153. Monath TP, Cropp CP, Muth DJ. Indirect fluorescent antibody test for the diagnosis of yellow fever. Trans R Soc Trop Med Hyg 75:282, 1981.
154. Theiler M, Casals J. The serological reactions in yellow fever. Am J Trop Med Hyg 7:585, 1958.
155. Porterfield JS. The haemagglutination-inhibition test in the diagnosis of yellow fever in man. Trans R Soc Trop Med Hyg 48:261, 1954.
156. Heinz FX. Epitope mapping of flavivirus glycoproteins. Adv Virus Res 31:103, 1986.
157. Sawyer WA. Persistence of yellow fever immunity. J Prev Med 5:413, 1931.
158. Bauer JH, Hudson NP. Duration of immunity in human yellow fever as shown by protective power of serum. J Prev Med 4:177, 1930.
159. Snijders EP, Postmus S, Schüffner W. On the protective power of yellow fever sera and dengue sera against yellow fever virus. Am J Trop Med 14:519, 1934.
160. Frederiksen H. Historical evidence for interference between dengue and yellow fever. Am J Trop Med Hyg 4:483, 1955.
161. Ashcroft MT. Historical evidence of resistance to yellow fever acquired by residence in India. Trans R Soc Trop Med Hyg 73:247, 1979.
162. Dudley SF. Can yellow fever spread into Asia? An essay on the ecology of mosquito-borne disease. J Trop Med Hyg 37:273, 1934.
163. Downs WG. A new look at yellow fever and malaria. Am J Trop Med Hyg 30:516, 1981.
164. Monath TP. The absence of yellow fever from Asia: Hypotheses. A cause for concern? Virus Inform Exch Newsletter 6:106, 1989.
165. Theiler M, Anderson CR. The relative resistance of dengue-immune monkeys to yellow fever virus. Am J Trop Med Hyg 24:115, 1975.
166. Henderson BE, Cheshire PP, Kirya GB, et al. Immunologic studies with yellow fever and selected African group B arboviruses in rhesus and vervet monkeys. Am J Trop Med Hyg 19:110, 1970.
167. Pincus S, Mason PW, Konishi E, et al. Recombinant vaccinia virus producing the prM and E proteins of yellow fever virus protects mice from lethal yellow fever encephalitis. Virology 187:290, 1992.
168. Gould EA, Buckley A, Barrett ADT, et al. Neutralizing (54K) and non-neutralizing (54K and 48K) monoclonal antibodies against structural and non-structural yellow fever virus proteins confer immunity in mice. J Gen Virol 67:591, 1986.
169. Brandriss MW, Schlesinger JJ, Walsh EE, et al. Lethal 17D yellow fever encephalitis in mice. I. Passive protection by monoclonal antibodies to the envelope proteins of 17D yellow fever and dengue 2 viruses. J Gen Virol 67:229, 1986.
170. Gollins SW, Porterfield JS. A new mechanism for the neutralization of enveloped viruses by antiviral antibody. Nature 321:244, 1986.
171. Schlesinger JJ, Chapman S. Neutralizing $F(ab')_2$ fragments of

protective monoclonal antibodies to yellow fever virus (YF) envelope protein fail to protect mice against lethal YF encephalitis. J Gen Virol 76:217, 1995.
172. Falconar AKI, Young PR. Production of dimer-specific and dengue group cross-reactive mouse monoclonal antibodies to the dengue-2 virus non-structural glycoprotein NS1. J Gen Virol 72:961, 1991.
173. Schlesinger JJ, Brandriss MW, Cropp CB, et al. Protection against yellow fever in monkeys by immunization with yellow fever virus nonstructural protein NS1. J Virol 60:1153, 1986.
174. Putnak JR, Schlesinger JJ. Protection of mice against yellow fever virus encephalitis by immunization with a vaccinia virus recombinant encoding the yellow fever virus non-structural proteins, NS1, NS2a and NS2b. J Gen Virol 71:1697, 1990.
175. Cane PA, Gould EA. Reduction of yellow fever virus mouse neurovirulence by immunization with a bacterially synthesized non-structural protein (NS1) fragment. J Gen Virol 69:1232, 1988.
176. Schlesinger JJ, Brandriss MW, Walsh EE. Protection against 17D yellow fever encephalitis in mice by passive transfer of monoclonal antibodies to the nonstructural glycoprotein gp48 and by active immunization with gp48. J Immunol 135:2805, 1985.
177. Schlesinger JJ, Foltzer M, Chapman S. The Fc portion of antibody to yellow fever virus NS1 is a determinant of protection against YF encephalitis in mice. Virology 192:132, 1993.
178. Lennette EH, Perlowagora A. Complement fixation test in the diagnosis of yellow fever; use of infectious mouse brain as antigen. Am J Trop Med 23:481, 1943.
179. Monath TP, Craven RB, Muth DJ. Limitations of the complement-fixation test for distinguishing naturally acquired from vaccine-induced yellow fever infection in flavivirus-hyperendemic areas. Am J Trop Med Hyg 29:624, 1980.
180. Schlesinger JJ, Brandriss MW. Antibody-mediated infection of macrophages and macrophage-like cell lines with 17D–yellow fever virus. J Med Virol 8:103, 1981.
181. Schlesinger JJ, Brandriss MW. Growth of 17D yellow fever virus in a macrophage-like cell line, U937: Role of Fc and viral receptors in antibody-mediated infection. J Immunol 127:659, 1981.
182. Halstead SB, O'Rourke EJ. Dengue viruses and mononuclear phagocytes. I. Infection enhancement by non-neutralizing antibody. J Exp Med 146:201, 1977.
183. Gollins SW, Porterfield JS. Flavivirus infection enhancement in macrophages: Radioactive and biological studies on the effect of antibody on viral fate. J Gen Virol 65:1261, 1984.
184. Cardosa MJ, Porterfield JS, Gordon S. Complement receptor mediates enhanced flavivirus replication in macrophages. J Exp Med 158:258, 1983.
185. Wisseman CL Jr, Sweet B. Immunological studies with group B arthropod-borne viruses. III. Response of human subjects to revaccination with 17D strain yellow fever vaccine. Am J Trop Med Hyg 11:570, 1962.
186. Bancroft WH Jr, Top FH Jr, Eckels KH, et al. Dengue-2 vaccine: Virological, immunological, and clinical responses of six yellow fever immune recipients. Infect Immun 31:698, 1981.
187. Scott RMcN, Eckels KH, Bancroft WH. Dengue 2 vaccine: Dose response in volunteers in relation to yellow fever immune status. J Infect Dis 148:1055, 1983.
188. Kurane I, Rothman AL, Bukowski JF, et al. T-lymphocyte responses to dengue viruses. New aspects of positive-strand RNA viruses. In Brinton MA, Heinz FX (eds). New Aspects of Positive Strand RNA Viruses. Washington, DC, American Society for Microbiology 1990, pp 301–304.
189. Kurane I, Hebblewaite D, Brandt WE, et al. Lysis of dengue virus–infected cells by natural cell-mediated cytotoxicity and antibody-dependent cell mediated cytotoxicity. J Virol 52:223, 1984.
190. Bukowski JF, Kurane I, Lai C-J, et al. Dengue virus–specific cross-reactive CD* human cytotoxic T lymphocytes. J Virol 63:5086, 1989.
191. Findlay GM. Yellow fever and the Anglo-Egyptian Sudan. Am Trop Med Parasitol 35:59, 1941.
192. Bensabath G, Pinheiro FP, Andrade AHP, et al. Exceptional achado em um caso humano de febre amarela. Isolamento de vírus a partir do sangue no 12° dia de doença. Rev Serv Esp Saude Publ 13:95, 1967.
193. Lhuillier M, Sarthou JL, Cordellier R, et al. Epidémie rurale de fièvre jaune avec transmission interhumaine en Côte d'Ivoire en 1982. Bull World Health Organization 63:527, 1985.
194. Varma MRG, Pudney M, Leake CL, et al. Isolations in a mosquito (*Aedes pseudoscutellaris*) cell line (Mos-61) of yellow fever virus strains from original field material. Intervirology 6:50, 1975.
195. Saluzzo JF, Monath TP, Cornet M, et al. Comparaison de différentes techniques pour la détection du virus de la fièvre jaune dans les prélièvements humains et les lots de moustiques: Intérêt d'une méthode rapide de diagnostic par ELISA. Ann Inst Pasteur Virol 136E:115, 1985.
196. Brown TM, Chang GJ, Cropp CB, et al. Detection of yellow fever virus by polymerase chain reaction. Clin Diagn Virol 2:41, 1994.
197. World Health Organization. Yellow fever—Kenya. Wkly Epidemiol Rec 70:169, 1995.
198. Monath TP, Hill LJ, Brown NV, et al. Sensitive and specific monoclonal immunoassay for detecting yellow fever virus in laboratory and clinical specimens. J Clin Microbiol 23:129, 1986.
199. Monath TP, Nystrom RR. Detection of yellow fever virus in serum by enzyme immunoassay. Am J Trop Med Hyg 33:151, 1984.
200. Piech KS, Shelburne JD, Connor DH et al. An electron microscopic study of a human case of yellow fever. Lab Invest 42:143, 1980.
201. De La Monte SM, Linhares AL, Travassos Da Rosa APA, et al. Immunoperoxidase detection of yellow fever virus after natural and expermental infections. Trop Geogr Med 35:235, 1983.
202. Filipe AR, Martins CMV, Rocha H. Laboratory infection with Zika virus after vaccination against yellow fever. Arch Ges Virusforsch 43:315, 1973.
203. Pettit A. Rapport sur la valeur immunisante des vaccins employés contre la fièvre jaune et la valeur thérapeutique du sérum antiamaril. Bull Acad Natl Med 105:522, 1931.
204. Pettit A, Stefanopoulo GJ, Frasey. Sérum anti-amaryllique. C R Seances Biol Fil 99:541, 1928.
205. US Army Medical Research Institute of Infectious Diseases, Annual Report. Washington, DC, unpublished report, 1972, p 246.
206. Gabrielsen B, Monath TP, Huggins JW, et al. Activity of selected Amaryllidaceae constituents and related synthetic substances against medically important RNA viruses. In Chu CK, Cutler HG (eds). National Products as Antiviral Agents. New York, Plenum, 1992, pp 121–135.
207. Gabrielsen B, Monath TP, Huggins JW, et al. Antiviral (RNA) activity of selected Amaryllidaceae isoquinoline constituents and synthesis of related substances. J Nat Prod 55:1569, 1992.
208. Sawyer WA, Whitman L. Yellow fever immunity survey of North, East and South Africa. Trans R Soc Trop Med Hyg 29:397, 1936.
209. Sawyer WA, Bauer JH, Whitman L. Distribution of yellow fever immunity in North America, Central America, West Indies, Europe, Asia and Australia, with special reference to the specificity of protection tests. Am J Trop Med 17:137, 1937.
210. Centers for Disease Control and Information. Health Information for International Travel 1996–97. Atlanta, GA, US Department of Health and Human Services, 1997, pp 1–208.
211. World Health Organization. International Travel and Health. Vaccination Requirements and Health Advice. Geneva, World Health Organization, 1997.
212. World Health Organization. Yellow fever in 1989 and 1990. Wkly Epidemiol Rec 67:245, 1992.
213. World Health Organization. Yellow fever in 1991. Wkly Epidemiol Rec 68:209, 1993.
214. World Health Organization. Yellow fever in 1992 and 1993. Wkly Epidemiol Rec 70:65, 1995.
215. World Health Organization. Yellow fever in 1994 and 1995. Wkly Epidemiol Rec 71:313, 1996.
216. Pan American Health Organization. Yellow Fever Conference. Pan American Health Organization Scientific Publ. No. 19, Washington, DC, Pan American Health Organization, World Health Organization, 1995. (Reprinted from Am J Trop Med Hyg 4:571–661, 1955.
217. Tikasingh ES (ed). Studies on the Natural History of Yellow

Fever in Trinidad. Pan American Health Organization/World Health Organization Caribbean Epidemiology Centre Monograph Series 1. Washington, DC, Pan American Health Organization, World Health Organization, 1991.

218. Monath TP. Epidemiology of yellow fever: Current status and speculations on future trends. In Saluzzo J-F, Dodet B (eds). Factors in the Emergence of Arbovirus Diseases. Paris, Elsevier, 1997, pp 143–156.
219. Aitken THG, Downs WG, Shope RE. *Aedes aegypti* strain fitness for yellow fever transmission. Am J Trop Med Hyg 26:985, 1977.
220. Tabachnick WJ, Wallis GP, Aitken THG, et al. Oral infection of *Aëdes aegypti* with yellow fever virus: Geographic variation and genetic considerations. Am J Trop Med Hyg 34:1219, 1985.
221. Lepiniec L, Delgarno L, Huong VTQ, et al. Geographic distribution and evolution of yellow fever viruses based on direct sequencing of genomic cDNA fragments. J Gen Virol 75:417, 1994.
222. Wang E, Weaver SC, Shope RE, et al. Genetic variation in yellow fever virus: Duplication in the 3′ noncoding region of strains from Africa. Virology 225:274, 1996.
223. Deubel V, Digoutte J-P, Monath TP, et al. Genetic heterogeneity of yellow fever virus strains from Africa and the Americas. J Gen Virol 67:209, 1986.
223a. Deubel V, Pailliez JP, Cornet M, et al. Homogeneity among Senegalese strains of yellow fever virus. Am J Trop Med Hyg 34:976, 1985.
224. Clarke DH. Antigenic analysis of certain group B anthropodborne viruses by antibody absorption. J Exp Med 111:21, 1960.
225. Theiler M, Downs WG. The Arthropod-Borne Viruses of Vertebrates. New Haven, Yale University Press, 1973.
226. Monath TP. Yellow fever: Victor, Victoria? Conqueror, Conquest? Epidemics and research in the last forty years and prospects for the future. Am J Trop Med Hyg 45:1, 1991.
227. DeCock KM, Monath TP, Nasidi A, et al. Epidemic yellow fever in eastern Nigeria, 1986. Lancet 19:630, 1988.
228. World Health Organization. Yellow fever, Kenya. Wkly Epidemiol Rec 68:77, 1993.
229. Sanders EJ, Borus P, Ademba G, et al. Sentinel surveillance for yellow fever in Kenya, 1993–1995. Emerg Infect Dis 2:236, 1996.
230. Pan American Health Organization. Present status of yellow fever: Memorandum from a PAHO meeting. Bull World Health Organ 64:511, 1986.
231. Sérié C, Casals J, Panthier R et al. Études sur la fièvre jaune en Éthiopie. 2. Enquête sérologique sur la population humaine. Bull World Health Organ 38:843, 1968.
232. Brès P, Cornet M, Ly C, et al. Une epidemie de fièvre jaune au Senegal en 1965. I. Charactéristiques de l'épidémie. Bull World Health Organ 36:113, 1967.
233. World Health Organization. Yellow fever in 1982. Wkly Epidemiol Rec 41:313, 1983.
234. Roux J, Baudon D, Robert V, et al. L'épidémie de fièvre jaune du sud-est de la Haute Volta (Octobre–Decembre 1983). Étude épidémiologique préliminaires. Med Trop (Mars) 44:303, 1984.
235. Vicens R, Robert V, Pignon D, et al. L'épidémie de fièvre jaune de l'extrême nort du Cameroun en 1990: Premier isôlement du virus amaril au Cameroun. Bull Organisation Mondiale de la Santé 71:173, 1993.
236. Monath TP, Smith EA, Onejeme SE, et al. Surveillance of yellow fever in Nigeria, 1970–71. Nigerian Med J 2:179, 1972.
237. Monath TP, Nasidi A. Should yellow fever vaccine be included in the Expanded Program of Immunization in Africa? A cost-effectiveness analysis for Nigeria. Am J Trop Med Hyg 48:274, 1993.
238. Murdock FF. The American Legation Guard, Managua, Nicaragua. US Naval Med Bull 14:684, 1920.
239. Warner RA. A case of yellow fever among personnel attached to the United States Naval Mission to Brazil. US Naval Med Bull 27:786, 1929.
240. Tomaszunas S. Przypadki Chorob Tropikalnych Wsrod Pacjentow Instytutu Medycyny Morskiej. Bull Inst Marine Med Gdansk 14:239, 1963.
241. Kirk R, Bayoumi A. Notes on a fatal case of yellow fever. Ann Trop Med Parasitol 38:205, 1944.
242. Elliot M. Yellow fever in the recently inoculated. Trans R Soc Trop Med Hyg 38:231, 1944.
243. Ross RW, Haddow AJ, Raper AB, et al. A fatal case of yellow fever in a European in Uganda. East Afr Med 30:1, 1953.
244. Bendersky N, Carlet J, Ricomme JL, et al. Deux cas de fièvre jaune observés en France et contractés au Sénégal (aspects épidémiologiques et cliniques). Bull Soc Pathol Exot 73:54, 1980.
245. Digoutte JP, Plassart H, Salaun JJ, et al. A propos de trois cas de fièvre jaune contractée au Sénégal. Bull World Health Organ 59:759, 1981.
246. Rodhain F, Hannoun C, Jousset FX, et al. Isôlement du virus de la fièvre jaune à Paris à partir de deux cas humains importés. Bull Soc Pathol Exot 72:411, 1979.
247. World Health Organization. Yellow fever in 1981. Wkly Epidemiol Rec 39:297, 1982.
248. World Health Organization. Yellow fever in 1985. Wkly Epidemiol Rec 61:377, 1986.
249. Nolla-Salas J, Sadalls-Radresa J. Imported yellow fever in vaccinated tourists. Lancet 2:1275, 1989.
250. McFarland JM, Baddour LM, Nelson JE, et al. Imported yellow fever in a United States citizen. Clin Infect Dis 25:1143–1147, 1997.
251. Barros ML, Boecken G. Jungle yellow fever in the central Amazon. Lancet 348:969, 1996.
252. Sawyer WA. Public health implications of tropical and imported diseases. Yellow fever and typhus and the possibility of their introduction into the United States. Am J Public Health 34:7, 1944.
253. Hughes JH, Porter JE. Measures against yellow fever entry into the United States. Public Health Rep 73:1101, 1958.
254. Coimbra TLM, Iversson LB, Spir M, et al. Investigação epidemiologica de casos de febre amarela na região noroeste do Esdade de São Paulo, Brasil. Rev Saude Publica 3:193, 1987.
255. Taylor RM. Epidemiology. In Strode GK (ed). Yellow Fever. New York, McGraw-Hill, 1951, pp 427–538.
256. Pinheiro FP, Travassos Da Rosa APA, Moraes MAP, et al. An epidemic of yellow fever in Central Brazil, 1972–1973. Am J Trop Med Hyg 27:125, 1978.
257. Soper FL. Present day methods for study and control of yellow fever. Am J Trop Med 17:655, 1937.
258. Cornet M, Chateau R, Valade M, et al. Données bioécologiques sur les vecteurs potentiels du virus amaril au Sénégal oriental. Rôles des différents espèces dans la transmission du virus. Cah ORSTOM Ser Entomol Med Parasitol 16:315, 1978.
259. Germain M, Cornet M, Mouchet J, et al. La fièvre jaune en Afrique: données récentes et conceptions actuelles. Med Trop (Mars) 41:31, 1981.
260. Germain M, Francy DB, Monath TP, et al. Yellow fever in The Gambia, 1978–1979: Entomological aspects and epidemiological correlations. Am J Trop Med Hyg 29:929, 1980.
261. Digoutte J-P, Cornet M, Deubel V, et al. Yellow fever. In Porterfield JS (ed). Exotic Virus Infections. London, Chapman & Hall 1995, pp 67–102.
262. Cordellier R. L'épidemiologie de la fièvre jaune en Afrique de l'Ouest. Bull World Health Organ 69:73, 1991.
263. Monath TP. Yellow fever and dengue—the interactions of virus, vector and host in the reemergence of epidemic disease. Semin Virol 5:133, 1995.
264. World Health Organization. Yellow fever virus surveillance in western Africa. Wkly Epidemiol Rec 69:93, 1994.
265. Reiter P. Weather, vector ecology and arboviral recrudescence. In Monath TP (ed). The Arboviruses: Ecology and Epidemiology. Vol I. Boca Raton, FL, CRC, 1988, pp 245–255.
266. Smith CEG. Human and animal ecological concepts behind the distribution, behaviour and control of yellow fever. Bull Soc Pathol Exot 64:683, 1972.
267. Koopman JS, Prevots DR, Marin MAV, et al. Determinants and predictors of dengue infection in Mexico. Am J Epidemiol 133:1168, 1991.
268. Pant CP, Yasuno Y. Field studies on the gonotrophic cycle of *Aedes aegypti* in Bangkok, Thailand. J Med Entomol 10:219, 1973.
269. Patz JA, Epstein PR, Burke TA, et al. Global climate change and emerging infectious diseases. JAMA 275:217, 1996.
270. Monath TP, Kemp GE. The importance of non-human primates in yellow fever epidemiology in Nigeria. Trop Geogr Med 25:28, 1973.
271. Taufflieb R, Robin Y, Cornet M. Le virus amaril et la faune

sauvage en Afrique. Cah ORSTOM Ser Entomol Med Parasitol 9:351, 1971.
272. Haddow AJ. The natural history of yellow fever in Africa. Proc R Soc Edinburgh 70:191, 1968.
273. Reiter P, Cordellier R, Ouma JO, et al. First recorded outbreak of yellow fever in Kenya, 1992–1993. II. Entomological investigations. Am J Trop Med Hyg: in press.
274. Walcott AM, Cruz E, Paoliello A, et al. An epidemic of urban yellow fever which originated from a case contracted in the jungle. Am J Trop Med Hyg 17:677, 1937.
275. Soper FL. Yellow fever: Present situation (October 1938) with special reference to South America. Trans Soc Trop Med Hyg 32:297, 1938.
276. Soper FL. The 1957 status of yellow fever in the Americas. Mosquito News 18:203, 1958.
277. Downs WG. Epidemiological notes in connection with the 1954 outbreak of yellow fever in Trinidad, BWI. In Boshell JM, Bugher J, Downs W, et al (eds). Yellow Fever. A Symposium in Commemoration of Carlos Juan Finlay. Philadelphia, Jefferson Medical College, 1955, pp 71–78.
278. Dutary BE, Leduc JW. Transovarial transmission of yellow fever virus by a sylvatic vector, *Haemagogus equinus*. Trans Soc Trop Med Hyg 75:128, 1981.
279. Fontenille D, Diallo M, Mondo M, et al. First evidence of natural vertical transmission of yellow fever virus in *Aedes aegypti*, its epidemic vector. Trans Soc Trop Med Hyg 91:533, 1997.
280. Germain M, Saluzzo J-F, Cornet JP, et al. Isôlement du virus de la fièvre jaune à partir de la ponte et larves d'une tique, *Amblyomma variegatum*. C R Acad Sci Paris Ser D 289:635, 1979.
281. Penna HA, Bittencourt A. Persistence of yellow fever virus in brains of monkeys immunized by cerebral inoculation. Science 97:448, 1943.
282. Gubler DJ, Trent DW. Emergence of epidemic dengue/dengue hemorrhagic fever as a public health problem in the Americas. Infect Agents Dis 2:383, 1994.
283. Low CG, Fairley NH. Laboratory and hospital infections with yellow fever in England. Br Med J 1:125, 1931.
284. Cook GC. Fatal yellow fever contracted at the hospital for tropical diseases, London, UK in 1930. Trans Soc Trop Med Hyg 88:712, 1994.
285. Miller WS, Demchak P, Rosenberger CR, et al. Stability and infectivity of airborne yellow fever and Rift Valley fever viruses. Am J Hyg 77:114, 1963.
286. Hearn HJ Jr, Chappel WA, Demchak P, et al. Attenuation of aerosolized yellow fever virus after passage in cell culture. Bacteriol Rev 30:615, 1966.
287. Findlay GM, MacCallum FO. Transmission of yellow fever virus to monkeys by mouth. J Pathol Bacteriol 49:53, 1939.
288. Bauer JH, Hudson NP. Passage of virus of yellow fever through skin. Am J Trop Med 8:371, 1928.
289. Sanarelli V. Immunity and serum therapy against yellow fever third report. Ann Inst Pasteur 11:753, 1897.
290. Marchoux E, Salimbeni I, Simond P-L. La fièvre jaune. Ann Inst Pasteur 17:665, 1903.
291. Burke AW, Davis NC. Notes on laboratory infections with yellow fever. Am J Trop Med Hyg 10:419, 1930.
292. Davis NC. On the use of immune serum at various intervals after the inoculation of yellow fever virus into rhesus monkeys. J Immunol 26:361, 1934.
293. Pettit A, Stefanopoulo GJ. Utilisation du sérum antiamaril d'origine animale pour la vaccination de l'homme. Bull Acad Natl Med 110:67, 1933.
294. Theiler M, Smith HH. Use of hyperimmune monkey serum in human vaccination against yellow fever. Bull Off Int Hyg Pub 28:2354, 1936.
295. Theiler M, Whitman L. Quantitative studies of the virus and immune serum used in vaccination against yellow fever. Am J Trop Med Hyg 15:347, 1935.
296. Hoskins M. Protective properties against yellow fever virus in the sera of the offspring of immune rhesus monkeys. J Immunol 26:391, 1934.
297. Soper FL, Beeuwkes H, Davis NC, et al. Transitory immunity to yellow fever in offspring of immune human and monkey mothers. Am J Hyg 19:549, 1938.
298. Stefanopoulo GJ, Laurent P, Wassermann R. Présence d'anticorps antiamarils dans le lait de femme immunisé contre la fièvre jaune. C R Seances Soc Biol Fil 122:915, 1936.
299. Hindle E. An experimental study of yellow fever. Trans R Soc Trop Med Hyg 22:405, 1928–1929.
300. Aragão H de B. Report upon some researches on yellow fever. Mem Oswaldo Cruz Inst Suppl 2:35, 1929.
301. Okell CC. Experiments with yellow fever vaccine in monkeys. Trans R Soc Trop Med Hyg 19:251, 1930.
302. Davis NC. Uso experimental de uma vaccina cloroformada contra a febre amarela. Brasil Med 45:368, 1931.
303. Gordon JE, Hughes TP. A study of inactivated yellow fever virus as an immunizing agent. J Immunol 30:221, 1936.
304. Sellards AW, Bennett BL. Vaccination in yellow fever with noninfective virus. Ann Trop Med Parasitol 31:373, 1937.
305. Theiler M. The susceptibility of white mice to virus of yellow fever. Science 71:367, 1930.
306. Findlay GM, Clarke LP. Infection with neurotropic yellow fever virus following instillation into the nares and conjunctival sac. J Pathol Bacteriol 40:55, 1935.
307. Lloyd W, Penna HA. Studies on the pathogenesis of neurotropic yellow fever virus in *Macaca rhesus*. Am J Trop Med 13:1, 1933.
308. Sellards AW. Behavior of virus of yellow fever in monkeys and mice. Proc Natl Acad Sci U S A 17:339, 1931.
309. Laigret J. Recherches expérimentales sur la fièvre jaune. Arch Inst Pasteur Tunis 21:412, 1933.
310. Laigret J. Sur la vaccination contre la fièvre jaune par le virus de Max Theiler. Bull Off Int Hyg Pub 26:1078, 1934.
311. Nicolle C, Laigret J. La vaccination contre la fièvre jaune par le virus amaril vivant, desséché et enrobé. C R Acad Sci 201:312, 1935.
312. Laigret J. Au sujet des réactions nerveuses de la vaccination contre la fièvre jaune. Bull Soc Pathol Exot 29:823, 1936.
313. Sorel F. La vaccination anti-amarile en Afrique occidentale française, mise en application du procédé de vaccination Sellards-Laigret. Bull Off Int Hyg Pub 28:1325, 1936.
314. Peltier M, Durieux C, Jonchère H, Arquié E. Pénétration du virus amarile neurotrope par voie cutanée: Vaccination contre la fièvre jaune et al variole, note préliminaire. Bull Acad Natl Med Paris 121:657, 1939.
315. Peltier M. Yellow fever vaccination, simple or associated with vaccination against smallpox, of the populations of French West Africa by the method of the Pasteur Institute of Dakar. Am J Public Health 37:1026, 1947.
316. Durieux C. Preparation of yellow fever vaccine at the Institut Pasteur, Dakar. In Smithburn KC, Durieux C, Koerber R, et al (eds). Yellow Fever Vaccination. Geneva, World Health Organization, 1956, pp 31–39.
317. Durieux C. Mass yellow fever vaccination in French Africa south of the Sahara. In Smithburn KC, Durieux C, Koerber R, et al. (eds). Yellow Fever Vaccination. Geneva, World Health Organization, 1956, pp 115–121.
318. Durieux C, Koerber R. Post-vaccination immunity with yellow fever vaccine of the Institut Pasteur, Dakar. In Smithburn KC, Durieux C, Koerber R, et al (eds). Yellow Fever Vaccination. Geneva, World Health Organization, 1956, pp 51–63.
319. Bonnel PH, Deutschman Z. La fièvre jaune en Afrique au cours des années récentes. Bull World Health Organ 11:325, 1957.
320. Kaplan M, Gluck AC. Méningo-encéphalite après vaccination anti-amarile. Soc Med Hop Paris 61:374, 1945.
321. Martin R, Rouesse G, Bonnefoi A. Cent cas de vaccination antiamarile (vaccin Laigret) pratiquée a l'Hôpital Pasteur. Bull Soc Pathol Exot 29:295, 1936.
322. Laigret J. Resultante de la vaccination contre la fièvre jaune après douze années de practique. Bull Acad Natl Med 13:131, 1947.
323. Husson RA, Koerber R. Le vaccin contre la fièvre jaune préparé par l'Institut Pasteur de Dakar. Ann Inst Pasteur 85:735, 1953.
324. Pellisier A, Trinquier E. Isolement d'un virus encephalomyélitique au cours d'une petite épidémie de "Poliomyélite clinique" à Brazzaville. Ann Inst Pasteur 85:316, 1953.
325. MacNamara FN. Reactions following neurotropic yellow fever vaccine given by scarification in Nigeria. Trans Am J Trop Med Hyg 47:199, 1953.
326. Stones PB, MacNamara FN. Encephalitis following neurotropic yellow fever vaccine administered by scarification in Nigeria: Epidemiological and laboratory studies. Trans R Soc Trop Med Hyg 49:176, 1955.

327. Eklund CM. Encefalitis infantil en Costa Rica y Honduras despues del empleo de la vacuna Dakar contra la fiebra amarilla. Bol San Panam 35:505, 1953.
328. Brès P, Lacan A, Diop I, et al. Des campagnes de vaccination antiamarile en République du Sénégal. Bull Soc Pathol Exot 64:1038, 1963.
329. Rey M, Satge P, Collomb H, et al. Aspects épidémiologiques et cliniques des encéphalites consécutives à la vaccination antiamarile (d'après 248 cas observés dans quatre services hospitaliers de Dakar à la suite de la campagne 1965). Bull Soc Med Afr Noire Lgue Fr 11:560, 1966.
330. Sankalé M, Bourgeade A, Wade F, et al. Contribution à l'étude des réactions vaccinales observées en dehors de Dakar. Bull Soc Med Afr Noire Lgue Fr 11:617, 1966.
331. Collomb H, Rey M, Dumas M, et al. Syndromes neuro-psychiques au cours des encephalites postvaccinales. Bull Soc Med Afr Noire Lgue Fr 3:575, 1966.
332. Ricosse JH, Albert JP. La vaccination antiamarile dats les états de l'OCCGE. Conférence sur l'épidémiologie et le contrôle de la fièvre jaune en Afrique de l'Ouest, Bobo Dioulasso, March 20–23, 1971. Unpublished document No. 266, OCCGE, Centre Muraz, Bobo Dioulasso, Haute Volta.
333. Brès P, Robin Y. Étude virologique. Considérations étiopathologéniques. Bull Soc Med Afr Noire Lgue Fr 11:610, 1966.
334. Dick GWA. A preliminary evaluation of the immunizing power of chick-embryo 17D yellow fever vaccine inoculated by scarification. Am J Hyg 55–56:140, 1952.
335. Hahn RG. A combined yellow fever-smallpox vaccine for cutaneous application. Am J Hyg 53–54:50, 1951.
336. Cannon DA, Dewhurst F, Meers PD. Mass vaccination against yellow fever by scarification with 17D strain vaccine. Ann Trop Med Parasitol 51–52:256, 1957–1958.
337. Cannon DA, Dewhurst F. The preparation of 17D virus yellow fever vaccine in mouse brain. Ann Trop Med Parasitol 49:174, 1955.
338. Cannon DA, Dewhurst F. Vaccination by scarification with 17D yellow fever vaccine prepared at Yaba, Lagos, Nigeria. Ann Trop Med Parasitol 47:381, 1953.
339. Meers PD. Combined smallpox-17D yellow fever vaccine for scratch vaccination. Trans R Soc Trop Med Hyg 53:196, 1959.
340. Meers PD. Further observations on 17D-yellow fever vaccination by scarification, with and without simultaneous smallpox vaccination. Trans R Soc Trop Med Hyg 54:493, 1960.
341. Draper CC, Knott EG. Failure to respond to vaccination with 17D yellow fever virus by scarification and its significance. West Afr J Med 13:78, 1964.
342. Fabiyi A, MacNamara FN. The effects of heterologous antibodies on the serological conversion rate after 17D yellow fever vaccination. Am J Trop Med Hyg 11:817, 1962.
343. Smith CEG, McMahon DA, Turner LH. Yellow fever vaccination in Malaya by subcutaneous injection and multiple puncture. Haemagglutinin-inhibiting antibody responses in persons with and without pre-existing antibody. Bull World Health Organ 29:75, 1963.
344. Smith CEG, Turner LH, Armitage P. Yellow fever vaccination in Malaya by subcutaneous injection and multiple puncture. Neutralizing antibody responses in persons with and without pre-existing antibody to related viruses. Bull World Health Organ 27:717, 1962.
345. Lloyd W, Theiler M, Ricci NI. Modification of the virulence of yellow fever virus by cultivation in tissues *in vitro*. Trans R Soc Trop Med Hyg 29:481, 1936.
346. Manso C deS. Mass vaccination against yellow fever in Brazil 1937–54. In Smithburn KC, Durieux C, Koerber R, et al (eds). Yellow Fever Vaccination. Geneva, World Health Organization, 1956, pp 123–140.
347. Fox JP, Penna HA. Behavior of 17D yellow fever virus in rhesus monkeys. Relation to substrain, dose and neural or extraneural inoculation. Am J Hyg 38:152, 1943.
348. Soper FL, Smith HH, Penna HA. Yellow fever vaccination: Field results as measured by the mouse protection test and epidemiological observations. In Proceedings of the Third International Congress of Microbiology; New York; Sept 2–9, 1939; pp 351–353.
349. Fox JP, Lennette EH, Manso C, et al. Encephalitis in man following vaccination with 17D yellow fever virus. Am J Hyg 36:117, 1942.
350. United Nations Relief and Rehabilitation Administration (UNRRA). Standards for the manufacture and control of yellow fever vaccine. Epidemiol Inform Bull 1:365, 1945.
351. Panthier R. À propos de quelques cas de réactions nerveuses tardives observées chez des nourrissons après vaccination antimarile (17D). Bull Soc Pathol Exot 49:478, 1956.
352. World Health Organization. Requirements for Yellow Fever Vaccine (Requirements for Biological Substances No. 3). Technical Report Series No. 136. Geneva, World Health Organization, 1957.
353. Monath TP, Kinney RM, Schlesinger JJ, et al. Ontogeny of yellow fever 17D vaccine: RNA oligonucleotide fingerprint and monoclonal antibody analyses of vaccines produced worldwide. J Gen Virol 64:627, 1983.
354. Dupuy A, Despres P, Cahour A, et al. Nucleotide sequence comparison of the genome of two 17D-204 yellow fever vaccines. Nucleic Acids Res 17:2989, 1989.
355. Brès P, Koch M. Production and testing of the WHO yellow fever primary seed lot 213-77 and reference batch 168-73. In WHO Expert Committee on Biological Standardization, 36th Report. Technical Report Series No. 745. Annex 6:113. Geneva, World Health Organization, 1987.
356. Gould EA, Buckley A, Cane PA, et al. Examination of the immunological relationships between flaviviruses using monoclonal antibodies. J Gen Virol 66:1369, 1985.
357. Post PR, Galler R. The use of yellow fever virus vaccine strain 17D in Brazil. Unpublished manuscript.
358. Marchevsky RS, Mariano J, Ferreira VS, et al. Phenotypic analysis of yellow fever virus derived from complementary DNA. Am J Trop Med Hyg 52:75, 1995.
359. World Health Organization Expert Committee on Biological Standardization. 46th Report. WHO Technical Report ser. No. 872. Geneva, World Health Organization, 1998.
360. Levenbook IS, Pelleu LJ, Elisberg BL. The monkey safety test for neurovirulence of yellow fever vaccines: The utility of quantitative clinical evaluation and historical examination. J Biol Stand 15:305, 1987.
361. Penna HA. Production of 17D yellow fever vaccine. In Smithburn KC, Durieux C, Koerber R, et al (eds). Yellow Fever Vaccination. Geneva, World Health Organization, 1956, pp 67–90.
362. Tannock GA, Wark MC, Hair CG. The development of an improved experimental yellow fever vaccine. J Biol Stand 8:23, 1980.
363. Lopes O de Souza, de Almeida Guimaràes SSD, de Carvalho R. Studies on yellow fever vaccine. I. Quality-control parameters. J Biol Stand 15:323, 1987.
364. Harris RJC, Dougherty RM, Biggs PM, et al. Contaminant viruses in two live virus vaccines produced in chick cells. J Hyg (Cambr) 64:1, 1966.
365. Waters TD, Anderson PS Jr, Beebe GW, et al. Yellow fever vaccination, avian leukosis virus, and cancer risk in man. Science 177:76, 1972.
366. World Health Organization. Requirements for Yellow Fever Vaccine. Addendum 1987. World Health Organization Technical Report Series No. 771. Annex 9. Geneva, World Health Organization, 1988, p 208.
367. World Health Organization. Yellow Fever Vaccines: Thermostability of freeze-dried vaccine. Wkly Epidemiol Rec 62:181, 1987.
368. Monath TP. Stability of yellow fever vaccine. Dev Biol Stand 87:219, 1996.
369. Barme M, Bronnaert C. Thermostabilisation du vaccin antiamaril 17D lyophilise. I. Essai de substances protectrices. J Biol Stand 12:435, 1984.
370. Barme M, Vacher B, Ryhiner ML, et al. Thermostabilisation du vaccin antiamaril 17-D lyophilisé. II. Lots-pilotes prepares dans les conditions d'une production industrielle. J Biol Stand 15:67, 1987.
371. Lopes O de Souza, de Almeida Guimaràes SSD, de Carvalho R. Studies on yellow fever vaccine II—stability of the reconstituted product. J Biol Stand 16:71, 1988.
372. Xie H, Cass A, Barrett ADT. Yellow fever 17D vaccine virus isolated from healthy vaccinees accumulates mutations at a very low frequency. Virus Res 55:93–99, 1998.

373. Mason RA, Tauraso NM, Ginn RK. Yellow fever vaccine. V. Antibody response in monkeys inoculated with graded doses of the 17D vaccine. Appl Microbiol 23:908, 1972.
374. Wheelock EF, Sibley WA. Circulating virus, interferon and antibody after vaccination with the 17-D strain of yellow-fever virus. N Engl J Med 273:194, 1965.
375. Actis DAS, Sa Fleitas MJ. Replaciones entre viremia y seroanticuerpos secundarious a la vacunacion antiamarilica de personsas vacunadas con "Cepa 17D-EP". Rev San Mil Argent 69:51, 1970.
376. Fox JP, Cabral AS. The duration of immunity following vaccination with the 17D strain of yellow fever virus. Am J Hyg 37:93, 1943.
377. Fox JP, Fonseca da Cunha J, Kossobudzki SL. Additional observations on duration of humoral immunity following vaccination with 17D strain of yellow fever virus. Am J Hyg 47:64, 1948.
378. Anderson CR, Gast Galvis A. Immunity to yellow fever five years after vaccination. Am J Hyg 45:302, 1947.
379. Dick GWA, Smithburn KC. Immunity to yellow fever six years after vaccination. Am J Trop Med 29:57, 1949.
380. Mason RA, Tauraso NM, Spertzel RO, et al. Yellow fever vaccine: Direct challenge of monkeys given graded doses of 17D vaccine. Appl Microbiol 25:539, 1973.
381. Smithburn KC. Immunology of yellow fever. In Smithburn KC, Durieux C, Koerber R, et al (eds). Yellow Fever Vaccination. Geneva, World Health Organization, 1956, pp 11–27.
382. Spector S, Tauraso NM. Yellow fever virus. I. Development and evaluation of a plaque neutralization test. Appl Microbiol 16:1770, 1968.
383. De Madrid AT, Porterfield JS. The flaviviruses (group B arboviruses): A cross-neutralization study. J Gen Virol 23:91, 1974.
384. Spector SL, Tauraso NM. Yellow fever virus. II. Factors affecting the plaque neutralization test. Appl Microbiol 18:736, 1969.
385. Poland JD, Calisher CH, Monath TP, et al. Persistence of neutralizing antibody 30–35 years after immunization with 17D yellow fever vaccine. Bull World Health Organ 59:895, 1981.
386. Tauraso NM, Coultrip RL, Legters LJ, et al. Yellow fever vaccine. IV. Reactogenicity and antibody response in volunteers inoculated with a vaccine free from contaminating avian leukosis viruses. Proc Soc Exp Biol Med 139:439, 1972.
387. Groot H, Ribeiro RB. Neutralizing and haemagglutination-inhibiting antibodies to yellow fever 17 years after vaccination with 17D vaccine. Bull World Health Organ 27:699, 1962.
388. Pond WL, Ehrenkranz NJ, Danauskas JX, et al. Heterotypic serologic responses after yellow fever vaccination; detection of persons with past St. Louis encephalitis or dengue. J Immunol 98:673, 1967.
389. Fox JP, Kossobudzki SL, Da Chuma JF. Field studies of the immune response to 17D yellow fever virus. Am J Hyg 38:132, 1943.
390. Freestone DS, Ferris RD, Weinberg A, et al. Stabilized 17D strain yellow fever vaccine: Dose response studies, clinical reactions and effects on hepatic function. J Biol Stand 5:181, 1977.
391. Lopes O de Souza, de Almeida Guimarães SSD, de Carvalho R. Studies on yellow fever vaccine III—dose response in volunteers. J Biol Stand 16:77, 1988.
392. Stuart G. Reactions following vaccination against yellow fever. In Smithburn KC, Durieux C, Koerber R, et al (eds). Yellow Fever Vaccination. Geneva, World Health Organization, 1956, p 143.
392a. Yellow Fever Vaccine: Recommendations of the Immunization Practices Advisory Committee (ACIP). MMWR Morb Mortal Wkly Rep 39(RR-6):1, 1990.
393. Connaught Laboratories Inc. Yellow fever vaccine YF-Vax® (package insert). Swiftwater, PA, 1997.
394. Wisseman CL Jr, Sweet B, Kitaoka M, et al. Immunological studies with group B arthropod-borne viruses. I. Broadened neutralizing antibody spectrum induced by strain 17D yellow fever vaccine in human subjects previously infected with Japanese encephalitis virus. Am J Trop Med Hyg 11:550, 1962.
395. Courtois G. Time of appearance and duration of immunity conferred by 17D vaccine. In Smithburn KC, Durieux C, Koerber R, et al (eds). Yellow Fever Vaccination. Geneva, World Health Organization, 1956, pp 105–114.
396. World Health Organization. International Health Regulations (1969) (3rd annotated ed). Geneva, World Health Organization, 1983.
397. Monath TP. Neutralizing antibody responses in the major immunoglobulin classes to yellow fever 17D vaccination of humans. Am J Epidemiol 93:122, 1971.
398. Boiron H. De l'influence des revaccinations antiamariles sur le taux de l'immunité humorale. C R Searces Soc Biol Fil 150:2219, 1956.
399. Calisher CH, Karabatsos N, Dalrymple JM, et al. Antigenic relationships among flaviviruses as determined by cross-neutralization tests with polyclonal antisera. J Gen Virol 70:37, 1989.
400. Omilabu SA, Adejumo JO, Olaleye OD, et al. Yellow fever haemagglutination-inhibiting, neutralising and IgM antibodies in vaccinated and unvaccinated residents of Ibadan, Nigeria. Comp Immunol Microbiol Infect Dis 13:95, 1990.
401. Schlesinger RW, Gordon I, Frankel JW, et al. Clinical and serologic response of man to immunization with attenuated dengue and yellow fever viruses. J Immunol 77:352, 1956.
402. Kayser M, Klein H, Paasch I. Human antibody response to immunization with 17D yellow fever and inactivated TBE vaccine. J Med Virol 17:35, 1985.
402a. Hacker UT, Jelinek T, Erhardt S, et al. In vivo synthesis of tumor necrosis factor-α in healthy humans after live yellow fever vaccination. J Infect Dis 177:774–778, 1998.
403. Rosenzweig EC, Babione RW, Wisseman CL Jr. Immunological studies with group B arthropod-borne viruses. Am J Trop Med Hyg 12:232, 1963.
404. Doherty RL. Effects of yellow fever (17D) and West Nile viruses on the reactions of human appendix and conjunctiva cells to several other viruses. Virology 6:575, 1958.
405. Brown RE, Katz M. Failure of antibody production to yellow fever vaccine in children with kwashiorkor. Trop Geogr Med 18:125, 1966.
406. Gandra YR, Scrimshaw NS. Infection and nutritional status. Am J Clin Nutr 9:159, 1961.
407. Bistrian BR, Winterer JC, Blackburn GL, et al. Failure of yellow fever immunization to produce a catabolic response in individuals fully adapted to a protein-sparing modified fast. Am J Clin Nutr 30:1518, 1977.
408. Bistrian BR, George DT, Blackburn GL, et al. The metabolic response to yellow fever immunization: Protein-sparing modified fast. Am J Clin Nutr 34:229, 1981.
409. Nasidi A, Monath TP, Vandenberg J, et al. Yellow fever vaccination and pregnancy: A four-year prospective study. Trans R Soc Trop Med Hyg 87:337, 1993.
410. Rojanasuphot S, Shaffer N, Chotpitayasunondh H, et al. Response to Japanese encephalitis vaccine among HIV-infected children. Unpublished manuscript, 1997.
411. Wolf HM, Pum M, Jager R, et al. Cellular and humoral immune responses in haemophiliacs after vaccination against tick-borne encephalitis. Br J Haematol 82:374, 1992.
412. Goujon C, Tohr M, Feuillie V, et al. Good tolerance and efficacy of yellow fever vaccine among subjects carriers of human immunodeficiency virus [abstract]. Fourth International Conference on Travel Medicine; Acapulco, Mexico; April 23–27, 1995.
413. Sibailly TS, Wiktor SZ, Tsai TF, et al. Poor antibody response to yellow fever vaccination in children infected with human immunodeficiency virus type 1. Pediatr Infect Dis J 16:1177, 1997.
413a. Wheelock EF, Toy ST, Stjenerholm RL. Lymphocytes and yellow fever. I. Transient virus refractory state following vaccination of man with the 17-D strain. J Immunol 105:1304, 1970.
414. Saenz AC. Yellow fever vaccines: Achievements, problems, needs. In Proceedings of the International Conference on the Application of Vaccines Against Viral, Rickettsial, and Bacterial Diseases of Man. Section A. Arbovirus Diseases. Pan American Health Organization Scientific Publ. No. 226. Washington, DC, Pan American Health Organization, World Health Organization, 1971, p 31.
415. Brès, P. Benefit versus risk factors in immunization against yellow fever. Dev Biol Stand 43:297, 1979.
416. Findlay GM, MacCallum FO. Hepatitis and jaundice associated with immunization against certain virus diseases. Proc R Soc Med 31:799, 1937.
417. Fox JP, Manso C, Penna HA, et al. Observations on the occur-

ence of icterus in Brazil following vaccination against yellow fever. Am J Hyg 36:68, 1942.
418. Sawyer WA, Meyer KF, Eaton MD, et al. Jaundice in Army personnel in western region of United States and its relation to vaccination against yellow fever. Am J Hyg 40:35, 1944.
419. Hargett MV, Burruss HW, Donovan A. Aqueous-base yellow fever vaccine. Public Health Rep 58:505, 1943.
420. Seeff LB, Beebe GW, Hoofnagle JH. A serologic follow-up of the 1942 epidemic of postvaccination hepatitis in the US Army. N Engl J Med 316:965, 1987.
421. Moss-Blundell AJ, Bernstein S, Wilma M, et al. A clinical study of stabilized 17D strain live attenuated yellow fever vaccine. J Biol Stand 9:445, 1981.
422. Pivetaud JP, Raccurt CP, M'Bailara L, et al. Clinique. Réactions post-vaccinales. A la vaccination anti-amarile. Bull Soc Pathol Exot 79:772, 1986.
423. Stefanopoulo GJ, Duvolon S. Réactions observées au cours de la vaccination contre la fièvre jaune par virus atténué de culture (souche 17D). A propos de 20.000 vaccinations pratiquées par ce procédé à l'Institut Pasteur de Paris (1936–1946). Bull Mem Soc Med Hop Paris 63:990, 1947.
424. Dick GWA, Horgan ES. Vaccination by scarification with a combined 17D yellow fever and vaccinia vaccine. J Hyg (Lond) 50:376, 1952.
425. Thomson WO. Encephalitis in infants following vaccination with 17D yellow fever virus: Report of a further case. BMJ 2:182, 1955.
426. Recommendations of the Immunization Practices Advisory Committee. Yellow fever vaccine. MMWR Morb Mortal Wkly Rep 18:189, 1969.
427. Louis JJ, Chopard P, Larbre F. Un cas d'encephalite après vaccination anti-amarile par la souche 17 D. Pediatrie 36:539, 1981.
428. Merlo C, Steffen R, Landis T, et al. Possible association of encephalitis and 17D yellow fever vaccination in a 29-year-old traveller. Vaccine 11:691, 1993.
429. Berge TO, Hargett MV. Anaphylaxis in guinea pigs following sensitization with chick-embryo yellow fever vaccine and normal chick embryos. Public Health Rep 57:652, 1942.
430. Cohen SG, Mines SC. Variations in egg white and egg yolk components of virus and rickettsial vaccines. J Allergy 29:479, 1958.
431. O'Brien TC, Maloney CJ, Tauraso NM. Quantitation of residual host protein in chicken embryo–derived vaccines by radial immunodiffusion. Appl Microbiol 21:780, 1971.
432. Sulzberger MB, Asher C. Urticarial and erythema multiforme–like eruptions following injections of yellow fever vaccine. US Naval Med Bull 40:411, 1942.
433. Swartz H. Systemic allergic reaction induced by yellow fever vaccine. J Lab Clin Med 43:1663, 1943.
434. Sprague H, Barnard J. Egg allergy, significance in typhus and yellow fever immunization. US Naval Med Bull 45:71, 1945.
435. Kouwenaar W. The reaction to yellow fever vaccine (17D), particularly in allergic individuals. Doc Med Geogr Trop 5:75, 1953.
436. American Academy of Pediatrics. Report of the Committee on Immunization Practices. (23rd ed). Elk Grove Village, IL, American Academy of Pediatrics, 1994.
437. Patterson R, DeSwarte RD, Greenberger PA, et al. Drug allergy and protocols for management of drug allergies. N Engl Reg Allergy Proc 7:325, 1986.
438. Mosimann B, Stoll B, Francillon C, et al. Yellow fever vaccine and egg allergy. J Allerg Clin Immunol 95:1064, 1995.
439. Miller JR, Orgel HA, Meltzer EO. The safety of egg-containing vaccines for egg-allergic patients. J Allerg Clin Immunol 71:568, 1983.
440. Vaccine Adverse Event Reporting System—United States. MMWR Morb Mortal Wkly Rep 39:730, 1990.
441. Receveur MC, Gabinski C, Le Bras M. Coma acidocétosique 4 jours après une vaccination antiamarile. Presse Med 24:41, 1995.
442. Martin L. Leucémie et vaccination antiamarile. Nouv Rev Fr Hematol 10:311, 1970.
443. Murgatroyd F, Findlay GM, MacCallum FO. Long-latent infection with *Plasmodium ovale* becoming manifest after yellow-fever vaccination. Lancet 1:1262, 1939.
444. Miller H, Cendrowski W, Schapira K. Multiple sclerosis and vaccination. BMJ 2:210, 1967.
445. Neumann HH. Herpes simplex and yellow fever vaccine. Lancet 2:250, 1977.
446. World Health Organization. Prevention and Control of Yellow Fever in Africa. Geneva, World Health Organization, 1986.
447. World Health Organization. Informal Discussions on the Use of Yellow Fever Vaccine in Africa. Unofficial report; May 10–11, 1985. Geneva, World Health Organization, 1985.
448. Oyelami SA, Oyaleye OD, Oyejide CO, et al. Severe post-vaccination reaction to 17D yellow fever vaccine in Nigeria. Rev Roum Virol 45:25, 1994.
449. Evans Medical Ltd. Yellow fever vaccine, Live BP (Arilvax). Package Insert. Liverpool, England, 1997.
450. Montenegro J. Gravidez e febre amarela. Rev Inst Adolfo Lutz 1:76, 1941.
450a. Sicé A, Rodallec B. Manifestations hémorragiques de la fièvre jaune (typhus amaril). Répercussions de l'infection maternelle sur l'organisme foetal. Bull Soc Pathol Exot 33:66, 1940.
451. Lewis MJ. Assessment of the yellow fever vaccination campaign in Trinidad, West Indies. In Tikasingh ES (ed). Studies on the Natural History of Yellow Fever in Trinidad. PAHO/WHO CAREC Monograph Series 1, 1991, p 125.
452. Tsai TF, Paul R, Lynberg MC, et al. Congenital yellow fever virus infection after immunization in pregnancy. J Infect Dis 168:1520, 1993.
452a. Nishioka SA, Nunes-Araujo FRF, Pires WP, et al. Yellow fever vaccination during pregnancy and spontaneous abortion: A case-control study. Trop Med Int Health 3:29, 1998.
452b. Marvin JA, Zvolanek EE, Nowosiwsky T, et al. Tuberculin sensitivity (Tine) in apparently healthy subjects after yellow fever vaccination. Am Rev Respir Dis 98:703, 1968.
452c. Starling KA, Falletta JM, Fernbach DJ. Immunologic chimerism as evidence of bone marrow graft acceptance in an identical twin with acute lymphocytic leukemia. Exp Hematol 3:244, 1975.
453. Ambrosch F, Fritzell B, Gregor J, et al. Combined vaccination against yellow fever and typhoid fever: A comparative trial. Vaccine 12:625, 1994.
454. Dukes C, Froeschle J, George J, et al. Safety and immunogenicity of simultaneous administration of Typhim Vi (TV), YF-VAX (YF) and Menomune (MV) [abstract]. 36th Interscience Conference on Antimicrobial Agents and Chemotherapy; New Orleans; American Society for Microbiology; Sept 15–18, 1996.
455. Mouchon D, Pignon D, Vicens R, et al. Étude de la vaccination combinée rougeole-fièvre jaune chez l'enfant Africain agé de 6 à 10 mois. Bull Soc Pathol Exot 83:537, 1990.
456. Meyer HM Jr, Hostetler DD Jr, Bernheim BC, et al. Response of Volta children to jet inoculation of combined live measles, smallpox and yellow fever vaccines. Bull World Health Organ 30:783, 1964.
457. Yvonnet B, Coursaget P, Deubel V, et al. Simultaneous administration of hepatitis B and yellow fever vaccines. J Med Virol 19:307, 1986.
458. Felsenfeld O, Wolf RH, Gyr K, et al. Simultaneous vaccination against cholera and yellow fever. Lancet 1:457, 1973.
459. Gateff C, Le Gonidec G. Boche R, et al. Influence de la vaccination anticholérique sur l'immunisation antiamarile associée. Bull Soc Path Exot 66:266, 1973.
460. Gateff C, Dodlin A, Wiart J. Comparaison des réactions sérologiques induites par un vaccin anticholérique classique et une fraction vaccinante purifiée associés ou non au vaccine antiamaril. Ann Inst Pasteur Microbiol 126A:231, 1975.
461. Kollaritsch H, Que JU, Kunz C, et al. Safety and immunogenicity of live oral cholera and typhoid vaccines administered alone or in combination with antimalarial drugs, oral polio vaccine, or yellow fever vaccine. J Infect Dis 175:871, 1997.
462. Kaplan JE, Nelson, DB, Schonberger LB, et al. The effect of immune globulin on the response to trivalent oral poliovirus and yellow fever vaccinations. Bull World Health Organ 62:585, 1984.
463. Tsai TF, Bolin RA, Lazuick JS, et al. Chloroquine does not adversely affect the antibody response to yellow fever vaccine. J Infect Dis 154:726, 1986.
464. Chambers TJ, Tsai TF, Pervikov Y, et al. Vaccine development against dengue and Japanese encephalitis: Report of a World Health Organization meeting. Vaccine 15:1494, 1997.
465. Pan American Health Organization. Modernization of yellow

fever production. Unpublished report. Washington, DC, PAHO, 1980.
466. Pan American Health Organization. Yellow fever vaccination in the Americas. PAHO Epidemiol Bull 4:7, 1983.
467. Calheiros LB. A febre amarela no Brasil. In Homma A, Da Cunha JF (eds). Simpósio Internacional sobre Febre Amarela e Dengue. Cinqüentenário da introdução da Cepa 17D no Brasil. Rio de Janeiro, Fundação Oswaldo Cruz, 1988, pp 74–85.
468. Meegan JM. Yellow Fever Vaccine. Unofficial report. WHO/EPI/GEN/91.6. Geneva, World Health Organization, 1991.
469. Robertson SE. The Immunological Basis for Immunization. 8. Yellow Fever. Document WHO/EPI/GEN/93.18. Geneva, World Health Organization, 1993.
470. World Health Organization. Expanded Programme on Immunization. Document WHO/EPI/GEN/97.02. Geneva, World Health Organization, 1997.
471. Robertson RL, Foster SO, Hull HF, et al. Cost-effectiveness of immunization in The Gambia. Am J Trop Med Hyg 88:343, 1985.
472. World Health Organization. Yellow-Fever Vaccinating Centres for International Travel. Geneva, World Health Organization, 1991.
473. Carey DE, Kemp GE, Troup JM, et al. Epidemiological aspects of the 1969 yellow fever epidemic in Nigeria. Bull World Health Organ 46:645, 1972.
474. Monath TP, Wilson DC, Lee VH. The 1970 yellow fever epidemic in Okwoga District, Benue Plateau State, Nigeria. 1. Epidemiological observations. Bull World Health Organ 49:113, 1973.
475. Addy PAK, Minami K, Agadzi VK. Recent yellow fever epidemics in Ghana (1969–1983). East Afr Med Jour 63:422, 1986.
476. World Health Organization. Yellow fever in 1987. Wkly Epidemiol Rec 64:37, 1989.
477. Baudon D, Robert V, Roux J, et al. L'épidémie de fievre jaune au Burkina Faso en 1983. Bull World Health Organ 64:873, 1986.
478. Roux J, Baudon D, Robert V, et al. L'epidemie de fièvre jaune du sud-est de la Haute-Volta. Med Trop (Mars) 44:304, 1984.
479. World Health Organization. Yellow fever in 1983. Wkly Epidemiol Rec 43:329, 1989.
480. Kurz X. Health planning and management for epidemic outbreaks. The yellow fever epidemic in Mali, September–November 1987. Unpublished report. Geneva, World Health Organization, 1988.
481. World Health Organization. Yellow fever in 1991. Wkly Epidemiol Rec 68:209, 1993.
482. World Health Organization. Yellow fever. Kenya. Wkly Epidemiol Rec 68:157, 1993.
482a. World Health Organization. Yellow fever. Wkly Epidemiol Rec 69:243, 1994.
483. Draper CC. A yellow fever vaccine free from avian leucosis viruses. J Hyg (Cambr) 65:505, 1967.
484. Tauraso NM, Myers MG, Nau EV, et al. Effect of interval between inoculation of live smallpox and yellow-fever vaccines on antigenicity in man. J Infect Dis 126:362, 1972.
485. Bancroft WH Jr, Scott R McN, Eckels KH, et al. Dengue virus type 2 vaccine: Reactogenicity and immunogenicity in soldiers. J Infect Dis 149:1005, 1984.
486. Georges AJ, Tible F, Meunier DMY, et al. Thermostability and efficacy in the field of a new, stabilized yellow fever virus vaccine. Vaccine 3:313, 1985.
487. Roche JC, Jouan A, Brisou B, et al. Comparative clinical study of a new 17D thermostable yellow fever vaccine. Vaccine 4:163, 1986.
488. Lhuillier M, Mazzariol MJ, Zadi S, et al. Study of combined vaccination against yellow fever and measles in infants from six to nine months. J Biol Stand 17:9, 1989.
489. Soula G, Sylla A, Pichard E. Étude d'un nouveau vaccin combiné contre la fièvre jaune et la rougeole chez des enfants agés de 6 a 24 mois au Mali. Bull Soc Pathol Exot 84:885, 1991.
490. Jackson J, Dworkin R, Tsai T, et al. Bioject® injection vs needle/syringe injection of yellow fever vaccine: Comparison of antibody response [abstract]. Third Conference on International Travel and Medicine; Paris; April 25–29, 1993.
491. Receveur MC, Quiniou JM, Delprat P, et al. Vaccination simultanée contre l'hepatite A et la fièvre jaune. Bull Soc Pathol Exot 86:406, 1993.
492. Coursaget P, Fritzell B, Blondeau C, et al. Simultaneous injection of plasma-derived or recombinant hepatitis B vaccines with yellow fever and killed polio vaccines. Vaccine 13:109, 1995.
493. Guerra HL, Sardinha TM, da Rosa APAT, et al. Efetividade de vacina antiamarilica 17D: Uma avaliação epidemiológica em serviços de saúde. Am J Public Health 2:115, 1997.
494. Dumas R, Forrat R, Lang J. Safety and immunogenicity of a new inactivated hepatitis A vaccine and concurrent administration with a typhoid fever vaccine or a typhoid fever + yellow fever vaccine. Adv Therapy 14:160, 1997.
495. Swift S. Encephalitis after yellow fever vaccination. BMJ 2:677, 1955.
496. Lartigaut M, Couteau M. Encéphalite bénigne après vaccination contre la fièvre jaune par le vaccine atténuée en tissu embryonnaire. J Med Bordeaux 121:506, 1954.
497. Smith JH. Encephalitis in an infant after vaccination with 17 D yellow fever virus. BMJ 2:852, 1954.
498. Haas L. Encephalitis after yellow-fever vaccination. BMJ 2:992, 1954.
499. Scott LG. Encephalitis after yellow fever vaccination. BMJ 2:1108, 1954.
500. Beet EA. Encephalitis after yellow fever vaccination. BMJ 1:226, 1955.
501. Lartigaut M, Lartigaut D. Encéphalite vaccinale du nourrisson après vaccination contre la fièvre jaune. J Med Bordeaux 131:1388, 1954.
502. De Castro Friere L. Meningoencephalite post vaccinação contra febre amarela. Rev Post Pediatr 18:65, 1955.
503. Feitel M, Watson EH, Cochran KW. Encephalitis after yellow fever vaccination. Pediatrics 78:956, 1960.
504. Schoub BD, Dommann CJ, Johnson S, et al. Encephalitis in a 13-year-old boy following 17D yellow fever vaccine. J Infect 21:105, 1990.
505. Drouet A, Chagnon A, Valence J, et al. Meningoencephalite après vaccination anti-amarile par la souche 17D: Deux observations. Rev Med Interne 124:257, 1993.
506. Ruben FL, Smith EA, Foster SO. Simultaneous administration of smallpox, measles, yellow fever, and diphtheria-pertussis-tetanus antigens to Nigerian children. Bull World Health Organ 48:175, 1973.
507. Gateff C, Relyveld EH, Le Gonidec G, et al. Étude d'une nouvelle association vaccinale quintuple. Ann Pasteur Paris Microbiol 124B:387, 1973.
508. Gil A, González A, Dal-Ré R, et al. Interference assessment of yellow fever vaccine with the immune response to a single-dose inactivated hepatitis A vaccine (1440 E.U.). A controlled study in adults. Vaccine 14:1028, 1996.

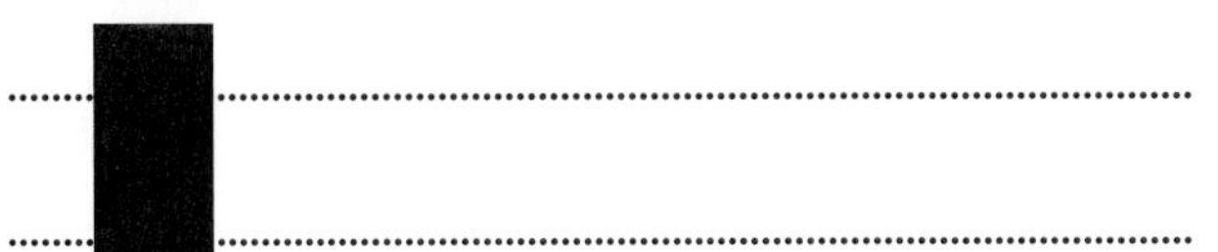

SELECTED VACCINES OF THE FUTURE

chapter

35 New Technologies for Making Vaccines

Ronald W. Ellis

The 1980s and 1990s have witnessed an explosion in the number of technological and immunological approaches for making new vaccines. These developments have flowed from major advances in a broad range of fields, including molecular biology and recombinant DNA (rDNA) technology, protein biochemistry, polysaccharide chemistry, analytical biochemistry, fermentation, macromolecular purification, virology, bacteriology, and immunology. Some of the earliest applications of the newer technologies were to previously existing vaccines, with the objective of increasing perceived safety (pertussis vaccine) or supply (hepatitis B vaccine). However, most of the applications have been directed toward the development of new vaccines for diseases not previously approachable. The traditional scope of vaccines has been the prevention (prophylaxis) of infectious diseases. However, new technologies have extended this scope to include vaccines for noninfectious diseases (e.g., fertility, autoimmune diseases, and cancer) and therapeutic vaccines (e.g., certain infectious diseases, cancer, and allergy).

There are two broad categories of vaccines, active and passive. An active vaccine stimulates the host's immune system to produce specific antibodies or cellular immune responses or both, which would protect against or eliminate a disease. A passive vaccine is a preparation of antibodies that neutralizes a pathogen and is administered before or around the time of known or potential exposure. Most references to the term *vaccine* refer to active vaccines, which are the subject of the majority of research and development activities in the field as well as the bulk of discussion in this chapter. Although in specific instances it is desirable or essential to administer a passive vaccine, particularly if no active vaccine is available or for immunocompromised individuals in some cases, establishing lasting immunity through the administration of an active vaccine is an important means of preventive medicine.

Vaccines are typically stored in liquid solution or in freeze-dried (lyophilized) form, depending on their physical and biological stability characteristics. Lyophilized vaccines are resuspended in diluent (resuspending fluid) at the time of administration. The liquid solution, lyophilized form, and diluent each may contain additional additives, such as (1) preservatives or antibiotics to prevent bacterial growth; (2) stabilizers, including proteins or other organic compounds, to extend the shelf-life or dating period for the vaccine; (3) adjuvants for enhancing immune responses to vaccines (see *Formulation of Antigens);* and (4) delivery systems for presenting the vaccine antigens to appropriate cells or preserving antigens in vivo (see *Formulation of Antigens).* The antigens and other added components together compose the vaccine formulation.

This chapter summarizes the major technologies, key issues, and immunological objectives for making different kinds of vaccines. Appropriate examples of specific vaccine types are given with accompanying references. The status of development of vaccines made by each approach is identified, whether licensed or in clinical or preclinical evaluations (Table 35–1). Although most common licensed vaccines are discussed, not every conceivable approach is documented in this chapter. In view of space limitations, only a few salient examples of each approach can be given with one or two accompanying references. Whereas most examples are for viruses and bacteria, there is also vaccine research for parasites, fungi, and noninfectious diseases. The technologies and examples presented should provide the reader with a strong framework for appreciating the diverse approaches being taken to the research and development of new vaccines.

ACTIVE VACCINES

The protective immunity elicited by an active vaccine ideally would be lifelong and robust after a single dose with no side effects (reactogenicity). Available vaccines as well as those under development fall short of this

Table 35–1. **STATUS OF DEVELOPMENT OF REPRESENTATIVE HUMAN VACCINES MADE BY DIFFERENT TECHNOLOGIES**

TYPE OF VACCINE*	STATUS OF DEVELOPMENT† Preclinical Evaluation‡	Clinical Evaluation§	Licensed Product‖	EXAMPLE¶	REFERENCE
Active					
Live					
Classical strategies: viral					
Attenuation in cell culture			X	Poliovirus	1
			X	Measles virus	2
			X	Mumps virus	3
			X	Rubella virus	4
			X	Varicella-zoster virus (VZV)	5
Variants from other species			X	Smallpox (vaccinia virus)	7
		X		Rotavirus	8, 9
Reassorted genomes		X		Rotavirus	10, 11
		X		Influenza virus	12
Temperature-selected mutants			X	Influenza virus	13
		X		Respiratory syncytial virus (RSV)	14
Recombinant virus		X		Herpes simplex virus (HSV)	15, 16
Recombinant viral vector		X		Vaccinia virus[a]	19, 20
		X		Adenovirus[b]	24
	X			VZV[c]	25
	X			HSV	15
	X			Poliovirus[d]	26, 27
Classical strategies: bacterial			X	Tuberculosis (bacille Calmette-Guérin [BCG])	29
			X	Typhoid fever (*Salmonella typhi*)	30, 31
Recombinant bacteria					
			X	Cholera (*Vibrio cholerae*)	32
		X		*Shigella flexneri*	34
Recombinant bacterial vector		X		*Salmonella typhi*[e]	35
		X		*V. cholerae*	36
	X			*S. flexneri*	37
	X			*Listeria monocytogenes*	38
	X			BCG	39, 40
	X			*Streptococcus gordonii*	41
Nonlive					
Whole-pathogen					
Inactivated bacteria			X	Pertussis (*Bordetella pertussis*)	43
			X	Cholera	44
		X		Enterotoxigenic *Escherichia coli*	45
Inactivated virus			X	Poliovirus	46
			X	Influenza virus	47
			X	Rabies virus	48
			X	Japanese encephalitis virus	49
			X	Hepatitis A virus	50
Protein-based					
Natural			X	Hepatitis B virus (HBV)	56
			X	Pertussis	57–59
Chemically inactivated			X	Tetanus (*Clostridium tetani*)	60
			X	Diphtheria (*Corynebacterium diphtheriae*)	61
			X	Pertussis	62
Genetically inactivated			X	Pertussis	63
		X		Diphtheria	64
Recombinant polypeptide			X	HBV	65, 66
		X		Human papillomavirus	68
	X			Rotavirus	69
		X		Human immunodeficiency virus (HIV)	70, 71
		X		HSV	72
		X		Lyme disease (*Borrelia burgdorferi*)	73
	X			Schistosome	74
		X		Allergy	75
		X		Diabetes	76, 77
		X		Fertility[f]	78
		X		Yeast Ty[g]	80

Table 35–1. **STATUS OF DEVELOPMENT OF REPRESENTATIVE HUMAN VACCINES MADE BY DIFFERENT TECHNOLOGIES** *Continued*

	STATUS OF DEVELOPMENT†				
TYPE OF VACCINE*	Preclinical Evaluation‡	Clinical Evaluation§	Licensed Product‖	EXAMPLE¶	REFERENCE
Peptide based					
Fusin protein		X		Malaria[h]	83
Conjugate		X		Malaria[i]	85
	X			Fertility[i]	86
Complex peptide	X			HIV	87
	X			Malaria	88
Mimetope	X			HBV	89
	X			HIV	90
T-cell epitope		X		HBV	91
Polysaccharide-based					
Plain polysaccharide			X	*Haemophilus influenzae* type b (Hib)	92
			X	Meningococcal (*Neisseria meningitidis*)	93
			X	Pneumococcal (*Streptococcus pneumoniae*)	94
Conjugate			X	Hib[j]	95
		X		Pneumococcal[k]	96
		X		Group B streptococcal (*Streptococcus agalactiae*)[l]	97
Anti-idiotype (antibodies)	X			HBV	98
		X		Cancer[m]	99, 100
	X			Schistosome	101
DNA-based					
DNA—naked		X		Influenza	104
Facilitated DNA	X			Influenza	106
		X		HIV	108
Viral delivery	X			Fowlpox virus[n]	110
		X		Canarypox virus[o]	111
Bacterial delivery	X			*S. flexneri*	112
Passive (antibodies)					
Polyclonal					
Human immune globulin (IG)			X	HBV (HBIG)	127
			X	VZV (VZIG)	128
			X	Cytomegalovirus (CMVIG)	129
			X	Tetanus (TIG)	134
		X		RSV (RSVIG)	130
Monoclonal					
Natural human		X		*Pseudomonas aeruginosa*	131
		X		Cancer[p]	132
		X		CMV	129
Recombinant human	X			HIV	137
Recombinant humanized		X		RSV	140

*These categories are presented in the same order and outline as in the text.
†This denotes the single most advanced status achieved by each example.
‡Not yet evaluated in a human clinical trial.
§In clinical trial but not yet licensed.
‖Licensed in one or more major countries in the world.
¶These are representative examples for each vaccine strategy and not a comprehensive list of all examples. There are one or two key references illustrative of each example.
[a]Expressing more than 50 different foreign polypeptides.
[b]Expressing at least six different foreign polypeptides.
[c]Expressing Epstein-Barr virus gp350.
[d]Expressing an epitope in HIV-1 gp41 or gp120.
[e]Examples of foreign polypeptides include toxoids from *Escherichia coli, Vibrio cholerae, and Clostridium tetani.*
[f]Reported as nonrecombinant in this reference but would be developed as recombinant vaccine after cloning and expression in a heterologous host cell.
[g]Examples of foreign polypeptides include those encoded by HIV-1 *gag* and *env* genes.
[h]Fusion partner is HBsAg.
[i]Conjugate carrier is TT.
[j]Conjugate carriers are TT, DT, and CRM197, an outer membrane protein complex.
[k]Conjugate carriers are TT and CRM197, an outer membrane protein complex.
[l]Conjugate carrier is TT.
[m]Monoclonal antibody specificities are for human tumor carbohydrate and a human colorectal carcinoma antigen.
[n]Expressing proteins from SIV.
[o]Expressing rabies virus glycoprotein.
[p]Monoclonal antibody specificity is for human ganglioside GD_2 antigen.

ideal, which continues to stimulate new research in the field.

There are three general categories of active vaccines, whose salient features are outlined in Table 35–2. A *live* vaccine is a microorganism that can replicate on its own in the host or can infect cells and function as an immunogen without causing its natural disease. A *nonlive* (also called killed, inactivated, or subunit) vaccine is an immunogen that cannot replicate in the host. A *DNA-based* vaccine, which cannot replicate in humans, is taken up by cells, in which it directs the synthesis of vaccine antigens. Note that the term *immunogen* refers to the property of eliciting an immune response, whereas the term *antigen* denotes the property of in vitro immunological reactivity.

The strategic decision for developing a live, nonlive, or DNA-based vaccine should be made after considering the epidemiology, pathogenesis, and immunobiology of the infection or disease in question as well as the technical feasibility of the various approaches. Epidemiology dictates the target population for the vaccine. The age and state of health of this population usually favor certain strategies as more appropriate for eliciting protective immunity. For example, minimal reactogenicity is important for a vaccine intended for healthy infants, and certain types of vaccines are useless for infants because they do not elicit protective immunity (see *Polysaccharide-Based Vaccines).* However, the degree of reactogenicity is less important in cases such as a therapeutic cancer vaccine. Populations (e.g., healthcare providers, drug addicts) at high risk for a given disease (e.g., hepatitis B) may not be amenable to accepting or seeking vaccination. In such cases, an effective public health strategy has become the vaccination of groups (e.g., all children) that are readily accessible to widespread vaccination other than only the high-risk groups themselves. A knowledge of immunobiology can aid in identifying the types of protective immunity that should be elicited by the vaccine; certain immune responses may be protective and others useless, or even detrimental, to the prevention or treatment of a particular infection. For example, the clearance of the natural infection may correlate with the appearance of antibodies against a particular microbial antigen; this would define that antigen as an immunogen for a candidate vaccine. Alternatively, the study of immunobiology is greatly facilitated (in some cases actually made possible) by developing an experimental animal model, the availability of which enables candidate vaccines to be tested and optimized for protective efficacy before the best ones are brought forward for clinical evaluation. Historically, only a limited range of technical approaches has been feasible for a particular vaccine. Nevertheless, considering the expanding number of technical approaches, it seems that it will be possible in the future to custom-design many vaccines for optimal efficacy and tolerability.

Table 35–2. **COMPARATIVE PROPERTIES OF ACTIVE VACCINES**

Live Vaccines

Able to replicate in the host
Attenuated in pathogenicity
Advantages:
- May elicit broader immune responses
- May require fewer doses
- Generally longer lasting protection

Killed Vaccines

Unable to replicate in the host
Advantages:
- Cannot multiply or revert to pathogenicity
- Generally less reactogenic
- Nontransmissible to another person
- Usually more feasible technically

DNA-Based Vaccines

Stimulate synthesis of antigens in cells
Advantages:
- Elicit cellular immune responses
- Standardized method of production

Live Vaccines

Some live vaccines come close to meeting the criteria for an ideal vaccine by being able to elicit lifelong protection with minimal reactogenicity using only one or two doses. This may be possible in cases in which the natural infection confers lifelong protection on the host. Such vaccines consist of microorganisms (usually viruses) that replicate in the host in a fashion resembling that of the natural microorganism; hence, the vaccine can elicit an immune response similar to that elicited by the natural infection. The live vaccine is attenuated, meaning that its disease-causing capacity is virtually eliminated by biological or technical manipulations. Care needs to be taken to ensure that the live vaccine is neither overattenuated, such that it is no longer infectious enough to function as a vaccine, nor underattenuated, whereby it retains pathogenicity even to a limited extent. Live vaccines usually elicit both humoral immunity (antibodies) and cellular immunity (e.g., cytotoxic T lymphocytes [CTL]).

Although these properties might make it appear desirable that all active vaccines be live vaccines, this is not technically feasible for most vaccines currently under development. A live vaccine may be incompletely attenuated and consequently cause its natural disease at a low frequency or be completely attenuated and incompletely immunogenic. Because a live vaccine can replicate, it may be possible for it to revert to its more naturally pathogenic form. Moreover, some live vaccine strains can be transmitted from the vaccinee to an unvaccinated individual, which can be serious if the recipient has an immunodeficiency disorder (e.g., acquired immunodeficiency syndrome) or is undergoing cancer chemotherapy. In some cases, the natural viral infection fails to produce a protective immune response, such that an attenuated virus (without further molecular engineering) also would not be expected to produce a protective response.

Classical Strategies: Viral

The term *classical* refers to technical strategies that do not use rDNA technology. The production of live viral vaccines depends on efficiently propagating the virus in cell culture.

Attenuation in Cell Culture. The first classical strategy became possible during the 1950s with the advent of modern cell culture and the ability to propagate viruses in these cultures. The approach is empirical, in that the wild-type virus isolated from a natural human infection is passaged in vitro through one or more cell types that the virus ordinarily does not encounter in vivo with the goal of attenuating its pathogenicity. In such cases, there may be competitive pressure to produce less damage to cells. (In contrast, a strategy to increase pathogenicity is to passage a microorganism serially in vivo.) The mechanism by which mutations are introduced during the course of attenuation is not well understood. It has been possible in some cases (e.g., poliovirus[1]) to demonstrate attenuation in a primate species, whereas attenuation has been proved in most cases only through the course of extensive clinical trials. The success of this empirical approach, which has been applied both to an oral vaccine (oral poliovirus vaccine [OPV]) and to injected (parenteral) vaccines (measles,[2] mumps,[3] rubella,[4] varicella[5]), has been borne out by the number of available licensed vaccines. The reactogenicity of such vaccines has been low enough that some of them (poliovirus, measles) are widely accepted worldwide for routine pediatric use. By means of intensive immunization programs with OPV, poliomyelitis is well on its way to worldwide eradication. As a vivid example of the difficulty in proving attenuation, the attenuated Urabe strain of mumps virus was licensed after it showed apparent safety in clinical trials. After several years of use in millions of children, it was observed that immunization with this vaccine could cause aseptic meningitis at a rate of approximately 1:10,000[6]; given the availability of an alternative mumps vaccine without this effect, this strain was withdrawn from use in several countries.

Variants from Other Species. An animal virus that causes a veterinary disease similar to a human disease can be isolated and cultivated. The anticipated outcome is that the animal virus will be attenuated for humans yet will be sufficiently related immunologically to the natural human virus to elicit protective immunity to the human agent. Smallpox, the prototype of this vaccine type, was the first modern vaccine. Two hundred years ago, Jenner first appreciated that individuals intentionally exposed to cowpox were resistant to smallpox, so he used the cowpox agent (vaccinia virus) for human vaccination against smallpox (caused by variola virus). The immunization program was applied worldwide using vaccinia virus[7] and resulted in the complete eradication of smallpox worldwide by the mid-1970s, the only infectious disease ever eradicated. This program is a tribute to an effective control strategy and to the tireless efforts of countless individuals. As a result, this vaccine has the proud distinction of having been unlicensed, the ultimate goal for any vaccine!

On the basis of this model, first-generation vaccines for rotavirus consisted of viruses isolated from rhesus monkeys[8] and cows.[9] However, these rotavirus vaccines were not reproducibly efficacious as human vaccines.

Reassorted Genomes. A reassortant virus derived after coinfection of a culture with two different viruses with segmented genomes contains genes from both parental viruses. To improve the efficacy of animal rotaviruses, reassortant rotaviruses were isolated containing mostly animal rotavirus genes, which confer the attenuation phenotype for humans, as well as the gene for a human rotavirus surface protein, which elicits serotype-specific neutralizing antibodies for human rotavirus.[10, 11] These reassortant rotaviruses have elicited higher efficacy rates as vaccine candidates than their nonreassortant parental animal viruses. The same approach has been applied to influenza vaccines, in which a virulent human influenza virus provides the genes that encode the immunogenic surface glycoproteins (hemagglutinin and neuraminidase), and an attenuated virus provides all other genes and, with them, the attenuation phenotype.[12]

Temperature-Sensitive Mutants. Viral mutants can be selected according to their growth properties at different temperatures. These viruses have been referred to as temperature-sensitive *(ts)*, being unable to grow at elevated temperatures, or cold-adapted *(ca)*, having been selected for growth in vitro at lower than physiological (37°C) temperatures (i.e., down to 25°C). The idea behind this approach is that *ca* or *ts* viruses will be less vigorous in their in vivo growth than their wild-type parental virus, hence less virulent and phenotypically attenuated. A *ca* influenza vaccine has been used widely in Russia,[13] and a double *ts* respiratory syncytial virus vaccine has been tested clinically with some promise.[14] The use of this double *ts* mutant, that is, one that contains two independent *ts* mutations, is an additional refinement resulting in a much lower frequency of reversion to wild-type virulence than for a single *ts* mutant.

Recombinant Virus

Specific modifications or deletions can be made in viral genes so that the virus is more stably attenuated, that is, highly unlikely or unable to revert to virulence (Fig. 35–1). The increased stability of the attenuation phenotype results from making the modifications extensive enough that reversion through back-mutation is

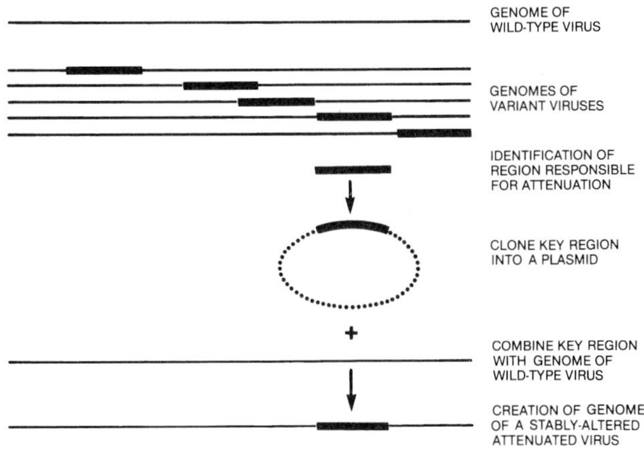

Figure 35–1. Attenuation of viruses using modern techniques in molecular biology.

impossible or highly unlikely. In contrast, attenuated viruses derived by classical strategies may have only point mutations and therefore have the capability to revert. Herpes simplex virus (HSV) has been genetically engineered[15] for the following functions: (1) to be attenuated with respect to both primary disease and reactivation of latent infection, (2) to provide for antibody markers of vaccination that are differentiable from those of wild-type HSV infection, and (3) to protect against the two serogroups HSV-1 and HSV-2. The attenuation of this recombinant HSV strain was demonstrated in both mice and owl monkeys. Deletions have also been introduced into HSV that make it unable to replicate; this recombinant virus is produced in vitro in a cell line that supplies the deleted gene in *trans*, and the resultant virus can initiate infection in vivo without being able to replicate further.[16] This deleted HSV thus functions in vivo as a DNA-based vaccine (see *DNA-Based Vaccines*). Similarly, the influenza virus genome can be engineered to reduce or prevent reversion to virulence, although this work is at an earlier stage of development.[17]

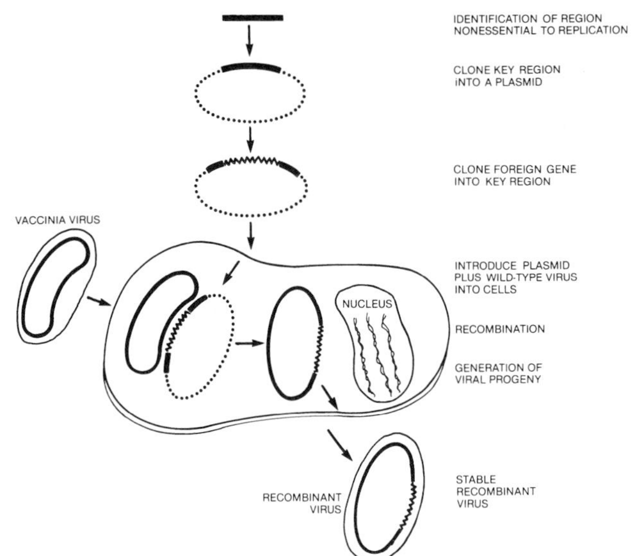

Figure 35–2. Creation of recombinant vaccinia viruses carrying genes that encode immunogens of other pathogens.

Recombinant Viral Vector

The second application of rDNA technology to the development of new live vaccines has been the engineering of viruses to become carriers or vectors of "foreign" recombinant polypeptides or peptide epitopes from other pathogens. The goal of creating such vectors is to present the recombinant antigen to the immune system in the context of a live virus infection so that the immune system responds to the antigen as a *live* immunogen and thereby develops broader immunity (humoral and cellular) to the corresponding human pathogen. As part of a live virus, the recombinant polypeptide is expressed within the infected cell and either is transported to the cell surface to stimulate antibody production or is broken down into peptide fragments that are transported to the cell surface where they elicit CTL responses. This strategy also has the potential advantage of amplification of the immunogenic signal when the live vector initiates multiple rounds of replication. If the vector virus is a commonly used vaccine, one could immunize simultaneously against the vector virus and another pathogen, ideally in a single dose. However, the nature of the immune response to the live viral vector may limit the effectiveness of revaccination.[18]

The prototype viral vector is vaccinia virus. A plasmid is created containing the gene for a recombinant polypeptide with adjoining sequences that direct its expression in cells, a combination referred to as an *expression cassette* (see *Protein-Based Vaccines, Recombinant Polypeptides*). The expression cassette is flanked by vaccinia viral sequences corresponding to a point in the viral genome at which one desires to place the expression cassette. Vaccinia virus and the expression cassette are taken up simultaneously into the cytoplasm, where they undergo a homologous recombinational event, thereby producing a recombinant vaccinia virus expressing the recombinant polypeptide (Fig. 35–2). Dozens of different recombinant polypeptides have been expressed in vaccinia virus.[19] In experimental animal models for infection, at least 25 models for different infections have shown that vaccination of animals can protect against the pathogen encoding the recombinant polypeptide. Recombinant vaccinia virus expressing the major envelope glycoprotein (gp120) of human immunodeficiency virus type 1 (HIV-1) has been tested clinically[20] for prophylactic and therapeutic applications. In addition, recombinant vaccinia viruses expressing tumor antigens have been shown to be protective in rodent tumor model challenge studies. Given the known sequelae to immunization for smallpox observed in the worldwide eradication program, which are more serious in immunocompromised individuals, vaccinia virus itself has been engineered to reduce its virulence without compromising its efficacy as a live viral vector.[21, 22] Cytokines can influence the nature or magnitude of the immune response (see *Formulation of Antigens*). To selectively manipulate the type of immune response to a vaccine antigen in the context of a live vector vaccination, a recombinant poxvirus vector has been constructed that expresses a cytokine as well as a recombinant vaccine antigen.[23]

Recombinant vaccinia virus has been referred to as "DNA in a tuxedo" (Enzo Paoletti). This description may be even more applicable to two other members of the poxvirus family, fowlpox and canarypox viruses, which are being developed as live virus vectors that can infect human cells but not produce infectious viral progeny. This inability to spread makes these viral vectors classifiable as DNA-based vaccines (see *DNA-Based Vaccines*).

Other mammalian viruses have been engineered into live vectors. Adenovirus strains, which have been used extensively as vaccines in military recruits to prevent acute respiratory disease, have been engineered to express foreign polypeptides and have elicited protective immunity in several viral challenge models in animals.[24] The Oka strain of varicella-zoster virus,[5] which has been developed as a routine pediatric vaccine for chickenpox and ultimately possibly for shingles as well, has been developed into a live recombinant vector.[25] As described before, HSV has also been engineered into a live vector.[15] For all these live viral vectors, optimizing recombinant polypeptide expression remains an important technical objective.

Poliovirus has been developed into a live vector for the expression of an epitope from another pathogen. The poliovirus RNA genome is small enough and the virion structurally constrained in a fashion whereby it is not straightforward to express a complete recombinant polypeptide in this virus. However, because the locations of the most antigenic sites in the VP1 protein on the surface of the virion have been mapped, it has been possible to substitute an epitope for these antigenic sites and still enable infectious virion formation to take place. A recombinant poliovirus expressing an epitope from the HIV-1 envelope glycoprotein gp41 elicits antibodies in rabbits that neutralize HIV-1 infectivity.[26] As another expression strategy, it is possible to exploit the expression of the poliovirus genome as a polyprotein that is proteolytically cleaved by the viral protease. Genes encoding polypeptides up to approximately 400 amino acids in length can be fused to the N terminus of the polyprotein and linked by a viral protease cleavage site, which then is proteolytically processed into infectious virus plus the recombinant polypeptide that is excluded from the virion. Animals (transgenic mice expressing the poliovirus receptor) infected with such a recombinant virus produce antibodies to the recombinant protein.[27]

Other RNA viruses can be engineered in similar fashion. Sindbis and other alphaviruses have received extensive attention because of their broad host range, ability to infect nondividing cells, and potential high-level expression per cell.[28] On this basis, Sindbis has been developed into a DNA-based vaccine (see *"Naked" DNA).*

Classical Strategies: Bacterial

It has not been readily possible to develop live attenuated bacterial vaccines by classical strategies, because there has been relatively little success with in vitro culture of bacteria for attenuation while maintaining immunogenicity and because of the proclivity of bacteria for reversion. There also may not be strong competitive or selective pressure for bacteria to become less virulent through genetic changes during in vitro passage; bacteria could stop expressing virulence factors in vitro, then turn their expression back on in vivo. The one widely available live bacterial vaccine based on serial in vitro passage is for tuberculosis. This vaccine consists of a live attenuated strain of *Mycobacterium bovis*, also known as bacille Calmette-Guérin (BCG).[29] Early in the 20th century, this bovine strain was attenuated by 231 successive in vitro subculturings during 13 years, some of these using unconventional growth media. There are many strains of BCG vaccine available worldwide that are derived from the original strain isolated in the early 20th century. These vaccines vary in terms of tolerability, immunogenicity, and rate of protective efficacy in clinical trials (range of 0 to 80% protection) for reasons that may relate to the actual vaccine strains used or to differences in study populations. BCG vaccines have been inoculated into more than 1 billion people worldwide and have generally acceptable tolerability profiles (in immunocompetent individuals). BCG vaccines have also been administered orally (see *Recombinant Bacterial Vector).*

Another technique for creating an attenuated strain has been chemical mutagenesis followed by selection. The Ty21a strain of *Salmonella typhi* was derived in this fashion[30] and was licensed for the prevention of typhoid fever on the basis of its record of safety and efficacy (about 60 to 70% for several years) after a regimen of three or four doses.[31]

One would anticipate that the techniques of rDNA technology now would be applied to attenuation of a new bacterial strain that had promise as a live attenuated vaccine. Therefore, by modern technical and regulatory standards, it seems unlikely that a new live bacterial vaccine attenuated by a classical strategy alone will be developed.

Recombinant Bacteria

The genetic engineering of bacteria for attenuation is much more complex than for viruses, given that bacterial genomes are about 100-fold larger than those of viruses. The technical focus has been directed toward the use of rDNA technology for attenuating live bacterial strains by applying methods similar to those currently used for viral strains. The strategy is to identify the gene responsible for the virulence of the bacteria or for their ability to colonize and survive in particular tissues in the host and to either eliminate the gene (preferred) or to abolish or modulate its in vivo expression. As is true for modification mutants of viruses, there can be a balance between the virulence of a bacterial strain and its activity as a vaccine, which means that it is possible to overattenuate a strain to the point that it no longer replicates sufficiently in vivo to elicit an effective immune response.

Given that an initial infection by *Vibrio cholerae* can protect against subsequent infections, *V. cholerae* strains have been developed as live cholera vaccines. Attenuation of these cholera strains (or of any bacterial strain in general) has been accomplished by the rDNA-directed deletion of genes that encode virulence factors (such as cholera toxin [CT], which is encoded within the *CTX* genetic element).[32] Live attenuated cholera vaccine candidates prepared in this fashion have been evaluated clinically, and one has been licensed. To ensure attenuation by reducing the probability of reversion, it is desirable to delete two or more independent genes or genetic loci that contribute to virulence. This appears important for *V. cholerae*, given the report that a strain deleted in its CT genes can reacquire the genes in vivo from a bacteriophage encoding the *CTX* element and become virulent.[33]

There have been attempts in the last three decades to develop *Shigella flexneri* strains into live *Shigella* vaccines. Recent work has focused on introducing mutating particular chromosomal or plasmid-based genes to reduce pathogenicity while retaining immunogenicity.[34]

Recombinant Bacterial Vector

Pathogenic bacteria can be engineered into live recombinant vectors for the expression of foreign polypeptides encoded by other microorganisms. The most common applications have been to engineer enteric pathogens so that they can induce mucosal immunity against the foreign polypeptide on oral delivery. In the field of developing live bacterial vectors, *S. typhi* has been the focus of the most effort in terms of strain development, immunology, and molecular development; clinical testing of recombinant *S. typhi* strains has been under way.[35] Similarly, *V. cholerae*,[36] *S. flexneri*,[37] and *Listeria monocytogenes*[38] have been engineered into orally administered recombinant vectors. The challenge for these live attenuated vectors is to retain sufficient virulence for replication in the gut and for the expression of appropriate levels of foreign polypeptides while achieving sufficient attenuation to ensure good tolerability. The BCG vaccine strain has also been engineered as a live vector to express foreign genes, including several from HIV-1.[39] The use of this strain as a parenteral vaccine vector (in immunocompetent individuals) has been considered acceptable on the basis of its excellent tolerability profile throughout decades of use worldwide in billions of doses. One aspect of the versatility of BCG is its efficacy in mice by different routes of administration, including oral, intranasal, and intradermal.[40] The ability of some of these bacterial species to replicate intracellularly may augment the ability of expressed foreign polypeptides to elicit cellular immune responses against their respective pathogens.

Streptococcus gordonii, a gram-positive commensal bacteria, has been engineered to express recombinant polypeptides on its surface by genetic fusion to surface attachment sequences of the *S. gordonii* surface M protein.[41] A potential advantage of this system is that the bacteria are not pathogenic. The challenges are whether the recombinant polypeptide will be sufficiently immunogenic on these bacterial cells, given that the bacteria do not elicit an immune response that clears them naturally, and whether the long-term persistence of the organism is of any biological concern.

Nonlive Vaccines

As discussed previously, live vaccines have several potential immunological advantages. Nevertheless, nonlive vaccines do have certain advantages that relate to their inability to multiply within the host (see Table 35–2). They are generally well tolerated, especially for the majority of nonlive vaccines that undergo purification to remove other macromolecules. Given the broad range of technological approaches available, it is also generally more feasible technically to produce a nonlive vaccine. The immunogenicity of a nonlive vaccine is usually enhanced by its administration with an adjuvant or delivery system (see *Formulation of Antigens).* Nevertheless, any development program for a nonlive vaccine should be undertaken with the realization that multiple doses, often followed by booster doses, are usually necessary for attaining long-term protective immunity; in some cases, short-term protection has been demonstrated after a single dose.[42] Nonlive vaccines usually function by stimulating humoral immune responses and by priming for immunological memory. In certain cases, especially when administered with certain adjuvants and delivery systems, nonlive vaccines may stimulate CTL immunity.

Whole-Pathogen Vaccines

The earliest approach to making nonlive vaccines relied on the inactivation of whole bacteria or whole viruses with the objective of eliciting the formation of antibodies to many antigens, some of which would neutralize the pathogen.

Bacteria. The initial inactivated bacterial vaccines were developed in the late 19th century at a time when there was little definition of bacterial antigens and their specific role in immunity. These vaccines are prepared by cultivating the bacteria (e.g., *Bordetella pertussis),* collecting the whole bacterial cells, and inactivating them with heat or with chemical agents such as thimerosal or phenol.[43] The final vaccine does not undergo further purification. Owing to their biochemically highly crude nature, which includes virtually all bacterial cellular components, the reactogenicity of such vaccines when they are given parenterally is usually greater than that of other types of vaccines. On the other hand, inactivated whole-cell *V. cholerae*[44] and enterotoxigenic *Escherichia coli* (ETEC)[45] vaccines have been well tolerated by the oral route. Given the number of alternative technologies available for preparing purified vaccines and the more exacting regulatory standards that have developed over time, it seems that new killed bacterial vaccines made in this fashion are less likely to become available in the future.

Virus. Inactivated viral vaccines likewise are prepared by an old technology, have been available for up to several decades, and are generally well tolerated. Because viruses are generally shed into the cell culture media when they are grown in vitro, cell-free media from infected cultures are collected. The large size of the virus particles relative to other macromolecules in the media enables the particles to be enriched readily by simple purification techniques. Examples include poliovirus,[46] influenza virus,[47] rabies virus,[48] and Japanese encephalitis virus.[49] Alternatively in the case of killed hepatitis A virus vaccine, infected cells are lysed, and virus particles are purified biochemically.[50] The virus particles are inactivated chemically, typically by treatment with formalin, and then adjuvanted by an aluminum salt. The key epitope on the surface of many nonenveloped small viruses that elicits a protective immune response (protective epitope) is often conformational, being formed by the highly ordered assembly of structural proteins into precise structures. For most of the listed viruses for which inactivated vaccines have been developed and licensed,[46–50] it may not be possible to mimic the conformation of such epitopes by other technologies (e.g., recombinant polypeptides). Inactivated viral vaccines tend to be highly potent immunologically. Thus, this classical strategy, which has had an excellent track record of producing well-tolerated and efficacious vaccines, remains the technology of choice for many viral vaccines.

Protein-Based Vaccines

Developing a (purified) protein-based vaccine is the strategy of choice for many pathogens in which a polypeptide contains protective epitopes, given the abovementioned issues regarding inactivated bacterial vaccines and assuming that an inactivated viral vaccine is technically infeasible. Protein-based approaches have relied on genetic, biochemical, and immunological techniques to identify the antigenic specificity of protective antibodies. Advances in such techniques have enabled protective epitopes and their corresponding polypeptides to be identified with fine specificity.

More recently, genomics technology has enabled the identification of new vaccine antigens in lieu of prior available biochemical or antigen data. Once the complete sequence of the genomic DNA or RNA or portions thereof are available, open reading frames are identified. The derived amino acid sequence can be inspected for structural features, such as homologies with proteins from other related pathogens that are vaccine candidates or a hydrophobic N-terminal sequence that suggests that the protein may be on the surface of the pathogen. The genes are expressed in a recombinant host cell (typically *E. coli*), and the recombinant polypeptide is purified and used to immunize animals to derive polyclonal antibodies. Alternatively, synthetic peptides from the hypothetical gene product are produced and used for immunizations. The polyclonal antisera are then used to identify whether the hypothetical protein is produced. Antisera can also be used in biological assays (neutralization of viruses, opsonization of bacteria, binding to surface of either) to see whether the protein may be an attractive vaccine candidate. The new protein can also be used for immunization and challenge in an animal model. Some of the earliest applications of genomics technology to viruses were to hepatitis C virus[51] and hepatitis E virus,[52] which were first identified by means of cloning the viral genomes. Since 1995, with the availability of the complete DNA sequence of *Haemophilus influenzae*,[53] the DNA sequences of many other bacterial genomes are becoming available. The DNA sequence of bakers' yeast *Saccharomyces cerevisiae* recently became available and points the way to availability of fungal genomic sequences.[54] For bacteria such as *Helicobacter pylori*, which have been analyzed previously at the protein level for surface proteins that might be vaccine candidates, this analysis can reveal new candidate antigens previously unrecognized.[55]

Natural. The first protein-based vaccines relied on natural (nonrecombinant) sources of antigens. In this regard, the first hepatitis B vaccine is unique among active vaccines in that it used a human tissue source (plasma) for the vaccine antigen. Liver cells of individuals chronically infected with hepatitis B virus (HBV) shed excess viral surface protein, that is, hepatitis B surface antigen (HBsAg), into blood. In the early 1970s, HBsAg was identified as a 22-nm lipoprotein particle antigen with protective epitopes. To develop a vaccine, plasma was harvested from long-term chronic carriers of hepatitis B, HBsAg purified, and the final preparation subjected to one to three inactivation techniques (depending on the manufacturer) to kill HBV and any other human virus that might have been present in the starting plasma.[56] This vaccine has enjoyed widespread use and is well tolerated and highly efficacious.

Proteins purified from cultures of *B. pertussis* can be combined to formulate acellular pertussis (P_{ac}) vaccines, which eventually should replace whole-cell pertussis vaccine for routine pediatric vaccinations in many developed countries. Depending on the number of different protein antigens, these P_{ac} vaccines are referred to as one-, two-, three-, four-, or five-component vaccines and have been licensed on the basis of recent efficacy studies.[57–59] These vaccines all contain pertussis toxoid (PT) as a component, whose preparation is described later.

Chemical Inactivation. Many bacteria produce protein toxins that are responsible for the pathogenesis of infection. It had been recognized for many decades that when a specific toxin was the chief mechanism of pathogenesis after infection by the causative bacteria, antitoxins (antisera enriched in toxin-specific antibodies) that were effective in neutralizing toxin activity in vivo could prevent or ameliorate symptoms of certain bacterial infections. This precedent established the basis for bacterial toxins to be formulated as active vaccines. The toxin molecules are purified from bacterial cultures, for example, *B. pertussis*, *Clostridium tetani* (T), and *Corynebacterium diphtheriae* (D), and then detoxified by incubation with a chemical such as formalin or glutaraldehyde. Detoxified toxins, referred to as *toxoids*, thus represent two of the vaccines in the diphtheria, tetanus, and pertussis (DTP) combination vaccine.[60, 61] PT[62] combined with other natural pertussis antigens composes the P_{ac} vaccines.

Genetic Inactivation. The chemical toxoiding procedure has several potential disadvantages, including the possible alteration of protective epitopes with ensuing reduced immunogenicity and the potential for the toxoid to revert to a biologically active toxin. The use of rDNA technology has been employed to produce a stable toxoid. As applied to pertussis, the toxin gene was cloned and sequenced, and codons for amino acids required for toxin bioactivity (adenosine diphosphate [ADP] ribosyltransferase) were mutated. The altered gene was substituted for the native gene in the parental organism (or heterologous organism, such as *E. coli*, if technically feasible to produce an immunogenic toxoid), which then produces immunogenic but stably inactivated PT. As a refinement of this strategy, two mutations were introduced into PT to ensure the inability to revert[63]; this double-mutant PT (which is also treated with formalin under milder conditions to improve its immunogenicity or stability) is a component of a P_{ac} vaccine.[56] A genetic approach to derive a D toxoid was also successful. Mutated cultures of *C. diphtheriae* were screened for the secretion of enzymatically inactive yet antigenic toxin molecules. Subsequent cloning and sequencing of one such mutated toxin gene identified a single amino acid mutation at the enzymatic active site (also an ADP-ribosyltransferase). This genetic toxoid (CRM_{197})[64] is the protein carrier for a licensed *H. influenzae* type b (Hib) conjugate vaccine (see *Polysaccharide-Based Vaccines*). This technology has also been applied to *V. cholerae* toxin and ETEC toxin to produce candidate mucosal adjuvants (see *Formulation of Antigens*).

Recombinant Polypeptides. The first application of rDNA technology to the production of a vaccine was for hepatitis B. Given the precedent of plasma-derived HBsAg as a well-tolerated and efficacious vaccine, the strategy employed in the late 1970s was to clone and sequence the HBV genome, identify the S gene encoding HBsAg, and express this gene in a heterologous host cell. The strategy for such foreign gene expression (Fig. 35–3) is to (1) construct an expression cassette with transcriptional initiation and termination sequences (directing formation of specific mRNA that can be translated into a polypeptide) immediately before and after the gene, (2) place the expression cassette into a larger DNA molecule (plasmid) capable of increasing its copy number in the host cell, (3) transform the plasmid into the host cell, and then (4) screen transformed cells with specific antibodies for expression of the desired polypeptide. Expression of the HBsAg gene in bakers' yeast *S. cerevisiae*[65] and in cultured mammalian cells[66] (Chinese hamster ovary [CHO] cells) resulted in the expression of 22-nm HBsAg particles, in the former case within cells and in the latter case in the culture media. HBsAg is a virus-like particle (VLP; Fig. 35–4) in that its surface is similar to that of HBV virions. Both sources of HBsAg have been isolated to a high level of purity and adjuvanted with aluminum salts for formulation as vaccines, which were licensed through the late 1980s. The yeast-derived vaccine, which is available worldwide in large

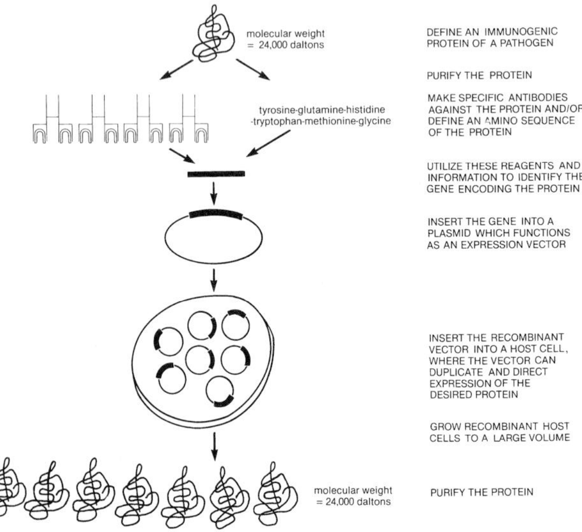

Figure 35–3. The use of recombinant DNA technology to express large amounts of a desired protein.

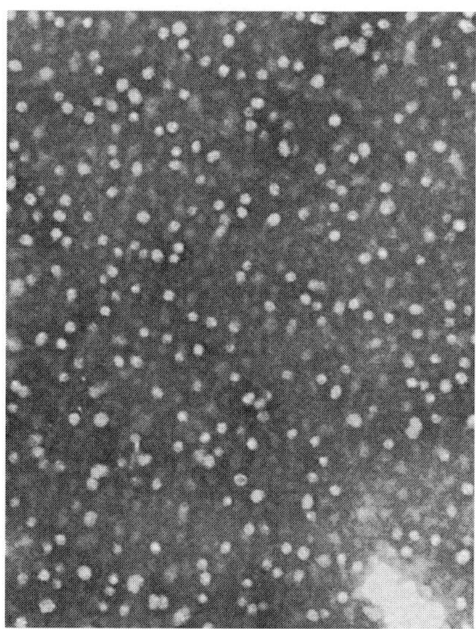

Figure 35–4. Electron micrograph of particles of hepatitis B surface antigen produced by recombinant yeast (× 165,000). (Courtesy of B. Wolanski, Merck Research Laboratories.)

supply, has largely supplanted the equally efficacious and well-tolerated plasma-derived vaccine. HBsAg has also been expressed in transgenic tobacco leaves and potato tubers; the purified HBsAg was immunogenic.[67]

Large particles are often more immunogenic than individual polypeptides. Furthermore, particles can elicit antibodies that recognize conformational epitopes on the particle, whereas isolated surface polypeptides of the particle might not elicit the production of such antibodies. Examples of such particle immunogens are hepatitis A virus particles (which are immunogenic in humans at dosage levels as low as 50 ng) and HBsAg particles (which are VLPs). Another recent example of the effective use of VLPs is for human papillomavirus (HPV). The HPV virion is a highly ordered structure whose major protein is L1. *E. coli*–expressed L1 is a polypeptide that after immunization elicits anti-L1 antibodies, which do not bind to papillomavirus virions or VLPs. However, expression of L1 in eukaryotic cells (e.g., *S. cerevisiae*) results in the formation of L1 VLPs that after immunization do elicit antibodies, which bind to the VLPs and to virions.[68] VLPs are currently in clinical trials. Similarly, recombinant rotavirus VLPs have been expressed as a potential parenteral vaccine.[69]

There are innumerable ongoing research and development applications of rDNA technology to produce proteins as vaccine candidates. HIV-1 gp120 elicits viral neutralizing antibodies. The gp120 gene has been expressed in *S. cerevisiae*, insect cells,[70] and CHO cells,[71] and the purified recombinant proteins (rgp120, rgp160) have been formulated into vaccines that are undergoing clinical evaluations. The insect cell–derived product is the first recombinant product from such cells to enter widespread clinical trials. Similarly, recombinant-derived HSV glycoproteins have been expressed in CHO cells and formulated as vaccines that are also in clinical trials.[72] The major surface protein, OspA, of *Borrelia burgdorferi* has been expressed in *E. coli* as a recombinant lipoprotein,[73] which has been in advanced clinical trials.

There are also experimental recombinant vaccines for parasites such as schistosomes.[74]

Especially noteworthy are recent vaccine applications outside the realm of infectious diseases. Because crude extracts from allergens such as ragweed can be used therapeutically for the amelioration of allergic symptoms, the gene encoding an allergen can be cloned and expressed in a heterologous host cell. As a further refinement, a recombinant dust mite allergen polypeptide has been engineered to reduce its capacity to induce in vivo skin test reactivity and in vitro histamine release from peripheral blood basophils of allergic patients while retaining T-cell epitopes essential for immunotherapy.[75] This approach can be extended to other major allergens, which eventually may result in a cocktail of defined allergens for formulation into a vaccine that could be more effective and better tolerated than currently available crude therapeutic vaccines.

Autoimmune diseases may be amenable to vaccine development. During the period before the development of clinical type I diabetes, autoantibodies become detectable to pancreatic β-cell autoantigens (e.g., insulin), after which destruction of β cells ensues. An appropriately formulated and delivered recombinant autoantigen can prevent the development of type I diabetes in a mouse model.[76] Furthermore, a small clinical trial showed that the subcutaneous injection of recombinant *E. coli*–derived insulin into prediabetic patients with detectable anti–β-cell autoantibodies resulted in a significant delay in the development of clinical type I diabetes.[77]

Another novel application is in the field of human fertility. A protein on the surface of guinea pig sperm was purified, adjuvanted, and then injected into female guinea pigs. Vaccinated animals were rendered sterile yet subsequently regained fertility after periods averaging 1 year following vaccination.[78] This result paves the way for the strategy of cloning and expressing the gene encoding the analogous human sperm protein for use as a reversible fertility vaccine.

Many host cells have been used for the expression of heterologous recombinant genes.[79] In addition to the previously mentioned *E. coli*, *S. cerevisiae*, insect, and CHO cell hosts, expression systems have been developed for cells from other bacterial and yeast species and other mammalian continuous cell lines (CCLs), such as African green monkey kidney (Vero). Whole animals and plants can also be employed as hosts for recombinant expression. In general, smaller proteins that do not require posttranslational modifications can be expressed efficiently in authentic form in microbial expression systems. Aside from the recombinant-derived hepatitis B vaccine made in yeast, other proteins produced in microbial expression systems have been developed and licensed for human therapeutic applications; such proteins include insulin, growth hormone, interferon, and interleukin-2. In contrast, polypeptides that require posttranslational modifications such as glycosylation, proteolysis, carboxylation, or hydroxylation for biological activity or desired pharmacokinetics are expressed in mammalian CCLs capable of correctly performing such modifications. Licensed therapeutic proteins produced in mammalian CCLs include tissue plasminogen activator and erythropoietin.

Carrier. A novel approach to recombinant vaccines is the use of yeast Ty particles as killed carriers for foreign proteins. Yeast Ty is a particle assembled in *S. cerevisiae* that cannot replicate in mammals. It is possible to express a gene encoding a foreign protein in conjunction with Ty genes such that the foreign proteins assemble with Ty proteins into mixed particles.[80] Because the foreign proteins are expressed on the surface of these large particles, their immunogenicity as vaccine antigens might be enhanced.

Peptide-Based Vaccines

In many cases, it has been possible to identify B-cell epitopes within a polypeptide against which neutralizing antibodies are directed (Fig. 35–5). The techniques of rDNA cloning and sequencing combined with serological studies have enabled some epitopes to be mapped to precise amino acid residues. In the preceding examples and others, a polypeptide or large peptide fragment is immunogenic and readily elicits neutralizing antibody directed against key epitopes on it. Many B-cell epitopes are conformational, being formed by the juxtaposition in three-dimensional space of amino acid residues from different portions of the polypeptide, which means that such epitopes require the full polypeptide for their proper immunogenic presentation. In contrast, other peptide epitopes are linear in nature, being fully antigenic as short linear sequences in the range of 6 to 20 consecutive amino acid residues in the polypeptide. Some linear epitopes are only weakly immunogenic when presented in the context of the full polypeptide. When neutralizing antibodies are directed against these weakly immunogenic epitopes, the full or partial poly-

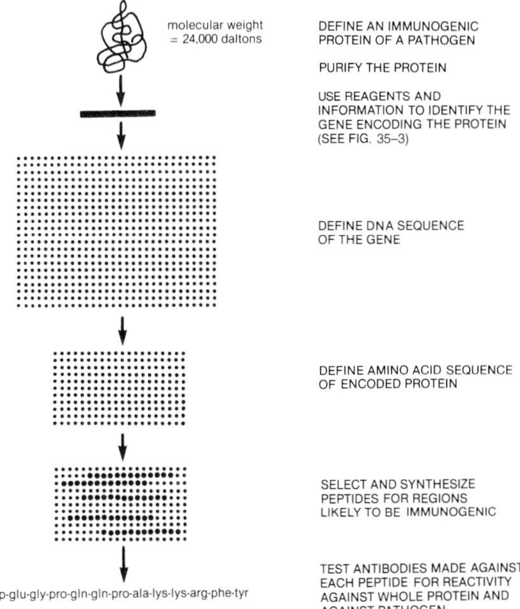

Figure 35–5. Defining immunogenic peptides from immunogenic proteins.

peptide containing the epitope might not be an effective immunogen for the vaccine. In other cases, natural peptides would be effective vaccine antigens if they were rendered more immunogenic than they are as native peptides.

There are several technologies for increasing the immunogenicity of such linear B-cell epitopes or of weakly immunogenic peptides to make them more suitable as vaccine antigens. Linear B-cell epitopes of this type have been defined for the malarial circumsporozoite protein (repetitive 4–amino acid sequence)[81] and for HIV-1 gp120 (within amino acid residues 301 to 336).[82] Both of these polypeptides contain linear epitopes that are recognized by antibodies that neutralize the respective pathogens, yet the whole polypeptides elicit such antibodies only weakly. It is interesting to speculate that this may represent a mechanism by which these and other pathogens have evolved to escape immunological surveillance by rendering their neutralization epitopes less immunogenic.

Fusion Protein. The immunogenicity of linear epitopes can be increased by making a genetic fusion of defined epitopes to a carrier protein that forms a large particle to improve the presentation of the peptide to cells of the immune system. Two commonly used protein fusion partners of this type are HBsAg[83] and hepatitis B core antigen,[84] a 28-nm particle encoded by HBV. The fusion can be at the N terminus, the C terminus, or the internal portion of the polypeptide sequence of the protein partner, depending on which location affords the best immunogenic presentation while maintaining efficient particle formation.

Conjugate. The peptide can be conjugated to a carrier protein, that is, chemically linked by a covalent bond. This technology was first shown in the 1920s to be effective in increasing the immunogenicity of a peptide. The peptide sequence is synthesized chemically with a reactive amino acid residue through which conjugation occurs to the carrier protein. The most commonly used carrier proteins in conjugates are bacterial proteins that humans commonly encounter, such as tetanus toxoid (TT), for which a conjugate with the malarial circumsporozoite epitope has been tested clinically.[85] Conjugation technology has also been applied to the formulation of a fertility vaccine based on human chorionic gonadotropin (hCG) or luteinizing hormone–releasing hormone (LH-RH). It has been demonstrated that antibodies to these hormones inhibit fertilization; however, LH-RH and hCG are only weakly immunogenic. Conjugates of hCG or LH-RH to TT are immunogenic and elicit antibodies that inhibit fertilization in laboratory animals. Such conjugate vaccines are in clinical evaluation as fertility vaccines.[86]

Complex Peptide. Multimers of the peptide sequence can be synthesized for linkage together in repeated arrays, as applied to the malarial circumsporozoite and HIV-1 gp120 peptide epitopes.[87, 88]

The application of these three strategies (fusion protein, conjugate, and complex peptide) to weakly immunogenic linear epitopes has resulted in immunogenic presentations that elicit substantially increased titers of neutralizing antibody compared with those elicited by the epitope presented in the context of its natural full-length polypeptide. Nevertheless, the most effective strategy in terms of ultimate clinical utility remains to be established.

Mimetopes. By screening recombinant-based peptide libraries with antisera, it is possible to identify small reactive peptides (mimetopes) that antigenically mimic the immunogen in question. Such sequences were identified in the HBV S polypeptide that would react with anti-HBs antibodies; these mimetopes, when fused with carrier proteins, could elicit anti-HBs antibodies.[89] Whereas this approach is not a sufficient substitute for the available highly immunogenic hepatitis B vaccines, it is a model for creating an antigen for an immunogen that cannot be readily produced by recombinant or synthetic methods. It has also been possible to use peptides that mimic carbohydrate epitopes on HIV-1 to elicit HIV-1–neutralizing antibodies.[90]

T-cell Epitopes. Peptide epitopes recognized by CTL may be useful immunogens for the prophylaxis of infections by agents such as HIV and *Mycobacterium tuberculosis* or immunotherapy for chronic diseases such as hepatitis B. CTL peptide epitopes are generally poor immunogens. Thus, for an immunotherapeutic hepatitis B vaccine, a CTL epitope from the HBV core protein was modified by covalent linkage to a T helper epitope (from tetanus toxoid) as well as two palmitic acid molecules.[91] This vaccine was shown in clinical studies to be immunogenic in a 500-mg dose for eliciting HBV-specific CTL and memory CTL.

Polysaccharide-Based Vaccines

There are many bacteria with an outer polysaccharide capsule. In many if not most of the encapsulated bacteria studied, antibodies directed against capsular polysaccharide are protective against bacterial infection. These observations have established capsular polysaccharides as vaccine antigens. In some cases, lipopolysaccharide, another abundant surface molecule on gram-negative bacteria, is a vaccine antigen.

Plain Polysaccharide. The natural capsular polysaccharide contains up to hundreds of chemically defined repeat units distinct for each bacterial species and antigenic subtype, in which each monomer consists of a combination of monosaccharides, phosphate groups, and small organic moieties. The polysaccharide is shed by the organism during its growth and is harvested and enriched from the culture medium. These polysaccharide preparations are usually immunogenic in adults and children older than 2 years. The polysaccharide elicits antibodies that may mediate the opsonization of the organism, thereby protecting against bacterial infection. Polysaccharide vaccines have been licensed for *H. influenzae* type b[92] (monovalent), *Neisseria meningitidis*[93] (quadrivalent), and *Streptococcus pneumoniae*[94] (23-valent). The shortcoming of these vaccines is that polysaccharides, being T-cell–independent immunogens, are poorly immunogenic or nonimmunogenic in children younger than 2 years owing to the immature status of their immune systems, and they do not elicit immunological memory in older children and adults.

Conjugate. Although infants and children younger than 2 years do not recognize T-cell–independent immunogens efficiently, they can recognize and respond immunologically to T-cell–dependent immunogens such as proteins. The chemical conjugation of polysaccharide to a carrier protein converts the polysaccharide from a T-cell–independent to a T-cell–dependent immunogen. As a consequence, polysaccharide-protein conjugate vaccines can elicit protective immunoglobulin G (IgG) and immunological memory in infants and young children. This strategy is particularly important for dealing with encapsulated bacteria such as *H. influenzae* type b (Hib) and *S. pneumoniae* (pneumococcus) owing to the preponderance of invasive diseases caused by these bacteria in children younger than 2 years, in whom a polysaccharide vaccine is ineffective. There are four different licensed Hib conjugate vaccines,[95] all with different carrier proteins (TT, DT, CRM_{197}, and an outer membrane protein complex from *N. meningitidis* type B) of different sizes and immunological character, distinct polysaccharide chain lengths, and distinct conjugation chemistries. Given these differences, the four conjugate vaccines display one or more differences in the following immunological properties: response of 2-month-old infants to the first dose of vaccine, response of 4- and 6-month-old infants to the second and third doses, response of children older than 1 year to a booster dose, kinetics of decay of antibody levels, peak of antibody titer, and age at which protection from clinical disease can first be shown. The polysaccharide-protein conjugates are also useful for increasing the immunogenicity of polysaccharide vaccines in adults.

The *H. influenzae* type b bacteria are a single serotype (b). Pneumococcal bacteria, on the other hand, consist of more than 80 serotypes, as reflected in distinct capsular polysaccharide structures. For designing a pediatric pneumococcal conjugate vaccine, eight serotypes have been recognized as responsible for 70 to 90% of the major pediatric pneumococcal diseases (acute otitis media, pneumonia, meningitis). Therefore, vaccines being tested in advanced clinical trials consist of a mixture of up to 11 individual pneumococcal polysaccharide conjugates.[96]

A conjugate of group B streptococcal polysaccharide can be used to immunize pregnant women,[97] with the goal that the IgG to group B streptococcal polysaccharide can cross the placenta for the prevention of neonatal group B streptococcal meningitis (in contrast to *H. influenzae* type b and pneumococcal invasive diseases, which are rare in children younger than 1 to 2 months).

Anti-idiotypic Antibodies

The *idiotype* (Id), that is, idiotypic determinant, is associated with the hypervariable region of the antibody molecule and represents its unique antigenic determinants. An antibody-1 (Ab-1) can be defined as an antibody recognizing a particular antigen, such as one that might be a vaccine candidate. The Id on Ab-1 itself can act as an antigen and elicit an immune response; the antibodies that bind to the Id on Ab-1 are referred to as *anti-idiotypic antibodies* (anti-Id) or Ab-2. The paratope is the site on Ab-1 that binds to the particular antigen; thus, the binding site of an antiparatope antibody is a molecular "mimic" of the antigen. If the Id and the paratope on Ab-1 represent the same or overlapping sites, then the particular antigen and Ab-2 both bind at that site and thus have similar conformations and are mimics (Ab-1 is the image of the antigen and Ab-2). By virtue of the antibody-binding site of Ab-2 mimicking the conformation of the particular antigen (which may be a vaccine candidate), Ab-2 molecules themselves can be used as nonlive vaccine candidates in which an epitope (mimicked by the Id on Ab-2) is presented on a carrier molecule (the whole Ab-2). An excellent demonstration that deriving anti-Id represents an effective vaccine strategy comes from studies in which it was shown that vaccination of chimpanzees with anti-Id that mimicked HBsAg protected the animals from infection with a pathogenic dose of HBV.[98] The strategy for the use of anti-idiotypic antibodies as vaccines is illustrated in Figure 35–6.

Numerous technologies exist for using an antigen as a vaccine candidate, either directly or by augmenting its immunogenicity as described earlier. Furthermore, an antibody molecule (Ab-2) is not necessarily a desirable immunological carrier for an antigen (anti-Id). Hence, the situations in which the use of anti-Id would be the preferred vaccine strategy are limited in number. Certain tumor antigens cannot be recognized immunologically by the host, because these antigens are self-antigens, often being expressed in low levels in the host. Nevertheless, the Ab-2 that is the mimic of the tumor antigen, yet not necessarily identical in structure to the antigen (hence not a self-antigen), can elicit an immune response

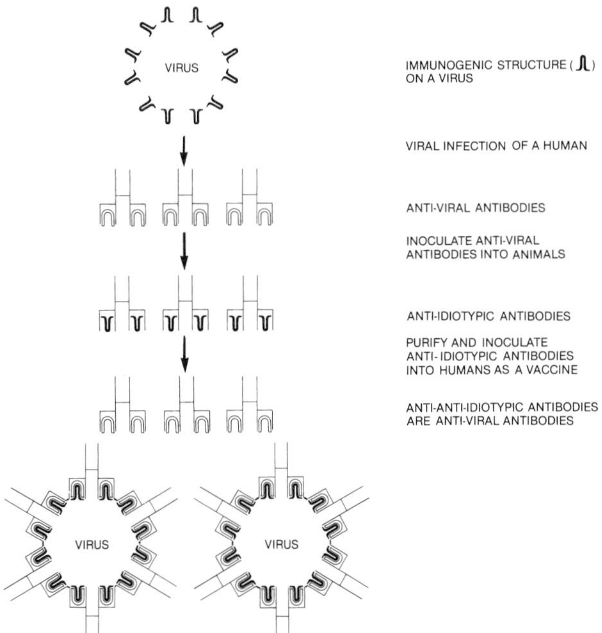

Figure 35–6. Strategy for the use of anti-idiotypic antibodies as vaccines.

against the tumor antigen.[99] When the tumor antigen is a defined polysaccharide that cannot be isolated or synthesized in quantities sufficient for vaccine studies, an anti-Id of the mimic of the polysaccharide can be a useful cancer vaccine candidate.[100] Similarly, an anti-Id for the parasite *Schistosoma mansoni* that is the mimic of a schistosome carbohydrate epitope has shown promise as a vaccine candidate,[101] whereas sufficient quantities of this carbohydrate could not be obtained. The ultimate utility of anti-Id as a vaccine strategy remains to be established. In particular, the degree to which the antigenic site in Ab-2 can structurally mimic the antigen in question to elicit a consistent protective immune response needs to be established. Furthermore, to obtain the highest degree of specificity as a vaccine candidate, one would derive a monoclonal antibody as an anti-Id and make it into a recombinant human or humanized monoclonal antibody (see *Monoclonal Antibodies)*.

DNA-Based Vaccines

A recent novel approach to a nonlive vaccine has been the use of DNA encoding a vaccine antigen. The in vitro paradigm for this approach lay in the transformation of mammalian cells in culture with a plasmid that directs the synthesis and secretion of a vaccine antigen from cells that take up the plasmid DNA. After cells in vivo take up DNA encoding vaccine antigens, the antigens can be secreted or can be associated with the cell surface in a way that would trigger a humoral or cellular immune response. Furthermore, the uptake of DNA can be facilitated by chemical formulation or delivery by a virus or bacteria. These approaches fit the definition of a DNA-based vaccine as one that cannot replicate in humans. "Naked," facilitated, and virally delivered DNA vaccines have recently entered clinical studies.

Immunization with DNA has been used as a new genomic technology, known as expression library immunization.[102] In this technique, a microbial DNA genome is cloned as a library of DNA expression plasmids, mixtures of which are used to immunize an animal that is then challenged with the microorganism of interest. By successive fractionation and testing in the challenge model, protective plasmids, hence genes encoding protective antigens, can be identified. This expression library immunization technique may be refined by cloning into the expression library open reading frames from the microorganism of interest, once its genomic sequence becomes available.

"Naked" DNA

One strategy has been to inject intramuscularly a solution of uncoated or "naked" DNA encoding a vaccine antigen.[103] Cells take up the DNA, transcribe its expression cassette, and synthesize the antigen, which may be processed in a way similar to a live viral infection. Humoral or cellular immune responses to the encoded antigen are elicited (Fig. 35–7). The advantages of using DNA are the relative technical ease of preparation and the ability to direct the synthesis of multiple copies of mRNA, hence an expected amplification of both antigen synthesis and immune response. Such vaccines have been shown to be effective in many animal models of infection, especially virus models.[104] Whereas naked DNA does elicit the production of specific antibodies, it is particularly proficient at eliciting cellular immune responses.

A variation on the design of the expression plasmid is to use a virus-based DNA expression system that can amplify the level of RNA and protein expression as occurs in a live virus infection. Such a system has been developed on the basis of Sindbis virus DNA vectors.[105]

Facilitated DNA

Facilitation can be at the level of cellular uptake, expression, or immunological activation. One strategy has been the incorporation of DNA into microprojectiles that then are "shot" directly into cells, which produce the encoded antigen that stimulates an immune response.[106] Whereas this "gene gun" technique has been reported to be potent at eliciting immune responses, it is cumbersome and not yet practical for broad clinical use. As another method for improving the efficiency of uptake, DNA has been coated with cationic lipids, lipospermines, or other molecules that neutralize its charge and have lipid groups for facilitating cellular uptake and membrane transfer.[107] Such formulations are also being researched for alternative routes of injection other than parenteral, which may elicit mucosal immunity. The anesthetic bupivacaine given in conjunction with DNA has been shown to enhance DNA uptake and expression.[108] The base composition of the DNA may affect its potency in that unmethylated CpG dinucleotides have been shown to induce B-cell proliferation and immunoglobulin secretion.[109]

Viral Delivery

The preceding DNA-based vaccines result in the deposition into a cell of a plasmid encoding only the vaccine antigen. For delivery of DNA by fowlpox or canarypox virus, the expression cassette for the recombinant protein is integrated into the viral genome (see *Recombinant Viral Vector)*. Although able to infect avian species and produce infectious virus, these avian poxviruses can infect mammalian (human) cells but not produce infectious virus[110, 111]; hence, this can be considered a DNA-based approach. This single round of self-limiting infection may be sufficient to elicit broad immunity to a pathogen whose recombinant polypeptide is expressed by these avian poxviruses in infected cells; at the same time, reactogenicity should be less than that associated with vaccinia virus given the inability of the virus to spread within the host. This paradigm of a live vaccine vector that efficiently infects cells without the capacity for replication in humans could prove to be immunologically useful and distinct from other approaches.

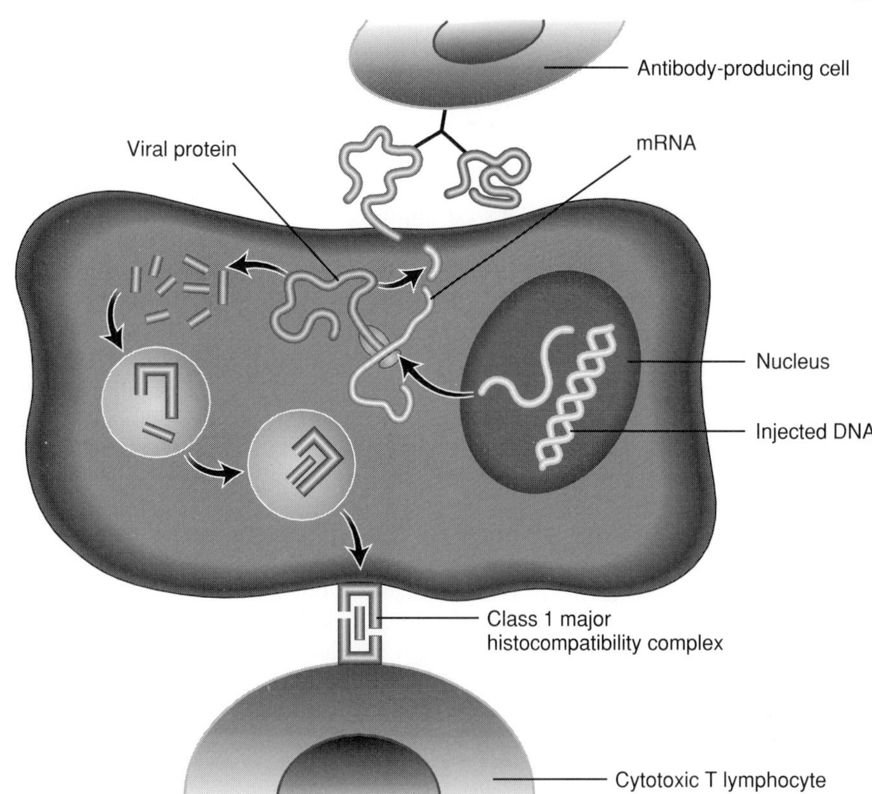

Figure 35–7. Injection of DNA encoding a foreign protein can elicit antibodies and cytotoxic T lymphocytes.

Bacterial Delivery

Bacteria that replicate intracellularly can be engineered to deliver plasmid DNA into cells for the expression of recombinant proteins.[112] *S. flexneri* has been attenuated by making a deletion mutant in the *asd* gene, an essential gene. Whereas such an attenuated strain can be propagated in vitro in the presence of diaminopimelic acid (DAP) and can invade cells (as long as it maintains a plasmid encoding invasion-associated polypeptides), it cannot replicate in vivo, where DAP is not available. A plasmid harboring a eukaryotic promoter and recombinant gene was transformed into this strain. The resultant recombinant *S. flexneri* strain was shown to be able to invade mammalian cells in vitro and to express the plasmid-encoded protein as a potential vaccine antigen. Because *S. flexneri* replicates in the intestine and stimulates mucosal immunity, this vector may be delivered orally and be effective for delivering DNA to cells where mucosal immunity is stimulated. Other bacterial species, such as attenuated *Salmonella typhimurium*,[112a] that can invade mammalian cells but not divide may also be able to deliver recombinant plasmids to different cell types for expressing recombinant proteins as vaccine antigens.

Formulation of Antigens

The immunological effectiveness of nonlive and DNA-based vaccines may be enhanced by their formulation, which refers to the final form of the vaccine to be administered in vivo. In addition to the vaccine "active substance" (antigen or DNA), the formulation contains excipients such as salts or other chemicals and also may contain an adjuvant or delivery system. The adjuvant is a protein or chemical that stimulates an increased humoral or cellular immune response to a coadministered antigen. The delivery system is a vehicle for ensuring the presentation of the vaccine in vivo to cells of the immune system or for stabilizing and releasing the antigen during an extended period of time. There may be overlap in structure and function between adjuvants and delivery systems. Many future vaccines are expected to contain new adjuvants and delivery systems. Because this topic has been addressed extensively in reviews by others,[113–116] this chapter provides an overview to the field and highlights a few key examples. These reviews also contain extensive bibliographies for the wide variety of available experimental adjuvants and delivery systems.

Adjuvants

Aluminum salts, such as hydroxide or phosphate, are currently the only adjuvants licensed for human use. This adjuvant has been used for decades in vaccines injected into more than 1 billion people worldwide. The vaccine antigen binds stably to the aluminum salt by ionic interactions and forms a macroscopic suspension in solution.[117] This adjuvant preferentially promotes a Th2-type immune response (i.e., antibody-based) and thus is not very useful in applications in which inducing a cell-mediated immune response is needed for protection. Whereas aluminum salts have been useful for certain vaccines (e.g., hepatitis B, pertussis), for other vaccine antigens they are not potent enough for inducing antibody responses that are high enough to be optimally effective. Aluminum salts have not been shown to be useful for presentation of vaccines by the oral or intranasal routes. Therefore, many chemicals, biochemicals from natural sources, and proteins with immune system activity (cytokines[118]) have been researched as potential adjuvants. The adjuvanticity of virtually all known formulations is associated with local or systemic side effects that may be mechanism based or nonspecific. The ideal adjuvant needs to achieve a balance between degree of side effects and immune enhancement.

Certain bacterial toxins with ADP-ribosylating activity have received considerable attention as mucosal adjuvants in terms of molecular engineering. In particular, CT was shown to be active as a mucosal adjuvant for a coadministered antigen[119] when presented by the oral, nasal, vaginal, or rectal routes, as was shown subsequently for the heat-labile toxin (LT) of ETEC. These toxins are composed of a catalytic A subunit and a pentameric B subunit that binds to GM_1 ganglioside on many cell types. However, both CT and LT are toxic in humans, especially by the oral route through which they induce diarrhea. To dissociate the toxicity and adjuvanticity of CT and LT, point mutations have been made that result in reduced or eliminated ADP-ribosylating activity, reduced toxicity, and the apparent retention of adjuvanticity in mice.[120] An alternative approach has been to eliminate the B subunit and substitute a synthetic dimeric peptide derived from *Staphylococcus aureus* protein A (DD) that binds to immunoglobulin. The fusion of the CTA subunit with the DD domain binds to immunoglobulin-positive cells, appears devoid of toxicity, retains ADP-ribosylating activity, and is active as an adjuvant in mice.[121] The tolerability and effectiveness of these engineered adjuvants need to be validated in humans.

Delivery Systems

Besides presenting an antigen or DNA to cells of the immune system, a delivery system may perform other key functions. There may be a depot effect whereby the antigen is maintained in an appropriate in vivo site for continual immune stimulation. There may be an enhancement of vaccine stability in vivo. For mucosally delivered vaccines, the delivery system may enable efficient presentation and uptake by M cells, followed by transcytosis into Peyer patches and presentation to lymphocytes for the induction of mucosal immunity. For certain formulations, the vaccine may be maintained in vivo inside a physical structure for a significant period of time, during which it is released slowly or in pulsatile fashion such that it may function as a one-dose vaccine. As for adjuvants other than aluminum salts, no delivery systems have been widely licensed. Gaining clinical and pharmaceutical experience with new delivery systems and adjuvants remains a key goal in the field.

Mixed Strategies

Vaccine development historically has focused on a vaccine made by a single technology delivered in one or more doses. More recently with increased appreciation of immunobiology, regimens have been developed that employ vaccines that are mixtures either of two different types of vaccines made by different technologies (mixed vaccines) or of different types of vaccines given during the dosing regimen (mixed regimens).

Mixed Vaccines

Oral inactivated whole-cell cholera (WCC) vaccine, which lacks CT (and its toxic effects), has been shown to be well tolerated and to have a rate of efficacy of approximately 60% for 3 years in a high-risk population.[44] To elicit antibodies that would neutralize CT, the recombinant B subunit of CT (CTB), which lacks toxin activity, is independently expressed, purified, and added back to the WCC vaccine. This combined WCC + rCTB vaccine was shown to have a somewhat higher rate of efficacy than WCC alone.[122] Moreover, because CTB cross-reacts immunologically with the B subunit of LT, the combined vaccine also shows some efficacy against ETEC.

Mixed Regimens

Several studies have examined immunization regimens involving a sequence of different vaccines to assess whether some immunogens are more efficient at priming immunological memory and others at boosting memory. Recombinant canarypox virus expressing HIV-1 gp160 or gp120 has been given in clinical studies in two priming doses followed by boosting with rgp160 protein.[123] This regimen induced higher levels of neutralizing antibodies than immunizing with gp160 alone. Likewise, clinical studies of two priming doses of rgp160 followed by boosting with a peptide from the major type-specific neutralization epitope[82] of gp160 demonstrated the production of higher levels of HIV-1 neutralizing antibodies than elicited by rgp160 alone.[124] Priming with adenovirus expressing HIV-1 gp160 followed by boosting with HIV-1 rgp120 elicited persistent titers of virus-neutralizing antibodies, CTL activity, and protection of chimpanzees from HIV-1 challenge.[125]

Given the different kinetics of immune responses of infants to different Hib conjugate vaccines (see *Polysaccharide-Based Vaccines, Conjugate)*, mixed regimens have been evaluated in an attempt to optimize the level of antibody response. It was found that immunization at 2 months with one particular Hib conjugate vaccine followed by boosting with another at 4 and 6 months of age elicited higher anti-Hib polysaccharide antibody levels after each dose than immunization with either vaccine separately in all three doses.[126]

These studies have demonstrated that the use of a vaccine with superior priming characteristics followed by boosting with a related vaccine more efficient at eliciting an antibody response may be an improved regimen for eliciting higher antibody titers. Whereas such a regimen is more complicated to develop technically and clinically and to license than a one-vaccine regimen, it may be useful in certain clinical settings.

PASSIVE VACCINES

In some situations, immediate immunological protection is necessary to treat an infectious disease. Because injection with an active vaccine can take 1 to 2 weeks to begin to elicit an antibody response, a preparation of antibodies with known protective effect against a pathogen could be efficacious if it were administered at or near the time of a known, suspected, or potential exposure to the pathogen. Examples include (1) postexposure prophylaxis for known or suspected exposure to HBV[127] or varicella-zoster virus[128] in individuals who are unvaccinated and with no known prior exposure to the virus, (2) preexposure prophylaxis for at-risk individuals with an underlying pathologic process (transplantees with cytomegalovirus,[129] infants with pulmonary diseases who have respiratory syncytial virus,[130] sepsis patients with *Pseudomonas aeruginosa*,[131] and people being treated for cancer[132]), and (3) administration to pregnant mothers who are viremic for cytomegalovirus[133] for the prevention of perinatal viral infection in newborns. The protective effect mediated by most of these antibody preparations is to neutralize the virus infectivity or bind to bacteria, which then are destroyed by phagocytic cells. In cases such as tetanus[134] and *P. aeruginosa*,[131] protection would be mediated by antibodies that bind to and neutralize toxin molecules elaborated by the pathogen. Such antibody preparations are referred to as *passive vaccines*.

Polyclonal Antibodies

The earliest preparations of antibody, or immune globulin, that were effective for antimicrobial therapy were made in species such as horses that had been injected with inactivated bacterial toxins. Although such antisera were therapeutically effective, the foreign antibody elicited serious side effects (e.g., serum sickness) in recipients. A more recently developed product, equine rabies globulin, is widely used in developing countries, giving less than 2% allergic reactions in recipients. Nevertheless, such antisera tend not to be widely used in humans, especially in developed countries, except in emergencies when no alternative therapy is available.

Human polyclonal immune globulins of different types have been available for more than 20 years. They are typically prepared by pooling plasma from normal healthy volunteers with known titers of the specific antibody desired. Such individuals would have acquired high titers by vaccination, recent natural infection, or remote infection and subsequent silent boosting by the pathogen, depending on the antibody under consideration. The pooled plasma is fractionated with alcohol to enrich for antibody. The preparations are heat treated under conditions that are known to destroy the infectivity of human pathogens, such as HIV-1. The final product is usually released on the basis of a minimal standardized specific antibody content. These products are generally efficacious.[127, 128, 130, 133, 134] However, the large injection volumes (normalized for body weight) and the high protein (antibody) content (as high as 1 g or more) result in frequent adverse reactions in recipients.

Monoclonal Antibodies

The use of monoclonal antibodies offers the prospects of avoiding human sources of immune globulins; of greatly improving the tolerability of passive vaccines by substantially reducing protein content and injection volume; and of providing an antibody source of unlimited supply with absolute standardization, high reproducibility, and unique specificity. These factors make monoclonal antibodies potential replacements for polyclonal human immune globulins as passive vaccines, although a mixture of monoclonal antibodies may be required to provide a multiple epitope immunological recognition more like that of polyclonal sera. The invention of hybridoma technology in the mid-1970s provided for a source of murine monoclonal antibodies that required only the availability of the specific immunogen for mice.[135] Many developments in rDNA technology in the 1980s and 1990s have enabled the expression of high levels of recombinant monoclonal antibodies in defined CCLs, the humanization of murine monoclonal antibodies, and the screening for specific human monoclonal antibodies from a "library" of monoclonal antibodies developed in lieu of an investigator's having enough immunogen in hand to immunize an animal or human volunteer as per traditional hybridoma technology.

Natural Human

The first licensed therapeutic monoclonal antibody was a murine monoclonal antibody, with specificity for a surface molecule on certain T cells, which inhibits rejection of certain transplanted organs. Given the technologies now available to produce natural human, recombinant human, or recombinant humanized monoclonal antibodies and in light of issues regarding the tolerability of nonhuman antibodies, it appears unlikely that additional murine monoclonal antibodies will become available for use as passive vaccines.

The technology for making human monoclonal antibodies was adapted from murine hybridoma technology in the 1980s and involves the creation and isolation of hybridomas secreting human monoclonal antibodies.[136] B lymphocytes are harvested from individuals recently infected with or vaccinated for the desired pathogen. Alternatively, B lymphocytes from healthy individuals are cultured in vitro in the presence of the desired pathogen or antigen. The B lymphocytes are then immortalized by transformation in vitro with Epstein-Barr virus or by fusion with a human or murine myeloma cell. The resultant cell population is cloned, and growth media from hundreds of clones are screened with specific antigens for the monoclonal antibody of the desired specificity. The positive cells are single-cell cloned, expanded, and preserved.

At this point, development of a human monoclonal antibody can take one of two paths. The immortalized cells (usually by fusion and called heterohybridoma cells) can be adapted to the desired growth medium[129, 132] and then expanded to the scale necessary to manufacture a product. Alternatively, the human monoclonal antibody genes can be cloned and expressed to derive a recombinant monoclonal antibody. Given the technical challenges of maintaining the stability and large-scale consistent growth characteristics of the heterohybridoma cells in contrast to the continuing increases in the level and stability of recombinant monoclonal antibodies secreted from defined CCLs, it appears likely that the recombinant route will be the preferred one as a source of product.

Recombinant Human

One starting point for deriving a recombinant monoclonal antibody is a heterohybridoma producing a human monoclonal antibody.[137] Starting with such heterohybridoma cells, the genes for the human monoclonal antibody heavy (H) and light (L) chains are cloned and coexpressed in a CCL, for example, non–antibody-producing myeloma cell with known capability for high levels of recombinant monoclonal antibody expression. Alternatively, one can harvest B lymphocytes from individuals without regard to the time of exposure to the pathogen or antigen of interest. The variable (V) regions of the IgG L and H chains are then cloned en masse to produce a "combinatorial library" of V regions expressed in *E. coli*, so named because all combinations of different H and L chains are coexpressed in individual *E. coli* cells.[138] This combinatorial expression library is screened for specific antigen binding by the reassembled V regions of the H and L chains. The identified V genes of interest are cloned from *E. coli*, reassembled with constant (C) regions into complete human H and L chain genes, and then coexpressed in a CCL, as are recombinant natural human monoclonal antibodies. Alternatively, it may be possible to use the identified V regions as less-than-complete antibody molecules. The efficiency of the combinatorial approach is continually increasing and does offer the advantage of flexibility of soliciting human B lymphocyte donors without the need for antigen for immunization as well as the ability to find antibodies of higher affinity than occur in nature.

Recombinant Humanized

Another novel rDNA technology has evolved whereby a murine monoclonal antibody can be changed into a humanized monoclonal antibody of the same antigenic specificity. The human immune system would not recognize the humanized monoclonal antibody as being foreign and therefore would not produce antibodies against it (other than anti-Id). The V regions of H and L chains contain three hypervariable regions or complementarily determining regions (CDRs) of 5 to 18 amino acid residues each. The six CDRs in an intact antibody molecule come together in three-dimensional space to form the specific antigen-binding region of the antibody molecule (note that this region contains the Id and paratope as discussed in *Anti-idiotypic Antibodies*). The three CDRs in each chain fall in linear sequence in the midst of four V region framework domains that are less variable. Humanization is accomplished by substituting on the DNA level the three CDRs from each murine H and L chain gene for the human CDRs in four human framework domains from individual H and L chain genes.[139] Often, human framework domains with sequence homology to the murine framework domains are chosen for recombination. The substituted H and L chain V regions are reassembled with human H and L chain C regions, which are coexpressed in a CCL for scaleup and development as for any recombinant human monoclonal antibody. The resultant humanized monoclonal antibody contains only human-derived polypeptide sequences except for the murine-derived CDRs and hence is nonimmunogenic other than for an anti-Id response that may be elicited by any antibody.[140]

CONCLUSION

Technological developments in the past decade have made it apparent that the number of general strategies for making new vaccines is rapidly expanding. I would foresee that in the next decade, the number of approaches will continue to expand and technical aspects will be further refined such that almost all antigens or epitopes can be presented in a highly immunogenic form in the context of a live or nonlive vaccine. Protein antigens alternatively can be expressed through a DNA-based vaccine. Further understanding of gene function in viral and bacterial pathogens should enable live vaccines to be more stably and predictably attenuated as vaccines and as live vectors for immunizing against other pathogens. Adjuvant technologies should advance to the point at which formulations that are more potent than aluminum salts, yet as well tolerated, gain widespread use for killed vaccines and oral delivery of purified proteins becomes feasible for immunization. Similarly, formulations of DNA may improve the potency of DNA and its ability to be delivered by routes that elicit mucosal immunity.

As all these technological advances proceed, it is likely that the limiting factor in developing new vaccines for human use will continue to be a more comprehensive understanding of immunology. Some areas in which increased knowledge would have a practical payoff for vaccine development are the immunobiology of pathogens, the precise type and specificity of immune response required for solid and persistent protection against infection and disease, the attainment of mucosal immunity, and the optimal vaccination strategy to achieve this protection. There should also be significant developments in applications to noninfectious diseases, such as cancer and autoimmune diseases.

REFERENCES

1. Sabin AB, Boulger LR. History of Sabin attenuated poliovirus vaccine. J Biol Stand 1:115–118, 1973.
2. Enders JF, Katz SL, Milovanovic MV, Holloway A. Studies on an attenuated measles-virus vaccine I. Development and preparation of the vaccine: Technics for assay of effects of vaccination. N Engl J Med 263:153–159, 1960.
3. Buynak EB, Hilleman MR. Live attenuated mumps virus vaccine. I. Vaccine development. Proc Soc Exp Biol Med 123:768–775, 1966.
4. Plotkin SA, Farquhar JD, Katz M, Buser F. Attenuation of RA27/3 rubella virus in WI-38 human diploid cells. Am J Dis Child 118:178–185, 1969.
5. Takahashi M, Okuno Y, Otsuka T, et al. Development of a live attenuated varicella vaccine. Biken J 18:25–33, 1975.
6. Miller E, Goldacre M, Pugh S, et al. Risk of aseptic meningitis after measles, mumps, and rubella vaccine in UK children. Lancet 341:879–882, 1993.
7. Henderson DA. Smallpox eradication. Proc R Soc Lond 199:83–97, 1977.
8. Vesikari T, Kapikian AZ, Delem A, Zissis G. A comparative trial of Rhesus monkey (RRV-1) and bovine (RIT 4237) oral rotavirus vaccines in young children. J Infect Dis 153:832–839, 1986.
9. Clark HF, Borian FE, Bell LM, et al. Protective effect of WC3 vaccine against rotavirus diarrhea in infants during a predominantly serotype 1 rotavirus season. J Infect Dis 158:570–587, 1988.
10. Rennels MB, Glass RI, Dennehy PH, et al. Safety and efficacy of high-dose Rhesus-human reassortant rotavirus vaccines—report of the national multicenter trial. Pediatrics 97:7–13, 1996.
11. Clark HF, Offit PA, Ellis RW, et al. The development of multivalent bovine rotavirus (strain WC3) reassortant vaccine for infants. J Infect Dis 174:S73–S80, 1996.
12. Maassab HF, DeBorde DC. Development and characterization of cold-adapted viruses for use as live virus vaccines. Vaccine 3:355–371, 1985.
13. Ghendon YZ, Klimov AI, Alexandrova GI, Polezhaev FI. Analysis of genome composition and reactogenicity of recombinants of cold-adapted and virulent virus strains. J Gen Virol 53:215–224, 1981.
14. McKay E, Higgins P, Tyrrell D, Pringle C. Immunogenicity and pathogenicity of temperature-sensitive modified respiratory syncytial virus in adult volunteers. J Med Virol 25:411–421, 1988.
15. Meignier B, Longnecker R, Roizman B. In vivo behavior of genetically engineered herpes simplex viruses R7017 and R7020: Construction and evaluation in rodents. J Infect Dis 158:602–614, 1988.
16. McLean CS, Challanain N, Duncan I, et al. Induction of a protective immune response by mucosal vaccination with a DISC HSV-1 vaccine. Vaccine 14:987–992, 1996.
17. Murphy BR, Chanock RM. Influenza virus. In Fields BN, Knipe DM, Chanock RM (eds). Virology. New York, Raven Press, 1989, pp 469–502.
18. Pincus S, Tartaglia J, Paoletti E. Poxvirus-based vectors as vaccine candidates. Biologicals 23:159–164, 1995.
19. Moss B. Vaccinia virus vectors. In Ellis R (ed). Vaccines: New Approaches to Immunological Problems. New York, Marcel Dekker, 1992, pp 345–357.
20. Perales MA, Schwartz DH, Fabry JA, Lieberman J. A vaccinia-gp160–based vaccine but not a gp160 vaccine elicits anti-gp160 cytotoxic T lymphocytes in some HIV-1 seronegative vaccinees. J Acquir Immune Defic Syndr Hum Retrovirol 10:27–35, 1995.
21. Lee MS, Roos JM, McGuigan LC, et al. Molecular attenuation of vaccinia virus: Mutant generation and animal characterization. J Virol 66:2617–2630, 1992.
22. Tartaglia J, Perkus ME, Taylor J, et al. NYVAC: A highly attenuated strain of vaccinia virus. Virology 188:217–232, 1992.
23. Leong KH, Ramsay AJ, Boyle DB, Ramshaw IA. Selective induction of immune responses by cytokines coexpressed in recombinant fowlpox virus. J Virol 68:8125–8130, 1994.
24. Graham FL, Prevec L. Adenovirus-based expression vectors and recombinant vaccines. In Ellis R (ed). Vaccines: New Approaches to Immunological Problems. New York, Marcel Dekker, 1992, pp 363–390.
25. Lowe RS, Keller PM, Keech BJ, et al. Varicella-zoster virus as a live vector for the expression of foreign genes. Proc Natl Acad Sci USA 84:3896–3900, 1987.
26. Evans DJ, McKeating J, Meredith JM, et al. An engineered poliovirus chimaera elicits broadly reactive HIV-1 neutralizing antibodies. Nature 339:385–389, 1989.
27. Andino R, Silvera D, Suggett SD, et al. Engineering poliovirus as a vaccine vector for the expression of diverse antigens. Science 265:1448–1451, 1994.
28. Schlesinger S. Alphaviruses—vectors for the expression of heterologous genes. Trends Biotechnol 11:18–22, 1993.
29. Weill-Halle B. Oral vaccination. In Rosenthal SR (ed). BCG Vaccination Against Tuberculosis. Boston, Little, Brown, 1957.
30. Germanier R, Furer E. Isolation and characterization of *galE* mutant Ty21a of *Salmonella typhi*: A candidate strain for a live, oral typhoid vaccine. J Infect Dis 131:553–558, 1975.
31. Levine MM, Black RE, Ferreccio C, Germanier R. Clinical Typhoid Committee. Large-scale field trial of Ty21a live oral typhoid vaccine in enteric-coated capsule formulation. Lancet 2:1049–1052, 1987.
32. Tacket CO, Losonsky G, Nataro JP, et al. Onset and duration of protective immunity in challenged volunteers after vaccination with live oral cholera vaccine CVD 103-HgR. J Infect Dis 166:837–841, 1992.
33. Waldor MK, Mekalanos JJ. Lysogenic conversion by a filamentous phage encoding cholera toxin. Science 272:1910–1914, 1996.
34. Kotloff KL, Noriega F, Losonsky GA, et al. Safety, immunogenicity, and transmissibility in humans of CVD 1203, a live oral *Shigella flexneri* 2a vaccine candidate attenuated by deletions in *aroA* and *virG*. Infect Immun 64:4542–4548, 1996.
35. Gonzalez C, Hone D, Noriega FR, et al. *Salmonella typhi* vaccine strain CVD 908 expressing the circumsporozoite protein of *Plasmodium falciparum:* Strain construction and safety and immunogenicity in humans. J Infect Dis 169:927–931, 1994.
36. Butterton JR, Beattie DT, Gardel CL, et al. Heterologous antigen expression in *Vibrio cholerae* vector strains. Infect Immun 63:2689–2696, 1995.
37. Noriega FR, Losonsky G, Wang JY, et al. Further characterization of ΔaroA ΔvirG *Shigella flexneri* as a mucosal *Shigella* vaccine and a live-vector vaccine for delivering antigens of enterotoxigenic *Escherichia coli*. Infect Immun 64:23–27, 1996.
38. Goosens PL, Montixi C, Saron M-F, et al. *Listeria monocytogenes:* A live vector able to deliver heterologous proteins within the cytosol and to drive a CD8-dependent T-cell response. Biologicals 23:135–143, 1995.
39. Stover CK, de la Cruz VF, Fuerst TR, et al. New use of BCG for recombinant vaccines. Nature 351:456–460, 1991.
40. Lagranderie M, Murray A, Gicquel B, et al. Oral immunization with recombinant BCG induces cellular and humoral immune responses against the foreign antigen. Vaccine 11:1283–1290, 1993.
41. Fischetti VA, Medaglini D, Pozzi G. Gram-positive bacteria for mucosal vaccine delivery. Curr Opin Biotechnol 7:659–666, 1996.
42. Werzberger WA, Mensch B, Kuter B, et al. A controlled trial of a formalin-inactivated hepatitis A vaccine in healthy children. N Engl J Med 327:453–457, 1992.
43. Cherry JD, Brunell PA, Golden GS, Karzon DT. Report of the task force on pertussis and pertussis immunization—1988. Pediatrics 81:939–945, 1988.
44. Clemens JD, Sack DA, Harris JR, et al. Field trial of oral cholera vaccines in Bangladesh: Results from three-year follow-up. Lancet 355:270–273, 1990.
45. Svennerholm A-M, Holmgren J, Sack DA. Development of oral vaccines against enterotoxigenic *Escherichia coli* diarrhoea. Vaccine 7:196–198, 1989.
46. Murdin AD, Barreto L, Plotkin S. Inactivated polio vaccines: Past and present experience. Vaccine 14:735–746, 1996.
47. Crawford CR, Faiza AM, Mukhlis FA, et al. Use of zwitterionic detergent for the preparation of an influenza virus vaccine. 1. Preparation and characterization of disrupted virions. Vaccine 2:193–198, 1984.
48. Plotkin SA. Rabies vaccine prepared in human cell cultures: Progress and perspectives. Rev Infect Dis 2:433–447, 1980.

49. Hoke CH, Nisalak A, Sangawhipa N. Protection against Japanese encephalitis by inactivated vaccines. N Engl J Med 319:608–614, 1988.
50. Provost PJ, Hughes JV, Miller WJ, et al. An inactivated hepatitis A viral vaccine of cell culture origin. J Med Virol 19:23–31, 1986.
51. Choo QL, Kuo G, Weiner AJ, et al. Isolation of a cDNA clone from a blood-borne non-A, non-B viral hepatitis genome. Science 244:359–362, 1989.
52. Tam AW, Smith MM, Guerra ME, et al. Hepatitis E virus: Molecular cloning and sequencing of the full-length viral genome. Virology 185:120–131, 1991.
53. Fleischmann RD, Adams MD, White O, et al. Whole-genome random sequencing and assembly of *Haemophilus influenzae* Rd. Science 269:496–512, 1995.
54. Goffeau A, Barrell BG, Bussey H, et al. Life with 6000 genes. Science 274:563–567, 1996.
55. Tomb J-F, White O, Kerlavage AR, et al. The complete genome sequence of the gastric pathogen *Helicobacter pylori*. Nature 388:539–547, 1997.
56. Hilleman MR, Bertland AU, Buynak EB, et al. Clinical and laboratory studies of HBsAg vaccine. In Vyas GN, Cohen SN, Schmid R (eds). Viral Hepatitis. Philadelphia, Franklin Institute Press, 1978, pp 525–541.
57. Greco D, Salmaso S, Mastrantonio P, et al. A controlled trial of two acellular vaccines and one whole-cell vaccine against pertussis. N Engl J Med 334:341–348, 1996.
58. Gustafson L, Hallander HO, Olin P, et al. A controlled trial of a two-component acellular, a five-component acellular, and a whole-cell pertussis vaccine. N Engl J Med 334:349–355, 1996.
59. Schmitt H-J, von König CH, Neiss A, et al. Efficacy of acellular pertussis vaccine in early childhood after household exposure. JAMA 275:37–41, 1996.
60. Jones FG, Moss JM. Studies on tetanus toxoid. I. The antitoxic titer of human subject following immunization with tetanus toxoid and tetanus alum precipitated toxoid. J Immunol 30:115–125, 1936.
61. Ramon G. Sur le pouvoir floculant et sur les proprietes immunisantes d'une toxin diphterique rendue anatoxique (anatoxine). C R Acad Sci 177:1338–1340, 1923.
62. Chazono M, Yoshida I, Konobe T. The purification and characterization of an acellular pertussis vaccine. J Biol Stand 16:83–89, 1988.
63. Nencioni L, Pizza MG, Bugnoli M, et al. Characterization of genetically inactivated pertussis toxin mutants: Candidates for a new vaccine against whooping cough. Infect Immun 58:1308–1315, 1990.
64. Giannini G, Rappuoli R, Ratti G. The amino-acid sequence of two non-toxic mutants of diphtheria toxin: CRM_{45} and CRM_{197}. Nucleic Acids Res 12:4063–4069, 1984.
65. Valenzuela P, Medina A, Rutter WJ, et al. Synthesis and assembly of hepatitis-B virus surface-antigen particles in yeast. Nature 298:347–350, 1982.
66. Burnette WN, Samai B, Browne J, Ritter GA. Properties and relative immunogenicity of various preparations of recombinant DNA-derived hepatitis B surface antigen. Dev Biol Stand 59:113–120, 1985.
67. Thanavala Y, Yang Y-F, Lyons P, et al. Immunogenicity of transgenic plant-derived hepatitis B surface antigen. Proc Natl Acad Sci USA 92:3358–3361, 1995.
68. Jansen KU, Rosolowsky M, Schultz LD, et al. Vaccination with yeast-expressed cottontail rabbit papillomavirus (CRPV) virus-like particles protects rabbits from CRPV-induced papilloma formation. Vaccine 13:1509–1514, 1995.
69. Crawford SE, Labbe M, Cohen J, et al. Characterization of virus-like particles produced by the expression of rotavirus capsid proteins in insect cells. J Virol 68:5945–5952, 1994.
70. Orentas RJ, Hildreth JE, Obah E, et al. Induction of $CD4^+$ human cytolytic T-cells specific for HIV-infected cells by a gp160 subunit vaccine. Science 248:1234–1237, 1990.
71. Berman PW, Gregory TJ, Riddle L, et al. Protection of chimpanzees from infection by HIV-1 after vaccination with recombinant glycoprotein gp120 but not gp160. Nature 345:622–625, 1990.
72. Langenburg AGM, Burke RL, Adair SF, et al. A recombinant glycoprotein vaccine for herpes simplex type 2: Safety and efficacy. Ann Intern Med 122:889–898, 1995.
73. Van Hoecke C, Comberbach M, De Grave D, et al. Evaluation of the safety, reactogenicity and immunogenicity of three recombinant outer surface protein (OspA) Lyme vaccines in healthy adults. Vaccine 14:1620–1626, 1996.
74. Pearce EJ, James SL, Hieny S, et al. Induction of protective immunity against *Schistosoma mansoni* by vaccination with schistosome paramyosin (Sm97), a nonsurface parasite antigen. Proc Natl Acad Sci USA 85:5678–5682, 1988.
75. Takai T, Yokota T, Yasue M, et al. Engineering of the major house mite allergen Der f 2 for allergen-specific immunotherapy. Nature Biotechnol 15:754–760, 1997.
76. Tian J, Clare-Salzler M, Hershenfeld A, et al. Modulating autoimmune responses to GAD inhibits disease progression and prolongs islet graft survival in diabetes-prone mice. Nat Med 2:1348–1353, 1996.
77. Keller, RJ, Eisenbarth GS, Jackson RA. Insulin prophylaxis of individuals at risk of type-1 diabetes. Lancet 341:927–928, 1993.
78. Primakoff P, Lathrop W, Woolman L, et al. Fully effective contraception in male and female guinea pigs immunized with the sperm protein PH20. Nature 335:543–546, 1988.
79. Prokop A, Bajpai PK, Ho C (eds). Recombinant DNA Technology and Applications. New York, McGraw-Hill, 1991, pp 3–152.
80. Kingsman SM, Kingsman AJ. Polyvalent recombinant antigens: A new vaccine strategy. Vaccine 6:304–306, 1988.
81. Zavala F, Cochrane AH, Nardin EH, et al. Circumsporozoite proteins of malaria parasites contain a single immunodominant region with two or more identical epitopes. J Exp Med 157:1947–1957, 1983.
82. Javaherian K, Langlois AJ, McDanal C, et al. Principal neutralizing domain of the human immunodeficiency virus-type 1 envelope protein. Proc Natl Acad Sci USA 86:6768–6772, 1989.
83. Vreden SGS, Verhave JP, Oettinger T, et al. Phase I clinical trial of a recombinant malaria vaccine consisting of the circumsporozoite repeat region of *Plasmodium falciparum* coupled to hepatitis B surface antigen. Am J Trop Med Hyg 45:533–538, 1991.
84. Schodel F, Peterson D, Hughes J, et al. Hybrid hepatitis B virus core antigen as a vaccine carrier moiety. I. Presentation of foreign epitopes. J Biotechnol 44:91–96, 1996.
85. Herrington DA, Clyde DF, Losonsky G, et al. Safety and immunogenicity in man of a synthetic peptide in malaria vaccine against *Plasmodium falciparum* sporozoites. Nature 328:257–259, 1987.
86. Nash H, Talwar GP, Segal SJ, et al. Observations on the antigenicity and clinical effects of a candidate anti-pregnancy vaccine: Beta subunit of human chorionic gonadotropin linked to tetanus toxoid. Fertil Steril 34:328–335, 1980.
87. Wang CY, Looney DJ, Li ML, et al. Long-term high-titer neutralizing activity induced by octomeric synthetic HIV-1 antigen. Science 254:285–288, 1991.
88. Tam JP, Clavijo P, Lu Y-A, et al. Incorporation of T and B epitopes of the circumsporozoite protein in a chemically defined synthetic vaccine against malaria. J Exp Med 171:299–306, 1990.
89. Meola A, Delmastro P, Monaci P, et al. Derivation of vaccines from mimetopes: Immunologic properties of human hepatitis B surface antigen mimetopes displayed on filamentous phage. J Immunol 154:3162–3172, 1995.
90. Agadjanyan M, Luo P, Westerink J, et al. Peptide mimicry of carbohydrate epitopes on human immunodeficiency virus. Nature Biotechnol 15:547–551, 1997.
91. Vitiello A, Ishioka G, Grey HM, et al. Development of a lipopeptide-based therapeutic vaccine to treat chronic hepatitis B infection. I. Induction of a primary cytotoxic T-lymphocyte response in humans. J Clin Invest 95:341–349, 1995.
92. Rodrigues LP, Schneerson R, Robbins JB. Immunity to *H. influenzae* type b I. The isolation, and some physicochemical, serologic and biologic properties of the capsular polysaccharide of *H. influenzae* type b. J Immunol 107:1071–1080, 1971.
93. Gotschlich EC, Liu TY, Artenstein MS. Human immunity to the meningococcus. III. Preparation and immunochemical properties of the group A, group B and group C meningococcal polysaccharides. J Exp Med 129:1349–1365, 1969.
94. Kass EG. Assessment of the pneumococcal polysaccharide vaccine. Rev Infect Dis 3:S1–S197, 1981.
95. Kniskern PJ, Marburg S, Ellis RW. *Haemophilus influenzae* type b conjugate vaccines. In Powell M, Newman M (eds). Vaccine

Design: The Subunit Approach. New York, Plenum Publishing, 1995, pp 673–694.
96. Klein D, Ellis RW. Pneumococcal conjugate vaccines. In Levine MM, Woodrow GC, Kaper JB, Cobon GS (eds). New Generation Vaccines. New York, Marcel Dekker, 1997, pp 503–526.
97. Wessels MR, Paoletti LC, Kasper DL, et al. Immunogenicity in animals of a polysaccharide-protein conjugate vaccine against type III group B *Streptococcus*. J Clin Invest 86:1428–1433, 1990.
98. Kennedy RC, Adler-Storthz K, Henkel RD, et al. Immune response to hepatitis B surface antigen: Enhancement by prior injection of antibodies to the idiotype. Science 221:853–855, 1983.
99. Herlyn D, Wettendorff M, Iliopoulos D, et al. Modulation of cancer patients' immune responses by administration of anti-idiotypic antibodies. Viral Immunol 2:271–276, 1989.
100. Diakun KR, Matta KL. Synthetic antigens as immunogens: III. Specificity analysis of an anti-anti-idiotypic antibody to a carbohydrate tumor-associated antigen. J Immunol 142:2037–2040, 1989.
101. Grzych JM, Capron M, Lambert PH, et al. An anti-idiotype vaccine against experimental schistosomiasis. Nature 316:74–76, 1985.
102. Barry MA, Wayne WC, Johnston SA. Protection against mycoplasma infection using expression-library immunization. Nature 377:632–635, 1995.
103. Wolff JA, Malone RW, Williams P, et al. Direct gene transfer into mouse muscle in vivo. Science 247:1465–1468, 1990.
104. Ulmer JB, Sadoff JC, Liu MA. DNA vaccines. Curr Opin Immunol 8:531–536, 1996.
105. Dubensky TW, Driver DA, Polo JM, et al. Sindbis virus DNA-based expression vectors: Utility for in vitro and in vivo gene transfer. J Virol 70:508–519, 1996.
106. Williams RS, Johnston SA, Riedy M, et al. Introduction of foreign genes into tissues of living mice by DNA-coated microprojectiles. Proc Natl Acad Sci USA 88:2726–2730, 1991.
107. Remy J-S, Sirlin C, Vierling P, Behr J-P. Gene transfer with a series of lipophilic DNA-binding molecules. Bioconjug Chem 5:647–654, 1994.
108. Coney L, Wang B, Ugen KE, et al. Facilitated DNA inoculation induces anti-HIV-1 immunity in vivo. Vaccine 12:1545–1550, 1994.
109. Krieg AM, Yi A-K, Matson S, et al. CpG motifs in bacterial DNA trigger direct B-cell activation. Nature 374:546–549, 1995.
110. Kent SJ, Stallard V, Corey L, et al. Analysis of cytotoxic T-lymphocyte responses to SIV proteins in SIV-infected macaques using antigen-specific stimulation with recombinant vaccinia and fowlpox viruses. AIDS Res Hum Retroviruses 10:551–560, 1994.
111. Fries LF, Tartaglia J, Taylor J, et al. Human safety and immunogenicity of a canarypox-rabies glycoprotein recombinant vaccine: An alternative poxvirus vector system. Vaccine 14:428–434, 1996.
112. Sizemore DR, Branstrom AA, Sadoff JC. Attenuated *Shigella* as a DNA delivery vehicle for DNA-mediated immunization. Science 270:299–302, 1996.
112a. Darji A, Guzman CA, Gerstol B, et al. Oral somatic transgene vaccination using attenuated *S. typhimurium*. Cell 91:765–775, 1997.
113. Cox JC, Coulter AR. Adjuvants—a classification and review of modes of action. Vaccine 15:248–256, 1997.
114. Gupta RK, Siber GS. Adjuvants for human vaccines—current status, problems and future prospects. Vaccine 13:1263–1276, 1995.
115. Stewart-Tull DES (ed). The Theory and Practical Applications of Adjuvants. Chichester, John Wiley & Sons, 1994.
116. Vogel FR, Powell MF. A compendium of vaccine adjuvants and excipients. In Powell MF, Newman MJ (eds). Vaccine Design. The Subunit and Adjuvant Approach. New York, Plenum Press, 1996, pp 141–228.
117. Shirodkar S, Hutchinson RL, White JL, Hem SL. Aluminum compounds used as adjuvants in vaccines. Pharm Res 7:1282–1288, 1990.
118. Lin R, Tarr PE, Jones TC. Present status of the use of cytokines as adjuvants with vaccines to protect against infectious diseases. Clin Infect Dis 21:1438–1449, 1995.
119. Elson CD, Falding W. Generalized systemic and mucosal immunity in mice after mucosal stimulation with cholera toxin. J Immunol 132:2736–2744, 1984.
120. Douce G, Turcottee C, Cropley I, et al. Mutants of *Escherichia coli* heat-labile toxin lacking ADP-ribosylating activity acts as non-toxic mucosal adjuvants. Proc Natl Acad Sci USA 92:1644–1648, 1995.
121. Agren LC, Ekman L, Lowenadler B, Lycke NY. A genetically-engineered nontoxic vaccine adjuvant that combines B-cell targeting with immunomodulation by cholera toxin A1 subunit. J Immunol 158:3936–3946, 1997.
122. Clemens JD, Sack DA, Harris JR, et al. Impact of B subunit killed whole-cell and killed whole-cell-only oral vaccines against cholera upon treated diarrhoeal illness and mortality in an area endemic for cholera. Lancet 1:1375–1379, 1988.
123. Pialoux G, Excler J-L, Riviere Y, et al. A prime-boost approach to HIV preventive vaccine using recombinant canarypox virus expressing glycoprotein 160 (MN) followed by recombinant glycoprotein 160 (MN/LAI). AIDS Res Hum Retroviruses 11:373–381, 1995.
124. Salmon-Ceron D, Excler J-L, Sicard D, et al. Safety and immunogenicity of a recombinant HIV type 1 glycoprotein 160 boosted by a V3 synthetic peptide in HIV-negative volunteers. AIDS Res Hum Retroviruses 11:1479–1486, 1995.
125. Lubeck MD, Ntuk R, Myagkikh M, et al. Long-term protection of chimpanzees against high-dose HIV-1 challenge induced by immunization. Nat Med 3:651–658, 1997.
126. Anderson EL, Decker MD, Englund JA, et al. Interchangeability of conjugated *Haemophilus influenzae* type b vaccines in infants. JAMA 273:849–853, 1995.
127. Gerety RJ, Smallwood LA, Tabor E. Hepatitis B immune globulin and immune serum globulin. N Engl J Med 303:529–532, 1980.
128. Zaia JA, Levine MJ, Wright GG, Grady GF. A practical method for preparation of varicella-zoster immunoglobulin. J Infect Dis 137:601–608, 1978.
129. Matsumoto Y, Sugano T, Miyamoto C, Masuho Y. Generation of hybridomas producing human monoclonal antibodies against human cytomegalovirus. Biochem Biophys Res Commun 137:273–280, 1986.
130. Siber GR, Leszczynski J, Pena-Cruz V, et al. Protective activity of a human respiratory syncytial virus immune globulin prepared from donors screened by microneutralization assay. J Infect Dis 165:456–463, 1992.
131. Teng NNH, Kaplan HS, Hebert JM, et al. Protection against gram-negative bacteremia and endotoxemia with human monoclonal IgM antibodies. Proc Natl Acad Sci USA 82:1790–1794, 1985.
132. Irie RF, Matsuki T, Morton DL. Human monoclonal antibody to ganglioside GM2 for melanoma treatment. Lancet 1:786–787, 1989.
133. Snydman DR, Werner BG, Heinze-Lacey B, et al. Use of cytomegalovirus immune globulin to prevent cytomegalovirus disease in renal-transplant recipients. N Engl J Med 317:1049–1054, 1987.
134. Rubbo SD, Suri JC. Passive immunization against tetanus with human immune globulin. Br Med J 2:79–81, 1962.
135. Kohler G, Milstein C. Continuous cultures of fused cells secreting antibody of predefined specificity. Nature 256:495–497, 1975.
136. Croce CM, Linnenbach A, Hall W, et al. Production of human hybridomas secreting antibodies to measles virus. Nature 288:488–489, 1980.
137. Gorny MK, Xu J-Y, Gianakakos V, et al. Production of site-selected neutralizing human monoclonal antibodies against the third variable domain of the human immunodeficiency virus type 1 envelope glycoprotein. Proc Natl Acad Sci USA 87:3238–3242, 1991.
138. Marks JD, Hoogenbaum HR, Bonnert TP, et al. By-passing immunization. Human antibodies from V-gene libraries displayed on phage. J Mol Biol 222:581–597, 1991.
139. Riechmann L, Clark M, Waldmann H, Winter G. Reshaping human antibodies for therapy. Nature 332:323–327, 1988.
140. Tempest PR, Bremner P, Lambert M, et al. Reshaping a human monoclonal antibody to inhibit human respiratory syncytial virus infection in vivo. Biotechnology 9:266–271, 1991.

chapter

36 Cytomegalovirus Vaccines

Stanley A. Plotkin

In developing a vaccine against the human cytomegalovirus (CMV), researchers must deal with a ubiquitous agent, immunity to which is influenced by the general immune status of the host. Nevertheless, substantial progress has been made.

Human CMV, one of the herpes viruses, is species specific, and replication occurs only in human cells.[1] In terms of public health, the most important effect of CMV is the damage caused to a fetus when primary infection of the mother occurs during the first half of pregnancy. Approximately 1% of all fetuses are infected in utero, of which 10 to 15% will suffer lasting damage, usually to the brain or organ of Corti.[2–4] Congenital CMV infection is occasionally manifest at birth in the form of microcephaly, hepatosplenomegaly, and other abnormalities, but the more usual situation is a silent infection, the result of which becomes evident later in life.[5] Although some infants born to seropositive mothers excrete CMV at birth, that type of fetal infection, which may be the result of reactivation in the mother, is less likely to cause damage.[2]

The consequences of congenital CMV infection to society are enormous: an estimated $1 billion in health care costs alone.[6]

A recent study from the University of Alabama group[7] concerned women with verified preconceptional immunity at the end of a previous pregnancy, whose progress was followed during a second pregnancy. They were compared with a group of pregnant women who had been seronegative at the end of the previous pregnancy but who had seroconverted in the interval. Congenital infection was demonstrated in 12.9% of the infants of mothers who had seroconverted. This percentage must be considered as the minimal risk for fetal transmission in pregnancy, as some of the women who seroconverted must have been infected before becoming pregnant the second time. Only 1.2% of the previously seroimmune mothers transmitted virus to their fetuses. Protection against infection of the infant afforded by prior seropositivity was calculated at 91%; protection against significant abnormality was even higher.

Adler studied CMV infections acquired by seropositive and seronegative mothers in contact with children excreting CMV in daycare centers.[8] Seropositivity after natural infection was unequivocally shown to protect against infection by contact with secretions. In contrast to the high rate of infection seen in seronegative mothers, infections in seropositive mothers were infrequent. Thus, the induction of immunity equivalent to natural infection should protect against both CMV infection and disease.

Recently, the possibility was raised that CMV infection leads to atherosclerosis, presumably through endoarterial injury resulting from CMV replication.[9–10b] A related complication of latent CMV infection may be the coronary artery restenosis that occurs with high frequency after endarterectomy.[11] Seropositive patients had a higher rate of restenosis than seronegative patients. The CMV IE2 protein has been shown to interact with the p53 tumor suppressor protein found in smooth muscle cells. According to one hypothesis, inactivation of p53 leads to smooth muscle hyperplasia and restenosis.[12]

The effects of human CMV on allograft recipients are dramatic. Seronegative kidney, liver, or heart transplant recipients are particularly likely to suffer severe disease or death when they receive kidneys from seropositive donors. Bone marrow transplant recipients are also prone to CMV disease, usually as a result of reactivation. CMV illness commonly takes the form of interstitial pneumonia, but hepatitis, nephritis, encephalitis, bone marrow depression, and potentiation of bacterial and fungal infections pose additional serious problems.[13–15a]

Patients with human immunodeficiency virus infection are also commonly coinfected with CMV, and CMV-induced retinitis is one of the most common opportunistic infections in such patients.[16] Although several antiviral agents are available to treat CMV infections, toxicity and viral mutations leading to resistance complicate treatment.

OBJECTIVES OF VACCINATION

The first objective of a human CMV vaccine is to prevent primary infections in women during pregnancy—the infections that are most likely to lead to fetal disease.[17] The second objective is to convert susceptible patients to an immune status before they face the challenge of transplantation with CMV-bearing organs under conditions of immunosuppression.

A CMV vaccine might also have a third therapeutic

objective if immune responses could be engendered to suppress reactivated infection. Infusion of donor lymphocytes capable of killing CMV-infected cells by $CD8^+$ human leukocyte antigen (HLA)–restricted cytotoxicity (CTL) protects bone marrow transplant patients against CMV pneumonia. This suggests that induction of CTL by a vaccine could help control the infection in patients undergoing transplant and in those with acquired immunodeficiency syndrome.[18]

IMMUNE GLOBULIN

Globulins containing high-titer antibodies to human CMV have been extensively studied. Although the results have been controversial, at least in bone marrow transplant patients,[19] the use of human CMV immunoglobulin (HCMV-IG) has become routine in solid organ transplant recipients, in whom good evidence for a preventive effect on CMV disease has been shown.[20–23]

Licensed products are now available in the United States and are indicated for use in recipients of kidney, liver, and heart transplants who initially are seronegative.[23, 24] Some centers use HCMV-IG in bone marrow recipients, together with antivirals.[25]

LIVE VIRUS VACCINES

Two live virus vaccines have been developed, one in the United Kingdom and one in the United States. Elek and Stern[26] used the AD-169 laboratory strain to immunize normal adults, but the strain has not been further developed. Plotkin and colleagues[27] and Plotkin and Huygelen[28] isolated and passaged a new isolate (Towne) from a congenitally infected infant in human embryo fibroblasts until the 125th passage, with three clonings by plaque purification; pools were prepared at the 129th passage for vaccine trials.[29, 30] Laboratory studies of the high-passage Towne virus indicated changes of in vitro markers that correlate with adaptation to cell culture.[29] Initial clinical trials were performed in healthy adult volunteers.[30–32] When the vaccine was given subcutaneously or intramuscularly, seroconversion was seen in nearly 100% of volunteers (Fig. 36–1), but intranasal administration was not successful. During the second week after immunization, a local reaction consisting of erythema and induration appeared at the site of inoculation and lasted approximately 1 week, but systemic reactions were absent. Suprisingly, no virus was excreted or recovered from the blood. Routine clinical laboratory tests also showed normal results.

Lymphocyte proliferation assays showed the important fact that cells had been sensitized to CMV antigens by vaccination. $CD8^+$ cell–mediated HLA restricted cytotoxicity of CMV-infected cells, thought to represent an important immune function,[33] was also elicited in the Towne vaccinees.[34, 34a] Towne virus thus induced cellular, as well as humoral, immunity to CMV.[35] However, tests of lymphocyte subsets failed to show the increase in suppressor cells and decrease in the helper-

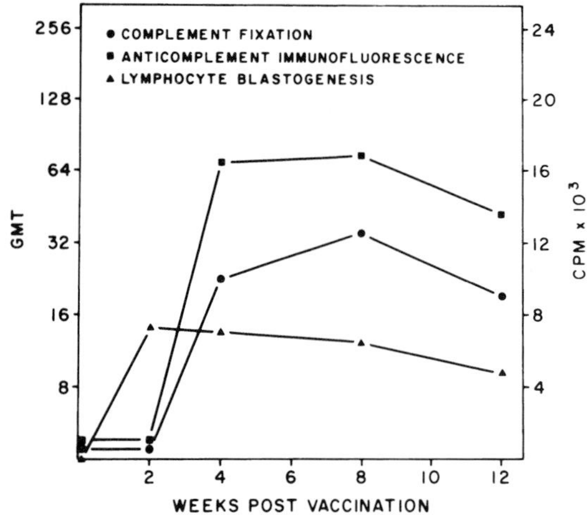

Figure 36–1. Typical immune responses to the Towne strain, live attenuated cytomegalovirus (CMV) vaccine showing the development of complement fixation antibodies, anticomplement immunofluorescence antibodies, and CMV-specific blastogenic responses.

to-suppressor ratio characteristic of acute CMV disease.[36]

Subsequent studies involved adult female pediatric nurses who were vaccinated with Towne and followed up for several years.[37] In related studies, sera of vaccinees were tested for antibodies to early antigen (EA) and immediate early antigens (IEA) of the virus.[38, 39] These are proteins not present in the virus particle and present only during replication. Most vaccinees developed IEA and EA antibodies, which signified limited replication of vaccine virus in the host. Biopsy and polymerase chain reaction studies revealed evidence of only transient production of virus.

Assessment of the data led to the conclusion that the Towne vaccine produces an abortive infection at the site of inoculation, which stimulates the same range of antibody and cellular responses that are noted after natural infection, including delayed-type hypersensitivity that is expressed as the local reaction described previously. However, no virus excretion or systemic reaction occurs after vaccination.[40]

Vaccine Efficacy in Transplant Patients

To demonstrate efficacy of Towne vaccine, advantage was taken of the high morbidity and mortality that CMV causes in seronegative renal transplant recipients who receive a kidney from a seropositive donor.[41–44] After a pilot study to demonstrate tolerance of the vaccine,[44] controlled double-blind trials were set up in prospective renal transplant recipients at the Hospital of the University of Pennsylvania and the Hospital of the University of Minnesota.

The seronegative patients were randomized to receive vaccine or placebo subcutaneously. After 6 weeks had passed, the patients were added to the transplant list, and they received kidneys as they became available, over periods ranging from weeks to months. Once transplantation was done, the patients were observed clinically, virologically, and serologically for CMV-associated disease by individuals blind to the patients' vaccine status. Clinical evaluation included an arbitrary scoring system that enabled one to judge retrospectively the seriousness of the CMV disease.

The results have been summarized in several articles[45–48] and are indicated in Figure 36–2. Despite the induction of relatively poor antibody and cellular immune responses due to the patients' uremia and dialysis, the vaccine appeared to provide partial protection similar to that of natural infection, which was also partly protective. Two additional studies in renal transplant patients, one of which was multicentric, reached the same conclusion.[49]

Vaccine Virus Latency

Because immunosuppression reactivates latent natural CMV in seropositive individuals, we reasoned that it should also reactivate vaccine virus in vaccinees. In fact, seronegative patients who received Towne vaccine followed by transplantation of a kidney from a seronegative donor did not excrete virus. Those who received kidneys from seropositive donors did excrete virus, but when the strains were examined by DNA restriction-endonuclease assays, they were not identical to Towne.[50] Presumably, they were strains that were latent in the donor kidneys that had been reactivated after transplantation.

Challenge of Normal Vaccinees

After this demonstration of safety and efficacy, normal volunteers were vaccinated to learn if they could be protected against an artificially administered challenge. Catholic priests who lived in a closed community and who were seronegative were vaccinated with Towne. One year later, they were challenged subcutaneously with varying doses of a different CMV strain, in company with unvaccinated seronegative and naturally seropositive priests. A dose of 1000 plaque-forming units (pfu) in cell culture caused illness, even in those who were naturally seropositive; therefore, this dose was not given to other groups.[51] At a 100-pfu dose, the challenge virus caused a mild infectious mononucleosis syndrome with virus excretion in seronegative individuals, but it did not affect naturally seropositive individuals.[52, 53] Vaccinees were also protected against disease caused by 100 pfu, but about half were asymptomatically infected. After injection of 10 pfu, CMV infection and symptoms were obvious in the seronegative individuals, whereas both vaccinated and seropositive individuals resisted the challenge. Thus, vaccination of normal individuals rendered them resistant to an artificial parenteral challenge but slightly less so than natural immunes. However, even natural immunity was imperfect if the challenge was large enough.

Despite the protection thus demonstrated against parenteral infection, Towne failed to prevent infection of mothers in contact with CMV-excreting children. A controlled trial[54] conducted in a daycare center showed no reduction in the infection rate of Towne-vaccinated mothers compared with placebo-inoculated mothers. The authors speculated that the 20-fold lower neutralizing antibody levels induced by Towne in comparison with natural seropositivity accounted for the failure. Studies continue to try to improve the immunogenicity of the Towne virus.

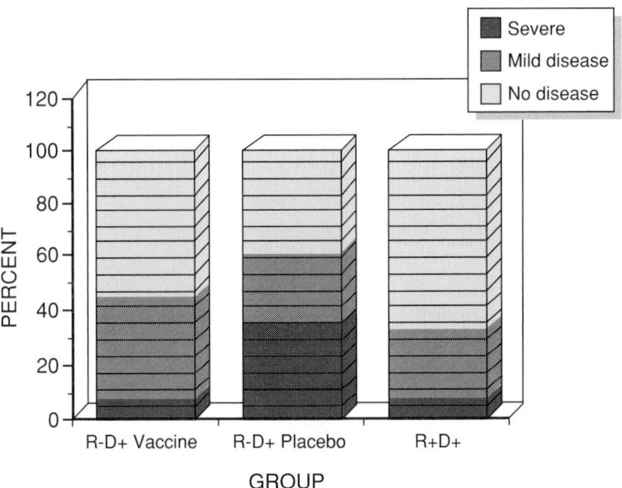

Figure 36–2. Results of a double-blind, placebo-controlled trial of the Towne strain, live attenuated cytomegalovirus (CMV) vaccine in renal transplant recipients. The *R-D+ Vacc.* column refers to the patients who were originally seronegative who received kidneys from seropositive donors and who had been vaccinated before the transplants. The *R-D+ Placebo* column refers to the control patients who received placebos before the transplants. The *R+D+* column represents the individuals who were naturally seropositive and received kidneys from seropositive donors. Thus, the second column shows the risk of mild and severe CMV disease in seronegative individuals, the first column shows the protective effect of prior vaccination, and the third column shows the protective effect of prior natural immunity.

Mutants of Towne

Scientists at the Aviron Company[54] discovered that Towne has genetic deletions in a particular part of its genome, called ULb′. A deletion of 13.5 kb was found in some lines of Towne virus, whereas in others, the orientation of the ULb′ section was reversed. This region, present in all low-passage clinical isolates, contains at least 19 genes not found in Towne. It was hypothesized that one or more of these genes code for proteins that would increase the replication and immunogenicity of Towne in vivo. Scientists at Aviron have prepared recombinant mutants of Towne, in which parts of the genome from the low-passage Toledo strain virulent virus have been inserted, and these mutant viruses will be tested for their safety and immunogenicity in humans.

NONLIVING AND VECTORED VACCINES

Alternative approaches to a human CMV vaccine have been pursued based on single or multiple proteins of the virus. The principal candidate proteins are listed in Table 36–1. For the production of antibodies, the most logical choices are the three major envelope glycopro-

Table 36–1. **CYTOMEGALOVIRUS PROTEINS THAT MIGHT BE INCLUDED IN A SUBUNIT VACCINE**

PROTEINS	MOLECULAR SIZE	HUMAN IMMUNE RESPONSES	
		Neutralizing Antibody	Cytotoxic T Cells
Envelope glycoproteins			
gB (gcl)	55–130 KDa	+	+
gH (gclll)	85–145 KDa	+	?
gcll	47–52 KDa	+	?
Structural proteins			
Lower matrix	65–71 KDa	−	+
Major nucleocapsid	150 KDa	−	+
28–32 kDa	28–32 KDa	−	−
Nonvirion			
IEl	72-KDa	−	+

teins of the virus that possess neutralizing epitopes,[55, 56] and all three have been studied. However, most attention has been directed toward the gB protein (so called because of its analogy with the herpes simplex gB). The reasons to base vaccine development on gB are given in Table 36–2. The gB protein appears to be immunodominant, as 50% or more of neutralizing antibody in the sera of seropositive individuals is directed against this protein.[57, 58] The glycoprotein analogous to gB has been purified from the guinea pig CMV and shown to protect pups whose mother had been immunized before pregnancy and subsequently challenged during gestation.[59]

The gB protein has been purified from the virus by immunoaffinity chromatography and inoculated into animals and then humans, with induction of neutralizing antibodies.[60–63] However, human CMV does not grow to sufficiently high titers to make native glycoprotein attractive as a vaccine source. Therefore, the gene for gB has been inserted into several expression vectors for use either for in vitro production of the protein or as a live vector. Chinese hamster ovary cells have been used to express whole or truncated gB.[64] Adenovirus 5, vaccinia, and canarypox deletion recombinants with the CMV gB gene inserted have been used in their living form to induce immune responses in animals, including neutralizing antibodies, lymphocyte proliferation to CMV virus, and human lymphocyte antigen–restricted T-cell cytotoxicity.[64–69]

Important progress toward the development of a gB-based vaccine has been made by scientists from the Chiron corporation, who have produced a truncated gB in Chinese hamster ovary cells, which was then purified

Table 36–2. **ARGUMENTS FOR GLYCOPROTEIN gB AS A CYTOMEGALOVIRUS VACCINE**

- gB bears neutralizing epitopes
- gB antibody accounts for about half of neutralizing activity in human convalescent sera
- Inoculation of gB elicits neutralizing antibody in animals and humans
- Proteins analogous to gB from mouse cytomegalovirus and guinea pig cytomegalovirus protect against acquired and transplacental infection

and combined with an oil-in-water emulsion called MF-59 for adjuvantation.[70] Inoculations of this material in concentrations of 100 μg induced anti-gB neutralizing antibodies after the third dose of a 0-, 1-, and 6-month schedule at a titer of approximately 1/60, similar to levels in natural seropositives.[71–73] A fourth dose at 12 months after the first boosted the titer to 1/115, falling back 6 months later to 1/67.[74] Toddlers were also vaccinated,[75] and after three doses at 0, 1, and 6 months, they achieved titers averaging 1/638, higher than in adults.

Interestingly, both mucosal IgG and secretory IgA antibodies were induced in many of the vaccinees. Presence of the former was correlated with a serum neutralizing antibody titer of over 1/64.[71]

A potential problem with gB-based vaccines is the discovery of four genotypes of this protein, based on sequencing of genomic DNA.[76] Although the genotypic differences do not appear to correlate with antigenic differences, there are associations of certain genotypes with specific clinical settings: Type 1 is most common in congenital infection,[77] whereas types 3 and 4 are associated with serious disease in transplant patients.[78, 79]

Whether a single protein will be sufficient as a vaccine is debatable. In the mouse, protection against murine CMV infection has been shown to depend on a $CD8^+$ cell–mediated cytotoxic T lymphocyte response directed against the IE1 protein of the virus.[80] Current research is attempting to identify the principal proteins of the human CMV that elicit cytotoxic T cells, and several candidates are listed in Table 36–1. Although IE1 is also one of the important proteins for human CTL, the lower matrix protein, pp65, appears to be more important,[81] and is the subject of current research seeking the best method to present the protein to the immune system. Ultimately, one or more of these proteins might be a component of a CMV vaccine also containing a surface glycoprotein. The proteins might be presented by like vectors in order to favor generation of CTL responses.[66, 67]

The recent discovery of DNA-based vaccination has been applied to CMV, with the demonstration of antibody and CTL responses in mice.[82]

The eventual success of one of these approaches to CMV vaccine is likely.[83, 84] Target groups for vaccination would be girls or women before they bear children and certain groups of seronegative potential transplant recipients.

REFERENCES

1. Weller TH. The cytomegaloviruses: Ubiquitous agents with protean clinical manifestations. N Engl J Med 285:214, 267–274, 1971.
2. Fowler KB, Stagno S, Pass RF, et al. The outcome of congenital cytomegalovirus infection in relation to maternal antibody status. N Engl J Med 326:663–667, 1992.
3. Stagno S, Pass RF, Cloud G, et al. Primary cytomegalovirus infection in pregnancy: Incidence, transmission to fetus, and clinical outcome. JAMA 256:1904–1908, 1986.
4. Williamson WD, Desmond MM, LaFevers N, et al. Symptomatic congenital cytomegalovirus: Disorders of language, learning, and hearing. Am J Dis Child 136:902, 1982.
5. Hanshaw JB. Congenital cytomegalovirus infection: A fifteen-year perspective. J Infect Dis 123:555–561, 1971.

6. Porath A, McNutt RA, Smiley LM, Weigle KA. Effectiveness and cost benefit of a proposed live cytomegalovirus vaccine in the prevention of congenital disease. Rev Infect Dis 12:31–40, 1990.
7. Fowler KB, Stagno S, Pass RF. Congenital cytomegalovirus (CMV) infection risk in future pregnancies and maternal CMV immunity [abstract 191]. 6th International Cytomegalovirus Workshop, Perdido Beach Resort. Orange Beach, AL; March 5–9, 1997.
8. Adler SP. Current prospects for immunization against cytomegaloviral disease. Infect Agents Dis 5:29–35, 1996.
9. Melnick JL, Adam E, DeBakey ME. Cytomegalovirus and atherosclerosis. BioEssays 17:899–903, 1995.
10. Nieto JF, Adam E, Sorlie P, et al. Cohort study of cytomegalovirus infection as a risk factor for carotid intimal-medial thickening, a measure of subclinical atherosclerosis. Circulation 94:922–927, 1996.
10a. Persoons M, Daemen M, Bruning J, et al. Active cytomegalovirus infection of arterial smooth muscle cells in immunocompromised rats. Circ Res 75:214–220, 1994.
10b. Berencsi K, Endresz V, Klurfeld D, et al. Early atherosclerotic plaques in the aorta following cytomegalovirus infection of mice. Cell Adhes Commun 5:39–47, 1998.
11. Zhou YF, Leon MB, Waclawiwq MA, et al. Association between prior cytomegalovirus infection and the risk of restenosis after coronary atherectomy. N Engl J Med 35:624–630, 1996.
12. Speir E, Modali R, Huang ES, et al. Potential role of human cytomegalovirus and p53 interaction in coronary restenosis. Science 265:391–394, 1994.
13. Glenn J. Cytomegalovirus infections following renal transplantation. Rev Infect Dis 3:1151–1178, 1981.
14. Falagas ME, Snydman DR, Griffith J, et al. Effect of cytomegalovirus infection status on first-year mortality rates among orthotopic liver transplant recipients. Ann Intern Med 126:275–279, 1997.
15. Winston DJ, Ho WG, Champlin RE. Cytomegalovirus infections after allogeneic bone marrow transplantation. Rev Infect Dis 12(suppl 7):S776–792, 1990.
15a. Zanten J, Leij L, Prop J, et al. Human cytomegalovirus: A viral complication in transplantation. Clin Transpl 12:145–158, 1998.
16. Mintz L, Drew W, Miner R, Braff E. Cytomegalovirus infections in homosexual men. Ann Intern Med 99:326–329, 1983.
17. Fowler KB, Stagno S, Pass RF, et al. The outcome of congenital cytomegalovirus infection in relation to maternal antibody status. N Engl J Med 326:663–667, 1992.
18. Riddell SR, Watanabe KS, Goodrich JM, et al. Restoration of viral immunity in immunodeficient humans by the adoptive transfer of T cell clones. Science 257:238–241, 1992.
19. Meyers JD. Critical evaluation of agents used in the treatment and prevention of cytomegalovirus infection in immunocompromised patients. Transplant Proc 23:139–143, 1991.
20. Snydman DR, Werner BG, Heinze-Lacey B, et al. Use of cytomegalovirus immune globulin to prevent cytomegalovirus disease in renal transplant recipients. N Engl J Med 317:1049–1054, 1987.
21. Werner BG, Snydman DR, Freeman R, et al. Cytomegalovirus immune globulin for the prevention of primary CMV disease in renal transplant patients: Analysis of usage under treatment IND status. Transplant Proc 25:1441–1443, 1993.
22. Snydman DR. Cytomegalovirus immunoglobulins in the prevention and treatment of cytomegalovirus disease. Rev Infect Dis 12:839–848, 1990.
23. Snydman DR. Prevention of cytomegalovirus-associated diseases with immunoglobulin. Transplant Proc 23:131–135, 1991.
24. Snydman DR, Werner BG, Dougherty NN, et al. Cytomegalovirus immune globulin prophylaxis in liver transplantation. Ann Intern Med 119:984–991, 1993.
25. Emanuel D, Cunningham I, Jules-Elysees K, et al. Cytomegalovirus pneumonia after bone marrow transplantation successfully treated with the combination of ganciclovir and high-dose intravenous immune globulin. Ann Intern Med 109:777–782, 1988.
26. Elek SD, Stern H. Development of a vaccine against mental retardation caused by cytomegalovirus infection in utero. Lancet 1:1–5, 1974.
27. Plotkin SA, Furukawa T, Zygraich N, Huygelen C. Candidate cytomegalovirus strain for human vaccination. Infect Immun 12:521–527, 1975.
28. Plotkin SA, Huygelen C. Cytomegalovirus vaccine prepared in WI-38. Dev Biol Stand 37:301–305, 1977.
29. Yamane Y, Furukawa T, Plotkin SA. Supernatant virus release as a differentiating marker between low-passage and vaccine strains of human cytomegalovirus. Vaccine 1:23–34, 1983.
30. Plotkin SA, Farquhar J, Hornberger E. Clinical trials of immunization with the Towne 125 strain of human cytomegalovirus. J Infect Dis 134:470–472, 1976.
31. Plotkin SA. Vaccination against herpes group viruses, in particular, cytomegalovirus. Monogr Paediatr 11:58–74, 1979.
32. Just M, Buergin-Wolff A, Emoedi G, Hernandez R. Immunization trials with live attenuated cytomegalovirus Towne 125. Infection 3:111–114, 1975.
33. Koszinowski UH, Del Val M, Reddehase MJ. Cellular and molecular basis of the protective immune response to cytomegalovirus infection. Curr Top Cell Regul 154:189–220, 1990.
34. Quinnan GV, Delery M, Rook AH, et al. Comparative virulence and immunogenicity of the Towne strain and a nonattenuated strain of cytomegalovirus. Ann Intern Med 101:478–483, 1984.
34a. Adler S, Hempfling SH, Starr SE, et al. Safety and immunogenicity of the Towne strain cytomegalovirus vaccine. Pediatr Infect Dis J 17:200–206, 1998.
35. Starr SE, Glazer JP, Friedman HM, et al. Specific cellular and humoral immunity after immunization with live Towne strain cytomegalovirus vaccine. J Infect Dis 147:585–589, 1981.
36. Carney WP, Hirsch MS, Iacoviello VR, et al. T-lymphocyte subsets and proliferative responses following immunization with cytomegalovirus vaccine. J Infect Dis 147:958, 1983.
37. Fleisher GR, Starr SE, Friedman HM, Plotkin SA. Vaccination of pediatric nurses with live attenuated cytomegalovirus. Am J Dis Child 136:294–296, 1982.
38. Friedman AD, Michelson S, Plotkin SA. Detection of antibodies to pre-early nuclear antigen and immediate-early antigens in patients immunized with cytomegalovirus vaccine. Infect Immun 38:1068–1072, 1982.
39. Friedman AD, Furukawa T, Plotkin SA. Detection of antibody to cytomegalovirus early antigen in vaccinated, normal volunteers and renal transplant candidates. J Infect Dis 146:255–259, 1982.
40. Plotkin SA. CMV vaccines. Bull World Health Organ 5:96–109, 1984.
41. Pass RF, Long WK, Whitley RJ, et al. Productive infection with cytomegalovirus and herpes simplex virus in renal transplant recipients: Role of source of kidney. J Infect Dis 137:556–562, 1978.
42. Burns RE, Brennan RB, Douglas RG, Talley TE. Clinical manifestations of renal allograft-derived primary cytomegalovirus infection. Am J Dis Child 131:759–763, 1977.
43. Suwansirikul S, Rao N, Downing JN, Ho M. Primary and secondary cytomegalovirus infection clinical manifestations after renal transplantation. Arch Intern Med 137:1026–1029, 1977.
44. Glazer JP, Friedman HM, Grossman RA, et al. Live cytomegalovirus vaccination in renal transplant candidates: A preliminary trial. Ann Intern Med 91:676–683, 1979.
45. Plotkin SA, Smiley ML, Friedman HM, et al. Prevention of cytomegalovirus disease by Towne strain live attenuated vaccine. Birth Defects 20:271–287, 1984.
46. Plotkin SA, Friedman HM, Fleisher GR, et al. Towne vaccine–induced prevention of cytomegalovirus disease after renal transplants. Lancet 1:528–530, 1984.
47. Balfour HH, Sach GW, Gehrz RC, et al. Cytomegalovirus vaccine in renal transplant candidates. Progress report of randomized placebo-controlled double-blind trial. In Plotkin SA, Michelson S, Pagano JS (eds). Cytomegalovirus: Pathogenesis and Prevention of Human Infection. New York, Alan R Liss, 1984, pp 289–304.
48. Plotkin S, Starr S, Friedman H, et al. Effect of Towne live virus vaccine on cytomegalovirus disease after renal transplant. Ann Intern Med 114:525–531, 1991.
49. Plotkin SA, Higgins R, Kurtz JB, et al. Multicenter trial of Towne vaccine in seronegative renal transplant recipients. Transplantation 58:1176–1178, 1994.
50. Plotkin SA, Huang E-S. Cytomegalovirus vaccine (Towne strain) does not induce latency. J Infect Dis 152:395–397, 1985.
51. Plotkin SA, Weibel RE, Alpert GA, et al. Resistance of seropositive volunteers to subcutaneous challenge with low-passage human cytomegalovirus. J Infect Dis 151:737–739, 1985.
52. Plotkin SA, Starr SE, Friedman HM, et al. Protective effects of

Towne cytomegalovirus vaccine against low-passage cytomegalovirus administered as a challenge. J Infect Dis 159:860–865, 1989.
53. Adler SP, Starr SE, Plotkin SA, et al. Immunity induced by primary human cytomegalovirus infection protects against secondary infection among women of childbearing age. J Infect Dis 171:26–32, 1995.
54. Cha TA, Tom E, Kemble GW, et al. Human cytomegalovirus clinical isolates carry at least 19 genes not found in laboratory strains. J Virol 70:78–83, 1996.
55. Pereira L, Hoffman M, Gallo D, Cremer N. Monoclonal antibodies to human cytomegalovirus: Three surface membrane proteins with unique immunological and electrophoretic properties specify cross-reactive determinants. Infect Immun 36:924–932, 1982.
56. Landini MP, La Placa M. Humoral immune response to human cytomegalovirus proteins: A brief review. Comp Immunol Microbiol Infect Dis 14:97–105, 1991.
57. Gonczol E, Plotkin SA. Progress in vaccine development for prevention of human cytomegalovirus infection. Curr Top Microbiol Immunol 54:255–274, 1990.
58. Britt WJ, Vugler L, Butfiloski EJ, Stephens EB. Cell surface expression of human cytomegalovirus (HCMV) gp55-116 (gB): Use of HCMV-recombinant vaccinia virus-infected cells in analysis of the human neutralizing antibody response. J Virol 64:1079–1085, 1990.
59. Harrison CJ, Britt WJ, Chapman NM, et al. Reduced congenital cytomegalovirus (CMV) infection after maternal immunization with a guinea pig CMV glycoprotein before gestational primary CMV infection in the guinea pig model. Infect Dis 172:1212–1220, 1995.
60. Furukawa T, Gonczol E, Starr S, et al. HCMV envelope antigens induce both humoral and cellular immunity in guinea pigs. Proc Soc Exp Biol Med 175:243–250, 1984.
61. Hudecz F, Gonczol E, Plotkin SA. Preparation of highly purified human cytomegalovirus envelope antigen. Vaccine 3:300–304, 1985.
62. Gonczol E, Hudecz F, Ianacone J, et al. Immune responses to isolated human cytomegalovirus envelope proteins. J Virol 58:661–664, 1986.
63. Gonczol E, Ianacone J, Ho WZ, et al. Subunit human cytomegalovirus vaccine induces humoral and cellular immune responses in human volunteers. Vaccine 8:130–136, 1990.
64. Spaete RR. A recombinant subunit vaccine approach to HCMV vaccine development. Transplant Proc 23:90–96, 1991.
65. Marshall GS, Ricciardi RP, Rando FR, et al. An adenovirus recombinant that expresses the human cytomegalovirus major envelope glycoprotein and induces neutralizing antibodies. J Infect Dis 162:1177–1181, 1990.
66. Gonczol E, Berencsi K, Pincus S, et al. Preclinical evaluation of an ALVAC (canarypox)–human cytomegalovirus glycoprotein B vaccine candidate. Vaccine 13:1080–1085, 1995.
67. Gonczol E, Berencsi K, Kauffman E, et al. Preclinical evaluation of an ALVAC (Canarypox)–human cytomegalovirus glycoprotein B vaccine candidate: Immune response elicited in a prime-boost protocol with glycoprotein B subunit. Scand J Infect Dis Suppl 99:110–112, 1995.
68. Gonczol E, Berencsi K, Pincus S, et al. Preclinical evaluation of an ALVAC (canarypox)-human cytomegalovirus glycoprotein B vaccine candidate. Vaccine 13:1080–1085, 1995.
69. Gonczol E, deTaisne C, Hirka G, et al. High expression of human cytomegalovirus (HCMV)-gB protein in cells infected with a vaccinia-gB recombinant: The importance of the gB protein in HCMV immunity. Vaccine 9:631–637, 1991.
70. Spaete RR, Saxena A, Scott PI, et al. Sequence requirements for proteolytic processing of glycoprotein B of human cytomegalovirus strain Towne. J Virol 64:2922–2931, 1990.
71. Wang JB, Adler SP, Hempling S, et al. Mucosal antibodies to human cytomegalovirus glycoprotein B occur following both natural infection and immunization with human cytomegalovirus vaccines. J Infect Dis 174:387–392, 1996.
72. Frey S, Harrison C, Pass R, et al. Biocine® CMV gB/MF59 vaccine induces antibody responses when given at two dosages and three immunization schedules [abstract 156]. 6th International Cytomegalovirus Workshop, Perdido Beach Resort, Orange Beach, AL; March 5–9, 1997.
73. Pass RF, Duliège AM, Boppana SB, et al. Immunogenicity of a recombinant CMV gB vaccine. Pediatr Res 37:185A, 1995.
74. Pass RF, Duliège AM, Sekulovich R, et al. Antibody response to a fourth dose of CMV gB vaccine in healthy adults [abstract 157]. 6th International Cytomegalovirus Workshop, Perdido Beach Resort, Orange Beach, AL; March 5–9, 1997.
75. Mitchell DK, Holmes SJ, Burke RL, et al. Immunogenicity of a recombinant human cytomegalovirus (CMV) gB vaccine in toddlers [abstract 745]. Ped Res 41:127A, 1997.
76. Chou S, Dennison KM. Analysis of interstrain variation in cytomegalovirus glycoprotein B sequences encoding neutralization-related epitopes. J Infect Dis 163:1229–1234, 1991.
77. Bale JF, Jr, Petheram SJ, Miller JE, Murph JR. Cytomegalovirus (CMV) glycoprotein B (gB) genotypes in child care environments [abstract 188]. 6th International Cytomegalovirus Workshop, Perdido Beach Resort, Orange Beach, AL; March 5–9, 1997.
78. Torok-Storb B, Gooley T, Leisenring W, et al. Marrow allograft failure is associated with specific cytomegalovirus (CMV) genotypes [abstract 33]. 6th International Cytomegalovirus Workshop, Perdido Beach Resort, Orange Beach, AL; March 5–9, 1997.
79. Lo CY, Woo PCY, Lo SKF, et al. The frequency and distribution of CMV-enveloped glycoprotein genotypes in bone marrow and renal transplant recipients with CMV disease [abstract 126]. 6th International Cytomegalovirus Workshop, Perdido Beach Resort, Orange Beach, AL; March 5–9, 1997.
80. Del Val M, Schlicht HJ, Wolkmer H, et al. Protection against lethal cytomegalovirus infection by a recombinant vaccine containing a single nonameric T-cell epitope. J Virol 65:3641–3646, 1991.
81. McLaughlin-Taylor E, Pande H, Forman SJ, et al. Identification of the major late human cytomegalovirus matrix protein pp65 as a target antigen for CD8 virus-specific cytotoxic T lymphocytes. J Med Virol 43:103–110, 1994.
82. Endresz V, Kari L, Berensci K, et al. Induction of human cytomegalovirus (HCMV)-glycoprotein B (gB)-specific neutralizing antibody and phosphoprotein 65 (pp65)-specific cytotoxic T lymphocyte responses by naked DNA immunization. Vaccine: in press.
83. Plotkin SA, Starr SE, Friedman HM, et al. Vaccines for the prevention of human cytomegalovirus infection. Rev Infect Dis 12:827–838, 1990.
84. Britt WJ. Vaccines against human cytomegalovirus: Time to test. Trends Microbiol 4:34–39, 1996.

chapter

37 Live Influenza Virus Vaccine

Hunein F. Maassab
M. Louise Herlocher
Martin L. Bryant

HISTORY

The human influenza viruses are members of the family *Orthomyxoviridae* and comprise three immunologically distinct types: A, B, and C. Influenza A and B are the most significant pathogens in terms of morbidity and mortality and therefore are best studied. For example, the influenza A pandemic of 1918 to 1919 caused the deaths of an estimated 20 million people. Analysis of the extensive contemporary observations of that episode and efforts to explain it have been a dominant concern of students of respiratory disease and epidemiology ever since, and the data have been exhaustively reviewed.[1] Modern knowledge of the causal agents of human influenza began in 1933 with the isolation in ferrets of a virus from patients with influenza.[2] In this study, it was also noted that sera of the convalescent patients contained neutralizing antibodies to the virus. The isolation of human virus was duplicated in 1934.[3] In 1940, a second etiological type, type B influenza virus, was identified during the epidemic at that time and retrospectively associated with earlier episodes.[4, 5] Both types A and B influenza have since been recognized in widespread outbreaks. A virus isolated from a patient in 1949[6] was found to be distinct from type A and B viruses, and in 1950 a second virus was isolated from an institutional outbreak of influenza and designated type C influenza.[7] Later, several small outbreaks of type C influenza virus were identified, and a high frequency of antibody was found in the general population.

In view of the multiple types and subtypes and their relative independence in distribution, specific causation of waves and recurrences noted in descriptions of past epidemics and pandemics is uncertain. However, one point is clear: Effective prophylaxis is unquestionably desirable in view of the recurrent and enormously widespread disease caused by influenza viruses.

The conclusion that vaccine development for the control of influenza is desirable is based on observations that recovery from infection is accompanied by antibody development that confers resistance to reinfection and that circulating antibody levels similar to those observed in convalescent patients can be obtained by vaccination and presumably reflect an accompanying immunity. The use of licensed inactive whole or subunit influenza vaccine in humans has been the subject of numerous studies, with an emphasis on providing an effective vaccine with minimal reactogenicity to all age groups. The results in field prophylaxis studies have been inconsistent, owing partly to transient protection related to the decline of vaccine-related homologous antibody and to constant changes in the two surface antigens of the virus. The use of vaccine for control of influenza has been shown to be effective when applied yearly to selected segments of the general population. The primary strategy for partial containment of influenza has been to concentrate efforts on prevention by vaccination of persons known to be at high risk. However, the problem of efficacy of the killed vaccine, duration of effect, adverse reactions on parenteral administration, inconvenience of annual vaccination, and failure to induce local or cellular immunity have stimulated research for alternative vaccination methods.

An approach to immunization using live-attenuated virus has obvious merit, and the design and testing of vaccines attenuated by various methods that may be administered by an easy, natural route (e.g., nasal spray) are now being enthusiastically pursued. It is the purpose of this chapter to review the research that may lead to the licensing of an acceptable live-attenuated influenza virus vaccine of types A and B for use in humans. The current status of live vaccines is summarized at the end of the chapter.

BACKGROUND—WHY THE DISEASE IS IMPORTANT

Influenza is the most common cause of lower respiratory tract infections. It was estimated that if one included all age groups, approximately 48 million cases of influenza occur in the United States each winter. However, this number varies depending on the susceptibility of the population to the virus and the infectiousness of the virus during an outbreak. Of the 48 million persons with influenza annually, approximately 3.9 million are hospitalized and 20,000 die.[8] During major influenza epidemics in the United States, more than 40,000 influenza-associated deaths have occurred. In recent decades, more than 90% of the deaths attributed to influenza occurred among persons 65 years or older.[8a] Influenza type A infection occurs most frequently and is responsible for the greatest amount of morbidity and mortality. Although influenza B has not caused a pandemic, it is responsible for regional epidemics that are less severe than influenza A epidemics. Influenza C rarely causes epidemics but has been associated with sporadic cases.[8, 9]

Clinical Description

The symptoms of influenza affect the patient and sufficient numbers of persons to interrupt the functions of a group or the community. The incubation period is ordinarily 1 to 2 days. The onset of illness is abrupt, with headache, sudden chills, fatigue, and generalized muscle aches. The temperature rises rapidly in 12 to 24 hours to a level of 101 to 104°F. Diffuse headache and severe muscular achiness of the back and the extremities are usual in adults but are generally less marked in children. The patient experiences a sense of fatigue and weakness, which builds rapidly to prostration. Ocular tension, conjunctival infection, and watery eyes are common, usually without photophobia. Although nasal or nasopharyngeal irritations may be noted early, constitutional symptoms are more prominent, with evidence of respiratory infection, sneezing, and mild discharge not uncommon. A hacking, unproductive cough is usual, but sore throat is uncommon. During the next 24 hours the fever reaches a sustained level. The nose may be obstructed, the throat feels dry, and laryngitis with hoarseness is frequent. Substernal soreness may be noted, probably reflecting the effect of the virus on lower respiratory mucosa. There is little appetite, and the patient is apathetic. Purulent exudate is not seen in the tonsils or the pharyngeal wall. Bacteriological examination of the throat has revealed no consistent bacterial accompaniment of influenza infection. Convalescence ordinarily proceeds rapidly, but annoying cough often persists. Despite the apparent recovery, distressing features of the disease may appear when the patient undertakes full activity too soon. Fatigue and weariness are often troublesome, but this is less pronounced in children and young adults. In older persons, they may be prolonged. Pulmonary complications are the most common serious consequence, especially if temperature and symptoms persist beyond the fourth and fifth days of illness. The clinical picture is essentially the same for influenza A and influenza B, whereas the clinical characteristics of influenza C are less clearly established but generally milder.[9, 10]

Virology

Because of the complexity of the subject, it is beyond the scope of this chapter to address all aspects of influenza virology. Therefore, this section presents a simple review emphasizing those areas relevant to the production and effectiveness of live-virus vaccines. For a comprehensive review of the biology of influenza viruses, the reader is directed to another text.[11]

Orthomyxoviruses have segmented, single-strand, negative-sense RNA genomes. Because they lack the proof-reading enzymes that maintain the fidelity of DNA replication, influenza viruses are subject to high rates of mutation during replication of their single-stranded RNA genome[12, 13] and to high-frequency gene reassortment during mixed infections because of their segmented genome.[14, 15] Because of these factors, influenza viruses undergo continual, and sometimes drastic, genetic changes that affect their growth in vitro and in vivo, their pathogenicity in humans and animals, and the epidemiology of the resultant disease.[13] New antigenic changes, occurring by one or both of these mechanisms, allow the virus to overcome existing immunity in previously infected hosts. The symptoms of influenza infection are as variable as viral antigenicity, probably because of mutations in the other viral proteins.[16] The explanation for this probably lies in the existence of both variable and conserved regions in the proteins of the virus.[17]

Soon after influenza viruses were isolated, their genetic variability was made apparent by their ability to adapt to laboratory animal hosts after serial passages[18] and by the conversion of amniotically grown O (original and filamentous in shape) virus to D (derived and spherical in shape) virus capable of growing allantoically in embryonated eggs.[19] The formal study of influenza virus genetics essentially started with the introduction of a limiting dilution technique in 1950.[20] The use of this "cloning" method, coupled with the use of embryonated eggs as a uniform substrate for the isolation and cultivation of influenza virus,[21, 22] enabled the discovery of the more important genetic mechanisms: reassortment[11] (then called recombination), multiplicity reactivation,[23] and phenotypic mixing[24] long before the advent of tissue culture and the tissue-culture plaquing methods that greatly enhanced the later genetic studies.[9]

Plaquing systems developed for influenza virus[25] and later modified by the addition of trypsin in the overlay medium[26] allowed the determination of reassortment, reversion, and reactivation rates. Plaquing provided a cloning system for influenza virus, enabling the isolation of temperature-sensitive (ts) mutants.[27, 28] These conditional lethal mutants, most of which varied from the parent by only a single mutational step, were used to map the influenza genome and dissect the viral replication cycle.[29] Biophysical analyses such as polyacrylamide gel electrophoresis were used to identify the genes having these mutations.[30, 31] Similar analyses were performed using reassortants made between strains of influenza viruses showing clear differences in the electrophoretic mobility of their RNA genome segments on polyacrylamide gels.[32–36] The ability to clone specific mutants, organize them into complementation groups, and then correlate these groupings with phenotype and the RNA segment containing the mutation has allowed researchers to map the influenza virus genome assigning each

Table 37–1. **PRODUCTS OF INFLUENZA A AND B VIRUS GENES**

RNA	GENE PRODUCTS	FUNCTIONS
1	PB2	Viral polymerase component involved in synthesis of capped messenger RNAs (mRNAs) and endonuclease, which cleaves host cell mRNA
2	PB1	Viral polymerase component with RNA transcription and replication activities
3	PA	Viral polymerase component involved in RNA replication
4	HA	Virion surface attachment and fusion glycoprotein, major antigenic determinant
5	NP	Major nucleocapsid structural component and type-specific antigen
6	NA	Virion surface glycoprotein with receptor-destroying enzyme activity, major antigenic determinant
	NB	Glycoptotein membrane ion channel (?) found only in type B
7	M1	Membrane matrix protein and type-specific antigen
	M2	Nonglycosylated membrane ion channel, found only in type A
8	NS1	Nonstructural protein—unique posttranscriptional regulator that inhibits the nuclear transport of poly A–containing mRNAs and inhibits pre-mRNA splicing by binding to a specific region of U6 small nuclear RNA
	NS2	Cellular and virion protein of unknown function

RNA segment to the encoded proteins and functions (Table 37–1).

More recent investigations have examined influenza virus using a variety of molecular biology techniques: monoclonal antibodies,[37–40] cloning of isolated genes and expression of the encoded proteins,[41] sequence analyses of cloned gene segments or direct sequencing of the virion RNA[42, 43] or sequencing using polymerase chain reaction techniques, and transfection of specifically modified genes.[44–49]

The mechanisms of antigenic drift and shift have been examined,[48] and the structure and function of the surface hemagglutinin and neuraminidase molecules and their antigenic and reactive sites have been elucidated.[48–51] Genes other than HA and NA also have been shown to change by the mechanisms similar to those responsible for antigenic shift and drift,[48] and sequence data have been compiled, allowing viral evolution and the rate of change of individual genes to be determined.[48, 52–54]

Methods of Attenuation

The segmented and single-stranded RNA genome of influenza virus has a direct and immediate impact on its antigenicity, epidemiology, and hence the manner in which this virus may be controlled. Influenza virus exhibits both antigenic drift[55] and antigenic shift,[48] whereas influenza B and probably influenza C viruses show only antigenic drift.[56] Antigenic drift is caused by the individual mutational changes in nucleotide sequence that occur because of the infidelity inherent in the replication of RNA genomes, with advantageous mutations becoming "fixed" in genomes of the replicating population. Although not subject to antigenic mediation, other genes also undergo this same mutational drift.[56] The rate of drift can vary among genes and viral types.[51, 57–61] Antigenic shift, however, requires complete replacement of one or both of the surface glycoprotein genes. The accepted explanation is that these new genes are acquired through reassortment between human and avian influenza A viruses.[51] Neither influenza B nor C virus has been shown to have a large active animal host population,[42] and neither exhibits antigenic shift.

After observing the conversion from the O to the D form of influenza virus, Burnet and Bull[19] suggested that attenuated live influenza virus suitable for vaccines might be produced by egg passage of the virus because of its inherent genetic instability. Thus, early on, investigators took advantage of the high mutation rate by passing the virus in nonhuman hosts, generating host range mutant (hr) viruses for use as live-virus vaccines. Vaccines made by this method have not been shown to be reliably attenuated[58] and could result in disease. Attempts to further attenuate hr viruses in the presence of heated guinea pig serum produced a vaccine strain that was clinically safe in adults[62, 63] but caused fever in children.[60] Thus, hr viruses have been abandoned as potential vaccine candidates.

The high rate of genetic reassortment in orthomyxoviruses can be employed to quickly generate vaccine strains containing the genes for the surface antigens (HA and NA) of newly emergent wild type (wt) viruses, while retaining other genes from attenuated strains.[64] Attenuated master strains must be shown to not cause significant illness in humans and to pass this property on to reassortants through the donation of genes other than the HA and NA genes.

Attenuated master strains have been made by several methods. They can be separated into three main classes: hr, ts, and cold-adapted (ca) mutants. Those master strains that have been used to generate live influenza reassortant vaccines for trials in humans are listed in Table 37–2.[63–98]

While hr mutants were abandoned as vaccine candidates, they have been used as master attenuated strains in reassortant vaccines. Live reassortant vaccines made using A/Puerto Rico/8/34 (H1N1) (PR8) as the attenuating master strain have proved unsatisfactory because the six nonsurface antigen genes of PR8 did not reliably confer attenuation in combination with some wt surface genes. There was no simple means of determining which reassortants were attenuated and which were not.[65] Similar problems were noted with A/Okuda/57 (H2N2) virus that had 280 passages in eggs and had been used in Japan.[66] Although experiments with avian master attenuated strains are ongoing, these strains appear to be unlikely candidates for human vaccines because some reassortants have required unrealistically high infectious doses to induce immunity. There is concern that avian

Table 37–2. **INFLUENZA A MASTER STRAINS USED IN THE PREPARATION OF LIVE REASSORTANT VIRUS VACCINES**

MASTER STRAIN	CURRENTLY IN USE	REFERENCES
	hr mutants	
A/PR/8/34 (H1N1)	No	63, 65–68
A/Okuda/57/ (H2N2)	No	68, 69
A/Mallard/6750/78 (H2N2)	No	70–74
A/Mallard/Alberta/88/76 (H3N8)	No	70, 72, 73, 91, 93–95
	ts mutants	
ts 1[E]	No	76
ts1A2	No	80
	ca mutants	
A/Ann Arbor/6/60 (H2N2)	Yes	79–81, 97, 98
B/Ann Arbor/1/66	Yes	82–89
A/Leningrad/134/17/57	Yes	85, 90, 92
A/Leningrad/134/47/57	Yes	86, 87

genes may lead to reassortants in vivo that might enhance virulence, and they have been more virulent in infants and children in studies comparing them with ca vaccines.

Ts master strains were generated by reassortment between A/Hong Kong/68 (H3N2) wt virus and ts mutants of A/Great Lakes/389/65 (H2N2) virus that had been grown in the presence of 5-fluorouracil.[76–80] Although several were shown to be attenuated in adults and children, some ts mutants reverted to virulence after passage in humans. Ts mutants have been abandoned because of this genetic instability.[99]

Cold adaptation has become the major means of generating live-virus vaccines in master attenuated viruses.[100] Several methods have been used for cold-adapting influenza A virus. A/Ann Arbor/6/60 (A/AA/6/60(H2N2)) virus has been grown at successively lowered temperatures in primary chick kidney cells until a virus has been derived that grows as well at 25°C as it does at 33°C. All three polymerase genes have been shown to contribute to the attenuated phenotype of the cold-adapted A/Ann Arbor/6/60 master strain.[101] The PA gene has been shown to be a major determinant of attenuation for the ca B/Ann Arbor/1/66 vaccine strain.[102] The ca A/AA/6/60 virus derived in this manner has been shown to be both ca and ts. (Whereas ca implies that the virus will grow well at a reduced temperature 25°/33°C, ts implies that the vaccine virus replication is reduced by at least 2 logs $TCID_{50}$ at the higher temperature 39°C for type A compared with growth at either 25°/33°C or 37°C.) In addition, owing to the serial passages in primary chick kidney (PCK) cells and embryonated eggs, the master strain may well contain hr mutations. Although few sequence differences have been found between the ca A/AA/6/60 virus and its wt progenitor,[97] sequencing evidence has been found for changes in all eight genes of the attenuated ca A/AA/6/60 virus from its virulent wt counterpoint.[98] There have been numerous human trials with reassortants made using ca A/AA/6/60 virus, and in all cases, attenuation, antigenicity, and genetic stability have remained unaltered and consistent.[82] Similar procedures have been used for influenza B viruses,[84] and vaccine lines using ca B/Ann Arbor/1/66 virus as a master strain are being produced and evaluated.[85, 86]

A ca master strain has also been used in Russia. Unlike the aforementioned ca A/Ann Arbor/6/60 virus, the Russian master strain, A/Leningrad/134/57 virus, was produced by multiple passages primarily at 25° or 26°C and not by a gradual lowering of incubation temperatures. The original ca master strain A/Leningrad/134/17/57[92, 103, 104] was passaged an additional 30 times in embryonated eggs at 25°C to generate a new ca master strain, A/Leningrad/134/47/57 virus.[88] Reassortants made between this latter ca master strain and wt A/Leningrad/322/79 H1N1 or A/Bangkok/1/79 H3N2 virus were shown to be nonreactogenic and immunogenic in children.[89] The A/Leningrad/134/47/57 master strain has been shown to contain changes in at least one of the polymerase genes as well as in the HA, NA, NP, and M genes.[105] A/Aichi/2/68 virus has been adapted to growth at 25°C in a manner similar to that used for the Russian master strain, but with fewer passages.[100] This virus has been tested in both ferrets and human volunteers and is also immunogenic and avirulent.[106–108]

New techniques, such as recombinant DNA cloning and the transfection of in vitro mutagenized gene segments, are providing new possibilities for the production of live-virus vaccines. The gene coding for the HA protein has been cloned into vaccinia virus and is expressed on the virus surface. Attenuated recombinant vaccinia viruses have been shown to provide protection to homologous wt virus challenge in hamsters.[109] If necessary, other influenza genes cloned into the vaccinia virus carrier could also be employed at the same time. Alternatively, future master strains might be composed of a number of selected genes with additional specific mutations.[99] CR43-3 virus is a cold reassortant whose genome contains an NS gene with a deletion in the NS1 protein coding region[110] and is restricted for growth both in Madin-Darby canine kidney cells and in ferrets.[111]

Deletions may also be generated through specific site mutagenesis in recombinant complimentary DNA (cDNA) clones. The ability to introduce RNA transcripts of specifically mutagenized cDNA clones into the influenza viruses as stable parts of the genome has opened new areas of research into vaccine development.[45, 46] It is now possible to conceive of "tailor-made" influenza vaccines engineered for specific purposes.

Pathogenesis as It Relates to Prevention

The pathology of influenza has been reviewed extensively.[112–115] Basically, the virus first contacts the mucous lining of the respiratory tract and then attaches to ciliated columnar epithelial cells after release from the mucous layer.[115, 116] The viral neuraminidase is probably involved in its release from the mucous receptors and the liquefaction of the mucous layer. The ciliated columnar epithelial cell is most likely the major site of infection.[116] Bronchitis and tracheitis also are common,[117] and there may be some lung involvement.[118] Viremia has been reported only sporadically[119, 120] amidst numerous negative reports.[121–123] Influenza B demonstrates pathology similar to that of type A, whereas influenza C generally causes an afebrile illness or subclinical infection of the upper respiratory tract.

Cleavage of the HA precursor protein into HA1 and HA2 proteins by posttranslational processing is necessary for the glycoprotein to become membrane fusion competent.[124, 125] In some cases, the NA gene can modulate infection by facilitating cleavage of the HA gene.[126] Neuraminidase activity is often complementary to HA receptor specificity, allowing the two to act in concert.[127]

Influenza in humans is usually restricted to infection primarily of the upper respiratory tract, although during severe pandemic periods, lung lesions may be present.[16] The amount of virus produced probably determines the extent and severity of symptoms.[99, 128] Useful live-virus vaccines therefore must be regulated to ensure sufficient growth to generate local and systemic immune responses yet must be attenuated so that they cause no serious symptoms.

Transmissability can be distinguished from virulence, as shown by genetic reassortment experiments,[129] but no one gene has been shown to be required, probably because this property is multigenic, as is viral pathogenicity.[114, 130, 131] Vaccine viruses should produce levels of virus shed during infection that are a minimum of 100 times lower than the 50% human infectious dose to make transmission of the vaccine strain unlikely.

Diagnosis

The most precise diagnosis of influenza is obtained by viral isolation in embryonated eggs or in cell cultures of nasopharyngeal or tracheal aspirates, or by using reverse transcriptase–polymerase chain reaction (RT-PCR). Serological diagnosis can be made by demonstrating four-fold rises in HA1 or CF antibodies.

EPIDEMIOLOGY OF INFLUENZA—HISTORICAL PERSPECTIVE

Influenza is unique among respiratory viral diseases for its recurring outburst of intense activity manifested by unusually high infection and morbidity rates in all age groups.[128, 132–134] In the northern hemisphere, influenza exhibits a distinct seasonal pattern, with influenza activity peaking during winter months. For instance, from 1967 to 1973, the number of documented influenza A infections peaked in January, February, or March, and influenza B infections peaked in March.[135] Environmental conditions during the winter may be important for the transmission of influenza because virus survival outside the body is favored by low relative humidity and ambient temperatures.[136–138] However, in the tropics, epidemic influenza commonly occurs during the monsoon season.[139] Thus, the principal effect of inclement weather can simply be to bring people together in enclosed shelters.[140] Although the great majority of disease attributable to influenza occurs during the annual activity peaks, sporadic outbreaks occur throughout the year, and endemic persistence between epidemics is well documented.[141–145]

The resultant pattern of influenza infection is generally one of high morbidity and low mortality, although outbreaks are also reflected in excess mortality from subsequent pneumonia and hence an increase of total mortality. An epidemic may be defined by both serology and virus isolation to determine the dates of incidence and prevalence[133] and the impact of health on families and communities.[141, 144]

By using excess mortality and morbidity due to influenza as an index, Collins[146] compiled an impressive record of influenza-associated mortality extending from 1887 through 1956. Over the period analyzed, the intervals between outbreaks and the sites affected varied greatly: After a decade of relative quiescence, the pandemic of 1889 to 1890 erupted violently and unexpectedly. The death toll between 1891 and 1892 was ever greater, and high, sharp peaks of excess mortality recurred through 1908. Afterward, the disease was apparently much less virulent until the catastrophic pandemic of 1918 to 1920, in which over 20 million lives were lost worldwide. Subsequently, moderate to severe outbreaks have been amply documented.[128, 147] Improved surveillance of influenza has been used as an accurate indicator and a valuable predictor of epidemic activity.[148]

Epidemic influenza tends to superimpose its profile on the existing pattern of respiratory disease, regardless of season. Influenza incidence rates vary with the nature of the epidemic virus strains and the population affected. Rates calculated from surveillance of individuals with upper respiratory illness suggest that influenza is responsible for roughly 10 to 20% of all respiratory illnesses per epidemic year,[141, 149] with rates for influenza A being somewhat higher than those for influenza B. Nevertheless, an illness rate of 83% was observed in one epidemic season during an influenza B outbreak in an isolated Alaskan village.[150] Using the National Health Survey analysis of 101 million medically attended respiratory illnesses for 1977 to 1978, it has been estimated that 20 million cases could be attributed to influenza.[133] Most studies have found infection rates in preschool- and school-aged children to be much higher than in adults, particularly during influenza B epidemics.[141, 142, 149, 151] Consequently, families with school-aged or younger children suffer disproportionately from influenza[133, 149] as the result of frequent primary introduction from family members younger than 20 years of age.[142, 152] These findings are consistent with the concepts that influenza is most likely to infect individuals with the least prior immunity and that children are a common source of influenza in the community. In epidemics, there appears to be relative uniformity in the manifestation of symptoms exhibited by the great majority of patients: abrupt onset with chills, aches, fever, and prostration without prominent respiratory signs and uncomplicated recovery beginning after 3 to 4 days of illness. Influenza can therefore be considered a disease possessing rather uniform basic characteristics that vary in amplitude and severity, since the causative agents differ qualitatively and quantitatively yet possess similar pathogenic potentials. Variation in severity and extent of disease can be related to differences among host populations and their immune status, primary causative agents, and environmental influences.

The epidemiology of influenza virus is complicated by the unique antigenic variability of virus when compared with that of other respiratory pathogens.[51] Antigenic shift and drift of type A influenza virus has come to be recognized as the cause of this epidemiological pattern. Various mechanisms have been offered to explain the emergence of these antigenic changes: (1) immunological pressure during passage of the virus in a population of differing immune status; (2) change resulting from mutation, deletion, or insertion in the genes coding for the surface glycoproteins; (3) reassortment among cocirculating human strains or among human and animal influenza viruses; and (4) recycling of viral strains.

Influenza virus type B was first isolated in 1940,[4] and data indicate that an antigenically similar strain was involved in the epidemic of 1936. Antigenic drift and heterogeneity among strains isolated in subsequent years have been widely recognized, but the degree of change has not been great enough to permit recognition and designation of subtypes.[152, 153]

Influenza virus type C was isolated during 1949 from a patient suspected to have influenza and was found to be unrelated antigenically to type A or type B.[6] Overt clinical disease incidence is low, but widespread infection can be demonstrated by the high frequency of antibodies in the general population. Sporadic cases and small local outbreaks have been identified in different countries. Findings suggest that antigenic change among type C strains has occurred over time, but, as with type B influenza, the degree of change does not warrant separation into subtypes.[154, 155]

ROLE OF IMMUNITY AS IT RELATES TO PREVENTION

The immune status of the population determines the incidence and prevalence of influenza infection. In the humoral antibody response, the factors that influence protection against infection are the specificity and the duration of antibody response.[156, 157] The type of antibody generated after infection, such as neutralizing, hemagglutination-inhibition (HI), and antineuraminidase antibodies, are the major determinants of humoral immunity. Following infection, the secretory immunoglobulin A (sIgA) or IgA immune response increases rapidly to a high titer and then declines. The rate of decline depends on each individual's base level of antibodies. There is now general agreement that the presence of sIgA in human nasal epithelium plays a major role in preventing influenza infection by inhibiting its spread or otherwise modifying the disease process.[156, 158, 159] Neutralization of the sIgA response has been thought to eliminate postinfection immunity.[158]

Immune protection against influenza involves both humoral and cell-mediated responses. Passive transfer of physiological amounts of IgG antibodies provides complete protection in mice from homologous infection in the absence of an active host response.[160, 161] Passive transfer of large amounts of neuraminidase (NA) antibody provides limited protection, whereas anti-NP or anti-M protein antibodies provide no protection. Thus, anti-HA antibodies play a major role in protection from influenza virus infection, whereas anti-NA antibodies play a lesser but potentially significant role. Protection from naturally occurring influenza due to preexisting anti-NA antibodies has been demonstrated in individuals who had N2 antibody but no relevant HA antibody immediately after the H2N2 to H3N2 antigenic shift.[161]

Evidence demonstrating that preseason HA inhibition titer and neutralizing antibody titer moderates susceptibility to infection and disease severity in humans has been obtained for both influenza A and influenza B.[160, 162] For influenza B, neutralizing antibody titers in excess of 3.5 $\log_2$ are 100% protective against illness and infection.[143] In this study, it was found that the mean titer rise after infection was correlated with the level of preinfection titer. Individuals with no preinfection titers demonstrated a mean rise of only 2.2 $\log_2$ neutralizing titer, which may help explain the relatively high rates of reinfection that occur during successive epidemics of influenza B.[150, 162]

Evidence is accumulating that cytotoxic T cells are involved in the recovery from influenza virus infections. Helper and suppressor T cells also play an important role in influenza virus infection through modulations of B cell and T cell responses.[162, 163]

Effective prophylaxis in the future requires the production and licensing of a live-virus vaccine that can mobilize multiple immunological functions for control of the disease.

ACTIVE IMMUNIZATION

All influenza live-virus vaccines currently being tested are reassortants that were prepared using wt virus human isolates crossed with attenuating master strains. The master strains in use are the ca and ts A/Ann Arbor/6/60 (H2N2) virus, the ca B/Ann Arbor/1/66 virus, and the ca and ts A/Leningrad/134/57 (H2N2) virus. The well-defined passage history for reassortant virus vaccines using A/Ann Arbor/6/60 and B/Ann Arbor/1/66 extends back through the reassortant experiments that produced the vaccine to the isolation of each parent, wt, and master strain.

HISTORY AND DEVELOPMENT

The ca and ts A/AA/6/60 virus was derived from a virus originally isolated in PCK cells that produced clinical symptoms in ferrets. This virus was adapted to growth at 25°C by passaging the virus at successively lower temperatures in PCK cells. After establishing a pool of virus that grew as well at 25°C as it did at 33°C, a clone was selected by seven repeated plaque-to-plaque purifications. This clone met the following criteria: high and equivalent virus yield in PCK cells and eggs at 33 and 25°C, retention of ca and ts markers in tissue culture, and attenuated behavior in ferrets. The ca B/AA/1/66 master strain was developed in the same manner, although it took fewer intermediate passages to achieve the final ca variant for type B virus than for type A.[84] The wt B/AA/1/66 influenza virus was restricted for growth at 36°C at the time of isolation, and therefore the ts phenotype is defined by a reduction in replication titer at 37°C compared with the achievable titer at 25°/33°C.[84, 89]

The ca and ts A/Leningrad/134/17/57 strain was derived from a wt virus that had been passaged in embryonated eggs at 32°C 20 or more times prior to cold adaptation.[84] This wt virus was passaged in embryonated eggs for 17 successive passages at 25 to 26°C, although it was twice passaged at 31°C during this procedure to amplify the existing viable virus to generate the A/Leningrad/134/17/57 master strain.[87, 104] A/Leningrad/134/47/57 virus was derived from this first master strain by 30 additional embryonated egg passages at 25°C.[79] It is important to note that differences do exist, notably between the phenotypic properties of the ca vaccines developed in the former Soviet Union[164] and those of the one developed in the United States.[82] The vaccine developed in the former Soviet Union is evaluated by using two type A donor strains with different passage history at suboptimal temperature and by comparing, in vitro, the donors of attenuation and their reassortants at 32°C (permissive) and 40°C (nonpermissive). In contrast, the ca donors A/Ann Arbor/6/60-H2N2 and B/Ann Arbor/1/66 grew equally well at 25 and 33°C with a shut-off temperature of 38°C for type A and 37°C for type B influenza viruses.

Selected wt viruses are cloned by one to two passages at 38 to 40°C in either embryonated eggs (former Soviet Union) or PCK cells (United States) to ensure that the wt virus is not ts.[104] Type B influenza wt viruses may require cloning at 37°C rather than at 38 to 40°C, the range used for type A influenza viruses. The wt viruses are then plaque purified in PCK cells (United States) or cloned by limiting dilution (former Soviet Union) in embryonated eggs.[104] The virulence of these cloned wt viruses may then be documented in the ferret animal model system.

An example of an influenza A ca reassortment experiment follows:

Derivation of Cold Reassortant (CR) Clones

Starting viruses:

Wild-type parent with relevant surface antigen(s)
Master strain cold-adapted variant A/AA/6/60 (H2N2) 7PI, SE3

Reassortment Steps

1. Pass at 25 or 33°C in PCK cells at a multiplicity of infection (MOI) of 5 plaque-forming units (PFU) per virus; incubate 72 hours; and freeze, thaw, centrifuge, and pass supernate.
2. Pass twice at 25 or 33°C in PCK cells in the presence of ferret immune serum to the cold variant.
3. Pass once at 25 or 33°C in PCK cells in the absence of immune serum (optional).
4. Pass once in SPAFAS embryonated hens' eggs at 33°C.
5. Titrate plaque at 25 or 33°C in PCK cells; select 20 clones for characterization.
6. Select clone(s) as seed vaccine on the basis that the six internal genes were derived from the master strain.
7. Perform plaque-to-plaque purification (three times) at 25 or 33°C in PCK cells.
8. Pass in SPAFAS embryonated hens' eggs for production of seed virus for distribution and for production of a volunteer pool.

The final choice of a cold-reassortant clone is based on its having the following:

a. Six internal genes from A/AA/6/60-master strain
b. Both ts and ca phenotypes
c. No reactogenicity in ferrets
d. High infectious yield at 33°C

The same procedure is followed to provide live, ca-reassortant vaccines for influenza B virus using the type B master strain. ca B/Ann Arbor/1/66-7PI-SE3 was used in the derivation of the type B 6/2 reassortant vaccine.

In the former Soviet Union, the wt virus is inactivated at 40°C for 24 hours prior to the reassortment procedure, which is performed at 25°C in embryonated eggs. Selected virus is then cloned three times by limited dilution passage in embryonated eggs at 25°C. If necessary, the product of the first mixed infection may be processed twice in the presence of antiserum to the A/Leningrad/134/57 ca and ts master strain.[104] All the vaccines are administered by an intranasal route. The American vaccines are currently being administered as nose drops and nasal spray, whereas the Russian vaccines are given as a spray.[104] The standard range of virus concentration is 10^6 to $10^{7.5}$ 50% tissue culture infectious dose ($TCID_{50}$) per mL. The 50% human infectious dose for the A/AA/6/60 reassortants ranges from $10^{5.5}$ to $10^{6.2}$ $TCID_{50}$ per mL.[165, 166]

STRATEGY AND ADVANTAGES OF THE ca-REASSORTANT VACCINES

Cold adaptation was found to be a reliable and efficient procedure for the derivation of live-attenuated influenza virus vaccines for humans. In addition, the process of genetic reassortment with the transfer of the six internal genes from a stable attenuated ca master donor strain of type A (A/Ann Arbor/6/60-H2N2) or type B (B/Ann Arbor/1/66) to the new prevailing wild-type epidemic strain has yielded consistently attenuated cold reassortant vaccines with the desired 6/2 gene profile for human use. These live ca reassortant vaccines for types A and B influenza viruses, developed at the University of Michigan, have been shown to have the proper level of attenuation, immunogenicity, and non-transmissibility combined with proven genetic stability and are produced in acceptable tissue culture substrates.[100]

In general, this live ca reassortant vaccine offers several advantages over the existing inactivated vaccines: (1) possible use of a single dose for all age groups, including children, annually; (2) administration by the natural route of infection (intranasally); (3) stimulation of a wide range of antibody responses; (4) induction of local and humoral immunity; (5) cost-effectiveness (from one embryonated egg one can harvest eight doses of the live vaccine, whereas it takes 12 embryonated eggs for one dose of the killed vaccine); (6) rapidity of production and updating in the event of antigenic changes; (7) availability of laboratory guidelines for the assessment of virulence (reactogenicity in ferrets); (8) reproducibility of attenuation; and (9) the presence of two phenotypic markers (the ts and ca phenotypes) for the evaluation of virulence and monitoring of the vaccine in the field.

RESULTS OF VACCINATION

Since 1976, the clinical development of the ca influenza virus vaccines has included the testing of multiple reassortant vaccines in over 7000 people between the ages of 4 months and 80 years or older (Table 37–3). These studies have consistently demonstrated the ca vaccines to be genetically stable, nontransmissible, and safe in all populations tested. More recently, studies on the ca vaccine have focused on three broad areas: (1) evaluating the range and extent of the immunological response; (2) determining the protective efficacy of this vaccine in the overall population as well as in targeted subsets; and (3) evaluating the immunological and efficacious consequences of combining and administrating all three ca influenza virus vaccines.

IMMUNE RESPONSES

The immunogenicity of the ca type A vaccine has been extensively evaluated in comparison with the trivalent inactivated vaccine (TIV) in both adults and children. In general, when ca vaccine is administered to volunteers who had previously been exposed to influenza virus (seropositives), the immunological responses observed are different from those seen in seropositive volunteers receiving TIV. Clements and colleagues[167] extensively analyzed the subset antibody response to TIV or ca vaccine administration in young adults and correlated that response with protection using artificial challenge to the homotypic wt virus. As predicted, in the seropositive TIV recipients, protection against influenza infection or illness correlated with the level of serum neuraminidase-inhibiting (NAI) antibody, serum hemagglutinin-inhibiting (HAI) antibody, and nasal IgG antibody to the viral HA. However, the protective correlates in seropositive adults receiving the ca vaccine were different. In this population, protection against virus infection and illness correlated with nasal IgA antibodies to the HA1 and serum NAI antibodies. Although in these studies no correlation was observed between protection and the level of HAI serum antibodies in ca vaccines, other studies have suggested that some relationship may exist.[168] Limited studies in T-cell response following TIV or ca vaccination of seropositive adults have also suggested differences in T-cell antibody response. In these studies, anti–influenza A virus cytotoxicity was evaluated in patients with chronic obstructive pulmonary disease following vaccination with a monovalent inactivated influenza A vaccine or a ca type A vaccine. In addition to inducing antigen-specific nasal IgA antibodies, volunteers receiving the ca vaccine also exhibited a broader stimulation of anti–influenza A cytotoxicity. The cytotoxicity observed in the ca vaccines was cross-reactive among heterologous strains of influenza A virus. No such cross-reactivity was observed in volunteers receiving monovalent inactivated vaccine.[169, 170]

Antibody profiles following TIV or ca vaccine administration in infants and children not previously exposed to influenza virus (seronegatives) are quite different from those seen in the seropositive population. In this population, significant serum HAI antibody responses are seen in the majority of children (60–100%) receiving the ca vaccine as well as those receiving TIV. However, serum and nasal IgA antibodies to influenza are almost exclusively found in ca vaccines, whereas antibody-specific serum IgM is more frequently seen in TIV recipients.[171, 172] Limited attempts to evaluate the T-cell response to ca vaccine in seronegative infants have suggested that ca vaccine may stimulate cytotoxic T lymphocyte response in this naive population, although the uniformity of that response is unclear (Cate and Mbawuike, personal communication, 1990).

PROTECTIVE EFFECT

Although the ca A vaccine has been repeatedly shown to be effective in placebo-controlled wt virus challenges and field studies,[172, 173] equivalent effectiveness of this vaccine, relative to the TIV, has only been suggested. To determine the relative efficacy of the ca vaccine and TIV, a large-field study was required. In 1985, a 5-year double-blind randomized study comparing the efficacy of the ca influenza A (H1N1 and H3N2) vaccine with that of TIV was initiated in Nashville, Tennessee. Edwards and colleagues designed a study that included the enrollment of a broad age range (1–65 years) of healthy individuals who would be vaccinated, on a yearly basis, with either the ca vaccine or TIV.[168] More than 5000 people were enrolled, and over 12,000 vaccinations were given. Vaccine efficacy was evaluated by several criteria, the strictest being culture confirmation associated with clinical illness and the broadest being a fourfold rise in HAI antibody titer approximately 1 month after vaccination. Compared with placebo, no clinically significant adverse reactions were observed in either vaccine group. Although statistically significant serological rises were observed in both vaccine groups when compared with placebo recipients, the serum IgG response in the ca vaccine group was lower than that observed in the inactivated vaccine group. Using the most stringent criteria

Table 37–3. **SUMMARY OF COLD-ADAPTED INFLUENZA VACCINES TESTED IN THE UNITED STATES**

COLD ADAPTED VACCINE		ATTENUATED	ANTIGENIC	GENETIC STABILITY
B/Hong Kong/73/, CR-7	Adults	+	+	+
	Children	ND	ND	ND
A/Victoria/75, (H3N2) CR-22	Adults	+	+	+
	Children	ND	+	+
A/Alaska/77, (H3N2) CR-29	Adults	+	+	+
	Children	+	+	+
A/Hong Kong/77 (H1N1) CR-35	Adults	+	+	+
	Children	+	+	+
A/California/78, (H1N1) CR-37	Adults	+	+	+
	Children	+	+	+
A/Washington/80, (H3N2) CR-48	Adults	+	+	+
	Children	+	+	+
A/Korea/82, (H3N2) CR-59	Adults	+	+	+
	Children	+	+	+
A/Dunedin/83, (H1N1) CR-64	Adults	+	+	+
	Children	+	+	+
B/Texas/84, CRB-87	Adults	+	+	+
	Children	+	+	+
A/Bethesda/85, (H3N2) CR-90	Adults	+	+	+
	Children	+	+	+
A/Texas/85, (H1N1) CR-98	Adults	+	+	+
	Children	+	+	+
A/Kawasaki/86, (H1N1) CR-125	Adults	+	+	+
	Children	+	+	+
B/Ann Arbor/86, CRB-117	Adults	+	+	+
	Children	+	+	+
A/Los Angeles/87, (H3N2) CR-149	Adults	+	+	+
	Children	+	+	+
A/Texas/36/91	Adults	+	+	+
	Children	+	+	+
A/Johannesburg/33/94	Adults	+	+	+
	Children	+	+	+
A/Wuhan/359/95	Adults	+	+	+
	Children	+	+	+
A/Shangdong/9/93	Adults	+	+	+
	Children	+	+	+
A/Shenzhen/227/95	Adults	+	+	+
	Children	+	+	+
B/Panama/25/90	Adults	+	+	+
	Children	+	+	+
B/Harbin/7/94	Adults	+	+	+
	Children	+	+	+
B/Yamagata/88	Adults	+	+	+
	Children	ND	ND	ND

ND, Not done.

Plus Implies the vaccine line exhibited the following: (1) proper level of attenuation with no reactogenicity when administered intranasally, (2) antigenic rise in humoral antibody response was demonstrated in volunteers receiving the vaccine, and (3) the vaccine was genetically stable because the shed virus from the vaccines retained the genetic markers of the live vaccine used. No reversion to virulence was evident.

for efficacy, however, both the ca and the inactivated vaccines were comparable and significantly greater ($P < 0.0001$) than the placebo controls. Other smaller efficacy studies have confirmed these results and have further suggested that in certain segments of the population, specifically young children, the ca vaccine may prove to be significantly more efficacious than the TIV.[172] The use of the ca vaccine as a challenge in children previously immunized with either the TIV or ca vaccine or in children previously infected with influenza virus has demonstrated an additional benefit of the ca vaccine. Specifically, like those volunteers who had been naturally infected, the ca vaccines shed less challenge virus than TIV vaccinees. This effect was due primarily to the high nasal IgA response in the children who had previously been vaccinated with TIV.[174] For ca vaccines, efficacy may include, in addition to protection from illness, a reduction in the carriage of influenza. Thus, vaccinating young children with ca vaccine may be an important strategy for controlling the spread of infection, especially for those in close contact with high-risk populations.

PERSISTENCE OF IMMUNITY

One of the theoretical benefits of a ca vaccine strategy has been the possibility of increasing the duration of immunity to homotypical, and perhaps heterotypical, influenza strains in a manner similar to that observed following natural infection. An example of long-term immunity following natural infection was seen following the reintroduction of the H1N1 virus between 1977 and 1978. This virus was similar to the H1N1 viruses that circulated prior to 1957 but had disappeared until the 1977 season. Epidemiological studies clearly demonstrated that although infection was common across all age groups, illness was rare in the population born before 1957.[133] The nature of that long-term memory is not entirely clear, although the role of infection-induced T-cell immunity appears to be of critical importance—specifically the role of cytotoxic T cells in the recovery from influenza virus infections and the use of helper and suppressor T cells as mediators for B-cell and cytotoxic T-cell responses.[163, 169, 170, 175] The ability of the ca vaccine to induce T-cell responses that appear to be comparable to those seen following natural infection suggests that the persistence of T-cell immunity following ca vaccine administration may be important in protection against influenza disease, especially in young children not previously exposed to influenza viruses.

The persistence of immunity has also been evaluated using the decay rate of influenza-specific HAI response in seronegative children. In this population, the influenza-specific IgG response in ca vaccine recipients has been significantly longer in duration than the IgG antibodies induced by TIV. In general, the serum HAI response is detected at 4 to 6 weeks after ca vaccine immunization and remains at approximately the same level over a 1- to 2-year period. In children receiving a single dose of TIV, a rapid fall in serum antibody levels has been observed between 6 weeks and 6 months after vaccination.[171] In adults having low levels of preexisting influenza antibodies, experimental challenges at various times after immunization have suggested that the duration of immunity may be comparable among recipients of inactivated and ca A vaccines.[167]

Attempts to evaluate the persistence of immunity in field studies have been limited. Couch and associates,[173] in a placebo-controlled trial, comparatively evaluated the efficacy of TIV and ca vaccination over a 2-year period (the 1983 and 1984 influenza seasons) following immunization of approximately 600 young adults having low preexisting antibody titers to influenza. During the first influenza season, two predominant influenza A strains circulated, A/Bangkok/79 (H3N2-like) and A/England/333 (H1N1-like), which were similar to the vaccine components for both the ca vaccines and the TIV. Infection rates were 19% in the placebo group, 7% in the ca vaccine group, and 1% in the TIV group. Rates of illness-associated infections were 10, 4, and 1%, respectively, in those same groups. During the 1989 season, the circulating influenza A strain, A/Victoria/89 (H1N1), was more distantly related to the H1N1 component of the vaccines received in 1983. Infection rates for that season were 30% in the placebo group, 16% in the ca vaccine group, and 16% in the TIV group. Infection and illness rates were 22, 9, and 7%, respectively, in those same groups. One analytical caveat was raised by the investigators in the interpretation of those results: specifically that infection was defined by virus isolation and/or antibody rise. Because antibody titers in TIV vaccinees were quite high following vaccination, it may not have been possible to identify additional antibody rises caused by virus infection in the TIV group. However, these results suggest that the duration of immunity for both the ca and the inactivated vaccines in adults having low preexisting antibody titers may be equivalent and may last at least 2 years.

SIMULTANEOUS ADMINISTRATION WITH OTHER VACCINES

Influenza vaccines, unlike other vaccines, are administered on a yearly basis just prior to the influenza season. Because of the limited yet flexible time window for vaccine administration, little work has been done to evaluate interference with other vaccines. More recent emphasis on the use of the ca vaccine in young children and infants has required a reconsideration of this issue. Currently, studies are being planned to evaluate the impact of ca vaccine administration when introduced in conjunction with other routine children's vaccines. However, one of the pressing needs for the development of the ca vaccine is to determine whether protective immunogenicity is compromised when a bivalent or trivalent preparation is administered and, if so, whether this interference can be overcome. Previous studies comparing monovalent and bivalent ca A vaccine (H1N1 and H3N2) administration in seronegative children demonstrated that the frequency of seroconversion was higher when vaccines were administered individually rather than simultaneously.[79, 176] Using simultaneous administration of 105 median ($TCID_{50}$), 50 of each of three ca vaccines (H1N1, H3N2, and B [less than 100 human infectious doses, HID_{50} per vaccine component]), Belshe and associates[177] evaluated the question of trivalent vaccine interference in infants. Among the seropositive children, few children shed vaccine virus, and few increases in antibody to any of the three vaccine components were observed. Within the triply seronegative infant group, 47% shed all three ca vaccine viruses, and 75% of these infants had a significant antibody rise to all three ca vaccine components. Of those who showed either shedding or antibody rise to two of the three ca vaccine components, no strain pair preference was observed. These results suggest that in infants and children not previously exposed to influenza, it may be possible to identify an appropriate dose (e.g., 100 HID_{50} per vaccine component) that could stimulate antibody response to all three components.

The question of serological and/or protective interference in the adult population has been raised but not answered, in relation to the bivalent ca A vaccine efficacy studies.[168, 176, 178] Trivalent vaccine administration has been evaluated in adults having low antibody levels to all three components. In the adult population, a reduction in virus shedding and a trend toward lower antibody responses has been observed in vaccinees receiving the trivalent ca vaccine when compared with either bivalent A or monovalent B controls.[179] Although these results do not answer the question of protective interference, they suggest that careful attention to optimization of the reassortant process and manufacturing processes (e.g., high PFU to particle ratios) will be needed to enhance the maximal response of each influenza vaccine component.

SIDE EFFECTS

Fever and Other Symptoms

The safety of the ca A vaccine has been repeatedly demonstrated when given at dosages that approximate 100 HID_{50}. In adults, some degree of reactogenicity, as measured by excess frequency of mild respiratory symptoms, is routinely seen in 8 to 10% of the adult ca vaccine recipients.[168] At dosages above the recommended level, fever and myalgia are observed in some vaccinees.[180] In infants and children receiving the recommended dosage of vaccine, no discernible clinical illness associated with ca A vaccine has been observed.[181–183] More recently, focus on the development of the ca B influenza virus vaccine also has confirmed observations made during the 1970s regarding the safety of the ca B vaccine in adults.[184–187] Although evaluations of the ca B vaccine in infants and children have not been as extensive, two studies using either the ca B/Ann Arbor/1/86 (CRB117) or the ca B/Texas/84 (CRB87) vaccine also have demonstrated an excellent safety profile when given at doses 100 times the HID_{50}.[187, 188]

Complications

Although ca vaccine virus isolates continue to be evaluated for reversion of the ca and ts phenotype to a wild or virulent phenotype, no such reversion has ever been observed. The possible spread of the attenuated virus to nonimmunized individuals also has been considered. In studies conducted by Wright and colleagues[189] in a vaccine clinic daycare setting, no virus transmission was observed among children who had received ca vaccine and nonimmunized seronegative children. Similarly, there has been no evidence of any severe or rare complication associated with the administration of ca vaccine. Although the safety experience with this vaccine has been outstanding in every population tested, it would be foolish to categorically state that rare complications or side effects could never occur with this vaccine.

INDICATIONS FOR IMMUNIZATION

Pediatric Populations

If one focuses on epidemiology of influenza virus epidemics in school-aged children, it is apparent that infection in this age group is skewed toward overrepresentation during the early phases of the epidemic, suggesting that this population is important in the subsequent spread of the disease.[164, 190] Annual influenza infection rates have been estimated to average 42 per 100 children younger than 5 years. The highest illness rates also are seen in this population (35%) and in elementary school-aged children (39%).[143, 144] Although the current Advisory Committee on Immunization Practices (ACIP) recommendations for influenza virus vaccination do not include the general use of influenza virus vaccine in this population,[147, 191] the potential health impact of this approach has encouraged clinical investigation in the young.

Several studies have been conducted to assess the relative efficacy of the ca vaccine and TIV in school-aged children. Clover and colleagues evaluated 191 children, 3 to 18 years of age, in a double-blind placebo-controlled study.[178] During the 1985 to 1986 influenza season, these volunteers experienced a heterotypic influenza outbreak (A/Taiwan/86 [H1N1]). An age-dependent difference in the efficacy of the vaccines was observed. In the 3- to 9-year-old category, only 1 of the 22 children (4.5%) receiving two doses of the ca vaccine was infected, compared with 8 of 33 children (24.2%) receiving two doses of TIV and 10 of 30 children (33.3%) in the placebo group. However, similar enhanced levels of protection in the ca vaccine group were not observed during the subsequent year's H3N2 outbreak.[192] The poor serological response to the H3N2 component of the ca vaccine (A/Bethesda H3N2) may explain these findings to some degree. During the 1985 to 1986 season, only 3.3% of the children vaccinated with the ca vaccine had a fourfold or greater neutralizing antibody rise. For the H3N2 vaccine component, the postvaccination geometric mean titer (GMT) of the TIV group in all age categories was significantly higher than the GMTs for children of comparable ages who had received the ca or placebo. Despite the poor serum IgG response to ca vaccination, protection was still evident in this age group. In the placebo group, 36% of children were infected, compared with 24% in the ca vaccine group and 11% in the TIV group. In addition, of the eight children infected in the ca vaccine group, only one had a febrile illness, compared with three of five in the TIV group and 8 of 18 in the placebo group.

High-Risk Populations

The development of the ca vaccine has increasingly focused on the safety, immunological response, and efficacy of the vaccine in high-risk populations. For influenza virus infections, high-risk populations are defined as those at increased risk of severe influenza-related disease and death. As defined by the ACIP,[147] groups at increased risk of influenza complications include the following:

1. Persons 65 years of age and older
2. Residents of nursing homes and other chronic-care facilities housing persons of any age with chronic medical conditions
3. Adults and children with chronic disorders of the pulmonary or cardiovascular systems, including children with asthma
4. Adults and children who have required regular medical follow-up or hospitalization during the preceding year because of chronic metabolic diseases (including diabetes mellitus), renal dysfunction, hemaglobinopathies, or immunosuppression (including immunosuppression caused by medications)
5. Children and teenagers (6 months–18 years of age)

who are receiving long-term aspirin therapy and therefore may be at risk of developing Reye syndrome after influenza.

Adults

The ca vaccine has been evaluated in several of these groups. Gorse and colleagues[193, 194] have shown the ca vaccine to be safe and immunogenic in a high-risk adult population having moderate to severe chronic obstructive pulmonary disease. As was seen by Clements and colleagues,[167] the antibody responses of these high-risk volunteers receiving ca vaccine were primarily secretory IgA, although very little difference in serum HAI response was observed in volunteers receiving either ca vaccine or TIV. Safety has been demonstrated in detailed evaluation of pulmonary functions in asthmatic adults receiving ca vaccine. No significant alterations in pulmonary function, as measured by spirometry and histamine bronchoprovocation in the first week following ca vaccination were detected.[194]

The use of this vaccine in high-risk children has also been evaluated and found to be safe.[195] Influenza ca vaccines were shown to be safe and immunogenic in cystic fibrosis patients.[196]

Perhaps the most extensively studied high-risk group has been the elderly. In an effort to improve the protective efficacy of the currently licensed inactivated influenza vaccine in the elderly population, Treanor and colleagues[197] conducted a randomized, double-blind, placebo-controlled trial in 662 elderly residents (mean age, 84.2 years) in long-term care units. The trial was designed to evaluate the protective efficacy of combined vaccination with intranasal ca influenza A vaccine and parenteral TIV compared with TIV alone. Volunteers who received combined vaccination and who were subsequently exposed to influenza A had significantly lower rates of influenza A infection than those who had received TIV alone. Although all 3 years of the study were associated with acute but mild influenza A infections, two cases of influenza A resulted in pneumonia and hospitalization, and one of those patients died. Both cases occurred in the TIV group. These results suggest a potential role of ca vaccine as an adjuvant in the elderly.

CONTRAINDICATIONS TO IMMUNIZATION

Immunosuppression or Preexisting Antibody

The possible risks associated with introduction of a live-attenuated virus in an immunocompromised patient have resulted in exclusion of this population from enrollment in clinical studies on ca vaccine. Because a good alternative to the ca vaccine exists—the inactivated influenza vaccine—it is unlikely that such studies would be considered. The presence of preexisting influenza antibody is not considered a contraindication. As discussed previously, the safety, immunogenicity, and protective efficacy of seropositive, immunosuppressed volunteers receiving the ca vaccine have been extensively evaluated, and no deleterious effects have ever been observed.

Pregnancy

Influenza infection of pregnant women in the second or third trimester has been associated with an increased risk of death.[198–200] This risk has led the ACIP to recommend that women who will be in the second or third trimester of pregnancy during the influenza season should be vaccinated, as the vaccine is considered safe for pregnant women.[147] The possible association of fetal malformations or childhood malignancies with congenital infection with influenza virus has been extensively evaluated by MacKenzie and Houghton,[200] with no consistent association found. This lack of association led the authors to suggest that vaccination with live attenuated influenza vaccines should present little risk to the fetus. This recommendation, however, was tempered with the reality that the experiences evaluated would not allow for a definitive conclusion; thus, attempts made in this direction should proceed with caution. To date, however, no such studies have been conducted.

CURRENT STATUS OF THE VACCINE

The live, attenuated, ca influenza vaccine technology of H. F. Maassab was licensed by Aviron in 1995 from the University of Michigan and the National Institutes of Health (NIH). Before 1995, over 90 clinical trials of ca vaccine strains, derived using the Maassab ca master strains, types A and B, were conducted by the Vaccine Treatment and Evaluation Units of the National Institute of Allergy and Infectious Diseases of the NIH, many of which were described in more detail earlier in the chapter.

The current clinical trial program being conducted by Aviron in collaboration with the NIH is designed to support application to the Food and Drug Administration for product approval in 1999 for use in children, adults, and the elderly.[201] The product is a trivalent formulation (two type A strains and one type B strain, each at a potency of $10^{7.0 \pm 0.5}$ $TCID_{50}$/dose) of the live, attenuated, ca influenza vaccine (CAIV-T) delivered intranasally as a spray. The current spray device is a needleless glass syringe fitted with a dose divider and a pressure-activated dispersion tip that delivers 0.25 mL of vaccine to each nostril as an aerosol mist (mean particle size, 62 μm). Its simple design and ease of use makes self-administration in adults and adult-assisted delivery in children possible. This vaccine provides an alternative to the injectable vaccine for healthy and high-risk children and adults and would be coadministered with the injectable vaccine in the elderly.

Aviron and the NIH initially conducted a double-blind, placebo-controlled study of CAIV-T to demonstrate efficacy of the intranasal trivalent formulation in healthy adults.[202] Volunteers were randomized to receive either CAIV-T, the inactivated injectable vaccine, or

Table 37–4. **EFFICACY OF ONE OR TWO DOSES OF LIVE ATTENUATED COLD ADAPTED INFLUENZA VACCINE FOR THE PREVENTION OF CULTURE-CONFIRMED INFLUENZA ILLNESS**

INFLUENZA TYPE	RANDOMIZED TO ONE DOSE			RANDOMIZED TO TWO DOSES AND TWO DOSES RECEIVED			ALL STUDY SUBJECTS*		
	Cases of Influenza			Cases of Influenza			Cases of Influenza‡		
	Vaccine *N = 189*	*Placebo* *N = 99*	**Efficacy (95% confidence interval)**	*Vaccine* *N = 849*	*Placebo* *N = 410*	**Efficacy (95% confidence interval)**	*Vaccine* *N = 1070*	*Placebo* *N = 532*	**Efficacy (95% confidence interval)**
Any influenza	3	14	89 (65–96)	10	74†	94 (88–97)	14	95†	93 (88–96)
A/H3N2	2	8	87 (47–97)	4	49†	96 (90–99)	7	64†	95 (88–97)
B	1	6	91 (46–99)	6	31†	91 (78–96)	7	37†	91 (79–96)

*Efficacy calculation in this category includes all children randomized to one dose, all children randomized to two doses and two doses received, and, in addition, children randomized to two doses but who had wild type influenza prior to dose two or for some reason did not receive dose two (see text). The latter children account for one additional case in the vaccinated children and seven additional cases in the placebo recipients.

†Six children had two influenza illnesses, with influenza A/H3N2 and influenza B isolated. These children are counted once for the "any influenza" efficacy calculation, and all six were in the two-dose cohort.

‡Includes febrile and nonfebrile disease.

placebo and then challenged 1 month later with the wt influenza virus, to which they were originally determined to be seronegative. The reduction in laboratory-documented influenza illness due to the wt H1N1, H3N2, or B strains compared with placebo was statistically significant for CAIV-T (85% [78–100% for all three strains; P = 0.001]) and the injectable vaccine (71% [60–100% for all three strains; P = 0.01]).

Following routine testing of the intranasal CAIV-T vaccine for safety, immunogenicity, and determination of dose in children,[203] Aviron and the NIH conducted a multicenter, randomized, double-blind, placebo-controlled field efficacy trial in 1602 children, 15 to 71 months of age, during the 1996 to 1997 influenza seasons. The trivalent formulation contained $10^{6.7}$ $TCID_{50}$/dose of each attenuated vaccine strain matching the hemagglutinin (HA) and neuraminidase (NA) antigens as recommended by the Food and Drug Administration for the 1996 to 1997 influenza season (A/Texas/36/91-like [H1N1], A/Wuhan/359/95-like [H3N2] and B/Harbin/6/94-like). No serious adverse events were associated with the vaccine; however, low-grade fever (mean, 100.7°F) was more common on day 2 following the first dose of vaccine. Rhinorrhea, or nasal congestion, was significantly more common among vaccinees on days 2, 3, 8, and 9 after the first dose. No significant differences between placebo and vaccine recipients were detected after the second dose. One dose of the vaccine stimulated a fourfold antibody rise to H3 (92%), B (88%), and H1 (16%) among seronegative children, and these rates increased to 96, 96, and 61%, respectively, after dose two (given 1–2 months apart). The vaccine was 93% efficacious (95% CI = 87–96%) against culture-confirmed influenza (Table 37–4). One or two doses of the vaccine were effective against A/H3N2 and B strains, which circulated in the 1996 to 1997 influenza season. The efficacy against A/H3N2 was 95%, and the efficacy against influenza B was 91%. In addition, there was a 30% reduction in febrile otitis media in the children vaccinated with CAIV-T.[203–205]

Of the 1602 children enrolled in year 1 of the randomized, placebo-controlled efficacy study, 1358 returned in year 2 (1997–1998 influenza season).[206] They remained in their randomized groups and were vaccinated with a single dose of CAIV-T or a placebo spray. During the second year of the study, CAIV-T provided 87% protection against all culture-confirmed influenza, including the A/Sydney strain, a strain with substantial antigenic drift from the A/Wuhan/359/95 (H3N2) strain in the vaccine. In the 1358 participants, there were five cases of influenza due to influenza strains included in the vaccine and 66 cases caused by the A/Sydney strain. Only 2% of the children vaccinated with CAIV-T (15 out of 917) experienced culture-confirmed influenza, all of which was attributable to the A/Sydney strain, whereas 13% of the placebo recipients (56 out of 441) experienced culture-confirmed influenza. The incidence of pneumonia and other lower respiratory tract diseases was also reduced in the vaccinees, compared with the placebo recipients. Eight children in the placebo group developed influenza-related wheezing, bronchitis, or pneumonia compared with no children who received CAIV-T. The year 2 data also showed that CAIV-T provided 94% protection against influenza-related otitis media (2 cases in the vaccine group vs 17 cases in the placebo group). These data suggest that the immunity induced by the CAIV-T was broad-based and that cold-adapted live attenuated vaccines have the potential to provide protection against heterologous influenza viruses.

Because the ca influenza vaccine is delivered as a nasal spray, it should provide the first practical way to immunize children on an annual basis. Children are an important target because, although the elderly experience the greatest mortality from the annual influenza epidemic, much of the morbidity and illness occurs in young children. Children are also thought to be important to the spread of influenza in the population. In addition to its proposed use in physician's offices, the nasal delivery of this vaccine should enable it to be administered by adults without special medical training, so that it will be practical to consider delivery in pharmacies, schools, daycare centers, and possibly in the home.

Clinical trials to obtain effectiveness data in healthy working adults and safety data in asthmatic children are in progress. Additional trials are planned for the 1998 to 1999 influenza season to study herd immunity in children and efficacy of coadministration in high-risk adults.

Of note, a novel method that uses the reverse genetics technology discovered by Dr. Peter Palese (Mt. Sinai Medical Center) to generate the vaccine strains each year (6:2 reassortants) has recently been developed.[206] It is now possible to selectively introduce the HA and NA gene segments of wt influenza A or B virus directly into the ca A and B master strains without in vitro propagation of wt influenza virus. This method should significantly shorten the time required to prepare 6:2 reassortants for the annual vaccine and improve reliability of the reassortment process by eliminating gene dominance that can occur using traditional methods. The vaccine virus prepared by the recombinant method has been shown to be safe, immunogenic, and protective in animal disease models. The antigenicity is identical to that of 6:2 reassortants derived using classical methods, and the nucleotide sequence of the HA and NA genes match the HA and NA of their respective wt influenza virus strains from which they were obtained. The safety of vaccine virus prepared using the recombinant methodology has been shown in a clinical trial completed this year.

Acknowledgments

The early research from this laboratory on ca viruses was supported in part by the U.S. Army Medical Research and Development Command, Department of the Army, contracts DA-49-193-MD-2066, DADA-17-70-C-0050, and DAD-17-C-3060. Since 1976, the research on influenza virus has been supported by contracts N01-AI-72521, N01-AI-52564, and N01-AI-05053; National Institute of Allergy and Infectious Diseases, Development and Application Branch, Bethesda, MD 20892; and the Aviron contract entitled "Roundtable Research Agreement," Mountain View, CA.

REFERENCES

1. Thomson D, Thomson R. Influenza with special reference to the complications and sequelae, bacteriology of influenzae pneumonia, pathology, epidemiological data, prevention and treatment. Ann Pickett-Thomson Research Lab 10:641–677, 1934.
2. Smith W, Andrewes CH, Laidlaw PO. A virus obtained from influenza patients. Lancet ii:66–68, 1933.
3. Francis T, Jr. Transmission of influenza by a filterable virus. Science 80:457–459, 1934.
4. Francis T, Jr. A new type of virus from epidemic influenza. Science 92:405–408, 1940.
5. Magill TP. A virus from cases of influenza-like upper respiratory infection. Proc Soc Exp Biol Med 45:73–164, 1940.
6. Taylor RM. Studies on survival of influenza virus between epidemics and antigenic variants of the virus. Am J Public Health 39:171–178, 1949.
7. Francis T, Jr., Quilligan JJ, Jr, Minuse E. Identification of another epidemic respiratory disease. Science 112:495–497, 1950.
8. Douglas RG, Edelson PJ. Respiratory viral infections. In Fishman A (ed). Pediatric pulmonary disease and disorders. New York, McGraw-Hill Book Company, 1988, pp 1583–1588.

8a. Centers for Disease Control and Prevention. Advisory Committee on Immunization Practices. Prevention and control of influenza. Morbidity and Mortality Weekly Report, 45:1–24, 1996.

9. Kilbourne ED. Influenza. New York, Plenum Book Company, 1987.
10. Frances JT, Maassab HF. Influenza viruses. In Harsfall FL, Tarуru I (eds). Viral and Rickettsial Infections of Man (4th ed). Philadelphia, JB Lippincott, 1965, pp 689–740.
11. Krug RM (ed). The Influenza Viruses. New York, Plenum Press, 1991.
12. Portner A, Webster RG, Bean WH. Similar frequencies of antigenic variation in Sendai vesicular stomatatis and influenza A viruses. Virology 104:235–238, 1980.
13. Holland J, Spindler K, Horodyski F, et al. Rapid evolution of RNA genomes. Science 215:1577–1585, 1982.
14. Burnet FM, Lind, PE. Recombination of characters between two influenza virus strains. Aust J Sci 12:109–110, 1949.
15. Hirst GK, Gotlieb T. The experimental production of combination forms of virus. II. A study of serial passage in the allantoic sac of agents that combine the antigens of two distinct influenza A strains. J Exp Med 98:53–70, 1953.
16. Shaw MW, Arden NH, Maassab HF. New aspects of influenza viruses. Clin Microbiol Rev 5:74–92, 1992.
17. Kilbourne ED. The influenza viruses and influenza—an introduction. In Kilbourne ED (ed). The Influenza Viruses and Influenza. New York, Academic Press, 1975, pp 319–350.
18. Andrewes CH, Laidlaw PP, Smith W. The susceptibility of mice to the viruses of human and swine influenza. Lancet ii:859, 1934.
19. Burnet FM, Bull DR. Changes in influenza virus associated with adaptation to passage in chick embryos. Aust J Exp Biol Med Sci 21:55–69, 1943.
20. Isaacs A, Edney M. Variation in laboratory stocks of influenza viruses: Genetic aspects of the variations. Br J Exp Pathol 31:209–216, 1950.
21. Burnet FM. Influenza virus infections of the chick embryo by the amniotic route. Aust J Exp Biol Med Sci 18:353–360, 1940.
22. Burnet FM. Growth of influenza virus in the allantoic cavity of the chick embryo. Aust J Exp Biol Med Sci 19:291, 1941.
23. Henle W, Liu OC. Studies on host-virus interactions in the chick embryo-influenza virus system. VI. Evidence for multiplicity reactivation of inactivated virus system. J Exp Med 94:305–322, 1951.
24. Fraser KB. Genetic interaction and interference between MEL and NWS strains of influenza A virus. Br J Exp Pathol 34:319, 1953.
25. Simpson RW, Hirst GK. Genetic recombination among influenza viruses. I. Cross reactivation of plaque-forming capacity as a method for selecting recombinants from the progeny of crosses between influenza A strains. Virology 15:436–451, 1961.
26. Appleyard G, Maber HB. Plaque formation by influenza viruses in the presence of trypsin. J Gen Virol 25:351–357, 1974.
27. Simpson RW, Hirst GK. Temperature-sensitive mutants of influenza A virus: Isolation of mutants and preliminary observations on genetic recombination and complementation. Virology 35:41–49, 1968.
28. Sugiura A, Tobita K, Kilbourne ED. Isolation and preliminary characterization of temperature-sensitive mutants of influenza virus. J Virol 10:639–647, 1972.
29. Mahy BWJ. Mutants of influenza virus. In Palese P, Kingsbury DW (eds). Genetics of Influenza Viruses. Vienna, Springer-Verlag, 1983, pp 194–254.
30. Almond JW, McGeoch D, Barry RD. Method for assigning temperature-sensitive mutations of influenza viruses to individual segments of the genome. Virology 81:62–73, 1977.
31. Almond JW, McGeoch D, Barry RD. Temperature-sensitive mutants of fowl plaque virus: Isolation and genetic characterization. Virology 92:416–427, 1979.
32. Palese P, Ritchey MB, Schulman JL. P1 and P3 proteins of influenza virus are required for complementary RNA synthesis. J Virol 21:1187–1195, 1977.
33. Palese P, Schulman JL. Mapping of the influenza virus genome: Identification of the hemagglutinin and the neuraminidase genes. Proc Natl Acad Sci U S A 73:2142–2146, 1976.
34. Schulman JL, Palese P. Selection and identification of influenza virus recombinants of defined genetic composition. J Virol 20:248–254, 1976.
35. Ritchey MB, Palese P, Schulman JL. Mapping of the influenza virus genome. III. Identification of genes coding for nucleoprotein, membrane protein, and nonstructural protein. J Virol 20:307–313, 1976b.
36. Ritchey MB, Palese P, Schulman JL. Differences in protein patterns of influenza A viruses. Virology 76:122–128, 1977.
37. Palese P, Ritchey MB, Schulman JL. Mapping of the influenza virus genome. II. Identification of the P1, P2 and P3 genes. Virology 76:114–121, 1977.
38. Laver WG, Air GM, Dopheide TA, Ward CW. Amino acid sequence changes in the hemagglutinin of A/Hong Kong (H3N2) influenza virus during the period 1968-77. Nature 283:454–457, 1980.
39. Van Wyke KL, Hinshaw VS, Bean WJ, Jr, Webster RG. Antigenic variation of influenza A virus nucleoprotein detected with monoclonal antibodies. J Virol 35:24–30, 1980.
40. Webster RG, Kendal AP, Gerhard W. Analysis of antigenic drift in recently isolated influenza A (H1N1) viruses using monoclonal antibody preparations. Virology 96:258–264, 1979.
41. Webster RG, Hinshaw VS, Berton MT, et al. Antigenic drift in influenza viruses and association of biological activity with the topography of the hemagglutinin molecule. In Nayak DP, Fox CF (eds). Genetic Variation Among Influenza Viruses. ICN-UCLA Symposia on Molecular and Cellular Biology. Vol. 21. New York, Academic Press, 1981, pp 243–251.
42. Gething M-J, Sambrook J. Expression of cloned influenza virus genes. In Palese P, Kingsbury DW (eds). Genetics of Influenza Viruses. Vienna, Springer-Verlag, 1983, pp 169–191.
43. Lamb RA. The influenza virus RNA segments and their encoded proteins. In Palese P, Kingsbury DW (eds). Genetics of Influenza Viruses. Vienna, Springer-Verlag, 1983, pp 26–59.
44. Air GM, Compans, RW. Influenza B and influenza C viruses. In Palese P, Kingsbury DW (eds). Genetics of Influenza Viruses. Vienna, Springer-Verlag, 1983, pp 280–304.
45. Enami M, Luytjes W, Krystal M, Palese P. Introduction of site-specific mutations into the genome of influenza virus. Proc Natl Acad Sci U S A 87:3802–3805, 1990.
46. Enami M, Palese P. High-efficiency formation of influenza virus transfectants. J Virol 65:2711–2713, 1991.
47. Luo G, Luytjes W, Enami M, Palese P. The polyadenylation signal of influenza virus mRNA involves a stretch of uridines followed by the RNA duplex of the panhandle structure. J Virol 65:2861–2867, 1991.
48. Webster RG, Bean WJ, Gorman OT, et al. Evolution and ecology of influenza A viruses. Microbiol Rev 56:152–179, 1992.
49. Wiley DC, Wilson IA, Skehel JJ. Structural identification of the antibody-binding sites of Hong Kong influenza hemagglutinin and their involvement in antigenic variation. Nature 238:373–378, 1981.
50. Wilson IA, Skehel JJ, Wiley DC. Structure of the hemagglutinin membrane glycoprotein of influenza virus at 3A resolution. Nature 289:366–373, 1981.

51. Webster RG, Laver WC, Air GM. Antigenic variation among type A influenza viruses. In Palese P, Kingsbury DW (eds). Genetics of Influenza Viruses. Vienna, Springer-Verlag, 1983, pp 309–322.
52. Colman, PM. Neuraminidase: enzyme and antigen. In Krug RM (ed). The Influenza Viruses. New York, Plenum Press, 1991, pp 175–210.
53. Young JF, Desselberger U, Palese P. Evolution of human influenza A viruses in nature. Sequential mutations in the genomes of new H1N1 isolates. Cell 18:73–83, 1979.
54. Krystal M, Young JF, Palese P, et al. Sequential mutations in the hemagglutinins of influenza B virus isolates. Definition of antigenic domains. Proc Natl Acad Sci U S A 80:4527–4531, 1983.
55. Burnet FM. Principles of Animal Virology (1st ed). New York, Academic Press, 1955.
56. Webster RG, Laver WG, Air GM, Schild GC. Molecular mechanisms of variation in influenza viruses. Nature 296:115–121, 1982.
57. Both GW, Sleigh MJ. Complete nucleotide sequence of the hemagglutinin gene from a human influenza virus of the Hong Kong subtype. Nucl Acids Res 8:2561–2757, 1980.
58. Beare AS, Bynoe ML, Tyrrell DAJ. Investigation into the attenuation of influenza viruses by serial passage. Br Med J 4:482, 1968.
59. Krystal M, Buonagurio D, Young JF, Palese P. Sequential mutations in the NS genes of influenza virus field strains. J Virol 45:547–554, 1983.
60. Hall CB, Douglas RG, Fralonardo SA. Live attenuated influenza virus vaccine trial in children. Pediatrics 56:991–998, 1975.
61. Palese P, Young JF. Molecular epidemiology of influenza virus. In Palese P, Kingsbury DW (eds). Genetics of Influenza Viruses. Vienna, Springer-Verlag, 1983, pp 321–336.
62. Minor TE, Dick EC, Dick RC, Inhorn SL. Attenuated influenza A vaccine (Alice) in an adult population: Vaccine-related illness, serum and nasal antibody production and intrafamily transmission. J Clin Microbiol 2:403, 1975.
63. Zaky DA, Douglas RG, Jr, Betts RF, et al. Safety and efficacy of "Alice" influenza virus vaccine in normal healthy adults. J Infect Dis 133:669–675, 1976.
64. Mackenzie JS. Virulence of temperature-sensitive mutants of influenza virus. BMJ 3:757–758, 1969.
65. Florent G. Gene constellation of live influenza A vaccines. Arch Virol 64:171–173, 1980.
66. Hay AJ, Bellamy AR, Abraham G, et al. Procedures for characterization of the genetic material of candidate vaccine strains. In International Symposium of Influenza Immunization, Vol. 2, Geneva 1977. Developments in Biological Standardization. Basel, Karger, 39:15–24, 1977.
67. Kilbourne ED. Future influenza vaccines and the use of genetic recombinants. Bull World Health Organ 41:643, 1969, pp 643–645.
68. Beare AS, Hall TS. Recombinant influenza-A viruses as live vaccines for man. Lancet 2:1271–1273, 1971.
69. Beare AS, Schild GC, Craig JW. Trials in man with live recombinants made from A/PR/*8/34 (H1N1) and wild H3N2 influenza viruses. Lancet 2:729–732, 1975.
70. Beare AS. Research into the immunization of humans against influenza by means of living viruses. In Beare AS (ed). Basic and Applied Influenza Research. Boca Raton, FL, CRC Press, 1982, pp 110–115.
71. McCahon D, Beare AS, Stealey VM. The production of live attenuated influenza A strains by recombination with A/Okuda/57. Postgrad Med J 52:389–394, 1976.
72. Steinhoff MC, Halsey NA, Wilson MW, et al. Comparison of live-attenuated cold-adapted and avian-human influenza A/Bethesda/85-H3N3 reassortant virus vaccines in infants and children. J Infect Dis 162:394–401, 1990.
73. Murphy BR, Sly DL, Tierney EL, et al. Influenza A reassortant virus derived from avian and human influenza A viruses is attenuated and immunogenic in monkeys. Science 218:1330–1332, 1982.
74. Steinhoff MC, Halsey NA, Fries LF, et al. The A/Mallard/6750/78 avian/human, but not the A/Ann Arbor/6/60 cold-adapted, influenza A/Kawasaki/86 (H1N1) reassortant virus vaccine retains partial virulence for infants and children. J Infect Dis 163:1023–1028, 1991.
75. Murphy BR, Snyder MH, Bucker-White AJ, et al. Avian-human influenza A virus reassortants as live virus vaccines in humans. In Mahy B, Kolakofsky D (eds). The Biology of Negative Strand Viruses. New York, Elsevier Science Publishers, 1987, pp 210–220.
76. Kim HW, Arrobio JO, Brandt CD, et al. Temperature-sensitive mutants of influenza A virus: Response of children to the influenza A/Hong Kong/68 ts-1 (E) (H3N2) candidate vaccine viruses and significance to neuraminidase antigen. Pediatr Res 10:238–242, 1976.
77. Murphy BR, Tolpin MD, Massicot JG, et al. Escape of a highly defective influenza A virus mutant from its temperature-sensitive phenotype by extragenic suppression and other types of mutation. Ann NY Acad Sci 354:172–182, 1980.
78. Murphy BR, Chanock RM. Genetic approaches to the prevention of influenza A virus infection. In Nayak DP (ed). Genetic Variation Among Influenza Viruses. New York, Academic Press, 1981, pp 601–616.
79. Wright PF, Okabe N, McKee KT, Jr, et al. Cold-adapted recombinant influenza A virus vaccines in seronegative young children. J Infect Dis 146:71–79, 1982.
80. Tolpin MD, Clements ML, Levine MM, et al. Evaluation of a phenotypic revertant of the A/Alaska/77/ts-1A1 reassortant virus in hamsters and in seronegative adult volunteers: Further evidence that the temperature-sensitive phenotype is responsible for attenuation of ts-1A2 reassortant viruses. Infect Immunol 36:645–650, 1982.
81. Maassab HF. Adaptation and growth characteristics of influenza virus at 25°C. Nature 213:612–614, 1967.
82. Maassab HF, Monto AS, DeBorde DC, et al. Development of cold recombinants of influenza virus as live virus vaccines. In Nayak D, Fox CF (eds). Genetic Variation Among Influenza Viruses. New York, Academic Press, 1981, pp 617–637.
83. LaMontagne JR, Wright PF, Clements ML, et al. Prospects for live, attenuated influenza vaccines using reassortants derived from the A/Ann Arbor/6/60 (H2N2) cold-adapted (ca) donor virus. In Laver WG (ed). The Origin of Pandemic Influenza Viruses. Amsterdam, Elsevier Science, 1983, pp 243–257.
84. Maassab HF. Development of variants of influenza virus. In Barry RD, Mahy BWJ (eds). The Biology of Large RNA Viruses. New York, Academic Press, 1970, pp 542–546.
85. Davenport FM, Hennessy AV, Maassab HF, et al. Pilot studies on recombinant cold-adapted live type A and B influenza virus vaccines. J Infect Dis 136:17–25, 1977.
86. Monto AS, Miller FD, Maassab HF. Evaluation of an attenuated, cold-recombinant influenza B virus vaccine. J Infect Dis 145:57–64, 1982.
87. Alexandrova GI, Smorodintsev AA. Obtaining of an additionally attenuated vaccinating cryophilic influenza strain. Rev Roum Inframicrobiol 2:179–189, 1965.
88. Ghendon YZ, Polezhaev FI, Lisovskaya KV, et al. Recombinant cold-adapted attenuated influenza A vaccines for use in children: Molecular genetic analysis of the cold-adapted donor and recombinants. Infect Immunol 44:730–733, 1984.
89. Alexandrova GI, Polezhaev FI, Budilovsky GN, et al. Recombinant cold-adapted attenuated influenza A vaccines for use in children. Reactogenicity and antigenic activity of cold-adapted recombinants and analysis of isolates from the vaccines. Infect Immunol 44:734–739.
90. Campbell D, Sweet C, Hay AJ, et al. Genetic composition and virulence of influenza virus: Differences in facets of virulence between two pairs of recombinants with RNA segments of the same parental origin. J Gen Virol 58:387–398, 1982.
91. Murphy BR, Clements ML, Tierney EL, et al. Dose response of influenza A/Washington/897/80 (H3N2) avian-human reassortant virus in adult volunteers. J Infect Dis 152:225–229, 1985.
92. Ghendon YZ, Klimov AI, Alexandrova GI, Polezhaev FI. Analysis of genome composition and reactogenicity of recombinants of cold-adapted and virulent virus strains. J Gen Virol 53:215–224, 1981.
93. Murphy BR, Hinshaw VS, Sly DL, et al. Virulence of avian influenza A viruses for squirrel monkeys. Infect Immunol 37:1119–1126, 1982.
94. Snyder MH, Clements ML, Betts RF, et al. Evaluation of live avian-human reassortant influenza A H3N2 and H1N1 virus

vaccines in seronegative volunteers. J Clin Microbiol 23:852–857, 1986.
95. Snyder MH, Clements ML, Herrington D, et al. Comparison of avian-human influenza A virus reassortants derived from different avian influenza virus donors: Studies in squirrel monkeys, chimpanzees, and adult volunteers. J Clin Microbiol 24:467–469, 1986.
96. Almond JW, Cann AJ. Attenuation. In Roitt IM (ed). Immune Intervention. Vol. 1. New Trends in Vaccines. New York, Academic Press, 1984, pp 13–49.
97. Herlocher ML, Maassab HF, Webster RG. Molecular and biological changes in the cold-adapted "master strain" A/AA/6/60 (H2N2) virus. Proc Natl Acad Sci U S A 90:6032–6036, 1993.
98. Herlocher ML, Clavo AC, Maassab HF. Sequence comparisons of A/AA/6/60 influenza viruses: Mutations which may contribute to attenuation. Virus Res 42:11–25, 1996.
99. Chanock RM, Murphy BR, Kai C-J, et al. Prospects for stabilization of attenuation. In Stuart-Harris CH, Potter CW (eds). The Molecular Virology and Epidemiology of Influenza. New York, Academic Press, 1984, pp 115–120.
100. Maassab HF, DeBorde DC. Development and characterization of cold-adapted viruses for use as live virus vaccines. Vaccine 3:355–369, 1985.
101. Snyder MH, Betts RF, DeBorde D, et al. Four viral genes independently contribute to attenuation of live influenza A/Ann Arbor/6/60 (H2N2) cold-adapted reassortant virus vaccines. J Virol 62:488–495, 1988.
102. Donabedian AM, DeBorde DC, Cook S, et al. A mutation in the PA protein gene of cold-adapted B/Ann Arbor/1/66 influenza virus associated with reversion of temperature sensitivity and attenuated virulence. Virology 163:444–451, 1988.
103. Alexandrova GI, Garmashova LM, Golubev DB, et al. Experience in selection of safe thermosensitive recombinants of influenza virus [in Russian]. Vopr Virusol 4:342–346, 1979.
104. Kendal AP, Maassab HF, Alexandrova GI, Ghendon YZ. Development of cold-adapted recombinant live, attenuated influenza A vaccines in the U.S.A. and U.S.S.R. Antiviral Res 1:339–365, 1981.
105. Cox NJ, Kendal AP, Shilov AA, et al. Comparative studies on A/Leningrad/134/57 wild-type and 47-times passages cold-adapted mutant influenza viruses: Oligonucleotide mapping and RNA-RNA hybridization studies. J Gen Virol 66:1694–1704, 1985.
106. Maassab HF. Biologic and immunologic characteristics of cold-adapted influenza virus. J Immunol 102:728–732, 1969.
107. Beare AS, Maassab HF, Tyrrell DAJ, et al. A comparative study of attenuated influenza viruses. Bull World Health Organ 44:593, 1971.
108. Davenport FM, Hennessy AV, Minuse E, et al. Pilot studies on mono and bivalent live attenuated influenza virus vaccines. Proc Symp Live Influenza Vaccine, Yugoslav Acad Sci Arts, Zagreb 6/7:105–113, 1971.
109. Smith GL, Murphy BR, Moss B. Construction and characterization of an infectious vaccinia virus recombinant that expresses the influenza virus hemagglutinin and that induces resistance to influenza virus infection in hamsters. Proc Natl Acad Sci U S A 80:7155–7159, 1983.
110. Buonagurio DA, Krystal M, Palese P, et al. Analysis of an influenza A virus mutant with a deletion in the NS segment. J Virol 49:418–425, 1984.
111. Maassab HF, DeBorde DC. Characterization of an influenza A host range mutant. Virology 130:342–350, 1983.
112. Douglas GR. Influenza in man. In Kilbourne ED (ed). The Influenza Viruses and Influenza. New York, Academic Press, 1975, pp 395–447.
113. Stuart-Harris CH. Influenza and Other Virus Infections of the Respiratory Tract. Baltimore, Williams & Wilkins, 1965.
114. Stuart-Harris CH. Influenza—the human disease. In Stuart-Harris CW, Schild GC (eds). Influenza, the Viruses and the Disease. Littleton, Mass, Publishing Sciences Group, 1976.
115. Klenk H-D, Rott R. The molecular biology of influenza virus pathogenicity. Adv Virus Res 34:247–281, 1988.
116. Tateno I, Suzuki S, Nakamura S, Kawamura A, Jr. Rapid diagnosis of influenza by means of fluorescent antibody technic. I. Some basic informations. Jpn J Exp Med 35:383, 1965.
117. Mulder J, Hers JF. Influenza. Groningen, Netherlands, Wolters-Noordhoff, 1972.
118. Smith H, Sweet C. Pathogenesis of influenza virus infection in ferrets, a model for human influenza. In Stuart-Harris CH, Potter CW (eds). The Molecular Virology and Epidemiology of Influenza. New York, Academic Press, 1984, pp 122–125.
119. Stanley ED, Jackson GG. Viraemia in Asian influenza. Trans Assoc Am Physicians 79:376, 1966.
120. Naficy K. Human influenza infection with proved viremia. N Engl J Med 269:964, 1963.
121. Minuse E, Willis PW III, Davenport FM, Francis T, Jr. An attempt to demonstrate viremia in cases of Asian influenza. J Lab Clin Med 59:1016, 1962.
122. Morris JA, Kasel JA, Saglam M, et al. Immunity to influenza as related to antibody levels. N Engl J Med 274:527, 1966.
123. Khakpour M, Saidi A, Naficy K. Proved viraemia in Asian influenza (Hong Kong variant) during incubation period. Br Med J 4:208, 1969.
124. Lazarowitz SG, Choppin PW. Enhancement of infectivity of influenza A and B viruses by proteolytic cleavage of the hemagglutinin polypeptide. Virology 68:440–454, 1975.
125. Klenk H-D, Rott R, Orlich M, Biodorn J. Activation of influenza A viruses by trypsin treatment. Virology 68:426–439, 1975.
126. Schulman JL, Palese P. Virulence factors of influenza A viruses. WSN virus neuraminidase required for productive infection in MDCK cells. J Virol 24:170–176, 1977.
127. Baum LG, Paulson JC. The N2 neuraminidase of human influenza virus has acquired a specificity complementary to the hemagglutinin receptor specificity. Virology 180:10–15, 1991.
128. Francis T, Jr, Maassab HF. Influenza viruses. In Horsfall FL, Jr, Tarur I (eds). Viral and Rickettsial Infections of Man. Philadelphia, JB Lippincott, 1965, pp 689–740.
129. Schulman JL, Kilbourne ED. Experimental influenza virus infection of mice. Proc First Intern Symp Aerobiol, Berkeley, University of California Press, 1963, pp 141–146.
130. Schulman JL. Experimental transmission of influenza virus infection in mice. IV. Relationship of transmissability of different strains of virus and recovery of airborne virus in the environment of infector mice. J Exp Med 125:479–488, 1967.
131. Schulman JL. The use of an animal model to study transmission of influenza virus infection. Am J Public Health 58:2092–2096, 1968.
132. Davenport FM. Influenza viruses. In Evans AS (ed). Viral Infections of Humans-Epidemiology and Control. New York, Plenum Medical Books, 1982, pp 110–120.
133. Glezen WP. Serious morbidity and mortality associated with influenza epidemics. Epidemiol Rev 4:25–44, 1982.
134. Stuart-Harris CH, Schild G. The epidemiology of influenza and the epidemiology of influenza. Part II. In Stuart-Harris CH, Schild G (eds). Influenza, the Viruses and the Disease. Littleton, MA, Publishing Sciences Group, 1976, pp 80–105.
135. Assad F, Cockburn WS. A seven-year study of W.H.O. Virus Laboratory reports on respiratory viruses. Bull World Health Organ 51:437–445, 1974.
136. Hemmes JH, Winkler KC, Kool SM. Virus survival as a seasonal factor in influenza and poliomyelitis. Nature 188:430–431, 1960.
137. Harper GJ. The influence of environment on the survival of airborne virus particles in the laboratory. Arch Ges Virusforsch 13:64–69, 1963.
138. Davey MI, Reid D. Relationship of air temperature to outbreaks of influenza. Br J Prev Soc Med 26:28–30, 1972.
139. Fox JP, Kilbourne ED. Epidemiology of influenza—summary of influenza workshop IV, from the National Institutes of Health. J Infect Dis 128:361–386, 1973.
140. Noble GR. Epidemiological and clinical aspects of influenza. In Beare AS (ed). Basic and Applied Influenza Research. Boca Raton, FL, CRC Press, 1982, pp 86–95.
141. Monto AS, Kioumehr F. The Tecumseh Study of Respiratory Illness. IX. Occurrence of influenza in the community, 1966–1971. Am J Epidemiol 102:553–563, 1975.
142. Fox JP, Hall CE, Cooney MK, Foy HM. Influenza virus infection in Seattle families, 1975–1979. I. Study design, methods and the occurrence of infections by time and age. Am J Epidemiol 116:212–227, 1982.
143. Hall CE, Cooney MK, Fox JP. The Seattle virus watch. IV. Comparative epidemiological observation of infection with influenza A and B viruses, 1965–1969, in families with young children. Am J Epidemiol 98:365–380, 1973.

144. Glezen WP, Six HR, Frank AL, et al. Impact of epidemics upon communities and families. In Kendal AP, Patriarca PA (eds). Options for the Control of Influenza; Proceedings of a Viratek–UCLA Symposium. New York, Alan R Liss, 1986, pp 63–75.
145. Murphy BR, Clements ML, Maassab HF, et al. The basis of attenuation of virulence of influenza virus for man. In Stuart-Harris CH, Potter CW (eds). The Molecular Virology and Epidemiology of Influenza. New York, Academic Press, 1984.
146. Collins SD. Influenza in the United States, 1887–1956. Public Health Monographs No. 48. Washington, DC, Government Printing Office, 1957.
147. Centers for Disease Control and Prevention. Prevention and control of influenza: recommendation of the Advisory Committee on Immunization Practices (ACIP). MMWR 46(No.RR-9):1–25, 1977.
148. Choi K, Thacker CB. Improved accuracy and specificity of forecasting deaths attributed to pneumonia and influenza. J Infect Dis 144:606–608, 1981.
149. Philip RN, Bell JA, Bean MO, et al. Epidemiologic studies on influenza in familial and general population groups, 1951–1956. II. Characteristics of occurrence. Am J Hyg 73:123–137, 1961.
150. Clark PS, Feltz ET, List-Young B, et al. An influenza B epidemic within a remote Alaskan community. JAMA 214:507–517, 1970.
151. Foy HM, Cooney MK, Allan I. Longitudinal studies of types A and B influenza among Seattle school children and families, 1969–1974. J Infect Dis 134:362–369, 1976.
152. Frank AL, Taber LH, Glezen PW, et al. Influenza B virus infections in the community and the family: The epidemics of 1976–1977 and 1979–1980 in Houston, Texas. Am J Epidemiol 118:313–325, 1983.
153. Schild GC, Pereira MS, Chakraverty P, et al. New antigenic variants of influenza B virus. BMJ 4:127–134, 1973.
154. Czekalowski JW, Prasad AK. Studies on influenza virus. I. Antigenic variations in influenza type C. Arch Ges Virusforsch 42:215–227, 1973.
155. Chakraverty P. Antigenic relationships between influenza C viruses. Arch Virol 58:341–348, 1978.
156. Couch RB, Kasel JA. Immunity to influenza. Ann Rev Microbiol 37:529–549, 1983.
157. Ada GL, Jones PD. The immune response to influenza virus infection. In Kendal A, Patriarca P (eds). Options for the Control of Influenza UCLA-ICN Symposia on Molecular and Cellular Biology, New Series. Vol 36. New York, Alan R Liss, 1986, pp 107–124.
158. Stuart-Harris CH, Schild G. Immunity in influenza. In Stuart-Harris CH, Schild G (eds). Influenza, the Viruses and the Disease. Littleton, MA, Publishing Sciences Group, 1976.
159. Benegar KB, Small PA. Immunoglobulin A mediation of murine anti-influenza virus immunity. J Virol 65:2146–2148, 1991.
160. Virelizier JL. Host defenses against influenza virus: The role of anti-hemagglutinin antibody. J Immunol 115:434–439, 1975.
161. Virelizier JL, Oxford JS, Schild GC. Mechanisms of immunity to influenza in experimental animals. The role of humoral immunity in host defense against influenza A infection in mice. Postgrad Med J 52:332–337, 1976.
162. Fox JP, Cooney MK, Hall CE, Foy HM. Influenza virus infections in Seattle families, 1975–1979. II. Pattern of infection in invaded households and relation of age and prior antibody to occurrence of infected and related illness. Am J Epidemiol 116:228–242, 1982.
163. Askonas BA, McMichael AJ, Webster RG. The immune response to influenza viruses and the problems of protection against infection. In Beare AS (ed). Basic and Applied Influenza Research. Boca Raton, FL, CRC Press, 1982, pp 70–85.
164. Zhdanov VM. Live influenza vaccines in USSR: Development of studies and practical application. In Kendal A, Patriarca P (eds). Options for the Control of Influenza UCLA-ICN Symposia on Molecular and Cellular Biology, New Series. New York, Alan R Liss, 1986, pp 193–206.
165. Clements ML, O'Donnell S, Levine MM, et al. Dose response of A/Alaska/6/77 (H3N2) cold-adapted reassortant vaccine virus in adult volunteers: Role of local antibody in resistance to infection with vaccine virus. Infect Immunol 40:1044–1051, 1983.
166. Murphy BR, Clements ML, Madore HP, et al. Dose response of cold-adapted, reassortant influenza A/California/10/78 virus (H1N1) in adult volunteers. J Infect Dis 149:816, 1984.
167. Clements ML, Betts RF, Tierney EL, et al. Serum and nasal wash antibodies associated with resistance to experimental challenge with influenza A wild-type virus. J Clin Microbiol 24:157–160, 1986.
168. Edwards KM, Dupont WD, Westrich MK, et al. A randomized controlled trial of cold-adapted and inactivated vaccines for the prevention of influenza A disease. J Infect Dis 169:68–76, 1994.
169. Gorse GJ, Belshe RB. Enhancement of anti-influenza A virus cytotoxicity following influenza A virus vaccination in older, chronically ill adults. J Clin Microbiol 28:2539–2550, 1990.
170. Gorse GJ, Belshe RB. Enhanced lymphoproliferation to influenza A virus following vaccination of older, chronically ill adults with live, attenuated viruses. Scand J Infect Dis 23:7–17, 1991.
171. Wright PF, Johnson PR, Karzon DT. Clinical experience with live, attenuated vaccines in children. In Kendal AP, Patriarca PA (eds). Options for the Control of Influenza; Proceedings of a Viratek–UCLA Symposium. New York, Alan R Liss, 1986, pp 243–254.
172. Clements ML, Betts RF, Tierney EL, Murphy BR. Comparison of inactivated and live influenza A virus vaccines. In Kendal AP, Patriarca PA (eds). Options for the Control of Influenza; Proceedings of a Viratek–UCLA Symposium. New York, Alan R Liss, 1986, pp 255–270.
173. Couch RB, Quarles JM, Cate TR, Zahradnik JM. Clinical trials with live, cold-reassortant influenza virus vaccines. In Kendal AP, Patriarca PA (eds). Options for the Control of Influenza; Proceedings of a Viratek-UCLA Symposium. New York, Alan R Liss, 1986, pp 223–241.
174. Johnson PR, Feldman S, Thompson JM, et al. Immunity to influenza A virus infection in young children: A comparison of natural infection, live cold-adapted and inactivated vaccines. J Infect Dis 154:121–126, 1986.
175. Mitchell DM, McMichael AJ, Lamb JR. The immunology of influenza. Br Med Bull 41:80–85, 1985.
176. Wright PF, Bhargava M, Johnson PR, et al. Simultaneous administration of live, attenuated influenza A vaccines representing different serotypes. Vaccine 3:305–308, 1985.
177. Belshe RB, Anderson EL, Newman F, et al. Immunization of infants and young children with live attenuated trivalent cold recombinant influenza A H1N1, H3N2 and B Vaccine. J Infect Dis 165:727–732, 1992.
178. Clover RD, Crawford S, Glezen WP, et al. Comparison of heterotypic protection against influenza A/Taiwan/86 (H1N1) by attenuated and inactivated vaccines to A/Chile/83-like viruses. J Infect Dis 163:300–304, 1991.
179. Keitel WA, Couch RB, Quarles J, et al. Trivalent live cold-adapted influenza virus vaccine: Evidence for virus interference in susceptible adults. J Infect Dis 167:305–311, 1993.
180. Betts RF, Douglas RG, Maassab HF, et al. Analysis of virus and host factors in a study of A/Peking/2/79 (H3N2) cold-adapted vaccine in which vaccine-associated illness occurred in normal volunteers. J Med Virol 126:175–183, 1988.
181. Anderson EL, Belshe RB, Bartram J, Maassab HF. Evaluation of cold-recombinant A/Korea (CR-59) virus vaccine in infants. J Clin Microbiol 27:909–914, 1989.
182. Belshe RB, Van Voris. Cold-recombinant influenza A/California/10/78 (H1N1) virus vaccine (CR-37) in seronegative children: Infectivity and efficacy against investigational challenge. J Infect Dis 149:735–740, 1984.
183. Wright PF, Karzon DT. Live attenuated influenza vaccines. Prog Med Virol 34:70–88, 1987.
184. Clements ML, Snyder MH, Sears SD, et al. Evaluation of the infectivity, immunogenicity, and efficacy of live cold-adapted influenza B/Ann Arbor/1/86 reassortant virus vaccine in adult volunteers. J Infect Dis 161:869–877, 1990.
185. Keitel WA, Couch RB, Cote TR, et al. Cold recombinant influenza B/Texas/1/84 vaccine virus (CRB87): Attenuation, immunogenicity, and efficacy against homotypic challenge. J Infect Dis 161:22–26, 1990.
186. Monto AS, Miller FD, Maassab HF. Evaluation of an attenuated, cold-recombinant influenza B virus vaccine. J Infect Dis 145:57–64, 1982.
187. Davenport FM, Hennessy AV, Maassab HF, et al. Pilot studies on recombinant cold-adapted live type A and B influenza virus vaccines. J Infect Dis 136:17–25, 1977.

188. Anderson EL, Newman FK, Maassab HF, Belshe RB. Evaluation of cold-recombinant influenza B/Texas (CRB-87) vaccine in young children. J Clin Micro 30:2230–2234, 1992.
189. Wright PF, Johnson PR, Karzon DT. Clinical experience with live, attenuated vaccines in children. In Kendal AP, Patriarca PA (eds). Options for the Control of Influenza; Proceedings of a Viratek–UCLA Symposium. New York, Alan R Liss, 1986, pp 243–254.
190. Glezen WP, Couch RB, Taber LH, et al. Epidemiologic observations on influenza B infections in Houston, Texas, 1976–1977. Am J Epidemiol 111:13–22, 1980.
191. Murphy BR, Phelan MA, Nelson DL, et al. Hemagglutinin-specific enzyme-linked immunosorbent assay for antibodies to influenza A and B viruses. J Clin Microbiol 13:554–560, 1981.
192. Couch R. Personal communication. Baylor College of Medicine, 1990.
193. Gorse GJ, Belshe RB, Munn NJ. Safety of and serum antibody response to cold-recombinant influenza A and inactivated trivalent influenza virus vaccines in older adults with chronic disease. J Clin Microbiol 24:336–342, 1986.
194. Gorse GJ, Belshe RB, Munn NJ. Superiority of live attenuated compared to inactivated influenza A virus vaccines in older, chronically ill adults. Chest 100:977–984, 1991.
195. King JC, Gross PA, Denning CR, et al. Comparison of live and inactivated influenza vaccine in high-risk children. Vaccine 5:234–238, 1987.
196. Gruber W, Campbell P, Thompson J, et al. Comparison of live attenuated and inactivated influenza vaccines in cystic fibrosis (CF) patients and their families. J Infect Dis 169:241–247, 1994.
197. Treanor JJ, Mattison R, Domyati G, et al. Protective efficacy of combined live intranasal and inactivated influenza A virus vaccines in the elderly. Ann Intern Med 117:625–633, 1992.
198. Schoebaum SC, Weinstein L. Respiratory infection in pregnancy. Clin Obstet Gynecol 22:293–299, 1979.
199. Greenberg M, Jacobziner H, Pakter J, Weisl BAG. Maternal morbidity in the epidemic of Asian influenza, New York City 1957. Am J Obstet Gynecol 76:897–902, 1958.
200. MacKenzie JS, Houghton M. Influenza infections during pregnancy: Association with congenital malformations and with subsequent neoplasms in children, and potential hazards of live virus vaccine. Bacteriol Rev 38:356–370, 1974.
201. Bryant ML, CAIV Research Team. Clinical progress and benefits of cold adapted influenza vaccine in children, adults, and elderly [abstract]. International Conference on Options for the Control of Influenza III. Cairns, Australia, May 4–9, 1996.
202. Treanor J, for P. Glasner. Update on clinical trials of safety an efficacy of trivalent cold-adapted influenza vaccine in children and adults [abstract]. IBC's International Industry Conference on Influenza and Other Respiratory Disorders: Latest Therapeutic and Vaccine Developments. Washington, DC, September 26–27, 1996.
203. King J, Belshe R, Bryant M, NIAID VEU Study Group. Safety and immunogenicity of intranasal live attenuated trivalent cold-adapted influenza vaccine (CAIV-T) given as drops or spray in children [abstract]. Am Soc Ped Res Washington, DC, May 2–6, 1997.
204. Belshe R, Iacuzio D, Mendelman P, Wolff M. Efficacy of a trivalent live attenuated intranasal influenza vaccine in children [abstract]. Infectious Disease Society of America 35th Annual Meeting, San Francisco, September 13–16, 1997.
205. Belshe RB, Mendelman PM, Treanor J, et al. The efficacy of live attenuated, cold-adapted, trivalent, intranasal influenza virus vaccine in children. N Engl J Med 338:1405–1412, 1998.
206. Belshe R, Iacuzio D, Mendelman P, Wolff M, for the NIAID. Efficacy of a trivalent live attenuated intranasal influenza vaccine in children (abstract S-116). 38th Interscience Conference on Antimicrobial Agents and Chemotherapy, San Diego, Sept 24–27, 1988.
207. Li S, Mo D, Bilsel P, Bryant M. Recombinant inactivated and cold-adapted vaccines [abstract]. Tenth International Conference on Negative Strand Viruses: Emergence and Re-emergence of Negative Strand Viruses. Dublin, Ireland, September 21–26, 1997.

chapter

38 Human Immunodeficiency Virus

Marc P. Girard

Jean-Louis Excler

The acquired immunodeficiency syndrome (AIDS) was first described in 1981 as an outbreak of *Pneumocystis carinii* pneumonia in a homosexual community.[1, 2] Serological and epidemiological studies have shown that the disease has spread to almost all countries in the world.[3, 4] It has been estimated that by the end of 1997, 30 million people were living with the human immunodeficiency virus (HIV) worldwide, among whom were more than 1 million children and 10 million women. The cumulative number of reported AIDS cases reached the 11 million mark at that time. Projections predict that by the year 2000, 40 million people in the world will be infected with HIV. UNAIDS, the United Nations AIDS agency, estimated in June 1998 that every day 16,000 people become infected with HIV, 90% of whom live in developing countries.[4a]

HIV is transmitted through contaminated blood or blood products, by use of contaminated needles or surgical instruments, or as a venereal infection. The spread of the epidemic could therefore be stopped or slowed down through simple measures such as screening of blood donations, use of disposable syringes, and use of condoms. However, these measures often meet with profound behavioral resistance or ignorance on the part of the individuals at risk.[5, 5a] A vaccine that would prevent infection with HIV is therefore urgently needed.

The development of effective HIV vaccines is hampered by the very properties of the virus (Table 38–1).

Table 38–1. **OBSTACLES TO THE DEVELOPMENT OF HIV VACCINES**

Antigenic diversity and hypervariability of the virus
Transmission of disease by mucosal route
Transmission of the virus by infected cells
Integration of the virus genome into the host cell chromosomes
Latency of viral infection
Sequestration of the virus in the central nervous system
No spontaneous recovery from natural infection in spite of high-level immune responses of the host
Progressive dysfunction and destruction of the immune system of the host

These properties constitute major differences from "ordinary" viruses, which explains why one doubts whether past successes in the development of vaccines can be easily duplicated in the case of HIV vaccines. Of particular concern is that HIV can persist in the host despite a vigorous and apparently normal immune response. In most individuals, at least during the early stages of infection, HIV elicits a comprehensive cell-mediated immune response that includes natural killer (NK) cell activity and cytotoxic T-lymphocyte (CTL) activity targeted to cells expressing a variety of HIV antigens. In addition, $CD8^+$ T lymphocytes are able to suppress the replication of HIV in vitro by a nonlytic mechanism[6, 7] and to secrete β-chemokines that can block the entry of macrophage-tropic HIV strains.[8, 9] Most individuals infected with HIV eventually mount an antibody response that is capable of neutralizing the infecting virus as well as mediating antibody-dependent cell-mediated cytotoxicity (ADCC) and complement-dependent lysis of infected cells. Why these antiviral mechanisms fail to clear the virus is still unknown. It has been suggested that the enormous turnover of $CD4^+$ T cells eventually exhausts the immune system[10, 11] and that overwhelming virus replication throughout the lymphoid system at the time of primary HIV infection leads to deletion or exhaustion of virus-specific CTL.[12] Progression to AIDS may be accelerated by gradual impairment of cellular immunity.[13] Whether immune mechanisms would be more efficacious if induced in response to vaccination is still to be proven. In spite of the encouraging success of vaccine-induced protection from simian immunodeficiency virus (SIV) in macaques,[14, 15, 15a] continuous efforts are still necessary before simple HIV vaccines can be made available for human use.[16–18a]

VIROLOGY

The etiological agent of AIDS, HIV,[19] was identified in 1983.[20–22] There are two well-defined viruses, HIV-1 and HIV-2,[23] both of which cause disease, but HIV-1 appears to be more aggressive and spreads more rapidly.[24] Both are nontransforming, cytopathic retroviruses belonging to the lentivirus subfamily. Lentiviruses produce characteristically slow, progressive infections, in which the virus causes disease after long periods of latency and persists in the host in spite of the host's active immune response.[25] Other lentiviruses are SIV, the feline immunodeficiency virus, the puma lentivirus, the bovine immunodeficiency virus, the Visna virus of sheep, the caprine arthritis-encephalitis virus, and the equine infectious anemia virus.

The genetic variability of HIV-1 is a major challenge in the development of a globally effective vaccine. A variety of HIV-1 genotypes or clades, designated A through J, and an outlier (O) group have been identified[26–28] (see later section). Recent data indicate that individuals can be infected with viruses belonging to different subtypes, which can result in the production of intersubtype recombinants.[28–30] The concern has been expressed that the amplification and diversification of HIV-1 during the last half-century is likely to be transcended in the next half-century.[30a]

The HIV virion consists of an internal core particle built from 1200 molecules of capsid (p24*gag*) protein (Fig. 38–1) surrounded by a lipid envelope spiked with some 75 oligomers of a highly glycosylated protein, gp160.[31] The core contains two copies of the RNA genome; several molecules of an associated reverse transcriptase; and internal viral proteins such as p1, p2, p6, and the p7*gag* nucleocapsid[32, 33] as well as cytoskeletal proteins such as cyclophilin A, nonmuscle and muscle actin, cofifin, ezrin, and moesin.[34] It also contains copies of viral proteins Vpr, Nef, and Vif, which play a role in early events in HIV replication. The gp160 spikes are made of two noncovalently linked polypeptide chains: the *trans*-membrane chain, gp41, which anchors the spikes in the lipid bilayer of the envelope, maintains their oligomeric structure,[31, 35, 36] and plays a major role in fusion of the virus and cell membranes[37–39]; and the external chain, gp120,[40] which carries the important antigenic determinants of the virus and binds the CD4 receptor and coreceptors[40a] (see later section). The 120-kDa gp120 molecule contains about 50 kDa of carbohydrate consisting of a mixture of high-mannose and complex sialic acid–containing carbohydrates.[40, 41] Folding, assembly, disulfide bond formation, glycosylation, and transport of the envelope protein to the cell surface have been studied in detail.[41–45] The envelope appears to be wrapped around a protein scaffold made of the matrix (p17*gag*) protein[46, 47] (see Fig. 38–1). There is also evidence that the envelope of HIV-1 contains numerous molecules of type II human leukocyte antigen (HLA)–DR and β_2-microglobulin borrowed from the host cell in which the virus last replicated.[48] Cellular components such as CD43, CD44, CD55, CD59, CD63, CD71, and adhesion molecules intercellular adhesion molecule 1 (ICAM-1) and lymphocyte function-associated antigen 1 (LFA-1) are also physically present on the virion surface.[49] This explains why the virus can

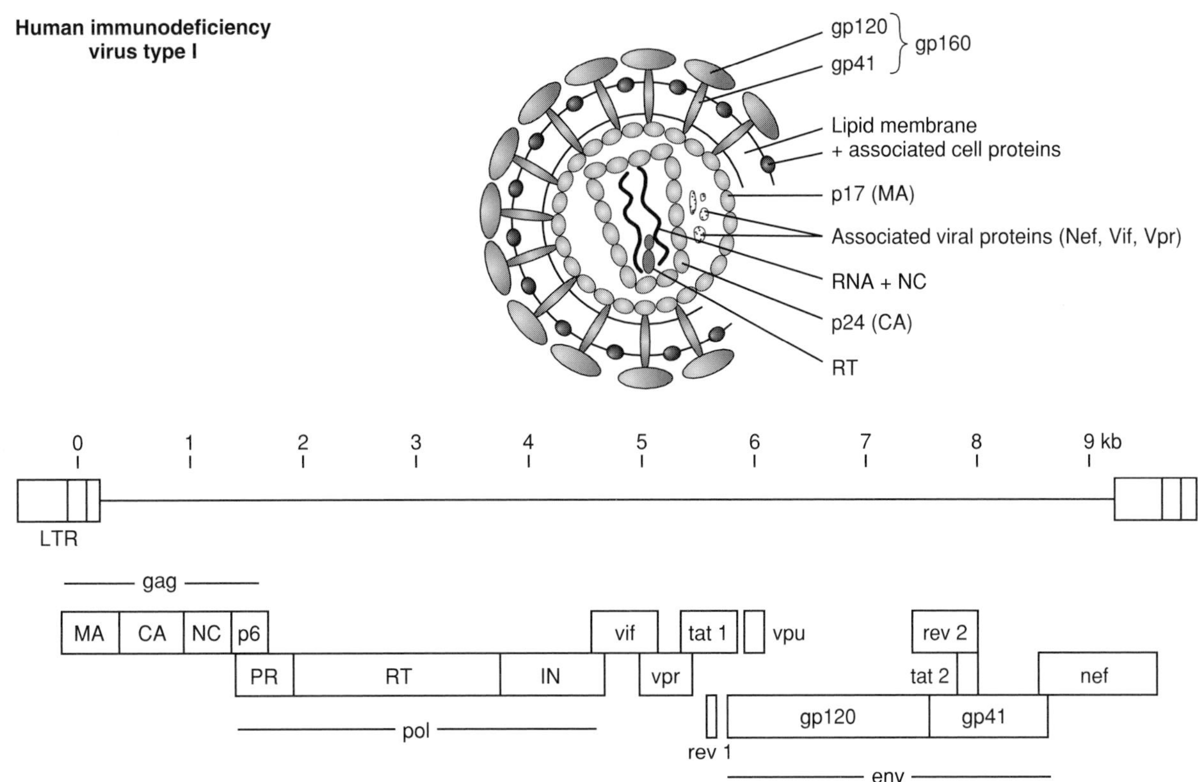

Figure 38–1. A schematic representation of the virion, depicting the viral envelope spiked with glycoprotein gp160 and associated cellular proteins and wrapped over a scaffold of matrix (MA) protein. The capsid, made of CA protein, encloses the dimeric genome RNA associated with the nucleocapsid (NC) protein, together with virion-associated proteins reverse transcriptase (RT), Vif, Vpr, and Nef. The diagram at the bottom represents the virus RNA as a straight line graded in kilobases (kb). The open boxes refer to the open reading frames (genes) on the RNA. IN, integrase; LTR, long terminal repeats; PR, protease.

be neutralized by antibodies to HLA-DR, to LFA-1, to β_2-microglobulin, or to ICAM-1.[50]

The genome of HIV is a single-stranded RNA molecule, 9.5 kilobases in length, that has been extensively studied at the molecular level.[26–28, 51–54] It is flanked by two regulator elements, the long terminal repeats, each containing a transcription promoter and terminator, a polyadenylation signal, and numerous regulatory elements that control the activity of the promoter and respond specifically to regulatory proteins from the host (Sp1, NF-κB, PRD-II factors) or from the virus (Tat protein). The RNA dimerizes through a "kissing loop" interaction involving a specific stem-loop element termed the dimer linkage structure.[55, 56]

The genes of HIV-1 fall into three categories[57]: the structural genes *gag* (core), *pol* (reverse transcriptase), and *env* (gp160), which are the basic genes found in all retroviruses; regulatory genes *tat* and *rev*, a unique feature of lentiviruses[58]; and "accessory" genes, the function of which is still little known, such as *nef*, *vpr*, *vpu*, and *vif*[59, 60, 60a] (Table 38–2). The mRNAs coding for the Gag-Pol, Env, Vif, Vpr, and Vpu proteins are unspliced or single-spliced, whereas those coding for the regulatory proteins are multispliced. This different property is used by the virus for the control of its expression.

The *tat* gene encodes a *trans*-activating protein that acts at the level of transcription by increasing viral mRNA production several hundred-fold through binding to a 59-residue stem-loop at the 5′ end of the nascent RNA molecules, called the transactivation responsive element. Tat thus prevents premature termination of mRNA transcription.[61] The Tat protein does not act alone but acts in conjunction with several host cell factors such as the Tat-associated kinase Cdk9 which phosphorylates RNA polymerase II.[60a, 62]

Table 38–2. **PRINCIPAL ROLES OF THE HIV ACCESSORY PROTEINS**

Vpr	Together with matrix protein, targets the viral preintegration complex to the nucleus through interaction with importin-α and nucleoporin Arrests dividing cells in G_2 of the cell cycle
Vpu	Down-regulates expression of CD4 molecules by targeting them to the proteosome, leading to their degradation in the endoplasmic reticulum Forms ion channels in the cell membrane, thus helping to promote the release of virions from infected cells
Vif	Plays a role in provirus formation and stabilizes newly synthesized DNA intermediates Associates with cytoskeleton intermediate filaments and helps transport incoming virions to the nucleus
Nef	Associates with cellular protein kinases (PAK65, p56tck, p59Hck) Stimulates viral DNA synthesis and enhances virus infectivity in primary T cells and macrophages Enhances virus replication in vivo, contributing to high viral loads and pathogenesis Binds CD4 molecules at the plasma membrane and mediates their rapid endocytosis and lysosomal degradation Down-regulates cell surface expression of major histocompatibility class I antigens, a cytotoxic T-lymphocyte escape mechanism

The *rev* gene encodes a protein that is required for efficient expression of the structural virus genes. The unspliced or single-spliced mRNAs contain multiple nuclear retention sequences, also called *cis*-acting repression sequences, that prevent them from migrating from the nucleus to the cytoplasm in the absence of Rev.[63] The Rev protein binds to a specific sequence element on these RNAs, the Rev-responsive element, and allows the mRNAs to migrate from the nucleus to the cytoplasm of the infected cell by interacting with nuclear export factors exportin-1 and Ran GTPase.[58, 60a, 63, 64] This, in turn, leads to virus assembly, maturation, and release of the virus particles through budding at the cell surface. At the same time, the expression of the regulatory proteins is down-regulated. The Rev protein thus controls the switch from an early phase of the virus cycle, when only regulatory viral proteins are synthesized, to a late phase, when structural proteins are made and virions assembled.[65]

The precise role and importance of *vif*, *vpu*, *vpr*, and *nef* are still not completely understood[59, 60, 60a, 66] (see Table 38–2). Vpr and Vpu are required for productive infection in macrophages. Vpr, Vif, and Nef are virion-associated proteins[67] and play a role in the transport of the proviral DNA into the resting host cell nucleus. Vpr arrests dividing cells in G_2 of the cell cycle through phosphorylation/dephosphorylation of several proteins required during mitosis ($p34^{cdc2}$). Vpu is a membrane-spanning protein that plays a role in the release of virus particles from the infected cells. HIV-2 and SIV lack a *vpu* gene but carry another accessory gene, *vpx*, which seems to be a duplication of *vpr*.[68] The *nef* gene, initially believed to code for a negative regulatory factor,[66] appears to be a major virulence factor.[14, 15, 69–72] Nef contributes to the maintenance of high virus loads and is required for pathogenesis, perhaps because it provides the virus with a mechanism for evading the host cellular immune response.[70, 71] Indeed, viruses expressing a fully functional *nef* gene have a strong growth advantage in vivo.[72–74]

Maturation of the core particle requires the proteolytic cleavage of the Gag and Gag-Pol precursor proteins Pr55*gag* and p160*gag-pol*, respectively, into matrix and an intermediate p40*gag* molecule, itself eventually cleaved to generate capsid, nucleocapsid, and the p1, p2, and p6 internal proteins.[33, 75, 76] HIV-1 nucleocapsid, which is at all times tightly associated with the RNA genome, contains two zinc finger motifs that are necessary for packaging of genomic RNA and infectivity.[77] The proteolytic cleavages take place during and after virion budding from the infected cell membrane and are catalyzed by a viral proteinase encoded by the virus *pol* gene. The HIV-1 viral proteinase belongs to the class of aspartyl proteinases. It is a homodimer, each subunit contributing the amino acid triplet DTG to form the active site. The *pol* gene also codes for other key viral enzymes: reverse transcriptase (associated with an RNase H activity) and an integrase that allows the integration of the virus cDNA into the host cell genome. These enzymes constitute prime targets for antiviral therapy.

The gag polyprotein binds to cyclophilin A and incorporates this cellular peptidyl prolylisomerase into virions. Viral isolates from HIV-1 group M require cyclophilin A for replication and are inhibited by cyclosporin A, but these reactions are not observed with isolates from group O.[77a]

VIRUS-CELL INTERACTIONS

The human immunodeficiency virus has been shown to infect cells that express the CD4 (OK-T4) receptor on their surface,[78–80] including helper T lymphocytes, monocytes-macrophages, lymph node follicular dendritic cells, Langerhans cells in the skin, and microglia in the central nervous system. The monocyte-macrophage tropism of HIV-1 strains depends on specific virus envelope determinants (see later) but is also controlled by viral genes *vpr* and *vpu*[59–60a] and cytokines such as transforming growth factor-β.[81] The virus can also infect $CD4^-$ cells, such as glial cells, mammary cells, NK cells, brain endothelial cells, and some gut epithelial cells in culture.[81–83] In several cases, the receptor molecule has been identified as a glycolipid, galactosylceramide.[81–84] Another HIV-1 receptor has been identified on human placenta; it belongs to the family of the C-type mannose-binding proteins.[85]

The CD4-binding domain of the gp120 molecule is a complex conformational motif made of discontinuous parts of the gp120 molecule.[40a, 86–88, 94a, 94b] CD4 binds in a recessed pocket of gp120 flanked by variable regions exhibiting considerable glycosylation, and makes extensive contacts over about 800 Å of the gp120 surface.[40a, 94a, 94b] After binding of gp120 to CD4, sequential conformational changes occur in the molecule[89] that ultimately result in the interaction with the host cell membrane of a fusogenic domain located at the amino terminus of the transmembrane gp41 molecule[37–39, 90, 91] (Fig. 38–2). The

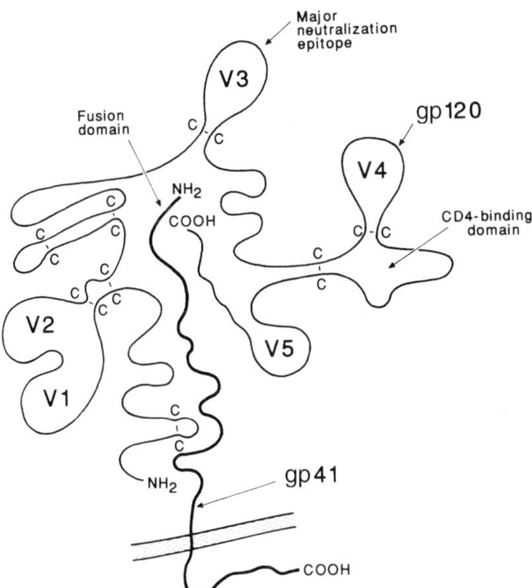

Figure 38–2. A diagrammatic two-dimensional representation of the gp120 molecule indicating the position of the disulfide bridges (C-C) and the five hypervariable domains (V1 to V5). The gp41 molecule has been drawn as a thick wavy line but actually shows extensive folding.[90, 138–140] (Modified from reference 40.)

coiled-coil formation of the leucine zipper domain in gp41[95] may allow the insertion of the fusion domain into the target cell membrane, as suggested for influenza virus hemagglutinin[96] (see later). HIV-1 envelope oligomerization is critical for virus adsorption and entry.[35] This process occurs during the processing and intracellular transport of gp160[43]; it is mediated through gp41.[31, 36, 92, 93]

Most primary HIV isolates obtained at the time of primary infection and during the asymptomatic period of the disease are macrophage-tropic (M-tropic): they replicate in peripheral blood mononuclear cells (PBMCs) but neither form syncytia in culture nor infect $CD4^+$-transformed T-cell lines.[97, 98] Emerging later in infection in association with $CD4^+$ T-cell decline and progression to AIDS are T lymphocyte–tropic (T-tropic) isolates.[99] These replicate in PBMCs as well as in immortalized T-cell lines and are syncytia inducing. A subset of T-tropic virus has been adapted to infect $CD4^+$-transformed T-cell lines, generating T-cell line–adapted (TCLA) virus strains that have lost their ability to replicate efficiently in PBMCs. The M-tropic and T-tropic phenotypes depend on specific envelope determinants located within or in the vicinity of the V3 region,[100–106] which constitutes the "principal neutralization determinant" of HIV-1 TCLA strains.[106–110] Formation of syncytia by TCLA virus strains depends on V3[101, 111] and can be aborted even after the CD4-binding step by V3-targeted neutralizing antibodies (see later section).

The V3 loop of HIV-1 can be cleaved by proteinases such as cathepsin E, tryptase TL-2, thrombin, or unidentified cellular proteinases.[112] This cleavage is greatly enhanced by prior binding to CD4[113] and is completely inhibited by binding of neutralizing antibodies to the V3 loop.[114] These observations have led to the suggestion that on binding of gp120 to CD4, the V3 loop undergoes endoproteolytic cleavage by a cell surface proteinase, which then allows the interaction of the gp41 fusion domain with the cell membrane. This hypothesis has not been confirmed, however.

It was found instead that two distinct chemokine receptors, CXCR-4 (fusin) and CCR-5, act as coreceptors for the T-tropic and M-tropic HIV-1 isolates, respectively.[9, 115–123] These receptors belong to the superfamily of G protein–coupled seven-transmembrane domain glycoproteins. TCLA HIV-1 strains use CXCR-4 as entry coreceptor, whereas M-tropic HIV-1 isolates use CCR-5. A subset of these isolates can also use CCR-3, depending on the sequence of the V1/V2 and V3 loops.[119, 120a] T-tropic primary isolates can use CXCR-4 as well as CCR-5, CCR-3, and CCR-2; they are therefore dual-tropic.[121, 122] Some HIV-2 isolates can use CXCR-4 as an alternative receptor, in the absence of CD4.[124] Unlike HIV-1, both M- and T-tropic SIV strains use CCR-5 but not CXCR-4.[125, 126] Specific SIV coreceptors have recently been identified.[127, 128] Gp120 from TCLA HIV strains can form a trimolecular complex with CD4 and CXCR-4 in vitro, whereas gp120 from M-tropic primary isolates physically interacts with CD4 and CCR-5.[129–131a] The affinity of gp120 for CCR-5 is greatly enhanced in the presence of CD4, suggesting that the latter not only provides a docking surface for gp120 but also triggers the exposure of the chemokine receptor–binding site, which is poorly exposed in the absence of CD4, in large part because of the overlying V2 and V3 loops.[40a] Thus, the real virus receptors are the chemokine receptors, whereas the CD4 receptor acts mostly as a facilitator. Anti-V3 antibodies block chemokine receptor binding.[129–131]

Confirming this model is the fact that CC chemokines RANTES, MIP-1α, and MIP-1β, the three known CCR-5 ligands, potently inhibit the intracellular entry of M-tropic HIV-1 isolates[8, 9] as well as the formation of CD4–gp120–CCR-5 trimolecular complexes in vitro,[130, 131] whereas stromal cell–derived factor 1 (SDF-1), a CXCR-4 ligand, blocks infection with TCLA virus strains.[132, 133] Progressive HIV-1 infection is characterized by the emergence of viruses resistant to inhibition by β-chemokines, which correspond to changes in coreceptor usage. The broadening of the host range may even enable the use of yet uncharacterized receptors.[134] The V3 domain is critical for the chemokine-mediated blockade of infection.[135–137] It is not known why some HIV-1 strains that can efficiently use the macrophage coreceptor CCR-5 nevertheless replicate poorly in primary macrophage cultures.[138]

Another confirmation of the model has come from the observation that individuals who suffer a homozygous defect in the gene encoding CCR-5 show high resistance to HIV-1 infection in vivo.[139] The genetic defect, a 32–base pair deletion that results in a frame shift mutation and generates a nonfunctional CCR-5 receptor, renders PBMCs from these individuals highly resistant to infection by M-tropic HIV-1 isolates in vitro.[138–141] The mutation is present on chromosome 3p21 at a frequency of 9 to 10% in the white population (about 1% *Δccr5/Δccr5* homozygotes) but is absent in black and Japanese populations.[141, 142] A few individuals who are homozygous for the *Δccr5* mutation have nonetheless been found to be infected with HIV-1[143]; the suspicion is that they probably were infected with a T-tropic virus strain that uses the CXCR-4 receptor.

Extensive conformational changes in the HIV envelope complex are thought to be involved during virus-cell fusion.[89] Binding of CD4 to gp120 exposes the chemokine receptor–binding site.[40a, 129–131] For TCLA virus strains, these changes are sufficient to cause gp120 to be "shed" from the virus surface, leaving the membrane-anchored gp41 subunit behind and inactivating the virus.[144] Primary isolates usually do not shed gp120 readily, although they also undergo conformational changes in both gp120 and gp41. These changes are thought to expose the hydrophobic, glycine-rich, N-terminal fusion peptide region of gp41 that is essential for membrane fusion activity.[37, 38] The oligomeric Env complexes on the surface of virus particles and infected cells have been variously described as dimers, trimers, and tetramers but are most likely trimeric.[35, 47, 94a, 94b, 145–147] Crystallographic analysis of the core structure of gp41 shows that it is a six-stranded helical bundle[145–147] with an interior coiled-coil trimer of three parallel helices corresponding to amino acid residues 540 to 590, around which three antiparallel helices corresponding to residues 624 to 665 pack in an oblique, antiparallel manner, in highly conserved, hydrophobic grooves on the surface of the trimer. The hydrophobic fusion peptide is immediately amino-terminal to the central three-stranded coiled-coil.[95, 145–147] This structure shows striking similarity to that of the low pH–induced conformation of the influenza HA2 subunit.[96] Activation of the envelope spike results in a release of the fusion peptide and extension of the coiled-coil structure. The new positioning of the fusion peptides at the tip of the stalk provides for easy contact with the target cell membrane.[146a] The prefusion conformation of gp41 is thought to mimic an "unsprung mousetrap."[147] Binding of HIV to the target cell triggers the gp41 mousetrap to snap closed, bringing into close proximity the transmembrane domain of gp41 and the N-terminal fusion peptide, thus facilitating the coalescence of the viral and cell membranes and, ultimately, membrane fusion.[147] It has been suggested that several gp120/gp41 trimers might assemble as an aster to create a fusion pore.[146] Peptides corresponding to the coiled-coil leucine zipper-like region of gp41, as well as an all D-amino acid fusion peptide,[146a] act as *trans*-dominant inhibitors of fusion.[39, 95, 148]

After the entry of the virus core into the cytoplasm of susceptible cells, the genomic RNA is transcribed by reverse transcriptase into a single-stranded DNA intermediate, then a double-stranded circular DNA that is eventually inserted into the DNA of the host cell as a provirus. In quiescent lymphocytes, this process occurs at a slow rate so that most of the virus is recovered as a labile, partial reverse transcript that is eventually degraded.[149] Unintegrated copies of viral DNA may persist for a long time in the cell cytoplasm. There is evidence that T cells in culture can accumulate up to 80 copies of unintegrated HIV-1 DNA per cell as a consequence of multiple reinfections.[150] In contrast, infected T cells in vivo contain a single copy of viral DNA.[151] Integration and subsequent expression of the provirus remain low-key as long as the host cell is not activated to begin differentiation or replication.[152, 153] Activation can occur in response to mitogens or antigens or in response to specific interleukins such as tumor necrosis factor-α (TNF-α), granulocyte-macrophage colony-stimulating factor, or interleukin (IL)–6.[153] At the molecular level, activation of the HIV-1 provirus results from the intervention of the cellular transcription activating factor NF-κB.[154] In resting cells, NF-κB is blocked in an inactive cytoplasmic complex with an inhibitor (IκB). On activation of the cell, the inhibitor is released and the factor migrates into the cell nucleus, where it binds specific cellular transcription activation sequences. Similar sequences are located upstream from the promoter on the HIV long terminal repeats. The human immunodeficiency virus thus uses for its own activation the activation machinery of the host cell.[154–157]

CLINICAL DISEASE

AIDS, a progressive deterioration of the immune status of the individual, is characterized by the progressive depletion of the CD4$^+$ T-lymphocyte population, which represents a major target of viral infection in vivo and profound perturbations of the cytokine network.[157] At the clinical level, this is characterized by a wide spectrum of clinical illnesses (lymphadenopathy, weight loss, chronic diarrhea, fevers, nephropathy, neuropathies) and the occurrence of opportunistic infections, such as *P. carinii* pneumonia, tuberculosis, *Mycobacterium avium-intracellulare* infections, toxoplasmosis, candidiasis, cryptosporidiosis, severe viral infections (cytomegalovirus, herpes simplex virus, Epstein-Barr virus), and cancers (Kaposi sarcoma and non-Hodgkin B-cell lymphomas of Epstein-Barr virus origin).

Within 2 to 6 weeks after infection, the patient experiences an acute febrile phase with disseminated lymphadenopathy, rash, arthralgia, and myalgia, which is reminiscent of an episode of infectious mononucleosis.[158] A transient decrease in the total lymphocyte count and an inversion of the CD4 to CD8 ratio are observed. Primary infection is accompanied by p24 antigenemia and high plasma viral loads (Fig. 38–3), with HIV-1 RNA levels typically in the range of 2×10^5 to 2×10^7 copies per milliliter (corresponding to 10^5 to 10^7 virions per milliter).[159–162] This burst of virus replication is accompanied by dissemination of the virus to lymphoid organs.[155, 163–166] The patient is highly contagious at this phase but cannot be diagnosed by usual serological procedures. Disappearance of clinical symptoms generally occurs within a few weeks together with down-regulation of viremia, as a consequence of the host's immune response.[161, 162] The major component of the immune response consists of HIV-1–specific $CD8^+$ CTL that are capable of eliminating a large number of virus-expressing cells.[167–170] A similar phenomenon has been observed in experimental SIV infection of rhesus monkeys.[171] In humans, a marked oligoclonal expansion of certain Vβ subsets of $CD8^+$ T cells occurs[167, 170] in association with increased expression of IL-10, TNF-α, and interferon (IFN)–γ,[172] but a significant number of HIV-specific CTL clones seem to rapidly disappear through clonal exhaustion.[12] A humoral immune response eventually follows,[166, 168, 173] and the patient becomes seropositive except in rare cases.[174, 175] In spite of the host's robust immune response, the virus almost invariably escapes from immune containment and establishes a state of chronic, persistent infection.

A long asymptomatic period of clinical latency follows, during which a slow but steady decline in the $CD4^+$ cell number is observed. The patient is infectious because HIV-1 replication continues throughout the course of infection.[151, 176–178] Although a high percentage of peripheral blood cells is actually infected and harbors HIV DNA, most are blocked at an early stage of HIV-1 infection.[149, 179–181] High antibody levels to all virus antigens (Env, Gag, and nonstructural virus proteins) are found in the patient's plasma together with circulating virions. Recent experiments studying the kinetics of viral turnover have estimated that 10^7 to 10^8 virions are produced per day, resulting in viral plasma loads of 10^4 to 10^7 RNA molecules per mL and in the destruction of approximately 2×10^9 $CD4^+$ T cells per day.[10, 11, 161, 180–183] Lymphoid organs tend to be the preferential site for replication as well as a reservoir of "trapped" extracellular virus on follicular dendritic cells.[163–165, 179, 184–188] In HIV-infected chimpanzees, active viral replication was detected in lymphoid organs; cells with transcriptionally silent but inducible HIV genomes circulated in the peripheral blood.[189] The contribution of latent genomes to the virus spread in vivo was thought to be relatively minor.[183] Recent evidence suggests, however, that in addition to the short-lived infected $CD4^+$ T cells, which have a $t_{1/2}$ of 1 to 6 days, long-lived infected cells with a $t_{1/2}$ of 1 to 4 weeks, which might be macrophages, also make a significant contribution to plasma viremia.[190] Indeed, tissue macrophages seem to constitute the major source of increasing viremia that characterizes the last phase of HIV disease, and a variety of opportunistic infections can dramatically increase their production of virus.[191] Infectious HIV-1 also persists latently in a postintegrated form in resting memory CD4 lymphocytes. This reservoir is small, generally

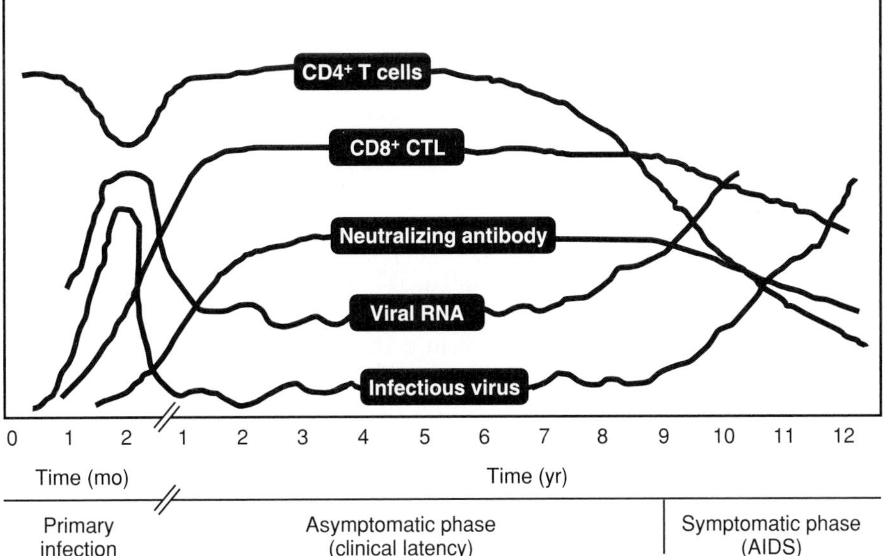

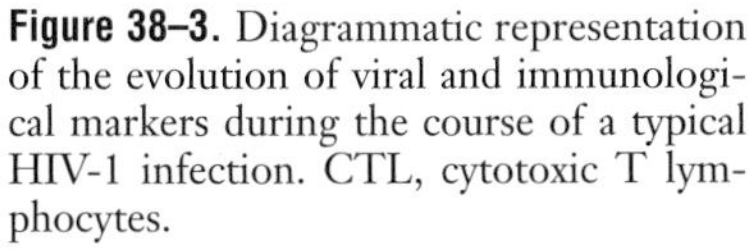
Figure 38–3. Diagrammatic representation of the evolution of viral and immunological markers during the course of a typical HIV-1 infection. CTL, cytotoxic T lymphocytes.

ranging from 10^4 to 10^6 cells per host. Its decay $t_{1/2}$ is about 3 to 5 months.[191a, 191b]

The asymptomatic phase can last from a few months to more than 16 years, after which symptoms appear. These have been classified according to severity and number[192] to define a series of successive stages in the evolution of the disease, such as the *lymphadenopathy syndrome*, the *AIDS-related complex*, and full-blown *AIDS*. The symptomatic phase of the disease is accompanied by p24 antigenemia, an accelerated decrease in the number of CD4+ T cells, a progressive loss of antibodies to Gag proteins and of HIV-specific CTLs, and a greatly increased virus load. Thus, the number of peripheral T4 cells producing HIV-1 can reach 1 in 100 and even 1 in 10 in the terminal stages of the disease, with production of up to 10^{10} virions per day.[10, 11, 161, 177, 178, 180–183] In industrialized countries, and before the advent of tri-therapies, death occurred with a median period of about 10 years, after the T4 cell number had dropped below 50 cells/mm^3, owing to fulgurant opportunistic infections. The survival time of adults and children with HIV infection is considerably shorter in subSaharan Africa, in part because of lack of adequate medical care but probably also because of persistent immune activation and high levels of cytokine secretion associated with chronic infections such as sexually transmitted and parasitic diseases.[155, 193] Studies of HIV infections in West Africa suggest that HIV-2 may induce a more benign form of disease than HIV-1.[23, 24]

Infection with HIV can also manifest itself as a purely cachectic disease, to which the name *slim disease* has been given in Africa. It can also affect the brain directly, causing purely neurological symptoms such as acute encephalitis or progressive dementia *(AIDS dementia complex)*. Virus strains isolated from brain biopsy specimens from deceased patients with neurological AIDS are M-tropic and use the coreceptors CCR-3 and CCR-5.[120]

The rate of progression to disease among people infected with HIV is highly variable among individuals. The reason that long-term nonprogressors remain devoid of symptoms more than 16 years after infection whereas others (the rapid progressors) develop a fatal disease within 2 years is unknown. These differences seem to depend on the age of the individual[194] and also on host and viral factors.[155–157a] Long-term nonprogressors typically show a polyclonal CTL response that is directed against multiple HIV-1 antigens and is maintained over time.[195] Survival analyses clearly show that disease progression is slower in Δ*ccr5* heterozygotes[141, 142] as well as in individuals with a mutation in CCR-2[196] and can vary with HLA alleles. Infections with parasites, bacteria (*Mycobacterium tuberculosis*), viruses (HHV-6, cytomegalovirus, HTLV-I), or mycoplasmas *(M. fermentans, M. penetrans, M. pirum)*[197, 198] have been implicated as possible cofactors. It was recently shown that human cytomegalovirus encodes a β-chemokine receptor, US28, that can serve as coreceptor for the entry of HIV-1 T-tropic as well as M-tropic isolates.[199] There is increasing evidence that the release of β-chemokines by primary PBMCs activated in vitro, including CD4+ cells, correlates with slow or absent progression to HIV disease.[199a–199c]

The steady-state level of plasma viral load from about 6 months after infection strongly predicts how fast the disease will progress.[200–202] Patients with more than 10^5 HIV RNA copies per milliliter of plasma within 6 months of seroconversion are 10-fold more likely to progress to AIDS during 5 years than are those with less than 10^5 copies per milliliter, and maintenance of plasma RNA levels below 10,000/mL in early disease appears to be associated with decreased risk of progression to AIDS. Similarly, plasma viremia levels in SIV-infected macaques are highly predictive of survival time.[203] Active replication of HIV-1 can also be estimated from the level of HIV-1 mRNA in PBMCs.[204] The level of plasma viremia probably depends on the vigor of the individual's immune response to primary infection.[167–170] Such vigor is reflected in the degree of diversity of the CD8+ Vβ repertoire that is mobilized in response to infection: T-cell receptor repertoire responses limited to only one or two Vβ families are associated with rapid disease progression, whereas broader CTL repertoire responses involving multiple Vβ families are associated with a clinically stable course and stable CD4+ T-cell counts.[205]

Patients with AIDS show increased levels of TNF-α; interleukins IL-1, IL-2, and IL-6; soluble IL-2 receptor; interferons IFN-α and IFN-γ; β_2-microglobulin; and neopterin (an interleukin produced by macrophages in response to TNF-α). Secretion of the proinflammatory cytokines TNF-α, IL-6, and IL-1β is increased in PBMCs and lymphoid tissues together with that of IFN-γ. TNF-α, which acts through activation of cellular transcription factor NF-κB, appears to be the most potent of the HIV-inducing cytokines. It has been said that AIDS is a tumor necrosis factor disease.[206] The level of HIV replication in CD4+ cells actually reflects the balance of the opposing effects of suppressive factors, such as the β-chemokines RANTES, MIP-1α, and MIP-1β,[8, 9] and HIV-1–inducing cytokines, such as TNF-α and IL-1β.[153, 155, 207] Another suppressor activity apart from that mediated by the β-chemokines was identified by Walker and colleagues[6, 7] in CD8+ T-cell culture supernatants. This activity is noncytotoxic, non–major histocompatibility complex (MHC) restricted, and mediated by soluble factors distinct from known cytokines.[208, 209]

CD4+ T cells are heterogeneous in their profile of cytokine secretion, designated Th1, Th2, and Th0.[210, 211] Th1 cells produce IL-2, TNF-β, and IFN-γ and promote cellular immunity (CTL), whereas Th2 cells produce IL-4, IL-5, and IL-10, promote humoral immunity, and suppress CTL activity. Th0 cells produce both Th1- and Th2-type cytokines. It has been observed that a shift from the Th1 to the Th2 cytokine profile,[212, 213] or, rather, to the Th0 profile,[214] occurs during the course of HIV infection, leading to AIDS. M-tropic HIV-1 isolates grow in primary CD4+ T cells irrespective of their Th subtype,[215] whereas T-tropic HIV-1 strains proliferate preferentially in Th2- and Th0-type cell clones.[214, 215] This might explain why M-tropic virus strains predominate during the asymptomatic phase of the disease, whereas T-tropic virus strains become dominant when AIDS develops.[99, 216, 217] β-Chemokines RANTES, MIP-1α, and MIP-1β, which inhibit the entry of M-tropic strains, stimulate the growth of T-tropic strains,[207] which would favor the transition to the latter. The extended dominance of M-tropic viruses in HIV-infected long-term nonprogressors[218, 219] argues strongly that host factors are important in controlling the virus population and that conditions favoring the replication of M- rather than T-tropic strains must be prevalent in these individuals.[153]

AIDS patients are anergic to recall antigens, as judged both by absence of delayed-type hypersensitivity (skin test) in vivo and by lack of T helper cell proliferation in vitro. The unresponsiveness to recall antigens could be the direct consequence of HIV infection of follicular dendritic cells, which severely impairs the ability of these cells to present antigens in T-cell responses in vitro.[220, 221] Engagement of T-cell receptors in the absence of a costimulatory signal, such as that provided by the B7-CD28 interaction at the contact between the antigen-presenting cell and the T cell, can lead to long-lived T-cell anergy. Destruction of the infected follicular dendritic cells, perhaps by virus-specific CTL, would lead to the observed destruction of lymph node follicles[184, 185, 188] and to profound immune suppression.[222] In addition, as demonstrated by use of the SCID-hu mouse implanted with human hematolymphoid organs, HIV-1 infection results in suppression of thymopoiesis, thereby precluding regeneration of the peripheral T-cell compartment.[223, 224] The selective loss of in vitro response to recall antigens in individuals who are positive for HIV could also result from active immunosuppression mediated by a soluble factor secreted by $CD8^+$ T cells.[225]

Another problem in the pathophysiology of AIDS is understanding the mechanism responsible for the continuous decline in the number of $CD4^+$ T cells.[155–157] It is not clear if direct killing of $CD4^+$ cells by HIV can explain the full spectrum of AIDS pathogenesis. Chimpanzee-adapted strains of HIV-1 are cytopathic for chimpanzee T cells, grow in chimpanzee macrophages-monocytes, and replicate efficiently in chimpanzees. However, these viruses do not induce AIDS in the animal,[226, 227] to the exception of one reported case.[228] Specific mechanisms have been suggested to account for the depletion of $CD4^+$ cells in HIV-infected humans, such as cytolytic attack by HIV-specific CTL of naive bystander $CD4^+$ cells that have bound virus-shed circulating gp120 molecules[229, 230]; T-cell alloactivation, as in graft-versus-host disease, due to antigenic mimicry of the MHC by the gp120 molecule[231–233]; superantigen-mediated deletion of specific $CD4^+$ T-cell subsets[234]; and apoptosis (programmed cell death),[235–241] perhaps induced by gp120[237] or, possibly, by the Tat protein.[238]

Apoptosis is due to the activation of a nuclear endonuclease that cleaves the DNA in internucleosomal regions, generating a ladder of low-molecular-weight DNA fragments. Apoptosis can be observed early after HIV infection. Interestingly, no apoptotic lymphocytes can be found in HIV-infected chimpanzees or in SIV-infected African green monkeys, which do not develop disease in spite of persistent infection, whereas apoptotic lymphocytes are readily detected in SIV-infected rhesus macaques, which develop a typical AIDS disease.[236, 239] In lymph nodes, apoptosis is found mostly in noninfected bystander cells and not in the productively infected cells, suggesting that apoptotic signals generated by the virus must be transmitted to uninfected cells.[240] Apoptosis can be blocked in vitro by Th1 cytokines IL-2 and IFN-γ and by IL-12, which favors cellular immune responses, whereas it is enhanced by Th2 cytokines IL-4 and IL-10.[241] The detailed mechanisms that lead to apoptosis still remain, however, to be unraveled.

Kaposi sarcoma is the leading neoplasm in AIDS patients. A direct effect of the HIV *tat* gene on the development of Kaposi sarcoma has been reported.[242, 243] However, this does not explain why most HIV patients do not get Kaposi sarcoma and why Kaposi sarcoma can occur in the absence of HIV infection. The involvement of another viral agent (KSHV/HHV-8) is most probable.[244, 245]

Interest has recently been focused on the individuals who remain uninfected and seronegative in spite of definite exposure to HIV-1 and who, in contrast to the *Δccr5* homozygotes,[139–141] have normal *ccr5* genes. These individuals seem to have developed a cellular immune response, including T helper cell proliferation and IL-2 secretion in response to envelope peptides,[246] or Env-specific CTL,[247] albeit in the absence of an antibody response. In addition, class I–restricted CTL activity has been detected against HIV-1 Pol or Nef in repeatedly exposed uninfected African commercial sex workers[248] as well as in uninfected children born to HIV-1–infected mothers[249] and in uninfected heterosexual partners of HIV-1–infected patients.[250] These findings are consistent with the hypothesis that these individuals experienced a silent HIV-1 infection that they were able to clear through a Th1-type cellular immune response and that their CTL activity represents protective immunity against HIV-1.[251] Other mechanisms, such as increased secretion of β-chemokines by $CD8^+$ lymphocytes,[199a–199c, 252] could also be involved. It has been reported that some of the uninfected African commercial sex workers show rare HLA haplotypes.[253] The fact that anti-HIV secretory immunoglobulin (Ig) A can be found in the cervicovaginal secretions of seronegative uninfected heterosexual partners of HIV-infected men[254] also suggests that a locally restricted B-cell response could contribute to protective mucosal immunity against sexual transmission of HIV.

VIRUS VARIABILITY

A remarkable feature of HIV is its genetic variability due to the error-prone nature of the viral reverse transcriptase, which lacks proofreading mechanisms and introduces mutations at the rate of about 3×10^{-5} changes per site per replication cycle.[255] A second factor is the high rate of virus production (up to 10^{10} viruses per day) and the large number of replication cycles (approximately 300 per year) that sustain HIV-1 infection in vivo.[10, 11, 256] The rapid emergence of drug-resistant viral escape mutants[11] illustrates the high rate at which virus variants can be generated.

Many different HIV-1 and HIV-2 strains and isolates have been described.[26, 27] Distinct variants are found within a single patient and can change over time, leading to a mini–evolutionary tree in each individual: HIV does not replicate as a unique molecular species but as a swarm of molecular clones[257–259] that form a "quasispecies."[260] In general, genetic diversity among virus clones within an individual is about 2 to 3%. Selective pressures within the microenvironments of different anatomic compartments result in the emergence in various tissues of anatomically distinct and independently evolving quasispecies.[260a] Because of the sequence variation of the virus, one notes the emergence of escape mutants that arise as a consequence of immune selection and can escape either neutralizing antibodies[261–263] or CTL.[264–268] Some of the virus clones may also be replication defective but are propagated through complementation with replication-competent clones.[269]

Longitudinal studies of individuals infected with HIV-1 show that at the time of primary infection and during the asymptomatic stage of the disease, the virus clones that predominate in the host are slow-growing, non–syncytia-inducing, M-tropic virus clones ("slow-low"), whereas the terminal, clinical phase of the disease sees the emergence of rapidly growing, syncytia-inducing, T-tropic viruses ("rapid-high").[97–99] Sexual transmission of non–syncytia-inducing, M-tropic viruses even in cases in which the donor harbored a syncytia-inducing, T-tropic virus has been well documented.[270] It has become evident that selection operates at the time of infection in favor of M-tropic viruses in each newly infected individual. On the basis of a detailed longitudinal phylogenetic analysis carried out on viral sequences from an HIV-1–infected hemophiliac cohort, it appears that all HIV genotypes in a given individual can be explained by progressive accumulation of mutations in the genotype found at seroconversion[271, 272]; there is no evidence for transmission of multiple genotypes.[273–276] However, owing to rapid diversification in the new host, virus isolates from two directly linked cases can vary by 4 to 7%.[275, 276] Several factors, such as duration of infection, host-immune pressure, disease stage, and therapy, may contribute to the degree and rate of HIV-1 genetic variation. Comparison between rapid and slow progressors shows that the latter develop a more diverse quasispecies over time, probably as a consequence of their more functional immune system.[277] Serial analysis of V3 sequences from epidemiologically linked individuals revealed a preponderance and accumulation of nonsynonymous rather than synonymous mutations in the V3 loop and flanking regions as they diverged over time in vivo, suggesting a dominant role for positive selection for amino acid changes.[278] The rate of evolution in the different individuals was different, suggesting that changes were host dependent. Nevertheless, HIV isolates from people with a common infection link, such as sex partners, mothers and their infants, or blood donors and recipients, show much closer genetic relatedness than do HIV isolates from people without a direct transmission link. Such genetic similarity can be used to investigate possible HIV transmission linkage, as was done in the case of transmission in a dental practice,[279] in the hospital,[280] and in a case of rape.[281]

The extraordinary diversity of the virus is readily apparent at the epidemiological level by the variation of the envelope glycoprotein among strains of HIV-1 from different geographical origins.[26–30, 282] Nucleotide distances of up to 30% in gp120 can be found among different strains. This is particularly true for the hypervariable parts of the molecule, including the V3 loop,[283–286] and constitutes a major problem in the development of an AIDS vaccine. Phylogenetic analysis of envelope sequences has revealed at least 10 genetically distinct HIV-1 subtypes or clades (designated A through J) within the main (M) group[26–28, 30a, 287] and an outlier (O) group in Cameroon and Gabon.[288–290] The two groups, M and O, differ by up to 47% in their Env protein sequences.

The prototype North American–European subtype B contains isolates from most continents because of the early spread of the virus from North America. In contrast, subtypes A and D are recovered mostly from central Africa; subtype C from South and East Africa, India, and China; subtype E from Thailand and neighboring countries in Southeast Asia but also from central Africa[286]; and subtype F from Romania and from Brazil. Progressive diffusion of non-B subtypes into new populations and new places is observed with time, however.[291–293] Phylogenetic classification of HIV-1 based on *gag* sequences shows the existence of seven subtypes, five of which correspond to five of the *env* subtypes.[294] Interestingly, all subtype E viruses thus far characterized fall within subtype A in the *gag* region[53, 54] and in the 3′ half of their gp41 coding region,[28] suggesting that they are the descendants of a hybrid virus generated by intersubtype recombination between subtype A and a no-longer existing subtype E ancestor.[54] Similarly, a high proportion of subtype C, D, and G viruses shows an intersubtype recombinant genome.[28–30, 295] Genetic characterization of a large number of HIV-1 isolates indicates that at least 10% of all strains have mosaic genomes generated by recombination between viruses of the same or different clades. In Africa, the frequency may be as high as 25%.[295, 296] This implies that dual HIV-1 infections and, possibly, superinfections are not rare.[297–299] That interclade recombination can occur in vivo after superinfection was demonstrated unequivocally in a chimpanzee.[300] Thus, intrasubtype and intersubtype recombination can generate yet more viral diversity, with important potential consequences for vaccine development.[28–30a]

In sharp contrast to the case with HIV-1, the region that corresponds to V3 in HIV-2 shows little variability.[301–303] Overall genetic variability among HIV-2 isolates is nevertheless as wide as that among HIV-1 isolates.[26, 27] HIV-1 and HIV-2 show only 40 to 50% genetic similarity, and their envelope glycoproteins are antigenically unrelated. HIV-1 is related to SIVcpz, isolated from a chimpanzee,[304, 305] whereas HIV-2 is closely related to SIVsm, isolated from sooty mangabeys, and to SIVmac from rhesus macaques.[306, 307] It has been suggested that HIV-2 and SIVmac are the result of cross-species transmission of SIVsm from mangabeys to humans and macaques, respectively.[27, 306–309] Sooty mangabeys in the wild remain healthy in spite of persistent SIV infection. Similarly, African green monkeys are chronically infected with another SIV, SIVagm, but do not develop an illness. SIVagm displays the highest genetic diversity of all animal lentiviruses, suggesting that it may be the oldest primate lentivirus.[308] Extensive cross-neutralization of HIV-2, SIVmac, and SIVagm occurs with high titer, reflecting the evolutionary relatedness of the *env* genes in these viruses.[301, 309]

EPIDEMIOLOGY

By the end of 1997, there were globally about 16,000 new HIV-1 infections each day, most of which were in developing countries.[4a] An increasing proportion (42%) were in women, and more than half were in people younger than 25 years.[4]

At the beginning of the epidemic in North America, Europe, and Australia, AIDS occurred principally among homosexual and bisexual men, intravenous drug users, blood transfusion recipients, and hemophiliacs who received contaminated clotting factor concentrates.[3, 4] HIV infections are now also being observed among heterosexual men and women with no other risk factors than multiple sexual partners.[4, 310] The overall incidence rate of new HIV infections has been decreasing recently in North America and western Europe owing to the success of prevention campaigns and antiviral therapy. Still, more than 1.2 million people are currently infected with HIV-1 in that part of the world. Prevalence as a whole is higher in minority communities, low-income groups, and inhabitants of large urban areas.[311] The use of intravenous drugs remains a major risk factor.

In sub-Saharan Africa, where an estimated 21 million people are infected with HIV-1, AIDS spreads mostly through heterosexual contacts. Prevalence surveys of HIV-1 infection among pregnant women in central and eastern African countries often show rates higher than 18%, with record highs of up to 40% in certain places. Similar figures have been reported in parts of South Africa. In groups at risk, such as female prostitutes, prevalence can reach 80%. Wars, social unrest, and political instability generating massive population movements are associated with large increases in incidence of sexually transmitted diseases, including HIV infection.

In Asia, the situation is potentially explosive, in view of the high prevalence in groups at risk, such as intravenous drug users and prostitutes.[312] During the year 1988, HIV rates in intravenous drug users in Bangkok increased from about 1% at the start of the year to more than 30%. A second epidemic began in female prostitutes and was followed by successive waves of transmission to their male clients who were not intravenous drug users and finally to the low-risk nonprostitute wives and girlfriends of these men.[312] A similar pattern of HIV-1 transmission has been observed in India, Laos, Malaysia, Vietnam, and southern China.[313] Because of active prevention campaigns and promotion of condoms, a decrease of HIV-1 incidence has been observed since 1995 in young adult men in Thailand.[5a] However, the epidemic is still progressing in other parts of the population. In India, as in many developing countries, HIV spreads from urban centers to rural areas through migration, labor, and trade. Prevalence of HIV in truck drivers can be as high as 10%.

Major sexual risk factors for homosexuals or heterosexuals include engaging in anal intercourse, increasing the number of sexual partners, having unprotected sexual relations with a partner or partners at an advanced stage of disease, engaging in sex with prostitutes, and contracting other sexually transmitted diseases.[314, 315] Risk of sexual transmission can be as high as 1:2 during the window period of primary infection or at the time of symptomatic stage but as low as 1:2000 with low virus loads. Lack of male circumcision is also a risk factor.[316] In addition, for heterosexuals, intercourse during menses poses a risk for both the uninfected man and the female partner. The presence of HIV and HIV-infected monocytes in semen has been well documented, as has transmission of HIV by vaginal intercourse[313–317] and the risk associated with genital ulcer disease.[317] Asymptomatic seropositive men appear to be fivefold more contagious to their female partners than are asymptomatic seropositive women to their male partners.[314] Possible reasons for the higher rate of heterosexual transmission of HIV in Africa compared with Europe and North America are the greater number of sexual relations, the prevalence of cervical ectopy, and the frequency of sexually transmitted diseases.

The vaginal mucosa of both human beings and macaques is susceptible to infection by primate lentiviruses. In situ polymerase chain reaction analysis has shown that the first cellular targets for genital SIV infection in female macaques are the Langerhans dendritic cells in the lamina propria of the cervicovaginal mucosa, immediately subjacent to the epithelium.[318] Dendritic cells rapidly migrate to the iliac-draining lymph nodes, where they presumably transmit infection. Progesterone implants, which mimic hormonally based contraceptives, enhance vaginal SIV transmission,[319] probably owing to the thinning of the epithelium. Paradoxically, isolated dendritic cells do not support a productive infection with HIV-1[320] because they lack Sp1 transcription factors. Unactivated T cells also do not support productive HIV-1 infection because they lack Rel proteins and NF-κB. HIV-1 infection induces the formation of dendritic cell–T cell syncytia[321] that coexpress NF-κB and Rel and Sp1 proteins and thus can replicate the virus efficiently. HIV-1 can also cross a tight human epithelial cell barrier by transcytosis to gain access to the basolateral side of the epithelium,[322] at least in vitro.

It has been extrapolated from in vitro work with dendritic cells that subtype E and C viruses could be transmitted with greater efficiency by the vaginal route than subtype B viruses, which would explain the rapid heterosexual spread of the HIV epidemic in developing countries.[323] However, subtype B, which is predominant in the Americas and Europe, is also the cause of major documented epidemics of heterosexually transmitted infections in Central America and the Caribbean. Moreover, studies have failed to confirm that non-B virus isolates show a preferential tropism for dendritic cells.[324, 325]

More than 300,000 infants worldwide become infected with HIV-1 each year through maternal-infant transmission. The major risk of maternal HIV-1 transmission appears to occur late during pregnancy or at delivery.[326] Transmission can also occur through breastfeeding, most often in mothers who experience primary infection after delivery.[327, 328] In North America and Europe, children born to mothers infected with HIV-1 run a 12 to 15% risk of being infected. This figure rises to 35 to 50% in African countries. It has been possible to lower the frequency of transmission by two thirds as a result of zidovudine therapy during pregnancy, during delivery, and to the newborn.[329] Risk of transmission from mother to infant increases with lower CD4$^+$ cell count and higher maternal viral load at delivery,[330, 331] although a high viral load seems insufficient to fully explain vertical transmission.[332]

Needles contaminated with HIV, such as those employed by intravenous drug users, are a major risk factor. Tattooing and other forms of exposure to contaminated instruments may also result in virus transmission. The most common route of infection in healthcare workers is through deep needle stick injuries. The risk of contracting HIV after accidental injection with HIV-infected blood is on the average 0.3%.[333]

Transmission of HIV-2 through sexual contact and from mother to infant is estimated at 3 times and 10 times lower, respectively, than that of HIV-1. Consequently, HIV-1 has spread much more rapidly than HIV-2. HIV-1 is encountered in every country in the world, whereas HIV-2 is located mostly in western Africa and a few other parts of the world.[334] Dual infections with both HIV-1 and HIV-2 have been reported, showing that infection with one type of virus does not protect against superinfection with the other type as well.[335] Contradictory results, namely, that preinfection with HIV-2 can protect from HIV-1 infection, have been reported in Senegal, however.[336]

ANTIGENIC DETERMINANTS AND EPITOPES OF INTEREST

The identification of the neutralization epitopes and of epitopes recognized by T helper cells and CTL in HIV antigens is of practical importance for the development of an HIV vaccine.[337]

Neutralizing Antibody Determinants

Neutralizing antibodies recognize both variable and conserved gp120 structures. The V2 and V3 loops contain epitopes for strain-specific neutralizing antibodies. Broadly neutralizing antibodies recognize conserved, conformational, discontinuous epitopes that have been mapped by x-ray to the crystal structure of the gp120 core.[40a, 94a]

The principal neutralizing antigenic determinant of HIV-1 TCLA strains has been mapped to the hypervariable V3 loop of gp120,[107–110] a continuous region of approximately 35 amino acids linked by a disulfide bond (see Fig. 38–2). Linear peptides with the sequence of the V3 loop elicit strain-specific neutralizing antibodies that do not interfere with CD4 binding but neutralize HIV-1 infectivity as a post-binding phenomenon by preventing fusion between virus envelope and cell membrane or between virus-infected and uninfected cells,[338, 339] probably by blocking interaction with the CXCR-4 coreceptor. The V3 loop is highly immunodominant; most HIV-1–infected or gp120/gp160-immunized individuals or animals produce antibodies to this epitope. V3-targeted neutralizing monoclonal antibodies have been demonstrated to protect chimpanzees passively from experimental infection with a TCLA strain of HIV-1.[340] The V3 domain features both hypervariable and relatively conserved neutralization epitopes. The variable sites are highly immunogenic and induce strain-specific neutralizing antibodies.[341–345] The more conserved regions map to the tip of the V3 loop (the GPGRAF motif in clade B viruses) and induce neutralizing antibodies that cross-neutralize HIV-1 TCLA strains with homology in that region.[346, 347]

In contrast to HIV-1, the V3 loops of HIV-2 and of SIV do not appear to constitute simple linear neutralization epitopes.[348, 349] Similarly, the V3 region of HIV-1 M-tropic strains is not a prime target for neutralizing antibodies; it is cryptic or hidden from blocking antibodies.[350–352] Primary HIV-1 isolates are relatively resistant both to sCD4 and to V3-specific neutralizing monoclonal antibodies, probably because of their three-dimensional envelope glycoprotein conformation in which access to the critical epitopes is restricted. Adaptation of primary HIV-1 to growth in permanent T-cell lines is accompanied by neutralization by both V3 monoclonal antibodies and anti-gp120 immune sera.[353–356] Depletion of V3-specific antibodies from HIV-1 sera results in significant reduction in the neutralizing efficiency of TCLA HIV-1 strains[352, 355, 355a] but not in that of primary, M-tropic isolates. Replacement of the V1, V2, or V3 loops of a TCLA strain with that of a primary isolate creates a neutralization-resistant virus. The V2 and V3 loops reside proximal to the chemokine receptor–binding site in gp120 and are thought to mask conserved gp120 epitopes from neutralizing antibodies while presenting potentially variable epitopes to the immune system.[40a] Differences in the observed neutralization profiles of TCLA viruses in T-cell lines versus primary strains in PBMCs[377] may be attributed not only to different coreceptor usage but also to possible differences of cellular components trapped in the envelope of the virion[50] or to differences in gp120 glycosylation.[354] The length and conditions of the virus-cell incubation period, the multiplicity of infection, and the use of resting versus activated T cells also influence neutralization efficiency.[356, 357]

A second important cluster of HIV-1–neutralizing epitopes has been identified in the V1/V2 region of gp120. Monoclonal antibodies specific for this region usually recognize conformational epitopes and can neutralize TCLA viruses as well as primary isolates.[358–360] A human monoclonal antibody to V2 was even found to neutralize primary but not TCLA virus strains.[361]

A group of monoclonal antibodies with discontinuous epitopes that overlap part of the CD4-binding site and competitively inhibit CD4 binding to monomeric gp120 neutralize a broad range of TCLA viruses with considerable potency but show only weak activity against primary viruses.[362–365] One exception in this group, IgG1b12, was obtained by recombinant technology.[366] It shows remarkably potent neutralization activity on primary virus isolates.[365–369] The b12 epitope is a major epitope on virions, as opposed to recombinant envelope gp160 or gp120 preparations,[370] suggesting that native envelope spikes from virions could have greater vaccine efficacy than recombinant Env molecules.[371] An HIV-1 escape mutant that resisted IgG1b12 neutralization showed two amino acid changes, one in V2 and the other in C3, immediately adjacent to amino acids implicated in CD4 binding.[40a, 372]

Another group of neutralizing monoclonal antibodies have been termed CD4-induced (CD4i) because they bind with enhanced efficacy to gp120 when it is complexed with CD4.[373] Although they are potent neutralizers of TCLA viruses, the activity of these monoclonal antibodies on primary virus isolates appears weak.[365]

Another epitope defined by a single human monoclonal antibody, 2G12, has been described at the base of the V3 loop and in close vicinity of the C4 region in gp120.[374] Monoclonal antibody 2G12 appears to be a remarkable neutralizer of primary virus isolates.[365, 369]

A few neutralization epitopes have also been described on gp41, but only one, the 2F5 epitope, which maps to the sequence LDKWA within the ectodomain of gp41 near the membrane-spanning domain, shows specific neutralizing activity.[375] Monoclonal antibody 2F5 neutralizes a broad range of primary isolates.[365, 369, 376]

Studies of monoclonal antibody binding to recombinant gp120 compared with gp120/gp41 oligomers have revealed that the majority of well-recognized epitopes on the monomer are poorly presented on the oligomer.[351, 371, 377–382] Neutralization of primary isolates correlates qualitatively with the relative affinity of the antibody for the oligomeric envelope glycoproteins[379] but not for monomeric gp120. Immunization with gp120 elicits neutralizing antibodies against TCLA but not against primary HIV-1 isolates[383, 384]; it is suspected that immunodominance in gp120 is for nonneutralizing epitopes or for neutralizing epitopes of restricted specificity, whereas the more important conformational neutralization epitopes are poorly immunogenic.[378, 382] Of potential interest is the observation that combinations of antibodies targeted to the V3 loop and the CD4-binding domain show synergistic neutralization of TCLA virus infectivity.[385–387] There might also be advantage in using vaccine preparations in which gp120 would be complexed to CD4.[388–390] A detailed map of the different epitopes on the HIV envelope has been constructed.[45, 382]

In the course of HIV-1 infection, neutralizing antibodies to the autologous virus strain in the patient develop slowly, appearing on the average only about 1 year after seroconversion, and titers remain low.[391] Heterologous neutralization of primary isolates seems to occur even later. It is not known why such a long maturation period is required for the appropriate type of antibodies to be produced by the immune system or why the titers remain so low. Similar observations have been made in the case of macaques immunized with live attenuated SIV vaccines or infected with chimeric simian/human immunodeficiency virus (SHIV),[391a] demonstrating the existence of a complex and lengthy maturation of the antibody response during the first 6 to 8 months after inoculation, as reflected in progressive changes in antibody conformational dependence, avidity, and neutralization activity.[392–394] It has been shown that mice infected with lymphocytic choriomeningitis virus rapidly develop specific CTL that selectively eliminate the infected B cells, which produce potent neutralizing antibodies.[395] Whether a similar mechanism might also operate in the case of HIV and SIV is still speculative at this time.

The possibility of classifying HIV-1 by neutralization serotypes has been tested in cross-neutralization studies using panels of virus isolates from genetic clades A through F and serum or plasmas from people infected with diverse HIV-1 subtypes. Data from several laboratories demonstrate that the pattern of neutralization of HIV-1 field isolates is not related to genetic subtype.[396–399] About one third of the plasma samples showed relatively broad, cross-clade neutralizing activity, whereas the other two thirds showed a full spectrum of neutralizing activity. Similarly, some of the virus isolates appeared to be most sensitive to neutralization, whereas others showed a broad spectrum of sensitivities.[396] With use of serum pools rather than individual sera, the B and E subtypes in Thailand could however be distinguished as two distinct neutralization serotypes.[400] In another study, HIV-1 isolates could be grouped by multivariate analysis in a few neutralization clusters not correlated with genetic clades.[397] Of note is that HIV-1 group M–infected sera could neutralize HIV-1 group O isolates. There is also extensive cross-neutralization between HIV-1 and SIVcpz isolates, reflecting their evolutionary origins, but only infrequent and low-titered cross-neutralization between HIV-1 and HIV-2.[401] Extensive cross-clade neutralization of HIV-1 primary isolates was observed with monoclonal antibodies to discontinuous epitopes, including IgG1b12 and 2G12,[369, 402] as well as with monoclonal antibody 2F5, the latter showing broad neutralization potency correlated with the presence of the LDKW motif in gp41.[375, 376] This suggests that a vaccine based on the induction of humoral immunity could be effective against multiple HIV-1 isolates, provided it would induce 2F5-, 2G12-, and b12-like antibodies.

Antigenic determinants that might induce the production of enhancing antibodies are of potential concern for the development of vaccines.[399] In the case of HIV infection, enhancing antibodies can be evidenced by use of either of two in vitro systems: complement-mediated enhancement was observed on MT-2 cells,[403, 404] and complement-independent enhancement in primary monocyte-macrophage cultures.[405, 406] Enhancing antibodies increase the infectivity of the virus for target cells by binding the virus to the Fc or the CR2 receptor at the cell surface. They were observed in sera from healthy human volunteers immunized with gp160.[407] Human monoclonal antibodies able to enhance HIV-1 infection in vitro were found to map to epitopes on gp41.[408] It was also observed that a V3 loop peptide from a given HIV-1 strain could elicit antibodies that enhanced infection by other HIV-1 strains.[344, 409] Enhancing antibodies were found after virus challenge in SIV-vaccinated macaques that happened not to be protected. However, these animals did not develop a more severe or accelerated disease compared with their unvaccinated controls. The role enhancing antibodies might play in facilitating infection with HIV or SIV or in aggravating disease therefore remains to be demonstrated.[410, 411]

HIV-1 gp120 has also been identified as a major target for ADCC, which might contribute to protective immunity against HIV-1.[412–414] Cytolysis by ADCC is independent of MHC restriction and could lead to rapid destruction of HIV-infected cells that are transmitted at the time of infection. Human neutralizing antibodies show ADCC and complement-mediated lysis activities.[414]

Cytotoxic T Lymphocytes

Experience shows that CTL are of major importance in eliminating virus-infected cells and controlling a variety of viral infections including AIDS.[247–252, 415, 416] Class I–restricted CD8$^+$ CTL from HIV-infected individuals can inhibit the replication of HIV in vitro either by direct killing or through local release of soluble inhibitory factors.[6–9, 208, 209, 417–421a] A clear HIV-1–specific CTL response has been detected at the time of primary infection and is maintained vigorously in long-term nonprogressors.[195, 422–425] A significant inverse correlation was observed between HIV-specific CTL frequency and plasma viral load.[425a] Cytotoxic activity specific for a variety of HIV-1 antigens has been described in HIV-infected people and may be detected in PBMCs without in vitro antigen-specific stimulation,[416, 419, 420] indicating a high frequency of in vivo activated CTL. Precursor CTL frequency in the blood of infected patients is usually as high as 1 per 10,000 and can eventually reach up to 1% of T cells.[420] Large numbers of SIV-specific CTL have also been found within vaginal intraepithelial lymphocytes[426] and intestinal intraepithelial lymphocytes[427] in SIV-infected macaques.

The HIV-1 Env glycoprotein can serve as a target antigen for CD8$^+$ MHC class I–restricted CTL, in association with HLA-A2, -A3, -B7, or -B17.[416, 428] The V3 loop contains a CTL epitope that is restricted by HLA-A2. Several other CTL epitopes have been identified in gp160, many of which appear to be relatively well conserved and several of which overlap on the molecule.[428, 429] Env-specific CD4$^+$, MHC class II–restricted CTL have also been evidenced in association with HLA-DR2 or HLA-DR4.[430]

Many HIV-1 CTL epitopes appear to be located in the Gag molecule, most particularly in highly conserved regions of p24*gag* (capsid), as well as in several regions of the highly conserved Pol protein, and in the central and carboxyl terminal regions of Nef, in which a continuum of epitopes is recognized by CTL in association with a variety of histocompatibility antigens.[428, 429, 431]

Emergence and positive selection of CTL escape virus variants have been described.[264, 265, 268] Some escape variants can actually antagonize the activity of CTL targeted to the wild-type epitopes, thus resulting in immune impairment and facilitating the persistence of virus strains that would otherwise be recognized by the existing CTL.[265–267] This might explain why diversification of the virus quasispecies is usually accompanied by maintenance of the original clones in the infected person.

Of major importance for vaccine development is the observation that CTL elicited in response to a clade B–based live recombinant canarypox HIV-1 vaccine were capable of recognizing primary HIV-1 isolates belonging to genetically diverse clades.[432] The number of antigens to include in a vaccine to induce broad cross-clade cellular immunity may, it is hoped, therefore be limited. This number is not known. Inclusion of several HIV-1 antigens in the same vaccine, such as Env, Gag, Nef, and Pol, is expected to broaden the CTL response. A CTL response with only a single epitope specificity was unable to provide protective immunity against a live SIV challenge in macaques.[433] Administration to an HIV-1–seropositive individual of a large number of autologous CTL to a single epitope in Nef resulted in the development of a virus strain missing that epitope.[268]

HIV antigens have also been studied for their ability to stimulate T helper cell proliferation or IL-2 production in vitro. T helper cell epitopes have been mapped using sets of synthetic peptides. A major T helper cell epitope, *env*T1, was identified in gp120,[434] and several T helper cell epitopes have been mapped to the p24*gag*[435] and to the Nef protein.[436]

CANDIDATE HIV VACCINES

The development of an HIV vaccine is a formidable challenge.[15a–18a, 437–439] Most classical vaccines prevent the development of disease but do not prevent infection; they allow a limited but controlled replication of the pathogen at the portal of entry. This raises the question of whether an HIV vaccine, if it is unable to prevent infection, could prevent development of disease and reduce HIV transmission. Because HIV-infected chimpanzees do not develop a disease, continued observation of vaccinated chimpanzees in which virus breakthrough has occurred cannot provide an answer to this question. Macaques infected with SIV do develop a disease similar to human AIDS. SIV-vaccinated and challenged macaques that became infected because of ineffective or insufficient immunization showed prolonged delay in the onset of disease and lived longer than unvaccinated control animals,[440–442] probably because of decreased initial virus loads. This suggests that HIV vaccines, even if they are unable to maintain sterilizing immunity, might delay disease onset and provide some protection against disease.

As discussed later, classical vaccine strategies based on attenuated live virus or whole inactivated virus have severe limitations. Most efforts to develop an HIV vaccine have therefore focused on newer vaccine approaches. Progress in antigen design and genetic manipulations of viral or bacterial vectors have considerably improved the diversity of antigen delivery systems. The following is a brief review of recent developments in the field.

Whole Inactivated Vaccines

Successful protection of macaques against pathogenic SIV challenge was observed in many experiments using whole inactivated SIV vaccines[440] or formalin-inactivated SIV-infected cell extracts. These vaccines were able to totally prevent infection in monkeys, but neutralizing antibody titers did not correlate with protection. The mechanism of protection unraveled when it was found that the relevant antigens in the vaccine preparations were not the SIV antigens but rather xenoantigens from the human cells used to grow the virus.[443] Indeed, macaques immunized with whole killed SIV vaccine were protected from challenge with SIV grown in human cells but not from challenge with SIV grown in macaque PBMCs.[444, 445] Monkeys could also be protected from challenge with SIV grown in human cells by immunization with purified HLA-DR,[446] entertaining the possibility of using alloimmunization to provide protection from HIV-1 infection in humans.[233] Whole inactivated HIV-1 vaccines have not so far been seriously considered as potential human vaccines, in part because of safety considerations and in part because of failure of an early approach in chimpanzees.[447]

Live Attenuated Vaccines

Several studies have demonstrated vaccine protection against SIV infection using live attenuated SIV vaccines. Rhesus monkeys infected with nonpathogenic molecular clones of SIVmac, such as 1A11 or BK28, developed persistent low-grade infection and were protected from infection with a low dose of pathogenic SIV and from disease, but not from infection with a high dose of SIV.[448] Attenuated strains of SIV induced a spectrum of antiviral immunity that was inversely associated with their degree of attenuation. Protection was directly related to induction of a CTL response.[449, 450] These observations suggested that avirulent virus mutant strains could be used as live attenuated vaccines.

A live SIVmac vaccine, attenuated by deletion of the *nef* gene, indeed demonstrated remarkable efficacy as a vaccine,[14] because macaques challenged more than 2 years after immunization were protected against 1000 animal infectious doses of pathogenic SIVmac grown in monkey PBMCs. Deletion of *nef*, alone or in combination with deletions in *vpr* and in the long terminal repeat region, showed no drastic effect on virus growth in cell culture.[451, 452] These results were confirmed using two molecular clones of SIVmac, J5, a full-length pathogenic molecular clone, and C8, which is attenuated because of a 12–base pair deletion in the *nef* gene.[15, 73, 453, 454] Immunization with C8 provided complete protection from infection with J5, including mucosal infection.[454]

However, SIVΔ*nef* establishes a state of indefinite persistence in the vaccinated host, it can revert to full-size *nef* virulence in some animals,[73] and it remains pathogenic to neonatal macaques, at least at a high dose.[455, 456] It can also cause disease in some adults.[457] Efforts to render the virus safer and more efficacious have included the construction of replication-competent SIVΔ*nef* that express human IFN-γ[458] or the herpesvirus thymidine kinase.[459, 460] Even if long-term safety testing of attenuated SIV in animals is successful, the prospect of using a live attenuated HIV-1 vaccine in humans would still meet with deep safety concerns, including the potential of promoting tumors through insertional oncogenesis.[459] Recently, a few individuals harboring HIV for long periods without any signs of AIDS were shown to be infected with *nef*-deleted viruses,[461–463] which have been presented as potential candidates for a live attenuated HIV-1 vaccine.

In the SIVmacΔ*nef*Δ*vpr* studies mentioned before, long-term protection against wild-type SIV was usually not observed before 6 to 8 months after inoculation[14, 392–394] and correlated with the strength of the replication of the live attenuated virus and with the development of conformation-dependent, high-avidity neutralizing antibodies.[392, 393, 464]

However, infection with attenuated SIVmacC8 also provided protection from infection with genetically divergent SIVsm[465] and with chimeric SHIV expressing an HIV-1 envelope[454, 466] against which no serological cross-reactivity could be detected. Similarly, live attenuated SIVΔ*nef*Δ*vpr* provided long-term protection against challenge strains with highly divergent envelope sequences, such as pathogenic SHIV-DH12.[466a] Vaccination of macaques with SIVΔ*nef* results in the induction of a vigorous CTL response that arises early in infection and persists for years after a single inoculation of virus.[466b] Macaques immunized with attenuated SIVmac showed a high-level CTL response in iliac, mesenteric, and rectal lymph nodes[454] and were protected from mucosal challenge. Similarly, macaques previously exposed to subinfectious doses of SIV or of HIV-2 demonstrated a virus-specific cellular immune response and were protected from SIV infection when challenged intrarectally, in spite of the absence of an SIV-specific antibody response.[467, 468] Therefore, activation of the cell-mediated arm of the immune system only, without antibody formation, might be able to prevent mucosal SIV transmission in macaques.[477a] Whether protection provided by the live attenuated SIV immunization depends on high-avidity neutralizing antibodies, CTL, other cellular immune mechanisms including the secretion of β-chemokines, or a combination of these different factors is still not clear.

Live Recombinant Vaccines

Live recombinant vaccines are made of a live attenuated viral or bacterial strain used as a vector to carry the gene or genes that encode the appropriate heterologous antigens (Table 38–3). Live recombinant vaccines have a number of attractive features, including the ability to stimulate both humoral and cell-mediated immunity.

Vaccinia virus vectors expressing a variety of HIV and SIV genes have been tested in animals and, in some

Table 38–3. **POTENTIAL VECTORS FOR LIVE RECOMBINANT HIV-1 VACCINES**

VIRUSES	BACTERIA
Vaccinia virus	Bacillus Calmette-Guérin
Canarypox virus	*Salmonella*
Fowlpox virus	*Lactobacillus*
Adenovirus	*Streptococcus*
Influenza virus	*Listeria*
VEEV	
Poliovirus	

VEEV, Venezuelan equine encephalitis virus.

cases, humans.[469–471] The results indicate that HIV-specific T-cell responses could be induced, including CTL, but anti-HIV antibody responses were usually weak and transient. The protective potential of recombinant vaccinia virus vaccines was demonstrated in the macaque/SIV model using a vaccinia virus expressing SIV Nef.[472] An inverse correlation was found between the vaccine-induced *nef*-specific CTL precursor frequency and virus load measured after challenge with pathogenic SIVmac. In the animal with the strongest CTL response, virus was not detectable at any time.[472] Recombinant poxvirus vectors have been used not only as live virus vaccines in vivo but also as an expression system for HIV antigens in vitro through infection of cells in culture.

The issue of safety of vaccinia virus recombinants in immunocompromised people has led to the development of new attenuated vaccinia virus strains such as the NYVAC strain[473] that should be safer to use than the classical vaccinia virus strains. An alternative is to replace vaccinia virus by canarypox (ALVAC) or avipox viruses.[474] The avian poxviruses do not replicate in mammalian cells and are therefore less immunogenic than vaccinia virus but show none of the potential risks of vaccinia virus in humans. The same applies to modified vaccinia virus Ankara (MVA),[475, 476] a highly attenuated, host range–restricted strain of vaccinia virus that grows to high titers in chick embryo fibroblasts but is restricted at the stage of virion formation in mammalian cells. A prolonged and marked suppression of replication of HIV-2 was observed after immunization of rhesus macaques with NYVAC- or ALVAC–HIV-1 expressing HIV-1 Gag, Pol, or Env and boosting with HIV-1 antigens or peptides.[477] Quite remarkably, an NYVAC vector expressing the *gag*, *env*, and *pol* genes of SIV provided protection from infection with SIVmac by the rectal route but not by the intravenous route, despite total absence of neutralizing antibodies.[477a] Extensive testing of ALVAC–HIV-1 constructs has been done in humans (see later section). Recombinant MVA were found to induce potent CTL responses in mice[478] and monkeys.[478a]

Human adenovirus types 4, 5, and 7 offer several potential advantages as vectors for live recombinant vaccines. They can be administered orally, in the form of gelatin-coated tablets from which the virus is released in the intestine, or intranasally, and they can induce both systemic and mucosal immunity. Recombinant adenoviruses expressing the Env or Gag antigens from HIV-1 or SIV have been tested in animals and shown to induce long-lasting protective immunity in chimpanzees.[479–481a]

Poliovirus can be used as a vector to express foreign antigenic determinants, such as the V3 loop, on the surface of its capsid, resulting in a chimeric virus particle.[482, 483] A chimeric influenza virus was similarly engineered by inserting an epitope from the V3 loop into antigenic site B in the hemagglutinin.[484] An influenza virus recombinant expressing the 2F5 epitope[375] was also engineered; it induced secretory antibody at the mucosal level but only low titers of circulating HIV-1–neutralizing antibodies.[485] A limitation of these chimeric virus systems is the small size of the HIV determinant that can be inserted into the virus particle without impairing stability.

Another type of viral recombinant can be engineered by substituting the sequence of the structural (capsid) proteins of the vector by that of the foreign antigen, resulting in a capsid-defective recombinant. The defective hybrid genome can be encapsidated by transcapsidation using a helper virus or a recombinant vaccinia virus that expresses the missing capsid proteins.[486] Poliovirus "replicons" that encode HIV-1 Gag,[486] SIV Gag, or SIV Env SU proteins[487] have been shown to generate immune responses to HIV or SIV antigens in animals. This approach has also been used in the case of Semliki Forest virus to generate defective recombinants that can be used to produce the HIV-1 envelope glycoproteins in cell culture[488] or as live recombinant vaccines.[442]

Live recombinant bacterial vaccines have also been developed using as a vector bacillus Calmette-Guérin (BCG, an attenuated *Mycobacterium bovis* strain)[489] or *Salmonella* strains[490] that have been attenuated by mutagenesis of genes involved in virulence and invasiveness. BCG is easy and inexpensive to manufacture, is heat stable, and can be administered as a single dose at birth. More than 2 billion people have been vaccinated with BCG without major side effects. Recombinant HIV-BCG strains have been engineered that expressed a variety of HIV antigens and induced good cell-mediated immune responses in mice[491, 492] and monkeys.[433] A BCG–HIV-1 recombinant was also described that induced HIV-1–neutralizing antibodies.[493]

A potential problem with live recombinant viral or bacterial vaccines is their relative lack of efficacy in individuals previously exposed to the vector. Such a restriction does not apply to the canarypox or avipox virus vectors but would apply to BCG, poliovirus, or adenovirus. It could also become a potential issue for any immunization regimen based on multiple booster injections.

Virus-like Particle Vaccines

This type of vaccine is made of virus-like, genomeless particles. Viral antigens in particulate form are more immunogenic and more likely to be stable than unassembled purified antigens. Several types of particle vaccines are under development. Among these are viral particles that are devoid of a genome as the consequence of a mutation in the packaging sequence of the genomic viral RNA. They have a normal protein content but lack detectable RNA.[494] Mutations of any of the cystein residues in either of the two zinc finger motifs of the p7*gag* (nucleocapsid) protein of HIV-1 also produce an RNA packaging defect.[495]

Virus-like particles can also be obtained by expressing the HIV-1 *gag* gene or *gag-pol* and *env* genes in cells infected with a recombinant baculovirus or vaccinia virus. The unprocessed Gag precursor protein expressed by recombinant *gag* baculovirus in insect cells spontaneously assembles into 100-nm particles that bud from the cell surface.[496] Double infection with recombinant vaccinia virus carrying the HIV-1 *gag-pol* and *env* genes, respectively, can be used to generate genomeless particles.[497]

Noninfectious HIV-1 pseudoparticles (pseudovirions) were also obtained from Vero cells that were stably transformed with the appropriate expression vector.[498] Immunization with these particles induced HIV-1–neutralizing, syncytium-inhibiting, and *env*-CD4–blocking antibodies.[499] The use of pseudovirions as a vaccine is attractive because they contain most of the HIV-1 protein components in a native conformation without the potential risks caused by the presence of the virus genome.

Another particulate vaccine of interest is made of hybrid particles in which the appropriate HIV antigenic determinants are exposed on particulate proteins as carriers. Epitopes in the V3 region of gp120 were inserted into poliovirus capsid,[483] hepatitis B virus core particles,[500] hepatitis B surface antigen particles,[501] or the yeast retrotransposon virus-like particles (Ty-VLP).[502] Hybrid HIV–Ty-VLP that expressed either HIV-1 Gag or Env V3 determinants[503, 504] showed good immune potency. When used in the absence of an adjuvant, such a particulate vaccine was also able to elicit a CTL response.[503] Owing to the particulate nature of the carriers and their high intrinsic immunogenicity, these approaches may be of interest in exposing a critical antigenic determinant such as the HIV-1 V3 loop or the 2F5 epitope[505] in an immunologically favorable environment. A limitation of this approach, however, is the small size of the determinant that can be inserted into the particle.

Subunit Vaccines

Many recombinant soluble HIV and SIV proteins have been produced for testing as subunit vaccines (Table 38–4). The observation that HIV-1 gp160, gp140 (a soluble form of gp160 resulting from the deletion of the transmembrane and intracytoplasmic domains), or gp120 induced only a transient response in primates has prompted the search for strong adjuvants or special delivery formulations that would be suitable for human use.[506] Thus, experimental vaccines have been developed in which the antigens were either formulated into liposomes[507] or complexed under the form of immunostimulating complexes with saponin derivative Quil A.[508, 509] Immunostimulating complexes are able to induce both neutralizing antibodies and MHC class I–restricted CTL. These responses were not, however, sufficient to protect macaques from challenge with the virulent SIVmac.[510]

Table 38–4. **EXPRESSION SYSTEMS USED FOR THE PRODUCTION OF HIV-1 ENVELOPE GLYCOPROTEINS**

ANTIGEN	CELL SUBSTRATE	VIRUS VECTOR
gp120	Transformed yeast	None
gp120	Transformed Chinese hamster ovary (CHO) cells	None
gp140	BHK-21 cells (hamster)	Vaccinia virus
gp160	Vero cells (monkey)	Vaccinia virus
gp160	Insect cells	Baculovirus

The immune response to recombinant HIV-1 gp140 or gp120 has also been under active investigation with use of more classical types of adjuvants such as alum or incomplete Freund adjuvant (IFA) and newer adjuvant formulations such as water-in-oil emulsions with saponin derivative QS21, enterobacteria cell wall derivatives, or muramyl dipeptide derivatives.[511] Specific adjuvant formulations such as SAF-1 or MF59[512] have been developed. These studies have underlined the importance of the conformational integrity of the envelope glycoprotein for the induction of neutralizing antibodies.[513] Current envelope vaccine candidates elicit high gp120-binding antibody titers with neutralizing activity against matched TCLA virus strains but not primary HIV-1 isolates.[378, 383, 384] Antibodies elicited by these vaccines are directed to linear epitopes exposed on denatured forms of gp120. In contrast, oligomeric gp160 in alum or monophosphoryl lipid A–containing water-in-oil emulsion elicited antibodies to native cell surface–expressed gp120/gp41 that were able to neutralize some primary HIV-1 isolates.[513] Immunization with virion-derived, native oligomeric gp140 from HIV-2 or SIV also protected macaques from challenge with pathogenic SIV.[514] These results suggest that the use of an oligomeric form of gp160 or gp140 might preserve some of the critical conformational epitopes in the molecule.[513]

The possibility of using soluble antigens for mucosal immunization has also been investigated. Encapsulation of the antigens in microspheres made of copolymers of lactide and glycolide protects them from degradation by low pH and proteolytic enzymes and allows them to be targeted through M cells into the Peyer patches[515, 516] or to be used as a controlled release system, thus reducing the number of immunizations required.[517]

Covalently cross-linked complexes of HIV-1 gp120 and CD4 receptor have also been increasingly viewed as potential subunit vaccines against HIV-1 infection.[389, 390]

The testing of subunit vaccines in animals has been extensively pursued and has yielded different results depending on the model. In the SIV/macaque model, a partial protective immune response was elicited with SIVmne gp160 given as a booster immunization after priming the animals with live recombinant vaccinia virus expressing the SIVmne gp160.[518, 519] No protection was obtained, however, when these experiments were repeated with the more virulent SIVmac.[520] Protection of cynomolgus monkeys against HIV-2 was achieved using a detergent-disrupted whole HIV-2 preparation in IFA or formulated in immunostimulating complexes and followed by boosting with V3 peptides.[521, 522] The importance of humoral immunity in protection was clearly demonstrated by showing that HIV-2 infection could be prevented in naive recipients by passive immunization with serum from the vaccinated, protected monkeys.[523]

Recently, the nature of protective immunity to SIVmne in the prime-boost immunized macaques was reexamined.[524] SIV-specific CTL were detected after challenge in the vaccine-protected animals, suggesting that undetected, low-level SIV infection had occurred after exposure to SIV but had been controlled by the immune system of the animals. These findings are of a paramount importance when they are related to the human situation.

Subunit SIVmac vaccines have also been shown to induce protection from intranasal challenge but not from vaginal challenge when they are targeted to the iliac lymph nodes.[525, 525a] Of interest was the observation that among the correlates of protection from intrarectal challenge in the vaccinated animals was the elevated level of secretion of β-chemokines RANTES and MIP-1β by iliac lymph node cells in response to immunostimulation in vitro. Female rhesus macaques could also be partially protected from vaginal infection with SIVmac by mucosal immunization with subunit vaccines combined with a live recombinant adenovirus.[526] Finally, high titers of neutralizing antibodies could be induced in rhesus macaques immunized with gp140 LAI that were boosted with a V3 peptide formulated in IFA or in SAF-1.[527] The testing of subunit HIV-1 vaccines in the chimpanzee model and in human volunteers is reviewed in a later section.

Synthetic Vaccines

Most attempts to use synthetic peptide immunogens have concentrated on the V3 loop. Sp10, a peptide with the sequence of part of the V3 loop from the HIV-1 MN strain, linked to that of *env*T1, a major T helper determinant of gp120, elicited long-lasting neutralizing antibody and T helper cell responses in a variety of animals without the need for coupling to a protein carrier.[528] Some of the animals even developed antibodies that could neutralize not only MN but also more distant TCLA HIV-1 strains, including IIIB (LAI). The *env*T1-V3 peptide was also able to induce a CD8$^+$ MHC class I–restricted CTL response.[529] The same peptide, linked to the sequence of the fusion domain of gp41, showed strong immune potency in goats and rabbits but was paradoxically tolerogenic in macaques and chimpanzees. Another type of peptide combining T-cell and B-cell epitopes was engineered that contained the HIV-1 MN V3 loop sequence linked to the sequence of one of the p24*gag* T-cell epitopes, p24E.[530] A high-titer neutralizing antibody response was elicited by the p24E-V3 combined peptide but not by the V3-p24E peptide, showing that epitope polarity can have a major effect on the quality of the immune response.[531]

Linked to branched polylysine molecules as a multiple antigen peptide system, V3 peptides induced a long-term high-titer neutralizing antibody response.[532] An octameric V3 multiple antigen peptide formulated in alum was found to be safe and immunogenic in pigtail macaques and human volunteers.[533] Adding a lipophilic membrane-anchoring moiety such as tripalmitoyl glyceryl cystein (P3C) at the carboxyl terminus of multiple antigen peptide systems enabled their inclusion into liposomes. An immunogen consisting of a tetrameric branched V3 peptide linked to P3C induced neutralizing antibody, CD4$^+$ T helper cell, and CD8$^+$ CTL responses in mice, even in the absence of an adjuvant.[534] The hydrophobic P3C "foot" served as an adjuvant and provided the V3 peptide with the ability to prime CTL in vivo. Although peptides and proteins usually do not induce a class I–restricted CD8$^+$ CTL response in vivo, lipopeptides have such a capacity[535, 536] and may represent an interesting formulation for boosting the CTL immune response to HIV.

The use of synthetic peptides as vaccines raises several issues,[537] however: peptides provide a limited base of CTL (or B-cell) epitopes for a population with wide HLA diversity; they generate a monospecific CTL (or antibody) response that can easily be dodged by the virus through emergence of antigenic escape variants[268]; and helper T cell epitopes, which are important for optimal generation of CTL responses, are not provided.

Anti-Idiotype Base Vaccines

Anti-idiotype antibodies can be used as a vaccine owing to the structural mimicry of the antigen by the anti-idiotype antibody. Indeed, primates immunized with a human anti-idiotype monoclonal antibody produced low-titer, broadly neutralizing anti–HIV-1 antibodies.[538] Whether such a procedure can lead to the development of an HIV-1 vaccine remains doubtful, however.

Naked DNA Vaccines

Injection into the muscle or the epidermis of an animal of a purified plasmid DNA that carries a gene encoding an antigen under the control of an appropriate mammalian transcription promoter leads to expression of the antigen in situ and triggers a strong immune response, mostly of the Th1 type.[539–547] The use of pure DNA offers many advantages, including ease of design, simplicity of preparation, and chemical stability. Vaccination with HIV-1 DNA can be substantially boosted with gp120,[548] gp160, or p24*gag* subunit vaccines, eliciting both neutralizing antibody and CTL responses. However, an initial attempt at protecting macaques from experimental SIVmac challenge through immunization with naked DNA failed, in spite of repeated immunizations.[543] Successful protection from SHIV infection in macaques[544, 545] and from HIV-1 infection in chimpanzees[546] has now been reported. In the latter case, two different DNA plasmids were used, one encoding the HIV-1 gp160 and Rev protein, and the other the HIV-1 Gag and Pol proteins; a total of eight immunizations was given. Codelivery of genes for IL-12 and granulocyte-macrophage colony-stimulating factor along with an HIV-1 DNA vaccine resulted in the reduction or the enhancement of specific antibody response, respectively.[547] In addition, coimmunization with the IL-12 gene led to a remarkable increase in the CTL response. The observation was also made that priming with a DNA vaccine followed by boosting with a recombinant poxvirus expressing the same antigen was more immunogenic than immunization with DNA alone.[537a, 537b]

DNA vaccine designs are promising candidates for an effective HIV-1 vaccine, but the concept merits careful and intensive evaluation, and the question of long-term safety still remains to be addressed.

HIV-1 VACCINE STUDIES IN ANIMALS

Primate models for AIDS vaccine development include the SIV/macaque model, the HIV-1/chimpanzee model, the HIV-2/macaque model, and the SHIV/macaque model.[549]

HIV-1 has been transmitted to chimpanzees,[226, 550] pigtail macaques (*Macaca nemestrina*),[551] and, in certain conditions, rabbits.[552, 553] It also replicates in immunodeficient mice engrafted with human fetal lymphoid tissue (SCID-hu mice)[554] or adult human peripheral blood leukocytes (hu-PBL-SCID mice).[555] Replication-competent chimeric viruses called SHIV that have the *gag, pol, vif,* and *nef* genes from SIVmac and the *env, tat,* and *rev* genes from HIV-1 replicate to high titers in cynomolgus and rhesus monkeys without causing disease.[556–559] Serial passages of the virus in macaques lead to the selection of pathogenic variants that induce CD4 lymphopenia and an AIDS-like disease in the animals[560–562] and should provide a valuable model for the study of HIV-1 vaccines.[544, 563]

Chimpanzees can be infected with some TCLA strains by the intravenous or intravaginal route; they usually do not develop symptoms of AIDS in spite of persistent infection,[226] although one chimpanzee was recently reported as susceptible to HIV-1–induced disease.[228]

The chimpanzee model has been widely used for the study of vaccine-induced protection against HIV infection. Several groups have shown that gp120- or gp140-based vaccines that induce neutralizing antibodies provide protection against experimental HIV-1 infection with either cell-free or cell-associated HIV-1 IIIB (LAI).[564–567] These studies showed strong correlation between protection against challenge and the titer of neutralizing antibody directed to the V3 loop domain of gp120. ADCC was also detected in the immunized animals.[568] Passive immunization of a chimpanzee with a V3-targeted, LAI-specific neutralizing monoclonal antibody protected the animal fully against challenge from cell-free HIV-1 LAI even when the antibody was administered after virus inoculation.[340, 569] Neutralizing antibodies therefore represent a surrogate marker for vaccine efficacy, at least in this experimental setting where the endpoint is infection with a TCLA strain.

Prince and colleagues[570] passively immunized chimpanzees with IgG prepared from a pool of HIV-1–seropositive human sera. Protection was achieved against challenge with a low dose of the HIV-1 LAI strain but not against a higher dose. This in itself is a remarkable result, in view of the fact that the V3 loop sequence of HIV-1 LAI is different from that of the virus isolates commonly encountered in the field, which implies that protection must have been achieved through broadly neutralizing antibodies. Preexposure infusion in two chimpanzees with monoclonal antibody 2F5 had a temporary prophylactic effect, delaying by a few weeks the multiplication of a primary HIV-1 isolate.[571] This suggests that the amount and timing of delivery of antibody are critical factors for the success of passive protection (see also a later section).

Protection from infection with a heterologous HIV-1 strain (HIV-1 SF2) was obtained by active immunization of chimpanzees with gp120 MN[572] and with hybrid gp140 MN/LAI and a V3 peptide formulated in IFA.[573] Protection from HIV-1 SF2 was also obtained with a live adenovirus expressing gp160 MN followed by boosting with gp120 SF2[481, 481a] or with a naked DNA vaccine.[546] In contrast, two chimpanzees that were primed with a low dose of ALVAC–HIV vCP125 that expresses gp160 MN, and boosted with gp140 MN/LAI, were not protected against challenge with SF2.[573] High neutralizing antibody titers against MN or LAI HIV-1 strains were detected in the protected chimpanzees compared with the unprotected ones. In the recombinant adenovirus-gp160 experiment, one chimpanzee with CTL was protected in the absence of neutralizing antibodies, whereas protection against high-dose challenge occurred only in chimpanzees with high-titer neutralizing antibodies.[481] The protected animals also showed neutralizing antibodies against a primary isolate close to HIV-1 SF2 (BZ187).[357, 481a] However, HIV-1 SF2 is not virulent in chimpanzees, and no virus could be isolated from the control immunized animals' PBMCs longer than 6 weeks after challenge, suggesting low virus burdens, even in control animals.

In the experiments by Girard and coworkers,[573] the protected animals were boosted again with gp140 and a V3 peptide, then challenged intravenously with a clade E HIV-1. All animals became infected, indicating that intraclade vaccine-mediated protection does not predict interclade protection, at least when vaccines are envelope based only and in the context of an intravenous challenge with clade B and E strains.

In another experiment, two chimpanzees were immunized with ALVAC–HIV vCP250, which expresses gp120 LAI/tm and *gag* and *protease* genes. The animal with the highest neutralizing antibody titer was protected against an intravenous HIV-1 IIIB (LAI) challenge.[574, 575] After a booster injection of vCP250, the protected animal was rechallenged with the HIV-1 DH012 primary isolate but this time was not protected. No neutralizing antibodies to DH012 were detected before challenge.

Female chimpanzees immunized repeatedly with vCP250 by different routes (intramuscular, intranasal, vaginal, and rectal) could be protected from a cervicovaginal homologous challenge with HIV-1 IIIB (LAI) without a subunit boost. In this case, however, protection did not correlate with the titer of neutralizing antibodies,[575] and one might speculate that other mechanisms such as secretion of β-chemokines or $CD8^+$ CTL were involved in protection at the mucosal level.[525] The observation was made in both female chimpanzees[575] and female macaques[576] that infection by the vaginal route with a low dose of virus was followed at times by transient viremia, but the infection never became established and seroconversion was not observed. This is reminiscent of the observations of Shearer and Clerici[577] in humans. The implication of these results is that a vaccine inducing partial decrease in virus infectivity at the site of entry might be sufficient to provide protection from infection by the genital route.

HIV-1 vaccines have also been studied in the SHIV/macaque model. Several chimeric SHIVs have been generated, including some with the envelope glycoprotein from clade B primary isolates.[556–559a] In vivo passage of SHIV in macaques generated pathogenic viruses that induced rapid $CD4^+$ T-cell depletion and AIDS-like illness in the animal.[560–563a] Recombinant subunit vaccines were successfully tested for protection against nonpathogenic SHIVs. Thus, vaccines based on the gp120 from a primary HIV-1 isolate were found to provide full protection from homologous challenge but not from a heterologous challenge with a SHIV based on another clade B strain.[577a, 577b] Macaques immunized with HIV-1 SF2 gp120 formulated in ISCOMS were similarly protected from challenge with a SHIV based on a related strain.[577c] Protection from infection with a nonpathogenic SHIV was also obtained using multiple homologous HIV-1 env DNA immunizations followed by boosts with the envelope protein,[544] or by HIV-1 env and SIV gag-pol DNAs alone.[545] However, there is as yet no report of successful protection of macaques against challenge with a pathogenic SHIV.

HUMAN CLINICAL TRIALS OF HIV-1 VACCINES

Between 1987 and 1997, more than 21 HIV-1 preventive vaccine candidates have been in phase I/II safety and immunogenicity studies involving nearly 3000 HIV-uninfected volunteers in the United States, France, the United Kingdom, Switzerland, and Japan.

Initial Trials

Initial trials tested envelope glycoproteins gp120 or gp140 derived from clade B TCLA HIV-1 strains IIIB, MN, or SF2 that were presented either in their soluble form or as related synthetic peptides (V3 loop) formulated with various adjuvants or expressed by live recombinant vectors (vaccinia virus, ALVAC) (Table 38–5). These envelope-based recombinant candidate vaccines were well tolerated, and to date there have been no important clinical or subclinical adverse immunological or neurological effects among the volunteers.[578] Results from these early studies[506, 579–582] have shown that soluble envelope glycoproteins or peptides are able to induce neutralizing antibodies against the homologous TCLA HIV-1 strain but not against primary HIV-1 isolates.[18a, 353, 377, 383, 384] Branched V3 peptides (multiple antigen peptides) failed to improve the quality and magnitude of the humoral response induced by recombinant envelope glycoproteins.[535, 582]

Initial candidate vaccines derived from the HIV-1 LAI strain were followed by vaccines based on HIV-1 MN. Emphasis was put on the use of mammalian cells for the production of recombinant envelope glycoproteins (because of better glycosylation) and of new adjuvants

Table 38–5. **HIV-1 VACCINE CANDIDATES TESTED IN HIV-UNINFECTED ADULT VOLUNTEERS**

TYPE OF VACCINE	ANTIGEN	SOURCE	ADJUVANT
Recombinant subunits	gp160 LAI	Baculovirus/insect cells	Alum
	gp 160 LAI	Vero cells	Deoxycholate
	gp 160 MN	Vero cells	Deoxycholate
	gp 140 MN/LAI	rVV/BHK-21 cells	Alum or IFA
	gp120 (env 2–3) SF2	Yeast	MF59, MTP-PE
	gp120 SF2	CHO cells	Alum, MF59, liposomes, MPL
	gp120 LAI	CHO cells	Alum
	gp120 MN	CHO cells	Alum, QS-21
	p24 gag SF2	Yeast	MF59
	p24 gag LAI	Ty-VLP hybrid particles	Alum
Synthetic peptides	V3 MN		Alum or IFA
	V3-MAPS MN, multi-clades	Octameric	Alum
	V3 MN, multi-clades	Conjugated to PPD	Alum
	V3 MN, multi-clades	Conjugated to *Pseudomonas aeruginosa* toxin A	Alum
	p17 gag LAI (HGP-30)	Peptide-KLH conjugate	Alum
Live recombinant viruses			
Vaccinia virus	gp160 LAI		
Canarypox virus (ALVAC-HIV)	vCP 125 (gp 160 MN)		
	vCP205 (gp120 MN tm/gag/protease LAI)		
	vCP300 (gp120 MN tm/gag/protease with pol and nef LAI CTL domains)		

rVV, recombinant vaccinia virus; CHO, Chinese hamster ovary; MTP-PE, muramyl tripeptide phosphatidylethanolamine; VLP, virus-like particles; KLH, keyhole limpet hemocyanin; IFA, incomplete Freund adjuvant; Ty, yeast retrotransposon; MAPS, multiantigen presentation system; PPD, purified protein derivative of *Mycobacterium tuberculosis;* MPL, monophosphoryl lipid A; QS-21, purified saponin from *Quillaria saponaria;* tm, transmembrane domain in gp41.

Table 38–6. **MAJOR RESULTS OF HIV-1 VACCINE IMMUNOGENICITY IN HIV-INFECTED VOLUNTEERS**

VACCINE	NEUTRALIZING ANTIBODIES[a]	CD8+ CTL[b]
rgp160 baculovirus	+	−
rgp160 mammalian	+	−
rgp120 yeast	+	−
rgp120 mammalian[c]	+/+ + +	±
rgp160 + V3 peptide	+ +	−
branched V3 peptides	+ +	−
rVV + rgp160	+	+
rVVgp160	±	+
vCP125 (10^6)	+	±
vCP125 (10^7)	+	+
vCP125 (10^6) + gp120 in alum/IFA	+/+ +	+ +
vCP125 (10^6) + gp120 in MF59	+ + +	+
vCP125 (10^7) + gp120 in MF59	+ + +[c]	+ + +
vCP205 ($10^{5.8}$)		
+ peptide p24E-V3MN	+	+ +
+ gp120 in MF59	+ + +[c]	+ + +

[a]Neutralization titer geometric means: +, <100; + +, <300; + + +, >300.
[b]Percentage responders with CTL: +, <10%; + +, <30%; + + +, >30%.
[c]Neutralizing antibodies against clade B syncytia-inducing primary isolate (BZ167) and antibody-dependent cell-mediated cytotoxicity activity to MN and SF2 were also detected in some of the vaccine recipients.

(in place of the standard aluminium hydroxide) (Table 38–6).

Injection of an LAI gp120 candidate vaccine in alum resulted in a dose-related induction of neutralizing antibodies against the homologous HIV-1 LAI strain and, to a lesser degree, against the heterologous HIV-1 SF2 strain. Maximum antibody levels were reached after three injections. A similar recombinant envelope subunit vaccine, based on HIV-1 MN (MN gp120), also induced antibodies that neutralized the homologous MN strain as well as other clade B TCLA virus strains (HIV-1 SF2 and LAI).

An SF2 gp120 candidate vaccine, combined with a novel adjuvant, MF59,[512] and administered with or without the immunomodulator muramyl tripeptide and dipalmitoyl phosphatidylethanolamine, induced gp120-binding antibodies that persisted for at least 24 weeks after the fourth injection. After three injections, all volunteers had developed neutralizing antibodies against the homologous HIV-1 SF2 strain, which in two thirds of them also cross-neutralized HIV-1 MN. A fully glycosylated HIV-1 LAI gp160 candidate vaccine, combined with alum and deoxycholate adjuvant, also resulted in a dose-related induction of neutralizing antibodies against the homologous HIV-1 LAI strain, however with lower titers than those observed with gp120.

Finally, vaccination with a chimeric MN/LAI gp140 molecule, consisting of HIV-1 MN gp120 and truncated LAI gp41, and boosting with a linear V3-MN synthetic peptide, resulted in high levels of neutralizing antibodies against the homologous MN strain. In about half of the volunteers, these antibodies also neutralized HIV-1 SF2 but not HIV-1 LAI. Two of the candidate vaccines described before (MN and SF2 gp120) have been evaluated in a phase II trial in the United States among 300 healthy volunteers, some of whom were at high risk of infection.[583] A phase III efficacy trial was launched in the United States in the early summer of 1998, involving 5000 volunteers. A similar study of 2500 volunteers in Thailand is expected to follow. The products tested will be HIV-1 gp120 from the MN clade B strain, supplemented by gp120 from primary isolates of either clade B or clade E.

Thus, a number of mammalian-derived subunit recombinant envelope candidate vaccines have been shown to be well tolerated and to induce neutralizing antibodies against the homologous TCLA strains and against a few other strains from the B clade. However, these neutralizing antibodies were active against TCLA-adapted strains but not against primary clinical HIV-1 isolates (see discussion later). Also, a CTL response (mainly mediated by $CD4^+$ T cells) was rarely detected in volunteers immunized with envelope subunits, although HIV-1–specific lymphoproliferative responses were constantly detected (see Table 38–6). In contrast, live recombinant vectors expressing Env induced little neutralizing antibodies but did induce a $CD8^+$ CTL response. These deficiencies led to the view that complementary immune responses might be elicited by using a prime-boost immunization regimen, combining the two types of vaccines[584] (Table 38–7).

Controversy has been raised by the occurrence of intercurrent HIV-1 infections in vaccinees.[583] Among the 2029 uninfected people enrolled by the AIDS Vaccine Evaluation Group (U.S.) in phase I and II trials of candidate AIDS vaccines between 1988 and 1996, 23 subjects were diagnosed with intercurrent HIV-1 infection. Seventeen infections were associated with high-risk sexual exposures and six with both intravenous drug use and unprotected heterosexual contact. Thirteen had received a complete immunization schedule (three or more injections), six were partially immunized (two or fewer injections), and four were placebo recipients. They were enrolled in nine different protocols including MN rgp120 with alum or QS-21, SF2 rgp120 in MF59 or MPL, recombinant vaccinia virus expressing LAI gp160 + LAI rgp160, and MN rgp160 with alum and deoxy-

Table 38–7. **PRIME-BOOST PROTOCOLS TESTED IN HIV-UNINFECTED ADULT VOLUNTEERS**

PRIMING	BOOSTING	ADJUVANT
rVV-gp160 LAI	gp160 LAI	Alum
	gp160 MN	Deoxycholate/alum
	gp120 SF2	MF59
	gp120 LAI	Alum
	gp120 MN	Alum
	peptides (V3, p18)	IFA
ALVAC-gp160 MN	gp140 MN/LAI	Alum/IFA
	gp120 SF2	MF59
ALVAC-gp120 MN	gp120 SF2	MF59
tm/gag/protease	p24E-V3 peptide	Alum/QS-21
LAI	lipopeptides	QS-21
ALVAC-gp120 MN	gp120 SF2	MF59
tm/gag/prot/pol/	lipopeptides	QS-21
nef LAI		
gp140 MN/LAI	V3 MN peptide	Alum/IFA

Modified from Excler JL, Plotkin S. The prime-boost concept applied to HIV preventive vaccines. AIDS 11(suppl A):S127–S137, 1997.

cholate. The incidence of HIV-1 infections in vaccine recipients was 0.38 per 100 person-years compared with 0.30 in placebo recipients. Overall incidence of HIV-1 infection was 0.20 in preassigned lower risk individuals and 1.97 in higher risk subjects. Virus load measured between 8 and 14 months after infection was lower in vaccine recipients than in nonvaccinated matched control subjects (7482 versus 16,696 RNA copies per milliliter, respectively), but this difference was not statistically significant. Syncytia-inducing viruses were isolated from two subjects who showed a rapid decline in $CD4^+$ lymphocyte counts, whereas the other 17 isolates obtained from the group were non–syncytia-inducing. The V3 loop amino acid sequence of the transmitted viruses was similar between vaccinees and control subjects. At 1 year after infection, $CD4^+$ lymphocyte counts were not significantly different between vaccine recipients and nonvaccinated matched control subjects (521 ± 249 versus 494 ± 236, respectively). The antibody responses before HIV infection in vaccinees were similar to those from the matched subjects who remained uninfected. Complement-mediated antibody-dependent enhancing activity (C-ADE) was not detected before infection in any of the subjects, and the C-ADE titer after infection was similar to that seen in other HIV-1–infected people. In summary, 13 fully vaccinated subjects (of a total of 1688 vaccine recipients) acquired HIV-1 infection during phase I and II trials, a relatively low number, but there was no indication that the vaccine-induced immune response had any effect on the genotypic or phenotypic characteristics of the transmitted virus or on the early clinical course of HIV-1 infection.[585]

The Prime-Boost Concept[584]

The first HIV-1 vaccine prime-boost regimen tested in humans, which included priming with recombinant vaccinia virus expressing gp160 followed by boosting with paraformaldehyde-fixed recombinant vaccinia virus–infected PBMCs and soluble gp160,[470, 586] was shown to induce both neutralizing antibodies to the homologous HIV-1 IIIB (LAI) strain and HIV-1–specific CTL. A simplified regimen using only recombinant vaccinia virus and soluble gp160 or peptides (V3, p18, *env*T1) (see Table 38–7) induced a transient neutralizing response after each boost, a long-lasting memory T-cell response (2-year follow-up), and memory $CD8^+$, HLA class I–restricted Env-specific CTL.[587] In a more systematic manner, vaccinia-naive volunteers first immunized with a recombinant vaccinia virus expressing HIV-1 gp160 IIIB (HIVAC-1e) were subsequently boosted with baculovirus-derived gp160 IIIB in alum.[588] Neutralizing and fusion inhibition activities against the homologous strain as well as CD4-blocking antibodies were detected in about 50% of the subjects. Cross-reactive neutralization activity against HIV-1 MN was also detected. Seventy-five percent of the vaccinees demonstrated T-cell proliferative responses in vitro that were 3- to 10-fold higher than those induced by either vaccine alone and sustained for more than 18 months. Moreover, both $CD8^+$ and $CD4^+$ CTL were detected.[589, 590] Some vaccine-induced $CD8^+$ CTL clones produced a soluble factor that inhibited HIV-1 replication in acutely infected autologous $CD4^+$ blasts.[590, 591] In a subsequent study, a longer interval between priming and boost and two HIVAC-1e inoculations were associated with significantly higher neutralizing and fusion-inhibition antibody titers after boosting.[592]

However, potential obstacles hinder the general use of recombinant HIV-1 vaccinia virus. Serious adverse effects have been reported in people given vaccinia virus for smallpox prevention, particularly in those with eczema or immunodeficiency.[593] Vaccinia virus caused severe local reaction and dissemination in an asymptomatic but severely immunodeficient HIV-1–infected person.[594] In subjects immunized with HIVAC-1e, generalized malaise as well as local pain and tenderness developed 9 to 12 days after vaccination. Lymphadenitis was observed in 50% of the vaccinated subjects, and the median time for complete healing of the vaccinia lesion was 25 days.[471]

The use of a live canarypox vector (ALVAC) offers significant potential advantages over conventional vaccinia virus vectors.[469, 473, 474] Recombinant canarypox vaccines administered intramuscularly have been well tolerated in adult volunteers,[595] including HIV-1–infected asymptomatic patients.[596] A prime-boost regimen including priming with ALVAC–HIV vCP125, which expresses HIV-1 MN gp160, followed by two booster immunizations with recombinant hybrid gp140 MN/LAI in alum or IFA was well tolerated.[597] Antibodies to gp160 and to V3 were not detected after the two vCP125 injections but developed after the first booster immunization with gp140. After the second booster dose of gp140, neutralizing antibodies against HIV-1 MN were induced in 90% of the volunteers and against HIV-1 SF2 in 50% of them. Lymphoproliferation to gp140 was detected in only 25% of the subjects after the injections of vCP125 but in 100% after the first gp140 boost. An envelope-specific CTL activity was also observed in 39% of the volunteers. This activity was mediated by MHC class I–restricted $CD8^+$ T cells and was still present 2 years after the initial immunization in some subjects.[598]

In contrast, three immunizations with gp140 MN/LAI alone elicited low-level neutralizing responses and lymphoproliferation to gp140 in 92% of the subjects but no CTL activity. Priming with gp140 MN/LAI followed by boosting with a synthetic V3 MN peptide induced high neutralizing antibody titers but no CTL,[599] again emphasizing the essential role of priming with a live recombinant vector for the induction of a CTL response.

The prime-boost regimen was next tested in vaccinia-naive and vaccinia-immune volunteers using ALVAC–HIV-1 vCP125 at either 10^6 or 10^7 median tissue culture infective doses, followed by boosting with a Chinese hamster ovary–derived gp120 SF2 in MF59 adjuvant. High-titer neutralizing antibodies were elicited against both HIV-1 MN and HIV-1 SF2 in 100% of the volunteers. Moreover, a neutralizing activity was detected in a resting cell neutralization assay[357] against an HIV-1 clade B primary isolate (BZ167) closely related to HIV-

1 SF2 and MN. ADCC against both MN and SF2 was also detected in 70% of the subjects. Although the dose of ALVAC-HIV used for priming did not significantly influence the final neutralizing antibody titers, the higher dose of ALVAC apparently resulted in better priming of the cellular response, because Env-specific CD8+ CTL were detected in 40% of the subjects. In contrast with the prime-boost regimen involving HIVAC-1e and gp120, the prior vaccinia-immune status of the volunteers did not appear to impair the ability of the volunteers to respond to ALVAC-HIV and gp120.[600–602]

ALVAC–HIV vCP205, which expresses gp120 MN with the anchor region of gp41 LAI together with the *gag* and *protease* genes, was able to induce low levels of neutralizing antibodies against MN in 33% of the volunteers and a CD8+ CTL activity directed against Gag (but also Env and protease) in 30 to 60% of the immunized subjects, depending on the time point chosen and on the assay used.[603] Booster injections with the synthetic tandem peptide p24E-V3MN did not enhance these immune responses (see Table 38–6).

Priming with a higher dose of ALVAC–HIV vCP205 and priming with ALVAC–HIV vCP300 that expresses *env* and *gag* together with *pol* and *nef* CTL domains, followed by booster immunizations with gp120 SF2 in MF59, are being evaluated in HIV-uninfected adults according to various immunization schedules. Also, a new generation of ALVAC vectors with potentially higher immune potency is under study in human volunteers.

The repertoire of antibodies induced by these prime-boost protocols in most volunteers included binding antibodies to the V3 loop, ADCC antibodies, and neutralizing antibodies to both TCLA strains MN and SF2 and to at least one primary (BZ167) HIV-1 isolate. However, the breadth of these responses remains to be ascertained. Three to four injections of ALVAC-HIV were required to induce antibodies as well as antigen-specific lymphoproliferation and CTL. Of major importance, CTL derived from recipients of ALVAC-HIV were found capable of lysing autologous CD4+ lymphoblasts infected with the TCLA HIV-1 LAI strain or with primary HIV-1 isolates from genetically diverse virus clades.[432] CTL from vCP125 recipients showed either a broad pattern of cytolysis in which viruses from all clades tested were recognized or a highly restricted pattern in which no primary isolates, including clade B, were lysed. In contrast to vCP125 vaccinees, CTL reactivities in recipients of ALVAC–HIV vCP205 were consistently directed against a spectrum of primary isolate–infected targets.

These studies demonstrate that clade B–based canarypox vaccines can elicit, at least in some volunteers, a broad CTL reactivity capable of recognizing viruses belonging to genetically diverse HIV-1 clades.[432] They also reinforce the importance of including viral core antigens in the vaccine. The prime-boost concept using a live recombinant vaccine followed by a recombinant subunit vaccine offers, at the moment, the best hopes in terms of combined HIV-1–specific neutralizing antibody and CTL responses, which explains why it is now in phase II study using ALVAC–HIV vCP205 mixed together with HIV-1 SF2 gp120.

Improved Concepts and Future Orientations

Current and future clinical studies are addressing several unresolved scientific issues. So far, the prime-boost protocols have been mostly aimed at enhancing immune responses to HIV-1 *env*. However, it is of major interest to know whether CTL responses targeted to Gag, Pol, or Nef could be enhanced by specifically designed booster subunits. In this regard, pseudovirions or pseudoparticles containing Env and Gag proteins[498, 499] are a logical booster for ALVAC-HIV expressing Env and Gag proteins. Other subunits are being considered, such as recombinant p24 capsid protein. Lipopeptides[535, 536, 604] could be administered as a booster immunization for CTL after priming with recombinant live vectors that express the corresponding genes. Naked DNA vaccination (nucleic acid vaccination) offers a new promising vaccine approach now being tested in humans.[539–546] The type and magnitude of the immune responses induced by DNA vaccines might be optimized and oriented toward a Th1- or a Th2-type response by the use of new adjuvants including cytokines.[547] Priming with naked DNA vaccines followed by boosting with recombinant poxvirus has been found to elicit high CTL responses in animals and should be tested soon in humans.[537a, 537b]

Protective efficacy has been achieved in animals with the prime-boost strategy under certain conditions, depending on the vaccine design and the challenge model used,[605] but it remains low compared with the efficacy of live attenuated SIVΔ*nef* vaccines.[14, 15, 605] Live attenuated SIV[448, 449, 451–454] induced potent CTL responses[450, 454] and neutralizing antibodies to primary and heterologous virus strains.[392, 393, 464] However, the prospect of using a live attenuated HIV-1 vaccine in humans is hampered by major safety concerns (see earlier) and appears highly unlikely in the near future.[457, 459, 606]

Other problems that have not been addressed yet are the long time needed to induce significant immune responses with the current immunization schedules (6 to 12 months) and the duration of the immune responses generated by currently available HIV vaccines. Shorter immunization schedules are under clinical investigation for their capacity to induce earlier specific immune responses. Little is known about the duration of the vaccine-induced immune response. This parameter is critical for protection and may vary with the type of vaccine and the immunization schedule.

Another important question is that of protection at mucosal sites of entry. The most important mode of transmission of HIV is, by far, through sexual intercourse.[4, 310] The fact that 80% of HIV transmission worldwide is heterosexual and that women have a significantly greater risk of acquiring the infection through heterosexual transmission than do men makes it urgent to address the question of vaccine-induced protection at the mucosal level. A vaccine-induced barrier of mucosal immunity might play an important role in tipping the balance in favor of the host and preventing the establishment of HIV infection. For example, although parenteral vaccination with a whole inactivated SIV vaccine successfully protected monkeys from SIV infection after intravenous challenge,[440, 607] it failed to provide protection against infection or ameliorate disease after genital tract challenge.[608] Animal studies have shown that immunization with microparticles containing killed SIV can protect against pathogenic SIV challenge by the vaginal route.[504, 516, 609] Although the role of secretory immunity to HIV is unclear,[610] induction of an immune response at the surface of the genital mucosa may be of added benefit in reducing HIV transmission.[254]

The observation that mucosal plasma cells can migrate to distant mucosal sites has generated the concept of a common mucosal immune system,[611–613] enabling the generation of an immune response at a mucosal surface distant from the mucosal site of antigen administration. It has been shown, for example, that not all the migrating lymphocytes that have been stimulated in the Peyer patches necessarily return to the intestinal mucosa. Certainly, the majority of these cells (70%) do recirculate to the intestine, but many are also found to colonize other mucosal surfaces, such as those of the respiratory and genital tracts.[612] To stimulate mucosal immunity, vaccines must therefore be administered by a mucosal route, although recent observations show that protective mucosal immunity can be induced by appropriate vaccination procedures,[525] independent of vaccination at mucosal surfaces. Further immunization experiments by the parenteral or mucosal routes (oral, nasal, vaginal, rectal), using live recombinant vaccines or DNA, possibly followed by boosting with subunit vaccines, are obviously required to address this important question.

A strong correlation has been established between low HIV-1 plasma virus load and long-term survival in humans.[201, 202] Even if HIV vaccines were unable to provide sterilizing immunity but led to diminished virus loads in subsequently infected individuals, they would bring a clear benefit by delaying onset of AIDS. Whether this is indeed the case with current vaccine candidates remains to be demonstrated.

POSTEXPOSURE VACCINATION

Because the progression of HIV disease seems to depend on the balance between viral replication and host immunity,[205a] either enhancement of host immunity or inhibition of viral replication could lead to long-term control of HIV disease. Studies of several candidate vaccines (envelope subunits, gp120-deleted inactivated HIV-1 preparations, and ALVAC-HIV expressing gp160 MN) have shown short-term safety but poor or no immunogenicity in HIV-infected individuals.[579, 596, 614, 615] A beneficial effect of HIV vaccines on the immunological and virological markers of HIV disease progression in seropositive patients has hardly been observed and remains controversial. However, these immune-based strategies have been tested in the absence of or in association with suboptimal combinations of antiviral therapy. In this regard, it should be underscored that antiviral therapy is essential for effective suppression of virus replication.

With regard to immune restoration in HIV-treated patients, the different immune-based strategies may have as objectives (1) the maintenance or potentiation of existing HIV-specific immune responses, (2) the restoration or potentiation of nonspecific immune responses, (3) the induction of de novo HIV-specific immune responses, and (4) the restoration of preexisting HIV-specific immunity lost during HIV disease. Active anti-HIV immunization, especially designed to induce cell-mediated immune responses, might be seen as a complement of antiviral therapy and cytokine immunomodulation[616, 617] and should deserve further clinical research.

PASSIVE IMMUNOTHERAPY

By analogy with the success of prophylactic and therapeutic regimens using passive immunization with specific hyperimmune globulin products derived from human plasma against bloodborne viral pathogens such as hepatitis B virus, the development of hyperimmune anti-HIV immune globulin preparations might be of help in prevention of HIV infection in laboratory workers and in newborns from HIV-infected mothers. Studies of possible correlations between levels and specificity of maternal HIV antibody and vertical transmission have shown conflicting results.[330–332] It is currently unclear whether increased levels of maternal anti-HIV antibodies achieved either by passive administration of anti-HIV immune globulins or by active vaccination could interrupt vertical transmission. In addition, it is unknown whether maternally derived anti-HIV antibodies can have beneficial therapeutic properties (by reducing viral replication and delaying disease progression) for infants who become infected.[618] Studies have indicated lower transmission rate from infected pregnant women with high-affinity/avidity antibody to conserved portions of HIV-1 gp41,[619] to the CD4 binding site,[620] or to the V3 loop of gp120.[621] Nontransmitting mothers frequently have neutralizing antibodies to their own virus; in contrast, transmitting mothers rarely have neutralizing antibody against their child's isolate. It has furthermore been reported that mothers with autologous neutralizing antibody frequently have antibodies that can neutralize heterologous primary isolates.[622] These data have prompted the search for human neutralizing monoclonal antibodies. However, few of them have been found that are able to neutralize HIV-1 primary isolates in vitro.[365, 369] Those that do, such as monoclonal antibodies 2F5,[376] b12,[366] and 2G12,[374] would certainly deserve further clinical studies. As in the hepatitis B model, passive immunotherapy could conceivably be coupled with active immunization, as was recently suggested by the protection of newborns against SIV infection through vaccination of the mothers during pregnancy followed by passive immunization of the offspring at birth.[623] Hyperimmune anti–HIV-1 immune globulins (HIVIG) in combination with monoclonal antibodies 2F5 and 2G12 have shown additive or synergistic neutralization of primary HIV-1 isolates.[624]

REMAINING OBSTACLES

Immune correlates of protection against HIV infection in humans are still unknown.[163, 359, 407, 483, 565, 565a] Although both the neutralizing antibody and the CTL arms of the immune response seem to be involved, other potential correlates are being investigated, such as secretion of chemokines,[8, 9, 252, 525] cytokines,[625] and the HIV-1 viral suppressive factor CAF.[6, 7, 208, 209]

With respect to neutralizing antibodies, the accessibility of gp120 to antibodies and its importance in early infection events have made it a key target for vaccine design. However, the question of how to induce antibodies able to neutralize primary HIV-1 isolates remains unsolved. Neutralization epitopes in gp120 are not immunodominant, except in the TCLA HIV-1 strains that have been passaged multiple times through T-cell lines. These strains are extremely sensitive to neutralization in vitro by sera from seropositive individuals and gp120 vaccinees, in contrast with primary HIV-1 isolates. The V3 loop of gp120, which was initially considered the principal HIV-1 neutralization determinant,[107–111, 338, 339] because of its immunodominance in HIV-1 TCLA strains, appears relatively inaccessible on the native envelope of primary isolates.[350–352] Antibodies that neutralize primary isolates have been mapped to three distinct conformational epitopes, defined by monoclonal antibodies b12, 2G12, and 2F5, but induction of this type of antibodies by candidate vaccines has been unsuccessful to date.

Another question for antibody-based vaccine design is whether neutralizing antibodies can protect against HIV-1 infection. Immunization-induced protection against HIV-1 challenge in chimpanzees was correlated with high neutralizing antibody titers, but these studies suffer from the fact that they were performed with easy-to-neutralize TCLA virus strains. Protection from infection with a primary HIV-1 strain was not obtained in chimpanzees infused with monoclonal antibody 2F5.[571] In contrast, hu-PBL-SCID mice were completely protected from infection with a primary HIV-1 isolate by injection of monoclonal antibody IgG1b12 before challenge.[371] However, the protective antibody serum concentration in vivo was found to be high, corresponding to that for which 100% neutralization was attained in an in vitro neutralization assay. Such a high concentration would be difficult to reach and even more difficult to maintain by vaccination.

Since the initiation of HIV vaccine trials in human volunteers, several recipients of gp120- or gp160-based vaccines have acquired HIV infection as a result of a high-risk behavior.[583] In contrast to nonvaccinated infected individuals, anamnestic HIV-specific B- and T-cell responses could be documented within 3 weeks in one of these individuals, showing that prior vaccination primed both memory B and T cells.[585] However, these responses were insufficient to protect against infection and subsequent CD4+ cell decline and dysfunction. There is, therefore, little hope that vaccines based on gp120 only may be protective against HIV-1 infection in humans. In that respect, results from the phase III clinical trial of gp120 begun recently in the United States will be of paramount importance.

A third question is why primary isolate-neutralizing antibodies appear so late and remain at so low levels in most HIV-1–infected individuals.[391, 391a] It was suggested recently that the antibody response in HIV-1 infection is elicited by viral debris and nonnative forms of the HIV-1 envelope rather than virions. Anti–HIV-1 envelope antibodies from long-term HIV-1–seropositive individuals show high-affinity binding to unprocessed gp160 but little significant binding to infected cells.[370, 371, 626] This inadequate response to conformation-dependent epitopes might reflect the phenomenon of the "original antigenic sin," according to which antibodies elicited in response to a secondary antigen (the native gp160 on virions) react more strongly with the primary antigen (the nonnative glycoprotein) against which the immune system was initially primed. This hypothesis leads to predict that to induce primary isolate-neutralizing antibodies, vaccines should contain native oligomeric gp120/gp41 complexes devoid of unprocessed gp160, monomeric gp120, or byproduct molecules.[626]

With respect to CTL, there is growing evidence that CTL may play an important role in controlling primary virus infection[422–425b] and in the protection of seronegative uninfected partners in discordant couples, commercial sex workers, and babies born to seropositive mothers.[247–252] In addition, induction of high-level CTL precursors was demonstrated to provide protection from SIV infection in macaques.[454, 466b, 472] As a natural consequence, emphasis has been put on the development of vaccine strategies that will maximize cellular immunity.[437, 439] However, the finding of high $CD8^+$ CTL activity targeted to many HIV-1 antigens in HIV-infected individuals raises the question of why CTL cannot naturally handle HIV.[16, 627] The sustained high rate of virus production from newly infected cells in HIV-infected persons[10, 11] strongly suggests that productively infected cells resist CTL-mediated lysis. A possible mechanism to explain such an escape is that these cells have down-regulated levels of MHC (HLA) class I molecules. The Nef protein has been shown to induce down-regulation of class I antigens.[70, 71] It has also been reported that the Tat protein could lead to repression of MHC class I gene promoter activity.[628]

The inability of CTL to contain HIV raises the question of whether a CTL-based vaccine can confer protective immunity against HIV. The answer can be found in the SIV protection results of Gallimore and colleagues,[472] who showed that to be efficacious, HIV vaccines should be designed to generate levels of virus-specific CTL precursors comparable to those found in HIV-infected humans or in SIVΔ*nef*-infected and protected macaques. So far, however, it has been extremely difficult to reliably achieve this result by immunization with available prototype vaccines, including live recombinant vaccines. Whether this will be possible using the combination of a DNA vaccine with a live recombinant vaccine such as a poxvirus recombinant remains to be demonstrated.[537–537b]

One of the major difficulties that was foreseen in the development of an efficacious HIV vaccine was that of the virus hypervariability. The existence of two virus groups and of a variety of virus subtypes and the emergence of intersubtype recombinants could be an insurmountable obstacle to a global HIV vaccine.[26–30a] This problem, however, might be partially overcome if it is confirmed that clade B antigens, particularly the Gag and regulatory proteins, can induce cross-clade CTL activity.[432, 628a] Furthermore, because all HIV-1 strains, independent of clades, must conserve binding sites on their gp120 molecule for both CD4 and CCR-5 (or CXCR-4), there must be a common three-dimensional structure to the envelope gp120/gp41 complexes of all HIV-1 strains that is conserved across the genetic subtypes. Indeed, a triple combination of monoclonal antibodies 2F5, 2G12, and IgG1b12 could neutralize primary HIV-1 isolates at a remarkably low concentration and showed broad neutralization potency across virus subtypes.[629] Raised by a vaccine, such a combination of antibodies would give true hope for prevention of HIV-1 transmission on a global scale.[369, 630] The problem of HIV-1 genetic variability may therefore be of lesser importance than once imagined, if one uses a prime-boost vaccine strategy combining an avipox vector or a DNA vaccine able to induce cross-clade CTL reactivity, followed by a booster immunization with novel immunogens such as oligomeric forms of Env from a primary isolate or, possibly, pseudovirions that could induce antibodies to the critical conformation-dependent neutralization epitopes.[370, 371, 630] These points will be important to address in clinical trials in both developed and developing countries.

The use of complex vaccine preparations including Env and Gag proteins may render more difficult the differentiation between vaccinees and HIV-infected individuals, especially in countries where a high frequency of indeterminate Western blots is found. To address this problem, the HIV-1 envelope expressed by ALVAC–HIV vCP205 was deleted of the immunodominant region in the ectodomain of gp41, to which most HIV-1 infected subjects react. Sera of vCP205 vaccinees were negative in Western blot for the gp41 band and tested negative in a peptide–enzyme-linked immunosorbent assay based on the immunodominant region of gp41. However, because the ectodomain of gp41 is involved in folding and oligomerization of the gp120/gp41 complex, such a deletion might render the construct unable to induce conformation-dependent neutralizing antibodies.

The design of HIV-1 efficacy trials will have to address several critical scientific, ethical, and feasibility issues.[17, 631] The different possible endpoints of an efficacy trial include protection against HIV-1 infection, protection against progression to disease, and reduction of the HIV transmission rate to others and to the offspring by decreasing the viral load in the host. The mode of transmission (homosexual, intravenous, heterosexual) in the population in which the vaccine will be tested, the availability of efficacious viral drugs (especially in developed countries), and the modification of behavior of vaccinees along the study could substantially influence the interpretation of the vaccine efficacy results. These points will have to be addressed in due time.

There is no doubt that an effective AIDS vaccine would be a major asset in a global AIDS program designed to stop the spread of HIV infection and that it warrants all our efforts. Unless we find a means to reverse the present trend, the AIDS epidemic will irreparably damage many societies and could turn into an epidemiological catastrophe.[4a, 631] However, there will be no "quick fix" to the HIV vaccine problem, and none should be expected.[18a]

Acknowledgments

The efficient assistance of Claude Avrameas with the manuscript preparation is gratefully acknowledged. We thank Andrew Borman for help with the figures and André Habel for helpful assistance with the bibliographical search.

REFERENCES

1. Gottlieb MS, Schroff R, Schanker HM, et al. *Pneumocystis carinii* pneumonia and mucosal candidiasis in previously healthy homosexual men. N Engl J Med 305:1425–1431, 1981.
2. Masur H, Michelis MA, Greene JB, et al. An outbreak of community acquired *Pneumocystis carinii* pneumonia. Initial manifestation of cellular immune dysfunction. N Engl J Med 305:1431–1438, 1981.
3. Chin J. Global estimates of AIDS cases and HIV infections. AIDS 5(suppl 2):S57–S61, 1991.
4. UNAIDS and WHO. VIH/SIDA: Le Point sur l'Épidémie Mondiale. Genève, OMS, December 1996.
4a. Piot P. The science of AIDS: A tale of two worlds. Science 280:1844–1845, 1998.
5. Sittitrai W, Brown T, Sterns J. Opportunities for over-coming the continuing restraints to behavioral change and HIV risk reduction. AIDS 4(suppl 1):S269–S276, 1990.
5a. Phaolcharoen W. HIV/AIDS prevention in Thailand: Success and challenges. Science 280:1873–1874, 1998.
6. Walker CM, Moody DJ, Stites DP, Levy JA. $CD8^+$ lymphocytes can control HIV infection in vitro by suppressing virus replication. Science 234:1563–1566, 1986.
7. Mackewicz C, Barker E, Levy JA. Role of beta-chemokines in suppressing HIV replication. Science 274:1393–1394, 1996.
8. Cocchi F, De Vico AL, Garzino Demo A, et al. Identification of RANTES, MIP-1 alpha and MIP-1 beta as the major HIV suppressive factor produced by $CD8^+$ T cells. Science 270:1811–1815, 1995.
9. D'Souza MP, Harden VA. Chemokines and HIV-1 second receptors. Nat Med 2:1293–1300, 1996.
10. Ho DD, Neumann AU, Perelson AS, et al. Rapid turnover of plasma virions and CD4 lymphocytes in HIV-1 infection. Nature 373:123–126, 1995.
11. Wei X, Gosh S, Taylor ME, et al. Viral dynamics in human immunodeficiency virus type 1 infection. Nature 373:117–122, 1995.
12. Pantaleo G, Soudeyns H, Demarest JF, et al. Evidence for rapid disappearance of initially expanded HIV-specific $CD8^+$ T cell clones during primary HIV infection. Proc Natl Acad Sci U S A 94:9848–9853, 1997.
13. Miedema F, Klein MR. AIDS pathogenesis: A finite immune response to blame? Science 272:505–506, 1996.
14. Daniel MD, Kirschhoff F, Czajak SC, et al. Protective effects of a live attenuated SIV vaccine with a deletion in the *nef* gene. Science 258:1938–1941, 1992.
15. Almond N, Kent K, Cranage M, et al. Protection by attenuated simian immunodeficiency virus in macaques against challenge with virus-infected cells. Lancet 345:1342–1344, 1995.

15a. Letvia NL. Progress in the development of an HIV-1 vaccine. Science 280:1875–1879, 1998.
16. Paul WE. Can the immune response control HIV infection? Cell 82:177–182, 1995.
17. Fauci A. Development of an HIV vaccine: A departure from the usual paradigms. In Vaccines, One Hundred Years After Louis Pasteur. Paris, Institut Pasteur, 1995, pp 177–180.
18. Girard M. Vaccin anti-VIH: Etat de la question. Virologie 1:191–194, 1997.
18a. Burton DR, Moore JP. Why do we not have an HIV vaccine and how can we make one. Nat Med 4:495–498, 1998.
19. Coffin J, Haase A, Levy JA, et al. What to call the AIDS virus? [letter] Nature 321:10, 1986.
20. Barré-Sinoussi F, Chermann JC, Rey F, et al. Isolation of a T-lymphocytropic retrovirus from a patient at risk for acquired immune deficiency syndrome (AIDS). Science 220:868–871, 1983.
21. Popovic M, Sarngadharan MG, Read E, Gallo RC. Detection, isolation and continuous production of cytopathic retroviruses (HTLV-III) from patients with AIDS and pre-AIDS. Science 224:497–500, 1984.
22. Levy JA, Hoffman AD, Kramer S, et al. Isolation of lymphocytopathic retroviruses from San Francisco patients with AIDS. Science 225:840–842, 1984.
23. Clavel F, Mansiho K, Chamaret S, et al. Human immunodeficiency virus type 2 infection associated with AIDS in West Africa. N Engl J Med 316:1180–1185, 1987.
24. Marlink R, Kanki P, Thior I, et al. Reduced rate of disease development after HIV-2 infection as compared to HIV-1. Science 265:1587–1595, 1994.
25. Narayan O, Clements JE. The biology and pathogenesis of lentiviruses. J Gen Virol 70:1617–1639, 1989.
26. Myers G, Korber B, Foley B, et al. Human retroviruses and AIDS: A compilation and analysis of nucleic acid and amino acid sequences. Theoretical Biology and Biophysics Group, Los Alamos National Laboratory, Los Alamos, NM, 1996.
27. Sharp PM, Robertson DL, Gao F, Hahn BH. Origins and diversity of human immunodeficiency viruses. AIDS 8(suppl 1):S27–S42, 1994.
28. Gao F, Morrisson SG, Robertson DL, et al. Molecular cloning and analysis of functional envelope genes from human immunodeficiency virus type 1 sequence subtypes A through G. J Virol 70:1651–1667, 1996.
29. Robertson DL, Sharp P, McCutchan FE, Hahn BH. Recombination in HIV-1. Nature 374:124–126, 1995.
30. Salminen MO, Carr JK, Robertson DL, et al. Evolution and probable transmission of intersubtype recombinant human immunodeficiency virus type 1 in a Zambian couple. J Virol 71:2647–2655, 1997.
30a. Korber B, Theiler J, Wolinsky S. Limitations of a molecular clock applied to considerations of the origin of HIV-1. Science 280:1868–1871, 1998.
31. Earl PL, Doms RW, Moss B. Oligomeric structure of the human immunodeficiency virus type 1 envelope glycoprotein. Proc Natl Acad Sci U S A 87:648–652, 1990.
32. Henderson CE, Sourder RC, Copeland TD, et al. Gag precursors of HIV and SIV are cleaved into six proteins found in the mature virions. J Med Primatol 19:411–419, 1990.
33. Henderson CE, Bowers MA, Sourder RC, et al. Gag proteins of highly replicative MN strain of human immunodeficiency virus type 1: Post-transcriptional modifications, proteolytic processing and complete amino acid sequences. J Virol 66:1856–1865, 1992.
34. Ott DE, Coren LV, Kane BP, et al. Cytoskeletal proteins inside human immunodeficiency virus type 1 virions. J Virol 70:7734–7743, 1996.
35. Lu M, Blacklow SC, Kim PS. A trimeric structural domain of the HIV-1 transmembrane glycoprotein. Nat Struct Biol 2:1075–1082, 1995.
36. Pombourios P, Wilson KA, Center RJ, et al. Human immunodeficiency virus type 1 envelope glycoprotein oligomerization requires the gp41 amphipathic alpha-helical/leucine zipper-like sequence. J Virol 71:2041–2049, 1997.
37. Bugge TH, Lindhardt BO, Hansen LL, et al. Characterization of the fusion domain of the human immunodeficiency virus type 1 envelope glycoprotein GP41. Proc Natl Acad Sci U S A 87:4650–4654, 1990.
38. Schaal H, Klein M, Gehrmann P, et al. Requirement of N-terminal amino acid residues of gp41 for human immunodeficiency virus type 1–mediated cell fusion. J Virol 69:3308–3314, 1995.
39. Chen C-H, Matthews TJ, Mc Danal CB, et al. A molecular clasp in the human immunodeficiency virus (HIV) type 1 TM protein determines the anti-HIV activity of gp41 derivatives: Implications for viral fusion. J Virol 69:3771–3777, 1995.
40. Leonard CK, Spellman MW, Riddle L, et al. Assignment of intra-chain disulfide bonds and characterization of potential glycosylation sites of the type 1 recombinant human immunodeficiency virus envelope glycoprotein (gp120) expressed in Chinese hamster ovary cells. J Biol Chem 265:1037–1038, 1990.
40a. Wyatt R, Sodroski J. The HIV-1 envelope glycoproteins: Fusogens, antigens, and immunogens. Science 280:1884–1888, 1998.
41. Ratner L. Glucosidase inhibitors for treatment of HIV-1 infection. AIDS Res Hum Retroviruses 8:165–173, 1992.
42. Earl PL, Moss B, Doms RW. Folding, interaction with GRP78-BIP, assembly, and transport of the human immunodeficiency virus type 1 envelope protein. J Virol 65:2047–2055, 1991.
43. Otteken A, Earl PL, Moss B. Folding, assembly and intracellular trafficking of the human immunodeficiency virus type 1 envelope glycoprotein analyzed with monoclonal antibodies recognizing maturational intermediates. J Virol 70:3407–3415, 1996.
44. Labranchie CC, Sauter MM, Haggarty BS, et al. A single amino acid change in the cytoplasmic domain of the simian immunodeficiency virus transmembrane molecule increases enveloped glycoprotein expression on infected cells. J Virol 69:5217–5227, 1995.
45. Moore JP, Sattentau QJ, Wyatt R, Sodroski J. Probing the structure of the human immunodeficiency virus surface glycoprotein gp120 with a panel of monoclonal antibodies. J Virol 68:469–484, 1994.
46. Cosson P. Direct interaction between the envelope and matrix proteins of HIV-1. EMBO J 15:5783–5788, 1996.
47. Hill CP, Worthylake D, Bancroff DP, et al. Crystal structure of the trimeric human immunodeficiency virus type 1 matrix protein: Implications for membrane association and assembly. Proc Natl Acad Sci U S A 33:3099–3104, 1996.
48. Arthur LO, Bess JW Jr, Sowder RC, et al. Cellular proteins bound to immunodeficiency viruses: Implications for pathogenesis and vaccines. Science 258:1935–1938, 1992.
49. Fortin JF, Cantin R, Lamontagne G, Tremblay M. Host-derived ICAM-1 glycoproteins incorporated on human immunodeficiency virus type 1 are biologically active and enhance viral infectivity. J Virol 71:3588–3596, 1997.
50. Rizzuto CD, Sodroski JG. Contribution of virion ICAM-1 to human immunodeficiency virus infectivity and sensitivity to neutralization. J Virol 71:4847–4851, 1997.
51. Ratner L, Haseltine W, Patarca R, et al. Complete nucleotide sequence of the AIDS virus, HTLV-III. Nature 313:277–284, 1985.
52. Wain-Hobson S, Sonigo P, Danos O, et al. Nucleotide sequence of the AIDS virus, LAV. Cell 40:9–17, 1985.
53. Carr JK, Salminen MO, Koch C, et al. Full-length sequence of a human immunodeficiency virus type 1 isolate from Thailand. J Virol 70:5935–5943, 1996.
54. Gao F, Robertson DL, Morrisson SG, et al. The heterosexual human immunodeficiency virus type 1 epidemic in Thailand is caused by an intersubtype (A/E) recombinant of African origin. J Virol 70:7013–7029, 1990.
55. Paillart JC, Skripkin E, Ehresman B, et al. A loop "kissing" complex is the essential part of the dimer linkage of genomic HIV-1 RNA. Proc Natl Acad Sci U S A 92:5572–5577, 1996.
56. Paillart JC, Berthoux L, Ottmann M, et al. A dual role of the putative RNA dimerization initiation site of human immunodeficiency virus type 1 in genomic RNA packaging and proviral DNA synthesis. J Virol 70:8348–8354, 1996.
57. Vaishnav YN, Wong-Staal F. The biochemistry of AIDS. Annu Rev Biochem 60:577–630, 1991.
58. Jeang KR, Chang YN, Berkhout B, et al. Regulation of HIV expression: Mechanisms of action of Tat and Rev. AIDS 5(suppl 2):S3–S14, 1991.
59. Trono D. HIV accessory proteins: Leading roles for the supporting cast. Cell 82:189–192, 1995.

60. Miller RH, Sarver N. HIV accessory proteins as therapeutic targets. Nat Med 3:389–394, 1997.
60a. Emerman M, Malim MH. HIV-1 regulatory/accessory genes: Keys to unraveling viral and host cell biology. Science 280:1880–1884, 1998.
61. Feinberg MB, Baltimore D, Frankel A. The role of Tat in the human immunodeficiency virus life cycle indicates a primary effect on transcriptional elongation. Proc Natl Acad Sci U S A 88:4045–4049, 1991.
62. Han XM, Laras A, Rounseville MP. Human immunodeficiency virus type 1 Tat-mediated transactivation correlates with the phosphorylation site of a TAR RNA stem-binding factor. J Virol 66:4065–4072, 1992.
63. Dayton AJ, Terwilliger EF, Potz J, et al. *Cis*-acting sequences responsive to the *rev* gene product of the human immunodeficiency virus. J Acquir Immune Defic Syndr 1:441–452, 1988.
64. Lu X, Heimer J, Rekosh D, Hammarskjold ML. U1 small nuclear RNA plays a direct role in the formation of a Rev-regulated human immunodeficiency virus *env* mRNA that remains unspliced. Proc Natl Acad Sci U S A 87:7589–7602, 1990.
65. Pomerantz RJ, Seshama T, Trono D. Efficient replication of human immunodeficiency virus type 1 requires a threshold level of Rev: Potential implications for latency. J Virol 66:1809–1813, 1992.
66. Harris M. From negative factor to a critical role in virus pathogenesis: The changing fortunes of Nef. J Gen Virol 77:2379–2392, 1996.
67. Pandori MW, Fitch NJS, Craig HM, et al. Producer-cell modification of human immunodeficiency virus type 1: Nef is a virion protein. J Virol 70:4283–4290, 1996.
68. Tritsen MC, Marshall AZ, Kapras J, et al. Origin of *vpx* in lentiviruses. Nature 347:341–342, 1990.
69. Brigino E, Haraguchi S, Koutsonikolis A, et al. Interleukin 10 is induced by recombinant HIV-1 Nef protein involving the calcium/calmodulin-dependent phosphodiesterase signal transduction pathway. Proc Natl Acad Sci U S A 94:3178–3182, 1997.
70. Schwartz O, Maréchal V, Le Gall S, et al. Endocytosis of major histocompatibility complex class I molecules is induced by the HIV-1 Nef protein. Nat Med 2:338–342, 1996.
71. Collins KL, Chen BK, Kalams SA, et al. HIV-1 Nef protein protects infected primary cells against killing by cytotoxic T lymphocytes. Nature 391:397–401, 1998.
72. Kestler HW, Ringler DH, Mori K, et al. Importance of the *nef* gene for maintenance of high virus loads and for development of AIDS. Cell 65:851–862, 1991.
73. Whatmore AM, Cook N, Hall GA, et al. Repair and evolution of Nef in vivo modulates simian immunodeficiency virus virulence. J Virol 69:5117–5123, 1995.
74. Deacon NJ, Tsykin A, Solomon A, et al. Genomic structure of an attenuated quasi species of HIV-1 from a blood transfusion donor and recipients. Science 270:988–991, 1995.
75. Mervis RJ, Ahmed N, Lillehof EP, et al. The *gag* gene products of human immunodeficiency virus type 1: Alignment within the *gag* open reading frame, identification of post-translational modifications and evidence for alternative *gag* precursors. J Virol 62:3993–4002, 1988.
76. Bryant M, Ratner L. Myristoylation-dependent replication and assembly of human immunodeficiency virus I. Proc Natl Acad Sci U S A 87:523–527, 1990.
77. Drummond JE, Mounts P, Gorelick RJ, et al. Wild-type and mutant HIV type 1 nucleocapsid proteins increase the propagation of long cDNA transcripts by viral reverse transcriptase. AIDS Res Hum Retroviruses 13:533–543, 1997.
77a. Braaten D, Franke EK, Luban J. Cyclophilin A is required for the replication of group M human immunodeficiency virus type 1 (HIV-1) and simian immunodeficiency virus SIV (CP2) GAB but not group O HIV-1 or other primate immunodeficiency viruses. J Virol 70:4220–4227, 1996.
78. Klatzmann D, Champagne E, Chamaret S, et al. T-lymphocyte T4 molecule behaves as the receptor for human retrovirus LAV. Nature 312:767–768, 1984.
79. Dalgleish AG, Beverley PCL, Clapham PR, et al. The CD4 (T4) antigen is an essential component of the receptor for the AIDS retrovirus. Nature 312:763–767, 1984.
80. Maddon PJ, Dalgleish AG, McDougal JS, et al. The T4 gene encodes the AIDS virus receptor and is expressed in the immune system and the brain. Cell 47:333–348, 1986.
81. Fantini J, Cook DG, Nathanson N, et al. Infection of colonic epithelial cell lines by type 1 human immunodeficiency virus is associated with cell surface expression of galactosylceramide, a potential alternative gp120 receptor. Proc Natl Acad Sci U S A 90:2700–2704, 1993.
82. Clapham P, Weber JM, Whitby D, et al. Soluble CD4 blocks the infectivity of diverse strains of HIV and SIV for T cells and monocytes but not for brain and muscle cells. Nature 337:388–390, 1989.
83. Clapham PR, McKnight A, Weiss RA. Human immunodeficiency virus type 2 infection and fusion of CD4-negative human cell lines: Induction and enhancement by soluble CD4. J Virol 66:3531–3537, 1992.
84. Harouse JM, Bhat S, Spitalnik SL, et al. Inhibition of entry of HIV-1 in neural cell lines by antibodies against galactosyl ceramide. Science 253:320–323, 1991.
85. Curtis BM, Scharnowske S, Watson AJ. Sequence and expression of a membrane-associated C-type lectin that exhibits CD4-independent binding of human immunodeficiency virus envelope glycoprotein gp120. Proc Natl Acad Sci U S A 89:8356–8360, 1992.
86. Lasky LA, Nakamura G, Smith D. Delineation of a region of the human immunodeficiency virus type 1 gp120 glycoprotein critical for interaction with the CD4 receptor. Cell 50:975–985, 1987.
87. Cordonnier A, Rivière Y, Montagnier L, Emerman M. Effects of mutations in hyper-conserved regions of the extracellular glycoprotein of human immunodeficiency virus type 1 on receptor binding. J Virol 63:4464–4468, 1989.
88. Olshevsky U, Helseth E, Furman C, et al. Identification of individual human immunodeficiency virus type 1 gp120 amino acids important for CD4 receptor binding. J Virol 64:5701–5707, 1990.
89. Sattentau QJ, Moore JP. Conformational changes in the human immunodeficiency virus envelope glycoproteins by soluble CD4 binding. J Exp Med 174:407–415, 1991.
90. Freed EO, Myers DJ, Risser R. Characterization of the fusion domain of the human immunodeficiency virus type 1 envelope glycoprotein gp41. Proc Natl Acad Sci U S A 87:4650–4654, 1990.
91. Freed EO, Myers DJ. Identification and characterization of fusion and processing domains of the human immunodeficienciy virus type 2 envelope glycoprotein. J Virol 66:5472–5478, 1992.
92. Center RJ, Kemp BE, Pombourios P. Human immunodeficiency virus type 1 and 2 glycoproteins oligomeric through conserved sequences. J Virol 71:5706–5711, 1997.
93. Earl PL, Moss B. Mutational analysis of the assembly domain of the HIV-1 envelope glycoprotein. AIDS Res Hum Retroviruses 9:589–594, 1993.
94. Moore JP, Willey RL, Lewis GK, et al. Immunological evidence for interactions between the first, second and fifth conserved domains of the gp120 surface glycoprotein of human immunodeficiency virus type 1. J Virol 68:6836–6847, 1994.
94a. Wyatt R, Kwong PD, Desjardins E, et al. The antigenic structure of the HIV gp120 envelope glycoprotein. Nature 393:705–711, 1998.
94b. Kwong PD, Wyatt R, Robinson J, et al. Structures of an HIV gp120 envelope glycoprotein in complex with the CD4 receptor and a neutralizing human antibody. Nature 393:648–659, 1998.
95. Shugars DC, Wild CT, Greenwell TK, Matthews TJ. Biophysical characterization of recombinant proteins expressing the leucine zipper-like domain of the human immunodeficiency virus type 1 transmembrane protein gp41. J Virol 70:2982–2991, 1996.
96. Wiley DC, Skehel JJ. The structure and function of the hemagglutinin membrane glycoprotein of influenza virus. Annu Rev Biochem 56:365–394, 1987.
97. Gartner S, Popovic M. Macrophage tropism of HIV-1. AIDS Res Hum Retroviruses 6:1017–1021, 1990.
98. Roos MT, Miedema F, Meinesz, et al. Viral phenotype and immune response in primary human immunodeficiency virus type 1 infection. J Infect Dis 165:427–432, 1992.
99. Schuittemaker H, Koot M, Kootstra NA, et al. Biological phenotype of human immunodeficiency virus type 1 clones at different

stages of infections: Progression of disease is associated with a shift from monocytotropic to T-cell-tropic populations. J Virol 66:1354–1360, 1992.
100. Shioda T, Levy JA, Cheng-Mayer C. Macrophage and T-cell-line tropism of HIV-1 are determined by specific regions of the envelope gp120 gene. Nature 340:167–169, 1991.
101. Grimaila RJ, Fuller BA, Rennert PD, et al. Mutations in the principal neutralization determinant of human immunodeficiency virus type 1 affect syncytium formation, virus infectivity, growth kinetics, and neutralization. J Virol 66:1875–1883, 1992.
102. Cheng-Mayer C, Quiroga M, Tung JW, et al. Viral determinants of human immunodeficiency virus type 1 T-cell or macrophage tropism, cytopathogenicity and CD4 antigen modulation. J Virol 64:4390–4398, 1990.
103. Hwang SS, Boyle TJ, Lyerly HK, Cullen BR. Identification of the envelope V3 loop as the primary determinant of cell tropism in HIV-1. Science 253:71–74, 1991.
104. Fouchier RA, Groenink M, Koostra NA, et al. Phenotype-associated sequence variation in the third variable domain of the human immunodeficiency virus type 1 gp120 molecule. J Virol 66:3183–3187, 1992.
105. Shioda T, Levy JA, Cheng-Mayer C. Small amino acid changes in the V3 hypervariable region of gp120 can affect the T-cell line and macrophage tropism of human immunodeficiency virus type 1. Proc Natl Acad Sci U S A 89:9434–9438, 1992.
106. Kuiken CL, de Jong J-J, Boan E. Evolution of the V3 envelope domain in proviral sequences and isolates of human immunodeficiency virus type 1 during transition of the viral biological phenotype. J Virol 66:4622–4627, 1992.
107. Putney SD, Matthews TJ, Rober WG, et al. HTLV-III/LAV neutralizing antibodies to an *E. coli* produced fragment of the virus envelope. Science 234:1392–1395, 1986.
108. Rusche JR, Javaherian K, McDanal CB, et al. Antibodies that inhibit fusion of human immunodeficiency virus–infected cells bind a 24–amino acid sequence of the viral envelope, gp120. Proc Natl Acad Sci U S A 85:3198–3202, 1988.
109. Javaherian K, Langlois AJ, McDanal CB, et al. Principal neutralizing domain of the human immunodeficiency virus type 1 envelope protein. Proc Natl Acad Sci U S A 86:6768–6772, 1989.
110. LaRosa G, Davide JP, Weinhold K, et al. Conserved sequence and structural elements in the HIV-1 principal neutralizing domain. Science 249:932–935, 1990.
111. Freed EO, Myers DJ, Risser R. Identification of the principal neutralizing determinant of human immunodeficiency virus type 1 as a fusion domain. J Virol 65:190–194, 1991.
112. Clements GJ, Price-Jones MJ, Stephens PE, et al. The V3 loops of the HIV-1 and HIV-2 surface glycoproteins contain proteolytic cleavage sites: A possible function in viral fusion? AIDS Res Hum Retroviruses 7:3–16, 1991.
113. Werner A, Levy JA. Human immunodeficiency virus type 1 envelope gp120 is cleaved after incubation with recombinant soluble CD4. J Virol 67:2566–2574, 1993.
114. Moore JP, Nara PL. The role of the V3 loop of gp120 in HIV infection. AIDS 5(suppl 2):S21–S33, 1991.
115. Feng Y, Broder CC, Kennedy PE, Berger EA. HIV-1 entry cofactor: Functional cDNA-cloning of a seven-transmembrane, G protein–coupled receptor. Science 272:872–877, 1996.
116. Dragic T, Litwin V, Allaway GP, et al. HIV entry into $CD4^+$ cells is mediated by the chemokine receptor CC-CKR-5. Nature 381:667–673, 1996.
117. Deng HK, Choe S, Ellmeier W, et al. Identification of a major co-receptor for primary isolates of HIV-1. Nature 381:661–666, 1996.
118. Alkatib G, Combadiere C, Broder CC, et al. CC-CKR5: A RANTES, MIP-1α, MIP-1β receptor as a fusion cofactor for macrophage-tropic HIV-1. Science 272:1955–1958, 1996.
119. Choe H, Farzan M, Sun Y, et al. The β-chemokine receptors CCR3 and CCR5 facilitate infection by primary HIV-1 isolates. Cell 85:1135–1148, 1996.
120. He L, Chen Y, Farzan M, et al. CCR3 and CCR5 are co-receptors for HIV-1 infection of microglia. Nature 385:645–649, 1996.
120a. Ross TM, Cullen BR. The ability of HIV type 1 to use CCR-3 as a coreceptor is controlled by envelope V1/V2 sequences acting in conjunction with a CCR-5 tropic V3 loop. Proc Natl Acad Sci U S A 95:7682–7686, 1998.
121. Simmons G, Wilkinson D, Reeves JD, et al. Primary, syncytium-inducing human immunodeficiency virus type 1 isolates are dual-tropic and most can use either Lestr or CCR5 as coreceptors for virus entry. J Virol 70:8355–8360, 1996.
122. Doranz BJ, Rucker J, Yi Y, et al. A dual-tropic primary HIV-1 isolate that uses fusin and the β-chemokine receptors CKR-5, CKR-3 and CKR-2b as fusion cofactors. Cell 85:1149–1158, 1996.
123. Berger EA. HIV entry and tropism: The chemokine receptor connection. AIDS 11(suppl A):S3–S16, 1997.
124. Endres MJ, Clapham PB, Marsh M, et al. CD4-independent infection by HIV-2 is mediated by fusin CXCR4. Cell 87:745–756, 1996.
125. Edinger AL, Amédée A, Miller K, et al. Differential utilization of CCR5 by macrophage- and T cell–tropic simian immunodeficiency virus strains. Proc Natl Acad Sci U S A 94:4005–4010, 1997.
126. Marcon L, Choe H, Martin KA, et al. Utilization of C-C chemokine receptor 5 by the envelope glycoproteins of a pathogenic simian immunodeficiency virus, SIVmac239. J Virol 71:2522–2527, 1997.
127. Alkhatib G, Liao F, Berger EA, et al. A new SIV coreceptor, STRL33 [letter]. Nature 388:238, 1997.
128. Deng HK, Unutmaz D, Kewal Ramani VN, Littman DR. Expression cloning of new receptors used by simian and human immunodeficiency virus. Nature 388:296–300, 1997.
129. Lapham C, Ouyang J, Chandrasekhar B, et al. Evidence for cell-surface association between fusin and the CD4-gp120 complex in human cell lines. Science 274:602–605, 1996.
130. Wu L, Gerard NP, Wyatt R, et al. CD4-induced interaction of primary HIV-1 gp120 glycoprotein with the chemokine receptor CCR5. Nature 384:179–183, 1996.
131. Trkola A, Dragic T, Arthos J, et al. CD4-independent antibody-sensitive interactions between HIV-1 and its co-receptor CCR-5. Nature 384:184–187, 1996.
131a. Verrier F, Charneau P, Altmeyer R, et al. Antibodies to several conformation-dependent epitopes of gp120/gp41 inhibit CCR5-dependent cell-to-cell fusion mediated by the native envelope glycoprotein of a primary macrophage-tropic HIV-1 isolate. Proc Natl Acad Sci U S A 94:9326–9331, 1997.
132. Oberlin E, Amara A, Bachelerie F, et al. The CXC chemokine SDF-1 is the ligand for LESTR/fusion and prevents infection by T-cell-line–adapted HIV-1. Nature 382:833–835, 1996.
133. Bleul CC, Farzan M, Choe H, et al. The lymphocyte chemoattractant SDF-1 is a ligand for LESTR/fusin and blocks HIV-1 entry. Nature 382:829–833, 1996.
134. Björndal A, Deng H, Jansson M, et al. Coreceptor usage of primary human immunodeficiency virus type 1 isolates varies according to biological phenotype. J Virol 71:7478–7487, 1997.
135. Cocchi F, DeVico A, Garzino-Demo A, et al. The V3 domain of the HIV-1 gp120 envelope glycoprotein is critical for chemokine-mediated blockade of infection. Nat Med 2:1244–1247, 1996.
136. Harrowe G, Cheng-Mayer C. Amino acid substitution in the V3 loop are responsible for adaptation to growth in transformed T cell–lines of a primary human immunodeficiency virus type 1. Virology 210:490–494, 1995.
137. Jansson M, Popovic M, Karlsson A, et al. Sensitivity to inhibition by β-chemokines correlates with biological phenotype of primary HIV-1 isolates. Proc Natl Acad Sci U S A 93:15382–15387, 1996.
138. Dittma MT, McKnight A, Simmons G, et al. HIV-1 tropism and co-receptor use. Nature 385:495–496, 1997.
139. Liu R, Paxton WA, Choe S, et al. Homozygous defect in HIV-1 coreceptor accounts for resistance of some multiply-exposed individuals to HIV-1 infection. Cell 86:367–377, 1996.
140. Samson M, Libert F, Doranz BJ, et al. Resistance to HIV-1 infection in Caucasian individuals bearing mutant alleles of the CCR-5 chemokine receptor gene. Nature 382:722–725, 1996.
141. Dean M, Carrington M, Winkler C, et al. Genetic restriction of HIV-1 infection and progression to AIDS by a deletion allele of the CKR5 structural gene. Science 273:1856–1862, 1996.
142. Rana S, Besson G, Cook DG, et al. Role of CCR5 in infection of primary macrophages and lymphocytes by macrophage-tropic strains of human immunodeficiency virus: Resistance to patient-derived and prototype isolates resulting from the Δ*ccr5* mutation. J Virol 71:3219–3227, 1997.

143. Biti R, French R, Young J, et al. HIV-infection in an individual homozygous for the CCR5 deletion allele. Nat Med 3:252–253, 1997.
144. Moore JP, McKeating JA, Weiss RA, Sattentau QJ. Dissociation of gp120 from HIV-1 virions induced by soluble CD4. Science 250:1139–1142, 1990.
145. Chan DC, Fass D, Berger JM, Kim PS. Core structure of gp41 from the HIV-1 envelope glycoprotein. Cell 89:263–273, 1997.
146. Weisenhorn W, Dessen A, Marrison SC, et al. Atomic structure of the ectodomain from HIV-1 gp41. Nature 387:426–430, 1997.
146a. Pritsker M, Jones P, Blumenthal R, Shai Y. A synthetic all D-amino acid peptide corresponding to the N-terminal sequence of HIV-1 gp41 recognizes the wild-type fusion peptide in the membrane and inhibits HIV-1 envelope glycoprotein-mediated cell fusion. Proc Natl Acad Sci U S A 95:7287–7292, 1998.
147. Binley J, Moore JP. The viral mousetrap. Nature 387:346–348, 1997.
148. Wild CT, Shugars, DC, Greenwell TK, et al. Peptides corresponding to a predicted α-helical domain of human immunodeficiency virus type 1 gp41 are potent inhibitors of virus infection. Proc Natl Acad Sci U S A 91:9770–9774, 1994.
149. Stevenson M, Stanwick TT, Dempsey MP, Lamonica CA. HIV-1 replication is controlled at the level of T-cell activation and proviral integration. EMBO J 9:1551–1560, 1990.
150. Robinson HL, Zinkus DM. Accumulation of human immunodeficiency virus type 1 DNA in T cells: Result of multiple infection events. J Virol 64:4836–4841, 1990.
151. Schnittman SM, Psallidopoulos MC, Lane HC, et al. The reservoir for HIV-1 in human peripheral blood is a T-cell that maintains expression of CD4. Science 245:305–308, 1989.
152. Kim S, Byrn R, Groopman J, Baltimore D. Temporal aspects of DNA and RNA synthesis during human immunodeficiency virus infection: Evidence for differential gene expression. J Virol 63:3708–3713, 1989.
153. O'Brien W, Zack JA, Chen ISY. Molecular pathogenesis of HIV-1. AIDS 4(suppl 1):S41–S48, 1990.
154. Leonardo MJ, Baltimore D. NF-κB: A pleiotropic mediator of inducible and tissue-specific gene control. Cell 58:227–229, 1989.
155. Fauci AS. Immunodeficiency virus: Infectivity and mechanisms of pathogenesis. Science 262:1011–1018, 1993.
156. McCune JM. HIV-1: The infective process in vivo. Cell 64:351–363, 1991.
157. Levy JA. Pathogenesis of human immunodeficiency virus infection. Microbiol Rev 57:183–289, 1993.
157a. Virelizier JL. Alternative, cytokine-mediated host defense mechanism against HIV infection: The concept of self-limitation of HIV replication. AIDS 12 (suppl A):S141–S146, 1998.
158. Niu MT, Jermano JA, Reichelderfer P, Schnittman SM. Summary of the National Institutes of Health workshop on primary human immunodeficiency virus type 1 infection. AIDS Res Hum Retroviruses 9:913–924, 1993.
159. Daar ES, Mougdil T, Meyer RD, Ho DD. Transient high levels of viremia in patients with primary human immunodeficiency virus type 1 infection. N Engl J Med 324:961–964, 1991.
160. Clark SJ, Saag MS, Decker WD, et al. High titers of cytopathic virus in plasma of patients with symptomatic primary HIV-1 infection. N Engl J Med 324:954–960, 1991.
161. Piatak M Jr, Saag MS, Yang LC, et al. High levels of HIV-1 in plasma during all stages of infection determined by competitive PCR. Science 259:1749–1754, 1993.
162. Graziosi C, Pantaleo G, Burini L, et al. Kinetics of human immunodeficiency virus type 1 (HIV-1) DNA and RNA synthesis during primary HIV-1 infection. Proc Natl Acad Sci U S A 90:6405–6409, 1993.
163. Pantaleo G, Graziosi C, Burini L, et al. Lymphoid organs function as major reservoirs for human immunodeficiency virus (HIV). Proc Natl Acad Sci U S A 88:9838–9842, 1991.
164. Chakrabati L, Cumont MC, Montagnier L, Hurtrel B. Variable course of primary simian immunodeficiency virus infection in lymph nodes: Relation to disease progression. J Virol 68:6634–6642, 1994.
165. Haase AT. Quantitative image analysis of HIV-1 infection in lymphoid tissue. Science 274:985–989, 1996.
166. Ferbas J, Daar ES, Grovit-Ferbas K, et al. Rapid evolution of human immunodeficiency virus strains with increased replicative capacity during the seronegative window of primary infection. J Virol 70:7285–7289, 1996.
167. Pantaleo G, Demarest JF, Soudeyns HH, et al. Major expansion of CD8+ T cells with a predominant Vβ usage during the primary immune response to HIV. Nature 370:463–467, 1994.
168. Koup RA, Safrit JT, Cao Y, et al. Temporal association of cellular immune responses with the initial control of viremia in primary human immunodeficiency virus type 1 syndrome. J Virol 68:4650–4655, 1994.
169. Borrow P, Lewicki H, Hahn B, et al. Virus specific CD8+ cytotoxic T-lymphocyte activity associated with control of viremia in primary human immunodeficiency virus type 1 infection. J Virol 68:6103–6110, 1994.
170. Haynes BF, Pantaleo G, Fauci AS. Towards an understanding of the correlates of immune protective imunity of HIV infection. Science 271:324–328, 1996.
171. Chen ZW, Kou ZC, Lekutis C, et al. T cell receptor V beta repertoire in acute infection of rhesus monkeys with simian immunodeficiency viruses and a chimeric simian-human immunodeficiency virus. J Exp Med 182:21–32, 1995.
172. Graziosi C, Gantt KR, Vaccarezzo M, et al. Kinetics of cytokine expression during primary human immunodeficiency virus type 1 infection. Proc Natl Acad Sci U S A 93:4386–4391, 1996.
173. Moore JP, Cao Y, Ho DD, Koup RA. Development of the anti-gp120 antibody response during seroconversion to human immunodeficiency virus type 1. J Virol 68:5142–5155, 1994.
174. Imagawa DT, Lee MM, Wolinsky SM, et al. Human immunodeficiency virus type 1 infection in homosexual men who remain seronegative for prolonged periods. N Engl J Med 320:1458–1462, 1989.
175. Montagnier L, Brenner C, Chamaret S, et al. Human immunodeficiency virus infection and AIDS in a person with negative serology. J Infect Dis 175:955–959, 1997.
176. McCune JM. Viral latency in HIV disease. Cell 82:183–188, 1995.
177. Ho DD, Moudgil T, Alam M. Quantitation of human immunodeficiency virus type 1 in the blood of infected persons. N Engl J Med 321:1621–1625, 1989.
178. Simmonds P, Balfe P, Pentherer JF, et al. Human immunodeficiency virus–infected individuals contain provirus in small numbers of peripheral blood mononuclear cells and at low copy number. J Virol 64:864–872, 1990.
179. Seshamma T, Bagasra O, Trono D, et al. Blocked early-stage latency in the peripheral blood cells of certain individuals infected with human immunodeficiency virus type 1. Proc Natl Acad Sci U S A 89:10663–10667, 1992.
180. Chun TW, Carruth L, Finzi D, et al. Quantification of latent tissue reservoirs and total body virus load in HIV-1 infection. Nature 387:183–188, 1997.
181. Sanchez G, Xu X, Chermann JC, Hirsch I. Accumulation of defective viral genomes in peripheral blood mononuclear cells of human immunodeficiency virus type 1–infected individuals. J Virol 71:2233–2240, 1997.
182. Perelson AS, Neumann AU, Markowitz M, et al. HIV-1 dynamics in vivo: Virion clearance rate, infected cell life-span, and viral generation time. Science 271:1582–1586, 1996.
183. Coffin J. HIV population dynamics in vivo: Implications for genetic variation, pathogenesis, and therapy. Science 267:483–489, 1995.
184. Fox CH, Tenner-Racz K, Racz P, et al. Lymphoid germinal centers are reservoirs for HIV-1 RNA. J Infect Dis 164:1051–1057, 1991.
185. Pantaleo G, Graziosi C, Desmarest JF, et al. HIV infection is active and progressive in lymphoid tissue during the clinically latent stage of disease. Nature 362:355–358, 1993.
186. Cameron PU, Freudenthal PS, Barker JM, et al. Dendritic cells exposed to human immunodeficiency virus type-1 transmit a vigorous cytopathic infection to CD4+ T cells. Science 257:383–387, 1992.
187. Embretson J, Zupancic M, Ribas JL, et al. Massive covert infection of helper T lymphocytes and macrophages by HIV during the incubation period of AIDS. Nature 362:359–362, 1993.
188. Heath SL, Tew JG, Tew JG, et al. Follicular dendritic cells and human immunodeficiency virus infectivity. Nature 377:740–744, 1995.

189. Saksela K, Muchmore E, Girard M, et al. High viral loads in lymph nodes and latent human immunodeficiency virus (HIV) in peripheral blood cells of HIV-1 infected chimpanzees. J Virol 67:7423–7427, 1993.
190. Perelson AS, Essunger P, Cao Y, et al. Decay characteristics of HIV-infected compartments during combination therapy. Nature 387:188–191, 1997.
191. Orenstein JM, Fox C, Wahl SM. Macrophages as a source of HIV during opportunistic infections. Science 276:1857–1861, 1997.
191a. Ho DD. Toward HIV eradication or revision: The tasks ahead. Science 280:1866–1867, 1998.
191b. Chun T-W, Stuyver L, Mizell SB, et al. Presence of an inducible HIV-1 latent reservoir during highly active antiretroviral therapy. Proc Natl Acad Sci U S A 94:13193–13197, 1997.
192. Centers for Disease Control. Revision of the CDC surveillance case definition for acquired immunodeficiency syndrome. MMWR Morb Mortal Wkly Rep 36(suppl):1S–15S, 1987.
193. Colebunders RL, Latif RS. Natural history and clinical presentation of HIV-1 in adults. AIDS 5(suppl 1):S103–S112, 1991.
194. Philips AN, Lee CA, Elford J, et al. More rapid progression to AIDS in older HIV-infected people: The role of CD4+ T-cell count. J Acquir Immune Defic Syndr 4:970–975, 1991.
195. Lubaki NM, Ray SC, Dhruva B, et al. Characterization of a polyclonal cytolytic T lymphocyte response to human immunodeficiency virus in persons without clinical progression. J Infect Dis 175:1360–1367, 1997.
196. Smith MW, Dean M, Carrington M, et al. Contrastic genetic influence of CCR2 and CCR5 variants on HIV-1 infection and disease progession. Science 277:959–965, 1997.
197. Lo SC, Tsai S, Benish JR, et al. Enhancement of HIV-1 cytocidal effects in CD4+ lymphocytes by the AIDS-associated mycoplasma. Science 251:1074–1076, 1991.
198. Lemâitre M, Hénin Y, Destouesse F, et al. Role of mycoplasma infection in the cytopathic effect induced by human immunodeficiency virus type 1 in infected cell lines. Infect Immun 60:742–748, 1992.
199. Pleskoff O, Tréboute C, Brelot A, et al. Identification of a chemokine receptor encoded by human cytomegalovirus as a cofactor for HIV-1 entry. Science 276:1874–1878, 1997.
199a. Zagury D, Lachgar A, Chams V, et al. C-C chemokines, pivotal in protection against HIV type 1 infection. Proc Natl Acad Sci U S A 95:3857–3861, 1998.
199b. Furci L, Scarlatti G, Burastero S. Antigen-driven C-C chemokine-mediated HIV-1 suppression by CD4(+) T cells from exposed uninfected individuals expressing the wild-type CCR-5 allele. J Exp Med 186:455–460, 1997.
199c. Garzino-Demo A, DeVico AL, Cocchi F, Gallo RC. β-chemokines and protection from HIV type 1 disease. AIDS Res Hum Retroviruses 14(suppl 2):S177–S184, 1998.
200. Connor RL, Mohri H, Cao Y, Ho DD. Increased viral burden and cytopathicity correlate temporally with CD4+ T lymphocyte decline and clinical progression in human immunodeficiency virus type 1–infected individuals. J Virol 67:1772–1777, 1991.
201. Mellors JW, Rinaldo CR, Gupta P, et al. Prognosis in HIV-1 infection predicted by the quantity of virus in plasma. Science 272:1167–1170, 1996.
202. O'Brien WA, Hartigan PM, Martin D, et al. Changes of plasma HIV-RNA and CD4+ lymphocyte counts and the risk of progression to AIDS. N Engl J Med 334:426–431, 1996.
203. Watson A, Ranchalis J, Travis B, et al. Plasma viremia in macaques infected with simian immunodeficiency virus: Plasma viral load early in infection predicts survival. J Virol 71:284–290, 1997.
204. Saksela K, Stevens C, Rubinstein P, Baltimore D. Human immunodeficiency virus type 1 mRNA expression in peripheral blood cells predicts disease progression independently of the number of CD4+ lymphocytes. Proc Natl Acad Sci U S A 91:1104–1108, 1994.
205. Pantaleo G, Desmarest JF, Schacker T, et al. The qualitative nature of the primary immune response to HIV infection is a prognosticator of disease progression independent of the initial level of plasma viremia. Proc Natl Acad Sci U S A 94:254–258, 1997.
205a. Graziosi C, Soudeyns H, Rizzardi GP, et al. Immunopathogenesis of HIV infection. AIDS Res Hum Retroviruses 14(suppl 2):S135–S142, 1998.
206. Matsuyama T, Kobayashi N, Yamamoto N. Cytokines and HIV infection: Is AIDS a tumor necrosis factor disease? AIDS 5:1405–1417, 1991.
207. Kinter A, Ostrowski M, Goletti D, et al. HIV replication in CD4+ T cells of HIV-infected individuals is regulated by a balance between the viral suppressive effects of endogenous β-chemokines and the viral inductive effects of other endogenous cytokines. Proc Natl Acad Sci U S A 93:14076–14081, 1996.
208. Rubbert A, Weissman D, Combadiere C, et al. Multi-factorial nature of noncytolytic CD8+ T cell–mediated suppression of HIV replication: β-chemokine–dependent and -independent effects. AIDS Res Hum Retroviruses 13:63–69, 1997.
209. Levy JA, Mackewicz CE, Barker E. Controlling HIV pathogenesis: The role of the noncytotoxic anti-HIV response of CD8+ T cells. Immunol Today 17:217–224, 1996.
210. Swain SL, Bradley M, Croft M, et al. Helper T-cell subsets: Phenotype, function and the role of lymphokines in regulating their development. Immunol Rev 123:115–144, 1991.
211. Romagnani S. The Th1/Th2 paradigm. Immunol Today 18:263–266, 1997.
212. Clerici M, Shearer GM. A TH1 → TH2 switch is a critical step in the etiology of HIV infection. Immunol Today 14:107–111, 1993.
213. Clerici M, Shearer GM. The TH1 → TH2 hypothesis of HIV infection: New insights. Immunol Today 15:575–581, 1994.
214. Maggi E, Mazzetti M, Ravina A, et al. Ability of HIV to promote a Th1 to Th0 shift and to replicate preferentially in Th2 and Th0 cells. Science 265:244–248, 1994.
215. Tanako Y, Koyanagi Y, Tanaka R, et al. Productive and lytic infection of human CD4+ type 1 helper T cells with macrophage-tropic human immunodeficiency virus type 1. J Virol 71:465–470, 1997.
216. Tersmette M, de Goede REY, Al BJ, et al. Differential syncytium-inducing capacity of human immunodeficiency virus isolates: Frequent detection of syncytium-inducing isolates in patients with acquired immunodeficiency syndrome (AIDS) and AIDS-related complex. J Virol 62:2026–2032, 1988.
217. Zhu T, Mo H, Wang N, et al. Genotypic and phenotypic characterization of HIV-1 in patients with primary infection. Science 261:1179–1181, 1993.
218. Pantaleo G, Menzo S, Vaccarezzo M, et al. Studies in subjects with long-term nonprogressive human immunodeficiency virus infection. N Engl J Med 332:209–216, 1995.
219. Cao Y, Qin L, Zahng L, et al. Virologic and immunologic characterization of long-term survivors of human immunodeficiency virus type 1 infection. N Engl J Med 332:201–208, 1995.
220. Macatonia SF, Grompels M, Pinching AJ, et al. Antigen presentation by macrophages but not by dendritic cells in human immunodeficiency virus (HIV) infection. Immunology 75:576–581, 1992.
221. Borrow P, Evans CF, Oldstone MBA. Virus-induced immunosuppression: Immune system–mediated destruction of virus-infected dendritic cells results in generalized immunosuppression. J Virol 69:1059–1070, 1995.
222. Odermatt B, Eppler M, Leist TP, et al. Virus-triggered acquired immunodeficiency by cytotoxic T-cell–dependent destruction of antigen-presenting cells with lymph follicle structure. Proc Natl Acad Sci U S A 88:8252–8256, 1991.
223. Bonyhadi ML, Rabin L, Salimi S, et al. HIV induces thymus depletion in vivo. Nature 363:728–735, 1993.
224. Kaneshima H, Su L, Bonyhadi ML, et al. Rapid-high, syncytium-inducing isolates of human immunodeficiency virus type 1 induce cytopathicity in the human thymus of the SCID-hu mouse. J Virol 68:8188–8192, 1994.
225. Clerici M, Roilides E, Via C, et al. A factor from CD8+ cells of human immunodeficiency virus–infected patients suppresses HLA self-restricted T helper cell responses. Proc Natl Acad Sci U S A 89:8424–8428, 1992.
226. Wanatabe M, Ringler DJ, Fultz PN, et al. A chimpanzee-passaged human immunodeficiency virus isolate is cytopathic for chimpanzee cells but does not induce disease. J Virol 65:3344–3348, 1991.
227. Heeney J, Boggers W, Buijs L, et al. Immune strategies utilized by lentivirus-infected chimpanzees to resist progression to AIDS. Immunol Lett 51:45–52, 1996.

228. Novembre FJ, Saucier M, Anderson DC, et al. Development of AIDS in a chimpanzee infected with human immunodeficiency virus type 1. J Virol 71:4086–4091, 1997.
229. Germain RN. Antigen processing and CD4+ T-cell depletion in AIDS. Cell 54:441–444, 1988.
230. Siliciano RF, Lawton T, Knall C, et al. Analysis of host-virus interactions in AIDS with anti-gp120 T-cell clones: Effect of HIV sequence variation and a mechanism for CD4+ depletion. Cell 54:561–575, 1988.
231. Habeshaw J, Hounsell E, Dalgleish A. Does the HIV envelope induce a chronic graft-versus-host–like disease? Immunol Today 13:207–210, 1992.
232. Zagury JF, Bernard J, Achour A, et al. Identification of CD4 as major histocompatibility complex functional peptide sites and their homology with oligopeptides from human immunodeficiency virus type 1 glycoprotein gp120: Role in AIDS pathogenesis. Proc Natl Acad Sci U S A 90:7573–7577, 1993.
233. Shearer GM, Clerici M, Dalgleish A. Alloimmunization as an AIDS vaccine. Nature 262:161–162, 1993.
234. Gougeon ML, Dadaglio G, Garcia S, et al. Is a dominant superantigen involved in AIDS pathogenesis? Lancet 342:50–51, 1993.
235. Ameisen JC, Capron A. Cell dysfunction and depletion in AIDS: The programmed cell death hypothesis. Immunol Today 12:102–105, 1991.
236. Gougeon ML, Garcia S, Heeney J, et al. Programmed cell death in AIDS-related HIV and SIV infections. AIDS Res Hum Retroviruses 9:553–563, 1993.
237. Laurent-Crawford AG, Krust B, Rivière Y, et al. Membrane expression of HIV envelope glycoproteins triggers apoptosis in CD4 cells. AIDS Res Hum Retroviruses 9:761–773, 1993.
238. Li CJ, Friedman DJ, Wang C, et al. Induction of apoptosis in uninfected lymphocytes by HIV-1 Tat protein. Science 268:429–431, 1995.
239. Estaquier J, Idziorek T, de Bels, et al. Programmed cell death and AIDS: Significance of T-cell apoptosis in pathogenic and nonpathogenic primate lentiviral infections. Proc Natl Acad Sci U S A 91:9431–9435, 1994.
240. Finkel TH, Tudor-Williams G, Banda NK, et al. Apoptosis occurs predominantly in bystander cells and not in productively infected cells of HIV- and SIV-infected lymph nodes. Nat Med 1:129–134, 1995.
241. Clerici M, Sarin A, Coffman RL, et al. Type 1/type 2 cytokine modulation of T-cell programmed cell death as a model for human immunodeficiency virus pathogenesis. Proc Natl Acad Sci U S A 91:11811–11815, 1994.
242. Ensoli B, Barillari G, Salahuddin SZ, et al. Tat protein of HIV-1 stimulates growth of cells derived from Kaposi sarcoma lesions of AIDS patients. Nature 345:84–86, 1990.
243. Ensoli B, Buonaguro L, Bavillari G, et al. Release, uptake, and effects of extracellular human immunodeficiency virus type 1 Tat protein on cell growth and viral transactivation. J Virol 67:277–287, 1993.
244. Moore PS, Chang Y. Detection of herpesvirus-like DNA sequences in AIDS-associated Kaposi's sarcoma. Science 265:1865–1891, 1994.
245. Renne R, Zhong W, Herndier B, et al. Lytic growth of Kaposi's sarcoma–associated herpesvirus (human herpesvirus 8) in culture. Nat Med 2:342–346, 1996.
246. Clerici M, Giorgi JV, Chou C-C, et al. Cell-mediated immune response to human immunodeficiency virus (HIV) type 1 in seronegative homosexual men with recent sexual exposure to HIV-1. J Infect Dis 165:1012–1019, 1992.
247. Pinto LA, Sullivan J, Berzofsky JA, et al. ENV-specific cytotoxic T lymphocyte responses in HIV seronegative health care workers occupationally exposed to HIV-contaminated body fluids. J Clin Invest 96:867–876, 1995.
248. Rowland-Jones S, Sutton J, Ariyoshi K, et al. HIV-specific cytotoxic T-cells in HIV-exposed but uninfected Gambian women. Nat Med 1:59–64, 1995.
249. Cheynier R, Langlade-Demoyen P, Marescot MR, et al. Cytotoxic T-lymphocyte response in the peripheral blood of children born to HIV-infected mothers. Eur J Immunol 22:2211–2217, 1992.
250. Langlade-Demoyen P, Ngo-Giang-Huang N, Ferchal F, Oskenhendler E. HIV nef-specific cytotoxic T lymphocytes in noninfected heterosexual contacts of HIV-infected patients. J Clin Invest 93:1293–1297, 1994.
251. Rowland-Jones SL, McMichael A. Immune responses in HIV-exposed seronegatives: Have they repelled the virus? Curr Opin Immunol 7:448–455, 1995.
252. Paxton WA, Martin SR, Yse D, et al. Relative resistance to HIV-1 infection of CD4 lymphocytes from persons who remain uninfected despite multiple high-risk sexual exposure. Nat Med 2:412–417, 1996.
253. Aunand VA, Luscher M, Wade JA, et al. Certain MHC class II DR alleles are associated with decreased susceptibility to HIV-1 infection [abstract 117]. Keystone Symposium on AIDS Pathogenesis; Silverthorne, CO; April 8–13, 1997, p 13.
254. Mazzoli S, Trabattoni D, Lo Capuco S, et al. HIV-specific mucosal and cellular immunity in HIV-seronegative partners of HIV-seropositive individuals. Nat Med 11:1250–1257, 1997.
255. Mansky LM, Temin MM. Lower in vivo mutation rate of human immunodeficiency virus type 1 than that predicted from the fidelity of purified reverse transcriptase. J Virol 69:5087–5094, 1995.
256. Perelson AS, Neumann AU, Markowitz M, et al. HIV-1 dynamics in vivo: Virion clearance rate, infected cell lifespan and viral regeneration time. Science 271:1582–1586, 1996.
257. Hahn B, Shaw GM, Taylor ME, et al. Genetic variation in HTLV-III/LAV over time in patients with AIDS or at risk for AIDS. Science 232:1548–1553, 1986.
258. Vartanian JP, Meyerhans A, Asjö B, Wain-Hobson S. Selection, recombination and G → A hypermutation of human immunodeficiency virus type 1 genome. J Virol 65:1779–1788, 1991.
259. Groenink M, Fouchier RAM, de Goede REY, et al. Phenotypic heterogeneity in a panel of infectious molecular human immunodeficiency virus type 1 clones derived from a single individual. J Virol 65:1968–1975, 1991.
260. Eigen M, McCaskill J, Schuster P. Molecular quasi-species. J Phys Chem 92:6881–6891, 1988.
260a. Wong JK, Ignacio CC, Torriani F, et al In vivo compartmentalization of human immunodeficiency virus: Evidence from the examination of *pol* sequences from autopsy tissues. J Virol 71:2059–2071, 1997.
261. Albert J, Abrahamson B, Nagy K, et al. Rapid development of isolate-specific neutralizing antibodies after primary HIV-1 infection and consequent emergence of virus variants which resist neutralization by autologous sera. AIDS 4:107–118, 1990.
262. Wolfs TFW, Zwart G, Bakker M, et al. Naturally occurring mutations within the HIV-1 V3 genomic RNA lead to antigenic variation dependent on a single amino acid substitution. Virology 185:195–205, 1991.
263. Arendrup M, Nielsen C, Hansen J, et al. Autologous HIV-1 neutralizing antibodies: Emergence of neutralization-resistant escape virus and subsequent development of escape virus neutralizing antibodies. J Acquir Immune Defic Syndr 5:303–307, 1992.
264. Phillips RE, Rowland-Jones S, Dixon DF, et al. Human immunodeficiency virus genetic variations that can escape cytotoxic T-cell recognition. Nature 354:453–459, 1991.
265. Price DA, Goulder PJR, Klenerman P, et al. Positive selection of HIV-1 cytotoxic lymphocyte escape variants during primary infection. Proc Natl Acad Sci U S A 97:1890–1895, 1997.
266. Kent SJ, Greenberg PD, Hoffman MC, et al. Antagonism of vaccine-induced HIV-1 specific CD4+ T cells by primary HIV-1 infection. J Immunol 158:807–815, 1997.
267. Klenerman PS, Rowland-Jones S, McAdam S, et al. Cytotoxic T-cell activity antagonized by naturally occurring HIV-1 Gag variants. Nature 369:403–407, 1994.
268. Koenig S, Conley AJ, Brewah YA, et al. Transfer of HIV-1 specific cytotoxic T lymphocytes to an AIDS patient leads to selection for mutant HIV variants and subsequent disease progression. Nat Med 1:330–336, 1995.
269. Li Y, Hui H, Burgess CJ, et al. Complete nucleotide sequence, genome organization, and biological properties of human immunodeficiency virus type 1 in vivo: Evidence for limited defectiveness and complementation. J Virol 66:6587–6600, 1992.
270. Zhu T, Mo N, Wang N, et al. Genotypic and phenotypic characterization of HIV-1 in patients with primary infection. Science 261:1179–1181, 1993.

271. Leigh-Brown AJ. Sequence variability in human immunodeficiency viruses: Pattern and process in viral evolution. AIDS 5(suppl 2):S535–S542, 1991.
272. Holmes EC, Zhang LQ, Simmonds P, et al. Convergent and divergent sequence evolution in the surface envelope glycoprotein of human immunodeficiency virus type 1 within a single infected patient. Proc Natl Acad Sci U S A 89:4835–4839, 1992.
273. Wolfs TFW, Zwart G, Bakker M, Goudsmit J. HIV-1 genome RNA diversification following sexual and parenteral virus transmission. Virology 189:103–110, 1992.
274. Wolinsky SM, Wike CM, Korber BTM, et al. Selective transmission of human immunodeficiency virus type 1 variants from mother-to-infants. Science 255:1134–1137, 1992.
275. McNearney T, Westervelt P, Thielan BJ, et al. Limited sequence heterogeneity among biologically distinct human immunodeficiency virus type 1 isolates from individuals involved in a clustered infectious outbreak. Proc Natl Acad Sci U S A 87:1917–1921, 1990.
276. Burger H, Weiser B, Flaherty K, et al. Evolution of human immunodeficiency virus type 1 nucleotide sequence diversity among close contacts. Proc Natl Acad Sci U S A 88:11236–11240, 1991.
277. McDonald RA, Mayers DL, Chung RC-Y, et al. Evolution of human immunodeficiency virus type 1 *env* sequence variation in patients with diverse rates of disease progression and T-cell function. J Virol 71:1871–1879, 1997.
278. Zhang L, Diaz RS, Ho DD, et al. Host-specific driving force in human immunodeficiency virus type 1 evolution in vivo. J Virol 71:2555–2561, 1997.
279. Ou CJ, Ciesielski CA, Myers G, et al. Molecular epidemiology of HIV transmission in a dental practice. Science 256:1165–1171, 1992.
280. Holmes EC, Zhang LQ, Smith Rogers A, Leigh Brown AJ. Molecular investigation of HIV infection in a patient of an HIV-infected surgeon. J Infect Dis 167:1411–1414, 1993.
281. Albert J, Wahlberg J, Leitner T, et al. Analysis of a rape case by direct sequencing of the human immunodeficiency virus type 1 *pol* and *gag* genes. J Virol 68:5918–5924, 1991.
282. McCutchan FE, Ungar BLP, Hegerich P, et al. Genetic analysis of HIV-1 isolates from Zambia and an expanded phylogenetic tree for HIV-1. J Acquir Immune Defic Syndr 5:441–449, 1992.
283. Putney SD, McKeating JA. Antigenic variation in HIV. AIDS 4(suppl 1):S129–S136, 1990.
284. Zwart G, Langeduk H, van der Hoek L, et al. Immunodominance and antigenic variation of the principal neutralization domain of HIV-1. Virology 181:481–489, 1991.
285. Cheingsong-Popov R, Lister S, Callow D, et al. Serotyping HIV type 1 by antibody binding to the V3 loop: Relationship to viral genotype. AIDS Res Hum Retroviruses 11:1379–1386, 1994.
286. Murphy E, Korber B, Georges-Courbot M-C, et al. Diversity of V3 region sequences of human immunodeficiency virus type 1 from Central African Republic. AIDS Res Hum Retroviruses 9:997–1006, 1993.
287. Kostrikis LG, Bagdades E, Cao Y, et al. Genetic analysis of human immunodeficiency virus type 1 strains from patients in Cyprus: Identification of a new subtype designated I. J Virol 69:6122–6130, 1995.
288. Charneau P, Borman AM, Quillent C, et al. Isolation and envelope sequence of a highly divergent HIV-1 isolate: Definition of a new HIV-1 group. Virology 205:247–253, 1994.
289. Van den Haesevelde M, Decourt JL, Deleys RJ, et al. Genomic cloning and complete sequence analysis of a highly divergent human immunodeficiency virus isolate. J Virol 68:1588–1596, 1994.
290. Loussert-Ajaka L, Chaix ML, Korber BTM, et al. Variability of human immunodeficiency virus type 1 group O strains isolated from Cameroonian patients living in France. J Virol 69:5640–5649, 1995.
291. Lukashov VV, Cornelissen MTE, Goudsmit J, et al. Simultaneous introduction of distinct HIV-1 subtypes into different risk groups in Russia, Byelorussia and Lithuania. AIDS 9:435–439, 1995.
292. Arnold C, Baslow KL, Parry JV, Clewley JP. At least five HIV-1 sequence subtypes (A, B, C, D, A/E) occur in England. AIDS Res Hum Retroviruses 11:427–429, 1995.
293. Louwagie J, Janssens W, Mascola J, et al. Genetic diversity of the envelope glycoprotein from human immunodeficiency virus type 1 isolates of African origin. J Virol 69:263–271, 1995.
294. Louwagie J, McCutchan F, Peeters M, et al. Phylogenetic analysis of *gag* genes from 70 international HIV-1 isolates provides evidence for multiple genotypes. AIDS 66:3602–3608, 1992.
295. Cornelissen M, Kampinga G, Zorgdrager F, et al. Human immunodeficiency virus type 1 subtypes defined by *env* show high frequency of recombinant *gag* genes. J Virol 70:8209–8212, 1996.
296. Kampinga GA, Simonon A, van de Perre P, et al. Primary infections with HIV-1 of women and their offspring in Rwanda: Findings of heterogeneity at seroconversion, coinfections, and recombinants of subtypes A and C. Virology 227:63–76, 1997.
297. Artenstein AW, VanCott TC, Mascola JR, et al. Dual infection with human immunodeficiency virus type 1 of distinct envelope subtypes in humans. J Infect Dis 171:805–810, 1995.
298. Zhu T, Wang N, Carr A, et al. Evidence for coinfection by multiple strains of human immunodeficiency virus type 1 subtype B in an acute seroconverter. J Virol 69:1324–1327, 1995.
299. Diaz RS, Salino EC, Mayer A, et al. Dual human immunodeficiency virus type 1 infection and recombination in a dually exposed transfusion recipient. J Virol 69:3273–3281, 1995.
300. Fultz P, Yue L, Wei Q, Girard M. Human immunodeficiency virus type 1 intersubtype (B/E) recombination in a superinfected chimpanzee. J Virol 71:7990–7995, 1997.
301. Robert-Guroff M, Aldrich K, Muldoon R, et al. Cross-neutralization of human immunodeficiency virus type 1 and 2 and simian immunodeficiency virus isolates. J Virol 66:3602–3608, 1992.
302. Boeri E, Giri A, Lillo F, et al. In vivo genetic variability of the human immunodeficiency virus type 2 V3 region. J Virol 66:4546–4550, 1992.
303. Schulz TF, Whitby D, Hood JG, et al. Biological and molecular variability of human immunodeficiency virus type 2 isolates from the Gambia. J Virol 64:5177–5182, 1990.
304. Huet T, Cheynier R, Meyerhans A, et al. Genetic organization of a chimpanzee lentivirus related to HIV-1. Nature 345:356–359, 1990.
305. Peeters M, Frausen K, Delaporte E, et al. Isolation and characterization of a new chimpanzee lentivirus (simian immunodeficiency virus isolate cpz-ant) from a wild captured chimpanzee. AIDS 6:447–451, 1992.
306. Hirsch VM, Olmsted RA, Murphey-Corb M, et al. An African primate lentivirus (SIVsm) closely related to HIV-2. Nature 339:389–392, 1989.
307. Myers G, MacInnes K, Korber B. The emergence of simian/human immunodeficiency viruses. AIDS Res Hum Retroviruses 8:373–386, 1992.
308. Johnson PR, Fomsgaaard A, Allan J, et al. Simian immunodeficiency viruses from African green monkeys display unusual genetic diversity. J Virol 64:1086–1092, 1990.
309. Gojobori T, Moriyama EN, Ina Y, et al. Evolutionary origin of human and simian immunodeficiency viruses. Proc Natl Acad Sci U S A 87:4108–4111, 1990.
310. Cameron DW, Podian NS. Sexual transmission of HIV and the epidemiology of other sexually transmitted diseases. AIDS 4(suppl 1):S99–S103, 1990.
311. Rosenberg PS, Levy MC, Brundage JF, et al. Population-based monitoring of an urban HIV/AIDS epidemic: Magnitude and trends in the District of Columbia. JAMA 268:495–503, 1992.
312. Brown T, Sittitrai W, Vanichseni S, Thisyakorn U. The recent epidemiology of HIV and AIDS in Thailand. AIDS 8(suppl 2):S131–S141, 1994.
313. Weniger BG, Brown T. The march of AIDS through Asia. N Engl J Med 335:343–345, 1996.
314. Plummer FA, Simonsen JN, Cameron DW, et al. Co-factors in male-female transmission of human immunodeficiency virus type 1. J Infect Dis 163:233–239, 1991.
315. European Study Group on Heterosexual Transmission of HIV. Comparison of female to male and male to female transmission of HIV in 563 stable couples. BMJ 304:809–813, 1992.
316. Moses S, Plummer FA, Bradley JE, et al. The association between lack of male circumcision and risk for HIV infection: A review of the epidemiological data. Sex Transm Dis 21:201–210, 1994.

317. Piot P, Laga M. Genital ulceration, other sexually transmitted diseases, and the sexual transmission of HIV. BMJ 298:623–624, 1989.
318. Spira AI, Marx PA, Patterson BK, et al. Cellular targets of infection and route of viral dissemination after an intravaginal inoculation of simian immunodeficiency virus into rhesus macaques. J Exp Med 183:215–225, 1996.
319. Marx PA, Spira AI, Gettie A, et al. Progesterone implants enhance SIV vaginal transmission and early virus load. Nat Med 2:1084–1089, 1996.
320. Pope M, Betjes MGH, Romani N, et al. Conjugates of dendritic cells and memory T lymphocytes from skin facilitate productive infection with HIV-1. Cell 78:389–398, 1994.
321. Granelli-Piperno A, Pope M, Inaba K, Steiman RM. Coexpression of NF-κB/Rel and Sp1 transcription factors in human immunodeficiency virus 1–induced, dendritic cell–T-cell syncytia. Proc Natl Acad Sci U S A 92:10944–10948, 1995.
322. Bomsel M. Transcytosis of infectious human immunodeficiency virus across a tight human epithelial cell line barrier. Nat Med 3:42–47, 1997.
323. Soto-Ramirez LE, Renjifo B, McLane MF, et al. HIV-1 Langerhans' cell tropism associated with heterosexual transmission of HIV. Science 271:1291–1293, 1996.
324. Dittmar MT, Simmons G, Hibbits S, et al. Langerhans cell tropism of human immunodeficiency virus type 1 subtype A through F isolates derived from different transmission groups. J Virol 71:8008–8013, 1997.
325. Pope M, Frankel SS, Mascola JR, et al. Human immunodeficiency virus type 1 strains of subtypes B and E replicate in cutaneous dendritic cell–T-cell mixtures without displaying subtype-specific tropism. J Virol 71:8001–8007, 1997.
326. Peckham C, Gibb S. Mother-to-child transmission of the human immunodeficiency virus. N Engl J Med 333:298–302, 1995.
327. Dunn DT, Newell ML, Peckham CS. Risk of human immunodeficiency virus type 1 transmission through breastfeeding. Lancet 340:585–588, 1992.
328. Van de Perre P, Simon A, Hitimana DG, et al. Infective and anti-infective properties of breastmilk from HIV-1 infected women. Lancet 341:914–918, 1993.
329. Connor EM, Sperling RS, Gelbert R, et al. Reduction of maternal-infant transmission of human immunodeficiency virus type 1 with zidovudine treatment. N Engl J Med 331:1173–1180, 1994.
330. Coll O, Hernandez M, Boucher CAB, et al. Vertical HIV-1 transmission correlates with a high maternal viral load at delivery. J Acquir Immune Defic Syndr Hum Retrovirol 14:26–30, 1997.
331. Pitt J, Brambilla D, Reichelderfer P, et al. Maternal immunological and virologic risk factors for infant human immunodeficiency virus type 1 infection: Findings from the women and infants transmission study. J Infect Dis 175:567–575, 1997.
332. Cao Y, Krogstad P, Korber BT, et al. Maternal HIV-1 viral load and vertical transmission of infection: The Ariel Project for the prevention of HIV transmission from mother-to-infant. Nat Med 3:549–552, 1997.
333. World Health Organization. Global programme on AIDS: HIV and HBV transmission in the health-care setting. Wkly Epidemiol Rec 26:189–191, 1991.
334. Pfützner A, Dietrich U, von Briesen H, et al. HIV-1 and HIV-2 infections in a high-risk population in Bombay, India: Evidence for the spread of HIV-2 and presence of a divergent HIV-1 subtype. J Acquir Immune Defic Syndr 5:972–977, 1992.
335. George JR, Ou CY, Parekh B, et al. HIV-2/HIV-1 mixed infections in Côte d'Ivoire. Lancet 340:337–339, 1992.
336. Travers K, M'boup S, Marlink R, et al. Natural protection against HIV-1 infection provided by HIV-2. Science 268:1612–1615, 1995.
337. Nixon DF, Brolinden K, Ogg G, Brolinden PA. Cellular and humoral antigenic epitopes in HIV and SIV. Immunology 76:515–534, 1992.
338. Nara PL. HIV-neutralization: Evidence for rapid binding/post-binding neutralization from infected humans, chimpanzees and gp120-vaccinated animals. Vaccine 89:137–144, 1989.
339. Nara PL, Garrity RR, Goudsmit J. Neutralization of HIV-1: A paradox of humoral proportions. FASEB J 5:2437–2455, 1991.
340. Emini EA, Schleif WA, Numberg JM, et al. Prevention of HIV-1 infection in chimpanzees by gp120 V3 domain–specific monoclonal antibody. Nature 355:728–730, 1992.
341. Scott CF, Silver S, Profy AT, et al. Human monoclonal antibody that recognizes the V3 region of human immunodeficiency virus gp120 and neutralizes the human T-lymphotropic virus type III_{MN} strain. Proc Natl Acad Sci U S A 87:8597–8601, 1990.
342. Gorny MK, Xu JY, Gianakakos V, et al. Production of site-selected neutralizing human monoclonal antibodies against the third variable domain of the human immunodeficiency virus type 1 envelope glycoprotein. Proc Natl Acad Sci U S A 88:3328–3342, 1991.
343. Ohno T, Terada M, Yoneda Y. A broadly neutralizing monoclonal antibody that recognizes the V3 region of human immunodeficiency virus type 1 glycoprotein gp120. Proc Natl Acad Sci U S A 88:10725–10729, 1991.
344. Kliks SC, Shiodo T, Haigwood NLO, Levy JA. V3 variability can influence the ability of an antibody to neutralize or to enhance infection by diverse strains of human immunodeficiency virus type 1. Proc Natl Acad Sci U S A 90:11518–11522, 1993.
345. Wolfs TP, Nara PL, Goudsmit J. Genotypic and phenotypic variation of HIV-1: Impact on AIDS pathogenesis and vaccination. Chem Immunol 56:1–33, 1993.
346. White-Sharf ME, Potts BJ, Smith LM, et al. Broadly neutralizing monoclonal antibodies to the V3 region of HIV-1 can be elicited by peptide immunization. Virology 192:197–206, 1993.
347. Nakamura GR, Byrn R, Rosenthal K, et al. Monoclonal antibodies to the extracellular domains of HIV-1 IIIB gp160 that neutralize infectivity, block binding to CD4, and react with diverse isolates. AIDS Res Hum Retroviruses 8:1875–1885, 1992.
348. Bjorling E, Broliden K, Bernardi D, et al. Hyperimmune sera against synthetic peptides representing the glycoprotein of human immunodeficiency virus type 2 can mediate neutralization and antibody-dependent cytotoxic activity. Proc Natl Acad Sci U S A 88:6082–6086, 1991.
349. Javaherian K, Langlois AJ, Schmidt S, et al. The principal neutralization determinant of simian immunodeficiency virus differs from that of human immunodeficiency virus type 1. Proc Natl Acad Sci U S A 89:1418–1422, 1992.
350. Bou-Habib DC, Roderiquez G, Ovarecz T, et al. Cryptic nature of envelope V3 region epitopes protects primary monocytotropic human immunodeficiency virus type 1 from antibody neutralization. J Virol 68:6006–6013, 1994.
351. Moore JP, Cao Y, Qing L, et al. Primary isolates of human immunodeficiency virus type 1 are relatively resistant to neutralization by monoclonal antibodies to gp120, and their neutralization is not predicted by studies with monomeric gp120. J Virol 69:101–109, 1995.
352. Vancott TC, Polonis VR, Loomis LD. Differential role of V3-specific antibodies in neutralization assays involving primary and laboratory-adapted isolates of HIV type 1. AIDS Res Hum Retroviruses 11:1379–1391, 1995.
353. Wrin T, Loh TP, Vennari JC, et al. Adaptation to persistent growth in the H9 cell line renders a primary isolate of human immunodeficiency virus type 1 sensitive to neutralization by vaccinee sera. J Virol 69:39–48, 1995.
354. Sawyer LS, Wrin MT, Crawford-Miksza L, et al. Neutralization sensitivity of human immunodeficiency virus type 1 is determined in part by the cell in which the virus is propagated. J Virol 68:1342–1349, 1994.
355. Vogel T, Kurth R, Norley S. The majority of neutralizing Abs in HIV-1–infected patients recognize linear V3 loop sequences. Studies using HIV-1MN multiple antigenic peptides. J Immunol 153:1895–1904, 1994.
355a. Morikita T, Maeda Y, Fujii S-I, et al. The V1/V2 region of human immunodeficiency virus type 1 modulates the sensitivity to neutralization by soluble CD4 and cellular tropism. AIDS Res Hum Retroviruses 13:1291–1299, 1998.
356. Hanson CV. Measuring vaccine-induced HIV neutralization: Report of a workshop. AIDS Res Hum Retroviruses 10:645–648, 1994.
357. Zolla-Pasner S, Alving C, Belshe R, et al. Neutralization of a clade B primary isolate by sera from human immunodeficiency virus–uninfected recipients of candidate AIDS vaccines. J Infect Dis 175:764–774, 1997.
358. McKeating JA, Shotton C, Cordell J, et al. Characterization of

neutralizing monoclonal antibodies to linear and conformation-dependent epitopes within the first and second variable domains of human immunodeficiency virus type 1 gp120. J Virol 67:4937–4944, 1993.

359. Wyatt R, Moore JP, Accola M, et al. Involvement of the V1/V2 variable loop structure in the exposure of human immunodeficiency virus type 1 gp120 epitopes induced by receptor binding. J Virol 69:5723–5733, 1995.
360. Wu Z, Kayman SC, Honnen W, et al. Characterization of neutralization epitopes in the V2 region of human immunodeficiency virus type 1 gp120: Role of glycosylation in the correct folding of the V1/V2 domain. J Virol 69:2271–2278, 1995.
361. Gorny MK, Moore JP, Conley AH, et al. Human anti-V2 monoclonal antibody that neutralizes primary but not laboratory isolates of human immunodeficiency virus type 1. J Virol 68:8312–8320, 1994.
362. Pinter A, Honnen WJ, Racho ME, Tilley SA. A potent, neutralizing monoclonal antibody against an unique epitope overlapping the CD4-binding site of HIV-1 gp120 that is broadly conserved across North American and African virus isolates. AIDS Res Hum Retroviruses 9:985–996, 1993.
363. Thali M, Furman C, Ho DD, et al. Discontinuous, conserved neutralization epitopes overlapping the CD4-binding region of human immunodeficiency virus type 1 gp120 envelope glycoprotein. J Virol 66:5635–5641, 1992.
364. McKeating JA, Thali M, Furman C, et al. Amino acid residues of the human immunodeficiency virus type 1 gp120 critical for the binding of rat and human neutralizing antibodies that block the gp120-sCD4 interaction. Virology 190:134–142, 1992.
365. D'Souza MP, Livnat D, Bradac JA, et al. Evaluation of monoclonal antibodies to human immunodeficiency virus type 1 primary isolates by neutralization assays: Performance criteria for selecting candidate antibodies for clinical trials. J Infect Dis 175:1956–1962, 1997.
366. Burton DR, Pyati J, Koduri R, et al. Efficient neutralization of primary isolates of HIV-1 by a recombinant human monoclonal antibody. Science 266:1024–1027, 1994.
367. Kessler JA II, McKenna PM, Emini EA, et al. Recombinant human monoclonal antibody IgG1b12 neutralizes diverse human immunodeficiency virus type 1 primary isolates. AIDS Res Hum Retroviruses 13:575–582, 1997.
368. McInerney TL, McLain L, Armstrong SJ, Dimmock NJ. A human IgG1 (b12) specific for the CD4 binding site of HIV-1 neutralizes by inhibiting the virus fusion entry process, but b12 Fab neutralizes by inhibiting a postfusion event. Virology 233:313–326, 1997.
369. Trkola A, Pomales AB, Yuan H, et al. Cross-clade neutralization of primary isolates of human immunodeficiency virus type 1 by human monoclonal antibodies and tetrameric CD4-IgG. J Virol 69:6609–6617, 1995.
370. Parren PWHI, Fisicaro P, Labrijn AF, et al. In vitro antigen challenge of human antibody libraries for vaccine evaluation: The human immunodeficiency virus type 1 envelope. J Virol 70:9046–9050, 1996.
371. Parren PWHI, Gauduin M-C, Koup RA, et al. Relevance of the antibody response against human immunodeficiency virus type 1 envelope to vaccine design. Immunol Lett 57:105–112, 1997.
372. Mo H, Stamatos L, Ip JE, et al. Human immunodeficiency virus type 1 mutants that escape neutralization by human monoclonal antibody IgG1b12. J Virol 71:6869–6874, 1997.
373. Thali M, Olshevsky U, Furman C, et al. Characterization of a discontinuous human immunodeficiency virus type 1 gp120 epitope recognized by a broadly reactive neutralizing human monoclonal antibody. J Virol 65:6188–6193, 1991.
374. Trkola A, Purtscher M, Muster T, et al. Human monoclonal antibody 2G12 defines a distinctive neutralization epitope on the gp120 glycoprotein of human immunodeficiency virus type 1. J Virol 70:1100–1108, 1996.
375. Muster T, Steindl F, Purtscher M, et al. A conserved neutralizing epitope on gp41 of human immunodeficiency virus type 1. J Virol 67:6642–6647, 1993.
376. Purtscher M, Trkola A, Gruber G, et al. A broadly neutralizing human monoclonal antibody against gp41 of human immunodeficiency virus type 1. AIDS Res Hum Retroviruses 10:1651–1658, 1994.
377. Moore JP, Ho DD. HIV-1 neutralization: The consequences of viral adaptation to growth on transformed T cells. AIDS 9(suppl A):S117–S136, 1995.
378. Poignard P, Klasse PJ, Sattentau QJ. Antibody neutralization of HIV-1. Immunol Today 17:239–246, 1996.
379. Fouts TR, Binley JM, Trkola A, et al. Neutralization of the human immunodeficiency virus type 1 primary isolate JR-FL by human monoclonal antibodies correlates with antibody binding to the oligomeric form of the envelope glycoprotein complex. J Virol 71:2779–2785, 1997.
380. Earl PL, Broder CC, Long D, et al. Native oligomeric human immunodeficiency virus type 1 envelope glycoprotein elicits diverse monoclonal antibody reactivities. J Virol 68:3015–3036, 1994.
381. Moore JP, Sattentau QJ, Wyatt R, Sodroski J. Mapping the topology of the human immunodeficiency virus surface glycoprotein gp120 with a panel of monoclonal antibodies. J Virol 69:469–484, 1994.
382. Moore JP, Sodroski J. Antibody cross-competition analysis of the human immunodeficiency virus type 1 gp120 exterior envelope glycoprotein. J Virol 70:1853–1872, 1996.
383. Mascola JR, Snyder SW, Weislow OS, et al. Immunization with envelope subunit vaccine products elicits neutralizing antibodies against laboratory-adapted but not primary isolates of human immunodeficiency virus type 1. J Infect Dis 173:340–348, 1996.
384. Van Cott TC, Bethke FR, Burke DS, et al. Lack of induction of antibodies specific for conserved, discontinuous epitopes of HIV-1 envelope glycoprotein by candidate AIDS vaccines. J Immunol 155:4100–4110, 1995.
385. Tilley SA, Honnen WJ, Racho ME, et al. Synergistic neutralization of HIV-1 by human monoclonal antibodies against the V3 loop and the CD4-binding site of gp120. AIDS Res Hum Retroviruses 89:461–467, 1992.
386. Buchbinder A, Karwowska S, Gorny MK, et al. Synergy between human monoclonal antibodies to HIV extends their effective biologic activity against homologous and divergent strains. AIDS Res Hum Retroviruses 8:425–427, 1992.
387. Laal S, Burda S, Gorny MK, et al. Synergistic neutralization of human immunodeficiency virus type 1 by combinations of human monoclonal antibodies. J Virol 68:4001–4008, 1994.
388. Denisova G, Stern B, Raviv D, et al. Humoral immune response to immunocomplexed HIV envelope glycoprotein gp120. AIDS Res Hum Retroviruses 12:901–909, 1996.
389. DeVico A, Silver A, Thornton APM, et al. Covalently crosslinked complexes of human immunodeficiency virus type 1 (HIV-1) gp120 and CD4 receptors elicit a neutralizing immune response that includes antibodies selective for primary virus isolates. Virology 218:258–263, 1996.
390. Kang C-Y, Hariharan K, Nara PL, et al. Immunization with a soluble CD4-gp120 complex preferentially induces neutralizing anti–human immunodeficiency virus type 1 antibodies directed to conformation-dependent epitopes of gp120. J Virol 68:5854–5862, 1994.
391. Moog C, Fleury HJA, Pellegrin C, et al. Autologous and heterologous neutralizing antibody responses following initial seroconversion in human immunodeficiency virus type-1 infected individuals. J Virol 71:3734–3741, 1997.
391a. Montefiori DC, Reimann KA, Wyand MS, et al. Neutralizing antibodies in sera from macaques infected with chimeric simian-human immunodeficiency virus containing the envelope glycoproteins of either a laboratory-adapted variant or a primary isolate of human immunodeficiency virus type 1. J Virol 72:3427–3431, 1998.
392. Wyand MS, Manson KH, Garcia-Moll M, et al. Vaccine protection by a triple deletion mutant of simian immunodeficiency virus. J Virol 70:3724–3733, 1996.
393. Cole KS, Rowles JL, Jagerski BA, et al. Evolution of envelope-specific antibody responses in monkeys experimentally infected or immunized with simian immunodeficiency virus and its association with the development of protective immunity. J Virol 71:5069–5079, 1997.
394. Cole KS, Rowles JL, Murphey-Corb M, et al. A model for the maturation of protective antibody responses to SIV envelope proteins in experimentally immunized monkeys. J Med Primatol 26:51–58, 1997.

395. Planz O, Seiler P, Hengartner H, Zinkernagel RM. Specific cytotoxic T cells eliminate cells producing neutralizing antibodies. Nature 382:726–729, 1996.
396. Weber J, Fenyö E-M, Beddons S, et al. Neutralization serotypes of human immunodeficiency virus type 1 field isolates are not predicted by genetic subtype. J Virol 70:7827–7832, 1996.
397. Nyambi PN, Nkengasong J, Lewi P, et al. Multivariate analysis of human immunodeficiency virus type 1 neutralization data. J Virol 70:6235–6243, 1996.
398. Moore JP, Cao Y, Leu J, et al. Inter- and intraclade neutralization of human immunodeficiency virus type 1 genetic clades do not correspond to neutralization serotypes but partially correspond to gp120 antigenic serotypes. J Virol 70:427–444, 1996.
399. Kostrikis LG, Cao Y, Ngal H, et al. Quantitative analysis of serum neutralization of human immunodeficiency virus type 1 from subtypes A, B, C, D, E, F and I: Lack of direct correlation between neutralization epitopes and genetic subtypes and evidence for prevalent serum-dependent infectivity enhancement. J Virol 70:445–458, 1996.
400. Mascola JR, Louder MK, Surman SR, et al. Human immunodeficiency virus type 1 neutralizing antibody serotyping using serum pools and an infectivity reduction assay. AIDS Res Hum Retroviruses 12:1319–1328, 1996.
401. Nyambi MN, Willems B, Janssens W, et al. The neutralization relationship of HIV type 1, HIV type 2, and SIVcpz is reflected in the genetic diversity that distinguishes them. AIDS Res Hum Retroviruses 13:7–17, 1997.
402. Moore JP, McCutchan FE, Poon S-W, et al. Exploration of antigenic variation in gp120 from clades A through F of human immunodeficiency virus type 1 by using monoclonal antibodies. J Virol 68:8350–8364, 1994.
403. Robinson WE Jr, Montefiori DC, Mitchell WM. Complement-mediated antibody-dependent enhancement of HIV-1 infection requires CD4 and complement receptors. Virology 175:600–604, 1990.
404. Boyer V, Desgranges C, Travaud M, et al. Complement mediates human immunodeficiency virus type 1–infection of a human T cell line in a CD4- and antibody-independent fashion. J Exp Med 173:1151–1158, 1991.
405. Takeda A, Tuazon CV, Ennis FA. Antibody-enhanced infection by HIV-1 via Fc receptor–mediated entry. Science 242:580–583, 1988.
406. Jouault T, Chapuis F, Olivier R, et al. HIV infection of monocytic cells. Role of antibody-mediated virus binding to Fc-gamma receptors. AIDS 3:125–131, 1989.
407. Dolin R, Graham BS, Greenberg SB, et al. The safety and immunogenicity of a human immunodeficiency virus type 1 (HIV-1) recombinant gp160 candidate vaccine in humans. Ann Intern Med 114:119–127, 1991.
408. Robinson WE Jr, Kawamura T, Gorny MK, et al. Human monoclonal antibodies to the human immunodeficiency virus type 1 (HIV-1) transmembrane glycoprotein gp41 enhance HIV-infection in vitro. Proc Natl Acad Sci U S A 87:3185–3189, 1990.
409. Jiang S, Neurath AR. Potential risks of eliciting antibodies enhancing HIV-1 infection of monocytic cells by vaccination with V3 loops of unmatched HIV-1 isolates. AIDS 6:331–332, 1992.
410. Homsy J, Meyer M, Levy JA. Serum enhancement of human immunodeficiency virus (HIV) infection correlates with disease in HIV-infected individuals. J Virol 64:1437–1440, 1990.
411. Montefiori DC, Pantaleo G, Fink LM, et al. Neutralizing and infection-enhancing antibody responses to human immunodeficiency virus type 1 in long-term nonprogressors. J Infect Dis 173:60–67, 1996.
412. Tyler DJ, Lyerly HK, Weinhold KJ. Anti–HIV-1 ADCC (mini-review). AIDS Res Hum Retroviruses 5:557–563, 1989.
413. Tanneau F, McChesney M, Lopez O, et al. Primary cytotoxicity against the envelope glycoprotein of human immunodeficiency virus-1: Evidence for antibody-dependent cellular cytotoxicity in vivo. J Infect Dis 162:837–843, 1990.
414. Posner MR, Elboim HS, Cannon T, et al. Functional activity of an HIV-1 neutralizing IgG human monoclonal antibody: ADCC and complement-mediated lysis. AIDS Res Hum Retroviruses 8:553–558, 1992.
415. Oldstone MBA, Tishon A, Eddleston M, et al. Vaccination to prevent persistent viral infection. J Virol 67:4372–4378, 1993.
416. McMichael AJ, Walker BD. Cytotoxic T lymphocyte epitopes: Implications for HIV vaccines. AIDS 8(suppl 1):S155–S173, 1994.
417. Mackewicz CE, Blackbourn DJ, Levy JA. $CD8^+$ T cells suppress human immunodeficiency virus replication by inhibiting viral transcription. Proc Natl Acad Sci U S A 92:2308–2312, 1995.
418. Blackbourn DJ, Mackewicz CE, Barker E, et al. Suppression of HIV replication by lymphocytic tissue $CD8^+$ cells correlates with clinical state of HIV-infected individuals. Proc Natl Acad Sci U S A 93:13125–13130, 1996.
419. Yang OO, Kalams SA, Trocha A, et al. Suppression of human immunodeficiency type 1 replication by $CD8^+$ cells: Evidence for HLA class I–restricted triggering of cytolytic and noncytolytic mechanisms. J Virol 71:3120–3128, 1997.
420. Moss PA, Rowland-Jones SL, Frodsham PM, et al. Persistent high frequency of human immunodeficiency virus–specific cytotoxic T cells in peripheral blood of infected donors. Proc Natl Acad Sci U S A 92:5773–5777, 1995.
421. Yang OO, Kalams SA, Rosenzweig M, et al. Efficient lysis of human immunodeficiency virus type 1–infected cells by cytotoxic T-lymphocytes. J Virol 70:5799–5806, 1996.
421a. Ferbas J. Perspectives on the role of $CD8^+$ cell suppressor factors and cytotoxic T lymphocytes during HIV infection. AIDS Res Hum Retroviruses 14(suppl 2):S153–S160, 1998.
422. Koup RA, Safrit JT, Cao Y, et al. Temporal association of cellular immune responses with the initial control of viremia in primary human immunodeficiency virus type 1 syndrome. J Virol 68:4650–4655, 1994.
423. Borrow P, Lewicki H, Hahn BH, et al. Virus-specific $CD8^+$ cytotoxic T-lymphocyte activity associated with control of viremia in primary human immunodeficiency virus type 1 infection. J Immunol 68:6103–6110, 1994.
424. Harrer T, Harrer E, Kalams SA, et al. Strong cytotoxic T-cell and weak neutralizing antibody responses in a subset of persons with stable non-progressing HIV type 1 infection. AIDS Res Hum Retroviruses 12:585–592, 1996.
425. Harrer T, Harrer E, Kalams SA, et al. Cytotoxic T-lymphocytes in asymptomatic long-term nonprogressing HIV-1 infection. J Immunol 156:2616–2623, 1996.
425a. Ogg GS, Jin X, Bonhoeffer S, et al. Quantitation of HIV-1 specific cytotoxic T lymphocytes and plasma load of viral RNA. Science 279:2103–2106, 1998.
425b. Matano T, Shibato R, Siemon C, et al. Administration of an anti-CD8 monoclonal antibody interferes with the clearance of chimeric simian/human immunodeficiency viruses during primary infection of rhesus macaques. J Virol 72:164–169, 1998.
426. Lohman BL, Miller CJ, McChesney MB. Antiviral cytotoxic T-lymphocytes in vaginal mucosa of simian immunodeficiency virus–infected rhesus macaques. J Immunol 155:5855–5860, 1995.
427. Couëdel-Courteille A, Le Grand R, Tulliez M, et al. Direct ex vivo simian immunodeficiency virus (SIV)–specific cytotoxic activity detected from small intestine intraepithelial lymphocytes of SIV-infected macaques at an advanced stage of infection. J Virol 71:1052–1057, 1997.
428. Autran B, Levine NL. HIV epitopes recognized by cytotoxic T-lymphocytes. AIDS 5(suppl 2):S145–S150, 1991.
429. Wilson CC, Kalams SA, Wilkes BM, et al. Overlapping epitopes in human immunodeficiency virus type 1 gp120 presented by HLA-A, -B and -C molecules: Effects of viral variation on cytotoxic T-lymphocyte recognition. J Virol 71:1256–1264, 1997.
430. Stanhope PE, Clements ML, Siliciano RF. Human $CD4^+$ cytotoxic T-lymphocyte responses to a human immunodeficiency virus type 1 gp160 subunit vaccine. J Infect Dis 168:92–100, 1993.
431. Koenig S, Fuerst TR, Wood L, et al. Mapping the fine specificity of cytolytic T-cell response to HIV-1 Nef protein. J Immunol 145:127–131, 1990.
432. Ferrari G, Humphrey W, McElrath MJ, et al. Clade B–based HIV-1 vaccines elicit cross-clade cytotoxic T-lymphocyte reactivites in uninfected volunteers. Proc Natl Acad Sci U S A 94:1396–1401, 1997.
433. Yasutomi Y, Koenig S, Woods RM, et al. A vaccine-elicited, single viral epitope-specific cytotoxic T-lymphocyte response does not protect against intravenous, cell-free simian immunodeficiency virus challenge. J Virol 69:2279–2284, 1995.

434. Cease KB, Margalit H, Cornette JL, et al. Helper T-cell antigenic site identification in the acquired immunodeficiency syndrome virus gp120 envelope protein and induction of immunity in mice to the native protein using a 16 residue synthetic peptide. Proc Natl Acad Sci U S A 84:4249–4253, 1987.
435. Mills KHG, Kitchin PA, Mahon BP, et al. HIV p24-specific helper T-cell clones from immunized primates recognize highly conserved regions of HIV-1. J Immunol 144:1677–1683, 1990.
436. Bahraoui E, Yagello M, Billaud JL, et al. Immunogenicity of the human immunodeficiency virus (HIV) recombinant *nef* gene product. Mapping of T-cell and B-cell epitopes in immunized chimpanzees. AIDS Res Hum Retroviruses 6:1087–1098, 1990.
437. Hilleman MR. Whether and when an AIDS vaccine? Nat Med 1:1126–1129, 1995.
438. Girard M. The challenge of HIV vaccines. Vaccine 9:781–783, 1991.
439. Schultz AM. Changing paradigms for an HIV vaccine. In Cohen S, Shafferman A (eds). Novel Strategies in Design and Production of Vaccines. New York, Plenum Press, 1996, pp 79–90.
440. Warren JT, Dolatshi M. First updated and revised survey of worldwide HIV and SIV vaccine challenge studies in non-human primates: Progress in first and second order studies. J Med Primatol 22:203–205, 1993.
441. Hirsch VM, Goldstein S, Hynes NA, et al. Prolonged clinical latency and survival of macaques given a whole inactivated simian immunodeficiency virus vaccine. J Infect Dis 170:51–59, 1994.
442. Mossman SP, Bex F, Berglund P, et al. Protection against lethal simian immunodeficiency virus SIVsmmPBj14 disease by a recombinant Semliki Forest virus gp160 vaccine and by a gp120 subunit vaccine. J Virol 70:1953–1960, 1996.
443. Stott EJ. Anti-cell antibody in macaques [letter]. Nature 253:393, 1991.
444. Le Grand R, Vaslin B, Vogt G, et al. AIDS vaccine developments [letter]. Nature 355:684, 1992.
445. Cranage MP, Ashworth LA, Greenaway PJ, et al. AIDS vaccine developments. Nature 355:685–686, 1992.
446. Arthur LO, Bess JW Jr, Urban RG, et al. Macaques immunized with HLA-DR are protected from challenge with simian immunodeficiency virus. J Virol 69:3117–3124, 1995.
447. Neidrig M, Gregerson JP, Fultz PN, et al. Immune responses of chimpanzees after immunization with the inactivated whole immunodeficiency virus (HIV-1), three different adjuvants and challenge. Vaccine 11:67–74, 1993.
448. Marthas ML, Sutjipto S, Higgins J, et al. Immunization with a live-attenuated simian immunodeficiency virus (SIV) prevents early disease but not infection in rhesus macaques challenged with pathogenic SIV. J Virol 64:3694–3700, 1990.
449. Lohman BL, McChesney MB, Miller CJ, et al. A partially attenuated simian immunodeficiency virus induces host immunity that correlates with resistance to pathogenic virus challenge. J Virol 68:7021–7029, 1994.
450. Johnson RP, Glickman RL, Yang JQ, et al. Induction of vigorous cytotoxic T-lymphocyte responses by live attenuated simian immunodeficiency virus. J Virol 71:7711–7718, 1997.
451. Desrosiers RC. HIV with multiple gene deletions as a live attenuated vaccine for AIDS. AIDS Res Hum Retroviruses 8:411–421, 1992.
452. Gibbs JS, Regier DA, Desrosiers RC. Construction and in vitro properties of SIVmac mutants with deletions in "nonessential" genes. AIDS Res Hum Retroviruses 10:607–616, 1994.
453. Rud EW, Cranage M, Yon J, et al. Molecular and biological characterization of simian immunodeficiency virus macaque strain 32H proviral clones containing *nef* size variants. J Gen Virol 75:529–543, 1994.
454. Cranage MP, Whatmore AM, Sharpe SA, et al. Macaques infected with live attenuated SIVmac are protected against superinfection via the rectal mucosa. Virology 229:143–154, 1997.
455. Baba TW, Jeong YS, Penninck D, et al. Pathogenicity of live, attenuated SIV after mucosal infection of neonatal macaques. Science 267:1820–1825, 1995.
456. Wyand MS, Manson KH, Lackner AA, Desrosiers RC. Resistance of neonatal monkeys to live attenuated vaccine strains of simian immunodeficiency virus. Nat Med 3:32–36, 1997.
457. Cohen J. Weakened SIV vaccine still kills. Science 278:24–25, 1997.
458. Giavedoni L, Ahmad S, Jones L, Yilma T. Expression of gamma interferon by simian immunodeficiency virus increases attenuation and reduces postchallenge virus load in vaccinated rhesus macaques. J Virol 71:866–872, 1997.
459. Chakrabarti BK, Maitra RK, Ma XZ, Kestler HW. A candidate live inactivatable attenuated vaccine for AIDS. Proc Natl Acad Sci U S A 93:9810–9815, 1996.
460. Smith SM, Markham RB, Jeang KT. Conditional reduction of human immunodeficiency virus type 1 replication by a gain-of-herpes simplex virus 1 thymidine kinase function. Proc Natl Acad Sci U S A 93:7955–7960, 1996.
461. Deacon NJ, Tsykin A, Solomon A, et al. Genomic structure of an attenuated quasi species of HIV-1 from a blood transfusion donor and recipients. Science 270:988–991, 1995.
462. Kirchhoff F, Greenough TC, Brettler DB, et al. Brief report: Absence of intact *nef* sequences in a long-term survivor with nonprogressive HIV-1 infection. N Engl J Med 332:228–232, 1995.
463. Mariani R, Kirchhoff F, Greenough TC, et al. High frequency of defective *nef* alleles in a long-term survivor with nonprogressive human immunodeficiency virus type 1 infection. J Virol 70:7752–7764, 1996.
464. Clements JE, Montelaro RC, Zinc MC, et al. Cross-protective immune responses induced in rhesus macaque by immunization with attenuated macrophage-tropic simian immunodeficiency virus. J Virol 69:2737–2744, 1995.
465. Putkonen P, Nilsson C, Mäkitalo B, et al. Immunization with live attenuated SIVmac can protect macaques against mucosal infection with SIVsm. In Channock RM, Lerner RA, Brown F, Ginsberg H (eds). Vaccines 96. Cold Spring Harbor, NY, Cold Spring Harbor Laboratory Press, 1996, pp 295–241.
466. Bogers WMJM, Niphuis H, ten Haaft P, et al. Protection from HIV-1 envelope bearing chimeric simian immunodeficiency virus (SHIV) in rhesus macaques infected with attenuated SIV. Consequences of challenge. AIDS 9:F13–F18, 1995.
466a. Shibata R, Siemon C, Czajak SC, et al. Live, attenuated simian immunodeficiency virus vaccines elicit potent resistance against a challenge with a human immunodeficiency virus type 1 chimeric virus. J Virol 71:8141–8148, 1997.
466b. Johnston RP, Glickman RL, Young JQ, et al. Induction of vigorous cytotoxic T-lymphocyte responses by live attenuated simian immunodeficiency virus. J Virol 71:7711–7718, 1997.
467. Clerici M, Clark EA, Polacino P, et al. T-cell proliferation to subinfectious SIV correlates with lack of infection after challenge of macaques. AIDS 8:1391–1395, 1994.
468. Putkonen P, Mäkitalo B, Böttiger D, et al. Protection of human immunodeficiency virus type 2–exposed seronegative macaques from mucosal simian immunodeficiency virus transmission. J Virol 71:4981–4984, 1997.
469. Tartaglia J, Pincus S, Paoletti E. Poxvirus-based vectors as vaccine candidates. Crit Rev Immunol 10:13–31, 1990.
470. Zagury D, Bernard J, Cheynier R, et al. A group-specific anamnestic immune reaction against HIV-1 induced by a candidate vaccine against AIDS. Nature 332:728–731, 1988.
471. Graham BS, Belshe RB, Clements ML, et al. Vaccination of vaccinia-naive adults with human immunodeficiency virus type 1 gp160 recombinant vaccinia virus in a blinded, controlled, randomized clinical trial. J Infect Dis 166:244–252, 1992.
472. Gallimore A, Cranage M, Cook N, et al. Early suppression of SIV replication by CD8^{+} *nef*-specific cytotoxic T cells in vaccinated macaques. Nat Med 1:1167–1173, 1995.
473. Tartaglia J, Perkus ME, Taylor J, et al. NYVAC: A highly attenuated strain of vaccinia virus. Virology 188:217–232, 1992.
474. Paoletti E. Two highly attenuated poxvirus vectors. In Girard M, Valette L (eds). Retroviruses of Human AIDS and Related Animal Diseases. 6ème Colloque des Cent Gardes. Lyon, Fondation Marcel Mérieux, 1992, pp 111–115.
475. Mayr A, Hochstein-Mintzel V, Stickl H. Abstammung, Eigenschaften und Verwendung des attenuierten vaccinia-stammens MVA. Infection 105:6–14, 1975.
476. Meyer H, Sutter G, Mayr A. Mapping of deletions in the genome of the highly attenuated vaccinia virus MVA and their influence on virulence. J Gen Virol 72:1031–1038, 1991.
477. Abimiku A, Franchini G, Tartaglia J, et al. HIV-1 recombinant poxvirus vaccine induces cross-protection against HIV-2 challenge in rhesus macaques. Nat Med 1:321–329, 1995.

477a. Benson J, Chougnet C, Robert-Guroff M, et al. Recombinant vaccine–induced protection against the highly pathogenic simian immunodeficiency virus SIV(mac251): Dependence on route of challenge exposure. J Virol 72:4170–4182, 1998.
478. Hanke T, Blanchard TJ, Schneider J, et al. Immunogenicities of intravenous and intramuscular administrations of modified vaccinia virus Ankara–based multi-CTL epitope vaccine for HIV type 1 in mice. J Gen Virol 79(pt 1):83–90, 1998.
478a. Hirsch VM, Fuerst TR, Sutter G, et al. Patterns of viral replication correlate with outcome in simian immunodeficiency virus (SIV)–infected macaques: Effect of prior immunization with a trivalent SIV vaccinia in modified vaccinia virus Ankara. J Virol 70:3741–3752, 1996.
479. Prevec L, Christie BS, Laurie KE, et al. Immune response to HIV-1 Gag antigens induced by recombinant adenovirus vectors in mice and rhesus macaque monkeys. J Acquir Immune Defic Syndr 4:568–576, 1991.
480. Lubeck MD, Natuk RJ, Chengalvala M, et al. Immunogenicity of recombinant adenovirus–human immunodeficiency virus vaccines in chimpanzees following intranasal administration. AIDS Res Hum Retroviruses 10:1443–1449, 1994.
481. Lubeck MD, Natuk RJ, Myagkikh M, et al. Long-term protection of chimpanzees against high-dose HIV-1 challenge induced by immunization. Nat Med 3:651–658, 1997.
481a. Zolla-Pazner S, Lubeck M, Xu S, et al. Induction of neutralizing antibodies to T-cell line–adapted and primary human immunodeficiency virus type 1 isolates with a prime-boost vaccine regimen in chimpanzees. J Virol 72:1052–1059, 1998.
482. Evans DJ, McKeating J, Meredith JM, et al. An engineered poliovirus chimaera elicits broadly reactive HIV-1 neutralizing antibodies. Nature 339:385–388, 1989.
483. Dedieu JF, Ronco J, van der Werf S, et al. Poliovirus chimaeras expressing sequences from the principal neutralization domain of human immunodeficiency virus type 1. J Virol 66:3161–3167, 1992.
484. Li S, Polonis V, Isobe H, et al. Chimeric influenza virus induces neutralizing antibodies and cytotoxic T cells against human immunodeficiency virus type 1. J Virol 67:6659–6666, 1993.
485. Muster T, Ferko B, Klima A, et al. Mucosal model of immunization against human immunodeficiency virus type 1 with a chimeric influenza virus. J Virol 69:6678–6686, 1995.
486. Morrow CD, Porter DC, Ansardi DC, et al. New approaches for mucosal vaccines for AIDS: Encapsidation and serial passages of poliovirus replicons that express HIV-1 proteins on infection. AIDS Res Hum Retroviruses 10:S61–S66, 1994.
487. Anderson MJ, Porter DC, Moldovean Z, et al. Characterization of the expression and immunogenicity of poliovirus replicons that encode simian immunodeficiency virus SIVmac239 Gag or envelope SU proteins. AIDS Res Hum Retroviruses 13:53–62, 1997.
488. Paul NL, Marsh M, McKeating JA, et al. Expression of HIV-1 envelope glycoproteins by Semliki Forest virus vectors. AIDS Res Hum Retroviruses 9:963–970, 1993.
489. Stover CK, de la Cruz FV, Fuerst TR, et al. New use of BCG for recombinant vaccines. Nature 351:456–460, 1991.
490. Steger KK, Pauza CD. Immunization of *Macaca mulatta* with *Aro*A attenuated *Salmonella typhimurium* expressing the SIVp27 antigen. J Med Primatol 26:44–50, 1997.
491. Aldovini A, Young RA. Humoral and cell-mediated immune responses to live recombinant BCG-HIV vaccines. Nature 351:479–482, 1991.
492. Lagranderie M, Balazuc AM, Gicquel B, Gheorghiu M. Oral immunization with recombinant *Mycobacterium bovis* BCG simian immunodeficiency virus *nef* induces local and systemic cytotoxic T-lymphocyte response in mice. J Virol 71:2302–2309, 1997.
493. Honda M, Matsuo K, Nakasone T, et al. Protective immune responses induced by secretion of a chimeric soluble protein from a recombinant *Mycobacterium bovis* bacillus Calmette-Guérin vector candidate vaccine for human immunodeficiency virus type 1 in small animals. Proc Natl Acad Sci U S A 92:10693–10697, 1995.
494. Aldovini A, Young RA. Mutations of RNA and protein sequences involved in human immunodeficiency virus type 1 packaging result in production of noninfectious virus. J Virol 64:1920–1926, 1990.
495. Gorelinck RJ, Nigida SM Jr, Bess JW Jr, et al. Non-infectious human immunodeficiency virus type 1 mutants deficient in genomic RNA. J Virol 64:3207–3211, 1990.
496. Gheysen DE, Jacobs E, DeForesta F, et al. Assembly and release of HIV-1 precursor Pr55Gag virus-like particles from recombinant baculovirus-infected insect cells. Cell 59:103–112, 1989.
497. Haffar OK, Smithgale MD, Moran PA, et al. HIV-specific humoral and cellular immunity in rabbits vaccinated with recombinant human immunodeficiency virus-like *gag-env* particles. Virology 183:487–495, 1991.
498. Haynes JR, Loo SX, Rovinski B et al. Production of immunogenic HIV-1 virus-like particles in stably engineered monkey cell lines. AIDS Res Hum Retroviruses 7:17–27, 1991.
499. Rovinski B, Rodriguez L, Cao SX, et al. Induction of HIV type 1–neutralizing and env-CD4 blocking antibodies by immunization with genetically engineered HIV type 1–like particles containing unprocessed gp160 glycoproteins. AIDS Res Hum Retroviruses 11:1187–1195, 1995.
500. Grene E, Mezule G, Borisova G, et al. Relationship between antigenicity and immunogenicity of chimeric hepatitis B virus core particles carrying HIV type 1 epitopes. AIDS Res Hum Retroviruses 13:41–51, 1997.
501. Schlienger K, Mancini M, Rivière Y, et al. Human immunodeficiency virus type 1 major neutralizing determinant exposed on hepatitis B surface antigen particles is highly immunogenic in primates. J Virol 66:2570–2576, 1991.
502. Adams SE, Dawson KM, Gull K, et al. The expression of hybrid HIV:Ty virus-like particles in yeast. Nature 329:68–70, 1987.
503. Layton GT, Harris SJ, Gearing AJH, et al. Induction of HIV-specific cytotoxic T lymphocytes in vivo with hybrid HIV-1 V3:Ty-virus-like particles. J Immunol 151:1097–1107, 1993.
504. Lehner T, Brookes R, Panagiotidi C, et al. T- and B-cell functions and epitope expression in non-human primates immunized with simian immunodeficiency virus antigen by the rectal route. Proc Natl Acad Sci U S A 90:8638–8642, 1993.
505. Eckart L, Rattlesberger W, Ferko B, et al. Immunogenic presentation of a conserved gp41 epitope of human immunodeficiency virus type 1 on recombinant surface antigen of hepatitis B virus. J Gen Virol 77:2001–2008, 1996.
506. Esparza J, Heyward WL, Osmanov S. HIV vaccine development: From basic research to human trials. AIDS 10(suppl A):S123–S132, 1996.
507. Alvin CR. Liposomes as carriers of antigens and adjuvants. J Immunol Methods 140:1–13, 1991.
508. Browning M, Reid G, Osborne R, Jarrett O. Incorporation of soluble antigens into ISCOMs: HIV gp120 ISCOMs induce neutralizing antibodies. Vaccine 10:585–590, 1991.
509. Osterhaus ADE, Vries P, Heeney J. AIDS vaccine developments. Nature 355:684–685, 1992.
510. Hulskotte EGJ, Geretti AM, Siebelink KHJ, et al. Vaccine-induced virus neutralizing antibodies and cytotoxic T-cells do not protect macaques from experimental infection with simian immunodeficiency virus SIVmac 32H (J5). J Virol 69:6289–6296, 1995.
511. Alving CR, Wassef NM, Richards RL. Use of adjuvants for enhancement of antibody responses. In Weir D, Blackwell C, Herzenberg L, Herzenberg L (eds). Handbook of Experimental Immunology. Vol 2A. Oxford, Blackwell Scientific Publications, 1996, pp 87.1–87.10.
512. Van Nest GA, Steimer KS, Haigwood NH, et al. Advanced adjuvant formulations for use with recombinant subunit vaccines. In Chanock RM, Lerner RA, Brown F, Ginsberg H (eds). Vaccines 92: Modern Approaches to New Vaccines. Cold Spring Harbor, NY, Cold Spring Harbor Laboratory, 1992, pp 57–62.
513. Van Cott TC, Mascola JR, Kaminski RW, et al. Antibodies with specificity for native gp120 and neutralization activity against primary human immunodeficiency virus type 1 isolates elicited by immunization with oligomeric gp160. J Virol 71:4319–4330, 1997.
514. Stahl-Hennig C, Coulibaly C, Petry H, et al. Immunization with virion-derived glycoprotein 130 from HIV-2 or SIV protects macaques against challenge virus grown in human or simian cells or prepared ex vivo. AIDS Res Hum Retroviruses 10(suppl 2):S27–S32, 1994.
515. Eldridge J, Stoas JK, Meulbroek JA, et al. Biodegradable micro-

spheres as a vaccine delivery system. Mol Immunol 28:287–294, 1991.
516. Marx PA, Compans RW, Gettie A, et al. Protection against vaginal SIV transmission with microencapsulated vaccine. Science 260:1323–1327, 1991.
517. Cleland JL, Powell MF, Lim A, et al. Development of a single-shot subunit vaccine for HIV-1. AIDS Res Hum Retroviruses 10(suppl 2):S21–S26, 1994.
518. Hu S-L, Klaniecki J, Dykers T, et al. Neutralizing antibodies against HIV-1 BRU and SF2 isolates generated in mice immunized with recombinant vaccinia virus expressing HIV-1 (BRU) envelope glycoproteins and boosted with homologous gp160. AIDS Res Hum Retroviruses 7:615–620, 1991.
519. Hu S-L, Abrams K, Barber GN, et al. Protection of macaques against SIV infection by subunit vaccines of SIV envelope glycoprotein gp160. Science 255:456–459, 1992.
520. Schultz AM, Stott EJ. Primate models for AIDS vaccines. AIDS 8(suppl 1):S203–S212, 1994.
521. Putkonen P, Thorstensson R, Walther L, et al. Vaccine protection against HIV-2 infection in cynomolgus monkeys. AIDS Res Hum Retroviruses 7:271–277, 1991.
522. Putkonen P, Björling E, Akerblom L, et al. Long-standing protection of macaques against cell-free HIV-2 with a HIV-2 Iscom vaccine. J Acquir Immune Defic Syndr 7:551–559, 1994.
523. Putkonen P, Thorstensson B, Ghavamzadeh L, et al. Prevention of HIV-2 and SIVsm infection by passive immunization in cynomolgus monkeys. Nature 352:436–438, 1991.
524. Kent SJ, Hu SL, Corey L, et al. Detection of simian immunodeficiency virus (SIV)–specific CD8+ T cells in macaques protected from SIV challenge by prior SIV subunit vaccination. J Virol 70:4941–4947, 1996.
525. Lehner T, Wang Y, Cranage M, et al. Protective mucosal immunity elicited by targeted iliac lymph node immunization with a subunit SIV envelope and core vaccine in macaques. Nat Med 2:767–775, 1996.
525a. Lu X, Kiyono H, Lu D, et al. Targeted lymph-node immunization with whole inactivated simian immunodeficiency virus (SIV) or envelope and core subunit antigen vaccines does not reliably protect rhesus macaques from vaginal challenge with SIVmac 251. AIDS 12:1–10, 1998.
526. Buge SL, Richardson E, Alipanah S, et al. An adenovirus-simian immunodeficiency virus *env* vaccine elicits humoral, cellular and mucosal immune responses in rhesus macaques and decreases viral burden following vaginal challenge. J Virol 71:8531–8541, 1997.
527. Ronco J, Dedieu JF, Marié FN, et al. High-titer HIV-neutralizing antibody response of rhesus macaques to gp160 and env peptides. AIDS Res Hum Retroviruses 8:707–713, 1992.
528. Haynes BF, Torres JV, Langlois AJ, et al. Induction of HIV MN neutralizing antibodies in primates using a prime-boost regimen of hybrid synthetic gp120 envelope peptides. J Immunol 151:1646–1653, 1993.
529. Hart MK, Weinhold KJ, Scearce RM, et al. Priming of anti-HIV CD8+ cytotoxic T-cells in vivo by carrier-free HIV synthetic peptides. Proc Natl Acad Sci U S A 88:9448–9452, 1991.
530. Sia DY. Structure and immunogenicity of synthetic HIV tandem epitopes. In Girard M, Valette L (eds). Retroviruses of Human AIDS and Related Animal Diseases. 6ème Colloque des Cent Gardes. Lyon, Fondation Marcel Mérieux, 1992, pp 105–109.
531. Cox JH, Ivanyi J, Young DB, et al. Orientation of epitopes influences the immunogenicity of synthetic peptide dimers. Eur J Immunol 18:2015–2019, 1988.
532. Wang CY, Looney DJ, Li ML, et al. Long-term high-titer neutralizing activity induced by octameric synthetic HIV-1 antigen. Science 254:285–288, 1991.
533. Kelleher AD, Emery S, Cunningham P, et al. Safety and immunogenicity of UBI HIV-1 MN octameric V3 peptide vaccine administered by subcutaneous injection. AIDS Res Hum Retroviruses 13:29–32, 1997.
534. Defoort JP, Nardelli B, Huang W, et al. Macromolecular assemblage in the design of a synthetic AIDS vaccine. Proc Natl Acad Sci U S A 89:3879–3883, 1992.
535. Deres K, Schild H, Wiesmüller KH, et al. In vivo priming of virus-specific cytotoxic T lymphocytes with synthetic lipopeptide vaccine. Nature 342:561–564, 1989.
536. Deprez B, Sauzet JP, Boutillon C, et al. Comparative efficiency of simple lipopeptide constructs for in vivo induction of virus-specific CTL. Vaccine 5:375–382, 1996.
537. Liu MA. The immunologist's grail: Vaccines that generate cellular immunity. Proc Natl Acad Sci U S A 94:10496–10498, 1997.
537a. Sedegah M, Jones TR, Kaur M, et al. Boosting with recombinant vaccinia increases immunogenicity and protective efficacy of malaria DNA vaccine. Proc Natl Acad Sci U S A 95:7648–7653, 1998.
537b. Schneider J, Gilbert SC, Blanchard TJ, et al. Enhanced immunogenicity for CD8+ T cell induction and complete protective efficacy of malaria DNA vaccination by boosting with modified vaccinia virus Ankara. Nat Med 4:397–402, 1998.
538. Kang C-Y, Nara P, Chaurat S, et al. Anti-idiotype monoclonal antibody elicits broadly neutralizing anti-gp120 antibodies in monkeys. Proc Natl Acad Sci U S A 89:2546–2550, 1992.
539. Wang B, Ugen KE, Srikantan V, et al. Gene inoculation generates immune response against human immunodeficiency virus type 1. Proc Natl Acad Sci U S A 90:4156–4160, 1993.
540. Lu S, Santoro JC, Fuller DH, et al. Use of DNAs expressing HIV-1 *env* and noninfectious HIV-1 particles to raise antibody responses in mice. Virology 209:147–154, 1995.
541. Yasutomi Y, Robinson HL, Lu S, et al. Simian immunodeficiency virus–specific cytotoxic T lymphocyte induction through DNA vaccination of rhesus monkeys. J Virol 70:678–681, 1996.
542. Wang B, Boyer J, Srikantan V, et al. Induction of humoral and cellular immune response to the human immunodeficiency type 1 virus in non-human primates by in vivo DNA inoculation. Virology 211:102–112, 1995.
543. Lu S, Arthos J, Montefiori DC, et al. Simian immunodeficiency virus DNA vaccination trial in macaques. J Virol 70:3978–3991, 1996.
544. Letvin NL, Montefiori DC, Yasutomi Y, et al. Potent, protective anti-HIV immune responses generated by bimodal HIV envelope DNA plus protein vaccination. Proc Natl Acad Sci U S A 94:9378–9383, 1997.
545. Boyer JD, Wang B, Ugen KE, et al. In vivo protective anti-HIV immune responses in non-human primates through DNA immunization. J Med Primatol 25:242–250, 1996.
546. Boyer JD, Ugen KE, Wang B, et al. Protection of chimpanzees from high-dose heterologous HIV-1 challenge by DNA vaccination. Nat Med 3:526–532, 1997.
547. Kim JJ, Ayyavoo V, Bagarazzi ML, et al. In vivo engineering of a cellular immune response by coadministration of IL-12 expression vector with a DNA immunogen. J Immunol 158:816–826, 1997.
548. Barnett SW, Rajasekar S, Legg H, et al. Vaccination with HIV-1 gp120 DNA induces immune responses that are boosted by a recombinant gp120 protein subunit. Vaccine 15:869–873, 1997.
549. Heeney JL. Primate models for AIDS vaccine development. AIDS 10(suppl A):S115–S122, 1996.
550. Fultz PN, Sancier M, Anderson DC, et al. Development of AIDS in a chimpanzee infected with human immunodeficiency virus type 1. J Virol 71:4088–4091, 1997.
551. Agy MB, Frumkin LR, Corey L, et al. Infection of *Macaca nemestrina* by human immunodeficiency virus type 1. Science 257:103–106, 1992.
552. Filice G, Cereda PM, Vanier OE. Infection of rabbits with human immunodeficiency virus. Nature 335:366–369, 1988.
553. Reina S, Markham P, Gard E, et al. Serological, biological, and molecular characterization of New Zealand white rabbits infected by retroperitoneal inoculation with cell-free human immunodeficiency virus. J Virol 67:5367–5374, 1993.
554. Namikawa R, Kaneshima H, Lieberman M, et al. Infection of SCID-hu mouse by HIV-1. Science 242:1684–1686, 1988.
555. Mosier DE, Gulizia RJ, Baird SM, et al. Human immunodeficiency virus infection of human PBL-SCID mice. Science 251:791–794, 1991.
556. Li JT, Lord CI, Haseltine W, et al. Infection of cynomolgus monkeys with a chimeric HIV-1/SIVmac virus that expresses the HIV-1 envelope glycoproteins. J Acquir Immune Defic Syndr 5:639–646, 1992.
557. Shibata R, Adochi A. SIV/HIV recombinants and their use in studying biological properties. AIDS Res Hum Retroviruses 8:403–409, 1992.

558. Li JT, Halloran M, Lord CI, et al. Persistent infection of macaques with simian human immunodeficiency virus. J Virol 69:7061–7071, 1995.
559. Reimann KA, Li JT, Voss G, et al. An *env* gene derived from a primary human immunodeficiency virus type 1 isolate confers high in vivo replicative capacity to a chimeric simian/human immunodeficiency virus in rhesus monkeys. J Virol 70:3198–3206, 1996.
559a. Bogers WM, Dubbes R, ten Haaft P, et al. Comparison of *in vitro* and *in vivo* infectivity of different clade B HIV-1 envelope chimeric simian/human immunodeficiency viruses in *Macaca mulatta*. Virology 236:110–117, 1997.
560. Reimann KA, Li JT, Veazuy R, et al. A chimeric simian/human immunodeficiency virus expressing a primary patient human immunodeficiency virus type 1 isolate *env* causes an AIDS-like disease after in vivo passage in rhesus monkeys. J Virol 70:6922–6928, 1996.
561. Joag SV, Li Z, Foresman L, et al. Chimeric simian/human immunodeficiency virus that causes progressive loss of CD4+ T cells and AIDS in pig-tailed macaques. J Virol 70:3189–3197, 1996.
562. Joag SV, Adamy I, Li Z, et al. Animal model of mucosally transmitted human immunodeficiency virus type 1 disease: Intravaginal and oral deposition of simian/human immunodeficiency virus in macaques results in systemic infection, elimination of CD4+ T cells, and AIDS. J Virol 71:4016–4023, 1997.
563. Lu Y, Salvato MS, Pauza CD, et al. Utility of SHIV for testing HIV-1 vaccine candidates in macaques. J Acquir Immune Defic Syndr Hum Retrovirol 12:99–106, 1996.
563a. Karlsson GB, Halloran M, Li J, et al. Characterization of molecularly cloned simian-human immunodeficiency viruses causing rapid CD4+ lymphocyte depletion in rhesus monkeys. J Virol 71:4218–4225, 1997.
564. Berman PW, Gregory TJ, Riddle L, et al. Protection of chimpanzees from infection by HIV-1 after vaccination with recombinant glycoprotein gp120 but not gp160. Nature 345:622–625, 1990.
565. Girard M, Kieny MP, Pinter A, et al. Immunization of chimpanzees confers protection against challenge with human immunodeficiency virus. Proc Natl Acad Sci U S A 88:542–546, 1991.
565a. Meeney JL, Bruck C, Goudsmit J, et al: Immune correlates of protection from HIV and AIDS. Immunol Today 18:4–8, 1997.
566. Fultz PN, Nara P, Barré-Sinoussi F, et al. Vaccine protection of chimpanzees against challenge with HIV-1 infected peripheral blood mononuclear cells. Science 256:1687–1690, 1992.
567. Bruck C, Thiriart C, Fabry L, et al. HIV-1 envelope-elicited neutralizing antibody titres correlate with protection and virus load in chimpanzees. Vaccine 12:1141–1148, 1994.
568. Belo M, Yagello M, Girard M, et al. Antibody-dependent cellular cytotoxicity against HIV-1 in sera of immunized chimpanzees. AIDS 5:169–176, 1991.
569. Emini EA, Nara PL, Schleif WA, et al. Antibody-mediated in vitro neutralization of human immunodeficiency virus type 1 abolishes infectivity for chimpanzees. J Virol 64:3674–3678, 1990.
570. Prince AM, Reesink H, Pascual D, et al. Prevention of HIV infection by passive immunization with HIV immunoglobulin. AIDS Res Hum Retroviruses 7:971–973, 1991.
571. Conley AJ, Kessler JA II, Boots LJ, et al. The consequence of passive administration of an anti–human immunodeficiency virus type 1 neutralizing monoclonal antibody before challenge of chimpanzees with a primary virus isolate. J Virol 70:6751–6758, 1996.
572. Berman PW, Murthy KK, Wrin T, et al. Protection of MN-2gp120–immunized chimpanzees from heterologous infection with a primary isolate of human immunodeficiency virus type 1. J Infect Dis 173:52–59, 1996.
573. Girard M, Meignier B, Barré-Sinoussi F, et al. Vaccine-induced protection of chimpanzees against infection by a heterologous human immunodeficiency virus type 1. J Virol 69:6239–6248, 1995.
574. Girard M, van der Ryst E, Barré-Sinoussi F, et al. Challenge of chimpanzees immunized with a recombinant canarypox–HIV-1 virus. Virology 239:98–104, 1997.
575. Girard M, Barré-Sinoussi F, Tartaglia J, et al. Protection from intravenous and genital HIV-1 challenge in chimpanzees by immunization with an HIV-1 canarypox recombinant [abstract 165]. Annual Meeting of the Institute of Human Virology; Baltimore, MD; September 7–12, 1996.
576. Miller CJ, Marthas M, Thorten J, et al. Intravaginal inoculation of rhesus macaques with cell-free simian immunodeficiency virus results in persistent or transient viremia. J Virol 68:6391–6400, 1994.
577. Shearer GM, Clerici M. Protective immunity against HIV infection: Has nature done the experiment for us? Immunol Today 17:21–24, 1996.
577a. Mooij P, van der Kolk M, Bogers WMJM, et al. A clinically relevant HIV-1 subunit vaccine protects rhesus macaques from *in vivo* passaged simian-human immunodeficiency virus infection. AIDS 12:F15–F22, 1998.
577b. Stott EJ, Almond N, Kent K, et al. Evaluation of candidate human immunodeficiency virus type 1 (HIV-1) vaccine in macaques: Effect of vaccination with HIV-1 gp120 on subsequent challenge with heterologous simian immunodeficiency virus–HIV-1 chimeric virus. J Gen Virol 79:423–432, 1998.
577c. Davis D, Morlein B, Åkerblom L, et al. A recombinant prime, peptide boost vaccination strategy can focus the immune response onto more than one epitope even though these may not be immunodominant in the complex immunogen. Vaccine 15:1661–1669, 1997.
578. Keefer MC, Wolff M, Gorse GJ, et al. Safety profile of phase I and II preventive HIV type 1 envelope vaccination: Experience of the NIAID AIDS vaccine evaluation group. AIDS Res Hum Retroviruses 13:1163–1177, 1997.
579. Walker MC, Fast PE. Clinical trials of candidate AIDS vaccines. AIDS 8(suppl 1):S213–S236, 1994.
580. Graham BS, Wright PF. Candidate AIDS vaccines. N Engl J Med 333:1331–1339, 1995.
581. Dolin R. Human studies in the development of human immunodeficiency virus vaccine. J Infect Dis 172:1175–1183, 1995.
582. Gorse GJ, Keefer MC, Belshe RB, et al. A dose-ranging study of a prototype synthetic HIV-1MN V3 branched peptide vaccine. J Infect Dis 173:330–339, 1996.
583. Graham BS, McElrath MJ, Connor RI, et al. Analysis of intercurrent HIV-1 infections in phase I and II trials of candidate AIDS vaccines. J Infect Dis 177:310–319, 1998.
584. Excler JL, Plotkin S. The prime-boost concept applied to HIV preventive vaccines. AIDS 11(suppl A):S127–S137, 1997.
585. McElrath MJ, Corey L, Greenberg PD, et al. Human immunodeficiency virus type 1–infection despite prior immunization with a recombinant envelope vaccine regimen. Proc Natl Acad Sci U S A 93:3972–3977, 1996.
586. Zagury D, Léonard R, Fouchard M, et al. Immunization against AIDS in humans. Nature 326:249–250, 1987.
587. Picard O, Achour A, Bernard J, et al. A 2-year follow-up of an anti-HIV immune reaction in HIV-1 gp160-immunized healthy seronegative humans: Evidence for persistent cell-mediated immunity. J Acquir Immune Defic Syndr 5:539–546, 1992.
588. Graham BS, Matthews TJ, Belshe RB, et al. Augmentation of human immunodeficiency virus type 1 neutralizing antibody by priming with gp160 recombinant vaccinia and boosting with rgp160 in vaccinia-naive adults. J Infect Dis 167:533–537, 1993.
589. Cooney EL, McElrath MJ, Corey L, et al. Enhanced immunity to human immunodeficiency virus (HIV) envelope elicited by a combined vaccine regimen consisting of priming with a vaccinia recombinant expressing HIV envelope and boosting with gp160 protein. Proc Natl Acad Sci U S A 90:1882–1886, 1993.
590. Hammond SA, Bollinger RC, Stanhope PE, et al. Comparative clonal analysis of human immunodeficiency virus type 1 (HIV-1)–specific CD4+ and CD8+ cytolytic T lymphocytes isolated from seronegative humans immunized with candidate HIV-1 vaccines. J Exp Med 176:1531–1542, 1992.
591. Bollinger RC, Quinn TC, Liu AY, et al. Cytokines from vaccine-induced HIV-1 specific cytotoxic T lymphocytes: Effects on viral replication. AIDS Res Hum Retroviruses 9:1067–1077, 1993.
592. Graham BS, Gorse GJ, Schwartz DH, et al. Determinants of antibody response after recombinant gp160 boosting in vaccinia-naive volunteers primed with gp160-recombinant vaccinia virus. J Infect Dis 170:782–786, 1994.
593. Goldstein JA, Neff JM, Lane JM, Koplan JP. Smallpox vaccina-

tion reactions, prophylaxis and therapy of complications. Pediatrics 55:342–347, 1975.
594. Redfield RR, Wright DC, James WD, et al. Disseminated vaccinia in a military recruit with human immunodeficiency virus (HIV) disease. N Engl J Med 316:673–676, 1987.
595. Plotkin SA, Cadoz M, Meignier B, et al. The safety and use of canarypox vectored vaccines. Dev Biol Stand 84:165–170, 1995.
596. Tubiana R, Gomard E, Fleury H, et al. Vaccine therapy in early HIV-1 infection using a recombinant canarypox virus expressing gp160 MN (ALVAC-HIV): A double-blind controlled randomized study of safety and immunogenicity. AIDS 11:819–841, 1997.
597. Pialoux G, Excler JL, Rivière Y, et al. A prime-boost approach to HIV preventive vaccine using a recombinant canarypox virus expressing glycoprotein 160 (MN) followed by a recombinant glycoprotein 160 (MN/LAI). AIDS Res Hum Retroviruses 11:373–381, 1995.
598. Fleury B, Janvier G, Pialoux G, et al. Memory cytotoxic T lymphocyte responses in human immunodeficiency virus type 1 (HIV-1)–negative volunteers immunized with a recombinant canarypox expressing gp160 of HIV-1 and boosted with a recombinant gp160. J Infect Dis 174:734–738, 1996.
599. Salmon-Céron D, Excler JL, Sicard D, et al. Safety and immunogenicity of a recombinant HIV type 1 glycoprotein 160 boosted by a V3 synthetic peptide in HIV-negative volunteers. AIDS Res Hum Retroviruses 11:1479–1486, 1995.
600. Egan MA, Pavlat WA, Tartaglia J, et al. Induction of human immunodeficiency virus type 1 (HIV-1)–specific cytolytic T lymphocyte responses in seronegative adults by a nonreplicating, host-range restricted canarypox vector (ALVAC) carrying the HIV-1MN *env* gene. J Infect Dis 171:1623–1627, 1995.
601. Clements ML, Corey L, Weinhold K, et al. HIV immunity induced by priming with canarypox or vaccinia–gp 160 recombinants and boosting with rgp120 [abstract 166]. Annual Meeting of the Institute of Human Virology; Baltimore, MD; September 7–12, 1996.
602. Lamhamedi-Cherradi S, Culmann-Penciolelli B, Guy B, et al. Qualitative and quantitative analysis of human cytotoxic T-lymphocyte responses to HIV-1 proteins. AIDS 6:1249–1258, 1992.
603. Excler JL, Salmon D, Sicard D, et al. Safety and immunogenicity of a live recombinant canarypox virus vaccine expressing gp120/gag/protease boosted by a p24E-V3 peptide [abstract 295]. AIDS Res Hum Retroviruses 11(suppl 1):S138, 1995.
604. Bourgault I, Chirat F, Tartar A, et al. Simian immunodeficiency virus as a model for vaccination against HIV. Induction in rhesus macaques of gag- or nef-specific cytotoxic T lymphocytes by lipopeptides. J Immunol 152:2530–2537, 1994.
605. Johnson RP. Macaque models for AIDS vaccine development. Curr Opin Immunol 8:554–560, 1996.
606. Haynes BF. HIV vaccines: Where we are and where we are going. Lancet 438:933–937, 1996.
607. Murphey-Corb M, Martin LN, Davison-Fairburn B, et al. A formalin-inactivated whole SIV vaccine confers protection in macaques. Science 246:1293–1297, 1989.
608. Miller C, Gardner MB. AIDS and mucosal immunity: Usefulness of the SIV macaque model of genital mucosal transmission. J Acquir Immune Defic Syndr 4:1169–1172, 1991.
609. Lehner T, Bergmeier LA, Panagiotidi C, et al. Induction of mucosal and systemic immunity to a recombinant simian immunodeficiency viral protein. Science 258:1365–1369, 1992.
610. Belec L, Georges AJ, Steenman G, Martin PM. Antibodies to human immunodeficiency virus in vaginal secretions of heterosexual women. J Infect Dis 160:385–391, 1989.
611. Mestecky J. The common mucosal immune system and current strategies for induction of immune responses in external secretions. J Clin Immunol 7:265–276, 1987.
612. McDermott MR, Bienenstock J. Evidence for a common immune system. I. Migration of B immunoblasts into intestinal, respiratory and genital tissues. J Immunol 122:1872–1898, 1979.
613. McDermott MR, Clark DA, Bienenstock J. Evidence for a common mucosal immunologic system. II. Influence of the estrous cycle on B immunoblast migration into genital and intestinal tissues. J Immunol 124:2536–2569, 1980.
614. Eron JJ, Ashby MA, Giordano MF, et al. Randomised trial of MN gp120 HIV-1 vaccine in symptomless HIV-1 infection. Lancet 348:1547–1551, 1996.
615. Levine AM, Groshen S, Allen J, et al. Initial studies on active immunization of HIV-infected subjects using a gp120-depleted HIV-1 immunogen: Long-term follow-up. J Acquir Immune Defic Syndr Hum Retrovirol 11:351–364, 1996.
616. Pantaleo G. How immune-based interventions can change HIV therapy. Nat Med 3:484–486, 1997.
617. Conors M, Kovacs JA, Krevat S, et al. HIV infection induces changes in $CD4^+$ T cell phenotype and depletion within the $CD4^+$ T-cell repertoire that are not immediately restored by antiviral or immune-based therapies. Nat Med 3:533–540, 1997.
618. Lambert JS, Mofenson LM, Fletcher CV, et al. Safety and pharmacokinetics of hyperimmune anti–human immunodeficiency virus (HIV) immunoglobulin administered to HIV-infected pregnant women and their newborns. J Infect Dis 175:283–293, 1997.
619. Ugen KE, Goedert JJ, Boyer J, et al. Vertical transmission of HIV infection: Correlation with reactivity of maternal sera with glycoprotein 120 and gp41 peptides from HIV type 1. J Clin Invest 89:1923–1930, 1992.
620. Khouri YF, McIntosh K, Cavacini L, et al. Vertical transmission of HIV-1. Correlation with maternal viral load and plasma levels of CD4 binding site anti-gp120 antibodies. J Clin Invest 95:732–737, 1995.
621. Rossi P, Moshese V, Broliden PA, et al. Presence of maternal antibodies to human immunodeficiency virus type 1 envelope glycoprotein gp120 epitopes correlates with the noninfective status of children born to seropositive mothers. Proc Natl Acad Sci U S A 86:8055–8058, 1989.
622. Scarlatti G, Albert J, Rossi P, et al. Mother-to-child transmission of human immunodeficiency virus type 1: Correlation with neutralizing antibodies against primary isolates. J Infect Dis 168:207–210, 1993.
623. Van Rompay KKA, Otsyula MG, Tarara RP, et al. Vaccination of pregnant macaques protects newborns against mucosal simian immunodeficiency virus infection. J Infect Dis 173:1327–1335, 1996.
624. Mascola JR, Louder MK, van Cott TC, et al. Potent and synergistic neutralization of human immunodeficiency virus (HIV) type 1 primary isolates by hyperimmune anti-HIV immunoglobulin combined with monoclonal antibodies 2F5 and 2G12. J Virol 71:7198–7206, 1997.
625. Zhou P, Goldstein S, Devadas K, et al. Human $CD4^+$ cells transfected with IL-16 cDNA are resistant to HIV-1 infection: Inhibition of mRNA expression. Nat Med 3:659–664, 1997.
626. Parren PWHI, Sattentau QJ, Burton DR. HIV-1 antibody—debris or virion? Nat Med 3:366–367, 1997.
627. Bevan MJ, Braciale TJ. Why can't cytotoxic T-cells handle HIV? Proc Natl Acad Sci U S A 92:5765–5767, 1995.
628. Howcroft TK, Strebel K, Martin MA, Singer DS. Repression of MHC class I gene promoter activity by two-exon Tat of HIV. Science 260:1320–1322, 1993.
628a. Wilson SE, Pedersen SL, Kuruch JC, et al. Cross-clade envelope glycoprotein 160-specific $CD8^+$ cytotoxic T lymphocyte responses in early HIV type 1 clade B infection. AIDS Res Hum Retroviruses 14:925–937, 1998.
629. Moore J, Trkola A. HIV type 1 co-receptors, neutralization serotypes, and vaccine development. AIDS Res Hum Retroviruses 13:733–736, 1997.
630. Burton DR. A vaccine for HIV type 1: The antibody perspective. Proc Natl Acad Sci U S A 94:10018–10023, 1997.
631. Mann JM. AIDS—the second decade: A global perspective. J Infect Dis 165:245–250, 1992.

chapter

39 Lyme Disease Vaccine

Janine Evans

Erol Fikrig

HISTORY

Lyme disease was first recognized as a distinct entity in 1975, when two concerned mothers contacted the Connecticut State Health Department about an unusual geographical clustering of inflammatory arthritis that had developed in a number of community children. The cases occurred in the sparsely populated, rural areas surrounding Lyme, Connecticut. Some of the children had been diagnosed with juvenile rheumatoid arthritis, an uncommon chronic disease that is not known to occur in epidemic fashion. The incidence of recently diagnosed juvenile rheumatoid arthritis was markedly higher than the expected attack rate for such a community. The observation prompted researchers to conduct a retrospective, community-based survey to determine whether the clinical and epidemiological features of this new illness could be characterized.[1]

The initial retrospective study conducted between December 1975 and April 1976 revealed 39 children and 12 adults from the contiguous Connecticut communities of Old Lyme, Lyme, and East Haddam who had arthritis typified by brief, recurrent episodes of swelling of one to a few large joints, most often the knee. The new syndrome was named Lyme arthritis because the first case had occurred in 1972 in Lyme.[2]

Epidemiological analysis revealed that most cases began in the summer months, and a significant number of affected individuals described an expanding annular skin lesion that appeared before the onset of arthritis, suggesting that the disease was transmitted by an arthropod. The skin lesion was similar in appearance to an entity erythema chronica migrans, an expanding skin lesion described earlier in the century by Afzelius in Sweden and by Lipschutz in Austria. Erythema chronica migrans was associated with bites from *Ixodes ricinus* ticks. Further studies uncovered that Lyme arthritis was part of the spectrum of a multisystem illness that affected primarily the skin, nervous system, heart, and joints. Hence, the name was changed to Lyme disease.[2]

In 1982, Burgdorfer and colleagues identified and isolated a previously unrecognized spirochete, now called *Borrelia burgdorferi*, from *Ixodes scapularis* ticks obtained from Shelter Island, New York.[3] Shortly thereafter, the same organism was isolated from blood, skin,and cerebrospinal fluid specimens from patients in the United States and Europe with Lyme disease.[4–7] Patients' immune responses were linked conclusively with the organism, and later a full antibody response was characterized by enzyme-linked immunosorbent assay (ELISA) and then Western blot analysis.[8]

Over the next 20 years, many of the gaps in knowledge about Lyme disease have been filled in, resulting in a more complete picture of the illness. Advances in research have uncovered the mechanisms underlying the specific interaction between the causative organism and the human host. Despite an improved understanding of the illness, many nagging questions remain regarding disease persistence and clinical variability. Clinicians often face difficult management decisions because of continued uncertainty about the disease, especially in its diagnosis and treatment.[9]

BACKGROUND

Clinical Description (Fig. 39–1, Table 39–1)

Lyme disease is a multisystem illness that primarily affects the skin, heart, joints, and nervous system. Clinical features vary during the course of infection and are frequently divided into general stages termed early localized, early disseminated, and late disease.[10] Early localized disease is manifested by the presence of a skin lesion, erythema migrans (EM). EM appears as an expanding erythematous papule or macule, often with a well-demarcated outer border and central clearing. The primary lesion occurs at the site of a deer tick bite. Typically, the lesion is flat, warm, and not painful. Sometimes, it becomes indurated, warm, and pruritic. With time, the lesion expands centrifugally and may become quite large (>5 cm). EM lesions occur approximately 1 to 36 days (median, 7 to 10 days) after a deer tick bite. Only 14 to 32% of patients with EM recall experiencing a tick bite. In untreated patients, the rash disappears without scarring several days to weeks after onset; in treated patients, resolution typically occurs faster. Up to 80% of patients with EM have associated systemic

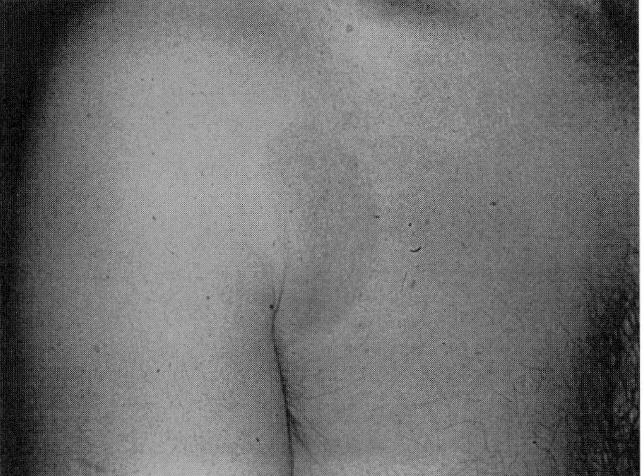

Figure 39–1. Erythema migrans (EM). EM, the pathognomonic skin lesion of Lyme disease, appears as an expanding erythematous lesion, often with central clearing, around the site of an *Ixodes* tick bite. EM is reported in 60 to 80% of patients. Common sites are the thigh, groin, trunk, and axilla. (Reproduced with permission from Steere AC, Bartenhagen NH, Craft JE, et al. The early clinical manifestations of Lyme disease. Ann Intern Med 99:76–82, 1983.)

complaints, including fatigue, myalgias, arthralgias, headache, fever and/or chills, and stiff neck. In early localized disease, these symptoms tend to be mild.[11]

In Europe, patients occasionally have a solitary cutaneous lesion with follicles resembling those seen in lymph nodes; this condition is termed *Borrelia* lymphocytoma. It has been reported to occur in less than 10% of individuals in most series.[2, 12] Lymphocytomas appear most often as a red or violaceous solitary lesion on the ear or nipple, but more widespread lesions sometimes occur. Patients usually have associated regional lymphadenopathy, but generalized symptoms are typically absent. Lesions promptly resolve with antibiotic therapy, although if untreated, they may last months and even years.[2]

Within days or weeks after inoculation, some patients

Table 39–1. **LYME DISEASE NATIONAL SURVEILLANCE CASE DEFINITION***

Disease definition

Lyme disease is a systemic, tick-borne disease with protean manifestations, including dermatologic, rheumatologic, neurologic, and cardiac abnormalities; the best clinical marker for the disease is the initial skin lesion, erythema migrans, which occurs in 60% to 80% of patients

Case definition

A person with erythema migrans *or*

A person with at least one late manifestation and laboratory confirmation of infection

General definitions

Erythema migrans: For purposes of surveillance, erythema migrans is a skin lesion that typically begins as a red macule or papula and expands over a period of days or weeks to form a large round lesion, often with partial central clearing; a solitary lesion must reach at least 5 cm in size; secondary lesions may also occur; annular erythematous lesions occurring within several hours of a tick bite represent hypersensitivity reactions and do not qualify as erythema migrans; in most patients, the expanding erythema migrans lesion is accompanied by other acute symptoms, particularly fatigue, fever, headache, mild stiff neck, arthralgias, or myalgias; these symptoms are typically intermittent; the diagnosis of erythema migrans must be made by a physician; laboratory confirmation is recommended for persons with no known exposure

Late manifestations (include any of the following when an alternate explanation is not found)

Musculoskeletal system: Recurrent, brief attacks (weeks or months) of objective joint swelling in one or a few joints; manifestations not considered as criteria for diagnosis include chronic progressive arthritis not preceded by brief attacks and chronic symmetric polyarythritis; additionally, arthralgias, myalgias, or fibromyalgia syndromes alone are not accepted as criteria for musculoskeletal involvement

Nervous system: Lymphocytic meningitis, cranial neuritis, particularly facial palsy (may be bilateral); radiculoneuropathy, or, rarely, encephalomyelitis alone or in combination; encephalomyelitis must be confirmed by showing antibody production against *Borrelia burgdorferi* in the cerebrospinal fluid, demonstrated by a higher titer of antibody in cerebrospinal fluid than in serum; headache, fatigue, paresthesias, or mild stiff neck alone are not accepted as criteria for neurologic involvement

Cardiovascular system: Acute-onset, high-grade (second or third degree) atrioventricular conduction defects that resolve in days to weeks and are sometimes associated with myocarditis; palpitations, bradycardia, bundle-branch block, or myocarditis alone are not accepted as criteria for cardiovascular involvement

Exposure: Exposure is defined as having been in wooded, brushy, or grassy areas (potential tick habitats) in an endemic county no more than 30 days prior to the onset of erythema migrans; a history of tick bite is not required

Endemic county: An endemic county is one in which at least two definite cases have been previously reported or one in which a tick vector has been shown to be infected with *Borrelia burgdorferi*

Laboratory confirmation: Laboratory confirmation of infection with *Borrelia burgdorferi* is established when a laboratory isolates the spirochete from tissue or body fluid, detects diagnostic levels of IgM or IgG antibodies to the spirochete in serum or cerebrospinal fluid, or detects a significant change in antibody levels in paired acute and convalescent serum samples; states may determine the criteria for laboratory confirmation and diagnostic levels of antibody; syphilis and other known causes of biologic false-positive serologic test results should be excluded as appropriate when laboratory confirmation has been based on serologic testing alone

From Centers for Disease Control. Case definitions for public health surveillance. MMWR Morb Mortal Wkly Rep 39(RR-13):19–21, 1990.

*It should be emphasized that this is an epidemiologic case definition intended for surveillance purposes only.

with Lyme disease experience lymphatic or hematogenous dissemination of the organism to multiple organs, such as the skin (multiple secondary skin lesions), the liver and spleen (mild hepatitis), the peripheral nervous system and brain (cranial and peripheral neuropathies, meningitis, encephalitis), the heart (heart block and myocarditis), and the joints (arthritis).[10] Constitutional systems, such as high fever, severe headache, stiff neck, significant arthralgias, and fatigue, are common and can be striking in such patients. Most individuals with early disseminated disease spontaneously recover over a period of several weeks to months, even if they are untreated.

After hematogenous spread, the host immune system is able to clear *B. burgdorferi* from most sites of infection. Incomplete eradication of the organism from certain immunologically privileged tissues, such as the central nervous system, eye, and joints, may result in late infection. In the United States, approximately 60% of untreated patients with Lyme disease acquire arthritis a mean 6 months after the onset of the disease.[13] Lyme arthritis is characterized by intermittent attacks of inflammatory arthritis in one or a few joints, typically in the knee. With time, episodes of arthritis often become longer, lasting months rather than weeks. After years of infection, most cases of Lyme arthritis tend to resolve. About 10% of patients have a chronic form of arthritis, defined as a year or more of continual joint inflammation. Chronic Lyme arthritis may lead to the erosion of cartilage and bone, causing permanent disability.

Late Lyme disease may involve both the central and the peripheral nervous systems. The spectrum of nervous system involvement includes progressive encephalomyelitis with spastic paraparesis, bladder dysfunction, ataxia, seventh- or eighth-cranial nerve deficits, and cognitive impairment, such as dementia. Additional syndromes, such as subacute encephalitis, demyelination, and distal paresthesia and radicular pain, have been reported.[14–16]

A late skin disorder, acrodermatitis chronica atrophicans, may occur after prolonged latency. Acrodermatitis chronica atrophicans begins insidiously with bluish-red discoloration and swollen skin on an extremity. The lesion's inflammatory phase may persist for many years or decades and gradually leads to atrophy of the skin. It has been observed primarily in European patients.[10]

Bacteriology (Fig. 39–2)

Borrelia species, along with the leptospira and the treponema, belong to the eubacterial phylum of spirochetes. As a group, *Borrelia* species are fastidious, microaerophilic bacteria that grow best at 33°C in a complex, liquid medium called Barbour-Stoenner-Kelly medium. *B. burgdorferi* can be cultured fairly easily from tick and skin biopsy specimens. In humans, it is rarely cultured from other sites of infection. *B. burgdorferi* grows slowly, elongating for 12 to 24 hours before dividing. After 10 to 15 passages in culture, it loses its pathogenicity and is no longer infectious.[10, 17]

Structurally, borrelia have a protoplasmic cylinder that

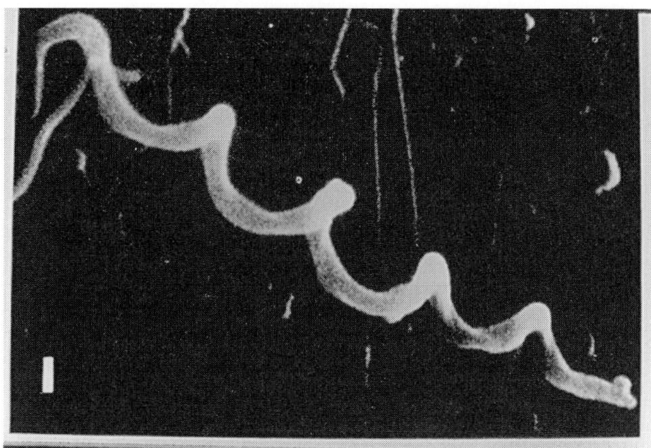

Figure 39–2. Scanning electron micrograph of the spirochete, *Borrelia burgdorferi*, the causative agent of Lyme disease. Note the left-handed coiling of the spirochete. Several strains of *B. burgdorferi* have been isolated throughout the world. (From Johnson RC, Hyde RW, Rumpel CM. Taxonomy of the Lyme disease spirochetes. Yale J Biol Med 57:529–537, 1984.)

is surrounded first by a cell membrane, then by flagella, and finally by an outer membrane. *B. burgdorferi* contains DNA that encodes for at least 30 different proteins, the functions of most of which are unknown. Many components of the outer membrane are encoded by genes theoretically located on extrachromosomal plasmids, allowing the organism to make antigenic changes more readily. Plasmids are also thought to code for proteins that are important in pathogenicity because the loss of infectivity of isolates after passage has been correlated with the loss of particular plasmids in culture.

Some of the genes of *B. burgdorferi* have been isolated and cloned. The protein products of some of the cloned genes have been characterized and include at least seven outer surface proteins termed OspA (31 kDa), OspB (34 kDa), Osp C (22 kDa), OspD (28 kDa), OspE (19 kDa), OspF (26 kDa), and a 66-kDa protein.[18–22] Many of the Osps are lipoproteins, and their expression by *B. burgdorferi* varies during the course of infection. A 41-kDa antigen is located on the flagellum and is similar to flagellar antigens of other spirochetes. Two heat-shock proteins from the Hsp60 and Hsp70 families have been identified and are cross-reactive with an equivalent antigen in other bacteria.[17] Additional antigens include the 39-kDa, 55-kDa (P55), 83-kDa, and 110-kDa proteins.[23–26]

Genetic analysis of borrelia isolated from North America, Europe, and Asia has led to the identification of distinct genospecies, such as *B. burgdorferi sensu stricto*, *B. afzelii*, and *B. garinii*, *B. japonica*, *B. andersoni*, and others.[27] *B. burgdorferi sensu stricto* has been reported to be the most prevalent species in ticks from North America, whereas *B. afzelii*, *B. sensu stricto*, and *B. garinii* are all commonly found in Europe. In some parts of Europe, all three species have been found in the same region, and mixed infections have been reported.[28] A new species of *Borrelia* has been isolated from three patients and from a soft tick, *Ornithodorus* species ticks in southern Spain.[29] The organism caused a relapsing spirochetemia with multiple organ involvement and was associated with predominately atypical clinical features of Lyme disease, such as fever and neurological symptoms in the absence of EM. It is likely that additional *Borrelia* organisms will be identified in the future.

Pathogenesis (Fig. 39–3)

Spirochetes are present in low copy number in the midgut of unfed nymphal ticks. Some studies have shown that on attachment of ticks to a host, the bacteria multiply quickly, with a doubling time close to 4 hours, and reach a maximum number after 72 hours of attachment, likely in response to the blood meal and changes in temperature.[30, 31] During an initial 15-hour period, the spirochetes appear restricted to the tick gut, but after 48 hours, they disseminate to the salivary glands, supporting previous data that indicated that the risk of infection before 36 hours of tick attachment is low.[32]

From its point of entry in the skin, *B. burgdorferi* spreads locally in 60 to 80% of patients and produces the characteristic early skin lesion EM. *B. burgdorferi* later disseminates through the blood and lymphatic system to invade distant organs after a period of spirochetemia. Although spread of an organism is the result of complex interactions between many bacterial and host factors, specific binding of host cells or extracellular matrix by the organism plays an important role. Movement of spirochetes through the skin or through the basement membranes of endothelium is likely to require the elaboration of proteases. *B. burgdorferi* does not produce collagenase, elastase, hyaluronidase, or other enzymes that digest extracellular matrix components.[33] Plasmin, a trypsin-like serine proteinase, was found to be important for tissue invasion by spirochetes.[34]

Some studies have demonstrated that on a receptor, *B. burgdorferi* binds human plasminogen, which leads to an accelerated formation of active plasmin in the presence of host-derived plasminogen activator. *B. burgdorferi* incubated with urokinase-type plasminogen activator was more infectious than control spirochetes, and binding of plasmin on the surface of *B. burgdorferi* resulted in greater invasion of endothelial cell monolayers grown on connective tissue substrates.[33–35] The cell surface–associated plasmin was able to degrade high molecular weight glycoproteins such as fibronectin, indicating that binding of plasmin onto its surface where exogenous urokinase-type plasminogen activator can generate plasmin is one mechanism by which *B. burgdorferi* disseminates. Glycosaminoglycan binding may also contribute to the attachment of the Lyme disease spirochete to host cells and matrix.[36]

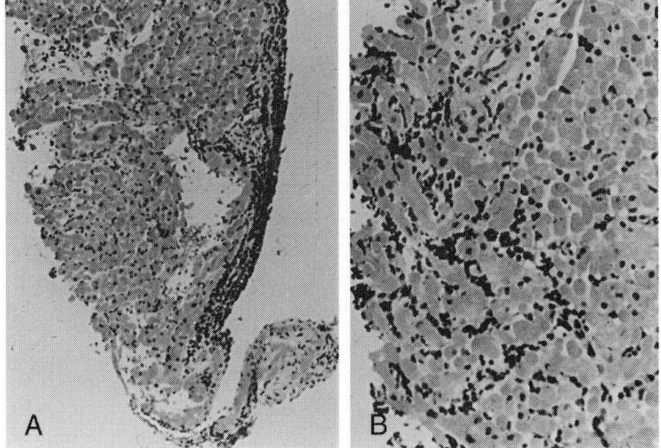

Figure 39–3. *A* and *B*, Endomyocardial biopsy specimen demonstrating Lyme myocarditis. A characteristic bandlike endocardial infiltration and diffuse interstitial infiltrates of lymphocytes, plasma cells, and some macrophages in the myocardium is seen. Spirochetes compatible with *Borrelia burgdorferi* have been demonstrated near lymphoid cells and in the endocardium (hematoxylin and eosin stain). (From Duray P, Steere AC. Clinical pathologic correlations of Lyme disease by stage. Ann NY Acad Sci 539:65–79, 1988.)

The presence of *B. burgdorferi* elicits strong host immune responses, with the subsequent release of inflammatory mediators. *B. burgdorferi* induces a host inflammatory response at least in part through activation of vascular endothelium.[37] Endothelial cell adhesion molecules mediate the attachment of circulating leukocytes to the blood vessel wall and direct inflammatory leukocytes to the site of spirochetal infection.

Histopathological studies have indicated that T and B lymphocytes and mixed, predominantly mononuclear cellular infiltrates with monocytes/macrophages are present in infected tissues.[38] It is likely that a combined effect of local spirochetal infection with an intense immunological reaction to the organisms is responsible for disease expression.

Diagnosis (Fig. 39–4)

The diagnosis of Lyme disease relies on the presence of characteristic clinical features and supporting serological test results. Although spirochetes have been isolated from a variety of patient specimens, culture or direct visualization of *B. burgdorferi* is difficult and frequently yields negative results. In response to the need of a uniform definition, the Centers for Disease Control and Prevention, in association with state health departments, developed a national surveillance case definition for Lyme disease. The criteria were intended to be used for epidemiological surveillance and for comparing the results of treatment in different trials.[9] Because the criteria are biased toward certainty in the diagnosis of Lyme disease, strict application in clinical practice may result in underdiagnosis and unnecessary delay in treatment. Serological confirmation is the most practical and widely used laboratory aid available. Serological testing should serve as an adjunct in diagnosis and should be applied only if clinical manifestations strongly suggest that Lyme disease is present.

Immunoglobulin M (IgM) antibodies usually develop within 2 to 4 weeks after the onset of infection, peak after 6 to 8 weeks of illness, and decline to the normal range after 4 to 6 months of illness in most patients. Antibodies of the immunoglobulin G (IgG) class are usually measured within 6 to 8 weeks after the onset of disease and peak after 4 to 6 months. In some patients, IgG levels remain elevated indefinitely.[39]

An immunological response can be detected within weeks of the onset of the disease by use of either an

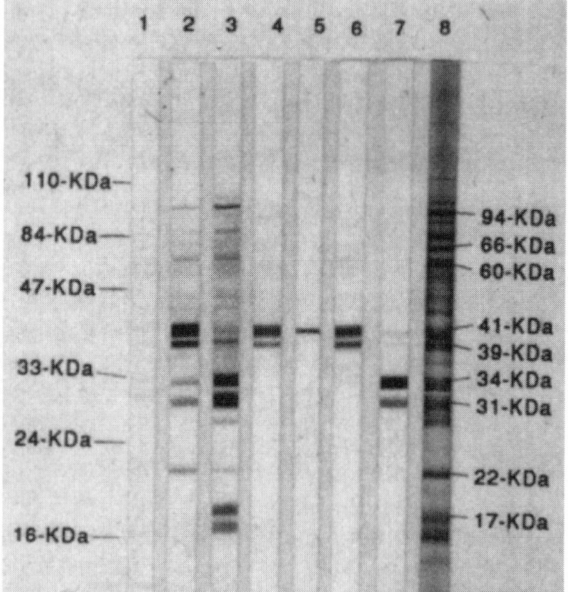

Figure 39–4. Immunoblots of *B. burgdorferi* strain B31 using several monoclonal antibodies, animal antisera, and human patient sera. Lane 1, amidoblack staining of *B. burgdorferi* sonicate; lanes 2–8, immunoblots using goat anti–*B. burgdorferi* sera (lane 2), rabbit anti–*B. burgdorferi* sera (lane 3), monoclonal antiflagellin antibodies (lane 4), anti–41-kD monoclonal antibody (lane 5), monoclonal antiflagellin antibody (lane 6), anti-OspA and -OspB antibodies (lane 7), and pooled human sera from patients with Lyme disease (lane 8). (From Ma B, Christen B, Leung D, Vigo-Pelfrey C. Serodiagnosis of Lyme borreliosis by Western immunoblot: Reactivity of various significant antibodies against *Borrelia burgdorferi*. J Clin Microbiol 30:370–376, 1992.)

indirect immunofluorescence assay or an ELISA.[40] ELISA tests are preferred because their sensitivity and reproducibility are better. Most ELISA assays use extracts of sonicated whole *B. burgdorferi* as antigen,[41] although purified *B. burgdorferi* proteins have also been used. Commercial tests vary in sensitivity and specificity; hence, identical serum samples sent simultaneously to different laboratories may yield different results. In even the best of circumstances, false-positive and false-negative results occur.

Immunoblotting has been advocated as a method of distinguishing true-positive from false-positive ELISA results. Antibodies directed against specific *Borrelia* proteins are identified. Because many proteins on *B. burgdorferi* are shared with other organisms, false-positive results may also occur with immunoblots. During the Second National Conference on Serologic Diagnosis of Lyme disease, a two-test approach for active disease and for previous infection that used serum enzyme immunoassay or immunofluorescent assay followed by a Western immunoblot was proposed.[41] It was recommended that an IgM immunoblot be considered positive if two of the following three bands are present: 24 kDa (OspC), 39 kDa (BmpA), and 41 kDa (Fla). IgG immunoblots were considered positive if five of the following 10 bands are present: 24 kDa (OspC), 28 kDa, 35 kDa, 39 kDa (BmpA), 41 kDa, 45 kDa, 58 kDa (not GroEL), 66 kDa, and 93 kDa.[42,43] The specificity of positive Western blot results for IgM was 92 to 94%, and that for IgG, after the first weeks of infection, was 95%. Use of different strains of *B. burgdorferi* as the antigen source in assays and different acrylamide gel concentrations for protein separation may lead to difficulty in matching protein bands. Monoclonal antibodies that are specific for certain *B. burgdorferi* proteins are available and can be used to assist in the proper interpretation of immunoblots to avoid confusion.

Sensitive and specific polymerase chain reaction (PCR) assays have been developed. The application of a PCR method on skin biopsy specimens resulted in a 80% positive result rate from patients with EM and a 92% positive result rate from those with acrodermatitis chronica atrophicans.[44] PCR of synovial fluid specimens has proved valuable in the study of patients with Lyme arthritis.[45] PCR techniques have also been applied to blood, urine, and cerebrospinal fluid specimens but have yielded disappointing results.[46–48] The major problem in using the PCR technique is the issue of false positivity, and proper handling of specimens is required to avoid contamination.[49] Interpretation of PCR results is reliable only when the test is performed in laboratories where appropriate precautions are taken.

Treatment and Prevention (Table 39–2)

Most *B. burgdorferi* infections are successfully cleared with appropriate antibiotic therapy. In early studies, treatment with penicillin, tetracycline, or erythromycin resulted in a shortened duration of EM lesions and reduced the incidence of major late sequelae of infection.[50] Tetracycline was the most efficacious in preventing late disease. At about the same time, high-dose intravenous penicillin was shown to be effective in the treatment of stage 2 neurological abnormalities.[51]

Subsequent studies resulted in the formation of treatment recommendations.[9, 52] In general, oral antibiotic regimens using doxycycline or amoxicillin are adequate for patients presenting with early Lyme disease. Doxycycline and amoxicillin have largely supplanted tetracycline and penicillin because these agents have easier dosing schedules and better tissue penetration. Intravenous penicillin or ceftriaxone is recommended in individuals with serious cardiac or neurological disease. Lyme arthritis can be treated orally or parenterally. Current recommendations (see Table 39–2) are considered guidelines for therapy and should be tailored in the treatment of individual patients—sicker patients require careful monitoring and a longer duration of antibiotic therapy. It is likely that some of the therapeutic regimens will be subject to modifications as our understanding of the disease process expands.

Despite adequate antibiotic therapy, some patients have late manifestations of Lyme disease.[53] These individuals usually respond to additional treatment; however, permanent tissue damage and subsequent disability may occur.

Prevention methods for Lyme disease include vector control, wildlife management, and personal protection.[54] Effective strategies for reducing tick populations have only recently been studied. Application of insecticides containing carbaril, diazinon, chlorpyrifos, and cyflu-

Table 39–2. **TREATMENT RECOMMENDATIONS**

Early Lyme disease*
- Amoxicillin, 500 mg three times daily for 21 d†
- Doxycycline, 100 mg twice daily for 21 d
- Cefuroxime axetil, 500 mg twice daily for 21 d
- Azithromycin, 500 mg daily for 7 d‡ (less effective than other regimens)

Neurologic manifestations
- Bell's palsy (no other neurologic abnormalities)
  - Oral regimens for early disease suffice
- Meningitis (with or without radiculoneuropathy or encephalitis)§
  - Ceftriaxone, 2 g daily for 14–28 d
  - Penicillin G, 20 million units daily for 14–28 d
  - Doxycycline, 100 mg twice daily (oral or intravenous) for 14–28 d||
  - Chloramphenicol, 1 g 4 times daily for 14–28 d

Arthritis¶
- Amoxicillin and probenecid, 500 mg 4 times daily for 30 d**
- Doxycycline, 100 mg twice daily for 30 d
- Ceftriaxone, 2 g daily for 14–28 d
- Penicillin G, 20 million units daily for 14–28 d

Carditis
- Ceftriaxone, 2 g daily for 14 d
- Penicillin G, 20 million units daily for 14 d
- Doxycycline, 100 mg orally twice daily for 21 d††
- Amoxicillin, 500 mg 3 times daily for 21 d††

Pregnancy
- Localized early disease
  - Amoxicillin, 500 mg three times daily for 21 d
- Any manifestation of disseminated disease
  - Penicillin G, 20 million units daily for 14–28 d
- Asymptomatic seropositivity
  - No treatment necessary

*Without neurologic, cardiac, or joint involvement. For early Lyme disease limited to single erythema migrans lesion, 10 days is sufficient.

†Some experts advise addition of probenecid, 500 mg, 3 times daily.

‡Experience with this agent is limited; optimal duration of therapy is unclear.

§Optimal duration of therapy has not been established. There are no controlled trials of therapy longer than 4 weeks for any manifestation of Lyme disease.

||No published experience in the United States.

¶An oral regimen should be selected only if there is no neurologic involvement.

**Amoxicillin is generally administered 3 times daily, but the only trial of this agent for Lyme arthritis used a 4-times-daily regimen.

††Oral regimens have been reserved for mild carditis limited to first-degree heart block with PR ≤ .30 seconds and normal ventricular function.

From Rahn DW, Malavista SE. Treatment of Lyme Disease. St Louis, MO, Mosby-Year Book, 1994, pp 21–36.

thrin have proved helpful in reducing deer tick populations in suburban residential areas. The insecticides should be applied in the early spring and fall to ensure adequate protection with minimal insecticide use. Insecticide use for controlling ticks in forested areas has not been successful.

The exclusion of deer as a host has had an impact on local tick populations. Experiments with deer exclusion by fencing resulted in a substantial reduction of nymphal ticks.[55, 56] In order to have lasting effect, such fences needed to be permanent and either 8 feet high or electrified. Deer exclusion is financially prohibitive and is not practical for most individuals.

Personal protection has been recommended for individuals living in endemic areas. Personal protection includes wearing light-colored clothing to make ticks more visible, tucking pant cuffs into socks to keep ticks from gaining access to exposed skin, and using tick or insect repellents. Repellents containing DEET (*N,N*-diethyl-*m*-toluamide) can be applied to skin and clothing. Permethrin repellents are also effective but can be applied only to clothing.[54]

Daily inspections for attached ticks also reduce the risk for developing Lyme disease. Ticks removed before 48 hours of attachment are unlikely to transmit the disease, even in highly endemic areas.[32]

EPIDEMIOLOGY (Fig. 39–5)

Incidence and Prevalence

Lyme disease occurs worldwide; however, most cases are reported from temperate regions and coincide with the distribution of the principal vector, ticks of the *Ixodes ricinus* complex, including *I. ricinus*, which is found in most of Europe; *Ixodes persulcatus*, which is found in eastern Europe and Asia; *Ixodes pacificus*, found in the Pacific northwestern United States; and *Ixodes dammini*, found in the eastern and central United States.[17] It is disputed whether *I. dammini* is the same species as *Ixodes scapularis*, the black-legged tick.[57]

In the United States, Lyme disease is the most common tick-borne disease. This is likely to be true for Europe as well. The number of reported cases of Lyme disease in the United States has increased steadily since 1982, the year that the Centers for Disease Control and Prevention initiated surveillance. In 1994, 13,083 cases of Lyme disease were reported to the Centers for Disease Control and Prevention by 44 state health departments, a 58% increase of cases than were reported in 1993.[58] Most (88% of nationally reported cases) were geographically restricted to the northeast, the upper midwest, and northern California, areas of established enzootic cycles of *B. burgdorferi*. Sporadic cases in states without established enzootic transmission of *B. burgdorferi* may have occurred in limited, unrecognized foci or during visits to endemic areas outside the state of residence, or they may have been due to misclassification or misdiagnosis.

Both OspA vaccines were effective against Lyme disease. Volunteers who received two doses obtained protection of about 50 to 70%. After the third dose was given 1 year later, protection obtained in the subsequent Lyme disease season was 80 to 100%. Younger volunteers were better protected than volunteers older than 65 years. Antibody correlates of immunity are under study. Comprehensive evaluations of these two studies should be published soon.

Lyme disease has been reported from almost all countries in Europe. It is particularly prevalent in European countries located in the temperate zones, including Sweden, Germany, Austria, and the central portion of the former Soviet Union extending from the Baltic Sea to the Pacific Ocean.[59] Results from a carefully designed, prospective, population-based study of Lyme disease in southern Sweden reported an annual incidence of 69 cases per 100,000 inhabitants (range, 26 to 160 cases per 100,000).[60] Similar findings have been reported from Germany and Slovenia,[61, 62] and France is not exempt from Lyme disease.[63]

Foci of *B. burgdorferi* are highly localized and depen-

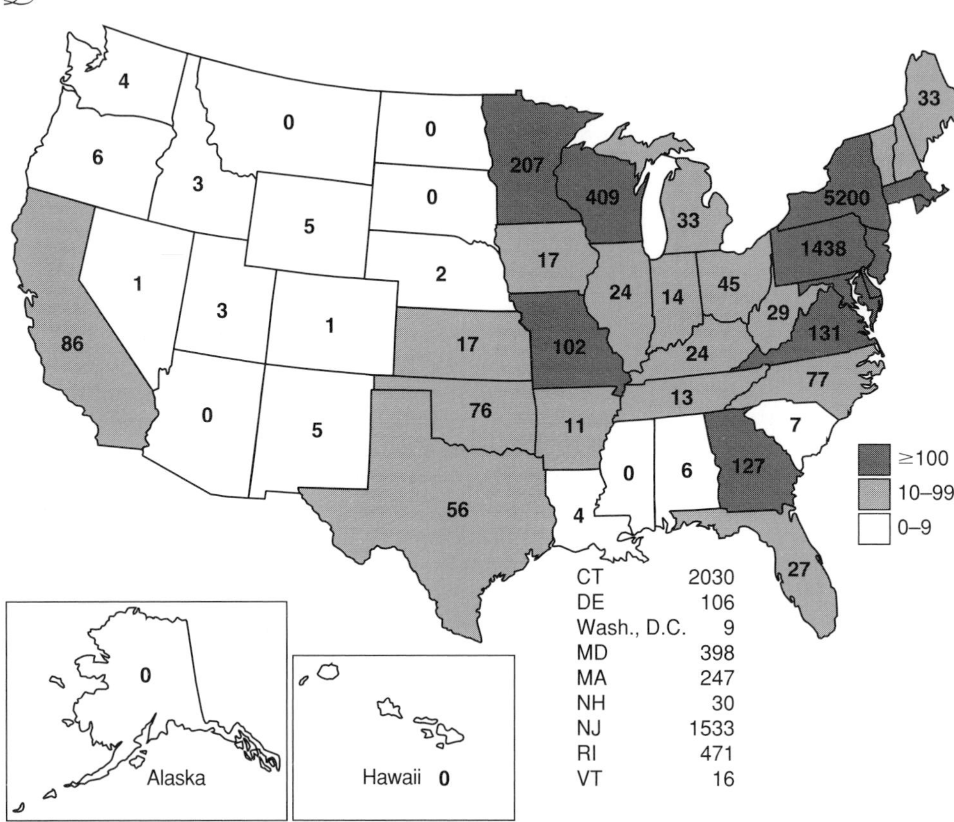

Figure 39–5. The number of reported cases of Lyme disease, by state, in the United States in 1995. Each case fulfilled the Centers for Disease Control surveillance criteria for the diagnosis of Lyme disease. (From Centers for Disease Control and Prevention. Lyme disease—United States, 1995. JAMA 276:274, 1996.

dent on environmental factors that are favorable to vector ticks, their maintenance hosts (especially deer), and animal reservoirs (especially rodents).[59, 64] Many mammalian and avian species are reservoir competent and are capable of infecting larval ticks with *B. burgdorferi*. All *Ixodes* ticks have four developmental stages: (1) egg, (2) larva, (3) nymph, and (4) adult. Each of the three motile stages feed only once before molting into the next stage. In the northeastern United States, where the epizootiology of Lyme disease has been most extensively studied, the white-footed mouse *Peromyscus leucopus* is the principal reservoir species, and the white-tailed deer is the preferred maintenance host of adult *I. scapularis* ticks. In this region, infection rates in nymphal ticks range from 10% to more than 50%. In the southern United States, immature *I. scapularis* feeds primarily on lizards, which are reservoir incompetent, resulting in infection rates of less than 1% in nymphal and adult ticks. In northern (*I. ricinus*) and eastern Europe (*I. persulcatus*), feeding cycles are similar to those in the northern United States, which accounts for the high infection rates in these tick species. The pattern of spread of Lyme disease and its vectors in the northeastern United States and Europe derives from the proliferation of deer, and the abundance of deer derives from the process of reforestation. Environmental and socioeconomic factors, such as the growth of suburban communities into farmland and wooded regions and the increasing exposure of humans to deer and deer ticks, contribute to the emergence of Lyme disease.

Lyme disease affects all age groups, although the greatest number of cases occur in children younger than 10 years and in middle-aged adults.[65] The incidence of early clinical manifestations peaks from June to August and tapers off in the early fall, coinciding with periods when nymphal ticks are feeding. Adult ticks, which are abundant during the early and late fall, are less likely to transmit the disease because they prefer deer as hosts and are more readily detected. Late manifestations of disease may occur at any time.

SIGNIFICANCE AS A PUBLIC HEALTH PROBLEM

It has been argued that the development of a vaccine for Lyme disease is of low priority because early disease is easily detected, effectively treated with a short course of oral antibiotics, and rarely, if ever, fatal. There is also concern that potential ill effects from the vaccine would outweigh the presumed minor benefit and would result in low public acceptance, not to mention a significant amount of litigation for harmful side effects. Despite these doubts, public and professional demand has driven efforts to develop a human vaccine. Proponents of a vaccine reason that Lyme disease is indeed a public health burden, the distribution of disease is expanding, late manifestations of Lyme disease are frequently disabling, and other prevention methods are inadequate or unacceptable.[66–68]

Lyme disease poses a significant public health threat in highly endemic areas. In some communities in coastal New England, as much as 16% of residents have been infected.[69] In one prospective assessment of school-aged children living in southeastern Connecticut, the incidences of clinical and asymptomatic *B. burgdorferi* infection were 10.1 and 3.8 cases/1000 person-years, respectively, indicating that Lyme disease is an important health problem in children living in Lyme endemic regions.[70]

Results of a cross-sectional survey of physicians in Maryland demonstrated that Lyme disease was underreported by 10- to 12-fold in that state and that there was significant discordance between the actual clinical treatment of patients and the recommended approach.[71] Much greater numbers of patients had been treated for presumptive Lyme disease, had been examined and given prophylaxis for tick bites, and had undergone diagnostic tests than were reported to the state department, indicating that real and perceived Lyme disease is a more extensive problem and uses more medical resources than official surveillance data suggest.

Economic considerations include the costs of diagnosing and treating the illness, days lost from work because of illness, diminished quality of life, and reduction of tourism and local real estate values in endemic regions as a result of fear of acquiring disease. It has been estimated that each case of Lyme disease may represent a cost of about $10,000 in the United States.[67]

The geographical distribution of disease continues to expand. In the northeastern United States, cases initially occurred along the northern side of the Connecticut River. Today, Lyme disease–endemic regions have extended to include much of the Atlantic seaboard.[72] Lyme disease appears to create a public health burden in other countries, especially in northern European and Asian temperate regions. In developing countries with a high transmission rate, early disease may go undetected and may result in chronic Lyme disease, a much more costly stage to treat.

A major concern prompting effective prevention methods pertains to long-term sequelae of the disease. Individuals treated for late manifestations of Lyme disease have a higher rate of persistent symptoms, permanent tissue injury, disability, and occasionally unresponsive disease.[73] The frequency of progression of disease in individuals who have asymptomatically seroconverted is uncertain.

IMMUNIZATION

Animal Models of Disease

The absence of an animal model that mimics human Lyme disease has hampered our understanding of the pathogenesis of Lyme disease and the development of effective strategies for prevention. Several laboratory animal species have been investigated as potential animal models of infection, including rabbits, hamsters, dogs, and mice.[74, 75] However, disease expression varies between animal species. Rabbits and guinea pigs develop cutaneous lesions of EM but do not display other signs of disease. Hamsters develop arthritis but only when they are inoculated in the footpad and irradiated. Infection in dogs produces fever, anorexia, fatigue, and, most commonly, limb and joint disorders. Monkeys infected with *B. burgdorferi* may develop EM and neurological disease.[75] Inoculation of *B. burgdorferi* into laboratory mice produces a disseminated infection, with acute inflammatory polyarthritis and carditis. The study of disease in mice is preferred because there is better characterization of immunological and genetic data in this species. Studies using different inbred strains of mice (C3H/He, SWR, C57BL, SJL, and Balb/c mice) have shown that disease severity is significantly influenced by mouse genotype and age.[76, 77] For example, immunocompetent C3H mice experienced severe joint and heart disease, whereas C57BL/6 mice displayed only mild disease. Severe combined immunodeficient mice have an overwhelming disseminated infection that is not seen in their immunocompetent counterparts.[78]

Passive Immunization

Antibody is essential for the killing of *B. burgdorferi*, suggesting that humoral immunity is an important host defense mechanism.[79, 80] The protective effect of antibody has been shown in animals. Passive immunization with *B. burgdorferi* antiserum protected hamsters from challenge with an intraperitoneal inoculation of spirochetes.[81] The role of specific *B. burgdorferi* antigens that elicit a protective response was not addressed in these studies. Passive immunization using polyclonal antiserum to *B. burgdorferi* in immunocompetent C3H and in immunodeficient severe combined immunodeficient mice was also protective against intradermal or intraperitoneal inoculation with *B. burgdorferi sensu stricto*.[82, 83]

After infection, borreliacidal activity was present at 7 days, peaked at weeks 3 to 5, and thereafter decreased.[84] *B. burgdorferi* activated the classical and alternate complement pathways but was resistant to the nonspecific bactericidal property of human serum.[84] Additional studies indicated that the complement-fixing IgG_2 immunoglobulin subclass played an important role in acquired resistance against infection and that depletion of complement abrogated the ability of immune serum to confer complete protection to irradiated hamsters challenged with *B. burgdorferi*.[85] Subsequent studies have shown that both complement-dependent and complement-independent antibody mechanisms are capable of conferring protection from infection.[86, 87]

Additional work investigated the roles of outer surface proteins A and B (OspA and OspB) in pathogenesis. As stated earlier, OspA (31-kDa protein) and OspB (34-kDa protein) are major surface components of the spirochete. The genes for OspA and OspB are on the same 49-kilobase linear plasmid, and both genes are transcribed from a common promoter.[88] Antibodies to OspA and OspB appear late in tick-transmitted murine infection and in human disease.[8] Patients with serum antibodies to OspA and OspB remain persistently infected. For these and other reasons, OspA and OspB were not considered to be candidates for a vaccine. However, Fikrig and colleagues have shown that passive immunization with monoclonal and polyclonal antibodies to recombinant and native forms of OspA or OspB confers protection in the C3H mouse model, indicating that antibodies to OspA or OspB are protective.[82, 89]

Active Immunization (Table 39–3)

Vaccine Development

In 1986, Johnson and associates performed the first immunization study.[80] Hamsters actively immunized with spirochetal lysates were effectively protected from infection from challenge using a homologous strain of *B. burgdorferi*. However, hosts challenged with a heterologous isolate were poorly protected.

Using the C3H/He mouse model, Fikrig and colleagues evaluated the capacity of recombinant *B. burgdorferi* proteins and fusion proteins to induce protection. Mice were immunized with *Escherichia coli* expressing OspA or with 20 μg of purified recombinant rOspA or rOspB glutathione transferase fusion proteins in complete Freund's adjuvant and were boosted twice at weekly intervals.[82, 90] Mice immunized with either recombinant protein, but not control subjects, developed strong IgG reactivity to these antigens 14 days after the last boost. Vaccinated mice challenged with an intradermal inoculum of either 10^2 or 10^4 low-passage virulent N40 strain spirochetes were fully protected from infection and disease, as determined by culture from internal tissues or by examination of histopathological specimens. OspA-immunized mice were protected against higher spirochete inoculums than in OspB-immunized mice. These studies have been confirmed by other laboratories.[91–93]

It was uncertain whether immunization with OspA would induce long-lasting protective immunity. *B. burgdorferi* can persist in its hosts for long periods of time: in human disease, spirochetes have been cultured from, or demonstrated in, tissue specimens years after initial infection,[7] and similar results have been observed in animal models. Studies addressing longevity of protection were performed in C3H mice. Mice sacrificed at later time points (up to 16 months) were shown to be free of infection. Furthermore, mice challenged with *B. burgdorferi* N40 up to 4 months after vaccination retained their immune status.[94]

The cross-protection afforded by vaccination with monovalent OspA and OspB proteins is unknown. Antigenic differences in OspA and in OspB have been documented between and within *B. burgdorferi* genospecies, including *B. burgdorferi sensu stricto*, *B. afzelii*, and *B. garinii*.[95–97] Moreover, spirochetes with mutations, frame shifts, or recombination between OspA and OspB have been isolated.[98, 99] These observations suggest that a single OspA or B antigen, cloned from a single isolate, may not be sufficient to provide broad cross-protective immunity.[100]

Studies attempting to define the degree of cross-protection conferred from single isolate proteins have indicated that *B. burgdorferi* with mutations in the Osp genes, in particular in regions that result in variability within the C-terminus of OspA or OspB, is able to produce disease in vaccinated hosts.[89, 101–103] Moreover, spirochete diversity can influence protective immunity in syringe-inoculation studies.[104–107] However, vaccination with OspA from a single isolate (*B. burgdorferi* N40) has been shown to protect mice against infection by ticks, even when those ticks carried *B. burgdorferi* that was antigenically heterogeneous.[108, 109]

Table 39–3. **PROTECTION OF EXPERIMENTAL ANIMALS FROM *Borrelia burgdorferi* INFECTION***

IMMUNIZATION	CHALLENGE	PROTECTION
B. burgdorferi	*B. burgdorferi*	+ + + + +
	B. afzelii	+ + +
	B. garini	+ + +
OspA	*B. burgdorferi*	+ + + + +
	B. afzelii	+ + +
	B. garini	+ + +
OspB	*B. burgdorferi*	+ + + +
OspC	*B. burgdorferi*	+ + +
OspD	*B. burgdorferi*	−
OspE	*B. burgdorferi*	−
OspF	*B. burgdorferi*	+
P35 and P37	*B. burgdorferi*	+ + + +
Flagellin	*B. burgdorferi*	−
P39	*B. burgdorferi*	+
P66	*B. burgdorferi*	+
P110	*B. burgdorferi*	+

The degree of protection is graded on a scale from (−) to (+ + + + +). (−) represents no protection and (+ + + + +) represents substantial (nearly complete) protection. Intermediate grades reflect mild-to-moderate protection.

*The data reflect the authors' interpretation of published studies. In general, animals were actively immunized with *B. burgdorferi* antigens, challenged with *Borrelia* by intradermal syringe or tick bite, and examined for infection. *B. burgdorferi* represents *B. burgdorferi sensu stricto*, and all the *B. burgdorferi*–specific antigens are from *B. burgdorferi sensu stricto* isolates.

Producers

Researchers at Fort Dodge Laboratories (Fort Dodge, Iowa) have produced a vaccine intended for use in dogs (*Borrelia burgdorferi* bacterin, Lymevax). It is composed of a high density of intact BSK (Barbour-Stoenner-Kelly)–cultivated killed *B. burgdorferi* of undisclosed origin suspended in bovine serum albumin and a proprietary adjuvant. It was conditionally licensed by the United States Department of Agriculture for use in dogs in 1980. The vaccine was given full licensure in 1992, despite limited published information on its effectiveness and safety.[110–112]

Two preparations of a recombinant human vaccine have been tested in clinical trials in the United States. SmithKline Beecham (Rixensart, Belgium) is using a purified, lipidated rOspA vaccine based on the German ZS7 strain of *B. burgdorferi*, an isolate with homology to North American *B. burgdorferi sensu stricto* isolates. Pasteur Mérieux Connaught Laboratories (Swiftwater, Pennsylvania) is using a lipidated and purified rOspA preparation that is based on the *B. burgdorferi* B31 isolate.[67]

Dosage and Route

In early safety trials, several regimens have been employed. In one study by Pasteur Merieux Connaught, two intramuscular doses of the OspA vaccine were given 30 days apart.[113] In a phase II ascending dose study with the Pasteur Mérieux Connaught OspA preparation, 330 healthy adult volunteers were randomly assigned to receive two intramuscular doses of 1, 5, 10, or 30 μg of OspA or placebo, 30 days apart.[110] A third study evaluated the safety and immunogenicity of the SmithKline Beecham OspA vaccine in patients with previous Lyme disease. Volunteers were given three intramuscular doses administered 30 days apart of 3, 10, and 30 μg.[114] With both preparations, 30 μg gave the best seroresponses, and this dose was chosen for further studies.

Vaccine stability is being evaluated.

Mode of Action (Fig. 39–6)

OspA vaccination appears to have a unique mode of action that is distinctive among human vaccines.[115] On examination of infected challenge ticks that fed on OspA-vaccinated mice, marked destruction and elimination of spirochetes within their midguts were observed.[116] Control ticks remained densely infected with *B. burgdorferi*. Further studies demonstrated that OspA is expressed in dormant ticks, but expression is later downregulated in response to a blood meal.[30] Thus, it is likely that protective OspA antibodies are ingested from a vaccinated host, are concentrate within the gut, and destroy the pathogens within, thereby preventing transmission of the spirochete.

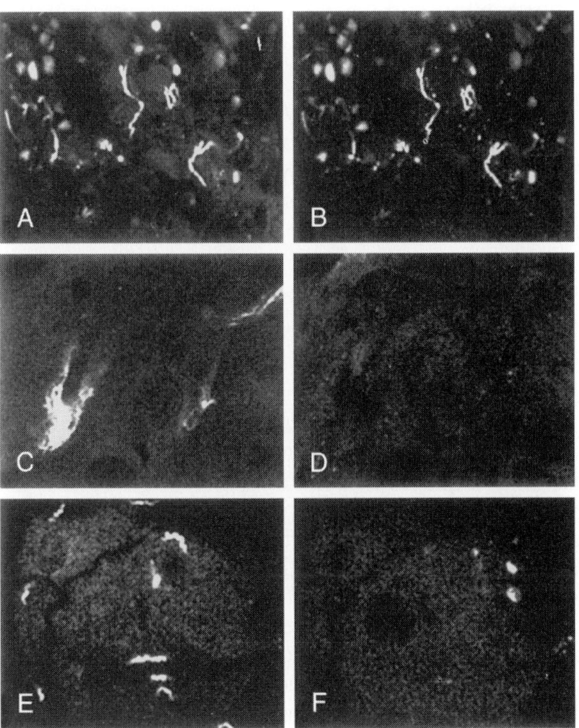

Figure 39–6. Confocal fluorescence images of *Borrelia burgdorferi* in tick organs stained for OspA expression. Immunofluorescence assays were performed on gut specimens of unfed and fed *Ixodes* ticks using polyclonal anti–*B. burgdorferi* (panels *A*, *C*, and *E*) and monoclonal polyclonal anti–*B. burgdorferi* (panels *B*, *D*, and *F*). Panels *A* and *B* are from an unfed infected nymph, panels *C* and *D* are from an infected nymph that fed for 60 hours, and panels *E* and *F* are a salivary acinus from a fed infected nymph. Note that OspA antibody staining was readily detected on spirochetes before tick feeding and disappeared during engorgement, indicating that OspA expression on *B. burgdorferi* diminishes in ticks shortly after a blood meal. (From deSilva AM, Telford DR, Brunet LR, et al. *Borrelia burgdorferi* OspA is an arthropod-specific transmission-blocking Lyme disease vaccine. J Exp Med 183:271–275, 1996.)

Results of Vaccination

Immune Responses

Data gathered from preliminary studies indicate that OspA preparations are immunogenic in humans. In the Connaught phase I study, vaccination with OspA resulted in an immune response in approximately 92% of recipients (a serological response was defined as a fourfold or greater increase over baseline titer).[113] Geometric mean titers of anti-OspA IgG increased approximately fivefold by 3 weeks after the first immunization. The second immunization, at week 4, produced IgG antibody titers reaching levels approximately 40-fold above baseline. The IgG titers decreased during the subsequent 4 months and were similar to levels observed before dose 2 was administered. Titers again rose approximately 10-fold within 1 month after administration of a third dose. Vaccine recipients also acquired antibodies capable of inhibiting growth of *B. burgdorferi* spirochetes in vitro. In one study, these in vitro inhibitory antibodies were shown to be short lived.[117]

The results of the ascending dose study with the Connaught OspA preparation showed a fourfold or greater rise in OspA antibody titer after the second dose was administered in 98% of volunteers who received the 30-μg dose, compared with 71%, 38%, 5%, and 2% in the groups receiving 10, 5, and 1 μg, respectively. In this study, overall, 93% of vaccine recipients developed high-titer OspA antibodies.[110]

In a safety and immunogenicity trial of the SmithKline preparation,[67] 300 subjects were given three doses of recombinant OspA with adjuvant at monthly intervals. Anti-OspA antibodies were detected by ELISA in more than 97% of subjects receiving vaccine; immunogenicity correlated with vaccine dose.

In another study, using the SmithKline preparation, of individuals with a previous history of Lyme disease, 93% acquired high-titer anti-OspA antibodies after vaccination with OspA.[114] Twenty-eight of 30 subjects were positive for antibodies to *B. burgdorferi* by whole-cell ELISA at the time of the first immunization. However, most did not have measurable antibodies to OspA. After the first immunization with OspA, the geometric mean antibody titer to OspA increased greater than 10-fold. Twenty-two of the subjects acquired very high titers of anti-OspA antibodies. People who received the 30-μg dose acquired higher mean titers than those who were given 3 or 10 μg. No significant adverse reactions were noted.

Antibodies reactive with a protective, conformational epitope of OspA, termed LA-2 equivalent antibody, were measured in a large, phase III, multicenter, safety and efficacy trial using the SmithKline Beecham vaccine preparation.[118] One month after the second injection,

95% of the vaccine recipients had positive test results for LA-2 equivalent antibodies, and the percentage increased to 99 1 month after the third injection. After the second injection of the vaccine, a geometric mean titer of 816 ng/mL was reached, which declined to approximately 150 ng per mL 10 months later. The booster dose generated strong anamnestic responses, elevating titers to more than 4000 ng per mL 1 month after the injection. At 8 months after the booster, the geometric mean titer was about 1600 ng/mL. Anti-LA-2 equivalent antibody titers were significantly lower in the vaccinated subjects with breakthrough cases of Lyme disease than in volunteers in the vaccine group in whom the diagnosis of Lyme disease was not confirmed, or in the general population of vaccinated subjects from one of the study sites.

Results of Controlled Trials of Protection Against Disease (Table 39–4)

SmithKline Beecham conducted a multicenter double-blind, placebo-controlled safety and efficacy trial of 10,936 subjects aged 15 to 70 years in endemic areas for Lyme disease.[118] Individuals received three doses of either vaccine (30 μg OspA) or placebo in a 0-, 1-, and 12-month dosing schedule and were monitored for clinical and/or laboratory evidence of Lyme disease. In the first year, after two injections, vaccine efficacy in preventing definite Lyme disease was 49%; it increased to 76% in the second year, after the third injection. Vaccine recipients were found to have a significantly reduced number of asymptomatic seroconversion compared with the placebo group. Overall, vaccine efficacy against definite Lyme disease and asymptomatic seroconversion was 80% after the third injection. Vaccine-related side effects were mild to moderate in severity and were typically self-limited.

The Pasteur Mérieux Connaught study enrolled 10,306 subjects aged 18 to 92 years in a double-blind, placebo-controlled safety and efficacy trial conducted in endemic areas for Lyme disease.[119] In the spring of the first year, recipients received two doses 1 month apart of either 30 μg of OspA lipoprotein or saline, with a booster dose 12 months later. Overall vaccine efficacy was 68% and increased to 92% after the third injection. Vaccinees older than 60 years were less well protected than younger vaccinees. The incidence of serious adverse events was similar in both the vaccine and placebo groups.

Table 39–4. **EFFICACY OF OspA-CONTAINING VACCINES AGAINST *Borrelia burgdorferi* INFECTION***

	PERCENT VACCINE EFFICACY (95% CI)	
	SmithKline Beecham	**Pasteur Mérieux Connaught**
First year, after two injections		
Definite cases	49 (15–69)	68 (36–85)
Asymptomatic	83 (32–97)	NA
Second year, after three injections		
Definite cases	76 (56–86)	92 (69–97)
Asymptomatic	100 (26–100)	NA
No booster dose given	NA	0 (0–60)

CI, confidence interval; NA, not available.
*Results are presented from two studies, each involving approximately 5000 vaccinees and 5000 control subjects.

Thus, human efficacy data bear out the results obtained in animal models.[120] Both OspA vaccines were effective against Lyme disease, as confirmed by laboratory tests. Vaccinees who received two doses obtained up to 70% protection during the first season of exposure, a result that varied with the vaccine and the subgroup of volunteers. After the third dose 1 year later, 80 to 95% protection was observed during the second season of exposure to ticks. Vaccinees older than 60 years were less well protected than younger vaccinees.

The majority of patients in these studies were diagnosed with erythema migrans. In the Pasteur Mérieux Connaught study, 6% of patients—the majority of whom were placebo recipients—did not have erythema migrans as the presenting feature. OspA vaccination did not appear to alter the clinical presentation or features of Lyme disease. In view of the differences in case ascertainment and the wide confidence limits of the estimates, it is likely that the two vaccines are equally efficacious.[120a]

Duration of Immunity

The length of protection acquired by vaccination with OspA preparations is unknown. Future studies will need to be performed to address the duration of immunity and the safety and the need for booster doses.

Adverse Events

Common Events

Mild local reactions were common in all trials published to date and appeared more often in vaccine recipients than in placebo recipients. The most common adverse reaction was local pain, tenderness, or both at the injection site, which occurred in up to 85% of subjects.[113, 114] Redness and swelling of the injection site was less common and reported in approximately 10 to 15% of individuals. Most local reactions were rated as mild, and local reactions rated moderate or severe were rare. Such reactions generally resolved spontaneously within 72 hours. The incidence of local reactions occurred more frequently in the higher-dose (10- and 30-μg) groups, but there was no associated increase with subsequent doses.

Systemic reactions were reported in up to 40% of the individuals for a given dose and group. Headache and fatigue were the most common systemic complaints; both occurred within 72 hours of vaccination and resolved spontaneously. Most systemic symptoms were rated as mild, and there was no increase in the incidence after each successive vaccine dose.[113, 114] Other, less common, systemic complaints included fever, rash, and arthralgias. In most cases, joint pain was transient, mild, and migratory; involved several large joints (including the shoulders, hips, elbows, and knees); and was not characteristic of Lyme arthritis.[108, 109] Joint pain typically did not require treatment. It did not appear to be causally related to vaccine and was not induced by revaccination.

The possible provocation of Lyme arthritis by inoculation with OspA was specifically studied for both experimental vaccines, in view of the suspicion that Lyme arthritis is in part an immunological phenomenon related to cross-reaction between OspA and host antigens (see later). In both phase III trials, adverse effects were more common in subjects who received the vaccine.[118, 119] The most frequently reported vaccine-related effects were mild and self-limited and included pain or tenderness at the injection site and local muscle pain. Systemic symptoms of myalgia, achiness, fever, or chills that were thought to be related or possibly related to vaccination were more commonly reported by vaccine recipients. Typically, such symptoms resolved within 7 days after injection. There were no significant differences between the groups in the frequency of severe side effects in either study.

Rare Adverse Events

Unanswered questions include the following: Does vaccination alter the clinical presentation of Lyme disease? Does it delay the onset of infection? Does it modify the initial infectious process? Preliminary analysis revealed no excess of serious or rare adverse events in the vaccinees when compared with results in placebo recipients.[118, 119]

Indications for Vaccine

Preliminary reports of two large safety and efficacy trials indicated that the human OspA vaccine is safe. Both trials enrolled more than 10,000 subjects. The vaccine was associated with local or general reactions, most of which were mild to moderate in severity and self-limited. Because the frequency of occurrence of serious adverse events was reported to be similar in both the vaccine and the placebo groups and because side effects were generally mild, Lyme vaccine appears to be acceptable for use in the high-risk population. Those who would benefit from vaccination include people who work, live, or engage in hobbies in highly endemic areas. Vaccination may also be considered, when appropriate, for people with significant transient exposures to the infection, such as travelers to, and individuals living near, high-risk endemic regions. Future studies will need to address the safety, immunogenicity, and effectiveness of vaccines in children.

A whole-cell animal vaccine, *Borrelia burgdorferi* Bacterin, has been approved by the United States Department of Agriculture for use in dogs. The experimental efficacy studies that have been performed suggest that the vaccine works, but the results were not conclusive.[110–112] The vaccine does appear to be safe, but the effects of multiple immunizations are not known. The manufacturer recommends that initially two doses be given a few weeks apart and that yearly booster immunizations be given thereafter. Further studies are needed to clarify issues regarding effectiveness, use in other animals, and long-term effects.

Contraindications and Precautions

In natural infection in humans, detectable OspA antibodies generally do not occur until late in the course of the illness and have been reported to appear at the onset of arthritis.[10] High-titer anti-OspA antibodies and the presence of major histocompatibility antigens HLA-DR4 and HLA-DR2 have been associated with antibiotic refractory cases of Lyme arthritis.[121, 122] These observations and results of animal studies have led researchers to postulate that OspA immune responses may play an etiological role in arthritis pathogenesis.[123–125] If so, there is concern that immunological responses to OspA vaccination may induce synovial inflammation in recipients. This concern has not been borne out by the results of early human studies, even in individuals with a previous history of Lyme arthritis or in those who carry the HLA-DR4 genetic allele, but larger studies are needed, since arthralgia and myalgia were seen more frequently in vaccinees.[113, 114]

Future Vaccines

Potential limitations with use of a single-protein recombinant OspA vaccine preparations include a lack of cross-protection for diverse *B. burgdorferi* strains and an evasion of the immune system by spirochetes that have truncated outer surface proteins and do not bind protective antibodies.[89, 103, 126–128] Multiple antigen vaccines may prove to be more effective.

Some work has identified other *Borrelia* proteins that are immunogenic, although they display strain heterogeneity that is similar to OspA. One such protein, outer surface protein C (OspC) has been identified as another possible vaccine candidate.[129] OspC is expressed in abundant amounts by *B. burgdorferi* and, in natural infections, induces a strong early immune response.[130] OspC expression appears to correlated negatively with OspA because it increases in response to tick feeding and contact with human tissues.[30, 131, 132] Animal studies have indicated that vaccination with recombinant OspC is also effective against challenge with limited strains of *B. burgdorferi*.[129, 133] Strain heterogeneity is likely to limit its usefulness.[20, 134] Human trials using OspC have not been performed.

Vaccinations using other *Borrelia* proteins have been explored. Potential candidates include OspB, OspF, a 110-kDa fusion protein containing a portion of a *B. burgdorferi* heat-shock protein (HSP70), and a live attenuated vaccine containing a flagella-less mutant of *B. burgdorferi*.[22, 90, 135, 136] Moreover, immunization with P35 and P37, two *Borrelia* proteins that are selectively induced in vivo provide protective immunity as well.[137] Vaccination experiments using OspD, OspE, or 39-kDa,

83-kDa, or P55 kDa *Borrelia* proteins did not appear to protect animals from infection.[22, 138, 139]

REFERENCES

1. Steere AC, Malawista SE, Snydman DR, et al. Lyme arthritis: An epidemic of oligoarticular arthritis in children and adults in three Connecticut communities. Arthritis Rheum 20:7–17, 1977.
2. Steere AC, Malawista SE, Craft JE, et al. Lyme disease: First International Symposium. Yale J Biol Med 57:445–713, 1984.
3. Burgdorfer W, Barbour AG, Hayes SF, et al. Lyme disease—a tick-borne spirochetosis? Science 216:1317–1319, 1982.
4. Steere AC, Grodzicki RL, Kornblatt AN, et al. The spirochetal etiology of Lyme disease. N Engl J Med 308:733–740, 1983.
5. Benach JL, Bosler EM, Hanrahan JP. Spirochetes isolated from the blood of two patients with Lyme disease. N Engl J Med 308:740–742, 1983.
6. Preac-Mursic V, Wilske B, Schierz G, et al. Repeated isolation of spirochetes from the cerebrospinal fluid of a patient with meningoradiculitis Bannwarth. Eur J Clin Microbiol 3:564–565, 1984.
7. Asbrink E, Hovmark A. Successful cultivation of spirochetes from the skin lesions of patients with erythema chronica migrans Afzelius and acrodermatitis chronica atrophicans. Acta Pathol Microbiol Immunol Scand 93:161–163, 1985.
8. Craft JE, Fischer DK, Shimamoto GT, Steere AC. Antigens of *Borrelia burgdorferi* recognized during Lyme disease: Appearance of a new immunoglobulin M response and expansion of the immunoglobulin G response late in the illness. J Clin Invest 78:934–939, 1986.
9. Rahn DW, Malawista SE. Lyme disease: Recommendations for diagnosis and treatment. Ann Intern Med 114:472–481, 1991.
10. Steere AC. Lyme disease. N Engl J Med 321:586–594, 1989.
11. Nadelman RB Wormser GP: Erythema migrans and early Lyme disease. Am J Med 98(suppl 4A):S15–S24, 1995.
12. Berglund J, Eitrem R, Ornstein K, et al. An epidemiologic study of Lyme disease in southern Sweden. N Engl J Med 333:1319–1324, 1995.
13. Steere AC, Schoen RT, Taylor E. The clinical evolution of Lyme arthritis. Ann Intern Med 197:725–731, 1987.
14. Logigian EL, Kaplan RF, Steere AC. Chronic neurologic manifestations of Lyme disease. N Engl J Med 323:1438–1444, 1990.
15. Finkel MJ, Halperin JJ. Nervous system Lyme borreliosis—revisited. Arch Neurol 49:102–107, 1992.
16. Halperin JJ, Logigian EL, Finkel MF, Pearl RA. Practice parameters for the diagnosis of patients with nervous system Lyme borreliosis (Lyme disease). Neurology 46:619–627, 1996.
17. Pfister H, Wilske B, Weber K. Lyme borreliosis: Basic science and clinical aspects. Lancet 343:1013–1016, 1994.
18. Barbour AG, Tessier SL, Todd WJ. Lyme disease spirochetes and *Ixodid* tick spirochetes share a common surface antigenic determinant defined by a monoclonal antibody. Infect Immun 41:795–799, 1983.
19. Barbour AG, Tessier SL, Hayes SF. Variations in a major surface protein of Lyme disease spirochetes. Infect Immun 45:94–100, 1984.
20. Wilske B, Preac-Mursic V, Jauris S, et al. Immunological and molecular polymorphisms of OspC, an immunodominant major outer surface protein of *Borrelia burgdorferi*. Infect Immun 61:2182–2191, 1993.
21. Norris SJ, Carter CJ, Howell JK, Barbour AG. Low passage associated proteins of *Borrelia burgdorferi* B31: Characterization and molecular cloning of OspD, a surface-exposed, plasmid-encoded lipoprotein. Infect Immun 60:4662–4672, 1992.
22. Nguyen TK, Lam TT, Barthold SW, et al. Partial destruction of *Borrelia burgdorferi* within ticks that engorged on OspE- or OspF-immunized mice. Infect Immun 62:2079–2084, 1994.
23. Scriba M, Ebrahim S, Schlott T, Eiffert H. The 39-kilodalton protein of *Borrelia burgdorferi*: A target for bactericidal human monoclonal antibodies. Infect Immun 61:4523–4526, 1993.
24. Feng S, Das S, Lam R, et al. A 55-kilodalton antigen encoded by a gene on a *Borrelia burgdorferi* 49-kilobase plasmid is recognized by antibodies in sera from patients with Lyme disease. Infect Immun 63:3459–3466, 1995.
25. LeFebvre RB, Perng GC, Johnson RC. The 83-kilodalton antigen of *Borrelia burgdorferi* which stimulates immunoglobulin M (IgM) and IgG responses in infected hosts is expressed by a chromosomal gene. J Clin Microbiol 28:1673–1675, 1990.
26. Caputa AC, Murtaugh MP, Bey RF, Loken KI. 110-kilodalton recombinant protein which is immunoreactive with sera from humans, dogs, and horses with Lyme borreliosis. J Clin Microbiol 29:2418–2423, 1992.
27. Barthold SW. Globalisation of Lyme borreliosis. Lancet 347:1603, 1996.
28. Busch U, Hizo-Teufel C, Boehmer R, et al. Three species of *Borrelia burgdorferi sensu lato* (*B. burgdorferi sensu stricto*, *B. afzelii*, and *B. garinii*) identified from cerebrospinal fluid isolated by pulsed-field gel electrophoresis and PCR. J Clin Microbiol 34:1072–1078, 1996.
29. Anda P, Sanchez-Yebra W, del Mar Vitutia M, et al. A new *Borrelia* species isolated from patients with relapsing fever in Spain. Lancet 348:162–165, 1996.
30. deSilva AM, Telford SR III, Brunet LR, et al. *Borrelia burgdorferi* OspA is an arthropod-specific transmission-blocking Lyme disease vaccine. J Exp Med 183:271–275, 1996.
31. Stevenson B, Schwan TG, Rosa PA. Temperature-related differential expression of antigens in the Lyme disease spirochete, *Borrelia burgdorferi*. Infect Immun 63:4535–4539, 1995.
32. Piesman J, Mather T, Sinsky R, Spielman A. Duration of tick attachment and *Borrelia burgdorferi* transmission. J Clin Microbiol 25:557–558, 1987.
33. Klempner MS, Noring R, Epstein MP, et al. Binding of human plasminogen and urokinase-type plasminogen activator to the Lyme disease spirochete, *Borrelia burgdorferi*. J Infect Dis 171:1258–1265, 1995.
34. Fuchs H, Wallich R, Simon MM, Kramer MD. The outer surface protein A of the spirochete *Borrelia burgdorferi* is a plasmin (ogen) receptor. Proc Natl Acad Sci USA 91:12594–12598, 1994.
35. Coleman JL, Sellati TJ, Testa JE, et al. *Borrelia burgdorferi* binds plasminogen, resulting in enhanced penetration of endothelial monolayers. Infect Immun 63:2478–2484, 1995.
36. Leong JM, Morrissey PE, Ortega-Barria E, et al. Hemagglutination and proteoglycan binding by the Lyme disease spirochete, *Borrelia burgdorferi*. Infect Immun 63:874–883, 1995.
37. Sellati TJ, Burns MJ, Ficazzola MA, Furie MB. *Borrelia burgdorferi* upregulates expression of adhesion molecules on endothelial cells and promotes transendothelial migration of neutrophils in vitro. Infect Immun 63:4439–4447, 1995.
38. Duray P, Steere AC. Clinical pathologic correlations of Lyme disease by stage. Ann NY Acad Sci 539:65–79, 1988.
39. Craft JE, Grodzicki RL, Steere AC. Antibody response in Lyme disease: Evaluation of diagnostic tests. J Infect Dis 149:789–795, 1984.
40. Shrestha M, Grodzicki RL, Steere AC. Diagnosing early Lyme disease. Am J Med 78:235–240, 1988.
41. Centers for Disease Control and Prevention. Recommendations for test performance and interpretation from the Second National Conference on Serologic Diagnosis of Lyme Disease. MMWR Morb Mortal Wkly Rep 44:590–591, 1995.
42. Engstrom SM, Shoop E, Johnson RC. Immunoblot interpretation criteria for serodiagnosis of early Lyme disease. J Clin Microbiol 33:419–427, 1995.
43. Dressler F, Whalen JA, Reinhardt BN, Steere AC. Western blotting in the serodiagnosis of Lyme disease. J Infect Dis 167:392–400, 1993.
44. Motor SE, Hofmann J, Wallich R, et al. Detection of *Borrelia burgdorferi sensu lato* in skin lesions of patients with erythema migrans and acrodermatitis chronica atrophicans by *ospA*-specific PCR. J Clin Microbiol 32:2980–2988, 1994.
45. Nocton JJ, Dressler F, Rutledge BJ, et al. Detection of *Borrelia burgdorferi* DNA of polymerase chain reaction in synovial fluid from patients with Lyme arthritis. N Engl J Med 330:229–234, 1994.
46. Goodman JL, Berger BW, Luger S, Johnson RC. Bloodstream invasion in early Lyme disease: Results from a prospective, controlled, blinded study using the polymerase chain reaction. Am J Med 99:6–12, 1995.
47. Karch H, Huppertz J, Bohme M, et al. Demonstration of *Borrelia burgdorferi* DNA in urine samples from healthy humans whose

sera contain *B. burgdorferi*-specific antibodies. J Clin Microbiol 32:2312–2314, 1994.
48. Christen HJ, Eiffert H, Ohlenbusch A, Hanefeld F. Evaluation of the polymerase chain reaction for the detection of *Borrelia burgdorferi* in cerebrospinal fluid of children with acute peripheral facial palsy. Eur J Pediatr 154:374–377, 1995.
49. Malawista SE, Barthold SW, Persing DH. Reply to the editor. J Infect Dis 171:1380, 1995.
50. Steere AC, Malawista SE, Newman JH, et al. Antibiotic therapy in Lyme disease. Ann Intern Med 93:108, 1980.
51. Steere AC, Pachner A, Malawista SE. Successful treatment of neurologic abnormalities of Lyme disease with high-dose intravenous penicillin. Ann Intern Med 99:767–772, 1983.
52. Rahn DW, Malawista SE. Treatment of Lyme disease. In Rogers DE, Bone RC, Cline MJ, et al (eds). Yearbook of Medicine. St. Louis, CV Mosby, 1994, pp 21–36.
53. Steere AC, Levin RE, Molloy PJ, et al. Treatment of Lyme arthritis. Arthritis Rheum 37:878–888, 1994.
54. Fish D. Environmental risk and prevention of Lyme disease. Am J Med 98(suppl 4A):S2–S9, 1995.
55. Stafford KC. Reduced abundance of *Ixodes scapularis* with exclusion of deer by electric fencing. J Med Entomol 30:986–996, 1993.
56. Daniels TJ, Fish D, Schwartz I. Reduced abundance of *Ixodes scapularis* and Lyme disease risk by deer exclusion. J Med Entomol 30:1043–1049, 1993.
57. Rich SM, Caporale DA, Telford SR, et al. Distribution of the *Ixodes ricinus*-like ticks of eastern North America. Proc Natl Acad Sci USA 92:6284–6288, 1995.
58. Centers for Disease Control and Prevention. Lyme disease-United States, 1994. JAMA 274:111, 1995.
59. Steere AC. Lyme disease: A growing threat to urban populations. Proc Natl Acad Sci USA 91:2378–2383, 1994.
60. Berglund J, Eitrem R, Ornstein K, et al. An epidemiologic study of Lyme disease in southern Sweden. N Engl J Med 333:1319–1324, 1995.
61. Spielman A. The emergence of Lyme disease and human babesiosis in a changing environment. J NY Acad Sci 140:146–156, 1995.
62. Strle F, Stantic-Pavlinic M. Lyme disease in Europe. N Engl J Med 334:803, 1996.
63. Christiann F, Rayet P, Petey O, Lafaix C. Epidemiology of Lyme disease in France: Lyme borreliosis in the region of Berry Sud: A six year retrospective. Eur J Epidemiol 12:479–483, 1996.
64. Barbour AG, Fish D. The biological and social phenomenon of Lyme disease. Science 260:1610–1616, 1993.
65. Shapiro ED. Lyme disease in children. Am J Med 98(suppl 4A):S69–S73, 1995.
66. Kantor FS. Disarming Lyme disease. Sci Am 271:34–39, 1994.
67. Telford SR, Fikrig E. Progress towards a vaccine for Lyme disease. Clin Immunother 4:49–60, 1995.
68. Wormser GP. A vaccine against Lyme disease? Ann Intern Med 123:627–628, 1995.
69. Steere AC, Taylor E, Wilson ML. Longitudinal assessment of the clinical and epidemiological features of Lyme disease in a defined population. J Infect Dis 154:295–300, 1986.
70. Feder HM, Gerber MA, Cartter ML, et al. Prospective assessment of Lyme disease in a school-aged population in Connecticut. J Infect Dis 171:1371–1374, 1995.
71. Coyle BS, Strickland GT, Liang YY, et al. The public health impact of Lyme disease in Maryland. J Infect Dis 173:1260–1262, 1996.
72. Centers for Disease Control and Prevention. Lyme disease—United States, 1995. JAMA 276:274, 1996.
73. Shadick NA, Phillips CB, Logigian EL, et al. The long-term clinical outcomes of Lyme disease. Ann Intern Med 121:560–567, 1994.
74. Simon M, Milward F, Lefebvre R, et al. Spirochetes: Vaccines, animal models and diagnostics. Res Microbiol 143:641–647, 1992.
75. Philipp MT, Johnson BJ. Animal models of Lyme disease: Pathogenesis and immunoprophylaxis. Trends Microbiol 2:431–437, 1994.
76. Barthold SW. Animal models for Lyme disease. Lab Invest 72:127–130, 1995.
77. Barthold SW, de Souza MS, Janotka JL, et al. Chronic Lyme borreliosis in the laboratory mouse. Am J Pathol 143:959–971, 1993.
78. Schaible U, Kramer M, Museteanu C, et al. The severe combined immunodeficient mouse: A laboratory model of Lyme arthritis and carditis. J Exp Med 170:240–247, 1989.
79. Kochi SK, Johnson RC. Role of immunoglobulin G in killing of *Borrelia burgdorferi* by the classical complement pathway. Infect Immun 56:314–321, 1988.
80. Johnson RC, Kodner C, Russell M, Duray PH. Active immunization of hamsters against experimental infection with *Borrelia burgdorferi*. Infect Immun 54:897, 1986.
81. Schmitz JL, Schell RF, Hejka AG, England DM. Passive immunization prevents induction of Lyme arthritis in LSH hamsters. Infect Immun 58:144–148, 1990.
82. Fikrig E, Barthold SW, Kantor FS, Flavell RA. Protection of mice against the Lyme disease agent by immunizing with recombinant OspA. Science 250:553–556, 1990.
83. Schaible UE, Wallich R, Kramer MD, et al. Protection against *Borrelia burgdorferi* infection in SCID mice is conferred by presensitized spleen cells and partially by B but not T cells alone. Int Immunol 6:671–681, 1994.
84. Schmitz JL, Schell RF, Lovrich SD, et al. Characterization of the protective antibody response to *Borrelia burgdorferi* in experimentally infected LSH hamsters. Infect Immun 59:1916–1921, 1991.
85. Schmitz JL, Schnell RF, Callister SM, et al. Immunoglobulin G2 confers protection against *Borrelia burgdorferi* infection in LSH hamsters. Infect Immun 60:2677–2682, 1992.
86. Bockenstedt LK, Barthold S, Deponte K, et al. *Borrelia burgdorferi* infection and immunity in mice deficient in the fifth component of complement. Infect Immun 61:2104–2107, 1993.
87. Ma J, Gingrich-Baker C, Franchi PM, et al. Molecular analysis of neutralizing epitopes on outer surface proteins A and B of *Borrelia burgdorferi*. Infect Immun 63:2221–2227, 1995.
88. Howe TR, Mayer LW, Barbour AG. A single recombinant plasmid expressing two major outer surface proteins of the Lyme disease spirochete. Science 227:645, 1985.
89. Fikrig ET, Tao H, Kantor FS, et al. Evasion of protective immunity by *Borrelia burgdorferi* by truncation of outer surface protein B. Proc Natl Acad Sci USA 90:4092–4096, 1993.
90. Fikrig E, Barthold SW, Marcantonio N, et al. Roles of OspA, OspB and flagellin in protective immunity to Lyme borreliosis in laboratory mice. Infect Immun 59:553–559, 1992.
91. Schaible UE, Kramer MD, Eichmann K, et al. Monoclonal antibodies specific for the outer surface protein A (OspA) of *Borrelia burgdorferi* prevent Lyme borreliosis in severe combined immunodeficiency (SCID) mice. Proc Natl Acad Sci USA 87:3768–3772, 1990.
92. Erdile LF, Brandt M, Warakomski DJ, et al. Role of attached lipid in immunogenicity of *Borrelia burgdorferi* OspA. Infect Immun 61:81–90 ,1993.
93. Chang Y, Appel MJG, Jacobson RH, et al. Recombinant OspA protects dogs against infection and disease caused by *Borrelia burgdorferi*. Infect Immun 63:3543–3549, 1995.
94. Fikrig E, Barthold SW, Kantor FS, Flavell RA. Long term protection of mice from Lyme disease by immunizing with recombinant OspA. Infect Immun 60:773–778, 1992.
95. Zumstein G, Fuchs R, Hofmann A, et al. Genetic polymorphism of the gene encoding the outer surface protein A (OspA) of *Borrelia burgdorferi*. Med Microbiol Immunol (Berl) 181:57–70, 1992.
96. Wilske B, Barbour AG, Bergstrom S, et al. Antigenic variation and strain heterogeneity in *Borrelia* spp. Res Microbiol 143:583–596, 1992.
97. Jonsson M, Noppa L, Barbour AG, Berstrom S. Heterogeneity of outer membrane proteins in *Borrelia burgdorferi*: Comparison of *osp* operons of three isolates of different geographic origins. Infect Immun 60:1845–1853, 1992.
98. Sadziene A, Rosa P, Hogan D, Barbour A. Antibody resistant mutants of *Borrelia burgdorferi*: In vitro selection and characterization. J Exp Med 176:799–809, 1992.
99. Fikrig E, Tao H, Barthold SW, Flavell RA. Selection of variant *Borrelia burgdorferi* isolates from mice immunized with outer surface protein A or B. Infect Immun 63:1658–1662, 1995.

100. Lovrich SD, Callister SM, DuChateau BK, et al. Abilities of OspA proteins from different seroprotective groups of *Borrelia burgdorferi* to protect hamsters from infection. Infect Immun 63:2113–2119, 1995.
101. Sears J, Fikrig E, Nakagawa T, et al. Molecular mapping of OspA-mediated protection against *Borrelia burgdorferi*, the Lyme disease agent. J Immunol 147:1995–2001, 1991.
102. McGrath BC, Dunn JJ, Gorgone G, et al. Identification of an immunologically important hypervariable domain of major outer surface protein A of *Borrelia burgdorferi*. Infect Immun 63:1356–1361, 1995.
103. Bockenstedt LK, Fikrig E, Barthold SW, et al. Inability of truncated recombinant OspA proteins to elicit protective immunity to *Borrelia burgdorferi* in mice. J Immunol 151:900–906, 1993.
104. Fikrig E, Barthold SW, Persing DH, et al. *Borrelia burgdorferi* strain 25015: Characterization of OspA and vaccination against infection. J Immunol 148:2256–2260, 1992.
105. Lovrich SD, Callister SM, Lim LCL, Schell RF. Seroprotective groups among isolates of *Borrelia burgdorferi*. Infect Immun 61:4367–4374, 1993.
106. Gern L, Schaible UE, Simon MM. Mode of inoculation of the Lyme disease agent *Borrelia burgdorferi* influences infection and immune responses in inbred strains of mice. J Infect Dis 167:971–975, 1993.
107. Roehrig JT, Peisman J, Hunt AR, et al. The hamster immune response to tick-transmitted *Borrelia burgdorferi* differs from the response to needle-inoculated, cultured organisms. J Immunol 149:3648–3653, 1992.
108. Telford SR, Fikrig E, Barthold SW, et al. Protection against antigenically variable *Borrelia burgdorferi* conferred by recombinant vaccines. J Exp Med 178:755–758, 1993.
109. Fikrig E, Telford SR, Wallich R, et al. Vaccination against Lyme disease caused by diverse *Borrelia burgdorferi*. J Exp Med 181:215–221, 1995.
110. Wormser GP. Lyme disease vaccine. Infection 24:203–207, 1996.
111. Levy SA, Lissman BA, Ficke CM. Performance of *Borrelia burgdorferi* bacterin in borreliosis-endemic areas. J Am Vet Med Assoc 202:1834–1838, 1993.
112. Chu HJ, Chavez LG, Blumer BM, et al. Immunogenicity and efficacy study of a commercial *Borrelia burgdorferi* bacterin. J Am Vet Med Assoc 201:403–411, 1992.
113. Keller D, Koster FT, Marks DH, et al. Safety and immunogenicity of a recombinant outer surface protein A Lyme vaccine. JAMA 271:1764–1768, 1994.
114. Schoen RT, Meurice F, Brunet CM, et al. Safety and immunogenicity of an outer surface protein A vaccine in subjects with previous Lyme disease. J Infect Dis 172:1324–1329, 1995.
115. Shih C, Spielman A, Telford SR. Short report: Mode of action of protective immunity to Lyme disease spirochetes. Am J Trop Med Hyg 52:72–74, 1995.
116. Fikrig EF, Telford SR, Barthold SW, et al. Elimination of *Borrelia burgdorferi* from vector ticks feeding on OspA-immunized mice. Proc Natl Acad Sci USA 89:5418–5421, 1992.
117. Padilla ML, Callister SM, Schell RF, et al. Characterization of the protective borreliacidal antibody response in humans and hamsters after vaccination with a *Borrelia burgdorferi* outer surface protein A vaccine. J Infect Dis 174:739–746, 1996.
118. Steere AC, Sikand VK, Meurice F, et al. Vaccination against Lyme disease with recombinant *Borrelia burgdorferi* outer-surface lipoprotein A with adjuvant. N Engl J Med 339:209–215, 1998.
119. Sigal LH, Zahradnik JM, Lavin P, et al. A vaccine consisting of recombinant *Borrelia burgdorferi* outer-surface protein A to prevent Lyme disease. N Engl J Med 339:216–222, 1998.
120. Telford SR, Kantor FS, Lobet Y, et al. Efficacy of human Lyme disease vaccine formulations in a mouse model. J Infect Dis 171:1368–1370, 1995.
120a. Steigbigel RT, Benach JL. Immunization against Lyme disease—an important first step. N Engl J Med 339:263–264, 1998.
121. Steere AC, Dwyer E, Winchester R. Association of chronic Lyme arthritis with HLA-DR4 and HLA-DR2 alleles. N Engl J Med 323:219–223, 1990.
122. Kalish RA, Leong JM, Steere AC. Association of treatment-resistant chronic Lyme arthritis with HLA-DR4 and antibody reactivity to OspA and OspB of *Borrelia burgdorferi*. Infect Immun 61:2774–2779, 1993.
123. Gondolf KB, Mihatsch M, Curschellas E, et al. Induction of experimental allergic arthritis with outer surface proteins of *Borrelia burgdorferi*. Arthritis Rheum 37:1070–1077, 1994.
124. Lim LCL, England DM, DuChateau BK, et al. Development of destructive arthritis in vaccinated hamsters challenged with *Borrelia burgdorferi*. Infect Immun 62:2825–2833, 1994.
125. Feng S, Barthold SW, Bockenstedt LK, et al. Lyme disease in human DR4Dw4-transgenic mice. J Infect Dis 172:286–289, 1995.
126. Sadziene A, Barbour AG. Experimental immunization against Lyme borreliosis with recombinant Osp proteins: An overview. Infection 24:195–202, 1996.
127. Lovrich SD, Callister SM, Lim LC, Schell RF. Seroprotective groups among isolates of *Borrelia burgdorferi*. Infect Immun 61:4367–4374, 1993.
128. Kramer MD, Wallich R, Simon MM. The outer surface protein A (OspA) of *Borrelia burgdorferi*: A vaccine candidate and bioactive mediator. Infection 24:190–194, 1996.
129. Preac-Mursic V, Wilske B, Patsouris E, et al. Active immunization with pC protein of *Borrelia burgdorferi* protects gerbils against *B. burgdorferi* infection. Infection 20:342–439, 1992.
130. Wilske B, Busch U, Fingerle V, et al. Immunological and molecular variability of OspA and OspC. Implications for *Borrelia* vaccine development. Infection 24:208–212, 1996.
131. Schwan TG, Peisman J, Golde WT, et al. Induction of an outer surface protein on *Borrelia burgdorferi* during tick feeding. Proc Natl Acad Sci USA 92:2909–2913, 1995.
132. Montgomery RR, Malawista SE, Feen KJM, Bockenstedt LK. Direct demonstration of antigenic substitution of *Borrelia burgdorferi* ex vivo: Exploration of the paradox of the early immune response to outer surface proteins A and C in Lyme disease. J Exp Med 183:261–269, 1996.
133. Gilmore RD, Kappel KJ, Dolan MC, et al. Outer surface protein C (OspC), but not P39 is a protective immunogen against a tick-transmitted *Borrelia burgdorferi* challenge: Evidence for a conformational protective epitope in OspC. Infect Immun 64:2234–2239, 1996.
134. Stevenson B, Barthold SW. Expression and sequence of outer surface protein C among North American isolates of *Borrelia burgdorferi*. FEMS Microbiol Lett 124:367–372, 1994.
135. Bey RF, Larson ME, Lowery DE, et al. Protection of C3H/He mice from experimental *Borrelia burgdorferi* infection by immunization with a 110-kilodalton fusion protein. Infect Immun 63:3213–3217, 1995.
136. Sadziene A, Thompson PA, Barbour AG. A flagella-less mutant of *Borrelia burgdorferi* as a live attenuated vaccine in the murine model of Lyme disease. J Infect Dis 173:1184–1193, 1996.
137. Fikrig E, Barthold SW, Sun W, et al. *Borrelia burgdorferi* P35 and P37 proteins, expressed in vivo, elicit protective immunity. Immunity 6:531–539, 1997.
138. Probert WS, LeFebvre RB. Protection of C3H/HeN mice from challenge with *Borrelia burgdorferi* through active immunization with OspA, OspB, or OspC, but not with OspD or the 83-kilodalton antigen. Infect Immun 62:1920–1926, 1994.
139. Feng S, Barthold SW, Telford SR, Fikrig E. P55, an immunogenic but nonprotective 55-kilodalton *Borrelia burgdorferi* protein in murine Lyme disease. Infect Immun 64:363–365, 1996.

chapter

40 Parasitic Disease Vaccines

Peter J. Hotez

Parasitic diseases caused by helminths and unicellular eukaryotes are major causes of human disease and misery in the less-developed nations of the tropics. Attempts to develop vaccines against these organisms have been hampered traditionally by the difficulties in maintaining the organisms in the laboratory. With a few exceptions, in vitro culture methods have not been adequate; frequently laboratory animals such as dogs and nonhuman primates have been necessary to propagate their complex life cycles. This problem has thwarted efforts to scale up production of large numbers of parasites in order to develop attenuated or killed vaccines. Within the last decade, investigators in academic and government laboratories have started to apply modern biotechnology to the study of parasitic helminths and protozoa, resulting in the cloning and expression of some promising recombinant protective antigens. However, there has been little commercial interest in the development of these protective antigens as human vaccines. Lack of enthusiasm for parasitic disease vaccines among the traditional large vaccine manufacturers has resulted from concerns about their markets in developing economies, as well as their scientific and technological complexities.[1]

ANTIPROTOZOAN VACCINES

Malaria

The World Health Organization estimates that malaria causes as many as 500 million clinical cases and 2.7 million deaths per year. Although there are four malarial species that cause human disease, most of the severe cases leading to cerebral malaria and death result from infection with *Plasmodium falciparum*. By some estimates, *P. falciparum* is the single leading killer of children younger than 5 years. Human infection occurs initially when infective sporozoites are inoculated into the blood through the bite of infected mosquitoes. On entry into the hepatic circulation, the sporozoites enter hepatocytes, where they reproduce into thousands of pre-erythrocytic parasites. On their release from hepatocytes, the parasites reenter the bloodstream, invade erythrocytes, and reproduce asexually. The predominant clinical and pathological features occur during the erythrocytic phase.[2] Transformation by some intraerythrocytic parasites into the sexual stages presages uptake by the mosquito before sexual reproduction in and transmission by the insect vector.

For vaccine development, most of the early attention has focused on the infective sporozoite stage *P. falciparum* malaria.[3] It was noted in the early 1970s by Ruth and Victor Nussenzweig at New York University Medical Center that human volunteers exposed to radiation-attenuated sporozoites were protected against subsequent challenge infections. Because it is not possible to produce sporozoites on a large scale, the proof of concept for the development of a sporozoite-based vaccine required the production of sporozoite antigens through genetic engineering. One of the first recombinant malarial vaccine antigens studied was one of the circumsporozoite proteins (CSPs), an immunodominant antigen from sporozoites. Initial test results in animals were encouraging both with the expressed recombinant protein and with selected multiple antigen peptides. However, inadequate levels of protective antisporozoite antibody titers were observed in vaccinated human subjects using an immunodominant B-cell CSP epitope conjugated to tetanus toxoid; protective efficacy against malaria was also low.[3]

In order to improve on the protection afforded by CSP or its peptide derivatives, Manuel Patarroyo and his colleagues from the Institute of Immunology in Bogota, Colombia, prepared a wholly synthetic peptide-based vaccine comprising two sequences containing a peptide repeat identified from CSP and three sequences from the erythrocytic stages of *P. falciparum*.[4, 5] Known as SPf66, the vaccine was designed to target both pre-erythrocytic and erythrocytic stages.[1] Under conditions of low transmission in Colombia, South America, the vaccine efficacy was estimated at 34% (95% confidence internal [CI] 19 to 46%). However, two double-blinded randomized studies in sub-Saharan Africa gave widely divergent estimates of efficacy as assessed by protection against a first attack of *P. falciparum* malaria following the complete immunization series.[6] An estimated 31% (95% CI zero to 52%) of Tanzanian children aged 1 to 5 years were noted to be protected under conditions of intense malarial transmission, but in Gambia the vaccine was not effective in infants aged 6 to 11 months. In a recent study with a power of 90% to detect an efficacy of 30%, defined as a reduction in the incidence of first cases of symptomatic falciparum malaria in 1221 children belonging to a Karen ethnic minority in northwestern Thailand, no protection was noted.[6]

Possibly, a more successful attempt to improve on the protection afforded by CSP immunization was conducted by scientists from the Walter Reed Army Institute of Research in Washington, D.C., in collaboration with industry.[7] The candidate vaccine antigen was a hybrid in which CSP was fused to hepatitis B surface antigen. Of the three vaccine formulations evaluated in an unblinded trial of 46 previously unexposed human volunteers, the one comprising the fused protein in an oil-in-water emulsion plus the immune stimulants monophosphoryl lipid A and QS21 was noted both to elicit high antisporozoite antibody titers and to reduce the relative risk of infection to 0.14 (95% CI 0.02 to 0.88; $P < 0.005$). Expanded safety studies are planned.

In addition to the CSPs, other pre-erythrocytic vaccine antigens are being developed in order to target the host immune responses against the infected hepatocyte. Numerous erythrocytic stage vaccine antigens are being developed.[1] Vaccines that target blood stage antigens offer the advantage of direct interference with the stages of *P. falciparum* responsible for anemia and cerebral malaria.[8] Antigens from the sexual stages of *P. falciparum* are also under evaluation as so-called altruistic vaccines that can potentially interrupt malarial transmission.[9] A successful transmission-blocking vaccine has the potential to enhance the efficacy of CSP and related antisporozoite vaccines, which may operate optimally in response to low sporozoite inoculation rates.[9] Several gametocyte and ookinete target antigens are undergoing clinical testing.

Hall has pointed out a number of difficulties anticipated in the evaluation of future malarial vaccines.[1] Among them are the appropriate endpoints in designing a clinical trial, and whether the goals are to prevent *P. falciparum* infection, clinical disease, or malarial transmission.

Leishmaniasis

Leishmania species are flagellated kinetoplastid protozoan parasites transmitted by the bite of a female sandfly. There are cutaneous (CL), mucocutaneous (MCL), and visceralizing (VL) forms of human leishmaniasis. CL and MCL in the Western Hemisphere (predominantly Central and South America) is caused by members of the *L. mexicana* and *L. braziliensis* complex, whereas CL in the Eastern Hemisphere (predominantly India, central Asia, and parts of Africa and the Middle East) is caused by members of the *L. tropica* complex. VL, also known as *kala-azar*, is caused by *L. donovani* in India, Bangladesh, Nepal, and China; *L. infantum* in central Asia, north Africa, and southern Europe; and *L. chagasi* in Latin America. Members of the *L. donovani* complex are important emerging opportunistic pathogens in patients with acquired immunodeficiency disease. Evidence in laboratory mouse experiments points strongly to the importance of helper T cell type 1 (Th1) immune responses in mediating protection against leishmaniasis. Partly for that reason, a number of clinical vaccine trials using bacille Calmette-Guérin (BCG) as an adjuvant are in progress. A first-generation vaccine that employs heat-killed *leishmania* parasites with BCG is under evaluation in endemic parts of Iran and Pakistan.[1]

ANTHELMINTIC VACCINES

Helminthic infections are among the most prevalent infections of humans. Up to 1 billion individuals harbor the nematodes *Ascaris lumbricoides*, *Trichuris trichiura*, and hookworms in their intestines. Hundreds of millions of people are infected with schistosomes and filarial worms. Children are particularly susceptible to heavy infections with intestinal nematodes and schistosomes; frequently they harbor heavier worm burdens than adults living in the same endemic area. There are two major consequences of increased "worminess" in children. First, because most helminths do not replicate in their human host, heavy worm burdens are associated with greater morbidity; for intestinal nematodes and schistosomes this is associated with deficits in physical, intellectual, and cognitive growth. Second, although a variety of anthelmintic drugs are available for reducing worm burdens and effecting cures, the effect is often temporary. Therefore, children re-acquire heavy worm burdens several months after the treatment.[10] This limits the usefulness of anthelmintic agents as a public health control measure.

Because of these unique features, the goals of anthelmintic vaccination are frequently different from those attached to more conventional antiviral and antibacterial vaccines. It is not likely that immunization with defined antigens will elicit sterilizing immunity against complex metazoan organisms. Instead the most important goal is to reduce the worm burden below the disease-causing threshold. The essential concept of anthelmintic vaccines is to attempt to immunize against *disease* rather than *infection*. Examples of this idea would be to reduce the hookworm burden below the threshold that results in significant intestinal blood loss or to reduce the schistosome burden below the threshold that results in significant egg deposition and subsequent granuloma formation in the liver, intestines, and bladder. An alternative approach to antidisease vaccination would be to directly block the action of parasite-induced pathogenic processes. In the case of hookworm this would require blocking parasite-derived virulence factors that cause blood loss, and for schistosomiasis blocking egg deposition. It is likely that anthelmintic vaccination will not be used in isolation, but rather in conjunction with other control efforts including conventional chemotherapy.[11, 12]

Hookworm Disease

Human hookworm infection is a leading cause of anemia and malnutrition among children in developing countries. An estimated 194 million cases occur in China alone. There are two major species, *Ancylostoma duodenale* and *Necator americanus*. The former causes greater blood loss and consequently more protein malnutrition and iron deficiency. Chronic hookworm infection during childhood has been linked to malnutrition, physical growth retardation, diminished intelligence, and diminished cognition. Humans become infected when third-stage larvae either penetrate through the skin (*N. americanus* and *A. duodenale*) or are ingested (*A. duodenale* only). On host entry, the larvae undergo extraintestinal migration in the vasculature and reach the heart and lungs. Hookworm larval lung migration is associated with a mild pneumonitis; the larvae ascend the airways and reach the larynx before they are coughed and swallowed. The larvae molt twice in the intestine to become adult hookworms that invade tissue and cause blood loss.

Early attempts at developing a hookworm vaccine relied on the observation that numerous small doses of living larvae could confer resistance against challenge hookworm infections. Resistance was measured by reductions in the worm burden, the worms' size, and the worms' fecundity. Immunity was seldom sterilizing. Later it was noted that larger doses of living larvae could be administered over shorter time periods if the larvae were first damaged by ionizing radiation. This provided the basis for commercial radiation-attenuated hookworm larval vaccines that could be administered to dogs in two doses. The canine hookworm vaccine was marketed first in Florida and later the eastern United States during the 1970s, but ultimately it failed as a commercial veterinary product.[13] Among the reasons for its lack of commercial success were the high production costs in harvesting living larvae, the limited shelf life of the product, and the misperceptions on the part of pet owners and veterinarians regarding an antidisease vaccine that reduced the worm burden but did not usually elicit sterilizing immunity.

It is not feasible to develop human antihookworm vaccines that use living larvae, damaged or otherwise. However, studies are in progress to identify vaccine antigens from the infective larval stages of hookworms that can reproduce the reduction in worm burdens afforded by the live vaccines.[14] One class of antigens under investigations is the *Ancylostoma*-secreted proteins (ASPs), which are released by host-stimulated infective hookworm larvae and contain amino acid sequence homologous to those of the major antigens from insect venoms.[15] Immunization of mice with an alum precipitate of recombinant ASP-1, a 45-kDa protein, reduces the worm burden on challenge with hookworm larvae.[16] Studies are also under way to genetically engineer hookworm immunodominant antigens that are recognized by mice immunized with living hookworm larvae.[17] Mice, however, are nonpermissive mammalian hosts, so testing in human volunteers may have to await the results of canine or even nonhuman primate challenge studies.

Schistosomiasis

Schistosomes are snail-transmitted, water-borne parasitic platyhelminths (order Trematoda). High rates of infection occur near bodies of fresh water such as tributaries of the Nile River in Egypt and Dongting and Boyang Lakes in China. The three major species groups of schistosomes, *Schistosoma mansoni*, *S. haematobium*, and the *S. japonicum* complex (including *S. japonicum* and *S. mekongi*), are typically distinguished by their unique snail vectors, location within the host vasculature, and egg morphology. Members of the *S. japonicum* complex also have important domestic animal reservoir hosts (pigs, cattle, water buffaloes). Asexual reproduction of the parasites occurs in freshwater snail intermediate hosts that release large numbers of free-swimming infective larval schistosomes, known as *cercariae*, into the water. The cercariae are attracted to linoleic acid and other skin components, causing them to attach and penetrate percutaneously with the aid of proteases. On host entry, the cercariae lose their characteristic tail and the migrating schistosomula spend the next few weeks migrating through the blood stream and lungs until they reach the liver. Here they differentiate into male and female schistosomes. Male and female worm pairs migrate through the portal vasculature until they reach their final destination in the mesenteric or bladder venules. The worm pairs release eggs, which exit from the body in feces or urine and then hatch in fresh water. Freshly hatched miracidia swim via the action of their cilia. They are pluripotent and potentially can give rise to thousands of progeny on their entry into a suitable snail host.

Most of the morbidity associated with schistosomiasis occurs when the eggs fail to exit from the definitive human host. Trapped in the intestinal or bladder wall, or in the liver as they are swept up by the portal circulation, the eggs elicit granulomas and host fibrosis. In the liver, the so-called Symmer pipestem fibrosis leads to portal hypertension and hepatosplenomegaly. Because of the location and greater numbers of eggs produced by *S. japonicum*, schistosomiasis japonica tends to be the most severe form. In addition, children with chronic schistosomiasis japonica (and possibly other forms as well) have deficits in physical growth.

A number of different approaches have been taken to design antischistosomal vaccines. As in other systems, the administration of radiation-attenuated cercariae results in the best protection to date. The mechanisms of resistance associated with the live cercarial vaccine have been worked out over the last 10 years using a mouse model.[18, 19] Briefly, the damaged cercariae successfully penetrate the skin, whenupon they enter skin-draining lymph nodes (SLNs). Antigens released by the damaged cercariae in the SLNs stimulate the proliferation of helper T cells with Th1 features, including the release of interferon-γ (IFN-γ) as a predominant cytokine. After induction of the primary immune response in the SLNs, lymphocytes mediating delayed-type hypersensitivity responses appear in the circulation. A proportion of attenuated parasites migrate from the skin to the lungs. The major site of immune elimination and parasite attrition occurs at this site. The arrival of schistosomula in the lungs provokes an infiltration of T lymphocytes, recruited from SLNs. Challenge of the vaccinated laboratory animals results in a second recruitment into the lungs of IFN-γ– and interleukin 3–secreting effector-memory T cells that have the capacity to block parasite migration. Thus, the mononuclear cell infiltrate triggered by the arrival of challenge parasites in the lungs aggregates into a dense pulmonary focus of cells that prevents worm migration. IFN-γ is a key cytokine in this process, since its neutralization results in a looser pulmonary focus that cannot impede the invading parasites.

In part based on this paradigm, vigorous attention has focused on potential vaccine antigens from the schistosomula stages. Vaccination with stage-specific schistosomula surface antigens has resulted in disappointing protection, usually less than 40%.[11] Somewhat better protection has been achieved in antigens shared between schistosomula and adult schistosomes including parasite-derived myosin (63 kDa), paramyosin (97 kDa), triose phosphate isomerase (28 kDa), gluathione *S*-transferases (GSTs, 26 and 28 kDa), a fatty acid–binding protein (14 kDa), and a 23-kDa surface protein.[11] Vaccine studies with these recombinant antigens have been conducted with numerous adjuvants including alum, BCG, saponin and *Bordetella pertussis*. Because of the suggested role of IFN-γ and Th1 cellular immune responses in mediating protection, there have been some efforts to bias the host cytokine profile at the time of vaccination. Some success has been reported in this regard using interleukin 12 as an adjuvant,[20] as well as with DNA immunizations.

A second approach to vaccination against schistosomiasis has been to target the fecundity of female adult schistosomes in order to diminish egg excretion into target host organs. Success with this approach has been reported by immunizing mice and large-animal reservoir hosts, including pigs and water buffaloes, with *S. japonicum* 26-kDa GST and other molecules.[21, 22] The possibility remains that if levels of egg excretion can be reduced by vaccination of animal reservoir hosts, then this approach might be sufficient to reduce schistosomiasis japonica transmission. Alternatively, it has been proposed that egg deposition and granuloma formation in the human host can be manipulated by immunotherapy since granuloma formation around the schistosome egg depends heavily on host cytokines including tumor necrosis factor and Th2-associated cytokines.[11, 23]

Bergquist and colleagues point out that the development of a schistosomiasis vaccine depends on the acquisition of immunity noted in adult humans living in endemic areas.[11] A major goal of a human schistosomiasis vaccine will be to accelerate this process through either immunization with a cocktail of recombinant antigens, DNA immunizations, or host cytokine manipulation through bioimmunotherapy.

REFERENCES

1. Hall BF. Vaccines for parasitic diseases of humans. In Ostriker R, and Savage L (eds). Vaccines: New Advances in Technologies and Applications. Southborough, MA, IBC Biomedical Library, 1996, pp 6.4.1–6.4.16.
2. Nussenzweig RS, Zavala F. A malaria vaccine based on a sporozoite antigen. N Engl J Med 336:128–130, 1997.
3. Nussenzweig V, Nussensweig RS. Rationale for the development of an engineered sporozoite malaria vaccine. Adv Immunol 45:283–334, 1989.
4. Patarroyo ME, Amador R, Clavijo P, et al. A synthetic vaccine protects humans against challenge with asexual blood stages of *Plasmodium falciparum*. Nature 332:158–161, 1988.
5. Moreno A, Patarroyo ME. Malaria vaccines. Curr Opin Immunol 7:607–611, 1995.
6. Nosten F, Luxembruger C, Kyle DE, et al. Randomised double-blind placebo-controlled trial of SPf66 malaria vaccine in children in northwestern Thailand. Lancet 348:701–707, 1996.
7. Stoute JA, Slaoui M, Heppner DG, et al. A preliminary evaluation of a recombinant circumsporozoite protein vaccine against *Plasmodium falciparum* malaria. N Engl J Med 336:86–91, 1997.
8. Greenwood B. What can be expected from malaria vaccines. In Hoffman SL (ed). Malaria Vaccine Development: A Multi-Immune Response Approach. Washington, DC, American Society for Microbiology, 1996, Chapter 11, pp 277–301.
9. Kaslow DC. Transmission-blocking vaccines. In Hoffman SL (ed). Malaria Vaccine Development: A Multi-Immune Response Approach. Washington, DC, American Society for Microbiology, 1996, Chapter 8, pp 181–227.
10. Albonico M, Smith PG, Ercole E, et al. Rate of reinfection with intestinal nematodes after treatment of children with mebendazole or albendazole in a highly endemic area. Trans R Soc Trop Med Hyg 89:538–541, 1995.
11. Bergquist NR, Hall BF, James S. Schistosomiasis vaccine development. Immunologist 2/4:131–134, 1994.
12. McCarthy JS, Nutman TB. Perspective: Prospects for development of vaccines against human helminth infections. J Infect Dis 174:1384–1390, 1996.
13. Miller TA. Industrial development and field use of the canine hookworm vaccine. Adv Parasitol 16:333–342, 1978.
14. Hotez PJ, Hawdon JM, Cappello M, et al. Molecular approaches to vaccinating against hookworm disease. Pediatr Res 40:515–521, 1996.
15. Hotez PJ, Ghosh K, Hawdon J, et al. Vaccines for hookworm infection. Pediatr Infect Dis J 16:935–940, 1997.
16. Ghosh K, Hawdon J, Hotez P. Vaccination with alum-precipitated recombinant *Ancylostoma*-secreted protein 1 protects mice against challenge infections with infective hookworm (*Ancylostoma caninum*) larvae. J Infect Dis 174:1380–1383, 1996.
17. Xiao SH, Ren HN, Yang YQ, et al. Protective immunity in mice elicited by living infective third-stage hookworm larvae (Shanghai strain of *Ancylostoma caninum*). Chin Med J 111:43–48, 1998.
18. Wilson RA. T cell derived cytokines in lung-phase immunity to *Schistosoma mansoni*. Mem Inst Oswaldo Cruz 87(suppl IV):105–110, 1992.
19. Richter D, Harn DA, Matuschka F-R. The irradiated cercariae vaccine model: Looking on the bright side of radiation. Parasitol Today 11:288–293, 1995.
20. Wynn TA, Jankovic D, Hieny S, et al. IL-12 enhances vaccine-induced immunity to *Schistosoma mansoni* in mice and decreases T helper 2 cytokine expression, IgE production and tissue eosinophilia. *J Immunol* 154:4701–4709, 1995.
21. Liu SX, Song GC, Xu XY, et al. Anti-fecundity immunity induced in pigs vaccinated with recombinant *Schistosoma japonicum* 26 kDa glutathione-*S*-transferase. Parasite Immunol 17:335–340, 1995.
22. Liu SX, Song GC, Xu YX, et al. Progress in the development of a vaccine against schistosomiasis in China. Int J Infect Dis 2:176–180, 1998.
23. Amiri P, Locksley RM, Parslow TG, et al. Tumor necrosis factor α restores granulomas and induces parasite egg-laying schistosome-infected SCID mice. Nature 356:604–607, 1992.

chapter

41 Rotavirus Vaccines*

H. Fred Clark

Roger I. Glass

Paul A. Offit

Rotaviruses are the leading cause of severe dehydrating diarrhea in infants and young children throughout the world. Virtually all children are infected by the time they reach 2 to 3 years of age.[1, 2] Even in developed nations, where standards of hygiene are high, rotavirus is the most common cause of infant diarrhea.[3]

In the United States, the most recent epidemiological studies estimate that rotavirus accounts for about 500,000 physician visits, 50,000 hospitalizations, and 20 to 40 deaths of children with diarrhea.[4, 5] The economic burden of disease is estimated to exceed $1 billion each year in medical and indirect costs.[4, 6, 7] In less developed countries, rotaviruses rank highest among the multiple microbial causes of severe gastroenteritis in children and contribute disproportionately to the mortality associated with the disease.[8–10] Rotavirus is estimated to cause 480,000 to 640,000 deaths in children each year (approximately 20% of the estimated 2.4 to 3.2 million deaths from diarrhea).[11–14] Whereas extensive global efforts to disseminate oral rehydration therapy in the developing world have undoubtedly contributed to a recent decline in diarrhea deaths,[15] the continuing mortality associated with rotavirus, 1600 to 2400 deaths per day, suggests that prevention through universal application of a safe, economical, and efficacious vaccine would be preferable. Because rotaviruses remain the most common cause of severe diarrhea in children in regions with high standards of health and sanitation, a rotavirus vaccine would have universal application as part of childhood immunization programs.

Several candidate rotavirus vaccines have proved to be safe and effective in clinical trials. One particular rotavirus vaccine was licensed by the U.S. Food and Drug Administration on Sept 1, 1998, while this book was in press. The Advisory Committee on Immunization Practices (ACIP) has already voted to recommend universal vaccination of infants, as described below. This review provides a description of the licensed vaccine as well as the candidate vaccines for the future.

BACKGROUND

The Virus

Rotavirus infection has been detected in most common species of domestic animals and in many species of wild mammals and birds. Whereas the great majority of human and animal rotaviruses share common group antigens (group A rotaviruses),[16] animal rotaviruses can generally be distinguished from human strains on the basis of type-specific surface antigens. Animals appear to be neither a reservoir for human strains nor a common source for transmission of rotaviruses to humans.

Certain rotaviruses of bovine or simian origin were propagated in cell culture to high titer before the more recent development of methods to propagate strains from humans.[17, 18] Therefore, the molecular structure of rotavirus was largely determined by studies of the bovine strain, Nebraska calf diarrhea virus,[19] and the simian strain, SA11.[20]

Rotaviruses are 70-nm icosahedral viruses that constitute a distinct genus of the family *Reoviridae*. The virus is formed by three shells (an outer capsid, inner capsid, and core) that encase the genome of 11 segments of double-stranded RNA. For the most part, each gene segment codes for a single protein. These segments can be separated on the basis of their molecular weight by migration, when subjected to polyacrylamide gel electrophoresis.[16] When mixed infections with distinct rotavirus strains occur under experimental conditions or in nature, the gene segments may reassort independently, producing progeny virus of mixed parentage. Analysis of such "reassortant" rotaviruses has led to identification of the gene segments encoding each of the structural polypeptides. This identification, in turn, has made possible techniques to intentionally reassort rotavirus strains and prepare candidate vaccine strains that incorporate desirable phenotypic characteristics of different parent strains.[21–23]

Four major structural and nonstructural proteins of rotavirus are of interest in vaccine development (Table 41–1). The outer shell of rotavirus contains two distinct proteins (VP4 and VP7), each of which bears type-specific antigenic determinants, elicits serotype-specific neutralizing antibodies, and induces serotype-specific protective immune responses in vivo.[24–26] Protein VP7 is coded by gene segment 7, 8, or 9 in different rotavirus strains; protein VP4 is coded by gene segment 4.[16] The VP7 molecule is glycosylated in the mature virion, but the carbohydrate residue is not essential for expression of its antigenic or immunogenic activity.[27] The most

*Recently licensed in the United States.

Table 41–1. **BIOLOGICALLY SIGNIFICANT STRUCTURAL AND NONSTRUCTURAL ROTAVIRUS PROTEINS**

DESIGNATION	PRODUCT OF GENE SEGMENT	APPROXIMATE MOLECULAR WEIGHT	VIRION LOCALIZATION	BIOLOGICAL SIGNIFICANCE
VP4*	4	88,000	Outer capsid	Type-specific antigen, hemagglutinin
VP6	6	44,000	Inner capsid	Major subgroup antigen
VP7	7, 8, or 9	38,000	Outer capsid	Type-specific antigen
NSP4	10	28,000	Nonstructural	Enterotoxin

*Trypsin treatment of virion leads to production of VP4 cleavage products designated VP5 (60,000 MW) and VP8 (27,000 MW).
From Estes MK, Cohen J. Rotavirus gene structure and function. Microbiol Rev 53:410–449, 1989; Bellamy AR, Both GW. Molecular biology of rotaviruses. Adv Virus Res 38:1–43, 1990; and Ball JM, Tian P, Zeng CQY, et al. Age-dependent diarrhea induced by a rotaviral nonstructural glycoprotein. Science 272:101–104, 1996.

highly represented viral structural protein is VP6, which is found in the internal capsid and bears group-specific antigenic determinants.[28] The nonstructural protein NSP4 has been shown to be an enterotoxin.[29] Three structural proteins (VP1, VP2, and VP3) form the viral core, and four other nonstructural proteins (NSP1, NSP2, NSP3, and NSP5) are made during infection.

Surface proteins VP7 and VP4 express distinct antigenic specificities that may vary independently.[24–26] Therefore, a new binomial antigenic nomenclature has been developed in which the VP7 types are designated G types (because VP7 is a glycoprotein) and the VP4 types are designated P types (because protease cleavage of VP4 is essential for virus infectivity).[30, 31] Whereas 10 G types and 7 P types have been found in rotavirus strains isolated from children worldwide, 4 major types predominate. P1aG1 appears to be the most common cause of disease worldwide; important incidence is also associated with P1bG2, P1aG3, and P1aG4. The current P designations and their usual G associations are listed in Table 41–2.

Historically, rotavirus serotypes were designated solely on the basis of G type specificities[32] (because the neutralizing antibody response to parenterally inoculated rotavirus in experimental animals is predominantly to the G antigen). However, contradictory results have been obtained in various evaluations of the relative magnitude of antibody responses to G and P antigens after natural infection or immunization of children.[33–35] Until this question is resolved, inclusion of both P and G proteins will have to be considered in attempts to design an ideal vaccine.

Table 41–2. **COMMON ASSOCIATIONS OF GROUP A ROTAVIRUS P (VP4) AND G (VP7) TYPES**

PHENOTYPE	VP4 SEROTYPE [GENOTYPE]	VP7 TYPE ASSOCIATIONS
Pathogenic	1a [8]	1, 3, 4, 9
Pathogenic	1b [4]	2
Asymptomatic (“nursery strains”)	2 [6]	1, 2, 3, 4
Pathogenic	3a	1 (strain K8)

From Gorziglia M, Larralde G, Kapikian A, Chanock RM. Antigenic relationships among human rotaviruses as determined by outer capsid VP4. Proc Natl Acad Sci U S A 87:7155–7159, 1990; Kobayashi N, Taniguchi K, Urasawa T, Urasawa S. Preparation and characterization of a neutralizing monoclonal antibody directed to VP4 of rotavirus strain K8 which has unique neutralization epitopes. Arch Virol 121:153–162, 1991; and The Rotavirus Nomenclature Working Group (M. Estes, personal communication).

Clinical Disease

Evaluation of children admitted to the hospital with rotavirus infection reveals a consistent pattern. The disease is characterized by the sudden onset of watery diarrhea, fever, and vomiting.[36–39] Most disease is mild, but about 1 of every 50 children infected with rotavirus[8, 11] will develop dehydration associated with severe loss of sodium and chloride in the stools and a compensated metabolic acidosis. In children admitted to the hospital with dehydration, fever and vomiting usually persist for 2 to 3 days and diarrhea for 4 to 5 days.[36–39]

Although excretion of rotavirus has been reported in association with other clinical entities such as aseptic meningitis,[40, 41] sudden infant death syndrome,[42] and Crohn disease,[43] there is no causal evidence implicating rotavirus in the pathogenesis of these diseases.

Pathogenesis

Studies of rotavirus pathology and pathophysiology in animals and humans have focused on several important questions: (1) In which intestinal and nonintestinal tissues do rotaviruses replicate and induce disease? (2) By what mechanism does rotavirus induce gastroenteritis? (3) Why is rotavirus-induced gastroenteritis primarily a disease of the young? and (4) What factors of the host determine why rotavirus disease is more severe in developing than in developed countries?

Studies of natural rotavirus infection indicate that rotavirus replication is restricted to mature villous epithelial cells in the mucosal surface of the small intestine.[44–49] Replication progresses from the proximal to distal small intestine.[47, 50] Rotaviruses do not appear to replicate in immature epithelial cells of the villous crypt or in M cells overlying Peyer patches.[51] In addition, rotaviruses have never been detected consistently in the blood or sites distant to the intestine. Although simian rotaviruses replicate in hepatic epithelial cells of inbred mice,[52] the relevance of these findings to human infection remains unclear.

Rotavirus replication in intestinal epithelial cells causes several physiological and morphological changes. Infected animals experience decreased absorption of sodium, glucose, and water and have decreased levels of intestinal lactase, alkaline phosphatase, and sucrase activity.[53, 54] These findings are consistent with an absorptive abnormality associated with an accelerated migration of immature epithelial cells toward the villous tip. Because no inflammatory changes occur in the lamina propria, in the Peyer patch, or at the intestinal mucosal surface,[44–49] it is unlikely that intestinal epithelial cell damage is mediated by the host immune response.

Rotavirus infections are more likely to be severe in infants and young children 3 to 24 months of age than in younger infants or older children and adults.[55–58] Several studies have attempted to explain these differences in age susceptibility. First, children of increasing age may be protected by a virus-specific immune response generated by repeated natural infections.[59] Protection of younger infants may be mediated by passively transferred maternal antibodies. Second, infant mice have been found to have a larger percentage than older mice do of intestinal epithelial cells with putative rotavirus-binding proteins on the surface,[60] an observation that correlates directly with the age susceptibility to disease. Third, rotavirus strains endemic in certain newborn nurseries ("nursery strains"), although of different G serotypes, have been found to contain homologous gene segments encoding the surface protein VP4.[61] Last, rotavirus entry into target cells is facilitated by cleavage of VP4,[62, 63] which occurs in the presence of trypsin, elastase, or pancreatin.[64] Quantities of these exopeptidases are decreased in intestinal fluid secretions of newborn infants compared with older infants and young children.[65]

A rotavirus nonstructural protein (NSP4) was recently shown to act as a viral enterotoxin.[29] Exposure of intestinal epithelial cells to NSP4 induced diarrhea in suckling mice in an age-dependent, dose-dependent, and specific manner. Disease was caused by excess chloride secretion by a calcium-dependent signaling pathway. This finding is consistent with studies using reassortant rotaviruses generated from pathogenic and nonpathogenic strains,[66] indicating that the genes which encoded VP3, VP4, VP7, and NSP4 were *all* required to reconstitute virulence. Because virus replication is required for generation of nonstructural proteins, it is not surprising that attenuation of rotavirus virulence can occur in the absence of attenuating NSP4 (R. L. Ward, personal communication).

Last, children in developing countries are more susceptible to severe rotavirus disease. This finding is probably based on poor medical access, poor nutrition, and concomitant infections with other viruses and enteropathogenic bacteria.[67] Several studies in animals support the hypotheses that poor nutrition[68, 69] or associated bacterial infections may enhance the severity of rotavirus-induced enteritis.[51, 70, 71]

Immunologic Factors Associated with Protection Against Disease

Protection against reinfection with rotavirus centers on two important questions. Which effector arm or arms of the immune response mediate protection? What is the importance of including different rotavirus serotypes in an optimal vaccine?

In 1983, the role of immunity to rotavirus was demonstrated by studies of natural infection in neonates.[72] Neonates infected in the first month of life were not protected against rotavirus reinfection but were protected against severe disease on reinfection. On the other hand, neonates free of rotavirus infection during the first month of life were fully susceptible to diarrheal disease associated with the first rotavirus infection. Since then, studies of natural infection in infants and young children indicate that first infections protect against severe disease on reinfection.[73, 74] Protection is mediated by the presence of virus-specific immunoglobulin A (IgA) at the intestinal mucosal surface[75, 76] and is predicted by the presence of virus-specific IgA in the serum or feces.[75–77]

Although natural rotavirus infection protects against moderate to severe disease caused by reinfection, some children experience repeated episodes of diarrhea with the same serotype during the following rotavirus season,[78–89] and a small number of children develop symptomatic rotavirus infection twice within the same season.[90] These observations are consistent with the fact that effector functions (such as production of virus-specific secretory IgA [sIgA]) at mucosal surfaces are usually short-lived and that rotavirus-specific IgA is often not detected at the intestinal mucosal surface within 1 year of symptomatic infection.[76]

The presence of rotavirus-specific IgA at the intestinal mucosal surface (as reflected in the feces) and in serum is predictive of protection against disease in studies of natural infection but not in vaccine trials. Consequently, after immunization of infants with simian × human reassortant rotaviruses (see later), virus-specific IgA in feces or serum does not predict protection against disease.[91–93] Several explanations for this phenomenon have been posited. In humans, protection against disease after immunization with animal rotaviruses may be mediated by virus-specific cytotoxic T lymphocytes (CTLs). Whereas the role of rotavirus-specific CTLs in protection against human disease is unknown, some evidence supports their importance in protection against disease in animals. First, rotavirus-specific CTLs are detected at the intestinal mucosal surface of mice acutely after infection.[94] Second, passive transfer of rotavirus-specific CTLs ameliorates disease or ablates rotavirus shedding in experimental animals.[95, 96] Third, rotavirus-specific CTLs have been found to protect against challenge in animals deficient in the capacity to make IgA heavy chain (J_HD knockout mice).[97] Alternatively, cytokines with antiviral activity may be generated either earlier or in greater quantities after immunization compared with primary infection.

A number of studies found that natural infection or immunization of children with one rotavirus serotype induced protection against challenge with a different serotype (heterotypic protection).[98, 99] Heterotypic protection may be mediated by antibodies directed against antigenically conserved inner capsid proteins that are actively transported through rotavirus-infected villous epithelial cells,[100] rotavirus-specific CTLs that broadly cross-react with cells infected with different rotavirus serotypes,[101] or antiviral cytokines generated by memory T cells.

Both outer capsid proteins (VP4 [P type] and VP7 [G type]) contain epitopes that evoke both serotype-specific and cross-reactive antibodies.[102] The relative importance of including both human P and G types in reassortant viruses containing simian or bovine rotavirus backgrounds remains undetermined. However, it is clear that after a primary, natural rotavirus infection, infants develop virus-specific neutralizing antibodies in serum directed against the infecting G type at levels greater than those directed against other G types.[103–107] Similarly, children are more likely to be protected against disease after reinfection with a G type to which the child has already been exposed.[77, 99] For these reasons, it may be of value for a rotavirus vaccine to contain all G types to which the child is likely to be exposed.

Diagnosis

Electron microscopy, which once served as the "gold standard" for diagnosis of rotavirus infections, has now been replaced by enzyme-linked immunosorbent assays (ELISAs). ELISAs, which use either polyclonal or monoclonal antibody preparations directed against the antigenically conserved inner capsid protein VP6, are as sensitive as electron microscopy but easier and less expensive to use.[108–110] However, false-positive ELISA results have been reported.[111]

More rapid detection of rotavirus antigens in fecal samples can be achieved by a latex agglutination assay.[112, 113] Latex agglutination can be completed in several minutes and does not require the use of special equipment. However, latex agglutination is somewhat less sensitive than an ELISA.

The detection of rotavirus by polyacrylamide gel electrophoresis, although not commercially available, offers several advantages over the ELISA and latex agglutination assays. Polyacrylamide gel electrophoresis is as sensitive as the ELISA but is absolutely specific for the presence of rotavirus. In addition, detection of specific migration patterns of segmented double-stranded RNA (electropherotypes) is of value in determining specific strains associated with community outbreaks or nosocomial infections.

EPIDEMIOLOGY

Rotavirus is a universal infection in young children.[2] All children are exposed to rotavirus and acquire antibodies by 3 to 5 years of age. Most rotavirus diarrhea occurs during the first 3 years of life. In the first 3 months of life, infections are generally asymptomatic, an observation that has not been fully explained but may in part be due to the protection afforded by maternal antibody (see earlier).[72] First infections after 3 months of age are generally associated with diarrhea that can be mild or severe, whereas subsequent exposures lead to milder illness or asymptomatic infections.[59, 73, 74] The observation that all children throughout the world are infected early in life suggests that rotavirus is not transmitted (like other bacterial and parasitic pathogens) through fecally contaminated water or food. Therefore, improvements in water, sanitation, and hygiene are unlikely to alter the incidence of disease. At the same time, the role of immunity in protecting against subsequent disease has been supported by the observations that the incidence and severity of disease decrease with increasing age, that neonatal infections protect children against subsequent disease,[72, 114] and that children observed from birth rarely have repeated disease and when they do, the illness is extremely mild.[59] The priority placed on the prevention of rotavirus by vaccination is predicated on the great global disease burden of rotavirus,[1, 115] the recognition that natural immunity is protective, and the expectation that alternative public health measures, including the provision of clean food and water, are unlikely to prevent disease.

Little is known about the exact mode of transmission of rotavirus. The inoculum size is likely to be small, which favors spread by airborne droplets or person-to-person contact. In a mouse model, airborne spread of epidemic diarrhea by a murine strain has been identified.[116] Furthermore, the disease has a distinct winter seasonality in temperate climates, similar to that seen for viruses spread by the respiratory route, such as influenza and measles. Annual epidemics in the United States begin in the Southwest and spread to the North and East (Fig. 41–1). Humans are believed to be the only reservoir of human strains, and transmission of animal strains to humans seems unlikely. Nevertheless, although classical epidemiology has failed to identify transmission of virus from animals to humans, reassortant strains composed of genomic segments from both human and animal rotaviruses have been identified, which indicates that some mixing of strains must occur in nature and that this reassortment may be important for virus evolution.[117–119]

Certain clues about immunity and transmission of rotavirus can be gained from epidemic investigations and special studies. Whereas immunity is believed to protect adults from disease, parents and caretakers of children with rotavirus diarrhea can get mild disease, perhaps because practices such as diaper changing ex-

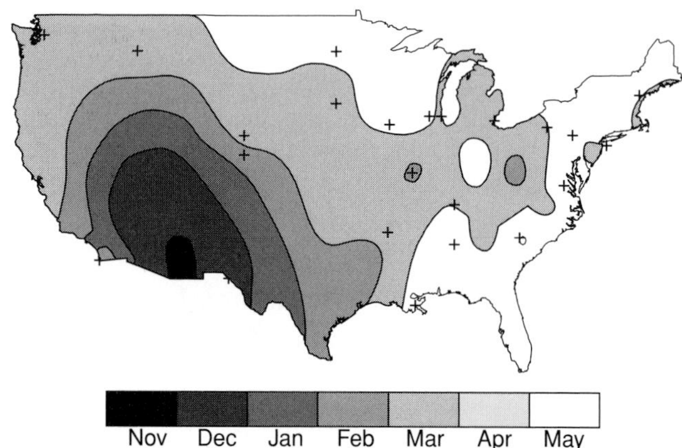

Figure 41–1. Month of peak rotavirus activity—United States, July 1996 to June 1997, plus participating NREVSS laboratories. (From Laboratory-based surveillance for rotavirus—United States, July 1996–June 1997. MMWR Morb Mortal Wkly Rep 46:1092–1094, 1997.)

pose them to a large infectious dose.[120] Outbreaks in daycare centers and hospitals can spread rapidly among nonimmune infants and young children presumably because of person-to-person contact, airborne or droplet spread, or contact with contaminated toys.[121–123] In the elderly, outbreaks have been described that may be linked to waning immunity. In travelers to developing countries, who would be expected to be immune, rotavirus has been identified as a cause of diarrhea, perhaps because the mode of transmission is different or the inoculum size is greater.[124] Finally, people immunocompromised by human immunodeficiency virus infection,[125] hereditary immunodeficiency,[126, 127] immunosuppression for organ transplantation,[128] or chemotherapy can develop rotavirus diarrhea with virus shedding that can persist for months.

Several differences in the epidemiology of rotavirus diarrhea between developed and developing countries may have an impact on future considerations concerning the use of vaccines.[129] The distinct winter seasonality of rotavirus hospitalizations in temperate climates stands in contrast to the year-round exposure seen in tropical settings.[10] This means that a child born in a temperate climate after the rotavirus season will have to wait a full year until the next exposure, whereas a child born in a tropical setting could be exposed any day of the year. Consequently, the average age at first infection is younger in developing countries in tropical areas, and most rotavirus diarrhea in such sites occurs during a child's first year of life, compared with the first 2 or 3 years of life in developed countries. This will have a direct impact on the timing of immunization; in a developing country, an effective vaccine program will require earlier and higher levels of coverage than programs in developed countries. In the laboratory, fecal specimens from children from developed countries have a simpler virological picture, typically with a single strain of virus drawn from one of the four common serotypes found globally.[130] In developing countries, the rate of mixed infections with two or more strains can reach 30% and the viruses can include uncommon serotypes not found in other parts of the world.[131–133]

The burden of rotavirus diarrhea for children in developing countries became evident when the first diagnostic tests were used to study the etiology of diarrhea in hospitalized children (Table 41–3). In more than 100 studies conducted around the world among children younger than 5 years hospitalized for diarrhea, rotavirus was the most common cause of diarrhea (detected in 20 to 60% of cases). Given that rotavirus is the most common cause of severe dehydrating diarrhea in children younger than 2 years and that an estimated 2.4 to 3.2 million children in this age group die each year of diarrhea, it has been estimated that between 480,000 and 640,000 children die each year of rotavirus diarrhea.[1, 115] Longitudinal studies of children observed from birth to 2 years of age suggest that the incidence of rotavirus diarrhea varies directly with the intensity of surveillance. These studies indicate that most children (i.e., 1 in 1.2 to 1.3) will have an episode of rotavirus diarrhea in their first 3 to 5 years of life and, depending on the locale,[134–136] require medical attention or treatment.

In developed countries, rotavirus was long considered to cause a mild diarrheal illness of children that was rarely if ever severe and never fatal. Whereas early studies documented a clear winter peak of hospitalizations (accounting for as much as 80% of cases), no child in the United States was known to have died with a diagnosis of rotavirus diarrhea. These findings suggested that rotavirus disease was more a nuisance than a severe problem.[3] However, a series of studies examining the national profile of diarrheal hospitalizations and deaths in the United States put national data in a different light.[6, 137, 138] Whereas no *International Classification of Diseases* code existed before 1993 that was specific for rotavirus diarrhea, the distinct winter peak in both hospitalizations and deaths for diarrhea among children 4 to 23 months of age was consistent with their being caused by rotavirus. Furthermore, in the United States, these peaks had a unique pattern that began in the Southwest in November and moved northeast, reaching New England in March and April. When laboratories were surveyed, rotavirus detections demonstrated the same temporal and geographical patterns.[139–141] On the basis of these data, the Centers for Disease Control and Prevention group developed national estimates for rotavirus diarrhea indicating that each year, 60 to 80% of the entire birth cohort of children will develop a mild diarrheal illness (~2.7 million episodes per year), 1 in 6.5 will seek medical attention, 1 in 72 (54,000 patients) will be hospitalized, and 1 in 200,000 (20 children) will die of rotavirus.[142] These data were similar to those developed by Matson and coworkers for the United States[143] and are lower than similar estimates made for

Table 41–3. **ESTIMATED DISEASE BURDEN OF ROTAVIRUS GASTROENTERITIS IN THE UNITED STATES AND WORLD (1995)**

	UNITED STATES		WORLD	
PARAMETER	**Total**	**Risk per Child**	**Total**	**Risk per Child**
Births	3.9 million	—	130 million	—
Episodes of rotavirus gastroenteritis	2.7 million	68 (1:1.4)	100 million	77 (1:1.3)
Physician or emergency department visits	600,000	15 (1:65)		
Hospitalizations	48,000	1.2 (1:81)		
Moderate-severe disease			16 million	13 (1:8)
Deaths	20	0.0005 (1:200,000)	600,000–873,000	0.4–0.6 (1:160–1:230)
Medical costs	$300 million		?	
Indirect and direct costs	$1.1 billion		?	

the United Kingdom[144] and Finland. The cost of medical care in the United States was estimated to be more than $400 million; indirect costs are estimated to be in excess of $1 billion.[7]

PASSIVE IMMUNIZATION

Amelioration of acute rotavirus infection in infants has been afforded by passive immunization with rotavirus-specific antibodies; sources of rotavirus-specific antibodies were either pooled, commercial preparations of human serum immune globulin or colostrum from cows parenterally immunized with rotavirus.[145–148] In both immunocompetent and immunocompromised children, oral inoculation with rotavirus-specific antibodies caused a decrease in the number of days with diarrhea as well as a decrease in the length of hospital stay.

ACTIVE IMMUNIZATION

Nonhuman Rotaviruses

Bovine Strain RIT4237

The first rotavirus vaccine to be evaluated in humans was the veterinary strain Nebraska calf diarrhea virus (P6G6),[19] adapted to primate cell culture and named RIT4237 for use in human trials.[149] This virus had previously been attenuated for calves by approximately 200 passages in bovine cell culture.[150] RIT4237 was administered to infants most often in a high dose of 10^8 tissue culture infective doses ($TCID_{50}$). Induction of immunity was apparently associated with minimal replication, because transient shedding of vaccine virus was noted in only 20%[151] or less[152] of vaccinees. Between 50 and 70% of vaccinees had a humoral immune response measured by rotavirus-specific ELISA for IgG or IgA or by virus neutralization.[152, 153] No adverse clinical effects were noted in infants as young as 2 weeks.

In two initial efficacy trials of RIT4237 in 6- to 12-month-old Finnish infants, 50% and 58%, respectively, were protected against all rotavirus diarrhea, but 88% and 82%, respectively, were protected against "clinically significant" disease.[153, 154] Protection was heterotypic because the bovine vaccine was effective against natural challenge with serotype G1 human rotavirus. In subsequent efficacy trials performed in Gambia, in Rwanda, and on a Native American reservation in the southwestern United States, little or no protection was observed.[151, 155, 156] In a three-dose trial in Lima, Peru, overall efficacy was 40%.[157] In a Finnish trial in which doses of RIT4237 were given once at birth and once at 7 months of age, the overall protection rate was 43% during a 28-month follow-up period.[158] Because of these disappointing results, RIT4237 was withdrawn from further development.

Several principles generally applicable to oral rotavirus vaccines in infants were established with RIT4237: (1) a live attenuated oral vaccine could protect children in some settings; (2) the highest rates of immune responses were achieved in infants 5 to 12 months of age, when prevaccination serum antibody titers (reflecting passively transferred maternal antibodies) were minimal[152, 153, 159]; (3) the specificity of serum virus-neutralizing antibody responses was primarily restricted to the homologous (G6) serotype in seronegative infants, but heterotypic booster responses were sometimes induced in seropositive infants; therefore, heterotypic immunity could protect children against human strains; (4) administration of infant formulas to buffer stomach acids before giving vaccine enhanced virus-specific immune responses[159, 160]; (5) coadministration of rotavirus vaccine with oral poliovirus vaccine (OPV) inhibited rotavirus-specific immune responses[161]; and (6) administration of multiple doses of vaccine did not lead to a dramatic increase in overall immune responses.[162]

Bovine Strain WC3

One possible explanation for the poor efficacy of the RIT4237 vaccine is that the strain was overattenuated by too many passages in cell culture. Consequently, another first-generation bovine rotavirus vaccine, strain WC3 (serotype P7G6), was evaluated as a vaccine after only 12 cell culture passages.[163] Like RIT4237, WC3 vaccine was given at high titers (10^7 PFU per child), was shed infrequently ($\leq$30% incidence) in feces, and caused no adverse reactions.[163, 164] Serum virus-neutralizing antibody responses occurred in 71 to 100% of infants in trials in the United States; neutralizing antibody responses were primarily homotypic, although approximately 50% of infants responded to simian (G3) rotavirus but not to human G3 rotavirus.

In an initial double-blind placebo-controlled efficacy trial performed in suburban Philadelphia, WC3 vaccine was associated with a 76% reduction in total rotavirus morbidity and 100% protection against "severe" rotavirus diarrhea[98] in a season when the natural challenge strain was G1. Only 71% of WC3-vaccinated infants exhibited virus-neutralizing antibodies in serum to the immunizing strain, but the lack of virus-neutralizing antibodies did not correlate with rotavirus illness in the vaccinated cohort. In a subsequent efficacy trial of WC3 conducted in Cincinnati,[165] 100% of infant vaccinees developed WC3-specific neutralizing antibodies in serum, but these infants were not protected against rotavirus disease. However, after immunization with WC3 vaccine, infants with evidence of prior infection with G1 rotavirus exhibited major booster responses in serum antibody titers to G1, G2, G3, and G4.[166] In an efficacy trial involving 472 infants in Bangui, Central African Republic,[167] vaccinees did not report fewer cases of rotavirus disease than placebo recipients did, although their disease was slightly but not significantly less severe. Only 60% of infants developed homotypic virus-neutralizing antibody responses. Finally, infants in Shanghai given two doses of WC3 at ages 4 and 10 weeks experienced a 50% decrease in cases of rotavirus diarrhea compared with control subjects (Guo et al., unpublished data). After these studies, WC3 was no longer considered a potential vaccine candidate.

Simian Strain RRV

The third of the first-generation animal-origin rotavirus vaccine candidates developed to the stage of clinical testing in infants was the rhesus rotavirus vaccine (RRV). The RRV strain MMU 18006 was isolated from a young monkey with diarrhea[169] and adapted to culture in fetal rhesus lung cells (FRhL-2) for use as a vaccine candidate in the 16th cell culture passage.[169] The neutralization phenotype of RRV is type G3,[168] but the G protein is not identical with human G3.[170]

RRV was safe and immunogenic in children 2 to 12 years of age,[169] but in a study of infants 5 to 20 months of age, a clustering of febrile responses was noted 3 to 4 days after inoculation.[171] In Finnish infants 6 to 8 months of age, significant clinical sequelae were associated with administration of RRV in a titer of 10^5 PFU. In the same study, infants administered RIT4237 vaccine exhibited a lower rate of serum antibody responses (RIT4237 = 75% and RRV = 88%) but had no adverse reactions.[172]

The increased incidence of fevers seen in vaccine trials in developed countries was frequently absent in RRV vaccine recipients in developing countries.[173] Reactivity was further reduced in younger infants (4 months of age or younger) inoculated with a lower dose of vaccine. The immunogenicity of the vaccine was less at lower doses ($\geq 10^4$ PFU) and in children who were breastfeeding or did not receive a buffer to protect the vaccine from stomach acid.[173–175] RRV at a dose of 10^4 PFU was nonreactogenic in a group of 40 newborn Venezuelan infants; a serum antibody response to the vaccine was shown by a serum IgA-specific ELISA test but not by other serum antibody assays.[176] Coadministration of RRV and OPV did not appear to lead to significant inhibition of the serum antibody response to either vaccine.[176, 177]

Results of clinical efficacy trials of RRV have varied. Clinical design has been similar: a single dose of 10^4 PFU of RRV given to infants between 2 and 12 months of age. Trials in Finland and Sweden identified modest protection (38% and 48%, respectively) against all cases of rotavirus diarrhea but greater efficacy against severe rotavirus diarrhea (67% and 80%, respectively).[178, 179] However, in three trials in the United States, no protection was observed in Rochester or Arizona,[180, 181] and only 29% protection was demonstrated in Maryland.[182] Surprisingly, in a second RRV trial conducted in Rochester 2 years after the first, the same RRV vaccine was associated with a 65% reduction in cases of rotavirus diarrhea.[183] In all of these trials, the natural challenge viruses identified were predominantly G1.

The greatest efficacy of RRV was observed in Venezuela, where the vaccine protected 65% of children from all rotavirus disease and all children from severe disease. In this trial, the natural challenge rotavirus was serotype G3.[184] For a time, this observation was cited as strong evidence that protection induced by rotavirus vaccine is serotype specific. However, a complete analysis of this Venezuelan clinical trial revealed that the vaccine-associated reduction in cases identified as G1, G2, or G4 (67%) was similar to the efficacy against G3 (70%).[185]

Animal × Human Reassortant Rotaviruses

A number of vaccine/challenge cross-protection studies performed in animals suggest that protection against disease caused by group A rotaviruses might be serotype specific. Therefore, vaccine developers have concluded that a recombinant (reassortant) rotavirus, bearing a human VP7 protein (to evoke human G type–specific neutralizing antibodies) and the remaining genes of an animal rotavirus (to attenuate rotavirus virulence for infants), might represent an ideal candidate vaccine. Such reassortant strains have been prepared by using both simian RRV and bovine strain rotaviruses as the parent strains.

Reassortants are prepared by coinfection of a human rotavirus strain with an animal rotavirus strain that is attenuated for humans. The first generation of reassortants, including those in the first licensed vaccine, are designed to contain the gene coding for VP7 of a human virus and 10 genes of the animal virus. To prepare a reassortant, susceptible cell cultures, usually derived from African green monkeys, are coinfected with a human virus and an animal virus. Reassortment occurs by chance in the culture, and a virus containing the desired VP7 is selected by suppressing the VP7 of animal origin with a monotypic antiserum against that protein. Only viruses with human VP7 will "break through," and those also containing 10 genes from the animal virus can be identified by gels showing the genomic segments of the reassortants. For further confirmation, sequencing of the genome can be done.

Simian (Strain RRV) × Human Reassortant Rotaviruses (Tetravalent Vaccine Under Consideration for License)

The reassortant rotavirus vaccine candidates that have been subjected to the most extensive clinical testing consist of simian × human rotavirus reassortants that contain a single human gene (i.e., VP7) and the remaining 10 genes from RRV. These reassortant viruses were prepared by the Laboratory of Infectious Diseases at the National Institutes of Health.[186] The vaccine, produced by Wyeth-Lederle Vaccines, contains the RRV strain of G3 serotype, designated G3 P5B RRV, and reassortants of G types 1, 2, and 4 with the RRV. In each case, the gene coding for VP7 of the human virus is incorporated into a virus containing all the other genes of RRV. The type 1 human virus was the D strain, and the reassortant is designated G1 P5B; the type 2 virus was DS-1, and the reassortant is designated G2 P5B; and the type 4 virus was ST-3, and the reassortant is designated G4 P5B.

The vaccine is supplied as a lyophilized product containing 10^5 of each of the four viruses, without preservative, but containing trace amounts of aminoglycosides and amphotericin B. The lyophilisate is reconstituted in 2.5 mL of buffer (see later). These reassortants have been tested both individually and as a "tetravalent" mixture containing rotaviruses with G type specificities 1,

2, and 4, respectively, and RRV itself as the G type 3 rotavirus (although some antigenic discrepancy has been shown between RRV VP7 and human VP7).[170]

Dosage and Route

Field trials of the tetravalent RRV × human reassortant vaccine (RRV-TV) were initiated at an inoculum of 10^4 PFU of each of the four viruses (i.e., 4×10^4 PFU) and completed at a dose of 4×10^5 PFU, the dose on the licensed vaccine.[186] In each of these trials, vaccine was administered orally in three doses, immunizations were separated by at least 3 weeks, and dosing was completed by the time a child reached 6 to 7 months of age. Outcomes included either episodes of rotavirus diarrhea reported through active surveillance by field workers during the rotavirus season or passive "catchment" surveillance of children attending a clinic or hospitalized for diarrhea confirmed to be rotavirus. In the United States, two separate but comparable multicenter trials using the low and high dose did not demonstrate a significant difference in efficacy.[187, 188] However, in Latin America, two trials conducted in Peru[189] and Brazil[190] with the lower dose of vaccine each demonstrated a lower efficacy against severe disease than a trial with the same low dose in the United States and a trial with the higher dose conducted in Venezuela.[191]

Rotaviruses are acid labile, and for maximum seroconversion, oral doses must be buffered with milk, formula, or antacids. The RRV-TV vaccine is reconstituted with 2.5 mL of citrate-bicarbonate (see also later section, *Factors Affecting Vaccine Immunogenicity and Efficacy).* Trace amounts of fetal bovine serum, neomycin sulfate, and amphotericin B are present in the vaccine.[191a]

Stability

RRV-TV is stable for 24 months between 20 and 25°C in its lyophilized state and for 60 minutes at room temperature or 4 hours in a refrigerator after reconstitution.[129]

Immunogenicity

RRV-TV vaccine was developed by using a cocktail of four strains with the hope that children will develop serotype-specific immunity to the four most common G types of rotavirus in global circulation. Whereas more than 90% of children develop an immune response, measured by the presence of virus-specific IgA or virus-neutralizing antibodies directed against the RRV parent strain of the vaccine, few children (<50%) develop specific neutralizing antibodies to each of the four human G serotypes. Table 41–4 summarizes the immunogenicity data from one of the RRV-TV studies performed in the United States.[188] Nonetheless, studies of efficacy of the quadrivalent RRV vaccine have consistently outperformed those using a single RRV × human reassortant (containing human G1) in seasons when strains other than G1 were circulating. This finding indicates that the strategy of using RRV-TV vaccine is correct even if we do not have adequate immunological markers to predict protection or a complete understanding of the mechanism of this protection.[187, 188, 192]

Efficacy

Seven efficacy trials of RRV-TV vaccine have been conducted to date, three using the vaccine in the lower dose and four using vaccine in the larger dose (Table 41–5). In all these trials, infants have been enrolled for immunization between 6 weeks and 2 months of age and three doses have been given: there are no data on efficacy among infants receiving fewer than three doses; efficacy has generally been greater against severe disease than against mild disease; and in those trials lasting 2 years, protection has endured for both years (with the exception of the trial conducted in Native American populations, where as in many developing countries, most of the disease occurred in the first year of life).[192]

In general, the efficacy of the vaccines has been lower in developing countries, an observation that has not been fully confirmed or completely explained. The protective efficacy of the low-dose vaccine was poorest in Peru,[189] intermediate in Brazil,[190] and best in the United States.[187] Similarly, the higher dose preparation performed least well among Native Americans,[180] better among Venezuelans[180] and Americans,[191] and best among Finns.[193]

In trials using high-dose RRV-TV vaccine, efficacy ranged from 48 to 68% against any rotavirus and from 64 to 91% against severe disease (see Table 41–5). Of particular note, the efficacy reported in Venezuela (48% for mild disease; 88% for severe disease) was not sig-

Table 41–4. **GEOMETRIC MEAN TITERS AND RATES OF SEROCONVERSION FROM A LARGE-SCALE CONSISTENCY LOT STUDY AND AN EFFICACY TRIAL OF RHESUS ROTAVIRUS VACCINE–TETRAVALENT[188]**

	ELISA	NEUTRALIZATION ANTIBODY ASSAYS*				
	Antirotaviral Serum IgA	RRV-3	G1 (Wa)	G2 (DS-1)	G3 (P)	G4 (ST-3)
Geometric mean titer						
RRV-TV (N = 142)	82.6	691.5	20.4	21.6	29.0	10.8
Placebo (N = 108)	17.7	7.1	10.4	6.6	7.6	6.3
% with 4-fold rise in antibody titer†						
RRV-TV (N = 185)	56	90	14	31	29	14
Placebo (N = 195)	2	2	1	0	1	2

*Strains include rhesus rotavirus serotype 3 (RRV-3) and human serotypes 1 to 4 (Wa, DS-1, P, and ST-3).
†All comparisons between vaccine and placebo recipients are statistically significantly different (P < 0.01).

Table 41–5. **EFFICACY OF RRV × HUMAN ROTAVIRUS REASSORTANT VACCINES**

DOSE (PFU)	COUNTRY	AGE GROUPS	N	CIRCULATING STRAINS	EFFICACY (%, CI) AGAINST All RV Disease	Severe RV Disease
4 × 10⁴	United States[92]	4–26 wk	662	G1, G3	57 (29, 74)	82 (−9, 97)
	Peru[189]	2–4 mo	428	G1, G2	24	60
	Brazil[190]	1–5 mo	540	G1, G2	57	NC
4 × 10⁵	United States[188]	5–25 wk	803	G1, G3	49 (31, 63)	80 (56, 91)
	Finland[193]	3–5 mo	2398	G1, G2	68 (57, 76)	91 (82, 96)
	Venezuela[191]	8–18 wk	2207	G1	48	88
	United States[192]	6–24 wk	695	G3	50 (26, 67)	69 (29, 88)

RRV, rhesus rotavirus vaccine; RV, rotavirus; CI, confidence interval; NC, not comparable.

nificantly different from that reported in the multicenter trial in the United States (57% and 82%), suggesting that RRV-TV might be well suited for use in developing countries. Furthermore, the observation that the higher dose worked in Venezuela, when a lower dose did not work in Peru or Brazil, suggests that in developing countries, vaccine dose may be critical. Only two trials were large enough to examine protection against hospitalization. In the trial in Finland, all 22 children hospitalized for rotavirus diarrhea were in the placebo group,[193] and in Venezuela, efficacy against hospitalization was 70%.[191]

Adverse Reactions

No major adverse reactions have been associated with administration of the RRV-TV vaccine among more than 17,000 children who have received it, but a significant increase in mild fevers has been observed 3 to 5 days after immunization. Low-grade fevers (temperature >38°C) have been most common (up to 15%) after the first dose, and a small group of children (1 to 2%) have had a higher temperature (>39°C).[187, 188, 192, 193] In the Finnish trial, fever was associated with diarrhea and abdominal cramping in about 3% of children.[193a] No increase in the incidence of vomiting has been associated with vaccination when it is given in the first 6 months of life. However, in earlier studies with RRV only, older children in Sweden did have an increased incidence of loose stools and fever, suggesting that replication of the virus in the older children without maternal antibody could lead to mild symptoms of diarrhea.[194]

Table 41–6 summarizes adverse events reported during placebo-controlled trials of RRV-TV.[129] Low-grade fever is the most prominent reaction.

Intussusception of the intestine has been reported after RRV-TV administration at a rate of 0.05% compared with 0% in placebo recipients. This difference is not statistically significant, and the rate in vaccinees does not appear to exceed the background rate of that syndrome (M. Rennels, personal communication, 1997).

Transmission

Rotavirus vaccine strains are excreted in the stool of infants, but the concentration appears to be too low to result in contact spread under usual hygienic conditions in industrialized countries, even in daycare. In Venezuela, however, nonvaccinated children did excrete vaccine virus.[191] In any case, contact infection does not appear to be pathogenic.[193, 195]

Bovine (Strain WC3) × Human Reassortant Rotaviruses

Type Gl, G2, G3, and G4 reassortants have been created containing at least the VP7 gene of a human rotavirus on a predominantly bovine WC3 rotavirus genome background. Reassortants of G1, G2, and G3 specificity have been administered to infants and demonstrated to be as safe as WC3 and, like WC3, to be shed in feces in low incidence (<20%) and at low concentration.[196–199]

WC3 × human reassortant rotaviruses appear to induce slightly lower rates of virus-specific immune re-

Table 41–6. **SUMMARY OF ADVERSE REACTIONS DURING PLACEBO-CONTROLLED TRIALS OF TETRAVALENT RHESUS ROTAVIRUS VACCINE†**

SYMPTOM	DOSE 1 RRV-TV	DOSE 1 Placebo	DOSE 2 RRV-TV	DOSE 2 Placebo	DOSE 3 RRV-TV	DOSE 3 Placebo
Temperature >38°C	461/2153 (21)**	124/2164 (6)	218/1983 (11)*	181/2002 (9)	273/1918 (14)	250/1920 (13)
Temperature >39°C	37/2153 (2)**	12/2164 (1)	22/1983 (1)	14/2002 (1)	42/1918 (2)	28/1920 (1)
Decreased appetite	375/2181 (17)**	238/2191 (11)	226/2017 (11)	236/2038 (12)	269/1954 (14)	236/1965 (12)
Irritability	541/1317 (41)**	428/1336 (32)	486/1272 (38)	507/1292 (39)	466/1232 (36)	433/1262 (35)
Decreased activity	436/2179 (20)**	292/2190 (13)	238/2018 (12)	244/2036 (12)	203/1952 (10)	212/1965 (11)

†Includes summary data supplied by Wyeth-Lederle Vaccines and Pediatrics; the data represent solicited symptoms observed at least once within 5 days after each dose for which differences between rates of symptoms between vaccine and placebo recipients were observed after any dose.

*P < .05; **P < .01; significance from placebo group (no.) = %.

sponses than WC3 alone; part of this reduction in immune responses is associated with infants seropositive to human-type rotaviruses.[196] Immune responses to the VP4 (P) protein of WC3 are generally more efficient than those to the VP7 (G) protein of the human parent virus. In phase I immunogenicity studies of three VP7 reassortant viruses of Gl, G2, or G3 specificity, the immune response rates to the VP4 specificity (bovine) after two doses varied from 40 to 69%, whereas immune responses to the VP7 rotavirus specificity (human) ranged from 40 to 55%.[196] Studies of the immune response to each of three doses of the G1 reassortant of WC3 revealed final immune response rates to the WC3 parent exceeding 90% and to G1 parent rotavirus of approximately 70%; most immune responses to WC3 (VP4) occurred after the first dose; the highest rate of immune response to G1 human rotavirus (VP7) occurred after the second dose (Clark et al., unpublished data). In numerous clinical trials of WC3 × human (VP7) reassortants and RRV × human (VP7) reassortants, a greater immune response (i.e., virus-neutralizing antibodies) was directed against the WC3 or RRV parent (represented by VP4) than to the human rotavirus parent (represented by VP7). Therefore, it was of interest to evaluate reassortants in which a human serotype VP4 was paired with a bovine VP7 surface protein. Initial concerns that a human VP4 protein would confer virulence on such a reassortant were alleviated after two studies in experimental animals suggested that rotavirus virulence is under multigenic control.[200, 201]

Two reassortants were constructed to contain a human type P1a VP4 gene with the remaining genome, including VP7 (G6), from WC3. These reassortants contained the VP4 (type P1a) from human P1aG1 (strain WI79) or from human P1aG9 (strain WI61). In phase I clinical trials in infants, these reassortants caused no detectable adverse effects at a dose of 10^7 PFU. However, the serum antibody response unexpectedly was of bovine rotavirus specificity. After two doses either of the reassortant containing WI79 P1a or of the reassortant containing WI61 P1a, the rate of serum antibody response to the human rotavirus parents was 28% and 47%, respectively, whereas the immune response rates to the WC3 (VP7) parent virus were 81% and 60%, respectively.[199]

A double reassortant containing both human VP4 (P1a) and human VP7 (G1) derived from human strain WI79 on a WC3 genome background gave a poor serum antibody response. After two doses of this reassortant, serum neutralizing antibody responses of infants were 35% to the parent human WI79 virus and 27% to bovine parent WC3. However, a mixture of two single WC3 reassortants containing equal amounts of the human G1 reassortant mixed with the human P1a reassortant was highly immunogenic. After two doses of this mixed vaccine, the serum neutralizing antibody response of infants was 71% to the human parent P1aG1 virus and 97% to the parent WC3 virus.[202] Three clinical efficacy trials of the G1 reassortant of WC3 and one efficacy trial of multivalent WC3 reassortant vaccine have been completed in the United States (Table 41–7). A small initial trial in Philadelphia revealed 100% protection against all rotavirus disease.[203] A second trial in Philadelphia and a larger trial in Rochester were characterized by levels of protection exceeding 60% for all disease and more efficient protection against severe disease (clinical score >8.0).[197] No adverse effects were associated with vaccine administration. Serum neutralizing antibody responses were near 100% to WC3 rotavirus in both Philadelphia trials; in the first trial, the antibody response rate specific to G1 rotavirus was only 21%, but in the second (three-dose) trial, the antibody response to G1 rotavirus was 70%.

A single multisite efficacy trial has been completed employing a vaccine that contains in each dose equal quantities (10^7 PFU) of WC3 reassortants of G1, G2, G3, and P1a specificity.[204] In this trial, protection was 67% against all rotavirus disease and 69% against severe rotavirus disease. There was a slight excess (8%) of mild diarrhea noted in the vaccine group after the first dose only. Evaluation of immune responses is in progress.

Bovine (Strain UK) × Human Reassortant Rotaviruses

Bovine × human reassortant rotaviruses have also been generated incorporating the genes for VP7 of either Gl, G2, G3, or G4 human serotypes and 10 genes from the bovine UK strain rotavirus, which (like strain WC3) is of serotype P7G6.[205] Phase I clinical studies of the G1 reassortant ($10^{5.8}$ PFU/dose) and of the G2 reassortant ($10^{5.3}$ PFU/dose) of UK indicated that this vaccine is tolerated in infants without adverse effects. Evidence of serum antibody response was observed in 10 of 20 infants after a single dose of the G1 reassortant; after two doses, all had responded.[206]

A quadrivalent vaccine incorporating G1–G4 serotype UK reassortants has been assembled. This is currently undergoing further clinical trials for efficacy.

Table 41–7. **EFFICACY OF WC3 × HUMAN ROTAVIRUS REASSORTANT VACCINES**

VACCINE	SITE	NUMBER OF DOSES	N	CIRCULATING STRAINS	EFFICACY (%) AGAINST	
					All RV Disease	Severe RV Disease
G1	Philadelphia, PA[203]	2	77	G1, G3	100	—
G1	Rochester, NY[197]	3	226	G1	64	84
G1	Philadelphia, PA[197]	3	86	G1	74	100
G1, G2, G3, P1a	United States[204]	3	405	G1	67	69

RV, rotavirus.

Attenuated Human Rotaviruses

Newborn Rotavirus Strain M37

"Newborn strains" have been studied as potential vaccines because (l) infants in neonatal nurseries in several locales worldwide have been found to be infected with rotavirus with high prevalence but little gastroenteritis[207]; (2) in neonatal nurseries in Melbourne and New Delhi, infants who were infected in the nursery experienced fewer and less severe subsequent episodes of rotavirus disease than did babies who escaped infection in the nursery[72]; and (3) a subclass of newborn rotavirus isolates obtained from nurseries in different countries was found to share the same antigenic phenotype of VP4, despite the fact that VP7 specificities were either G types 1, 2, 3, or 4.[31, 207]

Type G1 newborn strain M37, isolated in Venezuela,[207] has been given in doses of 10^4 PFU to infants as young as 1.5 months old. An increased incidence of fevers 3 to 4 days after administration was observed in Venezuela[208] and Finland[209] but not in Maryland.[210] Serum antibody response rates to rotavirus measured by ELISA (IgG or IgA) ranged from 50 to 74%. Virus-neutralizing antibody responses in serum to the immunizing M37 rotavirus ranged from 36 to 71%. However, G type 1–specific antibody responses were obtained in only 10 to 27% of vaccinees.[208–210]

In an efficacy trial of M37, administration of 10^4 PFU per dose was associated with no protection against rotavirus diarrhea when the natural challenge virus was predominantly G1.[209]

Rotavirus Strain 89–12

G1 rotavirus strain 89–12 was isolated from an infant with symptomatic disease in Cincinnati, Ohio, and attenuated by 33 serial passages in African green monkey kidney cells (Bernstein et al., unpublished data). When two doses of 89–12 vaccine (10^2 PFU per dose) were administered to 20 infants 6 to 26 weeks of age, no adverse clinical effects were noted. Vaccine virus was shed in the stools of 17 infants.

Nineteen (95%) of the vaccinated infants exhibited a rotavirus-specific serum IgA response, and 15 exhibited an intestinal mucosal (fecal) IgA response. However, serum neutralizing antibody responses to the vaccine virus were detected in less than half of the vaccinees. Evaluation of the efficacy of strain 89–12 in protection against rotavirus disease is currently under study.

Neonatal Rotavirus Strain RV3

Natural infection with RV3 (P6G3) in a neonatal nursery was reported by Bishop and colleagues[72] to protect infants from subsequent severe rotavirus disease. The virus was propagated in African green monkey kidney cell culture and evaluated as an oral vaccine in 3-month-old infants.[211]

Strain RV3 appeared to be safe, and fecal shedding of vaccine virus was not detected by ELISA. Rotavirus-specific serum antibody responses were not detected, but coproantibody responses were detected in some vaccinees. Protective efficacy data are not now available.[211]

Factors Affecting Vaccine Immunogenicity and Efficacy

The initial rotavirus vaccines to be licensed or proposed for licensure will be oral vaccines. Because of current recommendations to reduce the use of OPV, which will be rapidly implemented (at least in developed countries), rotavirus may soon be the only oral vaccine administered to infants. As such, its efficacy may be affected by a number of factors that do not influence the response to parenterally administered vaccines or that influence parenteral vaccines to a different extent. Among such factors are the dose administered (virus concentration and number of doses), approaches to reducing inactivation by stomach acid, and immune inactivation caused by feeding on breast milk containing rotavirus-specific antibodies. In areas where OPV continues to be administered, possible interference by OPV with the immune response to rotavirus vaccine may also have to be considered.

The effect of those factors on protective immune responses may be expected to vary to some extent for different vaccines with differing mechanisms of inducing immunity. The quadrivalent rhesus reassortant vaccine is given in lower dose than the WC3 bovine rotavirus reassortant vaccine and apparently replicates much more efficiently in the infant host. Neither the effective viable virus dose needed to contact the small intestinal mucosa nor the importance of subsequent replication of vaccine virus in the intestinal epithelium is known. Each of these factors may be completely reconsidered as novel approaches to rotavirus vaccination (for example, microcapsules or DNA vaccines) continue to be developed.

Virus Dose

RRV-TV has been administered in a low dose (10^4 PFU per reassortant)[212] to reduce reactogenicity and a higher dose (10^5 PFU)[188] to enhance immunogenicity. The differences in protective immune responses and induction of fevers have not been remarkable. A single, unbuffered dose of either 10^4 or 10^5 PFU of RRV-TV has been found to be poorly immunogenic.[213] Similarly, the effect of the number of doses on RRV efficacy is not clear (in a single study in Peru, Lanata and coworkers[189] found little advantage to multiple doses).

It has recently been reported that reactogenicity is not increased when infants are given a dose of 10^6 PFU per reassortant of RRV,[214] suggesting that reactions may be an "all or none" expression of presence or absence of a productive infection. RRV will be licensed to be administered in three doses of 10^5 PFU each per reassortant. Bovine (WC3) reassortant vaccine has been consistently administered at a concentration of 10^7 PFU per reassortant.[198] Few data are available for infants given lower doses, although it has been shown with WC3 rotavirus vaccine that serum antibody responses are reduced at doses below 10^3 PFU (unpublished data). The effect of number of doses on efficacy has not been shown, but the human G serotype–specific serum antibody response is greatly enhanced after the second and third doses of the G1 reassortant vaccine (Clark et al., unpublished data).

Buffering Stomach Acid

Paradoxically, although rotaviruses are spread by the fecal-oral route of transmission, they are rapidly inactivated at pH 3.0 or less, levels of acidity commonly found in the infant stomach.[215] Early studies with the RIT4237 vaccine indicated that immune responses were improved when infants were prefed infant formula.[159, 160] The majority of RRV trials involved prefeeding with buffer that was often fortified with additional bicarbonate. Prefeeding with formula was also performed in the reported WC3 bovine reassortant vaccine trials.

The requirement of prefeeding would be an impediment to the use of rotavirus vaccine in mass vaccination campaigns or in private pediatric practice. Ing and colleagues[216] demonstrated that RRV suspended in 2.5 mL of a citrate-bicarbonate buffer solution induces a serum antibody response that is clearly superior to that of RRV given in an unbuffered solution. This same buffer was employed in the largest U.S. prelicensure efficacy trial of "high-dose" (10^5 PFU per reassortant) RRV-TV, in which 49% protection was achieved against all rotavirus disease and 80% protection was obtained against severe episodes.[188]

Coadministration of Rotaviruses with OPV and with Parenteral Vaccines

Especially in developing nations, oral rotavirus vaccine may be coadministered with OPV. Data on the potential effects of this on rotavirus immune responses have been thoroughly reviewed by Rennels.[217] In a Thai trial, OPV given with "low-dose" RRV-TV vaccine led to depressed rotavirus-specific antibody responses to the initial rotavirus vaccine dose, but this inhibition was largely overcome by three doses.[218] OPV causes a dramatic inhibition of the immune response induced by RIT4237 bovine rotavirus in infants.[219, 220] There are no data available on OPV's possible interference with the immune response of infants to bovine (WC3 or UK) × human reassortant rotavirus vaccines.

RRV-TV does not interfere with responses to simultaneously administered DTP, inactivated polio vaccine, *Haemophilus influenzae* type b conjugate vaccine, or hepatitis B vaccine.[191a]

Maternally Acquired Antibodies and Breast-Feeding

Most infants possess maternally acquired serum antibodies to rotavirus that persist through the first few months of life. Although serum antibody cannot be demonstrated to be protective, seropositive infants are less likely to develop serum antibody responses to vaccine, and seronegative infants are more likely to develop adverse effects. Optimal immune responses have been obtained at 5 months of age and older. There has also been concern that breast-feeding may lead to inhibition of the immune response to oral rotavirus vaccine. Pichichero[175] performed a meta-analysis of studies involving the type 3 RRV strain and noted a significant adverse effect of breast-feeding on seroconversion: 48% versus 70% in non–breast-fed infants. However, the vaccine dose was low and only single doses were given. In a review of published data on the effect of breast-feeding, Rennels and coworkers[217] found that there was a "trend" toward lower titered antibody responses to rotavirus vaccine in breast-fed infants, but no demonstrable effect of breast-feeding on the protective effect of three doses of rotavirus vaccines has been reported.

Indications for RRV-TV Vaccine

These are summarized from the ACIP recommendations,[129] which relate to the use of the vaccine in the United States.

Vaccination is recommended universally for term infants, three oral doses being administered at 2, 4, and 6 months of age, simultaneously with other vaccines indicated at those ages. Because rotavirus gastroenteritis is a winter disease, an effort should be made to complete the three doses before the onset of annual epidemics in the particular region in which the child lives. The interval between doses of RRV-TV can be reduced to 3 weeks.

Infants older than 6 months may have more febrile reactions to rotavirus vaccine, because they will no longer have passive maternal antibodies, and initiation of RRV-TV is not recommended after 6 months of age.

Breast-feeding and simultaneous OPV administration may decrease immune responses to the first dose, but three doses will overcome those negative effects.

Contraindications

RRV-TV is not recommended for infants born earlier than 37 weeks of gestation; for infants with chronic vomiting, diarrhea, or other chronic gastrointestinal diseases; for infants with known or suspected immunodeficiencies including human immunodeficiency virus infection; or for infants with acute illnesses, primarily because clinical experience in these conditions is lacking.[129] The contraindication to vaccination of premature infants also relates to the concern that their deficiency in maternal rotavirus antibodies will make them more susceptible to febrile reactions.

As with other vaccines, transient respiratory illnesses with or without low-grade fever are not contraindications to rotavirus immunization.

Hypersensitivity to antibiotics in the vaccine is a contraindication.

Prior administration of blood products is not a contraindication.[129]

Limits of Present Candidate Vaccines and Approaches to Improved Vaccines

After either natural infection or immunization, production of rotavirus-specific sIgA by small intestinal lymphocytes in the lamina propria is usually short-lived. Therefore, one goal for future vaccines would be to prolong effector B-cell responses at the intestinal mucosal surface. Microencapsulation of rotaviruses, using a combination of aqueous anionic polymers (e.g., alginate or chondroitin sulfate) and aqueous amines (e.g., spermine), has been shown to enhance and prolong virus-specific IgA responses at the intestinal mucosal surface in mice.[221–223]

Another problem with using oral immunization of infectious virus to induce protection against challenge is the potential inhibitory effect of antibodies in breast milk and colostrum. There are two possible solutions to this problem. First, intramuscular immunization with rotavirus has been found to induce virus-specific antibodies in gut-associated lymphoid tissue and protection against challenge in animal studies.[224, 225] Second, microencapsulation has been shown to negate the inhibitory effects of passively transferred virus-specific antibodies in breast milk after oral inoculation of reovirus.[226]

Possible problems associated with the use of live attenuated virus vaccines are obviated by the use of virus-like particles[227] or rotavirus-specific naked DNA.[228]

PUBLIC HEALTH CONSIDERATIONS

The public health goal of the rotavirus vaccine program has been to develop a vaccine that could be administered to children as part of their routine program of immunizations and thus prevent this most common cause of severe diarrhea in children younger than 5 years. This vaccine would ideally have high efficacy, low reactogenicity, and affordable cost; its impact should be measurable within 1 year as a significant decline in diarrheal hospitalizations and possibly deaths. The first rotavirus vaccine is likely to be licensed in the United States in 1998, and at least seven other candidate vaccines are in different stages of development and testing.[229] Both national and international authorities have begun to consider recommendations for possible use of the vaccine and to identify ways to measure its impact in the future.[129, 230] Because all children are infected in the first few years of life, the first recommendations will be for the immunization of all children (i.e., universal immunization) with the possible exclusion of children with severe preexisting medical conditions. Whereas the first vaccine likely to be licensed (RRV-TV) has reasonably high efficacy against severe rotavirus diarrhea in Venezuela, the United States, and Finland, it provides only partial protection against mild disease, requires three doses, and induces some mild adverse reactions. Consequently, this vaccine may be viewed as a first-generation product that might be improved on in the future.[231, 232] In the United States, both the ACIP and the American Academy of Pediatrics' Red Book Committee are considering initial recommendations for use of rotavirus vaccines.[129] Given that the disease is rarely fatal in this country and leads primarily to hospitalizations, the burden of disease is partially measured in terms of cost to the healthcare system and society. The impact of the vaccination program needs to be assessed in terms of its cost-effectiveness. In the absence of information on price, preliminary estimates indicate that a vaccine that can be delivered at a cost of $30 per dose would have a positive cost-effectiveness ratio, provided that it could be administered at the time of a child's routine immunization visits (2, 4, and 6 months).[233] The effect of live oral rotavirus vaccines in severely premature or immunocompromised children is unknown, and although these children may experience prolonged shedding of vaccine strains, they might also get more severe disease if they are naturally infected. Postlicensure studies and special surveys will be needed to assess these problems as well as to identify possible adverse events that occur with low incidence. The impact of disease can be monitored through surveillance of children hospitalized or seen in other medical settings for diarrhea and should be evident within one season after vaccination. Theoretically, new rotavirus strains may appear with serotypes not included in the vaccine or with mutations that escape the vaccine's protection. Surveillance of rotavirus strains will be essential to detect these events, although their likelihood seems small. Because of the seasonal nature of rotavirus in temperate climates, vaccine coverage needs to be particularly encouraged and brought up to date in the fall, before the rotavirus season.

For developing countries, the vaccine has been tested in its final formulation only in Venezuela. More trials will be required in other countries where the epidemiology of rotavirus and the characteristics of the population may differ in ways that could have an impact on vaccine efficacy.[230] Past experience with the low immunogenicity of live OPV in tropical countries underscores the prudence in waiting for further testing of vaccines and administration schedules before the vaccine is introduced.[234] The high prevalence of neonatal rotavirus infections in India suggests the alternative possibility of immunizing during the neonatal period, at the same time as BCG.[114, 235] For the poorest countries, demonstration of efficacy alone will not lead to vaccine introduction because vaccine cost is a limiting factor. Efforts are needed first to determine whether new vaccines are effective in developing countries and then to ensure that they can be made available at a price that is affordable to expedite their introduction and use. Recent delays in introducing hepatitis B and *Haemophilus influenzae* type b vaccines into developing countries have demonstrated the bottleneck issues of vaccine economics and supply that need to be addressed early on so that rotavirus vaccine can be introduced expeditiously.

To date, only one trial of the RRV-TV vaccine has been conducted with the final titer of virus (4×10^5 PFU per dose) in a developing country. Consequently, a consensus conference held in Geneva recommended that this vaccine be tested further in Africa and Asia to determine whether it is equally effective in these settings with the recommended regimen.[230] Furthermore, many countries do not yet appreciate that rotavirus may be an important cause of hospitalization, and some surveillance will be required to assess the burden of disease, associated costs, and drains on local healthcare budgets.

REFERENCES

1. de Zoysa I, Feachem RG. Interventions for the control of diarrhoeal diseases among young children: Rotavirus and cholera immunization. Bull World Health Organ 63:569–583, 1985.
2. Kapikian AZ, Chanock RM. Rotaviruses. In Fields BN, Knipe DM, Howley PM, et al (eds). Fields Virology (3rd ed). Vol. 2. Philadelphia, Lippincott-Raven, 1996, pp 1657–1708.
3. Brandt CD, Kim HW, Rodriguez JO, et al. Pediatric viral gastroenteritis during eight years of study. J Clin Microbiol 18:71–78, 1983.
4. Glass RI, Kilgore PE, Holman RC, et al. The epidemiology of rotavirus diarrhea in the United States: Surveillance and estimates of disease burden. J Infect Dis 174(suppl 1):S5–Sll, 1996.
5. Kilgore PE, Holman RC, Clarke MJ, Glass RI. Trends of diarrheal disease–associated mortality in U.S. children, 1968 through 1991. JAMA 274:1143–1148, 1995.
6. Jin S, Kilgore PK, Holman RC, et al. Trends in hospitalizations for diarrhea in United States children from 1979–1992: Estimates of the morbidity associated with rotavirus. Pediatr Infect Dis J 15:397–404, 1996.
7. Smith J, Haddix A, Teutsch S, Glass RI. Cost effectiveness analysis of a rotavirus immunization program for the United States. Pediatrics 96:609–615, 1995.
8. Huilan S, Zhen LG, Mathan MM, et al. Etiology of acute diarrhoea among children in developing countries: A multicentre study in five countries. Bull World Health Organ 69:549–555, 1991.
9. Levine MM, Losonsky G, Herrington D, et al. Pediatric diarrhea: The challenge of prevention. Pediatr Infect Dis 5:S29–S43, 1986.
10. Cook SM, Glass RI, LeBaron CW, Ho M-S. Global seasonality of rotavirus infections. Bull World Health Organ 68:171–177, 1990.
11. Bern C, Martines J, de Zoysa I, Glass RI. The magnitude of the global problem of diarrhoeal disease: A ten year update. Bull World Health Organ 70:705–714, 1992.
12. Murray CJ, Lopez AD. Global mortality, disability, and the contribution of risk factors: Global burden of disease study. Lancet 349:1436–1442, 1997.
13. Walsh JA, Warren KS. Selective primary health care. An interim strategy for disease control in developing countries. N Engl J Med 301:967–974, 1979.
14. Snyder JD, Merson MH. The magnitude of the global problem of acute diarrhoeal disease: A review of active surveillance data. Bull World Health Organ 60:605–613, 1982.
15. Oral Rehydration Therapy: An Annotated Bibliography. Scientific Publication No. 445. Washington, DC, Pan American Health Organization, 1983.
16. Estes M. Rotaviruses and their replication. In Fields BN, Knipe DM, Howley PM (eds). Fields Virology (3rd ed). Vol. 2. Philadelphia, Lippincott-Raven, 1996, pp 1625–1655.
17. Sato K, Inaba Y, Shinozaki T, et al. Isolation of human rotavirus in cell cultures. Arch Virol 69:155–160, 1981.
18. Urasawa T, Urasawa S, Taniguchi K. Sequential passages of human rotavirus in MA-104 cells. Microbiol Immunol 25:1025–1035, 1981.
19. Mebus CA, Kono M, Underdahl NR, Twiehaus MJ. Cell culture propagation of neonatal calf diarrhea (scours) virus. Can Vet J 12:69–72, 1971.
20. Malherbe HH, Strickland-Cholmley M. Simian virus SA11 and the related O agent. Arch Ges Virusforsch 22:235–245, 1969.
21. Midthun K, Greenberg HB, Hoshino Y, et al. Reassortant rotaviruses as potential live rotavirus vaccine candidates. J Virol 53:949–954, 1985.
22. Clark HF, Offit PA, Dolan KT, et al. Response of adult human volunteers to oral administration of bovine and bovine/human reassortant rotaviruses. Vaccine 4:25–31, 1986.
23. Midthun K, Hoshino Y, Kapikian AZ, Chanock RM. Single gene substitution rotavirus reassortants containing the major neutralization protein (VP7) of human rotavirus serotype 4. J Clin Microbiol 24:822–826, 1986.
24. Hoshino Y, Sereno MM, Midthun K, et al. Independent segregation of two antigenic specificities (VP3 and VP7) involved in neutralization of rotavirus infectivity. Proc Natl Acad Sci U S A 82:8701–8704, 1985.
25. Offit PA, Blavat G. Identification of the two rotavirus genes determining neutralization specificities. J Virol 57:376–378, 1986.
26. Offit PA, Clark HF, Blavat G, Greenberg HB. Reassortant rotaviruses containing structural proteins VP3 and VP7 from different parents induce antibodies protective against each parental serotype. J Virol 60:491–496, 1986.
27. Sabara M, Gilchrist JE, Hudson GR, Babiuk LA. Preliminary characterization of an epitope involved in neutralization and cell attachment that is located on the major bovine rotavirus glycoprotein. J Virol 53:58–66, 1985.
28. Kalica AR, Greenberg HB, Wyatt RG, et al. Genes of human (strain WA) and bovine (strain UK) rotaviruses that code for neutralization and subgroup antigens. Virology 112:385–390, 1981.
29. Ball JM, Tian P, Zeng CQY, et al. Age-dependent diarrhea induced by a rotaviral nonstructural glycoprotein. Science 272:101–104, 1996.
30. Larralde G, Li B, Kapikian AZ, Gorziglia M. Serotype-specific epitopes present on the VP 8 subunit of rotavirus VP 4 protein. J Virol 65:3213–3218, 1991.
31. Gorziglia MKY, Green K, Nishikawa K, et al. Sequence of the fourth gene of human rotaviruses recovered from asymptomatic or symptomatic infections. J Virol 62:2979–2984, 1988.
32. Hoshino Y, Wyatt RG, Greenberg HB. Serotypic similarity and diversity of rotaviruses of mammalian and avian origin as studied by plaque reduction neutralization. J Infect Dis 149:694–702, 1984.
33. Svensson L, Sheshbaradaran H, Visikari T, et al. Immune response to rotavirus polypeptides after vaccination with heterologous rotavirus vaccines (RIT 4237, RRV-1). J Gen Virol 68:1993–1999, 1987.
34. Ward RL, Knowlton DR, Schiff GM, et al. Relative concentrations of serum neutralizing antibody to VP 3 and VP 7 proteins in adults infected with a human rotavirus. J Virol 62:1543–1549, 1989.
35. Ward RL, Knowlton DR, Greenberg HG, et al. Serum-neutralizing antibody to VP 4 and VP 7 proteins in infants following vaccination with WC3 bovine rotavirus. J Virol 64:2687–2691, 1990.
36. Tallett S, MacKenzie C, Middleton P, et al. Clinical, laboratory, and epidemiologic features of a viral gastroenteritis in infants and children. Pediatrics 60:217–222, 1977.
37. Carr M, McKendrick D, Spyridakis T. The clinical features of infantile gastroenteritis due to rotavirus. Scand J Infect Dis 8:241–243, 1978.
38. Kovacs A, Chan L, Hotrakitya C, et al. Rotavirus gastroenteritis: Clinical and laboratory features and use of the rotazyme test. Am J Dis Child 141:161–166, 1987.
39. Rodriguez W, Kim H, Arrobio J, et al. Clinical features of acute gastroenteritis associated with human reovirus-like agent in infants and young children. J Pediatr 91:188–193, 1977.
40. Salmi T, Arstila P, Koivikko A. Central nervous system involvement in patients with rotavirus gastroenteritis. Scand J Infect Dis 10:29–31, 1978.
41. Wong C, Price Z, Bruckner D. Aseptic meningitis in an infant with rotavirus gastroenteritis. Pediatr Infect Dis J 3:244–246, 1984.
42. Yolken R, Murphy M. Sudden infant death syndrome associated with rotavirus infection. J Med Virol 10:291–296, 1982.
43. Whorwell P, Beeken W, Phillips C, et al. Isolation of reovirus-like agents from patients with Crohn's disease. Lancet 1:1169–1171, 1977.

44. Mebus CA, Stair EL, Underdahl NR, Twiehaus MJ. Pathology of neonatal calf diarrhea induced by a reo-like virus. Vet Pathol 8:490–505, 1974.
45. Pearson GR, McNulty MS. Pathological changes in the small intestine of neonatal pigs infected with a pig reovirus-like agent (rotavirus). J Comp Pathol 87:363–375, 1977.
46. Snodgrass DR, Ferguson A, Allan F, et al. Small intestinal morphology and epithelial cell kinetics in lamb rotavirus infections. Gastroenterology 76:477–481, 1979.
47. Starkey WG, Collins J, Wallis TS, et al. Kinetics, tissue specificity and pathological changes in murine rotavirus infection of mice. J Gen Virol 67:2625–2634, 1986.
48. Holmes IH, Ruck BJ, Bishop RF, Davidson GP. Infantile enteritis viruses: Morphogenesis and morphology. J Virol 16:937–943, 1975.
49. Suzuki H, Konno T. Reovirus-like particles in jejunal mucosa of a Japanese infant with acute infectious non-bacterial gastroenteritis. Tohoku J Exp Med 115:199–211, 1975.
50. Sheridan JF, Eydelloth RS, Vonderfecht SL, Aurelian L. Virus-specific immunity in neonatal and adult mouse rotavirus infection. Infect Immun 39:917–927, 1983.
51. Torres-Medina A. Effect of rotavirus and/or *Escherichia coli* infection on the aggregated lymphoid follicles in the small intestine of neonatal gnotobiotic calves. Am J Vet Res 45:652–660, 1984.
52. Uhnoo I, Riepenhoff-Talty M, Dharakul T, et al. Extramucosal spread and development of hepatitis with rhesus rotavirus in immunodeficient and normal mice. J Virol 64:361–368, 1990.
53. Davidson GP, Gall DG, Petric M, et al. Human rotavirus enteritis induced in conventional piglets: Intestinal structure and transport. J Clin Invest 60:1402–1409, 1977.
54. Graham DY, Sackman JW, Estes MK. Pathogenesis of rotavirus-induced diarrhea: Preliminary studies in miniature swine piglet. Dig Dis Sci 29:1028–1035, 1984.
55. Kapikian AZ, Wha H, Wyatt RG, et al. Human reovirus-like agent as the major pathogen associated with "winter" gastroenteritis in hospitalized infants and young children. N Engl J Med 294:965–972, 1976.
56. Perez-Schael I, Daoud G, White L, et al. Rotavirus shedding by newborn children. J Med Virol 14:127–136, 1984.
57. Chrystie IL, Totterdell BM, Banatvala JE. Asymptomatic endemic rotavirus infections in the newborn. Lancet 1:1176–1178, 1978.
58. Wenman WM, Hinde D, Feltham S, Gurwith M. Rotavirus infection in adults: Results of a prospective family study. N Engl J Med 301:303–306, 1979.
59. Velazquez FR, Matson DO, Calva JJ, et al. Rotavirus infection in infants as protection against subsequent infections. N Engl J Med 335:1022–1028, 1996.
60. Riepenhoff-Talty M, Lee PC, Carmody PJ, et al. Age-dependent rotavirus-enterocyte interactions. Proc Soc Exp Biol Med 170:146–154, 1982.
61. Flores J, Midthun K, Hoshino Y, et al. Conservation of the fourth gene segment among rotaviruses recovered from asymptomatic newborn infants and its possible role in attenuation. J Virol 60:972–979, 1986.
62. Fukuhara N, Yoshie O, Kitaoka S, Konno T. Role of VP 3 in human rotavirus internalization after target cell attachment via VP 7. J Virol 62:2209–2218, 1988.
63. Kaljot KT, Shaw RD, Rubin DH, Greenberg HB. Infectious rotavirus enters cells by direct cell membrane penetration, not by endocytosis. J Virol 62:1136–1144, 1988.
64. Estes MK, Graham DY, Mason BB. Proteolytic enhancement of rotavirus infectivity: Molecular mechanisms. J Virol 39:879–888, 1981.
65. Lebenthal E, Lee PC. Development of functional response in human exocrine pancreas. Pediatrics 66:556–560, 1980.
66. Hoshino Y, Sereno MM, Kapikian AZ, et al. Genetic determinants of rotavirus virulence studied in gnotobiotic piglets. In Vaccines 93. Cold Spring Harbor, NY, Cold Spring Harbor Laboratory Press, 1993, pp 277–282.
67. Black REM, Merson MH, Rahman ASSM, et al. A two-year study of bacterial, viral and parasitic agents associated with diarrhea in rural Bangladesh. J Infect Dis 142:660–664, 1980.
68. Noble RL, Sidwell RW, Mahoney AW, et al. Influence of malnutrition and alterations in dietary protein on murine rotavirus disease. Proc Soc Exp Biol Med 173:417–426, 1983.
69. Morrey JD, Sidwell RW, Noble RL, et al. Effects of folic acid malnutrition on rotaviral infection in mice. Proc Soc Exp Biol Med 176:77–83, 1984.
70. Newsome PM, Coney KA. Synergistic rotavirus and *Escherichia coli* diarrheal infection of mice. Infect Immun 47:573–574, 1985.
71. Tzipori S, Makin T, Smith M, Krautil F. Enteritis in foals induced by rotavirus and enterotoxigenic *Escherichia coli*. Aust Vet J 58:20–23, 1982.
72. Bishop R, Barnes G, Cipriani E, Lund J. Clinical immunity after neonatal rotavirus infection: A prospective longitudinal study in young children. N Engl J Med 309:72–76, 1983.
73. Bernstein DI, Sander DS, Smith VE, et al. Protection from rotavirus reinfection: 2-year prospective study. J Infect Dis 164:277–283, 1991.
74. Ward RL, Bernstein D. Protection against rotavirus disease after natural infection. J Infect Dis 169:900–904, 1994.
75. Matson DO, O'Ryan ML, Herrera I, et al. Fecal antibody responses to symptomatic and asymptomatic rotavirus infections. J Infect Dis 167:577–583, 1993.
76. Coulson B, Grimwood K, Hudson I, et al. Role of coproantibody in clinical protection of children during reinfection with rotavirus. J Clin Microbiol 30:1678–1684, 1992.
77. O'Ryan ML, Matson DO, Estes MK, Pickering LK. Anti-rotavirus G type-specific and isotype-specific antibodies in children with natural rotavirus infection. J Infect Dis 169:504–511, 1994.
78. Yolken R, Wyatt R, Zissis G. Epidemiology of human rotavirus types 1 and 2 as studied by enzyme-linked immunosorbent assay. N Engl J Med 299:1156–1161, 1978.
79. Black R, Greenberg H, Kapikian A, et al. Acquisition of serum antibody to Norwalk virus and rotavirus in relation to diarrhea in a longitudinal study of young children in rural Bangladesh. J Infect Dis 145:483–489, 1982.
80. Bishop R, Barnes G, Cipriani E, Lund J. Clinical immunity after neonatal rotavirus infection: A prospective longitudinal study in young children. N Engl J Med 309:72–76, 1983.
81. Mata L, Simhon A, Urratia J, et al. Epidemiology of rotaviruses in a cohort of 45 Guatemalan Mayan Indian children observed from birth to the age of three years. J Infect Dis 148:452–461, 1983.
82. Chiba S, Nakata S, Urasawa T, et al. Protective effect of naturally acquired homotypic and heterotypic rotavirus antibodies. Lancet 1:417–421, 1986.
83. Linhares A, Gabbay Y, Mascarenhas J, et al. Epidemiology of rotavirus subgroups and serotypes in Belem, Brazil: A three-year study. Ann Inst Pasteur/Virol 139:89–99, 1988.
84. Georges-Courbot M, Monges J, Beraud-Cassel A, et al. Prospective longitudinal study of rotavirus infections in children from birth to two years of age in Central Africa. Ann Inst Pasteur/Virol 139:421–428, 1988.
85. Friedman M, Gaul A, Sarov B, et al. Two sequential outbreaks of rotavirus gastroenteritis: Evidence for symptomatic and asymptomatic reinfection. J Infect Dis 158:814–822, 1988.
86. Grinstein S, Gomez J, Bercovich J, Biscorn E. Epidemiology of rotavirus infection and gastroenteritis in prospectively monitored Argentine families with young children. Am J Epidemiol 130:300–308, 1989.
87. Reves R, Hossain M, Midthun K, et al. An observational study of naturally-acquired immunity in a cohort of 363 Egyptian children. Am J Epidemiol 130:981–988, 1989.
88. O'Ryan M, Matson D, Estes M, et al. Molecular epidemiology of rotavirus in young children attending day care centers in Houston. J Infect Dis 162:810–816, 1990.
89. DeChamps C, Laveran H, Peigue-Lafeville J, et al. Sequential rotavirus infections: Characterization of serotypes and electropherotypes. Res Virol 142:39–45, 1991.
90. Matson DO, O'Ryan ML, Herrera I, et al. Fecal antibody responses to symptomatic and asymptomatic rotavirus infections. J Infect Dis 167:577–583, 1993.
91. Madore H, Christy C, Pichichero M, et al. Field trial of rhesus rotavirus or human-rhesus rotavirus reassortant vaccine of VP7 serotype 3 or 1 specificity in infants. J Infect Dis 166:235–243, 1992.
92. Bernstein D, Glass R, Rodgers G, et al. Evaluation of rhesus rotavirus monovalent and tetravalent reassortant vaccines in US children. JAMA 273:1191–1196, 1995.

93. Ward R, Bernstein D. Lack of correlation between serum rotavirus antibody titers and protection following vaccination with reassortant RRV vaccines. Vaccine 13:1226–1252, 1995.
94. Offit PA, Dudzik KI. Rotavirus-specific cytotoxic T lymphocytes appear at the intestinal mucosal surface after rotavirus infection. J Virol 63:3507–3512, 1989.
95. Offit PA, Dudzik KI. Rotavirus-specific cytotoxic T lymphocytes passively protect against gastroenteritis in suckling mice. J Virol 64:6325–6328, 1990.
96. Dharakul T, Rott L, Greenberg HB. Recovery from chronic rotavirus infection in mice with severe combined immunodeficiency: Virus clearance mediated by adoptive transfer of immune $CD8^+$ T lymphocytes. J Virol 64:4375–4382, 1990.
97. Franco M, Tin C, Greenberg H. $CD8^+$ T cells can mediate complete short term and partial long term protection against reinfection by rotavirus. J Virol 71:4165–4170, 1997.
98. Clark HF, Borian FE, Bell LM, et al. Protective effect of WC3 vaccine against rotavirus diarrhea in infants during a predominantly serotype 1 rotavirus season. J Infect Dis 158:570–587, 1988.
99. Chiba S, Nakata S, Urasawa T, et al. Protective effect of naturally acquired homotypic and heterotypic rotavirus antibodies. Lancet 1:417–421, 1986.
100. Burns J, Siadet-Pajouh M, Krishnaney A, Greenberg HB. Novel anti-viral effect against murine rotavirus by an anti-VP6 IgA monoclonal antibody that lacks conventional in vitro neutralizing activity. Science 272:104–107, 1996.
101. Offit PA, Dudzik KI. Rotavirus-specific cytotoxic T lymphocytes cross-react with target cells infected with different rotavirus serotypes. J Virol 62:127–131, 1988.
102. Matsui S, Mackow E, Greenberg H. Molecular determinants of rotavirus neutralization and protection. Adv Virus Res 36:181–214, 1989.
103. Matson D, O'Ryan M, Pickering L, et al. Characterization of serum antibody responses to natural rotavirus infections in children by VP7-specific epitope-blocking assays. J Clin Microbiol 30:1056–1061, 1992.
104. Zheng B, Han S, Yan Y, et al. Development of neutralizing antibodies and group A common antibodies against natural infections with human rotavirus. J Clin Microbiol 26:1506–1512, 1988.
105. Puerto F, Padilla-Noriega L, Zamora-Chavez A, et al. Prevalent patterns of serotype-specific seroconversion in Mexican children infected with rotavirus. J Clin Microbiol 25:960–963, 1987.
106. Gerna G, Sarasini A, Torsellini M, et al. Group- and type-specific serologic response in infants and children with primary rotavirus infections and gastroenteritis caused by a strain of known serotype. J Infect Dis 161:1105–1111, 1990.
107. Clark H, Dolan K, Horton-Slight P, et al. Diverse serologic response to rotavirus infection of infants in a single epidemic. Pediatr Infect Dis 4:626–631, 1985.
108. Brandt CD, Kim HW, Rodriguez WJ, et al. Comparison of direct electron microscopy, immune electron microscopy and rotavirus enzyme-linked immunosorbent assay for detection of gastroenteritis viruses in children. J Clin Microbiol 13:976–981, 1981.
109. Rubenstein AS, Miller MF. Comparison of enzyme immunoassay with electron microscopy procedures for detecting rotavirus. J Clin Microbiol 15:938–944, 1982.
110. Chrystie IL, Totterdell BM, Banatvala JE. False positive Rotazyme tests on faecal samples from babies [letter]. Lancet 2:1028, 1983.
111. Doern GV, Herrman JE, Henderson P, et al. Detection of rotavirus with a new polyclonal antibody enzyme immunoassay (Rotazyme II) and commercial latex agglutination test (Rotalex): Comparison with a monoclonal antibody enzyme immunoassay. J Clin Microbiol 23:226–229, 1986.
112. Sanders RC, Campbell AD, Jenkins AF. Routine detection of human rotavirus by latex agglutination: Comparison with latex agglutination, electron microscopy and polyacrylamide gel electrophoresis. J Virol Methods 13:285–290, 1986.
113. Bridger JC. Novel rotaviruses in animals and man. In Diarrhea Viruses. Ciba Foundation Symposium 128. Chichester, England, John Wiley & Sons, 1987, pp 5–23.
114. Bhan MK, Lew JF, Sazawal S, et al. Protection conferred by neonatal rotavirus infection against subsequent diarrhea. J Infect Dis 168:282–287, 1993.
115. Institute of Medicine. The prospects of immunizing against rotavirus. In New Vaccine Development: Diseases of Importance in Developing Countries. Vol. 2. Washington, DC, National Academy Press, 1986, pp D13-1–D13-12.
116. Kraft LM. Studies on the etiology and transmission of epidemic diarrhea of infant mice. J Exp Med 106:743–755, 1957.
117. Alfieri AA, Leite JPG, Nakagomi O, et al. Characterization of human rotavirus genotype P[8]G5 from Brazil by probe-hybridization and sequence. Arch Virol 141:2353–2364, 1996.
118. Gentsch J, Das BK, Jiang B, et al. Similarity of the VP4 protein of human rotavirus strain 116E to that of the bovine B223 strain. Virology 194:424–430, 1993.
119. Nakagomi, T, Nakagomi O. RNA-RNA hybridization identifies a human rotavirus that is genetically related to feline rotavirus. J Virol 63:1431–1434, 1989.
120. Hrdy D. Epidemiology of rotaviral infection in adults. Rev Infect Dis 9:461–469, 1987.
121. Bartlett AV, Reves RR, Pickering LK. Rotavirus in infant-toddler day care centers: Epidemiology relevant to disease control strategies. J Pediatr 113:435–441, 1988.
122. Pickering LK, Bartlett AV, Reves RR, Morrow A. Asymptomatic excretion of rotavirus before and after rotavirus diarrhea in children in day care centers. J Pediatr 112:361–365, 1988.
123. Pickering LK, Evans DG, DuPont HL. Diarrhea caused by *Shigella*, rotavirus, and *Giardia* in day care centers: Prospective study. J Pediatr 99:51–56, 1981.
124. DuPont HL, Ericsson CD. Prevention and treatment of traveler's diarrhea. N Engl J Med 328:1821–1827, 1993.
125. Cunningham AL, Grohmann GS, Harkness J, et al. Gastrointestinal viral infections in homosexual men who were symptomatic and seropositive for human immunodeficiency virus. J Infect Dis 158:386–391, 1988.
126. Hindley F, McIntyre M, Clark B, et al. Heterogeneity of genome rearrangements in rotaviruses isolated from a chronically infected immunodeficient child. J Virol 61:3365–3372, 1987.
127. Saulsbury FT, Winkelstein JA, Yolken RH. Chronic rotavirus infection in immunodeficiency. J Pediatr 97:61–65, 1980.
128. Yolken RJ, Bishop CA, Towsend R. Infectious gastroenteritis in bone marrow transplant recipients. N Engl J Med 306:1009–1012, 1982.
129. Advisory Committee on Immunization Practices. Rotavirus vaccines for the prevention of rotavirus diarrhea in children (draft recommendations, dated June 3, 1998).
130. Gentsch JR, Woods PA, Ramachandran M, et al. Review of G and P typing results from a global collection of strains: Implications for vaccine development. J Infect Dis 174(suppl 1):S30–36, 1996.
131. Hoshino Y, Kapikian AZ. Rotavirus vaccine development for the prevention of severe diarrhea in infants and young children. Trends Microbiol 2:242–249, 1994.
132. Ramachandran M, Das BK, Vij A, et al. Unusual diversity of human rotavirus G and P genotypes in India. J Clin Microbiol 34:436–439, 1996.
133. Timenetsky M do C, Santos N, Gouvea V. Survey of rotavirus G and P types associated with human gastroenteritis in Šao Paulo, Brazil, from 1986 to 1992. J Clin Microbiol 32:2622–2624, 1994.
134. Gurwith M, Wenman W, Gurwith D, et al. Diarrhea among infants and young children in Canada: A longitudinal study in three northern communities. J Infect Dis 147:685–692, 1983.
135. Koopman JS, Turkish VJ, Monto AS, et al. Patterns and etiology of diarrhea in three clinical settings. Am J Epidemiol 119:114–123, 1984.
136. Rodriguez WJ, Kim HW, Brandt CD, et al. Longitudinal study of rotavirus infection and gastroenteritis in families served by a pediatric medical practice: Clinical and epidemiologic observations. Pediatr Infect Dis J 6:170–176, 1987.
137. Ho M-S, Glass RI, Pinsky PF, Anderson LJ. Rotavirus as a cause of diarrheal morbidity and mortality in the United States. J Infect Dis 158:1112–1116, 1988.
138. Ho M-S, Glass RI, Pinsky PF, et al. Diarrheal deaths in American children: Are they preventable? JAMA 260:3281–3285, 1988.
139. Ing D, Glass RI, LeBaron CW, Lew JF. Laboratory-based sur-

veillance for rotavirus in the United States, January 1989–May 1991. MMWR CDC Surveill Summ 41:47–56, 1992.
140. LeBaron CW, Lew J, Glass RI, et al, and The Rotavirus Study Group. Annual rotavirus epidemic patterns in North America: Results of a five-year retrospective survey of 88 centers in Canada, Mexico, and the United States. JAMA 264:983–988, 1990.
141. Torok TJ, Clarke MJ, Holman RC, Glass RI. Visualizing geographic and temporal trends in rotavirus activity in the United States, 1991–1996. Pediatr Infect Dis J 16:941–946, 1997.
142. Glass RI, Kilgore PE, Holman RC, et al. The epidemiology of rotavirus diarrhea in the United States: Surveillance and estimates of disease burden. J Infect Dis 174(suppl 1):S5–11, 1996.
143. Matson DO, Estes MK. Impact of rotavirus infection at a large pediatric hospital. J Infect Dis 162:598–604, 1990.
144. Ryan MJ, Ramsay M, Brown D, et al. Hospital admissions attributable to rotavirus infection in England and Wales. J Infect Dis 174(suppl 1):S12–S18, 1996.
145. Guarino A, Russo S, Castaldo A, et al. Passive immunotherapy for rotavirus-induced diarrhoea in children with HIV infection. AIDS 10:1176–1177, 1996.
146. Guarino A, Canani R, Russo S, et al. Oral immunoglobulins for treatment of acute rotaviral gastroenteritis. Pediatrics 93:12–16, 1994.
147. Guarino A, Guandalini S, Albano F, et al. Enteral immunoglobulins for treatment of protracted rotaviral diarrhea. Pediatr Infect Dis J 10:612–614, 1991.
148. Turner R, Kelsey D. Passive immunization for prevention of rotavirus illness in healthy infants. Pediatr Infect Dis J 12:718–722, 1993.
149. Delem A, Lobmann M, Zygraich N. A bovine rotavirus developed as a candidate vaccine for use in humans. J Biol Stand 12:443–445, 1984.
150. Mebus CA, White RG, Bass EP, Twiehaus MJ. Immunity to neonatal calf diarrhea virus. J Am Vet Med Assoc 163:880–883, 1973.
151. De Mol P, Zissis G, Butzler JP, et al. Failure of live, attenuated and rotavirus vaccine [letter]. Lancet 2:108, 1986.
152. Vesikari T, Isolauri E, Delem A, et al. Immunogenicity and safety of life oral attenuated bovine rotavirus vaccine strain RIT 4237 in adults and young children. Lancet 2:807–811, 1983.
153. Vesikari T, Isolauri E, Delem A, et al. Clinical efficacy of the RIT 4237 live attenuated bovine rotavirus vaccine in infants vaccinated before a rotavirus epidemic. J Pediatr 107:189–194, 1985.
154. Vesikari T, Isolauri E, D'Hondt E, et al. Protection of infants against rotavirus diarrhoea by RIT 4237 attenuated bovine rotavirus strain vaccine. Lancet 1:977–980, 1984.
155. Hanlon P, Hanlon K, Marsh V, et al. Trial of an attenuated bovine rotavirus vaccine (RIT 4237) in Gambian infants. Lancet 1:1342–1345, 1987.
156. Santosham M, Letson GW, Wolff M, et al. A field study of the safety and efficacy of two candidate rotavirus vaccines in a Native American population. J Infect Dis 163:483–487, 1991.
157. Lanata CF, Black RE, deAguila R, et al. Protection of Peruvian children against rotavirus diarrhea of specific serotypes by one, two, or three doses of the RIT 4237 attenuated bovine rotavirus vaccine. J Infect Dis 159:452–459, 1989.
158. Vesikari T, Ruuska T, Delem A, et al. Efficacy of two doses of RIT 4237 bovine rotavirus vaccine for prevention of rotavirus diarrhea. Acta Paediatr Scand 80:173–180, 1991.
159. Vesikari T, Isolauri E, D'Hondt E, et al. Increased "take" rate of oral rotavirus vaccine in infants after milk feeding [letter]. Lancet 2:700, 1984.
160. Vesikari T, Ruuska T, Bogaerts H, et al. Dose-response study of RIT 4237 oral rotavirus vaccine in breast-fed and formula-fed infants. Pediatr Infect Dis J 4:622–625, 1985.
161. Vodopija I, Baklaic Z, Vlatkovic R, et al. Combined vaccination with live oral polio vaccine and the bovine rotavirus RIT 4237. Vaccine 4:233–236, 1986.
162. Maldonado Y, Hestvik L, Wilson M, et al. Safety and immunogenicity of bovine rotavirus vaccine RIT 4237 in 3-month-old infants. J Pediatr 109:931–935, 1986.
163. Clark HF, Furukawa T, Bell LM, et al. Immune response of infants and children to low-passage bovine rotavirus (strain WC3). Am J Dis Child 140:350–356, 1986.
164. Garbag-Chenon A, Fontaine J-L, Lasfargues G, et al. Reactogenicity and immunogenicity of rotavirus WC3 vaccine in 5–12-month-old infants. Res Virol 140:207–217, 1989.
165. Bernstein DI, Smith VE, Sander DS, et al. Evaluation of WC3 rotavirus vaccine and correlates of protection in healthy infants. J Infect Dis 162:1055–1062, 1990.
166. Ward RL, Sander DS, Schiff GM, Bernstein DI. Effect of vaccination on serotype-specific antibody responses in infants administered WC3 bovine rotavirus before or after a natural rotavirus infection. J Infect Dis 162:1298–1303, 1990.
167. Georges-Courbot MC, Monges J, Siopathis MR, et al. Evaluation of the efficacy of a low-passage bovine rotavirus (strain WC3) vaccine in children in Central Africa. Res Virol 142:405–411, 1991.
168. Stuker G, Oshiro LS, Schmidt NH. Antigenic comparisons of two new rotaviruses from rhesus monkeys. J Clin Microbiol 11:202–203, 1980.
169. Kapikian AZ, Midthun K, Hoshino Y, et al. Rhesus rotavirus: A candidate vaccine for prevention of human rotavirus disease. In Lerner RA, Chanock RM, Brown F (eds). Molecular and Chemical Basis of Resistance to Parasitic, Bacterial, and Viral Diseases. Cold Spring Harbor, NY, Cold Spring Harbor Laboratory, 1985, pp 357–367.
170. Nishikawa K, Hoshino Y, Taniguchi K, et al. Rotavirus v.p. 7 neutralization epitopes of serotype 3 strains. Virology 171:503–515, 1989.
171. Losonsky GA, Rennels MB, Kapikian AZ, et al. Safety, infectivity, transmissibility and immunogenicity of rhesus rotavirus vaccine (MMU18006) in infants. Pediatr Infect Dis 5:25–29, 1986.
172. Vesikari T, Kapikian AZ, Delem A, Zissis G. A comparative trial of rhesus monkey (RRV-1) and bovine (RIT 4237) oral rotavirus vaccines in young children. J Infect Dis 153:832–839, 1986.
173. Perez-Schael I, Gonzalez M, Daoud N, et al. Reactogenicity and antigenicity of the rhesus rotavirus vaccine in Venezuelan children. J Infect Dis 155:334–338, 1987.
174. Pichichero ME, Losonsky GA, Rennels MB, et al. Effect of dose and comparison of measures of vaccine take for oral rhesus rotavirus vaccine. Pediatr Infect Dis J 9:339–344, 1990.
175. Pichichero ME. Effect of breast-feeding on oral rhesus rotavirus vaccine seroconversion: A metaanalysis. J Infect Dis 162:753–755, 1990.
176. Flores J, Daud D, Daud N, et al. Reactogenicity and antigenicity of rhesus rotavirus vaccine (MMV-18006) in newborn infants in Venezuela. Pediatr Infect Dis J 6:260–264, 1988.
177. Jalil F, Zaman S, Carlsson B, et al. Immunogenicity and reactogenicity of rhesus rotavirus vaccine given in combination with oral or inactivated poliovirus vaccines and diphtheria-tetanus-pertussis vaccine. Trans R Soc Trop Med Hyg 85:292–296, 1991.
178. Vesikari T, Rautanen T, Varis T, et al. Rhesus rotavirus candidate vaccine. Clinical trial in children vaccinated between 2 and 5 months of age. Am J Dis Child 144:285–289, 1990.
179. Gothefors L, Wadell G, Juto P, et al. Prolonged efficacy of rhesus rotavirus vaccine in Swedish children. J Infect Dis 159:753–757, 1989.
180. Santosham M, Letson GW, Wolff M, et al. A field study of the safety and efficacy of two candidate rotavirus vaccines in a Native American population. J Infect Dis 163:483–487, 1991.
181. Christy C, Madore HP, Pichichero ME, et al. Field trial of rhesus rotavirus vaccine in infants. Pediatr Infect Dis J 7:645–650, 1988.
182. Rennels MB, Losonsky GA, Young AE, et al. An efficacy trial of the rhesus rotavirus vaccine in Maryland. Am J Dis Child 144:601–604, 1990.
183. Christy C, Madore HP, Pichichero ME, et al. Field trial of rhesus rotavirus or human-rhesus reassortant rotavirus vaccine of VP7 serotype 3 or 1 specificity in infants. J Infect Dis 166:235–243, 1992.
184. Flores J, Perez-Schael I, Gonzalez M, et al. Protection against severe rotavirus diarrhea by rhesus rotavirus vaccine in Venezuelan children. Lancet 1:882–884, 1987.
185. Perez-Schael I, Garcia D, Gonzalez M, et al. A prospective study of diarrheal diseases in Venezuelan children to evaluate the efficacy of rhesus rotavirus vaccine. J Med Virol 30:219–229, 1990.
186. Kapikian AZ, Hoshino Y, Chanock RM, Perez-Schael I. Efficacy of a quadrivalent rhesus rotavirus–based human rotavirus vaccine

aimed at preventing severe rotavirus diarrhea in infants and young children. J Infect Dis 174(suppl 1):S65–S72, 1996.
187. Bernstein DI, Glass RI, Rodgers G, et al. Evaluation of rhesus rotavirus monovalent and tetravalent reassortant vaccines in US children. JAMA 273:1191–1196, 1995.
188. Rennels MB, Glass RI, Dennehy PH, et al. Safety and efficacy of high-dose rhesus-human reassortant rotavirus vaccines: Report of the national multicenter trial. Pediatrics 97:7–13, 1996.
189. Lanata CF, Midthun K, Black RE, et al. Safety, immunogenicity, and protective efficacy of one and three doses of the tetravalent rhesus rotavirus vaccine in infants in Lima, Peru. J Infect Dis 174:268–275, 1996.
190. Linhares AC, Gabbay YB, Mascarenhas JDP, et al. Immunogenicity, safety and efficacy of tetravalent rhesus-human, reassortant rotavirus vaccine in Belem, Brazil. Bull World Health Organ 74:491–500, 1996.
191. Perez-Schael I, Guntinas MJ, Perez M, et al. Efficacy of the rhesus-rotavirus based quadrivalent vaccine in infants and young children in Venezuela. N Engl J Med 337:1181–1187, 1997.
192. Santosham M, Moulton LH, Reid R, et al. Efficacy and safety of high-dose rhesus-human reassortant rotavirus vaccine in Native American populations. J Pediatr 131:632–638, 1997.
193. Joensuu J, Koskenniemi E, Pang XL, et al. Randomized placebo-controlled trial of rhesus-human reassortant rotavirus vaccine for prevention of severe rotavirus gastroenteritis. Lancet 350:1205–1209, 1997.
193a. Joensuu J, Koskenniemi E, Vesikari T. Clinical symptoms associated with rhesus-human reassortant rotavirus vaccine in Finland. Pediatr Infect Dis J 17:334–340, 1998.
194. Gothefors L, Wadell G, Juto P, et al. Prolonged efficacy of rhesus rotavirus vaccine in Swedish children. J Infect Dis 159:753–757, 1989.
195. Wright PF, King J, Araki K, et al. Simultaneous administration of two human-rhesus rotavirus reassortant strains of VP7 serotype 1 and 2 specificity to infants and young children. J Infect Dis 164:271–276, 1991.
196. Clark HF, Borian FE, Modesto K, Plotkin SA. Serotype l reassortant of bovine rotavirus WC3, strain WI79–9, induces a polytypic antibody response in infant. Vaccine 8:327–332, 1990.
197. Treanor J, Clark HF, Pichichero M, et al. Evaluation of the protective efficacy of a serotype l human-bovine rotavirus reassortant vaccine in infants. Pediatr Infect Dis J 14:301–307, 1995.
198. Clark HF, Offit PA, Ellis RW, et al. WC3 reassortant vaccines in children: Brief review. Arch Virol Suppl 12:187–198, 1996.
199. Clark HF, Offit PA, Ellis RW, et al. The development of multivalent bovine rotavirus (strain WC3) reassortant vaccine for infants. J Infect Dis 174(suppl l):S73–S80, 1996.
200. Hoshino Y, Saif LJ, Kang SY, et al. Identification of group A rotavirus genes associated with virulence of a porcine rotavirus and host range restriction of a human rotavirus in a gnotobiotic piglet model. Virology 209:274–280, 1995.
201. Broome RL, Vo PT, Ward RL, et al. Murine rotavirus genes encoding outer capsid proteins VP4 and VP7 are not major determinants of host range restriction and virulence. J Virol 67:2448–2455, 1993.
202. Clark HF, Welsko D, Offit PA. Infant responses to bovine WC3 reassortants containing human rotavirus VP7, VP4, or VP7 and VP4. 32nd Interscience Conference on Antimicrobial Agents and Chemotherapy; Anaheim, CA; October 11–14, 1992, p 343.
203. Clark HF, Borian FE, Plotkin SA. Immune protection of infants against rotavirus gastroenteritis by a serotype 1 reassortant of bovine rotavirus WC3. J Infect Dis 161:1099–1104, 1990.
204. Clark HF, White CJ, Offit PA, et al, and OHBRV Study Group. Preliminary evaluation of safety and efficacy of quadrivalent human-bovine reassortant rotavirus vaccine. Pediatr Res 37:172A, 1995.
205. Hoshino Y, Kapikian AZ. Rotavirus vaccine development for the prevention of severe diarrhea in infants and young children. Trends Microbiol 2:242–249, 1994.
206. Makhene M, Midthun K, Karron R, et al. Safety and immunogenicity of human–UK bovine rotavirus reassortants in adults and pediatric subjects [abstract SV39]. Program and abstracts of the Fifth Rotavirus Vaccine Workshop; Atlanta, GA; October 16–17, 1995.
207. Hoshino Y, Wyatt RG, Flores J, et al. Serotypic characterization of rotaviruses derived from asymptomatic human neonatal infections. J Clin Microbiol 21:425–430, 1985.
208. Flores J, Perez-Schael I, Blanco M, et al. Comparison of reactogenicity and antigenicity of M37 rotavirus vaccine and rhesus-rotavirus–based quadrivalent vaccine. Lancet 2:330–334, 1990.
209. Vesikari T, Ruuska T, Koivu H-P, et al. Evaluation of the M37 human rotavirus vaccine in 2- to 6-month-old infants. Pediatr Infect Dis J 10:912–917, 1991.
210. Midthun K, Halsey NA, Jett-Goheen M, et al. Safety and immunogenicity of human rotavirus vaccine strain M37 in adults, children and infants. J Infect Dis 164:792–796, 1991.
211. Barnes G, Bishop R, Lund J, et al. Phase 1 trial of a neonatal strain (RV3) rotavirus vaccine candidate [abstract SV-33]. Program and abstracts of the Fifth Rotavirus Vaccine Workshop; Atlanta, GA; October 16–17, 1995.
212. Bernstein DI, Glass RI, Rodgers G, et al, US Rotavirus Vaccine Efficacy Group. Evaluation of rhesus monovalent and tetravalent reassortant vaccines in US children. JAMA 273:1191–1196, 1995.
213. Pichichero ME, Marsocci SM, Francis AB, et al. A comparative evaluation of the safety and immunogenicity of single dose of unbuffered oral rhesus rotavirus serotype 3, rhesus/human reassortant serotypes l, 2 and 4 and combined (tetravalent) vaccines in healthy infants. Vaccine 11:747–753, 1993.
214. Dennehy PH, Rodgers GC, Ward RL, et al. Comparative evaluation of reactogenicity and immunogenicity of two dosages of oral tetravalent rhesus rotavirus vaccine. Pediatr Infect Dis J 15:1012–1018, 1996.
215. Weiss C, Clark HF. Rapid inactivation of rotaviruses by exposure to acid buffer or acidic gastric juice. J Gen Virol 66:2725–2730, 1985.
216. Ing DJ, Glass RI, Woods PA, et al. Immunogenicity of tetravalent rhesus rotavirus vaccine administered with buffer and oral polio vaccine. Am J Dis Child 145:892–897, 1991.
217. Rennels M. Influence of breast-feeding and oral poliovirus vaccine on the immunogenicity and efficacy of rotavirus vaccines. J Infect Dis 174(suppl 1):S107–S111, 1996.
218. Migasena S, Simasathien S, Samakoses R, et al. Simultaneous administration of oral rhesus-human reassortant tetravalent (RRV-TV) rotavirus vaccine and oral poliovirus vaccine (OPV) in Thai infants. Vaccine 13:168–174, 1995.
219. Vodopija I, Baklaic Z, Vlatkovic R, et al. Combined vaccination with live oral polio vaccine and the bovine rotavirus RIT 4237 strain. Vaccine 4:233–236, 1986.
220. Giammanco G, DeGrandi V, Lupo L, et al. Interference of oral poliovirus vaccine on RIT 4237 oral rotavirus vaccine. Eur J Epidemiol 4:121–123, 1988.
221. Offit PA, Khoury CA, Moser CH, et al. Enhancement of rotavirus immunogenicity by microencapsulation. Virology 203:134–143, 1994.
222. Brown KA, Moser CA, Khoury CA, et al. Enhancement by microencapsulation of rotavirus-specific intestinal immune responses in mice assessed by enzyme-linked immunospot assay and intestinal fragment culture. J Infect Dis 171:1334–1338, 1995.
223. Khoury CA, Moser CA, Speaker TJ, Offit PA. Oral inoculation of mice with low doses of microencapsulated, noninfectious rotavirus induces virus-specific antibodies in gut-associated lymphoid tissue. J Infect Dis 172:870–874, 1995.
224. Coffin SE, Klinek M, Offit PA. Induction of virus-specific antibody production by lamina propria lymphocytes following intramuscular inoculation with rotavirus. J Infect Dis 172:874–878, 1995.
225. Conner M, Crawford S, Barone C, Estes M. Rotavirus vaccine administered parenterally induces protective immunity. J Virol 67:6633–6641, 1993.
226. Periwal SB, Speaker TJ, Cebra JJ. Orally administered microencapsulated reovirus can bypass suckled, neutralizing maternal antibody that inhibits active immunization of neonates. J Virol 71:2844–2850, 1997.
227. Estes MK, Crawford SE, Penadanda ME, et al. Synthesis and immunogenicity of the rotavirus major capsid antigen using a baculovirus expression system. J Virol 61:1488–1494, 1987.
228. Herrmann JE, Chen SC, Fynan EF, et al. Protection against rotavirus infections by DNA vaccination. J Infect Dis 174:S93–S97, 1996.
229. Bresee J. Review of rotavirus vaccines [in press].

230. World Health Organization. Vaccine research and development. Rotavirus vaccines for developing countries. Wkly Epidemiol Rec 72:35–40, 1997.
231. Glass RI, Lang DR, Ivanoff BN, Compans RW. Introduction: Rotavirus—from basic research to a vaccine. J Infect Dis 174(suppl 1):S1–S2, 1996.
232. Lang DL, Glass RI, Compans RW. Summary of the Fifth Rotavirus Vaccine Workshop. J Infect Dis 174(suppl 1):S3–S4, 1996.
233. Tucker AW, Bresee JS, Haddix AC, et al. Rotavirus immunization program: Cost-effectiveness analysis in the US. JAMA 279:1371–1376, 1998.
234. Patriarca PA, Wright PF, John JT. Factors affecting the immunology of oral polio vaccine in developing countries: A review. Rev Infect Dis 13:926–939, 1991.
235. Cicirello HG, Das BK, Gupta A, et al. High prevalence of rotavirus infection among neonates born at hospitals in Delhi, India: Predisposition of newborns for infection with unusual rotavirus. Pediatr Infect Dis J 13:720–724, 1994.

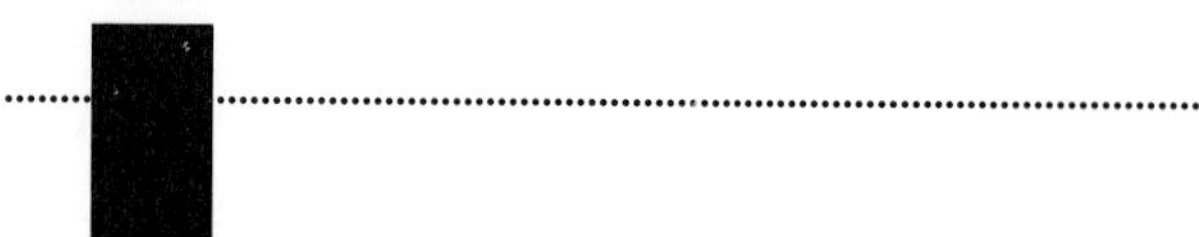

PUBLIC HEALTH AND REGULATORY ISSUES

chapter

42 Public Health Considerations—United States

Walter A. Orenstein
Alan R. Hinman
Lance E. Rodewald

Vaccines represent some of the most important tools available for the prevention of disease. In addition to protecting the vaccinated individual from developing a potentially serious disease, they help protect the community by reducing the spread of infectious agents. For diseases spread from person to person, if a high enough proportion of the population is immunized, transmission may be interrupted in the community, thus providing protection to those who are not themselves immunized. This indirect protection is often called *herd immunity*.[1, 2] From both theoretical and practical perspectives, disease usually disappears before immunization levels reach 100%, as has been seen with smallpox and poliomyelitis.[3–10]

With no intervention, the occurrence of a disease is affected only by the traditional considerations of host, agent, and environment (Fig. 42–1). As an intervention is applied, the incidence of the disease decreases, reaching an acceptable level of control. Further application of the intervention may lead to interruption of transmission of the agent and disappearance of the agent from the area under consideration, but with a threat of reintroduction large enough that continued application of the intervention is required. This stage, *elimination*, describes the current goals for measles and rubella in the United States. If enough areas achieve elimination, *regional eradication* may be achieved, in which the intervention can be halted. However, regional eradication is inherently unstable in this era of global transportation and is merely a way station on the road to true *eradication*, in which transmission of the agent has been halted throughout the world and continuation of the intervention is no longer needed.[11, 12]

In 1980, the world was declared free of smallpox, ending the centuries of disease and death brought about by that disease (see Chapter 6).[13] Eradication of smallpox was possible because there was a highly effective vaccine, no nonhuman reservoir to perpetuate circulation of virus, and no long-term carrier state to perpetuate potential for spread. Eradication was made simpler by the relatively low communicability of smallpox and by the fact that both disease and vaccine gave a readily visible marker of immunity, the scar. Eradication of smallpox has raised the possibility that other diseases might also be eradicated.[12, 14–22]

Elimination target dates have been set for various diseases in several different countries. The United States, Canada, and several countries in Europe have announced target dates to eliminate measles within this century.[23–29] In addition, the Pan American Health Organization (available at http://www.paho.org) has set a hemispheric goal of measles elimination by the year 2000.[30] Rubella elimination target dates have been set in the United States, Finland, Norway, and Sweden, and mumps elimination target dates have been set in Sweden and Finland.[22, 27–29, 31–33] Reflecting the difficulties in moving from control to elimination, the European Region of the World Health Organization has proposed a goal of eliminating indigenous measles transmission by 2007, rather than the year 2000 target set earlier.[34] The establishment of these elimination target dates indicates optimism that other diseases can be eradicated.

In May 1985, the Pan American Health Organization, speaking for the countries of North and South America, announced a hemispheric goal of eradicating wild polio virus transmission by the year 1990.[35] The last case

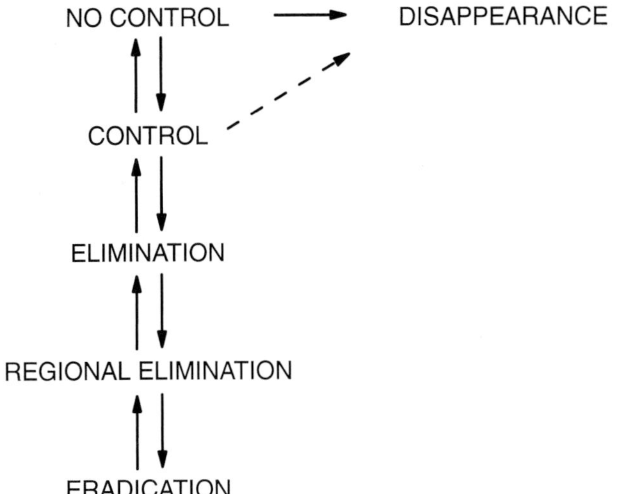

Figure 42–1. Spectrum of disease incidence.

of paralysis resulting from indigenously acquired wild poliovirus in the Americas had an onset in August 1991, and the Americas were certified free of poliomyelitis in 1994.[36, 37] The success of the polio eradication effort in North and South America[38, 39] spurred the World Health Assembly in 1988 to establish a goal of global eradication of polio by the year 2000.[40] The Western Pacific and European Regions of the World Health Organization established regional eradication goals for 1995.[41–43] Although these goals were not met in 1995, great progress is being made, and it appears that the goals will be reached by 1999.[44, 45] There is increasing support for establishment of a global measles eradication goal.[23, 46–53]

IMMUNIZATION RECOMMENDATIONS

The development of vaccine schedules and recommendations begins with prelicensure evaluation of a vaccine (available at http://www.fda.gov/cber). Prelicensure trials of vaccines are typically performed in controlled settings with relatively small numbers (i.e., thousands) of individuals involved. These trials provide important information on seroconversion following vaccination and on clinical efficacy of the vaccine in preventing disease after exposure. They also provide information about common adverse events following vaccination and contraindications to the use of the vaccines. Prelicensure evaluation also provides information on the number of doses required to achieve protection and may give an indication of the duration of immunity following vaccination. If the prelicensure trials indicate that the vaccine is safe and effective, it may be licensed for use in a particular population group. Information about the safety and efficacy of administering a vaccine simultaneously with other vaccines may be obtained either before or after licensure, but information about the safety and efficacy of combining vaccines is obtained before combinations are licensed.

Recommendations for use of a vaccine depend on the balance of benefits of vaccination (including duration of protection), risks of disease, and risks of vaccination. This balance must be assessed continually. As experience is gained with a particular vaccine, recommendations may be modified. Since the mid-1960s, recommendations in the United States about vaccination of children have traditionally been developed by two advisory bodies: (1) the Advisory Committee on Immunization Practices (ACIP) of the Public Health Service and (2) the American Academy of Pediatrics Committee on Infectious Diseases (the *Red Book* Committee).[54] The ACIP recommendations, which were originally geared primarily to providers in the public sector, have in recent years addressed providers in public and private sectors. The *Red Book* recommendations are directed mainly toward children served by pediatricians. Since 1995, the ACIP, the American Academy of Pediatrics, and the American Academy of Family Physicians have collaborated to issue a single childhood immunization schedule, which is published in the *Morbidity and Mortality Weekly Report*, *Pediatrics*, and *American Family Physician* annually.[55, 56] A continuously updated version of the harmonized schedule is available at http://www.aap.org/family/parents/immunize.htm or http://www.cdc.gov/nip/child.htm.

Recommendations of the ACIP are published in the "Recommendations and Reports" supplement of the *Morbidity and Mortality Weekly Report*; those of the *Red Book* Committee are published in the Report of the Committee on Infectious Diseases (the *Red Book*), which is revised every 2 to 4 years. New or revised recommendations of the *Red Book* Committee developed between editions of the *Red Book* are published as issued in *Pediatrics*. Appendix 1 of this text lists the published recommendations of the ACIP as of August 1998. The American College of Physicians and the Infectious Diseases Society of America have formed the Task Force on Adult Immunization, which has issued guidelines for adult immunization.[57] Recommendations for immunization of Armed Services personnel are developed by the Armed Forces Epidemiological Board.

The National Childhood Vaccine Injury Act of 1986 established a National Vaccine Program to coordinate all aspects of vaccine research, development, production, and use in both the private and the public sectors.[58] It also established a National Vaccine Advisory Committee to bring outside recommendations and advice to the National Vaccine Program.[59] Two important publications of the National Vaccine Advisory Committee have been the "measles white paper"[60] and the report on adult immunization.[61] In addition, the National Vaccine Advisory Committee played a critical role in the development of the "Standards for Pediatric Immunization Practices."[62] The National Vaccine Advisory Committee focuses most on programmatic policies and strategies, in contrast to the ACIP, which deals primarily with technical recommendations for vaccine use.

Sources of information about immunization recommendations include the following:

1. *Official package circular.* Manufacturers provide product-specific information with each vaccine; some of these circulars are reproduced in their entirety in the *Physicians' Desk Reference* (*Physicians' Desk Reference*, 52nd ed, 1998, Medical Economics Company, Montvale, NJ).

2. *Morbidity and Mortality Weekly Report.* This report is published weekly by the Centers for Disease Control and Prevention (CDC). ACIP statements are usually published in separate Recommendations and Reports Supplements to the weekly publication. Subscriptions are available through the Superintendent of Documents, US Government Printing Office, Washington, DC 20402-9235, and through MMS Publications, CSPO Box 9120, Waltham, MA 02254-9120, telephone: (800) 843-6356. The *Morbidity and Mortality Weekly Report* is also available online at http://www.cdc.gov/epo/mmwr/mmwr.html.

3. *Report of the Committee on Infectious Diseases of the American Academy of Pediatrics (Red Book).* The full report containing recommendations on all licensed vaccines is usually updated every 2 to 4 years. The most recent *Red Book* was published in 1997. It may be ordered from American Academy of Pediatrics, PO Box 927, Elk Grove Village, IL 60007.

4. *Red Book Update.* The Committee on Infectious Diseases of the American Academy of Pediatrics publishes its recent positions and specific recommendations in *Pediatrics,* the journal of the Academy. It may be ordered from American Academy of Pediatrics, PO Box 927, Elk Grove Village, IL 60009–0927.

5. *Guide for Adult Immunization.* This report was issued by the American College of Physicians in 1994 and can be ordered by calling (800) 523-1546, extension 2600; or from Subscriber Services, American College of Physicians, Independence Mall West, Sixth Street at Race, Philadelphia, PA, 19106-1572.

6. *Health Information for International Travel* (the Yellow Book). This booklet is published annually by CDC as a guide to requirements and recommendations for specific immunizations and health practices for travel to various countries.[63] It can be obtained from the Superintendent of Documents, United States Government Printing Office, Washington, DC 20402. A comprehensive and continuously updated resource for travel information is available at http://www.cdc.gov/travel/travel.html. This site includes the Yellow Book, the Blue Sheet of summary international travel information, and the Green Sheet of summary information for cruise ships.

7. *Advisory Memoranda.* Memoranda are published when necessary by CDC to advise international travelers or those who provide information to travelers about specific outbreaks of communicable diseases abroad. These memoranda include health information for prevention and specific recommendations for immunization. They may be obtained from the Division of Quarantine, Centers for Disease Control and Prevention, Atlanta, GA 30333; or at http://www.cdc.gov/travel/travel.html; or by telephone at (888) 232-3228.

8. *Control of Communicable Diseases Manual.*[64] This manual is published by the American Public Health Association at approximately 5-year intervals. The 16th edition (1995) is available now. The manual contains valuable information concerning infectious diseases, their occurrence worldwide, immunization, diagnostic and therapeutic issues, and up-to-date recommendations on isolation and other control measures for each disease presented. It may be ordered from The American Public Health Association, 1015 Fifteenth Street, NW, Washington, DC 20005.

9. *State and Local Health Departments, medical schools, and large hospitals.* Many of these agencies provide routine immunizations, immunization cards, and schedules to patients. They may also send out routine reports of disease incidence.

10. *The Task Force on Community Preventive Services* (available at http://web.health.gov/communityguide) is carrying out structured reviews of evidence for interventions to improve public health. One area being examined is universally recommended immunizations for children and adults.

The CDC National Immunization Program has established toll-free numbers for answering questions from both the general public and providers: (800) 232-2522 (English) and (800) 232-0233 (Spanish). Inquiries can also be addressed to CDC by E-mail (nipinfo@cdc.gov). The National Immunization Program operates an Internet site (available at http://www.cdc.gov/nip) that provides information for the general public, health departments, researchers, and providers.

Current Immunization Schedules

This section primarily addresses vaccines recommended for universal or widespread use in the United States. Selection of the age at which a vaccine should be administered depends on the ability of the vaccinee to respond to the vaccine, the risk of exposure to disease, and the age distribution of disease morbidity.[65–67] In general, the approach is to administer vaccine at the earliest possible age at which the vaccine is reliably effective. Sometimes, it is necessary to compromise if the risk of disease is great in young infants; for example, during the 1989 to 1991 measles resurgence, the recommended age for vaccination was temporarily lowered to 6 months in areas with a high measles incidence.[68]

Figure 42–2 shows the recommended immunization schedule for infants, children, and adolescents in the United States for 1999. As of January 1998, depending on the combination of vaccines used, a fully immunized child required 12 to 16 doses of vaccines by 18 months of age and 16 to 20 doses by 16 years of age.[56] The number of injections needed depends on whether inactivated polio vaccine is used in place of oral polio vaccine and on which combinations are selected. For a sequential inactivated polio vaccine/oral polio vaccine schedule, children would need 11 to 15 injections by 18 months of age and 14 to 18 injections by 16 years of age. With the licensure of rotavirus vaccine on August 31, 1998, three more doses of oral vaccine were added to the schedule during the first year of life at 2, 4, and 6 months of age. The United States schedule typically involves four to six visits in the first 2 years of life. Chapter 43 discusses the schedules for European countries, and Chapter 44, for developing countries. Table 42–1 summarizes recommendations for routine antigens for use in adults, and Table 42–2 outlines some recom-

Vaccines[1] are listed under the routinely recommended ages. Bars indicate range of acceptable ages for immunization. Any dose not given at the recommended age should be given as a "catch-up" immunization at any subsequent visit when indicated and feasible. Ovals indicate vaccines to be given if previously recommended doses were missed or given earlier than the recommended minimum age.

Age ▶ / Vaccine ▼	Birth	1 mo	2 mos	4 mos	6 mos	12 mos	15 mos	18 mos	4-6 yrs	11-12 yrs	14-16 yrs
Hepatitis B[2]	Hep B										
			Hep B		Hep B					(Hep B)	
Diphtheria, Tetanus, Pertussis[3]			DTaP	DTaP	DTaP		DTaP[3]		DTaP	Td	
H. influenzae type b[4]			Hib	Hib	Hib	Hib					
Polio[5]			Polio[6]	Polio		Polio[5]			Polio		
Rotavirus			*Rv*[6]	*Rv*[6]	*Rv*[6]						
Measles, Mumps, Rubella[7]						MMR			MMR[7]	(MMR[7])	
Varicella[8]							Var			(Var[8])	

Approved by the Advisory Committee on Immunization Practices (ACIP), the American Academy of Pediatrics (AAP), and the American Academy of Family Physicians (AAFP).

[1]This schedule indicates the recommended age for routine administration of currently licensed childhood vaccines. Combintion vaccines may be used whenever any components of the combination is indicated and its other components are not contraindicated. Providers should consult the manufacturers' package inserts for detailed recommendations.

[2]***Infants born to HBsAg-negative mothers*** should receive the 2nd dose of hepatitis B vaccine at least 1 month after the 1st dose. The 3rd dose should be administered at least 4 months after the 1st dose and at least 2 months after the 2nd dose, but not before 6 months of age for infants.
Infants born to HBsAg-positive mothers should receive hepatitis B vaccine and 0.5 mL hepatitis B immune globulin (HBIG) within 12 hours of birth at separate sites. The 2nd dose is recommended at 1–2 months of age and the 3rd dose at 6 months of age.
Infants born to mothers whose HBsAG status is unknown should receive hepatitis B vaccine within 12 hours of birth. Maternal blood should be drawn at the time of delivery to determine the mother's HBsAg status; if the HBsAg test is positive, the infant should receive HBIG as soon as possible (no later than 1 week of age).
All children and adolescents (through 18 years of age) who have not been immunized against hepatitis B may begin the series during any visit. Special efforts should be made to immunize children who were born in or whose parents were born in areas of the world with moderate or high endemicity of HBV infection.

[3]DTaP (diphtheria and tetanus toxoids and acellular pertussis vaccine) is the preferred vaccine for all doses in the immunization series, including completion of the series in children who have received one or more doses of whole-cell DTP vaccine. Whole-cell DTP is an acceptable alternative to DTaP. The 4th dose (DTP or DTaP) may be administered as early as 12 months of age, provided 6 months have elapsed since the 3rd dose and if the child is unlikely to return at age 15–18 months. Td (tetanus and diphtheria toxoids) is recommended at 11–12 years of age if at least 5 years have elapsed since the last dose of DTP, DTaP or DT. Subsequent routine Td boosters are recommended every 10 years.

[4]Three *H. influenzae* type b (Hib) conjugate vaccines are licensed for infant use. If PRP-OMP (PedvaxHIB and COMVAX [Merck]) is administered at 2 and 4 months of age, a dose at 6 months is not required. Because clinical studies in infants have demonstrated that using some combination products may induce a lower immune response to the Hib vaccine component, DTaP/Hib combination products should not be used for primary immunization in infants at 2, 4, or 6 months of age, unless FDA-approved for these ages.

[5]Two poliovirus vaccines currently are licensed in the United States: inactivated poliovirus vaccine (IPV) and oral poliovirus vaccine (OPV).
The ACIP, AAP, and AAFP now recommend that the first two doses of poliovirus vaccine should be IPV. The ACIP continues to recommend a sequential schedule of two doses of IPV administered at ages 2 and 4 months, followed by two doses of OPV at 12–18 months and 4–6 years. Use of IPV for all doses also is acceptable and is recommended for immunocompromised persons and their household contacts.
OPV is no longer recommended for the first two doses of the schedule and is acceptable only for special circumstances such as: children of parents who do not accept the recommended number of injections, late initiation of immunization which would require an unacceptable number of injections, and imminent travel to polio-endemic areas. OPV remains the vaccine of choice for mass immunization campaigns to control outbreaks due to wild poliovirus.

[6]Rotavirus (Rv) vaccine is shaded and italicized to indicate: (1) health-care providers may require time and resources to incorporate this new vaccine into practice; and (2) the AAFP feels that the decision to use rotavirus vaccine should be made by the parent or guardian in consultation with their physician or other health-care provider. The first dose of Rv vaccine should not be administered before 6 weeks of age, and the minimum interval between doses is 3 weeks. The Rv vaccine series should not be initiated at 7 months of age or older, and all doses should be completed by the 1st birthday.

[7]The 2nd dose of measles, mumps, and rubella vaccine (MMR) is recommended routinely at 4–6 years of age but may be administered during any visit, provided at least 4 weeks have elapsed since receipt of the 1st dose and that both doses are administered beginning at or after 12 months of age. Those who have not previously received the second dose should complete the schedule by the 11–12 year old visit.

[8]Varicella vaccine is recommended at any visit on or after the first birthday for susceptible children, i.e., those who lack a reliable history of chickenpox (as judged by a health-care provider) or who have not been immunized. Susceptible persons 13 years of age or older should receive 2 doses, given at least 4 weeks apart.

Figure 42–2. Recommended childhood immunization schedule, United States, January to December 1998. DTaP, diphtheria, tetanus, and acellular pertussis; DPT, diphtheria, pertussis, and tetanus; Hep B, hepatitis B; Hib, *Haemophilus influenzae* type b; Td, tetanus and diphtheria toxoids; MMR, measles, mumps, and rubella; Var, varicella. The schedule was published prior to licensure of rotavirus vaccine for administration at 2, 4, and 6 months.

Table 42–1. **VACCINES AND TOXOIDS RECOMMENDED FOR ADULTS, BY AGE GROUPS, UNITED STATES***

AGE GROUP (yr)	Td†	Measles	Mumps	Rubella	Varicella§	Influenza	Pneumococcal Polysaccharide
	VACCINE/TOXOID						
18–24	X	X	X	X	X		
25–64	X	X‡	X‡	X‡	X		
≥65	X				X	X	X

*Refer also to other chapters on specific vaccines or toxoids for indications, contraindications, precautions, dosages, side effects, adverse reactions, and special considerations.

†Td, tetanus and diphtheria toxoids, absorbed (for adult use), which is a combined preparation containing less than 2 flocculation units of diphtheria toxoid.

‡Varicella vaccination of susceptible adolescents and adults is desirable.

§Indicated for persons born after 1956, without evidence of immunity.

Modified from Centers for Disease Control and Prevention. Update on adult immunization: Recommendations of the Advisory Committee on Immunization Practices (ACIP). MMWR Morb Mortal Wkly Ref 40(RR-12):1–94, 1991; Prevention of Varicella, recommendations of the Advisory Committee on Immunization Practices. MMWR Morb Mortal Wkly Ref 45(No. RR-11): 1–36, 1996.

mendations for vaccine use in adults belonging to groups in the United States who are at particular risk because of lifestyle, occupation, or environment.[63, 69–71] Individual chapters on each of the vaccines should be consulted for detailed information. Continuously updated versions of the childhood and adult schedules are available at http://www.cdc.gov/nip/child.htm and http://www.cdc.gov/nip/adult.htm. Recommendations for immunization of adolescents have been developed (see under *Remaining Issues in Immunizations in the United States*).[72]

Special Groups for Whom Immunization Is Indicated

Certain groups of people are at increased risk for exposure to disease or for complications from disease

Table 42–2. **IMMUNOBIOLOGICS RECOMMENDED FOR SPECIAL OCCUPATIONS, LIFESTYLES, ENVIRONMENTAL CIRCUMSTANCES, TRAVEL, FOREIGN STUDENTS, IMMIGRANTS, AND REFUGEES, UNITED STATES***

INDICATION	IMMUNOBIOLOGICAL
Occupation	
Hospital, laboratory, and other health-care personnel	Hepatitis B, influenza, measles, rubella, mumps, varicella
Public-safety personnel	Hepatitis B, influenza
Staff of institutions for the developmentally disabled	Hepatitis B, varicella
Veterinarians and animal handlers	Rabies, plague
Selected field workers (those who come into contact with possibly infected animals)	Rabies, plague
Selected occupations (those who work with imported animal hides, furs, wool, animal hair, and bristles)	Anthrax
Lifestyle	
Men who have sex with men	Hepatitis B, hepatitis A
Injecting drug users	Hepatitis B, hepatitis A
Other illegal drug users	Hepatitis A
Heterosexual persons with multiple sexual partners or recently acquired sexually transmitted disease	Hepatitis B
Environmental situtation	
Long-term inmates of correctional facilities	Hepatitis B, varicella
Residents of institutions for the developmentally disabled	Hepatitis B, varicella
Household contacts of hepatitis B carriers	Hepatitis B
Homeless persons	Tetanus/diphtheria‡, measles, mumps, rubella, varicella, influenza
Travel†	Measles, mumps, rubella, polio, influenza, hepatitis B, hepatitis A, rabies, meningococcal polysaccharide, tetanus/diphtheria‡, yellow fever, typhoid, plague§, Japanese encephalitis, varicella
Foreign students, immigrants, and refugees	Measles, rubella, diphtheria, tetanus, mumps, hepatitis B, varicella

*Unless specifically contraindicated, the vaccines or toxoids recommended routinely for adults are also indicated.

†Vaccines needed for travelers will vary depending on individual itineraries; travelers should refer to Health Information for International Travelers, 1996–1997, for more detailed information.

‡If not received within 10 years.

§In or during travel to areas with enzootic or epidemic plague in which exposure to rodents cannot be prevented. From Update on adult immunization: Recommendations of the Advisory Committee on Immunization Practices (ACIP). MMWR Morb Mortal Wkly Rep 40(RR-12): 1–94, 1991; Prevention of varicella, recommendations of the Advisory Committee on Immunization Practices. MMWR Morb Mortal Wkly Rep 45(No. RR-11):1–36, 1996; Health Information for International Travel 1996–1997. Atlanta, GA, DHHS, 1997.

and are therefore particularly in need of immunization. In general, these concerns are addressed in the chapters on individual vaccines (see also Chapter 5); some issues are summarized in Table 42–2. Other groups require special consideration because of concern that their response to vaccines may be abnormal or that they may have unusually severe adverse events after immunization.

THE UNITED STATES IMMUNIZATION PROGRAM

History

In the United States, immunizations are provided through both the private and the public sectors. The public sector consists primarily of health departments but also includes other clinics, such as community and migrant health centers and public hospital–based clinics supported by public funds. The federal government has provided support to state and local health departments for maternal and child health programs since the 1920s, and some of that funding has been used to support immunizations.[73] However, there was no specific federal involvement in immunization activities until 1955, when the inactivated polio vaccine was licensed. Through the Polio Vaccination Assistance Act, Congress appropriated funds in 1955 and 1956 to the Communicable Disease Center (CDC, now the Centers for Disease Control and Prevention) to help states and local communities buy and administer vaccine. There was no further federal involvement until 1960, when Congress made a one-time appropriation of $1 million for a stockpile of oral polio vaccine to be used in combating epidemics. This was quickly used.

In February 1962, President John F. Kennedy sent the Vaccination Assistance Act of 1962 to Congress. The central thrust of this legislation was to allow the CDC to support mass immunization campaigns and to initiate maintenance programs, but no provision was made for a continuing program of support for immunizations. Two other important aspects of the bill were that it provided for vaccine instead of cash to be furnished directly to state and local health departments, and it also provided that personnel instead of cash could be furnished to grantees. These personnel were public health advisors and epidemiologists, who worked primarily in program coordination and surveillance. Direct delivery of immunization services (e.g., salaries of nurses, clinic supplies, expenses for increasing clinic hours) was not supported until 1992.

The first grants, authorized under section 317 of the Public Health Service Act, were made in June 1963. During the intervening 35 years, this grant program has thrived. There are now 64 grantees under what has become known as the "317" Immunization Grant Program: all 50 states, six large cities (including the District of Columbia), and eight territories and former territories.

The level of grant funding has varied greatly over the years. When the grant program began in 1963, the only vaccines available were diphtheria, tetanus, and pertussis (DTP), polio, and smallpox. Since that time, funding has been expanded to cover all vaccines routinely recommended for children.

During the 1960s and 1970s, grant funding fluctuated substantially. In 1966, a national effort to eradicate measles began.[15] By 1968, measles incidence had decreased by more than 90% compared with prevaccine era levels. With the licensure of the rubella vaccine in 1969 and the threat of a new epidemic of rubella, all federal funding for measles was shifted to rubella. A resurgence of measles occurred, peaking in 1971. In 1972, Congress appropriated additional funds that allowed the CDC to purchase vaccines other than rubella. Measles incidence decreased, reaching a low of 22,000 cases in 1974. During the mid-1970s, the overall budget for immunization grants decreased dramatically from the $8 to 10 million annually from 1963 to 1969 and the 1970 peak of $17 million to a low of only $5 million in 1976. A second resurgence of measles followed.[17, 18]

In 1976, a national election took place that led to significant changes in the immunization program. In the early 1970s, immunization programs around the country were in varying states of effectiveness. In Arkansas, it was apparent that much remained to be done. Mrs. Betty Bumpers, wife of the Governor, became personally interested in immunizations and succeeded in getting increased support for immunizations and improved immunization levels in Arkansas. Her husband, Dale Bumpers, was then elected to the U.S. Senate and became an important leader in the Congress on immunization. In November of 1976, Jimmy Carter was elected president. Subsequently, Mrs. Bumpers contacted the new administration and explained the deficiencies in the childhood immunization program in the United States and urged that something be done to improve the situation. As a result, in 1977, a national childhood immunization initiative was announced with two goals:

1. Attainment of immunization levels of 90% in the nation's children by October 1979
2. Establishment of a permanent system to provide comprehensive immunization services to the 3 million children born in America each year[74]

At the time, it was estimated that nearly 20 million American children needed at least one dose of a vaccine in order to be fully protected. The poor and the nonwhite populations were disproportionately represented among those needing protection.

Joseph A. Califano, Jr., the Secretary of the Department of Health, Education, and Welfare (now Health and Human Services) outlined a broad-based program involving increased federal support for immunizations, increased involvement of volunteers in all aspects of immunization activities, increased public awareness/public education activities, and increased cooperation between governmental agencies.[75]

Immunization grant funds increased dramatically from $5 million in 1976 to $17 million in 1977, $23 million in 1978, and $35 million in 1979. Intensive efforts began, concentrating on school-aged children, who experienced outbreaks of measles. A major effort was placed on reviewing immunization records of school children—in a 2-year period, more than 28 million records were reviewed, and children in need were immunized. Efforts were also expended to enact school immunization requirements in states that did not have them and to enforce those already in existence. As a result of these efforts, all 50 states soon had, and were enforcing, school entry immunization laws. Since 1981, 95% or more of children entering school have had documented immunization. Given these levels, even with lower levels in preschoolers, the overall immunization level in children of all ages in this country was 90% or greater. Thus, the first target of the initiative was met. Unfortunately, the second target of the 1977 initiative was not met.

Although the overall level of support for immunization grants rose rapidly in the late 1970s and throughout the 1980s (reaching $126.8 million in 1989), almost all of the increase was to meet the increasing cost of vaccines or the addition of new vaccines or additional doses of existing vaccines. In the 1980s, the level of federal support to grantees to carry out maintenance elements did not increase significantly, averaging $15.9 million but fluctuating between a low of $5 million in 1988 and a high of $26.1 million in 1989. Over the years, the federal government provided more of the same vaccines, as well as new ones, to a delivery system that was remaining static (at best) in the face of demands that were increasing. Investigations of the measles epidemics of 1989 to 1991, which especially affected unvaccinated preschool children, made it clear that the public sector delivery system was unequal to the challenge and that it required substantial assistance.

A part of the problem was that policies permitted immunization grant funds to be used to purchase vaccines and to carry out surveillance, investigation, education, and coordination but did not permit these funds to be used to support the delivery of vaccines (e.g., salaries of nurses, clinic supplies, expenses with increasing clinic hours). In 1991, President George Bush announced the federal government's support to accomplish a major health goal—namely, to raise immunization levels by the year 2000 so that 90% or more of the nation's children routinely completed their basic series of vaccinations by their second birthday.[76] The President announced that model immunization plans would be developed in several areas of the country as a beginning for the national effort to ensure adequate and timely immunization of infants and young children. This began a process that ultimately resulted in the preparation of Immunization Action Plans by all states and 28 metropolitan areas. Although there was great variation in needs reported from around the country, one theme common to virtually all plans was the need to increase the availability of immunization services. Consequently, for the first time, federal immunization grant funds were allowed to be used for the actual provision of immunization services.

President Bill Clinton's announcement of a Childhood Immunization Initiative (CII) in 1993[32, 77, 78] and the leadership and major infusion of funds associated with that initiative have brought the country to the point that it is now, finally, achieving 90% coverage in preschool children.[79] Grant support for immunization programs, including service delivery (but excluding vaccine purchase), rose to a peak of $237.3 million in 1995. The five components of the CII include (1) improving the quality and quantity of vaccination delivery services; (2) expanding access to vaccines, particularly for poor children; (3) enhancing community involvement, education, and building partnerships; (4) improving the measurement of immunization coverage and the detection of vaccine preventable diseases; and (5) simplifying the immunization schedule and improving vaccines.[80]

United States Immunization Program—1998

As described earlier, in the United States, immunizations are delivered by private physicians in their offices and through local health departments and other public-sector providers. Although vaccines are given in both private and public sectors, other important components of immunization programs in the United States are primarily coordinated by health departments and other public sector agencies, including surveillance and investigation of disease, outbreak control, promotion of immunization, adverse-events monitoring, assessment of immunization levels, and implementation of regulations and laws regarding immunization.[81, 82]

In an immunization delivery system, it is important to ensure that the recipient (or parent or guardian) is adequately aware of the risks and the benefits of vaccination and that the recipient has a record of all immunizations received.[83] The National Childhood Vaccine Injury Act of 1986 and subsequent changes (section XXI of the Public Health Service Act) requires that *all* vaccine providers formally notify patients and parents or guardians of the risks and benefits of specified vaccines (DTP or components; measles, mumps, rubella vaccine (MMR) or components; *Haemophilus influenzae* type b vaccine, hepatitis B vaccine, varicella, and poliomyelitis vaccines).[84] The use of standardized vaccine information sheets with these vaccines is now mandatory.[85] One of these forms is reproduced in Appendix 3. A series of "important information" sheets has been developed for use with other vaccines purchased with federal funds. This act also established a no-fault compensation mechanism for those who are injured by the vaccines specified in the act. Persons desiring further information about this program should contact the National Childhood Vaccine Injury Program at (800) 338-2382 if their questions are not answered at this Internet site: http://www.hrsa.dhhs.gov/bhpr/vicp. The National Childhood Vaccine Injury Act also requires providers to note in the patient's permanent medical record the date the vaccine was administered, the vaccine manufacturer, the vaccine lot number, and the name, address, and title of the person administering the vaccines, in addition to noting the provision of vaccine information materials. Finally, the act requires that providers report selected adverse events occurring after vaccination and events that would contraindicate further doses of vaccines to the Vaccine Adverse Event Reporting System (VAERS) (see Table 50–1 in Chapter 50 and http://www.hrsa.dhhs.gov/bhpr/vicp/table.htm). Providers are encouraged to report all serious adverse events following all vaccines, regardless of whether they believe that a vaccine caused the event.

Table 42–3. **CHANGES IN VACCINE COSTS FOR CHILDHOOD IMMUNIZATION 1987–1997, UNITED STATES**

YEAR					
1987*			**1997†**		
Vaccines	*CDC*	*Catalog*	*Vaccines*	*CDC*	*Catalog*
4 OPV	$5.72 ($1.43)§	$34.68 ($8.67)	2 OPV	$5.65 ($2.83)	$21.86 ($10.93)
			2 IPV	$12.42 ($6.21)	$30.84 ($15.42)
5 DTP	$15.05 ($3.01)	$56.10 ($11.22)	5 DTaP	‡$47.45–$53.50 ‡($9.49–$10.70)	‡$83.20–$85.60 ‡($16.64–$17.12)
1 MMR	$10.67	$17.88	2 MMR	$28.74 ($14.27)	$51.16 ($25.58)
1 Hib	$2.17	$6.68	3 Hib product	$20.58 ($6.86)	$50.25 ($16.75)
			4 Hib product	$26.88 ($6.72)	$63.52 ($15.88)
			3 HB	‡$25.11–$29.73 ‡($8.37–$9.91)	‡$50.76–$72.60 ‡($16.92–$24.20)
1 Td	$0.09	$0.65	1 Td	$1.64	$2.50
			1 Varicella	$34.40	$41.73
Total	$33.70	$115.99	Total	$175.99–$192.96	$332.30–$369.81

*Prices as of February 23, 1987 and October 31, 1997.
†Representative series, other choices possible, excise tax of $0.75 per dose per disease prevented (e.g., OPV = $0.75, DTaP = $2.25).
‡Range, taking all the highest-priced individual vaccines versus all the lowest-priced individual vaccines when there is more than one manufacturer for a product.
§Figures in parentheses are cost per dose.
CDC, Centers for Disease Control and Prevention; OPV, oral polio vaccine; DPT, diphtheria, pertussis, and tetanus; MMR, measles, mumps, rubella; Hib, *Haemophilus influenzae* type b; Td, tetanus and diphtheria toxoids; IPV, inactive polio vaccine; DTaP, diphtheria, tetanus, and acellular pertussis; HB, hepatitis B.

The Vaccine Adverse Event Reporting System forms can be obtained by calling (800) 822-7967, or through the Internet at http://www.fda.gov//cber/vaers.html. See Chapter 49 for further discussion of vaccine safety.

Vaccine Financing

The United States Immunization Program is a collaborative effort of public and private sectors. Public efforts have focused primarily on childhood immunizations. Approximately 60% of vaccines routinely recommended for children are purchased with public funds through federal contracts negotiated by the CDC with the vaccine manufacturers. These contracts allow state and local immunization programs to obtain vaccines at reduced prices (Table 42–3). The typical discount has been approximately 50% off the published catalog prices. Reasons for the reduced prices have included (1) the ability to ship large quantities of vaccines to only a limited number of sites within a state, with states taking responsibility for shipment to individual clinics and providers; (2) the absence of return privileges for expired or unneeded vaccines, a privilege common in contracts with the private sector; and (3) an interest on the part of manufacturers to provide vaccines at lower cost for poorer children, who tend to be served by the public sector.

Funds for purchase through the contracts are provided through the federal government and may be supplemented by funds from each of the 64 Federal Immunization Grant Recipients. There are two major sources of federal funds: (1) the Vaccines for Children (VFC) program and (2) the federal 317 grant program. The VFC program supplies vaccines to participating providers for children 18 years of age or younger who are (1) receiving Medicaid, (2) without any health insurance, or (3) Native American/Native Alaskan.[80, 86] In addition, children who receive their immunizations at federally qualified health centers who have health insurance that does not include vaccines (underinsured) can receive free vaccines through the VFC program.*

Funds for VFC are provided through the Medicaid Trust Fund, maintained by the Health Care Financing Administration. The VFC is an entitlement program that assures funds are available for eligible children each year. The ACIP establishes which vaccines are covered, the appropriate number of doses, and the schedule. An ACIP vote to include a vaccine in the VFC program or to increase the number of doses of a vaccine already in the program leads to immediate financing, allowing for rapid implementation of recommendations.

The 317 grant program provides federal funds for vaccines for children who are not eligible for VFC but who receive vaccines in state and local health department clinics, as well as for children served by private providers (in some states). Funds available under the 317 program must be appropriated each year by the Congress. The law establishing VFC provides for financing on the basis of ACIP recommendations without going through the usual annual congressional appropriations process.

State and local immunization grantees have the option to purchase vaccines through the VFC contracts with their own appropriated funds. Providers cannot charge parents or guardians for vaccines purchased through the federal contract, regardless of the funding source. Providers are permitted to charge a small administration fee. However, no one can be denied vaccines because of inability to pay the fee.

*Federally qualified health centers are centers determined to be eligible by the Bureau of Primary Health Care of the Health Resources and Services Administration and include community, migrant, and rural health centers (available at http://www.bphc.hrsa.dhhs.gov/fqhc).

Approximately 40% of vaccines are purchased through the private sector. Managed care plans generally provide recommended vaccines without charge beyond standard premiums for all covered services.[60, 87] In contrast, many traditional indemnity plans either do not cover routine childhood immunizations or cover them only after deductibles are paid. Vaccines not covered by insurance plans are usually purchased by parents or guardians.

The federal role for vaccines for adults is more limited. Medicare part B covers pneumococcal and influenza vaccination services for all persons 65 years of age and older who participate in part B (approximately 95% of all persons ≥65 years). State Medicaid programs, supported by federal contributions, may cover recommended vaccines for younger adults enrolled in Medicaid. State and local health departments may purchase limited quantities of influenza and pneumococcal vaccines with their own funds. The National Vaccine Advisory Committee estimated that public funds for vaccinations through health departments accounted for less than 10% of the financing of adult immunizations.[61] In 1996, public immunization grant programs reported purchasing less than 5% of all influenza and pneumococcal vaccines sold in the United States (CDC, unpublished data, 1996).

Vaccine Delivery

Most vaccines for children are administered by private sector providers. The 1994 National Health Interview Survey estimated that 68% of 19- to 35-month-old children (median age, 27 months) had obtained their vaccines from private health care providers.[88] Of the remainder, 22% were vaccinated in health department clinics, 5% in hospital-based clinics, and 5% in other clinics. Seventy-five percent received vaccines from one immunization provider, 22% from two providers, and 3% from three or more providers.

Vaccination delivery in the public sector is primarily a responsibility of state and local governments. Since 1992, federal 317 grant funds can also be used to support delivery, such as hiring of nurses and other clinic staff, vaccine promotion and education, and other delivery-related functions. In addition, federal funds that are part of state Medicaid resources and federal block grants to states can help support delivery.

Several changes in the US health care system should lead to increases in the percentage of children served by the private sector. The VFC program provides free vaccine to participating private providers in order to serve eligible children. Before VFC, parents of such children often had to pay for vaccines themselves or were referred to public clinics where vaccines were free.[89] Parental preference has been to have their children receive vaccines from their usual source of care.[90] Surveys have shown that providers enrolled in VFC are substantially more likely to immunize eligible children in their practices than are nonenrolled providers.[91]

An increasing proportion of children enrolled in Medicaid are in private managed care plans that cover all services for children, including vaccination.[92] In 1997, the new Title XXI of the Social Security Act, called the State Children's Health Insurance Program, was created. This program allows states to provide health benefits for uninsured, low-income children through expansion of the Medicaid program, through establishment of a separate child health care coverage program, or through provision of coverage with a combination of the Medicaid program and a new state program. This $24 billion program will be administered by the Health Care Financing Administration (available at http://www.hcfa.gov). Thus, through Medicaid or the Children's Health Insurance Program, the Health Care Financing Administration will provide health benefits to children up to 200% of the poverty level, or approximately 47% of the US population younger than 3 years of age. Providing full coverage for vaccination services, including administration costs, to previously uninsured children has been shown in one state to decrease health department clinic use by 67%, to increase primary care provider use by 27%, and to increase vaccination coverage levels by 5%.[93] The combination of VFC, managed Medicaid, and Children's Health Insurance Program is likely to result in fewer children being served in public clinics. Most vaccines for adults are administered by the private sector.

Disease Surveillance

The desired outcome of immunization is disease reduction or elimination. Reports of the occurrence of vaccine-preventable diseases are the major means of evaluating the impact of most of the vaccine-preventable disease programs.[94, 95] The Council of State and Territorial Epidemiologists, in consultation with CDC, establishes the list of nationally notifiable diseases. In the United States, most of the 10 vaccine-preventable diseases of childhood are reported to the National Notifiable Disease Surveillance System. Information is obtained through state health departments, which have authority for mandating reporting of selected diseases to the state level by physicians and other health care providers.[96]

Data collected weekly include date of report and county of residence for all notifiable diseases. In addition, for many of the vaccine-preventable diseases, supplemental data (e.g., date of onset, age, sex, race/ethnicity, vaccination status, whether the case was confirmed by a laboratory, and disease complications) are forwarded to CDC. For many of the vaccine-preventable diseases, reports by state of cases notified that week as well as the cumulative total for the year are published weekly in the *Morbidity and Mortality Weekly Report*. Case definitions have been established with Council of State and Territorial Epidemiologists that detail criteria for confirmation of a given illness as a case of a vaccine-preventable disease (see Appendix 4).[97]

The National Notifiable Disease Surveillance System is supplemented by a number of additional surveillance systems operated by CDC.[95] For example, a registry is maintained for congenital rubella syndrome; this registry collects comprehensive information on the clinical status of the baby, complications, laboratory data, vaccination status of the mother, and other information. The paralytic polio surveillance system collects extensive data on the clinical characteristics of suspected cases; these data are reviewed by experts to determine whether the illness is polio. Diphtheria surveillance is enhanced through monitoring requests to CDC for antiserum, which CDC has responsibility for distributing. Efforts to collect data beyond the National Notifiable Disease Surveillance System are made for measles, pertussis, tetanus, *H. influenzae* type b, and hepatitis B. Laboratory-based surveillance systems are used to monitor causes of bacterial meningitis, including *H. influenzae* type b and pneumococcal disease.[98] Other laboratory-based systems, as well as death certificate data, are utilized for influenza surveillance.

Where data are not available nationally, special sentinel surveillance systems in selected states and communities may be established.[94] Examples include the sentinel counties surveillance system for hepatitis B and a special varicella surveillance project in three sites (Los Angeles, CA; Travis County, TX; and Philadelphia, PA).[99–102]

Reporting sensitivity for each of the surveillance systems varies. An evaluation of measles surveillance during an outbreak revealed that 45% of cases seen and diagnosed at hospitals were reported.[103] Capture-recapture methods have been used to estimate the completeness of reporting for many different surveillance systems. A capture-recapture evaluation of the completeness of reporting of diagnosed cases of vaccine-associated polio found that 81% of cases were reported during the period 1980–1991.[104] The congenital rubella syndrome registry was estimated to receive reports on about 20% of cases in the past,[105] while only about 32% of pertussis hospitalizations were reported during the late 1980s.[106] Completeness of reporting varies by source of report and type of disease, with more complete reporting from hospitals and laboratories than from physicians for diseases such as *H. influenzae* type b.[107] In one varicella active surveillance project, there was more complete reporting by schools than by providers.[100]

Surveillance data are analyzed to determine whether expected reductions of disease occur with increasing vaccine coverage; to evaluate potential changing epidemiology of disease, such as a shift to a predominance of adult cases where there had been a childhood focus; and to determine whether cases are a result of failure of vaccine or of failure to vaccinate.[94] When a substantial proportion of cases occur in persons with a history of prior vaccination, an investigation is often undertaken to determine whether the rates of vaccine failure are within expected ranges. Several methods are used to evaluate vaccine effectiveness in the postlicensure setting, including cohort, case control, and other techniques.[108] Vaccine effectiveness is calculated as

$$(1 - \text{ARV/ARU}) \times 100,$$

where ARV is the attack rate in the vaccinated and ARU is the attack rate in the unvaccinated. When case-control studies are employed, the odds ratio is used to approximate the relative risk (ARV/ARU) (see Chapter 44 for a more detailed discussion on vaccine effectiveness).

When vaccine effectiveness is within expected limits yet disease transmission persists, new strategies may be considered. For example, investigations showed that measles transmission could persist despite a vaccine effectiveness of greater than 90% and high levels of coverage with a single dose of vaccine.[68] This information was critical in the decision to recommend a second dose of measles vaccine. When vaccine effectiveness is lower than expected, investigations are triggered into such causes as failure to maintain vaccine at the proper temperature (the "cold chain").

When most cases occur in unvaccinated persons, investigations can identify geographical and demographic characteristics to help guide future vaccination efforts. For example, a resurgence of measles in the United States during 1989 to 1991 was found to be caused by a failure to vaccinate young preschool children and led to a major national initiative to improve coverage.[60, 77, 78, 80]

Immunization Coverage

Immunization of preschool children is measured through the National Immunization Survey.[79] The National Immunization Survey consists of 78 random telephone surveys measuring immunization coverage of 19- to 35-month-old children (median age, 27 months). Approximately 1 million households are sampled annually to obtain data on about 33,000 children (J.D. Loft, personal communication, 1997). The National Immunization Survey provides a national estimate of coverage, usually with 95% confidence intervals within ± 1 percentage point of the point estimate, as well as comparable, statistically valid estimates for each of the 50 states and 28 of the largest urban areas. The survey is adjusted for households without telephones by use of data from the National Health Interview Survey, a national household probability sample that allows comparison at the national level of coverage of children residing in households with and without telephones. Attempts are made to collect immunization records from identified vaccine providers of each participant. Parental responses are adjusted on the basis of provider validation data. Further adjustments are made on the basis of demographic variables to give statistically valid estimates. The National Immunization Survey provides estimates by poverty status as well as by major racial and ethnic minority groups, including African Americans, Hispanics, Asian Pacific Islanders and Native Americans/Native Alaskans.[109]

A variety of techniques has been used to assess immunization coverage at the local level; these are primarily based on some form of cluster sample surveys.[110–116] The least expensive and easiest to perform surveys are retrospective. School immunization records of kindergarten or first grade students (5 to 6 years of age) are reviewed, and immunization status is determined retroactive to the second birthday.[116] Because these data are 3 to 4 years out of date (the interval between the time they were 2 years of age and the time they entered school), such retrospective surveys offer little help in monitoring ongoing immunization performance. Surveys of current preschool children are more difficult to perform and are usually costly.

Parental histories are frequently found to be inaccurate, particularly as the immunization schedule has gotten more complex.[117] When asked if immunizations for a given child are up to date, parents tend to overestimate coverage.[118–120] They tend to underestimate the number of doses received when asked about specific vaccines that are recommended to be given in multiple doses (e.g., DTP) and tend to overestimate coverage for vaccines recommended in a single dose for preschool children (e.g., MMR vaccine). On the basis of provider validation for the National Health Interview Survey, estimates for DTP and polio vaccines had to be adjusted upward, and estimates for measles-containing vaccines had to be adjusted downward.[121] Requiring provider validation for local surveys increases the complexity and cost, but the accuracy is greatly improved.

Techniques have been developed for measuring the performance of individual providers and clinics. The Clinic Assessment Software Application (CASA), which is available from the CDC, allows calculation of the coverage of children served by a given provider and can provide diagnostic information on reasons for low coverage, such as missed opportunities to provide all needed vaccines simultaneously. The CASA can be obtained through the Clinic Assessment Software Application Support Team, Mailstop E-62, National Immunization Program, CDC, or at http://www.cdc.gov/nip/casa. The most valid samples are taken randomly from all records, although limited data suggest that the immunization coverage of consecutive age-eligible children seen in a given practice, regardless of the reason for a visit, also gives a valid measure of coverage.[122]

A kit entitled "Make Every Visit Count" is available for self-assessment of immunization performance through state health departments or through the National Immunization Program at http://www.cdc.gov/nip/afix. The immunization status of 30 consecutive patients younger than 24 months of age is recorded on encounter forms. Information for children whose immunizations are not up to date that can be used to determine the reasons for not being adequately immunized is also recorded. Outputs include the proportion of children in compliance with the immunization schedule and information on the causes of low coverage, such as late start of the immunization series, reluctance to offer simultaneous immunizations, inability of the parent to pay, parental refusal, and contraindications.

The National Committee on Quality Assurance (NCQA) (available at http://www.ncqa.org) has established immunization performance measures for managed care organizations in the Health Plan Employer Data and Information Set (HEDIS). HEDIS 3.0 (1998) estimates immunization coverage for children who reached 2 years of age during the reporting year who were continuously enrolled in a specific managed care plan for the 12-month period preceding the 2nd birthday (including members who have had no more than one break in enrollment of up to 45 days during the 12 months preceding the 2nd birthday).[123, 124] Separate but comparable calculations are made for children enrolled in a plan covered by private funds and those covered by Medicaid.

The immunizations assessed through HEDIS 3.0 (1998) are shown in Table 42–4. For preschool immunization, coverage is assessed for each of the vaccines listed and for three progressively inclusive combinations of vaccinations. Coverage is estimated by the use of (1) claims or encounter data on individual children in the numerator and the entire plan membership in the denominator or (2) a random sample of 411 commercial and 411 Medicaid children, with chart review to determine their immunization status.

HEDIS 3.0 (1998) will also measure age-appropriate adolescent and older (≥65 years) adult vaccination coverage levels among plan members who were continuously enrolled for the previous 12 months (see Table 42–4).[123, 125, 126] Adolescent vaccination coverage has also been added to the 1996 National Health Interview Survey, but these results will not be available until 1998.

National Immunization coverage estimates for influenza and pneumococcal vaccinations and receipt of teta-

Table 42–4. **HEDIS 3.0 (1998) IMMUNIZATION PERFORMANCE MEASURES FOR PRESCHOOL CHILDREN, ADOLESCENTS, AND ADULTS**

2-YEAR-OLDS	ADOLESCENTS (13 YR)	ADULTS ≥65 YR
4 doses of DTaP*	Second dose of MMR	1 dose of influenza vaccine during the months September through December
3 doses of polio vaccine	3 doses of hep B	
1 dose of MMR	1 dose of varicella	
2 doses of Hib, with at least 1 during the second year of life		
2 doses of hep B, with 1 after 6 months of age but before 2 years of age		
1 dose of varicella†		
Combination one: 4 doses of DTaP; 3 doses of polio vaccine; 1 dose of MMR; 2 doses of hep B; 1 dose of Hib during the second year of life	Combination: second dose of MMR; 3 doses of hep B; 1 dose of varicella	
Combination two: combination one plus a second dose of Hib		
Combination three: combination two plus one dose of varicella		

*DTaP includes both DTP and DTaP.

†Varicella includes either documented vaccination with varicella vaccine or a history of chickenpox before the age of 13 years.

DTaP, diphtheria, tetanus, and acellular pertussis; DTP, diphtheria, tetanus, and pertussis; HEDIS, Health Plan Employer Data and Information Set; hep B, hepatitis B; Hib, *Haemophilus influenzae* type b; MMR, measles, mumps, and rubella; Td, tetanus and diphtheria toxoids.

From National Committee for Quality Assurance. HEDIS 3.0/1998—The Health Plan Employer Data and Information Set. Vol. 2: Technical specifications. Washington, DC, National Committee for Quality Assurance, 1997, pp 37–48.

nus toxoid among adults are obtained from the National Health Interview Survey.[127] State-specific data for influenza and pneumococcal vaccinations are collected through the Behavioral Risk Factor Surveillance System, a state-based telephone survey of the civilian, noninstitutionalized, adult (≥18 years of age) population.[128] In 1995, the system consisted of independent telephone surveys of all 50 states in which similar methods were used. Data are based on recall of the respondent.

Causes of Underimmunization in Children

Since the 1989 to 1991 measles resurgence, a great deal of research has been conducted to understand barriers that prevent timely immunization of preschool children. Several potential barriers were determined *not* to be significant barriers when they were examined closely. First, many investigators have speculated that parental attitudes toward vaccination can explain underimmunization; however, the evidence shows otherwise—most parents are very supportive of protecting their children through vaccination. Second, attitudes of providers have remained very positive toward routine vaccination. Third, most preschool children have access to an immunization provider. For example, according to the 1993 National Health Interview Survey, 93% of undervaccinated children who were 19 to 35 months of age had a usual source of primary care.[129] Having access to a primary care provider and using services are not the same, however.

Parental Factors

Many risk factors have been associated with low immunization coverage; these factors are primarily poverty related and include low educational level of parents, large family size, low socioeconomic status, nonwhite race or ethnicity, young parental age, lack of prenatal care, use of public clinics as a primary source of immunizations, and late start of the immunization series.[109, 130–138]

Some religious groups have opposed immunization, and a small percentage of parents have philosophical objections to immunizations. Although outbreaks of disease have been reported among persons who object to immunization, particularly because they may cluster in groups, persons opposed to immunization account for a small proportion of the population.[139–142] A survey of the United States showed that 42 states had less than 1% of the population claim any exemption between 1994 and 1996, including a medical contraindication under the school law.[143] Of the remaining states, none exceeded 2.5% exemptions, and their average was only slightly greater than 1%.

Although older studies tended to associate lower coverage with reliance on public clinics for immunization, the 1994 National Health Interview Survey provider record check shows that health department clinics and private providers have identical performance (73% vaccination coverage rates), even though the health department clinics serve over twice the proportion of impoverished children.[88]

Although children who are late in starting the immunization series often account for less than 50% of underimmunized children, almost all studies have shown that the failure to obtain any immunizations by 3 months of age has been associated with some of the highest relative risks of underimmunization at 24 months of age.[136, 138, 144–147] A child who appears at a vaccine provider at 3 months of age or older with no prior immunizations should be singled out for special tracking to ensure that the full series is completed before the 2nd birthday. Further, the information supports efforts to link every child with a vaccine provider at birth.

Parental health beliefs do not necessarily correlate with the immunization status of their children.[148] For example, Bates and coworkers queried mothers of poor urban infants in Indianapolis about their attitudes concerning vaccines and vaccine-preventable diseases 48 to 72 hours after they gave birth and evaluated the relationship of those beliefs to their child's immunization status at 7 months of age.[137] There were no significant differences in immunization status of children between parents who perceived vaccine-preventable diseases were serious and those who did not (28% vs. 32%) or between those who perceived their child was likely to be susceptible to disease and those who did not (30% vs. 29%). Paradoxically, children born to parents who believed there was great benefit to preventing disease were less likely to be immunized than those who saw less benefits from prevention (23% vs. 34%). Immunization levels were low in all groups. The lack of correlation of parental beliefs and immunization status of children has also been found in other studies.[133, 149, 150]

Most parents lack knowledge about the complexity of the immunization schedule and tend to overestimate coverage when asked if their child's immunizations are up to date. For example, Goldstein and colleagues found that more than one third of the children whose parents claimed that their child had received the recommended immunizations for his or her age were underimmunized according to clinic records.[118] Parents of more than half of all of the underimmunized children in the study thought their children's immunizations were up to date. These data and others suggest that immunization messages targeted to parents that stressed the importance of early childhood immunization may not have great impact on improving immunization levels, because many parents of underimmunized children believe that they have already adequately immunized their child. Few parents understand the complexity of the schedule and the fact that, with the licensure of rotavirus vaccine in August 1998, 15 to 19 doses of vaccines are recommended by 18 months of age to fully immunize a preschool child in the United States.

Several studies of parents have identified factors that parents believe contribute to underimmunization, such as long waiting times at clinics, difficulties obtaining appointments, lack of adequate transportation, and lack of understanding of the immunization schedule.[135, 151–153] However, the precise role of these factors in contributing to underimmunization is not clear. Some studies have shown that children with appointments for well-child care, including immunization, have high "no show rates," particularly if parents are poor, which can lead to failure to obtain timely immunization.[134, 154, 155] Employer practices that make it difficult for parents to get time off from work to get their children immunized may contribute to failure to obtain immunizations.[135] Parental beliefs that children with minor illnesses, such as upper respiratory illnesses, should not be vaccinated, even though the illnesses are not true contraindications, may also contribute to failure to keep appointments.[156]

The data taken together show that providers play a major, if not *the* major, role in the immunization status of their patients. Parents tend to want their children immunized, to look to their provider for guidance on immunization, and to rely on the provider for reminders about the schedule. Parents identify barriers in provider practices, such as long waits, that tend to discourage immunization.

Provider Factors

Underimmunized children appear to have substantially more access to the health care system than was previously assumed. Mustin and associates reported that 60% of infants who were not adequately vaccinated by 8 months of age had at least three well-child visits.[157] Almost all children have had at least one immunization by 2 years of age.[146, 147] Opportunities for immunization are being missed when children who are eligible for immunization visit health care providers but are not vaccinated.[158, 159]

Missed opportunities can be divided into two major categories: (1) a child seeks care in a setting in which immunizations are normally offered (e.g., well-child care) but is not adequately immunized, and (2) a child seeks care in a setting in which immunizations are not normally offered (e.g., an emergency department, an acute care clinic). The former generally occur because all needed immunizations are not offered simultaneously when they could be or because invalid contraindications are invoked to defer immunization. This type of missed opportunity also occurs if a child is not vaccinated at his or her usual source of care because of cost of vaccines and vaccine administration but is referred to a public clinic where vaccines are free.

A variety of studies has been performed to evaluate the impact of taking all opportunities to vaccinate.[132, 134, 146, 155, 160–174] Studies at the University of Rochester estimated that missed opportunities accounted for 13 to 60% of underimmunization time (time spent overdue for some immunizations during the first 2 years of life), depending on the practice type (the higher figure corresponds to the practice caring for the most impoverished patients).[175] Of the missed opportunities, 19 to 43% occurred in well-child settings, 9 to 36% occurred in follow-up appointments (e.g., ear rechecks), and 41 to 72% were attributable to failure to receive vaccinations in acute care settings. Studies in four inner cities documented that by the second birthday, DTP-4 coverage could have been 8 to 21% higher and MMR coverage could have been 6 to 9% higher if all opportunities to vaccinate had been taken.[160] Missed opportunities are not limited to inner city health care providers. A study of a large health maintenance organization documented that the immunization status of 30% of underimmunized children could have been brought up to date if simultaneous administration of all needed vaccinations were performed at each visit.[165] Most of the underimmunized population had made acute care visits, during which there were no discernible contraindications, yet they were not immunized.

Of the types of missed opportunities, the easiest to correct should be simultaneous immunization. Some work suggests that failure to provide simultaneous vaccination may be more a result of provider attitudes than parent attitudes. Woodin and coworkers reported that 60% of practicing physicians (compared with 40% of parents) had strong concerns about a 7-month-old receiving three injections. In fact, 64% of parents preferred that three injections be given simultaneously if it would decrease the need for an additional visit.[176] Similar findings were noted by Melman and colleagues, who reported that more than 90% of parents taking their children to an inner city clinic preferred two injections compared with two visits, 58% preferred three injections to two visits, and 42% preferred four injections to two visits.[177] A survey of health care providers at inner city clinics in Jersey City and Paterson, New Jersey showed that simultaneous immunization was not a concern of the public health providers but was a concern for 14 to 38% of private providers, depending on the number of injections given.[178]

Use of invalid contraindications in order to defer immunization is a common cause of missed opportunities. Gamertsfelder and associates reported that almost one fifth of doses delayed in a family practice residency clinic were due to invalid contraindications.[155] A national survey of practicing physicians reported that 28% would not give MMR to a well-hydrated 18-month-old child with afebrile, watery diarrhea, even though this is not a contraindication.[167] To combat the use of invalid contraindications, tables of valid contraindications and contraindication misperceptions have been prepared (see Chapter 5).

Most missed opportunities occur during acute care visits. Multiple factors play a role in the failure to take advantage of this opportunity. They include limited time for patient contact, use of invalid contraindications, desire to not potentially confuse the clinical course of the underlying illness with a vaccine reaction, inability to determine the true immunization needs of a patient (because immunization records are unavailable at the office or clinic and most parents do not bring home immunization records with them at the time of visits), and children being brought for visits by individuals who are not legally authorized to give consent. Reducing these kinds of missed opportunities can be particularly difficult. However, such interventions as screening nurses' reminding physicians that the patient about to be seen is in need of immunization can have some impact.[161, 179]

Concern has been raised that providing immunizations outside of well-child care, such as during acute care and emergency department visits, could adversely affect provision of well-child care.[171, 175, 180] Some view immunization as a parental incentive to make a well-child visit, and this incentive would be removed if immunization were provided in non–well-child care settings.[181] However, in a survey of 502 parents in Baltimore, Hughart and coworkers found that only 18% of parents were very likely to make a check-up visit if immunization were provided, but not if no immunizations were provided.[182] Further, in children of parents motivated primarily by immunizations, there was no difference between attendance at well-child clinic visits in which immunizations were usually provided (15- and 18-month visits) and visits normally without immunization (8- and 12-month visits). Joffe and Luberti also reported no difference in later well-child visits between children vaccinated during an emergency department visit and similar children seen in an emergency department who were not vaccinated.[183] Thus, although provision of immunization in the well-child setting along with other preventive services is ideal, providers should not fear that providing immunizations in other settings will be detrimental to well-child care.

Providers have other roles besides taking advantage of all opportunities to ensure that their patients are adequately immunized. Parents look to providers for education on the importance of vaccines and for reminders when immunizations are due or overdue.[151] Provider recommendations play an important role in parents' decisions about immunizing their children.[184] A survey of pediatricians, as part of market research conducted by Merck, showed that a provider recommendation against varicella vaccination was a strong deterrent to parental acceptance (30% vaccinated), a neutral recommendation resulted in fewer than half of parents accepting vaccination, and a strong recommendation for vaccination resulted in a high degree of parental acceptance (>85%).[185]

Despite the need for reminders for parents, few physicians operate reminder or recall systems. A national survey of pediatricians and family physicians in 1992 reported that only 13% of pediatricians and 10% of family physicians operated routine reminder systems.[186]

Cost as a Barrier

Another type of missed opportunity occurs when children seek other care from a private provider but are referred by that provider to public clinics for free vaccines. The need to make the extra visit may result in delayed immunization and increased time during which the child is susceptible to vaccine-preventable diseases. Private providers are more likely to refer children without insurance and children receiving Medicaid for vaccinations outside their practices, thus requiring an additional health care visit by the parent.[89, 168, 187–189] Providers who receive free vaccines, such as those offered through the VFC program, report substantially lower rates of referral than those who do not.[91]

The impact of providing free vaccines on the ultimate immunization coverage of young children has been the subject of debate. Immunization coverage has also been found to be low in populations in which cost is not a barrier. Only 65% of 2-year-old children of employees of a large corporation, who had medical insurance coverage for immunizations, had received the four DTP, three polio, and one MMR series, indicating that cost alone cannot account for all of the underimmunization.[135] One study comparing private practices in states that provide free vaccines for all children with practices in other states reported no differences in coverage between the two groups.[190] However, almost all the parents of children surveyed (in both types of states) were well educated, of moderate-to-high socioeconomic status, and therefore least likely to benefit from free vaccines from a private provider.

Parents who had previously paid out of pocket for immunization had substantial reductions in those costs when North Carolina began providing free vaccines to all children.[191] However, parents who previously had made an extra visit to a health department clinic and now wished to receive free vaccines from a private provider paid more because of vaccine administration charges, which were not assessed at the health department clinic. This cost might be smaller than the savings realized by not making extra visits, such as benefits received by not losing time from work. The fact that referrals to health departments decrease when free vaccines are provided suggests that some parents take advantage of the free vaccines to stay with their medical provider for immunization services.

Other studies have indicated that private provider referral for vaccination to a public clinic reduces immunization levels. Zimmerman and Janosky noted that children without insurance and those receiving Medicaid in Minnesota were more likely to be referred and to have had more time underimmunized than were insured patients.[192] Lieu and colleagues interviewed parents who came to public clinics; 63% would have preferred vaccination by their regular provider but came to the clinic because of cost.[90]

Determining whether free vaccines improve coverage levels of existing vaccines is only part of the issue raised by such a policy. Concern has been expressed that research and development of new and improved vaccines might be inhibited[193] if the government purchases a substantially higher proportion than occurs now of vaccines for children at reduced rates. Thus, any societal benefits from increased government purchase might be exceeded by the continuing costs of infectious diseases that are not yet preventable by vaccination.

In summary, free vaccines reduce referral of children to public clinics and allow them to be vaccinated by their primary provider, in their "medical home," and there is little controversy regarding the provision of free vaccines for poor children served by private providers. However, the debate is likely to continue regarding free vaccines for other children.

Provision of free vaccines addresses only one part of the cost issue. A survey by the American Academy of Pediatrics indicated that pediatricians, on average, charged approximately $15 per dose for vaccine administration.[194] Thus, administration costs are similar to vaccine costs. Several studies have shown that insurance coverage both for vaccines and for vaccine administration significantly increases immunization coverage levels.[93, 195]

One study evaluated the impact of (1) a marked increase in vaccine administration fees paid by Medicaid to private providers (from $2.00 per dose to $17.85 per dose) and (2) the provision of free vaccines through the VFC to private providers in New York City, who served primarily a Medicaid population.[196] Immunization of children in their practices increased significantly, along with increases in provision of other well-child services. It was not possible to evaluate the relative impacts of free vaccines versus increased administration fees. Federal purchase of vaccines through VFC freed up state funds that had been used for vaccine purchase and allowed them to be redirected toward increased reimbursements for administration.

The importance of cost is evolving because the cost of vaccinating a child continues to increase. The cost of vaccines (including excise taxes) to fully immunize a child is now more than $175 in the public sector and more than $330 in the private sector (see Table 42–3), up from $34 and $116, respectively, 10 years earlier. In addition, there are costs for visits to the physician and vaccine administration fees. As the immunization schedule gets more complex because of the addition of more doses of existing vaccines, new vaccines, excise taxes, and extra visits, all of which can add considerably to the cost of fully vaccinating a child, the importance of cost as a potential barrier may well increase. Thus, the financing of vaccines and their administration warrant continuing evaluation.

Important Strategies for Achieving and Maintaining High Levels of Immunization Coverage

Assessment and Feedback of Provider Immunization Performance

Most physicians and nurses want to ensure that their patients are immunized. In fact, when queried, they tend to overestimate the coverage of the children they serve. Bushnell asked physicians and nurses from both public and private sectors in Massachusetts what they believed to be the immunization coverage of their patient population. The range was 85 to 100%. Record reviews documented a median coverage of 61% and a range of 19 to 93%.[197] Other studies reported that physicians overestimated coverage by 10 to more than 40%.[180, 198] Such health care professionals are unlikely to be motivated to make improvements in their immunization practices because they mistakenly believe that their current efforts are adequate.

The purpose of assessment and feedback is to alert providers to the actual coverage in their patient populations and to help motivate them to improve that coverage. This method has been pioneered in the public clinics of the state of Georgia[164, 199] and includes four components:

1. *Assessment* of the immunization coverage of the preschool children served by a given clinic.
2. ***F***eedback of the results to persons in the clinic with the authority to make changes. Such feedback often includes potential problems identified during the review, such as failure to administer vaccines simultaneously
3. ***I***ncentives for improved performance. In the public sector, this often involves community recognition, plaques, and/or dinners rather than financial incentives.
4. E***x***change of information or comparing the performance of one clinic with others to stimulate competition to improve performance. Together, these spell *AFIX*, a slang expression denoting "a repair."

In Georgia, median immunization coverage for the four DTP, three polio, and one measles-containing vaccine series rose from 53% in 1988, early in the program, to 89% in 1994.[164] Further, the coverage level of the lowest clinic rose from less than 10% in 1988 to greater than 50% in 1994. Similar improvements have been seen in other states. Link implemented a similar system in private practices in Massachusetts and demonstrated increases in median coverage among two groups of private providers from 60 to 80% and from 52 to 77% over a 4-year period.[200]

Reminder and Recall Systems

Many studies have shown that reminders for immunizations that are due or recall systems for immunization appointments that are missed can significantly improve immunization coverage in a variety of settings.[201–207] In a health maintenance organization setting, computer-generated letters to families with children who had not received an MMR by 20 months of age improved coverage by 19% compared with similar children whose parents did not receive reminders (54% vs. 35%), at a cost of $4.04 per additional immunized child.[204] Computerized telephone reminders to families cared for in Georgia public clinics increased coverage for the fourth DTP vaccine, the third OPV vaccine, and/or MMR by 16% in the 30-day period after the reminder when compared with control subjects.[205] Despite the proven efficacy of reminder and recall systems, few physicians use them.[186]

Linkage with the Special Supplemental Food Program for Women, Infants, and Children

Approximately 44% of the US birth cohort is enrolled in the US Department of Agriculture's Special Supplemental Nutrition Program for Women, Infants, and Children (WIC), a federally supported, means-tested program that supplies vouchers for food for needy infants and young children.[208–210] Parents are required to make visits at 1- to 3-month intervals (depending on the policies of the local or state WIC program) to pick up vouchers that can be used to purchase food, such as infant formula. Infants and young children must be examined periodically. Because WIC eligibility is in part based on income and because low income is associated with underimmunization, WIC participants are at higher risk for underimmunization than non-WIC participants.[211, 212] During a resurgence of measles in the United States, 29 to 63% of preschool, unvaccinated, yet vaccine-eligible, children in five cities were enrolled in WIC.[213] State immunization programs are required to work with WIC to ensure that the children they serve are vaccinated.

A variety of WIC-based interventions has been proved effective without causing harm to WIC enrollment and have been well received by parents.[214–216] All require assessment of the child's immunization status, based on a written record and (at a minimum) a referral to a provider for vaccination. Other interventions have included outreach and education, escort of undervaccinated children to a provider site to ensure access to immunization, and use of voucher incentives that require parents of underimmunized children to pick up vouchers more often than parents of immunized children. Depending on the intervention used, immunization levels of children enrolled in WIC have been increased by as much as 40 percentage points through collaborative efforts of WIC and Immunization programs.[214, 217]

A recent large study in Chicago reported that use of voucher incentives (the high-risk protocol that WIC uses to see parents of children at higher risk of adverse outcomes, such as anemia, more frequently) had substantially greater impact than assessment and referral of underimmunized children without incentives.[215] The WIC clinics that used voucher incentives documented a 33% increase in age-appropriate immunization coverage (56 to 89%) compared to no improvement at sites using assessment and referral alone.

Standards for Pediatric Immunization Practices

In 1993, the National Vaccine Advisory Committee recommended a set of 18 standards to improve the immunization performance of providers who serve children (Table 42–5).[62] Many of the standards specifically address improving immunization coverage in children served, including removing barriers to immunization, taking advantage of all opportunities to vaccinate, simultaneously vaccinating and using only valid contraindications, establishing tracking systems to identify children who are underimmunized and to facilitate taking corrective actions, and semiannually auditing patients served by a given clinic or practice to evaluate performance and to determine whether improvements were needed. Other aspects call for working with communities and for providing education. Implementing the standards at a New Mexico clinic reduced dropout from DTP1 to DTP3 (the difference in the percentage of children who started the immunization series and those who finished the recommended three-dose series for infants) from 24% before the intervention to only 5% with the intervention.[218] In contrast, dropout at the control site increased from 39 to 51%. The Infectious Diseases Society of America has established 14 implementation standards that apply to both adults and children.[219]

The Role of Mass Immunization Campaigns

Campaigns attempting to vaccinate large numbers of children in 1 day or some other short period have been important in worldwide efforts to eradicate polio and eliminate measles.[30, 36, 220, 221] Such campaigns were useful in the United States for the introduction of new vaccines, such as the oral polio, measles, and rubella vaccines.[15, 222, 223] Those campaigns were generally nonselective, that is, everyone in the target age group received vaccine, regardless of prior vaccination or disease status. In contrast, today, most immunization campaigns in the United States are selective, attempting to vaccinate only a small proportion of the total population—children without a prior history of vaccination. Evaluation of the success of these campaigns is made difficult by the inability in most United States communities to estimate

Table 42–5. **STANDARDS FOR PEDIATRIC IMMUNIZATION PRACTICES**

Standard 1.	Immunization services are readily available.
Standard 2.	There are no barriers or unnecessary prerequisites to the receipt of vaccines.
Standard 3.	Immunization services are available free or for a minimal fee.
Standard 4.	Providers utilize all clinical encounters to screen and, when indicated, immunize children.
Standard 5.	Providers educate parents and guardians about immunization in general terms.
Standard 6.	Providers question parents or guardians about contraindications and, before immunizing a child, inform them in specific terms about the risks and benefits of the immunizations their child is to receive.
Standard 7.	Providers follow only true contraindications.
Standard 8.	Providers administer simultaneously all vaccine doses for which a child is eligible at the time of each visit.
Standard 9.	Providers use accurate and complete recording procedures.
Standard 10.	Providers coschedule immunization appointments in conjunction with appointments for other child health services.
Standard 11.	Providers report adverse events following immunization promptly, accurately, and completely.
Standard 12.	Providers operate a tracking system.
Standard 13.	Providers adhere to appropriate procedures for vaccine management.
Standard 14.	Providers conduct semi-annual audits to assess immunization coverage levels and to review immunization records in the patient populations they serve.
Standard 15.	Providers maintain up-to-date, easily retrievable medical protocols at all locations where vaccines are administered.
Standard 16.	Providers operate with patient-oriented and community-based approaches.
Standard 17.	Vaccines are administered by properly trained individuals.
Standard 18.	Providers receive ongoing education and training on current immunization recommendations.

From Ad Hoc Working Group for the Development of Standards. Standards for pediatric immunization practices. JAMA 269:1817–1822, 1993.

All material in this appendix is in the public domain.

accurately the target population and to determine the proportion reached in the campaign. Limited data suggest the campaigns have generally failed to immunize many of the children thought to be in need.[224, 225] Other information also suggests that these immunization campaigns are not likely to be effective. A high proportion of parents of underimmunized children mistakenly believe that their children's immunizations are up to date and would consequently not be motivated to participate in selective mass immunization campaigns for their children.[118–120] Further, the United States immunization schedule requires 15 to 19 doses of vaccines be given by 18 months of age, too many doses to be addressed in any one-time immunization campaign.[56] Thus, selective immunization campaigns cannot be recommended as a major means of improving overall immunization coverage. However, the publicity gained in such campaigns may be useful in improving the political and community support necessary for ongoing immunization efforts. The challenge is to conduct a campaign in such a way that the positive publicity is matched by achievable programmatic objectives, such as linking children to a medical home.

Laws and Regulations for Immunization

Laws requiring immunization in the United States date from the early 19th century.[226, 227] Massachusetts enacted a law in 1809 that required smallpox vaccination of the general population, and other jurisdictions followed during the course of the century. In 1905, the Supreme Court affirmed the right of states to pass and enforce compulsory immunization statutes. Laws requiring vaccination before school entry were affirmed by the Supreme Court in 1922. School entry laws were variably enforced, and the antigens covered varied considerably.[227] After measles vaccine was introduced in the mid-1960s, school entry requirements for measles vaccination became common because measles was a disease primarily of school-age children. It became apparent that states without laws were having more measles than those with laws (relative risk, 1.7 to 2.0 in 1973 to 1974), and, with the Immunization Initiative of 1977, considerable emphasis was placed on enactment and enforcement of school entry laws.[228, 229]

Laws requiring immunization before entry in school or day care are the safety net for the US immunization program. All 50 states and the District of Columbia have laws in effect, although the precise antigens, doses, and schedules may vary. The impact of those laws has been shown in the decreased incidence of measles and mumps in states with laws versus states without laws. For example, during the first 31 weeks of 1978, the incidence rate of measles was only 2.7/100,000 persons less than 18 years of age in six states that were strictly enforcing school laws, compared with 35.2/100,000 in the rest of the nation.[230] In a comparison of high-incidence and low-incidence areas of measles, the biggest difference found was the statewide enforcement of laws through exclusion of unvaccinated students from school until vaccinated.[231] Of the 13 low-incidence areas, 10 (77%) had such policies, compared with none of 10 high-incidence areas. A major resurgence of mumps during 1986 was shown to occur almost exclusively in states without comprehensive laws requiring mumps vaccination.[232]

In the United States, few parents object to immunization for their children. The laws serve primarily to enhance priority for immunization by requiring that children receive immunization for attendance at school or day care. Children who are not adequately immunized are not allowed to attend school or day care, although most states allow provisional attendance for children whose immunization status is not up to date as long as the children continue to obtain immunizations at recommended intervals. As of 1997, all state laws have exemptions for medical contraindications to vaccination, 48 have exemptions for religions that oppose immunization, and 15 have exemptions for philosophic objections to immunization. There is no evidence that school laws delay immunization until the child reaches school entry. In almost all areas studied, 80% or more of children have received at least one dose of a vaccine by 2 years of age.[79, 147]

Immunization coverage among children entering school or day care has been 95% or greater for all required vaccines since the 1981 to 1982 school year.

Regulations have also proved effective in protecting college students from vaccine-preventable diseases. Between 1988 and 1991, colleges with a state-mandated prematriculation immunization requirement had only one third the risk of measles outbreaks of other colleges.[233]

Causes of Underimmunization in Adults

Immunizing adults is a more complicated undertaking than is immunizing children. Vaccination recommendations for adults depend on a person's age, occupation, health status, and behavior (e.g., sexual activity and drug use). For example, for persons younger than 65 years of age, influenza and pneumococcal vaccines are targeted to persons at high risk for illness-related complications or death, most of whom are adults.[234, 235] This requires physicians and nurses to establish procedures to identify persons who are eligible, often from long lists of qualifying conditions, in contrast to childhood immunization, in which all are offered vaccine unless there are contraindications. Influenza vaccine must be given annually. The diseases to be prevented are often clinically indistinguishable from other causes of similar syndromes, making assessment of the impact of immunization difficult and potentially preventing both vaccinees and their vaccinators from seeing the benefits of immunization. Hepatitis B is exclusively targeted toward high-risk groups in the adult population.[236] Similarly, MMR vaccination of adults is primarily targeted to persons born since 1956, particularly health care workers, postsecondary school students (e.g., college, university students), international travelers, and women likely to become pregnant.[237]

Target Population Factors

A variety of factors have been linked to adults' failure to obtain vaccines. These include perceptions that adults are not susceptible to disease, the diseases are not severe, the vaccines are not effective, or the vaccines are not safe.[61, 238, 239] One of the major factors is failure of a strong recommendation for vaccination on the part of the individual's provider.[240–242] Cost, although a potential factor, is probably limited for influenza and pneumococcal vaccines. Although the cost may change, as of 1997, it was approximately $2 for influenza vaccine and $8 for pneumococcal vaccine, based on representative catalog prices. On the other hand, hepatitis B vaccine (with a cost of almost $55 per dose in 1997) can have substantial cost implications for the individual, particularly because many of the groups targeted for immunization, such as parenteral drug abusers, are unlikely to have insurance coverage.

Provider Factors

Missed opportunities are an important cause of failure to obtain adult immunizations.[243] Many of the patients who are at the highest risk for complications of influenza and pneumococcal disease have had a medical contact before disease onset and could have been vaccinated. About two thirds of patients hospitalized with pneumococcal bacteremia or pneumonia had a previous hospitalization within the preceding 5 years, when they could have been vaccinated.[244] A 1994 to 1995 study of Medicare beneficiaries in 12 states reported that opportunities to provide influenza vaccine and pneumococcal vaccine had been missed in 65% and 80% of hospitalized patients 65 years of age or older, respectively.[245]

Perhaps as important as missed opportunities is the responsibility patients give to providers for making immunization decisions. A study performed in Georgia reported that 75 and 76% of adults obtained influenza and pneumococcal vaccinations, respectively, if they were recommended by a provider, compared with 7 and 6% of adults if there was not a strong recommendation.[240] In fact, 70 and 33% of adults who were not favorable to vaccination were vaccinated against influenza and pneumococcal disease, respectively, if their provider recommended it.

Effective Strategies to Improve Adult Immunization

As with childhood immunization, improving the performance of physicians and nurses who treat adults appears to be the key to increasing coverage. In Rochester, New York, immunization staff reviewed the records of physicians and developed lists of patients (target populations) who were in need of influenza immunization and established graphing systems to track progress toward their targets.[246] Practices with the intervention had immunization coverage levels of 66%, compared with 50% in the control practices. Financial incentives can also improve coverage. In a second study, practices that were eligible to receive increased reimbursement if they achieved certain immunization coverage levels (providers received 10% more than the usual fee per patient immunized if they achieved a 70% coverage rate; they received 20% more than usual if they achieved an 85% coverage rate) had an average coverage of 73%, compared with 56% in control clinics that were not eligible for increased reimbursement.[247] Another intervention that has shown promise includes establishment of a "standing orders" system for immunization for hospitalized patients on discharge or for outpatients whereby immunization would be offered unless a physician specifically removed the vaccination from a patient's orders.[248–250] Nursing homes with written immunization policies or standing orders and which do not require written informed consent specifically for vaccination have higher rates of immunization than those that do not have such policies and procedures.[251] Reminder systems for high-risk groups can also significantly increase coverage.[252]

The National Coalition on Adult Immunization (available at http://www.medscape.com/Affiliates/NCAI), a group of more than 90 organizations dedicated to improving immunization coverage among adults, has issued a set of 10 standards for adult immunization (Table 42–6).[253] These standards encourage education, protection of health care providers themselves against vaccine-preventable diseases, routine screening of adults to determine immunization needs, use of all opportunities to vaccinate, adequate financing, and other measures.

The National Vaccine Advisory Committee has issued a comprehensive report on improving the protection of adults against vaccine-preventable diseases.[61] The report has five goals:

1. Increasing the demand for adult vaccination by improving provider and public awareness
2. Ensuring that the healthcare system has adequate capacity to deliver vaccines to adults
3. Ensuring adequate financing mechanisms to support expanded delivery of vaccines to adults
4. Monitoring and improving the performance of the nation's vaccine delivery system
5. Ensuring adequate support for research on
    a. Vaccine-preventable diseases of adults
    b. Adult vaccines
    c. Adult immunization practices
    d. New and improved vaccines
    e. International programs for adult immunization

Impact of Immunization Programs

Occurrence of Disease

The occurrence of most vaccine-preventable diseases is at or near record low levels. Table 42–7 shows the maximum level of disease reported or estimated for selected vaccine-preventable diseases. All diseases have been reduced by more than 95% from peak vaccine-era levels. The CII set seven goals for controlling or eliminating vaccine-preventable diseases by 1996.[33] In 1996, three of the seven goals were met. There were no cases of tetanus or wild virus–induced polio in persons

Table 42–6. **NATIONAL COALITION FOR ADULT IMMUNIZATION (NCAI) STANDARDS FOR ADULT IMMUNIZATION PRACTICE, 1990**

The NCAI

1. Encourages the promotion of appropriate vaccine use through information campaigns for healthcare practitioners and trainees, employers, and the public about the benefits of immunizations; and
2. Encourages physicians and other healthcare personnel (in practice and in training) to protect themselves and prevent transmission to patients by assuring that they themselves are completely immunized; and
3. Recommends that all health providers routinely determine the immunization status of their adult patients, offer vaccines to those for whom they are indicated, and maintain complete immunization records; and
4. Recommends that all healthcare providers identify high-risk patients in need of influenza vaccine and develop a system to recall them for annual immunization each autumn; and
5. Recommends that all healthcare providers and institutions identify high-risk adult patients in hospitals and other treatment centers and assure that appropriate vaccination is considered either prior to discharge or as part of discharge planning; and
6. Recommends that all licensing/accrediting agencies support the development by healthcare institutions of comprehensive immunization programs for staff, trainees, volunteer workers, inpatients, and outpatients; and
7. Encourages states to establish preenrollment immunization requirements for colleges and other institutions of higher education; and
8. Recommends that institutions that train healthcare professionals, deliver healthcare, or provide laboratory or other medical support services require appropriate immunizations for persons at risk of contracting or transmitting vaccine-preventable illnesses; and
9. Encourages healthcare benefit programs, third-party payers, and governmental healthcare programs to provide coverage for adult immunization services; and
10. Encourages the adoption of a standard personal and institutional immunization record as a means of verifying the immunization status of patients and staff.

From The public health burden of vaccine preventable diseases among adults: Standards for adult immunization practice. MMWR Morb Mortal Wkly Rep 39:725–729, 1990.

younger than 15 years of age. Only 751 cases of mumps were reported, down from a median of 4866 cases in the 5 years preceding CII. Although other diseases were not eliminated, they were close to elimination. Measles transmission within the United States was probably interrupted for periods of several weeks in 1993, 1995, and 1996, only to be periodically reestablished through importations.[33, 52, 254] There was a provisional total of only 138 cases in 1997, a record low. None of the cases was believed to be secondary to endemic circulating measles virus.[254a] Further gains in disease prevention will require improved international control to reduce the risk of importation, increased immunization levels not only in children but also in adults, as well as other measures.

Table 42–7. **COMPARISON OF MAXIMUM AND CURRENT MORBIDITY OF VACCINE-PREVENTABLE DISEASES**

	MAXIMUM CASES (YR)	1996	1997	PERCENT¶ CHANGE
Diphtheria	206,939 (1921)	2	5	−99.99
Measles	894,134 (1941)	508	135	−99.99
Mumps	152,209 (1968)	751	612	−99.59
Pertussis	265,269 (1934)	7796	5519	−97.92
Polio (paralytic)*	21,269 (1952)	0	0	−100.00
Rubella	57,686 (1969)	238	161	−99.72
Congenital rubella syndrome	20,000† (1964–65)	4	4	−99.98
Tetanus‡	1560‡ (1923)	36	43	−97.24
Haemophilus influenzae, invasive disease (<5 yr)	20,000†	273§	242	−98.79

*Wild virus caused.
†Estimated.
‡Deaths in 1923; cases in 1996.
§Also includes invasive disease due to non–type b *H. influenzae*.
¶In 1996, the immunization rates were higher than rates reported in any previous year (Table 42–8).[79]
1996 data from Summary of notifiable diseases: United States, 1996. MMWR 45:1–88, 1996; 1997 data from Summary of notifiable diseases: United States, 1997. MMWR Morb Mortal Wkly Rep 46:1265–1269, 1997.

Immunization Coverage

Preschool Immunization

The highest immunization rates ever documented in the United States were reported in 1996 (Table 42–8).[79] For children 19 to 35 months of age (median age, 27 months) who were born between February 1993 and May 1995, more than 90% had received three or more doses of DTP, polio, and *H. influenzae* type b vaccines; 91% had received a dose of a measles-containing vaccine; and 82% had received three or more doses of hepatitis B vaccine. All of the goals of the CII were achieved. The coverage for the four DTP, three polio, and one measles-containing vaccine series (4:3:1), a common measure of overall coverage, primarily DTP-4 coverage, which is the main determinant of the series coverage, was 78%. Varicella vaccination coverage for the last quarter of 1996 was 18%. In a comparison of coverage in 1996 with that in 1992, the year before the CII began, coverage increased by 8% for measles-containing vaccines and 74% for hepatitis B. Immunization coverage during 1997 was similar to coverage by 1996.[254b]

Immunization coverage was high in all racial and ethnic groups evaluated.[109] Levels exceeded 90% or were within 3% of 90% for three or more doses of DTP, polio, and *H. influenzae* type b and for one dose of a measles-containing vaccine for whites, African Americans, Hispanics, Asian and Pacific Islanders, and Native Americans/Native Alaskans. Poverty was the major predictor of underimmunization, with immunization among children below poverty levels being 4 to 11% lower than that of children at or above poverty levels. The greatest discrepancies were reported for DTP-4, which had the lowest immunization rate of any of the recommended vaccines and doses.

School-Age Immunization

As mentioned earlier, immunization levels for children entering school or day care are 95% or greater. As long

Table 42–8. **CHILDHOOD IMMUNIZATION INITIATIVE (CII) GOALS AND VACCINATION COVERAGE LEVELS AMONG CHILDREN AGED 19 TO 35 MONTHS, BY SELECTED VACCINES—UNITED STATES, 1992, 1996, AND 1997**

		1992 (NHIS*)		1996 (NIS†)		1997 (NIS†)	
VACCINE/DOSE	CII 1996 GOAL	%	(95% CI)	%	(95% CI)	%	(95% CI)
DTP/DT							
≥3 Doses	90%	83	(±2.2%)	95	(±0.4%)	95	(±0.4%)
≥4 Doses		59	(±2.9%)	81	(±0.7%)	81	(±0.7%)
Poliovirus							
≥3 Doses	90%	72	(±2.3%)	91	(±0.5%)	91	(±0.5%)
Hib							
≥3 Doses	90%	28	(±2.6%)	92	(±0.5%)	93	(±0.5%)
MCV‡							
≥1 Dose	90%	83	(±2.3%)	91	(±0.5%)	91	(±0.5%)
Hepatitis B							
≥3 Doses	70%	8§	(±1.7%)	82	(±0.7%)	84	(±0.6%)
Varicella	—	—	—	—	—	26	(±0.7%)
Combined series							
4 DTP/3 polio/1 MCV‖	—	55	(±2.8%)	78	(±0.8%)	78	(±0.7%)
4 DTP/3 polio/1 MCV/3 Hib¶	—	—	—	77	(±0.8%)	76	(±0.8%)

*National Health Interview Survey (NHIS), household data only. Children in this survey were born during February 1989–May 1991.
†National Immunization Survey (NIS), household and provider data. Children in this survey were born during February 1993–May 1995.
‡Vaccination coverage goals are specifically for measles-mumps-rubella vaccine.
§CDC, unpublished data, 1992.
‖Four or more doses of DTP/DT, three or more doses of poliovirus vaccine, and one or more doses of any MCV.
¶Four or more doses of DTP/DT, three or more doses of poliovirus vaccine, one or more doses of any MCV, and three or more doses of Hib.
CI, confidence interval; DTP/DT, diphtheria, tetanus, pertussis vaccine, diphtheria and tetanus toxoids; Hib, *Haemophilus influenzae* type b; MCV, measles-containing vaccine.
From Status report on the childhood immunization initiative: National, state and urban area vaccination levels among children aged 19–35 months in United States, 1996. MMWR Morb Mortal Wkly Rep 46:657–664, 1997; and National, state and urban area vaccination coverage levels among children aged 19–35 months—United States, 1997. MMWR Morb Mortal Wkly Rep 47:547–554, 1998.

as school laws remain in place and are enforced, these levels should continue.

Adult Immunization

Immunization levels for pneumococcal and influenza vaccines lag far behind the levels achieved for vaccines recommended routinely for children. Influenza immunization coverage in persons 65 years or older, determined from the 1994 National Health Interview Survey, reached 55%, the highest level ever reported but still well below childhood vaccine coverage levels.[127] Pneumococcal vaccination coverage was only 30%. Data from the Behavioral Risk Factor Surveillance System for 1997 suggest that the rates are continuing to rise, with 66% for influenza vaccine and 45% for pneumococcal vaccine in persons 65 years of age or older.[128] Immunization rates for members of racial and ethnic minority groups are substantially lower than for the white population, with African Americans tending to have the lowest rates.

REMAINING ISSUES IN IMMUNIZATIONS IN THE UNITED STATES

Remaining Disease Burden

There is no question that the vaccines recommended for universal or widespread use in infants and children address significant health problems and have had great impact. Table 42–7 indicated the maximum number of cases of some of these diseases before vaccines were available. Some of these conditions have been so well controlled by the use of vaccines that prospective recipients or their parents may not be aware of them, and many providers may not have seen cases themselves.

It is ironic that our success, which has given us very low levels of disease, might lead to a loss of awareness of the severity of these conditions if they do occur. This, in turn, could lead to a loss of political will to sustain immunization programs. It may be doubly ironic that we continue, as a society, to tolerate the level of mortality still seen in association with influenza and pneumococcal infection and do not mount major efforts to control it. More than 20,000 *excess* deaths regularly occur during influenza epidemics, and an annual average of 20,000 to 40,000 deaths are attributed to pneumococcal infection (CDC, unpublished data, 1997).[234]

Importations and Quarantine

Given the extent and rapidity of international travel, the risk of importation of vaccine-preventable diseases will remain until world-wide control or eradication occurs.[254–256] In 1997, most cases of measles reported in the United States were either imported from another country or directly attributable to importations. The countries that provided most of the importations were Brazil, Germany, Italy, Japan, and Switzerland.[254a]

Quarantine regulations have been used in the past to require, for example, smallpox vaccination of all persons entering a given country from infected countries. This approach resulted from international agreement (the International Sanitary Regulations) and was feasible because of the shared fear of smallpox and the limited extent of international travel at the time. In the absence of international accord and with the hundreds of millions of border crossings occurring in this country each year, vaccination requirements for all visitors (e.g., for measles) are not feasible. Monitoring and enforcement would be virtually impossible.

Registries

One of the most important components lacking at present in the US childhood immunization program is a system to track immunizations in individuals, recall them when they need additional doses, and remind providers to administer them. The pediatric standards call for such systems,[62] and similar systems are called for in the adult standards.[253]

Immunization registry systems should carry out five primary functions:

1. Monitor immunization status of individuals
2. Monitor immunization status of defined population groups
3. Remind individuals/parents of the need for immunization
4. Recall individuals in need of immunization
5. Remind practitioners to administer needed immunizations when they see patients who are due or overdue

Such systems also would provide a mechanism for identifying those who should receive new vaccines or additional doses of existing vaccines if recommendations change. It is likely that immunization registry systems may only be components of larger automated information systems about individuals' health status. Standards have been proposed for registry systems, particularly for childhood immunization registries.[257] They include automatic enrollment at birth (or arrival in the community) of all newborns or infants, registration of all doses of vaccines administered, regardless of the source of vaccination, and appropriate safeguards of confidentiality and restriction of access to information. Registries should be able to identify those in need of immunization, generate a recall message to them, remind the provider to administer vaccine, and provide summary information about the immunization status of those contained in the registry. They can be used to implement provider assessment and feedback systems, such as AFIX, and to help states and cities identify local populations in need of immunization. They can also generate reports for the HEDIS system. Registries could contain information about contraindications to vaccine and adverse events following immunization and could be used to generate the reports of adverse events mandated by the National Childhood Vaccine Injury Act. It seems clear that no single model will work throughout the country. What is essential is that there be agreement on the core data elements and that different systems be able to share information.[258]

All 50 states are now involved in development of immunization registries (but none is yet fully operational) encompassing all births and all doses of vaccine administered, regardless of the provider. Several jurisdictions, including Georgia and New York City, have legislation mandating registries, and these are now being implemented.

Adolescent Vaccination

There is a major new thrust to protect adolescents from vaccine-preventable diseases.[72] The strategy for protecting adolescents is targeted at children aged 11 to 12 years and includes (1) establishing a routine preventive care visit to the primary care provider, (2) vaccinating those without previous varicella vaccination or history of disease against varicella, (3) administering a second dose of MMR to those who have received only a single dose, (4) administering hepatitis B vaccine to those not previously vaccinated, (5) providing a booster dose of tetanus and diphtheria toxoids, (6) providing other vaccines (influenza, pneumococcal polysaccharide, and hepatitis A vaccines) indicated for certain high-risk adolescents, and (7) providing other preventive care measures as described in the Guidelines for Adolescent Preventive Services.[259]

Because of the CDC's recommendations for hepatitis B vaccination, adolescents are the largest group of young persons in need of one or more vaccinations.[72] Time is critical because as this cohort ages, it becomes more difficult to reach them through the health care system, and some members of this cohort will begin behavior patterns that place them at high risk for disease. More than 80,000 infections with hepatitis B would be expected over the lifetime of each cohort of 11- to 12-year-olds if they are not immunized.[260]

Some of the decisions regarding optimal strategies for reaching all adolescents will probably revolve around who should provide and pay for the vaccinations. School-based clinics have potential to vaccinate large groups of children. Managed care organizations and private providers have responsibility, however, for vaccinating their patients. A few states have adopted school entry regulations that require the initiation of hepatitis B vaccination before middle school entry, regardless of who provides the vaccinations; some states plan to conduct school-based vaccination clinics.

CONCLUSION

Development and use of vaccines in the United States represent a unique blend of public and private and federal, state, and local partnerships. Immunization programs have brought about dramatic reductions in the occurrence of disease in the United States and other countries. However, immunization of preschoolers has been inadequate, resulting in a resurgence of measles, a disease that had once been close to elimination. Efforts finally seem to be bringing about establishment of a permanent system to ensure full protection of US children at the earliest appropriate age. Programs to ensure appropriate immunization of adults and adolescents continue to be developed.

REFERENCES

1. Fine PEM. Herd immunity: History, theory, practice. Epidemiol Rev 15:265–302, 1993.
2. Fox JP, Elveback L, Scott W, et al. Herd immunity: Basic concept and relevance to public health immunization practices. Am J Epidemiol 94:179–189, 1971.
3. Hethcote HW. Measles and rubella in the United States. Am J Epidemiol 117:2–13, 1983.
4. Yorke JA, Nathanson W, Pianigiani G, Martin J. Seasonality and the requirement for perpetuation and eradication of viruses in populations. Am J Epidemiol 109:103–123, 1979.
5. Anderson RM, May RM. Directly transmitted infectious diseases: Control by vaccination. Science 215:1053–1060, 1982.
6. Schlenker TL, Bain C, Baughman AL, Hadler SC. Measles herd immunity. The association of attack rates with immunization rates in preschool children. JAMA 267:823–826, 1992.
7. Anderson RM, May RM. Immunization and herd immunity. Lancet 335:641–645, 1990.
8. Fenner F. Global eradication of smallpox. Rev Infect Dis 4:916–930, 1982.
9. Fenner F. Biological control, as exemplified by smallpox eradication and myxomatosis. Proc R Soc Lond 218:259–285, 1983.
10. Kim-Farley RJ, Bart KJ, Schonberger LB, et al. Poliomyelitis in the USA: Virtual elimination of disease caused by wild virus. Lancet ii:1315–1317, 1984.
11. Hinman AR. Prospects for disease eradication or elimination. NY State J Med 84:501–506, 1984.
12. Dowdle WR, Hopkins DR (eds). The Eradication of Infectious Diseases. Dahlem Workshop Report. Chichester, John Wiley & Sons, 1997, pp 1–218.
13. Fenner F, Henderson DA, Arita I, et al. Smallpox and its Eradication. Geneva, World Health Organization, 1988.
14. Stuart-Harris C, Western KA, Chamberlayne EC (eds). Can infectious diseases be eradicated? A report on the International Conference on the Eradication of Infectious Diseases. Rev Infect Dis 4:913–984, 1982.
15. Sencer DJ, Dull HB, Langmuir AD. Epidemiologic basis for eradication of measles in 1976. Public Health Rep 82:253–256, 1967.
16. Conrad JL, Wallace R, Witte JJ. The epidemiologic rationale for the failure to eradicate measles in the United States. Am J Public Health 61:2304–2310, 1971.
17. Hinman AR, Nieburg PI, Brandling-Bennett AD. The opportunity and obligation to eliminate measles from the United States. JAMA 242:1157–1162, 1979.
18. Hinman AR, Brandling-Bennett AD, Bernier RH, et al. Current features of measles in the United States: Feasibility of measles elimination. Epidemiol Rev 2:153–170, 1980.
19. Hinman AR, Kirby CD, Eddins DL, et al. Elimination of indigenous measles from the United States. Rev Infect Dis 4:538–545, 1983.
20. Frank JA, Orenstein WA, Bart KJ, et al. Major impediments to measles elimination: The modern epidemiology of an ancient disease. Am J Dis Child 139:881–888, 1985.
21. Atkinson WL, Orenstein WA, Krugman S. The resurgence of measles in the United States, 1989–1990. Annu Rev Med 43:451–463, 1992.
22. Orenstein WA, Bart KJ, Hinman AR, et al. The opportunity and obligation to eliminate rubella from the United States. JAMA 251:1988–1994, 1984.
23. White FMM. Policy for measles elimination in Canada and program implications. Rev Infect Dis 5:577–582, 1983.
24. Dittman S, Starke G, Ocklitz HW, et al. The measles eradication programme in the German Democratic Republic. Bull World Health Organ 53:21–24, 1976.
25. World Health Organization Expanded Programme on Immunization. Feasibility of elimination of vaccine-preventable diseases. Wkly Epidemiol Rec 59:143–145, 1984.
26. World Health Organization. Measles surveillance: Feasibility of measles elimination in Europe. Wkly Epidemiol Rec 58:229–230, 1983.
27. Christenson B, Bottiger M, Heller L. Mass vaccination programme aimed at eradicating measles, mumps, and rubella in Sweden: First experience. BMJ 287:389–391, 1983.
28. Rabo E, Taranger J. Scandinavian model for eliminating measles, mumps, and rubella. BMJ 289:1402–1404, 1984.
29. Bottiger M, Christenson B, Taranger J, Bergman M. Mass vaccination programme aimed at eradicating measles, mumps and rubella in Sweden: Vaccination of schoolchildren. Vaccine 3:113–116, 1985.
30. de Quadros CA, Olive JM, Hersh BS, et al. Measles elimination in the Americas. Evolving strategies. JAMA 275:224–229, 1996.
31. US Department of Health and Human Services, Public Health Service. Healthy people 2000. National health promotion and disease prevention objectives. Summary report, DHHS Publication No. (PHS) 91-50213. Washington, DC, US Government Printing Office, 1991, pp 121–123.
32. Centers for Disease Control and Prevention. Reported vaccine-preventable diseases—United States, 1993, and the Childhood Immunization Initiative. MMWR Morb Mortal Wkly Rep 43:57–60, 1994.
33. Centers for Disease Control and Prevention. Status report on the childhood immunization initiative: Reported cases of selected vaccine-preventable diseases—United States 1996. MMWR Morb Mortal Wkly Rep 46:665–671, 1997.
34. Begg N, Ramsay M. World Health Organization aims to eliminate measles in Europe by 2007. Eurosurveillance Wkly 1:971127, 1997. Available at http://www.eurosurv.org.
35. PAHO director announces campaign to eradicate poliomyelitis from the Americas by 1990. Bull Pan Am Health Organ 19:213–215, 1985.
36. de Quadros CA, Andrus JK, Olive JM, et al. Eradication of poliomyelitis: Progress in the Americas. Pediatr Infect Dis J 10:222–229, 1991.
37. Robbins FC, de Quadros CA. Certification of the eradication of indigenous transmission of wild poliovirus in the Americas. J Infect Dis 175(suppl 1):S281–S285, 1997.
38. Hull HF, Ward NA, Hull BP, et al. Paralytic poliomyelitis: Seasoned strategies, disappearing disease. Lancet 343:1331–1337, 1994.
39. Olive JM, Risi JB Jr, de Quadros CA. National immunization days: Experience in Latin America. J Infect Dis 175(suppl 1):S189–S193, 1997.
40. Wright PF, Kim-Farley RJ, de Quadros CA, et al. Strategies for the global eradication of poliomyelitis by the year 2000. N Engl J Med 325:1774–1779, 1991.
41. World Health Organization, Regional Office for the Western Pacific Region. Resolution WPR/RC39.R15. Manila, Regional Committee for the Western Pacific Region, September 1988.
42. World Health Organization, Regional Office for the Western Pacific Region. Eradication of poliomyelitis in the Western Pacific Region. Plan of Action for the period 1991–1995. Manila, Regional Office for the Western Pacific Region, July 1991.
43. World Health Organization, Regional Office for Europe. Resolution EUR/RC39/R5, Document EUR/RC39/9/7, Rev.1. Copenhagen, Regional Committee for Europe, September, 1989.
44. Centers for Disease Control and Prevention. Progress toward poliomyelitis eradication—Western Pacific Region, January 1, 1996—September 27, 1997. MMWR Morb Mortal Wkly Rep 46:1113–1117, 1997.
45. World Health Organization. Progress towards poliomyelitis eradication, WHO European Region, 1991—September 1997. Wkly Epidemiol Rec 72:321–327, 1997.
46. Hinman AR. World eradication of measles. Rev Infect Dis 4:933–936, 1982.
47. Hopkins DR, Hinman AR, Kooplan JP, Lan UM. The case for global measles eradication. Lancet i:1396–1398, 1982.
48. Henderson DA. Global measles eradication [letter]. Lancet ii:208, 1982.
49. Foege WH. The global elimination of measles. Public Health Rep 97:402–405, 1982.
50. Burgasov PN. Elimination of measles—the next task. J Microbiol Epidemiol Immunobiol (Russ) 6:3–6, 1983.
51. Hinman AR, Orenstein WA. Is measles eradicable? In Kurstak E (ed). Measles and Poliomyelitis: Vaccines and immunization. Springer-Verlag, Austria, 1993, pp 53–61.
52. Centers for Disease Control and Prevention. Measles eradication: Recommendations from a meeting cosponsored by the World Health Organization, the Pan American Health Organiza-

tion, and CDC. MMWR Morb Mortal Wkly Rep 46 (No. RR-11):1–20, 1997.
53. Advances in global measles control and elimination: Summary of the 1997 international meeting. MMWR Morb Mortal Wkly Rep 47(RR-11):1–23, 1998.
54. American Academy of Pediatrics, Peter G (ed). 1997 Red Book: Report of the Committee on Infectious Diseases (24th ed). Elk Grove Village, IL: American Academy of Pediatrics, 1997.
55. Centers for Disease Control and Prevention. Recommended childhood immunization schedule—United States, January 1995. MMWR Morb Mortal Wkly Rep 43(51–52):959–960, 1994.
56. Centers for Disease Control and Prevention. Recommended Childhood Immunization Schedule—United States, 1998. MMWR Morb Mortal Wkly Rep 47:8–12, 1998.
57. ACP Task Force on Adult Immunization and Infectious Diseases Society of America. Guide for Adult Immunization (3rd ed). Philadelphia, American College of Physicians, 1994.
58. Hinman AR. The National Vaccine Program and the National Vaccine Injury Compensation Program. In Proceedings of the 22nd Immunization Conference, San Antonio, TX, June 20–24, 1988. Atlanta, Centers for Disease Control, 1988, pp 9–12.
59. Dandoy S. The National Vaccine Advisory Committee: Mission/goals/progress. In Proceedings of the 23rd Immunization Conference, San Diego, CA, June 5–9, 1989. Atlanta, Centers for Disease Control, 1989, pp 21–22.
60. Anonymous. The measles epidemic. The problems, barriers, and recommendations. The National Vaccine Advisory Committee. JAMA 266:1547–1552, 1991.
61. Fedson DS. Adult immunization: Summary of the National Vaccine Advisory Committee Report. JAMA 272:1133–1137, 1994.
62. Ad Hoc Working Group for the Development of Standards. Standards for pediatric immunization practices. JAMA 269:1817–1822, 1993.
63. Centers for Disease Control and Prevention. Health Information for International Travel—1996–97. Atlanta, GA, DHHS, 1997.
64. Benenson AS (ed). Control of Communicable Disease Manual (16th ed). Washington, American Public Health Association, 1995.
65. Katzmann W, Dietz K. Evaluation of age-specific vaccination strategies. Theor Popul Biol 25:125–137, 1985.
66. Orenstein WA, Markowitz L, Preblud SR, et al. Appropriate age for measles vaccination in the United States. Dev Biol Stand 65:13–21, 1986.
67. Centers for Disease Control and Prevention. General recommendations on immunization: Recommendations of the Advisory Committee on Immunization Practices (ACIP). MMWR Morb Mortal Wkly Rep 43(No. RR-1):1–38, 1994.
68. Centers for Disease Control and Prevention. Measles prevention: Recommendations of the Immunization Practices Advisory Committee (ACIP). MMWR Morb Mortal Wkly Rep 38(No. S-9):1–13, 1989.
69. Centers for Disease Control. Update on adult immunization: Recommendations of the Immunization Practices Advisory Committee (ACIP). MMWR Morb Mortal Wkly Rep 40(RR-12):1–94, 1991.
70. Centers for Disease Control and Prevention. Prevention of varicella: Recommendations of the Advisory Committee on Immunization Practices (ACIP). MMWR Morb Mortal Wkly Rep 45(No. RR-11):1–36, 1996.
71. Centers for Disease Control and Prevention. Prevention of hepatitis A through active or passive immunization: Recommendations of the Advisory Committee on Immunization Practices (ACIP). MMWR Morb Mortal Wkly Rep 45(No. RR-15):1–30, 1996.
72. Centers for Disease Control and Prevention. Immunization of adolescents. Recommendations of the Advisory Committee on Immunization Practices, the American Academy of Pediatrics, the American Academy of Family Physicians, and the American Medical Association. MMWR Morb Mortal Wkly Rep 45(RR-13):1–16, 1996.
73. Hinman AR. Immunizations and CDC. Proceedings of the 30th Immunization Conference. Washington DC, US Government Printing Office, No. 1997, April 9, 1996, pp 7–13.
74. Hinman AR. A new U.S. initiative in childhood immunization. Bull Pan Am Health Organ 13:169–176, 1979.
75. Califano JA Jr. Address to Second National Immunization Conference, April 6, 1977. Washington, DC, Dept. Health, Education and Welfare, 1977.
76. Woods DR, Mason DD. Six areas lead national early immunization drive. Public Health Rep 107:252–256, 1992.
77. Robinson CA, Sepe SJ, Lin KF. The president's child immunization initiative—a summary of the problem and the response. Public Health Rep 108:419–425, 1993.
78. Robinson CA, Evans WB, Mahanes JA, Sepe SJ. Progress on the childhood immunization initiative. Public Health Rep 109:594–600, 1994.
79. Centers for Disease Control and Prevention. Status report on the childhood immunization initiative: National, state, and urban area vaccination levels among children aged 19–35 months—United States, 1996. MMWR Morb Mortal Wkly Rep 46:657–664, 1997.
80. Orenstein WA, Bernier RH. Toward immunizing every child on time. Pediatrics 94:545–547, 1994.
81. Centers for Disease Control. Vaccine Adverse Event Reporting System—United States. MMWR Morb Mortal Wkly Rep 39:730–733, 1990.
82. Ellenberg SS, Chen RT. The complicated task of monitoring vaccine safety. Pub Health Rep 112:10–20, 1997.
83. McCormick MC, Shapiro S, Starfield BH. The Association of Patient-Held Records and Completion of Immunizations. Clin Pediatr (Phila) 20:270–274, 1981.
84. Brink EW, Hinman AR. The Vaccine Injury Compensation Act: The new law and you. Contemp Pediatr 6:28–32, 35–36, 39, 42, 1989.
85. Department of Health and Human Services. New vaccine information materials. Federal Register 59:31888–31889, 1994.
86. Centers for Disease Control and Prevention. Vaccines for Children program, 1994. MMWR Morb Mortal Wkly Rep 43:705, 1994.
87. National Center for Health Statistics. Healthy People 2000 Review, 1997. Hyattsville, MD: Public Health Service, 1997, p 189.
88. Rodewald L, Peak R, Ezzati-Rice T, et al. Who are the Immunization Providers for U.S. Children: Findings from the 1994 National Health Interview Survey (NHIS) Provider Record Check (PRC). Ambulatory Child Health 3(1 Pt 2):168, 1997.
89. Ruch-Ross HS, O'Connor KG. Immunization referral practices of pediatricians in the United States. Pediatrics 94:508–512, 1994.
90. Lieu T, Smith M, Newacheck P. Health insurance and preventive care sources of children at public immunization clinics. Pediatrics 93:373–378, 1994.
91. Zimmerman RK, Medsger AR, Ricci EM, et al. Impact of free vaccine and insurance status on physician referral of children to public vaccine clinics. JAMA 278:996–1000, 1997.
92. Scholle SH, Kelleher KJ, Childs G, et al. Changes in Medicaid managed care enrollment among children. Health Aff (Millwood) 16:164–170, 1997.
93. Rodewald L, Szilagyi P, Holl J, et al. Health insurance for low-income working families. Arch Pediatr Adolesc Med 151:798–803, 1997.
94. Orenstein WA, Bernier RH. Surveillance-information for action. Pediatr Clin North Am 37:709–734, 1990.
95. Wharton M, Strebel PM. Vaccine preventable diseases. In Wilcox LS, Marks JS (eds). From Data to Action: CDC's Public Health Surveillance for Women, Infants, and Children. Atlanta, GA, US Department of Health and Human Services, Public Health Service, Centers for Disease Control and Prevention, 1994, pp 281–290.
96. Chorba TL, Berkelman RL, Safford SK, et al. Mandatory reporting of infectious diseases by clinicians. JAMA 262:3018–3026, 1989.
97. Centers for Disease Control and Prevention. Case definitions for infectious conditions under public health surveillance. MMWR Morb Mortal Wkly Rep 46(RR-10):1–55, 1997.
98. Schuchat A, Robinson K, Wenger JD, et al., the Active Surveillance Team. Bacterial meningitis in the United States in 1995. N Engl J Med 337:970–976, 1997.
99. Alter MJ, Mares A, Hadler SC, et al. The effect of under reporting on the apparent incidence and epidemiology of acute viral hepatitis. Am J Epidemiol 125:133–139, 1987.

100. Peterson CL, Maupin T, Goldman G, Mascola L. Varicella active surveillance: Use of capture-recapture methods to assess completeness of surveillance data. 37th Interscience Conference on Antimicrobial Agents and Chemotherapy; Toronto; September 28–October 1, 1997; Abstract H-111.
101. Goodnow KL, Watson B, Lutz J, et al. Epidemiology of varicella in an inner-city population. 31st National Immunization Conference; Detroit, MI; May 19–22, 1997; Abstract 280.
102. Luckey P, Gonzalez O, Howell B, et al. Varicella active surveillance project 1995 and 1996: Travis County, Texas. 31st National Immunization Conference; Detroit, MI; May 19–22, 1997; Abstract 284.
103. Davis SF, Strebel PM, Atkinson WL, et al. Reporting efficiency during a measles outbreak in New York City, 1991. Am J Public Health 83:1011–1015, 1993.
104. Prevots DR, Sutter RW, Strebel PM, et al. Completeness of reporting for paralytic poliomyelitis, United States, 1980 through 1991. Arch Pediatr Adolesc Med 148:479–485, 1994.
105. Cochi SL, Edmonds LE, Dyer K, et al. Congenital rubella syndrome in the United States 1970–1985. On the verge of elimination. Am J Epidemiol 129:349–361, 1989.
106. Sutter RW, Cochi SL. Pertussis hospitalizations and mortality in the United States, 1985–1988. Evaluation of the completeness of national reporting. JAMA. 267:386–391, 1992.
107. Standaert SM, Lefkowitz LB, Horan JM, et al. The reporting of communicable diseases: A controlled study of *Neisseria meningitidis* and *Haemophilus influenzae* infections. Clin Infect Dis 20:30–36, 1995.
108. Orenstein WA, Bernier RH, Hinman AR. Assessing vaccine efficacy in the field. Further observations. Epidemiol Rev 10:212–241, 1988.
109. Centers for Disease Control and Prevention. Vaccination Coverage by race/ethnicity and poverty level among children aged 19–35 months—United States, 1996. MMWR Morb Mortal Wkly Rep 46:963–969, 1997.
110. Morrow AL, Rosenthal J, Lakkis HD, et al. A population-based study of access to immunization among urban Virginia children served by public, private, and military health care systems. Pediatrics 101:e5, 1998.
111. Ewert DP, Thomas JC, Chun LY, et al. Measles vaccination coverage among Latino children aged 12 to 59 months in Los Angeles County: A household survey. Am J Public Health 81:1057–1059, 1991.
112. Ewert DP, Westman S, Ward B, et al. An increase in *Haemophilus influenzae* type B vaccination among preschool-aged children in inner-city Los Angeles, 1990 through 1992. Am J Public Health 84:1154–1157, 1994.
113. Lemeshow S, Stroh G Jr. Sampling techniques for evaluating health parameters in developing countries. Washington, DC, National Academy Press, 1988, pp 8–13.
114. Henderson RH, Sundaresan T. Cluster sampling to assess immunization coverage: A review of experience with a simplified sampling method. Bull World Health Organ 60:253–260, 1982.
115. Serfling R, Sherman I. Attribute sampling methods for local health departments. Public Health Service, Washington, DC, 1965.
116. Zell ER, Dietz V, Stevenson J, et al. Low vaccination levels of US preschool and school-age children. Retrospective assessments of vaccination coverage, 1991–1992. JAMA 271:833–839, 1994.
117. Suarez L, Simpson D, Smith D. Errors and correlation in parental recall of child immunizations: Effects on vaccination coverage estimates. Pediatrics 99:e3, 1997.
118. Goldstein KP, Kviz FJ, Daum RS. Accuracy of immunization histories provided by adults accompanying preschool children to a pediatric emergency department. JAMA 270:2190–2194, 1993.
119. Fierman A, Rosen C, Legano L, et al. Immunization and adolescent status as determined by patients' hand-held cards vs. medical records. Arch Pediatr Med 150:863–866, 1997.
120. Humiston SG, Rodewald LE, Szilagyi PG, et al. Decision rules for predicting vaccination status of preschool-age emergency department patients. J Pediatr 123:887–892, 1993.
121. Centers for Disease Control and Prevention. State and national vaccination coverage levels among children aged 19–35 months— United States, April—December 1994. MMWR Morb Mortal Wkly Rep 44:613, 619–623, 1995.
122. Darden PM, Taylor JA, Slora EJ, et al. Methodological issues in determining rates of childhood immunization in office practice. Arch Pediatr Adolesc Med 150:1027–1031, 1996.
123. National Committee for Quality Assurance. HEDIS 3.0—The Health Plan Data and Information Set. Vol. 2. Washington, DC, HEDIS 3.0:37–40, 1997.
124. National Committee for Quality Assurance. HEDIS 3.0—The Health Plan Employer Data and Information Set. Vol. 2: Childhood immunization status. HEDIS 3.0:19–25, 1997.
125. National Committee for Quality Assurance. HEDIS 3.0—The Health Plan Employer Data and Information Set. Vol. 2: Flu shots for older adults. HEDIS 3.0:28–29, 1997.
126. National Committee for Quality Assurance. HEDIS 3.0—The Health Plan Employer Data and Information Set. Vol. 2: Adolescent well-care visits. HEDIS 3.0:137–139, 1997.
127. Centers for Disease Control and Prevention. Influenza and pneumococcal vaccination coverage levels among persons ≥65 years—United States, 1993. MMWR Morb Mortal Wkly Rep 48:853–859, 1996.
128. Centers for Disease Control and Prevention. Influenza and pneumococcal vaccination levels among adults aged ≥65 years—United States, 1997. MMWR Morb Mortal Wkly Rep 47:797–802, 1998.
129. Tarande M, Dietz V, Lewin M, Zell E. Health care characteristics and their association with the vaccination status of children. Arch Pediatr Adolesc Med 150(4 suppl):a161, 1996.
130. Cutts FT, Orenstein WA, Bernier RH. Causes of low preschool immunization coverage in the United States. Ann Rev Public Health 13:385–398, 1992.
131. Orenstein WA, Atkinson W, Mason D, Bernier RH. Barriers to vaccinating preschool children. J Health Care Poor Underserved 1:315–330, 1990.
132. Williams IT, Milton JD, Farrell JB, Graham NM. Interaction of socioeconomic status and provider practices as predictors of immunization coverage in Virginia children. Pediatrics 96 (3 Pt 1):439–446, 1995.
133. Miller LA, Hoffman RE, Barón AE, et al. Risk factors for delayed immunization against measles, mumps, and rubella in Colorado two-year-olds. Pediatrics 94:213–219, 1994.
134. Hueston WJ, Mainous AG, Palmer C. Delays in childhood immunizations in public and private settings. Arch Pediatr Adolesc Med 148:470–473, 1994.
135. Fielding JE, Cumberland WG, Pettitt L. Immunization status of children of employees in a large corporation. JAMA 271:525–530, 1994.
136. Bobo JK, Gale JL, Thapa PB, Wassilak SGF. Risk factors for delayed immunization in a random sample of 1163 children from Oregon and Washington. Pediatrics 91:308–314, 1993.
137. Bates AS, Fitzgerald JF, Dittus RS, Wolinsky FD. Risk factors for underimmunization in poor urban infants. JAMA 272:1105–1110, 1994.
138. Wood D, Donald-Sherbourne C, Halfon N, et al. Factors related to immunization status among inner-city Latino and African-American preschoolers. Pediatrics 96(2 Pt 1):295–301, 1995.
139. Etkind P, Lett SM, Macdonald PD, et al. Pertussis outbreaks in groups claiming religious exemptions to vaccinations. Am J Dis Child 146:123–126, 1992.
140. Jackson BM, Payton T, Horst G, et al. An epidemiologic investigation of a rubella outbreak among the Amish of Northeastern Ohio. Public Health Rep 108:436–439, 1993.
141. Novotny T, Jennings CE, Doran M, et al. Measles outbreaks in religious groups exempt from immunization laws. Public Health Rep 103:49–54, 1988.
142. Centers for Disease Control and prevention. Poliomyelitis—United States, Canada. MMWR Morb Mortal Wkly Rep 46:1194–1199, 1997.
143. National Vaccine Advisory Committee. Report of the NVAC working group on philosophical exemptions. National Vaccine Program Office. Atlanta, GA, Centers for Disease Control and Prevention, 1998.
144. Guyer B, Hughart N, Holt E, et al. Immunization coverage and its relationship to preventive health care visits among inner-city children in Baltimore. Pediatrics 94:53–58, 1994.
145. Guyer B, Hughart N. Increasing childhood immunization coverage by improving the effectiveness of primary health care systems for children. Arch Pediatr Adolesc Med 148:901–902, 1994.

146. Dietz VJ, Stevenson J, Zell ER, et al. Potential impact on vaccination coverage levels by administering vaccines simultaneously and reducing dropout rates. Arch Pediatr Adolesc Med 148:943–949, 1994.
147. Cutts FT, Zell ER, Mason JD, et al. Monitoring progress toward US preschool immunization goals. JAMA 267:1952–1955, 1992.
148. Strobino D, Keane V, Holt E, et al. Parental attitudes do not explain underimmunization. Pediatrics 98(6 Pt 1):1076–1083, 1996.
149. Houtrouw SM, Carlson KL. The relationship between maternal characteristics, maternal vulnerability beliefs, and immunization compliance. Issues Compr Pediatr Nurs 16:41–50, 1993.
150. Taylor JA, Cufley D. The association between parental health beliefs and immunization status among children followed by private pediatricians. Clin Pediatr 35:18–22, 1996.
151. Lannon C, Brack V, Stuart J, et al. What mothers say about why poor children fall behind on immunizations. A summary of focus groups in North Carolina. Arch Pediatr Adolesc Med 149:1070–1075, 1995.
152. Salsberry PJ, Nickel JT, Mitch R. Why aren't preschoolers immunized? A comparison of parents' and providers' perceptions of the barriers to immunizations. J Community Health Nurs 10:213–224, 1993.
153. Hanson IC, Jenkins K, Spears W, Stoner D. Immunization prevalence rates for infants in a large urban center: Houston/Harris County, 1993. Tex Med 92:66–71, 1996.
154. Majeroni B, Cowan T, Osborne J, Graham R. Missed appointments and Medicaid managed care. Arch Fam Med 5:507–511, 1996.
155. Gamertsfelder DA, Zimmerman RK, DeSensi EG. Immunization barriers in a family practice residency clinic. J Am Board Fam Pract 7:100–104, 1994.
156. Abbotts B, Osborn LM. Immunization status and reasons for immunization delay among children using public health immunization clinics. Am J Dis Child 147:965–968, 1993.
157. Mustin HD, Hold VL, Connell FA. Adequacy of well-child care and immunizations in US infants born in 1988. JAMA 272:1111–1115, 1994.
158. Hutchins SS, Jansen HAFM, Robertson SE, et al. Studies of missed opportunities for immunization in developing and industrialized countries. Bull World Health Organ 71:549–560, 1993.
159. Grabowsky M, Orenstein WA, Marcuse EK. The critical role of provider practices in undervaccination. Pediatrics 97:735–737, 1996.
160. Centers for Disease Control and Prevention. Impact of missed opportunities to vaccinate preschool-aged children on vaccination coverage levels—selected U.S. sites, 1991–1992. MMWR Morb Mortal Wkly Rep 43:709–711, 717–718, 1994.
161. Christy C, McConnochie KM, Zernik N, Brzoza S. Impact of an algorithm-guided nurse intervention on the use of immunization opportunities. Arch Pediatr Adolesc Med 151:384–391, 1997.
162. Farizo KM, Stehr-Green PA, Markowitz LE, Patriarca PA. Vaccination levels and missed opportunities for measles vaccination: A record audit in a public pediatric clinic. Pediatrics 89:589–592, 1992.
163. Gindler JS, Cutts FT, Barnett-Antinori ME, et al. Successes and failures in vaccine delivery: Evaluation of the immunization delivery system in Puerto Rico. Pediatrics 91:315–320, 1993.
164. LeBaron C, Chaney M, Baughman A, et al. Impact of measurement and feedback on vaccination coverage in public clinics, 1988–1994. JAMA 277:631–635, 1997.
165. Lieu TA, Black SB, Sorel ME, et al. Would better adherence to guidelines improve childhood immunization rates? Pediatrics 98:1062–1068, 1996.
166. Szilagyi PG, Rodewald LE, Humiston SG, et al. Reducing missed opportunities for immunizations: Easier said than done. Arch Pediatr Adolesc Med 150:1193–1200, 1996.
167. Zimmerman RK, Schlesselman JJ, Baird AL, Mieczkowski TA. A national survey to understand why physicians defer childhood immunizations. Arch Pediatr Adolesc Med 151:657–664, 1997.
168. Zimmerman RK, Giebink GS, Street HB, Janosky JE. Knowledge and attitudes of Minnesota primary care physicians about barriers to measles and pertussis immunization. J Am Board Fam Pract 8:270–277, 1995.
169. Wood D, Pereyra M, Halfon N, et al. Vaccination levels in Los Angeles Public Health Centers: the contribution of missed opportunities to vaccinate and other factors. Am J Public Health 85:850–852, 1995.
170. Fairbrother G, Friedman S, DuMont KA, Lobach KS. Markers for primary care: Missed opportunities to immunize and screen for lead and tuberculosis by private physicians serving large numbers of inner-city Medicaid-eligible children. Pediatrics 97:785–790, 1996.
171. McConnochie KM, Roghmann KJ. Immunization opportunities missed among urban poor children. Pediatrics 89:1019–1026, 1992.
172. Szilagyi PG, Rodewald LE. Missed opportunities for immunizations: A review of the evidence. J Public Health Manage Pract 2:18–25, 1996.
173. Bell LM, Pritchard M, Anderko R, Levenson R. A program to immunize hospitalized preschool-aged children: Evaluation and impact. Pediatrics 100:192–196, 1997.
174. Holt E, Guyer B, Hughart N, et al. The contribution of missed opportunities to childhood underimmunization in Baltimore. Pediatrics 97:474–480, 1997.
175. Szilagyi PG, Rodewald LE, Humiston SG, et al. Missed opportunities for childhood vaccinations in office practices and the effect on vaccination status. Pediatrics 91:1–7, 1993.
176. Woodin KA, Rodewald LE, Humiston SG, et al. Physician and parent opinions. Are children becoming pincushions from immunizations? Arch Pediatr Adolesc Med 149:845–849, 1995.
177. Melman ST, Chawla T, Kaplan JM, Anbar RD. Multiple immunizations. Ouch! Arch Fam Med 3:615–618, 1994.
178. Askew GL, Finelli L, Lutz J, et al. Beliefs and practices regarding childhood vaccination among urban pediatric providers in New Jersey. Pediatrics 96:889–892, 1995.
179. Harper PG, Madlon-Kay DJ, Luxenberg MG, Tempest R. A clinic system to improve preschool vaccination in a low socioeconomic status population. Arch Pediatr Adolesc Med 151:1220–1223, 1997.
180. Szilagyi PG, Roghmann KJ, Campbell JR, et al. Immunization practices of primary care practitioners and their relation to immunization levels. Arch Pediatr Adolesc Med 148:158–166, 1994.
181. Siegel RM, Schubert CJ. Physician beliefs and knowledge about vaccinations. Are Cincinnati doctors giving their best shot? Clin Pediatr 35:79–83, 1996.
182. Hughart N, Vivier P, Ross A, et al. Are immunizations an incentive for well-child visits? Arch Pediatr Adolesc Med 151:690–695, 1997.
183. Joffe MD, Luberti A. Effect of emergency department immunization on compliance with primary care. Pediatr Emerg Care 10:317–319, 1994.
184. Lieu TA, Glauber JH, Fuentes-Afflick EF, Lo B. Effects of vaccine information pamphlets on parents' attitudes. Arch Pediatr Adolesc Med 148:921–929, 1994.
185. M. Keane, personal communication, Business Research, Merck Vaccine Division, December 1996.
186. Szilagyi PG, Rodewald LE, Humiston SG, et al. Immunization practices of pediatricians and family physicians in the United States. Pediatrics 84:517–523, 1994.
187. Bordley WC, Freed GL, Garrett JM, et al. Factors responsible for immunizations referrals to health departments in North Carolina. Pediatrics 94:376–380, 1994.
188. Schulte JM, Bown GR, Zetzman MR, et al. Changing immunization referral patterns among pediatricians and family practice physicians, Dallas County, Texas, 1988. Pediatrics 87:204–207, 1991.
189. Wright JA, Marcuse EK. Immunization practices of Washington State pediatricians—1989. Am J Dis Child 146:1033–1036, 1992.
190. Taylor J, Darden P, Slora E, et al. The influence of provider behavior, parental characteristics, and a public policy initiative on the immunization status of children followed by private pediatricians: A study from pediatric research in office settings. Pediatrics 99:209–215, 1997.
191. Freed GL, Clark SJ, Pathman DE, et al. Impact of a new universal purchase vaccine program in North Carolina. Arch Pediatr Adolesc Med 151:1117–1124, 1997.
192. Zimmerman R, Janosky J. Immunization barriers in Minnesota private practices: The influence of economics and training on vaccine timing. Fam Pract Res J 13:213–224, 1993.

193. Saldarini RJ. Putting prevention research at risk: Implementation of the Vaccines for Children programme. Vaccine 12:1364–1367, 1994.
194. Fleming G. Vaccine administration fee survey. Child Health Care11:6, 1995.
195. Lurie N, Manning WG, Peterson C, et al. Preventive care: Do we practice what we preach? Am J Public Health 77:801–804, 1987.
196. Fairbrother G, Friedman S, Hanson KL, Butts GC. Effect of the Vaccines for Children Program on inner-city neighborhood physicians. Arch Pediatr Adolesc Med 151:1229–1235, 1997.
197. Bushnell CJ. The ABC's of practice-based immunization assessments. Proceedings of the 28th National Immunization Conference. Atlanta, GA, US Department of Health and Human Services, 1994, pp 207–209.
198. Bordley WC, Margolis PA, Lannon CM. The delivery of immunizations and other preventive services in private practices. Pediatrics 97:467–473, 1996.
199. Dini EF, Chaney M, Moolenaar RL, LeBaron CW. Information as intervention: How Georgia used vaccination coverage data to double public sector vaccination coverage in seven years. J Public Health Manage Pract 2:45–49, 1996.
200. Link D. Chart audits to promote community-wide childhood immunization. Presented at the 31st National Immunization Conference; Detroit, MI; May 20, 1997.
201. Alemi F, Alemagno SA, Goldhagen J, et al. Computer reminders improve on-time immunization rates. Med Care 34(10 suppl):OS45–OS51, 1996.
202. Alto WA, Fury D, Condo A, et al. Improving the immunization coverage of children less than 7 years old in a family practice residency. J Am Board Fam Pract 7:472–477, 1994.
203. Dini EF, Linkins RW, Chaney M. Effectiveness of computer-generated telephone messages in increasing clinic visits. Arch Pediatr Adolesc Med 149:902–905, 1995.
204. Lieu TA, Black SB, Lewis EM, et al. Computer-generated recall letters for underimmunized children: How cost-effective? Pediatr Infect Dis J 16:28–33, 1997.
205. Linkins RW, Dini EF, Watson JG, Patriarca PA. A randomized trial of the effectiveness of computer-generated telephone messages in increasing immunization visits among preschool children. Arch Pediatr Adolesc Med 148:908–914, 1994.
206. Young SA, Haplin TJ, Johnson DA, et al. Effectiveness of a mailed reminder on the immunization levels of infants at high risk of failure to complete immunizations. Am J Public Health 70:422–424, 1980.
207. Tollestrup K, Hubbard BB. Evaluation of a follow-up system in a county health department's immunization clinic. Am J Prev Med 7:24–28, 1991.
208. Owen AL, Owen GM. Twenty years of WIC: A review of some effects of the program. J Am Diet Assoc 97:777–782, 1997.
209. Devaney BL, Ellwood MR, Love JM. Programs that mitigate the effects of poverty on children. Future Child 7:88–112, 1997.
210. Egan MC. Federal nutrition support programs for children. Pediatr Clin North Am 24:229–239, 1977.
211. LeBaron C, Birkhead G, Parsons P, et al. Measles vaccination levels of children enrolled in WIC during the 1991 measles epidemic in New York City. Am J Public Health 86:1551–1556, 1996.
212. Birkhead GS, Cicirello HG, Talarico J. The impact of WIC and AFDC in screening and delivering childhood immunizations. J Public Health Manage Pract 2:26–33, 1996.
213. Hutchins SS, Gindler JS, Atkinson WL, et al. Preschool children at high risk for measles: Opportunities to vaccinate. Am J Public Health 83:862–867, 1993.
214. Birkhead GS, LeBaron CW, Parson P, et al. The immunization of children enrolled in the Special Supplemental Food Program for Women, Infants, and Children (WIC). The impact of different strategies. JAMA 74:312–316, 1995 [erratum appears in JAMA 274:1762, 1995].
215. Hoekstra EJ, LeBaron CW, Megaloeconomou Y, et al. The impact of a large-scale immunization intervention in the Special Supplemental Nutrition Program for Women, Infants, and Children (WIC). JAMA 280:1143–1147, 1998.
216. Shefer A, Mezoff J, Caspari D, et al. What mothers in the WIC program feel about WIC-immunization linkage activities: A summary of focus groups in Wisconsin. Arch Pediatr Adolesc Med 152:65–70, 1998.
217. Hutchins SS, Rosenthal J. Results from WIC demonstration projects. Proceedings of the 29th National Immunization Conference. Atlanta, GA, US Department of Health and Human Services, 1994, pp 1–4.
218. Pierce C, Goldstein M, Suozzi K, et al. The Impact of the standards for pediatric immunization practices on vaccination coverage levels. JAMA 276:626–630, 1996.
219. Gershon AA, Gardner P, Peter G, et al. Quality standards for immunization. Clin Infect Dis 25:782–786, 1997.
220. Dietz V, Cutts F. The use of mass campaigns in the expanded program on immunization: A review of reported advantages and disadvantages. Int J Health Serv 27:767–790, 1997.
221. Sabin AB. Measles, killer of millions in developing countries: Strategy for rapid elimination and continuing control. Eur J Epidemiol 7:1–22, 1991.
222. Schonberger LB, Kaplan J, Kim-Farley R, et al. Control of paralytic polio in the United States. Rev Infect Dis 6:S424–S426, 1984.
223. Modlin JF, Brandlin-Bennett AD, Witte JJ, et al. A review of five years' experience with rubella vaccine in the United States. Pediatrics 55:20–29, 1975.
224. Fairbrother G, DuMont KA. New York City's 1993 child immunization day: Planning, costs, and results. Am J Public Health 85:1662–1665, 1995.
225. Centers for Disease Control and Prevention. Assessment of undervaccinated children following a mass vaccination campaign—Kansas, 1993. MMWR Morb Mortal Wkly Rep 43:572–573, 1994.
226. Jackson CL. State laws on compulsory immunization in the United States. Public Health Rep 84:787–795, 1969.
227. Orenstein WA, Hinman AR, Williams WW. The impact of legislation on immunisation in the United States. In Hall R, Richters J (eds). Immunisation: The Old and the New. Proceedings of the 2nd National Immunisation Conference, Canberra, May 27–29, 1991. Canberra, Public Health Association of Australia, 1992, pp 58–62.
228. Orenstein WA, Halsey NA, Hayden GF, et al. From the Centers for Disease Control: Current status of measles in the United States, 1973–1977. J Infect Dis 137:847–853, 1978.
229. Centers for Disease Control. Measles—United States. MMWR Morb Mortal Wkly Rep 26:109–111, 1977.
230. Centers for Disease Control. Measles and school immunization requirements—United States 1978. MMWR Morb Mortal Wkly Rep 27:303–304, 1978.
231. Robbins KB, Brandling-Bennett AD, Hinman AR. Low measles incidence: Association with enforcement of school immunization laws. Am J Public Health 71:270–274, 1981.
232. Cochi SL, Preblud SR, Orenstein WA. Perspectives on the relative resurgence of mumps in the United States. Am J Dis Child 142:499–507, 1988.
233. Baughman AL, Williams WW, Atkinson WL, et al. The impact of college prematriculation immunization requirements on risk for measles outbreaks. JAMA 272:1127–1132, 1994 [erratum appears JAMA 272:1822, 1994].
234. Centers for Disease Control and Prevention. Prevention and control of influenza: Recommendations of the Advisory Committee on Immunization Practices (ACIP). MMWR Morb Mortal Wkly Rep 46(No. RR-9):1–25, 1997.
235. Centers for Disease Control and Prevention. Prevention of pneumococcal disease: Recommendations of the Advisory Committee on Immunization Practices (ACIP). MMWR Morb Mortal Wkly Rep 46(No. RR-8):1–24, 1997.
236. Centers for Disease Control. Hepatitis B virus: A comprehensive strategy for eliminating transmission in the United States through universal childhood vaccination. Recommendations of the Immunization Practices Advisory Committee (ACIP). MMWR Morb Mortal Wkly Rep 40(RR-13):1–25, 1991.
237. Centers for Disease Control and Prevention. Measles, mumps, and rubella—vaccine use and strategies for measles, rubella, and congenital rubella syndrome elimination and mumps control: Recommendations of the Advisory Committee on Immunization Practices (ACIP). MMWR Morb Mortal Wkly Rep 47(RR-8):1–57, 1998.

238. Fiebach N, Beckett W. Prevention of respiratory infections in adults: Influenza and pneumococcal vaccines. Arch Intern Med 154:2545–2557, 1994.
239. Richardson JP, Michocki RJ. Removing barriers to vaccination use by older adults. Drugs Aging 4:357–365, 1994.
240. Centers for Disease Control. Adult Immunization: Knowledge, attitudes, and practices—DeKalb and Fulton Counties, Georgia, 1988. MMWR Morb Mortal Wkly Rep 34:657–661, 1988.
241. Fiebach NH, Viscoli DM. Patient acceptance of influenza vaccination. Am J Med 91:393–400, 1991.
242. Nichol KL, Lofgren RP, Gapinski J. Influenza vaccination: Knowledge, attitudes, and behavior among high-risk outpatients. Arch Intern Med 152:106–110, 1992.
243. Williams WW, Hickson MA, Kane MA, et al. Immunization policies and vaccine coverage among adults: The risk for missed opportunities. Ann Intern Med 108:616–625, 1988.
244. Fedson DS, Chiarello LA. Previous hospital care and pneumococcal bacteremia. Importance for pneumococcal immunization. Arch Intern Med 143:885–889, 1983.
245. Centers for Disease Control and Prevention. Missed opportunities for pneumococcal and influenza vaccination of Medicare pneumonia inpatients—12 western states, 1995. MMWR Morb Mortal Wkly Rep 46:919–923, 1997.
246. Buffington J, Bell K, LaForce F. A target-based model for increasing influenza immunizations in private practice. J Gen Intern Med 6:204–209, 1991.
247. Kouides R, Lewis B, Bennett N, et al. A performance-based incentive program for influenza immunization in the elderly. Am J Prev Med 9:250–255, 1993.
248. Fedson DS, Kessler HA. A hospital-based influenza immunization program, 1977–78. Am J Public Health 73:442–445, 1983.
249. Ratner ER, Fedson DS. Influenza and pneumococcal immunization in medical clinics 1978–1980. Arch Intern Med 143:2066–2069, 1983.
250. Fedson DS. Influenza and pneumococcal immunization in medical clinics, 1971–1983. J Infect Dis 149:817–818, 1984.
251. Setia U, Serrenti I, Lorenz P. Factors affecting the use of influenza vaccine in the institutionalized elderly. J Am Geriatr Soc 33:856–858, 1985.
252. Gyorkos TW, Tannenbaum TN, Abrahamowicz M, et al. Evaluation of the effectiveness of immunization delivery methods. Can J Public Health 85:S15–S30, 1994.
253. Centers for Disease Control. The public health burden of vaccine preventable diseases among adults: Standards for adult immunization practice. MMWR Morb Mortal Wkly Rep 39:725–729, 1990.
254. Centers for Disease Control and Prevention. Measles—United States, 1996, and the interruption of indigenous transmission. MMWR Morb Mortal Wkly Rep 46:242–246, 1997.
254a. Measles—United States, 1997. MMWR Morb Mortal Wkly Rep 14:273–276, 1998.
254b. National, state, and urban area vaccination coverage levels among children aged 19–35 months—United States, 1997. MMWR Morb Mortal Wkly Rep 47:547–554, 1998.
255. Vitek CR, Redd SC, Redd SB, Hadler SC. Trends in importation of measles to the United States. JAMA 277:1952–1956, 1997.
256. Rota JS, Heath JL, Rota PA, et al. Molecular epidemiology of measles virus: identification of pathways of transmission and implications for measles elimination. J Infect Dis 173:32–37, 1996.
257. All Kids Count National Childhood Immunization Initiative of the Robert Wood Johnson Foundation. Childhood Immunization Registry Systems: A General Definition of Terms, Scope and Components. Atlanta: All Kids Count National Program Office, 1994.
258. Cordero JF, Guerra FA, Saarlas KF (eds). Developing immunization registries: Experiences from the All Kids Count Program. Am J Prev Med 13(suppl):1–128, 1997.
259. American Medical Association, Elster A, Kuznets N (eds). AMA Guidelines for Adolescent Preventive Services (GAPS). Recommendations and Rationale. Baltimore, Williams & Wilkins, 1994.
260. Margolis HS, Coleman PJ, Brown RE, et al. Prevention of hepatitis B virus transmission by immunization. An economic analysis of current recommendations. JAMA 274:1201–1208, 1995.

chapter

43 Immunization in Europe

David M. Salisbury

Sieghart Dittmann

To many observers, immunization programs in Europe appear to be like a patchwork quilt, with almost as many immunization schedules as countries, a variety of legislative processes for surveillance or immunization, and little evidence of harmony. Indeed, a survey of immunization schedules revealed no two to be identical among forty-eight countries of the European region.[1] Many of these differences have come from historical influences, since much of immunization and public health has its roots in European countries. As different health service delivery mechanisms evolved, so each country adapted its immunization program in line with perceived epidemiological priorities, public health and primary care facilities, and vaccine availabilities. With immunization programs long established and accepted by health professionals and the public, reasons for change have to be balanced against consequential disruption without demonstrable public health benefit. Some of these concepts are coming under increasing challenge as national boundaries become less rigid, allowing unrestricted passage between countries, and the vaccine industry seeks to market its products on a regional rather than national basis.

Despite the multiplicity of countries and immunization programs, some generalizations can be made. The northern, western, and south central European countries have immunization programs that are independent of each other; among these programs lie the greatest differences in schedules, surveillance, vaccines used, and public health provisions. In the United Kingdom (UK), for example, all childhood vaccines and vaccinations are free, purchased by the government and provided by family practitioners. In France, pediatricians provide most childhood vaccines, and much of the cost incurred is reimbursed by the government. In Germany, reimbursement comes from insurance-based healthcare schemes. Vaccines and vaccinations are free in Scandinavian countries and are most often provided by primary care nurses.

Most former socialist countries in central and Eastern Europe had well-developed immunization programs, and many were able to maintain these programs effectively under the changed socioeconomic conditions of the 1990s. Until the breakup of the former Soviet Union, there was in effect a single immunization program in the 15 Soviet republics, surveillance requirements were the same, and the vaccines were produced in the Russian Republic. Since the dissolution of the former Soviet Union, the 11 newly independent states (excluding Russia) and the Baltic States have faced vaccine shortages, lack of "hard currency" to buy vaccines on the international markets, and a progressive shift to internationally recommended immunization policies. There has also been a move away from public sector– to private sector–based medical care.

POLICYMAKING PROCESSES IN EUROPEAN UNION COUNTRIES

Each European Union (EU) country has a national advisory committee on immunization that makes recommendations to the government. The effect of these recommendations varies according to the centralization of immunization programs and the balance of provision between the public sector and the private sector. In countries such as Germany, Spain, and Switzerland, the *Länder* (Germany) or the *autonomous regions* (Spain) or the *cantons* (Switzerland) have the responsibility for the protection of public health. Although each country has a national advisory committee, its recommendations can be modified at the local level, and the type of vaccines actually provided depends on the choice of private practitioners and reimbursement arrangements with insurance companies. In the UK, the Joint Committee on Vaccination and Immunisation makes recommendations to the government on immunization policy for England, Wales, Scotland, and Northern Ireland, and policy is implemented similarly in each country.

EU countries do not have a common immunization policy, although there are unified processes for vaccine registration, batch testing of vaccines, and coordinated networks for surveillance are developing. So far, immunization policy or practice has not been subject to European legislation for harmonization, although many relevant processes such as batch release are controlled through EU legislation. Under an EU directive, vaccines batch tested in one EU country cannot be retested if they are purchased for use in another country. Vaccine matters are included in the interests of several of the Directorates General (DGs). DG 3 is responsible for industry and is the DG most concerned with vaccines; it is responsible for all aspects of the regulation of medicines. Its Pharmaceutical Committee is an important forum for information exchange among member states. The remit of DG 5 (Employment, Industrial Relations, and Social Affairs) includes public health, disease prevention and monitoring, and health and safety at work. DG 12 (Science, Research, and Development) commissions research, particularly for which there is an EU-wide application.

In the past, individual countries licensed vaccines (and other medicinal products) according to local arrangements; not surprisingly, there were considerable differences in the registration requirements. Starting with medicinal products whose manufacture involved genetic manipulation, an EU centralized procedure has evolved such that any new product can now be licensed through a central clearinghouse—the European Medicines Evaluation Agency (EMEA), located in London. The EMEA is responsible for centralized licensing of biological or biotech medicines and mutual recognition of product licences and scientific advice through its Committee on Proprietary Medicinal Products (CPMP); it also has an equivalent veterinary committee. The CPMP has appropriate subcommittees; the Efficacy, Safety and Biotechnology Working Party gives the CPMP scientific advice on quality issues concerning specific products (those submitted for licensure or already licensed) and on more general scientific issues, such as transmissible spongiform encephalopathies and medicinal products. The CPMP and its working parties develop written *Notes for Guidance* for the pharmaceutical industry. These notes are usually specific to the EU but are sometimes developed in collaboration with U.S. and Japanese counterparts. Each member state has formal membership of all committees and working parties, but nominated rapporteurs from specific member states, with assistance from the EMEA secretariat, conduct procedures such as the licensure of specific products.

A wide range of techniques is employed to measure immunization coverage in the individual EU countries. In Denmark, the Netherlands, and the UK, public health data are fully computerized and actively managed. Thus, coverage is calculated by comparing the number of children who have completed immunization by a specified age with the number of children of the same age who reside in that community. In Austria, Belgium, Germany, Greece, and Spain, where private sector providers administer many vaccines, coverage is calculated by comparing the number of doses of vaccine imported or distributed with the estimated target population.[2] Allowance for wastage and inaccuracies in the target population makes these coverage estimates unreliable, however. In most countries, coverage is measured at 2 years of age, but in Germany, for example, it is measured at school entry at around 5 years of age. Because such different techniques for estimating coverage have been used and the accuracy of these estimations may differ considerably, comparisons among countries' coverage reports need to be made with caution. Nevertheless, some countries report very low coverage for certain vaccines.[3] Measles (Fig. 43–1) and pertussis coverages, for example, are estimated at around 50% in Italy, although the pertussis coverage is expected to rise with introduction of the acellular vaccine. A similar position pertains to Germany and Ireland, although coverage of measles, mumps, and rubella (MMR) vaccine is higher, at 75%. Other countries, particularly those in Scandinavia, the UK, the Netherlands, and Portugal, report high coverages for all antigens.

Apart from reporting of the incidence of vaccine-preventable diseases to the World Health Organization regional office for Europe, there is no formal centralized monitoring for the EU countries. However, the European Sero-Epidemiology Network was established in 1996 to coordinate and harmonize the serological surveillance of immunity to vaccine-preventable diseases in six countries (Denmark, England, France, Germany, Italy, and the Netherlands).[4] The diseases under surveillance are measles, mumps, rubella, pertussis, and diphtheria.

WIDER EUROPEAN POLICIES—THE WORLD HEALTH ORGANIZATION

The European office of the WHO has an overarching interest in developing immunization policies suitable for implementation in all 51 member states, and the WHO has been actively involved in immunization in Europe. The First European Technical Conference of the WHO, on the control of infectious diseases through vaccination programs, was held in 1959 in Rabat, Morocco. When the Expanded Programme on Immunization was launched in 1974 by the WHO, most countries of the European region had already successfully prevented serious childhood diseases such as poliomyelitis and diphtheria through countrywide immunization programs. Therefore, the European region considered participation in the Expanded Program on Immunization a low priority. This opinion changed in the early 1980s, when the member states of the European region were all signatories to the regional Health for All by the Year 2000 strategy.[5]

In 1984, the Second Conference on Immunization Policies in Europe was held in Karlovy Vary, Czechoslovakia. Here, participants reviewed the status of immunization programs in the region, established immunization targets, determined the actions necessary to reach the targets, and reinforced the commitment of member states to the goals and activities of the Expanded Programme on Immunization and to the regional targets. The conference became a turning point for strengthening regionwide coordinated immunization activities. The recommendations of the conference also strengthened the responsibility of the WHO regional office in Copenhagen, Denmark, whose Communicable Disease and Immunization Unit continues to coordinate regional activities.

A European Advisory Group was created in 1986 and

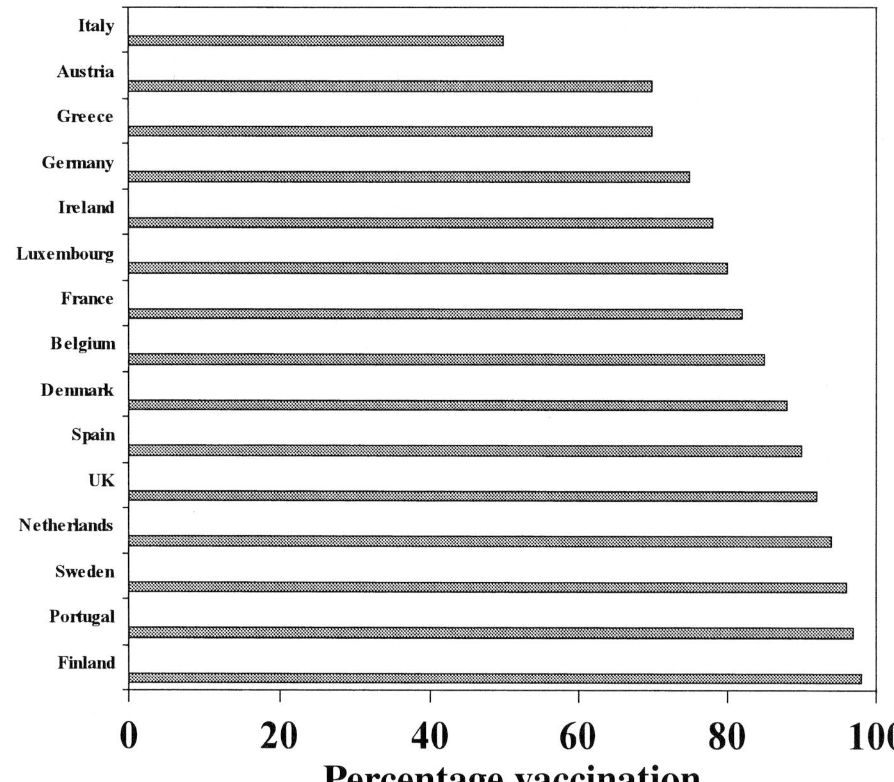

Figure 43–1. Reported coverage of measles vaccine in European Union countries, 1996. (From Guerin N, Roure C. Immunisation coverage in the European Union. Eurosurveillance 2(1):2–4, 1997.)

has met regularly since. The terms of reference of the group include the following:

- Periodically review the progress toward achieving the immunization targets, and consider constraints of immunization programs in European countries
- Recommend modifications and approaches of strategies based on new scientific or practical findings
- Provide technical recommendations to develop and foster national elimination programs
- Advise the WHO European office on priority areas for action to be taken, including proposals for submission to the WHO European office that might result in a resolution calling for action by member states and the European Office

In addition, program managers of the Expanded Program on Immunization's 51 European member states meet annually or biannually to better implement the recommendations of the European Advisory Group and to share experiences of achievements and constraints in approaching the regional targets.

The sudden and dramatic political and socioeconomic changes that followed the dissolution of the former Soviet Union have seriously compromised the ability of the newly independent states to produce or procure vaccines or to carry out disease control and immunization programs, resulting in a reemergence of epidemics of vaccine-preventable diseases. Initiated by the United States Agency for International Development and the Japanese government, an Interagency Immunization Coordinating Committee (IICC) was created in Kyoto, Japan, in 1994. The WHO European office provides the secretariat for and coordinates the activities of the IICC. The main objectives of the IICC are to support the newly independent states in the control of vaccine-preventable diseases, particularly the control of epidemic diphtheria and the eradication of poliomyelitis, and to help ensure primary immunization in children, with the ultimate goal of achieving sustainable immunization programs based on vaccine self-reliance. In addition to the cofounders, Japan and the United States, members of the IICC are Canada, Denmark, France, Germany, Turkey, the EU, the International Federation of Red Cross and Red Crescent Societies, Rotary International, the United Nations Children's Fund, and the WHO. Future work is targeted at achieving sustainability of immunization programs (financing, program management, quality control of vaccines and other supplies) in all newly independent states.

VACCINES USED IN EUROPEAN REGION COUNTRY PROGRAMS

Immunization schedules and the vaccines being used in the 51 member states of the WHO European Region are changing rapidly as new vaccines become available in the west of the region and as sociopolitical changes occur in the east of the region. Immunization schedules from EU countries and selected other European countries are shown in Tables 43–1 and 43–2. Use of individual vaccines is discussed here.

Polio Vaccine. Most (41) countries use oral polio vaccine (OPV). Inactivated polio vaccine (IPV) alone is

Table 43–1. **IMMUNIZATION SCHEDULES USED IN SELECTED COUNTRIES OF THE WORLD HEALTH ORGANIZATION EUROPEAN REGION, 1998 (WHO DATA)**

COUNTRY	VACCINE						
	BCG*	DTP	DTaP	DT/Td**	T	OPV	IPV
Austria	‡	3, 4, 5, 16–18 mo		7, 14–15 yr		4–5, 6–7, 16–18 mo; 7, 14–15 yr	
Belgium		3, 4, 5, 13 mo		6 yr		3, 5, 13 mo, 6 yr	
Bulgaria	Newb; 7, 12, 17 yr	2, 3, 4, 24 mo		7 yr/12, 17, 25, 35 yr		2, 3, 4, 24 mo; 7 yr	
Croatia	Newb; 2, 8, 13 yr	3, 4–5, 6 mo; 2, 4 yr		/7, 14, 19 yr		3, 4–5, 6 mo; 2, 4, 7, 14 yr	
Czech Republic	4 days–6 wk; 11 yr	3, 4, 5, 18 mo; 5 yr			15, 25 & every 10 yr	3–15, 5–17, 27–39, 29–41 mo†; 12 yr	
Denmark			3, 5, 12 mo	5 yr		2, 3, 4 yr	3, 5, 12 mo
Estonia	Newb; 8 yr	3, 4–5, 6 mo; 2 yr		/7, 12, 17 yr		3, 3–5, 6 mo; 2, 7 yr	
Finland	Newb	3, 4, 5, 20–24 mo		/11–13 yr			6, 12, 20–24 mo; 6, 11–13, 16–18 yr
France	6 yr‡	2, 3, 4, 16–18 mo		6, 11, 16–18 yr			2, 3, 4, 18 mo; 6, 11, 16–18 yr
Germany	‡		3, 4, 5, 12–15 mo	/6, 11–15 yr			3, 4, 5, 12–15 mo; 11–18 yr
Greece	5–6, 13–14, 20–25 yr	2, 4, 6, 18 mo; 4 yr				2, 4, 6, 18 mo; 4 yr	
Hungary	3–42 days	3, 4, 5, 36 mo; 6–7 yr		/11 yr		4, 5, 15, 36 mo; 6–7 yr	3 mo
Ireland	Newb; 12 yr		2, 4, 6 mo	5 yr		2, 4, 6 mo; 5 yr	
Italy			3, 5, 7, 15 mo; 6 yr			3, 4, 10 mo; 3 yr	
Latvia	Newb	3, 4–5, 6, 18 mo	Limited use	7 yr/14 & every 10 yr		18 mo; 7, 14 yr	3, 4–5, 6 mo
Lithuania	Newb; 11 mo§; 6–7 yr	3, 4–5, 6, 18 mo	Limited use	6–7 yr/15–16 yr		6–7, 12 yr	3, 4–5, 18 mo
Luxembourg		2, 3, 4, 18 mo		3 yr		3, 4, 10, 18 mo; 3 yr	
Netherlands	6 mo‡	3, 4, 5, 11 mo		4, 9 yr			3, 4, 5, 11 mo; 4, 9 yr
Norway	16 yr		3, 5, 12 mo	/11–12 yr			6, 8, 16 mo; 7–8, 16 yr
Poland	Newb; 12 mo§; 7, 12, 18 yr	2, 3–4, 5, 16–18 mo		6 yr/14, 19 yr		2, 3–4, 5, 16–18 mo; 6, 11 yr	
Portugal	Newb; 5, 11 yr	2, 4, 6, 18 mo; 5 yr				2, 4, 6 mo; 5 yr	
Romania	Newb; 14 yr	2, 4, 6, 12, 30–36 mo		7, 14 yr & every 10 yr		2, 4, 6, 12 mo; 9 yr	
Russia	Newb; 7, 14 yr	3, 4, 5, 18 mo		/6 yr, 11 yr,¶ 16–17 & every 10 yr		3, 4, 5, 18, 24 mo; 6 yr	
Slovakia	Newb; 10 yr	2, 3, 9 mo; 2, 5 yr			13 yr	3, 4, 14, 16 mo; 11 yr	
Slovenia	Newb; 14, 19 yr	3 doses between 3 and 12 mo; 4th dose at 2 yr	Limited use	/10 yr	18 yr	3–12 mo 3 doses, 2, 7, 14 yr	
Spain		3, 5, 7, 15–18 mo		6–7, 14 yr		3, 5, 7, 18 mo; 6, 14 yr	
Sweden			3, 5, 12 mo	/10 yr			3, 5, 12 mo; 5–6 yr
Ukraine	Newb; 7, 14 yr	3, 4–5, 6, 18 mo		6 yr/11, 14, 18 & every 10 yr		3, 4–5, 6, 18 mo; 3, 6, 14 yr	
United Kingdom	12 yr‡	2, 3, 4 mo		4, 15 yr		2, 3, 4 mo; 4, 15 yr	
Uzbekistan	Newb; 7, 15 yr	2, 3, 4, 16 mo		7, 16–17 yr		0, 2, 3, 4, 16 mo; 7 yr	

*Revaccination with BCG is mosly based on negative screening results after application of the Mantoux test.
†During campaigns in March and May, all children born during the previous year receive the first and second dose, and children born 2 years before receive the third and fourth dose.
‡Infants at risk.
§Or infants without vaccination scar.
¶Monovalent toxoid with reduced amount of toxoid (adult formulations).
**Ages to left of slash are for DT; ages to right of slash are for Td.
In western European countries, an increasing number of new combination vaccines are used, such as DTP-Hib, DTaP-Hib, DTaP-IPV, and DTaP-Hib-IPV.
BCG, bacille Calmette-Guérin; DTP, diphtheria, tetanus, and pertussis; DTaP, diphtheria and tetanus toxoids and acellular pertussis; DT, diphtheria and tetanus toxoids (pediatric formulation); Td, tetanus and diphtheria toxoids (adult formulation); T, tetanus toxoids; OPV, oral polio vaccine; IPV, inactivated polio vaccine; newb, newborn; and Hib, *Haemophilus influenzae* type b.

Table 43–2. **IMMUNIZATION SCHEDULES USED IN SELECTED COUNTRIES OF THE WORLD HEALTH ORGANIZATION EUROPEAN REGION, 1998 (WHO DATA)**

COUNTRY	VACCINE					
	MMR	Measles	Mumps	Rubella	Hib	Hep B
Austria	14 mo; 6 yr			13 yr (girls)	3, 4, 5, 14–18 mo	3, 4, 5 mo; 2 yr‡§
Belgium	15 mo; 11 yr				3, 4, 5, 13 mo	‡§
Bulgaria	13 mo	12 yr		12 yr (girls)		0, 1, 6 mo, and †
Croatia	2, 12 yr					
Czech Republic	15, 21–25 mo					
Denmark	15 mo; 12 yr				3, 5, 12 mo	‡§
Estonia	12 mo; 13 yr					
Finland	14–18 mo; 6 yr				4, 6, 14–18 mo	‡§
France	12 mo; 11–13 yr				2, 3, 4, 15 mo	2, 3, 4, 16–18 mo *‡§
Germany	12–15 mo; 6 yr				3, 4, 5, 12–15 mo	3, 5, 12–15 mo; and *
Greece	15 mo; 10 yr					‡§
Hungary	15 mo	11 yr				
Ireland	15 mo; 10 yr				2, 4, 6 mo	‡§
Italy	15 mo	15 mo		11 yr (girls)		3, 4, 10 mo*‡§
Latvia	15 mo	7 or 12 yr	7 yr	12 yr (girls)	3, 4–5, 6 mo	0, 1, 6–7 mo
Lithuania	15–16.5 mo; 12 yr				3, 4–5, 18 mo (optional)	3, 4–5, 18 mo (optional)
Luxembourg	15 mo; 12 yr				3, 5, 15 mo	‡§
Netherlands	14 mo; 9 yr				3, 4, 5, 11 mo	‡§
Norway	15 mo; 12 yr				3, 5, 12 mo	‡§
Poland		13–14 mo; 7 yr		13 yr (girls)		0, 2, 3–4, 12 mo
Portugal	15 mo; 11 yr					2, 4, 6 mo*‡§
Romania		9 mo; 7 yr				0, 2, 6 mo
Russia	12–15 mo; 6 yr¶	12–15 mo; 6 yr¶	12–15 mo; 6 yr¶	12–15 mo; 6 yr¶		
Slovakia	14 mo; 11 yr					2, 3, 9 mo**
Slovenia	2, 7 yr					7 yr 3 doses
Spain	15 mo; 11 yr					*‡§
Sweden	18 mo; 12 yr				3, 5, 12 mo	‡§
Ukraine		12 mo; 6 yr	12 mo	12 mo; 15–16 yr (girls)		
United Kingdom	13 mo; 4 yr				2, 3, 4 mo	†‡§

*Hep B (hepatitis B) immunization for adolescents not previously immunized.
†All students in medicine/dentistry/nursing.
‡Newborns of all HBsAg-positive mothers.
§Other individuals at risk.
¶Either monovalent or combination vaccine.
**Planned for 1998/1999
In western European countries, an increasing number of new combination vaccines are used, such as DTP-Hib, DTaP-Hib, DTaP-IPV, and DTaP-Hib-IPV.
MMR, measles, mumps, and rubella; Hib, *Haemophilus influenzae* type b; and HBsAg, hepatitis B surface antigen.

used in Iceland, Finland, France, the Netherlands, Norway, and Sweden, and a sequential schedule (IPV followed by OPV) is used in Denmark, Hungary, Israel, and Lithuania. Germany changed to an all IPV schedule in 1998.

Bacille Calmette-Guérin Vaccine. Immunization of newborns with Bacille Calmette-Guérin (BCG) vaccine is recommended in the majority of countries, although in some countries it is scheduled during school age. There is considerable variation in the recommendations for the number and timing of booster doses. A few countries immunize only those children who are considered to be at risk.

Haemophilus influenzae Type b Vaccine. Sixteen countries have implemented immunization against *Haemophilus influenzae* type b (Hib) infections, and the number of countries considering the use of Hib vaccine is increasing continuously. Apart from the UK, those countries using Hib vaccine recommend either a four-dose schedule or a three-dose regimen with the last dose close to the first birthday. In the UK, Hib vaccine is given combined with diphtheria, tetanus, and pertussis (DTP) vaccine at 2, 3 and 4 months of age, and no further booster doses are given.

Rubella and Mumps Vaccines. Owing to resource limitations, 15 countries have not yet been able to add rubella vaccine to their schedules, and 4 countries have not been able to add mumps vaccine to their schedules.

Measles, Mumps, and Rubella Vaccine. This preparation is the vaccine of choice in 28 countries; 13 countries recommend a second MMR immunization, usually around the fifth birthday, although this is given later in France, Sweden, Norway, Denmark, and Finland.

Hepatitis B Vaccine. Eight countries with a low (<2%) prevalence of hepatitis B surface antigen, and 5 with medium (2–8%) prevalence are already known to have implemented universal hepatitis B immunization of children (and/or adolescents). In some remaining countries, the implementation of universal hepatitis B immunization is under consideration or is already partially implemented, or immunization is recommended only for groups at risk. Hepatitis B immunization is urgently needed in countries of Central Asia and parts of the Russian Federation that have a high (>8%) prevalence of hepatitis B surface antigen. Implementation is under way in Kazakstan, Russia, and Uzbekistan.

Pertussis Vaccine. The timing and use of pertussis vaccine vary considerably. Since the late 1980s, when only whole-cell vaccines were available, Sweden did not use pertussis-containing vaccines. The vaccine was used in Italy only in a few provinces, and Germany had uneven usage: low coverage in western areas and high coverage in eastern areas. More recently, many western European countries have licensed acellular vaccines for booster immunization and for primary and booster immunizations. Pertussis immunization is now used in all European countries. However, where high quality whole-cell pertussis vaccine is available and high coverage is achieved, the impact is excellent: Countries such as Bulgaria, the Czech Republic, Hungary, Poland, and Slovakia, which have used whole-cell vaccine exclusively for many years, have registered incidence rates of pertussis less than 1 per 100,000 population. More than 60% of the countries of the European region use a primary series of three doses of diphtheria, tetanus, and pertussis (DTP) or acellular pertussis between ages 2 and 6 months. In a few countries, the third dose is recommended at a later age (10–18 months). In Ireland, Malta, Norway, Spain, and the UK, the primary three doses complete immunization against pertussis. Most countries recommend a fourth dose at the age of 2 years; others prefer to immunize before school entry. Croatia, Greece, Hungary, Italy, Slovenia, and Switzerland recommend a fifth dose of vaccine at ages 4 to 7 years.

IMMUNIZATION SCHEDULES IN NEWLY INDEPENDENT STATES

In general, immunization schedules in the newly independent states of the former Soviet Union include more booster doses, particularly for BCG and OPV. Following the recommendations by the WHO, schedules have been simplified during recent years. However, most countries still recommend at least one booster dose of BCG and, taking into account the current diphtheria epidemic, three diphtheria vaccine booster doses during the school-age years (i.e., at school entry, the middle school years, and before completing school).

CONTRAINDICATIONS

Recommendations on contraindications used in the majority of European countries correspond with the recommendations of WHO,[6] the UK Joint Committee on Vaccination and Immunisation,[7] or the U.S. Advisory Committee on Immunization Practices.[8] Some European countries still recommend lengthy lists of contraindications whose application may act as a disincentive for the successful implementation of immunization. The newly independent states of the former Soviet Union have continued to use elaborate lists of contraindications, but efforts are being made to reduce these. The increasing exchange of information with the WHO, the United Nations Children's Fund (UNICEF), other European countries, the United States, and Canada has helped give reassurance to health professionals that they can shorten an extensive list of contraindications without compromising safety.

IMMUNIZATION AGAINST EPIDEMIC DIPHTHERIA IN EASTERN EUROPE AND CENTRAL ASIAN REPUBLICS

Epidemic diphtheria has reemerged on a massive scale in the newly independent states and the Baltic countries of the former Soviet Union.[9] The recent epidemic began in the Russian Federation in 1990 and affected all 15 countries by the end of 1994. More than 150,000 cases and 4000 deaths have been reported to the European office of the WHO, representing more than 90% of all diphtheria cases reported worldwide from 1990 to 1996. A characteristic of this epidemic has been the high proportion of cases among adolescents and adults (38–82% in the various republics), whereas children were the predominant age group affected in the prevaccine era and in the massive epidemic in central and northern European countries during and after World War II. Exportations to other European countries (mainly to Finland, Germany, Poland, and the UK) and to Mongolia have been reported, causing an outbreak of diphtheria that affected more than 150 children, adolescents, and adults in Mongolia.

Reasons for this epidemic include the importation of toxigenic strains (possibly from Afghanistan); low DTP coverage among children during the 1980s and the first years of the 1990s; and a large gap of immunity among adults. The countrywide epidemic spread was caused by large population movements; the delay of aggressive anti-epidemic measures; inadequate information for physicians and the public; and inadequate supplies for prevention and treatment in the majority of the countries. Contributing factors were socioeconomic instability and, in some countries, deterioration of the healthcare infrastructure.

In close collaboration with the national authorities in countries with diphtheria epidemics, the IICC elaborated a plan for coordinated action.[10, 11] The three main components of the strategy were as follows[12]:

- Mass immunization of the whole population: at least one immunization for all, augmented by two additional doses for specific age groups (e.g., 30–50 years)
- Early detection and proper management of cases
- Early identification and proper management of close contacts

More than $US 25 million were provided by the international donor community, mainly the members of the IICC, to supply vaccines, antitoxin, antibiotics, syringes, needles, cold chain equipment, and other commodities.

After the implementation of control plans, most countries began reporting decreases in incidence by the end of 1995 that continued in 1996 and 1997. Whereas in 1994 and 1995 about 50,000 cases were reported annually, in 1996 the number decreased to 20,000 cases; about 7000 cases occurred in 1997. However, control of the diphtheria epidemic still requires intensified efforts by national health authorities, and some countries also require sustained aid from international organizations and agencies.

Based on epidemiological projections, it is estimated that the implementation of aggressive measures in the Russian Federation, in collaboration with the actions of the 14 other diphtheria epidemic countries and the international community, could have prevented more than 400,000 cases and 12,000 deaths (Fig. 43–2).

The main lessons learned[13] from reemerging epidemic diphtheria in the newly independent states[14] are the need for (1) maintenance of high coverage for primary and booster immunizations, (2) a comprehensive outbreak response strategy,[15] (3) modern diagnostic facilities,[16, 17] (4) refresher training of health workers, and (5) raising public awareness. Based on the experiences gained, in 1996 the European Advisory Group on Immunization made the following recommendations for all European countries[18]:

- In any country facing a diphtheria epidemic, mass campaigns should be implemented.
- A one-dose strategy should be implemented in the shortest possible period to all preschool children, schoolchildren, adolescents, and adults regardless of the immunization history (usually not known in adults).
- The achievement of very high (90–95%) coverage of primary immunization with DTP vaccine is of utmost importance; this immunization series should be completed before 6 months of age.
- Booster doses of tetanus and diphtheria vaccine should be given before school entry (DT) and at the completion of school (Td), with the timing of the first booster dose at 16 to 36 months of age.
- In a number of countries, especially those presently experiencing epidemic diphtheria or having recently experienced epidemic diphtheria, a further booster dose can be given in the middle period of school years.

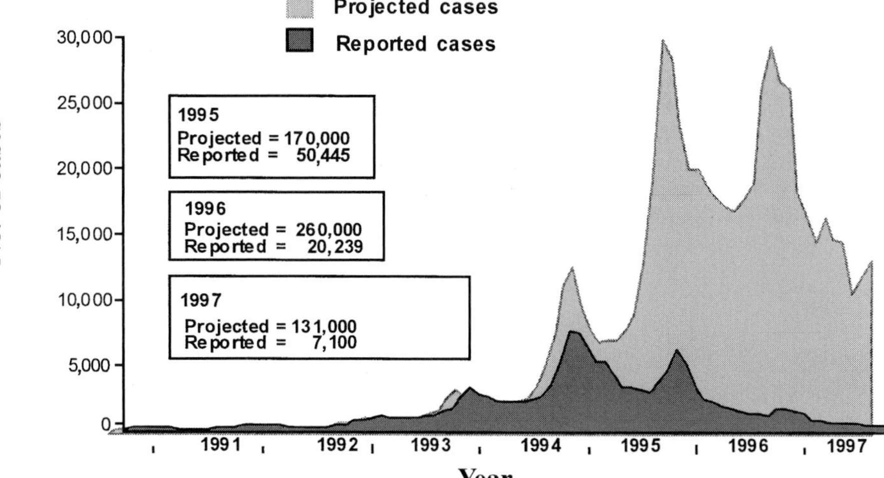

Figure 43–2. Projected and reported numbers of monthly cases of diphtheria in Europe, 1990 to 1997.

- Adults 30 to 50 years of age must receive a full primary immunization series in the absence of documented evidence of previous complete immunization against diphtheria. (Recommendations for adults were based on clinical trials undertaken in Georgia, Estonia, Latvia, Lithuania, and Ukraine,[19] in which vaccines were used that had different amounts of diphtheria toxoid (dosages ≥2 limit of flocculation) in different age groups. Protective antibody titers were achieved in less than 70% in certain distinct age bands (e.g., adults aged 30–50 years) after one dose and even after two doses of vaccine.)
- Where the risk of diphtheria is considered high, periodic booster doses for adults are necessary to prevent the resurgence of diphtheria in adults as immunity wanes.
- In other countries, adult diphtheria booster strategies need to be considered in light of the perceived risk of diphtheria, opportunities that exist for the provision of boosters, and the sensitivity of surveillance such that rapid responses can be implemented if diphtheria is introduced.

EXAMPLES OF EUROPEAN COUNTRY PROGRAMS

Examples of immunization programs in four countries, each representing a group of countries with similar programs, are described in this section. The account for the UK is expanded to describe in greater detail the particular operational changes that have been effected and that have been associated with significant improvements in program performance. Characteristics of the countries and their health programs are as follows:

- UK—an industrially highly developed western European country with a national health service in which the provision and financing of the childhood immunization program are entirely within the public sector
- Germany—an industrially highly developed western European country with services from both private and public organizations that are financed mainly from compulsory health insurance
- Slovenia—a new independent eastern European country that is in economic transition and that has a national health service in which the provision and financing of the immunization program are mainly within the public sector and national health insurance
- Republic of Moldova—a newly independent state of the former Soviet Union that is in economic transition and that has a national health service in which the provision and financing of health care and immunization are mainly within the public sector

United Kingdom

Since 1948, the UK has had a National Health Service that provides free health care for all UK residents. Every individual is registered with a general practitioner (GP) who provides primary care and, if appropriate, referral to appropriate specialists. All childhood immunizations and nationally recommended immunizations for adults, such as influenza vaccine, are provided free; only certain travel vaccines are paid for by the recipient. No immunizations are compulsory.

When a child's birth is reported, a duplicate notification alerts the local health authority, which in turn allocates the child to a GP, usually the same as that providing primary care for the mother. This process enrolls the child in the local health authority computerized database that schedules the immunizations, calculates local coverage, identifies defaulters, and arranges payments for the GPs. By the time a newborn child is 10 days old, the parents will have been visited by the Health Visitor, a nurse who provides community child health services. The Health Visitor discusses immunization arrangements with the parents and seeks their consent for the child to be entered into a computer-based program, thereby satisfying data protection requirements. Consent is almost universal. By the time the child is around 6 weeks old, the local health authority has issued a computer-generated invitation for the first immunization (which is mailed to the parents) and alerted the GP or local health clinic of the date and time scheduled for the child's immunizations and the antigens needed. Invitations for subsequent immunizations are issued in the same way. After attendance for immunization, the GP submits a completed form to the local computer unit, triggering the next step in the process. After two or three defaulted invitations (according to local practice), the GP and Health Visitor are alerted, allowing active follow-up to establish why the child has not attended for immunization. In some circumstances, especially for gypsy families, domiciliary immunization may be provided.

In 1987, as part of a review of immunization services in England, Peckham noted that coverage was among the lower third of levels reported by European countries.[20] In 1997, coverage for the UK (by the second birthday) was 96% for diphtheria, tetanus, polio, and Hib vaccines; 94% for pertussis vaccine; and 92% for MMR vaccine (Fig. 43–3).[21]

It remains difficult to identify the specific contributions that have led to these considerable improvements, since many aspects of the provision of immunization services have been changed during this decade.[22]

Improvements have included the following:

- Payment of GPs only when they reach coverage targets
- Improvements in the computerized tracking system to better identify and follow defaulters
- Widespread dissemination of updated guidelines on immunization theory and practice, sent free to all healthcare professionals involved in immunization
- Appointment of immunization coordinators in each health district
- Acceleration of the timing of scheduled immunizations
- Development of a national immunization communication strategy

Starting in 1986, efforts were made to ensure that every health district had an immunization coordinator.

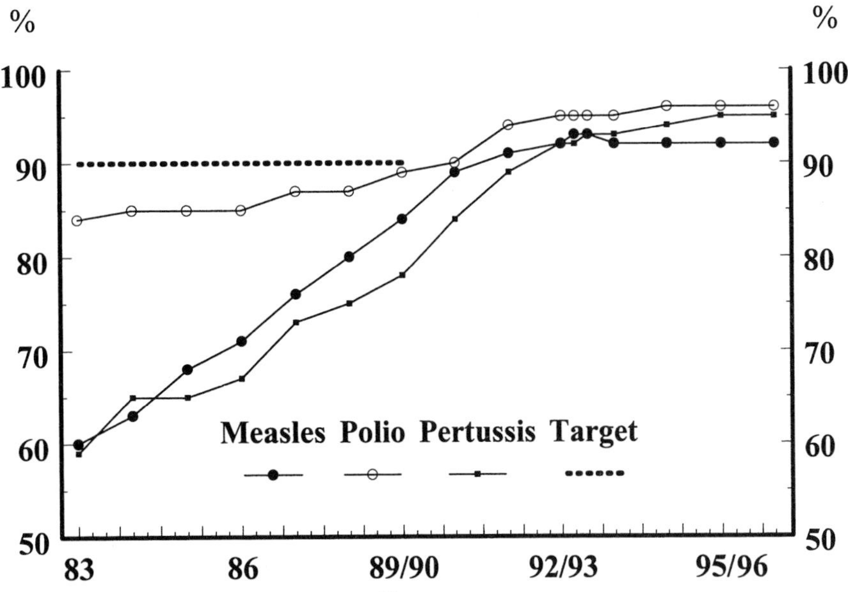

Figure 43–3. Immunization coverage by the second birthday in England, 1984 to 1997.

These health professionals were usually consultants in public health medicine, some were pediatricians, some nurses or administrators. The main requirement was the suitability of the individual to ensure the effective implementation of immunization services at local levels. Coordinators are expected to oversee the computerized immunization programs, the immunization training of health authorities and health professionals in primary care, and the production of quarterly statistical returns; they also take the local lead in introducing new strategies or new vaccines. The Department of Health in London maintains a database of coordinators and organizes regular national meetings to update coordinators, exchange experiences, and provide training.

Since 1986, at 2- to 3-year intervals, the Department of Health has issued a publication that provides updated national guidance on immunization. The publication—*Immunisation Against Infectious Disease*—is sent free to all medical practitioners (irrespective of speciality), all general practice nurses, health visitors, and nurses in community child health. The guidance covers practical immunization topics and also provides detailed information on individual vaccines. Special emphasis has been placed on reducing false contraindications and distinguishing causally related adverse events from those that are likely to occur by chance, unrelated to immunization. The publication is recognized as the standard reference for immunization policy and practice in the UK.[7]

After a detailed review of immunization services, undertaken by the British Market Research Bureau,[23] factors were identified that were contributing to a bias in the level of coverage among districts (i.e., the achievement of high coverage in some districts as opposed to low coverage in others with similar demographic features). Effective use of computerized services, training, and active participation of GPs were associated with high coverage, whereas social and demographic factors remained powerful influences in predicting low coverage. High mobility of young inner city families was notable, since this compounded any deficiencies in information services in tracking children. The schedule for primary immunization in place at the time (3, 4.5, and 8–11 months of age) was associated with high dropout rates, especially in inner cities. Based on an analysis of operational factors, the national schedule for DTP and polio (and subsequently Hib) immunization was accelerated to 2, 3, and 4 months of age, with no booster doses until school entry. This change, in May 1990, led to higher coverage achieved at an earlier age.[24]

In 1990, the Secretary of State for Health requested the development of a new scheme for payment of GPs that emphasized their responsibilities for disease prevention and health promotion. Before this time, GPs had been paid for immunization on an *item for service* basis: Each immunization attracted a payment after submission of an appropriate claim form. However, the payment for individual immunizations was relatively small, and the claim process was protracted. Because submission of the claim forms was sometimes used for scheduling and tracking purposes, any delays in claim processing obstructed the immunization program. The new scheme replaced the item for service payments with a target-based scheme. Now, each quarter, physicians are required to show that coverage targets have been reached for specified cohorts for all age-appropriate immunizations. The targets are 70 and 90% coverage for all immunizations by the age of 2 years, with similar targets for preschool booster immunizations. All children registered with a GP are included; the quarterly numerator is the number of fully immunized children, and the denominator is the number of resident children who reach their second birthday in the quarter. No exclusions from the denominator population are allowed, even children with valid contraindications. Despite many publicly voiced concerns at the outset of the scheme that the targets were unattainable, data from the payment records show that the majority of GPs regularly reach the higher target payments. For a GP with an average-sized population of children, the target payments, on an annual basis, are approximately $1100 for reaching 70% coverage by the second birthday for all primary series immunizations, and a further $3500 for reaching or exceeding 90% coverage. Matching payments for the preschool immunizations are $375 and 1100. These payments represent 5 to 7.5% of GP's salary.

Since the introduction of the scheme, there has been a continuous improvement in the proportion of GPs attaining coverage targets. Results show progressive shifts to higher proportions of GPs reaching the higher payment level targets (Fig. 43–4). Data for the first 2 years of the scheme show that the 10 localities that had the greatest increases in higher target attainment were predominantly in the inner city or were otherwise associated with high unemployment, poor housing, young families, or single parents. (These localities were Barking, Barnet, Bradford, Cleveland, Enfield, Gateshead, Lancashire, Manchester, Salford, and Sandwell.) A scheme that provided powerful motivation for immunization providers helped them overcome many of the obstacles to the achievement of high coverage.

The Department of Health collaborates with the Health Education Authority to implement a national immunization communication strategy. The Department of Health provides resources of around $2 million annually as baseline funding and increases this when necessary. For example, a high-profile advertising campaign in 1994 in advance of a nationwide measles rubella vaccination campaign cost an additional $1.5 million, most of which was spent on television advertising but which also funded newspaper and magazine materials. The annual funding provides for information materials on immunization that are given to every mother of a newborn infant as well as posters for public places and regular television advertising. The advertising materials are developed by commercial advertising agencies. Twice a year, using commercial market researchers, at least 1000 mothers of young children are interviewed to investigate their knowledge and attitudes about immunization and to examine their awareness of recent immunization advertising. The results of these studies[25] are fed back to coordinators and are used by the Department of Health and the Health Education Authority in shaping immunization promotion initiatives.

Before 1992, some vaccines were purchased centrally and provided free to users, central funding was disbursed to local authorities for some vaccine purchases against centrally negotiated prices, and other vaccines were purchased through local funds. After an internal review of these funding arrangements, agreement was reached that all vaccines would be purchased from central funds and provided free to all users. The financial savings from bulk purchasing were used to contract with a commercial distribution company that specialized in refrigerated delivery services. Since September 1992, all deliveries of vaccines are in cold chain–guaranteed conditions from the manufacturer to the end user. GPs now receive their vaccines on a weekly basis, thereby reducing the wastage caused by stocking unnecessary quantities of vaccines. Because the whole delivery system is computer controlled, detailed information on the cold chain is available continuously, and the whereabouts of every dose of vaccine can be accounted for, should any product recall be needed.

Germany

The Federal Republic of Germany is an industrially highly developed European country. Since its unification in 1990, the federal state has consisted of 16 *Länder*, each with its own legislature. Political authority is divided between the federal government and the governments of the Länder. Each Länder has legislative responsibility over matters such as education, culture, environmental protection, and police. The federal government maintains authority over foreign affairs, defense, finance, and others issues. The two levels of government share responsibility for social and health policy, with the federal government establishing general guidelines.[26]

The 1979 law on the prevention and control of communicable diseases distinguishes between the right of the Federal Minister of Health to make distinct immunizations compulsory for parts of the population threatened by severe, dangerous diseases and the right of the health authorities of the Länder to publicly recommend immunizations. In the case of vaccine injuries after a publicly recommended immunization, the Länder is responsible for providing necessary compensation. The health authorities of the Länder receive technical assis-

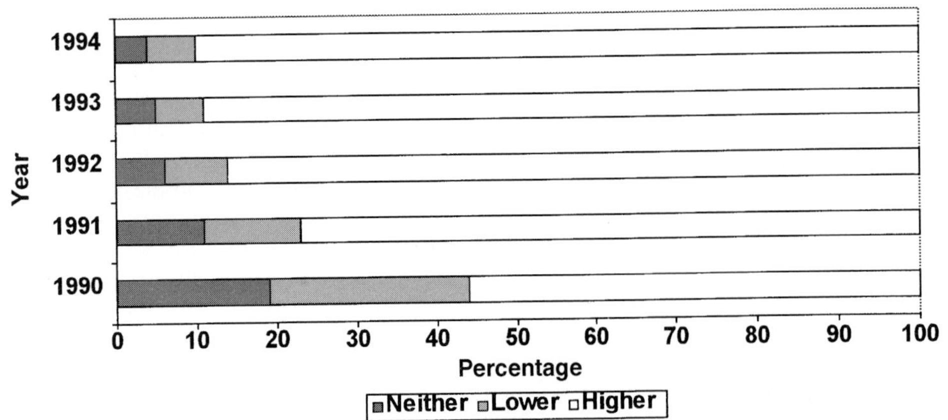

Figure 43–4. The proportion of United Kingdom general practitioners that reached target payment levels, 1990 to 1994. Neither indicates neither target payment; lower, lower target payment; and higher, higher target payment. (Data from the Department of Health, London.)

tance for their public recommendations through the Advisory Commission on Immunization of the Robert-Koch-Institut (Ständige Impfkommission). The Robert-Koch-Institut in Berlin is the federal institute on infectious and non-communicable diseases. The majority of the health authorities of the Länder implement the recommendations of the institute accordingly.

Ninety-five percent of all immunizations in Germany are carried out by private physicians, mainly pediatricians and general practitioners. Only a minority of immunizations is carried out by the public health service. Immunization is provided free of charge except those administered for private international travel. Germany's comprehensive social welfare system covers almost the entire population. The insurance companies reimburse immunizations that are carried out by private physicians.

Some of the vaccine-preventable diseases are reportable. Deaths due to measles, pertussis, and rubella are reportable but non-fatal cases are not. In some areas (e.g., Lower Saxony), sentinel surveillance systems (for measles, mumps, and rubella) are in place. There is a hospital-based surveillance system for Hib disease with the participation of more than 90% of all pediatric institutions in Germany.

Most of the Länder determine immunization coverage at school entry, and coverage sample surveys are also used. Many activities have been initiated to improve immunization coverage, particularly for MMR immunization. Based on estimations and surveys, the coverage rates in 1996 were more than 80% for diphtheria, tetanus, and poliomyelitis; more than 70% for Hib disease; 75% for measles and mumps; 35 to 60% for rubella; and 45% for pertussis.

At periodic intervals, the national reference center on poliomyelitis and enteroviruses determines the immunity of the population against poliomyelitis in large, randomized serosurveillance studies. Other reference laboratories (e.g., that for measles, mumps, and rubella) organize similar studies.

The last case of imported poliomyelitis occurred in 1992. Since 1994, 10 cases of diphtheria were reported, imported from Eastern Europe. Invasive Hib disease has been almost eliminated. The incidences of measles, mumps, rubella, and pertussis are still high, estimated at 15 to 75 per 100,000 population for measles and mumps and at 35 to 150 per 100,000 population for pertussis and rubella.

Slovenia

Slovenia is one of the smallest European countries, covering an area of 20,250 km^2 and bordering Austria, Croatia, Hungary, Italy, and the Adriatic Sea. Formerly a part of Yugoslavia, the country gained independence in 1991. Slovenia is divided administratively into 9 regions, about 240 communes, and 1203 communities and has a population of 1.99 million. In 1995, the gross domestic product per capita was approximately $US 13,132. In 1994, 7.9% of the gross domestic product was spent on health. Based on the criteria established by the Parliament, the Ministry of Health determines the services to be provided at the secondary and tertiary levels, whereas the city authorities and communities deal with primary care services. The privatization of physicians, dentists, and other services, such as diagnostic laboratories, is increasing rapidly.[27]

The main public health institutions responsible for infectious disease control and immunization are as follows:

- National Institute of Public Health—responsible for licensing of vaccines and immunoglobulins, importation of vaccines, data collection of reportable infectious diseases (including those preventable through immunization), immunizations and adverse events after immunization, and evaluation of collected data and feedback reporting
- Institute for Drug Control—the national control authority for pharmaceuticals and vaccines
- Institute of Blood Transfusion—the national control authority for biological products including immunoglobulins but excluding vaccines

A national Advisory Committee on Immunization proposes the national immunization program and the immunization schedule and provides recommendations on contraindications, immunization procedures, reporting of immunizations, target diseases, and adverse events after immunization. The director of the National Public Health Institute or one of the deputies acts as the national immunization program manager; at the regional level, regional public health institutes manage the immunization programs. Immunizations are carried out by physicians usually in public health centers or by private physicians.

Vaccines are provided free of charge, because the state purchases vaccines, other commodities, and the necessary logistics, including cold chain provision. Physicians are paid for immunizations through the health insurance system that covers the whole population. Immunization programs for people of all ages are specified in the mandatory health insurance regulations.

Slovenia does not manufacture vaccines, and thus all vaccines are imported. The National Institute of Public Health provides a central vaccine storage facility; in individual regions, vaccines are stored in the public health centers that are in turn responsible for the timely distribution of vaccines to health centers and private physicians.

The national immunization program aims to achieve Immunization Target 5 of the Health for All by the Year 2000 strategy of the European WHO.[28] Slovenia introduced a second dose of measles and mumps vaccine in 1979, and since 1990 MMR vaccine is administered at 12 months and 6 years of age. Hepatitis B immunization is compulsory for newborns of mothers who are positive for hepatitis B surface antigen. Immunization coverage has increased continuously and for 1995 was 96% for DTP, oral polio vaccine, and MMR vaccine and 98% for BCG vaccine.

Immunizations against Hib, hepatitis A, hepatitis B, influenza, meningococcal and pneumococcal disease, rabies, tick-borne encephalitis, typhoid fever, yellow fever, and varicella are recommended for people at professional or behavioral risk for these diseases (i.e., patients at risk, healthcare personnel, and travelers).

Immunizations included in the immunization schedule for children are compulsory, as is the reporting of 75 infectious diseases. Slovenia has a computer-based monitoring system for immunization and infectious diseases. The registry for immunizations is linked with the central population registry. The regional public health centers and the national Public Health Institute in Ljubljana are responsible for data collection, evaluation, and feedback.

The impact of a long-standing well-implemented immunization program is demonstrated by the fact that the last case of diphtheria occurred in the mid-1960s and of poliomyelitis in 1978. For many years, pertussis incidence has been below 2 per 100,000 population, and the same very low incidence levels are reported for measles (since 1988), mumps (since 1990), and rubella (since 1992). In 1994, however, the incidence of measles increased again with an epidemic particularly manifested among young adults.

Republic of Moldova

The Republic of Moldova is a small Eastern European, mainly rural country in economic transition. It was one of the republics of the former Soviet Union from 1940 to August 1992, when it became independent. Moldova borders Romania and Ukraine, and its population is approximately 4.35 million. In 1995, life expectancy for men was 62 years and for women 70 years. The infant mortality rate was 21.50 per 1000 live births (1995). Since 1990, the economy has shrunk every year and in 1994 the gross domestic product per capita was $US 1576. The percentage of the gross domestic product spent on healthcare was 3.1%.

The parliament, presidency and government of Moldova officially determine health policies and the broad parameters of interministerial coordination in the field of health services. The Law of Health Care adopted by the Parliament in 1995 regulates the organizational structure of the healthcare system. The Ministry of Health (MOH) formulates the health policy and takes a lead on healthcare issues. The MOH is not primarily involved in the delivery of healthcare at the district and municipal level and does not disburse the majority of health service funding. The MOH is responsible for the management and funding of republic-wide services and republican institutions. The private sector in healthcare is being developed as envisaged in the 1995 legislation; by 1997, more than 600 licenses for physicians, pharmacies, and opticians were issued.[29]

Preventive medicine, including state hygiene supervision, infectious disease prevention and control, and immunization, is the responsibility of the Department of Health Services and Health Care Reform of the MOH and the National Center for Scientific and Applied Hygiene and Epidemiology. A network of sanitary and epidemiological services with *San-Epid* stations in each district or municipality is responsible for the implementation of immunization programs. Immunizations are carried out as part of primary healthcare.

Moldova does not manufacture vaccines. Before the disintegration of the former Soviet Union, vaccines were provided by Russian manufacturers. When Moldova became independent, it began purchasing some vaccines and related commodities from traditional Russian suppliers and nearby republics. Humanitarian aid has been provided through UNICEF. Since 1995, and coordinated by the IICC, the country has received donated vaccines for primary immunizations of children. To control the large epidemic of diphtheria, vaccines containing diphtheria toxoid (DTP, DT, Td) were provided through UNICEF. The Japanese government has provided hepatitis B vaccine, syringes, needles, and cold chain equipment. The long-term intention of the government is to buy its vaccines through UNICEF. On behalf of the United States Agency for International Development, Basic Support for Institutionalizing Child Survival has provided training to the MOH on international purchase of vaccines. The annual vaccine bill amounts to approximately $US 740,000, representing more than 1% of the total health budget. Thus, support from the international community is needed until the current economic crisis has ended.

In 1994, the Moldovan government approved the national program on immunization. The program established coverage targets of 95% for primary immunizations against poliomyelitis, diphtheria, pertussis, and tetanus and 98% for primary immunization against measles, mumps, tuberculosis, and hepatitis B.

The immunization schedule includes one dose of measles vaccine recommended at 12 months of age, BCG vaccine for newborns and at school entry, and Td booster doses at school entry and school completion. Hepatitis B vaccine should be given at birth and 1 and 6 months of age. Plans have been made to provide booster doses of Td to adults at intervals of 5 to 10 years.

In 1996, the reported coverage rates for children younger than 2 years were 99% for oral poliomyelitis vaccine and 98% for BCG, diphtheria, tetanus, and measles vaccines.

Moldova faced problems similar to those of the other newly independent states regarding health professionals' application of lengthy elaborate lists of contraindications, which resulted in the achievement of low vaccine coverages. The recommendations of the MOH are now in line with WHO recommendations on contraindications and have been distributed to all pediatricians. Persistence of the pediatricians in applying false contraindications was one of the main reasons why coverage before 1996 remained low in some regions. The WHO has been informed that statistics for all children are now included in the denominators for coverage assessment, including children with contraindications.

The last case of poliomyelitis due to wild poliovirus was in 1993. During more recent years, the incidence of pertussis was fewer than 20 cases per 100,000 population, with a decreasing trend. The incidence of measles was 10 to 90 cases per 100,000 population, and the incidence of mumps was still high, between 100 and 200 cases per 100,000 population. The prevalence of hepatitis B surface antigen in Moldova is considered medium level: the incidence of reported acute hepatitis B is on average about 50 cases per 100,000 population.

Epidemic diphtheria started in 1990 in the Russian Federation and in 1991 in the Ukraine; thereafter, all republics of the former Soviet Union, including Moldova, developed epidemic diphtheria. In June 1995, a national diphtheria control plan was established and implemented with the assistance of the international community. The main activity was a full-scale national immunization campaign carried out in November and December of 1995.

The following statistics exemplify Moldova's ability to tackle such serious health challenges:

- Immunization coverage with vaccine containing diphtheria toxoid for the population aged 2 to 60 years reached 82%, and coverage for children younger than 2 years reached 96% by June 30, 1996.
- All diphtheria cases were treated with diphtheria antitoxin and antibiotics, and most primary contacts received a single injection of benzathine penicillin.
- In 1996, the diphtheria incidence decreased by almost 80% to 97 reported cases, from 418 cases reported in 1995; only 1 death from diphtheria occurred in 1996, as opposed to 23 in 1995.

Problems remain, however, including insufficient coverage in preschool children and adults aged 30 to 45 years, pockets of low immunization coverage, and sometimes lax surveillance and control measures.

THE FUTURE FOR IMMUNIZATION IN EUROPE

At present, there is little evidence of significant movement to harmonize immunization policies, where schedules are concerned, within EU countries. Changing schedules is disruptive and costly and is unlikely to be undertaken simply for cosmetic purposes when there would be no perceived gain to the countries. However, there are clear advantages to industry of a single market, and some harmonization may therefore occur as a consequence of the introduction of new vaccines. The immunization schedule used in Denmark, for example, was very different from that used anywhere else. After a change from whole-cell to acellular pertussis vaccine in 1997, the Danish schedule has been modified and is now similar to the schedule used in Sweden. Schedules and vaccines used in the northern and western countries are likely to reflect higher public health importance placed in antimeningitis vaccines, whereas southern countries have higher priority for hepatitis B vaccine combinations. It is possible, therefore, that some approximation of policies will follow the availability of new vaccines, but differences are likely to persist, reflecting different disease priorities and systems of healthcare provision.

There are already marked differences among the vaccines purchased in EU countries, those purchased in central European countries, and those purchased in countries of the former Soviet Union. For the most part, these differences reflect varied economic situations and may well become more exaggerated with the increasing prices for new vaccines set by multinational suppliers. Novel funding initiatives, such as the revolving fund mechanisms developed by the Pan American Health Organization,[30] may be needed to permit continuity in the provision of existing vaccines and the introduction of new vaccines for a number of European countries.

Activities to eliminate polio are already bearing fruit, with most of Europe presently polio free. Although there is some support for a measles elimination strategy,[31] there will be many challenges in finding the necessary resources in those countries that are presently experiencing difficulties in purchasing routinely used vaccines.

Acknowledgments

The authors are grateful to Dr. A. Kraigher, Institute of Public Health, Ljubljana, Slovenia, for information on immunization in Slovenia.

REFERENCES

1. Expanded Programme on Immunisation—Immunization schedules in the WHO European region. Wkly Epidemiol Rec 70:221–227, 1995.
2. Guerin N, Roure C. Immunisation schedules in the countries of the European Union. Eurosurveillance 0:5–7, 1995.
3. Guerin N, Roure C. Immunisation coverage in the European Union. Eurosurveillance 2(1):2–4, 1997.
4. Osborne K, Weinberg J, Miller E. The European Sero-Epidemiology Network. Euro Surveillance European Communicable Disease Bulletin 2(4):29–31, 1997.
5. Targets for Health for All. World Health Organization Regional Office for Europe. Copenhagen, 1985, pp 36–37.
6. Expanded Programme on Immunisation: Contraindications for vaccines used in EPI. Wkly Epidemiol Rec 37:279–281, 1988.
7. Salisbury DM, Begg NT (eds). Immunisation Against Infectious Disease. London, Her Majesty's Stationery Office, 1996.
8. Recommendations of the Advisory Committee on Immunization Practices (ACIP). Update: Vaccine side effects, adverse reactions, contraindications, and precautions. MMWR Morb Mortal Wkly Rep 45(RR-12):1–35, 1996.
9. Dittmann S, Roure C. Plan of Action for the Prevention and Control of Diphtheria in the European Region (1994–1995). Copenhagen, World Health Organization Regional Office for Europe, 1994, ICP/EPI 038(A).
10. WHO/UNICEF Strategy for Diphtheria Control in the Newly Independent States. Copenhagen, World Health Organization Regional Office for Europe, 1995.
11. Galazka AM, Robertson SE. Diphtheria: Changing patterns in the developing world and the industrialized world. Eur J Epidemiol 11:107–117, 1995.
12. Hardy IRB, Dittmann S, Sutter RW. Current situation and control strategies for resurgence of diphtheria in newly independent states of the former Soviet Union. Lancet 347:1739–1744, 1996.
13. Dittmann S. Epidemic diphtheria in the new independent states of the former USSR—situation and lessons learned. Biologicals 25:179–186, 1997.
14. Expanded Programme on Immunisation (EPI) Update: Diphtheria epidemic in the newly independent states of the former USSR, January 1995–March 1996. Wkly Epidemiol Rec 71:245–250, 1996.
15. Bass AG. Diphtheria control in Republic of Moldova. BASICS Assignment Report to World Health Organization Regional Office, Copenhagen, 1997.
16. Efstratiou A, George RC. Microbiology and epidemiology of diphtheria. Rev Med Microbiol 7:31–42, 1996.

17. Popovic T, Kombarova SY, Reeves MW, et al. Molecular epidemiology of diphtheria in Russia, 1985–1994. J Infect Dis 174:1064–1072, 1996.
18. Report of the 12th meeting of the European Advisory Group on the Expanded Programme on Immunization, Copenhagen, 1996. Copenhagen, World Health Organization Regional Office for Europe, 1997.
19. Hardy I, Kozlova I, Tchoudnaia L. Immunogenicity of Td vaccine in Ukrainian adults [abstract G25]. Abstracts of 35th Interscience Conference on Antimicrobial Agents and Chemotherapy. Washington, DC, American Society for Microbiology, 1995.
20. The Peckham Report: National Immunisation Study: Factors Influencing Immunisation Uptake in Childhood. Horsham, Sussex, UK, Action Research for the Crippled Child, 1989.
21. Vaccination and Immunisation: Summary Information for 1996–97, London, Department of Health Statistics Division, 1998.
22. White JM, Gillam SJ, Begg NT, Farrington CP. Vaccine coverage: Recent trends and future prospects. BMJ 304:682–684, 1992.
23. The Uptake of Pre-school Immunisation in England. Report on a National Study of Variation in Immunisation Uptake Between District Health Authorities. London, British Market Research Bureau, 1989.
24. White JM, Hobday S, Begg NT. 'COVER' (Cover of vaccination evaluated rapidly): 19. Commun Dis Rep CDR Rev 1(12):R140, 1991.
25. Gray R, Diba R. Childhood Immunisation Wave 12: A Report of the Tracking Survey, October 1991—March 1997. Publ. No. BMRB/BG/BW/1152-915. London, British Market Research Bureau International Limited, SRU Division, 1997.
26. Garcia-Barbero M, Goicoechea J. Health Care Delivery Profiles and Innovations in Selected European Countries. Copenhagen, World Health Organization Regional Office for Europe, 1996, pp 42–67.
27. Garcia-Barbero M, Goicoechea J. Health Care Delivery Profiles and Innovations in Selected European Countries. Copenhagen, World Health Organization Regional Office for Europe, 1996, pp 73–83.
28. European Health for All. Series 4, 1991. Copenhagen, World Health Organization Regional Office for Europe, 1991.
29. Health Care Systems in Transition: Republic of Moldova. Copenhagen, World Health Organization Regional Office for Europe, 1996.
30. EPI in the Americas. Benefits from Revolving Fund. WHO Chronicle 37(3):81–85, 1983.
31. Eliminating measles in Europe by 2007. Commun Dis Rep CDR Rev 7(48):425, 428, 1997.

chapter

44 Vaccination Programs in Developing Countries

Felicity T. Cutts

Jean-Marc Olivé

Since the late 1970s, a revolution has taken place in the delivery of vaccination to children around the world.[1] Globally, 80% of children are estimated to receive the primary childhood vaccination series of bacille Calmette-Guérin (BCG), oral poliovirus vaccine (OPV), diphtheria-tetanus-pertussis (DTP), and measles vaccines. More than 3 million deaths from measles, pertussis, and neonatal tetanus are estimated to be averted each year by vaccination[2] (Fig. 44–1). At current levels of coverage, diseases preventable by these vaccines are estimated to cause 10% of the global disease burden in terms of disability-adjusted life–years among children younger than 5 years (ranging from 15% in sub-Saharan Africa to less than 1% in established market economies).[2] Had immunization coverage levels remained at the low levels of the 1970s, these diseases would have caused 23% of disease burden in this age group.[2] In addition, with the certification of poliomyelitis eradication declared in 1994 in the Americas and the progress toward this in other regions, the goal to eradicate wild poliovirus from the world is well on its way. This achievement has renewed interest from countries and partner agencies in supporting immunization programs.[3]

Despite these successes, the recent resurgence of diphtheria in the former Soviet Union,[4–7] increasing spread of yellow fever in Africa,[8, 9] and continuing high morbidity and mortality from hepatitis B, measles, pertussis, and neonatal tetanus in the poorest countries of Africa and Southeast Asia[10, 11] emphasize the need for continued vigilance and support for vaccination programs. At the same time, an increasing range of vaccines against major infectious diseases is becoming available, but new vaccines are currently unaffordable in the poorest countries.

Vaccination programs in member states of the United Nations are coordinated internationally by the global

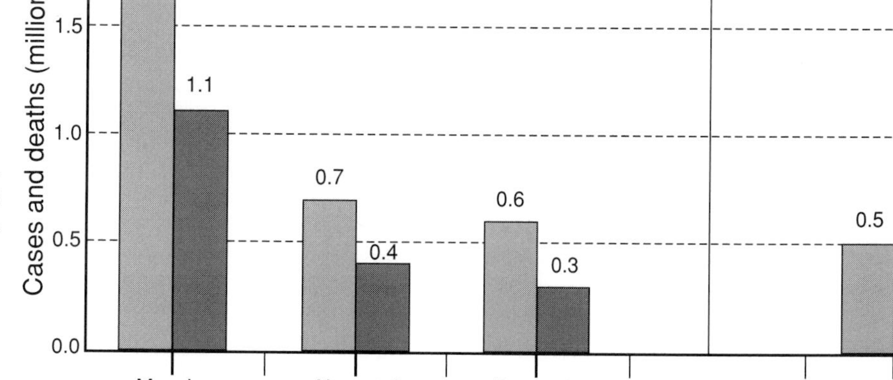

Figure 44–1. Cases and deaths occurring and prevented for selected diseases, developing countries, 1995.

Expanded Programme on Immunization (EPI), which was established in 1974.[1] The vaccines recommended by EPI for inclusion in routine childhood immunization schedules are BCG, OPV, DTP, hepatitis B, and measles vaccines; yellow fever vaccine is recommended in countries endemic for this disease. In certain developing countries, vaccines against diseases of local importance, such as Japanese encephalitis vaccine, are included in the national vaccination program,[12] whereas others such as rabies are used in special circumstances.

In this chapter, we first review policies and strategies relating to the vaccines included in the EPI. We discuss methods used to monitor and evaluate vaccination programs. We then summarize achievements, lessons learned, and techniques developed by and for the EPI. We discuss future trends in immunization services, and conclude with a summary of the major challenges to be faced, in light of the changing political, socioeconomic, and health services context of vaccination programs around the world.

POLICIES AND STRATEGIES FOR VACCINES INCLUDED IN THE EPI

Immunization programs in developing countries have traditionally been organized under a centralized system, predominantly through the public sector. Thus, Ministries of Health were responsible both for setting policies and norms and for managing programs. Donor support was given through the Ministries of Health that controlled the budget for immunization. Ministries of Health personnel, often with technical assistance from donors, trained and supervised peripheral health workers at district and health center levels.

This structure is, however, changing in many countries, and there is great diversity between countries and regions. Under health sector reforms promoted by international agencies, there is an increasing trend toward decentralization of implementation of health services and a burgeoning private sector. Countries vary in the degree to which health services have been decentralized. Where the process is most advanced, health services are under local government control, budgets are managed at district level, and the role of the Ministries of Health focuses on policymaking and advice. Donors may supply funds to, and work directly with, health managers at district level. There is also an increasing trend toward involvement of private organizations in health services delivery, including national and international not-for-profit agencies as well as private for-profit practitioners. A review of immunization in urban areas conducted in 1993 found that the private sector was providing as much as 40% of all immunizations in Lagos State, Nigeria; 25% in Teheran, Iran; and 30 to 45% in India.[13] This increases the need for effective coordination of the different service providers and for the dissemination of clear and practical policies.

Different groups of decision-makers are involved in ensuring that vaccines contribute effectively and efficiently to the disease control efforts of a country.[12] Decisions must be made about the goals of the vaccination program. Technical guidelines must be established regarding vaccine use, including selection of the optimal schedule and recommendations regarding contraindications to vaccines. Appropriate technology must be developed for vaccine storage (the "cold chain"), and appropriate strategies must be selected for delivery of vaccines.

Define Aims/Goals

Before 1974, vaccination programs in most developing countries were restricted to the urban elite (often the colonial power) and were modeled on programs in industrialized countries. Thus, vaccination services mainly targeted children of school age, despite the fact that the diseases occurred in younger children.[1]

The EPI was established in 1974, with the aims of making immunization available to every child in the world by 1990.[14] In the first 15 years of the program, efforts concentrated on establishing the physical and human resource infrastructure to deliver vaccination and monitoring vaccine coverage. In the last decade, the emphasis has shifted from a program with the goal of raising coverage to one with the aim of controlling disease.

With disease burden as the outcome, the choices of goals are eradication, elimination, or control.[15] Eradication refers to a situation in which the worldwide incidence of infection by a specific agent has been reduced to zero as a result of deliberate efforts and intervention measures are no longer needed.[16] The characteristics of an infection that make it theoretically eradicable are the absence of a nonhuman host, an easily recognizable illness with no subclinical or latent infection, low infectivity, and lifelong immunity after vaccination.[17] The only disease to have been eradicated globally by vaccination to date is smallpox. Elimination of disease or of infection means the reduction to zero of the incidence of a specified disease, or of infection caused by a specific agent, in a defined geographical area; continued intervention measures are required. Control, or containment, of a disease means the reduction of disease incidence, prevalence, morbidity, or mortality.

Current goals of the global EPI are that by the year 2000, at least 90% of children younger than 1 year will be immunized against diphtheria, pertussis, tetanus, measles, poliomyelitis, and tuberculosis; poliomyelitis will be eradicated; neonatal tetanus will be eliminated (incidence rate less than 1 case per 1000 live births in all districts); measles mortality and morbidity will be reduced respectively by 95% and 90% from the preimmunization era; and new hepatitis B virus carrier incidence (measured by the prevalence of hepatitis B surface antigen [HBsAg]) will be reduced by at least 80% (adapted from Ninth General Programme of Work, 1996–2001, World Health Organization, Geneva).

Selection of Vaccines and Schedules[18]

The World Health Organization (WHO) has encouraged countries to select vaccination schedules that are epidemiologically relevant, immunologically effective, operationally feasible, and socially acceptable.[1] Priority has been given to delivering the primary childhood immunization series and protecting adult women and their newborns against tetanus.

Routine Immunization of Infants. Recommendations for the age at which vaccines are administered are influenced by several factors[18]:

- age-specific risks of disease
- age-specific immunological response to vaccines
- potential interference with the immune response by passively transferred maternal antibody
- age-specific risks of vaccine-associated complications
- programmatic feasibility

The aim is to administer vaccines before the age at which children are at risk of disease. Vaccines are therefore generally given to children in the youngest age group that develops an adequate immune response to vaccination with minimal adverse effects from the vaccine. In addition to the need to protect infants before they encounter the wild disease-causing agents, administering vaccines early in life makes it easier to achieve high immunization coverage. To reduce the number of contacts required to complete the immunization series, as many antigens as possible are given at a single visit. All the EPI antigens are safe and effective when they are administered simultaneously.[18] The EPI does not, however, recommend mixing different vaccines in one syringe before injection or using a fluid vaccine for reconstitution of a freeze-dried vaccine. Such practices may lead to lower potency of both vaccines. If vaccines are not given on the same day, the main potential problem is interference between two live vaccines, which should then be spaced at least 4 weeks apart. Table 44–1 shows the immunization schedule recommended by the EPI for developing countries. The basis for the selection of this schedule has been reviewed in detail in a series of modules from WHO.[19]

Immunization of Women of Childbearing Age. The optimal program to protect newborns against neonatal tetanus by vaccination depends on the history of

Table 44–1. **THE IMMUNIZATION SCHEDULE FOR INFANTS RECOMMENDED BY THE WORLD HEALTH ORGANIZATION EXPANDED PROGRAMME ON IMMUNIZATION**

		HEPATITIS B VACCINE*	
AGE	VACCINES	Scheme A	Scheme B
Birth	BCG, OPV 0	HB 1	
6 wk	DTP 1, OPV 1	HB 2	HB 1
10 wk	DTP 2, OPV 2		HB 2
14 wk	DTP 3, OPV 3	HB 3	HB 3
9 mo	Measles, yellow fever†		

*In countries with carriage rates of HBsAg of ≥2%; scheme A is recommended in countries where perinatal transmission of hepatitis B virus is important (e.g., Asia), and scheme B in countries where perinatal transmission is less important (e.g., sub-Saharan Africa).

†In countries where yellow fever poses a risk.

BCG, bacille Calmette-Guérin; OPV, oral poliovirus vaccine; DTP, diphtheria-tetanus-pertussis; HB, hepatitis B.

Table 44–2. **TETANUS TOXOID (TT) IMMUNIZATION SCHEDULE FOR WOMEN OF CHILDBEARING AGE**

DOSE	WHEN TO GIVE	EXPECTED DURATION OF PROTECTION
TT 1	At first contact or as early as possible in pregnancy	None guaranteed
TT 2	At least 4 wk after TT 1	1–3 yr
TT 3	At least 6 mo after TT 2	5 yr
TT 4	At least 1 yr after TT 3 or during subsequent pregnancy	10 yr
TT 5	At least 1 yr after TT 4 or during subsequent pregnancy	All childbearing years

the use of vaccines containing tetanus toxoid (TT) in immunization programs. When most women of childbearing age have not previously been immunized with TT in their infancy or adolescence, implementation of a five-dose TT program for women of childbearing age is recommended (Table 44–2). Each country should define the age group to be included in the "childbearing age" category (e.g., 15 to 44 years, 15 to 35 years) according to local fertility patterns and the available resources. In practice, this scheme will also be used in areas where there is little or no documentation of past immunization with tetanus-containing vaccines, even if some women are likely to have received some doses in childhood.

In future, increasing numbers of women of childbearing age will have documentation of prior receipt of tetanus toxoid–containing vaccines in early childhood or school age. Other schemes of vaccination can then be considered, with progressively fewer doses of TT for adult women (see Chapter 18).

Booster Doses. The first priority of immunization programs is to ensure that infants are completely immunized against target diseases at the youngest age possible. Where resources are limited, the EPI suggests that booster doses should not be considered until coverage levels for fully immunized infants are above 80%.[18] Today, many developing countries have achieved such coverage levels and administer booster doses of various vaccines.

The number and frequency of booster doses depend on the epidemiological patterns of diseases in a particular country, the level of health services infrastructure, the level of resources available, and the relative priority of boosters compared, for example, with introduction of new vaccines into the primary vaccination schedule. The importance attached to booster doses has increased in recent years because of the resurgence of diphtheria in much of Europe[4–7, 20] and some developing countries[7, 21–23] and the recognition of the importance of adult pertussis as a contributor to community spread.[24–26]

Current WHO recommendations are that a booster dose of DTP should be given approximately 1 year after the primary series (at the middle or the end of the second year of life) in countries with successful routine immunization programs to maintain immunity against pertussis and diphtheria and contribute to the long-term strategy for neonatal tetanus control. Where disease is documented in schoolchildren, an additional preschool booster dose is appropriate. When the pattern shifts to mostly adult cases, a school-leaving booster of Td may be appropriate.

For BCG, there is much controversy over the effectiveness of repeated doses of the vaccine. There is no evidence that the degree of protection from BCG is related to scar formation or to tuberculin conversion.[27] On the other hand, there is evidence from some BCG trials that the protection afforded by BCG decreases with time after vaccination. Although some authors believe that repeating BCG vaccination increases its efficacy,[28, 29] a trial in Malawi showed no protective effect from either one or two doses of BCG.[30] For this reason, WHO does not recommend repeated BCG vaccination, but only administration of the vaccine at birth or in the first year of life.[31]

For measles, although high coverage with a single dose can achieve the mortality reduction targets,[32] more than one dose of vaccine is required for eradication. The second dose is not a true booster dose.[33] It is administered to protect children who failed to respond to the first dose and to provide another opportunity to reach children who did not receive a first dose of vaccine. In most developing countries, administration of additional doses is considered to be more effectively done through campaigns[34] than through a routine two-dose schedule.

The Cold Chain

The cold chain is a system necessary to ensure that vaccines are stored and transported at appropriate temperatures. In tropical countries with frequent logistics problems, a lack of refrigeration equipment and reliable power or fuel supply may raise the possibility of breaches in this system. Although the stability of EPI-recommended vaccines varies depending on the antigen, the required storage temperature at health facilities of 0 to 8°C has been determined by the thermolability of OPV and the sensitivity to freezing of DTP, diphtheria-tetanus (DT), and TT vaccines. The live virus vaccines against poliomyelitis, measles, and yellow fever can be stored long term at −20°C.[35, 36]

As soon as the WHO EPI was established, the program began to set operational standards and determine the characteristics of equipment needed for vaccine transport and storage at all the levels of the cold chain. The EPI team worked together with manufacturers to produce low-cost equipment for storing and transporting EPI vaccines.[37] Special refrigerators and freezers were developed to facilitate the storage of vaccine in areas where power supplies were intermittent.[38] Other equipment was tested and adapted, including kerosene, gas, and solar power refrigerators to cover areas where electricity was not available.[39, 40] Time and temperature vaccine monitor cards were developed to monitor vaccine potency along the cold chain.[41] The cold chain and associated logistics are major areas where appropriate technology developed for the EPI has benefited other areas of primary healthcare.

In the mid-1990s, success in the implementation of the cold chain has greatly reduced the chance of loss of potency of vaccines when they are used in the field. A different problem has, however, been recognized. It is estimated that half of the supplied vaccine is wasted.[42] Reasons for wastage may include discarding a multidose vial after use for one child; cold chain problems that lead to destruction of vaccine that has been exposed to excessive heat (especially OPV and measles vaccine) or freezing of toxoid vaccines; and poor stock control such that vaccine stocks accumulate and pass their expiration date. With the increasing cost of existing vaccines and the new ones soon to be introduced, it is important to reduce this wastage. To help in this process, new rules for handling vaccines have been introduced and chemical time-temperature indicators developed for OPV. These indicators enable the vaccines to be used with confidence up to their expiry date in the most difficult situations.[43, 44]

Select Strategies

Once the goals of vaccination programs have been decided, appropriate strategies must be designed to achieve them. The target population for the vaccine must be defined. Coverage targets must be set, according to the efficacy of the vaccine and the level of immunity needed in the population to achieve the stated aim of the program. For eradication or elimination, high coverage is required at an early age. For example, to eliminate measles, which is highly infectious, at least 90% of the population must be immune.[45] Assuming a vaccine efficacy of 95%, a minimum coverage of 95% is needed to achieve this.

Immunization programs require good management: vaccination must be accessible and available with minimal administrative barriers.[46–49] There must be reliable systems for the cold chain, logistics, and transport that include maintenance of equipment and a regular supply of fuel and vaccines. Health workers need to be trained and supervised in vaccination techniques, cold chain maintenance, logistics, the use of health information, and health education. Mothers need to be informed about the availability of vaccination and be motivated to bring their children.[14, 50, 51] Wherever vaccinations are offered, it is vital to use all opportunities to administer vaccines.[49, 52] For this, the immunization status of all children in the target age group should be screened routinely and immunization provided to eligible children and mothers. Health workers should be taught which are true and which are false contraindications, and supervisors should monitor compliance with recommendations, for example, using the EPI training module on missed opportunities.[53]

Delivery sites for vaccination range from fixed sites to mobile teams. Fixed sites are health facilities such as health centers and health posts that offer a range of primary healthcare activities or curative services. They may offer vaccination either daily or on specific days per week or per month, depending on patient load. The utilization of fixed sites is higher when good-quality curative care and an adequate supply of essential drugs are also available.[54, 55] To secure proper utilization of those fixed sites, the Bamako Initiative, combining provision of preventive care including immunizations with that of essential drugs, improvement of quality of basic curative care, and creation of local health committees to manage health center funds, was launched in many low-income countries. Countries such as Guinea and Benin reported that this initiative helped to raise and sustain coverage.[56]

In areas progressively further from a health facility, regular outreach services from the nearest health facility or district center or mobile teams (which involve stay of at least one night in a distant village) are used. Outreach and mobile services may be scheduled throughout the year, but in countries with poor communications and transport infrastructure, frequent postponement or cancellation of planned visits commonly leads to disruption and public loss of confidence in the program.[51] A "pulse immunization" strategy may be more appropriate in these situations[57–59] in which children are immunized in annual campaigns or "pulses" of vaccine. Each health institution is encouraged to assume responsibility for vaccination of all children in a specified geographical area. Voluntary institutions work jointly with the local government health service agency, pooling staff, vehicles, and other resources. Planning is carried out at district level; pulse campaigns are locally organized and conducted by primary healthcare staff, village health workers, and community volunteers. Where possible, the pulses are timed for the months preceding the seasonal peaks of diseases such as measles[59, 60] and whooping cough. Advantages for the health workers are easier management of vaccines, fuel, and equipment in a relatively concentrated period of activity each year and increased contact with the community. This strategy was used successfully in rural areas of Mozambique in the 1980s to provide immunization and maternal-child health services to villages, when direct and indirect effects of conflict precluded the year-round provision of services.[58]

Geographical proximity to a site providing vaccination is not in itself sufficient to ensure utilization of the service.[61, 62] Coverage in poor urban communities is often lower than in many rural areas.[63–67] Door-to-door canvassing[68] or channeling[69] has therefore been used to increase uptake among hard-to-reach groups that have geographical access to vaccination sites. In Mozambique, however, door-to-door canvassing accounted for more than 40% of human resource costs,[68] and in Khartoum, the sustainability of a system of follow-up birth registration and defaulter follow-up by midwives[70] was also questionable. It may be best reserved for tracking high-risk groups who are identified through operational research at the local level.

In addition to these strategies, which are part of regular immunization services and are predominantly under the control of local health authorities, periodic mass immunization campaigns at a national level are an increasing part of immunization programs. The experience with mass campaigns has been mixed.[71] In the region of the Americas, they have long been a major component of disease eradication programs and are implemented with a high degree of effectiveness and predominantly local funding.[34, 72] In low-income countries, early experience with campaigns that were conducted with the sole purpose of raising immunization coverage rapidly as part of the drive for universal child immunization was generally poor.[73–76] Such campaigns were seen as being imposed on countries or districts by donors, interrupting other health services and increasing donor dependency.[73, 77–80] Because there was rarely guaranteed donor support or coherent plans for follow-up after the campaigns, their effect on increasing coverage was short-lived in countries such as Guinea,[81] Ghana,[82] and Senegal.[83] In some instances, the quality of vaccination during campaigns was also low.[84, 85]

The mass campaign approach was also used with varying degrees of success to inform and motivate communities and families. In the drive for universal childhood immunization by 1990, "social mobilization" was promoted, predominantly with United Nations International Children's Emergency Fund (UNICEF) support. It was recognized that in many countries, the traditional health education delivered through the health sector would not reach large parts of the population who lacked access to health services for geographical, economic, or cultural reasons.[86] Social mobilization aimed to use individuals and organizations ranging from political, traditional, and religious leaders to governmental institutions, trade unions, teachers, revolutionary organizations,[87] or the military to deliver specific messages about immunization.[88–91] This was often done with a large amount of publicity and political attention. Like the campaigns conducted with the aim of improving coverage quickly, however, these large-scale media campaigns often failed to lead to sustained benefits in low-income countries.[73]

In the 1990s, campaigns are used much less with the sole aim of increasing coverage but more as a strategy to improve disease control or eradication (see later). Thus, current campaigns target all children, in an age group determined by disease epidemiology, irrespective of previous vaccination status, and usually do not attempt to update a child's vaccination status for the primary vaccination series. They are usually not conducted as an isolated event but are part of a medium-term plan of action to achieve the disease control or elimination goal.[92] The plans of action encompass all the necessary areas of activities including raising routine immunization coverage, development of surveillance, and strengthening of laboratory facilities. Targeted mass campaigns are also proposed in high-risk areas; for example, mass measles immunization campaigns may assist in controlling measles in the difficult environment of poor urban areas.[93]

No single strategy is likely to be appropriate for all circumstances and all diseases. The choice of strategy should depend on the epidemiology of the disease, the characteristics of the vaccine, the facilities available, the accessibility of the population and their cultural attitudes and practices, and the socioeconomic level of the country.[12, 50] The desire to extend coverage of immunization services rapidly and maintain international support for EPI needs to be balanced with the promotion of other health services.[76] The success of any approach to health service delivery depends on the context into which it is introduced. A vertical program added to a strong primary healthcare base can both reinforce it and benefit from it,[72] whereas in a weak system, it may disrupt priorities, undermine sustainability and local capacity, and fail to achieve even its own objectives.[73, 94] There is a need for continued capacity building for national and district-level managers to select strategies that are appropriate for their own context.[95–97]

Disease Elimination/Eradication Initiatives

As the efforts directed at the development of an infrastructure for immunization started to show impact on disease incidence, programs began to shift from an emphasis on raising coverage to one of controlling diseases.[98] In 1985, progress in controlling poliomyelitis in the Americas led that region, in which only 11 countries had endemic poliomyelitis, to adopt the goal of eradication of poliomyelitis from the Western Hemisphere by the year 1990.[99] Three years later, the 41st World Health Assembly ratified the goal of global eradication by the year 2000.[100] The last case of poliomyelitis due to wild virus in the Americas occurred on August 23, 1991, in Peru[34] (see also Chapter 16).

The achievement of poliomyelitis eradication requires special immunization strategies in addition to reaching and maintaining the highest possible routine immunization coverage of infants with OPV. National immunization days are recommended, in which all children in the target age, usually younger than 5 years, receive OPV during a short period with the aim of displacing the wild virus from communities by the mass circulation of the vaccine virus. Once transmission is reduced only to focal areas, "mopping up" operations consisting of door-to-door vaccination are conducted in areas at risk. The backbone of these strategies is high-quality surveillance, with investigation of every case of acute flaccid paralysis and collection of stool specimens for viral isolation.[101]

Several conditions must be met for these strategies to be implemented effectively. Political commitment is needed at global and national levels to advocate for and mobilize resources. Requirements of funds, personnel, equipment, and vaccines must be estimated realistically and with sufficient lead time for logistics and financial systems to be put in place. Interagency coordination is essential to ensure that resources are used efficiently. Laboratory support for surveillance must be made available. Personnel (including volunteers) must be trained appropriately and excellent communications established.

As of April 1997, substantial progress has been made toward the global goal.[3] Reported immunization coverage for three doses of OPV globally was 81% (1995, 83%). Reported coverage was above 80% in all regions except Africa, where OPV3 coverage increased from 32% in 1988 to 58% in 1995 and 60% in 1996. By the end of 1996, all poliomyelitis endemic countries in Asia and Europe had conducted national immunization days, and only 17 endemic countries in the world had not yet conducted national immunization days (15 of these were in Africa). National immunization days were increasingly coordinated between countries and WHO regions, to ensure that migrant populations in border areas were reached. Acute flaccid paralysis surveillance is now conducted in 126 (86%) of the 146 recently or currently endemic countries. However, such surveillance is still in its infancy in the South-East Asia and African Regions and requires substantial strengthening.[102] A total of 3997 cases of poliomyelitis were reported globally in 1996, with declines in all Regions. Activities will increasingly concentrate on countries affected by civil conflict and those with the weakest health service infrastructure.[3]

With use of the experience gained in the Western Hemisphere in designing an appropriate strategy for poliomyelitis eradication, measles was the next to be tackled[92] (see Chapter 12). The region of the Americas has adopted a measles elimination goal, and a goal of global eradication is under consideration.[103] In the measles elimination strategy, initial mass campaigns, targeting the age group in which most susceptibles have accumulated, are used to interrupt measles transmission. To prevent resurgence of measles transmission, programs must sustain high routine vaccination coverage of infants and conduct periodic supplemental campaigns when susceptibles (unvaccinated people and vaccine failures) accumulate. Surveillance of suspected measles cases with laboratory confirmation of cases is another key element of the strategy.[92] Similar initial mass campaign strategies have been implemented in industrialized countries with the aim of preventing predicted measles epidemics.[104–106] The impact of such strategies on interruption of measles has been impressive.[105, 107–109]

Another disease, neonatal tetanus, has been targeted for elimination[110] (see Chapter 18). In this case, the goal was defined as a reduction in the incidence of neonatal tetanus to less than 1 per 1000 live births in all districts of the world. The recommended strategies include routine immunization of pregnant women with TT, immunization of all women of childbearing age in high-risk areas, improvement of clean delivery and hygienic cord care practices, and effective neonatal tetanus surveillance. As of 1996, 102 countries of the world had claimed neonatal tetanus elimination. However, more than 370,000 cases are still estimated to occur each year, although only a small fraction are reported.

MONITORING AND EVALUATION OF IMMUNIZATION PROGRAMS

The definition of goals, strategies, and performance standards is likely to be ineffective unless systems to monitor compliance with performance standards and disease incidence are established and problem-oriented research is conducted.[51, 111, 112] Surveillance of vaccine-preventable diseases is a key component of disease control and elimination strategies, and reduced disease incidence and mortality are the ultimate indicators of program success.[111] It is also essential to monitor indicators of program performance to detect potential problems with the quality, uptake, and appropriateness of vaccination services quickly and identify appropriate so-

Table 44–3. **SELECTED INDICATORS TO MONITOR PROGRAM PERFORMANCE**

INDICATOR	DEFINITION
Fully vaccinated child	Proportion of children aged 12–23 mo who have received 1 dose of BCG 3 valid doses of DTP (minimum age 1st dose, 6 wk; minimum interval, 4 wk) 4 valid doses of OPV (as DTP + dose at birth) 3 valid doses of hepatitis B vaccine (HBV, if in schedule) 1 valid dose of measles vaccine (aged at least 9 mo) 1 valid dose of yellow fever vaccine (aged at least 6 mo if in schedule)
Access to services	Up-to-date (BCG + OPV0 and DTP1/OPV1) by age 2 mo
Tracking activities	Difference in percentage receiving DTP1/OPV1 and measles vaccines (indicator of dropout) Median age at receiving DTP1/OPV1, DTP3/OPV3, and measles
Missed opportunities	Percentage of children not receiving all vaccines for which they are eligible
Cold chain quality	Percentage of facilities storing vaccine at recommended temperatures Vaccine efficacy in expected range for each vaccine evaluated
Provider knowledge and practices	Proportion of providers who know and follow recommended guidelines, including those on simultaneous administration, contraindications, and safe injection procedures

BCG, bacille Calmette-Guérin; DTP, diphtheria-tetanus-pertussis; OPV, oral poliovirus vaccine; HBV, hepatitis B vaccine.

lutions[14, 47] (Table 44–3). These indicators provide information on outputs in the form of coverage of different vaccines and program quality, including dropout between vaccine doses (a measure of the degree of success of tracking and health education activities), missed immunization opportunities, cold chain maintenance, and provider information and education.

In this section, we review methods to monitor program performance. We briefly review additional operational research methods to determine reasons for incomplete vaccination. We then discuss the role of surveillance in the control of vaccine-preventable diseases. Finally, we review the role of economic analysis and mathematical modeling in program monitoring and planning.

Assessment of Vaccine Coverage

By monitoring coverage of different vaccines, insight can be gained not only into the overall program success in providing all vaccines to the target population (percentage of fully vaccinated children) but also into the areas of program failure. For example, high coverage of BCG/OPV0 may reflect a high coverage of hospital deliveries. High coverage of DTP1/OPV1 indicates high access to primary healthcare facilities. If DTP1/OPV1 coverage is high by age 2 months but coverage for the respective third doses is low, this high dropout needs further investigation to determine the cause (e.g., missed immunization opportunities, adverse events, poor patient education, poor tracking activities). As overall coverage of 12- to 23-month-old children increases, it becomes more important to monitor timeliness of vaccination to ensure that vaccines are received as close as possible to the recommended age.

Vaccine coverage is monitored through routine reports (the "administrative method") or community-based surveys.

The Administrative Method. Clinics participating report the numbers of each dose (e.g., OPV1, DTP3) administered to the target age group of 0 to 11 months, regularly (e.g., monthly) during the course of each year. The number of each of the doses administered is summed and divided by the population denominator of 0- to 11-month-olds. This method is easiest to perform in countries where the government health services deliver almost all immunizations, so that reports from government clinics reflect virtually all the doses administered. It is often more difficult to obtain cooperation from nongovernment clinics in submitting regular reports to the government health authorities, and where substantial numbers of doses are given in the private sector, falsely low coverage estimates may result. The accuracy of coverage estimates also depends on the accuracy of reports of vaccinations administered to 0- to 11-month-olds and of the population estimates.

The administrative method has the potential advantage of providing continuous information at the local level and being relatively inexpensive. Estimates of coverage can be compared between districts,[113, 114] ideally with a simultaneous comparison of program inputs, health service infrastructure, and socioeconomic characteristics in each district to assess the extent to which low coverage is related to inadequate resources, population characteristics, or poor health system performance.

The routine monitoring of TT coverage in pregnant women tends to underestimate achievements, because previous doses of TT are not taken into account, and pregnant women who have already received a full protective course are included as unvaccinated. The WHO is now recommending recording and reporting protection at birth when a mother brings her child for DTP vaccination. However, this approach requires that mothers retain records of vaccination during pregnancy.

From routine reports, the doses administered to children can also be compared with total doses distributed to estimate wastage rates. "Acceptable" wastage is difficult to define, because the cost of wasted vaccine must be balanced against the cost of missing an opportunity if a child is turned away from a health facility. However, if wastage is high, the causes should be determined (e.g., poor forecasting of vaccine demand so that vaccine expires before use, cold chain problems at different levels of the health system, or ongoing wastage at the health center level because multidose vials are discarded after use for one or two clients). Appropriate action can then be taken while trying to minimize the risk of missed opportunities.

Community Surveys. Because up-to-date and complete information on population denominators is often unavailable in developing countries,[114] the WHO EPI developed a modified cluster sampling survey method for the evaluation of vaccine coverage.[115–117] The survey was designed to estimate vaccine coverage with a precision of plus or minus 10 percentage points, that is, to provide a rough estimate of coverage in areas with no alternative reliable sources of data. The method is learned easily by midlevel health workers. Their participation in community surveys is in itself a good way to motivate them and increase their awareness of the constraints on obtaining vaccination that families face.[51, 62] Computer simulations have shown that the deviations in sampling methodology from classical cluster sampling do not greatly bias the estimates obtained.[118–120] However, bias may arise in the field because of practical problems, one major difficulty being low retention rates of home-based records so that vaccination status may be misclassified.[121, 122]

Cluster sample surveys provide more detailed information on vaccination than do routine reports, because the dates of each vaccination given to each child can be checked and compared. Thus, doses administered before the recommended age, or with too short an interval, are identified and discounted as invalid; a high proportion of invalid doses shows the need for specific in-service training of health workers about the schedule. Missed immunization opportunities through the failure to administer vaccines simultaneously can be identified, for example, by comparing dates of DTP and OPV vaccinations. Coverage surveys can be extended to include indicators of other programs, especially if home-based records include dates of visits to health facilities for curative care or growth monitoring.[51, 123] In that way, other sources of missed opportunities can be assessed. These analyses are facilitated by the use of COSAS, the computer software package developed for the EPI.[124]

Questionnaires to parents can also include information on reasons for failure to vaccinate the child[125–127] (see later); on the occurrence of adverse events, such as abscesses after vaccination[128]; and on other mother-child-health indicators, such as knowledge of oral rehydration therapy[129] and use of family planning. However, each addition to the survey has implications for interviewer training and quality control and potentially for the sample size.[117] The utility of additional questions should be closely scrutinized to avoid compromising the achievement of the main objective of the study.

As high coverage levels are reached, the EPI cluster survey becomes less helpful because the precision of the estimate is too low to detect smaller and smaller increases in coverage. It is also expensive and impractical to conduct surveys in every district, so surveys are rarely used for local program guidance (although in India, more than 900 district-level surveys have been conducted, providing audit information to compare with routine reports).[73]

Reviews of coverage data available from different sources and at different levels (e.g., government, WHO, UNICEF) have shown major discrepancies in data. In part, this may reflect the pressures that districts and countries face to demonstrate attainment of targets.[73] For example, in Uganda, a national coverage survey in 1991 showed that the reported coverage data exceeded survey data by one third to one half for every antigen. In the Philippines, the 1993 Demographic and Health Survey found the percentage of fully immunized children at 12 months was 62%, with 72% immunized against measles. This compared with a reported figure of 88% for measles. In India, in 1989, more than 70% of the antigen coverage figures were found in the surveys to be more than 25 percentage points lower than the values reported in the routine government figures.[73]

If coverage data are to guide program performance, it is important for every program to audit carefully the coverage estimates that are obtained. Programs must aim for complete and accurate routine reporting of vaccinations administered and better data on target populations, and the use of disease surveillance must be increased to guide the program.

Quality Assessment

Indicators of program quality can be assessed using relatively inexpensive studies based at health facilities.[61, 84, 130] Studies combine exit interviews with mothers, interviews with providers, and observation using checklists to evaluate timeliness of vaccination, dropout rates, and missed opportunities among children and mothers who attend vaccination sites and to assess provider knowledge and practices. Reasons for failure to immunize eligible children and causes of poor-quality services[130] can be identified quickly and inexpensively. Such studies can be combined with small surveys of households in the vicinity of the health facility to investigate reasons for failure to use accessible vaccination services.[61, 62]

Missed opportunities are easily monitored using health facility studies that can be included in routine supervisory visits.[53] A review of 79 missed opportunity studies from 45 countries found that a median of 32% of children and women of childbearing age who were surveyed (67% of those who were eligible for vaccines) had missed opportunities for immunization during visits to health facilities.[52] Among the children observed at health facilities, eliminating missed opportunities would have increased coverage by a median of 44%. The studies identified the following most important reasons for missed opportunities: (1) the failure to administer simultaneously all vaccines for which a child was eligible; (2) false contraindications to immunization; (3) health worker practices, including not opening a multidose vial for a small number of people to avoid vaccine wastage; and (4) logistical problems such as vaccine shortage, poor clinic organization, and inefficient clinic scheduling.[52]

Maintenance of the cold chain should be monitored through ongoing supervision and occasional surveys. As a routine procedure, any equipment storing vaccine (cold rooms, freezers, and refrigerators) should have its temperature monitored twice daily. To facilitate the monitoring of the cold chain from the vaccine producer to the health center, ensuring that no breaks occur,

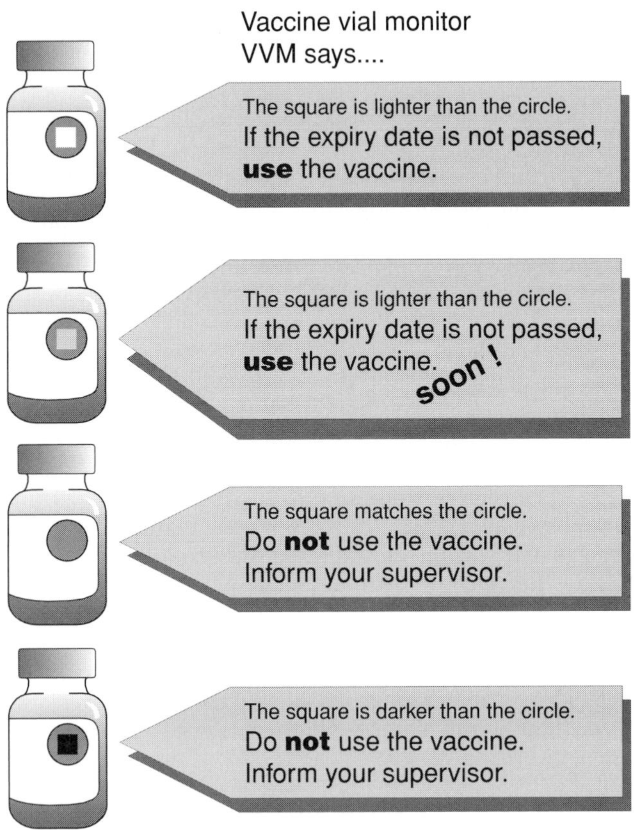

Figure 44–2. Vaccine vial monitor.

simple tools have been developed.[42] The cold chain monitor is one of the most successful ones, because it enables documentation of any problem that occurs during international transport. These indicators can also be used during transport of large quantities of vaccine within countries. For areas with very cold climates, where DTP, DT, and TT vaccines can be easily frozen, a "freeze watch" indicator has been developed. Vaccine vial monitors have recently been developed for OPV to enable vaccines to be used up to their expiry date[44] (Fig. 44–2).

To select units for study, the lot quality sampling technique has been found to be useful for assessing the quality and coverage of health services including vaccination.[131] It is designed to identify health centers or other health service units that are not meeting certain predefined standards of care. These standards may be immunization coverage among clinic attenders or standards of quality of care such as cold chain maintenance, safe injection techniques, use of all opportunities to vaccinate, and so on. The technique can also be used at the community level to identify variations between small areas in coverage of vaccination[132, 133] or other primary healthcare programs.[134, 135]

Vaccine Effectiveness

Vaccine effectiveness (VE) is the percentage reduction in disease incidence attributable to vaccination, calculated by means of the following equation:

$$\text{VE}\ (\%) = \frac{U - V}{U} \times 100$$

where U = the incidence in unvaccinated people and V = the incidence in vaccinated people.

Although vaccine effectiveness has traditionally been assessed with respect to prevention of the specific disease against which the vaccine is given, in the evaluation of vaccine effectiveness other outcome measures, such as all-causes mortality, may be preferable.[136] A vaccine may have unexpected beneficial effects; for example, measles vaccine has been reported to reduce mortality by a factor greater than that expected by the direct avoidance of measles illness.[137, 138] Conversely, there may be unanticipated adverse events. The unexpected finding of increased mortality among recipients of high-titer measles vaccines at 4 to 6 months of age was demonstrated in vaccine trials in West Africa only because mortality was one of the outcome measures in the trials.[139]

Methods to estimate vaccine effectiveness have been described in detail by Orenstein and colleagues.[140, 141] The most frequently used methods are the "screening method," outbreak investigations, and case-control studies. The simplest method to obtain an estimate of vaccine effectiveness is to use routine data on notifications of measles cases in vaccinated and unvaccinated children and to compare the proportion of cases vaccinated with the vaccine coverage among the same age group in the general population. If p is the proportion vaccinated in the population and c is the proportion of measles cases reported to be vaccinated, then

$$\text{VE} = (p - c)/p(1 - c) \times 100\%$$

Although this "screening test" seems a simple way to monitor vaccine effectiveness, estimates are susceptible to many sources of bias, because data are collected from many different, unsupervised, sources.[142]

Studies of vaccine effectiveness are commonly conducted during outbreaks, because the occurrence of an outbreak can both alert health authorities to a potential problem in the immunization program and provide large numbers of cases for investigation. In well-defined populations—for example, a village or a school—total population assessments may be conducted and attack rates calculated among the cohorts of individuals who were vaccinated and unvaccinated at the beginning of the outbreak.[143] Some authors recommend the determination of the secondary attack rate in families during outbreaks[144] to ensure uniform exposure of vaccinees and nonvaccinees.[145]

Case-control studies can be useful to facilitate field work when personal immunization records are not generally available but some other source such as records from one or more clinics can be obtained.[146] Case-control procedures have also been used within outbreak investigations to evaluate other risk factors, such as variation in vaccine effectiveness between vaccine providers.[147]

In practice, each approach has potential methodological problems that can lead to great difficulty in interpreting the estimates obtained in observational studies.[142] For example, an unpublished review of measles vaccine effectiveness studies in developing countries* found that the diagnosis of measles nearly always used clinical criteria only, leading to probable low specificity of diagnosis and an underestimate of effectiveness.[142, 148, 149] Vaccination status frequently relied on an undocumented maternal history.[150] Age at vaccination and age at disease onset were not always controlled for, and sample sizes were frequently small.

Despite potential methodological difficulties, in situations in which a high proportion of individuals have documented vaccination status and disease diagnosis is likely to be highly specific (e.g., because of laboratory confirmation or occurrence of a disease outbreak with epidemiological links between cases), assessment of vaccine effectiveness can highlight problems that may be of fundamental importance. For example, a case-control study of neonatal tetanus in Bangladesh showed that maternal receipt of two doses of tetanus toxoid vaccine had no protective effect (vaccine effectiveness adjusted for other risk factors: 24% [95% confidence interval, −29%, 55%]). Subsequent to the study, a reference laboratory reported no potency in three consecutive lots of tetanus vaccine from the production laboratory in Bangladesh.[151] The same study also showed the importance of missed immunization opportunities, because a history of neonatal tetanus in a previous child was a significant risk factor for neonatal tetanus in the most recent born child.

Operational Research to Identify Determinants of Nonvaccination or Incomplete Vaccination

In addition to monitoring the coverage and quality of vaccination programs, reasons for nonvaccination or incomplete vaccination should be investigated. Many of these will be identified during the studies and surveys described before or during supervision. Others may require special studies, particularly factors relating to community attitudes. To identify reasons for low immunization coverage, the following questions should be addressed[152]:

- Is the present vaccination system inadequate?
- Do the unvaccinated children and their families have special characteristics that can help identify them?
- Do parents lack accurate information?
- Do unfavorable attitudes among communities and families outweigh even a good vaccination system and good information?

As many data as possible are collected from secondary data sources (such as reports of previous program reviews, analysis of coverage data by health center) and by direct observation of vaccination practices and clinic organization during supervisory visits, discussions with experienced health workers, and community discussions.[153] Supplementary studies can then be conducted and designed to answer specific questions that remain. A number of methods are useful for studies of reasons for incomplete vaccination[154, 155]:

1. Qualitative methods to evaluate community and health professional knowledge and attitudes relating to vaccination.[154–156] These methods may be used alone,[156] as preliminary work to develop a quantitative data collection instrument,[157] or after quantitative surveys to study in depth the process through which risk factors operate and develop interventions.[158]
2. Interviews of mothers of incompletely vaccinated *or* of fully vaccinated children to describe their characteristics, but with no comparison group (case studies or case series).[159]
3. Quantitative studies of factors associated with incomplete vaccination, by comparing characteristics of "vaccinated" with "unvaccinated" groups—cross-sectional "knowledge, attitudes, and practice" surveys,[125, 128, 160] case-control studies,[161] or cohort studies.[162]
4. Intervention studies, in which communities are randomized to the intervention compared with a control group,[127] or in which a whole population receives the intervention and "before and after" comparisons of coverage are made.[58, 153, 163, 164]

Table 44–4 summarizes the factors that commonly affect vaccination uptake. In almost all studies, factors

Table 44–4. **CLASSIFICATION OF FACTORS AFFECTING RECEIPT OF VACCINES**

Immunization System	Family Characteristics
Distance	Education (maternal and paternal)
Security	Family size
Appropriateness of time	Income
Reliability (no cancellation of sessions)	Refugees
Availability of curative services	Recent migrants
Waiting time	Language
Use of all opportunities	Ethnic group
Health staff's motivation and attitude	**Parental Attitudes/Knowledge**
Cost and costing policies	Previous positive or negative experience at health services (e.g., turned away; postvaccination abscesses)
Coordination between different providers	Peer group pressure for or against vaccination
Quality of vaccination and other services	Family and social networks
Communications and Information	Perceived susceptibility to disease
Reception of information on "where and when" of vaccination	Perceived seriousness of disease
Person-to-person information from trusted health worker or community leader	Perceived safety of vaccine
Language compatibility between health workers and clients	Perceived efficacy of vaccine
Use of mass media according to levels of access and expertise	
Community involvement in planning and managing services and in social mobilization/channeling	
Action to dispel misconceptions	

*Flavia Bustreo. Reflections on the post-licensure assessment of measles vaccine efficacy in developing countries. Unpublished dissertation, MSc Communicable Disease Epidemiology, London School of Hygiene and Tropical Medicine, 1994.

relating to poor performance of the health system and inadequate information to parents about where and when vaccination is available have been identified as major determinants of undervaccination. Ease of access, in terms of distance to vaccination sites,[83, 125, 159] short waiting times,[125, 156] availability at the same site as curative services,[54, 55, 165] and cost,[81, 165] affects utilization. Missed immunization opportunities are important causes of low coverage, and asking mothers to return on another day for vaccination was associated with undervaccination in Mozambique[128] and Cameroon.[152] Lower socioeconomic status of families, particularly little parental education, is almost universally associated with lower vaccination uptake among children.[125, 128, 152, 160, 162, 165–168] Although it is difficult to change socioeconomic status in the short term, factors such as low educational level, recent migration,[128, 152] and large family size[161, 165, 169, 170] can be used to identify families that need extra support for their children to be fully immunized.

On the demand side, attitudes at community and individual levels should be assessed. The involvement of communities and local leaders in promoting immunization, planning immunization services, and informing families about the availability of vaccination services has been shown to be important particularly in rural areas.[96, 156, 165, 171–175] Families that have strong social networks in the local community[173, 176] and language and culture similar to those of health workers[152] are more likely to use health services. Adverse public opinion about vaccination has been documented when adverse effects occurred,[125, 159] including postvaccination abscesses.[128] Misconceptions about vaccination,[177] including associating tetanus toxoid vaccination with mass promotion of contraception,[178] have fortunately been reported relatively infrequently.

Determinants of immunization uptake are likely to vary between areas and perhaps at different phases of an immunization program. It is therefore important to investigate reasons for nonvaccination or incomplete vaccination in a variety of settings. There is no single "correct" research method, and qualitative and quantitative methods are complementary. Anthropological approaches yield information about health decision-making processes as well as an understanding of their specific cultural context but may not link that information to overall healthcare utilization patterns. Epidemiological surveys yield information about utilization rates and access to care factors but may not account for biases and assumptions implicit in Western constructs of disease and illness or take into account the context in which healthcare decisions are made.[158] There is increasingly consensus on the need to link the two approaches to contribute to the improvement of health services in developing countries.[154, 158, 179, 180] Use of a mix of methods[81] and feedback of results to decision-makers, health workers, and communities allow the continuous identification and solution of problems.

Disease Surveillance

Surveillance is primordial to measure the impact of immunization programs on vaccine-preventable diseases. As immunization programs move from a focus on raising coverage to one of controlling or eliminating diseases, the emphasis of surveillance moves from concentrating on measurement of coverage (a process measure) to measuring impact on disease incidence (a health outcome measure). Disease surveillance was a crucial component of the smallpox eradication program[111] and poliomyelitis elimination in the Americas,[34, 99, 181] but it remains one of the weak links in the cycle of program planning, implementation, and monitoring in the EPI. Weak, overstretched health systems that lack the infrastructure to implement programs similarly lack the personnel with skills, time, resources, and incentives to develop effective surveillance. Immunization programs, having simple measurable objectives, can nonetheless facilitate the development of surveillance of the target diseases, provided such surveillance is action oriented and complemented by adequate feedback to all reporting sites.

Different methods of surveillance have been used at different stages of immunization programs in the developing world (Table 44–5). Routine reports of cases of measles, neonatal tetanus, and poliomyelitis can be used to monitor program impact. Although disease incidence rates are frequently underestimated by routine reports, because only those cases that present to health facilities are detected, if the reporting system remains unchanged over time, disease trends can be monitored. Demonstration of the long-term reduction in disease incidence is especially important to convince policymakers of the effectiveness of EPI when an outbreak of a target disease occurs in an area with high immunization coverage.[182] Analysis of data from routine reports can also identify high-risk groups, which are then targeted for extra program efforts. For example, in western Cape Province, South Africa, measles notification rates among children younger than 2 years were 9 times higher in Cape Town than in the rest of the region and were 10-fold to 100-fold higher in blacks than in whites.[183]

The utility of surveillance based on routine reports from health facilities can be enhanced by reducing the number of diseases that must be notified (so that health workers have more time to focus on the important diseases), conducting active surveillance (e.g., regular visits or telephone calls to ask whether cases have occurred), and instituting "negative reporting" (i.e., reporting the absence of cases). Active surveillance in Kinshasa, Zaire, successfully identified neighborhoods with high incidence rates of paralytic poliomyelitis.[184]

Sentinel sites may substitute for routine systems where the latter are too poorly developed to detect trends in incidence.[185] In Maputo, Mozambique, one sentinel site for poliomyelitis reported an increase in the number of cases after expired poliomyelitis vaccine had been used, leading to revaccination of children in the affected age groups.[51] Sentinel sites can also complement routine systems by providing more detailed information on each case. Sites are selected on the basis of their geographical representativeness, case load, and willingness of staff to participate. A range of health facilities can be used for common and distinctive diseases such as

Table 44–5. **SURVEILLANCE METHODS FOR THE EXPANDED PROGRAMME ON IMMUNIZATION**

METHOD OF SURVEILLANCE	MAJOR FUNCTIONS	MAJOR DRAWBACKS
Routine	Usually a passive, relatively inexpensive system relying on reports from health centers of cases of target diseases Evaluate disease trends by age group, vaccination status, and so on Obtain general idea of impact on target diseases Identify remaining chains of transmission in diseases for which there is an elimination/eradication goal	Incomplete and delayed for most diseases, except if the system has been strengthened, e.g., because disease is targeted for elimination Usually too many diseases included in the reporting system, which discourages reporting and analysis at intermediate and operational levels Little or no action is taken at the local level based on reporting, and little feedback received from higher levels Difficult to include the private sector
Sentinel	Complements weak routine surveillance by providing more detailed information on each case Early warning for outbreaks Selection of sites depends on disease	Not representative Need close follow-up to ensure timeliness and completeness of reporting Not useful as vaccine-preventable diseases become rare Not sufficient for disease elimination/eradication programs
Special surveys	Conduct at the beginning of the program to identify disease burden and set priorities (lameness surveys, neonatal tetanus surveys)	Time-consuming and costly Problems with retrospective diagnoses Not practical to assess impact of immunization program Do not directly strengthen routine surveillance

measles, whereas specialist centers may be more suitable for diphtheria and pertussis.

Special surveys have been used to determine disease burden in areas where access to health facilities is low, particularly in the early years of immunization programs.[186, 187] They are relatively expensive, however, and unsuitable for monitoring disease incidence over time.

Whatever the source of data on target diseases, standard case definitions should be used and minimum data elements agreed on. Guidelines for surveillance of communicable diseases, including the EPI target diseases, are currently being updated and harmonized by WHO. Suggested case definitions are summarized in Table 44–6. Surveillance systems should be monitored through the use of quality indicators, the main three being the timeliness and completeness of reporting, the proportion of reported cases/outbreaks that are investigated in a timely manner (including laboratory confirmation of di-

Table 44–6. **CLINICAL CASE DEFINITIONS AND LABORATORY CONFIRMATION FOR TARGET DISEASES OF THE EXPANDED PROGRAMME ON IMMUNIZATION**

DISEASE	CLINICAL CASE DEFINITION	LABORATORY CONFIRMATION
Diphtheria	An illness characterized by laryngitis *or* pharyngitis *or* tonsillitis, *and* an adherent membrane of the tonsils, pharynx, or nose	Isolation of *Corynebacterium diphtheriae* from a clinical specimen *or* 4-fold or greater rise in serum antibody (both specimens before the administration of diphtheria toxoid or antitoxin)
Measles	Any person with fever *and* maculopapular rash *and* cough, coryza, or conjunctivitis	Presence of measles-specific IgM antibodies *or* At least a 4-fold rise in measles-specific IgG antibody level between acute and convalescent specimens *or* Isolation of measles virus
Pertussis	A person with cough lasting at least 2 wk *with one of the following:* Paroxysms of coughing Inspiratory "whoop" Vomiting immediately after coughing without other apparent cause	Isolation of *Bordetella pertussis or* Presence of IgG or IgA directed toward pertussis toxin or filamentous hemagglutinin antigen
Poliomyelitis	Any child <15 yr of age with acute flaccid paralysis or any person with paralytic illness at any age when polio is suspected*	Wild-type poliovirus isolated from stool†
Neonatal tetanus	**Suspect:** Any neonatal death between 3 and 28 d of age in which the cause of death is unknown; or any neonate reported as having neonatal tetanus but not investigated **Confirmed:** Any neonate with a normal ability to suck and cry during the first 2 d of life who between 3 and 28 d of age cannot suck normally and becomes still or has convulsions, *or* a hospital-reported case of neonatal tetanus	None

*A two-scheme classification is followed to investigate cases of acute flaccid paralysis according to the stage of the surveillance system in the country.

†A case is not discarded unless two adequate stool specimens have been collected (approximately 8 to 10 g collected 24 to 48 hours apart, within 14 days of onset of paralysis, in good condition with maintenance of the reverse cold chain for transport in cool conditions).

agnosis, where appropriate), and the proportion of investigated cases/outbreaks that are followed by an appropriate response.[185]

Outbreak investigations complement routine surveillance and can provide additional information on incidence and fatality by age and vaccine effectiveness. They provide an opportunity to identify reasons for the outbreak and to obtain reliable data on disease epidemiology that can assist in adjusting immunization strategies. By feeding back information from the outbreak investigation to personnel at the local level, they can lead to improvements in routine surveillance.

In addition to the difficulties in developing surveillance systems for the existing EPI vaccines, new candidates for inclusion in the program such as *Haemophilus influenzae* type b (Hib) and conjugate pneumococcal vaccines will present another challenge. The new vaccines tend to protect against diseases with less specific clinical manifestations, and special skills and technologies will be required for their differential diagnosis. Furthermore, for vaccines such as hepatitis B vaccine, included in the EPI since 1989, the desired outcome (prevention of liver disease) may not be measurable for many years or even decades after vaccination has begun, and other outcome measures—for example, the age prevalence of HBsAg—are useful to monitor program effectiveness in the shorter term.[188]

With the availability of low-cost, high-performance microcomputers, public health programs and services are automating the management and analysis of surveillance data. Computer systems, if properly designed, can support the three main functions of disease surveillance: (1) systematic collection of data; (2) consolidation, analysis, and evaluation of the data; and (3) feedback of the results.[189] To facilitate data analysis, computer software, such as Epi Info, has been developed using a combination of data base, statistical, and graphics packages. These systems are now of particular interest to immunization programs that are shifting toward the decentralization of data management (i.e., the monitoring of coverage and disease at the lowest geopolitical level). Finally, computer systems facilitate the basic objective of surveillance: the collection and timely analysis of data to identify those at risk, detect the changing pattern of the diseases, adjust strategies, and monitor the impact of immunization programs.

Laboratories play an essential role in the surveillance of most vaccine-preventable diseases, particularly once disease incidence decreases and clinical diagnosis may become less reliable. For the poliomyelitis eradication program, the setup of a laboratory network capable of detecting wild poliovirus has been an essential component of the process of eradication and its certification. For this purpose, the WHO has set up a Global Polio Laboratory network consisting of more than 60 national laboratories supported by 16 regional reference laboratories and assisted by 6 global specialized laboratories.[190, 191] Based on the establishment of this network, a similar network is being prepared for measles laboratory diagnosis worldwide and for yellow fever in the 33 countries of Africa endemic for yellow fever.[9]

Serological surveillance is a powerful tool used for monitoring the impact of vaccination programs and identifying populations at risk in industrialized countries,[192, 193] but it has been less used in developing countries because of a shortage of skilled personnel and adequately equipped laboratories. Simpler and less costly serological methods could enable developing countries to monitor current vaccination programs more accurately and to evaluate the impact of vaccines such as hepatitis B, rubella, and perhaps new candidate vaccines.[194] With the rapid growth of enzyme-linked immunoassay techniques, often in kit form, there is a great potential for wider use of serological surveillance. The detection of virus-specific antibody in saliva has been reported for human immunodeficiency virus (HIV), hepatitis,[195] and measles[196, 197] using the antibody capture format, and further development of this assay could greatly facilitate field surveys. Randomized age-structured serosurveys can provide useful background information by which to compare subsequent profiles of herd immunity, for example, of measles, rubella,[198, 199] and poliomyelitis; to identify groups with lower immunity levels before outbreaks occur among them[104, 192]; and to permit a greater understanding of the transmission characteristics of an infection in the community so that extra activities can be focused on the groups most important in transmission.[200]

Monitoring Adverse Events

Although modern vaccines are well tolerated and efficacious, no vaccine is totally safe. The more successful vaccination programs are in controlling disease, the higher the attention attracted to adverse events. In extreme cases when disease has been eliminated, the acceptance of even very rare adverse events becomes politically more and more difficult. For example, because of the interruption of the transmission of wild poliovirus, all cases of paralytic poliomyelitis occurring in the Western Hemisphere are now vaccine associated, and in the United States this has led to a change in policy to a combined schedule of inactivated and oral poliovirus vaccines.[201]

In developing countries, there is increasing recognition of the importance of adverse events that are due to program failure rather than inherent properties of the vaccine.[202] In some cases, vaccine caused side effects because it was reconstituted with the wrong diluent. Elsewhere, contaminated needles or syringes were used, or dangerous drugs were mistakenly administered instead of vaccines. In Zimbabwe, an outbreak of lymphadenitis after BCG immunization in 1982 was traced to a switch to a different strain of vaccine that was more reactogenic. The ensuing investigation also revealed problems with intradermal injection technique as a contributing factor.[203] Similar outbreaks of lymphadenitis have been reported in other countries.[204–207]

Adverse events relating to program failure are much more common than severe events that are related to inherent properties of the vaccine. They can be detected without the sophisticated systems needed for rare events. At a minimum, every country should report cases of abscesses, and severe events such as septicemia or death, that are temporally related to vaccination.[202, 208] Clinics and vaccine stores should note the manufacturer, lot number, and date of expiry of each vaccine received. Ideally the lot number should also be noted on the vaccination record, but this will require substantial improvement in record-keeping and would also increase time for administration. It may in itself, however, be useful to remind health workers of the potential for adverse events and the need for constant vigilance when biological preparations are administered to children and mothers.

Costs

Economic analysis can be used at a macro level to build up a vision of a cost-effective health service, for example, the World Bank (1993) World Development Report "Investing in Health."[209] In the World Development Report, the cost-effectiveness of different interventions was measured in terms of their cost per disability-adjusted life–year (DALY) gained.[209] Estimated costs were less than $10 per DALY gained (or about $300 per death averted) for measles immunization and less than $25 per DALY gained for a combination of OPV and DTP vaccines.[2] Cost analysis can also be used to demonstrate the savings that accrue to industrialized countries from global eradication programs and to promote investment in them.[210] Studies of costs can help program directors to manage their resources, compare different operational strategies, and decide how funds should be used.[211, 212]

The EPI developed costing guidelines in 1979 that were field tested in Indonesia, the Philippines, and Thailand[213] and subsequently developed spreadsheet software (EPICOST) to support costing studies. Operating cost components were defined as salaries of the immunization team and supervisors; vaccines and vaccine shipment; transport including fuel, allowances, and vehicle maintenance; maintenance of the cold chain, injection equipment, and running costs of health facilities (kerosene, electricity, stationery); and training costs. Capital costs included a portion of buildings and vehicles attributed to EPI plus costs of cold chain equipment and spare parts.

A review of costing studies done from 1979 to 1987 showed that the average cost of fully immunizing a child in low-income countries was $13, excluding technical assistance (1987 U.S. dollars), and $15 if technical assistance was included.[214] The cost ranged from $6 to more than $20, depending on the strategy used, the population density, and the prices of labor and other local inputs.[2, 213, 214] Although the relative costs of different strategies varied between countries, in general, routine services appeared more cost-effective than campaigns in the long term.[2] In Ecuador, for example, campaigns cost $66 per DALY gained compared with $30 for routine services.[215] However, in Thailand, increased use of mobile teams was more cost-effective in areas with a dispersed population.[213]

For all strategies, personnel costs accounted for the largest proportion, with supervision and management the second largest cost.[213] Vaccines represented approximately 10% of all costs. In general, costs of fully immunizing a child decreased as the number of children immunized increased.[213, 216] However, the studies included only coverage levels up to 65%, and the marginal costs are likely to increase in trying to reach the last 15 to 20% of infants.

The studies also showed the proportion of costs financed by donors for different strategies. On average, donors financed 43% (range, 4 to 73%) of the total cost of fixed facility strategies and 56% (range, 13 to 85%) of the campaign strategies in the developing countries that were assessed (predominantly those in sub-Saharan Africa).[214]

If costing is tailored to suit the client's needs and takes the context and goals of the immunization program into account, economic analysis can be a powerful tool to identify barriers to the implementation of cost-effective strategies at different levels of the health system.[79, 217] Economic analyses have helped to show problems in the process of disbursing funds, including irregular and delayed receipt of donor funds, poor accountability, overcentralization of management of funds so that there is no access to funds for running costs at the health center level, and nonstandardization of payments for daily allowances between different vaccination strategies or between agencies.[79] Monitoring the process of utilization of resources and establishing transparent and coordinated systems for accountability of donors as well as government health services could greatly improve efficiency.

Modeling

The choice of vaccination strategy requires an understanding of the dynamic effects of vaccination on disease transmission and knowledge of age-related changes in severity of disease, vaccine complications, and the probability of transmission of the infection.[45, 218] Mathematical models lend themselves to the task of measuring and comparing the merits of different strategies and improving our understanding of the observed impact of vaccination programs.[219]

Dynamic simulation models attempt to describe the dynamics of infections in populations and hence to predict their behavior under the altered conditions induced by a vaccination program.[45, 218–221] This approach has been used to explore the effects of different vaccination policies on measles,[222, 223] poliomyelitis,[224] and rubella.[198, 199, 225–227] It has also been used to compare different delivery strategies, for example, repeated pulse vaccination across a range of ages versus routine immunization at a single specified age.[228]

Modeling has been used to explore thresholds for elimination or eradication of infections from populations.[45, 218, 229] Immunization programs aim to interrupt transmission of infection by inducing herd immunity, which is the resistance of a group to attack by disease to which a large proportion of the members are immune because the chance of contact between an infectious person and a susceptible individual is low. Models have estimated the threshold level of population immunity that must be achieved for the incidence of the disease in question to decline toward zero.[45]

In terms of implications for policy, dynamic modeling has generally not considered the economic implications of the various scenarios. There is great scope, as yet little explored, for the combination of economic with dynamic modeling and for increasing the use of modeling in predicting the effects of different vaccination strategies.[221]

SUMMARY OF ACHIEVEMENTS: LESSONS AND TECHNIQUES LEARNED

For the last 20 years, the EPI has helped to create a global consensus on disease prevention and immunization. It helped in the establishment of a "culture of prevention" among politicians, health workers, and community members.[72] Global strategies for disease control and eradication have been implemented thanks to an unprecedented degree of commitment and cooperation among all partners within and outside the health sector, including national governments and international, national, and local organizations from the public and the private sectors. In these years, many tools have been developed to facilitate the implementation and delivery of immunization services (Table 44–7). Some of these tools were a pioneering development in their area and have been used for other applications outside immunization services.[72, 230]

The EPI quickly concentrated on developing effective training programs and modules for peripheral health workers and midlevel and senior-level managers. Countries were assisted in developing short- and medium-term plans of action, and as the number of donor agencies involved in supporting immunization services grew, interagency coordinating committees were encouraged. A series of clear guidelines on immunization practices were developed, and the strong field base of the EPI enabled WHO to update and clarify these guidelines to resolve questions raised by health workers, such as policies on simultaneous administration of vaccines, contraindications, minimum and maximum intervals between doses, and so on.[1] Guidelines were not just distributed to Ministries of Health but were followed up by supervision and monitoring through program reviews and ad hoc studies using simple protocols developed by the EPI.

In the area of the cold chain and safe injection practices, extensive innovative work was conducted to develop technology that was appropriate for the most extreme conditions of heat or cold. Standards were set not only for immunization policies but also for practical components of the program, such as the EPI product information sheets for immunization equipment. The ice-lined refrigerator enabled vaccines to be stored in situations where electricity is interrupted for up to 16 hours of each 24-hour period. This type of refrigerator is now used as a global standard in central and provincial

Table 44–7. **TECHNIQUES AND TOOLS DEVELOPED BY THE EXPANDED PROGRAMME ON IMMUNIZATION**

AREA	TOOL	PRINCIPLE
Planning	National EPI plan of action, including costs and sources of funds Interagency coordinating committees (regional and national levels)	Programming tool to help set priorities, monitor activities, and optimize donor contributions Created for advocacy and coordination; avoid duplication or competition between donors
Facilitating attainment of high coverage	Accelerated schedule Contraindications policy Missed opportunities protocol	Reduce number of immunization contacts and protect children before highest risk Take advantage of any visit to a health facility to immunize women and children
Management and training	Management training all levels Refrigerator repair technicians Driver and rider training Logistics for primary healthcare Program reviews EPI costing guidelines; EPICOST	Different sets of modules and training programs relating to all aspects of program, for adaptation at the local level Continuous in-service training to improve quality of services Methodology and software developed to estimate program costs
Monitoring coverage and disease surveillance	30 cluster methodology COSAS Lot quality sampling Surveillance guidelines Laboratory network and technology transfer	Simple sampling methodology to estimate immunization coverage, supported by computer software to assist in analysis Monitor impact on disease control; use surveillance as a guide for program planning
Cold chain	Range of appropriate refrigeration technology and spare parts kits EPI Product Information Sheets Cold chain monitors, vaccine vial monitors	Maintain correct temperatures in hot climates with erratic power supplies; use different power sources Inventory of equipment for immunization meeting standard specifications Monitor storage and transport of vaccine, and show whether or not vaccine is in appropriate condition for use
Injections	Plastic sterilizable syringes; steam sterilizers; hard-water pads and filters; autodestruct syringes; syringe safety boxes; prefilled injection devices	Appropriate technology to ensure that immunization injections are safe and free from risk of transmission of bloodborne infections

stores. The photovoltaic refrigerator, developed and tested with the U.S. National Aeronautics and Space Administration, enabled specifications to be issued to industry resulting in more than 5000 solar vaccine refrigeration systems installed and used globally today. Solar power is used not only for EPI but often also to provide energy for all health center needs. Extensive work was conducted to ensure adequate maintenance of equipment; universal spare parts kits were developed for refrigerator repair along with standard tool kits for the traveling repair technician, and cold chain technicians were trained in a series of national and regional courses. Similar effort was expended on developing appropriate technology for promoting adequate sterilization practices.[1] Again, all this work was followed through by developing protocols and simple methods for monitoring implementation in the field. Work on these areas of logistical support to the program expanded through the formation of TECHNET, a global network of cold chain and logistics experts who conduct applied research on logistics for primary healthcare.[230]

The pragmatic and field-based approach of the EPI, with its continuous cycle of planning, conducting applied research on priority problems, disseminating guidelines, monitoring closely all aspects of the program, and feeding back on progress through a wide range of communication methods, has provided an example for disease control programs throughout the world.

FUTURE TRENDS

In the past 20 years, a health services infrastructure has been developed through which immunization against many of the major causes of childhood mortality can be delivered. Although there are wide regional and national differences in the level of infrastructure and resources available for basic healthcare, immunization programs globally will continue to expand in any or all of the following ways:

- improving coverage levels of existing vaccines in the routine program;
- conducting additional activities to eliminate or eradicate disease using existing vaccines;
- improving the quality and safety of vaccines and injections; and
- adding new vaccines to the program.

Improving Coverage of Existing EPI Vaccines

Immunization coverage is a key indicator of access to and utilization of immunization services. In spite of continuous efforts to raise immunization coverage, since 1990 global figures for EPI vaccines have leveled off at around 80% for infants (Fig. 44–3), and considerable disparity remains both between and within countries (Fig. 44–4).

Of 165 countries for which 1990 and 1996 data are available, 106 have reported coverage of at least 80% for DTP3, whereas 36 countries have never achieved 80% coverage and 10 (of which 8 are in Africa) have not reached the 50% figure. Average coverage of DTP3 in the African region has not yet reached 60%. To improve coverage in the lowest-income countries, long-term, coordinated, and reliable investment by national governments and donors is required.[73, 78]

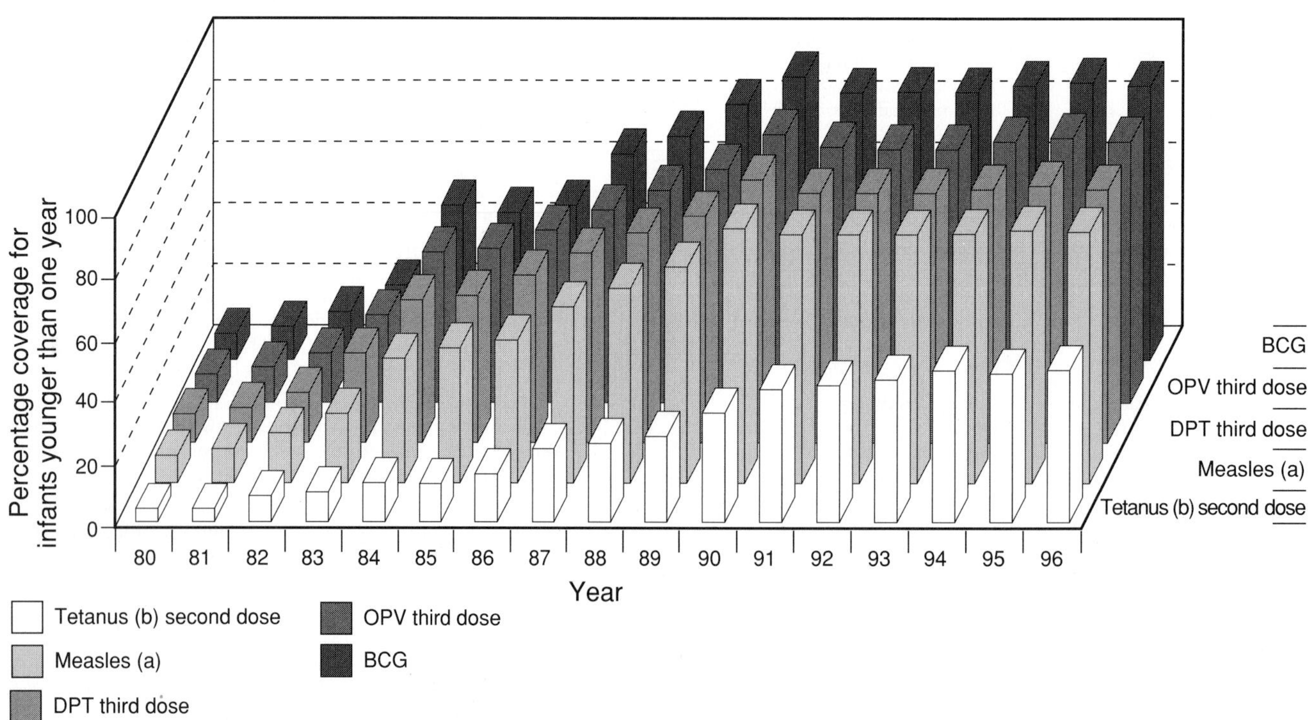

Figure 44–3. Expanded Programme on Immunization coverage, 1980 to 1996. Data before 1984 are estimated for (a) children up to 2 years of age and (b) tetanus toxoid (mothers). BCG, bacille Calumette-Guérin vaccine; DPT, diphtheria-pertussis-tetanus vaccine; OPV, oral poliovirus vaccine.

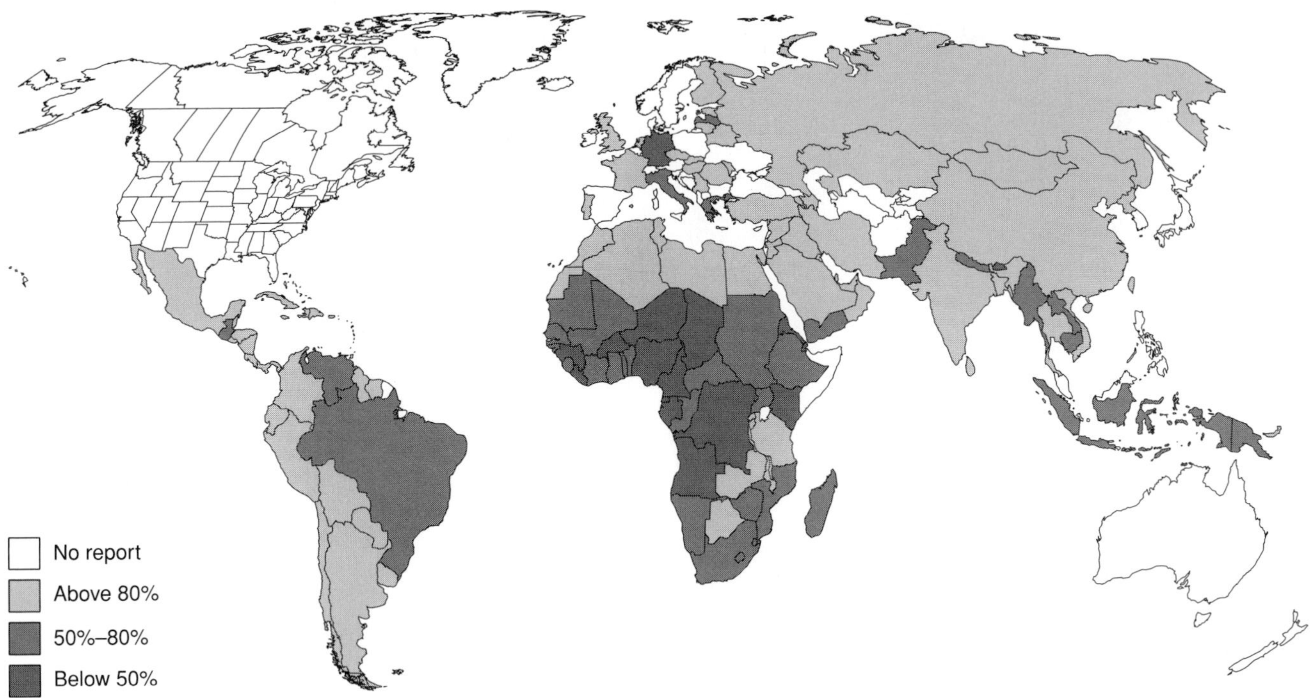

Figure 44–4. Percentage of 1996 immunization coverage with three doses of DTP in infants.

Hepatitis B is a major public health problem even though safe and effective vaccines have been available for more than 15 years. The WHO estimates that hepatitis B infection results in more than 1 million deaths every year worldwide.[231] Hepatitis B vaccine is estimated to be as cost-effective as measles vaccine in highly endemic countries (≥8% prevalence of carriage of HBsAg).[231] The high effectiveness of the vaccine has been demonstrated by reductions in the carrier rate from more than 8% to less than 2% in immunized cohorts of children in the Gambia, Singapore, Hong Kong, Taiwan, Alaska, Thailand, Indonesia, South Korea, and American Samoa.[232] In Taiwan, 10 years after implementation of a mass vaccination program, a fall in the annual incidence of hepatocellular carcinoma in children aged 10 to 14 years has already been documented.[232] In Singapore, 95% of infants complete the full immunization schedule, including hepatitis B. In the 1993 national seroepidemiological survey, HBsAg was detected in only 0.3% of vaccinated people, compared with 5.6% of unvaccinated people.[188]

Despite this, because complications occur many years after infection, donors and governments have been reluctant to invest in procurement of hepatitis B vaccine.[232] Delegates to the World Health Assembly in 1992 recommended that all countries should integrate hepatitis B vaccine into their national immunization programs by 1997. However, introduction of universal hepatitis B vaccination globally has been roughly inversely related to need (Fig. 44–5). Instead, it has been strongly determined by the economic status of the country and hence its ability to pay for the vaccine.

Since 1986, WHO has recommended that African countries at risk for yellow fever include this vaccine in their infant immunization programs. In the Gambia, adding yellow fever at the time of measles vaccine did not significantly increase the cost per dose of immunization delivered in the EPI.[233] As of March 1996, yellow fever vaccine has been available through UNICEF at a price of U.S. $0.18 per dose. However, a minority of the 33 African at-risk countries include yellow fever vaccine in their EPI (Fig. 44–6), and the Gambia is the only country to achieve high coverage and impact on disease. In 1994 and 1995, there was a resurgence of yellow fever across Africa with outbreaks reported in Ghana, Liberia, Nigeria, Sierra Leone, Gabon, and Kenya.[233]

Eradication/Elimination

Substantial progress has been achieved toward the goal of global eradication of poliomyelitis. The most notable progress in 1996 was the expansion of the number of countries conducting national immunization days, to cover almost two thirds of all children younger than 5 years globally with supplemental OPV immunization. Implementation of national immunization days in the remaining endemic countries and rapid improvements in surveillance are now the highest priority for the global eradication initiative. Poliomyelitis outbreaks in Albania, Greece, and the Federal Republic of Yugoslavia demonstrated that polio-free countries remain at risk from importations. Expansion of national immunization days and surveillance into war-torn or politically isolated countries including the Democratic Republic of the Congo (formerly Zaire), Somalia, and Sudan is crucial to final global eradication.[3] The total external funding support required for the period 1997 to 2005 is estimated at more than U.S. $1000 million.

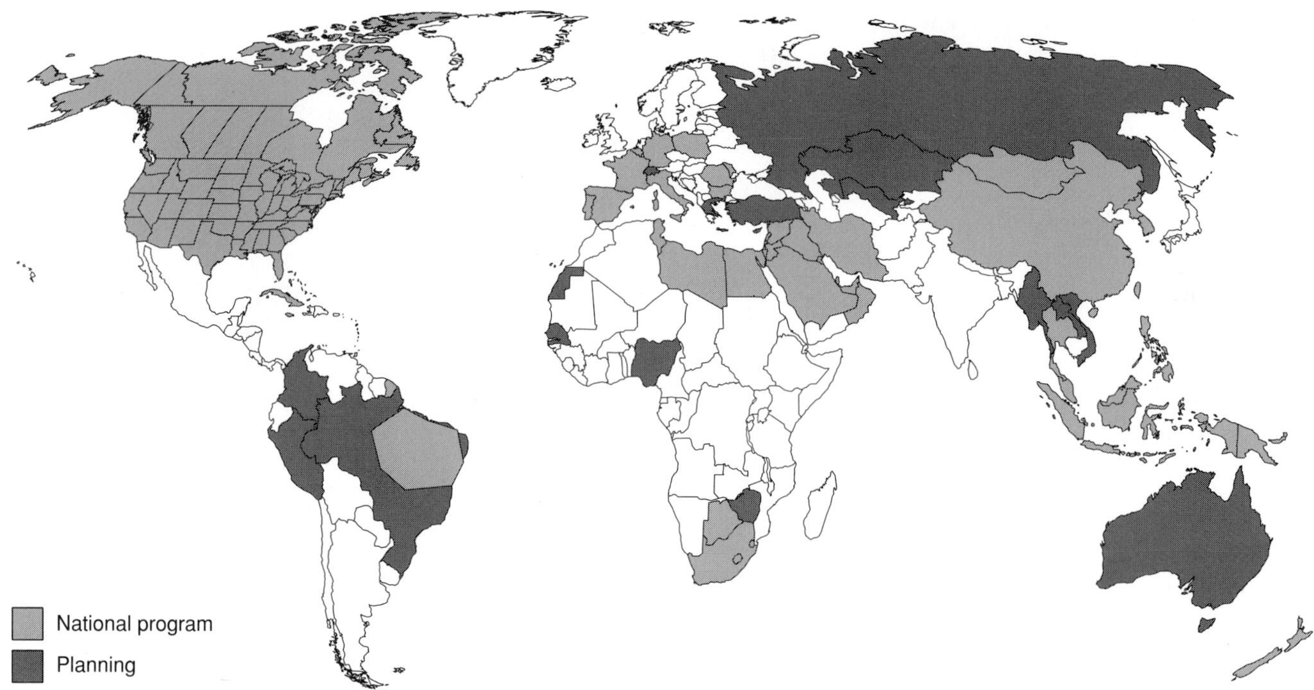

Figure 44–5. Hepatitis B vaccine: universal immunization policy, 1997.

Although much still remains to be done to achieve global poliomyelitis eradication, regions that have already eradicated poliomyelitis are keen to keep up the momentum of their immunization programs and are considering the eradicability of other diseases. In 1995, measles vaccination was estimated to have reduced measles-associated mortality worldwide by 88% from the prevaccination levels of as many as 5.7 million deaths per year.[234] In the region of the Americas, there was a 99% reduction in measles incidence and mortality compared with prevaccination levels. This accelerating progress in reducing measles incidence and mortality in many parts of the world has led to calls for its global eradication during the next 10 to 15 years.[235] Mass "catch-up" campaigns are being conducted, in some countries as a step toward interrupting transmission and in other countries as a means to increase measles immunization coverage rapidly.

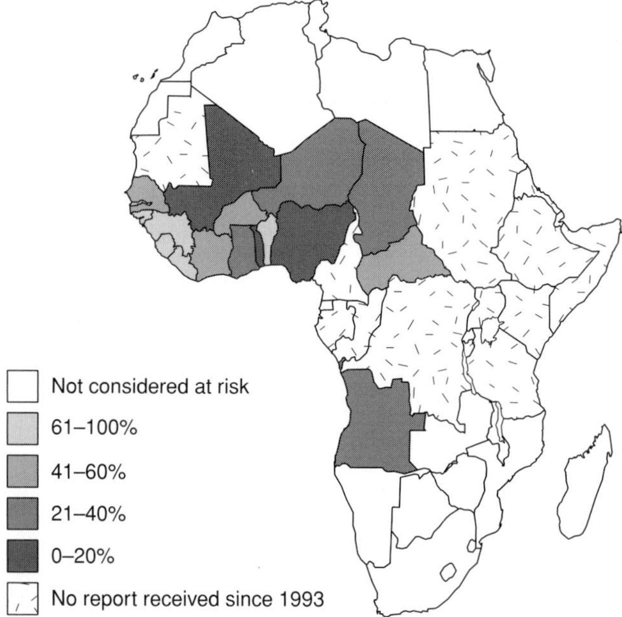

Figure 44–6. Reported yellow fever immunization coverage in countries at risk for outbreaks, 1993 to 1995.

The reduction of measles-associated mortality is a public health priority in developing countries. Measles eradication, defined as the interruption of measles transmission globally such that vaccination would not need to be continued,[235] is theoretically possible because there is no known animal reservoir and measles vaccine is highly effective.[236] In practice, the high infectivity of measles makes it difficult to eradicate, because more than 90% (and possibly more than 95%) of the population must be immune for incidence to decline toward zero.[45] The difficulties in reaching the required immunization coverage in developing countries and low public awareness about the seriousness of the disease in industrialized countries contribute to the practical difficulties.[17] Nonetheless, the recent success of measles elimination programs throughout the Americas[92] as well as in Finland,[237] Sweden,[238] and the United Kingdom[239] has shown that these practical problems can be overcome, given sufficient resources.

Several questions remain about the selection of the most appropriate strategies for measles control/eradication, fitting the national and local situation and priorities. Questions include the selection of the age range to vaccinate in campaigns, the ability to ensure maintenance of safe injection practices, and the feasibility and cost of reaching high enough coverage for eradication in the poorest countries. The marginal cost-benefit ratio of aiming for eradication rather than control needs to be assessed. Last, the effects of an eradication program on social development need to be considered.

Improving Vaccine Supply, Quality, and Injection Safety

In recognition of the increased amounts of vaccines needed to meet disease eradication and elimination goals and the increase in price of some vaccines, the Children's Vaccine Initiative's Task Force on Situation Analysis of Global Vaccine Supply was formed. The Children's Vaccine Initiative is a global coalition of organizations, from the public, nongovernmental, and private sectors, including the vaccine industry, that work together to develop and make available vaccines that are safe, effective, and easy to deliver. Launched at the World Summit for Children in 1990, the Children's Vaccine Initiative is cosponsored by UNICEF, the United Nations Development Programme, the World Bank, WHO, and the Rockefeller Foundation. The Task Force aims to enhance national self-sufficiency in vaccine supply, not only for the vaccines in use today but also for new, improved, and more expensive vaccines that will be available in the future.[240] Self-sufficiency is the ability of governments to take responsibility for the provision of adequate quantities of high-quality vaccines, through appropriate strategies directed toward more sustainable financing and procurement, local production, and quality-control practices.[240] The Task Force has encouraged the use of a grid that arrays countries according to their population and per capita income to define broad bands of countries for which different strategies are appropriate. The smaller, poorer countries will obtain vaccine by procurement, with substantial donor assistance for the foreseeable future. The larger countries, particularly those with higher per capita income, will increasingly be likely to produce their own vaccines.

A parallel initiative that arose from the experience in the Americas has been the promotion of revolving funds,[241] in which countries contribute funds in local currency to funds supported by international agencies such as UNICEF to procure vaccines.[242]

In addition to efforts to ensure the availability of adequate quantities of vaccines, concerns about the quality of many of the EPI vaccines produced in developing countries[151] led the Children's Vaccine Initiative's Task Forces of Global Vaccine Supply and Quality Control to examine the global status of vaccine production, supply, and quality in 43 vaccine-producing countries.[243] Six basic criteria were used to determine whether each national control authority was able to guarantee that a vaccine was of "known good quality" (appropriate legislation, clinical review, lot release, laboratory testing, inspections, and surveillance). Of the 43 countries surveyed, only 21 (including both industrialized and developing countries) had all six control functions in place. A second inventory assessed the quality of DTP production in 42 countries. Half the manufacturers were in countries without fully functional national control systems. About 10% of producers were failing to meet WHO minimum standards for the purity of the toxoids.[243] For tetanus toxoid, a total of 80 lots from 21 manufacturers in 14 countries reporting neonatal tetanus cases were tested for potency. Of these, 15 lots from eight manufacturers had potency values below WHO requirements.[244]

The Children's Vaccine Initiative's Task Force assessments identified the strengths and weaknesses of many vaccine producers and highlighted the need for improvements in production process, independent quality control, and national regulatory competence.[245] In a few cases, they even recommended closure of the production facilities pending needed improvements. On the other hand, these reports also served to increase general awareness that many vaccine producers in developing countries do, in fact, produce high-quality vaccines under acceptable quality-control conditions.[246]

To sustain the national, regional, and even global supply of the EPI vaccines, the most important areas of technology transfer for developing countries are those relevant to achieving and maintaining good manufacturing practice standards in vaccine production, establishing independent and credible national quality-control laboratories, and instituting national (or perhaps regional, if necessary) regulatory capability.[246] Facilitating successful and sustainable technology transfers is a challenge facing the international organizations that support the global EPI.

Vaccine quality must also be maintained once vaccines are distributed to the field. A new challenge facing vaccine storage is the global banning of chlorofluorocarbons by the first of January 1999 because of their damaging effect on the ozone layer. This gas is used as a refrigerant in most compression refrigerators and in all types of insulation foams. This ban will require the change of all equipment or repair tools, because new gas cannot be used in old appliances, nor should new refrigerators be contaminated by the old gas.

The last component of a high-quality vaccination service is ensuring that injection practices are safe. With more than 550 million injections administered in developing countries through the delivery of vaccines, representing only a small fraction of all injections performed, there is concern that safety is not always ensured.[247] EPI has had a long-standing policy of "a single sterile needle and a single sterile syringe should be used with each injection" and is continuing to develop and evaluate alternative injection technologies such as autodestruct syringes[248] and jet injectors to minimize the risk of unsafe injection practices.

Introduction of Additional Vaccines

A number of effective vaccines are available but not yet included in the EPI; still more are in the pipeline. Hib vaccine is a highly effective vaccine against a major pathogen. Its use has virtually eliminated invasive *H. influenzae* type b disease from much of the industrialized world.[249] It has recently been shown to have an efficacy of more than 90% in the developing-country setting of the Gambia,[250] where Hib vaccine also significantly reduced the incidence of radiologically defined pneumonia by 21% (95% confidence interval, 4.6 to 34.9%). This reduction in the overall incidence of pneumonia in vaccinees suggested that about 20% of episodes of pneumonia in young Gambian children were due to *H. influenzae* type b. If this is representative of the situation in other developing countries, the introduction of Hib vaccines could substantially reduce childhood mortality due to pneumonia as well as meningitis. Because pneumonia is estimated to underlie 18% of deaths in developing countries,[251] the development of mechanisms to make Hib vaccine affordable to children in the poorest countries is a major challenge for the international health community.

Rubella vaccine has been used for almost 30 years in industrialized countries. A review completed for the WHO in 1995 showed that 78 countries (92% of industrialized countries, 36% of countries in economic transition, and 28% of developing countries) include rubella vaccine in their national immunization programs.[252] There are many other countries in which rubella vaccine is used in the private sector only. The review also showed that seven developing countries have documented rubella outbreaks with congenital rubella syndrome incidence rates as high as those in industrialized countries before vaccination.[253] All seven countries now have national rubella vaccination policies. However, it remains difficult for health policymakers to determine the relative priority to give to control of congenital rubella syndrome because of inadequate data in many countries.[253] The collection of appropriate data and development of practical surveillance methods for low-income countries are urgently required if the opportunities presented by measles control and elimination programs are to be taken to control congenital rubella syndrome as well.[254] Similarly, data on the burden of disease from mumps are needed, as an increasing number of developing countries introduce the combined measles-mumps-rubella (MMR) vaccine.[252]

A wide range of new vaccines are expected to be licensed in the next decade. Lower respiratory infections and diarrheal diseases were among the top four causes of death worldwide in 1990,[11] and vaccines against these diseases thus have immense potential to improve health status. Some new vaccines will be licensed for the existing EPI target groups (e.g., rotavirus vaccine, conjugate pneumococcal and meningococcal vaccines), some will be targeted at adolescents (e.g., herpesvirus vaccines and HIV vaccines), and others will be indicated for people of all ages (e.g., dengue, malaria).[255] This means that the concept that the EPI target groups are only pregnant women and infants will be likely to change. Strategies to reach school-aged children, adolescents, and all adults will be needed,[254] giving further impetus to the drive to strengthen primary healthcare through the EPI.

Many factors influence the utility of new vaccines for developing countries,[256] including

- acceptability to the public and to the health authorities;
- affordability;
- heat stability;
- number of administrations (= contacts with health workers) of a vaccine required to induce lasting immunity;
- ability to be formulated as a component of a combination vaccine, such as DTP or MMR, or to be administered simultaneously with other vaccines; and
- route of administration, whether parenteral or mucosal (such as oral or respiratory).

Strategies to facilitate the introduction of new vaccines include actions in-country to define the disease burden, develop political will, and ensure that the infrastructure is adequate for sustainable financing, procurement, quality assurance, and delivery of vaccines and actions at the international level. The Children's Vaccine Initiative is working together with the Global Programme for Vaccines and Immunization to provide advice on strategic planning and analysis to help all collaborators in the development of new vaccines and their introduction into immunization programs.[254]

CONCLUSIONS

Immunization programs have spearheaded the development of public health worldwide. Through immunization, more than 3 million deaths are averted each year. Health professionals around the world have been trained to use a range of simple tools to plan, manage, and monitor their programs, and resources have been mobilized for the benefits of vaccines to reach most of the world's population. With the clear aim of controlling or even eradicating some of the most important childhood diseases, a pragmatic approach to making it as easy as possible for parents to get their children vaccinated, and a strong emphasis on continued training and supervision, EPI has led the way in infectious disease control. Lessons learned about simplifying immunization schedules,[257] providing protection as early in life as possible, establishing and disseminating clear guidelines for standards of care,[258–261] developing interagency coordinating committees,[260] and monitoring indicators of both process and impact[258, 262] have benefited industrialized countries as well as developing countries. Assessment tools such as the EPI cluster sample, missed opportunity, and cold chain monitor surveys have empowered peripheral health workers to evaluate their own programs. They have been modified for use in richer countries[61, 263–265] and for a wide range of public health programs.[117, 129] Nevertheless, the context in which immunization programs operate has changed markedly during the last decade,[266] and programs will need to respond flexibly and with innovation to these changes.

The health situation in nations is increasingly influenced by global determinants such as environmental threats and the expanded movement of people and goods that facilitates the spread of pathogens across national borders.[266] Global forces that affect health policies and systems in developing countries include the dominance of the market approach,[267] political systems around the world that condone increases in poverty and inequality,[266] and violent civil conflict within and between nations. Health systems in countries all over the world are undergoing intensive reforms, and international cooperation for world health faces unprecedented challenges.[266]

The diversity of health problems within and between countries means that national and international health systems must confront a vast array of needs. The populations of developing countries continue to suffer from infectious and parasitic diseases, maternal and perinatal disorders, and nutritional deficiences.[11] Worldwide, one third of deaths is from these causes, ranging from 65% in sub-Saharan Africa to 6% in established market economies and the former Socialist economies of Europe.[11] At the same time, developing countries have a high burden of noncommunicable diseases and injuries. Whereas much remains to be done to reduce the burden of communicable diseases (which represent 6 of the top 10 causes of mortality worldwide), increased attention is also needed for preventable causes of noncommunicable disease mortality, especially tobacco, alcohol, and injuries.

Healthcare systems worldwide absorb an increasingly large share of resources. In 1990, public and private expenditure on formal health services reached 8% of total world product. Industrialized countries spent almost 90% of this amount, with average per capita expenditure on healthcare of about $1500, yet official development assistance has declined to $0.3 per capita, its lowest level in real terms for 25 years.[268] In contrast, developing countries spent an average of only $41 per capita, and many of the poorest countries spent less than $5.[78] In the past 15 years, structural adjustment policies for economic reform, promoted by international banks, have cut government healthcare budgets by a third to a half in most sub-Saharan African countries.[269] Sizable sums of public money continue to be spent on tertiary-level hospitals at the expense of cost-effective interventions delivered at primary level. Access to basic health services remains low in many rural and dispersed communities. The involvement of the private sector (including for-profit services, missions, and nongovernmental agencies) in healthcare is increasing in all countries, raising challenges not only for equitable access to care but for coordination, standardization, and quality control of interventions.

There is a move toward radical reform of international organizations and national health systems. The function of international agencies will increasingly be to address core issues for which action at the national level is insufficient.[267] These include, at a minimum, surveillance and control of diseases that represent a global threat, promotion of research and development related to problems of global importance, development of standards and norms for international certification, protection of international refugees, and action as agents of assistance and advocacy for vulnerable populations. At the national level, the role of Ministries of Health is changing from implementation of health programs to leadership and coordination. Their functions and skills must include advocacy, consensus building, negotiation and mediation, formulating and advocating health policies, influencing the policies and monitoring the health effects of all sectors, and providing technical guidance.[267] Implementation of health programs will be increasingly decentralized and under local government control. This will require a shift from training programs that are oriented toward the delivery of specific interventions to capacity building in these broader policy and management skills.

There is increasing diversity between rich and poor countries in terms of the number of vaccines that can be included in the national schedule at an affordable price and the coverage that can be achieved and sustained. This disparity may be overcome for individual diseases in the short term through the supplementary efforts and resources invested in eradication programs. In the long term, however, countries need the capacity to devise appropriate policies based on sound evidence about local priorities, and communities must be involved in the planning and execution of immunization programs.

Against this changing background, immunization programs face a number of challenges, many of which require that the trend toward inequitable use of global resources be reversed. To reach the goals for poliomyelitis eradication, neonatal tetanus elimination, and measles control, politicians around the world must be dynamized to reverse the decline in assistance to the poorest countries. Measles continues to cause approximately half a million deaths per year in sub-Saharan Africa,[234] and of the 26 countries that account for 90% of globally estimated cases of neonatal tetanus, 16 are in Africa. Coverage for routine childhood immunizations and TT is below 50% in many countries of western and central Africa that do not yet have an adequate primary healthcare infrastructure. Campaigns can reach communities that lack access to routine services, but donors must be persuaded to invest not only in campaigns but also in strengthening the physical, human, and managerial infrastructures in those countries.[72] Poliomyelitis national immunization days are being implemented even in low-income countries, but acute flaccid paralysis surveillance lags behind, and the implementation of national campaigns in countries affected by civil conflict is a major challenge. Hepatitis B vaccine, which was to have been introduced in all highly endemic countries by 1997, is available in only a minority. Immunization services that are already highly cost-effective will become increasingly so as new vaccines are developed that can be delivered with use of the same contacts. Mobilizing governments in industrialized countries to help developing countries profit fully from these vaccines is a major challenge for public health professionals throughout the world.

Despite decades of sustained progress through development and targeted health interventions, 5 of the 10 leading causes of death are still communicable or perinatal disorders.[11] Further reduction of mortality from these conditions must remain one of the principal priorities for global public health action. The challenge for the 21st century is to develop health systems and services that are proactive and holistic.[267] The challenge for policymakers of immunization programs is to continue to expand services in ways that contribute to the development of comprehensive and sustainable health systems in the countries that need them most.

Acknowledgment

The authors thank Dr. Ana Maria Henao-Restrepo for assistance in compiling data from the World Health Organization.

REFERENCES

1. Henderson RH. Vaccination: Successes and challenges. In Cutts FT, Smith PG (eds). Vaccination and World Health. Chichester, England, John Wiley & Sons, 1995, pp 3–16.
2. Jamison DT, Saxenian H. Investing in immunization: Conclusions from the 1993 World Development Report. In Cutts FT, Smith PG (eds). Vaccination and World Health. Chichester, England, John Wiley & Sons, 1995, pp 145–160.
3. Expanded Programme on Immunization (EPI). Progress towards the global eradication of poliomyelitis, 1996. Wkly Epidemiol Rec 72:189–194, 1997.
4. Hardy I, Dittmann S, Sutter R. Current situation and control strategies for resurgence of diphtheria in newly independent states of the former Soviet Union. Lancet 347:1739–1744, 1996.
5. Rakhmanova A, Lumio J, Groundstroem K, et al. Diphtheria outbreak in St Petersburg: Clinical characteristics of 1860 adult patients. Scand J Infect Dis 28:37–40, 1996.
6. Galazka A, Robertson S, Oblapenko G. Resurgence of diphtheria. Eur J Epidemiol 11:95–105, 1995.
7. Galazka A, Robertson S. Diphtheria: Changing patterns in the developing world and the industrialized world. Eur J Epidemiol 11:107–117, 1995.
8. Roisin A. La fièvre jaune, une maladie toujours d'actualité en Afrique. Cah Sante 4:201–202, 1994.
9. Robertson SE, Hull BP, Tomori O, et al. Yellow fever, a decade of reemergence. JAMA 276:1157–1162, 1996.
10. Murray CJD, Lopez AD. Global Comparative Assessments in the Health Sector. Disease Burden, Expenditures and Intervention Packages. Geneva, World Health Organization, 1994, pp 1–196.
11. Murray CJL, Lopez AD. Mortality by cause for eight regions of the world: Global Burden of Disease study. Lancet 349:1269–1276, 1997.
12. Chunharas S. The role of epidemiology in the development of a vaccination programme. Discussion. In Cutts FT, Smith PG (eds). Vaccination and World Health. Chichester, England, John Wiley & Sons, 1995, pp 138–144.
13. Atkinson S, Cheyne J. Immunisation in urban areas: Issues and strategies. Bull World Health Organ 72:183–194, 1994.
14. Keja K, Chan C, Hayden G, Henderson RH. Expanded Programme on Immunization. World Health Stat Q 41:59–63, 1988.
15. Begg N, Cutts FT. The role of epidemiology in the development of a vaccination programme. In Cutts FT, Smith PG (eds). Vaccination and World Health. Chichester, England, John Wiley & Sons, 1995, pp 123–138.
16. Dowdle WR, Hopkins DR. The Eradication of Infectious Diseases. Dahlem Workshop Report. Chichester, England, John Wiley & Sons, 1998.
17. Centers for Disease Control and Prevention. Recommendations of the International Task Force for Disease Eradication. MMWR Morb Mortal Wkly Rep 42(RR-16):1–38, 1993.
18. Global Programme for Vaccines and Immunization, Expanded Programme on Immunization. Immunization Policy. WHO/EPI/GEN/95.03.REV.1, 1996.
19. Expanded Programme on Immunization. The Immunological Basis for Immunization. Module 1: General Immunology (A. Galazka); Module 2: Diphtheria (A. Galazka); Module 3: Tetanus (A. Galazka); Module 4: Pertussis (A. Galazka); Module 5: Tuberculosis (J. Milstien); Module 6: Poliomyelitis (S. Robertson); Module 7: Measles (F. Cutts); Module 8: Yellow Fever (S. Robertson). WHO documents WHO/EPI/GEN/93.12–93.19, 1993.
20. Galazka A, Robertson S. Immunization against diphtheria with special emphasis on immunization of adults. Vaccine 14:845–857, 1996.
21. Prempree P, Chitpitaklert S, Silarug N. Diphtheria outbreak—Saraburi province, Thailand. MMWR Morb Mortal Wkly Rep 45:271–273, 1996.
22. Khuri-Bulos N, Hamzah Y, Sammerrai S, et al. The changing epidemiology of diphtheria in Jordan. Bull World Health Organ 66:65–68, 1988.
23. Youwang Y, Jianming D, Yong X, Pong Z. Epidemiological features of an outbreak of diphtheria and its control with diphtheria toxoid immunization. Int J Epidemiol 21:807–811, 1992.
24. Cherry J. Acellular pertussis vaccines—a solution to the pertussis problem. J Infect Dis 168:21–24, 1993.
25. Cherry J. Pertussis: The trials and tribulations of old and new pertussis vaccines. Vaccine 10:1033–1038, 1992.
26. Edwards K. Acellular pertussis vaccines—a solution to the pertussis problem? J Infect Dis 168:15–20, 1993.
27. Comstock GW, Livesay VT, Woolpert SF. Evaluation of BCG vaccination among Puerto Rican children. Am J Public Health 64:283–291, 1974.
28. Kubit S, Czajka S, Olakowska T, Piasecki Z. Evaluation of the effectiveness of BCG vaccinations. Pediatr Pol 47:777–781, 1983.
29. Lugosi L. Analysis of the efficacy of mass BCG vaccination from 1959 to 1983 in tuberculosis control in Hungary. Bull Int Union Tuberc 16:15–34, 1987.
30. Fine P, Clayton D. Randomised controlled trial of single BCG, repeated BCG, or combined BCG and killed *Mycobacteruim leprae* vaccine for prevention of leprosy and tuberculosis in Malawi. Lancet 348:17–24, 1996.
31. Global Tuberculosis Programme and Global Programme on Vaccines. Statement on BCG revaccination for the prevention of tuberculosis. Wkly Epidemiol Rec 70:229–231, 1995.
32. Cutts FT, Monteiro O, Tabard P, Cliff J. Measles control in Maputo, Mozambique, using a single dose of Schwarz vaccine at age 9 months. Bull World Health Organ 72:227–231, 1994.
33. Markowitz LE, Preblud SR, Fine PEM, Orenstein WA. Duration of live measles vaccine–induced immunity. Pediatr Infect Dis J 9:101–110, 1990.
34. de Quadros CA. Strategies for disease control/elimination in the Americas. In Cutts FT, Smith PG (eds). Vaccination and World Health. Chichester, England, John Wiley & Sons, 1995, pp 17–34.
35. Expanded Programme on Immunization. Heat stability of vaccines. Wkly Epidemiol Rec 55:252–254, 1980.
36. Expanded Programme on Immunization. Stability of vaccines. Wkly Epidemiol Rec 30:233–235, 1990.
37. Lundbeck H, Hakansson B, Lloyd JS, et al. A cold box for the transport and storage of vaccines. Bull World Health Organ 56:427–432, 1978.
38. Expanded Programme on Immunization. Ice-lined refrigerators (ILR). Wkly Epidemiol Rec 59:63–64, 1984.
39. The cold chain for vaccine conservation: Recent improvements. WHO Chronicle 33:383–386, 1979.
40. World Health Organization, UNICEF. Product Information Sheets 1993/1994 (10th ed). Geneva, World Health Organization, 1993. WHO/UNICEF/EPI TS/93 1, 1993.
41. Expanded Programme on Immunization. Vaccine cold chain management indicators. Wkly Epidemiol Rec 55:145–147, 1980.
42. Zaffran M. Vaccine transport and storage: Environmental challenges. Dev Biol Stand 87:9–17, 1996.
43. Expanded Programme on Immunization. The use of open vials of vaccines in subsequent immunization sessions. World Health Organization Policy Statement. WHO/EPI/LHIS/95.01, 1995.
44. Expanded Programme on Immunization. Vaccine vial monitor and open vial policy. Questions and answers. WHO/EPI/LHIS/95.01, 1995.
45. Fine PEM. Herd immunity: History, theory, practice. Epidemiol Rev 15:265–302, 1993.
46. Hull D. Why children are not immunized. J R Coll Physicians Lond 21:28–31, 1987.
47. Cutts F, Orenstein W, Bernier R. Causes of low preschool immunization coverage in the United States. Annu Rev Public Health 13:385–398, 1992.
48. Foster SO. Immunization in 12 African countries 1982–1993. Centers for Disease Control; Africa Child Survival Initia-

tive—Combatting Childhood Communicable Diseases; USAID, WHO, UNICEF, 1993.

49. Foster S. Immunization opportunities taken and missed. Rev Infect Dis 11:S629–S630, 1989.
50. Poore P. A global view of immunization. J Roy Coll Physicians Lond 21:22–28, 1987.
51. Cutts F, Soares A, Jecque A, et al. The use of evaluation to improve the Expanded Programme on Immunization in Mozambique. Bull World Health Organ 68:199–208, 1990.
52. Hutchins S, Jansen H, Robertson S, et al. Studies of missed opportunities for immunization in developing and industrialized countries. Bull World Health Organ 71:549–560, 1993.
53. Expanded Programme on Immunization. Training for mid level managers. Identify missed opportunities. Geneva, World Health Organization. WHO/EPI/MLM/91.7, 1991.
54. Walley JD, McDonald M. Integration of mother and child health services in Ethiopia. Trop Doct 215:32–35, 1991.
55. Tandon B, Gandhi N. Immunization coverage in India for areas served by the Integrated Child Development Services programme. Bull World Health Organ 70:461–465, 1992.
56. Levy-Bruhl D, Soucat A, Diallo S, et al. Integration du PEV aux soins de santé primaires: l'Exemple du Benin et de la Guinée. Cah Santé 4:205–212, 1994.
57. John TJ, Steinhoff MC. Appropriate strategy for immunization of children in India. 3. Community-based annual pulse (cluster) immunization. Indian J Pediatr 48:677–683, 1981.
58. Cutts FT, Kortbeek S, Malalane R, et al. Developing appropriate strategies for EPI: A case study from Mozambique. H Pol Plann 3:291–301, 1988.
59. Foster SO, Spiegel RA, Mokdad A, et al. Immunization, oral rehydration therapy and malaria chemotherapy among children under 5 in Borni and Grand Cape Mount counties, Liberia, 1984 and 1988. Int J Epidemiol 22(suppl 1):S50–S55, 1993.
60. John TJ, Ray M, Steinhoff MC. Control of measles by annual pulse immunization. Am J Dis Child 138:299–300, 1984.
61. Gindler J, Cutts FT, Barnett-Antinori ME, et al. Successes and failures in vaccine delivery: Evaluation of the immunization delivery system in Puerto Rico. Pediatrics 91:315–320, 1993.
62. Malison MD, Sekeito P, Henderson PL, et al. Estimating health service utilization, immunization coverage, and childhood mortality: A new approach in Uganda. Bull World Health Organ 65:325–330, 1987.
63. Auer C, Tanner M. Childhood vaccination in a squatter area of Manila: Coverage and providers. Soc Sci Med 31:1265–1270, 1990.
64. Cutts F. Strategies to improve immunization services in urban Africa. Bull World Health Organ 69:407–414, 1991.
65. Kearney M, Yach D, van Dyk H, Fisher S. Evaluation of a mass measles immunisation campaign in a rapidly growing peri-urban area. S Afr Med J 74:157–159, 1989.
66. Fassin D, Jeannee E, Cebe D, Reveillon M. Who consults and where? Sociocultural differentiation in access to health care in urban Africa. Int J Epidemiol 17:858–864, 1988.
67. Fassin D, Jeannee E. Immunization coverage and social differentiation in urban Senegal. Am J Public Health 79:509–511, 1989.
68. Cutts F, Phillips M, Kortbeek S, Soares A. Door-to-door canvassing for immunization program acceleration in Mozambique: Achievements and costs. Int J Health Serv 20:717–725, 1990.
69. Romero MGG, Pizano ES, Lamo JA. Channelling, a new immunization strategy. Assoc Children 69/72:193–203, 1985.
70. Saeed H. Increasing vaccine coverage through new delivery systems: A Sudan approach. Rev Infect Dis 11:S644–S645, 1989.
71. Dietz V, Cutts F. The use of mass campaigns in the Expanded Programme on Immunization: A review of reported advantages and disadvantages. Int J Health Serv 27:767–790, 1997.
72. Pan American Health Organization. The impact of the Expanded Programme on Immunization and the polio eradication initiative on health systems in the Americas. Washington, DC, March 1995.
73. Taylor ME, Laforce FM, Basu RN, et al. Sustainability of achievements: Lessons learned from Universal Child Immunization. Report of a steering committee. New York, UNICEF, 1996, p 105.
74. Unger J-P. Can intensive campaigns dynamize front line health services? The evaluation of an immunization campaign in Thies health district, Senegal. Soc Sci Med 32:249–259, 1991.
75. Unger J-P, Killingsworth JR. Selective primary health care: A critical review of methods and results. Soc Sci Med 22:1001–1013, 1986.
76. Seaman J, Poore P. Good intentions, unfortunate consequences [letter]. Lancet 2:1334, 1987.
77. Poore P, Cutts F, Seaman J. Universal childhood immunisation: Is it sustainable? [letter] Lancet 341:58, 1993.
78. LaFond AK. When the money runs out. Lancet 343:371, 1994.
79. Waddington C, Goodman H. Does economic analysis affect vaccination policy? In Cutts FT, Smith PG (eds). Vaccination and World Health. Chichester, England, John Wiley & Sons, 1995, pp 163–173.
80. Banerji D. Hidden menace in the universal child immunization program. Int J Health Serv 18:293–299, 1988.
81. Cutts FT, Glik DC, Gordon A, et al. Application of multiple methods to study the immunization programme in an urban area of Guinea. Bull World Health Organ 68:769–776, 1990.
82. Godlee F. WHO's Special Program. Undermining from above. BMJ 310:178–182, 1995.
83. du Lou AD, Pison G. Barriers to universal child immunization in rural Senegal 5 years after the accelerated Expanded Programme on Immunization. Bull World Health Organ 72:751–759, 1994.
84. Bryce JW, Cutts FT, Saba S. Mass immunization campaigns and quality of immunization services. Lancet 335:739–740, 1990.
85. Anan A. India: Unhealthy immunization programme. Lancet 341:1402–1403, 1993.
86. Reid R. Political, economic, and administrative resources available for the control of vaccine-preventable diseases. Rev Infect Dis 11:S655–S658, 1989.
87. Williams G. Immunization in Nicaragua [letter]. Lancet 2:780, 1985.
88. Bassole A. Mobilisation générale en faveur de la "vaccination commando." Hygie 5:31–34, 1986.
89. Lasso HP, de Restrepo V, Munoz R. Influencia de los medios de comunicacion masiva en la cobertura de una campana de vacunacion. Bull Pan Am Health Organ 101:39–46, 1986.
90. Tweneboa-Kodua A, Obeng-Quaidoo I, Abu K. Ghana social mobilization analysis. Health Educ Q 18:125–134, 1991.
91. Duque LF, de Bello PV, Bejarano J, et al. The national vaccination crusade in Colombia. Assoc Children 65/68:159–178, 1984.
92. de Quadros CA, Olive JM, Hersh BS, et al. Measles elimination in the Americas. Evolving strategies. JAMA 275:224–229, 1996.
93. Global Programme for Vaccines of the World Health Organization. Role of mass campaigns in global measles control. Lancet 344:174–175, 1994.
94. Cairncross S, Peries H, Cutts F. Vertical health programmes. Lancet 349(siii):siii20–siii22, 1997.
95. Murugasampillay S. Who determines national health policies? In Cutts FT, Smith PG (eds). Vaccination and World Health. Chichester, England, John Wiley & Sons, 1995, pp 195–205.
96. Ndumbe PM. Do vaccines reach those who most need them? Cameroon. In Cutts FT, Smith PG (eds). Vaccination and World Health. Chichester, England, John Wiley & Sons, 1995, pp 225–238.
97. Chen L, Cash R. A decade after Alma Ata—can primary health care lead to health for all? N Engl J Med 319:946–947, 1988.
98. Expanded Programme on Immunization. Global Advisory Group—part I. Wkly Epidemiol Rec 3:11–15, 1992.
99. de Quadros CA, Andrus JK, Olive JM, de Macedo GC. Polio eradication from the Western Hemisphere. Annu Rev Public Health 13:239–252, 1992.
100. World Health Organization. Global eradication of poliomyelitis by the year 2000. Wkly Epidemiol Rec 63:161–162, 1988.
101. Hull HF, Ward NA, Hull BP, et al. Paralytic poliomyelitis: Seasoned strategies, disappearing disease. Lancet 343:1331–1337, 1994.
102. Expanded Programme on Immunization (EPI). Update: Progress towards poliomyelitis eradication, WHO South-East Asia Region, 1995–1997. Wkly Epidemiol Rec 72:157–162, 1997.
103. Centers for Disease Control. Measles eradication: Recommendations from a meeting cosponsored by the World Health Organization, the Pan American Health Organization, and CDC. MMWR Morb Mortal Wkly Rep 46(RR11):1–20, 1997.
104. Ramsay M, Gay N, Miller E, et al. The epidemiology of measles

in England and Wales: Rationale for the 1994 national vaccination campaign. Commun Dis Rep CDR Rev 4(R12):R141–R146, 1994.
105. Expanded Programme on Immunization. Progress towards measles elimination. Canada. Wkly Epidemiol Rec 72:223–226, 1997.
106. Tobias M, Christie S, Mansoor O. Predicting the next measles epidemic. New Zealand Public Health Report 4(1), 1997.
107. Pan American Health Organization. Special Programme for Vaccines and Immunization. Measles surveillance in the Americas. Weekly Bulletin 3(18), 1997.
108. Gay N, Ramsay M, Cohen B, et al. The epidemiology of measles in England and Wales since the 1994 vaccination campaign. Commun Dis Rep CDR Rev 7(R2):R17–R21, 1997.
109. Varughese P. Measles in Canada, 1996–1997 (as of February 15, 1997). Health Canada, Measles update 1(1), April 1997.
110. World Health Organization. WHA42 32. Forty-Second World Health Assembly; Geneva; May 8–19, 1989.
111. Henderson DA. Principles and lessons from the smallpox eradication programme. Bull World Health Organ 65:535–546, 1987.
112. Henderson R, Keja J. Global control of vaccine-preventable diseases: How progress can be evaluated. Rev Infect Dis 11:S649–S654, 1989.
113. Begg N, Gill O, White J. COVER (Cover of Vaccination Evaluated Rapidly): Description of the England and Wales scheme. Public Health 103:81–89, 1989.
114. Borgdorff MW, Walker GJA. Estimating vaccination coverage: Routine information or sample survey? J Trop Med Hyg 91:35–42, 1988.
115. Henderson RH, Sundaresan T. Cluster sampling to assess immunization coverage: A review of experience with a simplified sampling method. Bull World Health Organ 60:253–260, 1982.
116. Serfling RE, Cornell RG, Sherman IL. The CDC quota sampling technique with results of 1959 poliomyelitis vaccination surveys. Am J Public Health 50:1847–1857, 1960.
117. Bennett S, Woods T, Liyanage WM, Smith DL. A simplified general method for cluster-sample surveys of health in developing countries. World Health Stat Q 44:98–106, 1991.
118. Lemeshow S, Robinson D. Surveys to measure programme coverage and impact: A review of the methodology used by the Expanded Programme on Immunization. World Health Stat Q 38:65–75, 1985.
119. Lemeshow S, Tserkovnyi AG, Tulloch JL, et al. A computer simulation of the EPI survey strategy. Int J Epidemiol 14:473–481, 1985.
120. Lwanga SK, Abiprojo N. Immunization coverage surveys: Methodological studies in Indonesia. Bull World Health Organ 65:847–853, 1987.
121. Valadez JJ, Weld LH. Maternal recall error of child vaccination status in a developing nation. Am J Public Health 82:120–122, 1992.
122. Gareaballah ET, Loevinsohn BP. The accuracy of mothers' reports about their children's vaccination status. Bull World Health Organ 67:669–674, 1989.
123. Cutts FT, Zell ER, Soares AC, Diallo S. Obstacles to achieving immunization for all 2000: Missed immunization opportunities and inappropriately timed immunization. J Trop Pediatr 37:153–158, 1991.
124. Desve G. Les outils informatiques utilisés dans le PEV. Cah Santé 4:143–144, 1994.
125. Friede A, Waternaux C, Guyer B, et al. An epidemiological assessment of immunization programme participation in the Philippines. Int J Epidemiol 14:135–142, 1985.
126. Brugha F, Kevany J, Swan A. An investigation of the role of fathers in immunization uptake. Int J Epidemiol 25:840–845, 1996.
127. Brugha R, Kevany J. Maximizing immunization coverage through home visits: A controlled trial in an urban area of Ghana. Bull World Health Organ 74:18–20, 1996.
128. Cutts FT, Rodrigues LC, Colombo S, Bennett S. Evaluation of factors influencing vaccine uptake in Mozambique. Int J Epidemiol 18:427–433, 1989.
129. Cliff J, Cutts F, Waldman R. Using surveys in Mozambique for evaluation of diarrhoeal disease control. H Pol Plann 5:219–225, 1990.
130. Bryce J, Toole M, Waldman R, Voigt A. Assessing the quality of facility-based child survival services. H Pol Plann 7:155–163, 1992.
131. Global Programme for Vaccines and Immunization. Vaccine research and development. Monitoring immunization services using the Lot Quality Technique. WHO/VRD/TRAM/96.01, 1996.
132. Cutts F, Othepa O, Vernon A, et al. Measles control in Kinshasa, Zaire improved with high coverage and use of medium titre Edmonston Zagreb vaccine at age 6 months. Int J Epidemiol 23:624–631, 1994.
133. Lanata CF, Stroh G, Black RE, Gonzales H. An evaluation of lot quality assurance sampling to monitor and improve immunization coverage. Int J Epidemiol 19:1086–1090, 1990.
134. Rosero-Bixby L, Grimaldo C, Raabe C. Monitoring a primary health care programme with lot quality assurance sampling: Costa Rica, 1987. H Pol Plann 5:30–39, 1990.
135. Lanata CF, Black RE. Lot quality assurance sampling techniques in health surveys in developing countries: Advantage and current constraints. World Health Stat Q 44:133–139, 1991.
136. Hall AJ, Aaby P. Tropical trials and tribulations. Int J Epidemiol 19:777–781, 1990.
137. Clemens JD, Stanton BF, Chakraborty J, et al. Measles vaccination and childhood mortality in rural Bangladesh. Am J Epidemiol 128:1330–1339, 1988.
138. Aaby P, Samb B, Simondon F, et al. Non-specific beneficial effect of measles immunization: Analysis of mortality studies from developing countries. BMJ 311:481–485, 1995.
139. Garenne M, Leroy O, Beau J-P, Sene I. Child mortality after high-titre measles vaccines: Prospective study in Senegal. Lancet 338:903–907, 1991.
140. Orenstein WA, Bernier RH, Dondero TJ, et al. Field evaluation of vaccine efficacy. Bull World Health Organ 63:1055–1068, 1985.
141. Orenstein WA, Bernier RH, Hinman AR. Assessing vaccine efficacy in the field: Further observations. Epidemiol Rev 10:212–241, 1988.
142. Cutts FT, Smith PG, Colombo S, et al. Field evaluation of measles vaccine efficacy in Mozambique. Am J Epidemiol 131:349–355, 1990.
143. Hull HF, Williams PJ, Oldfield F. Measles mortality and vaccine efficacy in rural West Africa. Lancet 1:972–975, 1983.
144. McCormick JB, Halsey N, Rosenberg R. Measles vaccine efficacy determined from secondary attack rates during a severe epidemic. J Pediatr 90:13–16, 1977.
145. Top FH. Measles in Detroit, 1935. Factors influencing the secondary attack rate among susceptibles at risk. Am J Public Health 28:935–943, 1938.
146. Clarkson JA, Fine PEM. An assessment of methods for routine local monitoring of vaccine efficacy, with particular reference to measles and pertussis. Epidemiol Infect 99:485–499, 1987.
147. Wassilak SGF, Orenstein WA, Strickland PL, et al. Continuing measles transmission in students despite a school-based outbreak control program. Am J Epidemiol 122:208–217, 1985.
148. Cutts F, Brown D. The contribution of field tests to measles surveillance and control: A review of available methods. Rev Med Virol 5:35–40, 1995.
149. Dietz VJ, Nieburg P, Gubler DJ, Gomez I. Diagnosis of measles by clinical case definition in dengue-endemic areas: Implications for measles surveillance and control. Bull World Health Organ 70:745–750, 1992.
150. Sharma RS, Chawla U, Datta KK. Field evaluation of measles vaccine efficacy in Najafgarh Zone of Delhi. J Commun Dis 20:38–43, 1988.
151. Hlady G, Bennett J, Samadi A, et al. Neonatal tetanus in rural Bangladesh: Risk factors and toxoid efficacy. Am J Public Health 82:1354–1369, 1992.
152. Brown J, Djogdom P, Murphy K, et al. Identifying the reasons for low immunization coverage—a case study of Yaounde (United Republic of Cameroon). Rev Epidemiol Sante Publique 30:35–47, 1982.
153. Joseph A, Abraham S, Bhattacharji S, et al. Improving immunization coverage. World Health Forum 9:336–340, 1988.
154. Heggenhougen K, Clements J. Acceptability of childhood immunization. Social science perspectives. A study supported by the Expanded Programme on Immunization, World Health Organi-

zation. Evaluation and Planning Centre, London School of Hygiene and Tropical Medicine. EPC Publication No. 14, 1987.
155. Pillsbury B. Immunization: The Behavioural Issues. Washington, DC, The Office of Health, US Agency for International Development, Behavioural Issues in Child Survival Programs. Monograph 3, 1990.
156. Eng E, Naimoli J, Naimoli G, et al. The acceptability of childhood immunization to Togolese mothers: A sociobehavioral perspective. Health Educ Q 18:97–110, 1991.
157. Coreil J, Augustin A, Holt E, Halsey N. Use of ethnographic research for instrument development in a case-control study of immunization use in Haiti. Int J Epidemiol 18:S33–S37, 1989.
158. Glik D, Gordon A, Ward W, et al. Focus group methods for formative research in child survival: An Ivoirian example. Int Q Community Health Educ 8:297–316, 1987.
159. Belcher D, Nicholas D, Ofosu-Amaah S, Wurapa F. A mass immunization campaign in rural Ghana—factors affecting participation. Public Health Rep 93:170–176, 1978.
160. Cutts FT, Diallo S, Zell ER, Rhodes P. Determinants of vaccination in an urban population in Conakry, Guinea. Int J Epidemiol 20:1099–1106, 1991.
161. Selwyn BJ. An epidemiological approach to the study of users and non-users of child health services. Am J Public Health 68:231–235, 1978.
162. Zeitlyn S, Mahmudur Rahman A, Nielsen B, et al. Compliance with diphtheria, tetanus, and pertussis immunisation in Bangladesh: Factors identifying high risk groups. BMJ 304:606–609, 1992.
163. van Zwanenberg T, Hull C. Improving immunisation coverage in a province in Papua New Guinea. BMJ 296:1654–1656, 1988.
164. Zimicki S, Hornik RC, Verzosa CC, et al. Improving vaccination coverage in urban areas through a health communication campaign: The 1990 Philippine experience. Bull World Health Organ 72:409–422, 1994.
165. Brugha R, Kevany J. Immunization determinants in the Eastern Region of Ghana. H Pol Plann 10:312–318, 1995.
166. Cleland J, van Genneken J. Maternal education and child survival in developing countries: The search for pathways of influence. Soc Sci Med 27:1357–1368, 1988.
167. Streatfield K, Singarimbun M, Diamond I. Maternal education and child immunization. Demography 27:447–455, 1990.
168. Bhuiya A, Bhuiya I, Chowdhury M. Factors affecting acceptance of immunization among children in rural Bangladesh. H Pol Plann 10:304–311, 1995.
169. Sathe P, Shah U. Parental participation in poliovaccination programme. Indian J Public Health 9:107–110, 1965.
170. Akesode FA. Factors affecting the use of primary health care clinics for children. J Epidemiol Community Health 36:310–314, 1982.
171. Streatfield K, Singarimbun M. Social factors affecting the use of immunization in Indonesia. Soc Sci Med 27:1237–1245, 1988.
172. Henderson RH, David H, Eddins DL, Foege WH. Assessment of vaccination coverage, vaccination scar rates, and smallpox scarring in five areas of West Africa. Bull World Health Organ 48:183–194, 1973.
173. Hingson R. The impact of health beliefs on behavior during an immunization program in rural Haiti, 1972. Health Educ Monogr 2:505–507, 1974.
174. Ulin P, Ulin R. The use and non-use of preventive health services in a Southern African village. Int J Health Educ 24:45–53, 1981.
175. Expanded Programme on Immunization. Community participation and immunization coverage. Wkly Epidemiol Rec 59:117–124, 1984.
176. Lin N, Hingson R, Allwood-Paredes JA. Mass immunization campaign in El Salvador: Evaluation of receptivity and recommendation for future campaigns. Health Rep 86:1112–1121, 1971.
177. Bonilla JEZ, Gamarra JIM, Booth EM. Bridging the communication gap—how mothers in Honduras perceive immunization. Assoc Children 69/72:443–454, 1985.
178. Milstien J, Griffin PD, Lee J-W. Damage to immunization programmes from misinformation on contraceptive vaccines. Reproductive Health Matters 6:24–28, 1996.
179. Kroeger A, Franken H. The educational value of participatory evaluation of primary health care programmes: An experience with four indigenous populations in Ecuador. Soc Sci Med 15:535–539, 1981.
180. Kroeger A. Participatory evaluation of primary health care programmes: An experience with four Indian populations in Ecuador. Trop Doct 12:38–43, 1982.
181. de Quadros CA, Andrus JK, Olive J-M, et al. Eradication of poliomyelitis: Progress in the Americas. Pediatr Infect Dis J 10:222–229, 1991.
182. Cutts FT, Henderson RH, Clements CJ, et al. Principles of measles control. Bull World Health Organ 69:1–7, 1991.
183. Kettles AN. Differences in trends of measles notifications by age and race in the western Cape, 1982–1986. S Afr Med J 72:317–320, 1987.
184. Expanded Programme on Immunization. Poliomyelitis surveillance. Wkly Epidemiol Rec 66:81–88, 1991.
185. Cutts FT, Waldman RJ, Zoffman HMD. Surveillance for the Expanded Programme on Immunization. Bull World Health Organ 71:633–639, 1993.
186. Laforce FM, Lichnevski MS, Keja J, Henderson RH. Clinical survey techniques to estimate prevalence and annual incidence of poliomyelitis in developing countries. Bull World Health Organ 58:609–620, 1980.
187. Galazka A, Stroh G. Neonatal tetanus. Guidelines on the community-based survey on neonatal tetanus mortality. WHO/EPI/GEN/86/8, 1986.
188. Goh KT. Hepatitis B immunization in Singapore. Lancet 348:1385–1386, 1996.
189. Frerichs RR. Simple analytic procedures for rapid microcomputer-assisted cluster surveys in developing countries. Public Health Rep 104:24–35, 1989.
190. Hull BP, Dowdle WR. Poliovirus surveillance: Building the global laboratory network. J Infect Dis 175(suppl 1):S113–S116, 1997.
191. Expanded Programme on Immunization (EPI). Poliomyelitis eradication: The WHO Global Laboratory Network. Wkly Epidemiol Rec 72:245–249, 1997.
192. Gay NJ, Hesketh LM, Morgan-Capner P, Miller E. Interpretation of serological surveillance data for measles using mathematical models: Implications for vaccine strategy. Epidemiol Infect 115:139–156, 1995.
193. Morgan-Capner P, Wright J, Miller CL, Miller E. Surveillance of antibody to measles, mumps, and rubella by age. BMJ 297:770–772, 1989.
194. Cutts F, Nokes D. Immunization in the developing world: Strategic challenges. Trans R Soc Trop Med Hyg 87:353–354, 398, 1993.
195. Parry J, Perry K, Mortimer P. Sensitive assays for viral antibodies in saliva: An alternative to tests on serum. Lancet 2:72–75, 1987.
196. Perry K, Brown D, Parry J, et al. Detection of measles, mumps, and rubella antibodies in saliva using antibody capture radioimmunoassay. J Med Virol 40:235–240, 1993.
197. Ramsay M, Brugha R, Brown D. Surveillance of measles in England and Wales: Implications of a national saliva testing programme. Bull World Health Organ 75:515–521, 1997.
198. Azevedo-Neto RS, Silveira ASB, Nokes DJ, et al. Rubella seroepidemiology in a non-immunized population of São Paulo State, Brazil. Epidemiol Infect 113:161–173, 1994.
199. Massad E, Burattini MN, Azevedo-Neto RS, et al. A model-based design of a vaccination strategy against rubella in a non-immunized community of São Paulo State, Brazil. Epidemiol Infect 112:579–594, 1994.
200. Grenfell BT, Anderson RM. The estimation of age-related rates of infection from case notifications and serological data. J Hyg (Camb) 95:419–436, 1985.
201. Centers for Disease Control and Prevention. Poliomyelitis prevention in the United States: Introduction of a sequential vaccination schedule of inactivated poliovirus vaccine followed by oral poliovirus vaccine. MMWR Morb Mortal Wkly Rep 46(RR-3):1–25, 1997.
202. World Health Organization. Vaccine supply and quality. Surveillance of adverse events following immunization. Wkly Epidemiol Rec 71:237–241, 1996.
203. Expanded Programme on Immunization. BCG-associated lymphadenitis in infants. Wkly Epidemiol Rec 48:371–373, 1989.
204. Praveen KN, Smikle MF, Prabhakar P, et al. Outbreak of bacillus

Calmette-Guérin–associated lymphadenitis and abscesses in Jamaican children. Pediatr Infect Dis J 9:890–893, 1990.

205. Expanded Programme on Immunization. Lymphadenitis associated with BCG immunization. Mozambique. Wkly Epidemiol Rec 63:381–383, 1988.
206. Abdullah MA, Adam KA, Shagla A, Mahgoub. BCG lymphadenitis: A report of eight cases. Ann Trop Paediatr 5:77–81, 1985.
207. Helmick CG. An outbreak of severe BCG axillary lymphadenitis in Saint Lucia, 1982–83. West Indian Med J 35:12–17, 1986.
208. Expanded Programme on Immunization. Surveillance of adverse events following immunization: Field guide for managers of immunization programmes. Geneva, World Health Organization. WHO/EPI/TRAM/93.2, 1993.
209. World Bank. World Development Report 1993. Investing in Health. Oxford, Oxford University Press, 1993, pp 1–329.
210. Bart KJ, Foulds J, Patriarca P. Global eradication of poliomyelitis: Benefit-cost analysis. Bull World Health Organ 74:35–45, 1996.
211. Creese A. Cost effectiveness of alternative strategies for poliomyelitis immunization in Brazil. Rev Infect Dis 6:S404–S407, 1984.
212. Creese A, Dominguez-Uga M. Cost-effectiveness of immunization programs in Colombia. Bull Pan Am Health Organ 21:377–394, 1987.
213. Creese A, Sriyabbaya N, Casabal G, Wiseso G. Cost-effectiveness appraisal of immunization programmes. Bull World Health Organ 60:621–632, 1982.
214. Rosenthal G. The economic burden of sustainable EPI. Implications for donor policy. Resources for Child Health (REACH) project, 1990.
215. Shepard DS, Robertson RL, Cameron CSM III, et al. Cost-effectiveness of routine and campaign vaccination strategies in Ecuador. Bull World Health Organ 67:649–662, 1989.
216. Robertson R, Davis J, Jobe K. Service volume and other factors affecting the costs of immunizations in the Gambia. Bull World Health Organ 62:729–736, 1984.
217. Waddington C, Kello A, Wirakartakusumah D, et al. Financial information at district level: Experiences from five countries. H Pol Plann 4:207–218, 1989.
218. Anderson RM, May RM. Directly transmitted infectious diseases: Control by vaccination. Science 215:1053–1060, 1982.
219. Nokes DJ, Anderson RM. Application of mathematical models to the design of immunization strategies. Rev Med Microbiol 4:1–7, 1993.
220. McLean AR, Anderson RM. Measles in developing countries. Part II. The predicted impact of mass vaccination. Epidemiol Infect 100:419–441, 1987.
221. Fine PEM. The contribution of modeling to vaccination policy. In Cutts FT, Smith PG (eds). Vaccination and World Health. Chichester, England, John Wiley & Sons, 1995, pp 177–192.
222. McLean AR, Anderson RM. Measles in developing countries. Part I. Epidemiological parameters and patterns. Epidemiol Infect 100:111–133, 1988.
223. Foster SO, McFarland DA, John AM. Measles. In Jamison DT, Mosley WH, Measham AR, Bobadilla JL (eds). Disease Control Priorities in Developing Countries. New York, Oxford University Press, 1993, pp 161–187.
224. Anderson RM, May RM. Infectious Diseases of Humans: Dynamics and Control. Oxford, UK, Oxford University Press, 1991.
225. Anderson RM, May RM. Vaccination against rubella and measles: Quantitative investigations of different policies. J Hyg (Camb) 90:259–325, 1983.
226. Knox EG. Theoretical aspects of rubella vaccination strategies. Rev Infect Dis 7:S194–S198, 1985.
227. Massad E, Azevedo-Neto RS, Burattini MN, et al. Assessing the efficacy of a mixed vaccination strategy against rubella in São Paulo, Brazil. Int J Epidemiol 24:842–850, 1995.
228. Nokes DJ, Swinton J. The control of childhood viral infections by pulse vaccination. IMA J Math Appl Med Biol 12:29–53, 1995.
229. Anderson RM. The concept of herd immunity and the design of community-based immunization programmes. Vaccine 10:928–935, 1992.
230. Kim-Farley R and the Expanded Programme on Immunization team. Global immunization. Annu Rev Public Health 13:223–237, 1992.
231. Kane MA, Clements J, Hu D. Hepatitis B. In Jamison DT, Mosley WH, Measham AR, Bobadilla J (eds). Disease Control Priorities in Developing Countries. New York, Oxford University Press, 1993, pp 321–330.
232. Van Damme P, Kane M, Meheus A. Integration of hepatitis B vaccination into national immunization programmes. BMJ 314:1033–1037, 1997.
233. Expanded Programme on Immunization (EPI). Inclusion of yellow fever vaccine in the EPI. Wkly Epidemiol Rec 71:181–188, 1996.
234. Global Programme for Vaccines and Immunization. Progress of Vaccine Research and Development and Plan of Activities—1996. Geneva, World Health Organization, 1996, 45–47.
235. Expanded Programme on Immunization. Meeting on advances in measles elimination: Conclusions and recommendations. Wkly Epidemiol Rec 71:305–312, 1996.
236. Hopkins DR, Hinman AR, Koplan JP, Lane JM. The case for global measles eradication. Lancet 1:1396–1398, 1982.
237. Peltola H, Heinonen OP, Valle M, et al. The elimination of indigenous measles, mumps, and rubella from Finland by a 12-year, two-dose vaccination program. N Engl J Med 331:1397–1402, 1994.
238. Bottiger M, Christenson B, Romanus V, et al. Swedish experience of two-dose vaccination programme aiming at eliminating measles, mumps and rubella. BMJ 295:1264–1267, 1987.
239. Communicable Disease Report. The national measles and rubella campaign—one year on. Commun Dis Rep CDR Wkly 5:237, 1995.
240. Milstien JB, Evans P, Batson A. Vaccine production and supply in developing countries. Discussion. In Cutts FT, Smith PG (eds). Vaccination and World Health. Chichester, England, John Wiley & Sons, 1995, pp 60–66.
241. Carrasco P, de Quadros C, Umstead W. EPI in the Americas benefits from revolving fund. WHO Chronicle 37:81–85, 1983.
242. Casting off vaccine supply charity—the pace quickens. CVI Forum 10:9–13, 1995.
243. World Health Organization and UNICEF. State of the World's Vaccines and Immunization. Geneva, World Health Organization, 1996, pp 1–161.
244. Dietz V, Milstien J, van Loon F, et al. Performance and potency of tetanus toxoid: Implications for eliminating neonatal tetanus. Bull World Health Organ 74:619–628, 1996.
245. The Children's Vaccine Initiative and the Global Programme for Vaccines and Immunization. Recommendations from the Scientific Advisory Group of Experts. Part II. Vaccine quality and supply. Wkly Epidemiol Rec 72:249–251, 1997.
246. Shin Seung-il, Shahi G. Vaccine production and supply in developing countries. In Cutts FT, Smith PG (eds). Vaccination and World Health. Chichester, England, John Wiley & Sons, 1995, pp 39–60.
247. Aylward B, Lloyd J, Zaffran M, et al. Reducing the risk of unsafe injections in immunization programmes: Financial and operational implications of various injection technologies. Bull World Health Organ 73:531–540, 1995.
248. Marmor M, Hartsock P. Self-destructing (non-reusable) syringes. Lancet 338:438–439, 1991.
249. Steinhoff MC. *Haemophilus influenzae* type b infections are preventable everywhere. Lancet 349:1186–1187, 1997.
250. Mulholland K, Hilton S, Adegbola R, et al. Randomised trial of *Haemophilus influenzae* type-b tetanus protein conjugate for prevention of pneumonia and meningitis in Gambian infants. Lancet 349:1191–1197, 1997.
251. Garenne M, Ronsmans C, Campbell H. The magnitude of mortality from acute respiratory infections in children under 5 years in developing countries. World Health Stat Q 45:180–191, 1992.
252. Robertson SE, Cutts FT, Samuel R, Diaz-Ortega JL. Control of rubella and congenital rubella syndrome (CRS) in developing countries, Part 2: Vaccination against rubella. Bull World Health Organ 75:69–80, 1997.
253. Cutts FT, Robertson SE, Diaz-Ortega JL, Samuel R. Control of rubella and congenital rubella syndrome (CRS) in developing countries, part 1: Burden of disease from CRS. Bull World Health Organ 75:55–68, 1997.
254. The Children's Vaccine Initiative and the Global Programme for Vaccines and Immunization. Recommendations from the Special Advisory Group of Experts. Part II. Wkly Epidemiol Rec 71:269–273, 1997.

255. Ada GL. The development of new vaccines. In Cutts FT, Smith PG (eds). Vaccination and World Health. Chichester, England, John Wiley & Sons, 1995, pp 67–80.
256. de Quadros CA, Carrasco P, Olive J-M. The desired field performance characteristics of new improved vaccines for the developing world. Int J Tech Assoc Health Care 10:1–6, 1994.
257. Department of Health. 1996 Immunisation Against Infectious Disease. London, Her Majesty's Stationery Office, 1996, pp 1–290.
258. Orenstein WA, Bernier RH. Toward immunizing every child on time. Pediatrics 94:545–547, 1994.
259. Orenstein WA, Bernier RH. Crossing the divide from vaccine technology to vaccine delivery. The critical role of providers. JAMA 272:1138–1139, 1994.
260. The Interagency Committee to Improve Access to Immunization Services. The Public Health Service action plan to improve access to immunization services. Public Health Rep 107:243–251, 1992.
261. Ad Hoc Working Group for the Development of Standards for Pediatric Immunization Practices. Standards for pediatric immunization practices. JAMA 269:1817–1822, 1993.
262. Cutts FT, Zell ER, Mason D, et al. Monitoring progress towards US preschool immunization goals. JAMA 267:1952–1955, 1992.
263. Szilagyi P, Rodewald L, Humiston S, et al. Missed opportunities for childhood vaccinations in office practices and the effect on vaccination status. Pediatrics 91:1–7, 1993.
264. Bishai D, Bhatt S, Miller LT, et al. Vaccine storage practices in paediatric offices. Pediatrics 89:193–196, 1992.
265. Briggs H, Ilett S. Weak link in vaccine cold chain. BMJ 306:557–558, 1993.
266. Frenk J, Sepulveda J, Gomez-Dantes O, et al. The future of world health. The new world order and international health. BMJ 314:1404–1407, 1997.
267. Seventh Consultative Committee on Primary Health Care Systems for the 21st Century. Health care systems for the 21st century. BMJ 314:1407–1409, 1997.
268. Nelson EAS, Yu LM. Poverty focused assistance: New category of development aid. Lancet 348:1642–1643, 1996.
269. Evans I. SAPping maternal health. Lancet 346:1046, 1995.

chapter

45 Cost-Benefit and Cost-Effectiveness Analysis of Vaccine Policy

Mark A. Miller

Alan R. Hinman

Vaccination programs have greatly reduced morbidity and mortality worldwide. Although the development and introduction of new vaccines and the improved use of existing vaccines offer the prospect of further reductions in disease burden, policy makers are often constrained by limited public health resources. Studies involving the integration of epidemiological and economic data can be important in identifying the most judicious use of scarce public health resources to attain maximal health benefits.

A variety of quantitative techniques has been used to analyze policy decisions. The approaches used share the characteristics of explicit delineation of possible alternatives, estimation of probabilities or costs associated with each of the alternatives, and development of a summary statement of the implications of choosing a particular course of action. They also involve sensitivity analysis, in which estimated probabilities (or costs) are varied to determine how sensitive the conclusion is to particular variables. The summary statements are often couched in monetary terms. Four approaches are commonly used: decision analysis, cost-benefit analysis (CBA), cost-effectiveness analysis (CEA), and cost-utility analysis (CUA).

Decision analysis is an "explicit, quantitative, and systematic approach to decision making under conditions of uncertainty."[1] Decision analyses provide information about the likely outcomes of particular courses of action, often without putting a value (monetary or otherwise) on the outcomes. By contrast, the other techniques all use monetary terms to describe the inputs and outcomes of a particular course of action.

CBA is a technique that "attempts to value the consequences or benefits of an intervention program in monetary terms."[2] CBA involves assigning monetary value to all costs and benefits of a policy or program. Benefits are usually calculated by estimating the total cost of disease in the absence of an intervention and subtracting from that figure the total costs of residual disease occurring with a program. The costs of the program include vaccines, vaccine administration, costs of dealing with adverse events, and other program costs such as public education. In a CBA, results are usually presented as ratios of the benefits from the intervention divided by the costs of conducting the program (B-C ratio). By convention, the ratio is divided out to give a single figure, representing the ratio of benefits to a cost of 1. If the B-C ratio is greater than 1.0, the intervention is considered to be cost-saving; 1.0 is called the break-even point at which costs and benefits are equal. Because of the difficulties in estimating specific economic values for things such as human life, CBA is difficult to perform. However, because it is able to give a summary statement about whether the benefits of a program exceed its costs, irrespective of the character of the outcomes, it is a useful approach to compare health programs with nonhealth programs. CEA and CUAs are more useful for comparing different health programs.

In CEA, results are presented in terms of the cost required to achieve a particular health outcome (e.g., case or death prevented, year of life saved). Usually no attempt is made to assign an economic value to the prevented death. In general, interventions are considered cost-effective if the cost per year of life saved is less than or equal to the per capita gross domestic product, which may range, on average, from $500 for low-income countries to $25,000 for high-income countries. The relative cost-effectiveness of a death prevented may depend on the age of the individual and the consequent number of years of life saved. For example, an intervention that prevented death at an early age would generally be considered cost-effective even if the cost/death prevented was several times higher than the per capita gross domestic product. By contrast, a public health intervention with the same level of cost/death prevented might not be considered cost-effective in an elderly person with fewer potential years of life saved. CEA is particularly useful when there is a variety of options to achieve a single effect (e.g., delivering a second dose of measles vaccine in a campaign or as part of a routine schedule to prevent measles outbreaks). It is not useful when comparing investment in a health program to investment in a nonhealth program.[3]

CUA is a specific form of CEA in which outcomes are reduced to a common denominator such as the quality-adjusted life-year (QALY).[4] This permits comparisons to be made between interventions aimed at problems with different outcomes, such as acute illness and death versus prolonged disability. By measuring outcomes in terms of cost per QALY gained, it is possible to see whether, for example, investing in a measles prevention program would be a more effective use of resources than investing in a heart disease prevention program.

IMPORTANT CONSIDERATIONS IN CARRYING OUT A QUANTITATIVE POLICY ANALYSIS

Perspective. Those who benefit from immunizations are individuals, the health care system, and society at large. Analyses can be carried out from each of these perspectives.[5, 6] Given that immunization programs are often supported by governments and benefits accrue not only to those who are vaccinated but also to those who are not vaccinated (from the reduced likelihood of exposure), it seems most appropriate to take a societal perspective. Sometimes the most cost-effective intervention may not necessarily be the best choice to deal with a particular health problem. For example, if it dealt with only a part of the problem and a somewhat less cost-effective intervention dealt with the whole problem, the latter might be a better choice. Williams and colleagues found that the most cost-efficient use of hepatitis B vaccine in the United Kingdom would be to concentrate on high-risk populations. However, that would have only a small impact on the overall hepatitis B disease burden compared with the impact of a more costly universal infant or adolescent immunization strategy.[7]

Time Frame. Vaccines often protect against risks that may not occur for some time in the future. Programs such as eradication provide benefits that will accrue in perpetuity. Since the investment is made in a different time frame from the benefit, it often is necessary to discount future effects (both positive and negative) to take account of the implicit valuation that society has for health and financial costs and benefits over time. Even after accounting for inflation (which affects both costs and potential savings), there is an implicit difference in the value of an event which occurs today versus a future period. For example, it is generally felt that a child's death prevented today is worth more than a child's death prevented 50 years from now. There is general agreement among economists to discount both costs and benefits at the same rate, typically from 3 to 10% per year. Study results are often presented both discounted and undiscounted.

Disease Burden. Disease burden estimates are ideally based on specific studies, but it may be necessary to use approximations such as reported disease burden (usually an underestimate), results of mathematical modeling, or extrapolations from other representative populations. Analysis may need to be specific for age group, population/occupational group, risk for disease (e.g., healthcare workers), and outcome (including the timing of the outcome, e.g., death in the next year versus death 50 years in the future).

Measure Used for Health States. An outcome may be stated as the number of cases or deaths that occur or are prevented by an intervention. Years of potential life (YPL) represent a refinement of the death metric that quantifies the total years of life lost or prevented from being lost. It integrates the difference in an expected life span of each individual and the age at which death occurs. QALYs or disability adjusted life-years (DALYs) are further refinements of the YPL metric and integrate the YPL and a valuation of the disability from morbidity. These metrics defy simplicity, are derived by many subjective inputs, and may not be readily understood by some policymakers; however, they offer a common metric to compare all health outcomes.

Economic Valuation of Health Outcome States. This includes both direct and indirect costs and benefits. Direct costs include the costs of medical treatment and the costs of administering the vaccine. Indirect costs include wages lost by those who are ill and their caregivers. Intangible costs, such as pain and suffering or death, are difficult to measure. However, they may be captured in an unquantified way in the denominator of a CEA or CUA (e.g., as cost/death prevented), allowing the reader to imply their own value of death.

Vaccine Program Characteristics. This includes vaccine efficacy (performance of the vaccine under ideal conditions), vaccine effectiveness in the field setting, coverage of the program, adverse effects of the vaccine (or program), and the potential for benefits to accrue to those who are not vaccinated because of the vaccination of others (herd immunity).

Sensitivity Analysis. One of the most powerful tools of quantitative policy analysis is that it provides the opportunity to estimate the likely effects of different probabilities of events (or different costs) from those postulated in the "base case" analysis. This is particularly important when the true value of a parameter used in an analysis is not known and must be estimated. Testing a range of values for the uncertain assumption or assumptions can identify the factors to which the conclusion is most sensitive.

EXAMPLES OF USES OF QUANTITATIVE POLICY ANALYSIS

A large number of studies have been carried out. Most of those published in the literature regarding vaccines currently in use are summarized in Table 45–1. In reading the table, it should be kept in mind that the studies

Text continued on page 1083

Table 45–1. **COST-BENEFIT AND COST-EFFECTIVENESS ANALYSES OF VACCINES**

REFERENCE	TYPE	RESULTS	COMMENT
General			
Barnum and Setiady[14] (1980)	CEA	Indonesia—cost/death prevented 1979–1984 by BCG and DTP $130; cost/death prevented by BCG-only program $455, by DTP-only program $135	Considered only direct costs
Creese and Henderson[15] (1980)	CEA	Indonesia, Philippines, Thailand–BCG and DTP costs/fully immunized infant $2.86, $4.97, and $10.73, respectively	Considered only direct costs
Phonboon et al[16] (1989)	CEA	Thailand—DTP/BCG/OPV/measles average direct cost/fully immunized child $13.80 in hospitals, $11.80 in health centers; for fully immunized pregnant women (tetanus) $8.90 and $10.30, respectively	Also considered differential costs of fixed and outreach services
Shepard et al[17] (1989)	CEA	Ecuador—cost/fully immunized child $4.39 for routine services and $8.60 for mass vaccination campaign	Although campaign was less cost-effective, it significantly increased coverage of children missed by routine services
Bjerregaard[18] (1990)	CBA	Kenya—cost/fully EPI immunized child $12.39; cost/death prevented ≈$150	Used WHO EPICost software
Musgrove[19] (1992)	CBA	Americas—pneumonia, meningococcus type B, and typhoid vaccines would be economically justified if cost/vaccination (for 1 antigen) was $0.52–0.58 and benefits/disease prevented were $1000–2000	Considered only direct costs; 10% discount rate
Behrens and Roberts[20] (1994)	CBA	UK—B:C ratio 0.17, 0.06, and 0.06, respectively, for hepatitis A passive, active immunization and typhoid immunization of travelers	Results dependent on frequency of travel to endemic areas
Brenzel and Claquin[21] (1994)	CEA	Global—reviewed 30 studies; average cost to fully immunize a child $22, ranging from $8 (Tanzania, fixed site) to $33 (Cameroon, national campaigns)	All costs adjusted to 1992 dollars
Hadler[22] (1994)	CBA	US—significant cost savings ($90–150 million/year) would accrue from use of combination DTP-Hib or DTP-Hib-hepatitis B	Based on Hatziandreu studies
Shepard et al[23] (1995)	CUA	Global—rated cost/QALY of 13 candidate vaccines/vaccine strategies; range from $5 (measles vaccination <6 months of age) to $113,208 (acellular pertussis vaccines)	Projected likely research and development costs of new vaccines; 3% discount rate
Adenovirus			
Collis et al[24] (1973)	CBA	US—B:C ratio of 1.6 from using adenovirus vaccine types 4 and 7 in military recruits to prevent acute respiratory disease	Study included vaccine research and development costs
AIDS			
Cowley[25] (1993)	CBA	Ivory Coast—modeled range of break-even costs for a hypothetical vaccine; cost of each case of AIDS, $1500 (direct), $20,079 (total cost) per HIV infection	Wide range of assumptions for prevalence and vaccine efficacy
BCG			
Nettleman[26] (1993)	CBA	US—vaccinating persons attending homeless shelters would be cost saving if vaccines were 40% effective	5% discount rate; vaccine cost $10
Trnka et al[27] (1993)	CBA	Czech Republic—vaccine discontinuation in study region has B:C ratio 1 due to reduction in infection incidence in 0–6-yr-olds to <0.1%	Observed 80% vaccine efficacy
Cholera			
MacPherson and Tonkin[28] (1992)	CEA	Canada—routine vaccination against cholera for travelers to endemic areas would not be cost-effective; >CAN$28 million per case prevented	Vaccine cost CAN$28.67 per dose; persons traveling to regions with high transmission rates should be considered for vaccination
Cookson et al[29] (1997)	CBA	Argentina—assuming 75% coverage and 75% efficacy, the break-even cost of vaccine would be $1.81 per dose	5% discount rate
Diphtheria-Tetanus-Pertussis			
Hatziandreu et al[30] (1994)	CBA	US—B:C ratio 6.2 for direct costs; 30.1 for total costs	Reductions in diphtheria and pertussis contributed nearly equally to direct savings; diphtheria was major contributor to indirect savings
Pertussis			
Koplan et al[31] (1979)	CBA	US—B:C ratio 2.6 (direct costs only)	5% discount rate
Hinman and Koplan[32] (1984)	CBA	US—B:C ratio 11.1 (direct costs only)	5% discount rate
Hinman and Koplan[33] (1985)	CBA	US—B:C ratio 3.1 (direct costs only)	5% discount rate; recalculation following 90-fold increase in vaccine costs and newer estimates of serious adverse events
Tetanus			
Berggren[34] (1974)	CBA	Haiti—B:C ratio 9 for community-wide tetanus immunization (infants → adults)	Considered only direct hospital care costs; primary impact was in reduction of neonatal tetanus
Hutchison and Stoddart[35] (1988)	CEA	Canada—primary immunization of elderly would cost $1.9 million/case prevented, $7.1 million/death prevented, $810 thousand/life-year gained	5% discount rate

Carducci et al[36] (1989)	CBA	Italy—benefits of mass immunization of population older than 10 yr would exceed costs after 1 yr; gradual immunization also would exceed costs after 1 yr but would only reach total benefit of mass campaign after 9 yrs	Considered only direct costs
Berman et al[37] (1991)	CEA	Indonesia—compared routine TT administration to pregnant women with "crash" TT to all women 10–45; cost/woman immunized was comparable but cost/death averted was higher through "crash" program	
Balestra and Littenberg[38] (1993)	CEA	US—cost/year of life saved by decennial TT booster $143,138 compared with $4527 for single booster at age 65	However, decennial booster prevented four times as many cases as single booster
Haemophilus influenzae *Type b*			
Cochi et al[39] (1985)	CEA	US—routine use of polysaccharide vaccine would produce a net savings; two-dose vaccination beginning at 18 mo was most cost-effective for this vaccine	Study preceded current conjugate vaccines; projected vaccine cost $3/dose
Hay and Daum[40] (1987)	CBA CEA	US—routine use of polysaccharide vaccine would produce a net savings as compared with rifampin prophylaxis of appropriate contacts	Study preceded current conjugate vaccines; vaccine cost $8.13/dose
Hay and Daum[41] (1990)	CBA	US—vaccination with a single dose at 18 mo would have a B:C ratio 4.0 and would be cost beneficial to a vaccine efficacy of 22.7%; single dose estimated to prevent 11% of total cases	3% discount rate; assumed 81% vaccine efficacy; vaccine cost $14/dose
Martens et al[42] (1991)	CBA	Netherlands—break-even cost of vaccine would be $7 if administered with DTP-polio vaccines	
Ginsberg et al[43] (1993)	CBA	Israel—a four-dose program would have B:C ratio 0.3 for health services only; with chronic sequelae 1.3; with indirect costs and deaths valued 1.5; break-even vaccine costs are $2.24 when health service benefits only are considered and $11.21 when all benefits are included	Vaccine cost $7.74/dose
Levine et al[44] (1993)	CBA CEA	Chile—benefit/cost ratio 1.7; value of death prevented not included	Vaccine cost $1 for a three-dose regimen
Harris et al[45] (1994)	CEA CUA	Australia—cost/year life saved by three-dose conjugate vaccine AUS$3148; cost per QALY, AUS$1965; incremental analysis compared with single dose of conjugate vaccine at 18 mo AUS$5047/QALY saved; for aboriginal subpopulation, proposed vaccination program would be cost saving	Incidence 53 per 100,000, and 460 per 100,000 among non- and Aborigine populations, respectively; 5% discount rate; vaccine cost AUS$20 per dose
McIntyre et al[46] (1994)	CEA CUA	Australia—cost/QALY AUS $1231–9136 based on various dosing schedules	Based on disease incidence in non-Aboriginal children; vaccine cost $15 AUS/dose
Trolfors[47] (1994)	CBA	Sweden—B:C ratio 1.2 (direct and indirect costs); 1.6 if valuation of deaths included	Vaccine cost 125SEK/dose
Asensi et al[48] (1995)	CBA	Spain—B:C ratio 2.4–5.1 depending on public or private purchase of vaccine	Includes valuation of deaths; vaccine cost 3000 or 1800 pesetas per dose for private, public sectors, respectively
Hatziandreu and Brown[49] (1995)	CBA	US—B:C ratio 1.3–3.3 (direct costs), 2.2–5.1 (direct and indirect) for base case; B:C ratio of combined DTP–Hib vs. Hib alone 2.6 (direct), 4.0 (direct and indirect)	Vaccine cost $10.25/dose; combined products reduced overall costs of administering vaccines and are therefore more cost-beneficial
Hussey et al[50] (1995)	CBA	South Africa—vaccination in Cape Town would have B:C ratio 1.3–1.4	Direct and indirect costs assumed; based on vaccine price of $58 for three doses
Midani et al[51] (1995)	CA	US—cost of disease decreased from $27.5 to $0.9 million/year (97%) after vaccine introduction in Florida	
Hepatitis A			
Hinds et al[52] (1985)	CBA	US—B:C ratio 2.5 from conducting active vs. passive surveillance for hepatitis A with subsequent administration of immune globulin to contacts	Study preceded licensure of current hepatitis A vaccines
Tormans et al[53] (1992)	CEA	Belgium—passive immunization most cost-effective for travel to endemic areas <6 mo and < two times in a 10-yr period; results are sensitive to incidence, behavioral, and vaccine characteristics	Travelers from Europe to high-endemic countries; vaccine cost (including administration) $40, $24 for active and passive immunization, respectively
Bryan and Nelson[54] (1994)	CEA	US—passive immunization for postexposure prophylaxis or preexposure periods <6 mo is much less expensive than active immunization	Assumed hepatitis A vaccines to be priced at $10–25/dose
Jefferson et al[55] (1994)	CEA CBA	UK—for British Army, active immunization is more cost-effective (52,865 pounds per case prevented) than passive immunization (97,305 pounds per case prevented)	Study only assumed a 5 year four-exposure scenario; vaccine cost 11.7 pounds per dose
Jefferson et al[56] (1994)	CBA	UK—active vaccination of troops versus passive immunization for a single deployment is not cost-beneficial, B:C ratio 0.01–0.03	Vaccine cost $22.26/dose, immune serum globulin cost $6/dose
Van Doorslaer et al[57] (1994)	CEA	Belgium—passive immunization is most cost-effective for infrequent travelers, 7000 to 9000 pounds per infection prevented; active immunization becomes more cost-effective than passive for travel exceeding three times in 10 yr or for trips >6 mo duration (3500–7500 pounds per prevented infection)	5% discount rate; vaccine cost 15–22.5 pounds/dose; immune serum globulin cost 7 pounds/dose
Zuckerman and Powell[58] (1994)	CEA	UK—Screening prior to active immunization is cost-effective for travelers 40+ yr of age	Based on antibody prevalence in travelers attending London travel clinics

Table continued on following page

Table 45–1. **COST-BENEFIT AND COST-EFFECTIVENESS ANALYSES OF VACCINES** *Continued*

REFERENCE	TYPE	RESULTS	COMMENT
Hepatitis B			
Prevaccination Screening			
Corrao et al[59] (1987)	CEA	Italy—sequential testing of a single serum specimen for anti-HBc, anti-HBs and HBsAg prior to vaccination was most cost-effective of five possible screening protocols	Results particular to screening test and vaccine price at that time
Hankins et al[60] (1987)	CEA	US—screening paramedics for anti-HBs and HBsAg with subsequent prophylactic vaccination was not cost-effective compared with administering vaccine to all paramedics when expected prevalence is <2%	
Jacobson et al[61] (1987)	CBA CEA	US—prevaccination screening of dental workers would have B:C ratio 2.7	Screening only faculty with patient contact was most cost-effective
Arevalo and Washington[62] (1988)	CEA	US—routine serologic screening of pregnant women with subsequent immunization of infants of carrier mothers is cost-saving at a prevalence of 0.06%	4 and 6% discount rates; vaccine cost $50 for three doses
Tong et al[63] (1988)	CA	US—comparison between screening protocols; hepatitis B core antibody should be used for screening health care workers in hospitals with high prevalence	Prediction of high or low hepatitis B carriage prevalence may be based on the distribution of staff ethnicity
Thomas[64] (1990)	CEA	Australia—universal screening of public antenatal patients cost AUS$354/carrier identified	Sensitive to carrier prevalence
Audet et al[65] (1991)	CEA	Canada—universal screening of pregnant women with subsequent immunization of infants of carrier mothers would cost CAN$8915/prevented carrier	Costs/carrier prevented varied by ethnic origin from $540 (Asian to $126,279 (Canadian)
Schoub et al[66] (1991)	CEA	South Africa—prevaccination screening would be cost-beneficial in black nursing and laboratory personnel, but not their white counterparts	Seroprevalence 36–68% and 3–15% in black and white populations, respectively
Tormans et al[67] (1993)	CEA	Belgium—screening pregnant women would cost BEF583,581 per life-year saved	Carrier prevalence of .67% in this population; vaccine cost BEF1246/dose
Kwan-Gett et al[68] (1994)	CEA	US—vaccinating preadolescents without screening is more cost-effective than prevaccination screening in routine vaccination programs	
Yuan and Robinson[69] (1994)	CBA	Canada—combined HBV marker seroprevalence of at least 30–64% is required to justify screening prior to routinely vaccinating specific subpopulations	Vaccine cost CAN$20/dose
Ferraz et al[70] (1995)	CEA	Prevaccination screening of health care workers is more cost-effective at a seroprevalence greater than 11%; low-dose intradermal vaccination is more cost-effective than intramuscular injection	Vaccine cost $45.39 for three doses
Williams et al[7] (1996)	CEA	UK—antenatal screening and vaccination is most effective strategy; screening before vaccination is cost-effective for homosexually active persons but not for general population	Based on mathematical modeling of transmission dynamics
Fabrizi et al[71] (1996)	CEA	Italy—after the initial cost of vaccination, a savings of US$3272/year was realized by the elimination of frequent serologic screening of vaccine responders	45% prevalence in hemodialysis unit prior to institution of vaccination program
Vaccination			
Mulley et al[72] (1982)	CBA	US—routine vaccination would be cost-saving for populations with attack rates as low as 1–2% when indirect costs included	Based on costs from the early 1980s
Adler et al[73] (1983)	CBA	UK—net savings would be realized for a screening and vaccination program yielding a B:C ratio 1.5–7.4 for the homosexually active population	Only acute costs were considered
Hamilton[74] (1983)	CBA	US—vaccination of health care workers would have cumulative B:C ratio 1.2 over 10 yr	5% discount rate; vaccine cost $100 for three doses
Alter et al[75] (1983)	CBA	US—routine vaccination of patients and staff of hemodialysis units would be cost-saving compared with routine screening	Confirmed in the setting of reduced incidence in this population
Kirkman-Liff and Dandoy[76] (1984)	CA	US—cost per exposure in health care workers $109; $13,376/case	From hospital perspective
Lahaye et al[77] (1987)	CBA	Belgium—vaccination of health care workers is cost-saving	Not all future benefits included in analysis
Hicks et al[78] (1989)	CBA	US—average cost per case of HBV infection is $1990; vaccination of pediatric nurses would not be cost-effective at presumed attack rate of 1% and vaccine series price of $103	Vaccination would be cost-effective if attack rate were 2% of identified subpopulation or if vaccine series price were reduced from $103 to $27
Margolis et al[79] (1990)	CA	US—acute hepatitis $4855/case; acute fulminant hepatitis, $7000–8549/case; chronic hepatitis, $2905–7592/case	Study includes various costs (direct and indirect) for wide range of acute and chronic hepatitis B sequelae
Barboza et al[80] (1991)	CBA	Venezuela—cost per infection $1759; selective vaccination of hospital workers would be cost-saving	
Hatziandreu et al[81] (1991)	CEA	Greece—cost per case averted $970–7800 (with vaccine price $40/dose and incidence of 0.3–2%; cost saving at $8/dose or 11% annual incidence)	Plasma-derived hepatitis B vaccines from two manufacturers produced comparable results
Hayashi et al[82] (1991)	CEA	Japan—lower-dose intradermal injection was more cost-effective at eliciting antibody response than subcutaneous administration in a mentally handicapped population	Antibody titers were different between the study groups
Jönsson et al[83] (1991)	CBA	Spain—determined the threshold of attack rate in the target population to achieve cost-savings with routine hepatitis B vaccination; at a 5% attack rate, direct costs would be recouped; 1% for recoupment of direct and indirect costs	Target populations included health care workers, high-risk patients and intimate contacts of above
Leonard et al[84] (1991)	CEA	US—for screening and vaccination program in a mental health institution with 3-yr transmission rate of 27%, the cost per case prevented was $300; cost per death prevented, $12,100	Highly variable results depending on transmission rate

Vaccination			
Mauskopf et al[85] (1991)	CBA	US—a vaccine program for all workers with more than 11 exposures per year would have B:C ratio 2.1; if pain and suffering valued, B:C ratio would be 11.2	Assumes prescreening and vaccine costs of $133
Antoñanzas et al[86] (1992)	CEA	Spain—cost-effectiveness of alternative strategies compared with current screening of pregnant women with subsequent infant immunization; cost/case prevented for those living with carriers 115,000–310,000 pesetas; routine vaccination of pubescent youth, 30,000–130,000 pesetas; newborns, 400,000 pesetas; and accidental exposure, 500,000 pesetas	Used 4% and 7% discount rates
Demicheli and Jefferson[87] (1992)	CBA	Italy—routine infant vaccination is not cost-beneficial given declining incidence	Based on peak incidence of 6/100,000; 8% discount rate
Ginsberg et al[88] (1992)	CBA	Israel—neonatal vaccination program would have B:C ratio 1.6 (direct costs only) and 2.8 (direct and indirect costs)	7.5% discount rate; cost per pediatric dose $2.30
Ginsberg and Shoual[89] (1992)	CBA	Israel—vaccination program targeting all persons <16 would have B:C ratio 1.9 (direct costs only) and 2.8 (direct and indirect costs)	7.5% discount rate; cost per pediatric dose $2.19
Bloom et al[90] (1993)	CEA	US—screening newborns in combination with routine administration to 10-yr-old children is the most cost-effective strategy, $375 and $3695 (undiscounted, discounted) per life-year saved; vaccination (with or without screening) is a dominant strategy in adult high-risk populations	5% discount rate; vaccine costs $225, $160 for adults, newborns, respectively (including administration fees)
Hall et al[91] (1993)	CEA	The Gambia—cost to avert a death from liver cancer $150–200 (undiscounted); $1200–1500 (discounted)	6% discount rate; vaccine cost $1/dose
Krahn and Detsky[92] (1993)	CEA	Canada—cost-effectiveness of universal infant vaccination is CAN$30,347/life year; break-even vaccine price is $7/dose	
Oddone et al[93] (1993)	CEA	US—cost per case prevented $25,313 and $31,111, for predialysis and dialysis patients, respectively, due to lower immunogenicity among dialysis patients and low incidence 0.6%; break-even incidence 38%	5% discount rate; vaccine cost $152 for three doses plus booster dose
Zhuang and Xu[94] (1993)	CEA	China—vaccinating neonates and infants (aged 0–3 yr) is most cost-effective followed by vaccinating adults >25 yr of age	
Aggarwal and Naik[95] (1994)	CEA	India—cost per carrier prevented of universal vaccination and prenatal screening with vaccination is $126 and $495, respectively, compared with no program	Vaccine cost $1/dose; study did not account for any treatment savings
Bergus and Meis[96] (1995)	CEA	US—routine immunization program in Iowa would cost $2970 (undiscounted) and $41,906 (discounted) per life-year saved	5% discount rate; vaccine costs $26.25 and $86.40 for infant and adolescent series, respectively
Guillén Grima and Espín Rios[97] (1995)	CEA	Spain—cost/case prevented is 118,990, 64,476, and 82,840 pesetas, respectively, for universal vaccination of newborns, preadolescents, and universal vaccination of newborns with catch-up vaccination	
Kerleau et al[98] (1995)	CEA	France—cost of vaccinating young male adults is 36,000 F/case prevented; vaccination may be considered cost-beneficial for high-risk exposure groups with attack rates that approximate those of homosexually active men or are greater than those observed in drug users	
Liu et al[99] (1995)	CBA	China—B:C ratio 42.4–48.0 from routine infant immunization in Jinan City	
Mangtani et al[100] (1995)	CEA	UK—compared with no vaccination, cost per life-year saved for vaccination of infants, preadolescent children, and high-risk populations is 2568 pounds, 2824 pounds, and 8564 pounds (undiscounted), respectively; universal adolescent vaccination most cost-effective when benefits are discounted	6% discount rate; vaccine costs 22.08 pounds/child, 29.46 pounds/adult for three doses
Margolis et al[101] (1995)	CEA	US—cost per life-year saved (undiscounted) $164, $1522, and $3730 for perinatal HBV infection prevention, infant vaccination, and adolescent vaccination, respectively	Assumed 4.8% lifetime risk; vaccine price $20.01/infant, $40.02/adolescent for three doses
Van-Damme et al[102] (1995)	CEA	Europe—cost per infection prevented 6443 and 4745 pounds for routine neonate and adolescent vaccination, respectively	5% discount rate; vaccine cost 7.50 pounds/dose; 5 pounds for administration
Fenn et al[103] (1996)	CEA	UK—cost per life-year gained 188,015–301,365 pounds (discounted) or 5,234–13,034 pounds (undiscounted)	6% discount rate; vaccine cost 8.66 pounds, administration cost 10.63 pounds
Wiebe et al[104] (1997)	CEA	Canada—cost per life-year saved CAN$15,900, CAN$97,600 for universal infant and adolescent vaccination, respectively	5% discount rate; total vaccination costs are CAN$38.08 and CAN$55.31 for infants and 12-yr-olds, respectively
Influenza/Pneumococcal			
Rose et al[105] (1993)	CEA	US—cost/year of life saved for HIV-infected patients with CD4+ counts >500, 200–500, <200 for pneumococcal vaccine cost saving, cost saving, $2910, respectively; for influenza vaccine $101,201, $110,674, $105,588, respectively	5% discount rate
Influenza			
Kavet[106, 107] (1972, 1977)	CBA	US—annual immunization of high-risk population is cost-beneficial except in years with little influenza activity, which cannot be predicted	Model examined experience of 1960s, with five moderate epidemics, two large epidemics, and three years of little influenza activity
Klarman and Guzick[108] (1976)	CEA	US—cost/year of life gained for persons >65 is $700 if vaccine is 50% effective, $410 if vaccine is 70% effective	Estimates based on "composite" year in 1960s, taking into account cyclic nature of influenza and possibility of antigenic shift; generally followed Kavet's model
Schoenbaum et al[109] (1976)	CBA CEA	US—swine influenza immunization would be cost-beneficial if program restricted to those >25 yr of age and acceptance rates exceed 59%; cost/year of life saved ranged from $1,000–$13,200 in public sector and from $2,400–$12,600 in private sector for different population groups at acceptance rates of 20% and 100%	Assumed 10% probability of pandemic influenza and 6% discount rate. Included both direct and indirect costs

Table continued on following page

Table 45–1. COST-BENEFIT AND COST-EFFECTIVENESS ANALYSES OF VACCINES *Continued*

REFERENCE	TYPE	RESULTS	COMMENT
Influenza Continued			
Elo[110] (1979)	CBA	Finland—B:C ratio 0.9–1.8, 1.0–1.9, and 0.6–1.2, respectively, for vaccinating employed labor, health personnel, and medical risk groups with inactivated vaccine (range is for 30–60% vaccine efficacy)	Also considered other strategies including attenuated vaccine and drug prevention with amantidine
OTA[111] (1981) and Riddiough et al[112] (1983)	CEA	US—vaccination for all persons 65+ yr of age is cost-saving; cost/year of healthy life gained for those 65+ $1782	Also considered high-risk and non–high-risk persons of other age groups
Patriarca et al[113] (1987)	CEA	US—examined four strategies of vaccination/amantadine for prevention/control of influenza A in nursing homes; vaccination alone would be most cost-effective ($62/death averted) but also would allow higher rates of morbidity and mortality than other alternatives	Included only direct costs; giving amantadine continuously would result in least morbidity/mortality but would be most expensive ($786/death prevented)
Schoenbaum[114] (1987)	CBA	US—took individual's perspective and calculated that immunization in the fall of any given year would have B:C ratio >1 to the general population if it cost <$10 (<$45 for high-risk individuals)	In the face of an epidemic, benefits rise
Maucher and Gambert[115] (1990)	CBA	US—immunization of elderly would be cost-beneficial at vaccination cost (including vaccine and administration) as high as $61.46/person if infection rate was 10% and 30% of those ill required medical attention	Also examined break-even point if complications could be treated on ambulatory basis ($4.78/vaccination if infection rate was 10%)
Yassi et al[116] (1991)	CBA	Canada—B:C ratio 2.9 for immunization of hospital employees (direct costs)	B:C ratio derived from data presented; net benefit of $39.23/vaccinated employee
CDC[6] (1993)	CEA CBA	US—10 yr annual average B:C ratio 1.9 for immunization of Medicare beneficiaries	Considered only direct costs paid by Medicare; B:C ratio derived from data presented
Mullooly et al[117] (1994)	CEA	US—savings $6.11/vaccinee for vaccinating high-risk elderly; vaccinating non–high-risk elderly cost $4.82/vaccinee; overall, vaccination of elderly saved $1.10/vaccinee (direct medical costs)	HMO population
Nichol et al[118] (1994)	CBA	US—$117 in direct savings/year/vaccinee for vaccination of noninstitutionalized persons >65 yr, 1990–1993	Vaccinated persons had more illnesses at baseline than did nonvaccinated persons, thus true savings may have been higher
Campbell and Rumley[119] (1997)	CBA CEA	US—B:C ratio 2.5 for immunization of healthy textile workers; cost per saved lost workday $22.36	
Pneumococcal			
OTA[120] (1979) and Willems et al[121] (1980)	CEA	US—$1000/QALY for persons >65 yr of age; $5700/QALY for persons 45–64	Also considered high-risk and non–high-risk persons of other age groups; vaccination of elderly under a public program would be cost-saving
Patrick and Wooley[122] (1981)	CBA	US—B:C ratio 2.3 for immunizing those >50 yr of age or with chronic illness in an HMO population; 0.7 for all adults	
OTA[123] (1984) and Sisk et al[124] (1986)	CEA	US—$300/QALY for persons >65 yr of age	
Sisk et al[125] (1997)	CEA	US—vaccination of persons >65 yr of age cost saving if future medical costs (unrelated to pneumococcal disease) of survivors are excluded, cost/QALY $10,306–17,208 if future medical costs are included	$8.27 saved/person >65 yr of age vaccinated
Measles-Mumps-Rubella			
White et al[126] (1985)	CBA	US—MMR B:C ratio 14.1, including both direct and indirect costs	Also looked at individual vaccines B:C—measles 11.9, rubella 7.7, mumps 6.7
Bjerregaard[18] (1990)	CBA	Denmark—B:C ratio 3.2 for MMR two-dose program over 20 yr	
Wiedermann and Ambrosch[127] (1979)	CBA	Austria—measles/mumps B:C ratio 2.6 for direct costs; 4.4 for total costs	Also looked at individual vaccines—measles B:C ratio 1.7 and 2.9 for direct and total costs; mumps 1.9 and 3.6
Berger et al[128] (1990)	CBA	Israel—B:C ratio 1.1–1.2 for routine mumps/rubella immunization of 1-yr-olds based on reported cases; estimated >5.9 for true incidence	10% discount rate; also calculated with 5% discount rate
Ferson et al[129] (1994)	CEA	Australia—compared cost/person to vaccinate all health care workers ($3.14–$20.50); to serologically test all workers and vaccinate susceptibles ($5.11–$24.45); to vaccinate all with negative history ($2.56–$16.57), and to test all those with negative history and vaccinate susceptibles ($2.58–$15.49)	Study carried out in a population with >77% of those with negative history immune
Hatziandreu et al[130] (1994)	CBA	US—B:C ratio 16.3 for direct costs; 21.3 for total costs	Also considered B:C of individual components—measles 17.2, 17.2 for direct, total costs; mumps 6.1, 13.0; rubella 4.5, 11.1
Measles			
Axnick et al[131] (1969)	CBA	US—B:C ratio 4.9 for immunization 1963–1968	B:C ratio derived from data presented; 4% discount rate
Witte and Axnick[132] (1975)	CBA	US—B:C ratio ≈7.4 for immunization 1962–1972	B:C ratio derived from data presented; 4% discount rate
Albritton[133] (1978)	CBA	US—B:C ratio 10.3 for federal involvement 1966–1974	Used Box Tiao time series model to separate effect of federal funds from other efforts
Elo[110] (1979)	CBA	Finland—B:C ratio 3.9 (6% discount), 3.5 (9% discount) for vaccinating 1-yr-old children over 25-yr period	

Ponninghaus[134] (1980)	CBA	Zambia—B:C ratio positive in urban areas (>3.9 for lives saved) but not in rural areas	Not a standard B:C analysis
WHO[135] (1982)	CEA	Ivory Coast—$12.3/infant immunized; $13.9/case averted; $479/death averted; $10.4/year of life added	Estimated that 75% of all EPI costs were attributable to measles vaccine
Davis et al[136] (1987)	CEA	US—compared cost/case prevented of six different strategies in an outbreak setting; range from $56/case prevented by lowering recommended age of vaccination to 6 mo to $249/case prevented by vaccinating all residents 15 mo–28 yr of age	Specific results not generalizable but approach is
Ginsberg[137] (1990)	CBA	Israel—examined options of second dose of measles vaccine in Israel, West Bank, and Gaza: routine second dose at 6–7 yr (B:C ratio 4.5, 5.7, 9.5, respectively), routine second dose + mass vaccination of 7–17-year-olds (2.2, 2.0, 3.4), and routine second dose + mass vaccination of 7–17-year-olds (1.7, 1.5, 2.6)	Under any circumstance, addition of a second dose seemed justified
Mast et al[138] (1990)	CEA	US—compared cost/case prevented in an outbreak setting in schools—$3444/case prevented for revaccinating all students, $3166/case prevented for revaccinating those vaccinated before 1980, $2546/case prevented for revaccinating those vaccinated before 15 mo of age	43–53% of cases would not have been prevented by any of the strategies initiated after measles had appeared
Schlian et al[139] (1991)	CEA	US—compared cost/case prevented on college campus of various strategies; least expensive was to wait until an outbreak occurred before vaccinating; however, this would not be as effective as serologic screening of all students and vaccinating susceptibles or vaccinating all students	Recommended adopting mandatory immunization programs
Subbarao et al[140] (1991)	CEA	US—estimated that prevaccination serologic testing of health care workers would be cost-effective if screening cost <$12.75/test	86% of population studied had antibodies
Sellick et al[141] (1992)	CEA	US—compared cost/employee of screening all new employees serologically and vaccinating susceptibles ($2.42/employee) with "blind" immunization of all new employees ($8.30/employee)	Assumed susceptibles would require two doses of measles vaccine
Shepard[142] (1994)	CUA	Global—estimated $5/DALY for a measles vaccine that could be given as 1 dose at 6 mo of age compared with $17/DALY for current vaccines (given at 9 mo)	
Mumps			
Koplan and Preblud[143] (1982)	CBA	US—B:C ratio 7.4 using reported incidence of mumps; 39 using estimated actual incidence	Included both direct and indirect costs
Arday et al[144] (1989)	CBA	US—B:C ratio 0.2 for routine vaccination of Army recruits	Considered only marginal cost of adding mumps vaccine to existing measles, rubella vaccination; most recruits would already be immune
Rubella			
Schoenbaum et al[145] (1976)	CBA	US—B:C ratio 8 for vaccinating 2-yr-old children with monovalent rubella vaccine, 9 for 6-yr-old children, 27 for 12-yr-old girls, and 8 for vaccinating 2-yr-old children *and* 12-yr-old girls	Also estimated B:C ratio for use of combined measles and rubella
Farber and Finkelstein[146] (1979)	CBA	US—mandatory premarital rubella antibody screening B:C ratio <1 unless test cost ≈$0.55 and >37% of susceptible women were immunized	No place examined met both criteria
Elo[110] (1979)	CBA	Finland—B:C ratio 10.3, 3.3, and 5.8, respectively, for vaccinating all 13-yr-old girls and postpartum women, vaccinating all children 1–13 yr of age, followed by vaccination of 1-yr-old, and vaccinating 1-yr-olds only over 20 yr	Also considered other strategies
Stray-Pedersen[147] (1982)	CBA	Norway—B:C ratio 3 and 6, respectively, for vaccinating all 1-yr-old girls or all 13-yr-old girls with monovalent vaccine; 5 and 11 if using MMR	Also considered other strategies; none of which included vaccinating all 1-yr-olds, both male and female
Gudnadottir[148] (1985)	CEA	Iceland—serologic screening of women and teenage girls with vaccination of susceptibles would be more cost-effective than routine vaccination of all 1-yr-olds	Both strategies were cost-effective
Meningococcal			
Jackson et al[149] (1995)	CBA	US—routine vaccination of college students not cost-beneficial until incidence 6.5/100,000 (at least five times higher than the presumed endemic rate in this population)	
Polio			
Weisbrod[150] (1971)	CBA	US—annual "rate of return" on investment in polio vaccine research (both IPV and OPV) estimated at 11–12%	Benefits calculated based on present value of expected future earnings as well as treatment costs averted
Fudenberg[151] (1973)	CBA	US—B:C ratio 10 for IPV development over period 1955–1961	Also estimated net annual savings >$180 million from measles vaccination
Musgrove[152] (1988)	CBA	Americas—B:C ratio 5.8 over 15 yr for a 5-yr polio eradication campaign in the Americas if all cases received medical treatment and 1.4 if only ¼ of cases did	12% discount rate
Hatziandreu et al[153] (1994)	CBA	US—B:C ratio for OPV 3.4 for direct costs; 6.1 including indirect costs (total costs); B:C ratio for four-dose sequential IPV-OPV 3.0 for direct costs; 5.7 for total costs	Also considered 5- and 6-dose sequential schedules and B:C ratio of comprehensive program including OPV, DTP, and MMR (7.6 and 26.3 for direct and total costs under "intermediate case" scenario)
Bart et al[154] (1996)	CBA	Global—calculated net costs and benefits of polio eradication over the period 1986–2040. "Break-even" point reached in 2007 and total net savings by 2040 $13.6 billion	Did not consider indirect costs; used 6% discount rate
Miller et al[155] (1996)	CBA CEA	US—changing from OPV-only to IPV-only schedule would not be cost-beneficial; would cost $3.0 million/case of VAPP prevented; sequential IPV-OPV schedule would cost $3.1 million/case of VAPP prevented	National policy was changed to sequential IPV-OPV

Table continued on following page

Table 45–1. COST-BENEFIT AND COST-EFFECTIVENESS ANALYSES OF VACCINES *Continued*

REFERENCE	TYPE	RESULTS	COMMENT
Rabies			
Morrison et al[156] (1987)	CEA	US—intradermal administration of human diploid cell vaccine was more cost-effective than intramuscular in at-risk laboratory workers; savings of $120 per person vaccinated	Comparison of dosing regimens
Bernard and Fishbein[157] (1991)	CBA	Global—preexposure prophylaxis not cost-beneficial for long-term travelers (Peace Corps volunteers) to endemic areas	Analysis assumed exposed persons would receive follow-up care for possible rabies infections
Fishbein et al[158] (1991)	CBA CEA	Philippines—costs from rabies elimination program primarily through canine vaccination would be recouped in 4–11 yr; cost/death prevented = $2036 after 25 yr	Direct and indirect costs assumed in analysis
Uhaa et al[159] (1992)	CBA	US—B:C ratio 2.2–6.8 for oral vaccine bait for raccoons to prevent human rabies	
Rotavirus			
Griffiths et al[160] (1995)	CA	US—break-even costs for vaccine would be $11 per infant for tetravalent and $12 for serotype 1 vaccine	Based on hypothetical vaccine program
Smith et al[161] (1995)	CEA	US—at assumed disease incidence, 50% efficacy and $30/dose, routine infant immunization with a rotavirus vaccine would have B:C ratio 1.3 (direct costs) and 2.9 (total costs)	
Schistosomiasis			
Guyatt and Evans[162] (1995)	CEA	Hypothetical vaccine would need to cost no more than $3.50 to $4.30 above the current chemotherapy treatment to be cost-effective	Vaccine assumed to be added to existing national vaccination program
Varicella			
Preblud et al[163] (1985)	CBA	US—B:C ratio 6.9 with hypothetical vaccine	Assumed 90% lifelong efficacy
Preblud[164] (1988)	CA	US—estimated annual disease burden cost of $400 million	95% of cost due to lost wages for childcare
Weber et al[165] (1988)	CA	US—$56,000 spent in 1 yr in a 580-bed hospital for identification, prophylaxis and treatment of susceptible persons due to varicella exposure	Costs associated with hospital infection control
Kitai et al[166] (1993)	CBA	Canada—pretransplant vaccination program would have B:C ratio 8.3 (direct costs and benefits) and 9.5 (total costs and benefits)	Vaccine cost CAN$30/dose
Huse et al[167] (1994)	CBA	US—vaccination in routine schedules would have B:C ratio 0.34 (direct medical treatment costs only) or 2.0 (direct and indirect)	Vaccination cost-beneficial only if indirect costs included; 5% discount rate; vaccine cost $24/dose
Lieu et al[168] (1994)	CEA CBA	US—a one-dose program would cost $2500/life-year saved (medical costs only); if indirect costs were included B:C ratio 5	Vaccine cost $35/dose
Lieu et al[169] (1994)	CA	US—mean value of work lost because of chickenpox was $293/family or $183/chickenpox case; estimated costs of nonprescription medications were $20/family or $12.50/chickenpox case	
Ferson[170] (1995)	CA	Australia—universal infant vaccination will cause a greater proportion of varicella cases to occur in adults with associated serious complications; although economic costs resulting from lost time from work will fall dramatically, health costs may rise	
Lieu et al[171] (1995)	CEA	US—vaccinating all 6- to 12-yr-old children is more effective but more costly ($197/case prevented) than screening with subsequent vaccination if only direct costs are included; if indirect costs are included, vaccinating all is a dominant strategy (less costly and more effective); for 13- to 17-year-old children, testing all is most cost-effective but has a high cost	Vaccine cost $35; results highly sensitive to varicella prevalence among persons with uncertain histories; study addresses limitation of data concerning correlation of disease history with immune status
Beutels et al[172] (1996)	CBA CEA	Germany—adolescent vaccination is most cost-effective and had direct medical savings; vaccination at 15 mo would cost DM19,735/life-year (direct costs only) or DM6,915 if combined with adolescent catch-up vaccination at 12 yr	5% discount rate; vaccine cost DM75/dose
Strassels and Sullivan[173] (1997)	CBA	US—B:C ratio 0.9 and 5.4 for universal vaccination of persons without a history of infection from payers' and society's perspective, respectively	
Yellow Fever			
Monath and Nasidi[174] (1993)	CEA	Nigeria—although emergency response is more cost-effective than routine vaccination ($1904 vs. $3817/death prevented), routine vaccination would prevent seven times as many deaths	Valuation of deaths would greatly increase the benefits of routine immunization

AIDS, acquired immunodeficiency syndrome; BCG, bacille Calmette-Guérin; CA, cost analysis; CBA, cost-benefit analysis; CDC, Centers for Disease Control; CEA, cost-effectiveness analysis; CUA, cost-utility analysis; DALY, disability adjusted life-years; DTP, diphtheria, tetanus, and pertussis; EPI, Expanded Program of Immunization; Hib, *Haemophilus influenzae* type b; HBV, hepatitis B virus; HIV, human immunodeficiency virus; HMO, Health Maintenance Organization; IPV, inactived polio vaccine; MMR, measles, mumps, rubella; OPV, oral polio vaccine; OTA, Office of Technology Assessment; QALY, quality adjusted life-year; TT, tetanus toxoid; VAPP, vaccine-associated paralytic poliomyelitis; WHO, World Health Organization.

were carried out over a period of more than 20 years with varying assumptions and varying costs of vaccine, personnel, and medical care. Results are shown as presented in the report; no effort has been made to adjust expenditures or savings to present value. All results are presented in U.S. dollars unless otherwise specified, and the results shown are for the base case analysis. Unless otherwise specified, studies addressed both direct and indirect costs.

In addition to the studies shown in the table, a number of decision analyses and risk-benefit analyses have also been carried out, looking at, for example, approaches to evaluation of rubella susceptibility in pregnant women[8] or the likely outcome of different timing of administration of diphtheria, tetanus, and pertussis (DTP) vaccine.[9] These studies typically have not included economic valuations in outcomes and are not included in the table.

In general, CBA, CEA, and CUA have shown that immunization is an excellent investment (highly cost-effective and usually cost-saving) for vaccines that are currently recommended for universal use. Consideration of particular strategies in individual groups may show considerable variation, as demonstrated in Table 45–1 (particularly with respect to the use of hepatitis B vaccine in different risk groups). Brief comments for many of the vaccines are shown after the table.

General Immunization

Most of these studies addressed immunization in developing countries using "standard" Expanded Program of Immunization vaccines. They generally demonstrate low costs per immunized child and favorable benefit-cost ratios.

Diphtheria, Tetanus, and Pertussis and Components

Cost-benefit analyses of pertussis vaccine use in the United States consistently showed an excess of benefits over costs, even in the face of a dramatically increasing cost of vaccine. It is of interest that when considering combined DTP vaccine, reductions in diphtheria direct costs were essentially equal to reductions in pertussis direct costs, and diphtheria was the major contributor to savings in indirect costs. Analyses of tetanus toxoid varied from administration of toxoid to women who were pregnant (or of childbearing age), to mass immunization of the general population, to primary or booster vaccination of the elderly. Predictably, results varied greatly.

Haemophilus influenzae Type B

The first two analyses presented are for the original polysaccharide vaccines that have been replaced by conjugated polysaccharide vaccines. The conjugated vaccines have had a remarkable impact on disease incidence in all countries that have introduced it into routine schedules. Because of its cost, quantification of disease burden in economic terms may be necessary in middle- and low-income countries to demonstrate the utility of its incorporation into routine schedules.

Hepatitis A

Hepatitis A vaccines have been licensed recently and are more expensive than the older, routinely used vaccines. Analyses have been conducted in countries that can afford vaccine at current prices. Frequently, the analyses have compared routine vaccination of travelers to current practice of preexposure passive prophylaxis using immune serum globulin. Because of the relative costs of vaccine and screening tests, the screening protocols assessed in the analyses have been important determinants of the outcome, as has been the risk of infection in specific settings. As the cost of vaccine decreases over time, there will likely be more studies assessing routine use of this vaccine.

Hepatitis B

The hepatitis B vaccine was relatively expensive when first licensed, prompting many evaluations to identify its most efficient use. Table 45–1 presents studies broken into two categories: those that considered screening for immunity before vaccination and those that considered routine immunization without screening. Most early studies concentrated on subpopulations who were at greatest risk of infection, such as health care workers, injection drug users, and individuals at risk for sexually transmitted diseases. The relative costs of screening and vaccine and the specific prevalence of hepatitis B virus infection in the subpopulations studied were the most important determinants of outcome. Early studies also addressed prenatal screening to identify the most efficient approaches for screening, passive immunization, and active vaccination. As the cost of vaccines decreased, studies began to address costs, benefits, and effectiveness of routine vaccination of various age cohorts (infants, adolescents). Since vaccination is most easily delivered through an existing infant vaccination infrastructure, universal infant vaccination with hepatitis B vaccine has become a common practice for countries that can afford the vaccine. Many analyses have been conducted taking into account variations of vaccine price and prevalence of infection in different countries. Analyses of hepatitis B are complicated by the need to incorporate multiple outcomes that may occur over prolonged periods.

Influenza-Pneumococcal Disease

In spite of the frequently changing antigenic structure of the influenza virus, studies have consistently shown that the benefits of annual influenza immunization of the elderly and chronically ill are greater than the costs.

Similarly, studies of pneumococcal immunization of the elderly and chronically ill have demonstrated a reasonable cost per QALY.

Measles, Mumps, and Rubella and Components

Measles, mumps, and rubella vaccines as individual antigens have repeatedly been shown to be cost saving when administered to young children. The ratio of benefits to costs rises even higher when the vaccines are administered in combination, since the costs of administration are substantially lower. For measles vaccine, the B-C ratio for a single dose is high; it is of interest that the additional benefits derived from a second dose also outweigh the costs.

Polio

Polio is one of the few vaccines for which analyses have addressed global eradication. The two analyses that have been carried out indicate that the costs of eradication would be exceeded by the benefits within 12 to 15 years.

Varicella

As with other recently introduced vaccines, economic policies have been considered in the formulation of varicella vaccine policy. Although varicella vaccination has not been shown to be cost-saving when only direct medical costs are considered, it is clearly cost-saving when the indirect costs of lost income from caregivers are included in the analysis.

Other Vaccines

A number of studies have been conducted on hypothetical vaccines (e.g., acquired immunodeficiency syndrome, schistosomiasis) or unlicensed vaccines (e.g., rotavirus, varicella [prelicensure]). These studies help highlight and quantify economic and epidemiological assumptions regarding disease burden and the potential impact of vaccination. Vaccine characteristics such as cost and efficacy can be varied in the analysis to demonstrate the target values at which a vaccine would be cost-effective or cost-beneficial.

USES OF QUANTITATIVE POLICY ANALYSIS IN FORMULATING-MODIFYING IMMUNIZATION POLICY

Decision Analysis—Appropriate Polio Vaccine Strategy

A 1988 comparative analysis of benefits and risks of oral polio vaccine (OPV) and inactivated polio vaccine (IPV) supported the then-current U.S. policy placing primary reliance on OPV but noted that "the conclusion is heavily dependent on assumptions of risk of exposure to wild virus in the United States. Major declines in risk of exposure to wild virus could alter the balance significantly."[10] The risk of importation has declined dramatically since that time—the last case of paralysis due to indigenously acquired poliovirus in the Western Hemisphere (the primary source of U.S. importations) had its onset in August 1991. In 1996, the Advisory Committee on Immunization Practices and the American Academy of Pediatrics recommended a change in U.S. policy to favor a sequential schedule of IPV followed by OPV.[11]

Cost-Benefit Analysis—Varicella

A 1985 CBA of varicella immunization conducted by Preblud and associates found that universal immunization with varicella vaccine (at a presumed cost of $15 per dose) would have a benefit-cost ratio of 6.9.[163] The primary contribution to the savings was through reducing the need for parents to stay home and care for sick children, rather than in savings on medical care expenses. This analysis was carried out more than 10 years before varicella vaccine was licensed. Subsequent analyses have continued to show a positive benefit-cost ratio when considering both direct and indirect costs and have supported the decision to recommend universal vaccination of children.

Cost-Effectiveness—Influenza

Beginning with an early CBA by Kavet,[106, 107] a number of studies have demonstrated the positive ratio of benefits to costs of influenza immunization of the elderly or substantial cost-effectiveness of such immunization. Given these data as well as the clinical and public health data about the impact of influenza, Congress enacted legislation in 1987 to make influenza immunization reimbursable under Medicare unless it was shown not to be cost-effective.[12] In response, the Department of Health and Human Services implemented a demonstration at 10 sites, each of which included an intervention area and a comparison area. The resulting CEA led to the conclusion that among Medicare beneficiaries, "influenza vaccine would cost $145 per year of life gained, substantially below the cost of other preventive interventions. . . . Because of these generally favorable results, influenza vaccine was made a covered benefit . . ."[6]

Cost Utility—Basic Immunizations

The 1993 World Development Report (issued by the World Bank) addressed the burden of disease in countries around the world and carried out a cost-utility analysis of a variety of interventions to deal with major health problems.[13] The measure used to compare regions, conditions, and interventions is the DALY, a measure that combines healthy life-years lost because of premature mortality with those lost because of disability. The report assessed 52 interventions and found that basic immunizations (bacille Calmette-Guérin [BCG], DTP, OPV, and measles, as given in the Expanded Program on Immunization) were among the best investments to make in health. The report estimated that the cost per DALY gained by immunization in low-income countries was $12 to 17 ($25–30 in middle-income countries) compared with, for example, $200 to 350 per DALY for limited care, including assessment, advice, alleviation of pain, treatment of infection and minor trauma, and treatment of more complicated conditions as resources permit ($400–600 in middle income countries). The report described a limited package of five essential public health measures (including immunizations) and six clinical interventions that should be the highest priority for government financing. The findings of this study are being used to guide donor investments in developing countries.

CONCLUSION

Quantitative policy analysis techniques help rationalize the process of decision making in immunization by explicitly stating assumptions, costs, and benefits of different strategies and allowing, through sensitivity analysis, an indication of the most important determinants of program outcome. They are important tools to help evaluate options. When conducted appropriately, they help elucidate values and summarize data and knowledge gaps as well as the relative importance of epidemiologic and economic assumptions. However, it must be remembered that they are just tools and should not be the sole basis for making decisions about immunization policies or programs. Economic analyses of immunizations have shown them to be among the best investments in health.

REFERENCES

1. Snider DE, Holtgrave DR, Dunet DO. Decision analysis. In Haddix AC, Teutsch SM, Shaffer PA, Dunet DO (eds). Prevention Effectiveness: A Guide to Decision Analysis and Economic Evaluation. New York, Oxford University Press, 1996.
2. Clemmer B, Haddix AC. Cost-benefit analysis. In Haddix AC, Teutsch SM, Shaffer PA, Dunet DO (eds). Prevention Effectiveness: A Guide to Decision Analysis and Economic Evaluation. New York, Oxford University Press, 1996.
3. Haddix AC, Shaffer PA. Cost-effectiveness analysis. In Haddix AC, Teutsch SM, Shaffer PA, Dunet DO (eds). Prevention Effectiveness: A Guide to Decision Analysis and Economic Evaluation. New York, Oxford University Press, 1996.
4. Dasbach E, Teutsch SM. Cost-utility analysis. In Haddix AC, Teutsch SM, Shaffer PA, Dunet DO (eds). Prevention Effectiveness: A Guide to Decision Analysis and Economic Evaluation. New York, Oxford University Press, 1996.
5. Zalkind DL, Shachtman RH. A decision analysis approach to the swine influenza vaccination decision for an individual. Med Care 18:59–72, 1980.
6. Final results: Medicare influenza vaccination demonstration, selected states, 1988–1992. MMWR Morb Mortal Wkly Rep 42:601–604, 1993.
7. Williams JR, Nokes DJ, Medley GF, Anderson RM. The transmission dynamics of hepatitis B in the UK: A mathematical model for evaluating costs and effectiveness of immunization programmes. Epidemiol Infect 116:71–89, 1996.
8. Mann JM, Preblud SR, Hoffman RE, et al. Assessing risks of rubella infection during pregnancy: A standardized approach. JAMA 245:1647–1652, 1981.
9. Funkhouser AW, Wassilak SGF, Orenstein WA, et al. Estimated effects of a delay in the recommended vaccination schedule for diphtheria and tetanus toxoids and pertussis vaccines. JAMA 257:1341–1346, 1987.
10. Hinman AR, Koplan JP, Orenstein WA, et al. Live or inactivated poliomyelitis vaccine: An analysis of benefits and risks. Am J Public Health 78:291–295, 1988.
11. Poliomyelitis prevention in the United States: Introduction of a sequential vaccination schedule of inactivated poliovirus vaccine followed by oral poliovirus vaccine. Recommendations of the Advisory Committee on Immunization Practices (ACIP). MMWR Morb Mortal Wkly Rep 46:1–25, 1997.
12. Section 4071, PL100-203, Omnibus Budget Reconciliation Act of 1987. Washington, DC, US Congress, 1987.
13. World Bank. World Development Report 1993: Investing in health. Washington, DC, Oxford University Press, 1993.
14. Barnum HDT, Setiady I. Cost-effectiveness of an immunization program in Indonesia. Bull World Health Organ 58:499–503, 1980.
15. Creese A, Henderson RH. Cost-benefit analysis and immunization programmes in developing countries. Bull World Health Organ 58:491–497, 1980.
16. Phonboon K, Shepard DS, Ramaboot S, et al. The Thai expanded programme on immunization: Role of immunization sessions and their cost-effectiveness. Bull World Health Organ 67:181–188, 1989.
17. Shepard DS, Robertson RL, Cameron CS 3d, et al. Cost-effectiveness of routine and campaign vaccination strategies in Ecuador. Bull World Health Organ 67:649–662, 1989.
18. Bjerregaard P. Economic analysis of immunization programmes. Scand J Soc Med 46(suppl):115–119, 1990.
19. Musgrove P. Cost-benefit analysis of a regional system for vaccination against pneumonia, meningitis type B, and typhoid fever. Bull Pan Am Health Organ 26:173–191, 1992.
20. Behrens RH, Roberts JA. Is travel prophylaxis worth while? Economic appraisal of prophylactic measures against malaria, hepatitis A and typhoid in travelers. BMJ 309:918–922, 1994.
21. Brenzel L, Claquin P. Immunization programs and their costs. Soc Sci Med 39:527–536, 1994.
22. Hadler SC. Cost benefit of combining antigens. Biologicals 22:415–418, 1994.
23. Shepard DS, Walsh JA, Kleinau E, et al. Setting priorities for the Children's Vaccine Initiative: A cost effectiveness approach. Vaccine 13:707–714, 1995.
24. Collis PB, Dudding BA, Winter PE, et al. Adenovirus vaccines in military recruit populations: A cost-benefit analysis. J Infect Dis 128:745–752, 1973.
25. Cowley P. Preliminary cost-effectiveness analysis of an AIDS vaccine in Abidjan, Ivory Coast. Health Policy 24:145–153, 1993.
26. Nettleman MD. Use of BCG vaccine in shelters for the homeless. A decision analysis. Chest 103:1087–1090, 1993.
27. Trnka L, Dankova D, Svandova E. Six years' experience with the discontinuation of BCG vaccination. 2. Cost and benefit of mass BCG vaccination. Tuber Lung Dis 74:288–292, 1993.
28. MacPherson DW, Tonkin M. Cholera vaccination: A decision analysis. Can Med Assoc J 146:1947–1952, 1992.
29. Cookson ST, Stamboulian D, Demonte J, et al. A cost-benefit analysis of programmatic use of CVD 103-HgR live oral cholera vaccine in a high-risk population. Int J Epidemiol 26:212–218, 1997.
30. Hatziandreu E, Palmer CS, Brown RE, Halpern MT. A cost benefit analysis of the diphtheria-tetanus-pertussis (DTP) vaccine: Final report. Arlington, VA, Battelle, 1994.
31. Koplan JP, Schoenbaum SC, Weinstein MC, Fraser DW. Pertussis vaccine—an analysis of benefits, risks and costs. N Engl J Med 301:906–911, 1979.
32. Hinman AR, Koplan JP. Pertussis and pertussis vaccine—reanalysis of benefits, risks and costs. JAMA 251:3109–3113, 1984.

33. Hinman AR, Koplan JP. Pertussis and pertussis vaccine: Further analysis of benefits, risks, and costs. In Manclark CR (ed). Proceedings of the Fourth International Symposium on Pertussis. Dev Biol Stand 61:429–437, 1985.
34. Berggren W. Administration and evaluation of rural health services. I. A tetanus control program in Haiti. Am J Trop Med Hyg 23:936–949, 1974.
35. Hutchison BG, Stoddart GL. Cost-effectiveness of primary tetanus vaccination among elderly Canadians. Can Med Assoc J 139:1143–1151, 1988.
36. Carducci A, Avio CM, Bendinelli M. Cost-benefit analysis of tetanus prophylaxis by a mathematical model. Epidemiol Infect 102:473–483, 1989.
37. Berman P, Quinley J, Yusuf B, et al. Maternal tetanus immunization in Aceh Province, Sumatra: The cost-effectiveness of alternative strategies. Soc Sci Med 33:185–192, 1991.
38. Balestra DJ, Littenberg B. Should adult tetanus immunization be given as a single vaccination at age 65? J Gen Int Med 8:405–412, 1993.
39. Cochi SL, Broome CV, Hightower AW. Immunization of U.S. children with *Haemophilus influenzae* type b polysaccharide vaccine: A cost-effectiveness model of strategy assessment. JAMA 253:521–529, 1985.
40. Hay JW, Daum RS. Cost-benefit analysis of two strategies for prevention of *Haemophilus influenzae* type b infection. Pediatrics 80:319–329, 1987.
41. Hay JW, Daum RS. Economic analysis of *Haemophilus influenzae* type b vaccination. Pediatr Infect Dis J 9:246–252, 1990.
42. Martens LL, ten Velden GHM, Bol P. De kosten en baten van vaccinatie tegen *Haemophilus influenzae* type b. Ned Tijdschr Geneeskd 135:16–20, 1991.
43. Ginsberg GM, Kassis I, Dagan R. Cost benefit analysis of *Haemophilus influenzae* type b vaccination programme in Israel. J Epidemiol Commun Health 47:485–490, 1993.
44. Levine OS, Ortiz E, Contreras R, et al. Cost benefit analysis for the use of *Haemophilus influenzae* type b conjugate vaccine in Santiago, Chile. Am J Epidemiol 137:1221–1228, 1993.
45. Harris A, Hendrie D, Bower C, et al. The burden of *Haemophilus influenzae* type b disease in Australia and an economic appraisal of the vaccine PRP-OMP. Med J Aust 160:483–488, 1994.
46. McIntyre P, Hall J, Leeder S. An economic analysis of alternatives for childhood immunisation against *Haemophilus influenzae* type b disease. Aust J Public Health 18:394–400, 1994.
47. Trollfors B. Cost-benefit analysis of general vaccination against *Haemophilus influenzae* type b in Sweden. Scand J Infect Dis 26:611–614, 1994.
48. Asensi F, Otero MC, Pérez-Tamarit D, et al. Economic aspects of a general vaccination against invasive disease caused by *Haemophilus influenzae* type b (Hib) via the experience of the Children's Hospital La Fe, Valencia, Spain. Vaccine 13:1563–1566, 1995.
49. Hatziandreu EJ, Brown RE. A cost benefit analysis of the *Haemophilus influenzae* B (Hib) vaccine. Arlington VA, Battelle, 1995.
50. Hussey GD, Lasser ML, Reekie WD. The costs and benefits of a vaccination programme for *Haemophilus influenzae* type B disease. S Afr Med J 85:20–25, 1995.
51. Midani S, Ayoub EM, Rathore MH. Cost-effectiveness of *Haemophilus influenzae* type b conjugate vaccine program in Florida. J Fl Med Assoc 82:401–402, 1995.
52. Hinds MW, Skaggs JW, Bergeisen GH. Benefit-cost analysis of active surveillance of primary care physicians for hepatitis A. Am J Public Health 75:176–177, 1985.
53. Tormans G, Van Damme P, Van Doorslaer E. Cost-effectiveness analysis of hepatitis A prevention in travelers. Vaccine 10(suppl 1):S88–S92, 1992.
54. Bryan JP, Nelson M. Testing for antibody to hepatitis A to decrease the cost of hepatitis A prophylaxis with immune globulin or hepatitis A vaccines. Arch Intern Med 154:663–668, 1994.
55. Jefferson T, Demicheli V, Wright D. An economic evaluation of the introduction of vaccination against hepatitis A in a peacekeeping operation. Int J Technol Assess Health Care 10:490–497, 1994.
56. Jefferson TO, Behrens RH, Demicheli V. Should British soldiers be vaccinated against hepatitis A? An economic analysis. Vaccine 12:1379–1383, 1994.
57. Van Doorslaer E, Tormans G, Van Damme P. Cost-effectiveness analysis of vaccination against hepatitis A in travelers. J Med Virol 44:463–469, 1994.
58. Zuckerman JN, Powell L. Hepatitis A antibodies in attenders of London travel clinics: Cost benefit of screening prior to hepatitis A immunisation. J Med Virol 44:393–394, 1994.
59. Corrao G, Zotti C, Tinivella F, Moiraghi Ruggenini A. HBV pre-vaccination screening in hospital personnel: Cost-effectiveness analysis. Eur J Epidemiol 3:25–29, 1987.
60. Hankins DG, Ebert KD, Siebold CM, et al. Hepatitis B vaccine and hepatitis B markers: Cost effectiveness of screening prehospital personnel. Am J Emerg Med 5:205–206, 1987.
61. Jacobson JJ, La Turno DE, Jonston FK, Shipman C Jr. Cost effectiveness of prevaccination screening for hepatitis B antibody. J Dent Educ 51:94–97, 1987.
62. Arevalo JA, Washington AE. Cost-effectiveness of prenatal screening and immunization for hepatitis B virus. JAMA 259:365–369, 1988.
63. Tong MJ, Co RL, Marci RD, et al. A cost comparison analysis for screening and vaccination of hospital personnel with high- and low-prevalence hepatitis B virus antibodies in California. Infect Control Hosp Epidemiol 9:66–71, 1988.
64. Thomas IL. Cost effectiveness of antenatal hepatitis B screening and vaccination of infants. Aust NZ J Obstet Gynaecol 30:331–335, 1990.
65. Audet AM, Delage G, Remis RS. Screening for HBsAg in pregnant women: A cost analysis of the universal screening policy in the province of Quebec. Can J Public Health 82:191–195, 1991.
66. Schoub BD, Johnson S, McAnerney J, et al. Exposure to hepatitis B virus among South African health care workers: Implications for pre-immunisation screening. S Afr Med J 79:27–29, 1991.
67. Tormans G, Van Damme P, Carrin G, et al. Cost-effectiveness analysis of prenatal screening and vaccination against hepatitis B virus—the case of Belgium. Soc Sci Med 37:173–181, 1993.
68. Kwan-Gett TSC, Whitaker RC, Kemper KJ. A cost effectiveness analysis of prevaccination testing for hepatitis B in adolescents and preadolescents. Arch Pediatr Adolesc Med 148:915–920, 1994.
69. Yuan L, Robinson G. Hepatitis B vaccination and screening for markers at a sexually transmitted disease clinic for men. Can J Public Health 85:338–341, 1994.
70. Ferraz ML, de Oliveira PM, Figueiredo VM, et al. Otimizacao do emprego de recursos economicos para vacinacao contra hepatite B em profissionais da area de saude (Optimization of the use of economic resources for vaccination against hepatitis B in health professionals). Rev Soc Bras Med Trop 28:393–403, 1995.
71. Fabrizi F, Di Filippo S, Marcelli D, et al. Recombinant hepatitis B vaccine use in chronic hemodialysis patients. Nephron 72:536–543, 1996.
72. Mulley A, Silverstein M, Dienstag J. Indications for use of hepatitis B vaccine, based on cost-effectiveness analysis. N Engl J Med 307:644–652, 1982.
73. Adler MW, Belsey EM, McCutchan JA, Mindel A. Should homosexuals be vaccinated against hepatitis B virus? Cost and benefit assessment. BMJ 286:1621–1624, 1983.
74. Hamilton JD. Hepatitis B virus vaccine: An analysis of its potential use in medical workers. JAMA 250:2145–2150, 1983.
75. Alter MA, Favero MS, Francis DP. Cost benefit of vaccination for hepatitis B in hemodialysis centers. J Infect Dis 148:770–771, 1983.
76. Kirkman-Liff B, Dandoy S. Cost of hepatitis B prevention in hospital employees: Post-exposure prophylaxis. Infect Control 5:385–389, 1984.
77. Lahaye D, Strauss P, Baleux C, van Ganse W. Cost-benefit analysis of hepatitis B vaccination. Lancet 2:441–443, 1987.
78. Hicks RA, Cullen JW, Jackson MA, Burry VF. Hepatitis B virus vaccine. Cost-benefit analysis of its use in a children's hospital. Clin Pediatr 28:359–365, 1989.
79. Margolis HS, Schatz GC, Kane MA. Development of recommendations for control of hepatitis B virus infections: The role of cost analysis. Vaccine 8(suppl):S81–S85, 1990.
80. Barboza RF, Rivero D, Echeverria B, Machado IV. Costo beneficio de la vacunación contra la hepatitis B en trabajodores de hospitales de Venezuela. Bol Of Sanit Panam 111:16–23, 1991.
81. Hatziandreu EJ, Hatzakis A, Hatziyannis S, et al. Cost-effectiveness of hepatitis-B vaccine in Greece. A country of intermediate

HBV endemicity. Int J Technol Assess Health Care 7:256–262, 1991.
82. Hayashi J, Nakashima K, Noguchi A, et al. Cost effectiveness of intradermal vs. subcutaneous hepatitis B vaccination for the mentally handicapped. J Infect 23:39–45, 1991.
83. Jönsson B, Horisberger B, Bruguera M, Matter L. Cost-benefits analysis of hepatitis-B vaccination. A computerized decision model for Spain. Int J Technol Assess Health Care 7:379–402, 1991.
84. Leonard J, Holtgrave DR, Johnson RP. Cost-effectiveness of hepatitis B screening in a mental health institution. J Fam Pract 32:45–48, 1991.
85. Mauskopf JA, Bradley CJ, French MT. Benefit-cost analysis of hepatitis B vaccine programs for occupationally exposed workers. J Occup Med 33:691–698, 1991.
86. Antoñanzas F, Forcén T, Garuz R. Analysis de coste-efectividad de la vacunacion frente al virus de la hepatitis B (Cost-effectiveness analysis of vaccination against hepatitis B). Med Clin (Barc) 99:41–46, 1992.
87. Demicheli V, Jefferson TO. Cost-benefit analysis of the introduction of mass vaccination against hepatitis B in Italy. J Public Health Med 14:367–375, 1992.
88. Ginsberg GM, Berger S, Shouval D. Cost-benefit analysis of a nationwide inoculation programme against viral hepatitis B in an area of intermediate endemicity. Bull World Health Organ 70:757–767, 1992.
89. Ginsberg GM, Shouval D. Cost benefit analysis of a nationwide neonatal inoculation programme against hepatitis B in an area of intermediate endemicity. J Epidemiol Comm Health 46:587–594, 1992.
90. Bloom BS, Hillman AL, Fendrick AM, Schwartz JS. A reappraisal of hepatitis B virus vaccination strategies using cost-effectiveness analysis. Ann Intern Med 118:298–306, 1993.
91. Hall AJ, Robertson RL, Crivelli PE, et al. Cost-effectiveness of hepatitis B vaccine in the Gambia. Trans R Soc Trop Med Hyg 87:333–336, 1993.
92. Krahn M, Detsky AS. Should Canada and the United States universally vaccinate infants against hepatitis B? Med Decis Making 13:4–20, 1993.
93. Oddone EZ, Cowper PA, Hamilton JD, Feussner JR. A cost effectiveness analysis of hepatitis B vaccine in predialysis patients. Health Serv Res 28:97–121, 1993.
94. Zhuang GH, Xu HW. The use of decision making analysis for evaluating hepatitis B inoculation strategy. Chung Hua Yu Fang I Hsueh Tsa Chih 27:69–73, 1993.
95. Aggarwal R, Naik SR. Prevention of hepatitis B infection: The appropriate strategy for India. Natl Med J India 7:216–220, 1994.
96. Bergus G, Meis S. Hepatitis B vaccination: A cost analysis. Iowa Med 85:209–211, 1995.
97. Guillén Grima F, Espín Rios MI. Análisis coste-efectividad de las distinatas alternatives de vacunación frente a la hepatitis B en la región de Murcia (Cost-effectiveness analysis of the different alternatives of universal vaccination against hepatitis B in Murcia). Med Clin (Barc) 104:130–136, 1995.
98. Kerleau M, Flori YA, Nalpas B, et al. Analyse cout-avantage d'une politique de prevention vaccinale de l'hepatite virale B (Cost-benefit analysis of vaccinal prevention of hepatitis B policy). Rev Epidemiol Sante Publique 43:48–60, 1995.
99. Liu ZG, Zhao SL, Zhang YX. Cost-benefit analysis on immunization of newborns with hepatitis B vaccine in Jinan City. Chung Hua Liu Hsing Ping Hsueh Tsa Chih 16:81–84, 1995.
100. Mangtani P, Hall AJ, Normand CEM. Hepatitis B vaccination: The cost effectiveness of alternative strategies in England and Wales. J Epidemiol Commun Health 49:238–244, 1995.
101. Margolis HS, Coleman PJ, Brown RE, et al. Prevention of hepatitis B virus transmission by immunization. JAMA 274:1201–1208, 1995.
102. Van Damme P, Tormans G, Beutels P, Van Doorslaer. Hepatitis B prevention in Europe: A preliminary economic evaluation. Vaccine 13(suppl 1):54–57, 1995.
103. Fenn P, Gray A, McGuire A. An economic evaluation of universal vaccination against hepatitis B virus. J Infect 32:197–204, 1996.
104. Wiebe T, Fergusson P, Horne D, et al. Hepatitis B immunization in a low-incidence province of Canada: Comparing alternative strategies. Med Decis Making 17:472–482, 1997.
105. Rose DN, Schechter CB, Sacks HS. Influenza and pneumococcal vaccination of HIV-infected patients: A policy analysis. Am J Med 94:160–168, 1993.
106. Kavet J. Influenza and public policy. Unpublished dissertation. Harvard University, 1972.
107. Kavet J. A perspective on the significance of pandemic influenza. Am J Public Health 67:1063–1070, 1977.
108. Klarman H, Guzick D. Economics of influenza. In Selby P (ed). Influenza: Virus, Vaccine and Strategy. New York, Academic Press, 1976, pp 255–268.
109. Schoenbaum S, McNeil N, Kavet J. The swine-influenza decision. N Engl J Med 295:759–765, 1976.
110. Elo O. Cost-benefit studies of vaccinations in Finland. Dev Biol Stand 43:419–428, 1979.
111. Office of Technology Assessment. Cost effectiveness of influenza vaccination. Washington, DC, US Government Printing Office, December, 1981.
112. Riddiough MA, Sisk JE, Bell JC. Influenza vaccination. JAMA 249:3189–3195, 1983.
113. Patriarca PA, Arden NH, Koplan JP, Goodman RA. Prevention and control of type A influenza infections in nursing homes. Benefits and costs of four approaches using vaccination and amantadine. Ann Intern Med 107:732–740, 1987.
114. Schoenbaum SC. Economic impact of influenza. The individual's perspective. Am J Med 82:26–30, 1987.
115. Maucher JM, Gambert SR. Cost-effective analysis of influenza vaccination in the elderly. Age 13:81–85, 1990.
116. Yassi A, Kettner J, Hammond G, et al. Effectiveness and cost-benefit of an influenza vaccination program for health care workers. Can J Infect Dis 2:101–108, 1991.
117. Mullooly JP, Bennett MD, Hornbrook MC, et al. Influenza vaccination programs for elderly persons: Cost-effectiveness in a health maintenance organization. Ann Intern Med 121:947–952, 1994.
118. Nichol KL, Margolis KL, Wuorenma J, Von Sternberg T. The efficacy and cost effectiveness of vaccination against influenza among elderly persons living in the community. N Engl J Med 331:778–784, 1994.
119. Campbell DS, Rumley MH. Cost-effectiveness of the influenza vaccine in a healthy, working-age population. J Occup Environ Med 39:408–414, 1997.
120. Office of Technology Assessment. A review of selected federal vaccine and immunization policies based on case studies of pneumococcal vaccine. Washington, DC, US Government Printing Office 052-003-00701-1, September, 1979.
121. Willems JS, Sanders CR, Riddiough MA, Bell JC. Cost-effectiveness of vaccination against pneumococcal pneumonia. N Engl J Med 303:553–559, 1980.
122. Patrick KM, Wooley FR. A cost-benefit analysis of immunization for pneumococcal pneumonia. JAMA 245:473–477, 1981.
123. Office of Technology Assessment. Update of federal activities regarding the use of pneumococcal vaccine. Washington, DC, U.S. Government Printing Office, OTA-TM-H-23, May, 1984.
124. Sisk JE, Riegelman RK. Cost effectiveness of vaccination against pneumococcal pneumonia: An update. Ann Intern Med 104:79–86, 1986.
125. Sisk JE, Moskowitz AJ, Whang W, et al. Cost-effectiveness of vaccination against pneumococcal bacteremia among elderly people. JAMA 278:1333–1339, 1997.
126. White CC, Koplan JP, Orenstein WA. Benefits, risks and costs of immunization for measles, mumps and rubella. Am J Public Health 75:739–744, 1985.
127. Wiedermann G, Ambrosch F. Cost-benefit calculations of vaccinations against measles and mumps in Austria. Dev Biol Stand 43:273–277, 1979.
128. Berger SA, Ginsberg GM, Slater PE. Cost-benefit analysis of routine mumps and rubella vaccination for Israeli infants. Isr J Med Sci 26:74–80, 1990.
129. Ferson MJ, Robertson PW, Whybin LR. Cost effectiveness of prevaccination screening of health care workers for immunity to measles, rubella and mumps. Med J Aust 160:478–482, 1994.
130. Hatziandreu EJ, Brown RE, Halpern MT. A cost benefit analysis of the measles-mumps-rubella (MMR) vaccine: Final report. Arlington, VA, Batelle, 1994.
131. Axnick NW, Shavell SM, Witte JJ. Benefits due to immunization against measles. Public Health Rep 84:673–680, 1969.

132. Witte JJ, Axnick NW. The benefits from 10 years of measles immunization in the United States. Public Health Rep 90:205–207, 1975.
133. Albritton RB. Cost-benefits of measles eradication: Effects of a federal intervention. Policy Anal 4:1–22, 1978.
134. Ponninghaus J. Cost-benefit analysis of measles immunization: A case-control study from Southern Zambia. J Trop Med Hyg 83:141–149, 1980.
135. World Health Organization. Expanded Programme on Immunization. Cost-effectiveness: Ivory Coast. Wkly Epidemiol Rec 22:170–173, 1982.
136. Davis RM, Markowitz KE, Preblud SR, et al. A cost-effectiveness analysis of measles outbreak control strategies. Am J Epidemiol 126:450–459, 1987.
137. Ginsberg GM, Tulchinsky TH. Costs and benefits of a second measles inoculation of children in Israel, the West Bank, and Gaza. J Epidemiol Commun Health 44:274–280, 1990.
138. Mast EE, Berg JL, Hanrahan MS, et al. Risk factors for measles in a previously vaccinated population and cost-effectiveness of revaccination strategies. JAMA 264:2529–2533, 1990.
139. Schlian DM, Matchar D, Seymann GB. Cost-effectiveness evaluation of measles immunization strategies on a college campus. Fam Pract Res J 11:193–207, 1991.
140. Subbarao EK, Amin S, Kumar ML. Prevaccination serologic screening for measles in health care workers. J Infect Dis 163:876–878, 1991.
141. Sellick JA, Longbine D, Schifeling R, Mylotte JM. Screening hospital employees for measles immunity is more cost effective than blind immunization. Ann Intern Med 116:982–984, 1992.
142. Shepard DS. Economic analysis of investment priorities for measles control. J Infect Dis 170(suppl 1):S56–S62, 1994.
143. Koplan JP, Preblud SR. A benefit-cost analysis of mumps vaccine. Am J Dis Child 136:362–364, 1982.
144. Arday DR, Kanjarpane DD, Kelley PW. Mumps in the US Army 1980–86: Should recruits be immunized? Am J Public Health 79:471–474, 1989.
145. Schoenbaum SC, Hyde JN, Bartoshesky L, Crampton K. Benefit-cost analysis of rubella vaccination policy. N Engl J Med 294:306–310, 1976.
146. Farber ME, Finkelstein SN. A cost-benefit analysis of a mandatory premarital rubella-antibody screening program. N Engl J Med 300:856–859, 1979.
147. Stray-Pedersen B. Economic evaluation of different vaccination programmes to prevent congenital rubella. NIPH Ann (Norway) 5:69–83, 1982.
148. Gudnadottir M. Cost-effectiveness of different strategies for prevention of congenital rubella infection: A practical example from Iceland. Rev Infect Dis 7(suppl):S200–S209, 1985.
149. Jackson LA, Schuchat A, Gorsky RD, Wenger JD. Should college students be vaccinated against meningococcal disease? Am J Public Health 85:843–845, 1995.
150. Weisbrod B. Costs and benefits of medical research: A case study of poliomyelitis. J Polit Econ 79:527–544, 1971.
151. Fudenberg HH. Fiscal returns of biomedical research. J Invest Dermatol 61:321–329, 1973.
152. Musgrove P. Is polio eradication in the Americas economically justified? PAHO Bull 22:1–16, 1988.
153. Hatziandreu EJ, Palmer CS, Halpen MT, Brown RE. A cost benefit analysis of the OPV vaccine. Arlington, VA, Battelle, 1994.
154. Bart KJ, Foulds J, Patriarca P. Global eradication of poliomyelitis: Benefit-cost analysis. Bull WHO 74:35–45, 1996.
155. Miller MA, Sutter RW, Strebel PM, Hadler SC. Cost-effectiveness of incorporating inactivated poliovirus vaccine into the routine childhood immunization schedule. JAMA 276:967–971, 1996.
156. Morrison AJ Jr, Hunt EH, Atuk NO, et al. Rabies preexposure prophylaxis using intradermal human diploid cell vaccine: Immunologic efficacy and cost-effectiveness in a university medical center and a review of selected literature. Am J Med Sci 293:293–297, 1987.
157. Bernard KW, Fishbein DB. Pre-exposure rabies prophylaxis for travelers: Are the benefits worth the cost? Vaccine 9:833–836, 1991.
158. Fishbein DB, Miranda NJ, Merrill P, et al. Rabies control in the Republic of the Philippines: Benefits and costs of elimination. Vaccine 9:581–587, 1991.
159. Uhaa IJ, Dato VM, Sorhage FE, et al. Benefits and costs of using an orally absorbed vaccine to control rabies in raccoons. J Am Vet Med Assoc 201:1873–1882, 1992.
160. Griffiths RI, Anderson GF, Powe NR, et al. Economic impact of immunization against rotavirus gastroenteritis. Arch Pediatr Adolesc Med 149:407–414, 1995.
161. Smith JC, Haddix AC, Teutsch SM, Glass RI. Cost-effectiveness analysis of a rotavirus immunization program for the United States. Pediatrics 96:609–615, 1995.
162. Guyatt HL, Evans D. Desirable characteristics of a schistosomiasis vaccine: Some implications of a cost effectiveness analysis. Acta Trop 59:197–209, 1995.
163. Preblud SR, Orenstein WA, Koplan JP, et al. A benefit-cost analysis of a childhood varicella vaccination program. Postgrad Med J 61(suppl 4):17–22, 1985.
164. Preblud SR. Varicella: Complications and costs. Pediatrics 78:728–735, 1988.
165. Weber DJ, Rutala WA, Parham C. Impact and costs of varicella prevention in a university hospital. Am J Public Health 78:19–23, 1988.
166. Kitai IC, King S, Gafni A. An economic evaluation of varicella vaccine for pediatric liver and kidney transplant recipients. Clin Infect Dis 17:441–447, 1993.
167. Huse DM, Meissner HC, Lacey MJ, Oster G. Childhood vaccination against chickenpox: An analysis of benefits and costs. J Pediatr 124:869–874, 1994.
168. Lieu TA, Cochi SL, Black SB, et al. Cost-effectiveness of a routine varicella vaccination program for US children. JAMA 271:375–381, 1994.
169. Lieu TA, Black SB, Rieser N, et al. The cost of childhood chickenpox: Parents' perspective. Pediatr Infect Dis J 13:173–177, 1994.
170. Ferson MJ. Another vaccine, another treadmill. J Paediatr Child Health 31:3–5, 1995.
171. Lieu TA, Finkler LJ, Sorel ME, et al. Cost-effectiveness of varicella serotesting versus presumptive vaccination of school-age children and adolescents. Pediatrics 95:632–638, 1995.
172. Beutels P, Clara R, Tormans G, Van Doorslaer E. Costs and benefits of routine varicella vaccination in German children. J Infect Dis 174(suppl):S335–S341, 1996.
173. Strassels SA, Sullivan SD. Clinical and economic considerations of vaccination against varicella. Pharmacotherapy 17:133–139, 1997.
174. Monath TP, Nasidi A. Should yellow fever vaccine be included in the Expanded Program of Immunization in Africa? A cost effectiveness analysis for Nigeria. Am J Trop Med Hyg 48:274–299, 1993.

chapter

46 Vaccines for International Travel

Elizabeth Day Barnett

Robert T. Chen

Michel Rey

INTERNATIONAL TRAVEL

International travel is increasing by about 7% each year. Individuals travel for many reasons, including tourism, business, educational experiences, and to flee from war, famine, or other intolerable situations. The tourism business alone accounts for nearly 5 billion trips annually. Although Europe and the Americas have remained the most popular tourist destinations over the past three decades, Africa, East Asia, and the Pacific regions account for the largest increases in number of tourists, with more than 65 million tourist arrivals noted in 1990. International tourist arrivals are projected to more than double from 94 million in 1990 to 207 million in 2010. The largest increases are expected in East Asia and the Pacific and Africa. Estimates of business travel suggest that more than 50 million additional departures are undertaken by business travelers. Refugees and other displaced populations numbered more than 50 million individuals worldwide in 1996.[1]

The risk of travelers contracting infectious diseases depends on destination, duration of the trip, and nature and conditions of travel. The vaccine-preventable disease most commonly contracted by travelers is hepatitis A, which may occur as frequently as 20 cases per 1000 travelers per month for travelers who are exposed to conditions of poor hygiene. Diseases for which travelers are at low risk include paralytic polio, which is estimated to occur at a rate of 20 per million unimmunized travelers, and Japanese encephalitis, occurring at an estimated rate of less than 1 per million for the usual traveler.[2] The risk of specific diseases may be increased during periods in which outbreaks of disease are occurring, such as with meningococcal disease in Sub-Saharan Africa and diphtheria in the newly independent states of the former Soviet Union. Given the growth of international travel, it is likely that most health providers will be called on to offer advice about pretravel immunizations. Although clinics specializing in pretravel advice and immunization are present in many locations, it remains incumbent on primary care providers to be able to provide basic pretravel services and to be able to identify patients in need of specialized advice. Health information for international travel is now widely available via print and electronic media that is targeted toward both the professional and the consumer.

Information about disease epidemiology and vaccine characteristics are presented in detail in other chapters. This chapter focuses on disease risk specific to travelers and considerations taken in choosing whether a traveler is a candidate for specific vaccines. Because national standards for licensure differ, not all the vaccines are available in all countries. Similarly, vaccines against the same disease and recommended vaccine schedules may differ somewhat by manufacturer and the national authority.

GENERAL INFORMATION

Approach to Travel Immunizations

The two steps in immunizing travelers are to update routine immunizations and to provide travel-specific immunizations. To do the first, a knowledge of a patient's previous immunizations and medical history is necessary. For the second, detailed information about the patient's itinerary, living conditions during the journey, mode of travel (e.g., adventure travel or chaperoned luxury tour) and purpose of travel (e.g., medical or veterinary work, tourism, visiting relatives) is needed. Although sometimes mistakenly regarded as a rote selection of vaccines based on the destination country, the choice of vaccines more often requires thoughtful consideration based on details of the patient's medical history, knowledge of vaccine interactions with other vaccines or medications, timing of departure and nature of travel with regard to risk for vaccine-preventable diseases, and patient preferences.

Sources of Information on Travel Vaccines

Sources of health information for international travel include (1) International Travel and Health—Vaccination Requirements and Health Advice, published by the World Health Organization (WHO) in Geneva, Switzerland (phone 41-022-791-21-11 or via Internet at http://www.who.ch), and (2) Health Information for International Travel, published by the Centers for Disease Control and Prevention (CDC), Atlanta, Georgia. The CDC information (including how to order) is also available from the CDC hotline (404-332-4559), the Internet (http://www.cdc.gov), and the File Transfer Protocol server at ftp.cdc.gov. The CDC also publishes the biweekly Blue Sheets, which provide information about current travel issues. Many countries publish national guidelines regarding travel health information, and readers are encouraged to contact their local and national public health services. Several excellent sources of travel health information are also available in textbooks[3, 4] and in review articles.[5, 6] Most of these sources have excellent information about malaria prophylaxis, which is not covered here. Many sites on the Internet provide travel health information for health providers and the public.

Simultaneous Administration of Vaccines and Immunoglobulin

Scheduling of multiple vaccines for the traveler is challenging, especially when departures are imminent. Few travelers allow as long as a month for vaccines; many come for consultation only a few days before departure. Immunization schedules may need to be accelerated, or vaccines limited to those most appropriate to the infectious disease risks likely to be faced by the traveler. Although many patients as well as providers are concerned about the likelihood of adverse reactions to multiple vaccines administered simultaneously, a recent study reported that adverse events were generally minor and not incapacitating and therefore need not be a reason for withholding indicated vaccines.[7]

Most vaccines may be given simultaneously without concern for decreased immunogenicity. Inactivated vaccines can be given concurrently or at any interval before or after other inactivated or live vaccines. Live vaccines should be administered either simultaneously or 30 days apart, with two exceptions. Oral polio vaccine and measles, mumps, and rubella (MMR) may be given at any interval relative to each other, and cholera and yellow fever vaccines should be separated by 3 weeks or more.

Antibody responses to live vaccines may be impaired if live virus vaccines are given at the same time as immune globulin for prevention of hepatitis A. Live virus vaccines should be administered at least 2 weeks before, or at least 6 weeks after, immune globulin. Immune globulin has not been shown to interfere with responses to polio, yellow fever, or oral typhoid vaccines. For individuals who receive immune globulin at higher doses, more time may be required between immune globulin and vaccine administration. Information specific to this topic is available elsewhere.[8, 9] (See Chapter 5 and individual chapters on specific vaccines.)

Immunization of Individuals with Altered Immunocompetence

Detailed recommendations regarding immunization of immune-compromised individuals are published elsewhere.[10] In general, immunocompromised persons should not receive live viral vaccines. Information specific to travel vaccines is presented in the sections on individual vaccines.

Effect of Antimalarials and Antimicrobial Agents on Vaccine Response

When antimalarials in the chloroquine/mefloquine family are administered simultaneously with human diploid cell rabies vaccine and oral typhoid vaccine, they may interfere with immunogenicity of the vaccines.[56, 66, 67] Details of these interactions can be found in the sections devoted to individual vaccines. Antimicrobial agents taken concurrently with oral typhoid vaccine may also interfere with vaccine response.

Routine Childhood Immunizations and Modifications Needed for Travelers

Routine childhood immunizations should be brought up to date as part of preparation for international travel. Information is available from many sources about routine childhood immunizations. In the United States, a schedule is published every 12 months.[11] Readers are referred to country-specific schedules for this information. Some children will require accelerated schedules because of imminent departure dates or because of delays in receiving routine immunizations. The reader is referred to Chapter 5 for accelerated schedules and to the chapters on individual vaccines for detailed information on indications, contraindications, precautions, and expected adverse events. Children in the United States are immunized routinely against 10 diseases (Table 46–1). Most of the diseases are prevalent worldwide, although the risk of contracting these diseases may vary markedly depending on travel destination. For example, individuals traveling to the independent states of the former Soviet Union are at increased risk of diphtheria; those heading to many developing countries may be at greater risk for measles, mumps, and rubella; and those planning visits to areas of the world where hepatitis B remains endemic may be at greater risk for that disease. In contrast, travelers remaining within the Americas, where polio has been eradicated, do not need to receive polio immunization beyond a primary series, whereas those heading for destinations where polio still occurs should have one additional dose of vaccine. Risk for tetanus remains constant worldwide, and all adults should receive booster doses of toxoid every 10 years.

Routine Adult Immunizations

Pretravel consultation is an opportunity to update the immunization status of adults. Information about adult

Table 46–1. **VACCINATIONS RECOMMENDED ROUTINELY FOR CHILDREN AND ADULTS IN THE UNITED STATES WITH SPECIAL INDICATIONS FOR TRAVELERS**

DISEASE	VACCINE	AGE GROUPS	GREATEST AREAS OF RISK	SPECIAL INDICATIONS
Diphtheria	DTaP or DTP	<7 years	Developing world, countries of former Soviet Union	
	Td	≥7 years		
Tetanus	DTaP or DTP	<7 years	Worldwide	
	Td	≥7 years		
Pertussis	DTaP or DTP	<7 years	Worldwide circulation of organism	No vaccine available for ≥7 yr
Polio	IPV or OPV, or both	<18 years and previously vaccinated adults	Most of developing world except Americas	Extra dose of IPV or OPV (if previously fully immunized) for persons traveling to areas of risk
	IPV only	Unvaccinated adults and immunocompromised individuals		
Measles	MMR, MR, M	All ages for susceptible individuals	Most of the world	Second dose indicated if no prior history of two doses on or after second birthday; most persons born prior to 1957 can be considered immune and do not need vaccination
Mumps	MMR, Mu	All ages for susceptible individuals	Most of the world	
Rubella	MMR or MR, or R	All ages for susceptible individuals	Most of the world	Especially for nonpregnant females of childbearing age
Haemophilus influenzae type b	Hib	<5 yr	Most of the world	
Hepatitis B	Hep B	Routine childhood and adolescence; older ages with special risk	Most of the world See Figure 46–1 for areas most at risk	Stays of 6 mo or longer in developing countries or with occupational or behavioral risk factors for disease
Varicella	Varicella	All ages for susceptible individuals	Most of the world	
Influenza*	Influenza	1 dose annually in individuals ≥65 years; also younger special risk groups such as persons with chronic cardiopulmonary disease	Most of the world	Northern Hemisphere season December through March; Southern Hemisphere season April through September
Pneumococcal*	Pneumococcal	All adults ≥65 yr; also younger special risk groups such as persons with chronic cardiopulmonary disease	Most of the world	

*Vaccines routinely indicated for adults.

DTaP, diphtheria, tetanus, and acellular pertussis; DTP, diphtheria, tetanus, and pertussis; Hep B; hepatitis B; Hib; *Haemophilus influenzae* type b; IPV, inactivated polio vaccine; M, measles; MR, measles and rubella; MMR, measles, mumps, and rubella; OPV, oral polio vaccine; Td, tetanus and diphtheria; Mu, mumps; R, rubella.

immunization requirements are available from many sources.[12–14] Indications specific to travel are given in sections referring to individual vaccines. All adults 65 years or older should receive pneumococcal vaccine and annual influenza vaccination (see Table 45–1). Because influenza seasons vary between northern and southern hemispheres, the recommended time for influenza vaccination depends on itinerary and timing.

VACCINES FOR TRAVEL

Selected Routine Immunizations Especially Important for Travelers

Diphtheria

Recent epidemics of diphtheria in the newly independent states of the former Soviet Union[15] and in Thailand, Algeria, and Ecuador[16] underscore the need for attention to diphtheria immunization for travelers to these areas and for continuing to provide routine booster doses (supplied as a combination tetanus-diphtheria toxoid) throughout adulthood.

Although the risk of diphtheria is probably low, cases have been reported in travelers.[17, 18] Migrant populations may also be responsible for transmission of disease into populations in which immunity has waned because of a decrease in natural disease and lack of routine adult vaccine boosters. In the United States, 20 to 60% of adults older than 20 years of age are susceptible to diphtheria,[19, 20] and in western Europe serological surveys have shown immunity to diphtheria to be poor among adults, particularly women; men may be given boosters during military service.[21]

The travel consultation may be used as an opportunity to bring every individual up to date with diphtheria immunization, according to accepted schedules. A booster dose of combined tetanus-diphtheria toxoids every 10 years is acceptable in most countries.

Polio

The program for worldwide polio eradication is proceeding rapidly. The last case of paralytic polio due to wild poliovirus occurred in the Americas in 1991, and the Western Hemisphere was declared polio-free in 1994.[22] The goal of worldwide eradication by the year 2000 in most parts of the world or shortly thereafter seems attainable.

There remain areas of the world where polio occurs, and maintaining adequate levels of immunization against polio is important for travelers to these areas. The risk for polio in the traveler to developing countries has been estimated to be 0.002% for asymptomatic disease (unvaccinated individuals), and 0.0001% for paralytic disease.[23]

Individuals traveling to areas of the world where polio continues to occur should have their status with regard to polio immunization reviewed. If a full primary series cannot be documented, the series should be completed prior to departure, if possible. Inactivated polio vaccine (IPV) is indicated for unvaccinated adults; IPV or oral polio vaccine (OPV) can be used for children, although a sequential IPV/OPV schedule is now preferred in the United States.[23a] Children or adults who have been partially immunized may complete the series with either IPV or OPV. If time does not allow for full immunization prior to travel, the interval between doses of vaccine may be shortened to allow the maximal number of doses to be administered prior to departure. If a full series has been completed, a single additional dose of vaccine is indicated. Either OPV or IPV may be given, depending on the patient's individual situation. In some countries, a combination tetanus-IPV vaccine is available.

Hepatitis B

Hepatitis B is one of the most common serious vaccine-preventable diseases to affect travelers. Risk is increased with longer length of stay, contact with population groups with high carrier rates of hepatitis B (Fig. 46–1), occupations such as health care workers or laboratory workers, and behaviors such as injecting drug use and having multiple sex partners. For Swiss tourists traveling to developing countries, risk was reported to be 39 per 100,000 travelers for a stay of 1 month.[22] Long-term overseas workers are at greater risk; unimmunized U.S. missionaries serving in Africa were shown to have attack rates of 11% during the first 2 years of service and median annual attack rates of 1.2% over the next decade.[24] Professional workers in developing countries had a monthly incidence of symptomatic disease of 20 to 60 per 100,000.[25]

For travelers to countries where hepatitis B is prevalent, the three-dose series of vaccine is recommended for those whose stay will last 6 months or longer or those who have any of the risk factors indicated previously. The first two doses should be given 4 weeks apart and the third dose 4 to 12 months after the second. If insufficient time is available before departure, rapid seroconversion may be achieved by giving the third dose as early as 4 weeks after the second, with a fourth dose given 12 months from the first to ensure long-term protection. Hepatitis B vaccine is also indicated for travelers to all countries who may engage in high-risk behaviors.

Measles

Although cases of measles in the Americas have declined substantially in the last decade, measles continues to be an important cause of childhood morbidity and

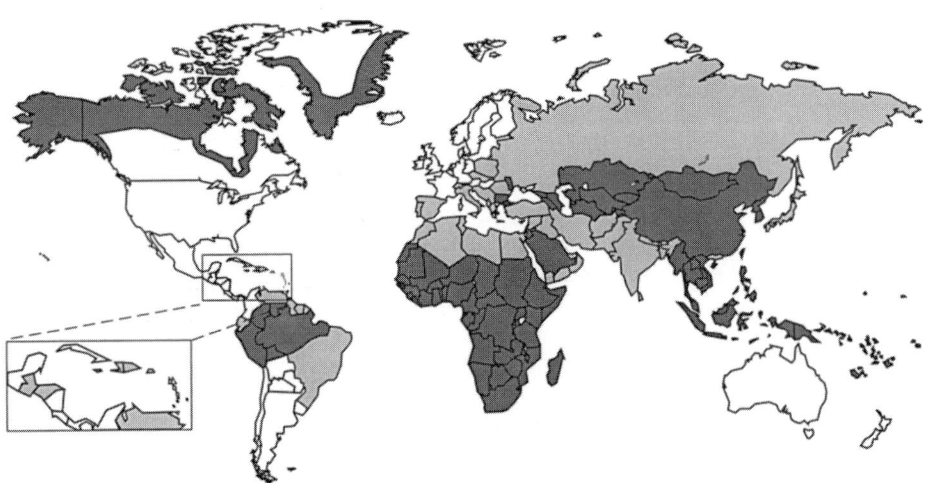

Figure 46–1. Geographical distribution of hepatitis B prevalence.

mortality worldwide. More than two thirds of cases of measles reported in the United States in 1996 were linked to international sources, primarily in Europe or Asia.[26] In the United States, 2 doses of vaccine are recommended for all school children and college students.[27]

Individuals who plan international travel to areas where measles remains prevalent should receive two doses of measles vaccine, preferably supplied as MMR vaccine, beginning at 12 months of age. MMR vaccine can be administered to children 6 to 12 months of age if traveling to areas where they will be at high risk of disease, but this dose of vaccine should not be counted toward the two-dose series. Monovalent measles vaccine may be given if available. Children younger than 6 months are likely to be protected by maternal antibody. Adults born before 1957 are assumed to have natural immunity; those born in 1957 or after without a history of vaccination who are traveling to endemic areas can receive a single dose of MMR vaccine, although two doses at least 1 month apart are preferable. Adults who received a dose in the past should receive a second dose.

Pertussis

Pertussis continues to be a disease of worldwide importance, affecting more than 50 million individuals and resulting in more than 500,000 deaths, despite widespread availability of vaccine.[28] Attack rates of pertussis are directly related to the use of vaccine; following declines in the use of vaccines in Japan, Sweden, and Britain, resurgence of disease was noted.[29] Acellular pertussis vaccines, now marketed in many areas, hold promise for equivalent or better efficacy than whole cell preparations, with fewer side effects.

The increased increment of risk for pertussis due to international travel is unknown. Children should complete as much of a primary series as possible, or be given any boosters due,[30] prior to international travel. Although there is substantial interest in protecting adults, currently adults are not candidates for pertussis vaccine.

Influenza

Influenza occurs worldwide; in the tropics transmission occurs throughout the year, whereas peaks of transmission occur from December through March in the northern Hemisphere and April through September in the Southern hemisphere.[31] Risk to travelers for contracting influenza depends primarily on season of travel; risk for serious disease depends on underlying health status. Individuals who travel during seasons of transmission are candidates for the current season's influenza vaccine, especially if at increased risk for complications.

TRAVEL VACCINES

Bacille Calmette-Guérin

Bacille Calmette-Guérin (BCG) vaccines are available in many countries but vary in efficacy. In the United States, a program of surveillance using tuberculin skin testing and early identification and treatment of infected individuals is preferred over universal immunization with BCG.[32]

Estimates of risk for tuberculosis (TB) among travelers are difficult to obtain. Studies of military personnel who served during the war in Vietnam cite skin test conversion rates of 4.7%, compared with rates of 1% per year for Army personnel who remained in the United States.[33] Risk to travelers is not felt to be high enough to warrant routine immunization for travel. For the rare circumstance in which BCG is indicated in the United States (a young child living in a household where exposure to active TB is unavoidable and where other preventive measures have failed or cannot be implemented) vaccine is available from Organon, Inc., West Orange, New Jersey. As the protective effect of BCG has been confirmed mainly in children, it is unlikely that there would be many indications for BCG for adults who are traveling.

BCG continues to be used in most countries of the world. Health care providers may be asked to provide BCG immunization to individuals who will be living for extended periods of time where BCG vaccine is used routinely. Risk of disease must be weighed against the loss of ability to test for infection using tuberculin skin testing. BCG might be considered for long-term residents of areas where the incidence of disease is high (more than 30 to 40 per 100,000) and where occupation or living conditions may result in significant exposures to infected individuals.

Side effects to vaccine occur in up to 10% of individuals and usually consist of local ulceration and inflammatory adenitis. BCG vaccine is contraindicated in immunocompromised individuals because of the risk of dissemination of infection. Decisions to immunize human immunodeficiency virus (HIV)-infected, but immunocompetent individuals is controversial; the bacteria are able to remain dormant for years and cause disease if an individual becomes immunocompromised. Risk of infection with TB, such as in infants in developing countries with high rates of tuberculosis, must be weighed against the risk of vaccination for those who may be at risk for HIV infection. The World Health Organization continues to recommend universal immunization with BCG for infants in areas where risk of TB is substantial.

Cholera

The risk of cholera is low for travelers; the disease is estimated to occur in 1 in 500,000 travelers.[34] The mainstay of protection against cholera remains avoidance of ingestion of high-risk foods, such as raw shellfish, and the use of precautions when making other food selections. Unchlorinated water is also a common source of infection.

Cholera occurring in the world today is due to *Vibrio cholerae* O-group 1 or O-group 139. The vaccine currently licensed in the United States probably provides virtually no protection against disease caused by *V. cholerae* O-group 139, and a two-dose series provides only about 50% effectiveness for 3 to 6 months against O-group 1. Because of low vaccine efficacy, low risk of disease, the ability to exercise precautions that can reduce risk of disease, and the treatable nature of disease, cholera vaccine is not recommended for travelers.[35] Newer oral vaccines and formulations that protect against *V. cholerae* O-group 139 are licensed in Europe and are likely to become more widely available; this development has not affected current recommendations for travelers.[36] For the rare individual traveling to areas of high risk and poor sanitary conditions (e.g., relief workers in the midst of cholera outbreaks), an initial series plus booster doses at 6-month intervals while the individual remains at risk may be considered. Food and water precautions continue to be crucial in view of the limited efficacy of vaccine.

According to World Health Organization recommendations, no country currently requires cholera immunization for entry. Occasionally travelers will report that they have been required to provide documentation of cholera immunization to obtain a visa despite these recommendations. If travelers are adamant about being immunized, a single dose documented on the International Certificate of Immunization is usually sufficient to satisfy authorities in these circumstances.

Vaccine dose depends on age and is indicated in Table 46–2. Serious adverse effects are rare, although immunization is often followed by local symptoms of pain, redness and swelling at the site of injection, which may be accompanied by fever, malaise, and headache. Children younger than 6 months should not be given vaccine; breast-feeding and good hand washing should be protective. Immunization is not recommended during pregnancy; specific safety information about the use of this vaccine during pregnancy is not available.

Antibody response to cholera and yellow fever vaccines may be impaired if these two vaccines are given simultaneously or separated by up to 3 weeks from each other; when possible, doses of these vaccines should be separated by at least 3 weeks.

Hepatitis A

Hepatitis A is the most common vaccine-preventable disease to affect travelers, and it may occur as much as 10 to 100 times as often as typhoid in unprotected American and European tourists who visit countries or areas of countries with poor hygienic conditions. For short-term travelers to areas of hepatitis A endemicity, risk has been estimated to range from 3 to 109 per 1000 travelers, for stays ranging from 2 weeks to 1 month.[37] For long-term travelers such as missionaries, attack rates were as high as 28% during the first 2 years of service.[38] Risk for disease depends on length of stay and conditions of travel, including frequency of exposure to contaminated food and water. Figure 46–2 shows the geographic distribution of risk for hepatitis A. Cases of hepatitis A, however, have been reported in tourists staying in luxury accommodations in countries where the risk of hepatitis A is high.[39] Despite the availability of both immunoglobulin and an effective vaccine, many travelers are not protected against hepatitis A.

Individuals born in Europe or North America since World War II have a low prevalence of immunity to hepatitis A. Rates of immunity are higher with increased age, history of jaundice, and birth or residence outside the United States. As many as 95% of individuals born and raised in developing countries with patterns of high endemicity for hepatitis A may be protected by naturally acquired antibody.[40]

Options for immunoprophylaxis of hepatitis A include intramuscular immunoglobulin and hepatitis A vaccine. Immune globulin was the mainstay of protection for many years and has been shown to be 85 to 90% protective. The major disadvantage of immune globulin is that it is short-acting and must be repeated for subsequent journeys, or additional doses must be given during prolonged residence in endemic areas. It does not offer effective protection against hepatitis B, C, or E. Adverse events are rare, although the large volume required may result in local discomfort. One advantage of this preparation is that it may be given immediately before departure.

Hepatitis A vaccines have been marketed in Europe since 1992 and in the United States since 1995. Three products, Havrix (SmithKline Beecham), VAQTA (Merck), and AVAXIM (Pasteur Mérieux Connaught) are now available, although the latter is not licensed in the United States as of October 1998. All three vaccines are highly immunogenic in adults, with protective antibody levels achieved in 95 to 100% of adults 1 month after the first injection, using the recommended adult doses of Havrix 1440 enzyme-linked immunosorbent assay (ELISA) units (EU) in 1.0 mL; VAQTA 50 units in 1.0 mL or AVAXIM 160 units in 0.6 mL. (It should be noted that as no international standardized reference exists for hepatitis A antigen content; each laboratory has expressed the antigen content using an in-house reference.) One month after the booster dose, given at 6 to 12 months, seroconversion rates of 100% were reported with all three vaccines.[41, 42] For last-minute

Table 46–2. **CHOLERA VACCINE**

	INTRADERMAL ROUTE*	SUBCUTANEOUS OR INTRAMUSCULAR ROUTE			
DOSES	5 Yr of Age and Older	6 Mo–4 Yr of Age	5–10 Yr of Age	Older than 10 Yr of Age	COMMENTS
Primary series: 1 and 2	0.2 mL	0.2 mL	0.3 mL	0.5 mL	Give 1 wk to 1 mo or more apart
Booster	0.2 mL	0.2 mL	0.3 mL	0.5 mL	1 dose every 6 mo

*Higher levels of protection (antibody) may be achieved in children less than 5 yr of age by the subcutaneous or intramuscular route.

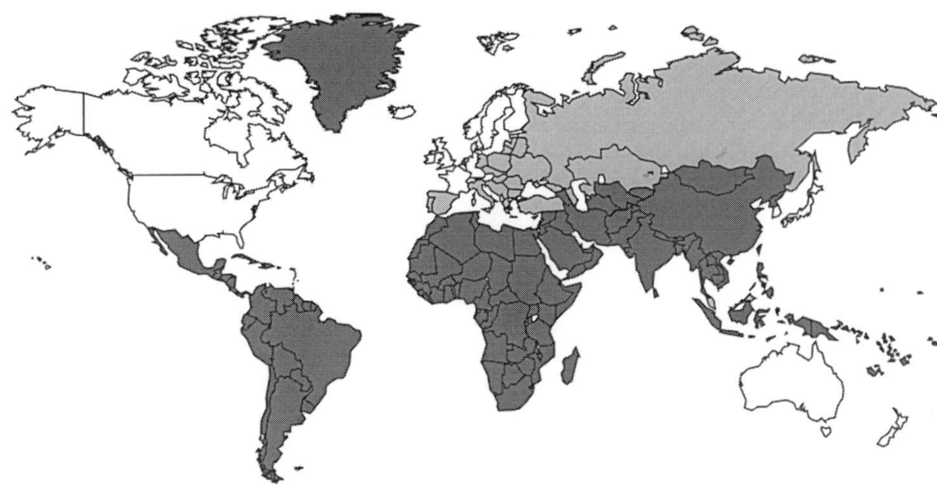

Figure 46–2. Geographical distribution of hepatitis A prevalence.

travelers, seroconversion rates of 87.1% (Havrix 1440 EU) and 95.7% (AVAXIM) were reported at 14 days in a comparative trial.[42a]

Efficacy studies have been performed in Thailand (Havrix) and during a hepatitis A epidemic in the United States (VAQTA), demonstrating clinical efficacy of 94% and 100%, respectively. Havrix and VAQTA also have a pediatric formulation for children 2 to 17 years (720 EU and 25 units, respectively). Similar protective levels of antibody have been reported in children as for adults.[43]

Individuals traveling to areas of intermediate or high endemicity are candidates for protection against hepatitis A. Ideally, vaccine should be given at least 4 weeks prior to initiation of travel because of the concern that neutralizing antibody is not optimal prior to this time. Travelers with earlier departure dates may receive, in addition to vaccine, an appropriate dose of immune globulin at a separate site. A booster dose 6 to 12 months after the initial dose is expected to provide long-term (at least 10 years) protection. Children younger than 2 years should receive immune globulin alone, since the safety and efficacy of vaccine have not been adequately evaluated in this age group. Doses of immune globulin may be given as close as possible to departure date; dose depends on weight and length of stay. Doses of vaccine and immune globulin are listed in Tables 46–3 through 46–5.

Hepatitis A vaccine is generally well tolerated. The most common vaccine side effects include soreness at the injection site, headache, and malaise. Serious adverse events appear to be rare. Vaccine should not be given to individuals with allergies to adjuvants or preservatives contained in the vaccine. Although the risk of vaccination during pregnancy should be low, risk of disease must be weighed against theoretical risk of immunization. Vaccine is inactivated and therefore may be used in immunocompromised individuals. Simultaneous administration of hepatitis A vaccine and diphtheria, oral and inactivated polio vaccines, tetanus, oral typhoid, cholera, Japanese encephalitis, rabies, or yellow fever vaccines does not impair immune response to either vaccine or increase adverse events.[44]

Serious adverse events following immune globulin are rare, although anaphylaxis has been reported in IgA-deficient individuals; immune globulin should not be used in these individuals.

Table 46–3. **IMMUNE GLOBULIN FOR PROTECTION AGAINST VIRAL HEPATITIS A**

LENGTH OF STAY	BODY WEIGHT		DOSE VOLUME*	COMMENTS
	lb	kg†		
Short-term travel (<3 mo)	<50	<23	0.5 mL	Dose volume depends on body weight and length of stay
	50–100	23–45	1.0 mL	
	>100	>45	2.0 mL	
Long-term travel (3–5 mo)	<22	<10	0.5 mL	
	22–49	10–22	1.0 mL	
	50–100	23–45	2.5 mL	
	>100	>45	5.0 mL	

*For intramuscular injection.
†kg = approximately 2.2 lb.

Table 46–4. **RECOMMENDED DOSES OF Havrix***

GROUP	AGE (YR)	DOSE (EU)†	VOLUME	NO. DOSES	SCHEDULE (MO)‡
Children and adolescents§	2–18	720	0.5 mL	2	0, 6–12
Adults	>18	1440	1.0 mL	2	0, 6–12

*Hepatitis A vaccine, inactivated, SmithKline Beecham Biologicals.
†EU = enzyme-linked immunosorbent assay (ELISA) units.
‡0 mo represents timing of the initial dose; subsequent numbers represent months after the initial dose.
§An alternate formulation and schedule (three doses) are available for children and adolescents and consist of 360 EU per 0.5 mL dose at 0, 1, and 6–12 months of age.

Immune globulin may interfere with response to certain live virus vaccines, such as measles, mumps, rubella, and varicella. It has been shown not to interfere with the immune response to oral polio or yellow fever vaccines. If travelers require both MMR or varicella vaccine and immune globulin, the vaccines ideally should be given 2 weeks (3 weeks for varicella vaccine) prior to giving immune globulin. If immune globulin for hepatitis A has been given, subsequent immunization with MMR or varicella vaccine should be delayed 5 months. If risk of multiple diseases is high, vaccine plus immune globulin may be given closer than 2 weeks apart, but the MMR and varicella vaccine doses should be repeated 5 or more months after immune globulin.

Testing for susceptibility to hepatitis A before offering vaccine or immune globulin may be cost-effective in specific situations. Candidates for testing may include individuals who were born and raised in high-endemicity areas and those with a history of jaundice. Other considerations include cost of testing compared with cost of immunization and assuring that testing will not delay ability to provide immunization if an individual is seronegative. It is estimated that if cost of screening is one third the cost of immunization, and the individual's likelihood of immunity is greater than 33%, testing should be cost-effective.[45]

Japanese Encephalitis

Japanese encephalitis is a leading cause of viral encephalitis in Asia and is transmitted by mosquitoes. Risk to travelers is low, with estimates of risk ranging from less than 1 per million to 1 in 5000 per month of exposure in rural endemic areas. Most travelers have no natural immunity to the disease. Although risk is highest for individuals who travel during the season of high transmission and remain in endemic areas for extended periods, cases have occurred in short-stay tourists.[46, 47] Detailed information about the risk of Japanese encephalitis by country, region, and season is listed in Table 46–6.

Japanese encephalitis vaccine has been licensed in Japan since 1954 and has been widely available in the United States since 1992.[48] Generalized urticaria and angioedema after vaccine have occurred within minutes to as long as 2 weeks after immunization. After a first vaccine dose, reactions occurred a median of 12 hours after immunization; 88% of reactions occurred within 3 days. The interval between a second dose and onset of symptoms was longer, with a median of 3 days, and extending to 2 weeks. Reactions have occurred after a second or third dose, even when earlier doses have been uneventful. Vaccinees should be observed for 30 minutes following immunizations and instructed about the possibility of these reactions; individuals with a previous history of urticaria may be at increased risk for these reactions. This risk plays a part in deciding whether individual travelers are candidates for vaccine.

Vaccine is not recommended for all travelers to endemic areas; protective measures for individuals who are not immunized include prevention of mosquito bites through the use of window screens, bed nets, and insect repellents. Vaccine is most appropriate for individuals who will spend a month or longer in endemic areas, especially in rural areas in the transmission season. Other travelers, such as those traveling to endemic areas during epidemic transmission or those whose occupation or living conditions will place them at increased risk of exposure, may be candidates for vaccine even if traveling for less than 1 month.

The primary series of Japanese encephalitis vaccine results in optimal immune response if given in three doses on days 0, 7, and 30 (Table 46–7). Time constraints may require abbreviated schedules of three doses on days 0, 7, and 14 or two doses on days 0 and 7; however, antibody response may be less. Ideally, the third dose of vaccine should be given at least 10 days

Table 46–5. **RECOMMENDED DOSES OF VAQTA* AND AVAXIM†**

GROUP	AGE (YR)	DOSE (UNITS)	VOLUME	NO. DOSES	SCHEDULE (MO)‡
VAQTA					
Children and adolescents	2–17	25	0.5 mL	2	0, 6–18
Adults	≥18	50	1.0 mL	2	0, 6
AVAXIM					
Adults	≥16	160	0.5 mL	2	0, 6–18

*Hepatitis A vaccine, inactivated, Merck & Company, Inc.
†Hepatitis A vaccine, Pasteur Mérieux Connaught.
‡0 months represents timing of the initial dose; subsequent numbers represent months after the initial dose.

Table 46–6. RISK OF JAPANESE ENCEPHALITIS BY COUNTRY, REGION, AND SEASON

COUNTRY	AFFECTED AREAS/JURISDICTIONS	TRANSMISSION SEASON	COMMENTS
Bangladesh	Few data, probably widespread	Possibly July–December, as in northern India	Outbreak reported from Tangail district, Dacca division; sporadic cases in Rajshahi division
Bhutan	No data	No data	
Brunei	Presumed to be sporadic-endemic, as in Malaysia	Presumed year-round transmission	
Cambodia	Probably endemic-hyperendemic country-wide	Presumed to be May–October	Cases from Phnom Penh recognized
India	Reported cases from all states except Arunachal, Dadra, Daman, Diu, Gujarat, Himachal, Jammu, Kashmir, Lakshadweep, Meghalaya, Nagar Haveli, Orissa, Punjab, Rajasthan, and Sikkim	*South India:* May–October in Goa; October–January in Tamil Nadu; August–December in Karnataka; second peak, April–June in Mandya district *Andrha Pradesh:* September–December *North India:* July–December	Outbreaks in West Bengal, Bihar, Karnataka, Tamil Nadu, Andrha Pradesh, Assam, Uttar Pradesh, Manipure, Maharashtra, and Goa; urban cases reported (e.g., Lucknow)
Indonesia	Kalimantan, Bali, Nusa Tenggara, Sulawesi, Mollucas, West Irian, Java, Lombok	Probably year-round risk; varies by island; peak risks associated with rainfall, rice cultivation, and presence of pigs; peak period of risk: November–March; June–July in some years	Hyperendemic on Bali; sporadic cases recognized elsewhere; vaccine not recommended if travel is to major cities only
Japan*	Rare-sporadic cases on all islands, except Hokkaido	June–September except Ryukyu Islands (Okinawa), April–October	Vaccine not routinely recommended if travel is to major cities only; enzootic transmission without human cases observed on Hokkaido
Korea*	*North Korea:* no data *South Korea:* rare sporadic cases	July–October	Last major outbreaks in 1982–1983; vaccine not recommended if travel is to major cities only
Laos	Presumed to be endemic-hyperendemic country-wide	Presumed to be May–October	No data
Malaysia	Sporadic-endemic in all states of Peninsula, Sarawak, and probably Sabah	No seasonal pattern; year-round transmission	Vaccine not recommended if travel is to major cities only
Myanmar	Presumed to be endemic-hyperendemic country-wide	Presumed to be May–October	Repeated outbreaks in Shan State in Chiang Mai Valley
Nepal	Hyperendemic in southern lowlands (Terai); sporadic cases now recognized in Kathmandu Valley	July–December	Vaccine recommended for travelers to lowlands
Papua-New Guinea	Sporadic cases (1956 and 1997–1998) reported from Western, Gulf, and South Highland Provinces	Unknown	Vaccine not routinely recommended
People's Republic of China	Cases in all provinces except Xizang (Tibet), Xinjiang, and Qinghai; hyperendemic in southern China; endemic–periodically epidemic in temperate areas; Hong Kong: rare cases in New Territories	*Northern China:* May–September *Southern China:* April–October (Guangshi, Yunnan, Gwangdong, and Southern Fujian, Szechuan, Guizhou, Hunan, and Jiangsi provinces)	Vaccine not routinely recommended for travelers to major cities only (including Hong Kong)
Pakistan	May be transmitted in central deltas	Presumed to be June–January	Cases reported near Karachi; endemic areas overlap those for West Nile virus
Philippines	Presumed to be endemic on all islands	Uncertain; speculations based on locations and agroecosystems *West Luzon, Mindoro, Negro Palowan:* April–November *Elsewhere:* Year-round; greatest risk, April–January	Outbreaks described in Nueva Ecija, Luzon, and Manila
Russia	Far Eastern maritime areas south of Khabarousk	Peak period, July–September	Rare human cases reported
Singapore	Rare cases—last indigenous case in 1992	Year-round transmission not detected recently	Vaccine not routinely recommended
Sri Lanka	Endemic in all but mountainous areas; periodically epidemic in northern and central provinces	October–January; secondary peak of enzootic transmission, May–June	Recent outbreaks in central (Anuradhapura) and northwestern provinces
Taiwan*	Sporadic cases except in central mountains	April–October; June peak	Cases in and around Taipei
Thailand	Hyperendemic in north; sporadic-endemic in south	May–October	Annual outbreaks in Chiang Mai Valley; sporadic cases in Bangkok suburbs
Vietnam	Endemic-hyperendemic in all provinces	May–October	Highest rates in and near Hanoi
Western Pacific and Australia	Discrete epidemics reported on Guam, Saipan (northern Mariana Islands); sporadic cases in Torres Strait and Cape York peninsula, Australia	Uncertain; possibly September–January in the Pacific; February–April in far northern Australia	Enzootic cycle may not be sustainable; epidemics may follow introductions of virus; single case reported on Australian mainland (Cape York peninsula) in 1998

*Reported human cases may not accurately reflect risks to nonimmune visitors because of high immunization rates in local populations. Humans are incidental to the transmission cycle. High levels of viral transmission may occur in the absence of human disease.

Notes:

1. Assessments are based on publications, surveillance reports, and personal correspondence.
2. Extrapolations have been made from available data.
3. Transmission patterns may change.
4. Consult the Centers for Disease Control and Prevention (970-221-6400) or other public health authorities for the latest trends.

From Tsai TF, Yu YX. Japanese encephalitis vaccines. Chapter 27, p 700.

Table 46–7. **JAPANESE ENCEPHALITIS VACCINE**

	SUBCUTANEOUS ROUTE		
DOSES	1–2 Yr of Age	3 Yr of Age or Older	COMMENTS
Primary series 1, 2, and 3	0.5 mL	1.0 mL	Days 0, 7, 30
Booster*	1.0 mL	1.0 mL	1 dose at ≥36 mo

*In vaccinees who have completed a three-dose primary series, the full duration of protection is unknown. Booster recommended at ≥36 months based on preliminary serologic data. Recommendations may change as more information is collected.

before commencement of travel to ensure optimal antibody response and to allow access to medical care should an adverse event occur. Children 1 to 2 years of age receive half the adult dose of vaccine given to individuals 3 years of age and older. Data are unavailable about safety and efficacy of vaccine in children less than 1 year of age; when possible, immunization should be deferred during the first year of life. Duration of immunity is unknown; at this time, booster doses are recommended after 3 years based on preliminary serologic data. Immunization during pregnancy is not generally recommended; no specific information is available about the safety and efficacy of the vaccine during pregnancy. Little information is available about immunization of immunocompromised individuals; a small study of such children did not reveal adverse outcomes or compromise of immune response.[49] Data regarding concurrent administration with diphtheria, tetanus, and pertussis vaccines suggest lack of compromise of immunogenicity or safety; concurrent administration with other vaccines or medications, such as antimalarials, has not been studied. Individuals receiving Japanese encephalitis vaccine should continue to receive other vaccines and antimalarials as appropriate for their destinations.

Meningococcus

Meningococcal disease occurs worldwide, but major epidemics occur more frequently in the meningitis belt of sub-Saharan Africa (Fig. 47–3). Isolated outbreaks have been described in Mecca, Saudi Arabia, Nepal, and other areas. Risk to travelers is low, estimated to be 0.4 per million travelers per month for a stay in a developing country, and up to 2000 per million in pilgrims to Mecca.[50] Outbreaks have occurred involving travelers, and travelers have become carriers of disease. American pilgrims who returned from Mecca, Saudi Arabia, following an epidemic of Group A meningococcal diseases in 1987 were more than 11 times as likely to carry the organism back to their home countries as travelers returning from other parts of Saudi Arabia.[51] Meningococcal vaccine is required by Saudi Arabia for pilgrims to Mecca and is recommended for travelers visiting an epidemic area. Individuals who will be traveling to countries within the meningitis belt of sub-Saharan Africa and who will have contact with the local population (individuals visiting friends and relatives, health care workers, long-term travelers such as missionaries and volunteer workers) are at higher risk and may benefit from immunization. Individuals who will travel to these areas and stay in tourist accomodations with little contact with the local population are at low risk and may elect not to be immunized. Immunization should be carried out, if possible, at least 10 to 14 days in advance of travel.

Serogroup A is the most common cause of outbreaks of meningococcal disease outside the United States and Europe but serogroups B and C can also cause disease. Currently available meningococcal polysaccharide vaccine in the United States contains the four serogroups A, C, Y, and W-135. In most other countries, bivalent A–C vaccines are used. Response to serogroup C is suboptimal in children less than 2 years of age, and response

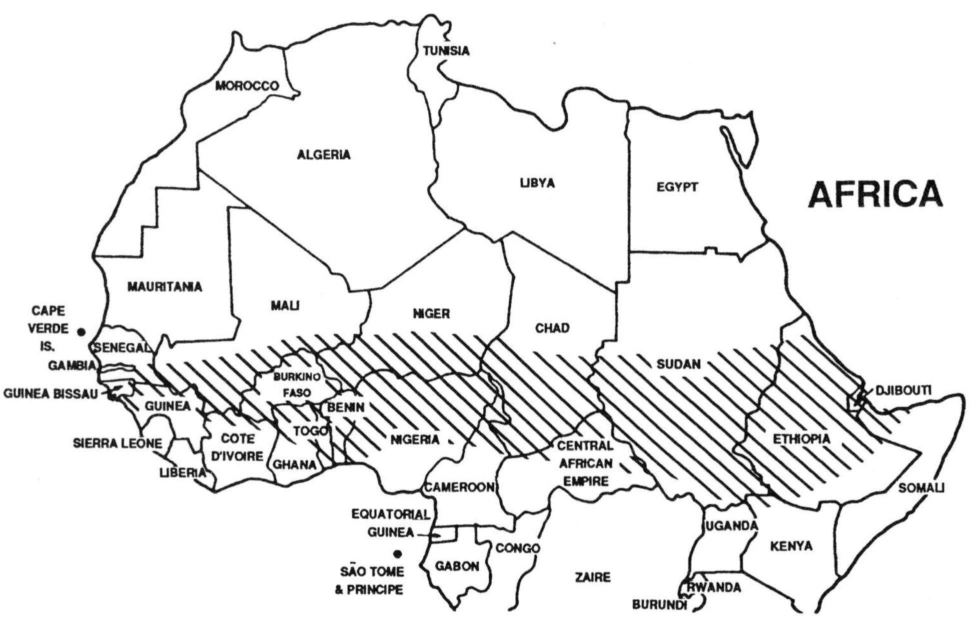

Figure 46–3. Areas with frequent epidemics of meningococcal meningitis.

to serogroup A may be reduced in children 3 to 11 months of age. Response to serogroups Y and W-135 polysaccharides is adequate in children 2 years of age or older, although clinical protection has not been documented.[52]

Duration of immunity is at least 3 years in individuals immunized when at least 4 years of age. Revaccination after 3 years can be considered in children who were immunized at 4 years of age or younger, especially if they remain at risk for disease. Since antibody titers decline rapidly in the 2 to 3 years following immunization, revaccination may also be considered for older children and adults within 3 to 5 years of the initial vaccination if they are at continued risk. Conjugate meningococcal vaccines, currently under development, hold promise for offering effective immunization of infants and young children.

The safety of this vaccine during pregnancy has not been established. When considering immunization during pregnancy, the theoretical risk of immunization must be balanced against the risk of disease.

Rabies

The risk of rabies to travelers is difficult to estimate. The vast majority of cases of rabies worldwide are due to dog bites sustained in countries where canine rabies remains endemic. A retrospective study of dog bites and licks experienced by travelers suggests that these are experienced by about 10% of travelers during an average stay of 17 days.[53] Rates of human rabies are highest in Asia, parts of Central and South America, and Africa.[54] Areas of the world that are reported to be rabies-free are listed in Table 46–8. Travelers should be informed about the risk of rabies in the region to which they will travel and be advised to avoid contact with animals that could be rabies carriers, especially dogs but also cats, skunks, raccoons, and bats.

Three inactivated rabies vaccines are licensed for use in the United States, with others available worldwide. In addition, rabies immunoglobulin preparations provide passive immune protection of short duration. Vaccines may be used to provide preexposure prophylaxis (termed *prophylaxis* rather than immunization to emphasize that receiving this product before exposure does not obviate the need for treatment if an exposure occurs) or postexposure prophylaxis. Travelers who will be spending 1 month or more in countries where canine rabies is endemic are candidates for preexposure vaccination, as are individuals whose purpose of travel includes relevant animal or laboratory work, those who are likely to be hiking or riding motorcycles, or those whose itineraries include remote destinations where prompt medical attention is impossible.[55] Preexposure vaccination does not remove the imperative to seek definitive treatment if an exposure occurs but does alter the postexposure prophylaxis regimen. Dosage schedules for the three vaccines licensed in the United States are listed in Table 46–9. Other vaccine preparations may be available in developing countries; these vaccines are produced locally and have unknown safety and efficacy. If bitten by a suspect animal, an individual should receive modern tissue culture vaccine preparations, even if this means receiving additional treatment once the individual has returned to the country of origin.

Adverse events such as local pain and swelling have been reported in 30 to 74% of recipients of the human diploid cell vaccine (HDCV). Systemic reactions may occur in up to 40% of individuals. Three cases of central nervous system disease have been reported following HDCV administration, but a causal relationship has not been established. Up to 6% of those receiving booster doses of HDCV may experience immune complex–like reactions. The newest vaccine available in the US (RabAvert, Chiron) is prepared in purified chick embryo cell culture. Although mild erythema, swelling, and pain may occur at the injection site, serum-sickness–like hypersensitivity reactions have not been reported following this vaccine.[55a] When given as postexposure prophylaxis, the series of doses should not be interrupted because of mild systemic or local reactions to vaccine; they can be managed with antiinflammatory agents.

Antimalarials such as chloroquine (and possibly mefloquine) may interfere with antibody response to HDCV rabies vaccine.[56] Other drugs (steroids or immunosuppressive agents) or conditions that affect the im-

Table 46–8. **COUNTRIES REPORTING NO CASES OF RABIES***

The following countries and political units stated that rabies was not present.

REGION	COUNTRIES
Africa	Mauritius,† Libya,† Djibouti,† Lesotho,† Seychelles†
Americas	**North:** Bermuda; St. Pierre and Miquelon **Caribbean:** Anguilla, Antigua and Barbuda, Bahamas, Barbados, Cayman Islands, Dominica, Guadeloupe, Jamaica, Martinique, Montserrat, Netherlands, Antilles (Aruba, Bonaire, Curacao, Saba, St. Maarten, and St. Eustatius), St. Christopher (St. Kitts) and Nevis, St. Lucia, St. Martin, St. Vincent and Grenadines, Turks and Caicos Islands, Virgin Islands (U.K. and U.S.). **South:** Uruguay†
Asia	Bahrain, Hong Kong, Japan, Republic of Korea,† Kuwait, Malaysia (Malaysia-Sabah†), Maldives, Singapore, Taiwan
Europe	Cyprus, Denmark, Faroe Islands, Finland, Gibraltar, Greece, Iceland, Ireland, Malta, Monaco, Norway (mainland), Portugal, Spain (except Ceuta/Melilla), Sweden, United Kingdom (Britain and Northern Ireland)
Oceania‡	American Samoa, Australia, Cook Islands, Fiji, French Polynesia, Guam, Indonesia (with exception of Java, Kalimantan, Sumatra, and Sulawesi), Kiribati, New Caledonia, New Zealand, Niue, Papua New Guinea, Solomon Islands, Tonga, Vanuatu

*Bat rabies exists in some areas that are free of terrestrial rabies.

†Countries whose classifications should be considered provisional.

‡Most of Pacific Oceania is "rabies-free." For information on specific islands not listed above, contact the Centers for Disease Control and Prevention, Division of Quarantine.

Data from World Health Organization: World Survey of Rabies 28, (for 1992); Veterinary Public Health Unit, Division of Communicable Disease, WHO, Geneva, 1994. WHO Collaborating Centre for Rabies Surveillance and Research: Rabies Bulletin Europe, 1994;18(2). Pan American Health Organization. Epidemiological surveillance of rabies in the Americas. 1992, 1993; Z4(1–12).

Table 46–9. **RABIES PREEXPOSURE IMMUNIZATION***

RISK CATEGORY	NATURE OF RISK	TYPICAL POPULATIONS	PREEXPOSURE REGIMEN
Frequent	Exposure usually episodic with source recognized, but exposure may also be unrecognized	Spelunkers, animal control and wildlife workers in rabies epizootic areas; certain travelers to foreign rabies epizootic areas	Primary preexposure immunization course; serologic examination or booster immunization every 2 yr
Infrequent (but greater than population at large)	Exposure nearly always episodic with source recognized	Animal control and wildlife worker in areas of low rabies endemicity; may include some travelers	Primary preexposure immunization course; no routine booster immunization or serologic examination

*Preexposure immunization consists of three doses of HDCV, RVA, or RabAvert, 1.0 mL, IM, one each on days 0, 7, and 21 or 28. Only HDCV may be administered by the intradermal (ID) dose/route (0.1 mL ID on days 0, 7, and 21 or 28). If the traveler will be taking chloroquine or mefloquine for malaria chemoprophylaxis, the three-dose series must be completed before initiation of antimalarials. If this is not possible, the IM dose/route should be used. Administration of routine booster doses of vaccine depends on exposure risk category as noted below. Preexposure immunization of immunosuppressed persons is not recommended.

HDCV, human diploid cell vaccine; IM, intramuscularly; RVA, rabies vaccine, adsorbed.

mune system may also impair the efficacy of vaccine. Individuals taking such agents or experiencing such conditions may be candidates for testing of serum antibody levels following immunization.

Pregnancy is not a contraindication to postexposure prophylaxis with rabies vaccine, and no harmful effects to the fetus from immunization have been noted. If risk of exposure is high, preexposure prophylaxis may be offered.[57]

Tickborne Encephalitis

Tickborne encephalitis is reported from limited areas of most countries in Europe except the United Kingdom, Ireland, Spain, Portugal, Belgium, the Netherlands, and Luxembourg. Risk depends on season of travel, exposure to forested areas, and tick activity, with highest transmission occurring from May to June and September to October. Risk may be focused in circumscribed areas within countries.

Although risk to travelers is difficult to assess, a study of American service members of a military unit that lived and trained in a highly endemic area found an infection rate of 0.9 per 1000 per month of exposure.[58] In the United States, vaccine is not available. Instead, measures to prevent exposures to ticks, such as the use of appropriate clothing and repellents containing N,N-diethyl-meta-toluamide (DEET) are encouraged. In many countries in Europe, vaccine is available and is recommended for high-risk individuals (such as forestry workers) and others who plan extended travels through endemic areas.

The vaccine is given as a three-dose series, with the first two injections 2 weeks to 3 months apart, and a third dose 9 to 12 months later. Boosters are recommended at 3-year intervals. Side effects of vaccine include local and mild systemic reactions. Individuals with egg allergy should not receive this vaccine.

Typhoid

Typhoid is the second most common vaccine-preventable disease affecting travelers. In the United States, 62% of cases reported between 1975 and 1984 occurred in international travelers.[59]

The risk of contracting typhoid depends largely on travel destination and living circumstances during travel. Estimates of risk for contracting typhoid for short-stay travelers have ranged from 1 in 30,000 to 10 in 30,000 for trips to North Africa, India, and Senegal.[60] Another study showed the risk of disease to be related inversely to receiving vaccine prior to travel: incidence rates per visit ranged from 16 per 100,000 North American tourists, 92% of whom had received typhoid vaccine prior to travel, to 216 per 100,000 in Israeli tourists, 6% of whom had been immunized.[61]

Several vaccines are available to protect travelers from disease, although none offers complete protection. Precautions against ingesting contaminated food and water must continue to be used to augment protection afforded by vaccine.

Parenteral whole-cell killed typhoid vaccine has been available since 1896. Limitations of this vaccine included the need for two doses of vaccine administered at least 4 weeks apart in order to induce adequate response, incidence of adverse events, and moderate vaccine efficacy, ranging from 51 to 76%.[62] In some countries, whole-cell killed vaccine is no longer distributed because of these limitations and because of the introduction of new products. Two vaccines have become available during the 1990s that, although they do not result in improved vaccine efficacy, do result in better ease of administration and fewer adverse events. An oral, live attenuated vaccine (Vivotif, Berna) manufactured from the Ty21a strain of *Salmonella typhi* is given in a series of four capsules taken every other day and has a vaccine efficacy of 67%.[63] It is not licensed for children younger than 6 years in the United States, and administration of this vaccine may be limited by the ability of small children to ingest capsules. Liquid preparations of vaccine hold promise for this age group. A capsular polysaccharide vaccine (Typhim Vi, Pasteur Mérieux Connaught), given in a single intramuscular dose, is available for individuals 2 years and older. Vaccine efficacy of this product ranges from 55 to 74%.[64, 65] Regardless of product given, booster doses are required within 2 to 5 years (Table 46–10).

Adverse events occur most commonly with the whole-cell preparation. Fever may occur in almost 25% of

Table 46–10. **DOSAGE AND SCHEDULES FOR TYPHOID FEVER VACCINATION**

VACCINATION	AGE	DOSAGE			
		Dose/Mode of Administration	No. of Doses	Interval Between Doses	Boosting Interval
Oral Live-Attenuated Ty21a Vaccine					
Primary series	≥6 yr	1 capsule*	4	48 hr	—
Booster	≥6 yr	1 capsule*	4	48 hr	Every 5 yr
Vi Capsular Polysaccharide Vaccine					
Primary series	≥2 yr	0.50 mL†	1	—	—
Booster	≥2 yr	0.50 mL†	1	—	Every 2 yr
Heat-Phenol-Inactivated Parenteral Vaccine					
Primary series	6 mo–10 yr	0.25 mL‡	2	≥4 wk	—
	≥10 yr	0.50 mL‡	2	≥4 wk	—
Booster	6 mo–10 yr	0.25 mL‡	1	—	Every 3 yr
	≥10 yr	0.50 mL‡	1	—	Every 3 yr
	≥6 mo	0.10 mL§	1	—	Every 3 yr

*Administer with cool liquid no warmer than 37°C (98.6°F).
†Intramuscularly.
‡Subcutaneously.
§Intradermally.
—Not applicable.

individuals, headache in up to 10%, and local pain or swelling in up to 35%. The capsular polysaccharide vaccine results in fever in 1% or fewer vaccine recipients, headache in up to 3%, and local reactions in about 7%. The oral vaccine results in fever or headache in about 5% of recipients. In general, either the oral vaccine or the Vi capsular polysaccharide vaccine is the option of choice for all individuals except for children between 6 months and 2 years of age, for whom the whole-cell vaccine is the only option available. Mothers of children younger than 6 months may be reassured that exclusive breast-feeding (reducing contact with contaminated food or water) offers protection for infants when careful hand washing is also carried out.

The oral typhoid vaccine is a live virus preparation and should not be given to immunocompromised individuals, including those with HIV infection. Concerns have been raised about the immunogenicity of this vaccine in individuals receiving antibiotics, immunoglobulin, antimalarials, or viral vaccines. Growth of the live Ty21a strain is inhibited by some antimicrobial agents and by the antimalarial agent mefloquine.[66, 67] Ideally, the oral typhoid vaccine series should be completed before beginning antimalarials, or doses of each should be separated by at least 24 hours. The antimalarial agent chloroquine does not inhibit the growth of Ty21a and may be given concurrently with vaccine. Ideally, oral typhoid vaccine should not be taken concurrently with antimicrobial agents; the vaccine should be taken 24 hours or more after the last dose of the antibiotic. Data are not available regarding concurrent administration of oral typhoid vaccine and other live virus vaccines. Vaccine may be administered at the same time as immune globulin. Safety of vaccines against typhoid has not been established during pregnancy, and immunization at this time should be avoided if possible.

Yellow Fever

A dramatic resurgence of yellow fever has occurred in the past decade, primarily in sub-Saharan Africa.[68] Outbreaks occurred in countries, such as Gabon, that had never previously had disease, and reemergence of disease was noted in Kenya, which had been yellow fever–free for nearly 50 years. In South America, the largest outbreak since the 1950s occurred in Peru in 1995, and cases were reported in Bolivia, Brazil, Colombia, Ecuador, and Peru from 1985 to 1994. Areas of current risk for disease are shown in Figures 46–4 and 46–5. Yellow fever can be a fatal disease and cases have occurred in travelers.

The vaccine against yellow fever offers high levels of protection, with seroconversion rates of greater than 95% in children and adults and duration of immunity of at least 10 years. Side effects are generally mild. Encephalitis has been reported in 22 patients among more than 200 million doses of vaccine distributed since 1945; most cases occurred in children younger than 4 months.

International efforts to prevent the spread of yellow fever include mosquito control at airports and shipping ports and the requirement of documentation of immunization against yellow fever for travelers arriving from areas where disease is occurring. Some affected countries, however, do not require immunization as a condition of entry, despite the presence of endemic or episodic disease. Yellow fever vaccine must be given at official yellow fever vaccine centers with an International Certificate of Vaccination, which is valid from 10 days through 10 years after the date of immunization.

Travelers are at risk for yellow fever through bites of vector mosquitoes. Largely because of international health regulations, many travelers to infected areas have received adequate immunization against yellow fever. Unimmunized individuals are at risk for serious disease, and fatal cases have been reported in travelers.[69]

Travelers to affected countries should receive a single dose of vaccine at least 10 days before departure. Vaccine is contraindicated in children less than 4 months of age and should be used cautiously in children less than 1 year of age. Individuals not protected by vaccine should

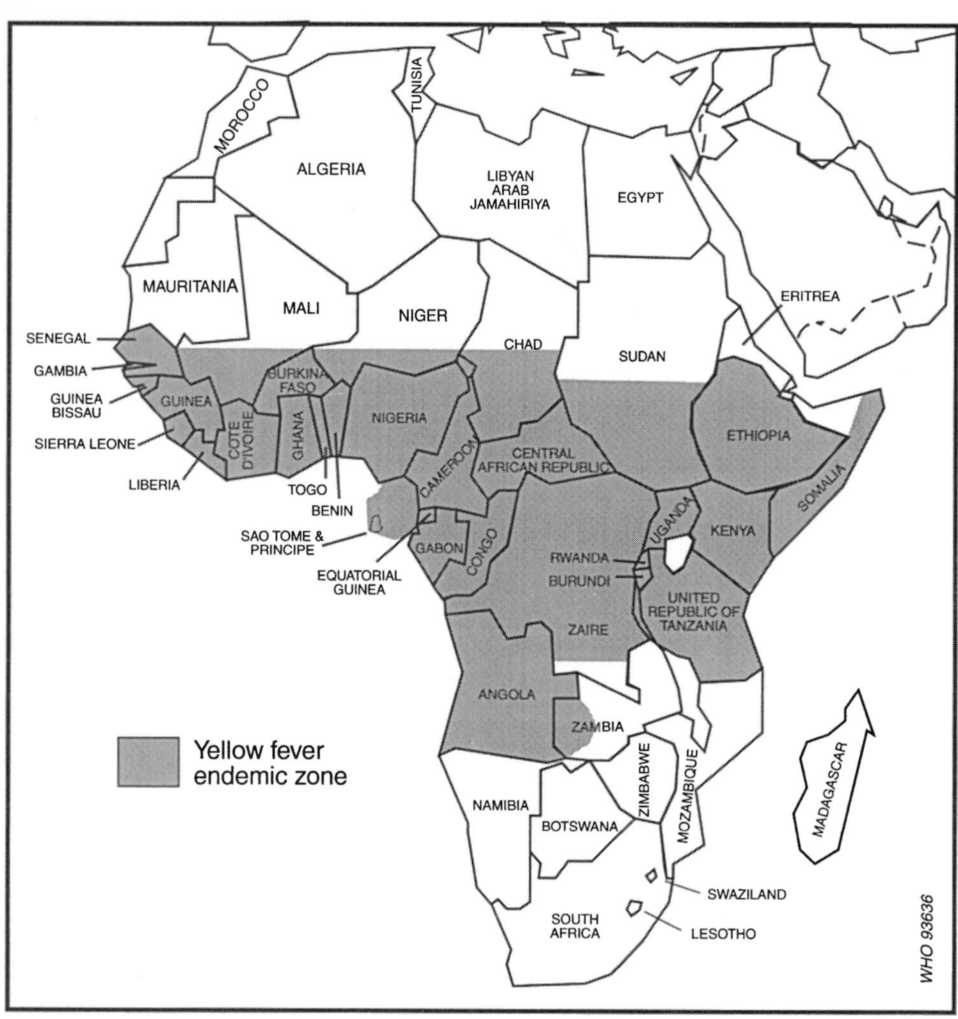

Figure 46–4. Yellow fever endemic zones in Africa.

use adequate personal protective measures to avoid mosquito bites.

Serologic response to yellow fever vaccine is not diminished by simultaneous administration of tetanus, diphtheria, pertussis, measles, polio, BCG, hepatitis A, hepatitis B, or the Vi antigen capsular polysaccharide vaccines. Immune globulin did not decrease the antibody response to yellow fever vaccine when given 0 to 7 days before immunization.[70] The antimalarial chloroquine has been shown not to adversely affect the antibody response to yellow fever vaccine.[71]

Yellow fever immunization is not recommended during pregnancy. A study that documented fetal infection in 1 of 41 infants exposed to maternal vaccination as well as the known neurotropism of the virus support this recommendation.[72]

Immunization with yellow fever vaccine is not recommended for immunocompromised individuals or those with symptomatic HIV infection. Vaccine has been administered with good tolerance and efficacy to asymptomatic HIV-infected individuals.[73]

Cost-Effectiveness of Travel Immunizations

Travel medicine experts have long noted the willingness of travelers to accept (and pay for) multiple vaccines for diseases for which they are at minimal risk, possibly analogous to purchasing travel insurance. In contrast, although well designed studies of cost-effectiveness of travel immunizations are few, most studies suggest that they probably are not cost-effective (relative to the costs of treating such illness), at least from a societal perspective (i.e., the costs of immunizing all travelers are greater than treating the illnesses in the few travelers who become ill in the absence of vaccination).[74, 75]

The most studied travel-associated vaccine in terms of cost-effectiveness is hepatitis A. In one study, which also examined the cost-effectiveness of typhoid immunization, neither of the two vaccines was found to be cost-effective; societal expenditures of more than £67 million were required to prevent a single death with either vaccine.[76] In contrast, a study from the Netherlands suggested that cost-effective choices are available with regard to hepatitis A immunization when frequency of travel, likelihood of prior immunity, and product used are taken into consideration.[77] Cost-effectiveness of preexposure rabies prophylaxis has been studied in Canada, with the conclusion that routine preexposure prophylaxis for most travelers is not indicated.[78]

Issues complicating the performance of studies of cost-effectiveness include difficulty in estimating with accuracy the risk of vaccine-preventable diseases to trav-

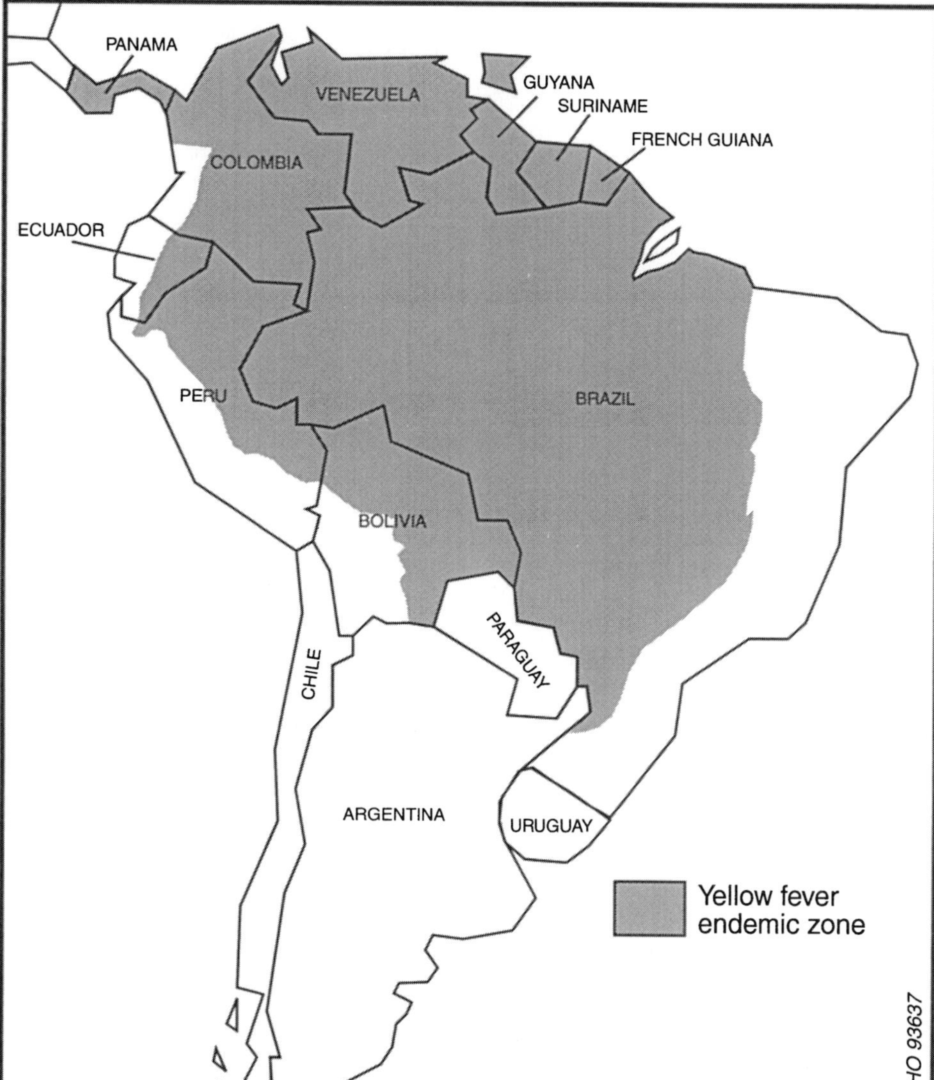

Figure 46–5. Yellow fever endemic zones in the Americas.

elers; difficulties in determining vaccine efficacy, especially for travelers who will have variable exposures in endemic areas; difficulties approximating costs associated with disease; and lack of sufficient experience with some newer vaccines to allow accurate estimation of incidence of vaccine-associated adverse events. Finally, some practitioners may be reluctant to omit any vaccine, no matter the risk of disease, for fear of liability. Until these issues are studied in greater detail, each travel medicine provider must continue to individualize recommendations for travel vaccination, taking into account the potential for adverse reactions to immunization and the patient's risk for the disease.

Rapid advances in biotechnology promise a potential revolution in the development of new vaccines using diverse approaches ranging from DNA vaccines to transgenic plant vaccines.[79] Vaccines against Lyme disease have recently been found to be safe and effective.[80] New-candidate vaccines show promise in protecting against diverse pathogens that cause diarrheal disease.[81] Optimism remains for the eventual development of vaccines against AIDS[82] and malaria.[83] In addition to the remaining technical hurdles, however, equally formidable economic hurdles remain in adequate funding of vaccine research and development against diseases that mostly afflict the poorest population in the poorest countries.[84] The increased interest in travel and travel immunizations by more affluent travelers may provide substantial assistance in making these much-needed vaccines a reality.

REFERENCES

1. Handszuh H, Waters SR. Travel and tourism patterns. In Dupont HL, Steffen R (eds). Textbook of Travel Medicine and Health. Hamilton, Ontario, 1997, pp 20–26.
2. Reid D, Keystone JS. Health risks abroad: General considerations. In Dupont HL, Steffen R (eds). Textbook of Travel Medicine and Health. Hamilton, Ontario, 1997, pp 3–9.
3. Dupont HL, Steffen R (eds). Textbook of Travel Medicine and Health. Hamilton, Ontario, 1997.
4. Wilson ME. World Guide to Infectious Diseases. New York, Oxford University Press, 1991.

5. Jong EC: Immunizations for international travel. Infect Dis Clin North Am 12:249–266, 1998.
6. Wolfe MS. Protection of travelers. Clin Infect Dis 25:177–186, 1997.
7. Falvo C, Horowitz H. Adverse reactions associated with simultaneous administration of multiple vaccines to travelers. J Gen Intern Med 9:255–260, 1994.
8. General recommendations on immunization: Recommendations of the Advisory Committee on Immunization Practices (ACIP). MMWR Morb Mortal Wkly Rep 43:1–38, 1994.
9. American Academy of Pediatrics, Committee on Infectious Diseases. Recommended timing of routine measles immunization for children who have recently received immune globulin preparations. Pediatrics 93:682–685, 1994.
10. Recommendations of the Advisory Committee on Immunization Practices (ACIP): Use of vaccines and immune globulins in persons with altered immunocompetence. MMWR Morb Mortal Wkly Rep 42:1–18, 1993.
11. Centers for Disease Control and Prevention: Recommended Childhood Immunization Schedule—United States, 1998. MMWR Morb Mortal Wkly Rep 47:8–12, 1998.
12. Update on adult immunization. MMWR Morb Mortal Wkly Rep 40:1–94, 1991.
13. Gardner P, Schaffner W. Immunization of adults. N Engl J Med 328:1252–1258, 1993.
14. Fedson DS. Adult immunization: Summary of the National Vaccine Advisory Committee report. JAMA 272:1133–1137, 1994.
15. Diphtheria epidemic—New independent states of the former Soviet Union, 1990–1994. MMWR Morb Mortal Wkly Rep 44:177–181, 1995.
16. Diphtheria outbreak—Saraburi Province, Thailand, 1994. MMWR Morb Mortal Wkly Rep 45:271–273, 1996.
17. Diphtheria acquired by US citizens in the Russian Federation and Ukraine—1994. MMWR Morb Mortal Wkly Rep 44:237–244, 1995.
18. Lumio J, Jahkosa M, Vuento R, et al. Diphtheria after visit to Russia. Lancet 342:53–54, 1993.
19. Crossley K, Irvine P, Warren JB, et al. Tetanus and diphtheria immunity in urban Minnesota adults. JAMA 242:2298–3000, 1979.
20. Koblin BA, Townsend TR. Immunity to diphtheria and tetanus in inner-city women of child-bearing age. Am J Public Health 79:1297–1298, 1989.
21. Christensson B, Bottiger M. Serological immunity to diphtheria in Sweden in 1978 and 1984. Scand J Infect Dis 18:227–233, 1986.
22. Certification of poliomyelitis eradication—the Americas, 1994. MMWR Morb Mortal Wkly Rep 43:720–722, 1994.
23. Steffen R, Rickenbach M, Willhelm U, et al. Health problems after travel to developing countries. J Infect Dis 156:84–91, 1987.
23a. Centers for Disease Control and Prevention: Poliomyelitis prevention in the United States: Introduction of a sequential vaccination schedule of inactivated poliovirus vaccine followed by oral poliovirus vaccine: Recommendations of the Advisory Committee on Immunization Practices (ACIP). MMWR Morb Mortal Wkly Rep 46(RR-3):1–25, 1997.
24. Lange WR, Frame JD. High incidence of viral hepatitis among American missionaries in Africa. Am J Trop Med Hyg 43:527–533, 1990.
25. Steffen R. Risks of hepatitis B for travelers. Vaccine 8:31–32, 1990.
26. Measles—United States, 1996, and the interruption of indigenous transmission. MMWR Morb Mortal Wkly Rep 46:242–246, 1997.
27. Centers for Disease Control and Prevention: Measles, mumps, and rubella—vaccine use and strategies for elimination of measles, rubella, and congenital rubella syndrome and control of mumps: Recommendations of the Advisory Committee on Immunization Practices (ACIP). MMWR Morb Mortal Wkly Rep 47(RR-8):1–25, 1998.
28. Ivanoff B, Robertson SE. Pertussis: A worldwide problem. Dev Biol Stand 89:3–13, 1997.
29. Gangarosa EJ, Galazka AM, Wolfe CR, et al. Impact of the anti-vaccine movements on pertussis control: The untold story. Lancet 351:356–361, 1998.
30. Pertussis Vaccination: Use of acellular pertussis vaccines among infants and young children: Recommendations of the Advisory Committee on Immunization Practices (ACIP). MMWR Morb Mortal Wkly Rep 46:1–25, 1997.
31. Prevention and control of influenza: Recommendations of the Advisory Committee on Immunization Practices (ACIP). MMWR Morb Mortal Wkly Rep 46:1–25, 1997.
32. The role of BCG vaccines in the prevention and control of tuberculosis in the U.S.: A joint statement by the Advisory Committee for Elimination of Tuberculosis and the ACIP. MMWR Morb Mortal Wkly Rep 45:1–18, 1996.
33. Crowley RG. Implication of the Vietnam War for tuberculosis in the United States. Arch Environ Health 21:479–480, 1970.
34. Wittlinger F, Steffen R, Watanage H, Handszuh H. Risk of cholera among Western and Japanese travelers. J Travel Med 2:154–158, 1995.
35. Cholera vaccine. MMWR Morb Mortal Wkly Rep 37:617–624, 1988.
36. Steffen R. New cholera vaccines—for whom? Lancet 344:1241–1242, 1994.
37. Christenson B. Epidemiological aspects of acute viral hepatitis A in Swedish travelers to endemic areas. Scand J Infect Dis 17:5–10, 1985.
38. Lange WR, Frame JD. High incidence of viral hepatitis among American missionaries in Africa. Am J Trop Med Hyg 43:527–533, 1990.
39. Steffen R, Kane MA, Shapiro CN, et al. Epidemiology and prevention of hepatitis A in travelers. JAMA 272:885–889, 1994.
40. Barnett ED, Holmes AH, Phillips SL, et al. Immunity to hepatitis A in travelers born and raised in hepatitis A endemic areas (abstract 280). Proceedings of the Fifth International Conference on Travel Medicine, Geneva, Switzerland, 1997, p 207.
41. Victor J, Knudsen JD, Nielsen LP, et al. Hepatitis A vaccine. A new convenient single-dose schedule with booster when long-term immunization is warranted. Vaccine 12:1327–1329, 1994.
42. Clemens R, Sarary A, Hepburn A, et al. Clinical experience with an inactivated hepatitis A vaccine. J Infect Dis 171(suppl 1):S44–S49, 1995.
42a. Vidor E, Fritzell B, Plotkin S. Clinical development of a new inactivated hepatitis A vaccine. Infection 24:447–458, 1996.
43. Nalin DR. VAQTA, hepatitis A vaccine, purified inactivated. Drugs Future 20:24–29, 1995.
44. Kruppenbacher J, Bienzle U, Bock HL, Clemens R. Co-administration of an inactivated hepatitis A vaccine with other travelers vaccines: Interference with the immune response (Abstract H115). In 1994 Interscience Conference on Antimicrobial Agents and Chemotherapy (ICAAC). American Society for Microbiology 1994, p 256.
45. Bryan JP, Nelson M. Testing for antibody to hepatitis A to decrease the cost of hepatitis A prophylaxis with immune globulin or hepatitis A vaccines. Arch Intern Med 154:663–668, 1994.
46. Macdonald WBG, Tink AR, Ouvrier RA, et al. Japanese encephalitis after a two-week holiday in Bali. Med J Aust 150:334–339, 1989.
47. Wittesjo B, Eitrem R, Niklasson B, et al. Japanese encephalitis after a 10-day holiday in Bali. Lancet 345:856, 1995.
48. Inactivated Japanese encephalitis virus vaccine. Recommendations of the Advisory Committee on Immunization Practices (ACIP). MMWR Morb Mortal Wkly Rep 42:1–15, 1993.
49. Yamada A, Imanishi J, Juang RF, et al. Trial of inactivated Japanese encephalitis vaccine in children with underlying diseases. Vaccine 4:32–34, 1986.
50. Koch S, Steffen R. Meningococcal disease in travelers: Vaccination recommendations. J Travel Med 1:4–7, 1994.
51. Moore PS, Harrison LH, Telzak EE, et al. Group A meningococcal carriage in travelers returning from Saudi Arabia. JAMA 260:2686–2689, 1988.
52. Centers for Disease Control and Prevention. Control and prevention of meningococcal disease: Recommendations of the Advisory Committee on Immunization Practices (ACIP). MMWR Morb Mortal Wkly Rep 46:1–10, 1997.
53. Phanuphak P, Ubolyam S, Sirivichayakul S. Should travelers in rabies endemic areas receive pre-exposure rabies immunisation? Ann Med Interne (Paris) 145:409–411, 1994.
54. Fishbein DB, Robinson LE. Rabies. N Engl J Med 329:1632–1638, 1993.
55. Rabies prevention—United States, 1991: Recommendations of the Immunization Practices Advisory Committee (ACIP). MMWR Morb Mortal Wkly Rep 40:1–19, 1991.

55a. A new rabies vaccine. Med Lett 40:64–65, 1998.
56. Pappaioanou M, Fishbein DB, Dreesen DW, et al. Antibody response to preexposure human diploid-cell rabies vaccine given concurrently with chloroquine. N Engl J Med 314:280–284, 1986.
57. Varner MW, McGuinness GA, Galask RP. Rabies vaccination in pregnancy. Am J Obstet Gynecol 143:717–718, 1982.
58. McNeil JG, Lednar WM, Stansfield SK, et al. Central European tickborne encephalitis: Assessment of risk for persons in the armed services and vacationers. J Infect Dis 152:650–651, 1985.
59. Ryan CA, Hargrett-Bean NT, Blake PA. *Salmonella typhi* infection in the United States, 1975–1984: Increasing role of foreign travel. Rev Infect Dis 11:1–8, 1989.
60. Taylor DN, Pollard RA, Blake PA. Typhoid in the United States and the risk to the international traveler. J Infect Dis 148:599–602, 1983.
61. Schwartz E, Shlim DR, Eaton M, et al. The effect of oral and parenteral typhoid vaccination on the rate of infection with *Salmonella typhi* and *Salmonella paratyphi* A among foreigners in Nepal. Arch Intern Med 150:349–351, 1990.
62. Typhoid immunization: Recommendations of the Immunization Practices Advisory Committee (ACIP). MMWR Morb Mortal Wkly Rep 39:1–5, 1990.
63. Ivanoff B, Levine MM, Lambert PH. Vaccination against typhoid fever: Present status. Bull WHO 72:957–971, 1994.
64. Acharya AIL, Lowe CU, Thapa R, et al. Prevention of typhoid fever in Nepal with the Vi capsular polysaccharide of *Salmonella typhi*. N Engl J Med 317:1101–1104, 1987.
65. Klugman KP, Gilbertson IT, Koornhof HJ, et al. Protective activity of Vi capsular polysaccharide vaccine against typhoid fever. Lancet 2:1165–1169, 1987.
66. Brachman PS, Metchock B, Kozarsky PE. Effects of antimalarial chemoprophylactic agents on the viability of the Ty21a vaccine strain [letter]. Clin Infect Dis 15:1057–1058, 1992.
67. Horowitz H, Carbonaro CA. Inhibition of the *Salmonella typhi* oral vaccine strain, Ty21a, by mefloquine and chloroquine [letter]. J Infect Dis 166:1462–1464, 1992.
68. Robertson SE, Hull BP, Tomori O, et al. Yellow fever: A decade of reemergence. JAMA 276:1157–1162, 1996.
69. Tsai TF, Niklasson B, Goujon C. Viral tropical infections. In Dupont HL, Steffen R (eds). Textbook of Travel Medicine and Health. Ontario, BC Decker, 1997.
70. Kaplan JE, Nelson DB, Schonberger LB, et al. The effect of immune globulin on the response to trivalent oral poliovirus and yellow fever vaccinations. Bull WHO 62:585–590, 1984.
71. Tsai TF, Bolin RA, Lazuick JS, Miller KE. Chloroquine does not adversely affect the antibody response to yellow fever vaccine [letter]. J Infect Dis 154:726–727, 1986.
72. Tsai TF, Paul R, Lynberg MC, Letson GW. Congenital yellow fever virus infection after immunization in pregnancy. J Infect Dis 168:1520–1523, 1993.
73. Goujon M, Tohr M, Feuillie V, et al. Good tolerance and efficacy of yellow fever vaccine among subject carriers of human immunodeficiency virus (abstract 32). Proceedings of the Fourth International Conference on Travel Medicine, Acapulco, 1995, p 63.
74. Wiedermann G. Is vaccination worthwhile before travel? In Steffen R, Lobel HO, Haworth J, Bradley DJ (eds). Travel Medicine. Berlin, Springer-Verlag, 1989, pp 208–215.
75. Beutels P, Van Damme P, Piper Jenks N, Hilton E. Economic evaluation in travel medicine. In Dupont HL, Steffen R (eds). Textbook of Travel Medicine and Health. Ontario, BC Decker, 1997, pp 276–286.
76. Behrens RH, Roberts JA. Is travel prophylaxis worth while? Economic appraisal of prophylactic measures against malaria, hepatitis A, and typhoid in travelers. BMJ 8:918–922, 1994.
77. Van Doorslaer E, Tormans G, Van Damme P. Cost-effectiveness analysis of vaccination against hepatitis A in travelers. J Med Virol 44:463–469, 1994.
78. LeGuerrier P, Pilon PA, Deshaies D, Allard R. Pre-exposure rabies prophylaxis for the international traveler: A decision analysis. Vaccine 14:167–176, 1996.
79. Liu MA. Vaccine developments. Nat Med 4(5 suppl):515–519, 1998.
80. Steigbigel RT, Benach JL. Immunization against Lyme disease—an important first step. N Engl J Med 339:263–264, 1998.
81. Sansonetti PJ. Slaying the hydra all at once or head by head? Nat Med 4(5 suppl):499–500, 1998.
82. Baltimore D, Heilman CL. HIV vaccines: Prospects and challenges. Sci Am 279:98–103, 1993.
83. Miller LH, Hoffman SL. Research toward vaccines against malaria. Nat Med 4(5 suppl):520–524, 1998.
84. Bloom BR, Widdus R. Vaccine visions and their global impact. Nat Med 5(5 suppl):480–484, 1998.

chapter

47 Vaccines for Healthcare Workers

David J. Weber

Kristen Weigle

William A. Rutala

Healthcare workers (HCWs) are commonly exposed to infectious agents. The risks and methods of preventing occupational acquisition of infection by HCWs have been reviewed.[1–17] Minimizing the risk of disease acquisition is based on strict adherence to three key recommended interventions: (1) handwashing,[18] (2) rapid institution of appropriate isolation precautions for patients with known or suspected communicable diseases,[19] and (3) appropriate immunizations. Laboratory personnel, including hospital personnel working in microbiology laboratories, are also at risk for acquiring infectious diseases.[20, 21] Prevention of laboratory-acquired infection requires adherence to recommended administrative protocols (e.g., no eating, drinking, or smoking in areas where microbiological or pathological samples are processed), engineering controls (e.g., containment hoods), personnel protective equipment (e.g., N-95 masks when culturing *Mycobacterium tuberculosis*), and appropriate immunizations.[22–25]

Vaccine-preventable diseases may be classified by their route of transmission and include airborne (e.g., influenza, varicella, measles), droplet (e.g., pertussis, meningococcal infection), contact (e.g., hepatitis A from contact with feces), and parenteral or mucosal exposure to blood or contaminated body fluids (e.g., hepatitis B).

Immunization of HCWs should be included by all healthcare facilities as part of a comprehensive occupational health program. Ensuring that HCWs are immune to vaccine-preventable diseases is important because it protects the HCW from infections with potentially serious complications when acquired as an adult (e.g., rubella, varicella, hepatitis B) and prevents the HCW from serving as a source for infecting patients, especially immunocompromised patients, which may lead to serious morbidity or even death (e.g., varicella). For this reason, all new employees should receive a prompt review of their immunization status for vaccine-preventable disease. Immunization status should also be reviewed yearly. Other important occupational health interventions include an accessible health service, periodic tuberculin skin tests, evaluation of ill employees with potential communicable diseases with appropriate treatment and work restrictions, evaluation of employees after infectious disease exposures for postexposure prophylaxis and work restrictions, and education of employees focusing on general infection control guidelines in addition to Occupational Safety and Health Administration (OSHA)–mandated training in the prevention of bloodborne pathogens[26] and tuberculosis.[27]

VACCINES RECOMMENDED FOR HEALTHCARE WORKERS: GENERAL GUIDELINES

General recommendations regarding vaccination of HCWs have been published by the Centers for Disease Control and Prevention (CDC),[1, 17] the Advisory Committee on Immunization Practices (ACIP),[28–30] the American College of Physicians (ACP),[31] the American Academy of Pediatrics,[32] and infectious disease experts.[33–37] It is recommended that all HCWs be immune to mumps, measles, rubella, and varicella (Table 47–1). All HCWs with potential exposure to blood or body fluids should be immune to hepatitis B. Influenza vaccine should be offered to all HCWs yearly. Detailed recommendations have been published regarding mumps,[38, 39] measles,[39, 40] rubella,[39, 41] varicella,[42–44] hepatitis B,[45–47] and influenza[48] vaccines. All HCWs should be included in these recommendations, including employees with direct patient care responsibilities (e.g., nurses, respiratory technicians, physical therapists, physicians, students), employees without direct patient care responsibilities (e.g., environmental service workers, security), contract workers, and emergency medical personnel. HCWs should be provided vaccines that are recommended for adults, including tetanus and diphtheria[49–50] and pneumococcal vaccines,[51–52] or referred to their local medical provider. In special circumstances, HCWs or laboratory personnel should be offered immunization with other vaccines, including polio,[53] quadrivalent meningococcal vaccine,[54–55] bacille Calmette-Guérin (BCG),[56] rabies,[57] plague,[58] typhoid,[59, 60] vaccinia (smallpox),[61] and hepatitis A[62] (Table 47–2).

Table 47–1. **VACCINES STRONGLY RECOMMENDED FOR ALL HEALTHCARE WORKERS**

VACCINE	DEMONSTRATION OF IMMUNITY*	INDICATIONS†	ADMINISTRATION†	MAJOR CONTRAINDICATIONS†
Measles	Born before 1957‡; physician-diagnosed disease*; laboratory evidence of immunity*; prior receipt of vaccine* (two doses of live vaccine on or after first birthday)§	All healthcare workers‖	0.5 mL SC¶; second dose at least 1 mo later	Pregnancy; history of anaphylactic reaction to gelatin or neomycin; immunocompromised state**; recent receipt of immunoglobulin; allergy to eggs for persons receiving MMR
Mumps	Born before 1957; physician-diagnosed disease*; laboratory evidence of immunity*; prior receipt of vaccine*	All healthcare workers‖	0.5 mL SC¶; no booster	As for measles (above) if provided as MMR
Rubella	Born before 1957††; laboratory evidence of immunity (if history negative or uncertain)*; prior receipt of vaccine*	All healthcare workers‖	0.5 mL SC¶; no booster	As for measles (above) if provided as MMR; monovalent rubella vaccine not produced in eggs and hence egg allergy not a contraindication
Varicella	Personal history of varicella-zoster virus infection or laboratory evidence of immunity*; laboratory evidence of immunity (if history negative or uncertain)*; prior receipt of 2 doses of vaccine (age ≥13 yr) separated by at least 1 mo*	All healthcare workers‖	0.5 mL SC; second dose 4–8 wk later if ≥13 yr of age	Pregnancy; history of anaphylactic reaction to neomycin or gelatin; immunosuppression**; recent receipt of immunoglobulin; avoid salicylate use for 6 wk after vaccination
Hepatitis B	Laboratory evidence of immunity*,‡‡; prior receipt of three doses of vaccine with an appropriate schedule*	All healthcare workers‖ with potential exposure to blood or body fluids	1.0 mL IM (deltoid) at 0, 1, 6 mo§§; booster doses not necessary	History of anaphylactic reaction to common baker's yeast; pregnancy should not be considered a contraindication
Influenza	Yearly reimmunization needed	All healthcare workers‖	0.5 mL IM annually (either whole- or split-virus vaccine)	History of anaphylactic reaction to eggs

*Written documentation should be required.

†The package insert and CDC/ACIP should always be consulted for specific recommendations regarding indications, storage, administration, precautions, and contraindications. Doses listed are for adults; CDC/ACIP guidelines should be consulted when providing vaccines for children.

‡Consideration should be given to immunizing or evaluating the immune status of all healthcare workers, including those born before 1957, because approximately 5 to 10% of nonimmunized healthcare workers born before 1957 may be serosusceptible. During an outbreak, immunity should be ensured by serological testing or immunization records.

§People vaccinated from 1963 to 1967 with a killed measles vaccine alone, with a killed vaccine followed by live vaccine, or with a vaccine of unknown type should be revaccinated with two doses of live measles virus vaccine.

‖People who provide healthcare to patients or who work in institutions that provide patient care (e.g., physicians, nurses, emergency medical personnel, dental professionals and students, medical and nursing students, laboratory technicians, hospital volunteers, and administrative and support staff in healthcare institutions).

¶MMR vaccine preferred.

**People immunocompromised because of immune deficiency diseases, human immunodeficiency virus infection, leukemia, lymphoma or generalized malignancy or immunosuppressed as a result of therapy with corticosteroids, alkylating drugs, antimetabolites, or radiation. Also see Table 47–3.

††Adults born before 1957 generally may be considered immune except for women of childbearing age. (Consideration should be given to serologically testing or immunizing all individuals born before 1957.)

‡‡Immunity is indicated by an anti-HBsAg titer of 10 mIU per mL or greater.

§§Immunity should be assessed 1 to 2 months after the third dose; if not immune, an additional three doses should be provided and immunity reassessed; if not immune, provide hepatitis B immune globulin as postexposure prophylaxis when indicated.

CDC/ACIP, Centers for Disease Control/Advisory Committee on Immunization Practices; HBsAg, hepatitis B surface antigen; IM, intramuscularly; MMR, measles-mumps-rubella; SC, subcutaneously.

Adapted from references 17 and 30.

Table 47–2. **VACCINES AVAILABLE FOR HEALTHCARE WORKERS AND LABORATORY PERSONNEL IN SPECIAL CIRCUMSTANCES**

VACCINE	INDICATION(S)*	ADMINISTRATION*	MAJOR CONTRAINDICATIONS*
BCG (for tuberculosis)	Healthcare workers in localities where (1) multidrug-resistant tuberculosis is prevalent; (2) a strong likelihood of infection exists; and (3) full implementation of infection control precautions have been inadequate in controlling the spread of infection	One percutaneous dose of 0.3 mL; no booster recommended	Immunocompromised state† or pregnancy
Meningococcal (A, C, Y, W135)	Not routinely indicated; may be useful during type C outbreaks	One dose in volume and route specified by manufacturer; need for boosters unknown	Safety not established in pregnancy; avoid in pregnancy unless risk of infection is high
Pneumococcal polysaccharide (23 valent)	Adults at increased risk of pneumococcal disease and its complications because of underlying health conditions; adults ≥65 yr old	One dose IM or SC; revaccination recommended for high-risk persons ≥5 yr after first dose	Safety not established in pregnancy; avoid in pregnancy unless risk of infection is high
Tetanus-diphtheria toxoids (Td)	All adults; additional tetanus prophylaxis may be required in wound management	Unimmunized adults: Two doses IM 4 wk apart; third dose 6–12 mo after second dose. Fully immunized adults: Booster dose as young adult and at age 50 (ACP) or every 10 yr (ACIP)	Avoid during first trimester in pregnancy; history of a neurologic reaction or anaphylaxis. Avoid for 10 yr after severe local (Arthus-type) reaction to a previous dose
Rabies	Personnel working with rabies virus or infected animals in diagnostic or research activities; postexposure prophylaxis boosters may be required despite primary immunization	Preexposure: HDCV, RVA, or PCEC IM on days 0, 7, 21, or 28 *or* HDCV ID on days 0, 7, 21, or 28. Follow standard guidelines for postexposure prophylaxis	—
Polio	Healthcare workers in close contact with people who may be excreting wild virus; laboratory personnel handling specimens that may contain wild virus	Unimmunized adults: Enhanced potency inactivated vaccine (IPV); two doses SC given 4–8 wk apart, followed by a third dose at 6–12 months after second dose; IPV should be used for a booster dose	History of anaphylaxis after streptomycin or neomycin; avoid in pregnancy
Typhoid‡	Laboratory personnel who frequently work with *Salmonella typhi*	One 0.5 mL dose IM (ViCPS); booster doses of 0.5 mL every 2 yr *or* Four oral doses (Ty21a) on alternate days§; as per manufacturer, revaccinate with the entire 4-dose series every 5 yr, *or* Two 0.5 mL doses SC (heat-phenol–inactivated vaccine), ≥4 wk apart; boosters of 0.5 mL SC or 0.1 mL ID every 3 yr if exposure continues	History of severe local reaction or anaphylaxis to a previous dose of typhoid vaccine
Vaccinia	Personnel who directly handle cultures or animals contaminated with recombinant vaccinia or orthopox viruses (monkeypox, cowpox) that infect humans	One dose administered with a bifurcated needle; boosters every 10 yr	Pregnancy; presence or history of eczema; immunodeficiency in vaccine recipient or household contact
Plague	Laboratory personnel who frequently work with *Yersinia pestis*	Three doses IM; first dose 1.0 mL; second dose 0.2 mL 1–3 mo after first dose; third dose 0.2 mL 5–6 mo after second dose; boosters 0.2 mL at 1–2 yr intervals if exposure continued	History of anaphylaxis to a previous dose
Hepatitis A	Not routinely indicated for healthcare workers; persons who work with HAV-infected primates or HAV in a laboratory setting	Two doses of vaccine IM either 6–12 mo apart (Vaqta) or 6 mo apart (Havrix)	History of anaphylaxis to a previous dose; safety not established in pregnancy; avoid in pregnancy unless risk of infection is high

*The package insert and Centers for Disease Control (CDC)/ACIP should always be consulted for specific recommendations regarding indications, storage, administration, precautions, and contraindications.

†Persons immunocompromised because of immune deficiency diseases, human immunodeficiency virus infection, leukemia, lymphoma, or generalized malignancy or immunosuppressed as a result of therapy with corticosteroids, alkylating drugs, antimetabolites, or radiation.

‡Typhoid vaccines include the following: ViCPS, Vi capsular polysaccharide vaccine; Ty21a, oral live-attenuated Ty21a vaccine; IP, heat-phenol-inactivated parenteral vaccine.

§Oral typhoid vaccine should probably be avoided in healthcare workers providing direct patient care.

ACIP, Advisory Committee on Immunization Practices; ACP, American College of Physicians; BCG, bacille Calmette-Guérin; HAV, hepatitis A virus; HDCV, human diploid cell rabies vaccine; IM, intramuscularly; IPV, inactivated polio vaccine; PCEC, purified chick embryo cell culture rabies vaccine; RVA, rabies vaccine adsorbed; SC, subcutaneously.

Adapted from reference 17.

Immunocompromised employees require special consideration in the provision of immunizations (Table 47–3).[63] First, live virus vaccines (e.g., mumps-measles-rubella [MMR], varicella, polio, BCG) may be contraindicated. Second, vaccines not routinely recommended may be indicated (e.g., pneumococcal, meningococcal, *Haemophilus influenzae* type b, and influenza vaccines). Third, higher antigen doses or postimmunization serological evaluation may be indicated (e.g., hepatitis B vaccine in people with renal failure) because immunization of immunocompromised people may elicit a lower antibody response. Finally, such employees should be individually evaluated for reassignment (with the consent of the employee) depending on their job duties.

Before the administration of any vaccine, the HCW should be evaluated for the presence of any condition(s) that is listed as a vaccine contraindication or precaution.[64] If such a condition is present, the risks and benefits of vaccination need to be carefully weighed by the healthcare provider and the employee. The most common contraindication is a history of an anaphylactic reaction to a previous dose of the vaccine or to a vaccine component. Factors that are not contraindications to immunization include the following: household contact with a pregnant woman; breast-feeding; reaction to a previous vaccination consisting only of mild-to-moderate local tenderness, swelling, or both, or fever less than 40.5°C; mild acute illness with or without low-grade fever; current antimicrobial therapy (except for oral typhoid vaccine) or convalescence from a recent illness; personal history of *allergies* except a history of an anaphylactic reaction to a vaccine component (e.g., people with a history of anaphylaxis to neomycin should not receive the MMR vaccine); and family history of *allergies*, adverse reactions to vaccination, or seizures.[31]

POSTEXPOSURE PROPHYLAXIS

All HCWs potentially exposed to a communicable disease should be evaluated by the institution's occupational health service. General guidelines for a postexposure evaluation of medical personnel have been published.[1, 17] In brief, the following steps should be undertaken: (1) confirm that the source has a communicable disease; (2) determine that potential transmission could have taken place (e.g., close contact for transmission of *Neisseria meningitidis* or *Bordetella pertussis*); (3) determine that the exposed employee was not protected by the use of personal protective equipment (e.g., N-95 respirator for airborne transmitted diseases); (4) determine that the exposed employee is susceptible to infection (i.e., may require laboratory evaluation); (5) determine if effective prophylaxis is available and recommended; (6) determine that the employee has no contraindications to use of the recommended prophylaxis; (7) if the employee has a contraindication to the recommended prophylaxis, determine if an alternative exists and is safe to use; (8) inform the employee of the risk of disease transmission, signs and symptoms of infection, and risks and benefits of prophylaxis; (9) obtain informed consent for prophylaxis; (10) obtain baseline laboratory tests, if indicated (e.g., anti–hepatitis B surface antigen [HBsAg] titer); (11) assess whether the employee should be restricted in his or her work activities or furloughed (e.g., days 8 to 21 after exposure to varicella-zoster in a susceptible employee); and (12) arrange follow-up evaluations.

Vaccines that may be indicated for postexposure prophylaxis include tetanus toxoid (tetanus-diphtheria [Td] toxoids preferred), hepatitis B, and rabies (Tables 47–4 and 47–5). The use of some newer vaccines for postexposure prophylaxis is currently being investigated, including hepatitis A vaccine and varicella vaccine. Several vaccines have been provided to individuals without known direct exposure to an infected case to help contain community-wide or institutional outbreaks, including hepatitis A, meningococcal vaccine, and pertussis vaccine. Immunoglobulin preparations may be indicated as part of postexposure prophylaxis for exposure to hepatitis A (immune globulin), hepatitis B (hepatitis B immune globulin [HBIG]), measles (immune globulin), rabies (rabies immune globulin), tetanus (tetanus immune globulin), and varicella (varicella-zoster immune globulin [VZIG]). All employees who are exposed to a communicable disease or with symptoms of an infectious disease should be evaluated with the consideration of whether work restriction or furlough is required to prevent secondary cases from developing among patients or staff (Table 47–6).

PROVIDING VACCINES FOR HEALTHCARE WORKERS

All HCWs new to a healthcare facility should be screened for immunity to vaccine-preventable diseases within 10 working days. Unless immune, the HCW should be appropriately immunized. In general, serological screening for immunity before immunization is neither necessary nor cost-effective. Each healthcare facility, however, needs to evaluate the cost-effectiveness of screening. Factors that determine the effectiveness of serologically screening employees for immunity include the cost of the screening test, the cost of the vaccine, and the prevalence of immunity in the population. The prevalence of immunity in the population likely depends on age, gender, race, place of birth, and socioeconomic status. In addition, the sensitivity and specificity of the screening test must be considered.

The immunization status of all HCWs should be recorded in their medical record, which should be maintained by the institution's Occupational Health Service. Each HCW should be provided the information required under the National Childhood Vaccine Injury Act of 1986 before receiving measles, mumps, rubella, polio, tetanus, diphtheria, hepatitis B, *H. influenzae* type b, or varicella vaccine.[65] Signed informed consent specific to each vaccine should be obtained before immunization. When vaccines are provided, appropriate information should be recorded in the employee's medical record (Table 47–7).

Table 47–3. **RECOMMENDATIONS ON IMMUNIZATION OF HEALTHCARE WORKERS WITH SPECIAL CONDITIONS**

VACCINE	PREGNANCY	HIV INFECTION	SEVERE IMMUNOSUPPRESSION*	ASPLENIA	RENAL FAILURE	DIABETES	ALCOHOLISM AND ALCOHOLIC CIRRHOSIS
BCG	UI	C	C	UI	UI	UI	UI
Hepatitis A	UI	UI	UI	UI	UI	UI	R
Hepatitis B	R	R	R	R	R	R	R
Influenza	R‡	R	R	R	R	R	R
MMR	C	R§	C	R	R	R	R
Meningococcus	UI	UI	UI	R†	UI	UI	UI
Polio, inactivated‖	UI	UI	UI	UI	UI	UI	UI
Polio, oral‖	UI	C	C	UI	UI	UI	UI
Pneumococcus†	UI	R	R	R	R	R	R
Rabies	UI	UI	UI	UI	UI	UI	UI
Tetanus/diphtheria†	R	R	R	R	R	R	R
Typhoid, inactivated and Vi¶	UI	UI	UI	UI	UI	UI	UI
Typhoid, Ty21a	UI	C	C	UI	UI	UI	UI
Varicella	C	C	C	R	R	R	R
Vaccinia	UI	C	C	UI	UI	UI	UI

R, recommended; C, contraindicated; UI, use if indicated.

*Severe immunosuppression can be the result of congenital immunodeficiency, HIV infection, leukemia, lymphoma, generalized malignancy, or therapy with alkylating agents, antimetabolites, radiation, or large amounts of corticosteroids.

†Recommendation is based on the person's underlying condition rather than occupation.

‡Recommended for women who will be in the second or third trimester of pregnancy during the influenza season.

§Contraindicated in persons with HIV infection and severe immunosuppression ($CD4^+$ levels ≤200 cells/mm^3).

‖Vaccination is recommended for unvaccinated healthcare workers who have close contact with patients who may be excreting wild polioviruses. Primary vaccination with IPV is recommended because the risk for vaccine-associated paralysis after administration of OPV is higher among adults than among children. Healthcare workers who have had a primary series of OPV or IPV who are directly involved with the provision of care to patients who may be excreting poliovirus may receive another dose of either IPV or OPV. Any suspected case of poliomyelitis should be investigated immediately. If evidence suggests transmission of wild poliovirus, control measures to contain further transmission should be instituted immediately, including an OPV vaccination campaign.

¶Capsular polysaccharide vaccine.

BCG, bacille Calmette-Guérin; HIV, human immunodeficiency virus; IPV, inactivated poliovaccine; MMR, measles-mumps-rubella; OPV, oral polio vaccine.

Adapted from references 17 and 30.

Table 47–4. **POSTEXPOSURE PROPHYLAXIS FOR VACCINE-PREVENTABLE DISEASES**

DISEASE	DEFINITION OF EXPOSURE	PROPHYLAXIS*	COMMENTS
Hepatitis A	Ingestion of contaminated food; contact with feces from a hepatitis A–infected patient	One dose IM of immune globulin 0.02 mL/kg given within 14 d of exposure in large muscle mass (gluteal or deltoid)	Avoid in people with IgA deficiency; do not administer within 2 wk of MMR vaccine or 3 wk of varicella vaccine unless benefits exceed risk (e.g., known exposure)
Hepatitis B	Contact with contaminated blood or body fluid via percutaneous, mucous membrane, or nonintact skin exposure	See Table 47–5	Employees who have ever demonstrated an anti-HBsAg titer ≥10 mIU/mL do not require postexposure prophylaxis
Influenza A	Cohabiting confined air space or face-to-face contact in an open area†	Amantadine or rimantadine 100 mg PO 2 × per day should be considered	
Measles	Cohabiting confined air space or face-to-face contact in an open area†	Susceptible personnel should receive immune globulin 0.25 mL/kg (maximum 15 mL) IM within 6 d of exposure *or* measles vaccine	Susceptible people should be furloughed from days 5–21 postexposure or for 7 d after the rash appears
Meningococcus	Direct contact with respiratory secretions from infected person (e.g., resuscitating, intubating, or closely examining the oropharynx of an infected patient)‡	Ciprofloxacin 500 mg PO × 1 or ceftriaxone 250 mg IM × 1 or rifampin 600 mg PO 2× per day for 2 d	Home contacts of exposed healthcare providers do not need to receive prophylaxis unless the employee develops infection; rifampin and ciprofloxacin not recommended in pregnancy
Pertussis	Direct contact with respiratory secretions or droplets from the respiratory tract of infected people‡	Exposed employees should receive erythromycin 500 mg 4× per day for 14 days‡; trimethoprim-sulfamethoxazole 1 PO 2× per day is an alternative in an erythromycin-intolerant person	Symptomatic people should be evaluated for infection with a nasopharyngeal culture plated on appropriate media, and they should be relieved from work
Varicella	Cohabiting confined air space or face-to-face contact in an open area† with a patient with active lesions or within 48 hr before the development of lesions	For susceptible employees, varicella-zoster immune globulin, 125 U/10 kg IM, maximum dose 625 U, is indicated for immunocompromised or pregnant adults (within 96 hr of exposure)	Susceptible employees should be furloughed from days 8–21 postexposure. Employees who receive VZIG should be furloughed from days 8–28 postexposure
Zoster	Cohabiting confined air space or face-to-face contact in an open area† with a patient with active lesions	As for varicella exposure	Same as varicella exposure

*The latest guidelines of the Centers for Disease Control and Prevention should always be consulted.
†Employee who was wearing a mask (surgical mask or N-95 respirator) is not considered exposed.
‡Some experts recommend the estolate preparation. In vitro and limited in vivo data suggest that azithromycin or clarithromycin may be effective (they are likely to produce fewer gastrointestinal side effects).
HBsAg, hepatitis B surface antigen; IM, intramuscularly; MMR, measles-mumps-rubella; PO, orally; VZIG, varicella-zoster immune globulin.
Adapted from reference 17.

Table 47–5. **POSTEXPOSURE HEPATITIS B PROPHYLAXIS AFTER EXPOSURE TO CONTAMINATED BODY FLUID**

EXPOSED PERSON	SOURCE HBsAg-POSITIVE	SOURCE HBsAg-NEGATIVE	SOURCE NOT TESTED OR UNKNOWN
Unvaccinated	HBIG × 1* and initiate HB vaccine	Initiate HB vaccine†	Initiate HB vaccine†
Previously vaccinated			
Known responder	No treatment	No treatment	No treatment
Known nonresponder	HBIG × 2 *or* HBIG × 1 and begin revaccination	No treatment	If known high-risk source, treat as if HBsAg-positive
Response unknown	Test exposed person for anti-HBs If adequate,‡ no treatment If inadequate, HBIG × 1 and booster	No treatment	Test exposed person for anti-HBs If adequate,‡ no treatment If inadequate, begin revaccination

* Hepatitis B immune globulin (HBIG) dose of 0.06 mL per kg administered intramuscularly.
† Hepatitis B (HB) vaccine dose—see text.
‡ Adequate anti-HBs is 10 mIU per mL or greater.
HBsAg, Hepatitis B surface antigen.
Adapted from reference 17.

IMPROVING VACCINE COVERAGE OF HEALTHCARE PERSONNEL

Despite recommendations regarding immunization of HCWs for vaccine-preventable diseases, studies continue to demonstrate that significant numbers of HCWs lacked evidence of immunity to these diseases and that many HCWs refuse immunization. A survey of 144 medical schools in the United States and Canada in 1988 revealed that 28% had no immunization requirements for matriculating medical students, 31% had no rubella immunity requirement, and 40% had no measles immunity requirement.[66] Not surprisingly, a survey in 1987 of arriving housestaff at Columbia Presbyterian Medical Center in New York revealed the following rates of potential susceptibility to vaccine-preventable diseases as determined by lack of known immunization or physician-diagnosed disease (measles, mumps) or serology (rubella, hepatitis B, varicella): measles, mumps, or rubella, 63%; hepatitis B, 37%; and varicella, 5%.[67] Other studies of hepatitis B and influenza vaccine coverage rates are shown in Table 47–8. A survey of 95 acute care hospitals in Los Angeles County conducted in 1992 revealed that 36, 60, and 22% lacked immunization requirements for measles, mumps, and rubella.[68]

Screening of hospital staff has consistently demonstrated that, in the absence of a policy requiring immunity, significant numbers of hospital staff are susceptible to vaccine-preventable diseases. For example, surveys of hospital employees between 1990 and 1991 revealed 5.3 to 10.3% were susceptible to measles despite a policy recommending measles immunity that did not include a requirement.[69, 70]

Surveys of physicians have reported high rates of failure to receive hepatitis B vaccine (see Table 47–8).[71–73] Similarly, surveys of HCWs have reported low rates of acceptance of influenza immunization.[74–76] Barriers to receiving influenza vaccine commonly reported by HCWs have included desire to avoid medications, inconvenient vaccine administration, concern about side effects, belief that influenza can be caused by the vaccine, and belief that the vaccine is ineffective.[74, 76, 77] Similar concerns are voiced about hepatitis B vaccine, including desire to avoid medications, perception that the HCW is at low risk for occupationally acquired hepatitis B virus (HBV) infection, and concern about side effects.[77] Interventions such as the use of a mobile cart vaccination program have been demonstrated to increase immunization rates with influenza vaccine but still to suboptimal levels.[78]

GUIDELINES FOR THE USE OF SELECTED VACCINES

Mumps-Measles-Rubella Vaccine

Epidemiology

The incidence of mumps, measles, and rubella has decreased dramatically since the widespread use of MMR vaccine. Cases reported to the CDC in 1996 were as follows (per 100,000 population): mumps, 751 (0.29); measles, 508 (0.20); rubella, 238 (0.10); and congenital rubella syndrome, 4.[79] All three diseases represent a significant health hazard for hospital personnel for the following reasons. First, all three are transmitted by the droplet route. Measles is also transmitted by the airborne route. Second, in all three diseases, people become infectious before developing a clinically recognizable illness. Third, a history of prior disease may be unreliable for determining whether employees actually suffered a vaccine-preventable disease in the past. Hence, many unimmunized employees may falsely believe themselves immune.

Rubella is of special concern because of its ability to cause congenital abnormalities in up to 90% of women with confirmed infection in the first trimester of pregnancy. Hospital workers are frequently female and of childbearing age. Infants with congenital rubella may be contagious until they are at least 1 year old.

Lessons from Hospital Outbreaks

Nosocomial outbreaks of mumps have been reported infrequently,[80–86] but transmission from patient to patient[80, 81, 85, 86] and from patient to healthcare provider

Table 47–6. **WORK RESTRICTIONS FOR VACCINE-PREVENTABLE DISEASES**

DISEASE	WORK RESTRICTION	DURATION
Hepatitis A	Relieve from direct patient contact and food handling	Until 7 d after onset of jaundice
Hepatitis B		
Acute	Relieve from direct patient contact	Until jaundice resolves
Chronic	No restriction unless demonstrated to transmit infection to patients	Counsel regarding need to follow standard precautions; if healthcare worker transmits hepatitis B despite practicing precautions, prohibit from performing invasive procedures and direct contact with patient equipment until hepatitis B antigenemia resolves
Measles		
Active	Furlough from healthcare facility	Until 4 d after rash appears
Postexposure (susceptible personnel)	Furlough from healthcare facility	From the 5th day after the first exposure through the 21st day after the last exposure or 4 d after the rash appears
Mumps		
Active	Furlough from healthcare facility	Until 9 d after onset of parotitis
Postexposure (susceptible personnel)	Furlough from healthcare facility	From the 12th day after the first exposure through the 26th day after the last exposure or until 9 d after onset of parotitis
Pertussis		
Active	Furlough from healthcare facility	From the beginning of the catarrhal stage through the third week after onset of paroxysms or until 5 d after start of effective antimicrobial therapy
Postexposure (asymptomatic personnel)	No restriction, on prophylactic antimicrobial therapy	—
Postexposure (symptomatic personnel)	Furlough from healthcare facility	Same as active pertussis
Rubella		
Active	Furlough from healthcare facility	Until 5 d after rash appears
Postexposure (susceptible personnel)	Furlough from healthcare facility	From the 7th day after the first exposure through the 21st day after the last exposure or 5 d after rash appears
Influenza A and B	Relieve from care of high-risk patients	Until acute symptoms resolve
Varicella		
Active	Furlough from healthcare facility	Until all lesions dried and crusted
Postexposure (susceptible personnel)	Furlough from healthcare facility	From the 8th day after the first exposure through the 21st day (28th day if VZIG given) after the last exposure, or if varicella occurs, until all lesions dried and crusted
Zoster		
Localized (nonexposed area of skin), in normal person	Cover lesions; relieve from care of high-risk patients	Until all lesions dried and crusted
Localized (exposed area of skin); localized in immunocompromised person; generalized	Furlough from healthcare facility	Until all lesions dried and crusted
Postexposure (susceptible personnel)	Furlough from healthcare facility	From the 8th day after the first exposure through the 21st day (28th day if VZIG given) after the last exposure, or if varicella occurs, until all lesions dried and crusted

VZIG, varicella-zoster immune globulin.
Adapted from reference 17.

has been reported.[83–86] In one case, it was suggested that a symptom-free immune carrier, a hospital nurse, introduced mumps into a children's hospital.[82] Community outbreaks are likely to lead to nosocomial exposures. For example, during the widespread epidemic of mumps in Tennessee from 1986 to 1987, six HCWs in three different hospitals developed mumps after nosocomial exposure.[85] Men, including male HCWs, are at higher risk of complications from mumps (such as orchitis) than are children.[87] Orchitis has been reported among male HCWs who developed mumps as a result of hospital exposure.[83]

Nosocomial measles is well documented in the literature[88–115] and may aid in the propagation of community outbreaks.[108–110] Analyses of measles cases reported to the CDC revealed acquisition in a medical setting for 241 people (1.1% of all cases) between 1980 and 1984[100] and 1209 people (3.5% of all cases) between 1985 and 1989.[111] Investigations of individual outbreaks, however, have reported that 17 to 53% of cases were acquired in a medical setting.[92, 94, 98, 101, 105, 109, 113] Acquisition of measles has occurred in outpatient settings, including emergency departments and physician offices, and has involved patient-to-patient, patient-to-staff, and staff-to-patient transmission. Transmission in the outpatient setting has occurred even though the index cases had left the waiting or examination room up to 75 minutes earlier.[91, 94, 96, 97, 104] Case-control studies have demon-

Table 47–7. **INFORMATION THAT SHOULD BE OBTAINED WHEN PROVIDING VACCINES TO HEALTHCARE WORKERS**

Employee name
Employee identification number
Date of birth or age
Date of immunization
Vaccine provided
Name of vaccine manufacturer
Lot number of vaccine
Site of immunization
Route of immunization
Date for additional immunizations, if required
Complications (if any)
Name, title, and address of person providing vaccine
Signed informed consent

strated that people who visited an emergency department had a 4.9-fold[115] to 5.2-fold[110] higher risk of developing measles one incubation period later compared with those who did not have such visits. In inpatient settings, transmission has also occurred among patients, from patients to staff and from infected staff to patients. Infected staff have most commonly been nurses, with other groups at high risk of infection being physicians and office or hospital clerical staff. Nosocomial outbreaks have led to hospitalization of infected staff,[112] severe complications in infected patients,[114] and occasionally death of patients.[108, 112] The cost of controlling a single outbreak has ranged from $28,000 to more than $100,000.[108, 112]

As with mumps and measles, nosocomial rubella is well documented in the literature.[116–132] Sources of rubella infection have not only included people with acute infection, but also infants with congenital rubella.[116, 124] Hospital-acquired infection of pregnant staff members has led to the termination of pregnancy.[123, 129]

Several valuable lessons have been learned from the outbreaks. First, it appears that mumps and rubella are acquired mainly via droplet transmission. Measles, however, may be acquired via airborne transmission. Further, measles transmission may occur for more than an hour after an infected case has left an enclosed area. Second, history of prior disease is unreliable for determining whether employees actually contracted measles in the past, and hence many employees falsely believe they are immune from past illness and fail to take appropriate precautions. Third, failure to institute a mandatory program requiring immunity results in a subpopulation of susceptible HCWs capable of propagating epidemics. In multiple outbreaks, three to more than five generations of disease transmission occurred. Fourth, the cost of outbreaks for these diseases is high in both monetary terms and human suffering. Fifth, patients with congenital rubella are capable of transmitting rubella to susceptible adults.

Preexposure Prophylaxis

All HCWs should be immune to mumps, measles, and rubella. Immunity may be demonstrated by meeting one of the following: (1) birth before 1957 (mumps, rubella except women with childbearing potential), (2) laboratory evidence of immunity (people with indeterminate levels are considered susceptible), (3) physician-diagnosed disease (measles, mumps), or (4) evidence of appropriate immunizations (see Table 47–1).[17] The Centers for Disease Control and Prevention/Hospital Infection Control Practices Advisory Committee (CDC/HICPAC) now recommends that measles vaccine be administered to all HCWs born before 1957 if they do not have evidence of measles immunity and are at risk of occupational exposure to measles.[17] This recommendation is based on data from outbreak investigations, which revealed that 4.0 to 9.0% of people born before 1957 were susceptible to measles.[102, 133, 134] Hospitals that do not implement this recommendation should assess the immunity of HCWs born before 1957, in the same manner as for younger HCWs, during a community or institutional outbreak of measles. The CDC/HICPAC recommends that rubella vaccine be administered to all female HCWs with childbearing potential if they do not have evidence of rubella immunity, including people born before 1957.[17] The American Academy of Pediatrics recommends that all HCWs, including those born before 1957, who are without serological evidence of immunity to rubella should be immunized regardless of gender.[32]

Two doses of measles vaccine are currently recommended to ensure immunity (see Table 47–1). Revaccination with MMR may also be indicated for mumps because studies have shown that mumps can occur in a highly vaccinated population.[135]

Postexposure Management of Exposed Healthcare Workers

No specific prophylaxis has been shown to be effective for mumps or rubella. Exposed susceptible people

Table 47–8. **VACCINE COVERAGE OF HEALTHCARE WORKERS IN RECENT SERIES**

AUTHOR	STUDY YEAR(S)	STUDY LOCATION	HEALTHCARE WORKERS	VACCINE	IMMUNIZATION FREQUENCY
Weingarten	1986–87	Los Angeles hospital	House staff and nurses	Influenza	3.5%
Shapiro	1991	3411 orthopedic surgeons	Orthopedics	Hepatitis B	65%
McArthur	1991	1270 extended-care facilities, Canada	All staff	Influenza	>75% in 3.7% of facilities
Panlilio	1991–92	21 hospitals	General surgery, orthopedics, gynecology	Hepatitis B	55%
Agerton	1992	150 hospitals, United States	All staff	Hepatitis B	51%
Nichol	1993–94	Minneapolis hospital	Physicians and nurses	Influenza	61.2%

should be furloughed from the hospital (see Table 47–6). Patients with incubating or active mumps or rubella should be placed on Droplet Precautions. Patients with measles should be placed on Airborne Precautions. Measles vaccine can be used to provide postexposure prophylaxis of susceptible personnel if administered within 72 hours of exposure. Immune globulin 0.25 mL/10 kg (maximum 15 mL) may be used for postexposure prophylaxis for susceptible personnel who are exposed to measles but must be provided within 6 days of exposure. It is especially recommended for pregnant women and immunocompromised people (dose, 0.5 mL/10 kg, maximum 15 mL).

Varicella Vaccine

Epidemiology

Varicella-zoster virus (VZV) is the causative agent of two diseases: varicella (chickenpox), the primary infection, and zoster (shingles), a secondary infection caused by reactivation of latent VZV.[136–141] Although varicella is generally a mild disease in children, serious morbidity and mortality are common if infection occurs in neonates, adults, or immunocompromised people. For these reasons, the CDC,[17] the American Academy of Pediatrics,[32] and infectious disease experts[37, 142–146] have published recommendations regarding the isolation of patients with VZV infection and the management of patients and HCWs exposed to VZV. With the licensure of a varicella vaccine, preexposure prophylaxis of HCWs for VZV is now possible.

In most cases, VZV appears to be transmitted from person to person by the droplet route and occurs most efficiently when there is close contact, but true airborne transmission may also occur. The secondary attack rate of varicella among susceptible people in the household setting has ranged from 61 to 87%.[147–149] Herpes zoster is also infectious, although analysis of households suggests that the risk of transmission is only a third that of varicella.

Lessons from Nosocomial Outbreaks

Control of varicella is important in healthcare facilities because varicella and zoster are highly contagious; infection in adults frequently results in complications, including hospitalization; infection in pregnant women may lead to the congenital varicella syndrome[150] or neonatal varicella[151]; and severe complications, including death, may occur in immunocompromised patients and employees. Importantly for hospitals, the risk of complications appears to be higher in neonates,[152, 153] adults,[152–154] and immunocompromised people.[154] Approximately 1 to 2% of adults who develop varicella become ill enough to require hospitalization.[152, 153] Among patients developing varicella while undergoing chemotherapy for malignancy or immunosuppressive therapy after organ or bone marrow transplantation, visceral dissemination or severe disease has been reported in 30 to 50% and death in 7 to 17%.[155–162] Current rates of morbidity and mortality are likely to be significantly lower because of prophylactic use of VZIG and availability of antivirals such as acyclovir.

Studies have noted that 60 to 86% (median, 78%) of U.S. HCWs report they have had varicella.[163–170] A report of prior varicella by an HCW has been demonstrated to be highly correlated with immunity as measured by serology. A history of prior household exposure to VZV, however, is not a reliable indicator of immunity in the absence of clinical illness.[163] Among HCWs with a negative or uncertain history of VZV infection, reported serosusceptibility has varied from 4 to 47% (median, 15%).[146, 163, 164, 166–172] Overall the susceptibility of HCWs to varicella has been reported to range from 1 to 7% (median, 3%).[164, 166, 167, 169–173] After nosocomial exposure to VZV infection, 2 to 16% of susceptible staff have developed clinical varicella.[146, 154, 167]

Nosocomial transmission of VZV has been well documented in the literature.[146, 149, 154, 163, 165, 167, 170, 173, 174–187] Varicella may be introduced into the hospital by infected patients, staff, or visitors. Several investigators have noted that the initial source case for an outbreak was in the incubating phase of varicella.[146, 148, 167] Nosocomial varicella has occurred among staff and patients who had no direct contact with the index case, supporting the airborne route as a mode of spread.[75, 184] Epidemiological studies using tracers[184] or measurement of VZV DNA[188] have provided definitive evidence to support airborne transmission. Exposure to dermatomal[146, 175, 180] or disseminated[165, 167] zoster in immunocompromised patients and to dermatomal zoster in immunocompetent hosts has led to transmission of VZV to susceptible HCWs via the airborne route or droplet route.[146, 184]

The CDC,[1, 19] the American Academy of Pediatrics,[32] and infectious disease clinicians[44, 142–146] have published guidelines or algorithms designed to aid clinicians in the control of nosocomial exposures. There are several areas of controversy among these various guidelines. First, the CDC suggests that exposed serosusceptible patients be placed on isolation and exposed serosusceptible employees be removed from work from days 10 through 21 postexposure, whereas the American Academy of Pediatrics[32] suggests isolation from days 8 through 21 postexposure. Second, the CDC continues to recommend that nonimmunocompromised patients with dermatomal zoster be placed on only contact isolation as opposed to airborne and contact isolation.[19] University of North Carolina Hospitals place patients with dermatomal zoster on airborne and contact isolation because of the difficulty of defining "immunocompromised patients" and reports of airborne or droplet transmission of varicella from nonimmunocompromised patients with dermatomal zoster.[146, 184] Third, the CDC has recommended that all patients with varicella or disseminated zoster and immunocompromised patients with dermatomal zoster be placed in rooms meeting engineering requirements suitable to house patients with tuberculosis (i.e., private room, negative pressure of room with respect to corridor, six or more air exchanges per hour, and air exhausted directly to the outside). The authors are unaware of any nosocomial outbreaks in which transmission was linked to recirculated air of infected patients placed in private rooms with negative pressure. Further, negative-pressure rooms have been reported to be adequate in preventing transmission of varicella from hospitalized patients.[183] Given the current incidence of varicella and tuberculosis, it is likely that many hospitals do not have adequate rooms meeting the OSHA tuberculosis requirements to use these rooms to isolate patients with VZV infections.

Preexposure Prophylaxis

The authors and other infectious disease specialists believe that all HCWs should be immune to VZV. There are several compelling reasons why HCWs should be immune. First, HCWs with incubating or clinical varicella have transmitted VZV infection to hospitalized patients. Such infections may lead to substantial morbidity in *high-risk* patients, such as pregnant women, neonates, and immunocompromised people. Second, HCWs are at risk of acquisition of VZV infection from patients with clinical varicella or zoster. Even healthy adults have a substantial risk of varicella complications. Further, secondary VZV infections may occur among their contacts. Finally, the presence of susceptible hospital staff results in significant costs for healthcare organizations. These costs are associated with the removal of susceptible staff from patient contact after VZV exposures, administration of VZIG to immunocompromised patients exposed to HCWs with incubating or clinical varicella, and time and effort of hospital staff in evaluating VZV exposures. Decision analysis has been used to demonstrate that immunization of HCWs susceptible to varicella is cost-effective for healthcare facilities.[189, 190]

HCWs should be screened for VZV immunity at the time of initial employment, as is currently recommended for mumps, measles, and rubella. Current employees may be screened at the time of their annual tuberculosis and immunization evaluation or via a special program. Employees with a history of VZV infection may be considered immune. Employees without a definitve history of VZV infection should undergo serological testing and, if negative, be considered for immunization. The preferred test for determining immunity is probably the latex agglutination test followed by an enzyme-linked immunosorbent assay (ELISA) test or radioimmunoassay. Employees without a vaccine contraindication or precaution should be immunized with two doses at least 4 weeks apart of varicella vaccine. Performing a postimmunization serology is not recommended because commercial tests may lack the sensitivity to detect the lower antibody levels associated with immunization compared with natural infection. Further, the gpELISA test (not commercially available) used by Merck Sharp & Dohme (West Point, PA) suggests a seroconversion rate of 99% in adults, making postimmunization serological testing not cost-effective.

There appears to be virtually no risk of transmission of the vaccine strain of virus from healthy people who do not develop a rash postimmunization. The risk of transmitting the vaccine strain even to immunocompromised people from HCWs who develop either a local rash or generalized rash is likely low but has not been precisely quantitated. The few employees who develop an injection site rash may continue to work with nonimmunocompromised patients, provided that the lesions are covered. Employees with a generalized rash should be furloughed until the rash is resolved. In the authors' experience, this has been approximately 5 days. The rash should not automatically be assumed to be due to vaccine, especially if exposure to a case of chickenpox has occurred in the preceding 3 weeks.

Management of Exposed Healthcare Workers

All employees potentially exposed to varicella or zoster should be evaluated as soon as feasible by the occupational health service. Employees with no history or an uncertain history (e.g., VZV infection in other family members) of varicella should be serologically tested for immunity. Employees with a positive test should be considered immune. All susceptible employees should be considered for postexposure prophylaxis with VZIG and removed from duty from days 8 through 21 postexposure. VZIG is indicated for employees who are pregnant or immunocompromised. Employees who develop varicella should be considered for antiviral therapy. Employees who develop varicella may return to work when clinically well and after all lesions are dried and crusted (usually about 5 days).

Insufficient data are available to provide definitive recommendations on the postexposure management of employees previously immunized with the varicella vaccine. One option[42] would be to test such employees serologically immediately postexposure. Serosusceptible employees would be retested for an anamnestic response 5 to 7 days postexposure. Employees testing nonimmune would be relieved from duty from days 8 though 21 postexposure. A second proposed option would be to examine employees daily and remove immunized employees only if they develop clinical varicella. If hospitals choose the latter option and an immunized employee develops varicella, it is unclear to what degree this employee would already have been a potential source case for patients or other staff.

Postexposure prophylaxis may be provided by administering VZIG or acyclovir. The latter measure should be considered experimental and requires additional prospective studies before adoption. Prophylactic acyclovir (20 mg/kg every 6 hours) from day 7 through day 17 postexposure has been successfully used to prevent disease in high-risk children.[191–193] The prophylactic use of acyclovir, however, was associated with a decreased rate of seroconversion; approximately 50% of the children remained serosusceptible.

The varicella vaccine is not Food and Drug Administration (FDA) approved for use as postexposure prophylaxis. Several studies, however, have investigated the ability of the Oka strain varicella vaccine to attenuate or prevent clinical varicella in healthy children when administered as postexposure prophylaxis.[194–202] The vaccine was most effective when administered within 3 days of exposure and is generally ineffective when administered more than 5 days after exposure. In a double-blind, placebo-controlled study, the Merck varicella vaccine was reported to be 67% effective in completely preventing illness and 100% effective in modifying varicella when administered within 5 days of exposure in children.[202] The efficacy of postexposure prophylaxis in adults is unknown.

VZIG is indicated for susceptible *high-risk* HCWs (i.e., leukemia or lymphoma, congenital or acquired immunodeficiency, immunosuppressive therapy, human immunodeficiency virus [HIV] infection) exposed to varicella.[32, 42] VZIG is most effective when administered within 72 hours of exposure; its efficacy when used more than 96 hours after exposure is unknown. The adult dose of VZIG is 125 U/10 kg (maximal dose, 625 U or 5 vials). VZIG should be administered intramuscularly or as directed by the manufacturer. It should *not* be administered intravenously. VZIG has been demonstrated to lead to attenuated disease in pregnant women and immunocompromised people but likely does not prevent congenital infection. VZIG may prolong the incubation period before disease; hence all employees treated with VZIG should be removed from duty from days 8 through 28.

All HCWs with VZV infection should be evaluated and after confirmation of infection should be offered recommended antiviral therapy, which should be initiated within 72 hours of the onset of clinical infection. Of the three drugs currently FDA approved for therapy of zoster in the normal adult (i.e., acyclovir, famcyclovir, valacyclovir), valacyclovir is the least expensive. Although the safety of acyclovir in pregnant women has not been firmly established, adverse fetal events have not been described. The American Academy of Pediatrics does not recommend the routine use of oral acyclovir for pregnant women with varicella. The Academy stated, however, that therapy with intravenous acyclovir should be considered for pregnant patients who develop serious varicella-associated complications.[32]

Hepatitis B Vaccine

Epidemiology

Exposure to bloodborne pathogens via parenteral or mucosal contact remains a major hazard for HCWs, especially those performing invasive procedures. Although more than 20 diseases have been transmitted by needle stick,[203] the agents of greatest concern are hepatitis B virus (HBV), hepatitis C virus, and HIV.[8, 204–207] Seroprevalence surveys conducted before the availability of the HBV vaccine in 1981 showed that HCWs had prevalence rates of past or present HBV infection threefold to fivefold higher than the general U.S. population.[208–211] The risk of infection was related to both the extent and the duration of blood contact. The CDC reported that in 1989 an estimated 12,000 American HCWs would become infected with HBV, which would result in 250 deaths.[212] With a decreasing incidence of hepatitis B, the CDC estimated that in 1994, 1012 HCWs became infected with HBV because of occupational exposures, leading to approximately 22 deaths.[213] The decline among HCWs is probably due to the use of hepatitis B vaccine, institution of Universal (now Standard) Precautions, and other preventive measures (e.g., needleless devices).

Lessons from Nosocomial Outbreaks

Hepatitis B acquisition represents a major hazard for HCWs for several reasons. First, HCWs have high rates of percutaneous blood contact. For example, a survey of New York City surgeons in 1988 reported that 86% had experienced at least one puncture injury in the preceding year.[214] A survey of American and Canadian orthopedic surgeons in 1991 revealed that 87.4% reported a blood-skin contact and 39.2% a percutaneous blood contact in the previous month.[215] Second, the virus is relatively stable in the environment, as demonstrated by its survival after drying and storage at 25°C and 42% relative humidity for 1 week.[216] Third, HBV is more transmissible than either HIV or hepatitis C virus with rates of disease transmission after a percutaneous injury with a contaminated sharp reported between 6 and 30%.[217–219] The risks of disease transmission via mucosal contact or contact with nonintact skin have not been quantitated but appear to be much lower than for percutaneous exposure. HBV infection has been acquired via ocular exposure[220] and has been transmitted to multiple patients by a respiratory therapist with severe exudative dermatitis while obtaining arterial blood gases.[221] The high frequency of hepatitis B among hospital personnel who did not recall a percutaneous exposure in the era before hepatitis B vaccine has been attributed to inapparent inoculation through mucous membranes or small breaks in the skin.[222] Fourth, a significant number of patients are infectious (i.e., HBsAg-positive) with their status unknown to the medical staff. For example, a study of consecutive blood samples submitted to the chemistry laboratory of an urban hospital in 1987 revealed that only 28% of HBsAg-positive specimens were labeled as per hospital protocol with a biohazard label.[223] Finally, many HCWs remain unimmunized.

Transmission of hepatitis B via contaminated medical instruments and environmental surfaces is well described. Nosocomial outbreaks of HBV infection have been associated with a blood-contaminated jet gun injector,[224] an endoscope,[225] multidose heparin vials,[226] and finger stick (i.e., capillary) blood-sampling devices.[227–231] Contamination of instruments or medication vials resulted in 67 of 243 cardiac transplant patients developing infection during transvenous endomyocardial biopsies.[232] Environmental surfaces in clinical laboratories were demonstrated to be positive for HBsAg in 34% of samples,[233] and contaminated file cards have been reported to lead to transmission among laboratory technicians.[234]

Transmission of hepatitis B in hemodialysis centers presumably via contaminated environmental surfaces, shared equipment, or common-dose medications continues to be a problem.[235–237] In addition to standard precautions, the following hemodialysis-specific infection control practices should be used: (1) Serum specimens from all susceptible patients should be tested monthly for HBsAg, and these results should be reviewed promptly. (2) HBsAg-positive patients should be isolated by room, machine, instruments, medications, supplies, and staff. (3) Instruments, medications, and supplies should not be shared between any patients. When sharing of multidose medication vials is necessary, medications must be prepared in a clean centralized area separate from areas used for patient care, laboratory work, or refuse disposal. (4) Routine cleaning and disinfection procedures should be followed. In addition, all serosusceptible hemodialysis patients should receive the hepatitis B vaccine. Because hemodialyzed patients have a diminished response to hepatitis B vaccine, higher doses and booster doses are recommended to maintain protection against HBV.

More than 35 outbreaks have been described of healthcare provider–to–patient transmission of hepatitis B.[238–241] The source has most commonly been a dentist, surgeon, or gynecologist performing invasive procedures.[239] The most important risk factors for transmission during an invasive procedure have been a hepatitis B e antigen (HBeAg)–positive source, degree of invasiveness of the procedure, lack of wearing gloves by the infected HCW, or injury to the infected HCW with a sharp object.[239] Guidelines for the management of the HBV-infected HCW have been published.[242]

Preexposure Prophylaxis

Because of the risks posed by bloodborne pathogens, OSHA has mandated since 1991 that all healthcare personnel undergo annual training in the prevention of bloodborne pathogen acquisition and use of personnel protective equipment (gloves, masks, gown, and eyewear) whenever exposure to blood or other potentially infectious body fluids is reasonably anticipated.[243] Despite the OSHA regulations and the introduction of new technologies, such as needleless devices, however, percutaneous, mucous membrane, and skin exposures to contaminated body fluids continue to occur at a high frequency. The OSHA standard also required that all healthcare facilities offer employees hepatitis B immunization. Employees may refuse immunization but must sign a declination form.

Protective serum titers of anti-HBsAg (≥10 mIU/mL) develop in 95 to 99% of healthy adults who receive a series of three intramuscular doses of hepatitis B vaccine.[244] The anti-HBsAg response, however, is reduced in people who are over 40 years of age or are otherwise immunocompromised.[244] Administering three doses on an accelerated schedule (e.g., 0, 1, 2 months) results in a more rapid antibody rise but may reduce peak titers.[245, 246] The two currently available hepatitis B vaccines, Recombivax HB and Engerix-B, are equally immunogenic and are interchangeable; either can be used (in its recommended dose) to complete an immunization series begun with the other.[244] Immunogenicity is not reduced when hepatitis B vaccine is given with other vaccines. Pregnancy is not a contraindication to hepatitis B vaccine. All injections should be provided in the deltoid because gluteal injection results in poor immunogenicity.

Most HCWs should receive vaccine on a 0, 1, and 6 month schedule. Consideration should be given to using a 0, 1, and 2 month or 0, 1, and 4 month schedule for unimmunized HCWs at high risk for HBV acquisition (e.g., hemodialysis workers, cardiac surgeons), but a fourth dose should be given at 12 months to ensure long-term protection. All HCWs should have an anti-HBsAg titer obtained 1 to 2 months after the third immunization. Because approximately half the people who do not develop a protective level of anti-HBsAg antibodies after a three-dose series do so after additional doses,[247] HCWs with an inadequate response to a three-dose series should receive up to three additional doses of hepatitis B vaccine. They may have their antibody response tested 1 to 2 months after each dose or at the end of a second three-dose series. Individuals who do not respond to these three additional doses should be considered nonresponders and should receive HBIG when indicated for postexposure prophylaxis.

Symptomatic hepatitis B is rare in immunized people who developed protective levels of antibody, even though there is eventual loss of detectable antibody in up to 50% of those people 5 to 10 years after immunization.[46] For this reason, there is currently no recommendation for periodic boosting of HCWs who have responded to hepatitis B vaccine.[17, 30, 207]

Postexposure Prophylaxis

All HCWs with potential exposure to blood or contaminated body fluids should be evaluated. Exposure is defined as parenteral, mucous membrane, or nonintact skin exposure to blood or contaminated fluids. In all cases, the source should be tested for HBsAg, hepatitis C, and HIV. If the source case is HBsAg-positive, postexposure prophylaxis may be indicated (see Table 47–5). HBIG has been shown to be effective when provided within 7 days. Immune globulin should not be used because of lack of efficacy. The simultaneous administration of HBIG and hepatitis B vaccine (at different sites) does not diminish the efficacy of the hepatitis B vaccine.[244]

Influenza Vaccine

Epidemiology

Influenza is characterized by the abrupt onset of fever, myalgia, sore throat, and nonproductive cough. Elderly people and people with underlying health problems are at increased risk for complications of influenza, including hospitalization and death. During major epidemics, the hospitalization rate for the elderly and people with chronic health problems may increase twofold to fivefold compared with nonepidemic periods.[248] During 9 of 20 influenza seasons (from 1972–1973 through 1991–1992), more than 20,000 influenza-associated excess deaths occurred each season; during four of these seasons, more than 40,000 deaths occurred.[249]

Influenza viruses are classified into subtypes on the basis of two surface antigens: hemagglutinin (H) and neuraminidase (N). Widespread human disease has been caused by three subtypes of hemagglutinin (H1, H2, and H3) and two subtypes of neuraminidase (N1 and N2). Immunity to these antigens, especially to hemagglutinin, reduces the likelihood of infection and lessens the severity of disease if infection occurs. Infection with a virus of one subtype confers little or no protection against viruses of other subtypes. Over time, antigenic variation (antigenic drift) within a subtype may be so marked that infection or immunization with one strain may not induce immunity to more distantly related strains of the same subtype. The antigenic characteristics of circulating strains provide the basis for selecting the viral strains included in each year's vaccine.

Influenza virus appears to spread from person to person by small particle aerosol transmission. Although aerosol transmission is well established, nosocomial transmission via fomites and contaminated hands remains possible. Influenza virus is shed for up to 5 days beyond the onset of illness in adults, but shedding may occur for up to 7 days in children. Humans are the primary reservoir of infection, but swine and avian (e.g., ducks) reservoirs are likely sources of new human subtypes thought to emerge through genetic reassortment.

Lessons from Nosocomial Outbreaks

Nosocomial acquisition of influenza has been well described.[250–263] Nosocomial transmission most commonly occurs during community influenza outbreaks when patients infected with influenza are admitted to the hospital. Because up to 25% of unimmunized HCWs may develop influenza during the winter months, however, infected staff may introduce infection into a healthcare facility.[264] Staff infected by patients have frequently served as the source for secondary transmission of influenza to patients and other staff.[252, 253, 258, 259] Acquisition of influenza by HCWs may cause absenteeism and significant disruption of healthcare.[253, 256, 259]

Nosocomial outbreaks have frequently involved extended-care facilities for the elderly.[265–280] Such outbreaks may cause significant morbidity and mortality.[268, 269, 277] High rates of influenza immunization among HCWs may lead to a decrease in the attack rate of influenza among patients. For example, patients in facilities in which greater than 60% of the staff had been immunized experienced less influenza-related mortality and illness compared with patients in facilities without immunized staff.[281] Nosocomial outbreaks have also been reported in other types of long-term care facilities, such as institutions caring for mentally challenged people.[282]

Important lessons from these outbreaks include the following. First, identification of all patients with influenza is problematic and incomplete.[259] Further, community indicators of influenza activity (e.g., visits to acute ambulatory care centers for upper respiratory illness) cannot be relied on to provide warning of influenza among hospitalized patients.[256] Second, influenza infection among staff is common during the winter season and results in significant absenteeism. Attack rates of 25 to 80% are often observed among both patients and staff during outbreaks. Third, failure to isolate patients treated with amantadine or rimantadine may result in the dissemination of drug-resistant strains.

Recommendations for prevention and control of nosocomial influenza have been published.[263, 283–289] The CDC recommends the following measures: (1) educate personnel about the epidemiology, modes of transmission, and means of preventing the spread of influenza; (2) establish mechanism(s) by which hospital personnel are promptly alerted of an increase in influenza activity in the local community; (3) arrange for laboratory tests to be available to clinicians, for use when clinically indicated, to confirm the diagnosis of influenza and other acute viral respiratory diseases promptly, especially during November through April; (4) offer vaccine to outpatients and inpatients at high risk of complications from influenza, beginning in September and continuing until influenza activity has begun to decline; (5) vaccinate HCWs before the influenza season each year, preferably between mid-October and mid-November; (6) isolate patients with known or suspected influenza in a private room, preferably under negative pressure; (7) institute masking of individuals who enter the room of a patient with influenza; (8) evaluate HCWs with febrile upper respiratory illnesses and consider removal from duties that involve direct patient care (use more stringent guidelines for staff working in *high-risk* areas, such as intensive care units, nurseries, or with severely immunocompromised patients); and (9) during community or hospital outbreaks, restrict hospital visitors who have a febrile respiratory illness.[287] During a nosocomial outbreak, the CDC recommends the following: (1) Early in the outbreak, obtain a nasopharyngeal swab or nasal-wash specimen from patients with recent-onset symptoms suggestive of influenza for virus culture or antigen detection; (2) administer current influenza vaccine to unvaccinated patients and staff; (3) administer amantadine or rimantadine for prophylaxis to all uninfected patients in an involved unit for whom it is not contraindicated; (4) administer amantadine or rimantadine for prophylaxis to all unvaccinated staff members for whom it is not contraindicated and who are in the involved unit or taking care of high-risk patients; (5) discontinue antiviral prophylaxis if laboratory tests confirm or strongly suggest that influenza type A is not the cause of the outbreak; (6) if the cause of the outbreak is confirmed or believed to be influenza type A *and* vaccine has been administered only recently to susceptible patients and personnel, continue antiviral prophylaxis until 2 weeks after the vaccination; and (7) to the extent possible, do not allow contact between those at high risk of complications from influenza and patients or staff who are taking amantadine or rimantadine for treatment of acute respiratory illnesses; prevent contact during and for 2 days after the latter discontinue treatment.

Preexposure Prophylaxis

Influenza vaccine is strongly recommended for any person aged 6 months or older who is at increased risk for complications of influenza because of age or underlying medical condition. People at increased risk for influenza-related complications include people aged 65 years or older; residents of extended-care facilities or long-term care facilities that house people of any age who have chronic medical conditions; adults and children who have required regular medical follow-up or hospitalization during the previous year because of chronic metabolic diseases (including diabetes mellitus), renal dysfunction, hemoglobinopathies, or immunosuppression; children and teenagers (aged 6 months to 18 years) who are receiving long-term aspirin therapy and therefore may be at risk for developing Reye syndrome after influenza; and women who will be in the second or third trimester of pregnancy during the influenza season.[48]

Influenza vaccine is also recommended for HCWs because when they are clinically or subclinically infected they can transmit influenza virus to people at high risk. The CDC specifically recommends immunization for the following HCWs: physicians, nurses, and other personnel in both hospital and outpatient care settings; employees of nursing homes and long-term care facilities who have contact with patients or residents; and providers of home care to people at high risk (e.g., visiting nurses and volunteer workers).[48] The CDC also recommends vaccine to any person who wishes to reduce the likelihood of becoming ill with influenza. A randomized, controlled trial in a general working population has demonstrated that providing influenza vaccine is cost-effective.[290]

Influenza immunization should not be provided to people known to have anaphylactic hypersensitivity to eggs or other components of the influenza vaccine.[48] People who have a history of anaphylactic hypersensitivity to vaccine components but who are also at high risk for complications of influenza, however, can benefit from vaccine after appropriate allergy evaluation and desensitization. Neither pregnancy nor breast-feeding is considered a contraindication to immunization, and, in fact, vaccine is specifically recommended for women who will be in the second or third trimester of pregnancy during the influenza season.

Chemoprophylaxis with amantadine or rimantadine has been used as both preexposure and postexposure prophylaxis to reduce the likelihood of developing influenza A infection. Adverse events have been noted in up to 33% of patients receiving amantadine leading to withdrawal of therapy in 6 to 11% more patients receiving active drug versus placebo.[288] Common side effects include anxiety, lightheadedness, ataxia, confusion, hallucinations, insomnia, nausea, and weakness. Rimantadine has been demonstrated to have equivalent efficacy and lower central nervous system toxicity but is substantially more expensive.[48] The recommended dose of either drug when used for prophylaxis is 100 mg twice daily. Dosage adjustment may be required for the following people: age 65 years or older, chronic liver disease, and chronic renal impairment. Physicians prescribing these drugs should be aware of drug interactions, including central nervous system stimulants, antihistamines, and anticholinergic drugs. Chemoprophylaxis is not a substitute for immunization.

Amantadine-resistant and rimantadine-resistant influenza A viruses can emerge when either of these drugs is administered for treatment. Amantadine-resistant strains are cross-resistant to rimantadine and vice versa.

Despite these recommendations, many HCWs choose not to take influenza vaccine.[67, 74, 290–293] Institutions should consider introducing innovative methods such as provision by mobile carts on hospital wards[288] or by offering vaccine to housestaff and students in clinics and conferences.[290]

Postexposure Prophylaxis

During community or nosocomial outbreaks, healthcare institutions should offer and strongly encourage the use of influenza vaccine among HCWs. If influenza A is the circulating virus, consideration should be given to providing chemoprophylaxis for 2 weeks to newly immunized HCWs who are at high risk of exposure to infected patients. Prophylaxis should be considered for all employees, regardless of immunization status, if the outbreak is caused by a variant strain of influenza A that might not be controlled by the vaccine. Only a few placebo-controlled trials have tested the possible efficacy of postexposure prophylaxis, an intervention that might be effective in controlling outbreaks or preventing the transmission of infection in households or other settings.[288] When the index case is treated concurrently with contacts, rapid selection and apparent transmission of resistant viruses to contacts has been reported.[288] The same problem has been noted in mass prophylaxis with amantadine in extended-care facilities.[275, 278] For this reason, all patients treated with an antiviral should be placed on isolation as recommended by the CDC. Amantadine and rimantadine can reduce the severity and shorten the duration of influenza A illness among healthy adults when administered within 48 hours of illness onset.

Hepatitis A Vaccine

Hepatitis A virus (HAV) is highly endemic in the United States with 31,582 cases (12.13 cases per 100,000) reported to the CDC in 1995. After the 1994 data, which noted 26,796 cases, were corrected for underreporting and asymptomatic infections, an estimated 80,000 cases and 134,000 infections occurred in 1994.[62, 294] The incidence of HAV varies by race and ethnicity (highest among Native Americans and Native Alaskans), location (highest in western United States), and age (highest in people 5 to 14 years of age). Sources of infection include household or sexual contact with a person with HAV (22 to 26%), with a child or employee in a daycare center (14 to 16%), or with an international traveler (4 to 6%) as well as food or waterborne outbreaks (2 to 3%).[295] In the United States, approximately 50% of people with HAV do not have an identified source of infection.[62, 294]

Hepatitis A results in substantial morbidity with significant costs caused by medical care and lost work time. Approximately 11 to 22% of people who develop hepatitis A require hospitalization.[294] In the United States, an estimated 100 deaths occur each year as a result of fulminant hepatitis A.

Lessons from Nosocomial Outbreaks

Nosocomial outbreaks from HAV have been relatively infrequent, especially when considering the large number of people hospitalized with this disease each year. Cohort studies reported in peer-reviewed journals have not demonstrated that HCWs are at increased risk for disease acquisition compared with control populations.[296–298] Further, a cohort study failed to find evidence of patient-to-patient transmission.[299] French and Belgium researchers, however, have reported in letters that HCWs had higher than expected rates of seropositivity to hepatitis A.[300, 301] Multiple nosocomial outbreaks of HAV have been reported.[302–317] Most outbreaks have occurred in one of the following settings. First, the source patient was not jaundiced and hepatitis was inapparent at the time of hospitalization. Second, the HAV-infected patient was fecally incontinent or had diarrhea. Nosocomial HAV has also been associated with contaminated blood transfusions[309, 312, 313] and contaminated food.[302, 303] Risk factors for HAV transmission to personnel have included activities that increase the risk of fecal-oral contamination, including caring for a person with unrecognized HAV infection[304–308, 310, 311, 314–317]; sharing food, beverages, or cigarettes with patients, their families, or the staff[307, 311, 312, 317]; nail biting; handling bile without proper precautions[317]; and not washing hands or wearing gloves when providing care to an infected patient.[312, 314, 315, 317]

Prevention of nosocomial HAV requires strict adherence to standard precautions, which suggest the use of gloves whenever dealing with secretions and excretions. Hand washing should precede and follow all patient contact. Several outbreaks would have been prevented by eliminating the eating of food in patient care areas.

Preexposure Prophylaxis

The current scientific literature supports the recommendation of the CDC that hepatitis A vaccine should not be routinely provided to HCWs. Although many outbreaks have involved neonates and children, even for these subgroups the likelihood of infection probably does not warrant a blanket recommendation of immunization. A cost-effectiveness study of providing hepatitis A vaccine to all medical students reported that the costs per life-year saved and quality adjusted life-year saved were $58,000 and $47,000. As with other special use vaccines, HCWs should be encouraged to review with their local medical provider their own risks and benefits for hepatitis A vaccine.

Postexposure Prophylaxis

Postexposure prophylaxis with hepatitis A vaccine may be indicated in community outbreaks of hepatitis A.[62, 294] The role for hepatitis A vaccine to control outbreaks in hospitals, daycare centers, and other institutions has not been evaluated.

Postexposure prophylaxis with immune globulin has been demonstrated to be effective in reducing secondary cases after exposure to a common source, such as contaminated food or close personal contact with an infected person. Immune globulin should not be routinely provided to HCWs after identification of a single infected patient in the hospital.[62, 294] Immune globulin should be administered to people who have close contact with index patients if an epidemiological investigation indicates HAV transmission has occurred between patients and staff.

Pertussis Vaccine

Epidemiology

In the United States, the highest recorded annual incidence of pertussis occurred in 1934, when greater than 260,000 cases were reported.[318] After the introduction of whole-cell diphtheria, tetanus, and pertussis (DTP) vaccine, the incidence declined more than 99%. Since the early 1980s, however, the reported pertussis incidence has increased steadily with 2719 to 6586 cases reported annually between 1988 and 1995. In addition to temporal trends, pertussis also exhibits a cyclical trend with 2- to 5-year cycles; peaks have occurred in 1983, 1986, 1990, and 1993.[319] In 1995, 5137 cases were reported (1.97 per 100,000 population). The highest attack rate of pertussis occurs in children less than 1 year of age, but approximately 20% of cases reported in 1995 were in people 15 years of age or older. Possible explanations for this increase in disease include (1) decreased vaccine efficacy, (2) decreased vaccine coverage, (3) waning immunity among adolescents and adults vaccinated during childhood, (4) increased diagnosis and reporting of pertussis because of greater awareness among physicians about the disease, and (5) enhanced surveillance and more complete reporting in some states.[320] Vaccine coverage levels, however, are higher than at any time in the past.

Adolescents and young adults play an important role in transmitting pertussis to susceptible infants because immunization-induced immunity to pertussis wanes with increasing age and because disease in adults is frequently not diagnosed or treated because it is often mild or atypical. Studies using serological methods have demonstrated that *B. pertussis* is a common cause of respiratory illness causing cough in adults.[321–323] Deville and colleagues[324] followed HCWs for 5 years and reported that 90% of subjects had a signficant antibody rise (immunoglobulin A [IgA] or IgG) to one or more *B. pertussis* antigens between two consecutive years; 55% had evidence of two infections, 17% had evidence of three infections, and 4% had evidence of four infections. Reinfection with *B. pertussis* may also follow native infection.[325]

Lessons from Nosocomial Outbreaks

At the University of North Carolina Hospitals, pertussis is the third most common source of infectious disease exposure evaluations with only varicella-zoster and tuberculosis more common (Weber, unpublished data). Multiple nosocomial outbreaks have been reported in the literature.[326–334] These most often have involved residential facilities for the mentally or physically impaired[329, 330, 332] or pediatric wards of acute care hospitals.[326–328] Although the source case most commonly was an infected patient in whom pertussis was unrecognized,[326, 327, 331] infected employees[329, 332] and the infected mother of a child with pertussis[328] also served as sources. Employees often served as vectors for additional nosocomial cases.[326, 327, 329, 332] In several instances, infected employees also infected members of their households.[327, 329] Nosocomial outbreaks have occurred for several reasons: (1) failure to recognize and appropriately isolate infected patients, (2) failure to give prophylaxis to exposed staff, and (3) failure to furlough symptomatic staff.[335]

Preexposure Prophylaxis

The primary means of preventing pertussis is via administration of pertussis vaccine to children at ages 2 months, 4 months, 6 months, 15 to 18 months, and 4 to 6 years. The DTaP (diphtheria-tetanus toxoid-acellular pertussis vaccine) is the preferred vaccine for all doses in the vaccination series because the new acellular pertussis vaccines are at least as effective as standard pertussis vaccine with significantly fewer side effects. Boosters are not currently recommended for adults. Because immunity wanes with time, many adults are susceptible to infection with *B. pertussis*.

The ability to boost immunity to *B. pertussis* among adults via immunization would aid in the prevention of nosocomial outbreaks and protect staff and their families from disease. In a study of 118 adults reimmunized with a vaccine containing acellular pertussis antigens in addition to diphtheria and tetanus toxoids, substantially enhanced antibody levels were noted without an increase in adverse reactions or diminution in response to the diphtheria and tetanus components.[336]

Postexposure Prophylaxis

B. pertussis is highly susceptible in vitro to erythromycin[337, 338] and the newer macrolides, azithromycin and clarithromycin.[339] *B. pertussis* is also susceptible to trimethoprim-sulfamethoxazole[338] and the quinolones, ciprofloxacin and ofloxacin.[338, 340, 341] *B. pertussis* is not susceptible to the first-generation cephalosporins.[342] Erythromycin has been shown to decrease the duration of illness when administered early in the course of pertussis and to eliminate *B. pertussis* from the nasopharynx. Erythromycin has also been successfully used to provide chemoprophylaxis of individuals exposed to *B. pertussis* and to aid in preventing secondary spread in households or terminating outbreaks in institutions.[325, 329, 334, 343–345] For these reasons, erythromycin is considered the drug of choice for the treatment and prophylaxis of pertussis.[335, 346–348] For clinical treatment, the estolate form is preferred by some clinicians because of its superior pharmacokinetics.[347] Trimethoprim-sulfamethoxazole is the recommended alternative for treatment and for chemoprophylaxis of individuals intolerant to erythromycin, although its efficacy as a chemoprophylactic agent has not been evaluated.[335, 346, 348] The evidence of trimethoprim-sulfamethoxazole's efficacy is based on small studies.[349, 350]

An erythromycin-resistant isolate of *B. pertussis* was reported in a 2-year-old child. None of the other strains isolated during the outbreak demonstrated erythromycin resistance.[351] The child was successfully treated with trimethoprim-sulfamethoxazole.

The administration of a half-dose of DTaP to adults was used as an adjunctive method to control a nosocomial outbreak of pertussis.[333] In the future, acellular pertussis vaccines may be used for preexposure prophylaxis either routinely or in an outbreak situation.

CONCLUSIONS

All susceptible HCWs, unless they have a contraindication to immunization, should be immunized against mumps, measles, rubella, and varicella. If HCWs have the potential for exposure to blood or contaminated fluids, they should be immunized against hepatitis B. In addition, HCWs should be immunized against influenza annually. HCWs should also receive tetanus-diphtheria and pneumococcal vaccines as recommended for the general public. If future studies reveal that HCWs are at higher risk for acquiring hepatitis A than the general public, use of the hepatitis A vaccine at institutional expense may be recommended. If future studies reveal that the acellular pertussis vaccine is safe and effective in adults, it is likely that boosting HCWs will be recommended to prevent nosocomial transmission. Selected HCWs may be candidates for other available vaccines, including polio, plague, typhoid, vaccinia, and rabies.

REFERENCES

1. Williams WW. CDC guideline for infection control in hospital personnel. Infect Control 4:326–349, 1983.
2. Omenn GS, Morris SL. Occupational hazards to healthcare workers: Report of a conference. Am J Ind Med 6:129–137, 1984.
3. Patterson WB, Craven DE, Schwartz DA, et al. Occupational hazards to hospital personnel. Ann Intern Med 102:658–680, 1985.
4. Gestal JJ. Occupational hazards in hospitals: Risk of infection. Br J Ind Med 44:435–442, 1987.

5. Moore RM, Kaczmarek RG. Occupational hazards to healthcare workers: Diverse, ill-defined and not fully appreciated. Am J Infect Control 18:316–327, 1990.
6. Hoffmann KK, Weber DJ, Rutala WA. Infection control strategies relevant to employee health. AAOHN J 39:167–181, 1991.
7. Valenti WM. Selected viruses of nosocomial importance. In Bennett JV, Brachman PS (eds). Hospital Infections (3rd ed). Boston, Little, Brown, 1992, pp 789–821.
8. Gerberding JL. Management of occupational exposures to bloodborne viruses. N Engl J Med 332:444–451, 1995.
9. Diekema DJ, Doebbeling BN. Employee health and infection control. Infect Control Hosp Epidemiol 16:292–301, 1995.
10. Clever LH, LeGuyader Y. Infectious risks for healthcare workers. Ann Rev Public Health 16:141–164, 1995.
11. Sepkowitz KA. Occupationally acquired infections in healthcare workers: Part I. Ann Intern Med 125:826–834, 1996.
12. Sepkowitz KA. Occupationally acquired infections in healthcare workers: Part II. Ann Intern Med 125:917–928, 1996.
13. Falk P. Infection control and the employee health service. In Mayhall CG (ed). Hospital Epidemiology and Infection Control. Baltimore, Williams & Wilkins, 1996, pp 1094–1099.
14. Sebazco S. Occupational health. In Olmsted R (ed). APIC—Infection Control and Applied Epidemiology. St. Louis, Mosby, 1996.
15. Doebbeling BN. Protecting the healthcare worker from infection and injury. In Wenzel RP (ed). Prevention and Control of Nosocomial Infections (3rd ed). Baltimore, Williams & Wilkins, 1997, pp 397–435.
16. Rogers B. Health hazards in nursing and healthcare: An overview. Am J Infect Control 25:248–261, 1997.
17. Bolyard EA, Tablan OC, Williams WW, et al. Guidelines for infection control in health care personnel. Am J Infect Control 26:289–354, 1998.
18. Larson EL. APIC guideline for handwashing and hand antisepsis in healthcare settings. Am J Infect Control 23:251–269, 1995.
19. Gardner JS, Hospital Infection Control Practices Advisory Committee. Guideline for isolation precautions in hospitals. Infect Control Hosp Epidemiol 17:53–80, 1996.
20. Buesching WJ, Neff JC, Sharma HM. Infectious hazards in the clinical laboratory: A program to protect laboratory personnel. Clin Lab Med 9:351–361, 1989.
21. Sewell DL. Laboratory-associated infections and biosafety. Clin Microbiol Rev 8:389–405, 1995.
22. National Committee for Clinical Laboratory Standards. Protection of laboratory workers from infectious diseases transmitted by blood, body fluids, and tissue: Tentative guideline. NCCLS Document M29-T2. 11(No. 14):1–214, 1991.
23. Biosafety in microbiological and biomedical laboratories. HHS Publication No. (CDC) 93-8395. Washington, DC, Government Printing Office, 1993.
24. Flemming DO, Richardson JH, Tulis JJ, Vesley D. Laboratory Safety (2nd ed). Washington, DC, ASM Press, 1995.
25. Turnberg WL. Biohazardous Waste: Risk Assessment, Policy, and Management. New York, John Wiley & Sons, 1996.
26. Occupational Safety and Health Administration. Occupational exposure to bloodborne pathogens: Final rule. 29 CFR Part 1910.1030. Fed Reg 56:54175–54182, 1991.
27. Occupational Safety and Health Administration. Occupational exposure to tuberculosis; proposed rule. 29 CFR Part 1910. Fed Reg 62:54160–54308, 1997.
28. Update on adult immunization: Recommendations of the Immunization Practices Advisory Committee (ACIP). MMWR Morb Mortal Wkly Rep 40(RR-12):1–94, 1991.
29. General recommendations on immunization: Recommendations of the Advisory Committee on Immunization Practices (ACIP). MMWR Morb Mortal Wkly Rep 43(RR-1):1, 1994.
30. Immunization of health-care workers: Recommendations of the Advisory Committee on Immunization Practices (ACIP) and the Hospital Infection Control Practices Advisory Committee (HICPAC). MMWR Morb Mortal Wkly Rep 46(No. RR-18):1–42, 1997.
31. ACP Task Force on Adult Immunization and Infectious Disease Society of America. Guide for Adult Immunization (3rd ed). Philadelphia, American College of Physicians, 1994.
32. Committee on Infectious Diseases, American Academy of Pediatrics. 1997 Red Book (24th ed). Elk Grove Village, IL, American Academy of Pediatrics, 1997.
33. Williams WW, Preblud SR, Reichelderfer PS, Hadler SC. Vaccines of importance in the hospital setting. Infect Dis Clin North Am 3:701–722, 1989.
34. Krause PJ, Gross PA, Barrett TL, et al. Quality standard for assurance of measles immunity among healthcare workers. Infect Control Hosp Epidemiol 15:193–199, 1994.
35. Poland GA, Haiduven DJ. Adult immunizations in the healthcare worker. In Olmsted R (ed). APIC Infection Control and Applied Epidemiology. St. Louis, Mosby, 1996, pp 24.1–24.34.
36. Beekmann SE, Doebbeling BN. Frontiers of occupational health: New vaccines, new prophylactic regimens, and management of the HIV-infected worker. Infect Dis Clin North Am 11:313–329, 1997.
37. Weber DJ, Rutala WA. Selection and use of vaccines for healthcare workers. Infect Control Hosp Epidemiol 18:682–687, 1997.
38. Mumps prevention: Recommendations of the Immunization Practices Advisory Committee (ACIP). MMWR Morb Mortal Wkly Rep 38:388–392, 397–400, 1989.
39. Measles, mumps and rubella—vaccine use and strategies for measles, rubella and congenital rubella syndrome: Recommendations of the Advisory Committee on Immunization Practices (ACIP). MMWR Morb Mortal Wkly Rep 47(RR-8):1–57, 1998.
40. Measles prevention: Recommendations of the Immunization Practices Advisory Committee (ACIP). MMWR Morb Mortal Wkly Rep 38(suppl 9):1–18, 1989.
41. Rubella prevention: Recommendations of the Immunization Practices Advisory Committee (ACIP). MMWR Morb Mortal Wkly Rep 39(RR-15):1–18, 1990.
42. Prevention of varicella: Recommendations of the Advisory Committee on Immunization Practices (ACIP). MMWR Morb Mortal Wkly Rep 45(RR-11):1–36, 1996.
43. Committee on Infectious Diseases. Recommendations for the use of live attenuated varicella vaccine. Pediatrics 95:791–796, 1995.
44. Weber DJ, Rutala WA, Hamilton H. Prevention and control of varicella-zoster infections in healthcare facilities. Infect Control Hosp Epidemiol 17:694–705, 1996.
45. Protection against viral hepatitis: Recommendations of the Immunization Practices Advisory Committee (ACIP). MMWR Morb Mortal Wkly Rep 39(RR-2):1–27, 1990.
46. Hepatitis B virus: A comprehensive strategy for eliminating transmission in the United States through universal childhood vaccination: Recommendations of the Immunization Practices Advisory Committee (ACIP). MMWR Morb Mortal Wkly Rep 40(RR-13):1–25, 1991.
47. Lemon SM, Thomas DL. Vaccines to prevent viral hepatitis. N Engl J Med 336:196–204, 1997.
48. Prevention and control of influenza: Recommendations of the Advisory Committee on Immunization Practices (ACIP). MMWR Morb Mortal Wkly Rep 46(RR-9):1–25, 1997.
49. Diphtheria, tetanus, and pertussis: Recommendations of the Immunization Practices Advisory Committee (ACIP). MMWR Morb Mortal Wkly Rep 40(RR-10):1–28, 1991.
50. Pertussis vaccination: Use of acellular pertussis vaccines among infants and young children—recommendations of the Immunization Practices Advisory Committee (ACIP). MMWR Morb Mortal Wkly Rep 46(RR-7):1–25, 1997
51. Pneumococcal polysaccharide vaccine: Recommendations of the Immunization Practices Advisory Committee (ACIP). MMWR Morb Mortal Wkly Rep 38:64–68, 73–76, 1989.
52. Prevention of pneumococcal disease: Recommendations of the Advisory Committee on Immunization Practices (ACIP). MMWR Morb Mortal Wkly Rep 46(RR-8):1–24, 1997.
53. Poliomyelitis prevention in the United States: Introduction of a sequential vaccination schedule of inactivated poliovirus vaccine followed by oral poliovirus vaccine: Recommendations of the Advisory Committee on Immunization Practices (ACIP). MMWR Morb Mortal Wkly Rep 46(RR-3):1–25, 1997.
54. Control and prevention of meningococcal disease: Recommendations of the Advisory Committee on Immunization Practices (ACIP). MMWR Morb Mortal Wkly Rep 46(RR-5):1–11, 1997.
55. Control and prevention of serogroup C meningococcal disease: Evaluation and management of suspected outbreaks: Recommendations of the Advisory Committee on Immunization Practices (ACIP). MMWR Morb Mortal Wkly Rep 46(RR-5):13–21, 1997.

56. The role of BCG vaccine in the prevention and control of tuberculosis in the United States: A joint statement by the Advisory Committee for the Elimination of Tuberculosis and the Advisory Committee on Immunization Practices. MMWR Morb Mortal Wkly Rep 45(RR-4):1–18, 1996.
57. Rabies prevention—United States, 1991: Recommendations of the Immunization Practices Advisory Committee (ACIP). MMWR Morb Mortal Wkly Rep 40(RR-3):1–19, 1991.
58. Prevention of plague: Recommendations of the Advisory Committee on Immunization Practices (ACIP). MMWR Morb Mortal Wkly Rep 45(RR-14):1–15, 1996.
59. Typhoid immunization: Recommendations of the Immunization Practices Advisory Committee (ACIP). MMWR Morb Mortal Wkly Rep 39(RR-10):1–5, 1990.
60. Typhoid immunization: Recommendations of the Immunization Practices Advisory Committee (ACIP). MMWR Morb Mortal Wkly Rep 43(RR-14):1–7, 1994.
61. Vaccinia (smallpox) vaccine: Recommendations of the Immunization Practices Advisory Committee (ACIP). MMWR Morb Mortal Wkly Rep 40(RR-14):1–10, 1991.
62. Prevention of hepatitis A though active or passive immunization: Recommendations of the Advisory Committee on Immunization Practices (ACIP). MMWR Morb Mortal Wkly Rep 45(RR-15):1–30, 1996.
63. Recommendations of the Advisory Committee on Immunization Practices (ACIP): Use of vaccines and immune globulin in persons with altered immunocompetence. MMWR Morb Mortal Wkly Rep 42(RR-4):1–18, 1993.
64. Update: Vaccine side effects, adverse reactions, contraindications, and precautions: Recommendations of the Advisory Committee on Immunization Practices (ACIP). MMWR Morb Mortal Wkly Rep 45(RR-12):1–35, 1996.
65. Public Law No. 99-660, 1986. Fed Reg 62:7685–7690, 1997.
66. Poland GA, Nichol KL. Medical schools and immunization policies: Missed opportunities for disease prevention. Ann Intern Med 113:628–631, 1990.
67. Lewy R. Immunization status of entering housestaff physicians. J Occup Med 30:822–823, 1988.
68. Ewert DP, Garcia D, George J, Mascola L. A comparison of hospital policies for measles, mumps, and rubella infection control in Los Angeles County, 1989 and 1992. Am J Infect Control 23:369–372, 1995.
69. Schwarcz S, McGraw B, Fukushima P. Prevalence of measles susceptiblity in hospital staff. Arch Intern Med 152:1481–1483, 1992.
70. Wright LJ, Carlquist JF. Measles immunity in employees of a multihospital healthcare provider. Infect Control Hosp Epidemiol 15:8–11, 1994.
71. Shapiro CN, Tokars JI, Chamberland ME. Use of the hepatitis-B vaccine and infection with hepatitis B and C among orthopedic surgeons. J Bone Joint Surg 78:1791–1800, 1996.
72. Panlilio AL, Shapiro CN, Schable CA, et al. Serosurvey of human immunodeficiency virus, hepatitis B virus, and hepatitis C virus infection among hospital-based surgeons. J Am Coll Surg 180:16–24, 1995.
73. Agerton TB, Mahoney FJ, Polish LB, Shapiro CN. Impact of the bloodborne pathogens standard on vaccination of healthcare workers with hepatitis B vaccine. Infect Control Hosp Epidemiol 16:287–291, 1995.
74. Weingarten S, Riedinger M, Bolton LB, et al. Barriers to influenza vaccine acceptance. Am J Infect Control 17:202–207, 1989.
75. McArthur MA, Simor AE, Campbell B, McGeer A. Influenza and pneumococcal vaccination and tuberculin skin testing programs in long-term care facilities: Where do we stand? Infect Control Hosp Epidemiol 16:18–24, 1995.
76. Nichol KL, Hauge M. Influenza vaccination of healthcare workers. Infect Control Hosp Epidemiol 18:189–194, 1997.
77. Christian MA. Influenza and hepatitis B vaccine acceptance: A survey of healthcare workers. Am J Infect Control 19:177–184, 1991.
78. Adal KA, Flowers RH, Anglim AM, et al. Prevention of nosocomial influenza. Infect Control Hosp Epidemiol 17:641–648, 1996.
79. Summary of notifiable diseases, United States, 1996. MMWR Morb Mortal Wkly Rep 45(53):1–87, 1996.
80. Thomson FH. The aerial conveyance of infection. Lancet 1:341–344, 1916.
81. Brunell PA, Brickman A, O'Hare D, Steinberg S. Ineffectiveness of isolation of patients as a method of preventing the spread of mumps. N Engl J Med 279:1357–1361, 1968.
82. Sparling D. Transmission of mumps. N Engl J Med 280:276, 1969.
83. Faoagali JL. An assessment of the need for vaccination amongst junior medical staff. N Z Med J 84:147–150, 1976.
84. Glick D. An isolated case of mumps in a geriatric population. J Am Geriatr Soc 18:642–644, 1970.
85. Wharton M, Cochi SL, Hutcheson RH, Schaffner W. Mumps transmission in hospitals. Arch Intern Med 150:47–49, 1990.
86. Fischer PR, Brunetti C, Welch V, Christenson JC. Nosocomial mumps: Report of an outbreak and its control. Am J Infect Control 24:13–18, 1996.
87. Reed D, Brown G, Merrick R, et al. A mumps epidemic on St. George Island, Alaska. JAMA 84:147–150, 1967.
88. Measles—Texas. MMWR Morb Mortal Wkly Rep 30:209–211, 1981.
89. Measles in medical settings—United States. MMWR Morb Mortal Wkly Rep 30:125–126, 1981.
90. Anonymous. Measles nearly eliminated, but still poses a nosocomial risk. Hosp Infect Control 9:133–136, 1982.
91. Imported measles with subsequent airborne transmission in a pediatrician's office—Michigan. MMWR Morb Mortal Wkly Rep 32:401–403, 1983.
92. Measles among children of migrant workers—Florida. MMWR Morb Mortal Wkly Rep 32:471–472, 477–478, 1983.
93. Interstate transmission of measles in a gypsy population—Washington, Idaho, Montana, California. MMWR Morb Mortal Wkly Rep 32:659–662, 1983.
94. Measles—Hawaii. MMWR Morb Mortal Wkly Rep 33:702, 707–711, 1984.
95. Measles—New Hampshire. MMWR Morb Mortal Wkly Rep 33:549–554, 559, 1984.
96. Remington PL, Hall WN, Davis IH, et al. Airborne transmission of measles in a physician's office. JAMA 253:1574–1577, 1985.
97. Bloch AB, Orenstein WA, Ewing WM, et al. Measles outbreak in a pediatric practice: Airborne transmission in an office setting. Pediatrics 75:676–683, 1985.
98. Measles—Puerto Rico. MMWR Morb Mortal Wkly Rep 34:169–172, 1985.
99. Dales LG, Kizer KW. Measles transmission in medical facilities. West J Med 142:415–416, 1985.
100. Davis RM, Orenstein WA, Frank JA, et al. Transmission of measles in medical settings: 1980 through 1984. JAMA 255:1295–1298, 1986.
101. Istre GR, McKee PA, West GR, et al. Measles spread in medical settings: An important focus of disease transmission. Pediatrics 79:356–358, 1987.
102. Watkins NM, Smith RP Jr, St. Germain DL, MacKay DN. Measles (rubeola) infection in a hospital setting. Am J Infect Control 15:201–206, 1987.
103. Sienko DG, Friedman C, McGee HB, et al. A measles outbreak at university medical settings involving healthcare providers. Am J Public Health 77:1222–1224, 1987.
104. Measles transmitted in a medical office building—New Mexico, 1986. MMWR Morb Mortal Wkly Rep 36:25–27, 1987.
105. Measles—Dade County, Florida. MMWR Morb Mortal Wkly Rep 36:45–48, 1987.
106. Measles—Los Angeles County, California, 1988. MMWR Morb Mortal Wkly Rep 38:49–52, 57, 1989.
107. Markowitz LE, Preblud SR, Orenstein WA, et al. Patterns of transmission in measles outbreaks in the United States, 1985–1986. N Engl J Med 320:75–81, 1989.
108. Raad II, Sherertz RJ, Rains CS, et al. The importance of nosocomial transmission of measles in the propagation of a community outbreak. Infect Control Hosp Epidemiol 10:161–166, 1989.
109. Measles—Washington, 1990. MMWR Morb Mortal Wkly Rep 39:473–476, 1990.
110. Farizo KM, Stehr-Green PA, Simpson DM, et al. Pediatric emergency room visits: A risk factor for acquiring measles. Pediatrics 87:74–79, 1991.
111. Atkinson WL, Markowitz LE, Adams NC, et al. Transmission

of measles in medical settings—United States, 1985–1989. Am J Med 91(suppl 3B):320S–324S, 1991.
112. Rivera ME, Mason WH, Ross LA, Wright HT Jr. Nosocomial measles infection in a pediatric hospital during a community-wide epidemic. J Pediatr 119:183–186, 1991.
113. McGrath D, Swanson R, Weems S, et al. Analysis of a measles outbreak in Kent County, Michigan in 1990. Pediatr Infect Dis J 11:385–389, 1992.
114. Freebeck PC, Clark S, Fahey PJ. Hypoxemic respiratory failure complicating nosocomial measles in a healthy host. Chest 102:625–626, 1992.
115. Miranda AC, Falcao JM, Dias JA, et al. Measles transmisson in health facilities during outbreaks. Int J Epidemiol 23:843–848, 1994.
116. Schiff GM, Dine MS. Transmission of rubella from newborns. Am J Dis Child 110:447–451, 1965.
117. Giles JW, Smith IM. The study of a rubella outbreak. J Iowa Med Soc 62:238–341, 1972.
118. Carne S, Dewhurst CJ, Hurley R. Rubella epidemic in a maternity unit. BMJ 1:444–446, 1973.
119. Baba K, Yabuuchi H, Okuni H, et al. Rubella epidemic in an institution: Protective value of live rubella vaccine and serological behavior of vaccinated, revaccinated and naturally immune groups. Biken J 21:25–31, 1978.
120. Exposure of patients to rubella by medical personnel—California. MMWR Morb Mortal Wkly Rep 27:123, 1978.
121. Rubella in hospital personnel and patients—Colorado. MMWR Morb Mortal Wkly Rep 28:325–327, 1979.
122. McLaughlin MC, Gold LH. The New York rubella incident: A case for changing hospital policy regarding rubella testing and immunization. Am J Public Health 69:287–289, 1979.
123. Polk BF, White JA, DeGirolami PC, Modlin JF. An outbreak of rubella among hospital personnel. N Engl J Med 303:541–545, 1980.
124. Nosocomial rubella infection—North Dakota, Alabama, Ohio. MMWR Morb Mortal Wkly Rep 29:629–631, 1981.
125. Gladstone JL, Millian SJ. Rubella exposure in an obstetric clinic. Obstet Gynecol 57:182–186, 1981.
126. Strassburg MA, Imagawa DT, Fannin SL, et al. Rubella outbreak among hospital employees. Obstet Gynecol 57:283–288, 1981.
127. Rubella in hospitals—California. MMWR Morb Mortal Wkly Rep 32:37–39, 1983.
128. Strassburg MA, Stephenson TG, Habel LA, Fannin SL. Rubella in hospital employees. Infect Control 5:123–126, 1984.
129. Heseltine PNR, Ripper M, Wohlford P. Nosocomial rubella—consequences of an outbreak and efficacy of a mandatory immunization program. Infect Control 6:371–374, 1985.
130. Storch GA, Gruber C, Benz B, et al. A rubella outbreak among dental students: Description of the outbreak and analysis of control measures. Infect Control 6:150–156, 1985.
131. Jacobson JT. Rubella: One hospital's experience. Am J Infect Control 15:136–137, 1987.
132. Poland GA, Nichol KL. Medical students as sources of rubella and measles outbreaks. Arch Intern Med 150:44–46, 1990.
133. Braunstein H, Thomas S, Ito R. Immunity to measles in a large population of varying age. Am J Dis Child 144:296–298, 1990.
134. Smith E, Wong VK. Measles susceptibility of hospital personnel. Arch Intern Med 153:1011, 1993.
135. Hersh BS, Fine PE, Kent WK, et al. Mumps outbreaks in a highly vaccinated population. J Pediatr 119:187–193, 1991.
136. Plotkin SA. Clinical and pathogenetic aspects of varicella-zoster. Postgrad Med J 61(suppl 4):7–14, 1985.
137. Straus SE, Ostrove JM, Inchauspe G, et al. NIH conference. Varicella-zoster virus infections: Biology, natural history, treatment, and prevention. Ann Intern Med 108:221–237, 1988 [published erratum appears in Ann Intern Med 109:438–439, 1988].
138. Brunell PA. Varicella-zoster infections. In Feigin RD, Cherry JD (eds). Textbook of Pediatric Infectious Diseases (3rd ed). Philadelphia, WB Saunders, 1992, pp 1587–1591.
139. Drwal-Klein LA, O'Donovan CA. Varicella in pediatric patients. Ann Pharmacother 27:938–949, 1993.
140. Whitley RJ. Varicella-zoster virus. In Mandell GL, Bennett JE, Dolin R (eds). Principles and Practice of Infectious Diseases (4th ed). New York, Churchill Livingstone, 1995, pp 1345–1351.
141. Arvin AM. Varicella-zoster virus. Clin Microbiol Rev 9:361–381, 1996.
142. Brunell PA. Contagion and varicella-zoster virus. Pediatr Infect Dis 1:304–307, 1982.
143. Brawley RL, Wenzel RP. An algorithm for chickenpox exposure. Pediatr Infect Dis 3:502–504, 1984.
144. Weitekamp MR, Schan P, Aber RC. An algorithm for the control of nosocomial varicella-zoster virus infection. Am J Infect Control 13:193–198, 1985.
145. Sayre MR, Lucid EJ. Management of varicella-zoster virus-exposed hospital employees. Ann Emerg Med 16:421–424, 1987.
146. Weber DJ, Rutala WA, Parham C. Impact and costs of varicella prevention in a University Hospital. Am J Public Health 78:19–23, 1988.
147. Simpson REH. Infectiousness of communicable diseases in the household (measles, chickenpox, and mumps). Lancet 2:549–554, 1952.
148. Ross AH. Modification of chickenpox in family contacts by administration of gamma globulin. N Engl J Med 267:369–376, 1962.
149. Josephson A, Karanfil L, Gombert ME. Strategies for the management of varicella-susceptible healthcare workers after a known exposure. Infect Control Hosp Epidemiol 11:309–313, 1990.
150. Gershon AA. Varicella-zoster virus: Prospects for control. Adv Pediatr Infect Dis 10:93–124, 1995.
151. Meyers JD. Congenital varicella in term infants: Risk reconsidered. J Infect Dis 129:215–217, 1974.
152. Wharton M. The epidemiology of varicella-zoster virus infection. Infect Dis Clin North Am 10:571–581, 1996.
153. Choo PW, Donahue JG, Manson JE, Platt R. The epidemiology of varicella and its complications. J Infect Dis 172:706–712, 1995.
154. Miller E, Marshall R, Vurdien J. Epidemiology, outcome and control of varicella-zoster infection. Rev Med Microbiol 4:222–230, 1993.
155. Feldman S, Hughes WT, Daniel CB. Varicella in children with cancer: Seventy-seven cases. Pediatrics 56:388–397, 1975.
156. Feldhoff CM, Balfour HH, Simmons RL, et al. Varicella in children with renal transplants. J Pediatr 98:25–31, 1981.
157. Locksley RM, Flournoy N, Sullivan KM, Meyers JD. Infection with varicella-zoster virus after marrow transplantation. J Infect Dis 152:1172–1181, 1985.
158. Meyers JD, MacQuarrie MB, Merigan TC, Jennison MH. Nosocomial varicella: Part 1. Outbreak in oncology patients at a children's hospital. West J Med 130:196–199, 1979.
159. Morgan ER, Smalley LA. Varicella in immunocompromised children. Am J Dis Child 137:883–885, 1983.
160. Whitley R, Hilty M, Haynes R, et al. Vidarabine therapy of varicella in immunosuppressed patients. J Pediatr 101:125–131, 1982.
161. Feldman S, Lott L. Varicella in children with cancer: Impact of antiviral therapy and prophylaxis. Pediatrics 80:255–262, 1987.
162. McGregor RS, Zitelli BJ, Urback AH, et al. Varicella in pediatric orthotopic liver transplant recipients. Pediatrics 83:256–261, 1989.
163. Myers MG, Rasley DA, Hierholzer WJ. Hospital infection control for varicella-zoster virus infection. Pediatrics 70:199–201, 1982.
164. Steele RW, Coleman MA, Fiser M, Bradsher RW. Varicella-zoster in hospital personnel: Skin test reactivity to monitor susceptibility. Pediatrics 70:604–608, 1982.
165. Hyams PJ, Stuewe MCS, Heitzer V. Herpes zoster causing varicella (chickenpox) in hospital employees: Cost of a casual attitude. Am J Infect Control 12:2–5, 1984.
166. Alter SJ, Hammond JA, McVey CJ, Myers MG. Susceptibility to varicella-zoster virus among adults at high risk for exposure. Infect Control 7:448–451, 1986.
167. Krasinski K, Holzman RS, LaCouture R, Florman A. Hospital experience with varicella-zoster virus. Infect Control 7:312–316, 1986.
168. Haiduven-Griffiths D, Fecko H. Varicella in hospital personnel: A challenge for the infection control practitioner. Am J Infect Control 15:207–211, 1987.
169. McKinney WP, Horowitz MM, Battiola RJ. Susceptibility of hospital-based healthcare personnel to varicella-zoster virus infections. Am J Infect Control 17:26–30, 1989.
170. Stover BH, Cost KM, Hamm C, et al. Varicella exposure in a neonatal intensive care unit: Case report and control measures. Am J Infect Control 16:167–172, 1988.

171. Shehab ZM, Brunell PA. Susceptibility of hospital personnel to varicella-zoster virus. J Infect Dis 150:786, 1984.
172. Haiduven DJ, Hench CP, Stevens DA. Postexposure varicella management of nonimmmune personnel: An alternative approach. Infect Control Hosp Epidemiol 15:329–334, 1994.
173. Gustafson TL, Shehab Z, Brunell PA. Outbreak of varicella in a newborn intensive care nursery. Am J Dis Child 138:548–550, 1984.
174. Evans P. An epidemic of chickenpox. Lancet 2:339–340, 1940.
175. McKendrick GDW, Emond RTD. Investigation of cross-infection in isolation wards of different designs. J Hyg Camb 76:23–31, 1976.
176. Morens DM, Bregman DJ, West CM, et al. An outbreak of varicella-zoster virus infection among cancer patients. Ann Intern Med 93:414–419, 1980.
177. Leclair JM, Zaia JA, Levin MJ, et al. Airborne transmission of chickenpox in a hospital. N Engl J Med 302:450–453, 1980.
178. Scheifele D, Bonner M. Airborne transmission of chickenpox [letter]. N Engl J Med 303:281–282, 1980.
179. Asano Y, Iwayama S, Miyata T, et al. Spread of varicella in hospitalized children having no direct contact with an indicator zoster case and its prevention by a live vaccine. Biken J 23:157–161, 1980.
180. Faizallah R, Green HT, Krasner N, Walker RJ. Outbreak of chickenpox from a patient with immunosuppressed herpes zoster in hospital. BMJ 285:1022–1023, 1982.
181. Gustafson TL, Lavely GB, Brawner ER, et al. An outbreak of airborne nosocomial varicella. Pediatrics 70:550–556, 1982.
182. Tsujino G, Sako M, Takahashi M. Varicella infection in a children's hospital: Prevention by vaccine and an episode of airborne transmission. Biken J 27:129–132, 1984.
183. Anderson JD, Bonner M, Schiefele DW, Schneider BC. Lack of nosocomial spread of varicella in a pediatric hospital with negative pressure ventilated patient rooms. Infect Control 6:120–121, 1985.
184. Josephson A, Gombert M. Airborne transmission of nosocomial varicella from localized zoster. J Infect Dis 158:238–241, 1988.
185. Morgan-Capner P, Wilson M, Wright J, Hutchinson DN. Varicella and zoster in hospitals. Lancet 335:1460, 1990.
186. Friedman CA, Temple DM, Robbins KK, et al. Outbreak and control of varicella in a neonatal intensive care unit. Pediatr Infect Dis J 13:152–153, 1994.
187. Faoagali JL, Darcy D. Chickenpox outbreak among the staff of a large, urban adult hospital: Costs of monitoring and control. Am J Infect Control 23:247–250, 1995.
188. Sawyer MH, Chamberlin CJ, Wu YN, et al. Detection of varicella-zoster virus DNA in air samples from hospital rooms. J Infect Dis 169:91–94, 1994.
189. Nettleman MD, Schmid M. Cost-effectiveness of varicella vaccination in hospital employees [abstract 70]. Program and Abstracts of the Sixth Annual Meeting of SHEA; Washington, DC; 1996.
190. Hamilton HA. A cost minimization analysis of varicella vaccine in healthcare workers. Thesis. Chapel Hill, Department of Epidemiology, University of North Carolina School of Public Health, 1996.
191. Asano Y, Yoshikawa T, Suga S, et al. Postexposure prophylaxis of varicella in family contact by oral acyclovir. Pediatrics 92:219–222, 1993.
192. Suga S, Yoshikawa T, Ozaki T, Asano Y. Effect of oral acyclovir against primary and secondary viraemia in incubation period of varicella. Arch Dis Child 69:639–642, 1993.
193. Abe C, Bradley J. Varicella in a pediatric convalescent hospital: Controlling clinical disease following widespread exposure [abstract S32]. Program and abstracts of the Fifth Annual Meeting of SHEA; San Diego; 1995.
194. Asano Y, Nakayama H, Yazaki T, et al. Protective efficacy of vaccination in children in four episodes of natural varicella and zoster in the ward. Pediatrics 59:8–12, 1977.
195. Udeda K, Yamada I, Goto M, et al. Use of a live varicella vaccine to prevent the spread of varicella in handicapped or immunosuppressed children including MSLC (muco-cutaneous lymph node syndrome) patients in hospitals. Biken J 20:117–123, 1977.
196. Katsushima N, Yazaki N, Sakamoto M, et al. Application of a live varicella vaccine to hospitalized children and its follow-up study. Biken J 25:29–42, 1982.
197. Asano Y, Hirose S, Iwayama S, et al. Protective effect of immediate inoculation of a live varicella vaccine in household contacts in relation to the viral dose and interval between exposure and vaccination. Biken J 25:43–45, 1982.
198. Katsushima N, Yazaki N, Sakamoto M. Effect and follow-up study of varicella vaccine. Biken J 27:51–58, 1984.
199. Sugino H, Tsukino R, Miyashiro E, et al. Live varicella vaccine: Prevention of nosocomial infection and protection of high risk infants from varicella infection. Biken J 27:63–65, 1984.
200. Naganuma Y, Osawa S, Takahashi R. Clinical application of a live varicella vaccine (Oka strain) in a hospital. Biken J 27:59–61, 1984.
201. Boda D, Bartyik K, Szuts P, Turi S. Active immunization of children exposed to varicella infection in a hospital ward using live attenuated varicella vaccine given subcutaneously or intracutaneously. Acta Paediatr Hung 27:247–252, 1986.
202. Arbeter AM, Starr SE, Plotkin SA. Varicella vaccine studies in healthy children and adults. Pediatrics 78(suppl):748–756, 1986.
203. Jagger J, Hunt Brand-Elnaggar J, Pearson RD. Rates of needlestick injury caused by various devices in a university hospital. N Engl J Med 319:284–288, 1988.
204. Gerderding JL. Risks to healthcare workers from occupational exposure to hepatitis B virus, human immunodeficiency virus, and cytomegalovirus. Infect Dis Clin North Am 3:735–745, 1989.
205. Weber DJ, Rutala WA. Hepatitis B immunization update. Infect Control Hosp Epidemiol 10:541–546, 1989.
206. Lanphear P. Trends and patterns in the transmission of bloodborne pathogens to healthcare workers. Epidemiol Rev 16:437–450, 1994.
207. Cardo DM, Bell DM. Bloodborne pathogen transmission in healthcare workers. Infect Dis Clin North Am 11:331–346, 1997.
208. Segal HE, Llewellyn CH, Irwin G, et al. Hepatitis B antigen and antibody in the U.S. Army: Prevalence in healthcare personnel. Am J Public Health 66:67–671, 1976.
209. Denes AE, Smith JL, Maynard JE, et al. Hepatitis B infection in physicians: Results of a nationwide seroepidemiologic survey. JAMA 239:210–212, 1978.
210. Dienstag JL, Ryan DM. Occupational exposure to hepatitis B virus in hospital personnel: Infection or immunization? Am J Epidemiol 115:26–39, 1982.
211. Hadler SC, Doto IL, Maynard JE, et al. Occupational risk of hepatitis B infection in hospital workers. Infect Control 6:24–31, 1985.
212. Guidelines for prevention of transmission of human immunodeficiency virus and hepatitis B virus to health-care and public-safety workers. MMWR Morb Mortal Wkly Rep 38(S-6):1–37, 1989.
213. Shapiro CN. Occupational risk of infection with hepatitis B and hepatitis C virus. Surg Clin North Am 75:1047–1056, 1995.
214. Lowenfels AB, Wormser GP, Jain R. Frequency of puncture injuries in surgeons and estimated risk of HIV infection. Arch Surg 124:1284–1286, 1989.
215. Tokars JI, Chamberland ME, Schable CA, et al. A survey of occupational blood contact and HIV infection among orthopedic surgeons. JAMA 268:489–494, 1992.
216. Bond WE, Favero MS, Peterson NJ, et al. Survival of hepatitis B virus after drying and storage for one week. Lancet 1:550–551, 1981.
217. Grady GF, Lee VA, Prince AM, et al. Hepatitis B immune globulin for accidental exposures among medical personnel: Final report of a multicenter controlled trial. J Infect Dis 138:625–638, 1978.
218. Seeff LM, Wright EC, Zimmerman HJ, et al. Type B hepatitis after needle-stick exposure: Prevention with hepatitis B immune globulin. Ann Intern Med 88:285–293, 1978.
219. Werner BG, Grady GF. Accidental hepatitis-B-surface-antigen-positive inoculations. Ann Intern Med 97:367–369, 1982.
220. Kew MC. Possible transmission of serum (Australia-antigen-positive) hepatitis via the conjunctiva. Infect Immun 7:823–824, 1973.
221. Syndman DR, Hindman SH, Wineland MD, et al. Nosocomial viral hepatitis B: A cluster among staff with subsequent transmission to patients. Ann Intern Med 85:573–577, 1976.
222. Ingerslev J, Mortensen E, Rasmussen K, Jorgensen J. Silent

hepatitis-B immunization in laboratory technicians. Scand J Clin Lab Invest 48:333–336, 1988.
223. Handsfield HH, Cummings MJ, Swenson PD. Prevalence of antibody to human immunodeficiency virus and hepatitis B surface antigen in blood samples submitted to a hospital laboratory: Implications for handling specimens. JAMA 258:3395–3397, 1987.
224. Hepatitis B assoicated with jet gun injection—California. MMWR Morb Mortal Wkly Rep 35:373–376, 1986.
225. Morris IM, Cattle DS, Smits BJ. Endoscopy and transmission of hepatitis B. Lancet 2:1152, 1975.
226. Oren I, Hershow RC, Ben-Porath E, et al. A common-source outbreak of fulminant hepatitis B in a hospital. Ann Intern Med 110:691–698, 1989.
227. Nosocomial transmission of hepatitis B virus associated with a spring-loaded fingerstick device—California. MMWR Morb Mortal Wkly Rep 39:610–613, 1990.
228. Douvin C, Simon D, Zinelabidine H, et al. An outbreak of hepatitis B in an endocrinology unit traced to a capillary-blood sampling device. N Engl J Med 322:57, 1990.
229. Polish LB, Shapiro CN, Bauer F, et al. Nosocomial transmission of hepatitis B virus associated with the use of a spring-loaded fingerstick device. N Engl J Med 326:721–725, 1992.
230. Stapleton JT, Lemon SM. Transmission of hepatitis B by a finger-stick device [letter]. N Engl J Med 327:497, 1992.
231. Nosocomial hepatitis B virus infection associated with reusable fingerstick blood sampling devices—Ohio and New York City, 1996. MMWR Morb Mortal Wkly Rep 46:217–221, 1997.
232. Drescher J, Wagner D, Haverick A, et al. Nosocomial hepatitis B virus infection in cardiac transplant recipients transmitted during transvenous endomyocardial biopsy. J Hosp Infect 26:81–92, 1994.
233. Lauer JL, VanDrunen NA, Washburn JW, Balfour HH Jr. Transmission of hepatitis B virus in clinical laboratory areas. J Infect Dis 140:513–516, 1979.
234. Pattison CP, Boyer DM, Maynard JE, Kelly PC. Epidemic hepatitis in a clinical laboratory: Possible association with computer card handling. JAMA 230:854–857, 1974.
235. Tanaka S, Yoshiba M, Iino S, et al. A common-source outbreak of fulminant hepatitis B in hemodialysis patients induced by precore mutant. Kidney Int 48:1972–1978, 1992.
236. Hardie DR, Kannemeyer J, Stannard LM. DNA single strand conformation polymorphism identifies five defined strains of hepatitis B virus (HBV) during an outbreak of HBV infection in an oncology unit. J Med Virol 49:49–54, 1996.
237. Outbreaks of hepatitis B virus infection among hemodialysis patients—California, Nebraska, and Texas, 1994. MMWR Morb Mortal Wkly Rep 45:285–289, 1996.
238. Weber DJ, Hoffmann KK, Rutala WA. Management of the healthcare worker infected with human immunodeficiency virus: Lessons from nosocomial transmission of hepatitis B virus. Infect Control Hosp Epidemiol 12:625–630, 1991.
239. Bell DM, Shapiro CN, Ciesielski CA, Chamberland ME. Preventing bloodborne pathogen transmission from health-care workers to patients. Surg Clin North Am 75:1189–1203, 1995.
240. Harpaz R, Von Seidlein L, Averhoff FM, et al. Transmission of hepatitis B virus to multiple patients from a surgeon without evidence of inadequate infection control. N Engl J Med 334:549–554, 1996.
241. Incident Investigation Team and Others. Transmission of hepatitis B to patients from four infected surgeons without hepatitis B "e" antigen. N Engl J Med 336:178–184, 1997.
242. AIDS/TB Committeee of the Society for Healthcare Epidemiology of America. Managament of healthcare workers infected with hepatitis B virus, hepatitis C virus, human immunodeficiency virus, or other bloodborne pathogens. Infect Control Hosp Epidemiol 18:349–363, 1997.
243. Occupational Safety and Health Administration. 29 CFR Part 1910.1030—Occupational Exposure to Bloodborne Pathogens; Final Rule. Fed Reg 56:64175–64182, 1991.
244. Lemon SM, Thomas DL. Vaccines to prevent viral hepatitis. N Engl J Med 336:196–204, 1997.
245. Jilg W, Schmidt M, Deinhardt F. Vaccination against hepatitis B: Comparison of three different vaccination schedules. J Infect Dis 160:766–769, 1989.
246. Hadler SC, de Monzon A, Lugo DR, Perez M. Effect of timing of hepatitis B vaccine doses on response to vaccine Yucpa Indians. Vaccine 7:106–110, 1989.
247. Hadler SC, Francis DP, Maynard JE, et al. Long-term immunogenicity and efficacy of hepatitis B vaccine in homosexual men. N Engl J Med 315:209–214, 1986.
248. Barker WH. Excess pneumonia and influenza associated hospitalizations during influenza epidemics in the United States, 1970–78. Am J Public Health 76:761–765, 1986.
249. Influenza surveillance—United States, 1992–93 and 1993–94. MMWR Morb Mortal Wkly Rep 46(No. SS-1):1–12, 1997.
250. Meibalane R, Sedmak GV, Sasidharan P, et al. Outbreak of influenza in a neonatal intensive care unit. J Pediatr 91:974–976, 1977.
251. Kapila R, Lintz DI, Tecson FT, et al. A nosocomial outbreak of influenza A. Chest 71:576–579, 1977.
252. Balkovic ES, Goodman RA, Rose FB, Borel CO. Nosocomial influenza A (H1N1) infection. Am J Med Tech 46:318–320, 1980.
253. Van Voris LP, Belshe RB, Shaffer JL. Nosocomial influenza B virus infection in the elderly. Ann Intern Med 96:153–158, 1982.
254. Rivera M, Gonzalez N. An influenza outbreak in a hospital. Am J Nurs 82:1836–1838, 1982.
255. Bean B, Rhame FS, Hughes RS, et al. Influenza B: Hospital activitity during a community outbreak. Diagn Microbiol Infect Dis 1:177–183, 1983.
256. Hammond GW, Cheang M. Absenteeism among hospital staff during an influenza epidemic: Implications for immunoprophylaxis. Can Med Assoc J 131:449–452, 1984.
257. Weingarten S, Friedlander M, Rascon D, et al. Influenza surveillance in an acute-care hospital. Arch Intern Med 148:113–116, 1988.
258. Suspected nosocomial influenza cases in an intensive care unit. MMWR Morb Mortal Wkly Rep 37:3–4, 9, 1988.
259. Pachucki CT, Pappas SAW, Fuller GF, et al. Influenza A among hospital personnel and patients. Ann Intern Med 149:77–80, 1989.
260. Grayston JT, Diwan VK, Cooney M, Wang S-P. Community- and hospital-acquired pneumonia associated with Chlamydia TWAR infection demonstrated serologically. Arch Intern Med 149:169–173, 1989.
261. Serwint JR, Miller RM. Why diagnose influenza infections in hospitalized pediatric patients? Pediatr Infect Dis J 12:200–204, 1993.
262. Whimbey E, Elting LS, Couch RB, et al. Influenza A virus infections among hospitalized adult bone marrow transplant recipients. Bone Marrow Transplant 13:437–440, 1994.
263. Evert RJ, Hanger HJC, Jennings LC, et al. Outbreaks of influenza A among elderly hospital inpatients. N Z Med J 109:272–274, 1996.
264. Odelin MR, Pozzetto B, Aymard M, et al. Role of influenza vaccination in the elderly during an epidemic of A/H1NI virus in 1988–1989: Clinical and serological data. Gerontology 39:109–116, 1993.
265. Serie C, Barme M, Hannoun C, et al. Effects of vaccination on an influenza epidemic in a geriatric hospital. Dev Biol Stand 39:317–321, 1977.
266. Hall WN, Goodman RA, Noble GR, et al. An outbreak of influenza B in an elderly population. J Infect Dis 144:297–302, 1981.
267. Goodman RA, Orenstein WA, Munro TF, et al. Impact of influenza A in a nursing home. JAMA 247:1451–1453, 1982.
268. Arroyo JC, Postic B, Brown A, et al. Influenza A/Philippines/2/82 outbreak in a nursing home: Limitations of influenza vaccination in the aged. Am J Infect Control 12:329–334, 1984.
269. Christie RW, Marquis LL. Immunization roulette: Influenza occurrence in five nursing homes. Am J Infect Control 13:174–177, 1985.
270. Horman JT, Stetler HC, Israel E, et al. An outbreak of influenza A in a nursing home. Am J Public Health 76:501–504, 1986.
271. Patriarca PA, Weber JA, Parker RA, et al. Risk factors for outbreaks of influenza in nursing homes. Am J Epidemiol 124:114–119, 1986.
272. Strassburg MA, Greenland S, Sorvillo FJ, et al. Influenza in the elderly: Report of an outbreak and a review of vaccine effectiveness reports. Vaccine 4:38–44, 1986.

273. Arden NH, Patriarca PA, Fasano MB, et al. The role of vaccination and amantadine prophylaxis in controlling an outbreak of influenza A (H3N2) in a nursing home. Arch Intern Med 148:865–868, 1988.
274. Gross PA, Rodstein M, LaMontage JR, et al. Epidemiology of acute respiratory illness during an influenza outbreak in a nursing home. Arch Intern Med 148:559–561, 1988.
275. Mast EE, Harmon MW, Gravenstein S, et al. Emergence and possible transmission of amantadine-resistant viruses during nursing home outbreaks of influenza A (H3N2). Am J Epidemiol 134:988–997, 1991.
276. Control of influenza A outbreaks in nursing homes: Amantadine as an adjunct to vaccine—Washington, 1989–90. MMWR Morb Mortal Wkly Rep 40:842–845, 1991.
277. Outbreak of influenza A in a nursing home—New York, December 1991–January 1992. MMWR Morb Mortal Wkly Rep 41:129–131, 1992.
278. Degelau J, Somani SK, Cooper SL, et al. Amantadine-resistant influenza A in a nursing facility. Arch Intern Med 152:390–392, 1992.
279. Taylor JL, Dwyer DM, Coffman T, et al. Nursing home outbreak of influenza A (H3N2): Evaluation of vaccine efficacy and influenza case definition. Infect Control Hosp Epidemiol 13:93–97, 1992.
280. Morens DM, Rash VM. Lessons from a nursing home outbreak of influenza A. Infect Control Hosp Epidemiol 16:275–280, 1995.
281. Potter J, Stott DJ, Roberts MA, et al. Influenza vaccination of healthcare workers in long-term-care hospitals reduces the mortality of elderly patients. J Infect Dis 175:1–6, 1997.
282. Atkinson WL, Arden NH, Patriarca PA, et al. Amantadine prophylaxis during an institutional outbreak of type A (H1N1) influenza. Arch Intern Med 146:1751–1756, 1986.
283. Fedson DS. Prevention and control of influenza in institutional settings. Hosp Pract 24:87–96, 1989.
284. Graman PS, Hall CB. Nosocomial viral infections. Semin Respir Infect 4:253–260, 1989.
285. Graman PS, Hall CB. Epidemiology and control of nosocomial viral infections. Infect Dis Clin North Am 3:815–841, 1989.
286. Gravenstein S, Miller BA, Drinka P. Prevention and control of influenza A outbreaks in long-term care facilities. Infect Control Hosp Epidemiol 13:49–54, 1992.
287. Tablan OC, Anderson LJ, Arden NH, et al. Guideline for prevention of nosocomial pneumonia. Infect Control Hosp Epidemiol 15:587–627, 1994.
288. Adal KA, Flowers RH, Anglim A, et al. Prevention of nosocomial influenza. Infect Control Hosp Epidemiol 17:641–648, 1996.
289. Gomolin IH, Leib HB, Arden NH, Sherman FT. Control of influenza outbreaks in the nursing home: Guidelines for diagnosis and management. J Am Geriatr Soc 43:71–74, 1995.
290. Nichol KL, Lind A, Margolis KL, et al. The effectiveness of vaccination against influenza in healthy, working adults. N Engl J Med 333:889–893, 1995.
291. Ohrt CK, McKinney WP. Achieving compliance with influenza immunization of medical house staff and students: A randomized controlled study. JAMA 267:1377–1380, 1992.
292. Nafziger DA, Herwaldt LA. Attitudes of internal medicine residents regarding influenza vaccination. Infect Control Hosp Epidemiol 15:32–35, 1994.
293. Watanakunakorn C, Ellis G, Gemmel D. Attitude of healthcare personnel regarding influenza immunization. Infect Control Hosp Epidemiol 14:17–20, 1993.
294. Centers for Disease Control. Hepatitis Surveillance Report No. 56. Public Health Service, CDC. Atlanta, US Department of Health and Human Services, 1996.
295. Shapiro CN, Coleman PJ, McQuillan GM, et al. Epidemiology of hepatitis A: Seroepidemiology and risk groups in the USA. Vaccine 10(suppl 1):S59–S62, 1992.
296. Kashiwagi S, Hayashi J, Ikematsu H, et al. Prevalence of immunologic markers of hepatitis A and B infection in hospital personnel in Miyazaki Prefecture, Japan. Am J Epidemiol 122:964–969, 1985.
297. Gibas A, Blewett DR, Schoenfield DA, et al. Prevalence and incidence of viral hepatitis in healthcare workers in the prehepatitis B vaccination era. Am J Epidemiol 136:1791–1800, 1992.
298. Abb J. Prevalence of hepatitis A virus antibodies in hospital personnel. Gesundheitswesen 56:377–379, 1994.
299. Papaevangelou GJ, Roumeliotou-Karayannis AJ, Contoyannis PC. The risk of hepatitis A and B virus infections from patients under care without isolation precaution. J Med Virol 7:143–148, 1981.
300. Germanaud J. Hepatitis A and health care personnel [letter]. Arch Intern Med 154:820, 1994.
301. Van Damme P, Cramm M, Van der Auwera J-C, Meheus A. Hepatitis A vaccination for healthcare workers. BMJ 306:1615, 1993.
302. Eisenstein AB, Aach RD, Jacobson W, Goldman A. An epidemic of infectious hepatitis in a general hospital: Probable transmission by contaminated orange juice. JAMA. 185:171–184, 1993.
303. Meyers JD, Romm FJ, Tihen WS, Bryan JA. Food-borne hepatitis A in a general hospital: Epidemiologic study of an outbreak attributed to sandwiches. JAMA 231:1049–1053, 1975.
304. Goodman RA, Carder CC, Allen JR, et al. Nosocomial hepatitis A transmission by an adult patient with diarrhea. Am J Med 73:220–226, 1982.
305. Krober MS, Bass JW, Brown JD, et al. Hospital outbreak of hepatitis A: Risk factors for spread. Pediatr Infect Dis J 3:296–299, 1984.
306. Klein BS, Michaels JA, Rytel MW, et al. Nosocomial hepatitis A: A multinursery outbreak in Wisconsin. JAMA 252:2716–2721, 1984.
307. Reed CM, Gustafson TL, Siegel J, et al. Nosocomial transmission of hepatitis A from a hospital-acquired case. Pediatr Infect Dis J 3:300–303, 1984.
308. Skidmore SJ, Gully PR, Middleton JD, et al. An outbreak of hepatitis A on a hospital ward. J Med Virol 17:175–177, 1985.
309. Azimi PH, Roberto RR, Guralnik J, et al. Transfusion-acquired hepatitis A in a premature infant with secondary nosocomial spread in an intensive care nursery. Am J Dis Child 140:23–27, 1986.
310. Baptiste R, Koziol DE, Henderson DK. Nosocomial transmission of hepatitis A in an adult population. Infect Control 8:364–370, 1987.
311. Drusin LM, Sohmer M, Groshen SL, et al. Nosocomial hepatitis A infection in a pediatric intensive care unit. Arch Dis Child 62:690–695, 1987.
312. Rosenblum LS, Villarino ME, Nainan OV, et al. Hepatitis A outbreak in a neonatal intensive care unit: Risk factors for transmission and evidence of prolonged viral excretion among preterm infants. J Infect Dis 164:476–482, 1991.
313. Lee KK, Vargo LR, Le CT, Fernando L. Transfusion-acquired hepatitis A outbreak from fresh frozen plasma in a neonatal intensive care unit. Pediatr Infect Dis J 11:122–123, 1992.
314. Watson JC, Flemming DC, Borella AJ, et al. Vertical transmission of hepatitis A resulting in an outbreak in a neonatal intensive care unit. J Infect Dis 167:567–571, 1993.
315. Doebbling BN, Li N, Wenzel RP. An outbreak of hepatitis A among healthcare workers: Risk factors for transmission. Am J Public Health 83:1679–1684, 1993.
316. Burkholder BT, Coronado VG, Brown J, et al. Nosocomial transmission of hepatitis A in a pediatric hospital traced to an anti-hepatitis A virus-negative patient with immunodeficiency. Pediatr Infect Dis J 14:261–266, 1995.
317. Hanna JN, Loewenthal MR, Negel P, Wenck DJ. An outbreak of hepatitis A in an intensive care unit. Anaesth Intensive Care 24:440–444, 1996.
318. Centers for Disease Control and Prevention. Pertussis vaccination: Use of acellular pertussis vaccines among infants and children: Recommendations of the Advisory Committee on Immunization Practices. MMWR Morb Mortal Wkly Rep 46(No. RR-7):1–25, 1997.
319. Cherry JD. The epidemiology of pertussis and pertussis immunization in the United Kingdom and the United States: A comparative study. Curr Probl Pediatr 14:1–78, 1984.
320. Cherry JD. Nosocomial pertussis in the nineties. Infect Control Hosp Epidemiol 16:553–555, 1995.
321. Mink C, Cherry JD, Christenson P, et al. A search for *Bordetella pertussis* infection in university students. Clin Infect Dis 14:464–471, 1992.
322. Rosenthal S, Strebel P, Cassiday P, et al. Pertussis infection

among adults during the 1993 outbreak in Chicago. J Infect Dis 171:1650–1652, 1995.

323. Wright SW, Edwards KM, Decker MD, Zeldin MH. Pertussis infection in adults with persistant cough. JAMA 13:1044–1046, 1995.
324. Deville JG, Cherry JD, Christenson PD, et al. Frequency of unrecognized *Bordetella pertussis* infections in adults. Clin Infect Dis 21:639–642, 1995.
325. von Konig CHW, Postels-Multani S, Block HL, Schmitt HJ. Pertussis in adults: Frequency of transmission after household exposure. Lancet 346:1326–1328, 1995.
326. Kurt TL, Yeager AS, Guenette S, Dunlop S. Spread of pertussis by hospital staff. JAMA 221:264–267, 1972.
327. Linneman CC, Ramundo N, Perlstein PH, et al. Use of pertussis vaccine in an epidemic involving hospital staff. Lancet 2:540–543, 1975.
328. Valenti WM, Pincus PH, Messner MK. Nosocomial pertussis: Possible spread by a hospital visitor. Am J Dis Child 134:520–521, 1980.
329. Steketee RW, Wassilak SGF, Adkins WN, et al. Evidence for a high attack rate and efficacy of erythromycin prophylaxis in a pertussis outbreak in a facility for the developmentally disabled. J Infect Dis 157:434–440, 1988.
330. Fisher MC, Long SS, McGowan KL, et al. Outbreak of pertussis in a residential facility for handicapped people. J Pediatr 114:934–939, 1989.
331. Addiss DG, Davis JP, Meade BD, et al. A pertussis outbreak in a Wisconsin nursing home. J Infect Dis 164:704–710, 1991.
332. Tanaka Y, Fujinaga K, Goto A, et al. Outbreak of pertussis in a residential facility for handicapped people. Dev Biol Stand 73:329–332, 1991.
333. Shefer A, Dales L, Nelson M, et al. Use and safety of acellular pertussis vaccine among adult hospital staff during an outbreak of pertussis. J Infect Dis 171:1053–1056, 1995.
334. Christie CDC, Glover AM, Willke MJ, et al. Containment of pertussis in the regional pediatric hospital during the greater Cincinnati epidemic of 1993. Infect Control Hosp Epidemiol 16:556–563, 1995.
335. Weber DJ, Rutala WA. Management of healthcare workers exposed to pertussis. Infect Control Hosp Epidemiol 15:411–415, 1994.
336. Edwards KM, Decker MD, Graham BS, et al. Adult immunization with acellular pertussis vaccine. JAMA 269:53–56, 1993.
337. Zackrisson G, Brorson J-E, Krantz I, Trollfors B. In-vitro sensitivity of *Bordetella pertussis*. J Antimicrob Chemother 11:407–411, 1983.
338. Kurzynski T, Boehm DM, Rott-Petri JA, et al. Antimicrobial susceptibilities of *Bordetella* species isolated in a multicenter pertussis surveillance project. Antimicrob Agents Chemother 32:137–140, 1988.
339. Hoppe JE, Eichhorn A. Activity of new macrolides against *Bordetella pertussis* and *Bordetella parapertussis*. Eur J Clin Microbiol Infect Dis 8:653–654, 1989.
340. Appleman ME, Hadfield TL, Gaines JK, Winn RE. Susceptibility of *Bordetella pertussis* to five quinolone antimicrobic drugs. Diagn Microbiol Infect Dis 8:131–133, 1987.
341. Hoppe JE, Simon CG. In vitro susceptibilities of *Bordetella pertussis* and *Bordetella parapertussis* to seven fluoroquinolones. Antimicrob Agents Chemother 34:2287–2288, 1990.
342. Hoppe JE, Haug A. Antimicrobial susceptibility of *Bordetella pertussis*: Part I. Infection 16:126–130, 1988.
343. Granstom G, Sterner G, Nord CE, Granstrom M. Use of erythromycin to prevent pertussis in newborns of mothers with pertussis. J Infect Dis 155:1210–1214, 1987.
344. Sprauer MA, Cochi SL, Zell ER, et al. Prevention of secondary transmission of pertussis in households with early use of erythromycin. Am J Dis Child 146:177–181, 1992.
345. De Serres G, Boulianne N, Dukval B. Field effectiveness of erythromycin prophylaxis to prevent pertussis within families. Pediatr Infect Dis J 4:969–975, 1995.
346. Anonymous. The choice of antimicrobial drugs. Med Lett Drugs Ther 38:25–34, 1996.
347. Hoppe JE, Haug A. Antimicrobial susceptibility of *Bordetella pertussis*: Part II. Infection 16:148–152, 1988.
348. Hoppe JE. Update of epidemiology, diagnosis, and treatment of pertussis. Eur J Clin Microbiol Infect Dis 15:189–193, 1996.
349. Henry RL, Dorman DC, Skinner JA, Mellis CM. Antimicrobial therapy in whooping cough. Med J Aust 2:27–28, 1981.
350. Hoppe JE, Halm U, Hagedorn H-J, Kraminer-Hagedorn A. Comparison of erythromycin ethylsuccinate and co-trimoxazole for treatment of pertussis. Infection 17:227–231, 1989.
351. Erythromycin-resistant *Bordetella pertussis*—Yuma County, Arizona, May–October 1994. MMWR Morb Mortal Wkly Rep 43:807–810, 1994.

chapter

48 Regulation and Testing of Vaccines*

Paul D. Parkman

M. Carolyn Hardegree

BACKGROUND

The need for regulation of vaccines is recognized worldwide. The developed countries of the world have established government agencies to conduct these regulatory activities. In the United States, the organization responsible for regulating such products is the Center for Biologics Evaluation and Research (CBER) of the Food and Drug Administration (FDA). These vaccine products are listed in Tables 48–1 and 48–2.

In addition to these national regulations, the World Health Organization (WHO), through its Expert Committee on Biological Standardization and its Biologicals Unit, provides guidance in the form of criteria for acceptability of products that move in international commerce.† More than 100 countries have adopted WHO requirements as their own national requirements. These standards have been particularly helpful to developing countries and have been useful in establishing a standard of acceptability for vaccines used by the international agencies involved in global immunization efforts. National standards are not required to be entirely consistent with the WHO criteria. However, international standardization efforts have been given special impetus by the formation of the European Community and this organization's attempts to harmonize the regulatory requirements of multiple European states. The efforts of the International Conference on Harmonization of drugs[1] have impacted vaccines less, but there is increasing global interest in additional harmonization of vaccine requirements.

The initial concepts used for the regulation of biologics in the United States were developed in 1902, modified in 1944, and expanded on in the 1950s. They stressed the need for a strong research base, an attitude of scientific problem solving, a keen familiarity with products, and an ability to deal with issues that arise in clinical testing of vaccines.

*All materal in this chapter is in the public domain, with the exception of any borrowed figures or tables.

†Reports of the World Health Organization's Expert Committee on Biological Standardization are published in the WHO Technical Report Series and may be obtained from the Distribution and Sales Office, World Health Organization, 1211 Geneva 27, Switzerland. Reprints of Requirements/Guidelines annexed to these reports can be obtained free of charge on request to Biologicals, World Health Organization, 1211 Geneva 27, Switzerland.

In addition to staff scientists and physicians, a regulatory organization needs continued exchange of information with the outside scientific community. To foster this interaction, the regulatory agency staff sponsor and participate in workshops, seminars, and international conferences. Also important are formal advisory committees, which include experts in the fields of vaccines, microbiology, infectious diseases, immunology, and clinical studies. These committees review and make recommendations on product development and approval. In addition, in the United States, the CBER works closely with its counterparts in other government agencies within the Public Health Service such as the Centers for Disease Control and Prevention (CDC), the National Institutes of Health (NIH), and Health Resources and Services Administration. The CDC is responsible, among other duties, for epidemiological surveillance of disease and for support of immunization programs. Its Advisory Committee on Immunization Practices (ACIP) makes recommendations for vaccine use. The National Vaccine Program Director, through the Director of the National Vaccine Program Office based at CDC, provides coordination of the Public Health Service's and other governmental agencies' vaccine efforts. The NIH conducts and funds biomedical research of all kinds.

The regulatory agencies responsible for controlling vaccines are faced with many difficult tasks, perhaps the greatest of which is assessing the safety and efficacy of products under development and, following product approval, continued monitoring.

In doing this, they must strive to oversee product approval in a way that neither hinders the availability of important new products nor permits the distribution of unsafe products. Thus, the regulatory agency has a key role to play in the overall immunization effort.

Historical Perspective

In the late 19th century, after the medical discoveries of Pasteur, Ehrlich, Koch, von Behring, Kitasato, and others, a number of vaccines and sera useful for the prevention or treatment of certain infectious diseases, such as rabies, diphtheria, and tetanus, were developed. These, together with smallpox vaccine, which had al-

Table 48–1. BACTERIAL VACCINES CURRENTLY LICENSED IN THE UNITED STATES

VACCINE	MANUFACTURER*
Anthrax vaccine, adsorbed	6
BCG vaccine	8
Cholera vaccine	11
Diphtheria and tetanus toxoids and pertussis vaccine, adsorbed	1, 3, 4, 6,† 11†
Diphtheria and tetanus toxoids and acellular pertussis vaccine, adsorbed	1, 3,‡ 12, 13
Diphtheria and tetanus toxoids and pertussis vaccine, adsorbed, and *Haemophilus* b conjugate (diphtheria CRM197 protein conjugate)	3
Diphtheria and tetanus toxoids, adsorbed	1, 2, 3, 4, 6, 11†
Diphtheria toxoid, adsorbed	6
Tetanus and diphtheria toxoids, adsorbed for adult use	1, 3, 4, 11
Tetanus toxoid	1, 2,† 3,
Tetanus toxoid, adsorbed	1, 3, 4,† 6,† 10, 11
Pertussis vaccine	1†
Pertussis vaccine, adsorbed	6
Haemophilus b conjugate vaccine (diphtheria CRM197 protein conjugate)	3
Haemophilus b conjugate vaccine (diphtheria toxoid conjugate)	1
Haemophilus b conjugate vaccine (meningococcal protein conjugate)	5
Haemophilus b conjugate vaccine (meningococcal protein conjugate) and hepatitis B recombinant vaccine	5
Haemophilus b conjugate vaccine (tetanus toxoid conjugate)	9
Haemophilus b polysaccharide vaccine	1†
Meningococcal polysaccharide vaccine, group A	1†
Meningococcal polysaccharide vaccine, group C	1†
Meningococcal polysaccharide vaccine, groups A and C combined	1†
Meningococcal polysaccharide vaccine, A, C, Y, W135 combined	1, 5
Plague vaccine	7
Pneumococcal vaccine, polyvalent	3, 5
Typhoid vaccine	11
Typhoid vaccine, live oral, Ty21a	10
Typhoid Vi Polysaccharide vaccine	9

*1, Connaught Laboratories, Inc.; 2, Connaught Laboratories, Ltd.; 3, Lederle Laboratories, Division American Cyanamid Co.; 4, Massachusetts Public Health Biological Laboratories; 5, Merck & Co., Inc.; 6, Michigan Biologics Products Institute; 7, Greer Laboratories, Inc.; 8, Organon Teknika Corporation; 9, Pasteur Mérieux Serums et Vaccins S.A.; 10, Swiss Serum and Vaccine Institute, Berne; 11, Wyeth Laboratories, Inc.; 12, SmithKline Beecham Biologicals; 13, North American Vaccine, Inc.

†Not in active production or distribution.

‡Licenses for the pertussis component of these two products are held by the Research Foundation for Microbial Diseases of Osaka University (Connaught Laboratories, Inc.) and Takeda (Lederle Laboratories, Division American Cyanamid Co.). These are the names of the license holders. Company names may be different.

ready been in use for about a century at that time, represented the first biological products. Although the need for special care in both preparing and testing of vaccines and antitoxins was foreseen early in their development, it was not until a major tragedy occurred in the United States that action was taken by the federal government to ensure public protection from unsafe products. Such an event occurred in 1901. Several children in St. Louis, Missouri, died of tetanus. It was discovered that they had received two doses of diphtheria antitoxin, later shown to have been prepared from horse serum contaminated with tetanus bacilli.[2] This event stimulated proposed legislation to regulate the sale of biologicals. On July 1, 1902, the Biologics Control Act was signed into law. During consideration of this legislation,[3] the following points were recognized:

1. There could be no assurance of purity if control was limited to inspections and tests of the final products, both because of the limitations of testing techniques and because such tests would need to include all materials, because the products varied owing to differences in the animals used in production. Therefore, an effective control would also need to include control of manufacturing establishments.
2. The products in question were generally administered directly into the circulatory system or the digestive tract, and there were few remedial measures available if the drugs were impure.
3. The control of potency was particularly important because, as was noted in the proceedings, if the first dose proves worthless, the loss of time may cost the patient his or her life.

These ideas formed an important start for ensuring

Table 48–2. VIRAL VACCINES CURRENTLY LICENSED IN THE UNITED STATES

VACCINE	MANUFACTURER*
Adenovirus vaccine, live oral, type 4	11†
Adenovirus vaccine, live oral, type 7	11†
Hepatitis A vaccine, inactivated	5, 9
Hepatitis B vaccine, recombinant	5, 9
Haemophilus b conjugate vaccine (meningococcal protein conjugate) and hepatitis B recombinant vaccine	5
Influenza virus vaccine	1, 3, 7, 11
Japanese encephalitis vaccine, inactivated	10
Measles virus vaccine, live	5
Mumps virus vaccine, live	5
Rubella virus vaccine, live	5
Measles, mumps, and rubella virus vaccine, live	5
Measles and mumps virus vaccine, live	5
Measles and rubella virus vaccine, live	5
Rubella and mumps virus vaccine, live	5
Poliovirus vaccine inactivated, human diploid cell	2
Poliovirus vaccine inactivated, monkey kidney cell	8
Poliovirus vaccine, live oral, trivalent	4
Poliovirus vaccine, live oral, type I	4‡
Poliovirus vaccine, live oral, type II	4‡
Poliovirus vaccine, live oral, type III	4‡
Rabies vaccine	2, 8, 12
Rabies vaccine, adsorbed	6
Rotavirus vaccine, live oral, tetravalent	11
Smallpox vaccine	11§
Varicella virus vaccine live	5
Yellow fever vaccine	1

*1, Connaught Laboratories, Inc.; 2, Connaught Laboratories, Ltd.; 3, Evans Medical, Ltd.; 4, Lederle Laboratories, Division American Cyanamid Co.; 5, Merck & Co., Inc.; 6, Michigan Department of Public Health; 7, Parke-Davis, Division of Warner-Lambert Co.; 8, Pasteur Mérieux Serums et Vaccins, S.A.; 9, SmithKline Beecham Biologicals; 10, The Research Foundation for Microbial Diseases of Osaka University; 11, Wyeth Laboratories, Inc.; 12, Chiron Behring GmbH & Co. These are the names of the license holders. Company names may be different.

†Limited distribution—United States military services only.

‡Released for further manufacturing use only.

§Not in active production or distribution.

Table 48–3. **CHRONOLOGY OF THE DEVELOPMENT OF BIOLOGICAL CONTROL AUTHORITY**

YEAR	LEGISLATION ENACTED	EXISTING ORGANIZATION
1902	Biologics Control Act (Virus, Serum, Toxin Law) of 1902	PHS Hygienic Laboratory
1930		Hygienic Laboratory renamed National Institutes of Health (NIH)
1937		Laboratory of Biologics Control (LBC) formed within NIH
1944	Enactment of USPHS Act 42 USC 262, 263	
1948		LBC incorporated into the National Microbiological Institute (later renamed the National Institute of Allergy and Infectious Diseases)
1955		Establishment of the Division of Biologics Standards (DBS) by the Surgeon General
1972		DBS transferred to FDA to become Bureau of Biologics (BoB)
1982–1983		BoB renamed Office of Biologics Research and Review (OBRR); joined with Office of Drugs Research and Review (ODRR) to form the Center for Drugs and Biologics (CDB)
1987		OBRR renamed Center for Biologics Evaluation and Research (CBER)
1997	Food and Drug Administration Modernization Act of 1997	

vaccine safety; they are used as the basis for ensuring safety and effectiveness throughout the world. The history of vaccine control organizations in developed nations has been one of increasing size and complexity. A chronology of the development of the U.S. Biologics Control Authority is summarized in Table 48–3.

In 1902, the U.S. Congress enacted another significant law that expanded the Public Health and Marine Hospital Service. For the first time, a federal agency was created in which public health matters could be coordinated. The Hygienic Laboratory, the principal research unit of the service, was located in Washington, DC. Within this organization the Biological Control Service assumed responsibility for the regulation of the three products then defined as biologicals, namely, smallpox vaccine, tetanus antitoxin, and diphtheria antitoxin. In 1930, the Hygienic Laboratory was reorganized and expanded, and its name was changed to the National Institutes of Health. In 1937, the Laboratory of Biologics Control was created within the Institutes, and in 1938 the NIH moved to its present location in Bethesda, Maryland. As the organization expanded, new institutes were added to study diseases other than those known to be caused by infectious agents.

In 1944, laws relating to the Public Health Service were revised and consolidated into the United States Public Health Service Act. This act incorporated the 1902 Biologics Control Act into Section 351.[4] Under this act, the federal government was empowered to license biological products as well as the establishments in which they are produced. The law prohibited interstate shipment for sale, barter, or exchange of "any virus, therapeutic serum, toxin, antitoxin, or analogous product . . . applicable to the prevention, treatment, or cure of diseases or injuries of man" without a license. A 1970 amendment added "vaccine, blood, blood component or derivative, [or] allergenic product" to the statutory list. Under the original act, government inspectors were authorized to inspect the manufacturing establishments and to determine whether products were correctly labeled with the name of the product; the name, address, and license number of the manufacturer; and the expiration date of the product, and to determine the manner in which the product was prepared. Section 352 of the act also permitted the PHS to manufacture biologic products should the need arise (i.e., if the product could not be obtained from already licensed establishments).[5] This authority has not been used to date. In 1948, the Laboratory of Biologics Control became part of the National Microbiological Institute (later renamed the National Institute of Allergy and Infectious Diseases).

The need for strengthening and expanding control of biologicals became evident in 1955. By this time, many biologicals (blood products as well as vaccines) had been licensed, including inactivated poliovirus vaccine prepared in monkey kidney cell cultures. Unfortunately, when several batches of the vaccine produced were used for immunization, a number of children developed poliomyelitis. The formaldehyde inactivation and safety test procedures employed were inadequate. It was determined in retrospect that 7 of 17 batches could be shown to contain living poliovirus. A later review indicated that a total of 79 cases of poliomyelitis occurred in vaccine recipients, with 105 cases among family contacts and 20 among community contacts.[6]

This much-publicized "Cutter incident" led to the expansion of the biologicals control function of the Public Health Service. Thus, the Division of Biologics Standards (DBS) was established within the NIH. In 1972, the DBS was transferred to the FDA. Since that time, it has undergone a series of reorganizations and has evolved into the current CBER.

Implementation

The CBER's legal authority derives primarily from Section 351 of the Public Health Service Act as well as from certain sections of the Federal Food, Drug, and Cosmetic Act.* One important mechanism for imple-

*During consideration of the 1944 legislation, there was agreement that a manufacturer would not have to get both an approved new drug application and an approved biologicals license application for the same product. However, the other applicable provisions of the Federal Food, Drug, and Cosmetic Act, such as those concerning drug or device adulteration or misbranding, would continue to apply to biologic products. See Division of Biologics Standards, National Institutes of Health, Legislative History of the Regulation of Biological Products, 19–21, 1971, and 42 U.S.C., Sec. 262(g).

menting these statutes is through regulations codified in the Code of Federal Regulations (CFR). The CFR contains a compilation of current regulations of all federal agencies. It is divided into 50 titles, and FDA regulations are located in Title 21.[7] Each title is further subdivided into chapters, subchapters, parts, and sections. Copies of these regulations may be ordered through the Superintendent of Documents, Attn: New Orders, P.O. Box 371954, Pittsburgh, PA 15250-7954. Parts 600 through 680 contain regulations specifically applicable to vaccines and other biologicals. In addition, because these vaccine products meet the legal definition of a drug, manufacturers must comply with the drug Current Good Manufacturing Practice Regulations (Parts 210 and 211), which describe requirements for personnel, buildings, equipment, production controls, records, and other aspects of the manufacturing process.[8] Those regulations applicable to vaccines and other biological products are summarized in Table 48–4. Other guidance documents that do not have the force of law but that provide useful and timely recommendations are listed in Table 48–5. These guidance documents are particularly useful in rapidly progressing areas of science and for specifying a degree of detail beyond what is included in the regulations. These documents can be obtained through the CBER FAX Information System (telephone number in the United States at 1-888-CBER-FAX and overseas at 301-827-3844) or through the CBER web page on the World Wide Web at http://www.fda.gov/cber/cberftp.html.

Table 48–4. **REGULATIONS APPLICABLE TO THE DEVELOPMENT, MANUFACTURE, LICENSURE, AND USE OF VACCINES**

TITLE 21, CODE OF FEDERAL REGULATIONS* CHAPTER 1—FDA, DHHS*	SUBJECT
Subchapter F—Biologics	
600–680†	
600	Biological products, general, definitions
	Establishment standards
	Establishment inspection
	Adverse experience reporting
601	Licensing
610	General biological product standards
Subchapter C—Drugs: General	
201	Labeling
202	Prescription drug advertising
210	Current good manufacturing practice in manufacturing, processing, packing, or holding of drugs, general
211	Current good manufacturing practice (GMPs) for finished pharmaceuticals
Subchapter D—Drugs for Human Use	
312	New drugs for investigational use
314	Applications for FDA approval to market a new drug on an antibiotic drug
Subchapter A—General	
25	Environmental impact considerations
50	Protection of human subjects
56	Institutional Review Boards
58	Nonclinical laboratory studies, good laboratory practice regulations

*Food and Drug Administration, Department of Health and Human Services.
†Parts 606, 607, 640, 660, and 680 apply to blood, blood products, diagnostic tests, and allergenics.

Table 48–5. **GUIDANCE DOCUMENTS APPLICABLE TO THE DEVELOPMENT, MANUFACTURE, LICENSURE, AND USE OF VACCINES***

NAME	DATE
Points to Consider	
Production and testing of new drugs and biologicals produced by recombinant DNA technology	1985
Computer-assisted submissions for license applications	1990
Supplement: Nucleic acid characterization and genetic stability	1992
Characterization of cell lines used to produce biologicals	1993
Plasmid DNA vaccines for preventive infectious disease indications	1996
Manufacture and testing of monoclonal antibody products for human use	1997
Guidelines	
Interpretive guidelines of the additional standards for source plasma (human)	1973
Interpretation of potency test results for all forms of adsorbed diphtheria and tetanus toxoids	1979
Meningococcal polysaccharide vaccines	1985
Submitting documentation for the stability of human drugs and biologicals	1987
Submitting documentation for packaging for human drugs and biologicals	1987
Guideline on general principles of process validation	1987
Sterile drug products produced by aseptic processing	1987
Validation of the limulus amebocyte lysate test	1987
Release of pneumococcal vaccine, polyvalent	1989
Test for residual moisture for biological products	1990
Guideline for adverse experience reporting for licensed biological products	1993
Guidance Documents	
CBER refusal to file (RTF) guidance for product and establishment license	1993
Guidance on alternatives to lot release for licensed biological products	1994
Changes to an approved application; draft guidance	1996
Draft guidance for industry; electronic submission of case report forms and case report tabulations	1996
Guidance for industry; providing clinical evidence of effectiveness for human drug and biological products	1997
Guidance for industry for the evaluation of combination vaccines for preventable diseases: production, testing and clinical studies	1997

*Available at no charge from the Office of Communication, Training and Manufacturers Assistance, HFM-40, 1401 Rockville Pike, Rockville, MD 20852-1448 (FAX Information System 1-888-CBER-FAX or 301-827-3844).

Before reviewing the various procedures involved in regulation of vaccines, it would be useful to examine several operational definitions[9] contained in the statute or regulations:

1. Section 351 of the Public Health Service Act defines a *biological product* as any virus, therapeutic serum, toxin, antitoxin, vaccine, blood, blood component or derivative, allergenic product, or analogous product applicable to the prevention, treatment, or cure of diseases or conditions of human beings. Thus, vaccines are clearly regulated as biological products.
2. *Safety* is defined as the relative freedom from harmful effect to people affected directly or indirectly by a

product when prudently administered, taking into consideration the character of the product in relation to the condition of the recipient at the time. Thus, the property of safety is relative and cannot be ensured in an absolute sense. For example, recombinant hepatitis B vaccine has been judged to be safe and effective. However, a rare but clearly causal relationship has been established between this vaccine and anaphylaxis.[10]

3. *Purity* is defined as the relative freedom from extraneous matter, regardless of whether it is harmful to the recipient or deleterious to the product. Usually, the concepts of purity and safety coincide; purity most often relates to freedom from such materials as pyrogens, adventitious agents, and chemicals used in manufacture of the product.

4. *Potency* is defined as the specific ability or capacity of the product, as indicated by appropriate laboratory tests or by adequately controlled clinical data obtained through administration of the product in the manner intended, to effect a given result. Potency as thus defined is equivalent to the concept that the product must be able to do what is claimed for it, and, if possible, this must correspond with some measurable effect in the recipient or be correlated with some quantitative laboratory finding.

5. *Standards* means specifications and procedures applicable to an establishment or to the manufacture or release of products that are designed to ensure the continued safety, purity, and potency of biological products. The word *standard* is also used with a secondary meaning, usually in the sense of a reference preparation, such as a bacterial or viral antigen that can be used in evaluating potency or, in some cases, safety and purity.

6. The regulations regarding biological products, in addition, define *effectiveness* as the reasonable expectation that, in a significant proportion of the target population, pharmacological or other effects of the biological product, when administered under adequate directions for use and warnings against unsafe use, will serve a clinically significant function in the diagnosis, cure, mitigation, treatment, or prevention of disease in humans.[11]

The CFR is published annually and contains any changes in regulations that have occurred during the previous year and that have been published in the *Federal Register.* Regulations are adopted in conformity with the Administrative Procedure Act.[12] Thus, before a regulation can be established, repealed, or changed, ordinarily it must be proposed and published in the *Federal Register* with an invitation to comment within a prescribed time, commonly a period of 1 to several months, to all interested people. Once comments have been received, they are taken into consideration by the FDA before publication of the final regulation in the *Federal Register.*

REGULATION OF BIOLOGICAL PRODUCTS

Premarketing Phase

The regulation of biological products covers both the premarketing phase, consisting of the investigational and licensing phases, and the postmarketing phase. Only licensed vaccines may be shipped from one state to another, except that during the premarketing phase the law and regulations allow interstate shipment of products for experimental purposes. These rules are spelled out in the Investigational New Drug (IND) regulations.[13] Before initiating the clinical investigation, a sponsor submits an IND application form.* In the application, the sponsor (1) describes the composition, source, and method of manufacture of the product and the methods used in testing its safety, purity, and potency; (2) provides a summary of all laboratory and preclinical animal testing; and (3) provides a description of the proposed clinical study and the names and qualifications of each clinical investigator. The sponsor must wait 30 days after submitting the IND application before starting the study. During this period, the application is reviewed by the FDA to determine that the study volunteers will not be exposed to unwarranted risks.

As part of the IND process, each clinical investigator files information describing his or her qualifications for performing clinical trials, details of the proposed study, and assurance that a number of conditions specified by the regulations will be met. A signed informed consent must be obtained from each study participant.[14] Approval for the study must be obtained in advance from a local institutional review board.[15] The regulations also deal with the preclinical laboratory animal studies undertaken to support the use of the product in humans.[16]

Clinical testing of experimental biologicals consists of three separate phases that may overlap (Fig. 48–1). It may be highly iterative in that multiple phase 1 or 2 trials may be performed as new data are obtained. Phase 1, initial testing in humans, begins with short-term studies in a small number of subjects (usually less than 20), primarily to test the safety of the biological. Testing is often initiated in adults. If the vaccine is designed to be used in infants or young children, as is commonly the case, the product is then evaluated in progressively younger age groups down into the first year of life. In phase 2, larger studies perhaps involving 50 to several hundred participants are performed to obtain preliminary information on the biological's effectiveness (immunogenicity) and additional safety data. In phase 3, more extensive testing is performed to provide a more thorough assessment of effectiveness and safety. Here the number of subjects may vary over a broad range.

In recent years, efficacy trials for various vaccines have involved from 1,000 to nearly 100,000 participants. The reason for this broad range is related to a number of interconnected variables. For efficacy, the more important are study design and the incidence of the disease to be prevented. For example, studies in which a new vaccine must be compared with an already existing product of the same type generally require larger numbers than one in which a new vaccine can be compared with another type of control. The incidence of the disease to

*Sponsors may be individual physicians, a university, a hospital, or a commercial firm as well as government agencies, such as one of the institutes of the NIH, the Department of Defense, or physicians within the FDA itself.

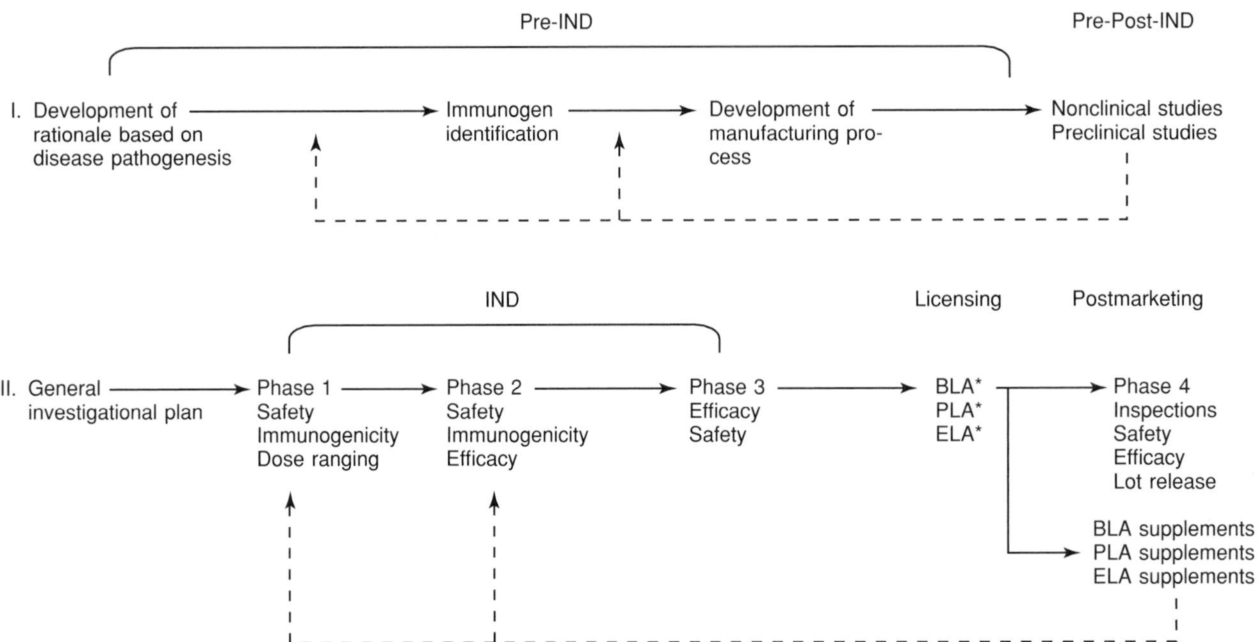

Figure 48–1. Stages of review and regulation of biological products: sequence of key events in product development through the premarketing experimental Investigational New Drug (IND) and licensing phases, and the postapproval marketing phase. *Dashed lines* indicate additional research/development submissions when significant changes are made in the product or its indications. *Historically both a Product License Application (PLA) and an Establishment License Application (ELA) have been required. In the future, only a Biologics License Application (BLA) will be required.

be prevented in the study population also is important. Convincing evidence for the effectiveness of the plasma-derived hepatitis B vaccine in a population at high risk required only 549 vaccinees and 524 placebo recipients. In contrast, a trial to show that Japanese encephalitis vaccine was successful in preventing this low incidence disease required more than 40,000 children divided approximately equally between the vaccinated and control groups. Immunogenicity studies may be requested to provide data on the immune response of target populations for the vaccine if they are different from those populations in whom the efficacy studies were done. These may be called "bridging" studies. Common reactions can be studied in hundreds of patients, but many thousands will be required to define low incidence adverse reactions. Additional controlled safety studies may be requested when the numbers of subjects included in the efficacy studies are deemed insufficient to provide adequate safety data. The studies need to be designed in such a way that statistical methods may be applied to their evaluation.

The internal review process in the CBER begins with an initial review for scientific content and compliance with the regulations. Reviewers are selected for their expertise with the type of product and its method of manufacture. For example, an IND application for a hepatitis B vaccine might be reviewed within several divisions in the CBER. Comments regarding the review are then communicated to the sponsor, usually in writing. Subsequently, correspondence from the sponsor concerning the results of studies or plans for new laboratory or clinical studies are ordinarily reviewed in the same fashion. Early in the process, the vaccine is assessed for immunological effects, toxicities, and, when appropriate, metabolic and pharmacological effects.

Sponsors are encouraged to avail themselves of a pre-IND meeting with the CBER reviewers in which the general experimental plan for the product is reviewed. Such a meeting is particularly important for new sponsors and for products that incorporate novel features. Other meetings also are encouraged at critical points throughout the IND review, including "end of phase 2" meetings to evaluate the safety of proceeding to phase 3 and the phase 3 plan. Continued participation by statisticians is important throughout the process. Use of well-defined study endpoints and appropriate analytical plans, including plans for interim analysis, is particularly important in producing interpretable results.

When the IND studies are nearing completion or have been completed and the sponsor believes that the product can be shown to be safe and effective for its intended use, the sponsor applies for a license to manufacture and distribute the product commercially. By this time, exact techniques of production should be developed, and the manufacturing process standardized. The manufacturer assumes the major role in documenting the safety and effectiveness of the specific product that is prepared by the described methods. Historically, two license applications have been required, one for the product and one for the establishment in which it is to be manufactured.[17]

However, as a result of the enactment of the Food and Drug Administration Modernization Act of 1997, only a biologics license application (BLA) is required. This application will continue to include detailed information about the product, but the information to be submitted about the establishment will be simplified. The prelicensing inspection will be used to provide some of the information previously detailed in the Establishment License Application.

In the BLA, information needs to be submitted that indicates that there is compliance with standards addressing requirements for (1) organization and personnel; (2) buildings and facilities; (3) equipment; (4) control of components, containers, and closures; (5) production and process controls; (6) packaging and labeling controls; (7) holding and distribution; (8) laboratory controls; and (9) records to be maintained. At this point in the product development, a prelicensing meeting is encouraged with the agency in which the sponsor's developmental plan is discussed.

The application contains (1) a complete description of all manufacturing and testing methods for the product; (2) the results of all laboratory tests performed on a specified number of lots (usually three to five), including stability testing; (3) a summary of the results of all clinical studies; and (4) proposed labeling, which includes the indications and directions for use of the product.

The scientific review of the application is performed by an internal FDA committee, with a chairperson selected on the basis of expertise with the specific product or similar products. The composition of the committee varies; members may be selected from several divisions, depending on the expertise required to review the application adequately. This process occurs for each license application or submission to a license in which significant changes are proposed. The application, as filed with the CBER, is intended to be complete and to contain all of the results of laboratory and clinical testing necessary to show safety and efficacy for the intended use of the product. During the review, there are discussions and correspondence between the sponsor and the CBER review committee, and sometimes with outside expert advisors and consultants, in which all the laboratory and clinical data are carefully reviewed.

Approval of a license application by the CBER is based on reviews of the data submitted by the applicant indicating that the product is safe and effective for its intended use. The standards to be applied for safety and efficacy are flexible. The benefit to risk ratio of a biological product is considered. The standards allow for a range of safety and efficacy, as is scientifically appropriate, as exemplified by the spectrum from typhoid vaccine to measles vaccine. Also important to this review are product labeling, including the printed material that accompanies the package and describes the indications for use, contraindications, dosage, and possible adverse effects; protocols for the manufacturing and testing of the number of product lots specified to establish the consistency of the process; and results of confirmatory testing within the CBER of samples of in-process material or product in final containers and conformance to existing regulations.

When the review of the license application is nearing completion, an announced prelicense inspection is performed after the manufacturer has informed the CBER that production has begun. This inspection is designed as an in-depth review of the facilities, records, total production process, methods, equipment, quality control procedures, and personnel. Reinspection may be necessary before a final decision about licensing is made.

The entire package of information is reviewed by the CBER, commonly with the assistance of its advisory committees and other consultants. The advisory committees are generally asked to comment on the adequacy of the data to support safety and efficacy in the target population. The committee's advice is taken into consideration in developing the recommendations for use to be given in the package insert. The committee may recommend additional studies to be performed either before or after approval. After the CBER determines that the data and information are satisfactory, the product is licensed.

Postmarketing Phase

Experimentation with the product may continue after licensure as the manufacturer seeks additional indications for product use (e.g., new target populations that would benefit from vaccination) or as experience leads to optimization of the production process. In some instances, at the time of approval the manufacturer commits to conduct so-called phase 4 studies; these are most often designed to collect additional safety data in large numbers of vaccine recipients.

If, as a result of continued research or acquisition of postmarketing surveillance data, the manufacturer wishes to significantly modify the manufacturing process or directions for vaccine use, approval must be obtained.[18] This is accomplished by the applicant's submitting an account of these changes to the appropriate license applications. For the past several years, efforts have been made to simplify and categorize these reporting requirements. Guidance documents that discuss the reporting requirements for changes in more detail are available.

After issuance of the license, there is continued surveillance of the product and of the manufacturer's production activities. For most vaccines, a protocol is submitted for each lot prepared by the firm that provides the details of production and a summary of test results. Samples of each lot also are submitted for release. Although not required by law or regulation, selected laboratory tests are often performed by the CBER. The type and extent of confirmatory testing performed by the CBER depend on several factors, such as the newness of the product or the difficulties that may have arisen with manufacture or use of the product. Release or rejection is based on a review of all test results, including those done by the manufacturer and those performed by the CBER.

An alternative schema to the traditional lot by lot release has been an option for extensively characterized products having a "track record" of continued safety, purity, and potency. For example, one of the hepatitis B vaccines met this standard and was the first vaccine product for which this exception was requested from the requirement for lot by lot release. New regulations have been developed that clearly specify the factors that are to be evaluated and include measures that allow additional products to be considered in this category. To be considered, the manufacturer must be able to produce a vaccine that repeatedly meets the standards for potency, purity, and stability of bulk and final container material while using a consistent process. Important factors to be considered are the nature of the product with respect to correlation between the measure of potency and biological activity and efficacy. Surveillance samples and protocols may be required to be submitted to the CBER at intervals.

Licensed establishments are inspected at least every two years. The purpose of the inspection is to determine that the product is manufactured and tested as described in the license application and in accordance with applicable regulations. Manufacturers who fail to meet product standards or who are not in compliance with the regulations may have their licenses suspended or revoked, depending on the nature of the potential health hazards created.[19]

Labeling changes are usually initiated by the manufacturer but may be initiated by the CBER. Historically, manufacturers have had to obtain prior approval from the CBER before the change is made. A recent regulatory change allows exceptions to this general rule for a change that adds or strengthens a contraindication, warning, precaution, or adverse reaction; adds or strengthens instructions about dosage and administration intended to increase safe use; or deletes false, misleading, or unsupported indications for use or effectiveness claims. Under this regulation, a manufacturer could effect such changes and, at the same time, submit them and the supporting data to the CBER without preapproval. In addition, minor changes (e.g., modification in analytical procedures with no change in the basic test methodology or release specifications) would not require prior approval but would be included for agency review in an annual report.

From time to time, manufacturers develop important improvements in their production processes, testing methods, equipment, or facility or make changes in personnel. Proposed changes in manufacturing methods that have a substantial potential to have an adverse effect on the safety or effectiveness of the product may not become effective until notification is given of the CBER's approval. A change has recently been implemented similar to that just outlined for labeling that would segregate such changes into those sufficiently significant with regard to safety, purity, potency, and efficacy of the product to require preapproval of a supplemental application before product distribution; those of lesser import for which the manufacturer must provide notification 30 days before distribution of product made using the change; and changes for which the manufacturer need only notify the agency by submission of an annual report.

Vaccine Testing

Laboratory testing of vaccines is conducted during both the experimental prelicensure phase and the postlicensure phase. The programs of vaccine testing are developed from a combination of the understanding of past adverse experiences and the best thinking regarding the potential for new ones. From past experience, a few highly important issues must receive special attention. For inactivated vaccines, a clear understanding of the kinetics of inactivation is key; this was the lesson of the so-called Cutter incident alluded to previously. For live vaccines, the agent must be at a stable level of attenuation; it must not become overattenuated or revert to virulence. The Brazilian experience, in which yellow fever vaccine appeared to revert to neurovirulence after multiple passages, demonstrated the need for a seed lot system in which the number of passages from the parent virus to the passage level used as vaccine is restricted.[20] For vaccines of any type, there must be an intensive search for extraneous contaminants. The experience in which human serum was used as a stabilizer for yellow fever vaccine and caused hundreds of cases of long-incubation hepatitis virus infection underscored this need.[21]

In the early 1960s, exogenous and endogenous contamination of both simian and avian cell cultures utilized in the production of several vaccines were reported. The issues related to cell substrates have been discussed in a variety of forums.[22, 23] The demonstration that viruses can be oncogenic in mammalian hosts produced an intense focus on cell-culture substrate safety. Despite these contamination episodes, no adverse effects on recipients have been documented to date.[24, 25] The issue continues to be discussed in national and international forums.[26, 27]

More recently, the epidemic of bovine spongiform encephalopathy and its possible relationship to human Creutzfeldt-Jakob disease has been of special concern. On this account, attention has been centered on the safety of substances derived from mammalian sources such as media components used for nurturing cell cultures and gelatins used as stabilizers.[28] In addition, the use of human blood components in manufacture or as excipients in vaccines has prompted discussions about potential substitutes. Whereas such risks remain entirely theoretical, the sources of such materials are being subjected to new restrictions, and the processing steps effective in eliminating scrapie used as a model agent are being evaluated.

At the inception of the recombinant DNA era, the possible risk of induction of transformation of cells of the recipient was a major concern. This issue has been approached by careful study of the constructs used and the stability of these constructs and by attempts to reduce extraneous DNA content to levels that are regarded as extremely unlikely to produce an adverse genetic event.[29–31] Currently, this issue is being evaluated anew in the context of possible future DNA vaccines. Each advance in vaccine technology has brought novel issues. The best that can be done is to attempt to devise testing schemes that will evaluate or predict potential adverse effects and then take action based on scientific consensus.

Preapproval test development may be conducted entirely by the sponsor or with involvement of the regulatory agency as well. The CBER is particularly likely to become involved if the product is new or represents a novel problem in testing. This involvement, bolstered by laboratory-based capability, has been one of the strengths of the vaccine regulatory program in the United States. As the product moves toward approval, the sponsor develops the testing program in greater detail. The final testing methods must be established before the major clinical trials undertaken to demonstrate efficacy and before the manufacture of batches of product that will be used to show a consistent ability to make a product of defined characteristics (i.e., a demonstration of "consistency of manufacture").

Among the very first efforts in product development should be explorations of a potency assay. Correlates are sought between the assay results and the preclinical and, later, the clinical testing results.

During the prelicensing phase, research testing results are evaluated to determine which tests under development need to be applied to every batch of product and which do not require such repetition. For example, with hepatitis B vaccines made using recombinant DNA technology, initial evidence for identity, purity, and genetic stability of the protein product was provided by physicochemical, immunological, and molecular biological test methods. These included protein characterization techniques (e.g., sodium dodecyl sulfate–polyacrylamide gel electrophoresis [SDS-PAGE], peptide mapping, amino acid composition analysis, amino-terminal sequencing, and high-performance size-exclusion chromatography [HPSEC]); immunological techniques (e.g., Western blotting for both hepatitis B surface antigen [HBsAg] and contaminating yeast proteins, radioimmunoassay [RIA], enzyme-linked immunosorbent assay [ELISA], and immunogenicity in mice); and techniques for assessing genetic stability (e.g., restriction endonuclease mapping of the expression construct, sequencing of the coding region of the product [from cells at the level of the master cell bank as well as at the end of the fermentation from at least one full-scale production run], and the percentage of host cells [yeast] retaining the expression construct and the copy number per cell). Once the consistency level of the results of these tests is validated for multiple lots produced during the IND application and product-licensing stage, a determination is made to routinely perform some of these tests, which will evaluate and ensure the consistent quality of the final product in each lot. In the case of the purified bulks or final containers of the recombinant hepatitis B vaccines, tests such as SDS-PAGE, Western blotting, HPSEC, ELISA, RIA, immunogenicity in mice, and the percentage of host cells carrying the expression construct were deemed sufficient (Table 48–6).

The regulation of biologicals includes requirements for testing of licensed products. Certain of these requirements are generally applicable to all products, whereas others are tailored to the specific vaccine. The tests, generally applicable to all products, include those for bacterial and fungal sterility, general safety, purity, identity, suitability of constituent materials, and potency.[32] Sterility testing is performed on both bulk- and final-container material, using media and conditions of incubation described in the regulations. In addition, cell culture–derived vaccines must be tested for mycoplasmas. The general safety test is usually performed by intraperitoneal inoculation of final container material into mice and guinea pigs to detect the possible presence of gross extraneous contaminants. Tests for purity are designed to determine that the product is free of extraneous material, except that which is unavoidable in the manufacturing process described in the approved license application, and may include tests for residual moisture and pyrogenic substances. Final container material must be identified by a test specific for each product (e.g., neutralization of each of the components of the live oral poliovirus vaccine with specific antisera). With regard to constituent materials, the manufacturer must ensure that all ingredients used in the product, such as diluents, preservatives, or adjuvants, meet generally accepted standards of purity. An adjuvant may not be used unless there is adequate proof that it does not adversely affect

Table 48–6. **TESTING REQUIREMENTS FOR THE RELEASE OF RECOMBINANT HEPATITIS B VACCINES**

	MERCK & CO., INC.		SMITHKLINE BEECHAM BIOLOGICALS	
TYPE OF TEST	**Test System**	**Stage of Production**	**Test System**	**Stage of Production**
Plasmid retention	Percentage of host cells with expression construct	Fermentation product	Percentage of host cells with expression construct	Fermentation product
Purity and identity	Formaldehyde	Bulk-adsorbed product	SDS-PAGE*	Nonadsorbed bulk
	Triton-X-100	Bulk-adsorbed product	DNA hybridization	Nonadsorbed bulk
	Protein (Lowry)	Bulk-adsorbed product		
	Gel electrophoresis	Sterile filtered product	Antigenic activity (RIA)	Nonadsorbed bulk
	HPSEC†	Sterile filtered product	Protein (SDS-PAGE*)	Nonadsorbed bulk and final container
Sterility	Thioglycollate medium	Final bulk	Thioglycollate medium	Final bulk
Sterility	Thioglycollate medium	Final container	Thioglycollate medium	Final container
General safety	Guinea pigs and mice	Final container	Guinea pigs and mice	Final container
Pyrogen	LAL‡	Final container	LAL‡	Final container
Purity	Aluminum	Final container	Total protein nitrogen	Final container
	Thimerosal	Final container	Aluminum	Final container
			Thimerosal	Final container
Potency	In vitro relative potency	Final container	Mouse potency	Final container

*SDS-PAGE, sodium dodecyl sulfate–polyacrylamide gel electrophoresis.
†HPSEC, high-performance size exclusion chromatography
‡LAL, limulus amebocyte lysate.

the safety or potency of the product. The only currently approved adjuvants are the aluminum salts, although others have been studied experimentally.

A potency test is applied to each product. The type of test varies depending on the product and is commonly based on studies of immunogenicity or protection from virulent challenge in laboratory animals. However, other in vitro tests can be involved, including virus titration (e.g., live vaccines such as polio, measles, mumps, and rubella), antigen content (e.g., influenza and inactivated poliovirus vaccines), and biochemical and biophysical measurements (e.g., meningococcal polysaccharide vaccines).

For cell culture–produced vaccines, extraneous proteins (e.g., serum or a serum derivative) cannot be present in the final product, or, if serum is used during production to stimulate growth of cultured cells, the calculated concentration in the final medium must not exceed one part per million. Antibiotics, except penicillin (and by analogy the β-lactam class) may be employed during the course of viral vaccine production in cell culture. Those antibiotics most commonly added in low concentrations are neomycin, streptomycin, and polymyxin. If antibiotics are present, the package circular must contain a statement concerning possible allergic reactions.

Other more specific tests designed to provide additional assurance of safety or purity may be required (e.g., neurovirulence testing and cell culture and animal tests for extraneous viruses applied to poliovirus vaccine).

Once the product is licensed, the manufacturer's testing must be conducted according to the exact specifications in the manufacturer's license application and the results of this testing must be within the prescribed limits specified. Tests performed for lot release of hepatitis B vaccines produced using recombinant DNA technology are listed in Table 48–6. Tests of a typical cell culture–produced viral vaccine and a polysaccharide conjugate bacterial vaccine are presented in Tables 48–7 and 48–8, respectively.

For the childhood vaccines covered, the National Childhood Vaccine Injury Act of 1986 (NCVIA) states explicit, extensive record-keeping requirements,[33] including identification of any significant problems encountered in the production, testing, or handling of the product. It also requires the reporting of any safety-test result indicating a health hazard. Any manufacturer of these vaccines who intentionally fails to report significant problems or test failures is subject to civil penalties, fines, or imprisonment.

Adverse Reaction Monitoring

An adverse biological product reaction or experience is defined as an event associated with the use of a biological product, regardless of whether it is considered product related, and any side effect, injury, toxicity, or sensitivity reaction or significant failure of pharmacological action (see Chapter 49 for more detail). Adverse reaction reports come from a variety of sources. The manufacturers of biologicals, the staff of the *United States Pharmacopoeia*, and other health-care professionals are the most common sources, but members of the lay public, including consumers and attorneys, are also free to report. The manufacturers also report data concerning adverse reactions from postmarketing studies, foreign sources, and both published and unpublished scientific literature. The results of reported reactions associated with vaccine use are compiled and entered into the Vaccine Adverse Event Reporting System (VAERS). Health-care providers are required, by the NCVIA, to report certain reactions to products containing diphtheria, tetanus, pertussis, measles, mumps, rubella, and poliomyelitis components. These adverse reaction reports are then entered into this monitoring system. Although compensation for injury after *Haemophilus* b, hepatitis B, and varicella vaccines may now be granted, no specific reporting requirement has been legislated. This list can be expected to be expanded in the future as additional vaccines are mandated for widespread use. The VAERS system is not limited to the listed vaccines; it also accepts voluntary reports of suspected adverse events occurring after administration of any vaccine.

Table 48–7. **TESTING REQUIREMENTS FOR THE RELEASE OF LIVE ORAL POLIOVIRUS VACCINE**

TYPE OF TEST	TEST SYSTEM	STAGE OF PREPARATION
Adventitious agents	Cell cultures*	Production culture fluids collected before virus inoculation
		Control culture fluids collected at time of virus harvest
		Control culture fluids collected 14 days after harvest
		Control cultures hemadsorbed 14 days after harvest
		Monovalent virus pools (prefiltration)
	Animals†	Monovalent virus pools (prefiltration)
	Sterility test media	Monovalent pools (prefiltration)
		Trivalent bulk
	Mycobacterium tuberculosis medium	Monovalent virus pools (prefiltration)
	Mycoplasma media	Monovalent virus pools (prefiltration)
		Control fluids
Safety	Monkeys (neurovirulence test)	Monovalent virus pools (postfiltration)
	In vitro markers	Monovalent virus pools (postfiltration)
	Guinea pigs and mice (toxicity test)	Final containers
Potency	HEp-2 cell cultures cytopathogenic effects (CPE) microassay	Monovalent virus pools (postfiltration)
		Final containers
Identity	Specific serum neutralization	Final containers

*Cell cultures from primary rhesus and *Cercopithecus* monkey kidney, rabbit kidney, human, and BS-C-1 (optional) cell cultures.
†Adult and suckling mice, rabbits, and guinea pigs.

Table 48–8. **TESTING REQUIREMENTS FOR THE RELEASE OF MENINGOCOCCAL POLYSACCHARIDE VACCINES**

TYPE OF TEST	TEST SYSTEM	STAGE OF PREPARATION
Moisture	Thermogravimetric analysis	Individual bulk powders
Purity	Biochemical determination	
	O-acetyl (group A)	Individual bulk powders
	Sialic acid (groups C, Y, W135)	Individual bulk powders
	Phosphorus	Individual bulk powders
	Protein (Lowry)	Individual bulk powders
	Nucleic acids (ultraviolet absorption)	Individual bulk powders
Serological specificity and identity	Rocket immunoelectrophoresis or equivalent method	Individual bulk powders
Quantitation	Polysaccharide content—chemical or immunochemical techniques (e.g., rocket electrophoresis or equivalent method)	Final container
Stabilizer content	Lactose determination	Final container
Pyrogenic substances	Rabbit pyrogen test	Final container
Molecular sizing	Sepharose gel filtration	Final container
Moisture	Thermogravimetric analysis	Final container
General safety	Guinea pigs and mice (toxicity test)	Final container
Adventitious agents	Sterility test media	Final container
Identity	Biochemical or immunochemical procedures (rocket immunoelectrophoresis or equivalent method)	Final container

The NCVIA also mandated the development of vaccine information materials for distribution by healthcare providers to each adult or to the legal representative of each child receiving any of the aforementioned vaccines.[34] This effort was made to ensure that sufficient written information about the risks from the diseases and the risks and benefits of the vaccines be provided.[35] The materials include information on the diseases, vaccine reactions, possible ways to reduce the risk of major adverse reactions, contraindications, information on groups at high risk for vaccination, availability of the National Vaccine Injury Compensation Program (see later), and federal recommendations about immunization schedules. The CBER collaborates with the CDC in the development of this information.

The vaccine information materials provided encourage the reporting of adverse reactions. In the event of a serious reaction or death, the parents or guardians are asked to have their physician or health department report the problem on a Vaccine Adverse Event Report form; if they think the problem was not reported, a toll-free number is provided for their own reporting.

If adverse reaction reports suggest a possible unexpected problem, a field or epidemiological (medical) investigation may be conducted, usually in collaboration with the CDC. In some instances, there may be an FDA field assignment that addresses product integrity and involves interviews with the manufacturer and the collection of records relating to adverse reaction reports as well as production and testing of the particular lot; samples may be collected for further testing by the CBER. The goal in this situation is to determine whether a cause-effect relationship can be established between use of the product and the observed unexpected adverse event. Depending on the extent and seriousness of the problem, a recall, or market withdrawal, of the product might be initiated by the manufacturer or by the CBER, or labeling might be changed to reflect the possible occurrence of a particular adverse reaction. The manufacturer might be requested to perform further testing or to conduct follow-up surveys to ensure that no problems continue to exist.

SPECIAL CONSIDERATIONS

Combination Vaccines

Since the early part of the 20th century, vaccine combinations and the simultaneous separate administration of different vaccines have been important as effective means of enhancing the efficiency of immunization programs. In the United States, combinations of diphtheria and tetanus toxoids, and these toxoids combined with pertussis vaccine, were licensed by the late 1940s. Since that time the number of additional combinations has grown steadily, including the individual types of live and killed poliomyelitis vaccines, the several combinations of measles, mumps, and rubella vaccines, and combinations of *Haemophilus* b conjugate vaccine with DTaP and hepatitis B vaccines. The current success in developing new vaccine products administered in the first years of life has complicated vaccine schedules and has put special pressure on the desire for additional combinations. Products for which this approach might be an option in future combinations include combinations of killed antigens already in use (i.e., *Haemophilus* b, hepatitis A and B, and the polioviruses). Perhaps even new products such as conjugate vaccines against pneumococcal and meningococcal infections might be added.

Among the live vaccines needed early in life are the trivalent oral poliovirus vaccines, measles-mumps-rubella, and varicella. In the future, rotavirus vaccines and perhaps others could be added to this list of products, some of which might be combined.

The manufacturing process and preclinical and clinical studies performed before approval of a new combination vaccine are all intensively scrutinized during product development. Vaccines are complex mixtures that include not only the viral or bacterial antigens but also other components, such as preservatives, adjuvants, stabilizers such as gelatin and sorbitol, and buffers and salts. These components may interact in the final combination. Particular care must be taken to ensure that a preservative that accompanies one component of the combined product does not have a deleterious effect on another component.[36] Similarly, when one or more of the components incorporates an adjuvant, the combination could affect antigen binding. Some of the bound antigen could be lost, or a previously unbound antigen could become adsorbed. Commonly, combinations raise issues related to successful potency, purity, identity, and sterility testing and may require alternative assay strategies. For example, vaccine components may have to be tested at an earlier bulk stage of manufacture rather than in the final container. The presence of adjuvants or residual antibiotics may require that adjustments be made in sterility test procedures.

Although reactions after combination vaccines have not been a major issue, safety needs to be carefully evaluated for each new product. However, it is not uncommon for combinations to unpredictably result in diminished immunogenicity. For example, depressed immune responses especially to *Haemophilus influenzae* type b polysaccharide were seen in one experimental *Haemophilus* b conjugate–acellular pertussis DTP combination.[37]

Interference may also occur with live vaccine combinations. A classic example of this is the interaction between the attenuated Sabin poliovirus strains, type 2 being dominant over types 1 and 3. To obtain seroconversion rates with the trivalent combination comparable to those of the three types given as a series of monovalents, it was necessary to administer sequential doses of trivalent vaccine spaced at 1- to 2-month intervals.[38]

Interactions between live vaccine components in combinations could, in theory, result in less safe progeny viruses. Recombination between attenuated poliovirus types occurs with regularity during multiplication in the human intestine.[39] The relationship of these altered viruses to the rare cases of vaccine-associated paralytic poliomyelitis (approximately one case to 2.4 million doses distributed, or one case to 750,000 children receiving their first dose of oral polio vaccine[40]) remains unclear.

In addition to approved combination vaccines, separate products are commonly administered simultaneously.[41] Reactions after simultaneously administered vaccines may be additive; but generally they have not been shown to be enhanced, although increased rates of systemic reactions have been reported after simultaneous immunization.[42]

Preclinical immunogenicity studies can be very useful in determining the characteristics of antibody induced (subclass, affinity, functionality, epitope recognition). Animal models may be helpful in comparing the responses to the combined product and the individual vaccines. Similarly, an appropriate challenge model can serve to bolster the human data collected later in development.

Whether the components of a new combination product have been previously licensed or not, clinical trials are needed. These studies are ordinarily randomized and controlled by comparisons between the new combination and the individual component or previously licensed combination vaccines. Clinical observations for safety in several thousands of subjects for reactions coupled with laboratory studies of immunogenicity are usually sufficient to assess the safety and effectiveness of the combination. (For additional discussion of these topics see Chapter 20.) Assessing the efficacy of combination vaccines made up of organisms having multiple serotypes (e.g., the pneumococcus) presents a particular challenge. Acceptable evidence for safety and effectiveness of such products has been derived from a combination of a direct showing of clinical effectiveness for the more common serotypes; by inference from immunogenicity using serological correlates from others; and by evidence from functional assays (in the pneumococcal example, opsonic assays).

Product Labeling and Advertising

As noted in earlier sections, in the United States the FDA regulates the format and content of labels for product containers and packages and the circulars that accompany them (package inserts). Promotional labeling and advertising are also regulated by the FDA using the same standards.

The initial labeling for a new vaccine is reviewed through the product licensing process described earlier. During this review, in addition to the draft labeling and clinical studies submitted by the manufacturer, the agency pays special attention to discussions of appropriate use for the product held by several non-FDA advisory groups, including the American Academy of Pediatrics' Committee on Infectious Diseases (the "Redbook Committee") and the CDC's committee, the ACIP.

Subsequently, significant changes in labeling, including new indications for use, new dosage forms or regimens, expanded patient populations who receive the product, and additional information regarding safety and effectiveness require that the manufacturer submit a supplemental filing for CBER review and approval.

All of these materials are reviewed to determine that they are not false and misleading, that is, that they comport with the scientific data the manufacturer developed in the application and data acquired subsequent to product approval. Unlike other product labeling, the promotional labeling and advertising are not subject to preclearance; however, they are similarly monitored for misleading claims. These documents must also meet the standard of "fair balance," that is, that claims of efficacy would be balanced with information about the product's adverse effects.

CONCLUSION

The regulatory agency, along with the vaccine manufacturer and the scientific community as a whole, must struggle with novel issues as they arise during the development of each new vaccine. New vaccine candidates must be evaluated using a blend of knowledge from the past and the best of current science in assessing their risks and benefits. The burden of these decisions is heavy, because vaccines are most often given to well individuals, commonly children. The risk-benefit ratio must be characterized by low risk and high benefit.

The effort to provide safe and effective vaccines is always fraught with a degree of uncertainty. As an example, today, follow-up of recipients of poliovirus vaccines extends only for 35 years (for live oral) to 42 years (for killed). Even after this period of use experience has elapsed, questions about the safety of these vaccines are currently debated. They probably will continue to be posed even after the disease which they were fashioned to prevent has been eradicated.

Acting on a broad scientific consensus after thorough review has been the mainstay of the effort to provide safe and effective vaccines. Although our knowledge is always imperfect, it is heartening that the experience with current vaccines has been overwhelmingly positive. The goal of disease eradication has been achieved in one instance, with the conquering of smallpox, and seems to be within near reach for poliomyelitis. It is within our present capability to extend this accomplishment to other infectious diseases through application of our current methods. Today's new technologies seem to presage an even brighter future.

Acknowledgments

We acknowledge Norman Baylor, Ph.D., Karen Chaitkin, Victoria Howard, and Mark Raza for their assistance in preparing sections of this manuscript and for their review and constructive comments.

REFERENCES

1. D'Arcy PF, Harron DWG. Proceedings of the First International Conference on Harmonization, Brussels, 1991. Antrim, Northern Ireland, Greystone Books, 1992.
2. Kondratas RA. Death helped write the biologics law. FDA Consumer 16:23–25, 1982.
3. Division of Biologics Standards, National Institutes of Health. Legislative History of the Regulation of Biological Products, 2nd printing, January 1968.
4. Public Health Service Act, July 1, 1944, Chap. 373, Title III, Sec. 351, 58 Stat. 702, currently codified at 42 U.S.C., Sec. 262.
5. Public Health Service Act, July 1, 1944, Chap. 373, Title III, Sec. 352, 58 Stat. 702, currently codified at 42 U.S.C., Sec. 263.
6. Paul JR. A history of poliomyelitis. New Haven, CT, Yale University Press, 1971.
7. Code of Federal Regulations, Title 21, Food and Drugs. Washington, DC, US Government Printing Office, 1997.
8. Code of Federal Regulations, Title 21, Part 211. Washington, DC, US Government Printing Office, 1997.
9. Code of Federal Regulations, Title 21, Sec. 600.3. Washington, DC, US Government Printing Office, 1997.
10. Vaccine Safety Committee Report, Institute of Medicine. Adverse Events Associated with Childhood Vaccines: Evidence Bearing on Causality. Stratton KR, Howe CJ, Johnston RB Jr (eds). National Academy Press, Washington, DC, 1994, p 230.
11. Code of Federal Regulations, Title 21, Sec. 601. 25(d)(2). Washington, DC, US Government Printing Office, 1997.
12. 5 United States Code, Sec. 551 et seq.
13. Code of Federal Regulations, Title 21, Part 312. Washington, DC, US Government Printing Office, 1997.
14. Code of Federal Regulations, Title 21, Part 50. Washington, DC, US Government Printing Office, 1997.
15. Code of Federal Regulations, Title 21, Part 56. Washington, DC, US Government Printing Office, 1997.
16. Code of Federal Regulations, Title 21, Part 58. Washington, DC, US Government Printing Office, 1997.
17. Code of Federal Regulations, Title 21, Secs. 601.10, 601.20. Washington, DC, US Government Printing Office, 1997.
18. Code of Federal Regulations, Title 21, Sec. 601.12. Washington, DC, US Government Printing Office, 1997.
19. Code of Federal Regulations, Title 21, Secs. 601.5, 601.6. Washington, DC, US Government Printing Office, 1997.
20. Fox JP, Lennette EH, Manso C, Souza Aguiar JR. Encephalitis in man following vaccination with 17D yellow fever virus. Am J Hyg 36:117–142, 1942.
21. Fox JP, Manso C, Penna HA, Parà M. Observations on the occurrence of icterus in Brazil following vaccination against yellow fever. Am J Hyg 36:68–116, 1942.
22. Brown F, Esber EC, Williams MH (eds). Continuous Cell Lines—An International Workshop on Current Issues. Dev Biol Stand 76:1–368, 1992.
23. World Health Organization Technical Report Series 747, Report of a WHO Study Group: Acceptability of Cell Substrates for Production of Biologicals. Geneva, World Health Organization, 1987.
24. Mortimer EA Jr, Lepow ML, Gold E, et al. Long-term follow-up of persons inadvertently inoculated with SV40 as neonates. N Engl J Med 305:1517–1518, 1981.
25. Waters TD, Anderson PS Jr, Beebe GW, Miller RW. Yellow fever vaccination, avian leucosis virus, and cancer risk in man. Science 177:76–77, 1972.
26. Lewis AM Jr, Egan W. Workshop on simian virus 40 (SV40): A possible human polyomavirus. Biologicals 25:355–358, 1997.
27. WHO Expert Committee on Biological Standardization. Highlights of the 45th Meeting. Weekly Epidemiologic Record. Geneva, World Health Organization, April 5, 1996.
28. Marwick, C. BSE sets agenda for imported gelatin. JAMA 227:1659–1660, 1997.
29. Points to Consider, Production and Testing of New Drugs and Biologicals Produced by Recombinant DNA Technology. Congressional, Consumer, and International Affairs Staff (HFB-142), Rockville, MD, 1985.
30. Points to Consider, Supplement to Production and Testing of New Drugs and Biologicals Produced by Recombinant DNA Technology, Nucleic Acid Characterization and Genetic Stability. Congressional, Consumer, and International Affairs Staff (HFB-142), Rockville, MD, 1990.
31. Points to Consider, in the Production and Testing of New Drugs and Biologicals Produced by Recombinant DNA Technology: Nucleic Acid Characterization and Genetic Stability. Congressional, Consumer, and International Affairs Staff (HFB-142), Rockville, MD, 1992.
32. Code of Federal Regulations, Title 21, Secs. 610.10–610.18. Washington, DC, US Government Printing Office, 1997.
33. United States Code, Sec. 300aa-28.
34. 42 United States Code, Sec. 300Aa-26.
35. New Vaccine Information Materials. Federal Register. Vol 59, No. 117, p 31888, 1994.
36. Pittman M. Instability of pertussis-vaccine component in quadruple antigen vaccine. JAMA 181:25–30, 1962.
37. Eskola J, Ölander RM, Hovi T, et al. Randomized trial of the effect of co-administration with acellular pertussis DTP vaccine on immunogenicity of *Haemophilus influenzae* type b conjugate vaccine. Lancet 348:1688–1692, 1996.
38. Sabin AB. Recent studies and field tests with a live attenuated poliovirus vaccine. In Live Poliovirus Vaccines: Papers Presented and Discussions Held at the First International Conference on Live Poliovirus Vaccines. Pan American Sanitary Bureau (special publication No. 44). Washington, DC, 1959.
39. Minor PD. Review article: The molecular biology of poliovaccines. J Gen Virol 73:3065–3077, 1992.
40. Recommendations of the Advisory Committee on Immunization Practices (ACIP). Poliomyelitis prevention in the United States: Introduction of a sequential vaccination schedule of inactivated poliovirus vaccine followed by oral poliovirus vaccine. MMWR 46:RR-3, 1997.
41. Recommendatons of the Advisory Committee on Immunization Practices (ACIP). General recommendations on immunization. MMWR 43:RR-1, 1994.
42. Olin P, Rasmussen F, Gottfarb P. Schedules and protection, simultaneous vaccination and safety: Experiences from recent controlled trials. Int J Infect Dis 1:143–147, 1997.

chapter

49 Safety of Vaccines

Robert T. Chen

Immunizations are among the most cost-effective and widely used public health interventions.[1] No vaccine is perfectly safe or effective,[2] however. As the incidence of vaccine-preventable diseases is reduced by increasing coverage with an efficacious vaccine, vaccine adverse events, both those caused by vaccines (i.e., *true* adverse reactions) and those associated with vaccination only by coincidence, become increasingly frequent and prominent (Fig. 49–1).[3] The number of both types of reports to the Vaccine Adverse Event Reporting System (VAERS) in the United States, approximately 10,000 per year, now exceeds the reported incidence of most vaccine-preventable childhood diseases combined (Table 49–1).

In such maturing immunization programs, close monitoring and timely assessment of suspected vaccine adverse events are critical to prevent loss of confidence, decreased vaccine coverage, and return of epidemic disease,[3, 4] as experienced with several countries for pertussis.[5] Similar concerns in the United States during the early 1980s led to substantial increases in the number of lawsuits and price of vaccines, the loss of vaccine manufacturers,[6] and the potential deterrence to the development of new vaccines.[7] In developing countries, the safety concerns are weighted toward inadequate control of vaccine production and programmatic errors, such as inadequate sterilization of injection equipment leading to transmission of bloodborne pathogens.[8] As nations in both developed and developing countries reach high vaccine coverages and lower their rates of vaccine-preventable diseases, vaccine safety issues may threaten the stability of their programs.[9] Accordingly the World Health Organization's (WHO)[10] *Expanded Programme on Immunization* (EPI) recommended in 1991 that all national programs implement surveillance for adverse events after immunizations.[11]

Recommendations for use of vaccines represent a dynamic balancing of risks and benefits. Vaccine safety monitoring is necessary to weigh this balance accurately. When diseases are close to eradication, data on complications secondary to vaccine relative to that of disease may lead to discontinuation or decreased use of the vaccine, as was done with smallpox vaccine[12] and with the shift to either inactivated polio[13] or sequential inactivated/live oral polio vaccine (OPV) schedules.[14] Few other vaccine-preventable diseases are likely to be eradicated in the near future, however. Most immunizations will therefore be needed indefinitely, with their attendant adverse reactions and potential for loss of public confidence. Research in vaccine safety can help to distinguish true vaccine reactions from coincidental events[15, 16]; estimate their attributable risk[17, 18]; identify risk factors that may permit development of valid contraindications[17, 19]; and, if the pathophysiological mechanism becomes known, develop safer vaccines.[20–23] Equally important, such research demonstrates a commitment to reducing disease from all causes, vaccine-preventable and vaccine-induced, and may help to maintain public confidence in immunizations and the credibility of immunization programs.

Despite two centuries of vaccinations, however, "substantial gaps and limitations" exist in knowledge and research infrastructure for vaccine safety.[2, 15, 16] Traditional prelicensure trials and passive surveillance have had limited utility in filling such gaps. Supplemental vaccine safety monitoring systems are only beginning to be developed.[18, 24, 25] In the meantime, vaccine safety remains a controversial issue.[26] If immunization programs are to take full advantage of the new vaccines made possible by biotechnology,[27] a Hippocratic willingness is required to understand both the risks and the benefits of immunizations. This chapter summarizes key policy and methodological issues on vaccine safety.

Table 49–1. **COMPARISON OF MAXIMUM AND CURRENT MORBIDITY, VACCINE-PREVENTABLE DISEASES**

	MAXIMUM CASES (YEAR)	1997	PERCENT CHANGE
Diphtheria	206,939 (1921)	5	−99.99
Measles	894,134 (1941)	135	−99.98
Mumps	152,209 (1968)	612	−99.60
Pertussis	265,269 (1934)	5519	−97.92
Polio (paralytic)*	21,269 (1952)	0	−100.00
Rubella	57,686 (1969)	161	−99.72
Congenital rubella syndrome	20,000† (1964–65)	4	−99.98
Tetanus‡	1560‡ (1923)	43	−97.24
H. influenzae, invasive disease (<5 yr)	20,000† (1984)	242§	−98.79
Vaccine adverse events		11,365	‖

*Wild virus caused.
†Estimated.
‡Deaths in 1923; cases in 1997.
§Includes invasive disease due to non–type b *H. influenzae*.
‖In contrast to disease reductions, adverse events have increased from 0 prevaccine to 11,365 in 1997.
Data from MMWR Morbid Mortal Wkly Rep 46:1265–1269, 1997, and the Vaccine Adverse Event Reporting System.

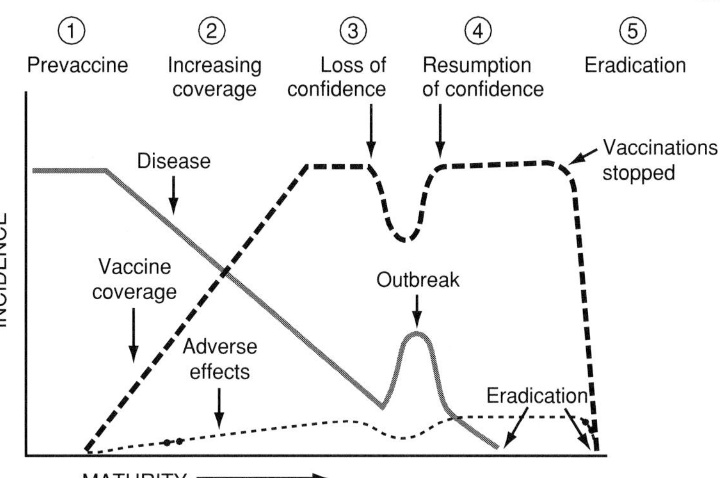

Figure 49–1. Evolution of immunization program and prominence of vaccine safety.

IMPORTANCE OF VACCINE SAFETY—FIRST DO NO HARM

A higher standard of safety is generally expected of vaccines than other medical interventions. In contrast to most pharmaceutical products, which are administered to ill people for curative purposes, vaccines are generally given to healthy people to prevent disease. Tolerance of adverse reactions to products given to healthy people—especially healthy infants—is substantially lower than to products administered to people who are already sick.[2] This lower risk tolerance for vaccines translates into a need to investigate the possible causes of much rarer adverse events after vaccinations than would be acceptable for other pharmaceutical products. For example, events occurring at approximately $1/10^5$ to $1/10^6$ doses (e.g., acute encephalopathy after whole-cell pertussis vaccine,[15, 17] Guillain-Barré syndrome [GBS] after swine influenza vaccine,[28] and OPV-associated paralytic polio[14]) are of concern for vaccinees, whereas side effects are essentially universal for cancer chemotherapy, and 10 to 30% of people on high-dose aspirin therapy experience gastrointestinal symptoms.[29]

The cost and the difficulty of studying events increase with their rarity, however. Furthermore, studies of rare events are less likely to provide definitive conclusions, while engendering much controversy. Attributable risks on the order of 1 per 10^5 to 1 per 10^6 are on the margin of resolution for epidemiological methods.[15, 30] Perhaps not surprisingly, the bulk of the published literature on vaccine safety to date has been in the form of case reports and case series rather than controlled studies with adequate power.[15, 16] To assess the possible association between pertussis vaccination and encephalopathy, the British organized a large case-control study.[17, 31] They enrolled all children 2 to 35 months of age in England, Scotland, and Wales who were hospitalized for a variety of neurological illnesses during a 36-month period (n = 1167). The finding of a significant association between vaccine and permanent brain damage was based on only seven exposed cases, however.[32] The validity of this study finding generated much controversy in and out of the courts.[15, 33] Despite considerably more robust data linking GBS with the swine influenza vaccine,[28] subsequent controversy[34, 35] resulted in a court-ordered independent reexamination of the data[36] and, ultimately, partial redo of the study confirming the initial findings.[37]

A higher standard of safety is also required of vaccines because of the large number of people who are exposed to vaccines, frequently on a compulsory basis for public health reasons.[38] The medical maxim "first do no harm" may apply even more in public health than in clinical medicine, where decisions affect fewer people. Inadequately inactivated polio vaccine was administered to about 400,000 people in the "Cutter incident," resulting in 260 polio cases.[39] There have been other incidents similar in tragedy if not in scope as a result of errors in production.[2] Concerns that polio vaccine contaminated by simian virus 40 may have been received by millions of people during the 1950s[40] and some vaccines may have contained gelatin stabilizers produced in cattle infected with bovine spongiform encephalopathy[41] further highlight the importance of ensuring the safety of relatively universal human-directed *exposures* like immunizations. These concerns are the basis for strict regulatory control of vaccines by the Food and Drug Administration (FDA),[42] for example, by banning use of bovine-derived products from countries with bovine spongiform encephalopathy.[41]

High standards of accuracy and timeliness are needed for vaccine safety studies because they have extremely narrow margins for error. In contrast to many classes of drugs for which other effective therapy may be substituted, vaccines generally have few alternative strains or types (oral and inactivated poliovirus vaccines being the best-known exception). The decision to withdraw a vaccine or switch between strains may also have wide ramifications. The circumstances surrounding the use and withdrawal of the 1976 "swine influenza" vaccine have been extensively documented,[34] as has the controversy surrounding the safety of whole-cell pertussis vaccines.[5] In 1992, the United Kingdom withdrew the license of mumps vaccines containing the Urabe strain after studies suggested a high rate of vaccine-associated meningitis.[43] The manufacturers subsequently withdrew this product worldwide. This left the countries where the Urabe strain had been the sole mumps vaccine licensed without an alternative vaccine.[44, 45] Therefore establishing associations of adverse events with vaccines and promptly defining the attributable risks are critical in placing adverse events in the proper risk-benefit perspective. An erroneous association or attributable risk can undermine confidence in a vaccine and have disastrous consequences for vaccine acceptance and disease incidence. However, denials of association despite accumulating evidence can backfire.[45, 46]

Finally, because many vaccinations are mandated for public health reasons and because no vaccine is perfectly safe, several countries have established compensation programs for people who may have been injured by vaccination.[47] Accurate assessment of whether adverse events can be caused by specific vaccines is essential to a fair, efficient vaccine injury compensation program.[48]

GAPS AND LIMITATIONS IN KNOWLEDGE OF VACCINE SAFETY

In 1967, the lack of scientific documentation of the risks of immunization moved Wilson,[2] former director of the Public Health Laboratory Service in the United Kingdom, to compile the first such review. He noted fear of compensation claims and inadvertent support for *anti-vaccinationists* as possible explanations for the incomplete record. Pursuant to the National Childhood Vaccine Injury Act of 1986, a Committee of the Institute of Medicine (IOM) in the United States was established to review the adverse consequences of childhood vaccines. This group still found severe limits in the knowledge and research capability on vaccine safety.[15, 16] For 50 (66%) of the 76 adverse events reviewed, there was either no or inadequate scientific evidence to judge for or against a causal link to vaccine. Specifically the IOM committee identified the following limitations: (1) inadequate understanding of biological mechanisms underlying adverse events, (2) insufficient or inconsistent information from case reports and case series, (3) inadequate size or length of follow-up of many population-based epidemiological studies, (4) limitations of existing surveillance systems to provide persuasive evidence of causation, and (5) few experimental studies published relative to the total number of epidemiological studies published.[15, 16]

Other factors may have also contributed to the scarcity of knowledge about vaccine safety. Vaccine safety research requires expertise in pharmacoepidemiology and *rare disease* epidemiology,[49] with its special set of methodological challenges.[50–52] Such studies are costly and difficult to organize, and the methods may be less familiar to most immunization experts with primary infectious disease background. Furthermore, interest and resource allocation for vaccine safety research have been severely handicapped by all too common characterization in narrow, negative terms of *adverse events* research (vs. larger, positive concepts of ensuring *vaccine safety*)—especially when competing against the positive *benefits and efficacy* side of vaccine research. Finally, similar to other areas of safety (e.g., blood, food, transport), vaccine safety cannot be studied directly but can be only inferred by the sum of its inverse: an absence of specific problems when appropriate surveillance and risk management systems are in place. This approach requires a systematic accumulation of *negative* findings, which may be more difficult to publish than *positive* findings. Scientifically, it is also more challenging to prove than disprove a concept, especially proving a negative concept.[53]

The IOM concluded that "if research capacity and accomplishments [are] not improved, future reviews of vaccine safety [will be] similarly handicapped." Although much remains to be done, much progress has been made in the last few years toward understanding these gaps and ameliorating the infrastructure to improve vaccine safety research.[3, 4, 18, 24, 25, 55, 56]

METHODS OF MONITORING SAFETY

Prelicensure

Vaccines, similar to other pharmaceutical products, undergo extensive safety and efficacy evaluations in the laboratory, in animals, and in phased human clinical trials before licensure.[42] *Phase 1* trials usually include fewer than 20 participants and can detect only extremely common adverse events. *Phase 2* trials generally enroll 50 to several hundred people. When carefully coordinated, as in the comparative infant diphtheria, tetanus, and acellular pertussis (DTaP) trials, important conclusions, such as the relationship between concentration of antigen, number of vaccine components, formulation technique, effect of successive doses, and profile of common reactions (i.e., *reactogenicity*), can be drawn. Such studies can affect the choice of the candidate vaccine chosen for *phase 3*.[57, 58] Sample sizes for phase 3 vaccine trials are principally based on efficacy considerations. Inferences on safety are drawn to the extent possible based on the sample size (approximately 10^2–10^5) and the duration of observation (often <30 days).[57] This usually means that only observations of common local and systemic reactions (e.g., injection site swelling, fever, fussiness) have been possible. Because of the *experimental* design of most phase 1 to 3 clinical trials, which (1) include a placebo group comparable to the vaccine group and (2) detect adverse events in a blinded fashion because neither physicians nor recipients know what they received, inferences on the causal relationship of an adverse event with the vaccine from such trials are relatively straightforward.[49]

Better standardization of safety evaluations in phase 3 trials is still needed so that safety data across trials and vaccines can be compared. In the phase 3 trials for infant DTaP, a standard case definition ironically was developed for efficacy but not for safety—the main reason for the development of DTaP.[59] For example, definitions of high fever across trials varied by the temperature (39.5 vs. 40.5°C), the mode of measurement (oral vs. rectal), and time after vaccination measured (48 vs. 72 hours).[60] Major differences in detected rates of hypotonic-hyporesponsive episodes after the same whole-cell pertussis vaccine used in the Swedish and Italian trials highlight the difficulty of standardizing assessment of rarer events across cultures and health systems, however.[61] The finding of delayed excess mortality in some recipients of high-titer measles vaccine has also raised difficult questions about design of future vaccine trials.[62, 63] Given the need to appreciate better safety of vaccines administered universally to healthy infants and the methodological difficulties of assessing safety postlicensure, some have argued that larger experimental trials to better assess vaccine safety prelicensure may be needed.[51, 64]

Fundamental to preventing safety problems is ensuring that any vaccines used are made under good manufacturing practices with prerelease lot testing for safety and potency.[42, 65] This evaluation usually occurs in parallel to the clinical trials before vaccine licensure. Immunization staff also need to be trained in appropriate vaccine storage, handling, and safe injection practices.[8]

Postlicensure

Because rare reactions, reactions with delayed onset, or reactions in subpopulations may not be detected before vaccines are licensed, postlicensure (also called postmarketing) evaluation of vaccine safety is critical. Historically, this evaluation has relied on passive surveillance and ad hoc epidemiological studies. More recently, phase 4 trials and preestablished large-linked databases (LLDBs) have been added to improve methodological capabilities to study rare risks of specific immunizations.[49] Variation in rates of adverse events (and immunogenicity) by manufacturer[66, 67] or even lot might be possible.[68] Postlicensure surveillance systems may detect potential manufacturer and lot-specific aberrations in a timely manner.

In contrast to the elegance of prelicensure randomized trials, however, postlicensure *observational* studies of vaccine safety pose a formidable set of methodological difficulties.[51, 52] Observational studies, for example, are prone to ascertainment bias because individuals are more likely to attribute any illness to a vaccine the more recently they have been vaccinated. *Confounding by contraindication* is also especially difficult to control for in nonexperimental designs; individuals who do not receive vaccine (e.g., because of contraindication or low socioeconomic group) may have a different risk for an adverse event than vaccinated individuals (e.g., background rates of seizures or sudden infant death syndrome may be higher in the unvaccinated). Teasing this issue out requires understanding of the complex interactions of multiple, poorly quantified factors.[51]

Passive Surveillance (Spontaneous Reporting Systems)

Informal or formal *passive surveillance or spontaneous reporting systems* (SRS) have been the cornerstone of most vaccine safety monitoring systems because of their relative low cost of operations.[69, 70] The national reporting of vaccine adverse events can be done through the same reporting channels as those used for other adverse drug reactions,[70] as is the practice in France,[71] New Zealand,[72] Sweden,[73] and the United Kingdom.[74] An increasing number of countries are collecting safety data specific to vaccinations either with reporting forms or surveillance systems different from the drug safety monitoring systems. These countries include Australia,[75] Canada,[4, 76] Denmark,[77] India,[78] Italy,[79] Mexico,[80] Netherlands,[81] Sao Paulo State in Brazil,[82] and the United States.[3] Vaccine manufacturers also maintain SRS for their products, which are usually forwarded subsequently to appropriate national regulatory authorities.[42, 80]

Because of their importance in infectious disease control, a significant proportion of vaccines in many countries are purchased or administered by national public health authorities. For example, the public sector (federal, state, and local governments), in coordination with the Centers for Disease Control and Prevention (CDC), purchases more than half of the childhood vaccines administered in the United States. In many developing countries, the Ministry of Health in conjunction with WHO's EPI administer almost all vaccines. Potential vaccine adverse events commonly are first reported to the healthcare providers who administered the vaccine. In many countries, such healthcare workers also participate in surveillance for other diseases. These health authorities (e.g., CDC) therefore commonly lead or collaborate with the vaccine licensure and regulatory agency (e.g., FDA) in developing vaccine adverse event reporting systems. A similar model is followed in Canada.[76]

U.S. Experience

The National Childhood Vaccine Injury Act of 1986 mandated for the first time that healthcare providers report certain adverse events after immunizations (see Table 50–1).[83] VAERS was implemented jointly by the CDC and FDA in 1990 to provide a unified national focus for collection of all reports of clinically significant adverse events, including, but not limited to, those mandated for reporting.[3] The creation of VAERS also provided an opportunity to correct some shortcomings of the predecessors, the CDC Monitoring System for Adverse Events Following Immunizations (MSAEFI) and the FDA Adverse Drug Reaction System.[84]

To increase sensitivity, the VAERS form is designed to permit narrative descriptions of adverse events (Fig. 49–2). All people, including patients or their parents (as of 1998, <5% of VAERS reports come from parents) and not just healthcare professionals, are permitted to report to VAERS, especially clinically significant events. There are no restrictions set on interval between vaccination and onset of illness or that a patient have medical care to be reported. Annual reminders about VAERS are mailed to physicians likely to administer vaccines. The form is preaddressed and postage paid so that after completion it can be folded and mailed. Report forms, assistance in completing the form, or answers to other questions about VAERS are available by calling a 24-hour toll-free telephone number (1-800-822-7967).

A contractor, under CDC and FDA supervision, dis-

VAERS

VACCINE ADVERSE EVENT REPORTING SYSTEM
24 Hour Toll-free information line 1-800-822-7967
P.O. Box 1100, Rockville, MD 20849-1100
PATIENT IDENTITY KEPT CONFIDENTIAL

For CDC/FDA Use Only
VAERS Number ______
Date Received ______

Patient Name: ______
Last First M.I.
Address ______
City State Zip
Telephone no. (____)______

Vaccine administered by (Name): ______
Responsible Physician ______
Facility Name/Address ______
City State Zip
Telephone no. (____)______

Form completed by (Name): ______
Relation to Patient ☐ Vaccine Provider ☐ Patient/Parent ☐ Manufacturer ☐ Other
Address *(if different from patient or provider)* ______
City State Zip
Telephone no. (____)______

1. State
2. County where administered
3. Date of birth __/__/__ mm dd yy
4. Patient age
5. Sex ☐ M ☐ F
6. Date form completed __/__/__ mm dd yy

7. Describe adverse event(s) (symptoms, signs, time course) and treatment, if any

8. Check all appropriate:
☐ Patient died (date __/__/__) mm dd yy
☐ Life threatening illness
☐ Required emergency room/doctor visit
☐ Required hospitalization (______days)
☐ Resulted in prolongation of hospitalization
☐ Resulted in permanent disability
☐ None of the above

9. Patient recovered ☐ YES ☐ NO ☐ UNKNOWN

10. Date of vaccination __/__/__ mm dd yy Time ______ AM PM

11. Adverse event onset __/__/__ mm dd yy Time ______ AM PM

12. Relevant diagnostic tests/laboratory data

13. Enter all vaccines given on date listed in no. 10

	Vaccine (type)	Manufacturer	Lot number	Route/Site	No. Previous doses
a.					
b.					
c.					
d.					

14. Any other vaccinations within 4 weeks prior to the date listed in no. 10

	Vaccine (type)	Manufacturer	Lot number	Route/Site	No. Previous doses	Date given
a.						
b.						

15. Vaccinated at:
☐ Private doctor's office/hospital ☐ Military clinic/hospital
☐ Public health clinic/hospital ☐ Other/unknown

16. Vaccine purchased with:
☐ Private funds ☐ Military funds
☐ Public funds ☐ Other /unknown

17. Other medications

18. Illness at time of vaccination (specify)

19. Pre-existing physician-diagnosed allergies, birth defects, medical conditions (specify)

20. Have you reported this adverse event previously? ☐ No ☐ To health department ☐ To doctor ☐ To manufacturer

Only for children 5 and under

22. Birth weight ____ lb. ____ oz.

23. No. of brothers and sisters

21. Adverse event following prior vaccination (check all applicable, specify)

	Adverse Event	Onset Age	Type Vaccine	Dose no. in series
☐ In patient				
☐ In brother or sister				

Only for reports submitted by manufacturer/immunization project

24. Mfr. / imm. proj. report no.

25. Date received by mfr. / imm. proj.

26. 15 day report? ☐ Yes ☐ No

27. Report type ☐ Initial ☐ Follow-Up

Health care providers and manufacturers are required by law (42 USC 300aa-25) to report reactions to vaccines listed in the Table of Reportable Events Following Immunization. Reports for reactions to other vaccines are voluntary except when required as a condition of immunization grant awards.

Form VAERS -1

Figure 49–2. The Vaccine Adverse Event Reporting System (VAERS) form.

tributes, collects, codes (using the Coding Symbols for a Thesaurus of Adverse Reaction Terms [COSTART]),[85] and enters VAERS reports in a database. Reporters of selected serious events receive written requests from VAERS (60 days after vaccination and 1 year after vaccination) for information about the patient's recovery. CDC and FDA have on-line access to the VAERS database and focus their efforts on analytical tasks of interest to the respective agencies. These data (without personal identifiers) are also available to the public. Since its inception in late 1990, approximately 10,000 VAERS reports have been received annually, 20% of which are defined as serious (death, life-threatening illness, disability, hospitalization) (Table 49–2).[86] Because of this volume, follow-up by a healthcare professional currently occurs on all reports of deaths and only selected serious events of interest.

Other National Experiences

Several other countries also have substantial experience with passive surveillance for vaccine safety. In 1987, Canada developed the Vaccine Associated Adverse Event (VAAE) reporting system.[76, 87] Reporting forms have checkoff boxes for specific events with accompanying case definitions. Provision is also made for *another* category. To supplement the VAAE, an active, pediatric hospital-based surveillance system that searches all admissions for possible relationships to immunizations known as *Immunization Monitoring Program—Active* (IMPACT) has been operational since 1990.[25] An Advisory Committee on Causality Assessment consisting of a panel of experts has also been formed to review the serious VAAE reports.[88] The Netherlands also convenes an annual panel to categorize their reports, which are then published.[81] The United Kingdom and most members of the former Commonwealth use the *yellow card* system, whereby a reporting form is attached to officially issued prescription pads.[70, 74] Data on adverse drug (including vaccine) events from about 40 nations are compiled by the WHO Collaborating Center for International Drug Monitoring in Uppsala.[89] Preliminary efforts are also underway to *harmonize* collection of postlicensure safety data across nations.[90]

A field guide for implementation of monitoring of

Table 49–2. **DISTRIBUTION OF REPORTS TO THE VACCINE ADVERSE EVENT REPORTING SYSTEM (VAERS), 1991 TO 1997**

YEAR	NET DOSES DISTRIBUTED (IN MILLIONS)	TOTAL REPORTS	SERIOUS REPORTS EXCLUDING DEATHS*	DEATH REPORTS*
1991	124	10,362	1095	163
1992	134	11,274	1127	225
1993	141	10,822	1087	227
1994	164	11,004	1189	226
1995	147	10,899	1120	140
1996	147	11,726	1006	128
1997	156	11,365	988	137

*Excluding duplicate and foreign reports.

Adverse Events Following Immunizations (AEFI) has been developed by the WHO EPI.[10] The primary focus is on detection of correctable programmatic errors, such as injection site abscesses (suggestive of inadequate sterilization), and development of a rapid response and assessment team for clusters of more serious events (e.g., toxic shock syndrome from contamination of vaccine vials[78] or deaths from confusing other medications for vaccines[9]). As of 1997, however, only 12 (14%) of 88 national EPIs had such a system in place.[65]

Classifications, Case Definitions, and Evaluative Protocols

Vaccine adverse events can be classified by frequency (common, rare), extent (local, systemic), severity (hospitalization, disability, death), causality, and preventability (intrinsic to vaccine, faulty production, faulty administration). Wilson[2] developed the first classification system with a focus on errors of production (e.g., bacterial, viral, toxin contamination) and administration (e.g., nonsterile apparatus). A more recent classification divides adverse events after vaccinations into[91, 92] (1) *vaccine-induced*—due to the intrinsic characteristic of the vaccine preparation and the individual response of the vaccinee; these events would not have occurred without vaccination (e.g., vaccine-associated paralytic poliomyeltis); (2) *vaccine-potentiated*—would have occurred anyway, but were precipitated by the vaccination (e.g., first febrile seizure in a predisposed child); (3) *programmatic error*—due to technical errors in vaccine preparation, handling, or administration; (4) *coincidental*—associated temporally with vaccination by chance or due to underlying illness.

Definitions of certain vaccine adverse events have been developed in Brazil,[82] Canada,[93] India,[78] and the Netherlands.[81] To improve comparability of data across reporting systems, the Workshop on Standardization of Definitions for Post-Marketing Surveillance of Adverse Vaccine Reactions was held in October 1991. Definitions for approximately 20 local, central nervous system, and other adverse reactions were adopted by the workshop participants.[93] These case definitions are printed on the Canadian VAAE form as guidance for what should be reported. The proportion of VAAE reports meeting the case definition criteria has increased from 69 to 87%.[87] Alternatively, in a more open reporting system such as VAERS, these definitions can be applied to reports to develop a case series for further investigation.

Because the simultaneous administration of vaccines is common and multiple adverse events may be reported, the Dutch system further classifies reports as (1) *simple*—a single vaccine injection and a single major reaction; (2) *compound*—a single vaccine injection and more than one major reaction (each major reaction is counted separately); (3) *multiple*—more than one vaccine injection in the same person and one major reaction; or (4) *compound-multiple*—more than one vaccine injection in the same person and more than one major reaction.[81]

To improve the quality of SRS data further and maximize its utility as a potential disease registry, protocols for the clinical evaluation of selected reported serious events of interest (e.g., deaths) can be developed. Such protocols could then be sent to the physicians who report such events to help standardize the evaluation of these patients. In time, a *case series* might then be available for further review that might aid understanding of the event.

Assessment of Causality

The formal process of assessing causality of an adverse event and an exposure (e.g., vaccine) is a complex process that can be considered in terms of the answers to three questions: (1) *Can It?* (2) *Did It?* (3) *Will It?*[94, 95] The answer to *Can It?* was the focus of the IOM reviews.[15, 16] It is usually based on population-level inferences drawn from epidemiological studies and the following considerations: (1) strength of association, (2) analytical bias, (3) biological gradient and dose-response, (4) statistical significance, (5) consistency, and (6) biological plausibility and coherence.[96]

For individual case reports, the *Did It?* question is more relevant. If the answer is yes, then *Can It?* is also answered in the affirmative. It is natural to suspect vaccine to be the cause when an adverse event occurs in temporal association after vaccination. To base causal inference purely on temporal association, however, is to fall for the logical fallacy of *post hoc ergo propter hoc* ("after this, therefore because of this").[16] Information useful for assessing causality in individual case reports includes (1) previous general experience with vaccine (e.g., duration of licensure, number of vaccinees, similar events observed among other vaccinees or nonvaccinees, existence of animal models to test vaccine as a cause); (2) alternative causes; (3) individual characteristics of the vaccinee that may increase the risk of the adverse event; (4) timing of events; (5) characteristics of the event (e.g., laboratory findings); and (6) rechallenge.[94, 95]

When a vaccine *can* cause an adverse event, the *Will It?* refers to the probability that an individual will experience the event or, for populations, the proportion that will experience it (i.e., the attributable risk). These data are critical for developing risk-benefit policy decisions for the population and valid contraindications for the individuals at high risk. The *Will It?* is usually difficult to answer, however, because it can be answered only on the basis of epidemiological studies.[16] Furthermore, the sample sizes of such studies may be large enough to establish whether vaccine can cause a given event yet inadequate to stratify by subgroups to examine risk factors that can help delineate potential contraindications.

Specific adverse events can usually be said to be caused by a specific vaccine if the event is associated with a unique (1) laboratory finding or (2) clinical syndrome. For example, Urabe mumps vaccine virus was implicated as a cause of aseptic meningitis because mumps virus isolated from the cerebrospinal fluid (a normally sterile body site) was shown to be vaccine and not wild strain by genetic sequencing.[97] Demonstration that severe local swelling after tetanus vaccination tended to occur in people with extremely high levels of circulating antitoxin (as a result of excessive tetanus boosters) supports the proposed mechanism of an Arthus reaction.[98] In countries such as the United States where wild polioviruses are unlikely to be circulating, someone who develops an illness clinically compatible with polio shortly after receipt (or contact with a recipient) of OPV is likely to have vaccine-associated paralytic polio.[14, 99] Causality also usually can be inferred if a specific clinical finding occurs after each vaccination (i.e., challenge-rechallenge), as in cases of alopecia after hepatitis B vaccination.[100]

If the adverse event is known to be associated with the wild vaccine-preventable disease (e.g., acute arthritis and idiopathic thrombocytopenic purpura after rubella), its association with the attenuated vaccine at a lesser frequency is not surprising.[15] This relationship is not universal, however, as pregnant women who receive rubella vaccine, in contrast to those exposed to wild rubella, have not been shown to have illness compatible with congenital rubella syndrome.[101] Clustering of events in time after vaccination can also suggest causation if *reporting bias* can be ruled out. Such bias may occur because parents and physicians are most likely to link adverse events with vaccinations the shorter the time interval between the two. Febrile seizures associated with killed bacterial vaccines tend to occur within a day of vaccination, whereas those due to live viral vaccines are delayed by about a week because of viral replication.[18, 24] Onset of GBS after the swine influenza vaccination was delayed up to 6 weeks because autoimmune demyelination is a slower process.[28]

Most serious reported vaccine adverse events lack these unique features that permit easy inferences on causality. Adverse events such as autism, chronic fatigue syndrome, sudden infant death syndrome, seizures, and GBS either have multiple or as yet unknown causes. For these outcomes, vaccination is clearly never the principal *cause* per se. Otherwise given the large number of vaccinations, many more such cases would be seen. The question is more whether the association with vaccination can either potentiate the outcome or induce it in a *high-risk* subpopulation; or, alternatively, is association purely coincidental and vaccination is blamed because it is a highly distinctive, painful, and memorable event usually followed by some true local and systemic vaccine reactions, such as injection site swelling and fever. For such adverse events, possible link with vaccination is usually based on a process of elimination, ruling out all other possible causes. Even after this is done, only a relatively unsatisfying nondefinitive conclusion can be drawn on any individual case report because other causes may not yet be discovered. The uncertainty in attributing vaccine as a cause of individual cases of illness has led to much confusion, controversy, and litigation.[47] With nonunique clinical syndromes or laboratory findings, epidemiological studies have to be relied on to ascertain likelihood of association and attributable fraction (see *Lessons Learned to Date*).

Another approach to causality is to assume that adverse events that occur within particular periods after vaccination are caused by the vaccine, regardless of whether they were truly causal or just coincidental. This approach to causality is used in some vaccine injury compensation programs to simplify the proceedings.[47]

In some countries, expert committees of specialists in relevant disciplines (e.g., pediatrics, infectious diseases, neurology) review reports. This *global introspection* approach[102] has been used in both Canada[88] and the Netherlands[81] to classify reports of adverse events in gradations of probable association to vaccination. Classifications are based on the reported symptoms, the interval between vaccination and onset of symptoms, and a set of case definitions. Because opinions of experts play such a major role in this form of causality assessment, the results are less satisfying than results obtained from rigorously conducted scientific studies.

The global introspection method can be improved by the use of branched logic tree algorithms[103] or the bayesian analysis.[104] In both, each expert's degree of belief in the key considerations of the plausibility of vaccine causation is made explicit and measured quantitatively. The algorithm requires the assessor to answer a series of questions, which are then scored. The bayesian analysis calculates the posterior probability of vaccine causation based on applying prior probability that the vaccine can cause the adverse event to the facts of an individual case. Advantages of these approaches include accountability and the possibility of recalculating the probability of causation if the quality of data improves. Disadvantages include the resources required and the frequent lack of information to construct the prior probabilities. This approach was piloted in a review of MSAEFI cases[91] and used by the IOM to review case reports[16] but has not yet been adopted for routine use.

Signal Detection

Identifying a potential new vaccine safety problem (*signal*) requires a mix of clinical intuition and epidemiological expertise.[105] Unusual clinical features and clustering by time or space usually tip off that something may be awry (see also under *Assessment of Causality*). For example, a report by a concerned mother of recurrent alopecia after successive hepatitis B vaccinations in her child led to a review of VAERS data that showed several other similar reports.[100] GBS was the only illness reported more commonly in the second and third week than in the first week after swine influenza vaccination. This unusual finding led to initiation of special validation studies.[28, 106]

Mass immunization campaigns may make it easier to detect adverse events after vaccination than routine immunization activities. The large number of doses administered over a well-defined short time result in more prominent clusters of vaccine adverse events. Absence of clusters following campaigns supports high levels of vaccine safety. Surveillance of vaccine adverse events around mass immunization campaigns has therefore been extremely useful in generating signals, either positive (e.g., GBS with swine influenza vaccine[28] or OPV,[107] allergic reactions after Japanese encephalitis vaccine,[108] neuropathy after rubella vaccine[109]) or negative (e.g., events after meningococcal vaccine,[110] GBS after measles[111]). Such signals still require validation, however, because some, after more careful scientific studies, turn out to be incorrect (e.g., GBS after OPV).[112] The aforementioned situations aside, ascertaining *signals* from SRS reports requires taking an epidemiological approach. Various means to automate *screening for signals* using SRS reports have been tried to date without great success,[113, 114] largely because of inherent methodological problems of SRS reports (see under *Lessons Learned to Date*).

Lessons Learned to Date

Several lessons are beginning to emerge from SRS, such as VAERS.[55, 115] VAERS has successfully detected unrecognized potential reactions and obtained data to evaluate whether these events are causally linked to vaccines.[100] VAERS has also successfully served as a source of cases for further investigation of idiopathic thrombocytopenic purpura after mumps, measles, and rubella (MMR),[116] encephalopathy after MMR,[117] and syncope after immunization.[118] VAERS has been of great value for answering routine public queries (e.g., Has adverse event *X* ever been reported after vaccine *Y*?). When denominator data on doses are available from other sources, VAERS can be used to evaluate changes in reporting rates over time or when new vaccines replace old vaccines. For example, VAERS showed that after millions of doses had been distributed, reporting rates for serious events such as hospitalization and seizures after DTaP in toddlers was one third that after diphtheria, tetanus, and pertussis (DTP).[119] VAERS is also currently the only surveillance system that covers the entire U.S. population with data available on a relatively timely basis. It is, therefore, the major means available currently to detect possible new, unusual, or extremely rare adverse events, including whether certain lots of vaccines are associated with unusually high rates of adverse events.[55, 80]

The reporting efficiency or sensitivity of SRS can be estimated if expected rates of adverse events generated from carefully executed studies are available. A higher proportion of serious events, such as seizures, that follow vaccinations are likely to be reported to VAERS than milder events, such as rash, or delayed events requiring laboratory assessment, such as thrombocytopenic purpura after MMR vaccination (Table 49–3).[120] Although formal evaluation has been limited, the probability that a serious event reported to VAERS has been accurately diagnosed (i.e., predictive value positive) is likely to be high. Of 26 patients reported to VAERS who developed GBS after influenza vaccination during the 1990–1991 season, and whose hospital charts were reviewed by an independent panel of neurologists blinded to immunization status, the diagnosis of GBS was confirmed in 22 (85%).[121]

Despite the aforementioned uses, SRS for drug and vaccine safety have a number of major methodological weaknesses. Underreporting, biased reporting, and incomplete reporting are inherent to all such SRS, and potential safety concerns may be missed.[105, 120, 122] Aseptic meningitis associated with the Urabe mumps vaccine strain, for example, was not detected by SRS in most countries.[18, 46] Most public health disease surveillance systems focus on one specific exposure (e.g., lead) or disease (e.g., measles), with a well-characterized laboratory diagnosis or case definition and well-characterized denominators (usually some type of population census). SRS, by contrast, have to examine multiple vaccine exposures and multiple medical events, assess rates of known risks, and detect new risks—all within one sur-

Table 49–3. **REPORTING EFFICIENCIES FOR SELECTED OUTCOMES, TWO PASSIVE SURVEILLANCE SYSTEMS FOR VACCINE ADVERSE EVENTS, UNITED STATES**

ADVERSE EVENT	VACCINE	REPORTING EFFICIENCY (%) MSAEFI	VAERS (Overall)	VAERS (Public Sector)
Vaccine-associated polio	OPV	72	68	*
Seizures	DTP	42	24	36
Seizures	MMR	23	37	49
Hypotonic-hyporesponsive episodes	DTP	4	3	4
Rash	MMR	<1	<1	5
Thrombocytopenia	MMR	<1	4	<1

DTP, diphtheria, tetanus, pertussis; MMR, measles, mumps, rubella; MSAEFI, Monitoring System for Adverse Events Following Immunizations; OPV, oral polio vaccine; VAERS, Vaccine Adverse Event Reporting System.
*Public and private sector information is missing on these cases.
Data from Rosenthal S, Chen RT. Reporting sensitivities of two passive surveillance systems for vaccine adverse events. Am J Public Health 85:1706–1709, 1995.

veillance system, a daunting task.[123] Perhaps the most important methodological weakness of SRS, however, is that such reports represent less than one fourth of the information necessary to complete an epidemiological analysis of a vaccine adverse event.

Such analyses require calculation of the rate of the adverse event after vaccination (a/(a + b) in Table 49–4) using SRS case reports (or other more complete sources; see later) for numerator and for denominator, if available, doses of vaccines administered (or, if unavailable, data on vaccine doses distributed or vaccine coverage survey data are used as surrogates). These rates are compared with the background rate of the same adverse event in the absence of vaccination if available (c/(c + d) in Table 49–4). Because SRS databases provide data only for cell *a* in Table 49–4, and, even then, only in a biased and underreported manner, they fundamentally lack the data in the other three cells needed to calculate rates and (1) generate accurate *signals* of potential vaccine safety problems or (2) make a rigorous epidemiological assessment of the role of vaccine in causation. Use of data from SRS are further complicated by lack of specific clinical syndromes being evaluated, absence of laboratory confirmation of many of the events, and simultaneous vaccinations that make determination of which vaccine might have caused the event difficult.

Current SRS are also prone to detecting increases in adverse events that are not true increases. Instead, they may be due to an increase in (1) reporting efficiency, (2) vaccine coverage, or (3) an adverse event due to other causes. SRS are usually unable to sort out causally related from coincidentally related adverse events because of inherent methodological weaknesses. For example, an increase in GBS reports after influenza vaccination during the 1993 to 1994 season was found to be largely due to improvements in vaccine coverage and increases in GBS independent of vaccination.[124] An increased reporting rate of an adverse event after one hepatitis B vaccine compared with a second brand was likely due to differential distribution of brands in the public versus private sectors, which have differential VAERS reporting rates (higher in the public sector).[125]

Table 49–4. **2 × 2 TABLE NECESSARY FOR EPIDEMIOLOGICAL ANALYSIS OF CAUSALITY BETWEEN VACCINE AND AN ADVERSE EVENT**

VACCINATED	ADVERSE EVENT Yes	No
Yes	a	b
No	c	d

Rate of adverse event after vaccination = a/a + b.
Rate of adverse event in the absence of vaccination = c/c + d.
Reports to passive surveillance systems for vaccine adverse events (e.g., Vaccine Adverse Event Reporting System) represent just partial information (because of underreporting and biased reporting) for cell *a* of the table. Epidemiological studies aim to gather information for all four cells of this table in an unbiased manner.

These studies highlight the crude nature of the signal generated by VAERS and the difficulty in ascertaining which vaccine safety concerns warrant further investigation. Not only are there problems with reporting efficiency and potentially biased reporting, but also precise denominators for calculating true rates are usually not available. Instead, crude measures, such as doses distributed, must often be used as surrogates for doses administered. Because of these difficulties, the requirement for manufacturers to notify the FDA whenever they receive an increased number of reports has been dropped.[90]

Historically, most countries have relied on SRS alone for postlicensure vaccine safety monitoring. The inadequacy of scientific information on vaccine safety found by IOM is related to these methodological weaknesses inherent to SRS. (The establishment of new population-based immunization registries in which all vaccines administered are entered may provide more timely submission of SRS reports as well as more accurate and specific denominators for doses administered, providing information necessary to calculate more accurate adverse event rates.[126, 127])

Postlicensure Clinical Trials

Immunization programs are in a dynamic relationship with their target diseases.[128] To optimize vaccine use, clinical trials may be conducted after vaccine licensure to assess the effects of changes in vaccine formulation,[129] vaccine strain,[130] age at vaccination,[131] the number and timing of vaccine doses,[132] simultaneous administration,[133] and interchangeability of vaccines from different manufacturers on vaccine safety and immunogenicity.[134] The importance of such trials was demonstrated when studies showed an unanticipated differential mortality among recipients of high and regular titer measles vaccine in developing countries,[63] albeit lower than among unvaccinated children.[135] This finding resulted in a change in recommendations by WHO for the use of such vaccines.[136] The development of large-linked databases (LLDBs, see later) may permit improved ability to monitor the safety of such postlicensure changes in vaccine use without necessarily conducting such clinical trials.

Phase 4 Surveillance Studies

To improve the ability to detect adverse events that are not detected during prelicensure trials, most recently licensed vaccines in developed countries have undergone formal phase 4 surveillance studies on populations with sample sizes of approximately 10^5. These studies usually have used cohorts in health maintenance organizations (HMOs) (see under *Large-Linked Databases*) supplemented by diary or phone interview. These methods were first extensively used after the licensure of polysaccharide and conjugated *Haemophilus influenzae* type b (Hib) vaccines.[137–139] Postlicensure studies on safety and efficacy of infant DTaP are also continuing.[59] Extensive phase 4 evaluation of varicella vaccine includes multiyear evaluation for disease incidence, herpes zoster, and a pregnancy registry.[140, 141] Requirements for phase 4 evaluation have even been extended to less frequently used vaccines, such as Japanese encephalitis vaccine.[142]

Ad Hoc Epidemiological Studies

Historically, ad hoc epidemiological studies have been employed to assess signals of potential adverse events detected by SRS, the medical literature, or other mechanisms. Traditional analyses of secular trends (ecological studies), cohort, and case-control studies have been used to gather information necessary to measure or compare risks of an adverse event after vaccination with risk in the absence of vaccination. Occasionally, data collected for other study outcomes may be reanalyzed to see if vaccine was causally related or not.[143, 144] Examples of ad hoc follow-up studies to signals of vaccine safety issues are the investigations of poliomyelitis after inactivated[39] and oral polio vaccines,[99] sudden infant death syndrome after DTP vaccination,[145–148] encephalopathy after DTP vaccination,[31, 149] meningoencephalitis after mumps vaccination,[45, 46] injection site abscesses postvaccination,[150] and GBS after influenza vaccination.[28, 121, 124] Many such studies have been compiled and reviewed by the IOM.[15, 16] Although LLDBs provide a more cost-effective and flexible framework for hypothesis testing, ad hoc epidemiological studies may still be needed in countries without LLDBs or where the power of the LLDB may be inadequate to answer a question in a timely manner.[24, 121, 124]

Large-Linked Databases

Ad hoc epidemiological studies of vaccine safety, although potentially informative about vaccine causality, are costly, time-consuming, and usually limited to assessment of a single event. The need to improve postlicensure monitoring of drug safety became widely recognized after the thalidomide disaster.[151] Faced with the methodological limitations in passive surveillance for adverse events from drugs, during the 1980s pharmacoepidemiologists began to turn to LLDBs linking computerized pharmacy prescription (and later immunization) and medical outcome records.[122] These databases derive from defined populations such as members of HMOs, single-provider healthcare systems, and Medicaid programs. Because the databases are usually generated in the routine administration of such programs and do not require completion of a vaccine adverse event reporting form, the problems of underreporting or recall bias are reduced. Because these programs have enrollees numbering from thousands to millions, large populations can be examined for relatively infrequent adverse events. Denominator data on doses administered and the ready availability of appropriate comparison groups are also useful. LLDBs therefore can potentially provide an economical and rapid means of conducting postlicensure studies of safety of drugs and vaccines.[18, 24, 56]

The CDC participated in two pilot vaccine safety studies using LLDBs in Medicaid and HMO populations during the late 1980s.[152–155] Although they validated this approach for vaccine safety studies and provided scientifically rigorous results, these studies were limited by their relatively small sample sizes, retrospective design, and focus on the most severe reactions.[15] These limitations, the constraints of VAERS, and the recognition of the need for improved monitoring of vaccine safety prompted the CDC to initiate the Vaccine Safety Datalink (VSD) project in 1990.[24] To help overcome the previously identified shortcomings, the VSD study prospectively collects vaccination, medical outcome (e.g., hospital discharge, outpatient visits, emergency department visits, and deaths), and covariate data (e.g., birth certificates, census) under joint protocol at multiple HMOs. Selection of staff model prepaid health plans also minimized potential biases for more severe outcomes resulting from data generated from fee-for-service claims. The VSD has conducted active surveillance on approximately 500,000 children from birth through 6 years of age (75,000 birth cohort, approximately 2% of U.S. population in these age groups) whose parents (or legal guardians) were enrolled in one of four staff model HMOs.[24] Expansion to include all age groups in the study is underway. Each site encodes patients' clinical data with unique study identifiers before sending data to CDC annually for merging and analysis, thereby preserving patient confidentiality. Depending on the background incidence of the medical event, the frequency of specific vaccinations, and their relative risk, events attributable to vaccinations as rare as 1 per 100,000 doses should be detectable within 5 years.

The VSD has focused its initial efforts on examining potential associations between immunizations and 34 serious neurological, allergic, hematological, infectious, inflammatory, and metabolic conditions. The VSD is also being used to test new ad hoc vaccine safety hypotheses. These may arise from the medical literature,[15, 16] from VAERS,[125] from changes in immunization schedules,[156] or from introduction of new vaccines.[137, 139] The diversity in vaccination practices at the four HMOs permits useful contrasts in safety experiences.[156] The size of the VSD population may also permit separation of the risks associated with individual vaccines from those associated with vaccine combinations, whether given in the same syringe or simultaneously at different body sites. Such studies are especially valuable in view of the new combined pediatric vaccines currently in development.[157]

Should the VSD identify an adverse event as being caused by vaccine, data on the incidence rate attributable to vaccine are available, permitting accurate risk-benefit assessment by both the public and policymakers.[158] Subgroup analyses may permit identification of risk factors for adverse events, which may be useful in identifying contraindications to vaccinations. Data from VSD should be useful in calculating background rates of illnesses in the absence of vaccination that can serve as expected rates when comparing rates of vaccine-associated events in SRS. Also, incidence rates of vaccine-associated adverse events derived from VSD can be used to evaluate the sensitivity of passive reporting systems. The VSD data can also aid the FDA in their evaluation of VAERS data[125] and the Vaccine Injury Compensation Program in determinations of what events should be compensated as vaccine *injuries*.[48] The cohort infrastructure created by the VSD project easily lends itself to a wide range of other vaccine-related studies beyond safety.[24]

Amid these promises, a few caveats are appropriate. Although diverse, the population in the four HMOs currently in the VSD is not wholly representative of the United States in terms of geography or socioeconomic status. More importantly, due to the high coverage attained in the HMOs for most vaccines, few nonvaccinated controls are available. The VSD must therefore rely predominantly on some type of *risk-interval* analysis (Table 49–5).[152–155] The capability of this approach to assess associations between vaccination and adverse events with delayed or insidious onset (e.g., autism) is limited. The VSD also cannot easily assess adverse events not currently captured in existing HMO databases, either because they do not result in a healthcare consultation (e.g., fever) or because the data are not automated (e.g., x-ray results).[24] The current VSD is also not large enough to examine the risk of extremely rare events, such as GBS, after each season's influenza vaccine. Finally, because the VSD relies on epidemiological methods, it may not successfully control for confounding and bias in each analysis,[50] and inferences on causality may be limited.[53]

Despite these potential shortcomings, the VSD provides a new, essential, powerful, and cost-effective complement to ongoing evaluations of vaccine safety in the United States. In view of the methodological and logistical advantages offered by LLDBs, the United Kingdom and Canada have also developed LLDBs linking immunization registries with medical files.[18, 56] Because of the relatively limited number of vaccines used worldwide and the costs associated with establishing and operating LLDBs, it is unlikely that all countries will be able to or need to establish their own LLDBs. These countries should be able to draw on the scientific base established by the existing LLDBs for vaccine safety and, if the need arises, conduct ad hoc epidemiological studies.

VACCINE RISK COMMUNICATIONS

Disease prevention, especially if it requires continuous near-universal compliance, is a formidable task. In the

Table 49–5. **EXAMPLE OF METHOD FOR RISK-INTERVAL ANALYSIS OF ASSOCIATION BETWEEN A UNIVERSALLY RECOMMENDED THREE-DOSE VACCINE (WITH FEW UNVACCINATED PERSONS FOR COMPARISON) AND AN ADVERSE EVENT**

1. Define biologically plausible *risk interval* for adverse event after vaccination (e.g., 30 days after each dose).
2. Partition observation time for each child in the study into periods within and outside of risk intervals, and sum respectively (e.g., for a child observed for 365 days during which 3 doses of vaccine were received, total risk interval time = 3 × 30 person-days = 90 person-days; total nonrisk interval time = 365 − 90 = 275 person-days).

```
0--------------x= = = =----------x= = = =------------x= = = =------//------>|
Birth        Dose 1            Dose 2              Dose 3        365 days
```

3. Add up (a) total risk interval and nonrisk interval observation times for each child in the study (= Person-Time Observed; for mathematical convenience, example below uses 100 and 1000 person-months of observation), and (b) adverse events occurring in each time period to complete 2 × 2 table (for illustration, example below uses 3 and 10 cases):

VACCINATED IN RISK INTERVAL	ADVERSE EVENT Yes	PERSON-TIME OBSERVED (MO)	INCIDENCE RATE
Yes	3	100	0.03
No	10	1000	0.01
TOTAL	13	1100	

Incidence rate adverse event $_{vaccinated}$ = 3/100 = 0.03
Incidence rate adverse event $_{unvaccinated}$ = 10/1000 = 0.01
Relative rate vaccinated:unvaccinated = 0.03/0.01 = 3.0
Probability finding due to chance: <5/100

Conclusion: There is a three-fold increase in risk for developing the adverse event within the interval after vaccination.

preimmunization era, vaccine-preventable diseases such as measles and pertussis were so prevalent that the risks and benefits of disease versus vaccination were readily evident. As immunization programs successfully reduced the incidence of vaccine-preventable diseases, however, an increasing proportion of healthcare providers and parents have little or no personal experience with vaccine-preventable diseases. For their risk-benefit analysis, they are forced to rely on historical and other more distant descriptions of vaccine-preventable diseases in textbooks or educational brochures. In contrast, some degree of personal discomfort and pain is generally associated with each immunization. For reasons discussed earlier, there may be uncertainty if vaccines can cause rare or delayed serious reactions (if only because the studies to demonstrate the negative have not or cannot be done). Combined with media that seek controversy,[26] the increasing popularity of alternative medicine, and the lack of standards for accuracy for many books or information posted on the Internet,[159] the art of handling vaccine safety concerns and vaccine risk communications has emerged as an increasingly important skill for managers of mature national immunization programs.

Risk Communication Principles

The science of risk perceptions and risk communications, developed initially for technology and environmental arenas,[160] has only recently been formally applied to immunizations.[161] Among the key principles and lessons are: (1) Individuals differ in their perceptions of risk depending on their personality, education, and life experience[162]; educational materials *tiered* for different needs are therefore likely to be more effective than a single tier. (2) Perceptions of risk may differ dramatically depending on whether the *stakeholder* is a member of the government, the industry, the average parent, or the parent of a vaccine-injured child. (3) *Voluntary* risks (e.g., driving a car) are usually more acceptable than involuntary risks (e.g., mandated immunizations); risk comparisons that fail to take the degree of voluntariness into account can be hazardarous. There are relatively few (if any) other infant experiences similar to immunizations in their risk profile that makes for easy comparisons. (4) For quantitatively equivalent risk that is due to action (e.g., vaccination reaction) versus inaction (e.g., vaccine-preventable disease caused by nonvaccination), many people have an *omission bias* in that they prefer the consequences of inaction to action.[163] (5) When there is uncertainty, patients frequently rely on the advice of their physician or other healthcare professional; continuing education of healthcare professionals on vaccine risk issues is therefore key.

In the United States, written information about the risks and benefits of immunizations developed by the CDC has been required to be provided to all people vaccinated in the public sector since 1978[158] and all recipients of routinely recommended childhood vaccinees since 1988.[164] More efforts have been devoted toward the use of focus groups and other research to assess and improve the effectiveness of such information materials.[165] In many countries, people who believe they or their children were injured by vaccine have organized to provide information that highlights the risks of and the alternatives to immunizations. These consumer activists argue that even if the vaccine risks are rare, if you are the person with the reaction, the risk is 100%. They have been increasingly successful in airing their views in both electronic and print media, frequently with poignant individual stories.[166] Materials to counter the misconceptions and allegations about immunizations are also beginning to be developed[167, 168] and made available via the internet (see http://www.cdc.gov/nip/vacsafe). Systems to develop and disseminate such materials to immunization providers in a timely manner and an oral history project for equally poignant tales of the impact of vaccine-preventable disease are urgently needed. This battle for the "hearts and minds" of the public in need of vaccination will clearly continue to be waged for some time.

Risk communication can be used for the purposes of advocacy, public education, or decision-making partnership.[160] People care not only about the magnitude of the risk, but also how the risks are managed and whether they participate in the risk management process, especially in a democratic society.[169] In medical decision making, this has resulted in a transition from more paternalistic models to increasing degrees of informed consent.[170] Some have argued that a similar transition to informed consent should also occur with immunizations.[171] Immunization is unlike most other medical procedures (e.g., surgery), however, in that the consequences of the decision affect not only the individual, but also others in the society. Because of this important distinction, many countries have enacted public health (e.g., immunization) laws that severely limit any individual's right to infect others. Without such mandates, a "tragedy of the commons" may occur when high vaccine coverage is reached and the individual risk-benefit ratio diverges from that of the society.[172, 173] People may attempt to avoid the risks of vaccination while being protected by the herd immunity resulting from others being vaccinated.[174] This commons provided by herd immunity may disappear if too many people avoid vaccination, with the resulting tragedy that outbreaks return. Debates in the United States have focused on whether philosophical (in addition to medical and religious) exemptions to mandatory immunizations should be allowed more universally and, if so, what standards for claim of exemption are needed.[171] Viewed largely, vaccine risk communications discusses not only the risks and benefits of specific vaccines, but also must inform the vaccinee regarding the delicate balance between societal and individual rights in a shared community.

Evaluating and Managing Vaccine Safety Concerns

A healthy dose of empathy, patience, scientific curiosity, and substantial resources may be needed in dealing with vaccine safety concerns. Although each evaluation is in some ways unique, judgment and some general principles may help. As with all investigations, the first step is objective and comprehensive data gathering with an open mind. Premature dismissal of new vaccine safety concerns as *unfounded* without gathering and weighing the evidence is unwise and unscientific. Novel reactions such as alopecia after hepatitis B vaccine were initially rejected,[100] sometimes even after substantial evidence had accumulated.[46] It is also important to gather and weigh evidence for causes other than vaccine. For individual cases or clusters of cases, a field investigation to gather data firsthand may be necessary.[10, 150] Advice and review from a panel of independent experts may be needed.[37, 63, 121] As discussed earlier, causality assessment at the individual level is difficult at best; further evaluation via epidemiological or laboratory studies may be required. Even if the investigation is inconclusive, sincere and honest search for the truth (vs. *protecting* the immunization program) can help dispel further allegations of a *cover-up*.[175]

Periodically, vaccine safety concerns may emerge in the media. Because the media frequently aim to present both sides of the story, the battle is to establish greater credibility to the audience while maintaining ethical and professional behavior.[176, 177] Factors that aid in such credibility include scientific expertise, prior relationship with the media based on prior experience with difficult issues, empathy, and ability to distill scientific facts and figures down to simple lay concepts. Statistics generally compete poorly with dramatic pictures of disabled children. Equally emotionally compelling firsthand accounts of people with vaccine-preventable disease may be needed. Clarifying the distinction between perceived and real risk for the concerned public is critical. If further research is needed, the degree of uncertainty (e.g., whether such rare vaccine reactions exist at all) should be acknowledged, but also what is certain (e.g., millions of people have received vaccine *X* and have not developed syndrome *Y*; even if vaccine causes *Y*, it is likely to be of magnitude *Z*, compared to the magnitude of known risks associated with vaccine-preventable diseases) should be noted.

SCIENTIFICALLY ACCEPTED RISKS OF COMMONLY USED VACCINES

Each chapter in this textbook on specific vaccines discusses the data on associated risks. The available scientific information on the risks associated with routine pediatric vaccines was systematically and exhaustively reviewed by the IOM in the early 1990s.[15, 16] The IOM classified the available evidence as a case report, case series, uncontrolled study, or controlled study, with increasing levels of validity. The total evidence for a causal relationship between vaccine and a specific adverse event was weighed then placed in one of five categories: (1) No evidence was available bearing on causality, (2) evidence was inadequate to accept or reject a causal relationship, (3) evidence favors rejection of a causal relationship, (4) evidence favors a causal relationship, and (5) evidence establishes a causal relationship.

As noted earlier, two thirds of the adverse events evaluated had either no (category 1) or inadequate evidence (category 2) for causality assessment, reflecting the need for additional research in vaccine safety. Relatively few associations were in either categories 4 or 5, in which the evidence either favored or established a causal relationship (Tables 49–6 and 49–7). In its update in 1996, the ACIP, while supporting the majority of IOM conclusions, reached different interpretations for some associations because of newly available evidence or different interpretations of the limited data reviewed by IOM.[178] Further revisions will occur as new evidence becomes available on these and newer vaccines. For example, the latest research cast doubts on the association between OPV and GBS[112] and RA27/3 rubella vaccine and chronic arthropathy.[179–181]

Comprehensive independent review of the risks associated with other routinely used vaccines, especially those used primarily by adults and travelers, is currently lacking. Relative to the IOM reviews, a review of these vaccines would be even more severely handicapped by the deficits of controlled studies with adequate power. The lack of accurate past vaccination histories among adults plus the range of locations in which adults may be vaccinated (e.g., occupational sites in addition to primary physician offices) also make future vaccine safety studies in older age groups especially difficult.

FUTURE CHALLENGES

Many people look to vaccines as the *magic bullet* solution to a number of public health problems that range from acquired immunodeficiency syndrome (AIDS) to malaria. Rapid advances in biotechnology have brought the promise of these new vaccines closer to reality.[182] Novel delivery technologies, such as DNA vaccines and new adjuvants, are being explored to permit more antigens to be combined, reducing the number of injections.[157, 183] These changes in vaccines and vaccine delivery, however, will continue to provide additional challenges in proving their safety to an increasingly skeptical and risk-averse public. Combined with methodological difficulties associated with studying rare, delayed, or insidious vaccine safety allegations,[49] well-organized antivaccine organizations,[166] media eagerness for controversy,[26, 176] and relatively rare individual encounters with vaccine-preventable disease, vaccine safety concerns are unlikely "to go away" in mature immunization programs.

Concomitantly, vaccine safety concerns have also emerged as an issue in EPIs developing countries.[9] The high-titer measles vaccine mortality experience highlighted the importance of improving the quality control and evaluating the safety of vaccines used in developing countries.[63, 130] Plans to eliminate neonatal tetanus and measles via National Immunization Days, during which millions of people receive parenteral immunizations over a period of days,[184] pose substantial challenges to ensuring injection safety,[8] especially given concerns about inadequate sterilization of reusable syringes and needles, recycling of disposable syringes and needles, and cross-

Table 49–6. **SUMMARIZED CONCLUSIONS OF EVIDENCE REGARDING THE POSSIBLE ASSOCIATION BETWEEN SPECIFIC ADVERSE EVENTS AND RECEIPT OF DIPHTHERIA AND TETANUS TOXOIDS AND PERTUSSIS VACCINE (DTP)* AND RA 27/3† RUBELLA-CONTAINING VACCINES, BY DETERMINATION OF CAUSALITY—INSTITUTE OF MEDICINE, 1991‡**

CONCLUSION, BY DETERMINATION OF CAUSALITY	ADVERSE EVENT REVIEWED	
	DTP Vaccine	RA27/3 Rubella Vaccine
1. No evidence was available to establish a causal relationship	Autism	None
2. Inadequate evidence to accept or reject a causal relationship	Aseptic meningitis Chronic neurological damage§ Erythema multiforme or other rash Guillain-Barré syndrome Hemolytic anemia Juvenile diabetes Learning disabilities and attention-deficit disorder Peripheral mononeuropathy Thrombocytopenia	Radiculoneuritis and other neuropathies Thrombocytopenic purpura
3. Evidence favored rejection of a causal relationship	Infantile spasms Hypsarrhythmia Reye syndrome Sudden infant death syndrome	None
4. Evidence favored acceptance of a causal relationship	Acute encephalopathy‖ Shock and unusual shock-like state	Chronic arthritis
5. Evidence established a causal relationship	Anaphylaxis Protracted, inconsolable crying	Acute arthritis

*The evidence differentiated only between components of DTP in the event of protracted, inconsolable crying, for which the evidence specifically implicated the pertussis vaccine component.

†Trivalent measles, mumps, rubella (MMR) vaccine containing the RA 27/3 rubella strain.

‡This table is an adaptation of a table published previously by the Institute of Medicine (IOM),[15] an independent research organization chartered by the National Academy of Sciences. The National Childhood Vaccine Injury Act of 1986 mandated that IOM review scientific and other evidence (e.g., epidemiological studies, case series, individual case reports, and testimonials) regarding the possible adverse consequences of vaccines administered to children. IOM comprised an expert committee to review and summarize all available information; this committee created five categories of causality to describe the relationships between the vaccines and specific adverse events.

§IOM reviewed this adverse event again in 1994.[16]

‖Defined in the controlled studies that were reviewed as encephalopathy, encephalitis, or encephalomyelitis.

Table 49–7. **SUMMARIZED CONCLUSIONS OF EVIDENCE REGARDING THE POSSIBLE ASSOCIATION BETWEEN SPECIFIC ADVERSE EVENTS AND RECEIPT OF CHILDHOOD VACCINES, BY DETERMINATION OF CAUSALITY—INSTITUTE OF MEDICINE, 1994***

DT/Td/TETANUS TOXOID†	MEASLES VACCINE‡	MUMPS VACCINE‡	OPV/IPV§	HEPATITIS B VACCINE	*HAEMOPHILUS INFLUENZAE* TYPE B (Hib) VACCINE
1. No Evidence Available to Establish a Causal Relationship					
None	None	Neuropathy Residual seizure disorder	Transverse myelitis *(IPV)* Thrombocytopenia *(IPV)* Anaphylaxis *(IPV)*	None	None
2. Inadequate Evidence to Accept or Reject a Causal Relationship					
Residual seizure disorder other than infantile spasms	Encephalopathy	Encephalopathy	Transverse myelitis *(OPV)*	Guillain-Barré syndrome	Guillain-Barré syndrome
Demyelinating diseases of the central nervous system	Subacute sclerosing panencephalitis	Aseptic meningitis	Guillain-Barré syndrome *(IPV)*	Demyelinating diseases of the central nervous system	Transverse myelitis
Mononeuropathy Arthritis Erythema multiforme	Residual seizure disorder Sensorineural deafness *(MMR)* Optic neuritis Transverse myelitis Guillain-Barré syndrome Thrombocytopenia Insulin-dependent diabetes mellitus	Sensorineural deafness *(MMR)* Insulin-dependent diabetes mellitus Sterility Thrombocytopenia Anaphylaxis‖	Death from SIDS¶	Arthritis Death from SIDS¶	Thrombocytopenia Anaphylaxis Death from SIDS¶
3. Evidence Favored Rejection of a Causal Relationship					
Encephalopathy** Infantile spasms (DT only)†† Death from SIDS (DT only)††,‡‡	None	None	None	None	Early-onset Hib disease (conjugate vaccines)

4. Evidence Favored Acceptance of a Causal Relationship					
Guillain-Barré syndrome§§ (ACIP Disagreed)‖‖	Anaphylaxis‖	None	Guillain-Barré syndrome *(OPV)* (ACIP Disagreed)‖‖	None	Early-onset Hib disease in children ages ≥18 mo whose first Hib vaccination was with unconjugated PRP vaccine
Brachial neuritis§§					
5. Evidence Established a Causal Relationship					
Anaphylaxis§§	Thrombocytopenia *(MMR)* Anaphylaxis *(MMR)*‖ Death from measles vaccine–strain viral infection¶,¶¶	None	Poliomyelitis in recipient or contact *(OPV)* Death from polio vaccine–strain viral infection¶,¶¶	Anaphylaxis	None

*This table is an adaptation of a table published previously by the Institute of Medicine (IOM),[16] an independent research organization chartered by the National Academy of Sciences. The National Childhood Vaccine Injury Act of 1986 mandated that IOM review scientific and other evidence (e.g., epidemiological studies, case series, individual case reports, and testimonials) regarding the possible adverse consequences of vaccines administered to children. IOM comprised an expert committee to review and summarize all available information; this committee created five categories of causality to describe the relationships between the vaccines and specific adverse events.

†DT, diphtheria and tetanus toxoids for pediatric use; Td, diphtheria and tetanus toxoids for adult use.

‡If the data derived from studies of a monovalent preparation, the causal relationship also extended to multivalent preparations. If the data derived exclusively from studies of the measles-mumps-rubella (MMR) vaccine, the vaccine is specified parenthetically in italics. In the absence of data concerning the monovalent preparation, the causal relationship determined for the multivalent preparations did not extend to the monovalent components.

§For some adverse events, the IOM committee was charged with assessing the causal relationship between the adverse event and only oral poliovirus vaccine (OPV) (i.e., for poliomyelitis) or only inactivated poliovirus vaccine (IPV) (i.e., for anaphylaxis and thrombocytopenia). If the conclusions for the two vaccines differed for the other adverse events, the vaccine to which the adverse event applied is specified parenthetically in italics.

‖The evidence used to establish a causal relationship for anaphylaxis applies to MMR vaccine. The evidence regarding monovalent measles vaccine favored acceptance of a causal relationship, but this evidence was less convincing than that for MMR vaccine because of either incomplete documentation of symptoms or the possible attenuation of symptoms by medical intervention.

¶This table lists weight-of-evidence determinations only for deaths that were classified as sudden infant death syndrome (SIDS) and deaths that were a consequence of vaccine-strain viral infection. If the evidence favored the acceptance of (or established) a causal relationship between a vaccine and a possibly fatal adverse event, however, the evidence also favored the acceptance of (or established) a causal relationship between the vaccine and death from the adverse event. Direct evidence regarding death in association with a vaccine-associated adverse event was limited to (1) Td and Guillain-Barré syndrome, (2) tetanus toxoid and anaphylaxis, and (3) OPV and poliomyelitis.

**The evidence derived from studies of DT. If the evidence favored rejection of a causal relationship between DT and encephalopathy, the evidence also favored rejection of a causal relationship between Td and tetanus toxoid and encephalopathy.

††Infantile spasms and SIDS occur only in an age group that is administered DT but not Td or tetanus toxoid.

‡‡The evidence derived primarily from studies of DTP, although the evidence also favored rejection of a causal relationship between DT and SIDS.

§§The evidence derived from studies of tetanus toxoid. If the evidence favored acceptance of (or established) a causal relationship between tetanus toxoid and an adverse event, the evidence also favored acceptance of (or established) a causal relationship between DT and Td and the adverse event.

‖‖The Advisory Committee on Immunization Practices (ACIP) concurred with the findings of the IOM except where noted because of new information that became available after IOM published this table.[178]

¶¶Deaths occurred primarily among persons known to be immunocompromised.

contamination resulting from the current generation of jet injectors.[185] Autodestruct syringes and needles and other new safer administration technologies are urgently needed.[8]

The increasing computerization and centralization of healthcare services may facilitate epidemiological studies to reassure the public about the safety of future vaccines.[24, 122] Similar to other arenas concerned with safety (e.g., aviation,[186] food,[187] blood[188]), a comprehensive *systems* design approach to minimize risk and promote vaccine safety is needed.[189] Developments in biotechnology may continue to offer better, safer vaccines.[182, 183] The availability of computerized immunization registries[127] may permit optimal implementation of immunization policies at the individual level, ensuring receipt of indicated vaccines, avoiding extravaccination, and appropriate observance of valid contraindications to vaccinations. On a longer horizon, vaccine safety research combined with genetic epidemiology may permit better characterization of risk groups for vaccine reactions.[190] Integrated with immunization registries for both children and adults, this may ultimately offer the possibility for better prevention of both vaccine-preventable and vaccine-induced diseases.

REFERENCES

1. World Bank. World Development Report 1993: Investing in Health. New York, Oxford University Press, 1993.
2. Wilson GS. The hazards of immunization. London, Athlone Press, 1967.
3. Chen RT, Rastogi SC, Mullen JR, et al. The Vaccine Adverse Event Reporting System (VAERS). Vaccine 12:542–550, 1994.
4. Duclos P. Surveillance des effets secondaires de la vaccination. Sante 4:215–220, 1994.
5. Gangarosa EJ, Galazka AM, Wolfe CR, et al. Impact of the anti-vaccine movements on pertussis control: The untold story. Lancet 351:356–361, 1998.
6. Orenstein WA. DTP vaccine litigation, 1988. Am J Dis Child 144:517, 1990.
7. Institute of Medicine. Liability for the production and sale of vaccine. In Sanford JP (ed): Vaccine Supply and Innovation. Washington, DC, National Academy Press, 1985, pp 85–122.
8. Zaffran M, Lloyd J, Clements J, Stilwell B. A drive to safer injections. Geneva, WHO/GPV/SAGE.97/WP.05, 1997.
9. World Health Organization. Vaccine supply and quality: Surveillance of adverse events following immunization. Wkly Epidemiol Rec 71:237–242, 1996.
10. World Health Organization. Surveillance of adverse events following immunization. Geneva, WHO/EPI/TRAM/93.02 Rev. 1, 1997.
11. Expanded Programme on Immunization: Report of the 13th Global Advisory Group Meeting. Geneva, WHO/EPI/GEN/91.3, 1991, pp 43–44.
12. Public Health Service recommendations on smallpox vaccination. MMWR Morb Mortal Wkly Rep 20:339–345, 1971.
13. Bottiger M. The elimination of polio in the Scandinavian countries. Public Health Rev 21:27–33, 1993–1994.
14. Poliomyelitis prevention in the United States: Introduction of a sequential vaccination schedule of inactivated poliovirus vaccine followed by oral poliovirus vaccine: Recommendations of the Advisory Committee on Immunization Practices (ACIP). MMWR Morb Mortal Wkly Rep 46(RR-3):1–25, 1997.
15. Howson CP, Howe CJ, Fineberg HV (eds), Institute of Medicine. Adverse Effects of Pertussis and Rubella Vaccines: A Report of the Committee to Review the Adverse Consequences of Pertussis and Rubella Vaccines. Washington, DC, National Academy Press, 1991.
16. Stratton KR, Howe CJ, Johnston RB (eds). Adverse Events Associated with Childhood Vaccines: Evidence Bearing on Causality. Washington, DC, National Academy Press, 1994.
17. Miller DL, Wadsworth J, Diamond J, Ross E. Pertussis vaccine and whooping cough as risk factors in acute neurologic illness and deaths in young children. Dev Biol Stand 61:389–394, 1985.
18. Farrington CP, Pugh S, Colville A, et al. A new method for active surveillance of adverse events from diphtheria/tetanus/pertussis and measles/mumps/rubella vaccines. Lancet 345:567–569, 1995.
19. Stetler HC, Orenstein WA, Bart KJ, et al. History of convulsions and use of pertussis vaccine. J Pediatr 107:175–179, 1985.
20. Robbins JB, Pittman M, Trollfors B, et al. Primum non nocere: A pharmacologically inert pertussis toxoid alone should be the next pertussis vaccine. Pediatr Infect Dis J 12:795–807, 1993.
21. Brown EG, Dimock K, Wright KE. The Urabe AM9 mumps vaccine is a mixture of viruses differing at amino acid 335 of the hemagglutin-neuraminidase gene with one form associated with disease. J Infect Dis 174:619–622, 1996.
22. Kew OM, Nottay BK. Molecular epidemiology of polioviruses. Rev Infect Dis 6:S499–S504, 1984.
23. Plotkin SA, Koprowski H. Rabies vaccine. In Plotkin SA, Mortimer EA, eds. Vaccines (2nd ed). Philadelphia, WB Saunders, 1994, pp 649–670.
24. Chen RT, Glasser J, Rhodes P, et al. The Vaccine Safety Datalink Project: A new tool for improving vaccine safety monitoring in the United States. Pediatrics 99:765–773, 1997.
25. Morris R, Halperin S, Dery P, et al. IMPACT monitoring network: A better mousetrap. Can J Infect Dis 4:194–195, 1993.
26. Freed GL, Katz SL, Clark SJ. Safety of vaccinations: Miss America, the media, and public health. JAMA 276:1869–1872, 1996.
27. Rabinovich NR, McInnes P, Klein DL, Hall BF. Vaccine technologies: View to the future. Science 265:1401–1404, 1994.
28. Schonberger LB, Bregman DJ, Sullivan-Bolyai JZ, et al. Guillain-Barré syndrome following vaccination in the national influenza immunization program, United States, 1976–1977. Am J Epidemiol 110:105–123, 1979.
29. McGoldrick MD, Bailie GR. Nonnarcotic analgesics: Prevalence and estimated economic impact of toxicities. Ann Pharmacother 31:221–227, 1997.
30. Marcuse EK, Wentz KR. The NCES reconsidered: Summary of a 1989 workshop. Vaccine 8:531–535, 1990.
31. Alderslade R, Bellman MH, Rawson NSB, et al. The National Childhood Encephalopathy Study. In Whooping Cough: Reports from the Committee on the Safety of Medicines and the Joint Committee on Vaccination and Immunisation. Department of Health and Social Security. London, HM Stationary Office, 1981, pp 79–169.
32. Miller D, Madge N, Diamond J, et al. Pertussis immunisation and serious acute neurological illnesses in children. Br Med J 307:1171–1176, 1993.
33. Wentz KR, Marcuse EK. Diphtheria-tetanus-pertussis vaccine and serious neurologic illness: An updated review of the epidemiologic evidence. Pediatrics 87:287–297, 1991.
34. Neustadt RE, Fineberg HV: The Swine Flu Affair: Decision-Making on a Slippery Disease. Washington, DC, U.S. Government Printing Office, 1978.
35. Kurland LT, Wiederholt WC, Kirkpatrick JW, et al. Swine influenza vaccine and Guillain-Barré syndrome: Epidemic or artifact?. Arch Neurol 42:1089–1090, 1985.
36. Langmuir AD, Bregman DJ, Kurland LT, et al. An epidemiologic and clinical evaluation of Guillain-Barré syndrome reported in association with the administration of swine influenza vaccines. Am J Epidemiol 119:841–879, 1984.
37. Safranek TJ, Lawrence DN, Kurland LT, et al. Reassessment of the association between Guillain-Barré syndrome and the receipt of swine influenza vaccine 1976–1977: Results of a two-state study. Am J Epidemiol 133:940–951, 1991.
38. Schumacher W. Legal/ethical aspects of vaccinations. Dev Biol Stand 43:435–438, 1979.
39. Nathanson N, Langmuir AD: The Cutter incident. Am J Hygiene 78:16–81, 1963.
40. Pennisi E. Monkey virus DNA found in rare human cancers. Science 275:748–749, 1997.

41. Food and Drug Administration. Bovine-derived materials: Agency letters to manufacturers of FDA-regulated products. Fed Reg 59:44591–44594, 1994.
42. Mathieu M (ed). Biologic Development: A Regulatory Overview. Waltham, MA, Paraxel, 1993.
43. Anonymous. Two MMR vaccines withdrawn. Lancet 340:922, 1992.
44. Schmitt HJ, Just M, Neiss A. Withdrawal of a mumps vaccine: Reasons and impacts. Eur J Pediatr 152:387–388, 1993.
45. Kimura M, Kuno-Sakai H, Yamazaki S, et al. Adverse events associated with MMR vaccines in Japan. Acta Paediatr Jpn 38:205–211, 1996.
46. Lloyd JC, Chen RT. The Urabe mumps vaccine: Lessons in adverse event surveillance and response [abstract]. Pharmacoepidemiol Drug Safety 5:S45, 1996.
47. Mariner WK. Compensation programs for vaccine-related injury abroad: A comparative analysis. St Louis Univ Law J 31:599–654, 1987.
48. Evans G. Vaccine liability and safety: A progress report. Pediatr Infect Dis J 15:477–478, 1996.
49. Chen RT. Special methodological issues in pharmacoepidemiology studies of vaccine safety. In Strom BL (ed). Pharmacoepidemiology. Sussex, UK, John Wiley & Sons, 1994, pp 581–594.
50. Fine PEM, Chen RT. Confounding in studies of adverse reactions to vaccines. Am J Epidemiol 136:121–135, 1992.
51. Fine PEM. Methodological issues in the evaluation and monitoring of vaccine safety. Ann N Y Acad Sci 754:300–308, 1995.
52. Farrington CP, Nash J, Miller E. Case series analysis of adverse reactions to vaccines: A comparative evaluation. Am J Epidemiol 143:1165–1173, 1996.
53. Rothman KJ (ed). Causal Inference. Chestnut Hill, MA, Epidemiology Resources, 1988.
54. Anonymous. Non-target effects of live vaccines. Langen, Germany, November 3–5, 1993. Proceedings of a workshop. Dev Biol Stand 84:1–281, 1995.
55. Ellenberg SS, Chen RT. The complicated task of monitoring vaccine safety. Public Health Rep 112:10–20, 1997.
56. Roberts JD, Roos LL, Poffenroth LA, et al. Surveillance of vaccine-related adverse events in the first year of life: A Manitoba cohort study. J Clin Epidemiol 49:51–58, 1996.
57. Rosenthal KL, McVittie LD. The clinical testing of preventive vaccines. In Mathieu M (ed). Biologic Development: A Regulatory Overview. Waltham, MA, Paraxel, 1993, pp 119–130.
58. Pinichiero ME. Acellular pertussis vaccines: Towards an improved safety profile. Drug Experience 15:311–324, 1996.
59. Chen RT. Safety of acellular pertussis vaccine: Follow-up studies. Dev Biol Stand 89:373–375, 1997.
60. Brown F, Greco D, Mastrantonio P, et al. Pertussis vaccine trials. Dev Biol Stand 89:1–410, 1997.
61. Heijbel H, Atti MC, Harzer E, et al. Hypotonic hyporesponsive episodes in eight pertussis vaccine trials. Dev Biol Stand 89:101–103, 1997.
62. Hall AJ, Cutts FT. Lessons from measles vaccination in developing countries. BMJ 307:1294–1295, 1993.
63. Fine PEM, Sterne J: High titer measles vaccine before nine months of age: Implications for child survival [working paper no. 13, 1992]. Presented at Consultation on Studies Involving High Titer Measles Vaccines Before Nine Months of Age; Atlanta; June 16–17, 1992.
64. Ray WA, Griffin MR. Confounding in studies of adverse reactions to vaccines [letter]. Am J Epidemiol 139:229, 1994.
65. Global Programme on Vaccines and Immunization. Quality: The first consideration. Geneva, WHO/GPV/SAGE.97/WP.03, 1997.
66. Steinhoff MC, Reed GF, Decker MD, et al. A randomized comparison of reactogenicity and immunogenicity of two whole-cell pertussis vaccines. Pediatrics 96:S567–570, 1995.
67. Baraff LJ, Cody CL, Cherry JD. DTP-associated reactions: An analysis by injection site, manufacturer, prior reactions, and dose. Pediatrics 73:31–36, 1984.
68. Baraff LJ, Manclark CR, Cherry JD, et al. Analyses of adverse reactions to diphtheria and tetanus toxoids and pertussis vaccine by vaccine lot, endotoxin content, pertussis vaccine potency and percentage of mouse weight gain. Pediatr Infect Dis J 8:502–507, 1989.
69. Rastogi SC, Wise RP. Exploring associations between vaccine lot potencies and human safety experience [abstract]. Pharmacoepidemiol Drug Safety 5:S75, 1996.
70. Wiholm BE, Olsoon S, Moore N, Wood S. Spontaneous reporting systems outside the U.S. In Strom BL (ed). Pharmacoepidemiology. Sussex, UK, John Wiley & Sons, 1994, pp 139–155.
71. Jonville-Bera AP, Autret E, Galy-Eyraud C, Hessel L. Thrombocytopenic purpura after measles, mumps and rubella vaccination. Pediatr Infect Dis J 5:44–48, 1996.
72. Mansoor O, Pillans PI. Vaccine adverse events reported in New Zealand 1990–1995. N Z Med J 110:270–272, 1997.
73. Taranger J, Holmberg K. Urgent to introduce countrywide and systematic evaluation of vaccine side effects. Lakartidningen 89:1691–1693, 1992.
74. Salisbury DM, Beggs NT (eds). 1996 Immunisation Against Infectious Disease. London, HMSO, 1996, pp 29–33.
75. Anonymous. Surveillance of serious adverse events following vaccination. Commun Dis Intelligence (Australia) 19:273–274, 1995.
76. Laboratory Centre for Disease Control. Adverse events temporally associated with immunizing agents—1989 report. Can Dis Wkly Rep 17:147–158, 1991.
77. Andersen MM, Ronne T. Side-effects with Japanese encephalitis vaccine. Lancet 337:1044, 1991.
78. Sokhey J. Adverse events following immunizations: 1990. Ind Pediatr 28:593–607, 1991.
79. Squarcione S, Vellucci L. Adverse reactions following immunization in Italy in the years 1991–93. Ig Mod 105:1419–1431, 1996.
80. Rastogi SC (ed). International Workshop: Harmonization of Reporting of Adverse Events Following Vaccination. Rockville, MD, FDA/CBER, 1993.
81. Health Council of the Netherlands. Committee on Adverse Reactions to Vaccinations. Adverse Reactions to Vaccines in the National Immunization Programme in 1993. The Hague, Health Council of the Netherlands, 1995; publication no. 1995/08E.
82. Brito GS. System of Investigation and Notification of Adverse Events Following Immunization, Preliminary Report. State of Sao Paolo, Brazil, Health Department, 1991.
83. Centers for Disease Control. National Childhood Vaccine Injury Act: Requirements for Permanent Vaccination Records and for Reporting of Selected Events after Vaccination. MMWR Morb Mortal Wkly Rep 37:197–200, 1988.
84. Stetler HC, Mullen JR, Brennan JP, et al. Monitoring system for adverse events following immunization. Vaccine 5:169–174, 1987.
85. Food and Drug Administration. COSTART—Coding Symbols for Thesaurus of Adverse Reaction Terms (3rd ed). Rockville, MD, FDA, 1989.
86. Braun MM, Ellenberg SS. Descriptive epidemiology of adverse events following immunization: Reports to the Vaccine Adverse Event Reporting System (VAERS), 1991–1994. J Pediatr 131:529–535, 1997.
87. Division of Immunization. Vaccine-associated adverse events in Canada, 1992 report. Can Commun Dis Rep 21:117–128, 1995.
88. Pless R, Duclos P. Reinforcing surveillance for vaccine-associated adverse events: The Advisory Committee on Causality Assessment. Can J Infect Dis 7:98–99, 1996.
89. Edwards IR, Biriell C. Harmonisation in pharmacovigilance. Drug Saf 10:93–102, 1994.
90. Food and Drug Administration. International Conference on Harmonisation: Guideline on clinical safety data management: Periodic safety update reports for marketed drugs; availability. Fed Reg 62:27470–27476, 1997.
91. Fenichel GM, Lane DA, Livengood JR, et al. Adverse events following immunization: Assessing probability of causation. Pediatr Neurol 5:287–290, 1989.
92. Wassilak SGF, Sokhey J. Monitoring of adverse events following immunization in the Expanded Programme on Immunization. WHO/EPI/GEN/91.2:1–29, 1991.
93. Laboratory Centre for Disease Control: Proceedings of a workshop on the standardization of definitions for post-marketing surveillance of adverse vaccine reactions, Ottawa, Canada, October 30–31, 1991. Ottawa, LCDC, 1992, pp 1–17.
94. Kramer MS, Lane DA. Causal propositions in clinical research and practice. J Clin Epidemiol 45:639–649, 1992.

95. Jones JK. Determining causation from case reports. In Strom BL (ed). Pharmacoepidemiology. Sussex, UK, John Wiley & Sons, 1994, pp 365–378.
96. Hill AB. The environment and disease: Association or causation. Proc Roy Soc Med 58:295–300, 1965.
97. Forsey T, Mawn JA, Yates PJ, et al. Differentiation of vaccine and wild mumps viruses using the polymerase chain reaction and dideoxinucleotide. J Gen Virol 71:987–990, 1990.
98. Edsall G, Elliot MW, Peebles TC, et al. Excessive use of tetanus toxoid boosters. JAMA 202:111–113, 1967.
99. Henderson DA, Witte JJ, Morris L, et al. Paralytic disease associated with oral polio vaccines. JAMA 190:153–160, 1964.
100. Wise RP, Kiminyo KP, Salive ME. Hair loss after routine immunizations. JAMA 278:1176–1178, 1997.
101. Rubella vaccination during pregnancy—United States, 1971–1988. MMWR Morb Mortal Wkly Rep 38:289–293, 1989.
102. Lane DA. A probabilist's view of causality assessment. Drug Inform J 18:323–330, 1984.
103. Venulet J (ed). Assessing Causes of Adverse Drug Reactions with Special Reference to Standardized Methods. London, Academic Press, 1982.
104. Lane DA, Kramer MS, Hutchinson TA, et al. The causality assessment of adverse drug reactions using a Bayesian approach. Pharmaceut Med 2:265–283, 1987.
105. Finney DJ. The detection of adverse reactions to therapeutic drugs. Stat Med 1:153–161, 1982.
106. Retailliau HF, Curtis AC, Storr G, et al. Illness after influenza vaccination reported through a nationwide surveillance system, 1976–77. Am J Epidemiol 111:270–278, 1980.
107. Uhari M, Rantala H, Niemelä M. Cluster of childhood Guillain-Barré cases after an oral poliovaccine campaign [letter]. Lancet 2:440–441, 1989.
108. Berg SW, Mitchell BS, Hanson RK, et al. Systemic reactions in U.S. Marine Corps personnel who received Japanese encephalitis vaccine. Clin Infect Dis 24:265–266, 1997.
109. Kilroy AW, Schaffner W, Fleet WF Jr, et al. Two syndromes following rubella immunization: Clinical observations and epidemiological studies. JAMA 214:2287–2292, 1970.
110. Yergeau A, Alain L, Pless R, Robert Y. Adverse events temporally associated with meningococcal vaccines. Can Med Assoc J 1154:503–507, 1996.
111. da Silveira CM, Salisbury DM, de Quadros CA. Measles vaccination and Guillain-Barré syndrome. Lancet 349:14–16, 1997.
112. Rantala H, Cherry JD, Shields WD. Epidemiology of Guillain-Barré syndrome in children: Relationship of oral polio vaccine administration to occurrence. J Pediatr 124:220–223, 1994.
113. Carson JL, Strom BL, Maislin G. Screening for unknown effects of newly marketed drugs. In Strom BL (ed). Pharmacoepidemiology. Sussex, UK, John Wiley & Sons, 1994, pp 431–447.
114. Chen RT. Proactive surveillance for vaccine safety. Pharmacoepidemiol Drug Safety 1998 (in press).
115. Lloyd JC, Singleton JA, Terracciano GJ, Chen RT. Evaluation of a surveillance system: Vaccine Adverse Event Reporting System (abstract). Pharmacoepidemiol Drug Safety 5:S44, 1996.
116. Beeler J, Varricchio F, Wise R. Thrombocytopenia after immunization with measles vaccines: Review of the vaccine adverse events reporting system (1990 to 1994). Pediatr Infect Dis J 15:88–90, 1996.
117. Weibel R, Glasser JW, Chen RT. Encephalopathy after measles vaccination: Accumulative evidence from four independent surveillance systems (abstract). Pharmacoepidemiol Drug Safety 6:S60, 1997.
118. Braun MM, Patriarca PA, Ellenberg SS. Syncope after immunization. Arch Ped & Adol Med 151:255–259, 1997.
119. Rosenthal S, Chen R, Hadler SC. The safety of acellular pertussis vaccine versus whole cell pertussis vaccine: A post-marketing assessment. Arch Pediatr Adolesc Med 150:457–460, 1996.
120. Rosenthal S, Chen RT. Reporting sensitivities of two passive surveillance systems for vaccine adverse events. Am J Public Health 85:1706–1709, 1995.
121. Chen RT, Kent JH, Rhodes PH, et al: Investigation of a possible association between influenza vaccination and Guillain-Barré syndrome in the United States, 1990–91 [abstract]. Postmarketing Surveillance 6:5–6, 1992.
122. Strom BL, Carson JL. Use of automated databases for pharmacoepidemiology research. Epidemiol Rev 12:87–107, 1990.
123. Chen RT. Surveillance for vaccine adverse events and public health disease: Similarities and differences [abstract]. Pharmacoepidemiol Drug Safety 5:S45, 1996.
124. Lasky T, Terracciano GJ, Magder L, et al. Association of the Guillain-Barré syndrome with the 1992–93 and 1993–94 influenza vaccines (abstract). Am J Epidemiol 145:S57, 1997.
125. Niu MT, Rhodes P, Salive M, et al. Comparative safety of two recombinant hepatitis b vaccines in children: Data from the Vaccine Adverse Event Reporting System (VAERS) and Vaccine Safety Datalink (VSD). J Clin Epidemiol 51:503–510, 1998.
126. Begg NT, Gill ON, White JM. COVER (cover of vaccination evaluated rapidly): Description of the England and Wales scheme. Public Health 103:81–89, 1989.
127. Cordero JF, Guerra FA, Saarlas KN (eds). Developing national immunization registries: Experience from the All Kids Count Program. Am J Prev Med 3(suppl 1):1–128, 1997.
128. Chen RT, Orenstein WA. Epidemiologic methods in immunization programs. Epidemiol Rev 18:99–117, 1996.
129. Patriarca PA, Laender F, Palmeira G, et al: Randomised trial of alternative formulations of oral poliovaccine in Brazil. Lancet 1:429–434, 1988.
130. Bhargava I, Chharparwal BC, Phadke MA, et al. Reactogenicity of indigenously produced measles vaccine. Ind Pediatr 33:827–831, 1996.
131. Orenstein WA, Markowitz LE, Preblud SR, et al. Appropriate age for measles vaccination in the United States. Dev Biol Stand 65:13–21, 1986.
132. Booy R, Aitken SJM, Taylor S, et al. Immunogenicity of combined diphtheria, tetanus, and pertussis vaccine given at 2, 3, and 4 months versus, 3, 5, and 9 months of age. Lancet 339:507–510, 1992.
133. Deforest A, Long SS, Lischner HW, et al. Simultaneous administration of measles-mumps-rubella vaccine with booster doses of diphtheria-tetanus-pertussis and poliovirus vaccines. Pediatrics 81:237–246, 1988.
134. Scheifele D, Law B, Mitchell L, et al. Study of booster doses of two Haemophilus influenzae type b conjugate vaccines including their interchangeability. Vaccine 14:1399–1406, 1996.
135. Aaby P, Samb B, Simondon F, et al. A comparison of vaccine efficacy and mortality during routine use of high titer EZ and Schwarz standard measles vaccines in rural Senegal. Trans Roy Soc Trop Med Hyg 90:326–330, 1996.
136. Expanded Programme on Immunization. Safety of high titer measles vaccines. Wkly Epidemiol Rec 67:357–361, 1992.
137. Black SB, Shinefield HR, and the Northern California Permanente Medical Care Program Department of Pediatrics Vaccine Study Group. b-CAPSA I Haemophilus influenzae, type b capsular polysaccharide vaccine safety. Pediatrics 79:321–325, 1987.
138. Meekison W, Hutcheon M, Guasparini R, et al. Post-marketing surveillance of adverse events following PROHIBIT vaccine in British Columbia. Can Med Assoc J 141:927–929, 1989.
139. Vadheim CM, Greenberg DP, Marcy SM, et al. Safety evaluation of PRP-D Haemophilus influenzae type b conjugate vaccine in children immunized at 18 months of age and older: Followup study of 30,000 children. Pediatr Infect Dis J 9:555–561, 1990.
140. Unintentional administration of varicella virus vaccine—United States, 1996. MMWR Morb Mortal Wkly Rep 45:1017–1018, 1996.
141. Coplan P, Black S, Guess HA, et al. Post-marketing safety of varicella vaccine among 44,369 vaccinees [abstract]. Am J Epidemiol 145:S76, 1997.
142. Inactivated Japanese Encephalitis Vaccine: Recommendations of the Advisory Committee on Immunization Practices (ACIP). MMWR Morb Mortal Wkly Rep 42(RR-1):1–15, 1993.
143. Jones P, Fine P, Piracha S. Crohn's disease and measles. Lancet 349:473, 1997.
144. Heijbel H, Chen RT, Dahlquist G. Cumulative incidence of childhood-onset IDDM is unaffected by pertussis immunization. Diabetes Care 20:173–175, 1997.
145. Bernier RH, Frank JA, Dondero TJ, Turner P. DTP vaccine and sudden infant deaths in Tennessee. J Pediatr 101:419–421, 1982.
146. Solberg LK. DTP vaccination, visit to child health center and sudden infant death syndrome (SIDS): Evaluation of DTP vaccination. Report to the Oslo Health Council 1985. Bethesda, MD, NIH Library Translation, 1985, pp 85–152.

147. Bouvier-Colle MH, Flahaut A, Messiah A, et al. Sudden infant death and immunization: An extensive epidemiologic approach to the problem in France—Winter 1986. Int J Epidemiol 18:121–126, 1989.
148. Mitchell EA, Stewart AW, Clements M, et al. Immunisation and the sudden infant death syndrome. Arch Dis Child 73:498–501, 1995.
149. Gale JL, Thapa PB, Wassilak SGF, et al. Risk of serious acute neurological illness after immunization with DTP vaccine: A population-based case-control study. JAMA 271:37–41, 1994.
150. Simon PA, Chen RT, Elliott JA, Schwartz B. Outbreak of pyogenic abscesses after diphtheria and tetanus toxoids and pertussis vaccination. Pediatr Infect Dis J 12:368–371, 1993.
151. Karch FE, Lasagna L. Adverse drug reactions. JAMA 234:1236–1241, 1975.
152. Walker AM, Jick H, Perera DR, et al. Diphtheria-tetanus-pertussis immunization and sudden infant death syndrome. Am J Public Health 77:945–951, 1987.
153. Walker AM, Jick H, Perera DR, et al. Neurologic events following diphtheria-tetanus-pertussis immunization. Pediatrics 81:345–349, 1988.
154. Griffin MR, Ray WA, Livengood JR, et al. Risk of sudden infant death syndrome following diphtheria-tetanus-pertussis immunization. N Engl J Med 319:618–623, 1988.
155. Griffin MR, Ray WA, Mortimer EA, et al. Risk of seizures and encephalopathy after immunization with the diphtheria-tetanus-pertussis vaccine. JAMA 263:1641–1645, 1990.
156. Davis RL, Marcuse E, Black S, et al. MMR2 at 4–5 years and 10–11 years of age: A comparison of adverse event rates in the Vaccine Safety Datalink (VSD) Project. Pediatrics 100:767–771, 1997.
157. Williams JC, Goldenthal KL, Burns DL, Lewis BP Jr (eds). Combined Vaccines and Simultaneous Administration: Current Issues and Perspective. New York, New York Academy of Science, 1995.
158. Hinman AR, Orenstein WA. Public health considerations. In Plotkin SA, Mortimer EA (eds). Vaccines (2nd ed). Philadelphia, WB Saunders, 1994, pp 903–932.
159. Carpl J. Can you trust your medical information? Books and web sites can be misleading, doctors warn. Investor's Business Daily 1997 June 23; Sect. A:1.
160. National Research Council. Improving Risk Communication. Washington, DC, National Academy Press, 1989.
161. Bostrom A. Vaccine risk communication: Lessons from risk perception, decision making and environmental risk communication research. Risk Health Safety Environment 8:173–200, 1997.
162. Slovic P. Perception of risk. Science 23:280–285, 1987.
163. Asch D, Baron J, Hershey JC, et al. Omission bias and pertussis vaccine. Med Decis Making 14:118–123, 1994.
164. National Childhood Vaccine Injury Act of 1986. Section 2125, Public Health Service Act, 42 U.S.C. §300aa-(Supp 1987).
165. Clayton EW, Hickson GB, Miller CS. Parent's responses to vaccine information pamphlets. Pediatrics 93:369–372, 1994.
166. Coulter HL, Fisher BL. DTP: A Shot in the Dark. Garden City Park, NY, Avery, 1991.
167. National Immunization Program. 6 Common Misconceptions About Vaccination and How to Respond to Them. Atlanta, Centers for Disease Control and Prevention, 1996.
168. Canadian Paediatric Society. Your Child's Best Shot: A Parent's Guide to Vaccination. Ottawa, Canadian Paediatric Society, 1997.
169. Lynn FM, Busenberg GJ. Citizen advisory committees and environmental policy: What we know, what's left to discover. Risk Anal 15:147–162, 1995.
170. Goldman A. The refutation of medical paternalism. In Arras JD, Steinbock B (eds). Ethical Issues in Modern Medicine. Mountain View, CA, Mayfield Publishing, 1995, pp 58–66.
171. Severyn KM, Jacobson V. Massachusetts: Impact on informed consent and vaccine policy. J Pharm Law 5:249–273, 1997.
172. Hardin G. The tragedy of the commons. Science 162:1243–1248, 1968.
173. Fine PEM, Clarkson JA: Individual versus public priorities in the determination of optimal vaccination policies. Am J Epidemiol 124:1012–1020, 1986.
174. Hershey JC, Asch DA, Thumasathit T, et al. The role of altruism, free riding, and bandwagoning in vaccination decisions. Organizational Behavior and Human Decision Processes 59:177–187, 1994.
175. Editorial. Betraying the public over nvCJD risk. Lancet 348:1529, 1996.
176. McNamee D. Communicating drug-safety information. Lancet 350:1646, 1997.
177. Wilkie T. Sources in science: Who can we trust? Lancet 347:1308–1311, 1996.
178. Update: Vaccine side effects, adverse reactions, contraindications, and precautions: Recommendations of the Advisory Committee on Immunization Practices (ACIP). MMWR Morb Mortal Wkly Rep 45(RR-12):1–35, 1996.
179. Slater PE, Ben-Zvi T, Fogel A, et al. Absence of an association between rubella vaccination and arthritis in underimmune postpartum women. Vaccine 13:1529–1532, 1995.
180. Tingle AJ, Mitchell LA, Grace M, et al. Randomised double-blind placebo-controlled study on adverse effects of rubella immunisation in seronegative women. Lancet 349:1277–1281, 1997.
181. Ray P, Black S, Shinefield H, et al. Risk of chronic arthropathy following rubella vaccination. JAMA 278:551–556, 1997.
182. Rabinovich RN, McInnes P, Klein DL, Fall FB. Vaccine technologies: View to the future. Science 265:1401–1404, 1994.
183. Russo S, Turin L, Zanella A, et al. What's going on in vaccine technology? Med Res Rev 17:277–301, 1997.
184. Olive JM, Risi JB, DeQuadros CA. National immunization days—experience in Latin America. J Infect Dis 175:S189–193, 1997.
185. Global Programme on Vaccines and Immunization. Steering Group on the Development of Jet Injection for Immunization, Geneva, 18–19 March 1997. Geneva, WHO/GPV, 1997.
186. Federal Aviation Administration. 1996 Strategic Plan. Washington, DC, Federal Aviation Administration, 1996.
187. Merrill RA. Food safety regulation: Reforming the Delaney Clause. Annu Rev Public Health 18:313–340, 1997.
188. Leveton LB, Sox HC, Stoto MA (eds). HIV and the Blood Supply: An Analysis of Crisis Decisionmaking. Washington, DC, National Academy Press, 1995.
189. Chen RT. A multi-faceted approach to improve vaccine safety in the United States. Proceedings of the 24th National Immunization Conference, May 21–25, 1990, Orlando, Florida. Atlanta, Centers for Disease Control, Division of Immunization, 1990, pp 107–109.
190. Khoury MJ, Risch N, Kelsey JL. Genetic epidemiology. Epidemiol Rev 19:1–185, 1997.

chapter

50 U.S. Law

Edmund W. Kitch
Geoffrey Evans
Robyn Gopin

In this chapter, we review liability for vaccine injuries under the common law; the rationale, development, and implementation of the national Vaccine Injury Compensation Program (VICP); and the program's current status. The first part of the chapter covers the development of the law in the United States up to 1986, the year of the passage of the National Childhood Vaccine Injury Act. The next two sections cover the administration of the VICP and the reported decisions relating to liability for the production and administration of vaccines after 1986, respectively.

VACCINE LIABILITY BEFORE 1986

U.S. courts have addressed two major legal issues related to vaccination. First, are participants in the vaccination program, such as vaccine producers and administering medical personnel, liable for the adverse reactions of vaccinees to the vaccination? The answer to this question has generally been no, unless the vaccine is defective or the personnel have failed to follow accepted medical procedures or to advise the vaccinee of the risks. Occasionally, the answer has been yes, even when the vaccine and the procedures were completely proper. Second, can the government compel vaccination? The answer is yes.

Manufacturers and administering medical personnel need not fear liability under U.S. law as the rules are usually stated, provided that two conditions are met: first, that the vaccine is properly made and administered in accordance with accepted medical procedures and, second, that the recipient has been warned of the risks associated with vaccination.

The risk of liability created by these two qualifications is important. If, for instance, a batch of vaccine is defective and causes disease in recipients because the disease-causing agent has not been sufficiently inactivated or because of contaminants, the manufacturer may be liable, whether or not the defect in the vaccine can be shown to be the manufacturer's fault. This happened with an early batch of Salk-killed poliovirus vaccine, and there were numerous and substantial recoveries by persons who acquired polio from the vaccine.* Or if a physician administers a vaccine when it is contraindicated—for instance, he or she administers Sabin oral poliovirus vaccine to a child known to be immunodeficient or administers a second dose of diphtheria-tetanus-pertussis (DTP) vaccine after a child has reacted strongly to the first—then the physician may be liable, if the adverse consequence risked by violating the indication occurs. Furthermore, if a physician administers a vaccine without warning the patient of the risks, the physician may be liable if the risks occur.

Court decisions that have imposed liability even if the vaccine was properly made and administered may be divided into three categories: the Reyes decision, the swine flu litigation against the government, and the 1980s decisions.

The cases discussed here are reported decisions in the appellate courts. An important aspect of the problem for the pharmaceutical houses was the number of cases filed. There is no systematic reporting of either pending or decided cases in the U.S. lower courts. *Reyes v. Wyeth Laboratories*, decided in 1974, held a producer of Sabin oral polio vaccine liable to a child who contracted polio after being administered the vaccine.* The facts on which the court based its opinion were that the manufacturer had sold the vaccine to the Texas Department of Public Health, accompanied by Food and Drug Administration (FDA) required package inserts containing a warning. The Texas Department of Public Health had then sent the vaccine on to the county health department without taking steps to ensure that the warning would actually be given to the vaccine recipients. The county public health nurse who administered the vaccine to the child had not warned the parents that there is a minute risk that a recipient or contact can contract the disease.

The general rule is that the manufacturer of prescription medicines, including vaccines, has no duty to directly warn the user of the product of risks. In contrast, the maker of an over-the-counter product sold directly to consumers does have a duty, on package labeling, to provide such warnings. These established rules would seem to have dictated a decision for the defendant phar-

**Gottsdanker v. Cutter Laboratories*, 182 Cal. App. 2d 602, 6 Cal. Reptr. 320 (Dist. Ct. App. 1960).

**Reyes v. Wyeth Laboratories*, 498 F.2d 1264 (5th Cir. 1974). Reyes was followed in *Givens v. Lederle*, 556 F.2d 1341 (5th Cir. 1977).

maceutical house. Instead, the court narrowed the exception for prescription drugs, holding that where a pharmaceutical house can reasonably be said to know that it was likely the vaccine would be administered in such a way that there would be no personalized medical advice provided, (e.g., in the context of a public health department immunization effort in which the patient had no direct contact with a physician), it was the manufacturer's responsibility to warn the consumer or ensure that warnings were given.

The next development was the unfortunate episode of the swine flu vaccine. In the spring of 1976, leading U.S. epidemiologists predicted that the United States would be afflicted the following winter with an unusually severe form of the flu, which would lead to numerous serious illnesses, the associated loss of work, and more serious consequences, including death, for some of those who contracted the disease. Such an epidemic never occurred, but the prediction of one led the government to recommend a campaign to immunize almost all U.S. adults, particularly the elderly, with the support of government funds.*

The *Reyes* decision, holding manufacturers liable for a duty to warn in a mass campaign, caused the manufacturers to refuse to provide the vaccine to the government at low cost (near the cost of production). In addition, the manufacturers, concerned about other unforeseen risks of liability in a program this large, did not want to accept any liability for vaccines that would be produced in accordance with FDA regulations. The result was a hastily drafted statute that imposed this liability on the federal government rather than on the vaccine producers and gave vaccine recipients who believed they had been injured the right to sue in federal district court for recovery.

The swine flu program was a considerable success as a matter of effective public health mobilization. The vaccine was successfully produced, distributed, and administered to more than 45 million people in a few months, with no notable mistakes. But when, in late fall, the feared swine flu epidemic had not yet appeared anywhere in the world and suspicions arose that there might be an association between the vaccine and Guillain-Barré syndrome (GBS), the program was suspended. With doubt and confusion in the air, numerous claims were filed. A Centers for Disease Control and Prevention (CDC)–sponsored study showed a statistically significant increase in the risk of GBS in the weeks after immunization compared with the risk in unvaccinated people. This finding caused the government to agree to accept liability for all cases of GBS with onset falling within the 10-week period for which the study showed a significant association. The government paid more than $90 million on the claims in these cases. (Unpublished data, the Torts Branch, Civil Division, U.S. Department of Justice). However, the government did not agree to accept liability for cases of GBS falling outside this interval nor for other illnesses not known to be caused by influenza vaccines and defended against such claims.

The defense of this litigation resulted in more than 100 judicial opinions on the subject and was almost entirely successful.* However, toward the very end of the litigation, three different courts of appeals wrote opinions in the *Reyes v. Wyeth* tradition that threatened increased liability for vaccine producers: *Hockett v. United States*, 730 F.2d 709 (11th Cir. 1984); *Unthank v. United States*, 732 F.2d 1517 (10th Cir. 1984); and *Petty v. United States*, 740 F.2d 1428 (8th Cir. 1984). The efforts of plaintiffs to establish common law, no-fault tort liability on the part of pharmaceutical houses (i.e., the manufacturer is liable even if adequate warnings are given and the vaccine is produced and handled in full compliance with FDA regulations), appeared to increase after *Reyes* and the swine flu episode. More often than not, plaintiffs lost. However, in the 1980s, plaintiffs also experienced some notable successes in the trial courts, which further confounded the producers and confused the law in this area. For instance, in *Johnson v. American Cyanamid Co.*,† a personal injury case was brought by the father of a vaccinated child who claimed to have contracted polio through contact with the child. The case was brought against both the manufacturer and administrator of the oral polio vaccine (OPV). A Kansas trial jury found that 100% of the fault was to be attributed to the manufacturer and imposed a verdict of $2 million compensatory and $8 million punitive damages in favor of the father. This verdict was reversed by the Kansas Supreme Court, which clearly held that the manufacturer's warning was adequate but implied that the physician, who testified that he did not warn the parents of the risk, might have been liable had the plaintiffs followed the right procedure.

In *Toner v. Lederle Laboratories*, a jury returned a verdict of $1,131,200 in favor of the recipient of a DTP vaccine who claimed that the vaccine caused transverse myelitis, a condition that had never been shown scientifically to be caused by any of the available DTP preparations.‡ The plaintiff's theory was that the DTP caused transverse myelitis and that the defendant could have marketed a safer vaccine, a vaccine once marketed by Eli Lilly and Company that was withdrawn from the market in the 1970s. The jury concluded that Lederle's failure to make a safer version of the vaccine was negligent. The verdict was appealed to the United States Court of Appeals for the Ninth Circuit, which in turn referred the issues to the Supreme Court of Idaho. The Supreme Court of Idaho held that because the jury had

*The episode is carefully summarized and evaluated in Silverstein AM. Pure Politics and Impure Science. Baltimore, Johns Hopkins University Press, 1981. A more partisan account is to be found in Neustadt R, Fineberg H. The Swine Flu Affair: Decision-Making on a Slippery Disease. Washington, DC, United States Department of Health, Education and Welfare, 1978.

*The litigation and the resulting opinions are summarized in detail in Institute of Medicine. Vaccine Supply and Innovation: Report of the Committee on Public-Private Sector Relations in Vaccine Innovation. Washington, DC, National Academy Press, 1985, pp 95–113.

†*Johnson v. American Cyanamid Co.*, Case No. 81 C 2470 (18th Jud. Dist., Sedgwick Co., Kansas), rev'd. 239 Kan. 279, 718 P.2d 1318 (1986).

‡*Toner v. Lederle Laboratories*, 779 F.2d 1429 (9th Cir. 1986), certified question answered by 112 Idaho 328, 732 P.2d 297 (1987), judgment affirmed 828 F.2d 510 (1988), cert denied. 485 U.S. 942 (1988).

determined that Lederle's design of DTP was negligent, the verdict should be affirmed.

The increased risk of liability in the courts for those who manufacture and administer vaccines, which became apparent in U.S. law after 1970, was but a footnote to the general movement in the law of many states toward greater liability for suppliers of goods and services to consumers. This general trend has had noted effects on the medical professions in numerous areas, many of which have been affected more dramatically than the area of vaccination. The reaction of the courts in the previously cited cases may have been related to the fact that the very success of vaccines has changed the way they are perceived by the public. Vaccines are no longer perceived as a miracle preventive measure against frightening disease but as a routine nuisance procedure to prevent disease that hardly anyone—including most young physicians—has actually experienced. It becomes all too easy to demand that a preventive measure against a disease that exists mostly as a historical memory not appear to injure any recipient.* Ironically, this attitude can retard the development of new vaccines against additional and currently threatening diseases. The material addressed here should remind medical experts and public health officials in charge of vaccination efforts that an effective vaccination program, no matter how justified medically and in relation to cost-benefit ratio, requires for its sustained success that its purposes and methods be well understood not only by medical personnel but by society in general. Lack of information, prejudice, and distrust in the larger community can operate to undermine perfectly rational and laudable public health objectives by leading to harmful legislation or ill-informed decisions by judges and juries. Patience and care in explaining what is being done and the reasons for it, no matter how tedious the process, can contribute importantly to the effectiveness of a vaccination program. The difficulties presented by the liability issues should not obscure the important fact that U.S. courts have in fact been very supportive of vaccination programs. That support reflects the judges' understanding of the importance of vaccination and their trust in public health professionals to carry out vaccination programs in a responsible and reasonable manner.

The Power to Compel Vaccination

U.S. courts have been deferential to public health judgments that mandatory vaccination is required. The leading case is *Jacobson v. Massachusetts.*† That case involved a Massachusetts statute that empowered local boards of health to require vaccination of the inhabitants "... if, in its opinion, it is necessary for the public health or safety." The statute demanded a penalty of $5.00 from anyone who failed to comply. The Board of Health of the city of Cambridge, Massachusetts, determined that all residents of Cambridge should be vaccinated against smallpox. Jacobson refused and was fined. Apparently, Jacobson had previously experienced adverse reactions to the vaccine. Jacobson appealed to the Supreme Court, challenging the constitutionality of the statute on the ground that a requirement that he submit to vaccination was an unreasonable infringement of his personal liberty. The Court unanimously rejected this argument.

Jacobson offered to prove in the lower courts that some medical opinion attaches ". . . little or no value to vaccination as a means of preventing the spread of smallpox," and that some physicians believe " . . . that vaccination causes other diseases of the body" (197 U.S. 30). The Court was content to rely on general belief, without hearing evidence. "What everybody knows the court must know, and therefore the state court judicially knew, as this court knows, that an opposite theory accords with the common belief and is maintained by high medical authority. We must assume that, when the statute in question was passed, the legislature of Massachusetts was not unaware of these opposing theories, and was compelled, of necessity, to choose between them. It was not compelled to commit a matter involving the public health and safety to the final decision of a court or jury" (197 U.S. 30).

In closing, the Court observed that "We are not prepared to hold that a minority, residing or remaining in any city or town where smallpox is prevalent, and enjoying the general protection afforded by an organized local government, may thus defy the will of its constituted authorities, acting in good faith for all, under the legislative sanction of the states. If such be the privilege of a minority then a like privilege would belong to each individual of the community, and the spectacle would be presented of the welfare and safety of an entire population being subordinated to the notions of a single individual who chooses to remain a part of that population" (197 U.S. 37–38).

Decisions of contemporary courts continue to be supportive of mandatory vaccination requirements. In *Maricopa County Health Department v. Harmon,** the health department sought an injunction that excluded unimmunized children from school. The health department had issued an emergency rule barring unimmunized children from attending school because of an outbreak of measles in the county. The purpose of the injunction was to enforce the health department rule. The trial court granted the injunction, and the appellate court affirmed. The families resisting exclusion from school argued that the health department had no authority to exclude children unless there had been a confirmed case of measles in the particular school. The court answered, "Appellants cite no authority for the proposition that there is no compelling state interest in taking limited and temporary steps to combat a reasonably perceived risk of the spread of measles absent a serologically confirmed

*Whether existing vaccines do in fact injure any recipient is a difficult question to answer, because the relative rarity of the phenomenon makes it difficult to study. The issues related to establishing actual causal connection are discussed in Ellenberg S and Chen R. The complicated task of monitoring vaccine safety. Public Health Rep 112:10–20, 1997.

†*Jacobson v. Massachusetts,* 197 U.S. 11 (1905).

**Maricopa County Health Department v. Harmon,* 156 Ariz. 161, 750 P.2d 1364 (Ariz. App. 1987).

case, and our research has revealed none" (750 P.2d 1369).*

Contemporary vaccination laws are not as sweeping as the law involved in *Jacobson*. All states require vaccination of children before their entry to school.† However, the recommended age of administration for these vaccines is during the first 2 years of life, and the vaccines are in fact administered to a high percentage of children at the recommended age. The laws may persuade reluctant parents that because vaccination will be required eventually, they might as well agree to vaccination at the recommended time. There are no requirements for adult vaccination in the United States.‡

The laws that require vaccination before school entry are congruent with the program operated by the Public Health Service under the provisions of the Public Health Service Act, 42 U.S.C. § 262. If a state or local government participates in a federally funded immunization program it must, among other things, have a " . . . plan to assure that children begin and complete their immunizations on schedule . . . " and a ". . . plan to systematically immunize susceptible children at school entry through vigorous enforcement of school immunization laws" (42 C.F.R. § 51b.204).

And in the *Matter of Christine M.*,* the court held that it was child neglect for an otherwise responsible and satisfactory parent to refuse to permit his or her 2-year-old child to be vaccinated for measles during a measles outbreak in New York City. However, the court, pointing out that vaccination would be required when the child entered school in any case and that the measles outbreak had ended by the time of the decision, refrained from ordering immediate vaccination.

*Whereas courts have upheld the right of individual states to mandate immunization, some states have voluntarily granted individuals exemptions from this requirement based on religious or personal beliefs. Although the court in *Brown v. Stone*, 378 So. 2d 218 (Mississippi, 1979), struck a religious exemption from the state statute on the grounds that it violated the equal protection clause of the Fourteenth Amendment, most courts have recognized the right of the state to allow religious exemptions. Instead, the courts have focused on the scope of the exemption. For example, in *Sherr v. Northport-East Northport Union Free School District*, 672 F. Supp. 81 (E.D.N.Y. 1987), the court held that limiting the religious exemption to "bona fide members of a recognized religious organization" whose doctrines oppose vaccinations violated the establishment clause and free exercise clause of the First Amendment. The court held that a deeply held religious belief in opposition to vaccination, regardless of whether the individual was part of an established religion, should satisfy the exemption. Other litigants have challenged the constitutionality of allowing religious exemptions and not philosophical exemptions. The courts have ruled that the First Amendment does not apply to philosophical exemptions and that there is no Constitutional right to such an exemption. As with religious exemptions, the courts have given the states the discretion to grant philosophical exemptions if they so choose. To date, less than one third of states allow philosophical exemptions. Other instances challenging mandatory vaccination include *Ritterband v. Axelrod*, 562 N.Y.S. 2d 605 (1990), in which a New York trial court upheld health department regulations that required, among other things, that hospital employees and medical staff have current rubella immunizations. The lawsuit was filed by a staff doctor who argued that the vaccination requirement was a violation of the Fourth Amendment protection against unreasonable searches and seizures.

†Some states do not require all of the standard pediatric vaccines for school entry. Six states (Idaho, Maine, New York, Oregon, Pennsylvania, and Texas) do not require pertussis vaccine. Requirements for daycare attendees for pertussis vaccine are in place in all states, and there is no exception to the law. Additionally, six others (Alaska, Arkansas, Iowa, South Carolina, Vermont, and West Virginia) do not require mumps vaccination. (United States Department of Health and Human Services, Centers for Disease Control and Prevention, National Immunization Program, State Immunization Requirements 1996–1997 [October 1997]). There is no indication that these vaccines are not widely administered to children even in those states that do not require them for school entry.

‡Vaccinations are required for entry into the military, but the United States no longer mandates any immunization for U.S. citizens who travel abroad. Although there are no federal mandates for adult vaccination, the Occupational Safety and Health Administration regulations require employers to make vaccination available to employees potentially exposed to bloodborne pathogens (e.g., healthcare workers must be offered hepatitis B immunization). An example of a nongovernment–related requirement is immunization for college entry.

*157 Misc. 2d 4, 595 N.Y.S. 2d 606 (Family Court, Kings County 1992).

NATIONAL CHILDHOOD VACCINE INJURY ACT

The National Childhood Vaccine Injury Act (NCVIA), was enacted in 1986.[1] Pleas to enact a federal statute date from *Reyes v. Wyeth*.†

The most dramatic development in the period after the *Reyes v. Wyeth* decision and its progeny was the withdrawal of a number of pharmaceutical houses from the activity of producing vaccines.‡

Vaccines were a stable, even declining, product market, with low profit margins even before concerns about product liability arose. For instance, the DTP vaccine was once sold for $0.10 a dose. With roughly 3 million children born each year in the United States during the early 1980s, even if all children received the recommended five doses, the total annual gross revenue generated by the vaccine at that price would be $1,500,000. If only a few of those children recovered $1,000,000, a not unreasonable amount for a young child suffering a lifetime of mental impairment, then the cost of the tort recovery would exceed not the profit, but the total revenue from the product. Considering that gross sales of DTP (not profit) were about $3 million in 1980 for all manufacturers, it is easy to understand withdrawal from the market in the face of increasing numbers of lawsuits with judgments that sometimes resulted in awards of millions of dollars. The difficulty of the cases was further compounded by the fact that under many state tort laws for children, the statute of limitations does not run out until some prescribed time period after they become adults. Thus, a case could be filed based on a vaccination given years before, with records lost and memories faded.

If the only problem presented by this liability was

†At the time of the swine flu program in 1976, the industry asked Congress to pass a statute dealing with the problem for all vaccines, but Congress passed a statute dealing only with the swine flu vaccine. The preamble to the statute stated that it was necessary ". . . in order to be prepared to meet the potential emergency . . . until Congress develops a permanent approach for handling claims arising under programs of the Public Health Service act." That "permanent approach" did not appear for another decade.

‡Information about these developments is presented in Institute of Medicine. Vaccine Supply and Innovation. Washington, DC, National Academy Press, 1985.

cost, then the producers could have dealt with it by simply raising their prices. To a large extent, that was what happened. For instance, DTP, which sold for $0.19 in 1980 increased to more than $12.00 by 1986. Although this strategy diverts scarce public health funds from other uses, it might be a stable long-term solution, except for the fact that the amount of the potential liability is completely unknowable. Aside from the uncertainty surrounding what the courts will do, the extent of the side effects actually caused by vaccines cannot be known precisely. The litigation has not arisen out of common adverse side effects, which occur with sufficient frequency that their rate of occurrence can be predicted, but from rare adverse side effects. Such events occur in a very small number of the population, and either are coincidental, chance events (i.e., "background rate") or are actually vaccine related, perhaps because there is something different about the immune systems of such people or their reactions to the attenuated disease-causing agent.

Even more troubling, the risk of liability is particularly threatening for any firm that contemplates vaccine research and development. Before a new vaccine can be introduced, it must, like any drug, be subjected to testing to establish its efficacy and safety. That process is very costly, and the cost can only be recovered after the vaccine has been marketed. Yet, it is simply impossible because of both cost and logistics to administer a new vaccine a sufficient number of times to detect adverse side effects that occur in only a few of 1 million administrations. What happens to a producer who, only after incurring all the costs of development and introduction, discovers that the vaccine has adverse side effects for a small number of recipients? The marginal commercial incentive to develop new vaccines was further reduced by the threat of tort liability.

Manufacturers in concert with the American Academy of Pediatrics (AAP) and the American Medical Association (AMA) argued that the unpredictable state of the law, combined with a rising tide of complaints, threatened continuation of an effective vaccination effort. Compelling evidence of this could be seen in the diminishing numbers of companies willing to continue production. Manufacturers of DTP declined from seven to two, of live oral poliovirus vaccine from three to one, and of measles vaccine from six to one. Both health organizations advanced proposals to ameliorate the disincentives created by the threat of tort liability.

The AAP and the AMA were concerned about both the continued availability of vaccines and the possibility that they were also at risk, because it is common for plaintiffs to join both the pharmaceutical house and the administering physician in the complaint, claiming that the physician did not adequately disclose the risk of the vaccine. This was dramatically demonstrated in North Carolina, when a federal jury found a leading pediatrician liable for more than $1 million for a routine pediatric immunization given years earlier. Although that verdict was overturned by the trial judge, it mobilized pediatricians in North Carolina to seek a statute protecting them from liability. The North Carolina legislature responded to the threat that North Carolina would no longer have an effective immunization program by passing a statute protecting all participants in the delivery of vaccines from liability and providing compensation to injured vaccinees. The statute passed unanimously, and the political message no doubt reached the members of Congress.*

National Vaccine Injury Compensation Program

Purpose and Goals

The VICP established by the NCVIA was authorized by Congress to address a variety of public policy needs.[2–4] First and most important, it is only simple justice that individuals inadvertently injured by properly produced and administered vaccines in public health programs should receive compensation. Because society mandates their use through state laws for school entry, it is not only reasonable but appropriate that society take responsibility for unavoidable adverse outcomes. Second, the delays and uncertainties of the tort system warranted a more reasonable, fair approach. Third, the vaccine production and supply situation would inevitably lead to serious outbreaks of otherwise preventable disease. Fourth, the unprecedented vaccine price increases were caused largely by the projected costs of litigation as calculated by the manufacturers. Fifth, the increasing scientific capability for the production of new and improved vaccines obviously required considerable interest and investment on the part of biological manufacturers, and, at the very least, the litigious climate surrounding the use of vaccines was detrimental to such efforts. Finally, there was no evidence that the problem was going to disappear, particularly in view of the attention devoted to it by the media.

Congress addressed these issues by creating the VICP, a federal "no-fault" compensation program under which awards can be made to vaccine-injured individuals quickly, easily, and generously. Persons injured through the receipt of a vaccine after the enactment of the legislation are required to file claims with the VICP before they are allowed to bring a civil suit. Rules of evidence, discovery, and other legal procedures are relaxed to accelerate the compensation process. Judgments (whether dismissing the claim or awarding compensation) must be expressly rejected by the petitioner prior to their seeking other remedies, such as filing a civil suit. Once a judgment is rejected, a person essentially forfeits any right to compensation under the program and can only seek remedies through other channels. Funding for the program is provided through a tax placed on designated childhood vaccines.

The existing controversy over vaccine causation played heavily in creating the VICP's framework and

*§§130A-422 to 130A-432 of the General Statutes of North Carolina, Senate Bill 859, passed July 15, 1986. This episode is described in the *American Medical News* for August 1, 1986. At the time of the swine flu program, two states passed statutes protecting administering personnel. California Health and Safety Code §§429.35 and 429.36; Maryland Code §18-401.

the Act's sweeping vaccine safety provisions. The federal government was essentially brought into a full-time vaccine safety role, with some viewing the legislation as perhaps more aptly named the National Childhood Vaccine Safety Act. The NCVIA included a mandate for the reporting of certain adverse events. Healthcare providers and vaccine manufacturers are now required to report the occurrence of any event set forth in the Vaccine Injury Table (Table 50–1), as well as any contraindicating reaction to a vaccine that is specified in the manufacturer's package insert. The report is to consist of the symptoms and manifestations of the illness or injury, how long after administration of the vaccine such symptoms occurred, and the manufacturer and lot number of the vaccine administered. These reports are to be made to what later became known as the Vaccine Adverse Event Reporting System (VAERS). Other vaccine safety mandates include office record keeping (documenting the date of vaccine administration, the manufacturer and lot number, and the name and address of administrator); development of risk-benefit information materials (currently known as Vaccine Information Statements); and Institute of Medicine (IOM) studies of adverse events for covered vaccines.

The NCVIA also provided for two advisory panels, the Advisory Commission on Childhood Vaccines (ACCV) and the National Vaccine Advisory Committee (NVAC). The ACCV is charged with monitoring the VICP and making recommendations to the Secretary of the U.S. Department of Health and Human Services (Secretary, HHS) regarding the program. A key responsibility is advising on changes to the Vaccine Injury Table. Other charges to the commission include responsibilities for monitoring vaccine safety and making recommendations for appropriate changes.

The NVAC has the much broader charge of reviewing and making recommendations concerning vaccine research, production, delivery, safety, and efficacy. Recommendations are forwarded to the Assistant Secretary for Health and have included ad hoc committee reviews of risks associated with each of the vaccines listed in the Injury Table. In response to the measles epidemic in the late 1980s, NVAC generated Congressional support for the much-needed funding and infrastructure to deal with this public health crisis. Both the *Measles White Paper*[5] and the *Standards for Pediatric Immunization Practice*[6] resulted from these efforts.

Structure and Process

The VICP is administered jointly by the Department of Health and Human Services, the U.S. Court of Federal Claims, and the Department of Justice (DOJ). The 10 vaccines designated by the CDC for "routine administration to children" are covered by the program. The vaccines include *Haemophilus influenzae* type b (Hib); diphtheria, tetanus, pertussis (DTP, DTaP [acellular pertussis], DTP-Hib, DT, Td, and TT [tetanus toxoid]); measles, mumps, and rubella (MMR, MR, M, R); polio (inactivated polio vaccine [IPV] and OPV); hepatitis B (HBV); and varicella-zoster virus (VZV) vaccines.

Under the Act, claims alleging injury for vaccines given on or after October 1, 1988 (the program's startup date, otherwise known as "post-1988 claims"), must first be filed under the VICP. Only if compensation is denied by the VICP or is refused by the claimant can civil litigation be undertaken. These so-called prospective claims must be filed within 36 months after the first symptom appeared following vaccination, and effects of the injury must have continued for at least 6 months. Death claims must be filed within 24 months of the death and within 48 months after the onset of the vaccine-related injury from which the death occurred. The Act provides for up to 14 months from the filing date for the court to issue a decision subject to extension. Awards are funded by a vaccine surtax levied on the manufacturers for each dose sold, which, of course, is passed on to the consumers. Compensation covers past and future unreimbursable vaccine-related medical costs. In addition, there is no statutory limitation on attorneys' fees or lost wages. Pain and suffering is limited to a maximum of $250,000.

Pre-1988 claims, also known as "retrospective claims," alleging injury from vaccines given before October 1, 1988, differ in several ways from those given on or after that date. First, these "retrospective" claims are no longer eligible for adjudication. The deadline for filing retrospective claims was January 31, 1991; until that point, petitioners had the option of seeking recourse under either the VICP or the tort system. Like prospective claims, the court had a statutory deadline for rendering a decision. Amendments subsequently gave petitioners the right to continue their vaccine claim in the federal system without a time limit for adjudication.[7] Awards are funded by an annual Congressional appropriation of $110 million, with compensation covering only future unreimbursable vaccine-related medical costs. Attorney's fees, pain and suffering, and lost wages are limited to a $30,000 combined cap.

Petitions (claims) are filed against the Secretary, HHS, as respondent on behalf of the government. Petitioners, either through an attorney or on their own, file a petition with the court, which begins the review and adjudication process. Supporting documents required by the court include medical records and affidavits of the parents (or other family members). Expert witness reports may also accompany the initial filing.

The VICP medical staff (currently four pediatricians and one neurologist) has 90 days in which to reach a recommendation on petitioners' entitlement to compensation, which is then forwarded to the court through the DOJ attorney assigned to the case.

Decision-making authority is vested in specially appointed attorneys called special masters (ranging from six to eight in number), who act in a capacity similar to administrative law judges. Proceedings are expedited by eliminating formal civil discovery and rules of evidence in favor of a more informal process. Court rules provide for regular telephone status conferences with both parties and informal review and even fact determinations by the master prior to hearing. These relaxed rules also seem to encourage and facilitate settlements.

The VICP medical staff recommendations are based

Table 50–1. NATIONAL CHILDHOOD VACCINE INJURY ACT REPORTING AND COMPENSATION TABLES*

Vaccine	Adverse Event	Interval from Vaccination to Onset of Event	
		For Reporting†	*For Compensation‡*
I. Tetanus toxoid–containing vaccines (e.g., DTaP, DTP, DT, Td, or TT)	A. Anaphylaxis or anaphylactic shock	0–7 days	0–4 hours
	B. Brachial neuritis	0–28 days	2–28 days
	C. Any acute complication or sequela (including death) of above events	No limit	No limit
	D. Events described in manufacturer's package insert as contraindications to additional doses of vaccine	No limit	Not applicable
II. Pertussis antigen–containing vaccines (e.g., DTaP, DTP, P, DTP-Hib)	A. Anaphylaxis or anaphylactic shock	0–7 days	0–4 hours
	B. Encephalopathy (or encephalitis)	0–7 days	0–72 hours
	C. Any acute complication or sequela (including death) of above events	No limit	No limit
	D. Events described in manufacturer's package insert as contraindications to additional doses of vaccine	No limit	Not applicable
III. Measles, mumps, and rubella virus–containing vaccines in any combination (e.g., MMR, MR, M, R)	A. Anaphylaxis or anaphylactic shock	0–7 days	0–4 hours
	B. Encephalopathy (or encephalitis)	0–15 days	5–15 days
	C. Any acute complication or sequela (including death) of above events	No limit	No limit
	D. Events described in manufacturer's package insert as contraindications to additional doses of vaccine	No limit	Not applicable
IV. Rubella virus–containing vaccines (e.g., MMR, MR, R)	A. Chronic arthritis	0–42 days	7–42 days
	B. Any acute complication or sequela (including death) of above event	No limit	No limit
	C. Events described in manufacturer's package insert as contraindications to additional doses of vaccine	No limit	Not applicable
V. Measles virus–containing vaccines (e.g., MMR, MR, M)	A. Thrombocytopenic purpura	0–30 days	7–30 days
	B. Vaccine-strain measles viral infection in an immunodeficient recipient	0–6 months	0–6 months
	C. Any acute complication or sequela (including death) of above events	No limit	No limit
	D. Events described in manufacturer's package insert as contraindications to additional doses of vaccine	No limit	Not applicable
VI. Polio live virus–containing vaccines (OPV)	A. Paralytic polio		
	In a nonimmunodeficient recipient	0–30 days	0–30 days
	In an immunodeficient recipient	0–6 months	0–6 months
	In a vaccine-associated community case	No limit	No limit
	B. Vaccine-strain polio viral infection		
	In a nonimmunodeficient recipient	0–30 days	30 days
	In an immunodeficient recipient	0–6 months	0–6 months
	In a vaccine-associated community case	No limit	No limit
	C. Any acute complication or sequela (including death) of above events	No limit	No limit
	D. Events described in manufacturer's package insert as contraindications to additional doses of vaccine	No limit	Not applicable
VII. Polio inactivated–virus containing vaccines (e.g., IPV)	A. Anaphylaxis or anaphylactic shock	0–7 days	0–4 hours
	B. Any acute complication or sequela (including death) of above event	No limit	No limit
	C. Events described in manufacturer's package insert as contraindications to additional doses of vaccine	No limit	Not applicable
VIII. Hepatitis B antigen–containing vaccines	A. Anaphylaxis or anaphylactic shock	0–7 days	0–4 hours
	B. Any acute complication or sequela (including death) of above event	No limit	No limit
	C. Events described in manufacturer's package insert as contraindications to additional doses of vaccine	No limit	Not applicable
IX. *Haemophilus influenzae* type b (Hib) polysaccharide vaccines (unconjugated vaccines)	A. Early-onset Hib disease	0–7 days	0–7 days
	B. Any acute complication or sequela (including death) of above event	No limit	No limit
	C. Events described in manufacturer's package insert as contraindications to additional doses of vaccine	No limit	Not applicable
X. Hib polysaccharide conjugate vaccines	A. No condition specified for compensation	Not applicable	Not applicable
	B. Events described in manufacturer's package insert as contraindications to additional doses of vaccine	No limit	Not applicable

Table continued on following page

Table 50–1. NATIONAL CHILDHOOD VACCINE INJURY ACT REPORTING AND COMPENSATION TABLES* *Continued*

Vaccine	Adverse Event	Interval from Vaccination to Onset of Event	
		For Reporting†	*For Compensation‡*
XI. Varicella-zoster virus–containing vaccine	A. No condition specified for compensation	Not applicable	Not applicable
	B. Events described in manufacturer's package insert as contraindications to additional doses of vaccine	No limit	Not applicable
XII. Any new vaccine recommended by the Centers for Disease Control and Prevention for routine administration to children, after publication by the Secretary of the Department of Health and Human Services of a notice of coverage.	A. No condition specified for compensation	Not applicable	Not applicable
	B. Events described in manufacturer's package insert as contraindications to additional doses of vaccine	No limit	Not applicable

QUALIFICATIONS AND AIDS TO INTERPRETATION

(1) *Anaphylaxis and anaphylactic shock* mean an acute, severe, and potentially lethal systemic allergic reaction. Most cases resolve without sequelae. Signs and symptoms begin minutes to a few hours after exposure. Death, if it occurs, usually results from airway obstruction caused by laryngeal edema or bronchospasm and may be associated with cardiovascular collapse. Other significant clinical signs and symptoms may include the following: cyanosis, hypotension, bradycardia, tachycardia, arrhythmia, edema of the pharynx and/or trachea and/or larynx with stridor and dyspnea. Autopsy findings may include acute emphysema which results from lower respiratory tract obstruction, edema of the hypopharynx, epiglottis, larynx, or trachea and minimal findings of eosinophilia in the liver, spleen, and lungs. When death occurs within minutes of exposure and without signs of respiratory distress, there may not be significant pathological findings.

(2) *Encephalopathy.* For purposes of the Vaccine Injury Table, a vaccine recipient shall be considered to have suffered an encephalopathy only if such recipient manifests, within the applicable period, an injury meeting the description below of an acute encephalopathy, and then a chronic encephalopathy persists in such person for more than 6 months beyond the date of vaccination.

(i) An *acute encephalopathy* is one that is sufficiently severe so as to require hospitalization (whether or not hospitalization occurred).

(A) *For children younger than 18 months* who present without an associated seizure event, an acute encephalopathy is indicated by a "significantly decreased level of consciousness" (see D, below) lasting for at least 24 hours. Those children younger than 18 months who present following a seizure shall be viewed as having an acute encephalopathy if their significantly decreased level of consciousness persists beyond 24 hours and cannot be attributed to a postictal state (seizure) or medication.

(B) *For adults and children 18 months of age or older*, an acute encephalopathy is one that persists for at least 24 hours and characterized by at least two of the following:

(1) A significant change in mental status that is not medication related; specifically a confusional state, or a delirium, or a psychosis

(2) A significantly decreased level of consciousness, which is independent of a seizure and cannot be attributed to the effects of medication

(3) A seizure associated with loss of consciousness

(C) Increased intracranial pressure may be a clinical feature of acute encephalopathy in any age group.

(D) A "significantly decreased level of consciousness" is indicated by the presence of at least one of the following clinical signs for at least 24 hours or greater (see paragraphs (2)(I)(A) and (2)(I)(B) of this section for applicable timeframes):

(1) Decreased or absent response to environment (responds, if at all, only to loud voice or painful stimuli)

(2) Decreased or absent eye contact (does not fix gaze upon family members or other individuals)

(3) Inconsistent or absent responses to external stimuli (does not recognize familiar people or things)

(E) The following clinical features alone, or in combination, do not demonstrate an acute encephalopathy or a significant change in either mental status or level of consciousness as described above: sleepiness, irritability (fussiness), high-pitched and unusual screaming, persistent inconsolable crying, and bulging fontanelle. Seizures in themselves are not sufficient to constitute a diagnosis of encephalopathy. In the absence of other evidence of an acute encephalopathy, seizures shall not be viewed as the first symptom or manifestation of the onset of an acute encephalopathy.

(ii) *Chronic encephalopathy* occurs when a change in mental or neurological status, first manifested during the applicable time period, persists for a period of at least 6 months from the date of vaccination. Individuals who return to a normal neurological state after the acute encephalopathy shall not be presumed to have suffered residual neurological damage from that event; any subsequent chronic encephalopathy shall not be presumed to be a sequela of the acute encephalopathy. If a preponderance of the evidence indicates that a child's chronic encephalopathy is secondary to genetic, prenatal or perinatal factors, that chronic encephalopathy shall not be considered to be a condition set forth in the Table.

(iii) An encephalopathy shall not be considered to be a condition set forth in the Table if in a proceeding on a petition, it is shown by a preponderance of the evidence that the encephalopathy was caused by an infection, a toxin, a metabolic disturbance, a structural lesion, a genetic disorder or trauma (without regard to whether the cause of the infection, toxin, trauma, metabolic disturbance, structural lesion, or genetic disorder is known). If at the time a decision is made on a petition filed under section 2111(b) of the Act for a vaccine-related injury or death, it is not possible to determine the cause by a preponderance of the evidence of an encephalopathy, the encephalopathy shall be considered to be a condition set forth in the Table.

(iv) In determining whether or not an encephalopathy is a condition set forth in the Table, the Court shall consider the entire medical record.

(3) *Residual seizure disorder.* A petitioner may be considered to have suffered a residual seizure disorder for purposes of the Vaccine Injury Table if the first seizure or convulsion occurred 5–15 days (not less than 5 days and not more than 15 days) after administration of the vaccine and two or more additional distinct seizure or convulsion episodes occurred within 1 year after the administration of the vaccine which were unaccompanied by fever (defined as a rectal temperature equal to or greater than 101.0°F or an oral temperature equal to or greater than 100.0°F). A distinct seizure or convulsion episode is ordinarily defined as including all seizure or convulsive activity occurring within a 24-hour period, unless competent and qualified expert neurological testimony is presented to the contrary in a particular case.

For purposes of the Vaccine Injury Table, a petitioner shall not be considered to have suffered a residual seizure disorder, if the petitioner suffered a seizure or convulsion unaccompanied by fever (as defined above) before the fifth day after the administration of the vaccine involved.

Table 50–1. NATIONAL CHILDHOOD VACCINE INJURY ACT REPORTING AND COMPENSATION TABLES* *Continued*

QUALIFICATIONS AND AIDS TO INTERPRETATION *(Cont.)*

(4) *Seizure and convulsion.* For purposes of paragraphs (2) and (3) of this section, the terms, "seizure" and "convulsion" include myoclonic, generalized tonic-clonic (grand mal), and simple and complex partial seizures. Absence (petit mal) seizures shall not be considered to be a condition set forth in the Table. Jerking movements or staring episodes alone are not necessarily an indication of seizure activity.

(5) *Sequela.* The term *sequela* means a condition or event which was actually caused by a condition listed in the Vaccine Injury Table.

(6) *Chronic arthritis.* For purposes of the Vaccine Injury Table, chronic arthritis may be found in a person with no history in the 3 years prior to vaccination of arthropathy (joint disease) on the basis of:

(A) Medical documentation, recorded within 30 days after the onset, of objective signs of acute arthritis (joint swelling) that occurred between 7 and 42 days after a rubella vaccination

(B) Medical documentation (recorded within 3 years after the onset of acute arthritis) of the persistence of objective signs of intermittent or continuous arthritis for more than 6 months following vaccination

(C) Medical documentation of an antibody response to the rubella virus

For purposes of the Vaccine Injury Table, the following shall not be considered as chronic arthritis: musculoskeletal disorders such as diffuse connective tissue diseases (including but not limited to rheumatoid arthritis, juvenile rheumatoid arthritis, systemic lupus erythematosus, systemic sclerosis, mixed connective tissue disease, polymyositis/dermatomyositis, fibromyalgia, necrotizing vasculitis and vasculopathies, and Sjögren's syndrome), degenerative joint disease, infectious agents other than rubella (whether by direct invasion or as an immune reaction), metabolic and endocrine diseases, trauma, neoplasms, neuropathic disorders, bone and cartilage disorders, and arthritis associated with ankylosing spondylitis, psoriasis, inflammatory bowel disease, Reiter's syndrome, or blood disorders.

Arthralgia (joint pain) or stiffness without joint swelling shall not be viewed as chronic arthritis for purposes of the Vaccine Injury Table.

(7) *Brachial neuritis* is defined as dysfunction limited to the upper extremity nerve plexus (i.e., its trunks, divisions, or cords) without involvement of other peripheral (e.g., nerve roots or a single peripheral nerve) or central (e.g., spinal cord) nervous system structures. A deep, steady, often severe aching pain in the shoulder and upper arm usually heralds onset of the condition. The pain is followed in days or weeks by weakness and atrophy in upper extremity muscle groups. Sensory loss may accompany the motor deficits, but is generally a less notable clinical feature. The neuritis, or plexopathy, may be present on the same side as or the opposite side of the injection; it is sometimes bilateral, affecting both upper extremities. Weakness is required before the diagnosis can be made. Motor, sensory, and reflex findings on physical examination and the results of nerve conduction and electromyographic studies must be consistent in confirming that dysfunction is attributable to the brachial plexus. The condition should thereby be distinguishable from conditions that may give rise to dysfunction of nerve roots (i.e., radiculopathies) and peripheral nerves (i.e., including multiple mononeuropathies), as well as other peripheral and central nervous system structures (e.g., cranial neuropathies and myelopathies).

(8) *Thrombocytopenic purpura* is defined by a serum platelet count less than 50,000/mm^3. Thrombocytopenic purpura does not include cases of thrombocytopenia associated with other causes such as hypersplenism, autoimmune disorders (including alloantibodies from previous transfusions), myelodysplasias, lymphoproliferative disorders, congenital thrombocytopenia, or hemolytic uremic syndrome. This does not include cases of immune (formerly called idiopathic) thrombocytopenic purpura (ITP) that are mediated, for example, by viral or fungal infections, toxins, or drugs. Thrombocytopenic purpura does not include cases of thrombocytopenia associated with disseminated intravascular coagulation, as observed with bacterial and viral infections. Viral infections include, for example, those infections secondary to Epstein-Barr virus, cytomegalovirus, hepatitis A and B, rhinovirus, human immunodeficiency virus (HIV), adenovirus, and dengue virus. An antecedent viral infection may be demonstrated by clinical signs and symptoms and need not be confirmed by culture or serological testing. Bone marrow examination, if performed, must reveal a normal or an increased number of megakaryocytes in an otherwise normal marrow.

(9) *Vaccine-strain measles viral infection* is defined as a disease caused by the vaccine strain that should be determined by vaccine-specific monoclonal antibody or polymerase chain reaction tests.

(10) *Vaccine-strain polio viral infection* is defined as a disease caused by poliovirus that is isolated from the affected tissue and should be determined to be the vaccine-strain by oligonucleotide or polymerase chain reaction. Isolation of poliovirus from the stool is not sufficient to establish a tissue specific infection or disease caused by vaccine-strain poliovirus.

(11) *Early-onset Hib disease* is defined as invasive bacterial illness associated with the presence of Hib organism on culture of normally sterile body fluids or tissue, or clinical findings consistent with the diagnosis of epiglottitis. Hib pneumonia qualifies as invasive Hib disease when radiographic findings consistent with the diagnosis of pneumonitis are accompanied by a blood culture positive for the Hib organism. Otitis media, in the absence of the above findings, does not qualify as invasive bacterial disease. A child is considered to have suffered this injury only if the vaccine was the first Hib immunization received by the child.

*Tables effective as of March 24, 1997.

†Taken from the Reportable Events Table (RET), which lists conditions reportable by law (42 USC 300aa-25) to the Vaccine Adverse Event Reporting System (VAERS), including conditions found in the manufacturer's package insert. In addition, individuals are encouraged to report *ANY* clinically significant or unexpected events (even if you are not certain the vaccine caused the event) for *ANY* vaccine, whether or not it is listed on the RET. Manufacturers are also required by regulation (21 CFR 600.80) to report to the VAERS program all adverse events made known to them for any vaccine. VAERS reporting forms and information can be obtained by calling 1-800-822-7967.

‡Taken from the Vaccine Injury Table (VIT) used in adjudication of claims filed with the National Vaccine Injury Compensation Program. Claims may also be filed for a condition with onset outside the designated time intervals or a condition not included in the Table. The Qualifications and Aids to Interpretation define conditions or injuries listed on the VIT. Information on filing a claim can be obtained by calling 1-800-338-2382 or through the Division of Vaccine Injury Compensation's Home Page: (http://www.hrsa.dhhs.gov/bhpr/vicp).

DTaP, diphtheria, tetanus, and acellular pertussis; DTP, diphtheria, tetanus, and pertussis; Hib, *Haemophilus influenzae* type b; OPV, oral polio vaccine; Td, tetanus and diphtheria toxoids; TT, tetanus toxoid.

on the medical records rather than the affidavits of family members, which are often generated (for purposes of litigation) months to years following the alleged injury. Eligibility for compensation is recommended if the VICP staff finds that the records fulfill the requirements of the Act. The court nearly always concurs with an entitlement recommendation, thereby obviating the need for a hearing. Damages are usually negotiated by the parties after future needs have been assessed by life-care planners and other consultants.

Those cases that are not conceded usually proceed to a hearing before a special master, at which point testimony on both sides is presented, including expert witnesses for each party. In some instances, the court may find the testimony of family members more persuasive than contemporaneously recorded events or give greater weight to the initial diagnosis of the treating physician over determinations made on subsequent clinical evaluations. Therefore, it is not uncommon for the court to award compensation after an entitlement hearing. In fact, a 1992 Office of Inspector General's report on the VICP found that slightly over half of the cases in which the VICP medical staff recommend against entitlement were later compensated in this manner.[8]

Injury awards are usually in the form of an initial lump sum plus an annuity providing a stream of benefits for the lifetime of the injured individual. Punitive damages and awards to others in the family for loss of companionship are not allowed. Compensation for death claims is awarded in a lump sum payment limited to $250,000, regardless of the date of vaccine administration. "Reasonable" attorneys' fees are paid whether or not petitioners are successful in obtaining compensation, providing the claim was brought in good faith. These fees are considerably less than those incurred under the civil tort system because of the abbreviated court procedures.

Special masters' decisions may be appealed by either party to a judge of the Court of Federal Claims and then to the Federal Circuit Court of Appeals. The Court of Appeals has issued approximately 64 published opinions in VICP-related cases, covering causation determinations, eligibility to file under the VICP, compensation type and amount, credibility of evidence determinations, and timelines and requirements for certain procedural steps in the adjudication process.[9] One VICP case decided by the Federal Circuit was eventually reviewed by the Supreme Court (see Whitecotton discussion, later).

A unique feature of the Act was creation of the Vaccine Injury Table and its definitional counterpart, the Qualifications and Aids to Interpretation. Individuals may become eligible to receive compensation if they can prove, by a preponderance of the evidence (more likely than not) that an injury listed on the Table occurred within the prescribed time frame. The government may rebut this with evidence of a definitive alternative cause. However, this "factor unrelated to the vaccine" can not include "any idiopathic, unexplained, unknown, hypothetical, or undocumentable injury, illness or condition." It can include "infection, toxins, trauma or metabolic disturbances."[10] This simplified approach greatly reduces the burden of proving causation. Not surprisingly, most VICP claims allege a Table condition, whether or not any records are able to verify the allegation.

One Federal Circuit Court of Appeals decision underscores the heavy burden placed on the government in rebutting a Table presumption. In *Koston v. Secretary, HHS*,* a child developed seizures within 12 hours after receiving her second DTP vaccination. The government originally conceded it as a Table-onset case for residual seizure disorder. However, a subsequent medical evaluation revealed that the child had Rett syndrome, a genetic condition associated with seizures. The government moved to withdraw the concession, stating that her condition was caused by a factor unrelated to the vaccine. The special master denied the motion, noting that the precise cause of Rett syndrome is unknown. In appealing the decision, the government argued that although the exact cause may be unknown, it is known to be present from birth and therefore cannot be related to the administration of the vaccine. The court held that under the Act's definition of factor unrelated, the cause of Rett syndrome was unknown and therefore could not be a factor unrelated.

If the injury is not listed on the Table or did not occur within the prescribed time frame, a petitioner may still gain entitlement by proof of causation, a standard that is more difficult than through a temporal association-based Table case. In *Grant v. Secretary, HHS*,† the Federal Circuit held that in causation cases, petitioners must show a logical sequence of cause and effect that is supported by a reputable medical or scientific explanation that the vaccination was the reason for the injury. Only a small percentage of VICP claims involve actual causation issues.

Petitioners may also receive entitlement based on a finding that the vaccine significantly aggravated a preexisting condition. The Act defines significant aggravation as "any change for the worse in a preexisting condition which results in markedly greater disability, pain, or illness accompanied by substantial deterioration of health." According to the legislative history, an example would be a child whose seizure frequency increased from one per month to one per day.[11]

Maggie Whitecotton was born with microcephaly in the second to third percentile for head size. She was developing normally at age 3 months, when she experienced seizures within 24 hours after receipt of her third DTP vaccination. Her seizures slowly increased over the next several years, and today she has cerebral palsy and mental retardation. Petitioners originally argued that Maggie suffered an on-Table encephalopathy and/or residual seizure disorder (rather than significant aggravation) as a result of her third DTP vaccination. The government argued that the first symptom of onset of her injury occurred prior to the vaccination and, in the alternative, that her condition was due to a factor unrelated, namely a chronic organic brain syndrome, as evidenced by the microcephaly that existed before the vaccination. The special master denied compensation. The Court of Federal Claims affirmed this decision.

***Koston v. Secretary, HHS*, 974 F.2d 157 (Fed. Cir. 1992).

†*Grant v. Secretary, HHS*, 956 F.2d 1144 (Fed Cir. 1992).

The Court of Appeals for the Federal Circuit reversed the decision, finding that the child was entitled to compensation. This decision was based on an interpretation of the language in the Act concerning when the first sign or symptom of the injury must occur.

The case was then taken to the Supreme Court, which unanimously reversed the Federal Circuit's decision. The Supreme Court found that the Federal Circuit misread the Act regarding the definition of "first symptom or manifestation" of an injury. However, Justice O'Connor, in a separate but concurring opinion, noted that the Federal Circuit opinion did not address the issue of significant aggravation of Maggie's preexisting condition (*Shalala v. Whitecotton**). The case was then remanded to the Federal Circuit, where the court addressed the "significant aggravation" standard. On remand, the Federal Circuit set forth a test specifying that the special master must (1) assess the person's condition prior to the administration of the vaccine, (2) assess the person's current condition, (3) determine if the person's current condition constitutes a significant aggravation of the person's condition prior to vaccination within the meaning of the statute, and, if the special master determines there has been a significant aggravation, then he or she must (4) determine whether the first symptom or manifestation of the significant aggravation occurred within the time period prescribed by the Table (*Whitecotton v. Secretary*†). Under this test, Maggie Whitecotton received compensation.

The Whitecotton decision appears to have set a new legal standard, although only six or seven claims relying on that standard have gone to hearing since that ruling, with decisions pending.

Implementation and Program Experience

Although the Act was landmark in design and scope, further legislation and program refinements were necessary. Funding of the VICP, not provided in the original legislation, was authorized by Congress in early 1987.[12] Additional protections for manufacturers defending "post-1988" Act claims were also written into the law at this time. These included the elimination of plaintiff allegations of vaccine misdesign or inadequate warning of risk, two common tort theories pursued in the 1980s, and the elimination of punitive damages unless it could be proven there was gross negligence in vaccine production.[13] At the same time, the limitation requiring claimants to pursue their claim through the VICP before filing a tort claim against manufacturers was expanded to include healthcare providers, a protection that was not offered to healthcare providers by the original Act.

In 1993, the Act's "sunset" provision terminated authorization for the program and the excise tax on vaccines. Concerns were voiced once again that physicians might be in jeopardy of civil litigation. Passage of the Omnibus Budget Reconciliation Act of 1993,[14] provided permanent reauthorization and a mechanism for adding vaccines. Those designated by CDC (usually on recommendation by the Advisory Committee on Immunization Practices) for routine administration to children would be added to the VICP. Congress would later enact an excise tax as a necessary second step before coverage could begin. The statute provided for 8 years retroactive coverage for those alleging injury from a newly added vaccine, with a 2-year window in which to file after enactment of coverage. Liability protection for future pediatric vaccines was now ensured, at least in principle.

Table 50–2 shows the numbers of claims filed by vaccine type and year of administration. These included hundreds given during the 1950s and 1960s, the oldest case dating back to 1918 for a death alleged to be associated with the pertussis vaccine. Ironically, the program processed many claims that were otherwise barred from the tort system by a state statute of limitations.

Table 50–3 shows the number of cases submitted as of December 31, 1997, including the number of cases pending, adjudicated, or dismissed and the dollars awarded.[15] Many were dismissed by the court on grounds of legal or medical insufficiency. Some, given the opportunity to obtain additional records, later refiled. Awards have ranged from $120 (reimbursement of the filing fee) to $7.5 million (an initial lump sum payment, with the remainder going toward purchase of an annuity) for an OPV-related paralytic polio claim in a young child.

**Shalala v. Whitecotton,* 514 U.S. 268 (1995).

†*Whitecotton v. Secretary, HHS,* 81 F.3d 1099 (Fed. Cir. 1996).

Table 50–2. **NATIONAL VACCINE INJURY COMPENSATION PROGRAM CLAIMS BY YEAR OF ADMINISTRATION AND VACCINE TYPE AS OF DECEMBER 31, 1997***

YEAR OF ADMINISTRATION	DTP, P DTP-Hib†	DT, Td, TT	MMR, MR, M	RUBELLA	OPV	IPV	Hib/HBV and VZV	TOTAL
1910–1919	1	—	—	—	—	—	—	1
1920–1929	1	—	—	—	—	—	—	1
1930–1939	1	0	1	—	—	—	—	2
1940–1949	63	1	2	0	1	1	—	68
1950–1959	178	4	3	1	5	211	—	402
1960–1969	376	5	104	6	76	52	—	619
1970–1979	823	6	120	43	53	0	—	1045
1980–1989	1864	34	199	100	78	0	1	2276
1990–present	459	42	143	25	48	0	3	720
Total	3766	92	572	175	261	264	4	5134

*(n = 5210). 75 claims for vaccines not covered or unspecified.

†One DTaP claim filed.

DTaP, diphtheria, tetanus, acellular pertussis; DT, diphtheria and tetanus for pediatric use; DTP, diphtheria-tetanus-pertussis; HBV, hepatitis B virus; Hib, *Haemophilus influenzae* type b; IPV, inactivated polio vaccine; M, measles or mumps; MMR, measles, mumps, and rubella; MR, measles and rubella; OPV, oral polio vaccine; P, pertussis; Td, diphtheria and tetanus for adult use; VZV, varicella-zoster virus.

Table 50–3. **STATUS OF THE NATIONAL VACCINE INJURY COMPENSATION PROGRAM AS OF DECEMBER 31, 1997**

	VACCINES ADMINISTERED BEFORE 10/1/88	VACCINES ADMINISTERED ON OR AFTER 10/1/88	TOTAL
Claims filed	4243	967	5210
Claims adjudicated	3683 (87%)	623 (64%)	4306 (83%)
Compensable	962 (26%)	281 (45%)	1243 (29%)
Dismissed	2721 (74%)	342 (55%)	3063 (71%)
Awards paid*	2126	450	2576
Dollars (millions)	$659.0	$185.9	$844.9

*Includes attorney fee awards. Some adjudicated claims above have not yet been processed for payment.

The majority (72%) of submissions allege DTP-related effects. The remaining claims break down as follows: 14% from MMR, given alone or in any combination (nearly one fourth involve adults alleging rubella vaccine–related injury); 5% from OPV; 5% from IPV (all before 1988); 2% from tetanus-containing vaccines; and 2% from vaccines either unspecified or not covered by the VICP. Because hepatitis B, Hib, and VZV vaccines were added just prior to publication, very few claims related to these vaccines have been submitted thus far. Although percentages vary slightly by vaccine, injuries account for 85% of claims; deaths, 15%.

The unexpected caseload far exceeded program resources in several respects. Efforts by staff and the court were increased, but the large caseload and the court's dual decision responsibility (entitlement and damages determinations) made timely adjudication impossible. Furthermore, funding soon became an issue, with exhaustion of the $80 million annual appropriation occurring by June 1992. Eventually, the appropriation was increased to $110 million, but not before the program had to twice shut down payments to successful claimants.

Without question, the biggest controversy (and challenge) has been the Vaccine Injury Table. Congress recognized that to ensure that cases of true vaccine injuries were compensated, the criteria for making awards would have to be quite broad; as a result, some persons with disorders that were clearly not vaccine related would receive awards. The legislative history noted the lingering controversy over what is and is not vaccine caused. The Table would serve as a compromise mechanism in the interim to facilitate recovery by individuals "thought" to be injured. Once the scientific studies by the IOM, called for by the Act, were completed, the Secretary, HHS, could make changes to the Table to bring it in line with current scientific thinking. However, change comes slowly, and program outcomes were increasingly at odds with what experts agreed should be attributed to vaccine effects.

For the most part, DTP injury claims are filed on behalf of children and adults with chronic encephalopathy of unknown cause. Overall, as many as 40% of these patients have no specific cause ever determined, with most thought to be due to migrational abnormalities of fetal brain development, or metabolic or "genetic" conditions not identifiable by current technology.[16] Many DTP claims reflect the onset of abnormal neurological signs during the first year of life (when vaccines are routinely given), ranging from the initial seizure of a child with incipient epilepsy to a case in which a child who may have experienced prolonged crying or irritability after vaccination has developmental retardation. Because a Table claim only requires the designated condition and time frame be satisfied to gain eligibility, within a few years, significant numbers of claims were being compensated for conditions thought to be non–vaccine related.

For example, more than one third of DTP injury claims reflect the onset of seizures during infancy as their first manifestation of neurological illness. Because DTP commonly causes fever, children with incipient epilepsy may experience the onset of their convulsive disorder secondary to this routine procedure. Naturally, many go on to have further seizures and developmental delay. Under the Table, residual seizure disorder afforded these children a Table presumption if their seizure onset and subsequent seizure episodes satisfied the Table and Aids. Because epilepsy is frequently idiopathic and the government could not meet its burden of showing an alternative cause, VICP staff routinely conceded these cases.

Another category often compensated was the 14% of DTP injury claims in children with infantile spasms. Those found by the court to have onset outside the Table interval or to be of known cause (i.e., symptomatic) were usually dismissed. However, those that fit the cryptogenic (idiopathic) category of infantile spasms, with onset within a table time frame, were often compensated by the court despite epidemiological studies showing the condition to be non–vaccine related. Court precedent soon led the VICP to choose not to expend resources defending these cases unless a non–vaccine-related cause could be determined.

Even more troublesome were program outcomes in many DTP death claims. Approximately half were due to Sudden Infant Death Syndrome (SIDS) with compatible histories and forensic findings in accordance with the 1989 National Institutes of Health consensus definition. However, because the cause of SIDS remains unknown, these cases are viewed as "idiopathic" by the court.

In hearings, the court would elicit the parents' description of events preceding the death in relation to the medical records to determine if a Table condition occurred. All available records were requested, including pediatric and emergency room records, police or ambulance reports, and the autopsy report. Some SIDS claims were compensated for encephalopathy, based on testimony of irritability or protracted crying, despite the absence of forensic findings of brain involvement. Others received entitlement based on descriptions of lethargy or sleepiness in the hours prior to death as evidence of shock collapse (hypotonic-hyporesponsive episode [HHE]). Unfortunately, "cardiovascular or respiratory arrest" was listed erroneously in the original Table as a manifestation of this DTP-related syndrome in the Aids to Interpretation. However, death for whatever reason is preceded by such terminal events, and it was on this basis that the government appealed several SIDS cases, ultimately reversing the compensation outcome in some.

In *Hellebrand v. Secretary, HHS,** the petitioners alleged HHE in a SIDS death that occurred within 24 hours of DTP vaccination. The special master denied compensation, which was later reversed by a judge of the Claims Court, who noted the respiratory and cardiac arrest language in the Aids. The Federal Circuit reversed this decision denying petitioners compensation, stating that the Aids were just that—"aids"—and therefore the Court did not have to rely on them solely. The ruling in *Hodges v. Secretary, HHS*† gave further support to this interpretation. Quoting from Hellebrand, the court established the standard that in SIDS cases with HHE, compensation requires petitioners to show that the child's death was a sequela of HHE and that although the symptoms of death, such as cardiac arrest or turning blue, are listed in the Aids to Interpretation as symptoms of HHE, those symptoms alone do not establish, by a preponderance of the evidence, that the vaccine caused the injury—in this case, death. If that were the case, the court would find all SIDS cases compensable. The Federal Circuit also noted that proximate temporal association of a death with vaccine administration does not in and of itself establish causation.

Beyond the statute and the court's adjudication approach lay criticisms that the Table was inaccurate, vague, or even misleading. Anaphylaxis was an easy target, with its time interval of 24 hours. By definition, this acute hypersensitivity reaction occurs within minutes to a few hours and is rare after DTP vaccine. (This was never a real issue, as few program cases were compensated for anaphylaxis alone.) Another complaint was the broad definition of encephalopathy in the Aids, which resulted in some claims being found on Table conditions based on the frequent, harmless, but unpleasant minor reactions to DTP, including fever, anorexia, excessive crying, and lethargy.[17]

Modifying the Vaccine Injury Table

By law, the Table can be modified or amended by the Secretary, HHS, in consultation with the Advisory Commission on Childhood Vaccines and after opportunity for public comment. Such changes apply only to cases filed after the effective date of the changes. (Retroactive changes in the Table can be made only by Congressional action.)

Two separate efforts by the VICP to modify the Table and Aids to Interpretation began with publication of the two Congressionally mandated IOM reviews in 1991 and 1994, respectively.[18–21] The first review called for under Section 312 of the Act covered adverse events after pertussis and rubella immunization. Proposed changes developed by VICP staff underwent extensive scientific review and public comment over the next 4 years, leading to publication of a final rule in the *Federal Register* effective March 10, 1995.[22] (Seventy-five claims were filed in the days and weeks prior to the effective date, no doubt trying to avoid adjudication under the more restrictive guidelines.)

The approach by VICP was straightforward: If the IOM concluded there was evidence that a condition was "causally related," it was added to the Table or left on. If, on the other hand, there was no proven evidence of an association, it was removed. The only exception was encephalopathy/encephalitis under DTP vaccine, which had been proposed for removal but was left on the Table in response to advice from the ACCV. The Commission argued that claims of acute encephalopathy of unknown etiology within 3 days of DTP vaccination should continue to receive a presumption of causation, but that the definition in the Aids needed to be more clinically precise. A subsequent 1994 analysis by the IOM[23] of a 10-year follow-up to the British National Childhood Encephalopathy Study[24] tried to answer, but fell short of answering, the ultimate question of whether DTP vaccine causes permanent brain damage.

The Section 312 modifications included adding chronic arthritis for rubella-containing vaccines and removing shock-collapse and residual seizure disorder under DTP vaccine (Table 50–4). Time intervals were changed for anaphylaxis (24 hours to 4 hours) and encephalopathy and residual seizure disorder under measles, mumps, and rubella vaccines (0–15 days to 5–15 days). Finally, clarifications in the definitions of conditions such as residual seizure disorder and encephalopathy were made in the Aids to Interpretation.

A legal challenge to the final rule was filed in federal court within 60 days of publication. The suit was brought by the family of a child who experienced the onset of seizures within 3 days of DTP vaccination and may have qualified for a Table presumption had residual seizure disorder not been removed from under DTP vaccine in March 1995.

In *O'Connell v. Shalala, Secretary, HHS,** petitioners challenged the Secretary's authority and the procedure used to publish the final rule. The Federal Court of Appeals decided in the government's favor on all issues, and the new regulation was allowed to stand.

It is still not clear how the court will apply the new Table and Aids in adjudicating seizure-onset, neurological disorders, or alleged encephalopathy occurring in children experiencing otherwise nonserious vaccine side effects (e.g., irritability, prolonged crying, or lethargy). Because of the removal of seizures and shock collapse from under DTP vaccine, petitioners must now prove that the vaccine caused their child's neurological sequelae. Only a small number had gone to hearing by December 1997 over issues such as the role of DTP in triggering the onset of seizures and the relevance of the recent British National Childhood Encephalopathy Study follow-up and IOM analysis to such cases. Only one reported case has addressed the new encephalopathy definition: In *Riggs v. Secretary, HHS,*† the Court deter-

**Hellebrand v. Secretary, HHS,* 999 F.2d 1565 (Fed. Cir. 1993).
†*Hodges v. Secretary, HHS,* 9 F.3d 958 (Fed. Cir. 1994).

**O'Connell v. Shalala, Secretary, HHS,* 79 F.3rd 170 (1st Cir. 1996).
†*Riggs v. Secretary, HHS,* Ct. Fed. Cl. No. 95-295 (1997).

Table 50–4. **NATIONAL VACCINE INJURY COMPENSATION PROGRAM SUMMARY OF VACCINE INJURY TABLE CHANGES***

TABLE VERSION	VACCINE	ADVERSE EVENT	TIME PERIOD
"Initial Table" (Effective: 10/1/88)	DTaP, DTP, DT, Td or TT	Anaphylaxis	24 hours
		Residual seizure disorder	3 days
		Hypotonic-hyporesponsive episode	3 days
		Encephalopathy	3 days
	MMR or any component	Anaphylaxis	24 hours
		Residual seizure disorder	15 days
		Encephalopathy	15 days
	OPV	Paralytic polio	30 days/6 months†
	IPV	Anaphylaxis	24 hours
"Section 312 Table" (Effective: 3/10/95)	DTaP, DTP, DT, Td or TT	Anaphylaxis	4 hours
		Encephalopathy	72 hours
	MMR or any component	Anaphylaxis	4 hours
		Residual seizure disorder	5–15 days
		Encephalopathy	5–15 days
	Rubella-containing	Chronic arthritis	42 days
	OPV	Paralytic polio	30 days/6 months†
	IPV	Anaphylaxis	4 hours
"Section 313 Table" (Effective: 3/24/97)	Tetanus-containing	Anaphylaxis	4 hours
		Brachial neuritis	2–28 days
	Pertussis-containing	Anaphylaxis	4 hours
		Encephalopathy	72 hours
	MMR or any component	Anaphylaxis	4 hours
		Encephalopathy	5–15 days
	Rubella-containing	Chronic arthritis	7–42 days
	Measles-containing	Thrombocytopenic purpura	7–30 days
		Vaccine-strain measles viral infection in an immunodeficient recipient	6 months
	OPV	Paralytic polio	30 days/6 months†
		Vaccine-strain polio viral infection	30 days/6 months†
	IPV	Anaphylaxis	4 hours
	HBV	Anaphylaxis	4 hours
	Hib (unconj)	Early-onset Hib disease	7 days
	Hib (conj)	No condition specified	Not applicable‡
	Varicella	No condition specified	Not applicable‡
	New vaccines¶	No condition specified	Not applicable‡

*The filing date of a claim determines which Table is used for adjudication.

†Time intervals for immunocompetent/immunodeficient individuals who receive oral poliovirus. Contact cases have no time limit.

‡No condition has been identified requiring inclusion on the Vaccine Injury Table, therefore, compensation for alleged injuries must be pursued on a causation in fact basis.

¶Any new vaccine recommended by the Centers for Disease Control and Prevention for routine administration to children after publication by the Secretary of the Department of Health and Human Services of a notice of coverage.

For abbreviations, see Tables 50–1 and 50–2.

mined that the child's symptoms did not satisfy the criteria for encephalopathy as defined in the Table.

The so-called Section 313 report reviewed adverse events after the administration of vaccines for diphtheria, tetanus, measles, mumps, and polio as well as for HBV and Hib, both of which are recommended for routine use in children. As with the 312 report, proposed changes developed by VICP staff were for the most part in accordance with the IOM conclusions for or against causation. There were, however, two exceptions: GBS following OPV and tetanus-containing vaccine.

The IOM's conclusion concerning OPV was based largely on a Finnish study following a national OPV campaign.[25] A subsequent U.S. study (therefore not considered by the IOM) showed no evidence of an increase in GBS after OPV administration.[26] Further doubt was cast when one of the Finnish study's coauthors wrote a letter noting that it was not their intention to claim that OPV was causally related to GBS, because the data could be interpreted more than one way.[27]

The question of GBS and tetanus-containing vaccines was even more difficult to decide. The IOM conclusion was based on case reports, particularly one regarding an individual who experienced GBS three times in the weeks following tetanus vaccination. The fact that he had other non–vaccine-related episodes made him immunologically unique. Population studies, on the other hand, showed no evidence that GBS incidence is higher in individuals receiving tetanus vaccine when compared with background rate.[27] Because there is no proven evidence of increased incidence overall, it was thought that GBS should continue to require proof of causation and therefore not be added to the Table. However, individuals who experience more than one episode of GBS temporally related to immunization will no doubt have strong causation arguments under the VICP. In fact, the program has compensated a claim involving a child who had two episodes of GBS, both within weeks of receiving tetanus-containing vaccines at ages 5 and 15 years.

The changes, published in February 1997 in the *Federal Register* became effective March 24, 1997 and included addition of brachial neuritis and removal of encephalopathy for tetanus-containing vaccines, addition of thrombocytopenia and vaccine-strain measles virus infection, and removal of residual seizure disorder for measles-containing vaccines, addition of vaccine-strain poliovirus infection for live polio virus vaccine, and a provision that any future vaccine recommended by the CDC for routine use in children also be added automatically to the VICP.[28]

Although most of the Table changes became effective on March 24, the date of coverage for adding three new vaccines—hepatitis B, Hib, and varicella—was delayed more than 4 months because an excise tax was required to make their coverage effective. (During rulemaking, the FDA licensed varicella vaccine, following which, the CDC recommended it for routine use in children.)

The original seven vaccines covered by the Act had excise tax levels set based on the estimated numbers and cost of claims that each would generate. This risk-based approach, however, had serious limitations. By 1996, the trust fund had exceeded anticipated needs, with $1 billion in holdings and annual receipts totaling $140 million against peak outlays in the $35 to $42 million range. Secondly, future licensure of multiple-antigen combination vaccines would make impossible the task of estimating the risk of adverse events for each antigen. An ideal solution was a flat-tax approach, which was sent by HHS to Congress in July 1995 as a legislative proposal. Vaccines currently covered under the VICP, as well as new vaccines added through rulemaking, would all have the flat rate per "dose" (disease prevented). Because the Omnibus Budget Reconciliation Act of 1993 mechanism of rulemaking and tax legislation required years to add new vaccines to the VICP, the legislative proposal also included an automatic tax provision.

Over the next 2 years, little progress was made. With passage of the Taxpayer Relief Act of 1997, the vaccine excise structure was revised, setting a 75-cents-per-"dose" (disease prevented) rate on all covered vaccines under the program, including the three vaccines added by rulemaking. The effective date of coverage was August 6, 1997.[29] The automatic tax provision was not included in the final legislation. Therefore, Congress will be required to assign an excise tax for each new vaccine added via the provision in the March 1997 final rule.

Medical Review of Claims

Nearly all claims filed under the VICP had some clinical outcome in temporal relation to vaccination, varying from the normal, expected side effects of crying, fever, or local swelling to much more serious acute illness. The claims represent an important database of possible vaccine-related events, although only a small percentage were thought to be on this basis after medical review. Some of the more relevant clinical diagnoses are reviewed here.

Diphtheria, Tetanus, and Pertussis Vaccine

Petitions filed for DTP vaccine (only one claim had been received alleging DTaP injury by December 31, 1997) for the most part involved cases in which primary series immunization was done in children younger than 12 months. Just over half of the injury claims involved initial onset seizures in various time intervals following vaccination, ranging from hours to several weeks or longer. Those with idiopathic epilepsy (31%) were the largest group, followed by those with infantile spasms (14%) and a small percentage with different convulsion types (e.g., absence, complex partial, psychomotor). Another significant category was the 20% of claimants who experienced developmental delay as their presenting neurological sign, with medical records rarely showing any significant effects following vaccination. However, parents might point to prolonged, inconsolable crying or extreme lethargy as a basis for assuming DTP-related outcomes. Only 11% of children demonstrated clinical signs of encephalopathy, and of those, approximately half had unknown etiology. The remaining claims comprised metabolic or genetic disorders and a variety of other non–vaccine-related conditions. Only a handful of HHE cases were identified on medical records review.

Tuberous sclerosis complex (TSC) is a genetic disorder characterized in many by classic skin lesions, growths (tubers), and other structural changes in the brain, causing seizures and mental retardation. Patients may be completely asymptomatic or have severe seizures and neurological deficits. Whereas TSC patients with seizures may or may not have mental retardation, the opposite is not true. TSC patients with mental retardation almost always have seizures—generally the earlier the onset, the worse the outcome.[30] Conventional thinking (prior to present-day neuroimaging) has been to avoid anything that may trigger the earlier onset of seizures, such as DTP vaccine. However, more recent magnetic resonance imaging scanning suggests that the number and location of cortical tubers is more determinant of clinical outcome than an earlier onset of seizures.[31]

Of 64 claims (all retrospective) involving TSC, 37 "off-Table" seizure-onset cases have been dismissed based on the recognition that TSC is non–vaccine related, or, in a few cases, for legal reasons. Twenty-seven claims await final adjudication, nearly all of which are on-Table seizure-onset cases. Of these, 22 claims were litigated as a group to determine whether DTP vaccine significantly aggravated the preexisting condition of the children. (The five remaining claims await fact determinations by the court as to the whether the onset of seizures occurred within a Table time frame.) Experts in neurology and epidemiology testified in special "omnibus" hearings held to decide this important question of vaccine aggravation. Several peer-reviewed articles by HHS consultants came from research generated by these efforts.[31–33]

In a ruling issued in September 1997, the court found that the Department of HHS had proven that the presence of tubers in the cerebral cortex leads to seizures in the majority of TSC patients, and that most of the TSC patients with seizures are mentally retarded. Furthermore, the epidemiological evidence "supports the view that DPT [sic] does not initiate seizures in [TSC] patients." The decision reflects the current state of scientific thinking and must now be applied to each of the remaining 27 cases.*

Approximately 50% of claims alleging DTP-related death had findings consistent with SIDS, verified by review of the records and autopsy reports. The next most frequent diagnostic category involved the 10% of patients with long-standing convulsive disorders (those who had severe, long-term seizures), followed by those with acute encephalopathy (9% [4%, known etiology; 5%, unknown etiology]), developmental delay onset (7%), and the remaining claims showing various non–vaccine-related conditions (e.g., choking, sepsis, congenital heart disease). Four deaths were due to anaphylaxis.

Tetanus-Containing Vaccines

Tetanus-containing vaccine claims (DT, Td, or TT) included at least seven cases of GBS and smaller numbers of patients with chronic inflammatory demyelinating polyneuropathy, multiple sclerosis, brachial neuritis, acute encephalopathy of unknown etiology, and other central and peripheral nervous system disorders.

Litigating GBS claims has been particularly challenging. Few were decided prior to the IOM report concluding that tetanus-containing vaccines could cause GBS if the onset was within 5 days to 6 weeks following immunization. Nevertheless, at least one GBS case was decided based on the IOM's conclusion. The court reached the opposite conclusion in the next case that went to hearing, based in large part on expert testimony challenging this conclusion. In deciding against causation, the court found that although Td can cause GBS, that does not mean it did cause GBS in any particular case. The case was appealed and affirmed by the Federal Circuit.†

Measles, Mumps, and Rubella Vaccines

The MMR vaccine is implicated in 14% of claims, most of which are events associated with immunization during the second year of life. Acute encephalopathy or encephalitis comprised 23% of injury claims ranging in onset from 1 day to several weeks after immunization. Most cases were of unknown cause. Although encephalopathy is known to result from natural measles infection, it is not clear if the vaccine can also cause central nervous system disease. Attempts to isolate vaccine virus in patients with acute illness have been unsuccessful, and there is no evidence of increased rates of acute central nervous system disease in vaccinees v. the background rate for this age group. Although the IOM found the evidence to be "insufficient" to determine whether measles vaccine can cause acute encephalopathy, there is some evidence of clustering of encephalopathy/encephalitis cases whose onset is 8 to 10 days following measles-containing immunization, with a recent VICP analysis of 48 claims showing similar results.[34]

The remaining diagnoses are seizure-onset cases (27%), most being febrile seizures in the 7- to 14-day time frame during which fever may accompany replication of vaccine virus. Those that fell within the 0- to 15-day time frame (now 5 to 15 days) for Table onset were usually recommended for entitlement by VICP staff.

Eighteen Subacute Sclerosing Panencephalitis (SSPE) claims have been identified, ten of them deaths. Early hearings resulted in a few being compensated due to the lack of participation by the HHS. Subsequent testimony by experts in infectious disease persuaded the court of the lack of any data supporting a causal connection, noting the tremendous decrease in SSPE incidence since licensure of the vaccine decades ago. Since then, claims of SSPE-related injury or death have been dismissed.

Included in the MMR analysis are 113 claims alleging injury from rubella vaccine. Most claims involve postpubertal women, usually healthcare workers or postpartum patients. Although 13 to 15% of susceptible (serology-negative) women may experience transient arthritis after the currently used rubella vaccine, with a higher percentage (up to 40%) reporting some type of musculoskeletal complaint, it is less clear what role, if any, the vaccine plays in causing recurrent or chronic arthropathy (i.e., arthralgia or arthritis).[18, 19] Forty-two percent of people making claims experienced acute arthritis within 6 weeks of immunization. Of these, 17% were diagnosed with chronic arthritis of unknown etiology, 4% with type-specific (non–vaccine-related) arthritis, and the remaining cases with chronic arthralgia (16%) and other subjective complaints (5%). Of the remaining claims without acute arthritis onset after immunization, 28% had chronic arthropathy or other generalized complaints similar to those of chronic fatigue syndrome, and 30% were diagnosed with a variety of non–vaccine-related conditions.

Based on the 1991 IOM report's finding that chronic arthritis may be caused by rubella vaccine, the court held a hearing to determine criteria necessary for proof of causation. Following the court's publication of these guidelines, the VICP added chronic arthritis to the Table in the 1995 final rule and more recently incorporated several of the court's criteria in the 1997 final rule. The main difference between the VICP and the court has been the latter's willingness to compensate arthralgia, a subjective symptom that is difficult to assess v. observable signs of arthritis. Adjudications to date have resulted in 39 claims being compensated by the court and 45 being dismissed. Additional research published since the IOM report has produced mixed results, including retrospective case reviews and a prospective double-blind study. If rubella vaccine does indeed cause chronic arthropathy, it would appear that the incidence is rare.[35–37]

Polio Vaccines

Polio vaccine–related claims totaled more than 500 of the retrospective case filings. Most involved vaccines given in the 1950s and 1960s, when polio was epidemic and endemic. It is reasonable to expect that some individuals acquired natural poliomyelitis in temporal relationship to receipt of IPV, particularly if only one or two doses were given. Although the Cutter incident, in which an estimated 260 cases of paralytic poliomyelitis

---

*_Barnes et al. v. Secretary, HHS_, 1997 WL 620115 (Fed. Cl. Spec. Mstr. Sep. 15, 1997).

†_Housand v. Secretary, HHS_, 114 F.3d 1206 (Fed. Cir. 1997).

were attributed to residual live virus in the vaccine, is well documented, no similar instances of killed vaccine-related poliomyelitis have been identified.[38] Of approximately 228 IPV claims, all but six have been dismissed by the court, with none being found to be secondary to Cutter vaccine administration. Decisions are pending on the few remaining claims yet to be adjudicated.

OPV claims were approached much differently, because paralytic polio is known to be a rare complication in vaccine recipients, as well as in contacts. Most claims arising since the early 1960s with confirmed paralytic polio were compensated by the program. Naturally, it is difficult to know which cases were vaccine related when polio was present in the community. Claims involving other conditions such as transverse myelitis and GBS have been rejected by the court based on the lack of proof of causation.

Public Policy Outcomes

Congress expected that the Act would once and for all address the liability and public health problems surrounding immunization. Few were certain it would work, given the continuing controversy over what solutions were appropriate. Success would be judged by some on how easily individuals were compensated. Others looked for marketplace stabilization first or how well manufacturers and administrators could go about the business of immunization as the primary success measure. How well has the VICP achieved these goals after 9 years of operation? One could say the report card shows high marks all around.

First, compensation awards have been made to over 1200 families and individuals apart from attorney's fees and costs. The average time overall from filing a post-1988 claim to payment is 2.5 years. Although the retrospective program experienced long delays getting claims processed, many petitioners were able to file claims otherwise banned by statutes of limitations under state law. One could argue that the delays were more than balanced by the unique opportunity afforded by the Act.

The no-fault approach, with limited rules of discovery and short, informal hearings eliminated or ameliorated many of the problems inherent in the tort system. Under the VICP, the majority of the hearings before the special masters are concluded within a day and are less adversarial than under the tort system. By HHS utilizing annuities, guardianships, and trusts, patients receiving compensation are ensured a lifetime stream of benefits.

Another program benefit has been the stabilization of the marketplace. Vaccine supply shortages of the past are a faint memory. Immunization rates are at an all-time high, with new vaccines being licensed annually (National Immunization Program data, Centers for Disease Control and Prevention). Annual Investigational New Drug requests to the FDA, a necessary step in beginning testing in human subjects, have more than doubled from 1986 to the present, signaling renewed confidence in vaccine research and development (Office of Vaccines Research and Review, Centers for Biologics Evaluation and Research, FDA, unpublished data). Dramatic price increases in childhood vaccines in the 1980s, which manufacturers associated with liability, have stopped. Vaccine prices today reflect public and private sector purchase trends and the effects of inflation rather than liability concerns or repercussions. Yet, some wonder why prices have not dropped to the level of the early 1980s now that the liability burden has been largely removed. Even the addition of the excise tax for MMR and DTP vaccines does not explain the pricing levels that exist today.

Perhaps the most important barometer is civil litigation. DTP claims against U.S. companies are at an all-time low and have remained so for the past 6 years (Fig. 50–1). More recent lawsuits involve cases already adjudicated by the VICP. Some have already been dismissed, whereas others are still pending adjudication. Although claims against healthcare providers are more difficult to track, there is no indication that their liability experience is any different than that of manufacturers.

A more indirect indicator is the number of petitioners who elect to reject the VICP judgment, thus preserving their rights to pursue civil litigation should they choose to do so. Of approximately 550 post-1988 adjudications through May 1997, only 47 petitioners had elected to reject their judgment, all of whom except one were unsuccessful in obtaining compensation under the Program. Previous surveys of petitioners' attorneys have shown that most petitioners had no plans to pursue further litigation (Office of the General Counsel, Department of HHS, unpublished data).

One policy question that some have raised is the need for "adult" vaccines to be included under the VICP. An NVAC review in 1996 found that there was little evidence to support the need, based on liability concerns by either manufacturers or health care providers.[39]

In conclusion, the VICP appears to have satisfied the critical public policy concerns that brought about passage more than 10 years ago. The uncertainty of the past is long gone, replaced by a healthy marketplace with the expectation of steady vaccine supplies and new, innovative products and technology. In addition to strong, capable administrative leadership by the governmental participants, guidance from the ACCV, and critical support from organizations such as the AAP and vaccine manufacturers, contributors to VICP success include Congress and its willingness to provide necessary fixes and process improvements as problems were identified and solved.

VACCINE LIABILITY SINCE 1986

The passage of the Act in 1986 did not have an immediate impact on the reported liability decisions of the courts. Reported opinions come almost exclusively from the appellate courts, and they tend to appear 5 or more years after the original filing of the case in the trial court. Because there had been a reported surge in liability case filings in the mid- to early 1980s, itself a factor in the passage of the Act, it would have been reasonable to expect an increase in the number of decisions in the late 1980s and early 1990s. In addition, the

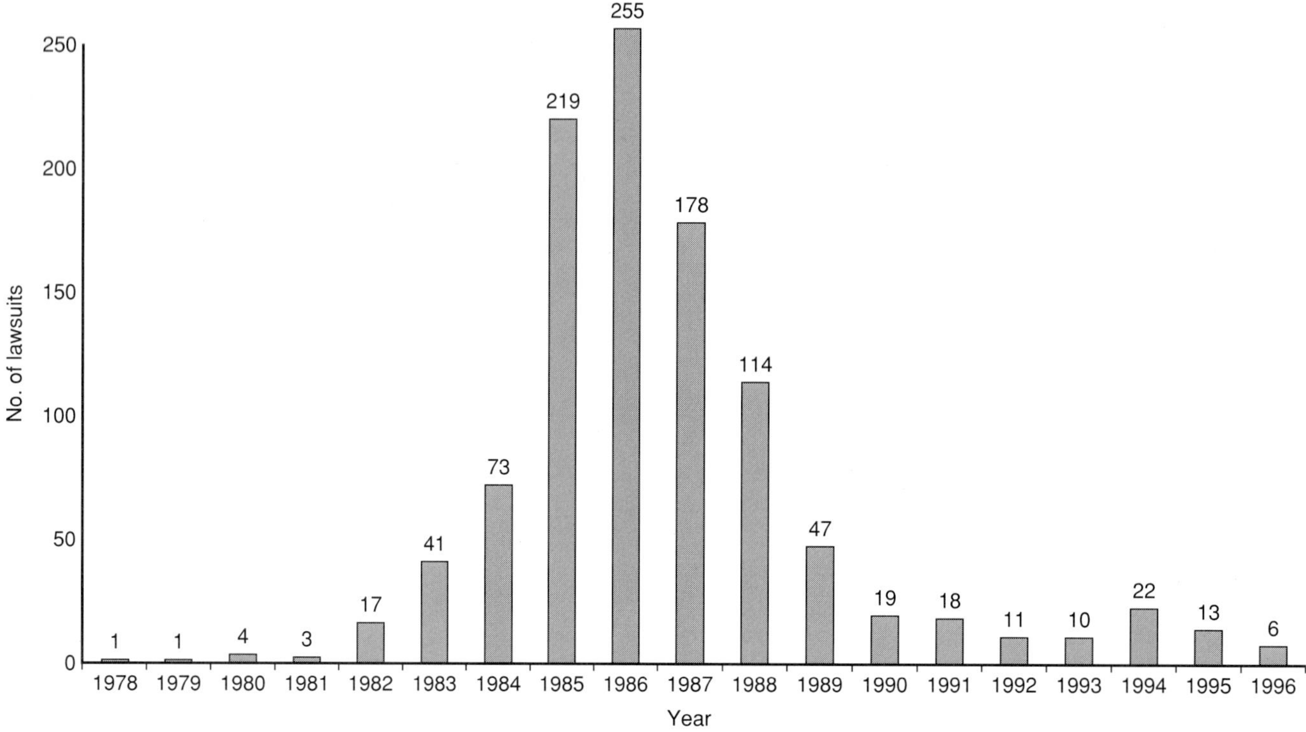

Figure 50–1. Number of diphtheria-tetanus-pertussis lawsuits against U.S. manufacturers, 1978 to 1996.

NCVIA gave claimants whose claims arose out of a vaccination administered prior to October 1, 1988 until January 31, 1991 to file claims under the Act. For a few years, retrospective claimants could continue to pursue their claims in court while preserving the option of making a claim under the program.

As a result of these factors, the number of reported opinions involving tort claims of vaccinees was greater in the period of 1987 to 1992, after the Act had been passed, than in any preceding 5-year period.*

Since 1992, the number of reported vaccine liability cases has declined sharply, which suggests that most claimants elected to file a claim under the Act and accept the judgment received. There is no indication that claimants unsuccessful under the Act have then successfully pursued claims in the courts. There is only one reported case involving an eligible claimant who either made a claim under the Act and rejected an award or made a claim under the Act and received no award, and then filed a claim in court. In that case (*Evans v. Lederle Laboratories*,†) the claimant, who suffered injury prior to 1988, had first filed several cases in court and then filed under the Act but did not receive an award, so then filed again in court. The renewed court claim was dismissed as barred by the state statute of limitations.

The tone of the post-1992 cases has changed as well. The tendency of the court appears to be much less sympathetic to plaintiffs. Even in instances in which the court has found liability, it appears to have gone out of its way to endorse vaccination. An interesting example of this is *In re Sabin Oral Polio Vaccine Products Litigation*,* in which the court held the U.S. government liable because the Divison of Biologic Standards (DBS) of the National Institutes of Health† had released some of the vaccine in violation of the standards established by its own regulations. The court went out of its way to emphasize that the finding of government liability was not meant to suggest that there was anything wrong with the vaccine:

> *"First, although I find DBS to have been negligent in the eyes of the law, I do not find DBS officials and consultants to have been derelict in the performance of their duties . . . Solely as a matter of public health administration, there was a sound basis for DBS's decision. By 1977, DBS had had fifteen years of experience with the OPV program. The experience had demonstrated that, regardless of its failure to perform satisfactorily (in comparison with the type 1 reference vaccine) on monkey neurovirulence tests, type 3 vaccine was safe (to the extent that a live vaccine can ever be said to be safe) when administered to humans."*‡

Most dramatically, claims based on the argument that the DTP vaccine was defective have not been successful. In *Jones v. Lederle Laboratories*,§ the court said of the

*This statement is true only if one does not count the large number of cases resulting from swine flu compensation claims filed against the federal government under the swine flu statute discussed and reported in the period of 1979 to 1986. The number of reported swine flu cases exceeded all of the other vaccine liability cases ever reported. It is now clear that the swine flu litigation episode was unique.

†*Evans v. Lederle Laboratories*, 904 F. Supp. 857 (C.D. I11. 1995).

**Sabin Oral Polio Vaccine Products Litigation*, 743 F. Supp. 410 (D. Md. 1990), 763 F. Supp. 811 (1991) 774 F. Supp. 952 (1991).

†Currently, the Center for Biologics Evaluation and Research of the FDA.

‡The decision has been affirmed by the United States Court of Appeals for the Fourth Circuit. In *re Sabin Oral Polio Vaccine Products Liability Litigation*, 984 F.2d 124 (4th Cir. 1993).

§*Jones v. Lederle Laboratories*, 785 F. Supp. 1123 (E.D.N.Y. 1992).

theory that the whole-cell vaccine is defective because of a possible acellular vaccine:

*"The case illustrates some of the strengths and weaknesses of the American system for marketing drugs. Requiring strict proof of safety—both to comply with FDA regulations and to avoid tort liability—slows the availability of new products. The result may well be that dangers will be enhanced during the necessarily extended developmental period. But these results are attributable to the way in which scientists usually solve problems—through incremental, peer-reviewed experiments—and to the regulatory system, not to any dereliction on the part of this defendant." (785 F. Supp. 1127.)**

Another theory involving both producers and administrators is the "duty to warn" theory. The theory, as applied by petitioners, is that the warning in the package insert (in cases involving producers) was inadequate or that the warning given by the administering health professional (in cases against the administrator) was inadequate. The Act itself resolves this issue for manufacturers. 42 U.S.C. Section 300aa-22 states that "[N]o vaccine manufacturer shall be liable in a civil action for damages arising from a vaccine-related injury or death associated with the administration of a vaccine after the effective date of this subpart solely due to the manufacturer's failure to provide direct warnings to the injured party . . . ." In addition, this section of the Act protects the manufacturer from liability for unavoidable adverse side effects as long as the vaccine is properly prepared and accompanied by proper directions and warnings. The Act also defines what constitutes proper directions and warnings. There are no such protections for administrators.

Risk to Healthcare Professionals

Assuming a petitioner rejects a VICP judgment in order to pursue civil litigation, the major risk for the health professional, outside of a breach in the accepted standard of care, revolves around the duty to warn. *Niemiera v. Schneider*,† which was a victory for the producer, also involved a claim against a health professional for failure to warn. This case occurred prior to the time when vaccine information materials, as stipulated by the Act were in effect. The trial court and the intermediate appellate court had found for the defendant doctor. The State Supreme Court reversed:

"DTP has an extraordinary potential for decreasing child-mortality rates, and the National Childhood Vaccinations Injury Act of 1986, 42 U.S.C. §§300aa-1 to -34, by providing a no fault remedy for some of the losses suffered by the one child in 100,000, may go a long way to eliminate the fitful dependency on tort litigation to provide human succor for the unfortunate few. But parents need to know the risks of the treatment and be prepared to use all the self-help they can to avert those consequences." (114 N.J. 567–68, 555 A.2d 1121–22).

Some plaintiffs argue that a warning that conveys the contents of the package insert is inadequate and incomplete, but the courts reject these arguments. The duty to give a warning and the threat of liability to the health professionals appear to be enhanced in some respects by the Act. 42 U.S.C. §300aa-26(d), provides that "each health care provider who administers a vaccine set forth in the Vaccine Injury Table shall provide to the legal representatives of any child or to any other individual to whom such provider intends to administer such vaccine a copy of the information materials developed [by the Secretary of Health and Human Services] . . . "* However, the fact that the Act gives responsibility to the federal government to develop information materials may reduce liability for any individual provider. Warnings provided, as long as the approved information materials are used, are likely to be considered adequate and the provider is not obligated to develop his or her own information.

The liability exposure of health professionals is further increased by the case law developments considered earlier that make producer liability less likely and by the provisions of the Act that limit producer liability for vaccines administered after the effective date of the Act.† These developments mean that injured recipients are unlikely to find recovery from the producers. The health professional will be left as the only available target. On the other hand, the healthcare provider is protected by the Act, in that persons who elect to accept judgments under the program cannot sue the healthcare provider.

Further protection for some healthcare professionals comes from the fact that some states have passed statutes that provide protection for health professionals and institutions that participate in the process of administering vaccines (e.g., North Carolina, discussed earlier). Although the Act preempts any state statute that bars an action against a vaccine manufacturer that is not barred by the other provisions of the Act, it does not explicitly preempt a state statute that bars an action against a person or institution involved in the administration of the vaccine.‡

The lesson for health professionals: It is important that offices involved in the administration of vaccines have a systematic procedure for delivering the approved warnings and preserving evidence that the warning has

---

*Other decisions suggesting no liability for DTP producers are *White v. Wyeth Laboratories*, 40 Ohio St.3d 390, 533 N.E.2d 748 (1988), affirming 1987 WL 14953 (Ohio App.) (defective design claim rejected) and *Miller v. Connaught Laboratories, Inc.*, 1995 WL 579969 (D. Kan. 1995) (defective design claim rejected). The opinion in *Miller* is most interesting, because it was written by a judge who in an earlier case had shown considerable sympathy to a plaintiff's DTP claim.

†*Niemiera v. Schneider*, 114 N.J. 550; 555 A. 2d 1112 (1989).

*The federal statutory obligation of healthcare providers to provide the information was, under the statute, to become effective not later than 6 months after the Secretary, HHS, published information materials in the *Federal Register.* This was first done, 56 FR 51798, on October 15, 1991, effective August 15, 1992. Criticism of their length and the long, mandatory review process led to amendment of section 2126 of the Public Health Service Act (42 U.S.C. §300aa-26). A "New Vaccine Information Materials: Notice" (59 FR 31888) was published in the *Federal Register* on July 20, 1994, effective October 1, 1994.

†Sections 22 and 23, 42 U.S.C. §§300aa-22, 300aa-23.

‡42 U.S.C. §300aa-22(e).

been given. A signature from the patient or the responsible adult in the case of a child may be the most clear evidence that the materials were given. However, the CDC does not require a signature that a parent or guardian has read and understood the vaccine information materials for vaccines purchased through federal contracts. The CDC does require the provider to note in the medical record that the relevant information materials were provided. The Act itself requires no signatures—only that the materials be provided.

Other Situations in Which Suits Are Not Barred by the Act

Although the trend in the reported decisions is consistent with the view that the Act has been successful in providing claimants with an alternative claim system that functions as a substitute for claims pursued in court, there are situations in which the Act does not bar suit against the manufacturers or healthcare providers even though the claim arises out of the administration of a vaccine. These are cases in which the claimant is ineligible to file a claim under the Act. Examples include claimants who cannot meet the requirement that they have at least $1000 in unreimbursable medical expenses or who do not file a claim within the time limitations set forth in the Act.* To date, neither category has shown much cause for concern. Regarding the former, only a small number of claims have been dismissed from the VICP, probably because the court gives petitioners every opportunity to meet the requirement. Designed by Congress to discourage frivolous claims, its value has been questioned increasingly. There is little evidence that it is needed, and a small number of otherwise sufficient claims have been dismissed under the VICP and may unnecessarily go to the tort system. Because of criticism, the ACCV in March 1997 recommended to the Secretary that the HHS propose legislation to Congress removing this requirement. The proposal is currently under consideration.

For those who have missed the filing deadline under the program, the recipient may be able to file a tort action under a longer state statute of limitations. Although the Act appears to preclude civil litigation in such cases, this issue has not yet been litigated. As a result, a health professional who observes that a patient may have suffered an adverse reaction to a vaccine should encourage that patient to seek compensation under the program immediately. If the patient does not do so but later attempts to sue in tort, the fact that the patient (or the patient's parents) failed to seek compensation at the time might be seen to be useful evidence on the question of whether there was in fact a reaction to the vaccine.

Another scenario is exemplified by two cases in which a person other than the injured party was allowed to recover in civil court, even though the injured party had already recovered under the Act. In *Schafer v. American Cyanamid*,* a mother became ill with polio subsequent to her child's receipt of OPV. The mother was compensated under the Act. Her husband and daughter sued the drug manufacturer for loss of consortium and companionship under state law. After the mother accepted her Act award, the defendant vaccine producer moved to dismiss the claim. The district court denied the motion, and the denial was appealed to the first circuit. The Court of Appeals affirmed, holding that the Act only bars claims by persons, either recipients or contacts, directly injured by the vaccine and who can make claims under the Act, and not claims by others arising out of the administration of the vaccine which cannot be compensated under the Act. The court held that if state law did provide an action for loss of consortium and companionship in this context, the Act did not bar the husband and daughter from pursuing it.

Another such scenario is reflected in *Abbott v. Secretary, HHS*.† David Abbott experienced the onset of seizures following DTP vaccination as an infant. Eventually he was placed in a residential care facility. At age 23, David was left unattended in the bathtub, where he then suffered a seizure and died. Ms. Abbott (David's mother) filed a wrongful death action against the group home and other state agencies, which resulted in a settlement. She then filed a claim with the VICP, claiming that David's death was a sequela of his vaccine-related injuries. The claim was dismissed by the special master because Ms. Abbott had already recovered in state court. The Federal Circuit Court of Appeals reversed and remanded the case to the special master, holding that the previous settlement covered only damages for injuries to David's beneficiaries and not for David's own injuries. VICP medical review then determined that a Table seizure disorder existed and that the death was a direct result of the vaccine-related seizure disorder, although David most probably would not have died had he been properly attended while having the seizure. The case was conceded, and the special master then awarded compensation in the statutory amount of $250,000.

To date, these appear to be the only two cases in which one family recovers two times for the same vaccine-related injury. Although, in theory, cases such as these might present a threat of liability to manufacturers and providers, there are only a handful of cases that are known to have been reported, and there is no sign that a majority of claimants who are ineligible under the Act have actually been able to advance successful claims against anyone.

SUMMARY, CONCLUSIONS, AND FUTURE IMPLICATIONS

There is clear evidence that the availability of compensation under the Act has given plaintiffs a sufficient incentive to abandon the pursuit of tort remedies against the producers and the administering health professionals. New court cases have nearly disappeared, which in

*See 42 U.S.C. Section 300aa-11(c)(1)(D)(I) and 42 U.S.C. Section 300aa-16(a), respectively.

**Schafer v. American Cyanamid*, 20 F.3rd 1 (1st Cir. 1994).

†*Abbott v. Secretary, HHS*, 19 F.3d 39 (Fed. Cir. 1994).

part can be explained by the fact that the Act requires claimants to first file for compensation under the Act. Only a small number of petitioners so far have chosen to reject their VICP judgment, with no indication that a significant percentage will choose civil action and no evidence that any claimant has yet done so successfully. This trend has been further reflected in the courts, in that recent decisions have shown a reluctance to consider vaccine-related cases, given the VICP's protective framework and operative success in compensating claimants.

The decrease of tort actions against manufacturers and administrators appears to be true for claims, regardless of vaccination date. The evidence seems to indicate that most pre-1988 claimants chose to file with the VICP and not pursue litigation in civil court. Post-1988 claims, once filed with the VICP, have the statute of limitations suspended by the Act. At the end of the petition process, the petitioner can choose whether to accept the compensation awarded or to file in court. Most who are unsuccessful under the more generous federal system so far seem to have chosen not to pursue further civil remedies.

The reported decisions are consistent with the conclusion that both producers and health professionals have no significant liability risk under tort law except for their own negligence. However, the protection is not absolute. Because the Act does not preclude an individual who is otherwise ineligible to file a claim under the VICP (e.g., family members of injured individuals) from pursuing civil litigation, liability exposure remains a possibility that seems small given the track record to date.

At a time when public confidence in government is mixed, it is reassuring that the public policy imperatives driving passage of the Act have been basically satisfied. The willingness to address weaknesses through almost yearly technical amendments proved critical in achieving success. The VICP's future seems bright, given its permanent reauthorization, an overly endowed trust fund, and, perhaps most importantly, the general recognition by its stakeholders (i.e., physicians, manufacturers, lawmakers and attorneys) that a successful immunization program can only be achieved with liability safeguards in place.

Since 1986, Congress has considered other variations on the tort reform theme. Most are familiar with the 1996 tort reform effort by the House and Senate, eventually leading to compromise legislation, only to be vetoed by the President.[40] Less known is a bill (H.R. 5893) called the AIDS Vaccine Development and Compensation Act of 1992, which proposed creation of a VICP-like compensation program to facilitate acquired immunodeficiency syndrome (AIDS) vaccine research and clinical trials. Should future AIDS vaccine research and development have liability problems, it is possible a companion system might be created or folded within the VICP.[41]

In preparation for the next influenza pandemic, the Public Health Service is developing a comprehensive plan based on some of the lessons learned from the swine flu experience. One of the six major areas addressed by the plan is creation of liability protection for both vaccine manufacturers and healthcare providers. Elements of the plan remain under discussion at present.[42]

Although the liability and vaccine supply uncertainty of the past have resolved, the vaccine safety focus remains. Due to media involvement and Internet access, the ability for misleading information to be disseminated has increased. As a result, effective vaccine risk communication becomes imperative, reminding patients of the risks of preventable disease, should immunization rates diminish, yet at the same time recognizing the difficult and confusing nature of risk assessment and decision-making for some.[43] Interwoven into vaccine safety awareness is the issue of state mandates for immunization and calls for all states to provide philosophical exemptions. The courts continue to uphold the state's police powers to mandate immunization for school entry, while allowing them to provide exemptions for medical, religious, or philosophical reasons as they see fit. Currently, 15 states allow philosophical exemptions for pertussis immunization, a level that has remained steady over the past several years.[44]

Memories of this nation's focus on vaccine adverse events and the secondary marketplace instability should serve as stark reminders of how uncertainty and fear come together when information is lacking. Today's providers administer vaccines in an atmosphere considerably changed, with a national surveillance system in place and two IOM reports basically confirming the safety of immunizations given routinely in this country. The reports went far beyond a focus point for changes to the VICP, helping repair the perception of risk that had so dominated thinking in the near past. Immunization must never be taken for granted, although most parents seem to believe in the wisdom of vaccination and use their healthcare providers as a key source of guidance in decision making. At the very least, the VICP's healthy presence should ensure that these efforts continue.

REFERENCES

1. Pub. L. No. 99~660 §§ 311 et seq., 100 stat 3755, codified at 42 U.S.C.A. §§ 300aa-1 et seq. (1989).
2. Pub. L. No. 99~660 §§ 311 et seq., 100 Stat. 3755, codified at 42 U.S.C.A. §§ 300aa-1 et seq. (1989).
3. Pub. L. No.100–203, §§ 4301 et seq. 101 Stat. 1330-221 (codified at 42 U.S.C.A. §§ 300aa-1 et seq. ([1989]).
4. Smith MH. National Childhood Vaccine Injury Compensation Act. Pediatrics 82:264–269, 1988.
5. National Vaccine Advisory Committee. The Measles Epidemic: The Problems, Barriers and Recommendations. JAMA 266:1547–1552, 1991.
6. Standards for Pediatric Immunization Practices. Ad Hoc Working Group for the Development of Standards for Pediatric Immunization Practices. JAMA 269:1817–1822, 1993.
7. Pub. L. No. 102–168, 105 Stat 1102 (1991).
8. Office of Inspector General, Department of Health and Human Services. The National Vaccine Injury Compensation Program: A Program Review. Washington, DC, December 1992.
9. Tandy, MK. Federal Circuit Review of Vaccine Compensation Cases under the National Childhood Vaccine Injury Act: 1990–1995. The Fed Cir Bar J 5:28–70, 1995.
10. 42 U.S.C. sec. §300aa-13(a)(2).
11. H.R. Rep. No. 99-908, 99th Cong., 2nd Sess., at 15 (1986), reprinted in 1986 U.S.C.C.A.N. 6344, 6356.

12. Pub. L. No. 100–203, 101 Stat 1330-221 (1987).
13. Clayton EW, Hickson GB. Compensation under the National Childhood Vaccine Injury Act. J Pediatr 116:508–513, 1990.
14. Pub. L. No. 103–66, 107 Stat 565, 567 (1993).
15. Division of Vaccine Injury Compensation, Bureau of Health Professions, Health Resources and Services Administration. Weekly Status Report. Rockville, MD, December 31, 1997.
16. Kinsbourne M. Disorders of mental development. In Menkes JH (ed). Textbook of Child Neurology. Philadelphia, Lea & Febiger, 1990, pp 763–770.
17. Cody CL, Baraff LJ, Cherry JD, et al. Nature and rates of adverse reactions associated with DTP and DT immunizations in infants and children. Pediatrics 68:650–660, 1981.
18. Howson CP, Howe CJ, Fineberg HV (eds). Adverse Effects of Pertussis and Rubella Vaccines. Institute of Medicine. Washington, DC, National Academy Press, 1991.
19. Howson CP, Fineberg HV. The ricochet of magic bullets: Summary of the Institute of Medicine report. Adverse effects of pertussis and rubella vaccines. Pediatrics 89:318–324, 1992.
20. Institute of Medicine. Stratton KR, Howe DJ, Johnston, RB (eds). Adverse events associated with childhood vaccines: Evidence bearing on causality. Washington, DC, National Academy Press, 1994.
21. Stratton KR, Howe CJ, Johnston RB. Adverse events associated with childhood vaccine other than pertussis and rubella. Summary of a report from the Institute of Medicine. JAMA. 271:1602–1605, 1994.
22. Health Resources and Services Administration. National Vaccine Injury Compensation Program. Revision of the vaccine injury Table. Fed Register 60:7678–7696, 1995.
23. Institute of Medicine, Stratton KR, Howe CJ, Johnston RB (eds). DPT Vaccine and Chronic Nervous System Dysfunction: A New Analysis. Washington, DC, National Academy Press, 1994.
24. Miller DL, Ross EM, Alderslade R, et al. Pertussis immunisation and serious acute neurological illness in children. Br Med J 307:1171–1176, 1993.
25. Kinnunen E, Farkkila M, Hovi T, et al. Incidence of Guillain-Barré syndrome during a nationwide oral poliovirus vaccine campaign. Neurology 39:1034–1036, 1989.
26. Rantala H, Cherry JD, Shields WD, Uhari M. Epidemiology of Guillain-Barré syndrome in children: Relationship of oral polio vaccine administration to occurrence. J Pediatr 124:220–223, 1994.
27. National Vaccine Advisory Committee. Report of the Ad Hoc Subcommittee on Childhood Vaccines. June 9, 1994.
28. Health Resources and Services Administration. National Vaccine Injury Compensation Program. Revisions and additions to the vaccine injury Table–II. Fed Register 62:7685–7690, 1997.
29. Pub. L. No. 105-34, 111 Stat. 251 (1997).
30. Berg BO. Neurocutaneous syndromes: Phakomatoses and allied conditions. In Swaiman KF (ed). Pediatric Neurology: Principles and Practice (2nd ed). St. Louis, MO, CV Mosby, 1994, pp 1050–1054.
31. Lamm SH, Goodman M, Engel A, et al. Cortical tuber count: A bio-marker indicating cerebral severity of tuberous sclerosis complex. J Child Neurol 12:85–90, 1997.
32. Goodman M, Lamm SH, Bellman MH. Temporal relationship modeling: DPT or DT immunizations and infantile spasms. Vaccine 16:25–31, 1997.
33. Jozwiak S, Goodman M, Lamm SH. Poor mental development in TSC patients: Clinical risk factors. Arch Neurol 55:379–385, 1998.
34. Weibel RE, Caserta V, Benor DE, Evans G. Acute encephalopathy followed by permanent brain injury or death associated with further attenuated measles vaccines: A review of claims submitted to the National Vaccine Injury Compensation Program. Pediatr 101:383–387, 1998.
35 Weibel RE, Benor DE. Chronic arthropathy and musculoskeletal symptoms associated with rubella vaccines. Arthritis Rheum 39:1529–1534, 1996.
36. Ray P, Black S, Shinefeld H, et al. Risk of chronic arthropathy among women after rubella vaccination. JAMA 278:551–556, 1997.
37. Tingle AJ, Mitchell LA, Grace M, et al. Randomized double-blind placebo-controlled study on adverse effects of rubella immunisation in seronegative women. Lancet 349:1277–1281, 1997.
38. Nathanson N, Langmuir AD. The Cutter incident: Poliomyelitis following formaldehyde-inactivated polio virus vaccination in the United States during the spring of 1955. Am J Hyg 78:29–60, 1963.
39. National Vaccine Advisory Committee. Expansion of VICP to Include Adult Immunizations, May 6, 1996.
40. Harris JF. Clinton vetoes product liability measure. Washington Post, May 3, 1996, p A14.
41. H.R. 5893: AIDS Vaccine Development and Compensation Act of 1992.
42. Patriarca PA, Cox NJ. Influenza pandemic preparedness plan for the United States. J Infect Dis 176(suppl 1):81–87, 1997.
43. Evans G, Bostrom A, Johnston RB, et al. (eds). Risk Communication and Vaccination: Workshop Summary. Washington, DC, National Academy Press, 1997.
44. National Immunization Program data, Centers for Disease Control and Prevention.

Acknowledgments

Dr. Evans and Ms. Gopin thank the following individuals for their assistance in preparing the manuscript: Vito Caserta, MD, MPH, Robert E. Weibel, MD, Marie Mann, MD, MPH, Michele A. Lloyd-Puryear, PhD, MD, Louis Offen, MD, MPH, and Linda Rozelle from the VICP, HHS; Deborah Harris and Ila Mizrachi from the Office of the General Counsel, HHS; Karen P. Hewitt, Mary H. Mason, Catherine Reeves, Vincent J. Matanoski, Mark W. Rogers, and Judith L. Bragdon, MS, RN from the Torts Branch, Vaccine Litigation Section, Department of Justice; and Skip Wolfe, Robert H. Snyder, and Joel Kuritsky, MD from the National Immunization Program, CDC.

Special recognition is given to Thomas E. Balbier, Jr., Director, VICP, HHS, and John Lodge Euler, JD, Deputy Director, Torts Branch, Department of Justice, for their leadership and management of the National Vaccine Injury Compensation Program, and David E. Benor, JD, Senior Attorney, Office of the General Counsel, HHS, for his editorial suggestions, as well as the guidance and wisdom he has provided to the Program over the years.

Epilogue

This book has concentrated for the most part on vaccines already in use or about to be licensed. In most chapters, however, indications were given of things to come, and Chapters 35 through 41 explicitly covered the future.

We close with a note concerning the major targets of vaccines that have yet to be developed. These are listed in the table (by no means comprehensive), which also gives an indication of the strategies being implemented to reach the goal of a successful vaccine for each disease. The reader will get some idea of the ferment of activity that engenders hope for the future emergence of successful vaccines against diseases that are now difficult to prevent.

PRINCIPAL TARGETS AND STRATEGIES FOR FUTURE VACCINES NOT COVERED IN THIS BOOK*

DISEASE OR ORGANISM	MAJOR STRATEGIES FOR EXPERIMENTAL VACCINES IN DEVELOPMENT
Bacteria	
Otitis	Attachment and surface proteins of nontypable *Haemophilus influenzae* and *Moraxella catarrhalis*
Streptococcus, group A	M proteins and polypeptides
Streptococcus, group B	Protein conjugation of polysaccharides
Escherichia coli, toxin producing	Killed bacteria plus cholera toxin subunit B Toxoids
Helicobacter pylori	Oral or parenteral administration of *H. pylori* urease, inactivated toxin, or other antigens
Neisseria gonorrhoeae	Outer membrane proteins Transferrin receptors
Mycobacterium tuberculosis	New attenuated strains BCG with added genes Secreted subunit proteins Nucleic acid of MTB genes
Chlamydia trachomatis	Major outer membrane protein
Chlamydia pneumoniae	Major outer membrane protein Nucleic acid
Mycoplasma pneumoniae	Outer membrane proteins
Viruses	
Respiratory syncytial	Attenuated strains F + G proteins
Parainfluenza 1–3	Attenuated strains HN + F proteins
Dengue 1–4	Attenuated strains Chimeric dengue strains Dengue E and NS1 genes in viral vectors
Epstein-Barr	EBV glycoprotein gene in viral vectors Glycoprotein subunit

Continued on following page

PRINCIPAL TARGETS AND STRATEGIES FOR FUTURE VACCINES NOT COVERED IN THIS BOOK* *Continued*

DISEASE OR ORGANISM	MAJOR STRATEGIES FOR EXPERIMENTAL VACCINES IN DEVELOPMENT
Viruses *Continued*	
Herpes simplex	Glycoprotein subunits
	Attenuated strains
Hepatitis C	Envelope proteins
	Nucleic acid of virus
	Nucleocapsid proteins
Hepatitis E	Structural proteins
Papilloma	Pseudovirions
	Nucleic acid of human papillomavirus genes
	Human papillomavirus genes in viral vectors
Lassa	Viral genes in vectors
Ebola	Viral genes in vectors
Fungi	
Cryptococcus sp.	Capsular polysaccharide
Coccidioides sp.	Inactivated organisms
	Subunit proteins
	Nucleic acid

*See also Chapters 29 and 35.

Appendix 1

Recommendations of the Advisory Committee on Immunization Practices*

Immunization of adolescents. MMWR Morb Mortal Wkly Rep 45(RR-13):1–16, 1996.

Update on adult immunization. MMWR Morb Mortal Wkly Rep 40(RR-12):1–94, 1991.

Recommended childhood immunization schedule—United States, 1998. MMWR Morb Mortal Wkly Rep 47:8–12, 1998.

General recommendations on immunization. MMWR Morb Mortal Wkly Rep 43(RR-1):1–38, 1994.

Use of vaccine and immune globulins in persons with altered immunocompetence. MMWR Morb Mortal Wkly Rep 42(RR-4):1–17, 1993.

The role of BCG vaccine in the prevention and control of tuberculosis in the United States: A joint statement by the Advisory Committee on Immunization Practices and the Advisory Committee for Elimination of Tuberculosis. MMWR Morb Mortal Wkly Rep 45(RR-4):1–18, 1996.

Cholera vaccine. MMWR Morb Mortal Wkly Rep 37(RR-40):617–624, 1988.

Diphtheria, tetanus, pertussis: Recommendations for vaccine use and other preventive measures. MMWR Morb Mortal Wkly Rep 40(RR-10):1–21, 1991.

Pertussis vaccination: Use of acellular pertussis vaccines among infants and young children. MMWR Morb Mortal Wkly Rep 46(RR-7):1–25, 1997.

Update: Vaccine side effects, adverse reactions, contraindications, and precautions. MMWR Morb Mortal Wkly Rep 45(RR-12):1–35, 1996.

Haemophilus b conjugate vaccines for prevention of *Haemophilus influenzae* type b disease among infants and children two months of age and older. MMWR Morb Mortal Wkly Rep 40(RR-1):1–6, 1991.

Haemophilus b conjugate vaccines and a combined diphtheria, tetanus, pertussis, and *Haemophilus* b vaccine. MMWR Morb Mortal Wkly Rep 42(RR-13):1–15, 1993.

Immunization of health-care workers. MMWR Morb Mortal Wkly Rep 46(RR-18):1–42, 1997.

Prevention of hepatitis A through active or passive immunization. MMWR Morb Mortal Wkly Rep 45(RR-15):1–30, 1996.

Hepatitis B virus: A comprehensive strategy for eliminating transmission in the United States through universal childhood vaccination. MMWR Morb Mortal Wkly Rep 40(RR-13):1–25, 1991.

Update: Recommendations to prevent hepatitis B virus transmission—United States. MMWR Morb Mortal Wkly Rep 44:574–575, 1995.

Prevention and control of influenza. MMWR Morb Mortal Wkly Rep 47(RR-6):1–26, 1998.

Inactivated Japanese encephalitis virus vaccine. MMWR Morb Mortal Wkly Rep 42(RR-1):1–15, 1993.

Measles, mumps, and rubella—vaccine use and strategies for elimination of measles, rubella, and congenital rubella syndrome and control of mumps. MMWR Morb Mortal Wkly Rep 47(RR-8):1–57, 1998.

Control and prevention of meningococcal disease and control and prevention of serogroup C meningococcal disease: Evaluation and management of suspected outbreaks. MMWR Morb Mortal Wkly Rep 46(RR-5):1–21, 1997.

Prevention of plague. MMWR Morb Mortal Wkly Rep 45(RR-14):1–15, 1996.

Prevention of pneumococcal disease. MMWR Morb Mortal Wkly Rep 46(RR-8):1–24, 1997.

Poliomyelitis prevention in the United States: Introduction of a sequential vaccination schedule of inactivated poliovirus vaccine followed by oral poliovirus vaccine. MMWR Morb Mortal Wkly Rep 46(RR-3):1–25, 1997.

Rabies prevention—United States, 1991. MMWR Morb Mortal Wkly Rep 40(RR-3):1–19, 1991.

Typhoid immunization. MMWR Morb Mortal Wkly Rep 43(RR-14):1–8, 1994.

Prevention of varicella. MMWR Morb Mortal Wkly Rep 45(RR-11):1–36, 1996.

Yellow fever vaccine. MMWR Morb Mortal Wkly Rep 39(RR-6):1–5, 1990.

Programmatic strategies to increase vaccination rates—assessment and feedback of provider-based vaccination coverage information. MMWR Morb Mortal Wkly Rep 45:219–220, 1996.

Programmatic strategies to increase vaccination coverage by age 2 years—linkage of vaccination and WIC services. MMWR Morb Mortal Wkly Rep 45:217–218, 1996.

Recommendations of the Advisory Committee on Immunization Practices, the American Academy of Pediatrics, and the American Academy of Family Physicians: Use of reminder and recall by vaccination providers to increase vaccination rates. MMWR Morbid Mortal Wkly Rep 47:715–717, 1998.

*As of Oct 20, 1998.

Appendix 2

Immunobiologicals and Their Manufacturers and Distributors

CURRENTLY AVAILABLE IMMUNOBIOLOGICALS IN THE UNITED STATES BY MANUFACTURER OR DISTRIBUTOR*

IMMUNOBIOLOGICAL	MANUFACTURER OR DISTRIBUTOR	PRODUCT OR BRAND NAME
Adenovirus vaccine	Wyeth Laboratories, Inc.	Adenovirus, live oral, type 4† Adenovirus, live oral, type 7†
Anthrax vaccine	Michigan Biologic Products Institute	Anthrax vaccine adsorbed‡
Bacille Calmette-Guérin	Organon Teknika Corporation	BCG vaccine
Cholera vaccine	Wyeth Laboratories, Inc.	Cholera vaccine
Cytomegalovirus immune globulin	Massachusetts Public Health Biologic Laboratories	Cytomegalovirus immune globulin, intravenous
Diphtheria and tetanus toxoids, adsorbed	Connaught Laboratories, Inc.	Diphtheria and tetanus toxoids, adsorbed (pediatric)
	Wyeth-Lederle Vaccines and Pediatrics	Diphtheria and tetanus toxoids, adsorbed (purogenated for pediatric use)
	Massachusetts Public Health Biologic Laboratories	Diphtheria and tetanus toxoids, adsorbed (pediatric)
	Michigan Biologic Products Institute	Diphtheria and tetanus toxoids, adsorbed (pediatric)‡
Diphtheria and tetanus toxoids and pertussis vaccine, adsorbed	Connaught Laboratories, Inc.	Diphtheria and tetanus toxoids and pertussis vaccine, adsorbed
	Wyeth-Lederle Vaccines and Pediatrics	Diphtheria and tetanus toxoids and pertussis vaccine, adsorbed (Tri-Immunol)
	Massachusetts Public Health Biologic Laboratories	Diphtheria and tetanus toxoids and pertussis vaccine, adsorbed
	Michigan Biologic Products Institute	Diphtheria and tetanus toxoids and pertussis vaccine, adsorbed‡
Diphtheria and tetanus toxoids and acellular pertussis vaccine, adsorbed	Connaught Laboratories, Inc.	Tripedia
	Wyeth-Lederle Vaccines and Pediatrics	Acel-Imune
	SmithKline Beecham Pharmaceuticals	Infanrix
	North American Vaccine, Inc.	Certiva
Diphtheria and tetanus toxoids with whole-cell pertussis combined with *Haemophilus influenzae* type b conjugate vaccine	Connaught Laboratories, Inc. and Pasteur-Mérieux Serums et Vaccins, S.A.	ActHIB DTP§
	Wyeth-Lederle Vaccines and Pediatrics	Tetramune
Diphtheria and tetanus toxoids and acellular pertussis vaccine adsorbed combined with *Haemophilus influenzae* type b conjugate vaccine	Connaught Laboratories, Inc. and Pasteur-Mérieux Serums et Vaccins, S.A.	TriHIBit
Haemophilus influenzae type b vaccine, polysaccharide-conjugate	Wyeth-Lederle Vaccines and Pediatrics	HibTITER
	Merck & Co., Inc.	PedvaxHIB
	Pasteur Mérieux Serums et Vaccins, S.A.§	ActHIB
	SmithKline Beecham Pharmaceuticals	OmniHIB
Hepatitis A vaccine	SmithKline Beecham Pharmaceuticals	Havrix
	Merck & Co., Inc.	Vaqta

CURRENTLY AVAILABLE IMMUNOBIOLOGICALS IN THE UNITED STATES BY MANUFACTURER OR DISTRIBUTOR* *Continued*

IMMUNOBIOLOGICAL	MANUFACTURER OR DISTRIBUTOR	PRODUCT OR BRAND NAME
Hepatitis B immune globulin	North American Biologicals, Inc.	Hepatitis B immune globulin (human) (H-BIG)
	Alpha Therapeutic Corporation	Hepatitis B immune globulin (human)
	Bayer Corporation	Hepatitis B immune globulin (human) (HyperHep)
Hepatitis B vaccine, recombinant	Merck & Co., Inc.	Recombivax HB
	SmithKline Beecham Pharmaceuticals	Engerix-B
Hepatitis B vaccine, recombinant, combined with *Haemophilus influenzae* type b vaccine, polysaccharide-conjugated	Merck & Co., Inc.	Comvax
Immune globulin	Bayer Corporation	Immune globulin, intravenous (Gamimune 5% and 10%)
	Central Laboratory Blood Transfusion Service	Immune globulin (human) (Gamastan) Immune globulin
	Swiss Red Cross	Intravenous (Sandoglobulin)
	Baxter Healthcare Corporation	Immune globulin, intravenous (human) (Gammagard)
	Massachusetts Public Health Biologic Laboratories	Immune serum globulin (human)
	Michigan Biologic Products Institute	Immune serum globulin (human)‡
	Centeon L.L.C.	Immune serum globulin, intravenous (human) (Gammar-P IV)
	V.I. Technologies, Inc.	Immune globulin (human)
	Oesterreichisches Institut fuer Haemoderivate Ges.m.b.H.	Immune globulin, intravenous (human) (Iveegam)
	Immuno-U.S., Inc.	Immune globulin (human)
Influenza vaccine	Connaught Laboratories, Inc.	Influenza virus vaccine (zonal purified) whole virion (Fluzone)
		Influenza virus vaccine (zonal purified) split virion (Fluzone)
	Evans Medical Ltd.	Influenza virus vaccine (split virion) (Fluvirin)
	Parkedale Pharmaceuticals	Influenza virus vaccine (split virion) (Fluogen)
	Wyeth Laboratories, Inc.	Influenza virus vaccine, subvirion type (Flushield)
Japanese encephalitis virus vaccine	Research Foundation for Microbial Diseases of Osaka University	JE-VAX
Measles, mumps, and rubella vaccine	Merck & Co., Inc.	Measles, mumps, and rubella virus vaccine, live (M-M-R II)
Measles and rubella vaccine	Merck & Co., Inc.	Measles and Rubella Virus Vaccine, Live (M-R-Vax II)
Measles vaccine	Merck & Co., Inc.	Measles virus vaccine, live attenuated (Attenuvax)
Meningococcal polysaccharide vaccine A, C, Y, and W-135	Connaught Laboratories, Inc.	Meningococcal polysaccharide vaccine (Menomune-A/C/Y/W-135)
Mumps vaccine	Merck & Co., Inc.	Mumps virus vaccine, live (Mumpsvax)
Pertussis vaccine, adsorbed	Michigan Biologic Products Institute	Pertussis vaccine adsorbed‡
Plague vaccine	Greer Laboratories, Inc.	Plague vaccine
Pneumococcal polysaccharide vaccine	Wyeth-Lederle Vaccines and Pediatrics	Pneumococcal vaccine, polyvalent (Pnu-Imune 23)
	Merck & Co., Inc.	Pneumococcal Vaccine Polyvalent (Pneumovax 23)
Poliovirus vaccine, inactivated	Connaught Laboratories, Ltd.	Poliovax
	Pasteur-Mérieux Serums et Vaccins, S.A.	IPOL
Poliovirus vaccine, live oral	Wyeth-Lederle Vaccines and Pediatrics	Poliovirus vaccine, live oral trivalent (Orimune)
Rabies immune globulin	Bayer Corporation	Rabies immune globulin (human) (Hyperab)
	Pasteur Mérieux Serums et Vaccins, S.A.‖	Rabies immune globulin (human) (Imogam)
Rabies vaccine	Chiron Behring GmbH & Co.	RabAvert
	Connaught Laboratories, Ltd.	Rabie-Vax
	Michigan Biologic Products Institute	Rabies vaccine adsorbed‡
	Pasteur Mérieux Serums et Vaccins, S.A.‖	Rabies vaccine, human diploid cell (Imovax, Imovax ID)

Table continued on following page

CURRENTLY AVAILABLE IMMUNOBIOLOGICALS IN THE UNITED STATES BY MANUFACTURER OR DISTRIBUTOR* *Continued*

IMMUNOBIOLOGICAL	MANUFACTURER OR DISTRIBUTOR	PRODUCT OR BRAND NAME
Respiratory syncytial virus immune globulin intravenous (human)	Massachusetts Public Health Biologic Laboratories	Respigam
Rho(D) immune globulin intravenous (human)	Cangene Corporation	WinRho SD
Rotavirus vaccine, live, oral	Wyeth Laboratories, Inc.	Rotavirus vaccine, live, oral, tetravalent (RotaShield)
Rubella vaccine	Merck & Co., Inc.	Rubella virus vaccine, live (Meruvax II)
Rubella and mumps vaccine	Merck & Co., Inc.	Rubella and mumps virus vaccine, live (Biavax II)
Tetanus immune globulin (human)	Centeon L.L.C.	Tetanus immune globulin (human)
	Alpha Therapeutic Corporation	Tetanus immune globulin (human)
	Immuno-U.S., Inc.	Tetanus immune globulin (human)
	Massachusetts Public Health Biologic Laboratories	Tetanus immune globulin (human)
	Bayer Corporation	Hyper-Tet
Tetanus and diphtheria toxoids, adsorbed	Connaught Laboratories, Ltd.	Tetanus and diphtheria toxoids, adsorbed (for adult use)
	Wyeth-Lederle Pediatrics and Vaccines	Tetanus and diphtheria toxoids, adsorbed (for adult use) (purogenated parenteral)
	Massachusetts Public Health Biologic Laboratories	Tetanus and diphtheria toxoids, adsorbed (for adult use)
	Wyeth Laboratories, Inc.	Tetanus and diphtheria toxoids, adsorbed (for adult use) (aluminum phosphate, ultrafined)
Tetanus toxoid, adsorbed	Connaught Laboratories, Inc., Wyeth-Lederle Vaccines and Pediatrics	Tetanus toxoid adsorbed, purogenated (aluminum phosphate, adsorbed)
	Massachusetts Public Health Biological Laboratories	Tetanus toxoid, adsorbed
	Michigan Biologic Products Institute	Tetanus toxoid, adsorbed‡
	Wyeth Laboratories, Inc.	Tetanus toxoid, adsorbed (aluminum phosphate, adsorbed, ultrafined)
	Swiss Serum and Vaccine Institute, Berne	Tetanus toxoid, adsorbed
Tetanus toxoid, fluid	Connaught Laboratories, Inc.	Tetanus toxoid (fluid)
	Connaught Laboratories Ltd.	Tetanus toxoid (fluid)
	Wyeth-Lederle Vaccines and Pediatrics	Tetanus toxoid (purogenated, tetanus toxoid, fluid)
Typhoid vaccine	Wyeth-Ayerst Laboratories, Inc.	Typhoid vaccine
	Wyeth-Ayerst Laboratories, Inc.	Typhoid vaccine† (acetone-killed and dried)
Typhoid vaccine, live oral/Ty21A	Swiss Serum and Vaccine Institute, Berne	Vivotif Berna
Typhoid vaccine, Vi polysaccharide	Pasteur Mérieux Serums et Vaccins, S.A.‖	Typhim Vi
Vaccinia immune globulin	Baxter Healthcare Corporation	Vaccinia immune globulin (human)
Vaccinia vaccine	Wyeth Laboratories, Inc.	Smallpox vaccine
Varicella vaccine	Merck & Co., Inc.	Varivax
Varicella-zoster immune globulin	Massachusetts Public Health Biologic Laboratories	Varicella-zoster immune globulin (human)¶
Yellow fever vaccine	Connaught Laboratories, Inc.	Yellow fever vaccine (live, 17D Virus) (YF-Vax)

* *Note:* In the preparation of this listing, every effort was made to ensure its completeness and accuracy. This listing was compiled from information obtained from manufacturers, the Food and Drug Administration, and the *Physicians' Desk Reference* (52nd ed), 1998, and to the best of our knowledge is an accurate and complete listing as of August 13, 1998. However, omissions and errors may have occurred inadvertently. This listing is intended to be a resource and does not replace the provider's obligation to remain otherwise current on the availability of vaccines, toxoids, and immune globulins.
Source identified for these products may or may not be the licensed manufacturer. See Tables 48–1 and 48–2 for licensed manufacturers. Appendix prepared by Karen Chaitkin, Center for Biologics Evaluation and Research, Food and Drug Administration; and Robert Snyder, National Immunization Program, Centers for Disease Control and Prevention.
† Available only to the U.S. Armed Forces.
‡ Outside Michigan, sold only to providers who will sign a "hold harmless" agreement.
§ Reconstitution of Pasteur Mérieux *Haemophilus influenzae* type b conjugate vaccine (PRP-T) with DTP vaccine (produced by Connaught Laboratories, Inc.).
‖ Pasteur Mérieux products distributed by Connaught Laboratories, Inc.
¶Varicella-Zoster Immune Globulin is available from selected blood banks in various locations in the United States. Consult Appendix 5 for a listing.

IMMUNOBIOLOGICAL MANUFACTURERS AND DISTRIBUTORS

Alpha Therapeutic Corporation
Los Angeles, CA 90032
(213) 227-7526
(800) 421-0008

Baxter Healthcare Corporation
Hyland Division
Glendale, CA 91203
(800) 423-2090

Bayer Corporation
Berkeley, CA 94701
(510) 705-5224

Centeon L.L.C.
King of Prussia, PA 19406
(610) 878-4048

Connaught Laboratories, Inc.
Swiftwater, PA 18370
(717) 839-7189
(800) 822-2463

Connaught Laboratories, Ltd.
North York, Ontario, Canada M2R 3T4
(416) 667-2779

Evans Medical Ltd.
Leatherhead, Surrey, KT22 7PQ, UK
U.S. contact, Medeva Americans, Inc.
(817) 545-7791

Greer Laboratories, Inc.
Lenoir, NC 28645
(704) 754-5327, x289

Massachusetts Public Health Biologic Laboratories
Boston, MA 02130
(617) 522-3700

Merck & Co., Inc.
West Point, PA 19486
(215) 652-5531
(800) 672-6372

Michigan Biologic Products Institute
Lansing, MI 48909
(517) 335-8119

New York Blood Center
Blood Derivatives
New York, NY 10021
(212) 570-3000
(800) 487-8751

North American Biologicals, Inc.
Boca Raton, FL 33487
(800) 458-4244

North American Vaccine, Inc.
Beltsville, MD 20705
(301) 419-8400

Organon Teknika Corporation
5516 Nicholson Lane
Kensington, MD 20895
(919) 620-2000

Parkedale Pharmaceuticals, Inc.
Briston, TN 37620
(800) 336-7783

Pasteur Mérieux Serums et Vaccins, S.A.
see Connaught Laboratories, Inc.

SmithKline Beecham Biologicals
Philadelphia, PA 19101
(215) 751-4912

Swiss Serum and Vaccine Institute, Berne
Coral Gables, FL 33146
(305) 443-2900

Wyeth-Ayerst Laboratories, Inc.
Philadelphia, PA 19101
(610) 688-4400
(800) 544-9871

Wyeth-Lederle Vaccines and Pediatrics
Philadelphia, PA 19101
(800) 572-8221

Appendix 3

Representative Vaccine Information Statement (VIS) That Must Be Given to Parents in the United States Before Immunization Against Diphtheria, Tetanus, and Pertussis

DIPHTHERIA, TETANUS, AND PERTUSSIS VACCINES

WHAT YOU NEED TO KNOW

1 Why get vaccinated?

Diphtheria, pertussis, and tetanus are serious diseases.

Diphtheria

- Diphtheria causes a thick covering in the back of the throat.
- It can lead to breathing problems, paralysis, heart failure, and even death.

Tetanus (Lockjaw)

- Tetanus causes painful tightening of the muscles, usually all over the body.
- It can lead to "locking" of the jaw so the person cannot open his mouth or swallow. Tetanus can lead to death.

Pertussis (Whooping cough)

- Pertussis causes coughing spells so bad that it is hard for infants to eat, drink, or breathe. These can last for weeks.
- It can lead to pneumonia, seizures (jerking and staring spells), brain damage, and death.

Diphtheria, tetanus, and pertussis vaccines prevent these diseases. Most children who get all their shots will be protected during childhood. Many more children would get these diseases if we stopped vaccinating.

2 Diphtheria, tetanus, and pertussis vaccines

DTP vaccine

- Protects against diphtheria, tetanus, and pertussis
- Used for many years

DTaP vaccine

- Protects against diphtheria, tetanus, and pertussis
- Newer than DTP

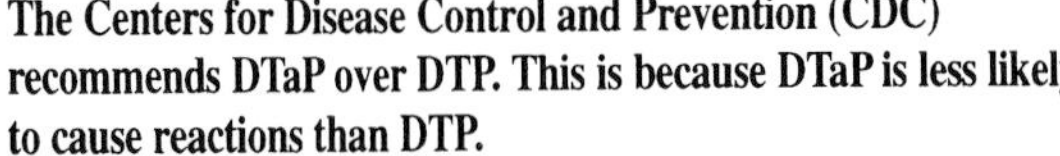

The Centers for Disease Control and Prevention (CDC) recommends DTaP over DTP. This is because DTaP is less likely to cause reactions than DTP.

Related vaccines

- **Combinations:** To reduce the number of shots a child must get, DTP or DTaP may be available in combination with other vaccines.
- **DT** protects against diphtheria and tetanus, *but not pertussis.* It only is recommended for children who should not get pertussis vaccine.

3 What are the risks from these vaccines?

- As with any medicine, vaccines carry a small risk of serious harm, such as a severe allergic reaction or even death.
- If there are reactions, they usually start within 3 days and don't last long.
- Most people have no serious reactions from these vaccines.

Possible reactions to these vaccines:

Mild Reactions (common)

- Sore arm or leg
- Fussy
- Tired
- Fever
- Less appetite
- Vomiting

Mild reactions are *much less likely* after DTaP than after DTP.

Moderate to Serious Reactions (uncommon)

Moderate to serious reactions have been uncommon with DTP vaccine:

- Non-stop crying (3 hours or more)........... 100 of every 10,000 doses
- Fever of 105° or higher................................30 of every 10,000 doses
- Seizure (jerking or staring)............................6 of every 10,000 doses
- Child becomes limp, pale, less alert..............6 of every 10,000 doses

With DTaP vaccine, these reactions are much less likely to happen.

Severe Reactions (very rare)

There are two kinds of serious reactions:

- Severe allergic reaction (breathing difficulty, shock)
- Severe brain reaction (long seizure, coma or lowered consciousness)

Is there lasting damage?

- Experts disagree on whether pertussis vaccines cause lasting brain damage.
- If they do, it is very rare.

Most experts believe serious reactions will be *more rare* after DTaP than after DTP.

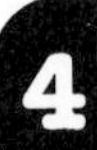

4 When should my child get vaccinated?

Most children should get a dose at these ages:

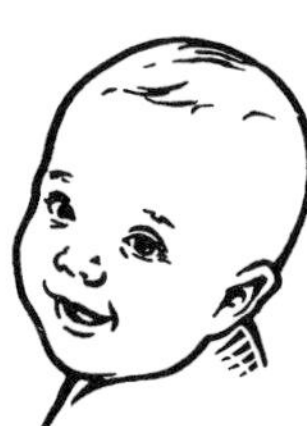

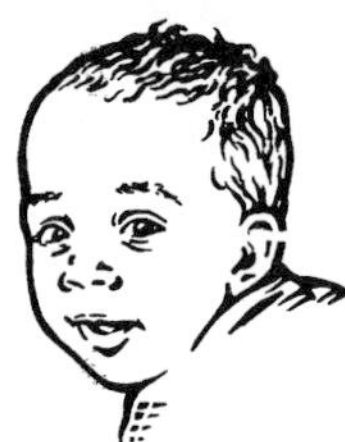

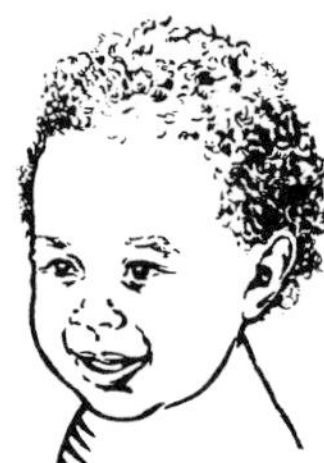

2 Months **4 Months** **6 Months**

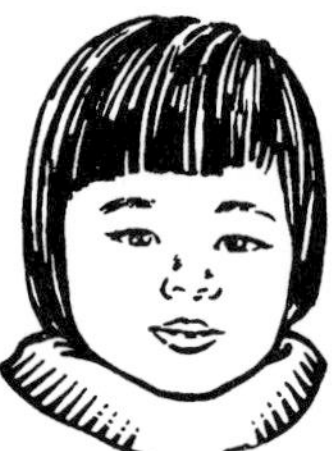

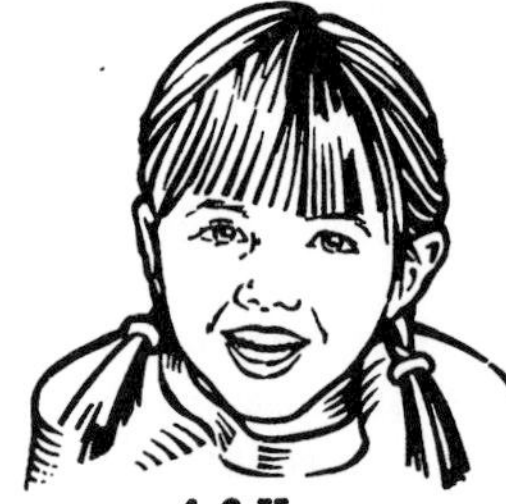

12-18 Months **4-6 Years**

At 11-12 years of age and every 10 years after that you should get a booster to prevent diphtheria and tetanus.

5 What can be done to reduce possible fever and pain after this vaccine?

Give your child an *aspirin-free* pain reliever for 24 hours after the shot.

This is important if your child has had a seizure or has a parent, brother, or sister who has had a seizure.

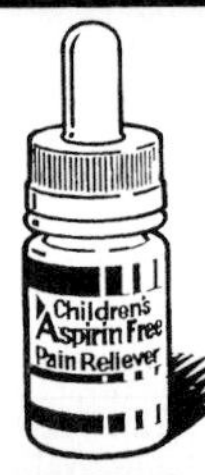

6 Some children should not get these vaccines or should wait

Tell your doctor or nurse if your child:

- Ever had a moderate or serious reaction after getting vaccinated
- Ever had a seizure
- Has a parent, brother, or sister who has had a seizure
- Has a brain problem that is getting worse
- Now has a moderate or severe illness

Your doctor or nurse has information on what to do in this case (for example, give one of these vaccines, wait, give medicine to prevent fever).

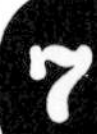

7 What if there is a moderate to severe reaction?

What should I look for?

- Any unusual conditions, such as those in item 3

What should I do?

- Call a doctor or get the child to a doctor right away.
- Tell your doctor what happened, the date and time it happened, and when the vaccination was given.
- Ask your doctor, nurse, or health department to file a Vaccine Adverse Event Report (VAERS) form, or call VAERS yourself at: **1-800-822-7967**

8 The National Vaccine Injury Compensation Program

The National Vaccine Injury Compensation Program is a federal program that helps pay for the care of those seriously injured by vaccines.

For details call **1-800-338-2382** or visit the program's website at **http://www.hrsa.dhhs.gov/bhpr/vicp/new.htm**

9 How can I learn more?

- Ask your doctor or nurse. They can give you the vaccine package insert or suggest other sources of information.
- Call your local or state health department. They can give you the *Parents Guide to Childhood Immunization* or other information.
- Contact the Centers for Disease Control and Prevention (CDC):

  Call **1-800-232-2522** (English)

  OR

  Call **1-800-232-0233** (Spanish)

  OR

  Visit the CDC website at **http://www.cdc.gov/nip**

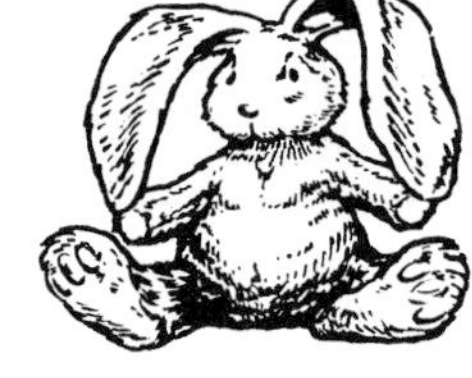

U.S. DEPARTMENT OF HEALTH & HUMAN SERVICES
Centers for Disease Control and Prevention
National Immunization Program

DTP/DTaP/DT (8/15/97)
Vaccine Information Statement
42 U.S.C. § 300aa-26

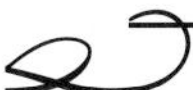

Appendix 4

Case Definitions for Selected Vaccine-Preventable Diseases Under Public Health Surveillance in the United States*

DIPHTHERIA

Clinical Description

An upper-respiratory tract illness characterized by a sore throat, low-grade fever, and an adherent membrane of the tonsil(s), pharynx, and/or nose.

Laboratory Criteria for Diagnosis

- Isolation of *Corynebacterium diphtheriae* from a clinical specimen *or*
- Histopathological diagnosis of diphtheria

Case Classification

Probable: a clinically compatible case that is not laboratory confirmed and is not epidemiologically linked to a laboratory-confirmed case
Confirmed: a clinically compatible case that is either laboratory confirmed or epidemiologically linked to a laboratory-confirmed case

Haemophilus influenzae (INVASIVE DISEASE)

Clinical Description

Invasive disease caused by *Haemophilus influenzae* may produce any of several clinical syndromes, including meningitis, bacteremia, epiglottitis, or pneumonia.

Laboratory Criteria for Diagnosis

Isolation of *H. influenzae* from a normally sterile site (e.g., blood or cerebrospinal fluid [CSF] or, less commonly, joint, pleural, or pericardial fluid).

Case Classification

Probable: a clinically compatible case with detection of *H. influenzae* type b antigen in CSF
Confirmed: a clinically compatible case that is laboratory confirmed

HEPATITIS B

Clinical Case Definition

An acute illness with discrete onset of symptoms and jaundice or elevated serum aminotransferase levels.

Laboratory Criteria for Diagnosis

- Immunoglobulin M (IgM) antibody to hepatitis B core antigen (anti-HBc) positive (if done) or hepatitis B surface antigen (HBsAg) positive
- IgM anti–hepatitis A virus negative (if done)

Case Classification

Confirmed: a case that meets the clinical case definition and is laboratory confirmed

PERINATAL HEPATITIS B VIRUS INFECTION ACQUIRED IN THE UNITED STATES OR IN U.S. TERRITORIES

Clinical Description

Perinatal hepatitis B in the newborn may range from asymptomatic to fulminant hepatitis.

Laboratory Criteria for Diagnosis

HBsAg positive

Case Classification

HBsAg positivity in any infant between the ages of 1 and 24 months who was born in the United States or in U.S. territories to an HBsAg-positive mother

MEASLES

Clinical Case Definition

An illness characterized by all the following:
- Generalized rash lasting 3 or more days
- Temperature of 101.0 F (38.3° C) or more
- Cough, coryza, or conjunctivitis

Laboratory Criteria for Diagnosis

- Positive serological test for measles IgM antibody *or*
- Significant rise in measles antibody level by any standard serological assay *or*
- Isolation of measles virus from a clinical specimen

Case Classification

Suspected: any febrile illness accompanied by rash
Probable: a case that meets the clinical case definition, has noncontributory or no serological or virological testing and is not epidemiologically linked to a confirmed case
Confirmed: a case that is laboratory confirmed or that meets the clinical case definition and is epidemiologically linked to a confirmed case; a laboratory-confirmed case does not need to meet the clinical case definition

*These case definitions are intended for use by public health authorities for classifying cases, which is often done retrospectively, for national reporting purposes. They should not be used as criteria for reporting by providers or for public health action. In most jurisdictions, state law or regulation requires prompt reporting by providers and others of suspected cases of specified infectious diseases; for more information of specific state reporting requirements, providers should contact the health department in their state.

Modified from Case definitions for infectious conditions under public health surveillance. MMWR, Morb Mortal Wkly Rep 46(RR-10):1–58, 1997.

MUMPS

Clinical Case Definition

An illness with acute onset of unilateral or bilateral tender, self-limited swelling of the parotid or other salivary gland, lasting 2 days, and without other apparent cause

Laboratory Criteria for Diagnosis

- Isolation of mumps virus from clinical specimen *or*
- Significant rise between acute- and convalescent-phase titers in serum mumps IgG antibody level by any standard serological assay *or*
- Positive serological test for mumps IgM antibody

Case Classification

Probable: a case that meets the clinical case definition, has noncontributory or no serological or virological testing, and is not epidemiologically linked to a confirmed or probable case
Confirmed: a case that is laboratory confirmed or that meets the clinical case definition and is epidemiologically linked to a confirmed or probable case; a laboratory-confirmed case does not need to meet the clinical case definition

PERTUSSIS

Clinical Case Definition

A cough illness lasting 2 weeks with paroxysms of coughing, inspiratory whoop, or posttussive vomiting, without other apparent cause

Laboratory Criteria for Diagnosis

- Isolation of *Bordetella pertussis* from clinical specimen *or*
- Positive polymerase chain reaction for *B. pertussis*

Case Classification

Probable: a case that meets the clinical case definition, is not laboratory confirmed, and is not epidemiologically linked to a laboratory-confirmed case
Confirmed: a case that is laboratory confirmed or one that meets the clinical case definition and is either laboratory confirmed or epidemiologically linked to a laboratory-confirmed case

POLIOMYELITIS, PARALYTIC

Clinical Case Definition

Acute onset of a flaccid paralysis of one or more limbs, with decreased or absent tendon reflexes in the affected limbs, without other apparent cause and without sensory or cognitive loss

Case Classification

Probable: a case that meets the clinical case definition
Confirmed: a case that meets the clinical case definition and in which the patient has a neurological deficit 60 days after the onset of initial symptoms, has died, or has unknown follow-up status
All suspected cases of paralytic poliomyelitis are reviewed by a panel of expert consultants before final classification occurs. Confirmed cases are then further classified based on epidemiological and laboratory criteria. Only confirmed cases are included in Table 1 in the *Morbidity and Mortality Weekly Report (MMWR).* Suspected cases are enumerated in a footnote to the MMWR table.

RUBELLA

Clinical Case Definition

An illness that has all the following characteristics:

- Acute onset of generalized maculopapular rash
- Temperature >99.0°F (>37.2°C), if measured
- Arthralgia/arthritis, lymphadenopathy, or conjunctivitis

Laboratory Criteria for Diagnosis

- Isolation of rubella virus *or*
- Significant rise between acute- and convalescent-phase titers in serum rubella IgG antibody level by any standard serological assay *or*
- Positive serological test for rubella IgM antibody

Case Classification

Suspected: any generalized rash illness of acute onset
Probable: a case that meets the clinical case definition, has no or noncontributory serological or virological testing, and is not epidemiologically linked to a laboratory-confirmed case
Confirmed: a case that is laboratory confirmed or that meets the clinical case definition and is epidemiologically linked to a laboratory-confirmed case

RUBELLA, CONGENITAL SYNDROME

Clinical Description

An illness usually manifesting in infancy resulting from rubella infection in utero and characterized by signs or symptoms from the following categories:

- (a) Cataracts or congenital glaucoma, congenital heart disease (most commonly patent ductus arteriosus or peripheral pulmonary artery stenosis), loss of hearing, and pigmentary retinopathy
- (b) Purpura, splenomegaly, jaundice, microcephaly, mental retardation, meningoencephalitis, and radiolucent bone disease

Clinical Case Definition

Presence of any defects or laboratory data consistent with congenital rubella infection

Laboratory Criteria for Diagnosis

- Isolation of rubella virus *or*
- Demonstration of rubella-specific IgM antibody *or*
- Infant rubella antibody level that persists at a higher level and for a longer period than expected from passive transfer of maternal antibody (i.e., rubella titer that does not drop at the expected rate of a twofold dilution per month)

Case Classification

Suspected: a case with some compatible clinical findings but not meeting the criteria for a probable case
Probable: a case that is not laboratory confirmed and that has any two complications listed in paragraph (a) under Clinical Description above or one complication from paragraph (a) and one from paragraph (b), and lacks evidence of any other etiology
Confirmed: a clinically compatible case that is laboratory confirmed
Infection only: a case that demonstrates laboratory evidence of infection but without any clinical symptoms or signs

TETANUS

Clinical Case Definition

Acute onset of hypertonia and/or painful muscular contractions (usually of the muscles of the jaw and neck) and generalized muscle spasms without other apparent medical cause

Case Classification

Confirmed: a clinically compatible case, as reported by a health-care professional

VARICELLA (CHICKENPOX)

Clinical Case Definition

An illness with acute onset of diffuse (generalized) papulovesicular rash without other apparent cause

Laboratory Criteria for Diagnosis

- Isolation of varicella virus from a clinical specimen *or*
- Significant rise in serum varicella IgG antibody level by any standard serological assay

Case Classification

Probable: a case that meets the clinical case definition, is not laboratory confirmed, and is not epidemiologically linked to another probable or confirmed case
Confirmed: a case that is laboratory confirmed or that meets the clinical case definition and is epidemiologically linked to a confirmed or probable case

Index

Note: Page numbers in *italics* refer to illustrations, page numbers followed by the letter t refer to tables.

ISBN 0-7216-7443-7